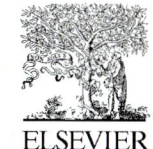

介入心脏病学

Textbook of Interventional Cardiology

第8版　8th Edition

中文精要·英文影印版

◎ 主编

[美] 埃里克·J. 托波尔（Eric J. Topol）
[美] 保罗·S. 泰尔斯坦（Paul S. Teirstein）

◎ 编译

吴永健
柳景华　编译委员会主任委员

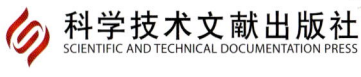

·北京·

图书在版编目（CIP）数据

介入心脏病学：第8版/（美）埃里克·J.托波尔（Eric J. Topol），（美）保罗·S.泰尔斯坦（Paul S. Teirstein）主编；吴永健，柳景华编译.—北京：科学技术文献出版社，2023.4
书名原文：Textbook of Interventional Cardiology 8th Edition
ISBN 978-7-5189-9610-0

Ⅰ.①介… Ⅱ.①埃…②保…③吴…④柳… Ⅲ.①心脏病—介入性治疗 Ⅳ.① R541.05

中国版本图书馆 CIP 数据核字（2022）第 177253 号
著作权合同登记号 图字：01-2022-5271
中文简体字版权专有权归科学技术文献出版社所有

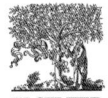

Elsevier (Singapore) Pte Ltd.
3 Killiney Road,
#08-01 Winsland House I,
Singapore 239519
Tel: (65) 6349-0200; Fax: (65) 6733-1817

Textbook of Interventional Cardiology, 8th Edition
Copyright © 2020 by Elsevier, Inc. All rights reserved.
ISBN-13: 9780323568142

This English Adaptation of Textbook of Interventional Cardiology, 8th Edition by Eric J. Topol and Paul S. Teirstein was undertaken by Scientific and Technical Documentation Press Co., Ltd. and is published by arrangement with Elsevier (Singapore) Pte Ltd.

Textbook of Interventional Cardiology, 8th Edition by Eric J. Topol and Paul S. Teirstein 由科学技术文献出版社进行改编影印，并根据科学技术文献出版社与爱思唯尔（新加坡）私人有限公司的协议约定出版。

《介入心脏病学》（第8版）（吴永健，柳景华编译）
ISBN: 9787518996100

Copyright © 2022 by Elsevier (Singapore) Pte Ltd. and Scientific and Technical Documentation Press Co., Ltd.

All rights reserved. No part of this publication may be reproduced or transmitted in any form or by any means, electronic or mechanical, including photocopying, recording, or any information storage and retrieval system, without permission in writing from Elsevier (Singapore) Pte Ltd. and Scientific and Technical Documentation Press Co., Ltd.

Online resources are not available with this adaptation. 本书不包含英文原版配套电子资源。

Notice

The adaptation has been undertaken by Scientific and Technical Documentation Press Co., Ltd. at its sole responsibility. Practitioners and researchers must always rely on their own experience and knowledge in evaluating and using any information, methods, compounds or experiments described herein. Because of rapid advances in the medical sciences, in particular, independent verification of diagnoses and drug dosages should be made. To the fullest extent of the law, no responsibility is assumed by Elsevier, authors, editors or contributors in relation to the adaptation or for any injury and/or damage to persons or property as a matter of products liability, negligence or otherwise, or from any use or operation of any methods, products, instructions, or ideas contained in the material herein.

Published in China by Scientific and Technical Documentation Press Co., Ltd. under special arrangement with Elsevier (Singapore) Pte Ltd. This edition is authorized for sale in the People's Republic of China only, excluding Hong Kong SAR, Macau SAR and Taiwan. Unauthorized export of this edition is a violation of the contract.

介入心脏病学（第8版）

| 策划编辑：张 蓉 | 责任编辑：张 蓉 段思帆 | 责任校对：张吲哚 | 责任出版：张志平 |

出 版 者	科学技术文献出版社
地　　址	北京市复兴路15号　邮编　100038
编 务 部	（010）58882938，58882087（传真）
发 行 部	（010）58882868，58882870（传真）
邮 购 部	（010）58882873
官方网址	www.stdp.com.cn
发 行 者	科学技术文献出版社发行　全国各地新华书店经销
印 刷 者	北京地大彩印有限公司
版　　次	2023年4月第1版　2023年4月第1次印刷
开　　本	889×1194　1/16
字　　数	2183千
印　　张	84.5
书　　号	ISBN 978-7-5189-9610-0
定　　价	880.00元

版权所有　违法必究

购买本社图书，凡字迹不清、缺页、倒页、脱页者，本社发行部负责调换

编译主任委员简介

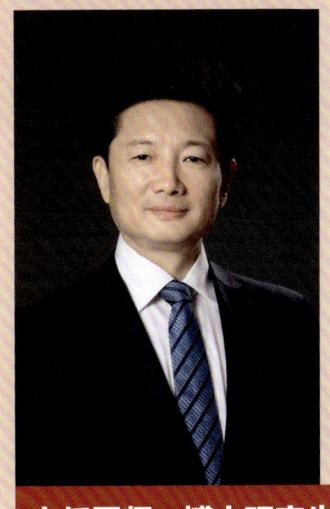

吴永健

主任医师，博士研究生导师，中国医学科学院北京协和医学院 长聘教授
中国医学科学院阜外医院冠心病中心主任，结构性心脏病中心副主任

【社会任职】

现任中华医学会心血管病学分会委员、中国医师协会心血管内科医师分会常务委员、中国医师协会心脏重症专业委员会副主任委员、世界中医药学会联合会心脏康复专业委员会主任委员、海峡两岸医药卫生交流协会心脏重症专家委员会副主任委员等；担任《中国循环杂志》《中国介入心脏病学杂志》编委，《中华心血管病杂志》、英国HEART杂志通讯编委等。

【专业特长】

主要从事冠心病和老年瓣膜性心脏病介入治疗及其相关研究，是我国最早开展不用开胸经导管进行主动脉瓣膜置换的专家之一，从零开始探索我国经导管主动脉瓣膜置换术体系，打造国内首个经导管主动脉瓣膜置换术影像学核心实验室；已完成经导管主动脉瓣膜置换术1000余例；推广标准化经导管主动脉瓣膜置换术体系在全国100多家医院应用。

【学术成果】

承担国家和省部级科研课题12项，横向课题10项；参与研发多款其他瓣膜，并获得专利30余项；参与制定我国首个《经导管主动脉瓣置换术中国专家共识》，在国际上首次提出CT"多平面评估体系"等。

编译主任委员简介

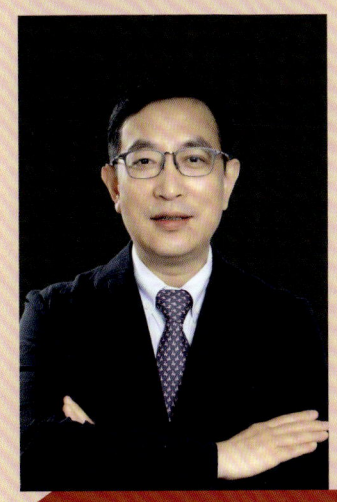

柳景华

主任医师，二级教授，博士研究生导师
首都医科大学附属北京安贞医院心脏内科医学中心副主任，冠心病中心主任

【社会任职】

现任中国医疗保健国际交流促进会常务理事、中华医学会心血管病学分会副主任委员、中国老年保健协会心脑血管疾病防治管理专业委员会名誉主任委员、中国医药教育协会血管微创医学专业委员会副主任委员、国际血管联盟心血管病专业委员会副主任委员、北京医师协会心血管专科医师分会副会长、北京医师协会胸痛专科医师分会副会长、北京市胸痛中心联盟副主席。

【专业特长】

擅长内科重症急救和心血管病介入性治疗。

【学术成果】

承担"973计划""863计划"、国家自然科学基金、北京市自然科学基金、北京市教育委员会科学研究基金和首都科学发展基金等科研课题；发表论文200余篇，主编论著5部，参编20部，获国家专利8项；获光华工程科技奖二等奖、部级科学技术进步奖三等奖；享受国务院政府特殊津贴。

原书编者名单

William T. Abraham, MD, FACP, FACC, FAHA, FESC, FRCP
Professor of Medicine, Physiology, and Cell Biology
College of Medicine Distinguished Professor
Division of Cardiovascular Medicine
The Ohio State University
Columbus, Ohio

Marcelo Abud, MD
Fellow
Interventional Cardiology and Endovascular Therapies
Cardiovascular Institute of Buenos Aires
Buenos Aires, Argentina

Jung-Min Ahn, MD
Associate Professor
Department of Cardiology
Asan Medical Center
University of Ulsan College of Medicine
Seoul, Republic of Korea

Takashi Akasaka, MD, PhD
Department of Cardiovascular Medicine
Wakayama Medical University
Wakayama, Japan

Ibrahim Akin, MD
Universitätsklinikum Mannheim
Fakultät Heidelberg
Abteilung Kardiologie
Mannheim, Germany

Waleed Alharbi, MD
Complex Coronary, Structural and Endovascular Interventional Cardiology Fellow
Prairie Heart Institute
Springfield, Illinois

David W. Allen, MD
Assistant Professor of Cardiology
Max Rady College of Medicine
University of Manitoba
Winnipeg, Manitoba, Canada

Alexandra Almonacid, MD
Associate Director
Beth Israel Deaconess Medical Center Cardiovascular Imaging Core Laboratory
Boston, Massachusetts

Dominick J. Angiolillo, MD, PhD
Professor of Medicine
Director, Cardiovascular Research
Program Director, Interventional Cardiology Fellowship
University of Florida College of Medicine
Jacksonville, Florida

Stephen Balter, PhD
Professor of Clinical Radiology (Physics) in Medicine
Radiology and Medicine
Columbia University
New York, New York

David T. Balzer, MD
Professor, Pediatrics
Division of Pediatric Cardiology
Director, Cardiac Catheterization Laboratory
Washington University School of Medicine
St. Louis, Missouri

Gregory W. Barsness, MD
Assistant Professor
Departments of Internal Medicine, Cardiovascular Medicine, and Radiology
Director, Cardiac Intensive Care Unit
Mayo Clinic
Rochester, Minnesota

Olivier F. Bertrand, MD, PhD
Quebec Heart-Lung Institute
Interventional Cardiology
Quebec City, Canada

Farzin Beygui, MD, MPH, PhD
Professor of Cardiology
Interventional Cardiology Unit
Caen University Hospital
Caen, France

John A. Bittl, MD
Interventional Cardiologist
AdventHealth Ocala
Ocala, Florida

Nyal Borges, MD
Department of Cardiovascular Medicine
Cleveland Clinic
Cleveland, Ohio

Vikram M. Brahmanandam, MD
Attending Cardiologist, Assistant Professor of Medicine
Cardiology
Montefiore-Einstein Center for Heart and Vascular Care
Bronx, New York

Éric Brochet, MD
Cardiology Department
Hopital Bichat
Paris, France

Sergio Buccheri, MD
Interventional Cardiologist
Cardiac-Thoracic-Vascular Department
Azienda Policlinico-Vittorio Emanuele
Associate Professor of Cardiology
University of Catania
Catania, Italy

Robert A. Byrne, MB BCh, PhD
Interventional Cardiologist
Deutsches Herzzentrum München
Technische Universität
Munich, Germany

Davide Capodanno, MD, PhD
Interventional Cardiologist
Cardiac-Thoracic-Vascular Department
Azienda Policlinico-Vittorio Emanuele
Associate Professor of Cardiology
University of Catania
Catania, Italy

Ivan P. Casserly, MD
Professor of Medicine
University College Dublin
Mater Misericordiae University Hospital
Dublin, Ireland

Matthews Chacko, MD
Assistant Professor of Medicine
Division of Cardiology
Johns Hopkins University and Hospital
Baltimore, Maryland

Derek P. Chew, MBBS, MPH, PhD FRACP, FACC, FESC, FCSANZ
Professor of Cardiology
Department of Cardiovascular Medicine
Flinders University
Network Director of Cardiology
Department of Cardiovascular Medicine
Southern Adelaide Health Service
Adelaide, Australia

Leslie Cho, MD
Section Head, Preventive Cardiology & Rehabilitation
Director, Womens Cardiovascular Center
Cleveland Clinic
Cleveland, Ohio

Michael L. Chuang, MD
Assistant Director
Beth Israel Deaconess Medical Center Cardiovascular Imaging Core Laboratory
Boston, Massachusetts

Antonio Colombo, MD
EMO-GVM Centro Cuore Columbus
San Raffaele Scientific Institute
Milan, Italy

Marco A. Costa, MD, PhD
University Hospitals Harrington Heart & Vascular Institute
Case Western Reserve University School of Medicine
Cleveland, Ohio

Alain Cribier, MD
Department of Cardiology
Rouen University Hospital
Rouen, France

Fernando Cura, MD, PhD
Director
Interventional Cardiology and Endovascular Therapies
Instituto Cardiovascular de Buenos Aires
Buenos Aires, Argentina

Ingo Daehnert, MD, PhD
Department of Pediatric Cardiology
University of Leipzig, Heart Center
Leipzig, Germany

Vishal Dahya, MD
Chief Fellow
Cardiovascular Medicine Fellowship
Summa Health Heart and Vascular Institute
Summa Health System
Akron, Ohio

Kimberly S. Delcour, DO, FACC
Director, Cardiac CT
Clinical Assistant Professor
Department of Internal Medicine, Division of Cardiology
Heart & Vascular Center
University of Iowa Hospitals & Clinics
Iowa City, Iowa

Robert S. Dieter, MD, RVT
Loyola University Medical Center/Hines VA
Maywood, Illinois

John S. Douglas, Jr., MD
Professor
Department of Medicine
Director, Interventional Cardiology Fellowship Program
Emory University School of Medicine
Emory University Hospital
Atlanta, Georgia

Helene Eltchaninoff, MD
Department of Cardiology
Rouen University Hospital
Rouen, France

Marvin H. Eng, MD
Center for Structural Heart Disease
Division of Cardiology
Henry Ford Hospital
Detroit, Michigan

Zaher Fanari, MD
Heartland Cardiology/Wesley Medical Center
University of Kansas School of Medicine
Wichita, Kansas

Vasim Farooq, MBChB, PhD
Newcastle upon Tyne Hospitals
NHS Foundation Trust
Newcastle, United Kingdom

Miroslaw Ferenc, MD
Head of Interventional Cardiology
Division of Cardiology and Angiology II
University Heart Center Freiburg - Bad Krozingen
Bad Krozingen, Germany

Kenneth A. Fetterly, PhD
Medical Physicist
Cardiovascular Diseases
Mayo Clinic and Foundation
Rochester, Minnesota

Peter J. Fitzgerald, MD, PhD
Professor Emeritus of Medicine and Engineering
Division of Cardiovascular Medicine
Stanford University School of Medicine
Director, Center for Cardiovascular Technology
Stanford University Medical Center
Stanford, California

Marat Fudim, MD
Duke University Medical Center
Duke Clinical Research Institute
Durham, North Carolina

Mario J. Garcia, MD
Chief of Cardiology
Medicine
Montefiore Medical Center
Bronx, New York

Baris Gencer, MD
Cardiology Division
Geneva University Hospital
Geneva, Switzerland

C. Michael Gibson, MD, MS
CEO of Baim and PERFUSE Research Institutes
Professor of Medicine
Cardiovascular Division, Department of Medicine
Beth Israel Deaconess Medical Center
Harvard Medical School
Boston, Massachusetts

Bryan H. Goldstein, MD
Associate Professor of Pediatrics
University of Cincinnati College of Medicine
The Heart Institute
Cincinnati Children's Hospital Medical Center
Cincinnati, Ohio

Jeffrey Goldstein, MD
Director of Cardiology Department
Prairie Heart Institute
Springfield, Illinois

Carlos A. Gonzalez Lengua, MD
Medicine-Cardiology
Mount Sinai St. Luke's Hospital
New York, New York

Mario J. Gössl, MD
Director, Transcatheter Research and Education, Center for Valve and Structural Heart Disease
Co-chair, Valve Science Center
Minneapolis Heart Institute
Abbott Northwestern Hospital
Minneapolis, Minnesota

Nilesh J. Goswami, MD, FACC, FSCAI, FSVM
Director of Cardiac Catheterization Laboratory
Director of Structural Heart Interventions
Prairie Heart Institute
Springfield, Illinois

Elliott M. Groves, MD, MEng, FACC, FSCAI
Director, Structural Heart Interventions
Department of Medicine, Division of Cardiology
University of Illinois at Chicago
Chicago, Illinois

Giulio Guagliumi, MD
Cardiovascular Department
ASST Papa Giovanni XXIII
Bergamo, Italy

Serge C. Harb, MD
Department of Cardiovascular Medicine
Cleveland Clinic
Cleveland, Ohio

Trent Hartshorne, MBBS, FRACP, FCICM, DDU
Cardiologist and Intensive Care Physician
Intensive Care Consultant
The Alfred Hospital
Melbourne, Australia

Grant Henderson, MD
Fellow, Cardiovascular Medicine
Cleveland Clinic
Cleveland, Ohio

Timothy D. Henry, MD, FACC, MSCAI
Medical Director, The Carl and Edyth Lindner Center for Research and Education at The Christ Hospital
The Carl and Edyth Lindner Family Distinguished Chair in Clinical Research
Director of Programmatic and Network Development Heart and Vascular Service Line
The Christ Hospital Health Network
Cincinnati, Ohio;
Professor of Medicine
University of Minnesota
Cedars-Sinai Heart Institute
University of California Los Angeles

Howard C. Hermann, MD
John W. Bryfogle Jr. Professor of Cardiovascular Medicine
Health System Director for Interventional Cardiology Program
Perelman School of Medicine, University of Pennsylvania
Philadelphia, Pennsylvania

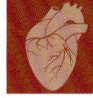

Dominique Himbert, MD
Cardiology Department
Hopital Bichat
Paris, France

Ravi S. Hira, MD, FACC, FAHA, FSCAI
Assistant Professor of Medicine
University of Washington
Seattle, Washington

Russel Hirsch, MD
Professor of Pediatrics
University of Cincinnati College of Medicine
The Heart Institute
Cincinnati Children's Hospital Medical Center
Cincinnati, Ohio

Kazuhiro Hisamoto, MD
Clinical Assistant Professor
Department of Cardiothoracic Surgery
NYU School of Medicine
New York, New York

Yasuhiro Honda, MD
Clinical Professor of Medicine
Division of Cardiovascular Medicine
Stanford University School of Medicine
Director, Cardiovascular Core Analysis Laboratory
Center for Cardiovascular Technology
Stanford University Medical Center
Stanford, California

Khalil Ibrahim, MD
Department of Cardiology
Johns Hopkins School of Medicine
Baltimore, Maryland

Bernard Iung, MD
Professor of Cardiology
University of Paris VII
Hospital Doctor
Cardiology Department
Hopital Bichat
Paris, France

Hani Jneid, MD, FACC, FAHA, FSCAI
Associate Professor of Medicine
Director, Interventional Cardiology Fellowship Program
Director, Interventional Cardiology Research
Baylor College of Medicine
Director, Interventional Cardiology
The Michael E. DeBakey VA Medical Center
Houston, Texas

James G. Jollis, MD, FACC
Professor of Medicine
Duke University
Durham, North Carolina

Michael A. Jolly, MD, FACC, RPVI
Interventional Cardiologist
OhioHealth Heart and Vascular
Columbus, Ohio

David E. Kandzari, MD, FACC, FSCAI
Director, Interventional Cardiology
Chief Scientific Officer
Piedmont Healthcare
Piedmont Heart Institute
Atlanta, Georgia

Samir R. Kapadia, MD
Professor of Medicine
Director, Sones Catheterization Laboratories
Director, Interventional Cardiology Fellowship
Department of Cardiovascular Medicine
Cleveland Clinic
Cleveland, Ohio

Adnan Kastrati, MD
Professor of Cardiology
Deutsches Herzzentrum and 1. Medizinische Klinik rechts der Isar
Technische Universität
Munich, Germany

Yuki Katagiri, MD
Department of Cardiology
Academic Medical Center
University of Amsterdam
Amsterdam, Netherlands

Athanasios Katsikis, MD, PhD
Department of Cardiology
General Military Hospital of Athens
Athens, Greece

Dean J. Kereiakes, MD, FACC, FSCAI
Medical Director, The Christ Hospital Heart and Vascular Center
Medical Director, The Christ Hospital Research Institute
The Christ Hospital Health Network
Cincinnati, Ohio
Professor of Clinical Medicine
Ohio State University

Morton J. Kern, MD
Chief of Medicine
Department of Medicine
VA Long Beach Health Care System
Long Beach, California

Ajay J. Kirtane, MD, SM, FACC, FSCAI
Associate Professor of Medicine, Columbia University Medical Center
Chief Academic Officer, Center for Interventional Vascular Therapy
Director, NYP/Columbia Cardiac Catheterization Laboratories
New York, New York

Serge Korjian, MD
PERFUSE Study Group
Cardiovascular Division, Department of Medicine
Beth Israel Deaconess Medical Center
Harvard Medical School
Boston, Massachusetts

Amar Krishnaswamy, MD
Program Director
Interventional Cardiology
Cleveland Clinic
Cleveland, Ohio

John M. Lasala, MD, PhD
Professor of Medicine
Director, Structural Heart Disease
Washington University School of Medicine
St. Louis, Missouri

Amir Lerman, MD
Professor
Department of Cardiovascular Medicine
Mayo Clinic
Rochester, Minnesota

Scott M. Lilly, MD, PhD
Associate Professor
Department of Medicine, Division of Cardiology
Ohio State University
Columbus, Ohio

Michael J. Lim, MD
Interim Director and Associate Professor of Medicine
Cardiology Division
Saint Louis University
St. Louis, Missouri

William L. Lombardi, MD, FACC, FSCAI
Director, Complex Coronary Artery Disease Therapies
University of Washington Medical Center
Seattle, Washington

Phillipp C. Lurz, MD, PhD
Department of Internal Medicine/Cardiology
Leipzig Heart Center, University Hospital
Leipzig, Germany

Kambis Mashayekhi, MD
Associate Head of Interventional Cardiology
Division of Cardiology and Angiology II
University Heart Center Freiburg - Bad Krozingen
Bad Krozingen, Germany

Roxana Mehran, MD
The Zena and Michael A. Wiener Cardiovascular Institute
Icahn School of Medicine at Mount Sinai
New York, New York

Adrian W. Messerli, MD, FACC, FSCAI
Associate Professor of Medicine
Director, Cardiac Catheterization Laboratories
Gill Heart Institute, University of Kentucky
Lexington, Kentucky

Rodrigo Modolo, MD, PhD
Department of Cardiology
Amsterdam University Medical Center
Amsterdam, Netherlands
Department of Internal Medicine
Cardiology Division
University of Campinas (UNICAMP)
Campinas, Brazil

Gilles Montalescot, MD, PhD
Pitié-Salpêtrière University Hospital
Institut de Cardiologie
Paris, France

Pedro R. Moreno, MD
The Zena and Michael A. Weiner
  Cardiovascular Institute
The Marie-Josée and Henry R. Kravis
  Cardiovascular Health Center
Icahn School of Medicine at Mount Sinai
New York, New York

Jeffrey W. Moses, MD
Interventional Cardiology
New York Presbyterian Hospital
Columbia University Medical Center
New York, New York

Debabrata Mukherjee, MD
Chairman, Department of Internal
  Medicine
Chief, Cardiovascular Medicine
Texas Tech University
El Paso, Texas

Dale J. Murdoch, MBBS
Centre for Heart Valve Innovation
St Paul's Hospital
University of British Columbia
Vancouver, Canada

Sahar Naderi, MD
Division of Cardiology
Kaiser Permanente, San Francisco
  Medical Center
San Francisco, California

Srihari Naidu, MD
Director, Cardiac Catheterization
  Laboratory
Division of Cardiology
Winthrop University Hospital
Mineola, New York
Associate Professor of Medicine
SUNY Stony Brook School of Medicine
Stony Brook, New York

Craig R. Narins, MD
Associate Professor of Medicine and
  Surgery
Divisions of Cardiology and Vascular
  Surgery
University of Rochester Medical Center
Rochester, New York

Nima Nasiri, MD
Research Fellow in Medicine
Division of Cardiovascular Medicine
Beth Israel Deaconess Medical Center
Boston, Massachusetts

Eliano P. Navarese, MD, PhD
Interventional Cardiology and
  Cardiovascular Medicine
Mater Dei Hospital and SIRIO
  MEDICINE Research Network
Bari, Italy;
Faculty of Medicine
University of Alberta
Edmonton, Canada

Gjin Ndrepepa, MD
Professor of Cardiology
Deutsches Herzzentrum München
Technische Universität
Munich, Germany

Franz-Josef Neumann, MD, PhD
Endowed Professor of Cardiovascular
  Medicine
University of Frieburg
Medical Director
Division of Cardiology and Angiology II
University Heart Center Freigurg - Bad
  Krozingen
Bad Krozingen, Germany

Christoph A. Nienaber, MD
Imperial College
The Royal Brompton & Harefield NHS
  Trust
Cardiology and Aortic Centre
London, England

Yoshinobu Onuma, MD, PhD
Thoraxcenter, Erasmus Medical Center;
Cardialysis
Rotterdam, Netherlands

Igor F. Palacios, MD
Associate Professor of Medicine
Director, Interventional Cardiology
  Fellowship Program
Director, Interventional Cardiology
  Research
Baylor College of Medicine
Director, Interventional Cardiology
The Michael E. DeBakey VA Medical
  Center
Houston, Texas

Tullio Palmerini, MD
Unità Operativa di Cardiologia
Dipartimento Cardio-Toraco-Vascolare
Policlinico S. Orsola
Bologna, Italy

Duk-Woo Park, MD, PhD
Associate Professor
Department of Cardiology
Asan Medical Center
University of Ulsan College of Medicine
Seoul, Republic of Korea

Seung-Jung Park, MD, PhD
Professor
Department of Cardiology
Asan Medical Center
University of Ulsan College of Medicine
Seoul, Republic of Korea

Manesh R. Patel, MD
Department of Medicine
Duke University Medical Center
Durham, North Carolina

Marc S. Penn, MD, PhD
Director of Research
Director of Cardiovascular Medicine
  Fellowship
Summa Health Heart and Vascular
  Institute
Summa Health System
Akron, Ohio;
Professor of Medicine
Integrative Medical Sciences
Northeast Ohio Medical University
Rootstown, Ohio

Jeffrey J. Popma, MD
Director, Interventional Cardiology
  Clinical Services
Medicine (Cardiovascular Division)
Beth Israel Deaconess Medical Center
Professor of Medicine
Harvard Medical School
Boston, Massachusetts

Matthew J. Price, MD
Assistant Professor
Director, Cardiac Catheterization
  Laboratory
Division of Cardiovascular Diseases
Scripps Clinic
La Jolla, California

Lorenz Räber, MD, PhD
Cardiology Department
Bern University Hospital
Bern, Switzerland

Vivek Rajagopal, MD
Staff Cardiologist
Piedmont Heart Institute
Atlanta, Georgia

Sunil V. Rao, MD
Duke Clinical Research Institute
Durham, North Carolina

Robert F. Riley, MD, MS, FACC, FAHA, FSCAI
Medical Director, Complex Coronary
  Therapeutics Program
Heart and Vascular Center
The Christ Hospital, Lindner Center for
  Research and Education
Cincinnati, Ohio

Madhur A. Roberts, MD
Interventional Cardiology Fellow
Cardiology
Westchester Medical Center
Valhalla, New York

Marco Roffi, MD
Cardiology Division
University Hospital
Geneva, Switzerland

Jason H. Rogers, MD
Division of Cardiovascular Medicine
University of California, Davis
Sacramento, California

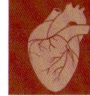

R. Kevin Rogers, MD, MSc, RPVI
Associate Professor
Program Director, Vascular Medicine & Intervention
Interventional Cardiology
University of Colorado
Aurora, Colorado

Jennifer A. Rymer, MD, MBA
Department of Medicine
Duke University Medical Center
Durham, North Carolina

Bruno Scheller, MD
Clinical and Experimental Interventional Cardiology
University of Saarland
Homburg/Saar, Germany

Beth A. Schueler, PhD
Professor of Medical Physics
Department of Radiology
Mayo Clinic
Rochester, Minnesota

Joshua Seinfeld, MD
Department of Neurosurgery
University of Colorado School of Medicine
Aurora, Colorado

Patrick W. Serruys, MD, PhD
National Heart and Lung Institute, Faculty of Medicine
Imperial College London
London, England

Margot M. Sherman Jollis, BS
Denison University
Granville, Ohio

Kunihiro Shimamura, MD
Department of Cardiovascular Medicine
Wakayama Medical University
Wakayama, Japan

Satya S. Shreeniva, MD
Interventional Cardiologist
The Lindner Research Center
Division of Cardiology
The Christ Hospital
Cincinnati, Ohio

Kevin H. Silver, MD
Director, Coronary Intensive Care Unit
Director, Cardiac Catheterization Lab
Summa Health Heart and Vascular Institute
Summa Health System
Akron, Ohio

Mitchell J. Silver, DO, FACC, FSVM, RPVI
Interventional Cardiologist
OhioHealth Heart and Vascular
Columbus, Ohio

Daniel I. Simon, MD
University Hospitals Harrington Heart & Vascular Institute
Case Western Reserve University School of Medicine
Cleveland, Ohio

Danielle N. Sin, MS
Senior Research Coordinator
Division of Adult Cardiac Surgery
NYU Langone Medical Center
New York, New York

Gagan D. Singh, MD
Division of Cardiovascular Medicine
University of California, Davis
Sacramento, California

Paul A. Sobotka, MD
Affiliated Clinical Professor
Medicine/Cardiology
The Ohio State University
Columbus, Ohio

Nishtha Sodhi, MD
Structural Heart Disease & Interventional Cardiology Fellow
Cardiovascular Department
Barnes Jewish Hospital of Washington University
St. Louis, Missouri

Paul Sorajja, MD
Roger L. and Lynn C. Headrick Chair, Valve Science Center Director
Center for Valve and Structural Heart Disease
Minneapolis Heart Institute, Abbott Northwestern Hospital
Minneapolis, Minnesota

Sabato Sorrentino, MD, PhD
The Zena and Michael A. Wiener Cardiovascular Institute
Icahn School of Medicine at Mount Sinai
New York, New York

Goran Stankovic, MD, PhD
Clinic for Cardiology
Department for Diagnostic and Catheterization Laboratories
Clinical Center of Serbia
Faculty of Medicine
University of Belgrade
Belgrade, Serbia

Curtiss T. Stinis, MD
Director, Peripheral Interventions
Program Director, Interventional Cardiology Fellowship
Division of Interventional Cardiology
Scripps Clinic
La Jolla, California

Matthew Summers, MD
Fellow Physician
Interventional Cardiology
Cleveland Clinic Foundation
Cleveland, Ohio

Paul S. Teirstein, MD
Interventional Cardiology
Scripps Clinic
La Jolla, California

On Topaz, MD, FACC, FACP, FSCAI
Professor of Medicine
Duke University School of Medicine
Chief, Division of Cardiology
Charles George Veterans Affairs Medical Center
Asheville, North Carolina

Mark K. Tuttle, MD
Fellow, Division of Cardiovascular Medicine
Beth Israel Deaconess Medical Center
Clinical Fellow, Harvard Medical School
Boston, Massachusetts

Alec Vahanian, MD, FESC, FRCP (Edin.)
Professor of Cardiology
University of Paris VII
Paris, France

Miguel Valderrábano, MD, FACC
Lois and Carl Davis Centennial Chair, Methodist DeBakey Heart and Vascular Center
Associate Professor of Medicine, Weill College of Medicine, Cornell University
Director, Division of Cardiac Electrophysiology
Department of Cardiology
Houston Methodist Hospital
Houston, Texas

Birgit Vogel, MD
The Zena and Michael A. Wiener Cardiovascular Institute
Icahn School of Medicine at Mount Sinai
New York, New York

Amit N. Vora, MD, MPH
Duke Clinical Research Institute
Durham, North Carolina

Robert Wagner, MD, PhD
Department of Pediatric Cardiology
University of Leipzig, Heart Center
Leipzig, Germany

John G. Webb, MD
Centre for Heart Valve Innovation
St Paul's Hospital
University of British Columbia
Vancouver, Canada

William S. Weintraub, MD
MedStar Heart & Vascular Institute
Georgetown University
Washington, DC

Sandra Weiss, MD
Christiana Care Health System
Newark, Delaware

Christopher J. White, MD, MSCAI, FACC, FAHA, FESC, FACP
Professor and Chairman of Medicine
The Ochsner Clinical School, University of Queensland
Chief of Medical Services
Ochsner Medical Center
New Orleans, Louisiana

Wendy Whiteside, MD
Assistant Professor of Pediatrics
University of Michigan Division of Pediatric Cardiology
C. S. Mott Children's Hospital Congenital Heart Center
Ann Arbor, Michigan

R. Jay Widmer, MD, PhD
Assistant Professor of Internal Medicine
Baylor Scott and White
Temple, Texas

Mathew R. Williams, MD
Associate Professor of Cardiothoracic Surgery & Medicine
Chief, Division of Adult Cardiac Surgery
Director, Interventional Cardiology
Director, CVI Structural Heart Program
NYU Langone Medical Center
New York, New York

Daaboul Yazan, MD
Research Fellow
PERFUSE Study Group
Cardiovascular Division, Department of Medicine
Beth Israel Deaconess Medical Center
Harvard Medical School
Boston, Massachusetts

Paul G. Yock, MD, MA, AB
Martha Meier Weiland Professor
Bioengineering and Medicine
Stanford University
Stanford, California

Katherine Yu, MD
Fellow
University of Southern California
Los Angeles, California

Alan Zajarias, MD
Associate professor of Medicine
Co-director, Center of Valvular Heart Disease
Cardiovascular Division
Washington University school of medicine
St. Louis, Missouri

Jeffrey D. Zampi, MD
Assistant Professor of Pediatrics
University of Michigan Division of Pediatric Cardiology
C. S. Mott Children's Hospital Congenital Heart Center
Ann Arbor, Michigan

Khaled M. Ziada, MD, FACC, FSCAI
Professor of Medicine
Clinical Chief of Cardiology
Director, Cardiovascular Interventional Fellowship Program
Gill Heart Institute, University of Kentucky
Lexington, Kentucky

David A. Zidar, MD, PhD
University Hospitals Harrington Heart & Vascular Institute
Case Western Reserve University School of Medicine
Cleveland, Ohio

Andrew A. Ziskind, MD
Senior Vice President, Premier's Academic Health System Strategy
Premier Inc.
Charlotte, North Carolina

编译委员会名单

丛书编译委员会顾问专家

高润霖（中国医学科学院阜外医院）
汪忠镐（首都医科大学宣武医院）

丛书编译委员会组长

吴永健（中国医学科学院阜外医院）
张　健（中国医学科学院阜外医院）

主任委员

吴永健（中国医学科学院阜外医院）
柳景华（首都医科大学附属北京安贞医院）

副主任委员（按姓氏笔画排序）

张洪亮（中国医学科学院阜外医院）
彭红玉（首都医科大学附属北京安贞医院）

委　员（按姓氏笔画排序）

丁　诚（中国医学科学院阜外医院）
丰德京（中国医学科学院阜外医院）
王　枞（首都医科大学附属北京安贞医院）
王　真（中国医学科学院阜外医院）
王　媛（首都医科大学附属北京友谊医院）
王　璨（中国医学科学院阜外医院）
王宇彬（首都医科大学宣武医院）
王玮玮（中国医学科学院阜外医院）
王彬成（中国医学科学院阜外医院）
见　闻（首都医科大学附属北京安贞医院）
牛冠男（中国医学科学院阜外医院）
叶蕴青（中国医学科学院阜外医院）
申学谦（首都医科大学附属北京安贞医院）
吕俊兴（中国医学科学院阜外医院）
刘严慈（首都医科大学附属北京安贞医院）
李　喆（中国医学科学院阜外医院）
李凡奇（首都医科大学附属北京安贞医院）
李子昂（中国医学科学院阜外医院）
李长江（首都医科大学附属北京安贞医院）
李英凯（首都医科大学附属北京安贞医院）
李秋忆（中国医学科学院阜外医院）
李秋雨（首都医科大学附属北京安贞医院）
杨　城（中国医学科学院阜外医院）
杨岚姝（中国医学科学院阜外医院）
何松原（首都医科大学附属北京安贞医院）
谷　喆（中国医学科学院阜外医院）
张　倩（中国医学科学院阜外医院）
张　斌（中国医学科学院阜外医院）
张而立（中国医学科学院阜外医院）
张宇轩（中国医学科学院阜外医院）
张宇超（首都医科大学附属北京安贞医院）
张洪亮（中国医学科学院阜外医院）
陈　阳（中国医学科学院阜外医院）
陈文杰（首都医科大学附属北京安贞医院）
陈思源（首都医科大学附属北京安贞医院）
苗旭光（首都医科大学附属北京安贞医院）
范　谦（首都医科大学附属北京安贞医院）
林小龙（首都医科大学附属北京安贞医院）
周　政（中国医学科学院阜外医院）
孟　真（中国医学科学院阜外医院）
赵天禄（首都医科大学附属北京安贞医院）
赵庆豪（中国医学科学院阜外医院）
赵宇昊（首都医科大学附属北京安贞医院）
赵振燕（中国医学科学院阜外医院）
胡祥铭（中国医学科学院阜外医院）
柳景华（首都医科大学附属北京安贞医院）
段振娅（中国医学科学院阜外医院）
姚　晶（首都医科大学附属北京安贞医院）
郭　帅（中国医学科学院阜外医院）
崔　松（首都医科大学附属北京安贞医院）
梁敬轩（首都医科大学附属北京安贞医院）
彭红玉（首都医科大学附属北京安贞医院）
程子超（首都医科大学附属北京安贞医院）
谢慕蓉（中国医学科学院阜外医院）
薄小雯（首都医科大学附属北京安贞医院）

原书前言

Textbook of Interventional Cardiology（8th Edition）的修订是本系列丛书出版以来最大的一次更新。本书充分涵盖近期介入心脏病学领域令人激动的进展，并强调严格的循证方法。本次修订新增的内容涉及冠状动脉微血管疾病的诊断和治疗、经皮三尖瓣修复和瓣中瓣介入。多年来，随着心脏支架技术的逐步成熟和药物治疗的进展，冠状动脉介入治疗的预后情况变得越来越可预测，而且在许多方面成为常规诊疗手段。在某些方面，介入心脏病学领域失去了一些开创性的火花，而这些火花从 20 世纪 80 年代开始就成为本学科最突出的特点。在那个激动人心的时代，在冠状动脉中行球囊血管成形术的结果往往是难以预测的，支架内血栓的风险相比如今也是难以预料的。介入心脏病学专家和科学家不仅要应对独特个案病例的挑战，而且要发现重要的创新，使该专业的突出地位和重要性得以延续。

如今，这些挑战仍在继续，但已今非昔比。接受冠状动脉介入治疗患者的复杂程度急剧增加，包括高龄、左主干病变、慢性闭塞病变，以及病情复杂到令医师望而却步的患者。A 型病变的患者到底发生过什么？经皮冠状动脉介入治疗在高 SYNTAX 积分的患者中应该怎样开展？同时，医疗经济方面的要求也给介入心脏学专家带来了更多的负担，包括时间、设备选择上的限制，以及履行对急性心肌梗死等紧急情况的全天候保障责任。此外，还有来自记分制措施和对手术适当性或过度使用的考核压力。但希望这些挑战都能被帮助有症状、生活质量受限的患者康复带来的巨大满足感所抵消。在医学界，这种感觉最普遍的莫过于经导管主动脉瓣置换术这一重大变革性领域。

本书旨在为介入心脏病学领域人士提供参考资料，其中不仅包括执业心脏病专家，还包括参与手术的团队、转诊医师，以及那些正在接受培训或有志于培训的人员。我们为许多章节邀请了新的作者，以提供一种全新的感受与视角，每一章的作者都是本领域中被广泛认可的专家学者。展望未来，我们充分认识到需要加强与心脏外科医师的合作——将介入与外科手术最擅长的方面进行交叉融合，在通力合作下使得心脏瓣膜手术日益普及，使更多患者受益。

我们想对来自世界各地的作者表示真诚和深切的感谢，他们为本书做出了巨大的贡献。他们共同组成了一个杰出的智囊团，我们在审核本书内容时从他们那里学到了很多。感谢 Elsevier 的 Mary Hegeler 对这项工作的专业支持，尤其特别感谢心血管读者群体，30 多年来他们一直支持本系列书使之成为主要的参考教材来源。这代表着我们要保持一种巨大的责任感，希望本书不负众望，甚至超出预期。

Eric J. Topol, MD
Paul S. Teirstein, MD
La Jolla, California, 2019

原书献词

感谢众多介入心脏病学专家、科学家和工程师，在过去的 40 年里，他们从根本上改变了心脏病的治疗方法，帮助了大量患者。

编译主任委员前言

介入心脏病学的产生和发展彻底改变了心血管疾病的治疗方式。在介入心脏病学出现之前，心血管疾病的治疗是以药物为主要形式的内科治疗和以开胸手术为主要形式的外科治疗，因此绝大多数医院将心血管疾病的诊疗科室分为心内科和心外科。介入心脏病学对于内科医师是创伤性治疗，而对于外科医师是微创治疗。介入心脏病学一经出现即显示出强大的生命力，患者因微创而乐于接受，更重要的是治疗效果逐渐接近外科手术，某些情况下甚至优于外科手术，如冠心病的介入治疗，早期只能治疗少数病变比较简单的患者，如今几乎可以治疗95%以上的患者，包括左主干病变、慢性闭塞病变、严重钙化病变等，而且随着药物洗脱支架和药物球囊的更新换代，效果越来越好。再如，老年瓣膜性心脏病、主动脉瓣狭窄的经导管主动脉瓣置换术早期，只能用于外科极高危手术或不能进行外科手术的患者。现今随着器械的改进和技术的提高，经导管主动脉瓣置换术可以用于外科低危患者、二叶式主动脉瓣狭窄的患者和单纯主动脉瓣反流的患者。介入心脏病学最初源于内科，目前部分外科医师也积极地投入进来，充分说明介入治疗技术的优势。

由Eric J. Topol和Paul S. Teirstein主编的*Textbook of Interventional Cardiology*（8th Edition）于2020年出版，虽然和中国读者见面晚了一些，但其内容和先进性依然具有可读性和吸引力。正如主编在其前言所说，第8版相较于以前的所有版本做了很大程度的调整。Eric J. Topol在美国心脏病学界是一位非常值得称道的杰出专家，他在心脏病多个领域成绩斐然，其*Textbook of Interventional Cardiology*作为教科书培育了一代又一代介入心脏病学专家，尤其是冠状动脉介入专家，我国很多介入专家均读过他的专著。本书中所有的作者都是该领域知名专家，而且绝大多数都是临床一线的术者，因此其内容非常具有实战性。第8版在冠心病介入治疗、周围血管介入治疗和结构心脏病介入治疗基础上增加了很多新的内容，如冠状动脉微循环、经皮三尖瓣修复和瓣中瓣介入。本书很多章节加入了新的作者，而且都是现阶段介入心脏病学的主流专家，体现了第8版的与时俱进。本书给读者的印象不再是一味地强调介入技术和循证医学的重要性，而是更多地侧重患者作为个体的特殊性和相应的治疗策略，以人为本的理念贯穿全书，体现了现代医学的进步和升华。

为了尽快将本书介绍给中国读者，玲珑医学经努力获得了本书在中国的 Elsevier 出版授权，并由科学技术文献出版社出版这部影印版的《介入心脏病学（第 8 版）》。所谓影印版即编译者对书中的每一章节进行中文导读的编撰，这样读者既可以快速了解该章节的主要内容，也可以对所感兴趣章节的英文原文进行详细阅读。这是在图书进口和翻译工作中的一次大胆尝试，主要考虑到我国读者的英文阅读能力普遍提高，且临床工作比较繁忙，使阅读成为一种奢侈，而本书可以满足读者的不同需求。参与本书的编译者是来自中国医学科学院阜外医院和首都医科大学安贞医院的两个团队，他们绝大多数都是临床一线的介入专家，具有丰富的临床经验，由衷期待能为大家带来切实的帮助。由于是首次尝试编译工作，个中问题和不足在所难免，还望读者朋友提出批评和指正。

吴永健　柳景华

2022 年 12 月

SECTION I Patient Selection, 1

1. **Individualized Assessment for Percutaneous or Surgical-Based Revascularization**, 5
   Vasim Farooq, Rodrigo Modolo, and Patrick W. Serruys

2. **Evidence-Based Interventional Practice**, 43
   Franz-Josef Neumann, Miroslaw Ferenc, and Kambis Mashayekhi

3. **Diabetes**, 65
   Marco Roffi and Baris Gencer

4. **Noninvasive Evaluation: Functional Testing, Multidetector Computed Tomography, and Stress Cardiac MRI**, 81
   Vikram M. Brahmanandam and Mario J. Garcia

5. **Intracoronary Pressure and Flow Measurements**, 103
   Morton J. Kern, Michael J. Lim, and Katherine Yu

6. **Contrast-Induced Acute Kidney Injury and the Role of Chronic Kidney Disease in Percutaneous Coronary Intervention**, 133
   Roxana Mehran, Birgit Vogel, and Sabato Sorrentino

7. **Radiation Safety During Cardiovascular Procedures**, 145
   Beth A. Schueler, Kenneth A. Fetterly, and Stephen Balter

8. **Coronary and Valvular Intervention Prior to Noncardiac Surgery**, 159
   Craig R. Narins

9. **Sex and Ethnicity Issues in Interventional Cardiology**, 173
   Matthew R. Summers, Sahar Naderi, and Leslie Cho

SECTION II Pharmacologic Intervention, 185

10. **Platelet Inhibitor Agents**, 189
    Matthew J. Price and Dominick J. Angiolillo

11. **Anticoagulation in Percutaneous Coronary Intervention**, 215
    Trent Hartshorne and Derek P. Chew

12. **Thrombolytic Intervention**, 229
    Matthews Chacko and Khalil Ibrahim

13. **Other Adjunctive Drugs for Coronary Intervention: Beta-Blockers, Calcium-Channel Blockers, and Angiotensin-Converting Enzyme Inhibitors**, 247
    David W. Allen and Vivek Rajagopal

SECTION III Coronary Intervention, 257

14. **Coronary Stenting: Practical Considerations, Equipment Selection, Tips and Caveats**, 261
    Elliott M. Groves and Curtiss T. Stinis

15. **Coronary Stenting**, 275
    Tullio Palmerini and Ajay J. Kirtane

16. **Bioresorbable Coronary Scaffolds**, 329
    Athanasios Katsikis, Rodrigo Modolo, Yuki Katagiri, Yoshinobu Onuma, and Patrick W. Serruys

17. **Drug-Eluting Balloons**, 343
    Bruno Scheller

18. **Elective Intervention for Stable Angina or Silent Ischemia**, 353
    Gregory W. Barsness, David E. Kandzari, and Eliano P. Navarese

19. **Intervention for Non-ST-Segment Elevation Acute Coronary Syndromes**, 373
    C. Michael Gibson, Serge Korjian, and Yazan Daaboul

20. **Percutaneous Coronary Intervention in Acute ST-Segment Elevation Myocardial Infarction**, 391
    Gjin Ndrepepa, Robert A. Byrne, and Adnan Kastrati

21. **Post-Percutaneous Coronary Intervention Hospitalization, Length of Stay, and Discharge Planning**, 439
    Amit N. Vora and Sunil V. Rao

22. **Interventions in Cardiogenic Shock**, 451
    Satya S. Shreenivas, Scott M. Lilly, and Howard C. Herrmann

23. **Bifurcations and Branch Vessel Stenting**, 461
    Antonio Colombo and Goran Stankovic

24. **Percutaneous Coronary Intervention for Unprotected Left Main Coronary Artery Stenosis**, 483
    Jung-Min Ahn, Duk-Woo Park, and Seung-Jung Park

25. **Complex and Multivessel Percutaneous Coronary Intervention**, 493
    Sergio Buccheri and Davide Capodanno

26. **Intervention for Coronary Chronic Total Occlusions**, 505
    Ravi S. Hira and William L. Lombardi

27. **Bypass Graft Intervention**, 519
    John S. Douglas, Jr.

28. **The Thrombus-Containing Lesion**, 537
    On Topaz

29. **Complications of Percutaneous Coronary Intervention**, 565
    Marvin H. Eng, Jeffrey W. Moses, and Paul S. Teirstein

30. **Periprocedural Myocardial Infarction and Embolism-Protection Devices**, 587
    Adrian W. Messerli, Khaled M. Ziada, and Debabrata Mukherjee

31. **Access Management and Closure Devices**, 613
    Fernando Cura and Marcelo Abud

32. **Transradial Access for Cardiovascular Catheterization and Intervention**, 629
    Farzin Beygui, Olivier F. Bertrand, and Gilles Montalescot

33 Role of the Cardiac Surgeon and the Heart Team, 645
Kazuhiro Hisamoto, Danielle N. Sin, and Mathew R. Williams

34 Restenosis, 657
David A. Zidar, Marco A. Costa, and Daniel I. Simon

35 Role of Adjunct Devices: Atherectomy, Cutting Balloon, and Laser, 671
John A. Bittl

36 Supported Percutaneous Intervention, 687
Srihari S. Naidu, Madhur A. Roberts, and Howard C. Herrmann

37 Regional Centers of Excellence for the Care of Patients With Acute Ischemic Heart Disease, 705
Robert F. Riley, Timothy D. Henry, and Dean J. Kereiakes

38 Diagnosis and Treatment of Coronary Microvascular Disease, 721
Amir Lerman and R. Jay Widmer

SECTION IV Peripheral Vascular Interventions, 729

39 Lower Extremity Interventions, 733
Debabrata Mukherjee

40 Upper Extremities and Aortic Arch, 753
Kimberly S. Delcour, Ivan P. Casserly, and Robert S. Dieter

41 Chronic Mesenteric Ischemia: Diagnosis and Intervention, 767
Christopher J. White

42 Renal Artery Stenosis, 773
Waleed Alharbi, Nilesh J. Goswami, and Jeffrey A. Goldstein

43 Device Therapy for Resistant Hypertension, 787
Marat Fudim, Marvin H. Eng, and Paul A. Sobotka

44 Aortic Vascular Interventions (Thoracic and Abdominal), 801
Christoph A. Nienaber and Ibrahim Akin

45 Venous Intervention, 819
Michael A. Jolly and Mitchell J. Silver

46 Carotid and Cerebrovascular Intervention, 841
R. Kevin Rogers, Joshua Seinfeld, and Ivan P. Casserly

47 Stroke Centers and Interventional Cardiology, 867
Christopher J. White

SECTION V Structural Interventions, 875

48 Imaging for Intracardiac Interventions, 879
Nyal Borges, Serge C. Harb, and Samir R. Kapadia

49 Percutaneous Closure of Patent Foramen Ovale and Atrial Septal Defect, 905
Nishtha Sodhi, Alan Zajarias, David T. Balzer, and John M. Lasala

50 Left Atrial Appendage Closure and Stroke: Local Device Therapy for Cardioembolic Stroke Protection, 929
Matthew J. Price and Miguel Valderrábano

51 Mitral Valvuloplasty, 951
Alec Vahanian, Dominique Himbert, Eric Brochet, and Bernard Iung

52 Percutaneous Mitral Valve Repair and Replacement, 963
Amar Krishnaswamy and Samir R. Kapadia

53 Balloon-Expandable Transcatheter Aortic Valve Replacement Systems, 981
Alain G. Cribier, Helene Eltchaninoff, and Alan Zajarias

54 Self-Expanding Transcatheter Aortic Valve Replacement, 1003
Mark K. Tuttle, Nima Nasiri, and Jeffrey J. Popma

55 Percutaneous Transcatheter Valve-in-Valve Implantation, 1029
Dale J. Murdoch and John G. Webb

56 Pulmonary Valve Interventions, 1039
Robert Wagner, Ingo Daehnert, and Philipp C. Lurz

57 Percutaneous Tricuspid Valve Repair, 1057
Gagan D. Singh and Jason H. Rogers

58 Hypertrophic Cardiomyopathy, 1077
Grant Henderson and Samir R. Kapadia

59 Percutaneous Balloon Pericardiotomy for Patients With Pericardial Effusion and Tamponade, 1095
Hani Jneid, Andrew A. Ziskind, and Igor F. Palacios

60 Transcatheter Therapies for Congenital Heart Disease, 1109
Bryan H. Goldstein, Wendy Whiteside, Jeffrey D. Zampi, and Russel Hirsch

61 Stem Cell Therapy for Ischemic Heart Disease, 1137
Vishal Dahya, Kevin H. Silver, and Marc S. Penn

62 Percutaneous Treatment of Paravalvular Leak, 1149
Mario J. Gössl and Paul Sorajja

63 Interventional Heart Failure, 1159
Scott M. Lilly and William T. Abraham

SECTION VI Evaluation of Interventional Techniques, 1167

64 Qualitative and Quantitative Coronary Angiography, 1171
Michael L. Chuang, Alexandra Almonacid, and Jeffrey J. Popma

65 Intravascular Ultrasound, 1193
Yasuhiro Honda, Peter J. Fitzgerald, and Paul G. Yock

66 The Dynamic Spectrum of Coronary Atheroma: From Atherogenesis to Vulnerable Plaque to Plaque Regression, 1213
Pedro R. Moreno and Carlos A. Gonzalez Lengua

67 Optical Coherence Tomography, 1247
Giulio Guagliumi, Lorenz Räber, Kunihiro Shimamura, and Takashi Akasaka

SECTION VII Outcome Effectiveness of Interventional Cardiology, 1275

68 Medical Economics in Interventional Cardiology, 1279
Zaher Fanari, Sandra Weiss, and William S. Weintraub

69 Quality of Care in Interventional Cardiology, 1297
Jennifer A. Rymer, Manesh R. Patel, and Sunil V. Rao

70 Volume and Outcome, 1323
James G. Jollis and Margot M. Sherman Jollis

中文目录

第一部分　患者的选择

第1章　冠状动脉血运重建的个体化评估 …………………………… 3

第2章　以循证医学为基础的介入治疗 …………………………… 41

第3章　糖尿病 …………………………… 63

第4章　无创性评估：功能学检查、多排CT和负荷心脏MRI ……… 79

第5章　冠状动脉内压力和流量测量 …………………………… 101

第6章　对比剂诱导的急性肾损伤和慢性肾脏疾病在经皮冠状动脉介入治疗中的影响 …………………………… 131

第7章　心血管手术中的辐射安全 …………………………… 143

第8章　非心脏外科手术前的冠状动脉/瓣膜介入治疗 …………… 157

第9章　介入心脏病学中的性别与种族问题 ……………………… 171

第二部分　药物治疗

第10章　血小板抑制剂 …………………………… 187

第11章　经皮冠状动脉介入治疗的抗凝治疗 …………………… 213

第12章　溶栓治疗 …………………………… 227

第13章　冠状动脉介入治疗的其他辅助药物：β受体阻滞剂、钙通道阻滞剂和血管紧张素转化酶抑制剂 ……………… 245

第三部分　冠状动脉介入治疗

第14章　冠状动脉支架置入：实践考虑、器械选择、手术技巧和注意事项 …………………………… 259

第15章　冠状动脉支架 …………………………… 273

第16章　生物可吸收冠状动脉支架 …………………………… 327

第17章　药物涂层球囊 …………………………… 341

第18章　稳定型心绞痛和无症状性心肌缺血的选择性干预 ……… 351

第19章　非ST段抬高型急性冠状动脉综合征的干预 …………… 371

第20章	急性ST段抬高型心肌梗死的介入治疗	389
第21章	经皮冠状动脉介入术后的住院治疗、住院时长及出院计划	437
第22章	心源性休克的干预	449
第23章	分叉和边支血管支架置入术	459
第24章	无保护左主干病变的经皮冠状动脉介入治疗	481
第25章	复杂多支病变	491
第26章	慢性完全闭塞病变的介入治疗	503
第27章	桥血管介入治疗	517
第28章	富含血栓病变	535
第29章	经皮冠状动脉介入治疗的并发症	563
第30章	围术期心肌梗死及栓塞保护装置	585
第31章	血管入路管理与血管闭合装置	611
第32章	经桡动脉途径的心血管诊疗	627
第33章	心脏外科医师及心脏团队的作用	643
第34章	再狭窄	655
第35章	辅助器械：切割球囊、激光、冠状动脉斑块旋切术	669
第36章	支持性经皮介入治疗	685
第37章	区域性急性缺血性心脏病救治中心	703
第38章	冠状动脉微血管疾病的诊断与治疗	719

第四部分　外周血管介入治疗

第39章	下肢血管介入	731
第40章	上肢和主动脉弓	751
第41章	慢性肠系膜缺血：诊断和治疗	765
第42章	肾动脉狭窄	771
第43章	难治性高血压的器械治疗	785
第44章	主动脉（胸腹）介入治疗	799
第45章	静脉介入	817
第46章	颈动脉及脑血管介入	839

第47章　卒中中心与介入心脏病学……………………………………… 865

第五部分　结构性心脏病介入治疗

第48章　心腔内介入手术的影像学评估…………………………………… 877

第49章　卵圆孔未闭及房间隔缺损的经皮封堵治疗……………………… 903

第50章　左心耳封堵与卒中：防止心源性卒中的局部器械治疗………… 927

第51章　二尖瓣成形术……………………………………………………… 949

第52章　经皮二尖瓣修复和置换…………………………………………… 961

第53章　球囊扩张式瓣膜经导管主动脉瓣置换术………………………… 979

第54章　自膨胀式瓣膜经导管主动脉瓣置换术…………………………… 1001

第55章　经导管瓣中瓣植入术……………………………………………… 1027

第56章　肺动脉瓣介入治疗………………………………………………… 1037

第57章　经皮三尖瓣修复…………………………………………………… 1055

第58章　肥厚型心肌病……………………………………………………… 1075

第59章　经皮球囊心包切开术治疗心包积液和心脏压塞………………… 1093

第60章　先天性心脏病的经导管治疗……………………………………… 1107

第61章　缺血性心脏病的干细胞治疗……………………………………… 1135

第62章　瓣周漏的经皮介入治疗…………………………………………… 1147

第63章　心力衰竭介入治疗………………………………………………… 1157

第六部分　介入治疗技术的评估

第64章　冠状动脉造影的定性、定量评估………………………………… 1169

第65章　血管内超声………………………………………………………… 1191

第66章　冠状动脉粥样硬化的动态演变：从动脉粥样硬化形成到
　　　　　易损斑块再到斑块消退……………………………………… 1211

第67章　光学相干断层成像………………………………………………… 1245

第七部分　介入心脏病学的疗效

第68章　介入心脏病领域的卫生经济学…………………………………… 1277

第69章　介入心脏病学医疗质量…………………………………………… 1295

第70章　手术量和预后……………………………………………………… 1321

SECTION I

第一部分

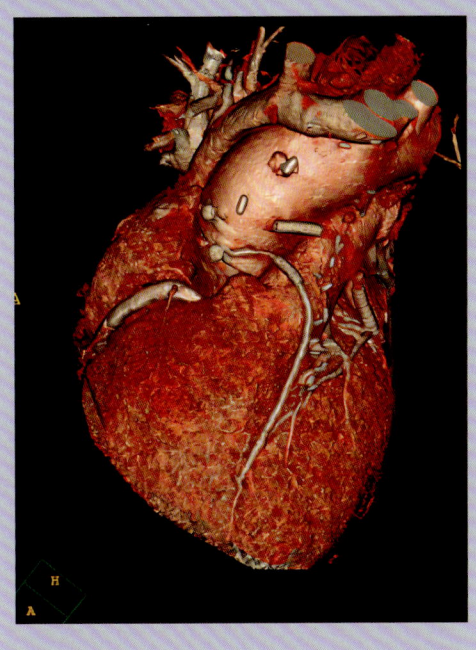

Patient Selection

患者的选择

中文导读

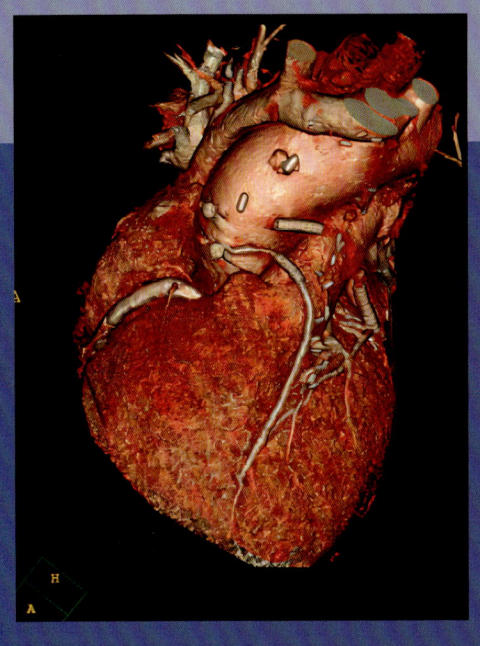

第1章
冠状动脉血运重建的个体化评估

　　自从经皮血管球囊成形术问世以来，冠心病血运重建策略取得了重大的进展，已从传统的、单一的冠状动脉旁路移植术，扩展到经皮冠状动脉介入治疗。无论是冠状动脉旁路移植术或经皮冠状动脉介入治疗，除了技术水平和个人意愿之外，临床和解剖因素会直接影响术后患者的临床预后和获益。因此，血运重建方式的选择（冠状动脉旁路移植术或经皮冠状动脉介入治疗）就成为心脏团队医师需要决策与回答的一个问题。而针对患者个体所做的术前评估，是获得个体化血运重建策略的基础和前提。

　　围绕个体化评估这一主题，本章节对现有临床评分工具做了概括性介绍，包括解剖评分工具（ACC/AHA病变评分等）、心肌风险评分工具（BRRI评分、APPROACH病变评分）、临床评分工具（EuroSCORE评分、NCDR CathPCI危险评分、New Mayo评分等）、综合解剖与临床危险因素的评分工具（EuroHeart PCI评分、NERS评分等）。此外，本章节重点介绍了具有里程碑意义的SYNTAX、FREEDOM和EXCEL研究，并介绍了SYNTAX所衍生出来的各种评分工具，包括解剖SYNTAX评分、临床SYNTAX评分、ACEF评分、SYNTAX Ⅱ评分、残余SYNTAX评分，以及冠状动脉旁路移植术后SYNTAX评分等。本章节还根据上述临床研究，初步阐明了冠状动脉旁路移植术或经皮冠状动脉介入治疗的适用范围。通过本章的介绍，将帮助临床医师合理应用这些评分工具对患者进行风险分层，并帮助临床医师选择患者个体化的血运重建策略。

李长江　彭红玉

章节要点

- 随着需要血运重建患者人群的变化、经皮和外科血运重建技术的进步、当代经皮与外科血运重建对比研究结果的公布，使得临床医师在选择治疗策略之前，必须对每一名患者都做个体化评估。

- 对于接受血运重建的患者，风险分层在患者评估中发挥着重要作用。

- 临床工具大体可分为基于临床并发症的评分工具、基于冠状动脉解剖的评分工具，或涵盖并发症与血管解剖的综合评分工具。这些临床评分工具可用来协助心脏团队对患者个体进行风险分层，并决定最佳的血运重建方式。

- 基于SYNTAX研究得出的临床评分工具，已经从最初的解剖SYNTAX评分（基于单纯的解剖因素）发展出SYNTAX Ⅱ评分（解剖因素联合临床变量），并衍生出可用于评估合理的不完全血运重建（这种不完全血运重建并不影响长期预后）程度的残余SYNTAX评分。目前正在验证这些新开发的临床评分工具的价值。

- 无论是外科或经皮血运重建术，患者的临床和解剖因素都会影响到术后短期和长期的并发症、发病率和死亡率。因此，心脏团队在与患者术前交流选择治疗策略时，应充分考虑到这些影响因素。

SECTION I Patient Selection

1 Individualized Assessment for Percutaneous or Surgical-Based Revascularization

Vasim Farooq, Rodrigo Modolo, Patrick W. Serruys

KEY POINTS

- Changes in the demographics of patients who present in need of revascularization, advances in percutaneous and surgical revascularization techniques, and results from contemporary studies of percutaneous versus surgical revascularization have made it essential that patients be assessed as individuals prior to selection of a treatment strategy.
- Risk stratification plays an important role in the assessment of patients undergoing revascularization.
- Clinical tools used to assist the heart team in risk stratifying patients and deciding the most appropriate revascularization modality can be broadly divided into assessments based on clinical comorbidities, coronary anatomy, or a combination of the two.
- Clinical tools based on the Synergy Between Percutaneous Coronary Intervention With Taxus and Cardiac Surgery (SYNTAX) trial have evolved from purely anatomic factors (anatomic SYNTAX score) to anatomic factors augmented by clinical variables (culminating in the development of the SYNTAX score II) and tools to assess a level of reasonable incomplete revascularization that would not have an adverse effect on long-term morbidity and mortality (residual SYNTAX score). Validation of many of these newly developed clinical tools is ongoing.
- Clinical and anatomic factors have an impact on short- and long-term morbidity and mortality following surgical or percutaneous revascularization and must be considered by the heart team in open dialogue with the patient during the decision-making process.

Revascularization of patients with coronary artery disease (CAD) has progressed exponentially since Andreas Grüntzig[1] performed the first balloon angioplasty in 1977. These developments, which have been fueled by new technology, have blurred the boundary between what was once considered exclusively surgical disease and what can be treated percutaneously. Consequently, there is a greater need than ever to tailor revascularization appropriately, taking into consideration a patient's comorbidities, coronary anatomy, personal preferences, and individual perception of risk. This chapter will explore the increasing requirement for a more individualized assessment of patients undergoing revascularization, and it will review the clinical tools currently available to assist in this decision-making process.

NEED FOR INDIVIDUALIZED PATIENT ASSESSMENT

A number of confounding factors have made it imperative that patients are assessed as individuals prior to the selection of revascularization strategy.

Patient Comorbidities

The demographics of patients presenting to tertiary care services in need of revascularization are constantly evolving. This has been largely the consequence of increased longevity of the general population, a lower threshold to investigate patients who present with symptoms suggestive of obstructive CAD, and increased resources that have made revascularization via percutaneous coronary intervention (PCI) or coronary artery bypass grafting (CABG) more accessible. Together with increased age, patients in need of revascularization are currently more likely to have comorbidities such as diabetes, hypertension, and hyperlipidemia.[2,3] These factors are all implicated in accelerating the progression of CAD, and consequently patients are more likely to present with more extensive CAD. The Arterial Revascularization Therapies Studies (ARTS) parts I and II were separated by a period of 5 years, and despite both studies having the same inclusion criteria, patients in ARTS-II had a significantly greater incidence of risk factors and overall increased disease complexity (Table 1.1).[4]

Patient comorbidities must be taken into consideration when assessing patients for revascularization because they have the potential to significantly influence patient outcomes; moreover, they may have a different impact depending on the underlying revascularization strategy selected. Notably in patients enrolled in the ARTS-I and II studies, patient age was shown to be a significant independent correlate of major adverse cardiovascular and cerebrovascular events (MACCEs) who were treated with CABG.[5] More recently, in the randomized all-comers SYNTAX trial, increasing age was shown to favor PCI over CABG when adjustments were made for other anatomic and clinical factors.[6–8] In addition, other anatomic and clinical factors were shown to have an impact on long-term mortality, and thereby decision making between CABG and PCI (SYNTAX score II[7,8]), and this topic is discussed later under "SYNTAX-Based Clinical Tools."

In a collaborative patient-level analysis of 10 randomized trials of patients with multivessel disease (MVD) treated with PCI using bare-metal stenting (BMS) and CABG, Hlatky and coworkers[9] demonstrated comparable rates of 5-year mortality between both treatment groups in patients without diabetes. Notably, when patients with diabetes were viewed as a whole, mortality was significantly higher in those treated with PCI, even after multivariate adjustment (Fig. 1.1). In the Future Revascularization Evaluation in Patients With Diabetes Mellitus: Optimal Management of Multivessel Disease (FREEDOM) trial,[10,11] it was shown that in patients with diabetes and advanced CAD, CABG was superior to PCI in that it significantly reduced rates

SECTION I Patient Selection

TABLE 1.1 Changing Baseline Demographics of Patients Enrolled in Drug-Eluting Stent Trials

	All-Comers Studies					
	SIRTAX[24]	Leaders[25]	Resolute[27]	Arts-I[28]	Arts-II[172]	SYNTAX[13]
Years of Enrollment	2003–2004	2006–2007	2008	1997–1998	2003	2005–2007
Stent Type	DES	DES	DES	BMS	DES	DES
DEMOGRAPHICS						
Age, years (mean ± SD)	62 ± 11	65 ± 11	64.4 ± 10.9	61 ± 10	63 ± 10	65 ± 10
Diabetes, %	20	24	23.5	19	26	26
Hypertension, %	61	73	71.1	45	67	69
Hypercholesterolemia, %	59	67	63.9	58	74	78
Previous myocardial infarction, %	29	33	28.9	44	34	32
Left ventricular function, % (mean ± SD)	57 ± 12	56 ± 12		61 ± 12	60 ± 12	59 ± 13
LESION CHARACTERISTICS (PER PATIENT)						
Multivessel disease, %	59	23	58.4	96	100	92
Bifurcation lesions, %	8	22	16.9	35	34	72
Total occlusions, %	19	12	16.3	3	17	24
SYNTAX score (mean ± SD)	12 ± 7	14 ± 9	15 ± 9	–	21 ± 10	28 ± 12
Mean number of diseased lesions	1.4	1.5	1.5	2.8	3.6	3.6[a]
PROCEDURAL CHARACTERISTICS (PER PATIENT)						
Mean number of stents	1.2 ± 0.5	1.3 ± 0.7[b]	11.9 ± 7.5	2.8 ± 1.3	3.7 ± 1.5	4.6 ± 2.3
Total stent length, mm (mean ± SD)	25.9 ± 15.5	24.7 ± 15.5[b]	34.4 ± 24.5	47.6 ± 21.7	72.5 ± 32.1	86.1 ± 47.9

[a]Treated lesions.
[b]Per lesion.
BMS, Bare-metal stent; *DES*, drug-eluting stent; *SD*, standard deviation; *SYNTAX*, Synergy Between Percutaneous Coronary Intervention with Taxus and Cardiac Surgery.

of death and myocardial infarction (MI) but at the expense of a higher rate of stroke (Fig. 1.2).[11] In addition, using the American College of Cardiology Foundation (ACCF) National Cardiovascular Data Registry (NCDR) and the Society of Thoracic Surgeons (STS) Adult Cardiac Surgery Database, Weintraub and colleagues[12] found that subjects who had elective intervention for MVD had a long-term survival advantage among patients who underwent CABG compared with PCI (Fig. 1.3). Findings have been corroborated in the randomized, all-comers SYNTAX trial,[13–16] as discussed later.

In addition, within the randomized Evaluation of the Xience Everolimus-Eluting Stent Versus Coronary Artery Bypass Surgery for Effectiveness of Left Main Revascularization (EXCEL) trial, in appropriately selected patients with left main (LM) CAD (low-intermediate anatomic SYNTAX scores), PCI with everolimus-eluting stents was shown to be noninferior to CABG with respect to the rate of the composite end point of death, stroke, or MI at 3 years (Fig. 1.4A).[17,18] Moreover, a substantially greater early benefit in quality of life (QOL) was evident with PCI at 1 month, with a similar QOL improvement at 36 months with both PCI and CABG (see Fig. 1.4B).[19] This corroborates findings originally made in the original landmark SYNTAX trial.[20] Conversely, in the randomized NOBLE[21] (Nordic-Baltic-British left main revascularisation study) and BEST (The Randomized Comparison of Coronary Artery Bypass Surgery and Everolimus-Eluting Stent Implantation in the Treatment of Patients with Multivessel Coronary Artery Disease) trials[22] investigating patients with unprotected LM and MVD, respectively, CABG was shown to offer superior long-term clinical outcomes compared with PCI with contemporary drug-eluting stents (DESs); notably in both trials, patients were not appropriately risk stratified and appropriately selected as occurred in EXCEL. Consequently, an urgent need exists for clinical tools that account for both anatomic and clinical factors and comorbidity to assist the heart team in decision making in regard to the most appropriate revascularization modality in patients with complex CAD.

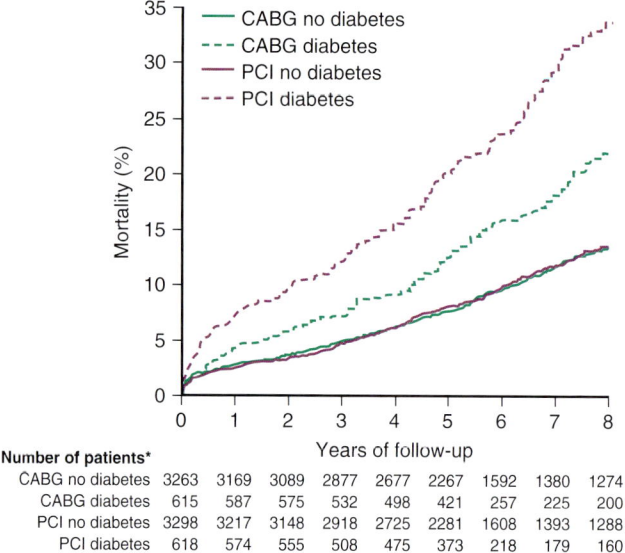

Fig. 1.1 Cumulative survival curve of long-term mortality stratified according to diabetic status among patients with multivessel disease randomized to treatment with percutaneous coronary intervention *(PCI)* or coronary artery bypass grafting *(CABG)*. The importance of diabetic status on outcomes are highlighted not only by the higher mortality among patients with diabetes compared with nondiabetics but also by the greater impact diabetic status had on patients treated with PCI compared with CABG. *Number of patients available for follow-up. (From Hlatky MA, Boothroyd DB, Bravata DM, et al. Coronary artery bypass surgery compared with percutaneous coronary interventions for multivessel disease: a collaborative analysis of individual patient data from ten randomised trials. *Lancet.* 2009;373[9670]:1190–1197.)

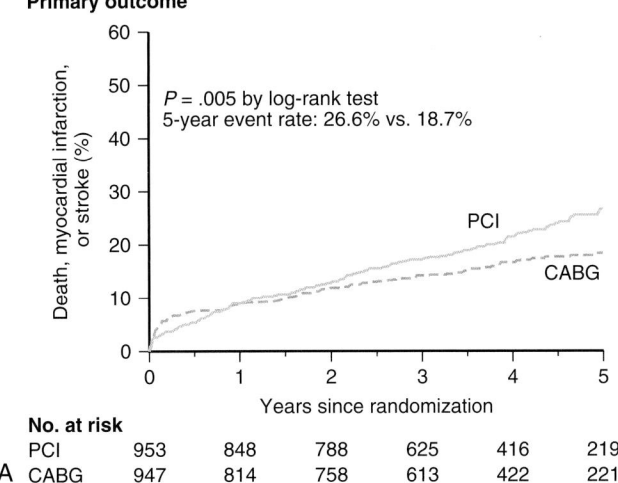
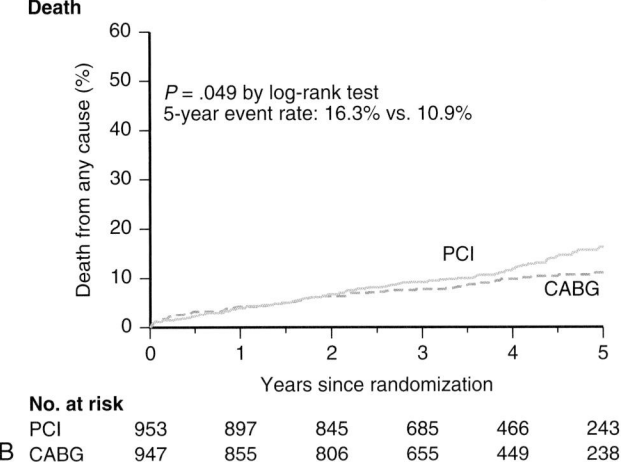

Fig. 1.2 Kaplan-Meier Estimates of the Composite Primary Outcome of death, myocardial infarction (MI), or stroke (A) and death from any cause (B) truncated at 5 years after randomization in the FREEDOM trial. In FREEDOM, patients with diabetes and multivessel coronary artery disease were assigned to undergo either percutaneous coronary intervention *(PCI)* with first-generation drug-eluting stents or coronary artery bypass grafting *(CABG)*. Patients were followed for a minimum of 2 years (median among survivors, 3.8 years), and CABG was shown to be superior to PCI with first-generation drug-eluting stents with significant reduced rates of death (10.9% vs. 16.3%, *P* = .049) and MI (6.0% vs. 13.9%, *P* < .001) but a higher rate of stroke (5.2% vs. 2.4%, *P* = .03). (From FREEDOM Trial Investigators. Strategies for multivessel revascularization in patients with diabetes. *N Engl J Med.* 2012;367(25):2375–2384.)

TECHNOLOGIC ADVANCES

The introduction in 2002 of DESs revolutionized the practice of interventional cardiology and was driven primarily through the dramatic reduction in rates of repeat revascularization.[23] The favorable results observed with DES use promptly resulted in an expansion of the indications for PCI, such that bifurcation lesions, chronic total occlusions (CTOs), and MVD were no longer in the exclusive domain of surgical revascularization, and these were increasingly treated with PCI. Evidence of this expansion can be seen in the changing baseline lesion characteristics of patients enrolled in all-comers PCI trials such as the Sirolimus-Eluting and Paclitaxel-Eluting Stents for Coronary Revascularization (SIRTAX) trial,[24] the Limus Eluted From a Durable Versus Erodable Stent Coating Study (LEADERS),[25,26] the Clinical Evaluation of the Resolute Zotarolimus-Eluting Coronary Stent System in the Treatment of De Novo Lesions in Native Coronary Arteries (RESOLUTE),[27] and in studies of complex three-vessel disease (3VD) and/or LM CAD, such as ARTS-I,[28] ARTS-II,[26] and the SYNTAX trial (see Table 1.1).[13–16] Further evidence in support of this change comes from assessments of real world clinical practice, which indicate that approximately one-third of patients with complex CAD are currently treated with PCI.[29] This practice has been coupled with the expanding use of PCI, driven largely through advances in PCI technology, with more deliverable newer-generation DESs, lower-profile balloons, new guidewires, adjunctive devices to aid stent delivery, crossing and reentry systems to aid total occlusion revascularization, functional assessment of lesions, intravascular ultrasound (IVUS) guidance to ensure adequate stent expansion, dedicated specialists for specific anatomic subsets including CTO operators with high successful revascularization rates, introduction of new adjunctive pharmacologic therapies, and the increasing availability of percutaneous extracorporeal circulatory support (eFig. 1.1).[30–36] From a technical perspective, a large subset of coronary lesions can currently be addressed with PCI; however, it is important to emphasize that the percutaneous approach to revascularization requires individual patient selection to ensure that it is appropriate.

HISTORIC (PRE-SYNTAX) CLINICAL TRIAL RESULTS

Historically, and prior to the publication of the SYNTAX trial,[13–16] randomized trials to compare CABG and PCI centered on two major patient groups: either isolated proximal left anterior descending (LAD) artery lesions or complex CAD (3VD and/or LM disease). Although results of these studies suggest no differences were found in the hard clinical outcomes of death and MI between patients treated with PCI or CABG at short- and long-term follow-up (Table 1.2),[9,37–41] there was profound selection bias in enrollment of patients prior to randomization. Specifically, between 2% and 12% of screened patients were randomized in most trials (Table 1.3), with patients with lesser comorbidities, such as impaired left ventricular function or coronary anatomy (predominantly single- or double-vessel disease) often "cherry-picked" prior to randomization.[42–44] Consequently, interpreting and extrapolating these results to routine and contemporary clinical practice has been challenging.

SYNTAX Trial

The landmark SYNTAX trial[13–16] represents the largest (and only) assessment of revascularization with PCI or CABG in all-comers with complex CAD. SYNTAX aimed to supply evidence to support the somewhat established but non–evidence-based practice of performing PCI in patients with complex CAD.[29] In addition, SYNTAX also sought to identify which patients should be treated with CABG only. Through an all-comers design, SYNTAX addressed the limitations of the earlier CABG versus PCI trials, which were plagued by profound selection bias as previously discussed (see Table 1.3),[43,44] and in doing so it was anticipated that the results would be more relevant to contemporary routine clinical practice. Specifically:

- To ensure results were applicable to routine practice, the study was designed as an all-comers trial such that there were no specific inclusion criteria other than the need to have revascularization of de novo 3VD or unprotected LM CAD (in isolation or with CAD). Exclusion criteria were limited to prior revascularization, ongoing MI, and patients requiring concomitant cardiac surgery.[16] In contrast to the earlier studies, 70.9% of eligible patients were enrolled.
- The previously indicated problem of reporting outcomes from all patients with complex CAD together, irrespective of disease severity, was addressed in the SYNTAX trial through the

SECTION I Patient Selection

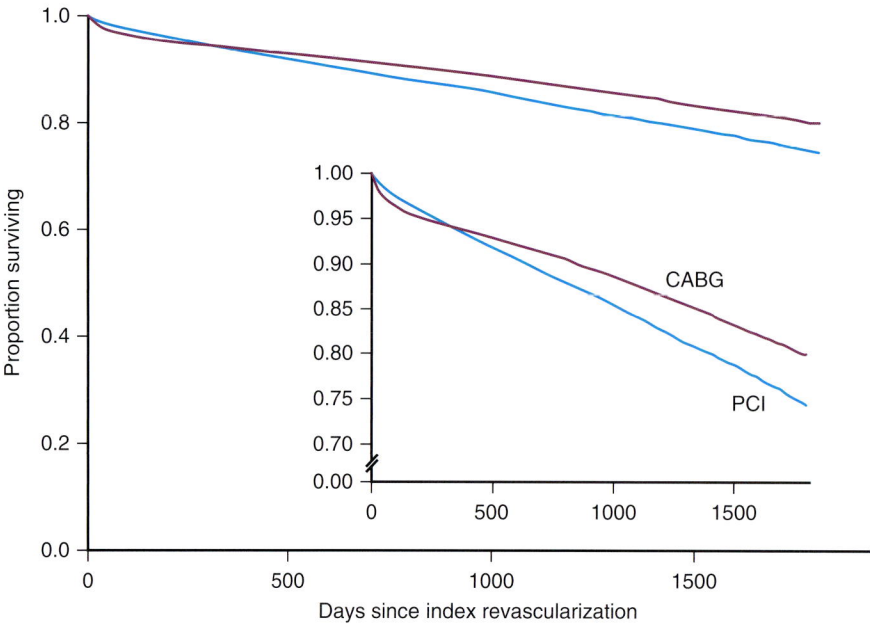

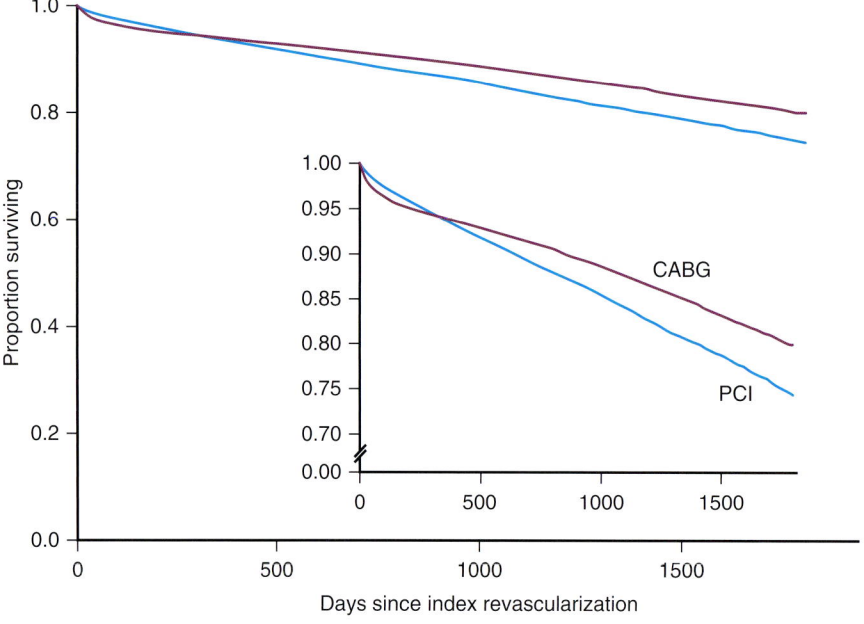

Fig. 1.3 Incidence of survival in the coronary artery bypass grafting *(CABG)* and percutaneous coronary intervention *(PCI)* cohorts, from unadjusted (A) and adjusted (B) analyses. Cumulative mortality with CABG and PCI and the relative risk of CABG compared with PCI are shown. Data from the American College of Cardiology Foundation and Society of Thoracic Surgeons Database Collaboration on the Comparative Effectiveness of Revascularization Strategies registry, the American College of Cardiology Foundation National Cardiovascular Data Registry, and the Society of Thoracic Surgeons Adult Cardiac Surgery Database from 2004 through 2008. (From Weintraub WS, Grau-Sepulveda MV, Weiss JM, et al. Comparative effectiveness of revascularization strategies. *N Engl J Med.* 2012;366[16]:1467–1476.)

use of the anatomic SYNTAX score (www.syntaxscore.com; Fig. 1.5),[13,45–49] which enabled CAD complexity to be objectively and prospectively quantified.

- To ensure assessment of patients on an individual level, all patients eligible for enrollment were discussed by the heart team.[50] An interventional cardiologist and cardiac surgeon carried out a careful and comprehensive review of the patient in terms of their anginal status, comorbidities, and coronary anatomy using the respective Braunwald score, European System for Cardiac Operative Risk Evaluation (EuroSCORE), and SYNTAX score (discussed under "SYNTAX-Based Clinical Tools"). The consensus reached from this meeting was subsequently used to allocate the patient into one of the three arms of the trial. In total, 3075 patients were enrolled into one of the following:
  1. Randomized group (n = 1800 [58.5%]; 897 CABG, 903 PCI): These patients had CAD and were equally suitable for revascularization with PCI or CABG. The mean SYNTAX score for this group was 26.1 and 28.8 in patients treated with CABG and PCI, respectively.
  2. Nested CABG registry (n = 1077 [35.0%]): These patients had CAD that was considered unsuitable for PCI, clearly reflected in the high mean SYNTAX score (37.8) for this group.
  3. Nested PCI registry (n = 198 [6.4%]): These patients were deemed unsuitable for CABG. The commonest reason for this decision was the presence of multiple comorbidities[13] reflected in the mean EuroSCORE, which was 2 points higher in this group than the mean in the randomized group (5.8 vs. 3.8).

Overall, SYNTAX failed to meet the prespecified primary end point of noninferiority in terms of 12-month MACCEs, a composite of death, stroke, MI, and repeat revascularization (17.8% vs. 12.4%, P = .002). Final 5-year reporting of SYNTAX demonstrated significantly higher incidence of MACCE

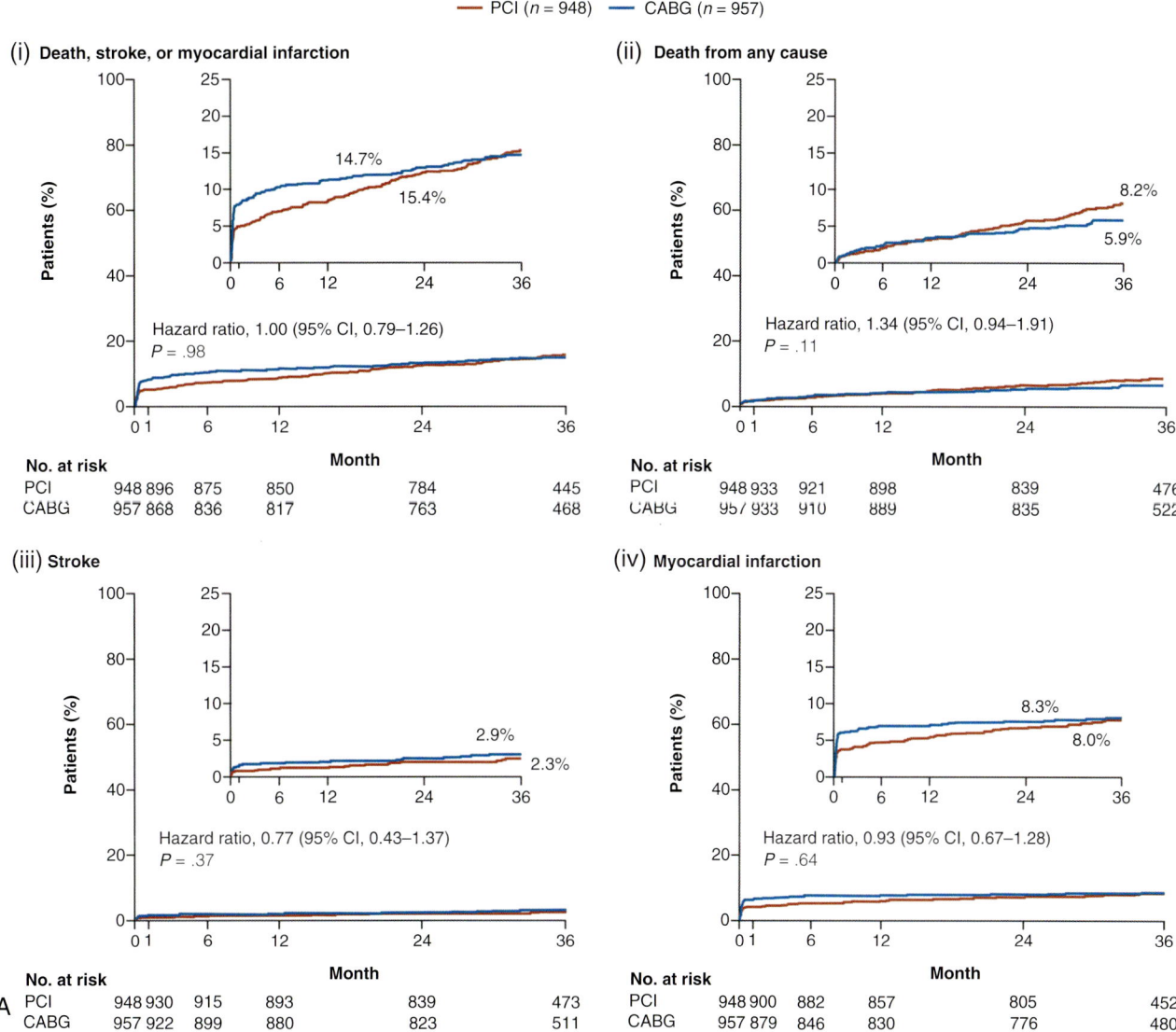

Fig. 1.4 Primary composite end point of death, stroke, or myocardial infarction and its components in the ongoing EXCEL trial at 3 years, indicating similar clinical outcomes (A).[17,18] In addition, both percutaneous coronary intervention *(PCI)* and coronary artery bypass grafting *(CABG)* result in similar quality of life (QOL) improvement at 36 months, with a substantially greater early benefit in QOL seen with PCI at 1 month (B).[19] *CI*, Confidence interval; *SAQ*, Seattle Angina Questionnaire. (Reproduced with permission from references 17 and 19.)

Continued

SECTION I Patient Selection

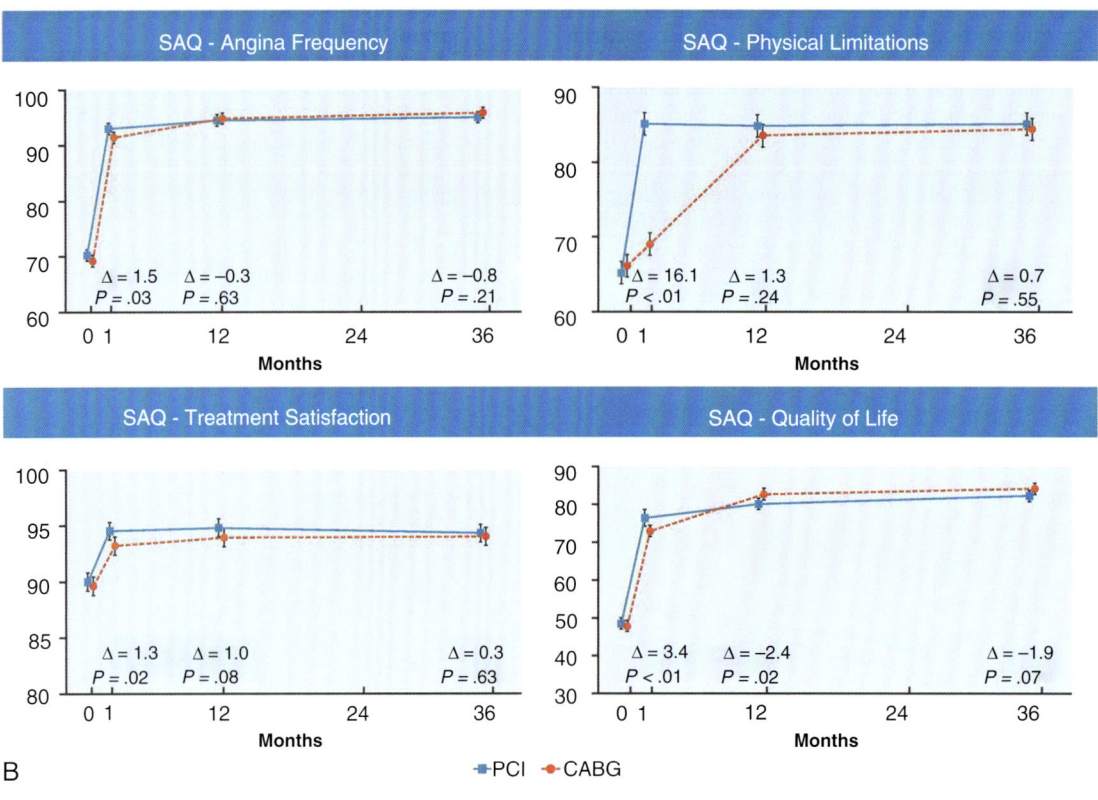

Fig. 1.4 cont'd

TABLE 1.2 Summary of Meta-Analyses Prior to Publication of the SYNTAX Trial Reporting Long-Term Outcomes in Patients With Isolated Proximal Left Anterior Descending Coronary Artery Disease or Multivessel Disease Randomized to Percutaneous or Surgical Revascularization

First Author	Number of Patients (PCI/CABG)	POBA/BMS/ DES (%)	Follow-Up (Months)	Death (PCI vs. CABG)	MI (PCI vs. CABG)	Stroke (PCI vs. CABG)	Repeat Revasc. (PCI vs. CABG)	MACCEs (PCI vs. CABG)
Isolated Proximal LAD								
Aziz[37]	1952 (1300/652)	0/91/9	34	2.9% vs. 3.4%	2% vs. 1.1%	2.4% vs. 3.5%	14.3% vs. 4.4%[a]	21.4% vs. 11.1%[a]
Kapoor[38]	1210 (633/577)	22/59/19	60	9.4% vs. 7.2%	NA	NA	33.5% vs. 7.3%[a]	NA
Multivessel Disease								
Hlatky[9]	7812 (3923/3889)	63/37/0	5.9	10.0% vs. 8.4%	16.7% vs. 15.4%[b]	–	24.5% vs. 9.9%[a,b]	36.4% vs. 20.1%[a]
Daemen[40]	3051 (1518/1533)	4/96/0	60	8.5% vs. 8.2%	2.5% vs. 2.9%	6.6% vs. 6.1%	25.0% vs. 6.3%[a]	34.2% vs. 19.6%[a]
Bravata[41]	9963 (5019/4944)	56/42/2	60	9.3% vs. 11.3%	0.6% vs. 1.2%[a]	11.9% vs. 10.9%	46.1% vs. 40.1% vs. 9.8%[a,c]	–

[a]$P < .001$.
[b]Composite with death.
[c]Balloon angioplasty versus PCI versus CABG.
BMS, Bare-metal stent; *CABG*, coronary artery bypass grafting; *DES*, drug-eluting stent; *LAD*, left anterior descending coronary artery; *MACCEs*, major adverse cardiovascular and cerebrovascular events (a composite of death, stroke, MI, and repeat revascularization); *MI*, myocardial infarction; *NA*, not available; *PCI*, percutaneous coronary intervention; *POBA*, plain old balloon angioplasty; *Revasc.*, revascularization.

TABLE 1.3 Summary of 15 Randomized Control Trials Comparing Coronary Artery Bypass Grafting Against Percutaneous Coronary Intervention in the Pre-SYNTAX Era

Trial	Number of Patients Screened	% Randomized	Stent	% 3VD	Proximal LAD	EF >50%	% Diabetes
MASS[39]	142	69	–	–	100	100	21
ERACI[173]	127	9	–	45	–	100	11
EAST[174]	392	4	–	40	70	100	25
GABI[175]	359	4	–	18	–	–	10
CABRI[176]	1054	3	–	40	–	100	12
BARI[177]	1829	12	–	41	36	100	24
SIMA[178]	121	–	–	–	100	100	11
LAUSANNE[179]	134	3	–	0	100	–	12
RITA[180]	1011	4	–	12	–	–	6
TOULOSE[181]	152	3	–	29	–	–	14
AWESOME[182]	454	–	+	45	–	–	–
ERACI-II[183]	450	2	+	56	–	–	17
ARTS[184]	1205	5	+	32	–	100	19
SOS[185]	988	5	+	38	45	100	14
MASS II[186]	408	2	+	41	–	–	–
Summary	**8826**	**5**		**35**	**41**	**100**	**16**

3VD, Three-vessel disease; *CABG*, coronary artery bypass grafting; *EF*, ejection fraction; *LAD*, left anterior descending artery; *PCI*, percutaneous coronary intervention. From Soran O, Manchanda A, Schueler, S. Percutaneous coronary intervention versus coronary artery bypass surgery in multivessel disease: a current perspective. *Interact Cardiovasc Thorac Surg.* 2009;8(6):666–671.

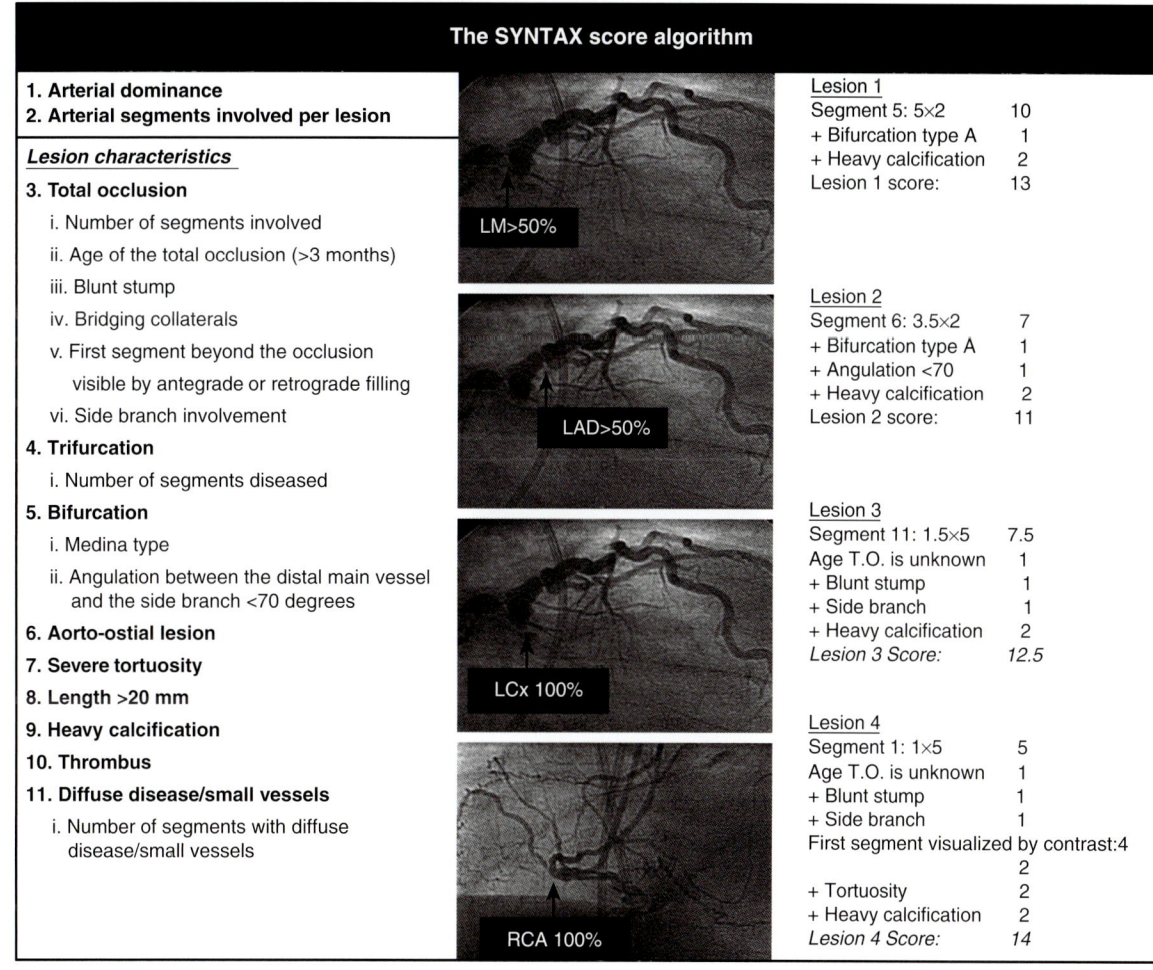

Fig. 1.5 The SYNTAX score algorithm is applied to each individual coronary lesion in a vessel larger than 1.5 mm in diameter that has a stenosis diameter greater than 50%; the individual lesion scores are added together to give the final SYNTAX score.[16,45-47] *LAD*, Left anterior descending; *LCx*, left circumflex artery; *LM*, left main; *RCA*, right coronary artery. (Modified from Serruys PW, Onuma Y, Garg S, et al. Assessment of the SYNTAX score in the SYNTAX study. *EuroIntervention.* 2009;5:50–56.)

SECTION I Patient Selection

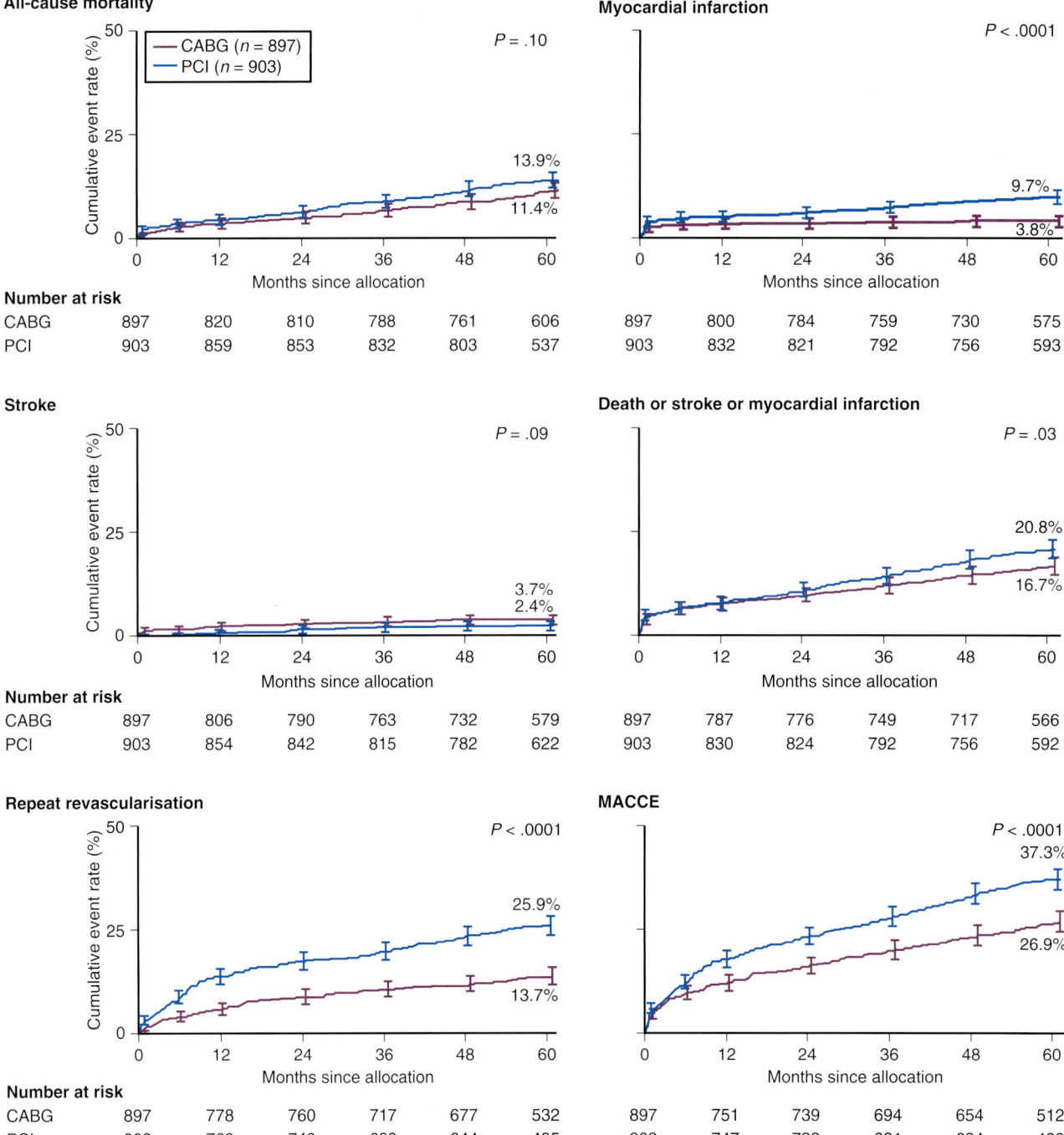

Fig. 1.6 Five-year Kaplan-Meier cumulative event curves of major adverse cardiovascular and cerebrovascular events (a composite of death, stroke, myocardial infarction and repeat revascularization) and its components among the 1800 patients randomized to percutaneous coronary intervention *(PCI)* or coronary artery bypass grafting surgery *(CABG)* in the SYNTAX trial. (From Mohr FW, Morice MC, Kappetein AP, et al. Coronary artery bypass graft surgery versus percutaneous coronary intervention in patients with three-vessel disease and left main coronary disease: 5-year follow-up of the randomised, clinical SYNTAX trial. *Lancet.* 2013;381[9867]:629–638.)

with PCI compared with CABG (26.9% vs. 37.3%, $P < .0001$; Fig. 1.6).[15]

As indicated earlier, analyses of all patients irrespective of disease severity does not provide adequate information for clinicians who are faced daily with patients who display a wide variety of CAD complexity. To address this limitation of earlier studies, patient outcomes in SYNTAX were stratified according to tertiles of the anatomic SYNTAX score. As shown in Fig. 1.7, clinical outcomes between patients treated with PCI and CABG in SYNTAX differed according to the presence of 3VD or unprotected LM CAD. With 3VD, a low SYNTAX score (<23) allowed for similar outcomes between CABG and PCI, whereas higher SYNTAX scores (particularly in the high SYNTAX score [>32] group) clearly favored CABG. With unprotected LM CAD, a low-intermediate SYNTAX score (<33) allowed for similar outcomes between CABG and PCI,

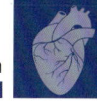

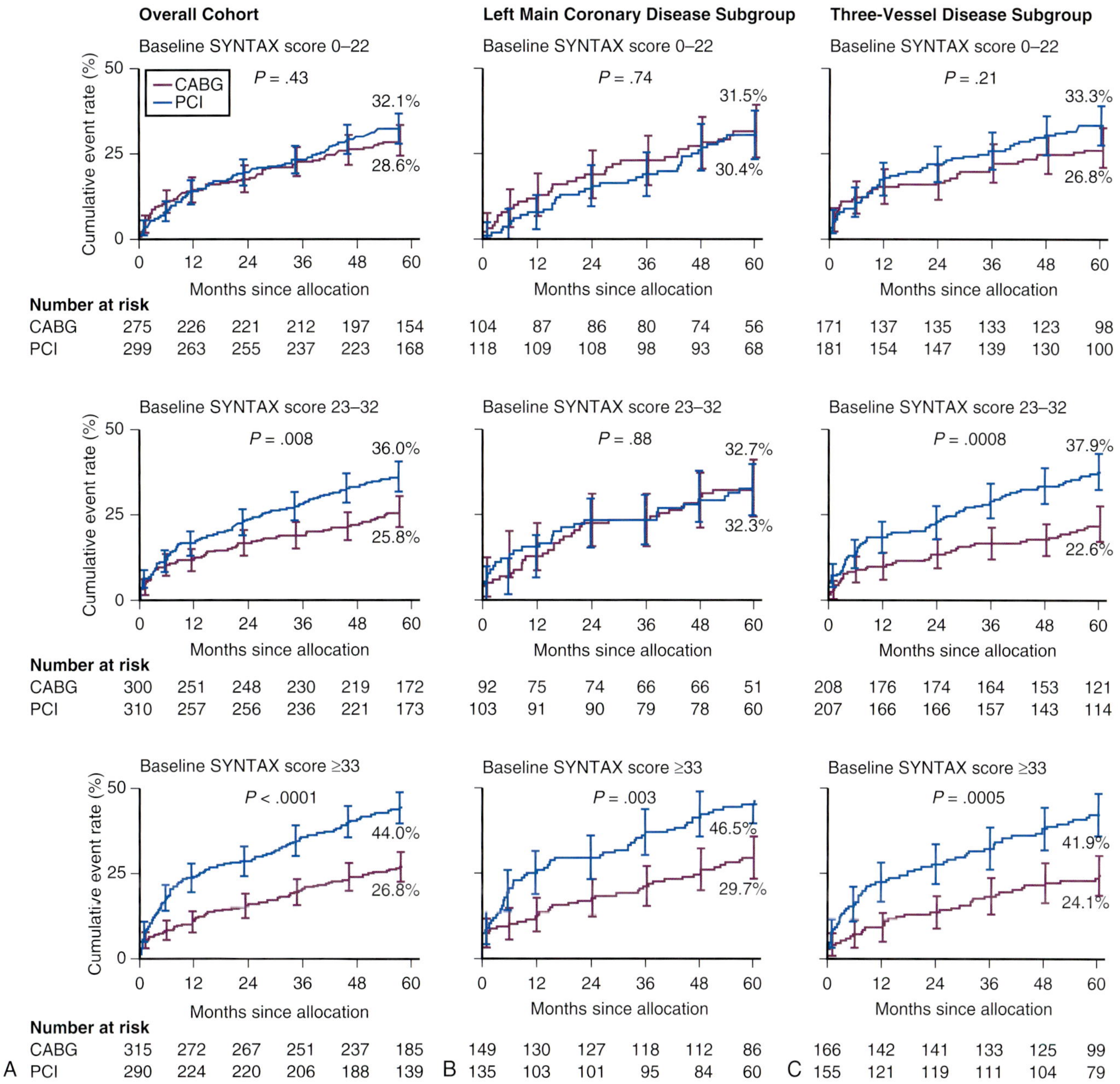

Fig. 1.7 The evidence supporting the use of the SYNTAX score as a tool to assist in revascularization decisions. Five-year Kaplan-Meier cumulative event curves of major adverse cardiovascular and cerebrovascular events (MACCEs; a composite of death, stroke, myocardial infarction and repeat revascularization) among the 1800 patients randomized to percutaneous coronary *(PCI)* or coronary artery bypass graft surgery *(CABG)* in the SYNTAX trial (A) and stratified by the presence of unprotected left main coronary artery disease (B) or de novo three-vessel disease (C). In patients with three-vessel disease (C), the incidence of MACCEs at 5-year follow-up was similar among patients treated with PCI and CABG for low SYNTAX scores (≤22); for all other SYNTAX scores (>22), outcomes were significantly better following CABG. (B) In patients with unprotected left main coronary artery disease, clinical outcomes were similar among patients treated by PCI or CABG for all low to intermediate SYNTAX scores (<33), whereas more complex disease (SYNTAX score >32) fared significantly better with CABG. (From Mohr FW, Morice MC, Kappetein AP, et al. Coronary artery bypass graft surgery versus percutaneous coronary intervention in patients with three-vessel disease and left main coronary disease: 5-year follow-up of the randomised, clinical SYNTAX trial. *Lancet.* 2013;381[9867]:629–638.)

whereas a high SYNTAX score (>32) clearly favored CABG. Furthermore, the SYNTAX score II,[7,8] essentially the anatomic SYNTAX score augmented with clinical variables shown directly to affect decision making between CABG and PCI, was developed in the randomized, all-comers SYNTAX trial and allowed for the identification of higher- and lower-risk subjects in all tertiles of the anatomic SYNTAX score who had a long-term mortality that favored either CABG, PCI, or both revascularization modalities (discussed under "SYNTAX-Based Clinical Tools").[7,8,13–16]

The results of SYNTAX reiterate the importance of assessing patients when selecting a revascularization strategy.

SYNTAX was able to identify those patients in whom either CABG or PCI was appropriate or in whom CABG or PCI was the optimal treatment. Considering the distribution of CAD in SYNTAX, overall one-third of patients with 3VD/LM disease were deemed to have CAD that could be treated safely and effectively with PCI or CABG, whereas in the remaining two-thirds, CABG remained the standard of care. Although these results helped further delineate the boundaries between a percutaneous and surgical revascularization approach in patients with complex CAD, the validation of the anatomic SYNTAX score and development of the SYNTAX score II notably facilitated a more objective assessment of patients by the heart team as discussed later under "SYNTAX-Based Clinical Tools."

INDIVIDUAL ASSESSMENT FROM A PHYSICIAN'S PERSPECTIVE

There is no disputing the need for and potential benefits of selecting a revascularization strategy following an individualized patient assessment or risk stratification. Risk stratification is performed routinely and subconsciously by physicians in everyday clinical practice and is in essence behind all clinical decisions made by a physician. Stratification of risk is vital when assessing patients for revascularization because this treatment is only considered appropriate when "the expected benefits, in terms of survival or health outcomes (symptoms, functional status, and/or QOL) exceed the expected negative consequences of the procedure."[51] However, it should be emphasized that the SYNTAX-pioneered heart team approach, consisting of at least an interventional/clinical cardiologist and a cardiac surgeon,[50] carries a class I recommendation in international guidelines for assessing risk and is subsequently the most appropriate revascularization modality in patients with complex CAD.[52-55]

Qualitative Versus Quantitative Risk Assessment

Qualitative risk stratification is subjective and relies on a clinician's experience. This subjective qualitative assessment also allows risk to be calculated and tailored to the expertise of the physician performing the procedure, as opposed to a clinician in another region who may use different techniques and who may have different equipment available. In addition, assessments of patient frailty can be made that are frequently not captured by conventional risk-scoring systems.[56] This assessment does not require a calculator or computer and can be "computed" subconsciously very quickly. The major disadvantages of this method of risk assessment are its dependence on the operator's prior experience, potential personal bias to undertake or withhold potential revascularization, and its high interobserver variability. In addition, influences of local practice often dominate clinical decision making, irrespective of the revascularization guidelines.

Quantitative risk stratification can be performed using a variety of risk scores that frequently incorporate clinical variables sourced from large patient registries,[57-64] with the exception of the SYNTAX score II,[7,8] which was developed in the all-comers randomized SYNTAX trial to reduce unavoidable (but often appropriate) selection bias inherent to all registries no matter their size. These risk scores largely incorporate objective variables to ensure adequate reproducibility of the score; however, those risk scores—such as the American College of Cardiology/American Heart Association (ACC/AHA) lesion score[65] or the anatomic SYNTAX score/newly developed SYNTAX score II,[7,8,46] which include angiographic variables—continue to have documented intraobserver and interobserver variability.[47,66] However, these tools do provide a more objective assessment of the patient risk and suitability for the most appropriate revascularization modality, which may be modified by the heart team consensus. In addition to their role in the risk stratification of individual patients, these quantitative risk scores have increasing use in the wider context of overall health care. They can provide a vital measure of overall patient care and can help to identify future directions to further improve outcomes. Clinical governance and the increasing requirement to publicly report clinical performance and complications have also propelled the need to risk stratify patients, thereby allowing a useful comparison of performance to be made between clinicians and institutions against the standards dictated by regulatory authorities.[67] In addition, calculation of risk using accepted risk scores may aid clinicians faced with an increasing need to be able to justify their clinical decisions to peers, regulatory bodies, and patients.

In comparison with the qualitative risk scores, the use of a finite number of variables results in these risk scores lacking the sensitivity to accurately predict risk in an individual, such that they are more apt at predicting risk for a population of patients with similar comorbidities. The number of variables included in the score must strike a balance between sufficient numbers to enable a meaningful prediction of risk to be calculated; however, the number must not be excessive so as to prevent use in routine practice. In addition, a minimal number of variables reduces the chances of colinearity between independent variables, which can result in redundant information being collected[62] while also increasing the chances of "overfitting" the score and thereby reducing the overall applicability and accuracy of the results to conventional clinical practice.[68]

The applicability of a risk score to contemporary practice must also take into consideration the time when the score was developed. Risk scores rely on large patient databases to derive appropriate weighting factors for variables in the score to enable the final calculation of risk. It follows that they are developed using retrospective information that may no longer be relevant in the era when the risk score is being used. For example, the EuroSCORE was developed in 1999; however, there have been calls for its recalibration because repeated evaluations indicate that it overestimates risk by a factor of 2 to 3, which has largely been attributed to improvements in surgical techniques and lower perioperative mortality in the decade following its construction.[69,70] The updated EuroSCORE II currently addresses many of the limitations of the original EuroSCORE.[71-73] The STS score is also derived from a large patient database and is periodically recalibrated to ensure its results are applicable to contemporary practice.[74]

Risk Scores in Contemporary Practice

Numerous risk scores are available to assist clinicians in stratifying risk among patients undergoing revascularization. Some scores are appropriate for patients prior to the selection of a revascularization strategy, whereas some have been validated only in patients undergoing one form of revascularization. Nevertheless, the various risk scores can largely be categorized according to the variables—clinical, angiographic, or a combination of both—used in the overall estimation of risk. Tables 1.4 and 1.5 summarize the different risk scores used in contemporary CABG and PCI practice (excluding SYNTAX-based tools), and Table 1.6 summarizes SYNTAX-based clinical tools. A selection of these is described in more detail later.

Clinical Scores

These risk scores incorporate only clinical variables and do not require any data from the angiogram. They offer the advantage of being able to be computed relatively quickly, usually at the bedside, and principally include variables that are not subject to user interpretation, thereby ensuring excellent reproducibility.

TABLE 1.4 Summary of Contemporary Risk Scores for Assessment of Risk in Patients Undergoing Surgical Revascularization With the Exception of the Anatomic SYNTAX Score

Risk Score	Number of Variables Used to Calculate Score		Validated in PCI/CABG	
	Clinical	Angiographic	PCI	CABG
EuroSCORE[13,57-59,75,76,80-84]	17	0	+	+
EuroSCORE II[71-73]	18	0	−	+
ACEF[62]	3	0	−	+
Society of Thoracic Surgery score[64,74,87,104]	40	2	−	+
Anatomic SYNTAX score[4,13,47,81,84,94,95,187-194]	0	11 (per lesion)	+	+

SYNTAX-based tools are shown in Table 1.6.
ACEF, Age, creatinine, and ejection fraction; *CABG,* coronary artery bypass grafting; *PCI,* percutaneous coronary intervention.

EuroSCORE and EuroSCORE II

The EuroSCORE is an established risk score that uses 17 clinical variables used in cardiothoracic surgical practice for predicting operative mortality, and it has been validated in many populations around the world.[58,75-77] In use since 1999, the score was derived from almost 20,000 consecutive patients from 128 hospitals in eight European countries. The additive EuroSCORE assigns an individual score to 17 clinical variables (Table 1.7) with a low-risk tertile that ranges from 1 to 2, an intermediate-risk tertile from 3 to 5, and a high-risk tertile of 6 and higher. However, early validation studies suggested that the additive EuroSCORE underestimated risk in those at highest risk; this led to the development of the logistic EuroSCORE, which uses the same clinical variables and requires use of an online calculator (available at www.euroscore.org) to quantify risk.[58,59,70,77] However, the logistic EuroSCORE has been shown to potentially overestimate observed mortality, and its accuracy at predicting risk varies in different surgical subgroups.[70,78]

In addition to the EuroSCORE's assessment and validation in patients undergoing surgical revascularization, Kim and colleagues[79] first demonstrated that the high-risk tertile of the additive EuroSCORE was an independent predictor of death/MI after unprotected LM intervention with sirolimus-eluting stents. Subsequently, Romagnoli and coworkers[80] applied the additive EuroSCORE to predict in-hospital mortality in 1173 consecutive patients undergoing PCI in a single high-volume center and correlated the higher-risk tertiles of the EuroSCORE with in-hospital mortality; the study population also included patients who had undergone unprotected LM PCI. The EuroSCORE has since been evaluated in numerous studies of patients undergoing PCI, the majority of which specifically enrolled patients with LM disease.[13,79,81-83] Notably, all studies, irrespective of disease severity, have demonstrated the EuroSCORE to be an independent predictor of mortality[81,82] and/or MACCE at follow-up ranging from 1 to 3 years.[13,79,81-83] Importantly, those studies that also included a surgical control group—such as the SYNTAX study, the Revascularization for Unprotected Left Main Coronary Artery Stenosis: Comparison of Percutaneous Coronary Angioplasty Versus Surgical Revascularization (MAIN-COMPARE) study, and the registry by Rodés-Cabau and colleagues[83]—also demonstrated the EuroSCORE to be an independent predictor of MACCE in surgical patients.[81,84] Only one study has examined the logistic EuroSCORE in PCI patients; however, little differences were found in stratifying risk when compared with the additive EuroSCORE.[80]

Specifically in the SYNTAX trial, which represents the only randomized study to assess the EuroSCORE, the additive EuroSCORE was shown to be an independent predictor of MACCE at 1-year follow-up irrespective of the method of revascularization (odds ratio [OR]: 1.21; 95% confidence interval [CI]: 1.12 to 1.32; $P < .001$) in 705 patients undergoing LM revascularization.[81]

Similarly, at intermediate follow-up of 23 months, Rodés-Cabau and colleagues[83] identified a EuroSCORE of 9 or higher as the best predictor of MACCE after PCI and CABG among 249 octogenarians with LM disease. In the MAIN-COMPARE registry, which enrolled more than 1500 patients with LM disease followed up for a median of 3.1 years, the EuroSCORE has been identified as an independent predictor of death, MI, and stroke irrespective of revascularization strategy.[84] In addition, in the same registry, a EuroSCORE of 6 or higher has been shown to be an independent predictor of mortality following either PCI or CABG.[82]

More recently, the EuroSCORE II (Table 1.8) was developed to improve the risk prediction of the original EuroSCORE. EuroSCORE II was developed on newer data to reflect more contemporary surgical practice given that cardiac surgical mortality has decreased significantly in the last 15 years, despite patients being older and sicker, and that the previous additive and logistic EuroSCOREs were suggested to be representative of outdated surgical practices.[71-73,85]

The EuroSCORE II was shown to have improved calibration (actual mortality 4.18%, predicted 3.95%) compared with the original EuroSCORE (actual 3.9%, additive predicted 5.8%, logistic predicted 7.57%) while preserving discrimination (area under the receiver operating characteristic [ROC] curve of 0.8095). However, it should be noted that regular revalidation of the EuroSCORE II will need to be continued to identify calibration drift or clinical inconsistencies seen in previous versions.[85,86]

In summary, while acknowledging that most of these studies have been nonrandomized observational studies, the findings do suggest that the EuroSCORE and EuroSCORE II are valuable tools in the individual assessment of risk prior to the selection of a revascularization strategy.

New Mayo Clinic Risk Score

The new Mayo Clinic Risk Score (MCRS) was designed to replace the original MCRS by predominantly excluding angiographic variables, namely the presence of LM or MVD, and a few of the interaction effects of specific clinical variables (see Table 1.5).

The new MCRS is based solely on baseline clinical and noninvasive assessments and incorporates seven preprocedural variables (age, serum creatinine, left ventricular ejection fraction [LVEF], MI within the past 24 hours, preprocedural shock, congestive heart failure, and peripheral vascular disease). The risk score had a C-statistic (area under ROC curve) of 0.74 and 0.89 for major adverse cardiovascular events (MACEs) and procedural death, respectively, in the population from whom the risk score was derived.[60,61] The risk score has since been validated for in-hospital mortality in the NCDR[61]; however, it has not been validated for MACEs. The new MCRS has also been demonstrated to be predictive of in-hospital mortality after CABG surgery.[87]

SECTION I Patient Selection

TABLE 1.5 Summary of a Selection of Established and Contemporary Risk Scores Categorized by Anatomic, Clinical, or Combined Types for the Assessment of Risk in Patients Proposing to Undergo Percutaneous Coronary Intervention

Clinical Risk Score	Number of Variables Used to Calculate Risk		PCI Outcomes (Surgical Outcomes in Italics)
	Clinical	Angiographic	
ANATOMIC SCORES			
ACC/AHA lesion classification[a]	0	11 (per lesion)	Pre-DES era: predictive of angiographic success of PCI and prognostic effect on early and late clinical outcomes. Conflicting results were yielded in the DES era.[93,95,195–197]
MYOCARDIAL JEOPARDY SCORES			
Duke Jeopardy Score	0		Coronary tree divided into six segments: LAD, diagonal, septal perforating branches, LCx, OM, and PDA; a segment distal to ≥70% is considered at risk. Each segment is assigned 2 points with a maximum of 12 points.[96,97b]
Myocardial Jeopardy Index (BARI)	0		Distal terminating portions of LAD, LCx, RCA, and major branch vessels (diagonals, OM, ramus, PDA and LV branches) assigned units of 1, 2, or 3 on the basis of length and vessel size. Septal perforators are arbitrarily assigned a maximum of 3 units. Extent of jeopardy defined by units jeopardized by ≥50% stenosis summated and divided by total LV territory.[97,98b]
APPROACH lesion score	0		Based on principle from autopsy studies that the LAD generally subtends 41% of the LV, with the LCx and RCA supplying the remainder, dependent on vessel dominance. Score is calculated by percent of myocardium supplied by a vessel or its branches and jeopardized territories supplied by vessels with ≥70% stenosis (≥50% in the LMS); the maximum score is 100.[97b]
CLINICAL SCORES			
New Mayo Clinic Risk Score[a]	7	0	Procedural death and MACEs for PCI; score has been externally validated for death[62,63] (in-hospital death with CABG).[87]
Parsonnet Score	14	0	Independent predictor of long-term MACEs after LMS PCI in two registry populations[198,199] (operative mortality after open-heart surgery)[200]
EuroSCORE (additive or logistic)	17	0	Evidence for predicting death or MACCEs in high-risk tertiles for PCI[79,80,83,201] (operative mortality for all forms of cardiothoracic surgery).[58,61]
NCDR CathPCI Risk Score[a]	8	0	Developed from 181,775 procedures performed in Medicare patients; incidence of in-hospital and 30-day mortality after all PCI patient types internally validated in two separate cohorts.[65]
ACEF score (age, creatinine, ejection fraction)	3	0	Predictor of cardiac death and MI at 1 year after PCI; inferior to the SYNTAX score at predicting overall MACEs and repeat revascularization in two separate populations[90,122] (operative mortality in elective cardiac operations).[62,88]
COMBINED (ANATOMIC AND CLINICAL) RISK SCORES			
EuroHeart PCI Score[a]	10	6	Developed from 46,000 patients from the Euro Heart Survey; in-hospital mortality in all PCI patient types; internally validated. The score has strong applicability for European practice.[105]
New Risk Stratification Score (NERS)	17	Angiographic: 33 Procedural: 4[c]	6-month cardiac death and cumulative MACEs after unprotected LMS PCI; although internally validated, application to larger all-comers population is required (see text).[106]
New York PCI Risk Score[b]	8	1	In-hospital death after PCI; developed based on data from 46,090 procedures in 2002 and validated from 50,046 procedures in 2003[202]; excellent predictive ability in validation cohort (C-statistic 0.905).
The Texas Heart Institute Risk Score[a]	8	Angiographic: 2 Procedural: 1[d]	Predictors of in-hospital MACEs after PCI or CABG; developed in 9494 patients (BMS era) and validated in 5545 patients (DES era).[203]
Mayo Clinic Risk Score[a]	6	2	In-hospital death, Q-wave myocardial infarction, emergent or urgent CABG or CVA after PCI; validated using the NHLBI registry.[204]

[a]Risk scores that include prediction of in-hospital mortality or MACEs. SYNTAX-based tools are shown in Table 1.6.
[b]All myocardial jeopardy scores were validated in one population-based cohort consisting of more than 20,000 patients and were predictive of 1-year mortality in patients treated with PCI or medically.[96–98]
[c]Need of intraaortic balloon pump, two-stent technique, intravascular ultrasound guidance.
[d]Number of stents.
ACC/AHA, American College of Cardiology/American Heart Association; *BMS,* bare-metal stent; *CABG,* coronary artery bypass grafting; *CVA,* cerebrovascular accident; *DES,* drug-eluting stent; *LAD,* left anterior descending artery; *LCx,* left circumflex artery; *LMS,* left main stem; *LV,* left ventricular; *MACCEs,* major adverse cardiovascular and cerebrovascular event; *MACE,* major adverse cardiovascular event; *MI,* myocardial infarction; *NCDR,* National Cardiovascular Data Registry; *OM,* obtuse marginal artery; *PCI,* percutaneous coronary intervention; *PDA,* posterior descending artery; *NHLBI,* National Heart, Lung, and Blood Institute; *RCA,* right coronary artery.

TABLE 1.6 Outline of the Anatomic SYNTAX Score and the Progression of SYNTAX-Based Tools

	Year	Structure	Remarks
Anatomic SYNTAX Score[4,13-15,48,55,60,64-72,166]	2006	Score of angiographic variables (i.e., anatomic complexity); developed during the design of the SYNTAX trial[13,47] as a tool to force the heart team to systematically analyze the coronary angiogram and agree equivalent anatomic revascularization (CABG and PCI) could be achieved	First reported to be useful for decision making between CABG and PCI in the SYNTAX trial in 2009[13]; categories of anatomic complexity (low, intermediate, and high), no clinical variables, no individual predictions; adding a functional component shown to improve accuracy[13]; noninvasive multislice computed tomography anatomic SYNTAX score in development,[36] with integration of a noninvasive functional component.[162]
DEVELOPMENT PHASE: AUGMENTING THE ANATOMIC SYNTAX SCORE WITH CLINICAL VARIABLES AND THE MOVE TOWARD INDIVIDUALIZED DECISION MAKING			
ACEF[163]	2009	Age, creatinine, ejection fraction	Predicted individual in-hospital operative mortality post CABG; shown to be at least comparable to the EuroSCORE (composed of 17 variables) in predicting operative risk[62,88,89]; shown to aid in long-term predictions of mortality after PCI or CABG.[62,89]
Clinical SYNTAX Score[127]	2010	Amalgamation of SYNTAX score with modified ACEF score (creatinine replaced with CrCl shown to be more predictive of mortality[121])	Similar to the SYNTAX score; categorized patient risk; could only identify a high-risk group in PCI-treated patients; provided little help in decision making between CABG and PCI; not individualized.
Global Risk[88,123]	2010	Amalgamation of SYNTAX score with surgical EuroSCORE (composed of 17 variables)	Similar to the SYNTAX score; categorized patient risk; could identify a low-risk group with comparable outcomes with CABG and PCI in LM and 3VD patients; not individualized; patients with a high EuroSCORE were found to have a prognostic benefit in undergoing CABG compared with PCI irrespective of the SYNTAX score provided an acceptable threshold of operative risk was not exceeded.
Logistic Clinical SYNTAX Score[126,127]	2011	Combination of age, SYNTAX score, CrCl, and LVEF shown to contain most of the prognostic data for 1-year mortality predictions after PCI	Individual 1-year mortality predictions in all PCI patients (STEMI, NSTEMI) irrespective of clinical presentation (except cardiogenic shock); not designed to help decision making between CABG and PCI; cross-validated in seven contemporary stent trials and more than 6000 patients and further externally validated.[123]
END RESULT OF THIS PROCESS LEADING TO THE DEVELOPMENT OF THE SYNTAX SCORE II			
SYNTAX Score II[124]	2012	Augmenting SYNTAX score with clinical variables; based on the principle that age, CrCl, LVEF, and SYNTAX score contain most of the long-term prognostic data in CABG and PCI patients; additional variables added that directly influenced decision making between CABG and PCI	Individualized approach; threshold of the SYNTAX score in guiding decision making between CABG and PCI shown to alter based on the presence of other risk factors; validated in the DELTA Registry[7,8] containing LM and 3VD (25% of the population) with almost a third (30%) with highly complex disease (SYNTAX scores ≥33); prospective validation studies are underway in the EXCEL trial (LM), and SYNTAX II trial is ongoing (de novo 3VD).
USE OF THE SYNTAX SCORE AS AN OBJECTIVE MARKER OF COMPLETENESS OF REVASCULARIZATION			
Residual SYNTAX Score[129]	2012	Recalculation of the SYNTAX score after PCI	Developed and validated in the ACUITY[146,147] and SYNTAX[146] trials; a residual SYNTAX score greater than 8 was shown to have an adverse effect on long-term prognosis at up to 5-year follow-up; further, prospectively run validation studies are awaited.
Post-CABG SYNTAX Score[147]	2013	Recalculation of the SYNTAX score after CABG with points deducted based on the importance of the diseased coronary artery segment (Leaman score[154,155]) that has a functioning bypass graft anastomosed distally	Pilot study in angiographic substudy of the SYNTAX trial demonstrated the feasibility of this approach in identifying subjects post CABG with an adverse long-term (5-year) prognosis[109]; validation studies are awaited.

3VD, Three-vessel disease; *CABG*, coronary artery bypass grafting; *CrCl*, creatinine clearance; *LM*, left main; *LVEF*, left ventricular ejection fraction; *NSTEMI*, non–ST elevation myocardial infarction; *PCI*, percutaneous coronary intervention; *STEMI*, ST elevation myocardial infarction.

Value of Age, Creatinine, and Ejection Fraction Score

Ranucci and colleagues[62,88] demonstrated in a relatively simple risk score consisting of only three clinical variables—age, preoperative serum creatinine value, and LVEF—a risk score for assessing operative mortality risk in elective cardiac operations. Notably, despite the simplicity of the score, the clinical performance of the Age, Creatinine, and Ejection Fraction (ACEF) score appeared to be comparable with either the additive or the logistic EuroSCORE.

The ACEF score is calculated using the following formula:

$$\text{ACEF} = [\text{Age}/\text{LVEF (\%)}] + [1 \text{ (if creatinine>2 mg/dL)}]$$

From ACEF, a mortality risk can be calculated from a graphical relationship of ACEF with an operative risk or an equation (Fig. 1.8).[62,88] ACEF was developed from an initial dataset of 4557 patients and a subsequent validation series of 4091 patients from a single institution. The results demonstrated a similar accuracy and calibration for the prediction of in-hospital mortality with ACEF when compared with other more complicated surgical risk scores such as the EuroSCORE and the Cleveland Clinic Score. Subsequent validation studies have shown ACEF to have an accuracy level at least comparable with that of the EuroSCORE for operative mortality risk

SECTION I Patient Selection

TABLE 1.7 Components of the EuroSCORE and Relevant Weighting Factors of the Additive and Logistic EuroSCOREs

Patient Characteristics	Additive		Logistic β Coefficient
Age	Per 5 years or part thereof over the age of 60 years	1	0.07
Sex	Female	1	0.33
Chronic pulmonary disease	Long-term use of bronchodilators or steroids for respiratory disease	1	0.49
Peripheral arteriopathy	Claudication, carotid stenosis >50%, previous or planned intervention on the abdominal aorta, limb arteries, or carotids[a]	2	0.66
Neurologic dysfunction	Severely affected mobility or day-to-day function	2	0.84
Previous cardiac surgery	Previous opening of the pericardium	3	1.00
Serum creatinine	Preoperatively greater than 200 μmol/L	2	0.65
Active endocarditis	Antibiotic therapy at time of surgery	3	1.10
Critical preoperative state	Preoperative cardiac arrest, ventilation, renal failure, inotropic support, intraaortic balloon pump use, ventricular arrhythmia[a]	3	0.91
CARDIAC-RELATED FACTORS			
Unstable angina	Rest pain that requires IV nitrates	2	0.57
Left ventricular function	Moderate (30%–50%)	1	0.42
	Poor (<30%)	3	1.09
Recent MI	Within 90 days	2	0.55
Pulmonary hypertension	Systolic pulmonary pressure greater than 60 mm Hg	2	0.77
OPERATION-RELATED FACTORS			
Emergency	Operation performed before the start of next working day	2	0.71
Other than isolated CABG	Major cardiac procedure other than or in addition to CABG	2	0.54
Surgery on thoracic aorta		3	1.16
Postinfarct septal rupture		4	1.46
Constant β_0			−4.79

[a]Any of these.
The logistic EuroSCORE can be calculated at www.euroscore.org.
CABG, Coronary artery bypass grafting; *IV*, intravenous; *MI*, myocardial infarction.
From Singh M, Rihal CS, Lennon RJ, et al. Bedside estimation of risk from percutaneous coronary intervention: the new Mayo Clinic Risk Scores. *Mayo Clinic Proc.* 2007;82:701–708; and Singh M, Peterson ED, Milford-Beland S, et al. Validation of the Mayo Clinic risk score for in-hospital mortality after percutaneous coronary interventions using the National Cardiovascular Data Registry. *Circ Cardiovasc Interv.* 2008;1:36–44.

stratification in a series of 29,659 patients undergoing elective cardiac surgery.[88,89]

In addition, ACEF was applied to PCI patients from the all-comers LEADERS population at 1-year follow-up.[90] Despite ACEF being demonstrated to be superior to the SYNTAX score alone as a predictor of cardiac death and MI after PCI, ACEF was found to be inferior to the SYNTAX score at predicting overall MACE rates and the risk of repeat revascularization. This reflects the observation that anatomic and clinical variables appear to be necessary requirements for a comprehensive risk score in predicting clinical outcomes after PCI.

National Cardiovascular Database Registry CathPCI Risk-Prediction Score

The NCDR CathPCI risk-prediction score is the most contemporary clinical risk score currently available. It incorporates information from nine clinical variables (Table 1.9), which are assigned appropriate weighted values and are then added together to give a final score that can be translated into risk of in-hospital mortality (Fig. 1.9).[63] The score was developed using data from more than 180,000 patients from the voluntary U.S. NCDR database and was validated in more than 400,000 patients from the same database who underwent PCI between March 2006 and March 2007. Notably, the C-statistic for the prediction of in-hospital mortality was consistently greater than 0.90 for in-hospital mortality, whereas a lower but nevertheless adequate C-statistic of 0.83 was seen for 30-day mortality.

Angiography-Based Scores

Two major angiography-based scores have been developed, both of which are independent of patient clinical variables, calculated using only angiographic data. As alluded to earlier, this introduces a subjective element to the assessment of risk[47,66] and consequently introduces a degree of intraobserver and interobserver variability, which is notably absent from the clinical scores described previously. In addition, these scores can be computed only after diagnostic coronary angiography has been performed, thereby moving assessment further down the treatment pathway.

American College of Cardiology/American Heart Association Lesion Classification System

The ACC/AHA lesion classification system was one of the first angiographic scoring systems developed. Initially devised in 1986 and modified in 1990, it uses 11 angiographic variables to categorize lesions into four groups: types A, B1, B2, and C (Table 1.10). Historic studies prior to the arrival of DESs indicated that that the ACC/AHA lesion classification did have a prognostic impact on early and late outcomes.[65,91,92]

However, registry data from the DES era has shown conflicting results. The German Cypher registry ($n = 6755$) failed to show any definite relationship between clinical outcomes and ACC/AHA lesion class at 6 months.[93] These results are at variance to the positive relationship identified between ACC/AHA lesion class and clinical outcomes in smaller studies of patients with more complex disease.[94,95]

TABLE 1.8 Final Risk Factors by Multivariate Regression for the EuroSCORE II

Risk Factor	Coefficient	Standard Error	z	P ≥ |z|	[95% Confidence Interval]
NEW YORK HOSPITAL ASSOCIATION (NYHA)					
II	0.1070545	0.1463849	0.73	0.465	[−0.1798547 to 0.3939637]
III	0.2958358	0.141466	2.09	0.037	[0.0185674 to 0.5731042]
IV	0.5597929	0.1697565	3.30	0.001	[0.2270763 to 0.8925095]
CCS4	0.2226147	0.1462888	1.52	0.128	[−0.0641061 to 0.5093356]
IDDM	0.3542749	0.145863	2.43	0.015	[0.0683887 to 0.6401611]
Age	0.0285181	0.0065954	4.32	0.000	[0.0155914 to 0.0414448]
Female	0.2196434	0.0953505	2.30	0.021	[0.0327599 to 0.4065269]
ECA	0.5360268	0.1106046	4.85	0.000	[0.3192458 to 0.7528079]
CPD	0.1886564	0.1232126	1.53	0.126	[−0.0528358 to 0.4301486]
N/M mob	0.2407181	0.1729494	1.39	0.164	[−0.0982564 to 0.5796927]
Redo	1.118599	0.1226272	9.12	0.000	[0.8782539 to 1.3589440]
RENAL DYSFUNCTION					
On dialysis	0.6421508	0.3083468	2.08	0.037	[0.0378021 to 1.2464990]
CC ≤ 50	0.8592256	0.1446758	5.94	0.000	[0.5756663 to 1.1427850]
CC 50–85	0.303553	0.1240518	2.45	0.014	[0.0604159 to 0.5466901]
Active endocarditis	0.6194522	0.2046001	3.03	0.002	[0.2184433 to 1.0204610]
Critical	1.086517	0.147657	7.36	0.000	[0.797115 to 1.3759200]
LEFT VENTRICULAR FUNCTION					
Moderate	0.3150652	0.1036182	3.04	0.002	[0.1119773 to 0.5181530]
Poor	0.8084096	0.1498233	5.40	0.000	[0.5147614 to 1.1020580]
Very poor	0.9346919	0.2917754	3.20	0.001	[0.3628227 to 1.5065610]
Recent MI	0.1528943	0.136257	1.12	0.262	[−0.1141646 to 0.4199531]
PULMONARY ARTERY SYSTOLIC PRESSURE					
31–55 mm Hg	0.1788899	0.1266713	1.41	0.158	[−0.0693812 to 0.4271611]
≥55	0.3491475	0.1676641	2.08	0.037	[0.0205318 to 0.6777632]
URGENCY					
Urgent	0.3174673	0.1174178	2.70	0.007	[0.0873326 to 0.5476020]
Emergency	0.7039121	0.1719835	4.09	0.000	[0.3668306 to 1.0409940]
Salvage	1.362947	0.33706	4.04	0.000	[0.7023221 to 2.0235730]
WEIGHT OF PROCEDURE					
1 non-CABG	0.0062118	0.1463574	0.04	0.966	[−0.2806434 to 0.2930670]
2	0.5521478	0.1268137	4.35	0.000	[0.3035975 to 0.8006980]
3+	0.9724533	0.1463969	6.64	0.000	[0.6855206 to 1.2593860]
Thoracic aorta	0.6527205	0.221183	2.95	0.003	[0.2192097 to 1.0862310]
Constant	−5.324537	0.1682446	−31.65	0.000	[−5.65429 to −4.9947830]

CABG, Coronary artery bypass grafting; *CC*, creatinine clearance; *CCS*, Canadian Cardiovascular Society; *CPD*, chronic pulmonary dysfunction; *Critical*, critical preoperative state; *ECA*, extracardiac arteriopathy; *IDDM*, insulin-dependent diabetes mellitus; *N/M mob*, neurologic or musculoskeletal dysfunction severely affecting mobility; *MI*, myocardial infarction; *Redo*, previous cardiac surgery.
Weight of procedure: 1, non-CABG, single major cardiac procedure (MCP) that is not isolated CABG; 2, two MCPs; 3+, three or more MCPs. For age, X_i = 1 if patient age is 60 or younger; X_i increases by one point per year thereafter (e.g., age 60 or less, X_i = 1; age 61, X_i = 2; age 62, X_i = 3, etc.).
From Nashef SA, Roques F, Sharples LD, et al. EuroSCORE II. *Eur J Cardiothorac Surg.* 2012;41(4):734–744.

Specifically, Valgimigli and colleagues[94] reported that a higher ACC/AHA lesion score (derived by assigning 1, 2, 3, and 4 points to type A, B1, B2, and C lesions, respectively) correlated with poor clinical outcomes among 306 patients with 3VD undergoing PCI with a DES. In addition, data from a small registry (n = 255) were potentially predictive of mortality and MACEs in unprotected LM stem PCI at 1-year follow-up.[95]

Anatomic SYNTAX Score

The anatomic SYNTAX score represents a comprehensive angiographic scoring system that allows the complexity of CAD to be objectively quantified. This is further discussed in the section on SYNTAX-based scoring tools.

Myocardial Jeopardy Scores

Myocardial jeopardy scores are a method of estimating the amount of myocardium at risk based on the assessment of both the severity of the coronary artery lesion and the volume of myocardium it supplies. Examples of such scores include the Duke Jeopardy Score, the Myocardial Jeopardy Index from the Bypass Angioplasty Revascularization Investigation (BARI) score, and the Alberta Provincial Project for Outcome Assessment in

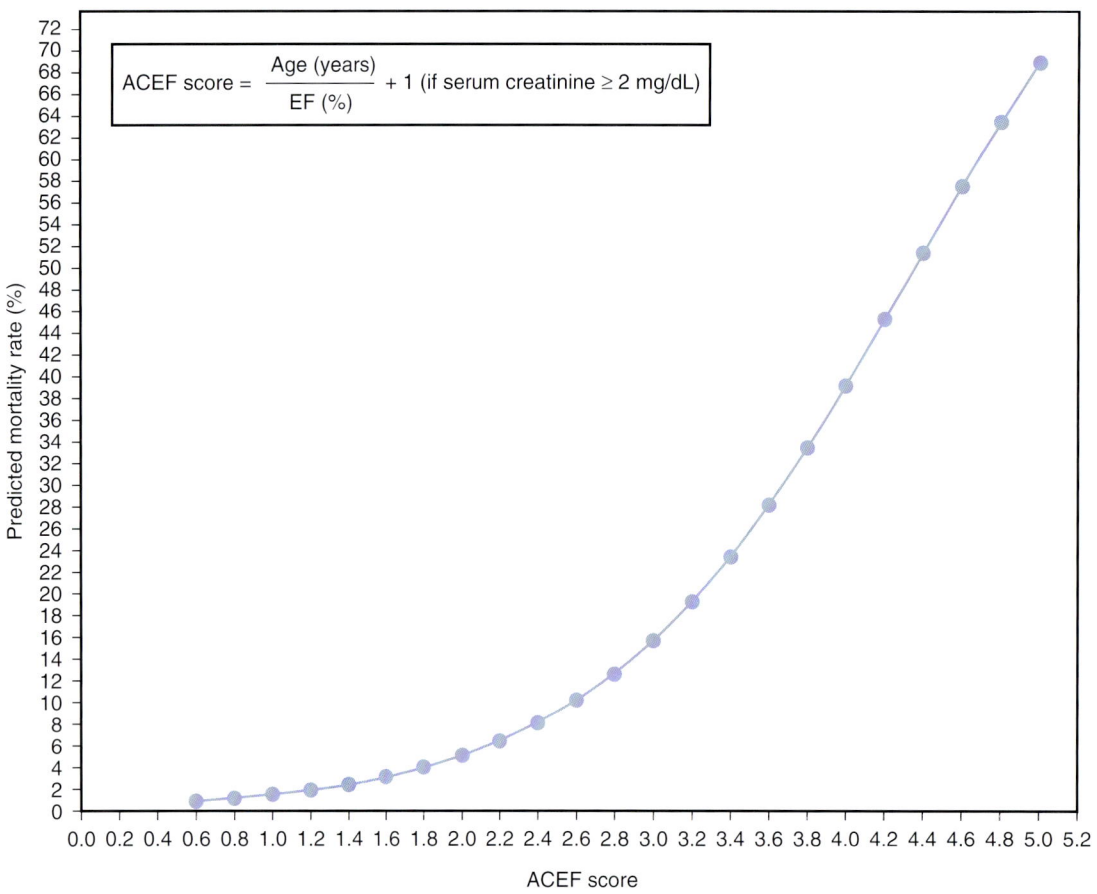

Fig. 1.8 Univariate association (logistic regression) between age, creatinine, and ejection fraction *(ACEF)* score—the value of age, creatinine, and ejection fraction—and mortality risk. (From Ranucci M, Castelvecchio S, Menicanti L, et al. Risk of assessing mortality risk in elective cardiac operations: age, creatinine, ejection fraction, and the law of parsimony. *Circulation.* 2009;119[24]:3053–3061.)

Coronary Heart Disease (APPROACH) score (Fig. 1.10; see Table 1.5). The Duke and BARI scores were developed and validated in relatively small populations. All three scores have since been validated in one population-based cohort consisting of more than 20,000 patients and were predictive of 1-year mortality in patients treated with PCI or treated medically; within this population, all three scores also had similar performance measures with only minor differences in C-statistics evident.[96–98]

It has since been shown that the Duke Jeopardy Score is an independent predictor of adverse clinical outcomes, namely death and MI, in medically treated patients with acute coronary syndromes (ACSs) at up to 1 year in a post hoc study of the Acute Catheterization and Urgent Intervention Triage Strategy (ACUITY) trial.[99]

The BCIS-1 (balloon pump-assisted coronary intervention study) Myocardial Jeopardy Score, a variant of the Duke Jeopardy Score that has been reported to be simpler to use, has recently been shown to have a strong correlation with the myocardial ischemic burden as assessed by cardiac magnetic resonance perfusion imaging.[100,101] A BCIS-1 Jeopardy Score of 10 to 12 and a revascularization index (preprocedural minus postprocedural jeopardy scores divided by preprocedural jeopardy score, with 1 indicating complete revascularization) of 0 to 0.33 were both shown to be highly predictive of mortality after contemporary PCI in a single U.K. center experience that involved over 600 patients.[102]

SYNTAX-based tools to assess completeness of revascularization (see Table 1.6) after CABG and PCI have been developed and are discussed in the section on SYNTAX-based tools.

Combined Risk Scores

The previous discussion has reviewed risk scores that rely on either clinical or angiographic variables (with the exception of SYNAX-based clinical tools). There is no disputing that for a complete individualized patient assessment, both factors must be taken into consideration. Moreover, current evidence indicates that clinical and angiography-based risk scores may be better suited to predict different patient outcomes. Clinical scores appear to be better at predicting clinical end points such as death or MI, whereas angiography-based scores appear to be superior for the prediction of angiographic success and the risk of repeat revascularization. Of note, Peterson and coworkers[63] observed only a minimal improvement in the ability of the NCDR CathPCI risk score to predict in-hospital mortality following the inclusion of angiographic variables. These findings are in line with previous reports, which demonstrated that the MCRS was superior to the ACC/AHA lesion classification in the prediction of death, stroke, MI, and emergent CABG but was inferior for the prediction of angiographic failure.[103]

TABLE 1.9 National Cardiovascular Database

Variable	Scoring Response Categories			
Age	<60	≥60, <70	≥70, <80	≥80
Weighted score	0	4	8	14
Cardiogenic shock	No	Yes		
Weighted score	0	25		
Prior CHF	No	Yes		
Weighted score	0	5		
Peripheral vascular disease	No	Yes		
Weighted score	0	5		
Chronic lung disease	No	Yes		
Weighted score	0	4		
GFR (mL/min)	<30	30 to 60	60 to 90	>90
Weighted score	18	10	6	0
NYHA Class IV	No	Yes		
Weighted score	0	4		
PCI Status (STEMI)	Elective	Urgent	Emergent	Salvage
Weighted score	12	15	20	38
PCI Status (no STEMI)	Elective	Urgent	Emergent	Salvage
Weighted score	0	8	20	42

CHF, Congestive heart failure; *GFR*, glomerular filtration rate; *NYHA*, New York Heart Association; *PCI*, percutaneous coronary intervention; *STEMI*, ST elevation myocardial infarction.
The risk of in-hospital mortality is derived using Fig. 1.11.
Registry risk score from Peterson ED, Dai D, DeLong ER, et al. Contemporary mortality risk prediction for percutaneous coronary intervention: results from 588,398 procedures in the National Cardiovascular Data Registry. *J Am Coll Cardiol*. 2010;55:1923–1932.

TABLE 1.10 American College of Cardiology/American Heart Association Characteristics of Type A, B, and C Lesions

TYPE A LESIONS (HIGH SUCCESS, >85%; LOW RISK)
Discrete (<10 mm length)
Concentric
Readily accessible
Nonangulated segment (<45 degrees)
Smooth contour
Little or no calcification
Less than totally occlusive
Not ostial in location
No major branch involvement
Absence of thrombus

TYPE B LESIONS (MODERATE SUCCESS, 60%–85%; MODERATE RISK)
Tubular (10–20 mm in length)
Eccentric
Moderate tortuosity of proximal segment
Moderately angulated segment, 45–90 degrees
Irregular contour
Moderate to heavy calcification
Ostial in location
Bifurcation lesions requiring double guidewires
Some thrombus present
Total occlusion less than 3 months old
Type B lesions are further subdivided into subtypes B1 (one type B characteristic) and B2 (two type B characteristics)

TYPE C LESIONS (LOW SUCCESS, <60%; HIGH RISK)
Diffuse (>2 cm length)
Excessive tortuosity of proximal segment
Extremely angulated segments (>90 degrees)
Inability to protect major side branches
Degenerated vein grafts with friable lesions
Total occlusion more than 3 months old

Krone RJ, Laskey WK, Johnson C, et al. A simplified lesion classification for predicting success and complications of coronary angioplasty. Registry Committee of the Society for Cardiac Angiography and Intervention. *Am J Cardiol*. 2000;85:1179–1184.

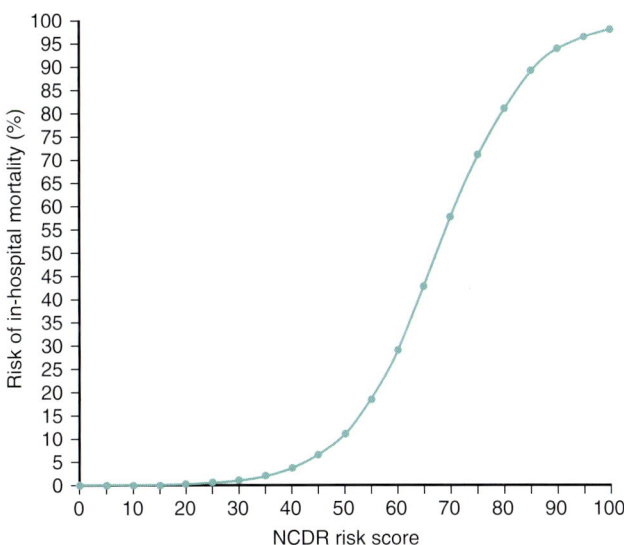

Fig. 1.9 The predicted risk of in-hospital mortality using the National Cardiovascular Database Registry *(NCDR)* risk score. (From Peterson ED, Dai D, DeLong ER, et al. Contemporary mortality risk prediction for percutaneous coronary intervention: results from 588,398 procedures in the National Cardiovascular Data Registry. *J Am Coll Cardiol*. 2010;55:1923–1932.)

According to the variables assessed in the risk score, these differential outcomes have raised interest in combined risk scores, which assess risk by considering both clinical and angiographic variables. In view of this, several combined clinical and angiographic risk scores have been developed. Other than the STS score, the newer combined scores have yet to be validated in large patient populations, such that outcome data are currently confined to small, retrospective studies with limited follow-up. The most prominent combined risk scores are discussed here.

Society of Thoracic Surgery Score
The STS score predicts the risk of operative mortality and morbidity after cardiac surgery and is calculated by means of an online calculator (www.sts.org) that requests information on 40 clinical and two angiographic variables (presence of LM lesion and number of vessels diseased).[64,74] As alluded to earlier, the STS score undergoes periodic recalibration, which is vital to ensure that its results remain applicable to contemporary practice. In comparison with other clinical risk scores in patients undergoing CABG, the STS score has been shown to be superior to both the MCRS[87] and the EuroSCORE.[104] However, notably, no evaluation has been done of the STS score in patients undergoing PCI, nor has any comparison been made between the STS score and angiography-based scores. Consequently, the role of the STS score in the assessment of patients undergoing revascularization is confined to those in whom surgical revascularization has already been selected.

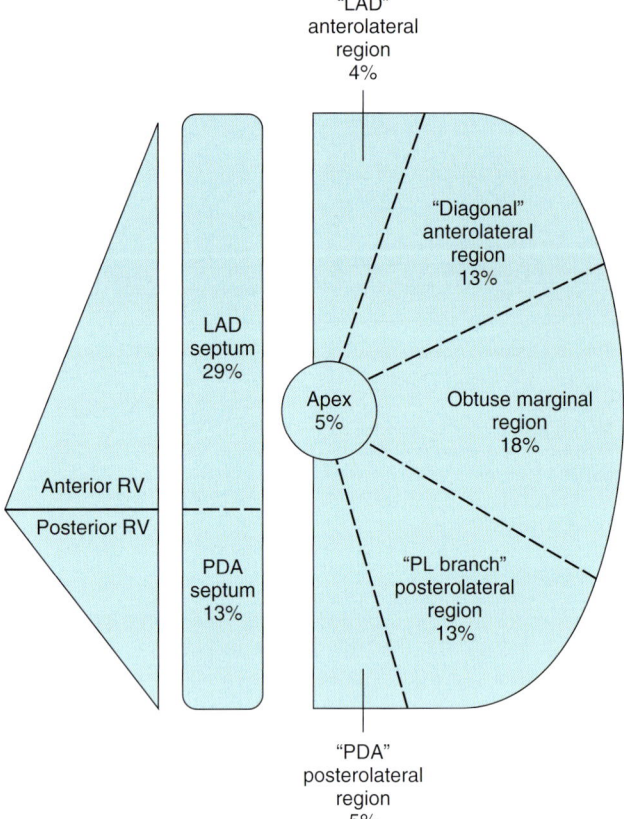

Fig. 1.10 An example of a Myocardial Jeopardy Score. The AP-PROACH lesion score illustrating the weighting factors for myocardial regions is illustrated. *LAD,* Left anterior descending artery; *PDA,* posterior descending artery; *PL,* posterolateral; *RV,* right ventricle. (From Graham MM, Faris PD, Ghali WA, et al. Validation of three myocardial jeopardy scores in a population-based cardiac catheterization cohort. *Am Heart J.* 2001;142[2]:254–261.)

EuroHeart Score
A logistic regression score comprising 10 clinical variables and 6 anatomic variables was developed based on the Euro Heart Survey, a European PCI registry consisting of more than 46,000 patients from 176 European centers who underwent PCI for differing indications (Fig. 1.11).[105] The risk score was shown to be highly predictive of in-hospital mortality (C-statistic 0.91); the strengths of this score were that it was internally validated within the registry population and that it retained its discriminatory power (C-statistic 0.90); the score was also sufficiently calibrated for the study and validation populations.

New Risk Stratification Score
The New Risk Stratification Score (NERS)[106] is a risk score developed to predict outcomes for unprotected LM stem PCI from four centers in China (*n* = 260). Reflecting the long time frame of this registry (approximately 10 years), the patients included either had bare-metal or DESs implanted. The NERS was subsequently validated in a different consecutive group of patients within the same registry, all treated with DESs (*n* = 337). The NERS consists of 54 variables (17 clinical, 4 procedural, and 33 angiographic features). A substantially higher C-statistic was evident for the NERS compared with the anatomic SYNTAX score (NERS 0.89 vs. SYNTAX score 0.69), indicating that it had an excellent discriminatory ability. When the NERS score was separated into two groups of risk (high and low) and clinical outcomes were assessed, the high-risk group was demonstrated to be significantly more predictive of MACE compared with the intermediate or high SYNTAX score tertiles (Fig. 1.12). However, in the low-risk NERS group, outcomes were similar to the low SYNTAX score group, suggesting at least from this study that anatomic variables alone may be sufficient to be predictive of clinical outcomes in the low-risk group. One of the main limitations of NERS is that patient comorbidity was significantly less prevalent compared with that of the all-comers SYNTAX population,[13,16] the latter of which was designed to overcome many of the limitations and selection bias inherent in small registries. A more simplified NERS II score consisting of 16 variables (seven clinical and nine angiographic) has been reported to have a predictive accuracy similar to that of the original NERS in a multicenter, prospective registry study in China.[107]

SYNTAX-Based Tools
The augmentation of the anatomic SYNTAX score with clinical variables, culminating in the development and validation of SYNTAX score II—in which objective and tailored decision making could be made for the individual patient—is detailed in the next section.

SYNTAX-BASED CLINICAL TOOLS

In this section we systematically examine the widening applications of tools for clinical decision making that are based on the SYNTAX score.

Anatomic SYNTAX Score

The anatomic SYNTAX score (www.syntaxscore.com) has emerged as an anatomic-based tool to objectively determine the complexity of CAD and to guide decision making between CABG and PCI.[45–48] Since the landmark SYNTAX trial[13–15] to compare CABG with PCI in patients with complex CAD (unprotected left main coronary artery [ULMCA] or de novo 3VD), numerous validation studies have confirmed the clinical validity of the SYNTAX score to identify higher-risk subjects and aid decision making between CABG and PCI in a broad range of patient types.[48,49] The SYNTAX score is currently advocated in both the European and U.S. revascularization guidelines[52,54,55] as part of the SYNTAX-pioneered heart team approach.[50] In addition, the U.S. Food and Drug Administration (FDA) mandates the SYNTAX score as entry criteria in ongoing contemporary stent and structural heart disease trials. Namely, the Evaluation of XIENCE PRIME or XIENCE V Everolimus-Eluting Stent System Versus Coronary Artery Bypass Surgery for Effectiveness of Left Main Revascularization (EXCEL) trial (ClinicalTrials.gov ID# NCT01205776),[108] and Safety and Efficacy Study of the Medtronic CoreValve System in the Treatment of Severe, Symptomatic Aortic Stenosis in Intermediate-Risk Subjects Who Need Aortic Valve Replacement (SURTAVI) trial (ID# NCT01586910).

The anatomic SYNTAX score was developed during the design of the SYNTAX trial as a tool to force the interventional cardiologist and cardiac surgeon to systematically analyze the coronary angiogram and to specify the number of coronary lesions that require treatment and assess their angiographic location and anatomic complexity.[13,45–49] The SYNTAX score combines the importance of a diseased coronary artery segment in terms of its severity (i.e., obstructive or occlusive), anatomic location, and importance in supplying blood to the myocardium (*vessel-segment weighting* based on the Leaman Score),[109] adverse lesion characteristics (ACC/AHA lesion classification),[110] bifurcation lesion characteristics (Medina classification),[111] and total occlusion characteristics from Recanalization of Total Coronary Occlusions Using a Laser

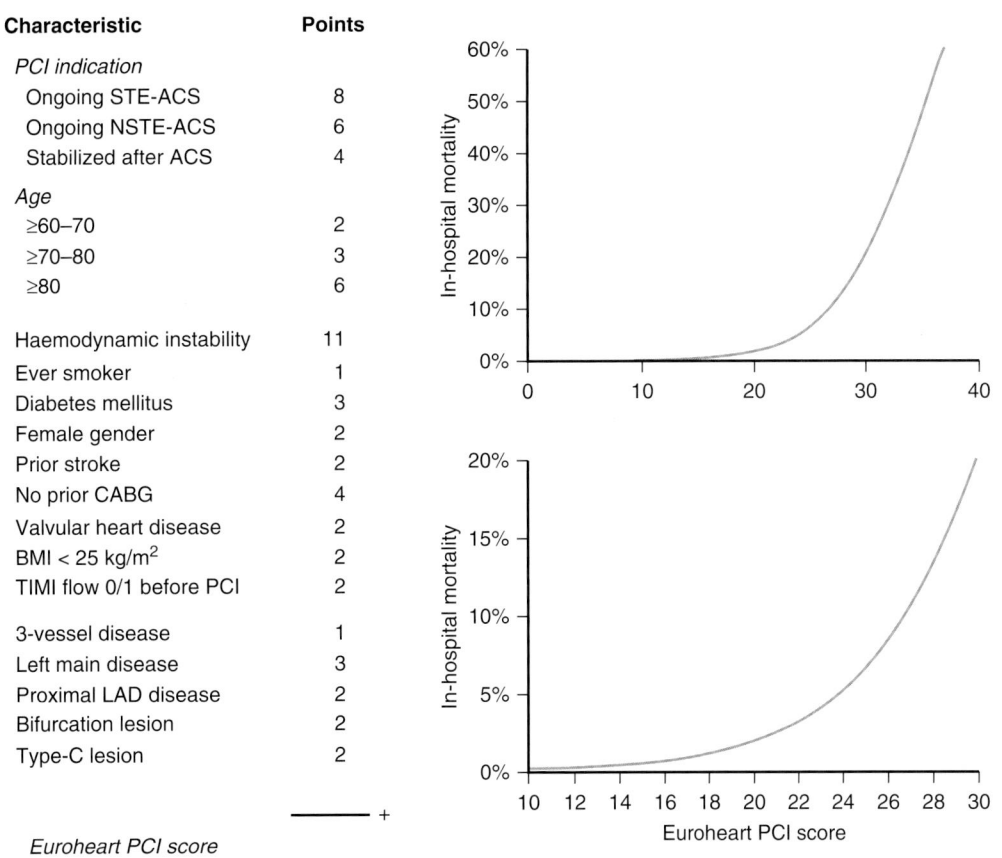

Fig. 1.11 EuroHeart PCI Score–assigned integer scores. *ACS,* Acute coronary syndrome; *BMI,* body mass index; *CABG,* coronary artery bypass grafting; *LAD,* left anterior descending; *NSTE,* non-ST elevation; *PCI,* percutaneous coronary intervention; *STE,* ST elevation; *TIMI,* thrombolysis in myocardial infarction. (From de Mulder M, Gitt A, van Domburg R, et al. EuroHeart score for the evaluation of in-hospital mortality in patients undergoing percutaneous coronary intervention. *Eur Heart J.* 2011;32[11]:1398–1408.)

Guidewire (the European TOTAL Surveillance Study).[112] Each vessel segment 1.5 mm in diameter or greater (Fig. 1.13, labeled 1 through 16) with a 50% or more diameter stenosis by visual estimation is awarded a multiplication factor related to coronary lesion location and severity (see Fig. 1.13A). Further characterization of the coronary lesions leads to the addition of more points (see Fig. 1.13B), which includes features of total occlusions (duration, length, blunt stumps, presence of bridging collaterals or side branch), bifurcation (Medina classification)[111] or trifurcation (number of diseased branches involved), side-branch angulation, aortoostial lesions, severe tortuosity, lesion length greater than 20 mm, heavy calcification, thrombus, and diffuse or small-vessel disease. An online SYNTAX score algorithm[45] automatically summates each of these features to calculate the total SYNTAX score.

Within the SYNTAX trial,[13] the distribution of the SYNTAX score was found to be normal (Gaussian) in the randomized PCI and CABG populations with the curves almost being superimposable on each other (eFig. 1.2). When the scores of the randomized SYNTAX population were divided into tertiles, the upper boundary of the lowest tertile was 22 (low risk), the second tertile ranged from 23 to 32 (intermediate risk), and the lower boundary for the highest tertile was equal to or greater than 33 (high risk).

Based primarily on the results of the SYNTAX trial,[13–15] current European revascularization guidelines[52] give subjects with 3VD and low SYNTAX scores (0 to 22) a class I recommendation, level of evidence (LOE) A, for CABG and a class IIa LOE B recommendation for PCI. In subjects with ULMCA disease and low to intermediate SYNTAX scores (<33), a class I LOE A recommendation is given for CABG and IIb B for PCI. Furthermore, U.S. guidelines currently give surgical revascularization for ULMCA disease a class I B recommendation[54,55] compared with a class I A recommendation in previous guidelines.[113]

Functional SYNTAX Score

PCI guided by the assessment of the functional significance of a lesion has been shown to improve clinical outcomes.[114–116] The functional SYNTAX score uses the principle of the functional assessment of coronary lesions to determine the SYNTAX score, rather than the angiographic determination of the SYNTAX score based on visual assessment, as is undertaken in conventional SYNTAX score calculations. In a retrospective subanalysis of almost 500 patients ($n = 497$) from the FFR-guided arm of the Fractional Flow Reserve Versus Angiography for Multivessel Evaluation (FAME) study, the primary benefit appeared in reclassifying higher-risk groups into lower-risk categories without any adverse sequelae in terms of MACEs and death or MI at 1 year.[36]

It should be emphasized that subjects in the FAME study had substantially less complex CAD (mean SYNTAX score 14.8 ± 6.0) compared with the PCI arm of the SYNTAX trial (mean SYNTAX score 28.4 ± 11.5) and that subjects with LM CAD were not investigated. Prospective validation studies of the functional SYNTAX score in complex CAD are ongoing

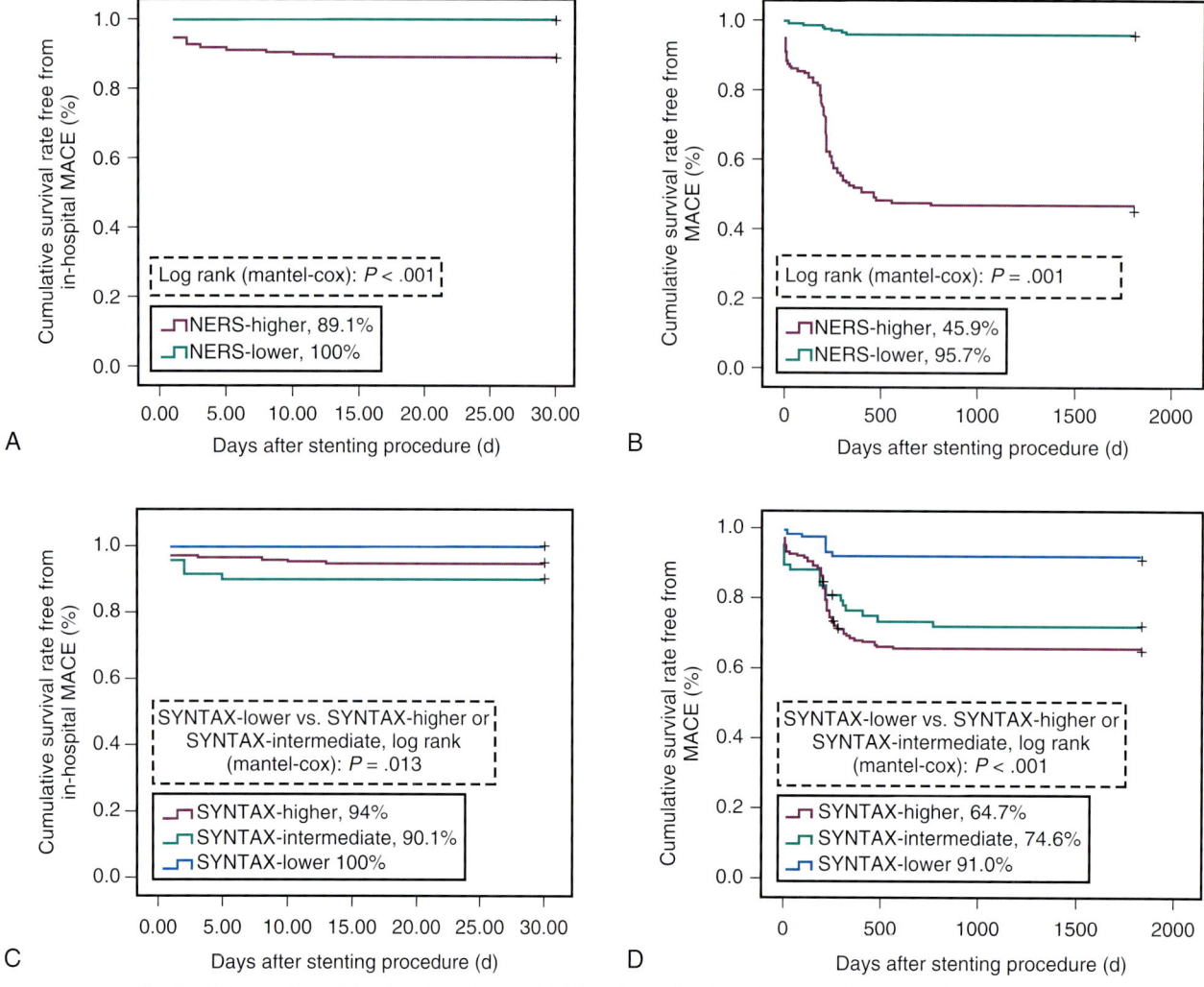

Fig. 1.12 Comparison of freedom from in-hospital (A) and overall major adverse cardiac events (*MACEs*, B) survival between New Risk Stratification *(NERS)* groups and in-hospital (C) and overall MACEs (D) survival among SYNTAX groups. (From Chen SL, Chen JP, Mintz G, et al. Comparison between the NERS [New Risk Stratification] score and the SYNTAX (Synergy Between Percutaneous Coronary Intervention With Taxus and Cardiac Surgery) score in outcome prediction for unprotected left main stenting. *JACC Cardiovasc Interv.* 2010;3[6]:632–641.)

at the time of writing. Namely the SYNTAX II trial, in which a noninvasive assessment of the functional SYNTAX is also being assessed with fractional flow reserve derived from computed tomography angiography,[117] and the FAME 3 trial [NCT02100722]).[118]

Augmenting the Anatomic SYNTAX Score With Clinical Factors and the Personalization of Decision Making: Development of SYNTAX Score II

Since the anatomic SYNTAX score was developed, limitations of this scoring system to aid decision making between CABG and PCI became evident—namely, the lack of clinical variables and lack of a personalized approach to decision making. Following is a brief overview of the "development phase" leading to SYNTAX score II, which was designed to overcome these limitations (see Table 1.6).

Age, Serum Creatinine, and Ejection Fraction

As described earlier, Ranucci and colleagues[62,88,89] developed a simple risk score that consisted of only three clinical variables—age, serum creatinine, and LVEF—for assessing operative mortality risk in elective cardiac operations (ACEF score, see Fig. 1.8). Based on the law of parsimony, or "Occam's razor," whereby a simple model can explain a phenomenon with the same level of accuracy as complex models, ACEF was shown to be least comparable to the EuroSCORE (composed of 17 variables)[58,59] in predicting in-hospital mortality after CABG.[62,89]

The three risk factors used in ACEF are natural continuous variables that are objectively defined and not subject to personal estimation (e.g., whether the patient has diabetes or extracardiac arteriopathy). In addition, the variables of ACEF were known independent risk factors for mortality, and it was subsequently shown that the end-organ manifestations of the risk factor as identified in ACEF were more important for predicting long-term prognosis rather than the actual presence of the risk factor.[6,88,119,120]

Clinical SYNTAX Score/Logistic Clinical SYNTAX Score

Based on the principle of ACEF, the clinical SYNTAX score[90,121,122] and subsequently the logistic clinical SYNTAX score (eFig. 1.3)[123,124] were developed and validated. Both the clinical SYNTAX score and logistic clinical SYNTAX score combined ACEF with the SYNTAX score and were shown to improve mortality predictions, compared with the SYNTAX score alone, in subjects with complex CAD.[90,121–124] Similar to the conventional SYNTAX score, the clinical SYNTAX score relied on categorization of risk into low, intermediate, and high groups and was able to only identify a high-risk group after PCI.[90,121,122] The logistic clinical SYNTAX score was designed to individualize risk and provide 1-year mortality predictions in an all-comers PCI population irrespective of clinical presentation (except cardiogenic shock).[123,124]

The logistic clinical SYNTAX score was developed and cross-validated (internal-external validation procedure[125]) in more than 6000 subjects from seven contemporary coronary stent trials[123] and was further externally validated in 2627 subjects presenting with non–ST elevation ACS and undergoing PCI from the ACUITY trial.[124] Notably, the addition of six clinical variables, including diabetes, to the logistic clinical SYNTAX score led to only a minor incremental benefit in improving risk predictions.[123,124] Thus the logistic clinical SYNTAX score was shown to follow the law of parsimony, as seen with the surgical ACEF score discussed previously,[62,88,89] and the end-organ manifestations of the risk factor were found to be more important for predicting prognosis than the actual presence of the risk factor.

Global Risk

In the SYNTAX trial, as well as the SYNTAX score in PCI subjects, it was shown that the EuroSCORE[58,59] is an independent predictor of MACEs in subjects undergoing surgical or percutaneous revascularization. Subsequently, it was hypothesized that the amalgamation of the anatomic SYNTAX score with the EuroSCORE could improve decision making between CABG and PCI (Fig. 1.14).[48] The feasibility of this "global risk" approach was demonstrated in a registry of 255 subjects with LM CAD using tertiles of the SYNTAX score and tertiles of the additive EuroSCORE that reflected the study population.[126] Subsequently, the global risk was validated in the SYNTAX trial using conventional tertiles of the SYNTAX score and EuroSCORE,[127] and compared with the SYNTAX score alone, it was shown to substantially enhance the identification of low-risk patients with ULMCA disease or de novo 3VD who could safely and efficaciously be treated with CABG or PCI.

One of the unexpected findings from the global risk was that higher-risk subjects (high additive EuroSCORE ≥6) in all tertiles of the SYNTAX score were shown to have a potential prognostic benefit from undergoing CABG compared with PCI irrespective of the baseline SYNTAX score, provided an acceptable threshold of operative risk was not exceeded.[127] For example, in the 3VD cohort of the SYNTAX trial, subjects with a low SYNTAX score (<23) and a high EuroSCORE (≥6) had a doubling of 3-year mortality when undergoing PCI (15.9%) compared with CABG (8.2%). Hypotheses to explain these findings included that the bypass graft would potentially "protect" the entire treated coronary vessel from future cardiac events for the life span of the graft in high-risk subjects compared with PCI, which would treat the individual lesion.[43] Based on these observations, it was hypothesized by the investigators that subjects of opposite risk concealed each other; for example, low-risk subjects were potentially concealed by high-risk subjects, and vice versa, in all tertiles of the SYNTAX score. This hypothesis is what prompted the investigators to develop a more individualized approach to decision making between CABG and PCI, and it is what subsequently led to the development of SYNTAX score II,[7] as detailed later.

SYNTAX Score II

As previously discussed, the combination of the anatomic SYNTAX score with ACEF contained most of the prognostic information in predicting mortality after CABG (excluding the anatomic SYNTAX score)[62,88,89,127] or PCI (including the anatomic SYNTAX score).[123] SYNTAX score II[7,8] augments the purely anatomic SYNTAX score with anatomic and clinical factors that were shown to alter the threshold value of the anatomic SYNTAX score for equipoise to be achieved between CABG and PCI for long-term mortality. This was accomplished through building SYNTAX score II on the ACEF "skeleton" with the addition of risk factors that were shown to directly affect decision making between CABG and PCI through interaction effects (i.e., a risk factor being more predictive of mortality in patients undergoing PCI compared with CABG, or vice versa; Fig. 1.15). For example, the anatomic SYNTAX score aids decision making between CABG and PCI because it is more predictive of clinical outcomes in patients undergoing PCI, compared with patients undergoing CABG, in whom it is not predictive. Based on this principle, younger age, female sex, and reduced LVEF favored CABG compared with PCI on long-term prognostic grounds (eFig. 1.4). Thus in such patients a *lower* anatomic SYNTAX score would be required for the long-term mortality risk to be similar between CABG and PCI. By contrast, older age, ULMCA, or chronic obstructive pulmonary disease (COPD) favored PCI compared with CABG (see eFig. 1.4), and thus, in this type of patient, a *higher* anatomic SYNTAX score would be needed for the long-term mortality risks to be similar.

By adopting the individualized approach of SYNTAX score II, augmented by clinical variables, it was shown that subsets of patients existed in all tertiles of the SYNTAX score in which CABG or PCI would confer a mortality benefit or offer a similar long-term prognosis (Fig. 1.16).[7] A nomogram was developed (Fig. 1.17) that allowed for an accurate individualized prediction of 4-year mortality in patients proposing to undergo CABG or PCI to objectively aid decision making. For example, a 60-year-old man with an anatomic SYNTAX score of 30, ULMCA disease, a creatinine clearance of 60 mL/min, an LVEF of 50%, and COPD would have 41 points (predicted 4-year mortality 16.3%) and 33 points (predicted 4-year mortality 8.7%) to undergo CABG and PCI, respectively. The same example, without COPD included, would lead to identical points (29 points) and identical 4-year mortality predictions (6.3%) for CABG and PCI. An online version of SYNTAX score II, version 2.11 using the 4-year data, is currently available as a download along with the original SYNTAX score calculator (www.syntaxscore.com).

Diabetics

Notably, diabetes was not included in the final SYNTAX score II despite medically treated diabetes being prestratified at randomization as a powered subgroup in the SYNTAX trial and present in more than a quarter of the study patients (26%), and in spite of diabetes being perceived as a specific high-risk group potentially warranting a differing treatment strategy compared with that considering other risk factors.[11,52,54,55] The primary reason was that diabetes was shown not to be important for decision making between CABG and PCI because it lacked an interaction effect (i.e., it was equally predictive of mortality in the CABG and PCI arms after adjustment for other risk factors) (see Fig. 1.15). As previously discussed in ACEF, the end-organ manifestations of diabetes are what affected long-term mortality in CABG and PCI populations.[6,51,88,89,123] The findings of the lack of inclusion of diabetes in SYNTAX score II are supported by epidemiologic data, in which nondiabetics with chronic kidney disease and proteinuria had a stronger association with risk of MI and a higher

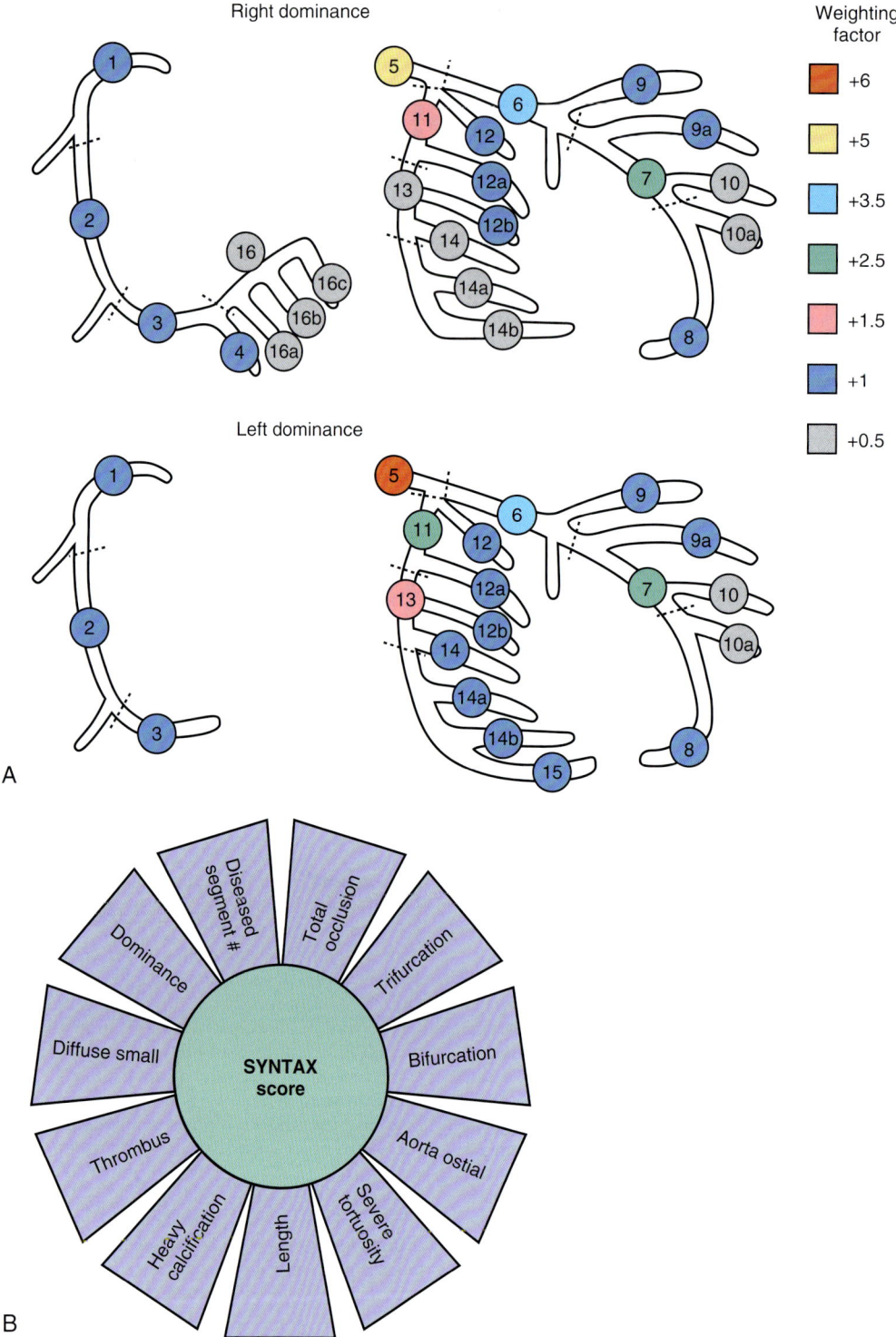

Fig. 1.13 Coronary tree segments and their importance in supplying blood flow to the left ventricle (vessel segment weighting factors; Leaman score[154,155]) based on the presence of a right or left dominant system (A).[109] A multiplication factor of two is used for nonocclusive lesions (50% to 99% diameter stenosis) and five for occlusive (100% diameter stenosis) lesions. For example, a nonocclusive stenotic proximal left anterior descending (LAD) coronary artery lesion (segment 6) would have a weighting factor of 3.5 × 2 (7 points) and an occlusive proximal LAD lesion a weighting factor of 3.5 × 5 (17.5 points). Other adverse lesion characteristics considered in the SYNTAX score have an additive value (B). #, Segment number. (Images courtesy the SYNTAX Trial Investigators.)

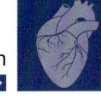

EuroSCORE	SYNTAX score		
	≤22	23–32	≥33
0–2	LOW	LOW	INT
3–5	LOW	LOW	INT
≥6	INT	INT	HIGH

LOW Global Risk: SYNTAX score <33 and EuroSCORE <6
Int Global Risk: SYNTAX score <33 and EuroSCORE ≥6
OR EuroSCORE <6 and SYNTAX score ≥33
High Global Risk: SYNTAX score ≥33 and EuroSCORE ≥6

Fig. 1.14 The Global Risk matrix. (From Serruys PW, Farooq V, Vranckx P, et al. A global risk approach to identify patients with left main or 3-vessel disease who could safely and efficaciously be treated with percutaneous coronary intervention: the SYNTAX Trial at 3 years. *JACC Cardiovasc Interv.* 2012;5[6]:606–617.)

rate of mortality compared with diabetics and that the relative risk of long-term mortality associated with chronic kidney disease was "much the same irrespective of the presence or absence of diabetes."[119,120]

Impaired Left Ventricular Ejection Fraction

Within SYNTAX score II, impaired LVEF favored CABG over PCI on long-term prognostic grounds, findings supported by a recent subanalysis of the Surgical Treatment of Ischemic Heart Failure (STICH) trial[128]; namely, that in subjects with more advanced ischemic cardiomyopathy with more extensive CAD and worse myocardial dysfunction and remodeling, a net longer-term prognostic benefit was seen for CABG compared with optimal medical therapy despite the short-term (30-day) mortality risk being higher with CABG.

Validation of SYNTAX Score II

Compared with existing revascularization guidelines using the anatomic SYNTAX score,[52,54,55] it was shown that if CABG or PCI was selected based on a higher or lower expected survival (irrespective of the margin of difference) with SYNTAX score II in the SYNTAX trial, SYNTAX score II would need to be used in only 110 patients to have one more patient alive at 4 years.[8]

External validation of SYNTAX score II[7] was performed in the multinational Drug-Eluting Stent for Left Main Coronary Artery Disease (DELTA) registry (14 centers in Europe, the United States, and South Korea)[129] composed of subjects with ULMCA disease with or without MVD (26% of the study population had 3VD). All variables in SYNTAX score II interacted in a similar way and therefore influenced decision making between CABG and PCI in the SYNTAX trial and DELTA registry with the exception of age and LVEF, which had minimal interactions in the DELTA registry—findings that may relate to the unavoidable selection bias inherent to all registries because decision making between CABG and PCI has already been made and would be difficult to control for.[130] Even randomized trials that lack an all-comers design, with restrictive inclusion and exclusion criteria, can potentially make application to clinical practice questionable.[43,44,131] This was exemplified in a recent meta-analysis of randomized trials undertaken prior to SYNTAX that compared PCI against CABG, where in most trials, 2% to 12% (see Table 1.3) of screened subjects were randomized due to the highly restrictive inclusion and exclusion criteria.[132] In this meta-analysis, CABG was shown to be favored in older subjects, and PCI was favored in younger subjects,[132] findings that have since been directly contradicted by SYNTAX score II in the all-comers SYNTAX trial in which the opposite was shown.[7] Hence "randomized" or prospective validation of SYNTAX score II was proposed[7] in which further validation would be conducted in randomized controlled trials or prospectively run studies.

Further retrospective validation of SYNTAX score II has recently been undertaken in 3896 patients with 3VD and/or ULMCA disease undergoing PCI ($n = 2190$) or CABG ($n = 1796$) from the Japanese Coronary Revascularization Demonstrating Outcome Study in Kyoto (CREDO-Kyoto) PCI/CABG multicenter registry.[133] In addition, the SYNTAX score II was externally validated in 1480 patients with multivessel and/or unprotected LM CAD in a pooled analysis of the BEST and PRECOMBAT (Premier of Randomized Comparison of Bypass Surgery versus Angioplasty Using Sirolimus-Eluting Stent in Patients with Left Main Coronary Artery Disease) randomized controlled trials.[134]

Prospective validation of SYNTAX score II is being evaluated in the ongoing EXCEL[17,18] and SYNTAX II[135–137] trials. In addition, prospective validation of decision making between CABG and PCI based on noninvasive (computed tomography derived) SYNTAX score II in patients with complex CAD is currently being undertaken in the randomized SYNTAX III Revolution trial and is discussed later under future directions.[138,139]

EXCEL Trial

The international multicenter EXCEL trial recently recruited 1905 patients with ULMCA disease and investigator-reported SYNTAX scores less than 33, randomized to CABG ($n = 957$) or PCI with contemporary stents ($n = 948$),[108] and reported the composite primary end point of death, stroke, or MI at 3 years (see Fig. 1.4).[17,18] As part of the prospective validation of SYNTAX score II, this tool was used to forecast and compare 4-year mortality in the PCI and CABG arms of EXCEL prior to the actual reporting of the primary outcome of EXCEL.[140] Based on 1000 4-year mortality simulations of the EXCEL trial using the SYNTAX score II, 77.9% of trial simulations ($n = 7790$) favored PCI and 22.1% of trial simulations ($n = 2210$) favored CABG (Fig. 1.18). Thus the SYNTAX score II indicated at least an equipoise for long-term mortality between CABG and PCI in subjects with ULMCA disease up to an intermediate anatomic complexity. Longer-term follow-up of EXCEL is awaited to allow validation of the SYNTAX score II.

SYNTAX II Trial

In the ongoing SYNTAX II trial (NCT02015832),[135] the SYNTAX score II is being used as a tool to recruit subjects with de novo 3VD (without LM involvement) on the grounds of patient safety (i.e., subjects with a similar long-term mortality between CABG and PCI) in conjunction with the heart team (Fig. 1.19). Notably, subjects from all tertiles of the SYNTAX score are eligible. The PCI procedure uses the state-of-art SYNTAX II PCI strategy of appropriate patient selection with the SYNTAX score II, newer-generation metal stent platform with a biodegradable polymer,[36] contemporary CTO revascularization strategies and functional and IVUS-guided PCI of all three vessels.[141,142] The PCI and CABG arms of the original SYNTAX trial[15,33] acted as control arms.

Notably, the use of functional guided PCI in SYNTAX II led to a deferral of almost one-third of lesions (31%), with two-thirds of lesions intervened on with PCI (69%) (Fig. 1.20A). In addition, 87% of attempted CTOs were successfully revascularized (compared with 53% in the original SYNTAX trial), and IVUS guidance was used in 84.1% of patients (compared with 4.8% patients in the original SYNTAX trial) (see Fig. 1.20B and C).

At 2-year follow-up of SYNTAX II, the SYNTAX II PCI strategy led to substantially improved clinical outcomes compared

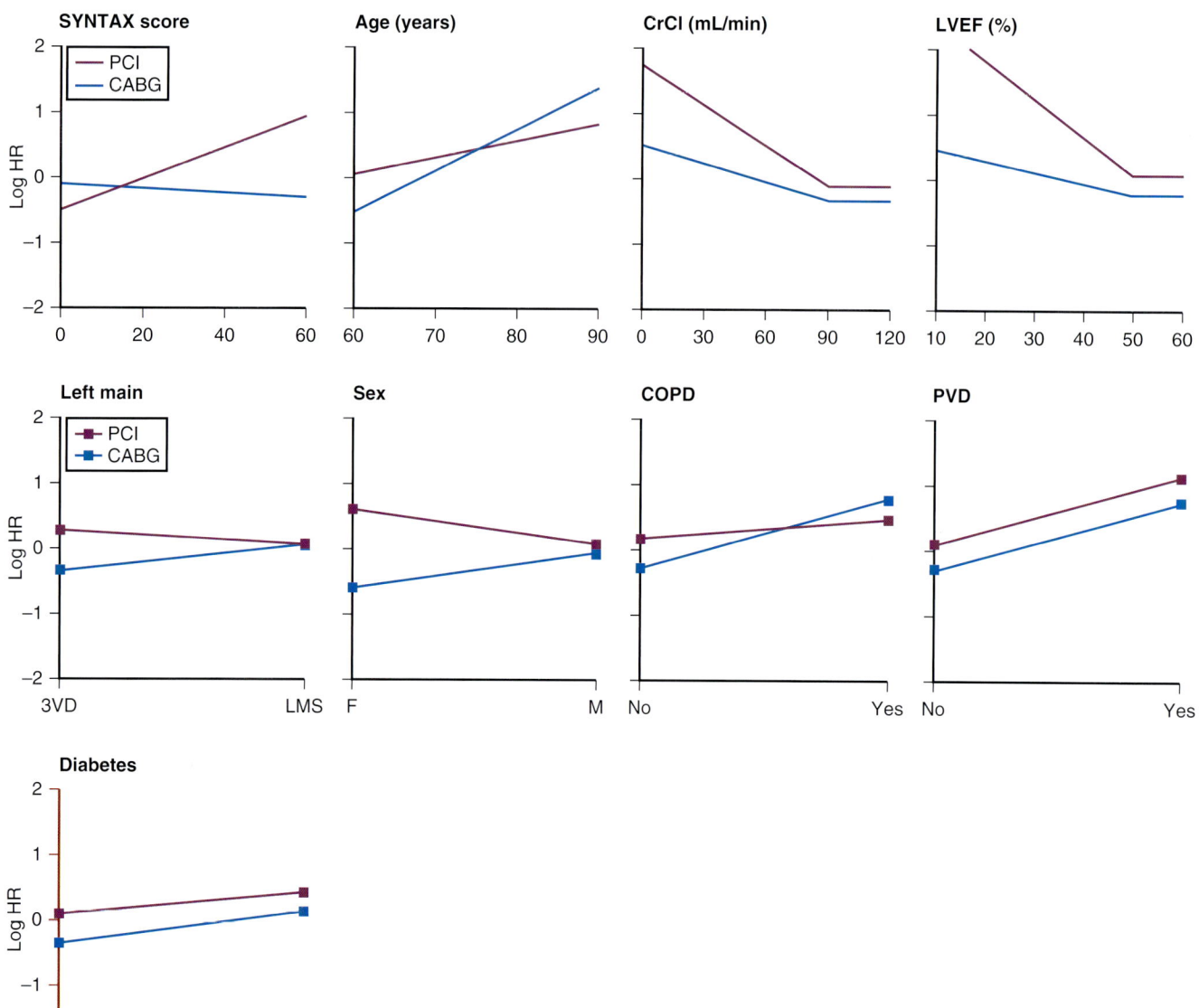

Fig. 1.15 Predictor effects for coronary artery bypass surgery *(CABG)* and percutaneous coronary intervention *(PCI)* in the SYNTAX score II. These are represented visually as a log hazard ratio *(HR)* for CABG and PCI on the y-axis for each predictor. Each predictor is expressed on the x-axis continuously *(upper)* or categorically *(lower)*, for a person of mean baseline characteristics. Diabetes is included *(highlighted in red)* to illustrate its absence of interaction when included in the analyses. Note the differing gradients of the hazards for PCI and CABG, leading to the hazards crossing at an anatomic SYNTAX score of 15. At this crossover point of hazards, the mortality risk is comparable between CABG and PCI. This threshold of crossover of hazards will vary according to the level of other variables, namely, being lower for female sex, reduced left ventricular ejection fraction *(LVEF)* and younger age, and higher for chronic obstructive pulmonary disease *(COPD)*, unprotected left main coronary artery disease, and older age. As both peripheral vascular disease *(PVD;* P = 1.00) and diabetes (P = .67) lacked an interaction effect, as indicated by almost parallel HRs (i.e., a comparable increase in mortality risk), their presence would have no impact on decision making between CABG and PCI. *CrCl,* Creatinine clearance. (From Farooq V, van Klaveren D, Steyerberg EW, et al. Anatomical and clinical characteristics to guide decision making between coronary artery bypass surgery and percutaneous coronary intervention for individual patients: development and validation of SYNTAX score II. *Lancet.* 2013;381[9867]:639–650.)

with the PCI strategy adopted in SYNTAX I (Fig. 1.21A). Moreover, clinical outcomes were similar in 3VD patients with a low anatomic SYNTAX score (≤22), in which revascularization guidelines currently support PCI or CABG-based revascularization[52–55]—compared with more anatomically complex 3VD (anatomic SYNTAX score >22), in which current revascularization guidelines support CABG (see Fig. 1.21B). In addition, the SYNTAX II PCI strategy demonstrated equipoise to CABG at 2-year follow-up for MACCE (exploratory end point) (see Fig. 1.21C). Longer (5 year) follow-up of SYNTAX II is awaited.

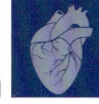

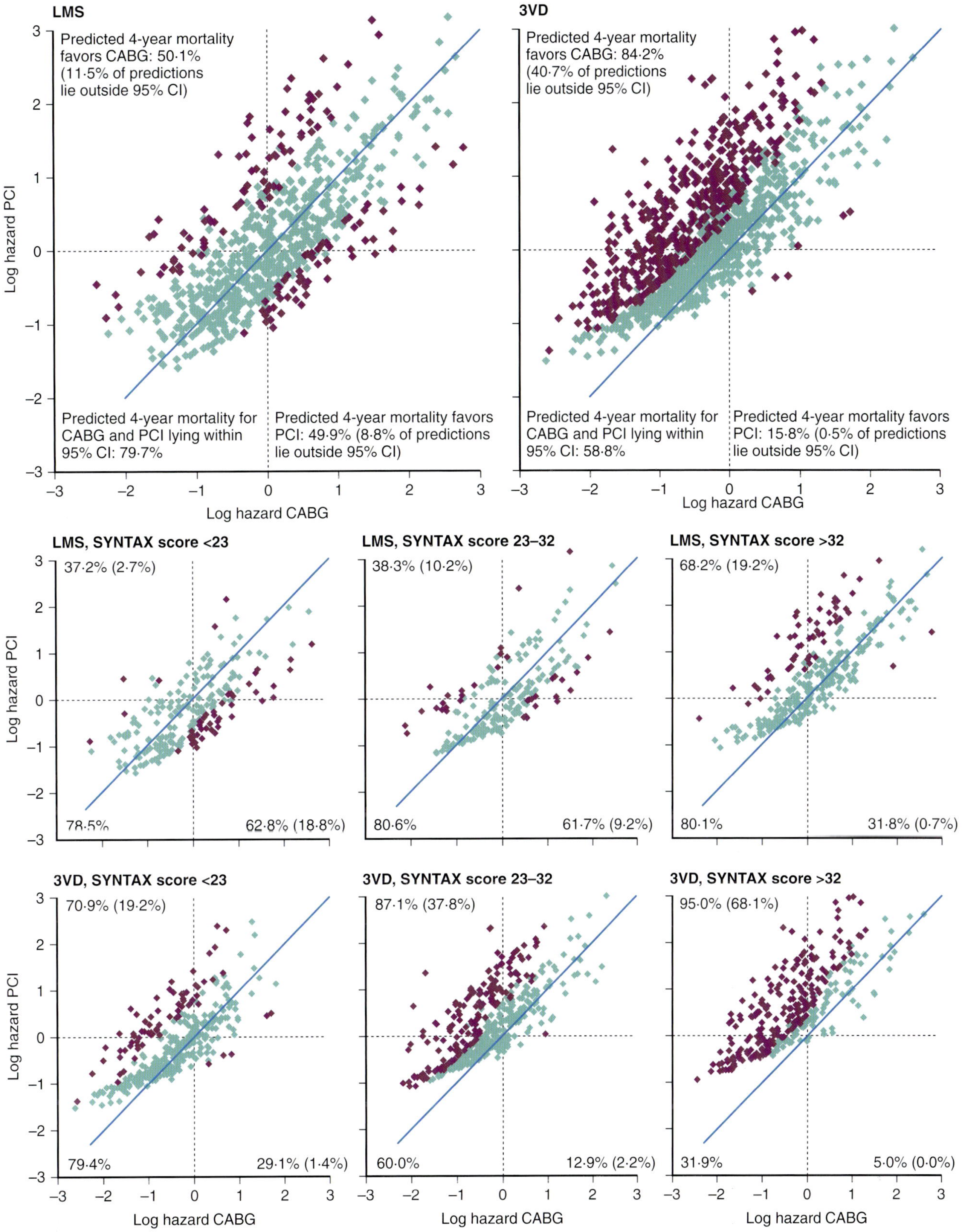

Fig. 1.16 Mortality predictions for coronary artery bypass grafting *(CABG)* versus percutaneous coronary intervention *(PCI)* for each individual patient in the randomized SYNTAX trial. The SYNTAX trial included 1800 participants, separated into left main stem *(LMS)* cohort and three-vessel disease *(3VD)* cohort *(upper panels)*, and by tertiles of the anatomic SYNTAX score *(lower panels)*. The diagonal line represents identical mortality predictions for CABG and PCI. Individual predictions plotted to the left of the diagonal line favor CABG (actual percentages shown in top left corner) and to the right favor PCI (actual percentages shown in bottom right corner). Individual mortality predictions for CABG or PCI that could be separated with 95% confidence ($P < .05$) are colored *blue* (actual percentage shown in parentheses in respective corners). Mortality predictions that could not be separated with 95% confidence ($P > .05$) are highlighted in *green* and identify patients with similar 4-year mortality. Percentages of patients in each category are shown. *CI*, Confidence interval. (From Farooq V, van Klaveren D, Steyerberg EW, et al. Anatomical and clinical characteristics to guide decision making between coronary artery bypass surgery and percutaneous coronary intervention for individual patients: development and validation of SYNTAX score II. *Lancet.* 2013;381[9867]:639–650.)

SECTION I Patient Selection

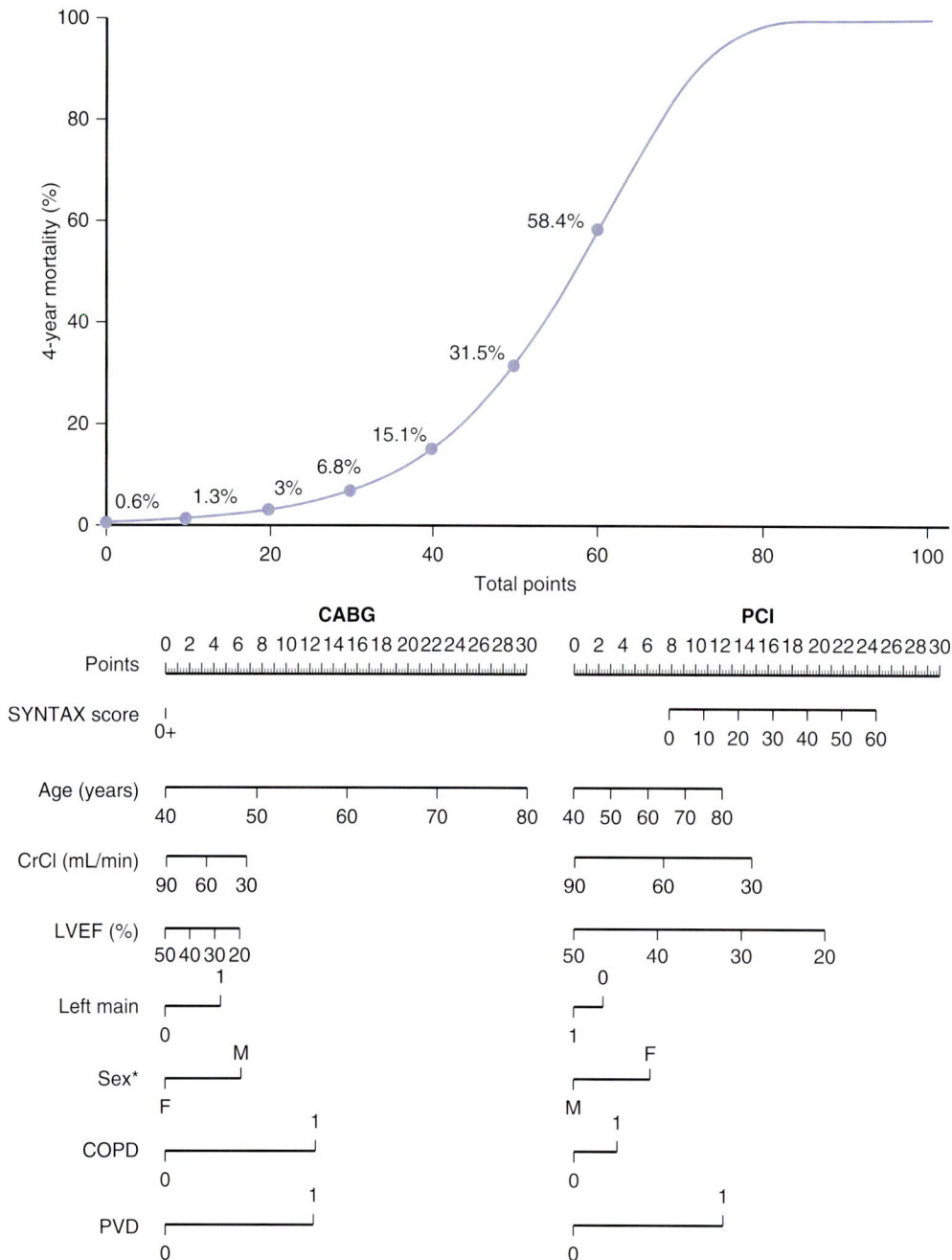

Fig. 1.17 The SYNTAX score II nomogram for bedside application. Total number of points for eight factors can be used to accurately predict 4 year mortality for the individual patient proposing to undergo coronary artery bypass grafting *(CABG)* or percutaneous coronary intervention *(PCI)*. *COPD,* Chronic obstructive pulmonary disease; *CrCl,* creatinine clearance; *LVEF,* left ventricular ejection fraction; *PVD,* peripheral vascular disease. *Because of the rarity of complex coronary artery disease in premenopausal women, mortality predictions in younger women are predominantly based on the linear relation of age with mortality. The differences in mortality predictions in younger women between CABG and PCI will therefore be affected by larger 95% CIs than those in older women. (From Farooq V, van Klaveren D, Steyerberg EW, et al. Anatomical and clinical characteristics to guide decision making between coronary artery bypass surgery and percutaneous coronary intervention for individual patients: development and validation of SYNTAX score II. *Lancet.* 2013;381[9867]:639–650.)

Tools for Assessment of Completeness of Revascularization

Interpreting the long-term prognostic impact of incomplete revascularization in patients with complex CAD has historically remained difficult.[143] The lack of standardized definitions of incomplete revascularization has confounded this issue and has made comparisons between studies difficult. In the SYNTAX trial, *complete revascularization* was defined as the treatment of any lesion with more than 50% diameter stenosis in vessels 1.5 mm or larger as estimated on the diagnostic angiogram during the local heart team conference and deemed appropriate for revascularization.[144,145] In SYNTAX, incomplete revascularization was shown to be linked to adverse long-term clinical outcomes, including mortality, in surgical and percutaneously treated patients (Fig. 1.22). The residual and post-CABG SYNTAX scores were

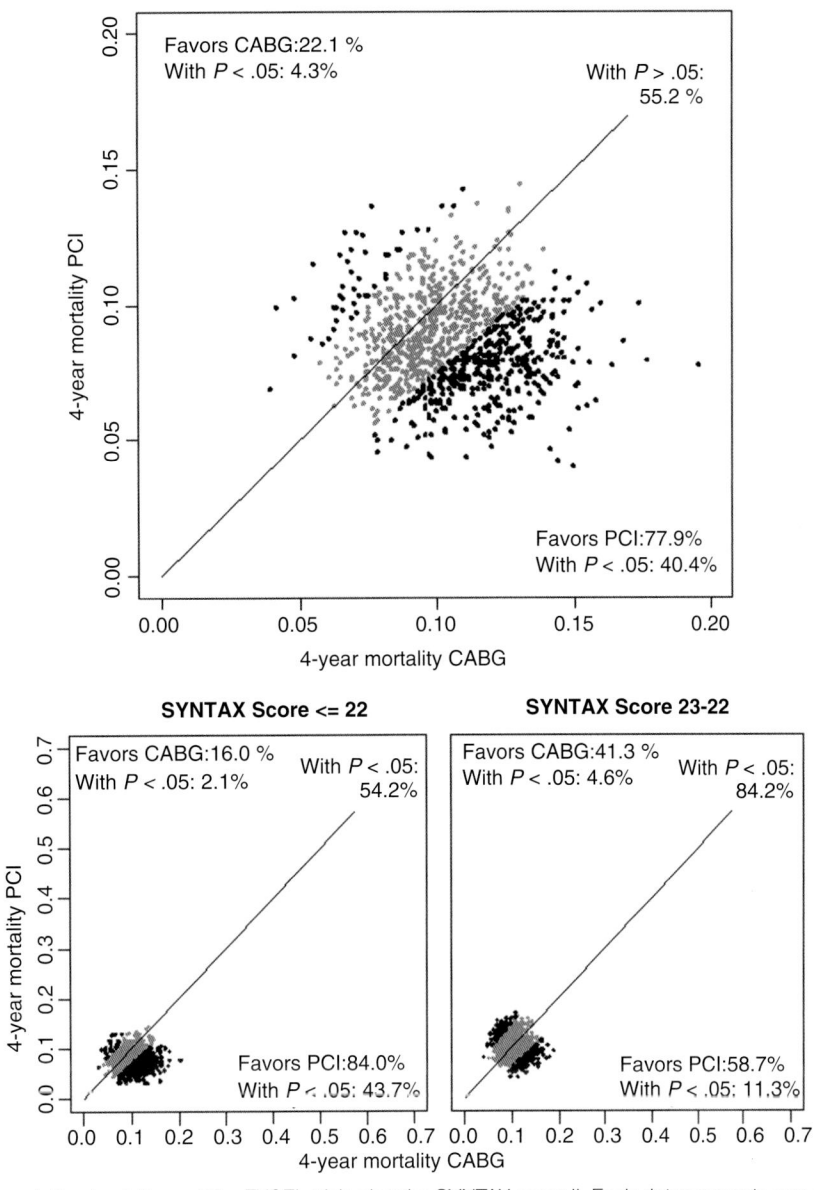

Fig. 1.18 First 1000 4-year mortality simulations of the EXCEL trial using the SYNTAX score II. Each dot represents one simulated trial mortality in both randomization arms based on individual predictions. The diagonal line represents identical mortality for coronary artery bypass grafting *(CABG)* and percutaneous coronary intervention *(PCI)*. A dot plotted to the left of the diagonal line favors CABG (actual percentages shown in top left corner), and to the right favours PCI (actual percentages shown in bottom right corner). Simulated trials with a significant ($P \leq .05$) mortality difference between CABG and PCI are colored *black* (actual percentage shown in parentheses in respective corners). Simulated trials with a nonsignificant ($P > 0.05$) mortality difference between CABG and PCI are colored *gray*. (Reproduced with permission from Campos CM, van Klaveren D, Farooq V, et al.; EXCEL Trial Investigators. Long-term forecasting and comparison of mortality in the Evaluation of the Xience Everolimus Eluting Stent vs. Coronary Artery Bypass Surgery for Effectiveness of Left Main Revascularization (EXCEL) trial: prospective validation of the SYNTAX Score II. *Eur Heart J.* 2015;36[20]:1231–1241.)

designed to quantify the degree of incomplete revascularization and allow for a threshold of incomplete revascularization that would not have a negative impact on long-term clinical outcomes (i.e., reasonable incomplete revascularization).

Residual SYNTAX Score

The residual SYNTAX score is based on the principle of being a measure of the myocardial ischemic burden dependent on the location of the coronary disease, its importance in supplying blood to the myocardium, and the anatomic complexity (e.g., calcification, bifurcation, long lesion) associated with the obstructive disease. The residual SYNTAX score is essentially the anatomic SYNTAX score recalculated after the PCI procedure, and it provides an objective quantitative measure of the degree and complexity of residual stenosis after revascularization. More proximal CAD scores higher on the residual SYNTAX score because this is dependent on the vessel segment weighting as previously discussed (see Fig. 1.13), particularly if the obstructive disease is more complex.[146,147]

Généreux and colleagues[146] first demonstrated that a residual SYNTAX score greater than 8 after PCI was associated with adverse 1-year mortality in a post hoc analysis of the ACUITY trial, which consisted of subjects with moderate to high-risk ACS undergoing PCI and substantially less complex CAD (median SYNTAX score 9.0, interquartile range [IQR] 5.0 to 16.0) compared with those in the SYNTAX trial (median SYNTAX score 28, IQR 20.0 to 36.0).

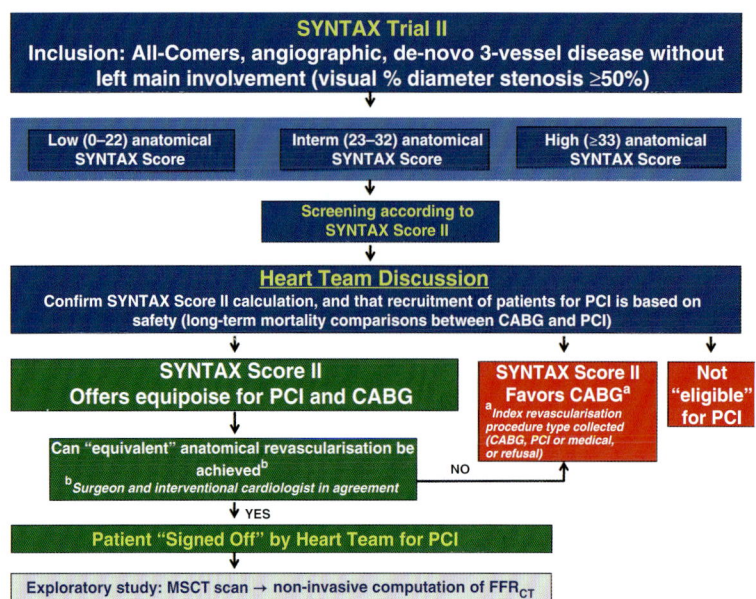

Fig. 1.19 Study flow chart of the SYNTAX II trial—using the state-of-art SYNTAX II percutaneous coronary intervention (PCI) strategy of appropriate patient selection with the SYNTAX score II, newer-generation stent platform with a biodegradable polymer, contemporary CTO revascularization strategies and functional and intravascular ultrasound–guided PCI. *CABG*, Coronary artery bypass grafting; *CTO*, chronic total occlusion; FFR_{CT}, fractional flow reserve derived from computed tomography; *MSCT*, multislice computed tomography. (From Escaned J, Banning A, Farooq V, et al. Rationale and design of the SYNTAX II trial evaluating the short to long-term outcomes of state-of-the-art percutaneous coronary revascularisation in patients with de novo three-vessel disease. *EuroIntervention*. 2016;12[2]:e224–e234.)

The residual SYNTAX score was subsequently validated in the randomized, all-comers SYNTAX trial, which comprised subjects with complex CAD (ULMCA or de novo 3VD) at the final 5-year follow-up.[147] The previous findings, of residual SYNTAX score greater than 8 being associated with adverse long-term clinical outcomes in the ACUITY trial,[146] were found to be of equal importance in SYNTAX patients who underwent 5-year follow-up. Notably, as the baseline SYNTAX score increased, the frequency of a residual SYNTAX score greater than 8 increased in unison, with an associated increase in long-term mortality (Fig. 1.23). In addition, progressively higher residual SYNTAX scores were shown to be a surrogate marker of sicker patients,[145] with greater baseline clinical comorbidity and anatomic complexity and consequent adverse long-term clinical outcomes, including all-cause mortality.

Stratified analyses in the powered subgroups of ULMCA disease and medically treated diabetes showed that a residual SYNTAX score greater than 8 was associated with adverse long-term clinical outcomes, including mortality. Stratified analyses in subjects with reduced LVEF also showed the results to be equally applicable, whereas in subjects with total occlusions, a more modest effect was shown that did not reach statistical significance. The latter perhaps implied that a higher level of a residual SYNTAX score was required in patients with total occlusions with MVD and/or that appropriate viability assessment was required to ensure that revascularization of the total occlusion was appropriate and clinically justified.[148]

Subsequently, several validation studies from registries have further supported the use of the residual SYNTAX score in complex CAD.[149–152] Specifically in one registry of 1043 patients with MVD and at least one CTO,[151] a higher cutoff value for the residual SYNTAX score (≤12) value was demonstrated, in which a reasonable level of incomplete revascularization was achieved that had similar outcomes to complete revascularization. These latter findings thus corroborated the effect of total occlusions on the residual SYNTAX score in the original SYNTAX trial as discussed in the last paragraph.

More recently, the prospect of a functionally guided incomplete revascularization has been proposed.[153] Notably in 385 patents who underwent three-vessel functional assessment following stent implantation, functionally incomplete revascularization was associated with a higher rate of 2-year MACEs compared with functional complete revascularization (functional incomplete revascularization vs. functional compete revascularization, 14.6% vs. 4.2%; hazard ratio: 4.09; 95% CI: 1.82 to 9.21; $P < .001$). In addition, functional incomplete revascularization was shown to be an independent predictor of MACEs (adjusted hazard ratio: 4.17; 95% CI: 1.85 to 9.44; $P < .001$), with the newly devised functional residual SYNTAX score appearing to better identify lower and high-risk patients. One of the main limitations of this study was that predominantly low anatomic complex disease patients were recruited, with only 28.8% having 3VD. At the time of writing, prospective validation of the functional residual SYNTAX score is awaited from further studies investigating more complex CAD, including the ongoing SYNTAX II trial.

In summary, the residual SYNTAX score (with possible functional assessment) allows for the quantification of the degree of revascularization and for determination of an objective level of reasonable incomplete revascularization,[143] whereby a threshold value could be determined that would not have a negative impact on long-term mortality and other clinical outcomes.

Post–Coronary Artery Bypass Grafting SYNTAX Score

The CABG equivalent of the residual SYNTAX score, the post-CABG SYNTAX score, has been shown to be linked to adverse 5-year clinical outcomes, including mortality, in the angiographic substudy of the SYNTAX trial (SYNTAX–LE MANS [Left Main Coronary Artery Stenting]; Fig. 1.24).[154,155] Because of the inherently differing mechanisms of treatment of CAD with CABG and PCI, calculation of the residual SYNTAX score (i.e., the burden of coronary disease removed by PCI) differs from that of the post-CABG SYNTAX score (i.e., coronary disease bypassed with a graft). The basic principle of the post-CABG SYNTAX score is that it deducts points from the "native" baseline SYNTAX score based on the level of "protection" conferred by the bypass grafts, through deduction of the vessel-segment weighting (Leaman score, see Fig. 1.13)[109] that the bypass graft provides (eFig. 1.5).

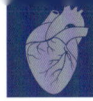

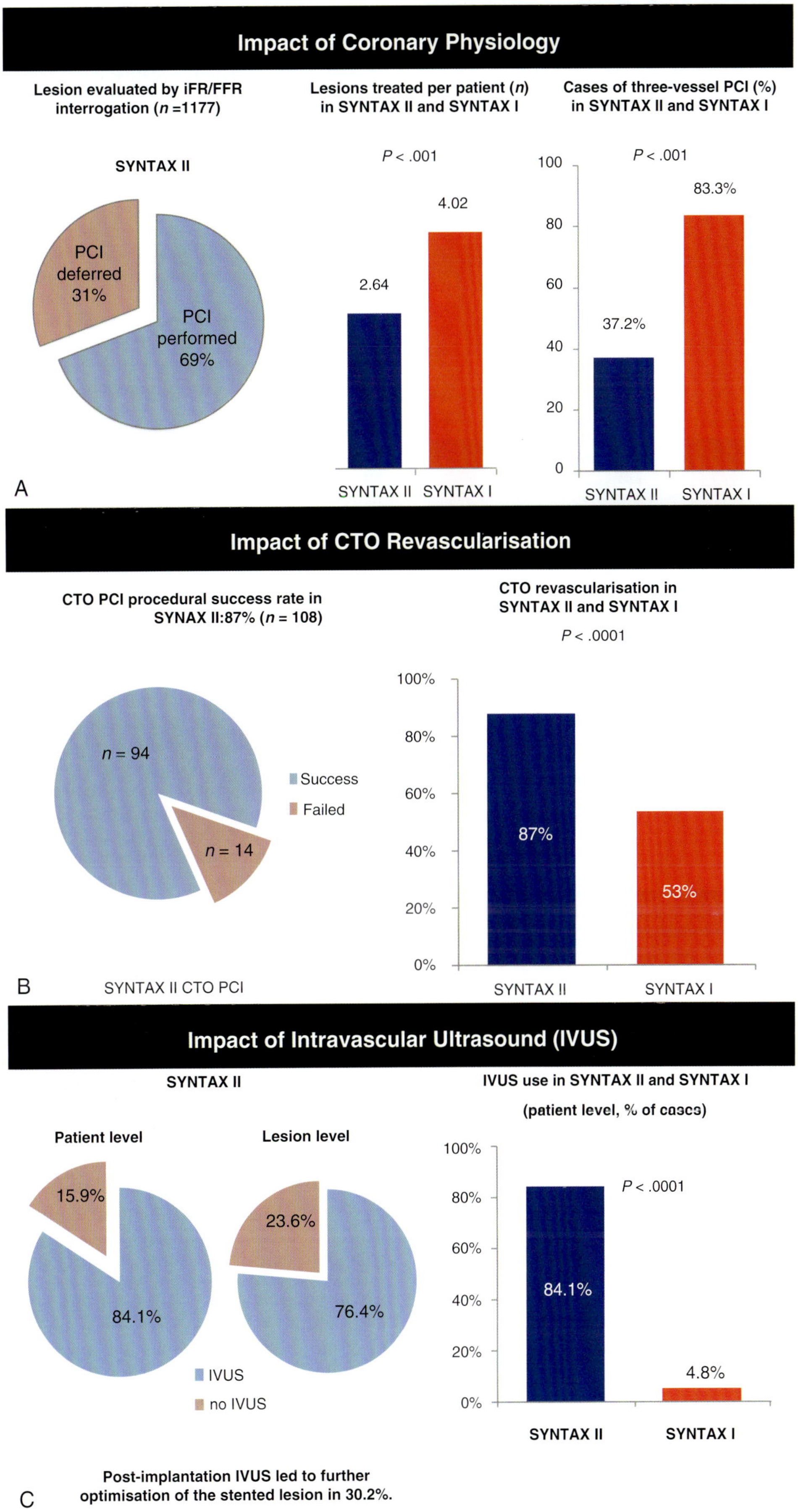

Fig. 1.20 Impact of the SYNTAX II PCI strategy—coronary physiology (A), chronic total occlusion *(CTO)* revascularization (B), and intravascular ultrasound *(IVUS)* (C)—in the SYNTAX II trial[135–137] compared with the original SYNTAX I trial. *FFR*, Fractional flow reserve; *PCI*, percutaneous coronary intervention.

SECTION I Patient Selection

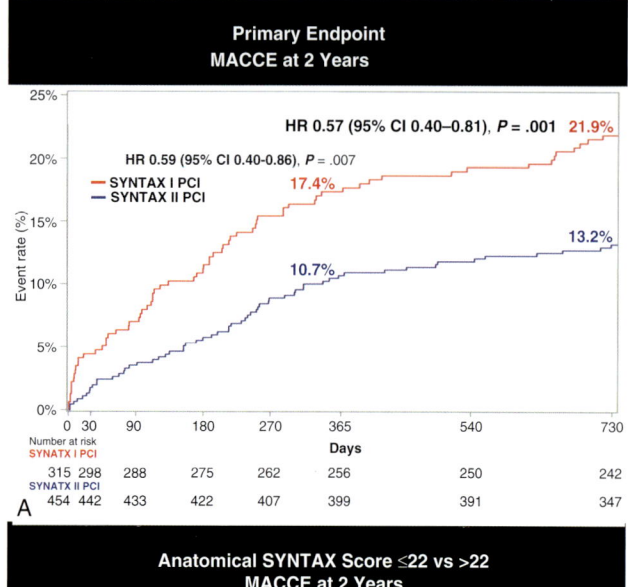

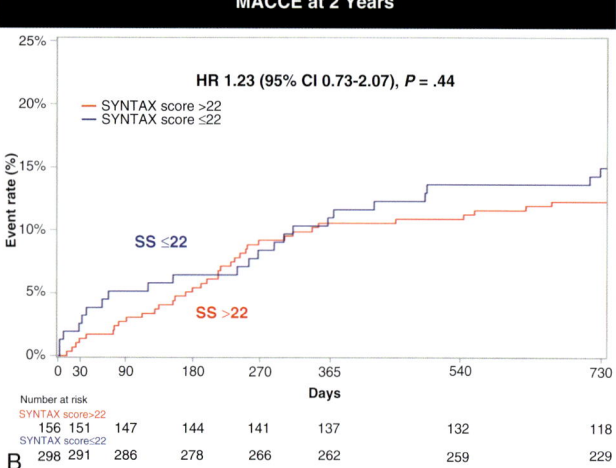

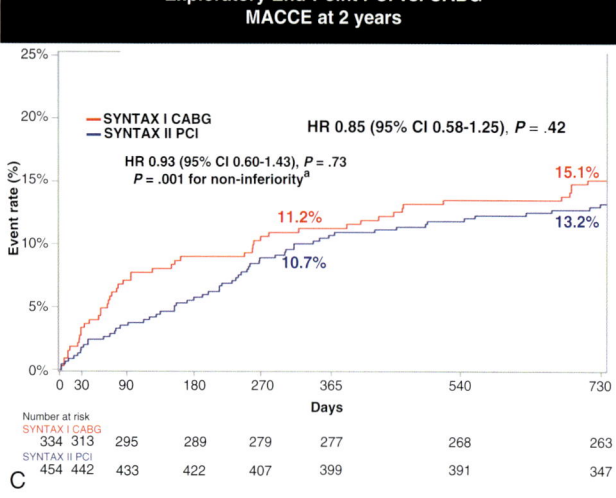

Fig. 1.21 Outcomes of the SYNTAX II trial, demonstrating superiority of the SYNTAX II PCI strategy compared with the PCI arm of the original SYNTAX I trial (primary end point) at 2 years (A); similar 2-year outcomes in patients stratified by low (≤22) and intermediate-high (>22) anatomic SYNTAX scores undergoing the SYNTAX II PCI strategy in the SYNTAX II trial (B); similar outcomes of the SYNTAX II PCI strategy compared with CABG in the SYNTAX I trial (exploratory end point) at 2 years (C).[135–137] *CABG*, Coronary artery bypass grafting; *CI*, confidence interval; *HR*, hazard ratio; *MACCE*, major adverse cardiovascular and cerebrovascular events; *PCI*, percutaneous coronary intervention.

Because the post-CABG SYNTAX score is based on validated physiologic principles of blood flow (Leaman score),[109] it does not arbitrarily deduct points for the type of bypass graft anastomosed. Points related to native coronary disease (e.g., bifurcation disease, calcification, total occlusions, long lesions, diffuse disease, etc.) remain unaltered.

Historical evidence to back the findings from the post-CABG SYNTAX score being linked to adverse long-term prognosis comes from the Coronary Artery Surgery Study (CASS)[156] and Rotterdam[157] registries. In both studies, more extensive preoperative CAD was linked to the higher prevalence and severity of other clinical risk factors and adverse long-term prognosis compared with subjects with less complex CAD. Furthermore, 5-year follow-up of the BARI trial demonstrated that native coronary disease progression, and not the extent of initial revascularization, was the predominant determinant of the recurrence of angina and jeopardized myocardium in percutaneous and surgically revascularized subjects.[158] Finally, coronary artery calcification has been linked to adverse all-cause mortality at 10 years independent of other risk factors.[159,160] An external validation study of the post-CABG SYNTAX score has recently been undertaken in Japan and it has shown to be a powerful prognostic factor after PCI in patients with previous CABG surgery.[161]

Future Directions

Papadopoulou and colleagues[162] first described the feasibility and reproducibility of a multislice computed tomography (MSCT)-derived SYNTAX score in 80 consecutive patients with symptomatic angina, using definitions of the angiographically defined SYNTAX score adapted for the MSCT capabilities. The underlying concept was to allow for the anatomic SYNTAX score to be calculated prior to the intervention to potentially aid decision making and optimize patient management. The addition of a noninvasive FFR component (HeartFlow; HeartFlow Inc., Redwood City, CA) has the potential to allow for the noninvasive calculation of a functional MSCT SYNTAX score (eFig. 1.6). This technology is based on using computational fluid-dynamic techniques applied to MSCT angiography.[162] Validation data of the noninvasive FFR MSCT has been reported in the Diagnosis of Ischemia-Causing Stenoses Obtained via Non-Invasive Fractional Flow Reserve (DISCOVER FLOW)[48,163] and multicenter Determination of Fractional Flow Reserve by Anatomic Computed Tomographic Angiography (DeFACTO) trials.[164] More recently in the SYNTAX II trial,[117] calculation of the noninvasive functional SYNTAX Score was shown to yield similar results to those obtained with invasive pressure-wire assessment.

SYNTAX III Revolution Trial Noninvasive Heart Team Assessment of Multivessel Coronary Disease With Coronary Computed Tomography Angiography

The SYNTAX III Revolution trial was designed to provide evidence in decision making by randomizing two heart teams—composed of a cardiac surgeon, radiologist, and interventional cardiologist—to come up with a virtual treatment decision (CABG or PCI) in patients with LM or de novo 3VD, using information received strictly from noninvasive means using multislice coronary computed tomography angiography with functional assessment (HeartFlow), or conventional (invasive angiography) means (Fig. 1.25).[138,139,165] The study was conducted in 223 patients over an 18-month period in six participating European centers. The Cohen's kappa statistic was used to indicate the level of agreement between the two heart teams in terms of their treatment decision between either CABG or PCI—based on the MSCT-first assessment or angiography-first

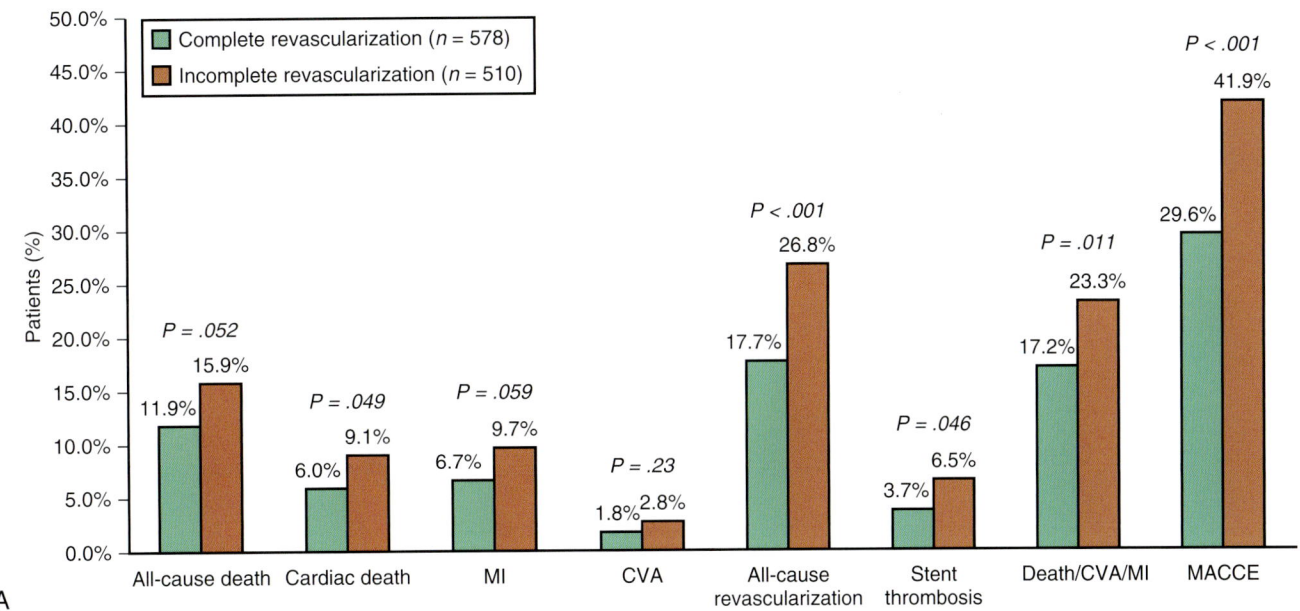

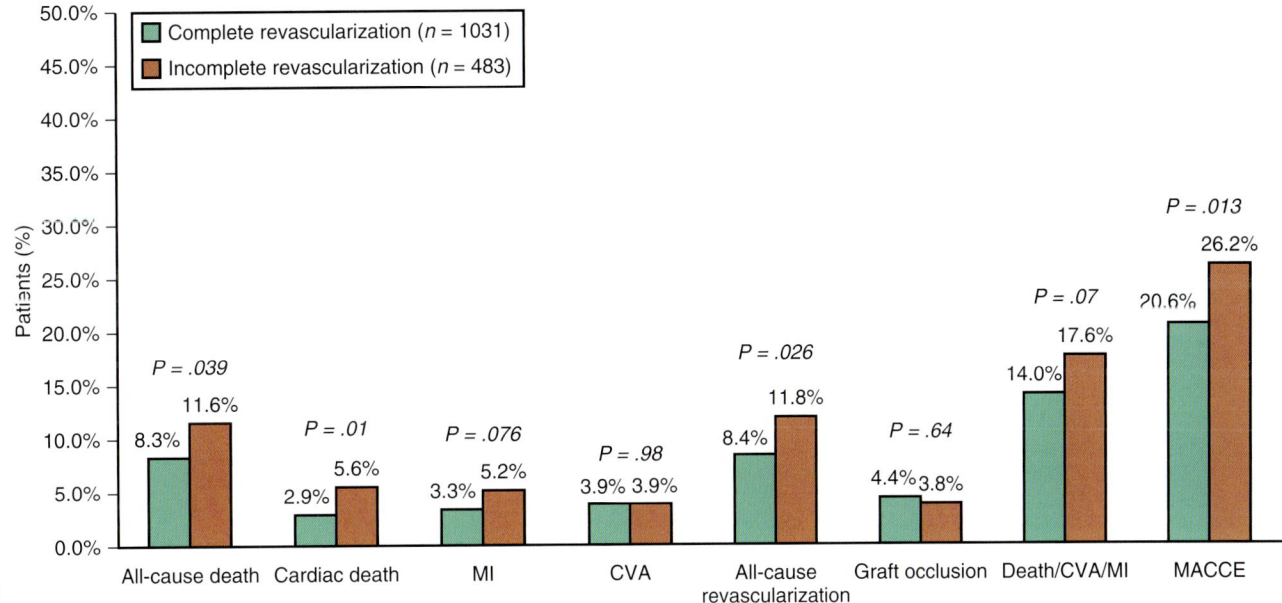

Fig. 1.22 Four-year clinical outcomes in patients by complete versus incomplete revascularization. Comparisons (Kaplan-Meier analyses) of 4-year clinical outcomes by completeness of revascularization in the all-comers percutaneous coronary intervention (A) and all-comers coronary artery bypass grafting (B) populations. *CVA*, Cerebrovascular accident; *MACCE*, major adverse cardiovascular and cerebrovascular events; *MI*, myocardial infarction. (From Farooq V, Serruys PW, Garcia-Garcia HM, et al. The negative impact of incomplete angiographic revascularization on clinical outcomes and its association with total occlusions: the SYNTAX [Synergy Between Percutaneous Coronary Intervention with Taxus and Cardiac Surgery] trial. *J Am Coll Cardiol.* 2013;61[3]:282–294.)

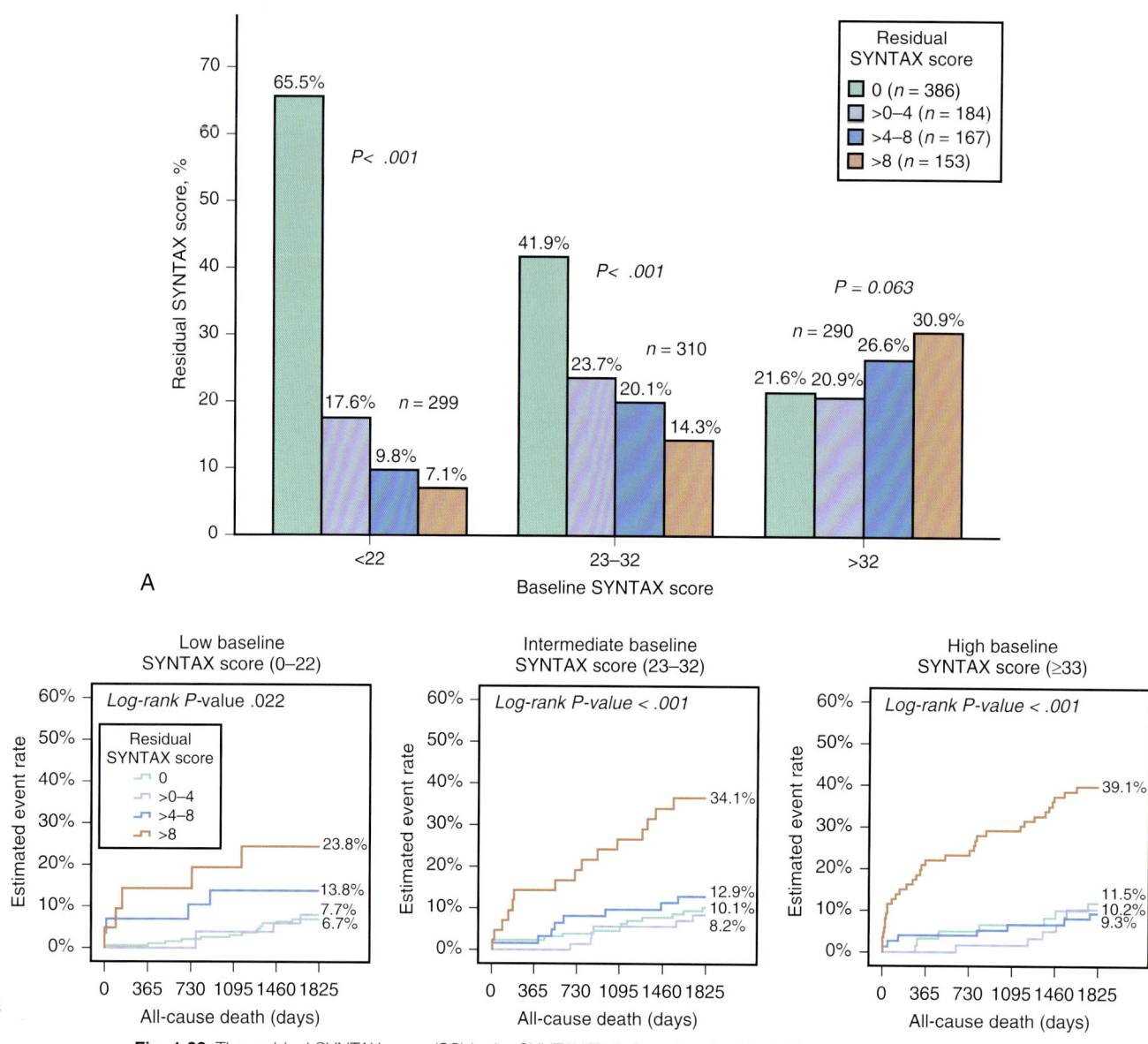

Fig. 1.23 The residual SYNTAX score (SS) in the SYNTAX Trial. Complete (residual SS = 0) and incomplete (tertiles of the residual SS [residual SS >0]) revascularization, stratified according to tertiles of the baseline SS (A). Kaplan-Meier curves show cumulative event rates through to 5 years, based on complete (residual SS = 0) and incomplete (tertiles of residual SS) revascularization, in the low (0 to 22), intermediate (23 to 32), and high (≥33) baseline SYNTAX scores (B). Note the progressive increase in the frequency of a residual SS above 8 across the tertiles of the baseline SS (A) and its association with adverse long-term mortality (B). *CVA*, cerebrovascular accident; *MACCE*, major adverse cardiovascular and cerebrovascular events; *MI*, myocardial infarction. (From Farooq V, Serruys PW, Bourantas CV, et al: Quantification of incomplete revascularization and its association with five-year mortality in the synergy between percutaneous coronary intervention with taxus and cardiac surgery [SYNTAX] trial validation of the residual SYNTAX score. *Circulation*. 2013;128[2]:141–151.)

evaluation. Treatment decisions were shown to be matched in 92.8% of patients with a high level of agreement evident on the diagnoses given by the two heart teams. (Cohen's kappa coefficient 0.82; 95% CI 0.73 to 0.91). In addition, functional based CT was shown to be feasible in 196/223 patients and changed the treatment decision in 7% of patients, mostly from CABG to PCI. Notably, the heart team agreed on the number of bypasses, how many stents should be used, and their location in the coronary circulation in 80% of cases. The next phase will be a first-in-man trial asking cardiac surgeons to treat patients based on multislice CT scan alone without looking at the invasive coronary angiography.

INDIVIDUAL ASSESSMENT FROM A PATIENT'S PERSPECTIVE

The previous discussions have focused entirely on the factors physicians must take into account when making revascularization decisions. However, in the era of increased patient choice and transparency and greater patient involvement in decision making, it is vital to also consider aspects from a patient's perspective through the assessment of health-related QOL.

Data on QOL from patients treated with a DES and CABG are limited to the 12-month results from the SYNTAX trial, 3-year results from the ARTS-II study, a minimum follow-up of 2 years

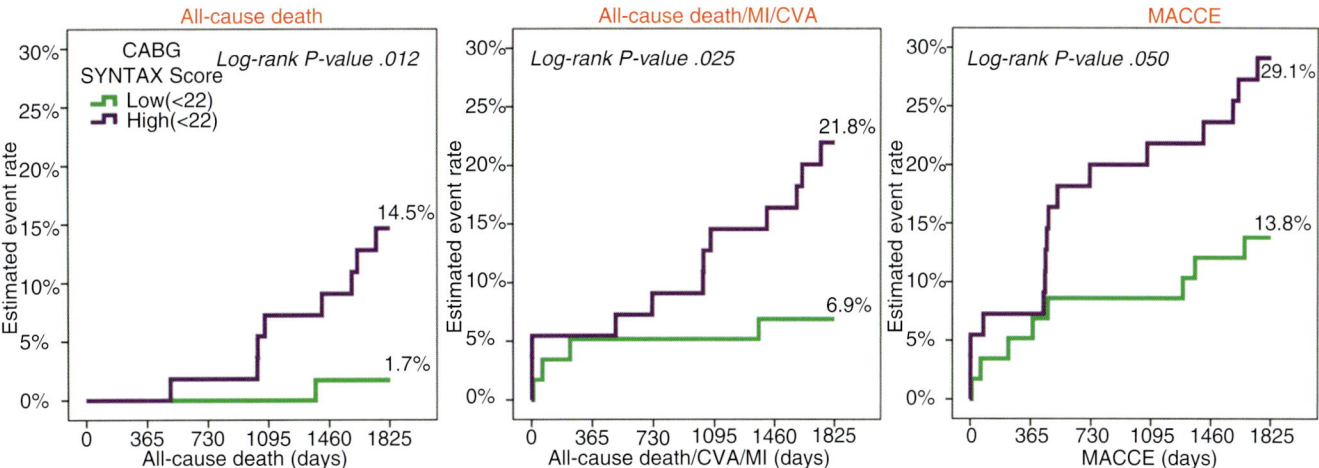

Fig. 1.24 The post–coronary artery bypass grafting (CABG) SYNTAX score in the angiographic substudy of the SYNTAX trial (SYNTAX-LE MANS). Outcomes (Kaplan-Meier curves) separated by the median of the post-CABG SYNTAX score into low (0 to 21, $n = 58$) and high (≥ 22, $n = 55$) score groups. At 5 years, significantly greater rates of all-cause mortality (left image), all-cause death/cerebrovascular accident (CVA)/myocardial infarction (MI; middle image), and major adverse cardiovascular and cerebrovascular events (MACCEs; right image) were evident in the post-CABG high SYNTAX score group compared with the low post-CABG SYNTAX score group. Note the peak in MACCEs at approximately 18 months secondary to patients undergoing scheduled coronary angiography, the findings of which triggered repeat revascularization. (From Farooq V, Girasis C, Magro M, et al. The CABG SYNTAX Score: an angiographic tool to grade the complexity of coronary disease following coronary artery bypass graft surgery: from the SYNTAX Left Main Angiographic (SYNTAX-LE MANS) substudy. *EuroIntervention.* 2013;8[11]:1277–1285.)

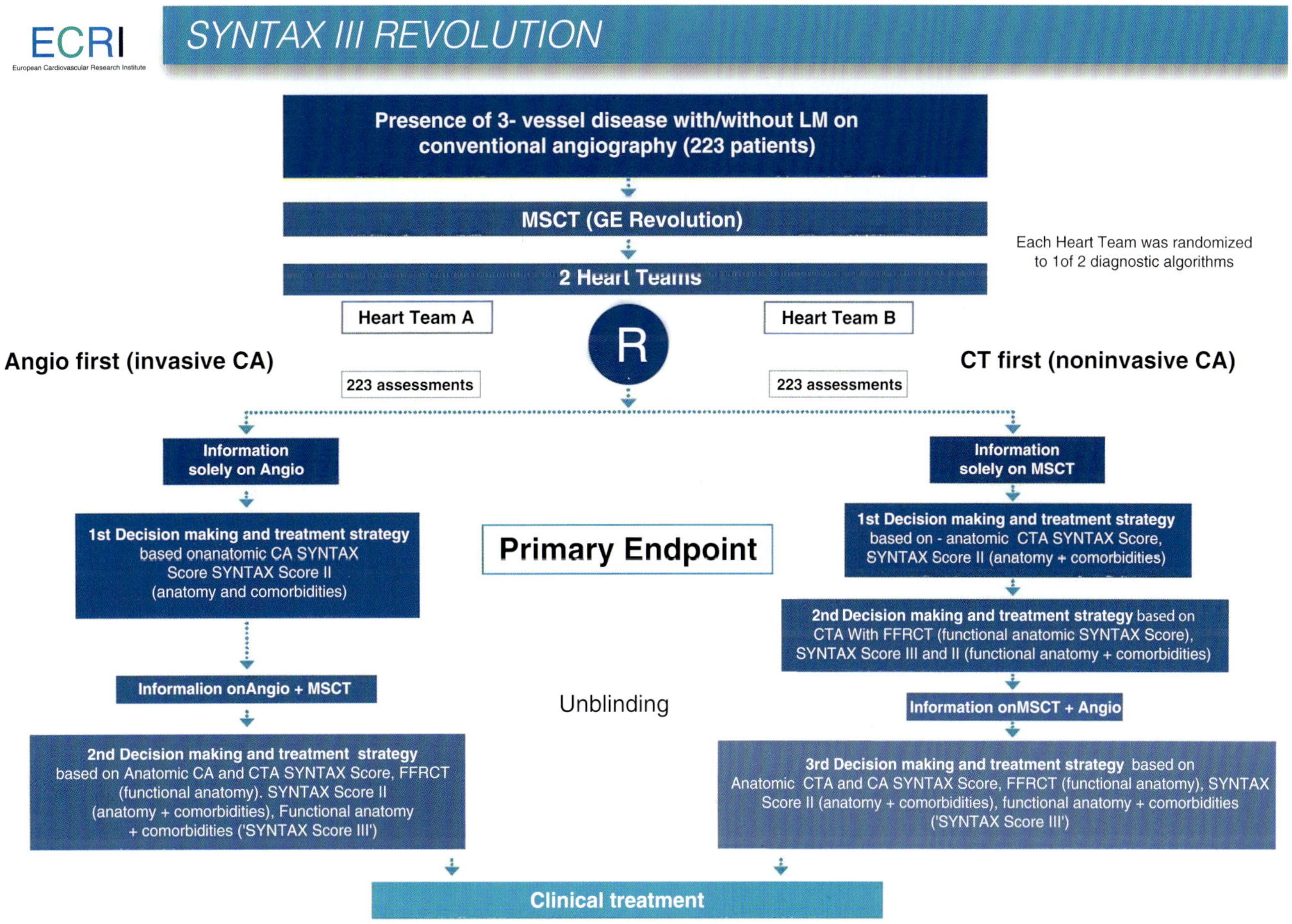

Fig. 1.25 Study design of the ongoing SYNTAX III Revolution trial.[138,139] *CA*, Cineangiography; *CT*, computed tomography; *CTA*, computed tomography angiography; *GE*, General Electric; *LM*, left main; *MSCT*, multislice computed tomography.

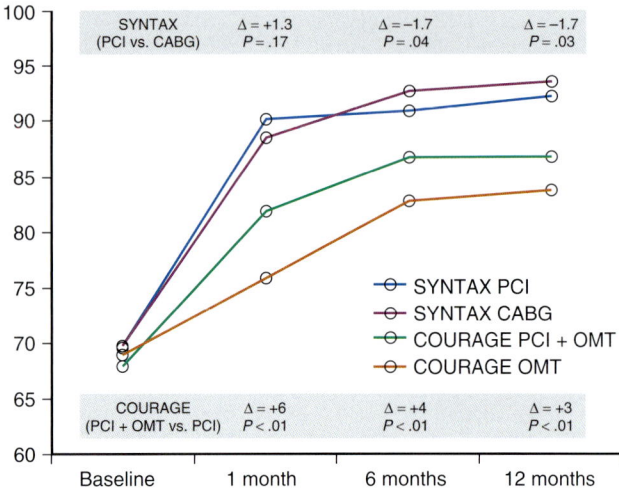

Fig. 1.26 The change in Seattle Angina Questionnaire angina frequency during follow-up of the SYNTAX and COURAGE studies.[166,169] All therapies lead to a reduction in angina frequency; however, the improvement is greatest following surgical revascularization. It is important to note that the difference between percutaneous coronary intervention *(PCI)* and coronary artery bypass grafting *(CABG)* in the SYNTAX study is not considered clinically significant; moreover, it is considerably less than the difference between PCI and optimal medical therapy *(OMT)* and OMT alone in the COURAGE study.

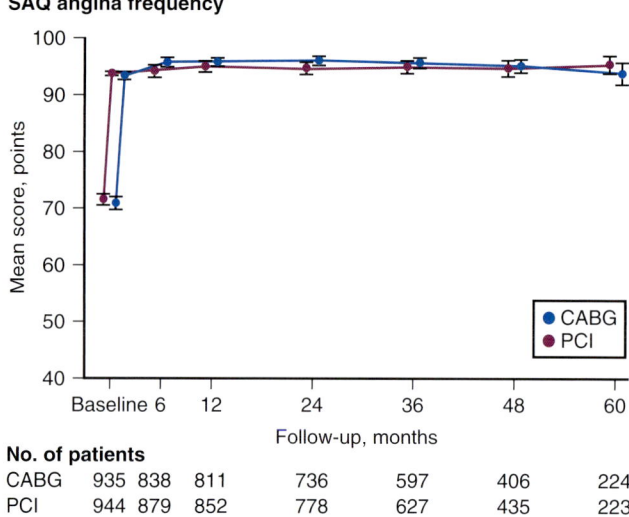

Fig. 1.27 Seattle Angina Questionnaire *(SAQ)* for angina frequency in FREEDOM. Mean scores are reported (error bars indicate 95% confidence intervals). Scores for each subscale range from 0 to 100 (reported by increments of 10) with higher scores representing better health status or quality of life. Note the benefits for coronary artery bypass grafting *(CABG)* at 12 to 24 months, without consistent differences beyond 24 months. *PCI*, percutaneous coronary intervention. (From Abdallah MS, Wang K, Magnuson EA, et al. Quality of life after PCI vs CABG among patients with diabetes and multivessel coronary artery disease: a randomized clinical trial. *JAMA*. 2013;310[15]:1581–1590.)

(median follow-up time of 3.8 years among survivors) from the FREEDOM trial, and 3-year follow up from EXCEL.[19,166-168] Results from the 12-month follow-up of SYNTAX indicate that treatment with PCI or CABG leads to a significant improvement in QOL compared with baseline measures (Fig. 1.26). In addition, the greatest improvement in QOL was seen in those treated with CABG. It is noteworthy that the difference in the Seattle Angina Questionnaire (SAQ) angina frequency between both groups, which was 1.7 at 6 and 12 months, is less than that deemed to be clinically relevant (with differences of 8 to 10 points suggested to be clinically meaningful for each of the SAQ subscales[10,168,169]) and also less than that observed in other studies such as SoS (Stent or Surgery) trial, which showed a 3-point difference at 12 months, and Clinical Outcomes Utilizing Revascularization and Aggressive Drug Evaluation (COURAGE), which showed a 3- to 6-point difference (see Fig. 1.26).[169]

Similarly, data from the ARTS-II study indicated the absence of any significant difference in angina status between patients treated with DES and CABG from as early as 1 month after the index procedure through to the 3-year follow-up; of note, treatment with a BMS in ARTS-II led to consistently higher rates of angina.[167] In the FREEDOM trial at 2-year follow-up, CABG provided a small benefit compared with PCI using a DES (mean treatment benefit [MTB] 1.3; 95% CI, 0.3 to 2.2), with CABG and PCI providing similar outcomes beyond 2 years (Fig. 1.27). However, it should be emphasized that the minimum follow-up of FREEDOM was 2 years, with a median follow-up time of 3.8 years among survivors, and although the benefits of CABG in FREEDOM were driven by significant reductions in all-cause mortality ($P = .049$) and MI ($P < .001$), the mortality benefit did not emerge until 4 to 5 years after the initial treatment where analyses appeared underpowered (see Fig. 1.2). Within the EXCEL trial, reflecting the fact that patients were appropriately selected based on the anatomical SYNTAX, both PCI and CABG result in similar QOL improvement at 36 months, with a substantially greater early benefit in QOL seen with PCI at 1 month (see Fig. 1.4B).[19]

However, it must be stressed that individual patients may have different concerns not captured in evaluations of QOL.

For example, some patients may be more willing to accept the increased chances of a repeat procedure with PCI because this treatment allows them to return to normal activity promptly after the procedure; conversely, others may be content with the longer convalescence from CABG because this offers a suitable trade-off with the subsequently lower risk of adverse clinical outcomes.[170] Of note, in the SYNTAX study, physical limitations, QOL, and treatment satisfaction were all significantly better with PCI compared with CABG at 1 month; however, by 6 months these differences were similar (Fig. 1.28). Similarly, in FREEDOM, measures of physical limitations and QOL outcomes were significantly better with PCI at 1 month (MTB, –8.1 [95% CI, –9.9 to –6.3] and –1.9 [95% CI, –3.6 to –0.2], respectively); in addition, measures of physical limitations were significantly better for PCI at 6 months (MTB, –2.3 [95% CI, –3.8 to –0.9] and 0.4 [95% CI, –1.1 to 1.8], respectively) and were slightly better with CABG at 2 years (MTB, 4.4 [95% CI, 2.7 to 6.1] and 2.2 [95% CI, 0.7 to 3.8], respectively).

Clearly, an individual patient's views on these issues cannot be captured in a questionnaire but rather through frank discussions among the patient, cardiologist, and cardiac surgeon. Consequently, the patient's thoughts, concerns, and individual perception of risk must be considered before deciding on the optimal revascularization strategy.

CONCLUSIONS

The face of revascularization is changing as a result of greater numbers of patients with comorbidities presenting with more extensive CAD in need of revascularization. Concurrent with this have been the advances in percutaneous and surgical technology, which have led to a blurring of the classical divisions between which patients and which coronary lesions are suitable exclusively for PCI or CABG. This welcome change has increased the importance of assessing patients as individuals and taking

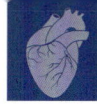

CHAPTER 1 Individualized Assessment for Percutaneous or Surgical-Based Revascularization

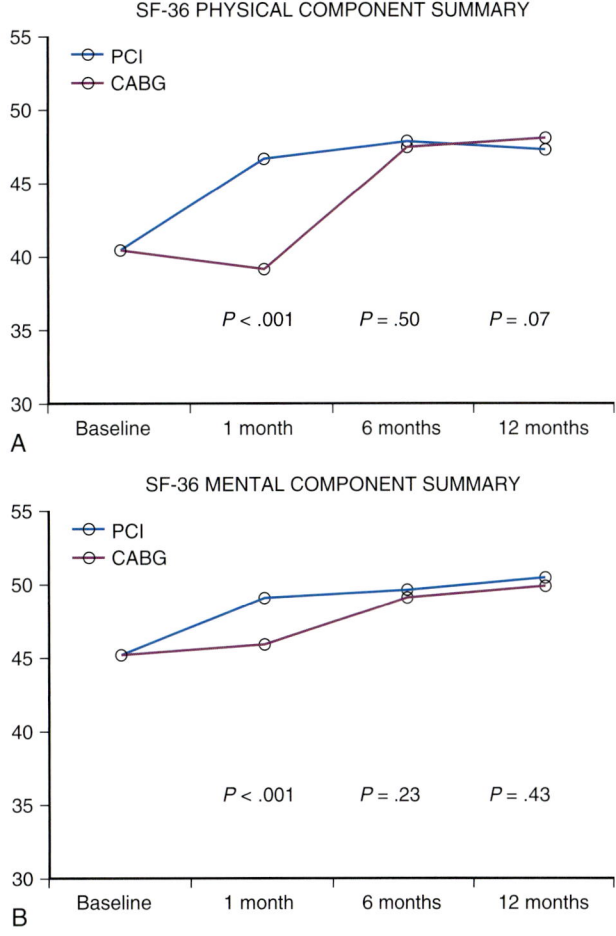

Fig. 1.28 The temporal change in the 36-Item Short Form Health Survey questionnaire *(SF-36)* physical (A) and mental (B) component during follow-up after revascularization with either percutaneous coronary intervention *(PCI)* or coronary artery bypass grafting *(CABG)* in the SYNTAX study. Of note, at 1 month, a significantly better outcome for both parameters was observed in those treated with PCI; however, by 12 months this difference had eroded such that both treatments were similar. (From Cohen DJ, Van Hout B, Serruys PW, et al. Quality of life after PCI with drug-eluting stents or coronary-artery bypass surgery. *N Engl J Med.* 2011;364[11]:1016–1026.)

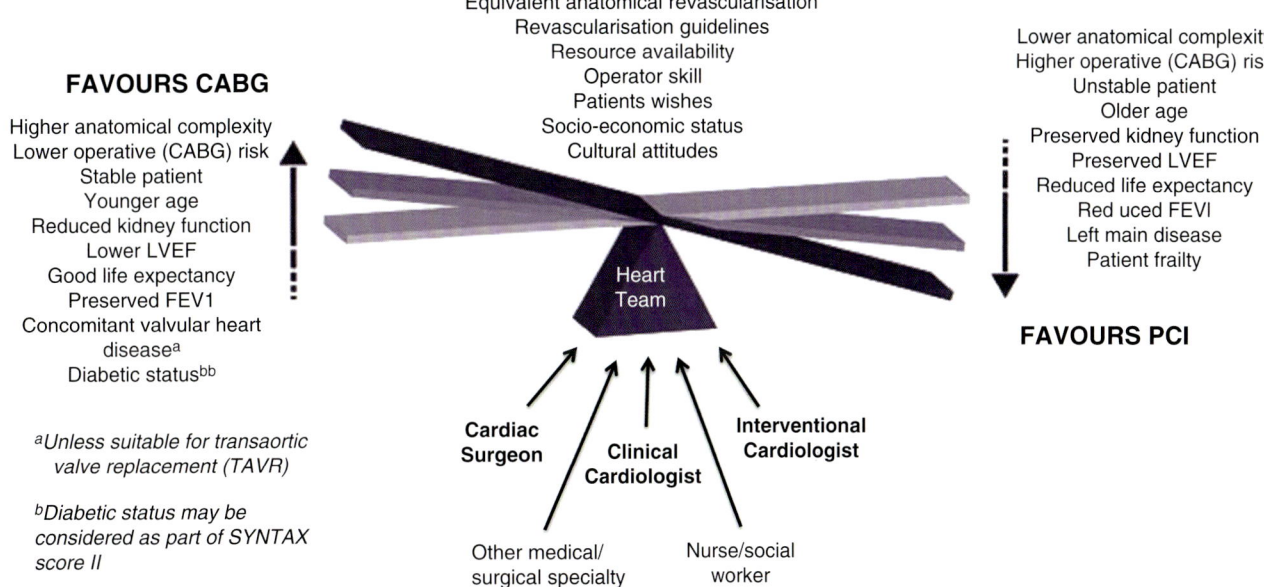

Fig. 1.29 The heart team and important factors that need to be considered in selecting the most appropriate revascularization modalities. As discussed in this chapter, clinical tools are required to simplify this process to aid the heart team in undertaking more objective, evidence-based decision making. *CABG,* Coronary artery bypass grafting; *FEV1,* forced expiratory volume in 1 second; *LVEF,* left ventricular ejection fraction; *PCI,* percutaneous coronary intervention. (Reproduced with permission from Farooq V, Di Mario C, Serruys PW. Balancing idealism with realism to safeguard the welfare of patients: The importance of Heart Team led decision-making in patients with complex coronary artery disease. *Indian Heart J.* 2016;68[1]:1–5.)

into consideration their comorbidities, angiographic findings, and ultimately, their personal preferences and individual perceptions of risk prior to establishing a treatment strategy[171] (Fig. 1.29). Unquestionably, SYNTAX, FREEDOM, and EXCEL have helped to delineate the boundaries on the appropriateness of each revascularization modality (CABG or PCI). To aid the heart team in quantifying levels of risk and to assist decision making between CABG and PCI, numerous clinical tools have been developed, each of which incorporates different clinical and angiographic parameters. The importance of these clinical tools in contemporary practice is in part currently emphasized by their inclusion in society guidelines on myocardial revascularization.

KEY REFERENCES

4. Serruys PW, Onuma Y, Garg S, et al. 5-Year clinical outcomes of the ARTS II (Arterial Revascularization Therapies Study II) of the sirolimus-eluting stent in the treatment of patients with multivessel de novo coronary artery lesions. *J Am Coll Cardiol.* 2010;55:1093–1101.
7. Farooq V, van Klaveren D, Steyerberg EW, et al. Anatomical and clinical characteristics to guide decision making between coronary artery bypass surgery and percutaneous coronary intervention for individual patients: development and validation of SYNTAX score II. *Lancet.* 2013;381:639–650.
9. Hlatky MA, Boothroyd DB, Bravata DM, et al. Coronary artery bypass surgery compared with percutaneous coronary interventions for multivessel disease: a collaborative analysis of individual patient data from ten randomised trials. *Lancet.* 2009;373:1190–1197.
11. Farkouh ME, Domanski M, Sleeper LA, et al. Strategies for multivessel revascularization in patients with diabetes. *N Engl J Med.* 2012;367:2375–2384.
12. Weintraub WS, Grau-Sepulveda MV, Weiss JM, et al. Comparative effectiveness of revascularization strategies. *N Engl J Med.* 2012;366:1467–1476.
15. Mohr FW, Morice MC, Kappetein AP, et al. Coronary artery bypass graft surgery versus percutaneous coronary intervention in patients with three-vessel disease and left main coronary disease: 5-year follow-up of the randomised, clinical SYNTAX trial. *Lancet.* 2013;381:629–638.
17. Stone GW, Sabik JF, Serruys PW, Investigators ET., et al. Everolimus-eluting stents or bypass surgery for left main coronary artery disease. *N Engl J Med.* 2016;375(23):2223–2235.
22. Park SJ, Ahn JM, Kim YH, et al. BEST Trial Investigators. Trial of everolimus-eluting stents or bypass surgery for coronary disease. *N Engl J Med.* 2015;372(13):1204–1212.
36. Nam CW, Mangiacapra F, Entjes R, et al. Functional SYNTAX score for risk assessment in multivessel coronary artery disease. *J Am Coll Cardiol.* 2011;58:1211–1218.
45. SYNTAX working-group. SYNTAX score calculator. http://www.syntaxscore.com; 2009.
48. Farooq V, Brugaletta S, Serruys PW. Contemporary and evolving risk scoring algorithms for percutaneous coronary intervention. *Heart.* 2011;97:1902–1913.
62. Ranucci M, Castelvecchio S, Menicanti L, et al. Risk of assessing mortality risk in elective cardiac operations: age, creatinine, ejection fraction, and the law of parsimony. *Circulation.* 2009;119:3053–3061.
81. Morice MC, Serruys PW, Kappetein AP, et al. Five-year outcomes in patients with left main disease treated with either percutaneous coronary intervention or coronary artery bypass grafting in the synergy between percutaneous coronary intervention with taxus and cardiac surgery trial. *Circulation.* 2014;129:2388–2394.
114. De Bruyne B, Pijls NH, Kalesan B, et al. Fractional flow reserve-guided PCI versus medical therapy in stable coronary disease. *N Engl J Med.* 2012;367:991–1001.
136. Escaned J, Collet C, Ryan N, et al. Clinical outcomes of state-of-the-art percutaneous coronary revascularization in patients with de novo three vessel disease: 1-year results of the SYNTAX II study. *Eur Heart J.* 2017;38(42):3124–3134.
140. Campos CM, van Klaveren D, Farooq V, EXCEL Trial Investigators, et al. Long-term forecasting and comparison of mortality in the Evaluation of the Xience Everolimus Eluting Stent vs. Coronary Artery Bypass Surgery for Effectiveness of Left Main Revascularization (EXCEL) trial: prospective validation of the SYNTAX Score II. *Eur Heart J.* 2015;36(20):1231–1241.
145. Farooq V, Serruys PW, Garcia-Garcia HM, et al. The negative impact of incomplete angiographic revascularization on clinical outcomes and its association with total occlusions: the SYNTAX (Synergy Between Percutaneous Coronary Intervention with Taxus and Cardiac Surgery) trial. *J Am Coll Cardiol.* 2013;61:282–294.
147. Farooq V, Serruys PW, Bourantas CV, et al. Quantification of incomplete revascularization and its association with five-year mortality in the Synergy Between Percutaneous Coronary Intervention With Taxus and Cardiac Surgery (SYNTAX) trial validation of the residual SYNTAX score. *Circulation.* 2013;128:141–151.
157. van Domburg RT, Kappetein AP, Bogers AJ. The clinical outcome after coronary bypass surgery: a 30-year follow-up study. *Eur Heart J.* 2009;30:453–458.
158. Alderman EL, Kip KE, Whitlow PL, et al. Native coronary disease progression exceeds failed revascularization as cause of angina after five years in the Bypass Angioplasty Revascularization Investigation (BARI). *J Am Coll Cardiol.* 2004;44:766–774.
165. Cavalcante R, Onuma Y, Sotomi Y, et al. Non-invasive Heart Team assessment of multivessel coronary disease with coronary computed tomography angiography based on SYNTAX score II treatment recommendations: design and rationale of the randomised SYNTAX III Revolution trial. *EuroIntervention.* 2017;12(16):2001–2008.

 Additional references available online at expertconsult.com

中文导读

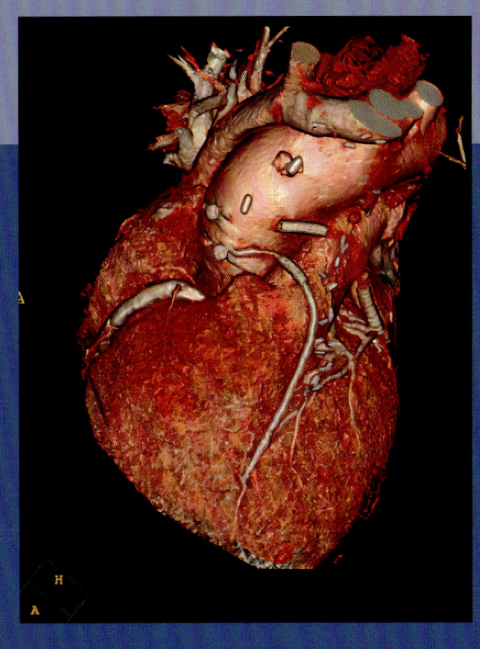

第2章
以循证医学为基础的介入治疗

随着药物涂层支架的普及，支架内再狭窄发生率明显降低，也使得越来越多的冠状动脉病变选择经皮冠状动脉介入治疗进行血运重建，而非选择冠状动脉旁路移植术。尽管如此，经皮冠状动脉介入治疗的预后能否与冠状动脉旁路移植术相当仍然是充满争议的问题，尤其是在多支血管病变或冠状动脉病变复杂度高的患者中。因此，依据相关循证证据制定血运重建方式的选择标准，将有利于临床决策，改善患者预后。

药物治疗和冠状动脉血运重建（经皮冠状动脉介入治疗或冠状动脉旁路移植术）是冠心病的主要治疗手段。这些治疗的主要目的是改善患者预后（预后改善的适应证）。另外一个目的是缓解症状，改善患者生活质量（症状缓解的适应证）。为实现这些目标，防止未来心肌梗死的发生是关键。在选择冠心病患者的最佳血运重建方式时，首先需要明确血运重建治疗是否存在预后或症状改善适应证［即能否改善预后和（或）缓解症状］，然后再选择最合适的血运重建策略。本章节介绍了临床决策时这两种策略的选择标准，其主要关注冠状动脉血运重建的预后适应证。在概括血运重建的一般标准的基础上，探讨了经皮冠状动脉介入治疗与冠状动脉旁路移植术相比较所具有的有效性和安全性；除此之外，还讨论了经皮冠状动脉介入治疗与单独药物治疗相比在稳定型冠心病治疗中改善症状的作用。

本章节主要围绕稳定型冠心病进行了阐述，条理清晰地总结了相关循证医学证据，并对血运重建方式选择标准进行了详细讨论，为临床决策提供了合理的依据，相信会带给读者全面的知识与收获。而对于急性冠状动脉综合征，具体内容将在其他章节分别阐述。

与单纯优化药物治疗相比，经皮冠状动脉介入治疗联合优化药物治疗可更有效缓解心绞痛症状，降低非计划性血运重建和自发性心肌梗死风险，还可改善稳定型心绞痛患者预后。改善预后的获益可能与大面积缺血区域的有效血运重建有关。因此，现有证据显示，心肌缺血面积超过左心室面积的10%、症状无法缓解或无法耐受药物治疗的患者，只要解剖条件适合，应该接受经皮冠状动脉介入治疗。稳定型冠心病患者接受抗心绞痛药物治疗后症状缓解，但缺乏相关区域残余可诱导心肌缺血，应接受保守治疗。

见 闻　柳景华

章节要点

- 当考虑进行冠状动脉血运重建时,需要区分预后改善适应证和症状改善适应证。
- 一般而言,对于单支病变,只有症状在术后预期得到改善或超过10%左心室面积的心肌缺血预期可得到缓解时,经皮冠状动脉介入治疗才是合理的策略。
- 对于多支血管病变或冠状动脉左主干狭窄病变时,血运重建方式选择经皮冠状动脉介入治疗或者冠状动脉旁路移植术,需取决于手术风险、能否获得完全血管重建、有无糖尿病,以及冠状动脉病变的复杂程度(可借助于SYNTAX评分加以判定)。
- 对于多支血管病变或冠状动脉左主干狭窄,若冠状动脉病变复杂度低(SYNTAX评分<23分)且无糖尿病,同时经皮冠状动脉介入治疗可获得完全性血运重建,那么经皮冠状动脉介入治疗的5年预后与冠状动脉旁路移植术相似。因此,在这种情况下,经皮冠状动脉介入治疗可以替代冠状动脉旁路移植术。
- 一般来说,对于多支血管病变,若冠状动脉病变复杂度为中高危(SYNTAX评分>22分),冠状动脉旁路移植术的预后优于经皮冠状动脉介入治疗。因此,在这种情况下,血运重建应选择冠状动脉旁路移植术。
- 对于冠状动脉左主干狭窄,尚缺乏充分的证据表明冠状动脉旁路移植术优于经皮冠状动脉介入治疗。因此,至少在SYNTAX评分为中危(23~32分)的冠状动脉左主干病变中,经皮冠状动脉介入治疗是一种可替代冠状动脉旁路移植术、合理的血运重建方式。
- 对于多支血管病变,糖尿病是冠状动脉旁路移植术预后优于经皮冠状动脉介入治疗的最强预测因子。因此,应选择冠状动脉旁路移植术治疗糖尿病合并多支血管病变。然而,对于SYNTAX评分较低的糖尿病患者,仍可以考虑经皮冠状动脉介入治疗。
- 在许多情况下,个体化治疗策略应该由心脏外科和心内科介入专家采用心脏团队(heart team)模式协商制定。

2 Evidence-Based Interventional Practice

Franz-Josef Neumann, Miroslaw Ferenc, Kambis Mashayekhi

KEY POINTS

- When coronary revascularization is considered, prognostic and symptomatic indications must be distinguished.
- In general, percutaneous coronary intervention (PCI) for single-vessel disease is justified only if an improvement of symptoms can be anticipated or ischemia that comprises more than 10% of the left ventricle can be relieved.
- With multivessel disease or left main coronary artery (LMCA) stenosis, the decision for PCI versus coronary artery bypass grafting (CABG) depends on the procedural risk, the ability to achieve complete revascularization, the presence or absence of diabetes mellitus, and the complexity of the coronary artery involvement, which can be gauged by the Synergy Between Percutaneous Coronary Intervention With Taxus and Cardiac Surgery (SYNTAX) score.
- With multivessel disease or LMCA stenosis and low anatomic complexity (i.e., SYNTAX score below 23) in the absence of diabetes mellitus, the 5-year outcome of PCI is similar to that after CABG, provided that complete revascularization can be achieved. Thus PCI can replace bypass surgery in this setting.
- In general, outcomes with CABG are superior to those with PCI in multivessel disease with intermediate-to-high anatomic complexity (i.e., SYNTAX score above 22) and CABG is the treatment of choice in this setting.
- In the subset of patients with LMCA stenosis, there is no compelling evidence for superiority of CABG over PCI. Thus at least in patients with intermediate SYNTAX-Scores (23 to 32), PCI is a reasonable alternative to CABG.
- In patients with multivessel disease, diabetes mellitus is the strongest predictor of superior outcomes with CABG. CABG is the treatment of choice in this setting. Nevertheless, PCI may be considered in selected patients with a low SYNTAX score.
- In many instances, individualized decisions must be made jointly by the cardiac surgeon and the interventional cardiologist at institutionalized meetings of the heart team.

OVERVIEW

Changing Paradigms of Coronary Revascularization

When the era of interventional cardiology began, with the pioneering work of Andreas Grüntzig on plain balloon angioplasty, percutaneous coronary intervention (PCI) was a treatment option only for isolated proximal coronary lesions that did not involve the ostium or the left main coronary artery (LMCA) stem. In the late 1980s, coronary stents were developed with the goal of reducing the risk of restenosis and achieving a more predictable acute result of angioplasty, thus avoiding the dreaded abrupt closure as a result of dissection. As shown subsequently, stents were successful in achieving this goal. Nevertheless, they created a new problem: subacute stent thrombosis. After intense research on periinterventional and postinterventional antithrombotic treatment, the concept of dual- or triple-antiplatelet therapy emerged, which significantly reduced the incidence of this complication. The use of coronary stents in conjunction with optimized antithrombotic treatment extended the spectrum of coronary lesions for which PCI was considered a reasonable treatment option and thereby led to a substantial expansion of interventional techniques. Because of the large number of patients who were being treated with coronary stents, restenosis as a result of neointima formation became a serious problem. Although various studies demonstrated that compared with plain balloon angioplasty, stents reduced the need for reintervention, restenosis rates continued to be relevant and ranged from just above 10% in the simplest lesions to more than 50% with diffuse disease in patients with diabetes.

Thus it is not surprising that the community of interventional cardiologists celebrated the advent of drug-eluting stents (DESs) as a major breakthrough, given that the initial studies suggested restenosis rates of zero. In the meantime, it has become clear that compared with bare-metal stents (BMSs), DESs reduce the need for target-vessel reintervention by around 80%, thus largely reducing—but not eliminating—the problem of restenosis. Subsequently, DESs led to another massive expansion of the proportion of patients treated with PCI. With the widespread use of these stents for PCI, reports appeared that pointed to a new problem that had not been seen with BMSs: late stent thrombosis. Yet a thorough reevaluation of the data from randomized studies—with uniform application of definitions for *definite*, *probable*, and *possible* stent thrombosis—failed to confirm these alarming initial reports.[1] Nevertheless, a meta-analysis of studies with first-generation paclitaxel- and sirolimus-eluting stents suggested a slight increase in the risk of very late (>1 year) stent thrombosis after the placement of DESs compared with BMSs.[2] In the meantime, DESs with improved design have replaced the first-generation paclitaxel- and sirolimus-eluting stents. For the most part, these next-generation DESs are more efficacious and safer than first-generation DESs.[3,4] Specifically, a network meta-analysis based on 49 trials that included 50,844 randomly assigned patients showed a 2-year risk of stent thrombosis for the everolimus-eluting stents that was even lower than that for BMSs.[3,4]

Despite the remaining problems of PCI, its use has increased exponentially over the past few decades. Initially, this increase has come at the expense of lone medical therapy. More recently, however, with the advent of DESs, a shift has been seen in patients with multivessel disease and other complex coronary anatomies from coronary artery bypass grafting (CABG) to PCI. This shift has been facilitated by both physician and patient preference for the supposedly easier approach to coronary revascularization, given the idea that the problem of restenosis has been largely solved. However, reasonable concern exists that this shift has led to the overuse of PCI and that in some patients, it may not yield the same outcome as CABG, which for a number of indications is an established treatment option with a well-documented survival benefit compared with that of medical therapy.

The Scope of This Chapter

In comparing PCI with medical treatment alone or with bypass surgery, it is important to scrutinize the available evidence that PCI offers at least as great a benefit as CABG on the one hand or a greater benefit than medical treatment alone on the other. This review summarizes and discusses the currently available evidence so as to present a rationale for clinical decision making.

Pharmacologic therapy and coronary revascularization, by either CABG or PCI, are the mainstays of treatment for coronary artery disease (CAD). The prime objective of such treatment is improved survival (prognostic indication); other reasonable treatment goals are relief of symptoms and improved quality of life (symptomatic indication). In pursuing these goals, the prevention of myocardial infarction (MI) is a key issue that pertains to both survival and quality of life. In deciding on the optimal revascularization strategy in a patient with CAD, it is necessary to determine first whether a prognostic or symptomatic indication for coronary revascularization exists and then to choose the most appropriate revascularization modality. This chapter presents criteria for both of these elements in clinical decision making and focuses primarily on the prognostic indication for coronary revascularization. Based on a review of the general criteria for revascularization, the efficacy and safety of PCI compared with CABG are discussed, and the role of PCI in symptomatic indications for coronary revascularization is also addressed, predominantly in comparison with medical therapy alone. The focus is on stable coronary disease. Acute coronary syndromes (ACSs) that include MI are discussed in depth in other chapters.

PROGNOSTIC INDICATIONS FOR MYOCARDIAL REVASCULARIZATION

Clinical Presentation

Several factors must be considered in regard to clinical presentation. Among these are ST-segment changes, cardiac troponin release, and ischemic area, which can help the clinician discern the appropriate treatment.

Myocardial Infarction and High-Risk Unstable Angina

The prognostic benefit of myocardial revascularization in patients with MI with or without ST-elevation or unstable angina with high-risk features is well established. The evidence is reviewed in detail in Chapters 18 and 19.

Among patients with chronic stable angina, those with severe angina, large or multiple perfusion defects on functional testing, or a low threshold for the induction of ischemia (Box 2.1) have a poor prognosis, with an annual mortality risk greater than 3%.[5] If these high-risk features are associated with double- or triple-vessel disease, patients benefit from revascularization irrespective of left ventricular (LV) function. In an analysis of 5303 patients in the Coronary Artery Surgery Study (CASS) registry, surgical benefit was greatest in patients who exhibited at least 1 mm of ST-segment depression and could exercise only into stage 1 or less. In the surgical group with triple-vessel disease and severe exercise-induced ischemia, 7-year survival was 81%, whereas it was 58% in the corresponding medical group.[6] Likewise, in another registry that included 2023 patients with severe angina and two-vessel disease, 6-year survival was 76% in patients treated medically and 89% in patients treated surgically ($P < .001$).[7] Cox multivariate analyses showed that surgical treatment was a beneficial independent predictor of survival for patients with two-vessel coronary disease and Canadian Cardiovascular Society (CCS) class 3 or 4 angina. The Asymptomatic Cardiac Ischemia Pilot (ACIP) is a more recent trial that was designed to compare the efficacy of medical therapy versus revascularization.[8] In ACIP, 558 patients with angiographically documented CAD, mostly multivessel disease, and stable CAD were randomly assigned to medical therapy, adjusted either to suppress angina or to suppress both angina and evidence of ischemia during ambulatory electrocardiogram (ECG) monitoring or revascularization with either PCI or CABG. Revascularization was significantly more effective in relieving ischemia than either of the medical strategies. During 1-year follow-up, the ACIP trial appeared to show better outcomes in patients treated with revascularization; mortality was 4.4% and 1.6% in the two conservative groups, whereas none of the patients in the revascularization group had died during the 1-year follow-up period. The apparent benefit of revascularization was largely confined to patients with double- or triple-vessel disease. Expanding the series done in 2003 and 2006,[9,10] a large observational study of patients who underwent exercise or adenosine myocardial perfusion single photon emission computed tomography (SPECT) analyzed the impact of the extent of inducible myocardial ischemia and of myocardial scar on the potential survival benefit of revascularization.[11] The study included 13,969 consecutive patients: 12,329 were treated medically, and 1226 underwent early revascularization (501 CABG, 725 PCI) in the first 90 days after scintigraphy. During a median follow-up of 8.9 years, 3893 patients (27.9%) died. Hazard ratios for all-cause death that compared early revascularization with medical treatment were derived from Cox models adjusted for logistic-based propensity scores for revascularization, extent of ischemia and scar, and baseline characteristics. In 11,880 patients without large myocardial scars (<10% fixed myocardial defect), a progressive decrease in the hazard ratios was found with increasing extent of inducible ischemia (Fig. 2.1). Thus the risk associated with conservative treatment increased as a function of percent myocardium ischemic, whereas the risk associated with revascularization decreased. Equipoise between revascularization and conservative treatment was reached at about 10% ischemic myocardium (see Fig. 2.1). Only in patients with extensive scar (≥10% fixed myocardial defect) was the ischemia treatment interaction not significant ($P = .469$), and an advantage of revascularization over conservative treatment could not be established. In summary, in the absence of extensive myocardial

> **BOX 2.1** Poor Prognosis in Stable Angina (Average Annual Mortality Risk >3%)
>
> High-risk treadmill score
> Stress-induced large or moderate-sized nuclear perfusion defect (particularly if in the anterior wall)
> Stress-induced multiple perfusion defects with left ventricle dilation or increased lung parenchymal uptake of thallium-201 isotope
> Echocardiographic wall-motion abnormality involving more than two segments, developing at a low dose of dobutamine (≤10 μg/kg/min) or at a low heart rate (120 beats/min)
> Stress-induced echocardiographic evidence of extensive ischemia

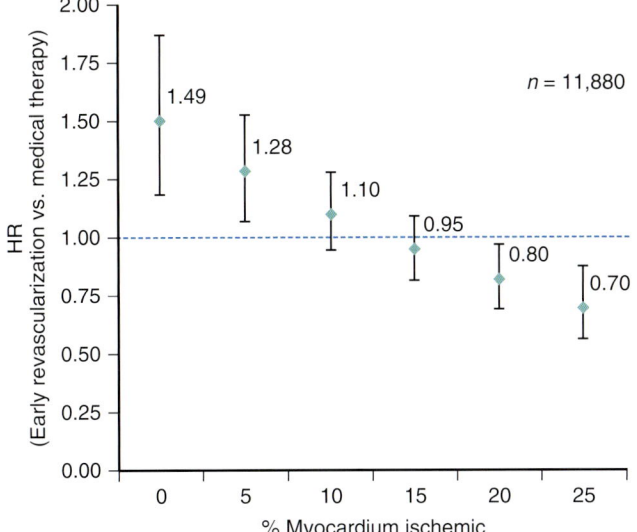

Fig. 2.1 Hazard ratio *(HR)* associated with early revascularization compared with medical therapy at specific values of percent myocardium ischemic in patients with less than 10% myocardial scar. *P* values per Cox proportional hazards model. (From Hachamovitch R, Rozanski A, Shaw LJ, et al. Impact of ischaemia and scar on the therapeutic benefit derived from myocardial revascularization vs. medical therapy among patients undergoing stress-rest myocardial perfusion scintigraphy. *Eur Heart J.* 2011;32[8]:1012–1024.)

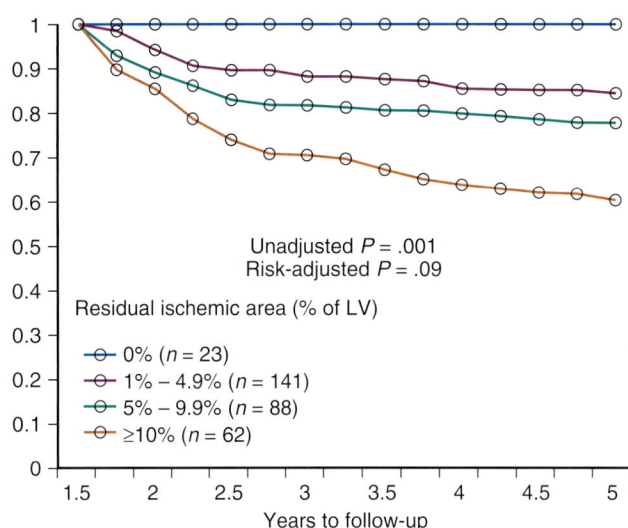

Fig. 2.2 Survival without myocardial infarction depending on residual ischemic area. *LV,* Left ventricle. (From Shaw LJ, Berman DS, Maron DJ, et al. Optimal medical therapy with or without percutaneous coronary intervention to reduce ischemic burden: results from the Clinical Outcomes Utilizing Revascularization and Aggressive Drug Evaluation [COURAGE] trial nuclear substudy. *Circulation.* 2008;117[10]:1283–1291.)

scars, myocardial revascularization compared with conservative treatment improved long-term survival in patients with significant (>10% myocardium) inducible ischemia. Early myocardial revascularization was, however, harmful in patients with minimal inducible ischemia.

Consistent results were obtained in a nuclear substudy on 314 patients in the Clinical Outcomes Utilizing Revascularization and Aggressive Drug Evaluation (COURAGE) trial.[12] In this substudy, the extent of residual posttreatment ischemia—assessed as a percentage of the left ventricle by myocardial perfusion SPECT—was a predictor of outcome: rates of death or MI ranged from 0% to 39% for patients with no residual ischemia to 10% or more residual ischemia despite treatment ($P = .001$ [risk-adjusted $P = .09$]; Fig. 2.2). With respect to treatment, a 5% or more reduction in ischemic myocardium lowered the risk of death or MI ($P = .037$ [risk-adjusted $P = .26$]), particularly if baseline ischemia was 10% or greater ($P = .001$ [risk-adjusted $P = .08$]). PCI on top of optimal medical therapy increased the likelihood of achieving this goal. The findings of this substudy suggest that revascularization is indicated if, in addition to optimal medical therapy, it affords at least a 5% reduction in myocardial ischemia.

Thus, although adequately powered randomized trials to address the impact of severe angina or large perfusion defects on outcome in patients with chronic stable angina are lacking, the bulk of the currently available evidence suggests that these patients benefit from revascularization, particularly if more than one vessel is affected.

Coronary Anatomy

Until now our understanding of the anatomic conditions that constitute a survival benefit from coronary revascularization compared with medical therapy alone has been largely based on milestone studies performed during the 1970s. Soon after CABG was introduced in 1969, three randomized trials compared surgical revascularization with lone medical therapy: the Veterans Administration (VA) Study, the European Coronary Surgery Study (ECSS), and CASS. Although these studies are outdated in many respects, including a low use of arterial conduits and limited means of pharmacologic risk-factor modification and platelet inhibition, it is unlikely that they will ever be replicated. In concert with analyses of large registry databases, these early studies established the conditions under which CABG improves survival compared with medical therapy (Box 2.2). A meta-analysis of the seven published randomized trials of CABG versus medical treatment alone for CAD identified left main CAD (diameter of stenosis ≥50%), multivessel disease, and involvement of the proximal left anterior descending coronary artery (LAD) as significant predictors of a survival benefit from CABG.[13] In the cumulative experience of the seven studies, the VA study being the first, surgical revascularization for left main CAD was associated with a 65% relative reduction in mortality compared with medical therapy alone.[13] Notably, in left main CAD, a survival benefit of surgery was reported irrespective of the presence or absence of spontaneous or inducible symptoms or signs of ischemia or reduced LV function. The same is also true for triple- or double-vessel disease involving the proximal LAD.[14]

In all other conditions, the indication for surgical coronary revascularization depends on a combination of anatomic and clinical criteria. If triple-vessel disease is associated with impaired LV function (LV ejection fraction <50%), surgical revascularization

---

BOX 2.2 Conditions in Which Coronary Artery Bypass Grafting Improves Survival Compared With Medical Therapy

Left main coronary artery disease
Triple- or double-vessel disease involving the proximal left anterior descending coronary artery
Triple- or double-vessel disease in the presence of severe angina or large areas of ischemia on functional testing
Triple-vessel disease associated with impaired left ventricle function

improves survival irrespective of LAD involvement.[15,16] In the presence of severe angina or large areas of ischemia on functional testing, surgical revascularization of triple- or double-vessel disease is also indicated for both symptomatic and prognostic reasons even in the absence of LV dysfunction.[6,7] Myocardial revascularization has never been shown to confer a survival benefit in patients with single-vessel disease. This is also true for isolated proximal LAD stenoses. Yusuf and colleagues' meta-analysis[13] that showed a survival benefit from surgery in patients with LAD involvement must be interpreted with the notion that this result was obtained in a cohort that had predominantly multivessel disease, and no dedicated subgroup analysis was undertaken for isolated LAD stenosis. More recently, the randomized Medicine, Angioplasty, or Surgery Study (MASS) trial compared medical treatment alone with plain balloon angioplasty or CABG in 214 patients with symptomatic, isolated, high-grade stenosis of the LAD.[17] During a 5-year follow-up, no appreciable difference was found among the three treatment arms with regard to either death or MI. Although the power to detect small differences in event rates was low in MASS, its results are consistent with the current judgment that no prognostic indication exists for coronary revascularization in stable single-vessel disease. No study ever demonstrated that in patients with stable angina, the risk of subsequent MI could be reduced by either bypass surgery or PCI. The degree of stenosis is a notoriously poor predictor of subsequent events. Although the risk of subsequent MI is higher with high-grade stenoses than with low-grade stenoses, the latter are far more frequent. Thus the majority of infarctions are triggered by low-grade stenoses. Despite advances,[18,19] our current means of identifying vulnerable plaques are limited.

Need for Complete Revascularization

Apart from the extent and distribution of CAD, the probability of achieving complete revascularization is an important criterion for the choice of the most appropriate revascularization strategy. In CABG, a number of studies have demonstrated that patients who are completely revascularized have better long-term outcomes than those with incomplete revascularization.[20] The same is also true for PCI. Several studies from the prestent era have confirmed better long-term outcomes after complete revascularization than after an incomplete procedure.[21,22] The reasons for not treating all diseased vessels may include technical obstacles such as heavy calcification, tortuous vessels or chronic total occlusions, the presence of serious concomitant disease, or the intention to treat only the "culprit lesion" thought to be responsible for the patient's symptoms. An analysis of a total of 21,945 patients with BMSs from New York State's Percutaneous Coronary Interventions Reporting System assessed the issue of incomplete revascularization with current practices of coronary revascularization. A follow-up period of 3 years was reported.[23] In this registry, 68.9% of the stent patients were incompletely revascularized. After adjustment for comorbidities and other baseline characteristics associated with increased risk, incompletely revascularized patients were significantly more likely to die at any time than completely revascularized patients (adjusted hazard ratio [HR], 1.15; 95% confidence interval [CI], 1.01 to 1.30). The risk associated with incomplete revascularization increased with the number of vessels that were not revascularized and was higher with nonrevascularized chronic total occlusions than in nonrevascularized nonocclusive lesions. Incompletely revascularized patients with total occlusions and two or more nonrevascularized vessels were at the highest risk compared with completely revascularized patients (HR, 1.36; 95% CI, 1.12 to 1.66). A more recent analysis from the same registry addressing CABG versus PCI with new generation everolimus-eluting stents revealed a similar incidence of subsequent MI after CABG or PCI with complete revascularization, whereas the risk of subsequent MI was increased after PCI with incomplete revascularization as compared with CABG ($P = .02$ for interaction).[24]

The first analysis of the role of completeness of revascularization with DESs was a post hoc analysis of the second Arterial Revascularization Therapies Study (ARTS-II), which failed to show a significant impact of incomplete revascularization on survival or survival without MI after placement of sirolimus-eluting stents.[25] However, this analysis was grossly underpowered. More recently, an analysis that included a substantially larger cohort of the Synergy Between Percutaneous Coronary Intervention with Taxus and Cardiac Surgery (SYNTAX) study appeared.[26] This analysis comprised the 899 patients randomized to PCI with paclitaxel-eluting stents, 890 patients randomized to CABG, and the patients who were deemed ineligible for randomization and who were included in the nested registries for PCI ($n = 198$) or CABG ($n = 649$). Consistent with previous studies, complete revascularization substantially reduced the risk of cardiac death during 4-year follow-up compared with incomplete revascularization both in the PCI group (HR, 0.64; 95% CI, 0.41 to 1.00; $P = .049$) and in the surgical group (HR, 0.50; 95% CI, 0.30 to 0.86; $P = .01$). Although the presence of a chronic total occlusion was independently associated with a higher incidence of incomplete revascularization, it showed no significant interaction with impact of completeness of revascularization on survival.

In a subsequent analysis, the same group quantitated the degree of incompleteness of revascularization in the randomized PCI cohort of the SYNTAX trial.[27] This analysis was based on the SYNTAX score that was developed prospectively to gauge the extent and complexity of CAD. To assess the degree of incompleteness of revascularization, the investigators calculated the SYNTAX score after PCI and thus obtained the residual SYNTAX score. A progressively higher residual SYNTAX score was shown to be associated with increased 5-year mortality.[27] Although patients with complete revascularization numerically had the lowest 5-year mortality, no significant differences were reported in 5-year mortality between patients with complete and those with minor incomplete revascularization (residual SYNTAX score 0, 8.5%; >0 to 4, 8.7%; >4 to 8, 11.4%; $P = .60$). In patients with a residual SYNTAX score greater than 8, however, 5-year mortality rose to 35.3% ($P < .001$; Fig. 2.3). Multivariable analysis confirmed the residual SYNTAX score as an independent predictor of 5-year mortality (HR, 1.65; 95% CI, 1.41 to 1.92; $P < .001$). Residual SYNTAX score was also associated with the composite of death, MI, and stroke and with major adverse cardiovascular and cerebrovascular events (MACCEs): death, MI, stroke, and target-vessel revascularization (TVR) (see Fig. 2.3).

The studies mentioned above have been based on anatomic criteria. In the intermediate range of stenoses, however, the anatomic degree—as judged by visual estimation or even quantitative computerized angiography—is poorly correlated with functional relevance, as assessed by noninvasive functional imaging or invasive functional testing, such as measurement of fractional flow reserve (FFR) or instantaneous wave-free ratio (iFR).[28-30] Recent studies with measurement of FFR or iFR have indicated that functional testing reliably discriminates between coronary stenoses that should be treated conservatively and those in need of revascularization.[29-33] Moreover, basing the PCI strategy on functional, rather than purely anatomic, criteria reduces the periinterventional risk[34] and improves the long-term outcome[35] of PCI as shown by the Fractional Flow Reserve Versus Angiography for Multivessel Evaluation (FAME) study.

A meta-analysis of the potential survival benefit of complete versus incomplete revascularization addressed not only the impact of the revascularization modality but also that of anatomic versus functional assessment.[36] This meta-analysis comprised 35 studies with 89,883 patients from subgroups of randomized trials or from observational studies. Irrespective of the revascularization modality, this meta-analysis confirmed a consistent survival benefit of complete

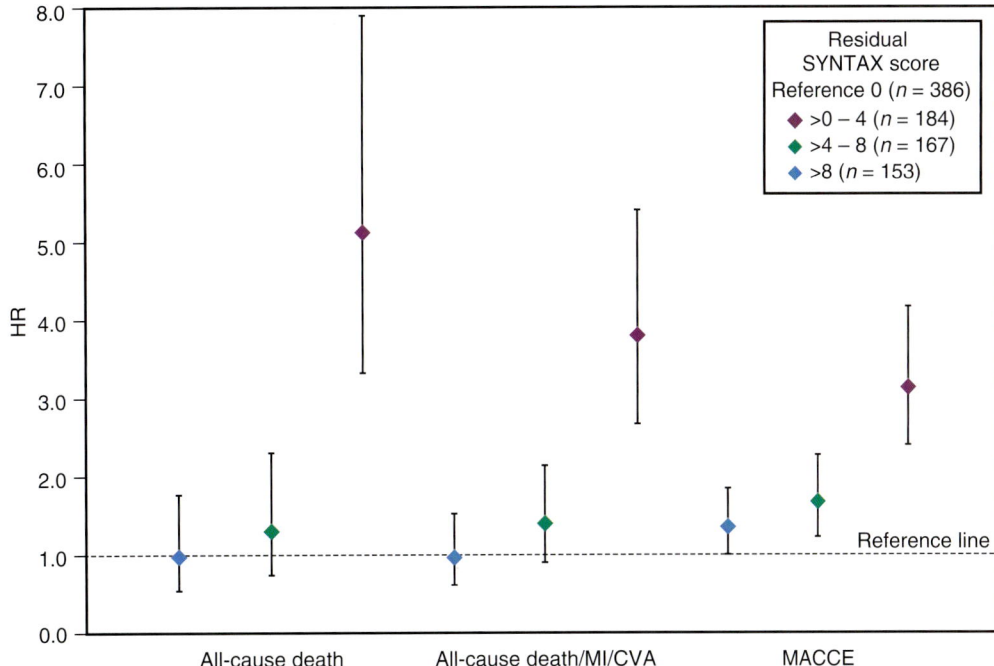

Fig. 2.3 Five-year clinical outcomes stratified by tertiles of the residual SYNTAX score. Hazard ratios *(HRs)* are relative to complete revascularization (reference line, residual SYNTAX score 0). HRs for tertiles of the residual SYNTAX score (>0) are shown. The error bars represent 95% confidence intervals. *CVA*, Cerebrovascular accident; *MACCE*, major adverse cardiovascular and cerebrovascular event; *MI*, myocardial infarction. (From Farooq V, Serruys PW, Bourantas CV, et al. Quantification of incomplete revascularization and its association with five-year mortality in the synergy between percutaneous coronary intervention with taxus and cardiac surgery [SYNTAX] trial validation of the residual SYNTAX score. Circulation. 2013;128[2]:141–151.)

versus incomplete revascularization with both anatomic and functional assessment (relative risk [RR] for mortality with complete revascularization, 0.73 [95% CI, 0.67 to 0.79; $P < .001$], with anatomic definition and RR, 0.57 [95% CI, 0.36 to 0.89; $P = .014$], with functional definition). Nevertheless, it is noteworthy that the point estimate of the relative risk of mortality, comparing complete with incomplete revascularization, was lower with functional complete revascularization than with anatomic complete revascularization.[36]

Given the major impact of the extent of revascularization on long-term survival, consideration must be given to the likelihood of achieving complete revascularization. When PCI is unlikely to achieve complete revascularization, surgery may offer better prospects, yet this may not always be the case; in some instances, poor target vessels for CABG may be treated by PCI with higher chances of success.

PROGNOSTIC INDICATION FOR REVASCULARIZATION: PERCUTANOUS CORONARY INTERVENTION VERSUS CORONARY ARTERY BYPASS GRAFTING

Multivessel Disease

From the late 1980s to the early 1990s, several studies compared plain balloon angioplasty with CABG. Among them were three larger trials—Randomized Intervention Trial of Unstable Angina (RITA; $n = 1011$), the Coronary Angioplasty Versus Bypass Revascularization Investigation (CABRI; $n = 1154$), and the Bypass Angioplasty Revascularization Investigation (BARI; $n = 1829$)—and three smaller trials—the German Angioplasty Bypass Surgery Investigation (GABI; $n = 358$), the Emory Angioplasty Versus Surgery Trial (EAST; $n = 392$), and the Toulouse monocentric study ($n = 152$). Since the early studies, major advances have been achieved in PCI, CABG, and medical treatment. Therefore, the results of randomized trials performed in the prestent era cannot be transferred to current practice.

Lessons From Studies With Bare-Metal Stents

Randomized Studies

Five randomized trials compared stenting with CABG for multivessel disease: ARTS,[37,38] Stent or Surgery (SoS),[39] the Argentine Randomized Trial of Percutaneous Coronary Angioplasty With Stenting Versus Coronary Bypass Surgery in Patients with Multiple-Vessel Disease (ERACI-II),[40,41] the MASS-II,[42] and Angina With Extremely Serious Operative Mortality Evaluation (AWESOME).[43] Four major studies were incorporated in a meta-analysis based on individual patient data, which confirmed the results of the majority of the individual studies.[44] This meta-analysis comprised ARTS, SoS, ERACI-II, and MASS-II but excluded AWESOME because the high-risk characteristics of the patients in this last trial were clearly different from those of the patient population of the other four trials. This meta-analysis confirmed that PCI with stent placement was associated with a 1-year incidence of death, MI, or stroke similar to that of CABG. Nevertheless, the need for repeat revascularization was considerably higher after PCI, although the observed gap with CABG surgery has narrowed from the approximately 30% reported in the prestent era to approximately 14%. Compared with PCI, CABG was associated with a slightly lower frequency of recurrent angina (77% vs. 82%; $P = .002$). Another meta-analysis based on aggregate data from ARTS,[37,38] SoS,[39] ERACI-II,[40,41] and Stenting Versus Internal Mammary Artery (SIMA)—a study on isolated proximal LAD stenosis—extended the analysis to a follow-up of 3 years.[45] The point estimates for both the 3-year incidence of death and nonfatal MI were lower after PCI than after CABG. However, a significant difference was found only for nonfatal MI. Moreover, this meta-analysis confirmed that the 1-year incidence of repeat intervention was 15% absolute higher after PCI than after CABG but did not demonstrate any significant further changes from 1 to 3 years. For ARTS, the largest trial to compare PCI with CABG for the treatment of multivessel disease,[37,38] 5-year results are available. ARTS included a total of 1205 patients with at least two de novo lesions located in different vessels and territories not including the LMCA. In this study, 600 patients were randomly assigned to stenting, and 605 were randomly assigned to bypass surgery; 67% of the patients had a double-vessel disease, and 32% had triple-vessel disease. At 5 years, the incidence of death was 8% in the stent group versus 7.6% in the CABG group (RR, 1.05; 95% CI, 0.71 to 1.55; $P = .83$). Likewise, no significant difference was found in cerebrovascular accident (3.8% vs. 3.5%; RR, 1.10; 95% CI, 0.62 to 1.97; $P = .76$), Q-wave MI (6.7% vs. 5.6%; RR, 1.19; 95% CI, 0.76 to 1.85; $P = .47$), non–Q-wave MI (1.8% vs. 0.8%; RR, 2.22; 95% CI, 0.78 to 6.35; $P = .14$), or the composite thereof (18.2% vs. 14.9%; RR, 1.22; 95% CI, 0.95 to 1.58; $P = .14$). However, a significant difference was reported in the incidence of repeat revascularization (30.3% vs. 8.8%; RR, 3.46; 95% CI, 2.61 to 4.60; $P < .001$). In the stent group, 10.5% of the revascularizations involved CABG, whereas in the CABG group 1.2% of the revascularizations involved CABG. In summary, the 5-year outcome with respect to the serious end points of death, MI, and cerebrovascular accident (CVA) with the surgical and nonsurgical approaches was similar. With the primarily catheter-based approach, the chance of avoiding CABG during the subsequent 5 years was 90%, with a similar outcome with respect to death, CVA, and MI as with the surgical approach but at the expense of a 20% higher incidence of repeat catheter interventions. Consistent with the long-term results of ARTS,[37,38] the 10-year results of MASS-II[42] showed no significant survival benefit of CABG over PCI (HR, 1.03; 95% CI, 0.69 to 1.53; $P = .88$), but a substantially increased need for repeat interventions was reported with PCI versus CABG (HR, 3.71; 95% CI, 1.82 to 7.52; $P < .0001$).

The studies described so far compared PCI with CABG in cohorts that were well suited for both procedures. The important question of whether patients at high risk for CABG surgery and refractory myocardial ischemia should undergo PCI as an alternative procedure was addressed in AWESOME.[43] This multicenter study included patients with myocardial ischemia refractory to medical management and the presence of one or more risk factors for adverse outcome with CABG, including prior open heart surgery, age greater than 70 years, LV ejection fraction less than 35%, MI within 7 days, or the need for intraaortic balloon pumping. Over a 5-year period, 2431 patients met the entry criteria. By physician consensus, 1650 patients formed a physician-directed registry assigned to CABG ($n = 692$), PCI ($n = 651$), or further medical therapy ($n = 307$), and 781 were angiographically eligible for random allocation. Of the patients who were angiographically acceptable, 454 consented to randomized assignment between CABG and PCI; the remaining 327 constituted a patient-choice registry. At all time points during the 5-year follow-up of the randomized study, an insignificant survival benefit of PCI over CABG was reported (97% vs. 95% at 30 days and 75% vs. 70% at 5 years).[46] Within the first 3 years after randomization, more patients randomized to PCI received a subsequent revascularization (37% vs. 18%, $P < .001$), whereas between 3 and 5 years of follow-up, repeat revascularization was similarly frequent in both the PCI group and the CABG group (6% vs. 4%). In the physician-directed subgroup, the 3-year survival rate was 76% for both CABG and PCI. In the patient-choice subgroup, the 3-year survival was 80% with CABG but 98% with PCI. The findings of the AWESOME registry[47] therefore support the findings of the main study. The AWESOME investigators specifically addressed the issue of whether PCI is the preferred option for repeat intervention in patients with previous CABG.[48] In the subgroup with previous CABG, 3-year survival rates were 73% and 76% with CABG or PCI, respectively, in the randomized patients; 71% versus 77% in the physician-directed registry; and 65% versus 86% ($P = .001$) in the patient-choice registry. The authors concluded that PCI is preferable to CABG for many post-CABG patients.

Registries
It has been argued that the randomized studies to compare PCI with CABG in multivessel disease comprised only a small proportion of the patients presenting at dedicated high-volume centers.[49] Therefore, it is claimed that the results of these trials may not be applicable to the vast majority of patients in need of coronary revascularization. It is thus an important question whether the absence of a substantial difference in survival between PCI and CABG can also be verified in large registries. Contrary to the randomized studies that compared PCI with BMSs to CABG, several large registry analyses from the Cleveland, New York, and Rotterdam databases found a significant difference in risk-adjusted survival that favored CABG over PCI.[50-52] Despite these statistically clear-cut results, the implications of the findings in these registries must be interpreted cautiously because several limitations derive from the nonrandomized nature of these comparisons. Adjustment by proportional hazard models cannot fully substitute for randomization because comprehensive inclusion of all confounders is impossible. One important confounder that was not included in any of the risk adjustment was subsequently published by the New York group[23]—that is, incomplete revascularization. These investigators noted that in their registry, 69% of the patients who received a stent had incomplete revascularization. In the same registry, incomplete revascularization after PCI had a statistically significant and clinically relevant impact on outcome, as discussed above. Between patients completely revascularized and those incompletely revascularized, a 2.1% survival disadvantage was reported in 3 years in the absence of a total occlusion, and a 2.7% difference was reported in the presence of a nonrecanalized total occlusion.[23] The difference between complete and incomplete revascularization within the stent group of the New York registry was on the same order of magnitude as the difference between the stent group and the CABG group in the entire registry. The comprehensive analysis from the Duke registry gives additional insight.[53] This registry comprised 18,481 patients with significant CAD between 1986 and 2000 who were assigned by physician preference to medical therapy ($n = 6862$), PCI ($n = 6292$), or CABG ($n = 5327$). Each group was categorized into three subgroups according to the baseline severity of CAD: *low severity* (predominantly single-vessel), *intermediate severity* (predominantly two-vessel), and *high severity* (all three vessels). Mortality was evaluated by Cox models adjusted for cardiac risk, comorbidity, and propensity for selection of a specific treatment. In all three anatomic subgroups, revascularization conferred a significant survival benefit compared with medical therapy. The extent of this survival benefit varied with the degree of CAD and ranged from an additional 8 months gained during 15 years in the low-severity group to 24 months gained in the high-severity group. In the low- and intermediate-severity groups, the benefit from revascularization was independent of the treatment modality, with similar results by CABG and PCI. In the high-severity subgroup, however, CABG was associated with a small but significant survival benefit of 8 months during 15 years. It is noteworthy that the impact of revascularization versus medical treatment is substantially larger than the impact of the choice of revascularization modality. In summary, registry data that compared PCI that used BMSs with CABG suggest a small survival benefit of surgery versus PCI in patients with multivessel disease. A large proportion of this survival benefit appears to be attributed to patients with the most

complex anatomy and to those who do not achieve complete revascularization with PCI.

Lessons From Studies With Drug-Eluting Stents
Registries
ARTS II[54]—a 45-center, 607-patient registry—intended to compare 1-year outcomes of the sirolimus-eluting stent against the historical results of the two arms of ARTS I.[37,38] To achieve the number of treatable lesions per patient comparable to ARTS I, patients were stratified to ensure that at least one-third had three-vessel disease. Compared with ARTS I, ARTS II comprised a higher-risk cohort: 53.5% had three-vessel disease, and diabetes was present in 26.2%. Mean stented length was 72.5 mm, with 3.7 stents implanted per patient. The 5-year incidence[55] of death, stroke, or MI was 12.9% in ARTS II, versus 14% in the CABG arm of ARTS I ($P = .1$), and it was 18.1% in the BMS arm of ARTS I ($P = .007$). The 5-year rate of MACCEs in ARTS II of 27.5% was significantly higher than that among patients in ARTS I who received CABG (21.1%, $P = .02$), and it was lower than that among ARTS I patients who received BMSs (41.5%, $P < .001$). The authors concluded that at 5 years, the sirolimus-eluting stent had a safety record comparable to that of CABG and superior to that of BMSs. Nevertheless, surgery still afforded a lower need for repeat revascularization, although overall event rates in ARTS II approached the surgical results in ARTS I.[37,38]

Two subsequent analyses based on larger registries subsequently challenged the promising results of ARTS II.[56,57] By linking several large databases, one study analyzed survival data of 185,793 patients 65 years of age or older who had two- or three-vessel CAD without acute MI.[56] Out of these patients, 86,244 had undergone CABG, and 103,549 had had PCI with a rate of DESs of 86%. To reduce treatment-selection bias, inverse-probability-weighting adjustment was performed with the use of propensity scores. At 4-year follow-up, mortality was significantly lower in the CABG group than in the PCI group (16.4% vs. 20.8%; RR, 0.79; 95% CI, 0.76 to 0.82), a finding that was consistent across multiple subgroups.[56] Similar results were obtained in an observational study based on New York State's reporting system.[57] Confirming and extending their earlier studies based on the same registry,[58] this analysis included patients undergoing the revascularization for two- or three-vessel disease without LMCA stenosis in the absence of acute MI.[57] To control for treatment-selection bias, patients were matched for several pertinent variables that included propensity of CABG. Thus 8121 pairs of matched patients were obtained. Compared with PCI patients, 5-year survival mortality was significantly lower in CABG patients (19.6% vs. 26.4%; HR, 0.71; 95% CI, 0.67 to 0.77; $P < .001$).[57] There was a significant interaction (P interaction [P_{int}] = .01) with age that indicated a greater survival benefit of CABG at younger ages, thereby contradicting the results of a meta-analysis of randomized studies that compared CABG with PCI using BMSs.[59] Despite this interaction, a significant survival benefit was found in both younger (<60 years) and older patients (>80 years), as well as in all other clinical and anatomic subsets investigated.

A more recent observational study analyzed 34,819 patients from registries of the New York State Department who underwent CABG or PCI with the use of everolimus-eluting stents. By propensity-score matching 9223 matched pairs could be compared.[24] At a mean follow-up of 2.9 years, all-cause mortality was similar with PCI using everolimus-eluting stents or CABG (3.1% per year and 2.9% per year, respectively; HR, 1.04; 95% CI, 0.93 to 1.17; $P = .50$). The risk of stroke was lower with PCI (0.7% per year vs. 1.0% per year; HR, 0.62; 95% CI, 0.50 to 0.76; $P < .001$), whereas the risk of MI was higher (1.9% per year vs. 1.1% per year; HR, 1.51; 95% CI, 1.29 to 1.77; $P < .001$). Yet, this increased risk of MI was confined to patients with incomplete revascularization; in the subset with complete revascularization the rates of MI after PCI were not significantly different from those after CABG (HR 1.02; 95% CI 0.71 to 1.47; $P = .93$; P_{int} = .02). Although the overall risk of repeat revascularization was low, it was significantly higher after PCI than after CABG (7.2% per year vs. 3.1% per year; HR, 2.35; 95% CI, 2.14 to 2.58; $P < .001$).

Although some of the registry data in the era of DESs continue to find a survival benefit of CABG over PCI, the same limitations apply as for the registry-based analyses with BMSs. Apart from unknown confounders, the issue of completeness of revascularization was not addressed, which obscures interpretation of the results. Moreover, none these registries stratified patients by state-of-the-art measures of anatomic complexity, such as the SYNTAX score.

Randomized Studies
The promising results of ARTS II had to be interpreted cautiously because this study does not account for advances in surgical technique that may have occurred since the days of ARTS I. Thus, randomized studies were needed to clarify the role of DESs compared with CABG for multivessel disease. This issue was the objective of the SYNTAX trial,[60] a randomized trial that compared PCI with paclitaxel-eluting stents and CABG for treating patients with previously untreated three-vessel or left main CAD or both. The study enrolled 1800 patients, in whom the local cardiac surgeon and interventional cardiologist determined that equivalent anatomic revascularization could be achieved with either treatment. At 1 year, the primary end point, MACCE, was significantly higher in the PCI group (17.8% vs. 12.4% for CABG; $P = .002$), in large part because of an increased rate of repeat revascularization (13.5% vs. 5.9%, $P < .001$). Apart from reintervention, no significant differences were found in any of the components of the primary end point or a combination thereof except for stroke, which was significantly more likely to occur with CABG (2.2% vs. 0.6% with PCI; $P = .003$). Five-year results of SYNTAX have been reported.[61] By 5 years, the primary end point, MACCE, was reached in 37.3% of the PCI group and in 26.9% of the CABG group ($P < .001$). This difference was largely caused by a difference in the need for reintervention (25.9% vs. 13.7%, $P < .001$). The composite risk of all-cause death, MI, and stroke was also significantly higher in the PCI group than in the CABG group (20.8% vs. 16.7%, $P = .03$). This difference was driven by significant difference in cardiac death (9.0% vs. 5.3%, $P = .003$) and MI (9.7% vs. 3.8%, $P < .001$) that favored CABG, whereas in the PCI group, a trend toward less frequent strokes prevailed (2.4% vs. 3.7%, $P = .09$). In SYNTAX, randomization was stratified according to LMCA involvement. In the 1095 patients who belonged to the subset defined by three-vessel disease without LMCA stenosis, PCI compared with CABG performed less well than in the entire SYNTAX study.[62] Five-year all-cause mortality after PCI in the three-vessel-disease stratum was significantly higher than that after CABG (14.6% vs. 9.2%, $P = .006$), as was the incidence of MI (10.6% vs. 3.3%, $P < .001$), but no significant difference was reported in stroke rate (3.0% vs. 3.4%, $P = .66$).[62] Thus both the 5-year composite of death, MI, and stroke—as well as 5-year MACCE after PCI—were significantly inferior to those after CABG (22.0% vs. 14.0%, $P < .001$; and 37.5% vs. 24.2%, $P < .001$, respectively).[62] The authors of the SYNTAX trial also prospectively stratified the study patients to tertiles of the SYNTAX score. In the lowest tertile of SYNTAX scores (those < 23), 3-year mortality in the three-vessel-disease subset after PCI was similar to that after CABG (10.2% vs. 9.3%, $P = .81$).[62] Likewise, only a statistically insignificant numerical increase was found in MACCE with PCI compared with CABG (33.3% vs. 26.8%, $P = .45$).[62] These results in the lowest tertile of SYNTAX scores in the three-vessel-disease subset were consistent with the results in the corresponding subset of the entire study (10.1% vs. 8.9% [$P = .64$] for death; and

32.1% vs. 28.6% [$P = .43$] for MACCE).[61] In the highest tertile of SYNTAX scores (>32), PCI was associated with excess 5-year mortality compared with CABG both in the three-vessel-disease subset and in the entire study cohort (17.8% vs. 8.8% [$P = .015$] and 19.2% vs. 11.4% [$P = .005$], respectively).[61,62] Similar to the finding in the entire subset with three-vessel disease, mortality in the middle tertile was also higher at 5 years after PCI than after CABG (16.3% vs. 9.6%, $P = .047$).[61,62] In the two highest tertiles of SYNTAX scores of the three-vessel-disease subset, major differences were also found in 3-year MACCE rates that favored CABG over PCI.[62]

When interpreting the results of SYNTAX, two caveats deserve consideration: First, 50 patients of the CABG group, but only 11 of the PCI group, were lost to follow-up because of withdrawal of consent.[61] The authors report that a sensitivity analysis showed that the primary end point analysis was not significantly affected by this imbalance of follow-up.[61] Nevertheless, it cannot be excluded that the effect size was affected. Second, the paclitaxel-eluting stent used in SYNTAX carries a higher risk of late stent thrombosis compared with the contemporaneous first-generation sirolimus-eluting stent[4,63] and, particularly, compared with modern, new-generation DESs.[4,64] Meta-analyses also suggest that the prevention of restenosis by paclitaxel-eluting stents is inferior to that of other DES types.[4,65] Therefore, it was speculated that the outcome of PCI, with modern new generation DESs as compared with CABG might be more favorable than what was found in the SYNTAX trial.

This hypothesis was tested in the multicenter Randomized Comparison of Coronary Artery Bypass Surgery and Everolimus Eluting Stent Implantation in the Treatment of Patients with Multivessel Coronary Artery Disease (BEST) trial.[66] This randomized noninferiority trial at 27 centers in East Asia compared PCI with everolimus-eluting stents to CABG in patients with multivessel coronary artery disease. Significant LMCA stenosis and acute ST-elevation myocardial infarction were exclusion criteria. After inclusion of 880 patients, enrollment was stopped due to slow recruitment. Of the patients included, 77% had three-vessel disease and 23% two-vessel disease; the mean SYNTAX score was 24. At a mean follow-up of 4.6 years the incidence of the primary end point, the composite of death, MI and TVR was higher in patients assigned to PCI than in patients assigned to CABG (15.3% vs. 10.6%; HR, 1.74; 95% CI, 1.01 to 2.13; $P = .04$). There were no significant differences between PCI and CABG with respect to death from any cause (6.6% vs. 5.0%, $P = .30$), MI (4.8% vs. 2.7%, $P = .11$), death or MI (9.8% vs. 7.7%, $P = .28$) or stroke (2.5% vs. 2.9%, $P = .72$). Thus, the significant difference in the primary end point between PCI and CABG was driven by a significant difference in the need for repeat TVR (11.1% vs. 5.4%; HR, 2.09; 95% CI, 1.28 to 3.41; $P = .03$). There was only a minor and statistically insignificant difference in target lesion revascularization between PCI and CABG (5.7% vs. 3.8%, $P = .19$). Yet CABG achieved complete revascularization more often than PCI (71.5% vs. 50.9%, $P < .001$) and less frequently required revascularization of new lesions (5.5% vs. 2.3%, $P = .01$). Hence, the difference in the need for repeat revascularization between PCI and CABG was caused predominantly by a difference in the need for nontarget lesion revascularization (5.3% vs. 1.6%, $P < .001$).

An individual patient data (IPD) meta-analysis of SYNTAX and BEST focused on patients with multivessel disease and proximal left anterior descending (LAD) involvement.[67] This meta-analysis comprised 1166 patients including 435 (37.3%) with diabetes mellitus. Primary end point of this analysis was the composite of all-cause death, MI, and stroke at 5 years. Consistent with the analysis in the absence of proximal LAD involvement, the primary end point in the entire cohort occurred more often in the PCI arm than in the CABG arm (16.3% vs. 11.5%; HR, 1.43; 95% CI, 1.05 to 1.95; $P = .026$). This difference was driven by significantly higher rates of cardiac death, MI, and all-cause revascularization after PCI. In the subset with low complexity of coronary disease (SYNTAX score ≤22) there were no significant differences in the primary end point (13.3% vs. 10.8%; HR, 1.21, 95% CI, 0.66 to 2.23; $P = .54$). In this subset, all-cause death (5.8% vs. 6.2%, $P = .81$) and the composite of death, MI, stroke, and repeat revascularization (24.9% vs. 18.2%; HR, 1.37, 95% CI, 0.87 to 2.17; $P = .17$) were also not significantly different between PCI and CABG. Thus, the main driver for the observed differences between PCI and CABG does not appear to be proximal LAD involvement but rather the overall anatomical complexity of coronary artery disease.

A more recent IPD meta-analysis takes an even broader view.[68] This meta-analysis summarizes the evidence as of July 2017 and, thereby, included 11,518 patients from 11 trials randomly assigning patients to PCI or to CABG. Mean follow-up was 3.8 years. The primary focus of this meta-analysis was all-cause mortality. In addition to the overall analysis, the treatment effect was explored in major subgroups defined by the presence or absence of LMCA stenosis, strata of SYNTAX score, as well as presence or absence of diabetes mellitus. A second publication also addressed the incidence of stroke.[69]

In the overall analysis 5-year all-cause mortality was 11.2% after PCI and 9.2% after CABG (HR 1.20, 95% CI 1.06 to 1.37; $P = .0038$). The 30-day incidence of stroke was significantly lower after PCI than after CABG (0.4% vs. 1.1%; HR = 0.33, 95% CI 0.20 to 0.53; $P < .001$), with no significant difference in stroke rate between the two treatment modalities during subsequent follow-up of up to 5 years.[69] With respect to all-cause mortality, the benefit of CABG over PCI increased significantly with strata of SYNTAX score (P for trend = .001). In the stratum with low SYNTAX score, there was no significant difference in mortality between CABG and PCI, whereas a significant survival benefit of CABG was found in the strata with intermediate or high SYNTAX scores (Fig. 2.4).

The survival benefit of CABG over PCI, as well as its dependence on the anatomical complexity as defined by the SYNTAX score, was even more prominent in the subgroup with multivessel disease without LMCA involvement (see Fig. 2.4). In this subgroup, 5-year all-cause mortality was 11.5% after PCI and 8.9% after CABG (HR 1.28, 95% CI 1.09 to 1.49; $P = .0019$). In patients with low SYNTAX score, the numerical difference in 5-year all-cause mortality was 2.1%, which did not reach statistical significance ($P = .57$), whereas in patients with intermediate and high SYNTAX score, the absolute differences in 5-year mortality were 4.9% ($P = .013$) and 6.8% ($P = .0094$), respectively (P for trend = .0006). This analysis of patients with multivessel disease comprised both patients with and without diabetes, as well as patients treated with BMSs or DESs.

In the era of DES, only two trials—BEST and SYNTAX—compared PCI with CABG in patients with multivessel disease. An IPD meta-analysis on the 1275 patients with multivessel coronary artery disease in the absence of diabetes mellitus in SYNTAX and BEST has been published.[70] Of these patients, 88% had three-vessel disease and the mean SYNTAX score was 28. During a median follow-up time of 61 months the risk of death from any cause was significantly lower after CABG than after PCI (5-year mortality 6.7% vs. 10.0%; HR, 0.65, 95% CI, 0.43 to 0.98; $P = .029$). In addition, CABG was associated with a lower risk of MI than PCI (3.4% vs. 8.9%; HR, 0.40; 95% CI, 0.24 to 0.65; $P = .001$) and the need for repeat revascularization was also significantly lower (HR, 0.55; 95% CI, 0.40 to 0.75, $P < .001$). Although there was no significant interaction between strata of SYNTAX score and treatment effect of PCI or CABG with respect to mortality, all-cause mortality was similar between CABG and PCI in patients with SYNTAX scores ≤22 (6.0% vs. 7.4%, $P = .66$), whereas a substantial survival benefit of CABG over PCI was found in patients with SYNTAX-Scores >22 (7.1%

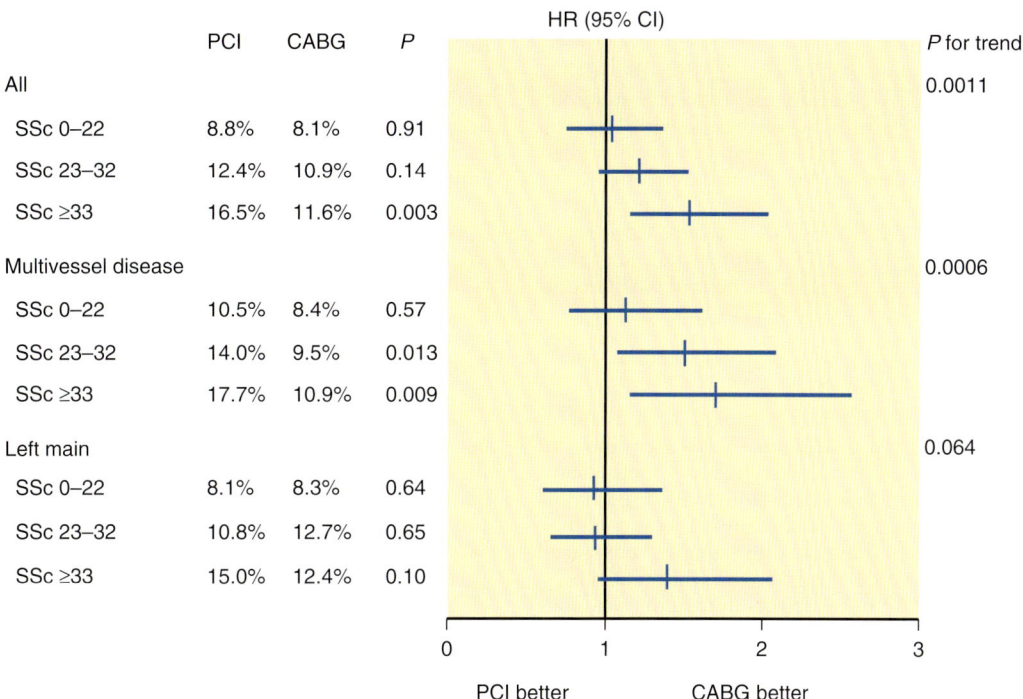

Fig. 2.4 Hazard ratios *(HRs)* with 95% confidence intervals *(CIs)* for all-cause mortality stratified by levels of SYNTAX score *(SSc)* in the individual patient data meta-analysis of randomized trials comparing percutaneous coronary intervention *(PCI)* with coronary artery bypass grafting *(CABG)* in the entire cohort as well as in the subgroups with multivessel disease or left main disease. Percent numbers are the estimated 5-year incidences for PCI or CABG. *P*-values are shown for the comparison between PCI and CABG and for trend of treatment effect with increasing level of SYNTAX score.[68] (From Windecker S, Neumann FJ, Jüni P, et al. Considerations for the choice between CABG and PCI as revascularisation strategies in major categories of patients with stable multivessel coronary artery disease—an accompanying article of the Task Force of the 2018 ESC/EACTS guidelines on myocardial revascularisation. *Eur Heart J.* 2019;40[2]:204–212.)

vs. 11.6%, *P* = .02). The pooled analysis of SYNTAX and BEST strengthens the message that in patients with intermediate to high anatomic complexity of CAD CABG is preferred to improve prognosis.

In summary, CABG is the preferred revascularization strategy in the majority of patients suffering from three-vessel disease without LMCA involvement. In this setting, compared with PCI, CABG improved survival and reduced the risk of MI and the need for reintervention. In patients with SYNTAX scores less than 23, however, PCI afforded similar outcomes with respect to survival and MACCEs. In this setting, PCI would be the treatment of choice because it is associated with less discomfort to the patient and less resource consumption.

Special Considerations in Patients With Diabetes Mellitus

Coronary revascularization in patients with diabetes mellitus differs in many respects from that in patients without diabetes. Thus, the indication for PCI in patients with diabetes deserves special attention.

Compared to patients without diabetes mellitus, those with diabetes often have a more advanced type of coronary atherosclerosis, with diffuse disease in small-lumen vessels. With any treatment modality for coronary revascularization, patients with diabetes have an inferior outcome compared with others. This was first shown for CABG. In patients with diabetes mellitus, CABG is associated with a more rapid progression of atherosclerosis in both grafted and nongrafted vessels and is also associated with an accelerated degeneration of venous bypass grafts. Nevertheless, the CASS researchers[71] demonstrated that in older patients with diabetes, coronary revascularization confers a substantial benefit compared with medical therapy alone. Likewise, PCI in patients with diabetes is associated with a substantially increased risk of adverse short- and long-term outcome compared with PCI in the absence of diabetes. In particular, the risk of restenosis after any type of PCI is substantially increased in patients with diabetes compared to patients without diabetes.[72,73] Moreover, whereas restenosis has little impact on survival in patients without diabetes, van Belle and coworkers[74] demonstrated that restenosis after plain balloon angioplasty in diabetics has a major impact on 10-year mortality, with a 45% relative increase for nonocclusive stenosis and more than a twofold increase with occlusive stenosis. The risk of periinterventional death and MI is also increased by about twofold after plain balloon angioplasty in patients with diabetes compared to patients without diabetes.[75] Comparing coronary bypass surgery with plain balloon angioplasty for multivessel disease, BARI reported 5- and 7-year mortalities in patients with diabetes of 34.5% and 44.3%, respectively, whereas after bypass surgery, the respective mortalities were 19.4% and 23.6% (*P* = .03 and .01, respectively).[76] The findings in BARI that were subsequently confirmed by the 8-year analysis of EAST[63] led to a clinical alert from the National Heart, Lung, and Blood Institute for the abandonment of plain balloon angioplasty as a treatment option for multivessel CAD. Given the major impact of restenosis on survival, it is plausible that compared with plain balloon angioplasty, stents may improve the long-term outcome of PCI substantially. Finally, the recently improved means of achieving tight metabolic control can further improve outcome after catheter intervention.[77,78]

Studies With Bare-Metal Stents

Of the studies that compared BMSs with CABG, the ARTS, AWESOME, and ERACI-II researchers reported subgroup analyses for patients with diabetes. Nevertheless, with less than 150 patients with diabetes randomized in any of these studies, numbers were too small to allow any meaningful conclusions.[79–81] The Alberta Provincial Project for Outcome Assessment in Coronary Heart Disease (APPROACH), the only large registry that addressed stent-supported PCI with bypass surgery in patients with diabetes, did not reveal any benefit of CABG compared with PCI.[82]

Studies With Drug-Eluting Stents

DESs are particularly appealing in patients with diabetes because they offer a solution to the most crucial problem of PCI in this patient subset—that is, restenosis. A meta-analysis of patients with diabetes in randomized studies that compared DESs with BMSs confirmed that in diabetes mellitus, DESs significantly reduce the risk of restenosis compared with BMSs[83–85] by 37% to 69% depending on the stent type.[84] Nevertheless, the excess risk of restenosis in patients with diabetes compared with patients without diabetes prevailed even with DESs.[83] No safety issues were reported with respect to the 1-year incidence of death or of the composite of death and nonfatal MI when DESs were compared with BMSs in patients with diabetes,[84] provided that dual antiplatelet therapy is pursued for at least 6 months.[85] Based on the older studies for PCI in patients with diabetes, it may be anticipated that the reduction in restenosis by DESs compared with BMSs may confer a survival benefit during longer-term follow-up in patients with diabetes.[74] Hence the role of PCI compared with CABG in the treatment of multivessel disease had to be reassessed in the era of DESs.

The Coronary Artery Revascularization in Diabetes (CARDia) trial was designed to compare PCI with CABG in patients with diabetes.[86] A total of 510 patients with diabetes and multivessel or complex single-vessel coronary disease were randomized to CABG or PCI with BMSs in the first 30% of the patients and subsequently with sirolimus-eluting stents. CARDia included a low-risk cohort: three-vessel disease accounted for only 62% of the cohort, and only 1% of the lesions treated by PCI in CARDia were bifurcations. The primary end point—the 1-year composite incidence of all-cause mortality, MI, and stroke—was 10.5% in the CABG group and 13.0% in the PCI group ($P = .39$); all-cause mortality rates were 3.2% and 3.2%; and the rates of repeat intervention were 2.0% and 11.8% ($P < .001$), respectively. Thus the 1-year rate of MACCEs after CABG was significantly lower than that after PCI (11.3% vs. 19.3%; HR, 1.77; 95% CI, 1.11 to 2.82; $P = .02$). With respect to the primary end point, as well as MACCEs, interactions occurred with the stent type that favored DESs over BMSs ($P = .076$ and $P = .131$, respectively). Nevertheless, the observed 1-year rate of MACCEs in the subgroup with sirolimus-eluting stents was 18.0% after PCI compared with 12.9% after CABG. In the meantime, 5-year outcomes of CARDia were reported.[87] Still, no significant differences were reported between CABG and PCI in all-cause mortality (12.6% vs. 14%; HR, 0.85; 95% CI, 0.53 to 1.37; $P = .53$) or the composite of all-cause mortality, MI, or stroke (20.5% vs. 26.6%; HR, 0.75; 95% CI, 0.52 to 1.06; $P = .11$). The need for repeat intervention was, however, higher after PCI than after CABG (22.2% vs. 9.2%; HR, 0.41; 95% CI, 0.26 to 0.65; $P = .11$). It remains unclear to what extent the increased need for intervention after PCI had to be attributed to the use of BMSs in some of the patients. CARDia suggested that in patients with diabetes and less complex CAD, PCI with DESs may be as safe as CABG but is associated with a higher need for intervention.

For patients with diabetes and multivessel CAD, the Future Revascularization Evaluation in Patients With Diabetes Mellitus: Optimal Management of Multivessel Disease (FREEDOM) trial was the landmark trial to assess the optimal revascularization strategy with contemporary state-of-the art surgical, interventional, and medical treatment.[88] With 1900 patients enrolled and a follow-up of 5 years, the study was adequately powered. The primary outcome, the 5-year composite incidence of death from any cause, nonfatal MI, and nonfatal stroke occurred less frequently in the CABG group than in the PCI group (18.7% vs. 26.6%, absolute difference of 7.9%; 95% CI, 3.3 to 12.5, $P = .005$).[89] This difference was driven by a significant 5-year survival benefit (10.9% vs. 16.3%, $P = .049$) and by a lower 5-year incidence of MI with CABG compared with PCI (6.0% vs. 13.9%, $P < .001$).[88] However, CABG was associated with a slight, but statistically significant, increase in the 5-year incidence of stroke (5.2% vs. 2.4%, $P = .03$). CABG also afforded a slightly better intermediate-term health status and quality of life than PCI.[90] The benefit of a CABG was similar in two-vessel and three-vessel disease.[88] There also was a post hoc assessment of SYNTAX score and a stratification to low (≤22), intermediate (23 to 32), and high (≥33) SYNTAX score. In the low range of SYNTAX score, the hazard ratio that compared CABG with PCI was close to unity and was statistically insignificant, whereas at SYNTAX scores above 22, a substantial and statistically significant benefit of CABG was found with respect to the primary end point. These findings are difficult to interpret, however, because the P value for interaction did not reach statistical significance ($P_{int} = .485$).[88] Thus the findings of FREEDOM demonstrate a substantial benefit of CABG over PCI in the majority of patients with diabetes and multivessel disease, particularly those with more complex coronary anatomies, but they do not completely rule out the option of PCI in patients with simple coronary anatomies, such as those with SYNTAX scores below 23.

The 5-year results of the diabetic subset of SYNTAX add relevant evidence.[91] In the PCI group, multivariate analysis identified diabetes as an independent predictor of MACCEs and of repeat revascularization but not of the composite of all-cause death, MI, or stroke. On the contrary, diabetes was not independently associated with any end point in the CABG group. In SYNTAX, randomization was stratified for diabetes. Among 452 patients with medically treated diabetes, 221 were assigned to CABG and 231 were assigned to PCI.[91] Concerning the 5-year incidence of MACCE, the primary end point of SYNTAX, CABG was superior to PCI (26.3% vs. 34.1%, $P = .002$).[91] To a large extent, this was due to a lower need for repeat revascularization (13.4% vs. 28.2%, $P < .001$). The differences in 5-year all-cause death (10.9% vs. 12.0%, $P = .048$) or the composite of all-cause death, MI, or stroke (15.9% vs. 19.8%, $P = .069$) were not significant between CABG and PCI. Nevertheless, significant differences that favored CABG were found for the 5-year incidence of cardiac death (4.9% vs. 7.7%, $P = .035$) and of MI (3.4% vs. 9.9%; $P < .001$). Stratifying the diabetic subgroup of SYNTAX to anatomic complexity as judged by tertiles of SYNTAX scores revealed diverse 5-year outcomes (Fig. 2.5): In the lowest tertile of SYNTAX scores (<23), the 5-year incidence of the composite of all-cause death, MI, or stroke was similar between CABG and PCI (20.1% vs. 19.4%, $P = .79$). Although there was a significantly lower need for reintervention after CABG versus PCI (18.5% vs. 38.5%, $P = .014$), it did not result in a significant difference in 5-year MACCE rates (33.7% vs. 42.5%, $P = .38$). The middle tertile of SYNTAX scores (23 to 32) exhibited a similar pattern of outcomes as the lowest tertile. In the highest tertile of SYNTAX scores (>32), however, 5-year MACCE rates were twice as high after PCI than after CABG (56.7% vs. 25.5%, $P < .001$). This comprised significant differences in the composite

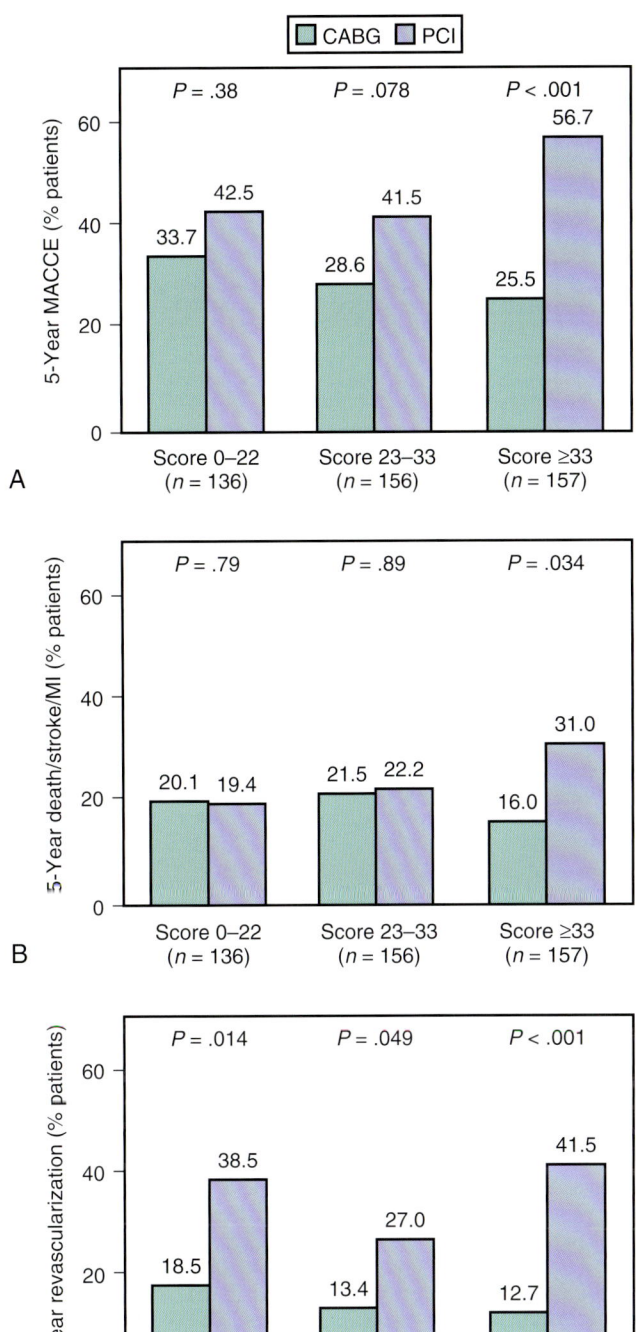

Fig. 2.5 Five-year outcomes for diabetic patients and nondiabetic patients, according to anatomic lesion complexity as measured by the SYNTAX score. Results from the SYNTAX trial comparing percutaneous coronary intervention *(PCI)* with coronary artery bypass grafting *(CABG)* in patients with three-vessel disease or left main coronary artery disease with or without distal coronary artery stenosis. Binary event rates of (A) major adverse cardiovascular or cerebrovascular event *(MACCE)*, (B) the composite end point of all-cause death/stroke/myocardial infarction *(MI)*, and (C) repeat revascularization in diabetic patients. Rates are separated according to SYNTAX score tertiles, indicating low (0 to 22), intermediate (23 to 32), and high (≥33) anatomic lesion complexity.[68] (From Kappetein AP, Head SJ, Morice MC, et al. Treatment of complex coronary artery disease in patients with diabetes: 5-year results comparing outcomes of bypass surgery and percutaneous coronary intervention in the SYNTAX trial. *Eur J Cardiothorac Surg.* 2013;43[5]:1006–1013.)

of all-cause death, MI, or stroke ($P = .034$) and in repeat revascularization ($P < .001$). In summary, the overall level of risk in the diabetic cohort of SYNTAX was higher than in the entire cohort, but on the whole, the findings are largely consistent with those in the entire study except for a higher risk of restenosis. Specifically, the subgroup analysis of diabetics suggests that the noninferiority of PCI compared with CABG in patients with SYNTAX scores less than 23, as found in the entire study, also applies to people with diabetes, at least as far as the hard end points are concerned.

These analyses from the SYNTAX trial are corroborated by a pooling with study-level data from the FREEDOM trial.[92] In patients with low and intermediate SYNTAX scores, this reveals insignificant differences in the composite risk of death, MI, and stroke between PCI or CABG (RR [95% CI] 1·32 [0·86 to 2·02] and 1·27 [0·96 to 1·68], respectively), but a higher risk with PCI (RR [95% CI] 1·73 [1·21 to 2·46]) in patients with high SYNTAX scores.

The Collaborative Atorvastatin Diabetes Study (CARDS) was another dedicated trial that compared CABG with PCI using DESs in diabetic patients. Although CARDS had a small size ($n = 198$) because of premature termination, 2-year follow-up revealed a survival benefit in patients with diabetes and severe CAD treated with CABG compared with those treated by PCI with DESs.[93]

Taken together, the four randomized controlled trials that compared CABG with PCI using DESs in diabetic patients—CARDia, FREEDOM, SYNTAX, and CARDS—show a survival benefit with CABG, as well as a reduction in the risk of MI and in the need for repeat revascularization.[94] In a meta-analysis of these trials, the relative risk of all-cause mortality comparing CABG with PCI was 0.65 (95% CI, 0.48 to 0.90; $P = .008$) at 5-year (or longest) follow-up.[94] However, some degree of heterogeneity was apparent ($I^2 = 49\%$), with the numerically lowest and insignificant benefit of CABG in CARDia and the largest in CARDS. The overall findings of the meta-analysis are reproducible in large, unselected patient cohorts. In a registry that comprised 2885 multivessel patients with diabetes, a propensity-matched comparison between patients treated by PCI and those treated by CABG revealed higher all-cause mortality with PCI (HR, 1.8; 95% CI, 1.4 to 2.2; $P < .0001$), as well as a higher risk of MI (HR, 3.3; 95% CI, 2.4 to 4.6, $P < .0001$) and of TVR (HR, 4.5; 95% CI, 3.4 to 6.1; $P < .0001$) during 5-year follow-up.[95]

Consistent results were obtained in the recently published comprehensive IPD meta-analysis. In this analysis, diabetes mellitus was the strongest modifier of treatment effect between PCI and CABG (P for interaction = .0077). In patients with diabetes, 5-year all-cause mortality after PCI was 15.7% as compared with 10.7% after CABG (HR 1.44, 95% CI 1.20 to 1.74; $P < .001$).[68] This difference was largely driven by a substantial survival benefit in patients with diabetes and multivessel disease (10.0% vs. 15.5%, $P < .001$) (Fig. 2.6).[68]

In summary, based on currently available evidence, CABG is the preferred method of revascularization for most diabetic patients with coronary multivessel disease. Nevertheless, the risk associated with PCI, as well as the benefit of CABG, is not uniform across the spectrum of complex CAD. This is suggested by the analysis of outcomes stratified to levels of SYNTAX score and also by the more favorable results of PCI in the lower-risk cohort of CARDia. Accordingly, PCI remains an option to be considered in low-complexity subsets of multivessel disease, such as those with a SYNTAX score less than 23.

Left Main Coronary Artery Disease

Since the early days of Andreas Grüntzig, plain balloon angioplasty has been considered contraindicated in unprotected left main stem lesions because of the almost inevitable fatality when

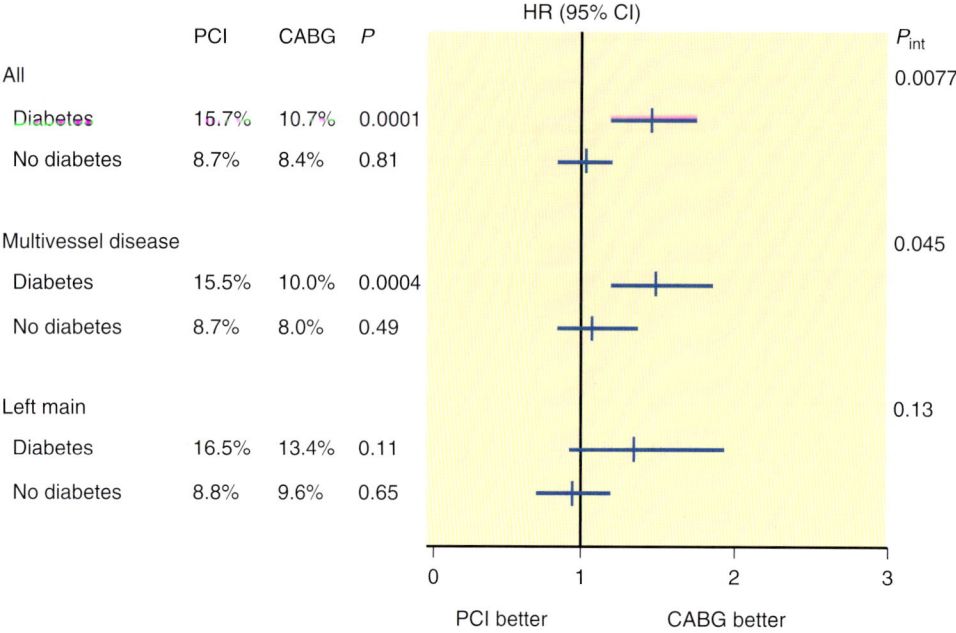

Fig. 2.6 Hazard ratios *(HRs)* with 95% confidence intervals *(CIs)* for all-cause mortality stratified by diabetes mellitus in the IPD meta-analysis of randomized trials comparing percutaneous coronary intervention *(PCI)* with coronary artery bypass grafting *(CABG)* in the entire cohort as well as in the subgroups with multivessel disease or left main disease. Percent numbers are the estimated 5-year incidences for PCI or CABG. *P*-values are shown for the comparison between PCI and CABG and for the interaction of treatment effect with diabetes. (From Windecker S, Neumann FJ, Jüni P, et al. Considerations for the choice between CABG and PCI as revascularisation strategies in major categories of patients with stable multivessel coronary artery disease—an accompanying article of the Task Force of the 2018 ESC/EACTS guidelines on myocardial revascularization. *Eur Heart J.* 2019;40[2]:204–212.)

the procedure fails and because CABG had been established as a therapy that reduced mortality compared with medical treatment alone. With the advent of coronary stents, however, the verdict against catheter treatment of LMCA stenosis was challenged. Stents are particularly attractive for percutaneous treatment of LMCA because they reduce acute complications and restenosis, especially in large-diameter vessels. Moreover, stents overcome the elastic recoil within the aortic wall, which represents a major problem with LMCA percutaneous transluminal coronary angioplasty (PTCA). It was thus not surprising that several groups reported favorable results of registries on BMS of unprotected LMCA stenosis.[96–100]

Registries with Drug-Eluting Stents

Several registries have addressed the efficacy and safety of DESs in the treatment of LMCA. In 2005, three key studies were published that comprised cohorts of 85 to 102 patients treated with DESs for unprotected LMCA and historic control groups with BMSs of 64 to 121 patients.[89,101,102] These studies suggested that DESs, compared with BMSs, may improve outcome—an assumption that was subsequently confirmed by nonrandomized comparisons and a small randomized study.[103–106] In the Intracoronary Stenting and Antithrombotic Regimen: DESs for Unprotected Left Main Stem Disease (ISAR-LEFT-MAIN) study, which comprised 607 patients treated with a drug-eluting stent, 2-year mortality was 9.7% and angiographic restenosis was 17.7%, with no significant difference between sirolimus- and paclitaxel-eluting stents.[107] Consistent results were reported from a multicenter registry.[108]

In 2006, the first two nonrandomized studies to compare implantation of DESs for unprotected LMCA with CABG were published.[109,110] With small sample sizes (*n* = 173 or 249) and short follow-up periods (6 or 12 months), these studies suggested similar outcomes of CABG or PCI with respect to survival and survival without MI and stroke, but somewhat higher rates of reintervention were reported after PCI than after CABG. Subsequently, several nonrandomized studies that compared PCI with DESs versus CABG reported consistent results.[111–120] The Revascularization for Unprotected Left Main Coronary Artery Stenosis: Comparison of Percutaneous Coronary Angioplasty Versus Surgical Revascularization MASS: Medicine, Angioplasty, or Surgery Study (MAIN-COMPARE) registry evaluated 2240 patients with unprotected LMCA who received coronary stents (*n* = 1102) or underwent CABG (*n* = 1138).[115] Among the PCI-treated patients, 318 received BMSs and 784 received DESs. Median follow-up was 5.2 years. The 5-year incidences after PCI versus CABG were 11.8% and 13.6% (*P* = .06) for death; 12.2% and 14.7% (*P* = .03) for the composite of death, Q-wave MI, or stroke; and 16.0% versus 4.0% (*P* < .001) for TVR. After adjustment for differences in baseline risk factors, the corresponding hazard ratios were 1.13 (95% CI, 0.88 to 1.44; *P* = .35) for death; 1.07 (95% CI, 0.84 to 1.37; *P* = .59) for the composite of death, Q-wave MI, or stroke; and 5.11 (95% CI, 3.52 to 7.42; *P* < .001) for TVR. Comparisons of BMSs with concurrent CABG and of DESs with concurrent CABG yielded similar results. Hence with respect to clinically important end points, CABG for unprotected LMCA did not afford a superior 5-year outcome compared with PCI. Yet a higher need for reintervention had to be faced when therapy was primarily based on PCI instead of CABG. After the results of the SYNTAX trial appeared, the investigators of MAIN-COMPARE performed a post hoc analysis of 5-year outcomes stratified to SYNTAX scores.[121] After multivariate adjustment, the hazard ratios for death (adjusted HR, 0.52; 95% CI, 0.21 to 1.28; *P* = .15) and for death, MI, or stroke (adjusted HR, 0.54; 95% CI, 0.22 to

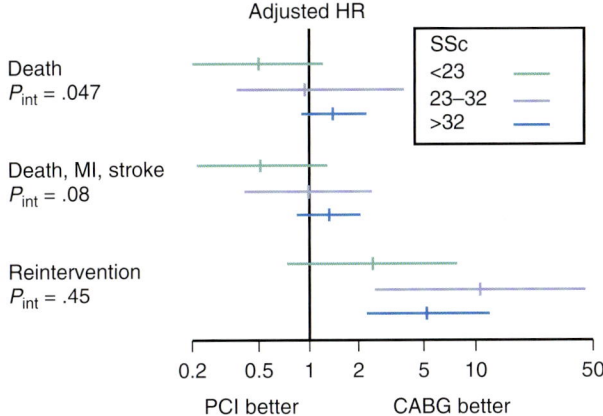

Fig. 2.7 Adjusted hazard ratios of percutaneous coronary intervention *(PCI)* versus coronary artery bypass grafting *(CABG)* in unprotected left main coronary artery stenoses stratified to levels of SYNTAX scores *(SSc)*. Point estimates and 95% confidence intervals for various outcomes are shown. *HR,* Hazard ratio; *MI,* myocardial infarction; P_{int}, interaction *P* value. (Data from Park DW, Kim YH, Yun SC, et al. Complexity of atherosclerotic coronary artery disease and long-term outcomes in patients with unprotected left main disease treated with drug-eluting stents or coronary artery bypass grafting. *J Am Coll Cardiol,* 2011;57[21]:2152–2159.)

1.34; *P* = .18) favored PCI with SYNTAX scores less than 23, whereas with SYNTAX scores greater than 32, they favored CABG (adjusted HR for death, 1.46; 95% CI, 0.92 to 2.30; *P* = .11; adjusted HR for the composite outcome, 1.36; 95% CI, 0.87 to 2.12; *P* = .18; Fig. 2.7). The interaction *P* was .047 for death and .08 for the composite outcome.

Another large registry in this field was the Multicenter Registry Evaluating Percutaneous Coronary Intervention Versus Coronary Artery Bypass Grafting for Left Main Treatment (DELTA), which included 1874 patients with unprotected LMCA stenosis treated with PCI and 901 treated with CABG.[118] At a median follow-up of 3.5 years, the adjusted analysis did not reveal any significant differences comparing PCI with CABG with respect to the primary composite end point of all-cause death, MI, and stroke (adjusted HR, 1.11; 95% CI, 0.85 to 1.42; *P* = .47) or with respect to all-cause mortality (adjusted HR, 1.16; 95% CI, 0.87 to 1.55; *P* = .32). Nevertheless, because of a higher incidence of TVR with PCI, the risk of the secondary end point, MACCE, was higher with PCI than with CABG (adjusted HR, 1.64; 95% CI, 1.33 to 2.03; *P* < .0001). Outcomes of the primary and the secondary end point were similar irrespective of sex.[122]

The largest registry to date is Interventional Research Incorporation Society-Left MAIN Revascularisation (IRIS-MAIN).[123] This registry included 5833 patients with relevant unprotected LMCA disease from 50 sites in Asia who were enrolled between 1995 and 2013. PCI was performed in 2866 patients and 2351 were treated with CABG. Three historical time periods were addressed: Wave 1 from 1995 to 2002 covering BMS, wave 2 from 2003 to 2006 covering first-generation DES, and wave 3 from 2007 to 2013 covering second-generation DES. Of note, the authors did not find any significant difference in death or the composite of death, MI, and stroke between PCI and CABG during any of the three waves. Specifically in wave 3, the adjusted risks of all-cause death or of the composite of death, MI, and stroke showed similar effectiveness of PCI as compared with CABG (HR [95% CI] 0.83 [0.60 to 1.15], *P* = .026 and 0.91 [0.68 to 1.21], *P* = .50, respectively). Nevertheless, throughout the three waves, there was a higher need for repeat revascularization after PCI as compared with CABG resulting in a significantly higher incidence of MACCE. These differences between PCI and CABG narrowed from wave 1 to wave 3. Finally in wave 3, the adjusted hazard ratio for MACCE comparing PCI with CABG was 1.50 (95% CI 1.17 to 1.92; *P* = .001).

In summary, the registry data do not support the concept that every LMCA stenosis should be treated surgically.

Randomized Studies With Drug-Eluting Stents

In SYNTAX, 705 patients belonged to the prespecified subset with LMCA.[124] During 5-year follow-up,[124] the incidence of MACCEs did not differ significantly between PCI and CABG (36.9% vs. 31.0%, *P* = .12). The composite of death, MI, and stroke to 5 years was also similar between the two groups (19.0% vs. 20.8%, *P* = .52), as were mortality (12.6% vs. 14.6%, *P* = .53) and rate of MI (8.2% vs. 4.8%, *P* = .10). At 5 years, reintervention was significantly more frequent in the PCI group (26.7% vs. 15.0%, *P* = .01), whereas stroke was significantly more frequent in the CABG group (1.5% vs. 4.3%, *P* = .03). The extent of CAD outside the LMCA had a major impact on outcome after PCI versus CABG. As in the entire study, the 5-year MACCE rate was excessive after PCI compared with CABG in the tertile with SYNTAX scores above 32 (46.5% vs. 29.7%, *P* = .003), which included a trend for higher mortality with PCI (20.9% vs. 14.1%, *P* = .11; Fig. 2.8). On the other hand, in the combined two lower tertiles of SYNTAX scores (5 through 32), all-cause mortality after PCI was significantly lower than that after CABG (7.9% vs. 15.1%, *P* = .02), and the 5-year MACCE incidence was almost identical between PCI and CABG (31.3% vs. 32.1%, *P* = .74; see Fig. 2.8). Moreover, only a clinically irrelevant and statistically insignificant numerical increase was found in the need for intervention after PCI compared with CABG (22.6% vs. 18.6%, *P* = .36). Thus the results of the SYNTAX study suggested that PCI is the treatment of choice for LMCA unless extensive disease is present, as judged by SYNTAX scores above 32.

The key results of SYNTAX left main are corroborated by the Leipzig left main multicenter trial, which randomized 201 patients with an unprotected LMCA to undergo sirolimus-eluting stenting (n = 100) or CABG using predominantly arterial grafts (n = 101).[125] Perioperative complications were higher after surgery (4% vs. 30%, *P* < .001). At 1 year, the primary clinical end point of major adverse cardiac events (MACEs)—comprising cardiac death, MI, and the need for TVR—was reached in 13.9% of patients after surgery as opposed to 19.0% after PCI (*P* = .19 for noninferiority). The combined rates for death and MI were comparable (surgery 7.9% vs. stenting 5.0%, noninferiority *P* < .001), but stenting was inferior to surgery for repeat revascularization (5.9% vs. 14.0%, noninferiority *P* = .35). Similar results were obtained during extended follow-up (median 37 months, interquartile range 24 to 61 months). Like SYNTAX, the Leipzig trial suggests equipoise between PCI and CABG with respect to prognostically relevant end points.

The Premier of Randomized Comparison of Bypass Surgery Versus Angioplasty Using Sirolimus-Eluting Stent in Patients With Left Main Coronary Artery Disease (PRECOMBAT)[126] trial randomly assigned 300 patients with unprotected LMCA stenosis to undergo CABG and 300 patients to undergo PCI with sirolimus-eluting stents. At 2-year follow-up, the primary composite end point of MACCE (death from any cause, MI, stroke, or ischemia-driven TVR) was reached in 12.2% of the PCI group versus 8.1% of the CABG group (HR, 1.50; 95% CI, 0.90 to 2.52; *P* = .12). The composite rate of death, MI, or stroke at 2 years was similar between PCI and CABG (4.4% vs. 4.7%; HR, 0.92; 95% CI, 0.43 to 1.96; *P* = .83). However, ischemia-driven TVR occurred more frequently in the PCI group than in the CABG group (9.0% vs. 4.2%; HR, 2.18; 95% CI, 1.10 to 4.32; *P* = .02). In line with the Leipzig left

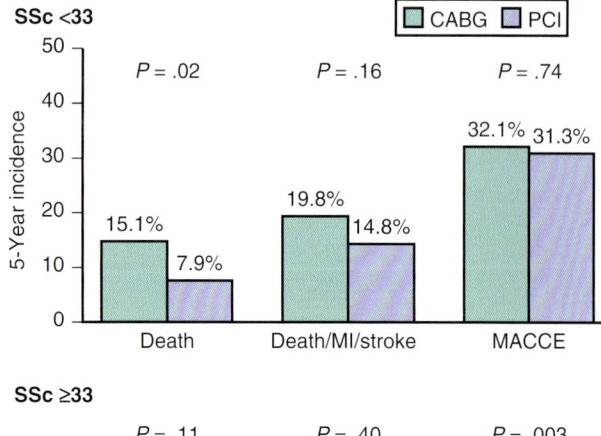

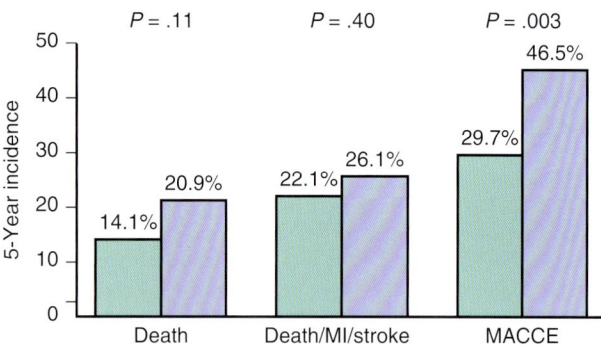

Fig. 2.8 Five-year incidences of all-cause death; of the composite of death, myocardial infarction *(MI)*, and stroke; and of major adverse cardiovascular or cerebrovascular events *(MACCEs)* after percutaneous coronary intervention *(PCI)* versus coronary artery bypass grafting *(CABG)* in patients with unprotected left main coronary artery disease of SYNTAX trial stratified to levels of SYNTAX score *(SSc)*. (A) SYNTAX score less than 33. (B) SYNTAX score 33 or greater. (Data from Morice MC, Serruys PW, Kappetein AP, et al. Five-year outcomes in patients with left main disease treated with either percutaneous coronary intervention or coronary artery bypass grafting in the synergy between percutaneous coronary intervention with taxus and cardiac surgery trial. *Circulation*. 2014;129[23]:2388–2394.)

main artery study and the left main artery cohort of SYNTAX, PRECOMBAT demonstrated that in terms of prognostically relevant end points, PCI is noninferior to CABG in the treatment of unprotected LMCA stenosis. Moreover, the need for repeat revascularization after PCI was low in PRECOMBAT with only a small, albeit statistically significant, surplus compared with CABG.

None of the above-mentioned randomized studies to compare CABG with PCI for unprotected LMCA were adequately powered. Thus, the need still existed for large randomized trials. This need was met by Evaluation of Xience Prime Versus Coronary Artery Bypass Surgery for Effectiveness of Left Main Revascularization (EXCEL) trial[127] and the Nordic-Baltic-British Left Main Revascularization Study (NOBLE).[128]

The multicenter EXCEL trial randomly assigned 1905 patients with angiographic significant LMCA disease and invasive or noninvasive evidence of ischemia to CABG or PCI with everolimus-eluting stents.[127] Primary end point was the composite of death, stroke, or MI at 3 years. The trial was powered for noninferiority with a noninferiority margin of 4.2 percentage points. Although high anatomical complexity with a SYNTAX score >32 was an exclusion criterion, post hoc core-lab evaluation revealed that 24% of the patients included had a high SYNTAX score. A primary end point event was incurred by 15.4% of the patients assigned to PCI and by 14.7% of the patients assigned to CABG ($P = .02$ for noninferiority, HR 1.00, 95% CI 0.79 to 1.28; $P = .98$ for superiority) (Fig. 2.9). There was no significant difference in any of the components of the primary end point. In the landmark analysis of events before and after 30 days, the incidence for periprocedural MI was significantly lower after PCI than after CABG (3.6% vs. 5.9%, $P = .02$) which included a lower incidence of ST-segment elevation MI (0.7% vs. 2.3%, $P = .005$). Conversely, the incidence of spontaneous MI was higher by trend after PCI as compared with CABG (4.3% vs. 2.7%, $P = .07$). PCI was associated with a significant increase in the need for repeat revascularization (12.6% vs. 7.5%, HR 1.72, 95% CI 1.27 to 2.33; $P < .001$). The findings were consistent across various subgroups. Although there was a trend toward a gradient of treatment effect with strata of SYNTAX score, this did not reach statistical significance.

The multicenter NOBLE trial included 1201 patients with unprotected LMCA disease presenting with stable or unstable angina pectoris or non–ST-elevation myocardial infarction.[128] Patients were randomly assigned to CABG or PCI with biolimus-eluting stents. Primary end point was MACCE, a composite of all-cause mortality, nonprocedural MI, stroke, and repeat coronary revascularization. The study was powered for noninferiority of PCI to CABG with a limit of 1.35 for the 95% CI of the hazard ratio during follow-up for up to 5 years. With a median follow-up of 3.1 years, a primary end point was reached in 29% of the PCI group as compared with 19% of the CABG group (HR 1.48, 95% CI 1.11 to 1.96; $P = .007$ for superiority). Thus, the trial failed to show noninferiority of PCI as compared with CABG for treatment of LMCA disease. Whereas periprocedural MI was neither included in the primary end point nor assessed as secondary end point, it was noted that nonprocedural MI was significantly more frequent after PCI than after CABG (7% vs. 2%; $P = .04$), as was repeat revascularization (16% vs. 10%; $P = .03$). There were no significant differences in all-cause death (11% vs. 9%; $P = .84$) (Fig. 2.10) or cardiac death (3% vs. 3%; $P = .82$) between PCI and CABG. With a mean SYNTAX score of 23% there was no appreciable association of treatment effect with strata of SYNTAX score.

Evidence from randomized trials comparing PCI with CABG in patients with LMCA disease has been reviewed in several meta-analyses. A meta-analysis that focused on trials with more than 3-year follow-up and exclusive use of DES included 4394 patients of SYNTAX, PRECOMBAT, EXCEL, and NOBLE.[129] During 5-year follow-up, PCI and CABG were associated with a similar composite risk of all-cause mortality, MI, or stroke (HR 1.06, 95% CI 0.90 to 1.24; $P = .48$). Likewise, there were no significant differences in all-cause or cardiac death (HR [95% CI 1.05] 1.05 [0.85 to 1.31]; $P = .65$ and 1.02 [0.76 to 1.36]; $P = .91$, respectively). Without reaching statistical significance, the incidence of MI was numerically higher with PCI as compared with CABG (1.21 [0.93 to 1.56]; $P = .15$), whereas the incidence of stroke was numerically lower (HR 0.86, 95% CI 0.56 to 1.32; $P = .49$). PCI was, however, associated with a significant increase in the need for repeat revascularization (HR 1.70, 95% CI 1.42 to 2.05; $P < .001$).

The comprehensive IPD meta-analysis of available data from randomized studies comparing PCI and CABG comprised 2231 patients with LMCA diseased assigned to PCI and 2245 patients assigned to CABG.[68] The 5-year estimates of all-cause mortality were similar between the two treatment modalities (10.7% after PCI vs. 10.5% after CABG; HR 1.07, 95% CI 0.87 to 1.33; $P = .052$). There was no significant interaction of the treatment effect with diabetes (P for interaction = .13) or with strata of SYNTAX score (P for trend = .064) (see Figs. 2.4 and 2.6). Nevertheless, it was conspicuous that mortality in the strata with low or intermediate SYNTAX score was numerically lower with PCI as compared with CABG, whereas it was numerically higher in patients with

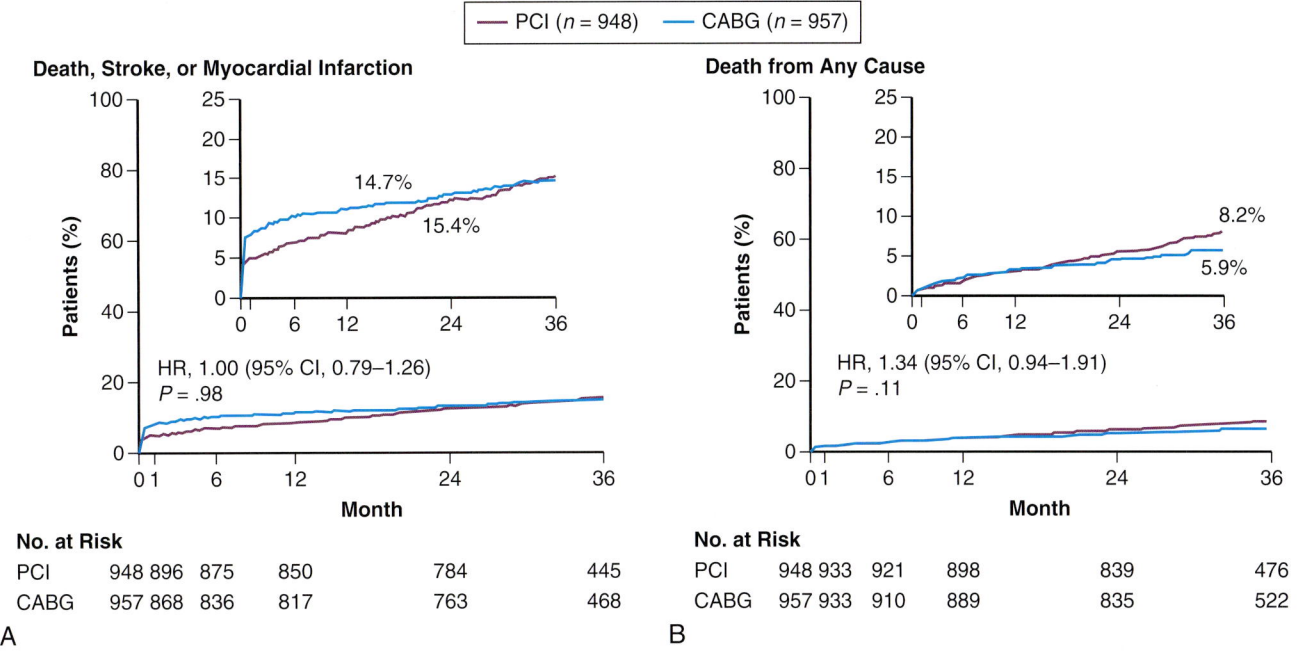

Fig. 2.9 Kaplan-Meier estimates of the composite primary outcome and death in the EXCEL trial comparing percutaneous coronary intervention *(PCI)* with coronary artery bypass grafting *(CABG)* in patients with left main coronary artery disease. *HR*, Hazard ratio. Shown are rates of the composite primary outcome of death, myocardial infarction, or stroke (A) and death from any cause (B) The *P* value was calculated by means of the log-rank test. (Reproduced with permission from Stone GW, Sabik JF, Serruys PW, et al. Everolimus-eluting stents or bypass surgery for left main coronary artery disease. *N Engl J Med.* 2016;375[23]:2223–2235.)

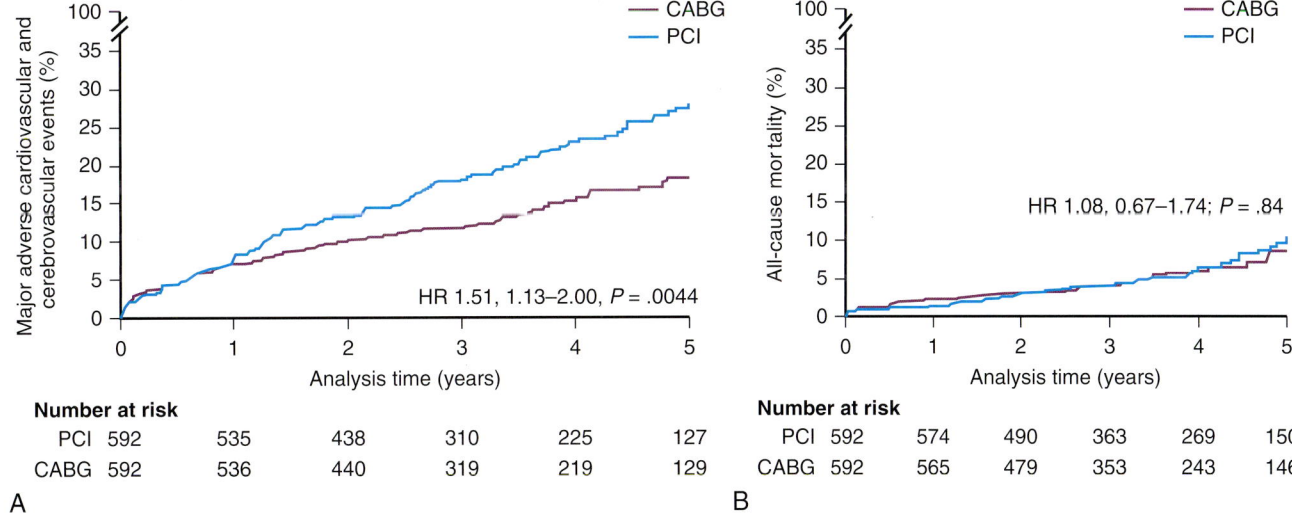

Fig. 2.10 Kaplan-Meier estimates of the composite primary outcome and death in the NOBLE trial comparing percutaneous coronary intervention *(PCI)* with coronary artery bypass grafting *(CABG)* in patients with left main coronary artery disease. Shown are rates of the composite primary outcome of all-cause death, nonprocedural myocardial infarction, repeat coronary revascularization and stroke (A) and death from any cause (B). The *P* value was calculated by means of the log-rank test. *HR,* Hazard ratio. (Reproduced with permission from Makikallio T, Holm NR, Lindsay M, et al. Percutaneous coronary angioplasty versus coronary artery bypass grafting in treatment of unprotected left main stenosis (NOBLE): a prospective, randomised, open-label, non-inferiority trial. *Lancet.* 388[10061]:2743–2752.)

high SYNTAX scores (15.8% vs. 12.4%; $P = .10$). Likewise, in patients with LMCA disease and diabetes mortality after PCI was numerically higher than after CABG (16.5% vs. 13.4%; $P = .11$).

In summary, currently available evidence suggests that PCI with DESs is a reasonable treatment option for many patients with unprotected LMCA. In general, survival and survival without MI or stroke are similar to those after surgery, and patients may thus decide whether they want to exchange the discomfort of surgery for the potential inconvenience of repeat revascularization procedures. With LMCA disease, the differential outcome of the two treatment strategies appears to be less dependent on the extent of concomitant CAD than with multivessel disease without LMCA involvement. Nevertheless, there remains reasonable concern that with widespread diffuse disease outside the LMCA, PCI may not achieve a similar prognostic benefit as CABG.

PERCUTANEOUS CORONARY INTERVENTION VERSUS MEDICAL THERAPY ALONE

Several studies of the present era compared PCI with medical therapy alone in single- or double-vessel disease without a prognostic indication for bypass surgery. A meta-analysis that included the Angioplasty Compared to Medicine (ACME), RITA 2, and Atorvastatin Versus Revascularization Treatments (AVERT) studies as well as MASS and one smaller German trial demonstrated a significant (30%) reduction in angina but found a significant increase in the need for CABG with PCI compared with medical treatment and trends toward increased risk of death, MI, and nonscheduled PCI.[130] This meta-analysis supported the concept that compared with medical therapy alone, PCI in patients with stable angina reduces symptoms but may be associated with a higher incidence of serious complications, such as death and MI. However, it must be considered that none of the studies included in this meta-analysis used contemporary interventional techniques, which includes the systematic use of stents with vigorous periinterventional and postinterventional antiplatelet treatment, or strict risk-factor modification, in particular the administration of statins. Modern periinterventional and postinterventional drug therapy would have reduced the risk of death and MI, and each of the three elements of modern interventional treatment—stents, statins, and antiplatelet drugs—would have reduced the need for subsequent unplanned revascularization procedures. Hence it may be anticipated that with modern interventional approaches, the complications of catheter intervention would have been substantially lower without corrupting the beneficial effect of this treatment on angina as compared with medical therapy alone. The role of PCI compared with medical therapy alone in patients without an established prognostic indication for coronary revascularization therefore needed reassessment in the light of contemporary interventional techniques and optimal periinterventional and postinterventional treatment.

This was the goal of the randomized COURAGE trial.[131] COURAGE involved 2287 patients who had objective evidence of myocardial ischemia and significant CAD; 1149 patients were assigned to undergo PCI with optimal medical therapy (PCI group), and 1138 were to receive optimal medical therapy alone (medical therapy group). Patients with persistent CCS class IV angina, a markedly positive stress test, unprotected LMCA, or hazardous PCI—as in ostial stenosis of the LAD—were not eligible for the study. COURAGE was highly successful in applying state-of-the-art preventive and antiischemic pharmacologic treatment. DESs, however, were not available except for the last 6 months of the study, thus only 2.7% of the COURAGE trial PCI patients received DESs. Among patients randomized to PCI, 6.4% did not have the procedure. On the other hand, 32% of the patients assigned to the medical therapy group crossed over to PCI during follow-up. Repeat PCI was also performed in 21% of the patients in the PCI group. During a median follow-up of 4.6 years, the cumulative primary event rates, the composite of death from any cause and nonfatal MI, were 19.0% in the PCI group and 18.5% in the medical therapy group (HR for the PCI group was 1.05; 95% CI, 0.87 to 1.27; $P = .62$).[131] Considering components of the primary end point, 85 deaths occurred in the PCI group and 95 occurred in the medical therapy group; spontaneous MIs numbered 108 and 109, and those of peri-PCI MI were 35 and 9, respectively. At 1 year and 3 years, but not at 5 years, a significantly higher proportion of patients in the PCI group were free of angina compared with the medical therapy group (66% vs. 58%, $P < .001$; 72% vs. 67%, $P = .02$; and 74% vs. 72%, $P = .35$; respectively). The striking 72%

angina-free status at 5 years in the medical therapy group may have been attributed to the fact that 43% of these patients began the trial with minimal (CCS class I) or no angina, and 32% went on to subsequent revascularization for relief of symptoms. Given the failure to reduce the risk of death and MI and the marginal symptomatic benefit of PCI plus optimal medical therapy (OMT) over OMT alone, it was concluded that an initial recommendation of PCI on top of OMT offers no important advantage over an initial recommendation of OMT alone.

More recently, results consistent with the COURAGE trial were reported from the Bypass Angioplasty Revascularization Investigation in Type 2 Diabetes (BARI 2D) trial,[132] which included 2368 patients with both type 2 diabetes and CAD. These patients were stratified as potential candidates for CABG ($n = 763$) or for PCI ($n = 1605$) and were then randomly assigned to prompt revascularization or intense medical therapy. Participants were also subrandomized to insulin-sensitization or insulin-provision therapy. At 5 years, rates of survival did not differ significantly between the revascularization group (88.3%) and the medical therapy group (87.8%, $P = .97$). The rates of freedom from major cardiovascular events also did not differ significantly among the groups: they were 77.2% in the revascularization group and 75.9% in the medical treatment group ($P = .70$). Taken together, COURAGE and BARI 2D suggest that with OMT, a conservative approach that reserves revascularization to patients with progression of angina, the development of an acute coronary syndrome, or severe ischemia is preferred over a strategy of prompt revascularization. Some caveats against an uncritical generalization of this concept must be considered. The first comes from the authors of the COURAGE trial. In their nuclear substudy of COURAGE, they demonstrated that the beneficial effect of therapy on prognosis is linked to a substantial reduction in stress-induced ischemia to a low residual level.[12] In their substudy, a reduction of the area of stress-induced ischemia of 5% or more and to 10% or less of the left ventricle was needed for a prognostic effect, especially if baseline ischemia was greater than 10%. Although this was achieved more frequently after PCI than after medical therapy alone, a substantial number of PCI patients fell short of this goal. This may not be considered an inherent limitation of PCI but rather a consequence of a PCI strategy that focused on the culprit lesion. Despite the fact that 69% of patients assigned to PCI had multivessel disease and 65% had multiple reversible perfusion defects on nuclear imaging, only 36% of the patients received more than one stent. Thus in a substantial proportion of patients, PCI resulted in incomplete revascularization. With respect to the overall outcome of the study, this will have diluted the beneficial effect of complete revascularization in some of the patients, as demonstrated in the nuclear substudy of COURAGE.[12] The findings of the BARI 2D trial also support the concept that revascularization will improve prognosis if a relevant area of the left ventricle can be relieved from ischemia. In this trial, the low-risk patients stratified as PCI candidates derived no benefit from revascularization compared with primarily medical treatment, whereas patients stratified as CABG candidates fared better with revascularization (major adverse events = 22.4% vs. 30.5%, $P = .01$; for interaction between stratum and study group, $P = .002$). Compared with PCI candidates, CABG candidates more often had three-vessel disease and a jeopardy score greater than 50% (odds ratios [ORs] were 4.4 and 4.1, respectively). Thus in BARI 2D, the larger reduction in ischemia in the CABG group, compared with that in the PCI group, resulted in a prognostic benefit. The second caveat comes from the observation of a 13% relative reduction in mortality by PCI plus OMT compared with OMT alone in the COURAGE trial. However, the trial was not sufficiently powered to establish the statistical significance of this finding.

A more contemporary trial to assess potential benefits of revascularization by PCI in patients with stable CAD was

FAME 2,[33] which included patients with stable angina in whom coronary angiography revealed at least one coronary artery stenosis of 50% or greater. All stenoses were interrogated by measurement of FFR. Patients with at least one functionally relevant stenosis (FFR ≤ 0.80) were randomly assigned to PCI with DESs plus the best available medical therapy (PCI group) or the best available medical therapy alone (medical-therapy group). Patients who did not have any functionally relevant stenoses were included in a registry. The study was designed to include 1632 randomized patients. The Data Safety Monitoring Committee, however, recommended a premature end to the study for a significant difference in event rates that favored PCI. Thus recruitment was halted prematurely after inclusion of 1220 patients. Out of these, 888 had undergone randomization, and 332 had entered the registry. With a mean duration of follow-up of 214 days, the primary end point—the composite of death, MI, or urgent revascularization—was reached in 4.3% of the PCI group and in 12.7% of the medical-therapy group (HR with PCI, 0.32; 95% CI, 0.19 to 0.53; $P < .001$).[33] This difference was driven by a lower need for urgent revascularization in the PCI group than in the medical therapy group (1.6% vs. 11.1%; HR, 0.13; 95% CI, 0.06 to 0.30; $P < .001$). However, no significant differences were reported in mortality (0.2% vs. 0.7%, $P = .31$) or in the incidence of MI (3.4% vs. 3.2%, $P = .89$). Yet PCI reduced the risk of death or MI beyond 7 days (HR with PCI, 0.42; 95% CI, 0.17 to 1.04; $P = .053$; $P_{int} = .003$ with 7-day landmark). Moreover, in the PCI group, fewer patients suffered from CCS class II to IV angina than patients in the medical therapy group (HR, 0.39; 95% CI, 0.28 to 0.53; $P < .001$ [at 30 days]; HR, 0.46; 95% CI, 0.28 to 0.74; $P = .002$ [at 6 months]). Confirming the validity of functional testing, the event rate was lowest in the registry (3% for the primary end point). Thus FAME 2 suggested some advantages of PCI with OMT over OMT alone, but it did not demonstrate better survival with PCI or better survival without MI.

One of the limitations of COURAGE, BARI 2D, and FAME 2 is the limited sample size. This problem may be overcome by meta-analyses. A meta-analysis of 17 randomized trials to compare a PCI-based invasive treatment strategy with medical treatment suggested that the PCI-based invasive strategy improves long-term survival compared with a strategy of medical treatment only (OR for all-cause death was 0.80 [95% CI, 0.64 to 0.99]; $P = .263$ for heterogeneity across trials).[133] Another group performed a meta-analysis of COURAGE and BARI 2D and six smaller trials (together, 7229 patients) and did not find any significant benefit of PCI over conservative treatment for prevention of death, MI, unplanned revascularization, and angina.[134] These researchers subsequently restricted their analysis to studies with objectively documented myocardial ischemia and with greater than 50% use of stents and statins. They also included FAME 2,[134] yet they reached essentially the same results. The most comprehensive recent conventional meta-analysis comprised 12 studies, including COURAGE and BARI 2D but not FAME 2, with 37,548 patient-years in 7182 patients.[135,136] PCI compared with conservative treatment was associated with a significantly lower incident rate ratio (IRR) for spontaneous nonprocedural MI (IRR, 0.76; 95% CI, 0.58 to 0.99) at the expense of a higher rate of procedural MI (IRR, 4.11; 95% CI, 2.53 to 6.88).[136] Finally, no significant difference was found in the total risk of MI (IRR, 0.96; 95% CI, 0.74 to 1.21). Consistent with the beneficial effect of PCI on spontaneous MI, all-cause mortality (IRR, 0.88; 95% CI, 0.75 to 1.03) and cardiovascular mortality (IRR, 0.70; 95% CI, 0.44 to 1.09) were lower after PCI than with medical treatment alone, and statistical significance was only just missed.[136] The point estimate for PCI versus conservative treatment for mortality paralleled that for spontaneous MI but not for procedural MI, indicating that procedural MIs

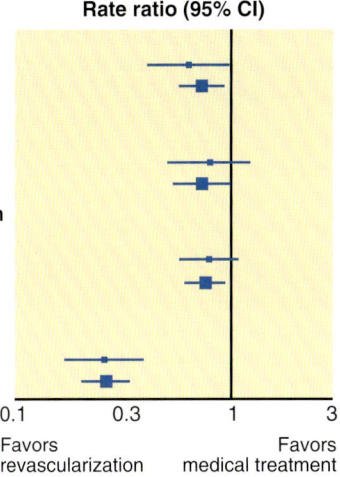

Fig. 2.11 Summary of a network meta-analysis based on 95 studies with 93,553 patients with stable coronary disease, assessing outcome after initial revascularization with new-generation drug-eluting stents or initial medical treatment without revascularization. Rate ratios of percutaneous coronary intervention with 95% confidence intervals (*CIs*) are shown for the everolimus-eluting stent *(EES)* and resolute zotarolimus-eluting stent *(R-ZES)* based on data closest to 5 years. (Adapted from Windecker S, Stortecky S, Stefanini GG, et al. Revascularization versus medical treatment in patients with stable coronary artery disease: network meta-analysis. *BMJ*. 2014;348:g3859.)

are less relevant for survival than spontaneous MIs. In addition to the reduction in spontaneous MI, the meta-analysis revealed a significantly higher freedom from angina after PCI than with medical therapy alone (RR, 0.83; 95% CI, 0.72 to 0.94).[135]

A common conundrum of studies that assess the benefits of PCI versus stable angina is the problem that within the spectrum of patients with stable angina, the higher-risk patients were underrepresented or not included at all. Specifically, this is true for patients with an accepted indication for CABG, in whom randomization would have been unethical. This means that patients who potentially derive the most benefit from revascularization by PCI hardly entered any of the studies that compared PCI with medical treatment alone. This problem in the assessment of the true benefit of PCI in stable angina may be overcome by network meta-analysis, as published recently. This network meta-analysis was based on 95 studies with 93,553 patients with stable coronary disease and assessed outcome data closest to 5 years (Fig. 2.11).[137] PCI with new-generation stents significantly reduced the risk of mortality with rate ratios of 0.75 (95% CI, 0.55 to 0.96) for everolimus-eluting stents and 0.65 (95% CI, 0.42 to 1.00) for zotarolimus-eluting stents.[137] With everolimus-eluting stents, a significant reduction of MI was also found compared with initial medical treatment (RR, 0.78; 95% CI, 0.63 to 0.96). Moreover, stent-supported PCI significantly reduced the need for subsequent revascularization compared with initial medical therapy, but to a variable degree. The largest reduction was found with new-generation DESs (RR, 0.27 [95% CI, 0.21 to 0.35] for everolimus-eluting stents and 0.26 [95% CI, 0.17 to 0.35] for zotarolimus-eluting stents). The findings of the network meta-analysis are consistent with a nonrandomized comparison between PCI and conservative therapy for stable angina using the New York State Cardiac Database.[138] Of 9586 patients, 8486 underwent PCI (71% with DESs) and 1100 were initially treated conservatively. By propensity matching through the use of 20 pertinent factors, 933 matched pairs were obtained. During 4-year follow-up, patients treated with PCI had an improved outcome compared with patients initially treated medically, with a significant reduction in mortality (10.2% vs. 14.5%; $P = .02$), MI (8.0% vs.

11.3%; *P* = .007), and subsequent revascularization (24.1% vs. 29.1%; *P* = .005). Adjusted hazard ratios of PCI compared with medical treatment were 0.67 (95% CI, 0.52 to 0.86) for death and MI and 0.68 (95% CI, 0.51 to 0.93) for death.

In the absence of an expected prognostic benefit of PCI, relief of symptoms that are unresponsive to the medical treatment tolerated by the patient is an accepted indication for PCI. Nevertheless, the efficacy of PCI in achieving this goal has recently been challenged by the Objective Randomised Blinded Investigation with optimal medical Therapy of Angioplasty in stable angina (ORBITA) trial.[139] ORBITA enrolled 213 patients with ischemic symptoms and a single ≥70% coronary artery stenosis. Over a 3-year period, 105 of the patients enrolled were assigned to PCI and 95 to a sham procedure. After enrollment antianginal medication was optimized for 6 weeks, patients then underwent pre-randomization assessment with symptom questionnaires, exercise testing, and dobutamine stress-echocardiography. This was repeated 6 weeks after PCI or sham procedure. The primary end point was the difference in exercise time between the two groups at follow-up. With an increment in exercise time of 16.6 sec (95% CI, −9.8 to 42.0) ORBITA did not reveal a significant difference in the primary end point between PCI or sham procedure (*P* = .20). Improvement in the symptoms reported by the patients was similar with PCI as with medical therapy alone. There was, however, a significantly larger improvement of the dobutamine stress-echocardiography peak stress wall motion score index with PCI as compared with the sham procedure (−0.07, 95% CI, −0.11 to −0.04; *P* < .0001). This finding challenges the imprecise estimate for the primary end point. Moreover, the short follow-up limits the clinical relevance of the findings. In this respect, it is important to note that after finishing the study, 85% of the patients in the placebo arm crossed over to PCI. Other limitations of the study as acknowledged by the investigators and outlined elsewhere[140] include the inclusion of patients with mild symptoms prerandomization with a background of only moderate symptoms to start with (CCS II in 59% of the patients) and additional optimization of antianginal medication before randomization (CCS 0/I in 23.5%, CCS III in only 28% of the patients), the group imbalance in ostial and proximal lesions (37% vs. 57%, *P* = .005), and the removal of patients after randomization. In addition, the imprecision of the estimate for the primary end point demonstrates that there was insufficient power to detect a clinically relevant difference between the groups. It is the merit of the ORBITA trial to demonstrate the value of optimal medical therapy in the management of stable angina. Nevertheless, it does not rule out a potential symptomatic benefit of PCI. Such benefit has been a consistent finding in various studies although not sham controlled. This includes improvement of symptoms in studies comparing DES with BMS,[140] the demonstration of a similar symptomatic benefit of CABG and PCI in the recent EXCEL trial,[141] as well as an early and sustained improvement of angina in FAME 2 (10.2% vs. 28.5% at 1 month, 5.2% vs. 9.7% at 3 years) in favor of PCI as compared with medical therapy.[33]

In summary, compared with OMT alone, OMT plus PCI with modern devices and interventional techniques more effectively relieves symptoms of angina, reduces the risk of unplanned revascularization procedures and of spontaneous MIs, and may even improve survival of patients with stable angina. The survival benefit appears to be linked to effective revascularization of large areas that demonstrate inducible ischemia. Hence currently available evidence suggests that patients who have an area of stress-induced ischemia involving more than 10% of the left ventricle[11] or who are not free of symptoms or do not tolerate medical therapy should undergo PCI if they are anatomically suited. Stable patients who are free of symptoms following antianginal medication and are free of relevant residual inducible ischemia should be managed conservatively.

SUMMARY

When coronary revascularization is considered, prognostic and symptomatic indications must be distinguished. With prognostic indications, PCI offers an alternative to CABG; with symptomatic indications, PCI competes with medical treatment. In the absence of an acute coronary syndrome, PCI for single-vessel disease is justified only if an improvement in symptoms can be anticipated or if there is a large area (>10% of the LV) of inducible ischemia.

In patients with multivessel disease, with or without LMCA stenosis, the choice of revascularization therapy will depend on the complexity of coronary artery involvement. With low complexity, such as with a SYNTAX score below 23, no current evidence suggests that CABG offers a relevant benefit over PCI with DESs. However, in patients with a higher complexity (e.g., SYNTAX score >22 in multivessel disease without LMCA), current evidence demonstrates a survival benefit of CABG over PCI. Moreover, surgery is preferred because of the lower risk of spontaneous MI after CABG. Patients must also be informed about the higher need for repeat procedures after PCI, which should be weighed against the discomfort of surgery.

LMCA stenosis is not a contraindication to PCI. In fact, at low-range SYNTAX scores, the outcome after PCI with LMCA involvement may be superior to that with CABG and there is no compelling evidence for superiority of CABG over PCI with LMCA and intermediate-range SYNTAX scores. In patients with diabetes mellitus, however, multivessel PCI does not achieve a prognostic benefit similar to that of CABG. Despite DESs, vigorous antiplatelet treatment, and tight metabolic control, diabetic patients continue to be at increased risk of death, MI, and reintervention if treated by PCI. Thus PCI in patients with diabetes may be considered only in low-complexity subsets of multivessel disease, such as with SYNTAX scores less than 23. Individualized decisions must consider the likelihood of complete revascularization, the risk associated with either approach, the patient's life expectancy based on age and comorbidities, and the patient's preference after thorough counseling. In many instances, decisions must be reached jointly by the cardiac surgeon and the interventional cardiologist at institutionalized meetings of the heart team.

KEY REFERENCES

27. Farooq V, Serruys PW, Bourantas CV, et al. Quantification of incomplete revascularization and its association with five-year mortality in the synergy between percutaneous coronary intervention with taxus and cardiac surgery (SYNTAX) trial validation of the residual SYNTAX score. *Circulation*. 2013;128(2):141–151.
28. Tonino PA, Fearon WF, De Bruyne B, et al. Angiographic versus functional severity of coronary artery stenoses in the FAME study fractional flow reserve versus angiography in multivessel evaluation. *J Am Coll Cardiol*. 2010;55(25):2816–2821.
29. Davies JE, Sen S, Dehbi HM, et al. Use of the instantaneous wave-free ratio or fractional flow reserve in PCI. *N Engl J Med*. 2017;376(19):1824–1834.
30. Gotberg M, Christiansen EH, Gudmundsdottir IJ, et al. Instantaneous wave-free ratio versus fractional flow reserve to guide PCI. *N Engl J Med*. 2017;376(19):1813–1823.
34. Tonino PA, De Bruyne B, Pijls NH, et al. Fractional flow reserve versus angiography for guiding percutaneous coronary intervention. *N Engl J Med*. 2009;360(3):213–224.
35. van Nunen LX, Zimmermann FM, Tonino PA, et al. Fractional flow reserve versus angiography for guidance of PCI in patients with multivessel coronary artery disease (FAME): 5-year follow-up of a randomised controlled trial. *Lancet*. 2015;386(10006):1853–1860.
36. Garcia S, Sandoval Y, Roukoz H, et al. Outcomes after complete versus incomplete revascularization of patients with multivessel coronary artery disease: a meta-analysis of 89,883 patients enrolled in randomized clinical trials and observational studies. *J Am Coll Cardiol*. 2013;62(16):1421–1431.

61. Mohr FW, Morice MC, Kappetein AP, et al. Coronary artery bypass graft surgery versus percutaneous coronary intervention in patients with three-vessel disease and left main coronary disease: 5-year follow-up of the randomised, clinical SYNTAX trial. *Lancet*. 2013;381(9867):629–638.

62. Head SJ, Davierwala PM, Serruys PW, et al. Coronary artery bypass grafting vs. percutaneous coronary intervention for patients with three-vessel disease: final five-year follow-up of the SYNTAX trial. *Eur Heart J*. 2014;35(40):2821–2830.

68. Head SJ, Milojevic M, Daemen J, et al. Mortality after coronary artery bypass grafting versus percutaneous coronary intervention with stenting for coronary artery disease: a pooled analysis of individual patient data. *Lancet*. 2018;391(10124):939–948.

69. Head SJ, Milojevic M, Daemen J, et al. Stroke following coronary revascularization: an individual patient-data pooled analysis of 11,518 patients from 11 randomized trials comparing CABG versus PCI. *J Am Coll Cardiol*. 2018;72(4):386–398.

70. Chang M, Ahn JM, Lee CW, et al. Long-term mortality after coronary revascularization in nondiabetic patients with multivessel disease. *J Am Coll Cardiol*. 2016;68(1):29–36.

71. Barzilay JI, Kronmal RA, Bittner V, et al. Coronary artery disease and coronary artery bypass grafting in diabetic patients aged > or = 65 years (report from the Coronary Artery Surgery Study [CASS] Registry). *Am J Cardiol*. 1994;74:334–339.

88. Farkouh ME, Domanski M, Sleeper LA, et al. Strategies for multivessel revascularization in patients with diabetes. *N Engl J Med*. 2012;367(25):2375–2384.

91. Kappetein AP, Head SJ, Morice MC, et al. Treatment of complex coronary artery disease in patients with diabetes: 5-year results comparing outcomes of bypass surgery and percutaneous coronary intervention in the SYNTAX trial. *Eur J Cardiothorac Surg*. 2013;43(5):1006–1013.

124. Morice MC, Serruys PW, Kappetein AP, et al. Five-year outcomes in patients with left main disease treated with either percutaneous coronary intervention or coronary artery bypass grafting in the synergy between percutaneous coronary intervention with taxus and cardiac surgery trial. *Circulation*. 2014;129(23):2388–2394.

127. Stone GW, Sabik JF, Serruys PW, et al. Everolimus-eluting stents or bypass surgery for left main coronary artery disease. *N Engl J Med*. 2016;375(23):2223–2235.

128. Makikallio T, Holm NR, Lindsay M, investigators Ns, et al. Percutaneous coronary angioplasty versus coronary artery bypass grafting in treatment of unprotected left main stenosis (NOBLE): a prospective, randomised, open-label, non-inferiority trial. *Lancet*. 2016;388(10061):2743–2752.

129. Giacoppo D, Colleran R, Cassese S, et al. Percutaneous coronary intervention vs coronary artery bypass grafting in patients with left main coronary artery stenosis: a systematic review and meta-analysis. *JAMA Cardiol*. 2017;2(10):1079–1088.

137. Windecker S, Stortecky S, Stefanini GG, et al. Revascularisation versus medical treatment in patients with stable coronary artery disease: network meta-analysis. *BMJ*. 2014;348:g3859.

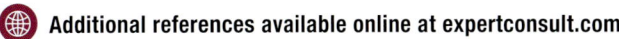 **Additional references available online at expertconsult.com.**

中文导读

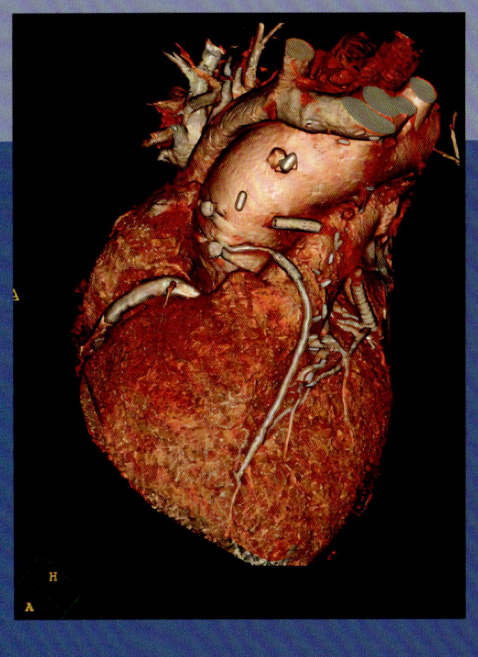

第3章
糖尿病

随着肥胖人群的迅速增加，以及老龄化社会的到来，糖尿病发病率也显著增加。更为重要的是，糖尿病易发生动脉粥样硬化，在临床中表现为冠心病发生年龄更为年轻、病情更为严重，临床表现更为隐匿（无症状性心肌缺血和无症状性心肌梗死），且冠心病死亡率及致残率也明显高于非糖尿病患者。因此，糖尿病合并冠心病患者是临床医师需要高度关注的一类特殊冠心病人群。

本章节对糖尿病动脉粥样硬化的病理生理学表现、糖尿病心肌缺血筛查、血运重建方式、药物治疗，以及预后等方面进行了多维度、全方位的概述，同时强调了循证医学证据对指导治疗的重要性。对于无心肌缺血症状的糖尿病患者，优化药物治疗和生活方式的改变仍然是至关重要的环节之一。现有证据不支持进行无选择的冠心病筛查，除非是具有极高危心血管疾病患病风险的糖尿病患者。对于血运重建策略的选择，需综合考虑冠状动脉病变的复杂程度、临床表现类型（急性冠状动脉综合征或稳定型冠心病）、患者健康状态、手术风险评估及并发症。伴有多支病变的糖尿病患者冠状动脉旁路移植术预后更好，而对于病变复杂度低的患者，经皮冠状动脉介入治疗可作为冠状动脉旁路移植术的替代血运重建方案。此外，患者是否为急性心肌梗死也影响策略的选择。长期的降糖治疗仍是改善糖尿病合并冠心病预后的重要方式。但控制血糖应遵循个体化方案，过度严格的血糖控制可能并不适合病程较长、病情严重的糖尿病合并冠心病患者。为了降低心血管事件风险，积极的抗血小板治疗，他汀类药物、血管紧张素转化酶抑制剂和血管紧张素受体阻滞剂的应用也是合理的选择。总而言之，对于糖尿病合并冠心病的患者，需要采用以循证医学证据为基础的综合治疗、精准治疗。只有这样，该类患者才能更多地获益。

见 闻 柳景华

章节要点

- 所有糖尿病患者都应被视为心血管风险高危患者。但若合并至少一个其他心血管危险因素或存在靶器官损伤,这类糖尿病患者则应被划分为心血管风险极高危患者。
- 糖尿病患者死于冠心病的风险是非糖尿病患者的两倍。
- 慢性高血糖状态、血脂异常、氧化应激和胰岛素抵抗与糖尿病中观察到的动脉粥样硬化加速形成有关,后者的特征表现包括促血栓形成、炎症增强和内皮功能障碍。
- 应选择性地对高危糖尿病患者进行无症状心肌缺血的筛查。但对于所有的无症状糖尿病患者,是否都需要进行常规冠心病筛查,目前尚无证据支持。
- 有证据显示,钠—葡萄糖协同转运蛋白2抑制剂——恩格列净、卡格列净可以减少糖尿病的大血管并发症。
- 糖尿病合并冠心病患者的血糖控制,应采取个体化方案。糖尿病病程越长、患者年龄越大、冠心病越严重,或者其他并发症越多/越严重,血糖控制越不宜过度严格。
- 糖尿病合并冠心病的患者,若症状稳定并且无高危特征(例如,大面积心肌缺血、左主干或近端左前降支严重狭窄病变),那么药物治疗可作为替代血运重建的一种有效治疗。
- 对于经皮冠状动脉介入治疗或冠状动脉旁路移植术这两种血运重建方案的选择,应基于患者的临床表现、并发症、冠心病的类型和严重程度、左心室功能,以及外科手术死亡的预测风险。
- 对于多支病变的稳定型冠心病合并糖尿病患者,若预测的死亡风险较低,且血管解剖条件为中等-复杂的冠状动脉病变,应推荐冠状动脉旁路移植术。而对于冠状动脉病变复杂程度低的患者,经皮冠状动脉介入治疗则可作为一种替代性血运重建方案。
- 糖尿病合并急性冠状动脉综合征的患者,其近期和远期的死亡率和致残率均高于非糖尿病患者。循证医学证据表明,包括早期介入策略在内的强化治疗,可使这类患者获益。
- 对于糖尿病合并冠心病的患者,除阿司匹林外,还应推荐血小板$P2Y_{12}$受体拮抗剂。为了降低该类患者的心血管事件风险,他汀类药物治疗、血管紧张素转化酶抑制剂或血管紧张素受体阻滞剂也应合理使用。

3 Diabetes

Marco Roffi, Baris Gencer

KEY POINTS

- Although all diabetic individuals should be considered at high cardiovascular (CV) risk, those with at least one additional CV risk factor or with target-organ damage should be considered at very high CV risk.
- Subjects with diabetes have twofold higher risk of dying from coronary artery disease (CAD) than do nondiabetic individuals.
- Chronic hyperglycemia, dyslipidemia, oxidative stress, and insulin resistance have been associated with the accelerated form of atherogenesis observed in diabetes, which is characterized by prothrombosis, enhanced inflammation, and endothelial dysfunction.
- Screening for silent myocardial ischemia may be considered in selected high-risk diabetic patients. The value of routine screening for CAD in asymptomatic diabetic individuals is not supported by the evidence.
- The glucose-lowering agents sodium glucose cotransporter 2 (SGLT2) inhibitors empagliflozin and canagliflozin have been found to reduce the macrovascular complications of diabetes.
- Glucose control in diabetic patients with CAD should be individualized. This depends on several factors: the longer the individual has been affected by diabetes and the older he or she is, as well as the more advanced the CAD and the more prevalent and/or advanced the comorbidities, the less stringent should be the glucose control.
- In diabetic patients with CAD, stable symptoms, and no high-risk features such as large areas of ischemia or significant left main or proximal left anterior descending (LAD) coronary artery disease, medical management is a valuable alternative to revascularization.
- The choice of revascularization modality—percutaneous coronary intervention (PCI) or coronary artery bypass grafting (CABG)—should be based on the individual's clinical presentation, comorbidities, pattern and severity of CAD, left ventricular (LV) function, and predicted surgical mortality.
- In stable diabetic patients with multivessel CAD, low predicted surgical mortality, and intermediate to high complexity of the coronary anatomy, CABG is recommended; PCI may represent an alternative for patients with low complexity of the coronary anatomy.
- Diabetic patients with acute coronary syndrome (ACS) have higher short- and long-term morbidity and mortality rates than their nondiabetic counterparts and benefit from intensive evidence-based treatments, including early invasive strategy.
- Platelet P2Y$_{12}$ receptor inhibition is recommended in patients with diabetes mellitus and CAD in addition to aspirin. Statin therapy, angiotensin converting enzyme inhibitors (ACE-I), or angiotensin receptor blockers (ARBs) are indicated in patients with diabetes mellitus and CAD to reduce the risk for CV events.

The prevalence of diabetes mellitus is increasing and parallels the growth of the elderly population and the rise in rates of obesity.[1] According to the International Diabetes Federation, 24.4 million Americans had diabetes in 2013, with an expected increase to 29.7 million by 2035.[2] It is estimated that cardiovascular (CV) disease represents two-thirds of deaths in subjects with diabetes mellitus, including approximately 40% related to coronary artery disease (CAD), 15% to congestive heart disease, and 10% to stroke.[3,4] Type 2 is by far the most frequent type of diabetes and is the focus of the present chapter. Because diabetes is one of the most important CV risk factors and individuals affected by diabetes may be asymptomatic or have had unspecific symptoms for several years before the diagnosis is made, screening for this condition is mandatory both for healthy individuals and for patients with established CV disease.[5]

The diagnostic criteria of diabetes according to the American Diabetes Association (ADA) are reported in Box 3.1.[6] Based on a combination of hemoglobin A$_{1C}$ (HbA$_{1c}$) and fasting plasma glucose, the diagnosis of diabetes can be made after two consecutive values are found to be above the diagnostic criteria. Several epidemiologic studies have shown that high postchallenge (2-hour oral glucose tolerance test) or postprandial glucose values were associated with greater CV risk independently of fasting plasma glucose.[7] However, oral glucose tolerance tests are cumbersome as well as costly and intervention trials failed to support the role of postprandial glucose as a risk predictor independent of HbA$_{1c}$. Therefore an oral glucose tolerance test should be considered only if the diagnosis of diabetes is inconclusive based on fasting plasma glucose and HbA$_{1c}$.[7]

PATHOPHYSIOLOGY OF ATHEROSCLEROSIS IN DIABETES

In patients with diabetes, CAD is more prevalent, more advanced, and occurs at a younger age than in nondiabetic counterparts. Several metabolic abnormalities—including chronic hyperglycemia, dyslipidemia, oxidative stress, and insulin resistance—have been associated with the accelerated atherogenesis observed in people with diabetes.[4] In addition to metabolic disturbances, diabetes alters the function of multiple cell lines, including endothelial cells, smooth muscle cells, and platelets.

Long-standing insulin resistance, characterized by elevated plasma glucose and compensatory hyperinsulinemia, has been associated with diabetic microvascular and macrovascular complications. The supposed link is via the development of (1) endothelial dysfunction and oxidative stress, (2) an inflammatory state, (3) a prothrombotic state, and (4) atherosclerotic plaque instability with subsequent risk of plaque rupture and occlusive thrombus formation.[4] These proatherogenic mechanisms observed in diabetic patients may be responsible for the higher rate of mortality and

> **BOX 3.1** Diagnosis of Diabetes Mellitus According to the American Diabetes Association
>
> HbA_{1C} (glycated hemoglobin) >6.5%[a]
> or
> fasting plasma glucose ≥126 mg/dL (7.0 mmol/L) with *fasting* defined as no caloric intake for at least 8 h
> or
> 2-h plasma glucose ≥200 mg/dL (11.1 mmol/L) during an oral glucose tolerance test performed as described by the World Health Organization using a glucose load containing the equivalent of 75 g anhydrous glucose dissolved in water
> or
> in a patient with classic symptoms of hyperglycemia, hyperglycemic crisis, or a random plasma glucose ≥200 mg/dL (11.1 mmol/L)
>
> [a]The test should be performed in a laboratory using a method that is certified by the National Glycohemoglobin Standardization Program (NGSP) and standardized to the Diabetes Control and Complications Trial (DCCT) assay.
> From the American Diabetes Association. Standards of medical care in diabetes—2014. *Diabetes Care*. 2014;37(suppl 1):S14–S80.

reinfarction in patients with CAD as well as for the higher rates of stent thrombosis and in-stent restenosis after percutaneous coronary intervention (PCI) observed in the diabetic population.[8]

CARDIOVASCULAR DISEASE IN DIABETES

A population-based study estimated that in patients older than 40 years, diabetes confers an equivalent CV risk to aging 15 years.[9] The 2013 American Heart Association (AHA)/American College of Cardiology (ACC) guidelines on cholesterol treatment considered the diabetic population as a group who were at higher risk and would benefit from intensive statin therapy in primary prevention, although the overall CV risk was considered to be lower than that of nondiabetic patients with established CV disease.[10] A meta-analysis has specifically studied whether patients with diabetes mellitus and without previous myocardial infarction (MI) had the same risk of CAD as nondiabetic patients with previous MI.[11] Based on findings from 13 studies involving 45,108 participants, subjects with diabetes without prior MI had a 43% lower risk of developing total CAD events compared with patients without diabetes with previous MI (odds ratio [OR] 0.56, 95% confidence interval [CI] 0.53 to 0.60).[11] Age-standardized rates of selected vascular diseases in individuals with diabetes have significantly decreased over time from 1990 to 2010 but are still higher compared with persons without diabetes (Fig. 3.1).[12] Autopsy and angiographic studies have shown that patients with diabetes more frequently have left main coronary artery lesions—multivessel as well as diffuse CAD—than their nondiabetic counterparts.[13] One angiographic study on patients with angina demonstrated that the greater the impairment of glucose metabolism (i.e., normal vs. impaired glucose tolerance vs. newly diagnosed diabetes vs. known diabetes), the smaller the average coronary artery diameter and the longer the lesions detected.[14] In addition, a retrospective study of 3805 patients with diabetes showed a significant association between the HbA_{1c} levels and the severity of the CAD according to the Synergy Between Percutaneous Coronary Intervention With Taxus and Cardiac Surgery (SYNTAX) score.[15]

MYOCARDIAL ISCHEMIA DETECTION IN DIABETIC PATIENTS

Diabetic patients have significantly higher rates of silent ischemia and silent MI than the general population.[16–18] Resting electrocardiography (ECG) may detect MI in 4% of patients with diabetes.[19] The sensitivity and specificity of exercise ECG to detect significant CAD in asymptomatic diabetic patients is estimated to be between 47% and 81%, respectively, and the addition of imaging significantly improves the diagnostic and prognostic values.[20] Stress nuclear imaging has the most extensive literature among the noninvasive modalities for both diagnostic and prognostic purposes in diabetes. With respect to stress echocardiography, several studies have addressed its prognostic accuracy in diabetes, although the data on its diagnostic value are scarce.[18]

Several studies have identified the coronary artery calcium score as a strong predictor of CV events and all-cause mortality in diabetic individuals. The Prospective Evaluation of Diabetic Ischemic Disease by Computed Tomography (PREDICT) study prospectively evaluated calcium score as a predictor of CV events in 589 asymptomatic individuals with type 2 diabetes.[21] The risk of a CV event increased with higher levels of calcium scores. In addition, the calcium score had greater predictive value for end points than a broad range of conventional and novel risk factors. Finally, a prospective cohort study in West London found that the calcium score was superior to established risk factors in predicting the presence of silent myocardial ischemia on perfusion scans.[22] The value of screening for CAD in asymptomatic diabetic patients is a source of controversy. In fact, it has not been demonstrated that implementation of this approach leads to better outcomes than strict CV risk-factor control alone. Cardiac testing may be considered in the presence of additional features of increased CV risk, such as peripheral or cerebrovascular disease, renal disease, albuminuria, abnormal resting ECG, microvascular diabetic complications, or additional CV risk factors.[23] In the Detection of Ischemia in Asymptomatic Diabetics (DIAD) study, 1123 diabetic participants with no symptoms of CAD were randomly assigned to adenosine stress radionuclide myocardial perfusion imaging or no screening in addition to optimal medical treatment.[24] At a mean follow-up of 4.8 years, the cumulative cardiac death or MI rate was 2.9% (0.6% per year), with no difference between the two groups. In the screened group, participants with normal results ($n = 409$) or small perfusion defects ($n = 50$) had lower event rates than the 33 patients with moderate or large defects on perfusion imaging (0.4% per year vs. 2.4% per year; hazard ratio [HR], 6.3; 95% CI, 1.9 to 20.1; $P = .001$) (Fig. 3.2).[24] Nevertheless, the positive predictive value (PPV) of having moderate or large defects on perfusion scans was only 12%. The overall rate of coronary revascularization was low in both groups (5.5% in the screened group and 7.8% in the unscreened group). The authors concluded that more aggressive screening for CAD did not improve the outcome of asymptomatic diabetic patients over optimal medical therapy and lifestyle modification. However, because the event rates were lower than estimated, the study was underpowered. In addition, among the 33 patients with moderate to large perfusion defects detected by screening, the rate of coronary angiography was only 15%. A meta-analysis including 10 prospective studies with 1360 asymptomatic patients with diabetes showed a prevalence of silent myocardial ischemia of 26.1%.[25] Patients with silent myocardial ischemia were at higher risk of cardiac death (risk ratio [RR] 4.60, 95% CI 1.78 to 11.84), nonfatal cardiac events (RR 3.48, 95% CI 2.30 to 5.28) and all-cause mortality (RR 2.20, 95% CI 1.14 to 4.35).[25] Another systematic review including five randomized controlled trials (RCTs) with 3299 asymptomatic diabetic patients suggested that noninvasive CAD screening significantly reduced cardiac events by 27% (RR 0.73, 95% CI 0.55 to 0.97, $P = .028$) but not cardiac death (RR 0.92, 95% CI 0.53 to 1.60).[26] Overall, evidence of benefit of preventive coronary revascularization in asymptomatic diabetic patients is lacking. In summary, although stress testing should be considered with a lower threshold in diabetic patients with suspected CAD than in nondiabetic individuals, especially if

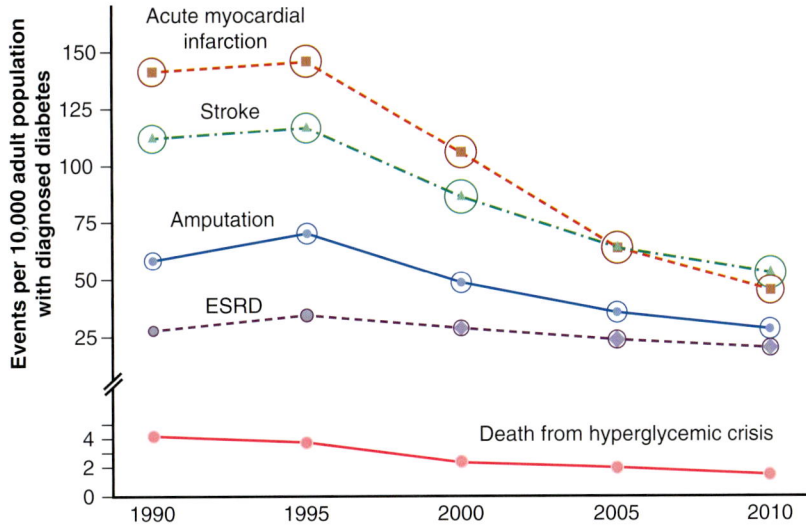

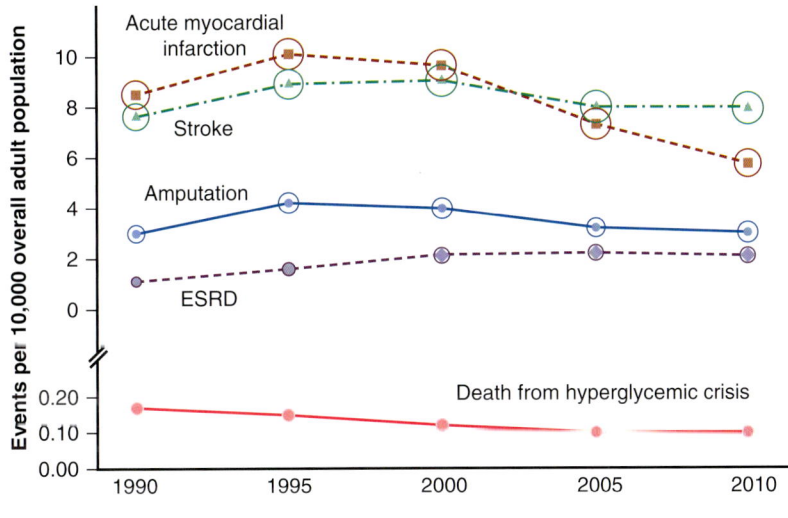

Fig. 3.1 (A and B) Trends in age-standardized rates of diabetes-related complications among US adults with and without diagnosed diabetes, 1990–2010. *ESRD,* End-stage renal disease. (Reproduced from Gregg EW, Williams DE, Geiss L. Changes in diabetes-related complications in the United States. *N Engl J Med.* 2014;371:286–287.)

associated with high-risk conditions, routine screening for CAD in asymptomatic diabetic patients is not indicated.[27]

Revascularization in Diabetic Patients With Stable Coronary Artery Disease

Despite improvements in the management of diabetic patients who undergo coronary revascularization—from a pharmacologic, interventional, as well as surgical standpoint—diabetes remains an independent predictor of CV events following both percutaneous and surgical revascularization.[28] In addition to RCTs, new meta-analysis designs—such as individual participant data analysis collaborations or network meta-analyses—have been developed to allow for both direct and indirect comparisons between PCI and CABG. These study designs have led to an increase in statistical power to address the diabetic population.[28]

Percutaneous Coronary Intervention

Whereas in-hospital and 30-day outcomes after PCI in diabetic patients were frequently found to be comparable with those of nondiabetic counterparts, diabetes has been invariably associated with increased target-vessel revascularization (TVR), major adverse cardiovascular and cerebrovascular events (MACCE), and late mortality at follow-up, even in the drug-eluting stent (DES) era.[28]

Accordingly, diabetic patients undergoing PCI have worse outcomes than nondiabetic individuals independently of the complexity of their coronary anatomy as defined by the SYN-TAX score.[29] A network meta-analysis of 35 RCTs compared DESs with bare-metal stents (BMSs) in 3852 diabetic patients and showed that DESs, although not affecting overall mortality or MI rates, were associated with a sizable reduction in target-lesion revascularization (TLR), with a relative risk reduction of 60% to 70%, depending on the type of stent used, and an absolute risk reduction of approximately 16% (Fig. 3.3).[30] Whereas first-generation DES use in diabetes was found to be an independent predictor of late stent thrombosis in several studies (Fig. 3.4), this does not seem to be the case with newer-generation DESs.[31] An individual participant data analysis from 18 prospective RCTs—which included 18,441 patients who underwent DES-based PCI, of whom 3467 were diabetic—reported significantly higher TLR in diabetic patients only in cases of complex lesions (type B2/C) and not in simple lesions (type A/B1; type B2/C according to ACC/AHA lesion classification and type A/B1 according to ACC/AHA lesion classification).[32]

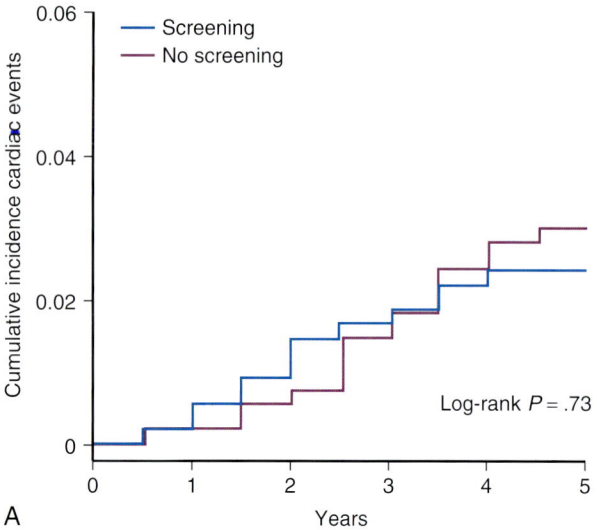

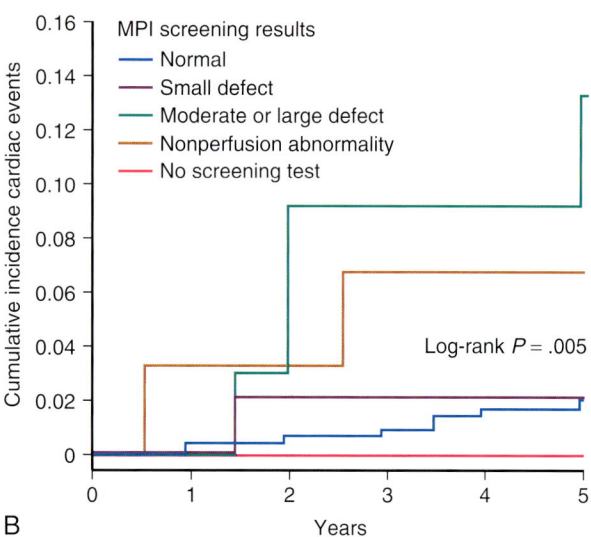

Fig. 3.2 (A) Cumulative incidence of cardiac events in 561 participants randomized to systematic baseline screening with stress myocardial perfusion imaging *(MPI)* and 562 participants randomized to receive no screening in the DIAD study. (B) Cumulative incidence of cardiac events according to results of systematic screening with stress MPI: normal, small defect, moderate or large defect, and nonperfusion abnormality. (From Young LH, Wackers FJ, Chyun DA, et al. Cardiac outcomes after screening for asymptomatic coronary artery disease in patients with type 2 diabetes: the DIAD study: a randomized controlled trial. *JAMA.* 2009;301:1547–1555.)

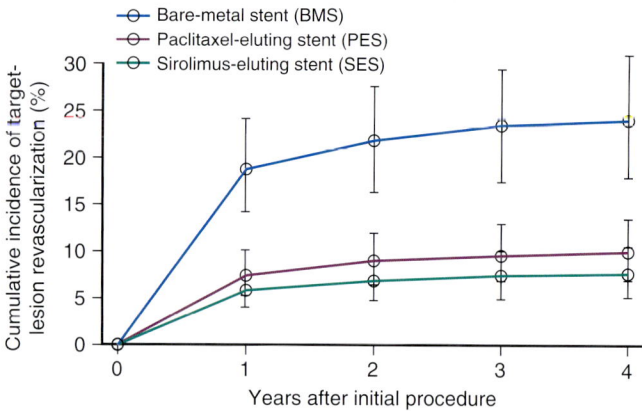

Fig. 3.3 Cumulative incidence of target-lesion revascularization and corresponding hazard ratios (95% confidence intervals) for three stent types estimated from a network meta-analysis for pairwise comparisons in patients with diabetes. *BMS,* Bare-metal stent; *PES,* paclitaxel-eluting stent (Taxus, Boston Scientific); *SES,* sirolimus-eluting stent (Cypher, Cordis). (From Stettler C, Allemann S, Wandel S, et al. Drug eluting and bare metal stents in people with and without diabetes: collaborative network meta-analysis. *BMJ.* 2008;337:a1331.)

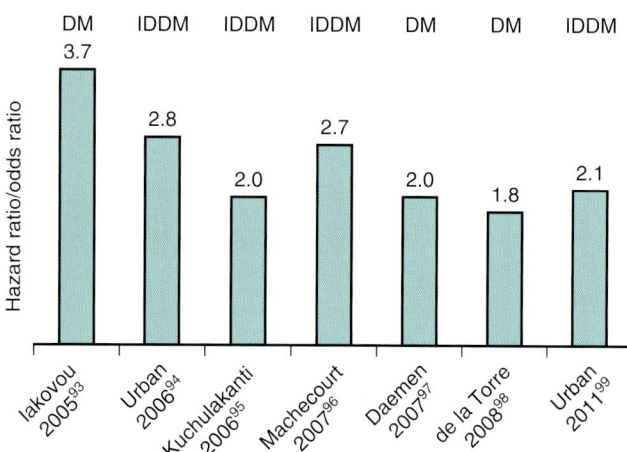

Fig. 3.4 Studies that have detected diabetes mellitus or insulin-dependent diabetes mellitus as an independent predictor of thrombosis associated with a drug-eluting stent. Reported is the hazard ratio or odds ratio of multivariate analyses. *DM,* Diabetes mellitus; *IDDM,* insulin-dependent diabetes mellitus. (From Roffi M, Angiolillo D, Kappetein AP. Current concepts on coronary revascularization in diabetic patients. *Eur Heart J.* 2011;32:2748–2757.)

With respect to newer-generation DESs, a subgroup analysis of the diabetic population ($n = 414$) in a head-to-head trial comparing the biolimus-eluting stent (Biomatrix, Biosensor) and the Cypher stent showed no difference in death, MI, or TVR at 9 months.[33] Similarly, a subgroup analysis for the diabetic population ($n = 1140$) of the head-to-head trial that allocated patients to either the everolimus-eluting stent (EES, Xience, Abbott) or the Taxus stent showed no difference in the target lesion failure at 1 year (6.4% vs. 6.9%).[34] A meta-analysis of 18 RCTs with 8095 patients compared the efficacy and safety of EES and zotarolimus-eluting stent versus first-generation DESs in patients with diabetes.[35] Use of the EES was associated with a significant reduction of major adverse CV events by 18% (RR 0.82, 95% CI 0.70 to 0.96), including MI, stent thrombosis, and TLR.

In summary, current evidence supports the contention that in diabetic patients, the use of DESs compared with BMSs dramatically reduced the risk of restenosis and repeat revascularization and had no harmful effect in terms of MI. Whereas with first-generation DESs diabetic patients had an increase in stent thrombosis rates compared with nondiabetic individuals, this does not seem to be the case with newer-generation devices. Current European Society of Cardiology (ESC) guidelines on myocardial revascularization recommend the DES as the device of choice for diabetic patients (class I, level of recommendation A).[36] US guidelines for PCI recommend the DES as the device of choice (class I, level of recommendation A) for patients at high risk of restenosis.[37]

Coronary Artery Bypass Surgery

Paralleling the observation for PCI, diabetes also negatively affects outcomes following CABG. The impact of diabetes on morbidity and mortality in patients undergoing surgical coronary

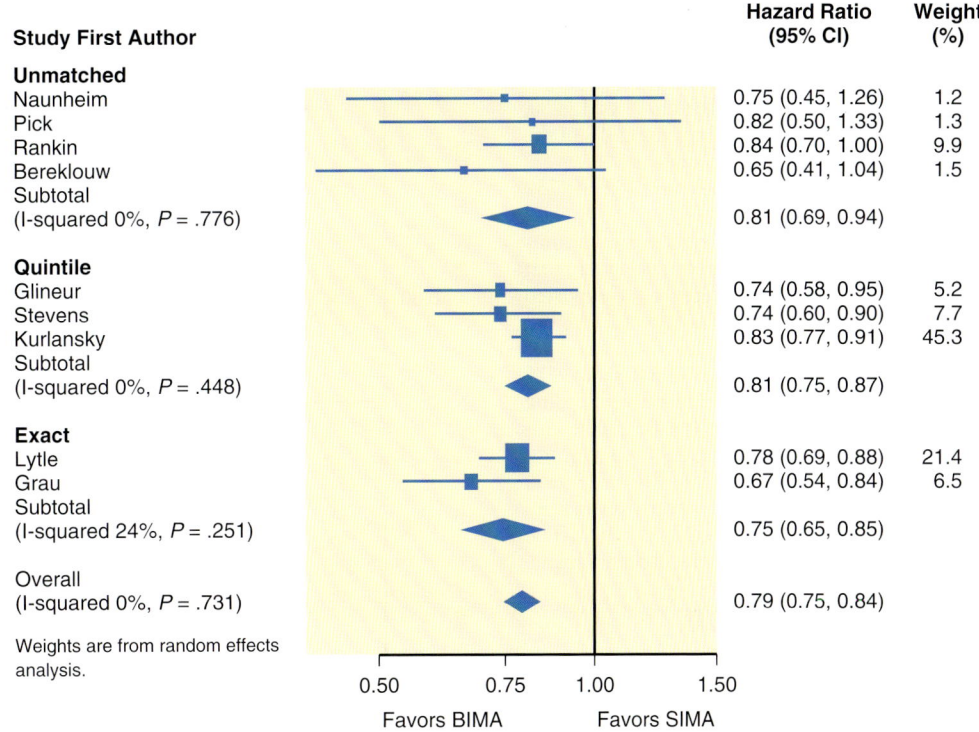

Fig. 3.5 Effects of bilateral internal mammary artery grafting on long-term survival. This random-effects meta-analysis is from nine studies. Horizontal lines indicate a 95% confidence interval (CI). The "unmatched" group included studies with no statistical matching method. The "quintile" group included studies that used a quintile-based stratification method with a propensity score. The "exact" group included studies with a propensity score–based exact (1:1) matching method. BIMA, Bilateral internal mammary artery; SIMA, single internal mammary artery. (From Yi G, Shine B, Rehman SM, et al. Effect of bilateral internal mammary artery on long-term survival: a meta-analysis approach. Circulation. 2014;130:539–545.)

revascularization was addressed in a retrospective analysis of the database of the Society of Thoracic Surgery and included 41,663 diabetic patients among a total population of 146,786 patients.[38] At 30 days, mortality was significantly higher in the diabetes group (3.7% vs. 2.7%). Looking into long-term mortality following CABG, a prospective cohort study that included 11,186 consecutive diabetic patients and 25,455 nondiabetic patients who underwent CABG from 1992 to 2001 detected a significantly higher annual mortality rate among diabetic patients (5.5%) compared with that of nondiabetic individuals (3.1%).[39] In addition to increased periprocedural morbidity and mortality as well as long-term mortality, diabetic patients require more frequent repeat revascularization following CABG than do their nondiabetic counterparts.[40]

The use of multiple arterial conduits, including bilateral internal mammary artery (BIMA) grafting, has been associated with improved long-term results following CABG and with reduced rates of repeat revascularization in the diabetic population. The Leipzig experience with 1515 consecutive patients who underwent BIMA grafting included 519 diabetic patients. Multiple regression analysis showed that, in addition to repeat operation (OR 12.7), both non–insulin-dependent (OR 4.6) and insulin-dependent diabetes (OR 6.9) were associated with a significantly increased risk of sternal infection.[41] An analysis of a population of 1107 consecutive patients with diabetes showed no difference in operative mortality (2.4% vs. 3.1%, $P = .28$), sternal wound infection (1.7% vs. 3.1%, $P = .18$), or total complications (17.1% vs. 17.1%, $P = 1.00$) using propensity score matching in the groups of single internal mammary artery (SIMA) or BIMA grafting. Late survival was significantly improved with the use of BIMA grafting after 13.1 years compared with SIMA grafting after 9.8 years.[42] A meta-analysis of nine observational studies with up to 10 years of follow-up that included 15,583 patients reported a reduction of mortality (HR, 0.79; 95% CI, 0.75 to 0.84) with BIMA compared with SIMA grafting (Fig. 3.5).[43]

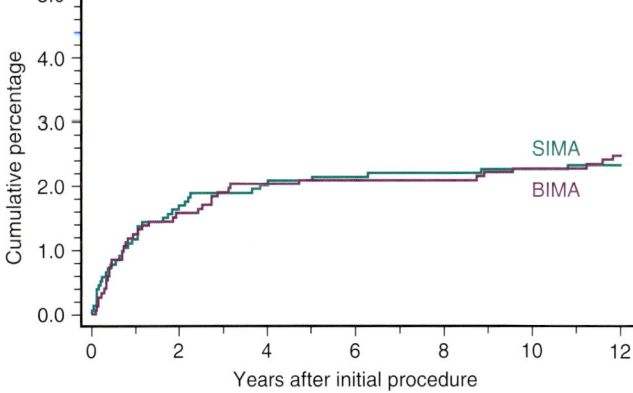

Fig. 3.6 All-cause mortality at 1 year in the Arterial Revascularisation Trial (ART). BIMA, Bilateral internal mammary artery; SIMA, single internal mammary artery. (From Taggart DP, Altman DG, Gray AM, et al. Randomized trial to compare bilateral versus single internal mammary coronary artery bypass grafting: 1-year results of the Arterial Revascularisation Trial [ART]. Eur Heart J. 2010;31:2470–2481.)

The Arterial Revascularisation Trial (ART) randomized 3102 patients to SIMA or BIMA with a primary outcome of survival at 10 years.[44] A mean of three grafts were applied in both groups, and 41% of the procedures were performed off pump. Mortality at 30 days was 1.2% in both groups, whereas at 1 year, it was 2.3% in the SIMA group and 2.5% in the BIMA group (Fig. 3.6). The rates of stroke, MI, and repeat revascularization were all 2% or less at 1 year and were similar between the two groups. Sternal wound reconstruction for infection was required in 0.6% and 1.9% of the SIMA and BIMA groups, respectively (RR, 3.2; 95% CI, 1.5 to 6.8). The results of the ART trial suggest that the use of BIMA grafts is feasible on a routine basis. The 5-year outcome analysis of the study did not show significant differences in either the SIMA or BIMA groups: the rate of death (8.4% vs. 8.7%, $P = .77$), the rate of a composite of death, MI, or stroke (12.7% vs. 12.2%, $P = .69$). In addition, in the subgroup of diabetic patients (24% of the total), no difference was observed between the two strategies.[45]

With respect to the impact of off-pump surgery, an RCT of 4752 patients (2253 with diabetes) treated with CABG compared the use of off-pump with on-pump surgery; the primary outcome was a composite of death, nonfatal stroke, nonfatal MI, or new renal failure that required dialysis at 30 days.[46] No significant difference was reported in primary end point (9.8% vs. 10.3%; HR, 0.95; 95% CI, 0.79 to 1.14); however, the use of off-pump CABG significantly reduced the rates of blood-product transfusion (50.7% vs. 63.3%; RR, 0.80; 95% CI, 0.75 to 0.85; $P < .001$), reoperation for perioperative bleeding (1.4% vs. 2.4%; RR, 0.61; 95% CI, 0.40 to 0.93; $P = .02$), acute kidney injury (28.0% vs. 32.1%; RR, 0.87; 95% CI, 0.80 to 0.l96; $P = .01$), and respiratory complications (5.9% vs. 7.5%; RR, 0.79; 95% CI, 0.63 to 0.98; $P = .03$), but it increased the rate of early revascularization (0.7% vs. 0.2%; HR, 4.01; 95% CI, 1.34 to 12.0; $P = .01$). The presence of diabetes did not significantly change the observations.

REVASCULARIZATION VERSUS MEDICAL MANAGEMENT

The Bypass Angioplasty Revascularization Investigation in Type 2 Diabetes (BARI 2D) trial randomly assigned 2368 diabetic patients with stable CAD in a two-by-two design to either prompt revascularization with intensive medical therapy or intensive medical therapy alone and to either insulin-sensitization or insulin-provision therapy.[47] Primary end points were the 5-year rates of death and of MACCE, defined as a composite of death, MI, or stroke. Randomization was stratified according to the choice of PCI or CABG as the more appropriate intervention. Survival did not differ between the revascularization group (88.3%) and the medical therapy group (87.8%). The rates of freedom from MACCE also did not differ significantly between the groups: at 77.2% in the revascularization group and 75.9% in the medical-treatment group. Whereas in the PCI stratum no significant difference was reported in primary end points between the revascularization group and the medical-therapy group, in the CABG stratum, the rate of MACCE was significantly lower in the revascularization group (22.4%) than in the medical therapy group (30.5%, $P = .01$; $P = .002$ for interaction between stratum and study groups).[47] Since BARI 2D did not compare PCI and CABG in terms of the comparative efficacy of these two revascularization modalities, no conclusion can be drawn from that trial.

Percutaneous Coronary Intervention Versus Coronary Artery Bypass Grafting in Stable Diabetic Patients With Multivessel Disease

An epidemiologic study assessed the clinical outcomes of patients with multivessel CAD who underwent revascularization with CABG ($n = 7437$) or with a DES ($n = 9963$) between the years 2003 and 2004 in New York State.[48] Patients who underwent CABG were older, more likely to be male and white, and had a lower ejection fraction, prior MI, other coexisting conditions, and three-vessel CAD. The outcomes of diabetic patients treated with CABG ($n = 2844$) did not differ from those who underwent PCI ($n = 3256$) with respect to the adjusted rate of death (HR, 0.97; $P = .75$) and death or MI (HR, 0.84; $P = .07$).

The Coronary Artery Revascularization in Diabetes (CARDia) trial compared PCI and CABG in 510 diabetic patients with symptomatic multivessel CAD. At 1 year of follow-up, the primary end point of death, MI, and stroke was 10.5% in the CABG group and 13.0% in the PCI group (HR, 1.25; $P = .39$). The need for repeat revascularization was 2.0% in the

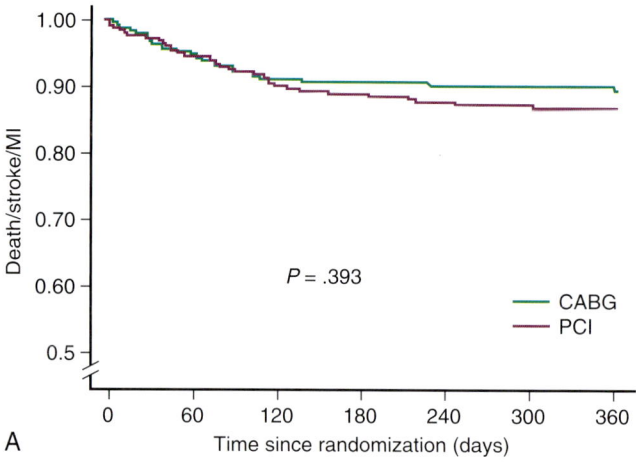

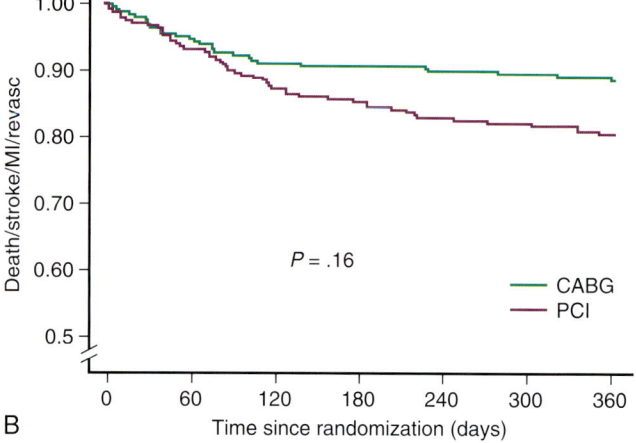

Fig. 3.7 One-year Kaplan-Meier event-free survival curves for coronary artery bypass grafting (CABG) and percutaneous coronary intervention (PCI). The primary outcomes were death, myocardial infarction (MI), or stroke (A) and death, MI, stroke, or repeat revascularization (revasc) in the CARDia trial (B). (From Kapur A, Hall RJ, Malik IS, et al. Randomized comparison of percutaneous coronary intervention with coronary artery bypass grafting in diabetic patients. 1-year results of the CARDia trial. *J Am Coll Cardiol.* 2010;55:432–440.)

CABG group and 11.8% in the PCI group (HR, 6.2; $P < .001$). All-cause mortality rates were the same, 3.2%, and the rates of death, MI, stroke, or repeat revascularization were 11.3% and 19.3%, respectively (HR, 1.77; $P = .16$) (Fig. 3.7).[49] In the first phase of the study, patients were randomized to either CABG or BMS implantation; thereafter, patients were randomized to CABG or DES implantation ($n = 350$). In the patient population randomized after the introduction of the DES, the death, MI, stroke, or repeat revascularization rates in the CABG and PCI groups were 12.9% and 18.0%, respectively (HR, 1.41; $P = $ nonsignificant [NS]).

The SYNTAX study randomly assigned 1800 patients (452 with diabetes) to receive paclitaxel DES-based PCI (Taxus) or CABG. The 1-year MACCE rate (death, stroke, MI, or repeat revascularization) was higher among diabetic patients treated with a DES (26.0%) than with CABG (14.2%; $P = .003$).[50] Conversely, no difference was observed in diabetic patients in the death, stroke, or MI rate (10.3% for CABG vs. 10.1% for PCI).[51] The presence of diabetes was associated with significantly increased mortality after either revascularization treatment. Mortality was higher after PCI than after CABG (13.5% vs. 4.1%, $P = .04$) for diabetic patients with highly complex lesions (i.e., SYNTAX

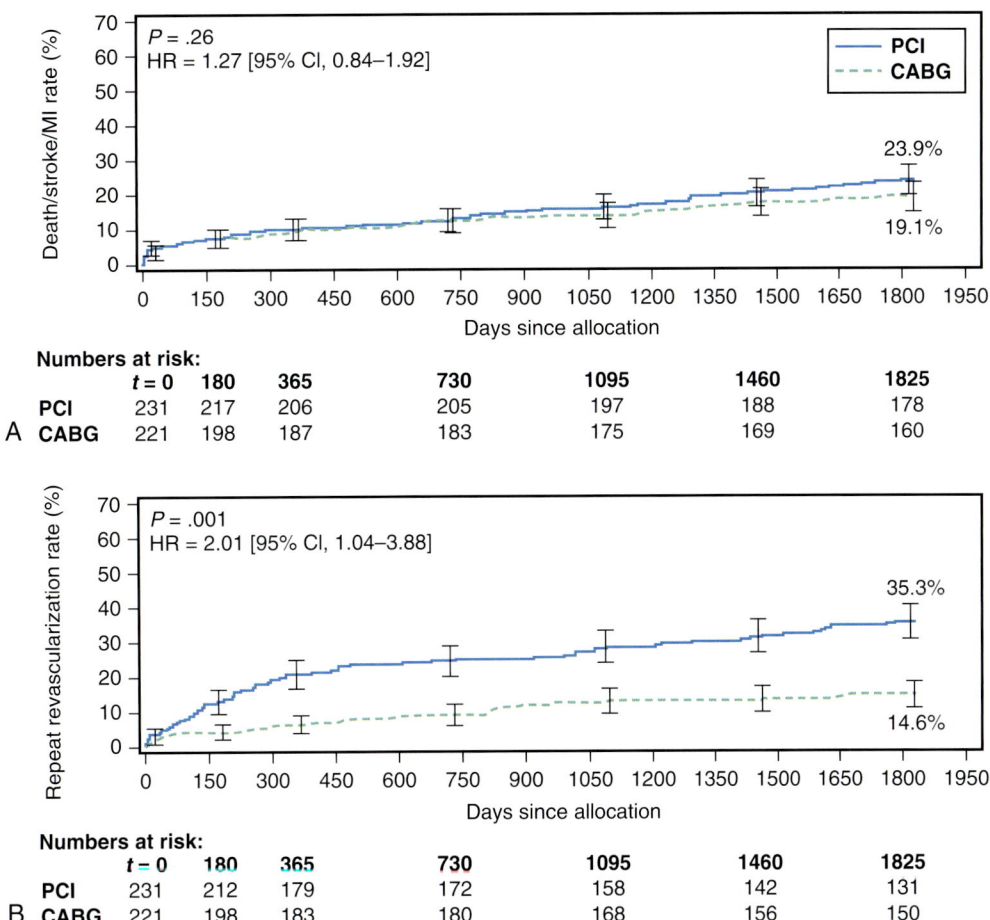

Fig. 3.8 Five-year outcomes of percutaneous coronary intervention *(PCI)* versus coronary artery bypass grafting *(CABG)* in diabetic and nondiabetic patients. (A) The composite end point of all-cause death, stroke, and myocardial infarction *(MI)* and (B) repeat revascularization in diabetic patients. *CI,* Confidence interval; *HR,* hazard ratio; *t,* time. (From Kappetein AP, Head SJ, Morice MC, et al. Treatment of complex coronary artery disease in patients with diabetes: 5-year results comparing outcomes of bypass surgery and percutaneous coronary intervention in the SYNTAX trial. *Eur J Cardiothorac Surg.* 2013;43:1006–1013.)

score ≥33). Treatment with PCI, rather than CABG, resulted in higher repeat revascularization rates for diabetic patients (6.4% vs. 20.3%, $P < .001$). The more complex the lesions according to the SYNTAX score, the greater the disadvantage of PCI in terms of MACCE, driven by an increased TVR rate. The 5-year follow-up of the SYNTAX trial in diabetic patients showed persistence of the benefit of CABG over PCI: the rates of MACCE were 29.0% in the CABG group versus 46% in the PCI group ($P < .0001$), mainly driven by repeat revascularization (35.3% for PCI vs. 14.6% for CABG, $P < .001$). However, no benefit of CABG was observed for the composite end point of death, MI, or stroke (23.9% vs. 19.1%, $P = .26$) (Fig. 3.8). The final 5-year follow-up of the SYNTAX trial in the total population showed persistence of the benefit of CABG over PCI: the rates of MACCE were 24.2% in the CABG group versus 37.5% in the PCI group ($P < .0001$). The benefit of CABG was observed for the composite end point of death, MI, and stroke (22.0% vs. 14.0%, $P < .001$), all-cause death (14.6% vs. 9.2%, $P = .006$), nonfatal MI (39.2% vs. 4.0%, $P = .001$), and the need for repeat revascularization (25.4% vs.12.6%, $P < .0001$). In the subgroup of patients with a low SYNTAX score (0 to 22 points), no differences in MACCE (26.8% vs. 33.3%, $P = .21$) were observed, but significantly more repeat revascularization was required (25.4% vs. 12.6%, $P = .038$). Differences were greater in diabetic patients (HR, 2.30; 95% CI, 1.50 to 3.55) compared with nondiabetic patients (HR, 1.51; 95% CI, 1.15 to 1.96).[52]

The Future Revascularization Evaluation in Patients With Diabetes Mellitus: Optimal Management of Multivessel Disease (FREEDOM) trial compared PCI (first-generation DES) with CABG in 1900 diabetic patients with multivessel CAD and showed an increased risk of MACCE in the PCI group (26.6% vs. 18.7%, $P = .005$) compared with the CABG group after 5 years of follow-up.[53] CABG was superior to PCI in terms of a reduced overall death rate (16.3% vs. 10.9%, $P = .049$) and a reduced rate of nonfatal MI (13.9% vs. 6.0%, $P < .001$), but CABG was inferior to PCI in terms of a higher rate of stroke at 5 years (2.4% in the PCI group and 5.2% in the CABG group, $P = .03$).

A mixed treatment comparison analysis of 68 RCTs in 24,015 patients with diabetes showed that PCI using cobalt-chromium EESs resulted in similar mortality compared with CABG (RR, 1.11; 95% CI, 0.67 to 1.84), whereas paclitaxel-eluting stents (RR, 1.57; 95% CI, 1.15 to 2.19) and sirolimus-eluting stents (RR, 1.43; 95% CI, 1.07 to 1.97) were associated with increased mortality. In addition, the excess repeat revascularization for PCI

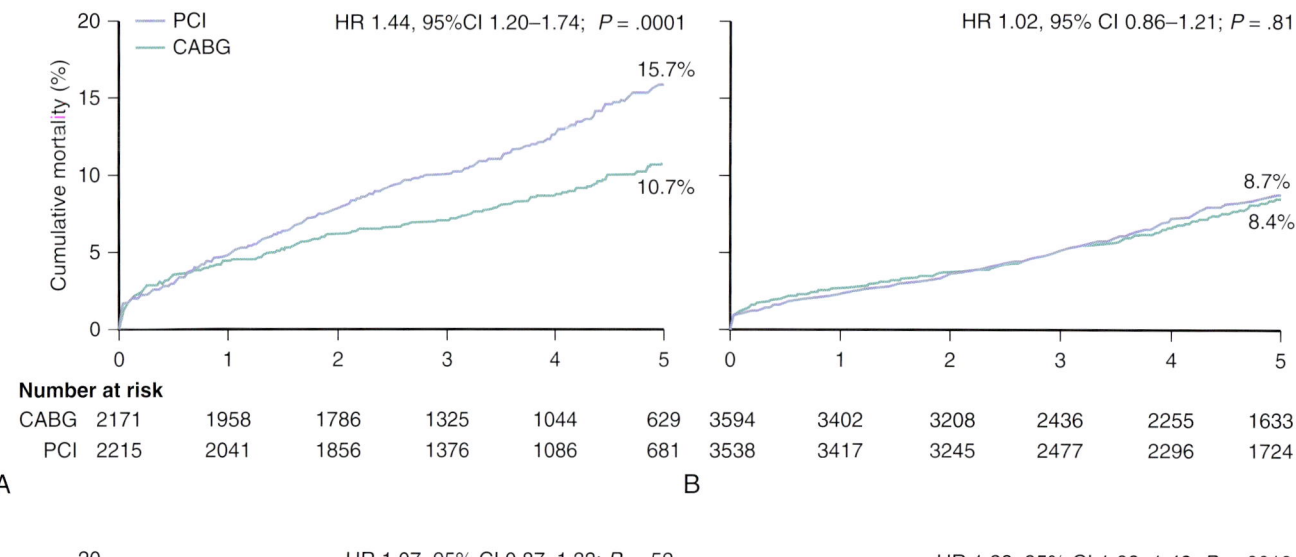
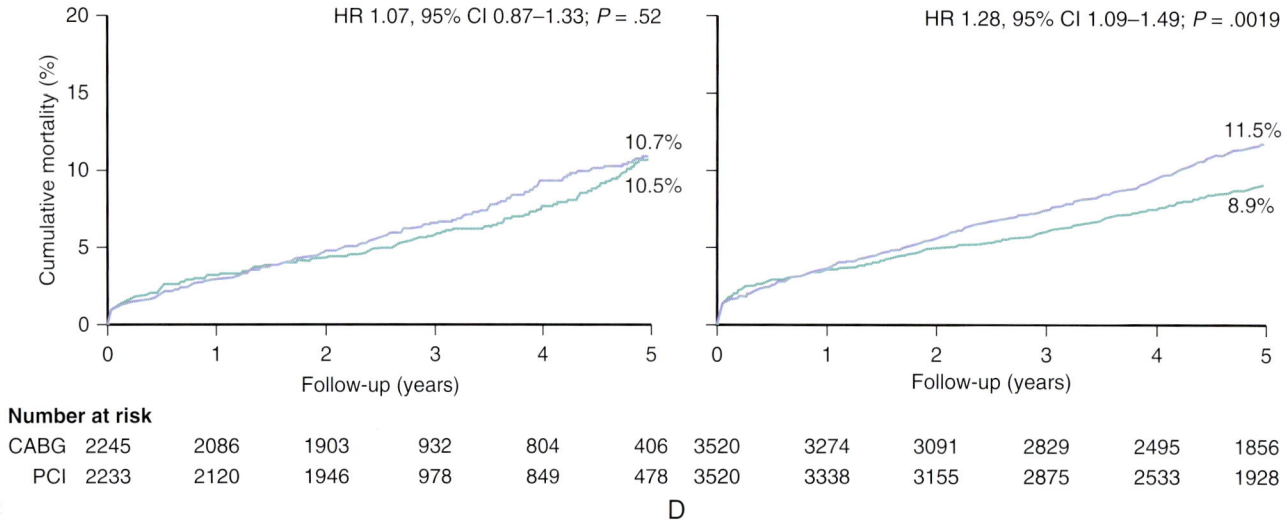

Fig. 3.9 Mortality after CABG versus after PCI during 5 years' follow-up of patients with (A) or without (B) diabetes and with left main disease (C) or multivessel disease (D). *CABG*, Coronary artery bypass grafting; *HR*, hazard ratio; *PCI*, percutaneous coronary intervention.

with cobalt-chromium EESs was not statistically significant (RR, 1.31; 95% CI, 0.74 to 2.29), although the point estimate favored CABG.[54]

Finally, a recent pooled individual participant data analysis including 11 RCTs and 11,518 patients (5753 allocated to PCI and 5765 to CABG) over a mean follow-up of 3.8 years assessed all-cause mortality at 5 years.[55] In the PCI group, 38.5% of patients (n = 2215) had diabetes, as did 37.7% (n = 2171) in the CABG group. The mean SYNTAX score was 26.0 (standard deviation 9.5), with 1798 (22.1%) having a SYNTAX score of 33 or higher. Significant differences between revascularization with PCI versus CABG were found in patients with multivessel diabetes and diabetes (15.5% for PCI vs. 10.0% for CABG, HR 1.48, 95% CI 1.19 to 1.84, P = .0004) (Fig. 3.9).[55] In contradistinction, no difference was observed in patients with no diabetes (8.7% vs. 8.4%, HR 1.02, 95% CI 0.86 to 1.21, P = .81). The observed results for PCI suggested that recent developments in stent techniques did not translate into a significant reduction of the gap between PCI and surgery in terms of long-term outcomes in the diabetic population.[55] In stable diabetic patients, the choice of revascularization modality should take into account multiple parameters that include coronary anatomy, left ventricular (LV) function, coexisting conditions, and estimated surgical risk (Fig. 3.10). A recent observational study focusing on patients with diabetes and LV dysfunction (n = 2837) suggested a lower risk for death in those treated with CABG compared with PCI both for LV ejection fraction between 35% and 49% and for less than 35%.[56]

Overall, surgery should be favored in diabetic patients with multivessel coronary disease and low surgical risk, and the threshold for surgery compared with PCI should be lower in diabetic patients compared with their nondiabetic counterparts.[28] According to the 2011 ACC Foundation/AHA/Society for Cardiovascular Angiography and Interventions (SCAI) guidelines, CABG is recommended for the revascularization of diabetic patients with complex (SYNTAX score >22) multivessel disease (class I, level B) or unprotected left main CAD (class I, level B).[37] The same guidelines recommend PCI as an acceptable alternative for patients with an unprotected left main coronary artery or multivessel disease with a low SYNTAX score (≤22 points) or for patients with a higher risk of adverse surgical long-term outcome (Society of Thoracic Surgeons [STS] predicted score of operative mortality ≥5%; class IIa, level B) and also for patients with multivessel disease and a low SYNTAX score (≤22 points; class

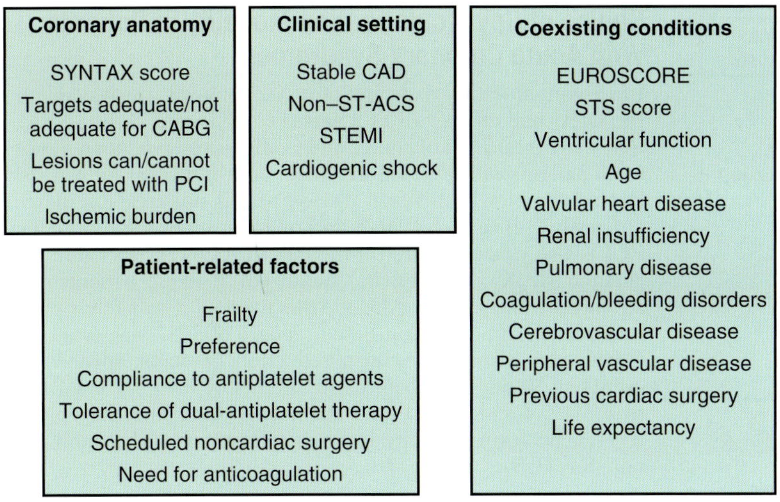

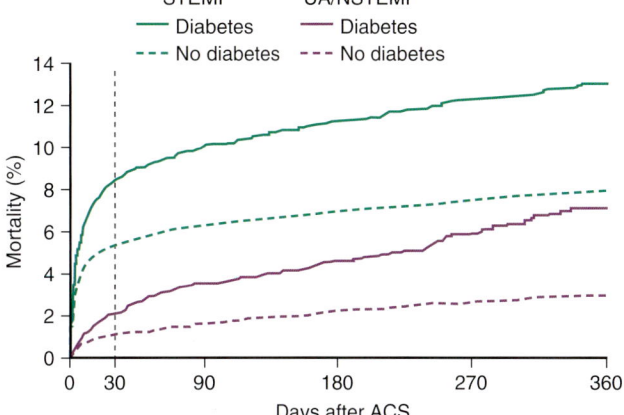

Fig. 3.10 Parameters guiding the choice of revascularization strategy in diabetic patients. *ACS,* Acute coronary syndrome; *CABG,* coronary artery bypass grafting; *CAD,* coronary artery disease; *EuroSCORE,* European System for Cardiac Operative Risk Evaluation; *PCI,* percutaneous coronary intervention; *STEMI,* ST-elevation myocardial infarction; *STS,* Society of Thoracic Surgery. (From Roffi M, Angiolillo D, Kappetein AP. Current concepts on coronary revascularization in diabetic patients. *Eur Heart J.* 2011;32:2748–2757.)

IIa, level B). ESC guidelines on stable CAD recommend CABG in patients with diabetes and multivessel or complex disease (SYNTAX score >22) to improve survival free from MACCE (class I, level A), whereas PCI may be considered for symptom control as an alternative to CABG in patients with diabetes and less complex multivessel disease (SYNTAX score ≤22; class IIb, level B).[36]

In conclusion, current evidence supports that in patients with diabetes and multivessel stable CAD, revascularization with CABG is superior to PCI in reducing the composite risk of death, MI, and stroke at follow-up. In patients with low complexity of the coronary anatomy (SYNTAX score ≤22), PCI is noninferior to CABG with respect to the same composite end point and may represent an alternative to CABG. For patients with intermediate-to-high anatomic complexity (SYNTAX score >22), CABG is recommended as the standard of care except for cases involving increased surgical risk. In these cases, it is recommended to select the appropriate revascularization method within the heart team.

DIABETES AND NON–ST-ELEVATION ACUTE CORONARY SYNDROMES

A high prevalence of abnormal glucose metabolism in patients with CAD—in particular among those with acute manifestations of the disease—has been detected in large-scale surveys on both sides of the Atlantic. In the American registry, Can Rapid Risk Stratification of Unstable Angina Patients Suppress Adverse Outcomes With Early Implementation of the ACC/AHA Guidelines (CRUSADE), the prevalence of diabetes was 33% among 46,410 patients who presented with non–ST-elevation acute coronary syndromes (non-ST ACS).[57] The prevalence of known diabetes in the Euro Heart Survey of patients with ACS was 32%, whereas use of an oral glucose tolerance test, impaired glucose tolerance or undiagnosed diabetes was detected in 36% and 22% of patients, respectively.[58] Diabetic patients more frequently than their nondiabetic counterparts have characteristics and comorbidities that may negatively affect outcomes in the setting of acute ACS. Nevertheless, even after accounting for imbalances in baseline characteristics, several studies have shown that diabetes remains an independent predictor of short-term morbidity and mortality in the setting of ACS.[59] As an example, in the CRUSADE registry, the in-hospital mortality rates were 6.8% for diabetic patients on insulin, 5.4% for diabetic patients not treated with insulin, and 4.4% for nondiabetic patients.[59] A pooled study of ACS patients enrolled in several randomized clinical trials comprised 46,577

Fig. 3.11 Patients with acute coronary syndrome *(ACS)* in 11 pooled independent Thrombolysis in Myocardial Infarction (TIMI) Study Group clinical trials from 1997 to 2006. This included 62,036 patients (46,577 with ST-segment elevation myocardial infarction *[STEMI]* and 15,459 with unstable angina/non–STEMI *[UA/NSTEMI]*), of whom 10,613 (17.1%) had diabetes. (From Donahoe SM, Stewart GC, McCabe CH, et al. Diabetes and mortality following acute coronary syndromes. *JAMA.* 2007;298:765–775.)

ST-elevation myocardial infarction (STEMI) patients and 15,459 non-ST ACS patients. The diabetic population (17% of the total) had a higher rate of mortality at 30 days compared with those who did not have diabetes, both in the setting of non-ST ACS (2.1% vs. 1.1%, $P < .001$) and STEMI (8.5% vs. 5.4%, $P < .001$).[60] Adjusted odds ratios for 30-day mortality in patients with diabetes after non-ST ACS were 1.78 (95% CI, 1.24 to 2.56), and 1.40 (95% CI, 1.24 to 1.57) for STEMI. At 1 year, diabetes at presentation with ACS was associated with a significantly higher mortality after unstable angina (UA)/non–ST-elevation myocardial infarction (NSTEMI; HR, 1.65; 95% CI, 1.30 to 2.10) or after STEMI (HR, 1.22; 95% CI, 1.08 to 1.38) (Fig. 3.11).[60]

EARLY INVASIVE VERSUS CONSERVATIVE STRATEGY

In diabetic patients with non–ST ACS, the positive impact of an early invasive strategy can be derived from a collaborative meta-analysis of nine RCTs that included 9904 subjects, 1789 of

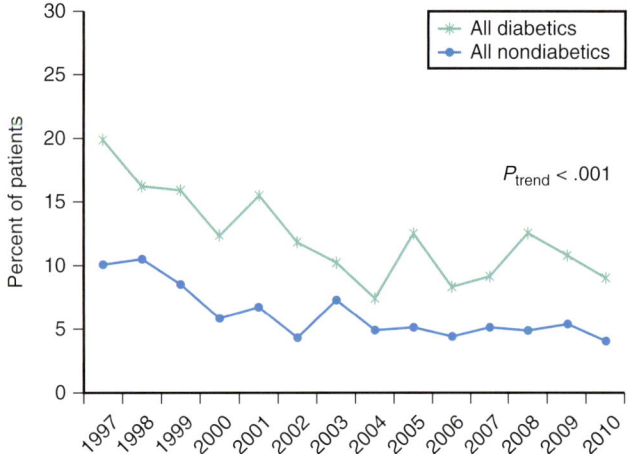

Fig. 3.12 Trends in in-hospital mortality stratified by diabetes status. (From Roffi M, Radovanovic D, Erne P, et al. Gender-related mortality trends among diabetic patients with ST-segment elevation myocardial infarction: insights from a nationwide registry 1997–2010. *Eur Heart J Acute Cardiovasc Care.* 2013;2:342–349.)

whom had diabetes. An early, routine invasive strategy compared with a selective invasive strategy was associated with a reduction of MI in diabetic patients (RR, 0.71; 95% CI, 0.55 to 0.92) but not in their nondiabetic counterparts (RR, 0.98; 95% CI, 0.74 to 1.29). The absolute risk reduction in MI was also significantly higher (3.7% vs. 0.1%, P = .02) in patients with diabetes compared with those without diabetes.[61] However, the relative risk for death, nonfatal MI, or rehospitalization with an ACS with routine invasive versus selective invasive strategies was similar between diabetic patients (RR, 0.87; 95% CI, 0.73 to 1.03) and nondiabetic patients (RR, 0.86; 95% CI, 0.70 to 1.06). In a more recent meta-analysis of eight RCTs and 5324 patients, the benefit in terms of mortality reduction of early invasive versus a delayed invasive strategy was more pronounced in patients with elevated cardiac biomarkers (HR 0.76, 95% CI 0.58 to 0.99), diabetes (HR 0.67, 95% CI 0.45 to 0.99), a Global Registry of Acute Coronary Events (GRACE) risk score more than 40 (HR 0.70, 95% CI 0.52 to 0.95), and those who were elderly (HR 0.65, 95% CI 0.45 to 0.93).[62]

The 2015 ESC guidelines on the management of non-ST ACS recommend an early invasive strategy for all diabetic patients who present with ACS.[63] The 2014 ACCF/AHA update for the management of patients with non–ST ACS considered diabetes as a criteria to favor an invasive strategy over a conservative one.[64]

DIABETES AND ST-ELEVATION MYOCARDIAL INFARCTION

Paralleling the observations for non-ST ACS, also in the setting of STEMI, diabetes is an independent predictor of morbidity and mortality. A retrospective study that evaluated admission glucose for 141,680 patients who presented with acute MI demonstrated an association between admission glucose levels and 30-day mortality in both diabetic and nondiabetic individuals.[65]

A retrospective analysis of a Swiss registry of 3565 diabetic and 15,531 nondiabetic patients hospitalized for STEMI showed that in-hospital mortality dramatically decreased from 19.9% in 1997 to 9.0% in 2010 among diabetic patients (P for trend < .001) (Fig. 3.12). However, mortality remained twice as high in diabetic patients compared with nondiabetic patients (12.1% vs. 6.1%, P < .001) and diabetes was identified as an independent predictor of mortality.[66] In terms of medical and revascularization strategies, the guidelines recommend that diabetic patients be managed the same as nondiabetic patients.[67]

Choice of Revascularization Modality in Patients With Acute Coronary Syndromes

Little contemporary data, and none randomized, are available on the safety and efficacy of PCI versus CABG in ACS. In STEMI, PCI is the treatment of choice and CABG is reserved for a minority of patients with PCI failure, major area of myocardium at risk, and/or complex multivessel disease that is not treatable percutaneously.[68] In non–ST ACS and ongoing myocardial ischemia, PCI is also clearly favored if the culprit lesion is accessible percutaneously. Conversely, in "stabilized" diabetic patients with advanced multivessel CAD, CABG may be a valuable option. Accordingly, a population-based registry of 2947 suggested that CABG was associated with a reduction of major adverse CV events at 30 days compared with PCI (OR 0.49, 95% CI 0.34 to 0.71).[69] Randomized data are needed to define the optimal revascularization modality for diabetic patients with "stabilized" non–ST ACS.

GLUCOSE-LOWERING THERAPY IN THE ACUTE PHASE OF ACUTE CORONARY SYNDROMES

In the Diabetes Mellitus, Insulin Glucose Infusion in Acute Myocardial Infarction 2 (DIGAMI 2) study, three glucose-lowering strategies were compared among 1253 diabetic patients with suspected acute MI: in group 1, acute insulin-glucose infusion was titrated to glucose levels for 24 hours, followed by insulin-based long-term glucose control; in group 2, insulin-glucose infusion was given for 24 hours, followed by standard glucose control; in group 3, routine metabolic management was undertaken according to local practice.[70] At 2 years, the mortality rates among the three groups were comparable and no significant differences in nonfatal MI or stroke were detected. Very recently, the 20-year follow-up of the DIGAMI 1 trial, which enrolled MI patients who presented with blood glucose concentrations higher than 11 mmol/L at hospital admission, showed that the median survival time was 7.0 years (interquartile range [IQR] 1.8 to 12.4) in the insulin-based intensified glycemic control group (n = 306) and 4.7 years (IQR 1.0 to 11.4) in the standard group (n = 314; HR, 0.83; 95% CI, 0.70 to 0.98).[71] The ESC guidelines recommend that in the setting of ACS, treatment of elevated blood glucose should avoid both hyperglycemia (>180 mg/dL) and hypoglycemia (<90 mg/dL).[7,63]

Long-Term Antidiabetic Therapy

For many years, the effect of lowering plasma glucose on major CV events in diabetic patients was far less defined than that of lowering blood pressure or treating dyslipidemia.[63] The Empagliflozin Cardiovascular Outcome Event Trial in Type 2 Diabetes Mellitus Patients-Removing Excess Glucose (EMPA-REG OUTCOME) trial showed that a glucose-lowering therapy with the sodium glucose cotransporter 2 (SGLT2) inhibitor empagliflozin reduced CV events—such as CV mortality, nonfatal MI, nonfatal stroke hospitalization for heart failure, and overall mortality—when given in addition to standard care in patients with diabetes at high CV risk.[72] The study was initially designed to assess the safety of empagliflozin, but prespecified in the design was the note that the superiority of empagliflozin would be tested if noninferiority was achieved. The primary composite outcome was CV death, MI, or stroke as analyzed in the pooled empagliflozin group versus the placebo group. The key secondary composite outcome was the primary outcome plus hospitalization for UA. The trial continued until a primary outcome occurred in at least 691 patients; the median duration of treatment was 2.6 years, and the median observation time was 3.1 years. The patient population had a mean age of 63 years and long-standing diabetes (>10 years in 57% of patients), and

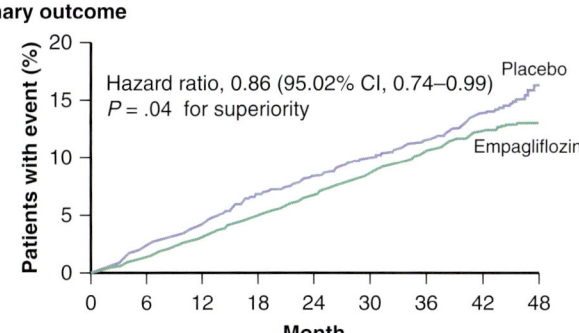
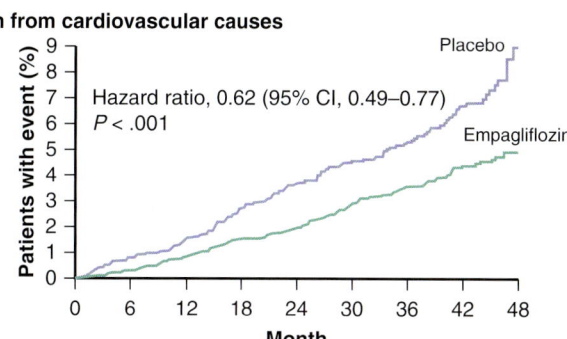
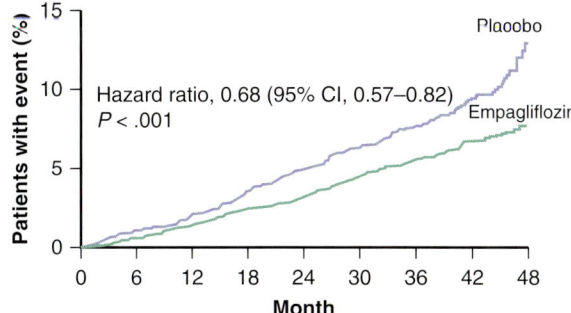
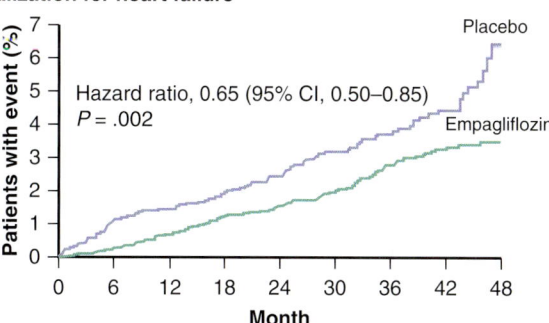

Fig. 3.13 Cardiovascular outcomes and death from any cause. Shown are (A) the cumulative incidence of the primary outcome (death from cardiovascular causes, nonfatal myocardial infarction, or nonfatal stroke), (D) the cumulative incidence of death from cardiovascular causes, (C) the Kaplan–Meier estimate for death from any cause, and (D) the cumulative incidence of hospitalization for heart failure. (From Zinman B, Wanner C, Lachin JM, et al. Empagliflozin, cardiovascular outcomes, and mortality in type 2 diabetes. *N Engl J Med.* 2015;373:2117–2128.)

more than 99% of patients had established CV disease. The primary end point occurred in 490 of 4687 patients (10.5%) in the empagliflozin arm (10- and 25-mg doses) and in 282 of 2333 patients (12.1%) in the placebo arm, resulting in a 14% relative risk reduction for the primary outcome (HR, 0.86; 95.02% CI, 0.74 to 0.99; $P < .001$ for superiority).[72] With no significant decrease in the relative risk of stroke or myocardial infarction, the CV event risk reduction was primarily driven by a 38% relative risk reduction in CV death (HR, 0.62; 95% CI, 0.49 to 0.77; $P < .001$). In addition, there was a 32% relative risk reduction in all-cause mortality (HR, 0.68; 95% CI, 0.57 to 0.82; $P < .001$) and a 35% relative risk reduction in the incidence of hospitalization for heart failure (HR, 0.65; 95% CI, 0.50 to 0.85; $P = .002$) (Fig. 3.13).

Another SGLT2 inhibitor, canagliflozin, was tested in the CANagliflozin cardioVascular Assessment Study (CANVAS) program integrating data from two trials involving 10,142 diabetic patients at high CV risk.[73] At baseline, 65.6% of the participants had a history of CV disease, the mean follow-up was 188.2 weeks, and the primary outcome was a composite of CV death, MI or stroke. The rate of primary outcome was lower with canagliflozin than with placebo (HR 0.86, 95% CI 0.75 to 0.97, $P < .001$ for noninferiority and $P = .02$ for superiority).[73]

Other trials currently ongoing are testing other glucose-lowering therapies (e.g., Dapagliflozin Effect on Cardiovascular Events [DECLARE-TIMI] for dapagliflozin, eValuation of ERTugliflozin effIcacy and Safety CardioVascular outcomes [VERTIS-CV] for ertugliflozin) in similar diabetic populations.[74]

Antithrombotic Therapy in Diabetes

Diabetes patients are characterized by enhanced platelet reactivity and a procoagulant state, which exposes them to an increased risk of atherothrombotic events.[8] Diabetic patients treated with antiplatelet agents such as aspirin and clopidogrel remain at higher risk of recurrent ischemic events in the setting of ACS and PCI. In part this may be related to a reduced responsiveness or resistance, defined as the failure of an antiplatelet agent to adequately block its specific target on the platelet (i.e., the cyclooxygenase 1 [COX-1] receptor for aspirin and the $P2Y_{12}$ receptor for clopidogrel).

Whereas data on the prevalence of aspirin resistance and its impact on CV outcomes in diabetic patients are sparse, most of the evidence supports the notion that inadequate response to clopidogrel in this patient population is more prevalent, both after a loading dose and at a maintenance dose, than in nondiabetic individuals.[75] Platelet reactivity on dual-antiplatelet therapy was found to be particularly elevated in diabetic individuals treated with insulin.[76] This may also explain why studies with first-generation DESs have repeatedly identified diabetes, and especially its insulin-requiring form, as an independent predictor of stent thrombosis (see Fig. 3.5).

ASPIRIN AND CLOPIDOGREL

Although the value of aspirin in a dose ranging from 75 to 325 mg/day as secondary prevention among diabetic patients has been well established, the benefit of aspirin in primary prevention is less well documented. The optimal antiplatelet therapy in the primary prevention of CV disease in patients with diabetes has still not been established. Based on available data, aspirin produces a modest reduction of ischemic events in the diabetic population; accordingly, the 2013 ESC guidelines on diabetes do not recommend antiplatelet therapy with aspirin in patients with diabetes who are at low risk by primary prevention of CV disease (class III, level of evidence A).[7]

The Clopidogrel for High Atherothrombotic Risk and Ischemic Stabilization, Management, and Avoidance (CHARISMA) trial investigated the safety and efficacy of long-term administration of aspirin (75 to 162 mg/day) and clopidogrel (75 mg/day) in comparison with aspirin alone in patients with established atherosclerotic disease or with multiple CV risk factors.[77] In the large diabetic population enrolled (n = 6556), mainly a primary prevention cohort, no benefit of the combination therapy was observed after a median follow-up of 28 months, and the bleeding rate increased. The Clopidogrel in Unstable Angina to Prevent Recurrent Events (CURE) trial randomized patients with ACS who were primarily managed medically to aspirin or aspirin and clopidogrel for 9 to 12 months. Diabetic patients (n = 2840) did not derive a significant benefit from the combined treatment.[78]

PRASUGREL AND TICAGRELOR

Prasugrel is a third-generation thienopyridine that inhibits the $P2Y_{12}$ receptor more rapidly and more consistently (i.e., with smaller individual variation) than standard and higher doses of clopidogrel, which is also true in diabetic individuals.[79] These properties may be particularly important for diabetic patients based on frequently encountered resistance to clopidogrel. The Trial to Assess Improvement in Therapeutic Outcomes by Optimizing Platelet Inhibition With Prasugrel–Thrombolysis in Myocardial Infarction (TRITON-TIMI 38) randomized 13,608 subjects with ACS (both STEMI and non-ST ACS) to clopidogrel or prasugrel for 6 to 15 months.[80] Among them, 3146 subjects had diabetes, and 776 were treated with insulin on admission. The primary end point—a composite of CV death, MI, or stroke—was significantly reduced with prasugrel among subjects without diabetes as well as those with diabetes (9.2% vs. 10.6%, HR 0.86, P = .02 for nondiabetic patients and 12.2% vs. 17.0%, HR 0.70, P < .001 for their diabetic counterparts) (Fig. 3.14). The beneficial effect of prasugrel was observed among diabetic subjects treated with insulin (14.3% vs. 22.2%, HR 0.63, P = .009) and those on oral hypoglycemic drugs (11.5% vs. 15.3%, HR 0.74, P = .009). Nonfatal MI was reduced by 18% with prasugrel among subjects without diabetes (7.2% vs. 8.7%, P = .006) and by 40% among subjects with diabetes (8.2% vs. 13.2%, P < .001). In the interaction analyses for treatment benefit, diabetic status showed a trend (P = .09) for the primary end point and was significant (P = .02) for MI, suggesting a preferential benefit of prasugrel in the diabetic population. Although TIMI major bleeds were increased among subjects without diabetes on prasugrel (1.6% vs. 2.4%,

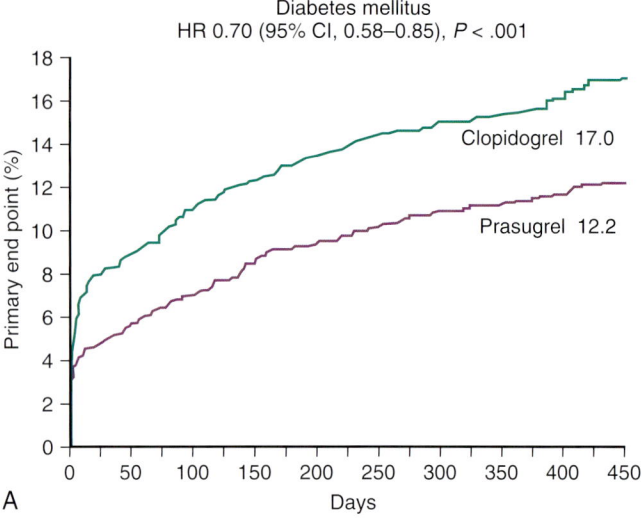

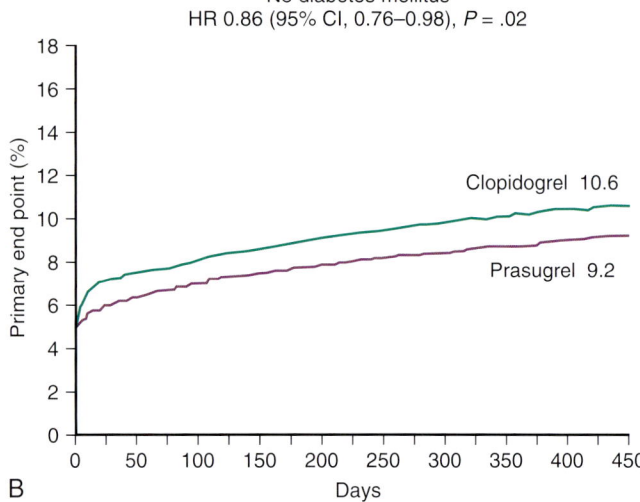

Fig. 3.14 Kaplan-Meier event-free survival curves; primary efficacy end point (cardiovascular death, nonfatal myocardial infarction, nonfatal stroke) stratified by diabetic status in the TRITON-TIMI 38 study. A greater clinical benefit of more intensive oral antiplatelet therapy with prasugrel was seen in patients with diabetes mellitus (A) compared to those with no diabetes mellitus (B). *CI*, Confidence interval. (From Wiviott SD, Braunwald E, Angiolillo DJ, et al. Greater clinical benefit of more intensive oral antiplatelet therapy with prasugrel in patients with diabetes mellitus in the trial to assess improvement in therapeutic outcomes by optimizing platelet inhibition with prasugrel-Thrombolysis in Myocardial Infarction 38. *Circulation.* 2008;118:1626–1636.)

HR 1.43, P = .02), the rates were similar among subjects with diabetes for clopidogrel and prasugrel (2.6% vs. 2.5%). Net clinical benefit with prasugrel was greater for diabetic patients (14.6% vs. 19.2%, HR 0.74, P = .001) than for nondiabetic individuals (11.5% vs. 12.3%, HR 0.92, P = .16; P interaction [P_{int}] = .05). Finally, the rate of stent thrombosis, both in the overall population and in the diabetic population, was significantly reduced by the allocation to prasugrel (0.9% vs. 2.0% and 2.0% vs. 3.5%, respectively).

Ticagrelor is an oral, reversibly binding $P2Y_{12}$ inhibitor with a plasma half-life of 6 to 12 hours. Like prasugrel, ticagrelor has a more rapid and consistent onset of action compared with clopidogrel, but it also has a faster offset of action with more rapid recovery of platelet function.[81] In the Platelet Inhibition

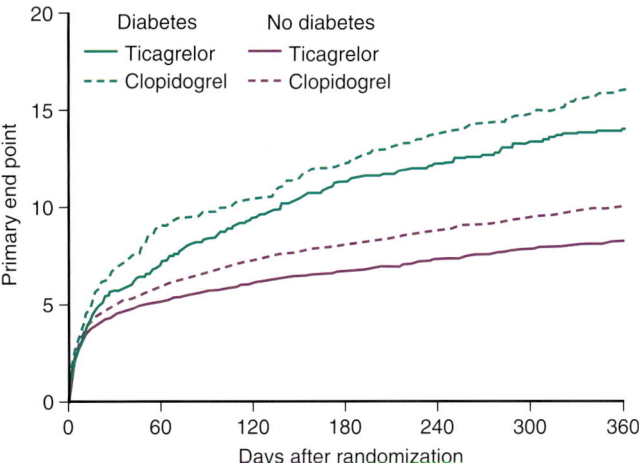

Fig. 3.15 Cumulative incidence of the primary composite of cardiovascular death, myocardial infarction, and stroke in the PLATO trial. Randomization was to ticagrelor (solid lines) or clopidogrel (dotted lines) and the presence (green lines) or absence (purple lines) of diabetes. (From James S, Angiolillo DJ, Cornel JH, et al. Ticagrelor vs. clopidogrel in patients with acute coronary syndromes and diabetes: a substudy from the PLATelet inhibition and patient Outcomes [PLATO] trial. *Eur Heart J.* 2010;31:3006–3016.)

and Patient Outcomes (PLATO) trial, ticagrelor reduced the primary composite end point of CV death, MI, or stroke but with similar rates of major bleeding compared with clopidogrel in 18,624 patients with ACS (both STEMI and non-ST ACS).[82,83]

In diabetic patients (n = 4662), including 1036 patients on insulin, the reduction in the primary composite end point (HR, 0.88; 95% CI, 0.76 to 1.03 [Fig. 3.15], all-cause mortality [HR, 0.82; 95% CI, 0.66 to 1.01], and stent thrombosis [HR, 0.65; 95% CI, 0.36 to 1.17] and no increase in major bleeding [HR, 0.95; 95% CI, 0.81 to 1.12]) with ticagrelor was consistent with the overall cohort and without significant diabetes status-by-treatment interactions.[83]

No heterogeneity in treatment efficacy was found among patients with or without ongoing insulin treatment. Because of the differences in protocols and populations enrolled in the TRITON-TIMI 38 and the PLATO studies, no comparisons with respect to safety or efficacy of the two molecules in diabetic patients can be made at this time. The 2015 ESC non-ST ACS guidelines recommended the newer $P2Y_{12}$ inhibitors as first choice of antiplatelet therapy.[63]

GLYCOPROTEIN IIB/IIIA RECEPTOR ANTAGONISTS AND ANTICOAGULANTS

In the pre–clopidogrel-loading era, the use of intravenous platelet glycoprotein (GP) IIb/IIIa receptor inhibitors and stents markedly reduced both the early hazard and the 1-year mortality in diabetic patients undergoing PCI.[84,85] However, the introduction of clopidogrel, and especially of prasugrel and ticagrelor, has markedly reduced the indication for those agents. Accordingly, the value of GP IIb/IIIa in the era of potent $P2Y_{12}$ inhibition and of newer anticoagulants, such as bivalirudin, still needs to be defined. Because no trial has specifically addressed the value of different anticoagulants in the PCI/ACS setting in diabetic patients, the same recommendations as for the nondiabetic population are valuable. Anticoagulants of choice have included unfractionated heparin, enoxaparin, fondaparinux (with the addition of unfractionated heparin at the time of PCI), or bivalirudin.

LONG-TERM DIABETES MANAGEMENT

Adequate glycemic control remains of paramount importance in the management of diabetic patients. A meta-analysis of five RCTs that included 17,267 participants who received intensive glucose control and 15,362 who received conventional therapy showed a significant reduction in MI (OR, 0.86; 95% CI, 0.78 to 0.93) but not of stroke (OR, 0.93; 95% CI, 0.81 to 1.07) or CV mortality (OR, 0.98; 95% CI, 0.77 to 1.23).[86] Although hyperglycemia has been associated with CV disease and epidemiologic evidence links lower blood glucose levels to a decrease in CV events, the impact of optimal glycemic control on macrovascular events remains controversial—especially following the publication of three large long-term clinical studies of glucose control and macrovascular disease in patients with type 2 diabetes—the Action to Control Cardiovascular Risk in Diabetes (ACCORD), Action in Diabetes and Vascular Disease: Preterax and Diamicron Modified Release Controlled Evaluation (ADVANCE), and the Veterans Affairs Diabetes Trial (VADT).[87–89] Overall, these trials suggested no significant reduction in CV outcomes with intensive glycemic control in these populations. However, in the ACCORD study, an unexplained increase in all-cause mortality in the intensive glycemic control group was detected. Hypothesized mechanisms include hypoglycemia, weight gain, rapid lowering of HbA_{1c} level, and medication interactions.[90] All three trials were carried out in participants with established diabetes (mean duration 8 to 11 years) and either known CV disease or multiple risk factors suggesting the presence of established atherosclerosis. Subset analyses suggest that a possible benefit from intensive glycemic control on CV outcomes may be observed in patients with a shorter duration of disease, better glucose control, younger age, no previous CV event, or fewer CV risk factors at the time of initiation of the intensified glucose control regimen.

Overall, the evidence—including subset analyses of ACCORD, ADVANCE, and VADT—of a CV benefit of intensive glycemic control rests primarily on long-term follow-up of study cohorts treated early in the course of type 1 and type 2 diabetes. However, the mortality findings in ACCORD and subgroup analyses of VADT suggest that the risks of very aggressive glycemic control may outweigh its benefits in some patients, such as those with a very long duration of diabetes, known history of severe hypoglycemia, advanced atherosclerosis, and advanced age or frailty. Certainly care providers should be vigilant in preventing severe hypoglycemia in patients with advanced disease and should not aggressively attempt to achieve near-normal HbA_{1C} levels in patients in whom such a target cannot be reasonably achieved easily and safely.[91]

Glucose control in diabetic patients with CAD should be according to a patient-centered approach: the longer the duration of the disease, the older the patient, the more advanced the CAD, and the more important the comorbidities, the less stringent the glucose control should be (Fig. 3.16).[91]

MULTIFACTORIAL INTERVENTION

Aggressive CV risk-factor modification—including optimal glycemic control, cessation of cigarette smoking, control of blood pressure and cholesterol levels, and weight reduction as well as exercise—is an essential part of diabetes care. According to the 2013 ACC/AHA guidelines on cholesterol treatment, individuals with diabetes belong to a clinical category in which statin therapy is strongly recommended in primary prevention for low-density lipoprotein cholesterol (LDL-C) greater than 70 mg/dL.[10]

Furthermore, a high-intensity statin drug regimen should be considered in patients with diabetes and a risk of CV disease of 7.5% or more over 10 years. In secondary prevention, a statin drug is strongly recommended, as it is in those without diabetes. A recently published pooled data analysis from 5034 diabetic patients across the Clinical Outcomes Utilizing Revascularization and

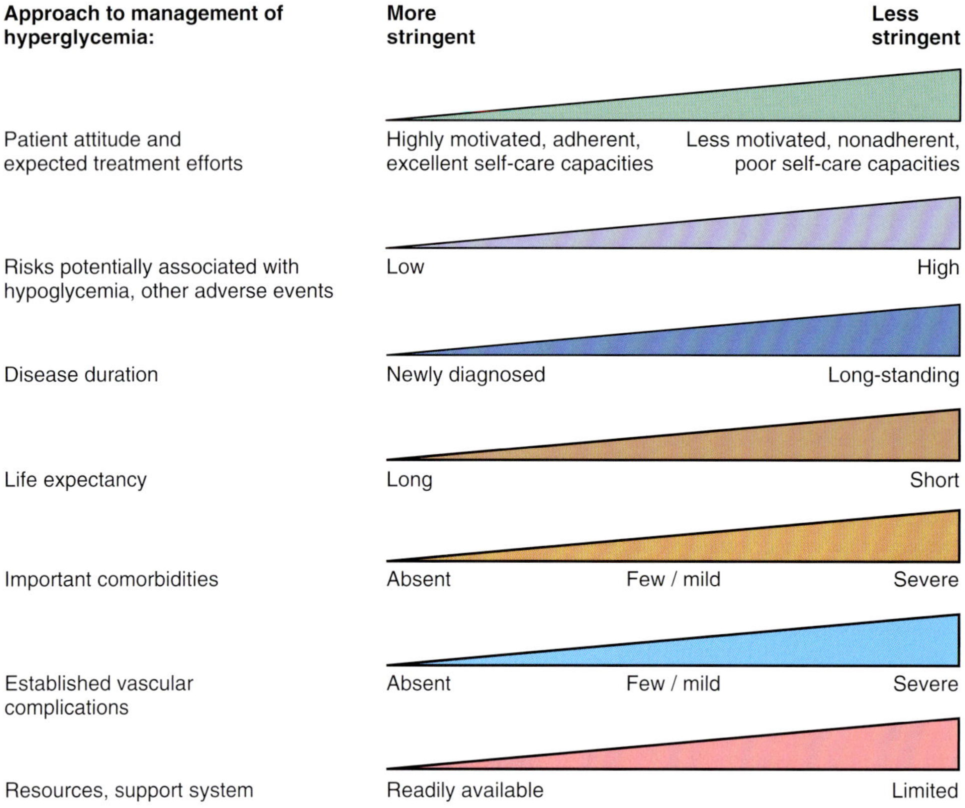

Approach to management of hyperglycemia:	More stringent	Less stringent
Patient attitude and expected treatment efforts	Highly motivated, adherent, excellent self-care capacities	Less motivated, nonadherent, poor self-care capacities
Risks potentially associated with hypoglycemia, other adverse events	Low	High
Disease duration	Newly diagnosed	Long-standing
Life expectancy	Long	Short
Important comorbidities	Absent · Few / mild · Severe	
Established vascular complications	Absent · Few / mild · Severe	
Resources, support system	Readily available	Limited

Fig. 3.16 Depiction of the elements of decision making used to determine appropriate efforts to achieve glycemic targets. Greater concerns about a particular domain are represented by the increasing height of the ramp. Thus characteristics/predicaments toward the left justify more stringent efforts to lower HbA_{1C}, whereas those toward the right are compatible with less stringent efforts. Where possible, such decisions should be made in conjunction with the patient, reflecting his or her preferences, needs, and values. (From Inzucchi SE, Bergenstal RM, Buse JB, et al. Management of hyperglycemia in type 2 diabetes: a patient-centered approach: position statement of the American Diabetes Association [ADA] and the European Association for the Study of Diabetes [EASD]. *Diabetes Care*. 2012;35:1364–1379.)

Aggressive Drug Evaluation (COURAGE), BARI 2D, and FREEDOM studies showed that a significant proportion of patients with CAD did not reach recommended secondary prevention targets: only 18% of the COURAGE patients with diabetes, 23% of the participants in BARI 2D, and 8% of patients with diabetes in the FREEDOM study had a combined achievement for systolic blood pressure, LDL-C, smoking cessation, and HbA_{1C} at 1 year of follow-up.[92] The ESC guidelines on diabetes made a strong recommendation for lifestyle modifications for the prevention of diabetes, such as smoking cessation, dietary counseling, an increased daily fiber intake, control of total and saturated fat intake, and moderate to vigorous physical activity of 150 minutes or more per week, including aerobic exercise and resistance training.[7]

KEY REFERENCES

7. Ryden L, Grant PJ, Anker SD, et al. ESC guidelines on diabetes, pre-diabetes, and cardiovascular diseases developed in collaboration with the EASD: the task force on diabetes, pre-diabetes, and cardiovascular diseases of the European Society of Cardiology (ESC) and developed in collaboration with the European Association for the Study of Diabetes (EASD). *Eur Heart J*. 2013;34:3035–3087.
30. Stettler C, Allemann S, Wandel S, et al. Drug eluting and bare metal stents in people with and without diabetes: collaborative network meta-analysis. *BMJ*. 2008;337:a1331.
31. Bangalore S, Kumar S, Fusaro M, et al. Outcomes with various drug eluting or bare metal stents in patients with diabetes mellitus: mixed treatment comparison analysis of 22,844 patient years of follow-up from randomised trials. *BMJ*. 2012;345:e5170.
36. Windecker S, Kolh P, Alfonso F, et al. 2014 ESC/EACTS Guidelines on myocardial revascularization: the task force on myocardial revascularization of the European Society of Cardiology (ESC) and the European Association for Cardio-Thoracic Surgery (EACTS) developed with the special contribution of the European Association of Percutaneous Cardiovascular Interventions (EAPCI). *Eur Heart J*. 2014;35:2541–2619.
47. Frye RL, August P, Brooks MM, et al. A randomized trial of therapies for type 2 diabetes and coronary artery disease. *N Engl J Med*. 2009;360:2503–2515.
53. Farkouh ME, Domanski M, Sleeper LA, et al. Strategies for multivessel revascularization in patients with diabetes. *N Engl J Med*. 2012;367:2375–2384.
54. Bangalore S, Toklu B, Feit F. Outcomes with coronary artery bypass graft surgery versus percutaneous coronary intervention for patients with diabetes mellitus: can newer generation drug-eluting stents bridge the gap? *Circ Cardiovasc Interv*. 2014;7:518–525.
55. Head SJ, Milojevic M, Daemen J, et al. Mortality after coronary artery bypass grafting versus percutaneous coronary intervention with stenting for coronary artery disease: a pooled analysis of individual patient data. *Lancet*. 2018;391:939–948.
58. Bartnik M, Ryden L, Ferrari R, et al. The prevalence of abnormal glucose regulation in patients with coronary artery disease across Europe. The Euro Heart Survey on diabetes and the heart. *Eur Heart J*. 2004;25:1880–1890.
61. O'Donoghue ML, Vaidya A, Afsal R, et al. An invasive or conservative strategy in patients with diabetes mellitus and non-ST-segment elevation acute coronary syndromes: a collaborative meta-analysis of randomized trials. *J Am Coll Cardiol*. 2012;60:106–111.
62. Jobs A, Mehta SR, Montalescot G, et al. Optimal timing of an invasive strategy in patients with non-ST-elevation acute coronary syndrome: a meta-analysis of randomised trials. *Lancet*. 2017;390:737–746.
63. Roffi M, Patrono C, Collet JP, et al. 2015 ESC Guidelines for the management of acute coronary syndromes in patients presenting without persistent ST-segment elevation: task force for the management of acute coronary syndromes in patients presenting without persistent ST-segment elevation of the European Society of Cardiology (ESC). *Eur Heart J*. 2016;37:267–315.
72. Zinman B, Wanner C, Lachin JM, et al. Empagliflozin, cardiovascular outcomes, and mortality in type 2 diabetes. *N Engl J Med*. 2015;373:2117–2128.
73. Neal B, Perkovic V, Mahaffey KW, et al. Canagliflozin and cardiovascular and renal events in type 2 diabetes. *N Engl J Med*. 2017;377:644–657.
92. Farkouh ME, Boden WE, Bittner V, et al. Risk factor control for coronary artery disease secondary prevention in large randomized trials. *J Am Coll Cardiol*. 2013;61:1607–1615.

 Additional references available online at expertconsult.com.

中文导读

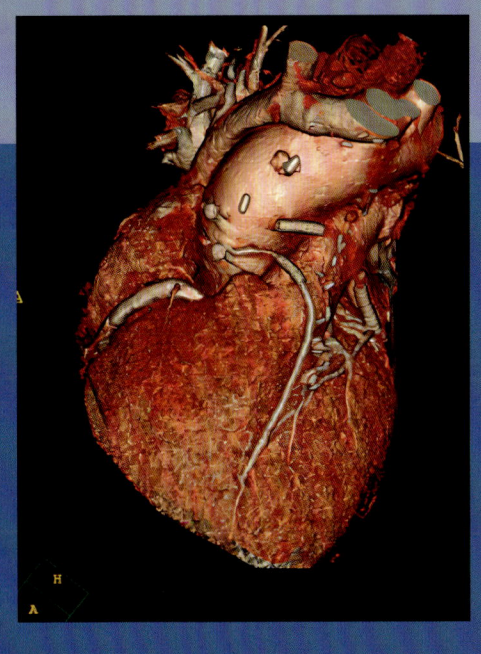

第4章
无创性评估：
功能学检查、多排CT和负荷心脏MRI

　　对已知或疑似冠心病患者进行心肌缺血相关无创性检查，其目的一方面是为了明确病因，另一方面也是为了评价患者的临床预后，尤其是有助于判断哪些患者能从药物治疗和（或）心肌血运重建治疗中获益，从而指导临床治疗决策。因此，无创性心脏影像学检查在临床实践中具有极其广泛的应用价值。

　　无创性心脏影像学检查包括无创性功能学检查和无创性解剖学检查。负荷心动图、负荷超声心动图、负荷闪烁法心肌灌注成像等这些无创性功能学检查是基于电异常、机械异常或灌注异常来对心肌缺血程度进行定量分析。心脏MRI灌注成像根据钆延迟增强，可用来识别瘢痕心肌、非存活心肌。而冠状动脉CT血管造影作为一种无创性解剖学检查方法，已经成为替代有创造影的一种评价方式，可用来直接评价冠状动脉血管解剖条件。一般而言，无创性解剖学检查方法在诊断冠心病方面具有很高的敏感性，而无创性功能学检查方法对于血运重建获益方面具有更高的预测价值。在临床实践中，临床医师需根据患者症状、冠心病患病危险分层、心电图，以及活动耐量情况、医院/医师经验等加以选择。

　　本章节分门别类地对现有的无创性心脏影像学检查方法及临床意义作了概括介绍。通过本章节的介绍，将有助于这些检查方法在临床中得到合理的使用。

梁敬轩　柳景华

章节要点

- 功能学检查如负荷心电图、负荷超声心动图和负荷核素灌注显像对于检测解剖性冠心病的准确度有限，但可提供重要的预后信息。
- 包括运动超声心动图和心肌灌注成像在内的功能学检查，其结果正常提示心脏事件发生风险极低。而负荷诱导的节段性室壁运动异常或灌注异常，其异常范围的大小有助于明确血运重建获益更大的人群，也有助于确定心血管事件风险增加的水平。
- 正电子发射断层显像是识别存活心肌最灵敏的方法之一。通过心脏MRI灌注成像检测钆延迟增强，这是识别瘢痕心肌、非存活心肌最灵敏的方法。
- 一项冠状动脉CT血管造影研究显示未发现冠状动脉钙化或狭窄，这几乎可排除冠心病。
- 各种影像学方法的合理使用取决于患者患病的可能性、医师个人偏好，以及医院影像学检查经验。
- 当医患双方根据当地医院条件和患者特定因素选择一种无创性检查方法时，ACC/AHA指南可为医患个体提供一个切实可行的实践标准，同时也能推动这些检查方法在大众人群中得到合理使用。

4 Noninvasive Evaluation: Functional Testing, Multidetector Computed Tomography, and Stress Cardiac MRI

Vikram M. Brahmanandam, Mario J. Garcia

KEY POINTS

- Functional tests such as stress electrocardiography (ECG), stress echocardiography, and stress nuclear perfusion imaging have limited accuracy for the detection of anatomic coronary artery disease but provide important prognostic information.
- Normal functional testing, including exercise echocardiography and myocardial perfusion imaging (MPI), is associated with a low risk of cardiac events. The extent of stress-induced segmental wall motion and perfusion abnormalities helps to define which populations of patients will benefit most from revascularization and their incremental levels of risk.
- Positron emission tomography (PET) is one of the most sensitive methods for the identification of viable myocardium. The detection of gadolinium-delayed enhancement by cardiac magnetic resonance (CMR) perfusion imaging is the most sensitive method for identifying scarred, nonviable myocardium.
- A coronary computed tomography angiogram (CCTA) study that shows no coronary calcification or stenosis virtually excludes the presence of coronary artery disease (CAD).
- Appropriate use of various imaging modalities depends on patient probability of disease, physician preference, and local imaging experience.
- American College of Cardiology/American Heart Association guidelines are intended to provide a practical standard to individual clinicians and patients when considering one of these procedures, based on any number of important local and patient-specific variables, while promoting optimal test utilization for the population at large.

Noninvasive testing for myocardial ischemia in patients with known or suspected coronary artery disease (CAD) is conducted to establish the diagnosis of obstructive coronary atherosclerosis as the cause of symptoms, and to determine whether a patient would benefit from medical therapy and/or myocardial revascularization. Functional tests, such as stress electrocardiography (ECG), stress echocardiography, and stress scintigraphic myocardial perfusion imaging (MPI), attempt to quantify the degree of ischemia based on electrical, mechanical, and perfusion abnormalities. Over the last decade, coronary computed tomography angiogram (CCTA) has evolved as a noninvasive alternative to invasive coronary angiography for the direct evaluation of coronary anatomy. In general, anatomic tests, such as CCTA, have greater sensitivity for the detection of CAD, whereas functional tests have a greater ability to predict benefit from revascularization. This chapter provides an overview of the methodology and interpretation of these tests with the main objective of providing guidelines for appropriate test selection and treatment.

STRESS TESTING

Angina in patients with obstructive CAD is caused by an imbalance between myocardial oxygen supply and demand. Asymptomatic patients with CAD have normal resting blood flow even in the presence of epicardial coronary artery stenosis as myocardial perfusion pressure and blood flow are maintained by compensatory dilation of the coronary arterioles. During stress, myocardial oxygen demand increases but myocardial blood flow does not increase proportionally, which leads to ischemia. The progressive metabolic and functional alterations that occur during ischemia, including electrical repolarization abnormalities and abnormal regional diastolic and systolic myocardial function, can be assessed by noninvasive testing. Stress may be accomplished by a number of methods that most commonly include exercise or pharmacologic agents. Whenever possible, exercise is the preferred stressor as the physiologic data obtained provides an assessment of a patient's functional status, and provides valuable prognostic information. The choice between ECG, echocardiography, or MPI is often determined by local availability, costs, and individual patient characteristics. In general, specificity has been reported to be higher with stress echocardiography, and sensitivity is higher with MPI. Accordingly, many clinicians prefer stress echocardiography for individuals with a lower pretest probability of obstructive CAD, and MPI for those with a higher probability. Although exercise ECG has lower sensitivity and specificity than stress imaging modalities, it is cost effective and provides comparable prognostic information in patients who have a normal resting ECG and are able to exercise. One disadvantage of exercise ECG is that it cannot localize ischemia, which renders it less useful as a guide for targeting revascularization. Stress cardiac magnetic resonance (CMR) perfusion imaging provides both perfusion and wall motion information with accuracy comparable to stress MPI in addition to myocardial viability, and it is growing in use. Exercise and dobutamine stress CMR are also in clinical use, but are less common outside of larger centers. Over the last two decades, the prognostic utility of stress testing has been increasingly recognized. Exercise physiologic parameters, ECG abnormalities, and imaging findings including wall motion and perfusion abnormalities are powerful predictors of outcome.

Exercise Stress Testing

Monitoring physiologic parameters during exercise such as heart rate, blood pressure, ventilatory capacity, and estimates of oxygen utilization help to define a patient's functional capacity and to objectively evaluate for limiting clinical symptoms including angina and dyspnea. One of the most important parameters to evaluate is the metabolic equivalents (METs) achieved, which refers to oxygen uptake during activity; 1 MET is equivalent to 3.5 mL O_2/kg/min of body weight and activities are estimated in multiples of METS. If a patient is able to jog at greater than 6 mph on level terrain, which would be approximately 10 METS, 20-year survival rates are significantly better than a patient who can only walk at 3 mph (3 METS).[1] If exercise capacity is known to be excellent, this information may obviate the need for further data collection such as ECG and imaging tests. Patients with chronotropic incompetence during exercise stress testing also have worse outcomes independent of other factors. Chronotropic incompetence may be a marker of impaired autonomic dysfunction, which has been associated with angiographic severity of CAD and increased mortality. Heart rate recovery, calculated as the difference in heart rate at peak exercise versus 1 minute into recovery, is another index that is related to autonomic tone. A value below 12 beats/min (bpm) is considered abnormal. Patients evaluated for suspected or known CAD with an abnormal heart rate recovery have a markedly increased mortality rate independent of other risk factors.[2] Although both impaired chronotropic response and heart rate recovery are powerful predictors of outcomes, it is unknown whether they are modifiable. Moreover, their association with mortality may be independent of the presence or severity of CAD.

Electrocardiography Stress Testing

Detection of ischemia by ECG stress testing relies on the development of abnormal repolarization that manifests as ST-segment depression during or immediately after exercise. Exercise ECG testing has modest diagnostic accuracy but remains a useful prognostic test. An index derived from the exercise ECG test that incorporates exercise time, magnitude of ST-segment deviation, and angina—known as the *Duke treadmill score*—has proven to be a powerful prognosticator of events. Exercise time is measured based on the Bruce protocol and appears to be the most important determinant of prognosis.[3] The 5-year survival rates among patients categorized as low, intermediate, and high risk were initially reported at 97%, 91%, and 72%, respectively.

Stress Echocardiography

The interpretation of stress echocardiography is based on the identification of regional wall motion abnormalities induced by ischemia in the presence of obstructive CAD. The test has gained increasing acceptance following the introduction of digital acquisition, harmonic imaging, and contrast agents, all of which have incrementally contributed to improved image quality, reproducibility, and accuracy. In stress echocardiography, regional wall motion is assessed from parasternal and apical images using a 17-segment model of the left ventricle (LV).[4] Each segment is described as either normal, hypokinetic, akinetic, or dyskinetic, and the results of the individual segments are averaged to calculate a global wall motion score. The diagnosis of CAD is based on the detection of either resting or stress-induced regional wall motion abnormalities (Figs. 4.1–4.3). In most cases, a *resting* regional wall motion abnormality implies a prior myocardial infarction (MI), whereas a *stress-induced* regional wall motion abnormality implies ischemia caused by obstructive CAD.

Exercise Echocardiography

Exercise stress may be performed with a treadmill, a supine or prone bicycle, and even arm ergometry. Treadmill stress echocardiography is by far the most commonly used modality in the United States. Both treadmill and bicycle ergometry allow the evaluation of important functional data such as exercise capacity, blood pressure response, hemodynamic responses to exercise (including the assessment of cardiac output and pulmonary pressures), and standard ECG ST-segment analysis. Several studies have reported sensitivities that range from 71% to 97% and specificities ranging from 64% to over 90%. The sensitivity of exercise echocardiography is lower for the detection of single-vessel CAD, in particular in the circumflex coronary artery distribution. Quite often, ischemia is only detected in the territory supplied by the most stenotic vessel in those patients with multivessel disease, especially if the test is discontinued at a submaximal workload typically defined as achieving less than 85% of the age-predicted maximum heart rate.

Of note, resting and/or exercise-induced wall motion abnormalities may occur in patients with cardiomyopathies, microvascular coronary disease, severe hypertension (increased afterload), or valvular disease, and they are often a cause of false positive interpretations. Several stress echocardiographic variables have important prognostic value in patients with known or suspected CAD. A low exercise wall motion score or a fall in exercise ejection fraction is highly predictive of an increased risk of adverse cardiac events. The rate of cardiac events in individuals with a normal exercise echocardiogram has been reported in several studies to be less than 1% per year. Videos 4.1–4.12 are an example of a typical exercise stress echocardiogram with resting, peak stress, and recovery views of the left ventricle from the long-axis, apical four-chamber (AP4), and apical three-chamber (AP3) views, suggestive of left main coronary artery disease or multivessel disease with corresponding coronary angiograms revealing diffuse coronary artery disease with a significant left main lesion.

Pharmacologic Stress Echocardiography

Intravenous (IV) dobutamine, dipyridamole, or adenosine may be used as pharmacologic stressors with echocardiography. Dobutamine is the most commonly used stressor in the United States. It is administered by continuous infusion at incremental rates starting from 5 up to 50 µg/kg/min. It is often complemented by handgrip exercise and/or IV atropine (0.5 to 2.0 mg) to increase the heart rate. Dobutamine increases myocardial oxygen demand by increasing contractility and the heart rate. The reported sensitivity and specificity of dobutamine echocardiography for the detection of obstructive CAD are equivalent to those reported for exercise echocardiography. The sensitivity is reduced in patients with concentric hypertrophy who experience cavity obliteration early during the test, as well as in those who do not achieve the target heart rate. Echocardiographic variables obtained during pharmacologic stress have also been shown to have significant prognostic value.[5] A normal dobutamine stress echocardiogram is associated with a low cardiac event rate while the presence of stress-induced regional wall motion abnormalities, particularly when detected at low heart rates, is a strong predictor of cardiac events. Low dose dobutamine stress echocardiography may be performed for risk assessment in patients after MI. In this setting, extensive resting regional wall motion abnormalities, stress-induced ischemia, absence of viability, and worsening LV ejection fraction (LVEF) with stress are associated with an increased risk of adverse events.

CONTRAST PERFUSION IMAGING

Adenosine and dipyridamole are used in many centers in Europe and South America, and they induce ischemia by creating a coronary steal in the setting of obstructive CAD, which can be assessed with the use of contrast agents. These agents consist of inert perfluorocarbon gases encapsulated in a biodegradable

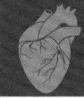

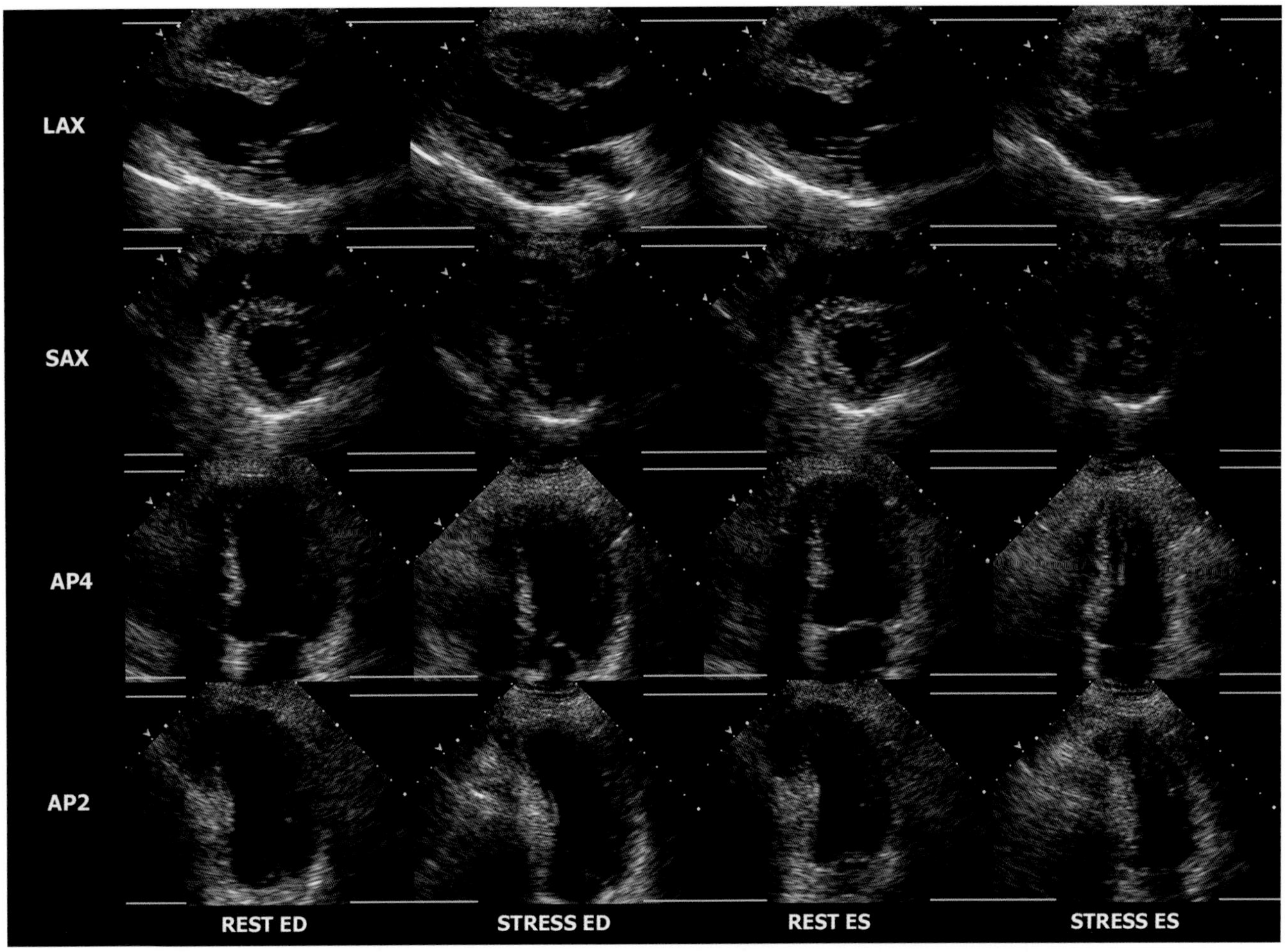

Fig. 4.1 Normal stress echo. Images obtained at end diastole *(ED)* and end systole *(ES)* at rest and immediately after exercise stress from the parasternal long-axis *(LAX)*, short-axis *(SAX)*, and apical four-chamber *(AP4)* and two-chamber *(AP2)* windows. Notice the decrease in end-systolic left ventricle cavity size after stress.

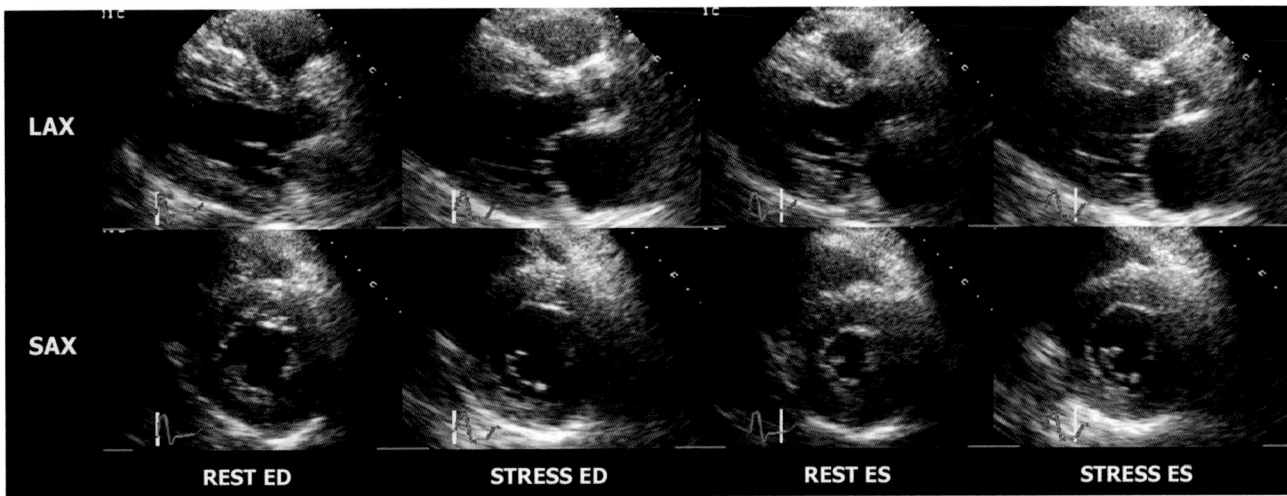

Fig. 4.2 Abnormal stress echo in a patient with severe multivessel coronary artery disease. Images obtained at end diastole *(ED)* and end systole *(ES)* at rest and immediately after exercise stress from the long-axis *(LAX)* and short-axis *(SAX)* windows. Notice the end-systolic dilatation of the left ventricle cavity.

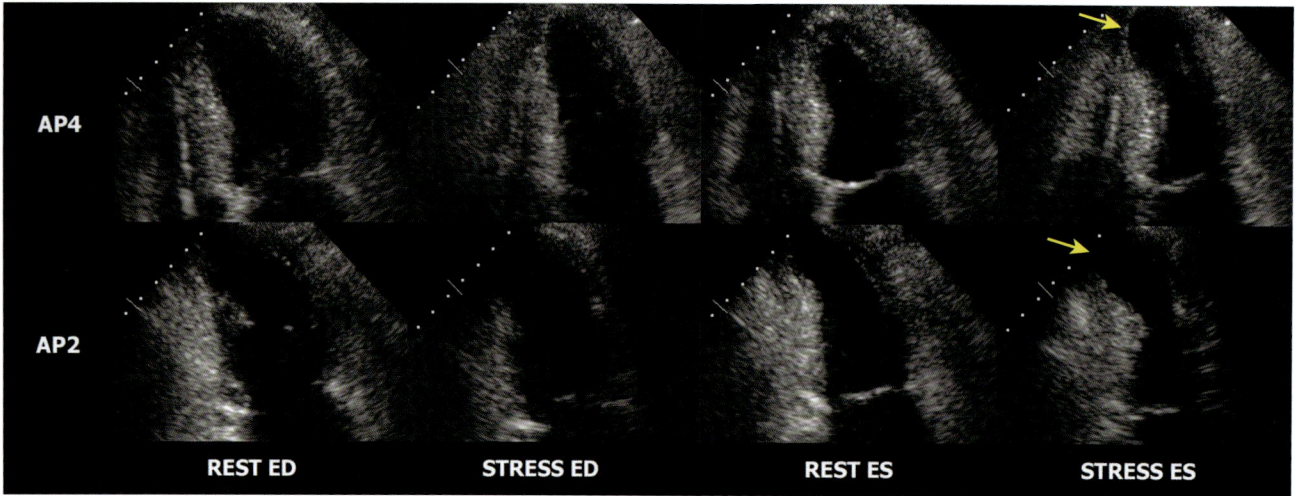

Fig. 4.3 Abnormal stress echo in a patient with severe stenosis of the mid–left anterior descending coronary artery. Images obtained at end diastole (ED) and end systole (ES) at rest and immediately after exercise stress from the apical four-chamber (AP4) and apical two-chamber (AP2) windows. Notice the relative end-systolic dilatation of the left ventricle apical segments (arrows).

shell, which remain as microbubbles when injected. The microbubbles have a small enough diameter (<10 μm) to cross the pulmonary capillary bed and enter the systemic circulation. When they are exposed to ultrasound, they act as strong reflectors and allow better endocardial border visualization in addition to an assessment of myocardial perfusion. As the LV myocardium has a dense capillary bed, the injection of contrast microbubbles results in myocardial enhancement proportional to the myocardial blood volume allowing for myocardial contrast echocardiography (MCE) to be clinical useful. During vasodilator stress in the presence of a flow-limiting coronary stenosis, capillary blood flow and myocardial blood volume is reduced in the segments supplied by the stenotic vessel. This may be detected as either a delay in myocardial enhancement following contrast injection or a relative reduction in enhancement in ischemic compared with normal segments (Fig. 4.4).

Although early studies demonstrated excellent sensitivity and specificity for MCE,[6,7] subsequent multicenter trials did not. The first of these demonstrated a sensitivity that ranged from 63% to 75% for MCE versus 63% to 76% for single-photon emission computed tomography (SPECT) and specificity of 47% to 59% for MCE versus 53% to 76% for SPECT.[8] The real-time assessment of myocardial perfusion (RAMP-1 and RAMP-2) trials studied a total of 662 patients and compared MCE to SPECT using coronary angiography as the gold standard. The overall accuracy of MCE was 66% to 71%, and it was noninferior to SPECT, with sensitivity that ranged from 50% to 77% and specificity that ranged from 55% to 88%.[9] The largest multicenter trial to date enrolled 628 patients, comparing MCE with SPECT again with coronary angiography as the gold standard. Higher sensitivity was obtained with MCE than with SPECT (75.2% vs. 49.1%), but specificity was lower (52.4% vs. 80.6%) for coronary stenosis of 70% or greater. Sensitivity for the detection of single-vessel disease and proximal disease with 70% or greater stenosis was higher for MCE, which may, in part, be due to the higher sensitivity of contrast echocardiography for the detection of microvascular abnormalities. These studies suggest that MCE demonstrates superior sensitivity but lower specificity for the detection of CAD compared with SPECT in a population with a high incidence of cardiovascular (CV) risk factors and intermediate to high prevalence of CAD.[10]

Stress Scintigraphic Myocardial Perfusion Imaging

The assessment of MPI by nuclear scintigraphic methods relies on the administration of a radionuclide isotope that accumulates in the myocardium in proportion to myocardial blood flow during rest and stress. MPI is performed with either single-photon–emitting or dual-photon–emitting isotopes using SPECT or positron emission tomography (PET). Thallium-201, technetium-99m sestamibi, and technetium-99m tetrofosmin are isotopes commercially available for SPECT imaging. Currently, technetium-99m–based isotopes are preferred for their higher photon energy, which results in higher image quality, and their shorter half-life, which results in lower radiation exposure. In the past few years, there have been substantial advances in gamma camera technology. New SPECT systems replace the traditional Anger camera with individual cesium iodide (CsI) scintillation crystals coupled to solid-state photodiodes or novel semiconductor-based detectors using cadmium–zinc telluride (CZT). They eliminate the need for conventional crystal and photomultiplier tubes by directly converting gamma radiation to an electronic pulse. CZT systems are significantly smaller than the traditional sodium iodide detectors and have shown improved efficiency, which makes it possible to obtain higher counts, thus improving signal-to-noise ratio and spatial resolution without increasing isotope dose or acquisition time. The most obvious direct benefit to patients is reduced radiation exposure without a sacrifice in image quality or an increase in acquisition time. Several studies have been performed to compare these new solid-state cameras to those acquired by conventional gamma cameras. All of them found comparable MPI quality with the benefit of significantly shorter image acquisition times. Some of these studies also evaluated LVEF and volumes and reported similar results between the two.[11–17]

PET imaging systems rely on the simultaneous detection of a pair of photons traveling in opposite directions. These photons travel toward detectors positioned around the subject, where they interact, become absorbed, and thus produce an electrical signal. The detector signals are processed by specialized coincidence circuitry. If the difference in the time of arrival of these photons is less than a predetermined value (typically <10 ns), a signal is recorded. Unlike SPECT imaging, PET imaging does not require collimation. Thus, the efficiency of PET is several

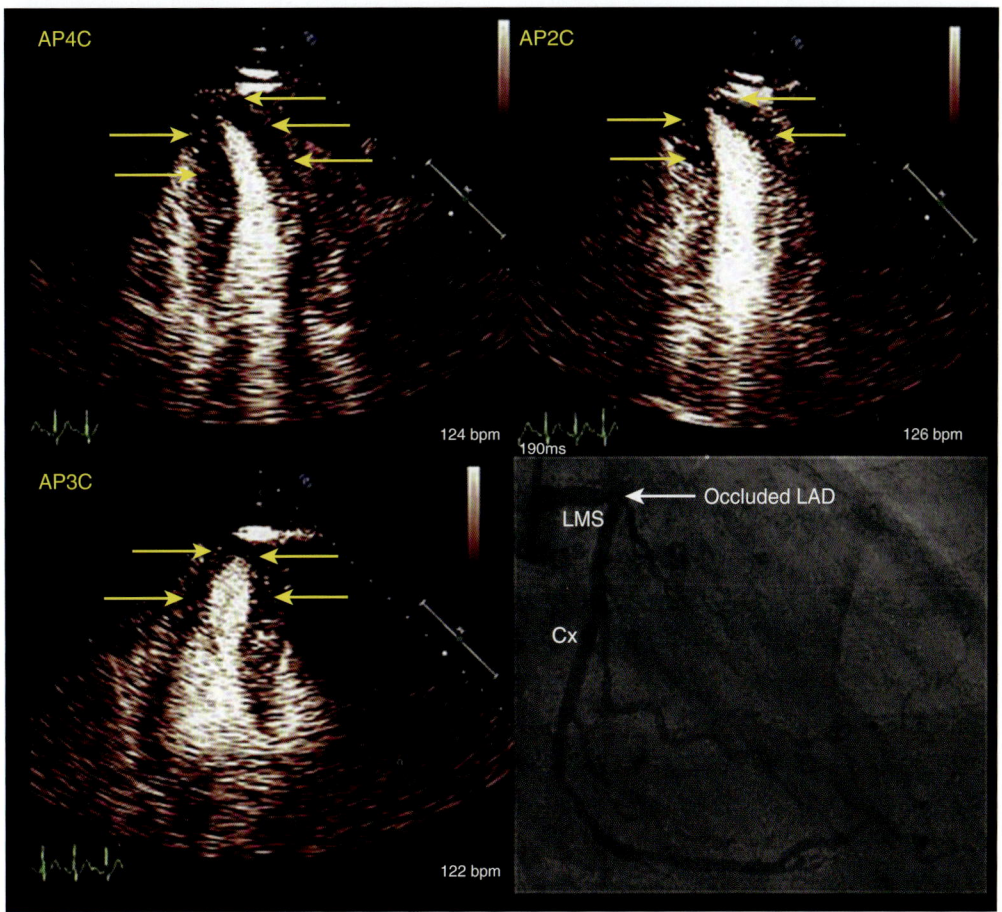

Fig. 4.4 A 56-year-old male smoker with hypertension who reported chest pain underwent standard echocardiography *(SE)* and myocardial contrast echocardiography *(MCE)*. SE showed a wall motion abnormality in only one segment (apical septum), but MCE revealed clear myocardium perfusion defects *(arrows)* in six segments in the apical four-chamber *(AP4C)*, apical two-chamber *(AP2C)*, and apical three-chamber *(AP3C)* views. Angiography *(bottom right)* revealed a completely occluded left anterior descending *(LAD)* coronary artery, which was successfully reopened. *Bpm,* Beats per minute; *Cx,* circumflex artery; *LMS,* left main stem. (From Shah BN, Chahal NS, Bhattacharyya S, et al. The feasibility and clinical utility of myocardial contrast echocardiography in clinical practice: results from the incorporation of myocardial perfusion assessment into clinical testing with stress echocardiography study. *J Am Soc Echocardiogr.* 2014;27[5]:520–530.)

magnitudes greater and provides higher resolution, lower noise, and lower radiation exposure.

With either SPECT or PET cardiac perfusion studies, images are obtained after stress and at rest. For segmentation of the left ventricle, a 17-segment model is applied. Images are interpreted visually or by using automated quantification based on normalized data. Myocardial scar is determined by the presence of a relative perfusion defect (compared with the segment with the highest counts), which persists on both stress and resting images. Ischemia is determined by the presence of a perfusion defect on stress images that improves or resolves on the resting images (Figs. 4.5–4.8).

Exercise Scintigraphic Myocardial Perfusion Imaging

Exercise stress is well suited for SPECT MPI. At peak exercise, either on a treadmill or bicycle ergometer, patients are injected with the radioisotope. Acquisition of the stress images is performed after a few minutes or up to 1 hour after exercise, depending on the radioisotope used. Resting images are obtained before or after the exercise images following the administration of a separate dose of the isotope at rest. Different isotopes may be used for resting and for stress imaging—for example, thallium-201 injected at rest and technetium-99m sestamibi injected at peak stress. The mean reported sensitivity and specificity for exercise SPECT is 86% and 74%.[18] However, most of the studies reported are potentially subject to verification bias. Accordingly, true sensitivity may be overestimated and specificity underestimated. Sensitivity and specificity are higher for the detection of multivessel disease, followed by single-vessel disease in the left anterior descending (LAD) artery distribution, right coronary artery (RCA), and left circumflex artery. False-positive results are often attributed to attenuation artifacts from large breasts in women and the diaphragm in obese individuals. Excessive bowel radioactivity may also result in false-positive or false-negative results. The introduction of ECG-gated SPECT imaging has allowed assessment of LV function in addition to perfusion. Studies have shown a good correlation for the assessment of LVEF between SPECT and other tomographic modalities.[19] However, LV volumes may be underestimated and ejection fraction overestimated in ventricles with a small LV cavity and hypertrophy of the walls because of partial volume effects. The accuracy of SPECT determination of LV volumes and ejection fraction is also limited in patients with extensive perfusion defects and LV aneurysms, where the entire geometry of the LV cavity

SECTION I Patient Selection

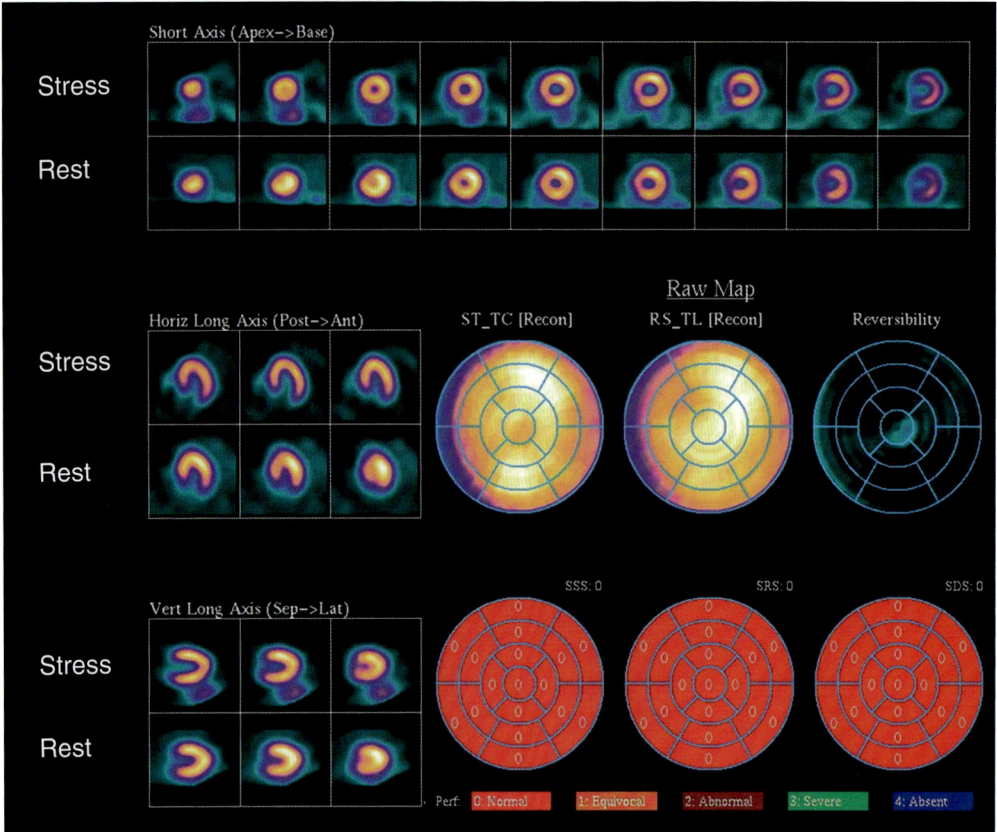

Fig. 4.5 Single-photon emission computed tomography technetium-99m sestamibi exercise stress study. Normal myocardial perfusion during stress and at rest are shown.

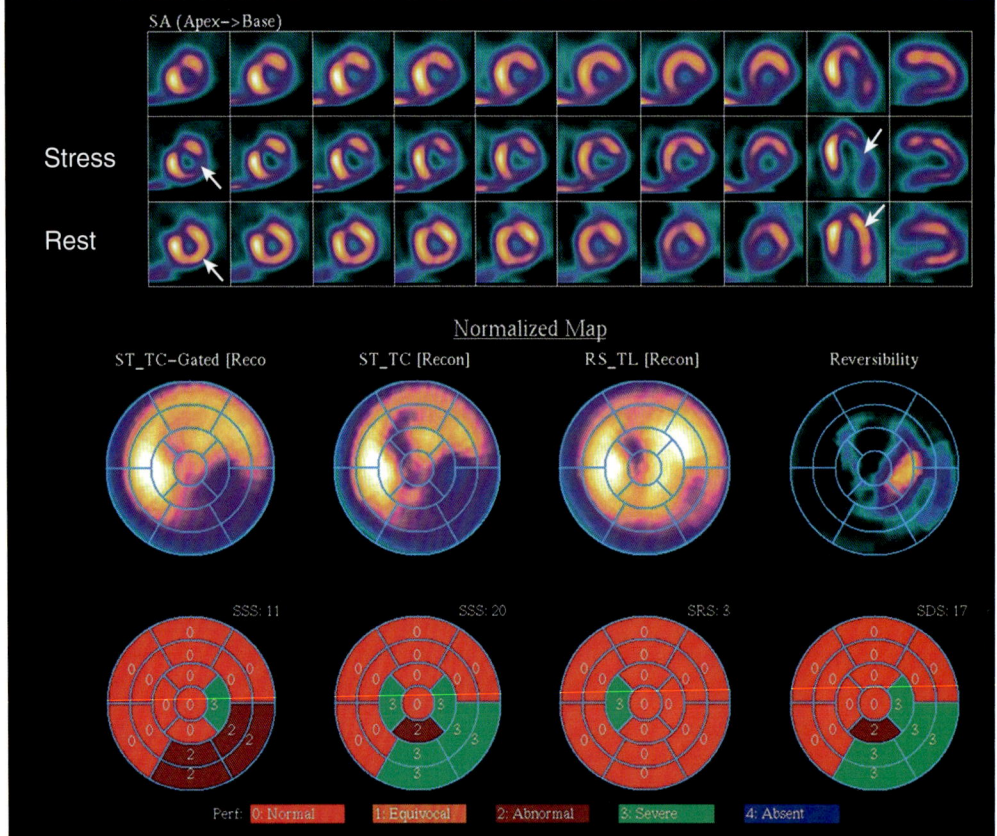

Fig. 4.6 Single-photon emission computed tomography technetium-99m sestamibi exercise stress study. A large myocardial perfusion defect is evident in the posterolateral walls during stress *(white arrows)* with complete reversibility on the resting study, indicating ischemia.

CHAPTER 4 Noninvasive Evaluation: Functional Testing, Multidetector Computed Tomography, and Stress Cardiac MRI

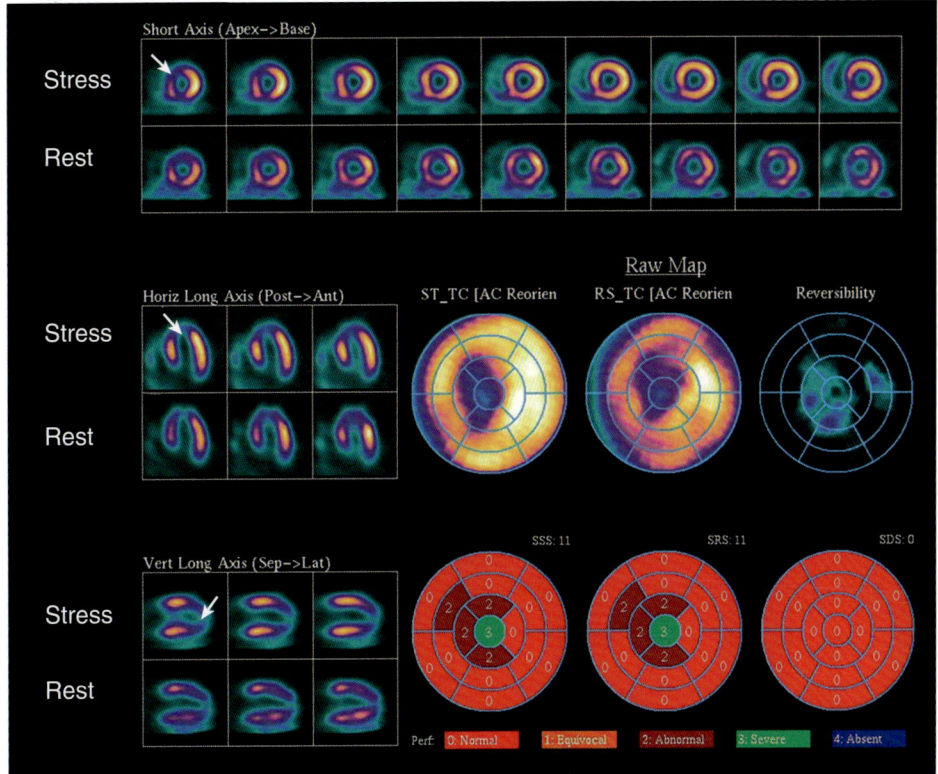

Fig. 4.7 Single-photon emission computed tomography technetium-99m sestamibi exercise stress study. A midsize myocardial perfusion defect is evident in the anteroseptal and apical walls during stress *(white arrows)* without reversibility on the resting study, indicating scar.

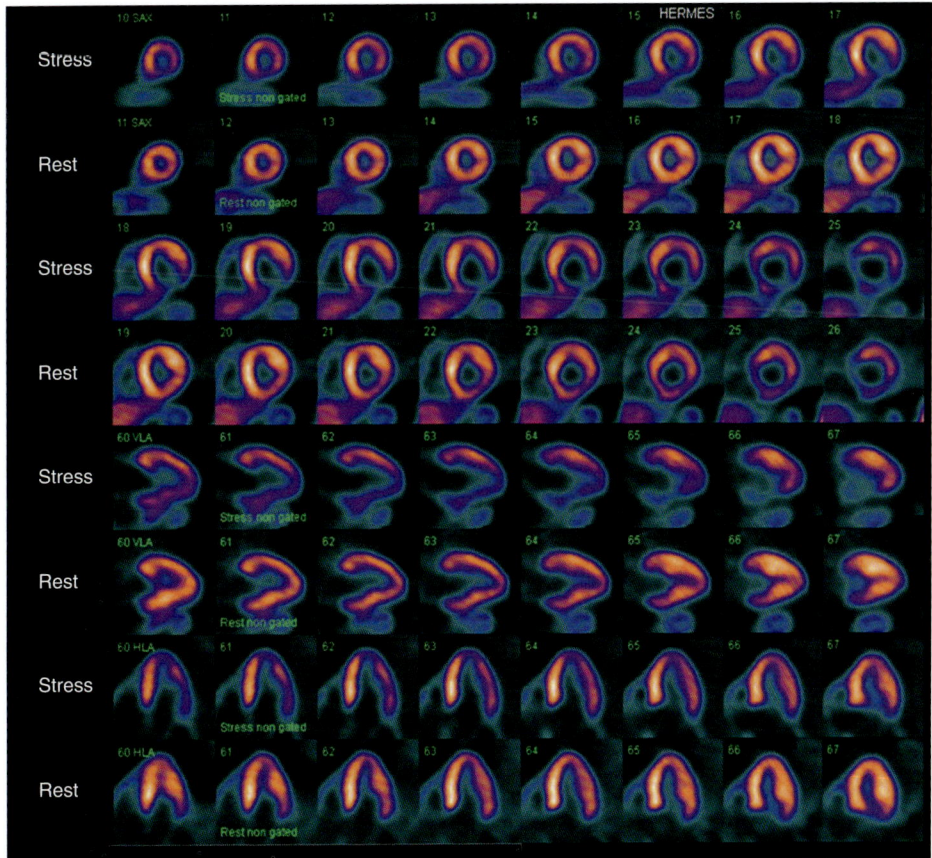

Fig. 4.8 Positron emission tomography cardiac perfusion study using nitrogen-13 ammonia. This study shows a moderate-sized myocardial perfusion defect in the inferior wall during stress with complete reversibility on the rest study, indicating ischemia.

cannot be defined. However, the additional information derived from regional systolic function in gated studies has improved the diagnostic accuracy of the test. Artifacts caused by soft tissue attenuation may be discriminated from true ischemia or scar by the demonstration of normal regional wall motion.

Another recent advancement in SPECT imaging has been the introduction of attenuation correction. Commercially available SPECT attenuation correction systems measure the nonhomogeneous attenuation distribution using external collimated radionuclide sources or computed tomography (CT). The application of attenuation correction in patients with excessive subdiaphragmatic activity corrects by enhancing the affected regions of the myocardium, such as the inferior and posterior LV walls. Several studies have shown significant improvements in specificity and modest improvements in sensitivity with the use of attenuation correction.[20,21]

Several studies have shown that a normal exercise stress SPECT study predicts a very low likelihood (<1%) of adverse events, such as cardiac death or MI, for at least 12 months, and that this level of risk is independent of sex, age, functional status, and even the presence of CAD. Therefore, in those patients with abnormal scans—with baseline clinical characteristics such as diabetes or severe, extensive SPECT perfusion abnormalities—it is possible to define incremental levels of risk and to define which populations of patients will benefit most from revascularization.

Pharmacologic Scintigraphic Myocardial Perfusion Imaging

In the United States, many patients who are referred for evaluation of suspected or known CAD are unable to exercise. Adenosine, regadenoson, and dipyridamole are vasodilator agents that, in the absence of epicardial coronary artery stenosis, increase myocardial blood flow three to five times over baseline. In the presence of a stenosis, a relative perfusion defect may be seen, indicating either failure to increase regional blood flow compared with myocardial segments supplied by a normal vessel or reduced myocardial blood flow due to coronary steal. For this reason, in some patients with multivessel disease and balanced ischemia, pharmacologic stress SPECT studies may appear normal. The average reported sensitivity and specificity of adenosine SPECT for the detection of CAD are similar to those of exercise SPECT studies, at 90% and 75%. With dipyridamole SPECT, sensitivity is similar (89%) but specificity is lower (65%). As previously discussed, verification bias may exaggerate true sensitivity and underestimate specificity. The sensitivities and specificities are also higher for multivessel than for single-vessel disease. Pharmacologic stress SPECT studies may also be performed with dobutamine. The mean reported sensitivity and specificity of this test are 82% and 75%. Unlike dobutamine echocardiography, the monitoring of ischemia-induced functional abnormalities is difficult during SPECT MPI. For this reason, dobutamine is not a preferred pharmacologic stressor in most clinical scenarios. Pharmacologic SPECT is a powerful prognosticator in populations of patients with suspected CAD and in at-risk patients being evaluated prior to noncardiac surgery. The risk of death in patients with normal scans has been reported to be low, but it is higher than in patients with a negative result from exercise SPECT (1% to 3% per year). This probably reflects higher comorbidities in selected populations of patients who cannot exercise. In patients undergoing noncardiac surgery, a pharmacologic stress test has a significant negative predictive value (NPV) but a low positive predictive value (PPV). For this reason, it has been recommended that this test be used in populations at moderate risk, such as those with anginal symptoms, prior infarction, or diabetes. The role of stress MPI is well accepted for the evaluation of symptoms but has not been clearly established for screening asymptomatic patients at risk. In the Detection of Ischemia in Asymptomatic Diabetics (DIAD) study, a randomized controlled trial (RCT) in which 1123 participants with type 2 diabetes and no symptoms of CAD were randomly assigned to be screened with adenosine stress MPI or not, the cardiac event rates were low and were not significantly reduced by MPI screening for myocardial ischemia over a follow-up period of 4.8 years.[22]

Pharmacologic stress imaging may also be performed with PET. Its higher spatial resolution, efficiency, and lower attenuation makes PET a superior method in certain groups, such as obese patients. Cardiac PET has also been validated for the quantitative assessment of regional myocardial perfusion, LV function, and viability. Current PET stress myocardial perfusion protocols require pharmacologic stress because of the short half-life of the commonly used radioisotope rubidium-82, which is preferred because it can be produced on site from a column generator and does not require a cyclotron. Two other radioisotopes approved for cardiac PET use in the United States are nitrogen-13 ammonia for perfusion and fluorine-18-2-fluoro-2-deoxyglucose (18F FDG) for viability. A new PET myocardial perfusion tracer, fluorine-18-flurpiridaz (Flurpiridaz F18), is undergoing investigation and is not currently in clinical use. Owing to its smaller kinetic positron energy and short positron range, it can take full advantage of PET's high spatial resolution. It also has a long half-life and therefore does not require an on-site cyclotron. Phase I and II clinical trials are complete and phase III trials are ongoing.[23] In a phase II trial, PET MPI with Flurpiridaz F18 was safe and was superior to SPECT MPI for radiation dose, image quality and interpretative certainty.[24]

In patients with suboptimal SPECT results, follow-up cardiac PET demonstrated superior accuracy. Most PET studies obtained in patients with a previous equivocal SPECT result are unequivocally classified as normal or mildly positive. PET is one of the most sensitive methods for the identification of myocardial viability in patients with ischemic LV dysfunction. PET defines *viable myocardium* as the presence of a perfusion/metabolism mismatch. Myocardial scar exhibits reduced uptake of both tracers, whereas ischemic viable myocardium shows preserved metabolic activity (Fig. 4.9). The extent of viability by PET has been shown in numerous studies to predict functional myocardial recovery after revascularization.

CARDIAC MAGNETIC RESONANCE IMAGING

CMR imaging has become a prominent modality because it provides both structural and functional assessment of the heart with accuracy. Furthermore, it is the only modality that directly characterizes the myocardium for acute injury, inflammation, infiltration, and scar. It allows for the determination of cardiac volumes, flow quantification, valve assessment, and wall motion analysis both at stress and at rest in addition to first-pass perfusion imaging to assess for myocardial ischemia and assessment of myocardial viability by imaging of scar tissue. An emerging role for CMR in the assessment of acute chest pain is to differentiate among the myriad etiologies including ischemia, myocarditis, pericarditis, aortic dissection, and pulmonary embolism. A recent study evaluating the use of stress CMR in a chest pain observation unit compared to routine care in patients with an intermediate risk for obstructive CAD found that a CMR guided approach reduced revascularization procedures, hospital readmission and downstream testing without an increase in cardiac events at 90 days follow-up.[25] Another advantage with CMR is that image quality is preserved even in obese patients, which makes it ideal compared to echocardiography and radionuclide MPI. Furthermore, obese patients with no evidence of myocardial ischemia or prior infarction have very low event rates.[26]

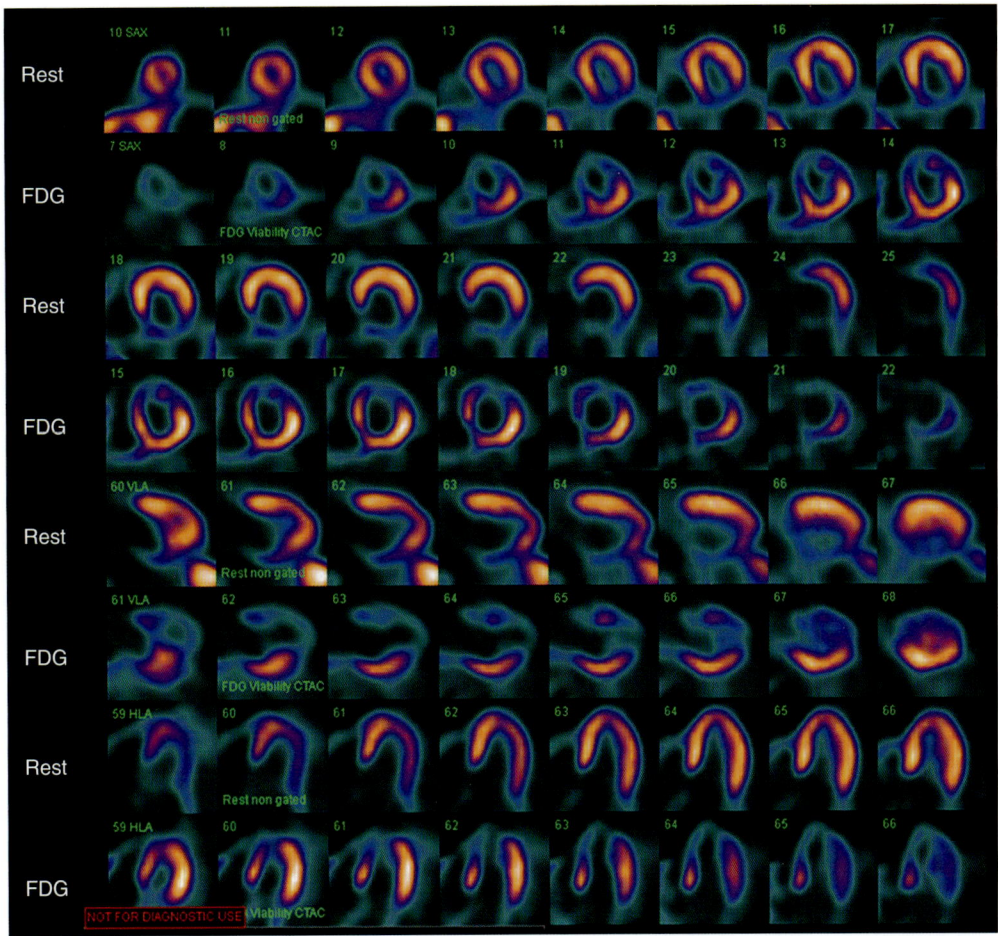

Fig. 4.9 Positron emission tomography myocardial viability study obtained in a patient with ischemic left ventricle dysfunction. Resting ammonia images show an extensive inferior perfusion defect. The fluorodeoxyglucose *(FDG)* images show matched preserved metabolic activity that indicates hypoperfused but viable myocardium.

Cardiac Magnetic Resonance Vasodilator Perfusion Imaging

The most common CMR protocol for the evaluation of myocardial ischemia is vasodilator perfusion imaging. Adenosine or regadenoson are the most widely used vasodilators and imaging of first pass perfusion after the IV administration of standard gadolinium-based magnetic resonance imaging (MRI) contrast agents is performed at rest and at stress. This method provides high spatial resolution images, which allows for the visualization of even small areas of subendocardial ischemia. Gadolinium based contrast agents are paramagnetic and remain extracellular, so during first pass they enhance the intravascular compartment and then deposit extracellularly. Using a fast imaging protocol with a steady state free precession (SSFP)-based sequence, the first pass enhancement of the myocardium may be visualized by CMR in near real time. CMR perfusion imaging makes it possible to identify areas of myocardial hypoenhancement at rest in the presence of severely reduced myocardial blood flow (Fig. 4.10); however, in most circumstances, resting blood flow is normal in segments supplied by stenotic vessels owing to compensatory arteriolar vasodilation. Therefore, vasodilator agents are utilized similar to SPECT and PET MPI to induce ischemia. In a recent multicenter study of patients undergoing cardiac catheterization, CMR perfusion imaging was compared with SPECT MPI. Based on receiver operating characteristic (ROC) analysis, CMR perfusion imaging performed much like SPECT.[27] However, in the CE-MARC trial, which was a large single center comparison of CMR perfusion imaging versus SPECT with invasive angiography as the gold standard in all patients, CMR had better sensitivity and NPV, and similar specificity to SPECT with the benefit of no additional radiation exposure to patients.[28] This trial supports the use of CMR in routine clinical practice and as centers gain experience with CMR, typical studies providing LV function, perfusion, and viability can be performed in approximately 30 minutes as compared to SPECT, which takes approximately 2 hours. The CE-MARC 2 trial found CMR and SPECT to be similar in terms of reducing unnecessary invasive coronary angiography procedures, however, again, CMR does not expose a patient to ionizing radiation.[29] CMR perfusion imaging is uniquely able to show microvascular dysfunction as well with diffuse subendocardial perfusion defects.[30] Videos 4.13–4.15 compare first pass perfusion at rest and post adenosine infusion in an AP2 view revealing diffuse subendocardial hypoperfusion consistent with microvascular coronary artery dysfunction in a patient with a normal coronary angiogram. Cine imaging displaying normal LV systolic function is also included. In addition, patients with a negative perfusion scan have a low likelihood (<1%) of a major cardiac event over the ensuing 2 years.[31–33]

Accumulating evidence dictates a shift away from purely anatomic assessment of CAD to an objective functional assessment. The Fractional Flow Reserve Versus Angiography for Multivessel Evaluation (FAME) and deferral versus performance of percutaneous coronary intervention (PCI) of functionally non-significant coronary stenosis (DEFER) trials have shown that patients who

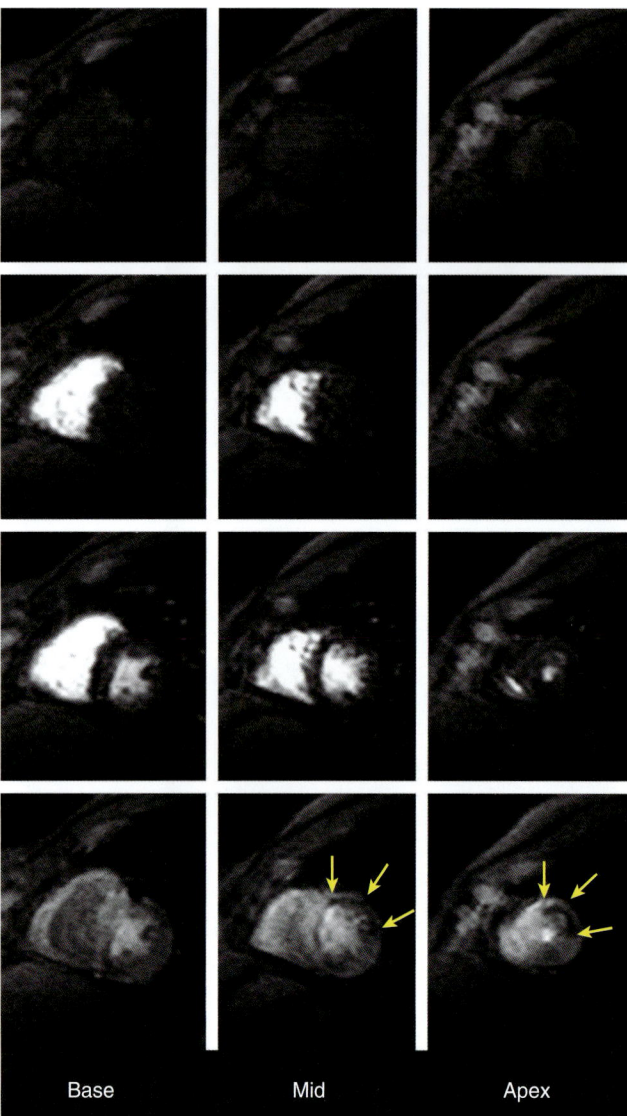

Fig. 4.10 First-pass gadolinium diethylene triamine pentaacetic acid myocardial perfusion study. *From top to bottom:* Sequential cross-sectional images obtained at the base *(left)*, middle *(center)*, and apex *(right)*. The first row of images was acquired before the arrival of contrast. The second row demonstrates the arrival of contrast in the right ventricle. The third row shows its arrival in the left ventricular cavity, and the fourth row shows enhancement of the myocardium. An area of subendocardial hypoenhancement is evident *(arrows)* in a patient with severe stenosis of a large marginal branch.

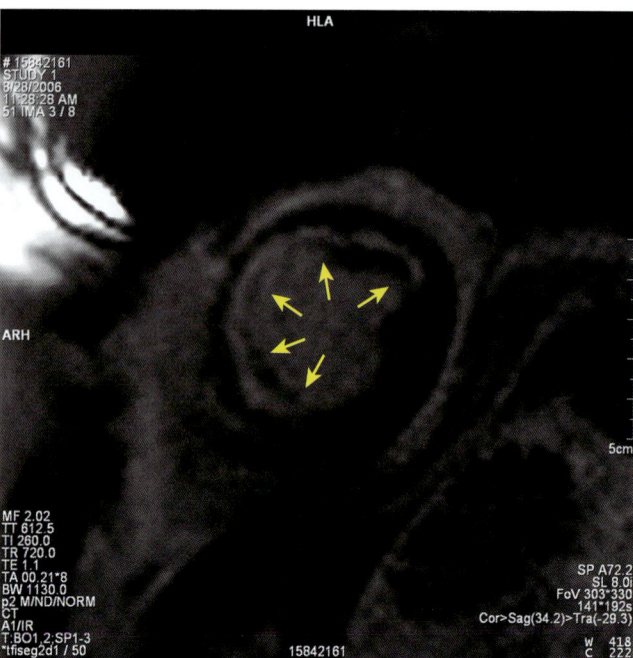

Fig. 4.11 Mid–left ventricle cross-sectional image obtained 20 minutes after injection of gadolinium diethylene triamine pentaacetic acid demonstrates a large area of subendocardial fibrosis (the white rim is indicated by *arrows*), which involves 50% of the transmural thickness in the septum and anterior walls.

undergo PCI of significantly stenotic lesions by fractional flow reserve (FFR) assessment have an improved outcome compared with those who have intervention solely based on a visual estimation of lesion severity. The 2-year follow-up of the FAME trial shows a significant reduction in major cardiac events in patients guided by FFR. CMR perfusion imaging is a well-established modality for accurately detecting significant coronary stenosis when validated against FFR.[34,35] Quantitative analysis of CMR perfusion images can be performed to determine the ratio of stress to rest blood flow and to assess myocardial perfusion reserve (MPR). Studies have shown that in patients with obstructive CAD, MPR increases after PCI.[36] New techniques to assess LV myocardial transmural perfusion gradients during CMR first-pass perfusion allow for semi-automated comparison of perfusion between the subendocardium and subepicardium. A transmural pressure gradient of 20% was identified as being as accurate as visual assessment and accurately predicts hemodynamically significant CAD as compared to FFR.[37] An additional and unique benefit of CMR is delayed gadolinium-enhanced imaging of the myocardium, which is a powerful technique for evaluating the presence of scar in patients with prior infarction, and the extent of infarct transmurality predicts functional recovery in patients referred for revascularization (Fig. 4.11).[38] CMR is the gold standard for the assessment of infarct scar. However, direct magnetic resonance coronary angiography also may be performed, and although the method is well established for the evaluation of congenital anomalies, it is less accurate for evaluating CAD. In a recent meta-analysis of 20 studies (989 patients) that comprised patients with suspected CAD assessed by MRI, mean sensitivity and specificity for the detection of obstructive CAD were 87.1% and 70.3%, respectively—considerably lower than the respective values found in a meta-analysis of 89 studies (7516 patients) assessed by CCTA (97.2% and 87.4%).[39]

Dobutamine and Exercise Stress Cardiac Magnetic Resonance

However, CMR may also be used to evaluate global and regional LV function at rest and during dobutamine or exercise stress similar to stress echocardiography, with higher spatial resolution and the advantage of the ability to perform delayed gadolinium-enhanced imaging to identify an infarct scar. The average reported sensitivity and specificity for the detection of obstructive CAD are 89% and 84%, respectively. One of the limitations of dobutamine CMR compared to echocardiography is the inability to obtain accurate ECG monitoring of ST-segment deviation during the test due to strong magnetic fields from the MRI machine. For this reason, many centers have favored the use of CMR vasodilator perfusion imaging protocols. CMR exercise stress protocols are limited to very few select centers and require an MRI compatible treadmill or bicycle; however, they are not widely used clinically. ECG monitoring is again limited with exercise protocols, however, the added benefit is the ability to assess a patient's functional status.

Evolving Noncontrast Imaging Techniques to Evaluate for Coronary Artery Disease and Ischemia With Cardiac Magnetic Resonance

While CMR offers comprehensive evaluation of patients with suspected or known CAD without exposing them to ionizing radiation, gadolinium-based contrast agents are generally avoided in patients with advanced renal disease, which limits CMR's widespread use. New techniques are in development that offer complete evaluation of CAD without the need for contrast. In a recent proof of concept study, T1 mapping—a technique that can be utilized to characterize myocardial water content and thus indirectly regional myocardial blood volume—was able to distinguish between healthy, ischemic, and infarcted myocardium during rest imaging and stress imaging post administration of adenosine.[40] Similarly, another study utilizing blood oxygen-level dependent CMR imaging which exploits the paramagnetic properties of deoxyhemoglobin in the blood pool, thus transforming it into a "natural" contrast agent, was able to identify regional myocardial ischemia post administration of adenosine, which correlated well with invasive coronary angiography.[41] Similar to CCTA's ability to characterize coronary plaques, noncontrast T1-weighted CMR imaging techniques can identify high intensity coronary plaques which are synonymous with low attenuation plaques and positive remodeling. A recent study of this technique found that high intensity plaques predict acute coronary syndrome (ACS).[42] As CMR develops, it may be able to offer the evaluation of LV function, myocardial ischemia and viability, coronary anatomy, and the identification of high risk plaques—all without the exposure to ionizing radiation and contrast.

MYOCARDIAL VIABILITY ASSESSMENT

Myocardial viability assessment is commonly sought prior to revascularization for ischemic heart disease to determine if restoration of blood flow will lead to improvement in myocardial function. Many imaging modalities are utilized for this purpose, including echocardiography, radionuclide imaging, and CMR. Echocardiographic assessment depends on incremental low-dose dobutamine protocols with real time monitoring for improvement in myocardial contractility or a lack thereof. Improvement in regional contractility at lower rates of dobutamine (5 to 10 μg/kg/min) in segments that are akinetic or hypokinetic at rest predicts functional recovery after revascularization, particularly when those same segments exhibit a reduction in contractility at high dobutamine rates (biphasic response). Patients with ischemic LV dysfunction and viable myocardium who undergo revascularization have better outcomes than those who are not revascularized or who have no evidence of viability regardless. The sensitivity with which dobutamine echocardiography predicts functional recovery ranges between 74% and 88%, and the specificity between 73% and 87%. Compared with radionuclide MPI, dobutamine stress echocardiography has a higher specificity but lower sensitivity and overall similar accuracy.[43] More recently, newer methods of characterizing ventricular function during stress echocardiography have been developed including measuring myocardial velocities and myocardial strain with tissue Doppler imaging (TDI) and speckle-tracking echocardiography (STE); however, neither are in widespread clinical use.[44-47]

In radionuclide viability imaging, a number of isotopes—including thallium and technetium—have been used. However, a combination of SPECT and PET imaging has gained popularity because it characterizes both perfusion (SPECT) and metabolism (PET). Studies have shown that a metabolism/perfusion mismatch threshold greater than 5% identified patients who had significantly improved survival if treated by revascularization rather than optimal medical therapy (OMT) alone. A limitation of this technique is that it requires two tests, which increases the radiation dose to the patient.[48]

CMR can determine myocardial viability via the accurate measurement of end-diastolic wall thickness (EDWT), contractile response to low-dose dobutamine, and transmural extent of infarction on late gadolinium imaging. A recent meta-analysis of 24 prospective studies (n = 698) evaluated these three CMR parameters and found that late gadolinium enhancement, using a 50% transmural extent of infarct, provided the greatest sensitivity and NPV, whereas low-dose dobutamine imaging yielded the highest specificity and PPV, as well as the greatest overall accuracy. EDWT showed good sensitivity but poor specificity.[49] The Prognostic Stratification of Patients With ST-Segment Elevation Myocardial Infarction (PROSPECT) trial revealed that CMR also has added value post-acute MI using non-stress–related parameters, including myocardial salvage index and microvascular obstruction, both of which improve risk stratification for future events compared to echocardiography and clinical parameters alone.[50] Overall, late gadolinium enhancement is the gold standard for the assessment of myocardial viability given its superior spatial resolution and direct imaging of infarct scar compared to other modalities.

In general, techniques that detect the presence of myocardial cellular integrity including SPECT, PET, MCE, and CMR scar imaging are more sensitive but less specific than techniques that detect contractile reserve including dobutamine stress echocardiography and CMR because a critical myocardial mass must be viable for a functional response to occur.

Despite our ability to assess myocardial viability, recent large trials, including the Heart Failure Revascularisation Trial (HEART),[51] Positron Emission Tomography and Recovery Following Revascularization (PARR-2) trial,[52] and the Surgical Treatment for Ischemic Heart Failure (STICH) trial,[53] have all questioned the superiority of revascularization over OMT. In the STICH trial, viability assessment was an inclusion criterion, but this was dropped secondary to poor recruitment. Subsequently, 50% of patients underwent viability assessment at the discretion of their physician. The main finding of this trial was that revascularization did *not* improve overall survival in ischemic cardiomyopathy compared with OMT. The viability sub study showed that survival of patients with viability was significantly longer than those without viability, but patients with viable myocardium who underwent coronary artery bypass grafting (CABG) did not show any survival benefit compared with those treated with OMT.[54] Although very informative, this trial had limitations. It only utilized SPECT and dobutamine stress echocardiography to assess myocardial viability as opposed to CMR. Furthermore, patients who underwent viability testing were less likely to benefit from revascularization because they had significantly greater LV dysfunction, LV dilatation, and incidence of previous MI. Each of the trials had limitations and considerable debate remains about the role of revascularization and viability testing in patients with ischemic cardiomyopathy.

Cardiac Computed Tomography

Cardiac computed tomography (CCT) is an accurate noninvasive method of evaluating the coronary anatomy and to assess for coronary atherosclerosis and has been extensively validated. Technical advances available in modern scanners now make it possible to obtain adequate image quality in most patients. Image acquisition and interpretation can be performed very rapidly, which makes this technology suitable for the evaluation of ambulatory patients.

Coronary Artery Calcium Scoring

Coronary artery calcium (CAC) scoring quantifies coronary calcification using a radiographic density-weighted volume of high attenuation regions (>130 Hounsfield units [HUs]). The prognostic value of CAC has been well established by Keelan and colleagues,[55] who demonstrated that a CAC Agatston score greater than 100 was an independent predictor (odds ratio [OR] 1.88) of adverse cardiovascular outcomes (death and nonfatal MI) at 7-year follow-up. Similarly, in a large MESA cohort, the addition of CAC to traditional clinical risk factors improved risk prediction for cardiac events. With the addition of CAC, 5.1% of the cohort was reclassified as high risk with an event rate of 16.4%, and 12.7% were reclassified as low risk with an event rate of 2.3%.[56] Recent studies have found that in asymptomatic nondiabetic patients, a CAC score of zero confers a 15-year warranty period against mortality and interestingly, patients with high clinical risk scores with a zero CAC score had a longer warranty period than those with low to intermediate clinical risk scores and a nonzero CAC score.[57] In asymptomatic diabetic patients, the warranty period is 5 years.[58]

Although CAC clearly adds value in terms of risk stratification by identifying atherosclerosis, it is unclear whether this information alters clinical outcomes. Also, it is important to recognize that a CAC score of zero in a symptomatic patient does not offer a similar high NPV as it does in asymptomatic patients. The COronary CT Angiography EvaluatioN For Clinical Outcomes: An InteRnational Multicenter (CONFIRM) registry found that 13% of symptomatic patients with a CAC score of zero had nonobstructive CAD and 3.5% had at least one > 50% stenosis as assessed by CCTA.[59] CAC improves risk stratification in the elderly as well in concert with their Framingham Risk Score. In the South Bay Heart Watch study,[60] a CAC greater than 300 was associated with increased cardiac event rates compared with that determined by the clinical score alone. These data again support the concept that CAC can improve risk prediction but has not been clearly shown to improve outcomes. Some studies suggest that wide implementation of CAC screening may in aggregate have a detrimental effect on the quality of life of those with nonzero scores.[61] Conversely, a recent systematic review found that patients with knowledge of CAC presence were more likely to follow lifestyle recommendations and pharmacologic interventions for the primary prevention of cardiac events.[62] CAC is also shown to be the strongest predictor of cardiovascular death, nonfatal MI, angina, and revascularization independent of race, and four major ethnic/racial groups were evaluated.[63] The addition of CAC to radionuclide MPI provides incremental value as well.[49,64] In patients with normal stress perfusion, adding CAC may improve the detection of CAD.[65] In summary, CAC is useful in identifying risk; however, it remains to be seen if it leads to changes in patient management which ultimately improve outcomes.

Contrast-Enhanced Computed Tomography Coronary Angiography

CCTA is a noninvasive alternative to invasive coronary angiography and offers detailed assessment of the coronary arterial wall and plaque characteristics, while invasive studies typically only assess the coronary lumen. Although the acquisition of CCTA takes less than 15 seconds, patient preparation and data interpretation require extensive training and attention to detail. Patient selection is important because dense coronary calcification, prior stents, and poor x-ray penetration in obese patients may compromise image quality. The frequency of artifacts related to diaphragmatic and/or cardiac motion has been significantly reduced with the newest wide detector coverage (128, 256, and 320 slice) scanners and dual-source imaging. However, most patients still require beta-blocker and nitrate administration and cooperation with breath-holding instructions during the acquisition.

Over the last few years, significant attention has focused on excessive radiation exposure with medical imaging.[66] In response, and in collaboration with medical imaging leaders, the industry has implemented several strategies to reduce radiation dose during CCTA. These include reduction in the volume of coverage, use of lower peak x-ray–tube currents, and wider adoption of prospective ECG-gated acquisition, which also allows for the upward modulation of the tube current. The use of prospective gating is very effective in reducing the radiation dose,[67] but limits CCTA image acquisition to a predetermined brief diastolic phase of the cardiac cycle. Thus, the analysis of LV function cannot be performed when this acquisition mode is being used. Patients in whom functional analysis is required, or those with rapid or irregular heart rates who may require reconstruction of multiple cardiac phases for coronary vessel examination, should be imaged using conventional retrospective ECG-gated acquisition. CCTA is very useful in assessing the origin and course of congenitally anomalous coronary arteries and the three-dimensional relationship of anomalous coronary arteries with the aorta and pulmonary arterial trunk.[68–70] Myocardial bridges and coronary arteriovenous fistulas are also well visualized by CCTA.

Cardiac Computed Tomography Angiography to Evaluate Coronary Luminal Stenosis

Figs. 4.12 and 4.13 are CCTA studies obtained from a patient with normal coronary arteries and another with severe multivessel disease. The corresponding invasive angiogram from the latter is shown in Fig. 4.14. Several single-center and multicenter studies have examined the accuracy of CCTA for establishing the diagnosis of obstructive CAD. Most of these studies have been performed in patients referred for diagnostic coronary angiography based on clinical indications. The prevalence of obstructive CAD in patients enrolled in these studies ranged anywhere from 35% to 80%. Accuracy was defined in these studies using segment-based, vessel-based, and/or patient-based analysis. *Segment-based analysis* has been restricted in many of these studies to segments greater than 1.5 mm or greater than 2 mm in diameter. In most studies, previously stented segments were excluded. Typically, either a greater than 50% or 70% reduction in luminal diameter on invasive coronary angiography was used as the reference standard to adjudicate a positive result. On *vessel-based analysis*, a positive result was defined as the presence of one or more abnormal segments in the specific vessel's distribution. On *patient-based analysis*, a positive result was defined as one or more abnormal segments anywhere in the coronary arterial tree.

In a multicenter study[71] that enrolled 187 patients with high or intermediate risk with a CAC score below 600, 71% of segments were deemed evaluable by CCTA. All non-evaluable segments were censored to be positive because in clinical practice, they would also lead to the performance of angiography. The sensitivity, specificity, PPV, and NPV for detecting greater than 50% luminal stenosis in segment-based analysis were 89%, 65%, 13%, and 99%, respectively. In a patient-based analysis, the sensitivity, specificity, PPV, and NPV were 98%, 54%, 50%, and 99%, respectively. The results of this study suggest that the clinical utility of CCTA, given its high NPV, lies primarily in the exclusion of obstructive CAD. Clinicians should be aware that extensive coronary calcification can substantially reduce the specificity of CCTA. In the Assessment by CCTA of Individuals Undergoing Invasive Coronary Angiography (ACCURACY) trial, sensitivity and specificity of CCTA were 95% and 83%, respectively; however, specificity decreased to 53% in those with CAC scores greater than 400.[72]

Prospective multicenter trials have demonstrated improved diagnostic characteristics of 64-slice CCTA in comparison to 16-slice.[73,74] The ACCURACY[75] trial was a U.S.-based

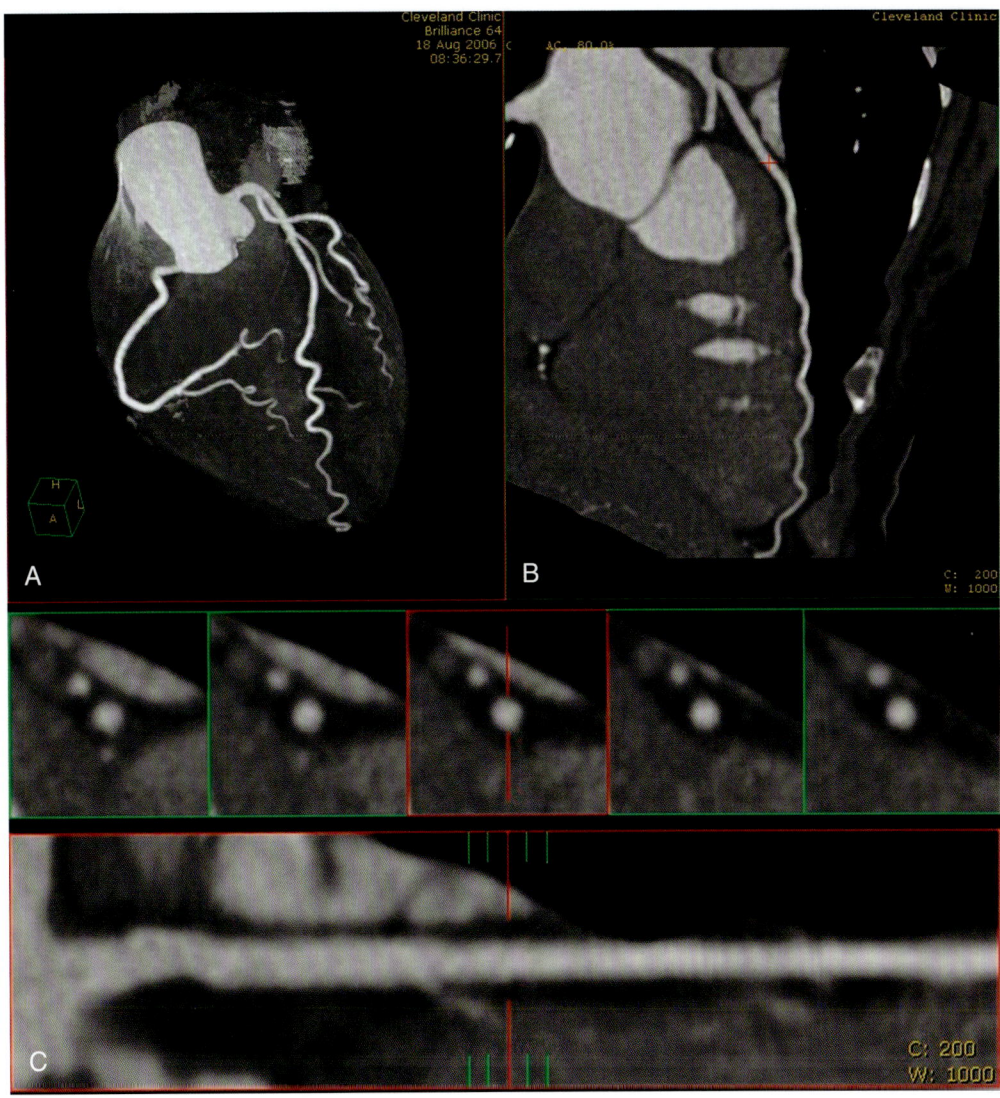

Fig. 4.12 Multidetector computed tomography coronary angiography of normal coronary arteries. (A) Volume-rendered maximum-intensity projection of the aortic root and coronary arteries. (B) Curved multiplanar reconstruction of the left anterior descending (LAD) coronary artery. (C) Series of cross-sectional images obtained from the mid-LAD at 1-mm intervals.

multicenter study that examined 230 patients who underwent CCTA prior to elective diagnostic coronary angiography. Researchers observed sensitivity, specificity, PPV, and NPV of CCTA to detect a 50% or greater stenosis of 95%, 83%, 64%, and 99%, respectively or a 70% or greater stenosis of 94%, 83%, 48%, and 99%, respectively. It is likely that a discrepancy will always exist between CCTA and invasive coronary angiography for the quantitative assessment of luminal stenosis. Unlike angiography, CCTA provides data on both the lumen and vessel wall plaque. In addition, CCTA provides an infinite number of projections with three-dimensional (3D) reconstruction that may allow better visualization of stenotic segments. In some cases, a presumed "false-positive" CCTA finding may represent a "false-negative" coronary angiogram, in which adequate projections were not obtained. The prognostic utility of CCTA has been examined in several single-center studies. Among 169 low- to intermediate-risk patients who underwent both exercise treadmill testing and CCTA, the presence of obstructive (≥70%) stenosis was associated with both ST-segment depression (adjusted OR, 3.38; 95% CI, 1.32 to 8.64; P = .001) and elevated-risk Duke treadmill scores (adjusted OR, 4.67; 95% CI, 1.97 to 11.03; P < .001). In this study, a graded relationship was found between the extent and severity of CAD and the exercise time, as well as the likelihood of ST-segment depression. In another study of 163 low- to intermediate-risk patients who underwent both MPI and CCTA, the extent and severity of CAD as measured by a modified Duke coronary artery jeopardy score was independently associated with a severely abnormal MPI result (OR, 2.25; 95% CI, 1.12 to 4.41; P = .02) for the highest risk group as compared with those without disease.[76] In a multicenter study of 541 intermediate-probability patients referred for symptoms or CAD risk factors who prospectively underwent both CCTA and MPI, the annualized hard event rate was 1.8% in those with mild or no CAD versus 4.8% in those with 50% or greater stenosis by CCTA, and it was 1.1% in those with a normal MPI versus 3.8% in those with an abnormal MPI.[77] In multivariate analysis, CCTA-visualized obstructive plaque and abnormal MPI were independent predictors of late events after adjustment for clinical risk factors, with significantly improved prediction by the combined use of CCTA and MPI compared with either modality

SECTION I Patient Selection

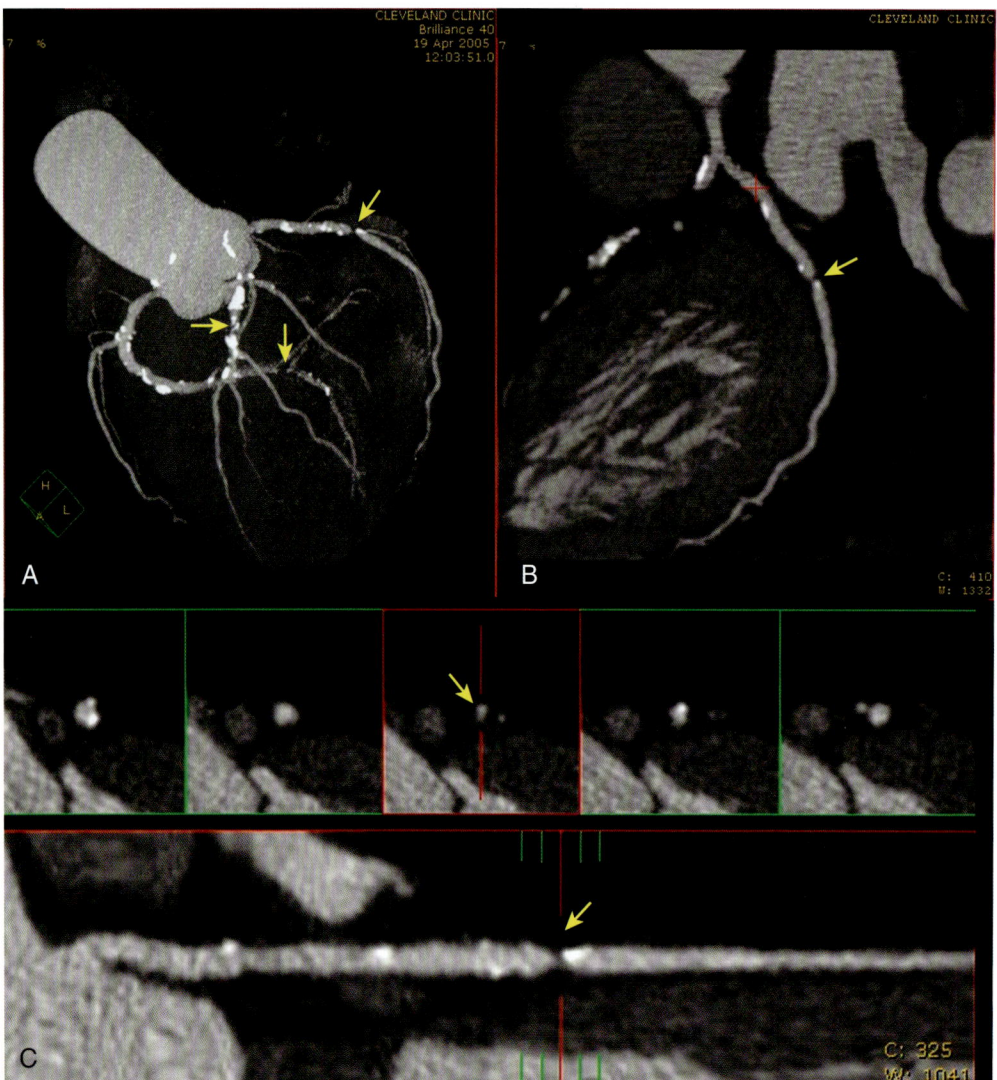

Fig. 4.13 Multidetector computed tomography coronary angiography of obstructive multivessel disease. (A) Volume-rendered maximum-intensity projection of the aortic root and coronary arteries. (B) Curved multiplanar reconstruction of the left circumflex *(LCX)* coronary artery. (C) Series of cross-sectional images obtained from the mid-LCX at 1-mm intervals. *Arrows* indicate areas of severe stenosis caused predominantly by noncalcified *(dark)* atherosclerotic plaques.

alone (log-rank test *P* value < .005). Over the study period, those with concordantly normal CCTA and MPI results had an annualized hard event rate of 1%; those with concordantly abnormal CCTA and MPI results had a hard event rate of 9.0%; and those with discordant CCTA and MPI results with either abnormal CCTA or abnormal MPI had event rates of 3.8% and 3.7%, respectively.

Second-generation 320-slice CT scanners enable the acquisition of a full cardiac dataset within a single cardiac cycle. Image acquisition time is reduced from approximately 12 seconds (64-slice CT) to 1 second. Such short image acquisition time allows the use of smaller contrast volumes and lower radiation, and it permits the inclusion of patient populations previously considered unsuitable for CCTA imaging, such as patients with cardiac arrhythmias. The Coronary Artery Evaluation Using 320-Row Multidetector CT Angiography (CORE-320) pilot study enrolled 64 subjects to assess radiation dose and image quality of the 320-row CT scanner. They found that only four subjects had limited image quality. Patient body mass index (BMI) was the strongest predictor of poor image quality.[78]

The PROspective Multicenter Imaging Study for Evaluation of chest pain (PROMISE) trial was a large multicenter trial comparing CCTA with usual-care functional stress testing. The trial enrolled over 10,000 patients to determine whether an initial anatomic testing strategy using CCTA could reduce the primary end point (all-cause death, nonfatal MI, major periprocedural complications, or hospitalization for unstable angina) by 20% when compared with an initial functional testing strategy over a follow-up of 2.5 years.[79] The trial ultimately found that in symptomatic patients with intermediate risk for CAD, an initial strategy of CCTA did not improve clinical outcomes or reduce radiation exposure and downstream testing; however, in the CCTA group there were fewer invasive coronary angiograms with no obstructive disease.[80] The CT Coronary Angiography in Patients With Suspected Angina Due to Coronary Heart Disease (SCOT-HEART) trial assessed patients with stable chest pain evaluated in an ambulatory setting comparing standard care with CCTA versus standard care alone with a primary endpoint of certainty of the diagnosis of angina secondary to CAD at 6 weeks follow-up. CCTA reclassified the diagnosis of angina due to CAD in a greater

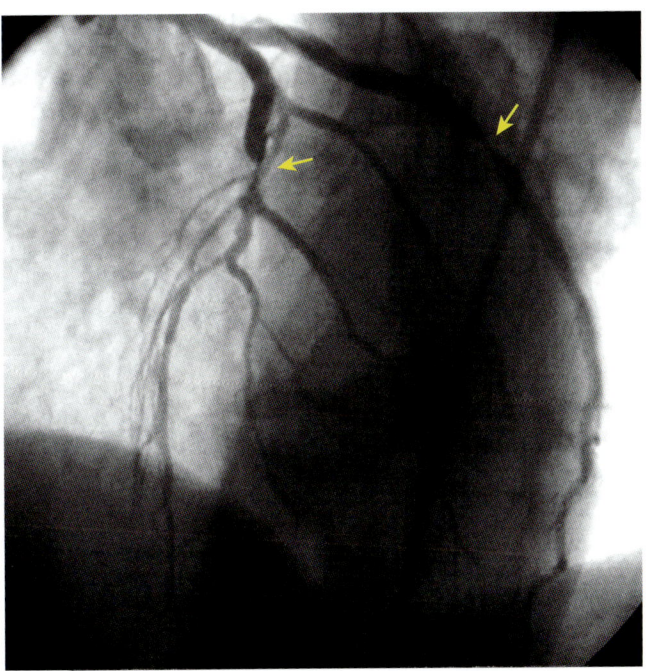

Fig. 4.14 Angiographic left anterior projection of the left coronary artery and branches obtained by catheterization in the patient in Fig. 4.13. *Arrows* indicate severe stenotic lesions in the left anterior descending and left circumflex coronary arteries.

proportion of patients than traditional noninvasive testing; however, at 1.7 years follow-up there was no significant difference in reduction of events defined as MI. CCTA did prove to be useful in specifically targeting interventions.[81] Both of these studies highlight the dilemma of using CCTA as an initial test for the evaluation of chest pain. Although CCTA provides detailed anatomic assessment of vessels, the lack of functional information including if stenoses are physiologically significant or not is important, and studies are ongoing evaluating CCTA with FFR techniques comparable to invasive FFR, and will be addressed in later sections.[82]

The benefit of CCTA in asymptomatic patients is not yet well established. In one study, 1000 asymptomatic patients underwent 64-slice CCTA as part of a general health evaluation; those with no plaque had no major adverse cardiac events (MACEs) over an average observation of 17 months, whereas 15 of the 215 individuals with any plaque developed unstable angina or underwent revascularization.[74,83] However, most events occurred within 90 days of the CCTA and were driven by revascularization procedures in this open-label trial. Furthermore, most events occurred in patients with an abnormal CAC, indicating that CCTA provided no significant incremental prognostic value in asymptomatic patients. In two studies including both asymptomatic and symptomatic patients, if coronary plaque was present by CCTA, specific plaque characteristics were predictive of future ACS events. In the first study, low attenuation plaque and positive vessel wall remodeling were both associated with higher risk of plaque rupture and clinical ACS.[84] In the second study, a napkin ring sign, which is defined as a ring of high attenuation surrounding a plaque suggesting a thin cap fibroatheroma prone to rupture, was also found to be associated with ACS.[85] Regardless of symptoms, CCTA offers insight into high risk plaques that may be nonobstructive and is an area of future research to determine if patient management can be altered to improve outcomes.

Accurate assessment of previously stented coronary vessels remains an important limitation of CCTA[86] and a noninvasive accurate test for in-stent restenosis would be invaluable. This is particularly true because the widespread use of drug-eluting stents reduces the incidence of in-stent restenosis, thus reducing the positive yield from repeated invasive coronary angiography. In a study that used 16-slice multidetector computed tomography (MDCT), only 126 of 232 stents (54%) could be evaluated.[76,87] Smaller stents in vessels less than 3 mm in diameter were harder to evaluate accurately, and internal luminal diameter is often underestimated. Studies performed with 64-slice scanners have shown improved sensitivity and specificity.[77,88] Nevertheless, the ability to evaluate the lumen of stented vessels depends on the type and diameter of the stent. Practical delineation of in-stent stenosis remains difficult in stents with a diameter less than 3 mm. New protocols utilizing prospective ECG-triggered imaging with low radiation dual source CT and iterative reconstruction have shown promise in evaluating coronary stents and will likely be utilized more widely in the near future.[89]

Coronary Computed Tomography Angiogram Is Useful in the Evaluation of Coronary Artery Bypass Grafts (Fig. 4.15)

In a study that used 64-slice scanners,[90] CCTA images of 138 grafts, native vessels, and anastomotic sites were compared with invasive coronary angiograms. The grafts included both venous and arterial bypass conduits. All the grafts were "evaluable" by CCTA, with sensitivity, specificity, PPV, and NPV of 100%, 94%, 92%, and 100%, respectively. Evaluation of the distal anastomosis site is often limited by surgical clips, and analysis of the native vessels is often more difficult in patients with previous CABG owing to poor runoff, extensive calcification, and smaller lumen size. This can potentially limit the diagnostic utility of CCTA; however, it remains a useful alternative to invasive angiography especially when direct catheterization carries significant risk, such as with suspected atheromas or when a high contrast load should be avoided. CCTA is also useful in defining the 3D location of preexisting coronary grafts in relation to the chest wall in patients undergoing repeated sternotomy to assist with surgical planning.

Guiding Interventions With Cardiac Computed Tomographic Angiography

Because of its 3D capabilities, CCTA has great potential to guide interventions. It can define the anatomic course, caliber, and length of a diseased segment and the extent of calcification in patients with chronic total occlusion (CTO) of a coronary vessel.[91] In addition, CCTA images may be projected side by side with the fluoroscopy images in the catheterization laboratory to guide the interventionalist.

Stress Myocardial Computed Tomography Perfusion Imaging

One major limitation of CCTA is the inability to detect whether lesions are physiologically or functionally significant as stress testing does. Stress myocardial CT perfusion (CTP) imaging is a novel application of coronary CT in which the examination can provide both anatomic and physiologic assessment. A combined CCTA/CTP approach has been shown to improve the diagnostic accuracy to detect functionally significant coronary lesions when compared with CCTA alone, at a radiation dose comparable to radionuclide MPI.[92] During this exam, contrast attenuation differences within the myocardium are measured and compared during rest and stress. A direct relationship exists between the amount of iodinated contrast within the myocardium and myocardial attenuation in HUs. As such, a relative difference in myocardial perfusion can be visualized as differing attenuations; areas of myocardium with decreased

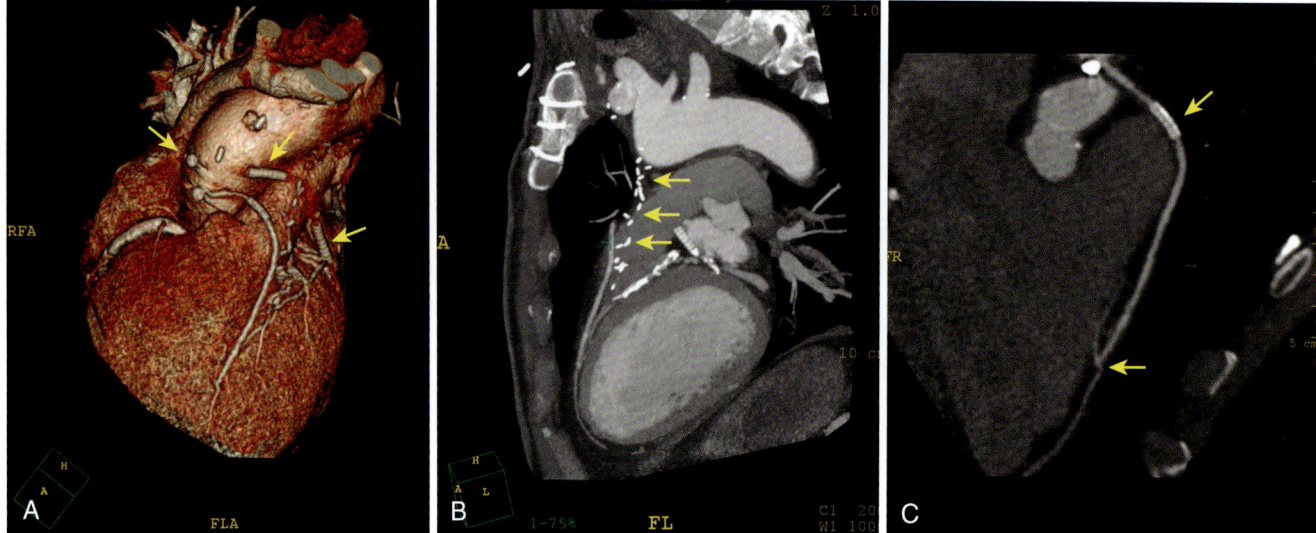

Fig. 4.15 Multidetector computed tomography coronary angiography obtained in a patient with previous coronary artery bypass grafts. (A) Volume-rendered projection of the heart shows the stump (arrows) of an occluded bypass to the circumflex coronary artery and stents previously deployed in this vessel. The graft is not visualized owing to the lack of contrast opacification. (B) Oblique sagittal maximum-intensity projection shows a series of staples (arrows) that correspond to an occluded left internal thoracic graft to the left anterior descending (LAD) coronary artery. (C) Curved multiplanar reconstruction of a saphenous vein bypass graft to the LAD. The arrows indicate a stent in the proximal segment and show the anastomosis to the distal LAD.

blood flow would have a lower attenuation—a perfusion defect. Single-center studies have established that myocardial CTP imaging can help accurately diagnose CAD compared with various reference standards that include SPECT, invasive coronary angiography, MRI, and FFR.[93–95] The combination of CCTA and CTP imaging was validated in the multicenter diagnostic accuracy CORE-320 study.[96] This prospective multicenter study also provided the opportunity to independently validate the diagnostic performance of CTP and SPECT in the diagnosis of anatomic CAD. Sixteen centers enrolled 381 patients, who underwent rest and adenosine stress CTP and either exercise or pharmacologic stress SPECT before and within 60 days of coronary angiography. The per-patient sensitivity and specificity for the diagnosis of CAD (stenosis ≥50%) were 88% (202 of 229 patients) and 55% (83 of 152 patients) for CTP and 63% (143 of 229 patients) and 67% (102 of 152 patients) for SPECT, with area under the ROC curve values of 0.78 (95% CI, 0.74 to 0.82) and 0.69 (95% CI, 0.64 to 0.74; P = .001). The sensitivity of CTP for single-vessel and multivessel CAD was higher than that of SPECT, with sensitivities for left main, three-vessel, two-vessel, and one-vessel disease of 92%, 92%, 89%, and 83%, respectively, for CTP, and 75%, 79%, 68%, and 41%, respectively, for SPECT.[96]

Coronary Fractional Flow Reserve Computed Tomography

At present, the gold standard assessment of the physiologic significance of coronary stenoses is invasive FFR. Recently, a series of innovations have allowed CCTA to be interpreted to calculate FFR (FFRCT), thereby creating the potential of this test to provide an integrated anatomic and physiologic assessment of CAD. This advance uses computational fluid dynamics to noninvasively calculate FFR from routinely acquired CCTA images. Three prospective multicenter clinical studies have been conducted thus far to evaluate the diagnostic performance of FFRCT using FFR as the gold standard. In these trials, FFRCT was demonstrated as superior to CCTA.[97–99] Furthermore, when comparing the susceptibility of FFRCT and CCTA visualized stenosis with respect to reduced diagnostic performance in the presence of common CT artifacts—such as poor contrast opacification, high calcium content, and motion artifact—FFRCT demonstrated a robustness in accuracy that was not observed with CCTA.

The multicenter Determination of Fractional Flow Reserve by Anatomic Computed Tomographic AngiOgraphy (DeFACTO) trial[100] investigated 407 vessels from 252 patients to determine the diagnostic performance of FFRCT for lesions of intermediate stenosis severity. In this study, FFRCT was compared with invasive FFR, and the researchers found that for these lesions accuracy, sensitivity, specificity, PPV, and NPV of FFRCT were 71%, 74%, 67%, 41%, and 90%, respectively, and with CCTA were 63%, 34%, 72%, 27%, and 78%, respectively. FFRCT possesses high diagnostic performance for identifying ischemic lesions of intermediate stenosis severity. Notably, the high sensitivity and NPV suggest the ability of FFRCT to effectively and noninvasively rule out ischemic intermediate lesions. The multicenter Prospective LongitudinAl Trial of FFRct: Outcome and Resource IMpacts (PLATFORM) trial evaluated patients with stable angina, comparing an FFRCT-guided strategy versus invasive coronary angiography, and found that FFRCT was associated with a lower rate of invasive coronary angiography revealing nonobstructive disease and provided improved information to guide revascularization with equivalent clinical outcomes and radiation exposure. Moreover, FFRCT was associated with lower resource utilization and overall cost.[101]

Coronary Computed Tomography Angiography in Acute Chest Pain

Acute chest pain is one of the leading presenting symptoms of patients who come to the emergency department (ED); responsible for more than 8 million annual visits in the United States. Only a minority of these patients will ultimately be diagnosed with myocardial ischemia, but most will be admitted to the hospital for investigations that cost $10 to $12 billion dollars annually.[102] Despite this effort and cost, up to 5% of ACS are missed.[103] To study the efficacy of CCTA in patients with acute chest pain, the Rule Out Myocardial Infarction/Ischemia Using Computer Assisted

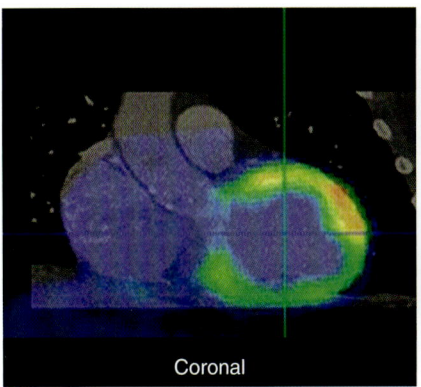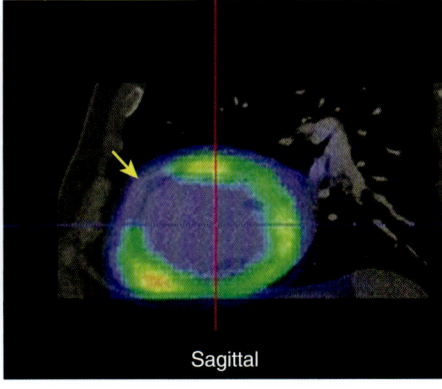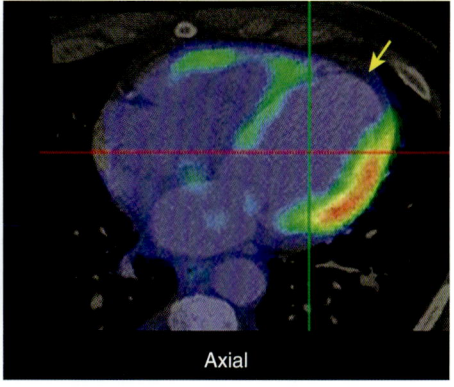

Fig. 4.16 Hybrid imaging. Fusion of anatomic multidetector computed tomography and functional images (positron emission tomography rubidium-82) in a patient with a large apical myocardial infarction *(arrows)*. Notice the thinning of the myocardium, which matches the lack of perfusion.

Tomography (ROMICAT) trial was conducted. CCTA was performed in ED patients with chest pain and negative cardiac biomarkers. The study found excellent sensitivity and NPV (both 100% for the presence of any atherosclerotic plaque) to rule out ACS in 368 subjects.[104] The effectiveness of CCTA in ruling out ACS in the ED was studied in three large, multicenter, randomized trials. The Coronary Computed Tomography Angiography for Systematic Triage of Acute Chest Pain Patients to Treatment (CT-STAT) study included 699 subjects with acute chest pain but an inconclusive ED evaluation, and patients were randomly allocated to CCTA or radionuclide MPI. CCTA resulted in a 54% reduction in time to diagnosis compared with radionuclide MPI, and costs of care were 38% lower compared with those of standard testing. The diagnostic strategies revealed no difference in MACE after normal index testing. The ROMICAT II trial[105] was a large multicenter randomized trial that enrolled 1000 patients with low to intermediate likelihood of ACS. The study was powered to a primary end point of length of stay in the hospital and secondary end points included time to diagnosis, rate of discharge from the ED, and resource utilization. Patients in the CCTA group had a shorter length of stay in the hospital, and almost four times as many patients were discharged directly from the ED without hospital admission (47% vs. 12%). These two studies, CT-STAT and ROMICAT II, also confirmed the 6-month absence of MACEs in patients who had a normal CCTA examination. A third, large, randomized, multicenter trial enrolled patients with a low (0 to 2) Thrombolysis in Myocardial Infarction (TIMI) score comparing CCTA with "traditional care." Similar to ROMICAT II, patients undergoing CCTA had a higher rate of discharge from the ED (50% vs. 23%) and a shorter length of stay in the hospital.[106] The CT-STAT and ROMICAT studies outlined above also confirmed the excellent safety profile of CCTA use in the ED, as well as the absence or very low incidence of MACE in patients who had a normal CCTA.

HYBRID IMAGING

Until the advent of CCTA, noninvasive imaging for the detection of CAD had mainly relied on functional imaging techniques to assess for indirect evidence of CAD. Functional imaging has been proven to be very valuable in determining prognosis and establishing the need for revascularization. However, neither echocardiography, radionuclide MPI, or CMR stress testing can establish the presence of mild to moderate CAD. Moreover, decisions regarding revascularization cannot rely solely on functional imaging without knowledge of the coronary anatomy. CCTA is capable of providing detailed information about the coronary anatomy that includes luminal stenosis and wall plaque. Because of the latter, it may establish the presence of atherosclerosis even earlier than invasive coronary angiography. However, the technique is limited in spatial and temporal resolution, making the differentiation between moderate and severe luminal stenosis difficult in most cases. In a study of 114 patients who underwent both radionuclide MPI and CCTA, 90% of patients with no visualized plaque by CCTA had normal MPI, 45% with any plaque visualized by CCTA had abnormal MPI results, and only 50% with any greater than 50% plaque by CCTA had abnormal MPI results.[91,107] The rationale for the development of PET-CT or SPECT-CT hybrid systems is that in many patients, knowledge of both coronary anatomy and the extent of ischemia are required to make management decisions. Hybrid systems consist of MDCT coupled with either a SPECT or PET camera. This facilitates the registration of functional and anatomic data in 3D space (Fig. 4.16). In oncology, Hybrid PET-CT imaging is now the standard because the benefits of integrating anatomic and functional data is clear, given the small size and large possible volume of distribution of metastatic tumors. However, in cardiology, the development of the technology has advanced before a clinical need has been clearly established.

APPROPRIATE USE CRITERIA

The unique clinical presentation of a patient is most often the deciding factor between anatomic and functional imaging. Anatomy is most helpful to exclude disease in asymptomatic or low-likelihood patients, whereas functional assessment may be most helpful in symptomatic patients. The American College of Cardiology, along with key specialty and subspecialty societies, conducted an appropriate use review of common clinical presentations for stable ischemic heart disease (SIHD) for which to consider the use of stress testing and anatomic diagnostic procedures. Tables 4.1 and 4.2 are intended to provide a practical guide to individual clinicians and patients when considering one of these procedures based on any number of important local and patient-specific variables, such as symptoms and global risk scores, while promoting optimal test utilization for the population at large.[108]

RADIATION EXPOSURE RELATIVE HEALTH RISKS

Over the last decade, the medical community has raised awareness about the potential health risks associated with radiation exposure from medical imaging. Even though most of the evidence that supports an increased lifetime incidence of cancer has been obtained from observational studies from overexposed children and adolescents, cardiac imaging organizations and the medical industry have introduced safer technologies and practices to reduce such risk. Table 4.3 provides a comparison of the typical radiation exposure and the estimated excess mortality risk attributed to the various tests discussed in this chapter. The reader

SECTION I Patient Selection

TABLE 4.1 Multimodality Detection and Risk Assessment of Ischemic Heart Disease Appropriate Use Criteria: Symptomatic Patients

	Indication Text	Exercise ECG	Stress RNI	Stress Echo	Stress CMR	Calcium Scoring	CCTA	Invasive Coronary Angiography
1	Low pretest probability of CAD, ECG interpretable, *and* able to exercise	A	R	M	R	R	R	R
2	Low pretest probability of CAD, ECG uninterpretable, *or* unable to exercise	–	A	A	M	R	M	R
3	Intermediate pretest probability of CAD, ECG uninterpretable, *and* able to exercise	A	A	A	M	R	M	R
4	Intermediate pretest probability of CAD, ECG uninterpretable, *or* unable to exercise	–	A	A	A	R	A	M
5	High pretest probability of CAD, ECG interpretable, *and* able to exercise	M	A	A	A	R	M	A
6	High pretest probability of CAD, ECG uninterpretable, *or* unable to exercise	–	A	A	A	R	M	A

A, Appropriate; *CAD,* coronary artery disease; *CCTA,* coronary computed tomography angiography; *CMR,* cardiac magnetic resonance; *ECG,* electrocardiogram; *Echo,* echocardiography; *M,* may be appropriate; *R,* rarely appropriate; *RNI,* radionuclide imaging.
From Wolk MJ, Bailey SR, Doherty JU, et al. ACCF/AHA/ASE/ASNC/HFSA/HRS/SCAI/SCCT/SCMR/STS 2013 multimodality appropriate use criteria for the detection and risk assessment of stable ischemic heart disease: a report of the American College of Cardiology Foundation Appropriate Use Criteria Task Force, American Heart Association, American Society of Echocardiography, American Society of Nuclear Cardiology, Heart Failure Society of America, Heart Rhythm Society, Society for Cardiovascular Angiography and Interventions, Society of Cardiovascular Computed Tomography, Society for Cardiovascular Magnetic Resonance, and Society of Thoracic Surgeons. *J Am Coll Cardiol*. 2014;63(4):380–406.

TABLE 4.2 Multimodality Detection and Risk Assessment of Ischemic Heart Disease Appropriate Use Criteria: Asymptomatic Patients

	Indication Text	Exercise ECG	Stress RNI	Stress Echo	Stress CMR	Calcium Scoring	CCTA	Invasive Coronary Angiography
7	Low global CHD risk regardless of ECG interpretability and ability to exercise	R	R	R	R	R	R	R
8	Intermediate global CHD risk, ECG interpretable *and* able to exercise	M	R	R	R	M	R	R
9	Intermediate global CHD risk, ECG uninterpretable *or* unable to exercise	–	M	M	R	M	R	R
10	High global CHD risk, ECG interpretable *and* able to exercise	A	M	M	M	M	M	R
11	High global CHD risk, ECG uninterpretable *or* unable to exercise	–	M	M	M	M	M	R

A, Appropriate; *CCTA,* coronary computed tomography angiography; *CHD,* coronary heart disease; *CMR,* cardiac magnetic resonance; *ECG,* electrocardiogram; *Echo,* echocardiography; *M,* may be appropriate; *R,* rarely appropriate; *RNI,* radionuclide imaging.
From Wolk MJ, Bailey SR, Doherty JU, et al. ACCF/AHA/ASE/ASNC/HFSA/HRS/SCAI/SCCT/SCMR/STS 2013 multimodality appropriate use criteria for the detection and risk assessment of stable ischemic heart disease: a report of the American College of Cardiology Foundation Appropriate Use Criteria Task Force, American Heart Association, American Society of Echocardiography, American Society of Nuclear Cardiology, Heart Failure Society of America, Heart Rhythm Society, Society for Cardiovascular Angiography and Interventions, Society of Cardiovascular Computed Tomography, Society for Cardiovascular Magnetic Resonance, and Society of Thoracic Surgeons. *J Am Coll Cardiol*. 2014;63(4):380–406.

TABLE 4.3 Estimated Radiation Exposure and Excess Lifetime Cancer Risk Attributable to Common Noninvasive Cardiac Diagnostic Studies

Modality	System	Protocol	Isotope	Isotope Dose (mCi)	Effective Dose (mSv)	Excess All-Cancer Risk (%)	Excess Fatal Cancer Risk (%)
SPECT-MPI	Anger	Rest-stress	Thallium-201	4.5	31.4	0.31	0.16
		Rest-stress	Thallium-201 Technetium-99m sestamibi	3.5/25	29.2	0.29	0.15
		Rest-stress	Technetium-99m sestamibi	37.5	11.3	0.11	0.06
		Stress only	Technetium-99m sestamibi	27.5	7.9	0.08	0.04
	Solid State	Rest-stress	Technetium-99m sestamibi	20	5.8	0.06	0.03
		Stress only	Technetium-99m sestamibi	12.5	3.6	0.04	0.02
PET-MPI		Rest-stress	Rubidium-82	100	13.5	0.14	0.07
		Rest-stress	13N-ammonia	30	2.5	0.03	0.01
		Rest-stress	Flurpiridaz-18F	10	7	0.07	0.04
PET-Metabolism			18F-FDG	10	7	0.07	0.04
						0.00	0.00
CT-CAC score		Retrospective			3	0.03	0.02
		Prospective			1	0.01	0.01
CT-CCTA		Nongated			18	0.18	0.09
		Retrospective			12	0.12	0.06
		Prospective			3	0.03	0.02

CAC, Coronary artery calcium; *CCTA*, cardiac computed tomography angiography; *CT*, computed tomography; *FDG*, fluorodeoxyglucose; *MPI*, myocardial perfusion imaging; *PET*, positron emission tomography; *SPECT*, single-photon emission computed tomography.
From Einstein AJ, Moser KW, Thompson RC, et al. Radiation dose to patients from cardiac diagnostic imaging. *Circulation.* 2007;116:1290–1305; Slomka PJ, Berman DS, Germano G. New cardiac cameras: single-photon emission CT and PET. *Semin Nucl Med.* 2014;44:232–251; and Contemporary Physics Education Project (CPEP). (2003). *Nuclear Science: A Guide to the Nuclear Science Wall Chart.* Available from: www2.lbl.gov/abc/wallchart/guide.html.

should understand that these estimates use data from atomic bomb survivors and assume a linear relationship between the level of exposure and the risk. The validity of the linear relationship theory has not been established; therefore the true risk associated with low levels of radiation exposure is unknown. Moreover, radiation dose estimates vary widely according to the equipment, protocol, isotopes, and patient characteristics involved.

CONCLUSIONS

The objectives of noninvasive cardiac imaging in patients with known or suspected CAD are to provide confirmatory evidence that CAD is the cause of symptoms, and to offer guidance for the appropriate selection of medical therapy and/or revascularization. In most cases, the extent of anatomic CAD is directly related to the extent and severity of stress-induced myocardial perfusion abnormalities. However, abnormal myocardial perfusion also may be associated with vascular dysfunction in the setting of nonobstructive CAD. Conversely, normal myocardial perfusion may be present in patients with obstructive CAD with increased collateral flow. Hence, because the objective of myocardial revascularization is to reduce myocardial ischemia, it may be concluded that the results of functional imaging tests are more important to guide therapeutic decisions than to direct anatomic imaging. In patients who have been evaluated by both radionuclide MPI and CCTA, the frequency of inducible ischemia is 0%, 5%, 33%, 54%, and 86% for CCTA stenosis of 0%, 0% to 60%, 60% to 70%, 70% to 80%, and greater than 80%, respectively.[75] Thus when severe ischemia is present and a false-positive result is unlikely, the likelihood of obstructive CAD is high. The additional information provided by CCTA in such cases is minimal in terms of dictating patient management. On the other hand, real-world experience has shown that a significant proportion of patients who are evaluated by functional tests have inconclusive, false-positive, or false-negative results. Thus, anatomic demonstration of CAD by CCTA may play an important role as a less expensive and safer alternative to diagnostic invasive coronary angiography.

A meta-analysis of comparative studies performed with 64-slice CCTA demonstrated diagnostic sensitivities and specificities of 94% (93% to 97%) and 85% (80% to 90%).[109] From these studies it is clear that the strengths of CCTA are its high sensitivity and high NPV, which exceeds 95%.[110] These characteristics suggest that CCTA would be most useful as a first diagnostic test for excluding obstructive CAD in low- to intermediate-risk patients. Furthermore, with technological advances in CCTA, FFRCT, and CMR to diagnose the functional significance of coronary lesions, these modalities are being used with more frequency and confidence.

In comparison with CCTA, radionuclide MPI has a lower sensitivity—in the range of 85% to 90%[111]—and it is even lower for the detection of single-vessel CAD. The rate of false-positive MPI scans has been reduced with the use of technetium-99m radioisotopes, attenuation-correction algorithms, and the incorporation of gated LVEF and regional wall motion analysis. The result has been improved specificity in the range of 80% to 90%.[111–113] Specificity is also very high with stress echocardiography. The sensitivity of CTP for single-vessel and multivessel

CAD was higher than that of SPECT, and studies have shown that MRI stress perfusion performs just as well. Therefore the strengths of functional stress imaging tests are their higher specificity and PPV. Accordingly, stress imaging would be most useful as a first diagnostic test for confirming obstructive CAD in intermediate- to high-risk patients. The clinical scenario is most often the deciding factor between anatomic and functional imaging, and appropriateness criteria have been established to guide clinicians when considering these tests. Several ongoing prospective multicenter trials seek to determine the utility of anatomic versus functional imaging tests in specific clinical scenarios.

KEY REFERENCES

1. Kokkinos P, Myers J, Kokkinos JP, et al. Exercise capacity and mortality in black and white men. *Circulation*. 2008;117(5):614–622.
5. Sicari R, Pasanisi E, Venneri L, et al. Stress echo results predict mortality: a large-scale multicenter prospective international study. *J Am Coll Cardiol*. 2003;41(4):589–595.
27. Schwitter J, Wacker CM, van Rossum AC, et al. MR-IMPACT: comparison of perfusion-cardiac magnetic resonance with single-photon emission computed tomography for the detection of coronary artery disease in a multicentre multivendor randomized trial. *Eur Heart J*. 2008;29(4):480–489.
28. Greenwood JP, Maredia N, Younger JF, et al. Cardiovascular magnetic resonance and single-photon emission computed tomography for diagnosis of coronary heart disease (CE-MARC): a prospective trial. *Lancet*. 2012;379(9814):453–460.
31. Jahnke C, Nagel E, Gebker R, et al. Prognostic value of cardiac magnetic resonance stress tests: adenosine stress perfusion and dobutamine stress wall motion imaging. *Circulation*. 2007;115(13):1769–1776.
51. Cleland JG, Calvert M, Freemantle N, et al. The Heart Failure Revascularisation Trial (HEART). *Eur J Heart Fail*. 2011;13(2):227–233.
53. Velazquez EJ, Lee KL, Deja MA, et al. Coronary-artery bypass surgery in patients with left ventricular dysfunction. *N Engl J Med*. 2011;364(17):1607–1616.
54. Bonow RO, Maurer G, Lee KL, et al. Myocardial viability and survival in ischemic left ventricular dysfunction. *N Engl J Med*. 2011;364(17):1617–1625.
60. Greenland P, LaBree L, Azen SP, et al. Coronary artery calcium score combined with Framingham score for risk prediction in asymptomatic individuals. *JAMA*. 2004;291(2):210–215.
79. Douglas PS, Hoffmann U, Lee KL, et al. PROspective Multicenter Imaging Study for Evaluation of chest pain: rationale and design of the PROMISE trial. *Am Heart J*. 2014;167(6):796–803.e1.
81. SCOT-HEART investigators. CT coronary angiography in patients with suspected angina due to coronary heart disease (SCOT-HEART): an open-label parallel-group multicentre trial. *Lancet*. 2015;385(9985):2383–2391.
82. Marwick TH, Cho I, Ó Hartaigh B, et al. Finding the gatekeeper to the cardiac catheterization laboratory: coronary CT angiography or stress testing? *J Am Coll Cardiol*. 2015;65(25):2747–2756.
84. Motoyama S, Sarai M, Harigaya H, et al. Computed tomographic angiography characteristics of atherosclerotic plaques subsequently resulting in acute coronary syndrome. *J Am Coll Cardiol*. 2009;54(1):49–57.
95. Bettencourt N, Chiribiri A, Schuster A, et al. Direct comparison of cardiac magnetic resonance and multidetector computed tomography stress-rest perfusion imaging for detection of coronary artery disease. *J Am Coll Cardiol*. 2013;61(10):1099–1107.
96. George RT, Mehra VC, Chen MY, et al. Myocardial CT perfusion imaging and SPECT for the diagnosis of coronary artery disease: a head-to-head comparison from the CORE320 multicenter diagnostic performance study. *Radiology*. 2014;272(2):407–416.
97. Koo BK, Erglis A, Doh JH, et al. Diagnosis of ischemia-causing coronary stenoses by noninvasive fractional flow reserve computed from coronary computed tomographic angiograms. Results from the prospective multicenter DISCOVER-FLOW (Diagnosis of Ischemia-Causing Stenoses Obtained Via Noninvasive Fractional Flow Reserve) study. *J Am Coll Cardiol*. 2011;58(19):1989–1997.
98. Min JK, Leipsic J, Pencina MJ, et al. Diagnostic accuracy of fractional flow reserve from anatomic CT angiography. *JAMA*. 2012;308(12):1237–1245.
101. Douglas PS, De Bruyne B, Pontone G, et al. 1-Year Outcomes of FFRCT-guided care in patients with suspected coronary disease: the PLATFORM study. *J Am Coll Cardiol*. 2016;68(5):435–445.
104. Hoffmann U, Bamberg F, Chae CU, et al. Coronary computed tomography angiography for early triage of patients with acute chest pain: the ROMICAT (Rule Out Myocardial Infarction using Computer Assisted Tomography) trial. *J Am Coll Cardiol*. 2009;53(18):1642–1650.
105. Hoffmann U, Bamberg F, Chae CU, et al. Coronary CT angiography versus standard evaluation in acute chest pain. *N Engl J Med*. 2012;367(4):299–308.
106. Litt HI, Gatsonis C, Snyder B, et al. CT angiography for safe discharge of patients with possible acute coronary syndromes. *N Engl J Med*. 2012;366(15):1393–13403.

Additional references available online at expertconsult.com.

中文导读

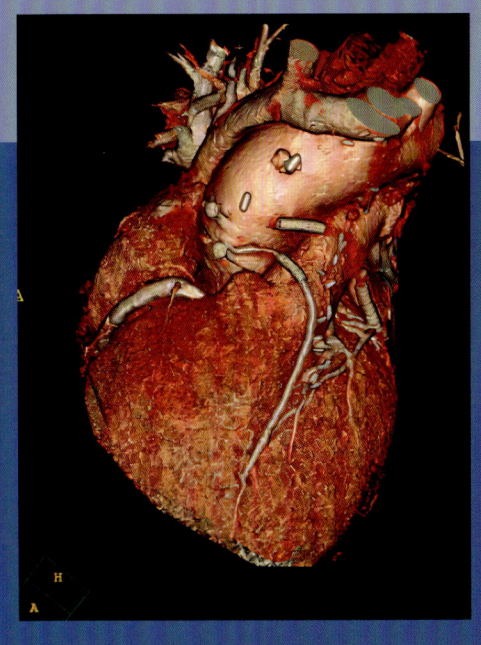

第5章
冠状动脉内压力和流量测量

　　冠状动脉内血流速度或流量可准确反映心肌获得的血流量。心肌血流量的明显减少决定冠心病患者的预后。荟萃分析显示，SPECT无心肌缺血冠心病患者的年死亡率或非致命性心肌梗死发生率仅0.6%，而这种事件的发生率在有SPECT缺血影像的患者中增加了7倍，达到了7.4%，且风险随缺血程度的增加而升高。因此，评估狭窄病变与心肌缺血的关系至关重要。

　　先前认为，冠状动脉造影对直径狭窄<30%或≥80%的病变功能严重程度可做出较为正确的判断，但对直径30%～70%的病变功能严重程度评价的准确性受到一定限制。血管内超声或光学相干断层成像能更准确地评价血管直径和管腔横截面积，但由于血管重构和微血管床的影响，准确评价狭窄生理功能的严重程度仍受限制。血流储备分数是一种基于冠状动脉内压力测量而间接评价冠状动脉内血流的方法，欧洲心脏病学会血运重建指南将血流储备分数作为ⅠA类适应证推荐用于缺血性相关血管不明确病变功能学的评价措施。基于血流储备分数而衍生出来的瞬时无波型比率也表现出了较好的临床应用价值。

　　在对经冠状动脉造影证实的临界病变行血运重建治疗时，需要了解这些病变是否诱发明显的心肌缺血？患者的临床症状是否与心肌缺血有关？干预这些病变能否改善患者的症状或预后？血流储备分数可以帮助我们回答这些问题。大规模的临床研究已经证实，非"缺血性"血流储备分数冠状动脉狭窄的延迟血运重建具有良好的长期预后。决定多支血管病变的"罪犯血管"及介入策略是对医师的一个挑战。在FAME研究中关于多支病变的结果表明，由血流储备分数指导策略选择的患者1年死亡或者心肌梗死风险明显低于血管造影指导的患者，2年随访结果与此相似，且心肌梗死的风险也显著降低，仅0.2%的未处理病变导致晚期心肌梗死，1.9%的病变进展需血运重建。血流储备分数应用于缺血性相关病变的确定，特别是对于多支血管病变、支架再狭窄病变、左主干病变和心肌梗死相关血管病变的精准评价，正发挥着越来越重要的作用。

李凡奇　范　谦

章节要点

- 仅靠血管造影往往不足以评估中等程度狭窄，甚至是重度狭窄的血管病变。
- 尽管附加的负荷试验存在着很多局限性，但血流储备分数可准确检测到与病变相关的特异性心肌缺血。
- 对于存在非"缺血性"血流储备分数的冠状动脉狭窄病变，延迟血运重建可获得良好的长期预后。
- 对于存在多支病变的冠心病患者，血流储备分数指导的经皮冠状动脉介入治疗无论在临床方面还是在经济方面都要优于血管造影指导的经皮冠状动脉介入治疗。
- 瞬时无波型比率在低危患者亚组中的表现不劣于血流储备分数。

5 Intracoronary Pressure and Flow Measurements

Morton J. Kern, Michael J. Lim, Katherine Yu

KEY POINTS

- Angiography alone is often insufficient to assess intermediate and, at times, severe stenoses.
- Although adjunctive stress testing has limitations, fractional flow reserve (FFR) provides an accurate detector of lesion specific myocardial ischemia.
- Deferring revascularization of a coronary stenosis with a non-"ischemic" FFR has a favorable long-term outcome.
- Percutaneous coronary intervention (PCI) guided by FFR is clinically and economically superior to angiography-guided PCI in patients with multivessel coronary artery disease.
- Instantaneous wave-free pressure ratio (iFR) demonstrated noninferiority to FFR in low-risk patient subgroups.

The goal of coronary revascularization is the relief of ischemia and restoration of coronary blood flow. The treatment of coronary stenosis with stenting improves exercise tolerance, reduces antiischemic medications, and improves survival in patients with ST elevation myocardial infarction (STEMI). However, in patients with stable coronary artery disease (CAD), stent placement is of no benefit if the angiographic stenoses are not responsible for ischemia.

The rationale for physiologic lesion assessment is simple: for lesions of intermediate severity, the angiogram cannot be relied on exclusively to direct coronary revascularization.[1] Coronary angiography produces two-dimensional (2D) luminograms, a silhouette image of the three-dimensional (3D) vascular lumen in a given projection. Angiography does not truly identify atherosclerosis, a disease within the vessel wall, but instead provides a "shadow" without intraluminal details sufficient to characterize a plaque. Furthermore, the eccentric shapes of plaques do not permit the observer to determine whether such an opening is limiting coronary blood flow. The accurate identification of both "normal" and "diseased" vessel segments by angiography further complicates the determination of a lesion's significance in the setting of diffuse CAD, which cannot easily be seen on an angiogram. Angiographic artifacts that include contrast streaming, branch overlap, vessel foreshortening, calcifications, and ostial origins further make the interpretation of some luminal narrowings unreliable. Despite numerous attempts to improve the angiographic imaging of complex anatomy, the angiographer is still confronted by a visual dilemma in which no single view or multiple views can provide an answer. Moreover, even sophisticated imaging modalities such as densitometry, rotational angiography, and computed tomography angiography (CTA) with 3D reconstruction (without the computational fluid-dynamic addition of fractional flow reserve computed tomography [FFRCT]) do not reliably reflect the physiologic significance of a given lesion.[2]

FUNDAMENTAL CONCEPTS OF CORONARY BLOOD FLOW

Coronary blood flow can increase from a resting level to a maximum (i.e., coronary reserve), depending on increases in myocardial oxygen demand or in response to neurogenic or pharmacologic hyperemic stimuli. Normally, large epicardial vessel resistance to blood flow is negligible. Most of the regulation of coronary flow occurs in the myocardial precapillary arteriolar resistance vessels. In a normal adult artery that supplies normal myocardium, coronary blood flow can increase more than threefold. However, several conditions—including left ventricular hypertrophy, myocardial ischemia, and diabetes—can affect the microcirculation, blunting the maximal absolute increase in coronary flow or increasing resting flow above the expected level for myocardial oxygen demand at rest. The regulation of coronary vasomotor tone and the influence of several mechanisms such as α-adrenoreceptor–mediated vasoconstriction have been extensively reviewed elsewhere and are beyond the scope of this chapter.[3] A significant atherosclerotic stenosis produces epicardial conduit resistance and, depending on flow, loss of distal pressure. In response to the loss of perfusion pressure and flow to the distal (poststenotic) vascular bed, the small resistance vessels dilate to maintain satisfactory basal flow appropriate for myocardial oxygen demand. Viscous friction, flow separation forces, and turbulence at the site of the stenosis produce energy loss at the stenosis (Fig. 5.1). Energy (heat) is extracted, which reduces pressure distal to the stenosis and thereby produces a pressure gradient between the proximal and distal arterial regions. The pressure loss or pressure gradient increases with increasing coronary flow in a curvilinear manner.[4] An absolute poststenotic myocardial perfusion pressure threshold exists, below which myocardial ischemia may be easily induced.

Coronary Flow and Flow Reserve

As the severity of an epicardial stenosis increases, maximal coronary flow becomes attenuated, and coronary flow reserve (CFR) decreases. CFR, the ratio of maximal to basal arterial flow, is a combined measure of the capacity of the major resistance components—the epicardial coronary artery and the supplied vascular bed—to achieve maximal blood flow in response to hyperemic stimulation. Although there is no true "normal CFR," a higher CFR implies that both epicardial and microvascular bed resistances are low (i.e., normally low resistance; Fig. 5.2). However, a lower CFR (<2.0) does not indicate which component is affected, a fact that limits the clinical applicability of this measurement for lesion assessment. Although early studies in animals and humans indicated an absolute "normal" range for CFR of 3.5 to 5, the CFR in adult patients undergoing cardiac catheterization with chest pain syndromes and CAD risk factors with "angiographically normal" vessels was 2.7 ± 0.6, suggesting a degree of patient variability and microvascular disease.

CFR may be reduced in patients with normal coronary arteries and either essential hypertension or aortic stenosis (AS), in part related to myocardial hypertrophy and an abnormal microvasculature. Furthermore, CFR can be altered by

SECTION I Patient Selection

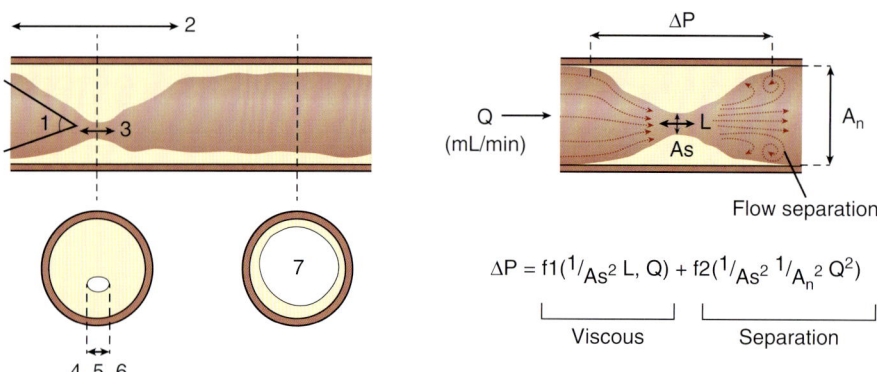

Fig. 5.1 Left: Diagram of coronary stenosis showing seven factors that produce resistance to flow: *(1)* entrance angle; *(2)* diseased segment length; *(3)* stenosis length; *(4–6)* shape factors of lumen area (minimum lumen diameter, minimum lumen area, eccentricity of stenosis); and *(7)* area of reference vessel. Right: Total pressure loss across a stenosis is derived from two sources: the frictional losses along the leading edge of the stenosis and the inertial losses stemming from the sudden expansion, which causes flow separation and eddies (exit losses). *Frictional losses* are linearly related to flow by Poiseuille's law, and *inertial losses* (exit losses) increase with the square of the flow (Bernoulli's law). The total change in pressure gradient (ΔP) is the sum of the two: the loss coefficients, *f1* and *f2*, are functions of stenosis geometry and rheologic properties of blood (viscosity and density). The graphic representation of this equation results in a quadratic relationship, in which the curvilinear shape demonstrates the presence of nonlinear exit losses. If no stenosis is present, the second term is zero, and the curve becomes a straight line (with a positive slope that depends on the diameter of the vessel, based on Poiseuille's law). A_n, Area of the normal segment; *As*, area of the stenosis; *L*, length; *Q*, flow. (Redrawn from Kern MJ, Samady H: Current concepts of integrated coronary physiology in the catheterization laboratory. *J Am Coll Cardiol*. 2010;55[3]:173–185.)

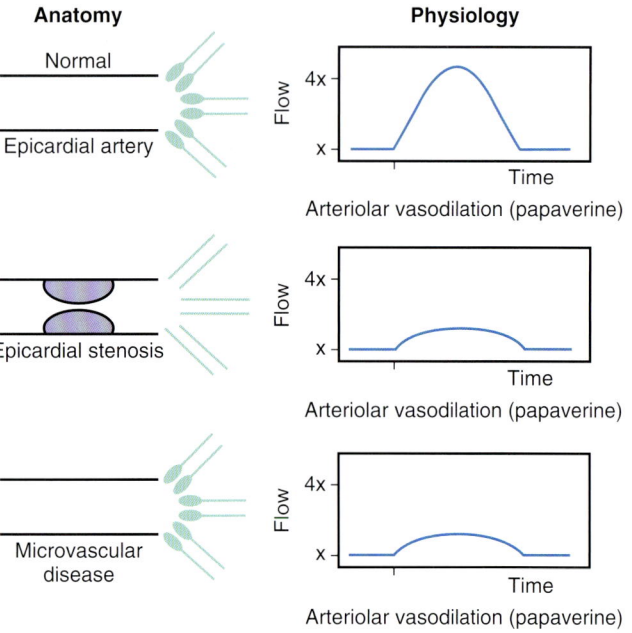

Fig. 5.2 Schematic representation of coronary flow reserve findings. Top panel: A normal artery without any epicardial stenosis or microvascular disease demonstrates the ability to significantly increase coronary flow when a hyperemic agent is given. Middle panel: An artery with significant epicardial stenosis that blunts the ability to increase flow over baseline. Bottom panel: The same finding of an artery unable to increase its flow rate. However, the reason in this case is not epicardial stenosis but severe microvascular disease. (Redrawn from Wilson RF, Lascon DD. A clinician's guide to assessing the physiologic significance of arterial stenoses. *Cathet Cardiovasc Diagn*. 1993;29:93–98.)

changes in basal and hyperemic flows, both of which are influenced by hemodynamics, loading conditions, and contractility. For example, tachycardia increases basal flow and decreases hyperemic flow, thus reducing CFR by 10% for each 15-beat increase in heart rate. In clinical terms, CFR is best used to assess the microcirculation in the absence of epicardial artery narrowings.

Intracoronary Pressure Measurements and Fractional Flow Reserve

As the limitations of invasive CFR were recognized, the development of pressure-sensor guidewires yielded a new concept of lesion assessment. As is the case from the earlier discussion regarding coronary flow, resistance to blood flow in a normal epicardial coronary artery is negligible, with virtually no energy loss as blood traverses the vessel. The aortic pressure thus remains constant throughout the conduit—including all branch vessels, regardless of their size—in the absence of epicardial disease. In the case of epicardial coronary narrowing, the resistance to flow and associated energy loss results in a pressure drop and is proportional to flow. To maintain resting myocardial perfusion at a constant level, a decrease in myocardial resistance compensates for any resistance of flow caused by the epicardial narrowing. The pressure ratio between normal and poststenotic pressure at constant maximal flow can represent an index of the physiologic consequences of a given coronary narrowing on the myocardium. Pressure measurements, made across a lesion during maximal hyperemia, are termed the *myocardial fractional flow reserve*, a concept introduced in 1993 by Pijls and colleagues.[5] FFR is the ratio of the maximal myocardial blood flow in the presence of a stenosis relative to expected normal flow in the absence of a stenosis, and it can be expressed as a fraction of its normal expected value if there were no lesion. Derived from pressure data alone for the myocardium, FFR measurement is based on several assumptions regarding translesional pressure measured during maximal hyperemia.[6] The proposed equations have been derived from a theoretic model of the coronary circulation and have been validated experimentally in instrumented dogs, and later in humans by comparison with myocardial flow measured by positron emission tomography (PET).[7] During maximal hyperemia (induced pharmacologically), coronary resistance is at the lowest level and remains constant, so that flow is directly related to the measured pressure. The total myocardial blood flow (Qn) in an area served by a coronary artery with a stenosis is the sum of the flow through the stenosis (Qs) and the collateral flow (Qc). *Fractional flow reserve* is then simply defined as the ratio of the measured flow (Qs) to the maximal flow that should be present without any stenosis (Qn):

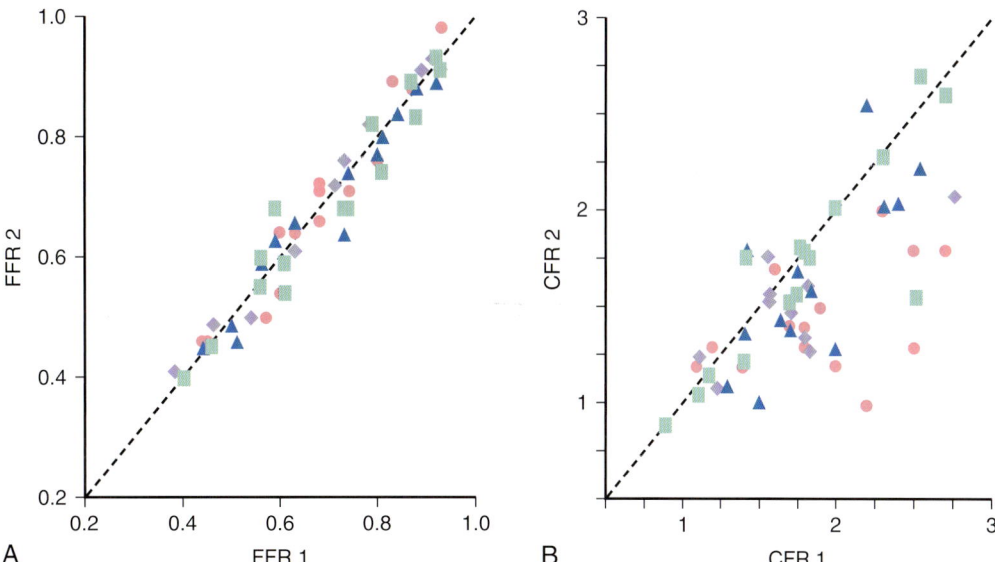

Fig. 5.3 (A) Reproducibility of fractional flow reserve *(FFR)* by serial measurements in a multicenter study of 325 patients in whom FFR was measured twice within a 10-minute interval. (B) Reproducibility of coronary flow reserve *(CFR)* in the same patients. *Blue boxes* represent baseline conditions. Violet diamonds represent changes in blood pressure induced by infusion of nitroprusside. *Blue triangles* represent changes in heart rate induced by pacing. *Pink circles* represent changes in contractility induced by infusion of dobutamine. Despite variations in heart rate of 40%, blood pressure of 35%, and contractility of 50%, FFR but not CFR was unaffected by these changes. (Data from De Bruyne B, Bartunek J, Sys SU, et al. Simultaneous coronary pressure and flow velocity measurements in humans: feasibility, reproducibility and hemodynamic dependence of coronary flow velocity reserve, hyperemic flow versus pressure slope index and fractional flow reserve. *Circulation.* 1996;94:1842–1849.)

$$Q_s = (P_d - P_v) \div R$$

and

$$Q_n = (P_a - P_v) \div R$$

where P_d is distal coronary pressure, P_a is aortic pressure, P_v is venous pressure (or right atrial pressure), and R is resistance of the myocardial vascular bed. In this model, P_v is assumed to be negligible, hence:

$$FFR = Q_s \div Q_n = [(P_d - P_v) \div R] \div [(P_a - P_v) \div R]$$

Given maximal hyperemia, resistance becomes constant and "near zero" in both the numerator and denominator, thus:

$$FFR = P_d \div P_a \text{ when measured at hyperemia}$$

FFR can thus be estimated as the ratio of the mean distal coronary blood pressure to the mean aortic blood pressure. Because each myocardial territory serves as its own control, FFR is a lesion-specific index. Furthermore, because FFR is measured only at maximal hyperemia, it is independent of microcirculation, heart rate, blood pressure, and other hemodynamic variables.

Unlike most other physiologic indexes, FFR has a normal value of 1.0 for every patient and every coronary artery. FFR has high reproducibility and low intraindividual variability (Fig. 5.3). Moreover, unlike CFR, FFR is independent of sex or CAD risk factors, such as hypertension and diabetes, and has less variability with common doses of adenosine. De Bruyne and associates[8] demonstrated that in humans, FFR is independent of hemodynamic conditions. Changes in heart rate affected by pacing, changes in contractility affected by dobutamine infusion, and changes in blood pressure affected by nitroprusside infusion did not alter FFR. The coefficient of variation between two consecutive measurements was 4.2%, which is lower than the 17.7% for CFR measured with a Doppler wire.

METHODOLOGY OF CORONARY PRESSURE MEASUREMENT
General Setup and Guidewire Manipulation

The measurement of coronary pressure is similar to performing an angioplasty in that a sensor guidewire is passed through an angioplasty Y-connector attached to a guiding catheter, with anticoagulation (intravenous [IV] heparin) given beforehand. To minimize measurement variability caused by vessel spasm, intracoronary (IC) nitroglycerin (100 to 200 μg) is given before the guidewire is advanced into the artery. For coronary pressure measurements, a guidewire with a pressure sensor can be used to measure distal coronary pressure. The angioplasty sensor guidewires (Fig. 5.4) have mechanical properties close to standard "workhorse" guidewires and have a pressure sensor located 3 cm from the tip, at the junction of the radiopaque and radiolucent portions of the wire. The wire tip can be shaped to facilitate delivery to the distal vessel. Recently, a novel 0.022-inch pressure-sensing monorail microcatheter has been made available to measure distal coronary pressure over any 0.014-inch standard guidewire of the operator's choice. The microcatheter has a pressure sensor associated with a marker that sends its signal via a fiberoptic pathway to the table-mounted analyzer (see Fig. 5.4).

All currently available systems have an "auto zero" feature that activates when the guidewire/catheter is connected to the analyzer. This signal should be zeroed against the "zero" from the guiding catheter transducer. The sensor is then introduced and positioned at the tip of the guiding catheter, where the guiding catheter and wire pressures are equalized (or normalized)—a step that electronically assimilates both pressure signals so that they are identical. Next, the sensor is advanced down the vessel and across the stenosis (or to the most distal part of the coronary artery for assessment of serial lesions or diffuse disease). A pharmacologic hyperemic stimulus (e.g., adenosine, discussed later) is then administered through the guiding catheter, or it can be

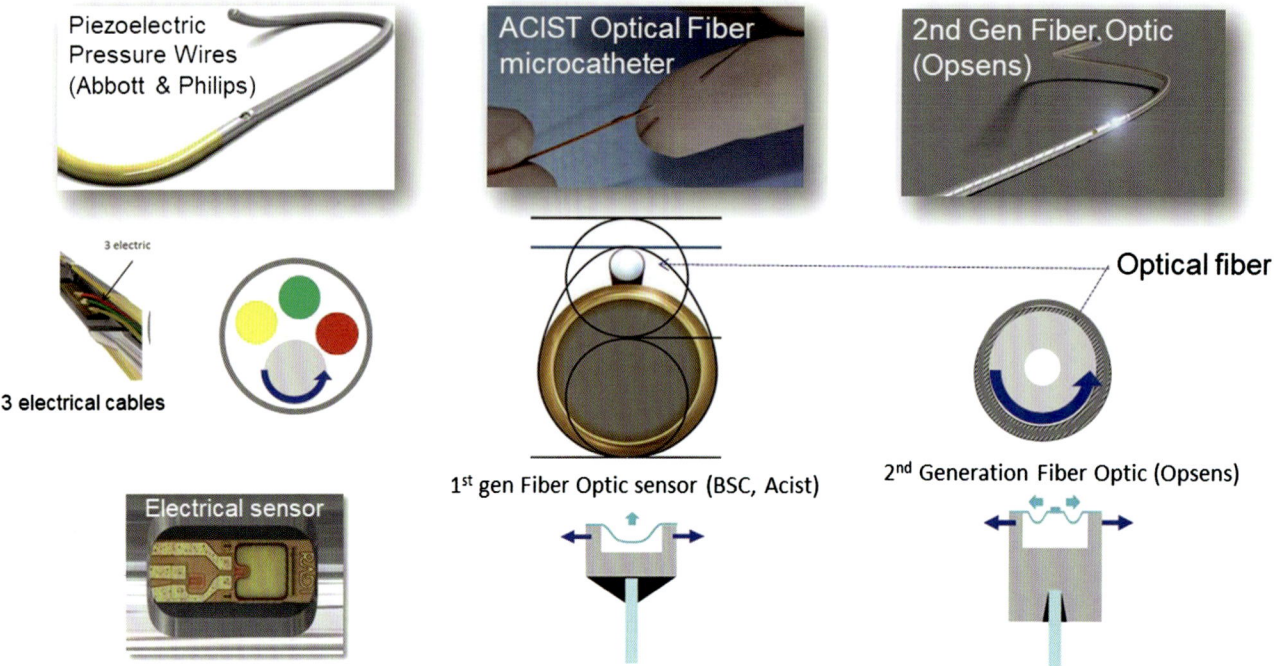

Fig. 5.4 **2019 Technology: new pressure sensor wires and microcatheter.** Top row: Piezoresistive sensor wires. *Left:* Abbott St. Jude, Philips Volcano Inc. *Middle:* Acist microcatheter. *Right:* Fiber optic Nitinol pressure wires from Opsens Inc, and Boston Scientific Co. Middle and bottom rows: *Left:* Wire construction with thin connecting wires to the electrical sensor. *Centre:* Cross section of Acist Rxi microcatheter which travels over any working 0.014" guidewire. It uses a first generation optical sensor. *Right:* Nitinol guidewires with central optical fiber provides improved torque function and employs a second generation (Opsens) pressure sensor.

given by IV infusion. The mean and phasic pressure signals are continuously recorded, and at peak hyperemia—represented by the steady-state nadir, or lowest, distal pressure once stable hyperemia is reached—the FFR is calculated as noted earlier (Fig. 5.5).

To study the distribution of abnormalities along a diseased coronary artery (with serial lesions or diffuse disease), the pressure sensor can be pulled back slowly during intravenously induced hyperemia. Simultaneously observing the location of the wire by fluoroscopy and the pressure tracings can pinpoint the location of hemodynamically significant atherosclerotic abnormalities. On pulling back the pressure sensor in a vessel with diffuse but not focal obstructions, gradual pressure recovery along the course of the vessel can be observed. In contrast, a vessel with a focal stenosis will demonstrate an abrupt increase in pressure proximal to the lesion. By moving the sensor back and forth, the exact location of a pressure drop, representing a focal obstruction to flow, can be determined. FFR is often measured using 6-Fr guiding catheters, but 5-Fr guides and diagnostic catheters as small as 4 Fr have been successfully used. In general, the smaller the lumen of the catheter, the greater care the operator must take at flushing the catheter to optimally achieve an accurate aortic pressure signal (Pa). As with any technique in the catheterization lab, attention to detail is required to reduce inaccuracies in the measurement of FFR. A more complete description of the application and nuances of coronary pressure measurements can be found elsewhere.[9]

Safety of Intracoronary Sensor Wire Measurements

Qian and coworkers[10] examined the safety of IC Doppler wire measurements in 906 patients. Of these, 15 patients (1.7%) had severe transient bradycardia after administration of IC adenosine, 14 in the right coronary artery (RCA) and 1 in the left coronary artery (LCA). Nine patients (1%) had coronary spasm during passage of the Doppler guidewire, five in the RCA and four in the left anterior descending (LAD) coronary artery. Two patients (0.2%) had ventricular fibrillation (VF) during the procedure. Hypotension with bradycardia and ventricular asystole occurred in one patient. Transplant recipients had more of these complications than did patients undergoing either diagnostic or interventional procedures. All complications were easily managed, and no long-term adverse consequences were observed. These data support the safe clinical practice of sensor-wire measurements with IC adenosine.

Pharmacologic Hyperemic Stimuli

Maximal coronary hyperemia is required for in-lab coronary physiologic lesion assessment (Table 5.1). The most widely used maximal vasodilator agent at this time is adenosine. Hyperosmolar ionic and low-osmolar nonionic contrast media do not produce maximal vasodilation. Nitrates increase volumetric flow, but because these agents also dilate the epicardial conductance vessels, the increase in coronary flow velocity is less than with adenosine or papaverine. IC nitroprusside has similar hyperemic effects compared with IC adenosine. Papaverine is no longer used for IC hyperemic stimulation because of the occasional QT interval prolongation and associated ventricular tachycardia (VT) or VF.

Adenosine

A principal advantage of adenosine is that it has a short half-life, with a return to basal flow within 30 to 60 seconds after cessation of infusion. Adenosine is benign in a wide range of dosages (IC and IV). Typically, IV adenosine will result in approximately a 10% drop in mean arterial pressure (MAP) and may be accompanied by symptoms of chest burning. IC adenosine down the dominant coronary artery will result in atrioventricular (AV) block at high enough doses that it will result in a significant, although transient, decline in MAP.

IV adenosine has the advantages of simplicity and weight-adjusted dosing (140 μg/kg/min) and is required for the evaluation

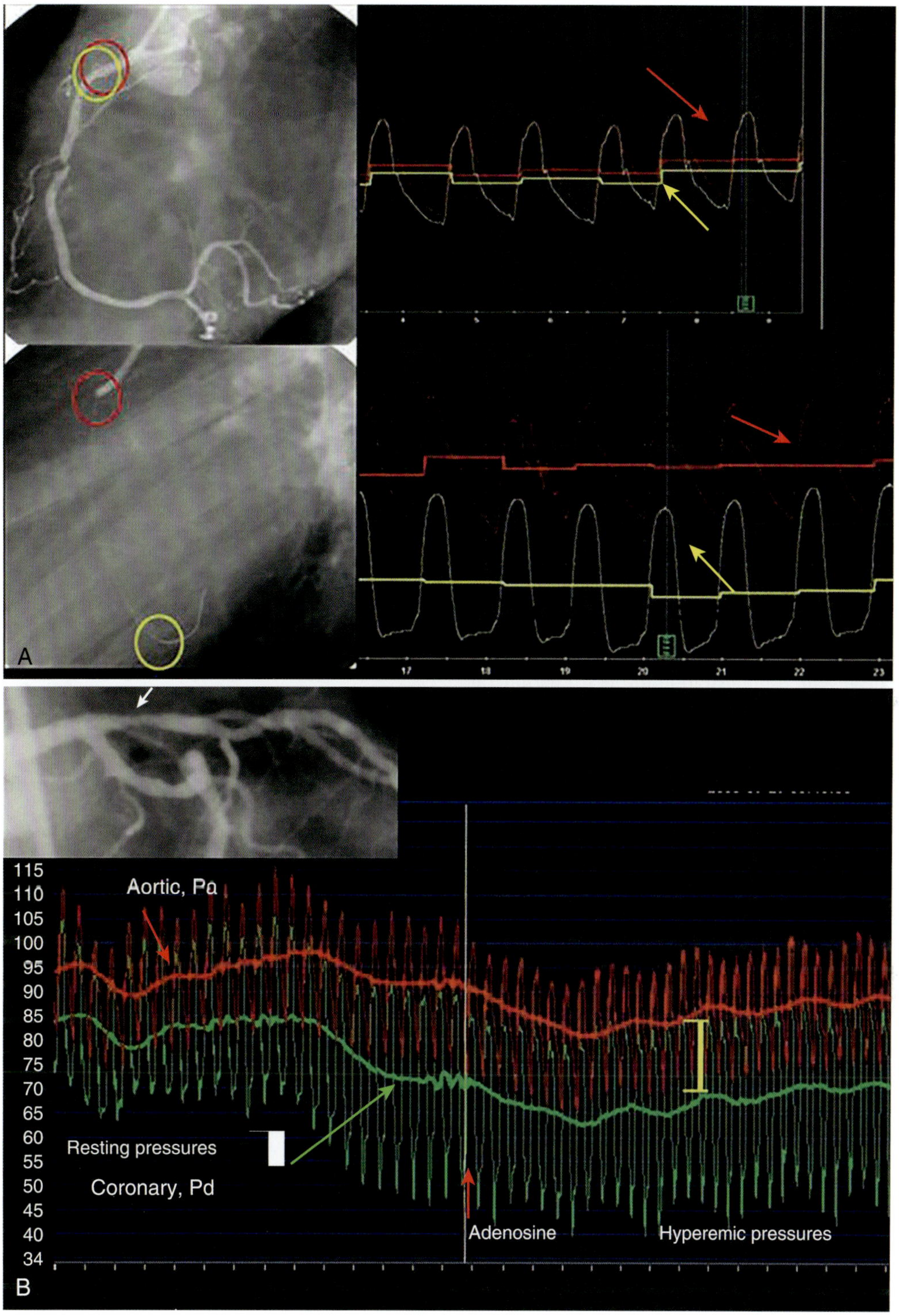

CHAPTER 5 Intracoronary Pressure and Flow Measurements

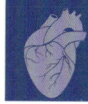

Fig. 5.5 (A) Top: The guidewire sensor and guide catheter *(red and yellow circles)* are shown in the proximal right coronary artery with corresponding pressures depicted on the right, showing "equalization" of pressures. Bottom: The guidewire has been advanced across the right coronary artery lesion and now is in the distal vessel with corresponding pressure loss as depicted on the right. (B) Fractional flow reserve (FFR) measurement across a proximal left anterior descending coronary artery lesion. The red pressure tracing is aortic guide catheter pressure, and the green tracing is coronary wire pressure. Adenosine is started, and the tracings from right to left reflect the changes over time. At the *yellow bar,* which reflects the lowest distal coronary pressure divided by aortic pressure (Pd/Pa) at steady state, the FFR is computed. FFR = Pd/Pa, or 65/90 (0.72). *Pa,* Aortic pressure; *Pd,* distal pressure.

TABLE 5.1 Pharmacologic Characteristics of Agents Used for Induction of Hyperemia

Drug	Dose	Plateau (s)	Half-Life (min)	Side Effects	Comments
Papaverine IC	15 mg LCA 10 mg RCA	30–60	2	Transient QT interval prolongation, torsades de pointes	Rarely used
Adenosine IV	140 µg/kg/min	60–120	1–2	Decreased blood pressure (10%–15%), chest burning	Avoid in patients with history of bronchospasm
Adenosine IC	100–200 µg LCA 50–100 µg RCA	5–10	0.5–1	Transient AV block when injected into the dominant artery	Must repeat with escalating doses to ensure that maximal hyperemia is reached
Dobutamine IV	20–40 µg/kg/min	60–120	3–5	Tachycardia, increase in blood pressure	May induce ischemia
Nitroprusside IC	0.3–0.9 µg/kg	20	1	Decreased blood pressure (20%)	
Regadenoson IV	0.4 mg	30	2–4[a]	Tachycardia	Exact length of hyperemia and ability to repeat bolus not studied in the cardiac catheterization lab for FFR

AV, Atrioventricular; *FFR*, fractional flow reserve; *IC*, intracoronary; *IV*, intravenous; *LCA*, left coronary artery; *RCA*, right coronary artery.
[a]Half-life is triphasic, with second phase lasting approximately 30 minutes and third phase lasting approximately 2 hours.

of ostial lesions or for the assessment of diffuse disease during pullback recordings. IV administration, however, tends to have a higher incidence of side effects such as flushing, chest tightness, bronchospasm, nausea, and transient AV block or bradycardia compared with IC dosing. It should also be noted that all the validation studies utilizing IV adenosine administered this infusion through a central vein. Administration through a peripheral vein may be accompanied by a long latent period before the onset of hyperemia without a clear-cut stability of the hyperemic phase.

IC adenosine appears to be equivalent to IV infusion for determination of FFR in most patients. Jeremias and colleagues[11] examined differences in FFR between IC adenosine (15 to 20 µg in the RCA or 18 to 24 µg in the LCA) and IV adenosine (140 µg/kg/min) in 52 patients with 60 lesions and found a strong linear relationship between IC and IV adenosine (regression coefficient [r] = 0.978, $P < .001$). The mean measurement difference for FFR was 0.004 (standard deviation [SD] ± 0.03). A small random scatter in both directions of FFR was noted in 8.3% of stenoses, where the IC adenosine FFR value was 0.05 greater than the IV adenosine FFR value, suggesting a suboptimal IC hyperemic response for which a repeated, higher IC adenosine dose may be helpful. Changes in heart rate and blood pressure were significantly greater with IV adenosine. Two patients with IV adenosine, but none with IC adenosine, had side effects such as bronchospasm and nausea. Despite these doses being correlated with hyperemic effects of IV adenosine, current dose recommendations are 50 to 100 µg in the RCA and 100 to 200 µg in the LAD to ensure maximal hyperemia is achieved.

Regadenoson

Regadenoson is a low-affinity α-2A adenosine receptor agonist that causes coronary vasodilation and increased myocardial blood flow and has been reported to be equivalent to adenosine. It selectively targets the α-2A receptor in coronary arteries and therefore has fewer adverse effects compared with adenosine. Regadenoson has a longer half-life of 2 to 3 minutes in the initial phase, 30 minutes in the intermediate phase, and 2 hours in the terminal phase, and it may prove to be easier to use. With a single infusion bolus of regadenoson (0.4 mg), maximum coronary hyperemia is achieved and maintained equivalent to that achieved with a constant infusion of adenosine. However, questions regarding the amount of time that hyperemia persists after this bolus and whether a similar hyperemic effect can be achieved with a second bolus demand further investigation. At this time, regadenoson is a useful agent for simple measurement of FFR (Fig. 5.6).[12–14]

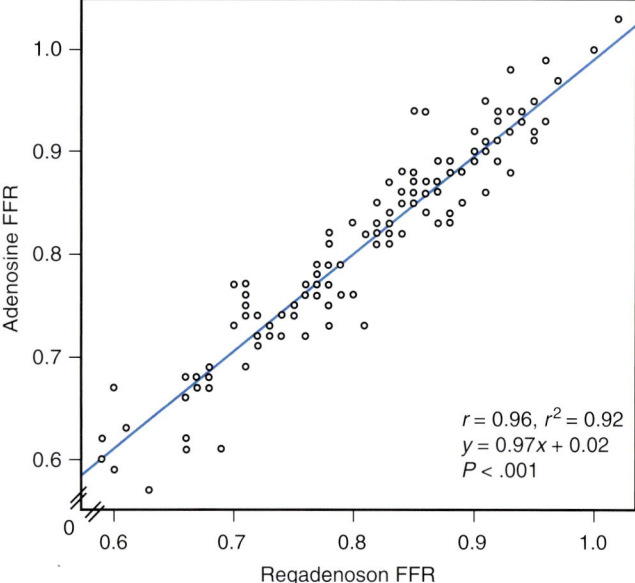

Fig. 5.6 Linear regression analysis of intrapatient fractional flow reserve *(FFR)* measured with an intravenous (IV) adenosine infusion and IV regadenoson bolus. *r,* Regression coefficient. (From Stolker JM, Guzman L, Zenni MM, et al. TCT-626 comparison of intravenous adenosine infusion and regadenoson bolus for calculating fractional flow reserve: results of a pooled analysis. *J Am Coll Cardiol.* 2013;62[18 S1]:B190.)

Dobutamine

Bartunek and associates[15] examined FFR in response to IC adenosine and IV dobutamine (10 to 40 µg/kg/min) in 22 patients with single-vessel CAD. Peak dobutamine infusion produced similar distal coronary pressures and pressure ratios (Pd/Pa, 60 ± 18 and 59 ± 18 mm Hg; FFR, 0.68 ± 0.18 and 0.68 ± 0.17, respectively; all P = not significant [NS]). An additional bolus of IC adenosine given at peak dobutamine in nine patients failed to change the FFR. As shown by angiography, high-dose IV dobutamine did not modify the area of the epicardial stenosis, and, much like adenosine, it fully exhausted myocardial resistance regardless of inducible left ventricular dysfunction.

Sodium Nitroprusside

IC nitroprusside may be an alternative to IC adenosine. Parham and associates[16] examined coronary blood flow velocity, heart rate, and blood pressure in unobstructed LAD arteries in 21 patients at rest, after IC adenosine (boluses of 30 to 50 μg), and after three serial doses of IC nitroprusside (boluses of 0.3, 0.6, and 0.9 μg/kg). IC nitroprusside produced equivalent coronary hyperemia with a longer duration (~25%) compared with IC adenosine. IC nitroprusside (0.9 μg/kg) decreased systolic blood pressure by 20% with minimal change in heart rate, whereas IC adenosine had no effect on these parameters. FFR measurements with IC nitroprusside were identical to those obtained with IC adenosine ($r = 0.97$). In doses commonly used for the treatment of the no-reflow phenomenon, IC nitroprusside can produce sustained coronary hyperemia without detrimental systemic hemodynamics. Sodium nitroprusside also appears to be a suitable hyperemic stimulus for coronary physiologic measurements.

Clinical Validation of Intracoronary Pressure Measurements

To define the threshold of FFR below which inducible ischemia is present, Pijls and colleagues[6] and De Bruyne and colleagues[17] conducted independent but parallel and complementary investigations. Pijls' group studied 60 patients accepted for single-vessel percutaneous transluminal coronary angioplasty (PTCA) who had a positive (abnormal or ischemic) exercise test in the preceding 24 hours. FFR was measured before and 15 minutes after PTCA, and the exercise test was repeated after 1 week. If the second exercise test had reverted to normal after PTCA, FFR values were associated with inducible ischemia. All except two FFR measurements greater than 0.74 were not associated with ischemia, and all FFR measurements of 0.74 or less were related to inducible ischemia. In normal coronary arteries, FFR was 0.98 (SD ± 0.03). De Bruyne's group studied FFR in 60 patients who each had one isolated lesion in one major coronary artery and a maximal exercise test 6 hours before catheterization. ST-segment depression was compared with FFR, APV_{max} (average peak velocity at maximal hyperemia), and APV_{rest}. Intersections of sensitivity and specificity curves were at 87%, 83%, and 75%, respectively, for FFR of 0.66, APV_{max} of 31 cm/s, and APV_{rest} of 12 cm/s. No abnormal test was present for FFR greater than 0.72. FFR has also been compared with the results of dobutamine echocardiography in 75 patients with normal left ventricular function and single-vessel CAD; the degree of dobutamine-induced dyssynergy correlated significantly with the quantitative coronary angiography (QCA) data, but the correlation was markedly better with FFR. All but one patient with an FFR greater than 0.75 had a normal stress test result.

Among the most important validations of FFR is that of Pijls and colleagues,[18] who compared FFR with a combined ischemic standard of common noninvasive testing modalities in 45 patients with moderate coronary stenoses and chest pain syndromes. When the FFR was less than 0.75 (21 patients), reversible myocardial ischemia was demonstrated unequivocally on at least one noninvasive test (bicycle exercise testing, thallium scintigraphy, stress echocardiography with dobutamine), and all these positive test results were reversed after PTCA or coronary artery bypass grafting (CABG). In 21 of 24 patients with an FFR greater than 0.75, all of the tests showed no demonstration of ischemia, and no revascularization procedure was performed. Importantly, no revascularization was required after 14 months of follow-up. The sensitivity of FFR in the identification of reversible ischemia was 88%, the specificity was 100%, the positive predictive value (PPV) was 100%, the negative predictive value (NPV) was 88%, and the accuracy was 93%.

Fractional Flow Reserve and Myocardial Perfusion Imaging

Magnetic resonance (MR) myocardial perfusion imaging (MPI) with IV adenosine (140 μg/kg/min) and a first-pass 0.1 mmol/kg gadolinium bolus has been shown to correlate well with FFR in detecting reversible ischemia. When tested against an FFR less than 0.75 in

TABLE 5.2 Summary of Correlation Between Noninvasive Stress Test Results and Physiologic Measurements

Index	Ischemic Test	N	Best Cutoff Value	Accuracy (%)
FFR	SPECT	763	0.74–0.78	75–95
	DSE	58	0.67–0.75	90
CFR	SPECT	704	1.7–2	75–92
	DSE	58	2	87–88
rCFR	SPECT	260	0.64–0.75	75–92
	DSE	28	0.75	81

BCV, Best cutoff value (defined as the value with the highest sum of sensitivity and specificity); *CFR*, coronary flow reserve; *DSE*, dobutamine stress echocardiography; *FFR*, fractional flow reserve; *N*, number of patients; *rCFR*, relative coronary flow reserve; *SPECT*, single-photon emission computed tomography.

103 patients with angina (300 coronary artery segments), MRMPI had a high sensitivity (91%), specificity (94%), PPV (91%), and NPV (94%) for detecting functionally significant coronary heart disease.[19]

PET-CT MPI shows poor concordance with FFR in identifying ischemic territories. In a study of 67 patients (201 vascular territories) with angiographic two-vessel or three-vessel coronary disease, PET-CT and FFR detected identical ischemic territories in only 42% of patients. In the remaining patients, PET-CT tended to significantly underestimate or overestimate the number of ischemic regions compared with FFR.[20]

Managing conflicting data when noninvasive stress imaging, such as nuclear perfusion imaging, and FFR produce different results creates uncertainty in the mind of the interventionalist. In such cases the operator must reevaluate his or her level of confidence in the accuracy of both test modalities. For nuclear perfusion imaging, a number of common conditions can produce false-positive and false-negative results. For FFR, certain rare situations produce false-positive results and almost none produce false-negative results. As recommended by the American College of Cardiology (ACC)/American Hospital Association (AHA)/Society for Cardiovascular Angiography and Interventions (SCAI) guidelines, use of FFR is a class III indication when the clinical scenario, angiogram, and ischemic test are concordant. Otherwise, the FFR serves to alleviate uncertainty when the clinical and testing data are at odds with one another. If the operator—for whatever reason—elects to use FFR, this decision should be based on FFR's ability to precisely define the ischemic potential of a stenosis in question.

Table 5.2 summarizes the comparison between ischemic stress testing and coronary physiologic measurements.

Fractional Flow Reserve and Angiography

Multiple studies have shown only a modest correlation between angiographic severity and FFR. In the largest study to date, Toth and associates[21] reported on more than 4000 intermediate lesions in which a slight yet statistically significant correlation was found between percent diameter stenosis as measured by QCA and FFR, with an r value of 0.38 ($P < .001$). A 50% or greater diameter stenosis had mediocre overall sensitivity (61%), specificity (67%), and diagnostic accuracy (64%) for predicting an FFR of less than 0.80. Using a stenosis diameter of 70% or greater, the measure became highly specific (98%) but poorly sensitive (13%), with a net decrease in the overall diagnostic accuracy for detecting functionally significant lesions. Their data also showed that the optimal diagnostic threshold of stenosis diameter was markedly lower in coronary segments that supply a larger myocardial area because FFR depends to some extent on the downstream mass. In particular, left main stenoses were often underestimated by the classical 50% diameter cutoff compared with FFR (Fig. 5.7).

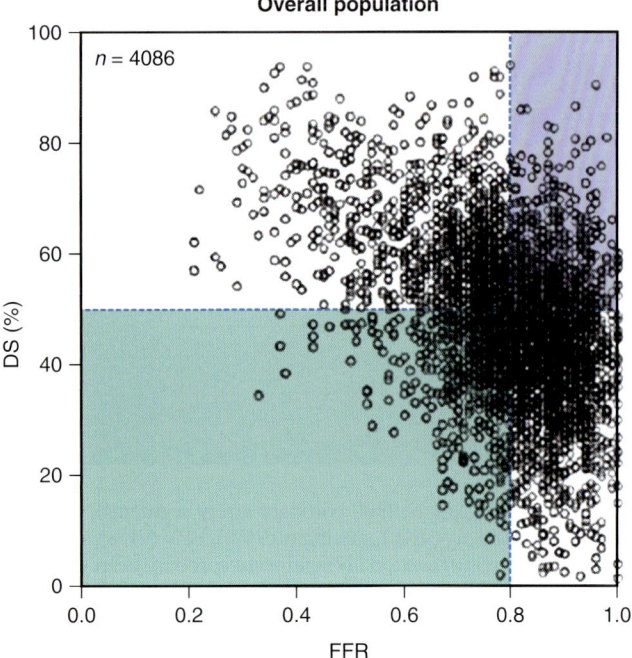

Fig. 5.7 Correlation between percent diameter stenosis *(DS)* and fractional flow reserve *(FFR)*. (From Toth G, Hamilos M, Pyxaras S, et al. Evolving concepts of angiogram: fractional flow reserve discordances in 4000 coronary stenoses. *Eur Heart J.* 2014;35[40]:2831–2838.)

Decision Making in the Fractional Flow Reserve "Gray Zone"

Clinical decision making in the "gray zone" FFR of 0.75 to 0.80 is controversial. Agarwal et al. found that in 238 patients having an FFR within the gray zone FFR, revascularization was associated with a significantly reduced risk of major adverse cardiovascular events (MACEs) compared with medical therapy alone.[22,23] On the other hand, in the Interventional Cardiology Research Incooperation Society Fractional Flow Reserve (IRIS-FFR), a large prospective, multicenter registry, the risk of MACE was not significantly different between deferred and revascularized lesions for FFR 0.76 or greater (including the gray zone).[24] In these situations, the decision to revascularize should be based on the clinical context.

Intracoronary Physiologic Measurements, Intravascular Ultrasound, and Optical Coherence Tomography Measurements

Intravascular ultrasound (IVUS) and optical coherence tomography (OCT) offer a high degree of anatomic detail that can aid the operator in making clinical decisions. The cross-sectional lumen area measured by these techniques (i.e., minimal luminal area [MLA]) has been proposed as a surrogate measurement of the functional significance of a given stenosis. However, in clinical practice, the anatomic measurements are more complementary than they are similar to FFR because FFR is a physiologic assessment, whereas IVUS and OCT are tools to measure vessel anatomy and lesion morphology. IVUS and OCT are highly accurate for vessel sizing and for confirming stent expansion and strut apposition.

A study to compare IVUS, QCA, and FFR in 42 patients with 51 stenoses also demonstrated that QCA alone was not accurate in determining physiologic lesion significance assessed by either IVUS or FFR.[25] A correlation was found between IVUS-MLA less than 3 mm² and stenosis cross-sectional area (CSA) greater than 60% with a measured FFR less than 0.75 (IVUS sensitivity 83%, specificity 92%). Several IVUS studies have compared FFR with IVUS measurements (e.g., MLA). Takagi and colleagues[26] found that most MLA values less than 4 mm² were associated with an FFR of less than 0.75, although several patients had a nonischemic FFR. The reason for this variance is that resistance to flow is based on various anatomic factors (entrance angle, length, MLA, eccentricity), of which MLA is only one. A 4-mm² MLA may limit flow in a large proximal vessel segment but will not impair flow in a smaller segment of the same artery. For assessment of the left main coronary artery (LMCA), unlike FFR, the IVUS threshold of "treat" or "do not treat" changes. Various IVUS MLAs have been reported to be the cutoff value, ranging from 5.9 to 7 mm² for treatment decisions.[27] Most IVUS thresholds are derived from clinical outcomes, with different areas from different studies. The poor correlation between MLA and FFR can be understood from a review of the factors that produce pressure loss across a stenosis. The loss of pressure across a stenosis can be computed from the two factors that produce the resistance to flow, viscous friction (factor 1 is coefficient of friction; factor 2 is coefficient of flow separation), and the energy loss in the coefficient of flow separation and reconstitution to laminar flow. Factor 1 (f1) is not only proportional to the inverse of the CSA squared but also directly proportional to the length of the narrowing:

$$\Delta P = \underbrace{f_1 (1/A_s^2 \ell, Q)}_{\text{Viscous}} + \underbrace{f_2 (1/A_s^2 1/A_n^2 Q^2)}_{\text{Separation}}$$

where ΔP is the pressure drop across a stenosis, A_s is the minimal stenosis CSA and Q is blood flow (velocity) through the tube. Unlike IVUS, FFR represents the net myocardial blood flow across the stenosis supplying the specific myocardial bed. For example, a 70% stenosis in a vessel subtending a small diagonal or a previously infarcted mid–anterior descending territory will have less physiologic impact compared with an identical lesion in a mid-anterior descending territory subtending a normal anterior wall region because of the significantly higher flow requirements. Thus it is not uncommon to encounter a visual-functional mismatch, wherein the angiography or IVUS measurements do not correspond with the FFR and the clinician's impression of lesion significance; in addition, the use of IVUS to determine lesion significance has not been shown to have a strong correlation with FFR or perfusion imaging.

Furthermore, the recent Fractional Flow Reserve and Intravascular Ultrasound Relationship Study (FIRST) demonstrated that using IVUS-MLA to guide intervention in intermediate lesions by calculation of the MLA was limited in accuracy (64% sensitivity and specificity) and highly variable based on reference vessel characteristics.[28] Previous work has varied greatly when defining an MLA that denotes functional significance, and currently the routine use of IVUS in place of FFR is not recommended.[29] Johnson and coworkers[30] summarize the results of 25 IVUS or OCT imaging studies correlated to FFR and note that the best cutoff value (BCV) for MLA ranged from 1.8 mm² to 4.0 mm² (excluding the left main BCVs of 4.8 to 5.9 mm²) with areas under the curve ranging from 0.63 to 0.90. However, although it is true that MLA greater than 4 mm² had an FFR greater than 0.8 in 91% of cases with a strong negative correlation, an MLA less than 4 mm² had poor correlation to FFR, with most studies reporting an approximately 50% chance of having an FFR less than 0.8 (Figs. 5.8 and 5.9).[31]

Given these caveats, operators should gain confidence in the higher-resolution anatomic data derived from modalities such as IVUS and OCT while using FFR (as discussed later) to determine the physiologic significance of a given epicardial coronary stenosis and guide treatment decision making.

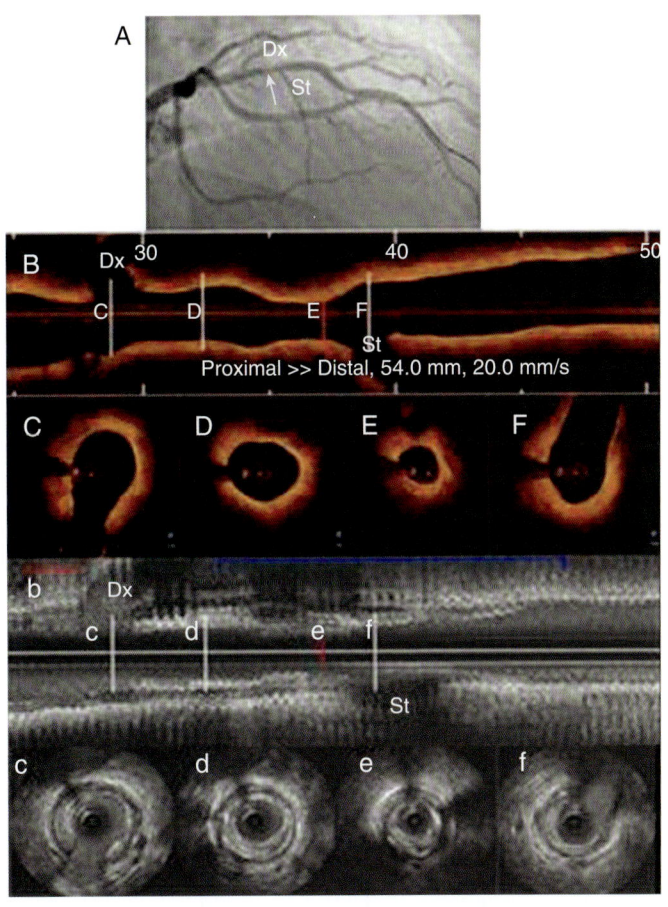

Fig. 5.8 Matching of optical coherence tomography (OCT) and intravascular ultrasound (IVUS) pullbacks. (A) Angiographic view shows an intermediate stenosis in the mid–left anterior descending coronary artery (arrow). Distal to the lesion is a septal branch (St), proximal to the lesion is a diagonal branch (Dx). (B) Longitudinal OCT and IVUS reconstructions show the two side branches (St and Dx) and the stenosis. Corresponding cross-sectional OCT and IVUS images: (C) Diagonal branch; (D) Reference cross section; (E) Minimum luminal area; (F) Septal branch. (From Gonzalo N, Escaned J, Alfonso F, et al. Morphometric assessment of coronary stenosis relevance with optical coherence tomography: a comparison with fractional flow reserve and intravascular ultrasound. *J Am Coll Cardiol.* 2012;59[12]:1080–1089.)

CLINICAL OUTCOMES WITH FRACTIONAL FLOW RESERVE–GUIDED PERCUTANEOUS CORONARY INTERVENTION

Three prospective randomized trials have demonstrated the safety and efficacy of using FFR to guide PCI, and these form the basis of the evidence that supports incorporating FFR into daily use in the catheterization lab. The first was Fractional Flow Reserve to Determine the Appropriateness of Angioplasty in Moderate Coronary Stenosis (DEFER) trial,[32] which randomized 325 patients with stable ischemic heart disease (SIHD) and an intermediate angiographic lesion. FFR was performed on all the lesions in question; those with an FFR less than 0.75 were treated with PCI and those with an FFR of 0.75 or greater were eligible for randomization to either PCI or medical therapy (i.e., deferral of angioplasty). The patients who received PCI for an FFR less than 0.75 comprised a reference group, and all patients were followed for 5 years. Outcomes are shown in Fig. 5.10.

The Fractional Flow Reserve Versus Angiography for Multivessel Evaluation (FAME) trial[33] was a prospective randomized trial that enrolled 1005 patients with multivessel CAD (at least two vessels with a 50% angiographic stenosis). Patients were randomized to a strategy of revascularization: the angiographically guided group had a drug-eluting stent (DES) placed in all prospectively identified lesions, and the FFR-guided group had a DES placed in only those lesions that produced an FFR of less than 0.80. The primary end point was a combined end point of death, nonfatal myocardial infarction (MI), and repeat revascularization at 1 year.

The Fractional Flow Reserve–Guided PCI Versus Medical Therapy in Stable Coronary Disease (FAME 2) trial[34] enrolled 1220 patients with angiographic disease in one, two, or three vessels that was suitable for PCI. After performing FFR, all patients with lesions that had an FFR less than 0.80 were randomized to either receive PCI or medical therapy. A composite of death from any cause, nonfatal MI, or unplanned hospitalization leading to urgent revascularization during a 2-year follow-up was the primary end point. Outcomes are shown in Fig. 5.11.

The following is a discussion of the major findings from these trials.

Deferring Percutaneous Coronary Intervention for Lesions With Nonsignificant Fractional Flow Reserve

From the DEFER study, we learned that at 5 years, the risk of death or MI was no different between the deferred and treated (performed) groups (3.3% vs. 7.9%).[32] Furthermore, the end point was much more frequently encountered in the group with the significant FFR and subsequent revascularization (15.7%), suggesting that lesions with an FFR of greater than 0.75 had a very good 5-year prognosis that was not improved with PCI. Specifically, in the group with deferred revascularization, three cardiac deaths and

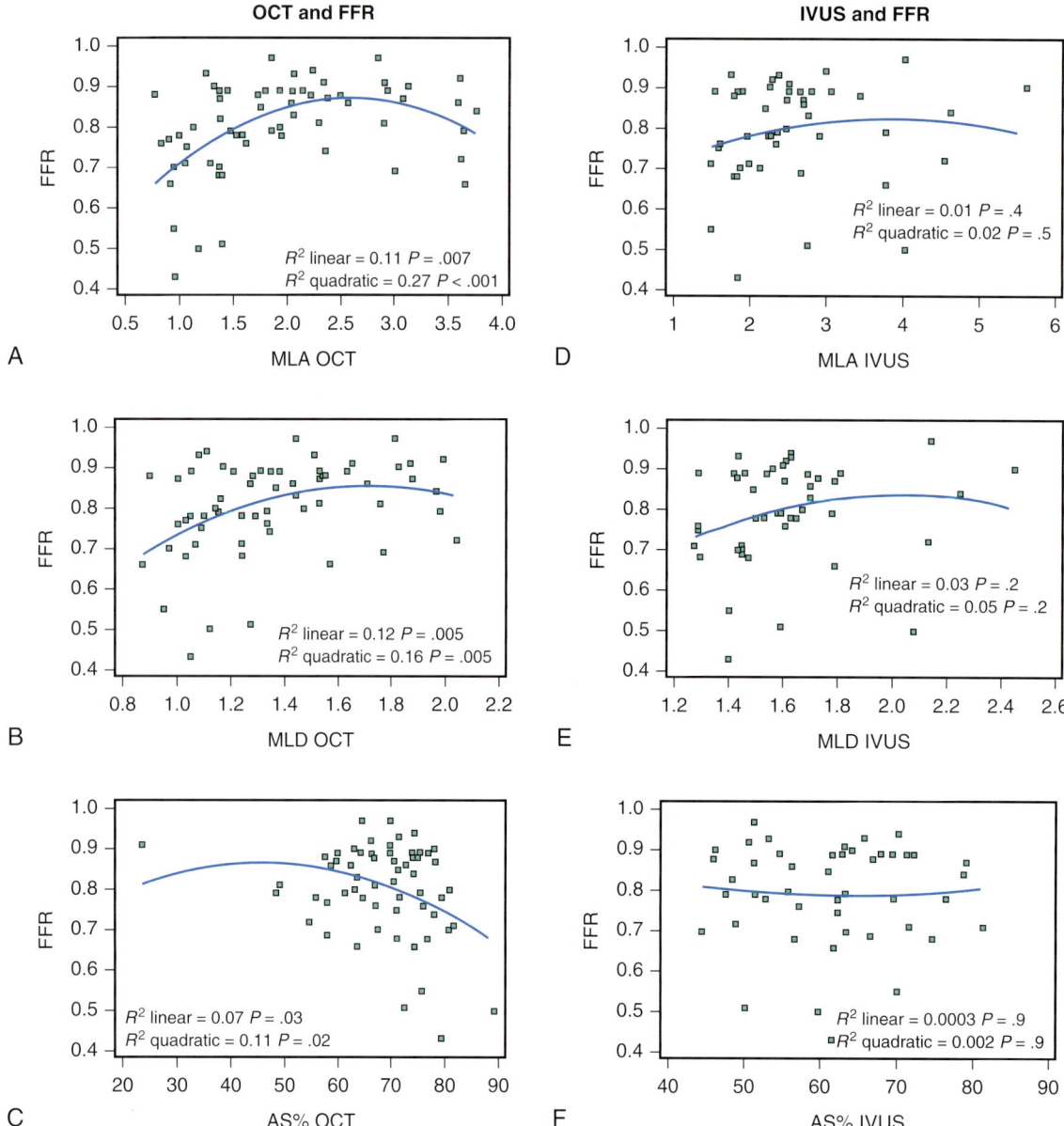

Fig. 5.9 Relation between fractional flow reserve *(FFR)* and optical coherence tomography *(OCT)* and intravascular ultrasound measurements *(IVUS)*. (A–C) FFR and OCT measurements. (D–F) FFR and IVUS measurements. *AS%,* Percent area stenosis; *MLA,* minimum lumen area; *MLD,* minimum lumen diameter. (From Gonzalo N, Escaned J, Alfonso F, et al. Morphometric assessment of coronary stenosis relevance with optical coherence tomography: a comparison with fractional flow reserve and intravascular ultrasound. *J Am Coll Cardiol.* 2012;59[12]:1080–1089.)

no MIs were reported over the course of the 5-year follow-up, and in the group that received PCI (despite an FFR > 0.75), two cardiac deaths and six MIs were reported during the same period.

In a more complex group of patients with multivessel lesions, in the FAME trial, there were 513 lesions with an FFR greater than 0.80 (i.e., deferred PCI) in 509 patients. In a 2-year follow-up, nine late MIs were reported, of which eight were related to either a stent in another lesion or a new lesion, and thus a 0.2% rate of late MI was reported in FFR-negative lesions that did not receive a stent. Furthermore, of those same 513 lesions in 509 patients, 53 repeat revascularizations were reported. However, 37 of those involved restenosis in a stent or a new lesion. This left only 10 lesions that had clearly progressed over the 2 years needing revascularization—a rate of 2%.

Finally, the FAME 2 trial had a registry arm that consisted of those lesions that had FFR values greater than 0.80. These patients had a low rate of the primary end point of death (0), MI (1.8%), or urgent revascularization (2.4%) throughout the follow-up period. This group represents one of the most recent randomized cohorts with no PCI and "modern" medical therapy, but it still reproduces consistent findings compared with patients enrolled in the DEFER trial in the late 1990s.

Taken together, these data strongly support the hypothesis that lesions in patients with stable CAD whose FFR is not physiologically significant (i.e., >0.80) have an exceptionally good prognosis without PCI, and the recommendation is that these lesions receive treatment with optimal medical therapy alone.

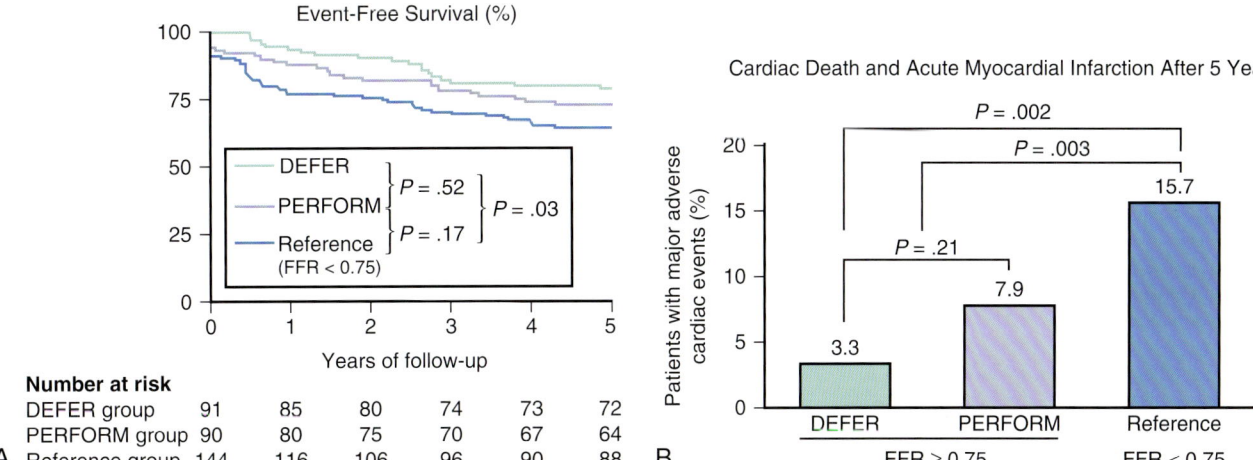

Fig. 5.10 Graphs showing the 5-year results from the *DEFER* trial. (A) Kaplan-Meyer freedom from events for three treatment groups. (B) Overall event rates for the three groups. The y-axis depicts the percentage of patients with major adverse cardiovascular events (MACEs): death, myocardial infarction, coronary artery bypass surgery, or percutaneous coronary intervention. The DEFER group (n = 91) consisted of those patients found to have an intermediate coronary stenosis in which the measured fractional flow reserve *(FFR)* was greater than 0.75, and no angioplasty was performed (MACE = 20%). The *PERFORM* group (n = 90) consisted of those patients with an intermediate coronary stenosis with FFR values greater than 0.75 in whom angioplasty was performed (MACE = 28%). The reference group (n = 144) comprised patients whose lesions had measured FFR values less than 0.75 in whom angioplasty was performed (MACE = 37%). (From Pijls NH, van Schaardenburgh P, Manoharan G, et al. Percutaneous coronary intervention of functionally nonsignificant stenosis: 5-year follow-up of the DEFER Study. *J Am Coll Cardiol.* 2007;49[21]:2105–2111.)

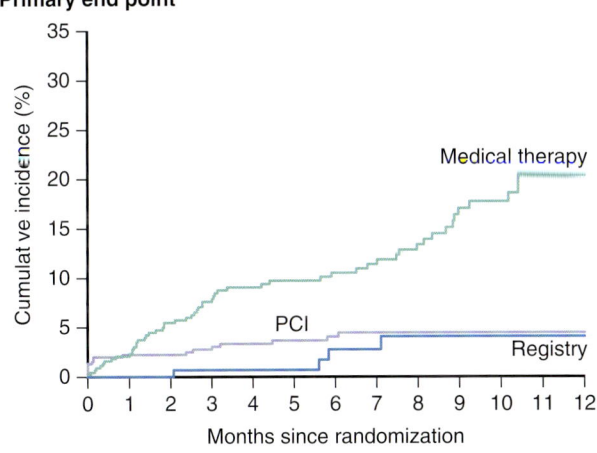

Fig. 5.11 FAME 2 asked the question, is optimal medical therapy (OMT) better than percutaneous coronary intervention *(PCI)* plus OMT for patients with abnormal fractional flow reserve (i.e., ischemia)? Kaplan-Meier curves for FAME 2 patients show that medical therapy had a more than 10-fold incidence of major adverse cardiovascular events compared with the PCI group, which was similar to the nonischemic registry group. (From De Bruyne B, Pijls NH, Kalesan B, et al. Fractional flow reserve-guided PCI versus medical therapy in stable coronary disease. *N Engl J Med.* 2012;367[11]:991–1001.)

Percutaneous Coronary Intervention Versus Medical Therapy for Significant Fractional Flow Reserve

FAME 2 studied 764 lesions with an angiographic stenosis of greater than 50% that had a corresponding FFR less than 0.80 (mean of 0.68 ± 0.15). Within this cohort were 3 deaths (0.7%), 14 MIs (3.2%), and 49 urgent revascularization (11.1%) end points. In the corresponding group that received revascularization for these FFR-significant lesions, only 1 death occurred (0.2%), 15 MIs were reported (3.4%), and 7 patients needed urgent revascularization (1.6%). A landmark analysis (Fig. 5.12) suggested a higher rate of acute coronary syndromes (ACSs) in the medical-therapy arm starting 1 week after randomization. These data strongly suggest that lesions with abnormal FFR values do not have the good long-term prognosis that those with normal FFR values have and that PCI of these lesions significantly improves patient outcomes.

Fractional Flow Reserve in Daily Clinical Practice

FFR optimizes the benefit of PCI by providing objective evidence of coronary ischemia for individual coronary lesions that require revascularization irrespective of each operator's threshold to revascularization by visual assessment. It is best used when decisions regarding the need for PCI are ambiguous based on the angiogram and available noninvasive data (i.e., intermediate angiographic stenosis). FFR is especially useful when noninvasive testing is absent, is equivocal, or does not provide objective evidence of ischemia in the myocardial segment subtended by the targeted lesion.

Studies have shown that routine use of FFR, even in those considered angiographically unambiguous, frequently leads to changes in the number and location of lesions that are functionally significant, and therefore it directs the clinician to what the appropriate treatment should be. In an analysis of the FAME trial, lesions with 50% to 70% diameter narrowing were hemodynamically significant based on FFR in only 35% of cases. In lesions with 71% to 90% narrowing, for which most operators would perform PCI, 20% were not hemodynamically significant by FFR. In two recently published studies of patients undergoing diagnostic angiography with routine FFR, clinicians were led to change their initial angiography-guided management decisions of medical therapy, PCI, or CABG in 26%[35] and 43%[36] of patients after taking the FFR data into consideration. Van Belle and coworkers[35] found that the 1-year rate of MACEs for those whose final FFR-based treatment had differed from the a priori angiography-based decision was as good (11.2%) as in patients in whom the FFR concurred with the a priori decision (11.9%, $P = .78$). In the prospective study by Curzen and colleagues[36] in

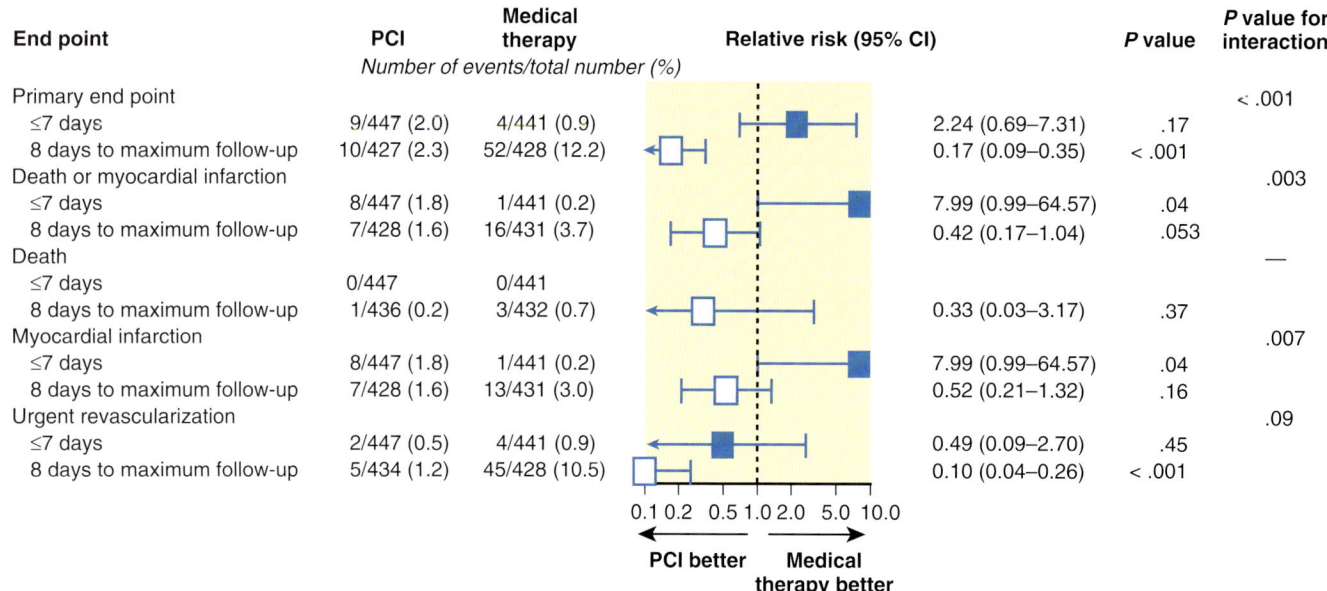

Fig. 5.12 Landmark analysis of FAME 2 outcomes shows outcomes of lesions with fractional flow reserve less than 0.80 over time. *CI*, Confidence interval; *PCI*, percutaneous coronary intervention. (From De Bruyne B, Pijls NH, Kalesan B, et al. Fractional flow reserve-guided PCI versus medical therapy in stable coronary disease. *N Engl J Med.* 2012;367[11]:991–1001.)

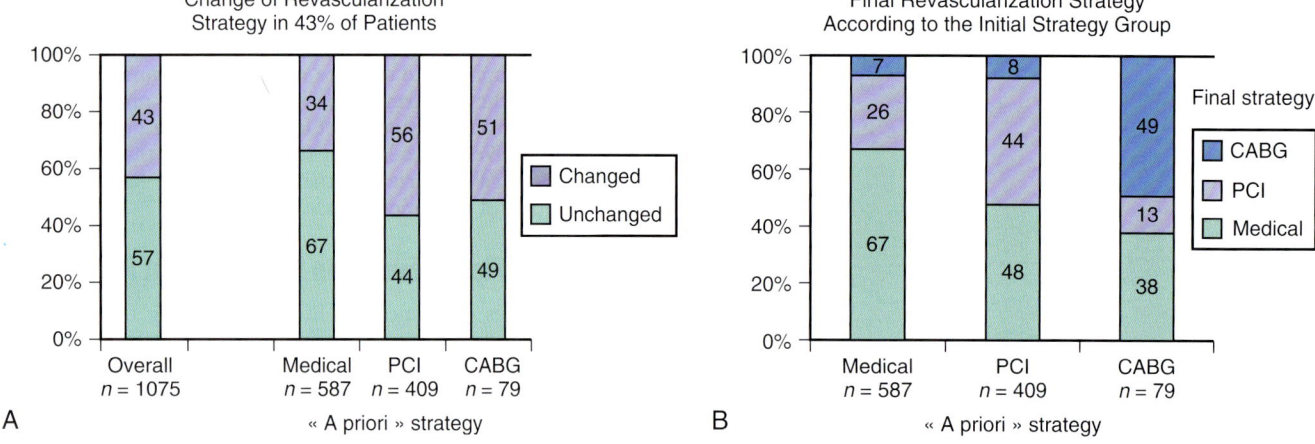

Fig. 5.13 Outcome impact of coronary revascularization strategy reclassification with fractional flow reserve (FFR) at time of diagnostic angiography: insights from a large French multicenter FFR registry. (A) Reclassification of the revascularization strategy according to the revascularization strategy a priori. Despite minor overall changes, a change in strategy has been observed in 43% of all patients (correlation statistic [κ], 0.22; 95% confidence interval, 0.17 to 0.27). (B) Details of the final revascularization strategy applied in each group a priori. *CABG*, Coronary artery bypass surgery; *PCI*, percutaneous coronary intervention. (From Van Belle E, Rioufol G, Pouillot C, et al. Outcome impact of coronary revascularization strategy reclassification with fractional flow reserve at time of diagnostic angiography: insights from a large French multicenter fractional flow reserve registry. *Circulation.* 2014;129[2]:173–185.)

which *all* patent coronary arteries had FFR measured, not just those with angiographic lesions, the number and localization of functional stenoses changed in 32% of patients. Van Belle et al. (Fig. 5.13) also show changes in strategy when FFR is used after angiography for decision making.

Implications for Fractional Flow Reserve in Patients With Multivessel Coronary Artery Disease and Coronary Artery Bypass Grafting

Although the surgical practice of grafting all vessels with angiographic stenosis of greater than 50% has been a long-standing standard, CABG of vessels with hemodynamically insignificant stenosis have a higher rate of graft closure compared with those vessels with severe stenoses. This was shown by Botman and colleagues,[37] who prospectively studied 525 lesions in 153 patients referred for bypass surgery on clinical grounds. FFR was performed on all lesions to be grafted, and the surgeon was blinded to the results. Repeat angiogram was performed 1 year after CABG, and at this early time, 21.4% of grafts on functionally insignificant lesions (FFR > 0.75) were occluded, compared with 8.9% of grafts on vessels with an FFR less than 0.75. As shown in Fig. 5.14, the rate of graft closure correlated with functional severity of the lesion. Although the highest percentage of occluded

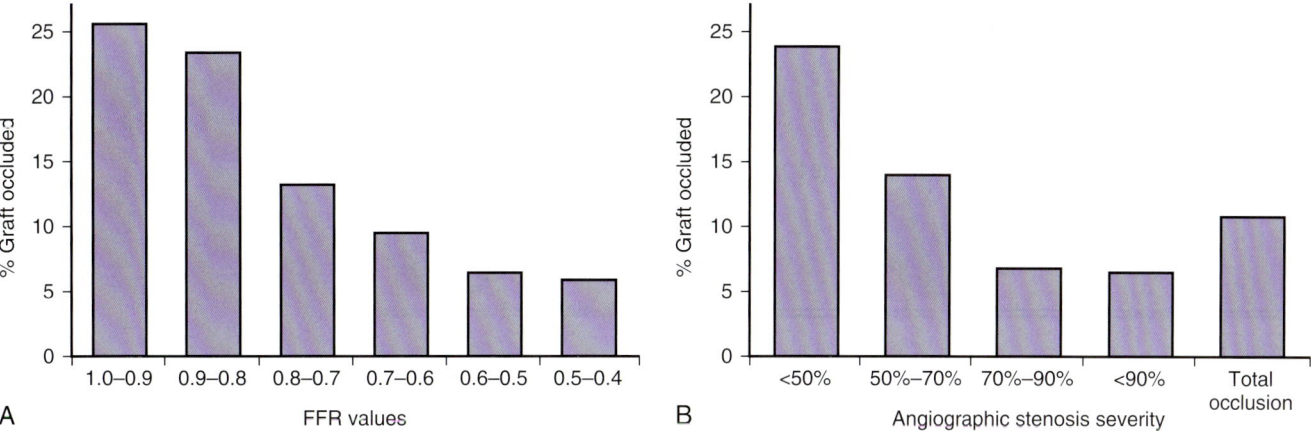

Fig. 5.14 (A) The relation between functional stenosis severity established by fractional flow reserve (FFR) measurements and graft failure at angiographic follow-up after 1 year. (B) The relation between angiographic stenosis severity prior to bypass grafting and graft failure after angiographic follow-up at 1 year. (From Botman CJ, Schonberger J, Koolen S, et al. Does stenosis severity of native vessels influence bypass graft patency? A prospective fractional flow reserve-guided study. *Ann Thorac Surg.* 2007;83[6]:2093–2097.)

grafts was found in the group placed on vessels with less than 50% stenosis, a high percentage of graft failure was still seen in the group with 50% to 70% stenosis. Thus FFR-guided bypass is a reasonable strategy to predict bypass graft patency and has superiority over the strategy of grafting all vessels with lesions with 50% or more stenosis.

In a prospective study of 150 patients with multivessel disease referred for CABG, FFR was performed on all vessels considered for bypass. If FFR proved functionally significant (FFR < 0.75) disease in three vessels or in two vessels with proximal LAD involvement, CABG was performed. Otherwise, patients underwent FFR-guided PCI. Ultimately, only 58% of patients underwent CABG and 42% received PCI. After a 2-year follow-up, no difference was found in event-free survival, including repeat revascularization, which shows that an individually tailored approach to patients with multivessel disease can be accomplished by determining the hemodynamic significance of each lesion.[38]

FFR-guided bypass was compared with angiography-guided bypass surgery in a retrospective review of 627 patients with stable CAD referred for CABG with at least one angiographically intermediate stenosis. In 31% of patients, FFR had been performed to determine whether an intermediate stenosis should be grafted or not.[39] In this group, the incidence of three-vessel disease was downgraded after FFR from 94% to 86%, and use of FFR was associated with a smaller number of anastomoses and rates of on-pump surgery. At 3 years, no difference in adverse events was found compared with those patients who underwent angiography-guided CABG, and the rate of angina was lower in the FFR group (31% vs. 47%, $P < .001$), possibly owing to a higher ratio of arterial-venous anastomosis (Fig. 5.15).

Although the Synergy Between Percutaneous Coronary Intervention With Taxus and Cardiac Surgery (SYNTAX) score has become incorporated into everyday practice as a useful tool to assist the decision making of how best to revascularize patients with multivessel disease, it remains solely dependent on angiographic determinants of coronary lesions. When the SYNTAX score was applied to those patients in the FAME trial, 497 patients were divided into tertiles based on their angiographic SYNTAX score (34% in the low-risk SYNTAX score group, 34% in the intermediate-risk SYNTAX score group, and 32% in the high-risk SYNTAX score group). When the functional data were then added to the SYNTAX score, lesions that had an FFR greater than 0.80 were no longer considered. This allowed a significant reclassification of patients to the same risk tertiles, with 59% of them now falling into the lowest-risk SYNTAX score group, 21% in the intermediate-risk group, and only 20% in the highest-risk group (Fig. 5.16).[40]

Together, these studies strongly support the utilization of routine measurement of FFR in patients with multivessel disease to provide optimal outcomes, best revascularization strategies, and best decision making.

Cost Effectiveness of a Routine Fractional Flow Reserve–Based Strategy

Measurement of FFR for any given coronary stenosis increases the utilization of materials within the lab. As costs for individual procedures become more important in the modern era, additive costs for a guide catheter, pressure wire/sensor, and pharmacologic stimuli for hyperemia may be a burden. Using a computer modeling algorithm that compared evaluating intermediate coronary lesions with nuclear stress testing, stenting, or FFR assessment, Fearon and associates[41] found that FFR was less expensive than either of the other strategies ($1795 less than nuclear stress testing and $3830 less than stenting). Leesar and colleagues[42] evaluated the cost effectiveness of using FFR in patients with unstable angina compared with a nuclear stress-testing strategy and found that an FFR strategy for these patients resulted in overall lower costs. Finally, using the FAME trial, an extensive economic evaluation was performed in a prospective manner.[43] In the patients with multivessel coronary disease, the FFR-guided revascularization strategy not only improved patient outcomes but also resulted in a significant decrease in resource utilization (Fig. 5.17). Thus FFR has consistently been shown to be a cost-effective strategy despite its increase in up-front expenses within the lab.

Left Main Coronary Artery Disease

LMCA stenosis may be among the most difficult angiographic subsets to interpret and carries the most significant clinical impact on the patient's life. LMCA stenosis may involve the aortic-ostial junction, midbody, or distal LMCA, which may involve the LAD or circumflex (CFX) ostium. From a technical perspective, when assessing ostial LM narrowings, FFR can be used if the operator works to avoid guide catheter damping by disengaging the guide from the ostium, using IV rather than IC adenosine to achieve consistent hyperemia. Specifically, before the guiding catheter is

SECTION I Patient Selection

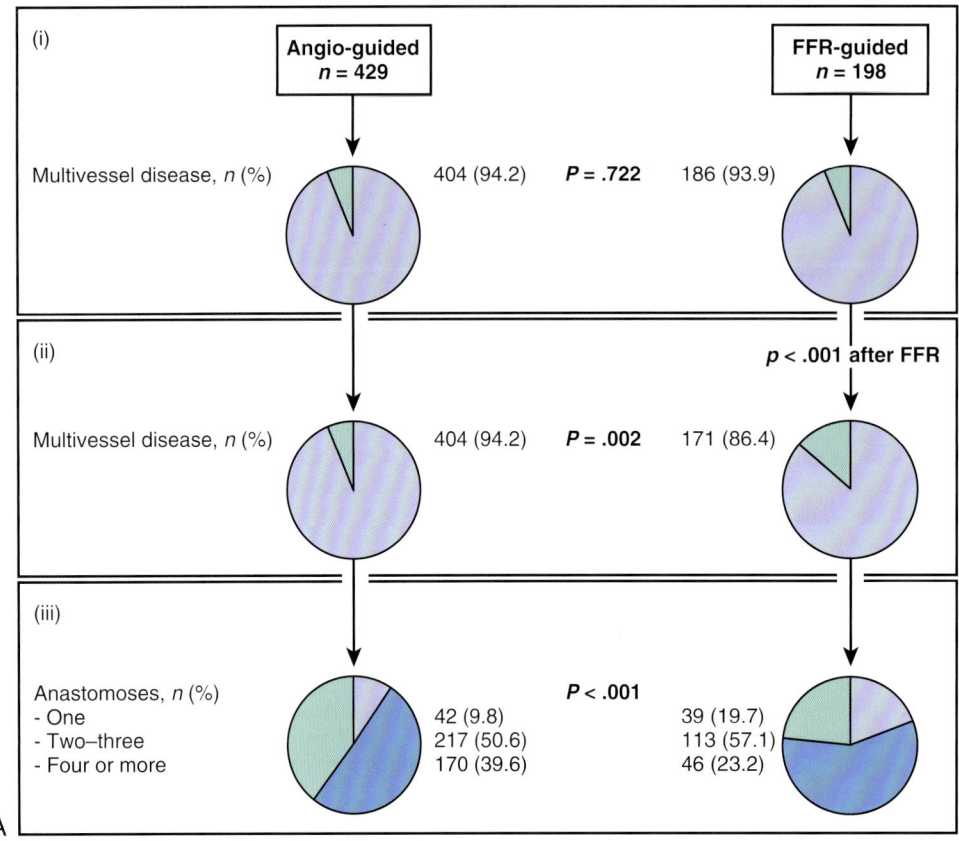

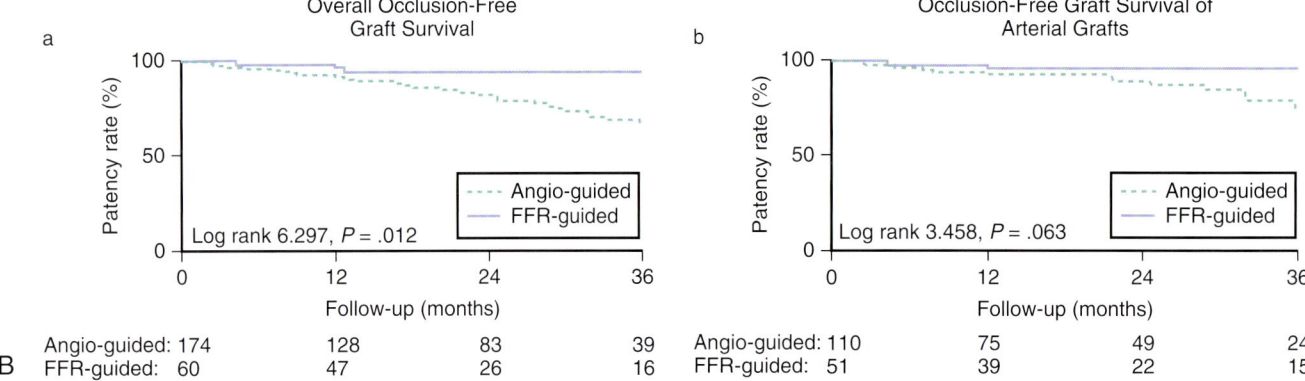

Fig. 5.15 (A) Fractional flow reserve *(FFR)*–guided versus angiography *(Angio)*-guided coronary artery bypass graft surgery. Rates of patients with multivessel disease before (i) and after (ii) FFR measurement and rates of patients with one, two to three, and four or more anastomoses (iii) are shown. (B) Occlusion-free survival of grafts with angiographic follow-up: occlusion-free survival of *all* grafts is shown in panel *a* (log rank, 6.297; *P* = .012); arterial grafts *only* is shown in panel *b* (log rank, 3.45; *P* = .063). (From Toth G, De Bruyne B, Casselman F, et al. Fractional flow reserve–guided versus angiography-guided coronary artery bypass graft surgery. *Circulation*. 2013;128[13]:1405–1411.)

seated, the guiding catheter and wire pressures should be matched (equalized) within the ascending aorta. Next, the guiding catheter is seated, and the pressure wire is advanced into the LAD or the CFX artery. The guiding catheter is then disengaged, and IV adenosine infusion is initiated. After 1 to 2 minutes, the FFR is calculated, and thereafter the wire can be pulled back slowly to identify the exact location of the pressure drop. In case of a distal narrowing of the LMCA, this procedure may be performed twice, once with the pressure wire in the LAD artery and then again in the CFX artery.

Numerous studies support FFR use for assessment of LMCA stenoses (Table 5.3). In the largest of such studies, Hamilos and coworkers[44] examined 5-year outcomes in 213 patients with an angiographically equivocal LMCA stenosis in whom revascularization decisions were guided by FFR. When FFR was 0.80 or greater, patients were treated medically or another stenosis was treated by coronary angioplasty (nonsurgical group; *n* = 138). When FFR was less than 0.80, CABG surgery was performed (surgical group; *n* = 75). The 5-year survival and event-free survival rates were similar, with 90% (74% in the nonsurgical [FFR ≥0.80]) group—and 85%

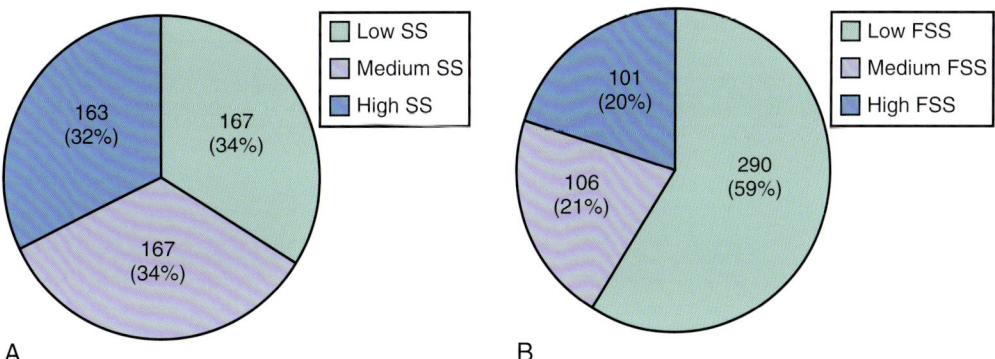

Fig. 5.16 (A) Percentage of patients from the FAME trial with corresponding SYNTAX scores based upon "traditional" angiographic SYNTAX score assessment. (B) When those lesions with a fractional flow reserve *(FFR)* greater than 0.80 were excluded from the calculations, a marked change was noted in the distribution of SYNTAX scoring with a marked increase in the number of patients in the lowest tertile and a corresponding decrease in the number of patients in the medium and high tertiles. *FSS,* Functional syntax score; *SS,* syntax score. (Modified from Nam CW, Mangiacapra F, Entjes R, et al. Functional SYNTAX score for risk assessment in multivessel coronary artery disease. *J Am Coll Cardiol.* 2011;58[12]:1211–1218.)

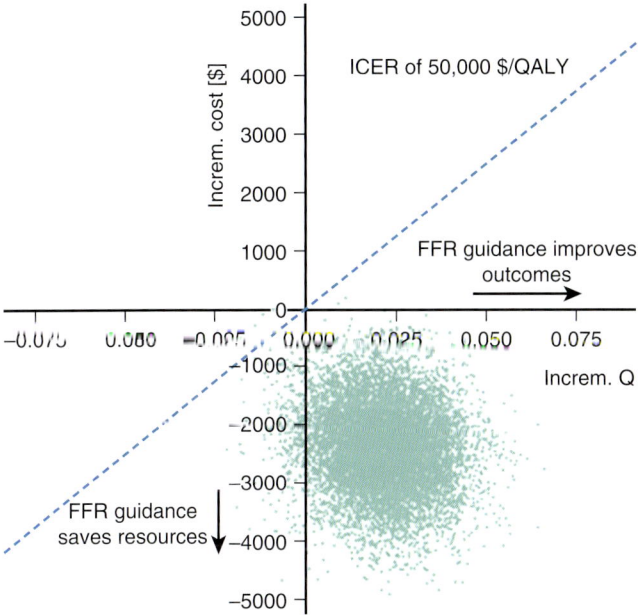

Fig. 5.17 Cost effectiveness of fractional flow reserve. The graph shows the improvement of patient-level outcomes on the x-axis and the costs on the y-axis. Each point represents a patient from the FAME trial; almost all points fall into the lower right quadrant, which reflects an improved outcome at a lower cost with fractional flow reserve *(FFR)*-guided multivessel revascularization as opposed to an angiographically guided strategy. *ICER,* Incremental cost-effectiveness ratio; *Increm.,* incremental; *Q,* quality; *QALY,* quality adjusted life years.

(82% in the surgical [FFR <0.80] group [*P* = .48; Fig. 5.18]). It is worth noting that only 23% of patients with LMCA narrowing >50% had hemodynamically significant FFR (i.e., <0.80).

Complex Left Main Coronary Artery Lesion Assessment (Left Main Coronary Artery Plus Downstream Lesions) With Fractional Flow Reserve

Although FFR of simple LMCA lesions has been shown to be predictive of clinical events, the measurement of FFR in complex LMCA lesions (LMCA plus downstream branch lesions) requires the operator to better understand the relationship between the multiple stenoses within the left coronary system and how they affect one another.

Basic tenets of FFR require maximal flow to be achieved across the target vessel. The LMCA transmits flow to the majority of the left ventricle through both the LAD and CFX branches and in proportion to the size of their associated viable myocardial beds. The myocardial bed for the LMCA is then the sum of both the LAD and LCX territories (Fig. 5.19). In the presence of a significant LAD stenosis, flow across the LAD may be reduced and could possibly limit maximal hyperemia, reducing total LMCA flow and hence LMCA FFR accuracy. This situation is the same as two lesions in series, which would be the LMCA and the LAD (or CFX) narrowing. The complex LMCA plus LAD stenosis could produce an "apparent" LMCA FFR (FFR_{app}) that is higher than the true LMCA FFR (FFR_{true}) because the LMCA bed flow is decreased as a result of the LAD stenosis. The same consideration would apply in the setting of a CFX narrowing. The higher LMCA FFR_{app} is not a concern if either the LAD or CFX are not hemodynamically significant. As Yong and colleagues[45] have shown (discussed later in this section), the apparent and true LMCA FFR will be very close to one another.

When measuring simple FFR across lesions in the LMCA and subsequent major vessel, it is simplest to measure the effect of both lesions by placing the pressure transducer distal to the most distal lesion in question. If the FFR at that level is greater than 0.80, neither lesion is physiologically significant. If the FFR is less than 0.80, a pressure pullback during hyperemia is performed, noting the largest pressure gradient (ΔP) and then the lesion in the LAD or LMCA with the largest ΔP is treated, and FFR is repeated on the remaining lesion. The downside of this approach is that once a significant LAD lesion is removed (i.e., stented), the LMCA FFR may become significant, which mandates further revascularization by stenting or CABG. Thus performing a PCI of a downstream lesion solely to measure the LMCA FFR may not be the best option.

Yong and colleagues[45] used balloon angioplasty catheters in an animal model to create variable stenoses in the LMCA and then in the LAD. Pressure guidewires were positioned in the LAD and CFX arteries. With increasing LAD severity, the difference between FFR_{true} in the LMCA alone and the LMCA FFR_{app} was greater than 0.03 units only when the epicardial FFR ($FFR_{epicardial}$) was less than 0.60, meaning that for practical

SECTION I Patient Selection

TABLE 5.3 Left Main Coronary Artery Revascularization Outcomes and Fractional Flow Reserve

	N			Fractional Flow Reserve Cutoff Value	Follow-Up Mean Duration (Months)	Overall Survival	
First Author	Total	DEFER Group	Surgical Group			DEFER Group (%)	Surgical Group (%)
Bech[77]	54	24	30	0.75	29 ± 15	100	97
Jasti[78]	51	37	14	0.75	25 ± 11	100	100
Jimenez-Navarro[79]	27	20	7	0.75	26 ± 12	100	86
Legutko[80]	38	20	18	0.75	24 ± 12	100	89
Suemaru[81]	15	8	7	0.75	33 ± 10	100	100
Lindstaedt[82]	51	24	27	0.75	29 ± 16	100	81
Hamilos[44]	213	138	75	0.80	35 ± 12	90	86
Total (or mean)	449	271	178	–	28 ± 13	95[a]	89

[a]P = nonsignificant compared with surgical group.
From Puri R, Kapadia SR, Nicholls SJ, et al. Optimizing outcomes during left main percutaneous coronary intervention with intravascular ultrasound and fractional flow reserve the current state of evidence. *J Am Coll Cardiol Interv.* 2012;5:697–707.

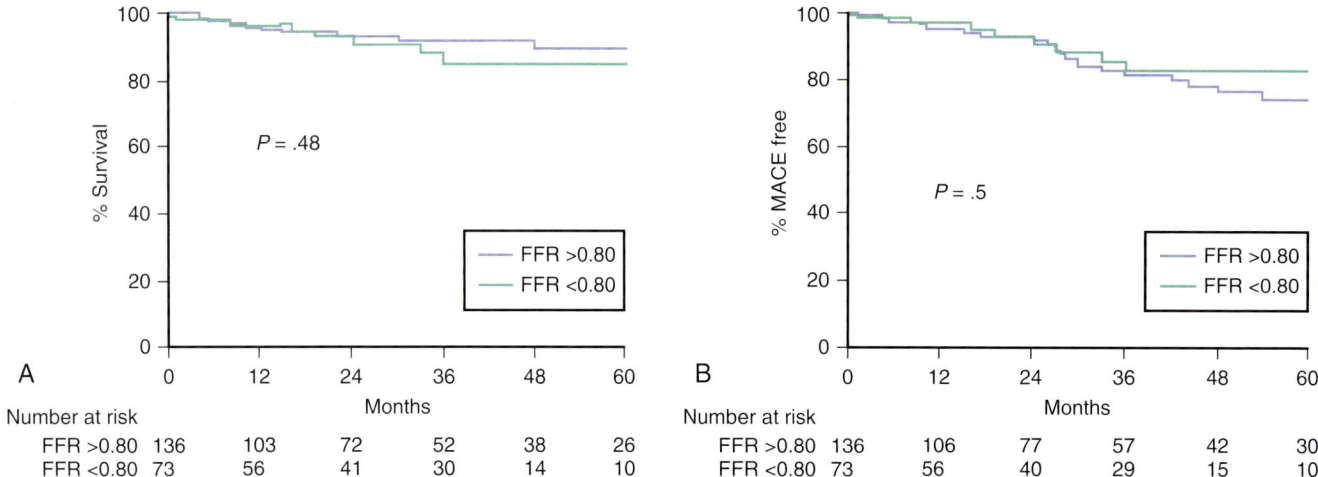

Fig. 5.18 Outcomes in patients with intermediate left main coronary artery disease based on treatment guided by fractional flow reserve *(FFR)* assessment. (A) Survival curves for patients who received medical therapy FFR > 0.80) and coronary artery bypass grafting (CABG; FFR <0.80) over 5 years. (B) Major adverse cardiovascular event *(MACE)* rates in patients treated with medical therapy (FFR >0.80) and CABG (FFR <0.80) over 5 years. (From Hamilos M, Muller O, Cuisset T, et al. Long-term clinical outcome after fractional flow reserve–guided treatment in patients with angiographically equivocal left main coronary artery stenosis. *Circulation.* 2009;120:1505–1512.)

purposes, only a severe and proximal LAD stenosis is likely to influence the true LMCA FFR. Subsequently, these observations were confirmed in a series of patients. In 16 patients post elective coronary intervention of either the LAD or CFX artery, an intermediate left main stenosis was created with variable LAD stenoses using a balloon inflated within the newly placed stent. Sixty-seven pairs of LMCA FFR assessments were obtained before and after an LAD balloon stenosis was created with a pressure wire in the nonstenosed downstream vessel. The investigators found that the FFR_{app} was modestly higher than the FFR_{true} in the absence of downstream stenosis (FFR 0.82 vs. 0.80, $P < .001$). The difference between FFR_{true} and FFR_{app} correlated with the FFR ($r = 0.36$, $P < .001$). This difference was only significant when FFR was very severely low. Among the 67 measurements, only two (3%) had a difference between FFR_{true} and FFR_{app} of greater than 0.05, and the FFR was less than 0.2 in both cases. From the studies by Yong and colleagues[45] for a complex LMCA with downstream disease, when FFR is less than 0.60, FFR_{app} may be questioned and IVUS assessment with a threshold of less than 6.0 mm² is recommended (Fig. 5.20).

Serial (Multiple) Lesions in a Single Vessel

If multiple stenoses are present in the same vessel, the hyperemic flow and pressure gradient through the first stenosis will be attenuated by the presence of the second one and vice versa. Each stenosis will mask the true effect of its serial counterpart by limiting the achievable maximum hyperemia. This fluid-dynamic interaction between two serial stenoses depends on the sequence, severity, and distance between the lesions, as well as the flow rate. If the distance between the two lesions is greater than six times the vessel diameter, the stenoses generally behave independently and the overall pressure gradient is the sum of the individual pressure losses at any given flow rate. When addressing two stenoses in series, equations have been derived to mathematically predict the FFR (FFR_{pred}) of each stenosis separately (i.e., as if the other one were removed), using arterial pressure (Pa), pressure between the two stenoses (Pm), distal coronary pressure (Pd), and coronary occlusive pressure (Pw). FFR_{app}, the ratio of the pressure just distal to that just proximal to each stenosis, and FFR_{true}, the ratio of the pressures distal and proximal to each stenosis but after removal of the other one, have been compared in instrumented

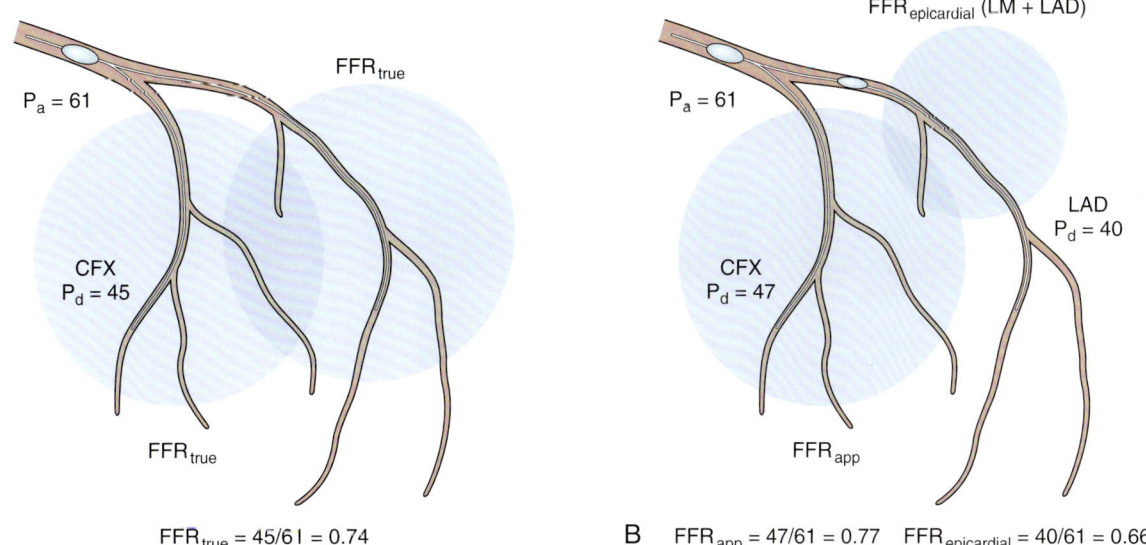

Fig. 5.19 Schematic example of physiologic measurements from an animal model of the left main (*LM*) coronary artery with or without left anterior descending (*LAD*) coronary artery stenosis. (A) True fractional flow reserve (*FFR$_{true}$*) of the left main coronary artery obtained during balloon inflation; no stenosis was evident in the LAD (FFR$_{true}$ = distal pressure [*Pd*] in the circumflex (*CFX*) artery divided by proximal arterial pressure (*Pa*). (B) FFR apparent (*FFR$_{app}$*) obtained during balloon inflation in the LAD (FFR$_{app}$ = CFX Pd/Pa during downstream balloon inflation). *FFR$_{epicardial}$* represents FFR of the LM plus the LAD (FFR$_{epicardial}$ = LAD Pd/Pa during LAD balloon inflation). (Modified from Yong AS, Daniels D, De Bruyne B, et al. Fractional flow reserve assessment of left main stenosis in the presence of downstream coronary stenosis. *Circ Cardiovasc Interv.* 2013;6[2]:161–165.)

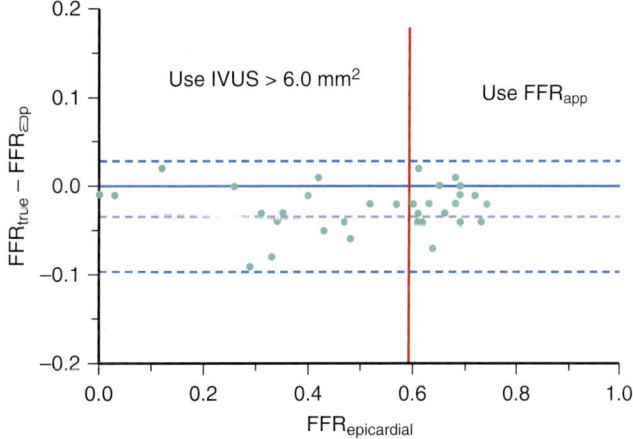

Fig. 5.20 Impact of downstream left anterior descending coronary artery on the left main coronary artery (LMCA) fractional flow reserve (FFR). A plot of the difference between true FFR (*FFR$_{true}$*) and apparent FFR (*FFR$_{app}$*) versus a composite FFR of the LMCA and stenosed downstream vessel (*FFR$_{epicardial}$*) is shown. *Dashed lines* and *dotted lines* indicate bias and 95% confidence interval of the agreement, respectively. *IVUS*, Intravascular ultrasound. (From Yong AS, Daniels D, De Bruyne B, et al. Fractional flow reserve assessment of left main stenosis in the presence of downstream coronary stenoses. *Circ Cardiovasc Interv.* 2013;6[2]:161–165.)

dogs and in humans.[46,47] FFR$_{true}$ was more overestimated by FFR$_{app}$ than by FFR$_{pred}$. It was clearly demonstrated that the interaction between two stenoses is such that the FFR of each lesion cannot be calculated by the equation for isolated stenoses applied to each separately; however, the FFR for each lesion can be predicted by more complete equations that take into account Pa, Pm, Pd, and Pw. Although calculation of the exact FFR for each lesion separately is possible, it remains largely academic. In clinical practice, the use of the pressure pullback recording is particularly well suited to identify the various regions of a vessel with large pressure gradients that may benefit from treatment. The one stenosis with the largest gradient can be treated first, after which the FFR can be remeasured for the remaining stenoses to determine the need for further treatment (see case examples in Figs. 5.21 and 5.22).

Diffuse Coronary Disease

A diffusely diseased atherosclerotic coronary artery can be viewed as a series of branching units that divert and gradually distribute flow along the longitudinally narrowing conduit length. The perfusion pressure gradually diminishes along this artery. FFR is reduced but is unassociated with a focal stenotic pressure loss. Therefore in the diffusely diseased vessel, mechanical therapy directed at a presumed "culprit" stenosis to reverse such abnormal physiology would be ineffective in restoring normal coronary

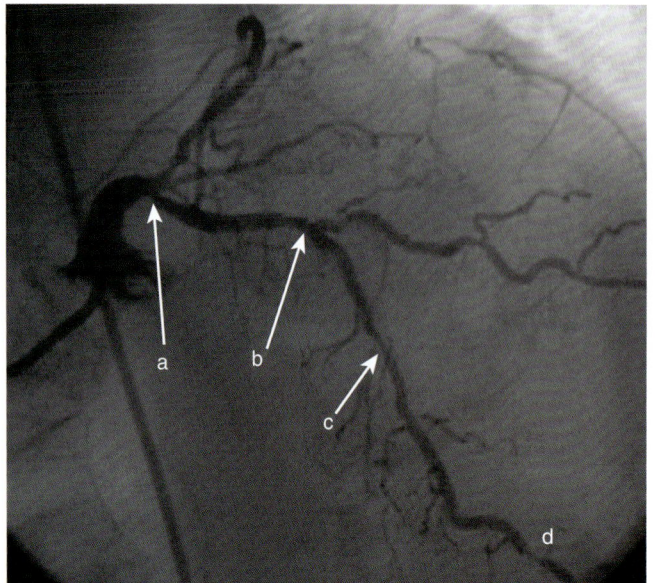

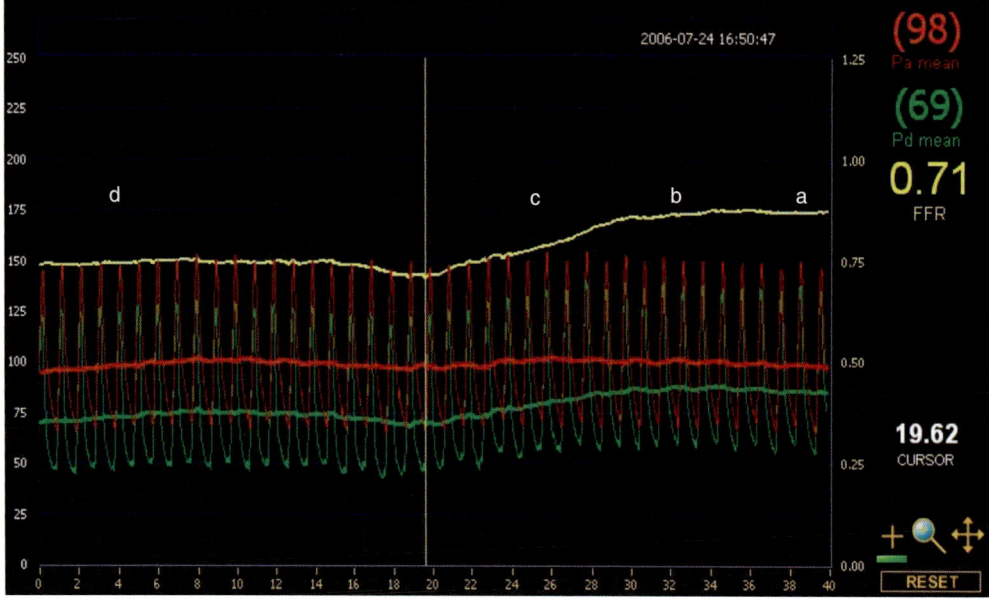

Fig. 5.21 Case example of a patient who presented to the catheterization laboratory complaining of angina-like symptoms. (A) *Top:* Right anterior oblique (RAO) cranial angiogram shows multiple lesions (*a* through *d*) within the left anterior descending (LAD) coronary artery. Bottom: A pullback curve through the LAD during intravenous adenosine administration (points *a* through *d* represent the lesions identified in *top panel*). (B) Top: RAO cranial angiogram after treatment of lesions *d* and *c* with stents. Bottom: Fractional flow reserve *(FFR)* of the LAD after stenting, with the wire distal to the last stent. The FFR of 0.86 reflects the fact that the ostial and middle lesions (*a* and *b*) did not need to be treated.

perfusion. A continuous-pressure pullback from a distal location to a proximal location will identify any specific area of focal angiographic narrowing and will confirm the presence of diffuse atherosclerosis. Diffuse atherosclerosis, as opposed to a focal narrowing, is characterized by a continuous and gradual pressure recovery without localized abrupt increase in pressure related to an isolated region. De Bruyne and coworkers[48] demonstrated the influence of diffuse atherosclerosis that often remains invisible at angiography. FFR measurements were obtained from 37 arteries in 10 individuals without atherosclerosis (group I) and from 106 nonstenotic arteries in 62 patients with arteriographic stenoses in another coronary artery (group II). In group I, the pressure gradient between the aorta and the distal coronary artery was minimal at rest (1 ± 1 mm Hg) and during maximal hyperemia (3 ± 3 mm Hg). Corresponding values were significantly larger in group II (5 ± 4 and 10 ± 8 mm Hg, respectively; both $P < .001$). The FFR was near unity (0.97 ± 0.02; range, 0.92 to 1) in group I, indicating no resistance to flow in truly normal coronary arteries; but it was significantly lower (0.89 ± 0.08; range, 0.69 to 1) in group II, indicating a higher resistance to flow. This resistance to flow contributes to myocardial ischemia and has consequences for decision making during PCI. As for patients with several discrete stenoses within one coronary artery, similar considerations can be applied for patients with diffuse CAD or long lesions. The

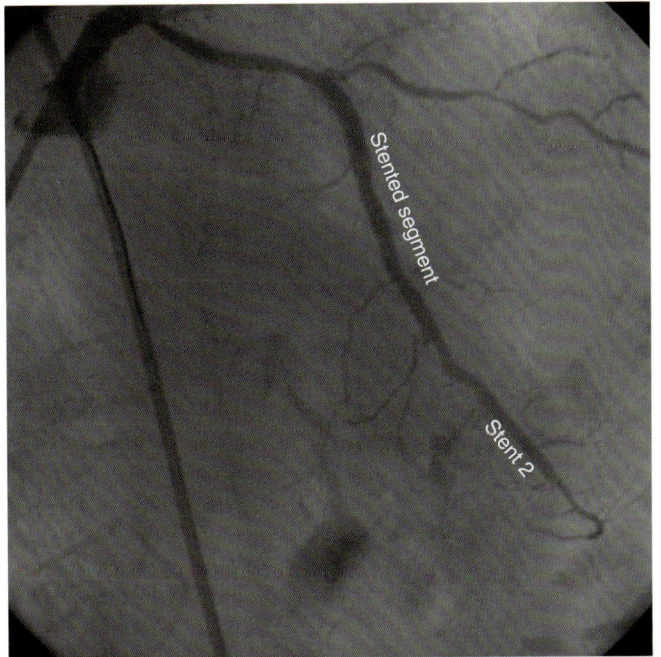

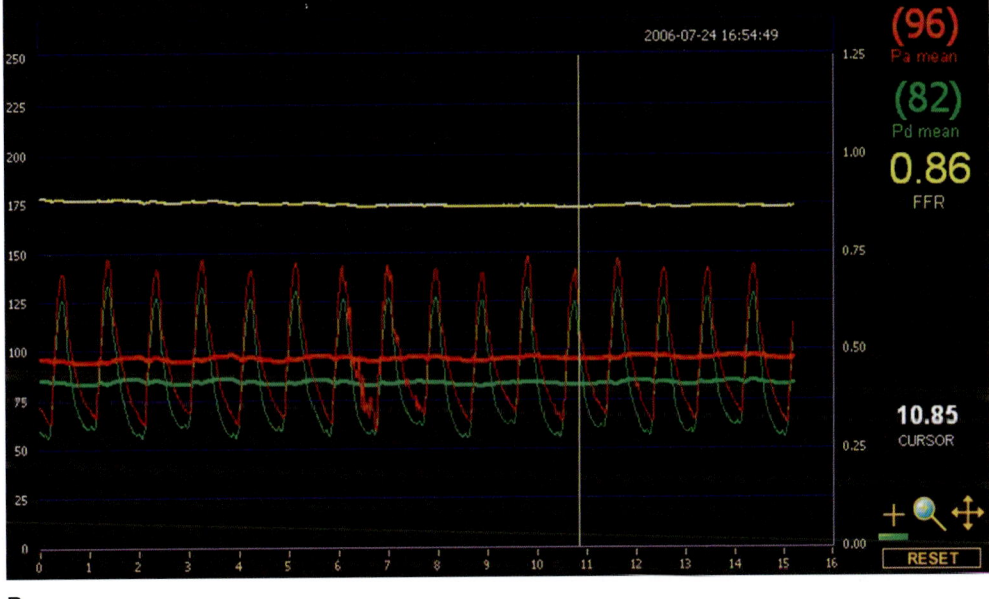

Fig. 5.21 cont'd

pressure pullback recording at maximum hyperemia provides the necessary information to decide whether and where stent implantation may be useful. The location of a focal pressure drop superimposed on the diffuse disease can be identified as an appropriate location for treatment. In some cases the gradual decline of pressure along the vessel occurs over a very long segment, such that interventional treatment is not possible (Fig. 5.23). Medical treatment (or CABG) can then be elected.

Ostial Lesions and Jailed Side Branches

The assessment of ostial narrowings, particularly in side branches "jailed" within stents, remains difficult with current angiographic techniques because of image foreshortening, the overlap orientation relative to the parent branch, and, in the case of jailed vessels, stent struts across the branch.

Koo and colleagues[49] compared FFR with the stenosis severity as measured by QCA for 94 jailed side-branch lesions. Only 20 (27%) of 73 lesions with 75% or greater stenosis were functionally significant by FFR. Reassuringly, no lesion with less than 75% angiographic stenosis had an FFR less than 0.75. These results suggest that most of these lesions do not have functional significance and thus may not need intervention. Similar findings have been reported for native ostial and branch stenoses found during routine coronary angiography.[50,51]

Fractional Flow Reserve in Acute Coronary Syndromes

After an acute MI, the predictive ability of FFR has some theoretic limitations because the microvascular bed in the infarct zone may not necessarily have a uniform and constant response to a

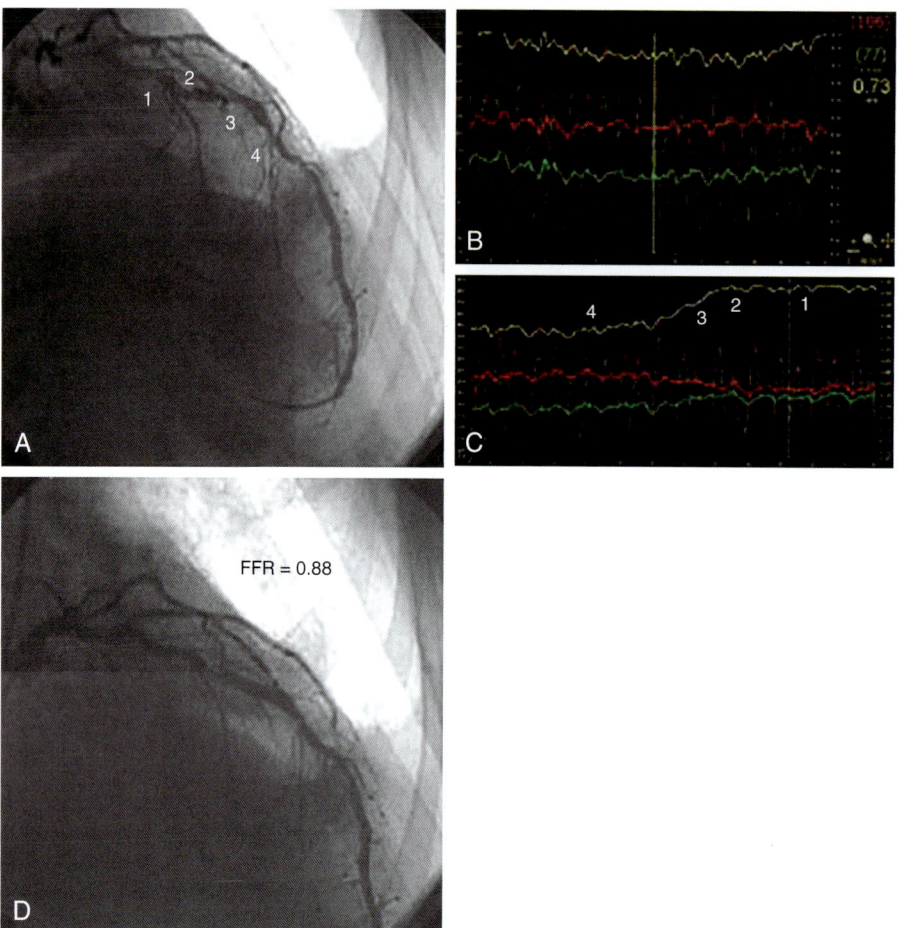

Fig. 5.22 Example of a patient with serial lesions in the left anterior descending coronary artery. (A) Multiple left anterior descending (LAD) artery lesions *(1–4)* were seen on angiography in a patient with a positive stress test for anterior ischemia. (B) Fractional flow reserve *(FFR)* assessment of the LAD beyond all the lesions show a physiologically significant gradient in the vessel (FFR = 0.73). (C) Pullback recording during continuous hyperemia demonstrates the relative changes in FFR at lesions 1 to 4. The largest change in the pressure gradient is seen to occur at lesion 3 only. (D) Right anterior oblique angiogram of the LAD following stenting of lesion 3 with a final FFR across all lesions of 0.88.

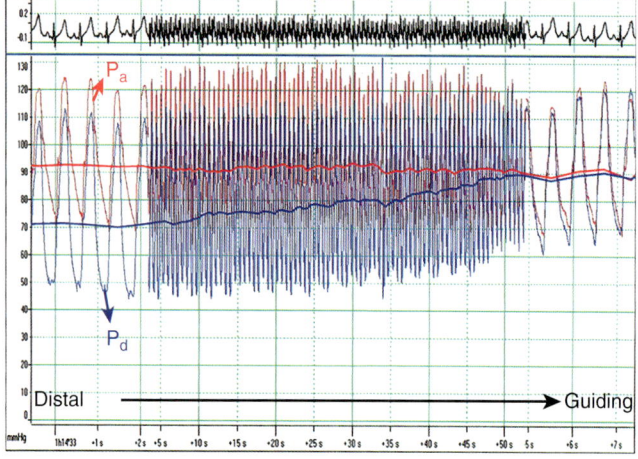

Fig. 5.23 A pullback curve created in a patient with diffuse disease throughout the left anterior descending coronary artery. The fractional flow reserve for this vessel is 0.67, which reflects ischemia-producing lesions. However, the gradual decrease in gradient from pressure distal to the stenosis (Pd) to arterial pressure (Pa) is reflective of severe, diffuse narrowing in the major portion of the vessel. This gradual change in the pressure curve shows that an extremely long segment is responsible for the ischemia and is most likely *not* best treated with multiple stents (i.e., "full metal jacket"). (Courtesy B. De Bruyne, Aalst, Belgium.)

pharmacologic hyperemic stimulus. Transient microvascular dysfunction impairs maximal coronary hyperemia to varying degrees, reducing the flow across a stenosis and elevating the measured FFR across lesions. It has been questioned to what extent this might affect the accuracy of FFR for both culprit and nonculprit lesions around the time of an ACS.

In an acute STEMI, FFR of most nonculprit lesions has been shown to be accurate, with the caveat that diffuse microvascular impairment may falsely elevate the apparent FFR. Therefore in this setting, a low FFR indicates hemodynamic significance of the nonculprit lesion, but a normal FFR may not be definitive. Ntalianis and associates[52] measured the FFR of 112 nonculprit lesions during an acute MI (75 patients with STEMI, 26 with non-STEMI [NSTEMI]) and again 35 (SD ± 24) days later. Only two lesions had a clinically meaningful change in which the FFR was greater than 0.80 during the acute episode and less than 0.75 at follow-up.

De Bruyne and associates[53] and Samady and colleagues[54] obtained FFR measurements of culprit vessels 3 or more days after acute MI and compared them with subsequent single-photon emission computed tomography (SPECT) imaging to identify true positives and negatives. Both studies showed that an FFR less than 0.75 had high sensitivity, specificity, and overall accuracy for detecting reversible ischemia on truly positive or negative SPECT imaging results, and they both reached the same BCV for FFR of 0.78. Furthermore, data from the FAME trial showed that among the 173 patients who had ACS prior to enrollment, an impressive 30% overall reduction in MACE was reported when FFR was applied to the revascularization decision making.[55] Trials that have evaluated the use of FFR in ACS are summarized in Table 5.4. Taken together, these studies strongly show that when used appropriately, FFR can be a useful tool in assessing patients after an acute MI.

Fractional Flow Reserve in ST Elevation Myocardial Infarction Patients

Traditional teaching has been to treat only the culprit vessel during STEMI because several meta-analyses and nonrandomized registry studies showed that treating all vessels at the same time as the STEMI culprit was associated with more adverse events. Up until the most recent 2015 update, the 2013 ACC/AHA/SCAI STEMI guidelines gave a class III recommendation against intervening on a noninfarct-related artery at the time of primary PCI in patients who are hemodynamically stable.[56] Since then, several studies have demonstrated the accuracy of FFR in ACS, including the Fractional Flow Reserve Versus Angiography in Guiding Management to Optimize Outcomes in Non-ST-Elevation Myocardial Infarction Cardiac Magnetic Resonance (FAMOUS NSTEMI CMR) substudy that showed an excellent accuracy of FFR less than 0.80 for predicting perfusion defects on cardiac MR.[57]

Furthermore, multiple trials including Preventive Angioplasty in Acute Myocardial Infarction (PRAMI), Complete Versus Lesion-Only Primary PCI Trial (CvLPRIT), and the Third Danish Study of Optimal Acute Treatment of Patients With STEMI: Primary PCI in Multivessel Disease (DANAMI-3–PRIMULTI) have shown that revascularizing nonculprit arteries, either at the time of primary PCI or later in a staged manner, reduce risk of MACE by a relative 44% to 65% compared with culprit-only PCI (Table 5.5)[58–60].

DANAMI-3–PRIMULTI was an open-label, randomized controlled trial that enrolled 627 patients with STEMI who had 1 or more clinically significant coronary stenosis in addition to the culprit lesion. After successful PCI to the culprit lesion, patients

TABLE 5.4 Fractional Flow Reserve and Acute Coronary Syndrome Trials

First Author	N	Vessel Assessed	Usefulness of Fractional Flow Reserve	Summary
Tamita[83]	33 STEMI	AMI	Culprit vessel	Unreliable	Mean FFR after successful PCI was higher (0.95 ± 0.04) than in the reference group of stable angina patients (0.90 ± 0.04, P = .002) despite identical IVUS parameters, likely reflecting microvascular stunning and dysfunction.
Ntalianis[52]	75 STEMI, 26 NSTEMI	AMI	Nonculprit vessel	Reliable	Nonculprit lesions (n = 112) were measured acutely and 35 ± 24 days later. Only two had clinically meaningful change (FFR > 0.80 during the acute episode and FFR < 0.75 at follow-up).
De Bruyne[53]	57 AMI with viable myocardium on left venogram	Recent MI	Culprit vessel	Reliable	FFR after acute MI (≥6 days, mean 20 days) was compared with SPECT before and after PCI. FFR < 0.75 had high sensitivity (87%) and specificity (100%) for detecting ischemia on true positive/negative SPECT (BCV for FFR, 0.78). An inverse correlation was found between FFR and LVEF; for a similar degree of stenosis, FFR depends on mass of viable myocardium.
Samady[54]	36 STEMI, 12 NSTEMI	Recent MI	Culprit vessel	Reliable	FFR after acute MI (STEMI ≥3 days, NSTEMI ≥2 days, mean 3.7 days) was compared with SPECT at 11 weeks. FFR ≤0.75 had high sensitivity (88%), specificity (93%), and overall accuracy (91%) for detecting reversibility on true positive/negative SPECT. BCV for FFR was 0.78.
Potvin[84]	125 ACS, 60 SIHD, 16 Atypical CP	Recent MI	Nonculprit vessel	FFR-guided PCI = good clinical outcomes	Patients (n = 201 consecutive, 62% UA, NSTEMI, or >24 h after STEMI) had ~50% stenosis in which PCI was deferred based on FFR ≥ 0.75; no differences were found in clinical outcomes between those with ACS and stable angina patients.
Fischer[85]	35 ACS	Recent MI		FFR-guided PCI = good clinical outcomes	FFR-guided PCI of intermediate lesions (50%–70%) was studied, deferring PCI for FFR ≥0.75 in patients with recent ACS; MACE rates were similar at 12 months compared with patients without ACS.
Leesar[42]	70 UA/NSTEMI	UA/NSTEMI	Culprit vessel	FFR-guided PCI = good clinical outcomes	Recent NSTE-ACS with intermediate single-vessel lesion was randomized to immediate FFR-guided PCI versus SPECT. FFR-guided treatment reduced hospital stay and cost with no increase in procedure time, radiation exposure, or clinical event rates at 1 year.
Sels[55]	326 UA/NSTEMI	UA/NSTEMI	Culprit + nonculprit vessel	FFR-guided PCI = good clinical outcomes	FAME studied FFR-guided PCI versus angiography-guided PCI for multivessel disease; in a subset of patients with recent NSTE-ACS, the MACE rate was significantly lower with FFR-guided PCI.

ACS, Acute coronary syndrome; *AMI*, acute MI; *BCV*, best cutoff value; *CP*, chest pain; *FFR*, fractional flow reserve; *IVUS*, intravascular ultrasound; *LVEF*, left ventricle ejection fraction; *MACE*, major adverse cardiovascular event; *MI*, myocardial infarction; *NSTE*, non–ST elevation; *PCI*, percutaneous coronary intervention; *SIHD*, stable ischemic heart disease; *SPECT*, single-photon emission computed tomography; *STEMI*, ST elevation myocardial infarction; *UA*, unstable angina.

TABLE 5.5 Key Trials of Fractional Flow Reserve in ST Elevation Myocardial Infarction and Other Acute Coronary Syndrome

	PRAMI	CvPRIT	DANAMI-3 PRIMULTI	Compare-Acute	PRIME-Fractional Flow Reserve
Study Design	Single-blind randomized	Randomized control trial	RCT	Prospective randomized trial	Prospective study
N	465	296	627	885	1983
Followed-up period	23 months	296 months	12 months	36 months	12 months
Long term mortality	Complete revascularization better	Complete revascularization better	Complete revascularization better	Complete revascularization better	Deferral based on FFR is safe in ACS
Assessment of nonculprit lesion	Angiography	Angiography	FFR	FFR	FFR
Timing	Immediate complete revascularization	Immediate complete revascularization or staged PCI	Staged PCI	Immediate complete revascularization or staged PCI	–

ACS, Acute coronary syndrome; *FFR*, fractional flow reserve; *PCI*, percutaneous coronary intervention; *RCT*, randomized control trial.

were randomized into no further invasive treatment or complete FFR-guided revascularization before discharge. A threshold of FFR less than 0.80 was used, and FFR was performed 2 days after primary PCI to avoid the risk of invalid FFR measurements inferred from acute changes in macrovascular tone or microvascular flow obstruction. The primary end point of a composite of all-cause mortality, nonfatal reinfarction, and ischemia-driven revascularization of lesions in noninfarct-related arteries was significantly lower in the complete revascularization group (13%) compared with the infarct-related only group (22%). The favorable effect was driven by significantly fewer revascularizations. A substudy of the DANAMI-3–PRIMULTI trial found that the benefit of staged FFR-guided complete revascularization was observed primarily in patients with three-vessel disease and at least one noninfarct-related stenosis with a 90% or greater diameter (Fig. 5.24).[61]

In the Fractional Flow Reserve-Guided Multivessel Angioplasty in Myocardial Infarction (COMPARE-ACUTE) trial, 885 patients with STEMI and multivessel disease who had undergone primary PCI of the infarct-related artery were randomized to undergo FFR-guided complete revascularization of noninfarct-related coronary arteries or no revascularization of noninfarct-related arteries. Unlike DANAMI-3–PRIMULTI, FFR of the noninfarct-related artery was done in the acute STEMI setting, during the time of primary PCI. At 1 year those who underwent FFR-guided complete revascularization of noninfarct-related arteries had a lower risk of death (1.4% vs. 1.7%), MI (2.4% vs. 4.7%), revascularization (6.1% vs. 17.5%), and cerebrovascular events (0.0% vs. 0.7%) compared with those who were treated for the infarct-related artery only.[62] Approximately half of the noninfarct-related artery lesions that were angiographically significant were not physiologically significant by FFR (≥0.80).

The ideal threshold for FFR in the ACS population has been debated. The FFR threshold of 0.80, which is used to determine functional significance in the SIHD population, was applied to the ACS population in the aforementioned studies. Hakeem et al. found that using FFR for clinical decision making in ACS patients using the standard FFR = 0.80 threshold was associated with a threefold increase in the risk of subsequent MI and target vessel failure compared with SIHD patients and advised caution in using FFR-derived values for clinical decision making in patients with ACS. They found that ACS patients had a higher FFR threshold of functional significance, and those with an FFR less than 0.85 had significantly higher event rates than those with FFR greater than 0.85.[63]

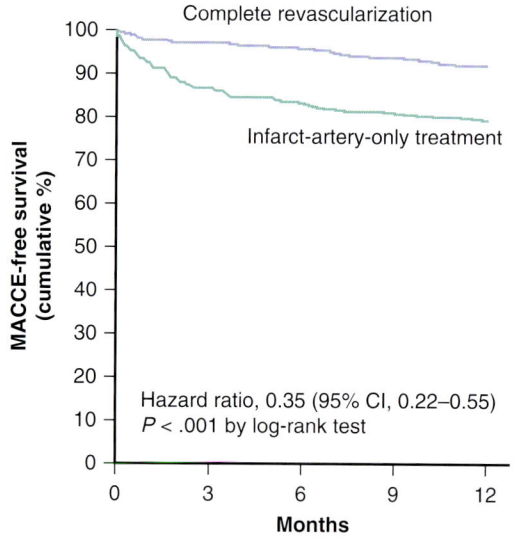

Fig. 5.24 In STEMI patients, the primary composite end point of all cause death, reinfarction, and ischemia-driven revascularization was lower in those who received fractional flow reserve-guided complete revascularization compared to infarct-related percutaneous coronary intervention alone. The primary end point was further reduced in patients with at least 1 noninfarct-related stenosis ≥90% compared to those with less than 90%. *MACCE,* Major adverse cerebral and cardiovascular events; *STEMI,* ST elevation myocardial infarction. (With permission from Smits PC, Abdel-Wahab M, Neumann FJ, et al. Fractional flow reserve-guided multivessel angioplasty in myocardial infarction. *N Engl J Med.* 2017;376[13]:1234–1244.)

Post–Percutaneous Coronary Intervention Fractional Flow Reserve

In contrast to pre-PCI FFR, the clinical implications of post-PCI FFR have not been as well demonstrated in large, randomized clinical trials. In a meta-analysis of 105 studies between 1995 and 2005 reporting on post-PCI FFR and evaluating the relationship between post-PCI and clinical outcomes post-PCI, Rimac et al. found that higher post-PCI FFR values are associated with significantly lower risks of repeat PCI and MACE during follow-up, and post-PCI FFR values of 0.90 or greater are associated with a relative risk reduction of repeat PCI of 55% and a relative risk reduction of MACE by 30%.[64] Results from the Randomized Study on Double Kissing

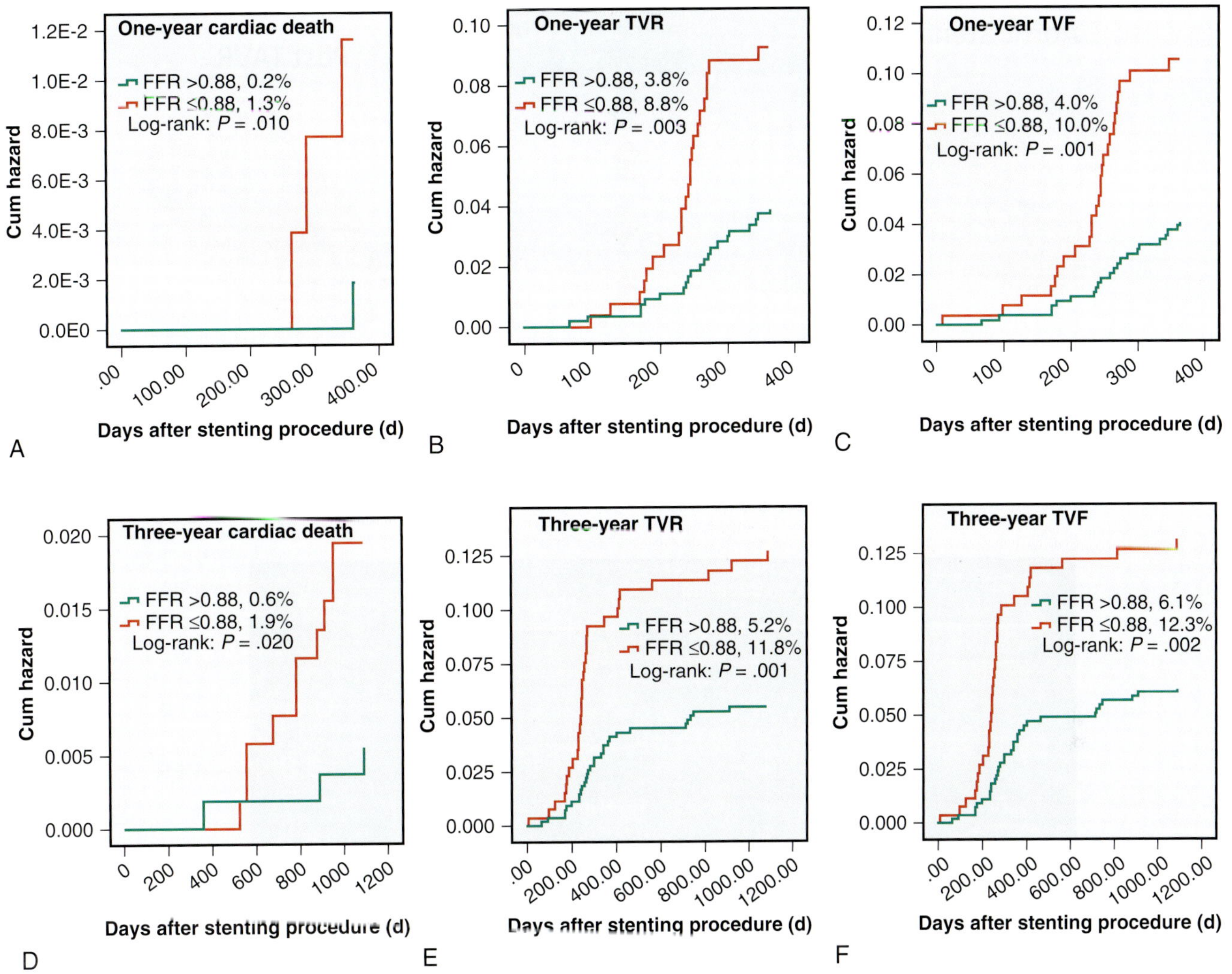

Fig. 5.25 Patients with a post-drug-eluting stent fractional flow reserve *(FFR)* greater than 0.88 had fewer rates of cardiac death, target vessel revascularization *(TVR)*, and target vessel failure *(TVF)* at 1 year compared with those with an FFR ≤0.88 (A–C). This beneficial trend continued at 3 years of follow-up (D–F). (From Li SJ, Ge Z, Kan J, et al. Cutoff value and long-term prediction of clinical events by FFR measured immediately after implantation of a drug-eluting stent in patients with coronary artery disease: 1- to 3-year results from the DKCRUSH VII Registry Study. *JACC Cardiovasc Interv.* 2017;10[10]:986–995.)

Crush Technique Versus Provisional Stenting Technique for Coronary Artery Bifurcation Lesions (DKCRUSH VII Registry Study) showed that a post-DES FFR of 0.88 or less strongly correlated with target vessel failure, and this was maintained after 3 years of follow-up (Fig. 5.25).[65] Impaired post-DES FFR may be influenced by several independent factors, including stent length, stent diameter, and disease in the LAD artery. In one study among patients receiving long stents (defined as 30 to 49 mm), only 12.2% were found to have an optimal post-PCI defined as an FFR greater than 0.95. Among patients who received ultralong stents (≥50 mm), none achieved an optimal post-PCI FFR.[66]

Fractional Flow Reserve and Transcatheter Aortic Valve Implantation for Aortic Stenosis

Many patients with severe AS have concomitant CAD, but there are no clearly established guidelines on revascularization management in patients undergoing transcatheter aortic valve implantation (TAVI). The utility of FFR in this patient population has been validated. In severe AS, there is increased microcirculatory resistance and reduced vasodilatory reserve, which may influence FFR. In a study of 54 patients with severe AS and CAD undergoing TAVI, 154 lesions were assessed by FFR both before and after TAVI. There were no ischemic complications related to the administration of IC adenosine during the FFR procedure or after 1 month of follow-up, demonstrating that an FFR evaluation is safe to perform in severe AS patients. Overall, there were only minor changes in FFR values before and after TAVI, confirming the validity of FFR in this clinical scenario. In approximately 15% of patients with CAD, the post-TAVI FFR assessment did change the indication to perform PCI, and this was mostly for angiographically intermediate lesions with unmasked functional significance (Fig. 5.26).[67]

Simultaneous Measurement of Flow Velocity and Transstenotic Pressure Gradient

Although the maximal flow and, consequently, the maximal transstenotic gradient are determined also by factors independent of

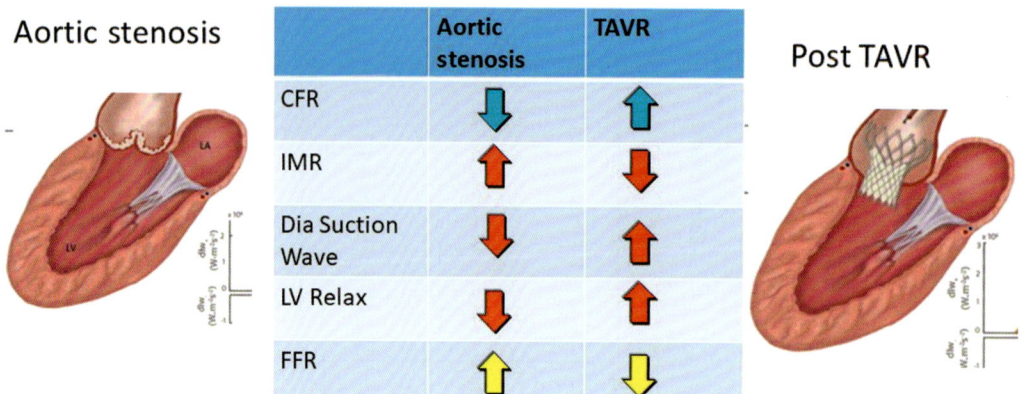

Fig. 5.26 Postulated changes in coronary flow reserve *(CFR)*, index of microvascular resistance *(IMR)*, diastolic suction by wave intensity analysis, left ventricle *(LV)* relaxation and FFR are shown for a patient before (A) and after (B) transcatheter aortic valve replacement *(TAVR)*. Aortic systolic and pulse pressures increased after TAVR. Wave intensity analysis was used to separate total wave intensity into contributions from the forward (dIw+) and backward (dIw−) traveling waves.

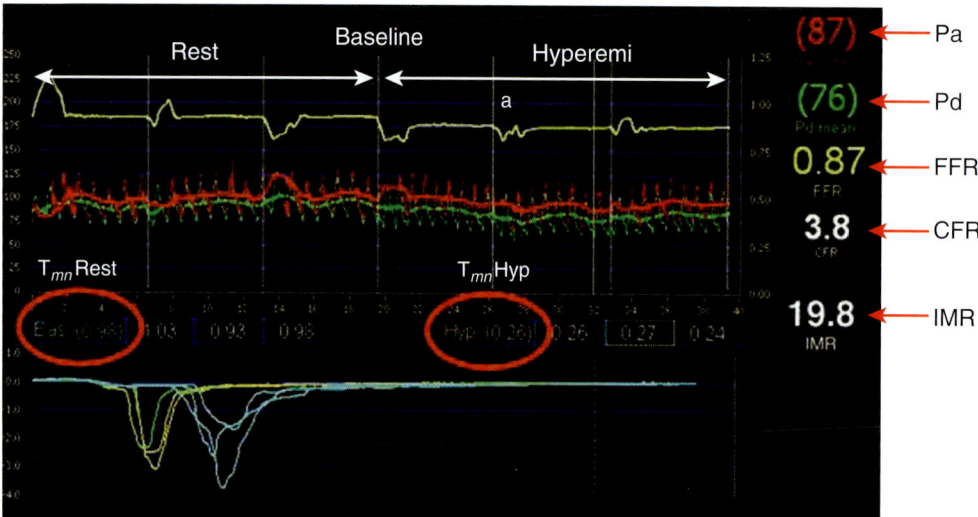

Fig. 5.27 Simultaneous measurement of pressure and flow (by thermodilution). The upper portion of the figure shows pressures proximal *(Pa)* and distal *(Pd)* at rest *(left)* and during hyperemia *(right)*. The lower portion of the figure depicts the thermodilution curves at rest and during hyperemia (Hyp) with the associated average transit times at baseline and at hyperemia *(circled)*. These values are used to calculate the coronary flow reserve *(CFR)* and the index of microcirculatory resistance *(IMR)*, as seen on the right side of the panel. FFR, Fractional flow reserve. (From Martin KC, Yeung AC, Fearon WF. Invasive assessment of the coronary microcirculation. Circulation. 2006;113[17]:2054–2061.)

the stenosis resistance, the pressure gradient-flow velocity relationship is intimately correlated with the stenosis hemodynamics. A method to assess the coronary vasculature that is easy to perform and currently poses the greatest clinical usefulness is the index of microcirculatory resistance (IMR). This index relies on using distal pressure and thermodilution flow, as assessed by the inverse of the arrival (transit) time of a room temperature saline bolus to the distal coronary artery segment. By measuring the mean transit time at rest and comparing it with the mean transit time at peak hyperemia, a thermodilution CFR can be calculated. The ability to measure distal pressure and estimate flow using the thermodilution technique (example shown in Fig. 5.27) with a single wire also allows independent assessment of the microvasculature by calculating the IMR. Although principally a research tool, assessment of IMR permits a unique characterization of the microcirculation, and this has been shown to be prognostic in patients after STEMI.[68,69]

Hyperemic microvascular resistance (HMR) is defined as the ratio of mean distal coronary pressure to flow velocity. Hyperemia is underestimated in the presence of coronary stenosis, compared with actual microvascular resistance, because of the lack of collateral flow contribution. To test whether HMR can accurately identify microvascular function abnormalities, the association between HMR and noninvasive testing was examined in 228 patients with 299 lesions.[70] IC distal pressure flow velocity assessed during IC adenosine hyperemia (20 to 40 μg) determined hyperemic stenosis resistance (HSR) and HMR. HMR values greater than 1.9 mm Hg/cm/s were defined as "high." The odds ratio (OR) for myocardial ischemia with high IMR compared with low IMR was 2.6 ($P < .001$). The authors concluded that increased risk of myocardial ischemia in the presence of high HMR is reflective of an increase in actual myocardial resistance, identifying pertinent pathophysiologic alteration in the microvasculature.

Periprocedural MI (PMI) may involve a significant number of patients after PCI and is associated with poor outcome. In the prediction of periprocedural events, no single laboratory test can be useful. Ng and colleagues[71] hypothesized that impaired baseline coronary microvascular reserve (IMR) results in the inability to tolerate ischemic insults (i.e., the IMR may predict the occurrence of PMI). The investigators used the pressure-temperature sensor wire to measure IMR before PCI in 50 patients, 10 of whom had PMIs. Univariate predictors of PMI included the pre-PCI IMR ($P = .003$) and the number of stents. A pre-PCI IMR of 27 units or more had 80% sensitivity and 85% specificity for PMI. The pre-PCI IMR was independently associated with a 23-fold risk of developing PMI. The authors indicated that the status of coronary microcirculation does play a role in determining susceptibility to PMI during elective PCI and may guide adjunctive preventive therapies.

Nonhyperemic Pressure Ratio Indices of Coronary Stenosis Significance

The use of resting, nonhyperemic translesional pressure gradients (aortic-distal poststenotic pressure, [Pa–Pd = ΔP]), or ratios (Pd/Pa) gave way to a hyperemic Pd/Pa (FFR) which better defined ischemia than resting indices. Although FFR has the most extensive record of clinical outcome studies, a revival of resting physiologic indices using a novel resting Pd/Pa taken during a specific diastolic interval, the iFR (instantaneous wave-free pressure ratio), has produced renewed interest but introduced controversy into the practice. However, there is little difference among the nonhyperemic pressure ratios (NHPRs) (iFR, diastolic pressure ratio [dPR] relative full cycle flow ratio [RFR], diastolic flow ratio [DFR]). Van Veer et al. found that all dPRs were nearly identical (Fig. 5.28).[72] iFR has been validated against FFR with an approximately 80% correspondence.[73] Recently, outcomes with iFR were found to be noninferior to those of FFR in the Functional Lesion Assessment of Intermediate Stenosis to Guide Revascularisation (DEFINE-FLAIR) and Instantaneous Wave-Free Ratio Versus Fractional Flow Reserve in Patients With Stable Angina Pectoris or Acute Coronary Syndrome Trial (iFR-SWEDEHEART) studies (see later).[74,75] However, application of NHPR indices to a wide variety of complex anatomy presentations, such as stenoses in series, must wait for clinical studies to fully support their use in daily practice.

Nonhyperemic Pressure Ratios

There are differences, albeit very small, among Pd/Pa and dPRs, and Pd/Pa is measured from the mean pressures over several cardiac cycles, whereas iFR is derived from a pressure ratio over the cardiac cycle's diastolic "wave-free" period, averaging individual values over five beats of data collection. iFR requires proprietary software, thus limiting real-time application to a specific pressure system and sensor wire (Philips Volcano, Verrata). The original iFR software required electrocardiographic (ECG) gating and was susceptible to poor ECG signals, whereas Pd/Pa is displayed continuously in real time and has fewer unacceptable artifacts. Both iFR and Pd/Pa are susceptible to transient hyperemia of contrast media, nitroglycerin, or saline flush and thus require some time before measurement to ensure a resting state. An iFR pullback recording can be coregistered with the angiogram, a feature yet to be developed for Pd/Pa.

Because iFR does not require hyperemia, it is an attractive alternative to FFR with a lower incidence of patient discomfort, side effects, and shorter procedural time. Utilization of a nonhyperemic pressure-derived index of coronary stenosis severity is a desirable feature among those working in the cardiac catheterization lab. Through the use of wave-intensity analysis, Sen and coworkers[73] found a period of diastole in which equilibration or balance is reached between pressure waves from the aorta and distal microcirculatory reflection; hence it

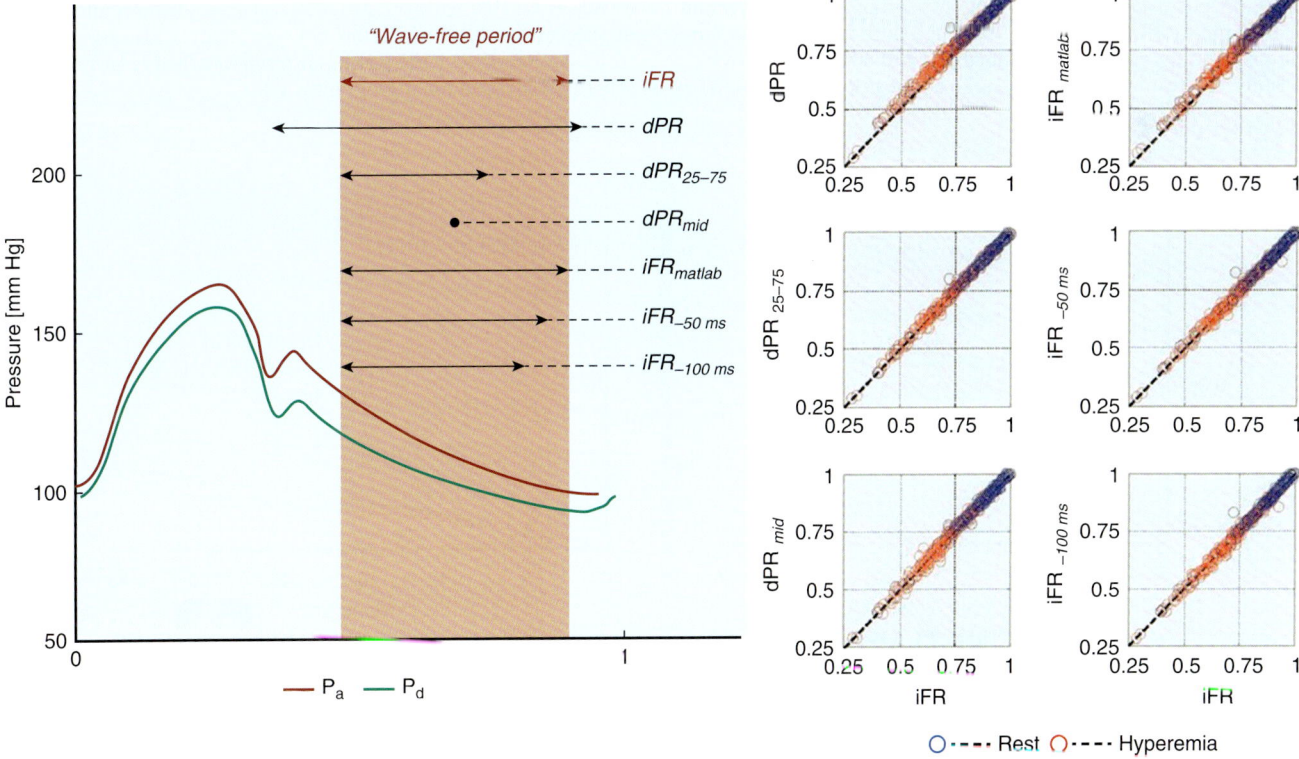

Fig. 5.28 Correlations among resting diastolic pressure ratios over various diastolic periods to iFR. *dPR*, Diastolic pressure ratio; *iFR*, instantaneous wave-free ratio. (Van't Veer M, Pijls NHJ, Hennigan B, et al. Comparison of different diastolic resting indexes to iFR: are they all equal? *J Am Coll Cardiol.* 2017;70:3088–3096.)

is wave free. This wave-free period (WFP) occurs 75% of the way through diastole to just before systole and is a period during which the resistance is fixed. In the Adenosine Vasodilator Independent Stenosis Evaluation (ADVISE) study, 157 stenoses were assessed with iFR and FFR to produce an 80% correspondence.

The Multicenter core laboratory comparison of the instantaneous wave-free ratio and resting Pd/Pa with fractional flow reserve (RESOLVE) study[76] compared the diagnostic accuracy of the iFR and resting coronary artery pressure with the aortic pressure ratio Pd/Pa with respect to the FFR in a core laboratory. The iFR, Pd/Pa, and FFR were measured in 1768 patients from 15 clinical sites. The core lab analyzed the data, and thresholds corresponding to 90% accuracy in predicting ischemic versus nonischemic FFR were then identified. In 1974 lesions, the optimal iFR to predict an FFR less than 0.8 was 0.92 with an accuracy of 80%. For the resting Pd/Pa ratio, the cutpoint was 0.92 with an overall accuracy of 92% with no significant differences between iFR and Pd/Pa. Both measures have 90% accuracy to predict positive or negative FFR in 65% and 48% of lesions, respectively. These data suggest that resting indices of lesion severity demonstrated an overall accuracy with FFR of approximately 80%, which can be improved to 90% in a subset of lesions.

Instantaneous Wave-free Pressure Ratio and Clinical Outcome

The DEFINE-FLAIR[74] (n = 2492) and the iFR-SWEDEHEART[73] (n = 2109) trials tested whether iFR-guided PCI was noninferior to FFR-guided coronary revascularization. The two trials had nearly identical trial designs and used the same primary composite end point of all-cause mortality, nonfatal MI, and unplanned revascularization. At 12 months, both studies demonstrated noninferiority to FFR (DEFINE-FLAIR 6.8% vs. 7.0% for iFR vs. FFR, noninferiority $P < .001$; iFR SWEDEHEART 6.7% vs. 6.1%, noninferiority $P = .007$) (Fig. 5.29). Because adenosine was avoided, iFR patients had shorter procedure times (<4.5 minutes) and fewer adenosine-related effects. There were also fewer positive lesions with iFR, translating to fewer referrals for PCI and CABG (Table 5.6). Although both trials had the limitations of studying low-risk populations and large noninferiority margins, the results have led many to adopt iFR in practice. The safety of using iFR instead of FFR in patients at increased risk (i.e., more severe ischemic lesions with low FFR) CAD is debatable because the average FFR in the two iFR studies was much higher than in FAME trials (FFR 0.83 vs. 0.71). Although iFR and FFR are concordant 80% of the time, discordance occurs in approximately 20% of patients and raises a clinical decision-making dilemma—which one is superior is an ongoing area of active research.

iFR also has the potential to simplify treatment of serial lesions by the use of pullback iFR measurements coregistered with the angiographic lesion locations (Fig. 5.30).[77a,b] This technology will likely be a vanguard of future research into the interaction of resting and hyperemic flow across serial stenoses. For the lower-risk patients tested in iFR outcome studies, the use of iFR reduced referrals for revascularization without increasing adverse events. For complex anatomy including serial or diffuse disease assessment, the iFR technique appears to be particularly helpful for pullback measurements as well as rapid multivessel testing. At this time, to replace FFR, iFR and other NHPR indices will need more long-term outcome studies, more independent validations versus ischemia testing, and greater experience in more diverse patient risk groups.

CONCLUSION

Coronary physiology is now recognized as a key part of the clinical decision making for interventional cardiologists. Exciting developments over the past few years have led to a renewed interest in the field. Future advances in coronary physiology will give practitioners the ability to evaluate the contribution of microvascular disease to a patient's symptoms, target therapies that can improve microvascular dysfunction, and evaluate endothelial dysfunction as a precursor to the atherosclerotic process. Conscientious operators use FFR and IVUS for appropriate decision making and improved outcomes in patients undergoing modern, complex PCI. With strong data showing favorable outcomes associated with the use of measuring coronary physiology in the cardiac catheterization lab, especially FFR and NHPRs (iFR, Pd/Pa, dPR, RFR, DFR), interventionalists can no longer rely on PCI based on angiography alone.

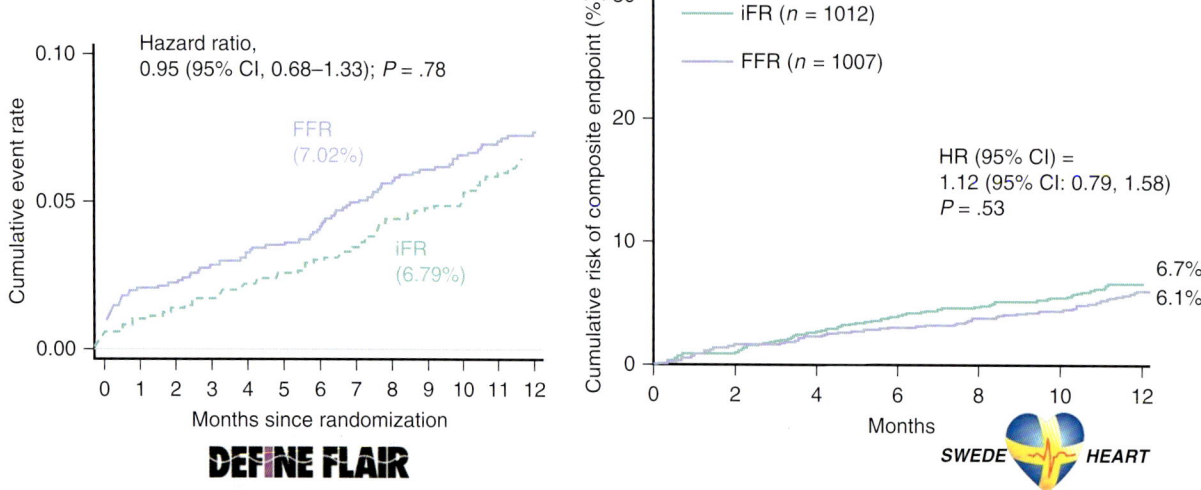

Fig. 5.29 DEFINE-FLAIR (left) and SWEDEHEART (right) studies. At 12 months, both studies demonstrated noninferiority to fractional flow reserve (FFR; DEFINE-FLAIR 6.8% vs. 7.0% for instantaneous wave-free ratio [iFR] vs. FFR, noninferiority $P < .001$; iFR SWEDEHEART 6.7% vs. 6.1%, noninferiority $P = .007$). (Left from Davies JE, Sen S, Dehbi HM, et al. Use of the instantaneous wave-free ratio or fractional flow reserve in PCI. N Engl J Med. 2017;376[19]:1824–1834. Right from Götberg M, Christiansen EH, Gudmundsdottir IJ, et al. Instantaneous wave-free ratio versus fractional flow reserve to guide PCI. N Engl J Med. 2017;376[19]:1813–1823.)

CHAPTER 5 Intracoronary Pressure and Flow Measurements

TABLE 5.6 Fractional Flow Reserve Versus Instantaneous Wave-Free Ratio Comparison

	Fractional Flow Reserve	Instantaneous Wave-Free Ratio
Quantity outcome data and length of experience	+++	++
Resistance to technical errors (damping, drift, equalization, changing basal flow)	++	+ Small equalization errors are more significant Administration of nitrates, contrast, saline or after PCI alters resting state
Procedure time (IC adenosine) (IV adenosine)	++ +	+++ +++
Avoidance of transient adenosine side effects	+ (Less with IC adenosine)	+++
Cost	++	+++ No adenosine, revascularization procedures
Pullback measurements	++ variability of hyperemic state	+++
Availability	+++ Can be performed with any of the five currently available systems and types of sensors/platforms	+ Requires use of Volcano/Philips technology

+++, favorable result; ++, average; +, less favorable.
IC, Intracoronary; *IV*, intravenous; *PCI*, percutaneous coronary intervention.

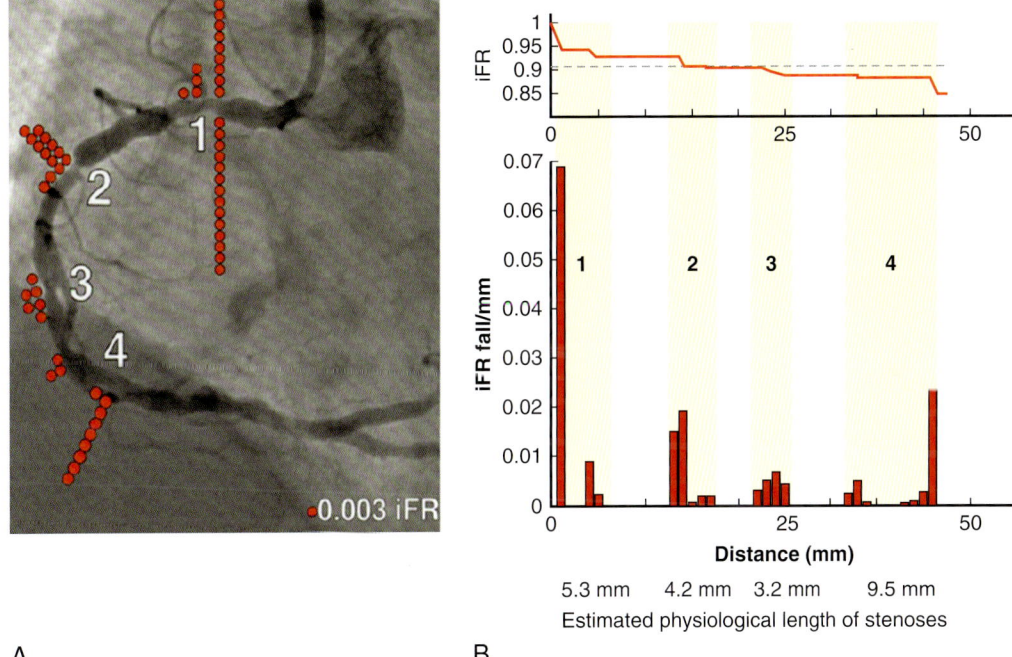

Fig. 5.30 (A) Shows a right coronary artery with four stenoses. (B) Shows an instantaneous wave-free ratio *(iFR)* intensity plot with sudden stepdowns that correspond to focal lesions, and gradual slopes that correspond to diffuse disease. (From Nijjer SS, Sen S, Petraco R, et al. Pre-angioplasty instantaneous wave-free ratio pullback provides virtual intervention and predicts hemodynamic outcome for serial lesions and diffuse coronary artery disease. *JACC Cardiovasc Interv.* 2014;7:12. https://doi.org/10.1016/j.jcin.2014.06.015.)

KEY REFERENCES

5. Pijls NH, van Son JA, Kirkeeide RL, et al. Experimental basis of determining maximum coronary, myocardial, and collateral blood flow by pressure measurements for assessing functional stenosis severity before and after percutaneous transluminal coronary angioplasty. *Circulation*. 1993;87(4):1354–1367.
8. De Bruyne B, Bartunek J, Sys SU, et al. Simultaneous coronary pressure and flow velocity measurements in humans. feasibility, reproducibility, and hemodynamic dependence of coronary flow velocity reserve, hyperemic flow versus pressure slope index, and fractional flow reserve. *Circulation*. 1996;94(8):1842–1849.
18. Pijls NHJ, De Bruyne B, Peels K, et al. Measurement of fractional flow reserve to assess the functional severity of coronary-artery stenoses. *N Engl J Med*. 1996;334(26):1703–1708.
21. Toth G, Hamilos M, Pyxaras S, et al. Evolving concepts of angiogram: fractional flow reserve discordances in 4000 coronary stenoses. *Eur Heart J*. 2014;35(40):2831–2838.
24. Ahn JM, Park DW, Shin ES, et al. Fractional flow reserve and cardiac events in coronary artery disease: data from a prospective IRIS-FFR Registry (Interventional Cardiology Research Incooperation Society Fractional Flow Reserve). *Circulation*. 2017;135(23):2241–2251.

32. Pijls NH, van Schaardenburgh P, Manoharan G, et al. Percutaneous coronary intervention of functionally nonsignificant stenosis: 5-year follow-up of the DEFER Study. *J Am Coll Cardiol*. 2007;49(21):2105–2111.
33. Tonino PA, Fearon WF, De Bruyne B, et al. Angiographic versus functional severity of coronary artery stenoses in the FAME study fractional flow reserve versus angiography in multivessel evaluation. *J Am Coll Cardiol*. 2010;55(25):2816–2821.
34. De Bruyne B, Pijls NH, Kalesan B, et al. Fractional flow reserve-guided PCI versus medical therapy in stable coronary disease. *N Engl J Med*. 2012;367(11):991–1001.
43. Fearon WF, Shilane D, Pijls NH, et al. Cost-effectiveness of percutaneous coronary intervention in patients with stable coronary artery disease and abnormal fractional flow reserve. *Circulation*. 2013;128(12):1335–1340.
44. Hamilos M, Muller O, Cuisset T, et al. Long-term clinical outcome after fractional flow reserve-guided treatment in patients with angiographically equivocal left main coronary artery stenosis. *Circulation*. 2009;120(15):1505–1512.
48. De Bruyne B, Hersbach F, Pijls NH, et al. Abnormal epicardial coronary resistance in patients with diffuse atherosclerosis but "Normal" coronary angiography. *Circulation*. 2001;104(20):2401–2406.
49. Koo BK, Kang HJ, Youn TJ, et al. Physiologic assessment of jailed side branch lesions using fractional flow reserve. *J Am Coll Cardiol*. 2005;46(4):633–637.
61. Lonborg J, Engstrøm T, Kelbæk H, et al. Fractional flow reserve-guided complete revascularization improves the prognosis in patients with ST-segment-elevation myocardial infarction and severe nonculprit disease: A DANAMI 3-PRIMULTI Substudy (Primary PCI in Patients With ST-Elevation Myocardial Infarction and Multivessel Disease: Treatment of Culprit Lesion Only or Complete Revascularization). *Circ Cardiovasc Interv*. 2017;10(4).
62. Smits PC, Abdel-Wahab M, Neumann F-J, et al. Fractional flow reserve-guided multivessel angioplasty in myocardial infarction. *N Engl J Med*. 2017;376(13):1234–1244.
74. Davies JE, Sen S, Dehbi M, et al. Use of the instantaneous wave-free ratio or fractional flow reserve in PCI. *N Engl J Med*. 2017;376(19):1824–1834.

Additional references available online at expertconsult.com.

中文导读

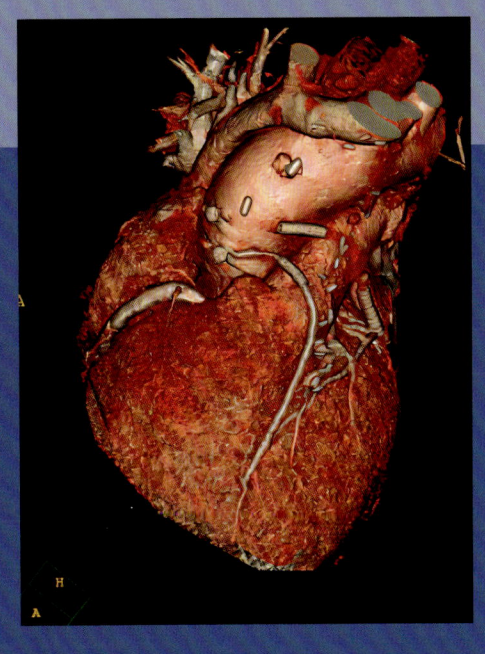

第6章
对比剂诱导的急性肾损伤和慢性肾脏疾病在经皮冠状动脉介入治疗中的影响

对比剂诱导的急性肾损伤通常定义为在使用碘对比剂之后48~72小时出现的急性肾损伤，且排除无其他原因所致。尽管新一代对比剂的出现降低了对比剂诱导的急性肾损伤的发生率，但仍然是一个值得关注的问题。基线肾功能是对比剂诱导的急性肾损伤最有力的预测因子。研究表明，sCyC、NGAL是对比剂诱导的急性肾损伤早期发现和预测主要不良反应的可靠标记物。慢性肾脏病是一种全球迅速增加的疾病，被认为是对比剂诱导的急性肾损伤最重要的预测因素之一。慢性肾脏病在冠心病患者中的患病率高，而慢性肾脏病与经皮冠状动脉介入治疗术后预后差相关。慢性肾脏病患者，特别是透析患者，再狭窄和再次靶血管重建的风险会增加，因此应谨慎为该类患者选择治疗方案，特别注意透析或接受肾移植的患者。降低对比剂引起的急性肾损伤风险是重要的，如前所述，碘对比剂的类型和使用剂量在对比剂诱导的急性肾损伤的发展中起着重要作用。建议选择低渗对比剂，并减少碘对比剂剂量，总剂量不应超过患者基线eGFR的2~2.5倍，减少碘对比剂剂量的策略包括使用更小的导管、双平面血管造影、诊断和治疗性血管造影分离至少72小时，以及避免左心室造影。在碘对比剂暴露前48小时停止可能增加对比剂诱导的急性肾损伤风险的药物，或使用"超低对比剂冠状动脉造影术"也是可行的。围手术期水化治疗可以预防对比剂诱导的急性肾损伤，指南建议在经皮冠状动脉介入治疗前3~12小时使用等渗生理盐水[1.0~1.5 mL/（kg·h）]，经皮冠状动脉介入治疗后6~24小时继续使用。另外，由于大多数接受冠状动脉造影术的患者都有他汀类药物的适应证，除非存在明确的禁忌证，否则使用他汀类药物可被视为预防高危患者对比剂诱导的急性肾损伤的常规策略。

梁敬轩　柳景华

章节要点

- 尽管新一代对比剂的出现降低了对比剂诱导的急性肾损伤的发生率，但这仍然是一个值得关注的问题，尤其是在接受心脏介入诊疗的患者中。
- 慢性肾脏病是对比剂诱导的急性肾损伤发生的一个极其重要的预测因子，其发病率在全球范围内正迅速增加。
- 一般而言，急性肾损伤与对比剂诱导的急性肾损伤在危险因素方面存在重叠，二者存在共同的危险因素。
- 区分真正的对比剂诱导的急性肾损伤与其他肾毒性原因所致的急性肾损伤，这是一件非常困难的事情。最近有研究显示，对比剂诱导的急性肾损伤的发生率可能被高估了。
- 目前需要新的策略来早期发现对比剂诱导的急性肾损伤，并能更好地将对比剂诱导的急性肾损伤与其他原因所致的急性肾损伤区分开来。因此，需要进一步的研究，包括关于新型生物标记物的研究。
- 降低经皮冠状动脉介入治疗术后对比剂诱导的急性肾损伤风险的策略包括使用低渗透压对比剂、减少对比剂量和围术期水化治疗。以研究预防策略为目的、具有充分检验效力的随机对照研究必不可少，同时还应关注具有对比剂诱导的急性肾损伤高危风险的经皮冠状动脉介入治疗患者。

6 Contrast-Induced Acute Kidney Injury and the Role of Chronic Kidney Disease in Percutaneous Coronary Intervention

Roxana Mehran, Birgit Vogel, Sabato Sorrentino

KEY POINTS

- Although the advent of new-generation contrast agents has resulted in a decreased incidence of contrast-induced acute kidney injury (CI-AKI), it remains a concern especially in patients undergoing cardiac catheterization.
- Chronic kidney disease (CKD) as one of the most important predictors of CI-AKI is rapidly increasing worldwide.
- Risk factors for AKI in general are common and overlap with risk factors for CI-AKI.
- Differentiating true CI-AKI from AKI due to other nephrotoxic causes is challenging, and recent reports suggest that the incidence of CI-AKI may have been overestimated.
- New strategies are needed for the early detection of CI-AKI and for better differentiation of CI-AKI from other forms of AKI. Further research is needed and should include the investigation of novel biomarkers.
- Strategies to minimize the risk of CI-AKI after percutaneous coronary intervention (PCI) include the use of low-osmolar contrast agents, minimizing the contrast volume and the administration of periprocedural hydration therapy. Adequately powered randomized controlled trials investigating prevention strategies are necessary and should focus on patients undergoing PCI at high risk for CI-AKI.

INTRODUCTION

Contrast-induced acute kidney injury (CI-AKI) is commonly defined as the occurrence of acute renal impairment within 48 to 72 hours after administration of iodinated contrast media (CM) in the absence of other causes for acute kidney injury (AKI).[1] Although the advent of new generation contrast agents has resulted in a decreased incidence of CI-AKI, it remains a concern especially in patients undergoing cardiac catheterization. The increasing volume of percutaneous coronary intervention (PCI) procedures, particularly in the elderly, also contributes to an increased number of patients at risk for CI-AKI. However, risk factors for AKI in general are common and overlap with risk factors for CI-AKI, especially in the elderly. Therefore, differentiating true CI-AKI from AKI due to other causes is challenging, and recent reports suggest that the incidence of CI-AKI may have been overestimated.[2] Data on the prevalence, risk factors, and risk assessment for CI-AKI in patients undergoing cardiovascular procedures including cardiac catheterization, PCI, and transcatheter aortic valve replacement (TAVR) are reviewed in this chapter. Furthermore, we will discuss the role of chronic kidney disease (CKD) as a condition that is rapidly increasing worldwide and is known to be one of the most important predictors of CI-AKI. Special considerations are described for patients on dialysis or who have undergone renal transplantation. Pharmacologic and nonpharmacologic strategies to prevent CI-AKI are discussed.

DEFINITION OF CONTRAST-INDUCED ACUTE KIDNEY INJURY

Varying terminology to describe CI-AKI has been used throughout the literature (e.g., contrast-induced nephropathy [CIN], contrast nephropathy, contrast-associated AKI). Several definitions of CI-AKI have also been proposed. Most commonly, CI-AKI is defined as an absolute serum creatinine (sCr) increase of ≥0.5 mg/dL (44 μmol/L) or a ≥25% relative increase in sCr from baseline within 48 to 72 hours of CM exposure.

Because many risk factors, preventive measures, and the prognosis of contrast-induced deterioration of renal function are similar to other forms of AKI, the Kidney Disease Improving Global outcomes (KDIGO) working group proposed a standardized definition with graded criteria for all forms of AKI. The term CI-AKI was introduced to describe patients with AKI secondary to CM exposure. The following criteria were developed and refer to its mildest stage: an increase in sCr ≥0.3 mg/dL (≥26.5 μmol/L) within 48 hours; or an increase in sCr ≥1.5 times the baseline value within 7 days; or a urine volume less than 0.5 mL/kg/h for 6 hours. Of note, this definition reflects functional assessment and considers urine output, combining elements from definitions previously proposed by the Acute Kidney Injury Network (AKIN)[3] and the Risk, Injury, Failure, Loss, and End-stage (RIFLE) criteria defined by the Acute Dialysis Quality Initiative (ADQI).[4] The severity of AKI is staged by the increase of sCr, reduction in urine output, and the need for renal replacement therapy (Fig. 6.1). Importantly, these criteria do not specify a time frame for the deterioration of kidney function after CM exposure. Most CI-AKI cases occur early after CM exposure but in a minority of patients the peak increase of sCr may occur as many as 5 days after the application of CM. The 2012 KDIGO practice guidelines strongly recommend to first rule out causes other than CM (e.g., drug toxicity, compromised hemodynamics) in patients who develop deterioration in kidney function after administration of CM.[5] The American College of Radiology Manual on Contrast Media uses an alternative approach and differentiates between post-contrast AKI (PC-AKI) and CIN.[6] PC-AKI may be due to any nephrotoxic cause including contrast application, whereas CIN is defined as a sudden deterioration in renal function that is specifically caused by the intravascular administration of iodinated CM. Hence, CIN or CI-AKI, respectively, are considered sub-entities of PC-AKI.

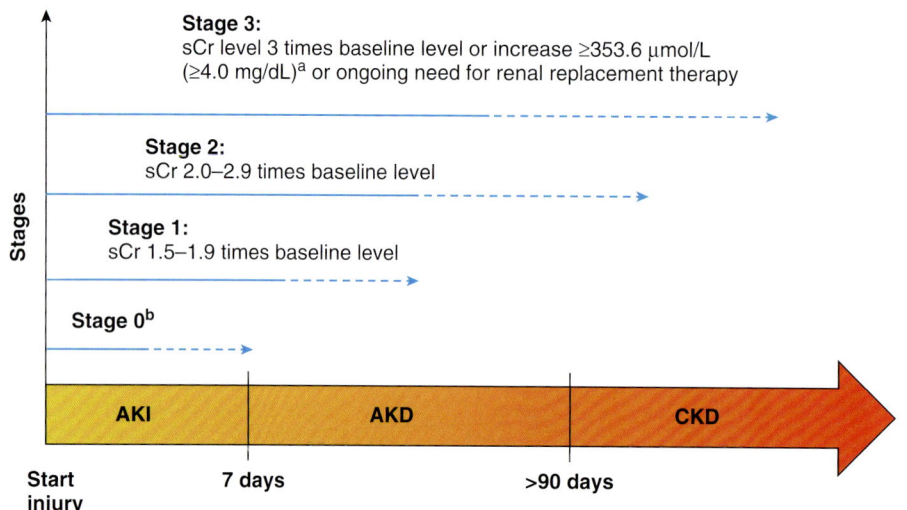

AKIN			RIFLE	
Serum creatinine (sCr)	Urine output (common to both)	Class	Serum creatinine or glomerular filtration rate (GFR)	
Stage 1: increase of ≥0.3 mg/dL or increase to 1.5 × to 2 × baseline sCr	<0.5 mL/kg/h for at least 6 h	Risk	Increase to 1.5 × baseline sCr or decrease in GFR by >25%	
Stage 2: increase to 2 × to 3 × baseline sCr	<0.5 mL/kg/h for >12 h	Injury	Increase to 2 × baseline sCr or decrease in GFR by >50%	
Stage 3: increased to >3 times baseline sCr or ≥4.0 mg/dL with an acute increase of ≥0.5 mg/dL or on RRT	<0.3 mL/kg/h for 24 h or anuria for 12 h	Failure	Increase to 3 × baseline or sCr >4 mg/dL with an acute increase of >0.5 mg/dL or decrease in GFR by >75%	
		Loss	Persistent acute renal failure or complete loss of kidney function for >4 wk	
		ESRD	ESRD for >3 months	

Fig. 6.1 Definition and classification of acute kidney injury *(AKI)* by AKIN, KDIGO, and ADQI.[3–5,50] Acute kidney disease *(AKD)* is defined as AKI stage 1 or greater that persists beyond 7 days after exposure. It may eventually result in chronic kidney disease, which is defined as abnormalities in kidney function that last greater than 90 days. The *blue arrows* reflect the risk to develop chronic kidney disease for each stage. [a]Assumes the baseline serum creatinine level is less than 353.6 μmol/L (<4.0 mg/dL), and that an episode of AKI has occurred. [b]Reflects that even when no apparent residual injury is present, the kidney might be vulnerable for some time after an episode of AKI. Stage 0 subtypes: C: SCr not back to baseline, B: Biomarker or loss of renal reserve indicates injury, A: No evidence of injury. *AKD,* Acute kidney disease; *AKI,* acute kidney injury; *AKIN,* acute kidney injury network; *CKD,* chronic kidney disease; *ESRD,* end-stage renal disease; *RIFLE,* risk, injury, failure, loss, and end-stage criteria; *RRT,* renal replacement therapy; *sCr,* serum creatinine.

PATHOPHYSIOLOGY

The pathophysiology of CI-AKI is complex, and the underlying mechanisms are not yet fully understood. Animal or laboratory studies suggest that CM is directly nephrotoxic to the tubular epithelium causing redistribution of membrane proteins, reduction of extracellular Ca^{2+}, DNA fragmentation, disruption of intercellular junctions, reduced cell proliferation, apoptosis, and altered mitochondrial function.[7,8] CM administration also indirectly promotes renal ischemic injury secondary to an imbalance between vasodilatory and vasoconstrictive mediators resulting in a decline in regional blood flow.[9,10] These effects, together with reactive oxygen species (ROS) formation, result in oxidative damage and cellular injury.[11,12] The hemodynamic effects of CM are greatest in the renal medulla, which is characterized by generally low blood flow to preserve osmotic gradients and enhance urinary concentration.[13] CKD plays a central role in the pathophysiology of CI-AKI because it is associated with fewer functional nephrons, which may increase the susceptibility for CM-induced toxicity.[14]

EPIDEMIOLOGY AND RISK FACTORS FOR CONTRAST-INDUCED ACUTE KIDNEY INJURY

The incidence of CI-AKI is highly dependent on the patient population studied and the diagnostic criteria used. Therefore, reported rates of CI-AKI among patients undergoing PCI vary significantly and range between less than 3% in patients with normal kidney function and up to 40% in patients with CKD.[15–17] Overall, the development of low-osmolar (mostly nonionic) iodinated contrast agents has resulted in a decrease of CI-AKI. Compared to earlier generation high-osmolar ionic CM, the newer agents are associated with reduced rates of CI-AKI and a decreased risk of other adverse effects.[18,19]

The volume of CM administered has also been shown to impact the risk of CI-AKI. High volumes of CM (>350 mL or >4 mL/kg) or previous administration of CM within 72 hours significantly increases the risk of CI-AKI.[20,21] However, even lower CM volumes (<100 mL) can place vulnerable patients at risk.[14] In this context, a CM volume to creatinine clearance ratio of greater

TABLE 6.1 Medications That May Increase the Risk of Contrast-Induced Acute Kidney Injury
MEDICATIONS THAT MAY INCREASE THE RISK OF CONTRAST-INDUCED ACUTE KIDNEY INJURY (CI-AKI)
Drugs That Influence Renal Hemodynamics
Nonsteroidal antiinflammatory drugs (NSAIDs)
Cyclooxygenase 2 (COX-2) inhibitors
Nesiritide
Angiotensin-converting enzyme (ACE) inhibitors
Angiotensin receptor blockers
Dipyridamole
Drugs That Cause Tubular Toxicity
Diuretics, including mannitol
Antibiotics, including aminoglycosides, vancomycin, amphotericin B
Immunosuppressants, including tacrolimus and cyclosporine

TABLE 6.2 Risk Factors for Contrast-Induced Acute Kidney Injury
RISK FACTORS FOR CONTRAST-INDUCED ACUTE KIDNEY INJURY
Patient-Related Factors
Chronic kidney disease
Diabetes mellitus
Advanced age
Anemia
Ejection fraction <40%
Peripheral vascular disease
Presenting Factors
Acute coronary syndrome
Hypotension
Heart failure
Volume depletion
Concomitant nephrotoxic medications
Procedural Factors
Contrast volume
Type of contrast medium
Multiple contrast media exposures within 72 h
Intraaortic balloon pump

than 3.7 is a significant and independent predictor of an early abnormal increase in sCr after PCI.[22]

The risk associated with CM is further confounded by other factors including concomitant medications, patient characteristics, and procedural details. Table 6.1 provides a summary of medications with a potential impact on the risk for CI-AKI. While some drugs may increase the risk of CI-AKI due to their influence on renal hemodynamics (e.g., nonsteroidal antiinflammatory drugs and angiotensin-converting enzyme inhibitors), others may cause direct tubular toxicity (e.g., diuretics and certain antibiotics).[23]

Among patient-related factors, baseline renal function is the most powerful predictor of CI-AKI. An analysis of 985,737 patients undergoing PCI from the National Cardiovascular Data Registry (NCDR) demonstrated that the risk of CI-AKI increased with declining baseline estimated glomerular filtration rate (eGFR).[17] Tsai et al. reported a 7.8% incidence of CI-AKI in patients with an eGFR ≥60 mL/min/1.73 m², 13.6% in patients with an eGFR of 45 to 60 mL/min/1.73 m², 23.1% in patients with an eGFR of 30 to 45 mL/min/1.73 m², and 36.9% in patients with an eGFR less than 30 mL/min/1.73 m².[17] Other patient-related risk factors that influence the risk of CI-AKI include age, diabetes, and anemia.[15–17,20,24]

Diagnostic cardiac catheterization and PCI, respectively, are the leading procedural causes of CI-AKI.[25] Patients receiving primary PCI for acute myocardial infarction (MI), especially in the setting of hemodynamic instability, are at the highest risk, followed by patients undergoing elective PCI and diagnostic cardiac catheterization.[26–28] These differences in risk may be attributed to insufficient time for preventive measures in MI patients undergoing urgent PCI, or the higher contrast load used for coronary interventions compared to diagnostic procedures. Patients presenting in an acute clinical setting may also have a higher risk profile compared to patients undergoing a diagnostic study. In patients with acute MI and hypotension or cardiogenic shock, hypoperfusion of the kidneys may directly lead to renal hypoxia and AKI, or it may increase the susceptibility for CI-AKI.[29] Overall, these findings underscore the complex and multifactorial etiology of CI-AKI and the challenge of identifying true CI-AKI.

Other forms of AKI after PCI may be misinterpreted as CI-AKI. Catheter manipulation may result in the release of atheroemboli from the aorta into the renal circulation, leading to AKI.[30] Authors of the recently published Acute Kidney Injury After Radial or Femoral Access for Invasive Acute Coronary Syndrome Management (AKI-MATRIX) trial hypothesized that a reduction of atheroemboli to the renal circulation may have been one of the contributing factors that led to the reduction of AKI associated with radial compared to femoral access.[31] The lower rate of AKI after PCI associated with a radial versus femoral approach was recently confirmed by data from a retrospective single-center cohort study of 2937 patients.[32]

PREDICTING THE RISK OF CONTRAST-INDUCED ACUTE KIDNEY INJURY

Risk Scores

A variety of scores have been developed to comprehensively assess the risk of CI-AKI. While most risk scores incorporate clinical and procedural variables to estimate the risk of CI-AKI and associated outcomes,[20,33–35] others only include pre-procedural variables to allow clinicians to evaluate the risks and benefits of PCI pre-procedure and plan for preventive strategies.[36] Table 6.2 summarizes the most common risk factors included in existing risk scores.

Biomarkers for Risk Prediction and Early Detection of Contrast-Induced Acute Kidney Injury

Changes in sCr have low sensitivity for rapidly detecting acute changes in renal function. sCr levels start to rise within 24 to 48 hours of CM administration, peak at 48 to 72 hours, and usually return to the baseline value within 2 weeks.[10] In addition, sCr levels are influenced by age, sex, muscle mass, nutritional status, and hydration.[37] Therefore, it was hypothesized that alternative biomarkers with faster kinetics could facilitate diagnosis and rapid detection of CI-AKI. Cystatin C (sCyC) and neutrophil gelatinase-associated lipocalin (NGAL) currently have the largest body of evidence. Studies suggest that sCyC increases earlier (as early as 8 hours after CM application) and is less influenced by non-renal factors compared to sCr.[38–40] While one study identified a 15% increase of sCyC as the optimal cutoff to predict CI-AKI,[41] another study reported that a sCyC increase of less than 10% at 24 hours is a reliable marker to rule out the risk for CI-AKI.[42] In both studies an increase of sCyC predicted major adverse events; patients with a rise in both sCyC and sCr had the highest risk.[41,42] Similarly, data suggest that NGAL is a reliable marker for the early detection of CI-AKI and prediction of 1-year major adverse events.[43] Serum and urine NGAL levels rise within 2 and 4 hours, respectively, after CM administration.[44,45] A serum/urine NGAL cutoff of 150 ng/mL has been used to diagnose CI-AKI.[46] In addition, urine NGAL less than 20 ng/mL and serum NGAL less than 179 ng/mL at 6 hours were identified as cutoffs to rule out CI-AKI.[43] Other biomarkers that have been investigated for the early detection and risk assessment of CI-AKI include serum liver fatty acid-binding protein (L-FABP), serum kidney injury marker 1 (KIM-1), and urine interleukin 18 (IL-18).[47] Despite promising results derived by several studies, further investigation is needed to validate threshold values and evaluate the role of these novel biomarkers in routine clinical practice.

PROGNOSIS OF CONTRAST-INDUCED ACUTE KIDNEY INJURY

In most cases, CI-AKI reflects a mild transient deterioration of renal function. A new requirement for dialysis occurs in less than 1% of patients.[48] In the analysis of the NCDR database by Tsai et al. the rate of new required dialysis was 0.3%.[17] While this rate within the overall population seems low, reported rates are higher in patients with certain clinical characteristics. The rate of new required dialysis was 4.3% in patients with CKD and 7.2% in patients with ST-segment elevation myocardial infarction (STEMI).[17] Numerous studies suggest an association between CI-AKI and worse clinical outcome, including a sustained deterioration of kidney function.[14,16,17,24,49] Compared to patients without AKI, the adjusted risk of a sustained decline in kidney function at 3 months following angiography increased more than 4-fold for patients with mild AKI to greater than 17-fold for those with moderate or severe stages of AKI.[49] The recently published consensus report of the ADQI 16 Workgroup concluded that resolution of an AKI episode within 48 hours is associated with better outcomes than longer durations of AKI.[50] Patients with AKI episodes persisting beyond 7 days are more likely to develop CKD. The ADQI proposed the term acute kidney disease for AKI stage 1 or greater that persists beyond 7 days after the exposure. It may eventually result in CKD, which is defined as abnormalities in kidney function that last greater than 90 days (see Fig. 6.1).[50]

In the NCDR analysis, MI, bleeding, and death rates were 3.8%, 6.4%, and 9.6%, respectively, in patients who developed AKI compared with 2.1%, 1.4%, and 0.5%, respectively, in patients who did not develop AKI.[17] The rates of MI (7.9%), bleeding (15.8%), and death (34.3%) were highest in patients who developed AKI requiring new dialysis.[17] A meta-analysis of 39 studies confirmed that CI-AKI was associated with an increased risk of end-stage renal disease (ESRD) as well as mortality, cardiovascular events, and prolonged hospitalization.[51] However, the association between CI-AKI and mortality was heavily confounded by baseline characteristics that increased risk for both AKI and mortality. The risk attributable to CI-AKI was much lower than that reported from unadjusted studies.[51] Indeed, the underlying mechanisms of the association between CI-AKI and future adverse events are uncertain. It is difficult to identify the risk attributable to CI-AKI alone since residual confounding in observational studies cannot be excluded even after comprehensive statistical adjustment. Hence, it remains uncertain whether the prevention of CI-AKI would result in improved clinical outcomes.

CHRONIC KIDNEY DISEASE

Epidemiology and Definition

CKD is one of the most important risk factors for CI-AKI, but it is also an independent predictor for cardiovascular events. In fact, the association between CKD and coronary artery disease (CAD)

TABLE 6.3 Criteria for the Diagnosis of Chronic Kidney Disease

CRITERIA FOR CHRONIC KIDNEY DISEASE (EITHER OF THE FOLLOWING PRESENT FOR >3 MONTHS)	
Markers of kidney damage (one or more)	Albuminuria (AER ≥30 mg/24 h; ACR ≥30 mg/g [≥3 mg/mmol])
	Urine sediment abnormalities
	Electrolyte and other abnormalities due to tubular disorders
	Abnormalities detected by histology
	Structural abnormalities detected by imaging
	History of kidney transplantation
Decreased GFR	GFR <60 mL/min/1.73 m^2 (GFR categories G3a–G5)

ACR, Albumin-to-creatinine ratio; AER, albumin excretion rate; GFR, glomerular filtration rate.
Adapted from Kidney Disease: Improving Global Outcomes (KDIGO) CKD Work Group. KDIGO 2012 clinical practice guideline for the evaluation and management of chronic kidney disease. Kidney Inter. Suppl. 2013;3:1–150.

is complex and bidirectional. The prevalence of CKD is drastically increasing in the aging population with the growing burden of risk factors such as obesity and diabetes.[52–54] A recent report suggested a prevalence of 14.8% for CKD in the U.S. population with an estimated 30 million American adults diagnosed with this condition.[55] The 2012 KDIGO Clinical Practice Guidelines define CKD as the presence of sustained abnormalities of kidney function for greater than 3 months with implications for health (Table 6.3).[56] Classification of CKD is based on cause, GFR category, and albuminuria category (Table 6.4).[56] However, GFR measurements have relevant limitations that should be considered in their interpretation. Direct measurement by calculation of the urinary clearance of creatinine (an endogenous filtration marker) from a timed urine collection (e.g., 24 hours) and blood sampling during the collection period is the most accurate method, but it is not feasible in routine clinical practice. Relying on sCr values is simple, but it is the least accurate approach. Therefore, the 2012 KDIGO guidelines suggest indirect measurement of GFR by incorporating sCr levels into formulas such as the Cockcroft-Gault, the Modification of Diet and Renal Disease (MDRD), or the Chronic Kidney Disease Epidemiology Collaboration (CKD-EPI) equation.[56–60] The former two equations were developed in patients with CKD and therefore underestimate measured GFR at higher values. All formulas have limitations inherent to sCr measurement itself, and from the underrepresentation of certain individuals in the study populations from which the equations were derived. Hence, the equations do not perform well in patients who (1) have very high or low muscle mass, weight, or age; (2) are severely ill or hospitalized; (3) ingest no meat or large amounts of meat; or (4) are from minority racial and ethnic groups, such as Asians or Hispanics.[61,62] Additional testing (e.g., sCyC) may be helpful in cases where the accuracy of eGFR based on sCr is uncertain.[56,63]

Chronic Kidney Disease in Patients Undergoing Percutaneous Coronary Intervention

The prevalence of CKD in patients with CAD is high with a reported rate of approximately 30%.[17,64,65] In addition, the number of patients with CKD referred for coronary catheterization is growing because the annual rates of PCI as the predominant means of coronary revascularization are increasing, especially in the elderly. However, CKD is associated with worse outcomes after PCI,[65,66] although the mechanisms are not completely understood. CKD is associated with several traditional cardiovascular risk factors, but this relationship does not fully explain the increased incidence of cardiovascular events and mortality in patients with CKD. CKD is also associated with several nontraditional risk factors, such as albuminuria, proteinuria, retention of uremic toxins, anemia, homocysteinemia, positive calcium balance, abnormalities in bone mineral metabolism, oxidative stress, increased inflammatory-poor nutrition state, endothelial dysfunction and insulin resistance, and conditions that promote coagulation, all of which accelerate atherosclerosis.[67-71] Finally, it is well documented that patients with CKD are less likely to receive guideline-recommended therapies, which might be associated with worse outcome.[53,72,73] The increased risk for both CI-AKI and bleeding complications may prevent patients with CKD from receiving PCI or antithrombotic therapy.[74-76] Balancing the risks of bleeding and thrombosis is particularly challenging in patients with CKD. The choice of antithrombotic therapy should be made carefully, and doses of agents such as eptifibatide, bivalirudin, enoxaparin, and fondaparinux should be appropriately adjusted for renal function.[77] Radial access may also reduce bleeding risk in patients undergoing PCI. The potential for radial access to decrease the risk of bleeding and CI-AKI compared to femoral access must be weighed against potential concerns that PCI via radial access could negatively impact the success of future arteriovenous fistulas and grafts in patients who progress to ESRD.[78] The risk of death from nonrenal causes and especially cardiovascular events is high, and most patients with CKD will not progress to ESRD. However, the number of patients who require maintenance dialysis or a kidney transplant is rapidly growing. In the United States, both the incidence and prevalence of ESRD have doubled in the past decade. In 2015, 124,111 new cases of ESRD were reported. Nearly 500,000 patients received maintenance dialysis and more than 200,000 were living with a kidney transplant.[55] However, data are limited in patients with ESRD undergoing PCI, and most of the evidence was derived from observational studies as clinical trials have largely excluded these patients. Nevertheless, an association between accelerated atherosclerosis and maintenance dialysis has long been recognized.[79] Cardiovascular death accounts for the greatest proportion of known cause-specific mortality in patients undergoing dialysis. More specifically, arrhythmia and cardiac arrest comprise 40% of known causes of death in patients receiving dialysis, followed by acute MI and atherosclerotic heart disease (17%) and heart failure (3%) according to data from the United States Renal Data System (USRDS).[55] Patients on dialysis who experience an acute MI have poor survival, although some data indicate survival trends are improving,[80] possibly due to increased use of PCI in STEMI. However, conflicting data exist on the impact of early revascularization in acute coronary syndrome (ACS) patients on dialysis. In an analysis from the Swedish Web-System for Enhancement and Development of Evidence-Based Care in Heart Disease Evaluated According to Recommended Therapies (SWEDEHEART) registry, early revascularization in non-ST segment elevation acute myocardial infarction (NSTEMI) patients with mild-to-moderate renal insufficiency was beneficial, but no effect was observed on survival of patients with stage 5 CKD and dialysis.[81] Conversely, a meta-analysis including patients with ACS and CKD suggested a beneficial effect across all stages of CKD including patients on dialysis.[82] These data suggest that early coronary revascularization may be an appropriate strategy, at least in patients with STEMI. Patients with CKD, especially those on dialysis, had an increased risk of restenosis and repeat target vessel revascularization (TVR), with reported rates of up to 80% in the pre-stent era.[83] Increased lesion complexity in patients with advanced CKD and ESRD may contribute to these findings. Patients with CKD, particularly those with ESRD, often have diffusely diseased coronary arteries with heavy atherosclerotic burden and severe calcification.[84] The use of high-frequency rotational atherectomy (HFRA) as the debulking procedure of choice might help, but it can also be challenging for the interventionalist.[84] Although HFRA, routine stenting, and the development of drug eluting stents (DES) have reduced the rates of restenosis and TVR in patients with CKD, the risk of adverse outcomes remains high, especially in those with ESRD.[85-91] An analysis of 23,033 dialysis patients from the USRDS has shown that coronary artery bypass grafting (CABG) was beneficial in terms of repeat revascularization and long-term survival compared to PCI with bare metal stents or DES, although the risk for in-hospital mortality was increased.[92] Therefore, surgery should also be considered in patients on dialysis suitable for both options. Overall, further studies are needed to identify the optimal treatment strategy for patients with CAD on dialysis. Of note, in patients with CKD not on dialysis, studies have shown that CABG was generally associated with higher rates of postprocedural AKI as compared with PCI.[93-95]

TABLE 6.4 Staging of Chronic Kidney Disease Based on Glomerular Filtration Rate and Albuminuria Category

GLOMERULAR FILTRATION RATE CATEGORIES IN CHRONIC KIDNEY DISEASE			
Glomerular Filtration Rate Category	Glomerular Filtration Rate (mL/min/1.73 m^2)		Terms
G1	≥90		Normal or high
G2	60–89		Mildly decreased[a]
G3a	45–59		Mildly to moderately decreased
G3b	30–44		Moderately to severely decreased
G4	15–29		Severely decreased
G5	<15		Kidney failure
ALBUMINURIA CATEGORIES IN CHRONIC KIDNEY DISEASE			
	AER	ACR (approximate equivalent)	
Category	(mg/24 h)	(mg/mmol)	(mg/g)	Terms
A1	<30	<3	<30	Normal to mildly increased
A2	30–300	3–30	30–300	Moderately increased
A3	>300	>30	>300	Severely increased

ACR, Albumin-to-creatinine ratio; *AER*, albumin excretion rate; *CKD*, chronic kidney disease; *GFR*, glomerular filtration rate.
[a]Relative to young adult level. In the absence of evidence of kidney damage, neither GFR category G1 nor G2 fulfill the criteria for CKD.
Adapted from Kidney Disease: Improving Global Outcomes (KDIGO) CKD Work Group. KDIGO 2012 Clinical Practice Guideline for the Evaluation and Management of Chronic Kidney Disease. *Kidney Inter.* 2013;(suppl 3):1–150.

In ESRD patients on maintenance dialysis in whom a PCI is planned, additional dialysis immediately after contrast application does not appear to be necessary. Studies have not shown benefits of this approach compared to maintenance of the routine dialysis schedule.[96–98] However, the studies were small, and individualized treatment may be needed for specific patients such as those with heart failure or with evidence of residual renal function. Preservation of the latter is vital for patients on peritoneal dialysis; once residual renal function is lost, these patients often require hemodialysis.

Whether patients evaluated for kidney transplantation should undergo routine screening for CAD is still a matter of debate. Guidelines based on expert opinion and limited observational data recommend noninvasive stress testing followed by coronary angiography if positive in patients at high risk for CAD (e.g., patients with diabetes).[99] Delaying coronary angiography due to concerns about the risk of CI-AKI in patients with stage 4 or 5 CKD may result in increased cardiovascular morbidity and mortality in the perioperative period and beyond. On the other hand, data on the benefits of coronary revascularization versus medical therapy in patients with significant CAD pre–kidney transplantation are limited and respective studies have shown mixed results.[100] Although patients have improved outcomes after kidney transplantation compared to those on dialysis, the risk for adverse cardiovascular outcomes remains high.[101–104]

Special considerations should be given to cardiac catheterization in patients post–kidney transplant. The location and laterality of the vascular anastomosis of the transplanted kidney should be identified to avoid injury of the transplanted organ. While the anastomosis is commonly at the level of the external iliac artery and vein, it can also be found at the internal iliac artery and vein or at the aorta and inferior vena cava. Fluoroscopy should be used to ensure that wires and catheters are steered away from the vascular anastomoses if instrumentation of the vessels that supply the transplanted kidney cannot be avoided. CM volume should be kept to a minimum since post-transplant patients are at high risk for CI-AKI.[105] Potential drug interactions between periprocedural therapy and immunosuppressants should be considered. Finally, indwelling arterial and venous catheters and vascular closure devices should be avoided because of the increased infection risk in patients receiving immunosuppressant therapy.

PREVENTION STRATEGIES TO MINIMIZE THE RISK OF CONTRAST-INDUCED ACUTE KIDNEY INJURY

The current recommendations for CI-AKI prevention strategies are summarized in Fig. 6.2. The following general strategies should be considered to minimize the risk of CI-AKI. As described above, the type and volume of CM plays an important role in the development of CI-AKI. Low-osmolar CM (LOCM)

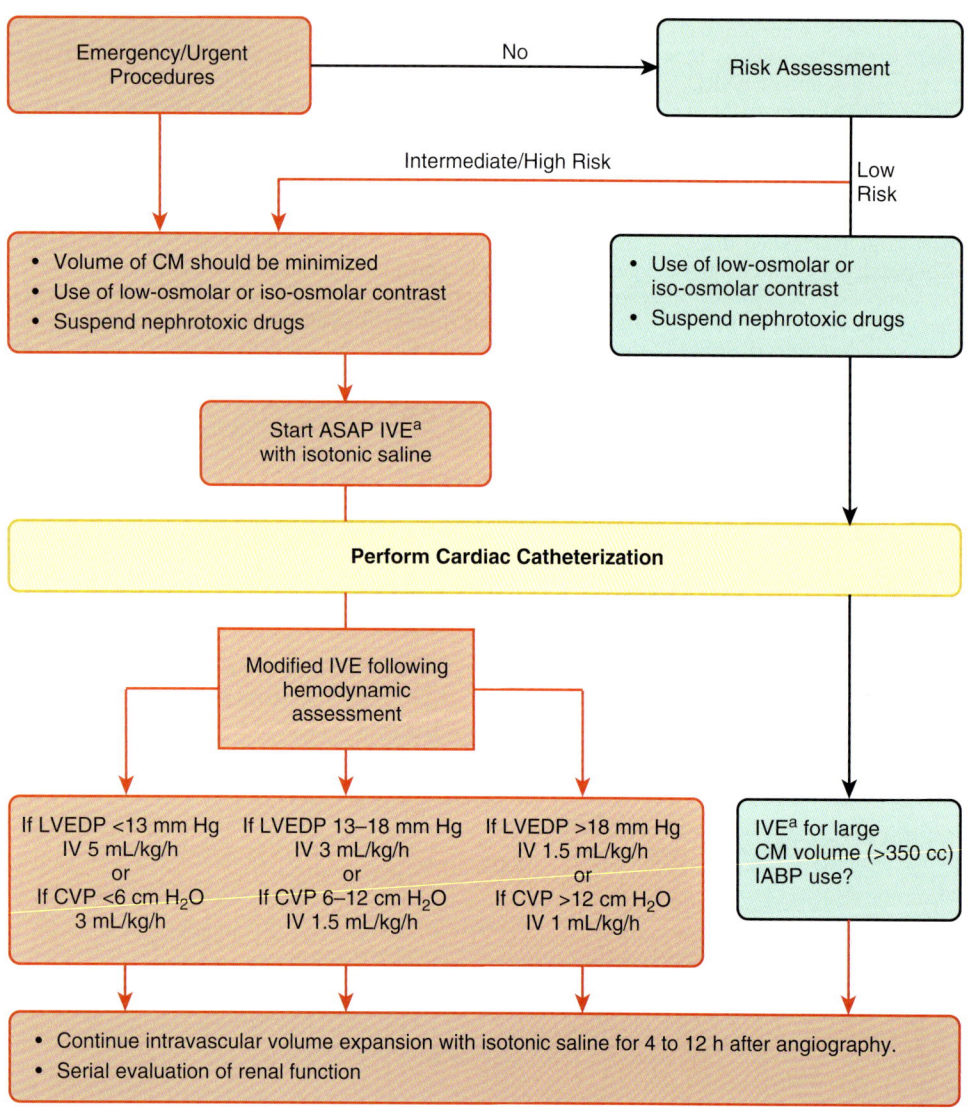

Fig. 6.2 Algorithm for risk assessment and prevention of contrast-induced acute kidney injury (CI-AKI). *Red lines*: patients undergoing urgent/emergent cardiac catheterization or at intermediate to high risk for CI-AKI. *Black Lines*: Patients at low risk for CI-AKI. [a]Isotonic saline at an infusion rate of 100 mL/h for 6 to 12 h before and 4 to 12 h after angiography. *ASAP*, As soon as possible; *CM*, contrast media; *CVP*, central venous pressure; *IABP*, intraaortic balloon pump; *IV*, intravenous; *IVE*, intravascular volume expansion; *LVEDP*, left ventricular end-diastolic pressure.

compared to high-osmolar CM (HOCM) has decreased the risk of CI-AKI regardless of pre existing CKD; therefore, LOCM is favored in current clinical practice.[19] A benefit of iso-osmolar CM (IOCM) over LOCM with regard to CI-AKI is uncertain due to mixed results of available studies on this topic.[106–109] International guidelines differ slightly with regard to the choice of IOCM or LOCM. While the European Society of Cardiology (ESC) favors IOCM over LOCM (Class IIa, Level of evidence A), the ACC/AHA recommends the use of either IOCM or LOCM.[110,111] A specific threshold for the CM volume that induces CI-AKI has not yet been identified. Recent analyses suggest that the total volume of CM should not exceed 2 to 2.5 times the patient's baseline eGFR.[36,112] Strategies to reduce the CM volume may include the use of smaller catheters, biplane angiography, separation of diagnostic and therapeutic angiograms by at least 72 hours, and the avoidance of left ventriculography.[113,114] A slight reduction in contrast volume was documented with the use of an automated contrast injector system, although it did not impact the occurrence of CI-AKI.[115] Discontinuing medications that may increase the risk of CI-AKI 48 hours before CM exposure is another measure that should be considered (see Table 6.1). One important and inexpensive method of reducing contrast exposure has been described. Called "ultra-low contrast coronary angiography," it uses meticulous contrast sparing techniques such as a small contrast syringe, avoidance of contrast "puffing," covering catheter side-holes with guide extension catheters during injections, liberal use of intravascular ultrasound, and use of previous angiograms side by side with the live fluoroscopy screen. These techniques can reduce contrast load during diagnostic and PCI procedures to under 10 to 20 cc and in some patients, contrast can be completely eliminated during PCI.[116–118] Further strategies have been investigated and are summarized in the following sections.

Periprocedural Hydration

Periprocedural hydration is the cornerstone of CI-AKI prevention. Hydration inhibits the renin-angiotensin-aldosterone system, reduces the release of vasoconstrictors and ROS formation, and downregulates tubuloglomerular feedback.[14,119] Guidelines recommend a regimen with isotonic saline (1.0 to 1.5 mL/kg/h) for 3 to 12 hours before and continuing for 6 to 24 hours after PCI.[110,120]

The greatest challenge associated with volume expansion for CI-AKI prevention is avoiding volume overload, especially in patients with heart failure and reduced left ventricular ejection fraction. Balancing the input and output of fluids is crucial to optimize the renal filtration rate and increase CM excretion while preventing volume overload. In the Renal Insufficiency After Contrast Media Administration II (REMEDIAL II) trial, a strategy of controlled forced diuresis using the RenalGuard system was investigated.[121] The concept of the RenalGuard system is based on measuring urine output by a Foley catheter and simultaneously infusing an equivalent volume of isotonic saline. After a 250 mL bolus of saline at 90 minutes prior to CM application, a continuous infusion of intravenous (IV) furosemide 0.25 to 0.5 mg/kg is started. The system automatically adjusts the rate of the continuous IV saline infusion to maintain a urine output rate greater than 300 mL/h throughout the procedure and for 4 hours thereafter. CI-AKI occurred in 16 of 146 patients in the RenalGuard group and in 30 of 146 patients in the control group (11% vs. 20.5%; odds ratio [OR] 0.47, 95% CI 0.24 to 0.92). In the majority of patients (93%) in the RenalGuard group, the target urine flow rate of ≥300 mL/h was reached with a limited furosemide dose and without significant impairment in electrolyte balance.[121] In the Prevention of Contrast Renal Injury with Different Hydration Strategies (POSEIDON) study, fluid administration to prevent CI-AKI was guided by the left ventricular end-diastolic pressure (LVEDP).[122] A total of 396 patients with an eGFR of 60 mL/min/1.73 m^2 and one additional risk factor were randomized to either a standard hydration protocol (1.5 mL/kg/h) or the LVEDP-guided strategy with isotonic saline at 5 mL/kg/h, 3 mL/kg/h, or 1.5 mL/kg/h for 4 hours after the procedure if LVEDP was less than 13 mm Hg, 13 to 18 mm Hg, or greater than 18 mm Hg, respectively. The overall rate of CI-AKI was significantly lower in the LVEDP-guided hydration group compared to the control (6.7% vs. 16.3%; relative risk 0.41; 95% CI 0.22 to 0.79; $P = .005$). Similar data were derived from a study that used central venous pressure to guide hydration.[123]

The randomized, single-center A MAastricht Contrast-Induced Nephropathy Guideline (AMACING) trial provides the most recent data on hydration as a strategy to prevent CI-AKI.[124] A total of 660 consecutive patients requiring CM administration who were at high risk for CI-AKI (eGFR 30–59 mL/min/1.73 m^2) were randomized (1:1) to periprocedural isotonic saline or no IV hydration. Patients undergoing elective procedures with intra arterial as well as IV CM administration were eligible for enrollment. CI-AKI was documented in 8 of 307 nonhydrated patients (2.6%) and in 8 of 296 hydrated patients (2.7%), resulting in an absolute risk difference (no hydration vs. hydration) of –0.10% (95% CI –2.25 to 2.06; $P = .4710$). No hydration was noninferior to hydration with regard to CI-AKI, and it was cost-saving. These results, however, should be interpreted with caution. The low proportion of intra arterial procedures (48%) and interventional procedures (16%) in this study does not allow assessment of the role of hydration in this subgroup of patients more prone to develop CI-AKI. The overall low rate of CI-AKI suggests that the study population may not have been at high risk for CI-AKI.[125] In addition, the volume of CM used in the study was low. Therefore, these results cannot be extrapolated to patients at high risk for CI-AKI or to those requiring high CM volume.

N-Acetyl Cysteine and Sodium Bicarbonate

N-acetyl cysteine (NAC) is assumed to limit CM-AKI by acting as a scavenger of ROS and promoting vasodilatory effects in the renal medulla. It has been widely investigated for the prevention of CI-AKI with mixed results. Earlier trials with small sample sizes suggested a potential benefit of NAC,[126–128] whereas larger studies failed to show a significant reduction in CI-AKI.[129–131] Similarly, isotonic sodium bicarbonate ($NaHCO_3$) was hypothesized to prevent CI-AKI due to inhibition of free-radical formation by alkalinizing the renal tubular fluid.[132] Although smaller studies suggested a benefit of $NaHCO_3$ administration for CI-AKI prevention, these findings were not confirmed in larger studies.[122] Additional studies evaluated the combination of NAC and $NaHCO_3$. In a randomized controlled trial of 720 patients with STEMI undergoing primary PCI, patients were randomized to one of four treatment groups: (1) standard treatment with IV saline alone; (2) standard treatment plus NAC; (3) standard treatment plus $NaHCO_3$; or (4) standard treatment plus NAC and $NaHCO_3$.[133] The rate of CI-AKI was not different for any of the treatment arms compared to standard treatment. However, a smaller proportion of patients in the combined NAC plus $NaHCO_3$ group experienced a greater than 25% increase in sCr from baseline to 30 days.[133] The most recently published Prevention of Serious Adverse Events Following Angiography (PRESERVE) trial is the largest randomized controlled trial to evaluate NAC and $NaHCO_3$ for the prevention of CI-AKI.[134] In a two-by-two factorial design, a total of 5177 high-risk patients undergoing elective angiography were randomized to receive either IV 1.26% $NaHCO_3$ or IV isotonic saline in matched 1-L bags and oral NAC capsules or matched placebo capsules. The study did not use a standardized protocol for fluid administration. The primary composite end point of death, need for dialysis, or persistent rise in sCr at 90 days did not differ between

TABLE 6.5 Definitions of Acute Kidney Injury Adopted by the Valve Academic Research Consortium (VARC)-1 and 2 Initiatives

Acute Kidney Injury Stages	Valve Academic Research Consortium-1	Valve Academic Research Consortium-2
Stages 1	Increase in serum creatinine to 150%–200% (1.5–2.0 × increase compared with baseline) OR Increase of ≥0.3 mg/dL (≥26.4 mmol/L)	Increase in serum creatinine to 150%–199% (1.5–1.99 × increase compared with baseline) OR Increase of ≥0.3 mg/dL (≥26.4 mmol/L) OR Urine output <0.5 mL/kg/h for >6 but <12 h
Stages 2	Increase in serum creatinine to 200%–300% (2.0–3.0 × increase compared with baseline) OR Increase between >0.3 mg/dL (≥26.4 mmol/L) and < 4.0 mg/dL (<354 mmol/L)	Increase in serum creatinine to 200%–299% (2.0–2.99 × increase compared with baseline) OR Urine output <0.5 mL/kg/h for >12 but <24 h
Stages 3	Increase in serum creatinine to 300% (3 × increase compared with baseline) OR Serum creatinine of 4.0 mg/dL (354 mmol/L) with an acute increase of at least 0.5 mg/dL (44 mmol/L) *Patients receiving renal replacement therapy are considered to meet Stage 3 criteria irrespective of other criteria*	Increase in serum creatinine to ≥300% (3 × increase compared with baseline) OR Serum creatinine of ≥4.0 mg/dL (≥354 mmol/L) with an acute increase of at least 0.5 mg/dL (44 mmol/L) OR Urine output <0.3 mL/kg/h for ≥24 h OR Anuria for ≥12 h

treatment groups (IV saline 4.4% vs. NaHCO$_3$ 4.7%, OR 0.93, 95% CI 0.72 to 1.22; P = .62; oral NAC 4.6% vs. placebo 4.5%, OR 1.02, 95% CI 0.78 to 1.33, P = .88). The secondary end point of CI-AKI also showed no effect.

Statins

Statins have been investigated for the prevention of CI-AKI because of their antioxidant and antiinflammatory properties. The Prevention of Radiocontrast-Medium-induced nephropathy using short-term high-dose simvastatin (PROMISS) trial investigated short-term pretreatment with high-dose simvastatin in patients with baseline renal insufficiency undergoing coronary angiography and did not show a benefit of this strategy with regard to deterioration of renal function.[135] However, the Protective Effect of Rosuvastatin and Antiplatelet Therapy On CI-AKI and myocardial damage in patients with Acute Coronary Syndrome (PRATO-ACS) trial showed that high-dose rosuvastatin (40 mg loading and 20 mg/day maintenance) compared to no statin significantly reduced CI-AKI and 30-day rates of cardiovascular and renal events (death, dialysis, MI, stroke, or persistent renal damage) in statin-naïve patients undergoing PCI.[136] The Rosuvastatin Prevent Contrast Induced Acute Kidney Injury in Patients With Diabetes (TRACK-D) study was the largest trial investigating the role of statins in CI-AKI prevention.[137] A total of 2998 statin-naïve patients with diabetes and CKD undergoing coronary or peripheral arterial angiography with or without percutaneous intervention were randomized to either rosuvastatin 10 mg/day for 2 days before and 3 days after the procedure or standard of care. A significant reduction of CI-AKI was reported for the statin group compared to the control (2.3% vs. 3.9%; P = .01). As most patients undergoing coronary angiography have an indication for statins, their use might be considered as a routine strategy to prevent CI-AKI in patients at risk unless a clear contraindication is present.

TRANSCATHETER AORTIC VALVE REPLACEMENT POPULATION

TAVR has become an established treatment approach for severe aortic stenosis (AS) in patients who are at high or prohibited risk for surgery.[138] Since its introduction in 2002, more than 200,000 procedures have been performed worldwide with remarkable improvement of the technique over time.[139,140] However, the high prevalence of comorbidities in this patient population increases the risk for periprocedural and postprocedural complications, including AKI. Although reported adverse event rates after TAVR are high, there is significant variation in the literature, which is partly due to differences in end point definitions. The Valve Academic Research Consortium (VARC) established an independent collaboration between academic research organizations and specialty societies to create standardized end point definitions and recommendations for TAVR clinical research programs. With regard to post-procedural AKI, the first VARC consensus statement recommended using a "modified" RIFLE classification.[3] The 2012 update recommended using the classification proposed by the KDIGO initiative that included urine output measurement.[141] Table 6.5 summarizes the definitions of AKI adopted by the VARC-1 and 2 initiatives. An analysis published by Nuis and colleagues evaluated the risk of AKI post-TAVR in 995 high-risk patients enrolled between November 2005 and January 2012. Using the VARC-1 criteria, CI-AKI stage 1 was documented in 15% of the population, whereas CI-AKI stage 2 or 3 were observed in 2% and 4%, respectively.[142] While a borderline association between contrast load and AKI was found in the univariate analysis, it was not confirmed as an independent predictor of AKI. The authors concluded that, unlike PCI, CM load only has a minor effect on the development of AKI in patients undergoing TAVR. Using the VARC-2 definition in a single-center study including 218 patients undergoing TAVR with a balloon expandable device, the rate of stage 2 or 3 AKI was 8.3%.[143] Of note, the mean CM volume in patients with significant AKI (stages 2 and 3) was not higher compared to those without significant AKI (stage 0 and 1). The rate of AKI stages 1, 2, and 3 post-TAVR were 14.0%, 2%, and 0%, respectively, in another study using the VARC-2 definition.[144] The relatively aggressive periprocedural hydration along with NAC administration, the long interval between angioplasty and TAVR, and the use of IOCM in all patients may have contributed to the low rate of AKI. Consistent with the findings of Nuis et al., contrast volume was not an independent predictor of AKI.

Table 6.6 summarizes risk factors for the development of AKI after TAVR reported in the literature.[144–155] Patient-related risk factors for AKI after TAVR are similar to those observed for CI-AKI after PCI. Contrast load may be less important for post-TAVR AKI than for CI-AKI after PCI, although data on CI-AKI in patients undergoing TAVR are lacking. A lower volume of CM is often used during TAVR procedures compared to PCI.

CHAPTER 6 Contrast-Induced Acute Kidney Injury and the Role of Chronic Kidney Disease in Percutaneous Coronary Intervention

TABLE 6.6 Risk Factors for Acute Kidney Injury After Transcatheter Aortic Valve Replacement

Risk Factors for Acute Kidney Injury After Transcatheter Aortic Valve Replacement
Patient-Related
Chronic kidney disease
Advanced age
Female sex
Diabetes mellitus
High operatory risk (EuroScore)
History of myocardial revascularization
Low ejection fraction
Hypertension
Procedural-Related
Intra-procedural
Contrast volume
Transapical approach
Bleeding transfusion
Post-procedural (follow-up)
Leukocytosis
Thrombocytopenia
Life-treating bleeding
Intraaortic balloon pump

Patients undergoing TAVR often have many additional risk factors for AKI, increasing the difficulty in identifying true CI-AKI post-TAVR. The PROphylactic effecT of furosEmide-induCed diuresis with matched isotonic IV hydraTion in Transcatheter Aortic Valve Implantation (PROTECT-TAVI) trial investigated the effect of the RenalGuard System on AKI prevention in 118 patients undergoing TAVR. The use of the RenalGuard system significantly decreased the risk of AKI ($n = 3$ [5.4%] vs. $n = 14$ [25.0%], respectively, $P = .014$), but the study was small, single-center, and open-label, thus the results are not definitive.[156] In the absence of specific investigation of CI-AKI prevention in TAVR, strategies studied in patients undergoing PCI may be extrapolated to TAVR. Time between CM administration during the TAVR work-up (including potential PCI) and the TAVR procedure should be planned. Intracardiac echocardiography to guide the TAVR procedure may also help to reduce the contrast load.[157] Finally, being aware of AKI risks and diligently avoiding excess contrast (reducing the number of contrast injections and contrast quantity) can vastly reduce contrast exposure during TAVR. Novel strategies, such as the placement of guidewires in two or all three aortic sinuses can provide fluoroscopic guidance without contrast injection during valve deployment, further limiting contrast exposure.

CRITICAL VIEW AND FUTURE DEMANDS

It is commonly acknowledged that CI-AKI is a leading cause of in-hospital AKI.[25] Recent data from computed tomography imaging have challenged this assumption, suggesting that the occurrence of CI-AKI may be lower than previously thought. Studies comparing outcomes of patients undergoing computed tomography with or without contrast have shown similar rates of AKI after propensity adjustment.[158] In addition, CM application was not an independent predictor of AKI, dialysis, or mortality, even in patients with CKD.[159] These findings suggest that a considerable number of patients diagnosed with CI-AKI may have AKI due to nephrotoxic causes other than CM administration. Since a randomized controlled experiment in this setting is not feasible, the studies comparing outcomes in patients undergoing imaging with versus without CM application is the best possible way to identify the risk of AKI attributable to CM. However, the decision to withhold CM is highly confounded and may result in a control group that is at excessively high risk for (CI-)AKI. Methods such as propensity score matching or multivariate adjustment may not fully account for this difference in risk between patients who received CM and those in whom CM was withheld. This confounding by risk might explain the results of an analysis from the Nationwide Inpatients Sample database on almost 6 million hospitalizations that showed an inverse relationship between CM application and AKI.[160] Additional limitations of these studies are inherent to their "big data approach" and include the use of discharge summaries to capture end point events (which may result in ascertainment bias), and the potential missingness of important variables. Finally, most of these data are derived from populations that underwent noninvasive procedures. Contrast volumes used in noninvasive procedures are lower than those used in PCI.

New strategies are needed for the early detection of CI-AKI and for better differentiation of CI-AKI from other forms of AKI. Further research is needed and should include the investigation of novel biomarkers. For prevention, adequately powered randomized controlled trials are necessary and should focus on patients undergoing PCI at high risk for CI-AKI.

KEY REFERENCES

1. Mehran R, Nikolsky E. Contrast-induced nephropathy: definition, epidemiology, and patients at risk. *Kidney Int Suppl.* 2006;69(suppl 100):S11–S15.
3. Mehta RL, Kellum JA, Shah SV, et al. Acute Kidney Injury Network: report of an initiative to improve outcomes in acute kidney injury. *Crit Care.* 2007;11(2):R31.
4. Bellomo R, Ronco C, Kellum JA, et al. Acute Dialysis Quality Initiative w. Acute renal failure—definition, outcome measures, animal models, fluid therapy and information technology needs: the Second International Consensus Conference of the Acute Dialysis Quality Initiative (ADQI) Group. *Crit Care.* 2004;8(4):R204–R212.
5. Kidney Disease Improving Global Outcomes (KDIGO). Clinical practice guideline for acute kidney injury. *Kidney Int Suppl.* 2012;2(1):1–138.
6. Manual on Contrast Media of the American College of Radiology (ACR) Committee on Drugs and Contrast Media.Version 10.2; 2016.
14. Azzalini L, Spagnoli V, Ly HQ. Contrast-induced nephropathy: from pathophysiology to preventive strategies. *Can J Cardiol.* 2016;32(2):247–255.
17. Tsai TT, Patel UD, Chang TI, et al. Contemporary incidence, predictors, and outcomes of acute kidney injury in patients undergoing percutaneous coronary interventions: insights from the NCDR Cath-PCI registry. *JACC Cardiovasc Interv.* 2014;7(1):1–9.
20. Mehran R, Aymong ED, Nikolsky E, et al. A simple risk score for prediction of contrast-induced nephropathy after percutaneous coronary intervention: development and initial validation. *J Am Coll Cardiol.* 2004;44(7):1393–1399.
25. Nash K, Hafeez A, Hou S. Hospital-acquired renal insufficiency. *Am J Kidney Dis.* 2002;39(5):930–936.
36. Gurm HS, Dixon SR, Smith DE, et al. Renal function-based contrast dosing to define safe limits of radiographic contrast media in patients undergoing percutaneous coronary interventions. *J Am Coll Cardiol.* 2011;58(9):907–914.
50. Chawla LS, Bellomo R, Bihorac A, et al. Acute kidney disease and renal recovery: consensus report of the Acute Disease Quality Initiative (ADQI) 16 Workgroup. *Nat Rev Nephrol.* 2017;13(4):241–257.
77. Capodanno D, Angiolillo DJ. Antithrombotic therapy in patients with chronic kidney disease. *Circulation.* 2012;125(21):2649–2661.
121. Briguori C, Visconti G, Focaccio A, et al. Renal Insufficiency After Contrast Media Administration Trial II (REMEDIAL II): RenalGuard System in high-risk patients for contrast-induced acute kidney injury. *Circulation.* 2011;124(11):1260–1269.
122. Brar SS, Aharonian V, Mansukhani P, et al. Haemodynamic-guided fluid administration for the prevention of contrast-induced acute kidney injury: the POSEIDON randomised controlled trial. *Lancet.* 2014;383(9931):1814–1823.

124. Nijssen EC, Rennenberg RJ, Nelemans PJ, et al. Prophylactic hydration to protect renal function from intravascular iodinated contrast material in patients at high risk of contrast-induced nephropathy (AMACING): a prospective, randomised, phase 3, controlled, open-label, non-inferiority trial. *Lancet.* 2017;389(10076):1312–1322.

133. Thayssen P, Lassen JF, Jensen SE, et al. Prevention of contrast-induced nephropathy with N-acetylcysteine or sodium bicarbonate in patients with ST-segment-myocardial infarction: a prospective, randomized, open-labeled trial. *Circ Cardiovasc Interv.* 2014;7(2):216–224.

134. Weisbord SD, Gallagher M, Jneid H, et al. Outcomes after Angiography with Sodium Bicarbonate and Acetylcysteine. *N Engl J Med.* 2017.

159. McDonald RJ, McDonald JS, Carter RE, et al. Intravenous contrast material exposure is not an independent risk factor for dialysis or mortality. *Radiology.* 2014;273(3):714–725.

 Additional references available online at expertconsult.com.

中文导读

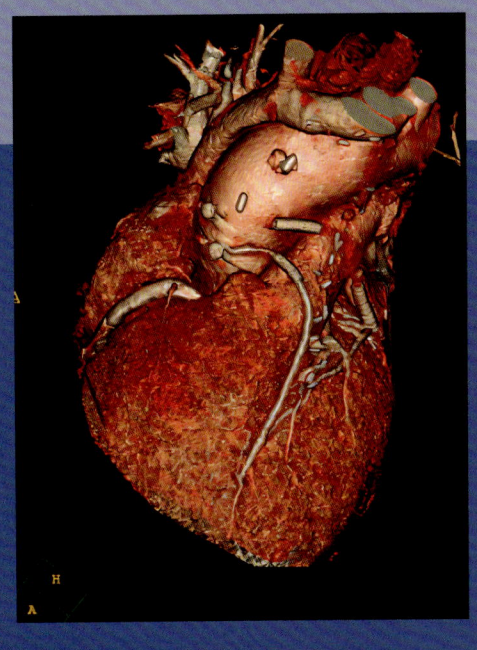

第7章
心血管手术中的辐射安全

　　透视引导下的介入心血管手术通过缓解症状、提高生活质量和取代开放手术的需要，为患者提供了实质性的好处。这些手术包括血管、电生理学和经皮心脏结构干预，手术风险也可能很大，包括脑卒中、心肌梗死、肾衰竭和死亡。在每一种类型的手术中，透视指导所需的电离辐射也有风险，特别是手术时间过长和肥胖的患者。这些辐射风险包括放射性致癌和皮肤损伤，尽管许多其他手术风险明显大于辐射风险。然而，重要的是要将医疗照射的辐射防护基本原则应用于患者。这些原则是正当的，即辐射的使用对患者的利大于弊，该原则应基于医学指导和优化，这意味着患者所接受的辐射剂量应纳入日常医疗管理中，并应避免不必要的辐射。同时，作为参与介入操作的医务人员，也会不可避免地接受辐射照射。辐射暴露水平与多种因素相关，包括荧光透视时间、摄像数目、X线摄入位置和角度等。在介入操作过程中，全面的质量保证体系可以降低患者和医务人员的辐射暴露，包括对设备的质量控制和对患者及医务人员的常规计量监测。如患者接受超过5 Gy的辐射暴露，医师应在病例中记载并告知患者可能发生的辐射皮肤效应，并提供适当的随访。为了避免不必要的辐射暴露，使用X线检查的从业人员应熟悉辐射风险，并应知道如何适当地管理辐射。

李凡奇　范　谦

章节要点

- 介入心脏病医师因需要使用X线透视，故应熟悉辐射风险，也应知晓如何合理地管理辐射。
- 介入术后患者的皮肤损伤事件已有报道。这些辐射所致的皮肤损伤很多是疏忽大意的结果，因为临床医师没有意识到辐射剂量及后果。
- 在选择适当的透视设备配置和剂量管理工具使用方面，介入心脏病医师必须接受相关培训。这种培训除了包括常规辐射剂量管理技术，还应包括关于其使用的透视设备型号和工作人员辐射防护工具的特定技术。
- 减少患者辐射剂量的策略包括使用低剂量率和低帧率的透视、保持影像接收器更靠近患者、使用准直和适度的X线光束角度、缩短透视时间和减少图像采集。
- 应利用透视设备所提供的累积辐射剂量来记录患者所接受的辐射剂量。
- 如果术中的参考点空气比释动能（在材料中释放的动能）超过5 Gy，介入心脏病医师应告知患者可能会发生辐射性皮肤损害效应，并对患者提供适当的随访。
- 在透视手术过程中的现场人员应采取X线防护措施，并在透视过程中远离患者，以减少其职业辐射暴露。

7 Radiation Safety During Cardiovascular Procedures

Beth A. Schueler, Kenneth A. Fetterly, Stephen Balter

KEY POINTS

- Interventional cardiologists who use fluoroscopy should be familiar with radiation risks and should know how to manage radiation appropriately.
- Incidents of patient skin injury following fluoroscopy-guided interventional procedures have been reported. Many reported skin effects resulting from fluoroscopic procedures were inadvertent, because the physician was unaware of the radiation dose and consequences.
- Interventional cardiologists must receive training in selection of appropriate fluoroscopic equipment configuration and utilization of dose-management tools. This training should include both general radiation dose-management practices and specific practices for the model of fluoroscopic equipment and personnel radiation protection tools they will use.
- Strategies for minimizing patient radiation dose include using a low dose rate and a low frame rate for fluoroscopy, keeping the image receptor close to the patient, using collimation and moderate x-ray beam angles, and minimizing fluoroscopy time and image acquisition.
- The cumulative radiation dose display provided by the fluoroscopic equipment should be utilized to keep track of patient dose.
- If reference point air *kerma* (kinetic energy released in material) exceeds 5 Gy for a procedure, the interventional cardiologist should inform the patient that a radiation skin effect may occur and provide appropriate follow-up.
- Personnel present during fluoroscopy procedures should use x-ray shielding and should move back from the patient during fluoroscopy to reduce their radiation exposure.

INTRODUCTION

Fluoroscopy-guided interventional cardiovascular procedures provide substantial benefit to patients by relieving symptoms, improving quality of life, and replacing the need for open surgical procedures. These procedures include vascular, electrophysiology, and percutaneous structural heart interventions. Procedure risks may also be substantial and include stroke, myocardial infarction (MI), renal failure, and death. The ionizing radiation required for fluoroscopic guidance in each of these types of procedures also carries risk, particularly for prolonged procedures and obese patients. These radiation risks include radiogenic cancer and skin injury, although many other procedural risks are significantly greater than the radiation risks. Nevertheless, it is important to apply the basic principles of radiation protection for medical exposure to patients. These principles are *justification*—that is, use of radiation should provide more benefit than harm to the patient, and the procedure should be medically indicated—and *optimization*, meaning the patient dose should be managed to be commensurate with the medical purpose, and unnecessary radiation exposure should be avoided.[1] To follow these principles, practitioners who use fluoroscopy should be familiar with radiation risk and should know how to manage radiation appropriately.

RADIATION RISK

Two types of health effects result from radiation exposure, stochastic and deterministic. *Stochastic effects* include cancer and genetic mutations. These effects are caused by damage to cell DNA. Because an effect may result from misrepair of a single cell, stochastic effects are independent of the amount of radiation exposure and are thought to have no lower threshold limit. *Deterministic effects* are tissue reactions from radiation exposure. The severity of tissue reactions increases with dose, and a minimum dose exists below which no observable effect occurs. Tissue reactions of concern related to fluoroscopy use include skin burns, hair loss, and cataracts.

Radiation-induced cancer risk has been studied extensively in many different exposed populations, including survivors of the atomic bomb detonations over Hiroshima and Nagasaki in World War II, patients receiving medical treatments, and workers exposed to radiation. Although the relationship between cancer induction and radiation exposure has been well established for high doses, cancer risk at low dose levels, such as those encountered in diagnostic imaging or from natural sources, is uncertain. Because the latent period for most cancers is long, and the natural incidence of cancer is high, it is difficult to determine cancer risk levels for whole-body doses less than approximately 100 mSv (which is equivalent to the radiation delivered during several complex percutaneous cardiac interventions [PCIs]). As a result, a model is used to estimate cancer risk at low doses from observed high-dose cancer rates. The commonly accepted linear nonthreshold model predicts a fatal cancer risk of 5% per Sv whole-body exposure for a working-age adult.[2] Typical effective dose values (estimation of whole-body dose from a partial body exposure) are 15 mSv for PCI, 7 mSv for diagnostic coronary angiography, 7 mSv for chest computed tomography (CT), and 0.1 mSv for a chest radiography exam.[3] For comparison, natural background radiation levels in the United States average about 3 mSv/year.[4]

Genetic mutations from radiation exposure have been found in animal studies, but no human study has demonstrated any effect. Although radiation-induced heritable effects were initially thought to be a significant radiation risk, it is now accepted that the genetic risk is minimal.

Skin injury from radiation exposure has been thoroughly characterized for radiation therapy patients. Although fluoroscopy x-ray energies are lower than high-energy radiation therapy x-ray beams, skin effects and threshold dose levels are similar to that of orthovoltage radiation therapy (50 to 250 kilovolt peak [kVp]; Table 7.1). Transient erythema may occur within 24 hours after a radiation dose of 2 Gy or more. Between 2 and 8 weeks from an exposure, epilation may occur with main erythema present for doses greater than 5 Gy, and desquamation may occur for doses greater than 10 Gy.

TABLE 7.1 Tissue Reactions From Single-delivery Radiation Dose to Skin of the Neck, Torso, Pelvis, Buttocks, or Arms

Band	Single-Site Acute Skin-Dose Range (Gy)[a,c,d]	NCI Skin Reaction Grade	Approximate Time of Onset of Effects[a,b]			
			Prompt <2 Weeks	Early 2–8 Weeks	Midterm 6–52 Weeks	Long-term >40 Weeks
A1	0–2	Not applicable	No observable effects expected at any time			
A2	2–5	1	Transient erythema	Epilation	Recovery from hair loss	None expected
B	5–10	1–2	Transient erythema	Erythema, epilation	Recovery; at higher doses, prolonged erythema, permanent partial epilation	Recovery; at higher doses, dermal atrophy or induration
C	10–15	2–3	Transient erythema	Erythema, epilation; possible dry or moist desquamation, recovery from desquamation	Prolonged erythema, permanent epilation	Telangiectasia,[e] dermal atrophy or induration, skin likely to be weak
D	>15	3–4	Transient erythema; after very high doses: edema and acute ulceration, long-term surgical intervention likely to be required	Erythema, epilation; moist desquamation	Dermal atrophy; secondary ulceration due to failure of moist desquamation to heal, surgical intervention likely to be required; at higher doses, dermal necrosis, surgical intervention likely to be required	Telangiectasia,[e] dermal atrophy, induration; possible late skin breakdown; wound can be persistent and may progress into a deeper lesion; surgical intervention likely to be required

[a]The dose range and approximate time period are not rigid boundaries. Also, signs and symptoms can be expected to appear earlier as the skin dose increases.
[b]Abrasion or infection of the irradiated area is likely to exacerbate radiation effects.
[c]Skin dose refers to actual skin dose (including backscatter). This quantity is *not* air kerma at the reference point ($K_{a,r}$).
[d]Skin dosimetry based on $K_{a,r}$ or air kerma area product (P_{KA}) is unlikely to be more accurate than ±50%.
[e]Refers to radiation-induced telangiectasia. Telangiectasia associated with an area of initial moist desquamation or the healing of ulceration may be present earlier.
This table is applicable to the normal range of patient radiosensitivities in the absence of mitigating or aggravating physical or clinical factors; this table does not apply to the skin of the scalp.
NCI, National Cancer Institute.
National Council on Radiation Protection and Measurements (NCRP). *Report 168: Radiation Dose Management for Fluoroscopically Guided Interventional Procedures*. Bethesda, MD: NCRP; 2010.

Longer term, for doses greater than 15 Gy, dermal atrophy and secondary ulceration may occur that may require surgical treatment.[5] Examples of fluoroscopic skin injuries are shown in Figs. 7.1 and 7.2. It should be noted that time intervals and dose thresholds given in Table 7.1 are approximate and will vary depending on the patient's health, location of the exposed area, and condition of the lesion. Other factors may also be associated with increased skin response to irradiation, including diseases such as diabetes mellitus and hyperthyroidism and also ataxia, telangiectasia, connective tissue diseases, and exposure to various chemotherapy agents.[6]

Although rare, skin injury following fluoroscopy-guided interventional procedures has been reported.[5,7] Many of these injuries involve complex cardiology procedures such as PCI for the recanalization of chronic total vascular occlusions and radiofrequency ablations. A rise in the number of reports to the U.S. Food and Drug Administration (FDA) in the early 1990s led to the release of a public health advisory in 1994.[8] Injury may also result from multiple procedures, even if individual sessions are below the threshold for skin effects. When exposure of the same skin location occurs over several episodes, injury threshold doses will depend on the dose level and the time interval between procedures.[5] It should be noted that many reported skin effects resulting from fluoroscopic procedures were inadvertent, and the physician was unaware of the radiation dose delivered.[9] As a result, patients were not made aware of the potential for skin injury, which caused a delay in the diagnosis of their wound.[7] Skin biopsy should not be performed in areas of suspected radiation skin injury because this leads to a delay in healing and/or to secondary infections.[6] Recording of patient dose, communication with the patient, and follow-up for significant dose levels are important radiation management methods that will be discussed later in this chapter.

RADIATION MANAGEMENT

Procedure optimization includes limiting radiation dose to a level that is as low as possible to accomplish the clinical task. This process requires attention to imaging equipment configuration and to radiation dose management practices. Interventional fluoroscopy systems contain many components that work together to form an image. For the most part, adjusting components to increase radiation dose will result in improved image quality. Although at first glance achieving excellent image quality may appear to be the aim of procedure optimization, this objective will generally result in an unnecessary dose. Instead, the appropriate image quality level that is clinically acceptable should be the goal so that an appropriate radiation dose can be used. Some tasks within an interventional procedure can be accomplished using an image with reduced radiation dose and image quality. Whenever possible, equipment configurations with a lower dose rate should be selected. This is best accomplished by adjusting initial settings to a low dose rate before a procedure begins, then selecting higher dose-rate settings as needed in a limited fashion for a specific imaging task, such as placing a guidewire or deploying a stent, where high spatial resolution and low image noise are needed. Further details about fluoroscopic equipment components will be covered in the next section of this chapter.

Staff training is an important component of procedure optimization. Operators of fluoroscopic systems are in charge of the

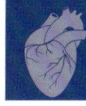

CHAPTER 7 Radiation Safety During Cardiovascular Procedures

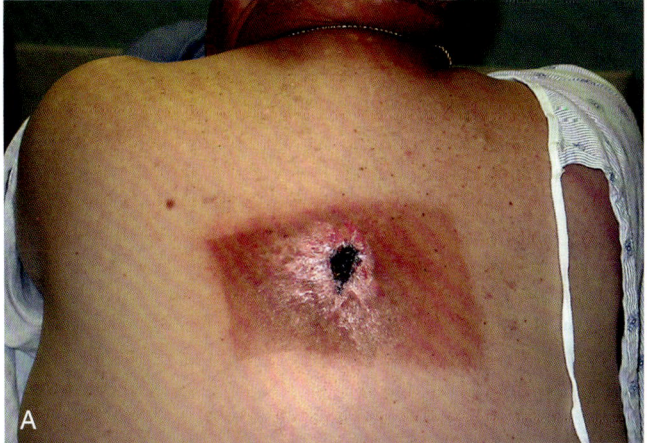

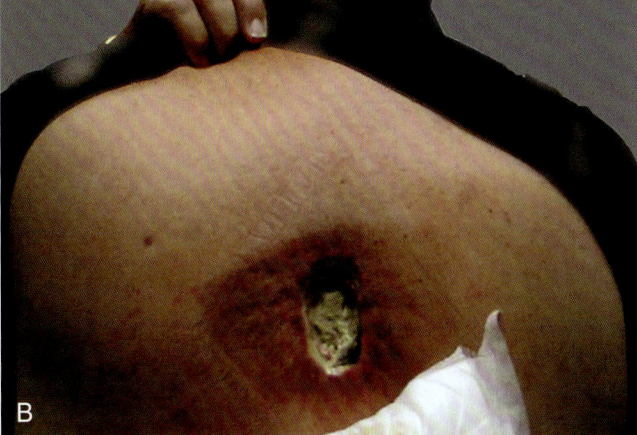

Fig. 7.1 Radiation injury in a 60-year-old man resulting from coronary angioplasty. Images show a time sequence of the injury. (A) At 30 weeks after exposure, a central area of deep necrosis surrounded by indurated and depigmented skin within an area of prolonged erythema is shown. (B) At 38 weeks after exposure, area of deep necrosis has increased in size. (From Balter S, Hopewell JW, Miller DL, et al. Fluoroscopically guided interventional procedures: a review of radiation effects on patients' skin and hair. *Radiology*. 2010;254[2]:326–341, Fig. 8A.)

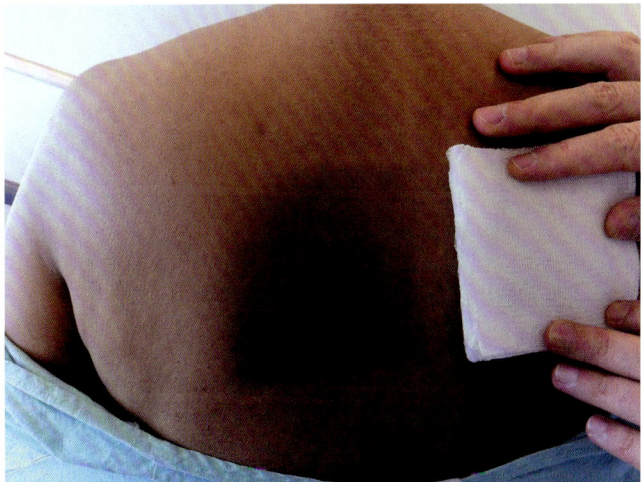

Fig. 7.2 Radiation injury in a 60-year-old woman resulting from a coronary angioplasty. At 18 months after exposure, erythema with dusky coloration is shown.

amount of radiation used during a procedure, which affects the dose to the patient, to themselves, and to other staff in the procedure room. It is important that operators receive training on how to select appropriate equipment configurations and how to utilize dose-management tools. Additional information regarding the components of this training are provided in this chapter.

FLUOROSCOPIC IMAGING EQUIPMENT

Because fluoroscopy-guided interventional procedures have the potential to deliver patient radiation dose levels that can cause skin injury, it is important that the fluoroscopic equipment used be suitable for the task. Several key equipment features are desirable to ensure proper management of patient and staff radiation dose. Some of these features include digital image acquisition, variable-rate pulsed fluoroscopy, added x-ray beam filtration, and patient radiation dose display.[10] Safe and effective patient care in complex interventional procedures is best realized when appropriate equipment is used. Fluoroscopy systems that comply with International Electrotechnical Commission (IEC)[11] standard IEC-60601-2-43 for interventional equipment include these and other elements appropriate for interventional procedures.

Image Chain Components

The basic components of a fluoroscopic imaging chain are an x-ray generator, tube, and beam filter; a collimator; the patient; a grid; and the image receptor, processor, and displays (Fig. 7.3). The operator controls the fluoroscopy system through the exposure foot switch, table-side controls, and configuration selection; the operator monitors the output of the system on the image display and on the radiation use display.

The x-ray generator provides electrical power to the x-ray tube that allows for adjustment of x-ray beam kilovolt peak and tube current (in milliamperes [mA]). The x-ray beam produced is generally pulsed at a rate of 1 to 30 pulses per second with pulse widths between 3 and 20 ms. Another important feature of an x-ray generator is automatic exposure rate control (AERC), which acts to keep the x-ray flux at the image receptor at a constant level as it is panned over body parts of differing thickness and attenuation. This is achieved by automatically adjusting the kilovolt peak, tube current, pulse width, and beam filtration settings through a feedback signal from the image receptor to maintain the x-ray exposure level at the entrance to the image receptor.

Within the x-ray tube, x-rays are produced by accelerating electrons emitted from a filament (cathode) toward a rotating tungsten disk (anode). The housing that surrounds the x-ray tube contains lead shielding that absorbs x-rays not directed out the exit port. The x-ray production process is relatively inefficient, with less than 1% of the energy input into the x-ray tube converted into x-rays; most of the energy is converted into heat, and x-ray tube heat can build up quickly during clinical procedures that require the capture of multiple images. To achieve a large heat capacity, angiography x-ray tubes are equipped with high-speed anode rotation (over 10,000 rotations/min) and a circulating water or oil heat exchanger with cooling fans. The instantaneous heat capacity of the x-ray tube may become a limiting factor for the selection of technique factors when imaging thick body parts and large patients, particularly when using mobile C-arm fluoroscopy systems. Many systems include an indicator of the thermal condition of the anode, which notifies the operator when the heat level is approaching threshold values.

X-ray tubes for fluoroscopy systems typically contain two focal spots: the *small focal spot* (SF) is selected for all fluoroscopy and image acquisition of thin body parts; the *large focal spot* (LF) is required for imaging thicker body parts, for which higher kilovolt peak and tube current are needed. The smaller the focal spot, the less geometric blur occurs for better spatial resolution (Fig. 7.4).

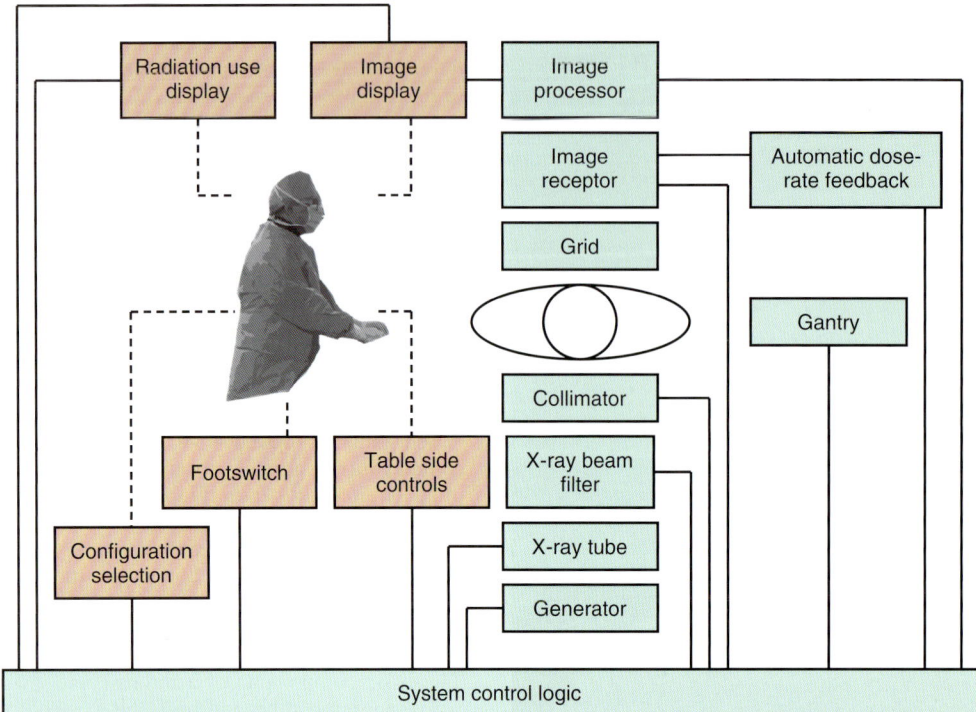

Fig. 7.3 Block diagram of a fluoroscopic imaging system. The imaging chain components (generator, x-ray tube, x-ray beam filter, collimator, image receptor, and gantry) are controlled by the operator through the configuration selection, footswitch, and table-side controls through system control logic via automatic dose-rate feedback. The radiation use display and image display are available for use by the operator.

Fig. 7.4 Focal spot size and geometric magnification effect on spatial resolution. Using a small focal *(SF)* spot and low geometric magnification *(Mag 1.5)* maximizes the visibility of the bars in this high-subject-contrast test pattern. The effects of using a large focal *(LF)* spot are seen in the lower left image, increasing geometric magnification *(Mag 2)* is seen in the upper right image, and the incorporation of both are shown in the lower right image.

However, concentrating the focal spot into a smaller area results in increased heat concentration that could reach temperatures hot enough to melt the anode material. Therefore the larger focal spot size is often needed for cine acquisition imaging.

The x-ray beam travels through a sheet of aluminum several millimeters thick before it exits the collimator assembly. This aluminum filtration material is present to attenuate low-energy x-rays from the beam, which are generally absorbed in the first few centimeters of patient tissue without being transmitted to the image receptor; this contributes to patient skin dose with little impact on image formation. Federal regulations specify a minimum thickness of filtration material be used for all fluoroscopy systems.[12] Additional filtration material, typically copper, is included in angiography and interventional fluoroscopy systems to further reduce patient skin dose. The filtration thickness may be fixed for a given program setting or it may be configured to vary automatically with changes in patient attenuation. Most modern x-ray angiography systems allow for use of additional x-ray beam filters for both fluoroscopic and angiographic imaging, and a minimum thickness equivalent to 0.1 mm Cu is recommended.

The collimator contains radiopaque shutter blades with two levels of control, primary and secondary, that define the shape of the x-ray beam. The *primary collimator control* automatically limits the x-ray beam field of view as operator changes are made in the magnification (zoom) mode selection or source-image receptor distance. The *secondary collimator control* allows the operator to further reduce the size of the x-ray beam to the area of clinical interest. Most fluoroscopy systems used for interventional procedures also contain equalization filters. These filters, also called *contour filters* or *wedge filters*, are partially radiolucent blades used to provide modest beam attenuation, which serves to reduce x-ray intensity in areas with low patient attenuation that may otherwise lead to areas of white glare in the images. Use of secondary collimation and equalization filters are an important tool to improve image quality and also reduce patient dose.

The image receptor used for most modern fluoroscopy systems is a flat-panel digital detector. A grid is mounted in front of the image receptor to reduce the scatter contribution to the image. Most detectors for fluoroscopy are of the indirect conversion type, in which a crystalline cesium iodide scintillator absorbs incident x-rays and produces light photons. The light photons are then detected and converted to a stored charge by a matrix array of photodiodes to create a digital image. Flat-panel fluoroscopy detectors are available in square or rectangular formats with sizes that range from 17 to 40 cm^2 typical pixel spacing is between 0.14 and 0.20 mm. Selection of magnification modes is also possible, although spatial resolution may not change. For large fields of view or high-frame-rate imaging, pixel binning (typically 2 by 2) may be used to reduce data transfer rates. However, pixel binning may reduce spatial resolution. Although spatial resolution is decreased, image noise is also decreased because of the large effective pixel size. Spatial resolution may also be limited by the resolution of the display monitor; if this is the case, a digital zoom can be used to better visualize detail.

Image processing is commonly applied to fluoroscopy and acquired images prior to display and archive. Processing is applied to increase image contrast, improve spatial resolution, and decrease the appearance of image noise. Adjustment of image-processing parameter settings allows for fine-tuning of image appearance to the clinical application and user preference. However, it should be noted that image quality improvements from image processing usually require a compromise in some other image quality characteristic. Most fluoroscopy systems acquire cine images with a pixel matrix size of approximately 1024 by 1024. However, when images are archived, the matrix size is typically decreased to 512 by 512. As a result, images viewed on the acquisition display monitor will generally provide the best spatial resolution.

Imaging Modes

Fluoroscopy systems used for interventional cardiovascular procedures typically have three imaging modes: (1) fluoroscopy, (2) acquisition or cine mode, and (3) digital subtraction angiography (DSA). *Fluoroscopy* is used for real-time visualization of moving structures or interventional devices for relatively long periods of time (seconds to minutes); therefore the dose rates with fluoroscopy are the lowest of all the imaging modes. Generally, the operator can select from several different dose rates and frame rates so that the lowest dose rate acceptable for the clinical task can be used. Federal regulations limit the maximum patient entrance air kerma rate to 88 mGy/min under test conditions.[12] Typical patient entrance air kerma rates for fluoroscopy can be highly variable but are generally 20 to 35 mGy/min[13] with a frame rate of 7.5 to 15 frames per second (fps).

Acquisition or *cine mode* is used to acquire quality images for diagnostic and archival purposes. Consequently, cine dose rates are typically 10 to 20 times higher than those used for fluoroscopy, with no maximum regulatory limit. Similar to fluoroscopy, many systems provide several different dose rates for cine acquisition to allow for dose reduction when possible. Cine acquisition frame rates are also selectable, with 15 fps being the typical rate and patient entrance air kerma rates between 150 and 250 mGy/min.[13] Note that the maximum air kerma rate for large patients can exceed 2000 mGy/min. Many systems permit retrospective storage of the last fluoroscopic sequence. Although the noise level is higher than cine, enough information is retained to keep the sequence for review instead of using a much higher dose cine sequence.

DSA is used for imaging noncardiac, stationary vessels. In DSA, a precontrast mask image is logarithmically subtracted from an image obtained at the same location after contrast media has been injected. The result is an image in which overlying bone and soft tissue are removed, leaving only vasculature. The process of subtracting images increases the appearance of noise, so DSA images require the highest air kerma rates, generally between 300 and 500 mGy/min using frame rates of 1 to 4 fps.

PATIENT RADIATION DOSE MANAGEMENT

Comprehensive patient radiation dose management requires consideration of both x-ray system technical parameters and the operator's procedural skills. As a result, formal training of physician and nonphysician staff should be considered essential. All staff should become familiar with concepts and practices that lead to a safe and effective clinical practice.[14–17] Staff education should include a combination of didactic and practical training. Practical, hands-on training in particular provides a controlled environment to teach and learn general concepts and specific practices that lead to safe radiation practices. All new staff should receive organized, formal, and documented training. All staff should receive incremental training when new x-ray equipment or features are introduced into the practice. Such training should broadly cover applicable x-ray imaging physics and image creation, best practices to ensure patient radiation safety, and best practices to ensure staff radiation safety, and it should be specific to the clinical practice and equipment.

Factors That Contribute to High Skin Dose

The two primary factors that determine skin dose are x-ray system output dose rate (air kerma rate) and duration of exposure. Each of these primary factors has several associated components. Dose rate is determined by a combination of x-ray system configuration, operator selection of operational mode, and patient thickness.[18] Exponential attenuation of the x-ray beam by the patient dictates that the x-ray tube output, and thereby the patient dose rate, increases rapidly as the x-ray beam path length through the patient increases. The instantaneous dose rate for large patients can be 10 or more times greater than that for small patients. Because x-ray intensity decreases as the square of the distance from the source increases, maintaining appropriate radiographic distances can significantly influence patient skin dose. The duration of x-ray exposure directly influences skin dose and varies substantially among patient procedures. X-ray duration varies greatly between procedure types and even among patients undergoing

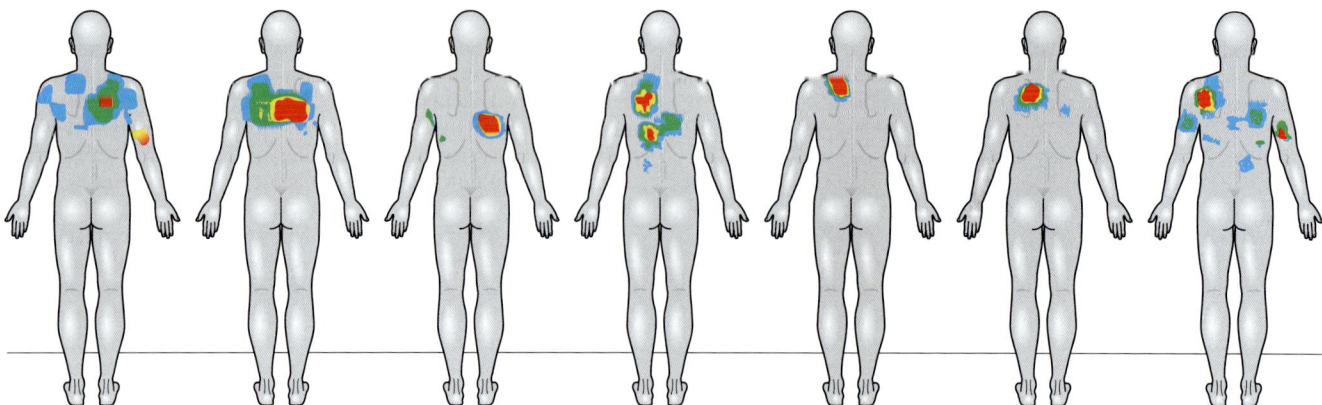

Fig. 7.5 Sample patient skin dose maps for seven different patient exams. The area of highest skin dose is shown in red. Decreasing skin dose is indicated by yellow, green, and light blue. (From Johnson PB, Borrego D, Balter S, et al. Skin dose mapping for fluoroscopically guided interventions, *Med Phys*. 2011;38[10]:5490–5499, Fig. 4.)

similar procedures.[19,20] It is critically important that nontarget anatomy is not in the x-ray beam. In particular, ensure that the patient's arms are never between the x-ray tube and the patient's thorax.

Radiation Dose Measurement

All modern interventional fluoroscopy systems display radiation dose metrics in the procedure room. These metrics include air kerma (K, in mGy) and air kerma area product (P_{KA}, in Gy cm^2, µGy m^2, cGy cm^2, or mGy cm^2). *Air kerma* is a measurement of primary x-ray beam intensity. In the procedure room, the air kerma is reported at a fixed point relative to the gantry that approximates, although not exactly, the location of the patient's skin. When the x-ray beam is on, the instantaneous air kerma rate is reported, and when the x-ray beam is off, the procedure's cumulative air kerma is reported. The *air kerma area product* is the integrated x-ray intensity over the field of view. It can be approximated as the product of the air kerma and the x-ray field area. Because the x-ray beam size is generally constant for cardiovascular procedures, air kerma and air kerma area product provide equivalent indicators of patient radiation burden. However, neither is a good indicator of actual patient skin dose, and neither should be used as such. Converting these metrics to an estimate of skin dose is an area of active academic research and implementation by the manufacturers (Fig. 7.5).[21] The newest interventional x-ray systems may offer advanced features that approximate actual patient skin dose during a procedure, thereby providing the operator some guidance to help avoid radiation skin injury during complex procedures. Traditionally, x-ray fluoroscopy time was used to monitor patient radiation burden. However, fluoroscopy time has important limitations for use as a dose metric. Specifically, it does not account for exposure from acquisition imaging or variation of fluoroscopy dose rate. Therefore fluoroscopy time is a poor indicator of patient radiation burden or skin dose and should not be used as a primary dose metric. Fluoroscopy time can be considered a useful secondary dose metric as a surrogate for procedure complexity or operator proficiency.

Best Practices for Patient Dose Management

Before starting a procedure, the patient record should be reviewed for prior instances of radiation exposure that could contribute to increased risk of radiation skin injury. No standard period of time exists over which the look-back should occur. Cellular injury from radiation commences immediately upon exposure, and repair mechanisms begin shortly thereafter.[22,23] If the radiation dose is sufficiently high, tissue damage can manifest over a period of several hours to several weeks after exposure.[5,24,25] Both cellular and tissue repair occur in the minutes, hours, days, and months following high exposure. When possible, multiple potentially high skin-dose procedures should be scheduled at least several weeks apart to minimize the potential for cumulative skin effects. When clinically necessary, repeat exposures over a period of a few days should be performed judiciously and should assume that the potential for radiation skin injury is cumulative.

Modern interventional x-ray systems include many features designed to result in a relatively low patient skin dose while still providing a clinically adequate image quality. System optimization for dose should be a collaborative effort between the clinical practice and the x-ray equipment manufacturer and should include a combination of a low detector-input dose, use of x-ray beam spectral filters, and a low frame rate.[26,27] Most invasive cardiac procedures can be performed using 7.5 fps fluoroscopy and 15 fps acquisition imaging. Operational modes should be created specifically for the variety of clinical tasks encountered in the invasive cardiology labs. Specific modes should be used for adult cardiac catheterization and ablation procedures, recognizing that the dose from catheterization procedures has approximately equal contributions from fluoroscopy and acquisition imaging and that the dose from ablation procedures is nearly entirely from fluoroscopy. Specific pediatric modes should be created with reduced detector input dose and should specify removal of the antiscatter grid for small patients (<20 kg).[28,29] System configuration and clinical use should recognize that some portions of procedures may require improved image quality. For these instances, it is useful to provide an operational mode that includes a higher radiation dose rate. As a matter of routine, the x-ray system should default to the lowest reasonable radiation dose rate mode, and the operator should be provided the option to temporarily switch to a higher dose-rate mode when improved image quality is required. Strategies for optimizing x-ray system settings to minimize patient radiation dose are summarized in Table 7.2.

For all x-ray imaging, it is important to minimize the time the x-ray beam is on to minimize the dose. Activate fluoroscopy only when necessary, and cease as soon as the live imaging is no longer needed clinically. For most cardiac operational modes, the dose rate associated with acquisition imaging is 10 to 20 times greater than that for fluoroscopic imaging. One method to reduce patient dose is to preferentially use and store fluoroscopic images obtained at a relatively low radiation dose rate, rather than acquisition imaging, when high-quality images are not required. Importantly, never use acquisition imaging to overcome poor fluoroscopic image quality.

If fluoroscopic image quality is clinically inadequate, switch to a fluoroscopy mode with a higher radiation dose rate.

Especially for large patients, use of relatively shallow (posteroanterior) x-ray projection angles can help minimize the x-ray path length through the patient and thereby reduce the dose rate.[31,32] To help minimize skin dose, ensure that the patient's skin is positioned as far as reasonably possible away from the x-ray source and that the image receptor is positioned as close as reasonably possible to the patient (minimize the "air gap" between the patient and the image detector; Fig. 7.6). For patient safety, it is particularly important to ensure that the patient's arms are not in the x-ray beam.

Particularly for complex procedures, including structural heart and ablation procedures, there is often a clinically preferred x-ray beam projection angle that is conducive to visualization of the anatomy. This can lead to high localized skin dose. When clinically possible, the effect can be reduced by using multiple x-ray projection angles such that the dose is distributed over a larger skin area. In this case, the projection angle must be changed enough (~15 degrees) to avoid overlap of the irradiated skin areas.

By default, x-ray systems are typically configured to modify the patient entrance air kerma rate with changes to the size of the primary field of view (magnification mode). Smaller fields of view (higher magnifications) are associated with increased patient skin-dose rates. Systems should be configured to operate using the most clinically useful x-ray beam size. This is typically a 20-cm diagonal field of view (at the image detector) for catheterization procedures and a 25-cm or larger field for structural heart and ablation procedures. Magnification modes should be used sparingly as necessary to support the clinical procedure. The operator should be familiar with and should use secondary collimator control. Secondary collimators reduce the x-ray beam area and thereby reduce patient dose and x-ray scatter to the operator and to the image receptor. Particularly for large patients, x-ray scatter to the image receptor contributes to reduced image contrast; therefore decreasing the size of the x-ray beam area with the secondary collimators can result in a notable improvement in image quality. Furthermore, systems equipped with a large-screen monitor may be configured to use the wide display mode for increased dose optimization. By using a larger field of view with collimation and zooming the image to a wide display, the use of magnification mode can be avoided.[33] Strategies to minimize patient radiation dose during a procedure are summarized in Table 7.3.

Active monitoring of the cumulative air kerma should be incorporated into the clinical practice for all procedures. Intraprocedure announcement of air kerma starting at 3 Gy and then in increments of 1 Gy thereafter is recommended.[10] After the procedure, air kerma and air kerma area product values should be included in the patient record for future reference. Each practice should routinely audit patient radiation dose metrics to recognize trends in patient dose and to facilitate relevant

TABLE 7.2 Strategies for Optimizing X-Ray System Settings to Minimize Patient Radiation Dose

Decrease frame rate	For at least most fluoroscopic imaging, 7.5 fps is adequate; for acquisition (cine) imaging, 15 fps is adequate.
Decrease detector target dose	Work with the x-ray system manufacturer to specify a lower dose target at the image receptor.
Increase use of x-ray spectral filtration	Ensure that both fluoroscopy and acquisition programs use x-ray beam spectral filters. A minimum of 0.1 mm copper should be used for acquisition imaging to reduce skin dose while maintaining image quality.[30]

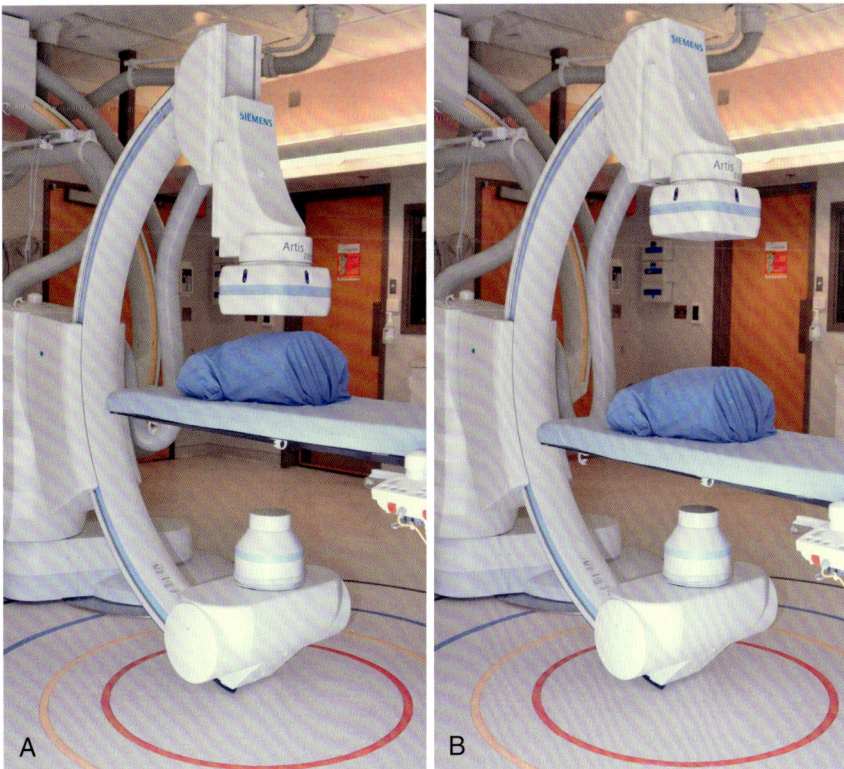

Fig. 7.6 (A) Good imaging geometry with the table elevated and a small air gap (<10 cm). (B) Poor imaging geometry with a short distance between the x-ray tube and patient (table too low) and a great distance between the patient and image receptor (air gap). (Photographs courtesy Mayo Clinic, Rochester, MN.)

quality improvement. Detailed recommendations for a facility's quality assurance–peer review (QA-PR) process and recommendations for administrative practices for the evaluation of known or suspected radiation injuries can be found in the reference section.[34]

Patients for whom the air kerma exceeded 5 Gy should receive post-procedure instruction and appropriate follow-up. Informing such patients that they received a substantial dose of radiation and asking them to have a family member check their back in 1 month are simple and effective first-level assessment steps. The patient should report the appearance of a red patch the size of a hand to the physician who performed the procedure. The physician should then arrange to see the patient to continue evaluation and management. Physicians should also consider prospectively contacting patients who received a substantial dose 1 to 2 months after the procedure. Physicians should regard any such signs as being of radiogenic origin until an alternative diagnosis is established.

Straightforward procedures, including diagnostic procedures, are typically not associated with a high skin dose that could lead to skin injury. However, it is important to practice low-dose radiation techniques during all procedures to master the skills necessary to maintain low skin dose during difficult procedures. It is important that all procedure room staff understand radiographic imaging and radiation safety principles, and physicians should foster a collaborative effort to ensure patient radiation safety.

STAFF RADIATION PROTECTION

Studies that report measurements of staff radiation dose during cardiac catheterization procedures show that high levels are possible.[35] Particular concern has been noted with regard to radiation doses to the lens of the eye,[36] the hands,[37] and lower extremities[38] of the operator. Recent reports have detected acute radiation-induced DNA damage in blood lymphocytes of physicians performing interventional fluoroscopy procedures.[39,40] It is possible for personnel to reduce occupational radiation exposure with careful attention to their actions during the procedure; such actions include knowledge of the sources of radiation exposure and methods that can be used to decrease exposure levels.

Occupational Dose Monitoring

Radiation monitors are worn by personnel who work in fluoroscopy procedure rooms to determine their individual occupational exposure level. In order to provide an estimate of personnel radiation risk when protective aprons are worn, the use of two radiation monitors is recommended.[10] One monitor is worn under the apron at the waist or chest level, and a second monitor is worn outside the apron at the neck. The values from both monitors are used to estimate effective dose, and the neck monitor provides an estimate of the dose to the lens and thyroid if protective glasses and a thyroid shield are not worn. Because the exposure reading under the apron will be much lower than the reading at the neck, it is essential that the monitors be clearly labeled to avoid accidental exchange.

Dose limits to personnel are set by regulatory agencies to prevent tissue reactions and to limit the risk of stochastic effects. Table 7.4 lists the current National Council on Radiation Protection and Measurements (NCRP) dose limits for occupational workers. When attention is paid to radiation safety and optimal work habits practices, a fluoroscopy operator's effective dose is likely to be between 2 and 4 mSv/year.[41]

Fluoroscopy operators should take special note of dose limits for the lens of the eye. Until recently, it has been generally accepted that radiation-induced cataracts do not form below a threshold lens dose of 2 to 5 Gy. This threshold provided the basis for the maximum permissible dose of 150 mSv/year for the lens. However, new data on the radiosensitivity of the eye indicate that the threshold dose may be significantly lower, and the International Commission on Radiological Protection (ICRP) has recommended a lower lens-dose limit of 20 mSv/year averaged over 5 years, with no single year exceeding 50 mSv.[42] Also, the NCRP has recently recommended an annual dose limit of 50 mSv.[43] Although U.S. regulatory agencies have not adopted a lower lens-dose limit, careful attention to radiation protection of the eye is warranted to minimize cataract risk. Protective shielding to reduce radiation exposure to the eye from scatter includes leaded eyewear and ceiling-suspended upper body shields. Additional information on lens-dose reduction is included later in this section.

For pregnant personnel, a lower dose limit is applied to minimize radiation exposure of the embryo/fetus. To monitor

TABLE 7.3 Intraprocedure Strategies to Minimize Patient Radiation Dose

Default to low-dose-rate fluoroscopy.	Configure the x-ray system to use the lowest reasonable fluoroscopy dose rate. Table-side controls provide access to modes with a higher dose rate when a higher-quality fluoroscopic image is required.
Be attentive to x-ray geometry.	Maintaining a long x-ray source–patient distance and a short patient–image receptor distance can substantially reduce patient skin dose.
Activate x-ray imaging judiciously.	Activate x-ray only when clinically indicated, and cease irradiation immediately after clinical utility has passed.
Use moderate x-ray beam angles.	When possible, use less x-ray beam angulation to decrease the path length through the patient, thereby decreasing x-ray attenuation and reducing dose rate.
Use secondary collimators.	The patient will receive less radiation, operator dose from scatter will go down, and the quality of images of large patients will improve.
Never use acquisition imaging to overcome poor fluoroscopic image quality.	Acquisition dose rates can be as much as 20 × greater than for fluoroscopy. When necessary to improve image quality, temporarily switch to a higher dose rate fluoroscopy mode.

TABLE 7.4 Occupational Dose Limits

Dose Quantity	Dose Limit
EFFECTIVE DOSE	
Annual[a]	50 mSv
Cumulative[a]	10 mSv × age in years
EQUIVALENT DOSE (ANNUAL)	
Lens of the eye[b]	50 mSv
Skin, hands, and feet[a]	500 mSv
Embryo and fetus, equivalent dose (monthly) once pregnancy is known[a]	0.5 mSv

[a]National Council on Radiation Protection and Measurements (NCRP). *Report 116: Limitation of Exposure to Ionizing Radiation*. Bethesda, MD: NCRP; 1993.
[b]National Council on Radiation Protection and Measurements (NCRP). *Commentary No. 26: Guidance on Radiation Dose Limits for the Lens of the Eye*. Bethesda, MD: NCRP; 2016.

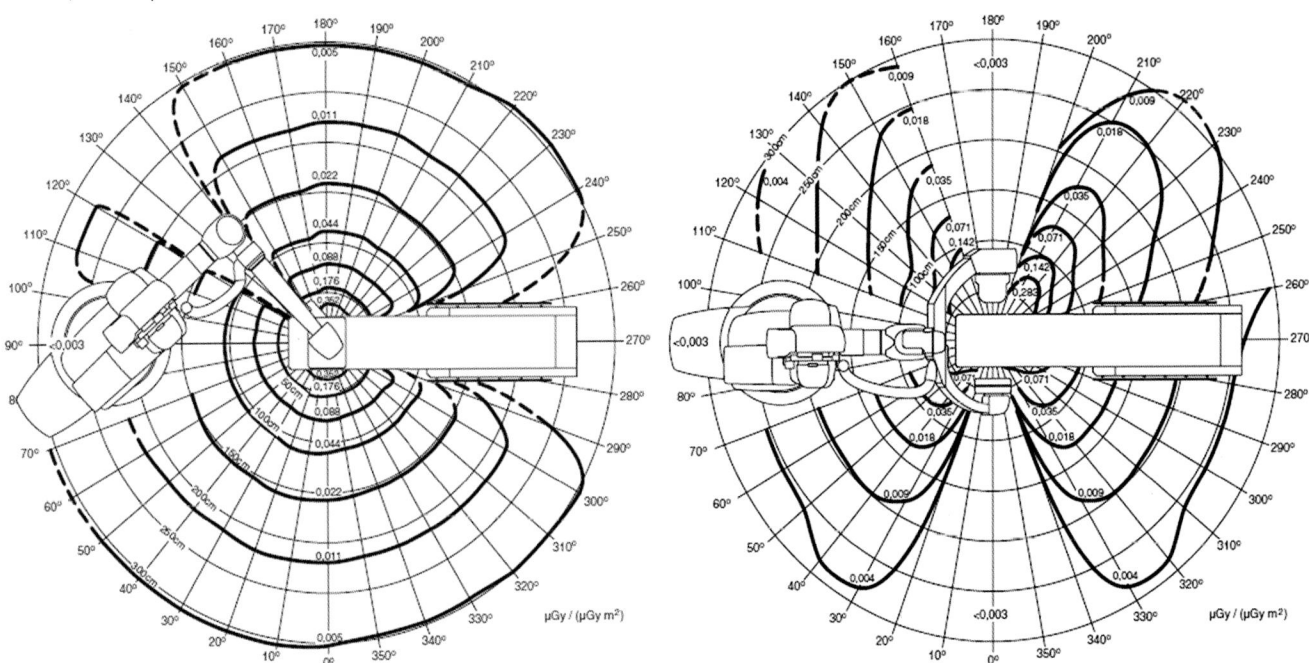

Fig. 7.7 Scatter isodose curves for a fluoroscopic system. Scatter levels at a height of 1 m is shown for a vertical *(left)* and lateral *(right)* orientation. Isodose lines are in units of μGy per μGy m² of patient air kerma area product as reported by the x-ray system. (Courtesy Siemens Medical Systems.)

the conceptus dose, a radiation monitor is provided when a worker has declared her pregnancy. This monitor is worn at the waist level under a protective apron and is exchanged on a monthly basis. Because current data do not suggest a significant increased risk to the fetus of pregnant personnel in the cardiac catheterization laboratory, it is not necessary—nor is it legal—to restrict pregnant workers from working in fluoroscopy procedure areas.[44] However, additional radiation safety precautions and monitoring of radiation exposure among pregnant personnel are warranted.

Sources of Personnel Radiation Exposure

Radiation exposure during fluoroscopy procedures comes from three sources: (1) the primary x-ray beam, (2) scattered x-rays, and (3) x-ray tube leakage x-rays. Occupational exposure to the *primary beam* may occur when the operator manipulates devices positioned within the imaging field of view. Dose rates in this region are in the range of 5 to 20 mGy/h at the surface, where the x-ray beam *exits* the patient during fluoroscopy. Dose rates to the operator's hands when they are placed in the unattenuated x-ray beam (patient-entrance side) can exceed 100 mGy/min for fluoroscopy and 2000 mGy/min for cine mode. *Scattered x-rays* are produced when tissue is exposed to the primary x-ray beam, and the rays travel in all directions from the point of origin. Scatter dose rates are typically 1 to 10 mGy/h at the operator's position. The third source of radiation is from *leakage x-rays* emitted from the x-ray tube in areas other than the primary beam port.

In general, scatter levels decrease in proportion to the inverse squared distance from the irradiated patient tissue volume. However, it should be noted that the radiation distribution surrounding the patient is not uniform. Fig. 7.7 shows a typical scatter isodose plot for a C-arm. For a lateral x-ray beam, note that radiation intensity is concentrated in the area near the x-ray tube. This distribution is caused by higher levels of scattered x-rays produced at the primary beam patient-input port. Forward scattered rays from the first few centimeters of tissue depth are heavily attenuated by the rest of the patient tissue, which results in higher radiation levels in the direction back toward the x-ray tube.

Personal Protective Equipment

X-ray scatter from the patient is the primary source of radiation dose to in-room personnel, and it should be minimized to reduce the likelihood of long-term health effects. Occupational radiation dose can be minimized through a combination of radiation safety devices and practices. These may be summarized by the concepts of reducing patient *dose rate*, reducing *time* duration of exposure, increasing *distance* from the scatter source (the patient), and use of *shielding* to block x-ray scatter. In addition, it is important to recognize that the occupational radiation dose *rate* that originates from the patient is directly proportional to dose rate to the patient. A primary step to reducing occupational dose is to reduce patient dose. For most interventional cardiac lab personnel, the amount of time spent in the procedure room is determined by the number and type of procedures performed and is not readily controlled on an individual basis. The inverse square law dictates that the intensity of radiation decreases in proportion to the square of the distance from the source. When the x-ray beam is on, personnel should position themselves as far as reasonably possible from the patient. It is recognized, however, that patient care necessitates that some personnel remain close to the patient during exposure. Therefore the most important concept for personnel radiation dose reduction is shielding.

Shielding refers to placement of any device between the patient and personnel with the purpose of absorbing x-ray scatter. All in-room personnel are required to wear a protective garment over the trunk of the body. A typical 0.5 mm lead-equivalent garment blocks about 98% of the x-ray scatter

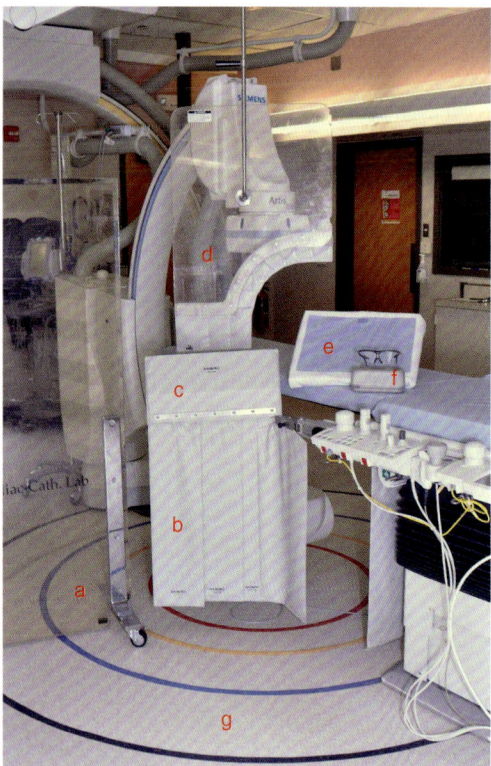

Fig. 7.8 Personnel radiation safety devices: *a*, portable leaded-glass shield; *b*, lower body shield; *c*, vertical extension to lower body shield; *d*, upper body shield with patient contour extensions; *e*, sterile, disposable radiation-absorbing drape; and *f*, leaded-glass safety glasses. The lines on the floor *g* indicate distance from the patient corresponding to 2× changes in scatter dose rate, providing a visual reminder of the protective effects of increased distance from the scatter source. Mandatory lead-equivalent garments and thyroid shield are not shown. (Photograph courtesy Mayo Clinic, Rochester, MN.)

TABLE 7.5 Strategies to Reduce Occupational Radiation Dose

Reduce patient dose.	Occupational radiation dose is proportional to patient dose. Efforts to reduce patient dose will positively affect occupational dose.
Use x-ray shields judiciously.	*Operators:* When properly used, the ceiling-mounted upper body shield can substantially reduce operator dose. *Nursing staff:* Remain behind a lead barrier when possible.
Wear your radiation monitoring badge.	Consistent use of the radiation monitoring badge is the best way to know how well your occupational dose-reduction efforts are working.
Maintain situational awareness.	*Operators:* Do not activate the x-ray unnecessarily when a nurse or technologist is tending to the patient. *In-room staff:* When possible, step back from the patient when the x-ray beam is on.
Wear leaded glasses.	Operators should wear leaded glasses with large side shields to reduce the dose to the lens of the eye and thereby reduce the lifetime risk of developing cataracts.

incident upon it. For a 0.35 mm lead-equivalent garment, attenuation is approximately 94%. Radiation shields or drapes attached to the patient table provide excellent protection of the lower body (Fig. 7.8). Shields are needed on both sides of the table when operators simultaneously work from both sides. Use of optional vertical extension of these drapes provides additional protection to the operator's midsection for femoral-access procedures, but they interfere with the patient for radial-access procedures. Ceiling-mounted, leaded-glass upper body shields can provide up to 80% protection of the upper body, including the otherwise unprotected neck and head.[20,45] For femoral artery–access procedures, the upper body shield should be positioned nominally perpendicular to the patient head-foot direction, tight to the patient abdomen, and just superior to the access point to minimize the angular size of the gap in protection under the shield occupied by the patient. For radial-access procedures, the upper body shield is best positioned nominally parallel to the patient's head-foot direction and close to the patient's arm. For upper body shields, flexible extensions attached to the bottom of the leaded-glass shield provide a soft and contoured contact between the shield and patient. A good guideline for use of the upper body shield is that the operator should have to look through the shield to see the volume of the patient being irradiated. Floor-mounted mobile shields should be available for protection of in-room personnel, particularly nursing staff. Physician operators should wear leaded glasses to reduce the dose to the lens of the eye and thereby minimize lifetime risk of radiation-induced cataracts.[40,46] Glasses with a large surface area, including side shields, are most effective.[47]

Disposable radiation-absorbing towels or drapes can provide up to 60% upper body protection in situations where the upper body shield cannot be readily used, including in the hybrid operating room.[20,48] These must be thoughtfully positioned to maximize protection. Other novel radiation protection devices are commercially available and may also be considered.[49,50] Generally, these novel systems are floor mounted or suspended and are designed to provide whole-body protection, thereby removing the weight burden of a protective garment.[51-53] Other novel technologies, such as robot-guided interventional systems, provide an opportunity for both operator radiation protection and ergonomic comfort.[54,55] Strategies to reduce occupational radiation dose are summarized in Table 7.5.

KEY REFERENCES

1. International Commission on Radiological Protection (ICRP). *The 2007 Recommendations of the International Commission on Radiological Protection.* ICRP Publication 103. Ann. ICRP. 2007;37(2–4).
5. Balter S, Hopewell JW, Miller DL, et al. Fluoroscopically guided interventional procedures: a review of radiation effects on patients' skin and hair. *Radiology.* 2010;254(2):326–341.
8. Food and Drug Administration (FDA). *Important Information for Physicians and Other Health Care Professionals. Avoidance of Serious X-Ray–Induced Skin Injuries to Patients During Fluoroscopically-Guided Procedures.* FDA; 1994. http://www.fda.gov/downloads/Radiation-EmittingProducts/RadiationEmittingProductsandProcedures/MedicalImaging/MedicalX-Rays/ucm116677.pdf. Accessed January 2, 2018.
10. National Council on Radiation Protection and Measurements (NCRP). *Report 168: Radiation Dose Management for Fluoroscopically-guided Interventional Procedures.* Bethesda, MD: NCRP; 2010.
14. Hirshfeld JW, Balter S, Brinker JA, et al. ACCF/AHA/HRS/SCAI clinical competence statement on physician knowledge to optimize patient safety and image quality in fluoroscopically guided invasive cardiovascular procedures. A report of the American College of Cardiology Foundation/American Heart Association/American College of Physicians Task Force on Clinical Competence and Training. *J Am Coll Cardiol.* 2004;44(11):2259–2282.
16. Chambers CE, Fetterly KA, Holzer R, et al. Radiation safety program for the cardiac catheterization laboratory. *Catheter Cardiovasc Interv.* 2011;77(4):546–556s.

34. National Council on Radiation Protection and Measurements (NCRP). *Statement 11 Outline of Administrative Policies for Quality Assurance and Peer Review of Tissue Reactions Associated with Fluoroscopically-guided Interventions*. Bethesda, MD: NCRP; 2014.
41. Miller DL, Vano E, Bartal G, et al. Occupational radiation protection in interventional radiology: a joint guideline of the Cardiovascular and Interventional Radiology Society of Europe and the Society of Interventional Radiology. *Cardiovasc Intervent Radiol.* 2010;33(2):230–239.
42. International Commission on Radiation Protection (ICRP). Statement on tissue reactions/early and late effects of radiation in normal tissues and organs—threshold doses for tissue reactions in a radiation protection context. ICRP Publication 118. Ann ICRP 2012;41(1–2).

Additional references available online at expertconsult.com.

中文导读

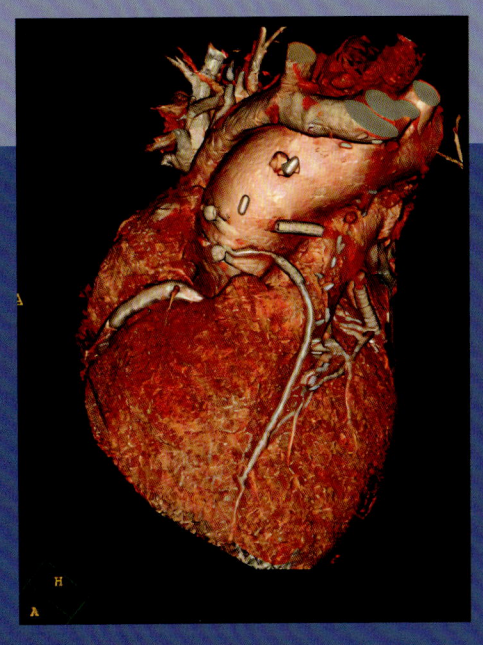

第8章
非心脏外科手术前的冠状动脉/瓣膜介入治疗

冠状动脉心脏病和瓣膜性心脏病患者，在进行非心脏外科手术时，往往需要面临极高的心脏不良事件风险，但是目前临床能够评估和预测手术风险和心脏不良事件风险的工具仍不够完善。本章节探讨了非心脏外科手术围手术期经皮冠状动脉介入治疗的指征、时机、手术方式和抗血小板治疗策略。

术前冠状动脉造影往往仅适用于具有高风险特征的冠心病患者，而对于需要行紧急非心脏外科手术的患者，不应该为了评估冠状动脉疾病而延迟外科手术治疗。在稳定型心绞痛患者中，CARP研究和DECREASE-V研究表明术前经皮冠状动脉介入治疗与保守治疗相比，并不能使患者明显获益。对于不稳定型心绞痛患者，术前经皮冠状动脉介入治疗适用于与非心脏外科手术无关的具有冠状动脉再通指征的情况，尤其是复发型心绞痛及近期急性心肌梗死等。在这些情况下建议多学科会诊共同做出权衡风险的医疗决策。术前经皮冠状动脉介入治疗干预技术的选择主要取决于非心脏外科手术的紧急性，经皮球囊扩张血管成形术、金属裸支架或药物洗脱支架置入术均在不同情境下可供选择。

经皮冠状动脉介入治疗术后行非心脏外科手术时机的选择，应权衡出血与血栓风险，采用个体化策略。若患者接受了球囊扩张血管成形术，那么非心脏外科手术应该延后2周。若是裸金属支架置入术，非心脏外科手术应推迟到1个月之后。药物洗脱支架置入术后，非心脏外科手术最好推迟3~6个月后再进行手术。

非心脏外科手术围手术期的抗血小板治疗同样是一个棘手的难题。需要认真评估出血并发症和支架血栓形成的风险，多学科参与、权衡利弊，制定个体化策略。一般来说，当正在进行双联抗血小板治疗的经皮冠状动脉介入治疗患者需要中断$P2Y_{12}$抑制剂以进行非心脏外科手术时，应尽可能继续使用阿司匹林，并在安全的情况下尽快重启$P2Y_{12}$抑制剂治疗。

最后，对于需要非心脏外科手术的严重症状性主动脉瓣狭窄患者，在非心脏外科手术前应尽快处理主动脉瓣膜病变。

李秋雨 范 谦

章节要点

- 围手术期心肌梗死通常发生在非心脏外科手术后的48~72小时，其即使无任何临床症状，也与患者真实早期和晚期死亡率相关。

- 对于未曾服用过β受体阻滞剂和（或）阿司匹林的患者，在非心脏外科手术前启动这些药物治疗会增加围术期不良事件的发生。因此，对这类患者不推荐在术前常规给予β受体阻滞剂和（或）阿司匹林。

- 在非心脏外科手术前，仅限于对具有不良心脏事件极高风险的患者选择性地进行冠状动脉造影。常规在非心脏外科手术前进行经皮冠状动脉介入治疗，其目的是让患者安全度过非心脏外科手术，但这种做法并未得到研究证实，甚至还可能是有害的策略。

- 支架置入后4~6周进行的非心脏外科手术，将明显增加支架血栓形成和主要不良心脏事件风险。如果可行，非心脏外科手术应适当延期。对于经皮球囊血管成形术的患者，非心脏外科手术可在术后2周进行；裸金属支架置入之后，非心脏外科手术可在介入术后1个月进行；而接受药物洗脱支架置入的患者，非心脏外科手术最好延迟到支架置入3~6个月后进行。

- 对于近期接受支架置入、随后需要非计划非心脏外科手术的患者，须决定是否继续或中止抗血小板治疗，这就需要权衡出血并发症与支架血栓风险，进行个体化评估。临床决策应该由心脏病医师、外科医师和其他相关专科医师进行多学科讨论后制定。

- 当正在进行双联抗血小板治疗的经皮冠状动脉介入治疗患者需要中断$P2Y_{12}$抑制剂以进行非心脏外科手术时，应尽可能继续使用阿司匹林，并在术后安全可行的情况下尽快重启$P2Y_{12}$抑制剂治疗。

- 及时识别和治疗非心脏外科手术后心脏并发症是改善患者预后的关键环节。

- 对于需要非心脏外科手术的严重症状性主动脉瓣狭窄患者，在择期非心脏外科手术前应强烈推荐先进行外科主动脉瓣置换术或经导管主动脉瓣置换术；如果是紧急非心脏外科手术，则应考虑在术前先行主动脉瓣球囊成形术。

8 Coronary and Valvular Intervention Prior to Noncardiac Surgery

Craig R. Narins

KEY POINTS

- Perioperative myocardial infarction typically occurs in the first 48 to 72 hours following noncardiac surgery (NCS) and, even if clinically silent, is associated with substantial early and late mortality.
- The initiation of β-blocker and/or aspirin therapy prior to NCS for patients not already taking these medications is associated with an increase in adverse perioperative events and is not recommended.
- The indications for performing coronary angiography prior to NCS are limited to a very select subset of patients at the highest risk for adverse cardiac events, and the routine use of percutaneous coronary intervention (PCI) to "get a patient through" NCS is unproven and potentially harmful.
- NCS performed within 4 to 6 weeks of stent implantation is associated with a substantial risk of stent thrombosis and major adverse cardiac events (MACEs). Surgery should be delayed if possible for 2 weeks after balloon angioplasty, 1 month after bare metal stenting, and ideally for 3 to 6 months following drug-eluting stent placement.
- When a patient with recent stent placement subsequently requires unanticipated NCS, the decision whether to continue or suspend antiplatelet therapy for surgery demands individualized assessment of the competing risks of bleeding complications and stent thrombosis. This decision should be made with multidisciplinary input from the cardiologist, surgeon, and other involved subspecialists.
- When patients with prior PCI on dual antiplatelet therapy require interruption of $P2Y_{12}$ inhibitor therapy for NCS, aspirin should be continued whenever possible and $P2Y_{12}$ inhibitor therapy should be restarted as soon as safely feasible postoperatively.
- Prompt recognition and treatment of postoperative cardiac complications following NCS is a critical element in optimizing patient outcomes.
- For patients with severe symptomatic aortic valve stenosis who require NCS, definitive therapy with surgical aortic valve replacement or transcatheter aortic valve replacement should be strongly considered prior to elective surgery, and preoperative balloon aortic valvuloplasty is a consideration if NCS is urgent.

INTRODUCTION

Noncardiac surgery (NCS) is associated with a considerable risk of adverse cardiac events among individuals with coronary artery or aortic valve disease. It has been noted that if perioperative mortality were categorized as a unique entity, it would constitute the third leading cause of death in the United States, with approximately one-third of such fatal complications related to cardiac events.[1] Using clinical prediction tools and sensitive biomarker assays including B-type natriuretic peptide (BNP), physicians have become more adept at stratifying surgical risk, yet measures to modify risk remain inadequate. Although the performance of percutaneous coronary intervention (PCI) prior to NCS to limit adverse perioperative events is generally neither advantageous nor clinically appropriate, selected patients at particularly increased risk may benefit from preoperative coronary revascularization. In addition, up to 10% of individuals who undergo coronary stenting require unanticipated NCS within the subsequent year. For these patients, decisions regarding the management of antiplatelet therapy can be complex and require careful consideration of the competing risks of perioperative stent thrombosis and bleeding. This chapter will provide a clinically oriented review of perioperative PCI including current indications for considering PCI prior to NCS, best approaches to performing angioplasty and stenting in the preoperative setting, strategies for managing antiplatelet therapy among patients with recent stent placement who require unanticipated NCS, and considerations for undertaking PCI in the early postoperative period when cardiac complications arise with NCS. In addition, principles regarding the use of transcatheter therapies for treatment of severe aortic valve disease prior to NCS will be reviewed.

PERIOPERATIVE MYOCARDIAL INFARCTION

As with myocardial infarction (MI) outside the context of surgery, perioperative myocardial infarction (PMI) can result either from atherosclerotic plaque rupture with thrombotic occlusion of the involved coronary artery (type 1 MI) or from a transient stress-induced mismatch of myocardial oxygen supply and demand, possibly in the setting of a fixed coronary artery stenosis or occlusion (type 2 MI).[2–4] Thrombosis of a previously implanted coronary stent represents another potential mechanism for PMI and is associated with particularly high mortality rates.[5–7] In the vast majority of instances, PMI does not occur during the surgical procedure but rather within the first 48 to 72 hours following surgery. This period is associated with multiple hemodynamic stresses and hematologic alterations that can predispose to plaque rupture, myocardial oxygen supply-demand mismatch, and a hypercoagulable state (Fig. 8.1).[8,9] The risk of MI can remain elevated for several weeks following major surgery.[10] The reported incidence of PMI varies considerably depending on the definition of MI and the risk profile of the population under study. The majority of infarcts in the postoperative period are clinically silent and remain unrecognized unless routine troponin testing is performed.[11] In the large Vascular Events in Noncardiac Surgery Patients Cohort Evaluation (VISION) study of 21,482 patients undergoing NCS, standardized high-sensitivity troponin T (hsTnT) testing detected the occurrence of PMI among 17.9% of participants, of whom 93.1% did not experience ischemic

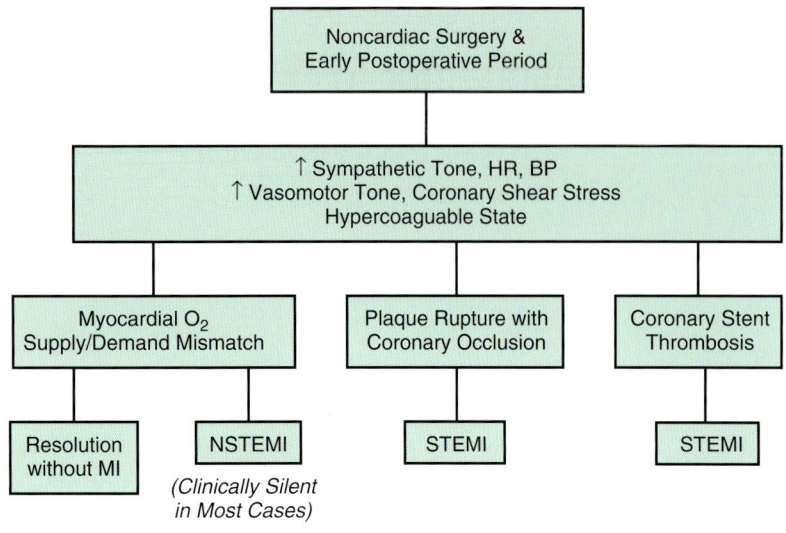

Fig. 8.1 Pathophysiologic events contributing to the genesis of perioperative myocardial infarction *(MI)*. *BP*, Blood pressure; *HR*, heart rate; *NSTEMI*, non–ST segment elevation myocardial infarction; *STEMI*, ST segment elevation myocardial infarction.

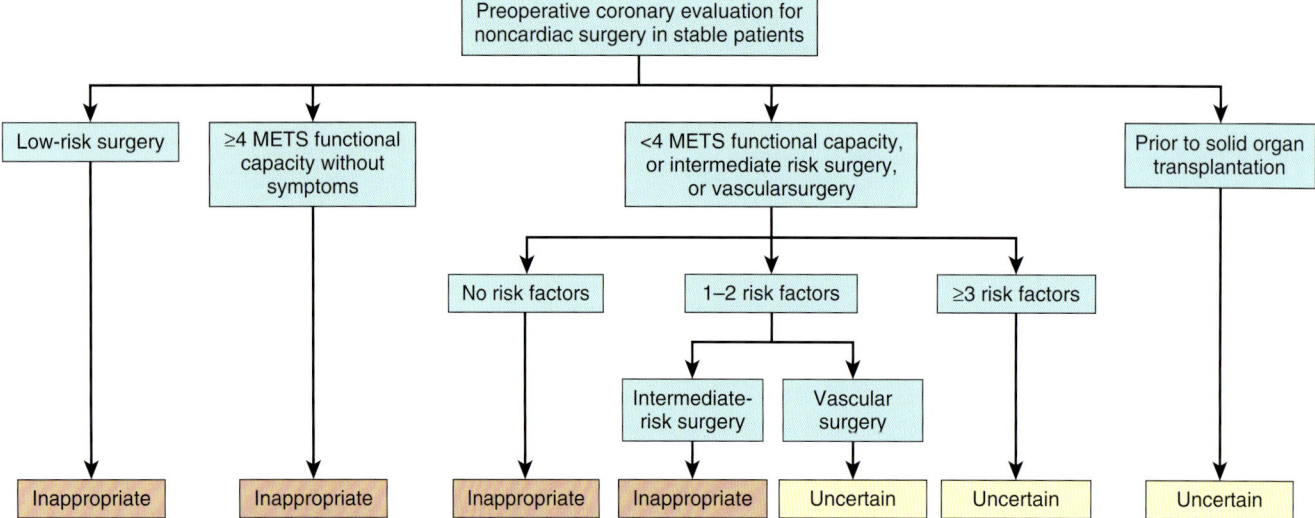

Fig. 8.2 Appropriate use criteria for preoperative coronary angiography for patients without prior noninvasive stress testing. *METS*, Metabolic equivalents. (From Patel MR, Bailey SR, Bonow RO, et al. ACCF/SCAI/AATS/AHA/ASE/ASNC/HFSA/HRS/SCCM/SCCT/SCMR/STS 2012 appropriate use criteria for diagnostic catheterization: a report of the American College of Cardiology Foundation Appropriate Use Criteria Task Force, Society for Cardiovascular Angiography and Interventions, American Association for Thoracic Surgery, American Heart Association, American Society of Echocardiography, American Society of Nuclear Cardiology, Heart Failure Society of America, Heart Rhythm Society, Society of Critical Care Medicine, Society of Cardiovascular Computed Tomography, Society for Cardiovascular Magnetic Resonance, and Society of Thoracic Surgeons. *J Am Coll Cardiol*. 2012;59[22]:1995–2027.)

symptoms.[12] In another large study, routine troponin testing after NCS was associated with a threefold greater detection rate of PMI compared with testing prompted by clinical suspicion alone.[13]

Thirty-day mortality rates following PMI are quite high, in the range of 10%, and even small or clinically silent infarcts are associated with considerably elevated intermediate- and late-term mortality independent of other clinical factors.[14] In a prospective study of 2018 consecutive patients undergoing NCS who were considered at increased cardiovascular risk, PMI detected by interval rise in hsTnT occurred after 16% of surgeries and was associated with a 30-day crude mortality rate of 8.9%, representing a sixfold increase compared with patients without PMI.[15] In a study of more than 15,000 patients undergoing NCS, small elevations in troponin T (0.02 ng/mL) were associated with a fourfold increase in 30-day mortality, and higher levels (≥0.30 ng/mL) were linked to a 16-fold escalation in 30-day death.[16] The same dose-dependent relationship holds true for the hsTnT assay, with a 30-day mortality rate approaching 30% among individuals whose postoperative levels exceeded 1000 ng/L in the VISION cohort.[12]

INDICATIONS FOR PREOPERATIVE CORONARY ANGIOGRAPHY

Despite the frequency and adverse implications of PMI, evidence that prophylactic coronary angiography and/or revascularization can mitigate the risk of perioperative cardiac events is lacking. The American College of Cardiology (ACC)/American Heart Association (AHA) consensus guidelines assert that preoperative coronary revascularization is "appropriate for only a small subset of patients at very high risk" and should be used sparingly if at all. It should be emphasized that, for patients who require emergency NCS, evaluation for coronary disease should not delay the necessary surgical procedure. For clinically stable patients, the current appropriate use criteria (AUC) for diagnostic catheterization offer limited indications for performing coronary angiography prior to NCS (Fig. 8.2).[17] Based primarily on expert opinion, specific instances when preoperative coronary angiography should be considered include[18,19]:

1. Noninvasive test results suggesting a high risk of adverse outcomes, such as extensive (multivessel distribution) MI, prior to high-risk surgery.
2. Canadian Cardiovascular Society (CCS) class III or IV angina not responsive to appropriate medical therapy.
3. Recent acute coronary syndrome or MI.
4. Moderate or severe aortic valve stenosis and anginal symptoms or heart failure.

PHARMACOLOGIC THERAPY FOR NONCARDIAC SURGERY

Although multiple medications, including β-blockers, aspirin, and statins, have been evaluated as means to reduce the frequency of adverse cardiovascular events with NCS, contemporary randomized controlled trial data do not support the routine preoperative initiation of any of these therapies. The large randomized Patients Undergoing Noncardiac Surgery (POISE) trial showed that extended-release metoprolol started 2 to 4 hours before NCS was associated with a reduction of cardiovascular death, MI, or cardiac arrest at 30 days; however, this advantage was offset by significantly increased frequencies of both all-cause mortality and stroke related to undesired bradycardia and hypotension among patients treated with β-blockers.[20] Current ACC/AHA guidelines recommend that "beta-blockers should be continued in patients undergoing surgery who are [already] receiving beta-blockers" for appropriate indications, but the routine initiation of high-dose β-blockers prior to surgery in the absence of dose titration is contraindicated (class III) for patients undergoing NCS who are not already taking β-blockers.[18] In the POISE-2 trial, aspirin therapy started immediately prior to NCS was associated with a significant increase in major bleeding events but not with a reduction in PMI or other cardiovascular events.[21] Consequently, current guidelines strongly recommend against the initiation or continuation of aspirin therapy to prevent perioperative events, except for patients with a recent coronary stent or those undergoing carotid endarterectomy.[22] Likewise, despite observational data supporting statin use for reducing perioperative complications,[23] the initiation of high-intensity statin therapy among statin-naïve patients undergoing NCS was not associated with a reduction in adverse cardiovascular events or all-cause mortality in the randomized Lowering the Risk of Operative Complications Using Atorvastatin Loading Dose (LOAD) trial.[24]

PREOPERATIVE PERCUTANEOUS CORONARY INTERVENTION

Stable Coronary Artery Disease

Two randomized trials have examined the role of coronary revascularization as a means to reduce the likelihood of perioperative events among individuals with stable coronary artery disease (CAD) scheduled to undergo vascular surgery.[25,26] Despite limitations including their modest size (<200 subjects in the two studies combined underwent PCI), use of older-generation stents, and documentation of investigator misconduct in one of the two studies,[27] these trials serve as the foundation for current recommendations that are critical of routine preoperative coronary revascularization.

The Coronary Artery Revascularization Prophylaxis (CARP) trial compared the strategy of preoperative coronary revascularization with that of stand-alone medical therapy for the reduction of early and late cardiac events following major vascular surgery.[25] The trial enrolled 510 patients scheduled for vascular surgery at one of 18 Veterans Affairs (VA) Medical Centers. Patients were eligible if angiography-proven CAD with a 70% or more stenosis in at least one major epicardial coronary artery was present, and they were randomized to either coronary

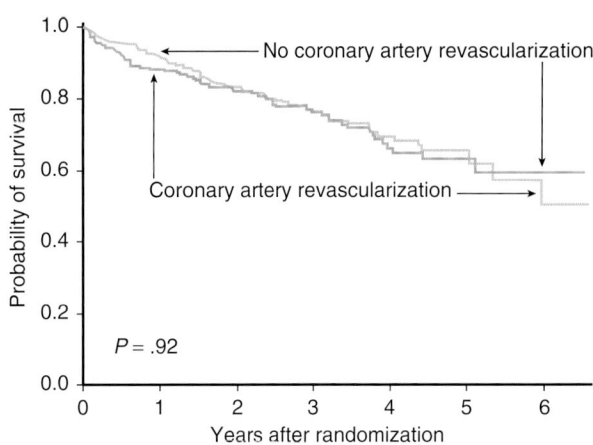

Fig. 8.3 Kaplan-Meier survival curve for patients enrolled in the coronary artery revascularization prophylaxis trial. There was no difference in early or late mortality following noncardiac surgery among patients with coronary artery disease who were randomized to undergo preoperative coronary revascularization rather than conservative therapy. (From McFalls EO, Ward HB, Moritz TE, et al. Coronary-artery revascularization before elective major vascular surgery. *New Engl J Med*. 2004;351[27]:2795–2804.)

revascularization followed by vascular surgery or to vascular surgery without preceding coronary revascularization. Among the group randomized to coronary revascularization, 41% of patients underwent coronary artery bypass grafting (CABG), and 59% were treated with PCI.

The majority of patients enrolled in the CARP trial were at low to intermediate rather than high risk for perioperative coronary events. The median age was 66 years, and whereas 42% had a prior MI, only 38% noted the presence of angina at the time of study entry, and less than 50% underwent a stress imaging study that documented moderate or severe ischemia prior to coronary angiography. Most patients had one- or two-vessel coronary disease with preserved left ventricular (LV) function, and those with left main stenosis of 50% or greater, a left ventricular ejection fraction (LVEF) of less than 20%, or severe aortic stenosis (AS) were excluded. The results of the CARP trial indicated that preoperative revascularization was not associated with any apparent benefit over conservative therapy. Although patients assigned to coronary revascularization had a significantly longer delay between randomization and vascular surgery (54 vs. 18 days), neither preoperative PCI nor CABG was associated with a reduction in the occurrence of adverse cardiac events or overall survival following vascular surgery at 30-day or 2.7-year follow-up (Fig. 8.3).

The Dutch Echocardiographic Cardiac Risk Evaluation Applying Stress Echocardiography (DECREASE-V) pilot study was designed to evaluate the effectiveness of prophylactic coronary revascularization prior to major vascular surgery among a higher-risk group of patients than those enrolled in the CARP trial.[26] A total of 101 patients with extensive myocardial ischemia on noninvasive stress imaging were randomized to either revascularization (65% had PCI, 35% had CABG) or no revascularization prior to vascular surgery. Within this small cohort, preoperative coronary revascularization was not associated with significant differences in the occurrence of death or MI either at 30 days or 1 year following NCS. Thus, despite their potential shortcomings, the CARP and DECREASE-V results lend support to the concept that performing prophylactic coronary revascularization in the setting of stable CAD for the purpose of "getting a patient through" NCS is rarely appropriate.

SECTION I Patient Selection

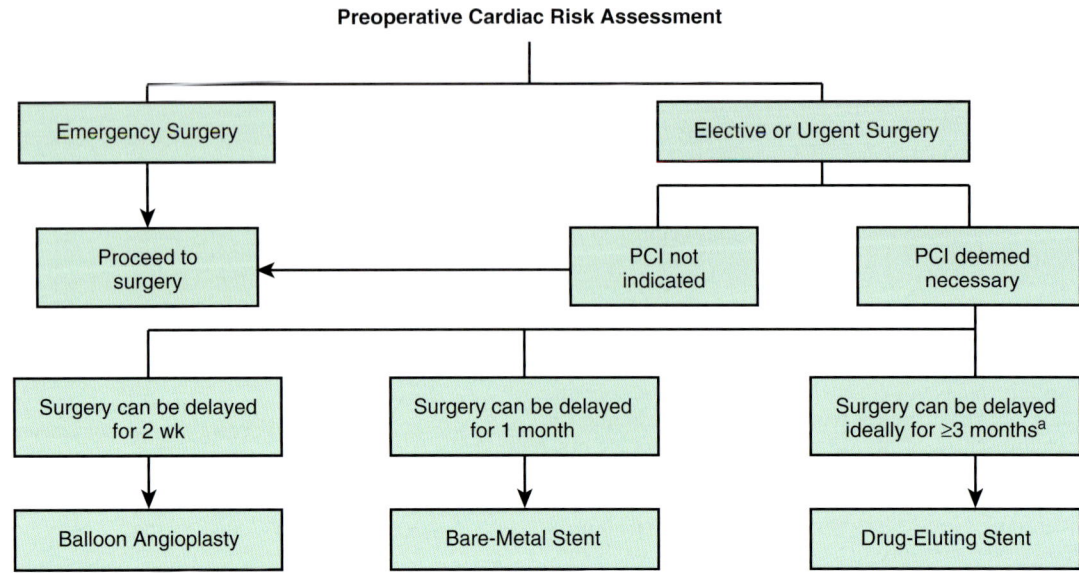

Fig. 8.4 Algorithm outlining device selection for preoperative percutaneous coronary intervention *(PCI)*. *DES*, Drug-eluting stent; *ESC*, European Society of Cardiology; *NCS*, noncardiac surgery.

Unstable Coronary Artery Disease

Currently, preoperative PCI should be considered only among patients who otherwise have an indication for coronary revascularization unrelated to NCS, particularly those with medically refractory angina, unstable angina, or recent MI. For these limited patient groups at the highest risk for adverse cardiac events, sufficient data regarding the efficacy and safety of preoperative revascularization are lacking, and the potential risks and benefits of preoperative revascularization need to be carefully weighed on an individual basis. Multidisciplinary communication involving the patient's primary care physician, cardiologist, cardiac surgeon, anesthesiologist, and surgeon intending to perform the noncardiac procedure is crucial in determining a rational preoperative strategy. Such a discussion can allow consideration of issues such as the anticipated risks and benefits of preoperative PCI or CABG; the risks, necessity, and urgency of the planned noncardiac surgical procedure; and the potential risks that antiplatelet agents such as aspirin or $P2Y_{12}$ receptor-blocker therapy may pose during the operation.

Revascularization Technique

When the decision has been made to perform preoperative PCI, a foremost consideration is the urgency of the surgical procedure, which often dictates whether stand-alone balloon angioplasty, bare-metal stenting (BMS), or drug-eluting stent (DES) implantation is performed (Fig. 8.4).

Balloon Angioplasty

Because of less reliable short- and long-term results, balloon angioplasty without stent placement is an infrequently used strategy for patients undergoing PCI in contemporary practice. However, because NCS performed within 1 month of coronary stent implantation is associated with substantial rates of adverse cardiac events, stand-alone balloon angioplasty may have a role in the preoperative setting because this approach does not introduce the possibility of perioperative stent thrombosis, permitting surgery with little delay following PCI. Among studies of preoperative balloon angioplasty performed in the pre-stent era, in-hospital mortality following subsequent NCS ranged from 0% to 2.7% for patients who underwent surgery following either recent (within 2 weeks) or remote preoperative angioplasty.[28–35] Current ACC/AHA guidelines recommend delaying surgery for at least 2 weeks following balloon angioplasty to allow for initial healing at the site of vessel injury and to overcome the usual time frame during which acute vessel closure and recoil typically occur. Surgery should not be delayed for more than 8 to 12 weeks following angioplasty because restenosis becomes a potential concern after this interval. Thus for a patient in whom PCI is deemed necessary prior to surgery but delaying surgery for more than 2 weeks is undesirable, balloon angioplasty without stenting may represent a reasonable option. However, it should be kept in mind that abrupt vessel closure or an inadequate angiographic result can occur in up to 10% to 20% of attempts at stand-alone balloon angioplasty and that unplanned stenting may become necessary.

Stent Placement

Despite advances in stent technology, major adverse cardiac event (MACE) rates remain considerable if NCS is performed early after stenting. Current guidelines recommend that NCS should be delayed for at least 30 days following BMS implantation, to allow completion of a full course of $P2Y_{12}$ receptor antagonist therapy. First-generation DESs were poorly suited for the preoperative setting, because stent thrombosis remained a concern for months to years following implantation,[36,37] leading to guideline recommendations that elective NCS be postponed when possible for at least 12 months following first-generation DES placement. The likelihood of stent thrombosis with newer-generation DESs appears similar to that with BMSs, and shorter dual antiplatelet therapy (DAPT) durations have become safe.[38–43] Nine large randomized controlled trials examining newer-generation DES platforms all demonstrated no difference in ischemic event rates following DES

CHAPTER 8 Coronary and Valvular Intervention Prior to Noncardiac Surgery

TABLE 8.1 Shorter Versus Longer DAPT Duration Following Stent Placement for Stable CAD in Randomized Trials Including Newer Generation DESs

Study	N	DAPT Duration (months)	Stent Type	Ischemic Events	Bleeding Events
SECURITY[44]	1399	6 vs. 12	Everolimus, zotarolimus or biolimus with biodegradable polymer	No difference	No difference
PRODIGY[45]	2013	6 vs. 24	Evrolimus (25%), zotarolimus (25%), paclitaxel (25%), or BMS (25%)	No difference	Increased in the longer duration group
OPTIMIZE[46]	3119	3 vs. 12	zotarolimus	No difference	No difference
EXCELLENT[47]	1443	6 vs. 12	Everolimus (75%) or sirolimus (25%)	No difference	No difference
RESET[48]	2055	3 vs. 12	zotarolimus	No difference	No difference
REDUCE[49]	1496	6 vs. 18	Sirolimus (abluminal surface) with endothelial progenitor cells (luminal surface)	No difference	No difference
ITALIC[50]	1850	6 vs. 12	Everolimus	No difference	No difference
NIPPON[51]	3773	6 vs. 18	Biolimus with biodegradable polymer	No difference	No difference
ISAR-SAFE[52]	4000	6 vs. 12	Variety (88% newer-generation DES)	No difference	No difference

BMS, Bare-metal stent; *CAD*, coronary artery disease; *DAPT*, dual antiplatelet therapy; *DES*, drug-eluting stent.

TABLE 8.2 Guideline Recommended Minimum Delays Between Percutaneous Coronary Intervention and Elective Noncardiac Surgery

	ACC/AHA[98] (2016 update)		ESC[99] (2017 update)	
PCI Method	Minimum Delay	Class & LOE	Minimum Delay	Class & LOE
POBA	14 days	IB		
BMS	30 days	IB	1 month	IIA
DES[a]	6 months	IB	1 month	IIA
	3 months[b]	IIB		

Note: Both the ACC/AHA and ESC guideline statements provide a class I recommendation that aspirin should be continued if possible during NCS when $P2Y_{12}$ inhibitor therapy must be stopped.

ACC, American College of Cardiology; *AHA*, American Heart Association; *BMS*, bare-metal stent; *DAPT*, dual antiplatelet therapy; *DES*, drug-eluting stent; *ESC*, European Society of Cardiology; *LOE*, level of evidence; *NCS*, noncardiac surgery; *PCI*, percutaneous coronary intervention; *POBA*, plain old balloon angioplasty.

[a]Second-generation DES.
[b]The ACC/AHA guidelines recommend that elective NCS should not be performed (class III) within 30 days of BMS or 3 months of DES implantation when DAPT will be discontinued perioperatively.

placement when DAPT was continued for only 3 or 6 months versus longer durations of 12 or 24 months (Table 8.1).[44–52] Although none of these trials specifically examined patients undergoing NCS, the safety of shorter DAPT durations following newer-generation DES placement is reflected in updates to perioperative guideline recommendations, which suggest that NCS can be performed much sooner after newer-generation DES implantation (Table 8.2). When preoperative PCI is performed, the completeness of revascularization may be of importance. Among 12,486 VA patients who underwent NCS within 2 years of coronary stent placement, those who had incomplete revascularization were at significantly increased risk for PMI and MACE compared with individuals with complete revascularization, especially if NCS was performed within 6 weeks of the PCI procedure.[53]

Coronary Artery Bypass Grafting

Although best suited for complex multivessel disease, CABG represents another consideration for patients undergoing coronary revascularization prior to NCS. Although a history of remote coronary bypass grafting may be protective during future surgical procedures, the role of CABG undertaken as a preemptive measure among patients discovered to have severe coronary artery prior to NCS remains uncertain.[54,55] Performance of CABG can substantially delay subsequent NCS and hence may not be feasible if the required noncardiac operation is urgent. Attempting to perform NCS very shortly after CABG may be associated with increased operative risks. For example, patients undergoing vascular surgery within 1 month of CABG in one observational study demonstrated a fivefold increase in operative mortality compared with matched controls who underwent vascular surgery without preceding CABG (20.6 vs. 3.9%, $P < .005$).[56] In a review of 211 patients who underwent NCS within 1 year of CABG, significant risk factors for adverse events included ejection fraction less than 45% and pulmonary artery systolic pressure greater than 40 mm Hg, and approximately two-third of adverse events occurred when NCS was performed within 90 days of CABG.[57]

UNANTICIPATED SURGERY AFTER STENTING

Even if elective stenting is avoided prior to known upcoming NCS, approximately 5% to 10% of patients who undergo PCI will require an unanticipated surgical procedure during the first year after stent placement.[5,40,58–61] For these individuals, the decision whether to continue or suspend antiplatelet therapy during NCS involves a presumptive trade-off between perioperative ischemic events and bleeding complications. The likelihood of ischemic events including those related to stent thrombosis is especially high if surgery is performed within the first 4 to 6 weeks following either BMS or DES placement. After 6 weeks, perioperative cardiac event rates fall substantially and appear to reach a stable nadir at 6 to 12 months after stent placement (Fig. 8.5).

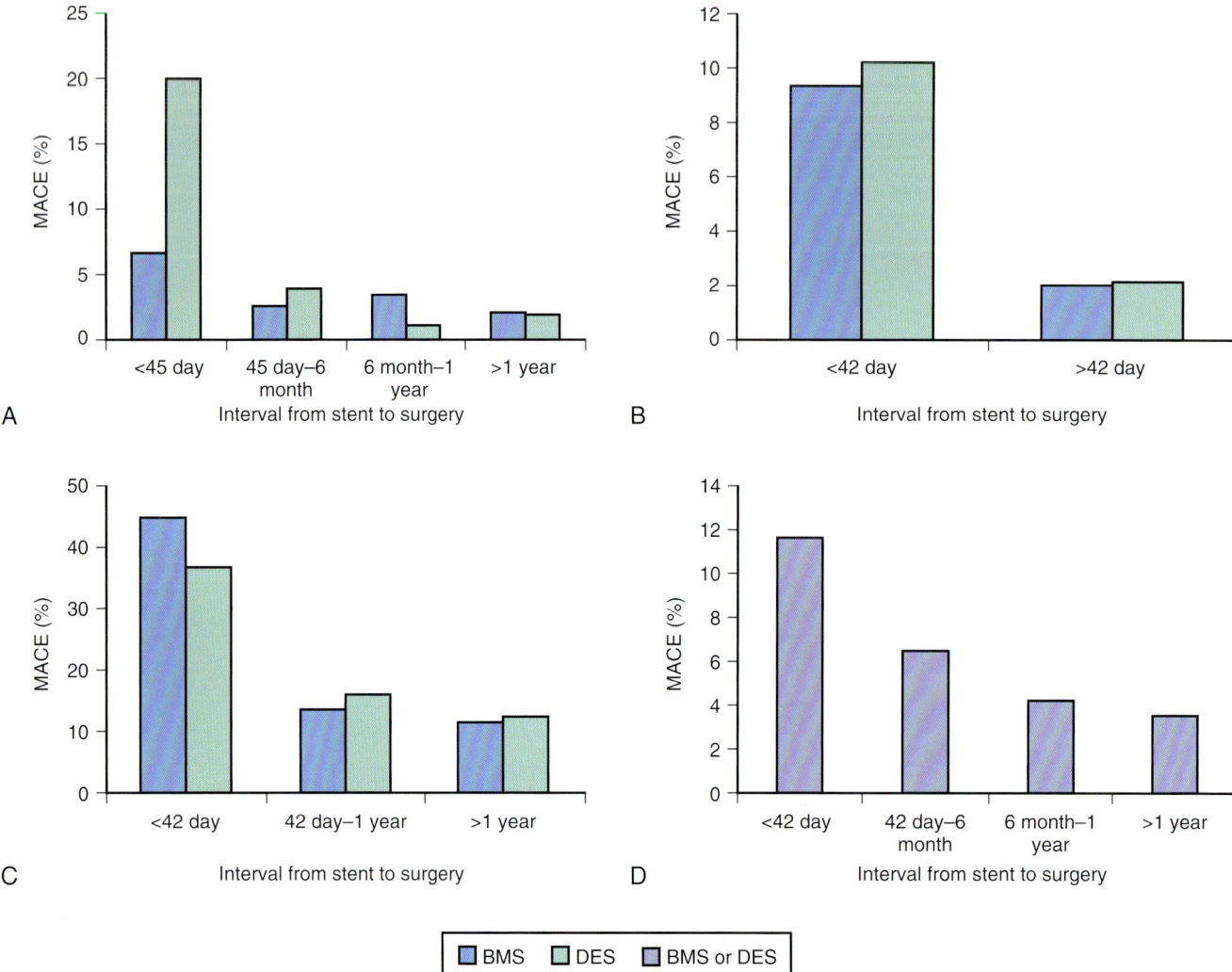

Fig. 8.5 Death and cardiac ischemic event rates by interval between stent placement and noncardiac surgery, as reported in several large registries. (A) Wijeysundera et al.[66] (B) CREDO-Kyoto PCI/CABG registry cohort-2 investigators.[78] (C) Cruden et al.[62] (D) Hawn et al.[64] *BMS,* Bare-metal stent; *CABG,* coronary artery bypass grafting; *DES,* drug-eluting stent; *MACE,* major adverse cardiac event; *PCI,* percutaneous coronary intervention.

In a Scottish registry of 1953 individuals who underwent NCS following coronary BMS or DES placement, when surgery was performed within 42 days of stenting, the incidence of perioperative death or cardiac ischemic events was quite high (42.4%, vs. 12.8% when surgery was performed after 42 days; $P < .001$).[62] Mortality rates fell after 6 weeks but remained fourfold greater when surgery was performed between 42 days and 1 year compared with after 1 year post PCI. Notably, no association was noted between stent type (BMS vs. DES) and adverse events. In a retrospective analysis of nearly 25,000 NCS procedures performed at Mayo Clinic, previous stent placement was associated with a greater than twofold increase in MACE and bleeding events when NCS was performed within 1 year of PCI, but the risk was not elevated after 1 year.[63] Among 41,989 VA patients who underwent NCS within 24 months of coronary stenting, MACE rates fell from 11.6% when surgery was performed within 6 weeks of stenting, to 6.4% when surgery was undertaken 6 weeks to 6 months after stent placement, and to 4.2% when surgery was delayed by more than 6 months.[64] The three factors most strongly associated with MACE were nonelective surgery, history of MI in the 6 months preceding surgery, and higher cardiac risk index score, and outcomes were not influenced by BMS versus DES use.

In a Danish study, the risk of perioperative MI and cardiac death was significantly higher among patients who underwent NCS following DES placement compared with matched controls but only when surgery was performed within 1 month of PCI.[65] In another large cohort of 2725 patients who underwent stent placement prior to NCS, MACE rates were likewise substantial when surgery was performed within 45 days of PCI (6.7% following BMS, 20.0% following DES).[66] Adverse event rates following BMS placement fell to 2.6% between 45 to 180 days post PCI and rose again after 180 days, possibly related to the occurrence of in-stent restenosis among some individuals. Following DES placement, surgical MACE rates remained greater than 3.0% until 180 days post PCI. Patients with recent MI as an indication for stent placement are at particularly high risk for perioperative events when NCS is performed early post PCI, demonstrating a fivefold increase in MACE in one observational study when NCS was performed within 3 months following stenting.[67]

Antiplatelet Drug Interruption

Although early cessation of antiplatelet therapy following PCI is among the strongest predictors of stent thrombosis, continuation of aspirin and/or P2Y$_{12}$ receptor–blocker therapy during NCS is associated with an increased likelihood of hemorrhagic complications.[68–71] If NCS can be delayed following DES placement, contemporary registries suggest that the risks associated with antiplatelet drug interruption prior to surgery may be acceptable.[72,73] In a registry of 4896 patients who received a zotarolimus-eluting stent, DAPT interruption within the first month was associated with a substantial rate of definite or probable stent thrombosis (3.6%) and cardiac death or target-vessel MI (6.8%); however, interruption after 1 month was not associated with an increased risk of stent thrombosis or MACE.[74] Likewise, in a pooled analysis of 11,219 patients enrolled in seven trials or registries of everolimus-eluting stent implantation, DAPT discontinuation before 30 days was strongly associated with the occurrence of stent thrombosis; however, after 90 days there was no association between DAPT interruption and stent thrombosis.[75] In the Patterns of Non-Adherence to Anti-Platelet Regimens in Stented Patients (PARIS) registry, 10.5% of patients had interruption of at least one antiplatelet drug (aspirin and/or a P2Y$_{12}$ receptor blocker) prior to a surgical procedure within 2 years of stent placement.[76] A nonsignificant trend toward increased MACE was observed among patients with DAPT interruption for surgery compared with the overall cohort (hazard ratio [HR], 1.41; 95% confidence interval [CI], 0.94 to 2.12; P = .10). Among a separate cohort of 1134 consecutive patients with coronary stents who underwent NCS at one of 47 French centers, 10.4% suffered a postoperative major adverse cardiac or cerebrovascular event, and such events were independently associated with cessation of antiplatelet therapy 5 or more days prior to surgery.[77] Conversely, in a Japanese registry of 2398 patients who underwent surgery within 3 years of coronary BMS or DES placement, continuation of DAPT during surgery was associated with neither a decrease in the rates of perioperative death, MI, or stent thrombosis nor an increase in bleeding events.[78] Although uncommon, it should be noted that very late stent thrombosis has been observed following cessation of DAPT for NCS months to years following second-generation DES placement.[79]

Antiplatelet Therapy and Surgical Bleeding Risk

The use of aspirin and/or P2Y$_{12}$ inhibitor therapy during NCS is associated with an increased risk of hemorrhagic events in most studies. In a large retrospective evaluation of nearly 50,000 patients who underwent a variety of surgical procedures, aspirin use was associated with a 1.5-fold increase in overall bleeding complications.[80] Despite the increase in overall bleeding, no increase was found in fatal bleeding among aspirin users except during intracranial surgery and transurethral prostatectomy. In a randomized trial of 220 high-risk patients undergoing NCS, perioperative aspirin therapy resulted in an 80% relative reduction in postoperative MACE compared with placebo, without an increase in bleeding events.[81] However, in the large POISE-2 trial which randomized 10,010 patients at risk for vascular complications to aspirin or placebo immediately prior to NCS, the administration of aspirin significantly increased the risk of major bleeding compared with placebo (HR, 1.23; 95% CI, 1.01 to 1.49) but had no significant effect on the rate of perioperative death or nonfatal MI (HR, 0.99; 95% CI, 0.86 to 1.15).[21] Smaller studies of clopidogrel use during noncardiac and cardiac surgery have demonstrated similar findings, with greater likelihoods of perioperative bleeding events and blood transfusions but no increase in bleeding-related mortality.[82–86]

A recent systematic review of studies focusing specifically on the perioperative management of DAPT among patients with coronary stents failed to identify an association between any particular antiplatelet strategy and the odds of either MACE or bleeding complications.[87] Consequently, substantial variability remains among physicians with respect to real-world perioperative antiplatelet drug management.[88–91] Because the excess bleeding that may occur with continuation of antiplatelet agents can render surgery more cumbersome and technically demanding, surgeons may strongly favor stoppage of antiplatelet drugs even if bleeding is not associated with increased surgical mortality rates.[92] Of interest, 68% of DAPT interruptions in the PARIS registry occurred for minor surgical procedures, which in many instances should not mandate cessation of antiplatelet therapy.[93] For "closed space" operations—including intracranial, spinal, and retinal surgery—even small amounts bleeding into a confined area can have devastating consequences, and cessation of all antiplatelet agents is typically considered mandatory. Other selected surgical procedures associated with high hemorrhagic risk are listed in Table 8.3. In an attempt to standardize decisions regarding perioperative DAPT, the Italian cardiology, surgical and anesthesiology societies developed consensus guidelines with detailed recommendations for the management of antiplatelet therapy among patients with coronary stents undergoing NCS, with an associated smartphone application for day-to-day clinical use.[94,95]

SUMMARY AND RECOMMENDATIONS

For patients with recently implanted coronary stents who require NCS, decisions regarding the timing of surgery and the

TABLE 8.3 Risk Factors for Bleeding and Thrombotic Complications With Noncardiac Surgery

NONCARDIAC PROCEDURES WITH HIGH RISK FOR BLEEDING
- Closed space surgery (intracranial, spine, eye)

OPEN THORACIC AND THORACOABDOMINAL
- Hepatic Resection
- Whipple procedure
- Urological surgery (including TURP, bladder or kidney resection, partial orchiectomy, percutaneous nephrostomy or lithotripsy)
- Major orthopedic surgery of the hip, pelvis, or proximal femur
- Certain GI endoscopic procedures (including dilation in achalasia, fine needle aspiration of pancreas, ampullectomy of ampulla of Vater and mucosectomy/submucosal resection)

HIGH-RISK CLINICAL VARIABLES FOR THROMBOTIC COMPLICATIONS WITH NCS AMONG PATIENTS WITH PRIOR PCI
- NCS performed early following PCI (within 2 weeks of POBA, 4 weeks of BMS, or 3 months of DES placement)
- NCS performed within 6 months of STEMI or acute coronary syndrome
- Complex PCI (long, multiple, bifurcation, or overlapping stents, smaller vessel)
- Incomplete revascularization
- History of stent thrombosis
- Diabetes mellitus
- Renal insufficiency

HIGH-RISK SITUATIONS IF STENT THROMBOSIS OCCURS
- Larger myocardial territory subtended by stent (e.g., unprotected LM)
- Low baseline LVEF
- Older patient age
- More comorbid conditions

BMS, Bare-metal stent; *DES,* drug-eluting stent; *GI,* gastrointestinal; *LM,* left main; *LVEF,* left ventricular ejection fraction; *NCS,* noncardiac surgery; *PCI,* percutaneous coronary intervention; *POBA,* plain old balloon angioplasty; *STEMI,* ST-segment elevation myocardial infarction; *TURP,* transurethral resection of the prostate.
Compiled from multiple sources including references [18,19,53,67,94,96,102–104].

TABLE 8.4 Considerations for Management of Antiplatelet Therapy Prior to Noncardiac Surgery for Individuals With a Coronary Stent

Favors Continuing Antiplatelet Therapy	Favors Interrupting Therapy
Recent stent placement (BMS within past 4 weeks, DES within past 3–6 months)	Remote stent placement
One or more clinical variables predisposing to thrombotic complications (see Table 8.3)	Minimal risk factors for stent thrombosis
Worse clinical consequences if stent thrombosis occurs	Consequences of bleeding are severe (e.g., "closed space" surgery)
Surgical procedure with low bleeding risk	Surgical procedure with higher likelihood of substantial bleeding

BMS, Bare-metal stent; *DES*, drug-eluting stent.

management of antiplatelet therapy in the perioperative period require an individualized approach in which the risks and consequences of bleeding and stent thrombosis are weighed (Tables 8.3 and 8.4).[94,96,97] Communication between the surgeon and cardiologist is crucial, and the following factors should be considered:

1. The amount of time that has elapsed since the stent was placed: The risk of stent thrombosis and cardiac events is substantial when NCS is performed within 1 month of stent placement. Elective NCS should be postponed for at least 1 month following BMS implantation. Current ACC/AHA guidelines recommend that elective NCS be delayed optimally for 6 months after second-generation DES placement when $P2Y_{12}$ inhibitor therapy will be interrupted but state that NCS can be considered after 3 months if the risk of further delay of surgery is greater than the expected risks of stent thrombosis. The guidelines further assert that elective NCS is contraindicated (class III) within 30 days of BMS or 3 months of DES implantation when DAPT will be interrupted.[98] Conversely, current European Society of Cardiology (ESC) guidelines advise that elective surgery requiring $P2Y_{12}$ inhibitor discontinuation can be considered 1 month after either BMS or DES placement if aspirin can be maintained throughout the perioperative period (see Table 8.2).[99] The more aggressive ESC guidelines cite observational studies that did not demonstrate an association between stent type and risk of adverse events among patients undergoing NCS.[65,67] All societal guideline statements strongly urge that aspirin be continued whenever possible following stenting if $P2Y_{12}$ inhibitor therapy is stopped for NCS.[18,19,94,98–100] A meta-analysis of multiple cases of late or very late DES thrombosis supports the concept that short-term discontinuation of $P2Y_{12}$ inhibitor therapy is likely safer if aspirin is continued.[101]
2. The patient-specific risk of stent thrombosis or adverse events: It should be determined whether the patient possesses any additional risk factors such as recent MI, renal insufficiency, diabetes, or stent use in complex coronary anatomy including long segment, overlapping, small vessel, or bifurcation stenting, all of which have been associated with an increased propensity for stent thrombosis.[67,102–104] If such risk factors exist, delaying elective NCS for at least 6 months may be prudent.
3. The potential consequences of stent thrombosis for the particular patient: For instance, stent occlusion may be especially devastating for patients with preexisting LV dysfunction or in circumstances when the stent is located in a vessel with a large territory of supply.
4. The potential risks and consequences of excess surgical bleeding for the proposed operation: For operations that have low bleeding risk, DAPT should be continued through surgery whenever possible. If bleeding risk is moderate, preoperative cessation of $P2Y_{12}$ inhibitor therapy with continuation of aspirin is typically recommended. For surgical procedures that involve closed spaces or those associated with a high risk of substantial blood loss, temporary cessation of all antiplatelet therapy is often compulsory.
5. For highly selected patients at particularly high risk of both perioperative stent thrombosis and surgical bleeding: A strategy of perioperative bridging can be considered, as discussed later. NCS following recent stent placement should be performed at a facility with availability of on-site 24/7 PCI availability, which would permit prompt treatment of stent thrombosis.

When the decision is made to discontinue $P2Y_{12}$ receptor–antagonist therapy for NCS, pharmacokinetic data suggest that clopidogrel and ticagrelor be stopped 5 days and prasugrel 7 days before the operation, to allow adequate time for recovery of platelet function.[105,106] However, two large clinical registries examining bleeding complications among patients undergoing CABG suggest that ticagrelor can safely be discontinued 3 days (instead of 5 days) before surgery without an increase in bleeding complications, whereas the bleeding risk with clopidogrel remains elevated out to 5 days.[107,108] When discontinued preoperatively, $P2Y_{12}$ inhibitors should be restarted with an appropriate bolus as soon as safely possible following surgery, ideally within 48 to 72 hours.

INVESTIGATIONAL STRATEGIES

Perioperative Bridging

Among patients receiving DAPT who are considered to be at particularly elevated risk for stent thrombosis but for whom antiplatelet agents must be stopped prior to surgery because of high bleeding risk, perioperative bridging—in which a short-acting parenteral platelet antagonist is administered during the interval between cessation of oral antiplatelet therapy and surgery—has been proposed as a means to reduce the risk of perioperative stent thrombosis (Fig. 8.6).[96,109–111] The small-molecule glycoprotein (GP) IIb/IIIa receptor antagonists eptifibatide and tirofiban both have relatively short physiologic half-lives with near complete recovery of platelet function within several hours of drug cessation, and represent suitable bridging agents.[112,113] Cangrelor, a reversible $P2Y_{12}$ receptor antagonist that is administered intravenously, has a very rapid onset of action and a half-life of only 3 to 6 minutes with recovery of platelet function within 60 minutes, which renders the drug a potentially attractive bridging agent.[114,115] In the Maintenance of Platelet Inhibition With Cangrelor After Discontinuation of Thienopyridines in Patients Undergoing Surgery (BRIDGE) trial, patients with either acute coronary syndrome or prior coronary stenting who were awaiting CABG were randomized to preoperative cangrelor or placebo infusion following cessation of theinopyridine therapy.[114] Cangrelor was effective in maintaining inhibition of platelet reactivity during the infusion, without an increase in major clinical bleeding events. Because a continuous intravenous (IV) infusion of drug is required, a bridging strategy necessitates hospitalization (Table 8.5).

Although theoretically attractive, published experience with perioperative bridging among patients with recent coronary stenting undergoing NCS is limited.[116–122] In a meta-analysis of eight studies of perioperative bridging that included 280 patients, the overall incidence of stent thrombosis was 1.3% with an in-hospital mortality rate of 3.5%, a major bleeding rate of 7.4%, and a need for blood transfusions among 13.9% of patients.[123] Thus stent thrombosis and bleeding events still can occur despite bridging, and given the absence of control groups in any of these studies, the relative efficacy and safety of this approach compared

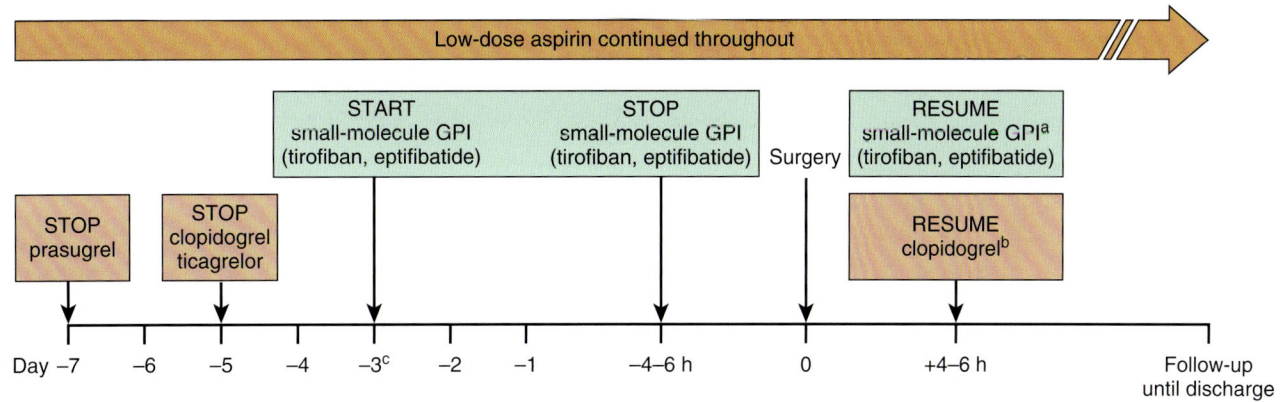

Fig. 8.6 Proposed bridging protocol for patients on dual-antiplatelet therapy with aspirin and a P2Y$_{12}$ receptor inhibitor referred for noncardiac surgery. [a]If oral administration is not possible. [b]With a 300- to 600-mg loading dose as soon as oral administration is possible; prasugrel and ticagrelor are discouraged. [c]Tirofiban: 0.1 µg/kg/min; if creatinine clearance <50 mL/min, adjust to 0.05 µg/kg/min. Eptifibatide: 2.0 µg/kg/min; if creatinine clearance is <50 mL/min, adjust to 1.0 µg/kg/min. Please note that the use of tirofiban and eptifibatide for periprocedural bridging represent off-label usages of these agents, and the safety and efficacy of a bridging strategy remains uncertain, as described in the text. −, Time before surgery; +, time after completion of surgery; *GPI*, Glycoprotein IIb/IIIa receptor inhibitor. (From Capodanno D, Angiolillo DJ. Management of antiplatelet therapy in patients with coronary artery disease requiring cardiac and noncardiac surgery. *Circulation*. 2013;128[25]:2785–2798.)

TABLE 8.5 Pharmacokinetics of Antiplatelet Agents

Drug	Route of Administration	Reversible Platelet Inhibition?	Time to Peak Activity After Loading Dose[a]	Elimination Half-Life[a]	Time to Platelet Recovery After Discontinuation[a]
Ticlopidine	Oral	No	3–4 days	4–5 days	5 days
Clopidogrel	Oral	No	2–6 h	8 h	5 days
Prasugrel	Oral	No	2–4 h	8 h	7 days
Ticagrelor	Oral	Yes	2–4 h	8 h	5 days[b]
Cangrelor	Intravenous	Yes	<10 min	3 min	<60 min
Tirofiban	Intravenous	Yes	<10 min	2 h	3–4 h
Eptifibatide	Intravenous	Yes	<10 min	2.5 h	4 h

[a]Times are approximate and demonstrate interindividual variability.
[b]Clinical studies suggest that discontinuation 3 days prior to surgery may be safe.[107,108]

with simply interrupting DAPT without bridging remains unknown. Pending further data, a bridging strategy might be considered for highly selected patients who are at particularly high risk for stent thrombosis, such as when surgery is required within 1 month of stent placement.

Platelet Function Testing

Because substantial individual variability exists in the degree of platelet inhibition and speed of platelet recovery following cessation of oral antiplatelet therapy, some patients are left vulnerable to ischemic events for a longer duration after discontinuation of antiplatelet drugs while awaiting surgery. In addition, a rebound state of hypercoagulability may occur shortly after cessation of antiplatelet therapy, which renders patients especially susceptible to thrombotic events, although this concept remains controversial.[124–128] A variety of assays are available to rapidly assess the level of platelet inhibition on a patient-specific basis and may be of value in determining the ideal timing for surgery following discontinuation of antiplatelet therapy.[129–131] To date, only a few small studies have examined the relationship of platelet function testing and operative bleeding events, all in CABG surgery.[132–134] Both the ESC and the Society of Thoracic Surgeons (STS) have given the premise of point-of-care testing of platelet inhibition for determining timing of surgery a class II recommendation; however, the ideal assay and specific platelet reactivity cutpoints to optimize clinical outcomes remain unknown.[135,136] Although intuitively attractive, the concept of using platelet function testing following antiplatelet therapy cessation to determine timing of surgery requires evaluation in larger scale clinical trials among post-PCI patients before its widespread use can be strongly recommended.

NOVEL DRUG-ELUTING STENT PLATFORMS

Evolving stent technologies, including polymer-free or bioabsorbable polymer DES platforms, offer the potential for shortened DAPT durations and may provide benefit for patients who require NCS soon after stent implantation. In one trial, 2466 patients undergoing PCI were randomized to receive a polymer-free biolimus A9–eluting stent versus a BMS, and both groups received only 1 month of DAPT post procedure. At 13-month follow-up, significant reductions in both the primary safety end point (cardiac death, MI, or stent thrombosis) and efficacy end point (target lesion revascularization) were observed in the DES group.[137] Likewise, in the Drug-eluting stents in elderly patients with CAD (SENIOR) trial, 1200 patients aged 75 years or older were randomized to bioabsorbable polymer DES versus BMS implantation. Following PCI, patients were treated with DAPT for only 1 month if they had presented with stable coronary disease or for 6 months following an unstable presentation. The primary composite end point of all-cause mortality, MI, stroke, or ischemia-driven target lesion revascularization at 1 year was significantly lower in the DES group, and similar stent thrombosis rates of 1% were observed in both treatment arms.[138]

Postoperative Care

Although prevention of operative complications through proper patient selection and management remains the cornerstone of achieving low surgical mortality rates, prompt recognition and treatment of postoperative complications when they do occur represents another critical element in optimizing outcomes following NCS. In a provocative multicenter study of more than 84,000 patients who underwent inpatient general or vascular surgery, major surgical complication rates were similar among the various hospitals included in the study. However, ultimate mortality rates among patients with major complications varied dramatically from 12.5% among hospitals in the lowest mortality quintile to 21.4% among hospitals in the highest mortality quintile.[139] These findings suggest that variations in mortality rates among hospitals may not result primarily from differences in initial surgical complication rates but from the care that patients receive after complications have occurred.

Because the vast majority of perioperative cardiac events occur within the first 72 hours following surgery, close surveillance of patients at increased risk is essential during this early postoperative period. If aspirin and/or $P2Y_{12}$ receptor–blocker therapy was suspended prior to surgery, these agents should be resumed as soon as safely possible because the prothrombotic milieu engendered by surgery persists into the postoperative period. Continuous telemetry monitoring is recommended in the early postoperative period for patients at risk for myocardial ischemia or MI. Because clinical symptoms are absent in the large majority of patients with PMI, routine daily postoperative troponin assessment for this first 48 to 72 hours is strongly recommended by the CCS perioperative guidelines for patients with a baseline greater than 5% risk for cardiovascular death or nonfatal MI at 30 days after NCS.[22]

If an acute ST segment elevation MI (STEMI) occurs early postoperatively, primary PCI is typically the treatment of choice, although the benefits versus the risks of intervention must be considered on a patient-to-patient basis. Thrombolytic therapy is contraindicated after all but the most minor surgical procedures because of the potential for hemorrhagic complications related to the surgical site. For this reason, patients at heightened risk for PMI—including those with prior stent placement in whom DAPT must be suspended prior to surgery—should have their surgical procedure performed at an institution with the on-site ability to perform primary PCI on a continuous basis. Among patients who require emergency PCI in the very early postoperative period, bleeding complications related to the surgical site remain a concern. Communication between the interventional cardiologist and the noncardiac surgical team regarding anticoagulant and antiplatelet therapy is essential. Urgent PCI following NCS is associated with a substantially increased risk of adverse events, hence the need for individualized decision making. Parasher et al. examined the outcomes of 281 patients who underwent PCI at their institution within 7 days of NCS and noted that mortality rates were quite high, with a 30-day death rate of 11.2% for all patients and 31.2% among those with STEMI.[140] Predictors of mortality included older age, renal insufficiency, vascular surgery as the index surgical procedure, and occurrence of a bleeding event after PCI.

Aortic Stenosis and Noncardiac surgery

With the widespread adoption of catheter-based therapies for AS, the prospect of interventional therapy for patients with severe aortic valve disease who require NCS has received increasing attention. Despite improved surgical outcomes with current anesthesia and operative techniques, the presence of symptomatic severe AS remains an important risk factor for adverse events with NCS.[141,142] Symptomatic status appears to represent a key factor in determining the risk for adverse perioperative events among patients with severe AS who undergo NCS. In a case-control study of 256 patients with severe AS undergoing NCS, asymptomatic patients were not at increased risk for 30-day MACE or mortality compared with matched controls, whereas the presence of symptoms (angina, dyspnea, or syncope) was associated with significantly elevated 30-day MACE and 1-year mortality rates.[142] A meta-analysis of three case-control studies examining patients with severe asymptomatic AS who underwent a moderate or high-risk noncardiac surgical procedure likewise indicated that the presence of severe asymptomatic AS was not associated with a significant increase in 30-day MACE.[143] Similarly, among 634 patients with moderate or severe AS who underwent NCS at the Cleveland Clinic, significant predictors of adverse outcomes included symptomatic severe AS, high-risk surgery, and coexistent mitral regurgitation or CAD.[144]

Although the presence of severe symptomatic AS is associated with increased adverse events during moderate or high-risk NCS, evidence regarding the optimal management of AS in the perioperative period is scant and guidelines are inconsistent. In determining whether to simply proceed with NCS or perform preemptive surgical aortic valve replacement (SAVR), transcatheter aortic valve replacement (TAVR), or balloon aortic valvuloplasty (BAV), a reasonable approach is to consider: (1) the urgency of the NCS procedure, (2) the risk of the proposed operation, (3) the severity of the AS, and (4) the symptomatic status of the patient. If emergency NCS is needed for an immediately life-threatening condition, the operation should not be delayed regardless of the underlying valve disease. Invasive perioperative monitoring using a right heart catheter and transesophageal echocardiography is generally recommended and aggressive measures should be undertaken to avoid and treat hypovolemia and hypotension and maintain sinus rhythm. Conversely, if surgery is elective and the patient otherwise has an indication for aortic valve replacement such as symptomatic severe AS, NCS is usually postponed until the aortic valve disease is addressed definitively, typically with SAVR or TAVR. If the patient is asymptomatic, lacks additional cardiac comorbidities, and is facing a low- or moderate-risk operation, surgery can typically be performed without need for preemptive valve intervention.

When surgery is considered urgent, such that there is insufficient time to prepare for, perform, or allow recovery from SAVR or TAVR, BAV represents a tenable option for patients with severe symptomatic AS.[145] BAV typically results in a modest improvement in aortic valve area, rarely to greater than 1.0 cm^2, which nevertheless may be sufficient to reduce the impact of hemodynamic stresses inherent to higher-risk NCS. BAV represents a temporizing measure, because restenosis of the aortic valve with return of clinical symptoms and severe stenosis is nearly universal at 6 to 12 months post procedure. With improved operator experience and better patient selection and equipment, adverse event rates with BAV have decreased in current practice; however, major and minor complications still are reported in up to 10% to 20% of procedures (including acute severe aortic regurgitation, stroke, MI, death, and vascular and hemorrhagic complications).[146] Mortality rates are significantly lower when higher-volume operators practicing in higher-volume centers perform BAV.[147] Given the reduced profile of current TAVR delivery systems, coupled with the more reliable and durable results of

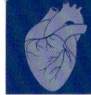

Fig. 8.7 Appropriate use criteria for the treatment of aortic stenosis among patients undergoing noncardiac surgery. (From Bonow RO, Brown AS, Gilliam LD et al: ACC/AATS/AHA/ASE/EACTS/HVS/SCA/SCAI/SCCT/SCMR/STS 2017 Appropriate Use Criteria for the Treatment of Patients With Severe Aortic Stenosis: A Report of the American College of Cardiology Appropriate Use Criteria Task Force, American Association for Thoracic Surgery, American Heart Association, American Society of Echocardiography, European Association for Cardio-Thoracic Surgery, Heart Valve Society, Society of Cardiovascular Anesthesiologists, Society for Cardiovascular Angiography and Interventions, Society of Cardiovascular Computed Tomography, Society for Cardiovascular Magnetic Resonance, and Society of Thoracic Surgeons, J Am Coll Cardiol. 2017,70[20]:2566–2508.)

TAVR and rapidity of patient recovery following the procedure, performance of TAVR rather than BAV prior to urgent NCS is a reasonable consideration, although whether a safe minimal waiting period should be observed between TAVR and NCS has not been studied. BAV generally should not be performed if moderate or greater aortic regurgitation is present because of the possibility of worsened regurgitation. Although BAV can provide temporary hemodynamic benefit among individuals with severe AS, only a few small case series have reported on its use prior to NCS, and no studies have examined whether the risks of preoperative BAV are outweighed by improved surgical outcomes.

Currently, recommendations for the management of AS among patients undergoing NCS are based on expert opinion and physiologic assumptions, which has produced variability among different guideline statements. For example, the ESC guidelines (2012) state that BAV can be considered in patients with symptomatic severe AS who require urgent NCS (class IIb indication, level of evidence C), whereas the ACC/AHA guidelines (2014) do not recommend BAV among patients undergoing urgent NCS.[148,149] Conversely, the more recently published ACC multidisciplinary AUC statement for the treatment of patients with severe AS (2017) provides strong support for interventional therapy among patients with symptomatic severe AS prior to elective or urgent NCS (Fig. 8.7).[150] Interestingly, the AUC statement also considers TAVR or SAVR "appropriate" (and no intervention as "may be appropriate") prior to elective NCS for patients with *asymptomatic* severe AS without obstructive coronary disease or signs of cardiac decompensation. Given the variability of guideline recommendations and the lack of comparative outcome data for the different treatment strategies, it is crucial to reemphasize the importance of an individualized patient-centered multidisciplinary heart-team approach to clinical decision making.

KEY REFERENCES

1. Devereaux PJ, Sessler DI. Cardiac complications in patients undergoing major noncardiac surgery. *N Engl J Med*. 2015;373:2258–2269.
18. Fleisher LA, Fleischmann KE, Auerbach AD, et al. 2014 ACC/AHA guideline on perioperative cardiovascular evaluation and management of patients undergoing noncardiac surgery: a report of the American College of Cardiology/American Heart Association Task Force on practice guidelines. *J Am Coll Cardiol*. 2014;64:e77–137.
22. Duceppe E, Parlow J, MacDonald P, et al. Canadian Cardiovascular Society Guidelines on Perioperative Cardiac Risk Assessment and Management for Patients Who Undergo Noncardiac Surgery. *Can J Cardiol*. 2017;33:17–32.
25. McFalls EO, Ward HB, Moritz TE, et al. Coronary-artery revascularization before elective major vascular surgery. *New Engl J Med*. 2004;351:2795–2804.

64. Cruden NL, Harding SA, Flapan AD, et al. Previous coronary stent implantation and cardiac events in patients undergoing noncardiac surgery. *Circ Cardiovasc Interv*. 2010;3:236–242.
76. Mehran R, Baber U, Steg PG, et al. Cessation of dual antiplatelet treatment and cardiac events after percutaneous coronary intervention (PARIS): 2 year results from a prospective observational study. *Lancet*. 2013;382:1714–1722.
94. Rossini R, Musumeci G, Visconti LO, et al. Perioperative management of antiplatelet therapy in patients with coronary stents undergoing cardiac and non-cardiac surgery: a consensus document from Italian cardiological, surgical and anaesthesiological societies. *EuroIntervention*. 2014;10:38–46.
96. Banerjee S, Angiolillo DJ, Boden WE, et al. Use of antiplatelet therapy/DAPT for post-PCI patients undergoing noncardiac surgery. *J Am Coll Cardiol*. 2017;69:1861–1870.
98. Levine GN, Bates ER, Bittl JA, et al. 2016 ACC/AHA Guideline Focused Update on Duration of Dual Antiplatelet Therapy in Patients With Coronary Artery Disease: A Report of the American College of Cardiology/American Heart Association Task Force on Clinical Practice Guidelines. *J Am Coll Cardiol*. 2016;68:1082–1115.
99. Valgimigli M, Bueno H, Byrne RA, et al. 2017 ESC focused update on dual antiplatelet therapy in coronary artery disease developed in collaboration with EACTS: The Task Force for dual antiplatelet therapy in coronary artery disease of the European Society of Cardiology (ESC) and of the European Association for Cardio-Thoracic Surgery (EACTS). *Eur Heart J*. 2017;39(3):213–260.
150. Bonow RO, Brown AS, Gillam LD, et al. ACC/AATS/AHA/ASE/EACTS/HVS/SCA/SCAI/SCCT/SCMR/STS 2017 Appropriate Use Criteria for the Treatment of Patients With Severe Aortic Stenosis: A Report of the American College of Cardiology Appropriate Use Criteria Task Force, American Association for Thoracic Surgery, American Heart Association, American Society of Echocardiography, European Association for Cardio-Thoracic Surgery, Heart Valve Society, Society of Cardiovascular Anesthesiologists, Society for Cardiovascular Angiography and Interventions, Society of Cardiovascular Computed Tomography, Society for Cardiovascular Magnetic Resonance, and Society of Thoracic Surgeons. *J Am Coll Cardiol*. 2017;70:2566–2598.

 Additional references available online at expertconsult.com.

中文导读

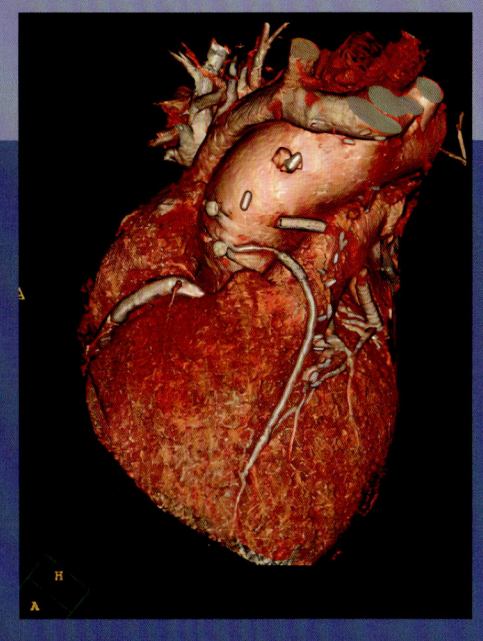

第9章
介入心脏病学中的性别与种族问题

　　冠状动脉粥样硬化性心脏病目前仍是导致男性和女性死亡的重要原因之一。现在越来越多的证据表明，不同性别、不同种族的心血管疾病的表现形式、预后、治疗效果、并发症都有明显的差异。女性罹患冠心病的年龄比男性延迟5~10年。女性更容易表现为非ST段抬高型急性冠状动脉综合征，在这部分非ST段抬高型急性冠状动脉综合征女性患者中，早期侵入性治疗获益较小。在这些情况下，应相应地考虑使用非侵入性检测进行风险分层。男性则更常见发生ST段抬高型心肌梗死。对于ST段抬高型心肌梗死的患者，无论是男性还是女性，均能从直接经皮冠状动脉介入治疗术中同等获益。但是，值得注意的是，ST段抬高型心肌梗死的女性患者，短期死亡率较男性患者更高。此外，与男性患者相比，接受经皮冠状动脉介入治疗的女性患者，存在更高的并发症发生率。即使在当今医疗环境下，女性发生血管并发症的概率是男性的1.5~4倍，尤其是在急性冠状动脉综合征的经皮冠状动脉介入治疗中有着更高的出血并发症。此外，女性也更容易受应激性心肌病、自发性冠状动脉夹层和微血管心绞痛的影响。

　　关于冠状动脉狭窄性病变与性别的研究数据目前较少，能够知晓的是在完全闭塞性病变经皮冠状动脉介入治疗手术中，男性所占的比例更高，而在左主干病变经皮冠状动脉介入治疗中，女性所占的比例更高。

　　在性别与治疗预后方面，无论是植入金属裸支架或药物洗脱支架的女性患者，与男性患者相比，其经皮冠状动脉介入治疗术后死亡率、短期预后、长期预后都相似。在药物治疗方面，女性和男性在急性冠状动脉综合征的辅助治疗和经皮冠状动脉介入治疗术后药物治疗中能够获益。

　　目前，针对种族的经皮冠状动脉介入治疗分析研究有限。然而，进行经皮冠状动脉介入治疗的非裔美国患者年龄更为年轻，更常表现为急性冠状动脉综合征，且并发症也更多。

李秋雨　范　谦

章节要点

- 女性接受经皮冠状动脉介入治疗时的年龄比男性更大，并发症也更多。无论是置入金属裸支架还是药物洗脱支架，女性患者与男性患者相比其短期和长期预后并无明显差别，包括经皮冠状动脉介入治疗术后死亡率也相近。定向冠状动脉粥样斑块切除术和准分子激光粥样斑块切除术等辅助经皮冠状动脉介入治疗术在女性患者中并发症发生率相对较高。

- 经皮冠状动脉介入治疗术后女性血管并发症和出血并发症发生率更高。尽管桡动脉入路可带来股动脉所不具有的潜在获益，而且女性经股动脉入路的风险也高于男性，但女性患者更可能通过股动脉入路进行经皮冠状动脉介入治疗，这可能与女性桡动脉入路所存在的技术挑战有关。

- 对于非ST段抬高型急性冠状动脉综合征女性患者，当存在低风险特征（心脏生物标记物阴性）时，她们可能并不能从早期干预策略中获益。在这些情况下，应考虑通过无创性检查对患者进行风险分层。然而，总体而言，女性发生非ST段抬高型急性冠状动脉综合征后出现住院期间并发症和长期并发症的风险更高，遵循指南治疗的获益则与男性相似。因此，如果女性患者并非低危患者时，无须关注性别，应按照指南给予治疗。数据显示，这些治疗的应用在性别上存在着差异。

- 对于ST段抬高型心肌梗死，女性和男性在直接经皮冠状动脉介入治疗中获益相似，但ST段抬高型心肌梗死女性患者的短期死亡率更高。

- 急性冠状动脉综合征和经皮冠状动脉介入治疗术后辅助药物治疗包括GPⅡb/Ⅲa抑制剂、$P2Y_{12}$抑制剂和直接凝血酶抑制剂。女性在这些辅助药物治疗中的获益与男性相近。

- 女性更容易受到应激性心肌病、自发性冠状动脉夹层和微血管心绞痛等特殊综合征的影响。

- 针对种族的经皮冠状动脉介入治疗分析研究极为有限。然而，接受经皮冠状动脉介入治疗的非裔美国患者更为年轻，而且女性可能更多，并发症也更多，更可能表现为急性冠状动脉综合征。

9 Sex and Ethnicity Issues in Interventional Cardiology

Matthew R. Summers, Sahar Naderi, Leslie Cho

KEY POINTS

- Women who present for percutaneous coronary intervention (PCI) are generally older and have more comorbidities compared with men. Women and men have comparable short- and long-term outcomes with bare-metal stents (BMSs) and drug-eluting stents (DESs), including similar mortality rates after PCI. Adjunctive PCI devices such as directional coronary atherectomy and excimer laser atherectomy are associated with higher complication rates in women.
- Women have higher rates of vascular complications and bleeding after PCI. Despite the potential benefits of transradial PCI and documented higher risks than men with femoral access, women are more likely to undergo transfemoral PCI, possibly based on presumed limiting technical challenges with transradial access.
- Women who present with non–ST-elevation acute coronary syndromes (NSTE-ACS) are less likely to benefit from an early-invasive strategy when they have low-risk features (i.e., negative cardiac biomarkers), and risk stratification with noninvasive testing should be considered accordingly in these situations. However, women have a higher risk of several in-hospital and long-term complications after NSTE-ACS overall and derive similar benefits from guideline-based therapies as men. As such, these therapies should be applied irrespective of sex when women are not at explicitly low risk. Data suggest sex-difference disparities in the application of these therapies.
- Women and men derive similar benefit from primary PCI for ST-elevation myocardial infarction (STEMI), but the short-term mortality after STEMI is higher among women.
- Women and men derive similar benefit from adjuvant acute coronary syndrome (ACS) and post-PCI medical therapies including glycoprotein (GP) IIb/IIIa inhibitors, $P2Y_{12}$ inhibitors, and direct thrombin inhibitors.
- Women are disproportionately affected by the unique syndromes of stress cardiomyopathy, spontaneous coronary artery dissection, and microvascular angina.
- Race-specific analyses of PCI are limited. However, African-American patients who present for PCI are younger and are more likely to be women, have more comorbidities, and are more likely to present with an ACS.

OVERVIEW

Cardiovascular disease (CVD) remains the leading cause of death regardless of sex and race. Historically, data extrapolated from large studies and registries have been applied to all populations irrespective of sex, race, or ethnicity. However, a growing body of literature shows sex and race differences in CVD manifestations, outcomes, and treatment effects. This chapter will explore these pertinent differences within the context of interventional cardiology.

SEX

CVD is the leading cause of morbidity and mortality among women in the United States.[1,2] It claims the lives of more women than the next five major causes of death combined.[1] CVD typically manifests approximately 5 to 10 years later in women than in men, which has in part contributed to the misconception that CVD is predominately a disease affecting men. Although overall rates of death attributable to CVD have declined over the past several decades, increasing data show a slower rate of decline and worse overall outcomes in women after a cardiovascular event, which may be explained by differences in comorbidities and pathophysiology and disparities in treatment.[1,3]

Characteristics and Outcomes of Women Undergoing Percutaneous Coronary Intervention

More than 1.3 million percutaneous coronary interventions (PCIs) are performed annually in the United States, with an estimated 35% performed in women.[1] Compared with men, women undergoing PCI are 5 to 10 years older and have a higher prevalence of hypertension, hyperlipidemia, diabetes, and other comorbidities such as smoking.[3,4] They are less likely to have a history of myocardial infarction (MI), PCI, or coronary artery bypass graft (CABG) surgery.[3,5] Women are more likely to present with non–ST-elevation acute coronary syndromes (NSTE-ACS), whereas men are more likely to present with an ST-elevation MI (STEMI).[5,6] Compared with men, women have similar lesion types but less multivessel disease and substantially smaller vessels.[5,7,8] Despite a lower prevalence of left ventricular dysfunction at baseline, women tend to have a higher incidence of congestive heart failure (CHF) and cardiogenic shock, and they have more functional impairment after revascularization than do men.[3,5]

Early reports of patients undergoing balloon angioplasty showed lower procedural success rates in women. In addition, early registry data found that women had higher in-hospital mortality after PCI even after adjusting for baseline comorbidities.[8] However, more recent studies report similar procedural success rates in both groups, with an increase in the number of women undergoing PCI over the past several decades.[5,9–11] Overall these studies demonstrate that both in-hospital and long-term mortality rates after PCI are similar between men and women despite women being older and having more complex lesion types (Tables 9.1 and 9.2).[11,12] This is likely due to heightened awareness of the effects of CVD on women, as well as advances within the field (i.e., newer-generation stents and balloons, smaller sheath sizes and catheters, and advances in adjunctive pharmacotherapies).[8,10,13] Controversy has surrounded the previously documented, less frequent use of diagnostic catheterization and delays in PCI in women compared with men.[14] These issues will be addressed further in the section on acute coronary syndromes (ACSs) later in the chapter.

TABLE 9.1 Odds of In-Hospital Death and Myocardial Infarction After Percutaneous Coronary Interventions, by Sex

Study	Women/Men (N)	Women (%)	Men (%)	Adjusted OR (95% CI)
PETERSON ET AL.[122]				
In-hospital death	35,571/74,137	1.8	1.0	1.07 (0.9–1.2)
In-hospital MI		1.5	1.2	1.25 (1.1–1.4)
JACOBS ET AL.[10]				
In-hospital death	895/1,629	2.2	1.3	1.6 (0.76–3.35)
In-hospital MI		0.2	0.7	
LANSKY ET AL.[18]				
In-hospital death	2,077/5,295	1.4	0.7	2.28 (1.15–4.55)
WATANABE ET AL.[59]				
In-hospital death	29,227/53,556	1.2	0.6	1.65 (1.33–2.04)
MALENKA ET AL.[8]				
In-hospital death	3,983/8,057	1.04	0.79	1.24 (0.96–1.60)
In-hospital MI		1.71	1.36	1.02 (0.85–1.24)
HEER ET AL.[41]				
In-hospital death	24,262/65,972	0.3	0.2	1.07 (0.83–1.41)
In-hospital MACE	24,262/65,972	0.7	0.4	1.37 (1.12–1.67)

CI, Confidence interval; *MACE*, major adverse cardiac event; *MI*, myocardial infarction.

TABLE 9.2 Long-Term Percutaneous Coronary Intervention Outcomes in Acute Coronary Syndrome Patients, by Sex

Study	Women/Men (N)	Women (%)	Men (%)	Adjusted OR (95% CI)
JACOBS ET AL.[10]				
1-Year death	895/1,629	6.5	4.3	1.26 (0.85–1.87)
1-Year death/MI		11.1	9.0	1.14 (0.86–1.50)
LANSKY ET AL.[18]				
1-Year death	2,077/5,295	4.4	3.3	No difference between sexes was noted; however, OR was not reported.
1-Year MACE		29.2	32.7	
MEHILI ET AL.[15]				
1-Year death	1,001/3,263	4.0	4.1	0.99 (0.54–1.13)
1-Year MACE		6.0	5.8	—
CHIU ET AL.[13]				
1-Year death	5,301/12,738	7	5	1.14 (0.93–1.41)
1-Year MACE		—	—	1.05 (0.97–1.13)
KUNADIAN ET AL.[11]				
1-Year death	3,938/7,448	8.1	5.6	1.44 (1.38–1.50)
BAVISHI ET AL.[57]				
1-Year death	4,391/4,132	8.5	8.0	1.01 (0.93–1.11)

CI, Confidence interval; *MACE*, major adverse cardiac event; *MI*, myocardial infarction; *OR*, odds ratio.

Sex and Percutaneous Coronary Devices and Adjuvant Therapies

No sex-based comparisons were made in the earlier randomized clinical trials comparing bare-metal stents (BMSs) with balloon angioplasty. Restenosis and revascularization rates were not well defined for women after bare-metal stenting because of the small sample of women in prospective trials with systematic angiographic follow-up. Even though women tend to have smaller vessel size, shorter lesions, and a higher prevalence of diabetes, some intriguing initial studies reported that women had similar or lower target-vessel revascularization (TVR) rates compared with their male counterparts after PCI.[15] However, systematic angiographic and clinical follow-up has not validated these findings. In the drug-eluting stent (DES) era, both sirolimus and paclitaxel stents have shown favorable outcomes in women. The Sirolimus-Eluting Stent in De-Novo Native Coronary Lesions (SIRIUS) trial and the TAXUS IV trial demonstrated the superiority of DESs with reduction in restenosis, TVR, and major adverse cardiac events (MACEs) at 1-year follow-up in women and men.[16,17] TAXUS IV randomized patients with severe coronary artery stenosis to DES (paclitaxel) versus BMS.[17] Women accounted for 27.9% of the study population. Restenosis rates were similar in women and men treated with the TAXUS stent (7.6% vs. 8.6%, $P = .80$), as were measurements of late luminal loss (0.23 mm vs. 0.22 mm, $P = .90$). Compared with BMSs, women treated with the TAXUS stent had a significant reduction in 9-month restenosis (29.2% vs. 8.6%, $P < .001$) and 1-year target-lesion revascularization (TLR) rates (14.9% vs. 7.6%, $P = .02$).[18] Of note, women had higher unadjusted TLR rates compared with men at 1 year; however, female sex was not an independent predictor of TLR (odds radio [OR], 1.72; 95% confidence interval [CI], 0.68 to 4.37; $P = .25$). A pooled analysis from four randomized sirolimus versus BMS trials was done to assess for sex differences.[19] In 1748 patients, 497 of whom were women, sirolimus-eluting stents were associated with a significant reduction in the rates of in-segment binary restenosis in women (6.3% vs. 43.8%) as well as in men (6.4% vs. 35.6%), which resulted in significant reduction in 1-year MACE rates ($P < .0001$). A pooled analysis of 11,557 women in 26 trials showed decreased mortality, MI, in-stent thrombosis, and TVR in those treated with a DES versus a BMS.[20] In addition, a significant benefit was found with newer-generation over early-generation DESs, including a lower risk of stent thrombosis at 12 months.[20,21] With respect to contemporary-generation, everolimus-eluting stents, women experience similar risk of 1-year MACEs (death, MI, TVR) but have higher adjusted risk of recurrent ischemic events related to nonstent-related MIs compared with men.[22]

Few sex-based studies on the efficacy of coronary atherectomy and adjuvant devices exist. Although directional coronary atherectomy (DCA) is no longer used, from a historical perspective, it appears to have been associated with lower procedural success and more bleeding complications in women.[12,23] Likewise, laser atherectomy with the excimer laser catheter was also associated with higher coronary perforation rates and increased morbidity in women.[12] Despite this demonstration, newer atherectomy techniques such as orbital atherectomy have not shown an increased rate of in-hospital or 30-day MACEs compared with men, despite higher baseline risks such as smaller vessels and older age.[24] Female sex is an independent risk factor for TVR after modern coronary brachytherapy with beta radiation for resistant DES in-stent restenosis (ISR).[25] Limited sex-specific data on rotational atherectomy, cutting or scoring balloon angioplasty, extraction atherectomy, or gamma brachytherapy are available. In smaller studies, sex has generally not been found to be an independent predictor of complications on the efficacy of these devices as a whole, although women have historically been underrepresented in earlier studies of adjuvant device therapies.

VASCULAR COMPLICATIONS

Women experience greater vascular and bleeding complications during PCI, particularly in the context of ACSs. Compared with men, they have an increased risk of major hematoma, retroperitoneal bleeding, bleeding that requires transfusion, and vascular injury that requires surgery after PCI.[13,26,27] Much of this may be explained by smaller vessel size, lower body mass index, and differences in platelet biology, drug distribution, and bioavailability. With the development of weight-adjusted heparin dosing, introduction of smaller sheath sizes, and early sheath removal, vascular complications have decreased.[26,28] However, even in the current era, women continue to have a 1.5 to 4 times higher risk of vascular complications compared with men.[26,27,29] Table 9.3 shows different vascular complication rates by sex as reported in recently published large studies.

Given that women have higher rates of vascular complications, they are seemingly ideal candidates for radial access. Data from the Study of Access Site for Enhancement of PCI for Women (SAFE-PCI) trial demonstrated significantly reduced bleeding and vascular complications in women undergoing cardiac catheterization or PCI with radial access as compared with femoral access (0.6% vs. 1.7%; OR 0.32; 95% CI, 0.12 to 0.90).[30] However, this trial did not show significant differences when limited to women undergoing PCI alone.[30] Of note was a significant access site crossover to the femoral approach, mostly as a result of radial artery spasm. In addition, in a subgroup analysis of the Radial Vs. femorAL access for coronary intervention (RIVAL) randomized trial, women undergoing coronary angiography and PCI had a significant reduction in major vascular complications when radial access was performed (3.1% vs. 6.1%; hazard ratio [HR] 0.5; 95%

TABLE 9.3 Vascular Complications by Sex

Study	Women/Men (N)	Women (%)	Men (%)	P Value
CHIU ET AL.[13]				
Blood transfusion	5,301/12,738	12	4	<0.001
Major hematoma		5	2	<0.001
Pseudoaneurysm		0.6	0.3	0.005
LANSKY ET AL.[29]				
Major hematoma	562/1,520	2.5	1.5	0.005
Retroperitoneal bleed		0.5	0.2	0.05
Surgical repair		3.8	2.4	0.001
WELTY ET AL.[123]				
Vascular injury	2,101/3,888	1.6	0.6	0.001
PETERSON ET AL.[122]				
Vascular injury	35,571/74,137	5.4	2.7	0.001

CI, 0.32 to 0.78; $P = .002$).[31] Despite the potential benefits from radial access in women, observational retrospective data from the National Cardiovascular Data Registry (NCDR) CathPCI registry suggest that women are still less likely to undergo radial access than men, presumptively because of ongoing concern for technical challenges involving spasm and tortuosity. These data notably suggest similar procedural success rates among women undergoing transradial PCI.[32]

Data are sparse on sex differences in vascular complications related to arterial vascular closure devices. However, subgroup analyses of a number of studies have shown that the odds of a vascular complication related to a closure device is 2 to 8 times higher in women than in men. Again, this is thought to be related to women's smaller arterial luminal diameter.[33]

Sex Differences in Lesion Subsets

Limited data exist on sex-based outcome differences for PCI by coronary lesion subsets as the primary trial and registry data for efficacy and safety of chronic total occlusions (CTOs), left main coronary disease (LM), and saphenous vein graft (SVG) interventions has historically underrepresented women. Older data indicated the possibility of higher MACEs in women undergoing PCI for CTOs, but these data were acquired between 1998 and 2007, after which techniques and understanding of CTO-PCI improved considerably.[34] More recent retrospective, single-center data demonstrate no discernable differences in procedural success and complication rates.[35] Men are much more likely to undergo CTO-PCI in published data.[34,35] Data on unprotected LM PCI of 2328 patients from the IRIS-MAIN registry demonstrated that ostial left main and ACS presentations of LM disease were more common in women, and that subsequent TVR was significantly higher in women than men (8.8% vs. 5.7%, $P < .05$). Women and men had similar frequency of the composite primary end point of all-cause death, MI, or cerebrovascular accident.[36] Sex appears to be a significant predictor of outcomes after SVG PCI. Women have higher 30-day cumulative mortality compared with men (4.4% vs. 1.9%, $P = .02$) but with notably higher incidence of vascular complications and postprocedural acute renal failure that may drive some of this effect.[37]

Sex Differences in Acute Coronary Syndrome

It is well known that the presentation, pathophysiology, diagnosis, treatment, and outcomes of ACSs differ among men and women. Although women usually present with typical symptoms of ACS, the frequency of atypical presentations of ACS is increased as

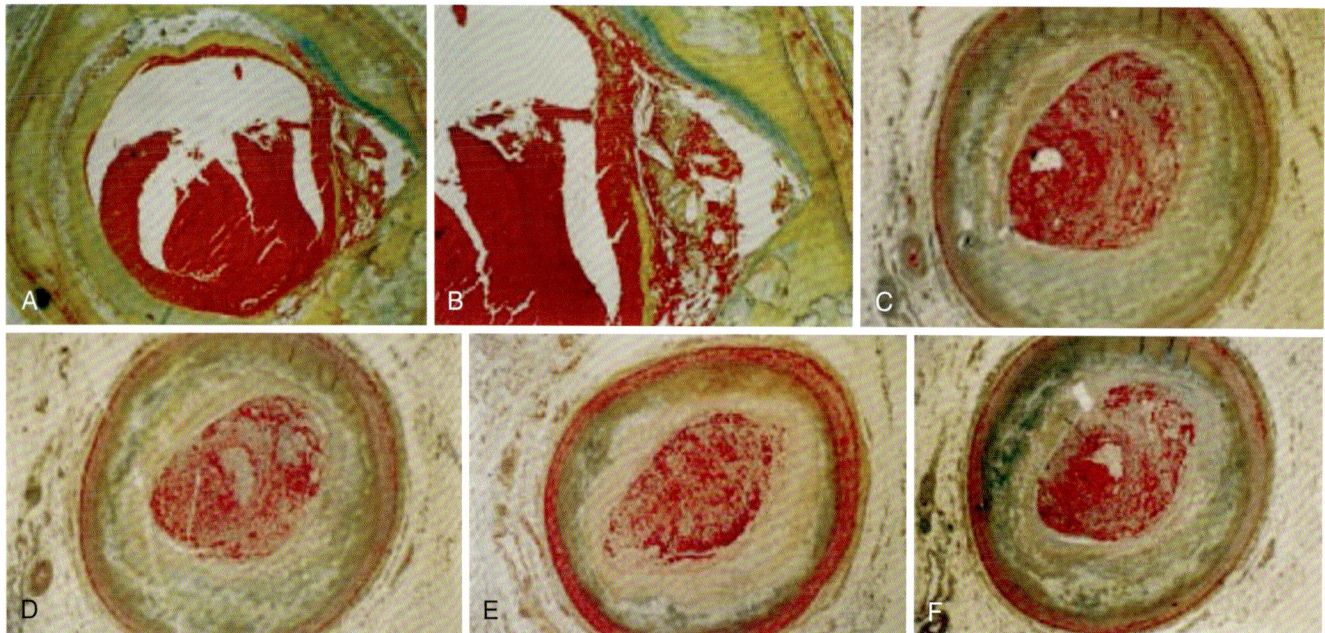

Fig. 9.1 (A and B) Plaque ulcer with hemorrhagic core. (C–F) Plaque erosion. Note the lack of continuity between the thrombus and the plaque. (From Arbustini E, Dall Bello B, Morbini P, et al. Plaque erosion is a major substrate for coronary thrombosis in acute myocardial infarction. *Heart.* 1999;82[3]:269–272.)

compared with men.[5,38,39] Women typically have higher Killip class and longer prehospital delays when presenting with ACS.[39] Women with suspected ACS are less likely than men to have obstructive or extensive epicardial coronary artery disease (CAD) and are more likely to have either a noncardiac cause or cardiac causes other than obstructive epicardial CAD.[5,39] Despite this, women with NSTE-ACS with no apparent obstructive epicardial disease still have a 2% 30-day mortality.[40] In fact, women of all ages have higher rates of in-hospital and long-term complications after NSTE-ACS than men including heart failure, cardiogenic shock, acute renal failure, recurrent MI, stroke, readmissions, and bleeding and vascular complications.[11,39,40] Data from more than 450,000 patients in the British Cardiovascular Intervention Society (BCIS) and Swedish Coronary Angiography and Angioplasty Registry (SCAAR) between 2007 and 2011 demonstrate significantly higher 30-day and 1-year mortality rates in women compared with men for both non–ST-elevation MI (NSTEMI) and STEMI. After multivariate regression, female sex was an independent predictor of all-cause mortality at 30 days and 1 year.[11] Further large registry data indicate higher in-hospital mortality for women with STEMI but not NSTEMI.[41] Women are also more likely to report preindex psychiatric symptoms including anxiety and depression.[4] Of pathobiologic interest, women who present with NSTE-ACS are more likely to have elevated C-reactive protein (CRP) and brain natriuretic peptide (BNP), whereas men are more likely to have elevated creatine kinase MB (CK-MB) and troponin.[42] Surprisingly, sex differences are apparent in acute MI plaque morphology as well. Autopsies reveal more plaque erosion than plaque rupture in women after fatal MI compared with men (Fig. 9.1A and B).[43] In addition, women appear to have more distal microvascular embolization compared with men during fatal MI.[44]

Women who present with an MI are less likely to undergo primary angioplasty within 90 minutes or to receive pharmacologic treatment on admission and are also less likely to be on evidence-based secondary prevention medical treatment upon discharge.[45–47] In numerous publications, median prehospital delays ranged from 1.8 to 7.2 hours for women versus 1.4 to 3.5 hours in men.[48] In the HORIZONS-AMI trial, symptom-onset-to-balloon time was longer, but this delay was largely driven by late arrival at the hospital.[49] Delays are partly due to the higher frequency of atypical presentations. Overall, women monitored by the National Registry of Myocardial Infarction (NRMI) were more likely than men to present without chest pain, particularly if younger. Women aged younger than 45 years were 30% more likely to present without chest pain than men of similar age.[50] This is an important discrepancy because the nature of presentation for ACS also prompts downstream diagnostic testing such as electrocardiographic (ECG) and biomarker testing, and the lack of symptoms may contribute to delays in diagnostic clarification even when women present to the hospital earlier in their course. Importantly, in studies of the most recent, high-sensitivity troponin assays, which improve diagnosis in both men and women, establishing sex-dependent thresholds doubles the diagnosis of MI in women without affecting the diagnosis rates in men.[51] Women diagnosed by these sex-specific thresholds were notably at a higher risk for death or recurrent MI at 12 months in the same study.[51].

In 2005, the Can Rapid Risk Stratification of Unstable Angina Patients Suppress Adverse Outcomes with Early Implementation of the American College of Cardiology/American Heart Association Guidelines (CRUSADE) investigators published data on sex differences in patients with NSTEMI from a large registry of more than 35,000 patients, of which 41% were women.[52] They found that women were less likely to receive guideline-based therapies such as heparin (adjusted OR, 0.91; 95% CI, 0.86 to 0.97) at presentation. Moreover, women were less likely to undergo diagnostic left heart catheterization (adjusted OR, 0.86; 95% CI, 0.82 to 0.91) or PCI (adjusted OR, 0.91; 95% CI, 0.86 to 0.96).[52] The CRUSADE registry confirms the unfortunate presence of continued treatment disparities between men and women. Another study that used the American College of Cardiology (ACC) NCDR looked at sex differences among patients with ACS (both NSTEMI and STEMI) and again showed disparities in treatment.[5] Of 199,690 patients, despite fewer high-risk criteria, the 55,691 women had greater in-hospital complications. For example, although the adjusted mortality among women and men was similar (OR, 0.97; 95% CI, 0.88 to 1.07; $P = .52$), women had higher rates of CHF (OR, 0.80; 95% CI, 0.69 to 0.92; $P = .002$), bleeding (OR, 0.55; 95% CI, 0.52 to 0.58; $P < .01$), and cardiogenic shock (OR, 0.82; 95% CI, 0.75 to 0.89; $P < .01$). Moreover, they found that women were less likely to receive aspirin (OR, 1.16; 95% CI, 1.13 to 1.20; $P < .01$) at admission and were less likely to be discharged on statins (OR, 1.10; 95% CI, 1.07 to 1.13; $P < .01$) or aspirin (OR, 1.17; 95% CI, 1.13 to 1.21; $P < .01$). Older age of female patients, symptom differences, and delay in presentation after acute MI have been suggested as possible explanations. Although these factors may explain initial treatment differences, they do not explain treatment disparities once the diagnosis has been made. These findings call for significant improvements in the care of ACS patients and highlight the importance of continued investigations into perceptual barriers that contribute to these differences.

Non–ST-Elevation Acute Coronary Syndromes

Numerous randomized trials have shown the benefit of an invasive strategy over conservative ("ischemia-guided") treatment in NSTE-ACS; however, the benefits for women in previous subgroup analyses have been less certain, and controversy exits over sex differences in revascularization benefits. A meta-analysis of eight large ACS trials that included 3075 women and 7075 men found that, similar to men, an invasive strategy was safe and effective in terms of the composite end point of death, MI, or rehospitalization (OR, 0.67; 95% CI, 0.50 to 0.88) in women who had positive biomarkers.[53] However, in women with negative biomarkers (unstable angina), an invasive strategy was associated with a trend toward higher rates of death and MI (OR, 1.35; 95% CI, 0.78 to 2.35; $P = .08$), suggesting potential harm. A more recent study of 46,455 patients in the Swedish Web-System for Enhancement and Development of Evidence-Based Care in Heart Disease Evaluated According to Recommended Therapies (SWEDEHEART) registry, which included 14,819 women—all of whom presented with NSTEMI and had positive biomarkers—showed a marked mortality reduction for both men and women treated with an invasive versus a noninvasive strategy (relative risk [RR], 0.46; 95% CI, 0.38 to 0.55).[54] However, a study of 184 women from the Fifth Organization to Assess Strategies in Acute Ischemic Syndromes (OASIS-5) trial randomized to a routine invasive strategy versus a selective invasive strategy—defined as catheterization for patients with refractory ischemia, hemodynamic instability, or new ST elevations—showed no difference in the rates of death, MI, or stroke (HR, 1.46; 95% CI, 0.73 to 2.94). A meta-analysis of 2692 women, which included this study group, showed no significant difference in the composite outcome of death or MI (OR, 1.18; 95% CI, 0.92 to 1.53) between the two treatment groups and demonstrated a trend toward higher mortality in those who received a routine invasive strategy (OR, 1.51; 95% CI, 1.00 to 2.29).[55] Overall, the 2014 ACC/American Heart Association (AHA) guidelines on NSTE-ACS specifically outline recommendations for women with NSTE-ACS and notably give a class III recommendation for an early-invasive approach in low-risk women (i.e., those with negative biomarkers) because of the lack of benefit and the possibility of harm.[40] Given the previously summarized data, the guidelines now specifically mention that women with NSTE-ACS should otherwise be managed with the same pharmacologic therapy as men and that women with high-risk features (i.e., positive troponin) should undergo an early invasive strategy (class I recommendations).

ST-Elevation Myocardial Infarction

The overall superiority of primary PCI (PPCI) over fibrinolytic therapy for women presenting with a STEMI has been demonstrated.[56] In fact, because of higher baseline comorbidities in women at presentation, the absolute benefit with PPCI is greater for women than for men.[12] An estimated 56 deaths are prevented for every 1000 women treated with PPCI compared with 42 deaths per 1000 men.[56,57] Sex-associated differences are also apparent in the amount of myocardial salvage after PPCI for STEMI, with greater salvage in women than in men.[58] This may be attributed to sex-specific tolerance of hypoxia demonstrated in a number of basic science experiments. From a historical perspective, sex-specific data regarding primary stenting versus primary balloon angioplasty in STEMI are also available. Women who presented with a STEMI benefitted from primary stenting with less reinfarction, TVR, and TLR. The Controlled Abciximab and Device Investigation to Lower Late Angioplasty Complications (CADILLAC) trial randomized 2082 patients, of whom 27% were women, to BMS versus primary balloon angioplasty with or without a glycoprotein (GP) IIb/IIIa inhibitor and found superior efficacy and safety with primary stenting, with or without abciximab, compared with balloon angioplasty.[29] In women, primary stenting resulted in a reduction in the 1-year composite of death, reinfarction, ischemia-driven TVR, or disabling stroke from 28.1% to 19.1% ($P = .01$) compared with percutaneous transluminal coronary angioplasty (PTCA) alone.

Much controversy surrounds potential differences in mortality rates between women and men after STEMI (Table 9.4). A higher in-hospital mortality is apparent among women undergoing PCI for STEMI compared with men. This is in contrast to NSTE-ACS, in which mortality differences are less apparent after adjusting for other factors. A large meta-analysis of 48 studies involving more than 100,000 patients undergoing PPCI for STEMI demonstrated significantly higher adjusted in-hospital and 30-day mortality in women compared with men at (RR 1.31, 95% CI, 1.08 to 1.65 and RR 1.19, 95% CI, 1.01 to 1.39, respectively). There was no difference in long-term mortality after adjustment.[57] A large study that used the Nationwide Inpatient Sample of 11,717 women and 24,028 men found a 5.2% in-hospital mortality rate in women compared with a 2.7% mortality rate in men. Even after adjusting for age, hypertension, institutional volume, and pulmonary disease, women had higher mortality (OR, 1.47; 95% CI, 1.23 to 1.75).[59] This has been replicated in a number of other studies.[47,60,61] However, no difference in mortality rates is apparent between the two groups at 30 days or 1 year (see Table 9.4). Of note, female sex is an independent risk factor for the development of cardiogenic shock as a complication of MI; however, no sex difference in mortality is apparent for patients with cardiogenic shock after adjustment for age. Thus the ACC/AHA STEMI guidelines recommend PCI or CABG for patients younger than 75 years who are in cardiogenic shock and have lesions amenable to revascularization regardless of sex.[40,62]

SEX DIFFERENCES IN ADJUNCTIVE PHARMACOTHERAPY

Antiplatelet Therapy

Various forms of antiplatelet therapy are recommended as first-line treatment of CAD in patients of both sexes. Variability in sex-specific responses and outcomes from these therapies exists.

Aspirin

Aspirin remains the mainstay of antiplatelet therapy in patients with CAD. It acts by irreversibly inactivating cyclooxygenase (COX), which causes inhibition of platelet thromboxane A2 synthesis and ultimately leads to inhibition of thromboxane-mediated platelet aggregation. Although its role in primary prevention in women is controversial, the efficacy of aspirin in secondary prevention has been well established. An early prospective primary-prevention cohort study of 87,678 healthy women aged 34 to 65 years found that 325 mg of aspirin one to six times a week was associated with a significant reduction in MI ($P = .005$).[63] However, a more recent randomized primary-prevention trial of 39,876 women who received 100 mg aspirin administered every other day found no cardiovascular risk reduction (RR, 0.91; 95% CI, 0.80 to 1.15).[64]

TABLE 9.4 Short-Term and Long-Term Percutaneous Coronary Intervention Outcomes in Patients With Myocardial Infarction by Sex

PCI-MI Studies	Women/Men (N)	Women (%)	Men (%)	Adjusted Rates OR (95% CI)
WATANABE ET AL.[59]				
In-hospital death	11,717/ 24,028	5.2	2.7	1.47 (1.23–1.75)
VAKILI ET AL.[60]				
In-hospital death	317/727	7.9	2.3	2.69 (1.4–5.2)
MEHILI ET AL.[15]				
30-Day death	502/1,435	8.4	8.5	—
1-Year death		13.8	12.9	0.65 (0.49–0.87)
LANSKY ET AL.[18]				
30-Day death	562/1,520	4.6	1.1	—
1-Year death		7.6	3.0	1.11 (0.53–2.36)
KUNADIAN ET AL.[11]				
30-Day death	1,861/3,482	3.8	2.6	1.46 (1.38–1.54)
1-Year death	3,938/7,448	8.1	5.6	1.44 (1.38–1.50)
BAVISHI ET AL.[57]				
30-Day death	3,072/1,861	7.1	4.3	1.19 (1.01–1.39)
1-Year death	4,391/4,132	8.5	8.0	1.01 (0.93–1.11)
HEER ET AL.[41]				
In-hospital death (STEMI)	9,156/23,830	6.3	3.6	1.19 (1.06–1.33)
In-hospital MACE (STEMI)	9,156/23,830	6.6	3.8	1.19 (1.07–1.34)
In-hospital death (NSTEMI)	14,336/33,879	2.4	1.8	1.02 (0.89–1.16)
In-hospital MACE (NSTEMI)	14,336/33,879	2.7	2.0	1.04 (0.91–1.18)

CI, Confidence interval; *MACE*, major adverse cardiac event; *MI*, myocardial infarction; *NSTEMI*, non–ST-elevation MI; *STEMI*, ST-elevation MI; *OR*, odds ratio; *PCI*, percutaneous coronary intervention.

However, aspirin did reduce the risk of ischemic stroke by 24%, and a subgroup analysis of women older than age 65 showed a consistent cardiovascular risk reduction with aspirin. A meta-analysis of six randomized controlled trials of primary prevention in 51,342 women and 44,144 men demonstrated sex-specific benefits. In women, aspirin decreased the rate of ischemic stroke (OR, 0.76; 95% CI, 0.63 to 0.93; $P = .0008$) but showed no benefit in reducing MI. In contrast, men had a reduction in MI (OR, 0.68; 95% CI, 0.54 to 0.86; $P = .001$), but no significant reduction in the incidence of stroke was observed.[65] The treatment variability has been attributed to baseline clinical differences and to unique sex-specific responses to aspirin therapy. Both men and women showed similar platelet inhibition in the COX-1 direct pathway after aspirin therapy. In aggregation assays that were indirectly dependent on the COX-1 pathway, compared with men, women had a modest increase in platelet reactivity after aspirin therapy.[66]

Aspirin resistance appears to be more common in women than in men. A study of 326 patients with CVD assessed the prevalence and clinical significance of aspirin resistance by optical platelet aggregation.[67] Of these patients, 17 were *aspirin resistant*, defined as having a mean platelet aggregation of 70% or more with 10 μM adenosine diphosphate (ADP) and 20% or greater with 0.5 mg/mL arachidonic acid. Women were more likely to be aspirin resistant. The much larger Heart Outcome Prevention Evaluation (HOPE) trial assessed the relationship between aspirin resistance and the risk of adverse cardiovascular outcomes.[68] Patients in the study had a history of CAD, stroke, peripheral vascular disease, or diabetes, in addition to at least one other cardiovascular risk factor. Aspirin resistance was determined by measuring urinary levels of 11-dehydro-thromboxane B2 (TXB2), a stable metabolite of thromboxane A2. Higher baseline urinary levels of 11-dehydro-TXB2 were associated with increased MI, stroke, and CVD mortality rates ($P = .01$). Female sex was independently associated with higher baseline levels of 11-dehydro-TXB2 level, indicating that women may be more aspirin resistant ($P = .0004$).

Despite these data, aspirin for secondary prevention in women has been well established, making underuse of aspirin in this group concerning. In a large secondary prevention trial in women, only 83% of those with established CAD or CVD received aspirin therapy.[69] Even among patients with unstable angina, women were less likely to receive aspirin therapy. These findings are replicated in large registries and speak to the treatment gap that still exists in practice.[70] Despite advances with proven medical therapy after PCI, aspirin, angiotensin-converting enzyme inhibitors (ACEi), β-blockers, and statins continue to be underused in all patients, particularly women.[70]

P2Y$_{12}$ Inhibitors

P2Y$_{12}$ inhibitors work by preventing activation of the P2Y$_{12}$ receptor, which promotes platelet aggregation. When given in addition to aspirin, these agents reduce the rates of subacute stent thrombosis after stent implantation. The PCI-Clopidogrel in Unstable Angina to Prevent Recurrent Events (CURE) study enrolled 2658 ACS patients treated with PCI, of whom 30.2% were women, and assigned them to either long-term or short-term clopidogrel plus aspirin. They found that clopidogrel for up to 12 months was superior to aspirin alone.[71] A trend toward benefit was seen in women (RR, 0.77; 95% CI, 0.52 to 1.15) compared with the statistically significant benefit seen in men (RR, 0.65; 95% CI, 0.48 to 0.87). In the Clopidogrel for Reduction of Events During Observation (CREDO) trial, 2116 patients were enrolled, of whom 29% were women, and long-term treatment with clopidogrel for up to 12 months after elective PCI compared with short-term clopidogrel was associated with a 27% RR reduction in the primary end point of death, MI, or stroke.[72] In women, a 32% RR reduction in the primary end point was reported; however, it did not reach statistical significance (RR reduction, 32.1%; 95% CI, 58.9 to 12.1). No sex-specific data are available with regard to clopidogrel loading dose. In the Intracoronary Stenting and Antithrombotic Regimen Rapid Early Action for Coronary Treatment (ISAR-REACT) trial, which enrolled 2159 low-risk patients for PCI pretreated with 600 mg of clopidogrel and assigned to either abciximab or placebo, no additional benefit to GP IIb/IIIa inhibition was found.[73] In this study, women composed 24% of the population. Patients with ACS, insulin-dependent diabetes, and other high-risk criteria were excluded from this trial. Death, MI, and TVR at 30 days did not differ between the abciximab and placebo groups in either the entire population (4.0% vs. 4.0%, P = nonsignificant [NS]) or in the female subset (3.0% vs. 3.0%, P = NS).

Data for the new $P2Y_{12}$ inhibitors, such as prasugrel and ticagrelor, also suggest similar efficacy in both men and women. In the Platelet Inhibition and Patient Outcomes (PLATO) trial, women appeared to have a similar benefit as men when comparing ticagrelor with clopidogrel in terms of the primary composite end point of cardiovascular death, MI, and stroke in women (11.2% vs. 13.2% [adjusted HR, 0.88; 95% CI, 0.74 to 1.06]) and in men (9.4% vs. 11.1% [adjusted HR, 0.86; 95% CI, 0.76 to 0.97]).[74] A benefit was also seen in terms of all-cause death in women (5.8% vs. 6.8% [adjusted HR, 0.90; 95% CI, 0.69 to 1.16]) and in men (4.0% vs. 5.7% [adjusted HR, 0.80; 95% CI, 0.67 to 0.96]) and definite stent thrombosis in women (1.2% vs. 1.4% [adjusted HR, 0.71; 95% CI, 0.36 to 1.38]) and in men (1.4% vs. 2.1% [adjusted HR, 0.63; 95% CI, 0.45 to 0.89]). No sex-specific difference was found in bleeding complications between women (adjusted HR, 1.01; 95% CI, 0.83 to 1.23) and men (adjusted HR, 1.10; 95% CI, 0.98 to 1.24).[74] In the Trial to Assess Therapeutic Outcomes by Optimizing Platelet Inhibition with Prasugrel–Thrombolysis in Myocardial Infarction (TRITON-TIMI) 38 trial, prasugrel was compared with clopidogrel in the management of patients who present with MI. A significant benefit of prasugrel over clopidogrel was seen in both men and women in terms of the combined primary end point of cardiovascular death, nonfatal MI, and nonfatal stroke.[75] A sex-specific meta-analysis of novel, potent $P2Y_{12}$ inhibitor trials (ticagrelor, prasugrel, and intravenous [IV] cangrelor) involving 14,494 women and 63,346 men demonstrated similar efficacy and safety (bleeding) between men and women.[76]

Glycoprotein IIb/IIIa Inhibitors

GP IIb/IIIa inhibitors prevent the interplatelet bridging mediated by fibrinogen. Many of the trials that show the efficacy of these drugs were performed prior to the development of the $P2Y_{12}$ agents.[26] With the advent of dual-antiplatelet therapy (DAPT) with aspirin and $P2Y_{12}$ inhibitors, the routine use of GP IIb/IIIa inhibitors in ACS has largely fallen out of favor given the excess bleeding risk and the lack of substantial benefit from triple-antiplatelet therapy. However, such therapies are still used in the modern era in certain high-risk patients. Even though GP IIb/IIIa inhibitors are associated with higher rates of both minor and major bleeding in women compared with men, the benefit derived is similar between the two groups.[26] The CRUSADE registry not only showed excess bleeding for women in the trial overall but also for women treated with a GP IIb/IIIa inhibitor (15.7% vs. 7.3%, P < .0001).[77] It also identified women as a vulnerable group more susceptible to excess dosing; therefore caution should be used when administering these agents to female patients.

Antithrombin Agents

Unfractionated Heparin

Unfractionated heparin (UFH) has long been used as the main anticoagulation therapy in PCI. In the early days of PCI, empiric heparin dosing was used. However, activated clotting time (ACT) levels after a fixed dose of UFH vary substantially because of differences in body size, concomitant use of other medications, and increased heparin resistance in ACS. Weight-based dosing is particularly essential in women given their higher risk of bleeding.[12] A weight-adjusted heparin dosing of 70 to 100 U/kg should be given to achieve an ACT of 250 to 300 seconds with the HemoTec device and 300 to 350 seconds with the Hemochron device.[78] The UFH bolus should be reduced to 50 to 70 U/kg when GP IIb/IIIa inhibitors are given, to achieve a target ACT of 200 seconds with either the HemoTec device or the Hemochron device.

Low-Molecular-Weight Heparin

The efficacy and safety of enoxaparin, a low-molecular-weight heparin (LMWH), in patients with an ACS undergoing PCI has been studied in two noninferiority trials.[79,80] The Aggrastat to Zocor (A-to-Z) study enrolled 3987 patients (29% women) and the Superior Yield of the New Strategy of Enoxaparin Revascularization and Glycoprotein IIb/IIIa Inhibitors (SYNERGY) study enrolled 9978 patients (34% women) and found no statistical benefit of enoxaparin over standard UFH in PCI. In the A-to-Z trial, no statistically significant difference was found in the primary composite end point of death, MI, or refractory ischemia in women treated with enoxaparin versus UFH.[79] In the SYNERGY trial, patients with ACS who were treated with an early invasive strategy were given either enoxaparin or UFH. At 30 days, no statistically significant difference in death or MI was found in women treated with enoxaparin versus UFH (13.5% vs. 12.9%, P = .59).[80] Some evidence suggests that LMWH causes more bleeding than UFH in women, but no difference is apparent in bleeding risk in men versus women treated with LMWH.

Direct Thrombin Inhibitors

The direct thrombin inhibitor bivalirudin has emerged as an alternative antithrombotic therapy during PCI. The Randomized Evaluation in PCI Linking Angiomax to Reduced Clinical Events (REPLACE-2) trial enrolled 6010 patients, of whom 1537 were women, and demonstrated that bivalirudin with a provisional GP IIb/IIIa inhibitor was equivalent to heparin and GP IIb/IIIa inhibition with regard to MACEs and was associated with less bleeding among patients undergoing PCI.[81] In a prospective analysis of sex, no difference was seen in the individual or composite end point of death, MI, or urgent revascularization at 30 days or 6 months between men and women with bivalirudin or heparin and a GP IIb/IIIa inhibitor.[27] No statistically significant difference was found in the composite of death, MI, or urgent revascularization at 30 days in women treated with heparin and a GP IIb/IIIa inhibitor versus bivalirudin (7.5% vs. 6.7%, P = .58). Major bleeding occurred in 5.9% of women in the heparin and GP IIb/IIIa inhibitor arm compared with 3.7% in the bivalirudin group (P = .04). Similarly, a decrease in minor bleeding (28.2% vs. 16.0%, P < .001) and access-site bleeding was reported with bivalirudin (4.1% vs. 1.6%, P = .003). Thus for female patients undergoing PCI, as in male patients, bivalirudin appears to provide lower bleeding events compared with heparin and a GP IIb/IIIa inhibitor.

Other Adjuvant Pharmacotherapy and Post–Acute Coronary Syndrome Treatments

As mentioned, variability exists in the post-ACS management of patients with regard to secondary prevention pharmacotherapy. Data from the HORIZONS-AMI trial and CRUSADE demonstrate that women are less likely to be discharged on guideline-based medical therapies such as aspirin (adjusted OR, 0.91; 95% CI, 0.85 to 0.98), ACEi (adjusted OR, 0.93; 95% CI, 0.88 to 0.98), and statins (adjusted OR, 0.92; 95% CI, 0.88 to 0.98).[49,52] Again, this is despite evidence that women derive the same benefit from

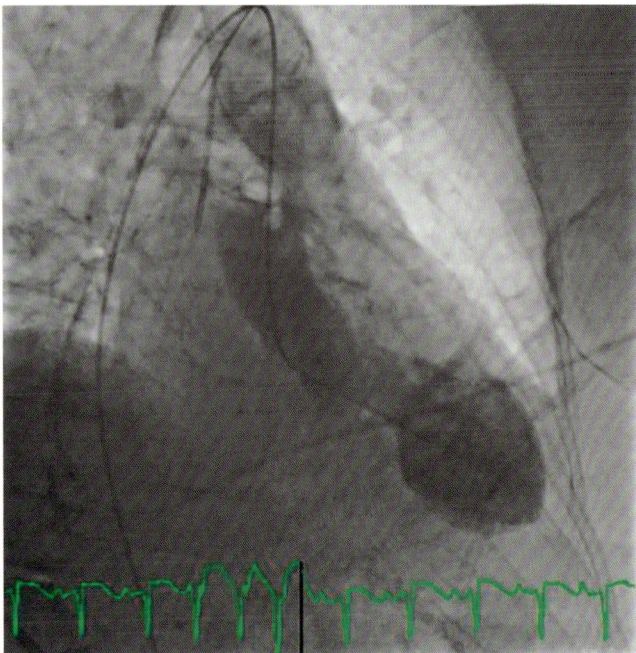

Fig. 9.2 Left ventriculogram of classic form of stress cardiomyopathy demonstrating "apical ballooning" with apical hypokinesis and basilar hyperkinesis.

these medications as men do. This is supported further by a subsequent study on Medicare Part D claims that found that women diagnosed with acute MI were less likely to be on active ACEi, angiotensin receptor blockers, β-blocker, and statin therapy at discharge and in follow-up.[82]

Sex-Specific Causes of Acute Coronary Syndromes

Stress Cardiomyopathy

Stress cardiomyopathy (SC), also known as takotsubo cardiomyopathy, apical ballooning syndrome, stress-induced cardiomyopathy, or "broken-heart" syndrome, is a unique, increasingly recognized form of transient, often severe, regional systolic left ventricular dysfunction that mimics an ACS and disproportionally affects postmenopausal women.[83–85] Commonly associated with sudden emotional or physical stress, patients typically present with clinical signs and symptoms of ACS (including severe chest discomfort and ST elevations on electrocardiograph) but have no demonstrable epicardial CAD culprits. The syndrome, initially reported in 1991 in Japan, is named after the round-bottomed and narrow-necked octopus trap that resembles the classic morphologic appearance of apical ballooning/akinesis and basal hypercontractility seen on left ventriculography (Fig. 9.2). Although there are morphologic variants, imaging characteristically demonstrates regional wall-motion abnormalities extending outside the perfusion territories of single epicardial vessels, and angiography subsequently shows no correlative obstructive epicardial disease.

The diagnostic criteria of SC require (1) transient hypokinesis, akinesis, or dyskinesis in the left ventricular midsegments with or without apical involvement; regional wall motion abnormalities that extend beyond a single epicardial vascular distribution; and frequently, but not always, a stressful trigger; (2) the absence of obstructive coronary disease or angiographic evidence of acute plaque rupture; (3) new ECG abnormalities (ST-segment elevation and/or T-wave inversion) or modest elevation in cardiac troponin; and (4) the absence of pheochromocytoma and myocarditis.[85] SC accounts for 1% to 2% of presentations of ACS, and among confirmed cases, nearly 89.9% are women at a mean age of 66.4 years.[86] The reason for a disproportionate involvement of postmenopausal women is unknown, but hormonal changes have been implicated, given that estrogen deficiency appears to attenuate the levels of cardioprotective substances in the body that in part regulate catecholamine surges. Estrogen deficiency may also increase the level of oxidative stress.[87]

The pathophysiology of SC is also unclear. Suggested etiologies have included multivessel epicardial coronary spasm or spontaneously resolved plaque rupture results in stunned myocardium. However, as mentioned, the regional distribution of wall motion abnormality is often out of proportion to the level of cardiac enzyme elevation observed, and in the case of plaque rupture, it is frequently inconsistent with a single coronary vessel.[87] A catecholamine surge causing myocardial and neurogenic stunning is likely involved.[88] Microvascular dysfunction has also been identified in a number of patients with this condition, but it is difficult to establish a causal relationship given that apical ballooning can result in microvascular dysfunction.[87] Complications can include cardiogenic shock, dynamic left-ventricular outflow tract obstruction, left ventricular thrombus and stroke, and, rarely, ventricular arrhythmias. Given that left ventricular dysfunction frequently resolves spontaneously within several weeks and recurrence is exceedingly rare, there is no standardized treatment for this condition.[86] There are no clear indications or evidence for other standard ACS therapies, such as aspirin and heparin, given the unclear mechanism of SC.

Spontaneous Coronary Artery Dissection

Spontaneous coronary artery dissection (SCAD) is an increasingly recognized cause of ACS identified predominantly in young (mean age, 30 to 45 years), healthy females. Nontraumatic dissection and separation of the coronary intimal or medial vessel layers or rupture and bleeding of the vasa vasorum can lead to intramural hematoma formation, which can ultimately result in various degrees of coronary occlusion.[89,90] The mid to distal vessel is most often involved. The possibility of SCAD should be raised in patients who present with ACS with features of (1) age younger than 50 years, (2) absence of traditional cardiovascular risk factors, (3) little or no typical atherosclerotic changes on angiography, (4) peripartum state, (5) history of fibromuscular dysplasia (FMD) or a connective tissue disorder, or (6) recent intensive exercise or emotional stress.[91] Approximately half of the patients in one series presented with STEMI, with the majority of the rest presenting with an NSTEMI.[90] Saw and colleagues[91] have classified SCAD into three types: *type 1* shows evident arterial wall staining; *type 2* shows diffuse stenosis of varying severity; and *type 3* mimics atherosclerosis. If the patient's presentation is clinically and angiographically consistent with type 1 SCAD, no further confirmatory test is necessary. If type 2 or type 3 SCAD is suspected, intravascular ultrasound (IVUS) or optical coherence tomography (OCT) can be used to better evaluate the vessel (Fig. 9.3).[89,91]

Although conservative management and CABG have resulted in minimal in-hospital morbidity, PCI has been complicated by technical failure in up to 35% of patients.[90] Experts currently recommend conservative management with standard ACS therapies. However, caution must be exercised with antithrombotic agents; although they can decrease thrombus burden, the risk of bleeding into the subintimal space is increased. If patients experience recurrent or ongoing ischemia despite conservative management, revascularization or referral for CABG may become necessary. OCT or IVUS should be considered to ensure proper stent alignment and positioning. Although the mortality rate is relatively low (95% survival at 2 years), the estimated risk of recurrent

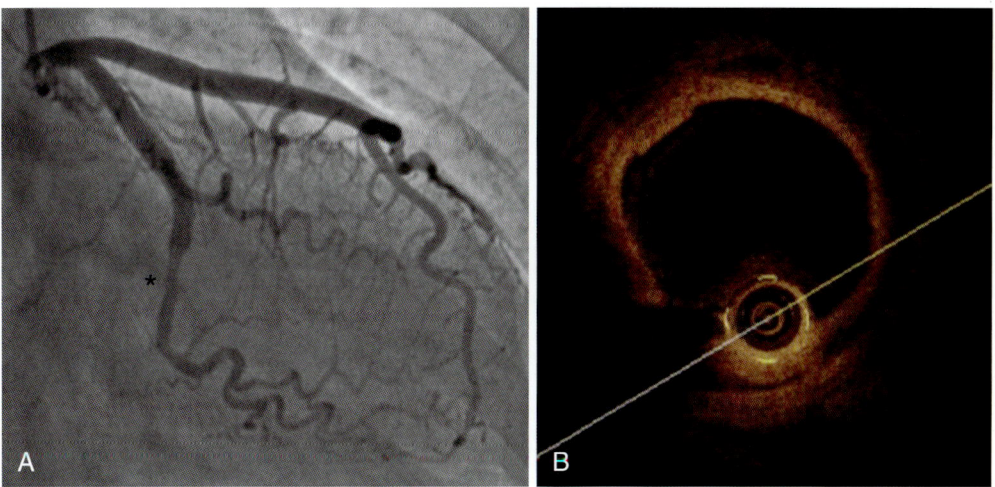

Fig. 9.3 (A and B) Coronary angiogram shows mild stenosis of the mid circumflex artery by spontaneous coronary artery dissection with intramural hematoma on optical coherence tomography. (From Saw J. Spontaneous coronary artery dissection. *Can J Cardiol*. 2013;29[9]:1027–1033. Image courtesy Dr. Deborah Kwon.)

SCAD at 10 years is approximately 30%.[89,91] Of interest, a sizeable number of SCAD patients have coexisting FMD, a nonatherosclerotic, noninflammatory vascular condition that can affect any vascular bed in the body, although a predilection for the renal and carotid arteries is apparent (Fig. 9.4). FMD disproportionately affects women and is seen almost exclusively in the female subset of patients with SCAD.[92] Imaging of the carotid and renal arteries of SCAD patients has revealed a number of cases of FMD[92]; therefore if a diagnosis of SCAD is made, patients should also be evaluated for FMD.

Microvascular Angina

The terms "microvascular angina," "cardiac syndrome X," and "chest pain with normal coronary arteries" have historically been used interchangeably in literature. Microvascular angina is a specific subset of chest pain with normal coronary arteries in which patients have anginal symptoms or evidence of myocardial ischemia with demonstration of coronary microvascular dysfunction and no significant angiographic evidence of obstructive atherosclerosis.[93] The condition is most commonly seen in perimenopausal and postmenopausal women younger than those who classically present with CVD and is often characterized by lingering, dull chest pain after exertion. Given the ECG changes commonly seen, the condition is thought to be caused by ischemia of the microvascular bed.[94] Microvascular dysfunction caused by insulin resistance, abnormal vasoconstriction and impaired vasodilation of the microvascular bed, increased systemic inflammation, and abnormal pain response have all been cited as potentially contributing to the etiology of microvascular angina.[93] Estrogen deficiency may play a central role in the significantly increased burden of microvascular disease seen in women. Some studies suggest relief of symptoms in women who receive hormone therapy (HT), although concerns for adverse cardiovascular outcomes in women who receive HT have limited further investigation. Studies have also shown worse cardiovascular outcomes, higher angina-related hospitalization rates, and repeat heart catheterizations in women with microvascular angina.[95] The diagnosis must be made by indirect means because no safe and minimally invasive technique exists by which to directly observe the microvasculature given that current coronary angiography techniques cannot visualize vessels smaller than 0.5 mm.[96] Because the coronary microvasculature controls total coronary resistance and therefore regulates myocardial blood flow, measuring myocardial blood flow at

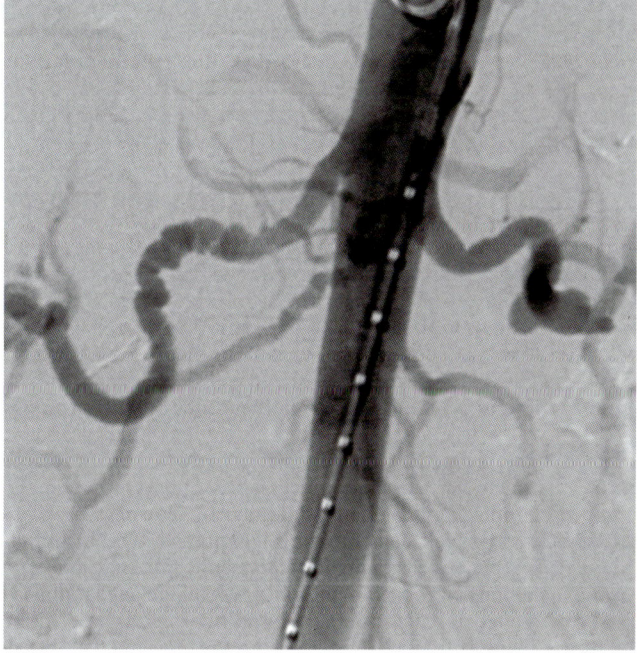

Fig. 9.4 Fibromuscular dysplasia of the renal arteries. (From Naderi S, Cho LS. Cardiovascular disease in women: prevention, symptoms, diagnosis, pathogenesis. *Cleve Clin J Med*. 2013;80[9]:577–587. Image courtesy Dr. Heather Gornik.)

maximum vasodilation via coronary flow reserve (CFR) can indirectly evaluate the degree of microvascular dysfunction.[97] CFR can be measured by invasive means in the catheterization lab after maximum hyperemia is induced by adenosine or another such vasodilatory agent.[98] It should be noted that CFR measurements performed in this invasive manner are greatly affected by hemodynamic changes and can have poor reproducibility.[97] In terms of noninvasive imaging, perfusion magnetic resonance imaging (MRI) or positron emission tomography (PET) is often performed (Fig. 9.5). Once a diagnosis has been made, lifestyle modification, antianginal agents, ACEi, and statins have been suggested for therapy.[96] Pain management techniques are also suggested given the increased pain sensitivity observed in women with this condition. More recently, ranolazine has shown promise in small groups of patients with this condition.[98]

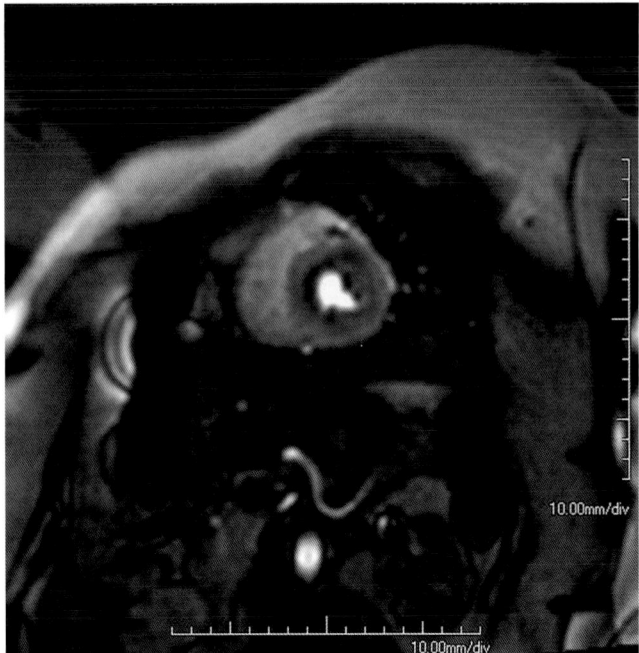

Fig. 9.5 Magnetic resonance imaging of a patient with microvascular disease. (From Naderi S, Cho LS. Cardiovascular disease in women: prevention, symptoms, diagnosis, pathogenesis. *Cleve Clin J Med.* 2013;80[9]:577–587. Image courtesy Dr. Deborah Kwon.)

SEX DIFFERENCES IN STRUCTURAL INTERVENTIONAL PROCEDURES

Given the very recent growth in the development of structural interventional procedure techniques, long-term data regarding sex-based differences in the outcomes are limited to small observational studies and subgroup analysis. Based on longitudinal data from the Transcatheter Valve Therapy (TVT) Registry, female patients undergoing transcatheter aortic valve replacement (TAVR) have a different risk profile compared with male patients, including older age, lower prevalence of CAD, atrial fibrillation, and diabetes melitus, a higher rate of porcelain aorta, worse renal function, and higher mean STS score (9.0% vs. 8.0%).[99] Women more commonly have alternative access (nontransfemoral; 45% vs. 34% in men), and had higher in-hospital vascular complications, with a trend towards higher bleeding (HR 1.19, CI, 0.99 to 1.44; P =.06). Despite these differences, 1-year mortality was significantly lower (21.3% vs. 24.5%; HR 073; CI, 0.63 to 0.85).

A meta-analysis of seven studies found that mortality, acute device success rates (mitral regurgitation reduction), and complications rates following transcatheter edge-to-edge mitral valve repair (TMVr) with MitraClip are similar for men and women. Men were more likely to report New York Heart Association class III or IV symptoms at 12 months and were more likely to require more than 1 clip.[100]

SEX DIFFERENCES IN PERIPHERAL INTERVENTIONAL PROCEDURES

Women suffer the consequences of peripheral arterial disease (PAD) at rates at least as high as those in men, but as with CAD, the effect of sex on PAD presentation, diagnostic testing, and outcomes has been historically understudied. Although the age-dependent prevalence of PAD in adult women is lower than for men, the total population burden appears to be higher in limited age-specific PAD prevalence studies.[101] Mortality and MACEs by sex also have not been well defined, but a trend exists that suggests higher event rates for women than for men when ankle-brachial index is less than 0.90 or greater than 1.40.[101,102] Parallel to CAD, asymptomatic or atypically symptomatic PAD is more common in women than men.[103] Women with PAD also have greater functional impairment than men with PAD and yet may be less likely to undergo lower extremity surgical revascularization than men.[104,105] However, associations between female sex and adverse outcomes with PAD revascularization (surgical and endovascular) are limited and likely confounded by age, comorbidity, and anatomic factors.[101]

RACE AND ETHNICITY

Currently, ethnic and racial minorities make up 37.8% of the U.S. population, and this is projected to increase to 47.5% of the population by 2050. Studies regarding race and ethnicity in medicine are fraught with difficulties, but numerous studies suggest disparities in cardiovascular care and outcomes.

Disparities in Coronary Artery Disease

Heart disease is the leading cause of death for all racial and ethnic groups in the U.S. population. African Americans, despite having an overall lower prevalence of CVD than whites, have the highest heart disease–related mortality, with a rate that is 1.6 times that of their white counterparts (Table 9.5).[1] Furthermore, disease onset is typically 5 years earlier in African Americans. Research indicates increasing rates of ischemic heart disease in other minority groups, namely Asian, Hispanic, and Native Americans.[106] Paradoxically, Hispanics, despite an increased burden of CVD risk factors and overall greater socioeconomic disadvantage, are less likely to have CVD and less likely to die from heart disease compared with nonHispanic whites.[106] The presence of obstructive epicardial CAD on angiography is seen less often in African Americans than in whites. Paradoxically, the prevalence of complications from atherosclerosis is greater in African Americans despite a lower incidence of obstructive CAD. This is most likely due to increased rates of hypertension, diabetes, and smoking and not to inherent differences in the pathophysiology of CAD.[106] The MESA cohort on coronary artery calcium (CAC) scores has produced many studies involving race and CAC scores and has noted that whites of both sexes consistently have higher likelihoods of detecting coronary calcium than other racial or ethnic minorities.[107] Of note, data from the National Health and Nutrition Examination survey showed that African Americans have a higher prevalence of PAD than their white counterparts (adjusted OR, 2.39; 95% CI, 1.11 to 5.12).[108] This finding was confirmed by the Genetic Epidemiology of Network Angiopathy (GENOA) study, which showed that this difference persisted in African American men and women despite adjusting for risk factors (adjusted OR was 4.7 [95% CI, 1.4 to 16] for African American men, and it was 2.2 [95% CI, 1.2 to 4.2] for African American women).[109]

Characteristics of Racial and Ethnic Minorities Undergoing Intervention

See Table 9.6.

African American patients undergoing PCI are younger, are more likely to be female, and have more comorbidities—such as hypertension, diabetes, and chronic renal insufficiency—than their white counterparts. They are more likely to undergo urgent, rather than elective, PCI, although immediate procedural success and short-term rates of death and MI appear similar between African and white Americans.[110,111] However, some have reported lower long-term survival after PCI in African Americans. In a large PCI registry, adjusted mortality rate was increased among African Americans at 2 years (OR, 1.87; 95% CI, 1.15 to 3.04),[112] findings consistent with another large, single-center PCI registry (OR,

TABLE 9.5 Cardiovascular Disease in the United States: American Heart Association 2017 Heart and Stroke Statistics

	Total	White Male	White Female	African American Male	African American Female	Hispanic Male	Hispanic Female
Prevalence	81.1 M	38.1%	34.4%	44.6%	46.9%	28.5%	34.5%
Mortality	831 K	340 K	372 K	47.9 K	50.9 K	—	—

M, Million; *K,* thousand.
From Writing Group Members. Heart disease and stroke statistics—2017 update: a report from the American Heart Association. *Circulation.* 2010;121: e46–e215.

1.45; 95% CI, 1.14 to 1.84).[110] These findings are likely multifactorial and are potentially due to a lack of access to quality health care for African Americans. Studies have shown that, in the United States, African Americans receive fewer preventive health services and less specialist care, and physicians treating African Americans have had less rigorous clinical training.[113] Another contributing factor is the high prevalence of left ventricular hypertrophy (LVH) together with increased endothelin-1 levels in African Americans.[114] Endothelin-1, a potent vasoconstrictor, is stimulated by transforming growth factor-β (TGF-β), which is increased in African Americans with hypertension. The combination of LVH and endothelial dysfunction in conjunction with CAD may contribute to greater mortality rates. It should be noted that despite the recent interest in the field, race-specific PCI analyses are still rare.

Acute Coronary Syndrome

African-American patients who present with ACS in the United States are likely to be younger and to have hypertension, diabetes, heart failure, and renal insufficiency. They are also less likely to have insurance coverage or specialist care.[115] The investigators of CRUSADE, a large NSTEMI registry, found that African-American patients were more likely to receive older ACS treatments such as aspirin, β-blockers, or ACEi but were significantly less likely to receive what was then considered newer ACS therapies such as GP IIb/IIIa inhibitors, clopidogrel, and statin therapy.[115] In addition, African Americans were less likely to receive cardiac catheterization, revascularization, or smoking-cessation counseling. In-hospital death and postadmission MI were similar between African American and white patients in the United States (adjusted OR, 0.92; 95% CI, 0.81 to 1.05), consistent with findings from the NRMI.[47] These data hold true when looking specifically at patients who present with a STEMI, and African Americans are less likely to undergo cardiac catheterization and revascularization following a STEMI.[116,117] The NRMI found that racial and ethnic minorities tended to be younger at presentation, and insurance status differed significantly among the groups studied.[116] They found that door-to-drug time and door-to-balloon time were significantly longer for minority patients. This finding persisted even after adjusting for age, sex, insurance status, clinical characteristics, time of arrival, time since symptom onset, and hospital characteristics. In the fully adjusted model, door-to-balloon time was 8.7 minutes longer in African Americans compared with whites ($P < .001$) and 3.7 minutes longer for Hispanics compared with whites ($P = .002$).[116] Similarly, a fully adjusted model of door-to-drug time showed a 5.1-minute increase in African Americans ($P < .001$), a 1.3-minute increase in Hispanic Americans ($P = .006$), and a 1.7-minute increase in Asian Americans ($P = .01$) compared with their white counterparts. Even though a substantial portion of the racial and ethnic disparities in time to treatment is accounted for by the hospital at which a patient is admitted, racial and ethnic treatment disparities persist despite adjusting for these factors. In a large fibrinolysis trial, the 30-day survival rates were similar between African Americans and whites, but African Americans had a higher rate of in-hospital stroke (OR, 1.75; 95% CI, 1.19 to 2.59) and more major bleeding events (OR, 1.32; 95% CI, 1.13 to 1.55).[118] According to the NRMI data, in-hospital mortality rates for STEMI patients are similar between African Americans and their white counterparts.[47] However, at 5 years, the death rate was significantly higher among African Americans despite their younger age (OR, 1.63; 95% CI, 1.41 to 1.90).[118] Several factors may explain the decreased rates of catheterization and revascularization in African Americans, and it certainly suggests that access to care may play a role, with evidence that African Americans with ACS are more likely to be treated in low-volume hospitals.[119] Although some race-specific data are available regarding differential antihypertensive medication response, to our knowledge, no such data exist on the efficacy of adjunctive PCI pharmacotherapy.

TABLE 9.6 Short-Term and Long-Term Percutaneous Coronary Intervention Outcomes in African Americans

Study	Total Patients (% African American)	Adjusted Event Rate Comparing African Americans With Whites (OR, 95% CI)
Maynard et al.[124]		
In-hospital death	24,625 (11%)	0.97 (0.83–1.12)
2-Year death		1.11 (1.05–1.17)
Leborgne et al.[125]		
1-year death	10,561 (12%)	1.35 (1.06–1.71)
Slater et al.[112]		
1-year death, MI, or CABG	4,618 (9.7%)	0.65 (0.36–1.14)
2-year death, MI, or CABG		1.47 (1.06–2.04)
Chen et al.[110]		
1-year death or MI	8,832 (8.0%)	1.45 (1.14–1.84)

CABG, Coronary artery bypass graft; *CI,* confidence interval; *MI,* myocardial infarction; *OR,* odds ratio.
Writing Group Members. Heart disease and stroke statistics—2010 update: a report from the American Heart Association. *Circulation.* 2010;121:e46–e215.

Social Aspects of Health Care Disparities

Disparities persist in health care because of complex social, political, physiologic, and genetic variation. Although it is important to note that patients from ethnic minority groups are more likely to be treated in low-volume hospitals and to refuse invasive procedures than their white counterparts, these factors do not fully account for the treatment disparities seen.[120] In reviewing more than 100 studies, the National Institute of Medicine's 2001 report[121] found that patients from minority groups are less likely to receive the needed services, compared with their white counterparts, even after accounting for issues related to access to health care. Assuming each group had similar comorbidities and access to health care, the committee considered three sets of factors as likely contributors to these treatment differences:

- Data suggest that minorities seek care later than their white counterparts and that they may refuse recommended care. It is thought that this might be due to a number of factors that include the patient's inability to relate to the provider, mistrust and poor prior interactions with the health care system, misunderstanding of instructions, and a lack of knowledge of how to use health care services. However, this does not fully explain racial and ethnic disparities and accounts for only a small proportion of the differences seen.

- Inherent stereotypes and discrimination exist in medicine, whether it is conscious or unconscious. A study of white and African American standardized patients revealed that cardiologists were more likely to refer white men and women and African American men for cardiac catheterization than African American women despite their exhibiting the same symptoms. In the report they concluded that even though a "myriad of sources contribute to these (treatment) disparities, some evidence suggests that bias, prejudice, and stereotyping on the part of the health care providers may contribute to differences in care."
- The organization and finances of the health care systems that minorities have access to have also been cited. For instance, a lack of interpretive services prevents many non–English speaking patients from adequately making decisions regarding their care. Fragmentation of health care with individuals receiving different tiers of care may also play a role. Although patients may have equal access to care, the quality of the care received may not be uniform.

To work toward eliminating disparities in care, the Institute of Medicine of the National Academies has recommended a comprehensive, multilevel strategy that includes training and educating health care providers, implementing policy and regulatory strategies that address health plans and health services, and promoting better use of clinical practice guidelines.

CONCLUSION

Much has been learned in the past few years regarding sex and racial differences in the presentation, management, and outcomes of patients with CAD. Much more remains to be learned regarding disparities in cardiovascular care, which requires ongoing research and education to bridge the divide.

KEY REFERENCES

2. Mosca L, Benjamin EJ, Berra K, et al. Effectiveness-based guidelines for the prevention of cardiovascular disease in women—2011 update: a guideline from the American Heart Association. *J Am Coll Cardiol*. 2011;57:1404–1423.
3. Hess CN, McCoy LA, Duggirala HJ, et al. Sex-based differences in outcomes after percutaneous coronary intervention for acute myocardial infarction: a report from TRANSLATE-ACS. *J Am Heart Assoc*. 2014;3:e000523.
4. Graham G. Acute coronary syndromes in women: recent treatment trends and outcomes. *Clin Med Insights Cardiol*. 2016;10:1–10.
5. Akhter N, Milford-Beland S, Roe MT, et al. Gender differences among patients with acute coronary syndromes undergoing percutaneous coronary intervention in the American College of Cardiology-National Cardiovascular Data Registry (ACC-NCDR). *Am Heart J*. 2009;157:141–148.
11. Kunadian V, Qiu WL, Lagerqvist B, et al. Gender differences in outcomes and predictors of all-cause mortality after percutaneous coronary intervention (data from United Kingdom and Sweden). *Am J Cardiol*. 2017;119:210–216.
12. Lansky AJ, Hochman JS, Ward PA, et al. Percutaneous coronary intervention and adjunctive pharmacotherapy in women—a statement for healthcare professionals from the American Heart Association. *Circulation*. 2005;111:940–953.
13. Chiu JH, Bhatt DL, Ziada KM, et al. Impact of female sex on outcome after percutaneous coronary intervention. *Am Heart J*. 2004;148:998–1002.
20. Stefanini GG, Baber U, Windecker S, et al. Safety and efficacy of drug-eluting stents in women: a patient-level pooled analysis of randomised trials. *Lancet*. 2013;382:1879–1888.
28. Ahmed B, Piper WD, Malenka D, et al. Significantly improved vascular complications among women undergoing percutaneous coronary intervention a report from the Northern New England Percutaneous Coronary Intervention Registry. *Circ Cardiovasc Inte*. 2009;2:423–429.
29. Lansky AJ, Pietras C, Costa RA, et al. Gender differences in outcomes after primary angioplasty versus primary stenting with and without abciximab for acute myocardial infarction—results of the Controlled Abciximab and Device Investigation to Lower Late Angioplasty Complications (CADILLAC) trial. *Circulation*. 2005;111:1611–1618.

 Additional references available online at expertconsult.com.

SECTION II

第二部分

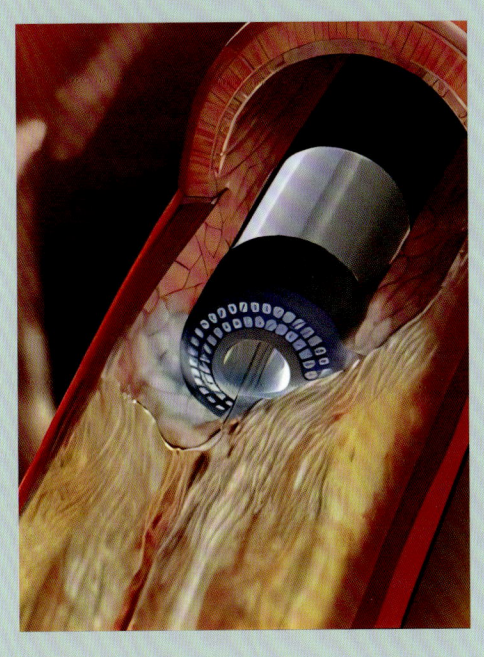

Pharmacologic Intervention

药物治疗

中文导读

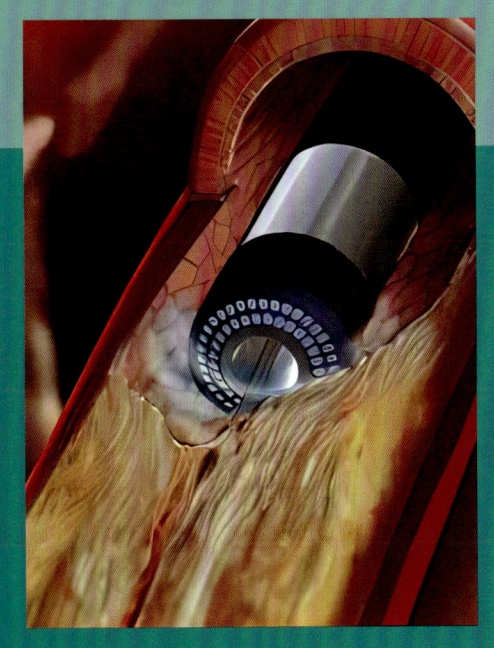

第10章
血小板抑制剂

血小板在止常止血和动脉粥样硬化性血栓性疾病的发病过程中起着关键作用。血小板在血管损伤部位提供最初的止血栓，促进病理生理性血栓形成，进而可导致心肌梗死、脑卒中和周围血管闭塞，因此，抗血小板药物是心血管疾病管理的关键和基石。理想的抗血小板治疗策略的主要目标是降低动脉粥样硬化血栓事件风险，同时不增加出血并发症尤其是大出血事件的发生。然而，由于血小板的病理和生理功能均是基于相同的机制，在临床中很难精准地去平衡抗血小板治疗的益处和潜在危害。阿司匹林联合$P2Y_{12}$受体拮抗剂的双联抗血小板治疗可改善冠状动脉支架置入术患者的预后。现在有越来越多的血小板抑制剂可用于经皮冠状动脉介入治疗围术期及术后，包括新型的噻吩并吡啶类药物，口服和静脉注射非噻吩并吡啶类药物，口服PAR-1拮抗剂——西洛他唑或静脉注射GPⅡb/Ⅲa抑制剂的三联用药，对这些药物的作用机制和试验数据的全面理解是获得最佳临床实践的必要前提。本章节介绍了阿司匹林、$P2Y_{12}$受体拮抗剂（包括噻吩并吡啶类药物中的氯吡格雷、普拉格雷，非噻吩并吡啶类药物中的替格瑞洛、坎格瑞洛）、凝血酶受体拮抗剂——沃拉帕沙、GPⅡb/Ⅲa抑制剂中的阿昔单抗和替罗非班等药物的药理作用，以及经皮冠状动脉介入治疗围术期应用的循证医学证据。通过上述内容介绍，相信读者会对现代抗血小板药物治疗形成一个全面、科学的理解，从而有助于这些药物在临床中得到合理的应用，进一步增加患者的临床净获益。

薄小雯 范 谦

章节要点

- 阿司匹林联合一种P2Y$_{12}$受体拮抗剂的双联抗血小板治疗是经皮冠状动脉介入患者的药物治疗基石。

- 噻吩并吡啶类药物，包括噻氯匹定、氯吡格雷和普拉格雷，均为P2Y$_{12}$拮抗剂的前体药物，因此需要转化为活性代谢物才能发挥抗血小板作用。这种活性代谢物不可逆地结合和拮抗血小板P2Y$_{12}$受体，以维持血小板寿命。

- 与氯吡格雷相比，普拉格雷可减少从未接受过噻氯吡啶类治疗的经皮冠状动脉介入治疗患者的缺血事件，但会增加出血风险。对于75岁以下、体重>60 kg、无卒中或短暂性脑缺血发作病史的患者，普拉格雷的临床净获益最大。对于非ST段抬高型急性冠状动脉综合征患者，与冠状动脉造影后应用普拉格雷相比，有创检查之前预先给予普拉格雷会增加大出血事件，但并未减少缺血风险。因此应避免过早启动普拉格雷治疗。

- 替格瑞洛是一种直接的、作用于可逆的非噻吩并吡啶类P2Y$_{12}$受体拮抗剂。在包括接受有创治疗的急性冠状动脉综合征患者中，替格瑞洛与氯吡格雷相比可降低缺血事件发生率和心血管死亡率。尽管替格瑞洛并不增加总体出血事件，但会使非冠状动脉旁路移植术的相关出血风险增加。

- 氯吡格雷抗血小板作用的个体差异极为显著。尽管采用氯吡格雷治疗，但血小板高反应性可识别出经皮冠状动脉介入治疗术后高缺血事件风险的患者。基于血小板功能测试采用个体化抗血小板策略，其临床获益尚未得到随机临床试验的证实。

- 一些基因多态性可降低CYP2C19酶活性，而后者是氯吡格雷转化为活性代谢物的关键。当接受氯吡格雷治疗时，与携带正常等位基因者相比，携带了可使CYP2C19酶功能降低的等位基因患者，尤其是携带有两种基因拷贝的患者（代谢不良者），其发生经皮冠状动脉介入治疗术后血栓事件的风险会更高。然而，普拉格雷或替格瑞洛的临床有效性却不受CYP2C19基因型的影响。

- 坎格瑞洛是一种经静脉使用的P2Y$_{12}$受体拮抗剂。对于从未接受过噻氯吡啶类治疗的经皮冠状动脉介入治疗患者，与传统的氯吡格雷相比，这种可快速起效和失效的P2Y$_{12}$受体拮抗剂可减少缺血事件的发生，这主要是因为来自全球定义的心肌梗死的支架内血栓事件的减少。同时，坎格瑞洛大出血并发症的发生率与安慰剂相似。

- 凝血酶是最有效的血小板激活剂，其作用主要通过PAR-1受体介导。沃拉帕沙是PAR-1拮抗剂，联合标准的抗血小板治疗，作为二级预防在既往发生过心肌梗死的患者中应用可获得净临床获益。但由于缺乏抗缺血有效性，且增加出血事件，PAR-1拮抗剂未获批准用于经皮冠状动脉介入治疗。

- 在使用P2Y$_{12}$受体抑制剂进行预处理的现状下，GPⅡb/Ⅲa抑制剂的益处似乎仅限于心脏生物标记物升高的急性冠状动脉综合征高危患者。

SECTION II Pharmacologic Intervention

10 Platelet Inhibitor Agents

Matthew J. Price, Dominick J. Angiolillo

KEY POINTS

- Dual-antiplatelet therapy (DAPT) with aspirin and a P2Y$_{12}$ receptor inhibitor is the cornerstone of therapy after percutaneous coronary intervention (PCI) with stents.
- The thienopyridines—ticlopidine, clopidogrel, and prasugrel—are P2Y$_{12}$ inhibitors that are prodrugs and therefore require conversion into an active metabolite to exert their antiplatelet effect. This active metabolite irreversibly binds and antagonizes the P2Y$_{12}$ receptor for the lifespan of the platelet.
- Compared with clopidogrel, prasugrel reduces ischemic events in thienopyridine-naïve patients undergoing PCI, but is associated with a higher risk of bleeding. Net clinical benefit is greatest in patients without a history of stroke or transient ischemic attack (TIA) who are younger than 75 years of age and weigh over 60 kg. Compared with prasugrel administered after coronary angiography, pretreatment with prasugrel in invasively managed patients with non–ST-elevation acute coronary syndrome (NSTE-ACS) increases major bleeding, does not reduce ischemia, and should be avoided.
- Ticagrelor is a direct, reversibly acting nonthienopyridine P2Y$_{12}$ antagonist. In patients with acute coronary syndrome (ACS), including those treated with an invasive strategy, ticagrelor reduced ischemic events and cardiovascular mortality compared with clopidogrel. Although overall bleeding was not increased with ticagrelor, the risk of non–coronary artery bypass grafting (CABG)-related bleeding was increased.
- Substantial interindividual variability is evident in the antiplatelet effect of clopidogrel. High on-treatment platelet reactivity despite clopidogrel therapy can identify patients at risk for ischemic events after PCI. The clinical benefit of individualized antiplatelet strategies based on platelet function testing has yet to be demonstrated in randomized clinical trials.
- Several genetic polymorphisms reduce the enzymatic activity of CYP2C19, which is critical for the conversion of clopidogrel to its active metabolite. When treated with clopidogrel, carriers of these alleles with reduced function, especially those with two copies (poor metabolizers), are at higher risk of thrombotic events after PCI compared with patients with normal alleles. The CYP2C19 genotype does not influence the clinical efficacy of prasugrel or ticagrelor.
- Cangrelor is an intravenous P2Y$_{12}$ antagonist with a rapid onset and offset of effect that reduces ischemic events compared with conventional clopidogrel therapy in thienopyridine-naïve patients undergoing PCI, driven by reductions in myocardial infarction (MI) according to the universal definition and in stent thrombosis, with major bleeding rates similar to placebo.
- The effects of thrombin, the most potent platelet activator, are mediated primarily through the protease-activated receptor 1 (PAR-1) receptor. The net clinical benefit of the PAR-1 antagonist, vorapaxar, is favorable in the setting of secondary prevention in patients with prior MI in combination with standard antiplatelet therapy but is not approved for use in the setting of PCI because of a lack of ischemic efficacy and increased bleeding.
- In the modern era of pretreatment with P2Y$_{12}$ inhibitors, the benefit of glycoprotein (GP) IIb/IIIa inhibition appears to be restricted to high-risk patients with ACS who have elevated cardiac biomarkers.

BASIC PRINCIPLES OF ANTIPLATELET THERAPY

Platelets play a critical role in normal hemostasis and in the pathogenesis of atherothrombotic disease processes. Platelets provide an initial hemostatic plug at the site of vascular injury and promote pathophysiologic thrombosis, which in turn precipitates MI, stroke, and peripheral vascular occlusion; therefore antiplatelet agents are key in cardiovascular disease management. In particular, the main goal of antiplatelet treatment strategies is to reduce the risk of recurrent atherothrombotic events without excessive bleeding complications. However, because both pathologic and physiologic functions of platelets are due to the same mechanism, it is difficult to separate therapeutic benefits from potential harmful effects.

Platelet plug formation at sites of vascular injury occurs in three stages: (1) the initiation phase involves platelet adhesion; (2) the extension phase includes activation, additional recruitment, and aggregation; and (3) the perpetuation phase is characterized by platelet stimulation and stabilization of clot.[1] Circulating platelets are quiescent under normal circumstances and do not bind to the intact endothelium. However, endothelial damage leads to the exposure of circulating platelets to the subendothelial extracellular matrix (ECM) and triggers platelet recruitment and adhesion (Fig. 10.1).[2] In the *initial phase* of primary hemostasis, the tethering of platelets at sites of vascular injury is mediated by the glycoprotein (GP) Ib-IX-V receptor complex, which binds von Willebrand factor (vWF). Subendothelial collagen exposed by damaged vessels engages platelets via GP VI and GP Ia/IIa receptors. These interactions allow the arrest and activation of adherent platelets. In the *extension phase*, additional platelets are recruited and activated via soluble agonists. These platelet-activating factors include adenosine diphosphate (ADP), thromboxane A2 (TXA$_2$), epinephrine, serotonin, collagen, and thrombin. Signaling via ADP receptors contributes to platelet activation during both protective hemostasis and pathologic thrombosis. Two ADP receptors are expressed by platelets: P2Y$_1$ couples to

SECTION II Pharmacologic Intervention

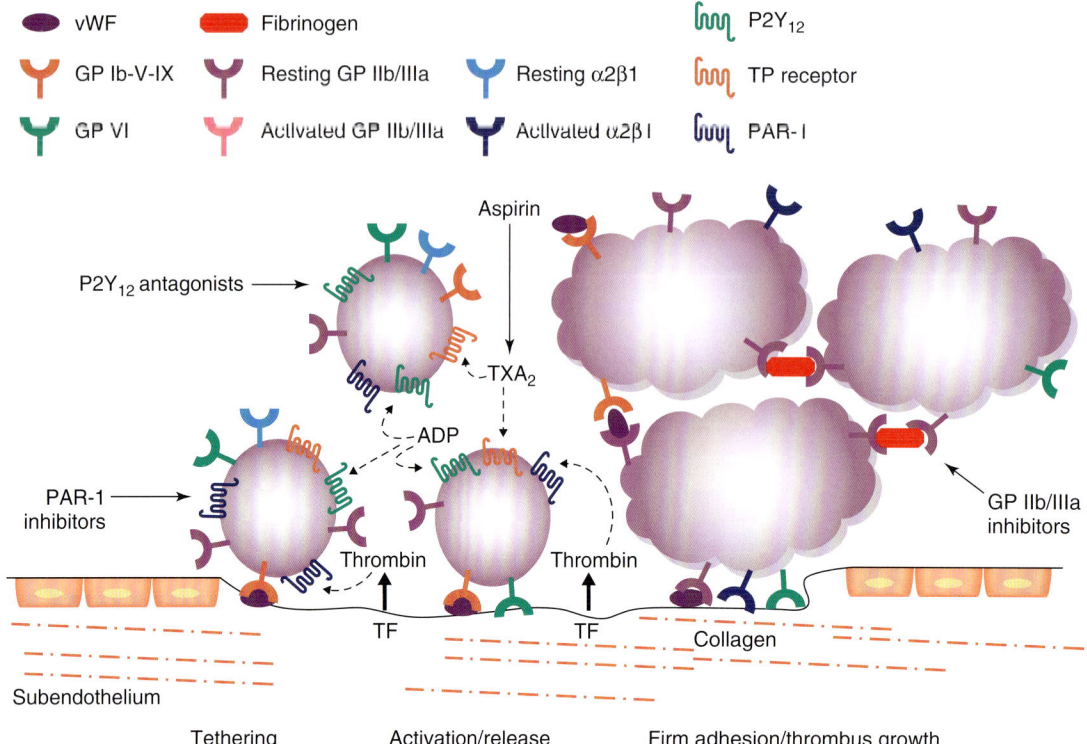

Fig. 10.1 Platelet-mediated thrombosis. The interaction between von Willebrand factor *(vWF)* and the platelet receptor glycoprotein *(GP)* Ib-V-IX mediates platelet tethering to the subendothelium at the sites of injury. GP VI binds collagen with low affinity, which triggers intracellular signals that shift platelet integrins to a high-affinity state and induce the release of the secondary mediators adenosine diphosphate *(ADP)* and thromboxane A2 *(TXA₂)*. In parallel, tissue factor *(TF)* locally triggers thrombin formation, which also contributes to platelet activation via binding to the platelet protease-activated receptor 1 *(PAR-1)*. Ultimately, the integrin GP IIb/IIIa, which is the final common pathway mediating platelet aggregation, transforms from a resting to an activated phase, which allows it to bind fibrinogen with high affinity and leads to platelet aggregates. In the perpetuation phase, the platelet-rich thrombus and coagulation cascades reinforce one another, which contributes to thrombus growth and culminates in the generation of a stable platelet-fibrin–rich plug at the sites of injury. (Adapted from Varga-Szabo D, Pleines I, Nieswandt B. Cell adhesion mechanisms in platelets. *Arterioscler Thromb Vasc Biol.* 2008;28:403–412.)

Gαq and contributes to initial aggregation, and $P2Y_{12}$ couples to $Gα_{12}$ and decreases cyclic adenosine monophosphate (cAMP), stabilizing the platelet aggregate.[3] $P2Y_{12}$ receptor signaling also stimulates surface expression of P-selectin and secretion of TXA_2, which is produced de novo and, like ADP, is released from adherent platelets. Generated from arachidonic acid through conversion by cyclooxygenase 1 (COX-1) and thromboxane synthase, TXA_2 binds platelet receptors TPα and TPβ; however, its effects in platelets are mediated primarily through TPα. ADP and TXA_2 are secreted from adherent platelets, contribute to the recruitment of circulating platelets, and promote alterations in platelet shape and granule secretion; thus platelet activation is amplified and sustained during the extension phase. Thrombin, generated at the site of vascular injury, represents the most potent platelet activator[4] and contributes to the formation of the hemostatic plug and platelet thrombus growth. Thrombin also directly activates platelets through stimulation of the protease-activated receptors (PARs). Human platelets express two PARs for thrombin, PAR-1 and PAR-4. Thrombin facilitates the production of fibrin from fibrinogen and thus contributes to the formation and stabilization of the hemostatic plug.[4] The final common pathway is activation of the integrin GP IIb/IIIa, which allows platelets to bind fibrinogen with high affinity, leading to platelet aggregates.[5] In the *perpetuation phase*, the platelet-rich thrombus and coagulation cascades reinforce one another and culminate in the generation of a stable platelet-fibrin–rich plug at the sites of injury.

The mechanisms by which antiplatelet drugs interfere with platelet function involve targeting enzymes or receptors critical for synthesis or targeting the action of important mediators of these functional responses. Current and investigational oral antiplatelet therapies target key platelet-signaling pathways (Fig. 10.2). This chapter reviews the mechanisms of action, efficacy, and safety of antiplatelet agents that inhibit key platelet-signaling pathways and their components—including the TXA_2 pathway, the $P2Y_{12}$ and PAR-1 receptors, phosphodiesterase III, and the GP IIb/IIIa receptor—and focuses on their roles in PCI.

ASPIRIN

Mechanism of Action

Aspirin irreversibly inactivates the cyclooxygenase activity of prostaglandin H (PGH) synthase 1 and 2, also referred to as *COX-1* and *COX-2*. PGH synthase 1 and 2 convert arachidonic acid to PGH_2, which acts as a substrate for the generation of several prostanoids, including TXA_2 and prostacyclin (PGI_2). Aspirin enters the COX channel and acetylates the amino acid serine at positions 529 and 516 of COX-1 and COX-2, respectively, thereby preventing arachidonic acid access to the catalytic site of the enzyme through steric hindrance. Mature platelets express only COX-1 and are the primary sources of TXA_2, which is released by the platelet in response to a variety

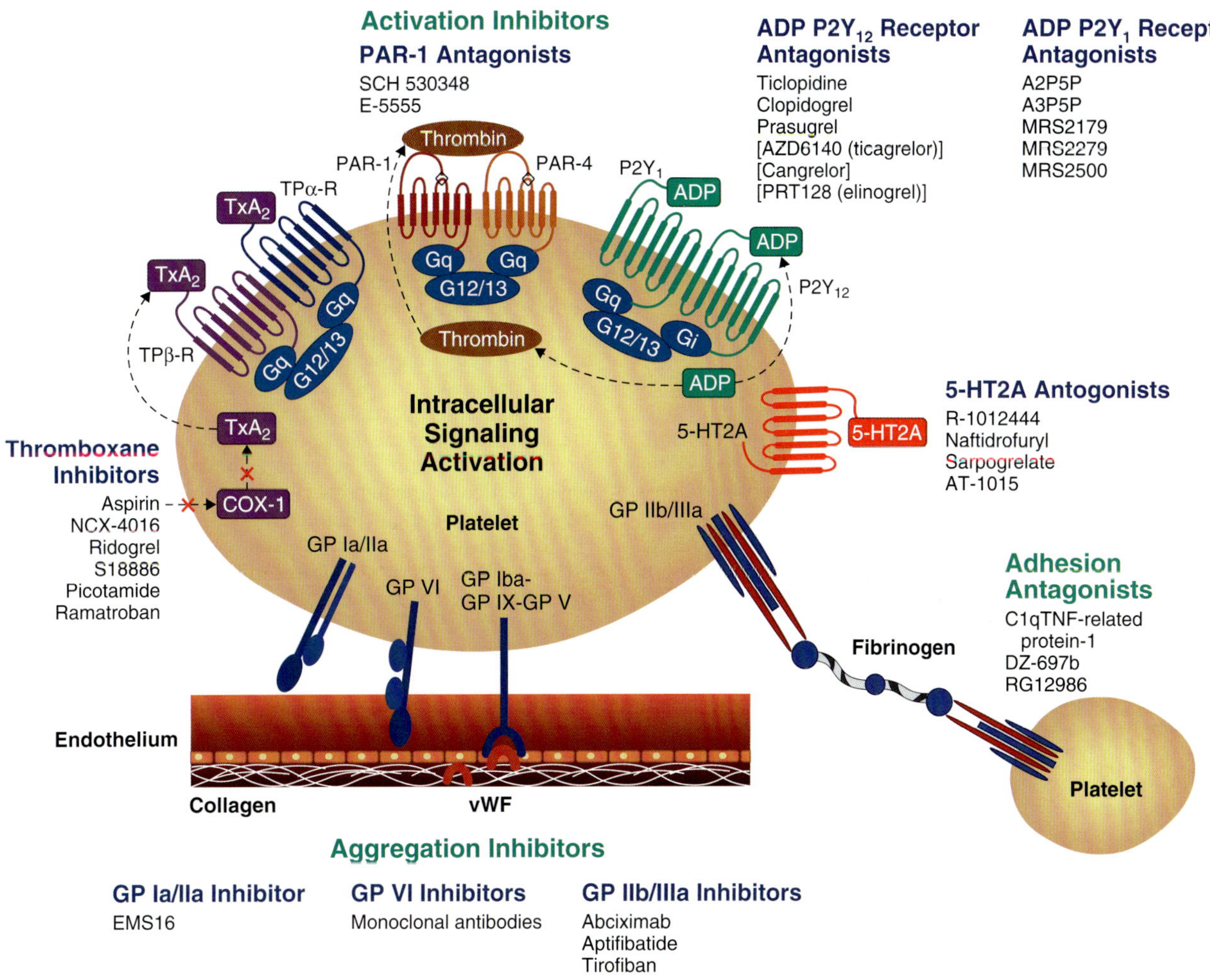

CHAPTER 10 Platelet Inhibitor Agents

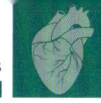

Fig. 10.2 Sites of action of current and emerging antiplatelet agents. Platelet adherence to the endothelium occurs at the sites of vascular injury through the binding of glycoprotein *(GP)* receptors to exposed extracellular matrix proteins (collagen and von Willebrand factor *[vWF]*). Platelet activation occurs via complex intracellular signaling processes and causes the production and release of multiple agonists, including thromboxane A2 *(TXA$_2$)* and adenosine diphosphate *(ADP)* and also causes local production of thrombin. These factors bind to their respective G protein–coupled receptors, mediating paracrine and autocrine platelet activation. Further, they potentiate each other's actions (P2Y$_{12}$ signaling modulates thrombin generation). The major platelet integrin GP IIb/IIIa mediates the final common step of platelet activation by undergoing a conformational shape change and binding fibrinogen and vWF, leading to platelet aggregation. The net result of these interactions is thrombus formation mediated by platelet-platelet interactions with fibrin. Current and emerging therapies that inhibit platelet receptors, integrins, and proteins involved in platelet activation include thromboxane inhibitors, ADP receptor antagonists, GP IIb/IIIa inhibitors, and the novel PAR antagonists and adhesion antagonists. Reversibly acting agents are indicated by brackets. *5-HT2A,* 5-Hydroxytryptamine 2A receptor; *COX,* cyclooxygenase; *PAR,* protease-activated receptor; *TNF,* tumor necrosis factor. (From Angiolillo DJ, Capodanno D, Goto S. Platelet thrombin receptor antagonism and atherothrombosis. *Eur Heart J.* 2010;31:17–28.)

of agonists and induces platelet aggregation through the G protein–coupled TXA$_2$ receptor, TP. Other cells, including the vascular endothelium, express both COX-1 and COX-2. COX-1 is responsible for the production of cytoprotective prostaglandins PGE$_2$ and PGI$_2$ in the gastric mucosa, and COX-2 is the main source of vascular PGI$_2$. Unlike mature platelets, gastric mucosal cells can synthesize COX-1 and therefore recover the ability to produce prostaglandins within hours after aspirin exposure. Compared with COX-1, higher levels of aspirin are required to inhibit COX-2; therefore low-dose aspirin is sufficient to inhibit platelet TXA$_2$ production but is insufficient to affect the generation of vascular PGI$_2$, which is a platelet inhibitor and vasodilator. In addition to its primary effect on platelet aggregation through inhibition of the PGH synthase COX-1 activity, it has been suggested that aspirin also exerts antiplatelet effects via COX-1–independent pathways.[6]

Pharmacokinetics and Pharmacodynamics

Aspirin is rapidly absorbed in the stomach and small intestine and achieves peak plasma levels in 30 to 40 minutes. Esterases in the gastrointestinal (GI) mucosa and liver hydrolyze aspirin into salicylic acid, which then interacts with platelets in the portal circulation. The half-life is short, approximately 20 to 30 minutes, but the pharmacodynamic effect is prolonged given the permanent inactivation of platelet COX-1 activity. Low-dose aspirin requires several days to effectively suppress TXA$_2$ production; therefore a loading dose (LD) is needed to quickly achieve effective platelet inhibition in aspirin-naïve subjects; however, LDs greater than 300 mg do not provide additional pharmacodynamic benefit at 2 hours after ingestion.

The American College of Cardiology Foundation (ACCF)/American Heart Association (AHA)/Society for Cardiovascular Angiography and Interventions (SCAI) 2011 percutaneous coronary intervention (PCI) guidelines state that patients not already taking daily long-term aspirin therapy should be administered 325 mg nonenteric aspirin before PCI (class I, level of evidence [LOE] B), and patients already on daily aspirin therapy should take 81 to 325 mg before PCI (class I, LOE B).

Aspirin Dose After Percutaneous Coronary Intervention

In healthy individuals, maintenance aspirin dosages as low as 30 mg daily are adequate to completely inhibit serum TXB_2 production, a marker of platelet thromboxane production. Collaborative meta-analyses of the clinical benefit of long-term aspirin regimens in high-risk patients show that dosages greater than 75 to 150 mg daily are no more effective in reducing ischemic events but are associated with a greater risk of bleeding. However, patients undergoing PCI and receiving stents are not represented in these studies. The ACCF/AHA/SCAI 2011 PCI guidelines[7] state that after PCI, it is reasonable to use aspirin 81 mg/day in preference to higher maintenance doses (MDs) (class IIa, LOE B).

The impact of different aspirin dosages on ischemia and bleeding in stented patients was examined in a post hoc observational analysis[8] of the PCI cohort of the Clopidogrel in Unstable Angina to Prevent Recurrent Ischemic Events (CURE) trial. This analysis suggests that doses of aspirin below 200 mg might be optimal after PCI with a bare-metal stent (BMS). The study stratified the 2658 patients who underwent PCI for acute coronary syndrome (ACS) in the CURE trial[9] into three groups: high-dose (≥200 mg), medium-dose (>100 to <200 mg), and low-dose aspirin (≤100 mg). No differences were found in the unadjusted or adjusted rates of death, myocardial infarction (MI), or stroke among the groups (high dose vs. low dose, adjusted hazard ratio [HR] 1.00; 95% confidence interval [CI], 0.67 to 1.48; medium dose vs. low dose, adjusted HR 1.09; 95% CI, 0.73 to 1.60). Unadjusted and adjusted rates of major bleeding were significantly greater with high-dose aspirin compared with low-dose aspirin (adjusted HR 2.03; 95% CI, 1.15 to 3.57).

The Clopidogrel and Aspirin Optimal Dose Usage to Reduce Recurrent Events—Seventh Organization to Assess Strategies in Ischemic Syndromes (CURRENT–OASIS 7)[10] examined the safety and efficacy of higher-dose aspirin (300 to 325 mg daily) compared with lower-dose aspirin (75 to 100 mg daily) in 25,086 patients with ACS treated with an invasive strategy. All patients received an aspirin LD of 300 mg or more the day of randomization, and patients were also randomized in a two-by-two factorial design to standard-dose or double-dose clopidogrel. In the overall cohort, the rate of cardiovascular death, MI, or stroke at 30 days was not different between higher-dose and lower-dose aspirin regimens (4.2% vs. 4.4%, HR 0.97; 95% CI, 0.86 to 1.09; $P = .61$). The incidence of major bleeding as defined by the trial was not different among groups (2.3% vs. 2.3%, HR 0.99; 95% CI, 0.84 to 1.17; $P = .9$). Minor bleeding was more frequent with higher-dose aspirin (5.0% vs. 4.4%, HR 1.13; 95% CI, 100 to 1.27; $P = .04$), as was GI bleeding (0.4% vs. 0.2%, $P = .04$). The findings were similar among those patients who underwent PCI, approximately 42% of whom received a drug-eluting stent (DES), and no difference was found in the incidence of stent thrombosis within the PCI cohort. Therefore a treatment strategy of lower-dose aspirin in invasively managed patients with ACS for 30 days appears to provide ischemic outcomes similar to higher-dose aspirin with less minor bleeding and less GI bleeding. However, longer treatment durations have not been examined in a randomized fashion.

$P2Y_{12}$ INHIBITORS

Basic Principles

The platelet $P2Y_{12}$ receptor plays a central role in amplifying the effect of various stimuli on platelet activation, and it promotes thrombus growth and stability. It is an inhibitory G protein–coupled receptor (Gα12) activated by ADP, which is released from dense granules after platelet activation from a variety of stimuli. ADP binding to the $P2Y_{12}$ receptor leads to a series of intracellular signaling events that result in further granule release and amplification of platelet activation, conformational changes of the GP IIb/IIIa receptor, and stabilization of the platelet aggregate. $P2Y_{12}$ activation further amplifies other responses to platelet activation including P-selectin expression, microparticle formation, procoagulant changes in the surface membrane, and potentiation of shear stress–induced platelet aggregation. The intracellular effect of $P2Y_{12}$ receptor activation is mediated by signal transduction via a secondary messenger system that activates phosphoinositide 3-kinase (PI3K) and inhibits adenylyl cyclase. PI3K activation leads to GP IIb/IIIa receptor activation through activation of a serine-threonine protein kinase B (PKB/Akt) and *RAP1B* guanosine triphosphate (GTP) binding protein. Inhibition of adenylyl cyclase decreases intracellular levels of cAMP, a key cofactor for the phosphorylation of vasodilator-stimulated phosphoprotein (VASP). Dephosphorylated VASP helps promote the conformational change of the GP IIb/IIIa receptor to its active state. Therefore through its action on cAMP levels, $P2Y_{12}$ activation drives the dephosphorylation of VASP and in turn drives GP IIb/IIIa activation (Table 10.1).

Thienopyridines

The thienopyridines—ticlopidine, clopidogrel, and prasugrel—are prodrugs that require biotransformation into an active metabolite to exert their antiplatelet effect. The active metabolite irreversibly binds and antagonizes the $P2Y_{12}$ receptor for the platelet's life span (7 to 10 days). Differences in the rapidity and magnitude of platelet inhibition between the thienopyridines are predominantly the result of differences in prodrug metabolism that affect the efficiency of active metabolite formation. Because the interaction between the active metabolite and the $P2Y_{12}$ receptor is irreversible, a substantial waiting period for platelet functional recovery is required after thienopyridine exposure, which appears to be related to the magnitude of the initial inhibition.[11-13]

Ticlopidine

Ticlopidine was the first thienopyridine to be introduced into clinical practice. It has a slow onset of action, is poorly tolerated, and its use is associated with blood dyscrasias. The incidence of neutropenia has been reported to be 2.4%, peaking at 4 to 6 weeks after the start of therapy; the incidence of aplastic anemia is 1 in 4000 to 8000 patients; and the incidence of thrombotic thrombocytopenic purpura is approximately 1 in 2000 to 4000 patients. The onset of hematologic disorders is rare after 3 months of therapy; therefore hematologic monitoring is required before initiation and for the first 3 months of exposure. The Stent Anticoagulation Restenosis Study (STARS)[14] demonstrated that the combination of aspirin and ticlopidine significantly reduced the rate of death, angiographically evident stent thrombosis, MI, or revascularization at 30 days by 85% compared with aspirin alone and by 80% compared with the combination of aspirin and warfarin. Ticlopidine has been widely replaced by clopidogrel, given its better tolerability and lack of blood-monitoring requirements.

CHAPTER 10 Platelet Inhibitor Agents

TABLE 10.1 Key Randomized Clinical Trials of P2Y$_{12}$ Inhibitors in Patients Undergoing Invasive Management for Acute Coronary Syndrome, Percutaneous Coronary Intervention, or Both

Trial Name	N	Population Studied	Intervention	Control	Primary End Point	F/U	Treatment Effect[b]
CLOPIDOGREL							
PCI-CURE[a]	2658	NSTE-ACS	Clopidogrel 300 mg LD, then 75 mg/day + ASA	Clopidogrel open-label for 28 days + ASA	CV death, MI, or revasc.	9 months	RR 0.70 [0.50–0.97] P = .03
CREDO	2116	Stable CAD and unstable angina	Clopidogrel 300 mg pre-PCI, then 75 mg/day + ASA	Clopidogrel 75 mg/day for 28 days + ASA	CV death, MI, or stroke	1 year	RRR 26.9% [3.9%–44.4%] P = .02
PCI-CLARITY[a]	1863	STEMI treated with fibrinolytics w/PCI 2–8 days later	Clopidogrel 300 mg before PCI, then 75 mg/day + ASA	Open-label clopidogrel starting at time of PCI + ASA	CV death, MI, or stroke	30 days	OR, 0.54 [0.35–0.85] P = .008
CURRENT-OASIS 7	25,807	NSTE-ACS and STEMI with intended PCI	Clopidogrel 600 mg before angiography, 150 mg/day for 6 days, then 75 mg/day + ASA	Clopidogrel 300 mg before angiography, then 75 mg/day + ASA	CV death, MI, or stroke	30 days	Overall cohort: HR 0.94 [0.83–1.06] P = .30 PCI cohort [a]: (n = 17,263) HR 0.86 [0.74–0.99] P = .04[a]
GRAVITAS	2214	Patients with high on-treatment reactivity to standard clopidogrel 12–24 hours after PCI	Clopidogrel 600 mg LD, then 150 mg/day + ASA	Clopidogrel 75 mg + ASA	CV death, nonfatal MI, stent thrombosis	6 months	HR 1.01 [0.58–1.76] P = .97
PRASUGREL							
TRITON–TIMI 38	13,608	NSTE-ACS and STEMI with planned PCI	Prasugrel 60-mg LD, then 10 mg/day MD + ASA	Clopidogrel 300-mg LD, then 75 mg/day MD + ASA	CV death, MI, or stroke	450 days	HR 0.81 [0.73–0.90] P < .001
ACCOAST	4003	NSTE-ACS planned for coronary angiography	Pretreatment with prasugrel 30-mg LD, additional 30-mg LD/10-mg MD if PCI performed	Pretreatment with placebo, 60-mg LD/10-mg MD if PCI performed	CV death MI, stroke, urgent revasc., or GP IIb/IIIa bailout at 7 days	30 days	HR 1.02 [0.84–1.25], P = .81
TICAGRELOR							
PLATO Invasive	13,400 (PCI in 77%)	NSTE ACS and STEMI, intended early invasive management	Ticagrelor 180-mg LD, then 90 mg bid + ASA	Clopidogrel 300- to 600-mg LD, then 75 mg/day + ASA	CV death, MI, or stroke	12 months	HR 0.84 [0.75–0.94] P = .0025
ATLANTIC	1862	STEMI	180-mg LD in the ambulance, 90 mg bid thereafter + ASA	Placebo in the ambulance, 180-mg LD in the catheterization laboratory, 90 mg bid thereafter + ASA	Co-primary: Lack of ST-segment resolution; TIMI flow <3 in infarct-related artery	In-hospital	ST-segment resolution: OR 0.93 [0.69–1.25], P = .63 TIMI flow: OR 0.97 [0.75–1.25], P = .82
				ASA + clopidogrel 600 mg post PCI	Death, MI, or revasc.	48 h	OR 0.87 [0.71–1.07] P = .17
				ASA + clopidogrel 600 mg pre-PCI	Death, MI, or revasc.	48 h	OR 1.05 [0.88–1.24] P = .59

[a]Postrandomization analysis of a larger clinical trial.
[b]Numbers in brackets represent 95% confidence intervals.

ACCOAST, Comparison of Prasugrel at the Time of Percutaneous Coronary Intervention or as Pretreatment at the Time of Diagnosis in Patients With Non-ST Elevation Myocardial Infarction; *ASA*, aspirin; *ATLANTIC*, Administration of Ticagrelor in the Cath Lab or in the Ambulance for New ST-Elevation Myocardial Infarction to Open the Coronary Artery; *CAD*, cardiovascular disease; *CLARITY*, Clopidogrel as Adjunctive Reperfusion Therapy; *CREDO*, Clopidogrel for the Reduction of Events During Observation; *CURE*, Clopidogrel in Unstable Angina to Prevent Recurrent Ischemic Events; *CURRENT–OASIS 7*, Clopidogrel and Aspirin Optimal Dose Usage to Reduce Recurrent Events–Seventh Organization to Assess Strategies in Ischemic Syndromes; *CV*, cardiovascular; *F/U*, duration of follow-up; *GP*, glycoprotein; *GRAVITAS*, Gauging Responsiveness With a VerifyNow Assay–Impact on Thrombosis and Safety; *HR*, hazard ratio; *LD*, loading dose; *MD*, maintenance dose; *MI*, myocardial infarction; *NSTE-ACS*, non–ST-elevation acute coronary syndrome; *OR*, odds ratio; *PCI*, percutaneous coronary intervention; *PLATO*, Platelet Inhibition and Patient Outcomes; *revasc.*, revascularization; *RR*, risk reduction; *RRR*, relative risk reduction; *STEMI*, ST-elevation myocardial infarction; *TIMI*, thrombolysis in myocardial infarction; *TRITON–TIMI 38*, Therapeutic Outcomes by Optimizing Platelet Inhibition with Prasugrel–Thrombolysis in Myocardial Infarction 38.

Clopidogrel

Metabolism

Clopidogrel is a prodrug that requires hepatic conversion into an active metabolite to exert its antiplatelet effect (Fig. 10.3). Approximately 85% of absorbed clopidogrel is hydrolyzed by human carboxylesterase[1] in the liver into an inactive carboxylic acid metabolite, so only a fraction of absorbed clopidogrel is available for conversion into the active metabolite by the cytochrome P450 (CYP) system. Hepatic biotransformation of absorbed clopidogrel into the active metabolite is thought to occur through a two-step process. The thiophene ring of clopidogrel is first oxidized to 2-oxo-clopidogrel, which is then hydrolyzed to a highly labile active metabolite (R-130964) that forms a disulfide bond with the $P2Y_{12}$ receptor as platelets pass through the liver. The first metabolic step involves the isoenzymes CYP2C19, CYP2B6, and CYP1A2; the second step involves the isoenzymes CYP2C19, CYP2B6, CYP3A4, CYP3A5, and CYP2C9. An alternative pathway for the oxidative biotransformation of clopidogrel that does not involve CYP2C19 has been suggested.[15] In this formulation, CYP-catalyzed oxidation of clopidogrel to 2-oxo-clopidogrel is mediated by CYP1A2, CYP2B6, and CYP3A, and conversion of 2-oxo-clopidogrel to the thiol active metabolite is mediated by the esterase paraoxonase 1 (PON-1). The catalytic activity of PON-1 is proposed to be the rate-determining step for the active metabolite formation of clopidogrel. However, this alternative pathway has not been independently validated; paraoxonase may catalyze the formation of a minor isomer of the active metabolite, rather than the major isomer, and several studies have shown no influence of genetic polymorphisms of *PON1* on clopidogrel active metabolite levels or on clopidogrel's antiplatelet effects.[16]

Pharmacodynamics

A daily dose of clopidogrel 75 mg requires 3 to 7 days to reach steady-state platelet inhibition, whereas an LD provides a rapid onset of action. However, the clinical benefit of a 300-mg LD may not be seen for 6 hours to as long as 15 hours after administration.[17,18] Larger doses provide higher circulating levels of active metabolite, more rapid onset, and more intense inhibition.[19,20] Peak inhibition after a 600-mg LD occurs at 4 to 6 hours after exposure.[19,21] A 900-mg LD may or may not provide more rapid and additional suppression of platelet function compared with a 600-mg dose because the intestinal absorption of clopidogrel may be limited at doses greater than 600 mg.[19,20] An MD regimen of 150 mg daily is associated with greater inhibition than a dose of 75 mg daily.[22,23] Variability is wide among individuals in regard to the antiplatelet effect of clopidogrel after either an LD or an MD. Higher doses of clopidogrel reduce, but do not eliminate, this variability. The pharmacodynamic response to clopidogrel has been associated with CYP2C19 genotype, age, diabetes mellitus, body mass index, sex, ACS presentation, active smoking, renal dysfunction, pretreatment reactivity, and concomitant therapy with calcium channel blockers or proton pump inhibitors (PPIs).[24–27] However, clinical characteristics and the CYP2C19 genotype only partly explain the variability in on-treatment reactivity.[16,25,28] The level of ADP-induced platelet reactivity measured by several ex vivo platelet function tests have been associated with clinical outcomes in clopidogrel-treated patients undergoing PCI.[29,30]

Clinical Studies

Non–ST-Elevation Acute Coronary Syndrome. The longer-term ischemic benefit of clopidogrel in patients who present with ACS was established by the CURE trial, which randomized 12,562 patients with NSTE ACS to aspirin and clopidogrel

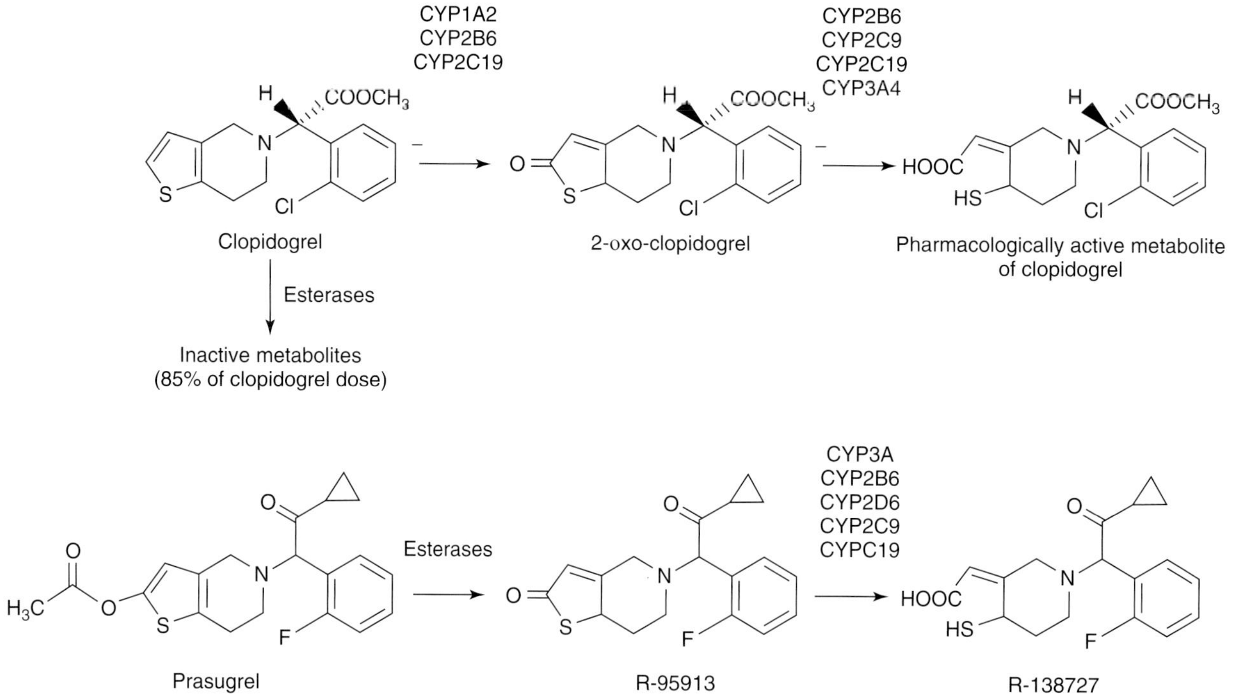

Fig. 10.3 Comparative metabolism of clopidogrel and prasugrel. Both are prodrugs that require biotransformation into their respective active metabolites to exert an antiplatelet effect. Clopidogrel undergoes a two-step process mediated by CYP450 isoenzymes with involvement of CYP2C19 and CYP2B6 in both steps. A substantial portion of absorbed clopidogrel is shunted into a dead-end pathway by esterases. Prasugrel undergoes a one-step oxidation after the formation of a thiolactone intermediate. The greater inhibitory effect of prasugrel compared with clopidogrel is believed to be attributable to differences in the efficiency of active metabolite formation. (From Giusti B, Abbate R. Response to antiplatelet treatment: from genes to outcome. *Lancet*. 2010;376:1278–1281.)

(300-mg LD followed by 75 mg daily) or aspirin alone for 3 to 12 months.[31] The composite end point of cardiovascular death, nonfatal MI, or stroke occurred in 9.3% of patients in the clopidogrel group and in 11.4% of patients in the placebo group ($P < .001$). Clopidogrel therapy was associated with an increased rate of major bleeding as defined by the trial (3.7% vs. 2.7%, $P = .001$). In the population of patients enrolled in CURE who underwent PCI (17% of the overall cohort, 82% of whom received a BMS), pretreatment with clopidogrel for a median of 6 days reduced the rate of cardiovascular death, MI, or urgent target-vessel revascularization within 30 days from 6.4% to 4.5% ($P = .03$).

ST-Elevation Myocardial Infarction. The Clopidogrel as Adjunctive Reperfusion Therapy–Thrombolysis in Myocardial Infarction (CLARITY–TIMI 28) trial[32] randomized 3491 patients 75 years of age and younger who received aspirin and fibrinolytic therapy within 12 hours of an ST-elevation MI (STEMI) to clopidogrel 300 mg followed by 75 mg daily or placebo. All patients underwent mandated angiography 2 to 8 days later. Clopidogrel significantly reduced the rates of occluded infarct-related artery, death, or recurrent MI before angiography (15.0% vs. 21.7%, $P < .001$) without increasing TIMI-defined major bleeding, minor bleeding, or intracranial hemorrhage. A prespecified analysis of patients who underwent PCI demonstrated that clopidogrel significantly reduced ischemic events from randomization through 30 days, from PCI through 30 days, and from randomization to PCI.[33] This trial supports the use of clopidogrel in patients 75 years and younger who present with STEMI and are treated with aspirin and fibrinolysis.

Pretreatment for Percutaneous Coronary Intervention
The rationale for clopidogrel pretreatment is based on the slow onset of a substantial pharmacodynamic effect even after a clopidogrel LD. The Clopidogrel for the Reduction of Events During Observation (CREDO) trial randomized 2116 patients with stable coronary artery disease (CAD), unstable angina (UA), or recent ACS to a clopidogrel 300-mg LD or placebo 3 to 24 hours before PCI. All patients received clopidogrel 75 mg daily for 28 days thereafter; patients in the control arm did not receive an LD. Pretreatment did not significantly reduce the primary composite end point of death, MI, and urgent target revascularization at 28 days (6.8% vs. 8.3%, $P = .23$). Post hoc analysis suggested that longer durations of pretreatment were associated with improved outcomes, but little benefit was achieved when the treatment duration was less than 12 hours.[18] A prospectively planned analysis of the 1863 patients in CLARITY–TIMI 28 who underwent PCI after mandated angiography showed that pretreatment for a median duration of 3 days in patients with STEMI treated with aspirin and fibrinolysis significantly reduced the incidence of cardiovascular death, MI, or stroke following PCI (3.6% vs. 6.2%, $P = .008$) and from randomization through 30 days (7.5% vs. 12.0%, $P = .001$).[33] Unfortunately, the use of a 300-mg LD in CREDO, PCI-CURE, and the Effect of Clopidogrel Pretreatment Before Percutaneous Coronary Intervention (PCI) in Patients With ST-Elevation Myocardial Infarction Treated With Fibrinolytics (PCI-CLARITY) studies and the prolonged duration of pretreatment in PCI-CURE and PCI-CLARITY limit their applicability to current practice patterns for both elective and urgent PCI. The ischemic benefit of a shorter pretreatment duration of high-dose clopidogrel before PCI has not been examined in a large, randomized, placebo-controlled trial. Post hoc analysis of the Intracoronary Stenting and Antithrombotic Regimen–Rapid Early Action for Coronary Treatment (ISAR-REACT) trial, which compared abciximab with placebo in elective PCI patients treated with clopidogrel 600 mg for at least 2 hours before intervention, showed no incremental benefit from durations of pretreatment greater than 2 to 3 hours.[34] The PRAGUE-8[35] study randomized 1028 patients undergoing coronary angiography and potential ad hoc PCI for stable angina to either clopidogrel 600 mg more than 6 hours before angiography or clopidogrel 600 mg in the catheterization laboratory only in the case of PCI. No differences were found in the rate of death, MI, stroke, or reintervention among groups at 7 days, not in the entire population or in the subgroup undergoing PCI (0.8% vs. 1.0%, $P = .7$; 1.3% vs. 2.8%, $P = .4$, respectively), but bleeding was increased in the pretreatment group (3.5% vs. 1.4%, $P = .025$). The findings of this small trial support a strategy of "on the table" clopidogrel loading before ad hoc PCI in elective patients, although the findings must be interpreted within the context of the relatively small sample size and very low event rates. The findings are supported by another smaller trial, Antiplatelet Therapy for Reduction of Myocardial Damage During Angioplasty (ARMYDA) PRELOAD, which randomized 409 patients (39% with ACS) to a 600-mg clopidogrel LD 4 to 8 hours before PCI or a 600-mg LD given in the catheterization laboratory after coronary angiography and before PCI.[36] The rates of major adverse cardiovascular events (MACEs) at 30 days were similar between groups and occurred in 10.8% of patients pretreated, compared with 8.8% in the patients receiving clopidogrel, in the laboratory ($P = .7$). No differences in the rates of bleeding were reported.

Dosing Strategies
Pharmacodynamic studies have demonstrated that higher clopidogrel LDs and MDs provide more rapid onset of action and greater levels of inhibition compared with a 300-mg LD and a 75-mg MD, respectively.[19–21,37] Two large randomized studies, CURRENT–OASIS 7 and GRAVITAS (Gauging Responsiveness With a VerifyNow Assay–Impact on Thrombosis and Safety), have examined the efficacy and safety of higher-dose clopidogrel in patients managed invasively or undergoing PCI.

The CURRENT–OASIS 7 trial[38] examined the ischemic benefit of a higher-dose strategy in 25,086 patients with NSTE-ACS and ST-elevation ACS undergoing an early invasive strategy, of whom 17,263 underwent PCI. Before angiography, patients were randomized to receive either a 600-mg LD, followed by 150 mg daily for 6 days and 75 mg daily thereafter, or a 300-mg LD followed by 75 mg daily thereafter. Patients were also randomized to high-dose aspirin or low-dose aspirin in a two-by-two factorial design. The primary end point—a composite of cardiovascular death, MI, or stroke at 30 days—was no different with double-dose clopidogrel or standard-dose clopidogrel (4.2% vs. 4.4%, $P = .30$). Major bleeding, as defined by the trial, was significantly greater in the patients randomized to double-dose clopidogrel (2.5% vs. 2.0%, HR 1.24; 95% CI, 1.05 to 1.46; $P = .01$); however, no differences were noted in fatal bleeding, coronary artery bypass grafting (CABG) related bleeding, or TIMI-criteria major bleeding. Within the subgroup of patients who underwent PCI, high-dose clopidogrel was associated with a 13% relative risk reduction in the primary end point (3.9% vs. 4.5%, $P = .04$).[39] However, the interaction test between patients who underwent PCI and those who did not failed to reach the prespecified threshold for statistical significance; therefore the possibility that the results of the PCI subgroup are a chance finding cannot be excluded.[38]

The GRAVITAS trial[40] tested whether an additional clopidogrel LD followed by a 6-month course of clopidogrel 150 mg daily would reduce thrombotic events compared with clopidogrel 75 mg daily in patients who had undergone PCI with a DES and displayed high on-treatment reactivity according to ex vivo platelet function testing (PFT) 12 to 24 hours after the intervention. Unlike the population examined by the CURRENT–OASIS 7 trial, the predominant indication for PCI in the enrolled population was stable CAD or low-risk UA. No difference was reported in the rate of cardiovascular death, nonfatal MI, or stent thrombosis at 6 months between groups (2.3% vs. 2.3%, $P = .9$). The incidence of severe or moderate bleeding per the Global Utilization of Streptokinase and t-PA for Occluded Coronary Arteries (GUSTO) criteria was not increased with the high-dose regimen (1.4% vs. 2.3%, $P = .10$). The higher-dose clopidogrel regimen had a significant but only modest effect on platelet inhibition in patients with high on-treatment reactivity to standard dosing, which may partly explain the similar outcomes of the two groups.

The Role of CYP2C19
The antiplatelet effect of clopidogrel is dependent on the generation of an active metabolite through the hepatic CYP450 system. Patients who are carriers for genetic polymorphisms that reduce the catalytic activity of CYP2C19 have lower clopidogrel active metabolite levels and diminished platelet inhibition with treatment. Approximately 5% to 12% of the variability in ADP-induced platelet reactivity appears to be explained by carriage of the reduced function CYP2C19*2 allele.[25,28] The sensitivity of active metabolite generation to changes in the catalytic activity of CYP2C19 may be attributed to the important contribution of this enzyme to both steps in clopidogrel biotransformation. Decreased CYP2C19 function could lead to a bottleneck at the level of hepatic activation, thereby shunting the prodrug into the pathway that leads to an inactive carboxylic acid metabolite.

Predicted Metabolic Phenotype
Patients can be classified on the basis of the predicted metabolic phenotype of the CYP2C19 genotype. The single-nucleotide polymorphisms that affect enzyme activity are described using the established "star allele" nomenclature. The CYP2C19*1 allele denotes the lack of known polymorphisms and therefore is considered to be wild type. CYP2C19*2 is the most common reduced-function allele, with an allelic frequency of approximately 13% in whites, 18% in blacks, and 30% in Asians. CYP2C19*3 is the second most common reduced-function allele; it has an allelic frequency of approximately 10% in Asians but is rare in other ethnicities. Much less common reduced-function alleles include *4, *5, *6, *7, *8, and *10. In addition, the *17 variant is associated with increased gene transcription and increased catalytic activity of the enzyme. The combination of two alleles (genotype) can be used to predict the metabolic phenotype of a particular individual (Table 10.2). Metabolic phenotype is associated with the pharmacokinetics and pharmacodynamics of clopidogrel. In a study of healthy volunteers, ultra-rapid metabolizers had the highest exposure to active metabolite and the greatest platelet inhibition, and poor metabolizers had the lowest exposure and least platelet inhibition with both loading and MDs.[41] The frequency of poor metabolizers is approximately 2% in the white population.

CYP2C19 and Clinical Outcomes
A collaborative meta-analysis of nine studies involving 9685 patients, 91% of whom had a PCI, reported a significantly increased risk of the composite end point of cardiovascular death, MI, or ischemic stroke in carriers of at least one reduced-function CYP2C19 allele (HR 1.57; 95% CI, 1.13 to 2.16; $P = .006$) and in patients with two reduced-function CYP2C19 alleles (HR 1.76; 95% CI, 1.24 to 2.50; $P = .002$). Carriers of at least one reduced-function CYP2C19 allele had an increased risk of stent thrombosis (HR 2.81; 95% CI, 1.81 to 4.37; $P < .0001$); this risk was especially strong in patients with two reduced-function alleles (HR 3.97; 95% CI, 1.75 to 9.02; $P = .001$). The influence of CYP2C19 genotype on outcomes is less apparent in populations treated with clopidogrel for indications other than PCI. In the genetic substudy of the Atrial Fibrillation Clopidogrel Trial With Irbesartan for Prevention of Vascular Events (ACTIVE A), a randomized comparison of aspirin and clopidogrel compared with aspirin alone for the prevention of thromboembolic events in atrial fibrillation (AF), the primary outcome was similar in carriers and noncarriers of the CYP2C19*2 reduced-function alleles. Similarly, in the CURE trial, in which only 14% of patients who presented with ACS underwent PCI, no difference was reported in ischemic outcomes according to CYP2C19 genotype.[42]

TABLE 10.2 Classification of Predicted Metabolic Phenotype According to CYP2C19 Genotype

CYP2C19 Genotype	Predicted Phenotype
*17/*17	Ultra-rapid metabolizer
*1/*17	Ultra-rapid metabolizer
*1/*1	Extensive metabolizer
*1/*2–*8	Intermediate metabolizer
*17/*2–*8	Intermediate metabolizer/unknown
*2–*8/*2–*8	Poor metabolizer

U.S. Food and Drug Administration's Boxed Warning
The U.S. Food and Drug Administration (FDA) mandated a warning in the clopidogrel package insert in the fall of 2009 that highlights the impact of CYP2C19 on the exposure to clopidogrel active metabolite, platelet inhibition, and clinical outcomes. This warning emphasizes that the effectiveness of clopidogrel is dependent on bioactivation by CYP2C19 and that poor metabolizers generate a less active metabolite and have less platelet inhibition with the recommended dosage of clopidogrel (i.e., 300-mg loading and 75-mg daily MDs). Furthermore, the warning states that compared with patients with normal CYP2C19 function, cardiovascular event rates are higher in poor metabolizers with ACS and those who are undergoing PCI when treated with recommended doses of clopidogrel. The warning goes on to state that tests are available to identify a patient's CYP2C19 genotype, that these tests can be used as an aid in determining therapeutic strategy, and that alternative treatment or treatment strategies should be considered in patients identified as poor metabolizers of CYP2C19. A subsequent ACCF/AHA Clopidogrel Clinical Alert stated that the evidence base was insufficient to recommend routine genetic testing, but testing to determine whether a patient is a poor metabolizer may be considered before starting clopidogrel therapy in patients believed to be at moderate or high risk for poor outcomes; for example, those undergoing elective high-risk PCI. The alert also noted that if genotyping identifies a poor metabolizer, other antiplatelet therapies, particularly prasugrel for coronary patients, should be considered, taking into account the balance of potential ischemic benefit with the known increased risk of bleeding.[43]

Other Genetic Polymorphisms
PON1. An alternative model for the bioactivation of clopidogrel posits a central role for the PON-1 enzyme in hydrolyzing 2-oxo-clopidogrel into the thiol active metabolite. A genetic variant that lowers the activity of PON-1 (Q192R) and may reduce the efficiency of clopidogrel bioactivation has been identified. Carriage of two *PON1* loss-of-function alleles was associated with definite stent thrombosis in a prospective cohort of 1982 patients with ACS (HR 10.20; 95% CI, 4.39 to 71.43; $P < .001$).[15] However, subsequent studies have raised the possibility that PON-1 is involved in the formation of a minor thiol metabolite isomer,[44,45] rather than the major clopidogrel active metabolite, and an association between *PON1* genotype and on-treatment platelet reactivity or clinical outcomes after PCI has not been confirmed in several other clinical studies.[16,46-48]

ABCB1. P-glycoprotein is an adenosine triphosphate (ATP)–dependent efflux pump encoded by the *ABCB1* gene. It is expressed in the intestinal epithelial cells, and its increased expression or function can influence the bioavailability of drugs that are its substrate. Healthy subjects homozygous for the 3435 C→T polymorphism have a decreased pharmacodynamic effect of clopidogrel.[49] The results of clinical outcomes studies are inconsistent. A genetic substudy of the Trial to Assess Improvement in the Therapeutic Outcomes by Optimizing Platelet Inhibition With Prasugrel–Thrombolysis in Myocardial Infarction (TRITON–TIMI 38) study reported that *ABCB1* 3435 TT homozygotes had a significantly increased risk of adverse cardiovascular events during treatment with clopidogrel after PCI for ACS, whereas event rates were highest in *ABCB1* 3435 CC homozygotes in the genetic substudy of the Platelet Inhibition and Patient Outcomes (PLATO) trial.[49,50]

Proton Pump Inhibitors

PPIs are extensively metabolized by CYP2C19 and CYP3A4. The different PPIs inhibit CYP2C19 activity to varying degrees. Omeprazole, lansoprazole, and esomeprazole demonstrate more potent inhibition by ex vivo assays, and lesser inhibition is observed with pantoprazole and rabeprazole.[51,52] A cross-over study in healthy volunteers showed that among the four PPIs evaluated, all decreased the peak plasma concentration of clopidogrel active metabolite by varying degrees (omeprazole > esomeprazole > lansoprazole > dexlansoprazole) and showed a corresponding order of interference with the effect of clopidogrel on platelet P2Y$_{12}$ reactivity.[53] In addition, a significant pharmacodynamic interaction does not appear to occur with pantoprazole.[52,54]

Large retrospective cohort and population-based studies have reported an association between concomitant PPI and clopidogrel use with an increased risk of recurrent cardiovascular events, including MI.[55,56] Although these analyses adjust for baseline differences among treatment groups, unmeasured confounders may, in part, explain these observations because patients treated with PPIs after PCI have substantially more comorbidities than those not treated with PPIs. Post hoc analysis of the TRITON–TIMI 38 randomized trial found no association between PPI use and the risk of cardiovascular death, MI, or stroke in patients treated with clopidogrel.[57]

The Clopidogrel and the Optimization of Gastrointestinal Events Trial (COGENT)[58] was a multicenter, randomized, phase III study of the safety and efficacy of a fixed-dose combination of clopidogrel 75 mg or omeprazole 20 mg in patients at high risk for GI bleeding who required aspirin and clopidogrel therapy for at least 12 months. The primary end point was the time to first occurrence of an upper GI clinical event; the primary cardiovascular end point was a composite of cardiovascular death, nonfatal MI, coronary revascularization, or ischemic stroke. The study was not powered a priori for the cardiovascular end point, and it was halted prematurely for lack of funding. A total of 3873 patients were randomized, of whom approximately 42% had a history of ACS. At 180 days, the rate of the composite GI end point was significantly lower in the combination clopidogrel-omeprazole group compared with the group who received clopidogrel alone (1.1% vs. 2.9%, HR 0.34; 95% CI, 0.18 to 0.63; $P < .001$), and no difference was apparent in the incidence of cardiovascular events (4.9% vs. 5.7%, HR 0.99; 95% CI, 0.68 to 1.44; $P = .96$). The cardiovascular end point was driven predominantly by the need for coronary revascularization (generally not a platelet-driven phenomenon); cardiovascular death or MI occurred in only 23 patients in the omeprazole group and in 20 patients in the placebo group. Given the possibility of a 44% increased hazard for cardiovascular events in the low-risk group that was studied, the COGENT results may not rule out a clinically meaningful difference in cardiovascular events with the use of omeprazole in patients administered clopidogrel for its labeled indications.[59] The findings of a meta-analysis of 13 studies involving 48,674 clopidogrel-treated patients suggested that the clinical impact of concomitant PPI use might be significant only in patients with high baseline cardiovascular risk.[60] In an analysis of the Assessment of Dual Antiplatelet Therapy with Drug-Eluting Stents (ADAPT-DES) study, PPI use was independently associated with high platelet reactivity on clopidogrel therapy (PRU >208), and was independently associated with an increased risk of post-discharge MACEs at 2-year follow-up (HR 1.21; 95% CI, 1.04 to 1.42; $P = .02$), with a strong trend toward mortality (HR 1.28; 95% CI, 1.00 to 1.63; $P = .51$).[61]

An ACCF/American College of Gastroenterology/AHA 2010 expert consensus document on the concomitant use of PPIs and thienopyridines states that clinical decisions regarding concomitant use of PPIs and thienopyridines must balance overall risks and benefits, considering both cardiovascular and GI complications.[62] Patients with ACS and prior upper GI bleeding are at substantial cardiovascular risk, so dual-antiplatelet therapy (DAPT) with concomitant use of a PPI may provide the optimal balance of risk and benefit.

Prasugrel

Metabolism

Prasugrel is a thienopyridine, like ticlopidine and clopidogrel, but its biotransformation into the active metabolite is substantially more efficient (see Fig. 10.3). Hydrolysis by human carboxylesterase 2 during absorption forms a thiolactone precursor, which is then oxidized in a single CYP-dependent step to the active metabolite. CYP3A4/5 and CYP2B6 are major contributors to this process, whereas CYP2C19 and CYP2C9 play a minor role; oxidation by intestinal CYP3A also occurs.[63] The biotransformation of prasugrel is more efficient than that of clopidogrel because of the lack of a competing metabolic pathway to an inactive metabolite. The greater magnitude of inhibition of platelet aggregation (IPA) achieved by prasugrel 60 mg compared with clopidogrel 600 mg is caused by differences in active metabolite exposure.[64] The area under the concentration-time curve of the prasugrel active metabolite is dose proportionate between 10 and 60 mg. Genetic polymorphisms that reduce the catalytic activity of CYP2C19 have no effect on active metabolite formation, the achieved level of platelet inhibition, or clinical outcomes in patients with ACS treated with PCI.[63,65]

Pharmacodynamics

Compared with clopidogrel, a prasugrel 60-mg LD followed by 10 mg daily provides a more rapid onset of action, significantly greater P2Y$_{12}$ inhibition, and less interindividual variability in the extent of inhibition. Prasugrel 60 mg achieves greater than twice the mean IPA at 4 hours after administration compared with a clopidogrel 300-mg LD in patients with stable CAD (ADP 5 mmol/L, 74% vs. 37%; ADP 20 mmol/L, 68% vs. 30%), and the stronger effect on IPA can be detected as early as 15 to 30 minutes after administration.[66] Prasugrel 10 mg daily provides a greater level of IPA compared with clopidogrel 75 mg daily (ADP 5 mmol/L, 59% vs. 31%; ADP 20 mmol/L, 58% vs. 31%).[66] A randomized pharmacodynamic study demonstrated that a prasugrel 60-mg load followed by 10 mg daily also provides a greater level of platelet inhibition than clopidogrel 600 mg followed by 150 mg daily.[67] The variability in inhibition among individuals is substantially less with prasugrel 10 or 60 mg compared with clopidogrel. However, prasugrel MDs of less than 10 mg daily are associated with greater degrees of interindividual variability in the extent of inhibition.[66]

Clinical Studies

The clinical efficacy and safety of prasugrel in ACS were examined in TRITON–TIMI 38.[68] In this phase III, randomized, active-control, time-to-event trial, 13,608 patients with moderate- to high-risk ACS undergoing treatment with PCI were assigned a prasugrel 60-mg LD followed by 10 mg daily or a clopidogrel 300-mg LD followed by 75 mg daily for 6 to 15 months. The primary efficacy end point was a composite of death from cardiovascular causes, nonfatal MI, or stroke. To be eligible, patients were required to be naïve to thienopyridine therapy. Randomization to the study drug occurred after diagnostic coronary angiography and determination that PCI was to be performed except in the case of STEMI, when randomization was allowed before the assessment of coronary anatomy. Over a median duration of therapy of 14.5 months, the primary composite end point occurred in 12.1% of the patients receiving clopidogrel and in 9.9% of patients receiving prasugrel ($P < .001$). The treatment effect of prasugrel was driven primarily by a reduction in the rate of nonfatal MI. The benefit of prasugrel was similar in patients with NSTE-ACS (HR 0.82; 95% CI, 0.73 to 0.93; $P = .002$) or STEMI (HR 0.79; 95% CI, 0.65 to 0.97; $P = .02$). The rate of definite or probable stent thrombosis was also significantly reduced with prasugrel (1.13% vs. 2.35%, HR 0.48; 95% CI, 0.36 to 0.64; $P < .001$). Key elements of the TRITON–TIMI 38 study design that may have impacted the findings were the timing of study drug administration and the clopidogrel dosing strategy to which prasugrel was compared (clopidogrel 300-mg LD at the time of PCI). Prespecified landmark analyses for efficacy were performed from randomization to day 3 and from day 3 to the end of the trial to separate the events that could be attributed to the LD of the study drug. These analyses demonstrated that in addition to an early benefit, prasugrel provided a significant reduction in the rates of MI and stent thrombosis after 3 days, supporting the hypothesis that prasugrel is superior to clopidogrel during the chronic phase of management after PCI (nonfatal MI: HR 0.69; 95% CI, 0.58 to 0.83; $P < .001$; stent thrombosis: HR 0.45; 95% CI, 0.32 to 0.64; $P < .001$).[69] Further, a landmark analysis[70] also showed that prasugrel reduced stent thrombosis both early (≤30 days, 0.64% vs. 1.56%, $P < .001$) and late (>30 days, 0.49% vs. 0.82%, $P = .03$). Although prasugrel provided a significant benefit with regard to ischemic outcomes, a significant hazard for major bleeding was also observed (HR 1.32; 95% CI, 1.03 to 1.68; $P = .03$), including fatal bleeding. A determination of net clinical outcome (combination of ischemic and bleeding events) may be helpful to assess the overall benefit of prasugrel for a particular patient, assuming that the components of this composite—death from any cause, nonfatal MI, stroke, and major non–CABG-related bleeding—can be considered of equivalent importance to the physician and the patient. In TRITON–TIMI 38, patients with a prior history of stroke or TIA experienced net harm from prasugrel because of a lack of ischemic benefit and a strong trend toward excessive major bleeding, including intracranial hemorrhage, and patients 75 years of age and older who weighed less than 60 kg experienced no net clinical benefit because of modest ischemic benefit balanced by an increased risk of bleeding; therefore prasugrel is contraindicated in patients with a history of stroke or transient ischemic attack (TIA). It can be considered in patients 75 years of age and older who have an increased ischemic risk (e.g., diabetes or prior MI) in whom the potential ischemic benefit may outweigh any increased risk of major bleeding, and an MD adjustment to 5 mg may be considered in patients who weigh less than 60 kg because pharmacokinetic modeling suggests that active metabolite exposure with this dose is similar to the 10-mg dose in heavier patients.

In TRITON–TIMI 38, subjects with prior exposure to a thienopyridine were excluded, and patients with NSTE-ACS received study drug (prasugrel LD or placebo) only after coronary anatomy was documented by angiography. The safety and efficacy of pretreatment with prasugrel prior to PCI were explored in the Comparison of Prasugrel at the Time of Percutaneous Coronary Intervention or as Pretreatment at the Time of Diagnosis in Patients With Non-ST Elevation Myocardial Infarction (ACCOAST) trial.[71] In this trial, 4033 patients with NSTE-ACS and elevated troponin who were scheduled for coronary angiography were randomly assigned to either pretreatment with prasugrel in a 30-mg LD or placebo. If PCI was indicated at the time of angiography, an additional prasugrel 30-mg LD was administered to the pretreatment group, and a prasugrel 60-mg LD was administered to the control group. Approximately one-quarter of the enrolled patients were at high risk (Global Registry of Acute Coronary Events [GRACE] score ≥140), and the time between pretreatment and coronary angiography was slightly greater than 4 hours. The primary end point—cardiovascular death, MI, stroke, urgent revascularization, or GP IIb/IIIa bailout at 7 days—was no different between study groups, whereas TIMI major bleeding was significantly increased in the pretreatment group (at day 7, HR 1.90; 95% CI, 1.19 to 3.02; $P = .006$). Therefore the results of the ACCOAST trial do not support pretreatment with prasugrel in the setting of NSTE-ACS.

Nonthienopyridines

Ticagrelor

Ticagrelor, a cyclopentyltriazolopyrimidine, is a reversibly binding oral $P2Y_{12}$ receptor antagonist (Fig. 10.4). It interacts with the $P2Y_{12}$ receptor at a ligand binding site separate from that for ADP or the thienopyridines and therefore antagonizes ADP-mediated $P2Y_{12}$ receptor activation noncompetitively.[72] In addition to $P2Y_{12}$ receptor antagonism, ticagrelor inhibits the adenosine transporter ENT-1 (type 1 equilibrative nucleoside transporter), thereby inhibiting cellular uptake of adenosine and increasing its concentration and biologic activity.[73,74]

Pharmacology and Metabolism
Unlike the thienopyridines, ticagrelor does not require metabolic conversion to an active form to antagonize the $P2Y_{12}$ receptor. Peak plasma concentration is attained at a median of 90 minutes after administration. The parent compound is metabolized primarily by CYP3A isoenzymes into a metabolite that has a similar potency in inhibiting the $P2Y_{12}$ receptor; this metabolite is present at approximately 40% of the parent concentration. Elimination of ticagrelor is mainly through hepatic metabolism, and the primary route of elimination of the active metabolite is likely through biliary excretion. CYP3A inhibitors such

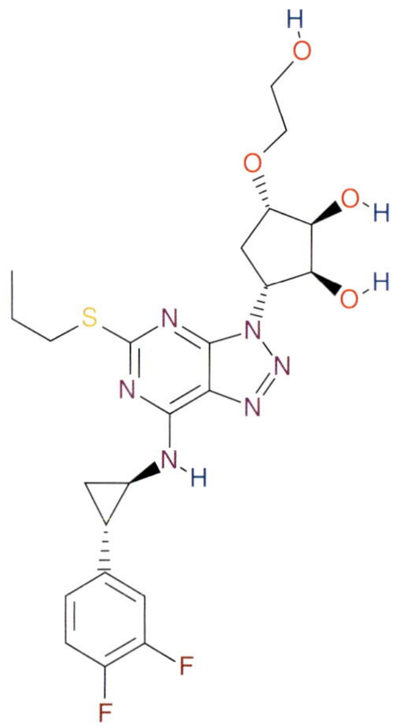

Fig. 10.4 Chemical structure of ticagrelor.

as ketoconazole or diltiazem increase plasma concentrations of ticagrelor, and ticagrelor increases the exposure to drugs that are CYP3A substrates, such as simvastatin. The CYP2C19 genotype has no effect on ticagrelor pharmacodynamics.[75] The mean half-lives of ticagrelor and its active metabolite are 7.2 hours and 8.5 hours, respectively.

Pharmacodynamics

Compared with clopidogrel, ticagrelor has a rapid onset of action, achieves more intensive $P2Y_{12}$ inhibition, and has a relatively faster offset of antiplatelet effect.[76] A ticagrelor 180-mg LD provides an IPA with ADP 20 mmol/L of 41% at 30 minutes and 88% at 2 hours after administration compared with 8% and 41% after a clopidogrel 600-mg LD, respectively. Maintenance-dose ticagrelor 90 mg twice daily provides an IPA with ADP 20 mmol/L of approximately 75% compared with 50% with clopidogrel 75 mg daily. The extent of inhibition is similar 24 hours after discontinuation of either clopidogrel or ticagrelor because of faster offset with ticagrelor, and the IPA for ticagrelor on day 3 after the last dose is comparable with that for clopidogrel at day 5.

Clinical Studies

The PLATO trial randomized 18,624 patients with ACS with or without ST-elevation to either ticagrelor or clopidogrel.[77] The primary efficacy end point was a composite of death from cardiovascular causes, MI, or stroke; the major safety end point was major bleeding as defined by the trial, which was more inclusive than TIMI-defined major bleeding. Initial patient management could be conservative or invasive, and patient randomization was stratified by the intent for early invasive management as indicated by the investigator. Unlike TRITON–TIMI 38, PLATO included both thienopyridine-naive patients and thienopyridine-treated patients. At 12 months, ticagrelor led to a significant reduction in the primary composite end point compared with clopidogrel (9.8% vs. 11.7%, HR 0.84; 95% CI, 0.77 to 0.92; $P < .001$). A similar relative reduction in the primary end point was observed in the 13,408 patients treated with a planned invasive strategy, 44% of whom had received clopidogrel before randomization and allocation to the study drug.[78] Ticagrelor significantly reduced cardiovascular mortality by an absolute risk reduction of 1.1% and reduced all-cause mortality by 1.4%; however, the statistical validity of this latter finding may be questioned because this end point was analyzed in a hierarchical fashion after the rate of stroke, which was not statistically significant between study arms. No increase in all-cause major bleeding was reported with ticagrelor. The rate of fatal intracerebral hemorrhage was significantly greater with ticagrelor therapy, but this was balanced by a higher rate of non-intracranial fatal bleeding with clopidogrel, resulting in an overall similar rate of fatal bleeding with the two therapies. Non–CABG-related TIMI major bleeding was significantly more frequent with ticagrelor (HR 1.25; 95% CI, 1.03 to 1.53; $P = .03$). In subgroup analyses according to region, ticagrelor did not provide an ischemic benefit in the North American cohort (HR 1.25; 95% CI, 0.93 to 1.67; P interaction $[P_{int}] = .045$). A potential explanation for this interaction was an observed attenuation of the treatment effect of ticagrelor with high-dose aspirin, which was more commonly used in North America.[79] To that end, the U.S. prescribing information for ticagrelor states that MDs of aspirin above 100 mg reduce the effectiveness of ticagrelor and should be avoided.

The timing of ticagrelor therapy in STEMI patients was further examined in the Administration of Ticagrelor in the Cath Lab or in the Ambulance for New ST-Elevation Myocardial Infarction to Open the Coronary Artery (ATLANTIC) trial, in which a total of 1862 STEMI patients were randomly assigned to receive a ticagrelor LD either upstream in the ambulance or in the hospital within the cardiac catheterization laboratory. The time from randomization to coronary angiography was rapid (48 min), and the mean duration of pretreatment for the in-ambulance group was 31 minutes. In-ambulance ticagrelor did not reduce the incidence of either of the coprimary end points (absence of ST-segment resolution and less than TIMI grade 3 flow in the infarct-related artery), nor did it affect the rates of MACEs or bleeding. The rate of early stent thrombosis was significantly lower with upstream treatment, but this finding must be considered exploratory and hypothesis generating because the results of the overall trial were negative.

The Prevention of Cardiovascular Events in Patients with Prior Heart Attack Using Ticagrelor Compared to Placebo on a Background of Aspirin–Thrombolysis in Myocardial Infarction 54 (PEGASUS-TIMI 54) trial evaluated the safety and efficacy of ticagrelor and aspirin compared with aspirin alone in 21,162 stable patients with prior MI.[80] Eligible patients had a spontaneous MI 1 to 3 years prior to enrollment, and had at least one additional risk factor placing them at higher ischemic risk. At a median duration of 33 months, ticagrelor 60 mg twice daily significantly reduced the risk of the primary composite end point of cardiovascular death, MI, or stroke compared with placebo (HR 0.85; 95% CI, 0.75 to 0.96; $P = .003$), driven by reduction in all components of the end point. Major bleeding according to the TIMI scale was significantly greater with ticagrelor 60 mg twice daily compared to placebo (HR 2.32; 95% CI, 1.68 to 3.21; $P < .001$). A ticagrelor 90 mg twice daily dose further increased the risk of bleeding compared with placebo, with no incremental efficacy over the 60 mg twice daily dose.

Adverse Effects

Ticagrelor has been associated with dyspnea, hyperuricemia, and ventricular pauses, possibly attributable to interference with adenosine degradation and inhibition of erythrocyte adenosine reuptake. The reversible interaction with the $P2Y_{12}$ receptor of sensory neurons may also contribute to the perception of breathlessness,[81,82] although this is speculative. Holter monitoring in a subgroup of patients in the PLATO trial demonstrated that ticagrelor led to an infrequent but greater rate of ventricular pauses of 3 or more seconds in the first week of therapy but did not result in significantly increased syncope or pacemaker implantation compared with clopidogrel. An increased rate of the complaint of dyspnea has been consistently observed in phase II and III studies. In the Dose Confirmation Study Assessing Anti-Platelet Effects of AZD6140 Versus Clopidogrel in Non–ST-Segment Elevation Myocardial Infarction (DISPERSE-2),[83] 10.5% of patients who received ticagrelor 90 mg twice daily reported dyspnea, compared with 6.4% of patients who received clopidogrel ($P = .07$). In PLATO, dyspnea was reported in 13.5% of ticagrelor-treated patients compared with 7.8% of clopidogrel-treated patients ($P < .001$). In a randomized, double-blind phase II study that actively monitored the complaint of dyspnea in 123 patients with stable CAD, 38.6%, 9.3%, and 8.3% of patients in the ticagrelor, clopidogrel, and placebo groups reported dyspnea, respectively ($P < .001$). Most cases of dyspnea occurred within 1 week of starting ticagrelor and were not associated with adverse changes in cardiac or pulmonary function.[84] "Real-world" data outside of clinical trials provide further insight into the frequency and clinical impact of ticagrelor-associated dyspnea. Among the 1209 ticagrelor-treated patients in the prospective Bern PCI registry, 31 patients discontinued the drug for dyspnea (2.6%), 7 of whom had no improvement in symptoms.[85]

Cangrelor

Pharmacology and Metabolism. Cangrelor is a nonthienopyridine ATP analogue.[86] It is administered intravenously and is a rapid and direct-acting reversible inhibitor of the $P2Y_{12}$ receptor that has a half-life of approximately 3 minutes (Fig. 10.5). Cangrelor is metabolized through dephosphorylation by ecto-endonucleatase (CD39) to form a nucleoside (AR-C69712XX), which is the major circulating metabolite. AR-C69712XX is further metabolized into several products and is primarily eliminated in the urine (58%) and to a lesser degree in the feces (35%). The pharmacokinetic/pharmacodynamic relationship for the parent compound and metabolites is unchanged in renal impairment. In healthy volunteers, a 30-µg/kg bolus followed by a 4-µg/kg/min infusion provided extensive IPA by 2 minutes after the bolus dose, and 80% of subjects returned to near-baseline platelet activity within 60 minutes.[87] In a phase II study of patients undergoing elective PCI, a dose of 4 µg/kg/min achieved greater than 95% IPA within 15 minutes of administration.[88]

Clinical Studies. Three randomized clinical trials have assessed the safety and efficacy of cangrelor during urgent and nonurgent PCI (Table 10.3). The Cangrelor Versus Standard Therapy to Achieve Optimal Management of Platelet Inhibition (CHAMPION)-PCI and CHAMPION-PLATFORM trials compared cangrelor with clopidogrel administered before or after PCI, respectively.[89,90] Cangrelor was not superior to clopidogrel in either trial with respect to the primary end point of death from any cause, MI, or ischemia-driven revascularization at 48 hours. The median times from hospital admission to PCI in CHAMPION-PCI and CHAMPION-PLATFORM were only 6.3 and 7.9 hours, respectively, which may have affected the ability to detect a periprocedural MI in those NSTE-ACS patients with elevated biomarkers at presentation; this is because increased biomarker levels may reflect the initial thrombotic event rather than being a result of the procedure. When the universal definition of MI was applied to a post hoc, pooled analysis of the CHAMPION-PCI and CHAMPION-PLATFORM trials, a significant reduction was reported in the primary end point of death, MI, and ischemia-driven revascularization with cangrelor (odds ratio [OR] 0.82, 95% CI, 0.68 to 0.99; P = .037).[91]

The CHAMPION-PHOENIX trial randomly assigned 11,145 patients with stable CAD or ACS undergoing PCI to receive either a bolus and infusion of cangrelor followed by transition to clopidogrel or a clopidogrel 300- or 600-mg LD at the time of PCI (see Table 10.3).[43] The primary end point was a composite of death, MI, ischemia-driven revascularization, or stent thrombosis at 48 hours. The definition of periprocedural MI involved an assessment of patients' baseline biomarker status, and if abnormal, additional clinical evidence of ischemia. Stent thrombosis included both intraprocedural stent thrombosis and definite stent thrombosis according to the Academic Research Consortium (ARC) definition. An independent and blinded angiographic core laboratory evaluated all procedures to determine any procedural complications. Cangrelor significantly reduced the primary efficacy end point (4.7% vs 5.9%, OR 0.78; 95% CI, 0.66 to 0.93; P = .005), driven by reductions in stent thrombosis and MI. The treatment effect of cangrelor was consistent across the subgroups of stable CAD, NSTE-ACS, STEMI, and whether the patient received clopidogrel in a 300-mg or 600-mg LD. With respect to safety, the rates of the primary safety end point—GUSTO severe bleeding—were not significantly different among the groups. In a pooled analysis of patient-level data from all three trials that compared cangrelor with clopidogrel, cangrelor significantly reduced the composite end point of death, MI according to the universal definition, ischemia driven revascularization, or stent thrombosis at 48 hours (4.7% vs. 3.8%, OR 0.81 [95% CI, 0.71 to 0.91], P = .0007).[92]

Adverse Effects. Pooled analysis of patient-level data from the CHAMPION trials demonstrated that cangrelor bolus and infusion during PCI does not increase GUSTO severe or TIMI major bleeding rates, nor does it increase the need for any blood transfusion. However, cangrelor was associated with increased bleeding according to more sensitive indices such as

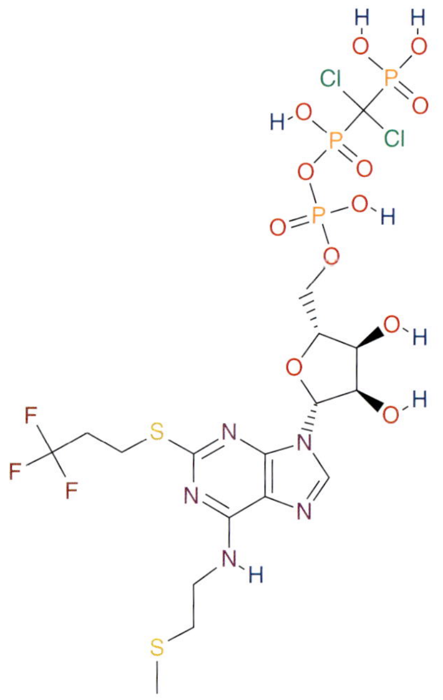

Fig. 10.5 Chemical structure of cangrelor.

TABLE 10.3 The Phase III Clinical Trials of Cangrelor

Trial	N	Prior Thienopyridine Exposure	Comparator	End Point	Duration	Outcome[a]
CHAMPION-PCI	8,877	Prior exposure allowed	Clopidogrel 600 mg within 30 min prior to PCI	Death, MI, or IDR	48 h	OR 0.87 [0.71–1.07] P = .17
CHAMPION-PLATFORM	5,362	Naïve patients only	Clopidogrel 600 mg at end of PCI	Death, MI, or IDR	48 h	OR 1.05 [0.88–1.24] P = .59
CHAMPION-PHOENIX	10,942	Naïve patients only	Clopidogrel 300 or 600 mg, dose and timing per operator	Death, MI (universal definition), IDR, or ST	48 h	OR 0.78 [0.66–0.93] P = .005

[a]Figures in brackets represent 95% confidence intervals. *CHAMPION,* Cangrelor Versus Standard Therapy to Achieve Optimal Management of Platelet Inhibition; *IDR,* ischemia-driven revascularization; *MI,* myocardial infarction; *OR,* odds ratio; *PCI,* percutaneous coronary intervention; *ST,* stent thrombosis.
Adapted from Walsh JA, Price MJ. Cangrelor for treatment of arterial thrombosis. *Expert Opin Pharmacother.* 2014;15:565–572.

Acute Catheterization and Urgent Intervention Triage Strategy (ACUITY) major bleeding (4.2% vs. 2.8%, $P < .0001$) and led to a greater rate of less severe bleeding events (GUSTO mild and TIMI minor bleeding). The rate of ACUITY major bleeding, excluding hematomas greater than 5 cm, was significantly more frequent with cangrelor, but the absolute difference was small (1.3% vs. 1.0%, $P = .007$). Cangrelor was associated with a higher rate of dyspnea compared with placebo (1.1% vs. 0.4%, $P < .0001$), which led to drug cessation in 0.1% of cases. Unlike GP IIb/IIIa inhibitors, cangrelor is not associated with acquired thrombocytopenia.[93]

In sum, cangrelor is a novel, intravenous (IV) ATP analogue that has been evaluated in several phase III studies involving over 25,000 patients undergoing PCI for stable CAD or ACS. The drug is well tolerated, although transient dyspnea may rarely occur. Cangrelor reduces ischemic events compared with conventional clopidogrel therapy in thienopyridine-naïve patients undergoing PCI, driven by reductions in MI according to the universal definition and in stent thrombosis, with rates similar to placebo of major bleeding and blood transfusions but at the cost of more minor bleeding events.[86] Cangrelor is currently approved for use by the FDA as an adjunct to PCI to reduce the risk of periprocedural MI, repeat coronary revascularization, and stent thrombosis in patients who have not been treated with a $P2Y_{12}$ platelet inhibitor and are not being given a GP IIb/IIIa inhibitor.

Thrombin Receptor Antagonists

Basic Principles

Thrombin exerts a multitude of effects on thrombosis, hemostasis, and inflammation. Generated at sites of vascular injury, it is the effector protease of the coagulation cascade, converting circulating fibrinogen to fibrin monomer, which polymerizes to form fibrin, the fibrous matrix of thrombus. Thrombin promotes edema by increasing the permeability of the vascular endothelium, induces vasoconstriction in the absence of the endothelium through its action on smooth muscle cells, and stimulates prostaglandin and cytokine production by endothelial cells. Thrombin is also the most potent agonist for platelet activation and provokes shape change, granule secretion, synthesis and release of TXA_2, mobilization of P-selectin and CD40 to the platelet surface, and activation of the GP IIb/IIIa receptor.[4] The cellular effects of thrombin are mediated primarily by the activation of PARs. The two platelet thrombin receptors in humans are PAR-1 and PAR-4, but PAR-1 is more important, mediating platelet activation at low thrombin concentrations, whereas PAR-4 mediates platelet activation only at high thrombin concentrations. PARs are unique in that each receptor carries its own ligand that is active only after cleavage. Thrombin binds the N-terminus of the PAR-1 receptor with high affinity at an extracellular, hirudin-like site and then cleaves the receptor between residues Arg 41 and Ser 42; this unmasks a new N-terminus beginning with the sequence *SFLLRN* (serine, phenylalanine, leucine, leucine, arginine, asparagine). This N-terminus functions as a tethered ligand that docks intramolecularly with the body of the receptor and activates it. The inability of PAR-4 to activate platelets at low thrombin concentrations is likely caused by the absence of an extracellular hirudin-like domain. The PAR-1 receptor is an attractive candidate for targeted inhibition in patients with cardiovascular disease. PAR-mediated signaling appears to be a more important contributor to thrombosis compared with hemostasis. In addition, platelet PAR antagonism maintains the fibrin-generating and protein-C functions of thrombin and does not appear to interfere with other platelet-signaling pathways such as those mediated by collagen and ADP (Fig. 10.6). Therefore, unlike other platelet receptor inhibitors, PAR-1 antagonists have been suggested to have a wider therapeutic window between ischemia reduction and bleeding risk. Although many PAR-1 antagonists have been developed and investigated in early phase clinical testing, only vorapaxar has been approved for clinical use.

Vorapaxar

Vorapaxar is a synthetic tricyclic 3-phenylpyridine analogue of himbacine (Fig. 10.7). It is a high-affinity, orally active, low-molecular-weight, nonpeptide competitive PAR-1 antagonist that is slowly eliminated, with a half-life of approximately 5 to 11 days. Recovery of platelet function to 50% or more of baseline occurred at 4 weeks after treatment discontinuation in healthy volunteers.

After the promising findings from early phase clinical investigations, vorapaxar was tested in two large-scale phase III clinical trials: Thrombin Receptor Antagonist for Clinical Event Reduction in Acute Coronary Syndrome (TRACER) and Thrombin Receptor Antagonist in Secondary Prevention of Atherothrombotic Ischemic Events–Thrombolysis in Myocardial Infarction (TRA 2P–TIMI 50).[94,95] After a safety review in January 2011, the Data and Safety Monitoring Board recommended halting the TRACER trial and discontinuing the drug in the ongoing TRA 2P trial in patients with prior stroke, in whom there was an observed excess of intracranial hemorrhage with vorapaxar.

TRACER tested the safety and efficacy of vorapaxar in combination with standard antiplatelet therapy in patients with NSTE-ACS.

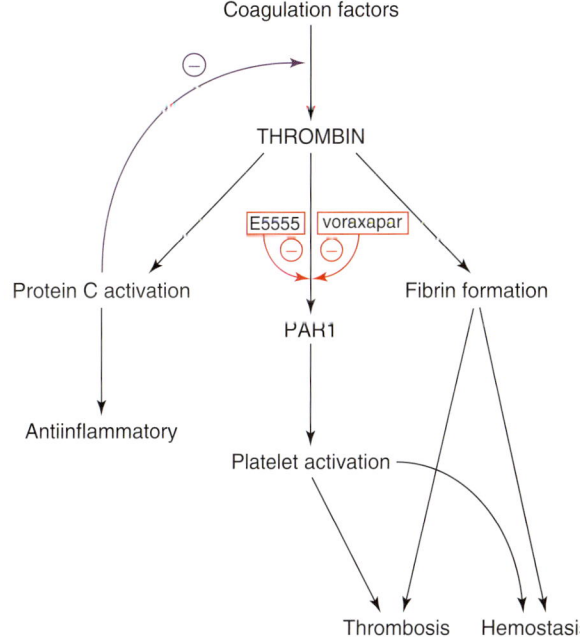

Fig. 10.6 Rationale for protease-activated receptor *(PAR)* inhibition in the treatment of cardiovascular disease. Thrombin acts as a platelet agonist through its activation of the platelet PAR-1 and PAR-4 receptors; it is the main effector protease of the coagulation cascade and triggers fibrin formation, and within the environment of the normal endothelium, it activates protein C to terminate its own production. Fibrin(ogen) appears to be more important than thrombin-induced platelet activation for hemostasis. PAR-1 is the primary mediator of thrombin-induced platelet activation, and PAR-1 antagonists may have a wide therapeutic window for platelet-dependent processes—such as acute coronary syndrome and stent thrombosis—by leaving the fibrin generation and protein-C functions of thrombin intact. Vorapaxar and atopaxar are PAR-1 inhibitors currently under clinical investigation. (From Angiolillo DJ, Capodanno D, Goto S. Platelet thrombin receptor antagonism and atherothrombosis. *Eur Heart J.* 2010;31:17–28.)

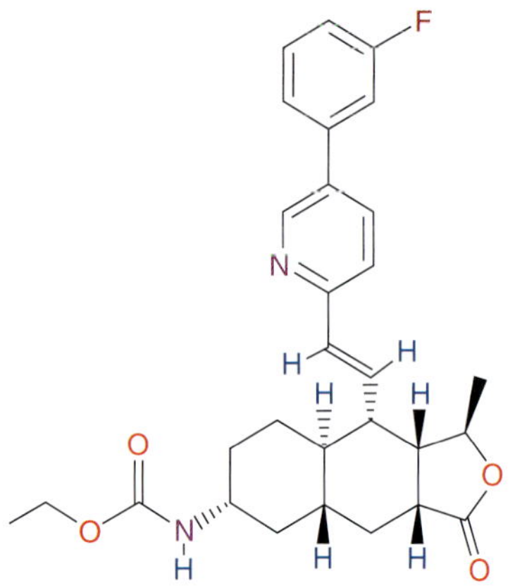

Fig. 10.7 Chemical structure of vorapaxar.

A total of 12,944 patients were randomly assigned to receive either vorapaxar (40-mg LD followed by 2.5 mg daily) or placebo in addition to standard antiplatelet therapy. Concomitant clopidogrel therapy was administered in 92%, and aspirin was administered in 99% of the enrolled patients.[94] The primary end point was a composite of death from cardiovascular causes, MI, stroke, recurrent ischemia with rehospitalization, or urgent coronary revascularization. In the patients assigned to vorapaxar, a nonsignificant decrease was found in the primary efficacy end point at 2 years (18.5% vs. 19.9%, HR 0.92; 95% CI, 0.85 to 1.01; $P = .07$) at the cost of a significant (35%) increase in the rate of GUSTO moderate or severe bleeding (7.2% vs. 5.2%, HR 1.35; 95% CI, 1.16 to 1.58; $P < .001$) and a threefold increase in the rate of intracranial bleeding (0.6% vs 0.2%, HR 3.39; 95% CI, 1.78 to 6.45; $P < .001$).

The TRA 2P–TIMI 50 trial evaluated the role of vorapaxar in the secondary prevention of cardiovascular events in patients with known atherothrombotic disease (i.e., history of prior MI, ischemic stroke, or peripheral arterial disease [PAD]).[95] A total of 26,449 patients were randomly assigned to receive either vorapaxar 2.5 mg daily or placebo in addition to standard-of-care therapy, including aspirin and/or a thienopyridine. Concomitant aspirin was administered in 94% of enrolled patients, and clopidogrel was given in a majority of the patients with a qualifying diagnosis of MI. After a median follow-up of 30 months, vorapaxar significantly reduced the primary end point (a composite of death from cardiovascular causes, MI, or stroke) compared with placebo (HR 0.87; 95% CI, 0.80 to 0.94; $P < .001$), driven by a 17% reduction in the rate of MI. However, vorapaxar increased the rate of GUSTO moderate or severe bleeding (HR 1.66; 95% CI, 1.43 to 1.93; $P < .001$), as well as intracranial bleeding (HR 1.94; 95% CI, 1.39 to 2.70; $P < .001$). In the subgroup of patients with prior stroke, vorapaxar was associated with higher rates of major bleeding and intracranial hemorrhage without any improvement in ischemic outcomes. The benefit of vorapaxar over placebo in reducing the primary end point was enhanced in the large subgroup of patients with prior MI (HR 0.80; 95% CI, 0.72 to 0.89; $P < .0001$) and was consistent across timing and types of MI.[96] Despite an increase in total bleeding (HR 1.61; 95% CI, 1.31 to 1.97; $P < .0001$), intracranial and fatal bleeding were not significantly higher in the vorapaxar group among patients with prior MI, and an overall benefit was seen in net clinical outcome.

The FDA approved vorapaxar for clinical use in 2014. Specifically, vorapaxar at a dose of 2.5 mg once daily is indicated for the reduction of thrombotic cardiovascular events in patients with a history of MI or with PAD, and it must be used in addition to antiplatelet therapy (aspirin and/or clopidogrel) as per the standard of care. Vorapaxar is contraindicated in patients with a history of stroke, TIA, or intracranial hemorrhage and in those with active pathologic bleeding.

Phosphodiesterase Inhibitors

Cilostazol

Cilostazol, a selective phosphodiesterase type 3 (PDE-3) inhibitor, increases cAMP levels in multiple cell lines—including platelets, endothelial cells, and smooth muscle cells—and results in both vasodilatory and antiplatelet effects. It was approved by the FDA in 1998 for the treatment of symptoms of intermittent claudication. Pharmacodynamic studies have shown that the addition of cilostazol to aspirin and clopidogrel (triple-antiplatelet therapy) results in greater ADP-induced platelet inhibition compared with aspirin and clopidogrel alone.[97] Adjunctive cilostazol therapy in addition to aspirin and clopidogrel has been associated with a reduced risk of stent thrombosis, restenosis, and MACEs without increased bleeding complications in patients undergoing PCI, including those treated with a DES.[98,99] These benefits have been more marked in complex settings such as in patients with diabetes mellitus and long lesions. The clinical studies of cilostazol in the PCI setting have been conducted primarily in Asia. The most common side effects of cilostazol include headache, tachycardia, palpitations, soft stools, and diarrhea, and these may lead to drug discontinuation in up to 15% of cases. Cilostazol should be avoided in patients with congestive heart failure of any severity, with or without preserved left ventricular systolic function, because of an increased mortality risk with PDE inhibitors.

Glycoprotein IIb/IIIa Inhibitors

The GP IIb/IIIa receptor is an integrin, a heterodimer consisting of noncovalently associated α and β subunits, which mediate the final common pathway of platelet aggregation. In specific, the GP IIb/IIIa receptor consists of the α_{IIb} and β_3 subunits. By competing with fibrinogen and vWF for GP IIb/IIIa binding, GP IIb/IIIa antagonists interfere with platelet cross-linking and platelet-derived thrombus formation (Fig. 10.8). Because the GP IIb/IIIa receptor represents the final common pathway leading to platelet aggregation, these agents are very effective in inhibiting platelets. Investigations of oral GP IIb/IIIa inhibitors have been stopped because of their lack of benefit and increased mortality in patients with ACS and in those undergoing PCI. The reasons for these negative outcomes remain elusive. Currently, only parenteral GP IIb/IIIa inhibitors are approved for clinical use and are recommended only in the setting of patients with ACS who are undergoing PCI. Although GP IIb/IIIa inhibitors have reduced MACEs (death, MI, and urgent revascularization) by 35% to 50% in patients undergoing PCI, their broad use has been limited because of their association with an increased risk of bleeding.[100]

Pharmacology

Three parenteral GP IIb/IIIa antagonists have been approved for clinical use: abciximab, eptifibatide, and tirofiban (Table 10.4).

Abciximab

Abciximab is a large chimeric monoclonal antibody with a high binding affinity that results in a prolonged pharmacologic effect. In particular, it is a monoclonal antibody that is a fragment antigen binding (Fab) fragment of a chimeric human–mouse genetic reconstruction of 7E3. The Fc portion of the antibody was removed to decrease immunogenicity, and the Fab portion was attached to the constant regions of a human immunoglobulin (Ig). Abciximab binding is specific for the β_3-subunit and explains its ability to bind other β_3-receptors such as vitronectin ($\alpha v \beta_3$). Unlike the small-molecule GP IIb/III inhibitors eptifibatide and tirofiban, abciximab interacts with the GP IIb/IIIa receptor at sites distinct from the ligand-binding RGD sequence site and exerts its inhibitory effect noncompetitively. Its plasma half-life is biphasic, with an initial half-life of less than 10 minutes and

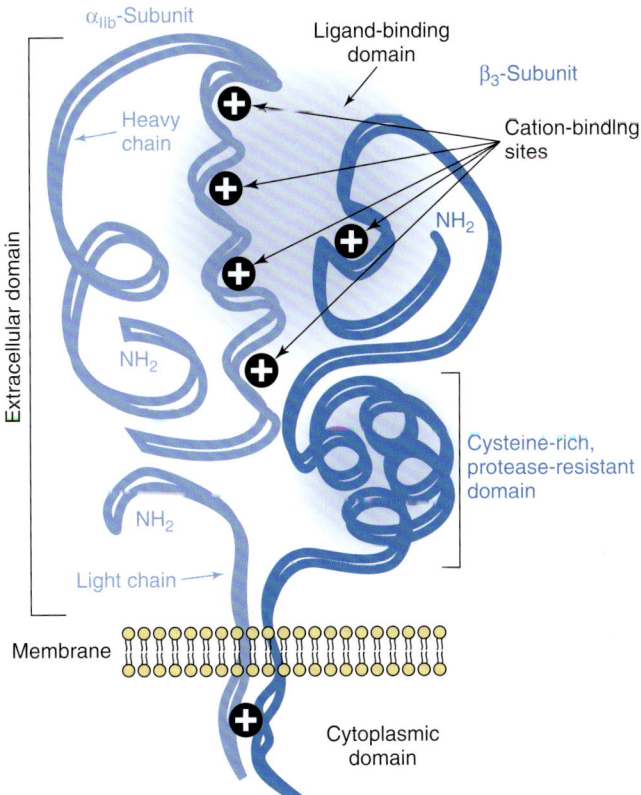

Fig. 10.8 Structure of the glycoprotein *(GP)* IIb/IIIa receptor. The GP IIb/IIIa receptor is an integrin, a heterodimer consisting of noncovalently associated α and β subunits that mediate the final common pathway of platelet aggregation. The GP IIb/IIIa receptor consists of the α_{IIb} and β_3 subunits. The α-subunit is a 136-kDa molecule with light and heavy chains; the light chain contains a short cytoplasmic tail, a transmembrane region, and a short extracellular domain, whereas the heavy chain is entirely extracellular. The β-subunit is an 84.5-kDa molecule with a short intracellular tail, a transmembrane region, and a large extracellular domain. Platelet activation leads to a conformational change in the GP IIb/IIIa receptor, which markedly increases its affinity for its ligands through its binding sites. On the GP IIb/IIIa receptor are two main binding sites: One recognizes the amino acid sequence arginine–glycine–aspartic acid (Arg-Gly-Asp, or *RGD*) found on multiple ligands (fibronectin, von Willebrand factor, and vitronectin) but most important on fibrinogen, the major GP IIb/IIIa ligand, in which the *RGD* sequence occurs twice. The other peptide sequence is the lysine–glutamine–alanine–glycine–aspartic acid–valine (Lys-Gln-Ala-Gly-Asp-Val [*KQAGDV*]) sequence, which is only located at the carboxyl terminus of the γ-chain of fibrinogen. (From Topol EJ, Byzova TV, Plow EF. Platelet GP IIB/IIIa blockers. *Lancet.* 1999;353:227–231.)

a second-phase half-life of approximately 30 minutes. However, because of its high affinity for the GP IIb/IIIa receptor, it has a biologic half-life of 12 to 24 hours; and because of its slow clearance from the body, it has a functional half-life of up to 7 days. Platelet-associated abciximab can be detected for more than 14 days after the infusion has been stopped. The recommended dose for abciximab is a 0.25 mg/kg bolus followed by an IV infusion with 0.125 μg/kg/min for 12 hours. No renal adjustments are required.

Epitifibatide

Unlike abciximab, the small-molecule agents eptifibatide and tirofiban do not induce an immune response and have a lower affinity for the GP IIb/IIIa receptor. Eptifibatide is a reversibly interacting and highly selective heptapeptide with a rapid onset and a short plasma half-life of 2 to 2.5 hours. Its molecular design is based on barbourin, a member of the disintegrin family, which contains a novel Lys-Gly-Asp (KGD) sequence, making it highly specific for the GP IIb/IIIa receptor. In the setting of PCI, a double-bolus and infusion regimen is recommended (180 μg/kg, followed by a second, 180 μg/kg bolus, followed by 2 μg/kg/min for a minimum of 12 hours); peak plasma levels are established shortly after the bolus dose, and a slightly lower concentration is subsequently maintained throughout the infusion period. Because eptifibatide is mostly eliminated through renal mechanisms, a lower infusion dose (1 μg/kg/min) is recommended in patients with creatinine clearance less than 50 mL/min. Recovery of platelet aggregation occurs within 4 hours of completion of the infusion.

Tirofiban

Tirofiban is a tyrosine-derived nonpeptide inhibitor that mimics the *RGD* sequence and is highly specific for the GP IIb/IIIa receptor. Tirofiban is associated with a rapid onset and a short duration of action, with a plasma half-life of approximately 2 hours. Like eptifibatide, substantial recovery of platelet aggregation is present within 4 hours of completion of infusion. Tirofiban was previously administered as a 10 μg/kg bolus followed by infusion 0.15 μg/kg/min for 18 to 24 hours. Several studies have documented that this treatment regimen achieves suboptimal levels of platelet inhibition for up to 4 to 6 hours, which likely accounted for its inferior clinical results in the PCI setting. For this reason, a high-dose bolus regimen (25 μg/kg) that achieves more optimal platelet inhibition has been tested and has shown antiplatelet efficacy comparable to the other GP IIb/IIIa inhibitors. The FDA has approved a high-bolus–dose tirofiban regimen, as well as a shorter duration of infusion, for patients undergoing PCI. Because tirofiban is mostly eliminated through renal mechanisms, dosage adjustment is required for patients with renal insufficiency.

Thrombocytopenia

Patients treated with GP IIb/IIIa inhibitors have a higher incidence of thrombocytopenia. Severe thrombocytopenia is more commonly associated with abciximab and requires immediate cessation of therapy. The mechanism of thrombocytopenia is unknown; however, regardless of its etiology, thrombocytopenia in patients undergoing PCI is associated with more ischemic events, bleeding complications, and mortality.[93] The platelet count typically falls within hours of GP IIb/IIIa administration. Readministration of abciximab, but not eptifibatide and tirofiban, is associated with a slightly increased risk of thrombocytopenia.

Pivotal Clinical Trials With Glycoprotein IIb/IIIa Inhibitors

Before the era of pretreatment with high LDs of clopidogrel, the safety and efficacy of GP IIb/IIIa inhibition was tested in several clinical studies that included patients with ACS and those with stable CAD. The landmark trial that demonstrated the efficacy of GP IIb/IIIa inhibition in the PCI setting was the Evaluation of IIb/IIIa Platelet Receptor Antagonist 7E3 in Preventing Ischemic Complications (EPIC).[101] In this study, high-risk patients undergoing balloon angioplasty were randomized to abciximab bolus and infusion, abciximab bolus alone, or placebo. The group treated with abciximab bolus and infusion had a 35% lower rate of death, MI, or unplanned urgent revascularization at 30 days compared with the placebo group. No significant benefit with abciximab bolus alone was observed, suggesting that a shorter duration of platelet inhibition was insufficient to favorably affect clinical outcomes. Major bleeding complications occurred in a very high proportion of patients treated with abciximab. A series of procedural modifications—including front-wall arterial puncture, reducing arterial sheath size (from 8 to 6 Fr), reducing heparin dosing (target activated clotting time [ACT] of 200 to 250 seconds rather

TABLE 10.4 Characteristics of the Glycoprotein IIb/IIIa Inhibitors

	Abciximab	Eptifibatide	Tirofiban
Molecule	Fab 7E3	Synthetic peptide	Nonpeptide mimetic
Molecular weight	~50,000	~800	~500
Stoichiometry (drug to GP IIb/IIIa)	~1.5:1	≫100:1	≫100:1
Binding	Noncompetitive	Competitive	Competitive
Half-life	Plasma: 10–15 h Biologic: 12–24 h	Plasma: 2–2.5 h Biologic = plasma	Plasma: 2–2.5 h Biologic = plasma
PCI dosing	Bolus: 0.25 mg/kg (10–60 min) Infusion: 0.125 µg/kg/min (12 h)	Bolus: 180 µg/kg (10 min) + 180 µg/kg Infusion: 2 µg/kg/min (24–48 h)	Bolus: 25 µg/kg (30 min) Infusion: 0.10 µg/kg/min (48 h)
Renal adjustment	No	Bolus: 180 µg/kg Infusion: 1 µg/kg/min (24–48 h)	Bolus: 12.5 µg/kg (30 min) Infusion: 0.10 µg/kg/min (48 h)

Fab, Fragment antigen binding; *GP,* glycoprotein; *PCI,* percutaneous coronary intervention.

than >300 seconds), early sheath removal, and abandoning the use of routine venous sheaths—markedly reduced major bleeding complications (~1% to 1.5% in later trials). After the EPIC trial, the Evaluation of Percutaneous Transluminal Coronary Angioplasty (PTCA) to Improve Long-Term Outcome With Abciximab GP IIb/IIIa Blockade (EPILOG)[102] was conducted in patients undergoing balloon angioplasty who were at a lower risk than the patients in EPIC. In EPILOG, abciximab was given with lower doses of weight-adjusted heparin and with weight-adjusted infusions of abciximab. This study was stopped prematurely because of a significant reduction in the incidence of death or MI in patients treated with abciximab and in the setting of acceptable bleeding rates. Similar results were reported in the Evaluation of Platelet GP IIb/IIIa Inhibition in Stenting (EPISTENT),[103] which was the first randomized trial to examine the use of GP IIb/IIIa inhibitors—in this case, abciximab—among patients undergoing stent placement. The Enhanced Suppression of the Platelet IIb/IIIa Receptor with Integrilin Therapy (ESPRIT)[104] trial conducted in patients undergoing coronary stenting using eptifibatide was also terminated early because of the superior efficacy of eptifibatide. Major bleeding was rare but occurred more frequently in eptifibatide-treated patients compared with placebo-treated patients. On the basis of these trials, GP IIb/IIIa inhibitors became a cornerstone in the treatment of patients undergoing PCI because of their ability to improve short- and long-term outcomes, mostly by reducing the occurrence of periprocedural MI. Subsequently, however, it was shown that a GP IIb/IIIa inhibitor may no longer benefit patients if they had been pretreated with high-dose clopidogrel, particularly those with stable CAD or in the absence of elevated cardiac enzymes. The first Intracoronary Stenting and Antithrombotic Regimen–Rapid Early Action for Coronary Treatment (ISAR-REACT) trial[105] showed that in 2159 low- to intermediate-risk patients undergoing elective PCI, all of whom had been pretreated for at least 2 hours with a 600-mg LD of clopidogrel, no benefit of abciximab therapy was found, compared with placebo, with respect to the incidence of death, MI, and urgent target-vessel revascularization at 30 days ($P = .8$). The findings were similar in the Intracoronary Stenting and Antithrombotic Regimen—Is Abciximab a Superior Way to Eliminate Elevated Thrombotic Risk in Diabetics? (ISAR-SWEET) trial,[106] the first dedicated randomized trial to evaluate GP IIb/IIIa blockade in patients with diabetes scheduled for elective PCI. Overall, these studies suggest that GP IIb/IIIa inhibitors offer no clinical benefit in low- to intermediate-risk patients scheduled for PCI, including those with diabetes, if they have been pretreated with clopidogrel. The ISAR-REACT 2 trial[107] assessed the incremental benefit of GP IIb/IIIa inhibitors for patients with ACS in the current era of treatment with a high LD of clopidogrel before PCI. This trial randomized 2022 patients with ACS pretreated with clopidogrel 600 mg for at least 2 hours to either abciximab or placebo in the catheterization laboratory at the time of PCI. Abciximab significantly reduced the incidence of the primary end point of death, MI, or target-vessel revascularization at 30 days, but the benefit of abciximab treatment was limited only to those patients who presented with elevated troponin. Overall, these findings, and those from retrospective analyses of other studies, suggest that in the modern era of interventional cardiology using high clopidogrel dosing regimens, GP IIb/IIIa inhibition should be reserved only for high-risk patients with ACS and elevated cardiac biomarkers.

Timing of Glycoprotein IIb/IIIa Administration

Two different timing strategies for the administration of GP IIb/IIIa inhibitors have been used in the large, randomized GP IIb/IIIa trials: before angiography *(upstream treatment)* or in the cardiac catheterization laboratory in patients about to undergo PCI *(provisional treatment)*. These two strategies were compared in the Early Glycoprotein IIb/IIIa Inhibition in Non–ST Segment Elevation Acute Coronary Syndrome (EARLY-ACS) trial,[108] which randomized 9492 invasively managed patients with NSTE-ACS to either routine upstream eptifibatide or placebo infusion and provisional eptifibatide after angiography. No differences were found between the groups in the primary end point, and patients in the early eptifibatide group had significantly higher rates of bleeding and transfusion. These findings do not support the routine use of upstream GP IIb/IIIa inhibition compared with ad hoc GP IIb/IIIa inhibition in patients with ACS undergoing PCI.

Glycoprotein IIb/IIIa Inhibitors in Primary Percutaneous Coronary Intervention

The use of GP IIb/IIIa inhibitors, in particular abciximab, in STEMI patients undergoing primary PCI is supported by a meta-analysis of 11 randomized trials that involved a total 27,115 patients. In this meta-analysis, the administration of abciximab was associated with a significant reduction in the rate of reinfarction, as well as mortality rates, at 30 days.[109] However, most of the studies included in the meta-analysis were conducted in patients who had not been pretreated with clopidogrel. In the Third Bavarian Reperfusion Alternatives Evaluation (BRAVE 3), 800 patients with acute STEMI within 24 hours from symptom onset, all of whom were treated with clopidogrel 600 mg, were randomly assigned to receive either upstream abciximab or placebo.[110] Abciximab was not associated with a reduction in the primary end point, infarct size, or ischemic end points at 30 days, which argued against the routine use of upstream abciximab in clopidogrel-pretreated patients undergoing primary PCI. Strategies of facilitated PCI have been developed on the basis of the premise that time to reperfusion is a critical determinant of outcome. A series of small pilot investigations with GP IIb/IIIa inhibitors that measured surrogate markers of ischemic benefit, such as angiographic flow or ST-segment resolution, showed promising results. This series set the basis for larger studies to clarify the safety and efficacy of different regimens of facilitated PCI using GP IIb/IIIa inhibitors alone or in combination with a reduced-dose fibrinolytic. In the Facilitated Intervention with Enhanced Reperfusion Speed to Stop Events (FINESSE) trial,[111] 2452 patients with STEMI who presented within 6 hours after symptom onset were randomized to receive PCI facilitated with early abciximab and half-dose reteplase (*combination facilitated*), PCI with early abciximab alone (*abciximab facilitated*), or primary PCI with abciximab at the time of the procedure. The primary end point—composite of death from all causes, ventricular fibrillation occurring more than 48 hours after randomization, cardiogenic shock, and congestive heart failure during the first 90 days after randomization—occurred in 9.8%, 10.5%, and 10.7% of the patients in the combination-facilitated, abciximab-facilitated, and primary PCI groups, respectively ($P = .55$) without significant differences in mortality. These results do not support the use of a facilitated pharmacologic strategy for reperfusion, with either abciximab alone or abciximab plus reduced-dose reteplase, in anticipation of urgent PCI for patients who present early with STEMI.[111]

Although the GP IIb/IIIa inhibitors are approved for IV use, several studies have assessed the efficacy of intracoronary (IC) administration in patients with STEMI undergoing primary PCI. A meta-analysis of small-sample studies[112] suggests a benefit of IC use of GP IIb/IIIa inhibitors; however, this finding was not supported by the large Abciximab Intracoronary Versus Intravenous Drug Application in ST-Elevation Myocardial Infarction (AIDA-STEMI) trial.[113] In this trial, a total of 2065 patients with STEMI undergoing primary PCI were randomly assigned to an IC or IV abciximab bolus during the PCI procedure, followed by an IV infusion. No difference was found between groups in the primary end point of all-cause mortality, recurrent infarction, or new congestive heart failure at 90 days, nor were there significant differences in the secondary end points of early ST-segment resolution, TIMI flow grade, or enzymatic infarct size. In the Intracoronary Abciximab and Aspiration Thrombectomy in Patients With Large Anterior Myocardial Infarction (INFUSE-AMI)[114] trial, IC abciximab delivered through a specialized drug-delivery catheter reduced infarct size compared with no abciximab in 452 patients with large, anterior MIs undergoing primary PCI with bivalirudin anticoagulation.

Duration of Oral Dual-Antiplatelet Therapy

The small but incremental risk of late thrombosis with DES use raised considerable uncertainty about the optimal duration of DAPT after PCI. Rates of late stent thrombosis appears to be lower with newer generation DES.[115] However, patients who have undergone PCI could possibly derive benefit from very long-term DAPT because of a reduction in atherosclerosis-mediated events rather than stent-mediated events. Indeed, randomized trials from the BMS era demonstrate the benefit of prolonged aspirin and clopidogrel over the first year after PCI.[17,116] The overall benefit of long-term DAPT after PCI likely depends upon the balance between bleeding and ischemic risk for the particular patient. For example, long-term DAPT reduces ischemic events in patients with prior MI and symptomatic peripheral arterial disease.[117]

DAPT was the first randomized, clinical trial to be adequately powered to test the safety and efficacy of prolonged dual-antiplatelet therapy on stent-related outcomes in patients treated with a DES.[118] A total of 9961 patients who had undergone DES placement and were MACE free at 12 months after the procedure and receiving DAPT with a thienopyridine and aspirin were randomly assigned to either continue the thienopyridine for an additional 18 months or to receive placebo; all patients continued to receive aspirin. Among the enrolled patients, 60% had been treated with a next-generation DES (47% everolimus-eluting and 13% zotarolimus-eluting stents). Continued DAPT significantly reduced the rate of the coprimary end point of definite or probable stent thrombosis (1.4% vs. 0.4%, HR 0.29; 95% CI, 0.17 to 0.48; $P < .001$), as well as definite stent thrombosis (1.2% vs. 0.3%, HR 0.26; 95% CI, 0.14 to 0.45; $P < .001$; Fig. 10.9). The treatment effect of continued DAPT on stent thrombosis was consistent across DES types (P_{int} = .79). The rate of MI was also significantly reduced by continued DAPT (4.1% vs. 2.1%, HR 0.47; 95% CI, 0.37 to 0.61; $P < .001$); MIs not related to stent thrombosis accounted for about 55% of this treatment effect. The second coprimary end point, a composite of major adverse cardiovascular and cerebrovascular events, was significantly reduced with continued DAPT (5.9% vs. 3.4%, HR 0.71; 95% CI, 0.59 to 0.85; $P < .001$). An increase in noncardiovascular mortality was observed (1.0% vs. 0.5%, HR 2.23; 95% CI, 1.32 to 3.78; $P = .002$), which the investigators suggest may have been because of the presence of a disproportionate number of patients with prior cancer

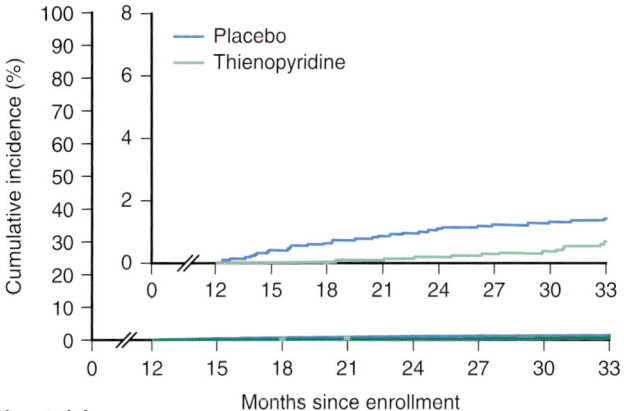

Stent thrombosis
12–30 months   Thienopyridine vs. placebo, 0.4% vs. 1.4%; hazard ratio, 0.29; $P < .001$
12–33 months   Thienopyridine vs. placebo, 0.7% vs. 1.4%; hazard ratio, 0.45; $P < .001$

Fig. 10.9 Cumulative incidence of definite or probable stent thrombosis in the Dual Antiplatelet Therapy Trial. At 12 months after drug-eluting stent implantation, continued aspirin and thienopyridine for an additional 18 months significantly reduced the rate of stent thrombosis compared with aspirin alone. (From the DAPT Study Investigators. Twelve or 30 months of dual antiplatelet therapy after drug-eluting stents. *N Engl J Med.* 2014;371[23]:2155–2166.)

in the placebo arm. A subsequent, large meta-analysis of randomized trials that assigned patients to extended thienopyridine use (>6 months), which included the DAPT trial, did not demonstrate any effect of thienopyridine treatment on noncardiovascular mortality.[119] Whereas continued thienopyridine therapy from 12 through 30 months after DES implantation reduced both stent-related and nonstent-related ischemic events in the DAPT trial, this was balanced by an increased risk in the primary safety end point, moderate or severe GUSTO bleeding (1.6% vs. 2.5%, $P = .001$), although no increase in fatal bleeding was reported. Therefore, the findings of the DAPT trial support continued thienopyridine treatment beyond 12 months in patients who receive a DES, irrespective of stent type, in those who are not at high risk for bleeding.

Meta-analysis of outcomes with second-generation DES suggest that a DAPT duration of less than 12 months may be associated with less bleeding and similar outcomes,[120] although these types of analyses are limited by methodological heterogeneity and lack of poolability of the included trials.[121] Since the totality of the data suggests that the risk of stent thrombosis is attenuated with newer generation DES, a major contributor to the risk/benefit calculus for extended therapy is the magnitude of the reduction in nonstent-related ischemic events with longer duration of DAPT. This may be of particular importance in ACS patients. In a randomized trial of 2712 patients with ACS, a shortened 6-month DAPT duration was associated with an increased risk of MI compared to the standard-of-care 12-month duration.[122]

Prediction Scores

Several scores have been developed to help guide the appropriate duration of DAPT for an individual patient. The DAPT score is a prediction rule derived from the DAPT trial, and focuses on patients who have tolerated 1 year of DAPT without major bleeding or ischemic events. This score may help differentiate patients who would derive a net clinical benefit from those that might suffer net harm with prolonged DAPT (i.e., beyond 12 months) (Box 10.1).[123] Factors incorporated into the DAPT score include clinical characteristics (elderly age, diabetes mellitus, smoking, prior MI, prior PCI, left ventricular dysfunction), clinical presentation (whether an MI was the index event that led to DES implantation), procedure-related characteristics (small reference vessel diameter, vein graft intervention), and type of DES (paclitaxel-eluting stent). The PRECISE-DAPT score was derived from pooled, patient-level data from eight randomized clinical trials. It incorporates 5 factors: age, creatinine clearance, hemoglobin level, white blood cell count, and previous spontaneous bleeding (see www.precisedaptscore.com).[124] Compared with shortened DAPT (3- to 6-month duration), prolonged DAPT (12 to 24 months) was associated with increased bleeding in patients with a high score (≥25) and decreased ischemic events in patients with a lower score.

Guideline Recommendations for Dual-Antiplatelet Therapy Duration

The recommendations laid forth in the 2016 ACC/AHA Focused Update on the Duration of Dual Antiplatelet Therapy in Patients With Coronary Artery Disease[125] are based on several fundamental principles. First, newer generation DES have a lower risk of stent thrombosis, and therefore the recommendations for DAPT duration after first-generation DES may not apply. Second, and most important, the bleeding and ischemic risk profile of the patient must be considered to individualize a management strategy. A longer-duration of therapy may be reasonable in patients with lower bleeding risk and higher ischemic risk, while a shorter duration of therapy may be reasonable in patients with higher bleeding risk and lower ischemic risk. Patients with ACS (non-STEMI [NSTEMI] or STEMI) should be given DAPT for at least 12 months, irrespective of BMS or DES implantation (class I, LOE B), and continuation of DAPT for longer than 12 months may be reasonable in ACS patients who have tolerated DAPT without a bleeding complication and who are not at high bleeding risk (class IIb, LOE A). In ACS patients treated with DAPT after DES of BMS implantation who develop a high risk of bleeding or significant overt bleeding, discontinuation of the oral $P2Y_{12}$ inhibitor at 6 months may be reasonable (class IIb, LOE C). In stable CAD patients treated with DES, DAPT should be given for at least 6 months (class I, LOE B); continuation of DAPT for longer than 6 months may be reasonable in patients treated with DES who have tolerated DAPT without a bleeding complication and who are not at high risk for bleeding (class IIb, LOE A); and discontinuation of the oral $P2Y_{12}$ inhibitor after 3 months may be reasonable in patients treated with DES who develop a high risk of bleeding or significant overt bleeding (class IIb, LOE C).

The recommendations detailed in the European Society of Cardiology (ESC) Focused Update on DAPT in Coronary Artery Disease[126] vary slightly from the American perspective. In patients with stable CAD, DAPT (aspirin and clopidogrel) is generally recommended for 6 months, irrespective of the stent type (class I, LOE A); DAPT for 3 months should be considered in patients at high bleeding risk (e.g., PRECISE-DAPT score ≥25) (class IIa, LOE B); and continuation of DAPT for >6 months and ≤30 months may be considered in patients who have tolerated DAPT without a bleeding complication and who are at low bleeding but high thrombotic risk (class IIa, LOE A). In patients with ACS, DAPT is recommended for 12 months unless there are contraindications such as excessive bleeding risk (e.g., PRECISE-DAPT ≥25) (class I, LOE A); discontinuation of the oral $P2Y_{12}$ inhibitor at 6 months should be considered in patients with high bleeding risk (class IIa, LOE B); and

---

BOX 10.1 Factors Used to Calculate Dual-Antiplatelet Therapy Score

Variable	Points
Age ≥75 years	−2
Age 65 to <75 years	−1
Age <65 years	0
Current cigarette smoker	1
Diabetes mellitus	1
MI at presentation	1
Prior PCI or prior MI	1
Stent diameter <3 mm	1
Paclitaxel-eluting stent	1
CHF or LVEF <30%	2
Saphenous vein graft PCI	2

A score of ≥2 is associated with a favorable benefit/risk ratio for prolonged DAPT while a score of <2 is associated with an unfavorable benefit/risk ratio.

CHF, Congestive heart failure; *DAPT*, dual antiplatelet therapy; *LVEF*, left ventricular ejection fraction; *MI*, myocardial infarction; *PCI*, percutaneous coronary intervention. Adapted from Yeh RW, Secemsky EA, Kereiakes DJ, et al. Development and validation of a prediction rule for benefit and harm of dual antiplatelet therapy beyond 1 year after percutaneous coronary intervention. *JAMA*. 2016;315:1735–1749.

continuation of DAPT longer than 12 months may be considered if DAPT has been tolerated without a bleeding complication (class IIb, LOE A).

Triple-Antithrombotic Therapy: Considerations for the Patient With Atrial Fibrillation Undergoing Percutaneous Coronary Infarction

AF represents the most common cardiac arrhythmia, and chronic oral anticoagulation (OAC) is strongly recommended to prevent cerebrovascular events among patients with high thromboembolic risk.[127] Notably, because the prevalence of both AF and CAD increase with age, these conditions frequently coexist. Nearly 30% of patients with AF have concomitant CAD; approximately 7% to 10% of AF patients undergo PCI. Management of these patients has become an emerging clinical problem given that they have the theoretical need for concomitant use of DAPT, including aspirin and a $P2Y_{12}$ receptor inhibitor in addition to OAC, also known as *triple-antithrombotic therapy* (TAT). However, the use of TAT comes at the expense of an increased risk of bleeding complications. Data are limited on the optimal antithrombotic treatment regimen for these patients, and the conundrum of the optimal antithrombotic treatment regimen for patients with AF undergoing PCI is further exacerbated by the introduction into clinical practice of the novel oral anticoagulants (NOACs).

Until recently, most information on clinical outcomes derive from studies using vitamin K antagonists (VKAs). Among these, the Use of Clopidogrel With or Without Aspirin in Patients Taking Oral Anticoagulant Therapy and Undergoing Percutaneous Coronary Intervention (WOEST) study,[128] was a landmark trial as it was the first to introduce the concept of stopping aspirin therapy as a strategy to reduce the risk of bleeding complications. In this study, patients undergoing PCI were randomly assigned to triple therapy or clopidogrel monotherapy and a VKA (double antithrombotic therapy). The double-therapy regimen was associated with significantly fewer bleeding events and improved ischemic outcomes compared with the triple-therapy regimen. However, the study size (573 patients) was rather small, and few patients in this trial were treated for complex disease: only one-quarter had a history of diabetes mellitus, approximately 70% had single-vessel disease, the mean target lesion reference vessel diameter was approximately 3.12 mm, one-third received a BMS, and one-third of patients were receiving an OAC for an indication other than AF. Larger studies are therefore warranted to support these findings. However, these findings set the foundation for further studies using the NOACs. Although the NOACs have shown favorable safety and efficacy profiles in patients with AF, data are limited on how to combine these agents with standard antiplatelet treatment regimens given that the use of DAPT was, for the most part, an exclusion criterion from enrollment in the pivotal trials leading to NOAC approval.

The results of two trials using the NOACs in AF patients undergoing PCI have been reported: A Study Exploring Two Strategies of Rivaroxaban and One of Oral Vitamin K Antagonist in Patients With Atrial Fibrillation Who Undergo Percutaneous Coronary Intervention (PIONEER AF-PCI) and Evaluation of Dual Therapy With Dabigatran vs. Triple Therapy With Warfarin in Patients With Atrial Fibrillation that Undergo a PCI with Stenting (REDUAL-PCI).[129,130] Both of these tested a NOAC (rivaroxaban or dabigatran) in combination with antiplatelet therapy in AF patients undergoing PCI. In brief, both studies support the concept that a NOAC in combination with single antiplatelet therapy using a $P2Y_{12}$ inhibitor (without aspirin), or double antithrombotic therapy, is superior to a strategy of triple therapy consisting

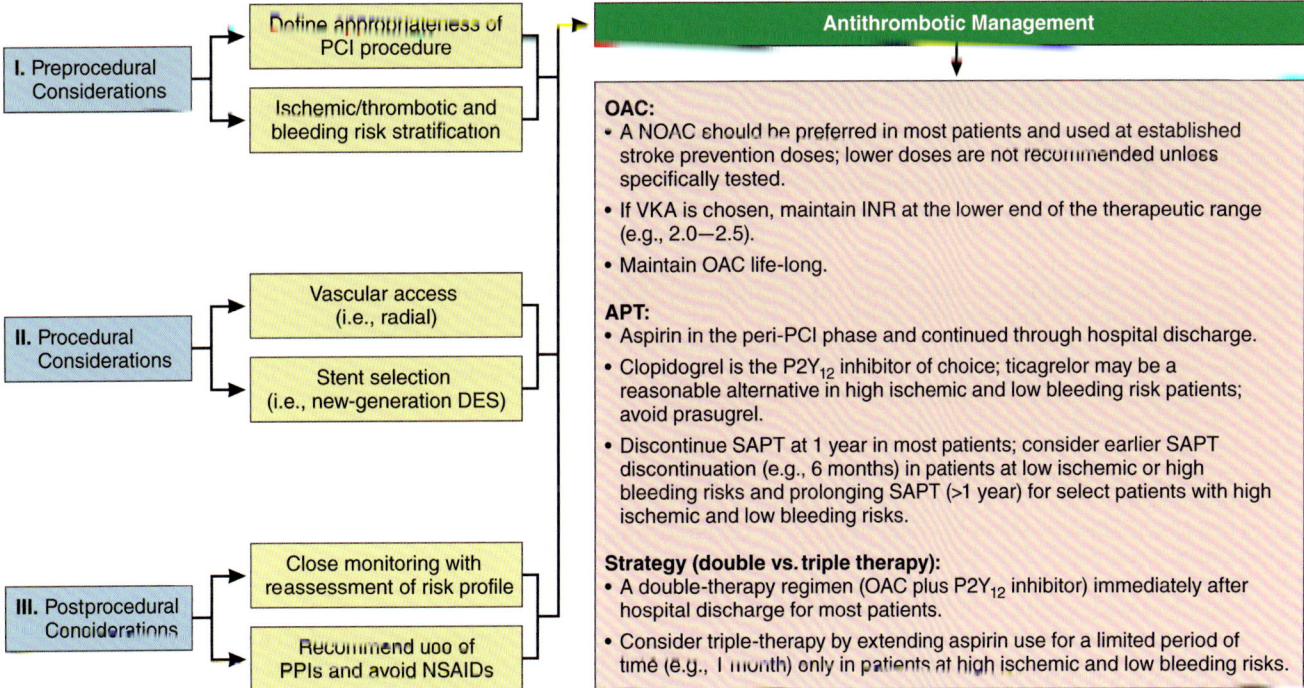

Fig. 10.10 Pragmatic algorithm for the management of patients with atrial fibrillation requiring oral anticoagulation (OAC) undergoing percutaneous coronary intervention (PCI). APT, Antiplatelet therapy; DES, drug-eluting stent; INR, international normalized ratio; NOAC, nonvitamin K antagonist oral anticoagulant; NSAID, nonsteroidal antiinflammatory drug; PPI, proton pump inhibitor; SAPT, single-antiplatelet therapy; VKA, vitamin K antagonist. (From Angiolillo DJ, Goodman SG, Bhatt DL, et al. Antithrombotic therapy in patients with atrial fibrillation treated with oral anticoagulation undergoing percutaneous coronary intervention: a North American perspective—2018 update. *Circulation*, 2018;138:527–536.)

of the combination of a VKA plus DAPT in reducing bleeding complications. The more favorable safety profile associated with a double antithrombotic treatment regimen occurred without any apparent trade-off in efficacy, with the caveat that the studies were not powered for efficacy outcomes. The outcome of all-cause mortality plus hospitalization is reduced as a consequence.[131] Meta-analysis showed halving of the odds of major and minor bleeding with double-therapy compared with triple-therapy (OR, 0.48; 95% CI, 0.34 to 0.68; $P < .001$) with no apparent increase in MACEs (e.g., death, MI, revascularization, thromboembolic events, or stent thrombosis) (OR, 0.91; 95% CI, 0.64 to 1.29; $P = .61$).[132]

In light of these most recent observation, expert consensus recommendations have been updated regarding antithrombotic management of AF patients who require the use of OAC and who are treated with stents (requiring antiplatelet therapy).[133] Results of these trials are summarized in Fig. 10.10. In particular, expert consensus recommend that a double-therapy regimen (OAC plus $P2Y_{12}$ inhibitor) immediately after hospital discharge should be considered for most patients. An NOAC should be preferred over a VKA. The dosing regimen of an NOAC should be that recommended for thromboembolic protection in AF patients, while the use of lower doses is not recommended, unless specifically studied in randomized trials (i.e., rivaroxaban 15 mg). Where different therapeutic dosing options (i.e., dabigatran 110 and 150 mg) are available, the intensity of anticoagulant treatment should be tailored according to the bleeding and thrombotic risk profile of the patient. In patients already on a VKA, continuing with the same agent after PCI may be reasonable, particularly if the patient has been compliant, with well-controlled international normalized ratio (INR), and has not experienced complications, targeting an INR in the lower therapeutic range (2.0 to 2.5). The intensity and duration of antiplatelet treatment should also be tailored according to the bleeding and thrombotic risk profile of the patient. The consistency of significantly lower risk of bleeding with double-therapy across major trials argues against the routine use of a triple-therapy regimen. Therefore, a double-therapy approach should represent the default strategy for most patients with a $P2Y_{12}$ inhibitor and an OAC, which should be started as soon as possible, including at hospital discharge. However, it is reasonable to extend low-dose aspirin therapy (i.e., triple-therapy) for a limited period of time (e.g., 1 month) post-PCI in selected patients at high ischemic/thrombotic and low bleeding risks. Clopidogrel remains the $P2Y_{12}$ inhibitor of choice, but ticagrelor may be considered in selected patients, particularly those at high ischemic/thrombotic risk and low bleeding risk. Discontinuation of single-antiplatelet therapy (SAPT) at 1 year should be considered for most patients who should continue treatment on OAC at the established dose for stroke prevention doses. However, it is reasonable to discontinue SAPT at 6 months post-PCI in patients at low ischemic/thrombotic risk and at high risk for bleeding, while continuation with SAPT (in addition to OAC) may be reasonable for select patients with high ischemic/thrombotic and low bleeding risks. These recommendations are summarized in Fig. 10.10.[133,134] Other large-scale randomized clinical trials are ongoing and include the use of other NOACs (apixaban and edoxaban) to better define the optimal antithrombotic treatment regimen in AF patients undergoing PCI.

Platelet Function Testing

The pharmacodynamic effect of an antiplatelet agent can be defined by the *response* before and after exposure (i.e., the IPA) or by the absolute level of platelet reactivity on therapy, termed *on-treatment reactivity* (Table 10.5). On-treatment reactivity has been proposed as a better measure of thrombotic risk because of the variability in platelet reactivity before treatment.[29] The results of several ex vivo platelet function tests have been associated with clinical outcomes after PCI in clopidogrel-treated patients (Table 10.6). Diagnostic cutoffs to identify at-risk patients using the various tests have been proposed using receiver-operator characteristic (ROC) curve analysis.[29] In a large, multicenter, observational study of more than 8500 patients undergoing PCI with DESs, patients with high on-treatment platelet reactivity despite clopidogrel therapy had a significantly greater 1-year risk of the primary end point of definite or probable stent thrombosis (adjusted HR 2.49; 95% CI, 1.43 to 4.1) and the secondary end point of MI (HR 1.42; 95% CI, 1.09 to 1.86), whereas the adjusted risk of clinically relevant bleeding was significantly decreased (HR 0.73; 95% CI, 0.61 to 0.89).[135]

The results of two small randomized trials suggested that intensified antiplatelet therapy with additional clopidogrel or adjunctive GP IIb/IIIa receptor antagonist therapy in patients with high on-clopidogrel reactivity, may reduce periprocedural ischemic events.[136,137] Two larger randomized trials have tested the hypothesis that adjustment of antiplatelet therapy around the time of PCI, based on PFT, may reduce ischemic events.

GRAVITAS

GRAVITAS trial was a multicenter, double-blinded, active control trial that randomly assigned 2214 patients with high on-treatment reactivity after PCI to either high-dose clopidogrel (additional 600-mg LD followed by a 150-mg daily MD) or standard-dose clopidogrel (75-mg MD).[138] Few patients enrolled in the trial had NSTEMI or STEMI. At 6 months, the rate of death from cardiovascular causes, MI, or stent thrombosis did not differ between the groups (2.3% vs. 2.3%, HR 1.01; 95% CI, 0.58 to 1.76; $P = .97$). High-dose therapy was not associated with increased GUSTO severe or moderate bleeding compared with standard-dose therapy (1.4% vs. 2.3%, HR 0.59; 95% CI, 0.31 to 1.11; $P = .10$). Lower-than-expected event rates reduced the power of the study to detect differences in outcomes between the study groups. Therefore a strategy of a clopidogrel 150-mg MD did not appear to provide therapeutic benefit in patients noted to have high on-treatment reactivity to standard dosing after PCI, particularly in patients with stable angina or ischemia. On pharmacodynamic analysis, the high-dose regimen provided only a 22% absolute reduction in the rate of high on-treatment reactivity. In a post hoc analysis, those patients who achieved lower levels of on-treatment reactivity after PCI or over follow-up ($P2Y_{12}$ reaction units [PRUs] <208) had a significantly lower adjusted risk of cardiovascular events.[139] Only a minority of patients who received a clopidogrel 150-mg MD achieved this threshold for reactivity, suggesting that an insufficient antiplatelet effect of the study intervention may in part have contributed to the lack of clinical efficacy observed in the overall trial.[140]

ARCTIC

The Conventional Antiplatelet Strategy Versus a Monitoring-Guided Strategy for Drug-Eluting Stent Implantation and of Treatment Interruption Versus Continuation One Year After Stenting (ARCTIC) trial[141] was a randomized, multicenter, open-label trial that tested whether the incorporation of PFT into antiplatelet therapy decision making would be superior to conventional management without PFT in reducing ischemic events in patients undergoing PCI. Patients in the PFT arm were assessed for both clopidogrel and aspirin responsiveness prior to PCI and again 2 to 4 weeks after the procedure. The choice of antiplatelet therapy in either the PFT or conventional management arms was according to operator discretion,

TABLE 10.5 Terminology Commonly Used to Describe the Antiplatelet Effect of $P2Y_{12}$ Inhibitors

Term	Sampling Requirements	Definition
High on-treatment reactivity High residual platelet reactivity High posttreatment reactivity	Single blood sample after $P2Y_{12}$ inhibitor exposure or on maintenance therapy	Platelet reactivity while on $P2Y_{12}$ inhibitor therapy (e.g., percent aggregation, PRU, PRI percent, AU·min) above a particular threshold
Nonresponsiveness	Blood sample before and after $P2Y_{12}$ inhibitor exposure	Change in platelet reactivity before and after $P2Y_{12}$ inhibitor exposure below a particular threshold

AU, Aggregation unit; *PRI*, platelet reactivity index; *PRU*, $P2Y_{12}$ reaction units.

TABLE 10.6 Methods to Measure the Effect of $P2Y_{12}$ Antagonists on Platelet Function

Assay	Methodology	Units of Measurement/Expression of Results
LTA	Transmission of light through platelet-rich sample compared with platelet-poor sample after exposure to ADP	• *Maximal aggregation* (%)—Measurement of on-treatment reactivity • *Final (late) aggregation* (%)—Aggregation 5–6 min after induction of ADP; measurement of on-treatment reactivity • *IPA* (%)—Relative change in aggregation before and after exposure • *Δ Platelet aggregation* (%)—Absolute change in aggregation before and after exposure)
VASP	Phosphorylation status of VASP measured by flow cytometry after incubation with ADP, PGE_1, or both	• *Platelet reactivity index* (%)—ratio of PGE_1-stimulated VASP phosphorylation to ADP– + PGE_1–stimulated VASP phosphorylation (i.e., a measure of the reduction of phosphorylated VASP induced by ADP)
VerifyNow	Agglutination of fibrinogen-coated beads by platelets in the presence of ADP (20 mmol) and PGE_1	• $P2Y_{12}$ *reaction units (PRUs)*—measurement of on-treatment reactivity • %—One minus the ratio of ADP-induced aggregation with iso-TRAP–induced aggregation; surrogate measure of IPA
Multiplate analyzer (MEA)	Change in electrical conductance between a pair of electrodes as platelets adhere after exposure to ADP	• AU—Measurement of on-treatment reactivity
Plateletworks	Ratio of single platelet counts by cell counter after stimulation with ADP versus baseline (no ADP)	• %—Measurement of on-treatment reactivity

Each test listed has been associated with clinical outcomes in clopidogrel-treated patients in at least one study.
ADP, Adenosine diphosphate; *AU*, aggregation unit; *IPA*, inhibition of platelet aggregation; *LTA*, light transmittance aggregometry; *MEA*, multiple electrode aggregometry; *PRI*, platelet reactivity index; *TRAP*, thrombin-receptor activating peptide; *VASP*, vasodilator-stimulated phosphoprotein phosphorylation analysis.

although general recommendations were provided for adjustment in the PFT group. Approximately three quarters of the enrolled patients presented with stable angina or ischemia. Among the patients with high on-treatment reactivity in whom the operators chose to adjust therapy, the most frequent interventions were administration of GP IIb/IIIa inhibitors at the time of the procedure and a clopidogrel 150-mg MD after the procedure. At 1-year follow-up, the rate of the primary end point—death, MI, stroke or TIA, urgent coronary revascularization, or stent thrombosis—did not differ between treatment groups (34.6% vs. 31.1%, HR 1.13; 95% CI, 0.98 to 1.29), driven by troponin-defined periprocedural MI (single troponin 3× the upper limit of normal [ULN] measured 6 hours after PCI). The rates of stent thrombosis were low and were similar between groups (0.7% vs. 1.0%, HR 1.34; 95% CI, 0.56 to 3.18).

Other Studies

Since the greatest benefit of intensive $P2Y_{12}$ inhibition occurs early after presentation of ACS managed with PCI, while the risk of bleeding is ongoing, PFT-guided de-escalation in the weeks following PCI may be of clinical benefit by identifying patients who are at the greatest ischemic risk with de-escalation.

The Testing Responsiveness to Platelet Inhibition on Chronic Antiplatelet Treatment for Acute Coronary Syndromes (TROPICAL-ACS) trial randomized 2160 patients after successful PCI for biomarker-positive ACS to one of two management strategies: standard treatment with prasugrel for 1 year, or guided de-escalation (prasugrel for 1 week, followed by clopidogrel for 1 week and PFT-guided maintenance therapy with clopidogrel or prasugrel from day 14 after hospital discharge depending on clopidogrel responsiveness).[142] The PFT-guided strategy was noninferior to standard prasugrel for the composite end point of cardiovascular death, MI, stroke, or Bleeding Academic Research Consortium (BARC) criteria grade 2 or higher. Notably, approximately 40% of patients in the PFT-guided group had to be re-escalated back to the intensive $P2Y_{12}$ inhibitor. Given these findings, PFT-guided de-escalation might be considered in selected cases where a standard 1 year course of intensive $P2Y_{12}$ inhibition is feasible but not preferred.

Synthesizing the Randomized Trials Incorporating Platelet Function Testing

Several tentative conclusions can be drawn from these trials. First, a clopidogrel 150-mg daily MD does not provide a

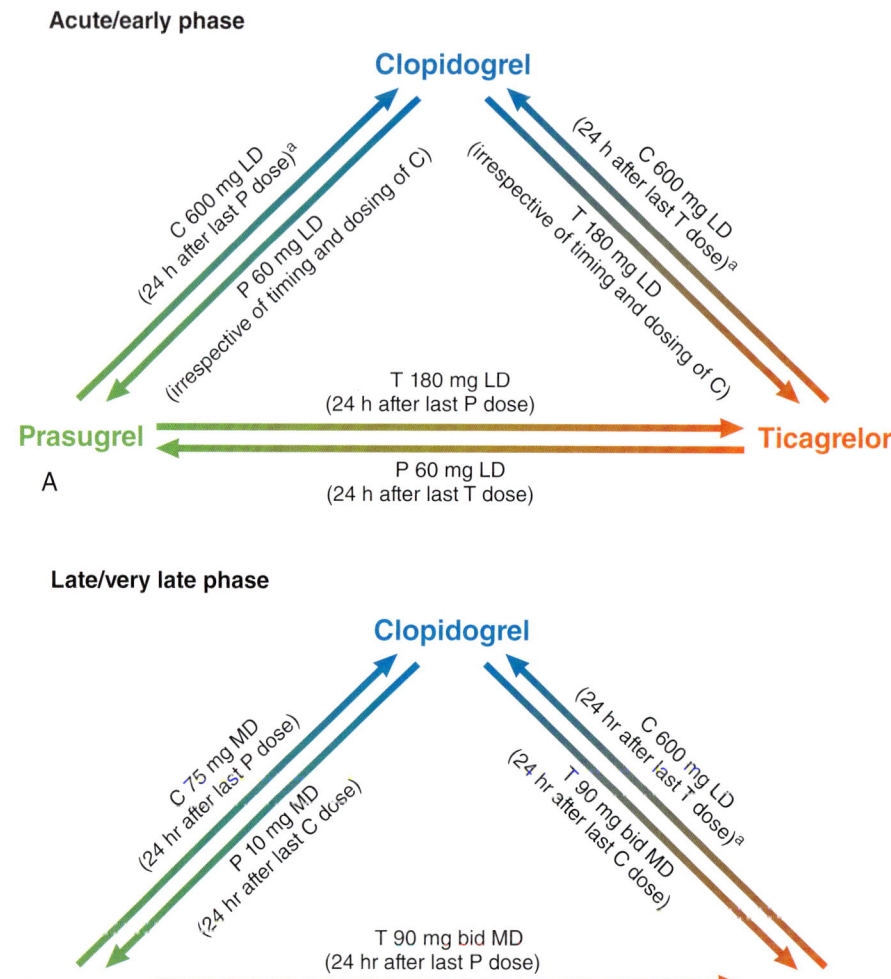

Fig. 10.11 Consensus recommendations on switching between oral P2Y$_{12}$ inhibitors. (A) Switching between oral agents in the acute/early phase. In the acute/early phase (≤30 days from the index event), switching should occur with the administration of a loading dose (LD) in most cases, with the exception of patients who are de-escalating therapy because of bleeding or bleeding concerns, in whom a maintenance dose (MD) of clopidogrel (C) should be considered. Timing of switching should be 24 hours after the last dose of a given drug, with the exception of when escalating to prasugrel (P) or ticagrelor (T), when the LD can be given regardless of the timing and dosing of the previous clopidogrel regimen. (B) Switching between oral agents in the late/very late phase. In the late/very late phase (>30 days from the index event), switching should occur with the administration of an MD 24 hours after the last dose of a given drug, with the exception of patients changing from ticagrelor to prasugrel therapy, for whom an LD should be considered. De-escalation from ticagrelor to clopidogrel should occur with administration of an LD 24 hours after the last dose of ticagrelor (but in patients in whom de-escalation occurs because of bleeding or bleeding concerns, an MD of clopidogrel should be considered). ªConsider de-escalation with clopidogrel 75-mg MD (24 hours after last prasugrel or ticagrelor dose) in patients with bleeding or bleeding concerns. (From Angiolillo DJ, Rollini F, Storey RF, et al. International expert consensus on switching platelet P2Y$_{12}$ receptor-inhibiting therapies. Circulation, 2017;136:1955–1975.)

sufficient pharmacodynamic effect in many patients with high on-treatment platelet reactivity after PCI.[143] Second, although high on-treatment reactivity is associated with cardiovascular outcomes after nonurgent PCI,[135] the absolute rate of post-discharge events is low irrespective of on-treatment reactivity, and routine intensification of antiplatelet therapy according to platelet function does not provide clinical benefit in this patient population. Third, patients who present with ACS—who have greater rates of recurrent thrombotic events—were not well represented in either GRAVITAS or ARCTIC, and the role of PFT in this patient population has not been fully addressed.[144]

Switching Antiplatelet Therapy

The availability of several P2Y$_{12}$ inhibitors raises the possibility to switch between agents. A variety of factors and clinical scenarios may contribute to the decision to switch. These include the clinical setting, patient characteristics, concomitant therapies, costs, social issues, development of side effects, medication adherence, and patient/physician preference.[145] The use of cangrelor, an IV P2Y$_{12}$ inhibitor that requires transition to an oral agent post-PCI, further adds to the settings in which switching therapies may occur. Most data on switching derive from pharmacodynamics studies.[145] Expert consensus recommendations have been developed to provide recommendations on when and how to switch between P2Y$_{12}$ inhibitors, taking into consideration the pharmacologic profiles of the oral and IV P2Y$_{12}$ inhibitors; data from clinical trials, clinical registries, and pharmacodynamic studies; as well as the potential for thrombotic complications based on the time elapsed from the index event leading to initiation of P2Y$_{12}$ inhibitor therapy.[146] In general, switching approaches that have shown to be possibly associated with drug–drug interactions (e.g., from a nonthienopyridine to a thienopyridine agent) should be avoided or minimized unless clinically necessary. Recommendations on switching vary depending on the timing from the index event; that is, early (<30 days) or late (>30 days). Switching between oral agents are classified as follows: *escalation* (switch from a less potent to more potent P2Y$_{12}$ inhibitor), *de-escalation* (switch from a more potent to a less potent P2Y$_{12}$ inhibitor), and *change* (switch between the newer generation oral P2Y$_{12}$ inhibitors). Switching from an oral agent to the IV cangrelor is defined as *bridging*, while switching from cangrelor to one of the oral agents is defined as *transition*. Specific recommendations on switching P2Y$_{12}$ inhibitors are summarized in Figs. 10.11 and 10.12.

CHAPTER 10 Platelet Inhibitor Agents

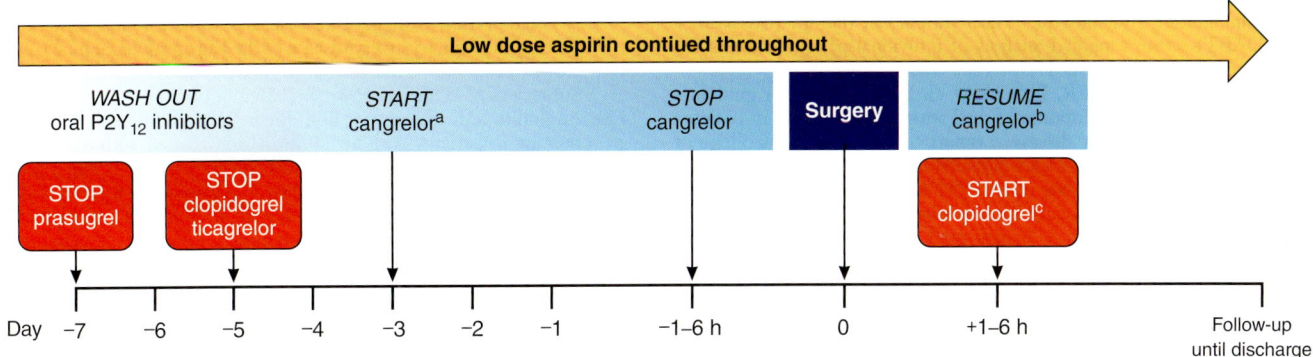

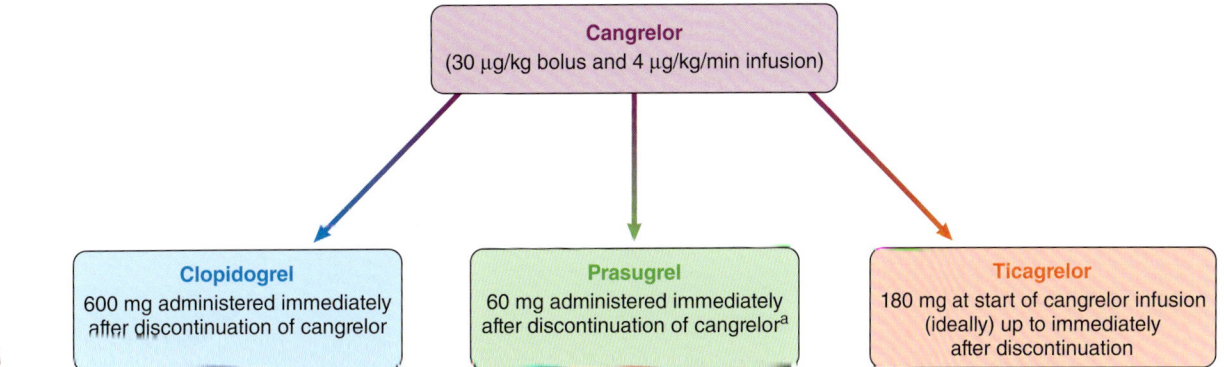

Fig. 10.12 Consensus recommendations on switching between oral and intravenous P2Y$_{12}$ inhibitors. (A) Bridging from oral to intravenous agents. For both cardiac and noncardiac surgery, if withdrawal of P2Y$_{12}$-inhibiting therapy is needed, clopidogrel and ticagrelor should be discontinued for 5 days and prasugrel for 7 days. It is reasonable to start cangrelor bridging up to 3 to 4 days after prasugrel discontinuation and 2 to 3 days of clopidogrel and ticagrelor discontinuation. Platelet function testing may be considered to help guide timing of starting cangrelor infusion. After surgery, regardless of bridging strategy, clopidogrel should be resumed with a loading dose (LD) as soon as oral administration is possible and the risk of severe bleeding is acceptable (prasugrel and ticagrelor administration should be discouraged). If the use of oral P2Y$_{12}$-inhibiting therapy is not possible, postsurgery bridging with an intravenous agent should be considered. (B) Transition from intravenous to oral agents. An LD should always be used when transitioning from cangrelor to an oral agent. In the case of thienopyridines (clopidogrel or prasugrel), this should be administered immediately after discontinuation of cangrelor infusion. Ticagrelor can be administered before, during, or immediately after cangrelor infusion, although earlier administration (e.g., at the time of percutaneous coronary intervention) should be considered. [a]According to the package insert of the European Medical Agency, but not that of the U.S. Food and Drug Administration, prasugrel may also be administered 30 minutes before infusion is stopped. Preliminary studies have shown that prasugrel given at the start of a 2-hour infusion of cangrelor results in sufficient platelet inhibition, but this strategy cannot be routinely recommended until more data are available. (From Angiolillo DJ, Rollini F, Storey RF, et al. International expert consensus on switching platelet P2Y$_{12}$ receptor-inhibiting therapies. *Circulation*, 2017;136:1955–1975.)

CONCLUSION

DAPT with aspirin and a P2Y$_{12}$ receptor antagonist improves outcomes in patients undergoing coronary stent implantation. There is now an ever-increasing array of options for platelet inhibitor therapy during and after PCI, including newer thienopyridines, oral and IV nonthienopyridines, and triple therapy with oral PAR-1 antagonists, cilostazol, or IV GP IIb/IIIa inhibitors. A comprehensive understanding of the mechanistic underpinnings and trial data for each of these agents and approaches is essential for best clinical practice.

KEY REFERENCES

1. Davi G, Patrono C. Platelet activation and atherothrombosis. *N Engl J Med*. 2007;357:2482–2494.
31. Yusuf S, Zhao F, Mehta SR, et al. Effects of clopidogrel in addition to aspirin in patients with acute coronary syndromes without ST-segment elevation. *N Engl J Med*. 2001;345:494–502.
124. Yeh RW, Secemsky EA, Kereiakes DJ, et al. Development and validation of a prediction rule for benefit and harm of dual antiplatelet therapy beyond 1 year after percutaneous coronary intervention. *JAMA*. 2016;315:1735–1749.

125. Costa F, van Klaveren D, James S, et al. Derivation and validation of the predicting bleeding complications in patients undergoing stent implantation and subsequent dual antiplatelet therapy (PRECISE-DAPT) score: a pooled analysis of individual-patient datasets for clinical trials. *Lancet.* 2017;389:1025–1034.
126. Levine GN, Bates ER, Bittl JA, et al. 2016 ACC/AHA guideline focused update on duration of dual antiplatelet therapy in patients with coronary artery disease: a report of the American College of Cardiology/American Heart Association task force on clinical practice guidelines: an update of the 2011 ACCF/AHA/SCAI guideline for percutaneous coronary intervention, 2011 ACCF/AHA guideline for coronary artery bypass graft surgery, 2012 ACC/AHA/ACP/AATS/PCNA/SCAI/STS guideline for the diagnosis and management of patients with stable ischemic heart disease, 2013 ACCF/AHA guideline for the management of ST-elevation myocardial infarction, 2014 AHA/ACC guideline for the management of patients with non-ST-elevation acute coronary syndromes, and 2014 ACC/AHA guideline on perioperative cardiovascular evaluation and management of patients undergoing noncardiac surgery. *Circulation.* 2016;134:e123–e155.
127. Valgimigli M, Bueno H, Byrne RA, et al. 2017 ESC focused update on dual antiplatelet therapy in coronary artery disease developed in collaboration with EACTS: the task force for dual antiplatelet therapy in coronary artery disease of the European Society of Cardiology (ESC) and of the European Association for Cardio-Thoracic Surgery (EACTS). *Eur Heart J.* 2018;39:213–260.
134. Angiolillo DJ, Goodman SG, Bhatt DL, et al. Antithrombotic therapy in patients with atrial fibrillation treated with oral anticoagulation undergoing percutaneous coronary intervention: a North American perspective—2018 update. *Circulation.* 2018;138:527–536.
139. Price MJ, Berger PB, Teirstein PS, et al. Standard- vs. high-dose clopidogrel based on platelet function testing after percutaneous coronary intervention: the GRAVITAS randomized trial. *JAMA.* 2011;205(11):1097–1105.
147. Angiolillo DJ, Rollini F, Storey RF, et al. International expert consensus on switching platelet $P2Y_{12}$ receptor-inhibiting therapies. *Circulation.* 2017;136:1955–1975.

Additional references available online at expertconsult.com.

中文导读

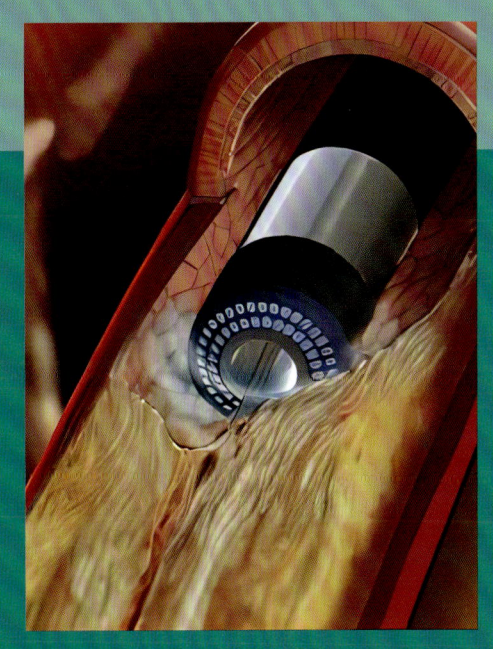

第11章
经皮冠状动脉介入治疗的抗凝治疗

在过去的20年中,已经见证了许多新型抗栓药物的出现,旨在改善经皮冠状动脉介入治疗患者的临床预后。在预防缺血事件的同时,最大限度地降低出血风险,仍然是当代抗栓治疗的理论基石。值得注意的是,随着桡动脉通路的使用、强效的抗血小板$P2Y_{12}$受体抑制剂的使用、出血风险计算器应用的普及、经皮冠状动脉介入治疗技术的发展,尤其是新型药物洗脱支架的出现,这些都不同程度地减少了经皮冠状动脉介入治疗术的出血和缺血风险。普通肝素、依诺肝素和比伐卢定是目前经皮冠状动脉介入治疗实践中使用最广泛的抗凝剂,它们形成了指南建议的主要基础。大量临床试验证据支持在接受经皮冠状动脉介入治疗的患者中使用抗凝剂以预防缺血性并发症。药物的选择最终是由包括临床试验结果、患者个体特征和医师熟悉度在内的综合因素所决定的。在本章节内容中,读者将学习到目前对于动脉粥样硬化血栓形成的生物学基础及其关键效应物凝血酶的回顾、目前使用的抗凝治疗的药理学作用基础,以及未来研究的方向。同时,本章节还将回顾支持在ST段抬高型心肌梗死、非ST段抬高型心肌梗死和择期经皮冠状动脉介入治疗中使用抗凝治疗的标志性试验。

薄小雯 范 谦

章节要点

- 血小板和凝血系统在血栓形成过程中发挥着协同作用。改进的抗凝血酶治疗可减少对抗血小板治疗的依赖以实现对缺血事件的抑制。
- 尽管缺血事件对晚期死亡率的影响已得到广泛认可,但出血事件和晚期死亡率之间的明确相关性是有据可查的。在权衡抗栓治疗的有效性和安全性时,应仔细考虑这些因素。
- 普通肝素、依诺肝素和比伐卢定是当代经皮冠状动脉介入治疗实践证实有效的抗凝药物。
- 从选择性经皮冠状动脉介入治疗到ST段抬高型心肌梗死,现在有大量关于上述不同临床情景下不同抗凝药物的对比临床试验数据。然而,这些研究的试验方案和纳入标准存在较大的异质性。因此,在选择药物时需要仔细考虑这些研究的局限性。
- 在选择药物时需要考虑多种因素,如经皮冠状动脉介入治疗的适应证、患者出血风险、肾功能状况、新型$P2Y_{12}$受体拮抗剂与GPⅡb/Ⅲa抑制剂的联合使用、对抗凝药物的熟悉程度、医院用药方案、目前ESC和ACC指南推荐。

11 Anticoagulation in Percutaneous Coronary Intervention

Trent Hartshorne, Derek P. Chew

KEY POINTS

- Platelets and coagulation play a synergistic role in the generation of thrombus. Improved antithrombin approaches reduce the dependence on antiplatelet therapy for achieving suppression of ischemic events.
- Although the impact of ischemic events on late mortality is well appreciated, a robust link between bleeding events and late mortality is evident. These factors bear careful consideration when weighing efficacy and safety considerations among antithrombotic therapies.
- Unfractionated heparin (UFH), enoxaparin, and bivalirudin are the anticoagulants with established efficacy in contemporary percutaneous coronary intervention (PCI) practice.
- A large collection of clinical trial data now exists that compares the different anticoagulants in various clinical settings, from elective PCI through to ST-elevation myocardial infarction (STEMI); however, substantial heterogeneity exists in the trial protocols and inclusion criteria, and these require careful consideration when choosing among agents.
- Multiple factors need to be considered when selecting an agent, such as indication for PCI, patient bleeding risk, renal function, concomitant use of the newer antiplatelet $P2Y_{12}$ agents and glycoprotein (GP) IIb/IIIa inhibitors, familiarity with the anticoagulant, hospital protocol, and current European Society of Cardiology and American College of Cardiology guidelines.

INTRODUCTION

The last two decades have witnessed the introduction of a number of new pharmacologic agents aimed at improving patient outcomes after percutaneous coronary intervention (PCI). Optimizing ischemic prevention while minimizing bleeding complications remains the cornerstone of contemporary pharmacologic practice. Notably, this period has seen improvements in PCI with the use of radial artery access, more potent antiplatelet $P2Y_{12}$ receptor inhibitors, and the availability of bleeding risk calculators (i.e., Can Rapid Risk Stratification of Unstable Angina Patients Suppress Adverse Outcomes with Early Implementation of the American College of Cardiology/American Heart Association Guidelines? [CRUSADE]); these advances, together with improvements in drug-eluting stent technology, have helped minimize the bleeding and ischemic risks during PCI.

Heparin, enoxaparin, and bivalirudin are the most widespread anticoagulant agents used in current PCI practice, and these form the basis of recommendations from major society guidelines. This chapter will discuss the current biologic basis of atherothrombosis and its key effector, thrombin; the pharmacology of the anticoagulant agents in current use; and the targets for future therapy. Also reviewed will be the landmark trials that support anticoagulant use in ST-elevation myocardial infarction (STEMI), non–ST-elevation myocardial infarction (NSTEMI), and elective PCI.

THE BIOLOGY OF ATHEROTHROMBOSIS

The coagulation cascade reflects the complex interplay among the coagulation proteins, platelets, and cellular phospholipid membranes of not only vascular endothelial cells but of a wide range of inflammatory cells that include monocytes and vascular smooth muscle cells.[1] The subsequent discussion will focus on the coagulation factors that serve as targets, although modern antithrombotic regimens, additional effects on platelet-mediated thrombosis, and vascular tissue function should not be ignored.

The Central Role of Thrombin

Disruption of endothelial integrity and expression of prothrombotic molecules such as tissue factor (TF) lead to the activation of the soluble coagulation proteins (Fig. 11.1). This amplifying cascade converges on the generation of activated factor X (FXa) and the prothrombinase complex, which leads to the conversion of thrombin from its parent molecule, prothrombin. Thrombin generation leads to multiple effects that influence the formation of thrombosis.[2] Specifically, thrombin catalyzes the conversion of fibrin from fibrinogen; this enables clot formation and also activates factors V, VIII, and X; thus it promotes its own generation. In addition, via its direct effects on protease-activated receptors (PARs) 1 and 4, thrombin promotes platelet activation that leads to the expression of CD40 ligand, P-selectin, and the glycoprotein (GP) IIb/IIIa receptor as well as to the secretion of vasoactive agents that include adenosine diphosphate (ADP), serotonin, and thromboxane A_2 (TxA_2). Direct effects of thrombin on endothelial cells and smooth muscle cells result in the expression of adhesion molecules that enables platelet and leukocyte attachment, and its effect on endothelial membrane permeability contributes to the transmigration of the cellular- and cytokine mediated inflammatory response within the vascular wall. Thrombin promotes vasodilation in the intact endothelium, and it contributes to vasoconstriction where the endothelium is damaged or denuded. Thrombin also appears to promote fibroblast cytokine production and is mitogenic (Fig. 11.2).[3]

However, thrombin has a short circulating half-life, and in the context of a normal endothelial barrier, the effects of thrombin are tightly controlled by a negative feedback mechanism. Antithrombin is a single-chain plasma glycoprotein produced by the liver. As an inhibitor of coagulation, this molecule has the ability to bind to thrombin and FXa and activated factor IX (FIXa) in equimolar concentrations. Antithrombin's action is increased over a thousand-fold by the binding of pentasaccharide-chain containing heparins. The pentasaccharide sequence enables the binding of heparins to antithrombin and augments the binding affinity for thrombin and the other clotting factors. Antithrombin is also activated by the glycosaminoglycan heparin sulfate found on the surface of endothelial cells. However, other pathways for the inhibition of thrombin exist and include the binding of thrombin to thrombomodulin and to protein C together with protein S. This inactivates the upstream coagulation proteins, factors Va and VIIIa, and promotes the release of tissue plasminogen activator (TPA).

Hence, thrombin plays a central effector role in the vascular response to balloon- and stent-induced vascular injury and remains an important therapeutic target for the prevention of ischemic complications during PCI. A schematic of the structure of the thrombin molecule is presented in Fig. 11.3. Separate substrate recognition sites are involved in the binding of heparin, fibrinogen, and thrombomodulin, and the catalytic site is responsible for the serine protease activity that is blocked by the direct thrombin inhibitors.[3,4]

ADVERSE EVENTS FOLLOWING PERCUTANEOUS CORONARY INTERVENTION

Improvements in interventional techniques and refinements in antithrombotic therapies have led to a substantial decline in the incidence of ischemic complications following PCI.[5] Hence further iterations in antithrombotic strategies can be considered a double-edged sword, with improved prevention of ischemic complications potentially leading to an increase in bleeding complications associated with increased mortality, stroke, nonfatal myocardial infarction (MI), and stent thrombosis. The contemporary definition of *PCI-related MI* includes a troponin elevation more than five times the 99th percentile in patients with normal values before PCI or a rise greater than 20% if the baseline values are elevated and are stable or falling (Table 11.1).[6] Accompanying the troponin elevation must be at least one of the following three factors: (1) new symptoms or electrocardiographic (ECG) changes, (2) angiographic findings consistent with a procedural complication, or (3) imaging findings consistent with new ischemia. This definition has limitations, however, because the levels of post-PCI troponin elevation whereby long-term prognosis is affected has not been well established. The troponin values in this definition are arbitrarily chosen and lack clinical utility to predict outcome.

More recently, definitions of *clinically meaningful postprocedural MI* have been proposed that are more in line with levels of myocardial injury used to define post-coronary artery bypass graft (CABG) MI.[7] These two unified clinically relevant values in patients with *normal baseline biomarkers* include a post-PCI creatinine kinase myocardial band (CK-MB) elevation 10 or more times the upper limit of normal (ULN) and a lower threshold five

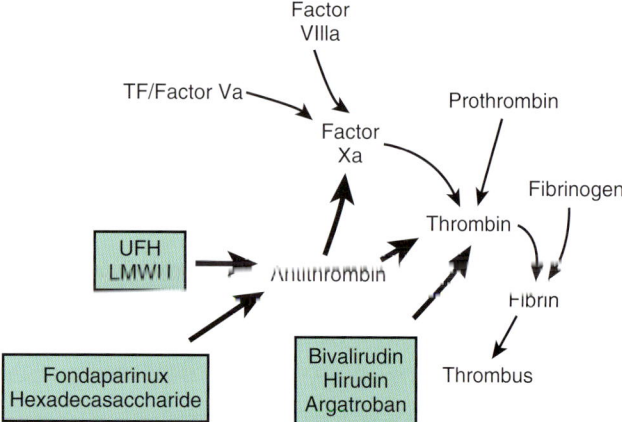

Fig. 11.1 Schematic representation of the relationship between coagulation and arterial thrombosis. Specific targets for therapy are highlighted. *LMWH*, Low-molecular-weight heparin; *TF*, tissue factor; *UFH*, unfractionated heparin.

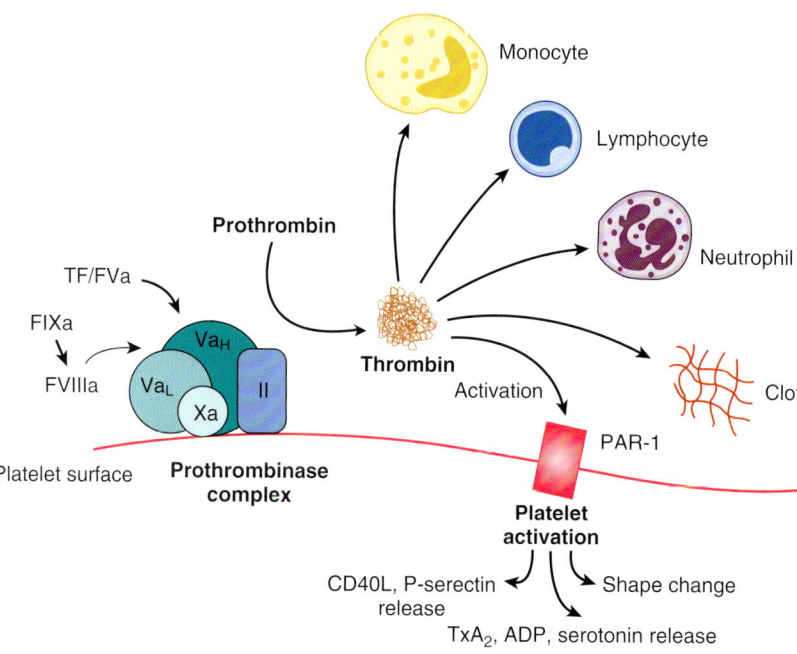

Fig. 11.2 The central role of thrombin in thrombosis and inflammation. *ADP*, Adenosine diphosphate; *FVa*, activated factor V; *PAR-1*, protease-activating receptor 1; *TF*, tissue factor; *TxA₂*, thromboxane A2.

or more times the ULN in the presence of new Q-waves or left bundle branch block (LBBB). For patients with elevated CK-MB prior to PCI that is either *stable or falling*, an increment 10 or more times the ULN from the most recent level is considered diagnostic. The definition for those whose CK-MB level is *not* stable or falling includes a further rise above the most recently measured value of 10 or more times the ULN plus new ST elevation or depression plus signs consistent with a clinically relevant MI, such as new or worsening heart failure or hypotension.

Historical definitions of PCI-related MI have included CK elevation (two times the ULN) but underestimated the incidence of periprocedural MI by 40% to 50%.[8] In an analysis of patients enrolled in the Randomized Evaluation in PCI Linking Angiomax to Reduced Clinical Events (REPLACE)-2 study, CK-MB elevation greater than or equal to three times the ULN was associated with a 3.5-fold excess risk of mortality at 12 months and accounted for 13.2% of all mortality seen by 12 months (Fig. 11.4).[9]

In one study, an isolated post-PCI troponin elevation, compared with no elevation, in patients with normal preprocedural values carried a small but increased risk of 30-day mortality (0.3% vs. 0.1%); however, this was not an independent predictor of long-term mortality.[8] Pre-PCI troponin elevation—as well as age, diabetes, and a history of congestive heart failure and stroke—were all independent predictors of long-term mortality.

Non–CABG-related bleeding within 30 days of PCI is strongly associated with increased mortality, stroke, nonfatal MI, and stent thrombosis (Table 11.2).[10,11] Factors that contribute to these outcomes include reduced myocardial oxygen delivery as a result of hypotension and anemia, cessation of anti-thrombotic and anti-ischemic agents, increased myocardial oxygen demand from the systemic inflammatory response syndrome, and the adverse effects of the storage lesion in the transfusion of red blood cells.[12,13] The bleeding rates after PCI in patients with acute coronary syndromes (ACSs) have been estimated to be as high as 10%, and various risk calculators have been developed.[10] However, the definition of *bleeding* in the major PCI trials has varied over the last 20 years, which makes comparisons among trials more difficult. Many trials use their own definitions of bleeding, along with the commonly used thrombolysis in myocardial infarction (TIMI) and global utilization of streptokinase and tissue plasminogen activator for occluded coronary arteries (GUSTO) definitions, both originally developed to monitor bleeding complications in fibrinolytic trials. This lack of uniformity has made it more difficult to judge the effectiveness of anticoagulant therapies among trials. More recently, however, an Academic Consortium definition of bleeding has been created in an attempt to standardize trial data and better evaluate the safety and efficacy of antithrombotic therapies (Table 11.3).[11]

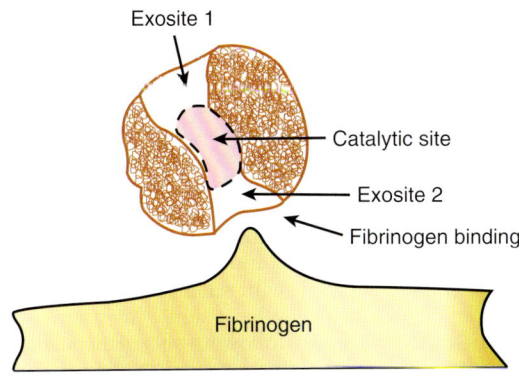

Fig. 11.3 Thrombin binding sites.

TABLE 11.1 End Point Definitions of Bleeding and Ischemia Commonly Used in Clinical Trials of Antithrombotic Agents in Percutaneous Coronary Intervention

End Point	Definition
Myocardial infarction (post PCI)	Troponin elevation more than five times the 99th percentile of the ULN in patients with normal baseline values or a rise more than 20% if baseline values are elevated. In addition, at least one of the following must accompany the troponin elevation: supportive symptoms, new ECG changes, angiographic findings, or imaging findings. SCAI definition: Clinically meaningful MI CK-MB rise more than 10 times the ULN or more than five times the ULN with new pathologic Q-waves in at least two contiguous leads or new persistent LBBB OR In the absence of baseline CK-MB, a cTn rise more than 70 times the ULN or a rise more than 35 times the ULN plus new pathologic Q-waves in at least two contiguous leads or new persistent LBBB
Myocardial infarction (post CABG)	Troponin elevation more than 10 times the 99th percentile in patients with normal baseline values; in addition, at least one of the following must accompany the troponin elevation: ECG changes (LBBB or new Q waves), angiographic findings, or imaging findings
Myocardial infarction (not periprocedural)	Detection of a rise and/or fall of a cardiac biomarker (preferably troponin) with at least one value above the 99th percentile with at least one of the following: symptoms, ECG changes, imaging findings, or angiographic findings
TIMI major bleeding	Intracerebral hemorrhage or any bleeding associated with a more than 5 g/dL fall in hemoglobin or a 15% absolute decrease in hematocrit[a]
TIMI minor bleeding	Any bleeding event associated with a more than 3 g/dL fall in hemoglobin or a 10% absolute decline in hematocrit or a more than 4 g/dL fall in hemoglobin or a 12% absolute decline in hematocrit in the absence of overt bleeding[a]
Major bleeding (REPLACE-2 definition)	Intracerebral hemorrhage or any bleeding event associated with a more than 3 g/dL fall in hemoglobin, a more than 4 g/dL fall in hemoglobin in the absence of overt bleeding, or any red cell transfusion of two or more units[a]
Severe or life-threatening bleeding (GUSTO definition)	Intracerebral hemorrhage or bleeding that causes hemodynamic compromise or requires intervention
Minor bleeding (GUSTO definition)	Bleeding that requires transfusion but does not cause hemodynamic compromise

[a]All calculations of drops in hemoglobin are adjusted for any transfusion by the Landefeld index.
CABG, Coronary artery bypass grafting; *CK-MB*, creatinine kinase myocardial band; *cTn*, cardiac troponin; *ECG*, electrocardiography; *GUSTO*, global utilization of streptokinase and tissue plasminogen activator for occluded coronary arteries; *LBBB*, left bundle branch block; *MI*, myocardial infarction; *PCI*, percutaneous coronary intervention; *REPLACE-2*, Randomized Evaluation in PCI Linking Angiomax to Reduced Clinical Events; *SCAI*, Society for Cardiovascular Angiography and Interventions; *TIMI*, thrombolysis in myocardial infarction; *ULN*, upper limit of normal.

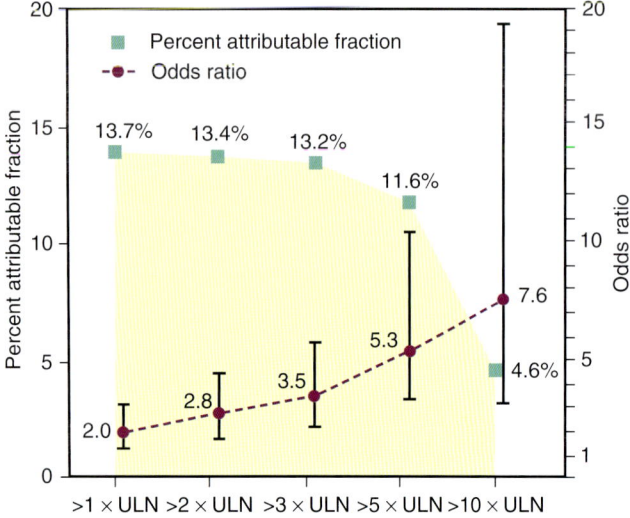

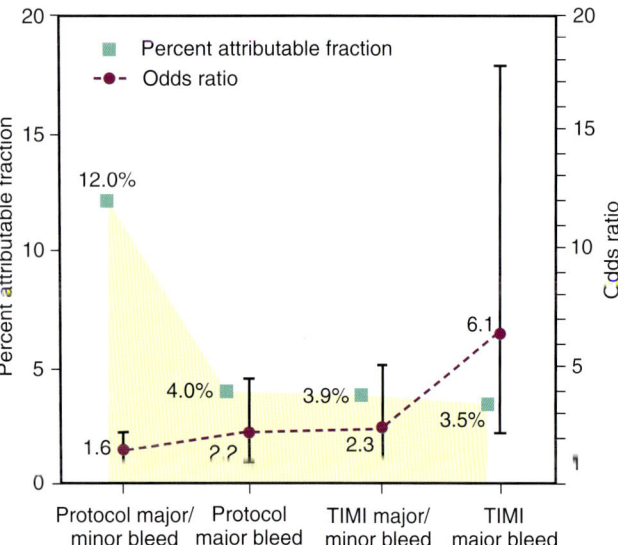

Fig. 11.4 The relationship among ischemic events, bleeding events, and late mortality. *TIMI*, Thrombolysis in myocardial infarction; *ULN*, upper limit of normal.

PHARMACOLOGY OF ANTICOAGULANT AGENTS USED IN CURRENT ERA PERCUTANEOUS CORONARY INTERVENTION

Unfractionated Heparin

Unfractionated heparin (UFH) is a heterogeneous group of glycosaminoglycans of various lengths (5000 to 30,000 Da) that exhibit a high affinity for antithrombin. This binding augments antithrombin's enzymatic inactivation of thrombin, FXa, and FIXa, but its effects on thrombin are the most pronounced.[14] UFH is considered an indirect antithrombin because its action requires the simultaneous binding to antithrombin and thrombin. Up to two-thirds of UFH preparations contain shorter molecules (<18 saccharides) that lack sufficient length to simultaneously span antithrombin and thrombin, and they do not exhibit antithrombin activity. However, the anti-FXa effects of heparin are not dependent on simultaneous binding of both antithrombin and FXa, and therefore antithrombin effects are observed across a wider range of saccharide chain lengths.

The elimination of UFH is initially through rapid but saturable metabolism within endothelial cells and macrophages (zero-order kinetics) followed by slower renal clearance (first-order kinetics). The plasma half-life depends on the dose administered and is approximately 1 hour at doses of 100 IU/kg. In the context of excessive dosing or bleeding, UFH can be reversed by the administration of protamine; however, the clinical efficacy and safety of this strategy has not been well established.

Limitations of UFH include the activation of platelets, a dependence on antithrombin levels, nonspecific binding to plasma proteins, and an inability to inhibit clot-bound thrombin. In addition, direct binding to platelet factor IV can contribute to heparin-induced thrombocytopenia (HIT) in 1% to 3% of treated patients. Platelet activation by heparin is evidenced by an increase in the expression of platelet surface adhesion molecules.[15]

Enoxaparin

The low-molecular-weight heparins (LMWHs) are produced by chemical or enzymatic depolymerization of UFH, which results in heparin fragments with a mean molecular weight approximately 30% of most UFH preparations. However, the molecular size of the heparin molecules still varies; therefore anticoagulant characteristics remain heterogeneous, although they are more predictable when compared with heparin.[16] The principal effect of the LMWHs is the inhibition of anti-FXa via antithrombin. In comparison with UFH, the LMWHs have a longer half-life and demonstrate a more consistent dose response. Reduced platelet activation and fewer platelet factor IV interactions result in less HIT. Clearance is by renal excretion, however, and the biologic half-life is increased in people with renal failure (Table 11.4).

In one study, adequate levels of anti-FXa where observed among patients 2 to 8 hours following subcutaneous dosing of enoxaparin 1 mg/kg twice daily, as well as in those receiving an additional 0.3 mg/kg intravenous (IV) dose 8 to 12 hours following subcutaneous dosing at 1.0 mg/kg.[17] Other investigators have suggested that doses as low as 0.5 mg/kg of IV enoxaparin may be safe and efficacious and may also enable easier sheath management, although a quarter of the patients in this study also received a GP IIb/IIIa inhibitor.[18] Some evidence suggests that enoxaparin may be reversed by the IV administration of protamine, but these data are limited.

Fondaparinux

Fondaparinux, a pentasaccharide, is a synthetic molecule that mimics the biologically active sequence of heparin in its interaction with antithrombin. Given that these molecules are short, their principal effect is the inactivation of FXa.[19] Similarly, these agents have relatively long half-lives and therefore offer once-daily dosing regimens. These agents are not reversed by protamine and require the administration of factor VII concentrates. Fondaparinux does not affect activated partial thromboplastin time (APTT), prothrombin time (PT), or activated clotting time (ACT), and routine monitoring is not performed. However, anti-FXa assays may be measured if monitoring is required, and fondaparinux may be used as the calibrator.

Direct Thrombin Inhibitors

The direct thrombin inhibitor hirudin, a 65–amino acid protein, is the prototypical molecule of this class.[19] Hirudin forms a stable noncovalent complex with thrombin by inhibiting the catalytic site and the anion binding exosite in a two-step process.[4] Generally the direct thrombin inhibitor molecules are smaller than the indirect thrombin inhibitors, and they demonstrate greater efficacy for the inhibition of clot-bound thrombin.[19]

The hirudin-thrombin interaction offers a method for categorizing the other direct thrombin inhibitors, which have been divided into univalent and bivalent molecules. The *univalent*

TABLE 11.2 Clinical Factors Associated With Myocardial Infarction and Non–Coronary Artery Bypass Grafting–Related Bleeding Within 30 Days Among Patients With Acute Coronary Syndrome Undergoing Early Invasive Management

Myocardial Infarction			Non-CABG Major Bleeding		
Clinical Factor	OR (95% CI)	P Value	Clinical Factor	OR (95% CI)	P Value
Biomarker elevation	1.66 (1.40–1.97)	<.001	Male sex	0.42 (0.36–0.50)	<.001
Family history of CAD	1.48 (1.27–1.73)	<.001	Anemia (Hct <39% in males and < 36% in females)	1.96 (1.63–2.36)	<.001
Age per 5 years	1.08 (1.04–1.11)	<.001	Age per 5 years	1.14 (1.10–1.19)	<.001
ST-segment deviation ≥1.0 mm	1.38 (1.18–1.61)	<.001	ST-segment deviation ≥1.0 mm	1.31 (1.10–1.54)	<.01
Prior MI	1.28 (1.08–1.50)	<.001	Prior PCI	0.70 (0.58–0.84)	<.01
			Creatinine per 0.1 mg/dL	1.08 (1.05–1.10)	<.001
			White cell count per 10^9/L	1.08 (1.05–1.11)	<.001
			Prior CVA	1.60 (1.21-2.10)	<.001

CABG, Coronary artery bypass grafting; *CAD,* coronary artery disease; *CI,* confidence interval; *CVA,* cerebrovascular accident; *Hct,* hematocrit; *MI,* myocardial infarction; *OR,* odds ratio; *PCI,* percutaneous coronary intervention.

TABLE 11.3 Academic Research Consortium Definition of Bleeding

Type	Definition
0	No bleeding
1	Bleeding that is not actionable (no investigations, treatment, or hospitalization is required); may include episodes of self-discontinuation of medical therapy by the patient
2	Any overt actionable sign of hemorrhage that does not fit criteria for type 3, 4, or 5 but does at least one of the following: (1) requires nonsurgical medical intervention, (2) leads to hospitalization or increased level of care, or (3) prompts evaluation
3	3a: Overt bleeding with Hb drop of 3-5 g/dL,[a] any transfusion with overt bleeding 3b: Overt bleeding with Hb of ≥5 g/dL,[a] cardiac tamponade, bleeding that requires surgical intervention or vasoactive agents 3c: Intracranial hemorrhage (does not include microbleeds or hemorrhagic transformation), intraocular bleed that compromises vision
4	CABG-related bleeding
5	5a: Probable fatal bleeding 5b: Definite fatal bleeding

[a]Provided Hb fall is related to the bleed.
CABG, Coronary artery bypass grafting; *Hb,* hemoglobin.

molecules—dabigatran, argatroban, and melagatran—inhibit only the catalytic site and inactivate only fibrin-bound thrombin. The *bivalent molecules*, recombinant hirudin and bivalirudin, bind to the catalytic site and to at least one of the exosites. Whereas the interaction between hirudin and thrombin is irreversible, the inhibition provided by bivalirudin is more transient. Bivalirudin is a synthetic 20–amino acid molecule with a shorter half-life than hirudin, and bivalirudin is the only direct thrombin inhibitor in current use for PCI (see Table 11.4). With the exception of argatroban, these agents are cleared renally, and clearance is attenuated in the setting of reduced renal function. In the setting of excessive dosing or bleeding, these agents can be removed by hemofiltration. Bivalirudin also undergoes proteolysis within the plasma, which contributes to its shorter half-life and relatively constant elimination characteristics even among patients with mild to moderate renal impairment. Nevertheless, dose attenuation is required among patients with creatinine clearance below 30 mL/min. These agents are not reversed by protamine and have no specific antidote. Nonspecific measures—such as transfusion of blood products, including fresh frozen plasma (FFP)—and local measures are recommended in the context of active bleeding. Monitoring is not routinely required with the use of bivalirudin; however, the ACT and PT are prolonged in a nonlinear fashion. If needed, however, the dose-linear escarin clotting time can be used to monitor bivalirudin's activity.

NEW PHARMACOLOGIC TARGETS

Multiple novel targets in the coagulation cascade have the potential for pharmacologic inhibition and prevention of thrombus formation, although few have reached phase III clinical trials for use in PCI; nevertheless, the potential for future development remains.

Agents that target the coagulation proteases in the amplification phase include FIXa inhibitors (pegnivacogin), FVIIa inhibitors (TB-402), and joint FVa/FVIIIa inhibitors (drotrecogin, recomodulin, and solulin).[14] Pegnivacogin is a first in its class of molecule, known as an *aptamer*.[20] Aptamers are oligonucleotide RNA molecules capable of not only binding target proteins with high affinity and specificity but also allowing complementary antidote binding that can reverse their pharmacologic activity.[21] The Effect of REG 1 anticoagulation system versus Bivalirudin on Outcome after Percutaneous Coronary Intervention (REGULATE PCI) trial was a randomized trial comparing REG1 (consisting of pegnivacogin and its reversal agent anivamersen) and bivalirudin in patients undergoing PCI. This trial was terminated prematurely due to REG1 being associated with severe allergic reactions, despite RNA aptamers being thought to be nonimmunogenic. The future role of the novel anticoagulant-reversal system is yet to be defined. The direct FXa inhibitor otamixaban was studied in the large phase III clinical trial Anticoagulation With Otamixaban and Ischemic Events in Non-ST Elevation Acute Coronary Syndromes (TAO).[22] This double-blind, active, controlled superiority trial randomized 13,229 patients with NSTEMI to either otamixaban or UFH plus downstream eptifibatide. No reduction was seen in the primary efficacy outcome; however, increased TIMI major and minor bleeding was noted with otamixaban (3.1% vs. 1.5%, P < .01), and otamixaban is no longer recommended based on the findings of this trial. The other orally active FXa inhibitors, rivaroxaban and apixaban, have been studied in patients after treatment for an ACS but have not been formally assessed in the peri-PCI setting.

TABLE 11.4 Pharmacokinetic Characteristics of Commonly Used Anticoagulants

Property	Unfractionated Heparin	Enoxaparin	Fondaparinux	Bivalirudin
Mean molecular weight (Da)	15,000	5000	1728	2180
Dependence on antithrombin	Yes	Yes	Yes	No
Anti-FXa, anti-FIIa activity	Yes	2–4	No anti-FXa activity	No anti-FXa activity
Half-life	~60 min	~240 min	17–21 h	25 min
Bioavailability	+ to +++	++++	++++ (Subcutaneous)	++++
Subcutaneous absorption	++	++++	++++	–
Binding to plasma proteins	+++	+	+	–
Binding to platelets/macrophages	++	+	–	–
Antigenicity/HIT	++	+	–/+ (Very rare)	–
Clearance	Renal	Renal	Renal	Renal/proteolysis
Protamine neutralization	++++	++	–	–

FIIa, Activated factor II; *FXa,* activated factor X; *HIT,* heparin-induced thrombocytopenia.

ANTICOAGULANT THERAPY IN STEMI, NSTEACS, AND ELECTIVE PERCUTANEOUS CORONARY INTERVENTION

ST-Elevation Myocardial Infarction

Heparin was the first antithrombotic agent used during PCI. This was followed by the addition of aspirin, and then clopidogrel to reduce ischemic complications. Furthermore, the use of GPIIb/IIIa inhibitors, when added to aspirin, clopidogrel, and heparin in patients with ACSs, has been shown to lower ischemic complications at the expense of increased bleeding complications.

This combination of agents in STEMI was challenged in the Harmonizing Outcomes with Revascularization and Stents in Acute Myocardial Infarction (HORIZONS-AMI) trial which found bivalirudin was superior to the combination of heparin and GPIIb/IIIa inhibitors, primarily due to a reduction in major bleeding outcomes, which drove a reduction in combined adverse events (a combination of ischemic and bleeding events). HORIZONS-AMI was a large randomized control trial of STEMI patients undergoing emergency angiography which preceded the introduction of more potent second-generation $P2Y_{12}$ inhibitors (prasugrel and ticagrelor), and mainstream use of radial artery vascular access. There was a statistically significant increase in early (<24 hours) stent thrombosis reported in the bivalirudin arm, although this did not translate to an increase in mortality or other cardiovascular end points. The open-label nature of the trial, along with approximately 65% of the bivalirudin arm receiving UFH prior to PCI, highlighted shortcomings of the trial design.

The introduction of radial-access PCI, the more potent $P2Y_{12}$ inhibitors ticagrelor and prasugrel, and a reduction in the use of GP IIb/IIIa inhibitors led to the European Ambulance Acute Coronary Syndrome Angiography (EUROMAX) trial.[23] This trial was a pre-PCI hospital-led protocol of ambulance or peripheral hospital initiation of either bivalirudin or UFH (with or without GP IIb/IIIa inhibitors) in 2198 patients with STEMI. GPIIb/IIIa use in the heparin group was 69.1% compared with 11.5% in the bivalirudin group. In contrast to HORIZONS-AMI, pre-enrollment use of heparin was only 2.2% in the bivalirudin group. The primary composite of death from any cause and non-CABG major bleeding at 30 days favored bivalirudin (5.1% vs. 8.5%, P = .001). As seen in HORIZONS-AMI, a statistically significant reduction in major bleeding (2.6% vs. 6.0%, P < .001) and an increase in early (<24 hours) stent thrombosis was seen with bivalirudin (1.6% vs. 0.5%, P = .02), but this did not translate to differences in death (either from cardiac or noncardiac causes) or major adverse cardiovascular or cerebrovascular events (MACCEs; a composite of death, reinfarction, ischemia-driven revascularization, or stroke) between the two groups.

These findings were challenged in the How Effective Are Antithrombotic Therapies in Primary Percutaneous Coronary Intervention? (HEAT-PPCI) trial, a single-center, open-label, delayed consent study of 1829 patients in which heparin was found to be superior to bivalirudin with reduced ischemic outcomes and no difference in bleeding rates. In this study GPIIb/IIIa use was 15% in the heparin group and 13% in the bivalirudin arm and only 1 patient in the bivalirudin arm received heparin. The primary efficacy outcome of 30-day major adverse cardiovascular events (MACE) rates were lower in the heparin group (8.7% vs. 5.7%, P = .01). HEAT-PPCI also found a statistically significant increase in the stent thrombosis rate, reinfarction rate, and unplanned target vessel revascularization (TVR) rate in patients receiving bivalirudin. This trial challenged the findings of HORIZONS-AMI and EUROMAX by questioning whether bivalirudin reduces bleeding when rates of GPIIb/IIIa use were low in the heparin arm. Again, there was an increased stent thrombosis risk with bivalirudin; however, in this trial it was associated with an increase in post PCI ischemic events. Notably, the trial design did not permit bivalirudin infusions to continue following PCI.

Further clinical data comes from the The Bivalirudin versus Heparin with or without Tirofiban During Coronary Intervention During Myocardial Infarction Trial (The BRIGHT RCT) which studied 2194 patients requiring primary PCI of which 87.7% had STEMI.[24] Patients were randomized to receive bivalirudin alone (735 patients), heparin alone (729 patients), or both heparin and tirofiban (730 patients) in an open-label design. Radial access was used in 78.5% of patients and the median duration of bivalirudin infusion post PCI was 180 minutes. Heparin use in the bivalirudin group was low (0.3%) and bailout GPIIb/IIIa use was around 5% in the bivalirudin- and heparin-only groups. Clopidogrel was the only $P2Y_{12}$ antagonist, and heparin use in the bivalirudin arm was low (0.2%). There was a significant reduction in the primary outcome (a composite of major adverse cardiac, cerebral, and bleeding events) at 30-days with bivalirudin (8.8%) compared with heparin (13.2%) or heparin/tirofiban (17.0%). This benefit was driven primarily by a reduction in bleeding with bivalirudin. There was no significant difference in the rates of stent thrombosis or ischemic events.

The Bivalirudin versus Heparin Monotherapy in Myocardial Infarction (VALIDATE-SWEDEHEART) was a large multicenter randomized control trial which included both STEMI (3005 patients) and NSTEMI patients.[25] There were high rates of radial access (90.3%), and GP IIb/IIIa use was low (around 2.5% in both groups); however, pre-enrollment administration of IV heparin occurred in 36.6% of patients. The mean duration of bivalirudin administration post PCI was 54 minutes. There were no major differences at 180 days in the primary end points (a composite of death, MI, and major bleeding), or secondary end points (individual components of the primary end points, stroke, and stent thrombosis). The most important limitation of this trial was the pre-enrollment administration of heparin in just over one-third of patients.

Despite multiple large-scale trials comparing bivalirudin and heparin, there is no definitive answer as to the agent of choice. Several trials have found both a reduced bleeding risk and increased rates of stent thrombosis with bivalirudin. How these affect net clinical benefit (a combination of ischemic and bleeding risk) appears to depend on factors (which are not consistent between trials) such as choice of $P2Y_{12}$ agent, concurrent use of GPIIb/IIIa inhibitors, duration of bivalirudin infusion post PCI, and single-dose heparin administration prior to commencing bivalirudin infusion.

With regard to the use of enoxaparin in STEMI, The Acute Myocardial Infarction Treated With Primary Angioplasty and Intravenous Enoxaparin or Unfractionated Heparin to Lower Ischemic and Bleeding Events at Short- and Long-Term Follow-Up (ATOLL) trial, which included 910 patients in an open-label trial design, is the largest randomized control trial.[26] Pre-PCI hospital or ambulance administration of either enoxaparin or UFH occurred in 71% of both study arms.

Patients who received enoxaparin were administered an IV bolus of 0.5 mg/kg, and if the procedure was prolonged by more than 2 hours or the clinician required stronger anticoagulation, an additional 0.25 mg/kg was administered. No dose adjustment was made for patients with renal failure, and patients who required ongoing anticoagulation for other reasons were given enoxaparin 1 mg/kg subcutaneously twice daily with a dose adjustment for renal failure. Radial access was used in approximately two-thirds of patients; however, 93% of patients received clopidogrel.

The primary composite end point of death, complication of MI, or major bleeding was nonsignificantly lower with enoxaparin (28% vs. 34%, P = .063); however, the main secondary end point—a composite of death, recurrent ACS, or urgent revascularization—was significantly reduced in the enoxaparin group (7% vs. 11%, P = .015). No difference in mortality or bleeding by 30 days was seen, and clopidogrel was the sole $P2Y_{12}$ antagonist. A subsequent per protocol analysis of ATOLL found that in the 87.4% of patients treated according to protocol, there was a statistically significant difference in the primary clinical end point in favor of enoxaparin (relative risk [RR] 0.76, 95% confidence interval [CI] 0.62 to 0.94, P = .001). These findings were also supported in a meta-analysis of 10,423 STEMI patients with reduced major bleeding and improved ischemic end points with the use of enoxaparin. It should be noted that pre-hospital anticoagulant administration may be challenging in certain hospital networks and the ease of administration of this agent in the context of patient transfer is appealing.

Since the Sixth Organization for the Assessment of Strategies for Ischemic Syndromes (OASIS-6) trial observed a numeric increased events in the fondaparinux group, this agent is not recommended in patients with STEMI and is not supported by major society guidelines.

SUMMARY

There remains clinical equipoise in the anticoagulant choice in STEMI due primarily to significant clinical trial heterogeneity. As a result, use of heparin, enoxaparin, or bivalirudin are acceptable options in patients with STEMI and are supported by major society guidelines.

Non–ST-Elevation Acute Coronary Syndrome

It is well recognized that anticoagulation should accompany antiplatelet agents in patients with non–ST-elevation acute coronary syndrome (NSTEACS) who present for invasive management, as seen in multiple small randomized trials and meta-analyses that predominantly compared UFH with placebo. The main agents in current clinical use with established efficacy are UFH, enoxaparin, fondaparinux, and bivalirudin.

Fondaparinux has a class 1 recommendation in the European Society of Cardiology (ESC) and American College of Cardiology (ACC) guidelines based on the OASIS-5 trial, which included 20,078 patients with unstable angina or NSTEMI who were randomized to receive fondaparinux or enoxaparin. In patients who underwent PCI, the key findings were that bleeding events were significantly lower in the fondaparinux group at 48 hours (enoxaparin, 3.4% vs. fondaparinux, 1.4%; $P < .001$), without any differences in ischemic end points. Significantly however, this study was performed before the widespread use of radial access and second generation $P2Y_{12}$ inhibitors. In addition, the trial protocol required amendment to include a heparin flush during PCI given a higher rate of catheter thrombus seen in the fondaparinux group. As a result, the optimal dose of adjunctive heparin for patients with NSTEMI undergoing PCI who receive fondaparinux was studied in the Fondaparinux Trial With Unfractionated Heparin During Revascularization in Acute Coronary Syndromes OASIS-8 (FUTURA OASIS-8), which compared standard-dose UFH (85 U/kg or 60 U/kg with GP IIb/IIIa use) or fixed low-dose UFH (50 U/kg) in 2026 patients.[27] The primary outcome of PCI-related major and minor bleeding was similar between the groups (standard dose, 5.8% vs. low dose, 4.7%; P = .27); however, the key secondary outcome of death, MI, and TVR was higher in the low-dose group (4.5% vs. 2.9%, P = .06). Standard heparin dosing is therefore recommended as adjunctive therapy during PCI for those anticoagulated with fondaparinux.

UFH and enoxaparin have been compared in several trials. Superior Yield of the New Strategy of Enoxaparin Revascularization and Glycoprotein IIb/IIIa Inhibitors (SYNERGY) was a prospective open-label trial of 10,027 patients with NSTEMI in which PCI was performed in about 47% of patients.[28] The primary end point of death or nonfatal MI was similar between enoxaparin and heparin (14.0% vs. 14.5%, P = .96). However, the increase in TIMI major (non-CABG related) bleeding events in the enoxaparin group was significant (2.4% vs. 1.8%, P = .03). Important limitations to the findings of SYNERGY were that 75% of patients received antithrombin therapy prior to enrollment. In the patients who did not receive pre-randomization antithrombin therapy or in whom the pre-randomization therapy was the same as the randomly assigned therapy, a reduction in the primary end point was reported with enoxaparin (13.3% vs. 15.9%,) along with similar rates of bleeding. This contrasts to the findings of a meta-analysis that included 13 trials of patients with NSTEMI and elective PCI which found no difference in all-cause mortality in those treated with enoxaparin compared with those treated with heparin.[29]

Bivalirudin in NSTEMI has been studied in several major trials. Acute Catheterization and Urgent Intervention Triage Strategy (ACUITY) was an open-label, randomized, multicenter trial that compared heparin plus a GP IIb/IIIa inhibitor, bivalirudin plus a GP IIb/IIIa inhibitor, and bivalirudin alone in patients with unstable angina (~42%) or NSTEMI (~58%) who were undergoing an early invasive strategy with planned PCI.[30] This trial comprised 13,819 patients enrolled across 450 centers in 17 countries, and 53% of patients underwent PCI. The main finding of ACUITY (Fig. 11.5) was that bivalirudin alone, compared with heparin plus a GP IIb/IIIa inhibitor, resulted in a significantly reduced rate of major bleeding (3.0% vs. 5.7%). This subsequently resulted in a superior net clinical outcome end point, defined as the composite ischemic end point and major bleeding (bivalirudin, 10.1%, vs. UHF/GP IIb/IIIa inhibition, 11.7%; $P = .02$; see Fig. 11.5).

In contrast to ACUITY, the Intracoronary Stenting and Antithrombosis Research Rapid Early Action for Coronary Treatment 4 (ISAR-REACT 4) was a trial that only enrolled NSTEMI patients. This double-blind randomized trial of 1721 patients compared bivalirudin with the combination of UFH and abciximab in patients with a planned early invasive approach. Notably, all patients received clopidogrel, and most coronary angiograms were performed through the femoral artery. The primary end point (a composite of death, recurrent MI, urgent TVR, or major bleeding at 30 days) was similar between both groups (10.9% vs. 11.0%; $P = .94$). However, a significant reduction in major bleeding was observed in patients treated with bivalirudin (2.6% vs. 4.6%; $P = .02$).

A more recent trial, The Bivalirudin versus Heparin Monotherapy in Myocardial Infarction (VALIDATE-SWEDEHEART), as previously discussed, was a large multicenter randomized control trial enrolling patients with ACSs which included 3001 NSTEMI patients.[25] As mentioned, this more contemporary trial had high rates of radial access, more potent second-generation P2Y$_{12}$ inhibitors, and low rates of GP IIb/IIIa use; however, its limitations included the pre-enrollment use of heparin in over one-third of patients and low event rates. In the NSTEMI sub-group, there were no major differences at 180 days in the primary end points (a composite of death, MI, and major bleeding), or secondary end points (individual components of the primary end points, stroke, and stent thrombosis).

These findings were supported in the Bivalirudin or Unfractionated Heparin in Acute Coronary Syndromes (MATRIX investigators) trial, a large randomized study of both STEMI and NSTEMI patients.[31] This trial found no differences between either agent with regard to net adverse clinical events; however, the NSTEMI sub-group was not reported.

Summary

A large body of heterogeneous, and at times conflicting, clinical trial evidence exists for the use of various anticoagulant agents in patients with NSTEMI in whom an invasive approach has been planned. UFH, enoxaparin, fondaparinux (with adjunctive heparin), and bivalirudin are all acceptable options for periprocedural anticoagulation and have been given a class 1 recommendation in the both the ESC and ACC guidelines.

Percutaneous Coronary Intervention for Stable Coronary Artery Disease

The rationale for anticoagulation in patients with stable angina presenting for elective PCI is to (1) prevent thrombus formation on the coronary guidewire and PCI catheter, (2) allow adequate

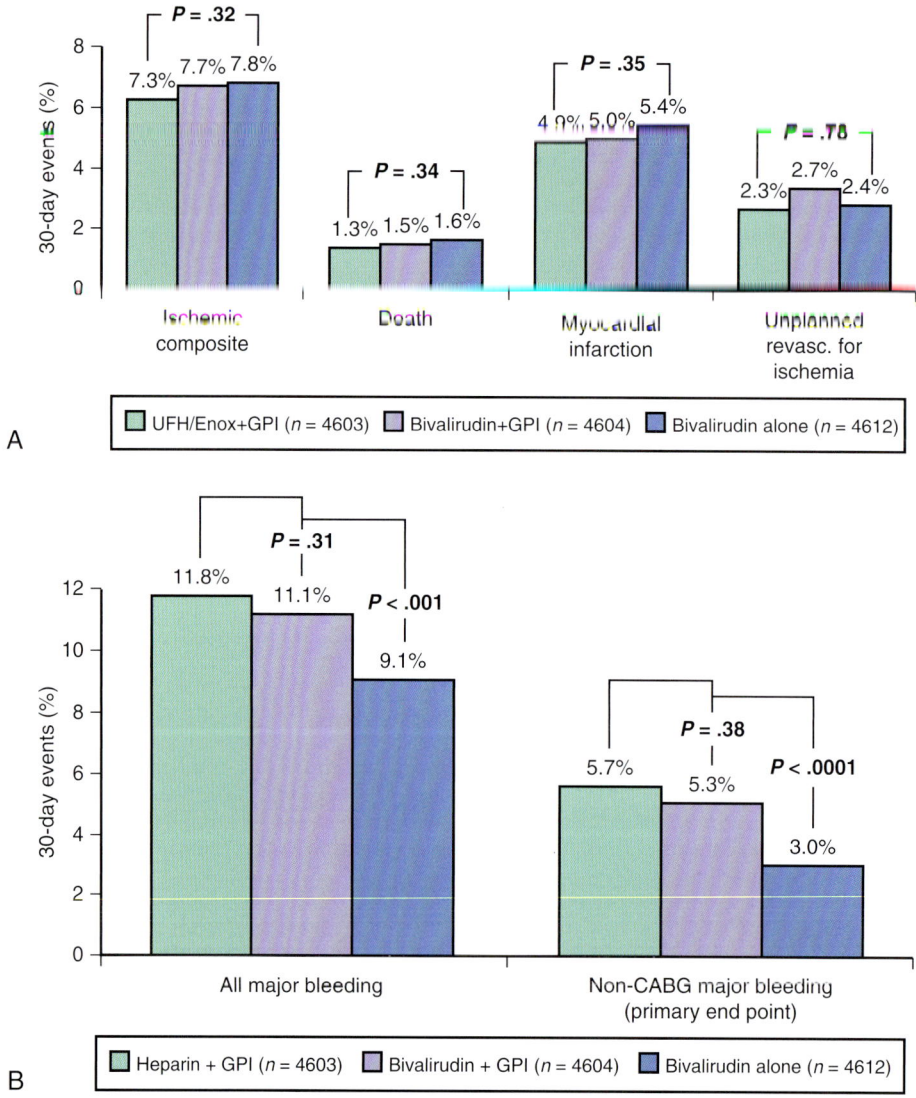

Fig. 11.5 Ischemic (A) and bleeding (B) outcomes with bivalirudin versus bivalirudin/glycoprotein IIb/IIIa inhibition *(GPI)* versus unfractionated heparin *(UFH)* or low-molecular-weight heparin/GPI in the ACUITY trial. *CABG,* Coronary artery bypass grafting; *Enox,* enoxaparin; *revasc.,* revascularization.

thrombin inhibition where intracoronary thrombus is present (seen in up to 65% of patients with stable angina), and (3) balance the prothrombotic and inflammatory responses of stenting.[14,20] Two moderate-sized randomized controlled trials (RCTs) have been undertaken that have challenged this dogma, both trials of heparin versus placebo in patients presenting for elective PCI.

The Efficacy and Safety of Triple Antiplatelet Therapy With and Without Concomitant Anticoagulation During Elective Percutaneous Coronary Intervention (REMOVE) trial randomized 159 patients undergoing elective PCI to eptifibatide alone or eptifibatide plus UFH. All patients received aspirin and clopidogrel.[32] The primary end point of bleeding (measured by the Landefeld bleeding severity index) was significantly reduced in the group who did not receive heparin (3.0% vs. 3.9%, P = .03). No difference was found in the composite end point of death and ischemic and bleeding end points. Limitations to REMOVE included the trial protocol having to be amended as a result of spontaneous thrombus formation during bifurcation-lesion PCI.

REMOVE was followed up by the larger Coronary Interventions Antiplatelet-Based Only (CIAO) trial.[33] This double-blind RCT compared the safety and efficacy of antiplatelet therapy alone versus use of UFH in 700 patients who presented for elective PCI of uncomplicated lesions. Of note, patients with high-risk angiographic characteristics such as calcification, long lesions, small vessels, bifurcation lesions, and vein graft lesions were excluded. Antiplatelet therapy consisted of aspirin and either ticlopidine or clopidogrel. All procedures were performed via femoral artery access, and GP IIb/IIIa inhibitors were not used. No difference was found in the 30-day primary end point (death, MI, or TVR) between the heparin and placebo groups (3.7% vs. 2.0%, respectively; P = .17), although less bleeding was reported in the placebo group; however, the absolute number of bleeding events was small, and significance was only reached in the Safety and Efficacy of Enoxaparin in PCI Patients, an International Randomized Evaluation (STEEPLE) bleeding-score assessment, not in TIMI, ACUITY, or GUSTO bleeding scores.

Given the pathobiologic basis for the important role of thrombin inhibition in elective PCI and the shortcomings of the REMOVE and CIAO trials, anticoagulation has become the standard of care for patients who present for elective PCI. The choice of agent is less clear because only one large RCT was specifically designed for patients undergoing elective PCI.

STEEPLE was an open-label multicenter trial that enrolled 3528 patients; it was designed to assess the safety of IV enoxaparin (0.75 or 0.5 mg/kg regardless of the use of GP IIb/IIIa inhibitors) versus UFH (IV bolus 70 to 100 IU followed by adjustment according to an ACT between 300 and 350 seconds).[34] The dose of UFH was reduced with the use of GP IIb/IIIa inhibitors (bolus IV dose of 50 to 70 IU and target ACT 200 to 300 seconds). Approximately 94% of patients had received a thienopyridine on the day of PCI. All arterial access was via the femoral artery, and sheath removal for the 0.75 mg/kg enoxaparin group occurred 4 to 6 hours after PCI but was done immediately for the 0.5 mg/kg enoxaparin group. Sheath removal for the UFH group occurred when the ACT was between 150 and 180 seconds. The primary end point of non–CABG-related major and minor bleeding within the first 48 hours was lowest in the 0.5 mg/kg enoxaparin group (5.9%); it was 6.5% in the 0.75 mg/kg enoxaparin group and 8.5% in the UFH group (Fig. 11.6). A statistically significant reduction was noted between the 0.5 mg/kg and UFH groups (P = .01), whereas the difference between the 0.5 mg/kg and 0.75 mg/kg enoxaparin groups met the prespecified criteria for noninferiority. In patients who did not receive GP IIb/IIIa inhibitors, even less bleeding was reported in the patients who received enoxaparin. No differences in ischemic end points were reported among the three groups, although the trial was not sufficiently powered to determine these effects.

Bivalirudin has been studied in elective PCI in a subgroup of ISAR-REACT 3 that comprised approximately 82% of the study population. This large trial of 4570 patients compared bivalirudin and UFH at high doses (140 U/kg) in patients pretreated with 600 mg clopidogrel and showed no difference in net clinical benefit between the two agents, although a significant reduction was seen in major bleeding with bivalirudin (3.1% vs. 4.6%, RR 0.66, 95% CI 0.49 to 0.90).

Summary

Anticoagulation remains the standard of care during elective PCI based on the atherothrombotic potential of stable plaque and the prothrombotic effect of stenting. This is despite two RCTs of REPLACE-2 and CIAO that challenged this assertion, although both trials have limitations. The choice of anticoagulation is more difficult because of the paucity of large RCTs with the currently available agents. Evidence from STEEPLE suggests that enoxaparin may be superior to heparin, and from ISAR REACT 3 that there is less bleeding with bivalirudin; however, radial arterial access and the newer-generation $P2Y_{12}$ antiplatelet agents were not in use, which limited these trials' applicability to current practice.

SPECIAL PATIENT GROUPS

With the broad array of therapies available, weighing the limitations and benefits of each approach is often difficult. In many patients, the use of UFH remains a safe and efficacious choice, especially in the context of pretreatment with a $P2Y_{12}$ inhibitor. However, in specific high-risk populations, the decision to use an alternative antithrombotic strategy may be considered.

Patients Transitioning From "Upstream" Management to the Catheterization Lab

Extrapolation of the clinical experience with UFH suggests that the degree of anticoagulation required during PCI is greater than that required during the medical management of ACS patients. As a result, strategies have evolved to optimize the antithrombin therapies among ACS patients proceeding to PCI while already receiving one of these agents. Among patients being treated with heparin, an ACT-guided approach is recommended, with an additional 20 to 50 U/kg IV administered to achieve an ACT greater than 200 to 250 seconds when concomitant GP IIb/IIIa inhibition is planned and more than 300 to 350 seconds when heparin is the sole agent. Data with enoxaparin suggest that PCI can proceed without additional dosing when the procedure is occurring within 8 hours of the subcutaneous dose, whereas an additional IV bolus of 0.3 mg/kg is recommended when the delay will be from 8 to 12 hours. Outside this window, a dose of 0.75 mg/kg by IV should be administered regardless of GP IIb/IIIa inhibition use based on the SYNERGY study. Among patients receiving infusions of bivalirudin, an additional bolus of 0.5 mg/kg and an increase in the infusion rate to 1.75 mg/kg was shown to be safe and efficacious in the ACUITY study, again regardless of GP IIb/IIIa use (Table 11.5). Observations from the ACUITY study also suggest that patients who receive bivalirudin after initial heparin or enoxaparin continued to experience a reduced rate of bleeding complications without compromise to ischemic benefits.

Patients With Renal Impairment

Increased ischemic and bleeding events are observed among patients with renal dysfunction. Analyses of the RCT experience with bivalirudin suggests the relative benefits of this agent are preserved in terms of bleeding complications and ischemic complications.[30,35,36] Hence in absolute terms, among patients with at least moderate renal dysfunction (creatinine clearance <60 mL/

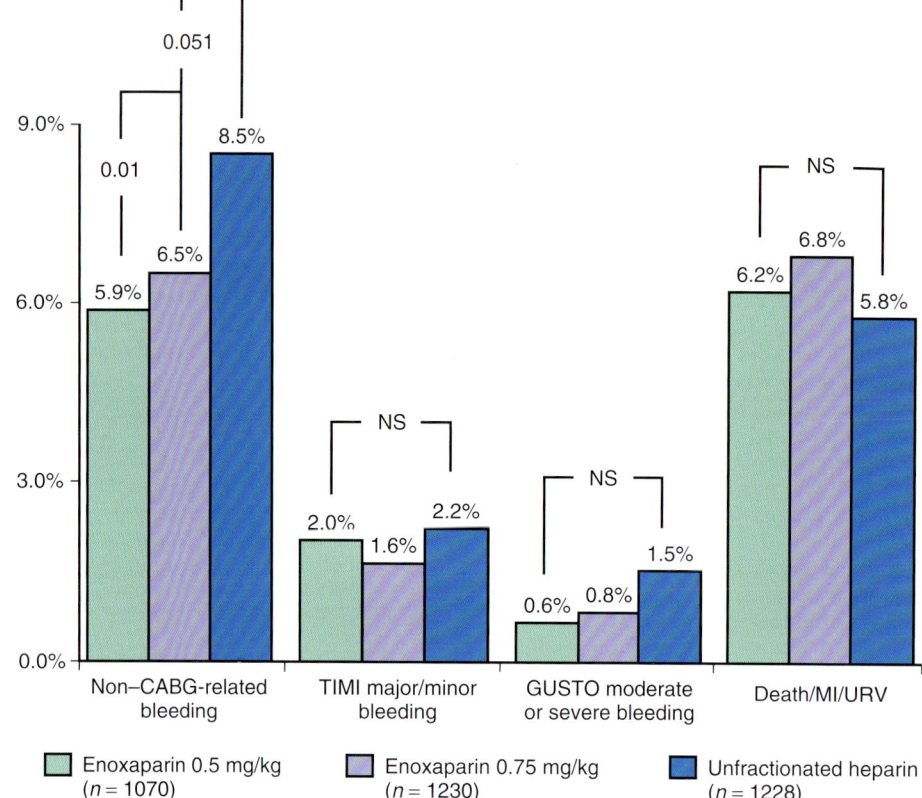

Fig. 11.6 Protocol-defined major bleeding and ischemic events in the STEEPLE trial. *CABG*, Coronary artery bypass grafting; *GUSTO*, global utilization of streptokinase and tissue plasminogen activator for occluded coronary arteries; *MI*, myocardial infarction; *NS*, nonsignificant; *TIMI*, thrombolysis in myocardial infarction; *URV*, urgent revascularization.

TABLE 11.5 Dosing of Currently Available Antithrombin Agents

	Unfractionated Heparin	Enoxaparin	Fondaparinux	Bivalirudin
No prior treatment	60–100 U/kg IV[a]	0.5–0.75 mg/kg IV	2.5 mg SC	0.75 mg/kg IV with 1.75 mg/kg/h infusion
Upstream ACS management	60 IU/kg IV and 800–1000 IU/h infusion	1.0 mg/kg SC BID	UFH bolus recommended (see text)	0.1 mg/kg IV with 0.25 mg/kg/h infusion
Additional bolus prior to PCI	20–50 IU/kg[a]	<8 h since last dose: None; 8–12 h since last SC dose: 0.3 mg/kg IV	2.5 mg IV with a GP IIb/IIIa inhibitor or 5 mg IV without a GP IIb/IIIa inhibitor	0.5 mg/kg IV bolus
Infusion during PCI	None	None	None	1.75 mg/kg/h infusion

[a]Targeting an activated clotting time (ACT) >200 s with concomitant glycoprotein IIb/IIIa inhibition or ACT >300–350 s without concomitant glycoprotein IIb/IIIa inhibition.
ACS, Acute coronary syndrome; *BID*, twice daily; *GP*, glycoprotein; *IV*, intravenous; *PCI*, percutaneous coronary intervention; *SC*, subcutaneous; *UFH*, unfractionated heparin.

min), bivalirudin is associated with a greater absolute benefit with respect to bleeding without an excess risk of ischemic events (Fig. 11.7). With enoxaparin and fondaparinux, limited data are available from small studies that have examined the relative risks and benefits in the context of renal impairment; however, reports of relative safety must be confirmed in larger studies.

Diabetic Patients

Subgroup analysis of RCTs appears to indicate that abciximab provides substantial benefits in terms of reduced repeat revascularization and mortality among diabetic patients, with comparable effects observed with tirofiban. Clinical trial evidence with bivalirudin supports similar conclusions. In the REPLACE-2 study, bivalirudin and provisional GP IIb/IIIa inhibition was compared with heparin and GP IIb/IIIa inhibition; bivalirudin-treated diabetic patients experienced a lower but nonsignificant (NS) rate of mortality at 12 months (2.3% vs. 3.9%, *P* = NS). No difference in the rate of 30-day bleeding and ischemic outcomes was observed.[37] Whereas the effects of enoxaparin-based strategies among diabetic patients have yet to be reported, a substantial rate of concomitant GP IIb/IIIa use in these studies will limit the interpretation of this data.

Patients With Heparin-Induced Thrombocytopenia

HIT precludes the use of UFH during PCI. Whereas the rate of HIT is less frequent with the LMWHs, cross-reactivity with these agents is observed and may be associated with increased rates of ischemic and bleeding complications. Fondaparinux has been used successfully to treat HIT, but the need for intraprocedural heparin with this agent precludes its use in PCI. Bivalirudin is well suited to the management of HIT patients who require PCI.[38] A registry of 52 HIT patients who received bivalirudin prior to PCI reported a 96% rate of freedom from death, Q-wave MI, and emergent CABG. Thrombocytopenia (platelet count <50 × 10^9/L) was not observed among these patients, which suggests

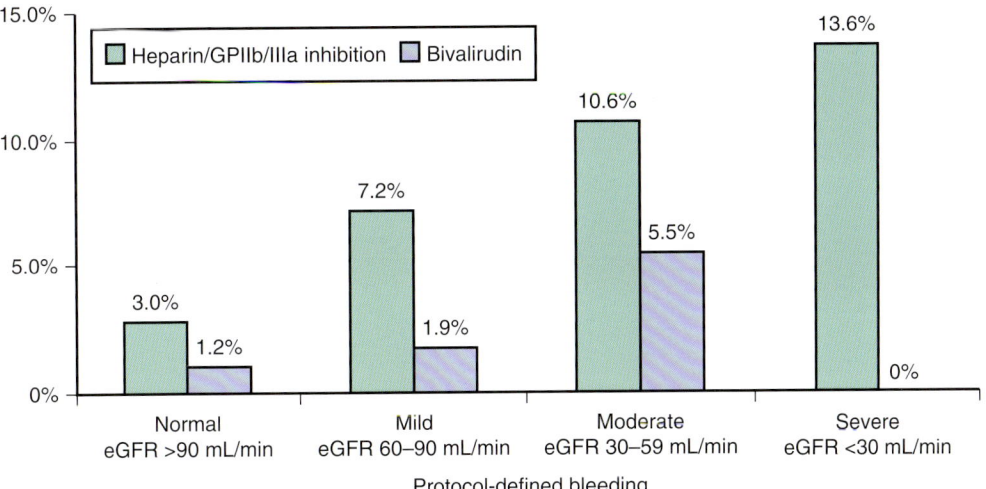

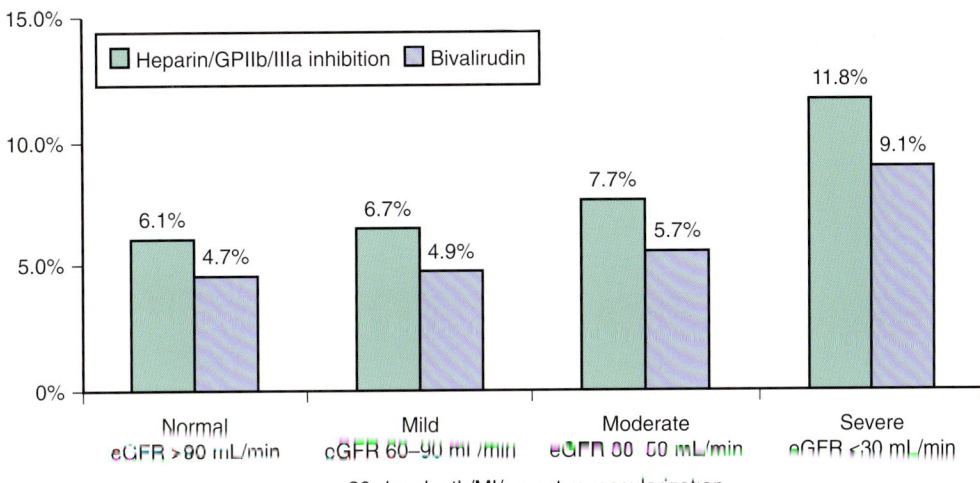

Fig. 11.7 Relationship between renal function and outcomes with bivalirudin. *eGFR*, Estimated glomerular filtration rate; *GP*, glycoprotein; *MI*, myocardial infarction.

bivalirudin is also an alternative anticoagulation strategy within this infrequent but high-risk subgroup.[39]

CONCLUSION

Substantial clinical trial evidence supports the use of anticoagulants among patients undergoing PCI to prevent ischemic complications. The choice of agent is ultimately guided by a combination of factors including clinical trial results, individual patient characteristics, and physician familiarity.

KEY REFERENCES

1. Schwartz RS, Borissoff JI, Spronk H. The hemostatic system as a modulator of atherosclerosis. *N Engl J Med*. 2011;364:1746–1760.
6. Thygesen K, Alpert JS, Jaffe AS, et al. Third universal definition of myocardial infarction. *J Am Coll Cardiol*. 2012;60:1581–1598.
7. Moussa ID, Klein LW, Shah B, et al. Consideration of a new definition of clinically relevant myocardial infarction after coronary revascularization: an expert consensus document from the Society for Cardiovascular Angiography and Interventions (SCAI). *J Am Coll Cardiol*. 2013;62(17):1563–1570.
11. Mehran R, Rao SV, Bhatt DL, et al. Standardized bleeding definitions for cardiovascular clinical trials: a consensus report from the Bleeding Academic Research Consortium. *Circulation*. 2011;123:2736–2747.
15. Lincoff A, Mehran R, Povsic T, et al. Effect of the REG1 anticoagulation system versus bivalirudin on outcomes after percutaneous coronary intervention (REGULATE-PCI): a randomized control clinical trial. *Lancet*. 2016;387:349–356.
23. Steg PG, van 't Hof A, Hamm CW, et al. Bivalirudin started during emergency transport for primary PCI. *N Engl J Med*. 2013;369:2207–2217.
24. Han Y, Guo J, Zheng Y, et al. Bivalirudin vs heparin with or without tirofiban during primary percutaneous coronary intervention in acute myocardial infarction. The BRIGHT randomised clinical trial. *JAMA*. 2015;313(13):1336–1346.
25. Erlinge D, Omerovic E, Frobert O, et al. Bivalirudin versus heparin monotherapy in myocardial infarction. *N Engl J Med*. 2017;377:1132–1142.
26. Montalescot G, Zeymer U, Silvain J, et al. Intravenous enoxaparin or unfractionated heparin in primary percutaneous coronary intervention for ST-elevation myocardial infarction: the international randomised open-label ATOLL trial. *Lancet*. 2011;378:693–703.
27. Steg PG, Jolly SS, Mehta SR, et al. Low-dose vs standard-dose unfractionated heparin for percutaneous coronary intervention in acute coronary syndromes treated with fondaparinux: the FUTURA/OASIS-8 randomized trial. *JAMA*. 2010;304:1339–1349.
28. Ferguson JJ, Califf RM, Antman EM, et al. Enoxaparin vs unfractionated heparin in high-risk patients with non-ST-segment elevation acute coronary syndromes managed with an intended early invasive strategy: primary results of the SYNERGY randomized trial. *JAMA*. 2004;292(1):45–54.
29. Silvain J, Beygui F, Barthelemy O, et al. Efficacy and safety of enoxaparin versus unfractionated heparin during percutaneous coronary intervention: systematic review and meta-analysis. *BMJ*. 2012;344:c553.
30. Stone GW, McLaurin BT, Cox DA, et al. Bivalirudin for patients with acute coronary syndromes. *N Engl J Med*. 2006;355:2203–2216.
31. Valgimigli M, Frigoli E, Leonardi S, et al. Bivalirudin or unfractionated heparin in acute coronary syndromes. *N Engl J Med*. 2015;373:997–1009.

Additional references available online at expertconsult.com

中文导读

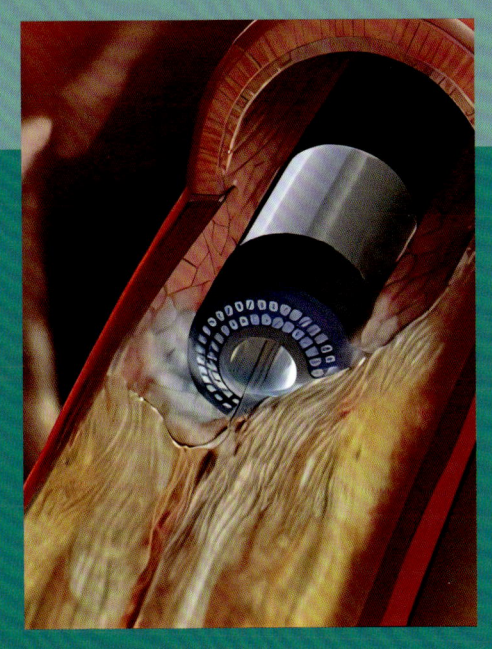

第12章
溶栓治疗

  溶栓治疗快速、简便。在不具备经皮冠状动脉介入治疗条件的医院或因各种原因使首次医疗接触至经皮冠状动脉介入治疗时间明显延迟时，对有适应证的ST段抬高型心肌梗死患者，静脉内溶栓仍是较好的选择。本章总结了溶栓常用药物及辅助药物治疗，并强调了其目前在ST段抬高型心肌梗死再灌注治疗中的作用证据，为该领域未来的发展奠定了基础。

  目前临床应用的主要溶栓药物包括非特异性纤溶酶原激活剂和特异性纤溶酶原激活剂两大类，全球范围内批准使用的溶栓药物（包括阿替普酶、瑞替普酶、替奈普酶等）在有效性和安全性方面无显著性差异。急性心肌梗死治疗的关键是再灌注治疗，需强调"时间就是心肌"的原则，发病2~3小时是挽救心肌的重要时机。因此，早期溶栓的效果明显优于晚期溶栓，并建议溶栓成功后的ST段抬高型心肌梗死患者均应尽早进行常规冠状动脉造影和经皮冠状动脉介入治疗。溶栓后的微循环再灌注也至关重要，通过使用有效的抗凝及抗血小板治疗以保证心外膜血管和微循环通畅。阿司匹林、氯吡格雷和肝素是目前证据级别最高的溶栓治疗后的抗栓方案，但也有试验结果证实血小板GPⅡb/Ⅲa拮抗剂和比伐卢定可减少再梗死的发生。

  现阶段依然存在中低等收入国家的多数患者和高收入国家的部分患者无法及时进行直接经皮冠状动脉介入治疗，而将溶栓作为初始的再灌注治疗策略，因此在今后相当长时间内溶栓治疗仍是ST段抬高型心肌梗死患者不可或缺的治疗方法。

王 枞　柳景华

章节要点

- 对于发病12小时内的急性ST段抬高型心肌梗死患者,当无法及时进行经皮冠状动脉介入治疗且无溶栓禁忌证时,溶栓治疗仍是首选的再灌注策略。
- 对于接受溶栓治疗的患者,辅助抗血小板和抗栓治疗在维持心外膜血管通畅和减少下游微血管阻塞方面至关重要。溶栓治疗后患者可从这些辅助治疗中得到明确的生存获益。
- 尚无临床证据支持可在直接经皮冠状动脉介入治疗过程中常规使用溶栓药物作为辅助治疗,一般应避免使用。
- 溶栓成功后的ST段抬高型心肌梗死患者,尤其是高危患者,均应尽早进行常规冠状动脉造影和经皮冠状动脉介入治疗。
- 尽管直接经皮冠状动脉介入治疗的应用越来越广泛,但鉴于全球心血管疾病的负担日益加重,特别是在发展中国家,溶栓治疗仍将是其最为常用且重要的再灌注策略。

12 Thrombolytic Intervention

Matthews Chacko, Khalil Ibrahim

KEY POINTS

- Thrombolytic therapy remains the preferred reperfusion strategy in patients with ST-elevation myocardial infarction (STEMI) who present within 12 hours of symptom onset when timely primary percutaneous coronary intervention (PCI) is not available and no contraindications to thrombolysis are present.
- Adjunctive antiplatelet and antithrombotic therapies are critical to the maintenance of epicardial vessel patency and to the reduction of downstream microvascular obstruction in patients treated with thrombolytics, and they offer proven survival benefits.
- The routine use of thrombolytics as adjunctive therapy in primary PCI is not supported by clinical evidence and should generally be avoided.
- Early routine coronary angiography and PCI following primary thrombolytic therapy for STEMI should be performed in all high-risk patients, and it should be considered in all patients following successful thrombolysis.
- Despite the growing availability of primary PCI, thrombolytic therapy will be the most common and important reperfusion strategy for STEMI given the growing burden of cardiovascular disease worldwide, particularly in developing nations.

INTRODUCTION

Atherosclerotic plaque rupture with subsequent thrombus formation through an intricate series of interactions among the coronary artery endothelium, exposed subendothelium, circulating platelets, and coagulation factors that lead to occlusion of an epicardial coronary artery are the pathophysiologic underpinnings of ST-elevation myocardial infarction (STEMI). The "open artery" hypothesis postulates that early reperfusion of the occluded artery translates into myocardial salvage and ultimately improved survival, and this is the basis of reperfusion therapy. The evidence for the benefit of thrombolytic therapy as a reperfusion strategy in STEMI is indisputable. Pivotal placebo-controlled randomized trials of patients with STEMI from the 1980s, beginning with the *Gruppo Italiano per lo Studio della Sopravvivenza nell'Infarto Miocardico* (GISSI) study and the Second International Study of Infarct Survival (ISIS-2), proved the value of early thrombolysis by reducing mortality by approximately 30% (Table 12.1).[1] These studies catalyzed the acceptance of thrombolysis as standard therapy for reperfusion in patients with acute myocardial infarction (AMI) and ushered in the *thrombolytic era*, a term that characterized the revolution in attitude among the medical community toward this disease. Although primary percutaneous coronary intervention (PCI) has superseded thrombolysis as the preferred reperfusion strategy in most patients presenting with STEMI, the most recent American College of Cardiology Foundation/American Heart Association (ACCF/AHA) STEMI guidelines continue to favor thrombolytic therapy over primary PCI as the primary reperfusion strategy in patients who (1) present within 12 hours of symptom onset, (2) have no invasive option (i.e., a catheterization laboratory is unavailable, vascular access issues are present) or face a delay of more than 120 minutes from first medical contact to primary PCI, (3) are not in cardiogenic shock, and (4) have no contraindications to thrombolytic therapy (Table 12.2).[2] However, because of concerns about bleeding complications, incomplete patency, and early reocclusion rates with thrombolytic therapy—combined with the fact that more primary PCIs are safely and successfully being performed at smaller hospitals without on-site cardiac surgery backup—thrombolytic therapy has been surpassed by primary PCI as the treatment modality for STEMI associated with better clinical outcomes (Fig. 12.1).[3-6] Whereas PCI has evolved into the preferred reperfusion strategy, particularly at high-volume experienced centers, it is not universally available. From 2003 to 2011 there was a 21% increase in PCI centers in the United States; however, most of this growth has occurred in population centers that already had preexisting PCI facilities.[7] Only 79.9% of the U.S. population lived within a 60-minute drive of a PCI-capable hospital in 2006.[8] Though the door-to-balloon (DTB) time has decreased significantly over the past few years with a median time of 96 minutes in 2005 down to 64 minutes in 2010, 9% of patients still had a DTB time greater than 90 minutes.[9] These two points indicate that a substantial number of patients still experience an inordinate delay in mechanical reperfusion therapy in current practice. This was further evidenced by a cohort study of 68,439 patients who presented to PCI-capable hospitals with STEMI between 1999 and 2002, which suggested that most STEMI patients received reperfusion therapy (68.7% PCI and 54.2% fibrinolysis) during off hours (weekdays 5 p.m. to 7 a.m. and weekends) and that these patients experienced significant delays in PCI but not in thrombolytic therapy.[10] Moreover, De Luca and colleagues[11] showed that every 30 minutes of delay in primary PCI results in a 7.5% increase in 1-year mortality. Therefore, thrombolytic therapy remains an important tool in the therapeutic armamentarium for treating STEMI, albeit with significant limitations. This chapter reviews the historic basis of thrombolytic intervention, summarizes current thrombolytic agents and adjunctive therapies, and highlights the evidence for its current role in reperfusion therapy for STEMI, laying the groundwork for future progress in this field.

THROMBOLYTIC AGENTS

Thrombolytic therapy was born in 1933, when Tillett and Garner[12] described the fibrinolytic activity of β-hemolytic streptococci, which led to the first therapeutic attempt by Tillett and Sherry[13] in 1948 to dissolve a fibrinous pleural effusion. Over 20 years later, in 1971, the

TABLE 12.1 Summary of Initial Randomized Clinical Trials for Thrombolytic Therapy in ST-Elevation Myocardial Infarction

Trial (n)	No. of Sites	Agent	Dose/Duration	Enrollment Dates	Placebo/Blinding	Age Criteria (Years)	Symptom Duration (h)
GISSI-1 (11,806)	176	SK	1.5 MU/1 h	2/84–6/85	No	All	<12
ISIS-2 (17,187)	417	SK	1.5 MU/1 h	3/85–12/87	Yes	All	<24
AIMS (1,258)	39	APSAC	30 U/5 min	9/85–10/87	Yes	<75	<6
ASSET (5,011)	52	tPA	100 mg/3 h	11/86–2/88	Yes	<75	<6

AIMS, Anistreplase Intervention Mortality Study; *APSAC,* anisoylated plasminogen streptokinase activator complex; *ASSET,* Anglo-Scandinavian Study of Early Thrombolysis; *GISSI-1,* Gruppo Italiano per lo Studio della Sopravvivenza nell'Infarto Miocardico; *ISIS-2,* Second International Study of Infarct Survival; *MU,* million units; *SK,* streptokinase; *tPA,* tissue plasminogen activator.
Modified from Kiernan TJ, Gersh BJ. Thrombolysis in acute myocardial infarction: current status. *Med Clin North Am.* 2007;91(4):617–637, table 2.

TABLE 12.2 Contraindications to Thrombolytic Therapy in Patients With ST-Elevation Myocardial Infarction[a]

ABSOLUTE CONTRAINDICATIONS
1. Any prior intracerebral hemorrhage
2. Known structural cerebral vascular lesion (e.g., arteriovenous malformation)
3. Known malignant intracranial neoplasm (primary or metastatic)
4. Ischemic stroke within 3 months, except acute ischemic stroke within 4.5 hours
5. Suspected aortic dissection
6. Active bleeding or bleeding diathesis (excluding menses)
7. Significant closed-head or facial trauma within 3 months
8. Intracranial or intraspinal surgery within 2 months
9. Severe uncontrolled hypertension (unresponsive to emergency therapy)
10. For streptokinase, prior treatment within the previous 6 months

RELATIVE CONTRAINDICATIONS
1. History of chronic, severe, poorly controlled hypertension
2. Systolic blood pressure >180 mm Hg or diastolic blood pressure >110 mm Hg on presentation
3. History of ischemic stroke more than 3 months prior
4. Dementia
5. Known intracranial pathology other than those in absolute contraindications
6. Traumatic or prolonged (>10 min) cardiopulmonary resuscitation
7. Major surgery within the prior 3 weeks
8. Internal bleeding within the prior 2–4 weeks
9. Noncompressible vascular punctures
10. Pregnancy
11. Active peptic ulcer
12. Oral anticoagulant therapy

[a]This table should be used only for assistance in clinical decision making and may not be all inclusive.
From O'Gara PT, Kushner FG, Ascheim DD, et al. 2013 ACCF/AHA guideline for the management of ST-elevation myocardial infarction: a report of the American College of Cardiology Foundation/American Heart Association Task Force on Practice Guidelines. *J Am Coll Cardiol.* 2013;61(40):e78–e140, table 6.

results of the first randomized controlled trial demonstrating the benefit of thrombolytic therapy using streptokinase in AMI were published.[14] In 1981, Rentrop and colleagues[15] showed that intracoronary streptokinase was effective in the lysis of coronary thrombi with the use of coronary angiography, and Markis and coworkers[16] demonstrated myocardial salvage with the same therapy, thus providing proof of the validity of the concept. Shortly thereafter, human tissue plasminogen activator (tPA) was isolated from a melanoma cell line[17] and was demonstrated to be effective in reducing mortality in AMI.[18] Current thrombolytic therapy comprises a class of agents known as *plasminogen activators*, which directly or indirectly convert the proenzyme plasminogen into plasmin. Plasmin is a nonspecific serine protease that catalyzes the degradation of fibrin, fibrinogen, prothrombin, and factors V and VII, thus disrupting the coagulation cascade and thrombus generation.[19] Plasminogen activators include the fibrin-specific agents such as *alteplase* (tPA), *single-chain urokinase plasminogen activator* (scu-PA), *tenecteplase* (TNK), and *staphylokinase* (SAK)—which enzymatically converts plasminogen into plasmin—as well as the non–fibrin-specific agents such as *streptokinase*, *anistreplase* (anisoylated plasminogen streptokinase activator complex [APSAC]), *urokinase*, *reteplase* (recombinant plasminogen activator [r-PA]), and *lanoteplase* (novel plasminogen activator [n-PA]) which have intermediate fibrin specificity. Currently, four thrombolytic agents are approved for use by the U.S. Food and Drug Administration (FDA) and are used most commonly worldwide: *streptokinase*, *alteplase*, *reteplase*, and *tenecteplase*. The last three agents were developed via recombinant deoxyribonucleic acid (DNA) technology to improve fibrin specificity and to increase the duration of activity to enable bolus dosing.[19] The major thrombolytic agents are briefly reviewed with regard to mechanism of action and thrombolytic profile (Table 12.3). Several novel fibrin-specific agents, *monteplase* (MT-PA), *palmiteplase* (YM866), *amediplase* (K[2]tu-PA), and *forteplase* (recombinant nonimmunogenic staphylokinase)—as well as a novel thrombin-activated plasminogen analogue, BB-10153, which would theoretically be activated only at the site of a developing thrombus—were evaluated in preclinical studies and small-scale human trials, but the efficacy of these agents has yet to be evaluated in larger phase III studies.

MAJOR HISTORICAL COMPARATIVE THROMBOLYTIC TRIALS

The GISSI-2/International trial with 20,891 patients with STEMI within 6 hours of symptom onset randomly assigned to either alteplase or streptokinase demonstrated no difference in mortality between streptokinase and alteplase with or without subcutaneous heparin (intravenous [IV] heparin was rarely used in this trial) but showed a higher rate of ischemic stroke in the alteplase group.[20] The ISIS-3 trial with 41,299 patients randomized to alteplase, streptokinase, or anistreplase demonstrated equivalence in mortality reduction among the three agents but found that streptokinase was associated with the lowest overall rates of stroke (1.1%) and intracerebral hemorrhage (0.3%).[21] IV heparin was not used in this trial; however, it has been borne out collectively through other studies of the fibrin-specific plasminogen activators that adjunctive heparin, although not critical to achieve thrombolysis, is important to sustain infarct vessel patency through the avoidance of recurrent thrombosis. The Global Utilization of Streptokinase and Tissue Plasminogen Activator for Occluded Coronary Arteries I (GUSTO-I) trial with 41,021 patients promulgated the benefit of "accelerated" alteplase plus IV heparin in STEMI, leading to a 15% relative and 1% absolute reduction in mortality (or 1 life saved per 100 patients treated).[22] This study included an angiographic component, which led to the major finding that early and complete infarct vessel patency was tightly linked to a reduction in mortality.[23] The Reteplase (r-PA) Angiographic Phase I International Dose-Finding Study (RAPID-I) suggested a

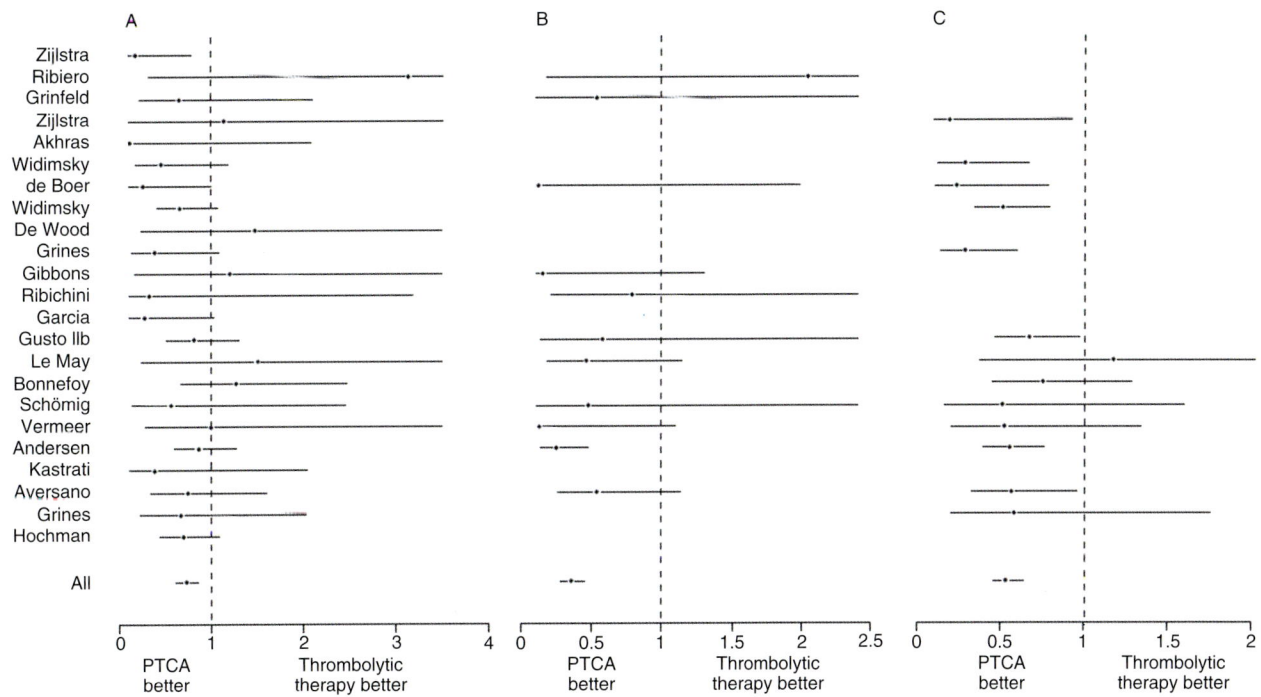

Fig. 12.1 Odds ratios (95% confidence interval) of short-term death (A), nonfatal reinfarction (B), and combined death, nonfatal reinfarction, and stroke (C) for patients treated with percutaneous coronary intervention (also known as percutaneous transluminal coronary angioplasty [PTCA]) versus thrombolytic therapy for ST-elevation myocardial infarction. (From Keeley EC, Boura JA, Grines CL. Primary angioplasty versus intravenous thrombolytic therapy for acute myocardial infarction: a quantitative review of 23 randomised trials. *Lancet.* 2003;361[9351]:13–20.)

TABLE 12.3 Characteristics of Thrombolytic Agents

	Streptokinase	Tenecteplase	Alteplase	Reteplase
Source	Group C streptococci	Recombinant, human	Recombinant, human	Recombinant, human mutant tPA
Molecular weight (kDa)	47	57[a]	63 to 70	39
Fibrin specificity	No	Yes	Yes	Yes
Metabolism	Hepatic	Hepatic	Hepatic	Renal
Half-life (min)	18–23	20–24	3–4	14
Mode of action	Activator complex	Direct	Direct	Direct
Antigenicity	Yes	No	No	No
Estimated hospital cost per dose (USD)[b]	$300/1.5 MU	$2200	$2200/100 mg	$2200/20 MU

[a]Turcasso NM, Nappi JM. Tenecteplase for treatment of acute myocardial infarction. *Ann Pharmacother.* 2001;35(10):1233–1240.
[b]Costs list U.S. prices of usual dose.
MU, Million units; *tPA,* tissue plasminogen activator; *USD,* United States dollars.
Modified from Granger CB, Califf RM, Topol EJ. Thrombolytic therapy for acute myocardial infarction. A review. *Drugs.* 1992;44(3):293–325.

nonsignificant 30-day mortality benefit with reteplase compared with alteplase (1.9% vs. 3.9%), and the RAPID-II trial showed a significant improvement in coronary artery patency defined as thrombolysis in myocardial infarction (TIMI) grade 2 flow within 90 minutes that favored reteplase over alteplase (85.2% vs. 77.2%, $P = .03$).[24,25] The GUSTO-III trial involved 15,021 patients but failed to show true equivalence of reteplase to "accelerated" alteplase, although it demonstrated a trend toward equivalence, especially for death and disabling stroke. These findings, combined with the more convenient double-bolus administration, rendered reteplase a viable option for thrombolysis.[26] The Assessment of the Safety and Efficacy of a New Thrombolytic 2 (ASSENT-2) trial of 16,949 patients randomized to receive either tenecteplase or alteplase found similar mortality rates, but the highly fibrin-specific tenecteplase was notable for significantly less bleeding compared with alteplase.[27] Although this result was tempered by a relatively high rate of intracerebral hemorrhage in both groups, lower rates of overall bleeding (26.1% vs. 28.4%, $P < .0003$) and blood transfusions (4.3% vs. 5.5%, $P = .0002$) were observed with tenecteplase compared with alteplase. Currently, thrombolytic agent selection at most hospitals in the United States is guided by hospital formulary and drug availability given the lack of any striking differences in the efficacy or safety of the approved thrombolytic agents.

SECTION II Pharmacologic Intervention

TIMING OF THROMBOLYTIC THERAPY

Early Treatment

The degree of myocardial salvage following AMI is clearly related to timely reperfusion, reinforcing the "time is myocardium" principle with the 2- to 3-hour time point representing the critical window to minimize morbidity and mortality (Fig. 12.2).[28,29] A meta-analysis of six randomized controlled trials of pre-hospital and in-hospital thrombolysis for AMI that included 6434 patients showed reduced time to thrombolysis (104 vs. 162 min, P = .007) and reduced all-cause hospital mortality (odds ratio [OR], 0.83; 95% confidence interval [CI] 0.70 to 0.98) with pre-hospital fibrinolysis.[30] Subsequent randomized trials have reproduced these findings in populations in the United States and in Europe and have demonstrated the feasibility of safe and effective pre-hospital fibrinolysis administered by paramedics.[31–33] Current ACCF/AHA guidelines for STEMI management recognize the potential benefit of pre-hospital fibrinolysis by appropriately trained personnel,[2] but logistical challenges that include implementation of systems for rapid pre-hospital diagnosis and training of personnel in the appropriate administration of thrombolytic agents and adjunctive therapies have limited the widespread acceptance and adoption of pre-hospital fibrinolysis.[34,35] Therefore the 2013 ACCF/AHA guidelines for STEMI management endorse the need for further research regarding the implementation of pre-hospital thrombolysis but stop short of recommending its use.[2]

There appears to be an early and sustained difference in favor of primary PCI versus thrombolysis as a function of time to reperfusion. A pooled analysis of 22 randomized clinical trials that included 6763 patients with STEMI who presented within 12 hours of symptom onset showed a 37% reduction in 30-day mortality (adjusted OR 0.63; 95% CI, 0.42 to 0.84) in patients randomized to primary PCI compared with those randomized to thrombolysis regardless of presentation delay up to 12 hours or a PCI-related delay up to 2 hours (Fig. 12.3).[5] Furthermore, the absolute mortality reduction in the PCI group increased from 1.3% in those who presented within an hour after symptom onset to 4.2% for those who presented 6 to 12 hours after symptom onset. Primary PCI is also superior to both pre-hospital and in-hospital thrombolysis with regard to 30-day mortality, 1-year mortality, reinfarction, and myocardial salvage.[36,37] In addition, long-term follow up of the Swedish Early Decision Reperfusion Strategy (SWEDES) trial showed that the benefit of primary PCI over fibrinolysis with respect to cardiac death or recurrent AMI persisted out to 5 years (hazard ratio [HR] 0.40; 95% CI, 0.19 to 0.82).[38] Even if transfer to another facility is required, the benefit of PCI over thrombolysis with regard to the combined reduction

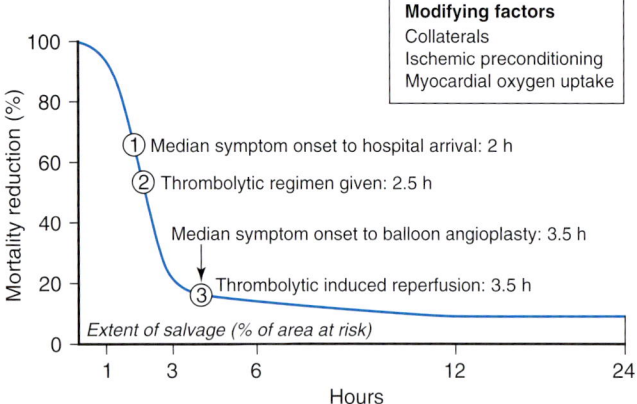

Fig. 12.2 Mortality reduction as a function of time with reperfusion therapy and the potential for myocardial salvage. This illustrates that unless patients present very early in the course of an ST-elevation myocardial infarction, thrombolysis before percutaneous coronary intervention would have little benefit. (Adapted from Stone GW, Gersh BJ. Facilitated angioplasty: paradise lost. *Lancet.* 2006;367[9510]:543–546.)

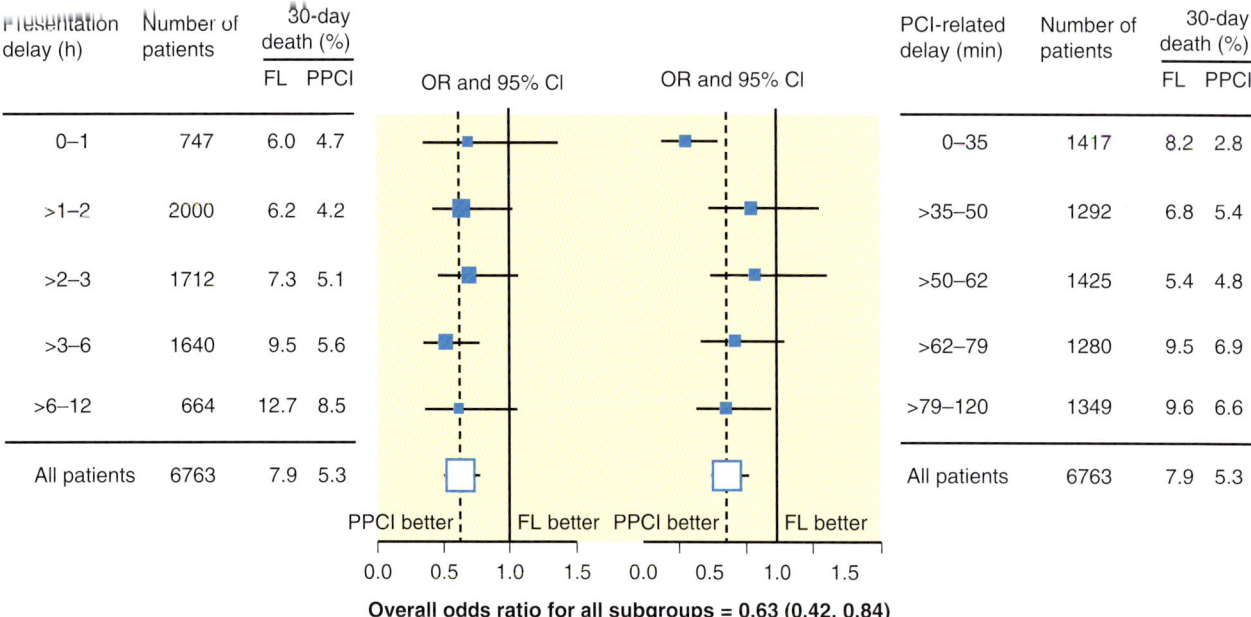

Fig. 12.3 Odds ratios *(ORs)* for 30-day death in a pooled analysis of 22 randomized trials of primary percutaneous coronary intervention *(PPCI)* compared with fibrinolysis *(FL)* according to presentation delay *(left panel)* and PCI-related delay *(right panel)*. *CI*, Confidence interval. (From the Primary Coronary Angioplasty vs. Thrombolysis Group. Does time matter? A pooled analysis of randomized clinical trials comparing primary percutaneous coronary intervention and in-hospital fibrinolysis in acute myocardial infarction patients. *Eur Heart J.* 2006;27[7]:779–788.)

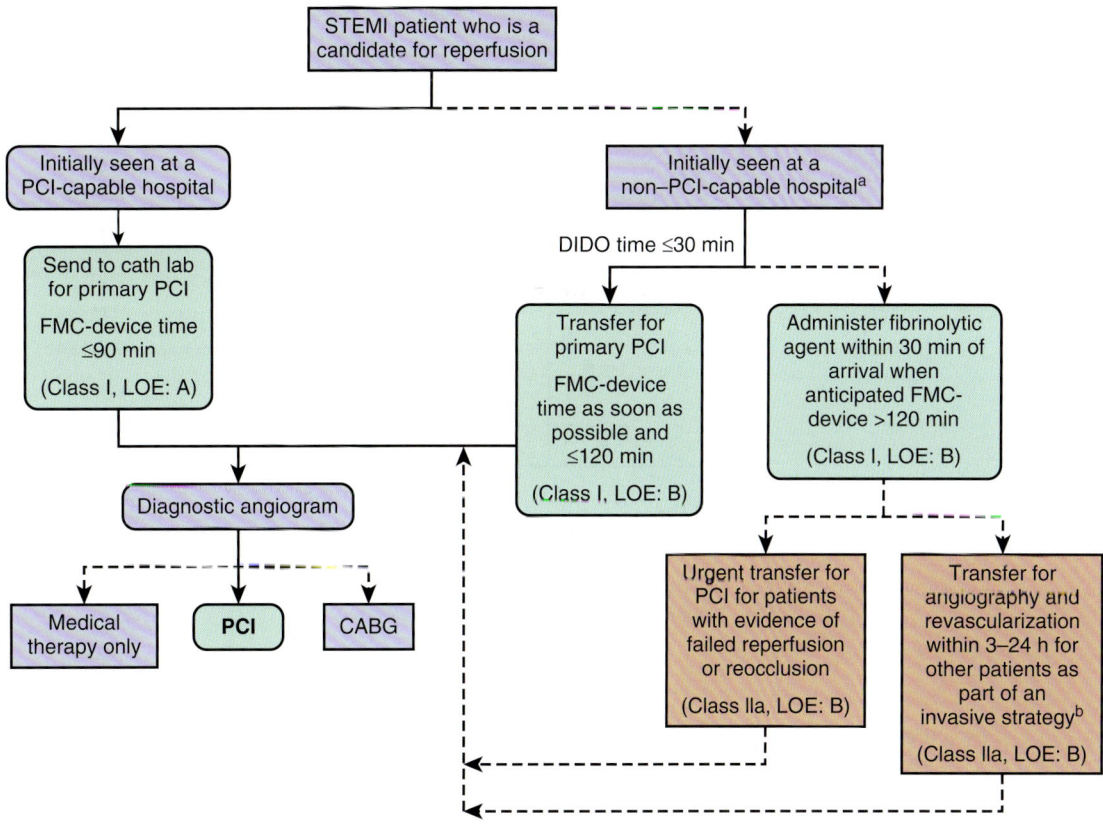

Fig. 12.4 Reperfusion therapy for patients with ST-elevation myocardial infarction (STEMI). The bold arrows and boxes are the preferred strategies. Performance of percutaneous coronary intervention (PCI) is dictated by an anatomically appropriate culprit stenosis. CABG, Coronary artery bypass graft; DIDO, door-in-door-out; FMC, first medical contact; LOE, level of evidence. (From O'Gara PT, Kushner FG, Ascheim DD, et al. 2013 ACCF/AHA guideline for the management of ST-elevation myocardial infarction: a report of the American College of Cardiology Foundation/American Heart Association Task Force on Practice Guidelines. J Am Coll Cardiol. 2013;61[4]:e78–e140.)

in death, reinfarction, and disabling stroke at 30 days (driven primarily by reinfarction) is sustained in those patients with STEMI who present within 12 hours of symptom onset.[3,39] Furthermore, in the referral hospital substudy of the Danish Trial in Acute Myocardial Infarction 2 (DANAMI-2), patients with STEMI transferred to a PCI-capable hospital for primary PCI within 120 minutes had improvements in reinfarction (13% vs. 18.5%, HR 0.66; 95% CI, 0.49 to 0.89) and mortality (26.7% vs. 33.3%, HR 0.78; 95% CI, 0.63 to 0.97) out to 8 years of follow-up.[40] However, the net benefit of primary PCI over thrombolysis may be neutralized if the DTB time for PCI is 60 minutes longer than door-to-needle (DTN) time for thrombolysis, given that every 30-minute delay in the interval from symptom onset to balloon inflation is associated with a 7.5% increased risk of death at 1 year.[11] Hence the 2013 ACCF/AHA STEMI guidelines recommend that in-hospital thrombolytic therapy should be administered to those patients who present to a non–PCI-capable hospital within 12 hours of symptom onset *if* transfer for primary PCI (the preferred reperfusion strategy) cannot be completed in a timely fashion—that is, time from arrival at the non–PCI-capable hospital to leaving for the PCI-capable hospital (door-in-door-out [DIDO] time) of 30 minutes or less or anticipated first medical contact to device time of 120 minutes of less—and there is no evidence of severe heart failure or cardiogenic shock (Fig. 12.4).[2]

In 30% to 40% of patients who fail thrombolysis (<70% ST-segment resolution at 90 min or ongoing chest pain), rescue PCI should be performed, given the benefit of this strategy (Fig. 12.5).[41–43] Accumulating evidence also supports the benefit of performing routine cardiac catheterization and PCI within 24 hours or earlier regardless of the success of thrombolysis (Fig. 12.6).[44–47] This pharmacoinvasive approach is discussed in more detail later in this chapter. The facilitated PCI approach, with early administration of a thrombolytic agent in anticipation of mechanical revascularization, is also discussed later in this chapter.

Late Treatment

Large mega-trials have suggested that most of the benefit of thrombolytic therapy is largely confined to the first 12 hours following symptom onset and that many of the complications, such as serious bleeding and latent myocardial rupture, occur with late

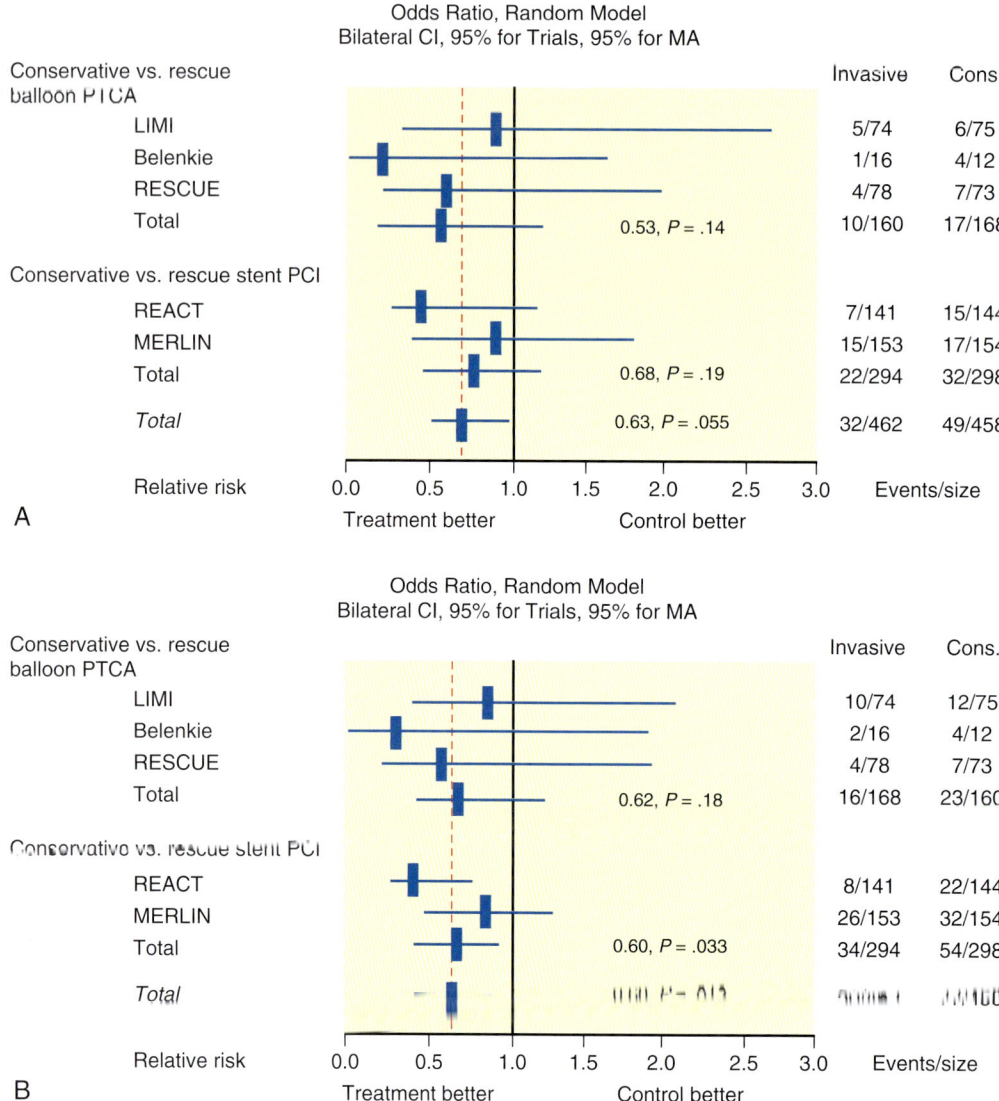

Fig. 12.5 Odds ratios for death (A) and death or reinfarction (B) with rescue percutaneous coronary intervention (*PCI*) versus conservative (*Cons.*) management of ST-elevation myocardial infarction at 30 days. *CI*, Confidence interval; *LIMI*, Limburg Myocardial Infarction Trial; *MA*, meta-analysis; *MERLIN*, Middlesborough Early Revascularization to Limit Infarction; *PTCA*, percutaneous transluminal coronary angioplasty; *REACT*, Rescue Angioplasty Versus Conservative Therapy or Repeat Thrombolysis Trial; *RESCUE*, Randomized Evaluation of Salvage Angioplasty with Combined Utilization of Endpoints. (From Collet JP, Montalescot G, Le May M, et al. Percutaneous coronary intervention after fibrinolysis: a multiple meta-analyses approach according to the type of strategy. *J Am Coll Cardiol.* 2006;48[7]:1326–1335.)

thrombolysis. Two specific trials, the *Estudio Multicentrico Estreptoquinasa Republica Americas Sud* (EMERAS [South American Multicenter Streptokinase Study])[48] and the Late Assessment of Thrombolytic Efficacy (LATE) trial,[49] addressed the issue of late thrombolysis and showed no demonstrable survival benefit beyond the 12-hour mark with streptokinase or alteplase, respectively, with excessive serious bleeding complications in the latter trial. The Fibrinolytic Therapy Trialists' Collaboration performed a pooled analysis of 52,892 patients enrolled into eight placebo-controlled trials (excluding LATE) and showed significant benefit up to but not beyond 12 hours from symptom onset.[50] The available data provide convincing evidence that there is a golden first hour and an ominous twelfth hour after symptom onset, illustrating the narrow therapeutic window for thrombolytic therapy (Fig. 12.7). Accordingly, health care systems should aim to develop and implement plans to minimize the delays in patient triage and facilitate timely initiation of reperfusion therapy.

ADJUNCTIVE THERAPIES

One of the remaining challenges of contemporary reperfusion therapy is to achieve tissue-level perfusion rather than simply restoring the patency of the infarct-related coronary artery. Microcirculatory reperfusion after thrombolysis is critical, and strategies to reduce platelet aggregation, maintain endothelial integrity, and prevent the downstream effects of an embolized thrombus and atherosclerotic debris through the use of potent anticoagulant, antithrombotic, and antiplatelet agents have led to several important clinical trials. To that end, adjunctive therapies aimed at improving epicardial and microcirculatory patency while preserving myocardial function are discussed below.

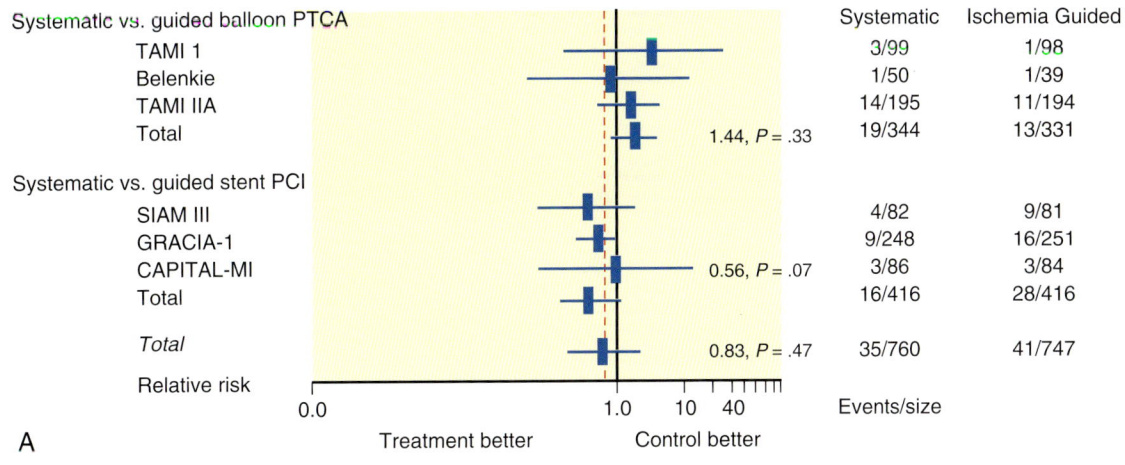

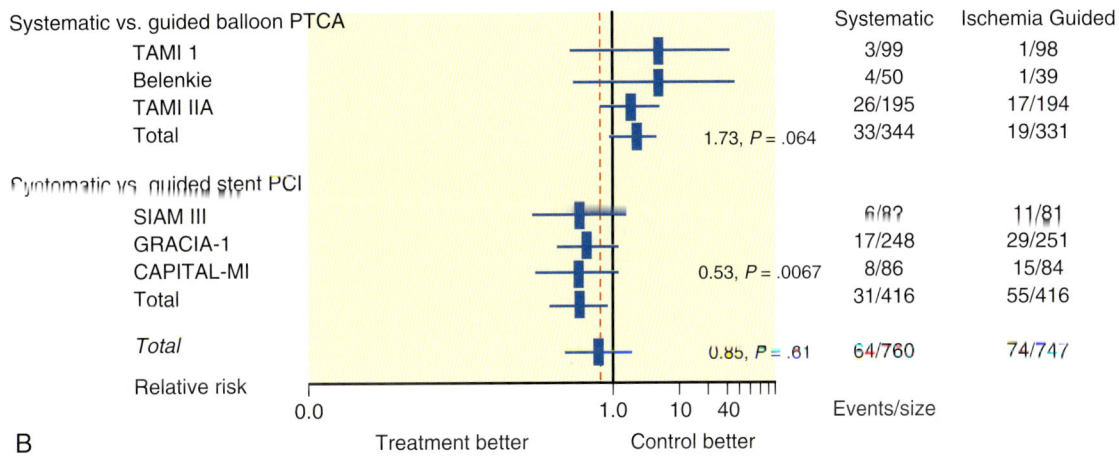

Fig. 12.6 Odds ratios for death (A) and death or reinfarction (B) with systematic versus ischemia-guided percutaneous coronary intervention *(PCI)* after ST-elevation myocardial infarction. *CAPITAL-MI,* Combined Angioplasty and Pharmacologic Intervention Versus Thrombolytics Alone in Acute Myocardial Infarction; *CI,* confidence interval; *Cons.,* conservative; *GRACIA-1,* Randomized Trial Comparing Stenting Within 24 Hours of Thrombolysis Versus Ischemia-Guided Approach to Thrombolyzed Acute Myocardial Infarction With ST-Segment Elevation; *MA,* meta-analysis; *PTCA,* percutaneous transluminal coronary angioplasty; *SIAM,* Comparison of Invasive and Conservative Strategies After Treatment With Streptokinase in Acute Myocardial Infarction; *TAMI,* Thrombolysis and Angioplasty in Myocardial Infarction. (Reproduced from Collet JP, Montalescot G, Le May M, et al. Percutaneous coronary intervention after fibrinolysis: a multiple meta-analyses approach according to the type of strategy. *J Am Coll Cardiol.* 2006;48[7]:1326–1335.)

Aspirin

The standard adjuvant pharmacotherapy for all patients with AMI undergoing thrombolysis should include a loading dose of 162 to 325 mg of aspirin in the absence of a documented allergy.[2,21,51,52] The benefit of aspirin therapy in ISIS-2 resulted in 25 lives saved per 1000 patients treated, as well as 10 prevented nonfatal reinfarctions and three strokes prevented per 1000 patients treated.[53] These findings appeared to be durable at 10 years of follow-up, making the duration of aspirin therapy in this setting indefinite.[54] Furthermore, in the CURRENT-OASIS 7 trial,[55] a maintenance dose of 81 mg/day was noninferior to 300 to 325 mg/day with regard to the composite end point of cardiovascular (CV) death, myocardial infarction (MI), or stroke at 30 days in patients with acute coronary syndromes (ACS) undergoing early PCI. On the basis of this study and others the 2016 ACC/AHA Guideline Focused Update on Duration of Dual Antiplatelet Therapy in Patients with Coronary Artery Disease provide a class I recommendation to an aspirin maintenance dose of 81 mg/day.[56]

P2Y$_{12}$ Receptor Antagonists

Clopidogrel, an oral P2Y$_{12}$ receptor antagonist, given at a loading dose of 300 mg (or 75 mg in patients ≥75 years of age) at or before the time of thrombolysis followed by 75 mg daily for a minimum of 1 year is standard adjuvant therapy (along with aspirin) in STEMI patients treated with thrombolytic therapy, and it likely serves to

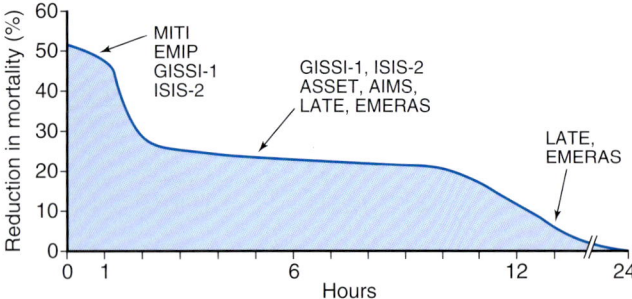

Fig. 12.7 Percent mortality reduction derived from thrombolytic therapy as a function of time from symptom onset to initiation of therapy with clinical trials noted from which these data are extrapolated. A greater than 50% reduction in mortality is noted during the first "golden hour," after which the mortality benefit declines to a plateau of approximately 25% reduction until 12 hours, after which there is no apparent survival benefit with thrombolytic therapy. *AIMS,* Anistreplase Intervention Mortality Study; *ASSET,* Anglo-Scandinavian Study of Early Thrombolysis; *EMERAS,* Estudio Multicentrico Estreptoquinasa Republicas de America Del Sur; *EMIP,* European Myocardial Infarction Project; *GISSI-1,* Gruppo Italiano per lo Studio della Sopravvivenza nell'Infarto Miocardico; *ISIS-2,* Second International Study of Infarct Survival; *LATE,* Late Assessment of Thrombolytic Efficacy; *MITI,* Myocardial Infarction and Triage Intervention Project. (Lincoff AM, Topol EJ. The illusion of reperfusion. Does anyone achieve optimal reperfusion during acute myocardial infarction? *Circulation.* 1993;88[3]:1361–1374.)

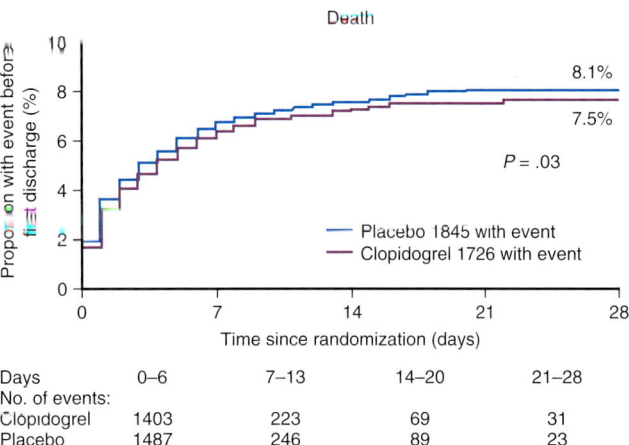

Fig. 12.8 Death rates from the Clopidogrel and Metoprolol in Myocardial Infarction Trial (COMMIT) with the addition of clopidogrel to aspirin in 45,852 patients with ST-elevation myocardial infarction. (From Chen ZM, Jiang LX, Chen YP, et al. Addition of clopidogrel to aspirin in 45,852 patients with acute myocardial infarction: randomised placebo-controlled trial. *Lancet.* 2005;366[9497]:1607–1621.)

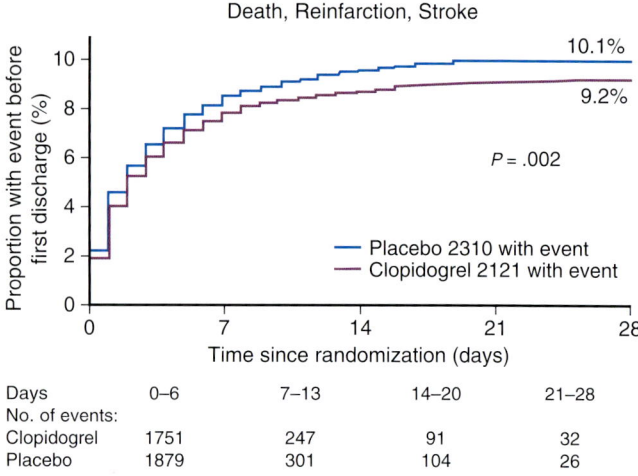

Fig. 12.9 Combined end point of death, reinfarction, and stroke from the Clopidogrel and Metoprolol in Myocardial Infarction Trial (COMMIT) with the addition of clopidogrel to aspirin in 45,852 patients with ST-elevation myocardial infarction. (From Chen ZM, Jiang LX, Chen YP, et al. Addition of clopidogrel to aspirin in 45,852 patients with acute myocardial infarction: randomised placebo-controlled trial. *Lancet.* 2005;366[9497]:1607–1621.)

help maintain patency of the infarct-related artery after thrombolysis.[2] In the Clopidogrel and Metoprolol in Myocardial Infarction Trial (COMMIT)[57] of 45,852 patients, clopidogrel was shown to significantly reduce death (7.5% vs. 8.1%, P = .03; Fig. 12.8) and the combined end point of death, reinfarction, and stroke (9.2% vs. 10.1%, P = .002) when given to aspirin-treated patients before thrombolytic therapy for STEMI (Fig. 12.9). The Clopidogrel as Adjunctive Reperfusion Therapy (CLARITY)–TIMI 28 trial[58] also supported the benefit of clopidogrel pretreatment before thrombolysis in patients aged 75 years or younger with STEMI and demonstrated reduced rates of death and recurrent MI or ischemia at 30 days and significant improvement in coronary blood flow at 48 hours with no excess bleeding with clopidogrel. Furthermore, in the subset of patients undergoing PCI within 2 to 8 days after thrombolysis, pretreatment with clopidogrel (300 mg loading dose followed by 75 mg daily thereafter) at the time of thrombolysis compared with placebo significantly reduced the combined end point of CV death, MI, and stroke through 30 days (7.5% vs. 12%, P = .001) with no significant increase in bleeding.[59] The Harmonizing Outcomes With Revascularization and Stents in Acute Myocardial Infarction (HORIZONS-AMI)[60] and Clopidogrel Optimal Loading Dose Usage to Reduce Recurrent Events/Optimal Antiplatelet Strategy for Interventions (CURRENT–OASIS 7)[55] trials have demonstrated the efficacy and safety of a 600-mg loading dose of clopidogrel in the treatment of ACS managed with an invasive reperfusion strategy, but no studies to date have evaluated this dosing strategy in combination with thrombolytic therapy. Based on the COMMIT and CLARITY-TIMI 28 trial, the 2016 ACC/AHA Guideline Focused Update on Duration of DAPT in Patients with Coronary Artery Disease provides a class I recommendation for clopidogrel to be continued for a minimum of 14 days and ideally at least 12 months in patients presenting with STEMI and treated with thrombolytic therapy. In patients who have tolerated dual-antiplatelet therapy (DAPT) without bleeding complications, continuation of DAPT for longer than 12 months may be reasonable (Class IIb recommendation).[56] This is largely based on data involving patients with PCI including the large DAPT study which randomized patients who had been treated with DAPT for 12 months without bleeding complications to an additional 18 months of DAPT or to aspirin monotherapy and found that prolonged DAPT therapy resulted in a 0.7% absolute reduction in very late stent thrombosis, a 2.0% absolute reduction in MI, and a 1.2% absolute increase in moderate to severe bleeding.[61]

Prasugrel, another oral $P2Y_{12}$ receptor antagonist with more potent platelet inhibition than clopidogrel, was shown to reduce the rate of CV death, nonfatal MI, and nonfatal stroke at 1 year compared to clopidogrel (9.9% vs. 12.1%, P < .001) in the Trial to Assess Improvement in Therapeutic Outcomes by Optimizing Platelet Inhibition With Prasugrel (TRITON)–TIMI 38 trial,[62] which included 13,608 patients with moderate- to high-risk ACS managed with PCI. Notably, higher rates of bleeding were also observed with prasugrel compared to clopidogrel (2.4% vs. 1.8%,

$P = .03$); however, no difference in mortality was observed. Other important findings of this study included net harm with prasugrel in patients with a history of cerebrovascular disease, those aged 75 years and older, and in patients weighing less than 60 kg and it should be avoided in those populations. Although the FDA approved prasugrel for use in the management of ACS with PCI, it has not been studied as an adjunct to thrombolytic therapy.

Ticagrelor is another oral $P2Y_{12}$ receptor antagonist that reversibly inhibits adenosine diphosphate (ADP)–stimulated platelet activation with more rapid and potent platelet inhibition than clopidogrel.[63] The Platelet Inhibition and Patient Outcomes (PLATO) study,[64] a randomized controlled trial that included 18,624 patients, showed a benefit of ticagrelor compared to clopidogrel in the management of ACS with PCI, with a reduction in vascular death, MI, and stroke at 12 months (9.8% vs. 11.7%, $P = .001$). While there was no difference in overall bleeding, a higher rate of nonprocedural bleeding was observed with ticagrelor (4.5% vs. 3.8%, $P = .03$), which included intracerebral hemorrhage. Ticagrelor is FDA approved for the treatment of ACS and to prevent stent thrombosis with PCI but has not been evaluated as adjuvant therapy with thrombolytic therapy.

Cangrelor is an intravenous reversible $P2Y_{12}$ receptor antagonist that causes almost complete inhibition of ADP-induced platelet aggregation and does not require conversion to an active metabolite. The Safety, Tolerability, and Effect on Patency in Acute Myocardial Infarction (STEP-AMI) angiographic trial[65] of 92 patients with STEMI randomized patients to aspirin and heparin with either cangrelor, full-dose alteplase, or half-dose alteplase with one of three doses of cangrelor. Although stopped early by the sponsor because of a change in the priority of drug development, cangrelor with half-dose alteplase appeared to result in a similar rate of complete reperfusion compared with full-dose alteplase. Whether cangrelor is more effective and/or safe than the oral $P2Y_{12}$ receptor antagonists as an adjuvant to thrombolytic therapy awaits further study.

Ticlopidine is an indirect $P2Y_{12}$ receptor antagonist and works by inhibiting ADP-induced platelet binding; however, no meaningful studies have looked at ticlopidine as adjunctive therapy in STEMI patients undergoing thrombolysis. The Ticlopidine Versus Aspirin After Myocardial Infarction (STAMI)[66] trial did address the role of ticlopidine in secondary prevention of CV events in STEMI patients treated with thrombolysis but found no difference compared with aspirin monotherapy.

Heparin

In the absence of heparin-induced thrombocytopenia or known allergy to heparin, unfractionated heparin (UFH), low molecular-weight-heparin (LMWH), or fondaparinux should also be part of the standard adjuvant pharmacotherapy for patients with AMI treated with thrombolysis, given the thrombin-mediated pro-thrombotic state that is engendered. All are given for a minimum of 48 hours and a maximum of 8 days or until revascularization. The 2013 ACCF/AHA STEMI guidelines recommend UFH given as a weight-adjusted IV bolus followed by an infusion titrated to keep the activated partial thromboplastin time (aPTT) between 1.5 and 2.0 times control (class I recommendation).[2]

LMWH is an alternative to UFH as adjunctive therapy for thrombolysis and is given as an IV bolus followed 15 minutes later by subcutaneous injection, with the dose adjusted according to age, weight, and renal function.[2] Several clinical trials have shown the noninferiority of LMWH compared with UFH with regard to death and nonfatal reinfarction. The ASSENT-3 trial[67] assessed two different combination strategies: (1) half-dose tenecteplase plus low-dose UFH and abciximab and (2) full-dose tenecteplase plus enoxaparin; the investigators compared these strategies with standard tenecteplase with UFH in 6095 patients. This study demonstrated an impressive reduction in reinfarction in both tenecteplase combination-therapy groups, confirming both the potency of the half-dose thrombolytics–abciximab combination and the efficacy of enoxaparin in this setting. However, this benefit was tempered by an increased rate of bleeding complications that required blood transfusions in both of the combination-therapy groups compared with the tenecteplase-plus-heparin group. Also disconcerting was the relatively high rate of intra-cerebral hemorrhage in all three groups of the study (0.8% to 0.9%), particularly in older individuals. The trial did provide encouraging data for the use of tenecteplase plus enoxaparin, rather than heparin, to reduce the short-term outcome of reinfarction, even though long-term follow-up at 1 year showed no difference among the treatment groups in terms of mortality.[68]

The Enoxaparin as Adjunctive Antithrombin Therapy for ST-Elevation Myocardial Infarction (ENTIRE)–TIMI 23 trial[69] evaluated ST-segment resolution at 180 minutes and early angiographic patency in 483 patients with AMI using (1) full-dose tenecteplase plus either UFH or enoxaparin or (2) half-dose tenecteplase with abciximab plus either UFH or enoxaparin. This study demonstrated a reduction in death and nonfatal MI at 30 days in the full-dose tenecteplase-plus-enoxaparin group compared with the full dose tenecteplase plus UFH group (4.4% vs. 15.9%, $P = .005$) without any difference in TIMI major hemorrhage (1.9% vs. 2.4%). Furthermore, no difference was reported in death or nonfatal MI at 30 days in the group that received tenecteplase plus abciximab and enoxaparin compared with those that received tenecteplase plus abciximab and UFH, although bleeding in both combination-therapy groups was higher than in the full-dose tenecteplase groups.

Validating the benefit of enoxaparin in reducing reinfarction, the Enoxaparin and Thrombolysis Reperfusion for Acute Myocardial Infarction Treatment (ExTRACT)–TIMI 25 trial[70] compared enoxaparin with UFH in 20,506 patients with STEMI undergoing fibrinolysis and demonstrated a 17% relative risk reduction in the primary end point of death or nonfatal reinfarction at 30 days (9.9% in the enoxaparin group vs. 12.0% in UFH group, $P < .001$). This observed benefit was driven primarily by a reduction in nonfatal reinfarction and was sustained at 1-year follow-up with no significant reduction in mortality.[71] However, this benefit occurred at the cost of a significant increase in major bleeding in those treated with enoxaparin (2.1% in the enoxaparin group vs. 1.4% in the UFH group, $P < .001$). The Clinical Trial of Reviparin and Metabolic Modulation in Acute Myocardial Infarction Treatment Evaluation (CREATE)[72] of more than 15,000 patients with STEMI treated with thrombolytic therapy randomized to the adjunctive use of the LMWH reviparin or placebo demonstrated benefit in favor of reviparin in the primary composite end point of death, reinfarction, or stroke at 7 days (9.6% vs. 11%, $P = .005$), although this too was offset by a small but significant increase in severe bleeding.

In their meta-analysis of randomized trials of LMWH versus UFH with thrombolytic therapy in STEMI, Eikelboom and colleagues[73,74] suggested a benefit of LMWH in terms of preventing reinfarction at 30 days, although no benefit was appreciated with regard to death (Fig. 12.10). These findings were confirmed by a subsequent meta-analysis by De Luca and Marino[75] of eight randomized trials that showed a reduction in reinfarction at 30 days with LMWH compared with UFH (3.2% vs. 4.8%, OR 0.65; 95% CI, 0.58 to 0.64). However, as highlighted earlier, this must be weighed against the risk of bleeding with caution in approaching older patients (>75 years old) and those with significant renal dysfunction, both of whom are more likely to bleed. Eikelboom and colleagues[73] found no increase in major bleeding with LMWH compared with UFH (3.3% vs. 2.5%, OR 1.30; 95% CI, 0.98 to 1.72), although the increase in minor bleeding was significant (22.8% vs. 19.4%, OR 1.26; 95% CI, 1.12 to 1.43), and De Luca and Marino[75] found a higher risk of major bleeding complications

SECTION II Pharmacologic Intervention

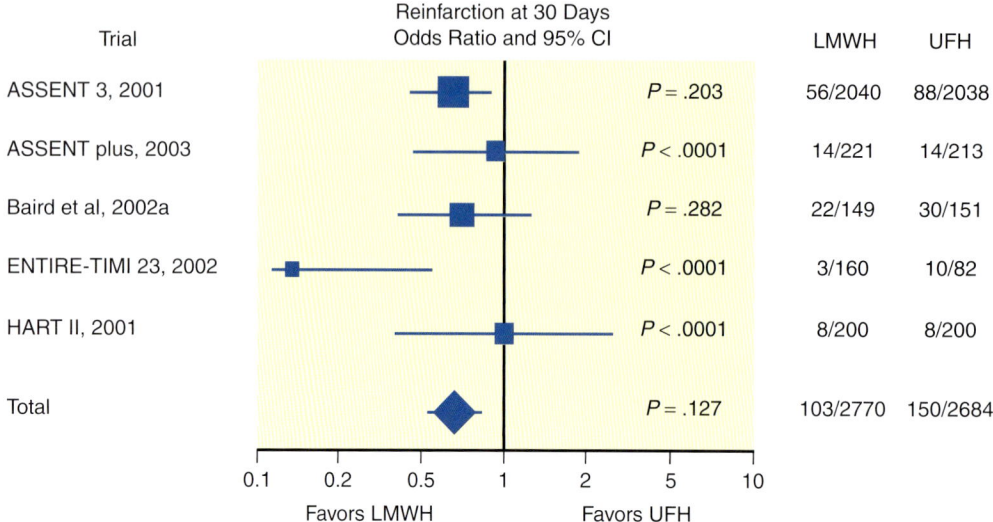

Fig. 12.10 Rates of reinfarction in patients treated with unfractionated heparin *(UFH)* versus low-molecular-weight heparin *(LMWH)* as adjuncts to thrombolysis in ST-elevation myocardial infarction *(STEMI)*. *CI,* Confidence interval. [a]Baird SH, Menown IBA, McBride SJ, et al. Randomized comparison of enoxaparin with unfractionated heparin following fibrinolytic therapy for acute myocardial infarction. *Eur Heart J.* 2002;23: 627– 632. (From Ejkelboom JW, Quinlan DJ, Mehta SR, et al. Unfractionated and low-molecular-weight heparin as adjuncts to thrombolysis in aspirin-treated patients with ST-elevation acute myocardial infarction: a meta-analysis of the randomized trials. *Circulation.* 2005;112[25]:3855–3867.)

(2.4% vs. 1.8%, OR 1.37; 95% CI, 1.16 to 1.61). Furthermore, increasing evidence underscores the importance of bleeding that adversely affects the prognosis of patients with ACS, as reflected by the directly proportional relationship observed between risk of death and severity of bleeding in these patients.[74] Accordingly, the decision to use LMWH instead of UFH should be individualized to the patient and their bleeding risk.

Direct Thrombin Inhibitors

The deficiencies of UFH and LMWH have led to studies of direct thrombin inhibitors such as hirudin and its synthetic peptide congener bivalirudin as adjuncts to thrombolytic therapy. The clot-bound thrombin is quarantined from the inhibition of heparin, where it amplifies its own generation through a positive feedback loop and activates platelets through thromboxane-independent mechanisms, making it an important effector of thrombus formation. Unlike heparin and LMWH, which potentiate the inhibitory effect of antithrombin III on soluble thrombin and can be highly variable from patient to patient (and even within the same patient), direct thrombin inhibitors directly bind and inactivate both soluble and bound thrombin.

A meta-analysis including five trials of thrombolytic therapy in STEMI (*n* = 9947) showed that bivalent direct thrombin inhibitors, including hirudin (lepirudin) and bivalirudin, reduced the rates of recurrent MI but not mortality, with no such benefit observed with univalent agents such as argatroban.[76] Hirudin was tested against UFH in two thrombolytic regimens, including streptokinase and alteplase, in the Global Use of Strategies to Open Occluded Coronary Arteries in Acute Coronary Syndromes (GUSTO IIb) trial[77] with 4000 STEMI patients; hirudin demonstrated a favorable interaction with streptokinase (but not alteplase) in reducing 30-day death or reinfarction. This study illustrated the crucial role of thrombin generation after streptokinase administration and its relationship to outcomes. The largest dedicated trial using a direct thrombin inhibitor was the Hirulog and Early Reperfusion or Occlusion 2 (HERO-2) trial,[78] in which 17,073 patients with STEMI were treated with streptokinase plus either heparin or bivalirudin. This multicenter international trial demonstrated a relatively high overall mortality (10.9% in the streptokinase-plus-heparin group vs. 10.8% in the streptokinase-plus-bivalirudin group). The reason for this remains unclear but may have been related to the use of streptokinase as the thrombolytic agent, the relatively late entry of patients from the time of symptom onset, and underutilization of reperfusion therapies for reinfarction across multiple study sites.[79] Whereas it did show a significant reduction in reinfarction (1.6% in the streptokinase-plus-bivalirudin group vs. 2.3% in the streptokinase-plus-heparin group, *P* = 0.001), a trend toward increased intracerebral hemorrhage and blood transfusions was noted in the streptokinase-plus-bivalirudin group. According to the 2013 ACCF/AHA STEMI guidelines, bivalirudin is an acceptable alternative to UFH as adjunctive therapy to thrombolysis in patients with heparin-induced thrombocytopenia.[2] Although recent trials have established the safety and efficacy of bivalirudin as adjunctive therapy to PCI in the management of ACS, no studies have evaluated this agent in combination with newer-generation thrombolytic agents in the treatment of STEMI.[80,81]

Glycoprotein IIb/IIIa Inhibitors

The rationale for more potent adjunctive therapies for thrombolysis originated from angiographic studies of thrombolysis monotherapy that showed incomplete clot dissolution. This is thought to occur because of platelet activation in the setting of fibrinolysis, which results in residual platelet-rich thrombus that is resistant to pharmacologic thrombolysis. Hence maximal platelet inhibition remains an important target for adjunctive therapy to thrombolysis in the management of STEMI. The combination of a thrombolytic agent at a half dose with a full-dose glycoprotein (GP) IIb/IIIa inhibitor was attractive in light of a number of studies that indicated better infarct vessel patency, more complete angiographic clot dissolution, and more ST-segment resolution.

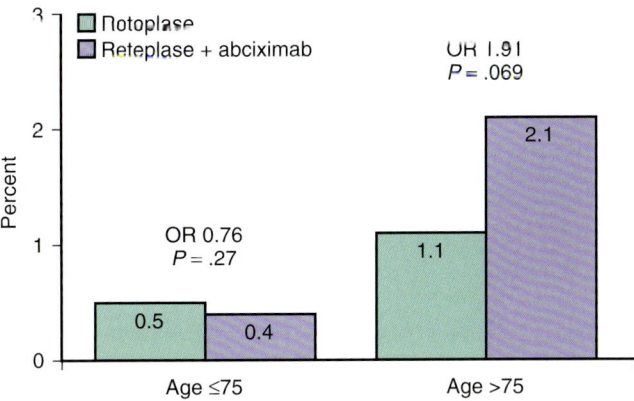

Fig. 12.11 GUSTO V trial data. Intracranial hemorrhage and treatment by age interaction. *OR,* Odds ratio. (From the GUSTO V Investigators. Reperfusion therapy for acute myocardial infarction with fibrinolytic therapy or combination reduced fibrinolytic therapy and platelet glycoprotein IIb/IIIa inhibition: the GUSTO V randomised trial. *Lancet.* 2001;357[9272]:1905–1914.)

Most of the available data for the use of the GP IIb/IIIa inhibitors as adjunctive therapy in STEMI involve abciximab and are demonstrated by the GUSTO V trial,[82] which evaluated the combination of half-dose reteplase plus abciximab compared with full-dose reteplase in 16,588 patients. The primary end point of 30-day mortality was slightly better with combination therapy (5.6% vs. 5.9%, $P = .45$), which fulfilled noninferiority criteria and represented the first combination reperfusion strategy validated as "at least as good as" full-dose thrombolytic therapy. However, an increase in bleeding complications required blood transfusions in 4% of the patients treated with full-dose reteplase and in 5.7% of the combination-treated patients, and most of this bleeding occurred in older patients who also had a significantly increased risk of intracerebral hemorrhage (Fig. 12.11). The main findings of the trial suggested that combination therapy may be useful in younger patients (<75 years old), particularly in those with anterior MI. Disappointingly, long-term data highlighted that there was no difference in 1-year mortality between the two strategies.[83] A meta-analysis by De Luca and colleagues[84] summarized the use of abciximab in this context and showed that as adjunctive therapy for thrombolysis for STEMI, it had no mortality benefit at 30 days or long term compared to primary angioplasty for STEMI. They also showed that although there were similar reductions in reinfarction at 30 days, the bleeding trade-offs with abciximab were significant.

Regarding the small-molecule GP IIb/IIIa inhibitor tirofiban, in the small, randomized dose-finding study Fibrinolytic and Aggrastat for ST-Elevation Resolution (FASTER)–TIMI 24,[85] the combination of tenecteplase plus tirofiban versus tenecteplase alone demonstrated more rapid and complete ST-segment resolution without an increase in major bleeding. The Safety and Efficacy of a Conjunctive Strategy for Reperfusion Enhancement (SASTRE)[86] investigators demonstrated higher rates of TIMI grade 3 flow and TIMI grade 3 myocardial perfusion, which translated to better clinical outcomes and no increased bleeding risk, when tirofiban was used as an adjunct to reperfusion therapy both with half-dose thrombolysis (alteplase) and with primary PCI in 144 patients. The Integrilin and Tenecteplase in Acute Myocardial Infarction (INTEGRITI)[87] trial evaluated tenecteplase with combinations of eptifibatide in STEMI and showed that double-bolus eptifibatide plus half-dose tenecteplase improved arterial patency and ST-segment resolution over tenecteplase monotherapy. However, this was at the expense of increased major bleeding and blood transfusions, which limits this as a useful strategy. Furthermore, the dose-confirmation arm of the Integrilin and Low-Dose Thrombolysis in Acute Myocardial Infarction (INTRO AMI) trial randomized 305 patients with STEMI to half-dose alteplase plus double-bolus eptifibatide with 30 minutes between boluses and low-dose infusion (group I) or half-dose alteplase plus double-bolus eptifibatide with 10 minutes between boluses (group II) and high-dose infusion versus full-dose alteplase (group III).[88] Group II had improved arterial flow with no differences in ST-segment resolution, death, reinfarction, need for revascularization, TIMI major bleeding, or intracranial hemorrhage.

Therefore large-scale trials showing a survival benefit with the adjunctive use of the small molecule GP IIb/IIIa inhibitors with thrombolysis as primary reperfusion therapy are still lacking. Limited data are available with regard to the role of the GP IIb/IIIa inhibitors in rescue PCI following failed full-dose thrombolytic therapy; the excessive bleeding (despite lower heparin doses) seen in the subjects in the GUSTO-III subgroup who underwent rescue angioplasty with abciximab is of particular concern.[89] A small series from the stenting era suggests that short-term clinical outcomes may be improved with this strategy with no significant trade-offs in terms of bleeding complications, although caution is certainly warranted.[90]

Factor Xa Inhibitors

The OASIS-6 trial[91] evaluated the adjunctive use of a selective factor Xa inhibitor, fondaparinux, versus UFH in 12,092 patients with STEMI and found no benefit in those undergoing primary PCI. However, this study did demonstrate a significant reduction in death and reinfarction at 30 days and at 3 to 6 months in those undergoing thrombolysis treated with fondaparinux and found no increase in severe bleeding after 9 days of therapy.[91,92] Unfortunately, an increased frequency of guide catheter thrombosis was observed with fondaparinux. Combined with the OASIS-5 trial in the non-STEMI population, in whom a mortality benefit was seen at 3 and 6 months with less major bleeding with fondaparinux compared with enoxaparin, there appears to be promise for fondaparinux across the spectrum of patients with ACS.[93] The available evidence has garnered a class I recommendation for the use of fondaparinux as adjunctive antithrombotic therapy in thrombolysis-treated patients as an alternative to UFH or LMWH.[2] However, fondaparinux should not be used as the sole anticoagulant for PCI given the increased incidence of guide catheter thrombosis, and it is contraindicated in patients with a creatinine clearance below 30 mL/min.

FACILITATED PERCUTANEOUS CORONARY INTERVENTION

Considerable attention has been given to the concept of facilitated PCI, which refers to the use of upstream pharmacologic therapy to serve as a "bridge" to primary PCI, given that survival is improved if TIMI grade 3 flow is present before mechanical reperfusion.[94] The use of full-dose thrombolytic therapy before PCI for STEMI was unhelpful and even harmful in the early major trials that combined thrombolytic therapy with immediate angioplasty.[95] This was thought to be largely because of the pro-thrombotic effect of plasminogen activators and the showering of platelet-rich microthrombi into the microcirculation, leading to poorer outcomes. Notably, these early trials were conducted before the routine use of intensive antiplatelet therapy (including GP IIb/IIIa inhibitors and $P2Y_{12}$ antagonists) and stents, which have improved outcomes with contemporary PCI for STEMI. One of the largest facilitated PCI trials to date, the Assessment of the Safety and Efficacy of a New Treatment Strategy for Acute Myocardial Infarction (ASSENT-4),[96] assessed the role of full-dose tenecteplase with primary PCI. This study was stopped prematurely because of higher in-hospital mortality in the facilitated PCI group compared with the primary PCI group (6% vs. 3%, $P = .01$), with the occurrence of significantly more frequent ischemic complications such as reinfarction and repeat target-vessel revascularization in the facilitated PCI group. The strategy of using half-dose thrombolytic therapy plus a full-dose GP IIb/IIIa inhibitor before PCI would seem especially attractive, given the benefit of the GP IIb/IIIa inhibitor in those undergoing primary PCI. The prematurely terminated (because of lack of enrollment) trial Addressing the Value of Facilitated Angioplasty After Combination Therapy or Eptifibatide Monotherapy in Acute Myocardial Infarction (ADVANCE MI)[97] tested this strategy by comparing eptifibatide plus half-dose tenecteplase to eptifibatide plus placebo before primary PCI for STEMI. This study suggested that eptifibatide plus half-dose tenecteplase was associated with adverse clinical outcomes and higher bleeding rates despite demonstrating improved pre-PCI coronary flow. The Bavarian Reperfusion Alternatives Evaluation (BRAVE) trial[98] addressed the use of upstream abciximab plus half-dose reteplase versus abciximab monotherapy in 253 patients undergoing PCI for STEMI. This trial found no reduction in infarct size by single-photon emission computed tomography (performed between 5 and 10 days after randomization), with non-significant trends toward more adverse cardiac events at 6 months and more major bleeding in the abciximab-plus-reteplase group. The more recent Leipzig Immediate Prehospital Facilitated Angioplasty in ST-Segment Myocardial Infarction (LIPSIA-STEMI)[99] trial failed to show a benefit of facilitated PCI with full-dose tenecteplase pretreatment versus primary PCI alone with regard to the primary end point of infarct size by magnetic resonance imaging, infarct size by biomarker release, resolution of ST-segment elevation, or clinical end points among 162 patients with long transfer delays to PCI (median overall symptom onset to first balloon inflation times of 158 minutes in the facilitated PCI group and 131 minutes in the primary PCI group).

The Facilitated Intervention with Enhanced Reperfusion Speed to Stop Events (FINESSE) trial[100] is the largest study to date to evaluate facilitated PCI using thrombolytic therapy. This double-blind international placebo-controlled trial randomized 2452 patients with STEMI undergoing PCI to half-dose reteplase plus abciximab pretreatment (combination-facilitated PCI), abciximab pretreatment (abciximab-facilitated PCI), or abciximab started at the time of PCI (primary PCI). The combination-facilitated PCI group demonstrated more rapid ST-segment resolution compared with the abciximab-facilitated PCI and primary PCI groups (43.9% vs. 33.1% and 31.0%, $P = .01$ and $P = .003$, respectively). However, at 90 days of follow-up, no differences were observed between the three groups with regard to the primary composite end point of all-cause death, ventricular fibrillation within 48 hours, and new-onset congestive heart failure (9.8%, 10.5%, and 10.7%, respectively, $P = .55$) or mortality (5.2%, 5.5%, and 4.5%, respectively, $P = .49$). Significantly higher rates of all bleeding, intracerebral hemorrhage, and transfusions were observed in the facilitated PCI groups. Specifically, TIMI major or minor bleeding occurred in 14.5% of the combination-facilitated group compared with 10.1% in the abciximab-facilitated group and 6.9% in the primary PCI groups ($P < .001$ for combination-facilitated PCI vs. primary PCI). A 1-year follow-up analysis of the FINESSE trial recapitulated the outcomes observed at 90 days.[101] Notably, a retrospective post hoc analysis of this study suggested a mortality benefit of the combination-facilitated PCI in high-risk patients as defined by a TIMI risk score of 3 or higher who presented to non-PCI hospitals within 4 hours of symptom onset.[102] This suggested a possible role for facilitated PCI in carefully selected patients.

A meta-analysis of 17 trials of 4504 patients with STEMI by Keeley and coworkers[103] and a more recent meta-analysis of six trials that included 2684 patients by De Luca and Marino[104] (including the FINESSE trial) summarized the lack of benefit of the facilitated PCI strategy and demonstrated that despite achieving initial improvements in early metrics of reperfusion, short-term outcomes are not improved, and rates of target-vessel revascularization, reinfarction, stroke, bleeding, and death may be increased with the facilitated approach (Figs. 12.12 and 12.13). In light of these observations, the 2013 ACCF/AHA STEMI guidelines recommend that, because of an increased bleeding risk, very early catheterization (within 2 to 3 hours) with intent to perform revascularization after thrombolytic administration should be limited to rescue PCI; that is, it should be attempted in those patients who fail thrombolysis and have significant myocardial territory in jeopardy.[2]

PHARMACOINVASIVE STRATEGY

A growing body of evidence supports the role of routine systematic coronary angiography with PCI following primary thrombolytic therapy for STEMI in selected patients. This pharmacoinvasive strategy is distinct from facilitated PCI in that thrombolytic therapy is not administered as adjunctive or facilitative therapy at reduced doses in combination with other adjunctive pharmacologic agents when primary PCI is planned and available in a timely fashion. Instead, thrombolytic therapy is routinely administered as the primary reperfusion strategy when timely primary PCI is not available, and routine early (more than 2 to 3 hours after thrombolytic administration) coronary angiography with provisional PCI is implemented to avoid recurrent ischemia related to incomplete recanalization and propagation of platelet-rich thrombus following fibrinolysis. This strategy is appealing given that many patients with STEMI do not have access to primary PCI within 120 minutes of their first contact with medical care, and it may be important in the management of STEMI patients who may live some distance from PCI-capable centers.

The Combined Abciximab Reteplase Stent Study in Acute Myocardial Infarction (CARESS-in-AMI) trial[45] compared routine coronary angiography and immediate PCI with ischemia-guided coronary angiography following treatment with half-dose reteplase and adjunctive abciximab, UFH, and aspirin in 600 patients with STEMI who presented to non–PCI-capable hospitals with at least one high-risk feature, defined as extensive ST-segment elevation, new-onset left bundle branch block, previous MI, a Killip class greater than 2, or a left ventricular ejection fraction (LVEF) of 35% or less. The mean time from symptom onset to thrombolysis was 165 minutes for both groups. PCI was performed in 85.6% of patients in the immediate PCI group compared with 30.3% in the standard care or rescue PCI group, with median times from thrombolysis to angiography of 125 and 200 minutes, respectively ($P < .0001$). The primary end point of all-cause death, reinfarction, or refractory ischemia at 30 days occurred in 4.4% of the immediate PCI group versus 10.7% of the standard care group, with no difference in bleeding (3.4% vs. 2.3%, $P = .47$) or stroke (0.7% vs. 1.3%, $P = .50$) between the two groups. This observed benefit was driven primarily by reductions in reinfarction and recurrent ischemia, with a trend toward reduced mortality in the immediate PCI group (Fig. 12.14).

The Trial of Routine Angioplasty and Stenting After Fibrinolysis to Enhance Reperfusion in Acute Myocardial Infarction (TRANSFER-AMI) study[105] randomized 1059 patients with STEMI with at least one high-risk feature, who presented to non–PCI-capable hospitals to undergo immediate transfer and PCI within 6 hours of thrombolytic therapy (routine PCI group) or standard treatment with rescue PCI (standard group) following primary reperfusion therapy with full-dose tenecteplase and adjunctive aspirin and UFH or enoxaparin; clopidogrel loading therapy was also encouraged.[44] High-risk features for enrollment into this trial were defined as 2 mm or more of ST-segment elevation or depression in two anterior leads, systolic blood pressure below 100 mm Hg, heart rate greater than 100 beats/min, Killip class 2 to 3, or 1 mm or more ST-segment elevation in right-sided lead V_4 indicative of right ventricular involvement for inferior MIs. The median time from onset of symptoms to

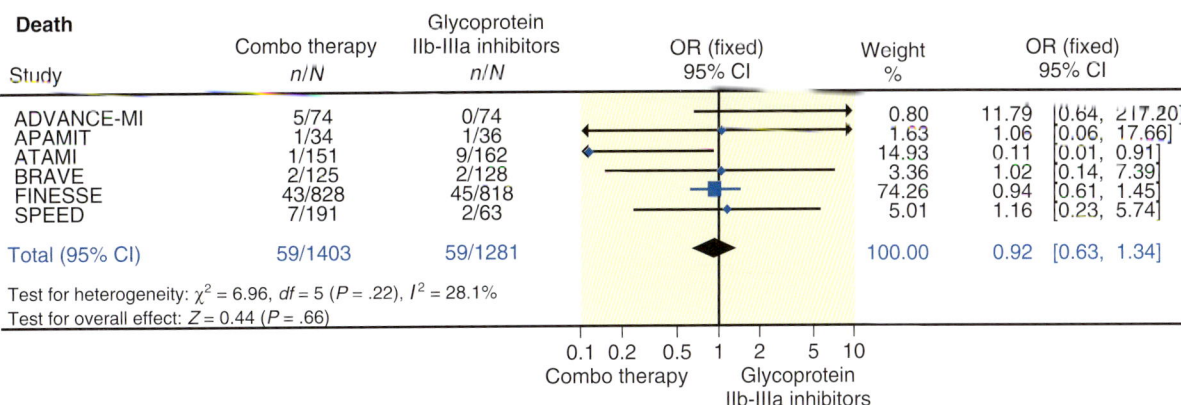
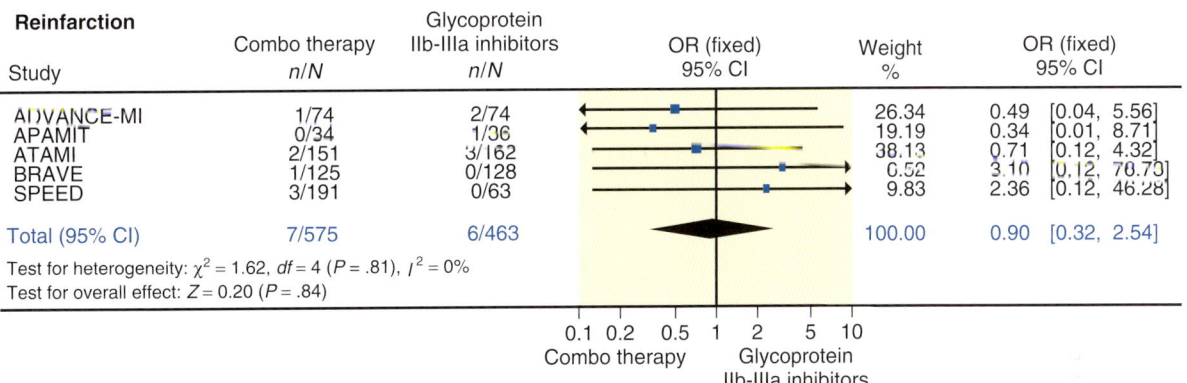

Fig. 12.12 Combination facilitated percutaneous coronary intervention (PCI) and benefits in mortality (*upper graph*) and reinfarction (lower graph) at 30-day follow-up compared with early glycoprotein IIb/IIIa inhibitor administration from a meta-analysis of trials of facilitated PCI with odds ratios (*ORs*) and 95% confidence intervals (*CIs*). The size of the data markers (*squares*) is approximately proportional to the statistical weight of each trial. (Adapted from De Luca G, Marino P: Facilitated angioplasty with combo therapy among patients with ST-segment elevation myocardial infarction: a meta-analysis of randomized trials. *Am J Emerg Med.* 2009;27[6]:683–690.)

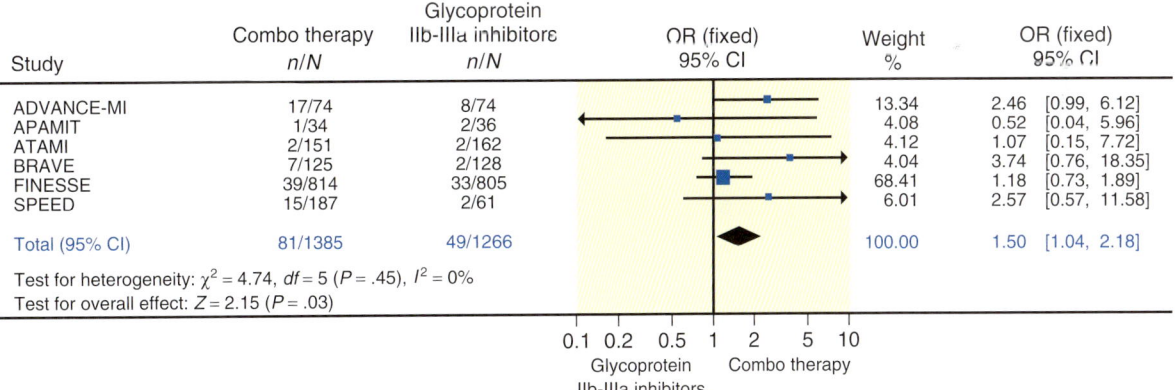

Fig. 12.13 Combination facilitated percutaneous coronary intervention (PCI) and risk of major bleeding complications compared with early glycoprotein IIb/IIIa inhibitor administration from a meta-analysis of trials of facilitated PCI with odds ratios (*ORs*) and 95% confidence intervals (*CIs*). The size of the data markers (*squares*) is approximately proportional to the statistical weight of each trial. (Adapted from De Luca G, Marino P. Facilitated angioplasty with combo therapy among patients with ST-segment elevation myocardial infarction: a meta-analysis of randomized trials. *Am J Emerg Med.* 2009;27[6]:683–690.)

thrombolysis was approximately 2 hours in both groups, whereas the median time from tenecteplase administration to angiography was 2.8 hours in the routine PCI group and 32.5 hours in the standard treatment group ($P < .001$). PCI was performed in 84.9% of the routine PCI group versus 67.4% of the standard treatment group, and more patients in the routine PCI group received clopidogrel (90.3% vs. 81.4%, respectively; $P < .001$) and β-blockers (90.1% vs. 85.4%, respectively; $P = .02$). The primary end point—a composite of death, reinfarction, recurrent ischemia, new or worsening heart failure, or cardiogenic shock at 30 days—occurred in 11.0% of the routine early PCI group and in 17.2% of the standard treatment group ($P = .004$), with no

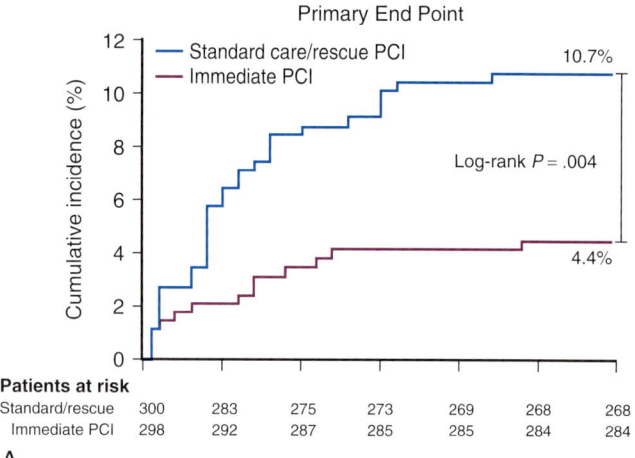
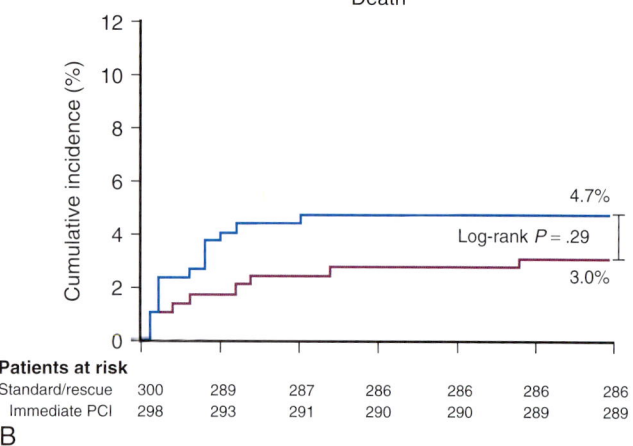
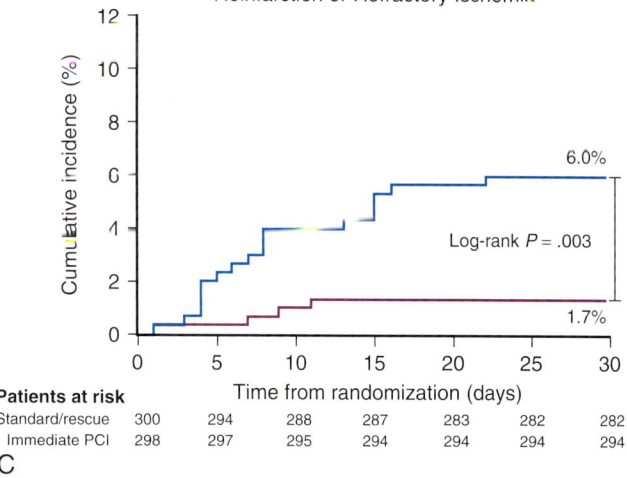

Fig. 12.14 Kaplan-Meier curves for the primary composite end point (A), death (B), reinfarction or (C) refractory ischemia in the CARESS-in-AMI trial. *PCI,* Percutaneous coronary intervention. (From Di Mario C, Dudek D, Piscione F, et al: Immediate angioplasty versus standard therapy with rescue angioplasty after thrombolysis in the Combined Abciximab REteplase Stent Study in Acute Myocardial Infarction [CARESS-in-AMI]: an open, prospective, randomised, multicentre trial. *Lancet.* 2008;371[9612]:559–568.)

significant difference in significant bleeding between the two groups. Reduction in reinfarction was also observed in the routine PCI group at 6 months of follow-up. No difference was reported in the rates of death or reinfarction (10.3% vs. 11.6%, P = .50), hospital readmission (15.4% vs. 16.5%, P = .64), or subsequent revascularization with either PCI or coronary artery bypass grafting (CABG) after index hospitalization (6.9% vs. 8.7%, P = .30) between the two groups at 1 year with excellent (98%) follow-up. An economic analysis also showed no difference in costs between the two treatment strategies.[105]

The Norwegian Study on District Treatment of ST-Elevation Myocardial Infarction (NORDISTEMI)[106] compared a strategy of immediate transfer for PCI with an ischemia-guided approach after thrombolysis with full-dose tenecteplase in 276 patients with long transfer distances to PCI (expected delay from first medical contact to PCI of >90 min). This study showed a reduction in the primary combined end point of death, reinfarction, stroke, or new myocardial ischemia in the immediate PCI group at 30 days (relative risk [RR] 0.49; 95% CI, 0.27 to 0.89; P = .03) with a nonsignificant trend toward benefit with this approach at 12 months (HR 0.72; 95% CI, 0.44 to 1.18; P = .19). No difference in bleeding was found between the two treatment groups. Notably, this study demonstrated a benefit for immediate PCI following thrombolysis despite allowing for more liberal use of coronary angiography and PCI in the ischemia-guided group, with 95% of subjects in this group undergoing angiography (mean of 5.5 days after receiving tenecteplase) compared with 99% in the immediate-PCI group (mean of 130 min after receiving tenecteplase). Additionally, use of clopidogrel loading and enoxaparin was universal, with no difference in the use of other evidence-based therapies between the two treatment groups.

The most recent trial examining the pharmacoinvasive approach was the 2013 Strategic Reperfusion Early After Myocardial Infarction (STREAM) study,[47] which randomized 1892 patients who presented with STEMI within 3 hours of symptom onset and were unable to undergo PCI within 60 minutes of symptom onset to prehospital thrombolysis with full-dose tenecteplase followed by routine coronary angiography within 6 to 24 hours or to primary PCI. The median delay from symptom onset to arrival in the cardiac catheterization laboratory was 600 minutes in the thrombolysis group and 170 minutes in the primary PCI group; the median time from symptom onset to tenecteplase infusion in the thrombolysis group was 100 minutes. The composite primary end point of death from any cause, shock, congestive heart failure, or reinfarction at 30 days occurred in 12.4% of patients in the thrombolysis group and in 14.3% of patients in the primary PCI group (RR 0.86; 95% CI, 0.68 to 1.09; P = .21). More strokes occurred in the thrombolysis group (1.6% vs. 0.5%; P = .03), driven primarily by an excess in intracranial hemorrhage among older adult subjects at the start of the trial (1.0% vs. 0.2%; P = .04). This resulted in a protocol amendment mandating a 50% tenecteplase dose reduction in patients over the age of 75. Thereafter, no difference was observed in the occurrence of intracranial hemorrhage between the two study groups (0.5% vs. 0.3%; P = .45). No differences in extra-cranial bleeding were noted between the groups. Of interest, whereas the vast majority of patients in both groups were treated with PCI, more patients in the thrombolysis group were ultimately treated with surgical revascularization (4.7% vs. 2.1%; P = .002). This study suggests that the pharmacoinvasive strategy of early full-dose thrombolysis followed by routine coronary angiography is an effective reperfusion strategy, with a statistically nonsignificant trend toward benefit versus delayed primary PCI, but it is associated with an increased risk of intracranial bleeding.

Two contemporary systematic reviews and meta-analyses of randomized trials to compare thrombolysis coupled with a routine invasive strategy with ischemia-guided provisional coronary angiography following thrombolysis have demonstrated a consistent benefit for the pharmacoinvasive approach in reducing the combined end point of mortality, reinfarction, and ischemia at 30 days (Fig. 12.15) and both reinfarction and death at 6 months and 1 year.[107,108] One study of 197 patients with a mean follow-up time

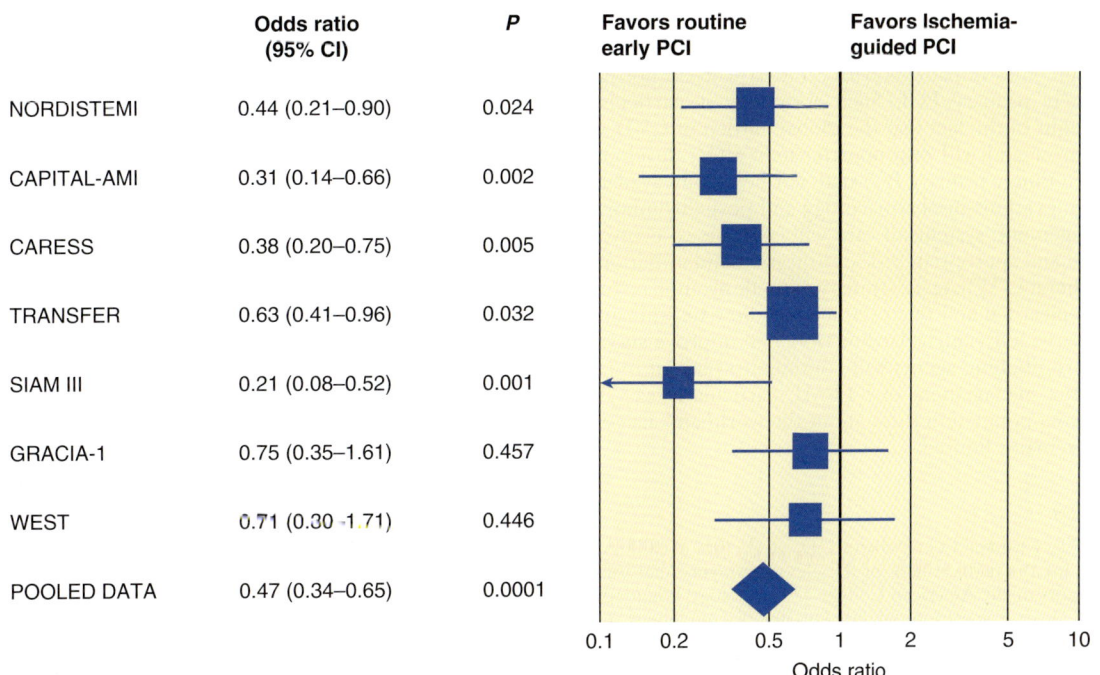

Fig. 12.15 Thirty-day combined end point of mortality, reinfarction, and ischemia with odds ratio favoring routine early percutaneous coronary intervention (PCI) following thrombolysis (P < .0001, significant). CAPITAL-AMI, Combined Angioplasty and Pharmacologic Intervention Versus Thrombolytics Alone; CARESS, Combined Abciximab Reteplase Stent Study; CI, confidence interval; GRACIA-1, Randomized Trial Comparing Stenting Within 24 Hours of Thrombolysis Versus Ischemia-Guided Approach to Thrombolyzed Acute Myocardial Infarction With ST-Segment Elevation; NORDISTEMI, Norwegian Study on District Treatment of ST-Elevation Myocardial Infarction. SIAM, Comparison of Invasive and Conservative Strategies After Treatment With Streptokinase in Acute Myocardial Infarction; TRANSFER, Trial of Routine Angioplasty and Stenting After Fibrinolysis to Enhance Reperfusion; WEST, Randomized trial of Tenecteplase with/without timely coronary intervention vs. primary percutaneous intervention after ST-Elevation Myocardial Infarction. (From D'souza SP, Mamas MA, Fraser DG, et al. Routine early coronary angioplasty versus ischaemia-guided angioplasty after thrombolysis in acute ST-elevation myocardial infarction: a meta-analysis. Eur Heart J. 2010;32[8]:972–982.)

of 7.9 years (±3.4 years; maximum, 11.2 years) showed a persistent and significant reduction in the composite of death, reinfarction, target-lesion revascularization, and ischemic events with the pharmacoinvasive approach (HR 0.61; 95% CI, 0.42 to 0.88; P = .008).[109] In aggregate, these data support the use of a pharmacoinvasive strategy with primary thrombolysis followed by routine early angiography and PCI in high-risk STEMI patients who present to non–PCI-capable hospitals. This strategy may also enable more rapid reperfusion with initiation of prehospital therapy in cases that may require prolonged transport times to PCI-capable centers.[110] The pharmacoinvasive strategy was given a class IIa recommendation in the 2013 ACCF/AHA STEMI guidelines.[2]

INTERNATIONAL PERSPECTIVE

Cardiovascular disease (CVD) remains a major cause of mortality and morbidity globally, and the burden of CVD is only expected to increase in the future. The World Health Organization estimates that by 2030, 23.3 million people will die from CVD. Low-income and middle-income countries are disproportionately affected by the global CVD epidemic, with more than 80% of all CVD deaths around the world occurring in these nations. Many individuals will die younger, often in their productive years, which will result in a significant economic impact, both at the individual family level and at the national level, hampering ongoing economic development.[111] Given that STEMI will continue to account for a significant proportion of the growing international CVD burden, and most patients in low-income and middle-income countries—as well as significant numbers in the high-income nations—will not have timely access to primary PCI, thrombolysis will serve as the primary reperfusion strategy for the majority of patients with STEMI worldwide. Developing systems for the early recognition and triage of these patients with prompt administration of thrombolytic therapy (unless timely primary PCI is available) and appropriate post-thrombolytic therapy care will be critical in reducing the tremendous global burden of CVD.

SUMMARY

Despite a deeper understanding of the pathophysiology of AMI, as well as the vast improvements in both the pharmacologic and mechanical reperfusion tools available, outcomes with STEMI remain suboptimal. Thrombolytic therapy revolutionized the management of STEMI and ushered in the modern era of reperfusion therapy as the primary treatment modality in AMI. Whereas thrombolytic therapy was once the mainstay of reperfusion therapy in STEMI, timely primary PCI has evolved to become the favored and recommended reperfusion strategy. However, many patients with STEMI do not have access to primary PCI within the critical time interval in which outcomes are maximally preserved with mechanical reperfusion, which underscores the continued importance of thrombolytic therapy in the management of STEMI. Outcomes with thrombolytic therapy will only improve as new thrombolytic agents are engineered with greater specificity for the actively forming thrombus, potentially reducing the risk of bleeding; more potent adjunctive antiplatelet and antithrombotic therapies will possibly reduce thrombolytic-mediated platelet aggregation and distal embolization of thrombus. Furthermore, a pharmacoinvasive approach using thrombolytic therapy as the primary reperfusion strategy with routine subsequent coronary angiography has the potential to improve outcomes in patients with STEMI who do not have access to timely primary PCI. Such a strategy is particularly attractive in light of the fact that the global burden of CVD will continue to grow and will disproportionately affect developing nations, where timely primary PCI may not be readily available. Along with innovations in pharmacology and post-thrombolytic therapy management, systems of care will continue to evolve to facilitate rapid and appropriate risk stratification and initiation of reperfusion therapy. Whatever strategy is used, prompt restoration of both epicardial and micro-circulatory flow to limit myonecrosis, preserve left ventricular function, and improve survival is crucial. Thrombolytic agents will continue to play an important role in the management of STEMI, particularly as CVD affects a growing population throughout the world and access to primary PCI remains limited.

KEY REFERENCES

2. O'Gara PT, Kushner FG, Ascheim DD, et al. 2013 ACCF/AHA guideline for the management of ST-elevation myocardial infarction: a report of the American College of Cardiology Foundation/American Heart Association task force on practice guidelines. *J Am Coll Cardiol*. 2013;61(4):e78–e140.
14. European Working Party. Streptokinase in recent myocardial infarction: a controlled multicentre trial. *BMJ*. 1971;770:325–331.
21. ISIS-3 (Third International Study of Infarct Survival) Collaborative Group. ISIS-3: a randomised comparison of streptokinase vs tissue plasminogen activator vs anistreplase and of aspirin plus heparin vs aspirin alone among 41,299 cases of suspected acute myocardial infarction. *Lancet*. 1992;339(8796):753–770.
22. The GUSTO Investigators. An international randomized trial comparing four thrombolytic strategies for acute myocardial infarction. *N Engl J Med*. 1993;329(10):673–682.
30. Morrison LJ, Verbeek PR, McDonald AC, et al. Mortality and prehospital thrombolysis for acute myocardial infarction: a meta-analysis. *JAMA*. 2000;283(20):2686–2692.
40. Nielsen PH, Maeng M, Busk M, et al. Primary angioplasty versus fibrinolysis in acute myocardial infarction: long term follow-up in the Danish acute myocardial infarction 2 trial. *Circulation*. 2010;121(13):1484–1491.
45. Di Mario C, Dudek D, Piscione F, et al. Immediate angioplasty versus standard therapy with rescue angioplasty after thrombolysis in the Combined Abciximab REteplase Stent Study in Acute Myocardial Infarction (CARESS-in-AMI): an open, prospective, randomised, multicentre trial. *Lancet*. 2008;371(9612):559–568.
47. Armstrong PW, Gershlick AH, Goldstein P, et al. Fibrinolysis or primary PCI in ST-segment elevation myocardial infarction. *N Engl J Med*. 2013;368(15):1379–1387.
50. Fibrinolytic Therapy Trialists' (FTT) Collaborative Group. Indications for fibrinolytic therapy in suspected acute myocardial infarction: collaborative overview of early mortality and major morbidity results from all randomised trials of more than 1000 patients. *Lancet*. 1994;343(8893):311–322.
53. ISIS-2 (Second International Study of Infarct Survival) Collaborative Group. Randomised trial of intravenous streptokinase, oral aspirin, both, or neither among 17,187 cases of suspected acute myocardial infarction: ISIS-2. *Lancet*. 1988;2(8607):349–360.
56. Levine GN, Bates ER, Bittl JA, et al. 2016 ACC/AHA guideline focused update on duration of dual antiplatelet therapy in patients with coronary artery disease: a report of the American College of Cardiology/American Heart Association task force on clinical practice guidelines: an update of the 2011 ACCF/AHA/SCAI guideline for percutaneous coronary intervention, 2011 ACCF/AHA guideline for coronary artery bypass graft surgery, 2012 ACC/AHA/ACP/AATS/PCNA/SCAI/STS guideline for the diagnosis and management of patients with stable ischemic heart disease, 2013 ACCF/AHA guideline for the management of ST-elevation myocardial infarction, 2014 AHA/ACC guideline for the management of patients with non–ST-elevation acute coronary syndromes, and 2014 ACC/AHA guideline on perioperative cardiovascular evaluation and management of patients undergoing noncardiac surgery. *Circulation*. 2016;134(10):e123–e155.
58. Sabatine MS, Cannon CP, Gibson CM, et al. Addition of clopidogrel to aspirin and fibrinolytic therapy for myocardial infarction with ST-segment elevation. *N Engl J Med*. 2005;352(12):1179–1189.
67. The Assessment of the Safety and Efficacy of a New Thrombolytic Regimen (ASSENT)-3 Investigators. Efficacy and safety of tenecteplase in combination with enoxaparin, abciximab, or unfractionated heparin: the ASSENT-3 randomised trial in acute myocardial infarction. *Lancet*. 2001;358(9282):605–613.
95. Topol EJ, Califf RM, George BS, et al. A randomized trial of immediate versus delayed elective angioplasty after intravenous tissue plasminogen activator in acute myocardial infarction. *N Engl J Med*. 1987;317(10):581–588.
100. Ellis SG, Tendera M, de Belder MA, et al. Facilitated PCI in patients with ST-elevation myocardial infarction. *N Engl J Med*. 2008;358(21):2205–2217.
105. Bagai A, Cantor WJ, Tan M, et al. Clinical outcomes and cost implications of routine early PCI after fibrinolysis: one-year follow-up of the Trial of Routine Angioplasty and Stenting after Fibrinolysis to Enhance Reperfusion in Acute Myocardial Infarction (TRANSFER-AMI) study. *Am Heart J*. 2013;165(4):630–637. e632.
106. Bohmer E, Hoffmann P, Abdelnoor M, et al. Efficacy and safety of immediate angioplasty versus ischemia-guided management after thrombolysis in acute myocardial infarction in areas with very long transfer distances results of the NORDISTEMI (NORwegian study on DIstrict treatment of ST-elevation myocardial infarction). *J Am Coll Cardiol*. 2010;55(2):102–110.

 Additional references available online at expertconsult.com.

中文导读

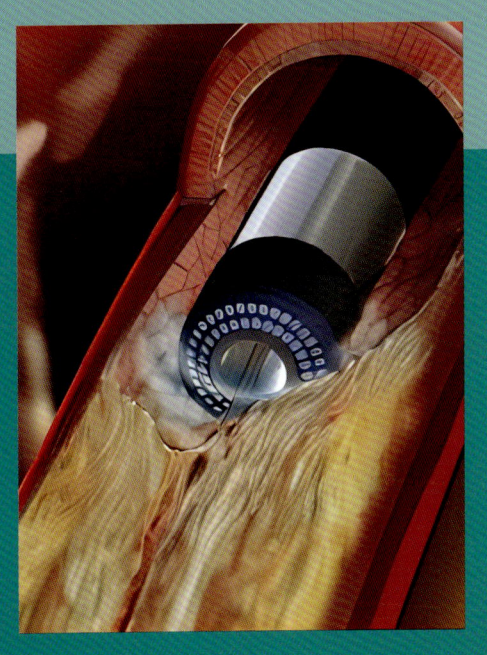

第13章
冠状动脉介入治疗的其他辅助药物：β受体阻滞剂、钙通道阻滞剂和血管紧张素转化酶抑制剂

几十年来，β受体阻滞剂、钙通道阻滞剂和血管紧张素转化酶抑制剂已广泛应用于冠心病的药物治疗。自20世纪80年代以来，大量临床试验已经证实了这些药物的获益。本章将简要介绍这些药物的药理学基础并深入探讨相关的随机临床试验，以及正在进行的研究，以提供治疗建议。

β受体阻滞剂通过直接与儿茶酚胺竞争结合β肾上腺素受体而发挥作用，其中对冠心病的疗效主要取决于β1受体的拮抗能力。由于β受体阻滞剂可以降低心肌耗氧，因此在冠心病人群中具有保护作用。尤其是在心肌梗死患者中，β受体阻滞剂可显著降低再梗死及心室颤动的发生率。尽管如此，COMMIT研究建议在心肌梗死早期应谨慎经静脉应用β受体阻滞剂，但研究结果同样表明了心肌梗死亚急性期和慢性期应用β受体阻滞剂的获益，并且建议所有心肌梗死后的患者长期应用β受体阻滞剂。

钙通道阻滞剂包括二氢吡啶类、苯烷基胺类和苯二氮䓬类，苯烷基胺类和苯二氮䓬类可减慢房室和窦房结传导，而二氢吡啶类血管扩张作用更显著。目前钙通道阻滞剂尚不作为急性冠状动脉综合征患者的常规推荐用药，但对于存在β受体阻滞剂明确禁忌证的部分患者，非二氢吡啶类的钙通道阻滞剂可作为首选。对于稳定的心肌梗死后患者，加用钙通道阻滞剂可用于高血压和心绞痛的有效治疗。

血管紧张素转化酶抑制剂可减少血管紧张素Ⅱ的产生，从而降低血压，增加每搏量和心排血量，促进良好的心室重塑。在心肌梗死后的患者中，特别是合并左心室功能障碍的患者，应用血管紧张素转化酶抑制剂已证实具有显著获益，而ARB类药物（如缬沙坦）可作为血管紧张素转化酶抑制剂的替代治疗。

将β受体阻滞剂、钙通道阻滞剂、血管紧张素转化酶抑制剂与其他已明确的药物治疗（如抗血小板药物和他汀类药物等）联合应用有利于患者获益最大化。

王枞　柳景华

章节要点

- β受体阻滞剂可降低心肌梗死后远期死亡率。
- 尽管应用β受体阻滞剂存在获益，但在心肌梗死早期应谨慎使用，以避免耐受性差的患者出现心源性休克。
- 对于少数β受体阻滞剂有明确禁忌证的心肌梗死患者，可选择钙通道阻滞剂作为替代方案。
- 血管紧张素转化酶抑制剂可降低心肌梗死患者的死亡率，在伴有左心室功能障碍的患者中尤为显著。
- 基因组学证实了一些特定人群对这些药物存在不同反应，进一步的研究有助于学者们在未来制定个体化药物治疗方案。

13 Other Adjunctive Drugs for Coronary Intervention: Beta-Blockers, Calcium-Channel Blockers, and Angiotensin-Converting Enzyme Inhibitors

David W. Allen, Vivek Rajagopal

KEY POINTS

- β-Blockers provide long-term mortality reduction after myocardial infarction (MI).
- Although β-blockers are beneficial, they should be used carefully immediately after MI to avoid cardiogenic shock in susceptible patients.
- Calcium-channel blockers are reasonable alternatives to β-blockers after MI in the few patients with strong contraindications to β-blockers.
- Angiotensin-converting enzyme (ACE) inhibitors reduce mortality in patients after MI, especially in those with left ventricular (LV) dysfunction.
- Genomic studies have demonstrated differential response of some populations to these agents, and further studies might help us target individuals with specific agents in the future.

INTRODUCTION

For several decades, β-blockers, calcium-channel blockers, and angiotensin-converting enzyme (ACE) inhibitors have been beneficial in a wide spectrum of coronary artery disease (CAD)—stable and unstable angina, ST-elevation myocardial infarction (STEMI), and non–ST-elevation myocardial infarction (NSTEMI). Multiple clinical trials since the 1980s have demonstrated benefits of these agents, which work either by reducing myocardial oxygen demand or by promoting favorable myocardial remodeling.

This chapter will discuss the basic pharmacology of these agents, followed by an in-depth discussion of randomized trials that have used them. Finally, we will discuss ongoing research and will also provide treatment recommendations.

β-ADRENERGIC RECEPTORS

β-Receptors belong to a well-characterized family of receptors known as *G protein-coupled receptors*.[1] The pathway involves binding of an agonist, such as catecholamines for β-receptors, to an extracellular receptor. Receptor activation causes a coupled G protein to stimulate adenylyl cyclase, which increases intracellular concentrations of cyclic adenosine monophosphate (cAMP). In turn, cAMP activates several AMP-dependent protein kinases, which phosphorylate other proteins and result in a cellular response.

The cellular response for β-receptors differs according to three major subtypes: β_1, β_2, and β_3. Whereas stimulation of β_2-receptors causes bronchodilation and peripheral vasodilation, stimulation of β_1-receptors predominantly affects the heart, increasing contractility, heart rate, and lipolysis. The β_3-receptor increases heat production in brown adipose tissue and increases lipolysis in both brown and white adipose tissue.[2,3] Notably, the β_3-receptor likely plays a role in obesity and insulin resistance and may promote endothelial nitric oxide synthase and nitric oxide bioavailability.[3–15]

β-Adrenergic Receptor Blockers

β-Blockers act by directly competing with binding of catecholamines to β-adrenergic receptors. These agents differ in their selectivity, lipid solubility, metabolism, and partial-agonist ability (intrinsic sympathomimetic ability [ISA]; Table 13.1). Although some data suggest that these differences might impact efficacy in certain conditions, such as chronic congestive heart failure (CHF), these differences mainly affect side effects, contraindications, and frequency of dosing. For example, nonselective agents may increase bronchospasm in asthmatic patients, whereas lipophilic agents may have more central nervous system (CNS) effects such as sedation and depression. Type of metabolism will affect plasma half-life in patients with renal or hepatic insufficiency. β-Blockers with ISA slow heart rate less than β-blockers without ISA; also, β-blockers with ISA are less likely to decrease high-density lipoprotein cholesterol (HDL-C) or to increase triglycerides.

Despite these pharmacokinetic differences, efficacy in CAD arises primarily from β_1-receptor antagonism. In acute MI, for example, the catecholamine storm decreases the fibrillation threshold, increases myocardial oxygen consumption, and promotes myocardial necrosis. By decreasing heart rate and contractility, blockade of the β_1-receptor lowers myocardial stress, which decreases necrosis. β-Blockade also raises the fibrillation threshold. By antagonizing lipolysis, β-blockers reduce concentrations of free fatty acids and cause greater use of glucose and less use of oxygen. Although controversial, β-blockers—in particular, carvedilol and nebivolol—may also inhibit platelet aggregation, but the mechanism could be membrane interaction instead of β-receptor antagonism.[16,17]

Given these beneficial effects, it is not surprising that numerous clinical trials have demonstrated the benefits of β-blockers in acute coronary syndromes (ACSs). Nonetheless, prudence is still required because β-blockers decrease inotropy and slow atrioventricular conduction, which can harm certain subgroups of patients.

Unstable Angina Pectoris

Because β-blockers potently reduce myocardial oxygen demand and possibly reduce inflammation in ACSs,[18] treating unstable angina with β-blockers has much intuitive appeal. A few small randomized trials have supported this. Gottlieb and

TABLE 13.1 β-Blockers

Type	Dose (mg)	Frequency (Q)	Excretion	Lipid Solubility	ISA
SELECTIVE β₁					
Acebutolol	200–600	12 h	Kidney	Moderate	Low
Atenolol	25–200	24 h	Kidney	None	None
Betaxolol	20–40	24 h	Kidney	Moderate	Low
Metoprolol	50–400	12 h	Liver	Moderate	None
Long-acting metoprolol		24 h			
NONSELECTIVE β					
Labetalol (α, β₁, β₂)	600–2400	6–8 h	Liver	None	None
Nadolol	80–240	24 h	Kidney	Low	None
Pindolol	15–45	8–12 h	Kidney	Moderate	Moderate
Propranolol	80–320	4–6 h	Liver	High	None
Long-acting propranolol		12 h			
Timolol	15–45	12 h	Liver	Moderate	None

ISA, Intrinsic sympathomimetic ability.
Adapted from Griffin B, Topol E, Nair D, et al. *Manual of Cardiovascular Medicine*. 3rd ed. Philadelphia: Lippincott Williams & Wilkins; 2008.

colleagues[19] randomized patients with unstable angina to 4 weeks of propranolol or placebo. All patients received calcium-channel blockers and/or nitrates. Although incidence of death, myocardial infarction (MI), or need for urgent coronary artery bypass grafting (CABG) did not differ between the groups, propranolol significantly reduced frequency and severity of recurrent ischemia. In the Holland Interuniversity Nifedipine and Metoprolol Trial (HINT),[20] 338 patients with unstable angina not pretreated with a β-blocker randomly received nifedipine alone, metoprolol alone, or nifedipine and metoprolol. The odds ratios (ORs) for recurrent ischemia or MI by 48 hours were 1.15 for nifedipine (95% confidence interval [CI], 0.83 to 1.64), 0.76 for metoprolol (95% CI, 0.49 to 1.16), and 0.80 for both (95% CI, 0.53 to 1.19). Not surprisingly, small numbers limited the power of this study, and these differences were not statistically significant. Hohnloser and associates[21] examined effects of esmolol, a short-acting (half-life 9 minutes) intravenous (IV) β-blocker in a randomized, placebo-controlled trial of 113 patients. Investigators increased esmolol until they reduced the double-product by about 25%; thereafter, the esmolol infusion continued for up to 72 hours. Acute MI or urgent revascularization occurred in 9 patients treated with placebo compared with 3 patients treated with esmolol ($P = .06$). In a more recent randomized trial, Brunner and colleagues[22] randomized 116 patients with unstable angina to placebo or carvedilol at 25 mg twice a day. Patients received 48-hour Holter monitoring to document ischemia. Carvedilol reduced ischemic time by 76% (204 vs. 49 minutes, $P < .05$) with a 66% reduction in number of ischemic episodes (24 vs. 8, $P < .05$).

Some retrospective data from recent studies also demonstrate benefit of β-blockers in unstable angina. Ellis and associates[23] pooled data from five randomized trials of abciximab during percutaneous coronary intervention (PCI): Evaluation of the 7E3 for the Prevention of Ischaemic Complications (EPIC) trial, Evaluation in percutaneous transluminal coronary angioplasty (PTCA) to Improve Long-Term Outcome With Abciximab GP IIb/IIIa Blockade (EPILOG), Evaluation of Platelet IIb/IIIa Inhibitor for Stenting (EPISTENT), c7E3 FAB Antiplatelet Therapy in Unstable Refractory Angina (CAPTURE), and ReoPro and Primary PTCA Organization and Randomized Trial (RAPPORT). Except for RAPPORT, which had STEMI patients, the other four trials included patients with unstable angina or NSTEMI. All-cause mortality by 30 days occurred in 0.6% of patients receiving β-blockers compared with 2.0% for patients who did not receive β-blockers. After adjusting for baseline characteristics and propensity score to receive β-blockers, β-blockers remained predictive of lower mortality (hazard ratio [HR], 0.25; 95% CI, 0.11 to 0.57; $P = .001$). This mortality difference persisted at 6 months (1.7% vs. 3.7%; adjusted HR, 0.53; 95% CI, 0.29 to 0.94; $P = .03$). Among patients with unstable angina, β-blockers reduced mortality at 3 months (1.6% to 0.6%, $P = .029$) and at 6 months (3.1% to 1.4%, $P = .009$).

Similarly, investigators found a mortality benefit of β-blockers in patients enrolled in the Can Rapid Risk Stratification of Unstable Angina Patients Suppress Adverse Outcomes with Early Implementation of the American College of Cardiology (ACC)/American Heart Association (AHA) Guidelines (CRUSADE) initiative.[24] In 72,054 patients with NSTEMI at 509 U.S. hospitals from 2001 through 2004, acute β-blocker use was associated with a lower hospital mortality (adjusted OR, 0.66; 95% CI, 0.60 to 0.72; $P < .01$). Notably, nearly all patient subgroups benefited, including patients aged 80 years and older.

Percutaneous Coronary Intervention

Although trials have evaluated adjunctive β-blockade in patients with unstable angina or MI undergoing PCI, fewer data exist for effect of β-blockade as a specific adjunct to PCI. In fact, most data for adjunctive benefit arise from nonrandomized registries.

Sharma and colleagues[25] evaluated 1675 consecutive patients undergoing PCI, none of whom had a previous MI; the authors did not specify how many patients presented with unstable angina. Creatine kinase myocardial band (CK-MB) elevation occurred in 13.2% of patients on β-blockers before the procedure compared with 22.1% of patients not on β-blockers ($P < .001$). On multivariate analysis, β-blockers remained an independent predictor of lower CK-MB release. Over a mean 15 months of follow-up, patients on preprocedural β-blockers had a mortality of 0.8% compared with 2.0% for patients not on preprocedural β-blockers ($P = .04$). Chan and colleagues[26] evaluated 4553 consecutive patients without acute or recent MI who underwent PCI according to whether they had been treated with β-blockers at the time of the PCI. Of these patients, 2056 (45%) were on β-blockers at the time of the intervention. Mortality was lower at 30 days for patients who received β-blockers (1.3% vs. 0.8%, $P = .13$) and at 1 year (6.0% vs. 3.9%, $P = .0014$). After adjusting for differences in the baseline characteristics by propensity analysis, β-blocker therapy remained independently predictive of 1 year survival (HR, 0.63; 95% CI, 0.46 to 0.87; $P = .0054$).

Along with these mortality data, other data suggest a benefit of β-blockers on restenosis. Jackson and colleagues[27] followed 4840 people who underwent PCI according to whether they received β-blockers on discharge. Patients treated with β-blockers had a 5-year clinical restenosis rate of 12% versus 14% (adjusted OR, 0.83; $P = .046$). These data are controversial, however, because a small randomized trial of adjunctive carvedilol failed to reduce restenosis in patients undergoing atherectomy.[28]

In another small randomized trial, Wang and colleagues[29] examined the effect of intracoronary (IC) propranolol during PCI. In this trial, investigators randomized 150 patients undergoing PCI to placebo or propranolol (15 μg/kg) injected into the distal coronary artery via the balloon catheter positioned across the stenosis. CK-MB elevation occurred in 17% of propranolol patients compared with 36% of placebo patients ($P = .01$). The incidence of death, MI, or urgent revascularization by 30 days occurred in 18% of propranolol patients compared with 10% of placebo patients ($P = .004$). The relative risk (RR) of MI did not differ between patients on prior β-blocker therapy and those not on prior therapy.

Uretsky and colleagues[30] also examined the effect of IC β-blockers during PCI by randomizing 400 patients to IC propranolol or placebo combined with systemic eptifibatide. At 1 year, the composite end point of death, postprocedural MI, urgent target-lesion revascularization (TLR), or MI after hospitalization occurred in 21.5% of propranolol patients and in 32.5% of placebo patients ($P < .01$), driven primarily by lower postprocedural MI (12.5% propranolol vs. 21.5% placebo; RR reduction 0.45; 95% CI, 0.08 to 0.65; $P = .018$).

In a unique study design, Park and colleagues[31] randomly assigned 70 patients undergoing elective PCI to either placebo or the short-acting β-blocker landiolol as a 1-minute IC infusion before and after first balloon inflation, followed by a 6-hour IV infusion. The troponin I (TnI) level at 24 hours trended lower in the landiolol group compared with placebo (0.5 ± 1.14 vs. 1.27 ± 2.48, $P = .07$), although it is unclear whether this difference, if verified in a larger cohort, would be clinically meaningful.

Acute Myocardial Infarction

Early Trials: The MIAMI and ISIS-1 Trials

The data for β-blockade in acute MI come from 26 small trials and two large trials: the First International Study of Infarct Survival (ISIS-1) trial[32] and the Metoprolol in Acute Myocardial Infarction (MIAMI) trial.[33]

The MIAMI Trial
Patients with acute MI within 24 hours of symptom onset ($n = 5778$) were randomized to receive IV metoprolol (15 mg) or placebo followed by oral metoprolol (200 mg daily) or placebo for 15 days. β-blockade reduced Q-wave infarction significantly, from 53.9% to 50.9% ($P = .024$), with a nonsignificant reduction in mortality (4.9% to 4.3%, $P = .29$). However, the MIAMI trial was significantly limited in its applicability to the modern era; patients enrolled in MIAMI were low risk (e.g., all Killip class I), and the trial occurred in the pre-reperfusion era before routine ACE inhibition and statin treatment.

The ISIS-1 Trial
Although ISIS-1 was similarly limited by lack of reperfusion, its larger size and power are important. ISIS-1 randomized 16,207 patients with suspected acute MI (mean 5-hour symptom onset) to control or to IV atenolol (5 to 10 mg) followed by 100 mg oral atenolol daily for 7 days. Treatment with atenolol significantly reduced vascular mortality from 4.57% to 3.89% ($P < .04$) from day 0 to day 7. Atenolol-treated patients also had a significantly lower vascular mortality by 1 year (10.7% vs. 12.0%, $P < .01$), although much of this late difference might have arisen because patients randomized to atenolol were more likely to be discharged on β-blockers compared with controls.

COMMIT and Other Trials
Given that most data for β-blockade in acute MI are several decades old, benefit for β-blockade in the current era—with aggressive use of antiplatelet therapy, thrombolysis, or primary angioplasty, statin therapy, and antialdosterone therapy—has remained uncertain, and physicians have hoped for trials with modern background therapy to assess the true value of β-blockade. This uncertainty has remained relevant because of persistent fears that β-blockers may exacerbate the condition of some acute MI patients, particularly those with signs and symptoms of CHF.

Ibanez and colleagues[34] randomized 270 patients of Killip class II or less with anterior STEMI to receive an IV β-blocker or a placebo before primary PCI. In this small group of selected patients, infarct size estimated by creatine kinase curves was smaller in the IV β-blocker group.

More definitive data come from the large-scale randomized trial Clopidogrel and Metoprolol in Myocardial Infarction Trial (COMMIT).[35] In fact, COMMIT was the largest trial ever to investigate β-blockers in acute MI. As such, it is exceptionally important to understand the trial in depth and its implications for period of management of

The COMMIT trial, also known as the Second Chinese Cardiac Study (CCS-2), was a placebo-controlled randomized trial with a two-by-two factorial design that randomized acute MI patients to metoprolol or placebo, as well as to clopidogrel or placebo, with a background therapy of aspirin, anticoagulant therapy (mostly unfractionated heparin [UFH]), and thrombolysis.

Patient Selection
The scale of the trial was impressive. Between August of 1999 and February of 2005, COMMIT enrolled 45,852 patients in 1250 Chinese hospitals. Inclusion criteria comprised left bundle branch block (LBBB, presumably new), ST-segment elevation, or ST depression within 24 hours of ischemic symptoms. Exclusion criteria comprised patients scheduled for primary PCI (because of combined aspirin and clopidogrel use that would have interfered with the other study arm) or those with conditions considered high risk for β-blocker therapy: systolic blood pressure less than 100 mm Hg or heart rate below 50 beats/min, heart block, or cardiogenic shock. Notably, moderate heart failure (Killip class II or III) was not a contraindication, unlike trials such as MIAMI.[33]

Study Protocol
Patients randomized to metoprolol received a 5 mg IV dose followed by second and third dose as long as systolic blood pressure was above 90 mm Hg and heart rate was above 50 beats/min after each dose. Patients then received 50 mg metoprolol 15 minutes after the last IV dose, repeated every 6 hours for 24 hours, followed by 200 mg controlled-release metoprolol once daily for up to 4 weeks.

End Points
The COMMIT trial had two primary end points: all-cause mortality until discharge or until day 28 and the composite of death, reinfarction, or cardiac arrest. Secondary end points included cardiogenic shock, cardiac arrest, and reinfarction. Prespecified subgroup analyses included effects of metoprolol on primary outcomes according to hospital days and the following subgroups: age, sex, time from

symptom onset, fibrinolysis, Killip class, heart rate, systolic blood pressure, and shock risk index (absolute risk of shock calculated from a Cox regression model using baseline prognostic characteristics).

Results

Not surprisingly, the large sample size of COMMIT ensured that baseline characteristics between groups were similar (Fig. 13.1). The mean age was 61 years; 26% were older than 70, and 72% were male. ST-segment elevation occurred in 87%, LBBB in 6%, and ST depression in 7%. Time from symptom onset to treatment was evenly distributed over 24 hours, and approximately one-third of patients were treated within 6 hours, one-third within 6 to 13 hours, and one-third within 13 to 24 hours. Although most patients had no signs or symptoms of CHF, a sizable percentage (24%) were Killip class II or III on presentation. Again, this contrasts with early β-blocker trials that enrolled lower-risk patients with no evidence of CHF. In COMMIT, 54% of patients received thrombolysis, and most of these patients received urokinase. Of those who presented within 12 hours, 68% received thrombolysis; it is unknown how many of the remaining patients did not receive thrombolytics because of clear contraindications. Notably, slightly fewer metoprolol-treated patients received ACE inhibitors (67.2% vs. 69.3%, $P < .0001$).

The primary composite outcome of death, reinfarction, or cardiac arrest did not differ between metoprolol-treated patients (9.4%) and placebo-treated patients (9.9%; OR, 0.96%; 95% CI, 0.90 to 1.01; $P = .10$; Fig. 13.2). Similarly, the co-primary outcome of death did not differ between metoprolol (7.7%) and placebo (7.8%) patients (see Fig. 13.1). Given the prior clinical data that support early β-blockade in acute MI, reasons for these counterintuitive results require a careful dissection. Specifically, did β-blockade reduce any particular clinical events, and did β-blockade benefit some patients much more than others?

β-Blockade significantly reduced any reinfarction (2.0% for metoprolol vs. 2.5% for placebo, $P = .001$) and risk of ventricular fibrillation (2.5% vs. 3.0%, $P = .001$). Treatment, however, increased risk of cardiogenic shock by 30% (5.0% vs. 3.9%, $P < .0001$). Therefore, although β-blockade significantly reduced arrhythmic death by 22% (1.7% for metoprolol vs. 2.2% for placebo, $P = .0002$), it significantly increased death secondary to cardiogenic shock by 29% (2.2% vs. 1.7%, $P = .0002$). Therefore, benefit in reducing arrhythmic death was counteracted by harm in increasing cardiogenic shock. In absolute terms, metoprolol prevented five episodes of ventricular fibrillation and five episodes of reinfarction per 1000 treated, but it caused 11 episodes of cardiogenic shock per 1000 treated. Of interest, these effects had differential time courses. Specifically, a 10 per 1000 excess risk for cardiogenic shock was noted within the first 24 hours. By contrast, reductions in risk of reinfarction and ventricular fibrillation began approximately 48 hours after treatment initiation.

Propensity of metoprolol to cause cardiogenic shock differed according to baseline characteristics. Metoprolol caused a much higher excess of cardiogenic shock in the various subgroups: 56.9 per 1000 for patients in Killip class III; 34.6 per 1000 for patients who presented with a heart rate greater than 110 beats/min; 23.3 per 1000 for patients presenting with systolic blood pressure below 120 mm Hg; and 23.1 per 1000 for patients aged 70 years or older. Not surprisingly, these differences translated into a much higher risk of cardiogenic shock with metoprolol according to baseline risk of shock: 1.7 per 1000 (low risk) versus 16.2 per 1000 (medium risk) versus 56.9 per 1000 (high risk; $P < .0001$).

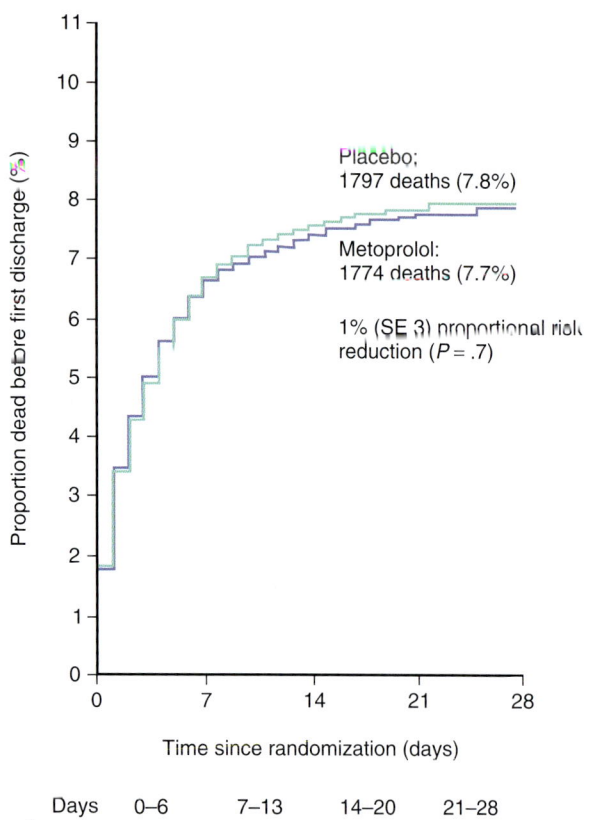

Fig. 13.1 Death, reinfarction, or cardiac arrest in COMMIT. *COMMIT*, Clopidogrel and Metoprolol in Myocardial Infarction Trial; *SE*, standard error.

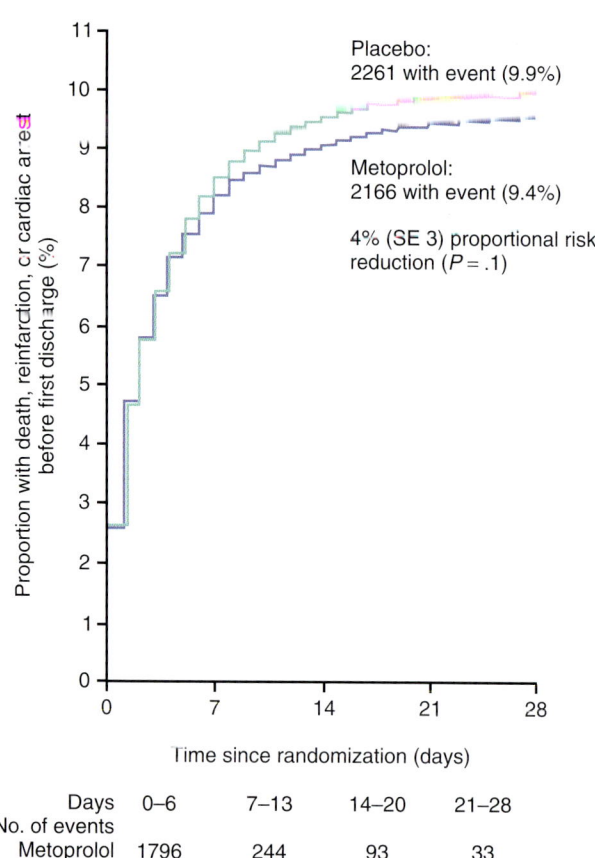

Fig. 13.2 Death in COMMIT. *COMMIT*, Clopidogrel and Metoprolol in Myocardial Infarction Trial; *SE*, standard error.

This differential effect on cardiogenic shock translated into a differential effect on mortality according to patients' baseline risk of shock. For patients at high risk of cardiogenic shock, metoprolol caused an absolute increase of 24.8 deaths per 1000 treated. Conversely, treatment caused an absolute *decrease* of 4.2 and 4.3 deaths per 1000 for medium-risk and low-risk patients, respectively.

Meta-Analysis Using COMMIT Patients

As the COMMIT investigators mentioned, patients in COMMIT had a significantly higher risk of shock and mortality compared with patients enrolled in prior trials. Therefore, the investigators examined the effect of β-blockade on patients in COMMIT comparable to the low-risk patients enrolled in MIAMI (i.e., heart rate >65 beats/min, Killip class I, systolic blood pressure >105 mm Hg). They also pooled these patients with patients from MIAMI, ISIS-1, and 26 small trials (Fig. 13.3). The magnitude of benefit in low-risk COMMIT patients (6.4% to 5.7%) was similar to that of MIAMI patients (4.9% to 4.3%). In the analysis of pooled patients (~52,000), β-blockade significantly reduced cardiac arrest (3.1% vs. 3.6%, $P = .002$), reinfarction (2.3% vs. 2.8%, $P = .0002$), and mortality (4.8% vs. 5.5%, $P = .0006$).

Recommendations for β-Blockade During Acute Myocardial Infarction

Given COMMIT's applicability to the modern era and its enormous size—almost twice as many patients as all others combined—the COMMIT data must form the core basis for any recommendations. Accordingly, early IV β-blocker therapy for acute MI cannot be recommended for all patients. Nevertheless, the neutrality of the primary end points was driven by excess of cardiogenic shock in patients at increased baseline risk of developing shock. Therefore, it is rational to consider early β-blockade in patients at low risk for shock: age younger than 70 years, heart rate below 110 beats/min, systolic blood pressure above 120 mm Hg, and Killip class I. This is, of course, not supported on a strict scientific basis because such a group was not prespecified, although a recent analysis from the Global Registry of Acute Coronary Events (GRACE) also confirms some hazard of indiscriminate early IV β-blockers.[36] A stronger recommendation can be made for waiting at least 24 hours to determine clinical stability before beginning β-blockade. Because the cardiogenic shock hazard arises within 24 hours, it is possible that waiting could circumvent this hazard because it would allow those who are fittest for β-blockade to emerge, thus giving these patients the reinfarction and cardiac arrest benefits, which emerge more slowly over the hospital course.

Chronic Therapy After Myocardial Infarction

ISIS-1 demonstrated a sustained benefit of β-blockade for patients with acute MI; 1-year mortality for atenolol-treated patients was 10.7% versus 12.0% for placebo patients ($P < .01$). Given that patients randomized to atenolol in this trial were more likely to be discharged on atenolol, the further separation in survival curves at 1 year suggests a beneficial effect of β-blockade given regularly after MI. Pooled data from all long-term trials of β-blockade after MI also show a significant protective effect.[37] Long-term β-blockade reduced sudden death from 5.2% to 3.6% ($P < .0001$),

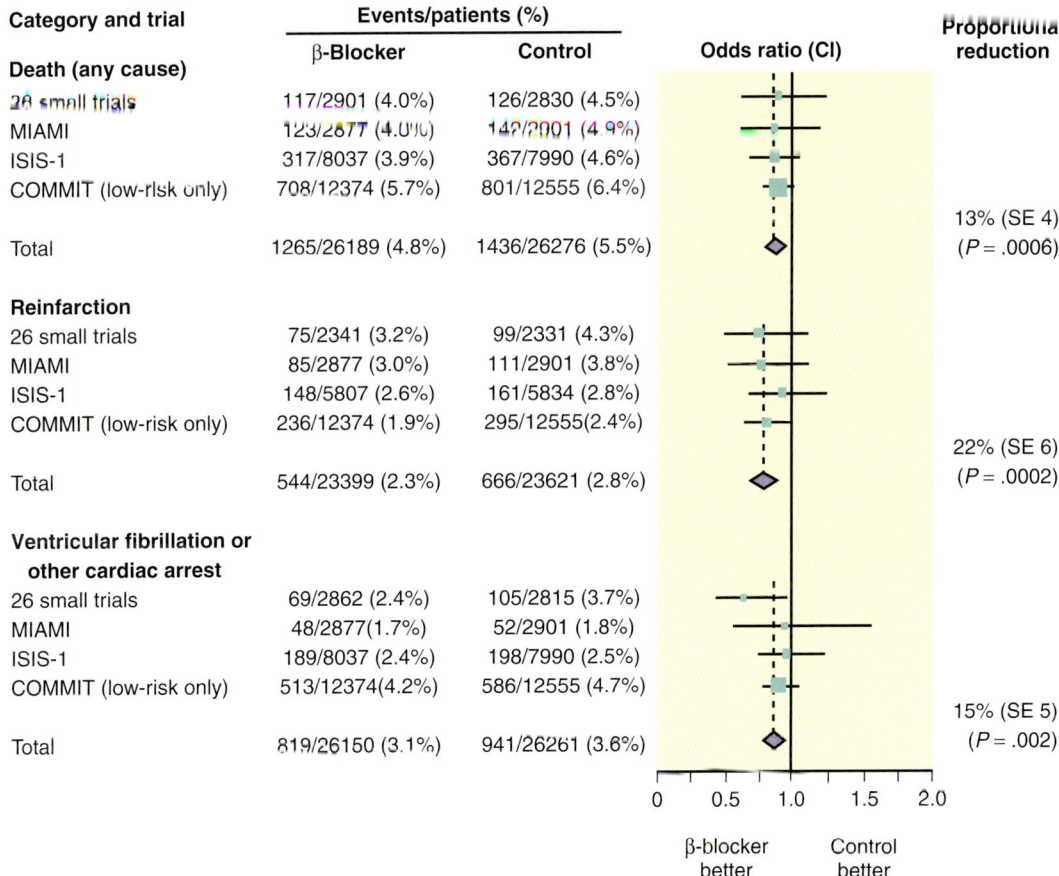

Fig. 13.3 Meta-analysis using COMMIT data. *CI*, Confidence interval; *COMMIT*, Clopidogrel and Metoprolol in Myocardial Infarction Trial; *ISIS*, International Study of Infarct Survival; *MIAMI*, Metoprolol in Acute Myocardial Infarction; *SE*, standard error.

reinfarction from 7.3% to 5.5% ($P < .0001$), and mortality from 9.5% to 7.5% ($P < .0001$) over a follow-up period of 1 to 3 years.

The Effect of Carvedilol on Outcome After Myocardial Infarction in Patients With Left-Ventricular Dysfunction (CAPRICORN) trial supported this benefit for patients with recent MI and systolic dysfunction.[38] CAPRICORN randomized 1959 patients with acute MI and left ventricular ejection fraction (LVEF) of 40 or less to carvedilol 6.25 mg twice daily (starting during hospitalization) or placebo. Carvedilol was titrated up to 25 mg twice daily over 4 to 6 weeks. After a mean follow-up of 15 months, carvedilol treatment reduced all-cause mortality from 15% to 12% (HR, 0.77; 95% CI, 0.60 to 0.98; $P = .03$). Importantly, the CAPRICORN trial represented modern therapy with aggressive reperfusion, antiplatelet therapy, and anticoagulation; furthermore, all patients received ACE inhibitors for 48 hours prior to randomization. Similarly, an analysis of the Valsartan in Acute Myocardial Infarction Trial (VALIANT)—which randomized 14,703 MI patients with heart failure to valsartan, captopril, or both—demonstrated a long-term survival advantage to patients on β-blockers.[39]

Patient Selection: Role of Genomics

Because β-blockade does not uniformly benefit patients after MI, as the COMMIT trial demonstrated, β-blockers may harm certain subgroups while benefiting others. Therefore, clinical trials remain blunt and crude instruments at best. Suppose, for example, a condition has 100% mortality, and a treatment demonstrates a large absolute reduction in mortality—for example, 40%. Thus, 4 of 10 patients given the treatment survive compared with 0 of 10 patients given placebo. That means that six treated patients did not receive benefit. This conundrum presented by clinical trials argues for a finer instrument to determine which patients will benefit.

Given recent advances in pharmacogenomics, characterization of patients' genetic polymorphisms may be a useful instrument to select the best candidates for β-blocker therapy. Lanfear and colleagues[40] studied polymorphisms in the $β_1$- and $β_2$-receptors among patients ($n = 597$) on β-blocker therapy after an ACS. No relationship existed between $β_1$-receptor polymorphisms and mortality in patients treated and not treated with β-blockers. Polymorphisms in $β_2$-receptors, however, correlated significantly to mortality in patients discharged on β-blockers. In particular, Kaplan-Meier 3-year mortality rates were 6%, 11%, and 16% for three different polymorphisms (GG, CG, and CC genotypes, respectively, for polymorphism Gln27Glu with HR 0.24 [95% CI, 0.09 to 0.68] for GG vs. CC, $P = .004$). Similarly, Cresci and colleagues[41] recently described differential effects of polymorphisms in the *ADRB1*, *ADRB2*, *ADRA2C*, and the *GRK5* genes in ACS patients in a race-specific manner. A $β_2$-receptor polymorphism, Gly16Arg, displayed a relationship between genotypes and mortality: 3-year Kaplan-Meier mortality rates of 10% for the GG and GA genotypes compared with 20% for the AA genotype (HR 0.44 [95% CI, 0.22 to 0.85] for GG vs. AA and 0.48 [95% CI, 0.27 to 0.86] for GA vs. AA, $P = .005$ for overall comparison). Significantly, these polymorphisms did not correlate with mortality in patients not treated with β-blockers, indicating a specific interaction of the polymorphisms with β-blocker treatment. Although the mechanism of this interaction is unknown, it is possible that these polymorphisms alter LV remodeling in response to β-blockade, as has been described for $β_1$-receptor polymorphisms.[42,43] Similarly, polymorphisms in the peroxisome proliferator activated receptor-α (PPARα) gene, which can alter LV remodeling, can interact with β-blocker therapy, affecting rehospitalization rates after an ACS.[44]

Polymorphisms can also interact differentially with β-blockers in the presence of diabetes. Beitelshees and colleagues[45] followed ACS patients ($n = 468$) with the -866G>A polymorphism in the mitochondrial uncoupling protein 2 (UCP-2) gene. Among diabetic patients with the GG genotype, β-blocker use reduced cardiac rehospitalization by 80%, whereas β-blocker use *increased* cardiac rehospitalization elevenfold among A-carrier patients with diabetes.

Although small, these studies suggest that genomic profiling might help tailor β-blocker therapy in patients with ACSs, thereby maximizing benefit and reducing risk. Furthermore, advances in high-throughput genotyping suggest that widespread application is feasible.

CALCIUM CHANNELS

Intracellular calcium concentrations are tightly regulated by calcium exchangers, ion pumps, and channels. At baseline, cytoplasmic calcium ion concentrations exist at very low levels (<100 nM) compared with extracellular concentrations (>1 mM). When calcium channels open at the plasma membrane or endoplasmic reticular level, intracellular concentrations of calcium rapidly rise; adenosine triphosphate (ATP)-dependent ion pumps and sodium/calcium exchangers restore equilibrium.

Calcium channels exist as three major subgroups: voltage dependent, stretch operated, and receptor operated. The *voltage-dependent* receptors exist as three subtypes: N type, L type, and T type. The *L-type* and *T-type* channels are important to cardiovascular medicine and are inhibited by calcium-channel blockers. L-type channels exist throughout the cardiovascular system in cardiac and smooth muscles; they mediate the slow inward current (plateau phase) of the action potential and might play a role in activation of pathologic hypertrophy.[46] T-type channels are found mainly in sinus nodal tissue, and few are found in ventricular myocardium.

Calcium-Channel Blockers

The three main classes of calcium-channel blockers include dihydropyridines, phenylalkylamines, and benzothiazepines (Table 13.2). These classes differ in their vasodilatory and chronotropic effects. In particular, phenylalkylamines (e.g., verapamil) and benzothiazepines (e.g., diltiazem) decrease atrioventricular and sinoatrial conduction, whereas dihydropyridines (e.g., amlodipine) do not. On the other hand, dihydropyridines are more potent vasodilators. Nifedipine, in particular, can cause profound peripheral vasodilation, resulting in reflex tachycardia. Despite these differences, all classes of calcium-channel blockers have been shown to reduce infarct size in animal models. Some have speculated that calcium-channel blockers protect myocardium via coronary vasodilation and decreased ischemic calcium overload.

Acute Myocardial Infarction

Obviously, most data for calcium-channel blockade after acute MI are more than a decade old. The pivotal trials for early treatment of MI include the Secondary Prevention Reinfarction Israeli Nifedipine Trial (SPRINT-II), the First Danish Study Group on Verapamil in Myocardial Infarction Trial (DAVIT), and three small diltiazem trials.[47] None of these trials showed any significant difference in reinfarction or mortality with calcium-channel blockade; in fact, SPRINT-II was stopped prematurely because of increased mortality in the nifedipine group.

Data are limited and are only usable to generate hypothesis. In a Japanese trial, investigators randomized 1090 patients after acute MI to β-blocker or calcium-channel blocker therapy.[48] At a mean follow-up of 455 days, patients treated with calcium-channel blockers did not have a different incidence of cardiovascular death (1.1% vs. 1.7%), reinfarction (1.3% vs. 0.9%), or nonfatal stroke (0.2% vs. 0.7%). Interestingly, the calcium-channel group had a

TABLE 13.2 Calcium Channel Blockers

Type	Vasodilatory Effects	Conduction Effects	Negative Inotropy
PHENYLALKYLAMINE			
Verapamil	+++	++++	+++
BENZOTHIAZEPINE			
Diltiazem	++	+++	++
DIHYDROPYRIDINE			
Amlodipine	+++	+	+
Felodipine	++++	+	0
Isradipine	+++	++	0
Nicardipine	++++	+	0
Nifedipine	++++	+	+
Nisoldipine	+++	+	+

0, No activity; ++++, most potent.

significantly lower incidence of CHF (1.1% vs. 4.2%, P = .001) and coronary spasm (0.2% vs. 1.2%, P = .027). Obviously, more data in other populations are required to verify these differences.

Recommendations for Acute Coronary Syndromes

Given the lack of large trials that demonstrate benefit in acute MI, calcium-channel blockers should not be administered routinely, particularly for patients presenting with STEMI. A prominent exception is the patient who presents with ST segment elevation following cocaine intoxication. Given the prominent role of coronary vasospasm after cocaine use and the possible exacerbation with β-blockade, it is reasonable to administer calcium-channel blockers for these patients.

For patients with unstable angina or NSTEMI, the ACC/AHA guidelines[49] endorse a class I recommendation for some with ACS: "patients with continuing or frequently recurring ischemia when β-blockers are contraindicated, a nondihydropyridine calcium antagonist (e.g., verapamil or diltiazem), followed by oral therapy, as initial therapy in the absence of severe LV dysfunction or other contraindications (Level of Evidence: B)." Furthermore, these guidelines endorse a class IIa recommendation for other ACS patients with recurrent ischemia already on β-blockers and nitrates: "oral long-acting calcium antagonists for recurrent ischemia in the absence of contraindications and when β-blockers and nitrates are fully used (Level of Evidence: C)." The guidelines also clearly indicate that short-acting dihydropyridines (e.g., nifedipine) are contraindicated because of their propensity to decrease blood pressure abruptly and worsen ischemia/infarction.

Chronic Therapy After Myocardial Infarction

Early Trials

Like the data for acute treatment, many studies that have investigated chronic treatment are limited by being more than a decade old. These trials started calcium-channel blockade weeks to months after MI and continued these agents long term. Data for nifedipine suggest harm, and trials evaluating verapamil and diltiazem show a nonsignificant reduction in noninfarction, although one large diltiazem trial showed this trend only in patients without CHF.[50] Taken together, the nifedipine trials demonstrate excess mortality with treatment; it is important to note that these trials had small numbers of events and used short-acting nifedipine, not controlled-release

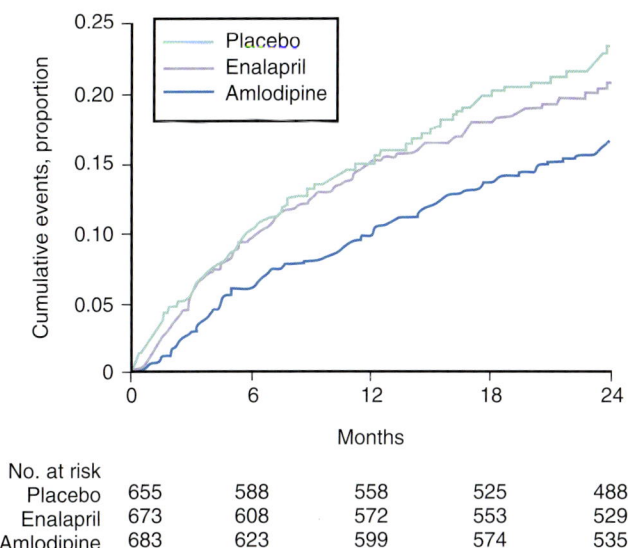

Fig. 13.4 Cumulative events in the CAMELOT trial. CAMELOT, Comparison of Amlodipine Versus Enalapril to Limit Occurrences of Thrombosis.

nifedipine. When the verapamil and diltiazem data are combined, treatment reduced reinfarction by 22% (95% CI, 33 to 0.8; P < .01).[51]

More Recent Trials

Several antihypertensive trials of calcium-channel blockers have demonstrated similar outcomes with calcium-channel blockers compared with other agents. Some of these trials have enrolled patients with a history of MI and provide reassuring data.

The CAMELOT Trial

The Comparison of Amlodipine Versus Enalapril to Limit Occurrences of Thrombosis (CAMELOT) study randomized 1991 patients with angiographically documented CAD (>20%) to amlodipine 5 to 10 mg daily, enalapril 10 to 20 mg daily, or to placebo.[52] Uniquely, these patients had "normal" blood pressure at baseline (~129/77). The primary outcome was incidence of adverse cardiovascular and cerebrovascular events that included cardiovascular death, resuscitated cardiac arrest, nonfatal MI, coronary revascularization, hospitalization for CHF, hospitalization for angina pectoris, stroke or transient ischemic attack (TIA), and any new diagnosis of peripheral vascular disease. The trial had an intravascular ultrasound (IVUS) substudy with the end point being percent change in atheroma volume. The mean age of the patients was about 57 years, and 38% of the entire population had a history of MI.

The primary end point occurred in 23.1% of placebo patients compared with 20.2% of enalapril patients and 16.6% of amlodipine patients, with significant differences between both the enalapril and amlodipine groups compared with placebo (Fig. 13.4). The amlodipine group had a statistical trend for fewer cardiovascular events compared with the enalapril group (HR, 0.81; 95% CI, 0.63 to 1.04; P = .10), and amlodipine treatment resulted in significantly fewer hospitalizations for angina (HR, 0.59; 95% CI, 0.42 to 0.84; P = .003). Of interest, amlodipine also displayed a trend for reduced atheroma progression compared with placebo (P = .12); also, amlodipine-treated patients with baseline blood pressures above mean had significantly reduced atheroma progression compared with placebo (P < .001).

The INVEST Trial

The International Verapamil-Trandolapril Study (INVEST) compared a calcium-channel blocker strategy to a non–calcium-channel blocker strategy for treatment of hypertension in CAD patients.[53] The trial randomized patients to baseline therapy of long-acting verapamil or atenolol. Patients not meeting Joint National Committee VII (JNC-7) blood pressure goals received trandolapril and/or hydrochlorothiazide. The primary end point was incidence of death, MI, or stroke.

The 22,576 enrolled patients all had documented CAD, and about 32% had a history of MI. Because secondary hypertensive therapy was not specified, secondary agents differed between the groups. The verapamil arm received more trandolapril than the atenolol arm (62.9% vs. 52.4%, $P < .001$) but received less hydrochlorothiazide (43.7% vs. 60.3%, $P < .001$). At a mean follow-up of 2.7 years, the primary end point did not differ between verapamil and atenolol arms (9.93% for verapamil vs. 10.17% for atenolol; RR, 0.98; 95% CI, 0.90 to 1.06; $P = 0.57$). Also, the primary end point did not differ according to treatment arm for patients with a history of MI (13.67% for verapamil vs. 14.38% for atenolol; RR, 0.95; 95% CI, 0.85 to 1.07).

Thus, the INVEST and CAMELOT trials confirm that long-term calcium-channel blockade is safe and efficacious in high-risk patients, even those with a history of MI. The JNC-7 guidelines recommend that post-MI patients receive ACE inhibitors and β-blockers; calcium-channel blockers have been given a "compelling indication" for patients with diabetes or high CAD risk. Most patients, of course, require multiple medications for blood pressure control, and all these data suggest that calcium-channel blockers are a reasonable part of the treatment plan.[54] Moreover, any concerns about an interaction with other agents, such as clopidogrel via the cytochrome P-450 enzymes, appear unfounded.[55]

Percutaneous Coronary Intervention

As an adjunct to PCI, calcium-channel blockers have shown beneficial effects on myocardial perfusion, particularly during a no-reflow state, and on restenosis. No-reflow phenomenon is slow epicardial flow and inadequate myocardial perfusion despite a patent epicardial vessel. Although the mechanisms of the no-reflow phenomenon are incompletely understood, many investigators believe that it occurs because of widespread microvascular dysfunction from overwhelming thromboembolism and reperfusion injury.

Because calcium-channel blockers are potent coronary vasodilators, investigators have used these agents in no-reflow states in hopes of opening the plugged microvasculature. Small studies support this idea. In a single-center, nonrandomized study, Hang and colleagues[56] administered IC verapamil to 50 acute MI patients undergoing primary PCI and compared these patients with 50 historic controls. Myocardial perfusion, as measured by thrombolysis in myocardial infarction (TIMI) perfusion grade, significantly differed with verapamil administration. Specifically, 42% of verapamil-treated patients had TIMI grade 3 flow compared with only 14% of control subjects ($P = .004$). Moreover, verapamil treatment was an independent predictor of TIMI grade (OR, 0.26; 95% CI, 0.12 to 0.58; $P = .001$).

Umemura and colleagues[57] confirmed this benefit of verapamil in patients with acute MI undergoing primary PCI. They performed Tc99m tetrofosmin single photon emission computed tomographic (SPECT) imaging before, immediately after, and 1 month after PCI in 101 acute MI patients. A no-reflow state occurred in 32 patients (31%). Verapamil administration independently predicted not only post-PCI TIMI grade 3 flow (OR, 22.4; $P = .002$) but also lower infarct size by 1 month according to SPECT imaging.

Corroborating both these studies, Huang and colleagues[58] randomized 102 patients with no-reflow phenomenon in primary PCI to receive IC diltiazem, verapamil, or nitroglycerin and found more complete ST-segment resolution at 3 hours and a lower peak troponin T level with diltiazem or verapamil compared with nitroglycerin. Finally, a recent meta-analysis found a lower 30-day wall motion index score and 2-month major adverse cardiac event (MACE) rate in ACS patients given IC verapamil during PCI.[59]

In addition to improving no-reflow states, calcium-channel blockers might also lower the incidence of restenosis. Although thus far the most effective agents for reducing neointimal hyperplasia have been sirolimus and paclitaxel, some data do exist for a beneficial effect of calcium-channel blockers in reducing restenosis. For example, recent data for benidipine, a dihydropyridine calcium-channel blocker, showed that proliferation of vascular smooth muscle cells (VSMCs) in culture was significantly reduced by benidipine.[60]

The reduction in VSMC proliferation may lead to less neointimal hyperplasia. Yamazaki and colleagues[61] showed this by randomizing 63 patients after successful coronary intervention with bare-metal stents to amlodipine 5 mg/day or quinapril 10 mg/day. Investigators performed quantitative coronary angiography before and immediately after stenting and 3 to 6 months later. Approximately 50% of each group also received IVUS at follow-up. Amlodipine-treated patients had a significantly larger minimal lumen diameter at follow-up (1.52 ± 0.53 vs. 1.88 ± 0.64 mm, $P < .01$) and a significantly smaller neointimal area (1.9 ± 0.5 vs. 2.7 ± 0.8 mm^2, $P < .01$).

This reduction in neointimal proliferation appears to lead to fewer clinical events, as demonstrated by the most recent clinical trial of calcium-channel blockade after PCI, the Verapamil Slow-Release for Prevention of Cardiovascular Events After Angioplasty (VESPA) trial.[62] The VESPA investigators randomized 700 patients after PCI using bare-metal stents to verapamil 240 mg twice daily for 6 months or placebo. Most patients (83%) received stents, and follow-up was excellent: 95% had complete clinical follow-up, and 94% received angiography at 6 months. The primary end point—a composite of death, MI, or target-vessel revascularization (TVR) by 1 year—was 19.3% for placebo patients compared with 29.3% for verapamil patients (RR, 0.66; 95% CI, 0.48 to 0.89; $P = .002$). The end point was driven by a lower risk of TVR (26.2% for placebo vs. 17.5% for verapamil; RR, 0.67; 95% CI, 0.49 to 0.93; $P = .006$). Furthermore, verapamil reduced the incidence of restenosis by 75% or more (13.7% vs. 7.8%; RR, 0.57; 95% CI, 0.35 to 0.92; $P = .014$). Despite these promising animal and clinical data, they are limited, and VESPA is a single small trial; furthermore, the advent of drug-eluting stents has significantly dampened enthusiasm for systemic therapies such as calcium-channel blockade.

Angiotensin-Converting Enzyme

ACE plays an important role in the renin-angiotensin-aldosterone system. When the kidneys sense a decrease in blood volume, the juxtaglomerular apparatus secretes renin, which catalyzes the conversion of angiotensinogen (hepatically produced) to angiotensin I. ACE, secreted by pulmonary and renal endothelial cells, converts angiotensin I to angiotensin II and also degrades bradykinin and other vasoactive peptides. Angiotensin II increases sympathetic activity, promotes aldosterone and antidiuretic hormone (ADH) release, and increases arteriolar vasoconstriction. Although these actions are helpful counterregulatory mechanisms (e.g., acute blood loss), chronic activation of this system promotes atherosclerosis, cardiomyopathy, and nephropathy.[63]

Angiotensin-Converting Enzyme Inhibitors

ACE inhibitors decrease the production of angiotensin II and prevent the degradation of bradykinin. Reduction of angiotensin II lowers arteriolar resistance, which lowers blood pressure and increases stroke volume and cardiac output. In addition to direct hemodynamic effects, ACE inhibitors have pleiotropic actions that promote favorable ventricular remodeling. For example, ACE-I inhibition prevents hypertrophy and apoptosis of cardiac myocytes and decreases myocardial fibrosis through lower collagen type 1 production and altered matrix metalloproteinase activity.[64]

Percutaneous Coronary Intervention

As an adjunctive agent to PCI, ACE inhibitors might reduce periprocedural injury according to some small trials. For example, Mangiacapra and colleagues[65] randomly assigned 40 patients undergoing elective PCI to IC enalaprilat or placebo. Patients pretreated with enalaprilat had lower peak troponin T levels. However, the small scale of this trial limits generalizing the findings.

Experimental animal models suggest that ACE inhibitors might reduce restenosis after coronary intervention with bare-metal stents,[66] although few clinical data exist to support this benefit. For example, Okimoto and colleagues[67] randomized 253 patients after coronary intervention to quinapril or placebo. Binary angiographic restenosis occurred in 34.3% of the quinapril group compared with 47.7% of the placebo group ($P < .05$). Similarly, Deftereos and colleagues[68] randomized 86 patients to quinapril or placebo after PCI and found a reduction in restenosis (9.3% vs. 25.6%, $P = .047$). Conversely, in the largest randomized trial of ACE inhibition after PCI, investigators found no reduction in restenosis.[69] With the introduction of drug-eluting stents, quality evidence regarding the true efficacy of ACE inhibitors in reducing restenosis will remain elusive.

Acute Myocardial Infarction

Numerous trials have demonstrated benefit of ACE inhibitors after MI. More than two decades ago, several investigators provided evidence that ACE inhibitors greatly attenuate unfavorable remodeling after MI. For instance, Pfeffer and colleagues[70] showed decreased end-diastolic volumes and pressures in patients given captopril after anterior MI, and large clinical trials confirmed benefit in a wide range of patients after MI.

The Survival and Ventricular Enlargement (SAVE) trial[71] randomized 2231 patients with an LVEF of 40% or less to captopril or placebo within 3 to 16 days of MI. Captopril significantly reduced recurrent MI (RR, 25%; 95% CI, 5 to 40; $P = .015$), severe heart failure (RR, 22%; 95% CI, 4 to 37; $P = .019$), and all-cause mortality (20% vs. 25%, $P = .019$). The Chinese Cardiac Study (CCS-1) also randomized patients ($n = 14,962$) after acute MI to captopril or placebo.[72] Captopril significantly reduced death or heart failure (21.5% vs. 23.1%, $P = .02$). Confirming a class effect for ACE inhibitors, the Acute Infarction Ramipril Efficacy (AIRE) trial demonstrated that ramipril reduced mortality (RR, 27%; 95% CI, 11 to 40; $P = .002$).[73] Similarly, the Gruppo Italiano per lo Studio della Sopravvivenza nell'infarto Miocardico (GISSI-3), Survival of Myocardial Infarction Long-Term Evaluation (SMILE), and Trandolapril Cardiac Evaluation (TRACE) trials demonstrated comparable benefits of lisinopril, zofenopril, and trandolapril, respectively.[74–76]

Complementing these trials was the largest and most definitive trial, ISIS-4. In this extraordinary trial, 58,050 patients within 24 hours of MI (median 8 hours) were randomized in a 2 × 2 × 2 factorial study to controlled-release mononitrate versus placebo, IV magnesium versus placebo, and 1 month of oral captopril (6.25 mg titrated up to 50 mg twice daily).[77] At 5 weeks, captopril reduced mortality significantly (7.19% vs. 7.69%, $P = .02$). Although the absolute benefit for the entire cohort was modest, higher-risk groups, such as those presenting with heart failure or a history of previous MI, benefited more (up to 10 fewer deaths per 1000 treated).

Although ACE inhibitors remain the first-line therapy in the angiotensin pathway to treat patients after MI, angiotensin-receptor blockers (ARBs) are important alternatives. In the VALIANT trial, 14,808 patients with recent MI and LV dysfunction were randomized to captopril, the ARB valsartan, or both. The primary end point, all-cause mortality, did not differ between captopril and valsartan, and combining the two conferred no additional benefit.[78]

CONCLUSION

Although the COMMIT trial suggests caution for acute IV β-blockade after MI, the data are strong for the benefit of β-blockers in the subacute and chronic treatment of patients with MI. Indeed, strong recommendations can be made for using β-blockers in all post-MI patients, particularly those with LV dysfunction. Similarly, in stable patients after MI, calcium-channel blockers can be a useful adjunct for hypertension and angina treatment. Finally, overwhelming evidence supports routine administration of ACE inhibitors after MI, particularly in those with LV dysfunction. Coupling these therapies with other well-established ones, such as antiplatelet agents and statins, is important for maximizing benefit for the patient and the public.

KEY REFERENCES

23. Lilli K, Tchong JE, Sapp S, et al. Mortality benefit of beta blockade in patients with acute coronary syndromes undergoing coronary intervention: pooled results from the Epic, Epilog, Epistent, Capture and Rapport Trials. *J Interv Cardiol*. 2003;16:299–305.
24. Miller CD, Roe MT, Mulgund J, et al. Impact of acute beta-blocker therapy for patients with non-ST-segment elevation myocardial infarction. *Am J Med*. 2007;120:685–692.
35. Chen ZM, Pan HC, Chen YP, et al. Early intravenous then oral metoprolol in 45,852 patients with acute myocardial infarction: randomised placebo-controlled trial. *Lancet*. 2005;366:1622–1632.
36. Park KL, Goldberg RJ, Anderson FA, et al. Beta-blocker use in ST-segment elevation myocardial infarction in the reperfusion era (GRACE). *Am J Med*. 2014;127:503–511.
37. Freemantle N, Cleland J, Young P, et al. beta Blockade after myocardial infarction: systematic review and meta regression analysis. *BMJ*. 1999;318:1730–1737.
38. Dargie HJ. Effect of carvedilol on outcome after myocardial infarction in patients with left-ventricular dysfunction: the CAPRICORN randomised trial. *Lancet*. 2001;357:1385–1390.
71. Pfeffer MA, Braunwald E, Moye LA, et al. Effect of captopril on mortality and morbidity in patients with left ventricular dysfunction after myocardial infarction. Results of the survival and ventricular enlargement trial. The SAVE Investigators. *N Engl J Med*. 1992;327:669–677.
78. Pfeffer MA, McMurray JJ, Velazquez EJ, et al. Valsartan, captopril, or both in myocardial infarction complicated by heart failure, left ventricular dysfunction, or both. *N Engl J Med*. 2003;349:1893–1906.

Additional references available online at expertconsult.com.

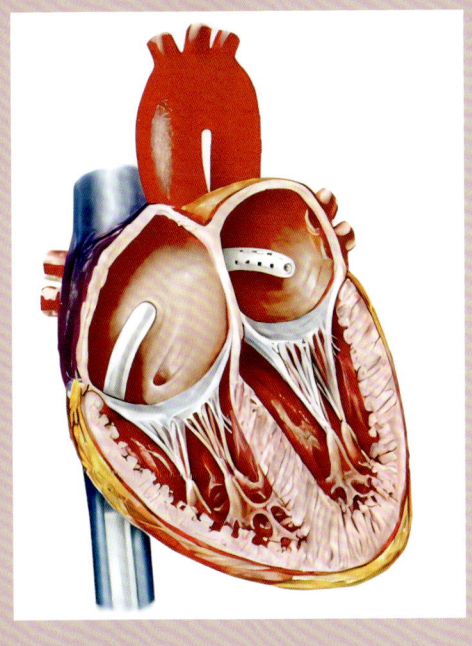

SECTION III
第三部分

Coronary Intervention

冠状动脉介入治疗

中文导读

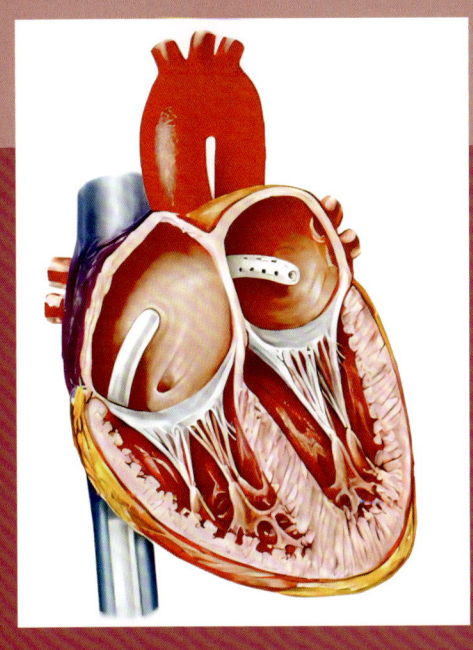

第14章
冠状动脉支架置入：实践考虑、器械选择、手术技巧和注意事项

经皮冠状动脉介入治疗是急性冠状动脉综合征患者血管重建的首选方法。此外，经皮冠状动脉介入治疗在复杂解剖病变、多支血管疾病、无保护左主干病变，以及慢性完全闭塞病变中的应用逐渐增加。而支架置入是经皮冠状动脉介入治疗常用的治疗手段。本章概述了经皮冠状动脉介入治疗手术尤其是支架置入术的实践考虑和操作技巧。

首先，正确的入路选择是支架置入术的第一步。股动脉通路曾经是介入心血管医师首选的血管入路。然而，桡动脉入路因并发症相对更少，并得到了大量临床证据的支持，目前已成为经皮冠状动脉介入治疗常用的血管入路，尤其是在女性等特定人群中。

其次，手术器械的选择对于冠状动脉支架置入术也至关重要。本章节详细讲述了指引导管、经皮冠状动脉介入治疗导丝、延长导管、微导管等手术器械的选择要点，同时阐述了支架选择，以及支架输送过程的操作重点。

最后，本章还介绍了经皮冠状动脉介入治疗相关并发症的预防，以及相关处理措施，包括冠状动脉穿孔、冠状动脉内血流受限/夹层、急性支架血栓形成、支架膨胀不良和无复流等。

刘严慈　柳景华

章节要点

- 手术入路的选择十分关键，应考虑到患者的舒适度，但最终取决于手术复杂程度，以及术者信心。
- 选择正确的指引导管以确保良好的支撑力，这是所有经皮冠状动脉介入治疗的关键。应用延长导管和改变导管形状技术，可以克服支撑力不足的问题。
- 选择冠状动脉导丝应考虑其通过病变的能力，还应考虑到达远端后导丝所能提供的支撑力。了解不同导线家族的特性，对手术成功也至关重要。
- 对于重度钙化过度和（或）迂曲的病变，包括冠状动脉粥样硬化斑块切除术在内的病变预处理至关重要。各种高级手术技术可用来协助支架的顺利输送。
- 对比剂用量最小化对患者安全至关重要。手术中可以使用各种技术减少对比剂用量，例如，使用小容量注射器、借助血管内超声指导、冠状动脉造影时利用延长导管覆盖指引导管侧孔并进行选择性造影。
- 冠状动脉支架置入的并发症并不常见，但后果很严重。然而，及时处理可以减轻并发症给患者所带来的有害影响。

SECTION III Coronary Intervention

14 Coronary Stenting: Practical Considerations, Equipment Selection, Tips and Caveats

Elliott M. Groves, Curtiss T. Stinis

KEY POINTS

- Access selection is a key decision that should encompass patient comfort, but ultimately be driven by the complexity of the case and operator confidence.
- Proper guide selection to ensure good support is key to any percutaneous coronary intervention. A lack of guide support can be overcome by the use of guide extensions and a variable guide technique.
- Coronary wire choice should encompass the ability of the wire to pass through the lesion, and the support provided by the wire after passing distally. Understanding the characteristics of wire families is also critical to success.
- For lesions with excessive calcification and/or tortuosity, proper lesion preparation including atherectomy is paramount. Stent delivery can be facilitated by several advanced procedural techniques.
- Minimizing contrast is important for patient safety. Several techniques, such as small manifold syringes, reliance on intravascular ultrasound (IVUS), and guide extensions that cover side-holes during coronary injection and can also provide selective injections, can be used.
- Complications are rare, but serious; however, proper management can mitigate any deleterious effects on the patient.

INTRODUCTION

Percutaneous coronary intervention (PCI) is the preferred modality for revascularization in patients with acute coronary syndromes. Additionally, the use of PCI in complex anatomy, multivessel disease, unprotected left main disease and chronic total occlusions (CTOs) is increasing. Due to the breadth of cases, highly variable coronary anatomy, and differing clinical scenarios, various challenges can present themselves. Fortunately, a multitude of techniques and equipment have been developed to overcome challenges and complete successful procedures. Outlined in this chapter are practical tips and techniques that can significantly improve the rate of procedural success for the interventional cardiologist.

ACCESS SITE SELECTION

The femoral artery has been the preferred access site for interventional cardiologists for decades. However, more recently, radial access has gained a significant foothold due to the reduction in access site complications and evidence of clinical benefit in ST-elevation myocardial infarction (STEMI) PCI.[1,2] However, radial artery access can present specific anatomical challenges. These challenges can be overcome, but if radial access is problematic, the femoral approach can be used to overcome many issues. Proper decision-making regarding access is critical to success.

Radial Access

Radial artery access has many advantages, though there are several possible limitations. The ultimate result of many of these limitations is the not infrequent difficulty in passing a wire and/or catheters into the aortic root. This challenge can result from a variety of circumstances including calcified radial arteries, small radial arteries, radial loops, subclavian tortuosity, heavy aortic and subclavian calcification, lack of dedicated radial equipment, and radial spasm.

Proper access to the radial artery is paramount. Anterior wall micro puncture is the most commonly used technique. With this technique, a low angle of puncture can be helpful in facilitating wire passage and sheath insertion. An additional access technique that is popular is a classic double-wall Seldinger technique using a dedicated "through and through" access system with a microcatheter over an access needle, similar in design to an angiocatheter. This technique allows for easier and more consistent passage of the wire. However, while uncommon (similar to femoral access), it can lead to hematoma formation in the radial artery due to posterior wall bleeding. Regardless of the technique used, it should be perfected and consistently applied to all cases in a repetitive manner.

The access location in the radial artery is important (Fig. 14.1). Accessing the artery too distally, over the styloid process of the radius, can result in difficult wire passage given the introduction of some tortuosity in that segment of the artery. Additionally, punctures in this area can make it difficult to apply a radial artery compression band. Punctures of the radial artery that are too proximal can also lead to difficulties and complications. Proximal punctures tend to result in sheath passage through increased soft tissue and decrease the efficacy of radial artery compression bands, resulting in an increased rate of bleeding. Optimal access is obtained approximately 1 to 2 cm proximal to the styloid process. This allows for easy wire passage, smooth sheath insertion, and optimal effectiveness of the radial artery compression band.

Frequently, operators will encounter calcified radial arteries that can present access issues. For example, the artery may deflect the needle when access is attempted. Using the radius to pin the artery with the left index finger can allow for puncture into the true lumen. This technique is also useful in mobile radial arteries. Once a calcified artery is punctured, passage of a micro puncture

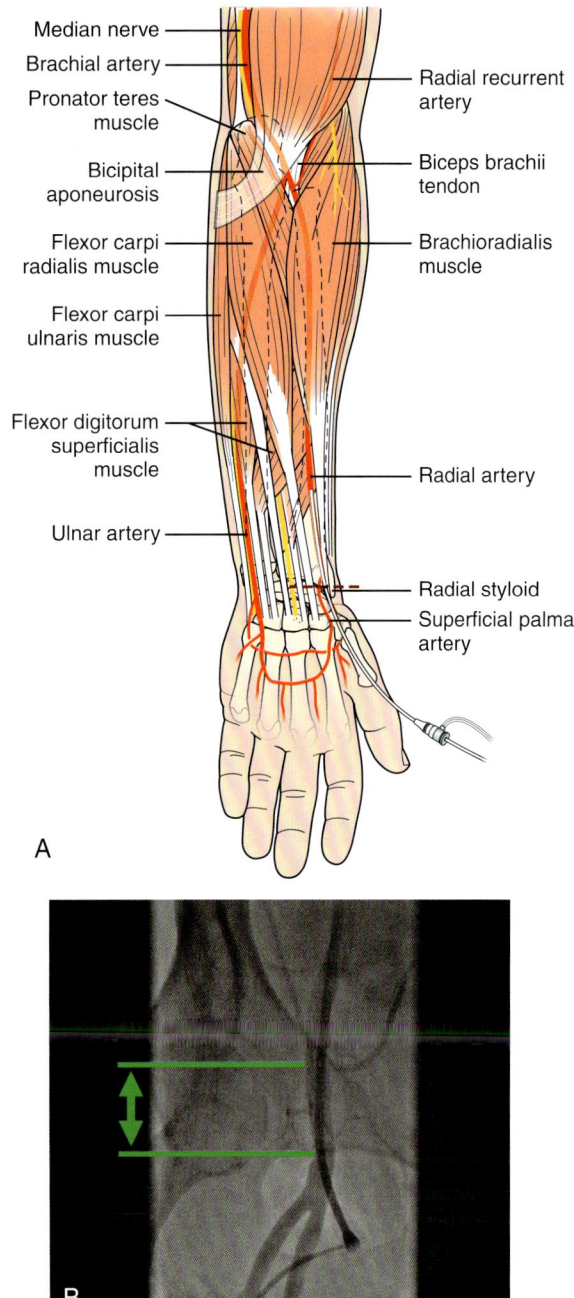

Fig. 14.1 Optimal sites of access. (A) Radial access: Optimal access site is proximal to the radial styloid. (B) Femoral access: Optimal access is within the portion of the common femoral artery (CFA), which directly overlies the pubis (defined by *green arrows*) to allow for adequate manual compression.

0.018–0.025-inch sheath wire can be difficult, as the wire is generally hydrophobic and not particularly flexible. An alternative can be the use of a 0.014-inch coronary guidewire. Typically, a workhouse wire will be able to navigate the calcification; however, under some circumstances, a polymer-jacketed wire is necessary. Operators should be careful to choose a wire with at least moderate support to facilitate sheath insertion and to avoid wire fracture. Once the sheath is inserted, the operator can either pass a small diagnostic catheter (4 or 5 Fr) over the wire (OTW) until a larger lumen is encountered, or balloon assisted tracking (BAT) can be used. Alternatively, after sheath insertion, the wire can be pulled out and a soft and steerable 0.035-inch (Wholey

[Medtronic Inc., Minneapolis, MN], Versacore [Abbott, Abbott Park, IL], or Bentson [Cook Medical, Bloomington, IN]) can be used with a Judkins Right (JR) diagnostic catheter.

Small radial arteries can be challenging. The Slender Glidesheaths (Terumo Medical, Somerset, NJ) can be very useful when adequate diagnostic images are needed, without using a sheath with a large outer diameter (OD). Alternatively, using a smaller sheath, such as 4 Fr, can be helpful. A complex intervention can be staged; alternatively, simple interventions can be completed with a 5 Fr system. Fractional flow reserve (FFR) can be completed through most diagnostic catheters if a wire-based system is used.[3] Aggressive use of antispasmodics and sedation can make a patient with a small radial artery more comfortable.[4]

Radial loops present a unique challenge. They generally can be straightened; however, even passing a wire through a loop can be difficult. A steerable soft tip 0.035-inch wire (Wholley, Versacore, Bentson) can navigate a loop, though these wires are hydrophobic and may not be able to traverse a loop. Alternatively, a coronary 0.014-inch wire can be used. Once a coronary wire has been used, it is recommended to use BAT to pass diagnostic or guide catheters into the aorta.[5] BAT is accomplished by placing a rapid exchange, semi compliant balloon halfway in and halfway out of the catheter on the wire. With the balloon inflated, the system is advanced OTW. This is analogous to the "torpedo technique" used with guide extensions (discussed later in this chapter). A 2-mm balloon can be used for 6 Fr catheters.

Subclavian tortuosity, like radial tortuosity, is challenging. Usually, the tortuosity can be navigated with either a steerable soft tip 0.035-inch wire (Wholley) or a standard angled glide wire. A multipurpose or JR diagnostic catheter will usually pass OTW into the aortic root. If the catheter will not pass, the operator can pass a small hydrophilic exchange catheter such as a CXI (Cook Medical) into the root and exchange for a stiff J-tip exchange length wire such as an Amplatz wire. In most cases, the tortuosity will straighten, and the operator can easily pass any catheter to the root. If this is not the case, there are commercially available hydrophilic diagnostic and guide catheters that will pass into the root. It is useful in these cases to use a universal catheter to minimize exchanges.

While the equipment dedicated for radial use is improving, many components still commonly used were designed for femoral use. An example of this is guide catheters. This is not an issue that can be resolved by the operator, but what can be understood is that sizing, particularly from the right radial, is generally smaller than from the femoral artery. For instance, a Judkins Left (JL) 3.5 as opposed to a JL 4 is usually a better fit from the radial, and for Contralateral Left Support (CLS; Boston Scientific, Marlborough, MA), Extra Back-Up (EBU; Medtronic Inc.) and Extra Back-Up (XB; Cordis Medical, Milpitas, CA) guides, a half size down for radial access is appropriate.

Radial spasm can make an ordinary case painful for the patient and the operator. Antispasmodics can be very helpful when given immediately after sheath insertion and between catheter exchanges. However, there is evidence that adequate moderate sedation is paramount.[6] Using 4 Fr or 5 Fr catheters also improves patient comfort.

Ultimately, radial catheterization has a steep learning curve, but with practice and using the techniques described above, it can be safely completed. Transitioning to a radial-first approach will reduce access site bleeding and hospital time for your patients.

Femoral Access

While radial access has taken a foothold, most cases in the United States are still completed via femoral access.[7] While typically devoid of many of the challenges of the radial approach, such as spasm and lack of dedicated equipment, there are many additional challenges that must be overcome. Femoral and iliac arteries can be prone to significant vascular disease, calcification, and tortuosity. Additionally, body habitus can greatly influence femoral artery access in a much more significant manner than radial access.

Accessing diseased and calcified femoral arteries must be done with care. A combination of palpation, fluoroscopy, and ultrasound can be used. With a strong femoral pulse, the operator can identify the anterior pelvis using fluoroscopy. The artery can then be accessed using a modified Seldinger technique. As opposed to using the wire provided with the sheath kit, the operator can utilize a steerable soft tip 0.035-inch wire (Wholley), with a bend that is commensurate with the size of patient's femoral artery. This allows more wire purchase and the ability to navigate through disease proximal to the access site. Polymer-jacketed wires (such as a Glidewire) should not be passed through needles because the polymer coating can be stripped off. Once the wire is safely in the true lumen of the aorta, the sheath should be inserted; however, not infrequently, the sheath may not pass through the calcified artery. The operator can pass the sheath dilator and then the full sheath and dilator, or the dilator can be used to pass a stiff wire into the aorta, then pass a long or short sheath. If there is a weak or no pulse, then ultrasound in conjunction with fluoroscopy is useful. With ultrasound, there is evidence for a reduction in complications, as one can identify a less calcified segment and ensure an anterior wall puncture.[8] It must be noted that regardless of the technique, fluoroscopy must be used to identify the anterior pubis. For optimal femoral access, the objective is to obtain a site of access which is overlying the pubis (see Fig. 14.1). This is critical in order to allow compression of the artery after sheath removal. A low puncture is not defined by the common femoral artery bifurcation, but by a puncture below the pubis. Additional common mistakes with access include a "through and through" technique which results in posterior wall bleeding and puncturing the artery with the local anesthetic needle, which also results in another non-controlled arterial puncture, even if it is small.

Iliac artery tortuosity is best navigated with a steerable soft tip 0.035-inch wire. A catheter can be used to exchange the wire for a stiff wire such as an Amplatz wire. Following this, a long sheath can be passed into the aorta. This minimizes friction and ensures that the operator does not need to repeatedly traverse the iliac artery or use an exchange length wire. When placing a long sheath, it is helpful to upsize by 1 Fr size. For example, if a 6 Fr system is desired, then pass a long 7 Fr sheath and use a 6 Fr catheter. This adds another layer of protection against friction and improves the ability to complete the procedure.

Overcoming large patient body habitus can be difficult. Use of a combination of palpation, fluoroscopy, and ultrasound is recommended. It is critical in the obese patient to access the common femoral artery over the anterior pubis. This allows the operator to have a host of hemostasis options including closure devices and manual pressure. Fluoroscopy is used to identify the pelvis, and ultrasound is then used to identify the femoral artery. Importantly, a femoral angiogram should be obtained immediately after access has been obtained, rather than performing it at the conclusion of the procedure. The rationale behind this is to expeditiously discover any acute problems that could contraindicate the use of anticoagulation or require urgent intervention (i.e., active bleeding at the access site) or possibly even require the operator to abort the PCI procedure (i.e., vascular perforation).

Ultimately, femoral artery access skills are essential even for radial operators. There will be cases where radial access is not possible. For example, if large systems, 8 Fr and above, are needed, then typically femoral access is preferred. In many CTO interventions, at least one femoral access is needed. Therefore, safe technique and proper understanding of the anatomy can improve outcomes and patient safety.

GUIDE CATHETER SELECTION

Proper selection of a guide catheter can significantly improve the chances of success with coronary interventions (Fig. 14.2). This is particularly relevant if the lesion or lesions are calcified, tortuous, or distal. Typically, guide support is dictated by the shape of the guide and the French size of the guide. Most interventions are undertaken with 5, 6, 7, or 8 Fr guides. Special consideration must also be taken for interventions that involve bifurcations or require atherectomy.

The French size (i.e., outside diameter) of a guide catheter correlates with the amount of support offered by the guide. Thus, a 7 Fr Amplatz (AL) 1 guide is typically more supportive than a 6 Fr AL 1. In addition to support, multiple other considerations must be considered. Access also dictates guide catheter selection. Radial access limits the operator somewhat. Radial sheaths come in many sizes, up to 7 Fr, which allow for 7 Fr guide catheters. However, sheath-less guides are also available, up to 7.5 Fr in most shapes, and 8.5 Fr in a limited number of shapes. What must be considered, however, is the patient's artery size and the ability for it to accommodate a large guide. For instance, a small elderly female patient would likely not be able to comfortably accommodate a 7.5 or 8.5 Fr guide in her radial artery. Larger radial guides are also associated with a significantly higher rate of radial artery occlusion. Sheath-less systems can also be cumbersome and if the wrong guide size or shape is selected, the exchange for an alternative guide is both difficult and significantly increases cost compared to the use of a second standard guide.

Beyond support, larger guide catheters are required for certain interventional techniques. When treating a bifurcation lesion, techniques such as a classic crush, simultaneous kissing stents (SKS), or V stenting require the insertion of two stents in the guide at the same time. Two simultaneous stents require a 7 Fr or larger system. Two simultaneous balloons or a stent and a balloon can be completed with a 6 Fr system allowing for a culotte, step crush, double kissing (DK) crush, or T and protrusion (TAP) to be successfully completed. Atherectomy must also be considered when choosing the size of the guide catheter. Rotablator (Boston Scientific) burr sizes range from 1.25 to 2.5 mm. The 1.25, 1.5, 1.75, and 2 mm burrs are commonly used in coronary interventions; 1.25 and 1.5 mm burrs fit through 6 Fr guides, while larger burrs usually require larger guide catheters. On the other hand, the laser (Spectranetics, Colorado Springs, CO) and orbital atherectomy (CSI, St Paul, MN) systems fit through 6 Fr guides. Orbital atherectomy systems allow for larger diameter atherectomy with the same crown by changing the speed of rotation.[9] However, this benefit is somewhat mitigated by a significant cost increase compared to the other atherectomy systems.

As important as the size of the guide is the shape of the guide. Guide catheters generally come in the same shapes as all diagnostic catheters and many more. Right-sided guide choice depends on the complexity of the intervention and the takeoff of the right coronary ostium. The anatomically straight takeoff in the left anterior oblique (LAO) projection can be amenable to multiple guides. For simple interventions and acute coronary syndrome cases, a JR guide is usually sufficient and generally very safe with a low dissection rate. With more complex cases and a typical ostium, the AL 0.75 and AL 1 guides are very supportive. These guides allow the operator to deliver devices through calcification and tortuosity. If the right coronary artery (RCA) has a standard position in the root, but quickly angles upward in the LAO projection (i.e., Shepherd's Crook), the AL guides perform best but if they cannot be manipulated into the RCA ostium, then an Internal Mammary (IM) guide or Hockey Stick guide can be very useful. An RCA with a straight anterior takeoff is best engaged with an AL

SECTION III Coronary Intervention

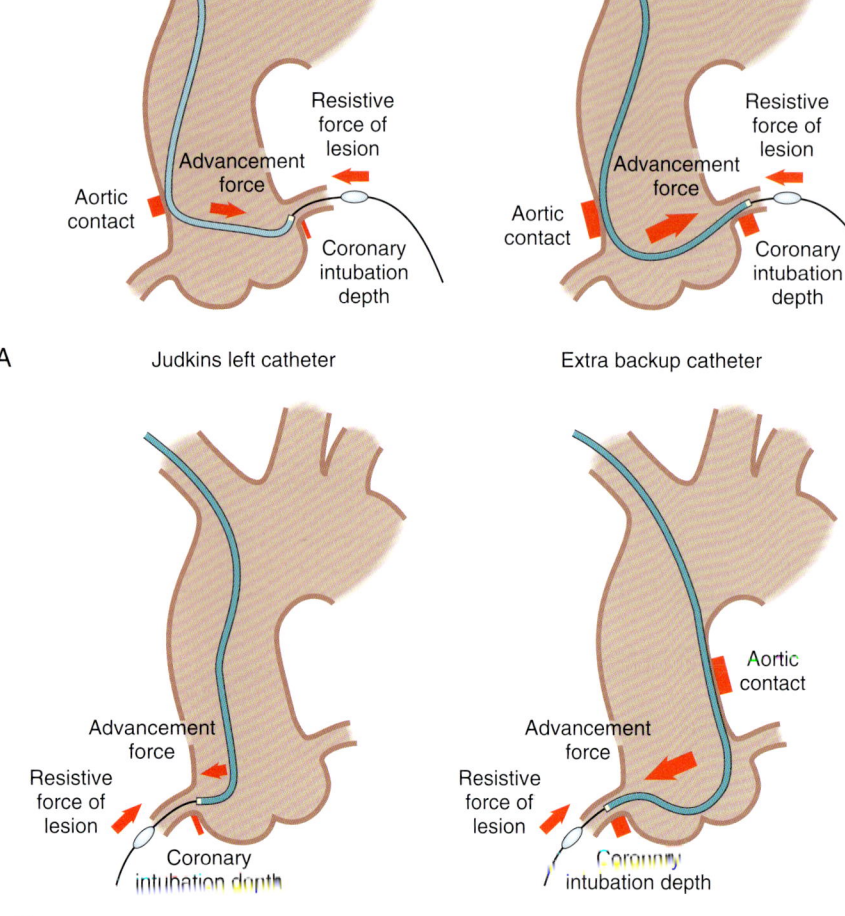

Fig. 14.2 Guide catheter selection. (A) Left Coronary System: For the left coronary system, extra backup catheter shapes (i.e., XB, CLS, EBU) allow larger advancement force due to a larger aortic contact surface area and a deeper and less angulated coronary intubation. (B) Right Coronary System: For the right coronary system, the Amplatz left catheter allows larger advancement force due to a larger aortic contact surface area and a deeper coronary intubation.

guide, while a down-going anterior takeoff can also be engaged with an multi-purpose A curve (MPA) guide in addition to an AL. There are many other guides that can be useful in certain select circumstances but should not be first-line choices. Side holes in a right-sided guide are typically useful if contrast limits allow. This results in reduced damping and can significantly reduce complications.

Left-sided guides are, again, available in many shapes. However, by far the most supportive guides are the backup support guides (XB, EBU, and CLS shapes). Using a JL or another non-supportive guide is a mistake that can lead to complications and increased case time and cost. Ultimately, in any complex case, the use of a JL instead of a backup support guide will likely lead to the need for a guide extension, which is an expensive addition to any case. In extreme circumstances, a custom guide can be created with the use of a heat gun or a sterile hot water bath. However, this should be limited to the most experienced operators.

Proper guide choice is an important aspect of a coronary intervention and many factors need to be taken into consideration. However, using a systematic approach and understanding the complexities of the case will lead to proper choices and success. Operator familiarity with a selection of guides will also lead to improved success and decision making.

GUIDE EXTENSIONS

Despite the proper selection of a supportive guide that is coaxial and well engaged, there will be cases where delivery of devices, particularly stents, is difficult. While there are many techniques that will be discussed to overcome this issue, few are more useful or successful than the addition of a guide extension. A guide extension is essentially a tube that is smaller than the guide with an atraumatic tip controlled with a metal extension that come in a variety of sizes and lengths (6 Fr, 7 Fr, 8 Fr, 145 cm, and 150 cm). The guide extension can be passed either into the proximal artery to create more aortic back support or can be passed via several techniques into the mid to distal vessel to serve ostensibly as a "highway" for device delivery. Additionally, when a guide cannot quite reach the coronary ostium and multiple attempts have failed, the operator can free-wire the vessel and then pass a guide extension OTW to create a custom guide. An important caveat to use of guide extensions is that, when used, the guide size has been decreased. A 6 Fr guide extension means it fits in a 6 Fr guide, but it functions as a 5 Fr guide or smaller. Therefore, some intravascular ultrasound (IVUS) catheters will not fit through them, using multiple wires is difficult, and delivering multiple devices is nearly impossible.

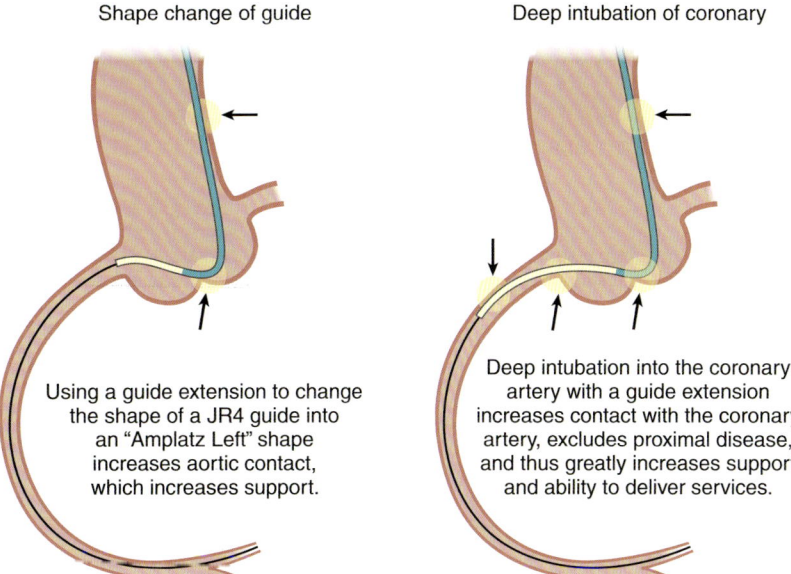

Fig. 14.3 The "Variable Guide Technique." Example of the "Variable Guide" technique using a Judkins Right 4 (JR4) catheter and a guide extension catheter.

Most commonly, the guide extension is used to create a variable guide (Fig. 14.3). This can be as simple as extending a JR guide into the RCA when engagement is poor, or to push the guide to the back wall of the aorta to create backup support. More advanced variable guide techniques include the "inchworm" and "torpedo." When distal delivery is difficult despite adequate pre-dilation and even atherectomy, a guide extension can be advanced using serial proximal-to-distal balloon inflations. Typically, for the "inchworm," a 2.5–mm- or 3–mm-compliant balloon is inflated to nominal pressure in the proximal vessel and then deflated.[10] While the balloon is deflating, the guide extension is tracked over the balloon to its distal tip, but not past, while the balloon stays stationary. The balloon is then advanced a balloon length once the guide extension is at its distal tip, and the process is repeated until the guide extension is adequately distal. Following this, stents can either be unsheathed or more easily delivered. Unless the operator plans on stenting the entire section of proximal vessel, this technique must be approached with great caution, as the proximal vessel will be undergoing angioplasty without stenting and may suffer dissection as a result.

A second effective and safe technique for advancement of a guide extension is the "torpedo."[10] This is very similar to BAT discussed earlier, except in the coronary artery. A 2- to 2.5- mm balloon is inflated halfway into the distal tip of the guide extension to lower than nominal pressures. The entire system is then advanced as a unit until an adequate distal position is achieved. This avoids balloon dilation of large sections of ultimately unstented vessel. However, this technique is typically more difficult in proximally diseased vessels.

The anchor technique is defined by a distal balloon inflation and then the passage of the guide extension over the shaft of the balloon while the balloon remains inflated.[10] This technique is by far the most dangerous and is not generally recommended. Although technically easier, if there is any tortuosity in the vessel, the guide extension can cause a large flow limiting dissection, and therefore if this technique is utilized, the operator should be prepared to extensively stent the proximal vessel. In addition, a distally positioned guide extension has the benefit of allowing excellent visualization of the vessel with lower contrast administration. One should take care, however, not to perform a high-volume and/or high-pressure injection through a distally positioned guide extension catheter; otherwise, extensive vessel dissection and/or perforation can occur.

One additional use of a guide extension is to close guide side-holes during contrast injection. The guide extension is pulled back during equipment manipulations to allow coronary flow via the side-holes and extended prior to each coronary injection to cover the side-holes.

Being facile with guide extensions is critical for any operator who performs complex interventions. They can be invaluable for device delivery. However, they must be used with care, and distal insertion can result in complications when care and proper technique is not utilized.

CORONARY GUIDEWIRE SELECTION

Coronary guide wires are a very personal choice among operators; however, particularly when a workhorse wire is insufficient, it is important to make proper wire choices moving forward. First-line wire choices or workhorse wires are typically wires with a hydrophobic low gram tip (<1.5 g) that is spring coiled. Modern workhorse wires usually have a hydrophilic body past the first 3 cm, which allows the body of the wire to pass easily through lesions once the tip of the wire has successfully navigated into the true lumen distal to the lesion. Using a polymer-jacketed hydrophilic wire or high gram tip wire for frontline use is not recommended. These wires have a much higher rate of perforation and dissection. It is very difficult to dissect or perforate with an appropriately chosen workhorse wire.

Workhorse and Specialty Crossing Wires

In a non-CTO lesion, there can occasionally be difficulty passing a workhorse wire distal to the lesion. When this difficulty is encountered, it is typically due to excessive tortuosity, a high grade or subtotal occlusion, or extensive calcification. After attempting and failing to wire with a workhorse wire, escalating to an alternative wire is necessary. Different scenarios require differing choices. When excessive tortuosity is encountered, the spring coils of the workhouse wire and the body arc likely causing friction; therefore, a polymer-jacketed hydrophilic wire will typically work well. However, excess penetrating force is not needed. Therefore, a low gram tip, hydrophilic wire works well; examples

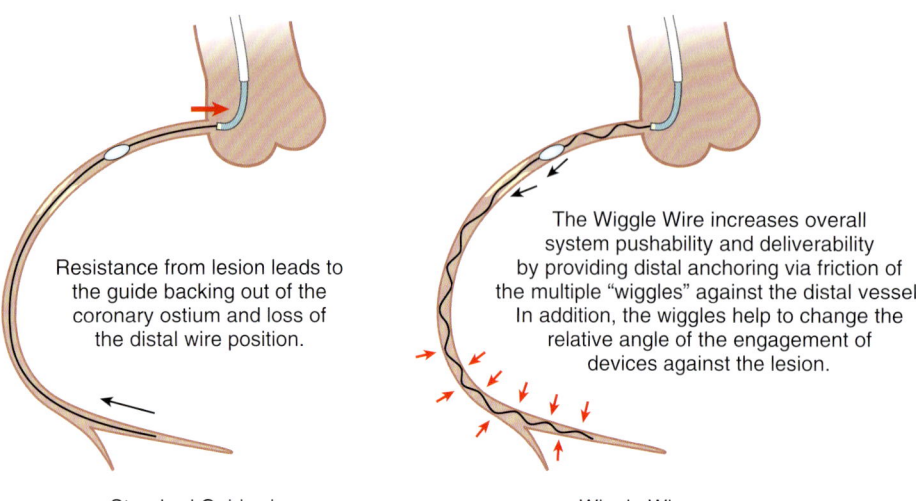

Fig. 14.4 The Wiggle Wire.

are the Pilot 50 (Abbott), Whisper (Abbott), Sion Black (Asahi Intecc, Aichi, Japan), and Fielder FC (Asahi Intecc). These wires all have a gram tip ≤1.5 g and thus have a lower risk of perforation or dissection while allowing smooth passage distally.

If a subtotal occlusion or long high-grade calcified lesion is not amenable to passage of a workhorse wire, a hydrophilic wire is also an excellent choice. In this case, however, the selection varies slightly. With a small channel, a tapered tip wire with a low gram tip can be used in lieu of a wire with a higher gram tip. These wires will typically pass through most non-CTO lesions with antegrade flow. Examples include the Fielder XT (Asahi Intecc), Fielder XT-A (Asahi Intecc), and the Fighter (Boston Scientific). By utilizing a lower gram tip, perforation is far less likely while achieving the required results. However, if more penetrating force is needed, there are several wires with a moderate tip load which can be used. It should be noted that it is usually still necessary to use a polymer-jacketed wire such as a Pilot 150 (2.7 g) (Asahi Intecc) or PT2 (2.9 g) (Boston Scientific). Typically, wires with a higher gram tip load are reserved for CTO lesions, which are discussed separately.

Occasionally, a wire can pass into branches just proximal to or at the primary lesion in a non-CTO case; however, it will not pass through the lesion. This can facilitate the progressive true lumen technique, where the wire is used to deliver a small balloon for gentle dilation in hopes of facilitating passage of a new wire into another more distal branch for further dilation, or into the distal true lumen. Once a branch in the lesion is dilated, an OTW system can be used to exchange for a highly angulated hydrophilic wire to reach the distal true lumen, then exchange for a workhorse or extra support wire.

Extra Support Wires

Once a lesion is crossed with a wire of the operator's choice, this wire is typically used to deliver devices into the coronary artery for treatment of the lesion or lesions. However, on occasion, device delivery is difficult. In this case, as previously discussed, guide extensions can be very helpful. However, there are many circumstances where an alternative strategy is preferred, given the potential complications of distal passage of a guide extension. In these cases, the use of an extra support wire can accomplish the goal.

Extra support wires (Ironman [Abbott], Grandslam [Asahi Intecc], Mailman [Boston Scientific]) are wires with a low gram hydrophobic tip and a stiff body that provides a strong rail for delivery. Due to the nature of these wires, they are very difficult to pass primarily; thus, an exchange must be made. If difficulty is anticipated before primary wiring, then the operator can insert his or her workhorse or specialty wire into a microcatheter or OTW balloon, wire the lesion, and then use this OTW device to exchange for an extra support wire. Alternatively, if this difficulty is not anticipated, but arises and a short (190 cm) wire has been used, a trap balloon can be inserted into the guide catheter to facilitate passage of a microcatheter or OTW balloon. Another strategy is the use of a wire extension, which extends the wire to 300 cm, but is ultimately removable. Of note, the Trapper (Boston Scientific) exchange device allows for using the trap technique in a 6 Fr guide. Once the extra support wire has been delivered distally, the exchange catheter is removed by either using a 300 cm extra support wire, a hydroplane technique, wire extension, or trapping. Repeat intervention is then attempted with likely improved results.

An alternative to a classic extra support wire is the Wiggle Wire (Abbott) (Fig. 14.4). The Wiggle Wire has a low gram hydrophobic tip and a moderately stiff body. The Wiggle Wire is unique in that mechanistically the "wiggles" in the wire contact the walls of the distal vessel in multiple locations, providing friction and anchoring of the distal portion of the wire, and it also reduces wire bias by changing the angle of delivered devices to the vessel wall over its course. This wire is very useful and overcomes one of the main criticisms of the classic support wires, which is wire bias. The Wiggle Wire can be inserted in the same manner as other extra support wires and cannot be used for primary wiring. Of note, when being removed, the Wiggle Wire can draw the guide into the coronary; thus, care must be taken.

CORONARY MICROCATHETERS AND OVER THE WIRE BALLOONS

Coronary microcatheters and OTW balloons were briefly discussed above. Here we will discuss their use as exchange devices. The OTW balloon is also used as a balloon dilation system by some operators, although this technique is less popular since the introduction of rapid exchange systems. These devices can both be used for wire exchanges; however, the coronary microcatheters are a superior option. Wire exchanges are necessary as discussed above when an extra support wire is needed. They are also necessary when a specialty wire is to be used, or when primary wiring with a Rotawire (Boston Scientific) or Viperwire (CSI) is not possible prior to atherectomy.

Microcatheters are low profile, hydrophilic coated devices with an internal metal braid and a soft, atraumatic, typically

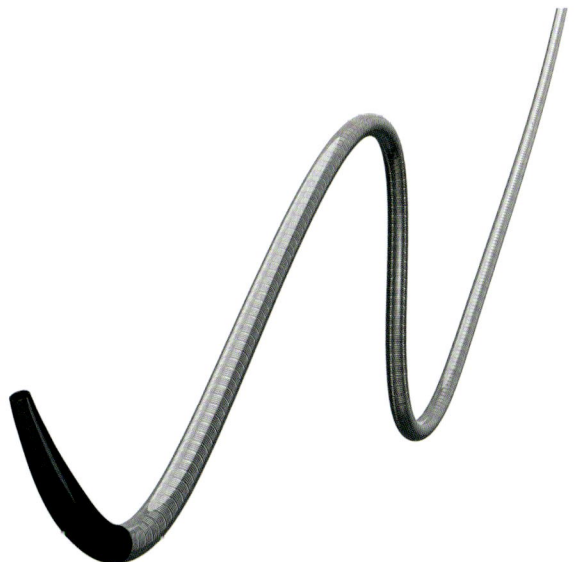

Fig. 14.5 Microcatheters. Asahi-Intecc Corsair Pro, an example of a commonly used micro catheter. This micro catheter shares many characteristics with other micro catheters, including a tapered tip, hydrophilic coating, and internal braiding. (With permission from Asahi Intecc USA.)

tapered tip. Examples are the Asahi Corsair and Corsair Pro (Asahi Intecc), Turnpike and Turnpike LP (Teleflex Inc, Wayne, PA), and the Finecross (Terumo Medical) (Fig. 14.5). These devices are specifically designed to cross through tortuosity, calcifications, and most coronary lesions, even a CTO. Due to the internal braid, the device can be advanced by both pushing and catheter rotation. These design characteristics make these devices superior to OTW balloons, which can only be pushed across lesions. However, if the exchange is simple, an OTW balloon can be considered and is certainly lower in cost.

Ultimately, the operator must assess the need for microcatheters and become familiar with their use. As with any equipment choice, it is in the operator's best interest to choose a specific microcatheter, familiarize his- or herself with its characteristics, and master its use.

STENT SELECTION

There is an extensive discussion in this text elsewhere regarding the currently available stent platforms. Thus, this section will focus on imparting some techniques that can be helpful in stent delivery that are specific to the stent itself. Stent delivery is the ultimate goal of any coronary intervention; therefore, delivery is imperative. Many techniques discussed here can facilitate that delivery, in addition to those techniques discussed previously and in the forthcoming sections.

Each stent platform has different characteristics, but also share many properties as well. One such shared characteristic is the longer the stent, the more difficult it will be to deliver when compared directly to a shorter stent from the same manufacturer. Every coronary operator has attempted to pass a long stent distally, only to have the leading 20 mm of the stent deliver, but the remaining length will not pass. A simple technique is to place multiple short stents as opposed to one long stent when a long stent will not pass. For instance, two 22 mm stents will cover the same lesion that a 38 mm stent will cover with a short overlap. Using shorter stents can allow an operator to finish a case without employing more advanced techniques. Of course, this technique is a more expensive solution and is only relevant if a longer stent of reasonable length will deliver (i.e., placing four or five overlapping 8 mm-stents is not appropriate).

One significant source of variability between stent platforms is the flexibility of the stent itself. Radial strength can be sacrificed for a more open cell stent design that is more deliverable, particularly through a tortuous vessel. If the operator has access to multiple stent platforms and one does not deliver, then another platform with different characteristics can be considered. Using a different platform is also relevant when considering vessel tapering, or bifurcation lesions. Understanding that many stents of the same platform are the same metal scaffold mounted on different balloon sizes can help the operator plan for proximal optimization and vessel tapering. For instance, in some platforms such as the Synergy stent (Boston Scientific), the 2.25, 2.5, and 2.75 mm stents are the same small vessel stent, whereas in the Resolute Onyx (Medtronic Inc.), the 2.75 mm stent is the same as the 3 mm stent and larger than the 2.25 and 2.5 mm. This allows a 2.75 mm Resolute Onyx to be post dilated to a larger diameter (4.4 mm) than a 2.75 mm Synergy (3.6 mm). However, this may also make the 2.75 mm Onyx less deliverable. The important take away from this point is that the operator must understand the individual characteristics of each stent platform he or she uses, as there are many important differences.

Stent selection is a critical aspect of coronary interventions and thus it is discussed in detail in this text. Here we provide a few useful tips for completing stent deployment based on stent characteristics. However, there are many more important aspects of stents of which interventionalists who do complex procedures should be aware.

FACILITATED STENT DELIVERY

When the use of a supportive wire or a guide extension fails to aid in stent delivery, there are additional techniques that can be used. These involve the use of additional coronary wires and balloons to either improve support or reduce bias. The first of these techniques and the simplest is the use of a buddy wire, or the placement of a wire in the coronary artery parallel to the wire that is being used for device delivery (Fig. 14.6).[11] A buddy wire is a low-cost method to increase guide support and reduce bias. Buddy wiring can reduce balloon movement during angioplasty as well, particularly in restenosis cases. The technique is particularly useful in cases with poor guide support, lesions with proximal tortuosity/angulations, distal lesions, anomalous coronaries, and lesions distal to previously placed stents.

If a buddy wire is insufficient, the use of a buddy balloon can facilitate stent delivery distally.[11] Again, this technique reduces bias and improves guide support in a similar manner to the buddy wire, but with a bulkier device. A secondary balloon can also be inflated for support. This is referred to as an anchor balloon.[12] To use this technique, a secondary wire is typically passed into a different branch of the artery than where the stent is to be delivered, and a balloon is passed over it. This balloon is then inflated to stabilize the guide and provide excellent support to either deliver a stent or a balloon to the target lesion. An anchor balloon can be useful in a host of circumstances such as when a TAP stent is being delivered into the side branch, or when a balloon will not pass through a CTO or subtotal occlusion for pre-dilation. In certain circumstances, the balloon can be inflated in the same vessel distal to where stent delivery is desired. When doing this, it is safest if the balloon is in an area that either will be stented or has been stented.

Familiarization with facilitated stent delivery techniques can make the difference between completing a successful PCI and failure. The use of buddy wires and buddy balloons, including an anchoring balloon, are relatively simple techniques that are very effective and should be in the armamentarium of all coronary operators.

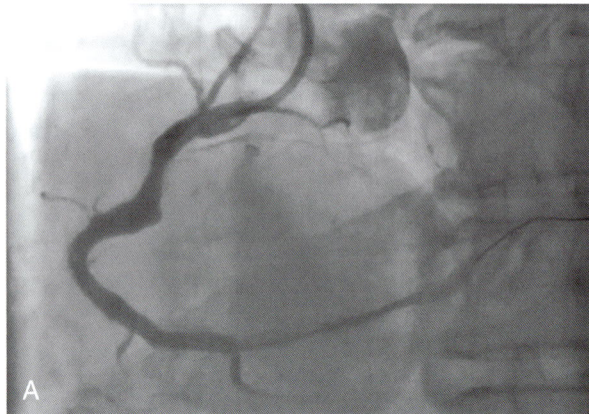
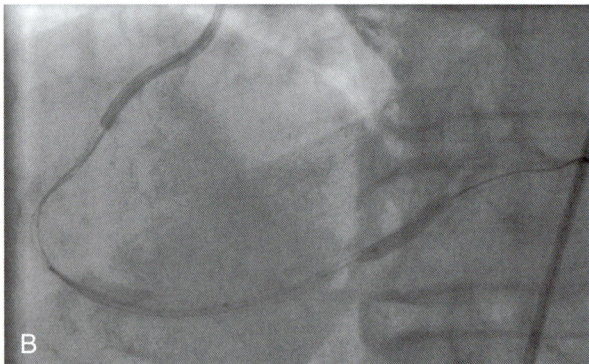
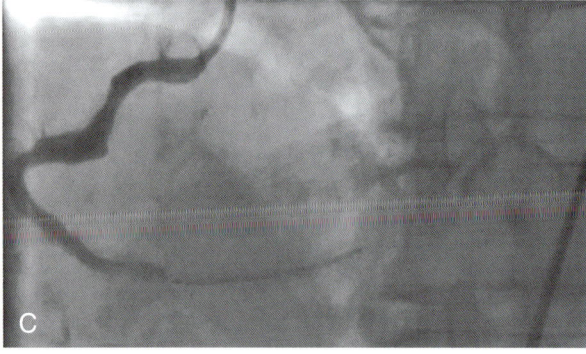

Fig. 14.6 Buddy wire and anchor balloon technique. Example of the buddy wire and anchor balloon technique. (A) A stent could not be advanced through the tortuous mid right coronary artery (RCA) lesion despite adequate guide support with an Amplatz Left 1 (AL1) guide. (B) A buddy wire was subsequently inserted, and a buddy balloon inserted and inflated across the diseased segment while a stent was advanced simultaneously over the first wire through the mid RCA. (C) Once the stent passed through the mid RCA, the buddy wire and balloon were removed, and the stent successfully deployed.

CORONARY ATHERECTOMY

Guide catheter selection with respect to atherectomy devices has already been previously discussed; however, there are several more practical aspects of its use that will be reviewed here, given that lesion preparation in complex coronary intervention is critical. In many cases, balloon pre-dilation affords inadequate lesion preparation, and stent under-expansion is associated with increased rates of in-stent restenosis; thus, atherectomy serves an important role in complex PCI.

Understanding the properties of each atherectomy system is important. Laser atherectomy is a focused beam that projects directly forward (Fig. 14.7). Although it is the most cost-effective atherectomy system, it is also felt to be the least efficacious and should only be used in select circumstances such as under-expanded stents and impenetrable proximal caps of CTOs. The specific laser technique used to treat an under-expanded stent will be discussed later. Rotational atherectomy is the most versatile of the atherectomy devices, given its leading-edge cutting ability and range of burr sizes. As mentioned previously, one needs to consider the guide catheter size when using rotational atherectomy if large burr sizes are needed. However, in most cases, a 1.5 mm burr is sufficient. One important caveat of Rotablator is the burr shape. The 1.25 mm burr is shaped differently than the other burrs, with a blunt back end, and this can lead to a higher risk of burr entrapment, so it should be used with caution. If only a wire can be passed into the distal lumen and atherectomy is needed, rotational atherectomy is the best choice since orbital atherectomy crowns may not pass. Also, it is important to remember that rotational atherectomy is only ablating plaque while moving proximally to distally and not in reverse.

Orbital atherectomy is the most recent addition to coronary atherectomy. A crown is mounted on a catheter and spins in an orbit, providing radial cutting.[13] The leading edge has no cutting surface, so if nothing will pass distal to the lesion, the crown will likely not pass, either. However, in other circumstances, the system can be useful and provides excellent results. As the crown can be adjusted to differing speeds, the radius of atherectomy achieved with a 6 Fr guide is the largest of any system. Additionally, the device performs atherectomy while passing distally and when returning toward the guide. In some cases, it is advantageous to pass the crown distal to the lesion and perform the first run coming back proximally. This can provide the ability to only treat a more precise area of the vessel, which could minimize complications. There has also been the suggestion of a lower rate of dissection with orbital atherectomy, although this is anecdotal since there has been no head-to-head comparison done with other atherectomy systems.

Atherectomy is increasing in popularity as the complexity of coronary disease treated with PCI increases. Diffusely calcified lesions, and lesions which prevent the passage of standard balloons, are ideal targets for atherectomy.[14] Although atherectomy is used somewhat infrequently, it is a complex modality, and understanding the systems and their strengths is important.

CONTRAST AND RADIATION SPARING

In an age of increasing complexity and CTO PCI, it is critical to remember the deleterious effects of excessive contrast and radiation on the patient. Contrast is necessary to define the anatomy; however, it does not need to be used with reckless abandon. Once the anatomy is defined, a careful plan for the procedure with placement of a roadmap in the lab will serve to minimize contrast on its own. However, this is frequently insufficient by itself. One frequently used technique in patients with chronic kidney disease (CKD) or acute kidney injury (AKI) is the use of a 3-mL syringe on the manifold setup. This precludes the injection of more than 3 mL at a time and can greatly reduce the total contrast use. It should also be noted that in patients with CKD or AKI, a manifold is far more effective at reducing contrast when compared to a power injector. In addition, or in place of a small syringe, a guide extension can be advanced OTW into the branch being intervened upon. For instance, if the left anterior descending (LAD) is being treated, a guide extension can be advanced into the proximal LAD to avoid the wasted contrast spilling into the left circumflex and aorta. IVUS can also be very useful to minimize contrast. After one setup image, the IVUS can then be used to define the distal and proximal landing zones and for vessel sizing.[15] Once stents have been deployed, IVUS can be used

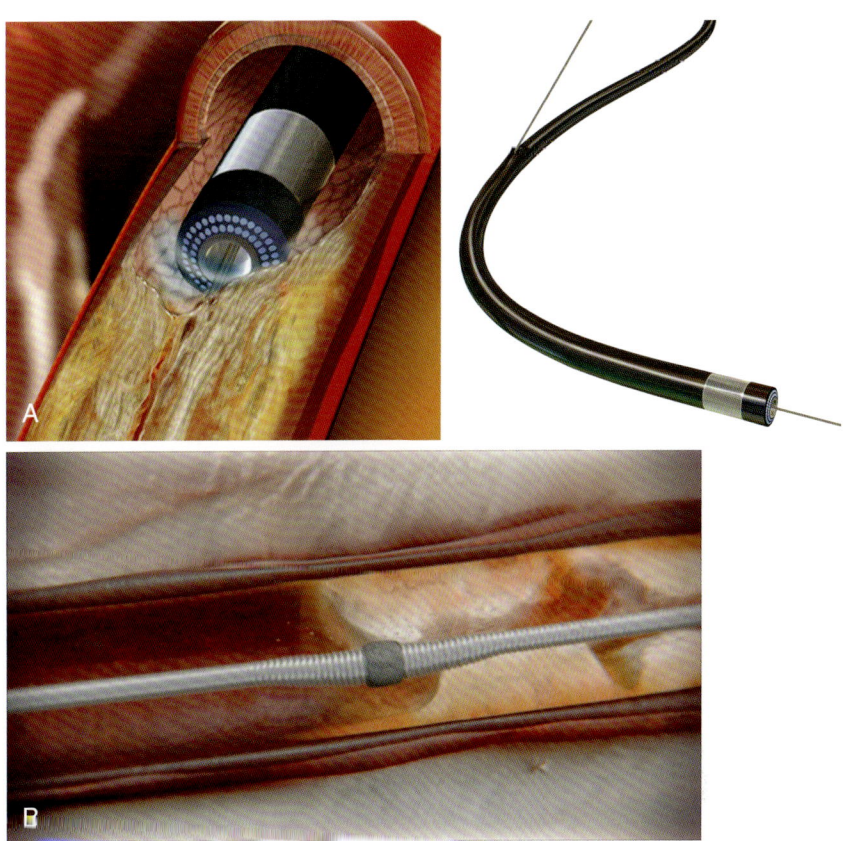

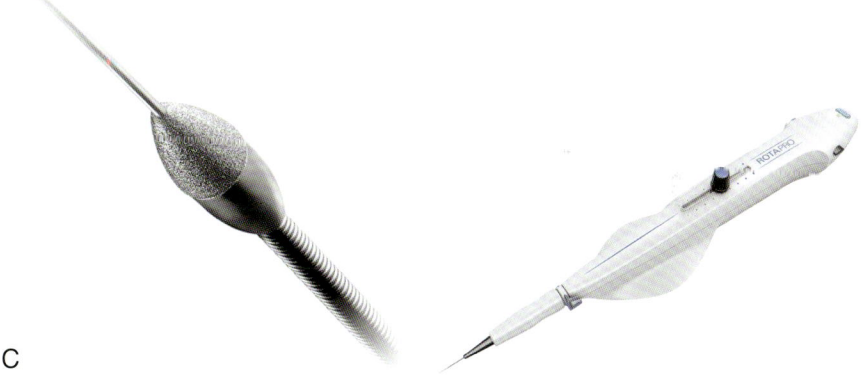

Fig. 14.7 Currently available coronary atherectomy devices. (A) Spectranetics Laser Atherectomy System, (B) CSI Atherectomy System. (C) Boston Scientific Rotablator Atherectomy System. ([A] Courtesy of Royal Philips. [B] ©2018 Cardiovascular Systems, Inc. CSI®, Diamondback 360®, GlideAssist®, ViperWire Advance® and ViperSlide® are registered trademarks of Cardiovascular Systems, Inc., and used with permission. [C] Image provided courtesy of Boston Scientific. © 2018 Boston Scientific Corporation or its affiliates. All rights reserved.)

to determine if there is proper expansion and if post dilation is needed, and whether the proximal and distal edges have any evidence of dissection or hematoma. A final image can be then be obtained to ensure nothing is missed and to exclude perforation. An entire PCI can be completed with only two or three low-contrast angiograms.

Radiation reduction is a topic important to both the patient and the operator. Standard techniques are critical and well defined (Table 14.1). Using low frame rate and low detail fluoroscopy/cine, utilizing fluoroscopy store as opposed to cine, minimizing the use of extreme angles, and ensuring the detector is as close to the patient as possible are techniques that can help minimize radiation exposure with respect to the fluoroscopy equipment. Personal safety is also important for the operator. Lead aprons should be frequently checked for cracks and be stored properly. All operators should wear radiation badges and monitor their exposure. Radiation pads placed on the patients and proper positioning of the radiation shields are also important steps to protect the operator. Finally, there are new radiation minimizing systems that can be purchased and should be explored by institutions who have out dated equipment.

MANAGEMENT OF COMPLICATIONS

Complications are an unfortunate consequence of any invasive procedure. However, the acute management is of critical importance. The most commonly encountered complications are coronary perforation, flow limiting dissections, acute stent thrombosis, no reflow phenomena, and stent under-expansion/regret.[1] Dealing with complications expeditiously prevents morbidity and mortality to the patient and can become routine with a systematic approach.

TABLE 14.1 Radiation Reduction Techniques		
Reduction to Patient	**Reduction to Operator**	**Reduction to Both**
Increase table height	Protective garments	Limit radiation usage
Vary beam angle	Increase distance from source	Decrease cine use
Keep extremities out of beam	Optimize shielding	Minimize steep angles
	Keep hands/arms out of beam	Keep detector close to patient
	Robotic cath lab	Decrease frame rate
		Collimate
		Real-time dose monitoring

Coronary perforations can be rapidly fatal due to the development of cardiac tamponade; however, rapid exclusion of the perforation can stop the development of an effusion and in many cases render pericardiocentesis unnecessary (Fig. 14.8). In a patient with normal renal function, it is good practice to at least give a 1 or 2 mL injection of contrast after any arterial dilation or stent placement. The angioplasty balloon or the stent balloon should be withdrawn into the guide and the contrast administered. This allows rapid identification of a perforation. Once a perforation is identified, the balloon should be rapidly inserted into the coronary and inflated across the perforation for several minutes. Operators should be very hesitant to reverse anticoagulation, particularly if stents have been placed, as this can lead to guide and stent thrombosis, which can be fatal. Either immediately in the case of a large perforation, or in case of a small perforation, after it has been identified that balloon tamponade is insufficient, a second access point should be obtained. The primary guide should then be withdrawn over the shaft of the inflated balloon several centimeters into the aorta to make room for a new guide to be passed from the secondary access and engaged in the coronary. A new wire is then passed to the inflated balloon, the balloon is quickly deflated, the second wire is quickly passed distally, and then the balloon is reinflated. With the tamponade balloon inflated, a covered stent can be passed from the second guide to the level of the perforation. The tamponade balloon is then deflated, the covered stent is then quickly positioned, the tamponade balloon and its wire are removed, and the covered stent is then quickly deployed. Aggressive post dilation of a covered stent can be required to be sure an adequate seal has been obtained. Once it has been confirmed that the perforation has been sealed, the case can be finished or aborted, depending on the clinical circumstances. This technique is referred to as "ping pong guides."[16]

Flow limiting dissections can occur as a result of overly aggressive pre-dilation, oversized stents, atherectomy and guide, or wire dissection. With a wire distally in the true lumen, a balloon should be rapidly inserted and used for gentle angioplasty and restoration of flow. The dissection can then be assessed and treated with PCI. It is important to not inject contrast excessively in the setting of a dissection, as it can hydraulically propagate the dissection plane. Edge dissection is easily treated with another stent, presuming the wire has not been removed. If it has, careful wiring and re-stenting is the treatment. Guide and wire dissections which become flow limiting are the most difficult to treat, as the true lumen is not secured distally. As mentioned previously, no further contrast should be injected, and prompt wiring is critical. A workhouse wire may pass distally; however, the spring coils on typical workhorse wires tend to bunch in the dissection and will not pass distally. Therefore, the use of a polymer-jacketed wire is typically needed. Extreme caution must be used, as, although the wire will pass between the membranes into the distal true lumen, it will also rapidly propagate dissections with less feedback if passed into the dissection plane. Another option is to use a guidewire with a very floppy distal segment, like the Sion guide wire (Asahi-Intecc) that is less likely to extend the dissection. Once the distal lumen is secured, angioplasty followed by stenting is the definitive treatment.

Acute stent thrombosis can also be rapidly fatal and must be treated with expediency. With a wire distally, balloon angioplasty should rapidly be performed to restore flow, followed by imaging to determine if there is a mechanical cause. Anticoagulation status should be reassessed, and the operator should consider administration of Cangrelor (Chiesi USA, Cary, NC) or a glycoprotein IIb IIIa inhibitor if adequate antiplatelet therapy is lacking. If the thrombosis presents after completion of the case and the patient has left the catheterization lab, then the situation should be treated as a STEMI with the exception of the fact that intravascular imaging is imperative. The operator must identify if there is any mechanical issue with the stent or vessel that prompted the thrombosis. In some cases, re-stenting may be required.

No reflow is a result of micro or occasionally macro emboli that congest the micro circulation and impair runoff.[17] Most commonly seen in vein graft interventions and ACS cases, it can also be seen after atherectomy. No amount of treating the large epicardial coronary vessels will solve the problem—proper treatment requires local delivery of agents to dilate the microvasculature. Either an OTW balloon, microcatheter, or Twin Pass catheter (Teleflex Inc.) should be passed distally, and verapamil, nitroprusside, or adenosine should be locally administered. A second dose can be given if full resolution is not achieved. Administering these agents through the guide catheter is not sufficient, since the lack of flow in the coronary vessel will prevent the drugs from reaching the microcirculation.

Stent under-expansion, also known as "stent regret," can be troublesome to deal with. The first-line treatment should be high pressure non-compliant balloon inflation. A balloon which is particularly useful in this regard is the Chocolate balloon (QT Vascular, Singapore), since it can be taken to very high pressures without rupturing (off label). If these techniques do not work, the laser atherectomy catheter can be set at 80/80 (fluence/repetition rate) and laser atherectomy can be performed within the stent with a contrast injection as opposed to saline. While the exact mechanism is unclear, this technique seems to direct the laser energy radially instead of longitudinally due to scatter against the iodine atoms within the contrast medium and this improves compliance of the surrounding coronary tissue. Repeating a high-pressure inflation then allows for expansion of the stent in many cases. This technique should be used with extreme caution since it can lead to vessel perforation and/or no reflow due to distal embolization of particles or of nitrogen gas bubbles which are released from the interaction of blood with laser energy.

Complications can arise during PCI procedures even in the best of hands. Of paramount importance is the treatment of any complication in an expeditious and organized way in order to minimize harm to the patient. Many of the techniques described herein can help achieve proper management in these challenging situations.

CONCLUSION

With an aging population and increasing complexity of disease being treated with PCI, there is a need for the dissemination of

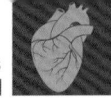

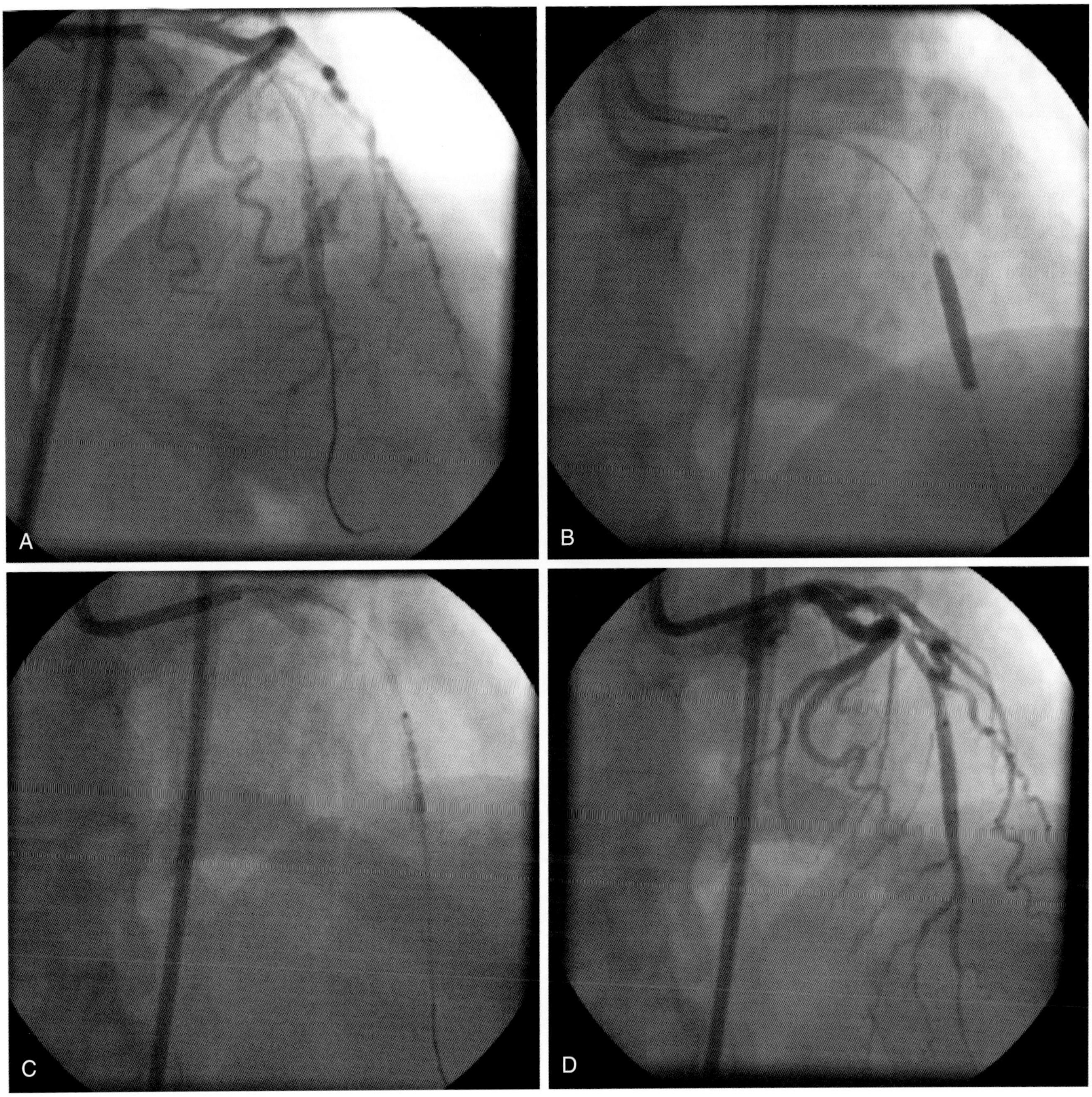

Fig. 14.8 Coronary perforation management. (A) Coronary perforation was noted after deployment of a stent in the mid left anterior descending coronary artery (LAD). The stent deployment balloon was immediately inserted and inflated to tamponade the perforation. (B) A second access site was obtained in the contralateral femoral artery and a second guide inserted. The stent balloon was deflated briefly, and a wire was passed into the LAD from the second guide, then the tamponade balloon was reinflated. (C) A Jomed covered stent (Abbott Vascular) was advanced from the second guide using the tamponade balloon to anchor the wire and facilitate delivery. Once the Jomed stent was advanced near the site of perforation, the original guidewire and balloon were quickly withdrawn and the Jomed stent deployed. (D) Angiography demonstrates resolution of the perforation after successful Jomed stent deployment.

practical considerations, guidance for proper equipment selection, tips, and caveats. Extensive, calcified, and complex disease can be effectively treated using what has been presented here. Modifications and progression of these techniques will surely arise. If one masters what is described here for practical use, the breadth of cases that can be successfully completed should increase considerably.

KEY REFFRENCES

1. Jolly SS, Yusuf S, Cairns J, et al. Radial versus femoral access for coronary angiography and intervention in patients with acute coronary syndromes (RIVAL): a randomised, parallel group, multicentre trial. *Lancet*. 2011;377(9775):1409–1420.
3. Legalery P, Seronde MF, Meneveau N, et al. Measuring pressure-derived fractional flow reserve through four French diagnostic catheters. *Am J Cardiol*. 2003;91(9):1075–1078.

4. Kiemeneij F, Vajifdar BU, Eccleshall SC, et al. Evaluation of a spasmolytic cocktail to prevent radial artery spasm during coronary procedures. *Catheter Cardiovasc Interv*. 2003;58(3):281–284.
6. Deftereos S, Giannopoulos G, Raisakis K, et al. Moderate procedural sedation and opioid analgesia during transradial coronary interventions to prevent spasm: a prospective randomized study. *JACC Cardiovasc Interv*. 2013;6(3):267–273.
8. Seto AH, Abu-Fadel MS, Sparling JM, et al. Real-time ultrasound guidance facilitates femoral arterial access and reduces vascular complications: FAUST (Femoral Arterial Access With Ultrasound Trial). *JACC Cardiovasc Interv*. 2010;3(7):751–758.
9. Lee MS, Park KW, Shlofmitz E, et al. Comparison of rotational atherectomy versus orbital atherectomy for the treatment of heavily calcified coronary plaques. *Am J Cardiol*. 2017;119(9):1320–1323.
10. Fabris E, Kennedy MW, Di Mario C, et al. Guide extension, unmissable tool in the armamentarium of modern interventional cardiology. A comprehensive review. *Int J Cardiol*. 2016;222:141–147.
13. Chambers JW, Feldman RL, Himmelstein SI, et al. Pivotal trial to evaluate the safety and efficacy of the orbital atherectomy system in treating de novo, severely calcified coronary lesions (ORBIT II). *JACC Cardiovasc Interv*. 2014;7(5):510–518.
14. Safian RD, Feldman T, Muller DW, et al. Coronary angioplasty and Rotablator atherectomy trial (CARAT): immediate and late results of a prospective multicenter randomized trial. *Catheter Cardiovasc Interv*. 2001;53(2):213–220.
17. Rezkalla SH, Stankowski RV, Hanna J, et al. Management of no-reflow phenomenon in the catheterization laboratory. *JACC Cardiovasc Interv*. 2017;10(3):215–223.

Additional references available online at expertconsult.com.

中文导读

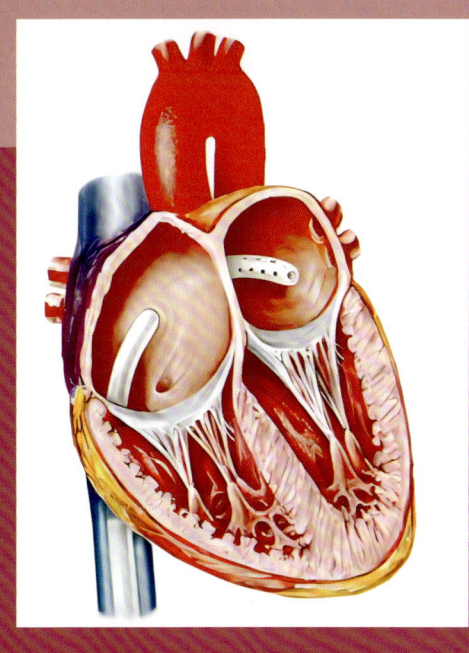

第15章
冠状动脉支架

　　经皮冠状动脉介入治疗的发展不断进步，从引入冠状动脉球囊血管成形术开始，经历了一系列飞跃性的技术突破。金属支架的出现，使经皮冠状动脉介入治疗成为绝大多数冠状动脉疾病患者所依赖的血运重建方式，并被心血管医师所接受和掌握。从最初的金属裸支架，到第一代、第二代药物洗脱支架的出现，直至出现完全可吸收支架（可能是非金属支架），冠状动脉支架的发展历程实际上就是专业人员试图解决支架再狭窄（有效性）、支架血栓（安全性）两大难题的过程。

　　本章节按照支架发展历程，逐一介绍了不同时期支架产品的设计、特点及具有里程碑意义的重要临床试验。此外，该章节还对在特定情况下应用支架尤其是第二代药物洗脱支架的安全性和有效性做了概述，这些特定情况包括急性心肌梗死、分叉病变、慢性完全闭塞病变、合并糖尿病患者和大隐静脉桥血管等。为了平衡出血与血栓风险，合理的双联抗血小板治疗对于经皮冠状动脉介入治疗术后患者也至关重要。个体化抗血小板治疗可能会使患者从第二代药物洗脱支架置入中得到更多的临床净获益。

　　最后，该章节讲解了支架置入失败的相关机制及处理措施，并对支架未来发展及辅助药物治疗做出了展望。

刘严慈　柳景华

章节要点

- 金属裸支架克服了球囊血管成形术的许多缺陷，但再狭窄限制了它的使用。金属裸支架再狭窄发生率为20%～40%。

- 药物洗脱支架由金属支架平台、携带药物的载体涂层（通常是聚合物）构成。该载体涂层能够控制抗增殖药物洗脱的剂量和时间。抗增殖药物已被证明可以显著减少支架内晚期管腔丢失，从而降低造影和临床再狭窄率。

- 第一代药物洗脱支架，包括西罗莫司洗脱药物支架和紫杉醇药物洗脱支架。在不同的患者和病变人群中，第一代药物洗脱支架所致的死亡率和心肌梗死发生率与金属裸支架相近；然而，由于对晚期支架血栓发生率增加的担忧使得第一代药物洗脱支架术后双联抗血小板治疗时间延长。有研究显示，在第一代药物洗脱支架置入1年之后，其支架血栓和心肌梗死的发生率增加。

- 第二代药物洗脱支架的问世是为了克服上一代产品的缺陷，其主要对支架平台做了更多改进。与第一代药物洗脱支架相比，其支架梁更薄，输送性也更佳，且聚合物生物相容性更好或使用了生物可吸收聚合物涂层。

- 既往研究已经证明，第二代药物洗脱支架不仅比第一代药物洗脱支架更安全、更有效，也比金属裸支架更安全。在特定的高危患者和复杂病变中（包括急性心肌梗死、分叉病变、慢性完全闭塞病变、合并糖尿病患者和大隐静脉桥血管等），第二代药物洗脱支架安全性的提升表现得尤为出色。与冠状动脉搭桥术相比，药物洗脱支架已被接受可用于某些特定左主干和多支血管病变患者。

- 第二代药物洗脱支架安全性的改善对支架置入后延长双联抗血小板治疗的观念提出了挑战。有证据表明，在接受第二代药物洗脱支架置入的低风险患者中，术后使用3个月或6个月的双联抗血小板治疗可能与持续1年的双联抗血小板治疗方案一样有效，但在安全性上可能更安全。然而，对于低危出血风险、冠状动脉粥样硬化血栓事件风险高危的患者，延长至术后数年甚至更长时间的双联抗血小板治疗可降低极晚期支架血栓发生风险，并能预防未干预的动脉粥样硬化斑块相关心肌梗死。

- 尽管新一代药物洗脱支架得到了改进，但由于新生动脉粥样硬化、支架梁断裂、支架与血管顺应性不匹配和局部血管生理学改变，支架置入部位相关的不良缺血事件在晚期随访时仍会持续增加。因此，完全生物可吸收支架可能会进一步改善远期预后，然而一些完全生物可吸收支架产品已被发现会增加支架血栓事件，这也引起了人们对其安全性的担忧。

15 Coronary Stenting

Tullio Palmerini, Ajay J. Kirtane

KEY POINTS

- Bare-metal stents (BMS) overcome many of the drawbacks of balloon angioplasty but are limited by restenosis, which develops in 20% to 40% of cases.
- Drug-eluting stents (DES)—which consist of a metallic stent coated with a drug carrier vehicle (usually a polymer) that controls the dose and timing of the elution of an antiproliferative agent—have been shown to significantly reduce in-stent late loss, resulting in reduced rates of angiographic and clinical restenosis.
- First-generation DES, including sirolimus-eluting and paclitaxel-eluting stents, have resulted in similar rates of mortality and myocardial infarction (MI) as BMS in a broad spectrum of patients and lesions; however, concern over an increased rate of late stent thrombosis led to reliance on extended dual antiplatelet therapy (DAPT), and studies have demonstrated an increase in stent thrombosis and MI beyond 1 year with these devices.
- Second-generation DES have been developed to overcome the drawbacks of their predecessors, principally by using improved stent platforms with thinner struts and enhanced deliverability, and more biocompatible or bioabsorbable polymers compared with first-generation devices.
- Second-generation DES have been shown to be safer and more effective than not only first- generation DES, but also may be safer than BMS. The enhanced safety of second-generation DES is especially apparent in specific high-risk and complex situations, including acute MI, bifurcation lesions, chronic total occlusions (CTO), diabetic patients, and saphenous vein grafts. The utility of DES compared with bypass surgery has also become accepted in some but not all cases of left main and multivessel disease.
- The improved safety profile of second-generation DES has challenged the notion of prolonged DAPT after DES implantation. Evidence has emerged that in low-risk patients, 3- or 6-month DAPT after second-generation DES implantation may be as effective as and safer than DAPT continued for 1 year. However, in patients with a low risk of bleeding and high risk of atherothrombotic events, prolonged DAPT for several years or longer after stent implantation may reduce the ongoing risk of very late stent thrombosis and prevent MI arising from untreated atherosclerosis.
- Even with the improvements with current-generation DES, adverse ischemic events arising from the stent site continue to accrue at late follow-up due to neoatherosclerosis, strut fractures, compliance mismatch, and altered vascular physiology. In this regard, fully bioresorbable vascular scaffolds (BVS) may further improve chronic outcomes, but the increased rates of stent thrombosis observed with some of these devices has raised concern over their safety.

INTRODUCTION

The history of percutaneous coronary intervention (PCI) may be described as a series of transformative steps, beginning with the introduction of coronary balloon angioplasty. Development of the implantable metallic stent enabled PCI to become a durable approach for the vast majority of patients with coronary artery disease, and one that most operators can apply safely. From balloons to atherectomy to lasers to bare-metal stents (BMS) and now drug-eluting stents (DES), the evolution of interventional cardiology has progressively and uncompromisingly advanced through the insights and inventions of thousands of physicians and scientists, coupled with the recognition of the importance of optimal adjunctive pharmacotherapy, on the foundation of thousands of randomized trials and registries performed around the world which provide an unparalleled evidence base for daily clinical decision making. The present chapter will trace the evolution and development of the coronary stent from its initial applications to treat balloon angioplasty failures to its widespread global adoption for the treatment of patients with ischemic coronary heart disease.

BARE-METAL STENT OVERVIEW

Limitations of balloon angioplasty and development of the coronary stent

The performance of the first successful balloon angioplasty by Andreas Gruentzig on September 16, 1977, in Zurich, Switzerland, was a landmark event heralding the inception of percutaneous management of obstructive coronary artery disease. Although this initial procedure set the stage for the millions of PCI procedures that have since taken place, stand-alone balloon angioplasty was a highly unpredictable experience. While the majority of vessels tolerate the focal plaque dissections caused by balloon dilatation and heal sufficiently to result in an adequate lumen, the injury to the vessel wall may unpredictably result in severe dissections, which along with acute recoil and chronic constrictive remodeling, result in balloon angioplasty's two major limitations: abrupt closure (occurring acutely, or within the first several days after angioplasty) and restenosis (occurring later, within months, and, rarely, years after the procedure). The coronary stent was thus devised as an endoluminal scaffold to create a larger initial lumen, to seal dissections, and to resist recoil and late vascular remodeling, thereby improving upon the early and late results of balloon angioplasty.

The first implantation of stents in human coronary arteries occurred in 1986 when Ulrich Sigwart and Jacques Puel and colleagues placed the Wallstent-sheathed self-expanding metallic mesh scaffold (Medinvent, Lausanne, Switzerland) in the peripheral and coronary arteries of eight patients.[1] Further experience with this device demonstrated high rates of thrombotic occlusion and late mortality,[2] although patients without thrombosis had a 6-month angiographic restenosis rate of only 14%, suggesting for the first time that stenting could improve late patency in addition to stabilizing the acute results obtained after conventional balloon angioplasty. Contemporaneously, Cesare Gianturco and Gary Roubin developed a balloon-expandable coil stent consisting of a wrapped stainless steel wire resembling a clamshell. Completion of a phase II study using the Gianturco-Roubin stent to reverse postangioplasty acute or threatened vessel closure[3] led to United States Food and Drug Administration (FDA) approval for this indication in June 1993. However, high rates of restenosis with this device relegated its use mainly for bailout of occlusive dissections and recoil after balloon angioplasty.

While these stents were being developed and tested, in 1984 Julio Palmaz designed a balloon-expandable stainless steel "slotted tube stent." In this stent design, rectangular slots were cut into a 15-mm-long, thin-walled stainless steel tube, such that balloon inflation within the stent deformed these rectangular slots into diamond-shaped windows or cells. While this design allowed for relatively straightforward deployment (and greater resistance to recoil than the clamshell design), the rigidity of this stent made it difficult to deliver in the coronary vasculature. In 1989, a design modification was suggested by Richard Schatz, consisting of the placement of a 1-mm central articulating bridge connecting two rigid 7-mm slotted segments,[4] creating the 15-mm Palmaz Schatz stent (Johnson and Johnson Interventional Systems, Warren, NJ) (Fig. 15.1). The first coronary Palmaz–Schatz stent was placed in a patient by Eduardo Sousa in São Paulo, Brazil, in 1987. The Palmaz–Schatz stent was subsequently investigated in two landmark randomized trials comparing balloon angioplasty to elective stenting. In the STent REStenosis Study (STRESS) and Belgian Netherlands Stent study (BENESTENT) 1 studies, routine use of the Palmaz–Schatz stent was associated with a 20% to 30% reduction in clinical and angiographic restenosis within 6 to 12 months compared with conventional balloon angioplasty (Fig. 15.2).[5,6] The Palmaz–Schatz stent also resulted in markedly improved initial angiographic results, with a larger postprocedural minimal luminal diameter and fewer residual dissections, which translated into a lower rate of subacute vessel closure. These results led to approval of the Palmaz–Schatz Stent by the FDA in 1994. Long-term follow-up up to 15 years has subsequently demonstrated a low (but not zero) rate of clinical angiographic recurrences from years 1 to 5 after coronary stent implantation,[7,8] with slight and progressive decrements in luminal size thereafter extending beyond 10 years.[9] The mechanisms of this late progression of disease are not entirely known, but, as discussed later, is usually described as atherosclerotic transformation of neointimal hyperplasia, known as neoatherosclerosis.

Despite the success of the Palmaz–Schatz stent in improving the early and late results of conventional balloon angioplasty, widespread adoption of stent technology was initially hindered by high rates of subacute stent thrombosis necessitating an intense antithrombotic and antiplatelet regimen (consisting of aspirin, dextran, dipyridamole, heparin, and warfarin). Further refinements in the stent procedure and periprocedural pharmacotherapy regimens were thus required. Antonio Colombo and colleagues demonstrated reduced rates of stent thrombosis with more aggressive intravascular ultrasound (IVUS)-guided deployment techniques including routine high-pressure adjunctive dilatation (>14 atmospheres),[10] along with the use of aspirin and a second antiplatelet agent (thienopyridine ticlopidine) rather than

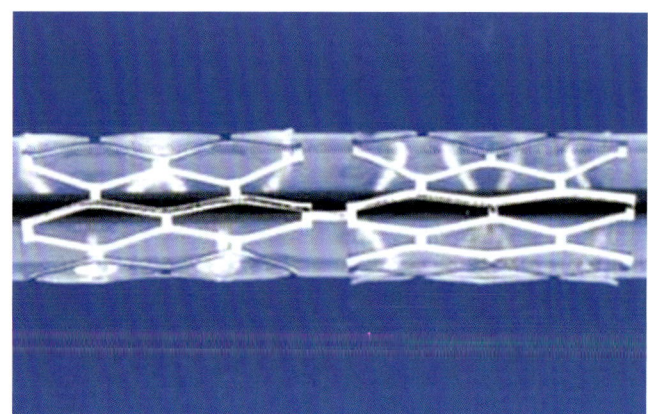

Fig. 15.1 The Palmaz–Schatz stent. Note the articulation between the two slotted tubes.

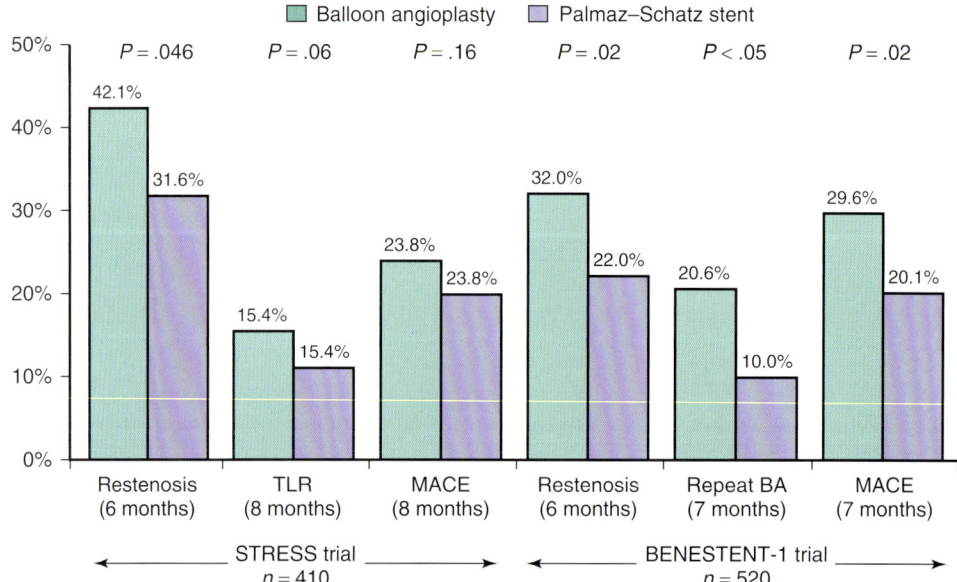

Fig. 15.2 The pivotal early stent versus PTCA studies. *BA*, Balloon angioplasty; *MACE*, major adverse cardiac events; *PTCA*, percutaneous transluminal coronary angioplasty; *TLR*, target-lesion revascularization.

prolonged warfarin therapy. These modifications significantly reduced the incidence of stent thrombosis to ~1% to 2%, along with a marked reduction in bleeding and femoral arterial complications.[11] The confirmation of these initial findings in several randomized clinical trials definitively established the superiority of dual antiplatelet therapy (DAPT) (with aspirin and ticlopidine) over anticoagulation with warfarin for prevention of stent thrombosis, and facilitated widespread adoption of coronary stenting by the late 1990s.[12–15]

Stent Design: Impact on Performance and Clinical Outcomes

Classification

Coronary stents may be classified based on their composition (e.g., metallic or polymeric), configuration (e.g., slotted tube vs. coiled wire), bioabsorption (either inert [biostable or durable] or degradable [bioabsorbable]), coatings (either none, passive [such as heparin or polytetrafluoroethylene {PTFE}], or bioactive [such as those eluting rapamycin or paclitaxel]), and mode of implantation (e.g., self-expanding or balloon expandable). In theory, the ideal coronary stent would be made of a nonthrombogenic material and have sufficient flexibility in its unexpanded state to allow passage through small guiding catheters and tortuous vessels. It would also have an expanded configuration that provides uniform scaffolding of the vessel wall with low recoil and maximal radial strength, while at the same time being conformable on bends. In addition, the stent should be sufficiently radiopaque to allow fluoroscopic visualization to guide accurate placement and management if restenosis occurs, but not so opaque as to angiographically obscure important vascular details.

Stent Composition

In the early stent experience, the most widely used stent material was 316 L stainless steel. More recently, cobalt chromium and platinum chromium alloys have been employed to allow lower-profile thin stent struts (60 to 82 μm vs. 100 to 150 μm in most stainless steel stents) that maintain strength and visibility. Most self-expanding stents utilize nitinol, a nickel-titanium alloy, which, after being baked at a high temperature, maintains shape memory for a predetermined size and configuration.

Other than gold (which has been shown to increase restenosis), there is little evidence that thrombosis or restenosis rates vary with the specific stent metal, though the final stages of surface finishing, smoothing, and purification or passivation may affect early thrombotic and late restenotic processes.[16] While a meta-analysis including nine randomized trials and 11,313 patients reported a better safety profile with DESs that use cobalt chromium platforms compared to stainless steel platforms, due to a significant reduction in the 30-day rates of myocardial infarction (MI), comparisons such as these may also take into account different polymers used in specific DES, thereby making stent-material-specific comparisons difficult to interpret.[17] There is a growing interest in polymeric and metallic fully biodegradable stents (bioresorbable scaffolds), which theoretically offer the advantages of increased longitudinal flexibility, compatibility with noninvasive imaging, and complete bioresorption over a period of months to a year or longer, with the potential to restore underlying vascular reactivity (see Chapter 16).

Stent Configuration and Design

Stents can be assigned to one of three distinct subcategories, based on construction/design elements: wire coils, slotted tubes/multicellular, and modular designs. The vast majority of stents in current use are either slotted tube/multicellular or modular in design. Within these subcategories, stents are often classified as having open cells or closed cells, based upon the design of connecting links between adjacent stent struts. Open-cell designs tend to have varying cell sizes and shapes, which provide increased flexibility, deliverability, and side branch access, with staggered cross-linking elements to provide radial strength. Closed-cell designs typically incorporate a repeating, unicellular element that provides more uniform wall coverage with less tendency for plaque prolapse, but at the expense of flexibility and side branch access.

Stent design may significantly impact acute and late vascular responses. Stents that possess better conformability, less rigidity, and greater circularity experimentally produce less vascular injury, thrombosis, and neointimal hyperplasia.[18,19] Clinical studies have suggested that thin stent struts may be associated with reduced neointimal hyperplasia and lower rates of restenosis.[20] In addition, an experimental study using an ex vivo modified Chandler loop generating pulsatile flow found that thick strutted stents (162 μm) are significantly more thrombogenic than otherwise identical thin-strutted stents (81 μm).[21] Stent design may also significantly impact longitudinal integrity of the stent, which principally depends on the number of connectors between hoops.[22] Longitudinal distortion may manifest as length change, strut overlap, or strut separation which may obstruct the lumen, predisposing to stent thrombosis or restenosis.[23]

Stent Coatings

A variety of coatings have been used to attempt to reduce the thrombogenicity or restenosis of metallic stents (Table 15.1). Experimental studies have demonstrated that coating stents with inert polymers may reduce surface reactivity and thrombosis,[24] though until recently, most polymers used were found to provoke intense inflammatory reactions.[25] With the advent of DES came a renewed interest in the study of stent coatings, primarily to act as drug-carrier vehicles. However, concerns regarding the long-term safety of DES and the requirement for extended-duration DAPT have led to the development of new stent coatings, which are either more biocompatible or bioabsorbable. Specifically, fluorinated copolymers have been shown in vitro to have thromboresistant properties, due to preferential absorption and retention of albumin, which passivates the stent surface.[26] Finally, covered stents (metallic stents covered by a distensible microporous PTFE membrane) are of unquestioned clinical utility in treating life-threatening perforations. They are also used

TABLE 15.1 Stent Coatings Designed to Reduce Thrombogenicity

Heparin
    Multiple formulations incorporating heparin bonding through covalent bonding, ionic bonds, or heparin complexes (Carmeda BioActive Surface [CBAS] covalently heparin-bonded Palmaz–Schatz and BX Velocity stents, Jomed Corline Heparin Surface [CHS] heparin-coated Jostent)

Carbon
    Turbostratic (Sorin Carbostent)
    Silicon carbide (Biotronik Tenax)
    Diamond-like films (Phytis Diamond and Plasmachem Biodiamond)

Phosphorylcholine
    Biocompatibles BiodivYsio stent
    Medtronic Endeavor drug-eluting stent

Ionic oxygen penetration into stent (Iberhospitex Bionert)

CD34 antibody to capture endothelial progenitor cells (Orbus–Neich Genous)

Trifluoroethanol (polyzene-F coated stent)

Nanolayer protein coating (SurModics Finale coating on Protex stent)

Nitric oxide scavengers including titanium-nitric oxide (Hexacath Titan stent)

Single Knitted PET Fiber Mesh (MGuard)

Biolinx polymer (Medtronic Resolute drug-eluting stent)

Abciximab and other glycoprotein IIb/IIIa inhibitors

Activated protein C

Hirudin and bivalirudin

Prostacyclin

Gold

for excluding giant aneurysms, pseudoaneurysms, and clinically significant fistulae (see Chapter 29). More recent is the application of polyethylene terephthalate (PET) mesh-covered stents (MGuard, Inspire MD, Tel Aviv, Israel) to minimize the risk of distal embolization in patients with ST-segment elevation myocardial infarction (STEMI) (see Chapter 20).

Balloon-Expandable Versus Self-Expanding Stents

Balloon-expandable stents are mounted onto a delivery balloon and delivered into the coronary artery in their collapsed state. Once the stent is in the desired location, inflation of the delivery balloon expands the stent against the arterial wall, following which the stent delivery system is removed. Almost all stents implanted in human coronary arteries are balloon-expandable. Self-expanding stents incorporate either specific geometric designs or nitinol shape-retaining metal to achieve a preset diameter, and are released from a resisting sheath once placed in position. While self-expanding stents are more flexible than their balloon-expandable counterparts, greater rates of restenosis have been observed with this design, presumably from chronic ongoing vascular injury, limiting their use in coronary arteries.[27] Recently, a renewed interest in self-expanding stents with reduced outward expansion force for the treatment of patients with acute coronary syndromes or vulnerable plaque has surfaced.[28-30]

Stenting after failed balloon angioplasty. Stents may be used either on a routine (planned) basis or after failed balloon angioplasty for acute or threatened vessel closure ("bail-out" stenting). One of the major benefits of stenting (indeed, the initial reason for the genesis of stents) is the ability to reverse abrupt closure due to dissection and recoil, thus eliminating the need for high-risk emergency bypass surgery.[31] These data, coupled with the fact that routine stent implantation compared to balloon angioplasty provides superior acute results and greater event-free survival in almost every patient and lesion subtype studied to date, has for the most part relegated balloon dilation to the rare lesion that is too small (<2.0 mm) for stenting, or to which a stent cannot be delivered because of excessive vessel tortuosity or calcification, or in patients in whom thienopyridines cannot be taken or are contraindicated.

Routine Stenting During Percutaneous Coronary Intervention

The utility of routine stent implantation as a modality to reduce acute vessel closure and late restenosis was first demonstrated in the STRESS and BENESTENT-1 trials, which enrolled patients undergoing PCI of discrete, focal lesions.[5,6] As a result, the types of lesions treated in these trials (discrete de novo lesions coverable by one stent, with reference vessel diameter [RVD] 3.0 to 4.0 mm) became known as "Stress/Benestent" lesions, to differentiate them from more complex stenoses. Despite initial concerns regarding diminished safety and efficacy of coronary stents (which were also more costly than balloon angioplasty alone) with more generalized use of these devices,[32] numerous randomized trials and observational studies comparing stenting to balloon angioplasty demonstrated an advantage to coronary stenting over conventional balloon angioplasty across a wide range of patient and lesion subsets.[33-35]

DRUG-ELUTING STENTS OVERVIEW

Limitations of Bare-Metal Stents

By the late 1990s, stent implantation became the predominant treatment for most patients with coronary artery disease as a result of more predictable acute and late angiographic results compared with conventional balloon angioplasty, atherectomy, and laser therapy. Improvements in procedural technique (including IVUS and optical coherence tomography [OCT] guidance), more effective antiplatelet regimens, and the introduction of increasingly lower profile, more flexible and deliverable devices additionally contributed to the ascendancy of stenting. With improvements in stent deliverability and reductions in rates of subacute stent thrombosis to less than 1%, restenosis emerged as the major persistent limitation of coronary stenting. While coronary stents increase acute luminal diameters to a greater extent than balloon angioplasty (greater acute gain), the greater vascular injury caused by stent implantation compared to balloon angioplasty elicits an exaggerated degree of neointimal hyperplasia, resulting in greater decreases in luminal diameter (late loss).[5,6] Importantly, however, comparing stents to balloon angioplasty, the mean incremental gain in luminal dimensions with stenting is statistically greater than the mean incremental increase in late loss, resulting in a larger net gain in minimal luminal dimensions. This observation led Kuntz and Baim to formulate the "bigger is better" concept: the greater the acute gain, the greater the late gain and the lower the ultimate rate of restenosis.[36,37] Nonetheless, even with optimal stent implantation, restenosis after BMS implantation still occurred in approximately 20% to 40% of patients within 6 to 12 months, in part due to stenting more complex patient and lesion subsets than in the balloon angioplasty era. As such, coronary restenosis became known as the "Achilles' heel" of coronary stenting, with significant resources devoted to its prevention and treatment (see Chapter 34).

DES, which maintain the mechanical advantages of BMS while delivering an antirestenotic pharmacologic therapy locally to the arterial wall, have been shown to effectively and safely reduce the amount of in-stent tissue that accumulates after stent implantation, resulting in significantly reduced rates of clinical and angiographic restenosis. These devices were designed specifically to prevent the neointimal hyperplasia resulting after conventional BMS placement, and have been highly successful in this regard. In numerous randomized trials, the reduction in neointimal hyperplasia that occurs with DES compared to BMS has been shown to result in a 50% to 75% reduction in binary angiographic restenosis and target lesion revascularization (TLR).[38-40] The initial results of the pivotal randomized trials that led to device approval have been replicated and validated in numerous subsequent trials and real-world registries across the spectrum of disease and lesion subtypes.[41,42]

Components of Drug-Eluting Stents

The three critical components of a DES that must be optimized to ensure its safety and efficacy are (1) the stent itself (including its delivery system); (2) the pharmacologic agent being delivered; and (3) the drug carrier vehicle, which controls the drug dose and pharmacokinetic release rate (Fig. 15.3).

Drug-Eluting Stents Stent Designs

The stent component of early DES platforms was typically that of the predicate BMS without design modifications (i.e., relatively thick strut designs composed of stainless steel). Indeed, first-generation DES designs often appropriated approved and "off-the shelf" stent designs in order to expedite device development and regulatory approval. Subsequent DES have incorporated newer materials, thinner struts, and more flexible designs, with resultant improvements in device delivery and performance.[43,44] Additionally, newer dedicated DES designs have included modifications aimed at either optimizing local drug delivery while reducing total drug dose (e.g., drug delivery limited to the abluminal direction), or modifying the stent surface to facilitate direct drug delivery and/or arterial healing following implantation

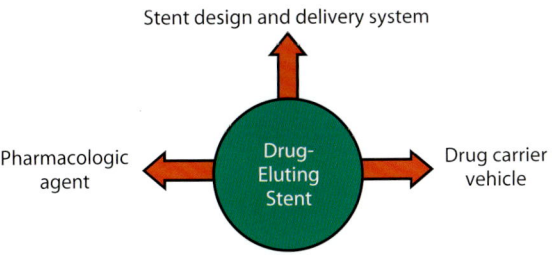

Fig. 15.3 Components of drug-eluting stent.

(without a drug carrier vehicle per se). The latest evolution has been the introduction of drug-eluting fully bioresorbable scaffolds (BRS), wherein the stent frame is composed of a bioabsorbable polymer or metal that provides a scaffolding function for 6 to 12 months and then completely resorbs over the next 1 to 3 years, recapitulating the underlying vessel anatomy and physiology.

Basic Drug-Eluting Stents Pharmacology

Following promising cell culture and in vitro development, the antirestenotic properties of a wide range of pharmacologic agents have been tested in humans (Fig. 15.4). Among these, the two most clinically effective classes of agents are the "rapamycin-analog family" of drugs and paclitaxel. The principal mechanism of action of rapamycin (also known as sirolimus), and its analogs (including zotarolimus, everolimus, biolimus A9, and novolimus) is inhibition of the mammalian target of rapamycin (mTOR), which prevents cell cycle progression from the G1 to S phase.[45] mTOR is also localized on platelet membranes where it mediates platelet activation and aggregation. Inhibition of mTOR by sirolimus analogs has been shown to prevent platelet spreading on fibrinogen coating cover slips, can inhibit platelet aggregation, and produce platelet disaggregation under shear flow conditions.[46] In addition, rapamycin or rapamycin analogs are able to inhibit mTOR-dependent clot retraction.[47] Although somewhat varying in lipophilicity and potency, most rapamycin analogs have been clinically comparable in their safety and efficacy effects. Two other rapamycin analogs that in the past (but not present) have been used on DES platforms—tacrolimus and pimecrolimus—have a different mechanism of action, binding directly to FKBP506, thereby inhibiting the calcineurin receptor with downregulation of cytokines and inhibition of smooth muscle cell activity[48]; unlike the mTOR inhibitors, these agents have not shown significant antirestenotic potential.

The other agent that has been used effectively not only in DES but also on drug-eluting balloons is paclitaxel. By interfering with microtubule function, paclitaxel has multifunctional antiproliferative and antiinflammatory properties, prevents smooth muscle migration, blocks cytokine and growth factor release and activity, interferes with secretory processes, is antiangiogenic, and impacts signal transduction.[49–51] At low doses (similar to those in DES applications), paclitaxel affects the G0 to G1 and G1 to S phases (G1 arrest) resulting in cytostasis without cell death.[49–52]

Drug-Eluting Stents Polymers and Drug Carrier Systems

The inability to predictably deliver a specific dose of active drug over the right time frame to the arterial wall led to the failure of early DES programs.[53] To ensure accurate drug dosing, a *drug delivery vehicle* became necessary, which for most first-generation stents was a durable (nonerodable) polymer. A wide range of polymer systems have since been developed, and are DES-specific (discussed in subsequent sections of this chapter). While the polymer is instrumental in regulating the pharmacokinetics of drug delivery to the arterial wall

Antiinflammatory, immunomodulators	Antiproliferative	Smooth muscle cell migration inhibitors, extracellular matrix modulators
Sirolimus (and analogs)	Sirolimus (and analogs)	Batimastat
Paclitaxel, Taxane	Paclitaxel, Taxane	Prolyl hydroxylase inhibitors
Dexamethasone	Actinomycin D	Halofuginone
M-prednisolone	Methotrexate	C-proteinase inhibitors
Interferon γ-1b	Angiopeptin	Probucol
Leflunomide	Vincristine	
Tacrolimus	Mitomycin	
Mycophenolic acid	Statins	
Mizoribine	MYC antisense	
Cyclosporine	RestenASE	
Tranilast	2-Chloro-deoxyadenosine	
Biorest	PCNA ribozyme	

Fig. 15.4 Potential antirestenotic agents for use with drug-eluting stent. (Adapted from Moscucci M, ed. *Grossman & Baim's Cardiac Catheterization, Angiography, and Intervention*. 8th ed. Philadelphia, PA: Lippincott Williams & Wilkins; 2013.)

(which is necessary for reduced neointimal hyperplasia), the polymer may elicit deleterious vascular responses. Specifically, histopathologic studies have demonstrated hypersensitivity and eosinophilic inflammatory reactions and delayed endothelialization with DES that were not previously seen with BMS.[54–56] Whether these maladaptive vascular responses are directly related to the polymer and/or to toxic reactions from the drug itself is speculative, but in animal models these effects can be attenuated by modification of the polymer vehicle.[57] It is believed that in selected patients, excessive inflammation and delayed endothelialization play a role in the development of late stent malapposition, aneurysm formation, and stent thrombosis and restenosis.[54–58] For these reasons, there has been great interest in developing inert and biocompatible polymers, bioabsorbable polymers (BP), and even polymer-free DES. For example, fluorinated copolymers coating some second-generation DES have been shown to possess thromboresistant properties in blood contact applications, and have been shown to reduce platelet adhesion compared to an otherwise identical BMS.[21,59] On the other hand, optimizing BP performance entails consideration of biocompatibility, composition, and degradation time of the polymer, which can be affected by the use of long polymer chains, decreased polymer hydrophobicity, and greater polymer crystallinity.[60] Polymer degradation can also be associated with significant inflammatory reactions and a persistent immune-mediated response to monomer breakdown product.[61]

Generational Classification of Drug-Eluting Stents

Given the rapid evolution of DES technologies, DES are often classified into several generations of development (Table 15.2). First-generation devices include the two DES that were initially approved for clinical use by most regulatory bodies, each of which utilized an early thick strut stainless steel stent platform (suboptimal by today's standards) with a durable polymer not specifically designed for biocompatibility (and prone to inflammation) to deliver either sirolimus or paclitaxel. Second-generation devices (currently used in the majority of DES procedures) have incorporated more deliverable, thinner-strut stents (most made from cobalt chromium or platinum chromium alloys) with more

TABLE 15.2 Generational Classification of Major Durable Polymer-Based Drug-Eluting Stents

Generation	Drug	Polymer	Stent
First	**Sirolimus or Paclitaxel**	**Not Specifically Designed for Biocompatibility**	**Early BMS Platforms**
Cypher	Sirolimus	Bio-stable mix of poly-n-butyl methacrylate and polyethylene–vinyl acetate	Bx-Velocity (stainless steel)
TAXUS Express	Paclitaxel	Styrene-isobutylene-styrene (SIBS)	Express (stainless steel)
TAXUS Liberté	Paclitaxel	Styrene-isobutylene-styrene (SIBS)	Liberté (stainless steel)
Second	**Rapamycin Analogus**	**Biocompatible Polymers**	**More Flexible, Thinner Strut BMS**
Endeavor	Zotarolimus	Phosphorylcholine	Driver (cobalt-chromium alloy)
Resolute, Resolute Onyx	Zotarolimus	Biolinx polymer (hydrophobic and hydrophilic trilayer)	Integrity (cobalt-chromium alloy)
Xience V, Xience Prime, Xience Expedition; Xience alpine, Xience Sierra	Everolimus	vinylidene fluoride and hexafluoropropylene	Vision (cobalt-chromium alloy)
Promus Element, Promus Premier	Everolimus	vinylidene fluoride and hexafluoropropylene	Omega (platinum-chromium alloy)

BMS, Bare-metal stents.

biocompatible polymers eluting (in most cases) rapamycin-analogs. In addition, a variety of BP-based DES have been developed, which are widely used in Europe and Asia, and have recently been approved for use in the United States. Future generation DES will continue to undergo iteration, with further modifications of the base stent, delivery polymers, and use of biodegradable/bioabsorbable or polymer-free drug delivery vehicles. Finally, more than 50,000 patients outside the United States have undergone implantation of an everolimus-eluting stent with a poly-L-lactic acid (PLLA) backbone, with large-scale trials, some of which are still ongoing, comparing these devices to metallic DES.

First-Generation Drug-Eluting Stents

First-generation DESs include The Cypher sirolimus-eluting stent (SES) (Cordis, Johnson and Johnson) and the Taxus paclitaxel-eluting stent (PES) (Boston Scientific, Natick, MA). Although the introduction of first-generation DES has heralded the inception of a new era in the percutaneous treatment of coronary artery disease, the interest of these devices is mainly historical due to discontinuation of Cypher and Taxus manufacturing in 2011 and 2016, respectively.

The Cypher Sirolimus-Eluting Stent

The Cypher SES was initially approved in Europe in 2002 and the United States in 2003. Sirolimus is a highly lipophilic, naturally occurring macrocyclic lactone, which was first isolated from *Streptomyces hygroscopicus* found in a soil sample from Easter Island, and was initially developed as an antifungal agent. Shortly thereafter, it was discovered that sirolimus also possessed potent immunosuppressive properties, and was initially approved by the FDA as Rapamune for prevention of renal transplant rejection in 1999. The primary mechanism of action of sirolimus's inhibition of neointimal hyperplasia is thought to be related to its ability to bind to FK binding protein-12 (FKBP-12) in cells; the sirolimus-FKBP-12 complex then binds to and inhibits activation of mTOR, preventing progression in the cell cycle from the late G1 to S phase.[45] The SES was demonstrated to have a marked effect on suppression of neointimal hyperplasia with low toxicity following implantation in initial small and large animal studies.[62,63]

The base stent platform for the Cypher SES was the Bx-Velocity stent, a slotted tube with a closed cell design constructed from 316 L stainless steel. Human experience with the Cypher SES was first reported from the first-in-man (FIM) study initiated in 1999 in 45 patients with symptomatic de novo lesions less than 18 mm in length with RVD 3.0 to 3.5 mm in native coronary arteries at the Institute Dante Pazzanese of Cardiology in São Paulo, Brazil, and the Thoraxcenter, Rotterdam, The Netherlands. In this study, SES demonstrated marked suppression of neointimal hyperplasia measured by IVUS and quantitative coronary angiography at 4 months, and 1, 2, and 4 years.[64] Serial angiography and IVUS have now been performed at 7 years, showing continued vessel patency without further late loss (Fig. 15.5).

Following the success of SES in this initial study, several randomized controlled trials (Table 15.3),[38,39,65] meta-analyses,[41] and observational registries[66] comparing Cypher with its BMS counterpart have been performed across a wide range of patient indications and lesion subsets. In April 2003, following the completion of the pivotal randomized Study of Sirolimus-Coated BX VELOCITY Balloon-Expandable Stent in Treatment of de Novo Native Coronary Artery Lesions (SIRIUS) trial,[39] the Cypher SES became the first DES approved by the FDA. To date, this stent has been one of the most studied devices in modern history, with at least 20 randomized trials performed comparing the commercialized Cypher SES to BMS, PES, or other second-generation DES across a range of patient indications and lesion subsets. Collectively, these trials demonstrated that the Cypher SES resulted in a near abolition of in-stent late loss (averaging ~0.15 mm across studies, compared to 0.8 to 1.0 mm with most BMS), with an approximate 70% to 80% reduction in angiographic restenosis and clinical recurrence (TLR) compared to bare-metal comparators. Longer-term follow-up with this device has extended to 5 years and beyond, particularly from the four major SES trials (Randomized Study With Sirolimus-Coated BxVelocity Balloon Expandable Stent [RAVEL] SIRIUS, C-SIRIUS, and E-SIRIUS). In these analyses, treatment with SES has resulted in sustained reductions in clinical restenosis end points with similar rates of death and MI found in both SES and BMS arms,[67] although as discussed below, subsequent studies have shown an ongoing propensity for very late (>1 year) stent thrombosis with the Cypher DES.[68,69] This led to the development of safer second-generation DES, and ultimately the discontinuation of the Cypher stent.

The Taxus Paclitaxel-Eluting Stent

Paclitaxel, a highly lipophilic diterpenoid compound, was first isolated in 1963 from the pacific yew tree (Taxus brevifolia), and was subsequently developed for its potent antineoplastic properties.

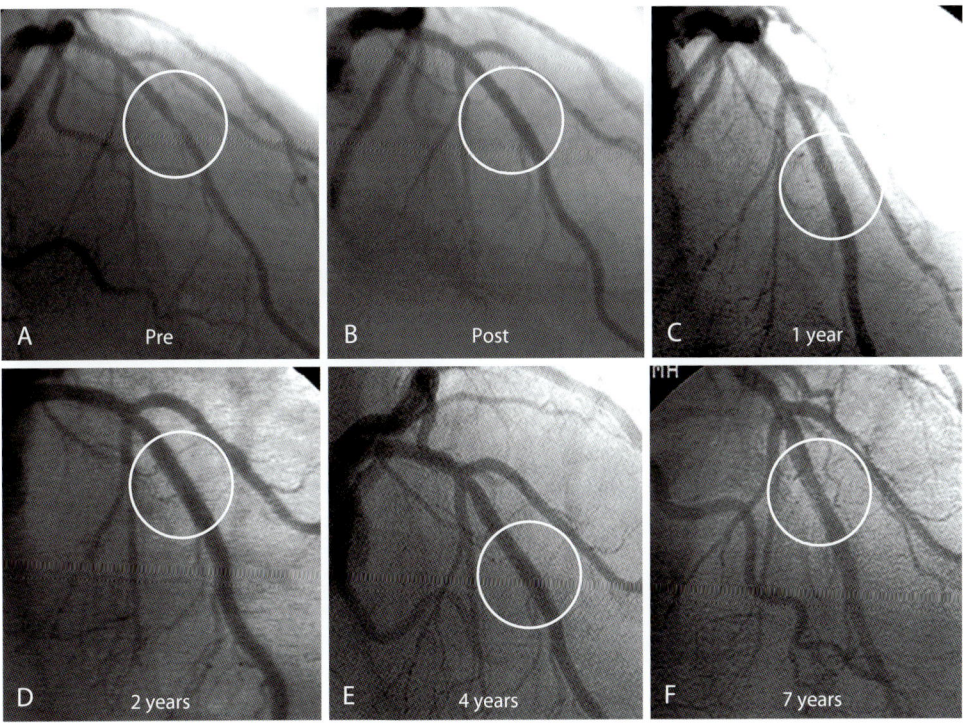

Fig. 15.5 Seven-year follow-up of one of the initial sirolimus-eluting stent implantations from Institute Dante Pazzanese of Cardiology in São Paulo, Brazil. (A) Severe stenosis of mid left anterior descending artery before stenting; (B) final result at the end of the procedure; (C) angiographic follow up at 1 year; (D) at 2 years; (E) at 4 years; and (F) at 7 years.

TABLE 15.3 Randomized Controlled Trials Comparing Sirolimus-Eluting Stents to Bare-Metal Stents

Trial Name and Reference	Study Cohort	Number Randomized (Planned Angiographic Follow-Up)	Latest Follow-Up to Date	Principal Findings
RAVEL[38]	Single de novo native coronary lesions	238 (all)	5 years	The 6-month late loss was significantly lower with SES vs. BMS (0.01 vs. 0.80 mm, $P < .001$); no restenosis was seen in the SES group at 6 months.
SIRIUS[39]	Single de novo native coronary lesions	1058 (approximately 850)	5 years	The 9-month rate of TVF was significantly reduced with SES vs. BMS (8.6% vs. 21.0%, $P < .001$), driven by a reduction in TLR. At 5 years, there was a maintained reduction in TLR with SES (9.4% vs. 24.2%, $P < .001$), with similar rates of death, MI, and stent thrombosis.
C-SIRIUS[65]	Single de novo native coronary lesions	100 (all)	5 years (in pooled analyses)	SES was associated with greater 8 month in-stent minimum lumen diameter (2.46 mm for SES vs. 1.49 mm with BMS, $P < .001$).
E-SIRIUS[495]	Single de novo native coronary lesions	352 (all)	5 years (in pooled analyses)	8-month minimum lumen diameter was greater with SES vs. BMS (2.22 vs. 1.33 mm, $P < .001$)
MULTI-STRATEGY[495]	STEMI	745 (none)	8 months	At 8 months, SES was associated with a reduction in TVR compared to BMS (3.2% vs. 10.2%, $P < .001$), with no differences observed between stent types in death or MI.
TYPHOON[230]	STEMI	712 (200)	1 year	One-year TVF was lower with SES vs. BMS (7.3% vs. 14.3%, $P = .004$). There were no differences between SES and BMS with respect to death, MI, or stent thrombosis.
MISSION![235]	STEMI	310 (all)	3 years	SES was associated with lower in-segment late lumen loss at 9 months than BMS (0.12 vs. 0.56 mm, $P < .001$). At 3 years, differences in TLR were attenuated (6.3% vs. 12.5%, $P = .06$).
SESAMI[227]	STEMI	320 (all)	3 years	SES was associated with lower 1-year binary restenosis compared to BMS (9.3% vs. 21.3%, $P = .032$). TLR was lower at 3 years, with no differences in death, MI, or stent thrombosis.

Continued

TABLE 15.3 Randomized Controlled Trials Comparing Sirolimus-Eluting Stents to Bare-Metal Stents—cont'd

Trial Name and Reference	Study Cohort	Number Randomized (Planned Angiographic Follow-Up)	Latest Follow-Up to Date	Principal Findings
PASEO[236]	STEMI	270 including 90 PES (none)	4 years	SES was associated with lower TLR at 1 year compared to BMS (3.3% vs. 14.4%, $P = .016$), which was maintained at 4 years
STRATEGY[233]	STEMI	175 (all)	5 years	At 8 months, TLR was lower with SES compared to BMS (6% vs. 20%, $P = .006$). This benefit was maintained at 5-year follow-up with no excess in stent thrombosis with SES.
Seville[496]	STEMI	120 (none)	1 year	SES was associated with a nonstatistically different rate of the primary end point of cardiac death, MI, or TLR compared to BMS (6.7% vs. 11.%, $P = .40$).
SCORPIUS[497]	Diabetic patients	200 (all)	1 year	In-segment late lumen loss was lower with SES compared to BMS (0.18 vs. 0.74 mm, $P < .001$), with lower rates of MACE.
DIABETES[498]	Diabetic Patients	160 (all)	2 years	SES was associated with lower late lumen loss at 9 months (0.06 vs. 0.47 mm, $P < .001$). At 2 years, SES was associated with a lower rate of TLR compared to BMS (7.7% vs. 35.0%, $P < .001$).
DECODE[499]	Diabetic patients	83 (all)	1 year	Mean in-stent late lumen loss at 6 months was lower with SES compared to BMS (0.23 vs. 1.10 mm, $P < .001$).
SCANDSTENT[500]	Complex CAD	322 (all)	3 years	SES was associated with greater MLD at 6 months than BMS (2.48 vs. 1.65 mm, $P < .001$). At 3 years TLR was significantly reduced with SES (4.9% vs. 33.8%, $P < .001$).
PRISON II[311]	CTO	200 (all)	4 years	SES had significantly lower 6-month binary in-segment restenosis than BMS (7% vs. 36%, $P < .001$). At 4 years, significant reductions in TLR were maintained with SES.
SES SMART[501]	Small Vessels	257 (all)	2 years	Eight-month binary in-segment restenosis was lower with SES compared to BMS (9.8% vs. 53.1%, $P < .001$). At 2 years, lower rates of TLR and MI were observed with SES compared to BMS.
RRISC[338]	SVG	75 (all)	3 years	Six-month in-stent late lumen loss was lower with SES compared to BMS (0.38 vs. 0.79 mm, $P = .001$). At 3 years, similar rates of TVR were observed with both stent types, with 11 deaths observed with SES vs. 0 deaths with BMS.
Pache et al.[502]	Unselected	500 (all)	1 year	SES had lower angiographic restenosis than a thin-strut BMS (8.3% vs. 25.5%, $P < .001$) with a lower incidence of TVR.
Ortolani et al.[503]	Unselected	104 (all)	1 year	SES had lower in-stent late loss compared to a thin-strut cobalt-chromium BMS (0.18 vs. 0.51 mm, $P < .001$). At 1 year, rates of TLR were lower with SES, but not statistically different.

BMS, Bare-metal stent; *CAD*, coronary artery disease; *CTO*, chronic total occlusion; *MACE*, major adverse cardiac event; *MI*, myocardial infarction; *MLD*, minimal lumen diameter; *SES*, sirolimus-eluting stent; *STEMI*, ST-segment elevation myocardial infarction; *SVG*, saphenous vein grafts; *TLR*, target-lesion revascularization; *TVF*, target-vessel failure (cardiac death, MI or TVR); *TVR*, target-vessel revascularization.

Paclitaxel is insoluble in water, and thus was combined with an intravenous oil-based cremophor for intravenous injection as the oncologic compound Taxol. The principal action of paclitaxel is to interfere with microtubule dynamics, preventing depolymerization. As microtubules are ubiquitous, paclitaxel has widespread multicellular and multifunctional activities, with dose-dependent effects. Paclitaxel has antiproliferative and antiinflammatory properties, prevents smooth muscle migration, blocks cytokine and growth factor release and activity, interferes with secretory processes, is antiangiogenic, and impacts signal transduction.[33,49–51] Although cytotoxic at high doses, at low doses (similar to those in DES applications), paclitaxel affects the G0 to G1 and G1 to S phases (G1 arrest) resulting in cytostasis without cell death (probably via induction of p53/p21 tumor suppression genes).[49,52] Systemic paclitaxel was shown to inhibit restenosis in a rat carotid injury model at levels more than 100-fold lower than that required for tumor cytotoxicity.[50] Neointimal area was greatly reduced in a rabbit balloon injury experiment using local paclitaxel administration,[49] and stent-based paclitaxel elution from polymer-based systems has been shown to profoundly reduce intimal hyperplasia in rabbit iliac arteries for up to 6 months with dose-dependent efficacy and toxicity.[70,71]

The TAXUS PES (Boston Scientific, Natick, MA) consisted of paclitaxel contained within a polyolefin derivative biostable polymer (styrene-isobutylene-styrene, referred to as SIBS [Translute]), originally coated on the Nir stent and subsequently on the Express open-cell slotted tube stainless steel stent platform (the device from which most of the randomized clinical trial data for this stent was derived). The base BMS of the last generation of TAXUS stent was the Liberté stent, a more flexible, thinner strutted open-cell stainless steel slotted tube stent. Depending on the relative ratio of paclitaxel to polymer, the stent could be formulated with varying release kinetics. The clinically available formulation of the TAXUS PES was the slow-release (SR) formulation, although the moderate-release (MR) formulation had also been tested in clinical trials. The SR stent used to have relatively more polymer-to-drug (paclitaxel concentration of 1 µg/mm^2), with a coat thickness 18 µm, and approximately 8% in vivo paclitaxel elution in 30 days. The drug was eluted in a rapid burst phase over the initial 48 hours, followed by a slow, sustained release for the next 10 to 30 days, with >90% of the drug sequestered in the bulk of the polymer matrix below the surface without pathways to the external environment (thus permanently retained on the stent). In a series of porcine experiments at 30, 90, 180, and 360 days involving a total of 350 swine and 800 stents, both SR and MR TAXUS stent formulations were shown to be vasculocompatible, with early development of a thin, mature neointima with low levels of inflammation, microthrombi and peristent amorphous material deposition, no evidence of cytotoxicity, and with complete healing and endothelialization within 90 days (data on file, Boston Scientific).

The clinical safety and efficacy of the TAXUS PES compared to BMS has been tested in at least 12 randomized trials (Table 15.4). Collectively, these trials have demonstrated consistent reductions in measures of neointimal hyperplasia (assessed by angiography and IVUS), with resultant reductions in clinical restenosis end points with PES compared to BMS. Longer-term follow-up with this device has extended to 5 years and beyond, particularly for the four major PES trials of the SR stent (TAXUS I, II, IV, and V). In these analyses, treatment with PES resulted in sustained reductions in clinical restenosis end points, with similar rates of death and MI found in both PES and BMS arms.[72] However, like Cypher, these and other studies have demonstrated an ongoing risk of stent thrombosis beyond the first year after Taxus stent implantation.[68,69,73] The introduction of safer (and more effective) DES resulted in a marked decrease in Taxus use, which eventually led to discontinuation of the manufacturing of this device.

Comparisons of First Generation DES
Following the approval of the TAXUS PES for commercial use, a series of comparisons between the two approved devices (Cypher SES and TAXUS PES) ensued, in order to determine whether superiority could be established for a particular DES. A total of 21 randomized comparisons of different sizes have been performed to date in numerous patient and lesion cohorts, and have included a variety of IVUS, angiographic, and clinical end points (Table 15.5). In summary, the totality of evidence appeared to indicate similar performance of SES and PES in routine de novo coronary artery lesions, despite less neointimal hyperplasia with SES as assessed by IVUS and angiography.[74–77] Among pooled analyses of more complex or "higher-risk" lesion subsets, there could be a clinical benefit to the Cypher SES due to its more potent suppression of neointimal hyperplasia, but validation of these findings would have required large-scale, adequately powered clinical trials before being considered definitive.[78]

Limitations of First-Generation Drug-Eluting Stents
Although individual pivotal trials did not raise major safety issues related to first-generation DES, subsequent studies revealed an ongoing propensity of these devices for an increased risk of very late stent thrombosis.[79,80] This safety concern was initially raised by a report of four cases of angiographically confirmed stent thrombosis late after elective implantation of SES or PES,[81] and then ignited by a meta-analysis performed on aggregate data presented in 2006 during the European Society of Cardiology annual meeting in Barcelona.[82] That meta-analysis, in which data from trial programs comparing SES or PES versus BMS were pooled, suggested an increased risk of mortality and MI with first-generation DES compared to BMS.[82] This concern was further fuelled by additional real-world studies which showed an increased risk of late stent thrombosis and MI in patients treated with first-generation DES after discontinuation of DAPT,[79] and a steady accrual of stent thrombosis at a rate of 0.6% per year with no evidence of plateau after 4-year follow-up.[69] In addition, human autopsy studies and pathologic studies in animal models suggested that the permanent polymer coating first-generation DES could be associated with chronic inflammation, chronic fibrin deposition, late hypersensitivity reactions, and delayed arterial healing, potentially increasing the risk of very late stent thrombosis in some patients.[56,83] These findings entailed a dramatic reduction of DES utilization in the U.S., which dropped from 90% before 2006 to 64% in the following years.[84]

In view of the rare incidence of stent thrombosis and the conflicting evidence, several pooled analyses and meta-analyses were performed to address the safety of first-generation DES (Table 15.6).[85–89] These studies collectively did not suggest an increased risk of mortality or MI with DES compared to BMS, but some of them confirmed an increased risk of late or very late stent thrombosis with both SES and PES compared to BMS.[85–89] Of note, SES but not PES was associated with a reduction of stent thrombosis during the first year compared to BMS, which was offset by an increased risk of very late stent thrombosis with SES after the first year.[87] The slightly increased risk of stent thrombosis with first-generation DES likely offset any potential long-term benefit of these devices in improving MI and survival by reducing restenosis.[90]

Second-Generation Drug-Eluting Stents

Following the initial development and approval of the SES and PES, further iterations in DES technology resulted from a desire to improve upon both the deliverability and efficacy of first-generation DES, as well as to address some of the safety limitations of these devices. In general, most second-generation DES have incorporated superior stent platforms and more biocompatible durable polymers or BP, principally with rapamycin-analog drugs in comparison with first-generation DES. Polymer-free stents have also been developed, which offer the potential of controlled drug release without the vascular toxicity associated with the presence of the polymer. Finally, the introduction of BRS represents a new paradigm in the treatment of coronary artery disease, providing drug-elution and a temporary vascular scaffolding function for 6 to 12 months, followed by complete bioresorption within the next 1 to 3 years depending on the device, theoretically restoring the underlying coronary anatomy and physiology, preventing very late (>1 year) adverse reactions from polymer reactions, neoatherosclerosis, and other mechanisms. However, concern has been raised over the increased propensity for stent thrombosis of these devices compared to metallic DES.[91]

Durable Polymer-Based Second-Generation Drug-Eluting Stents
Pivotal randomized trials have been completed with four second-generation permanent polymer-based DES: Xience V/Xience Prime/Xience Expedition/Xience Alpine (Abbott Vascular, Santa Clara, CA), which are cobalt-chromium stents eluting everolimus from a fluorinated copolymer (CoCr-EES); Promus Element and Promus Premier (Boston Scientific, Natick, MA), which are platinum-chromium stents eluting everolimus from a fluorinated copolymer (PtCr-EES); Endeavor (Medtronic, Santa Rosa, CA), a phosphorylcholine polymer-based stent that elutes zotarolimus relatively rapidly, mostly over several weeks (PC-ZES); and

TABLE 15.4 Randomized Controlled Trials Comparing Paclitaxel-Eluting Stents to Bare-Metal Stents

Trial Name and Reference	Study Cohort	Number Randomized (Planned Angiographic Follow-Up)	Latest Follow-Up to Date	Principal Findings
TAXUS I[504]	Single de novo or restenotic lesions	61 (all)	5 years (in pooled analyses)	Six-month percent diameter stenosis was lower with PES compared to BMS (13.6% vs. 27.3%, $P < .001$), with improvements in IVUS findings with PES as well.
TAXUS II[505]	Single de novo native coronary lesions	536 (all)	5 years	Six-month net volume obstruction was lower with PES slow release vs. BMS (7.9% vs. 23.2%, $P < .001$) as well as PES moderate release (MR) compared to BMS. Reductions in TLR were maintained at 5 years with both PES formulations, with no differences in death, MI, or stent thrombosis.
TAXUS IV[72]	Single de novo native coronary lesions	1314 (732)	5 years	PES was associated with lower TLR compared to BMS at 9 months (4.7% vs. 12.0%, $P < .001$) as well as lower rates of angiographic restenosis. Reductions in TLR were maintained at 5 years with no differences in death, MI, or stent thrombosis.
TAXUS V[506]	Single lesions, including complex lesions	1156 (all)	5 years	PES reduced 9-month TVR compared to BMS (12.1% vs. 17.3%, $P = .02$), with reductions in angiographic restenosis overall and among patients with complex disease. At 5 years, reductions in clinical restenosis have been maintained with similar death, MI, and stent thrombosis.
TAXUS VI[507]	Single long complex lesions	448 (all)	5 years	Nine-month TVR was lower with PES MR compared to BMS (9.1% vs. 19.4%, $P = .0027$), with lower rates of angiographic restenosis. At 5 years, TVR rates were similar between both stents, although TLR was lower with PES MR.
HORIZONS-AMI[231,508]	STEMI	3006 (1800)	3 years	PES was associated with lower rates of TLR compared to BMS at one year (4.5% vs. 7.5%, $P = .002$), and lower binary restenosis at 13 months (10.0% vs. 22.9%, $P < .001$). The reduction in TLR was maintained at 3 years, with no significant differences in death, MI, or stent thrombosis observed.
PASSION[?]	STEMI	619 (none)	2 years	PES and BMS were associated with nonstatistically different rates of the primary end point of TLF (8.8% vs. 12.8%, $P = .09$) at 1 year, a finding that was maintained at 2 years.
PASEO[236]	STEMI	270 including 90 SES (none)	4 years	PES was associated with lower TLR at 1 year compared to BMS (4.4% vs. 14.4%, $P = .023$), which was maintained at 4 years.
HAAMU-STENT[232]	STEMI	164 (all)	1 year	Angiographic end points were improved with PES compared to BMS, with a trend toward lower TVR at one year (3.7% vs. 11%, $P = .07$).
SELECTION[225]	STEMI	80 (all)	7 months	Volume of neointimal hyperplasia by IVUS was lower with PES compared to BMS (4.6% vs. 20%, $P < .01$) with no differences in late malapposition seen between the stent types.
Erglis et al.[291]	Left main stenosis	103 (all)	6 months	PES was associated with a lower rate of binary angiographic restenosis at 6 months compared to BMS (6% vs. 22%, $P = .021$). IVUS measures were also improved with PES.
SOS[337]	SVG	80 (all)	Median 1.5 years	Binary angiographic restenosis was lower with PES compared to BMS (9% vs. 51%, $P < .001$). Similar rates of MI and death were observed.

BMS, Bare-metal stent; *IVUS*, intravascular ultrasound; *MI*, myocardial infarction; *PES*, paclitaxel-eluting stent (slow-release); *SES*, sirolimus-eluting stent; *STEMI*, ST-segment elevation myocardial infarction; *SVG*, saphenous vein grafts; *TLR*, target-lesion revascularization; *TVF*, target-vessel failure (cardiac death, MI or TVR); *TVR*, target-vessel revascularization.

TABLE 15.5 Randomized Controlled Trials Comparing Sirolimus-Eluting Stents and Paclitaxel-Eluting Stents

Trial Name and Reference	Study Cohort	Number Randomized (Planned Angiographic Follow-Up)	Latest Follow-Up to Date	Principal Findings
REALITY[74]	1–2 de novo coronary lesions	1386 (all)	1 year	Despite lower late loss with SES, rates of binary angiographic restenosis were similar with SES and PES (9.1% vs. 11.1%, $P = .31$), with similar rates of MACE at 1 year.
Zhang et al.[509]	De novo coronary lesions	673 including 224 Firebird stent (none)	1 year	At 1 year, rates of MACE were similar between SES and PES (8.4% vs. 11.2%).
SORT OUT II[76]	Unselected	2098 (none)	1.5 years	There were no significant differences between SES and PES in MACE (9.3% vs. 11.2%) or other end points, including death, MI, or stent thrombosis.
SIRTAX[510]	Unselected	1012 (approximately half)	5 years	SES was associated with a lower rate of MACE at 9 months compared to PES (6.2% vs. 10.8%, $P = .009$). However, at 5 years, the rates were similar with an accrual of events in both stent groups.
TAXi[511]	Unselected	202 (none)	3 years	Six-month MACE was similar with SES and PES (6% vs. 4%, $P = .8$) with similar findings at 3 years.
DES-DIABETES[75]	Diabetic patients	400 (all)	2 years	Six-month in-segment restenosis was lower with SES compared with PES (3.4% vs. 18.2%, $P < .001$). At 2 years, TLR remained lower with SES (3.5% vs. 11.0%, $P = .004$).
ISAR-DIABETES[259]	Diabetic patients	250 (all)	5 years (in pooled analyses)	In-segment late lumen loss was lower with SES compared with PES (0.43 vs. 0.67 mm, $P = .002$), with nonstatistically different rates of TLR at 9 months (6.4% vs. 12.0%, $P = .13$).
Kim et al.[512]	Diabetic patients	169 (all)	6 months	Late lumen loss was similar with SES and PES (0.26 vs. 0.39 mm, $P = .36$); rates of TLR were similar at 6 months.
DiabeDES[513]	Diabetic patients	153 (all)	8 months	In-stent late lumen loss was lower with SES compared with PES (0.23 vs. 0.52 mm, $P = .025$). The rates of TLR and MACE were similar with both stents.
CORPAL[514]	Lesions at "high-risk for restenosis"	652 (all)	15 months	Angiographic restenosis rates were similar with SES and PES, with similar rates of TLR.
ISAR LEFT MAIN[292]	Left main stenosis	607 (all)	2 years	Similar rates of angiographic restenosis were observed with SES and PES (19.4% vs. 16.0%, $P = .30$), with no differences observed in death, MI, or TLR.
LONG DES II[515]	Long lesions	500 (all)	9 months	In-segment binary restenosis was lower with SES compared to PES (3.3% vs. 14.6%, $P < .001$), with lower 9-month TLR.
Han et al.[516]	Multivessel CAD	416 (all)	19.5 months	Rates of MACE were similar with SES and PES over the follow-up period (6.4% vs. 8.8%), with no differences in minimum lumen diameter.
ISAR-SMART 3[517]	Small vessels	360 (all)	5 years (in pooled analyses)	Late lumen loss at 6–8 months was greater with PES compared to SES (0.56 vs. 0.25 mm, $P < .001$), with greater TLR (14.7% vs. 6.6%, $P = .008$).
Pan et al.[518]	Bifurcation lesions	205 (all)	2 years	SES was associated with lower rates of binary angiographic restenosis, less late lumen loss, and lower TLR at 2 years compared to PES (4% vs. 13%, $P < .021$).
Petronio et al.[77]	Complex lesions	100 (all)	9 months	By IVUS, the area of neointimal hyperplasia was significantly lower with SES than PES (7.4% vs. 15.4%, $P < .001$) at 9 months.
Cervinka et al.[519]	Complex CAD	70 (all)	6 months	IVUS-assessed neointimal hyperplasia volume was lower with SES compared with PES (4.1 vs. 17.4 mm^3, $P = .001$).
ISAR-DESIRE[475,519]	BMS restenosis	300 including 100 balloon angioplasty patients (all)	5 years (in pooled analyses)	Angiographic restenosis was lower with both SES (14.3%) and PES (21.7%) compared to balloon angioplasty at 6 months (44.6%). TVR was lower with SES compared to PES (8% vs. 19%, $P = .02$).
ISAR-DESIRE 2[485]	SES restenosis	450 (all)	1 year	There were no differences in late lumen loss (0.40 vs. 0.38, $P = .85$) or other angiographic or clinical end points with SES or PES for the treatment of SES-restenosis.

Continued

TABLE 15.5 Randomized Controlled Trials Comparing Sirolimus-Eluting Stents and Paclitaxel-Eluting Stents—cont'd

Trial Name and Reference	Study Cohort	Number Randomized (Planned Angiographic Follow-Up)	Latest Follow-Up to Date	Principal Findings
PROSIT[520]	STEMI	308 (all)	1 year	In-segment restenosis was lower with SES compared to PES (5.9% vs. 14.8%, $P = .03$), with similar rates of TLR and MACE.
PASEO[236]	STEMI	270 including 90 BMS (none)	4 years	Similar reductions in TLR were seen with SES and PES (relative to BMS), this was maintained throughout the follow-up period.

BMS, Bare-metal stent; *CAD,* coronary artery disease; *IVUS,* intravascular ultrasound; *MACE,* major adverse cardiac event; *MI,* Myocardial infarction; *PES,* paclitaxel-eluting stent; *SES,* sirolimus-eluting stent; *TLR,* target lesion revascularization; *TVR,* target vessel revascularization.

TABLE 15.6 Meta-Analyses Comparing First-Generation Drug-Eluting Stents With Bare-Metal Stents

First Author	Stent Comparators	Number of Trials	Number of Patients	Principal Findings
Ellis et al.[85]	PES vs. BMS	4	3445	No significant difference was apparent in the 3-year rates of death, MI, or stent thrombosis between PES and BMS. However, in the period between 6 months and 3 years, PES was associated with significantly higher rates of stent thrombosis
Kastrati et al.[86]	SES vs. BMS	14	4958	No significant difference was apparent in the risk of death, MI, or stent thrombosis between SES and BMS after a follow-up ranging from 12 to 58 months.
Spaulding et al.[88]	SES vs. BMS	4	1748	No sence was apparent in the 4-year rates of death, MI, or stent thrombosis between PES and BMS. Compared to BMS, SES was associated with an increased risk of mortality in diabetic patients
Stone et al.[89]	SES vs. BMS PES vs. BMS	4 5	1748 3513	No significant difference was apparent in the 4-year rates of death, MI, or stent thrombosis between PES vs. BMS or SES vs. BMS. Rates of very late stent thrombosis were higher with PES and SES compared to BMS
Mauri et al.[87]	SES BMS	4 4	1748	PES vs. BMS or SES
Stettler et al.[521]	SES vs. PES vs. BMS	38	18,023	No difference in rates of morality or stent thrombosis was apparent between any DES and BMS. PES was associated with higher rates of late definite stent thrombosis compared to SES or BMS. SES was associated with lower rates of MI compared to PES or BMS.
Kirtane et al.[41]	DES vs. BMS	22 RCT 34 observational studies	9470 18,2901	In RCTs, no significant difference in mortality or MI was apparent between DES and BMS at long-term follow-up. However, in observational studies, DES were associated with significantly lower rates of death or MI compared to BMS.

BMS, Bare-metal stents; *DES,* drug-eluting stents; *MI,* myocardial infarction; *PES,* paclitaxel-eluting stent; *SES,* sirolimus-eluting stents; *RCT,* randomized controlled trial.

Resolute/Resolute Onyx (Medtronic), which uses a composite Biolinx polymer possessing hydrophilic and hydrophobic properties to release zotarolimus slowly over 4 months (Re-ZES). All four polymer-based stents release a rapamycin-analog which binds to cytosolic FKBP12 and subsequently mTOR, thereby blocking the stimulatory effects of growth factors and cytokines which are released after vascular injury. However, the underlying stent platform and polymers vary significantly, as do the drug pharmacokinetics and pharmacodynamics, which has resulted in unique angiographic and clinical profiles of these devices.

Cobalt-Chromium Everolimus-Eluting Stents (Xience)

In the CoCr-EES, everolimus (100 µg/cm^2) is released from a thin (7.8 µm), nonadhesive, durable, biocompatible fluorinated copolymer consisting of vinylidene fluoride and hexafluoropropylene monomers, coated onto a low-profile (81 µm strut thickness), flexible cobalt chromium stent (which has additionally undergone several iterations). The release kinetics are similar to that seen with sirolimus from the SES (~80% of the drug released at 30 days, with none detectable after 120 days). The polymer is elastomeric, and experiences minimal bonding, webbing, or tearing upon expansion. Fluoropolymers have been demonstrated to resist platelet and thrombus deposition in blood-contact applications.[59,92] This property is likely related to the capacity of fluoropolymer to attract and bind albumin which passivates the stent surface, avoiding fibrinogen binding.[26] The EES fluoropolymer has also been demonstrated to be noninflammatory in porcine experiments. The low profile stent struts facilitate rapid re-endothelialization[93] and are fracture resistant. Preclinical studies have demonstrated more rapid coverage of the stent struts with functional endothelialization with CoCr-EES compared to SES, PES, or PC-ZES.[57]

To date, CoCr-EES has been the second-generation DES that has received the most extensive investigation with at least 43 randomized controlled trials performed, and 61,228 randomized patients included (Table 15.7). The CoCr-EES has been compared with PES in six trials with 7313 randomized patients,[44,94–98] with SES in 10 trials with 11,931 randomized patients,[99–108] with Re-ZES in three trials with 4333 randomized patients,[109–111] with PtCr-EES in two trials with 4515 randomized patients,[112,113] and with BMS in four trials with 3037 patients.[103,114–116] In addition, CoCr-EES was used in 82.3% (66.8% PROMUS, 15.5% Xience) of patients enrolled in the DES arm of the randomized controlled Norwegian Coronary Stent Trial (NORSTENT) trial comparing BMS versus DES,[117] and it was compared with the ABSORB bioabsorbable vascular scaffold (BVS) in seven randomized controlled trials including 5583 patients.[91] Finally, CoCr-EES has been compared with BP-based DES in randomized controlled trials powered for clinical end points, including three trials with 8233 patients in which CoCr-EES has been compared with BP-based biolimus-eluting stents (BP-BES),[118–120] and six trials with 7437 patients in which CoCr-EES has been compared with different types of BP-based SES.[121–125]

Cobalt-Chromium Everolimus-Eluting Stents Versus First-Generation Drug-Eluting Stents

Among the six trials in which CoCr-EES has been compared to PES (see Table 15.7),[44,95–98,125] two large-scale trials sufficiently powered for clinical end points have been conducted.[44,95] In the large-scale Clinical Evaluation of the XIENCE V Everolimus Eluting Coronary Stent System (SPIRIT IV) trial, 3687 patients with stable coronary artery disease undergoing PCI of up to three lesions in three vessels were randomized to CoCr-EES versus PES (Express platform).[44] The primary end point of target-lesion failure (TLF; composite of cardiac death, target-vessel MI or ischemia-driven TLR) at 1 year was reduced by 39% (3.9% vs. 6.6%, $P = .0008$). CoCr-EES compared with PES also reduced the 1-year rates of stent thrombosis (0.3% vs. 1.1%, $P = .003$), MI (1.9% vs. 3.1%, $P = .02$), and TLR (2.3% vs. 4.5%, $P = .0008$). These results have been sustained at 3 years' follow-up.[126] In the Trial of Everolimus-Eluting Stents and Paclitaxel-Eluting Stents for Coronary Revascularization in Daily Practice (COMPARE) trial,[95] 1800 unrestricted "all-comer" patients were randomized to CoCr-EES versus PES (Liberté platform). The primary end point of major adverse coronary events (MACEs) at 1 year (death, MI, or TVR) was reduced by 31% with CoCr-EES (6.2% vs. 9.1%, $P = .02$), driven by reductions in stent thrombosis (0.7% vs. 2.6%, $P = .002$), MI (2.8% vs. 5.4%, $P = .007$), and TLR (1.7% vs. 4.8%, $P = .0002$). These results have been sustained up to a 5-year follow-up.[127]

Among the 10 randomized trials comparing CoCr-EES with SES (see Table 15.7),[99–104,106–108,128] three large-scale trials have been conducted.[102,103,128] In the Scandinavian Organization for Randomized Trials with Clinical Outcome IV (SORT OUT IV) trial,[102] 2774 unselected patients in Denmark were randomized to CoCr-EES versus SES and followed through the Danish Civil Registration System and Western Denmark Heart Registry. The primary 9-month end point of the composite of cardiac death, MI, definite stent thrombosis, or TVR occurred in a comparable proportion of patients in both groups, although the overall event rates were lower than expected. Definite stent thrombosis occurred in fewer CoCr-EES than SES patients (0.1% vs. 0.7%, $P = .05$). At 5-year follow-up, CoCr-EES were associated with significantly lower rates of MACE (4.8% vs. 7.0%, $P = .02$) and definite stent thrombosis (0.4% vs. 2.0%, $P = .0004$) compared to SES.[129] In the large-scale REal Safety and Efficacy of 3-month dual antiplatelet Therapy following Endeavor zotarolimus-eluting stent implantation (RESET) trial, 3197 unselected patients were randomized to CoCr-EES versus SES.[128] At 1-year follow-up, CoCr-EES resulted in nonsignificantly different rates of the primary end point of TLR (4.3% in the CoCr-EES group vs. 5.0% in the SES group). The cumulative incidence of definite stent thrombosis was similarly low between the two groups (0.32% vs. 0.38%, $P = .77$). Finally, in the Evaluation of Late Clinical Events After Drug-eluting Versus Bare-metal Stents in Patients at Risk (BASKET PROVE) trial, 2314 "all comer" patients with a lesion in coronary arteries with diameters greater than or equal to 3 mm were randomly allocated to receive CoCr-EES, SES, or BMS.[103] At 2-year follow-up, no significant difference was apparent between CoCr-EES and SES in the rates of the primary end point (a composite of death or MI) as well as in the rates of TVR or stent thrombosis.

In summary, in a broad cross-section of patients undergoing PCI, CoCr-EES have shown marked improvements in safety and efficacy outcomes compared with PES, and modest improvements compared with SES. In view of the limited power of these randomized trials in detecting differences in low-frequency end points, several meta-analyses have been performed. In a meta-analysis in which 13 randomized control trials (RCTs) with 17,101 patients were included, CoCr-EES use was associated with significant reductions in MI, TVR, and definite/probable stent thrombosis compared to pooled PES, SES, and Re-ZES after a median follow-up of 21 months.[130] However, the treatment effects for each end point varied by DES comparator, with the largest difference being apparent for CoCr-EES versus PES, intermediate for CoCr-EES versus Re-ZES, and smallest for CoCr-EES versus SES. In another meta-analysis including 11 trials with 16,775 patients and focusing on time-related differences in the risk of definite stent thrombosis, CoCr-EES was associated with significantly lower rates of early, late, 1-year, and 2-year definite stent thrombosis compared with pooled PES, SES, and Re-ZES, with no interaction apparent between the overall relative risk of definite stent thrombosis and any DES comparator.[131,132] These findings have been corroborated in a meta-analysis including eight trials with 11,167 patients followed for a follow-up ranging from 9 to 36 months.[132]

The reduced risk of stent thrombosis with CoCr-EES compared with first-generation DES apparent in these meta-analyses has since been confirmed in "real-world" observational studies. Specifically, in 1342 propensity score-matched pairs of patients followed for a median follow-up of 1.5 years, CoCr-EES was associated with significantly lower rates of definite stent thrombosis and MI compared to SES.[133] Moreover, in a large all-comers study including 12,339 patients, CoCr-EES was found to have significantly lower rates of definite stent thrombosis than either SES or PES up to a 4-year follow-up, with differences in stent thrombosis being most pronounced beyond the first year after stent implantation.[134]

Cobalt-Chromium Everolimus-Eluting Stents Versus Bare-Metal Stents

When second-generation DES reached the clinical arena, the natural comparator of these new devices was first-generation DES. As a consequence, few studies have compared second-generation DES with BMS. However, CoCr-EES has been compared with BMS in four randomized controlled trials: SPIRIT FIRST, BASKET PROVE, Xience or Vision Stents for the Management of Angina in the Elderly (XIMA), and Everolimus-Eluting Stents Versus Bare-Metal Stents in STEMI (EXAMINATION).[103,114–116] In addition, CoCr-EES has been compared with BMS in the Prolonging Dual Antiplatelet Treatment After Grading Stent-Induced Intimal Hyperplasia (PRODIGY) trial, in which 2013 patients were randomly assigned to receive 6-month DAPT versus 12-month DAPT and either CoCr-EES, BMS, PES, or PC-ZES,[135] and in the NORSTENT trial in which 82.3% of patients enrolled in the DES arm received CoCr-EES (66.8% PROMUS, 15.5% Xience).[117] SPIRIT FIRST was a small randomized trial showing significantly lower rates of restenosis and in-stent late loss with CoCr-EES compared to BMS at 6-month angiographic follow-up.[116] In the large-scale randomized BASKET PROVE trial, 2-year rates of the primary end point of death/MI were 3.2% with CoCr-EES and 4.8% with BMS ($P = .37$).[103] However, rates of TVR were significantly higher with BMS than CoCr-EES (10.3% vs. 3.7%, respectively, $P = .002$). The XIMA trial was a prospective randomized clinical trial comparing CoCr-EES with BMS in 800 patients aged greater than or equal to 80 years.[114] The primary end point, which was a composite of death, MI, cerebrovascular accident, TVR, or major hemorrhage, occurred in 18.7% of patients treated with BMS versus 14.3% of patients treated with CoCr-EES ($P = .09$). There was no difference in the risk of death (7.2% vs. 8.5%, respectively; $P = .50$), major hemorrhage (1.7% vs. 2.3%; $P = .61$), or cerebrovascular accident (1.2% vs. 1.5%; $P = .77$). In contrast, MI (8.7% vs. 4.3%; $P = .01$) and TVR (7.0% vs. 2.0%; $P =$

TABLE 15.7 Randomized Controlled Trials With Food and Drug Administration-Approved Second-Generation Drug-Eluting Stents

Study	Study Cohort	Latest Follow-Up to Date	Principal Findings
CoCr-EES vs. PES			
COMPARE[95,127]	All-comers	1800	5 years	CoCr-EES vs. PES resulted in lower 1-year rates of the primary end point, a composite of death, MI, or TVR (6.2% vs. 9.1%, $P = .02$). CoCr-EES also resulted in lower rates of MI, stent thrombosis, and TLR (see text). At 5 years the primary composite end point occurred in 18.4% of CoCr-EES patients vs. 25.1% of PES patients ($P = .0005$).
EXECUTIVE[96]	MVD, otherwise noncomplex CAD	200	9 months	CoCr-EES vs. PES resulted in lower 9-month rates of angiographic in-stent late loss (0.11 ± 0.27 mm vs. 0.36 ± 0.39 mm, $P = .008$).
SPIRIT II[97,522]	Noncomplex CAD; up to two lesions	300	5 years	CoCr-EES vs. PES resulted in lower 6-month rates of angiographic in-stent late loss (0.11 ± 0.27 mm vs. 0.36 ± 0.39 mm, $P < .0001$).
SPIRIT III[98,434]	Noncomplex CAD; up to two lesions	1002	5 years	CoCr-EES vs. PES resulted in lower 8-month rates of angiographic in-segment late loss (0.14 ± 0.41 mm vs. 0.28 ± 0.48 mm, $P = .004$), noninferior 9-month rates of TVF (7.2% vs. 9.0%, $P = .31$), and reduced rates of MACE at 1 year (5.7% vs. 9.9%, $P = .01$) and 5 years (13.2% vs. 20.7%, $P = .007$).
SPIRIT IV[44,126]	Noncomplex CAD; up to three lesions	3687	3 years	CoCr-EES vs. PES resulted in lower 1-year rates of TLF (3.9% vs. 6.6%, $P = .0008$) and ischemia-driven TLR (2.3% vs. 4.5%, $P = .0008$), with noninferior rates of cardiac death or target-vessel MI (2.2% vs. 3.2%, $P = .09$). CoCr-EES also resulted in lower rates of MI and stent thrombosis (see text). At 3 years TLF occurred in 9.2% of CoCr-EES patients vs. 11.7% of PES patients ($P = .02$).
SPIRIT V DIABETIC[94]	Diabetes mellitus	324	1 year	CoCr-EES vs. PES resulted in lower 9-month rates of angiographic in-stent late loss (0.19 ± 0.37 mm vs. 0.39 ± 0.49 mm, $P = .0001$).
CoCr-EES vs. SES			
CIBELES[106,105]	Chronic total occlusion	207	9 months	Noninferiority was present for the primary end point of in-segment late loss at 9 months (CoCr-EES 0.19 ± 0.69 mm vs. SES 0.29 ± 0.60 mm, $P_{NI} < .01$). Binary restenosis occurred in 10.0% of patients treated with SES and 9.1% of patients treated with CoCr-EES
EXCELLENT[105]	Noncomplex CAD	1443	9 months	Noninferiority was present for the primary end point of in-segment late loss at 9 months (CoCr-EES 0.10 ± 0.36 mm vs. SES 0.05 ± 0.34 mm, $P_{NI} = .02$). MACE occurred in only ~3.0% of patients in both groups at 9 months.
ESSENCE DIABETES[104]	Diabetes	300	1 year	CoCr-EES vs. SES resulted in lower 8-month angiographic in-segment late loss (mean 0.23 vs. 0.37 mm, $P = .02$) and lower binary restenosis (0.9% vs. 6.5%, $P = .04$).
ISAR TEST IV[a,100,523]	Simple and complex CAD	1304	3 years	CoCr-EES vs. SES resulted in nonsignificantly different rates of in-segment late loss at 24 months (0.29 ± 0.51 mm vs. 0.31 ± 0.58 mm, $P = .59$). TLF at 3 years was not significantly different between CoCr-EES and SES (19.6% vs. 22.3%, $P = .26$), although TLR tended to be less frequent with CoCr-EES (12.8% vs. 15.5%, $P = .15$).
LONG DES III[107]	Long lesion (≥25 mm)	450	9 months	In-segment late loss was significantly greater with CoCr-EES than SES (0.17 ± 0.41 mm vs. 0.09 ± 0.30 mm, P for noninferiority = .96, P for superiority = .04). However, in-stent late loss (0.22 ± 0.43 mm vs. 0.18 ± 0.28 mm, $P = .29$) were similar among the two groups. The incidence of death, MI, stent thrombosis, and TLR was not statistically different between the two groups.
RESET[524]	All-comers	3197	3 years	CoCr-EES vs. SES resulted in nonsignificantly different rates of TLR at 1 year (4.3% vs. 5.0%, $P_{NI} = .0001$). Definite stent thrombosis was similar between the two groups (0.32% vs. 0.38%, $P = .77$). At 3 years, the incidence of TLF was significantly lower with CoCr-EES vs. SES (8.8% vs. 11.4%, $P = .01$).

TABLE 15.7 Randomized Controlled Trials With Food and Drug Administration-Approved Second-Generation Drug-Eluting Stents—cont'd

	Study	Study Cohort	Latest Follow-Up to Date	Principal Findings
SEASIDE[99]	Bifurcations	150	18 months	CoCr-EES vs. SES resulted in similar procedural results in the main vessel and better results in the side branch. At 18 months the incidence of MACE (death, MI, TVR) was 12% with CoCr-EES and 9% with SES ($P = .60$)
SORT OUT IV[102,129]	All-comers	2774	5 years	CoCr-EES resulted in nonsignificantly different 9-month rates of MACE (cardiac death, MI, definite stent thrombosis, or TVR) compared to SES (4.9% vs. 5.2%, $P = .71$). At 5 years MACE were 14.1% with CoCr-EES vs. 17.4% with SES ($P = .02$). Definite stent thrombosis was 0.4% with CoCr-EES vs. 2.0% with SES ($P = .0004$).
XAMI[101]	STEMI	625	1 year	CoCr-EES vs. SES resulted in significantly lower 1-year rates of the primary composite end point of cardiac death, MI or TVR (4.0% vs. 7.7%, $P = .048$). One-year incidence of definite/probable stent thrombosis was 1.2% for CoCr-EES vs. 2.7% for SES ($P = .21$).
CoCr-EES vs. Re-ZES				
RESOLUTE All Comers[172,525]	All-comers	2292	5 years	CoCr-EES vs. RE-ZES resulted in nonsignificantly different 12-month rates of the primary end point of TLF defined as cardiac death, MI, or TLR (8.2% vs. 8.3%, $P = .94$). After 5 years of follow-up both stents showed similar results for the composite primary end point (17% vs. 16.2%, $P = .61$).
TWENTE[111,171]	All-comers with the only exception of patients with STEMI	1391	2 years	CoCr-EES vs. RE-ZES resulted in nonsignificantly different 12-month rates of the primary composite end point of TVF (8.2% vs. 8.1%, $P = .94$), MI (4.6% vs. 4.6%, $P = .99$), cardiac death (1.0% vs. 1.4%, $P = .46$), clinically driven TVR (3.3% vs. 2.7%, $P = .54$). After 2 years of follow-up both stents showed similar results for the composite primary end point (10.8% vs. 11.6%, $P = .65$).
ISAR LEFT MAIN II[109]	Left main	750	1 year	CoCr-EES vs. RE-ZES resulted in nonsignificantly different 12-month rates of the primary composite end point death, MI, and TLR (17.5% vs. 14.3%, $P = .25$).
CoCr-EES vs. BMS				
Prodigy[d,526]	All-comers	1003	2 years	CoCr-EES vs BMS resulted in significantly lower rates of the composite of death, nonfatal MI or TVR ($P < .01$).
BASKET PROVE[b,103]	All-comers with lesions in coronary arteries with diameter ≥3 mm	2314	2 years	CoCr-EES vs. BMS resulted in nonsignificantly different 2 years rates of cardiac death or MI (3.2% vs. 4.8%, $P = .37$).
EXAMINATION[115,239]	STEMI	1498	5 years	CoCr-EES vs. BMS resulted in nonsignificantly different 2 years rates of the primary composite end point of all-cause death, MI, any revascularization, TLR, and stent thrombosis (14.4% vs. 17.3%, $P = .11$). CoCr-EES was superior to BMS after 5 years of follow up (21% vs. 26%, $P = .033$).
XIMA[114]	Elderly patients	800	1 year	CoCr-EES vs. BMS resulted in nonsignificantly different 1-year rates of the primary end point of death, MI, cerebrovascular accident, TVR or major bleeding (14.3% vs. 18.7%, $P = .09$).
SPIRIT I[116,527]	Noncomplex CAD	60	5 years	CoCr-EES was superior to BMS for in-stent late loss after 6 months (16% vs. 29%, $P < .001$). The same results were clinically confirmed after 5 years of follow-up.
NORSTENT[c]	Noncomplex CAD	9013	6 years	CoCr-EES vs. BMS resulted in nonsignificantly different 6 years rates of the primary end point of death, MI (16.6% vs. 17.1%, $P = .66$).
CoCr-EES vs. PtCr-EES				
PLATINUM[113,147]	Noncomplex CAD; up to 2 lesions	1530	3 years	CoCr-EES vs. PtCr-EES resulted in nonsignificantly different 1-year reates of the primary composite end point of cardiac death, MI, and TLR (4.9% vs. 5.9%, $P = .97$). This result was confirmed after 3 years of follow-up (7.1% vs. 5.4%, $P = .4$).
PLATINUM PLUS[112]	All-comers	2980	1 year	PtCr-EES was noninferior to CoCr-EES for the primary composite end point of cardiac death, MI, TVR (4.6% vs. 3.2%, $P = .012$) at 1-year follow-up.

Continued

TABLE 15.7 Randomized Controlled Trials With Food and Drug Administration-Approved Second-Generation Drug-Eluting Stents—cont'd

Study	Study Cohort	Latest Follow-Up to Date	Principal Findings
RE-ZES VS. PTCR-EES			
DUTCH PEERS[144]	All-comers	1811	2 years	Re-ZES was noninferior to PtCr-EES for the primary composite end point of cardiac death, MI, TVR (6% vs. 5%, $P = .42$).
HOST ASSURE[172]	All-comers	3750	1 year	PtCr-EES was noninferior to CoCr-ZES for the primary composite end point of cardiac death, MI, TLR (2.9% vs. 2.9%, $P = .025$) at 1-year follow-up.
RE-ZES VS. SES			
ESSENCE DIABETES II[528]	Diabetes mellitus	256	9 months	Re-ZES was noninferior to SES for the primary end point of in-segment late loss (0.34-0.30 vs. 0.39-0.43 mm; $P < .001$ for noninferiority).

[a]In this trial CoCr-EES was compared with PES and SES.
[b]In this trial CoCr-EES was compared with BMS and SES.
[c]In This trial CoCr-EES was used in 82.3% of patients randomized to the DES arm of the trial and consisted in 66.8% of cases in PROMUS and 15.5% of cases in Xience.
[d]In this trial CoCr-EES was compared with BMS, ZES, and PES.
BMS, Bare-metal stent; *CAD*, coronary artery disease; *CoCr-EES*, cobalt-chromium everolimus-eluting stents; *MACE*, major adverse cardiac events (cardiac death, MI or TLR); *MI*, myocardial infarction; *MVD*, multivessel disease; *PES*, paclitaxel-eluting stents; *PtCr-EES*, platinum-chromium everolimus-eluting stents; *Re-ZES*, Resolute zotarolimus-eluting stents; *SES*, sirolimus-eluting stents; *STEMI*, ST-segment elevation myocardial infarction; *TLF*, target-lesion failure (cardiac death, target-lesion MI or TLR); *TLR*, target-lesion revascularization; *TVF*, target-vessel failure (cardiac death, target-vessel MI or TVR); *TVR*, target-vessel revascularization.

.001) occurred more often in patients in the BMS group than in the CoCr-EES group. The EXAMINATION trial was a prospective, multicenter trial randomly assigning 1498 patients with STEMI to either CoCr-EES or BMS.[115] Detail of this study will be discussed in the section Acute ST-Segment Elevation Myocardial Infarction. These five trials have been recently pooled in an individual patient level meta-analysis including 4896 randomized patients.[136] After a median follow-up of 2 years, CoCr-EES were associated with significantly lower rates of cardiac mortality (hazard ratio [HR] 0.67, 95% confidence interval [CI] 0.49 to 0.91), MI (HR 0.71, 95% CI 0.55 to 0.92), definite/probable stent thrombosis (HR 0.48, 95% CI 0.31 to 0.73), and TVR (HR 0.29, 95% CI 0.20 to 0.41) compared to BMS, demonstrating that best-in-class second-generation DES may have improved safety, including survival, compared to BMS. Finally, in the NORSTENT trial, 9013 patients with stable or unstable coronary artery disease were randomly assigned to receive either a BMS or a DES, which was CoCr-EES in 82% of cases or ZES in 12% of cases.[117] At 6-year follow-up, there was no significant difference in the primary end point, which was a composite of death or MI, between BMS and DES (17.1% vs. 16.6%, respectively, $P = .66$). However, compared to BMS, DES were associated with lower rates of any repeat revascularization (19.8% vs. 16.5%, $P < .001$) and lower rates of stent thrombosis (1.2% vs. 0.8%, $P = .0498$).

Cobalt-Chromium Everolimus-Eluting Stents Versus Second-Generation Drug-Eluting Stents
There have been at least 12 randomized trials comparing CoCr-EES with other second-generation DES.[a] The details of these trials are included under the subsections below describing each of these second-generation DES.

Platinum-Chromium Everolimus-Eluting Stents (Promus Element/Premier)
The PtCr-EES is made of a platinum chromium alloy with 81 µm strut thickness, with high radial strength and moderate radiopacity (somewhat greater than CoCr-EES). PtCr-EES uses the same durable, biocompatible, inert fluorocopolymer (~7 µm thick) and antiproliferative agent (everolimus at 100 µg/cm² concentration) as CoCr-EES but with a modified scaffold design that aims to provide improved deliverability, vessel conformability, side-branch access, radial strength, and fracture resistance. The PtCr-EES provides comparable everolimus-release kinetics, arterial tissue levels, and vascular responses as CoCr-EES in a nondiseased porcine coronary artery model.[139] The vascular response to the PtCr-EES was assessed in a small clinical study recruiting 73 patients with a single coronary lesion with RVD greater than or equal to 2.5 mm and lesion length less than or equal to 24 mm.[140] Surveillance coronary angiography performed at 9 months after PCI showed an in-stent late loss of 0.17 ± 0.25 mm, which was comparable with that of CoCr-EES reported in the SPIRIT trial program (0.10 ± 0.21 mm at 6 months in SPIRIT I[116]; 0.11 ± 0.27 mm at 6 months in SPIRIT II[97]; and 0.16 ± 0.41 mm at 8 months in SPIRIT III).[98] The percentage of volume obstruction determined by IVUS with PtCr-EES at 9-month follow-up was 7.2 ± 6.2%, also comparable to that reported with the CoCr-EES (8.0 ± 10.4% at 6 months in SPIRIT I,[116] 2.5 ± 4.7% at 6 months in the SPIRIT II trial,[97] and 6.9 ± 6.4% at 8 months in the SPIRIT III trial).[98]

The safety and efficacy of PtCr-EES were assessed in seven randomized controlled trials comparing this device with CoCr-EES (PLATINUM, PLATINUM plus, and PEXIP),[113,141,142] Re-ZES (DUTCH PEERS and HOST ASSURE, see below),[143,144] BES (LONG DES V, see below),[145] and with the EES bioabsorbable scaffold and the BES in the EVERBIO II trial (see Chapter 16).[146] PLATINUM was a large-scale, international, multicenter, prospective, single-blind randomized trial in which 1530 patients with up to 2 de novo coronary lesions were randomized to either PtCr-EES or CoCr-EES.[113] At 1-year follow-up, rates of TLF (target vessel-related cardiac death, target vessel-related MI, or ischemia-driven TLR) were 2.9% in patients assigned to CoCr-EES versus 3.4% in patients assigned to Pr-Cr-EES ($P_{noninferiority}$ [P_{NI}] = .001). In addition, no significant differences were observed between CoCr-EES and PtCr-EES in cardiac death or MI (2.5% vs. 2.0%, respectively, $P = .56$), TLR (1.9% vs. 1.9%, $P = .99$), or definite/probable stent thrombosis (0.4% vs. 0.4%, $P = 1$). Similar results were apparent when follow-up was extended up to 3 years, with no significant differences between CoCr-EES and PtCr-EES in the risk of mortality (4.3% vs. 3.7%, respectively, $P = .62$), cardiac mortality (1.9% vs. 1.2%, $P = .27$), MI (2.5% vs. 2.3%, $P = .81$), ischemia-driven TLR (4.9% vs. 3.5%, $P = .21$), or definite/probable stent thrombosis (0.5% vs. 0.7%, $P = .76$).[147]

PLATINUM PLUS was a prospective, multicenter noninferiority trial enrolling 2980 all-comer patients to either PtCr-EES or CoCr-EES.[141] At 1-year follow-up, the primary end point of

[a]References 100,109–113,120,122,123,125,137,138

TVF (a composite of cardiac death, target vessel MI, or TVR) was 4.6% of patients in the PtCr-EES group as compared to 3.2% of patients in the CoCr-EES group (P_{NI} = .01), with similar rates of the individual components of the primary end point in both groups. Definite/probable stent thrombosis was 0.8% in the PtCr-EES group and 0.5% in the CoCr-EES group (P = .44). However, in the per protocol analysis, the primary end point was significantly more common in the PtCr-EES compared to CoCr-EES (HR 1.64, 95% CI 1.05 to 2.55; P = .03). Finally, PEXIP was a small, all-comers randomized trial assigning 300 patients to either CoCr-EES (n = 150) or PtCr-EES (n = 150).[142] At 18 months, no significant difference was apparent in any clinical end point between the two groups of patients. These trials have been recently collected in a meta-analysis including 11,036 patients and comparing PtCr-EES (n = 6613) versus combined CoCr-EES (n = 1940), ZES (n = 2158), or BES (n = 325).[148] After a median follow-up of 1 year, there were no significant differences in any ischemic end point between PtCr-EES and pooled DES. However, PtCr-EES was associated with a higher risk of longitudinal stent deformation compared with other DES (0.4% vs. 0%, respectively, P = .02).

Several reports suggested that the Promus Element stent platform is particularly susceptible to longitudinal stent deformation,[23] an infrequent complication after stent placement appearing as a reduction or increase in stent length with strut overlap, strut separation, malapposition, and/or luminal obstruction.[22] When longitudinal stent deformation occurs, it can predispose to stent thrombosis or restenosis, and may obstruct passage of devices.[23] Stent distortion may occur after stent deployment, during positioning of a postdilation balloon, thrombectomy device, IVUS catheter, or due to guide catheter compression when the stent is deployed in an ostial or proximal location. Stent deformation may be more frequent with Promus Element than other second-generation DES due to fewer connectors between hoops, a design intended to confer great longitudinal flexibility and deliverability of this device.[149] Bench testing has demonstrated that Promus Element platform (Omega) has less longitudinal strength compared to platforms of SES, PES, or CoCr-EES.[22] Subsequently, the design of the Promus Element was modified by the addition of connectors between the hoops in the proximal segment of the stent (the most common site of longitudinal deformation), leading to a new PtCr-EES design (Promus Premier). In bench testing, deformation with Promus Premier was significantly less than Promus Element, and similar to other stent platforms[150]; in practice, longitudinal stent deformation has infrequently been reported with this device.

Zotarolimus-Eluting Stent (Endeavor)

PC-ZES elutes zotarolimus (10 μg/mm stent length) from a thin layer (5.3 μm) of the biocompatible polymer phosphorylcholine from a flexible, low-profile (91 μm strut thickness) cobalt chromium stent. Phosphorylcholine is a naturally occurring phospholipid found in the membrane of red blood cells, and is resistant to platelet adhesion.[151] The potencies of zotarolimus, everolimus, and sirolimus are roughly comparable, and zotarolimus is somewhat more lipophilic. However, the release rate of zotarolimus from Endeavor (~90% within 7 days, 100% within 30 days) is significantly faster than everolimus and sirolimus released from Xience V and Cypher stents, respectively.

In the Endeavor I FIM study,[152] PC-ZES was implanted in 100 patients with noncomplex coronary lesions. Although TLR was required in only 1% of patients at 1 year, mean in-stent late lumen loss was 0.33 mm at 4 months and 0.61 mm at 12 months. While significantly less than the 0.8 to 1.0 mm mean in-stent late loss typically experienced with BMS, this degree of late loss would be expected to result in greater rates of binary restenosis and TLR compared to greater potency DES such as SES, CoCr-EEs, and Re-ZES, which achieve greater suppression of neointimal hyperplasia.[153,154] PC-ZES was subsequently compared to an otherwise identical BMS in the ENDEAVOR II trial[155,156] in 1197 randomized patients with noncomplex coronary artery disease. As described in Table 15.8, compared to BMS PC-ZES, this trial resulted in significantly reduced rates of TVF and TLR at 9 months, results that were sustained for 5 years.[157] Although the 9-month rate of angiographic in-stent late loss was 0.61 ± 0.46 mm, this was sufficient to reduce in-segment binary restenosis to 13.2% from 35.0% with BMS (P < .0001).

In order to assess whether this degree of late loss suppression was sufficient to prevent clinical restenosis, a series of trials have been performed in which the PC-ZES was compared to other DES (see Table 15.8). In the ENDEAVOR III trial, the rates of late loss and restenosis were significantly greater with PC-ZES than SES; indeed, in this trial the PC-ZES failed to meet its primary end point.[158] However, at 5-year follow-up, PC-ZES was associated with lower rates of all-cause death (a trend was apparent for cardiac death), and significantly lower rates of MI compared to SES. In contrast, no significant difference was apparent between PC-ZES and SES in the rates of TVR and definite stent thrombosis. These findings were corroborated in the Intracoronary Stenting and Angiographic Results: Test Efficacy of Three Limus-Eluting Stents (ISAR-TEST II) trial, which found no significant difference between SES and PC-ZES in the rates of death, MI, or definite stent thrombosis.[159] The ENDEAVOR IV trial randomized 1548 to either PC-ZES or PES. In this trial, PC-ZES was associated with a greater late loss and angiographic restenosis compared to PES, although 9-month rates of TVF were comparable between the two devices.[43] However, and similar to the ENDEAVOR III experience, at 5-year follow-up, PC-ZES was associated with similar rates of TLR and significantly lower rates of cardiac death or MI compared with PES.

While the results of these trials ultimately led to device approval of PC-ZES, these studies were insufficiently powered to identify differences in hard clinical end points, and several other trials have been conducted with mixed results, specifically regarding the safety of PC-ZES. No significant differences in cardiac mortality, MI, TVR, and stent thrombosis were apparent between SES, PES, and PC-ZES in the Korean Multicentre Endeavor (KOMER) trial,[160] whereas significantly higher rates of MACE and significantly higher rates of definite stent thrombosis trial were apparent with PC-ZES compared to SES in the Novel Approaches for Preventing or Limiting Events (NAPLES) trial[161] and in the Zotarolimus-Eluting Stent Versus Sirolimus-Eluting Stent and PacliTaxel-Eluting Stent for Coronary Lesions (ZEST) trial,[162] respectively (see Table 15.8). Although these trials led to potential concerns regarding the overall performance of PC-ZES, two larger trials have examined these issues in more detail. The 2332 patient SORT OUT III trial reported significantly lower rates of all-cause mortality, MI, and definite stent thrombosis with SES compared to PC-ZES at shorter-term follow-up (1 year).[163] However, at 5-year follow-up, rates of MACE were similar between the two devices (17% with PC-ZES vs. 15.6% with SES, P = .40) due to time-related differences in clinical outcomes which favored SES during the first year of follow-up (8.0% with PC-ZES vs. 3.9% with SES, P < .0001), but favored PC-ZES between 1 and 5 years (9.0% vs. 11.6%, P = .07).[164] As shown in Fig. 15.6, definite stent thrombosis was more frequent with PC-ZES than SES at 1-year follow-up (1.1% vs. 0.3%, P = .036), whereas the opposite result was apparent in the period between 1 and 5 years (0.1% with PC-ZES vs. 1.8% with SES, P = .03).

Considered collectively, these trials demonstrate that despite greater late loss in the period of angiographic surveillance, PC-ZES is safe and effective over long-term follow-up compared to first-generation DES, and more effective than BMS. In this regard, early angiographic measures might be less predictive of late term outcomes, as suggested by several studies which have shown a better safety and efficacy profile with PC-ZES compared to first-generation DES after the first year of follow-up. With this background, a large-scale, multicenter trial was recently reported in

TABLE 15.8 Randomized Controlled Trials of Endeavor Zotarolimus-Eluting Stents

Trial Acronym and Reference	Study Cohort	PC-ZES vs.	Number Randomized (Planned Angiographic Follow-Up)	Latest Follow-Up to Date	Principal Findings
CATOS[529]	Chronic total occlusion	SES	160 (all)	9 months	PC-ZES resulted noninferior to the SES with respect to the primary end point of in-segment binary restenosis (14.1% vs. 13.7%, P_{NI} < .001) There were no significant between-group differences in TVF rates (10.0% vs. 17.5%; P = .17) nor in-stent thrombosis rates (0.0% vs. 1.3%; P = .32).
DIABEDES III[530]	Diabetes mellitus	SES	127 (105)	10 months	PC-ZES was associated with significantly higher 10-month late loss compared to SES (0.74 ± 0.45 mm vs. 0.14 ± 0.37 mm, P < .001). Neointimal hyperplasia determined by IVUS was significantly greater with PC-ZES compared to SES (0.0 mm² vs. 16.5 mm², P < .001).
Endeavor II[157,253]	Noncomplex CAD	BMS	1197 (600)	5 years	Compared to BMS, PC-ZES reduced the 9-months rates of TVF (the primary end point; 15.1% vs. 7.9%, P < .0001), TLR (11.8% vs. 4.6%, P < .0001), in-stent late loss (1.03 ± 0.58 to 0.61 ± 0.46 mm, P < .001) and in-segment binary restenosis (35.0% vs. 13.2%, P < .0001). The rate of stent thrombosis was 0.5% with PC-ZES vs. 1.2% with BMS (P = .22). At 5 years TLR was reduced with PC-ZES[531] (16.5% vs. 7.4%, P < .0001).
Endeavor III[158,532]	Noncomplex CAD	SES	436 (all)	5 years	Compared to SES, PC-ZES had higher 8-month rates of in-stent late loss (0.60 ± 0.48 vs. 0.15 ± 0.34, P < .001) and in-segment binary restenosis (11.7% vs. 4.3%, P = .04). At 5 years, MACE rates were 14.0% with PC-ZES vs. 22.2% with BMS (P = .05).
Endeavor IV[531,533]	Noncomplex CAD	PES	1548 (328)	5 years	Compared to PES, PC-ZES was noninferior for the primary end point of TVF at 9 months (6.6% vs. 7.1%, respectively) (P_{NI} < .0001, PSu P = .69). PC-ZES compared to PES resulted in higher rates of angiographic in-stent late loss (0.67 ± 0.49 vs. 0.42 ± 0.50 mm, P < .001) and a trend toward greater in-segment restenosis (15.3% vs. 10.4%; P = .28) at 8 months, but comparable rates of TLR at 1 (4.5% vs. 3.2%; P = .23) and 5 years (7.7% vs. 8.6%; P = .70). The rates of cardiac death or MI in PC-ZES vs. PES patients was 2.1% vs. 3.1% respectively at 1 year (P = .20) and 6.4% vs. 9.2% respectively at 5 years (P = .049). Definite/probable stent thrombosis after 5 years occurred in 1.4% of PC-ZES patients vs. 1.9% of PES patients (P = .42).
EXCELLA II[534]	Noncomplex CAD	NES	210 (All)	9 months	PC-ZES resulted in significantly higher rates of in-stent late lumen loss compared to NES (0.63 ± 0.42 mm vs. 0.11 ± 0.32 mm, P < .0001). There was no significant difference between stent groups in the device orientated composite end point of cardiac death, MI, and clinically indicated TLR (5.6% vs. 2.8%, P = .45).

TABLE 15.8 Randomized Controlled Trials of Endeavor Zotarolimus-Eluting Stents—cont'd

Trial Acronym and Reference	Study Cohort	PC-ZES vs.	Number Randomized (Planned Angiographic Follow-Up)	Latest Follow-Up to Date	Principal Findings
KOMER[159,160]	STEMI	SES and PES	611 (348)	1 year	For the primary composite end point of cardiac death, MI, and ischemia-driven TLR, no significant difference was apparent between PC-ZES, SES, and PES at 1-year follow-up (5.9% vs. 3.4% vs. 5.7%, respectively; $P = .46$). There was a trend toward lower 1-year rates of ischemia-driven TLR in the SES group (0.0%) compared to PC-ZES (2.5%) and PES (1.5%) groups ($P = .09$).
ISAR-TEST 2[159,424]	Simple and complex CAD	SES	674 (all)	2 years	PC-ZES vs. SES resulted in higher 6–8 month rates of late loss (0.58 ± 0.55 mm vs. 0.24 ± 0.51 mm, $P < .001$) and binary restenosis (19.3% vs. 12.0%, $P < .01$), and higher 1-year rates of TLR (19.3% vs. 7.2%, $P < .01$). At 2 years there was greater late loss with SES compared to PC-ZES such that the differences in binary restenosis (20.9% vs. 18.6%) and TLR (14.3% vs. 10.7%) were not as pronounced as the first year. The rates of death, MI, and stent thrombosis were not significantly different between the two stents at 9 months or 2 years.
NAPLES[161]	Diabetes mellitus	SES and PES	226 (none)	3 years	At 3 years, PC-ZES was associated with significantly higher rates of death, MI, or clinically driven TVR compared to both SES and PES (35.6% with PC-ZES, 13.2% with SES, 17.5% with PES, $P = .006$). No significant difference was apparent between SES and PES in any clinical end point.
PROTECT[165,166]	All-comers with no more than 4 lesions	SES	8800 (none)	5 years	For the primary end point of definite/probable stent thrombosis, no evidence of superiority of PC-ZES vs. SES was apparent at 3 years (1.4% with PC-ZES vs. 1.8% with SES, $P = .22$). However, PC-ZES was associated with significantly lower rates of definite/probable stent thrombosis compared to SES when follow-up was extended at 5 years (1.67% vs. 2.83%, $P = .0007$).
SORT OUT III[163,164]	All-comers	SES	2333 (none)	5 years	PC-ZES vs. SES resulted in higher 9-month and 18-month rates of cardiac death, MI, or TVR (6% vs. 3%, $P = .0002$, and 10% vs. 5%, $P < .0001$), MI (2% vs. <1%, $P = .006$, and 2% vs. 1%, $P = .03$), stent thrombosis (1% vs. <1%, $P = .048$, and 1% vs. 1%, $P = .13$) and TLR (4% vs. 1%, $P < .0001$, and 6% vs. 1%, $P < .0001$). Mortality was higher at 18 months after PC-ZES (4% vs. 3%, $P = .035$). However, between 1 and 5 years MACE (9.0% vs. 11.6, $P = .07$) and stent thrombosis (0.1% vs. 1.8%, $P = .003$) were lower with PC-ZES than SES, such that at 5 years no significant difference in clinical events was apparent between the two devices.

Continued

TABLE 15.8 Randomized Controlled Trials of Endeavor Zotarolimus-Eluting Stents—cont'd

Trial Acronym and Reference	Study Cohort	PC-ZES vs.	Number Randomized (Planned Angiographic Follow-Up)	Latest Follow-Up to Date	Principal Findings
ZEST[535,536]	Simple and complex CAD	SES and PES	2645 (all)	2 years	For the primary end point of TVF at 12 months, PC-ZES was noninferior to SES (10.2% vs. 8.3%, P_{NI} =.01, PSu P = .17) and superior to PES (10.2% vs. 14.1%, P = .01). In-segment binary restenosis at 9 months occurred in 12.1%, 2.4%, and 12.4% of PC-ZES, SES, and PES (P < .001). At 24 months the rates of TVF with PES, PC-ZES, and SES were 15.3%, 11.2%, and 9.9% (P = .43 and .01 for PC-ZES vs. SES and PES, respectively). There were no significant differences in the rates of death, MI, or stent thrombosis at 2 years between the three stents, although there was in TVR (8.6% vs. 6.0% vs. 3.1%, P = .03 and .01 for PC-ZES vs. SES and PES, respectively).
ZEST AMI[162]	STEMI	SES and PES	328 (all)	1 year	For the primary composite end point of death, MI, and ischemia-driven TVR, no significant difference was apparent between PC-ZES, SES, and PES at 1-year follow-up (11.3% vs. 8.2% vs. 8.2%, respectively, P = .83). In-segment late loss was 0.28 ± 0.42 mm with SES vs. 0.46 ± 0.48 mm with PC-ZES vs. 0.47 ± 0.50 mm with PES (P = .029). At 8-month follow-up, restenosis rates were 2.7% with SES vs. 15.9% with PC-ZES vs. 12.3% with PES (P = .027).

BMS, Bare-metal stent; *CAD,* coronary artery disease; *IVUS,* intravascular ultrasound; *MACE,* major adverse cardiac event; *MI,* myocardial infarction; *NES,* novolimus-eluting stents; *PC-ZES,* zotarolimus-eluting stents (Endeavor platform); *PES,* paclitaxel-eluting stents; *PSu,* primary sampling unit; *SES,* sirolimus-eluting stents; *STEMI,* ST-segment elevation myocardial infarction; *TLR,* target-lesion revascularization; *TVF,* target-vessel failure (death, MI or TVR); *TVR,* target-vessel revascularization.

which 8791 patients with coronary artery disease were randomized to either PC-ZES or SES, representing the only comparative DES trial prospectively powered to show differences in stent thrombosis.[165] At 3-year follow-up, no significant difference was apparent between the two devices with regard to the primary end point of definite/probable stent thrombosis (1.4% for PC-ZES vs. 1.8% for SES, P = .22). There were no significant differences between the two devices in the 3-year rates of death or MI, but there was a significant difference in the risk of TLR favoring SES (3.5% with SES vs. 5.6% with PC-ZES, P < .0001). However, at 5-year follow-up, definite/probable stent thromboses continued to accrue in the SES arm, such that PC-ZES was associated with significantly lower 5-year rates of definite/probable stent thrombosis compared with SES (1.7% vs. 2.8%, respectively, P = .0007).[166] As shown in Fig. 15.6, landmark analyses suggested time-related differences in stent thrombosis between the two devices such that PC-ZES was associated with slightly greater rates of definite/probable stent thrombosis during the first year (1.1% with PC-ZES vs. 0.7% with SES, P = .056), but with significantly lower rates of definite/probable stent thrombosis in the period between 1 and 5 years (0.6% with PC-ZES vs. 2.1% with SES, P < .001). In addition, PC-ZES was associated with significantly lower 5-year rates of overall MI (5.0% vs. 6.6%, P = .002) and target-vessel MI (4.2% vs. 5.5%, P = .027) compared with SES.

Re-ZES (Resolute)

In the Re-ZES, zotarolimus is eluted from the thin-strut cobalt-alloy BMS platform (which has undergone several iterations to increase deliverability and flexibility). Instead of the phosphorylcholine coating of the Endeavor stent, the Resolute stent employs a proprietary BioLinx tri-polymer coating (4.1 μm thickness), consisting of a hydrophilic endoluminal component and a hydrophobic component adjacent to the metal stent surface. This polymer serves to slow the elution of zotarolimus relative to the Endeavor phosphorylcholine polymer, such that 60% of the drug is eluted by 30 days and 100% by 180 days, making this the slowest rapamycin analog-eluting DES.

In the RESOLUTE trial, the Re-ZES stent was implanted in 139 patients with noncomplex coronary artery disease.[167]

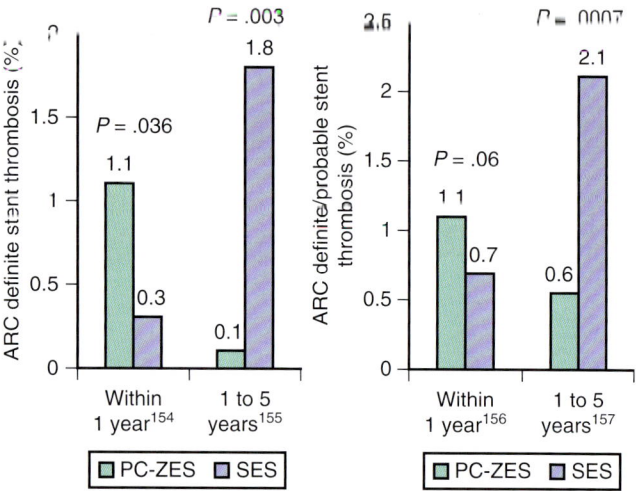

Fig. 15.6 Stent thrombosis rates before and after 1 year in the SORT OUT III trial *(left panel)* and in the PROTECT trial *(right panel).* *ARC,* Academic Research Consortium; *PC-ZES,* zotarolimus-eluting stents (Endeavor platform); *SES,* sirolimus-eluting stents.

The primary end point of in-stent late lumen loss at 9-months was 0.22 ± 0.27 mm, and the in-segment binary restenosis rate was 2.1%, both significantly less than seen with its bare-metal comparator platform. MACE, TLR, and Academic Research Consortium (ARC) definite/probable stent thrombosis at 12 months occurred in 8.7%, 0.7%, and 0% of patients, respectively. Following these favorable results, the efficacy and safety of Re-ZES were investigated in six randomized controlled trials comparing this device with CoCr-EES (RESOLUTE all-comers, TWENTE, and ISAR LEFT MAIN),[109–111] PtCr-EES (DUTCH PEERS and HOST ASSURE),[143,144] versus BES (SORT OUT VI see below),[168] or versus SYNERGY (Boston, MA) and ORSIRO (Biotronik, Swizerland) in the BIORESORT trial (see below).[169]

In the RESOLUTE all-comers trial, 2292 unselected patients were randomized to Re-ZES versus CoCr-EES (see Table 15.7).[110] Angiographic follow-up was planned in a subset of 460 patients at 13 months, after the 12-month assessment of the major clinical end points. Re-ZES compared to CoCr-EES was noninferior for the primary 1-year end point of TLF (8.2% vs. 8.3%, $P_{NI} < .001$). There were no significant differences between the two devices in the 1-year rates of death, cardiac death, MI, or TLR. However, CoCr-EES did result in significantly lower 1-year rates of definite (0.3% with CoCr-EES vs. 1.2% with Re-ZES, $P = .01$) and definite or probable stent thrombosis (0.7% with CoCr-EES vs. 1.6% with Re-ZES, $P = .05$) (see Table 15.7). At 13 months, restenosis occurred infrequently with both stents, although in-segment late loss was slightly greater with Re-ZES compared to CoCr-EES (0.15 ± 0.43 mm vs. 0.06 ± 0.40 mm, $P = .04$). When clinical follow-up was extended to 5 years, the results between the two stents were similar.[170] Specifically, the rates of TVF (20.0% with Re-ZES vs. 19.1% with CoCr-EES, $P = .69$), cardiac death (6.5% vs. 5.7%, $P = .48$), target-vessel MI (5.7% vs. 5.7%, $P = 1.00$), and clinically indicated TLR (7.0% vs. 7.1%, $P = .58$) were similar between Re-ZES and CoCr-EES. In addition, the difference in definite stent thrombosis which was apparent at 1 year was no longer statistically significant, although a trend was still maintained (0.8% with CoCr-EES vs. 1.6% with Re-ZES, $P = .08$). In the TWENTE trial, 1391 patients were randomly assigned to either CoCr-EES or Re-ZES.[111] At 1-year follow-up, rates of TVF (cardiac death, MI, or clinically driven TVR), the primary end point of the study, were 8.1% in the CoCr-EES group and 8.2% in the Re-ZES group ($P_{NI} = .001$). There was no significant difference in the rate of TVF components between the two devices. Definite/probable stent thrombosis rates were relatively low and similar for Re-ZES and CoCr-EES (0.9% and 1.2%, respectively, $P = .59$). Definite stent thrombosis rates were also low in both stent groups (0.58% with Re-ZES and 0% with CoCr-EES, $P = .12$). At 2-year follow-up, no significant difference was apparent between the two stent groups with respect to the primary end point of TVF (10.8% for Re-ZES vs. 11.6% for CoCr-EES, $P = .65$), despite fewer TLR in patients treated with CoCr-EES (4.9% vs. 2.6%, $P = .03$).[171] Similar results were apparent in the ISAR LEFT MAIN II trial, discussed further in the subsection on left main and multivessel disease (see Chapters 24 and 25).[109]

Two randomized controlled trials have compared Re-ZES with PtCr-EES.[143,144] In the 1811-patient DUTCH PEERS trial,[144] the primary end point of TVF (cardiac death, target-vessel MI, or TVR) at 1 year was 6% in the Re-ZES group and 5% in the PtCr-EES group, thus meeting the established criteria of noninferiority of Re-ZES vs. PtCr-EES ($P_{NI} = .006$). No significant difference was apparent in individual components of the primary end point or in the rate of definite stent thrombosis (0.3% vs. 0.7%, $P = .34$, respectively). In the HOST ASSURE trial, 3750 all-comers patients were randomized to either Re-ZES or PtCr-EES.[172] At 1-year follow-up, Re-ZES was noninferior to PtCr-EES for the primary end point of TLF (cardiac death, target-vessel MI, and ischemia-driven TLR), which was 2.9% for both Re-ZES and PtCr-EES ($P_{NI} = .02$). No significant difference was apparent in individual components of the primary end point, and definite stent thrombosis rates were (0.3% vs. 0.2%, $P = .34$). More recently, Re-ZES has been compared with the BioNIR stent (Medinol, Tel Aviv, Israel), a novel cobalt-alloy based coronary stent with a permanent elastomeric polymer eluting ridaforolimus, in the BIONICS trial, a prospective, multicenter, randomized noninferiority trial including 1919 patients with broad inclusion criteria. At 1-year follow-up, the primary end point of TLF, a composite of cardiac death, target-vessel–related MI, or TLR, was 5.4% with both devices ($P_{NI} = .001$). Definite probable stent thrombosis rates were 0.4% with BioNIR and 0.6% with Re-ZES ($P = .75$).[173]

In summary, these trials have collectively established overall similar efficacy and safety profiles of Re-ZES, CoCr-EES, and PtCr-EES. All these trials, however, have been insufficiently powered to detect small differences in low frequency end points such as stent thrombosis. In addition, four out of the five randomized trials comparing Re-ZES with the other second-generation DES (ISAR LEFT MAIN II, TWENTE, DUTCH PEERS and HOST ASSURE) turned out to be insufficiently powered also in relation to their respective primary study end points due to lower than expected observed event rates. Nonetheless, the current amalgamation of data regarding Re-ZES supports its use as a consistently high-performing second generation durable polymer DES platform.

BP-based second-generation DES. Through drug elution and complete bioabsorption of the polymer, BP-DES offer the potential to couple DES efficacy with the late safety profile of BMS. In most BP-based DES, the polymer is co-released with the drug, leaving behind a bare platform (or only a basecoat) that is potentially free of inflammatory stimuli triggered by permanent polymers coating first-generation DES. Most BP coatings are composed of PLLA or polyglycolic acid (PLGA) that are absorbed over a variable period of time. A variety of BP-DES has been recently developed, which differ by the stent platform, the composition/structure of the polymer and the kinetics of polymer bio absorption, and the eluted drug (Fig. 15.7). Among these devices, the one that has received the most extensive investigation so far is the biolimus-eluting bioabsorbable polymer stent (BES-BP). However, a new generation of such devices has recently reached the clinical arena, which have thinner struts compared with BP-BES, such as the BP-EES Synergy stent (Boston Scientific), BP-SES Orsiro (Biotronik), and BP-SES Ultimaster (Terumo).

BP-BES (Biomatrix/NOBORI) and Comparisons with First-Generation Drug-Eluting Stents

The BP-BES, which is manufactured as either BioMatrix (Biosensors, Newport Beach) or Nobori (Terumo Clinical Supply, Kakamigahara, Japan), elutes biolimus A9 (concentration 15.6 μg/mm), a semi-synthetic rapamycin analog with similar potency but greater lipophilicity than sirolimus, from the stainless steel S-Stent platform (120 to 125 μm strut thickness). Biomatrix and Nobori have similar stent platforms, polymers, and drugs, with slight differences in the delivery system, delivery balloon, and the stent coating process. The delivery polymer is made of PLLA, which is applied solely to the abluminal stent surface (11 to 20 μm thick), and is metabolized via the Krebs cycle into carbon dioxide and water after a 6-to-9 month period. Conceptually, such a stent might not be prone to late inflammatory reactions, as are occasionally seen with durable polymers, and thus result in improved outcomes after 1 year.

As shown in Table 15.9, the Biomatrix BP-BES has been investigated in the Limus Eluted From A Durable Versus ERodable Stent Coating (LEADERS) trial[174] and in the Biolimus-Eluting Stents With Biodegradable Polymer Versus Bare-Metal Stents in Acute Myocardial Infarction (COMFORTABLE AMI) trial,[175] including a total of 2864 randomized patients. In the LEADERS trial, 1707 "all-comer" patients (55% of whom had acute coronary syndromes) were randomized to BP-BES versus SES.[174]

Stent	Orsiro	Inspiron	Elixir DESyne	Elixir Myolimus	Infinnium	Supralimus	Firehawk	Biomatrix	Nobori	Excel stent	Axxess
Company	Biotronik	Scitech	Elixir Medical Corp	Elixir Medical Corp	Sahajanand Medical Technologies	Sahajanand Medical Technologies	MicroPort Medical	Biosensors	Terumo	JW Medical Systems	Devax Inc
Eluted drug	Sirolimus	Sirolimus	Novolimus	Novolimus	Paclitaxel	Sirolimus	Paclitaxel	Biolimus A9	Biolimus A9	Sirolimus	Biolimus A9
Stent platform	CoCr	CoCr	CoCr	CoCr	SS	SS	CoCr	SS	SS	SS	Nitinol
Strut thickness (μm)	60	75	80	80	80	80	86	112	112	119	152
Polymer	PLLA	PLA, PLGA	Abluminal PLA	Abluminal PLA	PLLA, PLGA, PCL, PVP	PLLA, PLGA, PVP	PLA	Abluminal PLA	Abluminal PLA	PLA	Abluminal PLA
Time of polymer degradation (months)	7	6–9	6–9	6–9	7	7	6–9	6–9	6–9	6–9	6–9

A

Stent	MiStent	Sparrow limus-eluting stent	Synergy	Ultimaster DES	Noya	Eucatax	Yukon Choice PC	Combo	Jactax	Coracto
Company	Micell Technologies	Cardiomind	Boston Scientific	Terumo	Medfavour Medical	Eucatech Medical	Translumina	Orbusneich Medical	Boston Scientific	Alvimedica
Eluted drug	Sirolimus	Sirolimus	Everolimus	Sirolimus	Sirolimus	Paclitaxel	Sirolimus	Sirolimus	Paclitaxel	Sirolimus
Stent platform	CoCr	Nitinol	PtCr	CoCr	CoCr	SS	SS	SS	SS	SS
Strut thickness (μm)	64	67	74	80	81	85	87	90	97	100
Polymer	PLGA	Dl-lactide, glycolide, ε-caprolactone and polyethylene-glicol copolymer	PLGA rollcoat abluminal	PDLLA-PCL copolymer	PDLLA	PLGA	PLA and shellac	Abluminal Dl-lactide, glycolide, ε-caprolactone and polyethylene-glycol with CD34 antibody layer	Abluminal (PLA)	PLGA
Time of polymer degradation (months)	2	6	3–4	3–4	4	2	2	3	4	2

B

Fig. 15.7 Main characteristics of drug-eluting stents coated with bioabsorbable polymers with a kinetics of bioabsorption (A) longer or (B) shorter than 6 months. *CoCr*, Cobalt-chromium; *DES*, drug-eluting stent; *PCL*, polycaprolactone; *PDLLA*, poly-D,L-lactide; *PLA*, polylactic acid; *PLGA*, poly lactic-co-glycolic acid; *PLLA*, poly-L-lactic acid; *PtCr*, platinum-chromium; *PVP*, polyvinylpyrrolidone; *SS*, stainless steel.

BP-BES was noninferior to SES for the primary 9-month composite end point of cardiac death, MI, or TVR, and demonstrated similar rates of TLR and stent thrombosis. A total of 427 patients were allocated to angiographic follow-up at 9 months, which demonstrated that BP-BES was noninferior to SES for the primary angiographic end point of in-stent diameter stenosis (mean 20.9% vs. 23.3%, P_{NI} = .001, P for superiority [P_{Sup}] = .26). At 5-year follow-up, not only did BP-BES maintain noninferiority compared to SES, it was also associated with a significant reduction in the more comprehensive patient-orientated composite end point of all-cause death, any MI, and all-cause revascularization (35.1% vs. 40.4%, P_{Sup} = .023). In addition, BP-BES was associated with significantly lower rates of very late definite stent thrombosis from 1 to 5 years (0.7% vs. 2.5%, P = .003).[176] These findings were confirmed in a meta-analysis[177] of patient-level data from the LEADERS,[174] ISAR-TEST III,[178] and ISAR TEST IV trials[100] comparing different types of BP-DES (BP-BES and the Yukon Choice PC-SES, Translumina, Germany) with first-generation SES. At 4-year follow-up, the risk of TLR and definite stent thrombosis were significantly lower with BP-DES compared to SES. Of note, BP-DES were associated with a significant reduction of very late stent thrombosis compared to SES, with a significant reduction also in the risk of late MI.

TABLE 15.9 Randomized Controlled Trials of Bioabsorbable Polymer-Based Drug Eluting Stents

Trial Acronym and Reference	Study Cohort	Stent Comparators	Number Randomized	Latest Follow-Up to Date	Brand	Results of the Primary End Point
BASKET PROVE II[118]	All-comers with lesions in coronary arteries ≥3 mm	BP-BES/BMS/CoCr-EES	2291	2 years	Nobori/ProKinetic/Xience	BP-BES resulted noninferior to CoCr-EES with respect to the primary end point of cardiac death, MI, or clinically indicated TVR at 2-year follow-up in the intention to treat analysis, but not in a per protocol analysis.
BIOFLOW II[125,123]	Noncomplex CAD	BP-SES/CoCr-EES	452	9 months	Orsiro/Xience	BP-SES resulted noninferior to CoCr-EES with respect to the primary end point of in-stent late lumen loss (0.10 ± 0.32 vs. 0.11 ± 0.29 mm, respectively, $P_{NI} < .0001$) There were no significant between-group differences in the rate of TLF (6.5% vs. 8.0%; $P = .58$). There were no episodes of stent thrombosis in both groups.
BIOFLOW V[191]	Noncomplex CAD in patients with no more than three lesions in a maximum of two native coronary arteries	BP-SES/CoCr-EES	1334	12 months	Orsiro/Xience	BP-SES resulted superior to CoCr-EES with respect to the primary end point of TLF (6% vs. 10%, $P = .04$).
BIORESORT[169]	All-comers	BP-EES/BP-SES/Re-ZES	3514	12 months	Synergy/Orsiro/Resolute	Both BP-EES and BP-SES were noninferior to Re-ZES for the primary end point of TVF (incidence rates 5% in all treatment arms).
BIOSCIENCE	All-comers with minimal exclusion criteria	BP-SES/CoCr-EES	2119	12 months	Orsiro/Xience	BP-SES resulted noninferior to CoCr-EES with respect to the primary end point of TLF (6.5% vs. 6.6%, respectively; $P_{NI} < .0004$).
CARE II[537]	Noncomplex CAD	BP-Sparrow SES/Sparrow-BMS/Driver	138	9 months	Sparrow limus/Sparrow BMS/MicroDriver	Sparrow SES resulted superior to both Sparrow-BMS and Driver with respect to the primary end point of in-stent late lumen loss at 6 months (0.29 ± 0.45 mm with Sparrow SES vs. 0.86 ± 0.54 mm with Sparrow BMS vs. 0.94 ± 0.39 mm with Driver, $P < .0001$).
CENTURI II[124]	Noncomplex CAD	BP-SES/CoCr-EES	1123	9 months	Ultimaster/Xience	Ultimaster resulted noninferior to CoCr-EES for the primary end point of TLF (4.1% with BP-SES vs. 5.4% with CoCr-EES, $P_{NI} < .0001$).
COMFORTABLE AMI[175]	STEMI	BP-BES/BMS	1157	1 year	Biomatrix/Gazelle	BP-BES resulted superior to BMS with respect to the primary end point of cardiac death, target vessel MI, or ischemia-driven TLR at 1 year (4.3% with BP-BES vs. 8.7% with BMS, $P = .004$). Rates of cardiac death were not significantly different between the two devices, whereas BP-BES was associated with significantly lower rates of target-vessel MI and ischemia-driven TLR.
COMPARE II[120,538]	All-comers	CoCr-EES/BP-BES	2707	3 years	Nobori/Xience	BP-BES resulted noninferior to CoCr-EES for the primary end point of cardiac death, MI, or TVR at 1 year (5.2% with BP-PES vs. 4.8% with CoCr-EES, $P_{NI} <.0001$). No significant difference was apparent in the individual components of the primary end point. Similar results were apparent at 3 years.

Continued

TABLE 15.9 Randomized Controlled Trials of Bioabsorbable Polymer-Based Drug Eluting Stents—cont'd

Trial Acronym and Reference	Study Cohort	Stent Comparators	Number Randomized	Latest Follow-Up to Date	Brand	Results of the Primary End Point
CORACTO[539]	Chronic total occlusion	BP-SES/BMS	95	2 years	Coracto/ Constant	BP-SES resulted superior to BMS for the primary end point of in-stent late lumen loss at 6 months (0.77 ± 0.63 mm with BP-SES vs. 1.82 ± 0.82 mm with BMS, $P < .0001$). In-segment restenosis was 17.4% wit BP-SES vs. 60.0% in BMS ($P < .0001$). There was no significant difference in the risk of death or MI between the two stents.
DESSOLVE II[198,540]	Noncomplex CAD	BP-SES/PC-ZES	184	2 years	MiStent/ Endeavor	BP-SES resulted superior to PC-ZES for the primary end point of in-stent late lumen loss at 9 months (0.27 ± 0.46 mm vs. 0.58 ± 0.41 mm, $P < .001$). There was no significant difference in the risk of death, MI, or TVR between the two stents at 2-year follow-up.
EUCATAX[541,542]	Noncomplex CAD	BP-PES/BMS	422	2 years	Eucatax/ Equivalent BMS	BP-PES resulted superior to BMS for the primary end point of cardiac death, MI, or TVR at 1 year (9.5% with BP-PES vs. 17.1% with BMS, $P = .02$).
EVOLUTION[543,544]	Noncomplex CAD	BP-SES/SES	1923	2 years	Excel/Cypher	BP-SES resulted noninferior to SES for the primary end point of cardiac death, MI, or ischemia-driven TVR at 1 year (0.89% with BP-SES vs. 1.34% with SES, $P = .25$). No significant difference was apparent in the rates of the individual components of the primary end point.
EVOLVE I[137]	Noncomplex CAD	HD BP-EES / LD BP-EES/ PtCr-EES	291	6 months	Synergy HD/ Synergy LD/ Promus Element	BP-EES resulted noninferior to PtCr-EES for the primary end point of cardiac death, target-vessel MI, or TVR at 30 days (0.0% with PtCr-EES, 1.1% with Synergy HD, and 3.1% with Synergy LD, $P_{NI} < .0001$). At 6 months, in-stent late lumen loss was 0.15 ± 0.34 mm for PtCr-EES, 0.10 ± 0.25 mm for Synergy HD, and 0.13 ± 0.26 mm for Synergy LD ($P_{NI} < .01$).
EVOLVE II[195]	Noncomplex CAD	BP-EES/PtCr-EES	1684	5 years	Synergy/Promus Element	BP-EES resulted noninferior to PtCr-EES for the primary end point of TLF (6.7% with BP-EES vs. 6.2% with PtCr-EES; $P_{NI} = .0003$). Similar results were apparent at 5 years.
EXCELLA BD[534]	Noncomplex CAD	BP-NES/PC-ZES	146	6 months	Elixir DESyne/ Endeavor	BP-NES resulted superior to PC-ZES for the primary end point of in-stent late lumen loss at 9 months (0.11 ± 0.32 mm with BP-NES vs. 0.63 ± 0.42 mm with PC-ZES, $P < .0001$). There was no significant difference in the risk of death, MI, or TVR between the two devices.
INSPIRON I[545]	Noncomplex CAD	BP-SES/BMS	58	2 years	Inspiron/ Cronus[451]	Inspiron resulted superior to Cronus for the primary end point of in-stent late loss at 6 months (0.22 mm with Inspiron vs. 0.84 mm with Cronus, $P < .001$). At 2 years, Inspiron was associated with lower rates of TLR compared to Cronus (0.0% vs. 21.1%, $P = .02$).

Continued

TABLE 15.9 Randomized Controlled Trials of Bioabsorbable Polymer-Based Drug Eluting Stents—cont'd

Trial Acronym and Reference	Study Cohort	Stent Comparators	Number Randomized	Latest Follow-Up to Date	Brand	Results of the Primary End Point
ISAR-TEST III[121,178]	Noncomplex CAD	BP-SES/SES/ polymer free-SES	404	2 years	Yukon C/Cypher/ Yukon[119]	BP-SES, resulted noninferior to SES for the primary end point of in-stent late lumen loss at 8 months (0.17 ± 0.45 mm with BP-SES vs. 0.23 ± 0.46 mm with SES, P_{NI} < .001). PF-SES did not meet the pre-specified criteria for noninferiority (in-stent late lumen loss = 0.47 ± 0.56 mm, P_{NI} = .94).
ISAR-TEST IV[100,523]	Noncomplex CAD	BP-SES/CoCr-EES/SES	2603	3 years	Yukon C/Xience/ Cypher	BP-SES resulted noninferior to pooled CoCr-EES and SES for the primary end point of cardiac death, MI, or TLR at 1 year (13.8% vs. 14.4%, respectively, P = .005). There were similar rates of cardiac death, MI, TLR and stent thrombosis between the three stent groups.
LEADERS[174,176,546]	All comers	BP-BES/SES	1707	5 years	Biomatrix/ Cypher	BP-BES resulted noninferior to SES for the primary end point of cardiac death, MI, or clinically indicated TVR at 9 months (9% with BP-BES vs. 11% with SES, P_{NI} = .003). Noninferiority was sustained at 5 years, with significantly lower rates of very late stent thrombosis with BP-BES compared to SES (0.7% vs. 2.5%, P = .005).
LONG DES[ ]	Long coronary lesions (≥25 mm)	BP-BES/PtCr-EES	500	9 months	Nobori/Promus Element	BP-BES was noninferior to PtCr-EES for the primary end point of late lumen loss (0.14 ± 0.38 vs. 0.11 ± 0.37; P_{NI} = .03)
NEXT[119,138]	All-comers	BP-BES/CoCr-EES	3235	2 years	Nobori/Xience	BP-BES resulted noninferior to CoCr-EES for the primary end point of TLR at 1 year (4.2% in both groups, P_{NI} < .0001). There were similar rates of cardiac death, MI, or stent thrombosis between the two stent groups. Noninferiority was sustained at 2-year follow-up.
NOBORI I phase I[179,547]	Noncomplex CAD	BP-BES/PES	120	5 years	Nobori/Taxus	BP-BES-resulted noninferior to PES for the primary end point of in-stent late lumen loss at 6 months (0.15 ± 0.27 mm vs. 0.32 ± 0.33 mm, respectively, P = .06). No significant difference was apparent between the two stents in the risk of death, MI, or TVR up to 5-year follow-up.
NOBORI I phase II[180,548]	Noncomplex CAD	BP-BES/PES	243	3 years	Nobori/Taxus	BP-BES resulted superior to PES for the primary end point of in-stent late lumen loss at 9 months (0.11 ± 0.30 mm vs. 0.32 ± 0.50 mm, respectively, P = .001). There were no significant differences in the risk of death, MI, TLR, or stent thrombosis between the two devices up to 3-year follow-up.
NOBORI JAPAN[105,524]	Noncomplex CAD	BP-BES/SES	326	3 years	Nobori/Cypher	BP-BES resulted noninferior to SES for the primary end point of cardiac death, MI, or TVR at 9 months (7.4% vs. 6.3%%, respectively, P_{NI} < .001). Similar results were apparent at 3 years.

Continued

TABLE 15.9 Randomized Controlled Trials of Bioabsorbable Polymer-Based Drug Eluting Stents—cont'd

Trial Acronym and Reference	Study Cohort	Stent Comparators	Number Randomized	Latest Follow-Up to Date	Brand	Results of the Primary End Point
NOYA I[549,550]	Noncomplex CAD	BP-SES/SES	300	2 years	Noya/Firebird 2	BP-SES resulted noninferior to SES for the primary end point of in-stent late lumen loss at 9 months (0.11 ± 0.18 mm vs. 0.14 ± 0.23 mm, respectively, $P_{NI} < .001$). No significant difference was apparent in the risk of cardiac death, MI, TLR, or stent thrombosis between the two devices at 2 years.
OCTDESI[551]	Noncomplex CAD	BP-PES/PES	60	6 months	HD Jacktax/ LD Jacktax/Taxus Libertè	JACTAX (both HD and LD) resulted in similar strut coverage as TAXUS Libertè at 6 months (7.0 ± 12.2% for JACTAX HD, 4.6 ± 7.3% for JACTAX LD, and 5.3 ± 14.7% for Taxus Libertè, $P = .81$). There were no deaths, MI, or stent thrombosis through 1 year in either stent group.
PAINT[552]	Noncomplex CAD	BP-PES/BP-SES/BMS	274	1 year	Infinnium/ Supralimus/ Milennium Matrix	BP-PES and BP-SES resulted superior to BMS for the primary end point of in-stent late lumen loss (0.54 ± 0.44 mm with BP-PES vs. 0.32 ± 0.43 mm with BP-SES vs. 0.90 ± 0.45 mm with BMS, $P < .001$). There was no significant difference in the risk of death or MI between the three stents, whereas TVR was significantly lower with BP-PES and BP-SES than BMS (5.6% with BP-PES, 5.8% with BP-SES, and 17.6% with BMS, $P < .01$).
PRISON IV[190]	Chronic total occlusion	BP-SES/CoCr-EES	330	9 months	Orsiro/Xience	BP-SES compared to CoCr-EES did not achieve noninferiority for the primary end point of in-segment late lumen loss (0.13 ± 0.63 mm vs. 0.02 ± 0.47, $P = .08$). TVF rates were comparable between the two groups.
REMEDEE[198]	Noncomplex CAD	BP-SES-CD34 ab/PES	183	9 months	Combo/Taxus Libertè	BP-SES-CD34 ab resulted noninferior to SES for the primary end point of in-stent late lumen loss (0.39 ± 0.45 mm vs. 0.44 ± 0.56 mm, respectively, $P_{NI} = .001$). At 1 year, there was no significant difference in the risk of death, MI, TLR, or stent thrombosis between the two devices.
SENIOR[196]	Noncomplex CAD	BP-EES/BMS	1200	1 year	Synergy/Omega or rebel	At 1 year, BP-EES resulted superior to BMS for the primary end point of all-cause death, MI, stroke or ischemia driven TLR.
SORT OUT V[181,182,553]	All-comers	BP-BES/SES	2468	5 years	Nobori/Cypher	BP-BES failed to achieve noninferiority compared to SES for the primary end point of cardiac death, MI, definite stent thrombosis, or TVR at 9 months (4.1% with BP-BES vs. 3.1% with SES, $P_{NI} = .06$). In addition, BP-BES were associated with significantly higher 1-year rates of definite stent thrombosis than SES (0.7% vs. 0.2%, respectively, $P = .03$). However, no significant differences were apparent in MACE and stent thrombosis between the two devices at 5-year follow-up.

Continued

TABLE 15.9 Randomized Controlled Trials of Bioabsorbable Polymer-Based Drug Eluting Stents—cont'd

Trial Acronym and Reference	Study Cohort	Stent Comparators	Number Randomized	Latest Follow-Up to Date	Brand	Results of the Primary End Point
SORT OUT VI[168]	Minimal exclusion criteria	BP-BES/Re-ZES	2999	1 year	Nobori/Resolute	At 1 year BP-BES was noninferior to Re-ZES for the primary end point of cardiac death, MI, or TLR (5.0% vs. 5.3%, P_{NI} = .004)
SORT OUT VII[183]	Minimal exclusion criteria	BP-SES/BP-BES	1261	1 year	Orsiro/Nobori	At 1 year, the Orsiro stent was noninferior to the Nobori stent for the primary end point of TLF (3.8% vs. 4.6%, P_{NI} < .0001. In addition, the Orsiro stent had significantly lower rates of definite stent thrombosis (0.5% vs. 1.2%, P = .03).
TARGET I[122,554]	Noncomplex CAD	BP-SES/CoCr-EES	460	2 years	Firehawk/Xience	BP-SES resulted noninferior to CoCr-EES for the primary end point of in-stent late lumen loss at 9 months (0.13 ± 0.24 mm vs. 0.13 ± 0.18 mm, respectively, P_{NI} < .0001). There was no significant difference in the rates of TLF between the two devices up to 2-year follow-up.

ab, Antibody; *BES*, biolimus-eluting stents; *BMS*, bare-metal stent; *BP*, bioabsorbable polymer; *CAD*, coronary artery disease; *CoCr-EES*, cobalt-chromium everolimus-eluting stents; *DES*, drug-eluting stents; *HD*, high dose; *LD*, low dose; *MACE*, major adverse cardiovascular events (death, MI, TVR); *MI*, myocardial infarction; *NES*, novolimus-eluting stents; *PC-ZES*, zotarolimus-eluting stents (Endeavor platform); *PES*, paclitaxel-eluting stents; *PtCr*, platinum chromium; *SES*, sirolimus-eluting stents; *TVR*, target-vessel revascularization; *TLF*, target-lesion failure (cardiac death, target lesion MI, or TLR); *TLR*, target-lesion revascularization; *TVF*, target-vessel failure (cardiac death, target vessel MI, or TVR).

Overall, these findings are consistent with the notion that bioabsorption of the polymer after the elution of the antiproliferative drug may minimize the risk of late adverse events. BP-BES were also studied in the COMFORTABLE AMI trial, a prospective, multicenter trial randomly assigning 1161 patients with STEMI to either BP-BES or BMS. The results of this trial are discussed below (see Chapter 20).[173]

The Nobori BP-BES has been investigated in six randomized trials (Nobori I phase I,[179] Nobori I phase II,[180] Nobori Japan,[105] SORT OUT V,[181] COMPARE II,[120] and NEXT[138]) with 9099 randomized patients. In the small-sized Nobori I phase I (120 patients) and phase II trials[180] (243 patients), BP-BES was shown to be noninferior compared to PES for the primary end point of 9-month late lumen loss, with demonstration of superiority in Nobori I phase II. Similarly, in the somewhat larger Nobori Japan trial recruiting 326 patients, Nobori was shown to be noninferior compared to SES for the composite primary end point of cardiac death, MI, or TVR at 9-month follow-up.[105] However, in the SORT OUT V trial, a large-scale prospective, randomized trial comparing Nobori (n = 1229) versus Cypher (n = 1239),[181] Nobori failed to reach the primary hypothesis of noninferiority for the primary end point of cardiac death, MI, definite stent thrombosis, or TVR at 9 months (4.1% with BP-BES vs. 3.1% with SES, P_{NI} = .06). In addition, a significant difference in the risk of stent thrombosis in favor of SES was apparent at 1 year (0.7% with BP-BES vs. 0.2% with SES, P = .03). These early differences were mitigated at 5-year follow-up, when no significant differences in MACE (14.8% with Nobori vs. 15.8% with Cypher, P = .53), or stent thrombosis (1.9% with Nobori vs. 1.5% with Cypher, P = .40).[182] There were 15 episodes of definite stent thrombosis between 1 and 5 years with Cypher and 13 with Nobori.

In summary, Nobori and Biomatrix have been compared with first-generation DES in a total of five randomized controlled trials, and although some of them have shown improved safety with similar efficacy of BP-BES compared to either PES or SES, others have not confirmed this association.

BP-BES (Biomatrix/Nobori) and Comparisons with Second-Generation Drug-Eluting Stents

BP-BES has been compared with CoCr-EES in three randomized controlled trials (COMPARE II,[120] NEXT,[138] and BASKET-PROVE II),[118] with Re-ZES in one randomized trial (SORT OUT VI),[168] with PtCr-EES in one randomized trial, (LONG DES V),[145] and with ORSIRO in one randomized trial (SORT OUT VII).[183] COMPARE II was a prospective, multicenter, controlled, randomized trial comparing BP-BES with CoCr-EES in 2707 all-comer patients.[120] At 1-year follow-up, BP-BES was shown to be noninferior to CoCr-EES for the primary end point of cardiac death, MI, or TVR (5.2% with BP-BES vs. 4.8% with CoCr-EES, P_{NI} < .0001). There was no significant difference between the two devices in the rates of the individual components of the primary end point, with similar rates of stent thrombosis (0.4% vs. 0.7%, respectively; P = .37). Similar results were apparent at 5-year follow-up.[184] NEXT was a controlled, multicenter, noninferiority trial randomly assigning 3235 patients to either BP-BES or CoCr-EES.[138] At 1-year follow-up, BP-BES was noninferior compared to CoCr-EES for the primary end point of TLR (4.2% with BES vs. 4.2% with CoCr-EES, P_{NI} < .0001). Episodes of stent thrombosis were rare in both groups, but they were numerically higher with BP-BES than CoCr-EES (0.25% with BES vs. 0.06% with CoCr-EES, P = .18). BP-BES was also noninferior to CoCr-EES for the primary angiographic end point of in-segment late loss (0.03 ± 0.39 mm vs. 0.06 ± 0.45 mm, respectively, P_{NI} < .0001). These results were sustained at 3 years.[185] Data from COMPARE II and NEXT trials have recently been pooled in an individual patient data meta-analysis including 5942 patients and showing similar rates of death, TLR, and stent thrombosis, but higher rates of target-vessel MI with BP-BES versus CoCr-EES (5.6% vs. 4.5%, P = .02).[186] Finally, in BASKET-PROVE II, 2291 patients requiring coronary stents greater than or equal to 3.0 mm in diameter were randomized to biolimus-A9-eluting BP-DES, CoCr-EES, or BMS.[118] The primary composite end point of cardiac death, MI, or clinically indicated TVR within 2 years occurred in 6.8% of patients with CoCr-EES, in 7.6% with BP-BES, and in 12.7% with BMS. BP-BES was noninferior to CoCr-EES by intention-to-treat (P_{NI} = .042), but not in a per protocol analysis (P_{NI} = .09). The 3 stent groups did not differ in event rates beyond 1 year.

In summary, although no major differences emerged between BP DES and CoCr-EES in these three trials, there was no evidence that BP-DES provided any late safety advantages compared to CoCr-EES. In contrast, in a pooled analysis of COMPARE II and NEXT trial, BP-BES had significantly higher rates of target-vessel MI compared to CoCr-EES. Larger trials are required to determine the relative safety and efficacy of these two devices.

SORT OUT VI was an open-label, multicenter, noninferiority randomized trial comparing BP-BES versus Re-ZES in 1502 patients. At 1-year follow-up, no significant difference was apparent between the two stents for the composite primary end point of cardiac death, MI, or TLR (5.0% vs. 5.3%, P_{NI} = .004).[168] Similar results were apparent at 3-year follow-up, with no significant difference in safety and efficacy outcomes.[187] In LONG DES V, 500 patients with long lesions (≥25 mm) were randomized to either BP-BES or PtCr-EES.[145] At 9-month follow-up, the primary end point of the study, in-segment late luminal loss, was comparable between the two groups (BP-BES, 0.14 ± 0.38 vs. PtCr-EES, 0.11 ± 0.37 mm; P_{NI} = .03). The incidence of in-segment (6.1% vs. 4.9%; P = .63) and in-stent (3.7% vs. 4.9%; P = .59) binary restenosis was also similar between the groups. Finally, in the large-scale registry-based randomized, multicenter, single-blind, 2-arm, noninferiority SORT OUT VII trial, 2525 patients were randomized to receive either Orsiro or Nobori. At 1-year follow-up, Orsiro was noninferior to Nobori for the primary end point of TLF, which was a composite of cardiac death, MI, or TLR (3.8% vs. 4.6%, P_{NI} = .0001). In addition, definite stent thrombosis was significantly lower with Orsiro compared to Nobori (0.4% vs. 1.2%, P = .03). These results were sustained at 2 years, but the difference in stent thrombosis between the two stents was not significant (NS) anymore (1.4% with Nobori vs. 0.8% with Orsiro, P = .14).[188]

Novel BP-BASED Drug-Eluting Stents: Orsiro and Synergy

Orsiro is a novel bioabsorbable polymer-based DES releasing sirolimus from biodegradable poly-l lactic acid polymer, which completely degrades during a period of 12 to 24 months. The metallic stent platform consists of ultrathin (60 μm) cobalt-chromium struts covered with an amorphous silicon carbide layer. The passive coating seals the stent surface and reduces interaction between the metal stent and the surrounding tissue by acting as a diffusion barrier. Orsiro has been compared with CoCr-EES in four randomized controlled trials (BIOFLOW II,[189] BIOSCIENCE,[123] PRISON IV,[190] and BIOFLOW V),[191] with Re-ZES and Synergy in the BIORESORT trial,[169] with Re-ZES in the ORIENT trial,[192] and with Nobori in the SORT OUT VII trial.[188] The BIOFLOW II trial was a small randomized trial of 452 patients showing noninferiority of Orsiro compared to CoCr-EES for in-stent late lumen loss at 9 months.[189] In the large-scale BIOSCIENCE trial, 2119 patients with few exclusion criteria were randomly allocated to receive either Orsiro or CoCr-EES.[123] At 1-year follow-up, TLF was 6.5% with Orsiro and 6.6% with CoCr-EES (P_{NI} < .0004), with stent thrombosis rates of 0.9% versus 0.4% (P = .16). In a prespecified analysis of the primary end point, Orsiro was associated with significantly lower rates of TLF compared to CoCr-EES in patients presenting with STEMI. PRISON IV was a multicenter, noninferiority randomized trial in which 330 patients with successful recanalization of chronic total occlusion (CTO) were assigned to either Orsiro or CoCr-EES.[190] The primary noninferiority end point, in-segment late lumen loss, was not met for Orsiro versus CoCr-EES (0.13 ± 0.63 mm vs. 0.02 ± 0.47 mm; P_{NI} < .11). In addition, the incidence of in-segment binary restenosis was significantly higher with Orsiro versus CoCr-EES (8.0% vs. 2.1%; P = .028). Clinically indicated TVR (9.2% vs. 6.0%, P = .33), TVF (9.9% vs. 6.6%, P = .35), and definite or probable stent thrombosis (0.7% vs. 0.7%; P = 1) were comparable between the two stents. More recently, the BIOFLOW V trial randomized 1334 patients undergoing elective or urgent PCI to either Orsiro or CoCr-EES.[191] At 1-year follow-up, Orsiro was associated with significantly lower rates of the primary end point TVF, a composite of cardiac death, target vessel MI, or TLR compared to CoCr-EES (6% vs. 10%, P = .039).

In a pooled analysis of BIOFLOW II, BIOFLOW IV, and BIOFLOW V, the Bayesian posterior probability was 100% for noninferiority and 96% for superiority of Orsiro versus CoCr-EES. However, most of the difference between the two stents was due to periprocedural MI, a finding likely related to the platform and not to the bioabsorbable polymer. In addition, there were several imbalances in baseline angiographic and procedural characteristics between the two randomized groups such that thrombus-containing lesions, calcified lesions, and tortuous vessels were numerically higher and number of stents per patients, overlapping stents, and total stent length were significantly higher with CoCr-EES versus Orsiro. After adjusting for these possible confounders, the difference between Orsiro and CoCr-EES was of borderline significance (odds ratio [OR] 0.66, 95% CI 0.42 to 1.01; P = .06). ORIENT is a small trial randomizing 372 patients with noncomplex coronary artery disease to either Orsiro or Re-ZES.[192] At 9-month follow-up, Orsiro was noninferior to Re-ZES for the primary end point of in-stent late lumen loss (0.06 mm with Orsiro vs. 0.12 with Re-ZES, P_{NI} < .001). However, percent diameter stenosis was significantly lower with Orsiro compared with Re-ZES (15% vs. 20%, P = .002). In a recent meta-analysis from 8 randomized trials and 11,176 patients, there were no significant differences in clinical outcomes between Orsiro versus pooled contemporary DES including CoCr-EES, ZES, and BP-BES.[193] In contrast, a subsequent meta-analysis from 10 trials and 11,658 patients showed reduced rates of target-vessel failure (TVF) and any stent thrombosis with ultra-thin strut DES including Orsiro (60 μm), MiStent (64 μm), and BioMime (65 μm) versus thicker-strut second-generation DES including CoCr-EES, ZES, and BP-BES.[194]

The PtCr PLGA-based everolimus-eluting Synergy stent (Boston Scientific Corporation) is characterized by very thin struts (74 μm) and a 4 μm thick abluminal coating of PLGA polymer which is completely absorbed within 4 months. In the Noninferiority Trial to Assess the Safety and Performance of the Evolution Coronary Stent (EVOLVE) trial, in which 291 patients were randomized, this stent (at both full- and half-concentration doses of everolimus) was shown to be noninferior to durable polymer PtCr-EES for the primary end point of angiographic late lumen loss (mean 0.10, 0.13, and 0.15 mm, respectively).[137] In addition, at 6-month follow-up, clinical event rates were comparable between the three stent groups. EVOLVE II trial is a 1684-patient multicenter randomized trial in which the Synergy stent (100 μg everolimus/cm²) was compared with the durable polymer PtCr-EES (Promus Element).[195] At 1 year, Synergy and Promus Element demonstrated similar rates of TLF (6.5% vs. 6.7% respectively, P_{NI} = .0005), with similar rates of the individual components of this end point. Stent thrombosis rates were similarly low with both stents, and no stent thromboses were observed with the Synergy stent beyond 30 days. Longer-term follow-up from this trial and additional studies in higher-risk patients than those enrolled in EVOLVE II will allow a more complete assessment of the safety and efficacy profile with this stent compared to a durable polymer EES.

The BIORESORT trial was a multicenter, assessor- and patient-blinded, three-arm, noninferiority trial randomizing 1:1:1 3514 patients to either Orsiro, Synergy, or Re-ZES.[169] Noninferiority of both Synergy and Orsiro compared with Re-ZES was achieved (both −0.7% absolute risk difference, 95%

CI −2.4 to 1.1; upper limit of one sided 95% CI 0.8%, $P_{NI} \le$ .0001). However, 44% of eligible patients were not randomized and observed event rates were 42% lower than expected, limiting the statistical power of the study. Finally, SENIOR was a multicenter, single blind trial randomizing 1200 patients aged 75 years or older to either Synergy or a similar thin-strut BMS (Omega or Rebel, Boston Scientific).[196] The duration of DAPT was recommended according to patient clinical presentation: 1 month in stable patients and 6 months in unstable patients. At 1 year, the primary end point of the study, a composite of all-cause death, MI, stroke, or ischemia-driven TLR, occurred in 12% of patients treated with Synergy and 16% of patients treated with BMS (RR = 0.71, 95% CI 0.52 to 0.94; P = .02). Bleeding complications and stent thrombosis at 1 year were infrequent in both groups.

Other BP-Based Drug-Eluting Stents

A variety of other BP-DES have been designed and studied to varying degrees (see Fig. 15.7). Some BP-DES are no longer manufactured (CoStar, Conor Med System, CA; XTENT, Menlo Park, CA; NEVO, Cordis), either due to disappointing clinical results[197] or for commercial reasons. As shown in Table 15.9, most of these devices have undergone small-sized randomized controlled trials powered for angiographic end points. With respect to sirolimus-based BP-DES, the COMBO and MiStent SES have shown promising angiographic outcomes.[198,199] The Yukon Choice PC SES has been studied in the ISAR TEST III and IV trials, and has been demonstrated to be noninferior to either CoCr-EES or SES for the composite end point of cardiac death, target-vessel MI, or TLR (see above).[100,178] Finally, in the recently reported CENTURI II trial, 1123 patients were randomly allocated to either CoCr-EES or the Ultimaster stent, a BP-based SES.[131] At 9 months, the primary end point, a composite of cardiac death, target-vessel MI, and TLR did not significantly differ between the two stents (4.14% with BP-SES vs. 5.38% with CoCr-EES, P = .66).

SAFETY AND EFFICACY OF DRUG-ELUTING STENTS AND BARE-METAL STENTS: SYNTHESIZING THE DATA THROUGH META-ANALYSES

DES are among the most-studied devices used in medicine today, and abundant assessments of comparative device efficacy have been performed through a multitude of randomized trials adequately powered for both surrogate and clinical end points. However, with the one exception of the Patient Related OuTcomes with Endeavor versus Cypher stenting Trial (PROTECT) trial,[165] these trials have been insufficiently powered to detect differences in infrequent safety end points such as death, MI, or stent thrombosis. In addition, several large head-to-head trials of DES have had lower than expected clinical event rates, further limiting their ability to reliably discriminate differences between stent types.[a] Furthermore, few studies have directly compared second-generation DES to each other or with BMS. In recognition of these issues, network meta-analyses have been performed to investigate relative differences in safety and efficacy between devices. Network meta-analysis and mixed treated comparisons are novel research methods capable of comparing different therapies using a common reference treatment.[200]

In an analysis of 49 randomized controlled trials in which 50,844 patients were enrolled and assigned to receive FDA approved stents, Palmerini et al. reported that: (1) At 1-year and 2-year follow-up, the risk of definite stent thrombosis was significantly lower with CoCr-EES than BMS, a result not apparent with other DES; (2) the reduction in stent thrombosis

[a]References 109,111,112,120,138,143,144.

with CoCr-EES compared to BMS was apparent both at 30 days and between 31 days and 1 year; and (3) CoCr-EES were also associated with significantly lower 1-year rates of definite stent thrombosis compared with other first- and second-generation DES, including PES, SES, PC-ZES, and Re-ZES (Fig. 15.8).[201] In a broader network meta-analysis including 77 RCTs with 117,762 patient-years of follow-up, study selection was not restricted to FDA-approved devices, nor to RCTs reporting stent thrombosis using the ARC criteria. Bangalore et al. reported comparable mortality rates with first-generation DES, second-generation DES, and BMS.[202] However, rates of MI were significantly lower with SES, Re-ZES, and CoCr-EES (but not with PES) compared with BMS. Data on stent thrombosis were consistent with the previous network meta-analysis, finding the lowest rates with CoCr-EES. In addition, each DES reduced long-term TVR compared with BMS, but the magnitude of the effect varied in relation to the type of DES, such that CoCr-EES, SES, and Re-ZES had greater efficacy in reducing TVR than PES or PC-ZES.

Several network meta-analyses have also investigated the relative safety and efficacy of BP-based DES versus other second-generation DES and BMS.[203–206] With the potentially large caveat that there may be differences between BP-based DES in not only base stent type, but polymer degradation times and release kinetics, these analyses can help to identify similarities among BP-based DES types. In an analysis including 89 randomized trials with 85,490 patients, the major findings were: (1) BP-BES were associated with significantly lower 1-year rates of cardiac death or MI, MI, and TVR compared to BMS, lower 1-year rates of TVR compared to PC-ZES, and improved long-term outcomes compared to BMS and PES; (2) BP-BES were associated with higher rates of 1-year and long-term definite stent thrombosis compared to CoCr-EES, with a trend suggesting lower rates of MI with CoCr-EES compared to BP-BES; and (3) significant time-related differences in stent thrombosis were apparent between different stent types, with CoCr-EES being associated with the lowest rates of stent thrombosis in the early and late periods, and PES and SES having the highest risk of very late stent thrombosis (Fig. 15.9).[206] In another network meta-analysis including 126 randomized trials with 258,544 patient-years of follow-up, pooled BP-DES showed similar efficacy as second-generation DES in reducing TVR, but had higher rates of stent thrombosis than CoCr-EES.[203] Similar findings have been observed in two other network meta-analyses.[204,205] As the benefit of BP-DES is expected to emerge at long-term follow-up, a network meta-analysis has been performed comparing BP-BES with other second-generation DES in trials with at least 3-year follow-up.[207] That meta-analysis, including 51 trials and 52,158 patients, reported lower rates of stent thrombosis with CoCr-EES compared with BP-DES (HR 0.58, 95% CI 0.38 to 1.00) after a median follow-up of almost 4 years.

A subsequent pairwise meta-analysis including 16 randomized trials and 19,886 patients compared pooled permanent polymer DES (CoCr-EES, PtCr-EES, ZES, and Re-ZES) versus pooled bioabsorbable polymer DES (BES, Orsiro, Ultimaster, MiStent, Synergy, Yukon choice, Firehawk, and Tivoli).[208] After a mean follow-up of 26 months, there were no significant differences in TVR (P = .62), cardiac death (P = .46), MI (P = .98), or stent thrombosis (P = .19) between the two stent groups. Of note, there was no difference in very late stent thrombosis (P = .62) between permanent polymer DES versus bioabsorbable polymer DES. More recently, a pairwise aggregate meta-analyses including eight randomized trials and 11,176 patients compared the safety and efficacy of Orsiro versus other contemporary DES.[209] Orsiro had similar clinical outcomes compared to EES, to all permanent polymer DES, or to all DES included in the meta-analysis (EES, Re-ZES, or BES), with a trend toward a reduction in MI, TLF, or stent thrombosis in favor of Orsiro. Large-scale randomized

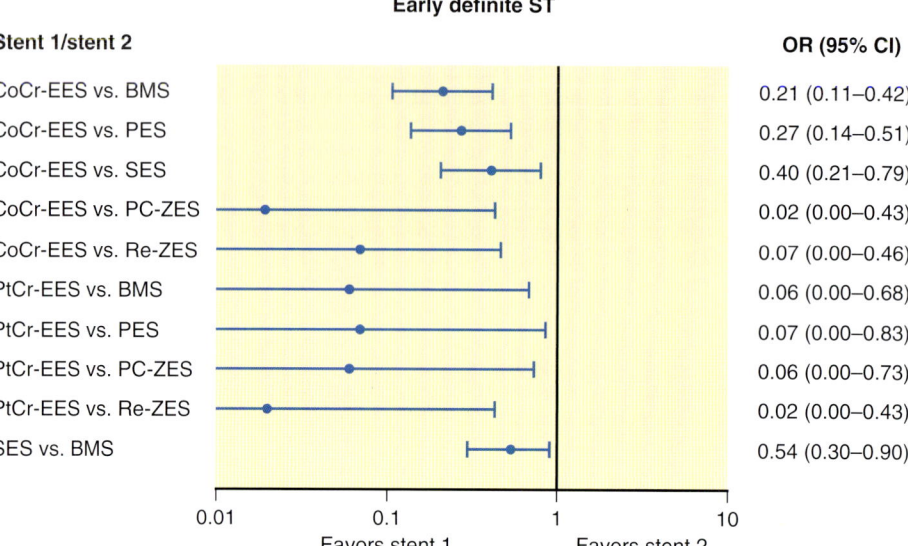
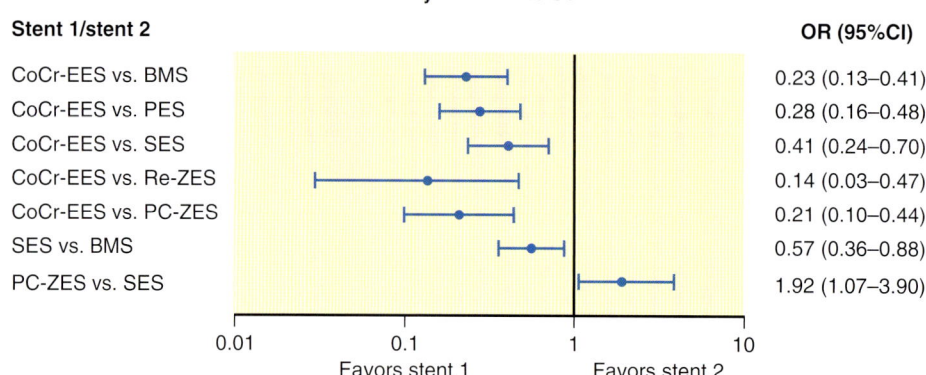
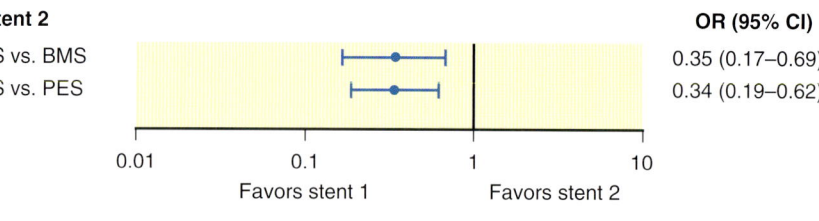

Fig. 15.8 Network meta-analysis including 49 randomized controlled trials and 50,844 patients showing time-related differences between various drug-eluting stents and bare-metal stents. Only statistically significant differences are shown. *BMS*, Bare-metal stents; *CI*, confidence interval; *CoCr-EES*, cobalt chromium everolimus-eluting stents; *OR*, odds ratio; *PC-ZES*, phosphorylcholine polymer-based zotarolimus-eluting stents; *PES*, paclitaxel-eluting stents; *PtCr-EES*, platinum-chromium everolimus-eluting stents; *Re-ZES*, Resolute zotarolimus-eluting stents; *SES*, sirolimus-eluting stents; *ST*, stent thrombosis.

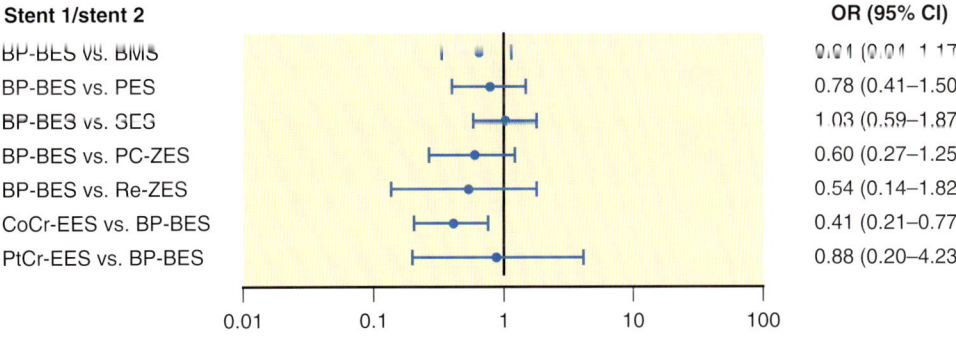

Fig. 15.9 Network meta-analysis including 89 randomized controlled trials and 85,490 patients showing time-related differences between biolimus-eluting stents versus other drug-eluting stents and bare-metal stents. *BMS*, Bare-metal stents; *BP-BES*, bioabsorbable polymer-based biolimus-eluting stents; *CI*, confidence interval; *CoCr-EES*, cobalt chromium everolimus-eluting stents; *OR*, odds ratio; *PC-ZES*, phosphorylcholine polymer-based zotarolimus-eluting stents; *PES*, paclitaxel-eluting stents; *PtCr-EES*, platinum-chromium everolimus-eluting stents; *Re-ZES*, resolute zotarolimus-eluting stents; *SES*, sirolimus-eluting stents; *ST*, stent thrombosis.

trials are needed to demonstrate the potential superiority of Orsiro versus other contemporary DES.

In summary, while most individual studies have not been adequately powered to assess overall DES safety, network meta-analyses have confirmed that second-generation durable polymer-based DES are both highly efficacious and have demonstrable safety advantages over first-generation DES platforms, and even over BMS. Meta-analyses to date have not demonstrated a safety advantage of BP-based DES over second-generation durable polymer-based DES, although stent-specific differences may be present. Longer-term follow-up from many of the conducted studies will provide important additional data in this regard.

POLYMER-FREE DRUG-ELUTING STENTS

Polymer-free DES feature the attractive combination of antiproliferative drug elution without a polymer coating. Polymer-free elution mechanisms include use of a nonpolymeric coating intermediate, surface modification techniques to adhere the drug onto the stent, with or without covalent bonding or chemical precipitation, use of reservoirs (grooves or wells) within the stent struts, and filling the inside of a hollow stent with drug which can diffuse out through holes drilled in the struts. As shown in Fig. 15.10, several polymer-free DES have been developed with different characteristics and novel mechanisms to control drug elution. However, clinical studies with these devices have been of limited size, have been underpowered for clinical end points, and have reported conflicting results (Table 15.10). In view of these limitations, a meta-analysis including eight randomized controlled trials with 6178 patients comparing pooled polymer-free DES versus SES, PES, or Re-ZES was recently reported.[210] In that meta-analysis, polymer-free DES appeared safe and effective, but did not provide any advantages compared to the other permanent polymer-based DES.

Renewed interest in this technology has recently been fostered by the Biofreedom stent, a polymer-free and carrier-free drug-coated stent which elutes the highly lipophilic biolimus in the vessel wall over a 1-month period. In the BIOFREEDOM FIM trial, Biofreedom was shown to be noninferior to PES for the primary end point of 1-year late lumen loss, showing safety and efficacy at 5-year follow-up, and prompting the investigation of this device in large-scale clinical trials.[211] In the LEADERS FREE trial, randomizing 2466 patients at high bleeding risk to either Biofreedom or the BMS Gazzelle (both Biosensors, Europe) followed by 1-month DAPT, Biofreedom was superior to the BMS for the primary end point of cardiac death, MI, or stent thrombosis.[212] In addition, Biofreedom was associated with lower rates of TVR compared to BMS. Thus, this trial established for the first time the superiority of a DES over a BMS with a 1-month DAPT regimen. However, the patient population included in the LEADERS FREE was heterogeneous including elderly patients (64% of the total population), patients on anticoagulant therapy (36%), patients with renal failure (20%), anemia or recent transfusion (16%), cancer (10%), or hospitalization for bleeding (3%), leaving undetermined which category of patients could benefit the most from Biofreedom stent and the 1-month DAPT regimen. In addition, 1-year stent thrombosis with the Biofreedom stent was 2.1%, due to high rates of early stent thrombosis (1.0%) as well as late stent thrombosis (1.1%). Finally, there were significantly lower rates of spontaneous MI not related to the target vessel in the Biofreedom group compared to the Gazzelle group, possibly inflating the difference in the overall rates of MI between the two stents.

Cre8 stent (Alvimedica, Saluggia, Italy) is another novel polymer-free DES that has shown promising results in the diabetic population.[213] Cre8 is a balloon-expandable stent with an 80-μm CoCr platform coated by an ultra-thin passive carbon coating (i-Carbofilm). The amphilimus formulation, constituted by sirolimus (0.9 μg/mm) and a mixture of long-chain fatty acids, is released from reservoirs located on the stent's abluminal surface. In the NEXT trial randomizing 323 patients with noncomplex coronary artery disease to either Cre8 or PES, Cre8 was superior to PES for the primary end point of in-stent late lumen loss.[214] In a propensity-matched pooled analysis of two multicenter national registries (ASTUTE[215] and INSPIRE-1[216]) including 1330 patients, Cre8 had similar safety and efficacy in nondiabetic patients, but better clinical outcomes in diabetic patients compared to BES.[213] Finally, in the multicenter, assessor blind RESERVOIRE trial, 112 patients with diabetes mellitus were randomized to receive either Cre8 or CoCr-EES.[217] At 1-year follow-up, Cre8 was noninferior to CoCr-EEs for the primary end point of in-stent neointimal volume obstruction assessed by OCT. In addition, a significant interaction between stent type and glycemic control was apparent, such that neointimal hyperplasia was significantly lower with Cre8 compared to CoCr-EES in the group of patients with higher HbA1C. Further studies are ongoing to establish the relative safety and efficacy of this stent compared to other DES.

Conclusions

In summary, significant progress has been made with second-generation DES compared to their first-generation counterparts in terms of enhanced deliverability, antirestenotic efficacy, and safety. Nonetheless, progressive iterations of stent platforms, drug delivery systems (including the absence of polymer), and drugs are being explored in an attempt to further improve on clinical outcomes with these devices.

STENTS IN SPECIFIC SITUATIONS

Acute ST-Segment Elevation Myocardial Infarction

Acute STEMI is caused in most cases by rupture of a thin-cap fibroatheroma, a lesion consisting of a lipid-rich necrotic core and an overlying thin (<65 μm), inflamed fibrous cap.[218] Tissue factor and other pro-thrombotic constituents are released, resulting in thrombotic occlusion of the coronary vessel and subsequent myocardial necrosis. Timely reperfusion with PCI results in improved myocardial salvage and reduced rates of recurrent ischemia, reinfarction, stroke, and death compared to fibrinolytic therapy.[219] As shown in Fig. 15.11, compared to balloon angioplasty, implanting BMS in STEMI further reduces subacute vessel closure and restenosis, but not death or reinfarction.[220] Stent implantation within or adjacent to a fibroatheroma may result in delayed endothelialization,[221] and the highest rates of stent thrombosis have been reported after stent implantation in STEMI, although this risk can be somewhat ameliorated with more potent antiplatelet agents.[222,223]

The safety and efficacy of DES in STEMI have been reported from at least 20 randomized trials in 11,924 patients and from at least 18 registries in 26,521 patients (Table 15.11). Considering that in five trials, three or more different DES have been compared to each other or versus BMS,[103,135,160,162,224] collectively there have been 15 randomized controlled trials comparing first-generation DES with BMS,[103,135,224–235] seven comparing first-generation DES to each other,[a] four comparing second-generation DES with BMS,[103,115,135,175] and six comparing second-generation DES versus first-generation DES.[95,101,103,135,160,162] In general, these studies have established the efficacy and safety of DES compared with BMS, with lower rates of TVR, and similar rates of death and MI. However, these individual studies were insufficiently powered to detect differences in safety end points across stent platforms, and therefore several meta-analyses have been performed to pool data. In the Drug-Eluting Stent in Primary Angioplasty (DES-ERT) cooperation, individual patient data were collected from 11

---

[a] References 75,103,135,160,162, 236, 237.

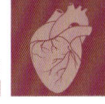

DES System	Platform	Antiproliferative Agent	Drug Carrier
Drug-filled stent Medtronic	Novel cobalt alloy platform	Sirolimus 1.1 µg/mm²	Drug elution controlled by diffusion
Amazonia Pax (Minvasys)	Amazonia Croco (L605) cobalt-chromium (Co-Cr) stent with strut thickness of 0.0028 inches (73 µm)	Paclitaxel ~2.5 µg/mm² of stent length	Abluminal coating (5 µm) applied on crimped stent
BioFreedom (Biosensors)	Bioflex II stent (316 L) stainless steel stent with a strut thickness of 0.0047 inches (119 µm)	Biolimus A9 (dose under investigation)	Modified microstructured abluminal stent surface
Optima (CID)	316 L stainless steel stent with strut thickness of 0.0054 inches (137 µm)	Tacrolimus ~2.3 µg/mm² of stent length	Integrated turbostratic carbon coating (Carbofilm) with multiple grooves (reservoirs) on its external surface
VESTAsync (MIV therapeutics)	GenX stainless steel (316 L) stent with strut thickness of 0.0026 inches (65 µm)	Sirolimus ~2.9 µg/mm² of stent length	Microporous hydroxyapatite coating
Yukon Choice (Translumina)	Yukon Choice 316 L stainless steel stent with strut thickness of 0.0034 inches (87 µm)	The largest successful experience was with a combination of sirolimus (120 µg/cm²) and probucol (100 µg/cm²)	Modified microporous stent surface

Fig. 15.10 Main characteristics of polymer-free drug-eluting stents *(DES)*.

TABLE 15.10 Randomized Controlled Trials of Polymer-Free Drug Eluting Stents

Trial Acronym and Reference	Study Cohort	Stent Comparators	Number Randomized	Latest Follow-Up to Date	Brand	Results of the Primary End Point
BIOFREEDOM First In Man[211]	Noncomplex CAD	PF-BES low dose/ PF-BES standard dose/PES	182	5 years	Bifreedom/ Taxus	The PF-BES standard dose, but not PF-BES low dose, demonstrated noninferiority versus PES in terms of in-stent LLL at 1year. At 5 years, clinical event rates were similar, between PF-BES an PES.
Carriè et al.[214]	Noncomplex CAD	PF-AES/PES	323	1 year	Cre8/Taxus Libertè	PF-AES resulted superior to PES for the primary end point of in-stent late lumen loss at 6 months (0.14 ± 0.36 mm vs. 0.34 ± 0.40 mm, respectively, $P < .000$t 1 year, cardiac death, MI, TLR or stent thrombosis did not significantly differ between the two devices.
Dang et al.[556]	STEMI	PF-PES/SES	105	1 year	Yinyi/Partner	At 1 year PF-PES and SES had similar rates of cardiac death, MI, or TLR. The two groups had also comparable angiographic outcomes, with similar rates of in-stent restenosis (8.6% for PF-PES vs. 5.0% for SES).
DEMONSTRATE[557]	Noncomplex CAD	PF-AES/BMS	38	3 months	Cre8/Vision	PF-AES was noninferior to BMS for the primary end point of strut coverage determined by OCT.

Continued

TABLE 15.10 Randomized Controlled Trials of Polymer-Free Drug Eluting Stents—cont'd

Trial Acronym and Reference	Study Cohort	Stent Comparators	Number Randomized	Latest Follow-Up to Date	Brand	Results of the Primary End Point
ISAR test[558,559]	Noncomplex CAD	PF-SES/PES	450	5 years	Yukon/Taxus Liberté	PF-SES resulted noninferior to PES for the primary end point of in-stent late lumen loss at 9 months (0.48 ± 0.61 mm vs. 0.48 ± 0.58 mm, respectively, P_{NI} = .02). At 5 years, cardiac death, MI, TLR or stent thrombosis did not significantly differ between the two devices.
ISAR test 2[159,424]	Noncomplex CAD	PF-Dual-DES[a]/SES/PC-ZES	1007	2 years	Yukon platform/Cypher/Endeavor	Six-month rates of binary restenosis in the Dual-DES group were significantly lower compared to PC-ZES (11.0% vs. 19.3%, respectively, P = .002), and similar compared to SES (12.0%, P = .68). Similarly, TLR with Dual-DES was significantly lower compared to PC-ZES and similar compared to SES. Between 1 and 2 years, Dual DES was associated with significantly lower rates of TLR compared to SES, but not to y
ISAR test 3[121,178]	Noncomplex CAD	PF-SES/BP-SES/SES	605	2 years	Yukon C/BP-Yukon/Cypher	PF-SES did not meet the criteria of noninferiority of late lumen loss at 6 months compared to SES (0.47 ± 0.56 mm vs. 0.23 ± 0.46 mm, respectively, P_{NI} = .94). There were no differences in safety outcomes between the three stent groups up to 2 years.
ISAR test 5[560]	Minimal exclusion criteria including patients with unprotected left main disease, or cardiogenic shock	Dual-DES/PC-ZES	3002	1 year	Yukon platform/Endeavor	Dual-DES resulted noninferior to ZES for the primary end point of cardiac death, MI or TLR at 1 year (13.1% vs. 13.5%, respectively, P_{NI} = .006). Rates of in-stent binary angiographic restenosis were similar between the two stent groups.
LEADERS FREE[212]	High bleeding risk patients	PF-BES/BMS	2466	1 year	Biofreedom/Gazzelle	PF-SES was superior to BMS for the primary end point of cardiac death, MI or stent thrombosis
LYPSIA YUKON[561,562]	Diabetes mellitus	PF-SES/PES	240	5 years	Yukon/Taxus	PF-SES did not meet the criteria of noninferiority of late lumen loss at 9 months compared to PES (0.63 ± 0.62 mm vs. 0.45 ± 0.60 mm, respectively). There were no significant differences between groups in the risk of death, MI, TLR, or stent thrombosis up to 5 years.
Zhang et al.[563]	Minimal exclusion criteria including patients with unprotected left main disease	PF-PES/BP-SES/SES	989	2 years	Yinyi/Excel/Partner	PF-PES and BP-SES resulted noninferior to SES for the primary end point of cardiac death, MI, TVR at 2 years (6.2% with PF-PES vs. 6.6% with BP-SES vs. 7.2% with SES). There were no significant differences between groups in the risk of stent thrombosis.

[a]This stent elutes both sirolimus and probucol.

AES, Amphilimus-eluting stents; *BMS*, bare-metal stent; *BP*, bioabsorbable polymer; *CAD*, coronary artery disease; *DES*, drug-eluting stents; *LLL*, late lumen loss; *MI*, myocardial infarction; *OCT*, optical coherence tomography; *PES*, paclitaxel-eluting stents; *PF*, polymer-free; *SES*, sirolimus-eluting stents; *STEMI*, ST-segment elevation MI; *TLR*, target-lesion revascularization; *TVR*, target-vessel revascularization.

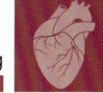

CHAPTER 15 Coronary Stenting

	Bare-metal stents	Balloon angioplasty	RR [95% CI]	RR [95% CI]	P Value
30-day events					
Mortality	2.9%	3.0%		0.97 [0.74–1.27]	.83
Reinfarction	2.0%	2.2%		0.92 [0.66–1.27]	.61
TVR	3.1%	5.1%		0.60 [0.47 0.77]	.0001
6- to 12-month events					
Mortality	5.1%	5.2%		0.98 [0.79–1.10]	.82
Reinfarction	3.7%	3.9%		0.94 [0.74–1.20]	.61
TVR	11.3%	18.4%		0.62 [0.55–0.69]	< .0001

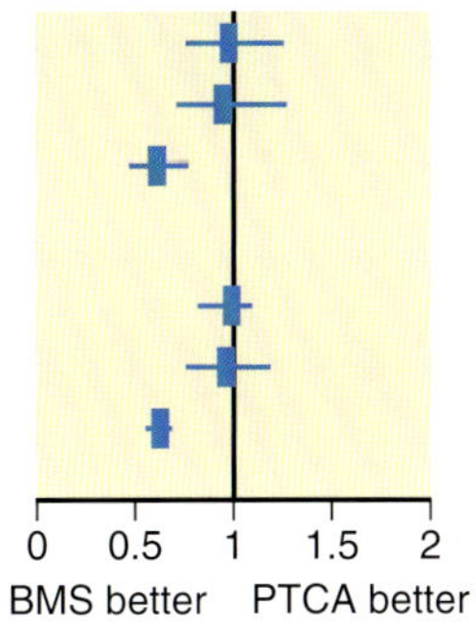

Fig. 15.11 Meta-analysis from 13 randomized controlled trials of bare-metal stents *(BMS)* compared to balloon angioplasty in acute myocardial infarction in 6922 patients. *CI*, Confidence interval; *PTCA*, percutaneous transluminal coronary angioplasty; *RR*, relative risk; *TVR*, target-vessel revascularization.

TABLE 15.11 Comparative Randomized Trials of Drug-Eluting Stents in ST-Segment Elevation Acute Myocardial Infarction

Study	Stent Comparators	Number Randomized	Latest Follow-Up	Results of the Primary End Point
Diaz de Llera[496]	SES/BMS	114	1	SES was associated with a trend towards reduced 1 year rates of TVR compared to BMS (0.0% with SES vs. 5.7% with BMS, *P* = .064)
EXAMINATION[115,239]	CoCr-EES/BMS	1504	2 years	CoCr-EES and BMS had similar rates of the primary end point of all-cause death, MI, or any revascularization at 1 year (11.9% with CoCr-EES vs. 14.2% with BMS, *P* = .19). CoCr-EES was associated with significantly lower 1-year rates of definite stent thrombosis compared to BMS (0.5% vs. 1.9%, respectively, *P* = .019). Similar results were apparent at 2 years.
GRACIA-3[229]	PES/BMS	419	1 year	There was no significant difference in the risk of in-segment binary restenosis between PES and BMS at 1 year (10.1% vs. 11.3%; respectively; *P* = .89). In-segment late lumen loss was significantly lower with PES compared to BMS (0.04 ± 0.05 mm vs. 0.27 ± 0.05 mm, *P* = .003)
HAAMU[209]	PES/BMS	164	1 year	PES was associated with a significantly lower late lumen loss compared to BMS at 6 months (0.26 ± 0.45 mm vs. 0.73 ± 0.56 mm, *P* < .001).
HORIZONS AMI[231,508]	PES/BMS	3006	3 years	PES was associated with significantly lower 1-year rates of ischemia-driven TVR (5.8% vs. 8.7%; *P* = .006). There was no significant difference in the risk of death, reinfarction or stent thrombosis between the two devices.
Juwana[237]	PES/SES	397	1 year	SES was associated with a significantly lower late lumen loss compared to PES at 1 year (0.01 ± 0.42 mm vs. 0.21 ± 0.50 mm, *P* = .001). There was no significant difference in the risk of death, MI, or stent thrombosis between the two devices.
KOMER[160]	PES/SES/PC-ZES	611	18 months	There was no significant difference in the risk of death, MI, or stent thrombosis between PES, SES, and PC-ZES (5.7% vs. 3.4% vs. 5.9%, respectively; *P* = .46) There was a trend towards lower rates of ischemia-driven TLR with SES compared to either PES or PC-ZES at 18 months (0.5% with SES vs. 1.5% with PES vs. 3.4% with PC-ZES, *P* = .09).
MISSION[235,564]	SES/BMS	310	5 years	SES was associated with a significantly lower late lumen loss compared to BMS at 9 months (0.12 ± 0.43 mm vs. 0.68 ± 0.57 mm, *P* < .001). There was no significant difference in the risk of death, MI, or stent thrombosis between the two devices.
MULTISTRATEGY[234,565]	SES/BMS	744	3 years	SES was associated with significantly lower 1 year rates of all-cause death, MI, and clinically driven TVR (7.8% vs. 14.5%, *P* = .004). There was no significant difference in the risk of stent thrombosis between the two devices.

Continued

TABLE 15.11 Comparative Randomized Trials of Drug-Eluting Stents in ST-Segment Elevation Acute Myocardial Infarction—cont'd

Study	Stent Comparators	Number Randomized	Latest Follow-Up	Results of the Primary End Point
Pasceri et al.[228]	SES/BMS	65	1 year	There was no significant difference in the risk of death, MI, TVR, or stent thrombosis between SES and BMS at 1 year.
PASEO[236,566]	PES/SES/BMS	270	4 years	PES and SES were associated with significantly lower 1-year rates of TLR compared to BMS (4.4% with PES vs. 3.3% with SES vs. 14.4% with BMS, $P = .03$ for PES vs. BMS, and $P = .016$ for SES vs. BMS). There was no significant difference in the risk of death, MI, or stent thrombosis between the three devices.
PASSION[226,567,568]	PES/BMS	619	5 years	There was a trend toward lower rates of cardiac death, MI, or TLR with PES compared to BMS (8.8% vs. 12.8%; $P = .09$). There was no significant difference in the risk of stent thrombosis between the two devices.
PROSIT[520,569]	PES/SES	308	3 years	There was a trend toward lower rates of all-cause death, MI, stent thrombosis, or TLR with SES compared to PES at 1 year (5.8% vs. 11.7%; $P = .07$). In-segment late lumen loss was 0.09 ± 0.45 mm with SES vs. 0.33 ± 0.68 mm with PES; ($P = .002$) on 6-month follow-up angiography. Similar results were apparent at 3 years.
SELECTION[225]	PES/BMS	76	7 months	The percentage of the stent volume obstruction by neointimal hyperplasia measured by intravascular ultrasound was significantly lower with PES compared to BMS at 7 months (4.6% vs. 20%; $P < .01$). PES was also associated with significantly lower rates of death, MI, and TLR compared to BMS.
SESAMI[227,570,571]	SES/BMS	320	5 years	SES was associated with significantly lower 1-year rates of binary restenosis (9.3% vs. 21.3%, $P = .032$), and TLR (4.3% vs. 11.2%; $P = .02$) compared to BMS. There was no significant difference in the risk of death, MI, or stent thrombosis between the two devices up to 5 years.
STRATEGY[233,572]	SES/BMS	175	5 years	SES plus high-dose bolus of tirofiban was associated with significantly lower 1-year rates of death, MI, stroke, or binary restenosis compared to BMS plus abciximab (19% vs. 50%, $P < .001$). Similar results were apparent at 5 years, but the difference between the two groups tended to be attenuated (29.9% with SES vs. 43.2% with BMS, $P = .067$).
TYPHOON[230,573]	SES/BMS	712	4 years	The rate of the primary end point, a composite of cardiac death, MI, or TVR, was significantly lower with SES than BMS (7.3% vs. 14.3%, $P = .004$). There were no significant differences in the risk of death or MI between the two stent groups, but lower rates of TVR with SES compared to BMS (5.6% vs. 13.4%, respectively; $P < .001$). Similar results were apparent at 4 years.
XAMI[101]	CoCr-EES/SES	625	1 year	CoCr-EES resulted noninferior to SES for the primary end point of cardiac death, MI, or TVR at 1 year (4.0% vs. 5.3%, respectively, $P_{NI} = .048$).
ZEST-AMI[162]	PES/SES/PC-ZES	328	1 year	At 1 year, the incidence of the primary end point, a composite of death, MI, or TVR was 11.3% with PC-ZES, and 8.2% both for SES and PES ($P = .83$). Individual components of the primary end point did not differ between the three groups.

BMS, Bare-metal stent; *CoCr-EES*, cobalt-chromium everolimus-eluting stents; *MI*, myocardial infarction; *PC-ZES*, phosphorylcholine polymer based zotarolimus-eluting stent; *PES*, paclitaxel-eluting stents; *SES*, sirolimus-eluting stents; *TLR*, target-lesion revascularization; *TVR*, target-vessel revascularization.

randomized trials including 6298 patients randomized to either first-generation DES (n = 6298) or BMS (n = 2318).[238] Compared with BMS, first-generation DES were associated with similar rates of death, MI, or stent thrombosis, but lower rates of TVR at a mean follow-up of 1201 days. However, first-generation DES were associated with higher rates of very late stent thrombosis and reinfarction.

Given the safety concerns of first-generation DES, particularly in the high-risk cohort of patients undergoing STEMI PCI, several studies have examined whether second-generation DES have further improved the outcomes of patients with STEMI. In the EXAMINATION trial, 1498 patients presenting with STEMI within 48 hours from symptom onset were randomized to either CoCr-EES (n = 751) or the equivalent BMS (n = 747).[115] At 1-year follow-up, the primary composite end point of all-cause death, MI, or any revascularization did not differ between the two groups (11.9% in the CoCr-EES group vs. 14.2% in the BMS group, P = .19). However, CoCr-EES resulted in significantly lower rates of both TVR and definite stent thrombosis compared with BMS. Similar results have been confirmed at 2-year follow-up.[239] At 5-year follow-up, patients treated with CoCr-EES had significantly lower rates of the composite of all-cause death, MI, or any revascularization compared with BMS (21% vs. 26%, respectively; P = .03).[240] There was also a significant reduction of all-cause mortality with CoCr-EES compared to BMS (9% vs. 12%; P = .047). In the XAMI trial, 625 patients with STEMI were randomized to either CoCr-EES (n = 404) or SES (n = 221).[101] At 1 year, CoCr-EES were noninferior to SES for the primary end point of cardiac death, MI, or any TVR, with a MACE rate of 4% for CoCr-EES versus 7.7% for SES. PC-ZES has been compared with both PES and SES in the Zotarolimus-Versus Sirolimus-Versus Paclitaxel-Eluting Stent for Acute Myocardial Infarction Patients (ZEST-AMI)[162] and KOMER trials.[160] Similar results were apparent in the Randomized comparison of everolimus-eluting stents and sirolimus-eluting stents in patients with STEMI (RACES-MI) trial, in which 500 patients were randomized to either CoCr-EES or SES. At 3-year follow-up, CoCr-EES was noninferior to SES for the primary end point of cardiac death, MI, definite probable stent thrombosis, or TVR. In addition, CoCr-EES was associated with significantly lower rates of stent thrombosis compared to SES (1.6% vs. 5.2%, P = .035).[241] Different results were apparent at a long-term follow-up (mean of 2132 days), when CoCr-EES was associated with lower rates of MACE (23.8% vs. 34.1%, P = .028) and lower rates of stent thrombosis (2.5% vs. 7.7%, P = .09) compared to SES.[242] ZEST-AMI trial included 328 patients who were randomly assigned to PC-ZES (n = 108), SES (n = 110), or PES (n = 110).[162] At 1-year follow-up, the primary end point, a composite of cardiac death, MI, and ischemia-driven TVR did not differ between the three groups. Similar results were apparent in the KOMER trial, in which 611 patients with STEMI undergoing primary PCI were randomized to PC-ZES (n = 205), SES (n = 204), or PES (n = 202).[160] The cumulative 1-year rate of MACE was 5.9% in the PC-ZES group, 3.4% in the SES group, and 5.7% in the PES group.

Among the bioabsorbable polymer-based DES, BP-BES is the only one that has been extensively investigated in patients with STEMI. In the COMFORTABLE AMI trial, 1157 patients presenting with STEMI within 24 hours from symptom onset were randomized to either BP-BES (n = 575) or to the equivalent BMS (n = 582).[175] Compared with BMS, BP-BES resulted in a significantly lower 1-year rate of the primary end point, a composite of cardiac death, MI, or ischemia-driven TLR (4.3% in the BP-BES group vs. 8.7% in the BMS group, P = .04). The difference was largely driven by a lower risk of target-vessel reinfarction and ischemia-driven TVR. No differences in stent thrombosis were noted. These results were confirmed at 2-year follow-up.[243]

Of interest, in a prespecified stratified analysis of the primary end point in the BIOSCIENCE trial, Orsiro was associated with significantly lower rates of TLF compared to CoCr-EES in patients with STEMI (3.3% vs. 8.7%, P = .024).[123] The potential superiority of Orsiro versus CoCr-EES in patients with STEMI is currently investigated in the BIOSTEMI trial (NCT02579031). More recently, in the ISAR TEST V, 311 patients with STEMI were randomized to either sirolimus and probucol-eluting stents or Re-ZES.[244] At 5-year follow-up, there was no difference between the two stents in the primary end point, a composite of cardiac death, target-vessel related MI, or TLR (18.3% with sirolimus and probucol-eluting stent versus 20.1% with Re-ZES, P = .62). Finally, the relative safety and efficacy of Absorb bioresorbable scaffold versus CoCr-EES in STEMI patients has been investigated in the TROFI II trial, a single-blind noninferiority randomized trial including 191 patients.[215] The primary end point of the study, the 6-month optical frequency domain imaging healing score based on the number of uncovered or malapposed stent struts, was lower in the scaffold arm compared to CoCr-EES (1.74 vs. 2.80, P_{NI} < .001). Device-oriented composite end point including cardiac death, target-vessel MI, or clinically driven TLR, was comparable between the two groups (1.1% with Absorb vs. 0% with CoCr-EES).

Given the availability of multiple studies examining the performance of different DES and BMS in STEMI, the relative safety and efficacy of these devices has been further investigated in two network meta-analyses. In a meta-analysis combining 22 trials including 12,453 randomized patients treated with CoCr-EES, PES, SES, and PC-ZES, CoCr-EES were associated with significantly lower rates of cardiac death or MI and stent thrombosis than BMS.[246] The difference in stent thrombosis was apparent as early as 30 days and was maintained up to 2 years. CoCr-EES were also associated with significantly lower rates of 1-year stent thrombosis than PES. SES were associated with significantly lower rates of cardiac death or MI than BMS at 1 year, but not at long-term follow-up. CoCr-EES, PES, and SES had significantly lower rates of 1-year TVR than BMS, with SES also showing lower rates of TVR than PES. Similar results were found in a confirmatory network meta-analysis.[247] In summary, although first-generation DES have significantly improved the outcomes of patients with STEMI by significantly reducing the risk of TVR, they have been associated with increased rates of very late stent thrombosis and reinfarction.[238] By reducing both TVR and stent thrombosis, second-generation DES have further improved the outcomes of patients with STEMI, with a possible benefit also in terms of cardiac mortality and reinfarction compared to PES and BMS.

Stents to Reduce Distal Embolization in STEMI

Beyond the use of DES in STEMI, several novel STEMI-specific stent devices are currently under investigation. These devices aim to reduce the impact of distal embolization of thrombus during STEMI PCI, an event that has been associated with a higher incidence of periprocedural complications as well as infarct size and mortality.[248] A novel BMS covered with a polyethylene terephthalate micronet mesh (MGuard, Inspire MD, Tel Aviv, Israel) may trap friable thrombotic and atheromatous material between the micronet and vessel wall, thereby preventing distal embolization.[249] This device was investigated in the MASTER trial in which 433 patients with STEMI presenting within 12 hours from symptom onset were randomized.[250] The MGuard resulted in increased rates of post-PCI Thrombolysis In Myocardial Infarction (TIMI)-3 flow and a significant improvement in the primary end point of complete ST-segment resolution compared to commercially available BMS or DES. A larger multicenter clinical study (MASTER II) was initiated to further evaluate the efficacy and safety of this device for patients undergoing PCI in STEMI, but unfortunately was prematurely terminated after 310 of 1114 planned patients were recruited due to slow enrollment. A drug-eluting version of this device is under development.

One other device that is actively undergoing investigation in STEMI PCI is a self-expanding BMS (Stentys Corporation, Paris, France) that, compared with balloon-expandable stents, aims to reduce deployment pressure and improve acute and late stent apposition (as thrombus between the vessel wall and the stent resolves). In the 80-patient randomized APPOSITION II trial comparing this device with a BMS, a lower number of malapposed stent struts was observed at 3 days with the self-expanding device, with a similar frequency of MACE at 6 months.[30] Unfortunately, the larger APPOSITION V trial was prematurely terminated after only 300 of 880 patients were enrolled because of slow enrollment. The failure to complete recruitment in both MASTER II and APPOSITION V reflect the increasing use of DES and declining use of BMS in STEMI.

Diabetes Mellitus

Patients with diabetes have higher rates of angiographic and clinical restenosis after BMS than those without diabetes.[251,252] In general, the pivotal trials in which DES were compared to BMS revealed comparable relative safety and efficacy with DES in patients with diabetes compared to those without diabetes, although with greater absolute reductions in TLR and TVR in diabetic patients given their higher baseline risk.[253–255] Most prior studies have shown comparable rates of in-stent late loss with PES in patients with versus without diabetes,[256] suggesting that the multiple pathways with which paclitaxel interferes with restenosis (by affecting microtubular function) makes its action relatively independent of the diabetic state.[257] Considerable controversy has existed, however, whether the greater suppression of late loss from stents which elute potent rapamycin analog-eluting stents (such as SES or EES) is preserved in patients with diabetes, given that the effect of rapamycin in interfering with the cell cycle is regulated by glycosalation-dependent enzymes.[258] In this regard, several small- to moderate-sized studies have provided conflicting results. For example, among 379 patients with diabetes randomized to SES versus PES in the REALITY trial, the rates of restenosis and clinical events were comparable with both stents.[74] In contrast, in the randomized 250-patient ISAR-Diabetes trial, SES compared to PES resulted in a greater reduction in late loss at 6 months, but nonsignificantly different rates of TLR at 9 months.[259]

This issue has been comprehensively addressed by a pooled patient-level analysis from the SPIRIT II, SPIRIT III, SPIRIT IV, and COMPARE trials, in which 6789 patients were randomized to CoCr-EES versus PES (Express or Liberté platforms). A total of 1869 patients (25%) had diabetes. In patients without diabetes, CoCr-EES were associated with a marked reduction in the 1-year composite rate of cardiac death, MI, or ischemia-driven TLR when compared with PES.[260] CoCr-EES also markedly reduced the individual rates of MI, stent thrombosis, and TLR compared with PES. In contrast, among patients with diabetes, the rates of composite adverse events at 1-year (and their components) were almost identical between the two stent types, with a significant interaction observed between diabetes and stent platform. In a network meta-analysis including 42 trials with 22,844 patient-years of follow-up, all DES (SES, PES, CoCr-EES, and Re-ZES) significantly reduced the risk of TVR compared with BMS in diabetic patients, but the magnitude of this effect varied with the type of stent.[261] In fact, SES and CoCr-EES appeared more efficacious than PES and Re-ZES in reducing the risk of TVR, with an 87% probability that CoCr-EES was associated with the lowest rate of TVR. There was no increased risk of death or MI with any DES compared to BMS. Finally, CoCr-EES had a 62% probability to be the stent associated with the lowest risk of any stent thrombosis. More recently, the Taxus Element versus Xience Prime in a Diabetic Population (TUXEDO) trial randomly assigned 1830 patients with diabetes mellitus to receive either PES or CoCr-EES.[262] At 1-year follow-up, CoCr-EES was associated with significantly lower rates of TVF (5.6% vs. 2.9%, P = .005), spontaneous MI (2.1% vs. 0.4%, P = .002), stent thrombosis (2.1% vs. 0.4%, P = .002), and TVR (3.4% vs. 1.2%) compared to PES. These benefits of CoCr-EES versus PES were maintained at 2 years.[263]

Promising results in diabetic patients have been shown with a novel polymer-free DES, Cre8, which uses an amphilimus formulation of sirolimus and fatty acid that elutes from laser-dug wells on the stent abluminal surface. In diabetic patients, glucose uptake and oxidation are impaired, and adenosine triphosphate generation relies mainly on fatty acid metabolism. Thus, it is possible that the use of fatty acid as carrier could improve the penetration of sirolimus in the vessel wall, optimizing the efficacy of the drug. As discussed in the previous section (see Polymer-free DES), observational studies and small randomized trials have supported this hypothesis. In particular, Cre8 has been shown to be superior to BES in diabetic, but not in nondiabetic patients,[213] and superior to CoCr-EES in patients with diabetes and impaired glycemic control.[217] Large-scale randomized trials are warranted to confirm these results.

Beyond stent selection during PCI in diabetic patients, the most critical revascularization decision in patients with diabetes mellitus is the mode of revascularization itself (i.e., whether to perform PCI or coronary artery bypass grafting [CABG]). Prior studies have demonstrated higher rates of repeat revascularization procedures among diabetic patients treated with BMS compared with CABG, although the rates of death, MI, and stroke have been similar.[264] The use of DES for diabetic patients was examined in the Coronary Artery Revascularization in Diabetes (CARDia) trial, which randomized 510 patients with diabetes mellitus and multivessel disease to PCI with either SES (69% of patients) or BMS (31% of patents) versus CABG.[265] The primary end point of all-cause death, MI, or stroke at 1 year occurred in 10.5% of patients with CABG versus 13.0% with PCI (P = .39); among the SES subgroup, the 1-year event rates were 12.4% vs. 11.6%, respectively (P = .82). Whereas CARDia was too underpowered to be definitive, the FREEDOM trial enrolled 1900 patients with diabetes mellitus and multivessel coronary artery disease to CABG versus PCI with first-generation DES

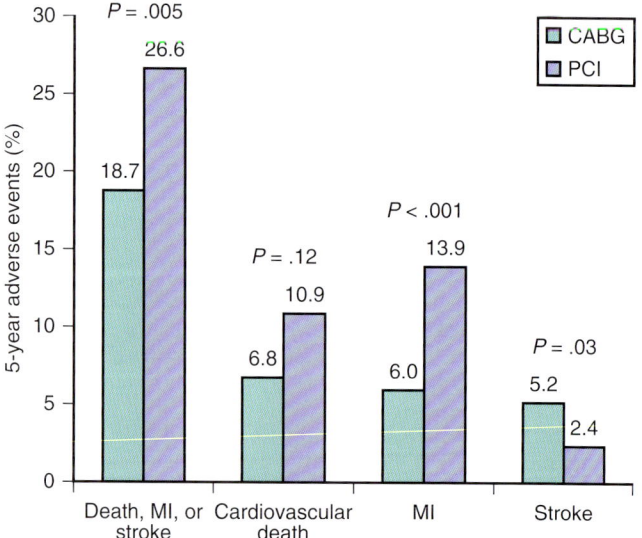

Fig. 15.12 Five-year results from the FREEDOM trial in which 1900 patients with diabetes mellitus and multivessel coronary artery disease were randomized to percutaneous coronary intervention *(PCI)* vs. coronary artery bypass graft surgery *(CABG)*. *MI*, Myocardial infarction.

(SES or PES).[266] As shown in Fig. 15.12, the 5-year rate of the primary end point was significantly higher among PCI patients compared with CABG patients (26.6% vs. 18.7%, respectively, P = .005). This difference was driven by a significant reduction in the risk of all-cause death (P = .049) and MI (P < .001) with CABG compared with PCI. However, stroke rates were significantly higher in the CABG group (5.2% vs. 2.4% in the PCI group, P = .03), a finding consistent with other reports not restricted to a diabetic population.[267,268] The relevance of these findings, given the improved outcomes with currently used second-generation DES platforms, is uncertain.

No RCTs have in fact been performed so far comparing newer-generation DES versus CABG in patients with diabetes mellitus, although three large observational registries have recently been reported.[269-271] In a large-scale population-based dataset from British Columbia, 4661 patients with multivessel coronary artery disease and diabetes mellitus undergoing either PCI using first- or second-generation DES or CABG between 2007 and 2014 were included.[271] As the proportional hazard assumption was not met over the 5-year follow-up period, outcomes were reported as early (from revascularization to 30 days) and late (31 day to 5 years). At 30-day follow-up, CABG was associated with a significantly lower adjusted risk of major adverse cardiac or cerebrovascular events (MACCE), a composite of all-cause mortality, MI, or stroke compared to PCI (OR 0.60, 95% CI 0.43 to 0.84). Interestingly, a significant interaction between clinical presentation and the strategy of revascularization was apparent ($P_{interaction}$ < .01), such that CABG significantly reduced clinical events in patients with acute coronary syndromes, but not in those with stable coronary artery disease. In the late period, CABG again was associated with a significantly lower adjusted risk of MACCE (HR 0.63, 95% CI 0.53 to 0.74), with 52% lower rates of death (HR 0.48, 95% CI 0.39 to 0.59), 60% lower rates of MI (HR 0.40, 95% CI 0.31 to 0.51), 72% lower rates of repeat revascularization (HR 0.28, 95% CI 0.23 to 0.35), and no interaction apparent between clinical presentation and the strategy of revascularization. Similar results were apparent in the SWEDEHEART registry, in which 2546 patients with type 1 diabetes mellitus underwent either CABG (n = 683) or any type PCI (n = 1863), thus including first- and second-generation DES.[270] After a mean follow-up of 10 years, CABG was associated with lower rates of cardiac mortality (HR 1.45, 95% CI 1.21 to 1.74), MI (HR 1.47, 95% CI 1.23 to 1.78), and repeat revascularization (HR 5.64, 95% CI 4.67 to 6.82).

These results differ from another large population-based registry including 16,089 patients with diabetes and multivessel coronary artery disease from New York State who underwent PCI with EES or CABG.[269] Therefore, this registry is the only study to compare exclusively second-generation DES with CABG. At short-term follow-up, EES was associated with a lower adjusted risk of death (HR 0.58, 95% CI 0.34 to 0.98), and stroke (HR 0.14, 95% CI 0.06 to 0.30), but higher risk of MI (HR 2.44, 95% CI 1.13 to 5.31). At long-term follow-up, EES was associated with a similar adjusted risk of death (HR 1.12, 95% CI 0.96 to 1.30), a lower risk of stroke (HR 0.76, 95% CI 0.59 to 0.99), but a higher risk of MI (HR 1.64, 95% CI 1.32 to 2.04) and repeat revascularization (HR 2.42, 95% CI 2.12 to 2.76). Interestingly, the higher risk of MI with EES versus CABG was not apparent in the subgroups of EES patients achieving complete revascularization (HR 1.37, 95% CI 0.76 to 2.47).

Therefore, whether diabetes independently modifies the relative outcomes after revascularization with second-generation DES compared with CABG still remains a matter of debate. Of note, even in the randomized SYNTAX trial using the first-generation PES versus CABG in patients with triple vessel and/or left main coronary artery disease, patients with versus without diabetes were at higher risk for 4-year mortality after both PCI and CABG. However, the presence of diabetes did not discriminate between the relative benefits of CABG versus PCI after considering other clinical and anatomic features.[272] In addition, in a patient-level pooled analysis from SYNTAX, PRECOMBAT, and BEST trials, including 1068 patients with diabetes mellitus, no significant difference was apparent in the 5-year rates of the composite of death, MI, or stroke between PCI and CABG among patients with low-intermediate (≤32) SYNTAX score (15.1% vs. 14.9%, respectively; P = .93), while a significant difference was present in those with SYNTAX score >32 (24.5% with PCI vs. 13.2% with CABG, P = .018).[273]

Left Main and Multivessel Disease

Although they are distinctly different conditions, revascularization decisions for patients with left main and multivessel disease are often considered together because historically the default strategy has been CABG. Patients with multivessel disease treated with PCI have higher restenosis and stent thrombosis rates than those with single-vessel disease, especially when diffuse disease, small vessels, and bifurcation lesions requiring treatment are present. In contrast, while restenosis and thrombosis are relatively rare after stenting the relatively short, large-caliber left main segment, PCI failure in the left main jeopardizes a sufficiently large amount of myocardium to entail a high risk of mortality.

Prior to introduction of DES, meta-analyses of PCI versus CABG trials in patients with multivessel disease demonstrated similar rates of death, MI, or stroke with PCI (using BMS or balloon angioplasty alone), but higher rates of repeat revascularization.[274] However, BMS were used in only 4 of these trials in 3051 patients,[275-278] and no study utilized DES. In light of the demonstrable efficacy of DES in reducing revascularization procedures compared with BMS, the SYNTAX trial was undertaken, randomizing 1800 patients with triple vessel disease (n = 1095) and/or left main disease (n = 705) to either PES or CABG, using broader inclusion criteria compared to previous trials.[279] The primary end point of the SYNTAX trial, the 1-year composite rate of all-cause mortality, stroke, MI, or unplanned repeat revascularization, occurred significantly less commonly with CABG than with PES (Fig. 15.12, left), largely due to greater rates of repeat revascularization with PCI compared to CABG. Conversely, the 1-year rate of stroke was lower with PCI, and the composite rates of death, MI, or stroke were similar in both arms at 1 year. However, as shown in Fig. 15.13 (right panel), 5-year follow-up from the SYNTAX trial demonstrated a more marked advantage favoring CABG with respect to the primary composite end point (26.9% in the CABG group vs. 37.3% in the PCI group, P < .0001). In addition, rates of MI (3.8% in the CABG group vs. 9.7% in the PCI group, P < .0001) and TVR (13.7% vs. 25.9%, P < .0001) were significantly lower with CABG compared to PCI, whereas the risk of death or stroke was not significantly different between the two treatment strategies. A borderline interaction (P_{int} = .10) was present such that the primary 5-year MACCE end point in the three-vessel disease subgroup was 50% higher in patients assigned to PCI compared to those assigned to CABG (24.2% in the CABG group vs. 37.5% in the PCI group, P < .0001), whereas no significant difference was apparent between the two strategies of revascularization in the subgroup of patients with left main disease (31.0% in the CABG group vs. 36.9% in the PCI group, P = .12).

Further substratification of the SYNTAX results based upon angiographically assessed lesion complexity has been performed. In these analyses, 5-year rates of the primary end point did not significantly differ between treatment groups in patients in the lower SYNTAX score tertile (SYNTAX score ≤22), but were significantly higher with PCI than CABG in patients in the intermediate (SYNTAX score 23 to 32) and upper (SYNTAX score ≥33) SYNTAX score tertiles, driven by a better survival, lower MI rates, and less TVR with CABG compared to PCI. As shown in Tables 15.12

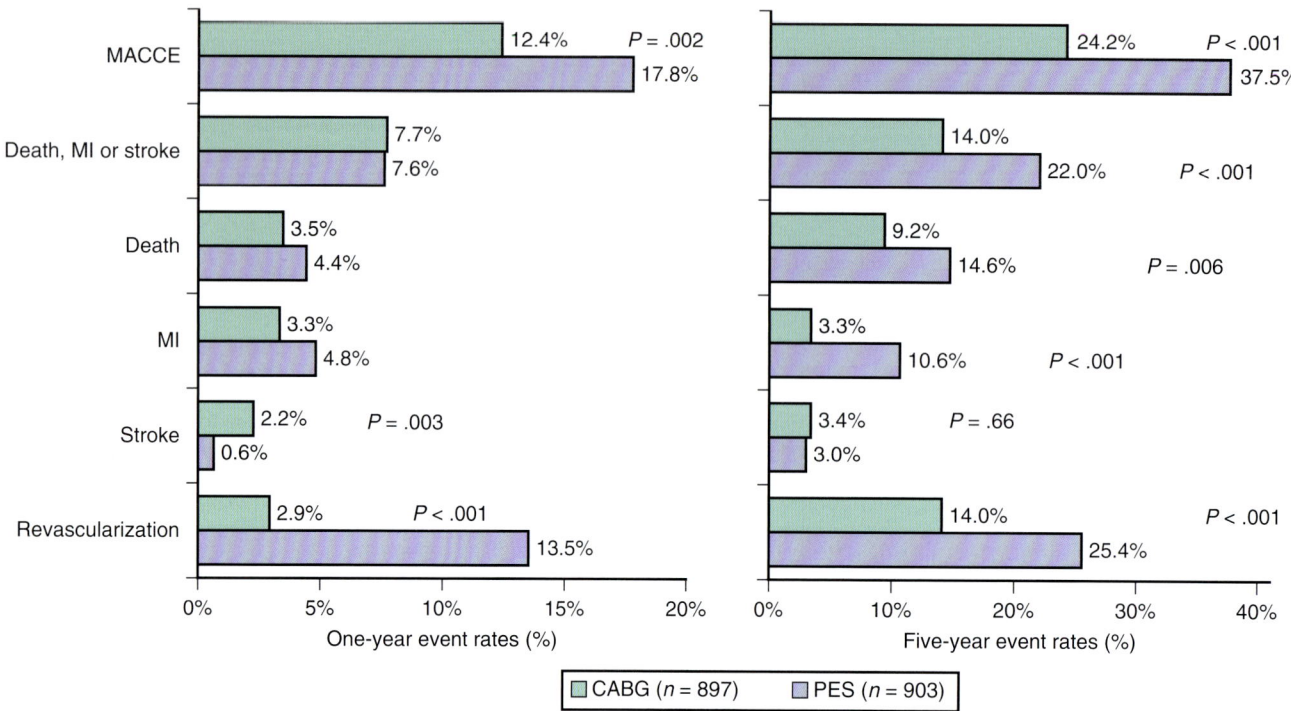

Fig. 15.13 One-year *(left)* and five-year *(right)* results from the SYNTAX trial in which 1800 patients with triple-vessel and/or left main disease were randomized to paclitaxel-eluting stents *(PES)* vs. coronary artery bypass graft surgery *(CABG)*. MACCE denote major adverse cardiac or cerebrovascular event; death, myocardial infarction *(MI)*, stroke or unplanned repeat revascularization. *P* = NS unless otherwise noted.

TABLE 15.12 Five-year Outcomes From the SYNTAX Trial in Patients With Triple Vessel Disease Stratified by SYNTAX Score Tertiles

	Low SYNTAX Tertile (≤22)			Intermediate SYNTAX Tertile (23–32)			High SYNTAX Tertile (≥33)		
	PES (n = 181)	CABG (n = 171)	P Value	PES (n = 207)	CABG (n = 208)	P Value	PES (n = 155)	CABG (n = 166)	P Value
MACCE	33.3%	26.8%	.21	37.9%	22.6%	<.001	41.9%	24.1%	<.001
Death, MI, or stroke	17.5%	14.8%	.56	23.2%	14.7%	.035	26.2%	12.5%	.02
Death	10.2%	9.3%	.81	16.3%	9.6%	.047	17.8%	8.8%	.5
MI	8.8%	4.9%	.	13.8%	3.1%	<.001	8.7%	1.9%	.008
Stroke	1.8%	3.9%	.24	2.5%	3.6%	.53	5.1%	2.6%	.31
Revascularization	23.1%	14.9%	.038	25.1%	11.0%	<.001	28.2%	12.6%	<.001

CABG, Coronary artery bypass graft surgery; *MACCE*, major adverse cardiac or cerebrovascular events (death, MI, stroke or revascularization); *MI*, myocardial infarction; *PES*, paclitaxel-eluting stents.

TABLE 15.13 Five-year Outcomes From the SYNTAX Trial in Patients With Left Main Disease Stratified by SYNTAX Score Tertiles

	Low and Intermediate SYNTAX Tertile (≤32)			High SYNTAX Tertile (≥33)		
	PES (n = 221)	CABG (n = 196)	P Value	PES (n = 135)	CABG (n = 149)	P Value
MACCE	31.3%	32.1%	.74	46.5%	29.7%	.003
Death, MI, or stroke	14.8%	19.8%	.16	26.1%	22.1%	.40
Death	7.9%	15.1%	.02	20.9%	14.1%	.11
MI	6.1%	3.8%	.33	11.7%	6.1%	.13
Stroke	1.4%	3.9%	.11	1.6%	4.9%	.13
Revascularization	22.6%	18.6%	.35	34.1%	11.6%	<.001

CABG, Coronary artery bypass graft surgery; *MACCE*, major adverse cardiac or cerebrovascular events (death, MI, stroke, or revascularization); *MI*, myocardial infarction; *PES*, paclitaxel-eluting stents.

and 15.13, however, the threshold of the SYNTAX score beyond which CABG improved outcomes relative to PCI varied depending on whether patients presented with triple-vessel disease or left main disease, with greater equipoise seen among patients with left main disease and those with less extensive disease as a whole.[280,281] However, given the modest sample sizes of these post hoc subgroups, these findings should be considered hypothesis-generating only. Recently, a new score for risk stratification of patients with multivessel or left main coronary artery disease has been developed by fitting multivariable models to the 4-year mortality results of the SYNTAX trial: the SYNTAX score II.[272] This individualized score demonstrates how the threshold of SYNTAX score favoring CABG rather than PCI can vary in relation to the presence or absence of additional clinical and angiographic variables that modify the overall trial observations favoring one or the other revascularization modality. Specifically, in the presence of variables that favors CABG, such as young age, female gender, and low left ventricular ejection fraction, lower SYNTAX scores are required to achieve equipoise in mortality between the two revascularization strategies, whereas in the presence of variables that favor PCI, such as old age, presence of left main disease, or chronic obstructive pulmonary disease, equipoise between the two treatments is achieved with higher SYNTAX scores.

An updated meta-analysis of CABG versus PCI in multivessel disease including a total of six trials with 6055 randomized patients has been reported.[282] To reflect current practice, only randomized trials with one or more arterial graft used in at least 90% of patients, and one or more stents used in at least 70% of cases, were included. After a median follow-up of 4.1 years, CABG was associated with significantly lower rates of mortality compared to PCI (risk ratio = 0.73, 95% CI 0.62 to 0.86, $P < .01$). In addition, CABG was also associated with significantly lower rates of MI (risk ratio = 0.58, 95% CI 0.48 to 0.72, $P < .001$), and TVR (risk ratio = 0.29, 95% CI 0.21 to 0.41, $P < .001$). In contrast, rates of stroke were significantly higher with CABG compared to PCI, as suggested by other recent meta-analyses.[267,268] Currently, most guidelines generally recommend CABG rather than PCI for patients with multivessel disease and a SYNTAX score of >22.[283,284] However, a major limitation of the current evidence base is the fact that all prior randomized trials compared CABG to first-generation DES. In SYNTAX, 10% of patients treated with PES had stent thrombosis by 5 years, and MACE in 8.1% of patients was attributable to stent thrombosis.[285] As previously discussed, second-generation DES have markedly improved the safety profile of DES, and CoCr-EES in particular may reduce stent thrombosis by 70% compared to PES.[98,201]

In addition, improved pharmacotherapy, coronary physiology-guided revascularization, IVUS-guided stent implantation, and improvement in techniques to treat CTO have fueled a renewed interest on the relative safety and efficacy of contemporary PCI compared to CABG in patients with multivessel coronary artery disease. In this regard, the SYNTAX II trial is a multicenter, all-comers, single arm, open label study that investigated the impact of a contemporary PCI strategy on clinical outcomes of selected patients with de novo 3-vessel coronary artery disease.[286] The strategy of PCI in the SYNTAX II study entailed patient selection based on equipoise 4-year mortality between PCI and CABG using the SYNTAX score II, use of the Synergy stent, physiology-guided revascularization, IVUS-guided stent implantation to optimize stent expansion, revascularization of CTO performed by experienced operators, and guideline-directed medical therapy. At 1-year follow-up, PCI with the SYNTAX II strategy was associated with significantly lower rates of the composite of death, MI, stroke, or any revascularization compared to a similar PCI cohort of patients selected from the original SYNTAX I trial (10.6% vs. 17.4%, $P = .006$), driven by lower rates of MI (HR 0.27, 95% CI 0.11 to 0.70, $P = .007$) and repeat revascularization (HR 0.57, 95% CI 0.37 to 0.90, $P = .015$). Rates of definite stent thrombosis were also lower in the SYNTAX II compared to the SYNTAX I PCI cohort (HR 0.26, 95% CI 0.07 to 0.97, $P = .045$). In addition, no significant difference was apparent for the 1-year rate of MACCE between the SYNTAX II PCI cohort and a comparable group of CABG-treated patients selected from SYNTAX I trial (10.6% vs. 11.2%, $P = .68$).

The only existing randomized trial that has compared a second-generation DES with CABG is the BEST trial.[287] BEST is a prospective, multicenter, open-label randomized trial conducted at 27 sites in South Korea, China, Malaysia, and Thailand comparing the relative safety and efficacy of CoCr-EES versus CABG in patients with multivessel coronary artery disease. The study was designed as a noninferiority trial of CoCr-EES versus CABG for the 2-year rates of the composite primary end point of death, MI, or TVR. Due to slow recruitment, the study was interrupted prematurely after 880 of the initially planned 1776 patients had been enrolled in the trial. At 2-year follow-up, rates of the primary end point were 7.9% with CABG versus 11.0% with CoCr-EES (P_{NI} = .32). After a median follow-up of 4.6 years, CABG was associated with significantly lower rates of the primary end point compared to CoCr-EES (10.6% vs. 15.3%, $P = .04$), with no significant difference between the two strategies of revascularization in the individual rates of death, any MI or stroke, but higher rates of TVR or spontaneous MI with CoCr-EES compared to CABG. In view of the several limitations of this trial, including the reduced statistical power due to early termination, insufficient statistical power for individual end points, rates of cross-over from CABG to PCI, and randomization of only 20% of the screened patients, further study is warranted to establish the relative safety and efficacy of newer-generation DES versus CABG in patients with multivessel coronary artery disease. Of note, recent findings have suggested that complete revascularization is a necessary requisite for PCI to achieve equipoise in mortality with CABG.[288]

Prior to the introduction of DES, there had been no randomized trials of PCI versus CABG in patients with unprotected left main disease, because observational studies had shown a high rate of procedural failure and late sudden cardiac death with balloon angioplasty,[289] and unacceptably high restenosis and MACE rates with BMS in this anatomic subgroup.[290] Erglis et al.[291] subsequently randomized 103 patients with left main disease to BMS versus PES, and demonstrated that PES resulted in significantly lower 6-month rates of binary restenosis (6% vs. 22%, $P = .02$) and MACE (13% vs. 30%, $P = .04$). Additional comparisons between stent types have been performed in the ISAR Left Main and ISAR Left Main II trials. ISAR Left Main randomized 650 patients with left main disease to PES versus SES,[292] and found comparable 1-year rates of composite death, MI, or TLR (13.6% vs. 15.8%, $P = .44$), definite stent thrombosis (0.3% vs. 0.7%, $P = .57$), and restenosis (16.0% vs. 19.4% $P = .30$) with the two stent types. In the ISAR Left Main II trial,[109] 650 patients with left main disease were randomized to either Re-ZES or CoCr-EES. At 1-year follow-up, the cumulative incidence of the primary end point, a composite of death, MI, and TLR was 17.5% in the Re-ZES group and 14.3% in the CoCr-EES group ($P = .25$). Three patients in the Re-ZES group (0.9%) and 2 patients in the CoCr-EES group (0.6%) experienced definite/probable stent thrombosis ($P = .99$). These results, in addition to the SYNTAX subgroup analyses demonstrating comparable outcomes with PCI and CABG for patients with left main disease (particularly those with lesser degrees of coexistent disease), have fueled a renewed interest in the percutaneous treatment of left main disease.

Following the promising results of three registries showing similar rates of death, MI, or stroke, but higher rates of TVR with PCI compared to CABG,[293–295] four randomized trials comparing CABG versus PCI with first-generation DES were performed in patients with left main disease (including the left main subset analysis from SYNTAX).[281,296–298] In a meta-analysis of these four trials (1611 randomized patients),[299] with data reported to 1 year, no significant differences in the risk of death or MI were apparent between the two strategies of revascularization. PCI, however, was associated with significantly higher rates of TVR (11.4% vs. 5.4%, $P < .001$) but significantly lower rates of stroke (1.7% vs. 0.1%, $P = .01$) compared to CABG. In the SYNTAX trial left main cohort ($n = 705$), with results to 5 years, there was no significant difference in the rate of the composite primary end point of death, MI, stroke, or clinically driven repeat revascularization (36.9% with PES vs. 31.0% with CABG, $P = .12$).[300] However, the results with PES were at least as good as CABG in patients with a low or intermediate SYNTAX score (≤ 32), whereas the results with CABG were superior in those with a high SYNTAX score (≥ 33).

In 2016, two landmark trials comparing DES versus CABG for the treatment of unprotected left main coronary artery disease have been reported: EXCEL and NOBLE.[301,302] EXCEL is an international, open-label, multicenter randomized trial comparing PCI with CoCr-EES versus CABG in 1905 patients with unprotected left main coronary artery disease and a site-adjudicated SYNTAX score less than or equal to 32.[302] The trial had a noninferiority design for the primary end point, which was the 3-year rates of the composite of death, MI, or stroke, with a noninferiority margin of 4.2%. Use of intravascular ultrasonographic imaging was strongly recommended and it was used in nearly 80% of patients in the PCI group. On the other hand, off-pump surgery, arterial revascularization, and transesophageal ultrasonography in the CABG group were used more frequently than in the SYNTAX trial. At 3-year follow-up, PCI was noninferior to CABG for the primary end point, which occurred in 15.4% of the PCI-treated patients and in 14.7% of the CABG-treated patients ($P_{NI} < .02$). Compared to CABG, PCI was associated with lower rates of death, MI, or stroke at 30 days (4.9% vs. 7.9%, $P = .008$), but higher event rates in the period between 31 days and the end of follow-up (11.5% vs. 7.9%, $P = .02$). In addition, symptomatic graft occlusions occurred more frequently than definite stent thrombosis after PCI (5.4% vs. 0.7%, $P < .001$). Finally, PCI was associated with higher 3-year rates of ischemia-driven revascularization (12.6% vs. 7.5%, $P < .01$).

The NOBLE trial was different from EXCEL in that it did not have restrictions of enrollment based on the SYNTAX score, it used both first- and second-generation DES, was performed in 36 centers in Northern Europe, it did not include periprocedural MI in the composite end point, and it included repeat revascularization as a component of the primary end point.[301] The study had a noninferiority design for the combined primary end point of death, stroke, nonindex treatment-related MI, and new revascularizations at 2-year follow-up with an HR = 1.36 for PCI versus CABG and 1186 patients needed to declare noninferiority. To accommodate lower than expected event rates, time to follow-up was extended up to 5 years for each patient, but then, due to changes in forecasting, a decision was made to report results after a median follow-up of 3 years based on roughly 75% of the total number of events expected to occur after the full 5-year follow-up. Between December 2008 and January 2015, 1201 patients were randomly assigned to either PCI ($n = 598$) or CABG ($n = 603$). After a median follow-up of 3.1 years, CABG was associated with significantly lower rates of the primary end point compared to PCI (19% vs. 29%, HR 1.48, 95% CI 1.11 to 1.96), exceeding the limit of noninferiority (HR 1.35), and achieving superiority ($P = .006$).

Besides differences in methodology, end point definition, and study design, EXCEL and NOBLE also demonstrated similarities in that they both reported no significant difference in mortality between the two strategies of revascularization, no significant difference in stroke rate, although in NOBLE it trended toward a higher risk with PCI, and a higher risk of spontaneous MI and repeat revascularization with PCI compared to CABG. However, none of the study had sufficient statistical power to determine differences in individual end points, and therefore several meta-analyses have been performed. In the meta-analysis by Nerlekar et al., including five randomized trials and 4594 patients, no significant difference was apparent between PCI and CABG in the individual end point of death (OR = 1.03, 95% CI 0.78 to 1.35), MI (OR = 1.46, 95% CI 0.88 to 2.45), or stroke (OR = 0.80, 95% CI 0.09 to 1.97).[303] However, PCI was associated with a higher risk of repeat revascularization (OR = 1.85, 95% CI 1.53 to 2.23). In the meta-analysis by Palmerini et al., including six randomized trials and 4686 patients, a significant interaction between the strategy of revascularization and the SYNTAX score for the risk of cardiac mortality was apparent after a median follow-up of 39 months, such that the relative risk for mortality tended to be lower with PCI compared with CABG among patients in the lower SYNTAX score tertile, similar in the intermediate tertile, and higher in the upper SYNTAX score tertile.[304] Moreover, PCI compared with CABG was associated with a similar long-term composite risk of death, MI, or stroke (HR = 1.06, 95% CI 0.82 to 1.37), with fewer events within 30 days after PCI offset by fewer events after 30 days with CABG ($P_{interaction} < .0001$).

The results of the recently reported randomized trials and meta-analyses challenge the most updated American Guidelines, which give PCI for the treatment of unprotected left main coronary artery disease a class IIa or IIb recommendation, depending on the relative risk and complexity of PCI versus CABG.[305] Current evidence suggests that PCI with newer-generation DES is an acceptable or even preferred alternative to CABG in selected patients with unprotected left main coronary artery disease. The optimal revascularization strategy should be decided after discussion with members of the heart team, taking into consideration patient characteristics and preferences. Longer follow-up of the EXCEL and NOBLE trials is eagerly awaited.[44,283,284,306–308]

Chronic Total Occlusions

Clinical and angiographic restenosis rates after both balloon angioplasty and stent implantation are increased following PCI of CTO compared to nonoccluded stenoses, due principally to an increased incidence of diabetes, greater lesion length, plaque mass, and calcification (see Chapter 26).[309,310] As such, it has been hypothesized that the benefits of DES in reducing clinical restenosis compared to BMS would be strongly evident in the treatment of CTO lesions. In a 200-patient randomized trial of SES versus BMS, the use of SES resulted in significant reductions in binary angiographic restenosis (7% vs. 36%, $P < .001$) and TLR (4% vs. 19%, $P < .001$), with reductions in clinical restenosis maintained at up to 4 years of clinical follow-up.[311] A large number of retrospective, nonrandomized and historically controlled comparisons of DES and BMS have similarly demonstrated approximately 60% reductions in clinical restenosis end points with DES compared to BMS. However, despite similar hazards of mortality and MI with DES compared to BMS in a meta-analysis aggregating this data, a trend toward increased stent thrombosis was observed with first-generation DES (RR 2.79, 95% CI 0.98 to 7.97, $P = .06$), meriting concern.[312] More recently, 207 patients with CTO lesions were randomized to either CoCr-EES or SES.[106] In-stent late loss at 9 months was 0.29 ± 0.60 mm in patients treated with SES versus 0.13 ± 0.69 mm in patients with CoCr-EES ($P_{NI} < .01$). There was also a trend toward lower 1-year rates of major adverse events (15.9% vs. 11.1%, $P = .33$), as well as lower rates of definite probable stent thrombosis (3.0% vs. 0.0%, $P = .07$) with CoCr-EES compared to SES. Similarly, observational studies have shown improved outcomes with second-generation DES compared to first-generation DES for the treatment of CTO lesions.[313]

More recently, CoCr-EES has been compared with Orsiro in 330 patients with CTO included in the multicenter, randomized PRISON IV trial (see paragraph "Novel BP-BASED DES: Orsiro and Synergy" in this chapter).[190] At 9-month follow-up, the noninferiority primary end point, in-segment late lumen loss, was not met for Orsiro versus EES. In addition, the incidence of in-stent and in-segment binary restenosis was significantly higher with Orsiro versus EES.

Although techniques and success rates for CTO have significantly improved in the last 10 years, it is uncertain whether CTO-PCI improves survival or even the quality of life compared to optimal medical therapy. In fact, most of the evidence supporting CTO-PCI has mainly relied on observational studies, which have residual treatment bias even after adjusting for possible confounders. For this reason, four randomized trials have been reported in the last two years comparing CTO-PCI versus optimal medical therapy. In the EXPLORE trial, 304 patients with STEMI referred for primary PCI who also had a concomitant CTO were randomized to either optimal medical therapy or CTO-PCI after treatment of the culprit artery.[314] The success rate of CTO was 77%. At 4-month follow-up, mean left ventricular ejection fraction, the primary end point of the study, was similar in the two treatment arms (44.1 ± 12.2% in the CTO-treated patients versus 44.8 ± 11.9% in the conservative-treated patients, P = .60). There were no significant differences in the 4-month rates of MACE (5.4% in the CTO group vs. 2.6% in the medically treated group, P = .25), although cardiac mortality trended toward higher rates in the CTO-treated group (2.7% vs. 0, P = .056). Similar results were apparent in the DECISION CTO trial, a prospective, multicenter, open-label randomized trial including 834 patients with de novo CTO located in a proximal-to-mid epicardial coronary artery with a reference diameter of greater than or equal to 2.5 mm.[315] At 3-year follow-up, optimal medical therapy was noninferior to CTO-PCI for the primary end point of the study, a composite of death, MI, stroke, or repeat revascularization (19.6% vs. 20.6%, P = .008). In addition, measures of health-related quality of life in the two groups were comparable throughout the follow-up period. However, several caveats of this study should be acknowledged. First, the study was prematurely interrupted when 834 of the initially planned 1284 patients were recruited due to slow enrollment, and therefore it is underpowered for its primary end point. Second, cross-over rates from one treatment to the other were relatively high (18.1% from medical therapy to CTO-PCI and 15.6% from CTO-PCI to medical treatment), and in the "per protocol analysis" as well as in the "as treated analysis," optimal medical therapy did not achieve noninferiority compared to CTO-PCI. Finally, the use of IVUS in treating CTO was only 6%. EURO CTO is a prospective, open-label, multicenter, randomized trial including 403 patients with stable coronary artery disease and at least one CTO in a major artery with a reference diameter greater than or equal to 2.5 mm.[316] At 1-year follow-up, the primary efficacy end point of the study, the health status of patients as assessed by the Seattle Angina Questionnaire, was significantly better with CTO-PCI compared to medical therapy. However, also this study was interrupted prematurely due to slow recruitment. In addition, the study was not powered for clinical end point, which tended to be numerically higher in the CTO-PCI group. Finally, REVASC was a multicenter trial randomizing 204 patients to either CTO-PCI or optimal medical therapy.[317] At 6-month follow-up, compared to optimal medical therapy, CTO PCI did not improve regional or global left ventricular function, the primary end point of the study. At 1-year follow-up, CTO PCI was associated with significantly lower rates of MACE (18.2% vs. 5.9%, P = .02), with similar rates of death, similar rates of MI, but lower rates of clinically driven revascularization with CTO-PCI compared to optimal medical therapy (3.0% vs. 13.5%, respectively).

The ongoing SHINE CTO trial is a multicenter, double-blind, sham-controlled trial that will randomize symptomatic patients with a CTO to CTO-PCI or a sham procedure. All patients will receive optimal medical therapy (NCT02784418). The primary end point of the study is improvement in disease-specific health status, as assessed by the 7-item Seattle Angina Questionnaire Summary Score at 1-month follow-up.

In summary, although four randomized trials comparing CTO-PCI versus medical therapy have recently been reported, these studies were all underpowered for their primary end point due to insufficient numbers of patients recruited, reported discordant results, and were hampered by high rates of cross-over. Comparing CTO-PCI versus optimal medical therapy in a well-designed randomized trial powered for meaningful clinical end point is a difficult task because recruitment of these patients is difficult. Appropriate patient selection based on careful evaluation of symptoms and ischemia burden remains of paramount importance when selecting patients for CTO-PCI.

Bifurcation Lesions

Bifurcation lesions represent 20% or more of stenoses undergoing angioplasty, and PCI of coronary bifurcation lesions is associated with increased procedural complications and worsened long-term outcomes (see Chapter 23). Due to the higher rates of clinical restenosis at bifurcation lesions, the use of DES for the main vessel of a bifurcation lesion has become standard of care for bifurcation disease. A strategy of provisional stenting of the side branch is the generally accepted current approach to bifurcation disease unless there is significant high-grade and lengthy disease within the side branch, especially in case of distal left main disease.[318,319] In unprotected distal bifurcation left main disease, a two-stent strategy may be more appropriate as suggested by the recently reported DKCRUSH-V trial, which randomized 482 patients with true distal left main bifurcation lesions to either double-kissing crush 2-stent technique or provisional stenting.[320] At 1-year follow-up, the double-kissing crush technique was associated with significantly lower rates of TLR compared to provisional stenting (5.0% vs. 10.7%, P = .02).

A variety of strategies for the treatment of bifurcation disease with drug-eluting balloons are also currently undergoing evaluation,[321,322] but current data using drug-eluting balloons in native coronary stenoses have been mixed (see Chapter 17). The strategy of implanting a DES in the main branch with the use of a drug-eluting balloon in the side branch is of interest. In the DEBSIDE study, enrolling 50 patients with bifurcations treated with DES in the main branch and the DANUBIO paclitaxel-eluting balloon (Minvasys; Gennevillers, France) in the side branch, rates of TLR were 10% in the main branch and 2% in the side branch.[323] Even better results were apparent in the BIO-LUX I trial, which reported no binary restenosis both in the main branch treated with CoCr-EES and in the side branch treated with the Pantera Lux paclitaxel-eluting balloon (Biotronik, Baar, Switzerland).[324] In contrast, rates of restenosis were 40% in the main branch and 6% in the side branch in the SARPEDON trial, which used several types of first- and second-generation DES in the main branch and the Pantera Lux paclitaxel-eluting balloon in the side branch.[325]

Several dedicated drug-eluting bifurcation stent systems have been designed and are under investigation. Bifurcation stent systems can be classified as those that facilitate access to the side branch to simply the PCI procedure, versus novel stents designed to address the unique geometric challenges of the bifurcated stenosis. Initial experiences with the Devax self-expanding nitinol stent (coated with the bioabsorbable polymer PLLA eluting the antiproliferative rapamycin analog Biolimus A9) have demonstrated low rates of restenosis of both the main vessel and side branch in both true bifurcation lesions as well as in the distal bifurcation of the left main coronary artery.[326,327] This "reverse cone" stent is designed to adapt to and cover the main parent vessel and the bifurcation carina, and is used in conjunction with dedicated DES of one or both branches when necessary. Preliminary data has also been published on the use of the Stentys paclitaxel-eluting side branch access stent[328] and the Taxus Petal dedicated bifurcation stent.[329] The BiOSS LIM (Balton; Warsaw, Poland) is a coronary, dedicated balloon-expandable bifurcation stent. The platform is made of 316L stainless steel and is coated with a biodegradable polymer that elutes sirolimus. The BiOSS LIM consists of two parts, proximal and distal, joined with two connection struts at the middle zone. BiOSS LIM was compared to a mixture of first- and second-generation DES in the randomized POLBOS II trial, in which 202 patients with stable or non-ST segment elevation acute coronary syndrome were recruited.[330] At 1-year follow-up, BiOSS LIM was associated with similar rates of the composite of cardiac death, MI, or TLR as regular DES (11.8% vs. 15.0%, respectively, $P = .08$). Finally, the results of the TRYTON trial, in which 704 patients with true bifurcation lesions were randomized to either the TRYTON bifurcation two-stent approach versus a provisional one-stent approach, have been recently presented.[331] The TRYTON BMS, made from a cobalt chromium alloy, provides scaffolding within the side branch with minimal coverage in the main vessel. After deployment of the TRYTON stent system, a conventional DES is placed in the main vessel and the procedure is completed with a final kissing balloon inflation (facilitated culotte technique). At 9-month follow-up, the primary end point of the study, a composite of cardiac death, target vessel MI, and ischemia-driven TVR, was 17.4% in the TRYTON group versus 12.8% in the provisional group ($P = .11$), which did not meet criteria for noninferiority because of a greater rate of periprocedural MI with the TRYTON. However, side branch diameter stenosis was significantly lower in the TRYTON group versus the provisional group (31.6% vs. 38.6%, respectively, $P = .002$), and outcomes tended to be improved with the Tryton in large side branches. A post hoc analysis revealed that the trial inadvertently enrolled patients with too small side branches (<2.25 mm), and that it would have reached the primary end point, had the intended population been enrolled.[332] Thus, the TRYTON Confirmatory Study, which was a prospective, single-arm extension of the TRYTON Pivotal RCT, enrolled an additional 133 patients to confirm the safety of the TRYTON stent in bifurcation with side branch diameter greater than or equal to 2.25 mm.[333] Periprocedural MI occurred in 10.5% of patients, which was numerically lower than in the provisional group of the TRYTON Pivotal RCT (11.9%), thus confirming the safety of the TRYTON stent in bifurcations with side branch diameters greater than or equal to 2.25 mm. Further clinical data are awaited in order to determine whether the use of dedicated bifurcation stents (compared to a provisional single-stent approach) offer long-term advantages for the treatment of bifurcation disease.

Saphenous Vein Grafts

PCI of saphenous vein graft (SVG) has traditionally been associated with higher early and late adverse ischemic events compared with PCI of native coronary arteries.[334] The most common cause of recurrent ischemia following CABG surgery is atheromatous degeneration within the body of a SVG, and BMS have been associated with improved outcomes compared to balloon angioplasty in SVG intervention.[335,336] While DES have the potential to further lower rates of restenosis of the target lesion within SVGs, the "tolerated late loss" within SVG lesions is typically greater than native coronary vessels (due to the large caliber of most SVGs), and disease progression at nontarget sites within SVGs is frequent (see Chapter 27). Two small randomized trials of DES versus BMS for critical SVG stenoses have been conducted in patients with SVG lesions, and demonstrated lower rates of angiographic restenosis with DES.[337,338] With extended follow-up to a median of 32 months in one of these studies, however, the antirestenotic advantage of SES compared to BMS was lost, and SES was associated with higher morality.[339] In the larger ISAR-CABG trial, 610 patients were allocated to either DES (PES, SES, or BP-SES) or BMS.[340] At 1-year follow-up, the primary end point, a composite of death, MI, or TLR, was significantly reduced with DES compared with BMS (15% vs. 22%, respectively, $P = .02$). The difference in the primary end point was driven by a significant reduction of TLR with DES compared to BMS (7% vs. 13%, $P = .01$), whereas no significant difference in the risk of death or MI was apparent between treatment groups. Two more randomized trials comparing BMS versus DES have recently been reported at the annual meeting of the European Society of Cardiology in 2016 and 2017, the BASKET SAVAGE and the DIVA trial,[341,342] which reported conflicting results. In the BASKET SAVAGE trial, randomizing 173 patients to either PES or BMS, a significant reduction in the 1-year rate of MACE (cardiac death, MI, or TVR) was apparent with PES compared to BMS (2.3% vs. 17.9%, $P < .001$).[342] In contrast, the DIVA trial, which enrolled 599 patients with SVG, reported no significant difference between a mixture of first- and second-generation DES versus BMS for the 1-year rate of the primary end point of TLF (17% vs. 19%, respectively, $P = .67$).[341] These data have been summarized in a recent meta-analysis including all these five randomized trials with a total of 1535 patients.[343] After a mean follow-up of 24.5 months, no significant difference was apparent between DES and BMS in the rates of MACE (22.7% vs. 33.5%, $P = .20$), or the individual component of all-cause death (9.5% vs. 5.6%, $P = .33$), MI (7.1% vs. 11.7%, $P = .20$), TVR (11.7% vs. 24.4%, $P = .07$), or stent thrombosis (2.5% vs. 6.1%, $P = .55$). These findings suggest that further study is needed to develop better strategies of treating SVG lesions.

Finally, a small pilot study of prophylactic "sealing" of moderate, noncritical SVG lesions with PES in order to prevent disease progression within SVGs was superior to medical therapy alone, suggesting a possible preventive role for DES in degenerating SVG lesions prior to their becoming critical.[344] A large randomized trial is required, however, before such an approach can be recommended in less severe SVG stenoses.

STENT FAILURE MECHANISMS AND MANAGEMENT

Stent Thrombosis

The most feared complication following stent placement is stent thrombosis, which in more than 40% of patients presents as a large MI and results in death within 30 days in 10% to 25% of patients.[345,346] While it was initially believed that stent thrombosis with BMS was largely confined to the first 30 days following PCI, more recent analyses confirm that stent thrombosis (even with BMS) can occur years after the initial stent implantation.[347] Treatment for stent thrombosis is almost always emergent repeat PCI, although optimal reperfusion is only achieved in two-thirds of patients.[348] Moreover, approximately 20% of patients with a first-stent thrombosis experience a recurrent stent thrombosis episode within 2 years.[349] Thus, understanding and preventing this complication is of paramount importance. Of note, the PRESTIGE registry recently reported increased platelet reactivity in patients presenting with STEMI for stent thrombosis, despite treatment with chronic DAPT with aspirin and a $P2Y_{12}$ inhibitor, suggesting maintenance antiplatelet therapy was inadequate.[350]

The most widely utilized definition and timing classification of stent thrombosis was developed by the ARC,[351] with definite or probable stent thrombosis considered by most to represent the best tradeoff between sensitivity and specificity (Table 15.14). Stent thrombosis is considered acute if it occurs within the first 24 hours, subacute if between 1 and 30 days, early if within the first 30 days, late if between 30 days and 1 year, and very late if after 1 year. Stent thrombosis is also classified as primary if it is directly related to an implanted stent, or secondary if it occurs at the stent site after an intervening TLR procedure for restenosis. The ARC definitions specifically pertain to out-of-laboratory stent thrombosis; intraprocedural stent thrombosis (IPST)—stent thrombosis occurring within the cardiac catheterization laboratory during or immediately after the index PCI procedure itself—are not captured within the ARC definitions. IPST has been strongly associated with major ischemic events,[352] and should be considered and tracked as a separate entity. In the prospective, double blind, multicenter, randomized CHAMPION PHOENIX trial comparing cangrelor to clopidogrel in patients undergoing PCI, patients with IPST had significantly higher rates of death (5.6% vs. 0.3%, $P < .0001$), MI (25.8% vs. 4.0%, $P < .0001$), ischemia-driven revascularization (4.6% vs. 0.6%, $P < .0001$), and out-of-lab ARC definite stent thrombosis (3.4% vs. 0.3%, $P < .0001$).[353]

The mechanisms underlying stent thrombosis are multifactorial, and include patient-, lesion-, procedural-, and stent-related factors. Stent thrombosis occurs more frequently in complex patients and complex lesions, especially in patients with acute coronary syndromes and thrombotic lesions (possibly due to stent implantation within or adjacent to necrotic core),[354] diabetes and renal insufficiency, and diffuse disease, small vessels, and bifurcation lesions requiring multiple stents.[345,346,355–358] A recent study has suggested an independent association between the risk of stent thrombosis and the SYNTAX score.[359] Different mechanisms are involved in the risk of early, late, and very late stent thrombosis.

Early stent thrombosis is in general related to procedural factors, such as stent underexpansion, edge dissection, and residual disease at the stent margins.[360–362] In this regard, the routine use of intravascular imaging such as IVUS may help in optimizing the procedural results, further decreasing the risk of stent thrombosis. This is consistent with the results of a large nonrandomized propensity-adjusted study suggesting lower 30-day and 1-year rates of stent thrombosis with IVUS guidance compared to angiography guidance,[363] and with the results of a substudy of the ADAPT-DES trial, a prospective, multicenter, nonrandomized "all-comers" study in 8582 consecutive patients designed to determine the frequency, timing, and correlates of stent thrombosis and adverse clinical events after DES implantation.[364] Specifically, in a propensity-adjusted analysis from ADAPT DES, IVUS guidance compared with angiographic guidance was associated with significantly lower propensity adjusted 1-year rates of definite/probable stent thrombosis (0.6% vs. 1.0%, $P = .003$), MI (2.5% vs. 3.7%; $P = .004$), and MACE (3.1% vs. 4.7%; $P = .002$).[365]

Late and very late stent thrombosis (Fig. 15.14), in contrast, have been associated with delayed arterial healing, chronic inflammation with chronic fibrin deposition, and neoatherosclerosis,[56,58] as well as late strut fractures[366] and late acquired stent malapposition (reflecting underlying vascular toxicity from the drug and/or polymer).[367,368] Although late and very late stent thrombosis also occurs with BMS,[347] for many years the ongoing and increased risk of stent thrombosis after first-generation DES has remained a concern.[68,69,82] In contrast, emerging data from randomized trials,[115] observational studies[134] and meta-analyses[201,202] suggest that second generation DES may be as safe if not safer than BMS, representing a major paradigm shift.[369] In particular, durable fluoropolymer-coated CoCr-EES may be associated with the lowest rates of stent thrombosis not only compared to other DES, but even to BMS.

Dual Antiplatelet Therapy and Stent Thrombosis

Five randomized trials have demonstrated that stent thrombosis and MACE within 30 days of BMS implantation is markedly reduced by addition of the thienopyridine ticlopidine to aspirin,[12–15,370] and in this regard clopidogrel has comparable efficacy compared to ticlopidine with an enhanced safety profile.[371] In patients with acute coronary syndromes, the rates of stent thrombosis have also been reduced with more potent thienopyridines such as prasugrel and ticagrelor.[222,223] While observational studies have uniformly documented that premature thienopyridine discontinuation (generally <3 months) after DES placement is strongly associated with stent thrombosis,[372,373] whether prolonged DAPT beyond this time will enhance freedom from stent thrombosis and/or death and MI is controversial, with some studies in support of this hypothesis[79,374] and others against.[372,375]

On this background, 18 randomized trials comparing different DAPT durations after stent placement have been reported in the last 5 years including a total of 40,419 patients (Table 15.15).[135,376–390] These studies varied in design, DAPT duration, end point definition, and sometimes have reported conflicting results. In summary, there have been three randomized trials comparing 3-month versus 1-year DAPT,[378,385,390] seven trials comparing 6-month versus

TABLE 15.14 Academic Research Consortium Definitions of Stent Thrombosis

Classification	
Definite	An acute coronary syndrome with angiographic or autopsy evidence of thrombus or occlusion within or adjacent to a stent.
Probable	Unexplained death within 30 days after stent implantation or acute myocardial infarction involving the target-vessel territory without angiographic confirmation.
Possible	Any unexplained death beyond 30 days after the procedure.
Timing	
Acute	Within 24 h (excluding events within the catheterization laboratory)
Subacute	1–30 days
Early	Within 30 days (excluding events within the catheterization laboratory)
Late	30 days to 1 year
Very late	After 1 year

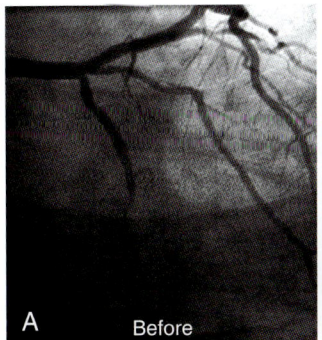
A Before

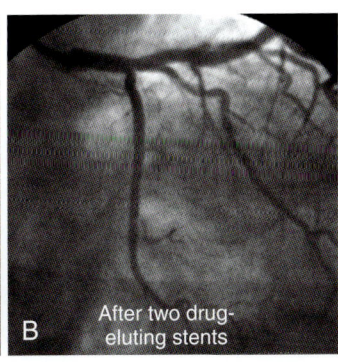
B After two drug-eluting stents

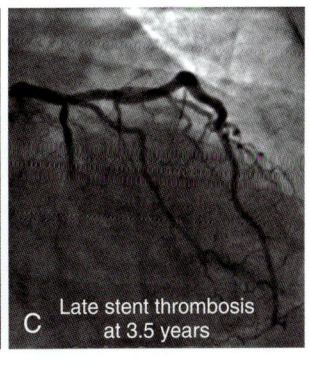
C Late stent thrombosis at 3.5 years

Fig. 15.14 A high-grade stenosis is present in the mid portion of the left circumflex artery (A). An excellent angiographic result was obtained after placement of two 15-mm long 2.5-mm diameter sirolimus-eluting stents (B). The patient was asymptomatic until 3.5 years later when he presented with acute myocardial infarction due to thrombotic occlusion within the prior implanted stents (C).

TABLE 15.15 Main Characteristics of the Randomized Trials Performed on Dual Antiplatelet Therapy Duration After Coronary Stenting

Study	N° Patients in Each Treatment Arm	Primary End Point	Design and Randomization	Follow-Up Duration After Randomization	Results of the Primary End Point
ARCTIC-Interruption[376]	12 months ($n = 624$) 18–24 months ($n = 635$)	Death/MI/ST/CVA/TVR	Superiority Randomization at DAPT discontinuation	Median of 17 months	Superiority of >12-month DAPT not demonstrated
DAPT[386]	12 months ($n = 4941$) 30 months ($n = 5020$)	Death/MI/ST/CVA/bleeding	Superiority Randomization at DAPT discontinuation	18 months	Superiority of 30-month DAPT demonstrated
DAPT STEMI[384]	6 months ($n = 433$) 12 months ($n = 437$)	Death/MI/CVA/any revascularization/TIMI major bleeding	Noninferiority Randomization at DAPT discontinuation	18 months	Noninferiority demonstrated
DES-LATE[574]	12 months ($n = 2514$) 36 months ($n = 2531$)	Cardiac death/MI/CVA	Superiority Randomization at DAPT discontinuation	24 months	Superiority of 24-month DAPT not demonstrated
EXCELLENT[108]	6 months ($n = 722$) 12 months ($n = 721$)	Cardiac death/MI/ischemia-driven TVR	Noninferiority Randomization at the time of PCI	1 year	Noninferiority demonstrated
I LOVE IT[381]	6 months ($n = 909$) 12 months ($n = 920$)	Cardiac death/target vessel MI/ischemia-driven TLR	Noninferiority Randomization at the time of PCI	1 year	Noninferiority demonstrated
IVUS XPL[457]	6 months ($n = 699$) 12 months ($n = 701$)	Cardiac death/MI/stroke/TIMI major bleeding	Noninferiority Randomization at the time of PCI	1 year	Noninferiority demonstrated
ISAR-SAFE[389]	6 months ($n = 1997$) 12 months ($n = 2003$)	Death/MI/ST/CVA/Bleeding	Noninferiority Randomization at DAPT discontinuation	9 months	Noninferiority demonstrated
ITALIC[393]	6 months ($n = 953$) 24 months ($n = 941$)	Death/MI/CVA/TVR/Bleeding	Noninferiority Randomization at the time of PCI	1 year	Noninferiority demonstrated
NIPPON[387]	6 months ($n = 1654$) 18 months ($n = 1653$)	Death/MI/stroke/Major bleeding	Noninferiority Randomization at the time of PCI	18 months	Noninferiority demonstrated
OPTIDUAL[382]	12 months ($n = 690$) 36 months ($n = 695$)	Death/MI/stroke/Major bleeding	Superiority Randomization at DAPT discontinuation	36 months	Superiority of extended DAPT over short DAPT not demonstrated
OPTIMA C[392]	6 months ($n = 684$) 6-months ($n = 684$)	Cardiac death/MI/TLR	Noninferiority Randomization at the time of PCI		Noninferiority demonstrated
OPTIMIZE[378]	3 months ($n = 1563$) 12 months ($n = 1556$)	Death/MI/CVA/Major bleeding	Noninferiority Randomization at the time of PCI	1 year	Noninferiority demonstrated
PRODIGY[526]	6 months ($n = 983$) 24 months ($n = 987$)	Death/MI/CVA	Superiority Randomization 1 month after PCI	24 months	Superiority of 24-month DAPT not demonstrated
REDUCE[390]	3 months ($n = 751$) 12 months ($n = 745$)	Death/MI/ST/CVA/TVR/Bleeding	Noninferiority Randomization at the time of PCI	12 months	Noninferiority demonstrated
RESET[524]	3 months ($n = 1059$) 12 months ($n = 1058$)	Cardiac death/MI/ST/TVR/Major bleeding	Noninferiority Randomization at the time of PCI	1 year	Noninferiority demonstrated

TABLE 15.15 Main Characteristics of the Randomized Trials Performed on Dual Antiplatelet Therapy Duration After Coronary Stenting—cont'd

Study	N° Patients in Each Treatment Arm	Primary End Point	Design and Randomization	Follow-Up Duration After Randomization	Results of the Primary End Point
SECURITY[377]	6 months ($n = 682$) 12 months ($n = 717$)	Cardiac death/MI/CVA/ST/Bleeding	Noninferiority Randomization at the time of PCI	1 year	Noninferiority demonstrated
SMART-DATE[391]	6 months ($n = 1357$) 12 months ($n = 1355$)	All-cause death, MI, or stroke	Noninferiority Randomization at the time of PCI		Noninferiority demonstrated. However, shorter DAPT was associated with higher rates of MI compared to longer DAPT.

ARCTIC, Assessment by a double Randomization of a Conventional antiplatelet strategy versus a monitoring-guided strategy for drug-eluting stent implantation and of Treatment Interruption versus Continuation 1 year after stenting trial; *CVA*, cerebrovascular accident; *DAPT*, the dual antiplatelet therapy; *DES-LATE*, Optimal Duration of Clopidogrel Therapy With DES to Reduce Late Coronary Arterial Thrombotic Event trial; *EXCELLENT*, Efficacy of Xience/Promus Versus Cypher to Reduce Late Loss After Stenting; *ISAR-SAFE*, The Intracoronary Stenting and Antithrombotic Regimen: Safety And Efficacy of 6 Months Dual Antiplatelet Therapy After Drug Eluting Stenting study; *ITALIC*, Is There A Life for DES after discontinuation of Clopidogrel trial; *MI*, myocardial infarction; *OPTIMA C*, OPTIMAl duration of Clopidogrel after implantation of second-generation drug-eluting stents; *OPTIMIZE*, Optimized Duration of Clopidogrel Therapy Following Treatment With the Zotarolimus-Eluting Stent In Real World Clinical Practice; *PCI*, percutaneous coronary intervention; *PRODIGY*, The Prolonging Dual Antiplatelet Treatment After Grading Stent-Induced Intimal Hyperplasia Study; *RESET*, REal Safety and Efficacy of a 3-month dual antiplatelet Therapy following E-ZES implantation; *SECURITY*, SEcond Generation Drug-Eluting Stent Implantation Followed by Six-Versus Twelve-Month Dual Antiplatelet Therapy trial; *SMART-DATE*, Safety of 6-Month Duration of Dual Antiplatelet ThErapy after percutaneous coronary intervention in patients with acute coronary syndromes; *ST*, stent thrombosis; *TIMI*, Thrombolysis in Myocardial Infarction; *TLR*, target-lesion revascularization; *TVR*, target-vessel revascularization.

1-year DAPT,[a] four trials comparing 6-month versus longer than 1-year DAPT,[135,384,387,393] and four trials comparing 1-year versus longer than 1-year DAPT.[376,382,386,388] In general, trials comparing less than or equal to 6-month DAPT versus greater than or equal to 1-year DAPT have not reported significant differences in the risk of ischemic events between the two treatment arms,[b] but some of them have shown increased rates of bleeding with longer compared to shorter DAPT.[135] In addition, although in the SAMART-DATE trial enrolling patients with acute coronary syndrome 6-month DAPT was noninferior to 1-year DAPT for the primary end point of all-cause death, MI, stroke, 6-month DAPT was associated with increased rates of MI compared to 1-year DAPT.[391] None of these trials, however, had sufficient statistical power for low-frequency events such as stent thrombosis, and many of them enrolled low-risk patients,[377–381,385] were prematurely interrupted for slow recruitment,[377,379,389] considered as primary end point a combination of ischemic and bleeding events,[377–379,382,385,387,389,390] and were underpowered because of lower than expected event rates.[377,378,380,385,389] In addition, the majority of these trials randomized patients at the time of PCI and not at the time of DAPT discontinuation in the short-term arm.[c]

In view of these limitations, several meta-analyses were performed.[394–397] Palmerini et al. amalgamated four trials comparing less than or equal to 6-month versus 1-year DAPT in an individual patient level meta-analysis with a total of 8180 patients.[396] At 1-year follow-up, short-term DAPT was associated with similar rates of the composite of cardiac death, MI, or definite probable stent thrombosis (HR 1.11; 95% CI 0.86 to 1.43; $P = .44$), but significantly lower rates of bleeding (HR 0.66; 95% CI 0.46 to 0.94; $P = .03$) compared to prolonged DAPT. Similar results were apparent in the landmark period between DAPT discontinuation and 1-year follow-up. A subsequent individual-patient data and network meta-analysis including six trials with 11,473 comparing 3 versus 6 versus 1-year DAPT analyzed the relation between DAPT duration and clinical presentation.[395] In acute coronary syndrome patients, less than or equal to 6-month DAPT was associated with nonsignificantly higher 1-year rates of MI or stent thrombosis compared with 1-year DAPT (HR 1.48, 95% CI 0.98 to 2.22; $P = .059$), whereas in stable patients rates of MI and stent thrombosis were similar between the two DAPT strategies (HR 0.93, 95% CI 0.65 to 1.35; $P = .71$; $P_{interaction} = 0.02$). By network meta-analysis, 3-month DAPT, but not 6-month DAPT, was associated with higher rates of MI or stent thrombosis in acute coronary syndrome patients, whereas no significant difference was apparent in stable patients. Short DAPT was associated with lower rates of major bleeding compared with 1-year DAPT, irrespective of clinical presentation.

Among the four randomized trials comparing 1-year versus longer than 1-year DAPT, discrepant results were reported.[376,382,386,388] Specifically, although no significant difference in the rate of the primary end point was apparent between the two DAPT strategies in the DES-LATE, ARCTIC-Interruption, and the OPTIDUAL trials,[376,382,388] different results were apparent in the DAPT TRIAL.[386] DAPT is the largest randomized trial to examine the issue of prolonged DAPT duration, randomizing 9961 DES patients free from MACE and bleeding events 1 year after SES, PES, EES, or ZES implantation to aspirin alone or aspirin plus a thienopyridine (either clopidogrel or prasugrel) for an additional 18 months. Among DES-treated patients, continuance of DAPT was associated with reductions in stent thrombosis (0.4% vs. 1.4%, $P < .001$), as well as MI (2.1% vs. 4.1%, $P < .001$). Of note, 45% of the benefit in reducing MI was by prevention of stent thrombosis, whereas 55% of the benefit derived from preventing MI from nontreated sites (secondary prevention). The reduction in stent thrombosis with prolonged DAPT was present with all stents, although the absolute reduction was least with CoCr-EES (0.4% absolute reduction over 18 months), and there was no reduction in MACCE with CoCr-EES. The ischemic benefits of prolonged DAPT in this trial were offset by increases in moderate/severe bleeding complications (2.5% vs. 1.6%, $P = .001$). Additionally, there was a strong trend toward increased all-cause mortality among patients randomized to extended duration DAPT (2.0% vs. 1.5%, $P = .05$), which was explained by an excess of bleeding-related, trauma-related, and cancer-related deaths among patients randomized to extended duration of DAPT. Finally, the reduction in MACCE with prolonged DAPT was greater for patients presenting with MI (3.9% vs. 6.8%; $P < .001$) compared with those with no MI (4.4% vs. 5.3%; $P = .08$; interaction $P = .03$).[398]

---
[a]References 377,380,381,383,389,390,392
[b]References 135,377,379–381,383–385,387,389,390
[c]References 377,378,380,381,385,387,390

To investigate more in depth the association between prolonged DAPT and mortality, several meta-analyses have been performed.[394,397,399] In a meta-analysis including 10 trials and 31,666 patients, shorter DAPT was associated with significantly lower all-cause mortality compared with longer DAPT (HR 0.82, 95% CI 0.69 to 0.98; $P = .02$), with no significant heterogeneity apparent across trials.[397] The reduced mortality with shorter compared with longer DAPT was attributable to lower noncardiac mortality (HR 0.67, 0.51 to 0.89; $P = .006$), with similar cardiac mortality (HR 0.93, 0.73 to 1.17; $P = .52$). Shorter DAPT was also associated with a lower risk of major bleeding, but a higher risk of MI and stent thrombosis. In a subsequent larger meta-analysis including 12 randomized trials and 34,880 patients with an individual patient data substudy of six trials and 11,473 patients, a significant association between prolonged DAPT and bleeding-related death was reported.[400]

Taken together, these trials show that although prolonged DAPT is not absolutely mandatory beyond 3 to 6 months, there may be some benefit to continuing DAPT for several years in preventing late stent thrombosis and MI (arising both from the stent site and elsewhere), especially in patients with acute coronary syndromes, although such therapy should be utilized only in patients in whom the benefits of reducing long-term atherothrombotic complications would be expected to outweigh the increased risks of bleeding.[401] In this regard, several risk scores have been developed to assist clinical decision making on the optimal DAPT duration after DES implantation in individual patients.[402–404] Details of these scores are reported in Table 15.16.

The DAPT score was created as a clinical decision tool to identify patients expected to derive benefit versus harm from continuing thienopyridine beyond 1 year after PCI.[404] The score was derived from the DAPT trial and then validated via internal bootstrap, and by using the data of the Patient Related OuTcomes with Endeavor versus Cypher stenting Trial (PROTECT) trial.[165] The score assigns positive integers to variables associated with ischemic risk and negative integers to variables associated with bleeding risk. In patients with DAPT score greater than or equal to 2, the balance between ischemic versus bleeding events tips towards prolonged DAPT, whereas in patients with DAPT score <2, shorter DAPT is more appropriate. This score, however, has several limitations: it has a limited discrimination power, it does not include several important variables associated with bleeding, such as baseline anemia, previous bleeding, thrombocytopenia, anticoagulant therapy, it includes PES as a risk factor for ischemic events, which is not used any longer, and it is not applicable to patients using ticagrelor or prasugrel.

The PARIS score was developed using data from 4190 patients treated with DES and enrolled in the PARIS registry.[402] Separate risk scores were developed to predict ischemic events (stent thrombosis or MI) and type 3 or 5 bleeding according to the Bleeding Academic Research Consortium definition. External validation was performed using the ADAPT-DES dataset.[364] Using the probability-based estimates from each model, absolute risk differences between ischemic versus bleeding events were calculated for individual patients to define each individual global risk profile. Although no recommendation is provided on how to integrate these two scores in clinical practice, the PARIS double score represents an initial attempt for global risk stratification to determine the optimal DAPT duration after DES placement.

Finally, PREdicting bleeding Complications In patients undergoing Stent implantation and subsEquent DAPT (PRECISE DAPT) is a five-item score which was developed to predict the risk of bleeding events from a pooled dataset of individual patient data from eight randomized trials including a total of 14,963 patients.[403] The score showed a good discrimination power in the derivation cohort (c index = 0.73), and in the validation cohort (c index = 0.70), which included patients enrolled in the PLATO trial.[405] Prolonged DAPT (≥1 year) significantly increased the risk of bleeding in patients with PRECISE DAPT score greater than or equal to 25, but not in those with score <25 ($P_{interaction} = 0.007$), who also received a significant clinical benefit in terms of prevention of ischemic events from prolonged DAPT.

Although risk scores may be useful tools in clinical practice, they have several limitations because they do not factor all variables associated with the outcome of interest, they somewhat imply dichotomy in risk stratification (high vs. low risk) and therapy recommendation (short vs. long DAPT), and hold a constant risk of events through follow-up. Thus, the use of these scores should always be guided by a more comprehensive appraisal of the patient's clinical profile, choosing different DAPT durations (3 vs. 6 vs. 12 vs. longer than 1 year) depending on patient clinical characteristics and the nuances of balancing ischemic versus bleeding risk in individual patients. Other trials currently ongoing comparing different DAPT duration are summarized in Table 15.17.

Restenosis

By increasing acute luminal gain[36,37] and eliminating late recoil and negative vessel remodeling,[406] BMS reduce the rates of restenosis

TABLE 15.16 Risk Scores for Determining Dual Antiplatelet Therapy Duration

Risk Score	Variables	Points
DAPT	Age	
	≥75	−2
	65–<75	−1
	<65	0
	Cigarette smoking	+1
	Diabetes mellitus	+1
	MI at presentation	+1
	Prior PCI or prior MI	+1
	Paclitaxel-eluting stent	+1
	Stent diameter <3 mm	+1
	CHF or LVEF <30%	+2
	Vein graft stent	+2
PRECISE—DAPT	Hemoglobin	
	White blood cell count	
	Age	
	Creatine clearance	
	Prior bleeding	
PARIS	Age	
	<50	0
	50–59	+1
	60–69	+2
	70–79	+3
	80	+4
	BMI, kg/m²	
	<25	+2
	25–34.9	0
	35	+2
	Current smoking	
	Yes	+2
	No	0
	Anemia	
	Present	+3
	Absent	0
	Creatine clearance <60 mL/min	
	Present	+2
	Absent	0
	Triple therapy on discharge	
	Yes	+2
	No	0

BMI, Body mass index; *CHF,* chronic heart failure; *DAPT,* dual antiplatelet therapy; *LVEF,* left ventricular ejection fraction; *MI,* myocardial infarction; *PARIS,* Patterns of Non-Adherence to Anti-Platelet Regimen in Stented Patients; *PCI,* percutaneous coronary intervention; *PRECISE-DAPT,* PREdicting bleeding Complications In patients undergoing Stent implantation and subsEquent Dual Anti Platelet Therapy.

TABLE 15.17 Ongoing Randomized Controlled Trials Comparing Different Duration of Dual Antiplatelet Therapy After Drug-Eluting Stent Implantation

Study	Number of Patients	DAPT Duration	Type of Stent	Primary End Point	Duration of Follow-Up
EDUCATE	2500	12 vs. 30 months	ZES	Cardiac death, MI, stent thrombosis, or bleeding	36 months
MASTER DAPT	4300	1 vs. 12 months	Ultimaster	All-cause death, MI, stroke, or bleeding defined as BARC 3 or 5	12 months
ISAR DAPT	906	3 vs. 6 months	Coroflex ISAR stent	Cardia death, MI, target-lesion revascularization	12 months
GLOBAL LEADERS	16,000	1-month ASA+ ticagrelor followed by ticagrelor monotherapy up to 24 months vs. 12-month ASA + clopidogrel (stable patients) or ticagrelor (ACS) followed by 12-month ASA	BP-BES	All-cause death or MI	24 months
TWILIGHT	9000	3-month ASA + ticagrelor followed by ticagrelor monotherapy up to 12 months vs. 12-month ASA + ticagrelor	Any DES	Superiority of ticagrelor monotherapy for bleeding defined as BARC type 2, 3, or 5, and noninferiority for ischemic events.	12 months

ACS, Acute coronary syndrome; *ASA*, aspirin; *BARC*, Bleeding Academic Research Consortium; *BES*, biolimus-eluting stent; *BP*, bioabsorabable polymer; *DAPT*, dual antiplatelet therapy; *DES*, drug-eluting stent; *MI*, myocardial infarction; *ZES*, zotarolimus-eluting stent.

compared to balloon angioplasty.[5,6] However, stents induce more arterial injury than balloon angioplasty, which results in a greater absolute amount of neointimal hyperplasia developing over the first 6 to 12 months after the procedure,[407] thereby resulting in binary angiographic restenosis in 10% to more than 50% of lesions (depending on patient and lesion complexity). While restenosis most commonly presents with stable angina and exercise induced ischemia within 1 year of stent implantation, it has become increasingly recognized that restenosis presents as an acute coronary syndrome in as many as 25% of patients, occasionally even with STEMI.[407,408] In the SYNTAX trial, patients who underwent repeat revascularization had significantly higher rates of MACE compared to those not undergoing repeat revascularization.[409] After adjustment for possible confounders, repeat revascularization remained an independent predictor of MACE after both initial PCI and initial CABG.

The prognostic implications of restenosis and repeat revascularization have recently been the objective of a large pooled analysis including 21 PCI trials with 32,524 patients treated with either BMS or DES.[410] After a median follow-up of 37 months, nonemergent, uncomplicated TLR was an independent predictor of mortality (HR 1.23, 95% CI 1.04 to 1.45, $P = .02$). In a restricted dataset including 12 trials and 19,732 patients that reported data on any repeat revascularization, TLR was again an independent predictor of mortality (HR 1.33, 95% CI 1.08 to 1.64, $P = .006$), while non-TLR (including non-TLR TVR and non-TVR) was not significantly associated with mortality. These data suggest that efforts aiming at reducing restenosis may translate in improved survival as well.

Numerous studies have demonstrated that the most reproducible determinants of restenosis after BMS implantation are the presence of diabetes mellitus (especially if insulin is required), small RVD, and long lesion length.[251,252,411–414] Other factors associated with restenosis are treatment of ostial and/or calcified lesions, true bifurcation lesions requiring main vessel and side branch stents, CTOs, and SVGs.[415] The same factors are associated with higher rates of DES restenosis. However, angiographic and clinical restenosis (as well as death, MI, and stent thrombosis) after DES occurs less frequently in FDA-approved "on-label" lesions (generally noncomplex lesions for which safety and efficacy has been established in large-scale randomized trials) than in less-well studied and more complex "off-label" lesions,[416,417] although in nearly all cases DES have been shown to reduce TLR compared to BMS,[41,418,419] including SVG lesions, with a recent randomized trial showing lower rates of restenosis with DES compared to BMS in this subset of lesions.[340]

The timing of early angiographic restenosis after BMS peaks within approximately 6 months; thereafter, continued organization of the extracellular matrix results in slight luminal enlargement, and serial angiographic and IVUS studies have rarely shown late restenosis.[420–422] However, during 10-year follow-up after BMS, the minimal luminal diameter continues to slowly decrease,[422] and late neoatherosclerosis with plaque rupture can present as restenosis years after BMS implantation.[423] A monotonically increasing amount of angiographic late loss has also been described for several years after SES and EES, although perhaps somewhat less with PES.[424–428] These observations imply the existence of low-grade chronic vascular inflammation from either the polymer or lack of healing. In the largest randomized trial examining this issue (SIRTAX), 1012 patients were randomized to PES versus SES and followed for 5 years, with angiographic follow-up performed systematically at 8 months and 5 years.[429] Incremental late loss between these two time periods occurred with both stents, although more so with SES than PES. At 1 year, the rate of TLR was less with SES than PES; this benefit was somewhat mitigated at 5 years. The degree to which routine angiographic follow-up triggered late TLR procedures and therefore confounded the clinical results is unknown.[430] As a result of this ongoing late loss, BMS, PES, and SES demonstrate an incrementally increasing rate of stent-site specific TLF events during long-term follow-up.[69,424,429,431–433] The same observations have been made with the best second-generation DES, such as CoCr-EES.[126,434]

The causes of restenosis after stents are multifactorial. In addition to excessive late neointimal hyperplasia, restenosis after BMS and DES has been associated with stent under-expansion,[435–437] edge dissections and residual untreated disease,[438,439] geographic miss,[440] and strut fractures.[441–443] Some[444] but not all[445,446] studies

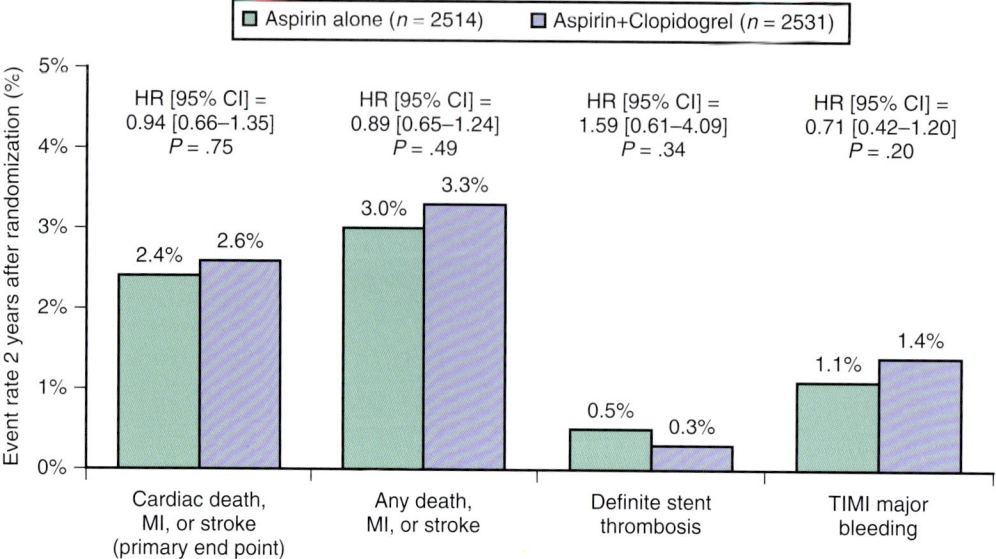

Fig. 15.15 Outcomes in the drug-eluting stent (DES)-LATE randomized trial 2 years after randomizing 5045 patients free from adverse cardiovascular events at least 1 year after DES implantation to aspirin alone vs. aspirin plus clopidogrel. *CI*, Confidence interval; *HR*, hazard ratio; *MI*, Myocardial infarction; *TIMI*, Thrombolysis In Myocardial Infarction.

have found an association between nickel allergy and restenosis after BMS or DES. Genetic mutations in the genes encoding mTOR or polymorphisms in the genes encoding proteins involved in paclitaxel metabolism may result in resistance to SES and PES, respectively.[447,448] Other genetic polymorphisms have also been associated with restenosis.[449,450] Excessive inflammation from first-generation DES polymers (specifically eosinophilic reactions to PES and granulomatous reactions to SES) may provoke late restenosis.[55,451] And of course, the antiproliferative effects of DES depend on both the drug (with rapamycin-analogs being inherently more potent than paclitaxel) and the release kinetics (with extended release of rapamycin-analogs beyond 1 month being necessary for maximal efficacy). The role of neoatherosclerosis as a cause of restenosis has been previously discussed.[336,365,423,452] As discussed above, newer-generation stents have been shown to have enhanced efficacy and safety. In addition, by facilitating the operator's ability to achieve larger lumen areas, IVUS may reduce restenosis and improve clinical outcomes after BMS and DES.[453–455] No single randomized trial, however, has been adequately powered to demonstrate a reduction in TLR with IVUS after DES implantation, although the Angiography Versus IVUS Optimization (AVIO) trial demonstrated that the postprocedural minimal luminal diameter was significantly greater in DES with IVUS guidance.[456] Two randomized trials in complex lesion subsets (long lesions and in CTO) have demonstrated the superiority of an IVUS-guided approach to PCI with DES compared with an angiography-guided approach.[118,457] More recently, a randomized trial comparing OCT-guided versus IVUS-guided versus angiography-guided PCI in 450 patients undergoing DES implantation was reported.[458] Post-PCI minimum stent area, the primary end point of the study, was 5.79 mm² with OCT guidance, 5.89 mm² with IVUS guidance, and 5.49 mm² with angiography guidance. OCT guidance was noninferior to IVUS guidance, but also not superior. In addition, OCT guidance was also not superior to angiography guidance. These data warrant large-scale randomized trials to establish whether an OCT- or IVUS-guided strategy translate in better clinical outcomes compared to an angiography-guided strategy.

Patients who develop in-stent restenosis are at high risk for recurrence after percutaneous treatment, especially if the pattern of restenosis is diffuse.[459,460] IVUS imaging is highly useful in patients with restenosis to differentiate neointimal hyperplasia from stent underexpansion, geographic miss, strut fracture, and other rare occurrences such as chronic recoil and stent embolization which require directed approaches to successfully manage.[461] Radiofrequency-IVUS, OCT, and near infrared spectroscopy can identify neoatherosclerosis as a cause of restenosis (or stent thrombosis), either with or without plaque rupture.[462–464]

Treatment of Restenosis

Isolated restenosis at the stent edge can often be effectively treated with balloon angioplasty only or with an additional short stent. Treatment options for diffuse BMS restenosis due to neointimal hyperplasia have been extensively studied. In the BMS era, neither cutting balloons, directional or rotational atherectomy, or repeat BMS proved better than balloon angioplasty for diffuse in-stent restenosis.[465] Vascular brachytherapy with either locally applied beta or gamma radiation was effective in reducing recurrent restenosis within 1 year,[466,467] but was logistically complex, and the resultant vascular toxicity with prolonged inflammation and obliteration of normal cell lines resulted in high rates of late stent thrombosis (especially when new BMS were implanted) and restenosis.[468,469] Subsequently, two multicenter randomized trials demonstrated that SES and PES significantly reduce angiographic restenosis and improve event-free survival at 9 months compared to either beta or gamma vascular brachytherapy in patients with BMS restenosis (Fig. 15.15, left).[470,471] With follow-up to 2 to 3 years, event-free survival was reduced with PES and noninferior with SES compared to brachytherapy in these two trials (Fig. 15.15, right).[472,473] Thus, the use of brachytherapy fell short to treatment with DES for in-stent restenosis, and logistically issues have limited its use to a few centers in the United States. The only current indication to vascular brachytherapy is recurrent DES restenosis. Negi et al. have recently reported clinical outcomes of 186 patients with recurrent DES restenosis treated with brachytherapy using the Beta Cath system (Best Vascular Inch, Springfield, Virginia).[474] Results were acceptable with TLR rates of 3.3% at 6 months, 12.1% at 1 year, 19.1% at 2 years, and 20.7% at 3 years. There were no episodes of subacute stent thrombosis and one episode of late stent thrombosis during 3-year follow-up.

In the ISAR-DESIRE trial, 300 patients with BMS restenosis were randomized to balloon angioplasty alone versus SES versus PES.[475] Angiographic follow-up at 6 months showed recurrent restenosis after balloon angioplasty in 44.6% of patients, versus 14.3% for SES ($P < .001$) and 21.7% for PES ($P = .001$), with TVR rates of 33%, 8%, and 19%, respectively ($P < .001$ and $P = .02$ compared to balloon angioplasty, respectively). Based on the results of these trials, DES have supplanted brachytherapy and other approaches for treatment of nearly all cases of BMS restenosis due to intimal hyperplasia, except possibly isolated edge stenoses.

Implanting a second stent, even a DES, to treat BMS restenosis is not inherently desirable because of the obligate reduction in luminal diameter with layered devices. As a result, drug-eluting balloons have been investigated as a treatment for BMS ISR (see Chapter 17). Three small randomized trials with angiographic end points suggested the Paccocath paclitaxel-eluting balloon was more effective than balloon angioplasty alone and at least as effective as PES for the treatment of BMS restenosis.[476–478] In the RIBS V trial, 189 patients with BMS restenosis were randomized to CoCr-EES versus the Sequent Please paclitaxel-eluting balloon. The mean in-segment diameter stenosis at 9 months was less with CoCr-EES than drug-eluting balloon (DEB) (13% ± 17% vs. 25% ± 20%, $P < .001$), and restenosis tended to be reduced with EES, although there was no difference in the 1-year rate of MACE, which was low in both arms.[479] At 3 years, rates of cardiac death (2% vs.1%), MI (4% vs. 5%), and TVR (9% vs. 5%) were similar between DEB and CoCr-EES.[480] However, rates of TLR were significantly lower with CoCr-EES compared with DEB (2% vs. 8%; $P = .04$). Rates of late TVR were low and similar in the two groups (3.2% in both groups). Given the superior angiographic results in this trial which was under-powered for MACE, most cases of BMS restenosis should be treated with a potent second-generation DES, unless the RVD is very small, in which case a DEB may be a preferable first choice.

Compared to BMS restenosis, DES restenosis tends to be focal, and is diffuse in less than one-quarter of patients. However, recurrence rates after treatment of DES restenosis are higher than after treatment of BMS restenosis.[481,482] If the DES (re)stenosis is isolated to the margin of the stent, or is focal within the stent, either balloon angioplasty or implantation of a short DES of the same type is often selected. Management of diffuse DES restenosis has been less well studied. In the CRISTAL trial, 197 patients with diffuse restenosis (mean length ~14 mm) of either a SES or PES were randomized to treatment with SES versus balloon angioplasty.[483] Follow-up at 12 months demonstrated a significantly larger minimal lumen diameter (MLD) with SES compared to balloon angioplasty only (2.14 ± 0.62 mm vs. 1.71 ± 0.55 mm, $P < .0001$), with a trend toward less TLR (5.9% vs. 13.1%, $P = .10$). Many operators consider diffuse in-stent restenosis after DES (if IVUS demonstrates adequate stent expansion) to represent "drug failure" and will treat with a different class of agent (e.g., PES after SES failure). Consistent with this hypothesis are the data of the RIBS III trial, a nonrandomized, multicenter registry including 363 patients with DES restenosis who were treated with either a different DES (switch strategy) or a conventional strategy including balloon angioplasty, BMS, or the same DES.[484] After a median follow-up of 2 years, the switch strategy was associated with significantly lower restenosis rates compared to the conventional strategy. Interestingly, the use of second-generation DES compared to first-generation DES as well as IVUS guidance compared to angiography guidance resulted in better long-term outcomes. These findings were not, however, confirmed in the ISAR-DESIRE-2 trial, in which 450 patients with SES restenosis were randomized to SES versus PES.[485] At 6- to 8-month follow-up, there were no differences between SES and PES in late loss (0.40 ± 0.65 mm vs. 0.38 ± 0.59 mm; $P = .85$), binary restenosis (19.6% vs. 20.6%; $P = .69$), or TLR (16.6% vs. 14.6%; $P = .52$).

DES restenosis has also been treated with DEB. In a small study including 50 patients with DES restenosis, DEB were superior to plain balloon angioplasty for angiographic and clinical outcomes.[486] The efficacy of DEB for the treatment of DES restenosis has been subsequently confirmed in a multicenter randomized trial including 110 patients.[487] More recently, the ISAR DESIRE III trial randomized 402 patients with DES restenosis 1:1:1 to PES, Sequent Please paclitaxel-eluting balloons, or plain balloon angioplasty.[488] At 8-month follow-up, paclitaxel-eluting balloons were superior to BMS, and noninferior to PES for the primary end point of diameter stenosis (38.0% with paclitaxel-eluting balloons vs. 54.1% with plain balloon angioplasty vs. 37.4% with PES, $P_{Sup} < .0001$ and $P_{NI} = .007$). Finally, in the RIBS IV study, 309 patients with DES restenosis were randomized to Sequent Please paclitaxel-eluting balloons or CoCr-EES.[489] At 9-month angiographic follow-up, the in-segment diameter stenosis was significantly lower with EES ($P = .009$), and a strong trend was present for less binary restenosis with EES (11% vs. 19%, $P = .06$). At 1 year, the rates of TLR (4% vs. 13%, $P = .008$) and MACE (cardiac death, MI, or TVR; 10% vs. 18%, $P = .04$) were significantly lower with EES, establishing a potent second-generation DES as the treatment of choice for most patients with restenosis of previously implanted DES. However, a pooled analysis of RIBS IV and RIBS V including 249 randomized patients treated with CoCr-EES suggested less satisfactory results in patients with DES ISR than in patients with BMS ISR.[490]

Finally, a network meta-analysis comparing and ranking different percutaneous strategies for the treatment of in-stent restenosis has recently been reported.[491] The meta-analysis included 27 randomized clinical trials with 5923 patients with follow-up ranging from 6 to 60 months. PCI with CoCr-EES was the most effective treatment for the primary angiographic end point of percent diameter stenosis 6 to 12 months after the intervention, with an absolute mean difference of −9.0% compared to DEB, −9.4% versus SES, −10.2 versus PES, −19.2% versus vascular brachytherapy, −23.4% versus BMS, −24.2% versus plain balloon angioplasty, and −31.8% versus rotablator. DEB ranked as the second-most effective treatment, but without significant difference versus SES or PES. CoCr-EES was also associated with the lowest risk of further TLR during follow-up. Significant inconsistencies were apparent across trials for death and for MI, with imprecise estimates of risk. Thus, current evidence suggests that the two most effective strategies to treat in-stent restenosis are CoCr-EES, which is associated with the best angiographic and clinical outcomes, and DEB, which provides favorable results without adding further layers of metal.

CONCLUSIONS AND FUTURE DIRECTIONS

The development and evolution of the coronary stent has resulted in remarkable progress in the lesser invasive treatment of coronary artery disease. The evolution from BMS to first-generation DES further reduced restenosis at the cost of an increased rate of very late stent thrombosis and MI, and a dependence on longer-term DAPT. Best-in-class second-generation DES have eliminated these very late risks, resulting in devices more effective and possibly even safer than BMS, although the optimal duration of DAPT after all stents is still debated. Novel DES are under active development to enhance the rate and completeness of endothelialization to further reduce reliance on DAPT and enhance long-term safety,[492] as are polymer-free systems. Initial experience with these devices has been promising and large-scale randomized trials are warranted to investigate their relative safety and efficacy in comparison to permanent polymer and bioabsorbable polymer-based DES. Dual-agent DES may also confer improved safety and/or efficacy. Fully bioabsorbable vascular scaffolds[493,494] may represent the greatest opportunity for further major improvement in outcomes, offering the potential to reduce or eliminate the problems which may arise from a permanent metallic cage and durable polymers, including neoatherosclerosis, late strut fractures, compliance mismatch, altered vascular physiology, and the inability of the vessel to remodel to accommodate plaque progression (see Chapter 16). However, concern has been raised over the increased propensity for stent thrombosis of ABSORB compared to CoCr-EES. In addition, data regarding other fully bioabsorbable vascular scaffolds are scant and large-scale randomized trials are needed before these devices can be used in a broad population. In the future, stents will continue to improve in deliverability and ease of use, and further advances in adjunctive drugs and devices will enable PCI for the most complex patients and coronary anatomies.

KEY REFERENCES

201. Palmerini T, Biondi-Zoccai G, Della Riva D, et al. Stent thrombosis with drug-eluting and bare-metal stents: evidence from a comprehensive network meta-analysis. *Lancet*. 2012;379:1393–1402.
212. Urban P, Meredith IT, Abizaid A, et al. Polymer-free drug-coated coronary stents in patients at high bleeding risk. *N Engl J Med*. 2015;373:2038–2047.
222. Cannon CP, Harrington RA, James S, et al. Comparison of ticagrelor with clopidogrel in patients with a planned invasive strategy for acute coronary syndromes (PLATO): a randomised double-blind study. *Lancet*. 2010;375:283–293.
223. Montalescot G, Wiviott SD, Braunwald E, et al. Prasugrel compared with clopidogrel in patients undergoing percutaneous coronary intervention for ST-elevation myocardial infarction (TRITON-TIMI 38): double-blind, randomised controlled trial. *Lancet*. 2009;373:723–731.
272. Farooq V, van Klaveren D, Steyerberg EW, et al. Anatomical and clinical characteristics to guide decision making between coronary artery bypass surgery and percutaneous coronary intervention for individual patients: development and validation of SYNTAX score II. *Lancet*. 2013;381:639–650.
279. Serruys PW, Morice MC, Kappetein AP, et al. Percutaneous coronary intervention versus coronary-artery bypass grafting for severe coronary artery disease. *N Engl J Med*. 2009;360:961–972.
302. Stone GW, Sabik JF, Serruys PW, et al. Everolimus-eluting stents or bypass surgery for left main coronary artery disease. *N Engl J Med*. 2016;375:2223–2235.
364. Stone GW, Witzenbichler B, Weisz G, et al. Platelet reactivity and clinical outcomes after coronary artery implantation of drug-eluting stents (ADAPT-DES): a prospective multicentre registry study. *Lancet*. 2013;382:614–623.
369. Palmerini T, Biondi-Zoccai G, Della Riva D, et al. Stent thrombosis with drug-eluting stents: is the paradigm shifting? *J Am Coll Cardiol*. 2013;62:1915–1921.
386. Mauri L, Kereiakes DJ, Yeh RW, et al. Twelve or 30 months of dual antiplatelet therapy after drug-eluting stents. *N Engl J Med*. 2014;371(23):2155–2166.
395. Palmerini T, Della Riva D, Benedetto U, et al. Three, six, or twelve months of dual antiplatelet therapy after des implantation in patients with or without acute coronary syndromes: an individual patient data pairwise and network meta-analysis of six randomized trials and 11 473 patients. *Eur Heart J*. 2017;38:1034–1043.
452. Otsuka F, Vorpahl M, Nakano M, et al. Pathology of second-generation everolimus-eluting stents versus first-generation sirolimus- and paclitaxel-eluting stents in humans. *Circulation*. 2014;129:211–223.

Additional references available online at expertconsult.com.

中文导读

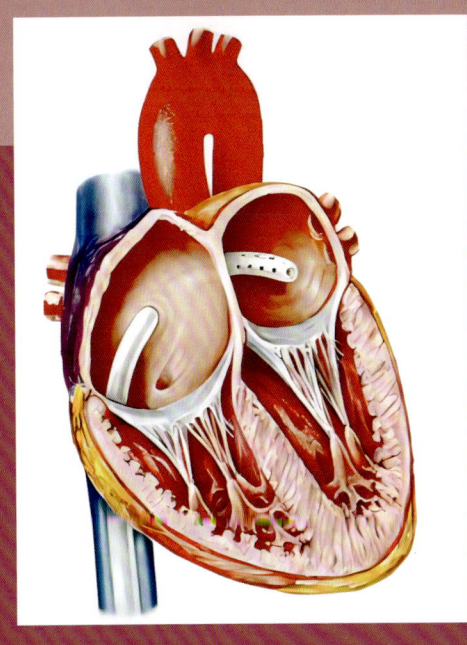

第16章
生物可吸收冠状动脉支架

　　临床上初次使用球囊血管成形术后，经皮冠状动脉重建术的发展主要以3个器械为标志，按照时间顺序分别是裸金属支架、药物洗脱支架、生物可吸收支架。支架设计旨在克服球囊血管成形术的一些主要缺陷，尤其是急性血管闭塞和弹性回缩。

　　生物可吸收支架理念最初的提出始于20世纪80年代末，即"支架在起作用（为血管提供短暂的物理支持并抑制早期收缩性重塑）后完全消失"。但是，最初的临床前研究结果差强人意。之后的研究发现，可降解的高分子聚合物或可侵蚀的金属材料可以满足生物可吸收支架理念的需要，已成为生物可吸收支架最为常用的材料。与新一代药物洗脱支架相比，生物可吸收支架提供了许多理论上的优势。这些优势是在生物降解的基础上所获得的：①可恢复血管生理学特性和功能，包括血管搏动性、血管舒缩和血管机械-化学转导（血管将血流动力学的机械力转换为化学刺激或信号通路），并保持血管进行外向重塑的能力；②可恢复血管解剖结构，减少血管角度和曲率的变化；③血管局部没有永久性异物存在，这可减少以往金属支架异物对血管内皮细胞的慢性刺激，避免血流紊乱及血栓形成；④扩大了冠状动脉支架的适应证，除了治疗具有功能学意义的狭窄病变，生物可吸收支架还可用于包括易损斑块的稳定钝化治疗及儿童等特殊人群。尽管已有临床试验并未得出令人鼓舞的结果，但生物可吸收支架的未来前景仍然值得我们期待。

　　本章节系统地介绍了生物可吸收支架的原理、材料的选择，以及各种生物可吸收支架的临床试验成果，这有助于我们对这个新兴领域进行更全面的认识。

赵宇昊　柳景华

章节要点

- 生物可吸收支架可提供临时的血管支架，然后被降解吸收，这可能将克服新一代药物洗脱支架尚未解决的缺陷。
- 生物可吸收支架由可降解的聚合物或可侵蚀的合金所组成。当代生物可吸收支架最常用的材料是聚左旋乳酸，其次是镁。
- 截至2017年5月，有5种生物可吸收支架已获得欧洲CE认证标志，包括Absorb、DESolve、ART Pure、Fantom和Magmaris，其中只有Absorb获得美国FDA和日本PMDA批准。
- Absorb支架是目前唯一一种在随机临床试验中与新一代药物洗脱支架进行对比，并至少完成中期随访的生物可吸收支架产品。然而，随着这些试验数据的积累，结果却显示这种生物可吸收支架可异常增加血栓风险，因此生产厂家最终停止了Absorb的商业化生产。
- 目前，许多其他的生物可吸收支架产品正处于与新一代药物洗脱支架对照临床试验阶段，同时在全球范围内也正在进行更深入地研究和开发，以推进这项技术，并且有望达到生物可吸收支架预期目标。

16 Bioresorbable Coronary Scaffolds

Athanasios Katsikis, Rodrigo Modolo, Yuki Katagiri, Yoshinobu Onuma, Patrick W. Serruys

KEY POINTS

- Bioresorbable scaffolds (BRS) have the potential to overcome the remaining limitations of new generation drug eluting stents (DES) by providing temporary vessel scaffolding and then disappearing.
- They are composed of either polymer or corrodible metal-based alloys and the most frequently used material in the current generation of BRS is poly(L-lactic) acid (PLLA) followed by magnesium.
- As of May 2017, five BRS—Absorb, DESolve, ART Pure, Fantom, and Magmaris—have acquired the Conformité Européenne (CE) mark, while Absorb has also been approved by the Food and Drug Administration (FDA) and the Pharmaceuticals and Medical Devices Agency (PMDA) in Japan.
- Absorb is presently the only BRS that has been tested against a new generation DES in randomized trials with at least mid-term follow-up. However, with the accumulation of data from these trials, a paradoxically increased thrombotic risk of this scaffold emerged and the manufacturing company eventually stopped its commercial production.
- Numerous other BRS are currently in the phase of clinical trials against a new generation DES while intensive research and developments are ongoing globally to advance this technology and hopefully meet its expectations.

INTRODUCTION

The evolution of percutaneous coronary revascularization, after its introduction in clinical practice with balloon angioplasty,[1] has been characterized by three device-based landmarks; chronologically, these are the bare metal stents (BMS), the drug-eluting stents (DES), and the bioresorbable scaffolds (BRS). BMS were designed to overcome some of the major drawbacks of balloon angioplasty, most importantly acute vessel closure and recoil. Two landmark trials, the comparison of balloon-expandable-stent implantation with balloon angioplasty in patients with coronary artery disease (BENESTENT) trial[2] and STent REStenosis Study (STRESS),[3] demonstrated the superiority of BMS over balloon angioplasty and introduced BMS as the new standard of practice in percutaneous revascularization in the early 1990s. BMS, however, were still plagued by significant rates of in-stent restenosis.[2,3] To address this problem, DES were developed by coating BMS with polymers containing antiproliferative drugs. First-generation DES significantly reduced in-stent restenosis and target lesion revascularization (TLR) compared with BMS,[4] but there were remaining concerns of late or very late stent thrombosis (ST).[5,6] To overcome this limitation, DES were further developed with more biocompatible or biodegradable polymers, thinner struts, and new antiproliferative drugs. These developments led to the current generation DES that are associated with both excellent efficacy and improved safety profile.[7–9] New-generation DES represent the latest revolution in percutaneous coronary intervention and are considered the best currently available technology in the field, but room for improvement still exists. This room is associated with the permanent implant that is left in the coronary arteries and has been the driving force for the development of BRS. The concept of a device that "does the job (i.e., provides short-term vessel support and inhibits early constrictive remodeling) and disappears" is very appealing and due to their intriguing features, BRS have the potential to become not only another revolution, but literally the "holy grail" of percutaneous coronary revascularization.[10] The currently available evidence does not yet support this optimistic view; however, intensive research and developments are ongoing globally to advance this technology and hopefully meet its expectations.

TERMINOLOGY: STENTS, SCAFFOLDS, BIODEGRADATION, BIOABSORPTION AND BIORESORPTION

The word "*Stent*," now used in many medical disciplines, derives from the name of an English dentist born in 1807, Charles Thomas Stent. Jacques Puel and Ulrich Sigwart are to be credited for introducing and popularizing this term in percutaneous coronary intervention, substituting previously used terms such as intravascular prostheses or grafts. In their landmark 1987 work,[11] the researchers described the first use of intracoronary stents in humans, which at that time were called "Wallstents" after its inventor, Hans Wallstén. *Scaffold* is a newer term that implies temporary arterial support and was introduced in the interventional cardiology field to distinguish these devices from permanent stents. It has been widely used in peer-reviewed medical literature over the last years and has become the preferred term to designate this bioresorbable device. The scientific community also recommends that the term bioresorbable instead of bioabsorbable or biodegradable is used in conjunction with the word scaffold.[12] *Bioabsorption* refers to the disappearance of the compound into another substance but does not necessarily equate to degradation and, even less, to elimination of the polymer from the body. Indeed, even if a "bioabsorbable" polymeric device is no longer visible as a result of degradation ("bioabsorption"), high molecular mass molecules can still be trapped between skin and mucosa without passing physiological barriers. *Bioresorption* indicates the total elimination of polymers from the body via natural routes (like kidney or lungs) by dissolution, assimilation, and excretion.[12] The words "*degradation*" and "*bio-degradation*" are also confusing and should be restricted to cases of unknown or abiotic mechanisms ("degradation") or cell-mediated in vivo mechanisms ("biodegradation").

TABLE 16.1 Mechanical and Physical Properties of Bioresorbable Scaffolds and Metallic Stents Materials

Material	Strength	Elasticity	Phase Behavior		Deformation	Degradation
	Tensile Strength (MPa)	Young's or Tensile Modulus (GPa)	T_g (°C)	T_m (°C)	Elongation at Break (%)	Degradation Rate (Months)
PLA	65	2–4	60	180–190	2–6	18–30
PLLA	60–70	2.7–4	60–65	175–180	2–6	>24
PDLLA	45–55	1.9–3.7	55–60	Amorphous	2–6	12–16
PCL	23	0.34–0.36	−54	55–60	>4000	24–36
PGA	90–110	6.0–7.0	35–40	225–230	1–2	6–12
PC	55–75	2–2.4	≈147	225	80–150	>14
Mg alloy (WE43)	220–330	40–50	NA	540–640	2–20	3–12
Stainless steel 316L	668	193	NA	1371–1399	40+	Biostable
Cobalt chromium	1449	210–235	NA	≈1454	≈40	Biostable

NA, Not applicable; *PC*, Tyrosine-derived polycarbonates; *PCL*, Polycaprolactone; *PDLLA*, poly(D,L-lactic acid); *PGA*, Poly(glycolic acid); *PLA*, pure poly(lactic acid); *PLLA*, poly(L-lactic) acid.
Adapted from Ang HY, Bulluck H, Wong P, et al. Bioresorbable stents: Current and upcoming bioresorbable technologies. *Int J Cardiol*. 2017;228:931–939.)

RATIONALE AND PROMISES OF BIORESORBABLE SCAFFOLD

BRS provide a number of theoretical advantages over new-generation DES. These advantages become established after biodegradation is completed, liberating the vessel from its "cage," and can be grossly classified as follows: **(1) Restoration of vessel physiology and functionality,** including vessel pulsatility, vasomotion, and vascular mechano-transduction (conversion of hemodynamic forces to chemical stimuli or signaling pathways) and preservation of the vessel's ability to undergo positive, outward remodeling. **(2) Restoration of vessel anatomy**, producing less alteration in angulation and curvature.[13] In addition to limiting vascular straightening, any area/diameter mismatch causing step-up or step-down regions is also expected to subside following scaffold degradation. **(3) Absence of a permanent foreign-body implant** which serves as a nidus for chronic irritation, flow disturbances, and thrombosis, especially when full endothelial coverage is not achieved and/or sustained endothelial dysfunction or late acquired strut malapposition is observed. At the vessel level, a disappearing stent could also result in avoidance of side branch "jailing" and "overhanging" in bifurcation and/or ostial lesions, as well as overcoming the inability to graft the stented segments. The latter is particularly pertinent to complex, multi-vessel coronary artery disease, where the use of multiple long stents and the need for repeat revascularization are common. Furthermore, the use of noninvasive imaging modalities like computed tomography (CT) and magnetic resonance imaging (MRI) for stent assessment could be facilitated by eliminating the metal-related blooming artefact. **(4) Expansion of indications for coronary stenting** beyond the treatment of a functionally significant stenosis, to include passivation of vulnerable plaques regardless of their hemodynamic significance and treatment of special populations, like pediatric patients.[14] Finally, since the duration of biodegradation is modifiable, a tuned elution of multiple drugs from the different components of the scaffold could become feasible, targeting multiple mechanisms of restenosis.

HISTORIC DEVELOPMENT

The efforts to create BRS started 30 years ago[15] and during the '90s, research groups from the Thorax Centre, Mayo clinic, Cleveland clinic, and the Kyoto University performed a number of experimental studies attempting to elucidate the properties of various different polymers. The first preclinical studies performed were disappointing,[16] but ongoing research indicated that polymer molecular weight was a major determinant of the observed vascular responses,[17] and subsequent studies with high-molecular-weight poly(L-lactic) acid (PLLA) showed more promising results.[17,18] However, although the idea of a BRS had been present since the early days of stent development, the technology failed to develop at that stage for the lack of an ideal polymer and the advent of metallic DES,[12] and matured long after DES had become the golden standard in percutaneous revascularization. In 2000, the Igaki-Tamai PLLA-based scaffold became the first BRS to be implanted in humans and aliphatic polyesters have dominated the field as scaffold materials ever since, despite the compromises that had to be made in various mechanical performance properties. The first investigations of magnesium alloy-based scaffolds for cardiovascular interventions started in 2003 and the first clinical trial of magnesium-based BRS for intracoronary use was published in 2007.[19]

MATERIALS AND PROPERTIES

New-generation DES are typically made of stainless steel, cobalt-chromium, or platinum-chromium. The current BRS, on the other hand, are composed of either polymer or corrodible metal-based alloys. The physical properties of the different materials used for stent and scaffold manufacturing are compared in Table 16.1. The most frequently used material in the current generation of BRS is PLLA, followed by magnesium.

Polymers

The term "polymer" originates from the Greek words «πολύ» (many or much = poly) and «μέρος» (part = mer) and refers to a macro-molecule that is composed of multiple repeated sub-units. Polymers have specific characteristics that define their mechanical properties which in turn define their suitability to be used as materials for scaffold development. Copolymerization of polymers with different properties has been widely employed in BRS fabrication to overcome the individual weaknesses of each polymer. The key polymer characteristics, beyond their type, include molecular weight, crystallinity, and hydrophobicity, while the key mechanical properties are tensile strength, elasticity, phase behavior, and biodegradation rate. The weight-averaged molecular weight of the polymer affects its processability whereas the number-averaged molecular weight influences its mechanical strength and elasticity.[20,21] *Crystallinity* is determined by the degree of monomers' linear arrangement and affects both tensile strength and degradation rate; in general, higher crystallinity results in longer degradation time and higher tensile strength.[22] *Hydrophobicity*, from the Greek word «ύδωρ» = hydro (water) and «φόβος» = phobia, is the property of repelling water rather than absorbing it or dissolving in it and is also a regulating factor of the degradation rate. *Tensile strength* quantifies the amount of stress that a material can endure before suffering permanent deformation. Good radial strength allows for thinner struts and lower profile, hence better deliverability. *Elasticity*, from the Greek word «ἐλαστός» = ductible, is defined as the ability of a body to resist a distorting/deforming influence or force and return to its original size and shape when the latter is removed. For polymers, their elastic properties are quantified by the Young's or tensile modulus of elasticity which is highly dependent on temperature. In the case of PLLA, increasing crystallinity is expected to increase its strength but at the expense of reducing its elasticity,[23] limiting the amount of expansion that a polymer scaffold can endure during deployment without fracturing. The *phase behavior* of polymers is defined by their glass transition temperature (T_g) (= the temperature that the polymer starts to display rubbery behavior) and melting point temperature (T_m).

Poly(Aliphatic-Esters)

Pure poly(lactic acid) *(PLA)* has unfavorable mechanical properties for BRS production but exists as two stereo-isomers that result in four distinct polymers, namely PLLA, poly(D-lactic acid) or PDLA, poly(D,L-lactic acid) or PDLLA, and meso-PLA. The first three have favorable characteristics for BRS fabrication. *PLLA* is a semi-crystalline material that consists of highly ordered segments with high concentrations of polymer, termed crystal lamellae, bound together by less dense, amorphous polymer tie chains. It has high tensile strength, although still inferior to the durable metals used in conventional stent fabrication, while the additional methyl group makes it more hydrophobic, leading to slower absorption rates than non-PLA-related polymers.[24] Furthermore, it is less inflammatory and has the highest T_g among the general biodegradable polymers, well above the body temperature of 37°C, so that the scaffold is dimensionally stable in its deployed size under physiological conditions. For these reasons, PLLA is the most commonly used polymer for BRS fabrication. The degradation of PLLA takes place in three steps. First, hydrolysis of the amorphous regions, which are less packed and therefore more accessible to water, occurs. The molecular weight decreases, with little effect on mechanical performance and a slight reduction in crystallinity. In the second phase, continuous cleavage of the amorphous tie chains occurs, which causes a decrease in mechanical strength (due to scission of the amorphous tie chains) and polymer fragmentation into low-weight oligomeric poly-lactic acid molecules. This results in further mass loss and visible structural discontinuities. Finally, the oligomers hydrolyze to lactic acid monomers which de-protonate to lactate. Lactate is then converted to pyruvate and enters the Krebs cycle, where it is further metabolized in CO_2 and H_2O excreted through the lungs and kidneys, respectively.[12] Remaining particles smaller than 2 μm are phagocytosed by macrophages.[25] In practice, since the degradation rate depends on a number of more or less interrelated factors, there is not one PLLA but a number of polymers having the same basic chemical structure but different behaviors depending on the synthesis route. *PDLA* is a crystalline material with similar physico-chemical and hydrolytic properties to PLLA, although somewhat lower tensile strength and stiffness. However, the derived polymer has not been exploited so far, primarily because the D-lactic acid precursor is less accessible than the L-isomer. *PDLLA* is an amorphous polymer, due to the random distribution of the two isomeric forms of PLA that it contains, it and has a lower tensile strength and a shorter degradation rate than PLLA. *Poly(glycolic acid) (PGA)* is the simplest linear aliphatic polyester and one of the first biodegradable polymers ever investigated for medical use. It has the highest tensile strength among the polymers used for BRS fabrication, but it also has a rapid degradation rate and an increased inflammatory trend. *Polycaprolactone (PCL)* is a semi-crystalline polymer with very high elongation at break but very low in vivo degradation rate. The structural changes during the bioresorption process of three characteristic BRS based on aliphatic polyesters are shown in Fig. 16.1.

Non-Poly(Aliphatic-Esters)

Tyrosine-derived polycarbonates (PC) are a class of polymers that contain amino acid-like backbones connected by carbonate bonds, resulting in strong mechanical properties with preservation of the biocompatibility of their degradation products. Their resorption pathway is similar to PLLA (see Fig. 16.1). **Polyanhydrides** have the unique property that the degradation of the anhydride bond is dependent on backbone polymer chemistry, thus allowing for precise tuning of payload release, but have poor mechanical properties.

Corrodible Metals

Magnesium Alloys

In its pure form, magnesium has low strength and rapid biodegradation. Therefore, in BRS it is used in alloy forms with a variety of other elements to adjust the mechanical and physical properties of magnesium-based implants. A wide range of methods have been described for this purpose. Precipitation-hardened magnesium alloys have a high strength-to-weight ratio,[26] enhanced biocompatibility, and low thrombogenicity. However, magnesium-based scaffolds have overall physical properties intermediate between classical metallic stents and polymeric scaffolds and suffer from very low radiopacity and elasticity. This leads to difficulty in forming mesh-like tubular scaffolds and susceptibility to strut fractures when over-expanded, which is further aggravated by the susceptibility to localized corrosion. Magnesium bioresorption occurs via corrosion, which means the degradation of metals by chemical surface reactions with aggressive components of the environment. The degradation process takes place in two steps (see Fig. 16.1). The first step is the anodic reaction of the magnesium alloy in water, resulting in magnesium hydroxide. The second, is the conversion of magnesium hydroxide to magnesium phosphate and subsequent replacement by amorphous calcium phosphate. Magnesium is removed by diffusion from the amorphous matrix and is absorbed by the body. The by-product in the vessel is hydroxyapatite, which is eventually digested by macrophages.

Iron Alloys

Iron has good mechanical properties and radiopacity, which make it another attractive candidate material for BRS fabrication. However, it has a very slow degradation rate and in addition, interference with MRI imaging and special production and storage conditions make its use problematic. The process of iron bioresorption involves oxidation of ferrous ion to ferric ion or interaction with nearby cells. A variety of methods have been described to accelerate the resorption process[27] and adjust the mechanical strength of iron-based BRS alloys. The IBS (Lifetech Scientific, China) ultrathin (53 μm) sirolimus-eluting scaffold, composed of nitrided iron with PDLLA coating, is the most mature sample in this category, though still at preclinical level of testing.[28]

CURRENT LANDSCAPE OF CLINICALLY TESTED BIORESORBABLE SCAFFOLD

Numerous manufacturing companies have developed scaffolds that, after favorable outcomes in preclinical testing, have transitioned to clinical studies (Table 16.2). The front-runner in

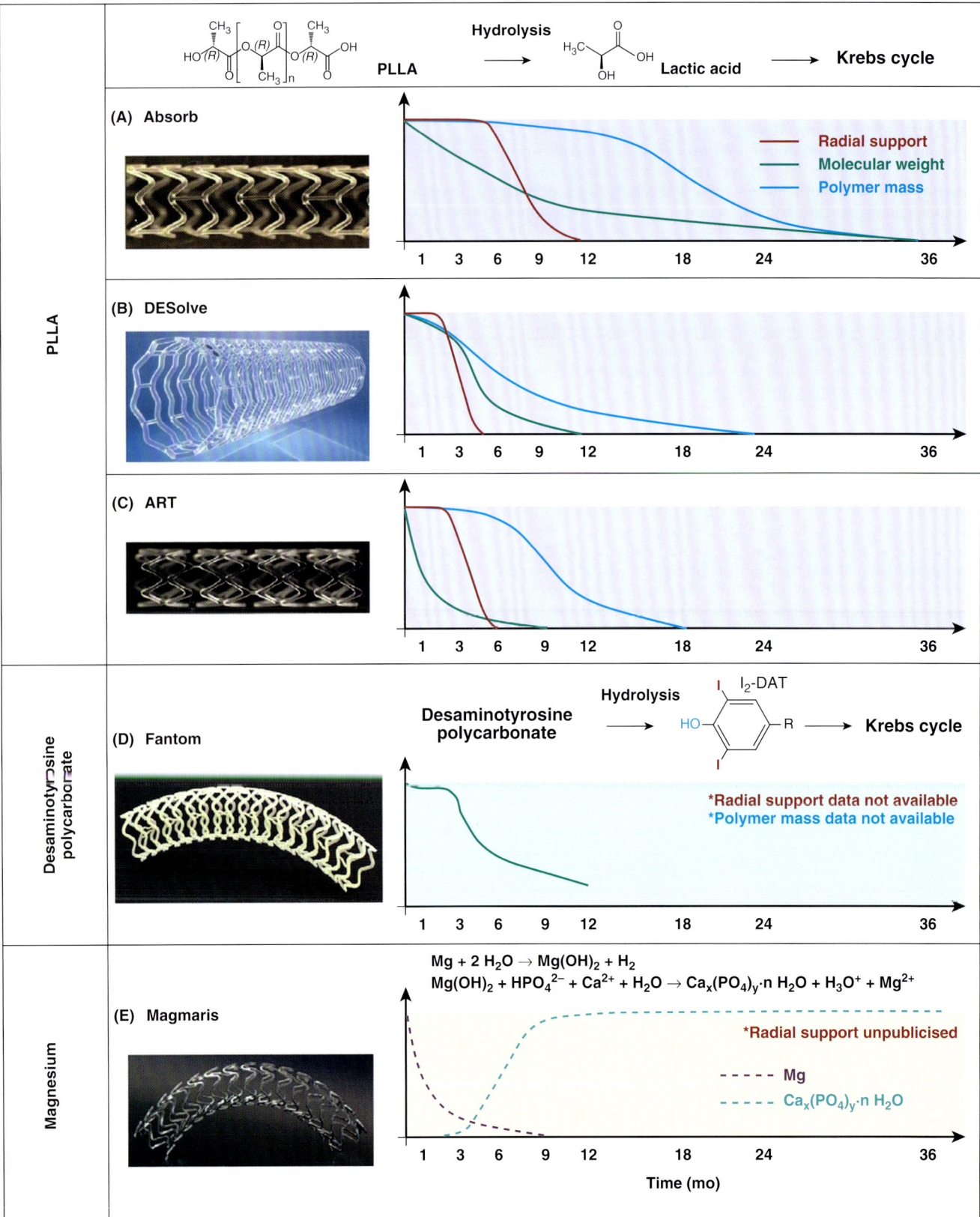

Fig. 16.1 Biodegradation process of CE-mark approved bioresorbable stent. (Reprinted from Katagiri Y, Stone GW, Onuma Y, et al. State of the art: the inception, advent and future of fully bioresorbable scaffolds. *EuroIntervention*. 2017;13[6]:734–750; with permission from Europa Digital and Publishing)

CHAPTER 16 Bioresorbable Coronary Scaffolds

TABLE 16.2 Summary Characteristics of Bioresorbable Scaffold With Published Clinical Data That Have Either CE Mark or Ongoing Follow-Up in a Human Trial

Scaffold	Manufacturer	Strut Material	Coating Material	Eluted Drug	Strut Thickness (µm)	Crossing Profile	Radiopacity	Resorption Time (Months)	Drug Dose and Release Kinetics	Current Status
Igaki-Tamai	Igaki Medical Planning	PLLA	None	None	170	NA	Gold markers	24-36	NA	First generation, first human implantation CE mark only for peripheral use
BVS 1.1 (Absorb GT1)	Abbott Vascular	PLLA	PDLLA (2-4 µm)	Everolimus	156	1.4 mm	Platinum markers	24-36	75% of drug eluted within 30 days Drug dose: 100 µg/cm²	First generation, sales discontinued CE mark, FDA approval
DESolve (first generation)	Elixir	PLLA	BD polymer and drug matrix (<3 µm)	Novolimus	150	1.5 mm	Metallic markers	12-24	>85% of drug eluted within 30 days Drug dose: 5 µg/mm	First generation CE mark
DESolve Cx (second generation)					120	1.3 mm				Second generation CE mark
Fantom	Reva Medical	Iodinated, desamino-tyrosine polycarbonate	Same as backbone (NA)	Sirolimus	125	1.3 mm	Intrinsic radiopacity	36	80% of drug eluted within 90 days Drug dose: 115 µg (for 3.0 × 18 mm scaffold)	Second generation CE mark
ART Pure	ART	PDLLA	None	None	170	6-Fr compatible	None	24	NA	First generation CE mark but development terminated
Fortitude	Amaranth Medical	Ultra-high-molecular-weight PLLA	PDLLA (NA)	Sirolimus	150ᵃ	6-Fr compatible	None	10	Drug release profile: N/A Drug density: 96 µg/cm²	First generation
Aptitude					115ᵃ		None	>24		Second generation CE mark approval submitted
Magnitude					<100ᵃ		None	NA		Second generation FIM trial results awaited in 2018
MeRes	Meril Life Sciences	PLLA	PDLLA (3-4 µm)	Sirolimus	100	1.2 mmᵇ	Platinum markers	up to 24	100% of drug eluted within 90 days Drug dose: 1.25 µg/mm²	Second generation
Mirage	Manli Cardiology	PLLA	PLLA (NA)	Sirolimus	125 (≤3 mm) 150 (≥3.5 mm)	1.12–1.47 mm	Metallic markers	14	NA	Second generation Further development on-going
Firesorb	Shanghai MicroPort Medical	PLLA	PDLLA (<5 µm)	Sirolimus	100–125	NA	Metallic markers	36	Drug dose: 4 µg/mm	Second generation
Xinsorb	Shandong Huaan Biotechnology	PLA, PCL, PGA	PDLLA & PLLA (NA)	Sirolimus	160	NA	Platinum markers	24-36	80% of drug eluted within 28 days Drug dose: 140 µg/mm²	First generation
DREAMS-2 (Magmaris)	Biotronik	93% Mg, 7% rare earth elements	PLLA (1 µm)	Sirolimus	150	1.7 mm	Tantalum markers	9-12	100% of drug eluted in 3-6 months Drug dose: 1.4 µg/mm²	Second generation CE mark
NeoVas	Lepu	PLLA	PDLA (NA)	Sirolimus	170	NA	Platinum markers	24	Drug dose: 15.3 µg/mm	First generation 1 year RCT data vs. Xience reported

ᵃAll scaffold sizes.
ᵇAverage profile for 3 mm.

BD, Biodegradable; FIM, first-in-man; NA, not available; PCL, polycaprolactone; PDLA, poly(D,L-lactic acid); PGA, polyglycolic acid; PLLA, poly(L-lactic) acid; RCT, randomized controlled trials.

this process is the Absorb scaffold, which is presently the only BRS that has been tested against a new-generation DES in randomized trials with at least mid-term follow-up and has an estimated number of devices implanted at the order of >200,000.[29] However, following the negative results of the clinical trials (discussed later), the manufacturer decided on a worldwide halt to sales of the Absorb scaffold as of September 14, 2017.

Igaki-Tamai

Igaki-Tamai (Igaki Medical Planning Company, Kyoto, Japan), a PLLA-based BRS with no antiproliferative drug elution, was the first device of its kind to be evaluated in humans. This system was self-expanding but required a second balloon inflation with contrast heated at 70°C to 80°C. The first-in-man (FIM) trial of this scaffold ($n = 15$) was reported in 2000 and showed angiographic restenosis rates of 10.5% and major adverse cardiac event (MACE) rates of 6.7% at 6 months.[30] The long-term-follow-up results ($n = 50$) were fully reported in 2012 and demonstrated TLR rates of 28% with one cardiac death (CD), four myocardial infarctions (MI), and two definite scaffold thromboses (ScT) at 10 years.[31] Despite this good safety profile and the potential for further improvement with the addition of an antiproliferative drug, the device fell out of favor for use in coronary arteries because of concerns about the intracoronary use of heated contrast and is now only of historic value. However, it has achieved and retains Conformité Européenne (CE) mark for peripheral use.

ABSORB

The ABSORB BRS has a PLLA-based backbone with a PDLLA coating. The latter contains everolimus with a coating-to-drug ratio of 1:1 and controls its release in a purely diffusion-related fashion.[25] There have been two iterations of this device. The first generation, 1.0, was tested in the FIM ABSORB A trial ($n = 30$), demonstrating very late lumen enlargement (from 6 months to 2 years) and restoration of vasomotion and endothelial function at 2 years,[32,33] with a MACE rate of 3.4% and no ScT at 5 years.[34] At 6-month follow-up, the angiographic in-stent late lumen loss (LLL) was 0.44 mm, attributed mainly to a mild reduction of the stent area (–11.8%) as measured by intravascular ultrasound (IVUS) (chronic recoil). The neointimal area was small (0.30 mm^2), with a minimal area obstruction of 5.5%, demonstrating effective suppression of restenosis by everolimus.[35] In the second-generation device, 1.1, the design of the hoops and the manufacturing process of the polymer were modified to achieve a more uniform and increased radial support, preservation of mechanical integrity for a longer period,[36] better stent security, and the convenience of storage at room temperature. Absorb 1.1 was tested in the FIM ABSORB cohort B trial, enrolling 101 patients who were split in two parts, undergoing multimodality invasive imaging at different follow-up periods, ranging from 6 months to 5 years after the index procedure. In the entire cohort B, the rates of MACE and ischemia driven (ID) TLR were 11% and 8%, respectively, at 5 years, while no cases of ScT were observed.[37] After the encouraging results of ABSORB B, a number of large registries were initiated[38–40] to evaluate results in real world patients, but most importantly, a series of randomized controlled trials (RCTs) comparing the Absorb BRS versus a CoCr-based, everolimus-eluting stent (Xience, Abbot Vascular) were conducted, with ongoing follow-up. Currently, 2-year interim analysis results are available for all these trials and for most, even longer follow-up results have been presented. The planned follow-up extends to 5 years for all ABSORB RCTs, except for ABSORB Japan (4 years) and the Comparison of the Everolimus Eluting Bioresorbable Vascular Scaffold System With a Drug-Eluting Metal Stent in Acute ST-Elevation Myocardial Infarction (ABSORB-STEMI TROFI II)(3 years). In general, these trials included relatively simple lesions. Intravascular imaging guidance was used only in 23.9% of the BRS-treated patients[41] with no collection of the manner in which it was applied to guide device implantation.[42] The latest available results of these trials are presented in Table 16.3. In ABSORB China, enrolling 480 patients (1:1) with a primary end point of angiographic in-segment LLL at 12 months, Absorb BRS was noninferior to Xience with regard to the primary end point,[43] while at 3 years there were no statistically significant differences between the two devices with respect to all clinical end points.[44] In ABSORB Japan, enrolling 400 patients (2:1) with a primary end point of target lesion failure (TLF) at 12 months (a composite of CD, target-vessel MI [TV-MI], and ID-TLR), Absorb BRS was demonstrated to be noninferior to Xience,[45] while TLF rates were not significantly different between the two devices at both 2 and 3 years of follow-up.[46,47] ABSORB II enrolled 501 patients in a 2:1 fashion and the primary end point was superiority of the Absorb BRS versus the Xience DES in angiographic vasomotor reactivity at 3 years with a coprimary end point being the noninferiority of angiographic LLL. The trial, which is the longest randomized comparison to date, did not meet its coprimary end points. More troubling, however, was the fact that although the study was not powered for clinical end points, the Absorb BRS demonstrated significantly higher rates of the secondary TLF end point at 3 years (10% vs. 5%, $P = .04$), driven by increased rates of TV-MI (6% vs. 1%; $P = .01$),[48] despite similar rates of this end point at shorter follow-ups: 1[49] and 2[50] years. Patient-oriented composite end point and definite ScT rates were not statistically different between the two devices, but rates of definite or probable ScT were higher for Absorb (3% vs 0%, $P = .03$).[48] Interestingly, the recently published 4 years' data in 428 patients documented nonsignificantly different rates of TLF (11.5% vs. 6.0%, $P = .06$), while no new events of ScT were observed in the landmark analysis from 3 to 4 years.[51]

ABSORB III is the largest RCT reported today and the pivotal trial of U.S. premarket approval of the Absorb BRS. It enrolled 2008 patients randomized in a 2:1 fashion and its primary end point was TLF (CD, TV-MI or ID-TLR) at 1 year. Although Absorb was noninferior to Xience in both intention-to-treat and as-treated analyses with regard to the primary end point[52] at 2 years, TLF rates were significantly higher for Absorb BRS (11.0% vs. 7.9%, $P = .03$) and this result was driven by the higher rates of TV-MI (7.3% vs. 4.9%, $P = .04$).[53] At 3 years, TV-MI rates remained significantly higher for Absorb BRS and additionally, the numeric higher tendency in device thrombosis against Absorb observed at 2 years (1.9% vs. 0.8%) became a statistically significant difference (2.3% vs. 0.7%; $P = 0.01$). However, TLF rates were nonsignificantly higher both through 3 years (13.4% vs. 10.4%, $P = .06$) and between 1 and 3 years (7.0% vs. 6.0%, $P = .39$).[54] Patients with thrombotic events in both treatment periods were taking dual antiplatelet therapy (DAPT) at the time of the events, the majority of which occurred in appropriately sized vessels. However, in BRS-assigned patients, treatment of vessels with a diameter less than 2.25 mm was an independent predictor of 3-year TLF and ScT, driven by the relationship at 1 year. The Amsterdam Investigator-initiateD Absorb Strategy All-comers (AIDA) trial enrolled 1845 patients in a 1:1 fashion and was designed to evaluate the noninferiority of Absorb versus Xience at 2 years with regard to TLF (a composite of CD, TV-MI or TLR). The data and safety monitoring board of the trial recommended early reporting of the study results, due to safety concerns, after a median follow-up of 707 days. By then, no significant differences in the rates of the primary end point were observed (11.7% vs. 10.7%, $P = .43$) and this was also the case for CD and TLR. However, a higher incidence of TV-MI (5.5% vs. 3.2%, $P = .04$) was observed, driven by increased rates of definite or probable ScT for the Absorb BRS (3.5% vs. 0.9%, $P < .001$). Furthermore, no major predictors of ScT were found.[55] The Comparison of Everolimus- and Biolimus-Eluting Coronary Stents with Everolimus-Eluting Bioresorbable Vascular Scaffold (EVER-BIO II) trial had the most liberal inclusion criteria in the ABSORB RCTs family. In this single-center study, a total of 240 patients were randomized in a 1:1:1 fashion to Absorb BRS, everolimus-eluting persistent polymer DES (EES), and biolimus-eluting bioabsorbable

TABLE 16.3 Summary Characteristics and Latest Available Results of the ABSORB Randomized Controlled Trial Series

Trial	N	Inclusion Criteria	Key Exclusion Criteria	Primary End Point	% Pre-Dilatation	% Post-Dilatation	%B2/C Lesions	In Segment LLL (mm) (BRS vs. DES)	TLF, CD, MI, ID-TLR (BRS vs. DES)	Device Thrombosis (BRS vs. DES)
ABSORB China[43,44]	480	Evidence of myocardial ischemia De novo coronary lesions (n ≤2) RVD: ≥2.5 and ≤3.75 mm Lesion length ≤24 mm	Acute or recent (≤7 days) MI Left main or ostial stenosis Bifurcation lesion with SB-D >2.0 mm Previous PCI in the target vessel ≤1 year	12-Month angiographic in-segment LLL	99/98	63/54	75/72	At 1 year: 0.19 ± 0.38 vs. 0.13 ± 0.38 (P noninferiority = 0.01)	At 3 years: TLF: 5.5% vs. 4.7% (P = .68) CD: 0.4% vs. 1.3% (P = .37) TV-MI: 2.5% vs. 0.9% (P = .28) D-TLR: 4.2% vs. 2.6% (P = 0.31)	At 3 years (definite/probable): 0.9% vs. 0% (P = .5)
ABSORB II[48,51]	501	Evidence of myocardial ischemia De novo coronary lesions (n ≤ 2)	Acute or recent (≤ 7 days) MI Left main or ostial stenosis Bifurcation lesion with SB-D >2.0 mm Re-stenotic lesions	1. 36-Month Vasomotion 2. Δ MLD	100/99	61/59	46/49	At 3 years: (0.37 [0-45] vs. 0.25 [0-25]; P noninferiority = 0.78)	At 4 years: TLF: 11.5% vs. 6% (P = .06) TV-MI: 4.6% vs. 1.3% (P = .07)[a] CD: 1.3% vs. 2.7% (P = .28) CI-TLR: 3.9% vs. 2% (P = .4)[a]	At 4 years (definite/probable):3% vs. 0% (P = .03)
ABSORB III[54]	2008	Evidence of myocardial ischemia De novo coronary lesions (n ≤2) RVD: ≥2.5 and ≤3.75 mm Lesion length ≤24 mm	Acute or recent (≤7 days) MI Left main or ostial stenosis Bifurcation lesion with SB-D >2.0 mm Previous PCI in the target vessel ≤1 year	12-Month TLF	100/100	65/51	69/72	Not applicable No angiographic follow-up	At 3 years: TLF 13.4% vs. 10.4% (P = .06) TV-MI: 8.6% vs. 5.9% (P = .71) ID-TLR: 7.2% vs. 5.9% (P = .27)	At 3 years (definite/probable): 2.3% vs. 0.7% (P = .01)
ABSORB Japan[47]	400	Evidence of myocardial ischemia De novo coronary lesions (n ≤2) RVD: ≥2.5 and ≤3.75 mm Lesion length ≤24 mm	Acute or recent (≤72 hours) MI Left main or ostial stenosis Bifurcation lesion with SB-D >2.0 mm Previous PCI in the target vessel ≤1 year	12-Month TLF	100/100	82/77	76/76	At 3 years: 0.29 ± 0.54 vs. 0.16 ± 0.4 (P = .007)	At 3 years: TLF: 8.9% vs. 5.5% (P = .23) CD: 0.4% vs. 0% (P = 1) TV-MI: 5.4% vs. 3.1% (P = .31) ID-TLR: 7% vs. 3.9% (P = .23)	At 3 years (definite/probable): 3.6% vs. 1.6% (P = .35)
AIDA[55]	1845	Stable IHD, UA, STEMI & NSTEMI RVD: ≥2.5 and ≤4 mm Lesion length ≤70 mm	Left main stenosis Bifurcation lesions (≥1 stent planned) In-stent restenosis	24-Month TVF	97/91	74/49	55/51	Not applicable No angiographic follow-up	At 2 years: TLF: 11.7% vs. 10.7% (P = .43) CD: 2% vs. 2.7% (P = .43) TV-MI: 5.5% vs. 3.2% (P = .04) ID-TLR: 7.0% vs. 5.2% (P = .15)	At 2 years (definite/probable): 31 vs. 8 (P < .001)
EVERBIO II[56,57]	240	Stable IHD, UA, STEMI & NSTEMI RVD <4.0 mm	The study protocol defined no limit for lesion length, number of target lesions, or number of vessels	9-Month angiographic in-device LLL	97/86	34/31	30/35	At 9 months: BRS vs. EES/BES = 0.28 ± 0.39 vs. 0.25 ± 0.36 (P = .3)	At 2 years for BVS vs. EES + BES: DOCE: 21% vs. 13% (P = .12) CD: 1% vs. 1% (P = .55) TV-MI: 3% vs. 0% (P = .11) CI-TLR: 14% vs 8% (P = .16)	At 2 years (definite, for BVS vs. EES + BES): 1 vs. 0 (P = .33)
TROFI II[58,59]	191	STEMI ≤24 h RVD ≥2.25 and ≤3.8 mm	Unprotected left main stenosis Cardiogenic shock	6-Month OFDI-HS	56/51	50/25	100/100	At 6 months: 0.14 ± 0.23 vs. 0.06 ± 0.29 (P = .09)	At 3 years: DOCE: 5.3% vs. 3.1% (P = .47) CD: 2.1% vs. 0 (P = ns) TV-MI: 2.1% vs. 3.1% (P = .68) CI-TLR: 3.2% vs. 1.0% (P = .33)	At 3 years (definite/probable): 2 (2.1%) vs. 1 (1.0%) (P = .55)

[a]Excluding patients with device thrombosis.[116] Rates of pre- and post dilatation and B2/C lesions are given for BRS/DES.

BES, Biolimus-eluting bioabsorbable polymer DES; *BRS*, bioresorbable scaffolds; *CD*, cardiac death; *CI-TLR*, clinically indicated target lesion revascularization; *DES*, drug eluting stents; *DOCE*, device-oriented composite end point; *EES*, everolimus-eluting persistent polymer DES; *ID-TLR*, ischemia driven target lesion revascularization; *IHD*, ischemic heart disease; *LLL*, late lumen loss; *MI*, myocardial infarctions; *MLD*, minimum lumen diameter; *NSTEMI*, non ST-elevation MI; *OFDI-HS*, optical frequency domain imaging healing score; *PCI*, percutaneous coronary intervention; *RVD*, reference vessel diameter; *SB-D*, side branch diameter; *STEMI*, ST-elevation MI; *TLF*, target lesion failure; *TVF*, target vessel failure; *TV-MI*, target-vessel myocardial infarctions; *UA*, unstable angina.

polymer DES (BES) with the primary end point being angiographic in-device late loss at 9 months. The rates of the primary end point were similar for BRS vs. EES/BES, while a post hoc noninferiority analysis showed noninferiority ($P < .001$) of the BRS for the same end point.[56] Overall, event rates were very low and the study was underpowered regarding clinical end points. However, in the comparison between BRS and BES, device-related adverse events at 2 years were significantly higher for Absorb.[57] TROFI II was another relatively small RCT ($n = 191$) whose importance lies in the fact that it included only patients with STEMI undergoing primary percutaneous coronary revascularization. The primary end point of the 6-month optical frequency domain imaging healing score (HS) was based on the presence of uncovered and/or malapposed stent struts and intraluminal filling defects and was lower in the Absorb arm ($P_{noninferiority} < .001$).[58] At 3 years, the rates of all clinical secondary end points were similar between the two devices.[59] Again, event rates were too low to allow any meaningful statistical comparisons or clinical correlations.

DESolve

The DESolve family of PLLA-based BRS (Elixir Medical, Sunnyvale, CA) includes the first-generation device with 150 μm strut thickness and the second-generation device with a strut thickness of 120 μm and elutes novolimus, an active metabolite of sirolimus. In both iterations, the scaffold is coated with a matrix of polylactide-based biodegradable polymer and antiproliferative drug, which is applied using a proprietary technique.[25] The important features of the DESolve BRS are intrinsic self-correcting deployment properties that become operative in the event of minor strut malapposition and an ability to over-expand across a wide range of diameters without risk of strut fracture.[60] The first iteration was initially tested as a myolimus- eluting device, in the small ($n = 16$) FIM DESolve I trial, which showed encouraging imaging and clinical results at 6 and 12 months, respectively.[61] Subsequently, the novolimus-eluting version was tested in the larger ($n = 126$) single arm DESolve NX trial, in which the primary end point of in-stent LLL at 6 months was 0.21 ± 0.32 mm (113 patients with paired analysis) with 98.7% struts coverage at the same time point. At 5 years, the rates of MACE, TV-MI, CD, and clinically indicated TLR (CI-TLR) were 9%, 1.6%, 3.3%, and 4.1%, respectively. No cases of definite ScT were observed.[62] A single, retrospective, comparative analysis between this device and the Absorb BRS using propensity-score matching is also available, showing similar outcomes between the two devices with regard to 1-year rates of TLF, TLR, CD, and definite ScT.[63] The second iteration was tested in the relatively small ($n = 50$) single arm DESolve Cx trial, showing in-scaffold LLL of 0.19 ± 0.25 mm at 6 months and no MACE at 12 months' follow-up.[64] Both iterations have CE mark and the company is currently developing a third-generation device (Desolve NXT plus) with 120 strut thickness and a contoured strut design for enhanced acute performance.

Reva Medical Bioresorbable Scaffolds

The first two iterations of the first generation of the Reva Medical (San Diego, CA) BRS showed high TLR and low technical success rates in the Reva Endovascular Study of a Bioresorbable Coronary Stent (RESORB) FIM trial (bare form)[65] and the RESTORE I trial (sirolimus-eluting version, ReZolve BRS), respectively.[65] A third iteration, ReZolve BRS 2, is being tested in the RESTORE II trial. Preliminary results in 67 patients at 6 months showed 3 MACE cases and the trial is ongoing.[66] However, the problematic deliverability of the device pushed the company to feature a conventional balloon-expandable system for its next and current iteration of the scaffold, named Fantom. The most characteristic feature of the Fantom BRS is that it contains iodine covalently bound to its desaminotyrosine PC backbone, which makes it intrinsically radiopaque and may decrease the need for intravascular imaging during follow-up. Furthermore, it has a wide expandability range, and although the time required for full reabsorption is significantly longer compared to PLLA-based scaffolds (3 years), more than 80% molecular weight loss takes place within the first year. Clinically, the Fantom BRS was initially tested in a small FIM trial[67] and subsequently in the FANTOM II trial which included 240 patients split in two cohorts. Acute technical and procedural success was observed in 95.8% and 99.1%, respectively, of the cohort A patients. The 6 months' angiographic and clinical primary end points for cohort A have been formally published.[68] Recently, 12 months' results for the entire cohort showing a MACE rate of 4.2% with a single ScT (subacute)[69] and 24 months' results for 125 patients showing a MACE rate of 5.6% and a single very late ScT were reported.[70] In addition to the latest clinical follow up, a 25-patients' subset in the trial underwent angiographic imaging, showing a final in-scaffold LLL of 0.25 mm, which is in the desired range of 0.2 to 0.4 mm. CE mark approval for the Fantom scaffold was received in April 2017, while cohort C of the FANTOM II trial is currently enrolling patients with more complex lesions. Reva has also announced a new iteration, named Fantom Encore, with a strut thickness of 95 μm in 2.5 mm diameter; its performance results are awaited.

Art Pure

The ART Pure (Arterial Remodeling Technologies, Terumo) is a PDLLA-based, nondrug eluting BRS. It was tested in the FIM ART-DIVA trial ($n = 30$), with 6 months' MACE as a primary end point. No cases of CD or MI were observed, while the ID-TLR rate was 3.3% (in total 3 [10%] patients had TLR but only one was ischemia-driven).[71] The scaffold received CE mark in May 2015, but was never marketed in Europe and in February 2017 Terumo announced the termination of the product's co-development with ART.

Amaranth Bioresorbable Scaffolds

The Amaranth scaffold family includes BRS with unique polymer production features that result in enhanced radial force and over-expansion capabilities with increased fracture resistance. The first-generation device in this group is the Fortitude scaffold (150 μm), which was initially tested as a nondrug eluting version in the MEND I ($n = 13$) trial and subsequently as a sirolimus-eluting version with encouraging results in the RENASCENT-I, MEND II[72] and FORTITUDE ($n = 63$) trials,[73,74] with the latter showing 5.3% TLF and 1.8% ScT rates at 2 years. It was then further miniaturized, leading to two newer iterations, the Aptitude and Magnitude scaffolds, with strut thickness of 115 and 98 μm, respectively. The single arm RENASCENT-II trial enrolled 60 patients treated with the Aptitude scaffold and has reported on its primary end points of safety and efficacy at 9 months.[75] In-scaffold LLL was 0.34 ± 0.36 mm, TLF rates were 3.4% driven by two cases of TV-MI, while no ScT were observed. Clinical success was 98.3%, while optical coherence tomography (OCT) demonstrated 97% strut coverage and low rate of malapposition. CE mark approval has been submitted. The ongoing FIM RENASCENT-III trial with complete enrollment of 70 patients will address the outcomes of the Magnitude scaffold, the world's first clinically tested sub-100-μm BRS, and the results regarding its 9-month primary end point are expected in May 2018. Preliminary results at 30 days for the entire cohort have shown three target vessel failure (TVF) cases and no ScT.[74]

IDEAL BioStent

The backbone of the IDEAL BioStent (Xenogenics Corp, Canton, MA) is made of polylactide anhydride mixed with a polymer of salicylic acid with a sebacic acid linker. A salicylate coating controls the elution of sirolimus at a dose of 8.3 μg/mm while the scaffold also elutes approximately 10 μg of salicylic acid. The unique design of this thick struts (200 μm) BRS is thought to provide additional antiinflammatory properties to the antiproliferative action of the macrocyclic lactone.[76] This device was tested in 2009 in the FIM WHISPER study (n = 11). Although the trial has not been fully reported, IVUS and OCT showed higher-than-expected intimal hyperplasia that was attributed to the too-rapid elution and the too-low surface area dose of the antiproliferative drug.[77] A new iteration has been developed with higher dose and slower release kinetics of the drug and also thinner struts. It is currently undergoing preclinical evaluation.

MeRes

MeRes BRS (Meril Life Sciences, Vapi, Gujarat, India) is a PLLA-based, sirolimus-eluting BRS with hybrid geometry structure that provides high radial strength, thin struts, and tri axial radiopaque markers. MeRes I FIM study (n = 108) was performed in 16 medical centers of India (58) and showed in-scaffold LLL of 0.15 ± 0.23 mm with "virtually complete" strut coverage (99.3%) at 6 months and very low MACE rates at 1 year (0.93%, 1 ID-TLR with no ST). Based on the impressive results of the FIM trial, the company has initiated an ambitious program of further trials being performed in non U.S. centers, but with worldwide participation, including MeRes-I extend and MeRes-100 China, a pivotal RCT of MeRes versus Xience (1:1) with a goal of enrolling 470 patients.

Mirage

Mirage (Manli Cardiology, Singapore) is a PLLA-based sirolimus-eluting scaffold that incorporates a unique helix coil design for high flexibility, has relatively short bioresorption time, high scaffold dislodging force, and high radial strength, and it can be stored at room temperature (as long as it is below 25°C) and has been shown to be "MR conditional."[78] Clinically, it was evaluated in a single-blinded, randomized clinical trial of 60 patients who were randomized to either the Mirage (n = 31) or the Absorb (n = 29) BRS. The primary end point of in-scaffold LLL at 12 months (0.48 ± 0.49 mm for Mirage), as well as the rates of all clinical end points, were similar between the two study groups, despite the fact that diameter stenoses 1 year after implantation on angiography and OCT were significantly higher with Mirage.[79] Clinical follow-up of this trial is scheduled yearly for 5 years, but the company will begin a new study, incorporating small changes to further enhance the performance of this device.

Firesorb

Firesorb (Shanghai MicroPort Medical, Shanghai, China) is a sirolimus-eluting BRS with similar structure to the Absorb BRS but significantly lower strut thickness and antiproliferative drug dose (60%). It has been tested in the FIM FUTURE I trial, a single-center Chinese study in 45 patients randomly assigned to 2 cohorts (2:1) undergoing multimodality intravascular imaging at 6 months and 1 year, respectively. TLF and ScT rates were 0% both at 30 days (primary end point) and at 1 year, with only 1 patient undergoing revascularization for a nontarget MI the day after the index procedure. At 6 months, in-scaffold LLL was 0.15 ± 0.11 mm and struts coverage 98.4%. At 12 months, the latter was significantly increased to 99.0%, while there were no other significant differences between the two cohorts in terms of imaging findings.[80] In September 2017, the manufacturing company announced the enrollment of the first patient in the FUTURE II RCT, which is designed to enroll 610 patients and test the Firesorb BRS against the Xience stent (NCT02890160).

Xinsorb

The Xinsorb BRS (Shandong Huaan Biotechnology Co., Ltd., Hangzhou, Zhejiang, People's Republic of China) is a sirolimus-eluting BRS with a backbone composed of a mixture of PLA, PCL, and PGA and a coating of PDLLA mixed with PLLA. The device is stored at 4°C.[81] The manufacturing company has completed a small (n = 30) FIM trial in China, in which imaging findings at 6 months were favorable[82] and no MACE were observed, but extended clinical follow-up to 30 months demonstrated a MACE rate of 3.3%, with one confirmed case of ScT and 2 cases of ID-TLR.[83] Based on the encouraging initial results of the FIM trial, an RCT versus a biodegradable-polymer DES of 400 patients and a single-arm registry of 800 patients were subsequently initiated. Both these trials have completed enrollment in June 2016 and are currently in the data collection phase.

Magmaris

Three iterations of this magnesium device have been tested in the clinical arena. Absorbable Mg Scaffold (AMS 1) (BIOTRONIK, Berlin, Germany) was the initial bare version with a strut thickness of 165 μm and was tested in the PROGRESS AMS FIM in 63 patients showing disappointing TLR rates of 45% at 1 year, despite the absence of ST, leading to the redesign of this device. The second iteration, AMS 2 (DREAMS 1), used a refined, WE43 alloy (93% magnesium and 7% rare earth elements) with slower bioresorption time (9 to 12 months), higher radial strength, 125 μm struts with rectangular shape, and paclitaxel elution for 3 months. It was tested in BIOSOLVE I study, which demonstrated angiographic in-stent LLL of 0.52 ± 0.49 mm at 1-year,[84] while at 3 years TLR rates reached 6.6%, with no cases of CD, TV-MI, or ScT.[84] A newer iteration (second-generation DREAMS, marketed as Magmaris) made of the same alloy and design but with a strut thickness of 150 μm has been recently developed. This device elutes sirolimus instead of paclitaxel, has tantalum radiopaque markers at both ends, and a modified, electropolished strut cross-sectional profile. These modifications result not only in slower dismantling and resorption rate but also improved visibility, higher flexibility, increased deployment diameter, and higher acute radial force and fracture resistance compared to the previous generations. Magmaris was evaluated in the international multicenter FIM BIOSOLVE II trial (n = 123). In-scaffold LLL was 0.27 ± 0.37 mm at 6 months (primary end point) and 0.39 ± 0.27 mm at 12-months' follow-up. TLF, a composite of CD, TV-MI, CI-TLR, and coronary artery bypass grafting, occurred in 4 patients (3%), consisting of one CD, one TV-MI, and two CI-TLR.[85] Long-term results of the Magmaris BRS have been recently published in 184 patients, including pooled follow-up data at 24 months from BIOSOLVE II and at 6 months from the pilot BIOSOLVE III trial (n = 61), demonstrating TLF rates of 5.6% at 2 years.[86] Most importantly, up to now no cases of definite or probable ScT have been reported in patients treated with any of the three iterations of this magnesium-based BRS.

NeoVas

This sirolimus-eluting, PLLA-based BRS with relatively thick struts (NeoVas, Lepu Medical, Beijing, China) was initially tested in an FIM study of 31 patients that at 6 months reported TLF rates of 3.2%, no ScT, and in-scaffold LLL of 0.26 ± 0.32 mm[87] and subsequently in a 1:1 design RCT of 560 patients versus the Xience stent. In February 2018, Han et al. reported the 1-year clinical and imaging results of the latter study,[88] making the NeoVas the first BRS to present controlled data after Absorb. According to these data, NeoVas was noninferior to Xience for the primary end point of 1-year angiographic in-segment LLL (0.14 ± 0.36 mm vs. 0.11 ± 0.34 mm, $P_{noninferiority}$ < .0001), and resulted in comparable 1-year clinical outcomes, including TLF

(1.1% vs. 0.7%, $P = .64$) and definite or probable device thrombosis (0.4% vs. 0%, $P = .31$). Furthermore, OCT demonstrated a higher proportion of covered struts (98.7% vs. 96.2%; $P < .001$) and less strut malapposition (0% vs. 0.6%; $P < .001$) with NeoVas. These results are promising; however, it should be noted that the trial was not powered to detect differences in clinical outcomes, it included predominantly simple lesions, and although the primary noninferiority end point was met, the 1-year follow-up showed a smaller minimal lumen area for NeoVas compared with Xience (4.71 ± 1.64 vs. 6.00 ± 2.15 mm^2; $P < .001$).

FROM INITIAL TRIALS AND PROMISES TO CURRENT STATUS AND FUTURE OUTLOOK

Seventeen years after the first implantation of a BRS in human, there are still few data to support the theoretical advantages of these devices. Although improvements in vasomotion within the treated coronary segment were documented using physiological testing in observational studies,[37,84] in ABSORB B at 5 years the improvement in vasomotion did not reach the functionality of the native vessels[89] and the randomized controlled ABSORB II trial failed to show this improvement at 3 years for the Absorb BRS against the Xience stent.[48] The latter trial, on the other hand, demonstrated that expansive vessel wall remodeling was more frequent and intense with Absorb at 3 years,[90] supporting: (1) previous, nonrandomized observations that showed that at 6 to 12 months after BRS implantation, coronary geometry tends to revert to its pre implant level,[91] and (2) recent observations showing persistence of in-scaffold late lumen enlargement with normalization of the fractional flow reserve (FFR)$_{CT}$ up to 6 years.[92] It should be noted however, that LLL was generally larger in the Absorb compared to the Xience group. Although the altered vessel geometry and biomechanics can result in chronic irritation and flow disturbances that may contribute to neointimal proliferation and adverse events,[93,94] the clinical impact of these observations remains uncertain. This is also the case for the scarce data showing late increases in scaffold-free ostial area in jailed side branches[95]—despite initial higher post procedural incidence of side-branch occlusion compared to DES[96]—and facilitation of noninvasive surveillance imaging with CT.[97] On the contrary, sufficient mid-term clinical data are now available to support the fact that Absorb BRS is inferior to new generation DES[48,53,55] and both FDA[98] and European Society of Cardiology-European Association of Percutaneous Cardiovascular Interventions[29] have issued documents reflecting on this position. Paradoxically, the greatest promise turned out as the Achilles heel of this emblematic first-generation BRS. In all ABSORB RCTs, published rates of device thrombosis were numerically higher for Absorb, regardless of the statistical significance of this difference, while a meta-analysis of the first six trials reported a two fold increase in the risk of device thrombosis with Absorb at just 1 year of follow-up, despite similar rates of all other clinical end points.[99] Moreover, several recent meta-analyses summarizing mid-term outcomes at 2 years, and one also at 3 years,[41,100-104] reported concordant findings, with a higher risk of both thrombosis and TLF for the Absorb BRS, the latter driven mainly by increased rates of TV-MI and ID-TLR. Current evidence also suggests no late advantage in terms of clinical efficacy, including relief of angina pectoris.[48]

It should be emphasized that the advantages of BRS are not fully demonstrated until bioresorption is complete and long-term results (i.e., >3 years) are still needed to complete the picture. In this regard, the 4 years' results of ABSORB II, although they do not represent the beginning of a clinical benefit, may be interpreted at least as the end of the increased mid-term thrombotic risk. The ultimate judge of the Absorb BRS will probably be the ongoing ABSORB IV trial that has recently reported 30 days' results in 2604 patients.[105] Since ABSORB III and IV will be pooled together for a landmark clinical end point analysis between 3 and greater than 5 (7 to 10) years, we still need to wait many years before understanding if a long-term clinical benefit can come from BRS. However, even if such a final benefit can be reached for Absorb, it will have to pass through the "Symplegades" of increased mid-term thrombotic risk. This risk was concordant across the early (<30 days), late (30 days to 1 year), and very late (>1 year) periods,[100,101,104,106] an observation in favor of an inherent thrombogenicity of the scaffold. The latter is partially supported by the results of the AIDA trial and seems to originate from the rather thick struts of this first-generation device, although issues inherent to the mechanical disintegration of the scaffold during the resorption process may also contribute.[101,104,107] Whether the risk of ScT can be mitigated by a specific implantation technique, by avoiding very small vessels, or by prolonging DAPT is subject to debate. Extension of DAPT duration until BRS resorption is completed is widely recommended; however, this is based more on expert's consensus[108] rather than on solid evidence[109] and is subject to a potential offset of its beneficial effect by the accompanying increased bleeding risk. Regarding the effects of meticulous adherence to good implantation techniques, briefly summarized in the acronym PSP (predilate, sizing, post dilate),[42] there are indeed data suggesting improved outcomes.[40,110,111] However, these data were derived from post hoc analyses and have not been prospectively validated. In ABSORB-IV, where pre- and post dilatation were performed in 99.8% and 82.6% of the lesions, respectively, overall rates of device thrombosis at 30 days were markedly lower compared to ABSORB III at the same time point (0.6% vs. 1.1% for Absorb BRS) and Absorb was noninferior to Xience with regard to the primary end point of TLF, but again with numerically higher rates of ScT. Furthermore, it has been estimated that only half of patients with late or very late ScT might benefit from meticulous implantation techniques,[112] which in addition result in a significant lengthening of the procedure.[113] Finally, small vessel diameter, which was an exclusion criterion in the ABSORB RCTs series, has consistently shown to be a predictor of adverse events,[41,111] but the effect of this observation in the results of these trials can only be speculated. It is conceivable that even if the aforementioned solutions become accepted as a necessary short-term price to pay in order to achieve the potential long-term benefits of BRS, it will be a "Pyrrhic victory" for Absorb in an era where DES are both "operator-friendly" in terms of implantation and related with very short DAPT durations. Reflecting on this, Abbott has discontinued the sales of Absorb in both the U.S. and Europe and restricted its use in Europe in registries, maintaining a rigorous follow-up of the ongoing RCTs in the hope of more favorable long-term results.[114] For the BRS technology overall, however, at present hope seems to lie more on the development of second- generation devices, and even Abbott is developing a new generation, sub-100 μm scaffold named Falcon.[114] Currently, the distinction between first- and second-generation devices is based predominantly on strut thickness, although a number of other characteristics still need improvement to achieve an ideal BRS platform, including over-expansion capability, visibility, deliverability, and storage conditions. A number of second-generation devices have shown encouraging results in clinical trials[115] and coupled with clear differences in material technology from the archetypical Absorb BRS challenge the class effect of its so-far unfavorable results. The evaluation of these devices will not be possible until randomized data from mid-term follow-up studies become available and many experts doubt if an appropriate challenger is currently available to go against a mature technology with solid results, like DES.[113] In spite of this, a number of companies worldwide have initiated ambitious RCTs for their products that will determine if BRS evolutional history will follow the pattern of DES in terms of success through further development, or another scenario will prevail.

KEY REFERENCES

29. Byrne RA, Stefanini GG, Capodanno D, et al. Report of an ESC-EAPCI Task Force on the evaluation and use of bioresorbable scaffolds for percutaneous coronary intervention: executive summary. *EuroIntervention*. 2018;13(13):1574–1586.
40. Puricel S, Cuculi F, Weissner M, et al. Bioresorbable coronary scaffold thrombosis: multicenter comprehensive analysis of clinical presentation, mechanisms, and predictors. *J Am Coll Cardiol*. 2016;67(8):921–931.
41. Ali ZA, Serruys PW, Kimura T, et al. 2-Year outcomes with the Absorb bioresorbable scaffold for treatment of coronary artery disease: a systematic review and meta-analysis of seven randomised trials with an individual patient data substudy. *Lancet*. 2017;390(10096):760–772.
48. Serruys PW, Chevalier B, Sotomi Y, et al. Comparison of an everolimus-eluting bioresorbable scaffold with an everolimus-eluting metallic stent for the treatment of coronary artery stenosis (ABSORB II): a 3 year, randomised, controlled, single-blind, multicentre clinical trial. *Lancet*. 2016;388(10059):2479–2491.
51. Chevalier B, Cequier A, Dudek D, et al. Four-year follow-up of the randomised comparison between an everolimus-eluting bioresorbable scaffold and an everolimus-eluting metallic stent for the treatment of coronary artery stenosis (ABSORB II trial). *EuroIntervention*. 2018;12:1561–1564.
52. Ellis SG, Kereiakes DJ, Metzger DC, et al. Everolimus-eluting bioresorbable scaffolds for coronary artery disease. *N Engl J Med*. 2015;373(20):1905–1915.
54. Kereiakes DJ, Ellis SG, Metzger C, et al. 3-Year clinical outcomes with everolimus-eluting bioresorbable coronary scaffolds: the ABSORB III trial. *J Am Coll Cardiol*. 2017;70(23):2852–2862.
55. Wykrzykowska JJ, Kraak RP, Hofma SH, et al. Bioresorbable scaffolds versus metallic stents in routine PCI. *N Engl J Med*. 2017;376(24):2319–2328.
58. Sabate M, Windecker S, Iniguez A, et al. Everolimus-eluting bioresorbable stent vs. durable polymer everolimus-eluting metallic stent in patients with ST-segment elevation myocardial infarction: results of the randomized ABSORB ST-segment elevation myocardial infarction-TROFI II trial. *Eur Heart J*. 2016;37(3):229–240.
86. Haude M, Ince H, Kische S, et al. Sustained safety and clinical performance of a drug-eluting absorbable metal scaffold up to 24 months: pooled outcomes of BIOSOLVE-II and BIOSOLVE-III. *EuroIntervention*. 2017;13(4):432–439.
88. Han Y, Xu B, Fu G, et al. A randomized trial comparing the NeoVas sirolimus-eluting bioresorbable scaffold and metallic everolimus-eluting stents. *JACC Cardiovasc Interv*. 2018;11(3):260–272.
90. Serruys PW, Katagiri Y, Sotomi Y, et al. Arterial remodeling after bioresorbable scaffolds and metallic stents. *J Am Coll Cardiol*. 2017;70(1):60–74.
100. Montone RA, Niccoli G, De Marco F, et al. Temporal trends in adverse events after everolimus-eluting bioresorbable vascular scaffold versus everolimus-eluting metallic stent implantation: a meta-analysis of randomized controlled trials. *Circulation*. 2017;135(22):2145–2154.
102. Ali ZA, Gao RF, Kimura T, et al. Three-year outcomes with the absorb bioresorbable scaffold: individual-patient-data meta-analysis from the ABSORB randomized trials. *Circulation*. 2018;137(5):464–479.
111. Stone GW, Abizaid A, Onuma Y, et al. Effect of technique on outcomes following bioresorbable vascular scaffold implantation: analysis from the ABSORB trials. *J Am Coll Cardiol*. 2017;70(23):2863–2874.

Additional references available online at expertconsult.com.

中文导读

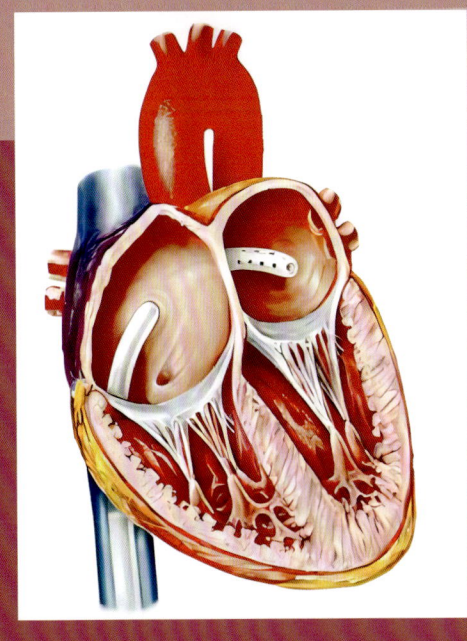

第17章
药物涂层球囊

在冠状动脉介入治疗领域中一项重要的进展是支架的出现。通过药物洗脱支架对紫杉醇、西罗莫司及其相关类似物进行局部血管内药物输送，一定程度上解决了血管再狭窄的问题。但支架并不完美，其带来了血管局部异物存留及慢性炎症的新问题。药物涂层球囊可能是替代药物洗脱支架用于局部血管内药物输送的一种方法。

本章节首先介绍了药物涂层球囊发展历程及前期研究结果。2001年药物涂层球囊概念得以被提出，即将紫杉醇等抗增殖药物涂在用于扩张狭窄病变的传统球囊表面，这在理论上可以实现局部药物输送——随着球囊扩张，药物也随之转移到扩张的血管节段。这种方式在非常低的全身暴露情况下，就能达到有效的局部药物浓度，同时还无其他异物的长期存留。在美国，已有3种药物涂层球囊产品批准上市。而在欧洲，获得上市批准的药物涂层球囊更多。但不同药物涂层球囊所携带的药物载体、药物及剂量并不完全相同，因此不同药物涂层球囊缺乏类效应，不推荐将一个药物涂层球囊产品的研究证据拓展到其他药物涂层球囊产品。

基于临床研究结果，本章节还重点介绍了药物涂层球囊的临床适应证。目前，药物涂层球囊主要用于治疗冠状动脉支架内再狭窄，也可用于治疗股浅动脉的新生，以及非支架术后的血管再狭窄病变。药物涂层球囊的其他可能适应证，尚需临床研究进一步证实。

赵宇昊　柳景华

章节要点

- 药物涂层球囊导管已被证明可替代药物洗脱支架，用于局部血管内药物输送。
- 基础研究数据表明，药物涂层球囊可以有效抑制血管再狭窄；然而，不同药物涂层球囊之间缺乏一致的类效应。
- 药物涂层球囊在治疗冠状动脉支架内再狭窄、股浅动脉的新生（de novo）病变，以及非支架术后的血管再狭窄病变方面的有效性和安全性，已得到随机临床试验证实。
- 对于其他适应证，例如，冠状动脉de novo病变、股浅动脉支架内再狭窄病变、膝关节以下外周动脉病变，药物涂层球囊的作用仍需进一步证实。

17 Drug-Eluting Balloons

Bruno Scheller

KEY POINTS

- Drug-coated balloon (DCB) catheters are the most advanced proven alternative to drug-eluting stents for local intravascular drug delivery.
- Preclinical data indicate effective inhibition of restenosis; however, there is no uniform class effect on drug-coated balloons.
- Randomized clinical trials have shown the efficacy and safety of these devices in the treatment of coronary in-stent restenosis (ISR) and treatment of de novo and nonstented restenotic lesions in the superficial femoral artery (SFA).
- The role of DCBs in other indications such as coronary de novo disease, SFA ISR, and below the knee must be further determined.

INTRODUCTION

Coronary angioplasty was introduced into clinical use by Andreas Grüntzig in 1977.[1] In the field of coronary intervention, the most important advance has been the introduction of stents. Stenting overcomes the weaknesses of balloon angioplasty alone, which include acute recoil and dissection, and longer term negative vessel remodeling, but not restenosis because of continued or increased neointimal proliferation with stents. Local intravascular drug delivery by drug-eluting stents (DESs) that elute paclitaxel, sirolimus, and their associated analogues have successfully addressed this cellular basis of restenosis in the coronary territory. However, stents cannot be implanted or may be suboptimal at coronary sites where neointimal proliferation may limit the long-term benefit of angioplasty, such as in small vessels and bifurcations. Moreover, DESs that use sirolimus and its analogues have not been found to be effective in the treatment of atherosclerotic disease of the femoropopliteal territory. In the coronary arteries, sometimes delayed or incomplete reendothelialization with the need for long-term dual-antiplatelet therapy (DAPT) to reduce the risk of late stent thrombosis can limit the use of this technology in certain patients at risk for hemorrhagic complications, or it can limit the need for planned surgery. Sustained drug release seems to be essential for stent-based local drug delivery because of the inhomogeneous drug distribution from DESs to the arterial wall,[2] the time course of the inflammation related to the initial trauma of the procedure, and the provocation of neointimal hyperplasia due to the implanted prosthesis and any associated polymeric coating. About 75% to 85% of the stented vessel wall area is not covered by the stent struts, resulting in low tissue levels of the antiproliferative agent in these areas. Cell culture experiments indicate that low drug concentrations require much longer exposure times to achieve sufficient inhibition of cell proliferation than do higher concentrations.[3] Therefore high drug concentrations on the stent struts, including a controlled and sustained release, are mandatory for stent-based local drug delivery,[4] with the consequence of delayed and incomplete reendothelialization of the stent struts. Autopsy studies show that even beyond 40 months, some DESs can demonstrate incomplete endothelial coverage.[5] Furthermore, the polymeric matrices on the stent that are meant to control the release kinetics of the antiproliferative drug can induce inflammation and thrombosis.[6] On the other hand, incomplete suppression of neointimal hyperplasia at the stent margins or between the struts may limit the efficacy of DESs.[2]

Alternative approaches to overcome the limitations of DESs have included modifying the sustained drug release from stent struts to allow for earlier reendothelialization, using bioerodable polymers or nonpolymeric release mechanisms (such as surface-modified stent struts), and using thinner struts that require less coverage.

Antiproliferative taxanes, such as paclitaxel, seem to be suitable for the prevention of local intravascular restenosis because of their high lipophilicity and tight binding to various cell constituents compared with sirolimus and its analogues; this results in effective local retention at the site of delivery.[3] The addition of a contrast agent surprisingly resulted in a solubility of taxanes far beyond the concentrations applied in previous investigations.[7] In the porcine coronary model, the intracoronary bolus administration of a taxane–contrast medium formulation led to a significant reduction of neointimal formation after experimental coronary stent implantation despite the short application time.[8,9] Paclitaxel in a contrast agent was better tolerated and led to higher local tissue concentrations than diluted Taxol, indicating the impact of additional compounds for local drug transfer.[10] The surprising discovery was that sustained drug release is not a precondition for long-lasting restenosis inhibition. In 2001, the basic premise of a more lesion- than vessel-specific method of intramural drug delivery became embodied in the concept of a drug-coated balloon (DCB).[11] By coating paclitaxel onto the surface of a conventional angioplasty balloon used to dilate the stenotic artery, an exclusively local effect could theoretically be achieved, with the drug transferred to the dilated segment as the balloon was inflated. In this way, an effective local drug concentration is achieved with very low systemic exposure. However, several properties of the balloon coating are crucial for ensuring effective drug delivery to the target site: (1) its form on the balloon surface; (2) the homogeneity of distribution along the surface of the balloon; (3) its stability during production, handling, and storage; (4) the degree of premature loss while transiting to the target vessel segment; (5) the ability to release during balloon expansion; (6) the transfer efficiency to the vessel wall; and (7) the amount of particulate material released to the distal circulation.

PRECLINICAL DATA

Using various coating procedures, Speck and colleagues coated conventional coronary balloon catheters with different doses of paclitaxel and studied their pharmacokinetics in a porcine coronary model.[10] The paclitaxel dose was variable on the coated balloons, between 1.3 and 3 µg/mm², which corresponded to a total dose of approximately 220 to 650 µg of paclitaxel, depending on the balloon size. About 10% of the initial amount of paclitaxel on the balloon was lost while the catheter was being advanced to the lesion through the hemostatic valve and the guiding catheter, and about 80% of the dose was released during inflation. Most of the dose released at the target site was distributed as particulate distally in the bloodstream, with less than 20% being directly taken up into the vessel wall. In this way, paclitaxel-coated balloons deliver drug to the target site in a very short time, and the dosing is higher than that released by stents over the course of several weeks' elution. At 5-week follow-up, the implantation of bare-metal stents (BMSs) premounted on paclitaxel-coated balloons was found to have caused a marked dose-dependent and statistically significant reduction in late lumen loss (LLL) and an equally impressive statistically significant increase in minimal lumen diameter (MLD) compared with controls. Quantitative coronary angiography revealed no edge effects or signs of malapposition or aneurysm. Histomorphometry showed a statistically significant increase in lumen diameter and lumen area and a corresponding decrease in maximal neointimal thickness and neointimal area in the vessels treated with paclitaxel-coated balloons (a reduction of neointimal area by 63% in the paclitaxel-coated balloon group vs. the uncoated balloon group).[11] Furthermore, the drug was more evenly distributed on the vessel surface compared with that delivered by a DES.[12] However, studies suggest that the amount of paclitaxel in the arterial tissue varies widely depending on the dose of drug on the balloon and particularly on the coating formulation. An adequate inhibition of neointimal proliferation was observed when balloons were coated with paclitaxel mixed with the contrast agent iopromide dissolved in acetone; the effect was markedly lower when ethyl acetate was used as a solvent without iopromide. The difference in efficacy of these two coating formulations may be primarily explained by the presence of the hydrophilic iodinated contrast medium in the case of the acetone version, thus suggesting that a proper solubilizing agent is important.[13]

Paclitaxel admixed with a small amount of the hydrophilic contrast medium iopromide has also been registered under the name Paccocath (Charite University Hospital, Berlin, Germany). These balloons were standard angioplasty balloons coated with a more uniform paclitaxel dose of 3 µg/mm² of balloon surface. The situation in the peripheral arteries is not directly comparable with that in the coronary arteries, and treatment is much more complex in several respects. Specifically, the incidence of restenosis in the superficial femoral artery (SFA) is considerably higher and can reach up to 50% within the first 6 months after intervention in longer lesions.[14] Given the clinical need, it was very encouraging when Albrecht and colleagues[15] developed early preclinical data that demonstrated local intraarterial administration of paclitaxel using DCBs or an admixture of paclitaxel and contrast medium could inhibit in-stent stenosis of peripheral arteries in the porcine overstretch model: in-stent stenosis in the control group was 38% (±20%, uncoated balloons). In the treatment groups, it was reduced: treatment group I used balloons coated with 330 µg paclitaxel, and in-stent stenosis was 18% (±22%); treatment group II used balloons coated with 480 µg paclitaxel, and the rate was 12% (±18%); and treatment group III used 6.4 mg paclitaxel dissolved in 50 mL iopromide 370 + 5 mL ethanol), and the rate was 18% (±20%; $P < .05$). Cremers and coworkers subsequently evaluated the effects of various inflation times (10, 60, and 2 × 60 seconds) on the efficacy of restenosis inhibition and the safety of different doses (5 µg; 2 × 5 µg paclitaxel/mm² balloon surface) in pigs. Treatment with a DCB (5 µg paclitaxel/mm² balloon surface with iopromide) for 10 seconds reduced the neointimal area to the same extent as contact with the vessel wall for 2 times 60 seconds (by 57% and 56%, respectively, compared with control). Furthermore, neointimal proliferation and all other parameters that characterize in-stent restenosis (ISR) were not further decreased by inflating two drug-coated balloons (each containing 5 µg paclitaxel/mm² balloon surface) in the same vessel segment for 60 seconds each. These results suggest that balloons coated with the paclitaxel-iopromide formulation release most of the drug rapidly during the first seconds of inflation. Thus the initial contact of the coated balloon membrane with the vessel wall appears to produce the desired effect of inhibiting neointimal proliferation. The results of this study indicate that it may be sufficient to inflate the balloon for a few seconds only to achieve adequate protection from restenosis. The results also show that doses of up to 10 µg paclitaxel/mm² balloon surface applied by the inflation of two DCBs does not appear to be linked with clinical toxicity, such as increasing the risk of thrombosis or aneurysm.[16] In addition, persistence of detectable drug in the vessel has been demonstrated to at least 30 days.[17]

Since this initial research was published, several manufacturers have started commercializing or developing DCBs. Currently, paclitaxel is the drug of choice, the typical dosage being 3 µg/mm² of balloon surface. The critical factor enabling successful drug transfer is the formulation used to coat the balloon. Current products range from those with no additive and very tight binding of the drug to the balloon membrane, to those applied in conjunction with contrast agents or other beneficial additives. A number of these developers have undertaken extensive research into this issue with the assumption that the formulation will be critical to successful product performance and adoption (Table 17.1). The matrix coating of the SeQuent Please balloon catheter (B. Braun Melsungen AG, Germany) for percutaneous transluminal coronary angioplasty (PTCA) consists of a mixture of paclitaxel and iopromide, identical in composition to Paccocath. The preclinical data compare very well with the results from the Paccocath program. Buszman and colleagues reported histologic results showing the Cotavance coating (Bayer-Schering, Berlin, Germany), an iterative coating formula based on Paccocath, to be superior to an uncoated balloon in treating coronary artery and SFA lesions in pigs. In an additional pilot study, single or overlapping Cotavance balloons were compared with single nonoverlapping balloons coated with a contrast medium (iopromide) without paclitaxel in a healthy porcine iliofemoral stent model. Balloon angioplasty was followed by self-expandable BMS implantation. After 28 days, Cotavance balloons decreased neointimal proliferation in a dose-dependent manner when assessed by quantitative angiography (LLL with Cotavance single 1.5 ± 0.7 mm vs. Cotavance overlap 0.7 ± 0.6 mm compared with contrast-coated control 1.7 ± 0.4 mm).[18,19] Unfortunately, this balloon is no longer produced, nor is it available for use.

FreePac (Medtronic Invatec, Italy) is a proprietary hydrophilic coating formulation in which urea serves as the matrix substance. Urea is a nontoxic, ubiquitous endogenous compound commonly used in pharmacy; it is meant to enhance the release of paclitaxel during the short time of contact with the vessel wall. In the porcine coronary model, similar amounts of paclitaxel were transferred to the vessel wall with the Paccocath coating (214 ± 106 µg paclitaxel) and the FreePac coating (175 ± 101 µg paclitaxel) 15 to 25 minutes after stent implantation. Twenty-eight days after balloon dilation, the original Paccocath coating caused the known strong inhibition of neointimal formation in the porcine coronary model (MLD: 2.7 ± 0.3 mm; LLL, 0.3 ± 0.2 mm). The FreePac coating was equally efficacious and equally well tolerated (MLD: 2.7 ± 0.2 mm; LLL, 0.4 ± 0.2 mm).[20] The aim of another preclinical study was to determine the minimum effective dose and local toxicity at extremely high doses of the FreePac formulation. The balloons were coated with 1 to 9 µg paclitaxel/mm² balloon surface. In the highest-dose group, three balloons, each coated with 9 µg paclitaxel/mm² balloon surface, were expanded in the same vessel segment. FreePac paclitaxel-coated balloon catheters efficaciously inhibited neointimal proliferation starting with the lowest dose tested (1 µg/mm²) and were well tolerated up to 3 times the preferred dose of 3 µg/mm². Stent occlusions observed at the highest dose level and repeated treatment (3 × 9 µg/mm²) indicate that the limit of tolerance was reached.[21]

TABLE 17.1 Paclitaxel-Coated Balloons Currently on the Market

Company	Device	Additive and Substance class		Dose [μg/mm^2]	Vessel territory
Bard Lutonix, USA	Moxy	Polysorbate + sorbitol	Surfactant + sugar alcohol	2	peripheral
Boston Scientific, USA	Agent	Acetyl tributyl citrate	Plasticizer	2	coronary
	Ranger	Acetyl tributyl citrate	Plasticizer	2	peripheral
Spectranetics, USA	Stellarex	Polyethylene glycol	Synthetic polymer	2	peripheral
Aachen Resonance, Germany	Elutax SV	none	-	2.2	coronary/peripheral
Minvasys, France	Danubio	n-Butyryl tri-n-hexyl citrate	Plasticizer	2.5	coronary
Acotec, China	Orchid	Magnesium stearate	Salt of stearin acid	3	peripheral
B.Braun, Germany	SeQuent Please	Iopromide	X-ray contrast medium	3	coronary
	SeQuent Please OTW	Resveratrol	Antioxidant	3	peripheral
Biotronik, Germany	Pantera Lux	n-Butyryl tri-n-hexyl citrate	Plasticizer	3	coronary
	Passeo Lux	n-Butyryl tri-n-hexyl citrate	Plasticizer	3	peripheral
Cardionovum, Germany	Legflow	Shellac	Varnish	3	peripheral
	Restore	Shellac	Varnish	3	coronary
Spectranetics, USA	AngioSculptX	Nordihydroguaiaretic acid	Antioxidant	3	coronary
QT Vascular, Singapore	Chocolate Touch	undisclosed	-	3	coronary/peripheral
Cook Med., USA	Advance PTX	none		3	peripheral
Eurocor, Germany Biosensors, Switzerland	Dior II, BioStream	Shellac	Varnish	3	coronary
	Freeway	Shellac	Varnish	3	peripheral
iVascular, Spain	Essential	undisclosed	-	3	coronary
	Luminor	undisclosed		3	peripheral
Medtronic Vascular, USA	IN.PACT (Admiral, Pacific, Falcon)	Urea	Endogenous metabolite	3.5	coronary/peripheral

As early as 2007, a paclitaxel-coated balloon catheter, Dior (Eurocor GmbH, Bonn, Germany), received approval in Europe (Conformité Européenne [CE] mark). A study of first-generation Dior balloon catheters reported a tissue paclitaxel concentration of the dilated segment in porcine arteries 1.5 hours after dilation of 1.82 μmol/L (±1.60), which decreased significantly to 0.73 (±0.27; P = .03), 0.62 (±0.34), and 0.44 μmol/L (±0.31) at 12, 24, and 48 hours, respectively.[21] In a direct comparison with the Paccocath balloon, the roughened Dior balloon failed to produce statistically significant effects on angiographic measures of stenosis or morphometric parameters such as maximal neointimal thickness and luminal area. Use of the matrix-coated Paccocath balloon led to a highly significant (P < .01) reduction in all parameters, indicating improved neointimal proliferation compared with both the uncoated control and Dior balloons at 28-day follow-up.[22] Only about 50% of the drug coating was released from the roughened balloons during the recommended balloon inflation time of 45 to 60 seconds. In contrast, the iopromide matrix was found to release the full amount of the drug (4.5% ± 0.7 % of the total paclitaxel dose on balloons after the procedure), which may contribute to its superiority in inhibiting restenosis. The second-generation Dior II balloon is a coronary dilation balloon for human use with a paclitaxel coating of 3.0 μg/mm^2 on the balloon surface, which is applied using a completely different coating technique: the drug is mixed with shellac composed of a network of hydroxy fatty acid esters and sesquiterpene acid esters with a molecular weight of about 1000. The 1:1 mixture of paclitaxel and shellac is coated onto regular balloon catheters. A balloon inflation time dependency study in the porcine model of coronary artery overstretch showed almost maximal tissue paclitaxel concentrations after balloon inflation times of 30 seconds and demonstrated release of 75% of the drug from the balloon surface, which resulted in an up to 20-fold higher tissue concentration compared with the first-generation Dior. Two weeks after overstretch injury, histomorphometry showed significantly smaller neointimal hyperplasia and neointimal thickness in the Dior group compared with the conventional uncoated balloon group. As a result, the area of the coronary artery lumen was larger in the Dior-treated arteries compared with those treated with the conventional balloon (1.20 ± 0.27 mm^2 vs. 0.5 ± 0.22 mm^2, P < .001).[23]

Elutax (Aachen Resonance, Germany) uses pure paclitaxel without a matrix coated on a structured balloon surface, and preclinical data on the Moxy paclitaxel-coated balloon catheter (Lutonix Inc., New Hope, MN) were recently published. It has a paclitaxel dose of 2 μg/mm^2 using polysorbate and sorbitol as excipients, resulting in paclitaxel tissue concentrations of 58.8 ng/mg at 1 hour and 0.3 ng/mg at 30 days. The treated arteries showed a long-term dose-dependent drug effect.[24]

Pantera Lux (Biotronik AG, Berlin, Germany) uses butyryltrihexyl citrate (BTHC) as a carrier for paclitaxel. BTHC is used in different medical devices and cosmetics and is approved for blood contact in blood bags.[25] The same excipient is used with lower paclitaxel doses for the Danubio (Minvasys, Paris, France) and the Ranger DCB (Boston Scientific, Marlborough, MA).

A different, alternative mode of local drug delivery into the target artery segment has been developed using the Genie balloon (Acrostak Corp., Winterthur, Switzerland). Paclitaxel is delivered by a system consisting of a balloon with a distal and proximal occlusive segment and a central segment that allows transfer of paclitaxel to the vessel wall by infusion of paclitaxel solution into the vascular chamber created between the balloons.[26] Preclinical investigations in the coronary arteries of pigs demonstrated that the administration via Genie of 10 μM paclitaxel (Taxol, diluted paclitaxel in a mixture of 50% cremophor and 50% ethanol [2.9 ± 1.6 mL 10 μM paclitaxel in this study equals 24.8 ± 13.7 μg paclitaxel]) markedly reduced LLL (0.9 ±

0.1 mm) compared with controls (2.2 ± 0.2 mm, $P < .001$). The histologic examination showed a statistically significant increase in the lumen area (5.2 ± 1.0 mm^2) and a corresponding decrease in maximal neointimal thickness (0.1 ± 0.01 mm) and neointimal area (1.0 ± 0.1 mm^2) in the stented artery treated with paclitaxel versus the control group (3.0 ± 0.3 mm^2, 0.3 ± 0.04 mm, 2.4 ± 0.2 mm^2).[25] These preclinical results suggest that a solid form (crystalline or amorphous) of paclitaxel is not a requisite for effectiveness.

Preclinical data with a paclitaxel-coated scoring balloon (AngioScore, Fremont, CA) showed increased luminal areas of 6.8 (±1.6) mm^2 compared with uncoated scoring balloons (2.3 ± 1.5 mm^2; $P = .001$).[27] This concept of drug-coated specialty balloons dedicated to plaque modification may allow for better initial lumen gain and a reduced risk of dissections, leading to less stent usage.

Paclitaxel is a suitable drug for balloon coating due to its irreversible binding to the microtubes[28] resulting in long persistence in the vascular cells[10,17] and favorable cell-specific effects.[29] Sirolimus and its analogues reversibly bind to FKBP 12, forming a complex with the mammalian target of rapamycin (mTOR), thus blocking cell cycle progression at the juncture of the G1 and S phases.[30] In the case of DES, sirolimus must be released for a period of several weeks for effective inhibition of neointimal proliferation.[31]

Balloon-based delivery of sirolimus should also include some kind of delayed release technology to overcome this reversible binding. Few studies have indicated neointimal inhibition by limus-coated balloons in animals,[32] especially for zotarolimus.[33,34] Different sirolimus coatings on balloons showed a rapid decrease of tissue concentration.[32,35] In contrast, a crystalline sirolimus coating was associated with persistent vessel concentrations of up to 50% of the initial concentration at 1 month.[36] First clinical evidence was reported from 50 patients with ISR treated with sirolimus in a liquid formulation delivered by a porous balloon (Sirolimus Angioplasty Balloon for Coronary In-Stent Restenosis [SABRE] trial). In this patient population, in-segment LLL at 6 months was 0.31 ± 0.52 mm.[37]

CLINICAL DATA ON DRUG-COATED BALLOONS

At the time of this publication, three DCB devices have been approved for human use in the United States. In Europe, regulatory approval currently exists for several coronary and peripheral devices. In spite of multiple device approvals, there is a comparative paucity of data in the literature regarding the clinical safety and utility of DCBs as a standalone therapy or in combination with other modalities. The use of DCBs in combination with BMSs or debulking devices has both positive and negative potential: the potential for a better, more secure initial patency comes with questions of efficacy, given the potential for edge effect, geographic miss, and safety.

Human Pharmacokinetics of Current Drug-Coated-Balloon Technology

Data on the current first generation of DCBs suggest that the amount of drug delivered by the coated balloon to the vessel wall is a minor fraction of the total dose loaded and that the majority of the drug is distributed into the bloodstream either before or during balloon inflation. Therefore, defining the possible systemic dose of drug delivered with this technology is important, especially given the requirement to use larger, longer, and possibly multiple coated balloons in certain peripheral vascular applications. In a pharmacokinetic study,[38] 14 patients treated at two sites for femoropopliteal disease with DCB had blood sampling at multiple time intervals before and after treatment with balloons ranging up to 10 cm, with monitoring of vital signs and electrocardiography (ECG) analysis, which demonstrated no untoward effects. Mean blood levels of paclitaxel in the immediate postintervention phase were roughly an order of magnitude less than the mean chemotherapeutic levels, and blood levels at 2 hours in more than half the samples were below the lower limit of quantification. Although the study was small, with a considerable heterogeneity of both patients and balloon sizes, a reasonable safety margin of systemic paclitaxel was demonstrated. Still to be determined is what, if any, systemic effects the use of longer or multiple balloons in more extensive SFA disease will have.

Data From the Coronary Application of Drug-Coated Balloons

Although a DES is overwhelmingly the device of choice for most coronary lesions, and their efficacy and safety continue to improve to remarkable degrees, specific challenges remain to their delivery and use in specific coronary territories such as bifurcations, small vessels, saphenous vein grafts, long lesions, and diabetic disease, all of which have less robust outcomes with DES use than do simpler lesions. In addition, the current need for prolonged DAPT can be clinically challenging for some patients with medication intolerance or bleeding tendencies. Although improved antiplatelet medication duration appears to be shortening and is also available to address the possible consequences for those patients who do not respond to clopidogrel, antiplatelet efficacy is often traded for increased bleeding risk. DCBs have the potential to improve outcomes for difficult vascular stent territories with a more limited duration of DAPT.

Although all of the mechanisms of DCB efficacy have yet to be determined, several randomized clinical studies suggest the efficacy of the technology in both coronary and peripheral territories. However, it is important to note that not all DCBs have the same formulation, and this can have implications for clinical effectiveness.[22] In the following discussion of clinical trial results, specifics as to the formulations used are designated for the DCB tested to the extent that they are known.

Coronary In-Stent Restenosis

DCB use in humans was first described in a 2006 publication.[39] In this multicenter study, 52 patients with coronary ISR were randomized to receive angioplasty with either an uncoated balloon or a 3-µg/mm^2 iopromide-paclitaxel–coated balloon (Paccocath); aspirin and clopidogrel were given for 1 month, followed by aspirin alone. Baseline demographics, angiography, and short-term procedural outcomes were not different between the two groups. As determined by angiography at 6 months, the Paccocath group demonstrated a clear advantage in the primary end point of less in-segment LLL (0.74 ± 0.86 vs. 0.03 ± 0.48 mm; $P = .002$), as well as in the 6-month secondary end points of MLD and binary restenosis. An additional 56 patients with coronary ISR were randomized, and the combined cohort of 108 patients was followed for 5 years.[40] The primary end point of 6-month angiographic in-segment LLL was similar to that in the original report, with in-segment binary restenosis of only 6% for the DCB group compared with 51% for the standard balloon group; no differential effects were found by gender or diabetes mellitus. Further, a sustained clinical effect of Paccocath was noted up to 5 years, as manifested by a significant reduction in target-lesion revascularization (TLR); no subacute thrombosis or other safety issues were seen in the DCB group.[41] Another group of investigators initiated a series of studies called PEPCAD (Paclitaxel-Eluting PTCA Catheter in Coronary Disease) to test the same DCB Paccocath formulation (SeQuent Please, licensed by B. Braun) using a variety of coronary therapy comparisons. PEPCAD II was a multicenter, randomized trial of the SeQuent Please DCB versus the Taxus Liberté DES in 131 patients with coronary

ISR.[42] In the two groups of patients with reference vessels averaging 3.0 mm in diameter, the primary end point of 6-month in-segment LLL was significantly less with the DCB compared with the DES (0.17 ± 0.42 vs. 0.38 ± 0.61 mm; $P = .03$). At 12 months, TLR trended in favor of the DCB (6% vs. 15%; $P = 0.15$), suggesting that the DCB was at least as effective as the DES for coronary ISR and without the need for repeat stent implantation.[42,43] Subsequently, eight randomized trials have been published studying the SeQuent Please DCB in BMS ISR[41,42,44] and DES ISR.[45–49] Based on these trials, the 2014 European Society of Cardiology (ESC)/European Association for Cardio-Thoracic Surgery (EACTS) guidelines on myocardial revascularization state, with a class I level A recommendation, that DCBs are recommended for the treatment of ISR (within a BMS or DES).[50]

Later, the original "Paccocath" coating was improved for coronary use (SeQuent Please; B.Braun) and studied in different clinical trials[39,42,45,47–49,51–54] leading to a class I level A recommendation for the treatment of coronary ISR in the 2014 European guidelines.[50]

In contrast to other randomized studies, the Spanish RIBS IV trial showed a significant advantage of everolimus-DES (EES) versus DCB for the treatment of DES ISR in angiographic end points and TLR.[53] However, DCB treatment avoids several layers of metal,[55] reduces the need for prolonged DAPT therapy, allows for repeatability of the procedure,[56] and could positively influence hard clinical end points on longer follow-up.[57,58] For example, after 3 years in ISAR DESIRE 3 (Intracoronary Stenting or Angioplasty for Restenosis Reduction - Drug-Eluting Stents for In-Stent Restenosis), the hazard ratio for overall mortality was 0.38 (6.0% vs. 15.3%; $P = .02$) and 0.27 for cardiac mortality ($P = .03$) in favor of DCB versus first-generation DES in the treatment of DES-ISR. Important to note, this benefit was not related to reintervention rates.[57] This finding might be explained by an elevated stent thrombosis risk with multiple layers of DES.[59]

Lesion preparation before DCB use is mandatory to assure sufficient initial lumen gain. Because it is hard to achieve stent-like results with balloon angioplasty alone, the German DCB consensus group proposed the term "acceptable result" after lesion preparation. Acceptable results exclude flow-limiting dissections (type A and B are allowed), a reduced thrombolysis in myocardial infarction (TIMI) flow, and a diameter stenosis of more than 30%. If the requirements of an acceptable result are fulfilled, "DCB-only" seems to be feasible[60] and is associated with a significant reduction of TLR at 1 year compared to an angioplasty-only result.[61] Lesion preparation with scoring balloons before DCB may further improve angiographic outcomes.[62] Drug-coated scoring balloons could improve lumen gain and facilitate drug transfer.[63]

Coronary De Novo Disease

Initial concepts for the use of DCB in de novo coronary disease included the combination with a BMS to create a "polymer-free" DES. However, results from the PEPCAD III trial to compare such a BMS-DCB combination with the Cypher sirolimus-eluting stent (Cordis/Johnson & Johnson, Miami Lakes, FL) revealed this concept as an inferior approach. The primary angiographic end point of 9-month in-stent LLL was significantly better for the DES compared with the BMS-DCB combination (0.16 ± 0.39 vs. 0.41 ± 0.51 mm; $P = .001$), although there was less difference for in-segment LLL. The 9-month clinical efficacy end points of TLR and target-vessel revascularization (TVR) favored the DES approach; however, the difference in total major adverse cardiovascular events (MACEs) was not significant (15% vs. 18%).[64,65] Other approaches that combined BMS and DCB as standalone devices in the same lesion also failed.[66–69] These results have been partially explained by suboptimal percutaneous coronary intervention (PCI) technique and inferior DCB coatings.[22,70] Nevertheless, even with optimized PCI technique and mature coatings, no benefit was found compared with current-generation DESs.[71,72] A Prospective, Randomized Trial Evaluating a Paclitaxel-Eluting Balloon in Patients Treated With Endothelial Progenitor Cell Capturing Stents for De Novo Coronary Artery Disease (PERfECT STENT)[72] randomized 120 patients with implantation of the CD34 antibody–coated Genous stent (OrbusNeich, Hong Kong). In-segment LLL was reduced from 0.61 mm to 0.16 mm by postdilation with a longer SeQuent Please DCB ($P < .001$). Furthermore, binary restenosis (23.2% vs. 5.1%), TLR (15.5% vs. 4.8%), and MACE (17.2% vs. 4.8%) were significantly less frequent.

PEPCAD I was a nonrandomized study that investigated the safety and efficacy of the SeQuent Please DCB with provisional BMS implantation in small-vessel (mean reference vessel diameter, 2.36 mm) de novo lesions in 120 patients.[73] At the 6-month follow-up, in-segment LLL was significantly less with DCB alone compared with DCB plus a stent (0.18 and 0.73 mm, respectively); the majority of the restenosis was noted at the stent edges, ostensibly where DCB coverage was inadequate. Although this trial was not adequately powered to assess stent thrombosis, vessel thrombosis occurred less frequently in the DCB-alone group despite a shorter duration of DAPT (1 vs. 3 months). In patients with additional BMS implantation, geographic mismatch between coated-balloon dilation and stent implantation was frequently associated with the occurrence of restenosis.[64,74]

As a consequence of these findings, a DCB-only strategy has been proposed that includes a rigorous approach to establish the concept of leaving nothing behind. It includes careful lesion preparation with a balloon/vessel ratio of 0.8:1.0. Depending on the result after predilation, the operator can decide whether to proceed with the DCB only, if there is an acceptable angiographic result, or use a stent or scaffold in case of a major dissection (type C or higher), significant residual stenosis, or reduced flow. The strengths of this concept include a low need for stent implantation and a shortening of DAPT (4 weeks in DCB standalone procedures).[60,75]

This strategy has been investigated successfully in two large registries[51,76] and in the randomized Balloon Elution and Late Loss Optimization (BELLO) study,[77] in which 182 patients with small coronary vessel disease were treated with either an In.Pact Falcon balloon, applying the DCB-only approach, or with a Taxus stent. The primary end point, LLL at 6 months, was significantly lower in the DCB arm (0.08 ± 0.38 mm vs. 0.29 ± 0.44 mm; $P = .001$), demonstrating superiority of the DCB-only approach over DES implantation in terms of angiographic end points.

A recently published propensity score matched comparison in small vessel disease (SVD) indicated similar clinical outcomes of DCB when compared with EES (MACE rate at 1 year 12.2% with DCB and 15.4% with EES).[78] Lesion preparation before DCB in SVD with a scoring balloon (NSE Alpha, Nipro, Japan), leads to significantly larger MLD postintervention and a significant reduction of bailout stenting or a residual stenosis of more than 50%.[79] A small randomized study that compared a scoring balloon followed by DCB versus EES showed no difference in angiographic outcomes at 6 months. Target lesion reintervention was 0 after scoring balloon + DCB versus 6% with EES ($P = NS$).[80] Patient inclusion in the large-scale randomized Basel Stent Kosten Effektivitäts Trial Drug Eluting Balloons vs. Drug Eluting Stents in Small Vessel Interventions (BASKET SMALL 2) trial comparing EES with DCB in SVD was completed in February 2017 [https://clinicaltrials.gov/ct2/show/NCT01574534]; the primary clinical end point at 1 year will be presented in 2018.

The role of DCB in bifurcations may be a pluralistic approach with DCB-only in main and side branch[81] or a limus-DES in the main branch and DCB in the side branch. Two randomized studies showed a significant reduction of LLL and binary restenosis in the side branch by DCB (primary end point LLL in PEPCAD-BIF 0.13 mm in the DCB vs. 0.51 mm in the conventional balloon group; $P = .013$).[82,83]

Clinical Data From the Peripheral Vascular Application of Drug-Coated Balloons

There are a variety of vascular beds for which the DCB technology could be applied, but the focus has largely been on the femoropopliteal and, more recently, the infrapopliteal territories. These vascular territories are the most relevant, with the greatest demonstrated need for reduced restenosis rates. The contiguous SFA and popliteal artery (femoropopliteal) are responsible for most lifestyle-limiting claudication. Taken together, these vessels are the longest nonaortic conduits in the body (at times >300 mm in length) and carry a significant atherosclerotic burden; they are often significantly calcified and chronically occluded throughout their length. As important as their biologic descriptors are their physical ones: the vessel is subject not only to the potential for external compression but also other complex forces during hip and knee flexion (bending, torsion, and axial elongation/shortening). Balloon angioplasty has proved to be inferior to stent implantation for moderate-length lesions (<13 cm),[84,85] but 1-year patency rates even with stents are still suboptimal at 63% and are worse for longer lesions. Until recently, DESs have not proved to be effective in reducing restenosis in the femoropopliteal territory; at least two trials with self-expanding nitinol stents coated with either sirolimus[86] or everolimus using a durable polymer failed to show efficacy.[87] However, a third trial evaluated the Zilver PTX stent, which uses paclitaxel without a polymer, and demonstrated effectiveness compared with angioplasty alone (percutaneous transluminal angioplasty [PTA]) and BMS, but in a relatively constrained (~5- to 6-cm) lesion length.[88] Many involved in this field believe that among the explanations for the failure to date of most of the attempts at DES placement in the femoropopliteal region is the tendency for stents to fracture because of the forces mentioned earlier; this appeared to be associated with restenosis in an early nonrandomized analysis,[89] the ongoing irritant of a rigid stent interacting with a vessel constantly in motion, and the lack of the correct "formula" of drug dose and duration when accounting for stent provocation of intimal hyperplasia in this unique vessel. However, the 24-month patency data for the Zilver PTX treatment cohort did show a durable effect with this device.[88]

The development of DCB technology holds the promise of improved outcomes without a permanent stent prosthesis. The first human examination of a DCB in a noncoronary territory was the Local Taxane With Short Exposure for Reduction of Restenosis in Distal Arteries (THUNDER) trial, a multicenter European study. This study involved the three-way randomization of 154 patients with lesions of the femoropopliteal segment to standard balloon angioplasty (control), an iopromide-paclitaxel–coated (3 µg/mm², Paccocath) balloon, or to paclitaxel mixed with iopromide contrast (0.171 mg/cm³) and used for a standard balloon procedure up to a maximum dose of 17.1 mg.[90] With a moderate mean lesion length of about 7.5 cm, a marked reduction was seen in the iopromide-paclitaxel balloon group for the primary end point of 6-month angiographic LLL compared with both the control balloon and paclitaxel in contrast groups (0.4 ± 1.2 vs. 1.7 ± 1.8 vs. 2.2 ± 1.6 mm; $P < .001$ for DCB vs. control). TLR at 6 months was reduced in the DCB group compared with the control group (4% vs. 29%; $P = .001$); again, no effect was seen with the paclitaxel and contrast groups (29%; $P = .41$). Notably, vis-à-vis the prior DES concerns, the comparative benefits of DCBs were sustained at 24-month and 5-year follow-ups.[91] A second study using the same coating technology produced remarkably similar results. In the Femoral-Paclitaxel (Fem-Pac)[92] trial, 87 patients underwent 1:1 randomization between control balloon angioplasty and iopromide-paclitaxel–coated balloon angioplasty in relatively short (~6 cm) lesions in the femoropopliteal arteries. For the primary end point of LLL, the coated balloon arm showed results that were superior to those of the control balloon at 6 months (0.5 ± 1.1 vs. 1.0 ± 1.1 mm; $P = .031$), with significantly fewer TLR events (6.7% vs. 33%; $P = .002$); this difference in TLR was sustained beyond 18 months. Of note, no safety issues related to the balloon coating were manifest in either study.

In the Lutonix Paclitaxel-Coated Balloon for the Prevention of Femoropopliteal Restenosis (LEVANT I)[93] study, 101 patients with femoropopliteal disease were assigned to either a balloon-only strategy or a stent-assisted strategy if it was felt that a bail-out stent would be required after initial PTA predilation. Thereafter, each group was randomized to treatment with either the Lutonix DCB coated with 2 µg/mm² paclitaxel and a polysorbate/sorbitol carrier or standard PTA balloon. With a reasonable mean lesion length of about 8 cm, at 6 months, the DCB groups—both PTA and stent—demonstrated significantly better primary end point LLL compared with that of the PTA group (0.46 ± 1.13 mm vs. 1.09 ± 1.07 mm; $P = .016$).

In the United States, 543 patients were enrolled in the Lutonix/Bard LEVANT II pivotal trial aimed at U.S. Food and Drug Administration (FDA) approval; in this trial, 476 subjects were randomized 2:1 to Lutonix DCB ($n = 316$) and PTA ($n = 160$). Target lesion length was 6.1 cm, including 21% total occlusions. At 1 year, freedom from the primary safety end point—perioperative death, index limb amputation or reintervention, or limb-related death—was 84% for DCB and 79% for PTA ($P = .005$ intention to treat [ITT]; $P = .08$ per protocol). Primary patency (freedom from target lesion binary restenosis defined by Doppler ultrasound plus TLR) was 65.2% for DCB and 52.6% for PTA ($P = .015$ ITT; $P = .11$ per protocol). Of interest, no difference in target lesion reintervention was observed at 1 year (38.0% vs. 37.5%; $P = .5$).[94]

In the Paclitaxel-Coated Balloons in Femoral Indication to Defeat Restenosis (PACIFIER) trial,[95] patients with symptomatic femoropopliteal atherosclerotic disease were randomized to In.Pact Pacific or uncoated balloons ($n = 91$). Average lesion length was 7.0 (±5.3) and 6.6 (±5.5) cm for DCB and control arms, respectively. At 6 months, LLL was –0.01 mm for DCB versus 0.65 mm for PTA ($P = .001$) with fewer binary restenoses (9% vs. 32%) and fewer major adverse events (7% vs. 35%).

In the Invatec/Medtronic In.Pact SFA trial aiming for FDA approval, 331 patients with claudication or rest pain due to superficial femoral lesions were enrolled with a mean lesion length of 8.9 cm (150 subjects at 13 European centers and 181 subjects at 44 U.S. sites). At 1 year, the DCB group was superior to PTA in terms of primary patency (82% vs. 54%), clinically driven TLR (2.4% vs. 21%), primary sustained clinical improvement (upgrade in Rutherford classification ≥1 class in amputation- and TVR-free surviving patients; 85% vs. 69%), primary safety end point (freedom from 30-day device- and procedure-related death and from target limb major amputation and clinically driven TVR through 12 months; 96% vs. 77%), and MACE (death, clinically driven TVR, target limb major amputation, and thrombosis; 6% vs. 24%).[91] At 2[96] and 3 years a sustained benefit with regard to primary patency and clinically driven TLR was reported. Other randomized studies confirmed those results including treatment of restenotic lesions.[97]

Although differences in outcomes between these two pivotal femoropopliteal trials are apparent, differences in patient and lesion complexity, end point determination and time point of reporting, effects of evaluator blinding, and so on, make direct comparison between trials problematic and should be taken with some circumspection.

Below-the-knee (BTK) intervention in patients with critical limb ischemia has been studied in small, single-center studies with and without randomization, all of which appeared to demonstrate benefit in terms of patency and/or TLR.[98,99] However a well-done large, multicenter, randomized, controlled European effort—the Invatec/Medtronic Study of IN.PACT Amphiron Drug-Eluting Balloon Versus Standard PTA for the Treatment of Below-the-Knee Critical Limb Ischemia (IN.PACT DEEP) trial[100]—failed to show a beneficial drug effect. Although there were some baseline differences in lesion length (favoring DCB), impaired inflow (favoring PTA), and prior target limb revascularization (favoring PTA), the groups appeared to be reasonably similar. The primary efficacy end points of clinically driven TLR (9.2% vs. 13.1%; P = NS) and LLL (0.61 ± 0.78 vs. 0.62 ± 0.78; P = NS) were no different between DCB and PTA. However, a small difference was reported in the primary safety end point (17.7% vs. 15.8%; P = .021), driven primarily by more frequent major amputations in the DCB arm (8.8% vs. 3.6%; P = .080). As a result of the outcomes in this trial, the In.Pact Deep DCB was voluntarily removed from the market in 2013. There is another trial in this population currently recruiting subjects by Lutonix/Bard in the United States. Until these results are known, the efficacy and safety of DCBs in infrapopliteal disease will remain speculative, as will the causes of the failure of In.Pact Deep.

THE FUTURE OF DRUG-COATED-BALLOON TECHNOLOGY

Although some data support the efficacy of DCBs in both the coronary and peripheral circulations, some of the coronary trial outcomes have been less than robust. It is becoming clearer that it is not only the specific coating formulation that is important in clinical efficacy but also the interaction of the DCB and newly implanted stents, which is still not well understood. Most of the current efforts in DCB development are focused on addressing the potential limitations of the technology. The safety and efficacy of these technologies in certain applications—such as overlapping balloons, visceral vessel applications, and in use with adjunctive therapies, including atherectomy and stents—need to be assessed. Notably, the risk of particulate embolization of the coating and any unintended effects need to be better elucidated, especially in visceral applications. In addition, as the mechanism of action of DCBs becomes better understood, the opportunities to modify various aspects of the technology will increase, including improvements in the antiproliferative agents used, which in combination with different carrier molecules might further extend the tissue residence of the agents and result in more directed deposition of drug into the vessel, with reduced wash-off and distal embolization. Despite the many devices and manufacturers involved with DCBs, a paucity of large-scale clinical datasets on the safety and effectiveness of this technology remains. Fortunately, multiple clinical studies are either underway or are being planned in the near future in Europe that involve coronary, femoropopliteal, and infrapopliteal applications.

SUMMARY

Both the preclinical and clinical data to date, albeit with some mixed results in selected coronary applications, support the early effectiveness and safety of DCBs in several vascular territories and validate the concept that the balloon delivery of a short burst of an antiproliferative agent to a targeted vessel segment is feasible. At the time of this publication, accepted indications for DCB are the treatment of coronary ISR and the treatment of de novo and restenotic lesions in the SFA.

KEY REFERENCES

 Additional references available online at expertconsult.com.

中文导读

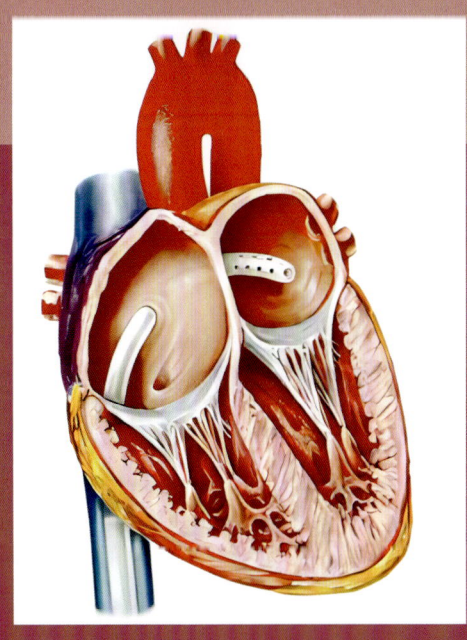

第18章
稳定型心绞痛和无症状性心肌缺血的选择性干预

心绞痛是冠状动脉粥样硬化性心脏病的典型症状。冠状动脉狭窄导致的心肌氧供需不匹配是冠心病相关症状发生的主要机制。冠状动脉粥样硬化病变直径为50%～79%的患者在心肌代谢需求增加时会表现出心肌缺血。无症状性心肌缺血的特征是在没有胸部不适或其他心绞痛症状的情况下，存在心肌缺血的客观证据。

尽管目前尚无治愈缺血性冠心病的方法，但通过利用现有药物、外科手术和冠状动脉介入治疗来改变疾病的进程是可行的策略。冠状动脉缺血的功能评估和临床风险分层工具，使冠心病患者能得到更精准的治疗策略。成功的疾病管理和症状缓解可以通过基于最佳药物治疗和通过饮食及锻炼改变风险因素的方法来实现。经皮冠状动脉介入治疗在改善生活质量和改善预后方面也发挥着重要作用，它可以直接通过减少缺血负担，以及症状控制和提高运动耐量间接有效地改善长期预后。但在卫生保健成本上升和有限资源的经济背景下，制定最适当的血运重建策略，将确保继续为越来越多可能受益的患者提供治疗。

本章详细地介绍了针对稳定型心绞痛及无症状心肌缺血的临床治疗策略，包括最佳药物治疗、经皮冠状动脉介入治疗及冠状动脉旁路移植术等相关研究进展，为临床医师决策提供了证据。

李英凯　柳景华

章节要点

- 慢性心绞痛是一个日益严重的世界性问题，造成了巨大的经济和社会代价。
- 通过减轻缺血负荷，经皮冠状动脉血运重建可为已确诊的阻塞性冠心病患者带来重要的临床获益。最明显的效果是迅速控制症状和提高运动耐量。但在大规模慢性、稳定型冠心病患者中，尚缺乏直接证据可证实介入治疗能改善生存率或明确减少主要心血管事件。对靶病变的生理学评估有助于指导血运重建决策。
- 对于已确诊的冠心病患者和存在冠心病风险的患者，最佳药物治疗是有效治疗的重要组成部分。
- 除了最佳药物治疗，心绞痛的治疗与合并高血压、高脂血症患者一样还应包括改变生活方式、降低心血管风险的药物治疗。戒烟、锻炼和节食是降低这一类人群心血管风险的有效措施。
- 不良事件风险较高的患者，包括左心功能不全、慢性肾病、糖尿病和广泛心肌缺血负荷。对于这些患者，除了最佳药物治疗，血运重建更可能让患者得到显著的预后获益。

18 Elective Intervention for Stable Angina or Silent Ischemia

Gregory W. Barsness, David E. Kandzari, Eliano P. Navarese

KEY POINTS

- Chronic angina is a growing worldwide problem with significant economic and societal costs.
- By reducing the ischemic burden, percutaneous coronary revascularization provides important clinical benefit in patients with established obstructive coronary artery disease (CAD). The foremost effect is prompt symptom control and improved exercise tolerance. Direct evidence for improvement in survival or definitive reduction of major cardiovascular events is lacking in the broad population of patients with chronic, stable symptomatic CAD. Physiologic assessment of the target coronary lesion is useful to guide decisions regarding revascularization.
- Optimal medical therapy (OMT) is an essential component of the successful treatment of patients with established CAD and those at risk.
- Along with OMT, management of angina should include lifestyle changes and pharmacotherapy to reduce cardiovascular risk, including those associated with high blood pressure and elevated lipid levels. Smoking cessation, exercise, and diet are effective measures to reduce cardiovascular risk in this population.
- Patients at elevated risk for adverse events—including those with left ventricular dysfunction, chronic kidney disease, diabetes mellitus, and an extensive ischemic burden—have greater potential for measurable prognostic benefit with revascularization in addition to OMT.

INTRODUCTION

Angina pectoris, caused by episodes of transient myocardial ischemia, is the dominant symptom of chronic ischemic heart disease. It affects approximately 9 million of the 16.3 million people with a diagnosis of coronary artery disease (CAD) in the United States, with 500,000 new cases of angina occurring every year (Figs. 18.1 and 18.2).[1,2] In combating this disease, U.S. physicians performed an estimated 6.8 million inpatient cardiovascular procedures in 2007, an increase of 27% over the previous decade, including approximately 622,000 percutaneous coronary revascularization procedures. Despite this measurable success in addressing established disease, the incidence and costs associated with symptomatic CAD continue to grow throughout the world and contribute an ever-increasing proportion to the overall morbidity, mortality, and lost economic productivity in both developed and developing regions. Revascularization is intuitively central to the treatment paradigm for CAD. The stable CAD population is a heterogeneous group of patients both for clinical presentations and for different underlying mechanisms. A mismatch between myocardial oxygen supply and demand due to a coronary stenosis is the predominant mechanism implicated in the development of symptoms associated with obstructive CAD. Patients with a fixed coronary atherosclerotic lesion of 50% to 79% diameter obstruction (70% to 90% by cross-sectional area measurement) show myocardial ischemia during increased myocardial metabolic demand as the result of a significant reduction in coronary flow reserve. Revascularization is intuitively pivotal to the treatment paradigm for CAD; when associated with clinical or objective evidence of ischemia, it offers the opportunity of symptom management.

The sphere of patients with symptoms or signs of ischemia is broad and may also include those with abnormal coronary endothelial function, coronary vasospasm, microvascular dysfunction, and even asymptomatic myocardial ischemia. In addition, symptoms reminiscent of ischemic angina may be a manifestation of a noncardiovascular process, such as gastrointestinal, musculoskeletal, or neuropsychiatric pathology—in general, anything from the navel to the nose—whereas other patients, especially women and older adults, may present with symptoms such as fatigue, chronic "soreness," or dyspnea, which may not be immediately recognized as an expression of cardiovascular disease (Table 18.1).

In addition to the decrease in myocardial blood supply due to increased coronary resistance in large and small coronary arteries, other causal factors of angina include increased extravascular forces, such as severe left ventricular hypertrophy caused by hypertension, aortic stenosis, or hypertrophic cardiomyopathy, reduction in the oxygen-carrying capacity of blood, such as severe anemia, and other processes (Table 18.2).[3] The pattern of clinical presentation of stable angina is also extremely heterogeneous: patients can be symptomatic for stable angina pectoris, or with a history of obstructive or non-CAD, who have become asymptomatic with treatment and need regular follow-up; alternatively symptoms can be described for the first time, with subjects presenting already in a chronic stable condition. The typical episode of angina pectoris starts gradually and reaches its maximum intensity over a time frame of minutes. Angina pectoris is usually aggravated by exertion or emotional stress and is relieved within minutes by rest or nitroglycerin. The location pattern is predominantly substernal and radiation may occur to the neck, jaw, arms, back, or epigastrium. Isolated epigastric discomfort or pain in the lower mandible may rarely be a symptom of myocardial ischemia or fatigue may occur. Individuals with significant ischemia may also remain apparently unaffected by symptoms because of self-regulation of activity, essentially avoiding activities that have previously caused discomfort. Careful attention to individual patient presentation and characteristics, then, is essential for proper diagnostic triage

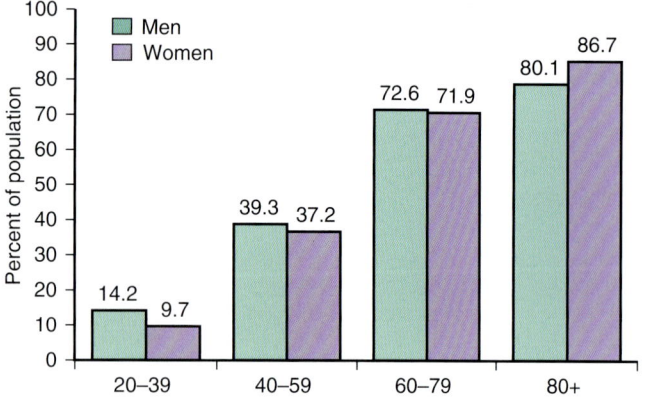

Fig. 18.1 U.S. prevalence of cardiovascular disease by age and sex. Data include coronary disease, heart failure, stroke, and hypertension. (From Roger VL, Go AS, Lloyd-Jones DM, et al. Heart disease and stroke statistics—2011 update: a report from the American Heart Association. *Circulation*. 2011;123[4]:e18–e209.)

TABLE 18.1 Potential Nonischemic Diagnoses in Patients With Chest Pain

NONISCHEMIC CARDIOVASCULAR	
Aortic dissection, pericarditis	
PULMONARY	
Embolus, pneumothorax, pneumonia, pleuritis	
GASTROINTESTINAL	
Esophageal, esophagitis, spasm, reflux, cholecystitis, choledocholithiasis, cholangitis, peptic ulcer, pancreatitis	
CHEST WALL	
Costochondritis, fibrositis, rib fracture, sternoclavicular arthritis, biliary herpes zoster	
PSYCHIATRIC	
Anxiety, hyperventilation, panic disorder, affective disorders, somatoform disorder	

From Gibbons RJ, Abrams J, Chatterjee K, et al. ACC/AHA 2002 guideline update for the management of patients with chronic stable angina: a report of the American College of Cardiology/American Heart Association Task Force on Practice Guidelines (Committee to Update the 1999 Guidelines for the Management of Patients with Chronic Stable Angina). *Circulation*. 2003;107:149–158.

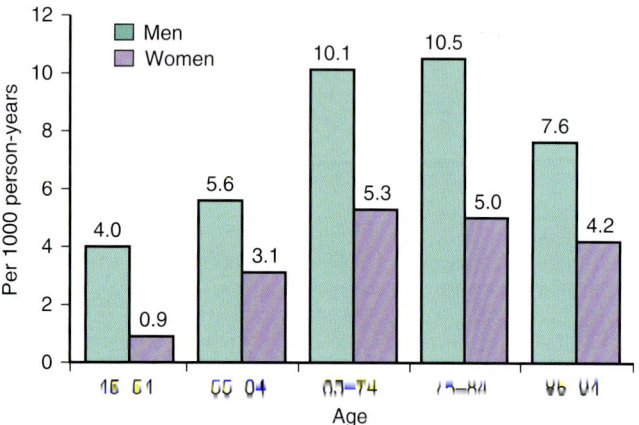

Fig. 18.2 Incidence of stable angina pectoris from the Framingham Heart Study (1980 to 2003) stratified by age and sex. (From Roger VL, Go AS, Lloyd-Jones DM, et al. Heart Disease and Stroke Statistics—2011 update: a report from the American Heart Association. *Circulation*. 2011;123[4]:e18–e209.)

TABLE 18.2 Ischemic Provocation or Exacerbating Factors

Increased Oxygen Demand	Decreased Oxygen Supply
NONCARDIAC CONDITIONS	
Hyperthermia	Anemia
Hyperthyroidism	Hypoxemia
Sympathomimetic toxicity (e.g., from cocaine)	Sickle cell disease
	Sympathomimetic toxicity
Hypertension	Hyperviscosity
Anxiety	Polycythemia
Arteriovenous fistula	
CARDIAC CONDITIONS	
Hypertrophic cardiomyopathy	Hypertrophic cardiomyopathy
Aortic stenosis	Aortic stenosis
Dilated cardiomyopathy	
Tachycardia	

From Gibbons RJ, Abrams J, Chatterjee K, et al. ACC/AHA 2002 guideline update for the management of patients with chronic stable angina: a report of the American College of Cardiology/American Heart Association Task Force on Practice Guidelines (Committee to Update the 1999 Guidelines for the Management of Patients with Chronic Stable Angina). *Circulation*. 2003;107:149–158.

and management. Once recognized, the goals and methods of treatment include reduction in both morbidity and mortality, although anticipated benefits depend on patient characteristics and the treatment modality used.

Percutaneous revascularization has, as its principal benefit, the relief of angina. Symptom relief is the direct effect of a reduction in ischemic burden, although additional complex factors no doubt play a role, especially in the setting of residual disease or incomplete abrogation of ischemia (Fig. 18.3).[4] Whereas improved survival and reduction of major cardiovascular events are important therapeutic objectives, limited data are available to support a major role for percutaneous revascularization in reducing adverse events in the broader population of patients with stable ischemic coronary disease (Fig. 18.4).[5] A clear survival advantage for revascularization over optimal medical therapy (OMT) in patients undergoing surgical revascularization with coronary artery bypass grafting (CABG) was found to occur in patients at high clinical or anatomical risk, based on location and severity of the lesion, the number of diseased vessels, and the presence of left ventricular dysfunction. Specifically, high-risk features associated with survival benefits following surgical revascularizations include symptomatic triple-vessel disease, concomitant left ventricular dysfunction; survival improvement is possible since the surgical intervention can modify the ischemic burden of a large amount of myocardium supplied by the diseased vessel(s) or the significant associated underlying left ventricular dysfunction.[5] The survival advantage of revascularization strategies over OMT in patients with CAD and reduced ejection fraction has been confirmed in a recent meta-analysis of current evidence (Fig. 18.5).[6]

REVASCULARIZATION IN PATIENTS WITH CHRONIC STABLE ANGINA

The principles and practice of modern coronary revascularization strategies are rooted in the conduct and results of studies performed in the 1970s and 1980s. These historic investigations set the framework for our current understanding of the role of both surgical and percutaneous coronary intervention (PCI) in the treatment armamentarium of chronic symptomatic ischemic CAD. Whereas these studies provided important insight into the outcome of revascularization and medical therapy using the methodology of the time, great strides have subsequently been made in all areas of treatment, thus decreasing the applicability of these trials to guide therapy in the prevailing health care environment. Today, OMT has been clearly established as the cornerstone of treatment for CAD. The impact of medical therapy has grown with the introduction of advanced antiplatelet therapy, statins, and angiotensin-converting enzyme (ACE) and receptor inhibition, among other established and evolving therapies, such as ranolazine, which diminishes myocardial ischemia by reducing calcium overload caused by inhibition of the late sodium current.[7] Indeed, correct application of evidence-based therapy has had important societal health implications, with a resultant measurable reduction in adverse cardiac events over the past several decades. Although appropriate revascularization in patients with chronic angina contributed an estimated 5% to this observed reduction in cardiac mortality between 1980 and 2002, a much larger 50% of the total reduction is attributed to improvement in the risk-factor profiles of those populations in jeopardy, largely thanks to improved agents and the greater application of this medical therapy.[2] Whereas PCI is an important adjunct for symptom control and has established value in reducing both subsequent morbidity and mortality after acute coronary syndromes (ACSs), both PCI and surgical revascularization are not curative, and lesion progression accounts for significant recurrent morbidity. Recent studies demonstrate the impact of lesion progression and the need for aggressive concomitant medical therapy in the setting of PCI. Park and colleagues[8] retrospectively studied 507 patients who underwent PCI and found that 16% of them underwent clinically driven repeat PCI to treat preexisting nonculprit coronary lesions during the 3-year study period. During the first year after initial PCI, 7.7% of patients in this cohort underwent nonculprit lesion PCI, with the rate increasing to 16% at 3 years. Greater extent of disease, as manifest by a larger baseline number of significant coronary lesions, independently predicted repeat PCI (odds ratio [OR], 2.29; 95% confidence interval [CI] 1.5 to 3.5; $P < .001$), as did the baseline risk factors of low levels of high-density lipoprotein (<40 mg/dL; OR, 2.01; 95% CI 1.01 to 3.98; $P = .046$), hypercholesterolemia (total cholesterol >200 mg/dL; OR, 1.46; 95% CI 1.22 to 1.97; $P = .04$), history of PCI (OR, 1.24; 95% CI 1.09 to 1.60; $P = .003$), and increased triglyceride levels (OR, 1.003; 95% CI 1.001 to 1.007; $P = .038$). An additional natural history study[9] of patients who underwent intravascular ultrasound evaluation after PCI for an ACS found that fully one-half of major subsequent adverse events at 3 years occurred at nonculprit sites. OMT is complimentary to revascularization with either PCI or CABG; however, it is still underused, particularly after CABG.[10] In the Euro Heart Survey, a significant number of patients with chronic stable angina, managed medically or invasively, were not on OMT, and this was related to worse outcomes.[11] A post hoc analysis of the SYNergy between percutaneous coronary intervention with TAXus and cardiac surgery (SYNTAX) trial has shown that prescription of OMT (combination of at least one antiplatelet drug, statin, β-blocker and ACE inhibitor) was only 41% at the time of discharge after revascularization (PCI or CABG), and at 5 years only one-third patients in both treatment groups were taking OMT

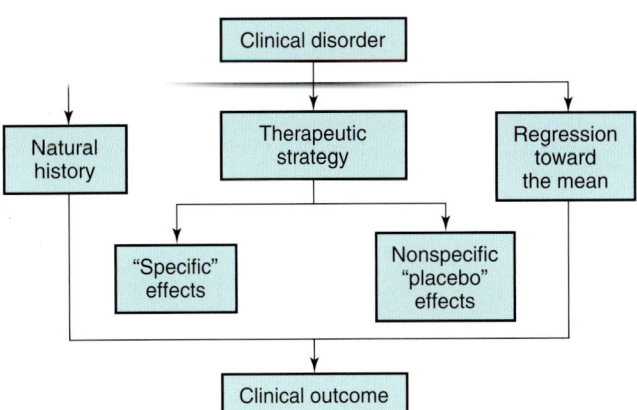

Fig. 18.3 Factors with potential influence on clinical response to treatment. These include *specific intended effects,* such as ischemia reduction after percutaneous coronary intervention, and *nonspecific effects,* often described as "the placebo effect." These effects occur within the context of the natural history of the clinical condition itself, along with the normal "moderation" of effects, or regression toward the mean outcome, that occurs within populations. (Adapted from Bonetti PO, Holmes DR, Lerman A, et al. Enhanced external counterpulsation for ischemic heart disease. What's behind the curtain? *J Am Coll Cardiol*. 2003;41[11]:1918–1925.)

(PCI 40% and CABG 36%).[12] Adequate medical therapy and risk modification are essential in the periinterventional and postinterventional setting to reduce subsequent mortality and morbidity, including symptom recurrence and the need for repeat procedures associated with lesion progression and new lesion development.

Percutaneous Coronary Revascularization: Efficacy on Symptom Improvement

The selection of treatment strategies in patients with chronic stable angina depends on symptom status, anatomic complexity, clinical comorbidity, and risk. The main indications for revascularization are to improve symptoms that persist despite OMT and to improve prognosis. Although they generally suggest a benefit for revascularization, most randomized trials that compare medical therapy with percutaneous revascularization are limited by their historical nature and entry bias. Clinical efficacy studies of PCI in patients with stable CAD have demonstrated an incremental benefit of alleviating angina symptoms over medical therapy. The medicine angioplasty or surgery study (MASS II) trial randomly assigned 611 patients with multivessel disease (MVD), preserved left ventricular systolic function, and stable angina to CABG, PCI (with bare-metal stenting in 72% and without stenting in 28%), or OMT.[13] The primary end point was freedom from all-cause death, myocardial infarction (MI), or refractory angina requiring revascularization. At 1 year, 88% of the patients in the CABG group, 79% in the PCI group, and 46% in the medical therapy group were free of angina ($P < .0001$). In addition, freedom from all-cause death, MI, or refractory angina requiring revascularization was significantly lower with PCI than with medical therapy or CABG (76 vs. 88%–93%, respectively). The central hypothesis is therefore that the benefit from PCI is symptom relief, a concept demonstrated in several trials and confirmed in a meta-analysis[14] of 14 trials that demonstrated a statistically significant benefit in angina relief with PCI compared with medical therapy (OR, 1.69; 95% CI 1.24 to 2.30). Notably, important heterogeneity was found across the trials, with substantially less

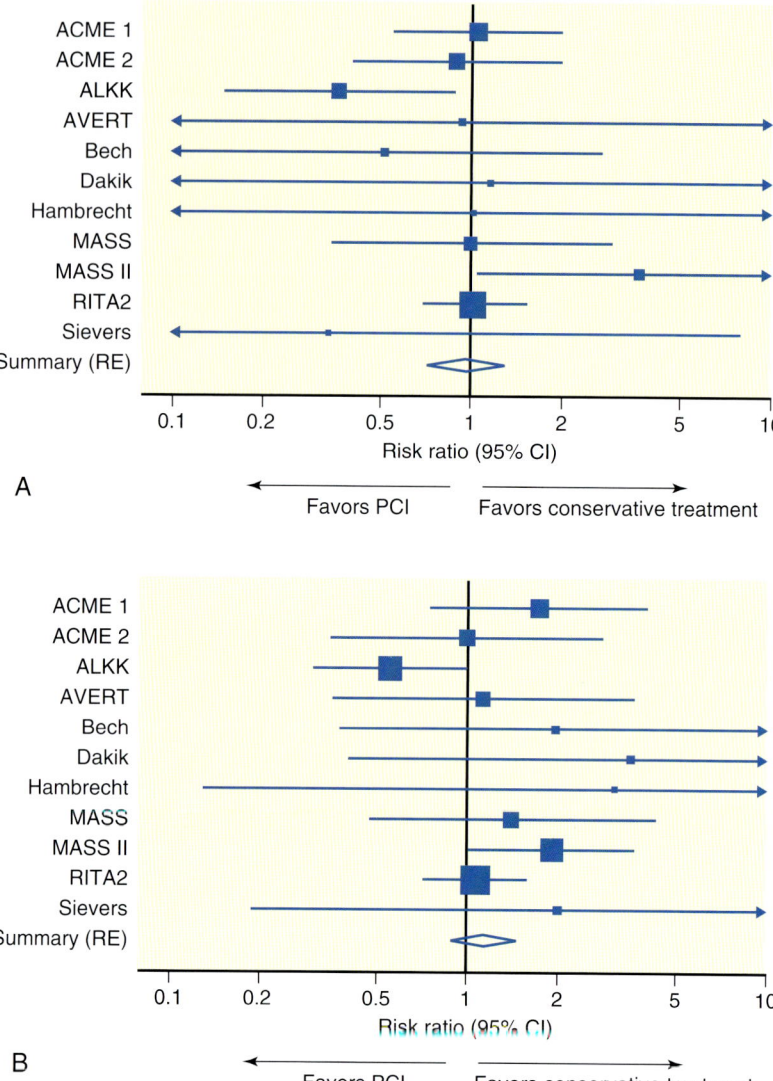

Fig. 18.4 Point estimates, 95% confidence intervals *(CIs)*, and summary statistics in 11 studies that enrolled patients from 1992 to 2001. (A) For risk of all-cause death after treatment with percutaneous coronary intervention *(PCI)* or medical therapy. (B) For risk of cardiac death or myocardial infarction after PCI or medical therapy. (From Katritsis DG, Ioannidis JPA. Percutaneous coronary intervention versus conservative therapy in nonacute coronary artery disease: a meta-analysis. Circulation. 2005;111[22]:2906–2912.)

benefit noted in more contemporary trials of PCI versus OMT, such as the Clinical Outcomes Utilizing Revascularization and Aggressive Drug Evaluation (COURAGE) trial,[15] published in 2007 (OR, 1.10; 95% CI 0.81 to 1.49), and the Occluded Artery Trial (OAT),[16] published in 2006 (OR, 0.83; 95% CI 0.47 to 1.47). Using metaregression analysis of the treatment effects of PCI relative to medical therapy, Wijeysundera and colleagues[14] were able to document an inverse relationship between freedom from angina and the number of "evidence-based" medications utilized during the conduct of a trial (Fig. 18.6). A subgroup analysis of the COURAGE trial[12] confirmed a diminution of angina benefit over time for patients treated with PCI as an initial strategy. Although a statistically significant difference was found in rates of freedom from angina between the OMT-alone and the OMT-plus-PCI groups at 3 months (42% vs. 53%, $P < .001$), this difference was no longer evident at 3 years (56% vs. 59%, $P = .30$). Although potential reasons for this convergence of angina rates during follow-up are numerous and include crossover to revascularization from the medical arm, ascertainment bias due to small follow-up populations, an important finding is that in both groups, patients with the most significant anginal burden at baseline obtained the greatest benefit from PCI. Therefore, for many stable angina patients, especially those unable or unwilling to comply with a rigorous and costly drug regimen, PCI is the more effective long-term therapy. In fact, COURAGE showed that those patients who underwent PCI experienced less chest pain and took fewer medications specifically to treat stable angina symptoms than patients on medication alone. In aggregate, these data support a robust, reliable antianginal benefit for PCI in patients with persistent symptoms despite medical therapy.

The recent percutaneous coronary intervention in stable angina (ORBITA) trial called into question the efficacy of percutaneous revascularization compared to placebo.[17] This was as a double-blind, randomized controlled trial that evaluated PCI versus sham control procedure for improved exercise capacity in patients with severe CAD who were receiving optimum medical therapy.

The investigators enrolled patients with severe (≥70%) single-vessel stenoses who were entered into a 6-week medication optimization phase. Then prior to randomization, patients underwent a cardiopulmonary exercise assessment, symptom questionnaire, and a dobutamine stress echocardiography. The primary end point was incremented in treadmill exercise time between the treatment arms at a follow-up of 6 weeks. A total of 200 patients were randomized (PCI: 105; Placebo: 95). At 6 weeks of follow-up, exercise time increased from baseline by a mean of 28.4 seconds in the PCI group ($P = .001$) and by 11.8 seconds in the sham group ($P = .235$). However, the primary end

Study name	Hazard ratio	Lower limit	Upper limit	Z-Value	P Value
ASAN-MAIN, TCT/JACC 2015	0.86	0.423	1.748	−0.418	.676
CREDO-Kyoto, Am J Cardiol 2014	0.73	0.506	1.044	−1.725	.085
IRIS-MAIN, TCT/JACC 2015	0.74	0.411	1.325	−1.018	.309
Toda et al., Ann Thorac Surg 2002	0.83	0.475	1.437	−0.676	.499
OVERALL	**0.76**	**0.594**	**0.983**	**−2.092**	**.036**

Statistics for each study

A

Study name	Hazard ratio	Lower limit	Upper limit	Z-Value	P Value
Ahn et al., JACC Abstract 2011	0.85	0.462	1.585	−0.522	.602
AWESOME-Registry, Am J Cardiol 2004	1.08	0.809	1.445	0.527	.598
Cleland et al., Eur J Heart Fail 2011	1.13	0.413	3.063	0.230	.818
CREDO-Kyoto, Am J Cardiol 2014	0.73	0.506	1.044	−1.725	.085
Gioia et al., Cath Cardiovasc Int 2007	1.39	0.604	3.205	0.776	.438
Nagendran et al., Ann Thorac Surg 2013	0.92	0.792	1.060	−1.173	.241
Toda et al., Ann Thorac Surg 2002	0.83	0.475	1.437	−0.676	.499
OVERALL	**0.92**	**0.821**	**1.035**	**−1.376**	**.169**

Statistics for each study

B

Study name	Hazard ratio	Lower limit	Upper limit	Z-Value	P Value
Ahn et al., JACC Abstract 2011	0.85	0.462	1.565	−0.522	.602
Bangalore et al., NEJM 2015	0.90	0.599	1.353	−0.507	.612
CREDO-Kyoto, Am J Cardiol 2014	0.64	0.390	1.050	−1.766	.077
Gioia et al ., Cath Cardiovasc Int 2007	1.38	0.602	3.142	0.755	.450
Hannan et al., NEJM 2008	0.77	0.591	1.002	−1.942	.052
Yang et al., Am J Cardiol 2013	0.88	0.621	1.191	−0.907	.365
OVERALL	**0.82**	**0.696**	**0.963**	**−2.415**	**.016**

Statistics for each study

C

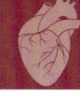

Fig. 18.5 Individual and summary hazard ratios for mortality of studies stratified by treatment comparison: (A) coronary artery bypass grafting *(CABG)* versus optimal medical treatment (OMT); (B) percutaneous coronary intervention *(PCI)* versus OMT; and (C) CABG versus PCI. (From Wolff G, Dimitroulis D, Andreotti F, et al. Survival benefits of invasive versus conservative strategies in heart failure in patients with reduced ejection fraction and coronary artery disease: a meta-analysis. *Circ Heart Fail*. 2017;10[1]:e003255.)

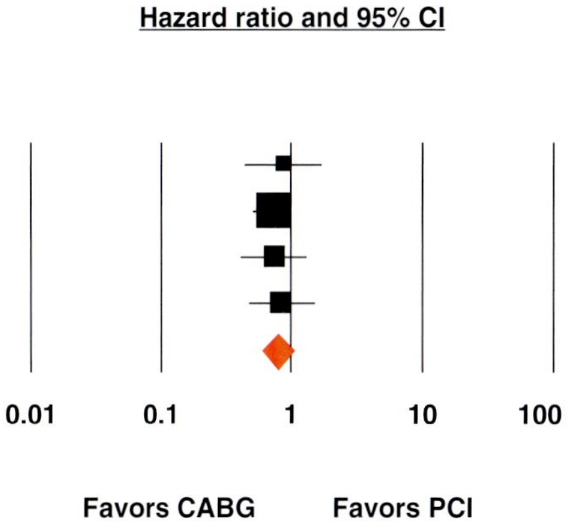

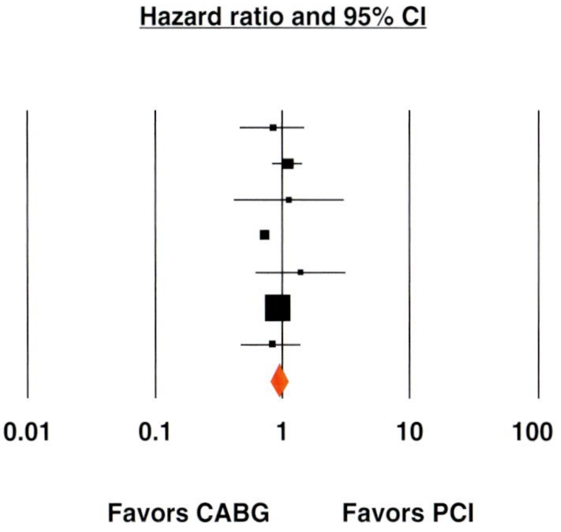

point of between-group change in exercise time based on a conservative estimate of 30 seconds was not significant: +16.6 seconds (P = .200). PCI was associated with a significant reduction in ischemia, assessed by dobutamine stress echocardiography change in wall-motion stress index (P = .0011). Although both groups had improved outcomes, there was no between-group difference in Seattle Angina Questionnaire angina frequency or physical-limitation scores or in quality of life. At enrollment, 98% of patients had Canadian Cardiovascular Society (CCS) class II or III angina, but by randomization 9% of PCI patients and 14% of sham patients were free of angina, improving at follow-up to 39% and 29%, respectively. The findings of the ORBITA study are in line with what was observed in the COURAGE trial, reinforcing the role of OMT in stable angina. These results raised the question of whether PCI is associated with any incremental improvement in angina relief compared with OMT. These negative findings associated with PCI should, however, be viewed with caution and might be explained by the lower risk profile of the enrolled patients who had very good functional capacity, infrequent angina, and a low burden

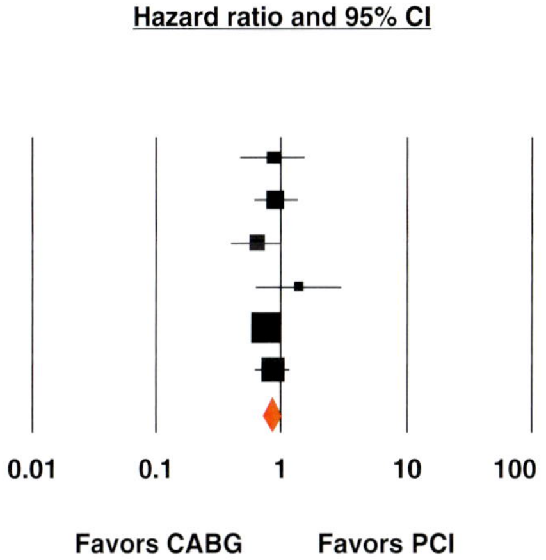

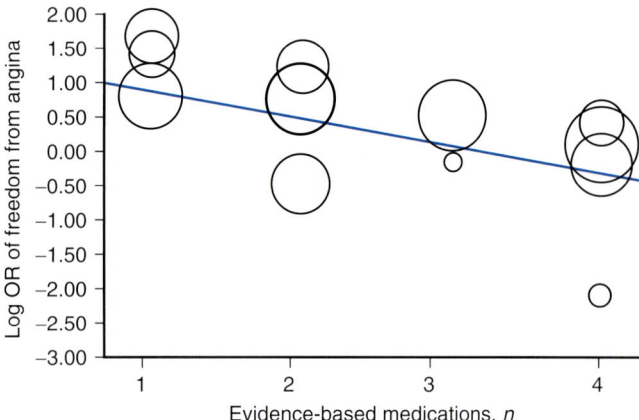

Fig. 18.6 Metaregression demonstrates an inverse relationship between freedom from angina and adherence to optimal evidence-based medical regimens within individual trial components of the meta-analysis. In more contemporary trials, evidence-based medication was used more frequently, and the measurable symptom-relief benefit of percutaneous coronary intervention was diminished. *OR,* Odds ratio. (From Wijeysundera HC, Nallamothu BK, Krumholz HM, et al. Meta-analysis: effects of percutaneous coronary intervention versus medical therapy on angina relief. *Ann Intern Med.* 2010;152[6]:370–379.)

of CAD. The potential benefits in the symptom relief associated with PCI might have been blunted due to lower ischemic risk of the selected population. Notably, the duration of follow-up after randomization (6 weeks) was extremely brief. At the end of the 6-week randomized treatment period, 85% of placebo patients received stents. This short duration of follow-up (6 weeks) was probably too brief to assess durable differences between the two treatment arms. Similar considerations apply to the potential lack of precision of the study, as reflected in its CIs that might have been inadequate to capture a true benefit with PCI due to small sample size. Attention should also be paid to the lesion severity assessment in the study; a sizeable number (28%–32%) of randomized subjects had either normal fractional flow reserve (FFR) or instantaneous wave-free ratio (IFR), and therefore did not have a physiologically significant, or flow-limiting stenosis. Notably, the mean number of antianginal medications in the PCI group was 0.90 at enrollment, 2.8 at prerandomization, and 2.9 at follow-up, compared with 1.0, 3.1, and 2.9, respectively, in the sham group. Therefore the high number of medications in the two groups might have also contributed to dilute the antianginal effect carried by PCI. Finally, all patients in ORBITA received maximal medical therapy ensured by physician to patient phone calls one to three times per week and urine drug testing. PCI patients remained on maximal medical therapy, including aggressive β-blockade despite stenting, which likely blunted differences in the primary end point (i.e., exercise time). The hypothesis that the background of maximal medical therapy in the randomized arms of the ORBITA trial might have decreased the efficacy of PCI for angina relief is supported by the observation of a previous metaregression of the treatment effects of PCI relative to medical therapy.[14] In this analysis, Wijeysundera and colleagues[12] reported an inverse relationship between freedom from angina and the number of "evidence-based" medications utilized during the conduct of a trial. Based on the metaregression findings, in more contemporary trials in which evidence-based medications were used more often, the benefit associated with PCI for symptom relief was diminished.[14] The controversy surrounding ORBITA has been blunted by the second ORBITA report published 7 months after the first, which documented patient reported angina, instead of physician reported angina, was significantly reduced by PCI (49.5% vs. 31.5%, *P* = .006).[18]

Percutaneous Coronary Revascularization: Effect on Clinical End Points

The benefit of percutaneous revascularization on the hard end points of death and MI is more controversial, and the complexities are greater. The selection of treatment strategies in patients with chronic stable angina depends on symptom status, anatomic complexity, clinical comorbidity, and risk. The relatively low event rates among stable patients with coronary disease, particularly those healthy enough and eligible to be enrolled in randomized prospective trials, limits the discriminatory ability of individual clinical trials to identify treatment effects. Even large meta-analytic studies, limited by significant heterogeneity of patient groups and inclusion of antiquated therapies (balloon angioplasty and limited medical options), have provided conflicting results. A meta-analysis by Katritsis and colleagues[19] incorporated data from 11 randomized trials of PCI compared with medical therapy in patients with documented CAD in the absence of a recent ACS. With 2950 patients included in the analysis, no significant difference could be identified between PCI and medical therapy in rates of overall death (see Fig. 18.4A), cardiac death and MI (see Fig. 18.4B), or subsequent revascularization. Another meta-analysis by Schömig and colleagues[20] of 17 trials involving 7513 patients with chronic stable angina randomized over a 17-year period to PCI or OMT alone again found no significant benefit for PCI over medical therapy with regard to rates of nonfatal MI (Fig. 18.7). However, with selection of cardiac mortality, rather than overall mortality, as an end point, this analysis did suggest a potential advantage for a PCI-based therapeutic strategy for improving long-term outcome (see Fig. 18.7A). Further analysis suggested that this benefit was most pronounced in patients who had suffered a recent MI (<4 weeks prior); they had about a 35% reduction in the odds of death compared with an estimated risk reduction of 17% for patients with truly stable coronary disease. Both of these meta-analyses, however, were limited by several factors, including significant heterogeneity of patient groups and treatments, inclusion of patients with recent ACSs, and significant variability in treatments across studies and time periods. Another meta-analysis[21] that compared revascularization (surgical or percutaneous) with medical therapy over a 30-year period from 1977 to 2007 confirmed a significant reduction in all-cause mortality associated with revascularization (OR, 0.74; 95% CI 0.63 to 0.88). When this study was stratified by revascularization type, the investigators were also able to show a reduction in mortality with both surgical (OR, 0.62; 95% CI 0.50 to 0.77) and percutaneous (OR, 0.82; 95% CI 0.68 to 0.99) revascularization approaches compared with OMT. However, this meta-analysis, like the others, included trials that encompassed a broad array of patient populations, including those with recent ACSs; it was also limited by the historic nature of treatment algorithms spanning the 30-year study period. In a 20-year network meta-analysis that took into account the evolution of interventional approaches over time, Trikalinos and colleagues[22] were unable to document a beneficial effect of PCI-based strategies on rates of death or MI compared with contemporaneous medical therapy. As previously noted, a major hurdle in the assessment of survival benefits associated with revascularization trials is the relatively low overall event rate. Whereas annualized mortality associated with chronic CAD remains approximately 1% to 3% in contemporary series,[11,21] the risk of adverse events increases with the degree of left ventricular (LV) dysfunction,[6] ischemic burden,[19] functional limitation, MVD, and calcium score by coronary computed tomography angiography (CTA; Table 18.3).[23,24] In addition, risk is increased in the presence of diabetes mellitus, chronic kidney disease, and greater severity of ischemic symptoms[16] and anatomic complexity.[21] It is not surprising then that a gradient of benefit can be

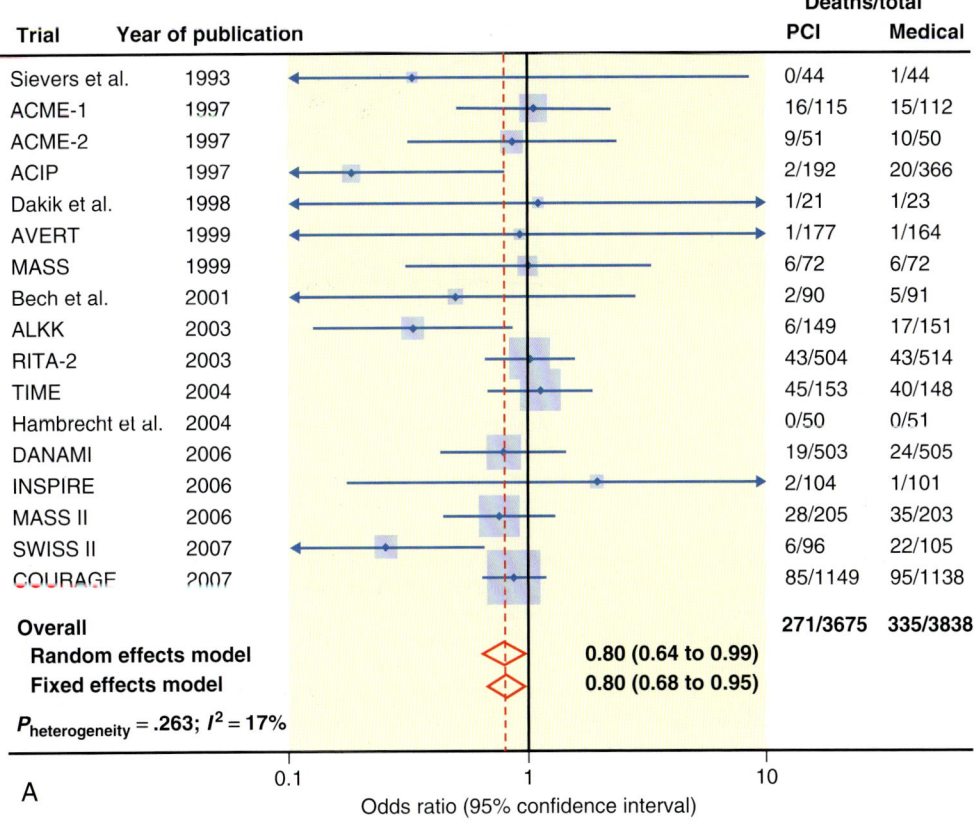
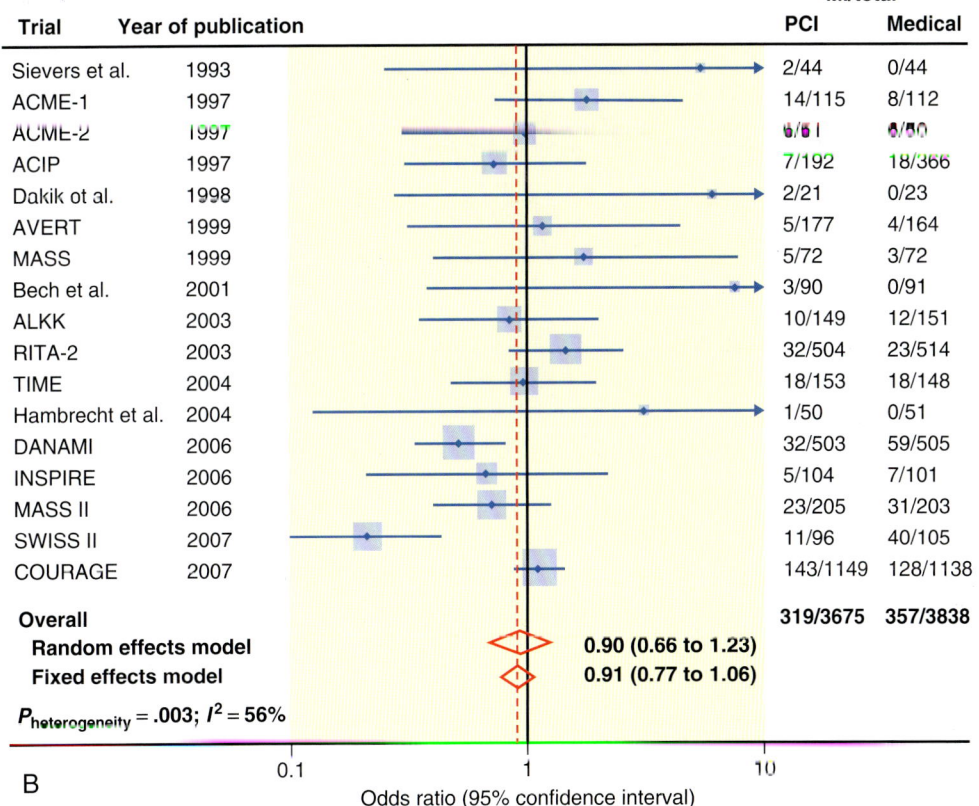

Fig. 18.7 Odds ratios with 95% confidence intervals among 17 randomized trials of percutaneous coronary intervention *(PCI)* or medical therapy with an average follow-up period of 51 months, along with summary statistics. (A) Risk of cardiac death. (B) Risk of nonfatal myocardial infarction *(MI)*. (From Schömig A, Mehilli J, de Waha A, et al. A meta-analysis of 17 randomized trials of a percutaneous coronary intervention-based strategy in patients with stable coronary artery disease. *J Am Coll Cardiol.* 2008;52[11]:894–904.)

observed for revascularization compared with medical therapy, with greater efficacy identified in those patients at greatest risk, whether due to anatomic complexity (Fig. 18.8)[25] or severity of ischemic substrate (Fig. 18.9).[26]

Recent prospective trials have helped elucidate the potential benefit of percutaneous revascularization across the spectrum of clinical and anatomic risk, along with the continued importance of OMT. The COURAGE trial[15] is the largest trial yet performed to evaluate whether PCI provides additional clinical benefit over OMT alone. This trial randomized 2287 patients to OMT or OMT with early PCI, utilizing predominantly baremetal stents (BMS). OMT was intended to include antiplatelet therapy, β-blockade with metoprolol, ACE inhibition or angiotensin receptor blocker (ARB) therapy, and antiischemic measures that included amlodipine and/or nitrate therapy. Diet, exercise, and smoking cessation were also encouraged. All patients underwent entry angiographic evaluation, and those with more than 70% diameter stenosis in at least one epicardial coronary artery with evidence of ischemia or more than 80% stenosis and typical anginal symptoms were eligible for inclusion if coronary anatomy was felt to be suitable for PCI. Exclusion criteria included persistent CCS class IV angina, markedly positive stress evaluation, significant heart failure symptoms, left ventricular ejection fraction (LVEF) below 30%, or revascularization within the previous 6 months. At a mean follow-up of 4.6 years, no significant difference was seen in the primary end point of death or MI between the PCI and medical treatment (MT) groups (OR, 1.05; 95% CI 0.87 to 1.27; $P = .62$), nor was any difference found in overall mortality (7.6% vs. 8.3%, $P = .38$) or freedom from angina (74% vs. 72%, $P = .35$). However, in patients treated with PCI in addition

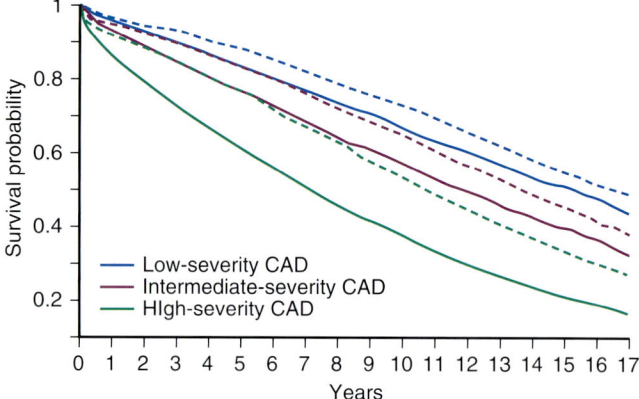

Fig. 18.8 Adjusted long-term survival estimates for patients treated with an initial medical revascularization *(solid lines)* or surgical or percutaneous revascularization *(dotted lines)* approach, stratified by extent of coronary artery disease *(CAD)* as defined by tertiles of the Duke Coronary Artery Disease Severity Index. High-severity CAD anatomy encompasses those patients with significant (50% to 75% stenosis) left main and/or three-vessel disease; low-severity CAD includes patients with single-vessel disease or noncritical (<95% stenosis) two-vessel disease; and intermediate-severity CAD comprises patients with critical proximal left anterior descending disease and the remaining two-vessel disease anatomic subgroups. (Adapted from Smith PK, Califf RM, Tuttle RH, et al. Selection of surgical or percutaneous coronary intervention provides differential longevity benefit. *Ann Thorac Surg.* 2006;82[4]:1420–1429.)

TABLE 18.3 Risk Stratification in Patients With Angina

HIGH RISK (>3% ANNUAL DEATH OR MYOCARDIAL INFARCTION)
1. Severe resting LV dysfunction (LVEF <35%) not readily explained by noncoronary causes
2. Resting perfusion abnormalities ≥10% of the myocardium in patients without prior history or evidence of MI
3. Stress ECG findings including ≥2 mm of ST-segment depression at low workload or persisting into recovery, exercise-induced ST-segment elevation, or exercise-induced VT/VF
4. Severe stress-induced LV dysfunction (peak exercise LVEF <45% or drop in LVEF with stress ≥10%)
5. Stress-induced perfusion abnormalities encumbering >10% myocardium or stress segmental scores indicating multiple vascular territories with abnormalities
6. Stress-induced LV dilation
7. Inducible wall motion abnormality (involving >2 segments or 2 coronary beds)
8. Wall motion abnormality developing at low dose of dobutamine (10 mg/kg/min) or at a low heart rate (<120 beats/min)
9. CAC score >400 Agatston units
10. Multivessel obstructive CAD (≥70% stenosis) or left main stenosis (≥50% stenosis) on CCTA

INTERMEDIATE RISK (1%–3% ANNUAL DEATH OR MYOCARDIAL INFARCTION)
1. Mild/moderate resting LV dysfunction (LVEF 35%–49%) not readily explained by noncoronary causes
2. Resting perfusion abnormalities in 5%–9.9% of the myocardium in patients without a history or prior evidence of MI
3. ≥1 mm of ST-segment depression occurring with exertional symptoms
4. Stress-induced perfusion abnormalities encumbering 5%–9.9% of the myocardium or stress segmental scores (in multiple segments) indicating 1 vascular territory with abnormalities but without LV dilation
5. Small wall motion abnormality involving 1–2 segments and only 1 coronary bed
6. CAC score 100–399 Agatston units
7. One vessel CAD with ≥70% stenosis or moderate CAD stenosis (50%–69% stenosis) in ≥2 arteries on CCTA

LOW RISK (<1% ANNUAL DEATH OR MYOCARDIAL INFARCTION)
1. Low-risk treadmill score (score ≥5) or no new ST segment changes or exercise-induced chest pain symptoms; when achieving maximal levels of exercise
2. Normal or small myocardial perfusion defect at rest or with stress encumbering <5% of the myocardium[a]
3. Normal stress or no change of limited resting wall motion abnormalities during stress
4. CAC score <100 Agatston units
5. No coronary stenosis >50% on CCTA

[a]Although the published data are limited; patients with these findings will probably not be at low risk in the presence of either a high-risk treadmill score or severe resting LV dysfunction (LVEF <35%). *CAC,* Coronary artery calcium; *CAD,* coronary artery disease; *CCTA,* coronary computed tomography angiography; *LV,* left ventricular; *LVEF,* left ventricular ejection fraction; *MI,* myocardial infarction; *VT/VF,* ventricular tachycardia/ventricular fibrillation.
From Patel MR, Calhoon JH, Dehmer GJ, et al. ACC/AATS/AHA/ASE/ASNC/SCAI/SCCT/STS 2017 appropriate use criteria for coronary revascularization in patients with stable ischemic heart disease: a report of the American College of Cardiology Appropriate Use Criteria Task Force, American Association for Thoracic Surgery, American Heart Association, American Society of Echocardiography, American Society of Nuclear Cardiology, Society for Cardiovascular Angiography and Interventions, Society of Cardiovascular Computed Tomography, and Society of Thoracic Surgeons. *J Am Coll Cardiol.* 2017;69(17):2212–2241.

to OMT, freedom from angina was significantly greater up to 3 years, and the medical therapy cohort exhibited a "catch-up" pattern only after the initial 2 years of follow-up (Fig. 18.10).[27] Additional early benefits associated with percutaneous intervention included a reduced need for follow-up revascularization during the first year (21% vs. 33%, $P < .001$) with a concomitant reduction in the need for antiischemic drug therapy. These results support the widespread use of OMT in patients with established CAD and suggest that in this setting, early PCI is not associated with reduced long-term event rates. Whereas an initial strategy of OMT alone was not associated with increased rates of death or MI, it was associated with a significant crossover rate of 30% within the first year of follow-up.[23] In addition, enrolled patients were at relatively low risk, with one-, two-, and three-vessel coronary disease rates of 31%, 39%, and 30%, respectively, and only a 31% incidence of proximal left anterior descending (LAD) disease. Patients also had relatively preserved LV function, and those with left main CAD were not included. Finally, compliance rates with medical therapy at 5 years ranged from 85% for β-blockade to 95% for aspirin or clopidogrel,[15] rates that far exceeded the less than 40% compliance noted in community-based registry studies such as the 40,000-patient "real world" Reduction of Atherothrombosis for Continued Health (REACH) registry.[28]

The COURAGE nuclear substudy[29] evaluated a small but relatively high-risk patient subset of the overall trial. Based on previous work that demonstrated the prognostic benefit of coronary revascularization in patients with a significant burden of ischemic myocardium,[26,30] the authors initiated an exploratory evaluation that involved 314 consecutive study patients who underwent serial rest/stress myocardial perfusion imaging (MPI) studies. Based on comparisons of pretreatment ischemic burden and studies performed at 6 to 18 months after randomization, patients in the PCI–plus-OMT group experienced a greater degree of ischemia reduction (≥5% reduction in ischemic myocardium) than those treated with OMT alone (33% vs. 19%, $P = .0004$). The degree of ischemia resolution was also greater in patients with more ischemia at baseline. Importantly, low levels of residual ischemia at follow-up were associated with improved symptom status and better unadjusted survival free of MI ($P = .037$), suggesting an important prognostic role for aggressive ischemia reduction in these patients. As with all large randomized trials, the generalizability of these findings is limited by the type of patients enrolled and the already outmoded forms of therapy provided (drug-eluting stents [DESs] were largely unavailable during recruitment, as were many novel medical therapeutics, including ranolazine). However, the results of this trial provide additional support for the importance of a foundation of OMT while providing confidence in the benefit of percutaneous revascularization as an adjunctive method of symptom and ischemia control. The Bypass Angioplasty Revascularization Investigation in Type 2 Diabetes (BARI 2D)[31] trial addressed a similar question; it enrolled 2368 patients with type 2 diabetes mellitus to early revascularization (CABG or PCI, at the discretion

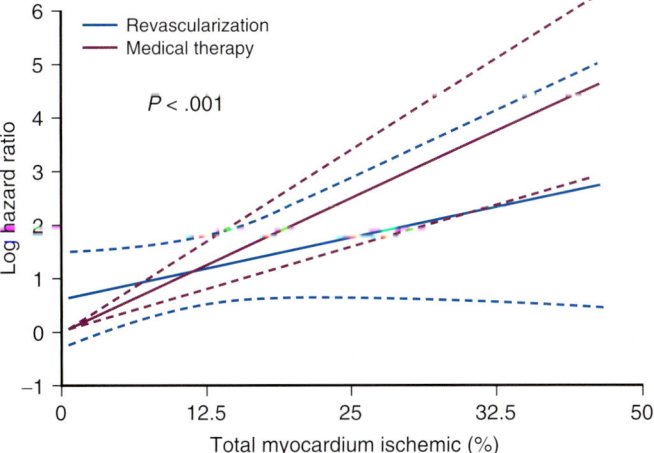

Fig. 18.9 Log hazard ratio for 10,627 patients undergoing revascularization or medical therapy for ischemic coronary artery disease as a function of extent of myocardial ischemia. The intersection of curves at an approximate point of inducible ischemia of 10% or more of the myocardium represents the retrospectively identified threshold for survival benefit associated with revascularization. (Adapted from Hachamovitch R, Hayes SW, Friedman JD, et al. Comparison of the short-term survival benefit associated with revascularization compared with medical therapy in patients with no prior coronary artery disease undergoing stress myocardial perfusion single photon emission computed tomography. *Circulation*. 2003;107[23]:2900–2907.)

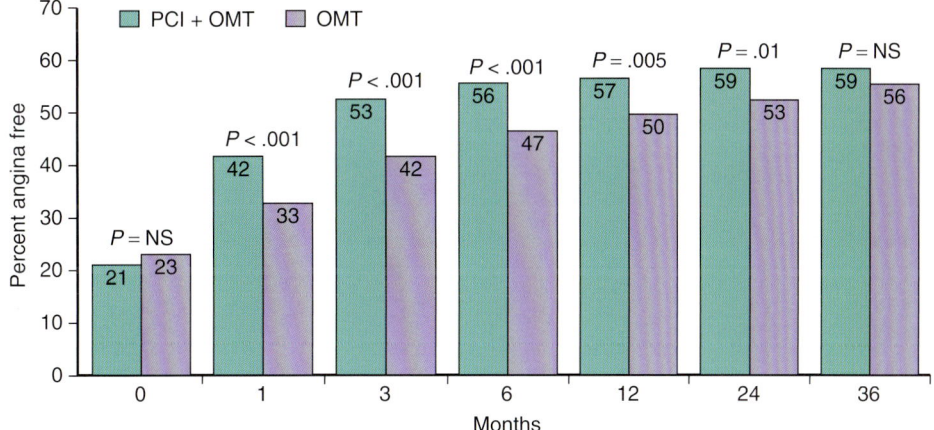

Fig. 18.10 Changes in the angina frequency scale of the Seattle Angina Questionnaire over time in the COURAGE Trial. Data shown are for the COURAGE trial cohorts of percutaneous revascularization with optimal medical therapy (percutaneous coronary intervention [PCI] plus optimal medical therapy [OMT]) and OMT alone. The early anginal benefit demonstrated with PCI plus OMT is reduced over time because patients in the OMT group experience progressively greater freedom from angina over the initial 3 years of follow-up. *NS*, Not significant. (Adapted from Weintraub WS, Spertus JA, Kolm P, et al. Effect of PCI on quality of life in patients with stable coronary disease. *N Engl J Med*. 2008;359[7]:677–687.)

of the treating physician) with OMT and later revascularization as needed for symptom relief. Along with OMT, patients were assigned exercise and risk-factor modification programs with frequent assessment and modification of glycemic control. Patients were included in the trial if they had stable CAD (CCS class I or II in 82%), a positive stress test, and coronary anatomy suitable for revascularization. Exclusion criteria included the need for immediate revascularization, left main CAD, significant heart failure, or prior revascularization within a year of study entry. Like the COURAGE trial, the primary end point of 5-year all-cause mortality was similar between the groups (hazard ratio [HR], 0.5; 95% CI –2.0 to 3.1; P = .97). Also reminiscent of the COURAGE results, 42% of patients originally assigned to OMT alone crossed over to subsequent revascularization, reinforcing the role of adjunctive revascularization in managing symptoms. Of interest, because the choice of revascularization was left to the discretion of the treating physician and patient, patients with more extensive disease were generally treated with surgical, rather than percutaneous, revascularization. In this group of high-risk patients with diabetes mellitus, surgical revascularization offered a significant reduction in nonfatal infarction, with no such advantage noted in those patients selected for PCI over pharmacologic therapy.[32] Of note, nearly 60% of patients enrolled in the COURAGE trial had either no ischemia or very mild ischemia on provocative testing. From the COURAGE trial, ischemia eligibility criteria included new resting ST-T wave changes, ≥1 mm exertional ST segment changes, or ≥1 ischemic imaging defect. Enrollment was also permitted for patients with angina and ≥70% stenosis without any stress test requirement. These criteria can be subquestioned, considering that electrocardiographic (ECG) changes and small amounts of ischemia are suboptimal in predicting event risk and obstructive CAD severity. Most of the stents used in COURAGE were BMS. Nowadays, current DES have appreciably improved safety and efficacy profiles in stable CAD compared with BMS and DES devices. More recently, Navarese and colleagues,[33] in an important large-scale network meta-analysis conducted in patients undergoing PCI with various DES generations, noted more modern permanent polymer second-generation DES were associated with significant reduction of MI (by 29% to 34%; Fig. 18.11) compared with first-generation paclitaxel-eluting stents. Thus the findings of neutral benefit from PCI versus OMT on hard clinical end points, as observed in the COURAGE trial, might less likely apply to a contemporary population of individuals treated with newer and more biocompatible generation DESs. A 2014 meta-analysis evaluated all-cause mortality in 95 trials (n = 93,553 patients) that compared one type of coronary revascularization (CABG or stenting) with another or placebo.[34] Compared with initial MT, newer generation DES were associated with reduced mortality (everolimus-eluting: rate ratio [RR] 0.75, 95% CI 0.59 to 0.96; zotarolimus-eluting [Resolute] RR 0.65, 95% CI 0.42 to 1.00). This network meta-analysis raises the question as to whether newer generation DES may be associated with improved survival compared to medical therapy. However, there are important limitations of this study, including only one direct comparison of a newer generation DES to OMT. The almost completed International Study of Comparative Health Effectiveness with Medical and Invasive Approaches (ISCHEMIA) trial (NCT01471522) will provide definitive data on the best management strategy for higher-risk patients with stable ischemic heart disease. ISCHEMIA is a multicenter randomized controlled trial with a planned enrollment of patients with moderate to severe ischemia on stress testing. Patients are randomized to a routine invasive strategy with cardiac catheterization followed by revascularization plus OMT or to a conservative strategy of OMT, with cardiac catheterization and revascularization reserved for those who fail OMT. Moreover, unlike prior trials, ISCHEMIA eligibility is not limited to stress nuclear imaging, but includes moderate-severe ischemia on stress echocardiography or magnetic resonance (MR) imaging. In addition, a patient may meet trial eligibility based on moderate-severe ischemia by exercise electrocardiography (without imaging). Blinded coronary CTA is performed to exclude patients with no obstructive stenosis or significant left main stenosis and to confirm the presence of obstructive CAD.

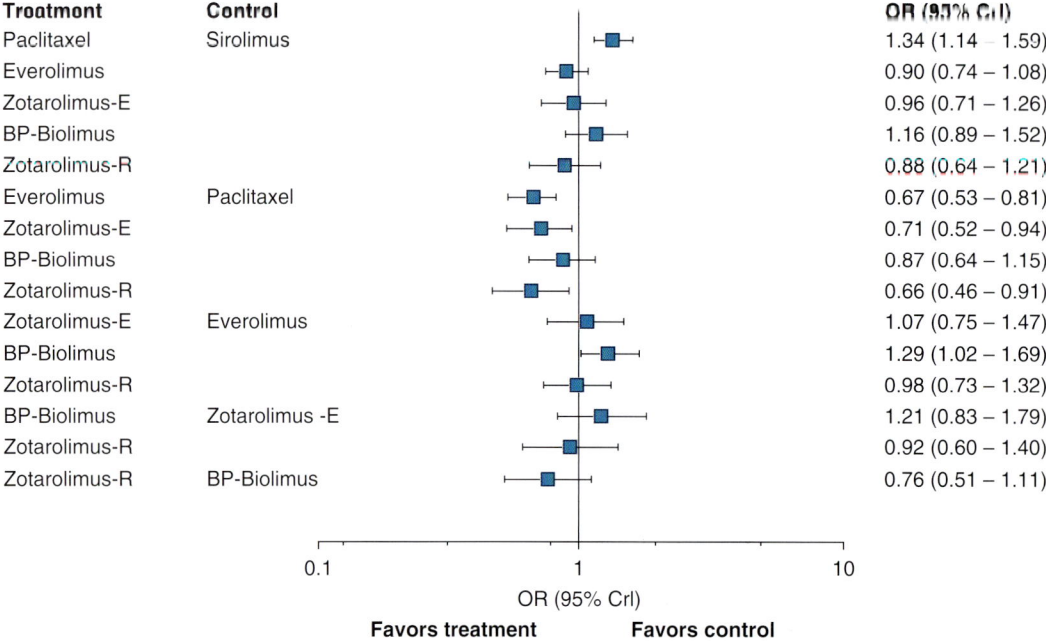

Fig. 18.11 Clinical outcomes with various types of drug-eluting stents compared to each other by network meta-analysis. Pooled odds ratio (*OR*) and 95% credible intervals (*CrI*) for myocardial infarction. *BP,* Biodegradable polymer; *E,* endeavor; *R,* resolute. (Adapted from Navarese EP, Tandjung K, Claessen B, et al. Safety and efficacy outcomes of first and second generation durable polymer drug eluting stents and biodegradable polymer biolimus eluting stents in clinical practice: comprehensive network meta-analysis. *BMJ.* 2013;[347]:f6530.)

SELECTION OF REVASCULARIZATION STRATEGY

Risk-factor control and adherence to guideline-based medical therapy are the cornerstones of treatment in patients with stable-CAD, and revascularization, either by PCI or by CABG, should be considered in patients who have persistent anginal symptoms despite OMT or high-risk features of CAD. The indication for revascularization should always be clearly defined on symptomatic and/or prognostic grounds. Patients with more complex stable-CAD should be discussed by a "Heart Team" comprising as a minimum a noninterventional as well as an interventional cardiologist and a cardiac surgeon. The selection of a specific revascularization strategy depends on numerous factors, including the extent and complexity of the coronary anatomy, presence and severity of comorbidities, patient and physician preference, and available scientific evidence. As technology has advanced in the application of both CABG and PCI, this discussion has evolved dramatically. However, whereas the goals of therapy for both PCI and CABG involve providing symptomatic and prognostic improvement, the methods of achieving these goals continue to be fundamentally different and help explain the major difference in outcome between the two strategies—that is, the need for more subsequent repeat revascularization in patients undergoing PCI. Because coronary disease is a progressive, incurable condition, both PCI and CABG provide only palliation. Surgical revascularization, however, addresses obstructive coronary disease by providing a perfusion conduit that circumvents a long segment of proximal disease. This allows greater protection from the inexorable development of new and progressive lesions compared with the focal treatment strategy associated with stent placement. In addition, surgical revascularization is associated with more extensive revascularization and a greater likelihood of successful revascularization of all affected territories (full anatomic revascularization),[35] with potential implications for improved survival at follow-up.[28,36] For patients with single-vessel, nonleft main CAD and indications for revascularization, few contemporary data are available to suggest the superiority of CABG over PCI. Revascularization in patients with single vessel disease generally entails less risk of major morbidity or mortality than that in patients with MVD, and outcomes with PCI have been as good as, or better than, those with surgical revascularization. Historically, however, proximal LAD disease has been considered the purview of the surgeon, with randomized and registry data suggesting a survival advantage with surgery in this group (Fig. 18.12).[37] However, more recent meta-analytic studies[31,32] and 10-year follow-up of one randomized trial[33] have failed to confirm a survival benefit for CABG over PCI for the treatment of LAD disease in the modern era. As with other lesion subsets, a PCI-based strategy is associated with increased subsequent repeat revascularization, even with the routine application of coronary stents.[33]

Now of largely historic interest, the 1980s and 1990s saw the initiation and completion of several multicenter randomized trials to compare percutaneous transluminal coronary angioplasty (PTCA) with CABG in patients with MVD. Among nearly 5000 patients with multivessel coronary disease amenable to either angioplasty or bypass surgery, no difference in death or MI, quality of life, or employment status was demonstrated in these trials; this suggests that the main disadvantage to a primary strategy of angioplasty was the increased need for repeat revascularization. PCI, then, was felt to be a reasonable initial revascularization choice in the setting of preserved ventricular function and technically favorable anatomy.[34] Retrospective database evaluations also confirmed the safety of both modes of revascularization in the majority of patients while documenting a gradient of benefit associated with PTCA or CABG that was dependent on, and correlated directly with, the extent and location of coronary stenoses.[30]

It appears of paramount relevance when judging upon benefits of PCI versus CABG to recognize the inherent trial limitations which, for the large majority, enrolled patients not representative of routine daily practice. Thus the complementary information from registries which provide information drawn from real world is relevant in this context. Moreover, the iteration of the coronary stent technology is an important factor that has further contributed to influence the outcome of the comparison between PCI and CABG strategy. Contemporary studies of revascularization in patients with MVD have compared a predominantly stent-based PCI strategy with contemporary surgical techniques, including the judicious use of internal thoracic arterial conduits. The initial equivalent prognostic impact of BMS placement or CABG for the treatment of MVD was confirmed in a pooled patient-level meta-analysis[38] of 5-year data from 3051 patients enrolled in the Arterial Revascularization Therapies Study (ARTS); the Argentine Randomized Trial of Coronary Angioplasty with Stenting Versus Coronary Bypass Surgery in Patients with Multivessel Disease (ERACI II); the Medicine, Angioplasty, or Surgery Study for Multivessel Coronary Artery Disease (MASS-II); and Stent or Surgery (SoS) trials. In this analysis, the 5-year cumulative incidences of death, MI, and stroke were similar among patients randomized to PCI with BMS compared with CABG (16.7% vs. 16.9%; HR, 1.04; 95% CI 0.86 to 1.27; $P = .69$). Repeat revascularization, however, occurred significantly more often in patients assigned to PCI (29.0% vs. 7.9%; HR, 0.23; 95% CI 0.18 to 0.29) compared with CABG, with a

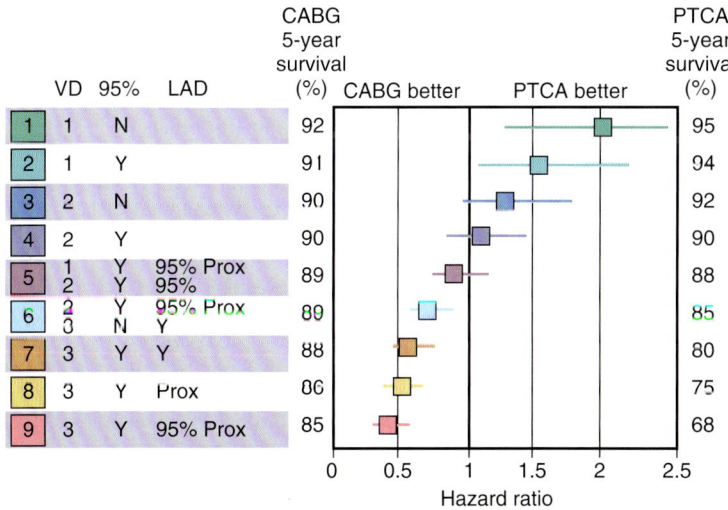

Fig. 18.12 Relationship of graded coronary anatomy. This includes the number of vessels with at least 75% stenosis (VD), severity of disease (≥95% stenosis), presence of left anterior descending (LAD) coronary artery disease (CAD), and differential mortality hazard after either coronary artery bypass grafting (CABG) or percutaneous transluminal coronary angioplasty (PTCA). A gradient of outcome effect is identified because increased severity of CAD is associated with improved outcome in CABG-treated patients compared with the outcome associated with percutaneous coronary intervention (PCI) in patients with similar high-severity disease. N, No; Prox, proximal; Y, yes. (Adapted from Jones RH, Kesler K, Phillips HR 3rd, et al. Long-term survival benefits of coronary artery bypass grafting and percutaneous transluminal angioplasty in patients with coronary artery disease. J Thorac Cardiovasc Surg. 1996;111[5]:1013–1025.)

persistent separation of the curves over time. Given the comparable safety of stent-based PCI and CABG in the broad population of patients who present for multivessel revascularization, the further evolution of DES technology has fueled the enthusiasm for the conduction of further comparative studies. The largest trial to compare PCI and CABG in patients with three-vessel disease after DES is the large Synergy Between Percutaneous Coronary Intervention with TAXUS and Cardiac Surgery (SYNTAX) trial.[39] The study randomized 1800 patients with three-vessel and/or left main CAD to paclitaxel-eluting stent placement or CABG. The trial was designed as an all-comers noninferiority trial to evaluate long-term outcomes in patients undergoing revascularization for severe CAD. Inclusion criteria comprised patients with previously untreated lesions of 50% or greater diameter stenosis with stable or unstable angina or atypical chest pain. If asymptomatic, patients were required to have positive evidence of myocardial ischemia. Exclusion criteria comprised previous PCI or CABG, acute MI, or the need for concomitant cardiac surgery. At 12 months, the primary end point of major cardiac and cerebrovascular events (MACCEs) was higher in the group of patients who underwent PCI (17.8% vs. 12.4%, P = .002), largely the result of an increased rate of repeat revascularization in the PCI arm (13.5% vs. 5.9%, P < .001), despite a mean of 4.6 stents (standard deviation [SD] ± 2.3) placed per patient. The trial therefore failed to demonstrate noninferiority for paclitaxel stent-based PCI compared with CABG in this high-risk cohort, although the safety end points were reassuringly similar between groups. In fact, no difference was found between the PCI and CABG groups for the composite of all-cause death, MI, and stroke at 12 months (7.6% vs. 7.7%), and no difference was noted in the individual components of death and MI. However, an excess of stroke was noted after CABG compared with PCI (2.2% vs. 0.6%). By 5 years of follow-up, MACCE rates remained higher in patients randomized to PCI (37.3% vs. 26.9%, P < .0001), due primarily to a persistent excess of repeat revascularization (25.9% vs. 13.7%, P < .0001) but also to a newly apparent excess of MI (9.7% vs. 3.8%, P < .0001). Differences in all-cause death (13.9% vs. 11.4%) and stroke (2.4% vs. 3.7%) were found to be statistically insignificant between PCI and CABG patients at 5-year follow-up. Potential weaknesses of this trial, in comparison to current understandings, are that neither PCI (that used first-generation DES, which are inferior to the current generation of DES) nor surgery (low use of bilateral internal mammary artery grafts, low use of secondary preventive medication) was optimal. Outcomes analysis in 1095 patients with three-vessel disease was a prespecified subset of the whole trial. At 5 years, CABG reduced absolute mortality (by 5.4%), MI (by 7.3%), and the need for repeat revascularization (by 12.8%). The outcome of MACCE depended on the complexity of coronary disease, as judged by the SYNTAX score. In patients with the lowest tertile SYNTAX score (0 to 22), there was no significant difference between CABG and PCI (33.3% vs. 36.8%). In contrast, as lesion complexity worsened, the patients randomized to CABG had markedly improved outcome (24.1% vs. 41.9%). One of the largest meta-analyses to address this issue included six recent trials of PCI versus CABG with 6054 patients,[40] although three of the trials (ARTS, SOS, MASS), involving 40% of the PCI patients, did not use DES. The authors reported that compared with PCI, CABG resulted in significant reductions in the risk ratios for total mortality (0.73 [95% CI 0.62 to 0.86]), MI (0.58 [95% CI 0.48 to 0.72]), and repeat revascularization (0.29 [95% CI 0.21 to 0.41]). The more recently reported Randomized Comparison of Coronary Artery Bypass Surgery and Everolimus-Eluting Stent Implantation in the Treatment of Patients with Multivessel Coronary Artery Disease (BEST) trial of an everolimus DES versus CABG was terminated early owing to slow recruitment.[41] Of 880 randomized patients, the primary end point (a composite of death, MI, or target-vessel revascularization at 2 years) had occurred in 11.0% of the PCI patients and in 7.9% of CABG patients. At longer-term follow-up (median: 4.6 years), the primary end point had occurred in 15.3% of the patients in the PCI group and in 10.6% of those in the CABG group (HR 1.47; 95% CI 1.01 to 2.13; P = 0.04). There were no significant differences between the two groups in the occurrence of a composite safety end point of death, MI, or stroke, but the rates of any repeat revascularization and spontaneous MI were significantly higher after PCI.

The application of catheter-based assessment of ischemia has become increasingly important and is now a central component of societal-based guidelines. FFR has been studied in multiple randomized trials and registries and is now widely used to assess a lesion for its functional significance in routine catheterization practice. The application of FFR in patients with more extensive or complex lesions has important implications for deciding on strategies for revascularization. Most recently, the 5-year results of the Fractional Flow Reserve Versus Angiography for Multivessel Evaluation (FAME) study confirmed that a strategy of FFR-guided PCI resulted in a significant decrease in major adverse cardiac events for up to 2 years[42] after the index intervention but that from 2 to 5 years, the risks were similar in both groups. This clinical outcome was achieved with a lower number of stented arteries and less resource utilization in the FFR-guided group, implying that FFR guidance in MVD should be the standard of care in most patients.[43] The choice of revascularization modality in unprotected left main stenosis is a separate realm. Among 705 patients with left main CAD in the SYNTAX trial, 38 1-year MACCE rates were similar among the PCI- and CABG-treated groups (15.8% vs. 13.7%, P = .44), including similar rates of death (4.2% vs. 4.4%, P = .24) or MI (4.3% vs. 4.1%); however, as in the overall trial, the rate of stroke was higher in the CABG group than in the PCI group (2.7% vs. 0.3%, P = .009). When scored for anatomic complexity (see the Tools for Selection of Therapy section), outcomes for those patients with low or intermediate SYNTAX scores were similar between the PCI and CABG groups. However, in patients in the highest tertile of SYNTAX score, adverse outcomes were significantly higher in those treated with PCI, driven primarily by increased requirements for repeat revascularization.

Two studies have recently entered the arena of revascularization of left main disease. In the EXCEL trial, patients with low- or intermediate-SYNTAX scores treated with an everolimus-eluting stent had comparable rates of death, stroke, or MI at 3 years when compared with patients treated with CABG surgery.[44] Investigators also found more periprocedural MI and ST-elevation MI (STEMI) in the CABG-treated patients at 30 days. In contrast, in the NOBLE trial,[45] treatment with PCI using predominantly a biolimus-eluting stent was associated with a significantly higher rate of MACCEs at 5 years when compared with CABG surgery. Individually, all-cause mortality was comparable between the two treatments, while nonprocedural MI and the need for a repeat coronary revascularization were higher among those treated with PCI. Stroke rates were higher among the CABG patients at 30 days but numerically higher among PCI patients at 5 years. The discordant conclusions of these trials (i.e., PCI was noninferior to CABG in EXCEL, whereas CABG was better than PCI in NOBLE) can be largely explained by disparities in study end points (i.e., EXCEL did not incorporate target-vessel revascularization in the primary composite end point, and used an MI definition that included periprocedural events), time of assessment (3 years in EXCEL, 5 years in NOBLE), and procedural characteristics (everolimus-eluting stents were used in EXCEL, biolimus-eluting stents were mostly used in NOBLE). Compared with previous trials, patients from EXCEL and NOBLE were more often selected (i.e., those with broader anatomical complexity were excluded) and procedure characteristics in the PCI and CABG arms were more reflective of current practice standards. The Future Revascularization Evaluation in Patients with Diabetes Mellitus: Optimal Management of Multivessel Disease (FREEDOM) trial[46] has provided further insight into revascularization strategies in diabetic patients with multivessel coronary disease. In this trial, 1900 patients were randomized to PCI or CABG to evaluate the primary end point of all-cause mortality, nonfatal MI, or nonfatal stroke over a median follow-up period of 3.8 years. At 5 years, the primary outcome occurred more frequently in the PCI group compared with the CABG group (26.6% vs. 18.7%, P = .005). The benefit of CABG was driven by differences in rates of both MI (P < .001) and death from any cause (P = .049). Stroke was more frequent in the CABG group, with 5-year rates of 2.4% in the PCI group and 5.2% in the CABG group (P = .03). In a secondary analysis, between 6 months and 2 years following index revascularization, CABG provided greater improvements in health status measured by angina relief, physical function, and overall quality of life than treatment with PCI. However, both revascularization strategies resulted in substantial and sustained improvements in quality of life and functional status, and the magnitude of benefit with CABG over PCI was modest. Beyond 2 years, no difference was seen in health status assessments, in part due to the higher rate of repeat revascularization with PCI.

The introduction of FFR has refined the assessment of coronary lesions for their functional significance prior to PCI. In the FAME-2 FFR-guided PCI was compared with medical therapy in patients with stable CAD. Functionally significant lesions were defined as an FFR ≤0.80.[47] Patients with abnormal FFR who were randomized to PCI plus best available medical therapy versus medical therapy alone had improved outcomes. Two-year follow-up data showed an ongoing reduction in the primary end point (8.1% vs. 19.5%; HR, 0.39; 95% CI 0.26 to 0.57; P < .001), which was driven by reduction in urgent revascularization.[48] There was high crossover, with 41% of the OMT group receiving a stent versus 8% in FFR receiving an additional stent.

The application of FFR in patients with more extensive or complex lesions has major implications when selecting the revascularization strategy. In patients with MVD, not all lesions are functionally significant and responsible for ischemia. Accordingly, patients considered to have significant angiographic three-vessel disease and therefore potentially better served by CABG, may have only one or two functionally significant lesions when measured by FFR, in which case they may be treated as well or even better by PCI. Another factor to drive to the selection for surgical or percutaneous revascularization in subjects with MVD is concomitant heart failure. Several studies and a recent important meta-analysis of current evidence have reported improved survival by revascularization with CABG compared with MT.[6,49,50]

Tools for Selection of Therapy

Risk benefit prediction models are important for decision-making in recommending specific therapeutic strategies and essential in counseling and educating patients. Several recently available comparative tools can assist physicians in deciding upon revascularization options. These tools provide guidance through the integration of certain anatomic, functional, and/or baseline clinical profile characteristics. The growing number and scope of prospective trials on revascularization has provided an important objective structure to guide general discussion of treatment algorithms. However, revascularization decisions for individual patients continue to rely on the subjective "read" by practicing physicians of what is best for the patient. Beyond the essential institution of OMT and risk-factor modification programs for all patients, determination of whether to offer revascularization—and if so, what type—is often based on the subjective compilation of baseline clinical characteristics and presentation features. Factors such as anginal status, age, sex, and risk-factor profile provide important clues regarding the selection of optimal treatment. In addition, individual patient desires and experience, as well as the bias of treating physicians, play a significant role in shading discussions and ultimate treatment choice. Several comparative tools are now available to assist physicians and patients in discussing revascularization options. These tools provide guidance through the integration of certain anatomic, functional, and/or baseline clinical components. Some scores, such as the Mayo Clinic risk score[51] and the National Cardiovascular Data Registry (NCDR) risk score,[52] were developed to aid in risk assessment after PCI, whereas others—such as the Society of Thoracic Surgeons (STS) score (see the online risk calculator at http://riskcalc.sts.org/STSWebRiskCalc273);[53] the EuroSCORE[54] (see the online risk calculator at www.euroscore.org/calc.html); and the age, creatinine, and ejection fraction (ACEF)[55] score—have been validated as independent predictors of adverse events in patients undergoing CABG. Although several of these scores have subsequently been evaluated for prognostic ability in patients who present for either PCI or CABG,[51,56] they have not proved useful in determining optimal treatment selection. The SYNTAX score,[57] on the other hand, was developed to provide prognostic information regarding outcome after either PCI or CABG in patients with MVD based on the functional impact of angiographically documented coronary disease. The SYNTAX score is a quantitative score that provides a cumulative measure of the extent and complexity of angiographically evident CAD, taking into account the number, location, and characteristics of lesions identified angiographically, as well as the extent of myocardium subserved. Among patients with three-vessel and/or left main CAD randomized in the SYNTAX trial,[39] those who were treated with paclitaxel-eluting stent PCI exhibited increasing MACCE rates at 2 years in direct relationship to increased disease complexity as defined by the baseline SYNTAX score. This effect was not identified in patients treated with an initial strategy of CABG. Although MACCE rates were not statistically different between patients treated in the PCI or CABG arms when the baseline SYNTAX score was low (0 to 22) or intermediate (23 to 32), patients with high SYNTAX scores (>32) experienced lower MACCE rates when treated with CABG compared with those who underwent PCI.[58] Because the SYNTAX score has not shown discriminative ability for risk prognostication among patients undergoing CABG, a mode of revascularization less affected by the complexity of disease, the primary impact of this score is to aid in the identification of patients at undue risk for MACCE after PCI who might therefore benefit from treatment with CABG. Given the importance of clinical variables on outcome, the initial angiographic SYNTAX score has been modified to include seven clinical factors (age, creatinine clearance, LVEF, left main disease, peripheral arterial disease, female sex, and pulmonary disease [SYNTAX II score]).[59] This score has been found to discriminate for the end point of 4-year mortality in both CABG and PCI patients. For example, to achieve similar 4-year mortality after CABG or PCI, younger patients, women, and patients with reduced LVEF required lower anatomical SYNTAX scores, while patients who were older, had left main disease, or had impaired lung function required higher anatomical SYNTAX scores.

An additional iteration of the SYNTAX score has been developed and studied in the PCI cohort of the SYNTAX trial.[60] This specific score (Residual Syntax score), which was shown to be a surrogate marker of increasing clinical comorbidity and anatomic complexity, defines the impact of the degree of incompleteness of revascularization achieved by PCI on subsequent outcome. Patients with residual SYNTAX scores ≤8 had comparable 5-year mortality (residual SYNTAX score: >0 to 4, 8.7%; >4 to 8, 11.4%; P = .60). In contrast, a residual SYNTAX score greater than 8 resulted in an all-cause mortality at 5 years of 35.3% (P < .001). This score can therefore be used in planning revascularization strategies so that if substantial degree of incomplete revascularization can be anticipated (e.g., a chronic occlusion that cannot be treated with PCI) then surgery should be favored. A recent meta-analysis indicated that revascularization strategies are superior to MT in patients with ischemic heart disease and reduced ejection fraction (see Fig. 18.5). In this analysis, revascularization with either CABG or PCI carried a significant improvement in long-term survival over OMT,

One-Vessel Disease

		Asymptomatic		Ischemic Symptoms					
		Not on AA Therapy or With AA Therapy		Not on AA Therapy		On 1 AA Drug (BB Preferred)		On ≥2 AA Drugs	
	Indication	PCI	CABG	PCI	CABG	PCI	CABG	PCI	CABG
No Proximal LAD or Proximal Left Dominant LCX Involvement									
1.	■ Low-risk findings on noninvasive testing	R (2)	R (1)	R (3)	R (2)	M (4)	R (3)	A (7)	M (5)
2.	■ Intermediate- or high-risk findings on noninvasive testing	M (4)	R (3)	M (5)	M (4)	M (6)	M (4)	A (8)	M (6)
3.	■ No stress test performed or, if performed, results are indeterminate ■ FFR ≤0.80[a]	M (4)	R (2)	M (5)	R (3)	M (6)	M (4)	A (8)	M (6)
Proximal LAD or Proximal Left Dominant LCX Involvement Present									
4.	■ Low-risk findings on noninvasive testing	M (4)	R (3)	M (4)	M (4)	M (5)	M (5)	A (7)	A (7)
5.	■ Intermediate- or high-risk findings on noninvasive testing	M (5)	M (5)	M (6)	M (6)	A (7)	A (7)	A (8)	A (8)
6.	■ No stress test performed or, if performed, results are indeterminate ■ FFR ≤0.80	M (5)	M (5)	M (6)	M (6)	M (6)	M (6)	A (8)	A (7)

Fig. 18.13 Appropriateness ratings for asymptomatic patients or with ischemic symptoms and one-vessel disease (no or proximal left anterior descending coronary artery/left circumflex artery) judged at low, intermediate or high risk. The number in parentheses next to the rating reflects the median score for that indication. [a]iFR measurements with appropriate normal ranges may be substituted for FFR. *A*, Appropriate; *AA*, antianginal; *BB*, β-blockers; *CABG*, coronary artery bypass graft; *FFR*, fractional flow reserve; *iFR*, instant wave-free ratio; *LAD*, left anterior descending coronary artery; *LCX*, left circumflex artery; *M*, may be appropriate; *PCI*, percutaneous coronary intervention; *R*, rarely appropriate. (From Patel MR, Calhoon JH, Dehmer GJ, et al. ACC/AATS/AHA/ASE/ASNC/SCAI/SCCT/STS 2017 appropriate use criteria for coronary revascularization in patients with stable ischemic heart disease: a report of the American College of Cardiology Appropriate Use Criteria Task Force, American Association for Thoracic Surgery, American Heart Association, American Society of Echocardiography, American Society of Nuclear Cardiology, Society for Cardiovascular Angiography and Interventions, Society of Cardiovascular Computed Tomography, and Society of Thoracic Surgeons. *J Am Coll Cardiol*. 2017;69[17]:2212–2241.)

with CABG showing a significantly improved survival compared with PCI, that persisted among patients with left main/proximal LAD disease and in studies conducted after the advent of DES, and CABG compared with PCI was associated with a significant reduction in the risk of MI or need for repeat revascularization, albeit with a numerically higher rate of strokes.

Risk scores can provide statistical insight into the population-based risks associated with percutaneous or surgical revascularization, but they are unable to identify specific risks for an individual patient. To provide additional assistance in risk stratification and treatment selection, some national bodies have recently undertaken an initiative to provide guidance through the publication of appropriateness criteria. These documents are essentially an extension of evidence-based guideline documents and serve to fill the gap between known scientific findings and individual patient variability; they assist in the selection of the proper patients for the procedure to minimize unnecessary risk while maximizing patient benefit. In 2009 the American College of Cardiology Foundation (ACCF), Society for Cardiovascular Angiography and Interventions (SCAI), STS, American Association for Thoracic Surgery (AATS), American Heart Association (AHA), and American Society of Nuclear Cardiology (ASNC) developed the Appropriate Use Criteria for Coronary Revascularization (AUC) to assess the quality of patient selection for coronary revascularization procedure. The AUC was intended to be a practical, quality improvement guide that applies published trial evidence and the generalized recommendations of practice guidelines to specific clinical scenarios likely to be encountered in everyday practice.[61] These scenarios are rated on a scale of 1 to 9, first by individual panelists and then collectively. Recently, revised criteria for coronary revascularization in stable ischemic heart disease have been issued.[24] This document uses the new terms "appropriate care (scores 7 to 9)," "may be appropriate care (scores 4 to 6)," and "rarely appropriate care (scores 1 to 3)," which were described in the updated AUC methodology paper. The current criteria continue to emphasize the use of more objective measures of ischemia within indications to stratify patients into low-risk or intermediate-/high-risk findings, as described in the Stable Ischemic Heart Disease guideline. The scenarios also expand the use of intracoronary physiologic testing, mainly with FFR. The structure of the AUC tables concerning the use of antianginal therapy has changed to reflect usual practice patterns rating patients on the basis of no antianginal therapy, use of one antianginal drug, or use of two or more antianginal drugs. It is assumed that all patients are being treated with optimal guideline-directed medical therapies to reduce risk. In general, in patients with a low burden of coronary disease (e.g., single-vessel disease), low-risk findings on noninvasive testing, and/or no antianginal therapy, revascularization by PCI or CABG surgery is thought to be rarely appropriate as the initial step. As disease burden progresses through two-vessel to three-vessel and left main disease, revascularization by PCI or CABG frequently becomes rated as "may be appropriate care" or "appropriate care," with CABG surgery consistently rated as "appropriate care" for intermediate or high disease complexity (SYNTAX score ≥22), even in patients with ischemic symptoms who are not on antianginal therapy. Of note, CABG surgery was consistently rated as "appropriate care" and PCI as "rarely appropriate care" for left main bifurcation disease with intermediate or high disease burden in other vessels. In this way, recommendations found in the appropriateness criteria can facilitate discussions with patients, family, and members of the medical team regarding the likely benefits of revascularization strategies (Figs. 18.13, 18.14, 18.15, 18.16).

Two-Vessel Disease

	Asymptomatic		Ischemic Symptoms					
	Not on AA Therapy or With AA Therapy		Not on AA Therapy		On 1 AA Drug (BB Preferred)		On ≥2 AA Drugs	
Indication	PCI	CABG	PCI	CABG	PCI	CABG	PCI	CABG
No Proximal LAD Involvement								
7. ■ Low-risk findings on noninvasive testing	R (3)	R (2)	M (4)	R (3)	M (5)	M (4)	A (7)	M (6)
8. ■ Intermediate- or high-risk findings on noninvasive testing	M (5)	M (4)	M (6)	M (5)	A (7)	M (6)	A (8)	A (7)
9. ■ No stress test performed or, if performed, results are indeterminate ■ FFR ≤0.80[a] in both vessels	M (5)	M (4)	M (6)	M (4)	A (7)	M (5)	A (8)	A (7)
Proximal LAD Involvement and No Diabetes Present								
10. ■ Low-risk findings on noninvasive testing	M (4)	M (4)	M (5)	M (5)	M (6)	M (6)	A (7)	A (7)
11. ■ Intermediate- or high-risk findings on noninvasive testing	M (6)	M (6)	A (7)	A (7)	A (7)	A (7)	A (8)	A (8)
12. ■ No stress test performed or, if performed, results are indeterminate ■ FFR ≤0.80 in both vessels	M (6)	M (6)	M (6)	M (6)	A (7)	A (7)	A (8)	A (8)
Proximal LAD Involvement With Diabetes Present								
13. ■ Low-risk findings on noninvasive testing	M (4)	M (5)	M (4)	M (6)	M (6)	A (7)	A (7)	A (8)
14. ■ Intermediate- or high-risk findings on noninvasive testing	M (5)	A (7)	M (6)	A (7)	A (7)	A (8)	A (8)	A (9)
15. ■ No stress test performed or, if performed, results are indeterminate ■ FFR ≤0.80 in both vessels[a]	M (5)	M (6)	M (6)	A (7)	A (7)	A (8)	A (7)	A (8)

Fig. 18.14 Appropriateness ratings for asymptomatic patients or with ischemic symptoms and two-vessel disease (low or proximal left anterior descending coronary artery with or without diabetes) judged at low, intermediate or high risk. The number in parentheses next to the rating reflects the median score for that indication. [a]iFR measurements with appropriate normal ranges may be substituted for FFR. *A*, appropriate; *AA*, antianginal; *BB*, β-blockers; *CABG*, coronary artery bypass graft; *FFR*, fractional flow reserve; *iFR*, instant wave-free ratio; *LAD*, left anterior descending coronary artery; *M*, may be appropriate; *PCI*, percutaneous coronary intervention; *R*, rarely appropriate. (From Patel MR, Calhoon JH, Dehmer GJ, et al. ACC/AATS/AHA/ASE/ASNC/SCAI/SCCT/STS 2017 appropriate use criteria for coronary revascularization in patients with stable ischemic heart disease: a report of the American College of Cardiology Appropriate Use Criteria Task Force, American Association for Thoracic Surgery, American Heart Association, American Society of Echocardiography, American Society of Nuclear Cardiology, Society for Cardiovascular Angiography and Interventions, Society of Cardiovascular Computed Tomography, and Society of Thoracic Surgeons. *J Am Coll Cardiol.* 2017;69[17]:2212–2241.)

Silent Myocardial Ischemia

Silent myocardial ischemia is characterized by the presence of objective evidence of myocardial ischemia in the absence of chest discomfort or another anginal equivalent symptom. Silent myocardial ischemia can become manifest through ambulatory ECG monitoring or cardiac stress testing. Although the precise mechanism responsible for silent myocardial ischemia has not been established, a number of possible reasons for a lack of anginal symptoms during some episodes of ischemia have been proposed and include lesser severity and shorter duration of episodes, higher threshold for pain and/or inability to reach pain threshold, impaired perception of painful stimuli, defective anginal warning system, and higher β-endorphin levels. Reports in the 1980s and 1990s documented that between 25% and 45% of patients with coronary heart disease have myocardial ischemia during daily life, and most (>75%) of these ischemic episodes are not associated with chest pain. Furthermore, most silent ischemic episodes, as assessed by ambulatory ECG monitoring, occur during minimal or no physical exertion.[62,63]

Indeed, substantial evidence supports the prognostic hazard associated with silent myocardial ischemia, which may be present in 2% to 4% of the general population and is associated with numerous risk factors and markers of adverse outcome. Patients with diabetes mellitus, prior MI or ACS, chronic renal failure, sudden death episodes, and typical/atypical anginal symptoms may all exhibit evidence of asymptomatic myocardial ischemia on Holter monitor or exercise treadmill testing; prognosis may be impaired in these groups of patients. Unfortunately, it remains unclear when or in whom it is appropriate to screen for silent ischemia. The epidemiology of silent myocardial ischemia may be viewed from the standpoint of two groups of patients: patients with or without a known history of CHD. The increased risk of coronary events and cardiac mortality in association with silent myocardial ischemia has been extensively documented in patients with CHD. In a study of 937 patients with stable CHD (prior MI, documented coronary stenosis of at least 50%, prior ischemia on stress testing, or prior coronary revascularization) who underwent exercise stress echocardiography at baseline and were followed for an average of 3.9 years, 188 patients (20%) had silent myocardial ischemia, which was associated with a significant increase in cardiac death or MI compared with patients without angina or ischemia (HR 2.2; 95% CI 1.4 to 3.5).[64] In a study of 107 patients with chronic stable angina who underwent

SECTION III Coronary Intervention

Three-Vessel Disease

Indication	Asymptomatic				Ischemic Symptoms			
	Not on AA Therapy or With AA Therapy		Not on AA Therapy		On 1 AA Drug (BB Preferred)		On ≥2 AA Drugs	
	PCI	CABG	PCI	CABG	PCI	CABG	PCI	CABG
Low Disease Complexity (e.g., Focal Stenoses, SYNTAX ≤22)								
16. ■ Low-risk findings on noninvasive testing ■ No diabetes	M (4)	M (5)	M (5)	M (5)	M (6)	M (6)	A (7)	A (7)
17. ■ Intermediate- or high-risk findings on noninvasive testing ■ No diabetes	M (6)	A (7)	A (7)	A (7)	A (7)	A (8)	A (8)	A (8)
18. ■ Low-risk findings on noninvasive testing ■ Diabetes present	M (4)	M (6)	M (5)	M (6)	M (6)	A (7)	A (7)	A (8)
19. ■ Intermediate- or high-risk findings on noninvasive testing ■ Diabetes present	M (6)	A (7)	M (6)	A (8)	A (7)	A (8)	A (7)	A (9)
Intermediate or High Disease Complexity (e.g. Multiple Features of Complexity as Noted Previously, SYNTAX >22)								
20. ■ Low-risk findings on noninvasive testing ■ No diabetes	M (4)	M (6)	M (4)	A (7)	M (5)	A (7)	M (6)	A (8)
21. ■ Intermediate- or high-risk findings on noninvasive testing ■ No diabetes	M (5)	A (7)	M (6)	A (7)	M (6)	A (8)	M (6)	A (9)
22. ■ Low-risk findings on noninvasive testing ■ Diabetes present	M (4)	A (7)	M (4)	A (7)	M (5)	A (8)	M (6)	A (9)
23. ■ Intermediate- or high-risk findings on noninvasive testing ■ Diabetes present	M (4)	A (8)	M (5)	A (8)	M (5)	A (8)	M (6)	A (9)

Fig. 18.15 Appropriateness ratings for asymptomatic patients or with Ischemic symptoms and three-vessel disease (low or intermediate/high disease complexity). The number in parentheses next to the rating reflects the median score for that indication. *A*, Appropriate; *AA*, antianginal; *BB*, β-blockers; *CABG*, coronary artery bypass graft; *M*, may be appropriate; *PCI*, percutaneous coronary intervention; *SYNTAX*, Synergy between PCI with Taxus and Cardiac Surgery trial. (From Patel MR, Calhoon JH, Dehmer GJ, et al. ACC/AATS/AHA/ASE/ASNC/SCAI/SCCT/STS 2017 appropriate use criteria for coronary revascularization in patients with stable ischemic heart disease: a report of the American College of Cardiology Appropriate Use Criteria Task Force, American Association for Thoracic Surgery, American Heart Association, American Society of Echocardiography, American Society of Nuclear Cardiology, Society for Cardiovascular Angiography and Interventions, Society of Cardiovascular Computed Tomography, and Society of Thoracic Surgeons. *J Am Coll Cardiol.* 2017;69[17]:2212–2241.)

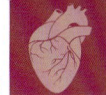

Left Main Disease

Indication	Asymptomatic		Ischemic Symptoms					
	Not on AA Therapy or With AA Therapy		Not on AA Therapy		On 1 AA Drug (BB Preferred)		On ≥2 AA Drugs	
	PCI	CABG	PCI	CABG	PCI	CABG	PCI	CABG
24. • Isolated LMCA disease • Ostial or midshaft stenosis	M (6)	A (8)	A (7)	A (8)	A (7)	A (9)	A (7)	A (9)
25. • Isolated LMCA disease • Bifurcation involvement	M (5)	A (8)	M (5)	A (8)	M (5)	A (9)	M (6)	A (9)
26. • LMCA disease • Ostial or midshaft stenosis • Concurrent multivessel disease • Low disease burden (e.g., 1–2 additional focal stenoses, SYNTAX score ≤22)	M (6)	A (8)	M (6)	A (9)	A (7)	A (9)	A (7)	A (9)
27. • Ostial or midshaft stenosis • Concurrent multivessel disease • Intermediate or high disease burden (e.g., 1–2 additional bifurcation stenosis, long stenoses, SYNTAX score >22)	M (4)	A (8)	M (4)	A (9)	M (4)	A (9)	M (4)	A (9)
28. • LMCA disease • Bifurcation involvement • Low disease burden in other vessels (e.g., 1–2 additional focal stenosis, SYNTAX score ≤22)	M (4)	A (8)	M (5)	A (8)	M (5)	A (9)	M (6)	A (9)
29. • LMCA disease • Bifurcation involvement • Intermediate or high disease burden in other vessels (e.g., 1–2 additional bifurcation stenosis, long stenoses, SYNTAX score >22)	R (3)	A (8)	R (3)	A (9)	R (3)	A (9)	R (3)	A (9)

Fig. 18.16 Appropriateness ratings for asymptomatic patients or with ischemic symptoms and left main disease. The number in parentheses next to the rating reflects the median score for that indication. *A*, Appropriate; *AA*, antianginal; *BB*, β-blockers; *CABG*, coronary artery bypass graft; *LMCA*, left main coronary artery; *M*, may be appropriate; *PCI*, percutaneous coronary intervention; *R*, rarely appropriate; *SYNTAX*, Synergy between PCI with Taxus and Cardiac Surgery trial. (From Patel MR, Calhoon JH, Dehmer GJ, et al. ACC/AATS/AHA/ASE/ASNC/SCAI/SCCT/STS 2017 appropriate use criteria for coronary revascularization in patients with stable ischemic heart disease: a report of the American College of Cardiology Appropriate Use Criteria Task Force, American Association for Thoracic Surgery, American Heart Association, American Society of Echocardiography, American Society of Nuclear Cardiology, Society for Cardiovascular Angiography and Interventions, Society of Cardiovascular Computed Tomography, and Society of Thoracic Surgeons. *J Am Coll Cardiol.* 2017;69[17]:2212–2241.)

ambulatory ECG monitoring and were followed for an average of 23 months, 46 patients (43%) had documented silent myocardial ischemia; patients with silent myocardial ischemia had a significantly greater likelihood of cardiac death.[65]

In the prospective "Heart and Soul Study," which enrolled 937 patients with stable CHD, the prevalence of "angina alone" was 14%, and the prevalence of "inducible ischemia without angina" (silent myocardial ischemia) was 20%. This study also demonstrated that inducible ischemia, in the absence of self-reported angina, predicts poor clinical outcomes. The Detection of Ischemia in Asymptomatic Diabetics (DIAD) trial[60] was a randomized trial to assess the clinical impact of screening for CAD in asymptomatic adults with diabetes mellitus. The study enrolled 1123 patients, of whom 522 were randomly assigned to adenosine-stress radionuclide myocardial perfusion imaging and 562 to routine care and follow-up. Of the screening group, 22% had documented silent myocardial ischemia, and 6% exhibited a significant degree of ischemia. At 5-year follow-up, the overall cardiac event rate was 2.9% (0.6%/year) and was not significantly different between the screened group and the group that was not screened (2.7% vs. 3.0%, P = .73). Among the small group of patients who underwent initial screening and had a significant degree of demonstrable ischemia, event rates were significantly higher than in the overall population (2.4%/year vs. 0.4%/year, P = .001). This trial demonstrated the low yield associated with screening asymptomatic patients, even those with high clinical risk profiles. In addition, although this trial was not intended to evaluate the benefit of revascularization for asymptomatic ischemia and did not regulate additional diagnostic or therapeutic measures beyond protocol-specified nuclear stress imaging, the impact of screening was very minor. Perhaps most remarkable was the dynamic nature of the documented ischemia. At 3-year follow-up, 79% of the patients identified as having asymptomatic myocardial ischemia at baseline no longer exhibited evidence of ischemia, but 10% of patients without previously documented ischemia had an abnormal study during that time.

The most direct evidence of a potential role for revascularization in patients with asymptomatic ischemia was documented in the Asymptomatic Cardiac Ischemic Pilot (ACIP) trial.[66] In ACIP, 558 patients with coronary disease suitable for revascularization, silent ischemia on Holter monitor, and ischemia on exercise testing were randomized to MT of angina, MT of angina and ambulatory ischemic episodes, or revascularization. At both 1- and 2-year follow-up, survival was best in the routine revascularization arm and was worst in the angina-guided arm, suggesting that amelioration of silent ischemia through prompt revascularization may provide important clinical benefit (Fig. 18.17).

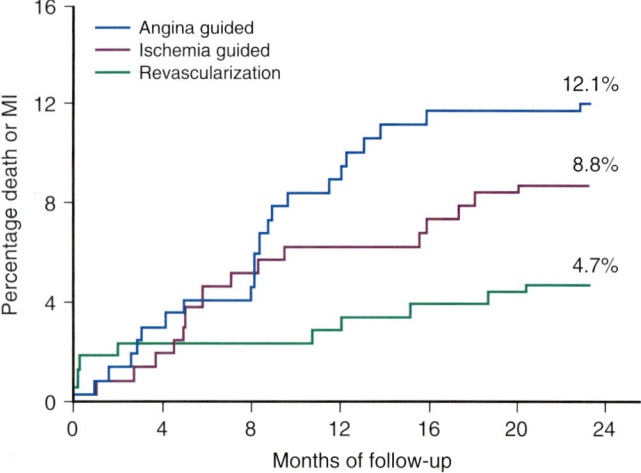

Fig. 18.17 Two-year cumulative rates of death or myocardial infarction. Data are from 558 patients with ischemia on ambulatory monitoring and stress testing treated with revascularization, revascularization in the presence of documented ischemia, or angina-guided revascularization. The outcome of the planned revascularization strategy was significantly different from that of the angina-guided strategy, with a 61% relative risk reduction ($P < .01$). The 27% relative risk reduction between the angina-guided and ischemia-guided arms was not significant, nor was the difference between the revascularization and ischemia-guided strategies. *MI*, Myocardial infarction. (From Davies RF, Goldberg AD, Forman S, et al. Asymptomatic Cardiac Ischemia Pilot [ACIP] study two-year follow-up: outcomes of patients randomized to initial strategies of medical therapy versus revascularization. *Circulation*. 1997;95[8]:2037–2043.)

SUMMARY

Symptomatic CAD is a growing problem throughout the world, with significant associated economic and societal costs. Although there is presently no cure for ischemic CAD, it is increasingly possible to alter the course of the disease through judicious utilization of the rapidly evolving medical, surgical, and percutaneous therapies currently available. Functional assessment of coronary ischemia and the current diagnostic tools to stratify clinical risk significantly contributed to the elaboration of more refined treatment algorithms of patients with CAD. Successful disease management and symptom palliation can be achieved by a robust regimen based on optimal medical management and risk-factor modification through diet and exercise. Percutaneous revascularization also plays an important role in achieving improved quality of life and, ultimately, prognosis. Indeed, percutaneous revascularization can effectively modulate long-term outcome directly through a reduction of ischemic burden, as well as indirectly through symptom control and improved exercise tolerance. As percutaneous technology continues to evolve, which it surely will, promising new indications will be discovered and added to the ever-expanding list of beneficial effects. In the setting of rising health care costs and the economic realities of delivering a finite resource, however, efforts to establish and clarify the most appropriate revascularization strategies and candidates will ensure the continued availability of these techniques for an ever-growing population of those who may benefit.

KEY REFERENCES

5. Barsness GW, Gersh BJ, Brooks MM, et al. Rationale for the revascularization arm of the Bypass Angioplasty Revascularization Investigation 2 Diabetes (BARI 2D) Trial. *Am J Cardiol*. 2006;97(12A):31G–40G.
9. Stone GW, Maehara A, Lansky AJ, et al. A prospective natural-history study of coronary atherosclerosis. *N Engl J Med*. 2011;364(3):226–235.
12. Iqbal J, Zhang YJ, Holmes DR, et al. Optimal medical therapy improves clinical outcomes in patients undergoing revascularization with percutaneous coronary intervention or coronary artery bypass grafting: insights from the Synergy Between Percutaneous Coronary Intervention with TAXUS and Cardiac Surgery (SYNTAX) trial at the 5-year follow-up. *Circulation*. 2015;131(14):1269–1277.
14. Wijeysundera HC, Nallamothu BK, Krumholz HM, et al. Meta-analysis: effects of percutaneous coronary intervention versus medical therapy on angina relief. *Ann Intern Med*. 2010;152(6):370–379.
15. Boden WE, O'Rourke RA, Teo KK, et al. Optimal medical therapy with or without PCI for stable coronary disease. *N Engl J Med*. 2007;356(15):1503–1516.
17. Al-Lamee R, Thompson D, Dehbi HM, et al. Percutaneous coronary intervention in stable angina (ORBITA): a double-blind, randomised controlled trial. *Lancet*. 2018;391(10115):31–40.
24. Patel MR, Calhoon JH, Dehmer GJ, et al. ACC/AATS/AHA/ASE/ASNC/SCAI/SCCT/STS 2017 appropriate use criteria for coronary revascularization in patients with stable ischemic heart disease: a report of the American College of Cardiology Appropriate Use Criteria Task Force, American Association for Thoracic Surgery, American Heart Association, American Society of Echocardiography, American Society of Nuclear Cardiology, Society for Cardiovascular Angiography and Interventions, Society of Cardiovascular Computed Tomography, and Society of Thoracic Surgeons. *J Am Coll Cardiol*. 2017;69(17):2212–2241.
31. Frye RL, August P, Brooks MM, et al. A randomized trial of therapies for type 2 diabetes and coronary artery disease. *N Engl J Med*. 2009;360(24):2503–2515.
39. Serruys PW, Morice MC, Kappetein AP, et al. Percutaneous coronary intervention versus coronary-artery bypass grafting for severe coronary artery disease. *New Engl J Med*. 2009;360(10):961–972.
40. Sipahi I, Akay MH, Dagdelen S, et al. Coronary artery bypass grafting vs percutaneous coronary intervention and long-term mortality and morbidity in multivessel disease: meta-analysis of randomized clinical trials of the arterial grafting and stenting era. *JAMA Intern Med*. 2014;174(2):223–230.
43. van Nunen LX, Zimmermann FM, Tonino PA, et al. Fractional flow reserve versus angiography for guidance of PCI in patients with multivessel coronary disease (FAME): 5-year follow-up of a randomised controlled trial. *Lancet*. 2015;386(10006):1853–1860.
44. Stone GW, Sabik JF, Serruys PW, et al. Everolimus-eluting stents or bypass surgery for left main coronary artery disease. *N Engl J Med*. 2016;375(23):2223–2235.
46. Farkouh ME, Domanski M, Sleeper LA, et al. Strategies for multivessel revascularization in patients with diabetes. *N Engl J Med*. 2012;367(25):2375–2384.
48. De Bruyne B, Fearon WF, Pijls NH, et al. Fractional flow reserve-guided PCI for stable coronary artery disease. *N Engl J Med*. 2014;371(13):1208–1217.
50. Velazquez EJ, Lee KL, Deja MA, et al. Coronary-artery bypass surgery in patients with left ventricular dysfunction. *N Engl J Med*. 2011;364(17):1607–1616.
56. Morice MC, Serruys PW, Kappetein AP, et al. Outcomes in patients with de novo left main disease treated with either percutaneous coronary intervention using paclitaxel-eluting stents or coronary artery bypass graft treatment in the Synergy Between Percutaneous Coronary Intervention with TAXUS and Cardiac Surgery (SYNTAX) trial. *Circulation*. 2010;121(24):2645–2653.
59. Farooq V, van Klaveren D, Steyerberg EW, et al. Anatomical and clinical characteristics to guide decision making between coronary artery bypass surgery and percutaneous coronary intervention for individual patients: development and validation of SYNTAX score II. *Lancet*. 2013;381(9867):639–650.

 Additional references available online at expertconsult.com.

中文导读

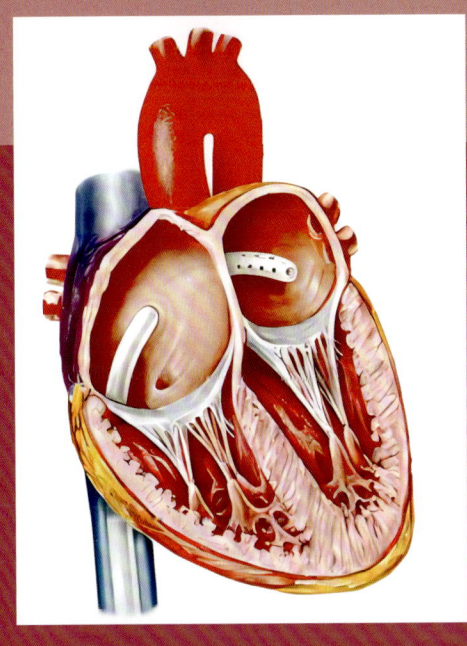

第19章
非ST段抬高型急性冠状动脉综合征的干预

  不稳定型心绞痛和非ST段抬高型心肌梗死属于急性冠状动脉综合征的范畴，但与ST段抬高型心肌梗死在病理生理、临床路径、总体预后等方面存在差异。虽然即刻冠状动脉再灌注治疗ST段抬高型心肌梗死明显优于非ST段抬高型急性冠状动脉综合征，但对于非ST段抬高型急性冠状动脉综合征的最佳治疗策略、时机和干预措施仍存在争议。尽管在药物和机械干预方面取得了进展，但非ST段抬高型急性冠状动脉综合征相关的短期和长期死亡率及并发症发生率仍然很高。因此，对于非ST段抬高型急性冠状动脉综合征的患者应进行充分评估，通过缺血（GRACE评分）、出血（CRUSADE评分）危险分层为不同患者制定更精准的治疗策略。非ST段抬高型急性冠状动脉综合征的辅助抗栓治疗，包括抗血小板、肠外抗凝治疗，以及GPⅡb/Ⅲa受体抑制剂的应用，这些治疗使缺血事件风险尤其是介入术后支架内血栓风险大大降低，但同时也应关注这些治疗所带来的出血风险。对于经皮冠状动脉搭桥术和冠状动脉旁路移植术的有效性和安全性的比较，尽管在过去的几十年里进行了多项随机临床试验，但除了在特定的亚群中，没有确凿的证据表明冠状动脉旁路移植术和经皮冠状动脉介入治疗之间的疗效有显著差异。对于特殊病变、特殊人群，如左主干病变、多支血管病变、糖尿病、左心室功能障碍的患者，应在利用评分工具充分评估后，进行血运重建策略的选择。对于多支血管病变，非ST段抬高型急性冠状动脉综合征患者可以在评估病变的解剖复杂性、冠状动脉血流动力学意义，以及对比剂诱导的肾病和其他并发症的风险基础上选择个体化经皮冠状动脉介入治疗策略。

  本章主要介绍了非ST段抬高型急性冠状动脉综合征患者的危险分层、血运重建策略、辅助抗栓治疗，以及非ST段抬高型急性冠状动脉综合征合并复杂病变和在特殊人群中的注意事项等，这对临床决策有一定的指导意义。

李英凯　柳景华

章节要点

- 所有非ST段抬高型急性冠状动脉综合征患者在诊断时都需要进行危险分层。风险分层可提供预后价值,并有助于指导治疗决策。

- 对于出现血流动力学不稳定、危及生命的心律失常或心肌梗死机械性并发症的非ST段抬高型急性冠状动脉综合征患者,建议在2小时内进行即刻冠状动脉造影。

- 与缺血指导的治疗相比,早期有创血运重建策略已证实可减少再发缺血事件发生率。对于非ST段抬高型急性冠状动脉综合征患者,尤其是具有高危特征(例如,ST段改变或生物标记物升高)的患者,支持进行早期有创治疗。

- 对于所有确诊为非ST段抬高型急性冠状动脉综合征的患者,建议采用阿司匹林联合$P2Y_{12}$抑制剂的方案进行双联抗血小板治疗。$P2Y_{12}$抑制剂的选择、用药时机和持续时间取决于患者因素及手术因素。

- 无须考虑治疗策略,所有诊断为非ST段抬高型急性冠状动脉综合征的患者,均推荐给予注射抗凝治疗。

- 所有GPⅡb/Ⅲa受体抑制剂均在经皮冠状动脉介入治疗时使用,对于具有高危特征的非ST段抬高型急性冠状动脉综合征患者应持续维持给药。

- 在非ST段抬高型急性冠状动脉综合征患者中,与股动脉相比,桡动脉是首选入路。已证实,非ST段抬高型急性冠状动脉综合征患者经桡动脉入路的大出血发生率更低。

- 在特殊人群中,如存在左主干病变、多支血管病变或糖尿病的患者,对于冠状动脉旁路移植术与经皮冠状动脉介入治疗的疗效差异,目前还存在相当大的争论。反映当代临床实践的新试验表明,经皮冠状动脉介入治疗可为这些特殊人群带来潜在的净获益,但这一证据仍然没有定论。

19 Intervention for Non–ST-Segment Elevation Acute Coronary Syndromes

C. Michael Gibson, Serge Korjian, Yazan Daaboul

KEY POINTS

- All patients with non–ST-segment elevation acute coronary syndromes (NSTE-ACS) need to undergo risk stratification at the time of diagnosis. Risk stratification provides prognostic value and helps guide the therapeutic decision-making process.
- Immediate angiography within 2 hours is recommended for NSTE-ACS patients who present with either hemodynamic instability or life threatening arrhythmias or mechanical complications of myocardial infarction.
- Compared with ischemia-guided management, an early invasive strategy for revascularization has been associated with a reduced rate of recurrent ischemic events and is favored among patients with NSTE-ACS, particularly among those with high-risk features, such as ST-segment changes or elevated biomarkers.
- Dual antiplatelet therapy with aspirin plus a $P2Y_{12}$ inhibitor is recommended for all patients diagnosed with NSTE-ACS. The choice, timing, and duration of the $P2Y_{12}$ inhibitor depends on individual patient (as well as procedural) factors.
- Irrespective of the treatment strategy, parenteral anticoagulant therapy is recommended for all patients diagnosed with NSTE-ACS.
- All GP IIb/IIIa inhibitors are administered at the time of percutaneous coronary intervention (PCI) and are reserved for NSTE-ACS patients with high-risk features.
- Radial access is preferred to femoral access and has been associated with a lower incidence of major bleeding among NSTE-ACS patients.
- There is considerable debate regarding the difference in efficacy between coronary artery bypass graft and PCI in special populations, such as those with left main coronary artery disease, multivessel disease, or history of diabetes. New trials that reflect contemporary practice suggest a potential net benefit with PCI, but this evidence remains inconclusive.

OVERVIEW

Unstable angina (UA) and non–ST-segment elevation myocardial infarction (NSTEMI) belong to the spectrum of acute coronary syndromes (ACSs), but are distinct from ST-segment myocardial infarction (STEMI) in their pathophysiology, clinical approach, and overall prognosis. While immediate coronary reperfusion is clearly superior in STEMI, controversy remains regarding the optimal strategy, timing, and interventions for non–ST-segment elevation acute coronary syndromes (NSTE-ACS). Despite advances in pharmacologic and mechanical interventions, the risks of short-term and long-term mortality and morbidity associated with NSTE-ACS remains elevated.

RISK STRATIFICATION

Ischemic Risk Stratification

Several risk stratification tools have been developed that can be applied at the time of the diagnosis of NSTE-ACS, which are associated with short-term and long-term outcomes, including death, recurrent myocardial infarction (MI), and need for urgent revascularization. In addition to providing prognostic value, risk stratification may help guide the therapeutic decision-making process, including recommendations regarding the use of antithrombotic and antiplatelet agents, and the need for early revascularization. The importance of early risk stratification has also been highlighted in cardiovascular society guidelines, and currently has a class I recommendation in the 2015 European Society of Cardiology (ESC) guidelines and a class IIa recommendation in the 2014 American Heart Association (AHA) and American College of Cardiology (ACC) guidelines.[1,2] While many risk scores have already been well validated, each is limited by its individual drawbacks and should be interpreted in the context of these limitations.

The Thrombolysis in Myocardial Infarction (TIMI) risk score utilizes seven clinical variables and is designed to be easily calculated at the bedside to predict the 14-day risk of all-cause mortality, MI, or recurrent ischemia requiring revascularization (C-statistic = 0.65) (Fig. 19.1).[3] The variables are: age ≥ 65 years, at least three coronary artery disease (CAD) risk factors, known CAD with stenosis on angiography of at least 50%, use of aspirin in the past 7 days, severe angina with two or more episodes within 24 hours, ST-segment changes of at least 0.5 mm, and positive cardiac biomarker. The TIMI risk score was initially derived from cohorts of two phase 3 randomized trials for unfractionated heparin (UFH) versus enoxaparin in NSTE-ACS. The test cohort included patients randomized to the UFH group in the TIMI 11B trial ($n = 1957$), whereas the three validation cohorts included the remainder of patients in the merged data; that is, patients randomized to the enoxaparin group in the TIMI 11B trial ($n = 1953$) and the two treatment groups in the ESSENCE trial (Efficacy and Safety of Subcutaneous Enoxaparin in Unstable Angina and Non–Q-Wave MI) ($n = 3171$). The presence of each risk factor corresponds to 1 point, and the simple arithmetic sum of the number of variables present correlates with clinical outcomes.[3] Accordingly, a TIMI risk score of 0 correlates with a 4.7% event rate through 14 days, whereas a ten-fold gradient event rate (40.9%) occurs among patients with a score of 6 to 7.

Following its internal validation, the TIMI score was then applied to other randomized clinical trials, and externally

- Age ≥65 years
- ≥2 anginal events in 24 h
- ST-segment deviation
- Elevated serum cardiac markers
- ≥3 risk factors for CAD
- Aspirin use (prior 7 days)
- Prior coronary stenosis (>50%)

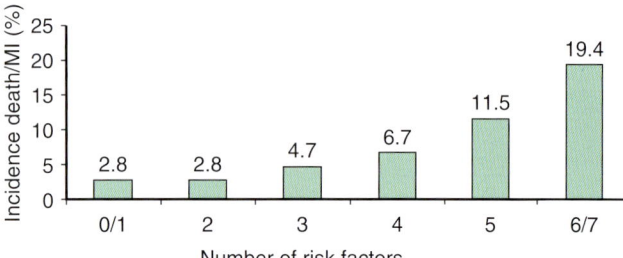

Fig. 19.1 The Thrombolysis in Myocardial Infarction (TIMI) risk score for death or myocardial infarction *(MI)* at 14 days. A score of 1 is assigned when a factor is present. *CAD,* Coronary artery disease.

validated in other real-world registries for long-term outcomes occurring through 30 days, 6 weeks, and 12 months.[4–8] In the platelet receptor inhibition for ischemic syndrome management in patients limited by unstable signs and symptoms (PRISM-PLUS) trial for tirofiban (*n* = 11,915), the TIMI risk score demonstrated a strong prognostic discriminatory capacity in identifying patients who were more likely to benefit from more aggressive pharmacologic therapy using platelet glycoprotein (GP) IIb/IIIa inhibitors in addition to heparin and aspirin.[4] The TIMI risk score modified the treatment effect, where patients with a TIMI risk score of 4 or greater were at higher risk of developing adverse events, and had a greater relative risk reduction as compared with those with lower TIMI risk scores. Similarly, in the TACTICS-TIMI 18 trial for tirofiban (Treat Angina with Aggrastat and Determine Cost of Therapy with an Invasive or Conservative Strategy), NSTE-ACS patients with either intermediate risk (TIMI score of 3 or 4) or high risk (TIMI score of 5 to 7) derived a significant 30-day benefit from the use of early invasive strategy for revascularization, whereas low-risk patients (TIMI risk score of 1 or 2) did not.[5]

In a similar fashion to the TIMI risk score, the PURSUIT risk score was developed using a cohort of patients who were randomized in the PURSUIT trial for eptifibatide (Platelet glycoprotein IIb/IIIa in UA: Receptor Suppression Using Integrilin (eptifibatide) Therapy) (*n* = 9461).[9] The risk models in PURSUIT identified seven patient characteristics that were associated with either all-cause death alone (C-statistic = 0.81) or the composite of all-cause death or MI (C-statistic = 0.67) through 30 days following hospital admission. These characteristics included patient age, gender, highest Canadian Cardiovascular Society (CCS)-class in the previous 6 weeks prior to admission, heart rate, systolic blood pressure, signs of heart failure, and ST-segment depression on presenting electrocardiogram (ECG). Points were given for each predictive factor that was present, which were then added to provide a final risk score. This score was then plotted on a graph that illustrated the variation of 30-day mortality (y-axis) as a function of the risk score (x-axis). Interestingly, the score relied heavily on patient age (i.e., age contributes to 8 to 14 points out of the total 20 points), whereas baseline biomarkers were not included.

In contrast to both TIMI and PURSUIT risk scores, the Global Registry of Acute Coronary Events (GRACE) risk score was developed using the patient cohort included in the GRACE registry (*n* = 43,810) (Fig. 19.2).[10] The GRACE risk score models predicted in-hospital risk, as well as the cumulative 6-month risk, of the same end points studied in the PURSUIT risk score: either all-cause death alone (C-statistic = 0.81) or the composite of all-cause death or MI (C-statistic = 0.73).[11] The score was then validated using the cohort of patients randomized in the GUSTO IIb trial (Global Use of Strategies to Open Occluded Open Arteries) (*n* = 12,142).[12] However, it was thought that the original risk models were too complex, consisting of 14 variables for the in-hospital all-cause death outcome and 12 variables for the composite outcome. Due to their complexity, a simplified nomogram was eventually developed that reduced the score to the most substantial eight variables that provided the highest predictive capacity for both the in-hospital and 6-month outcomes. These variables included patient age, heart rate, systolic blood pressure, serum creatinine, Killip class for heart failure, cardiac arrest at admission, ST-segment deviation on presenting ECG, and baseline elevation in cardiac biomarkers.

Afterwards, the GRACE 2.0 score was developed to evaluate risk of outcomes through longer periods of time, that is, 1 year and 3 years, and was then validated externally against the French Registry on Acute ST-Elevation and Non–ST-Elevation Myocardial Infarction (FAST-MI) registry.[13] Compared with the initial GRACE score, the GRACE 2.0 score excluded serum creatinine and Killip class, which might not be readily available at the time of clinical evaluation, and replaced them with renal failure and diuretic use, respectively. More importantly, GRACE 2.0 incorporated non linear statistical models that could estimate risks more accurately than the original GRACE models.[13] Notably, the robustness of the GRACE risk score remained strong even when outcomes were evaluated at the 5-year follow-up mark (C-statistic = 0.77 for all-cause mortality).[14]

More recently, the CRUSADE (Can Rapid Stratification of Unstable Angina Patients Suppress Adverse Outcomes with Early Implementation of the ACC/AHA Guidelines) risk score was developed using the CRUSADE registry data. The patient population specifically included older NSTE-ACS patients of at least 65 years of age, and risk modeling was performed based on long-term outcomes through 1, 2, and 3 years (*n* = 43,239).[15] In the validation cohort, a total of 13 baseline clinical variables were independently associated with the outcome of all-cause mortality through 1 year and were further evaluated in the validation cohort (C-statistic = 0.75). Variables included patient age, gender, heart rate, systolic blood pressure, weight, signs of heart failure on presentation, prior history of heart failure, history of stroke, history of diabetes mellitus, history of peripheral arterial disease, hematocrit, serum creatinine, and troponin on admission. The CRUSADE models identified age as the most significant predictor of mortality, a finding previously reported in the PURSUIT risk score. However, when compared to the 5-year GRACE cohort, the CRUSADE population was significantly older (mean age of 77 years in CRUSADE vs. 67 years in the GRACE).[14,15] The advantages of the CRUSADE risk score is its strong discriminatory capacity; nonetheless, it is newer than the TIMI, PURSUIT, and GRACE scores and is yet to be validated as extensively as the other scores in external cohorts.

When reconciling all these risk scores, it is evident that they are not only clinically useful, but also suffer from substantial limitations, as each has been individually criticized for fundamental design, statistical, and clinical pitfalls. Their predictive power is moderately good, where the C-statistic is reported to be low as 0.65 when the internal validation cohorts were evaluated, and occasionally lower with other external validations. The positive predictive value of these scores may also be modest. Despite their limitations, these tools—particularly the TIMI and GRACE scores—have withstood the test of time and proven useful when extensively validated in real-world observational studies, as well as when used as stratification methods for investigational therapies in randomized

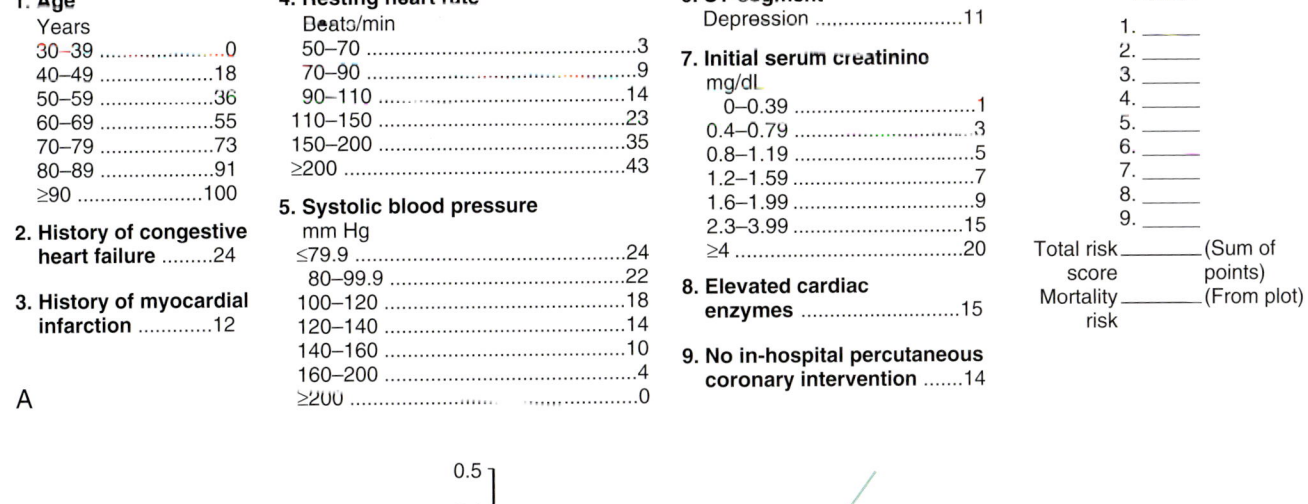

Fig. 19.2 (A) The Grace Risk Score for estimation of 6-month mortality in patients after hospitalization for acute coronary syndrome. (B) Plot of predicted all-cause mortality by total risk score.

clinical trials. Nonetheless, novel assessment models are under development in an effort to overcome these limitations, but these scores have so far been based on modest sample sizes and, albeit promising, will require extensive validation prior to becoming clinically useful.[16,17]

Bleeding Risk Stratification

Although patients with NSTE-ACS benefit from antithrombotic therapy at the time of diagnosis, antiplatelet and anticoagulant therapies are associated with an increased risk of bleeding. Balancing the risk of ischemia and the risk of bleeding is challenging, and there are no prediction models that simultaneously incorporate the two. Furthermore, bleeding scores have not been as extensively employed in the stratification of patients in clinical trials as ischemic scores. However, baseline prediction of the bleeding risk may complement the estimation of ischemic risk and may help guide a balanced approach to the risks and benefits of adjunctive pharmacologic therapies in NSTE-ACS.

The CRUSADE bleeding score was developed among 71,277 patients enrolled in the CRUSADE quality improvement initiative.[18] It is comprised of eight clinical variables that include baseline hematocrit, creatinine clearance, gender, signs of congestive heart failure on presentation, history of diabetes mellitus, history of prior vascular disease, heart rate, and systolic blood pressure (C statistic = 0.71). The score quantifies risk for in-hospital major bleeding and categorizes patients by quintiles of bleeding risk ranging from very low risk (3.1% risk of bleeding) to very high risk (19.5% risk of bleeding).[18,19] Remarkably, all eight variables in the CRUSADE bleeding score have been included in ischemic risk scores, highlighting that patients with high bleeding risk are also those with high risk of ischemia.

APPROACH TO REVASCULARIZATION

Once the diagnosis of NSTE-ACS is made, early risk assessment using risk scores is indicated for all patients and is used to assign patients to one of three strategies for revascularization: (1) immediate angiography, (2) invasive strategy; that is, revascularization without the need for prior non-invasive evaluation, or (3) ischemia-guided strategy; that is, referral for noninvasive evaluation followed by revascularization when indicated (Fig. 19.3).[1] The determination and implementation of the most appropriate revascularization strategy carries significant short-term and long-term prognostic implications.

Immediate Angiography

Immediate angiography within 2 hours is recommended for patients who present with at least one of the following features: hemodynamic instability due to either cardiogenic shock or mechanical complication of the MI event, overt heart failure, persistent angina despite pharmacologic therapy, or unstable ventricular arrhythmias. There are no randomized trials that compare a strategy of immediate angiography to other strategies in this subgroup of patients, and these recommendations are therefore based on expert opinion. Overall, the prognosis in these clinical scenarios is thought to be poor; and accordingly, these patients would likely benefit from immediate revascularization if they have no other severe life-threatening co-morbidities that would preclude either surgical or endovascular intervention.

Invasive Versus Ischemia-Guided Strategy

An early invasive strategy for revascularization is favored among patients with NSTE-ACS. Compared with an ischemia-guided strategy, an early invasive strategy has been associated with a reduced rate of recurrent ischemic events. Historically, prior to the

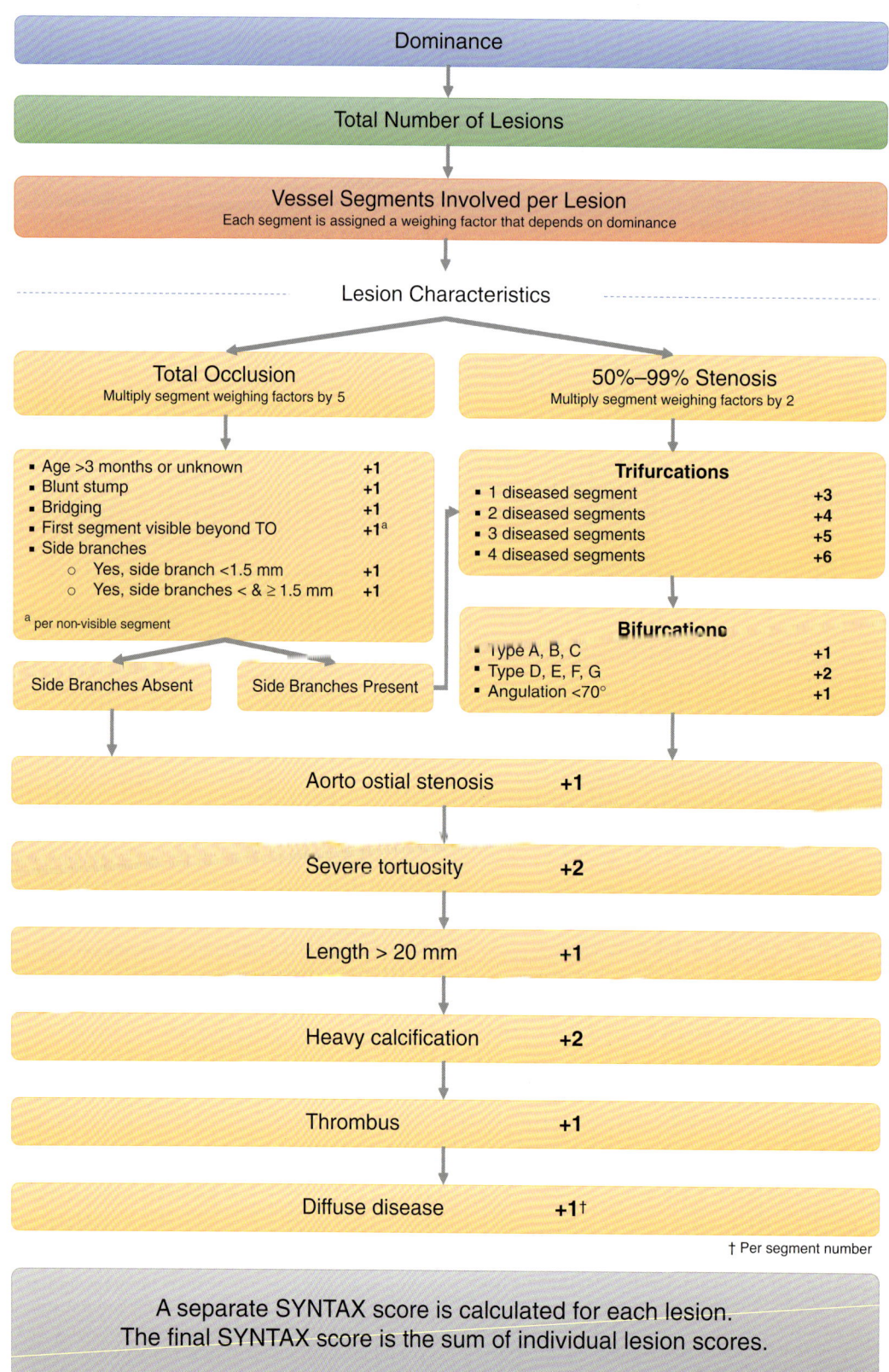

Fig. 19.3 Algorithm for the management of patients with NSTE-ACS. *TO*, Total Occlusion. (From Amsterdam EA, Wenger NK, Brindis RG, et al. 2014 AHA/ACC Guideline for the Management of Patients with Non-ST-Elevation Acute Coronary Syndromes: a report of the American College of Cardiology/American Heart Association Task Force on Practice Guidelines. *J Am Coll Cardiol.* 2014;64[24]:e139–e228.)

development of novel antithrombotic therapies and new devices, trials comparing invasive versus ischemia-guided strategies showed mixed, inconclusive results.[20-22] The FRISC-II study (Fragmin and Fast Revascularization during Instability in Coronary Artery Disease) was the first randomized trial to compare an early invasive strategy to ischemia-guided strategy in the era of stenting and GP IIb/IIIa inhibitors. An early invasive strategy within 7 to 10 days significantly reduced the composite of all-cause death or MI through 6 months (9.4% vs. 12.1%, $P = .031$) and 1 year (10.4% vs. 14.1%, $P = .005$) ($n = 2457$) as compared with a conservative strategy of heparin administration for 3 months. Although the 6-month analysis demonstrated no reduction in death at 6 months in the overall population, there was a significant 43% relative risk reduction in the rate of death when comparison was made at 1 year.[23,24] Further subgroup analysis also demonstrated a gender effect, where men derived the most benefit with an invasive strategy, an effect that was not observed among women (P-interaction = .012 for the composite end point of death and MI, and P-interaction = .029 for the end point of death alone).

More recently, additional pharmacologic and mechanical interventions have been introduced; since the introduction of the strategies, the balance between an invasive and ischemia-guided strategy has increasingly favored early intervention. In the TACTICS-TIMI-18 randomized trial (Treat Angina with Aggrastat and Determine Cost of Therapy with an Invasive or Conservative Strategy–Thrombolysis in Myocardial Infarction 18), NSTE-ACS patients were randomized to either early invasive strategy within 4 to 48 hours or conservative strategy ($n = 2220$). Only high-risk patients treated with the GP IIb/IIIa inhibitor tirofiban who also had either ST-segment or T-wave changes, elevated biomarkers, or history of CAD were enrolled. Compared with conservative strategy, early invasive strategy was associated with a significant reduction in ischemic outcomes through 6 months (15.9% vs. 19.4%, $P = .025$). Similarly, the rates of the composite of all-cause death or nonfatal MI were significantly lower with the invasive strategy when evaluated at 30 days (4.7% vs. 7.0%) and at 6 months (7.3% vs. 9.5%).[5]

As the definition of MI evolved, the relevance of TACTICS-TIMI-18 was questioned given its use of earlier definitions of MI. Subsequently, the RITA-3 trial (third Randomized Intervention Treatment of Angina) randomized NSTE-ACS patients to either early intervention or conservative strategy ($n = 1810$), but the definition of MI was consistent with the new third universal definition.[25] Early intervention in RITA-3 was likewise associated with reduction in the primary end point of all-cause death, nonfatal MI, or refractory angina through 4 months compared with ischemia-guided strategy (9.6% vs. 14.5%, 0.66, 95% confidence interval [CI] 0.51-0.85; $P = .001$). This reduction was driven mainly by differences in rates of refractory angina.[26]

In contrast to other contemporary trials, the ICTUS trial (Invasive Versus Conservative Treatment in Unstable Coronary Syndromes) showed no benefit with routine invasive strategy ($n = 1200$). ICTUS enriched for high-risk subjects and enrolled only NSTE-ACS patients with positive troponin and either a history of CAD or new ischemic ECG changes. Patients were randomized to either an early routine invasive strategy or a selective invasive strategy (i.e., medical management and subsequent revascularization only if persistent symptoms or life-threatening features).[27] Both strategies had similar rates of the primary end point of all-cause death, nonfatal MI, or rehospitalization for anginal symptoms at 1 year. Although an early invasive strategy was associated with a significantly reduced rate of rehospitalization (7.4% vs. 10.9%, $P = .04$), this was offset by a higher rate of nonfatal MIs (15.0% vs.10.0%, $P = .005$), particularly in the periprocedural timeframe. This high rate of MI was attributed to the protocol's definition of MI, which used a very low threshold for MI using creatine-kinase myocardial bands (CK-MB), as well as a substantially high sampling frequency for CK-MB of every 6 hours postpercutaneous coronary intervention (PCI). Although this definition was consistent with the contemporary society guidelines at the time, it was different from the definitions used in any of the other trials.[28]

Unfortunately, individual trials lacked statistical power to demonstrate efficacy. In a pooled meta-analysis of FRISC-II, ICTUS, and RITA-3 ($n = 5467$), a routine invasive strategy was associated with 19% reduced risk of the composite of cardiovascular (CV) death or nonfatal MI as compared with selective invasive strategy through 5 years (14.7% vs. 17.9%, hazard ratio [HR] = 0.81, 95% CI 0.71 to 0.93; $P = .002$).[24,27,29,30] This reduction was primarily driven by a 23% reduced rate of nonfatal MIs (10.0% vs. 12.9%), with numerical trends also favoring routine invasive strategy for CV death and all-cause death.[30] The benefit of an early invasive strategy did not attenuate over time among patients followed through 5 years.[30] In another pooled analysis of seven randomized trials including 8375 NSTE-ACS patients, the early invasive strategy was similarly associated with a 25% relative risk reduction for all-cause death (4.9% vs. 6.5%, HR = 0.75, 95% CI 0.63 to 0.90; $P = .001$) and 17% for nonfatal MIs (7.6% vs. 9.1%, HR = 0.83, 95% CI 0.72 to 0.96; $P = .012$) through 1 year.[31]

Among NSTE-ASC patients, an early invasive strategy is generally preferred over an ischemia-guided strategy. High-risk patients, namely patients with troponin elevation and ST-segment change, are the subgroup of patients most likely to benefit from an early invasive strategy.

Timing of the Intervention: Early Versus Delayed Invasive Strategy

While it was postulated that early angiography leads to early revascularization and resolution of tissue ischemia, delayed angiography beyond 24 hours was thought to result in stronger plaque stabilization, the onset of pharmacologic efficacy of orally administered antiplatelet agents, and a reduced rate of periprocedural thromboembolic events. Results from smaller trials were inconsistent, and data from larger trials were not helpful as the median timing of the PCI in these trials ranged widely between 19 hours in ICTUS and 96 hours in FRISC-II.[24,27] In small trials, namely VINO (Value of First Day Coronary Angiography/Angioplasty in Evolving Non-ST Segment Elevation Myocardial Infarction) ($n = 131$), ISAR-COOL (Intracoronary Stenting With Antithrombotic Regimen Cooling Off among NSTE-ACS patients) ($n = 410$), and RIDDLE-NSTEMI (Randomized study of Immediate versus Delayed Invasive Intervention in patients with NSTEMI) ($n = 323$), an early invasive strategy, when performed within 2 to 24 hours, was associated with a significant reduction in the rate of all-cause death or recurrent MI as compared with a delayed strategy.[32-34] In contrast, there was an increased rate of MI with immediate PCI in the OPTIMA trial ($n = 142$),[35] and no benefit with early angiography when performed within 24 hours in ABOARD (Angioplasty to Blunt the Rise of Troponin in Acute Coronary Syndromes Randomized for an Immediate or Delayed Intervention) ($n = 352$), enzyme-linked immunosorbent assay (ELISA) ($n = 220$), ELISA-3 ($n = 542$), and LIPSIA-NSTEMI (Leipzig Immediate versus early and late PercutaneouS coronary Intervention triAl in NSTEMI) ($n = 401$).[36-39]

All these trials were primarily limited by their small sample size, low event rates, and occasionally the use of surrogate measures assess clinical outcomes. The comparison between early intervention within 24 hours and delayed intervention beyond 36 hours was eventually performed in the adequately powered, large-scale TIMACS randomized trial (The Timing of Intervention in Acute Coronary Syndromes) ($n = 3031$). Early intervention did not reduce the primary end point of all-cause death, MI, or stroke, but was associated with a 28% relative risk reduction in the secondary outcome of death, MI, or refractory ischemia (9.5% vs. 12.9%, HR = 0.72, 95% CI 0.58 to 0.89; $P = .003$) and also appeared to be particularly superior among high-risk patients who had a GRACE score of more than 140 points on admission.[40]

Finally, a meta-analysis of eight randomized trials, including TIMACS, demonstrated that early intervention was associated with a numerical reduction in mortality, but this benefit did not reach statistical significance (HR = 0.81, 95% CI 0.64 to 1.03; $P = .088$). Patients with elevated biomarkers at baseline, history of diabetes, age of more than 75 years, and high GRACE score were identified as subgroups who derived significant benefit with an early invasive strategy within 24 hours.[41]

In conclusion, based on adequately sized randomized trials and meta-analyses of smaller trials, an early invasive strategy, preferably within 24 hours of diagnosis, is favored. This hypothesis may likely require periodic reevaluation with the introduction of earlier and more potent pharmacologic interventions in the future.

ADJUNCTIVE ANTITHROMBOTIC THERAPIES IN NSTE-ACS

Antiplatelet Therapy

Aspirin

Aspirin remains a mainstay of antiplatelet therapy for NSTE-ACS, and the recommendation for the use of aspirin has remained unchanged for several years. Based on the results of the landmark ISIS-2 trial (Second International Study of Infarct Survival) ($n = 17,187$), aspirin is administered at the time of diagnosis of NSTE-ACS at a dose of 162 to 325 mg once and is generally continued indefinitely with or without PCI at a maintenance dose of 81 to 162 mg daily.[1,42] However, despite its benefit, the efficacy of aspirin alone is suboptimal, particularly in the era of coronary stenting and the new risk of stent thrombosis.

Clopidogrel

Clopidogrel, a cytochrome P450-dependent prodrug and irreversible $P2Y_{12}$ inhibitor, in addition to aspirin remains the most extensively studied combination for the indication of NSTE-ACS. In the CURE trial (Clopidogrel in Unstable Angina to Prevent Recurrent Events Trial), NSTE-ACS patients were randomized to either aspirin monotherapy or dual antiplatelet therapy (DAPT) with aspirin plus clopidogrel ($n = 12,562$). The addition of clopidogrel to aspirin reduced the composite of death, MI, or stroke through 12 months (9.3% vs. 11.4%, HR = 0.80, 95% CI 0.72 to 0.90; $P < .001$).[43] Although the rate of major bleeding was significantly higher in the DAPT group, the rate of life-threatening bleeding was similar in the two arms. Following these favorable results, the efficacy of clopidogrel as pretreatment followed by long-term therapy after PCI was then evaluated in the CURE-PCI trial, which consisted of a subset of patients who were enrolled in the CURE trial and had undergone PCI ($n = 2658$).[44] Consistent with the results from CURE, long-term DAPT was associated with significantly lower rate of the primary end point of CV death, MI, or urgent target-vessel revascularization (TVR) within 30 days of PCI (4.5% vs. 6.4%, HR = 0.70, 95% CI 0.50 to 0.97; $P = .03$) with no associated increase in major bleeding.[44]

Accordingly, the administration of clopidogrel is recommended at a loading dose of 300 to 600 mg followed by a maintenance dose of 75 mg daily. Nonetheless, both the dose and the duration of clopidogrel therapy depend on whether patients undergo stent implantation or not. Among patients who undergo stenting, the 600 mg loading dose was associated with significant reduction in the rate of major ischemic events compared with the 300 mg loading dose.[45] In these patients—particularly those who did not experience a bleeding event in the first 12 months—therapy beyond 12 months is also reasonable due to the persistent benefits observed with DAPT in reducing stent thrombosis and major CV and cerebrovascular events when continued for an additional 18 months (i.e., for a total of 30 months).[46] In contrast, both the 300 mg and the 600 mg loading doses have similar efficacy in patients who do not undergo stenting. For those patients, clopidogrel may be continued for up to 12 months only.[1,2] For all patients, however, if the risk of bleeding is thought to outweigh its benefit, clopidogrel may be discontinued earlier.[1,2,46]

Following the success of clopidogrel, the use of DAPT for NSTE-ACS became the standard of care. Nonetheless, the rate of secondary atherothrombotic events remained high despite the use of aspirin plus clopidogrel, and more potent $P2Y_{12}$ inhibitors to further reduce the risk of secondary events remained an unmet need.

Prasugrel

Prasugrel is a thienopyridine that irreversibly binds and inhibits $P2Y_{12}$. The safety and efficacy of prasugrel among patients with confirmed ACSs who had already undergone PCI was compared with clopidogrel in the TRITON-TIMI-38 trial ($n = 13,608$). NSTE-ACS patients consisted of 74% of the overall randomized population ($n = 10,074$). Prasugrel reduced the rate of CV death, MI, or stroke (9.3% vs. 11.2%, $P = .002$) as compared with clopidogrel, but at the expense of increased rate of both major bleeding (2.4% vs. 1.8%, $P = .02$) and fatal bleeding events (0.4% vs. 0.1%, $P = .002$).[47] In particular, prasugrel was associated with reduced rates of stent thrombosis as compared with clopidogrel (1.1% vs. 2.4%, $P < .001$).[48] In contrast, a lack of efficacy was observed specifically among the subgroup of patients with a prior history of stroke or transient ischemic attack, patients aged 75 years or older, and those with low weight less than 60 kg. While all patients received therapy following PCI in TRITON-TIMI-38, the benefit of upfront therapy with prasugrel prior to PCI is not clear. In the ACCOAST trial (Pretreatment at the Time of Diagnosis in Patients with Non-ST Elevation Myocardial Infarction) ($n = 4033$), systematic pretreatment with prasugrel at the time of NSTE-ACS diagnosis was not associated with a reduced rate of major ischemic events as compared with selective administration in patients undergoing PCI, but instead significantly increased the rate of major bleeding complications.[49] When prasugrel was then evaluated among NSTE-ACS patients who had no plan for revascularization in the TRILOGY-ACS trial (The Targeted Platelet Inhibition to Clarify the Optimal Strategy to Medically Manage Acute Coronary Syndromes) ($n = 7243$), there was also no reduction in the primary end point with prasugrel, but additional analyses of the total number of events (i.e., time-to-multiple-events or time to any event analysis) nonetheless suggested a potential benefit with prasugrel.[50]

Based on these results, the administration of prasugrel is not recommended prior to PCI among patients with NSTE-ACS. If patients undergo PCI, prasugrel may then be chosen over clopidogrel for patients who are not at an increased risk of bleeding. A loading dose of 60 mg is administered at the time of the procedure, then maintenance therapy is continued at a dose of 10 mg daily for at least 12 months.[1,2] However, if the risk of bleeding is thought to outweigh its benefit, prasugrel may be discontinued before 12 months. Finally, based on the findings from TRITON-TIMI-38, prasugrel is contraindicated in patients with a prior history of stroke or transient ischemic attack, patients aged 75 years or older, and those with low weight less than 60 kg.

Ticagrelor

Ticagrelor is a reversible inhibitor of $P2Y_{12}$ characterized by a rapid onset of action and a short plasma half-life. The safety and efficacy of ticagrelor was evaluated in the PLATO trial (Study of Platelet Inhibition and Patient Outcomes) among ACS patients

(n = 18,624), of whom 59.5% had NSTE-ACS (n = 11,080).[51] Compared with clopidogrel, ticagrelor reduced the primary end point of the composite of CV death, MI, or stroke through 12 months (HR = 0.83, 95% CI 0.74 to 0.93; P = .001). When individual end points were further evaluated, ticagrelor was similarly associated with reduced rates of CV death (3.7% vs. 4.9%, P = .007) and all-cause mortality (4.3% vs. 5.8%, P = .002). This reduction was not met with an increase in the rate of fatal or life-threatening bleeds, but compared with clopidogrel, ticagrelor was associated with a higher rate of non-CABG TIMI major bleeding (4.8% vs. 3.8%, P = .014) and dyspnea is observed in approximately 20% of patients. Also, when patients who were planned for noninvasive management were evaluated alone (n = 3143), ticagrelor remained associated with reduced ischemic events (HR = 0.85, 95% CI 0.73 to 1.00; P = .04).[52] Unlike prasugrel, the optimal timing of ticagrelor administration among patients undergoing PCI (i.e., pretreatment vs. treatment following angiography) has not been formally investigated, and a recommendation for or against pretreatment with ticagrelor in this group of patients remains unclear. Although some patients were administered ticagrelor prior to cardiac catheterization in the Plato trial, this was at investigator discretion and the selection may be confounded.

Accordingly, among NSTE-ACS patients, ticagrelor is administered at a loading dose of 180 mg followed by a maintenance dose of 90 mg twice-daily. In patients who are not planned to undergo stenting, therapy may be continued for up to 12 months. In stented patients, ticagrelor is preferred over clopidogrel and may reasonably be continued beyond 12 months, with persistent benefits demonstrated through 3 years of therapy.[1,2,53] However, if the risk of bleeding is thought to outweigh its benefit, ticagrelor may be discontinued before 12 months.

Cangrelor

Cangrelor is a rapid- and short-acting, reversible $P2Y_{12}$ inhibitor that is administered intravenously. It is administered at the beginning of PCI as a bolus of 30 μg/kg then followed by an infusion of 4 μg/kg/min. The safety and efficacy of cangrelor has been evaluated in the CHAMPION trials (Cangrelor versus Standard Therapy to Achieve Optimal Management of Platelet Inhibition) comparing cangrelor to clopidogrel. In CHAMPION-PCI (n = 8877), 72.8% of patients had NSTE-ACS (n = 6464), whereas the remainder had either stable CAD or STEMI.[54] In CHAMPION-PLATFORM (n = 5352), patients with STEMI were excluded from the trial, and 94% of patients had NSTE-ACS (n = 5033).[55] Clopidogrel was administered at the end of the procedure, and cangrelor was administered at the beginning of the procedure and continued for 2 to 4 hours. In both trials, cangrelor did not reduce the rate of ischemic outcomes, but was associated in a significant reduction in secondary outcomes, including stent thrombosis, without an increase in bleeding.

Subsequently, the CHAMPION-PHEONIX trial was designed to evaluate the safety and efficacy of cangrelor in reducing PCI-related ischemic complications (n = 10,939).[56] In the trial, only 25% of enrolled patients had NSTE-ACS (n = 2810). While cangrelor reduced the rate of ischemic events in the overall population, sensitivity analysis by type of ACS (STEMI vs. NSTE-ACS) did not demonstrate a significant interaction with the treatment strategy that would alter outcomes. Given that the trial was not powered to evaluate NSTE-ACS patients alone, a consistent numerical reduction in events with cangrelor was observed among these patients, but it did not reach statistical significance (HR = 0.80, 95% CI 0.55 to 1.17).[56] In a meta-analysis of all three trials (n = 24,910), cangrelor was associated with reduced rates of PCI peri procedural ischemic complications in the subgroup of NSTE-ACS patients (2.9% vs. 3.5%, odds ratio [OR] = 0.82, 95% CI 0.68 to 0.99) (n = 14,282) and favorably a concomitant significant reduction in bleeding outcomes (0.4% vs. 0.7%, OR = 0.53, 95% CI 0.33 to 0.85) compared with clopidogrel.

In the ESC 2015 guidelines, cangrelor may be considered among $P2Y_{12}$ inhibitor-naive patients undergoing PCI (class IIb recommendation).[2] In contrast, its approval in the United States was made in 2015 and its use was not reflected in the preceding 2014 ACC/AHA guidelines for NSTE-ACS.[1]

Parenteral Anticoagulant Therapy

Unfractionated Heparin

Irrespective of the treatment strategy, parenteral anticoagulant therapy is recommended for all patients diagnosed with NSTE-ACS. Prior to the era of DAPT, the addition of intravenous UFH to aspirin was associated with a nonsignificant trend towards reduced risk of death and MI in patients with UA.[37–62] Despite the favorable results, the superiority of this combination therapy has not been established definitively in a large, adequately powered randomized trial.

Compared with fixed doses of UFH, weight-based doses of UFH (loading dose of 60 IU/kg for maximum of 4000 IU and infusion of 12 IU/kg/h) have been associated with higher rates of achieving target activated partial thromboplastin time (aPTT) ranges, and are preferred.[1,63] For patients undergoing an ischemia-guided strategy, anticoagulation with UFH is usually continued for at least 48 hours. For patients undergoing PCI, an additional bolus of UFH is administered following sheath insertion (to achieve target activated clotting time [ACT] of 250 to 300 seconds if GP IIb/IIIa inhibitors are not co-administered vs. target ACT of 200 to 250 seconds if a GP IIb/IIIa inhibitor is being co-administered). For uncomplicated procedures, UFH may generally be stopped immediately post-procedure. However, it may occasionally be continued among patients who undergo high-risk procedures or among those with a preexisting indication for long-term anticoagulation (e.g., atrial fibrillation).

Low Molecular Weight Heparin

Low molecular weight heparin (LMWH), namely enoxaparin, is a factor IIa and Xa inhibitor. It is administered subcutaneously at a dose of 1 mg/kg every 12 hours, with an initial intravenous loading dose of 30 mg, and continued for the duration of the hospitalization or the PCI procedure, whichever is sooner. Unlike UFH, it does not require monitoring, but is excreted renally and is thus contraindicated in severe renal impairment (i.e., creatinine clearance <30 mL/min). Early randomized trials comparing enoxaparin to UFH prior to the common use of DAPT and GP IIb/IIIa inhibitors demonstrated a consistent significant reduction in the rate of thrombotic events with enoxaparin. In the TIMI 11B trial, NSTE-ACS patients were randomized to intravenous UFH for at least 3 days and were then randomized to either subcutaneous placebo or enoxaparin (n = 3910). Enoxaparin reduced the primary end point of all-cause death, MI, or urgent revascularization through 43 days (17.3% vs. 19.7%, HR = 0.85 95% CI 0.72 to 1.00; P = .048).[64] There was no increase in major bleeding events, but more bleeding was observed when enoxaparin was continued postdischarge. In the ESSENCE trial (Efficacy and Safety of Subcutaneous Enoxaparin in Non-Q Wave Coronary Events) (n = 3171), enoxaparin similarly reduced the 1-year composite end point of all-cause death, MI, or recurrent angina as compared with UFH (32.0% vs. 35.7%, P = .022).[65]

The superiority of enoxaparin over UFH seems to have attenuated with the introduction of more advanced antithrombotic therapies. SYNERGY (Superior Yield of the New Strategy of

Enoxaparin, Revascularization and Glycoprotein IIb/IIIa Inhibitors) compared enoxaparin to UFH among high-risk NSTE-ACS patients planned for early invasive strategy (n = 10,027). Patients received GP IIb/IIIa inhibitor and underwent revascularization within 24 hours. Although enoxaparin was noninferior to UFH in the reduction of the composite of all-cause death or MI through 30 days (14.0% vs. 14.5%, HR = 0.96 (95% CI 0.86 to 1.06; P = .40),[66] this was offset by a significantly higher rate of TIMI major bleeding events (9.1% vs. 7.6%, P = .008). These results were also demonstrated in the A to Z trial (n = 3987), where no reduction in the composite of all-cause death, MI, or refractory ischemia was observed with enoxaparin as compared with UFH (8.4% vs. 9.4%, HR = 0.88, 95% CI 0.71 to 1.08; P = NS).[67]

When the combination of old and contemporary clinical trials for NSTE-ACS were collectively analyzed in a meta-analysis (n = 21,946), enoxaparin was found to be more efficacious than UFH in reducing the composite of death or MI at 30 days (10.1% vs. 11.0%, HR = 0.91, 95% CI 0.83 to 0.99) without an increase in the rate of major bleeding.[68] Although these differences were statistically significant, the clinical significance of these modest differences, particularly in light of the advances in pharmacologic therapies and stents, remains an area of debate.

Fondaparinux

Fondaparinux is an activated, selective factor X inhibitor that is administered subcutaneously at a dose of 2.5 mg daily. Similar to LMWH, fondaparinux does not require monitoring and is contraindicated in severe renal impairment of creatinine clearance less than 30 mL/min. The safety and efficacy of fondaparinux was compared to enoxaparin in the OASIS-5 trial (Organization to Assess Strategies in Ischemic Syndromes) (n = 20,078).[69] Fondaparinux was noninferior to enoxaparin in reducing the primary end point of death, MI, or refractory ischemia at 9 days. When additional long-term end points were compared, fondaparinux also reduced mortality at 30 days (2.9% vs. 3.5%, P = .02) and 180 days (5.8% vs. 6.5%, P = .05). Interestingly, these benefits were not at the expense of increased bleeding, whereby fondaparinux was associated with half the rate of bleeding events observed with enoxaparin (2.2% vs. 4.1%, P < .001). Based on these results, fondaparinux is thought to have the most favorable risk–benefit profile among all anticoagulants.

Of importance, subgroup analyses from OASIS-5 demonstrated that patients in the fondaparinux group had significantly higher rates of catheter-related thrombus formation (0.9% vs. 0.3%). However, this complication was eliminated by the use of UFH at the time of PCI, as confirmed by the FUTURA/OASIS 8 trial (The Fondaparinux Trial With UFH During Revascularization in Acute Coronary Syndrome) (n = 3235)[70] with no increase in bleeding when fondaparinux and UFH were combined.[70] These findings resulted in the recommendation to add UFH (50 to 100 U/kg adjusted to ACT) to fondaparinux for all patients who are planned to undergo PCI. On the other hand, among NSTE-ACS patients with no plan for angiography, fondaparinux without UFH should be continued for at least 48 hours up to a maximum of 8 days or until discharge, whichever is the sooner.[1]

Bivalirudin

Bivalirudin is a direct-acting intravenous thrombin inhibitor administered at a dose of 0.10 mg/kg loading dose followed by 0.25 mg/kg/h. The safety and efficacy of bivalirudin was studied among moderate- to high-risk NSTE-ACS patients receiving DAPT and planned for an early invasive strategy in the ACUITY trial (Acute Catheterization and Urgent Intervention Triage Strategy) (n = 13,819).[71] Patients were randomized in a 1:1:1 ratio to one of three treatment arms: (1) standard of care UFH/enoxaparin plus GP IIb/IIIa inhibitor, (2) bivalirudin plus GP IIb/IIIa inhibitor, or (3) bivalirudin alone (with provisional use of GP IIb/IIIa inhibitor during PCI). Patients receiving GP IIb/IIIa inhibitors were then randomized in a two-by-two factorial design to receive the GP IIb/IIIa inhibitor either immediately following randomization (upstream approach) versus deferred administration until the beginning of the PCI procedure. Both bivalirudin groups (i.e., plus GP IIb/IIIa inhibitor or alone) were noninferior in reducing the 30-day rate of the composite of all-cause death, MI, or unplanned revascularization for ischemia as compared with standard of care UFH/enoxaparin plus GP IIb/IIIa inhibitor (7.7% and 7.8% vs. 7.3%, respectively). However, the net clinical benefit was overall in favor of the bivalirudin only group, due to significant 47% relative risk reduction in the rate of major bleeding compared with the UFH/enoxaparin plus GPIIb/IIIa inhibitor group (3.0% vs. 5.7%, HR = 0.53, 95% CI 0.43 to 0.65; P < .001). In contrast, the bivalirudin plus GPIIb/IIIa inhibitor group and the UFH/enoxaparin plus GPIIb/IIIa inhibitor group had statistically similar rates of major bleeding. Paradoxically to the overall population, in patients not pretreated with clopidogrel prior to PCI, the bivalirudin only group was associated with a 29% increased rate of ischemic events as compared with the UFH/enoxaparin plus GPIIb/IIIa inhibitor group.[72,73]

Based on the results of ACUITY, the use of bivalirudin has been recommended only among intermediate- to high-risk NSTE-ACS patients who are anticipated to undergo angiography provided that they are pretreated with DAPT. It should be continued, with a provisional use of a GP IIb/IIIa inhibitor, for the duration of the procedure and stopped thereafter. There was no difference in ischemic outcomes between the upstream use of GP IIb/IIIa inhibitors versus their deferred administration, but the upstream approach was associated with significantly higher rates of major bleeding through 30 days (4.9% vs. 6.1%, P = .009).[74]

Glycoprotein IIb/IIIa Receptor Inhibitors

The GP IIb/IIIa receptor inhibitors, namely the chimeric monoclonal antibody abciximab and the high-affinity nonantibody receptor inhibitors tirofiban and eptifibatide, are small antiplatelet agents that inhibit platelet aggregation by binding reversibly to the glycoprotein IIb/IIIa receptor. All GP IIb/IIIa inhibitors are administered at the time of PCI and are reserved for NSTE-ACS patients with high-risk features (e.g., elevated troponin) irrespective of pretreatment with DAPT.[1]

Abciximab

Abciximab was extensively studied in the prestenting era of percutaneous transluminal coronary angioplasty (PTCA) and before the routine use of DAPT. In a meta-analysis of five randomized trials for abciximab in NSTE-ACS patients undergoing angiography, abciximab reduced the 30-day end point of all-cause death or MI (HR = 0.55, 95% CI 0.43 to 0.69; P < .001) without an increase in major bleeding and irrespective of the device category; that is, balloon angioplasty alone, elective stenting, bailout stenting, or directional coronary atherectomy.[75] In contrast, when administered among ACS patients not planned to undergo early revascularization (n = 7800), abciximab was not associated with reduction in ischemic events through 1 year.[76] The lack of benefit with abciximab in this patient population is unclear and is not consistent with other GP IIb/IIIa inhibitors, but has been attributed to either the inadequate abciximab dosing in these trials or to its unique properties of low drug-to-receptor ratio that potentially reduce its long-term efficacy. When later combined with UFH in NSTEMI patients undergoing PCI, abciximab also failed to reduce the rate of ischemic outcomes and increased the risk of major bleeding when compared with bivalirudin monotherapy (n = 1721).[77,78]

Over time, and with the introduction of stents and antithrombotic therapies, the use of abciximab has diminished. At present, it is only indicated as an adjunct to PCI at a dose of 0.25 mg/kg bolus over at least 1 minute, to be started 10 to 60 minutes before the start of PCI, followed by continuous infusion at a rate of 0.125 µg/kg/min for 12 hours (not to exceed infusion rate of 10 µg/min). Among UA patients, abciximab is started within 24 hours, continued for 1 hour after PCI or stopped in patients with failed PCI. Among patients with severe renal insufficiency, abciximab is preferred over the other agents in this class.

Tirofiban

Tirofiban is a nonpeptide reversible inhibitor of GP IIb/IIIa receptor that is characterized by a high drug-to-receptor ratio. The RESTORE trial (Randomized Efficacy Study of Tirofiban for Outcomes and Restenosis) evaluated the safety and efficacy of tirofiban in NSTE-ACS patients planned for revascularization and not pretreated with $P2Y_{12}$ inhibitors (n = 2139). Tirofiban was associated with a numeric, but nonsignificant, 16% relative risk reduction in the primary ischemic end point through 30 days compared with placebo (10.3% vs. 12.2%, P = .16).[79] However, in subsequent analyses the benefit with tirofiban was mostly apparent early within 2 days and 7 days following angioplasty (38% and 27% relative risk reduction, respectively), an effect mainly driven by the reduction in the rates of nonfatal MI and the need for repeat angioplasty.[79]

Notably, the failure of tirofiban to reduce the primary end point was thought to be related to the suboptimal dose of tirofiban used in the trial (i.e., bolus of 10 µg/kg over 3 minutes followed by 36-hour infusion of 0.15 µg/kg/min). Accordingly, a new higher dose of tirofiban was studied among high-risk patients undergoing PCI in the ADVANCE trial (n = 202). Compared with placebo, high-dose bolus tirofiban over 24 to 48 hours (i.e., bolus of 25 µg/kg over 3 minutes then followed by infusion of 0.15 µg/kg/min) was safe and significantly reduced the incidence of the composite of death, MI, TVR, and bailout use of GP IIb/IIIa inhibitors.[80]

PRISM (Platelet Receptor Inhibition in Ischemic Syndrome Management) then compared the infusion of tirofiban to heparin among UA patients when administered for 48 hours on a background of aspirin (n = 3232).[81] Tirofiban did not reduce the risk of the composite ischemic end point, but alternatively was associated with a reduced risk of all-cause death (2.3% vs. 3.6%, P = .02). Following these promising results, PRISM-PLUS then tested the safety and efficacy of multiple strategies of tirofiban in all NSTE-ACS patients with intermediate to high-risk features irrespective of whether they underwent angiography or not (n = 1915).[82] Patients were randomized within 24 hours of NSTE-ACS to one of three groups: (1) high-dose tirofiban only, (2) combination of lower-dose tirofiban plus heparin, or (3) heparin only. The combination lower-dose tirofiban plus heparin group was associated with a significant reduction in the primary end point of 7-day risk of ischemic events (12.9% vs. 17.9%, HR = 0.68, 95% CI 0.53 to 0.88; P = .004), as well as longer-term events through 30 days and 6 months. The reduction was primary driven by 47% reduction in nonfatal MI and 30% reduction in the risk of refractory ischemia. In contrast, there was a notably premature discontinuation of the higher-dose tirofiban only group, as it was associated with a fourfold significant increase in 7-day mortality (4.6%) when compared with either the heparin only group (1.1%) or the combination group (1.6%).

In conclusion, tirofiban is reserved for intermediate- to high-risk NSTE-ACS patients, and may be administered with or without pretreatment with DAPT and UFH. Due to its high drug-to-receptor ratio when administered, platelet infusion for patients who are bleeding with tirofiban is not as effective as it is for abciximab.

Eptifibatide

Eptifibatide is a cyclic heptapeptide that reversibly binds to GP IIb/IIIa inhibitor in a similar manner to tirofiban with a high drug-to-receptor ratio. In the phase II IMPACT trial (Integrilin to Minimize Platelet Aggregation and Coronary Thrombosis) (n = 150), eptifibatide was associated with a trend towards reducing the composite ischemic end point at the expense of more than two fold increase in bleeding.[83] Following the results from IMPACT, two lower doses of eptifibate were carried forward in the phase III IMPACT-II trial. However, neither of these new doses of eptifibatide significantly reduced the primary end point of 30-day risk of ischemic events despite a clear signal for efficacy.[84]

Accordingly, PURSUIT (Platelet Glycoprotein IIb/IIIa in Unstable Angina: Receptor Suppression Using Integrilin Therapy) evaluated the safety and efficacy of new eptifibatide doses among NSTE-ACS patients regardless of whether PCI was planned or not (n = 10,948).[85] Patients with either ischemic ECG changes or elevated biomarkers were randomized to eptifibatide versus placebo on a background of heparin plus aspirin. Notably, the study drug was administered as soon as possible following the occurrence of chest pain, without waiting for a decision to revascularize or not. Eptifibatide was associated with a 9.5% relative reduction in the 30-day risk of the composite end point of all-cause death or MI (14.2% vs. 15.7%, P = .04) without an increase in the rate of intracranial hemorrhage. Furthermore, there was no heterogeneity in effect when subsequent subgroup analyses were performed, including analysis of patients who underwent PCI versus those who were medically managed.[86]

As direct thrombin inhibition with bivalirudin alone was demonstrated to be noninferior to the combination of GPIIb/IIIa inhibitors plus full doses of UFH/enoxaparin in the ACUITY trial, it was uncertain if using the same combination at a reduced dose of UFH/enoxaparin would be associated with improved net clinical profile. This hypothesis was subsequently tested in the PROTECT-TIMI-30 trial (Randomized Trial to Evaluate the Relative Protection against Post-PCI Microvascular Dysfunction and Post-PCI Ischemia among Anti-Platelet and Anti-Thrombotic Agents–TIMI-30), and angiographic outcomes were compared (n = 857). The trial showed mixed results in favor of both arms. The primary end point of post-PCI coronary flow reserve (i.e., ratio of hyperemic to basal epicardial flow after PCI) was significantly greater with bivalirudin monotherapy. However, the combination of eptifibatide plus reduced UFH/enoxaparin improved myocardial perfusion, albeit at the expense of higher rates of minor bleeding and need for blood transfusions.

Eptifibatide is now recommended among NSTE-ACS patients at the doses studied in the PURSUIT trial; that is, bolus of 180 µg/kg over 1 to 2 minutes followed by a continuous infusion of 2 µg/kg/min for up to 72 hours. For patients who undergo PCI, another bolus dose of 180 µg/kg is administered following the first bolus dose, and the infusion is continued for at least 12 hours. The infusion rate of eptifibatide is reduced to 1 µg/kg/min among patients with renal impairment of creatinine clearance <50 mL/min.

RADIAL VERSUS FEMORAL APPROACH

Major bleeding is observed in approximately 2% of NSTE-ACS patients in the setting of potent anticoagulation and antiplatelet therapy and has been associated with increased mortality and adverse CV events.[87] Among NSTE-ACS patients whose management includes PCI, at least half of reported major bleeding events are postprocedural and related to the vascular access site.[88] Initial PCIs performed in the early 1970s were via femoral or brachial artery access.[89] In comparison, the radial artery is a smaller, more superficial, and compressible access site, which allows for better control of access site bleeding.[90]

Prior to 2011, observational data and small, single-center clinical trials suggested that radial access decreases the risk of procedure-related bleeding among patients with ACS and is associated with a similar and occasionally lower incidence of major adverse cardiovascular events (MACEs) when compared with femoral access. Additionally, the radial approach allowed for early patient ambulation and shorter overall hospital length of stay.[91–95] The RIVAL trial (radial versus femoral access for coronary angiography and intervention in patients with ACSs) was the first randomized, multicenter clinical trial to evaluate the transradial vs. transfemoral PCI among patients presenting with ACS (n = 7021). RIVAL demonstrated similar rates of the composite of death, MI, stroke, or noncoronary artery bypass graft (non–CABG)-related major bleeding at 30 days between radial and femoral approaches (3.7% with radial vs. 4.0% with femoral access). Although analysis of the subgroup of patients with STEMI showed a significant reduction in the primary end point with radial access, this was not observed among patients with NSTE-ACS. The discrepancy between the two subgroups was hypothesized to be related to the more potent antithrombotic therapies administered to patients with STEMI. The other principal finding of the RIVAL trial was a significantly lower rate of local major vascular complications with the radial approach in comparison with the femoral approach in the overall study population as well as in patients with NSTE-ACS (1.4% with radial access vs. 3.8% with femoral access; HR = 0.38; 95% CI 0.26 to 0.55; $P < .001$).

Given the findings of the RIVAL trial, the majority of studies focused on the evaluation of the radial approach among patients with STEMI rather than NSTE-ACS. Additional data on the optimal approach among patients with NSTE-ACS were provided by the MATRIX trial (Minimizing Adverse Haemorrhagic Events by TRansradial Access Site and Systemic Implementation of angioX), a randomized, multicenter, superiority trial comparing transradial against transfemoral access among patients with ACS (n = 8404). In contrast to the RIVAL trial, MATRIX enriched for high-risk NSTE-ACS patients (e.g., age 60 or older, positive biomarkers, dynamic ST shifts) to determine whether this select subpopulation had similar benefits observed among patients with STEMI. MATRIX also required operators with higher skill and greater case volumes than prior studies. The trial demonstrated that radial access was associated with a 16% relative risk reduction (1.9% absolute risk reduction) in net clinical outcomes (composite of MACE or Bleeding Academic Research Consortium major bleeding) with radial access compared to femoral access that was driven mostly by a reduction in major bleeding ($P = .0092$). All-cause mortality was also reduced among patients with a radial approach (1.6% vs. 2.2%; $P = .045$). Furthermore, a sensitivity analysis by the type of ACS on presentation (STEMI vs. NSTE-ACS), demonstrated no significant difference, but in contradistinction to prior data, showed marginally greater efficacy and safety among NSTE-ACS patients. MATRIX also demonstrated that outcomes with either approach were contingent on the proportion of radial-to-femoral PCIs performed at the participating centers. High-volume radial PCI centers were significantly more likely to have better outcomes via radial access compared with femoral access. In comparison, centers with intermediate-to-low proportion of radial PCIs had no difference in outcomes between radial and femoral approaches.[96]

Compared to femoral access, coronary angiography and PCI via radial access allows for early patient ambulation and shorter overall hospital stays. Based on the available evidence, a radial approach is associated with a lower incidence of major bleeding among NSTE-ACS patients. Additionally, there may be an associated reduction in mortality that is observed in high-volume radial PCI centers among high-risk NSTE-ACS patients (older patients, patients with positive biomarkers, patients with dynamic ECG changes). Radial access is thus preferred to femoral access for patients with NSTE-ACS, particularly in high-volume centers with skilled radial PCI operators.

CONSIDERATIONS IN PATIENTS WITH NSTE-ACS AND COMPLEX CORONARY DISEASE

Percutaneous Coronary Intervention Versus Coronary Artery Bypass Graft

Ever since the introduction of percutaneous techniques for coronary revascularization, the comparative efficacy and safety of PCI versus CABG has been of interest to interventional cardiologists and cardiac surgeons alike. Despite multiple randomized clinical trials over the past few decades, no definitive evidence exists to demonstrate a significant difference in efficacy between CABG and PCI, except in specific subpopulations. It is important to note that there exists an inherent difficulty in comparing PCI and CABG given that both PCI and CABG techniques are constantly evolving as newer methods, devices, and medical therapies become available. While PCI may fail early, CABG may fail later, and this must be kept in mind. In comparison to older trials, contemporary PCI involves improved assessment of coronary stenosis with instantaneous wave-free ratios and fractional flow reserves (FFRs), optimized stent placement with intravascular ultrasound and optimal coherence tomography and improved adjunctive antiplatelet and anticoagulant therapies. The CABG procedure has also evolved with greater usage of arterial conduits, improved myocardial protection techniques, and superior perioperative care. Furthermore, there are no contemporary randomized controlled trials that compare PCI and CABG specifically among patients with NSTE-ACS.

Multivessel Disease

Interest in comparing the long-term outcomes significantly increased in the 1990s as PCIs became more widely performed for treatment of medically refractory angina or UA. PCI is less invasive, provides more rapid revascularization of the culprit lesion, and carries a lower risk of stroke compared with CABG. However, early data from registries and observational studies suggested that complete revascularization rates with multivessel CAD were significantly lower with PCI compared with CABG, and long-term mortality rates and complications were higher. Accordingly, there developed a need for higher quality evidence to guide practice among patients with multivessel disease.

Historically, there have been three distinct generations of clinical trials comparing PCI to CABG among patients with multivessel disease that have mirrored the major timeframes in PCI history: the era of plain balloon angioplasty, the era of bare-metal stents (BMSs) and the era of drug-eluting stents (DESs). Although not temporally related, the CABG procedure has also significantly evolved over this time frame. Given the lack of clinical trials comparing PCI versus CABG among patients with multivessel disease and NSTE-ACS, the data presented in this section are from trials with populations of mixed stable CAD and NSTE-ACS.

The initial upsurge of clinical trials in the early to mid-1990s compared PCI to CABG among patient with angina and angiographically documented coronary heart disease who had a need for intervention. These trials were not uniform in their methods, with varying enrollment of patients with single or two-vessel disease, varying cutoffs for ejection fraction (EF), and varying durations of follow-up. However, these trials were all consistent and demonstrated no difference in mortality or recurrent MI among patients with multivessel disease, but demonstrated an increased risk of recurrent angina and repeat revascularization with PCI, which was four to seven times greater than with CABG. In the majority of trials, these differences could be observed as early as 1 year after the initial intervention. These differences highlighted the shortcomings of conventional balloon angioplasty, which was the preferred method at the time, and which is known to be associated with a higher risk of restenosis and stent thrombosis compared with stent placement.[26,97–100] The largest study among patients with multivessel disease in the 1990s was the BARI trial (Bypass Angioplasty Revascularization Investigation) that randomized patients with multivessel disease and angina requiring intervention to an initial treatment strategy of either CABG or PCI. BARI confirmed the results from earlier trials, but identified patients with diabetes as a population of interest with a very significant reduction in 5-year mortality observed among those treated with CABG vs. PCI (65.5% vs. 80.6%; $P = .003$).[101] BARI became the basis of contemporary trials that compared PCI with stent placement to CABG.

Although the first generation of trials helped identify populations of interest and outcomes for further evaluation, they are no longer considered in the evidence-based decision making for patients with multivessel disease given their outdated interventional techniques. The second generation of trials performed in the late 1990s and early 2000s compared PCI with BMS placement to CABG among patients with multivessel disease. Similar to preceding trials, the rate of repeat revascularization was significantly higher among patient who underwent PCI (three to five times compared with CABG), although the absolute rate of repeat intervention was halved compared with previously reported rates with plain balloon angioplasty.[102–104] The trials did not show a difference in the incidence of MI, and with the exception of one trial,[102] did not show a difference in mortality between PCI and CABG. Subgroup analyses from these trials further demonstrated that the presence of diabetes mellitus was an important predictor of outcome among patients who underwent PCI.[104]

With the advent of DESs in the mid-2000s, newer data were required given the improved outcomes and lower risk of restenosis with these stents compared with BMS. In addition, despite the lack of evidence in patients with complex coronary anatomy, PCI became more common in this patient population often excluded from clinical trials. The SYNTAX trial (Synergy between PCI with Taxus and Cardiac Surgery) was the first randomized trial to evaluate the safety and efficacy of PCI with the first-generation paclitaxel-eluting stent (Taxus) compared with CABG among patients with three-vessel or left main CAD using an all-comers approach to mimic clinical practice. The SYNTAX trial also tested the SYNTAX score, a grading system that combines multiple known identifiers of coronary anatomy complexity such as the Leaman score, the Duke and International Classification for Patient Safety classification systems for bifurcation lesions, and the chronic total occlusion classification system, as a predictor of outcomes among patients undergoing PCI (Fig. 19.4).[105] The trial demonstrated that PCI was associated with an increased risk of major adverse cardiac or cerebrovascular events (composite of death from any cause, stroke, MI, or repeat revascularization) among patients who had undergone PCI (17.8% vs. 12.4%; $P = .002$), despite an increased risk of stroke observed among patients who underwent CABG (0.6% vs. 2.2%; $P = .003$). There was no significant difference in mortality between the two groups. At 3 years, patients with multivessel disease had a lower risk of death, MI, and repeat revascularization with CABG compared with MI. The trial also demonstrated that high SYNTAX scores (≥33), indicating more complex coronary disease, were associated with an increased risk of major adverse cardiac or cerebrovascular events, and a nonsignificant trend towards an increased risk of the composite of death, MI, and stroke. Data from the 3-year follow-up period demonstrated that both intermediate and high SYNTAX scores were associated with higher major adverse cardiac and cerebrovascular event rates among patients who underwent PCI. In contrast, outcomes with CABG were not influenced by the SYNTAX score.[106,107] Beyond the SYNTAX trial, the SYNTAX score was validated using data from the ARTS II Study (Arterial Revascularization Therapies Study II), the first nonrandomized study to evaluate PCI with sirolimus-eluting stent (Cypher) placement versus CABG among patients with two- or three-vessel disease. The SYNTAX score was similarly shown to be an independent predictor of major adverse cardiac and cerebrovascular events among patients who had undergone PCI and had a SYNTAX score ≥33.[108] Despite the available evidence, the complexity and variable reproducibility of the SYNTAX score have limited its clinical use as a tool to guide decision making. The SYNTAX score has since been validated in other cohorts and expanded upon to include additional angiographic and clinical factors associated with adverse outcomes with PCI. Evidence supporting baseline and residual SYNTAX scores after intervention has also been compelling, but none of these scoring systems have had broad adoption in the clinical setting.

Significant advances in PCI techniques and newer generations of DESs have created a need for contemporary evidence regarding the efficacy and safety of PCI versus CABG for patients with multivessel disease. The BEST trial (The Randomized Comparison of Coronary Artery Bypass Surgery and Everolimus-Eluting Stent Implantation in the Treatment of Patients with Multivessel Coronary Artery Disease) is the only large-scale trial performed after SYNTAX to compare CABG with PCI employing second-generation everolimus-eluting stents among patients with multivessel disease. The trial demonstrated that PCI with everolimus-eluting stents was associated with a nonsignificant higher risk of MACEs (defined as death, MI, or TVR) at 2 years compared with CABG. With longer-term follow-up of a median of 4.6 years, this difference was statistically significant, driven mostly by an increase in repeat revascularization and spontaneous MI among patients who had undergone PCI.[109] The trial was difficult to apply to clinical practice given the lack of data on disease complexity, a higher than previously reported incomplete revascularization rate in the PCI group, and methods that mandated revascularization of all lesions greater than 70% irrespective of clinical or angiographic evidence of hemodynamically significant disease.

Based on available evidence, patients with multivessel disease and intermediate to high anatomic complexity by SYNTAX scoring may benefit from CABG over PCI, given lower major adverse cardiac and cerebrovascular event rates with CABG, as well as a lower risk of repeat revascularization. Given the lack of decisive evidence, decisions to proceed with PCI vs. CABG should involve a heart team given the considerations that need to be made and the individualization that is often required. Determination of surgical risk is essential and several validated risk scores may aid in risk stratification including the EuroSCORE, the Society of Thoracic Surgeons (STS) score, and the Cardiac Surgery Reporting System (CSRS) score. Other factors that play into the final decision include comorbidities, life expectancy, and patient preference. Until more conclusive evidence is available for PCI versus CABG in this patient population, additional factors such as the centers' and interventionalists' expertise with complex PCI may also play a role in decision making. Ultimately, the available evidence at this time does not reflect advances in PCI techniques, devices, and adjunctive medical therapies and newer trials are needed. Diabetic patients with multivessel disease have been evaluated in separate clinical trials and are discussed later (see *Special Populations*).

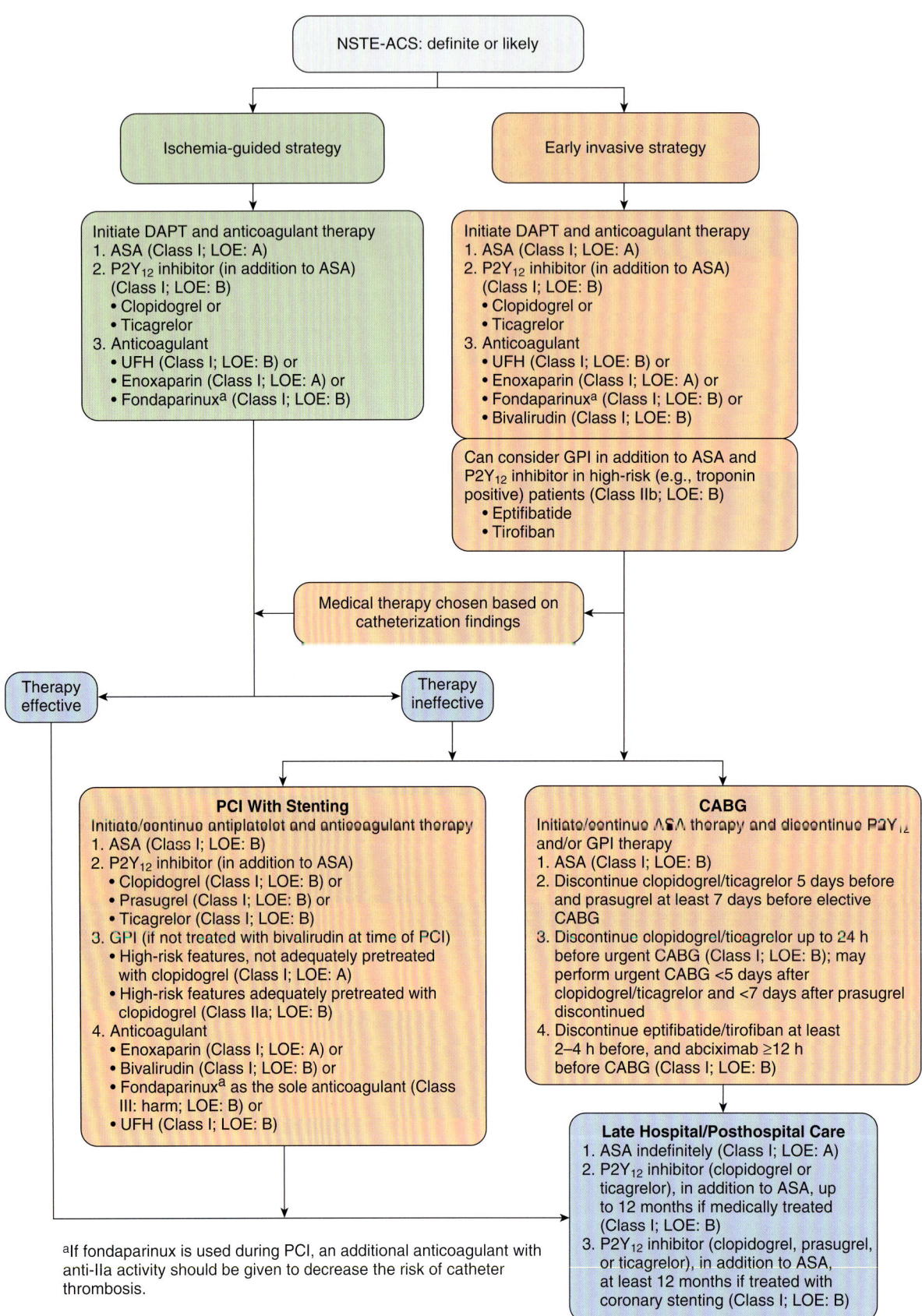

Fig. 19.4 The Synergy between PCI with Taxus and Cardiac Surgery (SYNTAX) Score Algorithm. *ASA*, Aspirin; *CABG*, Coronary artery bypass graft; *DAPT*, dual-antiplatelet therapy; *GPI*, glycoprotein IIb/IIIa inhibitor; *LOE*, level of evidence; *NSTE-ACS*, non–ST-elevation acute coronary syndrome; *PCI*, percutaneous coronary intervention; *UFH*, unfractionated heparin.

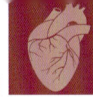

Left Main Coronary Artery Disease

Interventions involving the left main coronary artery (LMCA) have been associated with a higher risk of morbidity and mortality, owing to the substantial area of myocardium the LMCA supplies. Given the risk of abrupt closure or restenosis with unprotected LMCA angioplasty, initial trials comparing CABG to PCI with plain balloon angioplasty excluded patients with left main CAD, and CABG was the default intervention among these patients. However, with the introduction of stents, interventional cardiologists expanded the application of PCI to include patients with left main disease, despite lack of evidence for the long-term outcomes. Similar to trials for multivessel disease, there exist no trials that evaluate the efficacy and safety of PCI vs. CABG exclusively among patients with NSTE-ACS, and the data discussed in this section include a mixed population with stable CAD and NSTE ACS.

Initial data from registry studies comparing PCI with stent placement versus CABG for unprotected LMCA disease were inconclusive, but demonstrated an overall trend towards similar mortality rates between CABG and PCI after several years of follow-up. The first prospective data presented was a subgroup analysis of patients with unprotected LMCA disease in the SYNTAX trial. At 1 year, PCI and CABG were not significantly different in the rate of major adverse cardiac and cerebrovascular events; however, CABG was associated with a higher risk of stroke (2.7% vs. 0.3%; P = .009), and PCI was associated with higher risk of repeat revascularization (6.5% vs. 11.8%; P = .02). Comparable to the overall population, high baseline SYNTAX scores were associated with worse outcomes among patients with LMCA.[110] The first randomized clinical trial to evaluate PCI with DES placement was the PRECOMBAT trial (Premier of Randomized Comparison of Bypass Surgery versus Angioplasty Using Sirolimus-Eluting Stent in Patients with Left Main Coronary Artery Disease). PRECOMBAT enrolled 600 patients with unprotected LMCA disease involving at least 50% of the diameter of the LMCA who were eligible for either PCI or CABG. At 12 and 24 months, there was no significant difference in the composite of death from any cause, MI, stroke, and ischemia-driven TVR. Of the individual end points, ischemia-driven TVR was significantly more frequent among patients who had undergone PCI compared with CABG (9.0% vs. 4.2%; P = .02). A sensitivity analysis by presence or absence of ACS did not demonstrate any significant difference or treatment effect modification, indicating similar findings among patients with stable CAD and NSTE-ACS.[111] The NOBLE Study (Nordic-Baltic-British Left Main Revascularization Study) was the second trial to evaluate the efficacy and safety of PCI with DES placement versus CABG among patients with unprotected LMCA disease and at least three coronary lesions. Notably, the trial initially employed first-generation sirolimus-eluting stents (Cypher) then converted to a second-generation biolimus-eluting stent (BioMatrix Flex) with a higher strut thickness and higher risk of stent thrombosis compared to novel everolimus-eluting stents (Xience) and did not enroll patients based on SYNTAX score. The open-label trial demonstrated that at 5 years, CABG was superior to PCI for unprotected LMCA disease owing largely to a reduction in the composite of death from any cause, nonprocedural MI, repeat revascularization, or stroke. Individually, all-cause mortality was similar between the two groups; however, nonprocedural MI and repeat revascularization were higher with PCI compared with CABG. The trial also reported numerically higher rates of stroke in the PCI group, which was contradictory to the large body of evidence demonstrating a higher risk of stroke with CABG.[112] In comparison, everolimus-eluting stents (Xience) were evaluated in the EXCEL trial (Evaluation of XIENCE versus Coronary Artery Bypass Surgery for Effectiveness of Left Main Revascularization) among 1905 patients with unprotected LMCA disease and intermediate to low anatomic complexity by SYNTAX scoring. At 3 years, PCI was noninferior to CABG for the composite primary end point of death, stroke, or MI. PCI was also shown to be superior at 30 days for the same composite end point. Unlike prior data, PCI was noninferior to CABG for the composite of death, stroke, MI, or ischemia-driven revascularization, which is consistent with the lower risk of restenosis and stent thrombosis with the novel everolimus-eluting stents.[113] Data beyond 3 years are not available and would be essential to provide more robust evidence in this patient population.

Based on available data, among patients with unprotected LMCA disease and intermediate to low SYNTAX scores who are eligible for both PCI and CABG, it is reasonable to proceed with PCI with everolimus-eluting stent placement as opposed to CABG. Among patients with more complex anatomy, CABG remains the standard of care. Similar to cases of multivessel disease, a heart team is required to make the decision of PCI versus CABG given the multitude of factors that play into the decision. Additional clinical trials and long-term follow-up data are still required to further corroborate the available evidence.

Special Populations

Patients with Diabetes Mellitus

Approximately one in four patients with multivessel disease have diabetes mellitus. Based on findings from the BARI trial, diabetic patients with multivessel disease were identified as a population in whom CABG may be associated with a mortality benefit compared with PCI.[101] CABG became the standard of care for this patient population based on this data and despite the lack of dedicated large-scale clinical trials. In 2010, the CARDia (Coronary Artery Revascularization in Diabetes) trial became the first randomized trial that compared PCI with stenting versus CABG among diabetic patients with multivessel or complex single-vessel disease (n = 510). At 1 year, PCI was demonstrated to be noninferior to CABG for the composite end point of death, MI, and stroke. Patients who underwent PCI had a significantly higher rate of repeat revascularization.[114] The trial had a very short duration of follow-up and a combination of BMS and first-generation DES were used, which limited the interpretation and applicability of the results.

The primary evidence supporting the use of CABG over PCI among patients with diabetes and multivessel disease originated from the FREEDOM trial (Future Revascularization Evaluation in Patients with Diabetes Mellitus: Optimal Management of Multivessel Disease). FREEDOM enrolled 1900 patients with diabetes and angiographically confirmed multivessel disease and reported follow-up data of 5 years. CABG was superior to PCI with a lower incidence of the primary composite end point of death from any cause, MI, or stroke (18.7% vs. 26.6%; P = .005). The difference was driven by a significantly higher incidence of MI and a marginally significant increase in mortality with PCI. However, consistent with prior data, strokes were twice as common with CABG than with PCI.[115] Findings from FREEDOM provided additional evidence to support a recommendation for CABG among patients with diabetes and multivessel disease in place of PCI. Although available evidence still trails behind current practice in regard to techniques and stents employed, CABG will remain the standard of care in this patient population until newer evidence is available to support the use of PCI.

Patients with Left Ventricular Dysfunction

Impaired ventricular function is a marker of adverse outcomes among patients presenting with NSTE-ACS, particularly those with left main disease or multivessel CAD. Nonetheless, evidence is lacking to support the selection of an adequate revascularization strategy in this patient population. Practice patterns have generally mimicked those in the general NSTE-ACS population discussed previously. It is recommended that patients with reduced EF undergo invasive intervention with decisions on the strategy guided by anatomical and clinical considerations.

CULPRIT-VESSEL VERSUS MULTIVESSEL PERCUTANEOUS CORONARY INTERVENTION

Patients presenting with NSTE-ACS often have concomitant stenoses in nonculprit arteries that may be amenable to intervention. However, there are no randomized clinical trials that evaluate the efficacy and safety of culprit-vessel-only versus multivessel PCI among patients with NSTE-ACS with multivessel CAD. Limited data from observational studies and post hoc analyses have provided contradictory results; nonetheless, they suggest reduced repeat revascularization rates with multivessel compared to culprit-vessel-only PCI.[116-120] Accordingly, in the absence of shock, multivessel PCI can be performed among NSTE-ACS patients, and interventions should be guided by several factors including anatomic complexity of lesions, hemodynamic significance guided by FFR measurement, and the risk of contrast-induced nephropathy and other complications. Furthermore, until further evidence is available to guide decision making, both culprit-vessel-only and multivessel PCI are considered to be acceptable among patients with NSTE-ACS.

In contrast, among patients presenting with NSTE-ACS and cardiogenic shock, data from the CULPRIT-SHOCK trial (Culprit Lesion Only PCI vs. Multivessel PCI in Cardiogenic Shock) suggest differently. CULPRIT-SHOCK enrolled 706 patients presenting with ACS and cardiogenic shock and randomized them to either culprit-vessel-only PCI versus multivessel PCI with a primary composite end point of death or renal-replacement therapy at 30 days. Among patients who had culprit-vessel-only PCI, there was significantly lower incidence of the primary end point compared with multivessel PCI (45.9% vs. 55.4%, $P = .01$), as well as a reduction in all cause mortality. These findings apply to both STEMI and NSTE-ACS patients alike and suggest that among patients presenting with multivessel disease and cardiogenic shock, culprit-vessel-only PCI is strategy of choice.[121]

SINGLE-SITTING VERSUS STAGED MULTIVESSEL PERCUTANEOUS CORONARY INTERVENTION

Among patients presenting with NSTE-ACS and multivessel disease amenable to PCI, revascularization of hemodynamically significant nonculprit lesions may be performed in a single-setting along with the culprit lesion, or separately by multistage PCI. The SMILE trial (Impact of Different Treatment in Multivessel Non-ST Elevation Myocardial Infarction Patients: One Stage Versus Multistaged Percutaneous Coronary Intervention) is the only randomized trial to evaluate this question among patients presenting with NSTEMI (n = 584). The open-label study demonstrated a lower incidence of the composite of death, MI, rehospitalization for UA, TVR, and stroke at 1 year among patients randomized to single-sitting PCI compared with multistage PCI (second PCI within 3 to 7 days of index PCI). This finding was largely driven by an increase in the rate of TVR among patients who underwent multistage PCI (8.3% vs. 15.2%, $P = .01$).[122] Given the small sample size, open-label design, numerous individual end points used in the primary composite end point, and the unprecedently high rate of TVR in the multistage PCI group, it is difficult to interpret the findings as definitive evidence against the use of multistage PCI in NSTEMI patients. Further trials are required to guide decision making, and thus careful consideration of anatomic and patient risk-factors is essential for the selection of an appropriate revascularization strategy. Both single-setting and multistage PCI are considered acceptable among patients with NSTE-ACS.

KEY REFERENCES

3. Antman EM, Cohen M, Bernink PJ, et al. The TIMI risk score for unstable angina/non-ST elevation MI: a method for prognostication and therapeutic decision making. *JAMA*. 2000;284(7):835–842.
9. Boersma E, Pieper KS, Steyerberg EW, et al. Predictors of outcome in patients with acute coronary syndromes without persistent ST-segment elevation. Results from an international trial of 9461 patients. The PURSUIT Investigators. *Circulation*. 2000;101(22):2557–2567.
10. Fox KA, Dabbous OH, Goldberg RJ, et al. Prediction of risk of death and myocardial infarction in the six months after presentation with acute coronary syndrome: prospective multinational observational study (GRACE). *BMJ*. 2006;333(7578):1091.
13. Fox KA, Fitzgerald G, Puymirat E, et al. Should patients with acute coronary disease be stratified for management according to their risk? Derivation, external validation and outcomes using the updated GRACE risk score. *BMJ Open*. 2014;4(2):e004425.
18. Subherwal S, Bach RG, Chen AY, et al. Baseline risk of major bleeding in Non-ST-Segment-Elevation myocardial infarction: the CRUSADE (Can Rapid risk stratification of Unstable angina patients Suppress ADverse outcomes with Early implementation of the ACC/AHA guidelines) Bleeding Score. *Circulation*. 2009;119(14):1873–1882.
25. Thygesen K, Alpert JS, Jaffe AS, et al. Third universal definition of myocardial infarction. *Eur Heart J*. 2012;33(20):2551–2567.
41. Jobs A, Mehta SR, Montalescot G, et al. Optimal timing of an invasive strategy in patients with non-ST-elevation acute coronary syndrome: a meta-analysis of randomised trials. *Lancet*. 2017;390(10096):737–746.
43. Yusuf S, Zhao F, Mehta SR, et al. Effects of clopidogrel in addition to aspirin in patients with acute coronary syndromes without ST-segment elevation. *N Engl J Med*. 2001;345(7):494–502.
47. Wiviott SD, Braunwald E, McCabe CH, et al. Prasugrel versus clopidogrel in patients with acute coronary syndromes. *N Engl J Med*. 2007;357(20):2001–2015.
51. Wallentin L, Becker RC, Budaj A, et al. Ticagrelor versus clopidogrel in acute coronary syndromes. *N Engl J Med*. 2009;361(24):2385–2388.
54. Harrington RA, Stone GW, McNulty S, et al. Platelet inhibition with cangrelor in patients undergoing PCI. *N Engl J Med*. 2009;361(24):2318–2329.
55. Bhatt DL, Lincoff AM, Gibson CM, et al. Intravenous platelet blockade with cangrelor during PCI. *N Engl J Med*. 2009;361(24):2330–2341.
56. Bhatt DL, Stone GW, Mahaffey KW, et al. Effect of platelet inhibition with cangrelor during PCI on ischemic events. *N Engl J Med*. 2013;368(14):1303–1313.
69. Majure DT, Aberegg SK. Fondaparinux versus enoxaparin in acute coronary syndromes. *N Engl J Med*. 2006;354(26):2829–2830.
71. Stone GW, McLaurin BT, Cox DA, et al. Bivalirudin for patients with acute coronary syndromes. *N Engl J Med*. 2006;355(21):2203–2216.
75. Bhatt DL, Lincoff AM, Califf RM, et al. The benefit of abciximab in percutaneous coronary revascularization is not device-specific. *Am J Cardiol*. 2000;85(9):1060–1064.
79. Effects of platelet glycoprotein IIb/IIIa blockade with tirofiban on adverse cardiac events in patients with unstable angina or acute myocardial infarction undergoing coronary angioplasty. The RESTORE Investigators. Randomized Efficacy Study of Tirofiban for Outcomes and REstenosis. *Circulation*. 1997;96(5):1445–1453.
81. Platelet Receptor Inhibition in Ischemic Syndrome Management (PRISM) Study Investigators. A Comparison of Aspirin plus Tirofiban with Aspirin plus Heparin for Unstable Angina. *N Engl J Med*. 1998;338(21):1488–1497.
84. Randomised placebo-controlled trial of effect of eptifibatide on complications of percutaneous coronary intervention: IMPACT-II. *Lancet*. 1997;349(9063):1422–1428.

96. Valgimigli M, Gagnor A, Calabro P, et al. Radial versus femoral access in patients with acute coronary syndromes undergoing invasive management: a randomised multicentre trial. *Lancet*. 2015;385(9986):2465–2476.
100. First-year results of CABRI (Coronary Angioplasty versus Bypass Revascularisation Investigation). CABRI Trial Participants. *Lancet*. 1995;346(8984):1179–1184.
105. Sianos G, Morel MA, Kappetein AP, et al. The SYNTAX Score: an angiographic tool grading the complexity of coronary artery disease. *EuroIntervention*. 2005;1(2):219–227.
115. Farkouh ME, Domanski M, Sleeper LA, et al. Strategies for multivessel revascularization in patients with diabetes. *N Engl J Med*. 2012;367(25):2375–2384.
122. Sardella G, Lucisano L, Garbo R, et al. Single-staged compared with multi-staged PCI in multivessel NSTEMI patients: the SMILE trial. *J Am Coll Cardiol*. 2016;67(3):264–272.

Additional references available online at expertconsult.com

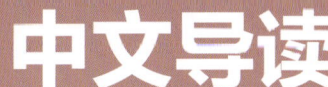

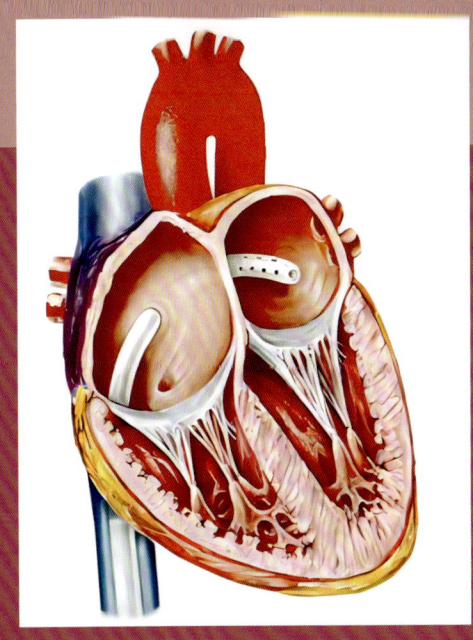

第20章
急性ST段抬高型心肌梗死的介入治疗

　　ST段抬高型心肌梗死是冠心病最严重的临床类型，主要是由急性血栓诱发的冠状动脉急性闭塞所致，具有较高的死亡率和致残率。早期、快速并完全地开通梗死相关动脉是改善ST段抬高型心肌梗死患者预后的关键。

　　再灌注治疗显著改善了ST段抬高型心肌梗死患者的预后和生活质量。直接经皮冠状动脉介入治疗适用于人群广、禁忌证数量少，对症状早期或晚期的患者疗效高、发症少，因此直接经皮冠状动脉介入治疗已成为ST段抬高型心肌梗死患者再灌注治疗的主流。而介入技术的进步、多种不同新型支架的研发（如新一代药物洗脱支架、生物可吸收支架、自膨胀支架等）、辅助装置的应用（如远端保护装置、血栓切除装置、IABP等）和新的抗血栓或抗凝药物增强了直接经皮冠状动脉介入治疗在ST段抬高型心肌梗死患者中的疗效。此外，经皮冠状动脉介入治疗不仅作为溶栓失败后的补救措施，而且是溶栓再灌注初始成功的重要辅助手段。尽管近年来接受经皮冠状动脉介入治疗的ST段抬高型心肌梗死患者比例稳步上升，但仍需做出重大努力，通过优化分诊和转诊系统，让所有ST段抬高型心肌梗死患者在症状出现后能够在短时间内接受这种治疗。除此之外，还需要进一步研究开发新的有效辅助疗法，通过预防或减轻远端栓塞、梗死面积和再灌注相关心肌损伤，并提供血流动力学支持，在直接经皮冠状动脉介入治疗手术期间进一步促进心肌挽救。与此同时，针对心肌细胞再生的深入实验和临床研究正在进行，并为改善ST段抬高型心肌梗死患者的预后和生活质量提供了新的前景。

林小龙　范　谦

章节要点

- 直接经皮冠状动脉介入治疗已成为ST段抬高型心肌梗死患者再灌注治疗的主要策略。
- 无论患者风险或是否需要转院进行经皮冠状动脉介入治疗，直接经皮冠状动脉介入治疗在减少ST段抬高型心肌梗死患者的死亡、再梗死、颅内出血、梗死相关动脉再闭塞和心肌缺血方面均优于溶栓治疗。
- 用来协调医院和急救医疗服务的区域医疗系统可缩短就诊至再灌注的时间，增加及时接受直接经皮冠状动脉介入治疗的患者数量，并降低ST段抬高型心肌梗死患者的死亡率。
- 与溶栓治疗相比，直接经皮冠状动脉介入治疗可在症状出现后更长的时间窗内去挽救心肌，并能改善临床结局。如果从首次医疗接触至器械时间≤120分钟，则直接经皮冠状动脉介入治疗是ST段抬高型心肌梗死患者的推荐治疗。
- 如经皮冠状动脉介入治疗相关延迟在120分钟以内，患者转运至直接经皮冠状动脉介入治疗中心的策略优于就地溶栓治疗。
- 症状出现≥12小时的ST段抬高型心肌梗死患者，进行直接经皮冠状动脉介入治疗获益的证据仍然十分有限。
- 对于所有预计首次医疗接触至器械时间超过120分钟限制的ST段抬高型心肌梗死患者，建议采用药物—有创策略，即先进行直接纤维蛋白溶解，然后进行冠状动脉造影和经皮冠状动脉介入治疗（支架植入）。初始直接纤维蛋白溶解后接受常规冠状动脉造影和经皮冠状动脉介入治疗（术后3~24小时）对于ST段抬高型心肌梗死患者是有益的。
- 对于ST段抬高型心肌梗死患者来说，支架植入是首选的经皮冠状动脉介入治疗方法，新一代药物洗脱支架应作为首选器械用于直接经皮冠状动脉介入治疗。
- 对于接受直接经皮冠状动脉介入治疗的ST段抬高型心肌梗死患者，推荐选择桡动脉作为血管通路。桡动脉入路可显著降低直接经皮冠状动脉介入治疗手术期间血管入路相关出血的风险。
- 纤维蛋白溶解失败后的挽救性经皮冠状动脉介入治疗可挽救缺血心肌，并改善临床结局。因此，对于溶栓失败的患者推荐进行挽救性经皮冠状动脉介入治疗。
- 在直接经皮冠状动脉介入治疗手术过程中，氯吡格雷、普拉格雷或替格瑞洛均可用于血小板抑制。普拉格雷和替格瑞洛能更快、更强地抑制血小板，但与氯吡格雷相比，其出血并发症的风险更高。
- 普通肝素、比伐卢定或依诺肝素可用于直接经皮冠状动脉介入治疗手术期间的围手术期抗凝。比伐卢定可降低出血风险，但会增加早期支架血栓形成风险。
- 对于ST段抬高型心肌梗死合并多支血管病变的患者，尽管支持多支血管干预的证据有所增加，但这些证据还不足以推荐在ST段抬高型心肌梗死患者中常规进行多支血管干预。有证据支持，对于非"罪犯病变"可利用血流储备分数去指导经皮冠状动脉介入治疗。
- 根据目前的证据，机械性血栓切除术、手动抽吸血栓切除术或远端保护装置不能改善甚至还会恶化临床结局，不推荐用于ST段抬高型心肌梗死患者。对于未合并心源性休克的ST段抬高型心肌梗死患者，没有证据支持使用机械循环支持设备。
- 在ST段抬高型心肌梗死患者直接经皮冠状动脉介入治疗手术期间，为减少微血管阻塞、梗死面积或再灌注损伤，以及促进心肌挽救而进行的药理学（或调节）干预仍在临床研究中。

20 Percutaneous Coronary Intervention in Acute ST-Segment Elevation Myocardial Infarction

Gjin Ndrepepa, Robert A. Byrne, Adnan Kastrati

KEY POINTS

- Catheter-based primary percutaneous coronary intervention (PPCI) has become the mainstay of reperfusion therapy in patients with ST-elevation myocardial infarction (STEMI).
- PPCI is superior to thrombolytic therapy in reducing death, reinfarction, intracranial bleeding, reocclusion of the infarct-related artery, and myocardial ischemia in patients with STEMI irrespective of the patient's risk or whether interhospital transfer for PCI is required.
- Regional systems of care coordinating hospitals and emergency medical services (EMSs) reduce the time-to-reperfusion, increase the number of patients undergoing PPCI in a timely manner, and can improve mortality in patients with STEMI.
- PPCI retains its myocardial salvaging capacity and its ability to improve clinical outcome over a wider time window after symptom onset than fibrinolysis and is the recommended therapy for patients with STEMI if performed ≤120 minutes from first medical contact (FMC)-to-device time.
- A strategy of patient transfer to a PPCI center is better than onsite fibrinolysis for PCI-related delays up to 120 minutes.
- The evidence on the benefits of PPCI for patients presenting ≥12 hours from the symptom onset remains limited.
- A pharmacoinvasive strategy consisting of primary fibrinolysis followed by coronary angiography and PCI (stenting) is recommended in all patients with STEMI in whom the FMC-to-device time is expected to exceed the 120-minute limit. Routine coronary angiography and PCI (3 to 24 hours after presentation) after an initial primary fibrinolysis strategy is beneficial in patients with STEMI.
- Primary stenting is the preferred PPCI approach for patients with STEMI, and newer-generation drug-eluting stents should be considered the preferred device for use in PPCI.
- Radial artery is recommended for vascular access in patients with STEMI who undergo PPCI. The approach markedly reduces the risk of access site bleeding during PPCI procedures.
- Rescue PCI after failed fibrinolysis salvages ischemic myocardium and improves clinical outcome and thus is the recommended treatment for these patients.
- Clopidogrel, prasugrel, or ticagrelor may be used for platelet inhibition during PPCI procedures. Prasugrel and ticagrelor cause faster and deeper platelet inhibition but are associated with a higher risk of bleeding complications compared with clopidogrel.
- Unfractionated heparin, bivalirudin, or enoxaparin may be used for periprocedural anticoagulation during PPCI procedures. Bivalirudin is associated with reduced risk of bleeding but with a higher risk of early stent thrombosis.
- Although evidence favoring the multivessel intervention in patients with STEMI and multivessel disease has increased, the evidence is not strong enough to recommend a routine use of this approach in patients with STEMI. Evidence supports a fractional flow reserve (FFR)-guided intervention in nonculprit coronary stenoses.
- Based on current evidence, mechanical thrombectomy, manual aspiration thrombectomy, or distal protection devices do not improve (or even worsen) clinical outcome and are not recommended in patients with STEMI. There is no evidence to support the use of mechanical circulatory support devices in patients with STEMI not complicated by cardiogenic shock.
- Pharmacological (or conditioning) interventions to reduce microvascular obstruction, infarct size, or reperfusion injury and promote myocardial salvage during PPCI procedures in patients with STEMI remain under clinical investigation.

INTRODUCTION

ST-segment elevation myocardial infarction (STEMI) represents the most malignant presentation of coronary artery disease (CAD) resulting from acute thrombus-mediated closure of a coronary artery with the exception of inaugural sudden cardiac death. Recent epidemiological evidence shows a steady decline in the acute myocardial infarction (MI) rates,[1-3] proportion of patients with STEMI,[4] and a reduction in STEMI-related in-hospital and 1-year mortality,[3] probably due to increased effectiveness of preventive strategies and better therapy (Fig. 20.1). The clinical characteristics of patients with STEMI seem also to have changed over time. A recent retrospective analysis of a nationwide inpatient database of 738,433 patients with STEMI admitted within 24 hours after pain onset who underwent primary percutaneous coronary intervention (PPCI) between 2004 and 2012 showed an increase in unadjusted in-hospital mortality from 3.9% to 4.7% over the study period. After adjustment, however, mortality decreased over time (a 5% reduction in the adjusted risk). Moreover, there was an increase in the proportion of patients with ≥3 comorbidities (from 14.8% to 29.0%) and those with intubation or cardiac arrest on presentation (from 3.2% to 7.8%) and both conditions had a strong independent association with mortality.[5] Notwithstanding these trends, STEMI still remains one of the most important causes of morbidity and mortality in developed countries, with an in-hospital and 1-year mortality in the range of 5% to 6% and 7% to 18%, respectively.[6]

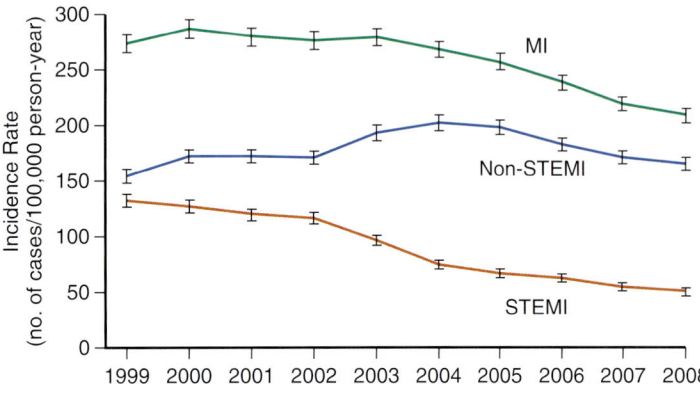

Fig. 20.1 Age- and sex-adjusted incidence rates of acute myocardial infarction (MI), 1999–2008. I bars represent 95% confidence intervals. *STEMI*, ST-segment elevation myocardial infarction. (From Yeh RW, Sidney S, Chandra M, et al. Population trends in the incidence and outcomes of acute myocardial infarction. *N Engl J Med*. 2010;362:2155–2165.)

In most cases, STEMI results from acute thrombotic occlusion of a large epicardial coronary artery, typically occurring as a consequence of atherosclerotic plaque disruption, erosion, or fissuring, which leads to exposure of thrombogenic material (plaque lipid content, collagen, and subendothelial extracellular matrix) to circulating blood with subsequent intraluminal thrombosis and acute vessel occlusion. Other causative factors of lesser importance include acute plaque expansion (such as occurring due to intraplaque hemorrhage leading to acute closure without or with minimal intraluminal thrombus formation), embolism, spontaneous dissection, coronary inflammation, and extracoronary factors. Interruption of coronary blood flow results in myocardial ischemia in the blood deprived myocardial area which, if severe enough and of sufficient duration, results in ischemic myocardial necrosis. As acute coronary thrombosis is often abrupt in onset and the ensuing ischemic damage progresses rapidly to necrosis following blood interruption, the rationale for prompt reperfusion therapy (pharmacological or mechanical removal of occlusive thrombi), aiming at early restoration of coronary blood flow to the infarct-related artery (IRA), is strong. Timely reperfusion results in myocardial salvage, increased electrical stability, and reduced incidence of fatal ventricular arrhythmias in the acute phase, as well as preservation of left ventricular function and improvement in short- and long-term patient survival. The evidence is definitive that reperfusion therapy with PPCI or fibrinolysis improves both survival and quality of life of patients with STEMI. PPCI refers to a strategy of emergent coronary angiography followed by coronary angioplasty with or without stenting of the IRA and without prior administration of fibrinolytic therapy. PPCI was introduced in the early 1980s as a reperfusion strategy in patients with STEMI. In the last decade, PPCI has become the dominant reperfusion strategy (and the standard of care) for STEMI and it continues to evolve.[7] Current guidelines recommend PPCI as the default reperfusion strategy for patients with STEMI presenting within the first hours from the symptom onset.[8,9]

Over the last two decades, considerable efforts have been made at the societal and medical community levels to improve the reperfusion therapy of patients with STEMI by working in three fields: (1) increased availability of centers capable of performing PPCI and building of triage and transfer systems of care to provide timely access to reperfusion in STEMI patients; (2) improvement of the PPCI equipment including new generations of coronary stents and their delivery systems and adjunct pharmacologic therapy (antithrombotic/anticoagulant drugs); and (3) development and evaluation of pharmacological or mechanical strategies to enhance myocardial salvage during PPCI procedures via optimizing acute procedural success, attenuation of distal embolization, microvascular obstruction (MVO) and reperfusion injury, and providing hemodynamic support.[10] The main focus of this chapter is to summarize recent developments in the field of PPCI in patients with STEMI.

GENERAL ASPECTS

Primary Percutaneous Coronary Intervention Versus Fibrinolysis as Reperfusion Strategy for ST-Elevation Myocardial Infarction

Restoration of coronary blood flow in the occluded coronary artery and the subtended myocardial tissue, as rapidly as possible, is the fundamental aim of early STEMI therapy. The introduction of fibrinolytic therapy represented an important development in the treatment of STEMI. The application of fibrinolytic agents early after symptom onset was associated with reduced mortality compared to no reperfusion. A meta-analysis of initial fibrinolytic trials demonstrated that the absolute mortality benefit at 5 weeks following fibrinolysis was 3% for patients presenting within 6 hours, 2% for patients presenting between 7 and 12 hours and 1% (statistically insignificant) for those presenting between 13 and 18 hours.[11] Despite the clear benefits of fibrinolysis compared with no reperfusion, it has serious limitations related to the high proportion of patients with relative or absolute contraindications to this therapy, life-threatening bleeding complications (disproportionately affecting elderly patients), a narrow window of therapeutic action after symptom onset due to rapid time-dependent loss of efficacy, limited ability to restore normal blood flow in the IRA even if applied in a timely fashion, and frequent reocclusions of the IRA resulting in recurrent ischemia or reinfarction within subsequent months. Apart from markedly attenuating these limitations, PPCI has other advantages over fibrinolytic therapy such as restoration of significantly higher rates of Thrombolysis in Myocardial Infarction (TIMI) flow grade 3 in the IRA (a finding that is both durable due to enhanced stability of the reopened vessel and relatively independent of time from symptom onset), salvage of greater amounts of myocardium, delineation of coronary anatomy and hemodynamic status resulting in improved risk stratification, and facilitation of patient care and earlier hospital discharge.[12] In earlier trials, balloon angioplasty (without stenting) was compared with fibrinolysis in terms of efficacy and safety. An earlier meta-analysis of 10 randomized trials of balloon angioplasty versus fibrinolysis showed a significant reduction of 30-day mortality (4.4% vs. 6.5%), lower rates of death or nonfatal reinfarction (7.2% vs. 11.9%) and stroke (0.7% vs. 1.1%) by balloon angioplasty.[13] Another meta-analysis of randomized trials that compared PPCI (with balloon angioplasty

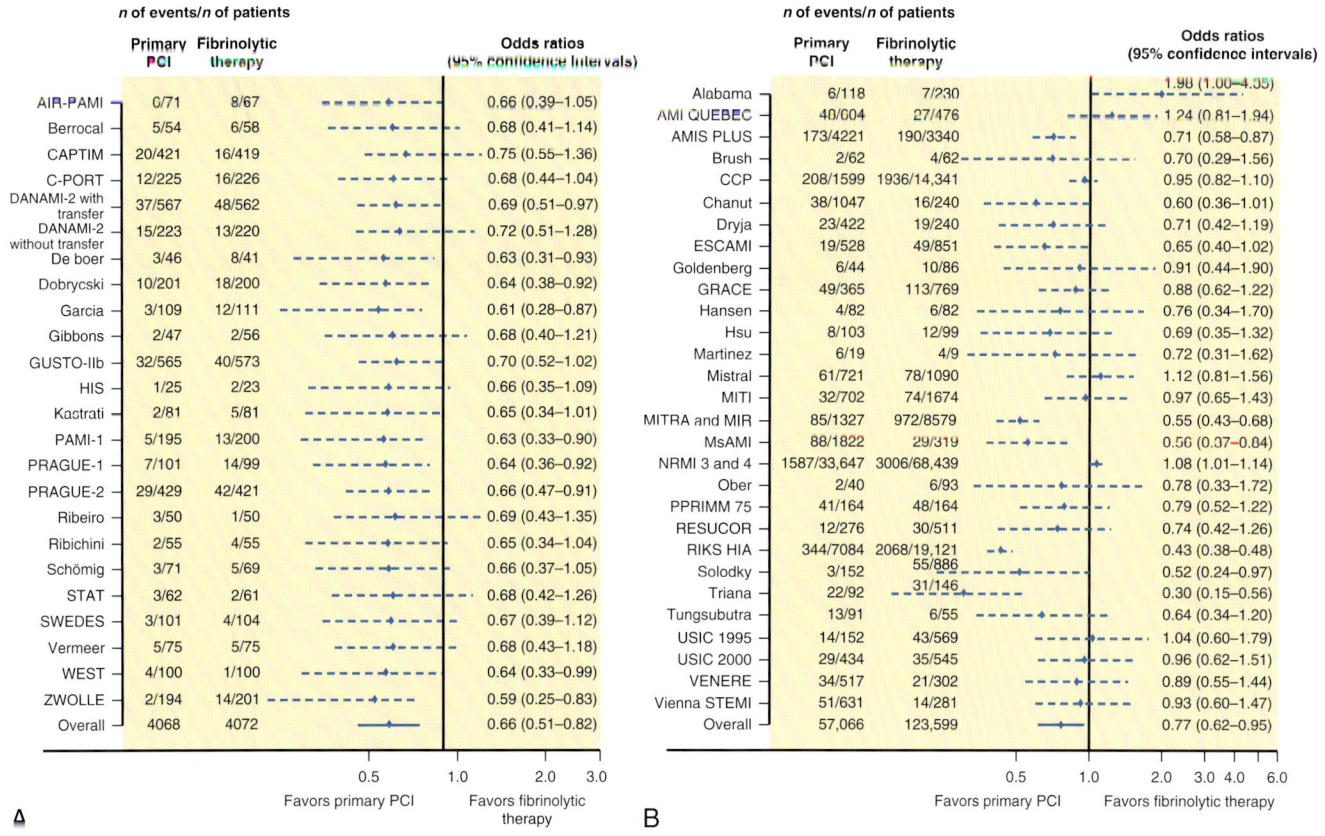

Fig. 20.2 Bayesian forest plot of all-cause short-term mortality rates in studies that have compared primary percutaneous coronary intervention *(PCI)* with fibrinolysis. (A) Bayesian forest plot of all-cause short-term mortality rates in randomized controlled trials. (B) Bayesian forest plot of all-cause short-term mortality rates in observational studies. (From Huynh T, Perron S, O'Loughlin J, et al. Comparison of primary percutaneous coronary intervention and fibrinolytic therapy in ST-segment-elevation myocardial infarction: Bayesian hierarchical meta-analyses of randomized controlled trials and observational studies. *Circulation* 2009;119[24]:3101–3109.)

only or coronary stenting) with fibrinolysis in patients with STEMI showed that PPCI is superior to fibrinolysis in terms of improving early and late survival as well as in reducing the incidence of reinfarction, intracranial bleeding, reocclusion of IRA, and recurrent myocardial ischemia.[12] Randomized trials have shown that coronary stenting has greater efficacy than fibrinolysis[14–18] or balloon angioplasty only[19–21] as reperfusion strategy in patients with STEMI.

PPCI improves survival even in patients with STEMI who have contraindications to fibrinolysis[22] or in patients presenting outside the therapeutic window of fibrinolysis.[23,24] Superiority of PPCI over fibrinolysis has been witnessed particularly in high-risk patients[25] and in centers without on-site cardiac surgery.[26] The DANish trial in Acute Myocardial Infarction-2 (DANAMI-2) trial demonstrated that the benefit of PPCI is largest in high-risk patients; in patients with TIMI risk score ≥5, there was a significant reduction in the mortality with PPCI versus fibrinolysis (25.3% vs. 36.2%; $P = .02$) which was not observed in the low-risk group (TIMI risk score 0 to 4).[25] The benefit of PPCI over fibrinolysis was maintained at long-term follow-up. A further report from the DANAMI-2 trial showed that 8-year composite of death or reinfarction was 34.8% in patients treated by PPCI versus 41.3% in patients treated with fibrinolysis ($P = .003$). Of note, PPCI reduced the risk of reinfarction (13% vs. 18.5%) and mortality (26.7% vs. 33.3%) among patients randomized at referral hospitals.[27] A large meta-analysis that included 23 randomized controlled trials (8140 patients) and 32 observational studies (185,900 patients) analyzed a series of outcomes of patients treated with PPCI or fibrinolysis (Fig. 20.2). In randomized trials, PPCI was associated with reductions of short-term (6-week) mortality by 34%, long-term (≥1 year) mortality by 24%, short-term reinfarction by 65%, long-term reinfarction by 51%, and stroke by 63% compared with fibrinolysis. In observational studies, PPCI was associated with reductions of short-term mortality by 23%, long-term mortality by 12% (statistically insignificant), short-term reinfarction by 53%, long-term reinfarction by 42% (statistically insignificant), and stroke by 61% compared with fibrinolysis. The differences in major bleeding between both reperfusion strategies did not reach the level of statistical significance in randomized trials or observational studies.[28] The study reinforced the recommendation that PPCI should be offered to STEMI patients if transport to invasive hospitals can be completed within 120 minutes. Evidence available also suggests that PPCI is cost-effective compared to fibrinolysis.[29,30]

The American College of Cardiology/American Heart Association (ACC/AHA) Guidelines define PPCI as a class 1 indication in patients with STEMI for 3 conditions: patients with STEMI with ischemic symptoms <12 hours (level of evidence A), patients with STEMI with ischemic symptoms <12 hours who have contraindications to fibrinolysis irrespective of time delay from the first medical contact (FMC; level of evidence B), and patients with

STEMI and cardiogenic shock or severe heart failure irrespective of the time delay from the STEMI onset (level of evidence B).[8] The recent guidelines of the European Society of Cardiology (ESC) for STEMI treatment recommend PPCI over fibrinolysis within the following timeframes: maximum expected delay from STEMI diagnosis to PPCI (wire crossing) of ≤120 minutes; maximal time from STEMI diagnosis to wire crossing in patients presenting at hospitals with PPCI of ≤60 minutes; and maximum time from STEMI diagnosis to wire crossing in transferred patients of ≤90 minutes (class 1, level of evidence A; Table 20.1).[9] Moreover, a strategy of PPCI is indicated in the absence of ST-segment elevation but with evidence on suspected ongoing ischemic symptoms suggestive of MI in the following situations: hemodynamic instability or cardiogenic shock, recurrent, or ongoing chest pain refractory to medical treatment, life-threatening arrhythmias or cardiac arrest, mechanical complications of MI, acute heart failure or recurrent dynamic ST-segment or T wave changes, particularly with intermittent ST-segment elevation (class I, level of evidence C).[9] If timely PPCI cannot be performed after STEMI diagnosis, fibrinolytic therapy is recommended within 12 hours of symptom onset in patients without contraindications (class 1, level of evidence A).[9] Of note, when FMS-to-device time is anticipated to be in excess of 120 minutes, guidelines recommend administration of fibrinolytic agents within 30 minutes of arrival[8] or within 10 minutes from STEMI diagnosis[9] followed by emergency transfer to PPCI centers for coronary angiography and percutaneous coronary intervention (PCI).

TIME-TO-REPERFUSION AND OUTCOME OF PRIMARY PERCUTANEOUS CORONARY INTERVENTION

Knowledge of the speed with which ischemic myocardium succumbs to necrosis following an abrupt occlusion of a coronary artery is important to understanding the time dependency of efficacy of reperfusion regimens and the degree of benefit from reperfusion in patients with STEMI. Reimer et al.[31] assessed the spatial and temporal progression of myocardial damage following coronary artery occlusion in anesthetized dogs. In this study, acute coronary artery occlusion resulted in myocardial ischemia that gradually progressed to necrosis, which was typically complete at ~6 hours after vessel occlusion. Following coronary occlusion, a rapid phase of cell death occurred mostly in the subendocardial layers, and about half of the ischemic myocardium that was necrotic at 24 hours was already dead 40 minutes after the occlusion. A second phase of cell death occurred more slowly in the midepicardial and subepicardial myocardium. This phase of myocardial necrosis was pretty much complete within 6 hours of coronary occlusion and about one-third of ischemic myocardium was still salvageable at 3 hours after the coronary occlusion.[31]

Time-to-reperfusion interval is an estimate of overall duration of myocardial ischemia that encompasses the time interval from the onset of symptoms of coronary occlusion to the initiation of reperfusion therapy—fibrinolysis or PPCI. It is a multi-component metric that includes: the interval from the symptom onset to the FMC by emergency medical service (EMS; patient delay); the interval from FMC to a PPCI hospital (prehospital system delay); and the time interval from hospital arrival to PPCI (door-to-balloon [DTB] time delay). In case of an initial referral to a hospital without PPCI in patients intended to be treated with PPCI, the prehospital system delay consists of the time interval from the FMC to the hospital without PCI, the in-hospital time (door-in-door-out [DIDO] time interval), and time interval from hospital without PCI to the hospital with primary PCI. The term system delay signifies the sum of the prehospital system and DTB time delays. Apart from its association with the duration of myocardial ischemia, time-to-reperfusion interval is an index of quality and readiness of the health care system to provide reperfusion therapy in a timely fashion.

Evidence available shows that time-to-reperfusion (or total ischemic time) is crucial for fibrinolysis and important for PPCI. Cardiac magnetic resonance (CMR) imaging studies demonstrated a close relationship between time-to-reperfusion and infarct size, amount of myocardium salvaged, or MVO. A prior study used contrast-enhanced CMR (performed 5 ± 3 days after PPCI) to assess extent of myocardial necrosis or severe MVO in 64 patients with first STEMI in relation to time-to-reperfusion interval.[32] The mean time-to-reperfusion was 190 ± 110 minutes and transmural necrosis and severe MVO was present in 65% and 23% of the patients, respectively. For patients without transmural necrosis or MVO, transmural necrosis only, or both conditions, the mean time-to-reperfusion was 90 ± 40 minutes, 110 ± 107 minutes, and 137 ± 97 minutes, respectively ($P < .001$). Importantly, for every 30-minute longer delay, the adjusted risk of transmural necrosis or MVO increased by 37% ($P = .032$) and 21% ($P = .021$), respectively. The finding of lower rates of transmural necrosis or MVO in patients with residual blood flow in the IRA suggested that establishing some blood flow in the IRA before PPCI (i.e., with prehospital fibrinolysis) could be beneficial.[32] A study of 70 patients with STEMI successfully treated with PPCI within 12 hours from the symptom onset showed significantly larger infarct size and MVO and reduced myocardial salvage (assessed by CMR 3 ± 2 days after hospital admission) with longer time-to-reperfusion delay.[33] Thus, for patients with symptom-to-balloon intervals of ≤90 minutes, >90 to 150 minutes, >150 to 360 minutes, and >360 minutes, the infarct size was 8%, 11.7%, 12.7%, and 17.9% of the left ventricle, respectively. Accordingly, salvaged myocardium markedly decreased when reperfusion occurred >90 minutes after coronary occlusion.[33] In another study that included 208 patients with STEMI undergoing PPCI within 12 hours from symptom onset and T2-weighted

TABLE 20.1 Time Targets in the Management of Acute STEMI

Time Intervals	Target
Maximum time from FMC to ECG and diagnosis[a]	≤10 min
Maximum expected delay from STEMI diagnosis to primary PCI (wire crossing) to choose primary PCI strategy over fibrinolysis (if this target time cannot be met, consider fibrinolysis)	≤120 min
Maximum time from STEMI diagnosis to wire crossing in patients presenting at primary PCI hospitals	≤60 min
Maximum time from STEMI diagnosis to wire crossing in transferred patients	≤90 min
Maximum time from STEMI diagnosis to bolus or infusion start of fibrinolysis in patients unable to meet primary PCI target times	≤10 min
Time delay from start of fibrinolysis to evaluation of its efficacy (success or failure)	60–90 min
Time delay from start of fibrinolysis to evaluation angiography (if fibrinolysis is successful)	2–24 h

[a]ECG should be interpreted immediately.
ECG, Electrocardiogram; *FMC*, first medical contact; *PCI*, percutaneous coronary intervention; *STEMI*, ST-segment elevation myocardial infarction.
Ibanez B, James S, Agewall S, et al. 2017 ESC Guidelines for the management of acute myocardial infarction in patients presenting with ST-segment elevation: The Task Force for the management of acute myocardial infarction in patients presenting with ST-segment elevation of the European Society of Cardiology (ESC). *Eur Heart J.* 2018;39(2):119–177.

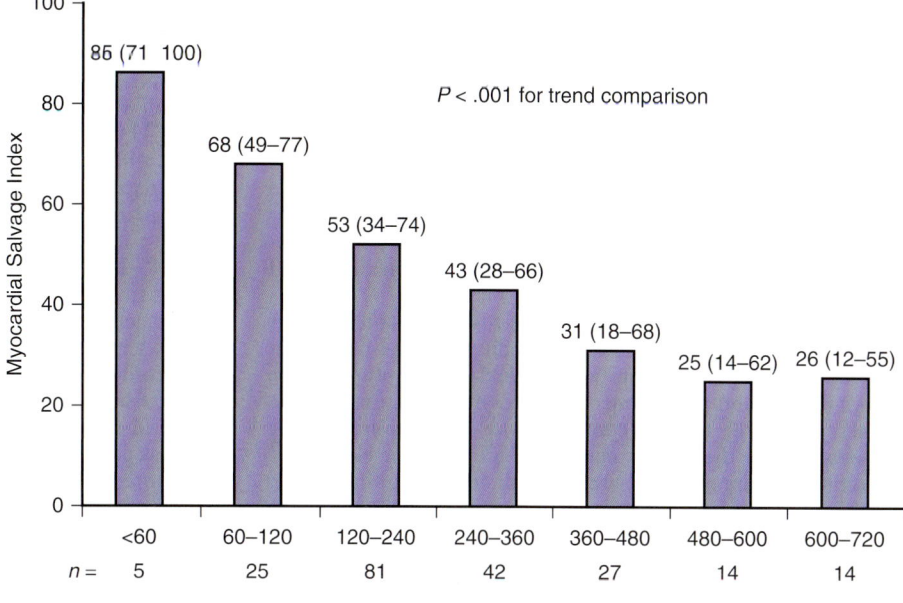

Fig. 20.3 Amount of myocardial salvage according to time from symptom onset to reperfusion. *PCI,* Percutaneous coronary intervention. (From Eitel I, Desch S, Fuernau G, et al. Prognostic significance and determinants of myocardial salvage assessed by cardiovascular magnetic resonance in acute reperfused myocardial infarction. *J Am Coll Cardiol.* 2010;55[22]:2470–2479.)

and contrast-enhanced CMR, there was a close relationship between myocardial salvage index, the proportion of area at risk salvaged, and the time-to reperfusion interval. Thus, myocardial salvage index was 85% (71% to 100%) in patients with symptom-to-balloon time <60 minutes and 26% (12% to 55%) in those with symptom-to-balloon time between 600 and 720 minutes (Fig. 20.3). However, only 5 of 208 patients (2.4%) were reperfused within the first hour from symptom onset.[34]

Large clinical studies mostly support an association between time-to-reperfusion and outcome after PPCI. The Zwolle cohort of 1791 patients with STEMI treated by primary angioplasty showed that the adjusted risk of 1-year mortality increased by 7.5% for each 30-minute increase in symptom-to-balloon time.[35] Data from the National Registry for Myocardial Infarction (NRMI) showed no association between symptom onset-to-balloon time and survival in a cohort of 27,080 consecutive patients with acute MI treated with primary angioplasty.[36] In this study, however, the DTB time (median 1 hour and 56 minutes) correlated with in-hospital mortality; the adjusted odds of mortality was significantly increased by 41% in patients with a DTB time between 121 and 150 minutes and by 62% in patients with a DTB time between 151 and 180 minutes. The authors suggested that DTB appears to be a valid quality-of-care indicator that should be considered when choosing a reperfusion strategy.[36] However the NRMI data should be interpreted in the context of very long DTB time (and consequently long symptom onset-to-balloon time) and impact of survival bias introduced by not considering patients who died before hospital arrival.[37] An analysis of 2635 patients enrolled in 10 randomized trials of primary angioplasty versus fibrinolysis demonstrated that with increasing time-to-presentation interval, major adverse cardiac event (MACE) rates increased after fibrinolysis but remained relatively stable after angioplasty.[38] A publication from the DANAMI-2 trial involving only the PPCI substudy showed that 3-year mortality did not differ among patients with symptom onset-to-balloon times <3 and 3 to 5 hours. However, mortality was significantly increased in patients presenting ≥5 hours from symptom onset (hazard ratio [HR] = 2.36; 95% confidence interval [CI] 1.51 to 3.67; *P* < .001) and the difference in mortality remained significant after adjustment for potential confounders. A shorter symptom onset-to-balloon interval was associated with higher rates of TIMI flow grade of 3 after PPCI and with a smaller proportion of patients with a left ventricular ejection fraction ≤40.[39] An analysis that included 2056 patients from the Harmonizing Outcomes with Revascularization and Stents in Acute Myocardial Infarction (HORIZONS AMI) trial showed that delay to reperfusion therapy was associated with greater injury to the microcirculation, assessed by myocardial perfusion grade or ST-segment resolution.[40] In patients with symptom-to-balloon onset times ≤2, >2 to 4, and >4 hours, 3-year unadjusted mortality rates were 2.6%, 4.4%, and 7.2%, respectively (log-rank test *P* = .007). A study of 3391 Japanese patients with STEMI undergoing PPCI showed a close association between symptom onset-to-balloon time and a composite of 3-year death or congestive heart failure (13.5% vs. 19.2%; risk reduction of 29.7% for symptom onset-to-balloon time <3 hours vs. >3 hours). The association remained significant after adjustment for potential confounders. No difference in the composite of 3-year death or congestive heart failure was found in subgroups of patients according to short (≤90 minutes) versus long (>90 minutes) DTB times (16.7% vs. 18.4%, risk reduction of 9.2%; *P* = .54). However, a DTB time of ≤90 minutes was associated with lower incidence of death or congestive heart failure only in patients presenting within the first 2 hours from symptom onset (11.9% vs. 18.1%; *P* = .01) but not in those presenting more than 2 hours from symptom onset (19.7% vs. 18.7%; *P* = .44). The study demonstrated a significant interaction (*P* for interaction = .01) between DTB time and time to presentation.[41]

Reasons for the reported inconsistencies with regard to the relationship between the ischemia time estimated by time-to-reperfusion interval and outcome remain unclear. One possibility may be that the reperfusion is offered in the relatively flat part of the ischemia time myocardial salvage curve, particularly in those presenting late after symptom onset. Thus, a short DTB time may be associated with a better clinical outcome (lower mortality) when it is a part of an overall short symptom-to-reperfusion time but may show a weaker (or no) association with mortality when placed at the end of a long ischemic time interval. Another important reason for the controversial findings may involve the inaccuracy of measurement of the time-to-reperfusion interval, particularly the patient-related delay component. It has been reported that patients with STEMI do not seek medical care for 1.5 to 2 hours after symptom onset and that this interval has remained fairly stable over time.[42,43] Other studies suggested that patient-related delay accounts for up to two-thirds of the overall ischemic time and it is greatest among women, older adults, patients with diabetes, patients of low socioeconomic status, and those presenting during night time.[44] Apart from being a large component, the patient delay is the most poorly estimated part of the total ischemic interval. In general, it is accepted that patients provide low credibility data regarding symptom onset due to recall bias (common in patients with STEMI, particularly under the effect of opiates) and stuttering course with intermittent preinfarction angina symptoms, obscuring the exact time of STEMI onset.

Risk distribution alongside the time-to-reperfusion is rather complex and of importance in understanding the time-dependent efficacy of PPCI in patients with STEMI. Prior studies have shown that patients presenting early after symptom onset have the highest risk score[45] which is consistent with observation that early presenters have the largest cumulated ST-segment elevation[46] reflecting the largest initial areas at risk and prompting urgent seeking of medical aid. This group of patients with STEMI benefit from PPCI mostly in terms of myocardial salvage, preservation of ventricular function, and survival due to early intervention of the ischemic lesion. Patients who present later after symptom onset may have smaller initial area at risk producing milder symptoms and their outcome may be influenced by the survivor-cohort effect, meaning that they have already survived the highest risk of death in the early hours after coronary occlusion. However, late presenters may have a more adverse cardiovascular risk profile. Prior reports showed that patients who presented later were older, more often women, diabetic, and had a past history of coronary bypass surgery. Adjusting for these factors considerably attenuates the association between time-to-reperfusion and mortality (from highly significant in univariable analysis to a borderline significance after adjustment in a multivariable model).[35] Patients with a greater delay on admission are also expected to present more frequently with additional adverse characteristics such as impaired renal function, peripheral arterial disease, and greater inflammatory burden, factors not accounted for in the multivariate model. Associated comorbidities and the less favorable cardiovascular risk profile may mask the benefits of mechanical reperfusion due to myocardial salvage and the unfavorable outcome after coronary intervention may erroneously be attributed solely to the longer time-to-reperfusion interval. Therefore, it is highly probable that a more adverse baseline risk profile of patients with longer delay to presentation may explain, at least in part, the apparent association between time-to-reperfusion interval and mortality. These considerations are important because the apparent reduction of benefit from PPCI with increased time to presentation may be interpreted as a poor incentive for a prompt intervention in patients with delayed presentation who benefit from this treatment.

DOOR-TO-BALLOON TIME AND OUTCOME OF PRIMARY PERCUTANEOUS CORONARY INTERVENTION

Time-to-reperfusion or total ischemic time is an important metric of reperfusion, yet concerns have been raised that this metric is hardly measurable and consequently inaccurate. Although DTB is only a part of total ischemic time, it has been the most commonly used quality-of-care metric in patients with STEMI. DTB is actionable and easy to measure, compare, and reproduce. DTB time is an important indicator of patient characteristics[46] and of the experience of the institution providing PPCI.[47] Comorbid conditions, absence of chest pain, delayed presentation after symptom onset, less-specific ECG findings, and hospital presentation during off-hours were associated with longer total DTB times.[46] Longer DTB times were encountered in patients of older age, female sex, nonwhite race, and those with complex medical histories.[48] DTB delay also depends heavily on hospital-related characteristics. Thus, presentation at night and treatment at lower-volume facilities were strong independent predictors of longer DTB interval.[48,49] A greater experience with PPCI is associated with shorter DTB times and lower in-hospital mortality in patients with STEMI treated with PPCI.[47] A pooled (patient-level) analysis of 22 trials with 6763 patients in the setting of the Primary Coronary Angioplasty Trialist versus Thrombolysis (PCAT)-2 Collaboration found that PPCI was superior to fibrinolysis irrespective of the DTB time the treating institution was able to achieve[50] or patient baseline risk.[51] The strength of association between DTB and mortality may depend on the patients' risk profile and the presentation delay. Thus, in a study of 2322 patients with STEMI followed up for a median of 83 months, delays in DTB time impacted late survival in high-risk but not low-risk patients and in patients presenting early but not late after the symptom onset.[52] A further study demonstrated that a combination of shorter DTB time (<90 minutes) with a shorter symptom onset-to-door time (<4 hours) was associated with lowest longer-term mortality.[53] Other studies have also demonstrated that short DTB times (≤90 minutes) were associated with a lower mortality in early presenters but not in late presenters.[54]

DTB has been the focus of considerable efforts and initiatives at regional and national levels aiming at its improvement. A 2006 survey that included 365 hospitals in the United States that have applied at least one strategy to decrease the DTB time in American hospitals showed that the mean of median DTB time of each hospital was 100.4 ± 23.5 minutes and 40% of hospitals had DTB times greater than 110 minutes.[55] The authors identified 28 strategies used by hospitals to reduce DTB times. After adjustment for eventual confounders, six strategies were associated with a positive impact on DTB times (Table 20.2). Although the association between these strategies and DTB times was significant, causality remains unproven and the evidence in support of the individual component strategies remains limited. Later, the DTB Alliance—a nationwide campaign initiated by the ACC and composed of clinicians, organizations, and hospitals working jointly to improve reperfusion in patients with acute MI—proposed two additional strategies to improve systems of care for patients with STEMI: senior management commitment and a team-based approach.[56] A report from the Acute Coronary Treatment and Intervention Outcomes Network (ACTION) - Get With the Guidelines registry showed that performance of prehospital electrocardiograms was associated with a 10-minute reduction in the FMC-to-balloon time.[57]

TABLE 20.2 Adjusted Associations Between Hospital Strategies and Door-to-Balloon Times

Strategy	Decrease in Door-to-Balloon Time (min)
Emergency physician activation of catheterization laboratory	8.2
Single call activation of the catheterization laboratory	13.8
Prehospital activation	15.4
Catheterization laboratory ready in 20 min (vs. more than 30 min)	19.3
Attending cardiologist on site	14.6
Real-time data feedback	8.6

Bradley EH, Herrin J, Wang Y, et al. Strategies for reducing the door-to-balloon time in acute myocardial infarction. *N Engl J Med*. 2006;355(22):2308–2320.

Moreover, data from the same registry showed that direct referral of patients to the catheterization laboratory, i.e., bypassing the emergency department, was associated with on average 20-minute reduction in the FMC-to-device time interval.[58] A recent report from a registry that included 33,901 transferred STEMI patients showed that the direct transfer of STEMI patients to the catheterization laboratory for PPCI was associated with significantly faster reperfusion (median DTB 116 vs. 191 minutes) and lower in-hospital mortality (4.6% vs. 11.2%; $P < .0001$) compared with transfer first to the emergency department/ward.[59] As a result of national efforts to decrease DTB time, the median DTB time was reduced from 96 minutes in 2005 to 64 minutes in 2010 and the proportion of patients with a DTB ≤90 minutes has increased from 44.2% to 91.4% over the 6-year period beginning in 2005.[60] However, it is widely accepted that there is a great variability and heterogeneity in using these strategies across various hospitals, regions, or countries.

Notwithstanding these characteristics, studies that have assessed the association of DTB or measures to reduce it with markers of reperfusion or outcome after PPCI have given conflicting results. An earlier study that included 1791 patients with STEMI from the Zwolle cohort found no association between DTB and 1-year mortality. However, the study found an association (even after adjustment) between symptom-to-balloon time and 1-year mortality which was stronger in low-risk patients.[61] A recent study of 786 patients with STEMI treated with PPCI between 2008 and 2013 also found no association between DTB categorized at <30, 30 to 59, 60 to 89, and ≥90 minutes time intervals and 30-day mortality.[62] Furthermore, in a subgroup of 262 patients, the DTB did not correlate with infarct size assessed by CMR 3 to 5 days after index event. Notably, the symptom onset-to-balloon time correlated closely with both outcomes.[62] Conversely, a 2009 report from the National Cardiovascular Data Registry that included 43,801 patients with STEMI reported a median DTB time of 93 minutes with 57.9% of patients treated within 90 minutes. Longer DTB times were associated with a higher adjusted risk of in-hospital mortality, which increased in a continuous nonlinear fashion (DTB interval 30 minutes, mortality 3.0%; 60 minutes, 3.5%; 90 minutes, 4.3%; 120 minutes, 5.6%; 150 minutes 7.0%; 180 minutes 8.4%; $P < .001$).[63] A recent meta-analysis of 32 studies involving 299,320 patients showed that patients with STEMI and longer (>90 minutes) DTB had higher risk of short-term (pooled odds ratio [OR] = 1.52 [1.40 to 1.65]) and mid-term (pooled OR = 1.53 [1.13 to 2.06]) mortality compared with patients with shorter DTB times. A nonlinear time-risk relationship was observed and the association between longer DBT and outcome was stronger for patients with shorter prehospital delays.[64]

Data on the impact of the improvements in the DTB times on mortality are also inconsistent. An earlier analysis from the NRMI registry reported a significant reduction in mortality, from 8.6% to 3.1%, associated with a decline in DTB times from 111 minutes in 1994 to 79 minutes in 2006.[65] Conversely, a study involving patients included in a quality improvement database in Michigan found no change in short-term mortality between 2003 and 2008 despite a decrease in DTB time from 113 minutes to 76 minutes.[66] A recent study of 96,738 admissions for PPCI between July 2005 and June 2009 (a period coinciding with national efforts to reduce DTB times) at 515 hospitals participating in the CathPCI Registry showed that median DTB times declined significantly, from 83 minutes in the first 12 months (2005–06) to 67 minutes in the last 12 months (2008–09) of the survey ($P < .001$). Despite improvements in DTB times, unadjusted in-hospital mortality (4.8% vs. 4.7%, $P = .43$), adjusted in-hospital mortality (5.0% vs. 4.7%, $P = .34$), and unadjusted 30-day mortality (9.7% vs. 9.8%, $P = .64$) remained unaffected.[67] Finally, a recent report from the National Cardiovascular Data Registry CathPCI Registry that included data from 423 hospitals and 150,116 PPCI procedures performed between January 2005 and December 2011 showed a significant reduction in DTB time from a median of 86 minutes in 2005 to 63 minutes in 2011 ($P < .0001$).[68] Although risk-adjusted mortality increased (from 4.7% to 5.3%; $P = .06$ for in-hospital mortality and from 12.9% to 14.4%; $P = .001$ for 6-month mortality) due to changing characteristics of patients undergoing PPCI over time, shorter DTB times were associated with lower in-hospital (adjusted OR = 0.92 [0.91 to 0.93] for each 10-minute decrease) and 6-month (adjusted OR = 0.94 [0.93 to 0.95]) mortality, with both risk estimates calculated per each 10-minute decrease in DTB.[68] Thus, although DTB remains an excellent process-of-care metric for expediting a patient's arrival in the cardiac catheterization laboratory, its association with the outcome after PPCI remains controversial. Concerns were raised that DTB is only one component of total ischemic time and once it is reduced to a certain level, the time before arrival at a hospital may become a more important factor. Consequently efforts with the intention to improve outcomes after PPCI should be directed throughout the ischemic time interval including increased patients' awareness of the STEMI symptoms, shortening of transfer times between medical facilities, or even improving in-hospital and post-discharge care to improve long-term outcome after PCI.[67] A short DTB may be closely correlated with improved outcomes after PPCI in the setting of short symptom-to-balloon times but not in the setting of long delays after symptom onset and measures that reduce DTB by a few minutes may not translate into large benefits if this reduction occurs at the end of prolonged total ischemic times. Furthermore, there is a possibility that low-risk STEMI patients are treated more quickly and that patients with complications may take longer to treat, which may dilute the impact of reduced DTB time on mortality.[69] Following the 2013 ACC/AHA guidelines for STEMI therapy, the FMC-to-device (in essence any type of device [wires, balloons, stents, aspiration catheters, or other]) time is increasingly being used instead of DTB. The FMC-to-device time interval is accurately measurable, encompasses a longer portion of ischemia time (by including prehospital delay), allows a better assessment of the impact of prehospital strategies aiming at reducing the interval itself and DTB (like prehospital ECG transmission, bypassing of hospitals without PCI facility or emergency departments) on time-to-reperfusion, and may be a suitable metric in the setting of regional network systems of STEMI care. A Danish study (a country that has implemented regional STEMI systems of care) of 6209 patients with STEMI undergoing PPCI within 12 hours from symptom onset showed an association and dependence of long-term (median 3.4 years) mortality on the system delay. Thus, for delays 0 to 60 minutes, 61 to 120 minutes, 121 to 180 minutes, and 181 to 360 minutes long-term mortality was 15.4%, 23.3%, 28.1%, and 30.8%, respectively (Fig. 20.4). Of note, in multivariable analysis adjusting for other potential correlates of mortality, the system delay was associated independently with mortality (a 10% increase in the adjusted risk for mortality per 1 h delay).[70] Although the FMC-to-device metric has advantages and is increasingly being used as a quality benchmark in the setting of STEMI systems of care, many hospitals still remain focused on DTB and use it as a public performance measure.

NETWORK SYSTEMS OPTIMIZING REPERFUSION IN PATIENTS WITH ST-ELEVATION MYOCARDIAL INFARCTION

PPCI is a preferred reperfusion strategy in patients with STEMI and its maximal benefit in terms of reduction of mortality and morbidity is achieved if this therapeutic strategy is offered in a timely manner, that is, as soon as possible following the symptom onset. The need for expedited reperfusion by PPCI has led to the development of STEMI systems of care with a

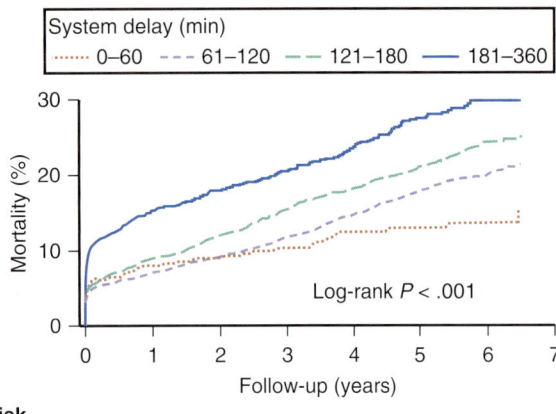

Fig. 20.4 Kaplan-Meier cumulative mortality estimates for patients with ST-segment elevation myocardial infarction treated with primary percutaneous coronary intervention, stratified according to intervals of system delay (time from contact with the health care system to the time of primary PCI). (From Terkelsen CJ, Sorensen JT, Maeng M, et al. System delay and mortality among patients with STEMI treated with primary percutaneous coronary intervention. *JAMA.* 2010;304[7]:763–771.)

TABLE 20.3 Essential Components of STEMI Systems of Care

- Single telephone emergency number
- Ambulances (vehicles, helicopters, planes) equipped with 12-lead ECGs and defibrillators and staffed with physicians or well-trained paramedics capable of basic and advanced life support
- Occasionally automatic ECG interpretation or ECG telemetry
- Direct telephone access to the catheterization laboratory
- Protocols for standardized care (diagnosis, therapy, and transfer)
- Cardiologist or intensive care specialist as a network leader
- Involvement of healthcare authorities
- Public information campaigns
- Regular meetings of involved parties
- Prospective registry

ECG, Electrocardiogram; *STEMI,* ST-segment elevation myocardial infarction.
Huber K, Gersh BJ, Goldstein P, et al. The organization, function, and outcomes of ST-elevation myocardial infarction networks worldwide: current state, unmet needs and future directions. *Eur Heart J.* 2014;35(23):1526–1532.

focus on prehospital diagnosis of STEMI, direct transfer to a center capable of performing PPCI, and 24/7 on-call services with activation times no longer than 30 minutes.[71] In order to reduce time to PPCI and increase the number of patients with STEMI reperfused in a timely manner by this preferred reperfusion strategy, several hospitals in the United States embarked on beyond-the-hospital initiatives to coordinate care for patients with STEMI.[72–76] Although the initial efforts were not fully developed systems and mostly included measures to coordinate the first and subsequent contacts of patients with STEMI with EMS and inter-hospital transport, they markedly reduced delays in achieving reperfusion and inspired efforts for more complete systems to optimize reperfusion in patients with STEMI.[77] In 2007, the AHA launched the initiative Mission: Lifeline encouraging communities to develop their own systems to optimize reperfusion therapy in patients with STEMI.[78] The goal of the initiative was implementation of urban, suburban, and rural ideal systems of care for patients with STEMI that allow the timely delivery of the appropriate lifesaving therapies to all patients in all places. A system is defined as an integrated group of entities within a region coordinating the provision of diagnostic and therapeutic services; a STEMI care system includes EMS providers, referral centers/non-PCI hospitals, and receiving centers/PPCI hospitals.[78] In general, the systems of care consist of a series of multidisciplinary, orchestrated, hospital-wide measures aiming at reduction of the time-to-reperfusion in patients with acute coronary syndromes, particularly STEMI. Recently, experts have proposed the essential components that a contemporary system of care for patients with STEMI should have (Table 20.3). Analysis of various regional systems of care for patients with STEMI across Europe, the United States, and Canada has shown that for most countries in Europe and many regions in North America, geographic conditions and availability of PPCI centers enable provision of PPCI given the systems of care are in place.[79]

Although regional STEMI treatment systems using standardized transfer protocols have been shown to improve the treatment times,[74,80] performance of these systems remains poorly investigated and, even in the most sophisticated systems, the treatment delays are relatively common. A recent prospective, observational study of 2034 patients transferred for PPCI in the setting of a regional STEMI system showed that treatment delays occur even in efficient STEMI systems of care.[81] Delays of the greatest magnitude were due to diagnostic dilemmas (median delay, 95.5 minutes) and nondiagnostic initial electrocardiograms (median delay, 81 minutes). Thus, up to 50% of patients with STEMI fail to meet the guideline recommended goals of FMC-to-device time of less than 120 minutes.[58,82–84] Furthermore, there are several barriers to system implementation including a highly fragmented health system comprising approximately 4750 acute care hospitals and >15,000 EMS agencies (in the United States) as well as remarkable heterogeneity in organization, protocols, and practices across systems, hospital or cardiology group competition, EMS transport and financial issues.[85] In 2012, the Duke Clinical Research Institute in collaboration with the AHA initiated the Mission: Lifeline STEMI Accelerator Project with the following goals: (1) comprehensively accelerate the implementation of STEMI care systems in 17 selected large metropolitan regions across the United States; (2) facilitate effective delivery of STEMI care in a timely, coordinated, and consistent manner; and (3) improve clinical outcomes of STEMI patients by broadly improving use and timeliness of reperfusion therapy.[86] The results of the project are encouraging. A report from the Accelerator Project involving 484 hospitals and 1253 EMS agencies in 16 regions in the United States with 23,809 patients presenting with STEMI between July 2012 and December 2013 showed a modest but significant increase in the proportion of patients meeting guideline goals of FMC-to-device time including patients presenting directly to a PCI hospital (50% to 55%) or transferred patients (44% to 48%). Of note, trends toward lower in-hospital mortality compared to national data toward the end of the measurement period were observed.[85] Another report from the project assessed whether implementing key care processes was associated with system performance improvement. In 167 hospitals with 23,498 patients surveyed between March 2012 and July 2014, uptake of four key care processes increased after intervention: prehospital catheterization laboratory activation (62% to 91%), single call transfer protocol from an outside facility (45% to 70%), emergency department bypass for EMS direct presenters (48% to 59%), and transfers (56% to 79%). The improvement of these indexes was associated with significant reductions in the FMC-to-device times.[87] The most recent report from the Mission: Lifeline Accelerator 2 project that included 10,730 STEMI patients in 12 metropolitan regions (in the United States) including 132 PCI hospitals

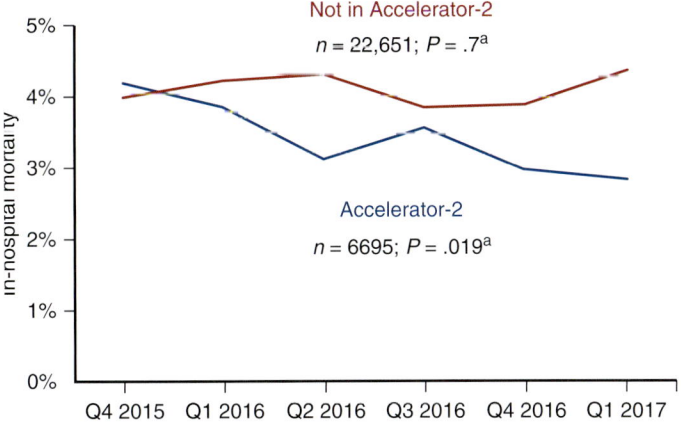

Fig. 20.5 In-hospital mortality according to hospital participation in the Accelerator-2 project. (From Jollis JG, Al-Khalidi HR, Roettig ML, et al. Impact of regionalization of ST elevation myocardial infarction care on treatment times and outcomes for emergency medical services transported patients presenting to hospitals with percutaneous coronary intervention: Mission: Lifeline Accelerator-2. *Circulation.* 2018;137:376–387.)

and 946 EMS agencies, surveyed between April 2015 and March 2017, showed a better cooperation between EMS and hospitals, improved reperfusion times, and reduced in-hospital mortality. More specifically the proportions of patients with a FMC-to-device time of ≤90 minutes (67% to 74%), a FMC-to-catheterization laboratory activation of <20 minutes (38% to 56%; $P < .0001$), and emergency department dwell time of <20 minutes (33% to 43%; $P < .0001$) were significantly increased. Notably these improvements corresponded to a significant reduction in in-hospital mortality from 4.4% to 2.3% (Fig. 20.5) which was not observed in hospitals not participating in the project during the same time period.[88] These studies clearly demonstrated that coordinated care of STEMI patients through regional-based systems coordinating hospitals and EMS systems can reduce the time-to-reperfusion and mortality of patients with STEMI. They offer support to the ACC/AHA STEMI guidelines recommendation that "all communities should create and maintain a regional system of STEMI care that includes assessment and continuous quality improvement of EMS and hospital-based activities."[8]

PRIMARY PERCUTANEOUS CORONARY INTERVENTION IN LATE PRESENTERS

Registry data have shown that between 9% and 31% of patients with STEMI present more than 12 hours from the symptom onset.[22,89] For patients with STEMI presenting beyond 12 hours from the symptom onset, fibrinolysis is associated with little or no benefit and may even be harmful and thus it is not recommended. On the other hand, PPCI remains a therapeutic option even though evidence available on the benefit of this therapeutic modality is limited or controversial. Registry-based studies have suggested a potential benefit of PPCI in patients with STEMI presenting >12 hours from the symptom onset. In the NRMI-2 registry, which included 7258 patients with STEMI presenting >12 hours from the symptom onset, 1631 patients (22%) received invasive treatment within 6 hours of admission, and 5727 patients received conservative therapy. Compared with those who received conservative therapy, patients who received invasive treatment had lower in-hospital mortality (3.4% vs. 6.6%), less recurrent ischemia or angina (10.7% vs. 13.8%), and a reduced incidence of recurrent MI (1.2% vs. 2.2%). After adjustment, invasive therapy was associated with a 33% reduction in the adjusted risk for mortality.[90] In another registry of 2036 patients with STEMI presenting 12 to 24 hours from symptom onset, without cardiogenic shock or pulmonary edema and not reperfused by fibrinolysis, 910 (44.7%) underwent invasive treatment. Patients with an invasive approach had lower mortality at 12 months than patients with a conservative approach (9.3% vs. 17.9%). The mortality benefit persisted after adjustment (a 27% reduction in the adjusted risk) or propensity matching (adjusted relative risk [RR] = 0.73, 95% CI 0.58 to 0.99).[91] Scintigraphic studies showed that substantial myocardial salvage by PPCI (more than 50% of initial area at risk salvaged) occurs in 41% of late comers (>12 hours from the symptom onset).[92]

Studies that have investigated the efficacy of PCI in late presenters on a randomized basis have given conflicting results, mostly because some studies addressed the late presenters, whereas other studies addressed the occluded vessel. The Beyond 12 hours Reperfusion AlternatiVe Evaluation (BRAVE-2) randomized 365 patients with STEMI presenting 12 to 48 hours from the symptom onset to invasive or conservative treatment. The study demonstrated a significant reduction of the scintigraphic infarct size (median infarct size 8% vs. 13% of the left ventricle, $P < .001$) and a trend toward a reduction of secondary end point of death, recurrent MI, or stroke at 30 days (4.4% vs. 6.6%) with invasive treatment.[24] A later update from the BRAVE-2 trial demonstrated a mortality benefit out to 4 years in patients assigned to invasive treatment (11.1% in patients assigned to invasive treatment vs. 18.9% in patients assigned to conservative therapy; $P = .047$; Fig. 20.6).[93] The DEsobstruction COronaire en Post-Infarctus (DECOPI) trial randomized 212 patients with first Q-wave MI and an occluded vessel to percutaneous revascularization or medical therapy 2 to 15 days after symptom onset. The primary end point was a composite of cardiac death, nonfatal MI, or ventricular tachyarrhythmia. At 6 months, left ventricular ejection fraction was 5% higher in the invasive group compared with the conservative therapy group ($P = .013$) and more patients had a patent artery (82.8% vs. 34.2%, $P < .0001$). At a mean of 34 months of follow up, there were no significant differences in the primary end point between patients assigned to invasive or conservative therapy (7.3% vs. 8.7%, $P = .68$) but the overall costs were higher for invasive treatment.[94] The Occluded Artery Trial (OAT) randomized 2166 stable patients who had an occluded IRA (by cardiac catheterization) to PCI with stenting or optimal medical therapy 3 to 28 days after acute STEMI. The primary end point was a composite of death, MI, or New York Heart Association class IV heart failure. At 4 years, the rate of the composite end point was not statistically different between the PCI and the medical therapy groups (17.2% and 15.6%, respectively; HR = 1.16; 95% CI 0.92 to 1.45; $P = .20$), with no interaction between treatment effect and any subgroup variable (age, sex, race or ethnic group, IRA, ejection fraction, diabetes, Killip class, and the time from MI to randomization). During a 6-year median survivor follow-up (longest 9 years), there was no significant difference between the two treatment strategies in the rates of either the primary end point or its individual components.[95] Due to the study size, the OAT trial had an important negative impact on the use of invasive treatment in the stable late presenters with STEMI. A meta-analysis of 10 randomized trials (OAT trial included) with 3560 patients with acute MI presenting between 12 hours and 60 days after symptom onset demonstrated significant reduction in long-term mortality (6.3% vs. 8.4%) with invasive treatment. Eight of 10 included studies showed improvements in long-term survival. There was a greater improvement in left ventricular ejection fraction over time in patients who received invasive treatment (+4.4% change in the left ventricular ejection fraction) compared to patients who received medical therapy.[23] However, the results of this meta-analysis need to be interpreted with caution, in light of the considerable heterogeneity across the studies.

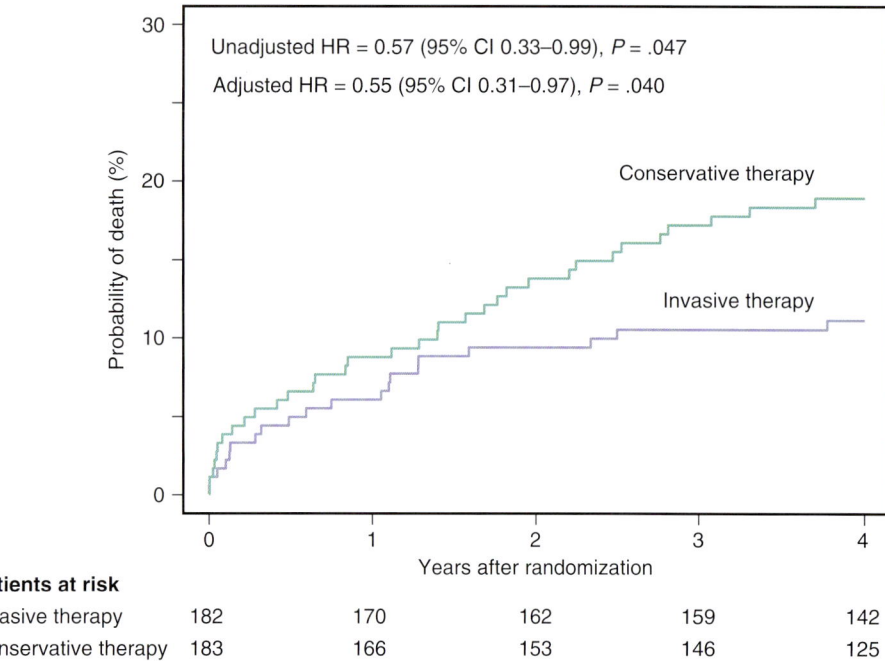

Fig. 20.6 Kaplan-Meier curves of 4-year mortality in the invasive and conservative therapy groups of the Beyond 12 hours Reperfusion Alternative Evaluation (BRAVE-2) trial. *CI,* Confidence interval; *HR,* hazard ratio. (From Ndrepepa G, Kastrati A, Mehilli J, et al. Mechanical reperfusion and long-term mortality in patients with acute myocardial infarction presenting 12 to 48 hours from onset of symptoms. *JAMA.* 2009;301[5]: 487–488.)

In aggregate, the benefit of PPCI in late presenters with STEMI lacks strong evidence. For patients with STEMI presenting between 12 and 24 hours, the current ESC guidelines give a class I (level of evidence: C) for the use of PPCI in patients with time from symptom onset >12 hours, in the presence of ongoing symptoms suggestive of ischemia, hemodynamic instability, or life-threatening arrhythmias; a class IIa (level of evidence: B) for a routine PPCI strategy in patients presenting 12 to 48 hours after symptom onset; and a class III (level of evidence: A) for the routine use of PPCI in asymptomatic patients and an occluded IRA >48 hours after onset of STEMI.[9] The ACC/AHA guidelines give a class IIa recommendation (level of evidence: B) for the use of PPCI in patients with STEMI presenting between 12 and 24 hours who have evidence of ongoing ischemia.[8] The consensus is, however, that patients with STEMI presenting late (>12 hours from the symptom onset) should undergo coronary angiography. Moreover, it is reasonable to perform PPCI in late presenters with STEMI who manifest severe heart failure or have electrical or hemodynamic instability or persistent ischemia. Some experts also recommend performing PPCI in these patients if subtotal occlusions in the IRA with collateral circulation in the territory distal to the occlusion were found in coronary angiography.

INTERHOSPITAL TRANSFER FOR PRIMARY PERCUTANEOUS CORONARY INTERVENTION

The lack of PCI facilities in hospitals that receive patients with STEMI, the wider therapeutic window, and the proven superiority of PPCI over fibrinolysis have led to the concept of emergency interhospital transfer for PPCI instead of initial fibrinolysis in the presenting hospital in patients with STEMI. Although the number of PCI-capable hospitals increased by almost 50% and 90% of Americans live within 60 minutes of a PCI-capable facility,[85] there are multiple scenarios in which patients with STEMI can end up in a hospital without a PCI facility. In case the diagnosis of STEMI is not immediately clear to the EMS or when patients with STEMI self-present to the nearest emergency department, these patients also may find themselves in hospitals without a PPCI facility. Earlier randomized trials of on-site fibrinolysis versus interhospital transfer plus PCI have confirmed that transfer of patients for PPCI is a better treatment than fibrinolysis at the initial hospital. The results of these trials have been summarized in two meta-analyses. The first meta-analysis of six randomized trials performed before 2003 including 3750 patients showed that a strategy of patient transfer plus PPCI was associated with a 42% reduction in the 30-day incidence of combined end point of death, reinfarction, and stroke compared with a strategy of on-site fibrinolysis.[96] The other quantitative review of studies that have involved patient's transfer for PCI have suggested that for every 100 patients treated, PPCI after interhospital transfer instead of on-site fibrinolysis prevented seven MACEs defined as death, nonfatal reinfarction, or nonfatal stroke.[97]

More recent studies provided further evidence on the benefits of transfer of patients for PPCI compared with on-site fibrinolysis. A prior study randomized 401 patients presenting to community hospitals to a strategy of on-site fibrinolysis or intravenous tirofiban and transport for PPCI. The delay to reperfusion defined as interval from admission to start of fibrinolysis or PPCI was 35 and 145 minutes, respectively. The composite end point of death, reinfarction, or stroke was lower in patients assigned to the transport plus PPCI strategy at 30 days (8.0% vs. 15.5%, $P = .019$) and 1 year (11.4% vs. 21.5%, $P = .006$).[98] A study of 850 patients with STEMI enrolled in the PRimary Angioplasty in patients transferred from General community hospitals to specialized PTCA Units with or without Emergency fibrinolysis (PRAGUE)-2 trial showed that the 5-year composite end point of death, reinfarction, stroke, or revascularization was 40% in patients assigned to a strategy of transfer plus PPCI versus 53% in patients assigned to on-site fibrinolysis in the presenting hospital ($P < .001$).[18] A large registry including 16,043 STEMI patients treated with in-hospital fibrinolysis, 3078 treated with prehospital fibrinolysis, and 7084 treated with PPCI indicated that transfer for PCI is better than prehospital fibrinolysis even in early presenters in whom the treatment is initiated within 2 hours.[99] A strategy of patient transfer for PPCI instead of on-site fibrinolysis inevitably incurs additional time delays imposed by transport, logistics, and organizational and technical aspects of PCI procedures. PCI-related time delay is an integral part of treatment algorithms for patients with STEMI. The recently published results from a prospective multicenter STEMI registry in Spain showed that in early STEMI patients assisted in noncapable PCI centers, in situ fibrinolysis

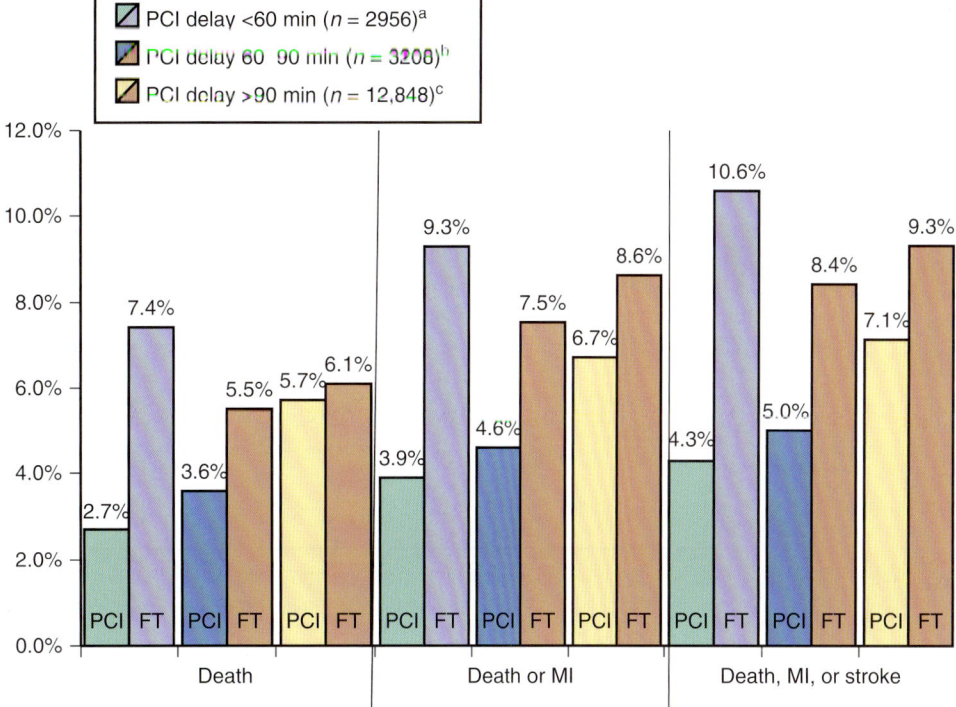

Fig. 20.7 Clinical outcomes among matched patients stratified by percutaneous coronary intervention (PCI)-related delay. [a]Standardized difference >10% for all outcomes. [b]Standardized difference >10% for only death or myocardial infarction (MI) and for death, MI, or stroke. [c]Standardized difference >10% for all outcomes. *FT,* Fibrinolytic therapy. (From Pinto DS, Frederick PD, Chakrabarti AK, et al. Benefit of transferring ST-segment-elevation myocardial infarction patients for percutaneous coronary intervention compared with administration of onsite fibrinolytic declines as delays increase. *Circulation.* 2011;124[23]:2512–2521.)

was associated with worse prognosis (a 1.91-fold increase in the adjusted risk for 30-day mortality) than the transferred patients and the study recommended transfer to a PCI-capable center for all patients with a FMC-to-device time <140 minutes.[100]

PCI-related delay has been the subject of intense investigation and, historically, many time intervals at which mortality rates of PCI after patients' transfer and on-site fibrinolysis are at equipoise have been proposed. In many studies, the PCI-related delay was calculated based on published summarized data and not on individual patient data. Consequently, several prior estimations were subsequently found to be flawed and corrected, in general, by expanding the metric. A report from the PCAT-2 Trialists' Collaborative Group demonstrated that for PCI-related delays up to 120 minutes, PPCI was associated with a 26% reduction in mortality compared to fibrinolysis or in 19 lives saved per 1000 patients treated. The absolute reduction in mortality with PPCI widened over time from 1.3% within the first hour to 4.2% after >6 hours after symptom onset. The most thorough time-based analysis that used individual patient data showed that PPCI is superior to fibrinolysis up to a PCI-related delay of 120 minutes.[50] In this study, even in the group of patients presenting within 1 hour, mortality was lower with PPCI (4.7% vs. 6.0%) indicating that even in early presenters with PCI-related delays of 60 minutes or less there is no reason to prefer fibrinolysis instead of PPCI as reperfusion strategy.[50] In 192,509 patients entered into the NRMI 2 to 4 registries, the mean PCI-related delay at which mortality benefits of PPCI and fibrinolysis were at equipoise was 114 minutes (95% CI 96 to 132 minutes).[101] Of note, the study showed that PCI-related delay was not static and varied considerably depending on the risk characteristics of patients, such as age, symptom duration, and infarct location. Thus, PCI-related delay varied from <1 hour for patients <65 years of age with anterior infarction who presented within <2 hours to almost 3 hours for patients >65 years of age, with nonanterior infarction who presented >2 hours from symptom onset. A regression analysis including 27 trials with 4399 patients randomized to PPCI and 4474 patients randomized to fibrinolysis found that the higher the risk of patients the larger the reduction in mortality achieved by PPCI. It was calculated that for each 10-minute increase of PCI-related delay, there was a 0.75%, 0.45%, and 0.0% mortality benefit in high-, medium-, and low-risk patients, respectively.[102] A report from the NRMI 2 to 5 registries assessed the impact of PCI-related delay in 107,028 patients with STEMI within 12 hours of pain onset: 11,662 patients undergoing PCI after transfer and 95,366 patients undergoing onsite fibrinolysis. In the whole sample, in-hospital mortality was 4.9% among patients treated with PCI and 8.1% among patients treated with onsite fibrinolysis. Among matched patients (9,506 patients in each treatment strategy), in-hospital survival was similar (4.8% vs. 6.2%) but the composite end points of death/MI or death/MI/stroke were lower with PCI. The PCI-related benefit was time dependent. The mortality was lower with PCI compared to onsite fibrinolysis for PCI-related delays <60 minutes and reduced for PCI-related delays 60 to 90 minutes and the difference was almost absent at PCI-related delays exceeding 90 minutes (Fig. 20.7). The number needed to treat to show superiority of PPCI over onsite fibrinolysis went from 23, to 44, and to 250 for PCI-related delays <60 minutes, 60 to 90 minutes, and >90 minutes, respectively. The regression analysis showed that mortality benefit of PCI over onsite fibrinolysis for PCI-related delays beyond 120 minutes (which occurred in 48% of the patients) was negated (Fig. 20.8). The equipoise for mortality for patients presenting within 2 hours from the symptom onset was longer (about 132 minutes). For the composite end point of death/MI/stroke, equipoise occurred at about 158 minutes.[103]

Although these studies showed that longer delays reduce the survival benefits of PPCI, a longer PCI-related delay could be acceptable and beneficial in high-risk STEMI patients, such as cardiogenic shock. In essence, a flexible PCI related delay according to the risk profile of STEMI patients is suggested. The assessment of the relationship between PCI related time delay and outcome provides helpful information for optimization of the PPCI network. In an attempt to shorten PCI-related time delay, direct transportation of patients to hospitals capable of performing PPCI rather than transporting them to the nearest hospital without PCI facility has also been suggested.[104] Concerns have

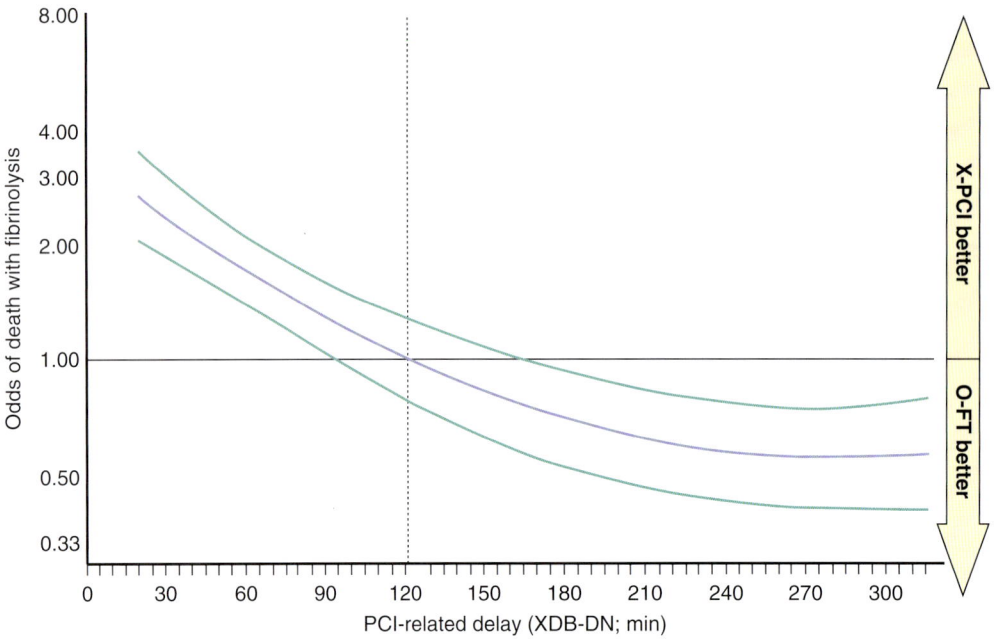

Fig. 20.8 Relationship between percutaneous coronary intervention *(PCI)*–related delay (minutes) and in-hospital mortality. *Dotted lines* represent 95% confidence interval. *O-FT*, On-site fibrinolytic therapy; *XDB-DN*, transfer delay (transfer door-to-balloon–door-to-needle time); *X-PCI*, transfer for primary percutaneous coronary intervention. (From Pinto DS, Frederick PD, Chakrabarti AK, et al. Benefit of transferring ST-segment-elevation myocardial infarction patients for percutaneous coronary intervention compared with administration of onsite fibrinolytic declines as delays increase. *Circulation.* 2011;124[23]:2512–2521.)

also been raised that transfer of patients for PCI may be associated with issues related to antithrombotic/anticoagulant adjunct therapy. Administration of low-molecular-weight heparin and glycoprotein IIb/IIIa inhibitors (GPI) at the STEMI-referring hospital was associated with longer delays to reperfusion compared with administration at the STEMI-receiving hospital, whereas early use of unfractionated heparin was not. The transferred patients who underwent treatment were more likely to receive excess doses of unfractionated or low-molecular-weight heparin (28% and 54% increase in the adjusted risk, respectively) and were at increased risk for major bleeding (a 10% increase in the adjusted risk for bleeding).[105]

For patients requiring interhospital transfer for PPCI, delays in the referral hospital are relatively frequent. To quantify the delays in the referral hospital a new performance measure, i.e., the DIDO time, has been introduced and a DIDO ≤30 minutes has been recommended. The performance of this metric was assessed in a retrospective cohort of 14,821 patients recruited in the ACTION—Get With the Guidelines registry. The study showed that the DIDO time was 68 minutes (interquartile range 43 to 120 minutes) and only 11% of the patients had a DIDO time ≤30 minutes. The study identified older age, female sex, off-hours presentation, and non-EMS transport to the first hospital as independently associated with a DIDO >30 minutes. Patients with a DIDO time of ≤30 minutes were significantly more likely to have a DTB time ≤90 minutes compared with patients with a DIDO >30 minutes (60% vs. 13%) and a significantly lower in-hospital mortality (2.7% vs. 5.9%; adjusted OR for in-hospital mortality =1.56 [1.15 to 2.12]). Thus, based on the results of this study, a DIDO time ≤30 minutes is rarely achieved and this parameter contributes to reperfusion delays and in-hospital mortality.[106] A recent study reported a DIDO median (25th to 75th percentile) time of 51 (35 to 82) minutes and that only 14.1% of the patients had a DIDO interval ≤30 minutes. The study also identified female sex, more comorbidities, longer symptom duration, arrival by means other than ambulance, arrival at a hospital not exclusively transferring patients for PPCI, arrival at a center with a low STEMI volume, and an ambiguous ECG as independent correlates of longer DIDO time. Moreover, when turnaround was timely, 70% of patients received timely PPCI (door-to-device time ≤90 minutes).[107]

Interfacility transfer for PPCI from referring facilities to PCI centers causes delay in treatment of patients with STEMI which may impact the efficacy of PPCI. In the CREDO-Kyoto acute MI registry that included 3820 patients with STEMI undergoing PPCI within 24 hours from symptom onset, the symptom onset-to-balloon time (median with 25th-75th percentiles) was 5.0 hours (3.5 to 9.1 hours) in patients undergoing PPCI after interfacility transfer (n = 1725 patients) and 3.6 hours [2.5 to 5.9 hours] in patients who underwent PPCI after direct transfer to a PPCI facility ($P < .001$). The cumulative 5-year incidence of death or hospitalization for heart failure was significantly higher in the interfacility transfer patients than in those with direct admission (26.9% vs. 21.2%; log-rank $P < .001$). After adjustment for potential confounders, there was a 22% increase in the adjusted risk for death or hospitalization for heart failure associated with interfacility transfer.[108] Along the same lines more than one-third of transferred U.S. STEMI patients fail to achieve first door-to-device time ≤120 minutes despite estimated transfer times <60 minutes. Delays were mostly related to process variables, comorbidities, and lower annual PCI hospital STEMI volumes.[82] A prospective nationwide Polish registry of 70,093 STEMI patients showed that 39,144 (56%) were admitted directly to a PCI center. As compared with patients directly admitted in PCI centers, transferred patients had longer symptom-to-admission time intervals (by 44 minutes; $P < .001$), longer total ischemic time (270 [180 to 420] minutes vs. 228 [156 to 378] minutes), and higher propensity-matched 12-month mortality (9.6% vs. 10.4%; $P < .001$).[109] Based on these data, transport of a patient with STEMI to a non-PCI hospital should be a "never event" except for rare instances when the patient is critically unstable and unlikely to survive longer transport.[110]

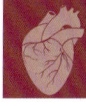

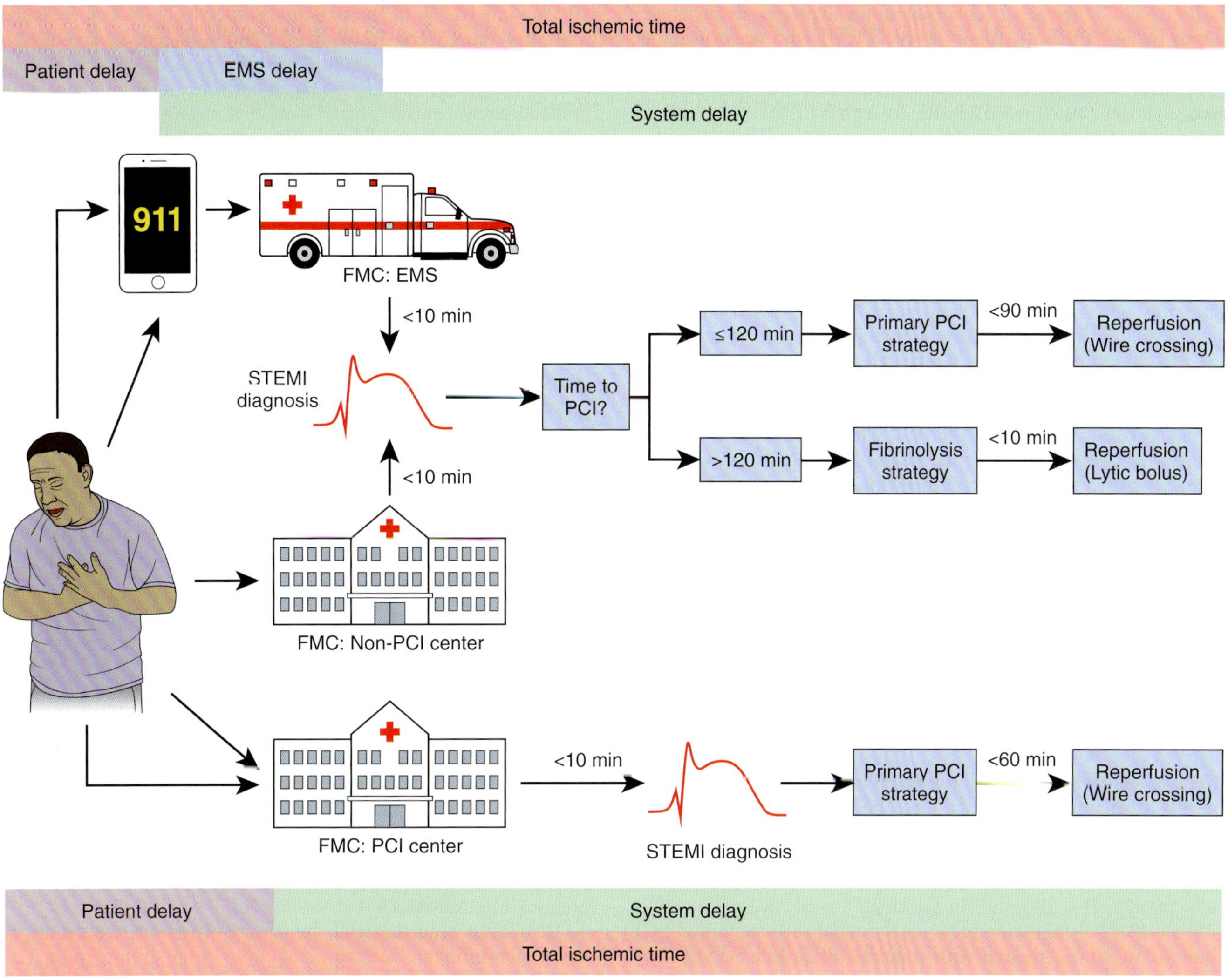

Fig. 20.9 Modes of patient presentation, components of ischemia time, and flowchart for reperfusion strategy selection in patients with ST-segment elevation myocardial infarction *(STEMI)*. *EMS,* Emergency medical system; *FMC,* first medical contact; *PCI,* percutaneous coronary intervention. (From Ibanez B, James S, Agewall S, et al. 2017 ESC guidelines for the management of acute myocardial infarction in patients presenting with ST-segment elevation: the task force for the management of acute myocardial infarction in patients presenting with ST-segment elevation of the European Society of Cardiology (ESC). *Eur Heart J.* 2018;39[2]:119–177.)

In summary, prompt referral of patients with acute MI to centers with PCI facilities should be the primary objective of first contact EMSs. This is currently feasible for the large majority of patients with STEMI in the United States and should be attempted in the future for all patients with STEMI seeking medical aid. Nearly 90% of the adult population in the United States lives within 60 minutes of a hospital with a PCI facility and even among those living closer to hospitals without a PCI facility, almost three-fourths would experience less than 30 minutes of additional delay related to direct referral to a hospital with a PCI facility.[85,111] The development of regional systems of STEMI care is a matter of utmost importance for improving the treatment of patients with STEMI. Current guidelines do not focus on relative PCI-related delay or specific DTB or DIDO times as quality-of-care metrics of reperfusion therapy. Instead they recommend the FMC-to-device metric and set a limit of ≤120 minutes. This corresponds to a PCI-related delay of 110 minutes (given that the recommended FMC-to-needle [fibrinolysis] is 10 minutes) which is in the range of the times identified in old studies and registries to choose PPCI as reperfusion strategy (Fig. 20.9).[9] A flexible consideration of what degree of PCI-related delay is acceptable for high-risk STEMI patients also seems justified.

FACILITATED PERCUTANEOUS CORONARY INTERVENTION

Facilitated PCI refers to a deliberate strategy of administration of pharmacological drugs aimed at restoring anterograde flow in the IRA prior to proceeding to definitive revascularization by PCI in patients with STEMI. It was conceived as an option for filling the time gap between patient presentation and performance of PCI. The pharmacological regimen consists of drugs known for their ability to restore flow such as full-dose or half-dose fibrinolysis, or a combination of half-dose fibrinolysis with GPI. As data about the ability of GPI to reopen the IRA is controversial, the isolated use of these drugs may or may not be part of the strategy of facilitated PCI. Two factors underpin the rationale behind the concept of facilitated PCI: first, ventricular function and prognosis have been found to be better in patients with STEMI who present at the time of PPCI with spontaneous TIMI flow grade 2 or 3 compared with those who have a TIMI flow grade of 0 and 1 in the IRA; second, a large proportion of patients with STEMI are unable to receive mechanical reperfusion without a certain time delay due to a variety of reasons. Facilitated PCI was hypothesized to offer a reduction in ischemia time, earlier reperfusion, higher TIMI flow rates in the IRA and facilitated guidewire/balloon passage, decreased clot burden, and lower incidence of distal embolization.

The Bavarian Reperfusion Alternatives Evaluation (BRAVE) trial was the first randomized trial to evaluate the impact of facilitated PCI with reteplase plus abciximab on left ventricular infarct size estimated by single photon emission computed tomography (SPECT). Although the study reported a higher rate of pre-PCI TIMI flow grade 3 in the IRA in the facilitated PCI group, no reduction in infarct size was observed in this group.[112] These results were confirmed by several subsequent clinical trials on this issue. The Assessment of the Safety and Efficacy of a New Treatment Strategy for Acute Myocardial Infarction (ASSENT)-4 PCI study was a randomized trial of patients with STEMI presenting within 6 hours from the symptom onset, scheduled to undergo PCI after an anticipated delay of 1 to 3 hours who were assigned to standard PCI (n = 838) or PCI preceded by administration of full-dose tenecteplase (n = 829).[113] All patients received aspirin and a bolus without an infusion of unfractionated heparin. The investigators of ASSENT-4 PCI planned to enroll 4000 patients, but the Data and Safety Monitoring Board recommended early cessation due to higher in-hospital mortality in the facilitated PCI group than in the group with standard PCI. The primary end point of ASSENT-4 PCI was death, congestive heart failure, or shock within 90 days from randomization. This occurred in 19% of patients in the facilitated PCI group and 13% in the group with standard PCI (RR = 1.39, [1.11 to 1.74]; P = .005). There were more in-hospital strokes (1.8% vs. 0%, P < .001) and a higher incidence of ischemic complications such as reinfarction (6% vs. 4%, P = .03) and repeat target-vessel revascularization (7% vs. 3%, P = .004) among patients treated with facilitated PCI than among those treated with standard PCI. The ASSENT-4 PCI trial concluded that a strategy of facilitated PCI consisting of full-dose fibrinolysis (tenecteplase) plus antithrombotic cotherapy and preceding PCI by 1 to 3 hours was associated with worse clinical outcome than a strategy of PPCI alone and cannot be recommended.[113] A meta-analysis by Keeley et al.[114] which included 17 trials of STEMI patients assigned to facilitated PCI (n = 2237) or PPCI (n = 2267) showed that facilitated PCI was associated with significantly worse short-term outcomes (up to 42 days) than PPCI alone: death (5% vs. 3%), nonfatal reinfarction (3% vs. 2%), urgent target-vessel revascularization (4% vs. 1%), major bleeding (7% vs. 5%), hemorrhagic stroke (0.7% vs. 0.1%), and total stroke (1.1% vs. 0.3%). The increased rates of adverse events were observed mainly when fibrinolytic therapy was used to facilitate PCI.[114] The Facilitated Intervention with Enhanced Reperfusion Speed to Stop Events (FINESSE) trial served to further confirm the inefficacy and even detrimental effects of facilitated PCI in patients with STEMI.[115] The study enrolled 2452 patients with STEMI presenting within the first 6 hours from the symptom onset who were randomly assigned to a strategy of facilitated PCI with half-dose reteplase plus abciximab versus abciximab alone versus conventional PCI with abciximab given in the catheterization laboratory. All patients received unfractionated heparin or enoxaparin before PCI and a 12-hour infusion of abciximab after PCI. The primary end point was the composite of death from all causes, ventricular fibrillation occurring more than 48 hours after randomization, cardiogenic shock, and congestive heart failure during the first 90 days after randomization. In the combination therapy-facilitated group, abciximab-facilitated group, and PPCI group, the primary end point occurred in 9.8%, 10.5%, and 10.7% of the patients, respectively (P = .55); 90-day mortality rates were 5.2%, 5.5%, and 4.5%, respectively (P = .49); early ST-segment resolution occurred in 43.9%, 33.1%, and 31.0% (P = .01 and P = .03, respectively). Overall, there was a graded increase in the rates of bleeding, intracranial hemorrhage, and transfusions in the PCI-facilitated groups.[115]

The evidence offered by the ASSENT-4 PCI trial,[113] the meta-analysis by Keeley et al.[114] and the FINESSE trial[115] discourages the use of fibrinolysis either at full- or half-dose combined with GPI as pharmacological facilitation of PCI. The reasons for the failure of facilitated PCI are not entirely clear. However, pre-PCI fibrinolysis may be associated with increased risks of bleeding and enhanced platelet activation.

ROUTINE USE OF PERCUTANEOUS CORONARY INTERVENTION AFTER FIBRINOLYSIS – PHARMACOINVASIVE STRATEGY

While the strategy of facilitated PCI was associated with worse outcomes, the pharmacoinvasive strategy—routine use of a fibrinolytic agent or GPI prior to subsequent, planned PCI—was associated with clinical benefit in patients with STEMI. As a rule, in the setting of this strategy, angiogram and planned PCI are performed after 2 to 24 hours of presentation (Fig. 20.10). This strategy is mostly applied in patients undergoing transfer from one hospital without PCI to a hospital with a PCI facility. The main reason for PCI following fibrinolysis is the suboptimal outcome of fibrinolysis, in terms of suboptimal and instability of blood flow restoration and clinical outcome.

The Grupo de Análisis de la Cardiopatía Isquémica Aguda (GRACIA) 2 and the Which Early ST-elevation myocardial infarction Therapy (WEST) randomized trials reported comparable efficacy and safety of pharmacoinvasive and PPCI strategies.[116,117] Both studies, however, included limited numbers of patients and consequently were underpowered for clinical end points. The GRACIA-1 trial randomized 500 patients with STEMI after receiving full-dose fibrinolysis with recombinant tissue plasminogen activator to either angiography plus PCI (within 24 hours of fibrinolysis) if indicated or ischemia-guided conservative approach. The primary end point was a composite of death, reinfarction, or revascularization at 12 months. The invasive therapy was associated with a significant reduction in the incidence of the primary end point (23% vs. 51%; risk ratio = 0.44 [0.28–0.70]; P < .001).[118] The Southwest German Interventional Study in Acute Myocardial Infarction (SIAM) III trial randomized 163 patients to immediate (transferred within 6 hours after fibrinolysis for angiography and stenting of the IRA) or to delayed stenting (elective angiography and stenting of the IRA 2 weeks after fibrinolysis). Immediate stenting was associated with a significant reduction in the 6-month composite end point of ischemic events, death, reinfarction, or target-lesion revascularization (25.6% vs. 50.6%, P = .001).[119] The Combined Abciximab REteplase Stent Study in Acute Myocardial Infarction (CARESS-in-AMI) trial included 600 patients ≤75 years of age with at least 1 high-risk feature (extensive ST-segment elevation, left bundle branch block of new onset, previous MI, Killip class >2, or left ventricular ejection fraction ≤35%) who presented within 12 hours from symptom onset and were treated initially in non-PCI hospitals with half-dose reteplase, abciximab, heparin, and aspirin.[120] Patients were randomized to immediate transfer for PCI (299 patients) or standard care with transfer for rescue PCI (301 patients). The primary outcome was a composite of 30-day death, reinfarction, or refractory ischemia. In the group assigned to immediate PCI, 97% (289 patients) of patients underwent angiography and 85.6% (255 patients) underwent PCI. In the group assigned to standard care, 30.3% (91 patients) underwent rescue PCI. The primary end point occurred in 4.4% of

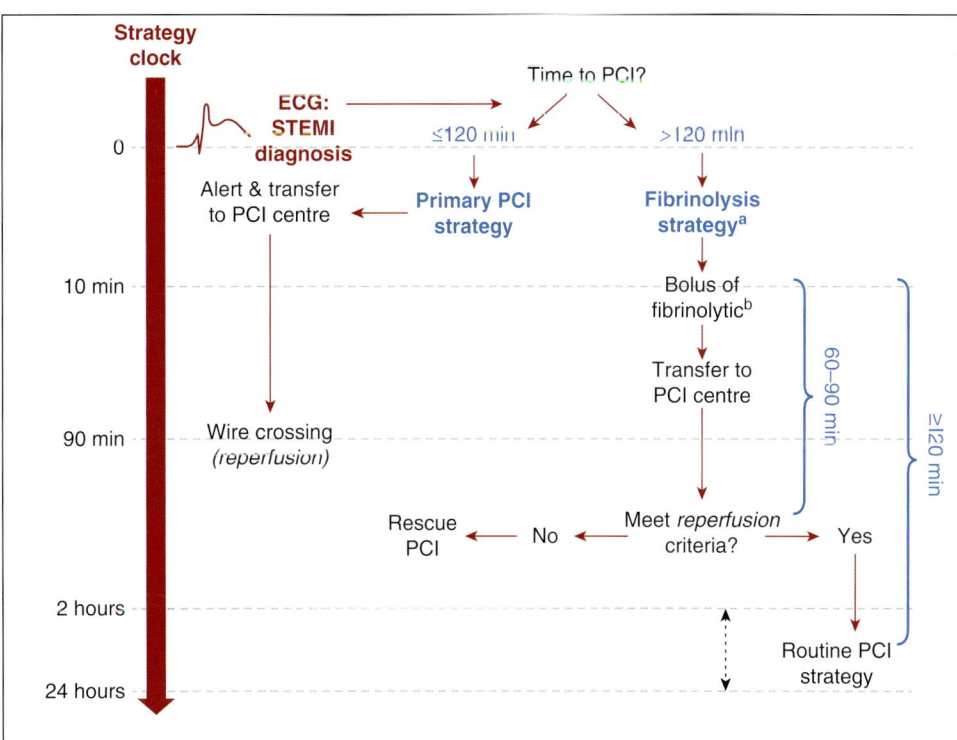

Fig. 20.10 Maximum target times according to reperfusion strategy selection in patients presenting via emergency medical service or in a non-percutaneous coronary intervention (PCI) center. *ECG,* Electrocardiogram; *STEMI,* ST-segment elevation myocardial infarction. [a]If fibrinolysis is contraindicated, direct for primary PCI strategy regardless of time to PCI. [b]10 min is the maximum target delay time from STEMI diagnosis to fibrinolytic bolus administration; however, it should be given as soon as possible after STEMI diagnosis (after ruling out contraindications); *IV,* intravenous. (From Ibanez B, James S, Agewall S, et al. 2017 ESC Guidelines for the management of acute myocardial infarction in patients presenting with ST-segment elevation: the task force for the management of acute myocardial infarction in patients presenting with ST-segment elevation of the European Society of Cardiology (ESC). *Eur Heart J.* 2018;39[2]:119–177.)

patients assigned to immediate PCI and 10.7% of the patients assigned to standard care with rescue PCI as required ($P = .004$) with no differences in major bleeding (3.4% vs. 2.3%, $P = .47$) or stroke (0.7% vs. 1.3%, $P = .50$). In the immediate PCI group the time interval from reteplase to angiography/PCI was 2.25 hours.[120] The Trial of Routine Angioplasty and Stenting after Fibrinolysis to Enhance Reperfusion in Acute Myocardial Infarction (TRANSFER-AMI) included 1059 high-risk patients with STEMI who presented to non-PCI hospitals within 12 hours from symptom onset.[121] Patients were randomized to standard treatment, including rescue PCI (522 patients) or a strategy of immediate transfer for PCI within 6 hours after fibrinolysis (537 patients). All patients received aspirin, tenecteplase, and heparin or enoxaparin; concomitant clopidogrel was strongly encouraged. The primary end point was the composite of death, reinfarction, recurrent ischemia, new or worsening congestive heart failure, or cardiogenic shock within 30 days. In the group assigned to transfer for PCI, 98.5% underwent coronary angiography and 84.9% received PCI (2.8 hours after randomization); in the group assigned to standard care, 88.7% underwent coronary angiography and 67.4% received PCI (32.5 hours after randomization). At 30 days, the primary end point occurred in 11.0% of the patients assigned to the immediate PCI and in 17.2% of the patients assigned to standard treatment ($P = .004$). Most of the benefit was due to a reduction in reinfarction or recurrent ischemia. The bleeding rates were similar in both groups.[121] A series of meta-analyses supported the pharmacoinvasive strategy for patients with STEMI. A meta-analysis that included seven trials with 2961 patients comparing early routine PCI after fibrinolysis with standard therapy in patients with STEMI found that early routine use of PCI after fibrinolysis reduced the 30-day rate of reinfarction (2.6% vs. 4.7%, $P = .003$), the combined end point of death or reinfarction (5.6% vs. 8.3%, $P = .004$), and recurrent ischemia (1.9% vs. 7.1%, $P < .001$) without affecting the rates of major bleeding (4.9% vs. 5.0%, $P = .70$) or stroke (0.7% vs. 1.3%, $P = .21$).[122] The benefits of routine use of PCI after fibrinolysis were maintained at 6 to 12 months of follow-up. Another meta-analysis of nine trials with a total of 3325 patients showed a 24% reduction in total mortality ($P = .06$), a 45% reduction in recurrent MI ($P < .001$), and a 65% reduction in recurrent ischemia ($P < .001$) with no significant difference in the incidence of major bleeding or stroke in patients managed with early or immediate PCI after fibrinolysis as opposed to standard care.[123] A more recent meta-analysis including 3195 patients (eight trials) showed that the composite end point of 30-day mortality reinfarction and ischemia was lower in the routine early PCI group compared with the ischemia-guided PCI group after fibrinolysis (7.3% vs. 13.5%; OR = 0.47 [0.32 to 0.68]; $P < .001$) driven by significant reduction in both reinfarction (OR = 0.62 [0.42–0.90]; $P < .011$) and ischemia (OR = 0.21 [0.10–0.47]; $P < .001$). The 30-day mortality or major bleeding rates were not significantly different between the strategies. This meta-analysis supported the use of routine early PCI within 24 hours of fibrinolysis when PPCI was not feasible.[124]

The Strategic Reperfusion Early after Myocardial Infarction (STREAM) study evaluated whether a fibrinolytic therapy approach (prehospital or early fibrinolysis with contemporary antiplatelet and anticoagulant therapy) coupled with timely angiography (urgent in case of reperfusion failure or routine at 6 to 24 hours) provides a clinical outcome similar to that with PPCI in patients with STEMI who present early after symptom onset.[125] In the STREAM trial, 1892 patients with STEMI (≥2 mm ST elevation in two contiguous leads) who presented within 3 hours of symptom onset and who could not undergo PPCI within 1 hour of FMC were assigned to a strategy of early fibrinolysis followed by coronary angiography in 6 to 24 hours or rescue PCI, if needed ($n = 944$), or standard PPCI ($n = 948$). The primary end point was a composite of death from any cause, shock, congestive heart failure, or reinfarction at 30 days. The early fibrinolysis group received tenecteplase, aspirin, clopidogrel, and enoxaparin in the ambulance or emergency room. Patients in the early fibrinolysis group were more likely to have TIMI-3 blood flow compared with the PPCI group (58.5% vs. 20.7%). The median time from symptom onset to the start of reperfusion therapy (tenecteplase or arterial sheath insertion) was 100 minutes in the early fibrinolysis group versus 178 minutes in the PPCI group. In the fibrinolysis group, emergency angiography was required in 36.3% of the patients; the remaining patients underwent angiography at a median of 17 hours after randomization. There were no significant differences in the primary end point between both treatment strategies (12.4% in the early fibrinolysis vs. 14.3% in the PPCI group; RR = 0.86 [0.68 to 1.09]; P = .21). The rates of intracranial hemorrhage were 1.0% in the fibrinolysis group and 0.2% in the PPCI group (P = .04); after protocol amendment (the tenecteplase dose was halved in patients ≥75 years of age at the 20% planned recruitment), the difference was no longer significant (0.5% vs. 0.3%, P = .45). The main conclusion of the STREAM trial was that prehospital fibrinolysis followed by routine angiography within 6 to 24 hours in stable patients (or immediate or rescue PCI in case of failed reperfusion or unstable patients) is a reasonable alternative to PPCI when expected treatment delay was more than 1 hour.[125] A recent report from the STREAM trial showed that the frequency of aborted MI (defined as ST-segment resolution ≥50%) was significantly higher among patients undergoing a pharmacoinvasive therapy than PPCI (11.1% vs. 6.9%, P < .01).[126] Some limitations of the STREAM trial are worth mentioning: exclusion of patients who could receive PCI within 60 minutes (potentially biases the study in favor of fibrinolysis) and the amendment of the trial protocol; also, more than one-third of patients were recruited in an expensive system of care designed to promote prehospital fibrinolysis, which may not be directly applicable to other systems of care. Moreover, the high rate of no (or poor) responders to fibrinolysis (36.3% rate of urgent angiography in the fibrinolysis group) may support a strategy of expedited transfer to a PCI-capable facility of every patient undergoing fibrinolysis after STEMI. Finally, 1-year rates of all-cause (6.7% vs. 5.9%, P = .49) or cardiac (4.0% vs. 4.1%, P = .93) mortality were similar in patients randomized to pharmacoinvasive or PPCI treatment strategies.[127]

Recent studies offer additional support for a pharmacoinvasive strategy, particularly in patients with STEMI with a prolonged PCI-related delay. In a prespecified analysis from the STREAM trial that included data from hospitals that randomized >10 patients, the 30-day clinical outcomes (a composite of death, congestive heart failure, cardiogenic shock, or MI) was analyzed according to PCI-related delays of ≤55, >55 to 97, and >97 minutes. The composite end point occurred in 10.6% versus 10.3% (≤55 minutes, P = .910); 13.9% versus 17.9% (>55 to 97 minutes, P = .148), and 13.5% versus 16.2% (>97 minutes, P = .470) of the patients assigned to a pharmacoinvasive or PPCI strategy. While there was no worsening of outcomes for the pharmacoinvasive strategy arm across the PCI-related delay spectrum, this occurred in the PPCI arm (P for trend = 0.038). When PCI-related delay was analyzed for every 10-minute increment, there was an increasing trend toward benefit among pharmacoinvasive strategy assigned patients (P for trend = .073).[128] The recently published Early Routine Catheterization After Alteplase Fibrinolysis Versus Primary PCI in Acute ST-Segment–Elevation Myocardial Infarction (EARLY-MYO) trial showed that for patients with STEMI presenting ≤6 hours after symptom onset and with an expected PCI-related delay, a pharmacoinvasive strategy with half-dose alteplase and timely PCI was associated with better epicardial and tissue reperfusion compared to PPCI. However, the 30-day clinical outcome including rates of all-cause mortality, reinfarction, heart failure, major bleeding, or intracranial bleeding differed little between both strategies; minor bleeding was more frequent among patients undergoing a pharmacoinvasive strategy.[129]

Some studies strongly suggest that transradial approach is particularly advantageous in patients undergoing a pharmacoinvasive strategy. In the British Cardiovascular Intervention Society Dataset that included 10,209 patients who received fibrinolysis and PCI between 2007 and 2014, transradial artery approach was used in 48% of the patients (n = 4959). Transradial artery approach was associated with a significant reduction of in-hospital mortality (41%), major bleeding (55%), MACEs (28%), and 30-day mortality (28%). The study strongly suggested the use of transradial artery approach for PCI in the setting of pharmacoinvasive strategy.[130] A recent report from the STREAM trial found that transradial approach was associated with improved clinical outcomes regardless of the use in the setting of PPCI or pharmacoinvasive therapy (P for interaction = .730).[131]

In aggregate, these studies demonstrated that the approach of routine catheterization and PCI after an initial primary fibrinolysis strategy is beneficial in patients with STEMI. Current guidelines recommend a pharmacoinvasive strategy in all patients in whom the FMC-to-device time is expected to exceed the 120-minute limit (see Fig. 20.10).[8,9] However, as recently reported, in the United States neither fibrinolysis nor PPCI is being optimally used to achieve guideline-recommended reperfusion targets.[132]

RESCUE PERCUTANEOUS CORONARY INTERVENTION

Despite confirmed superiority of PPCI over fibrinolysis, the latter remains an important therapeutic modality mostly due to limited availability of PPCI. Rescue PCI is defined as PCI performed within 12 hours after failure of fibrinolysis in patients with continuing or recurrent myocardial ischemia. In the absence of coronary angiography, partial (<50%) resolution of ST-segment resolution on the surface electrocardiogram, continuation of chest discomfort, and/or hemodynamic instability or heart failure, even though they are known to be imprecise, are used as markers of failed fibrinolysis. It has been reported that between 12% and 17% of patients with STEMI in the U.S. are treated with fibrinolytic therapy.[133,134] Even with the use of the most advanced fibrin-specific fibrinolytic agents, fibrinolysis restores optimal epicardial blood flow TIMI 3 in just over half of STEMI patients. Earlier reports have shown that 20% to 30% of patients with STEMI develop early recurrent acute ischemia, thrombotic coronary artery reocclusion, or reinfarction 2 to 4 days after an apparently successful fibrinolysis.[135–137] The less-than-optimal results with fibrinolysis are explained by time-dependent resistance to fibrinolysis, the plaque/thrombosis ratio at the site of coronary occlusion being 80% (plaque) to 20% (thrombotic material) on average,[138] and that not infrequently plaque expansion contributing more than acute thrombosis to the acute coronary occlusion.[139] In the presence of these and other factors, the establishment of TIMI flow grade 3 by fibrinolysis is less likely. Patients with an occluded IRA (TIMI flow grade 0 to 1) and those with suboptimal blood flow restoration (TIMI flow 2) have increased mortality compared to patients with restoration of TIMI flow grade 3 in the IRA.[140] In the past patients with failed fibrinolysis have been treated with conservative therapy and watchful waiting, repeat fibrinolysis, or rescue PCI.

The efficacy of rescue PCI for failed fibrinolysis has been assessed in a number of randomized trials (six trials in a 2007 meta-analysis).[141] Earlier trials included limited numbers of patients (from 28 to 151 patients) and underestimated the benefits of rescue PCI since it consisted of percutaneous transluminal coronary angioplasty (PTCA) without stenting. The superiority of coronary stenting over angioplasty in rescue PCI interventions has been shown in the Stent Or PTCA for Occluded Coronary Arteries after Failed Fibrinolysis in Patients with Acute Myocardial Infarction (STOPAMI)-4 trial, which showed a significantly higher salvage index (35% vs. 25% of the initial perfusion defect salvaged by rescue interventions) obtained by paired scintigraphic studies performed 7 to 10 days apart.[142] The most important randomized trials in the setting of rescue interventions for failed fibrinolysis have been the Middlesbrough Early Revascularization to Limit Infarction (MERLIN) trial[143] and the Rescue Angioplasty or Repeat Fibrinolysis (REACT) trial.[144] The MERLIN trial randomized 307 patients with STEMI and failed fibrinolysis (failure of ST-segment elevation in the lead with maximal elevation to resolve by 50%) to emergency coronary angiography with or without rescue PCI or conservative therapy. The primary end point was all-cause mortality at 30 days. It should be emphasized that coronary stents were used in just half of the patients. Thirty-day all-cause mortality was similar in the rescue and conservative groups (9.8% vs. 11%, $P = .7$). The combined incidence of MACE was reduced in the rescue PCI group (37.3% vs. 50.0%, $P = .02$) driven by less subsequent revascularization (6.5% vs. 20.1%, $P = .01$). Reinfarction (7.2% vs. 10.4%, $P = .03$) and congestive heart failure (24.2% vs. 29.2%, $P = .30$) were less common among patients undergoing rescue PCI. There was an increased incidence of stroke (4.6% vs. 0.6%, $P = .03$) and blood transfusion (11.1% vs. 1.3%, $P = .001$) among patients treated by rescue PCI versus those treated by conservative therapy.[143] The 3-year follow-up of patients of the MERLIN trial showed that rescue angioplasty compared with conservative treatment did not confer a survival benefit at 3 years (17.6% vs. 16.9%, $P = .90$) but was associated with fewer unplanned revascularization procedures (14.4% vs. 33.8%, $P < .01$).

The REACT trial included 427 patients with STEMI within 6 hours of symptom onset and 90-minute electrocardiographic criteria for failed fibrinolysis (less than 50% ST-segment resolution in the leads with previous maximal ST-segment elevation). Patients were randomly assigned to one of three options: rescue PCI ($n = 144$), repeat fibrinolysis ($n = 142$), or conservative therapy ($n = 141$). Coronary stents were used in 68.5% of patients and 43.4% of patients received a GPI. The 6-month probability of event-free survival was significantly higher in patients assigned to rescue PCI (84.6%) compared with patients assigned to conservative therapy (70.1%) or repeat fibrinolysis (68.7%, $P = .004$). A subsequent report from the REACT trial[145] showed that the 6-month advantage in the event-free-survival was maintained at 1 year of follow-up (81.5%, 67.5%, and 64.1% in rescue PCI, conservative therapy, and repeat fibrinolysis arms, respectively; $P = .004$) and that there was a significant reduction in mortality at a median of 4.4 years: mortality rates were 11.2% in the rescue PCI arm, 21.4% in the conservative therapy arm, 21.3% in the repeat fibrinolysis arm (HR = 0.43 [0.23 to 0.97] for rescue PCI vs. conservative therapy and HR = 0.41 [0.22 to 0.75] for rescue PCI vs. repeat fibrinolysis). Of importance was the finding that repeat fibrinolysis did not offer any benefit compared with conservative therapy.[145]

A 2007 meta-analysis of randomized trials showed that rescue PCI was associated with insignificant 31% reduction in the relative risk for all-cause mortality and significant reductions in the risk for heart failure (27%) and reinfarction (42%) compared with conservative treatment. Moreover, repeat fibrinolysis was not associated with improvements of mortality or reinfarction, but it increased the risk of minor bleeding by 84%.[141]

Patients with STEMI and failed fibrinolysis represent a high-risk group particularly for PCI-related bleeding complications. Recent studies have suggested that transradial approach is associated with better outcome and less bleeding complications compared with femoral artery approach in patients undergoing rescue PCI. An analysis from the STREAM trial in which the pharmacoinvasive arm included 379 patients (42.3%) undergoing rescue PCI showed that within the pharmacoinvasive therapy group, there was a trend for an advantage of transradial artery approach in terms of reduction of primary outcome (a composite of 30-day death, shock, congestive heart failure, or reinfarction) in the subgroup undergoing rescue PCI (13.4% vs. 26.3%; OR = 0.65 [0.39 to 1.07]). Moreover, within the group undergoing rescue PCI, radial approach was associated with less nonintracranial major bleeding compared with femoral artery approach (6.1% vs. 11.6%; $P = .064$).[131] Among 9494 patients with STEMI undergoing rescue PCI between 2009 and 2013 in the National Cardiovascular Data Registry's CathPCI Registry, transradial artery access was used in 14.2% of patients. In propensity-matched analyses, transradial artery approach rescue PCI was associated with significantly less bleeding (OR = 0.67 [0.52 to 0.87]; $P = .003$) and gastrointestinal bleeding (OR = 0.23 [0.05 to 0.98]; $P = .05$) but not mortality (OR = 0.81 [0.53 to 1.25]; $P = .35$) than transfemoral artery approach.[146]

In summary, rescue PCI improves clinical outcome and should be recommended in patients with STEMI after failed fibrinolysis. Current guidelines recommend rescue PCI (class I recommendation, level of evidence: A) immediately after failed fibrinolysis (<50% ST-segment resolution at 60 to 90 minutes) or at any time in the presence of hemodynamic or electrical instability, or worsening ischemia.[9]

TECHNICAL ASPECTS AND MECHANICAL STRATEGIES TO ENHANCE MYOCARDIAL SALVAGE DURING PRIMARY PERCUTANEOUS CORONARY INTERVENTION IN ST-ELEVATION MYOCARDIAL INFARCTION

From a technical point of view, PPCI is not substantially different to elective PCI. However, PPCI in the early phase of a STEMI can be more difficult and requires more expertise than routine PCI in a stable patient. PPCI is performed in conditions of increased risk due to hemodynamic and electrical instability, increased thrombogenicity associated with STEMI, and increased bleeding risk due to adjuvant treatments, particularly if PCI is performed following failed fibrinolysis and often complete occlusion of the stenotic coronary artery. The latter finding impedes visualization of the coronary artery, makes guidewire and/or balloon passage through the occluded lesion more difficult, and predisposes to distal embolization of thrombotic material with a potential for further worsening of microcirculation function. The presence of coronary artery thrombus increases the risk of distal embolization or side branch occlusion and suboptimal flow and tissue reperfusion after PPCI compared with elective PCI. Stent placement in acute thrombotic lesions has been reported to predispose for late stent malapposition after the bare-metal stent (BMS) or drug-eluting stent (DES) implantation,[147,148] potentially due to thrombus sequestration behind the struts, which subsequently resolves and leads to eventual vasoconstriction in the acute phase, predisposing to stent underdeployment, malapposition, and increased risk of stent thrombosis. Operators performing PPCI in STEMI must act rapidly to restore coronary blood flow in the IRA as early as possible in order to stop evolving ischemia and progression to necrosis, and to increase chances of myocardial salvage and infarct size reduction. Vascular access is achieved via the radial or femoral artery, though radial artery access is increasingly being preferred. Adjunct antithrombotic therapy is used periprocedurally (see section on Periprocedural Antithrombotic/Anticoagulant Therapy in Patients With STEMI Undergoing PPCI). After the procedure, the patient is monitored continuously and in the absence of complications, is discharged from the hospital within a few days. Over the last two decades many mechanical (Fig. 20.11) and pharmacological strategies have been developed to improve procedural success or boost myocardial salvage during PPCI procedures.

PRIMARY STENTING

In the early days of mechanical reperfusion for STEMI, balloon angioplasty was the mainstay of therapy. However, although superior to fibrinolysis, balloon angioplasty often produces suboptimal results mostly related to recurrent ischemia and reocclusion occurring within the first days and weeks after the procedure, as well as a high incidence of late vessel narrowing (restenosis).

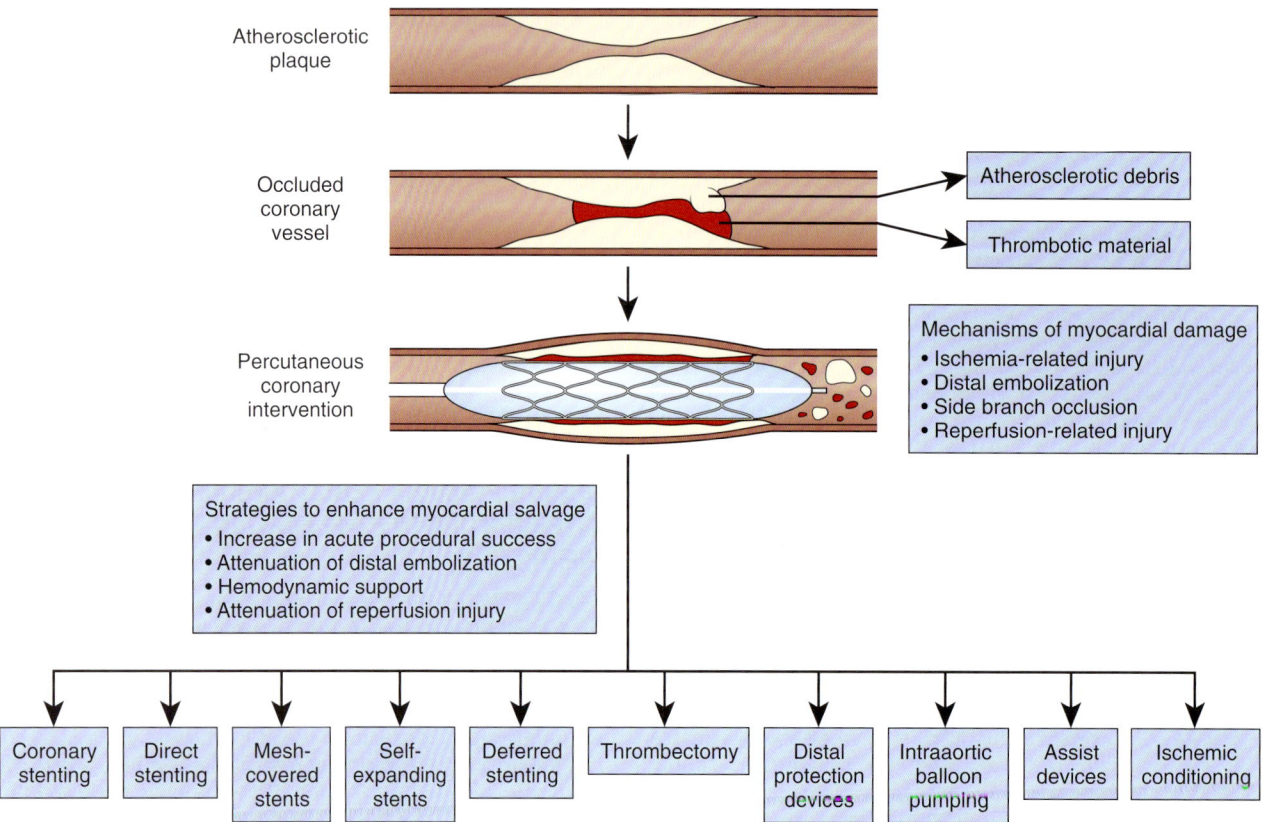

Fig. 20.11 Mechanical strategies to enhance myocardial salvage during primary percutaneous coronary intervention in patients with ST-segment elevation myocardial infarction. (From Ndrepepa G, Kastrati A. Mechanical strategies to enhance myocardial salvage during primary percutaneous coronary intervention in patients with STEMI. *EuroIntervention.* 2016;12[3]:319–328.)

Despite these limitations of balloon angioplasty, in the early days of mechanical reperfusion for STEMI, coronary stenting in the setting of STEMI was avoided due to the fear that implantation of a metallic structure within the highly thrombogenic milieu of the IRA (including thrombotic material and balloon-induced plaque disruption) would predispose to acute stent thrombosis and coronary reocclusion. Furthermore, in the early days of PCI the profound anticoagulation needed to protect from stent thrombosis markedly increased the risk of bleeding, posing additional risk for patients. Refinement in stent technology and advances in periprocedural and long-term antithrombotic therapy transformed primary stenting from an infrequently used therapeutic option, usually in bail-out situations, to the dominant form of PPCI in patients with STEMI.

Earlier studies showed superiority of balloon angioplasty over fibrinolysis and later the superiority of stenting over balloon angioplasty alone. The Stent versus Fibrinolysis for Occluded Coronary Arteries in Patients with Acute Myocardial Infarction (STOPAMI) trial showed that coronary stenting plus abciximab is safe and leads to a greater degree of myocardial salvage and a better clinical outcome than fibrinolysis with a tissue plasminogen activator. Final infarct size (estimated by repeat scintigraphic studies) was 14.3% in the group with stenting and 19.4% of the left ventricle in the group with fibrinolysis ($P = .02$); the salvage index (proportion of initial area at risk salvaged by reperfusion) was 57% in the stent group versus 26% in the fibrinolysis group ($P < .001$), and the cumulative 6-month incidence of death, MI, or stroke was lower among patients treated with stenting (8.5% vs. 23.2%, $P = .02$).[15] The STOPAMI trial offered mechanistic information that explains the superiority of stenting over fibrinolysis in patients with STEMI. A meta-analysis summarized the results of 13 trials, which randomized 6922 patients with acute MI to coronary stenting (3460 patients) or balloon angioplasty alone (3462 patients).[149] Five trials included patients with cardiogenic shock. In this meta-analysis, primary stenting reduced significantly the need for repeat revascularization at 1 year (11.3% vs. 18.3%) but had no effect on mortality (5.1% vs. 5.2%) or reinfarction (3.7% vs. 3.9%). The meta-regression analysis demonstrated a significant association between patients' risk profile and mortality benefits from primary stenting at 1 year.[149] These conclusions, however, are subject to limitations related to significant variations in the cross-over rates and possible confounding effects of thienopyridine treatment in patients treated with primary stenting. Against this, an analysis of the Primary Angioplasty in Myocardial infarction (PAMI) trial showed not only better angiographic results with primary stenting but also a sustained benefit in mortality out to 5 years after index event.[150] Mechanistically, coronary stents achieve better angiographic results (less residual stenosis), fewer early ischemic events because of the sealing of plaque rupture and dissection, and longer-term patency due to lessening of the elastic recoil and constrictive remodeling compared with balloon angioplasty alone. These studies and other evidence transformed coronary stenting from a feared therapeutic option to a default PPCI strategy in patients with STEMI.

Drug-Eluting Stents

The development of DES represented an important milestone in the evolution of PCI. Compared with BMS, DES has reduced the need for target-vessel revascularization by 60% to 70% in the setting of randomized clinical trials. In general, although the results of current research have been reassuring, there are still concerns about a possible excess of stent thrombosis (especially late events beyond 1 year) after DES implantation due to inhibition or delayed reendothelization of the stented segment.[151] Specifically, it has been postulated that the risk of stent thrombosis might be higher if DES are implanted in patients with STEMI. Putative mechanisms offered to explain higher rates of stent thrombosis after DES implantation in patients with STEMI include an increased risk of stent malapposition (thrombus jailing and subsequent dissolution as well as coronary spasm at culprit lesions during the acute event may increase the risk of stent undersizing), a modulation of drug release kinetics by superimposed thrombotic material, and uptake of lipophilic drugs by necrotic core material, which, due to very slow turnover, may lead to further prolongation of tissue exposure and exacerbate delayed healing.[151] Despite these still unresolved issues, recent evidence about the use of DES in STEMI has been mostly reassuring and DES implantation is increasingly being used in the setting of PPCI.

Recent information on the use of DES in patients with STEMI has emerged from registries, randomized trials, and meta-analyses. A series of randomized trials have investigated the efficacy and safety of first-generation DES versus BMS in patients with STEMI.[152–157] Their results have been summarized in multiple meta-analyses. Important comparative evidence comes from a recent patient-level meta-analysis (individual data obtained in 11 trials) with 6298 patients (3980 randomized to DES [99% sirolimus-eluting or paclitaxel-eluting stents] and 2318 randomized to BMS). At a mean follow-up of 3.3 years, DES implantation significantly reduced the occurrence of target-vessel revascularization (12.7% vs. 20.1%; HR = 0.57 [0.50 to 0.66]; $P < .001$) without any significant difference in all-cause mortality (8.5% vs. 10.2%, $P = .11$), cardiac mortality (5.7% vs. 6.8%, $P = .19$), reinfarction (9.4% vs. 5.9%, $P = .36$), or stent thrombosis (5.8% vs. 4.3%, $P = .38$). However, with regard to the occurrence of stent thrombosis or reinfarction, the assumption of proportionality was not met and the Cox model with time-varying regression coefficients showed an increase in the risk for these events over long-term follow-up. Thus, after 2 years from the beginning of the study, the rate of stent thrombosis (HR = 2.81 [1.28 to 6.19]; $P = .04$) and reinfarction (HR = 2.06 [1.22 to 3.49]; $P = .03$) increased significantly among patients with DES compared with those who had received a BMS.[158] Another meta-analysis that included 15 trials with 7867 patients comparing first-generation DES with BMS in patients with STEMI further evidenced an increased risk for very late stent thrombosis associated with DES. While the overall risk for definite stent thrombosis was similar for DES and BMS (risk ratio = 1.08 [95% CI 0.82 to 1.43]) there were time-dependent effects with risk ratio increasing from 0.80 (95% CI 0.58 to 1.12) in the first year to 2.10 (95% CI 1.20 to 3.69) in the subsequent years with an interaction between the time and risk ratio for stent thrombosis ($P = .009$). Of note, the study concluded that an early benefit in terms of reduction of target-vessel revascularization and a trend toward less definitive stent thrombosis with the use of first-generation DES in PPCI for STEMI was offset in subsequent years by an increased risk of very late stent thrombosis.[159] It has to be mentioned, however, that first-generation DES are now no longer used in current practice.

Second-generation DES incorporate a series of technical refinements compared to BMS or first-generation DES and are increasingly being used in patients with STEMI. Briefly, they consist of cobalt-chromium or platinum-chromium platforms, have thinner struts and improved biocompatibility making them more tissue friendly, and have a reduced thickness of durable or biodegradable polymer matrices. They release antiproliferative drugs such as sirolimus, everolimus, zotarolimus, biolimus, novolimus, or myolimus over weeks to months after implantation.[160] Several randomized trials and meta-analyses have investigated their efficacy and safety in patients with STEMI. The Comparison of Biolimus Eluted From an Erodible Stent Coating With Bare Metal Stents in Acute ST-Elevation Myocardial Infarction (COMFORTABLE AMI) trial randomized 1161 patients with STEMI with symptom onset within 24 hours to receive a biolimus-eluting stent ($n = 575$) or a BMS ($n = 582$). The biolimus was embedded in a biodegradable polymer. At 1 year, the primary end point—a composite of cardiac death, target-vessel–related reinfarction, or ischemia-driven target-lesion revascularization—occurred in 4.3% of the patients assigned to a biolimus stent and 8.7% of the patients assigned to a BMS (HR = 0.49 [0.30 to 0.80]; $P = .004$). The difference was driven by a lower risk of target-vessel–related reinfarction (0.5% vs. 2.7%) and ischemia-driven target-lesion revascularization (1.6% vs. 5.7%) in patients receiving a biolimus-eluting stent. There was a lower risk of definite stent thrombosis (0.9% vs. 2.1%) in patients treated with a biolimus-eluting stent, but the difference was statistically insignificant ($P = .10$).[161] A more recent publication from the COMFORTABLE AMI trial showed that the favorable results with biolimus-eluting stent were durable up to 2 years of follow-up.[162] The clinical Evaluation of the Xience-V stent in Acute Myocardial INfArcTION (EXAMINATION) trial randomized 1504 patients with STEMI up to 48 hours after symptom onset to receive an everolimus-eluting stent (with a durable fluoropolymer) or a BMS. The primary end point was a composite of all-cause death, recurrent MI, or revascularization at 1 year. The primary end point was similar in both groups (11.9% in everolimus stent group vs. 14.2% in the BMS group [$P = .19$]). The use of everolimus-eluting stents was associated with a lower risk of target-lesion revascularization (2.1% vs. 5.0%, $P = .003$) and definite stent thrombosis (0.5% vs. 1.9%, $P = .018$) and no difference in all-cause (3.5% vs. 3.5%) or cardiac (3.2% vs. 2.8%, $P = .76$) mortality.[163] The 5-year results of the EXAMINATION trial were recently published. The combined patient-oriented outcome of all-cause death, any MI, or any revascularization occurred in 159 (21%) patients in the Xience-V (everolimus-eluting stent) group versus 192 (26%) in the BMS group (HR = 0.80 [0.65 to 0.98]; $P = .033$; Fig. 20.12). The difference was mainly driven by a reduced rate of all-cause mortality (9% vs. 12%; HR = 0.72 [0.52–1.00]; $P = .047$). The device-oriented combined end point occurred in 12% of patients in the everolimus-eluting stent group and 15% of patients in the BMS group (HR = 0.75 [0.57–0.99]; $P = .043$; Fig. 20.13).[164] The Norwegian Coronary Stent (NORSTENT) trial did not show a significant difference in the incidence of all-cause death or nonfatal spontaneous MI (16.6% vs. 17.1%; HR = 0.98 [0.88 to 1.09], $P = .66$) over a 6-year follow-up in 9013 patients (26% with STEMI) randomized to a DES or BMS.[165] In this trial, the risk of stent thrombosis was lower with DES.

A network meta-analysis which included 22 trials with 12,453 randomized patients addressed the overall efficacy and safety of first- and second-generations of DES. At 1-year follow-up, cobalt-chromium everolimus-eluting stents were associated with significantly lower rates of all-cause death or MI (OR = 0.65 [0.46 to 0.90]), cardiac death or MI (OR = 0.63 [0.42 to 0.92]), target-vessel revascularization (OR = 0.45 [0.29 to 0.66]), and definite stent thrombosis (OR = 0.32 [0.11 to 0.78]) compared with BMS. Differences in stent thrombosis were apparent as early as 30 days and were maintained for 2 years. Cobalt-chromium everolimus stents were associated with lower rates of 1-year definite stent thrombosis than paclitaxel-eluting stents (OR = 0.33 [0.11 to 0.87]). Sirolimus-eluting stents were also associated with significantly lower rates of 1-year cardiac death/MI than BMS. Chromium-cobalt everolimus-eluting stents, paclitaxel-eluting stents, and sirolimus-eluting stents—but not zotarolimus-eluting stents—had significantly lower rates of 1-year target-vessel revascularization than BMS. Sirolimus-eluting stents showed lower rates of target-vessel revascularization compared with paclitaxel-eluting stents.[166] The results of this meta-analysis highlighted the steady improvements in clinical outcomes with the evolution from BMS to first-generation and second-generation DES.

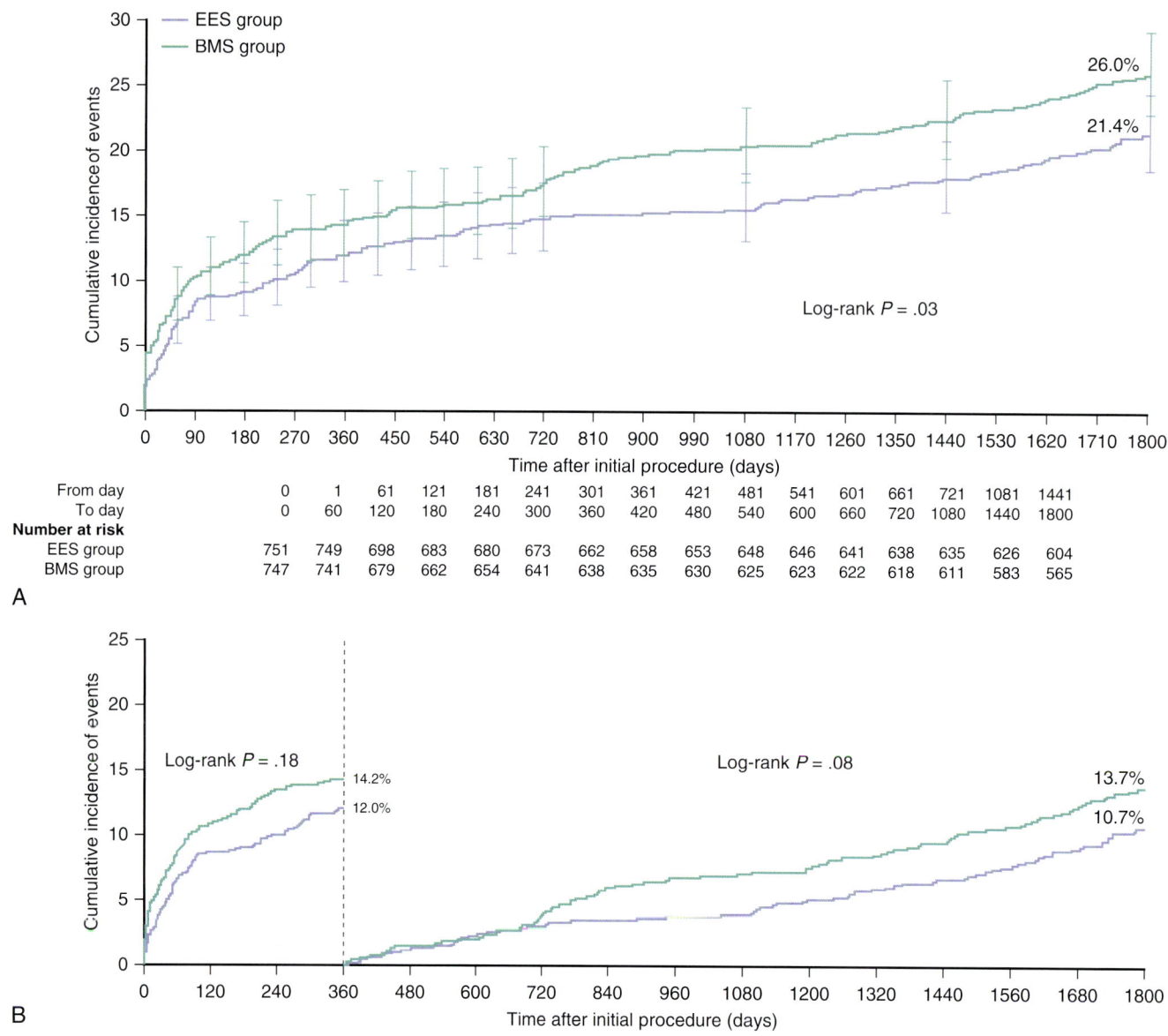

Fig. 20.12 Time-to-event analysis of the patient-oriented end point of all-cause death, any myocardial infarction, or any revascularization over 5 years. (A) Kaplan-Meier analysis of cumulative 5-year incidence. (B) Landmark analyses for 0 to 1 year and 1 to 5 years. Error bars indicate point-wise two-sided 95% CI with a complementary log-log transformation. Standard error was calculated with the Greenwood Formula. *BMS*, Bare-metal stent; *CI*, confidence interval; *EES*, everolimus-eluting stent. (From Sabate M, Brugaletta S, Cequier A, et al. Clinical outcomes in patients with ST-segment elevation myocardial infarction treated with everolimus-eluting stents versus bare-metal stents [EXAMINATION]: 5-year results of a randomised trial. *Lancet.* 2016;387[10016]:357–366.)

In summary, ample evidence from multiple sources proves a clear antirestenotic advantage of DES over BMS in patients with STEMI. Moreover DES, in particular second-generation DES, may also confer safety benefits versus BMS in the early phase after intervention. Although some concerns persist regarding very late adverse events, DES is considered the preferred approach for patients with STEMI undergoing PPCI.

Drug-Eluting Balloons

Due to an increased risk for very late stent thrombosis with DES (particularly with the first generation of these devices), the efficacy and safety of drug-eluting balloons in combination with BMS has been proposed as an alternative treatment strategy in patients with STEMI. Drug-eluting balloons are semicompliant angioplasty balloons coated with an antiproliferative drug, which is released into the vessel wall in high concentrations during short (30 to 60 seconds) balloon-vessel contact.[167] The putative advantages of drug-eluting balloons consist in the local delivery of antirestenotic agents and inhibition of intimal proliferation without delayed healing and prolonged inflammatory response related to implantation of metal/polymer platforms.[168] The efficacy of drug-eluting balloons is investigated in the Drug Eluting Balloon in Acute Myocardial Infarction (DEB-AMI) trial. In this trial, 150 patients were randomized to a strategy of a BMS, a drug-eluting balloon (paclitaxel) plus a BMS, or a paclitaxel-eluting DES. The primary end point was 6-month angiographic in-stent late-luminal loss. Secondary end points were in-stent binary restenosis and MACE (cardiac death, MI, target-vessel revascularization). In a subgroup of patients, stent (mal)apposition (by optical coherence tomography) and endothelial function (by acetylcholine infusion) was assessed. Procedural success was achieved in 96.7%. In

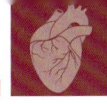

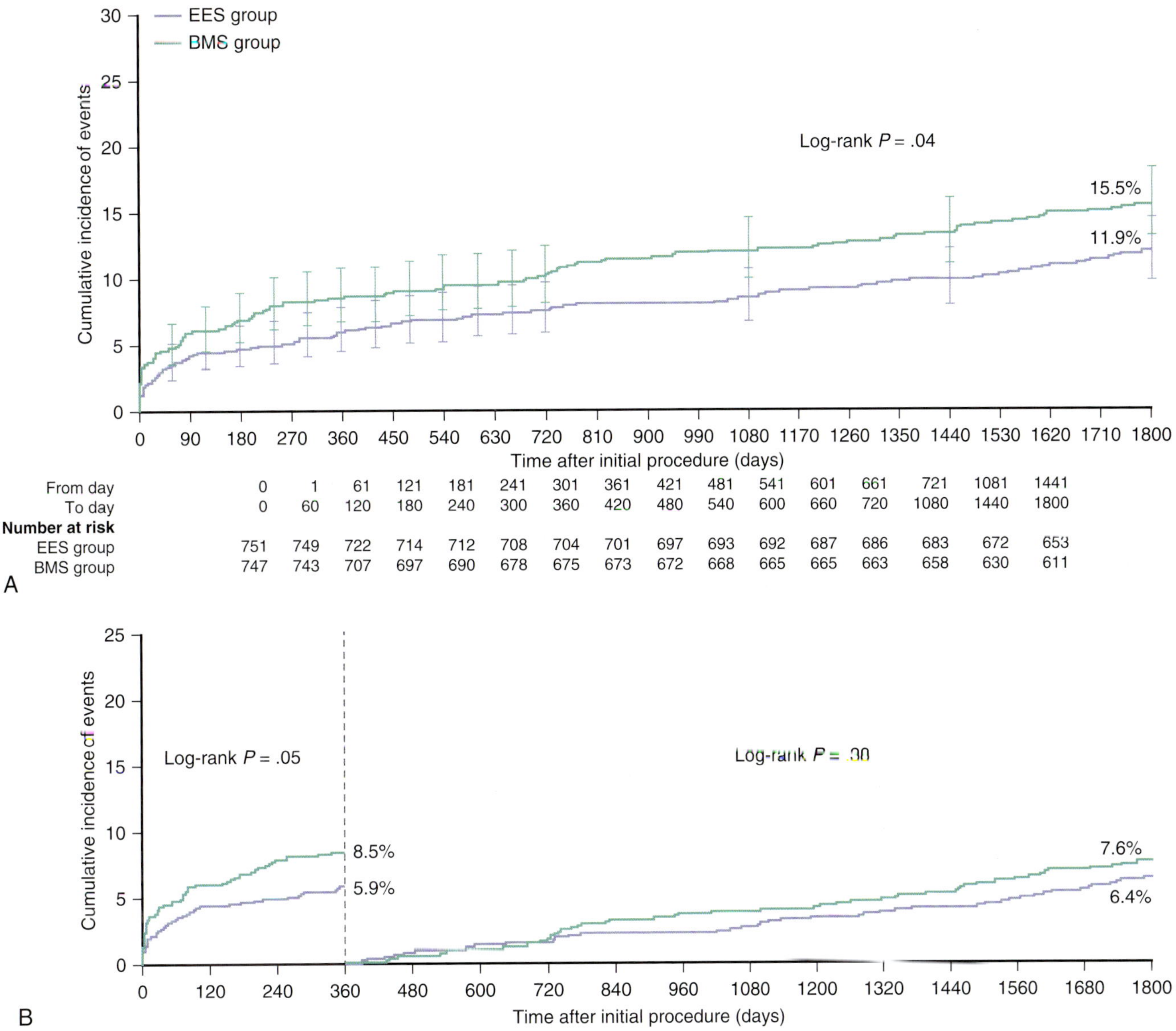

Fig. 20.13 Time-to-event curves for the device-oriented end point of cardiac death, target-vessel myocardial infarction, or target-lesion revascularization over 5 years. (A) Kaplan-Meier analysis of cumulative 5-year incidence. (B) Landmark analyses for 0 to 1 year and 1 to 5 years. Error bars indicate pointwise two-sided 95% CI with a complementary log-log transformation. Standard error was calculated with the Greenwood Formula. *CI,* confidence interval; *BMS,* Bare-metal stents; *EES,* everolimus-eluting stents. (From Sabate M, Brugaletta S, Cequier A, et al. Clinical outcomes in patients with ST-segment elevation myocardial infarction treated with everolimus-eluting stents versus bare-metal stents [EXAMINATION]: 5-year results of a randomised trial. *Lancet.* 2016;387[10016]:357–366.)

BMS, drug-eluting balloon plus a BMS, or a paclitaxel-eluting stent groups, late-luminal loss was 0.74 ± 0.57 mm, 0.64 ± 0.56 mm, and 0.21 ± 0.32 mm, respectively (P = .01); binary restenosis was 26.2%, 28.6%, and 4.7%, respectively (P = .01); and MACE rates were 23.5%, 20.0%, and 4.1%, respectively (P = .02). The median percentage (25th to 75th interquartile range) of uncovered and malapposed stent struts per lesion was 0 (0 to 0.35), 2.84 (0 to 6.63), and 5.21 (3.25 to 14.5), in the respective groups (P = .01). Significant paradoxical vasoconstriction was seen in groups with drug-eluting balloon (paclitaxel) plus a BMS, or paclitaxel-eluting DES. The study failed to show angiographic superiority of a strategy of drug-eluting balloon followed by BMS implantation compared to a BMS-only strategy.[169] The fourth nonrandomized treatment arm—a prospective registry of 40 patients with STEMI recruited using the same inclusion/exclusion criteria as in the DEB-AMI trial and implanted with a drug-eluting balloon only—showed that a drug-eluting–balloon-only strategy was associated with similar procedural success and yielded angiographic and clinical outcomes comparable to those of BMS or drug-eluting balloon followed by BMS strategies. No acute or late thrombotic events occurred in the drug-eluting–balloon-only strategy. The study suggested that drug-eluting balloons may represent a potential treatment alternative during PPCI in patients with contraindications to DES.[167] Despite these results, the evidence on the use of drug-eluting balloons in patients with STEMI remains rather limited. Furthermore, the role of drug-eluting balloons in patients with STEMI is uncertain due to the excellent results seen with current generation DES.

Bioresorbable Vascular Scaffolds

The use of first-generation DES resulted in reduced need for repeat revascularization compared with BMS and newer stent generations with improved biocompatibility of polymers may have improved clinical outcome (reduced the rate of adverse clinical events) after implantation of these devices. However, the permanent presence of a metallic structure within the coronary arteries is considered disadvantageous in many aspects including permanent caging and impairment of vessel vasomotion, side branch jailing and lack of possibility of late lumen enlargement, noninvasive imaging, and future surgical revascularization of stented segments.[170] Initial studies yielded encouraging results in terms of feasibility and safety of bioresorbable vascular scaffolds in patients with STEMI.[171-173] A prospective, single-arm, single-center study reported feasibility and safety of bioresorbable vascular scaffolds in 49 patients with STEMI. The study reported a procedural success of 97.9%, a TIMI flow after device implantation of 91.7%, and the postprocedure percentage diameter stenosis was 14.7 ± 8.2%. No patients had angiographically visible residual thrombus at the end of the procedure. Optical coherence tomography analysis performed in 31 patients showed that the postprocedure mean lumen area was 8.02 ± 1.92 mm^2, minimum lumen area 5.95 ± 1.61 mm^2, mean incomplete scaffold apposition area 0.118 ± 0.162 mm^2, mean intraluminal defect area 0.013 ± 0.017 mm^2, and mean percentage malapposed struts per patient 2.80 ± 3.90%. At 30-day follow-up, target-lesion failure rate was 0% and no cases of cardiac death or scaffold thrombosis were observed.[171] The PRAGUE-19 study reported similar results in 41 patients (with 49 bioresorbable vascular scaffolds) with STEMI including a procedural success of 98% and restoration of TIMI flow grade of 3 in 95% of the patients. The optical coherence substudy performed in 21 patients showed a 1.1% rate of scaffold strut malapposition. The 9-month event free survival was similar in bioresorbable vascular scaffold and control groups implanted with metallic stent structures (log-rank test $P = .674$).[172] The randomized multicenter ABSORB-STEMI TROFI II trial assigned 191 patients with STEMI to receive an everolimus-eluting bioresorbable vascular scaffold or a durable polymer everolimus-eluting metallic stent. The primary outcome was 6-month optical frequency domain imaging healing score based on the presence of uncovered and/or malapposed stent struts and intraluminal filling defects. The study found that stenting of culprit lesions with the bioresorbable vascular scaffold in the setting of STEMI resulted in a nearly complete arterial healing which was comparable with that of a durable polymer metallic stent at 6 months. The 6-month healing score (mean ± standard deviation) was lower in the bioresorbable vascular scaffold (Absorb) arm compared with everolimus-eluting stent arm (1.74 ± 2.39 vs. 2.80 ± 4.44; P for noninferiority <.001). Device-oriented composite end point was also comparably low between groups (1.1% vs. 0%).[174] Recent small nonrandomized studies have shown similar results in STEMI patients implanted with bioresorbable vascular scaffolds or everolimus-eluting stent in terms of patient- (or device-) oriented end points over short-term (up to 1 year) follow-up.[175,176]

Despite these results, concerns exist with current generation bioresorbable vascular scaffolds related to strut thickness, poor deliverability, lack of radial strength, and particularly in the setting of STEMI, requirement for predilatation, which may increase the risk of distal embolization of thrombotic material.[177] Moreover, the optimal duration of antithrombotic therapy after bioresorbable scaffold implantation is not clear. The general safety issues raised in recent studies, particularly those related to increased risk of device thrombosis,[177] and the decision by the manufacturer of the most widely-used device to withdraw the scaffold from the market, discourages the use of these devices in patients with various aspects of CAD including PPCI in STEMI.

Mesh-Covered Stents

The MGuard mesh-covered stent (InspireMD, Boston, MA)—a BMS with a polyethylene terephthalate MicroNet mesh covering—has been designed to prevent distal embolization by trapping and excluding embolism-prone material at the level of the culprit lesion in patients with STEMI or saphenous vein grafts, both conditions associated with abundant thrombotic material and increased risk of distal embolization and no-reflow after PCI. The porous net is effective as a mechanical barrier, decreasing or preventing thrombus protrusion and distal embolization. After small studies testing the feasibility and safety of the MGuard stent,[178] the Safety and Efficacy Study of MGuard Stent After a Heart Attack (MASTER) trial tested the efficacy of the stent in the setting of PPCI. The study randomly assigned 433 patients with STEMI presenting within 12 hours to receive the MGuard stent or a commercially available BMS or DES. The primary end point (ST-segment resolution ≥70%, 60 to 90 minutes after procedure) was significantly improved in patients randomized to the MGuard stent compared to control patients (57.8% vs. 44.7%, $P = .008$). TIMI flow grade of 3 was more frequent among patients who received the MGuard stent (91.7% vs. 82.9%, $P = .006$). In 59 patients (30 patients assigned to the MGuard stent), CMR was performed at 3 to 5 days; it did not show a significant difference in the infarct size expressed as mass (median: 17.1 g vs. 21.3 g, $P = .27$) or percentage of the left ventricular mass (median: 13.3% vs. 16.6%, $P = .48$) between patients assigned to the MGuard stent or controls. Mortality (0% vs. 1.9%, $P = .06$) and MACE at 30 days (1.8% vs. 2.3%, $P = .75$) did not differ significantly between patients assigned to the MGuard stent or controls.[179] At 1 year, the incidence of MACE (all-cause death, reinfarction, or ischemia-driven target-lesion revascularization) was higher among patients with the MGuard stent (9.1% vs. 3.3%, $P = .02$), driven by more frequent ischemia-driven target-lesion revascularization compared to patients with conventional stenting. One-year mortality tended to be lower with the MGuard stent (1.0% vs. 3.3%, $P = .09$). The binary restenosis rate (assessed in 38 patients with the MGuard stent) on 13-month angiography was 31.6%.[180] A recently published propensity matching analysis-based study of two groups of 79 patients with STEMI implanted with the MGuard Stent or BMS showed similar mortality (7.6% in each group); insignificant differences in cardiac mortality, stent thrombosis, nonfatal MI, or MACE (20.3% vs. 12.7%, $P = .198$); but significantly higher rates of target-vessel (11.4% vs. 1.3%, $P = .009$) and target-lesion (11.4% vs. 1.3%, $P = .009$) revascularization with the MGuard Stent over a mean follow-up of 321 days.[181] The MGuard stent may be useful to prevent distal embolization in patients with STEMI and high thrombus burden.[182] Notwithstanding these results, the use of mesh-covered stents in patients with STEMI is not well-supported. The development of drug-eluting mesh-covered stents may warrant further investigation.

Self-Expanding Stents

The presence of thrombus and epicardial vasoconstriction may lead to underestimation of the vessel size, which increases the risk of stent undersizing—a well-known factor for stent thrombosis.[183,184] The ability of the self-expanding stents to grow gradually in size may allow stent deployment at lower pressures, which may lead to less local trauma. Less local trauma could result in less plaque disruption and less distal embolization of thrombotic-atherosclerotic debris.[185,186] A feasibility study of 25 patients with STEMI showed that the use of STENTYS (STENTYS S.A., Paris, France) self-expanding stents is safe and feasible in these patients. Angiography and intravascular ultrasound or optical coherence tomography were performed immediately after stent deployment, after 3 days, and at 6 months. The imaging studies showed that, 3 days after the procedure, the stent expanded to the same extent as the epicardial vasodilatation and appeared completely apposed to the vessel wall. No death, reinfarction, or stent thrombosis occurred over 6 months of follow-up.[187] The Randomized Comparison Between the STENTYS Self-expanding Coronary Stent and a Balloon-expandable Stent in Acute Myocardial Infarction (APPOSITION II) study randomized 80 patients with STEMI undergoing PPCI to receive a self-expanding stent (STENTYS) (n = 43) or a balloon-expandable stent (VISION, Abbott Vascular, Santa Clara, CA; or Driver, Medtronic, Minneapolis, MN) (n = 37) at nine European centers. At 3 days after implantation, on a per-strut basis, a lower rate of malapposed stent struts was observed by optical coherence tomography in the self-expanding stent group than in the balloon-expandable group (0.58% vs. 5.46%, P < .001). On a per-patient basis, none of the patients in the self-expanding stent group versus 28% in the balloon-expandable group presented ≥5% malapposed struts (P < .001). The 6-month rates of MACE did not differ significantly between the groups (2.3% in the self-expanding stent group vs. 0% in the balloon expandable stent [P = NS]).[188] A recent optical coherence tomography-based subgroup analysis from the APPOSITION II study showed that both persistent and newly acquired incomplete stent apposition occurred less frequently with self-expanding stent than balloon expandable stents, 3 days after PPCI.[189] The most recent results from the APPOSITION III multicenter postmarketing registry that included 965 STEMI patients showed 2-year lower rates of MACE (11.2%), cardiac death (2.3%), target-vessel MI (2.3%), clinically-driven target-lesion revascularization (9.2%), and definite stent thrombosis (3.3%) with the self-expanding stent. Of note, the incremental rates between 1- and 2-year follow-up were 1.0% for target-vessel MI, 1.8% for clinically-driven target-lesion revascularization, and 0.5% for definite stent thrombosis.[190] In general, the study showed lower rates of adverse events with self-expanding stents in STEMI. The use of the self-expanding stents has been shown to be safe and feasible for the treatment of bifurcation culprit lesions in the setting of PPCI.[190] Despite these results, the experience with the use of self-expanding stents in the setting of PPCI remains limited. Furthermore, concerns have been raised on the optimal stent/vessel ratio, continuation of self-expansion after stent deployment predisposing for plaque prolapse, and arrest of self-expansion in calcified lesions.[191] The APPOSITION V has been designed as a randomized trial powered on clinical end points to directly compare the STENTYS self-apposing stent with a conventional balloon-expandable stent in patients presenting with STEMI undergoing PPCI.[192] However, a decision to discontinue recruitment at 2-year follow-up has been taken.

Direct Stenting

Evidence in favor of direct stenting, that is, stent implantation without predilation, comes from a limited number of small randomized trials.[193–195] A 2002 study randomized 206 patients with STEMI to direct stent implantation or stent implantation after balloon predilation. Although the postintervention TIMI flow or TIMI corrected frame count did not differ significantly between the 2 strategies, the composite angiographic (corrected TIMI frame count, slow-flow/no-reflow, or distal embolization) end point (11.7% vs. 26.9%, P = .01) or ST-segment resolution (79.8% vs. 61.9%, P = .01) were better in patients with direct stenting compared with patients who had stent implantation after predilation.[193] Other randomized trials reported better postprocedural TIMI flow grade or corrected TIMI flow count[194] or an improvement in cost/benefit ratio with direct stenting.[193] One randomized study reported no improvement in the 5-year clinical outcome and a higher incidence of in-stent restenosis at 1 year with direct stenting.[195] Support in favor of using direct stenting comes also from the HORIZONS-AMI trial in which 698 patients were treated with direct stenting. Direct stenting compared with conventional stenting (after predilation) was associated with better ST-segment resolution at 60 minutes after the procedure (median 74.8% vs. 68.9%, P = .01) and lower rate of all-cause death (1.6% vs. 3.8%, P = .01) and stroke (0.3% vs. 1.1%, P = .049) with nonsignificant differences in target-lesion revascularization, MI, stent thrombosis, and major bleeding.[196] Death at 1 year remained lower in patients with direct stenting (HR = 0.42 [0.21 to 0.86]; P = .02) after adjustment and in a propensity score–based analysis (HR = 0.92 [0.88 to 0.95]; P = .02). Recent observational studies have also suggested that direct stenting is associated with improved ST-segment resolution and better early and 1-year survival compared with conventional stenting after predilation.[197]

Two recent meta-analyses have summarized studies on direct stenting in patients with STEMI or acute coronary syndromes.[198,199] A 2015 meta-analysis that included 12 studies (three randomized studies) with a total of 9331 patients showed that direct stenting was associated with significantly lower rates of mortality (OR = 0.55 [0.33 to 0.94]) or MACE (OR = 0.71 [0.60 to 0.84]) in nonrandomized studies but not in randomized trials (OR = 0.56 [0.26 to 1.23] for mortality and OR = 0.99 [0.61 to 1.60] for MACE). ST-segment resolution, no reflow, final TIMI flow, and final TIMI myocardial perfusion grade were significantly better with direct stenting in nonrandomized studies and nonsignificantly better in randomized trials.[198] The other meta-analysis that included 12 studies with 8998 patients showed better results with direct stenting with respect to no-reflow (OR = 0.48 [0.31 to 0.75]), MACE rates (OR = 0.61 [0.46 to 0.80]), or 1-year mortality (OR = 0.40 [0.29 to 0.57]).[199] Direct stenting may be advantageous over stenting after predilation in several aspects including the use of fewer and shorter stents, shorter fluoroscopy time and less use of contrast media, and reduced microvascular dysfunction/obstruction and no-reflow by reduced distal embolization. Potential disadvantages of direct stenting may include: failure to reach and/or to cross the lesion, stent loss, erroneous estimation of stent length, difficulty with stent positioning (especially in case of persistent TIMI flow 0 to 1), underexpansion of the stent in an undilatable (i.e., calcified) lesion, and stent undersizing due to underestimation of vessel diameter because of reduced flow.[200] Notwithstanding these disadvantages, direct stenting is considered almost as a default strategy during PPCI. The combination of direct stenting with aspiration thrombectomy—hailed for the advantages of direct stenting in prior studies—has recently been questioned in light of suboptimal results with aspiration thrombectomy. Heavy calcification of the vessel or poor visualization of the distal edge are contraindications to this strategy. One recent study has suggested that restoration of anterograde blood flow in patients with STEMI and a TIMI flow grade <1 using a microcatheter allows downstream visualization of arteries and increased success rate of direct stenting, and was associated with less manual thrombectomy, or bailout GPI use, and lower peak levels of cardiac enzymes with no impact on final TIMI flow of 3 or the incidence of MACE (death, cardiogenic shock, or arrhythmias) or left ventricular ejection fraction.[201]

Another recent study that included 17,329 patients from three randomized studies showed that patients with direct stenting underwent thrombus aspiration more often (41% vs. 22%, P < 0.001), required less contrast (162 vs. 172 mL, P < .001), and had shorter fluoroscopy time (11.1 minutes vs. 13.3 minutes, P < .001). After propensity matching there were no differences in 30-day cardiovascular death (1.7% vs. 1.9%, P = .60) or 30-day stroke or transient ischemic attack (0.6% vs. 0.4%, P = .99) between direct and conventional stenting. One-year results were also similar.[202]

RADIAL ARTERY VERSUS FEMORAL ARTERY VASCULAR ACCESS FOR PRIMARY PERCUTANEOUS CORONARY INTERVENTION

Although vascular access via the femoral artery was previously considered almost as a default strategy for vascular access for PCI in general, including PPCI, evidence favoring the use of radial artery for vascular access is rapidly increasing. The most important argument for the use of radial artery comes from multiple sources showing significant reductions in bleeding complications with radial artery compared with femoral artery route. Recent randomized trials and large registries offer support for the use of radial artery approach in PPCI procedures. In a prespecified analysis of the RadIal versus femoRAL access for coronary intervention (RIVAL) trial that included 1958 patients with STEMI, the transradial artery approach was associated with significantly lower primary outcome of death, MI, stroke, or noncoronary artery bypass graft (CABG)-related major bleeding at 30 days (3.1% vs. 5.2%, $P = .026$).[203] However caution is always required in the interpretation of subgroup analysis particularly in a trial with an overall negative result. The two strategies were directly compared in the Radial Versus Femoral Randomized Investigation in ST-Elevation Acute Coronary Syndrome (RIFLE-STEACS) study, which randomized 1001 patients with STEMI to undergo primary or rescue PCI via transradial or transfemoral artery approaches. The primary end point was the 30-day rate of net adverse clinical events, defined as a composite of cardiac death, stroke, MI, target-lesion revascularization, and bleeding. The primary end point occurred in 13.6% of the patients in the transradial artery arm and 21.0% of the patients in the transfemoral artery arm ($P = .003$). The difference was driven largely by a reduction in cardiac mortality (5.2% vs. 9.2%, $P = .020$) with transradial artery access. However, radial compared to femoral artery access was also associated with significantly lower rates of bleeding (7.8% vs. 12.2%, $P = .026$) and shorter hospital stay (5 days vs. 6 days, $P = .03$).[204] Another recent randomized trial showed that transradial artery approach was superior to transfemoral artery approach in reducing the major bleeding/vascular complications (1.4% vs. 7.2%, $P < .001$), though the antithrombotic regimen used consisted of high-dose heparin (>100 IU/kg) and high rates of GPI use. Thirty-day net adverse clinical events, defined as death, MI, stroke, or major bleeding vascular complications was also lower with transradial artery access (4.6% vs. 11%, $P = .0028$) but not 6-month mortality (2.3% vs. 3.1%, $P = .64$).[205] A decision-analytic model that used the data from the RIVAL and RIFLE-STEACS trials suggested that a substantial delay in DTB time would need to be introduced during transradial artery PCI to eliminate the observed mortality benefits of a transradial approach.[206]

Two recent large registries in Italy and the United States offer additional support for the use of transradial artery approach during PPCI procedures. The REgistro regionale AngiopLastiche dell'Emilia-Romagna (REAL) registry that included 11,068 patients showed that the 2-year risk-adjusted mortality rates were lower for the transradial than for the transfemoral artery group (8.8% vs. 11.4%, $P = .0250$). The rate of vascular complications requiring surgery or need for blood transfusion were also significantly decreased in the transradial artery group (1.1% vs. 2.5%, $P = .0052$).[207] A recent report from the CathPCI Registry that included 294,769 patients undergoing PCI for STEMI between 2007 and 2011 showed that over a 5-year period the use of trans-radial PCI versus transfemoral PCI increased from 0.9% to 6.4% ($P < .001$).[208] Transradial PCI was associated with longer median DTB time (78 vs. 74 min, $P < .001$) but lower adjusted risk for bleeding (OR = 0.62 [0.53 to 0.72]; $P < .001$) and lower adjusted risk of in-hospital mortality (OR = 0.76 [0.57 to 0.99]; $P = .0455$).

In the setting of the Minimizing Adverse Haemorrhagic Events by TRansradial Access Site and Systemic Implementation of angioX (MATRIX) trial, 4010 patients with STEMI were randomized to radial ($n = 2001$) or femoral ($n = 2009$) access. The 30-day coprimary outcomes which were MACE (defined as death, MI, or stroke) and net adverse clinical events (defined as MACE or major bleeding) occurred in 6.1% and 6.3% (RR = 0.96 [0.75 to 1.24]) and 7.2% and 8.3% (RR = 0.86 [0.68 to 1.08]) in patients randomized to a transradial versus those randomized to a transfemoral artery approach, respectively (Fig. 20.14).[209]

There are at least 15 meta-analyses that have assessed efficacy and safety of PPCI via transradial artery approach versus transfemoral artery approach. One recent meta-analysis comprising data from 16 trials with a total of 9726 patients showed a reduction of all-cause mortality (RR = 0.68 [0.54 to 0.85]), major bleeding (RR = 0.56 [0.42 to 0.74]), access site bleeding (RR = 0.38 [0.29 to 0.50]), MACEs (RR = 0.80 [0.68 to 0.94]), and length of hospital stay (standardized mean difference −0.38 days [−0.46 to −0.31 days]) with the transradial compared with the transfemoral approach. The greatest reduction in the major bleeding rates was found in the subgroup with trials recruiting only PPCI patients compared with those that included varying proportions of rescue PCIs. GPI use and cross-over rates did not have a significant association with outcome measures in the subgroup analysis. Incidence of stroke was numerically greater with the transradial approach but did not achieve statistical significance (RR = 1.22 [0.56 to 2.66]).[210] In the current ESC guidelines, radial access is recommended over femoral access if performed by an experienced radial operator (class 1 recommendation; level of evidence: A).[9]

MULTIVESSEL INTERVENTION IN PATIENTS WITH ST-SEGMENT ELEVATION MYOCARDIAL INFARCTION

Between 40% and 65% of patients with STEMI have additional stenoses in noninfarct-related coronary arteries and the outcome of these patients after PCI is worse compared with patients with single-vessel CAD.[211,212] The increase in cardiovascular risk in patients with multivessel CAD is explained by a series of factors including impaired function of noninfarct zone, impact of extensive atherosclerotic disease, presence of stunned and hibernating myocardium, and slow flow in the critically narrowed non-infarct-related arteries. For patients not intended to undergo coronary artery bypass surgery, the revascularization strategy of nonculprit lesions in patients with STEMI consists of PCI of nonculprit lesions during the same session of PPCI, delayed planned PCI (staged approach), or PCI at a later time if driven by ischemia symptoms or strong evidence by positive ischemia tests. However, the most optimal revascularization strategy in these patients remains debatable.

Multivessel intervention during PPCI procedures has been investigated in observational and randomized studies and its overall effect has been investigated in a series of meta-analyses. A 2011 pairwise and network meta-analysis has compared three PCI strategies in patients with STEMI and multivessel disease: culprit-vessel-only PCI strategy; multivessel PCI strategy defined as PCI of culprit vessel as well as ≥1 nonculprit vessel lesions; and staged PCI strategy, defined as PCI confined to culprit vessel, after which ≥1 nonculprit vessel lesions are treated during staged procedures. Overall 18 studies (four prospective and 14 retrospective studies) with 40,280 patients were included. The meta-analysis showed that staged PCI was associated with lower short- and long-term mortality as compared with culprit PCI and multivessel-PCI strategies. Of note, multivessel-PCI strategy was associated with highest mortality rates at both short- and long-term follow-up.[213] Another meta-analysis that included 14 studies (11 cohort and three randomized controlled studies) compared the multivessel PCI with the IRA PCI-only strategies. The

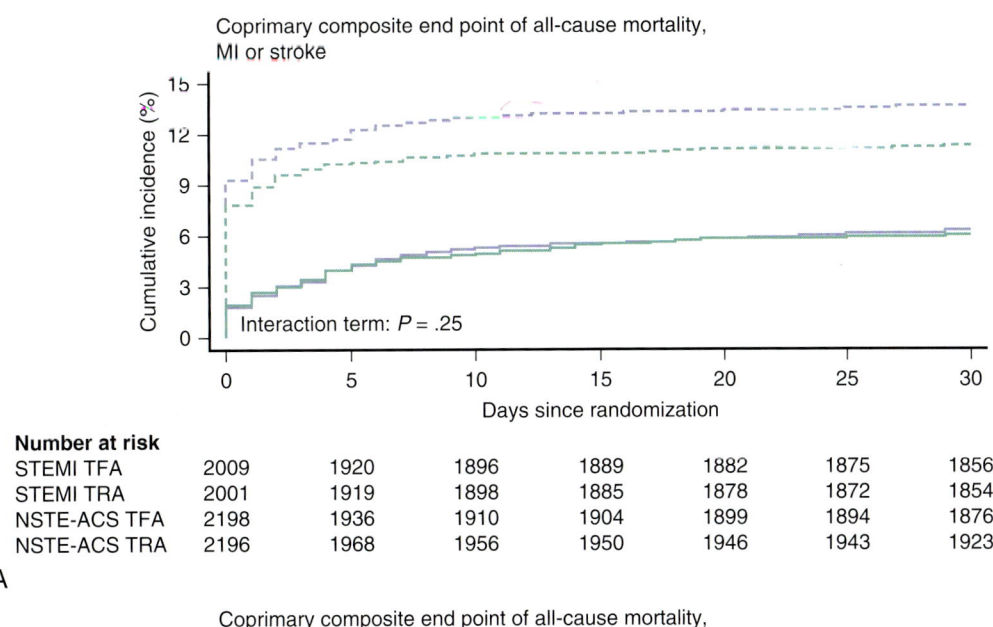

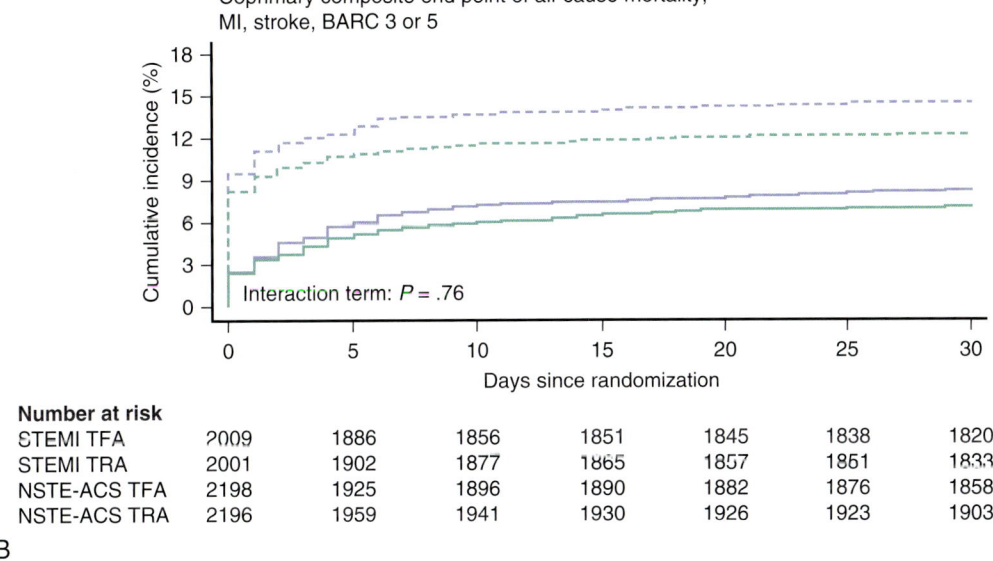

Fig. 20.14 (A) All-cause mortality, myocardial infarction, or stroke, and (B) all-cause mortality, myocardial infarction, stroke, or Bleeding Academic Research Consortium *(BARC)* 3 or 5 bleeding. *Lavender* lines illustrate patients randomized to femoral access and *blue* lines correspond to the patients randomized to radial access. *Dashed* lines correspond to the NSTE-ACS patients and *unbroken* lines stand for the STEMI population. *MI,* Myocardial infarction; *NSTE-ACS,* non–ST-segment elevation acute coronary syndrome; *STEMI,* ST-segment elevation MI; *TFA,* transfemoral access; *TRA,* transradial access. (From Vranckx P, Frigoli E, Rothenbuhler M, et al. Radial versus femoral access in patients with acute coronary syndromes with or without ST-segment elevation. *Eur Heart J.* 2017;38[14]:1069–1080.)

primary composite end point of death, MI, and revascularization was higher in the multivessel-PCI group in the short-term (OR = 1.63 [1.12 to 2.37]) and long-term (OR = 1.60 [1.18 to 2.16]) time interval. However, after excluding patients with shock, there was no difference in primary end point for the short- (OR = 1.33 [0.67 to 2.63]) or long-term (OR = 1.39 [0.80 to 2.42]) follow-up. In analyses limited to randomized controlled trials, the rate of the primary end point was similar during short-term (OR = 0.79 [0.19 to 3.28]) but significantly lower for multivessel-PCI group in the long-term (OR = 0.55 [0.34 to 0.91]) follow-up.[214] A 2014 meta-analysis that included 26 studies (23 nonrandomized and 3 randomized studies) with 46,324 patients showed that staged multivessel PCI improved short- and long-term survival and reduced the need for repeat PCI. Although overall there was no difference in in-hospital mortality with multivessel PCI or IRA PCI only (OR = 1.11 [0.98 to 1.25]; *P* = .10), multivessel PCI during index catheterization was associated with increased hospital mortality (OR = 1.35 [1.19 to 1.54]; *P* < .001). When multivessel PCI was performed as a staged procedure, hospital mortality was lower (OR = 0.35 [0.21 to 0.59]; *P* < .001). The risk of long-term mortality was reduced by 26% (*P* < .001) and the need for repeat PCI was reduced by 35% (*P* = .01) with multivessel PCI.[215]

Several recent randomized studies have assessed the efficacy and safety of multivessel intervention in the setting of PPCI. The Preventive Angioplasty in Acute Myocardial Infarction (PRAMI) trial gave support for a preventive strategy (multivessel intervention at the time of PPCI). The preventive strategy consisted of the same-time PCI on nonculprit coronary arteries with >50%

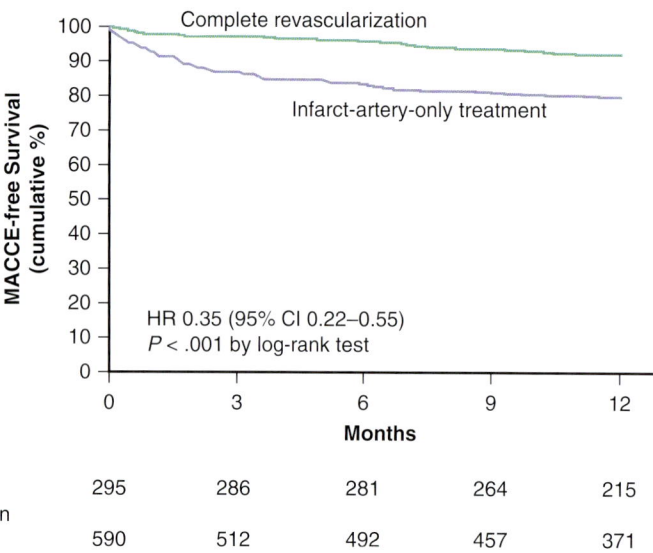

Fig. 20.15 Kaplan-Meier event curves of the combined primary outcome. MACCE denotes the composite of all-cause mortality, nonfatal myocardial infarction, any revascularization, and cerebrovascular events. *CI*, Confidence interval; *HR*, hazard ratio; *MACCE*, major adverse cerebrovascular and cardiovascular event. (From Smits PC, Abdel-Wahab M, Neumann FJ, et al. Fractional flow reserve–guided multivessel angioplasty in myocardial infarction. *N Engl J Med*. 2017;376[13]:1234–1244.)

diameter stenosis. The study randomized 465 patients with STEMI undergoing PPCI to a preventive PCI (234 patients) or no preventive PCI (231 patients). The trial was planned to include 600 patients but the data and safety monitoring committee prematurely terminated the trial after finding a significant difference in the primary end point (a composite of death from cardiac causes, nonfatal MI, or refractory angina). During a mean follow-up of 23 months, the primary outcome occurred in 21 patients assigned to preventive PCI and in 53 patients assigned to no preventive (infarct-artery only) PCI (HR = 0.35 [0.21 to 0.58]; *P* < .001). HRs for the three components of the primary outcome were 0.34 (0.11 to 1.08) for death from cardiac causes, 0.32 (0.13 to 0.75) for nonfatal MI, and 0.35 (0.18 to 0.69) for refractory angina.[216] Although the PRAMI trial offered support for a preventive PCI in patients with STEMI, the limited number of events, particularly limited number of deaths (4 and 10 deaths per group), the choice of control group (staged PCI strategy was not included as control), the lack of validation of the criterion for applying the preventive strategy (50% or greater diameter stenosis), and the premature termination of the trial potentially overestimating the benefit are limitations of this study.[216] The Complete versus Lesion-only Primary PCI trial (CvLPRIT) compared a strategy of complete revascularization at index admission (at the time of PPCI or before hospital discharge) with the treatment of the IRA only in 296 patients with STEMI. The primary end point—a 12-month composite of all-cause death, recurrent MI, heart failure, or ischemia-driven revascularization—occurred in 10.0% of patients in the complete revascularization group versus 21.2% of the patients in the IRA-only revascularization group (HR = 0.45 [0.24 to 0.84]; *P* = .009). No significant reduction in the rates of death or MI was observed. Moreover, there was no difference in ischemic burden on myocardial perfusion scintigraphy or in the safety end points of major bleeding, contrast-induced nephropathy, or stroke between the groups.[217] The CMR substudy that included 205 patients of the CvLPRIT trial showed no difference in the infarct size (median [interquartile range]) between the strategies (13.5% [6.2% to 21.9%] in the IRA-only revascularization group vs. 12.6% [7.2% to 21.6%] of the left ventricle in the complete revascularization group; *P* = .57).[217] The complete revascularization group had an increase in non-IRA MI on the predischarge CMR (22 of 98 vs. 11 of 105, *P* = .02). There was no difference in total infarct size or ischemic burden between treatment groups at follow-up CMR.[217] The DANAMI-3—PRIMULTI trial investigated the clinical outcome of patients with STEMI treated with fractional flow reserve (FFR)-guided complete revascularization versus treatment of the IRA only. The study enrolled 627 patients with STEMI and the primary end point was a composite of all-cause mortality, nonfatal reinfarction, and ischemia-driven revascularization of lesions in non-IRAs. Over a median follow-up of 27 months (range 12 to 44 months), the primary end point occurred in 22% of patients who had PCI of the IRA only and in 13% of patients who had complete revascularization (HR = 0.56 [0.38 to 0.83]; *P* = .004).[218] A recent publication from the DANAMI-3-PRIMULTI trial showed that the benefit from FFR–guided complete revascularization in patients with STEMI and multivessel disease depended on the presence of three-vessel disease and noninfarct diameter stenosis ≥90% and was particularly pronounced in patients with both of these angiographic characteristics.[219] The Comparison Between FFR Guided Revascularization Versus Conventional Strategy in Acute STEMI Patients With Multivessel DIsease (COMPARE-ACUTE) trial randomized 885 patients with STEMI and multivessel disease who had undergone PPCI of an IRA in a 1:2 ratio to undergo FFR-guided complete revascularization of non-IRAs (*n* = 295) or no revascularization of non–IRAs (*n* = 590). The primary end point was a composite of death from any cause, nonfatal MI, revascularization, and cerebrovascular events at 12 months. Clinically indicated elective revascularizations performed within 45 days after PPCI were not counted as events in the group receiving PCI for an IRA only. The primary end point occurred in 23 patients in the complete-revascularization group and in 121 patients in the IRA-only group that did not receive complete revascularization (HR = 0.35 [0.22 to 0.55]; *P* < .001; Fig. 20.15). Death (1.4% vs. 1.7%; HR = 0.80 [0.25 to 2.56]) or MI (2.4% vs. 4.7%; HR = 0.50 [0.22 to 1.13]) did not differ significantly between complete revascularization or IRA-only revascularization. Cerebrovascular events were low (0% vs. 0.7%). Notably, revascularization rate was significantly reduced by complete revascularization strategy (6.1% vs. 17.5%; HR = 0.32 [0.20 to 0.54]). The study showed that FFR-guided complete revascularization of non-IRAs in STEMI reduced the risk of composite cardiovascular outcomes mostly due to a reduction in subsequent revascularizations.[220] Finally, a recent randomized trial-only based meta-analysis showed that a strategy of complete revascularization in patients with STEMI and multivessel disease is associated with a reduced risk of MACE, cardiac death, and repeat revascularization with no benefit on all-cause mortality or nonfatal MI.[221]

At present current guidelines encourage performing multivessel PCI at the time of PPCI by giving a class IIa (level of evidence

A)[9] or class IIb recommendation[222] for routine revascularization of non-IRA lesions in STEMI patients with multivessel disease before hospital discharge.

DISTAL PROTECTION DEVICES IN PRIMARY PERCUTANEOUS CORONARY INTERVENTION

The strategy of distal protection during PPCI consists in the deployment of devices (distal filters, distal occluders, proximal occluders, or thrombus extraction devices) to restrict distal embolization of debris dislodged from the culprit lesions at the time of PPCI. Distal protection devices have improved clinical outcome when used to treat stenotic lesions in bypass graft vessels.[223] Despite ample evidence that distal protection devices can be safely deployed and that they effectively retrieve debris, most of the clinical research on the efficacy of these devices in patients with STEMI has been disappointing. The Enhanced Myocardial Efficacy and Recovery by Aspiration of Liberated Debris (EMERALD) trial randomized 501 patients with STEMI presenting within 6 hours who underwent primary or rescue PCI to receive PCI with a balloon occlusion and aspiration distal microcirculatory protection system or angioplasty without distal protection. ST-segment resolution (>70%) measured 30 minutes after PCI and infarct size measured by technetium (^{99m}Tc) sestamibi imaging at 5 to 14 days were coprimary end points. Visible debris was retrieved from 73% of the patients. ST-segment resolution (63.3% vs. 61.9%), infarct size (median: 12.0% vs. 9.5% of the left ventricle), and the 6-month composite end point of MACE (10.0% vs. 11.0%) did not differ significantly among patients assigned to distal protection or not.[224] The Drug Elution and Distal Protection in ST-Elevation Myocardial Infarction (DEDICATION) trial randomized 626 patients with STEMI referred within 12 hours for PPCI to distal protection with a filterwire system (FilterWire EZ; Boston Scientific, Marlborough, MA) or conventional stenting without distal protection. The primary end point was complete ST-segment resolution measured by continuous ST-segment monitoring. Peak values of cardiac troponin T and creatine kinase myocardial band were used as estimates of infarct size. There was no significant difference in ST-segment resolution (76% vs. 72%), peak cardiac troponin T (4.8 μg/L vs. 5.0 μg/L), or peak creatine kinase myocardial band (185 μg/L vs. 184 μg/L) among patients assigned to distal protection or not. There was a trend toward a higher rate of major adverse cardiac and cerebral events at 1 month after PPCI in patients with distal protection (5.4% vs. 3.2%, $P = .17$).[225] Another randomized trial came to similar conclusions regarding the efficacy of distal protection devices to improve reperfusion or reduce infarct size in patients with STEMI.[226]

Reasons for the failure of distal protection devices to improve reperfusion in the setting of PPCI remain unknown. However, the embolization caused by crossing the lesion with the device, impaired microcirculation by the device (nonembolic effects), dislodgement and embolization of vasoconstrictor material not halted by the device, and failure to protect downstream side branches have been proposed as putative mechanisms. Distal protection devices are not recommended to be used in the setting of PPCI.

MECHANICAL AND ASPIRATION THROMBECTOMY

Thrombectomy devices have been used in the setting of PPCI to reduce the chance (or extent) of distal embolization by removing thrombotic material from the occluded coronary arteries. Thrombus removal is enabled by mechanical or aspiration thrombectomy strategies. With regard to mechanical thrombectomy, randomized trials did not show a benefit in terms of clinical outcome. A meta-analysis that included seven trials with 1598 patients showed no difference between mechanical thrombectomy and conventional PPCI arms in the incidence of MACE (RR = 1.10 [0.59 to 2.05]), mortality ($P = .57$), recurrent MI ($P = .32$), target-vessel revascularization ($P = .19$), or final infarct size ($P = .47$). A benefit in ST-segment resolution at 60 minutes ($P = .007$) but not in the TIMI blush grade ($P = .48$) was also noted.[227] Based on these data mechanical thrombectomy is not recommended to be performed in the setting of PPCI in patients with STEMI.

Earlier randomized trials that used manual aspiration thrombectomy reported encouraging results in terms of improvement of markers of reperfusion or clinical outcomes with manual aspiration thrombectomy.[228,229] This led to an increased use of manual aspiration thrombectomy as an adjunctive therapy to PPCI. However, more recent research in the field of manual thrombectomy in the setting of PPCI did not offer evidence on the beneficial effects of this strategy in patients with STEMI. The Thrombus Aspiration in ST-Elevation Myocardial Infarction in Scandinavia (TASTE) trial did not show a benefit of manual aspiration thrombectomy compared to PPCI alone in terms of improved clinical outcome. The study included 7244 patients with STEMI undergoing PCI randomized to manual aspiration followed by PCI or to PCI only. The 30-day incidence of all-cause mortality (2.8% vs. 3.0%, $P = .63$), hospitalization for recurrent MI (0.5% vs. 0.9%, $P = .09$), and stent thrombosis (0.2% vs. 0.5%, $P = .06$) did not differ significantly among patients treated with manual aspiration plus PCI or PCI only.[230] Notably, the rates of stroke and neurologic complications at the time of discharge did not differ in groups with or without manual aspiration ($P = .87$). The outcome analysis at 1 year did not find any clinical benefit of manual aspiration irrespective of thrombus burden or coronary flow before PCI, ruling out any late benefit of this strategy in patients with STEMI.[231] The Trial of Routine Aspiration Thrombectomy with PCI versus PCI Alone in Patients with STEMI (TOTAL) study delivered another blow to the use of manual aspiration as an adjunct to PPCI.[232] The study randomized 10,732 patients with STEMI undergoing PPCI to a strategy of routine upfront manual thrombectomy versus PCI alone. The primary outcome—a composite of cardiovascular death, recurrent MI, cardiogenic shock, or New York Heart Association class IV heart failure within 180 days—occurred in 6.9% of patients in the thrombectomy versus 7.0% ($P = .86$) in the PCI-alone group. Stroke within 30 days (secondary outcome) occurred in 0.7% of patients in the thrombectomy group versus 0.3% of patients in the PCI-alone group (HR = 2.06 [1.13 to 3.75]; $P = .02$). Apart from confirming the lack of efficacy of manual thrombotic aspiration, the TOTAL trial was important in offering evidence on the increased risk of neurological complications, potentially due to an increased risk of systemic embolism by the procedure in the setting of PPCI.[232] The 1-year results of the TOTAL trial showed no efficacy of manual aspiration thrombectomy in terms of primary outcome (8% vs. 8%) or cardiovascular death (4% vs. 4%). The key safety outcome, stroke within 1 year, was more frequent among patients assigned to manual aspiration (1.2% vs. 0.7%; HR = 1.66 [1.10 to 2.51]; $P = .015$).[233]

Meta-analyses offered more evidence in terms of clinical futility or safety concerns related to manual aspiration in STEMI. A meta-analysis of seven studies with 950 patients assessed the impact of aspiration thrombectomy on infarct size estimated by CMR or SPECT. Infarct size did not differ between the aspiration thrombectomy and PCI-only arms (17.1% vs. 17.3% of the left ventricle; $P = .64$). When the analysis was restricted to CMR studies only, again there was no difference in the infarct size between the study arms ($P = .23$).[227] A recent meta-analysis of 17 randomized trials with 20,853 patients showed no significant difference in all-cause mortality (4.6% vs. 5.3%; RR = 0.88 [0.75 to 1.04]), cardiovascular mortality (3.0% vs. 3.7%; RR = 0.83 [0.68 to 1.01]), reinfarction (2.1% vs. 2.2%; RR = 0.96 [0.80 to 1.15]), or stent thrombosis (1.2% vs. 1.4%;

RR = 0.84 [0.65 to 1.07]) over a weighted mean follow-up of 9.3 ± 3.3 months between aspiration thrombectomy and PCI-only groups. However, stroke rates were more frequent with aspiration thrombectomy (0.84% vs. 0.52%; RR = 1.56 [1.09 to 2.25]).[234] However, the increased risk of stroke was not found in another recent meta-analysis.[235] In another meta-analysis that pooled individual patients' data from TAPAS, TASTE, and TOTAL trials (n = 18,306 patients), 30-day cardiovascular deaths occurred in 2.4% of patients randomized to thrombus aspiration and 2.9% of the patients randomized to PPCI alone (HR = 0.84 [0.70 to 1.01]; P = .06); stroke or transient ischemic attack occurred in 0.8% and 0.5% in patients randomized to thrombus aspiration or PPCI alone (OR = 1.43 [0.98 to 2.10]; P = .06). In the subgroup with high thrombus burden (TIMI thrombus grade ≥3), thrombus aspiration was associated with fewer cardiovascular deaths (2.5% vs. 3.1%; HR = 0.80 [0.65 to 0.98]; P = .03) but with more strokes or transient ischemic attacks (0.9% vs. 0.5%; OR = 1.56 [1.02 to 2.42]; P = .04). However, no significant interaction was observed (P for interaction were 0.32 and 0.34, respectively).[236]

In summary, routine thrombus aspiration during PPCI for STEMI did not reduce longer-term clinical outcomes and might be associated with an increase in the risk of stroke. As a result, thrombus aspiration can no longer be recommended as a routine strategy in STEMI. However, in patients with a large thrombus burden, thrombus aspiration may be considered (after initial opening of occluded vessel with a wire or small balloon).

DEFERRED STENTING

Deferred stenting refers to a two-step strategy of initial reperfusion by balloon angioplasty (or thrombus removal) followed by stent implantation hours (or days) after the initial procedure. A deferred stenting strategy has also been pursued following initial minimal interventions (small size balloons to avoid both large dissection and distal embolization sufficient to restore flow in the IRA which is sustained by maximized antithrombotic therapy)[237] or after spontaneous reperfusion with optimal TIMI flow and ST-segment recovery.[238] Mechanistically, a strategy of deferred stenting may reduce distal embolization of thrombotic and/or vasopressor material compared with a strategy of immediate stenting with or without balloon predilation. Observational studies have shown that a deferred stenting strategy is safe in the majority of patients with STEMI.[239] So far, four randomized studies have investigated the strategy of deferred stenting in patients with STEMI. The first randomized study was the Deferred Stenting Versus Immediate Stenting to Prevent No- or Slow-Reflow in Acute ST-Segment Elevation Myocardial Infarction (DEFER-STEMI) trial which randomized 101 patients with STEMI with ≥1 risk factors for no-reflow to a deferred stenting strategy (4 to 16 hours after initial reperfusion) or immediate stenting strategy. Aspiration thrombectomy was performed in 85.7% and 88.5% of the patients undergoing immediate and deferred stenting, respectively.[240] The primary outcome was the incidence of no-/slow-reflow defined as TIMI flow grade ≤2. The median time to the second procedure in the deferred stenting group was 9 hours. The primary end point (6% vs. 29%, P = .006), the frequency of no-reflow (2% vs. 14%, P = .052), and intraprocedural thrombotic events (10% vs. 33%, P = .010) were achieved in fewer patients assigned to a strategy of deferred stenting compared to immediate stenting. Myocardial salvage index (proportion of initial perfusion defect salvaged) at 6 months (measured with CMR) was greater in the deferred tenting group (median 68% vs. 56%, P = .031).[240] The Minimalist Immediate Mechanical Intervention (MIMI) trial randomized 140 patients with STEMI presenting ≤12 hours to immediate stenting (n = 73) or deferred stenting (n = 67) after TIMI grade 3 restoration by thrombus aspiration. The study showed a nonsignificant trend toward lower MVO (primary outcome) in the immediate stenting group compared with deferred stenting group (1.88% vs. 3.96% of the left ventricle; P = .051), which became significant after adjustment for the area at risk (P = .049). Median infarct weight, left ventricular ejection fraction, and infarct size or 6-month outcomes did not differ between groups.[241] The Impact of Immediate Stent Implantation Versus Deferred Stent Implantation on Infarct Size and Microvascular Perfusion in Patients With ST Segment–Elevation Myocardial Infarction (INNOVATION) trial did not show an impact of deferred stenting (following a median time of 72.8 hours) on CMR-estimated infarct size (15.0% vs. 19.4% of the left ventricle; P = .112) or MVO (42.6% vs. 57.4% of the left ventricle; P = .196) compared with a strategy of immediate stenting in 114 patients with STEMI. However, in anterior wall STEMI infarct size (16.1% vs. 21.7%, P = .017) and the incidence of MVO (43.8% vs. 70.3%, P = .047) were significantly reduced in the deferred stenting group. There was no urgent revascularization event during deferral period.[242] The DANAMI 3 DEFER trial randomized 1215 patients with STEMI presenting within the first 12 hours from chest pain onset to a strategy of standard PPCI (n = 612) or deferred stenting (n = 603). The primary end point was a composite of all-cause mortality, hospital admission for heart failure, recurrent infarction, and any unplanned revascularization of the target vessel within 2 years' follow-up. Over a follow-up of 42 months, the primary end point (18% vs. 17%; HR = 0.99 [0.76 to 1.29], P = .92) or procedure-related MI, bleeding requiring transfusion or surgery, contrast-induced nephropathy, or stroke (5% vs. 4%) did not differ in groups assigned to standard PPCI or deferred stenting strategy. The rate of any unplanned target-vessel revascularization was higher in patients assigned to deferred stenting (7% vs. 4%, P = .0345). The study concluded that a strategy of routine deferred stenting did not reduce the occurrence of death, heart failure, MI, or repeat revascularization compared with a strategy of conventional PPCI.[243] A recent subgroup analysis from the DANAMI-3-DEFER trial that included 510 patients with at least one CMR study showed that the strategy of deferred stenting did not reduce infarct size (9% vs.10%, P = .67) or presence of MVO (43% vs. 42%, P = .78) or increase myocardial salvage (myocardial salvage index: 66% vs. 67%, P = .80) compared with a strategy of conventional PPCI.[244]

The association of deferred stenting strategy with angiographic of clinical outcomes was assessed in a series of recent meta-analyses.[245–247] The most up-to-date meta-analysis that included all four randomized studies (overall 1570 patients) showed that a deferred stenting strategy was associated with a lower incidence of no-/slow reflow (RR = 0.49 [0.24 to 0.96]) and improved myocardial blush grade of 3 (RR = 1.42 [1.14 to 1.77]). However, at a mean follow-up of 34 ± 15 months, both strategies were associated with a similar risk of all-cause mortality (RR = 0.85 [0.58 to 1.24]), cardiovascular mortality (RR = 0.84 [0.48 to 1.45]), reinfarction (RR = 1.54 [0.43 to 5.49]), and stent thrombosis (RR = 0.35 [0.04 to 3.35]). The meta-analysis showed that in patients undergoing primary PPCI, deferred stenting is associated with improvement in surrogate outcomes, but does not appear to improve clinical outcomes.[247] Based on these data, a routine deferred stenting strategy should not be performed in the setting of PPCI.

MECHANICAL CIRCULATORY SUPPORT DEVICES DURING PRIMARY PERCUTANEOUS CORONARY INTERVENTION

Strategies to improve hemodynamics of patients with STEMI encompass several mechanical circulatory support devices (intraaortic balloon counterpulsation, Impella pump, TandemHeart, or extracorporeal membrane oxygenation [ECMO]) that are mostly used in patients with STEMI complicated by cardiogenic shock.

However limited and inconclusive evidence exists on the use of these strategies during PPCI procedures in patients with STEMI not complicated by cardiogenic shock. Among these, intraaortic balloon counterpulsation is most commonly used. Intraaortic balloon counterpulsation produces immediate hemodynamic effects that lead to increased diastolic pressure, increased coronary perfusion pressure, and reduced left ventricular afterload and all these effects are believed to be beneficial in patients with STEMI undergoing PPCI. The use of intraaortic balloon counterpulsation was associated with reduced infarct size in a canine infarction model[248] and it may prevent early infarct extension and ventricular remodeling in a clinical setting.[249] The Counterpulsation to Reduce Infarct Size Pre-PCI for Acute Myocardial Infarction (CRISP-AMI) trial assessed the impact of intraaortic balloon counterpulsation on infarct size (the primary outcome) measured with CMR 3 to 5 days after the procedure in 337 patients with anterior wall STEMI who were randomized to receive intraaortic balloon pumping, initiated before PCI and continued for ≥12 hours, plus PCI or PCI alone. Infarct size did not differ significantly in patients assigned to the intraaortic balloon counterpulsation plus PCI versus the PCI-alone (mean: 42.1% vs. 37.5% of the left ventricle; $P = .06$). At 30 days, there was no significant difference between the groups in terms of major vascular complications (4.3% vs. 1.1%, $P = .09$) or major bleeding or blood transfusion (3.1% vs. 1.7%, $P = .49$). The 6-month mortality was 1.9% among patients assigned to intraaortic balloon counterpulsation plus PCI and 5.2% among patients assigned to PCI alone ($P = .12$).[250] A meta-analysis of six earlier trials with 1054 patients (49.1% with intraaortic balloon counterpulsation) showed that intraaortic balloon counterpulsation did not reduce all-cause mortality (4.4% vs. 4.1%, $P = .80$), congestive heart failure (17.1% vs. 18.0%, $P = .83$), or reinfarction (5.3% vs. 7.7%, $P = .42$). Intraaortic balloon counterpulsation reduced recurrent ischemia (3.6% vs. 20.3%, $P < .001$) but it increased the risk of cerebrovascular accidents (2.0% vs. 0.3%, $P = .03$) and bleeding (21.4% vs. 16.1%, $P = .02$).[251] Two recent meta-analyses of randomized trials that stratified patients according to the presence of cardiogenic shock did not report any advantage of intraaortic balloon counterpulsation in terms of mortality reduction. One meta-analysis reported no difference in short-term (30-day mortality) between patients receiving intraaortic balloon counterpulsation or not (pooled OR = 0.98 [0.57 to 1.69]; $P = .95$),[252] whereas the other meta-analysis reported no difference according to intraaortic balloon counterpulsation in terms of short- (RR = 0.88 [0.60 to 1.29]) or long-term (RR = 0.73 [0.49 to 1.09]) mortality.[253] The latter also reported increased risk of hemorrhage (RR = 1.49 [1.09 to 2.04]; $P = .013$) and recurrent ischemia (RR = 1.85 [1.26 to 2.70]; $P = .002$).[253] Based on these data, the routine use of intraaortic balloon counterpulsation in patients with STEMI does not seem to be justified.

In analogy with intraaortic balloon counterpulsation, left ventricular assist devices unload the left ventricle and when used in addition to reperfusion therapy, may reduce infarct size and give the myocardium time to recuperate. These devices have mostly been used in patients with STEMI complicated by cardiogenic shock. The use of these devices in hemodynamically less compromised patients with STEMI is rather limited. The Academic Medical Center Mechanical support for Acute Congestive Heart failure in STEMI patients (AMC MACH) 2 study assessed the safety and feasibility of left ventricular unloading with the Impella LP2.5 (Abiomed Europe GmbH, Aachen, Germany) in patients with first anterior STEMI presenting within the first 6 hours from symptom onset and without cardiogenic shock. Immediately after PCI, 10 patients received 3 days of Impella support and 10 concurrent patients received routine care, including intraaortic balloon counterpulsation if indicated. Impella insertion was successful in all cases. In the Impella group, the left ventricular ejection fraction improved from 28% at baseline to 37% at 3 days ($P < .05$) and 41% at 4 months ($P < .05$). Nevertheless, support for these results is limited due to the rather small number of patients and the nonrandomized design of the study.[254] There is no evidence to support the use of other mechanical circulatory support devices in the setting of PPCI procedures in patients with STEMI not complicated by cardiogenic shock.

ANTITHROMBOTIC THERAPY IN PATIENTS WITH ST-ELEVATION MYOCARDIAL INFARCTION UNDERGOING PRIMARY PERCUTANEOUS CORONARY INTERVENTION

Platelet inhibition by various antithrombotic agents used before, during, and after PCI procedure is an integral part of PPCI in patients with STEMI. Main antiplatelet drugs and their mechanism of action are shown in Fig. 20.16.[255] In the current practice of PPCI, a combination of aspirin and a P2Y[12] receptor inhibitor is used to achieve platelet inhibition. Although the efficacy or optimal dosing of aspirin in the setting of PPCI remains poorly investigated, a loading dose of 162 to 325 mg of uncoated aspirin is used. There is no evidence that higher doses are more effective; however, they bear the risk of more gastric irritation or inhibition of cyclooxygenase-2-dependent prostacyclin synthesis. Aspirin tablets should be chewed or crushed to boost absorption. A recent randomized study showed that intravenous 250 to 500 mg of acetyl salicylic acid leads to faster and deeper inhibition of thromboxane A_2 generation and platelet inhibition and comparable bleeding complications compared with 300 mg of oral aspirin.[256] In the current practice of PPCI, clopidogrel, prasugrel, and ticagrelor are mostly used and current guidelines give all of them a class I recommendation for use during PPCI.

Although the efficacy or safety of clopidogrel in addition to aspirin versus aspirin only has never been investigated in patients with STEMI undergoing PPCI, the drug is commonly used during PPCI. The efficacy and safety of clopidogrel were investigated in the PCI-Clopidogrel as Adjunctive Reperfusion Therapy (CLARITY) study which consisted of a prospectively planned analysis of 1863 patients undergoing PCI after mandated angiography in CLARITY–TIMI 28 trial.[257] Patients received aspirin and were randomized to receive either clopidogrel (300 mg loading dose, then 75 mg once daily) or placebo initiated with fibrinolysis and given until coronary angiography, which was performed 2 to 8 days after initiation of the study drug. The primary outcome was a composite of cardiovascular death, recurrent MI, or stroke from PCI to 30 days after randomization. Pretreatment with clopidogrel significantly reduced the incidence of the primary end point (3.6% vs. 6.2%; adjusted OR = 0.54 [0.35 to 0.85]; $P = .008$) with no significant excess in the rates of TIMI major or minor bleeding (2.0% vs. 1.9%, $P > .99$). Based on the results of experimental and randomized trials, a 600 mg loading dose of clopidogrel is preferred to a 300 mg loading dose due to more rapid and extensive platelet inhibition and better clinical outcome with the 600 mg loading dose of the drug.[258] The impact of the timing of clopidogrel relative to PCI was investigated in several observational and randomized studies. A meta-analysis estimated the impact of clopidogrel timing on outcome in 37,814 patients (8608 patients, 25% with STEMI) obtained from randomized and observational studies. The analysis of the randomized studies showed that clopidogrel pretreatment as compared with treatment after catheterization was not associated with a reduction of death (absolute risk, 1.54% vs. 1.97%; OR = 0.80 [0.57 to 1.11]; $P = .17$) but was associated with a lower risk of the secondary composite end point of MI, stroke, or urgent revascularization (9.83% vs. 12.35%; OR = 0.77 [0.66 to 0.89]; $P < .001$). There was no significant association between pretreatment and major bleeding (3.57% vs. 3.08%, $P = .18$).[259]

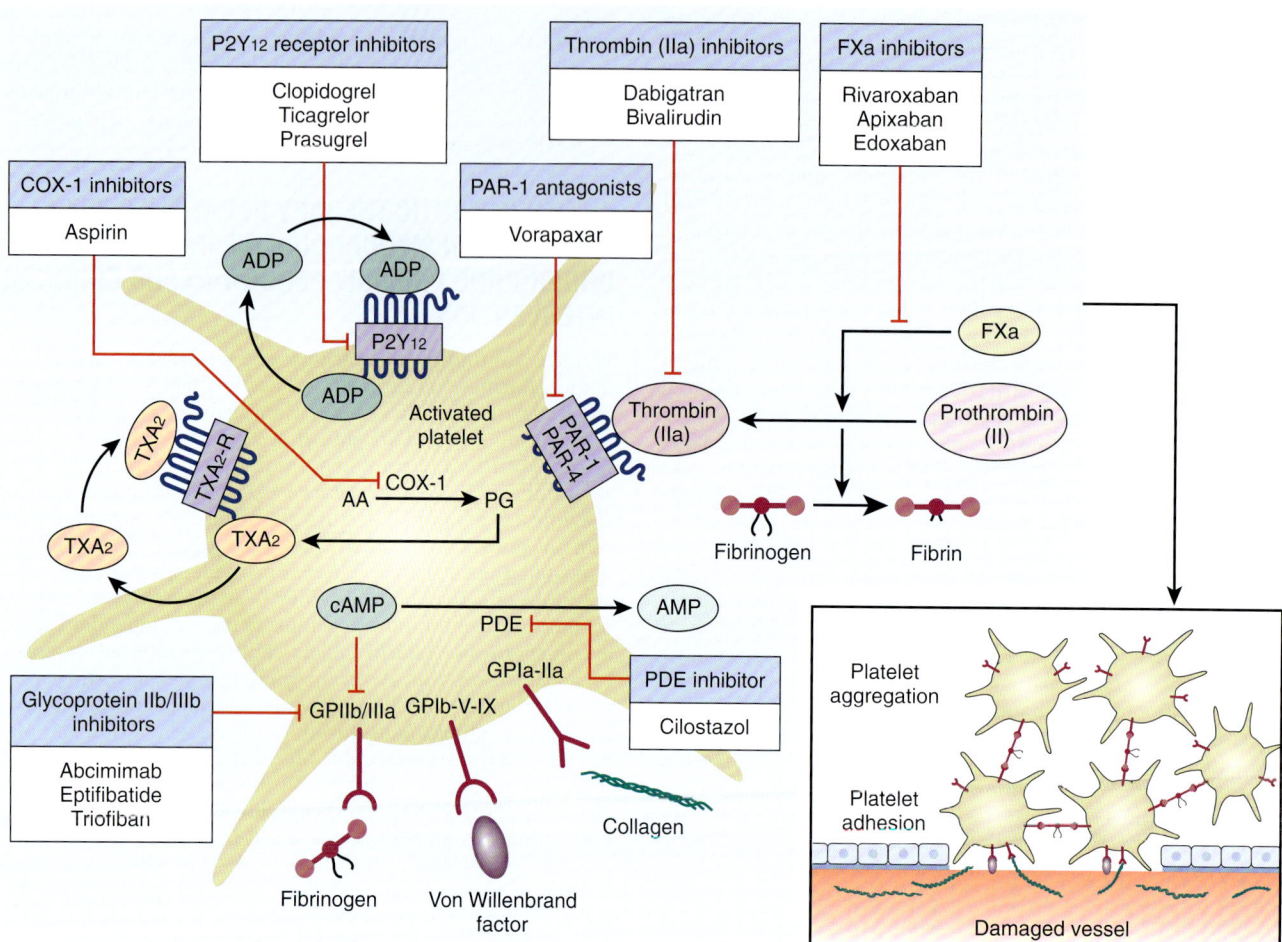

Fig. 20.16 Platelet activation and aggregation and sites of action of antiplatelet drugs. Platelet activation can occur via multiple pathways that include, among others, von Willebrand factor, collagen, thromboxane A2 *(TxA2)*, and ADP via P2Y^{12} receptors and thrombin via protease activated receptors *(PAR)* PAR-1 and PAR-4. Platelet activation results in conformational change, release of α and dense granule contents, and activation of glycoprotein *(GP)* IIb/IIIa leading to platelet aggregation. Cyclic adenosine monophosphate *(cAMP)* is an inhibitor of GPIIb/IIIa and therefore regulates platelet aggregation. Phosphodiesterase *(PDE)* converts cAMP to adenosine monophosphate *(AMP)*, which is the inactive compound. Cilostazol is a selective PDE3 inhibitor reducing platelet aggregation. *AA,* Arachidonic acid; *COX,* cyclooxygenase; *ADP,* adenine dinucleotide phosphate, FXa, factor Xa; *PG,* prostaglandine. (From Spinthakis N, Farag M, Rocca B, et al. More, more, more: reducing thrombosis in acute coronary syndromes beyond dual antiplatelet therapy-current data and future directions. *J Am Heart Assoc.* 2018. https://doi.org/10.1161/JAHA.117.007754.)

Prasugrel (a 60-mg loading dose) was compared with clopidogrel (a 300-mg loading dose) in the Therapeutic Outcomes by Optimizing Platelet Inhibition with Prasugrel–Fibrinolysis in Myocardial Infarction (TRITON–TIMI) 38 trial. Overall, the study found that in patients with acute coronary syndromes scheduled for PCI, prasugrel therapy was associated with significantly reduced rates of ischemic events, including stent thrombosis, but with an increased risk of major bleeding, including fatal bleeding.[260] A total of 3534 patients with STEMI (26%) were enrolled. Of these, 1769 patients received prasugrel and 1765 received clopidogrel. The primary end point of cardiovascular death, nonfatal MI, or nonfatal stroke at 30 days was 6.5% in patients assigned prasugrel and 9.5% in patients assigned clopidogrel (HR = 0.68 [0.54 to 0.87]; P = .0017). This effect was maintained at 15 months of follow-up (10.0% vs. 12.4%; HR = 0.79 [0.65 to 0.97]; P = .0221). The secondary end point of cardiovascular death, MI, or urgent target-vessel revascularization was reduced by prasugrel both at 30 days (6.7% vs. 8.8%; HR = 0.75 [0.59 to 0.96]; P = .0205) and 15 months (9.6% vs. 12.0%; HR = 0.79 [0.65 to 0.97]; P = .025). Stent thrombosis was reduced by prasugrel, both at 30 days (1.2% vs. 2.4%, P = .0084) and 15 months (1.6% vs. 2.8%, P = .0232). TIMI major bleeding unrelated to coronary-artery bypass graft surgery did not differ between the study drugs at 30 days (P = .3359) or 15 months (P = .6451). TIMI major bleeding after CABG surgery was significantly increased with prasugrel (P = .0033).[261] This study provided strong support for the use of prasugrel over clopidogrel in patients undergoing PPCI procedures. A small double-blind, randomized study of 62 patients with STEMI scheduled for PPCI to 60 mg of prasugrel or 600 mg of clopidogrel in the ambulance or emergency department showed that pre-PCI administration of prasugrel was associated with a faster platelet inhibition compared with clopidogrel.[262] Evidence from randomized studies also suggest that in STEMI patients undergoing PPCI, crushed prasugrel leads to faster drug absorption, and consequently, more prompt and potent antiplatelet effects compared with whole tablet ingestion.[263]

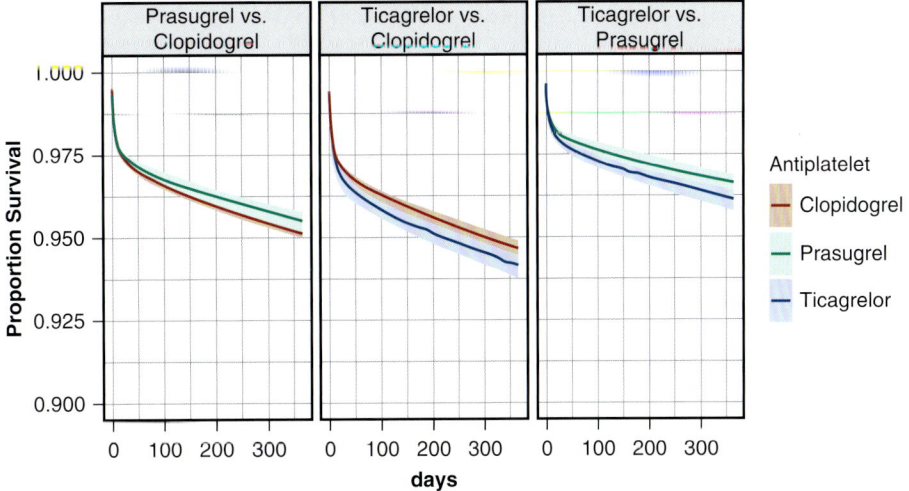

Fig. 20.17 Kaplan-Meier curves of survival based on the propensity-score-matched datasets. Survival analyses were performed using multivariate Cox regressions, in which the survival time outcome was censored at 1 year. Confidence intervals (CIs) are represented by colored shades. (From Olier I, Sirker A, Hildick-Smith DJ, et al. Association of different antiplatelet therapies with mortality after primary percutaneous coronary intervention. Heart. 2018;104(20). https://doi.org/10.1136/heartjnl-2017-312366.)

Ticagrelor differs from clopidogrel or prasugrel in that it reversibly binds to the platelet $P2Y^{12}$ receptor. As with prasugrel, ticagrelor has a more rapid onset of action and is associated with a more potent inhibition of platelets compared with clopidogrel. In the subset of 7544 patients with STEMI from the Platelet Inhibition and Patient Outcomes (PLATO) trial treated with PCI, ticagrelor (initial 180 mg loading followed by 90 mg twice daily) was compared with clopidogrel (300 to 600 mg loading followed by 75 mg daily). The primary end point of death from vascular causes, MI, or stroke occurred in 9.4% of the ticagrelor group and 10.8% of the clopidogrel group (P = .07). There were significant differences between ticagrelor and clopidogrel in all-cause mortality (5.0% vs. 6.1%, P = .05) with a trend for reduction in cardiovascular mortality (4.5% vs. 5.3%, P = .07) and definite stent thrombosis (1.6% vs. 2.4%, P = .03), MI (4.7% vs. 5.8%, P = .03) without a detectable difference in major bleeding (9.0% vs. 9.2%, P = .76).[264] The Administration of Ticagrelor in the Cath Lab or in the Ambulance for New ST Elevation Myocardial Infarction to Open the Coronary Artery (ATLANTIC) trial assessed the efficacy and safety of different timings of ticagrelor in patients with STEMI. The trial randomized 1862 patients with STEMI of <6 hours' duration to receive ticagrelor (loading dose of 180 mg) either during transfer for PPCI (in the ambulance) or immediately before angiography. The coprimary end points were the proportion of patients who did not have a 70% or greater resolution of ST-segment elevation before PPCI or the proportion of patients who did not have TIMI flow grade of 3 in the IRA at initial angiography. Secondary end points included the rates of MACE and definite stent thrombosis at 30 days. The median time from randomization to angiography was 48 minutes, and the median time difference between the two treatment strategies was 31 minutes. The two coprimary end points and the rates of MACE or major bleeding did not differ significantly between the prehospital and in-hospital groups. The rates of definite stent thrombosis were lower in the prehospital group than in the in-hospital group (0% vs. 0.8% in the first 24 hours; 0.2% vs. 1.2% at 30 days). The study showed that prehospital administration of ticagrelor in patients with acute STEMI was safe but did not improve pre-PCI coronary reperfusion.[265] Ticagrelor and prasugrel were directly compared in the PRAGUE-18 study which randomly assigned 1230 patients (90% with STEMI) to receive prasugrel (loading dose of 60 mg) or ticagrelor (loading dose of 180 mg). The study was stopped early for futility reasons. The primary end point—a composite of death, reinfarction, urgent target-vessel revascularization, stroke, or serious bleeding requiring transfusion or prolonging hospitalization at 7 days—did not differ between groups receiving prasugrel and ticagrelor (4.0% vs. 4.1%; OR = 0.98 [0.55 to 1.73]; P = .939). The key secondary end point of death from cardiovascular causes, nonfatal MI, or stroke (2.7% vs. 2.5%; OR = 1.06 [0.53 to 2.15]; P = .864) did not differ in patients assigned to prasugrel or ticagrelor.[266] The 1-year results were similar in patients who received prasugrel or ticagrelor: the combined end point of cardiovascular death, MI, or stroke at 1 year occurred in 6.6% of patients who received prasugrel versus 5.7% of patients who received ticagrelor (HR = 1.167 [0.742 to 1.835]; P = .503).[267] It has been suggested that ticagrelor (loading dose of 180 mg) is better than clopidogrel (loading dose of 600 mg) in reducing microvascular injury in STEMI patients undergoing PPCI.[268] A smaller infarct size has been reported with ticagrelor or prasugrel compared to clopidogrel.[269] Concerns have been raised about an impaired response to ticagrelor in the early hours after drug administration in patients with STEMI (due to a delay in drug absorption which cannot be overcome by increasing loading dose)[270] or that morphine delays and attenuates ticagrelor exposure and action in patients with MI.[271] The use of crushed ticagrelor tablets in patients with STEMI provides earlier platelet inhibition compared with standard integral tablets.[272] In a cohort of over 89,000 patients undergoing primary PCI for STEMI in the U.K. prasugrel is associated with a lower 30-day and 1-year mortality than clopidogrel and ticagrelor (Fig. 20.17).[273]

Cangrelor has been investigated in randomized trials including mixed groups of patients either against placebo or clopidogrel. A recent pooled analysis of all three trials that have compared cangrelor with clopidogrel (or placebo) showed that cangrelor reduced the primary outcome—a composite of death, MI, ischemia-driven revascularization, or stent thrombosis at 48 hours (3.8% vs. 4.7%, P = .0007), stent thrombosis (0.5% vs. 0.8%, P = .0008), and the odds of all-cause death, MI, or ischemia-driven revascularization (3.6% vs. 4.4%, P = .0014). The benefit was maintained at 30 days. There was no difference in the primary safety outcome—non–CABG-related GUSTO (Global Use of Strategies to Open Occluded Coronary Arteries) severe or life-threatening bleeding at 48 hours (0.2% in both groups), in GUSTO moderate bleeding (0.6% vs. 0.4%), or in transfusion (0.7% vs. 0.6%), but cangrelor increased GUSTO mild bleeding (16.8% vs. 13.0%, P < .0001). In 2884 STEMI patients (11% of participants in the pooled analysis), cangrelor was not associated with a better primary efficacy outcome (2.9% vs. 3.5%; OR = 0·84 [0.55 to 1·27]).[274]

In aggregate, these studies showed that newer P2Y[12] receptor inhibitors—prasugrel and ticagrelor—lead to extensive and rapid platelet inhibition and are superior to clopidogrel in terms of reduction of ischemic adverse events and potentially mortality in patients with acute coronary syndrome in general but also in subgroups presenting with STEMI.

ANTICOAGULANT THERAPY IN PATIENTS WITH ST-ELEVATION MYOCARDIAL INFARCTION UNDERGOING PRIMARY PERCUTANEOUS CORONARY INTERVENTION

Anticoagulant drug therapy is always used in patients with STEMI undergoing PPCI to prevent the subsequent thrombotic vessel closure. Although unfractionated heparin was never tested on a randomized basis in the setting of PPCI, the agent was and remains the most commonly used peri-PPCI anticoagulant. In general, the recommended initial bolus doses of unfractionated heparin during PPCI procedure vary between 70 and 100 U/kg of weight and there is no strong evidence in favor of monitoring unfractionated heparin with the activated clotting time test. Bivalirudin and enoxaparin are alternative drugs that seem to have a comparable efficacy in PPCI procedures.

Bivalirudin—a direct thrombin inhibitor—has been studied in several randomized trials of PPCI. In the HORIZONS-AMI trial, 3602 patients with STEMI who presented within 12 hours after the onset of symptoms were randomized to PPCI with heparin plus a GPI or bivalirudin alone.[275] Coprimary end points were major bleeding and net adverse clinical events (the combined end point of major bleeding, death, reinfarction, target-vessel revascularization, or stroke) at 30 days. Bivalirudin alone, as compared with heparin plus GPI, was associated with reduced 30-day rate of net adverse clinical events (9.2% vs. 12.1%, P = .005) and a lower rate of major bleeding (4.9% vs. 8.3%, P < .001). Of importance was the finding that treatment with bivalirudin alone reduced the 30-day incidence of cardiac (1.8% vs. 2.9%, P = .03) and all-cause mortality (2.1% vs. 3.1%, P = .047). The rate of stent thrombosis within the first 24 hours was higher following treatment with bivalirudin (1.3% vs. 0.3%, P < .001) though this did not persist at 30 days. The advantages of bivalirudin were sustainable up to 3 years after PCI. Thus, at 3 years after PCI, patients who received bivalirudin had lower rates of all-cause mortality (5.9% vs. 7.7%), cardiac mortality (2.9% vs. 5.1%), reinfarction (6.2% vs. 8.2%), and non–CABG-related major bleeding (6.9% vs. 10.5%) with no significant differences in the rates of ischemia-driven target-vessel revascularization, stent thrombosis, or composite adverse events.[276] The HORIZONS-AMI trial demonstrated that reduction of bleeding by bivalirudin was associated with significant improvements in the clinical outcome including reduction in early and long-term mortality. The HORIZONS-AMI trial strongly supported the use of bivalirudin as an anticoagulant/antithrombotic regimen in the setting of PPCI.

The European Ambulance Acute Coronary Syndrome Angiography (EUROMAX) trial randomly assigned 2218 patients with STEMI who were being transported for PPCI to prehospital administration of either bivalirudin or a heparin (either unfractionated or low molecular weight) with optional GPI.[277] The dose of bivalirudin was similar to that used in the HORIZONS AMI trial, but the drug was continued for 4 hours after procedure to reduce the risk of stent thrombosis observed in the HORIZONS-AMI trial. The primary outcome at 30 days was a composite of death or major bleeding not associated with CABG. Bivalirudin, as compared with the heparin group, reduced the risk of the primary outcome (5.1% vs. 8.5%; RR = 0.60 [0.43 to 0.82]; P = .001). Prehospital bivalirudin reduced the risk of major bleeding (2.6% vs. 6.0%), but it increased the risk of acute stent thrombosis (1.1% vs. 0.2%) with no impact on 30-day mortality (2.9% vs. 3.1%) or reinfarction (1.7% vs. 0.9%) compared with unfractionated (or low-molecular-weight) heparin plus optional GPI. Although there were differences between the trials regarding the route used for vascular access (radial artery was used in 47% of the patients in the EUROMAX trial), the use of newer antithrombotic drugs (prasugrel or ticagrelor were used in >50% of patients in the EUROMAX trial) or the use of thrombectomy (32% in the EUROMAX trial), the results of EUROMAX and HORIZONS AMI trials are mostly consistent. Bivalirudin compared with heparin decreased the risk of major bleeding but it increased the risk of acute stent thrombosis. A prespecified analysis from the EUROMAX trial showed that bivalirudin started during transport for PPCI reduced major bleeding compared with patients treated with heparin plus bail-out GPI or heparin plus routine GPI, but increased the risk of stent thrombosis.[278]

Although acute stent thrombosis is a serious, albeit rare, complication of PPCI and some patients (such as those with prior stent thrombosis) may be more prone to develop this complication, currently there are no validated risk stratification algorithms available. Nevertheless, if the risk for stent thrombosis is perceived as high, unfractionated heparin plus a GPI, a combination of bivalirudin with a more potent antiplatelet drugs, or prolonged postprocedural bivalirudin infusion may be seen as reasonable alternatives to reduce the risk of stent thrombosis associated with bivalirudin. The BRAVE 4 study tested whether a PCI strategy based on prasugrel plus bivalirudin is superior to a strategy based on clopidogrel plus unfractionated heparin in terms of net clinical outcomes. Owing to slow recruitment, the trial was stopped prematurely after enrollment of 548 of 1240 planned patients. At 30 days, the primary composite end point of death, MI, unplanned revascularization of the IRA, stent thrombosis, stroke, or bleeding was observed in 15.6% of patients randomized to prasugrel plus bivalirudin and 14.5% of the patients randomized to clopidogrel plus heparin (RR = 1.09; [one-sided 97.5% CI 0 to 1.79]; P = .68). The composite ischemic end point of death, MI, unplanned revascularization of the IRA, stent thrombosis, or stroke occurred in 4.8% of the patients in the prasugrel plus bivalirudin group and 5.5% of the patients in the clopidogrel plus heparin group (P = .89). Bleeding defined according to the HORIZONS-AMI criteria occurred in 14.1% of the patients in the prasugrel plus bivalirudin group and 12.0% of the patients in the clopidogrel plus heparin group (P = .54).[279] Results were consistent across various subgroups of patients. The study showed no evidence of advantage of a strategy of combining bivalirudin with prasugrel compared with a strategy of unfractionated heparin plus clopidogrel in terms of ischemic or bleeding complications. However, these data should be interpreted with caution due to premature termination of the trial, which markedly reduced the power of the study.

The How Effective Are Antithrombotic Therapies in PPCI (HEAT-PPCI) trial randomly assigned 1829 patients receiving PPCI at a single hospital in the United Kingdom to receive unfractionated heparin (a preprocedural bolus dose of 70 U/kg of weight) or bivalirudin (a bolus of 0.75 mg/kg, followed by infusion of 1.75 mg/kg/h for the duration of the procedure). At 4 weeks, the primary efficacy end point, a composite of all-cause mortality, cerebrovascular accident, reinfarction, or unplanned target-lesion revascularization, occurred in 8.7% of bivalirudin-treated patients and in

5.7% of heparin-treated patients (RR = 1.52 [1.09 to 2.13]; P = .01). Definite or probable stent thrombosis occurred in 3.4% of bivalirudin-treated patients and in 0.9% of heparin-treated patients (RR = 3.91 [1.61 to 9.52]; P = .001). Major bleeding occurred in 3.5% of bivalirudin-treated patients and in 3.1% of heparin-treated patients (RR = 1.15 [0.70 to 1.89]; P = .59). The study concluded that the use of heparin rather than bivalirudin was associated with reduced MACE, fewer stent thromboses and reinfarctions, no difference in bleeding complications, and the potential for substantial saving in drug costs.[280] The Bivalirudin in Acute Myocardial Infarction vs Heparin and GPI Plus Heparin Trial (BRIGHT) randomly assigned 2194 patients with acute MI undergoing PPCI to receive bivalirudin with a post-PCI infusion (n = 735), heparin alone (n = 729), or heparin plus tirofiban with a post-PCI infusion (n = 730). Among patients treated with bivalirudin, a postprocedure 1.75 mg/kg/h infusion was administered for a median (interquartile range) of 180 [148 to 240] minutes. The primary end point was 30-day net adverse clinical events, a composite of major adverse cardiac or cerebral events (all-cause death, reinfarction, ischemia-driven target-vessel revascularization, or stroke) or bleeding. Acquired thrombocytopenia at 30 days and stent thrombosis at 30 days and 1 year were also assessed. The primary outcome occurred in 8.8% of patients treated with bivalirudin, 13.2% of patients treated with heparin (RR = 0.67 [0.50 to 0.90]; P = .008), and 17% of patients treated with heparin plus tirofiban (RR = 0.52 [0.39 to 0.69]; P < .001 for bivalirudin vs. heparin plus tirofiban). The 30-day bleeding rate was 4.1% in bivalirudin, 7.5% in heparin, and 12.3% in heparin plus tirofiban (P < .001) treated patients. The 30-day rates of major adverse cardiac or cerebral events (5.0%, 5.8%, and 4.9%; P = .74), stent thrombosis (0.6%, 0.9%, and 0.7%; P = .77), acquired thrombocytopenia (0.1%, 0.7%, and 1.1%; P = .07), or acute (<24 hours) stent thrombosis (0.3% in each group) did not differ in patients assigned to bivalirudin, heparin, or heparin plus tirofiban. The BRIGHT trial showed that among patients with acute MI undergoing PPCI, bivalirudin with a median 3 hours postprocedure infusion decreased net adverse clinical events compared with both a heparin alone or heparin plus tirofiban regimen. This reduction was primarily due to a reduction in bleeding events with bivalirudin, without significant differences in major adverse cardiac or cerebral events or stent thrombosis.[281]

The recently published MATRIX trial randomized 7213 patients with an acute coronary syndrome (3010 patients with STEMI) and an anticipated PCI to receive either bivalirudin (bolus of 0.75 mg/kg of weight followed immediately by an infusion of 1.75 mg/kg of weight per hour until the end of procedure) or unfractionated heparin (70 to 100 U/kg of weight in patients not receiving GPI or at a dose of 50 to 70 U/kg of weight in patients receiving GPI). The primary outcomes were the occurrence of MACEs (a composite of death, MI, or stroke) and net adverse clinical events (a composite of major bleeding or MACE). The primary outcome for the comparison of a post-PCI bivalirudin infusion with no post-PCI infusion was a composite of urgent target-vessel revascularization, definite stent thrombosis, or net adverse clinical events. There was no significant difference between bivalirudin and unfractionated heparin with respect to MACE (10.3% vs. 10.9%; RR = 0.94 [0.81 to 1.09]; P = .44) or the rate of net adverse clinical events (11.2% vs. 12.4%; RR = 0.89 [0.78 to 1.03]; P = .12; Fig. 20.18). Post-PCI bivalirudin infusion, as compared with no infusion, did not significantly decrease the rate of urgent target-vessel revascularization, definite stent thrombosis, or net adverse clinical events (11.0% vs. 11.9%; RR = 0.91 [0.74 to 1.11]; P = .34; Fig. 20.19).[282] A recently published subgroup analysis from the MATRIX trial showed no interaction between the type of acute coronary syndrome and treatment with bivalirudin or clinical events (P for interaction = 0.73).[283] A recent SWEDEHEART registry-based randomized trial that included a total of 6006 patients (3005 with STEMI and 3001 with non-STEMI) found no difference between bivalirudin or heparin as monotherapy in terms of a composite end point of death from any cause, MI, or major bleeding during 180 days of follow-up (12.3% vs. 12.8%; HR = 0.96 [0.83 to 1.10]; P = .54). No significant differences between bivalirudin and heparin were observed with respect to individual end points of MI (2.0% vs. 2.4%), major bleeding (8.6% vs. 8.6%), definite stent thrombosis (0.4% vs. 0.7%), or death (2.9% vs. 2.8%).[284] A recent meta-analysis of five randomized trials (STEMI subsets from the MATRIX or SWEDEHEART registry trials were not included) with 10,350 patients showed comparable results between bivalirudin and heparin in terms of 30-day rates of all-cause death (2.8% vs. 2.7%; OR = 0.97 [0.74 to 1.28]; P = .84), cardiovascular death (2.0% vs. 2.5%; OR = 0.76 [0.56 to 1.0]; P = .07), reinfarction (1.9% vs. 1.2%; OR = 1.47 [0.94 to 2.30]), stroke (0.8% vs. 0.9%; OR = 0.87 [0.56 to 1.37]; P = .55), or revascularization (2.4% vs. 1.6%; OR = 1.46 [0.95 to 2.25]; P = .09). The risk of acute stent thrombosis (1.4% vs. 0.4%; OR = 3.55 [1.67 to 7.56]; P = .001) but not 30-day definite stent thrombosis (1.9% vs. 1.0%; OR = 1.71 [0.84 to 3.46]; P = .14) was higher with bivalirudin. A significant reduction of major bleeding was observed with bivalirudin (3.9% vs. 7.2%; OR = 0.58 [0.40 to 0.85]; P = .005).[285]

The efficacy and safety of enoxaparin compared with unfractionated heparin was tested in the open-label Acute Myocardial Infarction Treated with Primary Angioplasty and Intravenous Enoxaparin or Unfractionated Heparin to Lower Ischemic and Bleeding Events at Short- and Long-term Follow-up (ATOLL) trial which randomized 910 patients with STEMI to receive enoxaparin (intravenous bolus of 0.5 mg/kg) or unfractionated heparin (intravenous bolus of 70 to 100 U/kg of weight or 50 to 70 U/kg of weight with a GPI) before PPCI.[286] Patients received aspirin (75 to 500 mg/day), clopidogrel (93%), and a GPI (80%) according to local practice. Radial artery was used for vascular access in 67.4% of the patients. The primary end point was 30-day incidence of death, MI, procedure failure, or major bleeding. The null hypothesis was not rejected—the primary end point occurred in 28% of patients assigned to enoxaparin and 34% of patients assigned to unfractionated heparin (RR = 0.83 [0.68 to 1.01]; P = .06). The incidence of death (4% vs. 6%), complication of MI (4% vs. 6%), procedure failure (26% vs. 28%), or major bleeding (5% vs. 5%) did not differ in groups with enoxaparin or unfractionated heparin. However, the composite end point of death, recurrent acute coronary syndrome, or urgent revascularization was significantly reduced by enoxaparin (7% vs. 11%; RR = 0.59 [0.38 to 0.91]; P = .015). A recent meta-analysis addressed the efficacy and safety of enoxaparin versus unfractionated heparin during PCI procedures. Among 30,966 patients from 23 trials, 10,243 patients underwent PPCI for STEMI. In patients who underwent PPCI, enoxaparin as compared to unfractionated heparin reduced death (RR = 0.52 [0.42 to 0.64]; P < .001), death or MI (RR = 0.56 [0.42 to 0.76]; P < .001), and major bleeding (RR = 0.72 [0.56 to 0.93]; P = .01).[287] Thus based on these results, enoxaparin seems to be a reasonable alternative to unfractionated heparin for patients with STEMI undergoing PPCI via radial approach. Although intravenous enoxaparin may be a reasonable alternative to unfractionated heparin in patients with STEMI undergoing PPCI via femoral approach, the optimal dosing of the drug remains uncertain.

There are no properly designed studies on the value of factor Xa inhibitors in patients with STEMI treated with PPCI. A PCI subset analysis from the Organization for the Assessment of Strategies for Ischemic Syndromes (OASIS-6) trial could not show any benefit with the use of fondaparinux.[200]

Based on these data, unfractionated heparin, bivalirudin, or enoxaparin seem to have similar efficacy and should be considered as adjunct anticoagulant therapy for patients with STEMI undergoing PPCI. In patients with an increased risk of bleeding as well as in patients with heparin-induced thrombocytopenia, bivalirudin may be preferred as an anticoagulant during PPCI procedures.

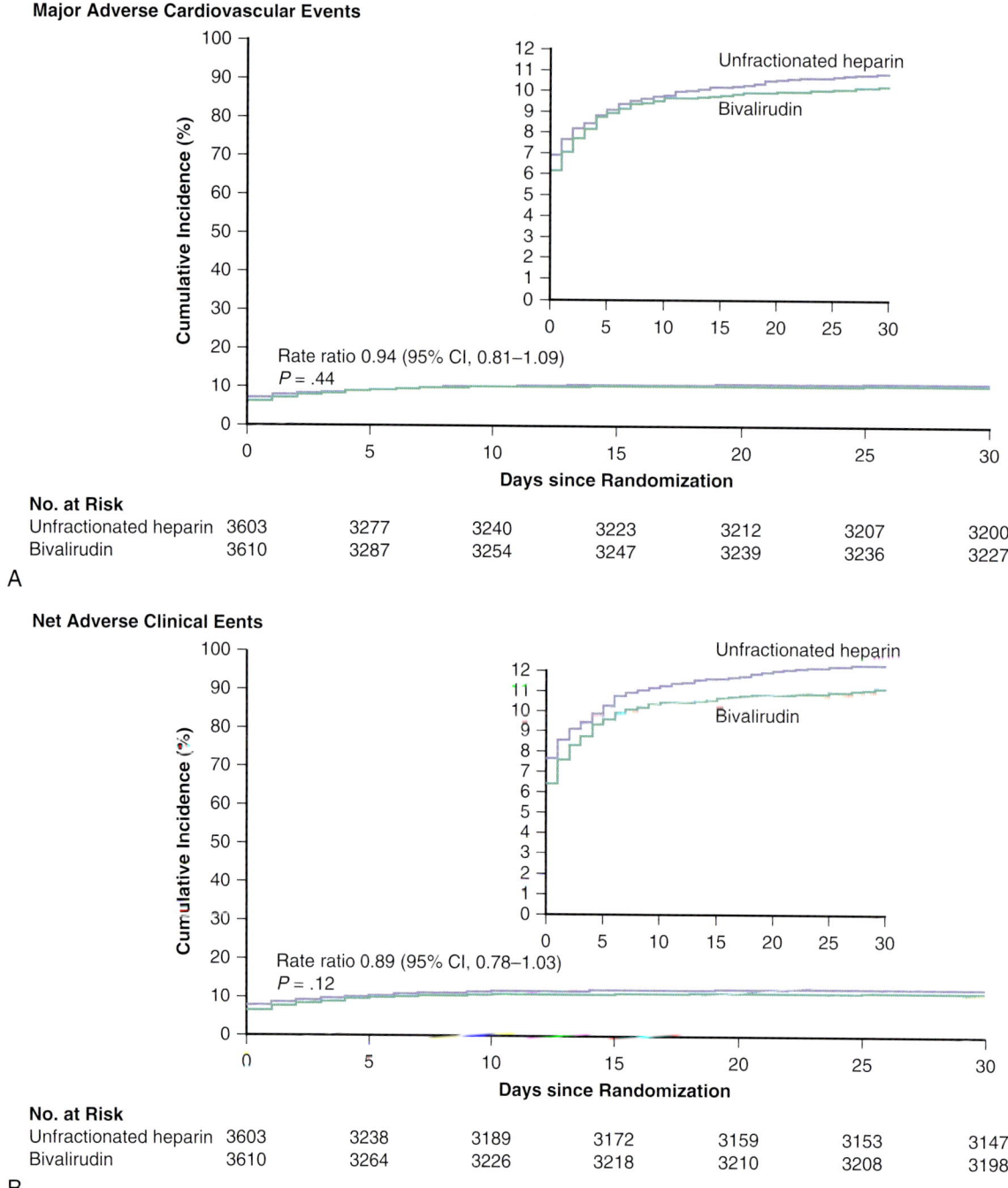

Fig. 20.18 Coprimary composite study outcomes at 30 days. Panel A shows the cumulative incidence of the coprimary outcome of major adverse cardiovascular events, which were defined as a composite of death from any cause, myocardial infarction, or stroke, up to 30 days, among patients receiving either bivalirudin or unfractionated heparin. Panel B shows the rate of net adverse clinical events, which were defined as a composite of major bleeding that was not related to coronary artery bypass grafting (Bleeding Academic Research Consortium [BARC] type 3 or 5) or major adverse cardiovascular events up to 30 days. The insets show the same data on an enlarged y axis. *CI*, Confidence interval. (From Valgimigli M, Frigoli E, Leonardi S, et al. Bivalirudin or unfractionated heparin in acute coronary syndromes. *N Engl J Med.* 2015;373[11]:997–1009.)

GLYCOPROTEIN IIB/IIIA INHIBITORS

Studies that have investigated the efficacy and safety of GPI inhibitors have been performed mostly in the era prior to modern potent oral $P2Y_{12}$-inhibitors and their relevance for current-day practice of PPCI is therefore limited. A meta-analysis of abciximab use in primary stenting, including high-risk patients with STEMI, showed a significant reduction in the composite end point of death or reinfarction with abciximab out to 3 years of follow-up (12.9% vs. 19.0%, $P = .008$); mortality alone was also reduced (10.9% vs. 14.3%, $P = .052$).[289] Another recent meta-analysis including 16 trials with 10,085 patients showed that GPI—mostly abciximab—did not reduce 30-day mortality (2.8 vs. 2.9%, $P = .75$) or reinfarction (1.5 vs. 1.9%, $P = .22$), but were associated with higher risk of major bleeding (4.1 vs. 2.7%, $P <$ .001).[290] An interaction between patient's risk and benefits from GPI in terms of mortality was observed ($P =$ .008).[290]

Abciximab is the most extensively investigated GPI in the setting of PPCI. A series of studies have also shown that abciximab, tirofiban, and eptifibatide seem to have an equivalent efficacy. The BRAVE-3 trial included 800 patients, all pretreated with a 600 mg loading dose of clopidogrel, who were randomized to abciximab or placebo. Infarct size measured with technetium (^{99m}Tc) sestamibi imaging at discharge (15.7% vs. 16.6%, $P =$ .47) or 30-day incidence of death, reinfarction, stroke, or urgent revascularization (5% vs. 3.8%, $P =$ .40) did not differ significantly among patients assigned to abciximab or placebo.[291] The trial raised doubt concerning the routine use of abciximab in the setting of PPCI after pretreatment with $P2Y^{12}$ inhibitors. The Ongoing Tirofiban In Myocardial infarction Evaluation (On-TIME 2) trial in which a high bolus dose of tirofiban was administered in the ambulance on top of unfractionated heparin (5000 U bolus), aspirin (500 mg), and clopidogrel (600 mg loading dose) came to different conclusions. MACE (a composite of death, recurrent MI, or urgent target-vessel revascularization at 30 days) were significantly reduced (5.8% vs. 8.6%, $P =$ .043) and there was a strong trend toward a decrease in mortality (2.2% vs. 4.1%, $P =$ .051) with tirofiban.[292]

Based on studies showing a beneficial effect of abciximab on the microcirculation level, the efficacy of direct intracoronary GPI was also tested. The Comparison of Intracoronary Versus Intravenous Abciximab Administration During Emergency Reperfusion of ST-Segment Elevation Myocardial Infarction (CICERO) study randomized 534 patients with STEMI to intravenous or intracoronary abciximab infusion.[293] In this trial, intracoronary administration of abciximab did not improve myocardial reperfusion as assessed by ST-segment resolution (the primary end point); however, it improved myocardial reperfusion as assessed by myocardial blush and reduced the enzymatic infarct size compared with intravenous administration. The Abciximab Intracoronary versus intravenous Drug Application in ST-Elevation Myocardial Infarction trial (AIDA STEMI) randomized 2065 patients to intracoronary abciximab ($n = 1032$) or intravenous abciximab ($n = 1033$). The primary end point was a composite of all-cause mortality, recurrent infarction, or new congestive heart failure within 90 days of randomization. Intracoronary, as compared with intravenous abciximab, resulted in a similar rate of the primary end point (7.0% vs. 7.6%; OR = 0.91 [0.64 to 1.28]; $P =$ .58.). The incidence of death (4.5% vs. 3.6%, $P =$ .36) and reinfarction (1.8% vs. 1.8%, $P =$ .99) did not differ significantly among patients in both treatment groups. However, less patients in the intracoronary abciximab group had new congestive heart failure (2.4% vs. 4.1%, $P =$ .04). The study concluded that in patients with STEMI undergoing PPCI, intracoronary as compared to intravenous abciximab did not result in a difference in the combined end point of death, reinfarction, or congestive heart failure.[294] The recently published CMR substudy of the AIDA STEMI did not show a benefit of intracoronary abciximab compared with intravenous abciximab in myocardial damage and/or reperfusion injury.[295] A 2011 meta-analysis of 10 randomized trials with 1590 patients showed that intracoronary GPI had favorable effects on TIMI flow, target-vessel revascularization, and short-term mortality after PCI with no difference in rates of bleeding compared with intravenous use of these agents.[296] Prehospital routine upstream use of GPI compared with the use in the catheterization laboratory offered no advantages but increased the risk of bleeding.[115,292] Moreover, a combination with unfractionated heparin did not have advantages compared

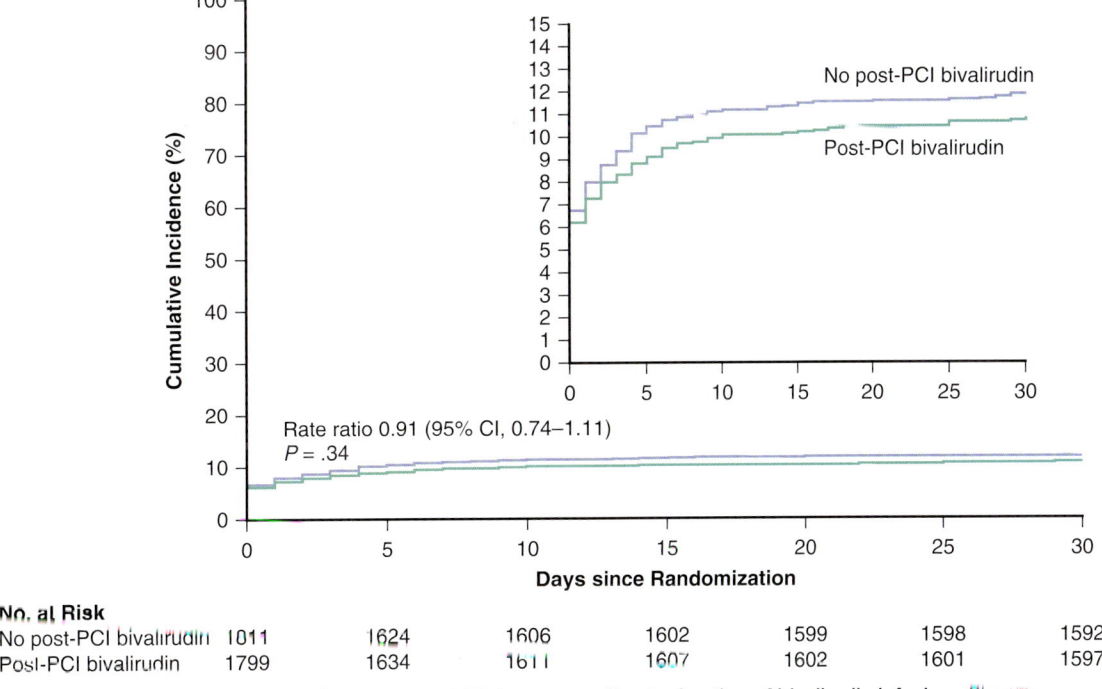

Fig. 20.19 Primary composite outcome at 30 days, according to duration of bivalirudin infusion. Shown is the cumulative incidence of the primary outcome for the treatment-duration subgroup of patients who were randomly assigned to receive an infusion of bivalirudin after percutaneous coronary intervention (PCI), as compared with those who were assigned not to receive a post-PCI infusion, which was a composite of urgent target-vessel revascularization, definite stent thrombosis, or net adverse clinical events up to 30 days. The inset shows the same data on an enlarged y axis. CI, Confidence interval. (From Valgimigli M, Frigoli E, Leonardi S, et al. Bivalirudin or unfractionated heparin in acute coronary syndromes. N Engl J Med. 2015;373[11]:997–1009.)

with bivalirudin.[275] Intracoronary abciximab may improve the efficacy of PPCI in diabetic patients with STEMI compared with the intravenous bolus.[297]

In aggregate, these studies showed that the role of GPI in the current practice of PPCI is markedly reduced due to availability of potent antiplatelet inhibitors. The use of GPI should be considered in the presence of no reflow or thrombotic complications during PPCI procedures (class 2a, level of evidence: C).[9]

THERAPIES TO REDUCE MICROVASCULAR OBSTRUCTION, REPERFUSION INJURY, AND INFARCT SIZE

MVO and no-reflow are frequent adverse events in patients with STEMI treated with PPCI and their presence is associated with reduced myocardial salvage, increased infarct size, impaired left ventricular function, and increased risk of short- and long-term mortality.[298] MVO is diagnosed immediately after PPCI by coronary angiography (a TIMI flow grade <3, or a TIMI flow grade of 3 with a myocardial blush grade ≤1), late gadolinium enhancement CMR, contrast echocardiography, scintigraphy, or positron emission tomography imaging. Although timely reperfusion is the most effective way of reducing infarct size, reperfusion per se may cause myocardial cell death and contribute to infarct size through so-called reperfusion injury. Although there are no tools to prove the existence or quantify reperfusion injury in clinical setting, on the basis of experimental studies, it is thought that reperfusion injury-related cell death contributes to almost 50% of final infarct size.[299] A brief description of events leading to reperfusion injury is summarized in Fig. 20.20.[300] Over the years various nonpharmacological (discussed earlier in this chapter) or pharmacological strategies have been used as adjunct therapy to PPCI to alleviate MVO or reperfusion injury and enhance myocardial salvage and improve the outcome in patients with STEMI.[10,300]

Pharmacological interventions to reduce myocardial injury during PPCI include a wide range of agents used to target a multitude of components involved in the genesis of reperfusion injury in patients with STEMI undergoing PPCI.[301] Encouraged by beneficial effects of bivalirudin on clinical outcome, the impact of the drug on infarct size compared to unfractionated heparin plus abciximab was investigated in a CMR substudy of the HORIZONS-AMI trial. Infarct size was not significantly different after treatment with bivalirudin compared with heparin plus abciximab either within 7 days (median: 9.3% vs. 20.0%, P = .28) or at 6 months (6.7% vs. 8.2%, P = .73).[302] In the Intracoronary Abciximab and Aspiration Thrombectomy in Patients

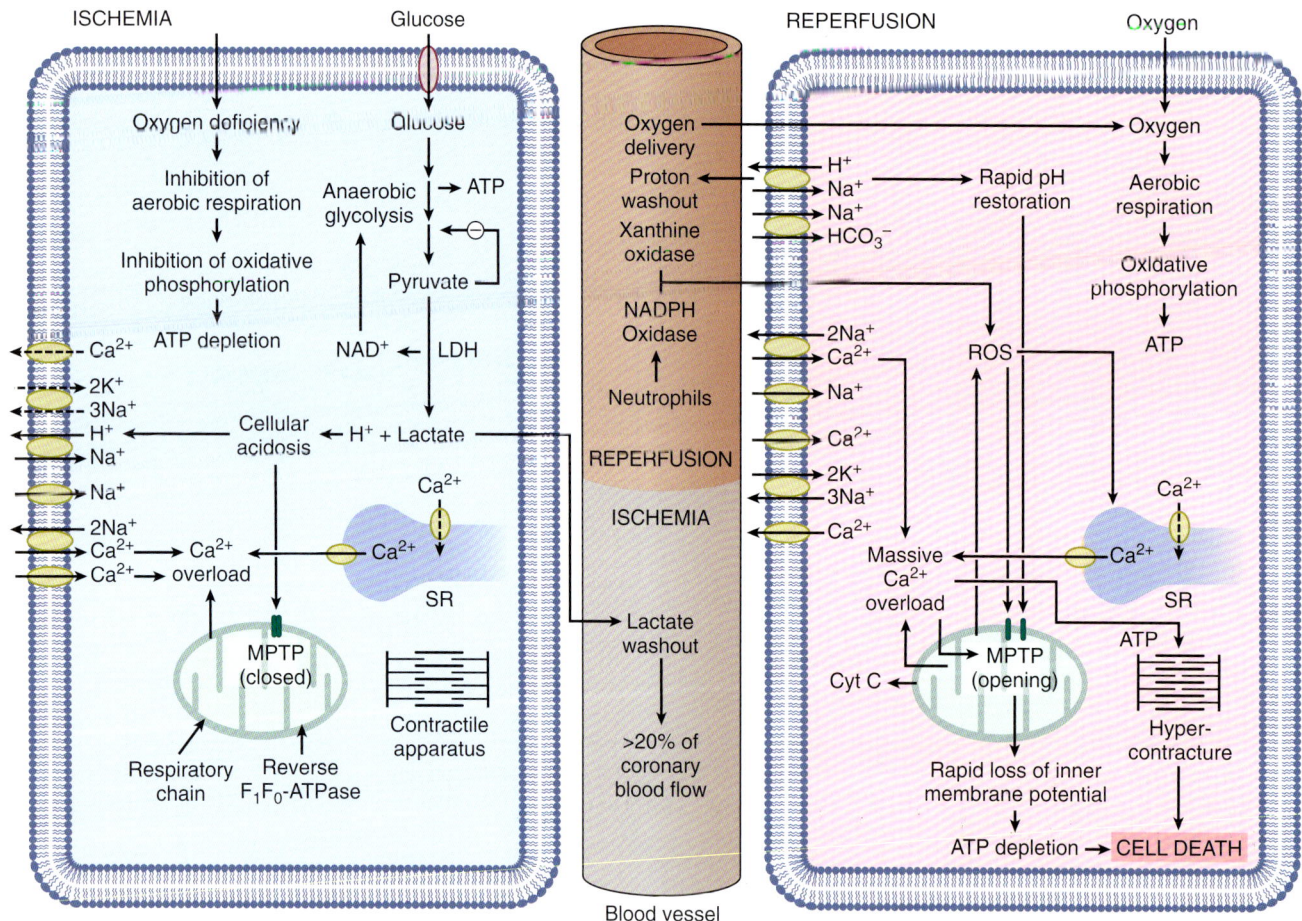

Fig. 20.20 Main metabolic events occurring during ischemia and reperfusion in cardiomyocytes. *Dashed arrows* show adenosine triphosphate *(ATP)*-dependent ionic pumps. *Cyt C,* Cytochrome C; *LDH,* lactate dehydrogenase; *MPTP,* mitochondrial permeability transition pore; *NAD,* nicotinamide adenine dinucleotide; *NADPH,* nicotinamide adenine dinucleotide phosphate; *ROS,* reactive oxygen species; *SR,* sarcoplasmic reticulum. (From Ndrepepa G, Colleran R, Kastrati A. Reperfusion injury in ST-segment elevation myocardial infarction: the final frontier. *Coron Artery Dis.* 2017;28[3]:253–262.)

With Large Anterior Myocardial Infarction (INFUSE-AMI) trial, patients randomized to intracoronary abciximab compared with no abciximab (aspiration thrombectomy was used in both arms) had a significant reduction in 30-day infarct size (median: 15.1% vs. 17.9%, P = .03).[302] In a small study of 39 patients with STEMI, upstream high-dose tirofiban did not reduce infarct size measured with CMR compared with conventional PPCI (mean: 21.1% vs. 25.2% of the left ventricle; P = .44), although tirofiban improved pre-PCI TIMI flow grade 2 to 3.[303] It has been demonstrated that aspirin[304] and clodidogrel[305] and prasugrel[306] reduce infarct size. These drugs are routinely used during PPCI procedures.

Over the last three decades a large number of pharmacological agents or therapeutic strategies have been used to reduce MVO, reperfusion injury, and infarct size and boost myocardial salvage during PPCI in patients with STEMI. Apart from antiplatelet and anticoagulant drugs used during routine PPCI procedures, the following drugs (or drug classes) have been tested: statins, angiotensin-converting enzyme inhibitors, calcium channel antagonists, β-blocking agents, antioxidants, neutrophil and complement system inhibitors, antidiabetic drugs, glucose–insulin–potassium infusion, antiischemic agents (like trimetazidine), inhibitors of mitochondrial permeability transition pore opening (like cyclosporine), nitric oxide donors, Na^+/H^+ ion exchanger inhibitors, Na^+/Ca^{2+} ion exchanger inhibitors, atrial natriuretic peptides, erythropoietin, adenosine, endothelin receptor inhibitors, protein kinase inhibitors, and therapeutic strategies of hypothermia, hyperoxemia, and ischemic conditioning.[301] Despite intensive research, no strategy or intervention has been shown to prevent reperfusion injury or enhance myocardial salvage and reduce infarct size in a consistent manner in the clinical setting. Among all pharmacological agents, adenosine, nitroprusside, β-blocking agents, and inhibitors of mitochondrial permeability transition pore opening have been considered as more promising drugs to alleviate MVO, reperfusion injury, and infarct size during PPCI.

Intracoronary and intravenous adenosine—a potent vasodilator of arterioles—has been tested as adjunctive therapy to PPCI in patients with STEMI. In experimental studies, adenosine reduces ischemia-reperfusion injury, limits infarct size, and improves left ventricular function. However, most of the recent research on the use of adenosine as adjunctive to PPCI was disappointing. A recent randomized study of intracoronary adenosine found no evidence that selective high-dose intracoronary administration of adenosine distal to the occlusion site of the culprit lesion in STEMI patients results in incremental myocardial salvage or a decrease in MVO.[307] The REperfusion Facilitated by LOcal adjunctive therapy in STEMI (REFLO-STEMI) trial did not find a significant difference in infarct size (assessed by CMR) or MVO in patients assigned to intracoronary high-dose adenosine, sodium nitroprusside, or controls. On per-protocol analysis, infarct size and the rate of 6-month MACEs were increased by intracoronary adenosine compared with control.[308] Recent meta-analyses have suggested an improvement in some markers of reperfusion, reduced risk of congestive heart failure but no impact on all-cause mortality or MI after PPCI by intracoronary adenosine.[309–311] Based on these results, there is no clear benefit with use of adenosine as adjunctive to PPCI.

Sodium nitrite—a selective nitric oxide donor—has multiple vascular functions including arteriolar vasodilatation, platelet inhibition, and antiinflammatory actions. Sodium nitrite was shown to markedly reduce infarct size in experimental settings and the agent is under investigation as a protective agent against reperfusion injury in the clinical setting. The recently published Nitrites in Acute Myocardial Infarction (NIAMI) trial—a randomized placebo-controlled study—did not demonstrate a reduction in infarct size (measured with CMR at 6 to 8 days and at 6 months) by sodium nitrite administered intravenously immediately prior to reperfusion in patients with acute STEMI.[312] In another recent study of 240 patients with STEMI with pre-PCI TIMI flow grade 0/1 undergoing PPCI and thrombus aspiration and randomized to receive adenosine, nitroprusside, or saline, ST-segment resolution greater than 70% was observed in 71% of patients assigned to adenosine, 54% of patients assigned to nitroprusside, and 51% of patients assigned to saline (P = .009 and 0.75 for adenosine versus saline and nitroprusside vs. saline, respectively).[313]

The impact of peri-PPCI β-blockade on infarct size remains controversial. The Effect of Metoprolol in Cardioprotection During an Acute Myocardial Infarction (METOCARD-CNIC) trial investigated whether early pre-reperfusion intravenous β-blocker therapy (up to three 5-mg intravenous boluses of metoprolol tartrate 2 minutes apart) reduces infarct size in 270 patients with STEMI of the anterior wall presenting within 6 hours from symptom onset. The primary end point was infarct size estimated by CMR. Infarct size calculated either in grams of infarcted tissue (25.6 ± 15.3 vs. 32.0 ± 21.2 g; P = .013) or as a percentage of the left ventricle (21.2 ± 11.5% vs. 25.1 ± 13.9% of the left ventricle; P = .029) was significantly reduced by metoprolol. Of note, 34.9% of the initial myocardial area at risk was salvaged in the metoprolol group compared with 27.7% in the control group (P = .028).[314] The left ventricular ejection fraction was slightly but significantly higher in the metoprolol group. However, the recently published Early-β blocker Administration before reperfusion primary PCI in patients with ST-elevation Myocardial Infarction (EARLY-BAMI) trial dampened the enthusiasm with respect to the use of β-blocking agents to boost myocardial salvage during PPCI. The trial randomized 683 patients with STEMI presenting within the first 12 hours in Killip class I to II without atrioventricular block to receive intravenous metoprolol (2 × 5 mg bolus) or placebo. The primary end point was infarct size assessed by CMR at 30 days. CMR was performed in 342 patients (54.8%). Infarct size (percent of left ventricle by CMR) did not differ between the metoprolol (15.3 ± 11.0%) and placebo groups (14.9 ± 11.5%; P = .616). Left ventricular ejection fraction by CMR was 51.0 ± 10.9% in the metoprolol group and 51.6 ± 10.8% in the placebo group (P = .68). The incidence of adverse events was not different between groups.[315]

Based on the central role of mitochondrial permeability transition pore in the cascade of events leading to reperfusion injury and cell death during ischemia/reperfusion, its inhibitors were considered very promising drugs to reduce reperfusion injury and infarct size during PPCI procedures. Cyclosporine A was the most commonly used inhibitor of mitochondrial permeability transition pore in experimental and clinical setting. The protective action of cyclosporine is hypothesized to involve reduced oxidative stress and calcium overload by inhibition of mitochondrial permeability transition pore opening preventing cell death (see Fig. 20.20). A small randomized trial of cyclosporine gave promising results in terms of reduced infarct size (assessed by creatine kinase or CMR) by the agent.[316] However, the recently published and larger randomized trials of cyclosporine did not confirm these results. The Does Cyclosporine Improve Clinical Outcome in ST Elevation Myocardial Infarction Patients (CIRCUS) trial randomized 970 patients with an anterior STEMI undergoing PPCI within 12 hours from the symptom onset and who had complete occlusion of the culprit coronary artery to receive a bolus injection of cyclosporine (administered intravenously at a dose of 2.5 mg per kilogram of body weight) or matching placebo before coronary recanalization. The primary outcome was a composite of death from any cause, worsening of heart failure during the initial hospitalization, rehospitalization for heart failure, or adverse left ventricular remodeling at 1 year. The rate of the primary outcome was 59.0% in the cyclosporine group and 58.1% in the control group (OR = 1.04 [0.78 to 1.39]; P = .77). Cyclosporine did not reduce the incidence of the separate clinical components of the primary outcome or other events, including recurrent infarction, unstable angina, and stroke. No significant difference in the safety profile was observed between the two treatment groups. The study showed that intravenous cyclosporine did not result in better clinical outcomes than those with placebo and did not prevent adverse left ventricular remodeling at 1 year.[317] The CYCLosporinE A in Reperfused Acute Myocardial Infarction (CYCLE) trial randomly assigned 410 patients, with large ST-segment elevation MI within 6 hours of symptom onset, a baseline TIMI flow grade of 0 to 1 in the IRA, and committed to PPCI to 2.5 mg/kg intravenous cyclosporine A ($n = 207$) or control ($n = 203$). The primary end point was incidence of ≥70% ST-segment resolution 60 minutes after TIMI flow grade 3. Secondary end points included high-sensitivity cardiac troponin T on day 4, left ventricular remodeling, and clinical events at 6-month follow-up. ST-segment resolution ≥70% was found in 52.0% of patients who received cyclosporine and 49.0% of controls ($P = .55$). Median high-sensitivity cardiac troponin T on day 4 was 2160 ng/L in cyclosporine A group and 2068 ng/L in controls ($P = .85$). The left ventricular ejection fraction at day 4 or 6 months did not differ in patients with cyclosporine or controls. Six-month mortality was 5.7% in cyclosporine group and 3.2% in controls ($P = .17$). The study concluded that a single intravenous cyclosporine bolus before PPCI had no effect on ST-segment resolution, high-sensitivity cardiac troponin T (an estimate of infarct size) and the drug did not improve clinical outcomes or left ventricular remodeling up to 6 months.[318] In out-of-hospital cardiac arrest patients presenting with nonshockable cardiac rhythm, intravenous bolus injection of cyclosporine, 2.5 mg/kg, at the onset of advanced cardiovascular life support did not prevent early multiple organ failure.[319]

Based on the hypothesis that hyperoxemia reduces formation of lipid peroxide radicals, alters nitric oxide synthase expression, and inhibits leukocyte adherence and plugging in the microcirculation,[320] this approach has been tested to reduce infarct size during PPCI procedures. However, the evidence is limited and the data are inconsistent. The Acute Myocardial Infarction with Hyperoxemic Therapy (AMIHOT) trial randomized patients with acute MI within 24 hours after primary stenting to intracoronary hyperoxemic reperfusion with aqueous oxygen or control.[321] Although the hyperoxemic reperfusion was safe and well-tolerated, it did not impart improvement in ST-segment resolution, regional wall motion by serial echocardiography, or reduction in SPECT infarct size. In post hoc analysis, however, patients with anterior MI reperfused <6 hours showed a greater improvement in regional wall motion and smaller infarct size (9.0% vs. 23% of the left ventricle; $P = .03$) with hyperoxemic reperfusion. At 30 days, the incidence of MACE was similar between the control and aqueous oxygen groups (5.2% vs. 6.7%, $P = .62$). The AMIHOT-II trial which included 301 patients with STEMI of anterior wall showed that intracoronary delivery of supersaturated oxygen reduced scintigraphic infarct size (20% vs. 26.5%; adjusted $P = .03$) with noninferior rates of MACE at 30 days, compared with placebo.[322] A recent SWEDEHEART registry-based randomized trial showed that routine supplemental oxygen did not reduce 1-year all-cause mortality in patients presenting with suspected acute MI and an oxygen saturation of ≥90%.[323]

Hypothermia during ischemia may reduce metabolic demand and inflammatory response.[320] A reduction in infarct size by therapeutic hypothermia has been reported if applied at the beginning or during ischemia but not during (or after) the reperfusion.[324,325] A pooled analysis of two small randomized trials has shown that hypothermia was associated with a 24% relative reduction (mean ± standard error: 10.7 ± 1.3% vs. 14.1 ± 1.6%, $P = .049$) in the infarct size estimated by scintigraphy or CMR.[326] However, the Rapid Endovascular Catheter Core Cooling combined with cold saline as an Adjunct to Percutaneous Coronary Intervention For the Treatment of Acute Myocardial Infarction (CHILL-MI) trial did not show a significant reduction in the infarct size (as a percent of myocardium at risk) assessed by CMR at 4 ± 2 days.[327] The trial randomized 120 patients with STEMI (<6 hours) scheduled to undergo PPCI to hypothermia induced by the rapid infusion of 600 to 2000 mL cold saline and endovascular cooling or standard of care. Hypothermia was initiated before PCI and continued for 1 hour after reperfusion. Median infarct size/myocardium at risk was 40.5% in patients assigned to hypothermia versus 46.6% in the control group ($P = .15$). The incidence of heart failure was lower with hypothermia at 45 ± 15 days (3% vs. 14%, $P < .05$). Exploratory analysis of early anterior infarctions (0 to 4 hours) found a reduction in infarct size/myocardium at risk end point of 33% ($P < .05$). A recent randomized trial showed that peritoneal hypothermia is feasible and achieves rapid cooling with only a modest increase in treatment times but it is associated with increased rate of adverse events without reducing infarct size.[328] A recent meta-analysis of 6 randomized controlled trials with 819 patients with STEMI showed no benefit of hypothermia in preventing MACEs, all-cause mortality, new MI, heart failure/pulmonary edema, or infarct size. Hypothermia did not increase the risk of bleeding, ventricular arrhythmias, or bradycardias (safety end point).[329]

Ischemic postconditioning (transient episodes of deliberate ischemia/reperfusion caused by repetitive inflation/deflation of an occluding balloon in the IRA) has been demonstrated to reduce infarct size in experimental studies. In small randomized human studies, the impact of postconditioning on infarct size has been controversial. A small randomized study of 50 patients with STEMI showed that postconditioning reduced infarct size and myocardial edema estimated with CMR.[330] Conversely, another recent study that randomized 76 STEMI patients to standard PCI or postconditioning did not show a reduction in the infarct size estimated with delayed enhancement CMR. However, infarct size was significantly reduced by postconditioning in patients with large initial areas at risk ($P < .001$).[331] It has to be mentioned, however, that many additional studies that have used biochemical markers of necrosis have shown a reduction of infarct size by postconditioning. Another randomized trial did not show an impact of ischemic postconditioning on infarct size or secondary study outcomes, which included markers of necrosis, myocardial salvage, ejection fraction, and adverse cardiac events.[332] In addition, a meta-analysis of 15 trials showed no improvement in surrogate or clinical outcomes with ischemic postconditioning at 5 months following PPCI.[333] The Third Danish Study of Optimal Acute Treatment of Patients With ST Elevation Myocardial Infarction–Ischemic Postconditioning (DANAMI-3–iPOST) trial randomized 1234 patients with STEMI presenting within 12 hours from pain onset and a baseline TIMI flow grade of 0 to 1 to conventional PPCI with stent implantation or postconditioning performed as four repeated 30-second balloon occlusions followed by 30 seconds of reperfusion immediately after opening of the IRA and before stent implantation. The main study outcome was a combination of all-cause death and hospitalization for heart failure. Over a median of 38 months (interquartile range 24 to 58 months) the primary outcome occurred in 11.2% of patients assigned to conventional PPCI and 10.5% of patients assigned to postconditioning (HR = 0.93 [0.66 to 1.30]; $P = .66$ for primary outcome; HR = 0.75 [0.49 to 1.14]; $P = .18$ for all-cause mortality and HR = 0.99 [0.60 to 1.64]; $P = .96$ for heart failure). The study showed that postconditioning failed to improve clinical outcome in patients with STEMI undergoing PPCI (Fig. 20.21).[334]

Remote ischemic conditioning, or repetitive cycles of ischemia in a tissue remote from the heart, has also been shown to significantly increase myocardial salvage when performed in patients with STEMI in the ambulance en route to a PPCI center.[335] Two recent meta-analyses have summarized the findings of the studies that have investigated remote postconditioning in patients with STEMI. One meta-analysis of 11 studies (nine randomized controlled trials) with a total of 1220 patients showed a higher myocardial salvage index (mean difference: 0.08) and reduced infarct size (mean difference: 2.46) with remote

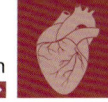

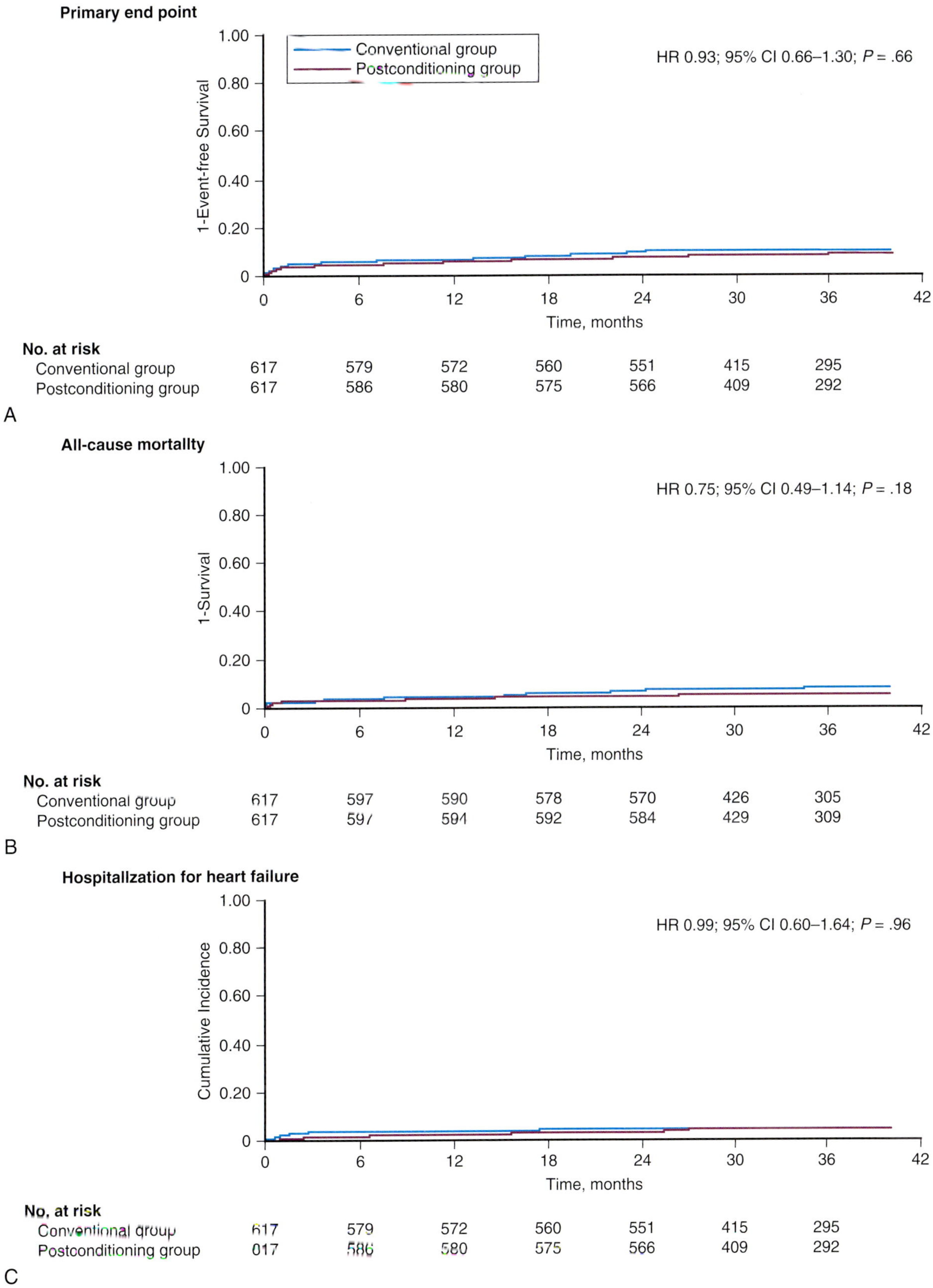

Fig. 20.21 Event rates in the Third Danish Study of Optimal Acute Treatment of Patients with ST Elevation Myocardial Infarction–Ischemic Postconditioning (DANAMI-3–iPOST) trial from the time of the primary percutaneous intervention to 40 months after the index treatment. (A) Combined primary outcome; (B) all cause mortality; and (C) hospitalization for heart failure. The Cox proportional hazards model was used to calculate hazard ratios *(HRs)*, 95% confidence intervals *(CIs)*, and *P* values. (From Engstrom T, Kelbaek H, Helqvist S, et al. Effect of ischemic postconditioning during primary percutaneous coronary intervention for patients with ST-segment elevation myocardial infarction: a randomized clinical trial. *JAMA Cardiol.* 2017;2[5]:490–497.)

postconditioning. MACEs were lower in patients who underwent remote postconditioning plus PCI versus the PCI alone group (9.5% vs. 17%; RR = 0.57 [0.40 to 0.82]).[336] The other meta-analysis of 8 trials with a total of 1083 patients showed that remote ischemic postconditioning was associated with reduced infarct size assessed by biomarker release, better rates of ST-segment resolution (54% vs. 30%; RR = 1.78 [1.35 to 2.34]; P < .001), and reduced major adverse cardiac and cerebrovascular events (11% vs. 20%; RR = 0.57 [0.39 to 0.83]; P = .003). However, infarct size estimated by cardiac imaging techniques was not reduced by remote ischemic conditioning.[337] Despite these results, the clinical benefit of postconditioning remains largely unexplored and additional high-quality research is required before a change in practice can be considered with respect to the use of this potential therapeutic modality in patients with STEMI undergoing PPCI.

In summary, although there is still interest in a variety of adjunctive pharmacological (or conditioning) interventions directed at enhancing myocardial reperfusion and reducing infarct size by limiting no-reflow, MVO, and reperfusion injury, available evidence is not strong enough to recommend any of these interventions for routine use as an adjunct to PPCI in patients with STEMI.

CELL-BASED THERAPY AND REGENERATIVE AGENTS AFTER ST-ELEVATION MYOCARDIAL INFARCTION

Reperfusion therapy has proven to be life-saving in patients with STEMI; however, progression of the disease toward chronic myocardial dysfunction still remains a real challenge. Due to insufficient regeneration of lost myocardial cells, intuitively, patients with STEMI may be considered as prime candidates for application of cell-based cardiac repair techniques to enhance myocardial recovery after MI by replacing lost cardiomyocytes. Animal studies of MI have reported that stem cell and progenitor cell transplantation has resulted in neoangiogenesis and myogenesis and improved contractile function. Although the exact mechanisms of the beneficial effect from stem cells remain unclear, a series of putative mechanisms have been proposed.[338]

A number of recent meta-analyses have summarized the results of these trials. One meta-analysis included 29 randomized controlled trials with 1830 patients.[339] The pooled analysis of trials showed that intracoronary bone marrow stem cell therapy resulted in an overall improvement in left ventricular ejection fraction of 2.70% ([1.48 to 3.92]; P < .001) in the short term and 3.31% ([1.87 to 4.75]; P < .001) over the longer term. The meta-regression suggested a dose–response relationship between quantity of CD34+ cells delivered and increase in the left ventricular ejection fraction (P = .007). Another recent meta-analysis of randomized trials has shown a sustained improvement in the left ventricular function and significant reductions in the rate of recurrent MI and readmission for heart failure in patients who received intracoronary cell therapy.[340] Along the same lines, another recent meta-analysis included 16 studies with 1641 patients (984 patients with intracoronary bone marrow cell therapy and 657 controls). The absolute improvement in the left ventricular ejection fraction was greater among cell-treated patients compared with controls (2.55% increase, [1.83–3.26]; P < .001). Treatment benefit in terms of left ventricular function improvement was more pronounced in younger patients (age <55 years: 3.38% vs. age ≥55 years: 1.77%, P = .03). Patients with left ventricular ejection fraction <40% derived more benefit from cell therapy than those with left ventricular ejection fraction ≥40% (5.30% increase vs. 1.45% increase, P < .001).[341] Timing of application of cell therapy was thought to be important. However, the Timing In Myocardial infarction Evaluation (TIME) trial showed that among patients with STEMI treated with PPCI, intracoronary bone marrow cells infused at either 3 days or 7 days after the event had no significant effect on recovery of global or regional left ventricular function compared with placebo.[342] A recent publication from the TIME trial showed that intracoronary bone marrow cells did not improve recovery of left ventricular function over 2 years.[343] The most recent meta-analysis that included 42 randomized controlled trials performed over 15 years with 3365 STEMI patients showed that bone marrow stem cell therapy did not significantly decrease mortality (risk ratio = 0.71 [0.45 to 1.11]). Bone marrow stem cell therapy had no effect on secondary outcomes of cardiac death, heart failure, arrhythmias, repeat MI, target-vessel revascularizations, health-related quality of life, left ventricular ejection fraction, or infarct size.[344]

The ability of granulocyte colony stimulating factor (G-CSF) to mobilize stem cells from bone marrow (CD34+ mononuclear blood stem cells) and to increase their circulating levels has led to its use (G-CSF injection) for stem cell mobilization in patients with STEMI and for harvesting stem cells for intracoronary delivery. Recent data with this agent has shown conflicting results. A meta-analysis of 10 randomized trials with 445 patients demonstrated no significant improvement of left ventricular ejection fraction in the groups treated with G-CSF injection versus placebo with a mean difference of 1.32% (P = .36), no significant difference in infarct size (P = .17), target-vessel revascularization rates, or mortality at follow-up.[345] A recent Cochrane review concluded that limited evidence from small trials suggests a lack of benefit of G-CSF therapy in patients with acute MI.[346] Based on source studies and on the results of these meta-analyses, G-CSF does not represent a useful therapy in patients with STEMI undergoing PCI.

Based on these data, the impact of cell therapy or agents used to mobilize stem cells form bone marrow on clinical outcome of patients with STEMI treated with PPCI remains largely unproven.

SPECIAL ISSUES IN PRIMARY PERCUTANEOUS CORONARY INTERVENTION

Out-of-Hospital Cardiac Arrest

Cardiac arrest is not an uncommon presentation of STEMI. Between 4% and 11% of PPCI procedures are performed in patients with STEMI after being resuscitated due to out-of-hospital cardiac arrest[72,347] and cardiac arrest is an independent predictor of in-hospital-mortality.[347] According to one study, of 714 patients presenting with out-of-hospital cardiac arrest, 435 patients had no obvious extracardiac causes of the condition and a significant coronary lesion was found in 304 of them (70%). STEMI was found in 134 patients (31%). The hospital survival rate was 40% and multivariable analysis showed that successful PCI was an independent correlate of improved survival (OR = 2.06 [1.16 to 3.66]). The study strongly recommended coronary angiography in patients presenting with out-of-hospital cardiac arrest and no obvious extracardiac cause.[348] In 2010, the International Liaison recommended that immediate angiography and subsequent PCI should be considered in patients with STEMI upon the return of spontaneous circulation after out-of-hospital cardiac arrest.[349] In the same vein, a consensus document from the European Association for Percutaneous Cardiovascular Interventions recommends immediate coronary angiography (within 2 hours) for all patients presenting with out-of-hospital cardiac arrest in the absence of an obvious noncoronary cause with immediate PCI if a culprit lesion is identified.[350] For comatose patients or those deeply sedated, mild therapeutic hypothermia is also recommended (target temperature between 32°C and 36°C for at least 24 hours).[9] In a recent study, 484 out of 4118 patients with STEMI (11.8%) had cardiac arrest. The overall in-hospital mortality in patients with cardiac arrest was 20.5%. Those sustaining cardiac arrest before ambulance arrival had the highest unadjusted mortality (29.7%) compared to those who had cardiac arrest after ambulance arrival (12.0%), in hospital (16.1%), and in the catheterization room (23.8%, $P = .03$). Multiple logistic regression analysis showed that age (OR = 1.05 [1.02 to 1.08]; $P = .0009$ for each year increment of age), female gender (OR = 2.42 [1.17 to 4.99]; $P = .0173$), previous PCI (OR = 7.59; [1.72 to 33.53]; $P = .0075$), asystole/electromechanical dissociation (OR = 13.43; [5.34 to 33.80]; $P < .0001$), and patient location at arrest (OR = 5.77 [2.55 to 13.07]; $P < .0001$ for before ambulance arrival) were independent correlates of in-hospital mortality.[351] According to a recent meta-analysis of 8 studies of patients with out-of-hospital cardiac arrest, early coronary angiography was associated with reduced short-term and long-term mortality and improved neurological outcome at discharge and over follow-up even in patients without ST-segment elevation.[352] Recent research suggests that although the use of coronary angiography and PCI in patients presenting with out-of-hospital cardiac arrest has increased, which parallels with an increasing trend in survival, a significant portion of these patients do not undergo coronary angiography and revascularization.[353] Regional systems and admission to invasive centers was also associated with improved survival of patients with out-of-hospital cardiac arrest.[354] Some studies have reported comparable 1-year survival rates in patients older than 65 years of age presenting with or without out-of-hospital cardiac arrest.[355] Current guidelines on the treatment of patients with STEMI recommend that immediate angiography and PCI should be performed in resuscitated patients whose initial electrocardiogram shows evidence of STEMI.[9]

Cardiogenic Shock

Cardiogenic shock occurs in approximately 6% to 10% of patients with STEMI.[356] Cardiogenic shock is not a mere decrease in cardiac contractile function, but also a multiorgan dysfunction syndrome (MODS) resulting from peripheral hypoperfusion with microcirculatory dysfunction, often complicated by a systemic inflammatory response syndrome (SIRS) and sepsis.[357] Cardiogenic shock is a serious complication and major cause of death in patients with STEMI. Despite use of acute revascularization and circulatory support devices, improved medical therapy, and significant advances in cardiac intensive care medicine, mortality attributed to shock in patients with STEMI remains at 40%.[357] In a recent survey that included 1,990,486 patients aged ≥40 years with STEMI from 2003 to 2010, cardiogenic shock occurred in 157,892 patients (7.9%). The overall incidence of cardiogenic shock increased from 6.5% in 2003 to 10.1% in 2010 ($P_{trend} < .001$). During the same time period, early mechanical revascularization rates (30.4% to 50.7%, $P_{trend} < .001$) and intraaortic balloon counterpulsation use (44.8% to 53.7%, $P_{trend} < .001$) also increased. In-hospital mortality decreased significantly (44.6% to 33.8% [$P_{trend} < .001$]; adjusted OR = 0.71 [0.68 to 0.75]). However, the average hospital costs increased from $35,892 to $45,625 ($P_{trend} < .001$) during the study period. There was no change in the average length of stay ($P_{trend} = .394$).[358] A recent survey of 5782 patients with an acute MI admitted to 11 hospitals in central Massachusetts (between 2001 and 2011) showed declines in the death rates associated with early and late cardiogenic shock but an increase in the deaths related to prehospital cardiogenic shock. Overall the shock frequency was 5.2%.[359]

Emergency revascularization by PPCI (if coronary anatomy is suitable) or by CABG surgery (if coronary anatomy is not suitable for PCI, or PCI has failed) is a class 1 recommendation in patients with STEMI who develop cardiogenic shock irrespective of time delay from STEMI onset.[8,9] The Should We Emergently Revascularize Occluded Coronaries for Cardiogenic Shock (SHOCK) trial was important in establishing the place of early mechanical reperfusion in patients with STEMI complicated by cardiogenic shock. The trial randomized 302 patients with acute MI complicated by cardiogenic shock to receive early revascularization (mostly PCI, $n = 152$) or initial medical stabilization ($n = 150$) treatment.[360] At 1 year of follow-up there was an absolute 13% difference in survival rates favoring patients assigned to early revascularization approach. This benefit in survival remained almost unchanged at 3 and 6 years of follow-up (13.1% and 13.2%, respectively). The 6-year survival rates for hospital survivors were 62.4% in those assigned to early revascularization and 44.4% in those assigned to initial medical stabilization with annual rates of death of 8.3% and 14.3%, respectively. For 1-year survivors, the annual rates of death were 8.0% versus 10.7%, again favoring patients assigned to early revascularization. The SHOCK trial demonstrated that almost two-thirds of hospital survivors with cardiogenic shock complicating acute MI who were treated with early revascularization survived a 6-year follow-up.[360] The trial strongly recommended early revascularization in patients with acute MI complicated by cardiogenic shock. The TRIUMPH (Tilarginine Acetate Injection in a Randomized International Study in Unstable MI Patients With Cardiogenic Shock) trial tested the impact of nitric oxide inhibition with tilarginine—a nitric oxide synthase inhibitor—in patients with STEMI who developed cardiogenic shock, 96% of them treated with PCI. The study randomized 398 patients to tilarginine (1-mg/kg bolus and 1-mg/kg/h 5 hours infusion) or placebo. The 30-day (48% vs. 42%, $P = .24$) and 6-month (58% vs. 59%, $P = .80$) all-cause mortality did not differ among patients assigned to tilarginine or placebo.[361] The study was terminated before completion for reasons of futility. Apart from failure of nitric oxide inhibition to improve outcome, the study showed that early mortality in patients with cardiogenic shock remains high despite recent advances in mechanical and pharmacological therapy.

The multivessel PCI has been performed in patients with STEMI and cardiogenic shock based on the belief (or limited evidence) that complete revascularization is advantageous to patients with STEMI and cardiogenic shock. However, the currently published Culprit Lesion Only PCI versus Multivessel PCI in Cardiogenic Shock (CULPRIT-SHOCK) gave a blow to this strategy.[362] The study randomized 706 patients who had multivessel disease, acute MI, and cardiogenic shock to a strategy of PCI of the culprit lesion only with the option of staged revascularization of nonculprit lesions or immediate multivessel PCI. The primary end point was a composite of death or severe renal failure leading to renal-replacement therapy (dialysis, hemofiltration, or hemodiafiltration) within 30 days after randomization. Safety end points included bleeding and stroke. At 30 days, the primary end point occurred in 45.9% of patients in the culprit-lesion-only PCI group and 55.4% of the patients in the multivessel PCI group (RR = 0.83 [0.71 to 0.96]; $P = .01$). The individual end points of death (RR = 0.84 [0.72 to 0.98]; $P = .03$) and renal replacement therapy (RR = 0.71 [0.49 to 1.03]; $P = .07$) were less frequent in patients assigned to culprit-lesion-only PCI (Fig. 20.22). The time to hemodynamic stabilization, the risk of catecholamine therapy and the duration of such therapy, the levels of troponin T and creatine kinase, and the rates of bleeding and stroke did not differ significantly between the two groups.[362] The current ESC guidelines (published before the CULPRIT-SHOCK trial) give a class IIa (level of evidence: C) for complete revascularization during the index procedure in patients with STEMI and cardiogenic shock.[9] Whether this recommendation will further be downgraded as a consequence of poor results of complete revascularization in the setting of the CULPRIT-SHOCK trial remain to be seen.

Despite weak evidence, until very recently intraaortic balloon counterpulsation has been a standard treatment in patients with STEMI complicated by cardiogenic shock. This therapeutic strategy offers mechanical support by left ventricular pressure

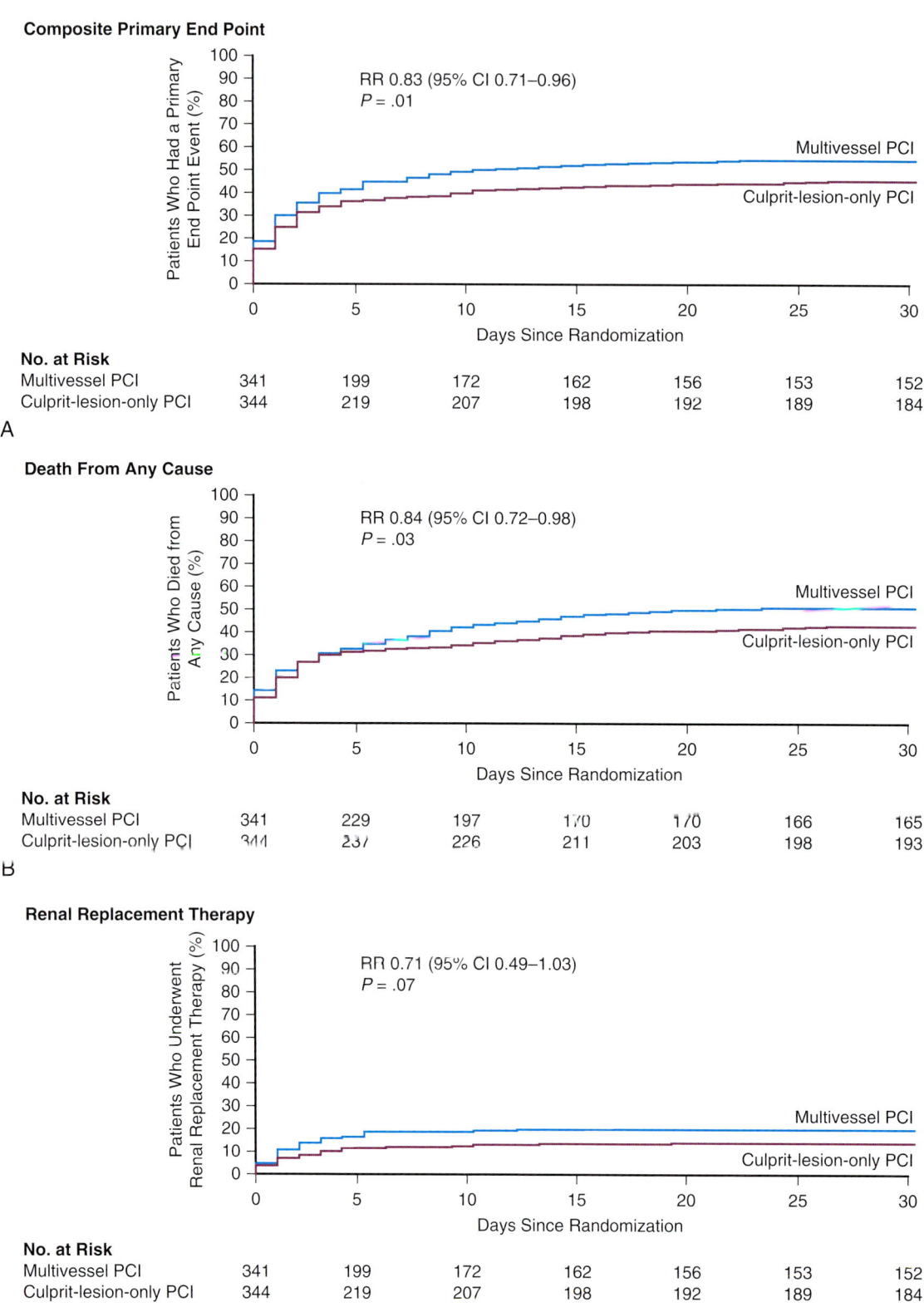

Fig. 20.22 Event rates of the primary end point and its components at 30 days. Shown are Kaplan–Meier time-to-event curves for the primary end point of a composite of death from any cause or severe renal failure leading to renal-replacement therapy (A), as well as the individual components of death from any cause (B) and renal replacement therapy (C), within 30 days after randomization. *CI*, Confidence interval; *PCI*, percutaneous coronary intervention; *RR*, relative risk. (From Thiele H, Akin I, Sandri M, et al. PCI strategies in patients with acute myocardial infarction and cardiogenic shock. *N Engl J Med.* 2017;377[25]:2419–2432.)

unloading. The Intraaortic Balloon Pump in cardiogenic shock II (IABP-SHOCK II) trial randomized 600 patients with STEMI complicated by cardiogenic shock undergoing early mechanical revascularization to intraaortic balloon pump counterpulsation (301 patients) or control (299 patients). All-cause mortality at 6 months (48.7% vs. 49.2%, P = .91) or 12 months (51.8% vs. 51.4%, P = .91) did not differ among patients assigned to intraaortic balloon counterpulsation or control. There were also no differences among patients assigned to intraaortic balloon counterpulsation or control regarding 12-month incidence of reinfarction (9% vs. 3%, P = .05), recurrent revascularization (20% vs. 22%, P = .77), or stroke (2% vs. 1%, P > .99). In general, data available are not strong enough in favor or against the use of intraaortic balloon pumping in patients with STEMI complicated by cardiogenic shock. A 6% increase in mortality by intraaortic balloon pumping in PCI trials has been reported.[363] Current guidelines give a class IIa (level of evidence: C) for the use of intraaortic balloon counterpulsation in patients with hemodynamic instability/cardiogenic shock due to mechanical complications but discourage routine use of this therapeutic modality in patients with cardiogenic shock (class III recommendation).[9] Apart from the intraaortic balloon counterpulsation, other devices provide mechanical support via left ventricular volume unloading (the Impella Recover LP micro-axial rotary pump or the TandemHeart), mechanical biventricular support (a combination of right ventricular circulator support using a modified TandemHeart and an Impella pump), or mechanical biventricular support with ECMO.[357] A recent small randomized study that compared percutaneous mechanical circulatory support device Impella (Impella CP, Abiomed, Danvers, MA) with intraaortic balloon counterpulsation with 24 patients with cardiogenic shock in each group showed no difference between the treatment arms in 30-day mortality (50% vs. 46%; HR = 0.96 [0.42 to 2.18]) or 6-month mortality (50% in each group; HR = 1.04 [0.47 to 2.32]).[364] Along the same lines, a recent meta-analysis of three rather small randomized trials showed no difference in mortality or left ventricular ejection fraction in patients with cardiogenic shock treated with Impella versus those treated with intraaortic balloon counterpulsation.[364]

Primary Percutaneous Coronary Intervention During Presentation Off-Hours

The relationship between time of day during which patients with STEMI present to the hospital and outcomes after PPCI has been assessed in several studies. This issue has been addressed in a 2014 meta-analysis and systematic review of 48 studies with fair quality with 1,896,859 patients. Of them, 36 studies reported mortality outcomes for 1,892,424 patients with acute MI, and 30 studies reported DTB times for 70,534 patients with STEMI. In patients with acute MI, off-hour presentation was associated with higher short-term mortality (OR = 1.06 [1.04 to 1.09]). Patients with STEMI presenting during off-hours were less likely to receive PCI within 90 minutes (OR = 0.40 [0.35 to 0.45]) and had longer DTB time by 14.8 (10.7 to 19.0) minutes. Apart from suggesting an association between the off-hour presentation and the increased risk of mortality, the meta-analysis also suggested that increased risk of mortality, at least partially, may be attributed to longer DTB times in patients with STEMI presenting off-hours.[365] The Mayo Clinic Percutaneous Coronary Intervention registry that included 3422 and 2664 patients with acute MI admitted during off-hours and regular hours, respectively, showed that patients admitted during off-hours were more likely to have STEMI (56% vs. 48%, P = .001), cardiogenic shock at presentation (6% vs. 4%, P = .002), and develop shock after presentation (6% vs. 5%, P = .004). After multivariable analyses, off-hour admission was not significantly associated with in-hospital mortality (OR = 1.12 [0.84 to 1.49]), 30-day mortality (OR = 1.12 [0.87 to 1.45]), or 30-day readmissions (OR = 1.01 [0.84 to 1.20]) but the composite end point of major complications and any of emergent CABG surgery, ventricular arrhythmia, stroke/transient ischemic attack, and gastrointestinal/retroperitoneal/intracranial bleeding was more frequent among patients with off-hours admission (OR = 1.27 [1.05 to 1.55]; P = .015).[366] More recent studies, however, suggest that differences in the outcome between STEMI patients admitted during off-hours (weekends, nights, and holidays) compared to those admitted during regular hours are attenuated or even abolished following regional systems of care for STEMI patients. The REAL (Registro Regionale Angioplastiche dell'Emilia-Romagna) registry assessed in-hospital and 1-year cardiac mortality among 3072 consecutive STEMI patients treated with PPCI in the setting of a regional STEMI network. The proportion of patients presenting off-hours was 53%. Patients presenting off-hours had longer pain-to-balloon (195 [140 to 285] minutes vs. 186 [130 to 280] minutes; P = .03) and DTB (88 [60 to 122] vs. 77 [48 to 116] minutes; P < .001). However, in-hospital (5.8% vs. 7.2%, P = .11) or 1-year mortality (8.4% vs. 10.3%, P = .08) did not differ significantly between patients presenting off-hours versus those presenting during regular hours. The findings remain consistent after adjustment in multivariable analysis for overall population or patients presenting to an interventional center. The study demonstrated that when PPCI is performed in the setting of an efficient regional STEMI network of reperfusion, the clinical effectiveness of PPCI performed either off-hours or regular hours is comparable.[367] This finding is congruent with recent studies that have shown no difference in the outcome of patients admitted during off-hours versus those admitted during regular hours, if PPCI is performed in the setting of STEMI networks of reperfusion.[368,369]

Primary Percutaneous Coronary Intervention in Elderly

Elderly patients represent an increasing proportion of patients admitted to hospital with STEMI and advanced age is an important correlate of poor outcome after both PCI and fibrinolysis. It is widely accepted that PPCI in elderly is more challenging for a variety of reasons, such as more complex coronary anatomy (multivessel disease, calcified and tortuous coronary arteries with lower rates of TIMI flow grade 3 postprocedure), increased rate of bleeding complications, increased rate of vascular complications due to a higher prevalence of peripheral vascular disease, increased prevalence of comorbidities such as impaired renal function predisposing to contrast nephropathy, delayed presentation, and atypical symptoms. The optimal management of patients with STEMI is still unclear, at least in part due to under-representation of elderly and very elderly patients in trials that have established the therapeutic value of PPCI. Interestingly the PCAT-2 pooled analysis reported that the absolute reduction of mortality with PPCI increased with advancing age, from 1% at an age <65 years to 6.9% at an age ≥85 years.[50] Three randomized trials have assessed the efficacy of PPCI in elderly. A small study that included 87 patients ≥75 years of age showed that PPCI was superior to fibrinolysis with streptokinase in reducing the composite end point of death, reinfarction, or stroke at 1 year (13% vs. 44%, P = .001).[370] In the Senior Primary Angioplasty in Myocardial Infarction (SENIOR PAMI) trial 481 patients ≥70 years of age were randomized between PCI and fibrinolysis. In patients 70 to 80 years of age, there was a trend toward reduced 30-day mortality with PPCI (7.1% vs. 11.3%, P = .17) and a significant reduction in the composite end point of death, reinfarction, or stroke (7.7% vs. 17.0%, P < .01) with PPCI compared to fibrinolysis. However, none of these end points differed between the two treatment options in patients >80 years of age.[371] The TRIANA (TRatamiento del Infarto Agudo de miocardio eN Ancianos, or Treatment of Acute Myocardial Infarction in the Elderly) study included 266 patients ≥75 years of age who were randomized to PPCI (134 patients) or fibrinolysis (132 patients). The trial reported a trend toward reduction in the 30-day composite end point of death, reinfarction, or disabling stroke with PPCI (18.9% vs. 25.4%, P = .21).[372] Nonsignificant reductions were found in the incidence of death (13.6% vs. 17.2%, P = .43), reinfarction (5.3% vs. 8.2%, P = .35), or disabling stroke (0.8% vs. 3.0%, P = .18). Recurrent ischemia was encountered less commonly in PPCI-treated patients (0.8% vs. 9.7%, P = .001). It is notable that both Senior-PAMI and TRIANA trials were terminated before completion due to slow recruitment. The findings of the individual trials were reinforced by a meta-analysis of all three studies.[372] The study strongly supported the use of PPCI in older patients with STEMI.

A survey from the 2001 to 2010 United States Nationwide Inpatient Sample (NIS) database reported temporal trends in STEMI, use of PCI for STEMI, and outcomes among patients aged 65 to 79 and ≥80 years. Among 4,017,367 patients aged ≥65 years with acute MI, 1,434,579 (35.7%) had STEMI. During the study period, in patients aged 65 to 79 and ≥80 years, STEMI decreased by 16.4% and 19%, respectively and the use of PCI for STEMI increased by 33.5% and 22%, respectively (P_{trend} < .001). There was a significant decrease in age-adjusted in-hospital mortality in patients aged ≥80 years (P_{trend} = 0.02) but not in patients aged 65 to 79 years (P_{trend} = .886). In multivariable analysis, intraaortic balloon pump use, acute renal failure, acute cerebrovascular disease, age ≥80 years, peripheral vascular disease, gastrointestinal bleeding, female gender, congestive heart failure, chronic lung disease, weekend admission, and multivessel PCI were independent correlates of increased in-hospital mortality among patients ≥65 years of age who underwent PCI for STEMI.[373] A recent study of 2225 STEMI patients ≥70 years (72.8% were ≥70 to 79 years of age and 27.2% were ≥80 years of age) admitted in the network of the International Registry of Acute Coronary Syndromes registry study in Transitional Countries (ISACS-TC) registry reported 30-day rates of mortality of 13.4% in patients ≥70 to 79 years of age and 23.9% in patients ≥80 years of age. Importantly PPCI was associated with reduced risk of mortality in patients ≥70 to 79 years of age (OR = 0.32 [0.24 to 0.43]) and in patients ≥80 years of age (OR = 0.45 [0.30 to 0.68]). The study showed that PPCI offers beneficial effects and should be performed in elderly patients with STEMI.[374]

The recently published Short Duration of Dual antiplatElet Therapy With SyNergy II Stent in Patients Older Than 75 Years Undergoing Percutaneous Coronary Revascularization (SENIOR) trial randomly assigned 1200 patients 75 years or older (127 patients with STEMI) to receive a DES or a similar BMS. The primary outcome was a composite of all-cause mortality, MI, stroke, or ischemia-driven target-lesion revascularization at 1 year in the intention-to-treat population. The primary end point occurred in 12% of patients in the DES group and 16% of patients in the BMS group (RR = 0.71 [0.52 to 0.94]; P = .022). Bleeding complications (5% vs. 5%) and stent thrombosis (1% vs. 1%) at 1 year did not differ between the groups. The study suggested that a strategy of combination of a DES to reduce the risk of subsequent repeat revascularizations with a short dual-platelet therapy regimen (similar to the strategy used after BMS implantation) to reduce the risk of bleeding event is an attractive option for elderly patients who have PCI.[375] A recent publication from a French registry that included 3389 elderly patients (≥75 years of age) with acute MI showed that early mortality after hospital admission decreased from 25.0% to 8.4% and 1-year mortality decreased from 36.2% to 20.0% (adjusted HR = 0.47 [0.39 to 0.57] for 2010 vs.1995; Fig. 20.23). The reduction in 1-year mortality was for STEMI (36.8% to 21.1%) and non-STEMI (34.8% to 19.1%).[376]

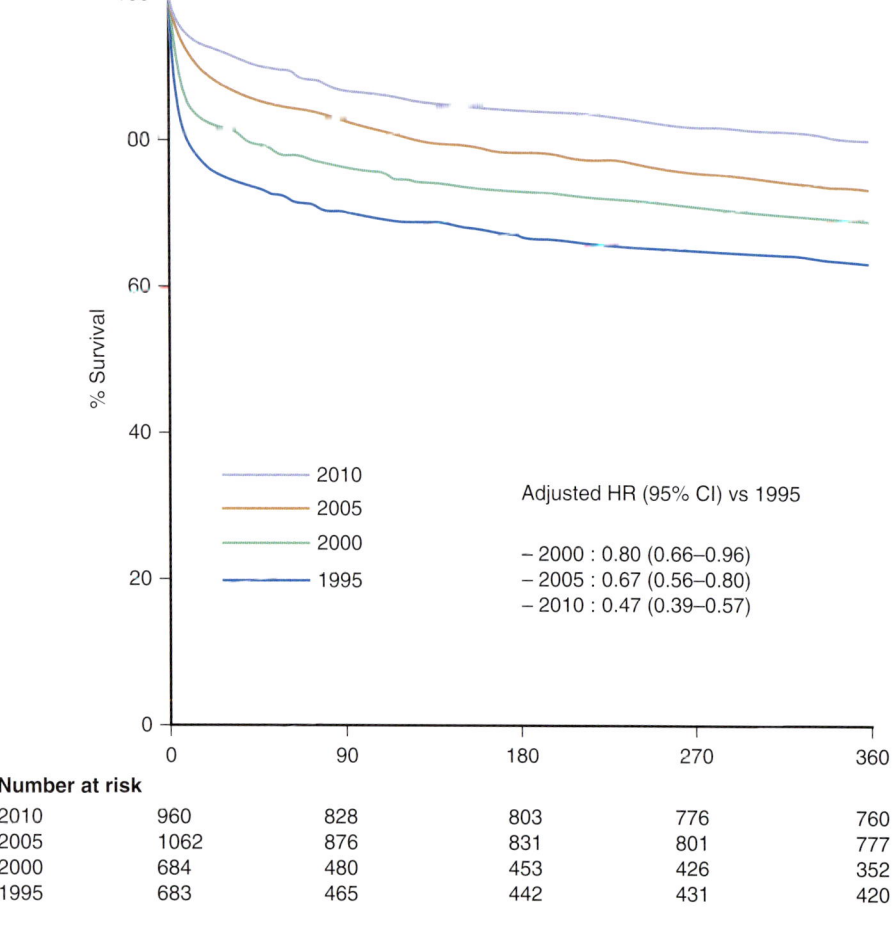

Fig. 20.23 One-year mortality in acute myocardial infarction in elderly patients (≥75 years of age). The survival curves are unadjusted, and the hazard ratios (HR) adjusted for baseline characteristics are provided with their 95% confidence intervals (CI). (From Puymirat E, Aissaoui N, Cayla G, et al. Changes in one-year mortality in elderly patients admitted with acute myocardial infarction in relation with early management. Am J Med. 2017;130:555–563)

Primary Percutaneous Coronary Intervention in Women

Numerous studies have demonstrated that mortality rates after acute MI are higher for women than men. Several factors have been linked with the poorer prognosis in women: older age; more comorbidities; higher prevalence of cardiovascular risk factors, including arterial hypertension, diabetes, and prior congestive heart failure; longer time-to-hospitalization interval; and undertreatment in the early phase of acute MI, with women less likely than men to undergo coronary angiography, PPCI, or CABG. Although there are no gender-based differences in the efficacy or indications to perform PPCI in patients with STEMI, there may be gender-based differences in the outcome after PPCI. A recent meta-analysis of 21 studies (between 2001 and 2013) comprising 47,439 men and 16,927 women showed that women were older (mean age: 67.9 vs. 61.0), were more likely to have diabetes (24% vs. 15%) and arterial hypertension (58% vs. 45%), and had longer symptom-to-balloon times (266 vs. 240 minutes) and less use of GPI (51% vs. 57%) than men. The in-hospital (8% vs .4%, $P < .001$), 30-day (8% vs. 6%, $P < .001$), and 1-year (12% vs. 8%) mortality was significantly higher in women than in men.[377] The increased risk of mortality following PPCI in women may be related to a disadvantageous risk profile and delayed presentation leading to a postponed treatment in women. Recent data from the National Cardiovascular Data Registry that included 102,515 patients showed that women had longer FMC-to-device time (80 [65 to 97] vs. 75 [61 to 90] minutes, $P < .001$) and a higher frequency of cardiogenic shock (5.8% vs. 4.0%, $P < .001$) and heart failure (5.8% vs. 3.4%, $P < .001$) and in-hospital mortality (4.1% vs. 2.0%, $P < .001$) than men.[378] The existence of these differences in mortality after PPCI should invigorate efforts to optimize reperfusion therapy and secondary prevention measures in women with STEMI.

Primary Percutaneous Coronary Intervention in Hospitals with and Without Onsite Coronary Artery Bypass Graft Surgery

The answer to the question whether PPCI should be performed only in hospitals with CABG or whether it should be expanded to hospitals without cardiac surgery is of importance because of the expanding number of hospitals performing PPCI and the potential for worse outcomes due to lower volumes and lack of cardiac surgery backup. Since seven studies and two meta-analyses of PPCI showed no difference for in-hospital or 30-day mortality between sites with and without on-site surgery, concerns about the risks of performing PPCI in centers without onsite surgery have abated.[379] A meta-analysis of PPCI studies for STEMI of 124,074 patients did not show an increase in in-hospital mortality in centers without versus centers with on-site surgery (4.6% vs. 7.2%; OR = 0.96 [0.88 to 1.05]). The meta-analysis showed that sites without on-site surgery had a lower occurrence of emergency CABG after PPCI (OR = 0.53 [0.35 to 0.79]).[380] Another meta-analysis identified nine PPCI studies (106,089 patients) and found no increase in in-hospital mortality (OR = 0.93 [0.83 to 1.05]) or early CABG (6.1% vs. 7.6%; OR = 0.87 [0.68 to 1.11]) in centers without on-site surgery compared with centers with on-site surgery.[381] The message from these studies is that PPCI can be performed in hospitals without cardiac surgery onsite.

CONCLUSION

Reperfusion therapies have dramatically improved prognosis and quality of life of patients with acute STEMI. PPCI is superior to thrombolytic therapy in reducing death, reinfarction, intracranial bleeding, reocclusion of the IRA, and myocardial ischemia in patients with STEMI irrespective of the patient's risk or whether interhospital transfer for PCI is required. Its advantages are conferred by the extremely low number of contraindications, high efficacy in patients presenting early or late after onset of symptoms, and low number of complications. Regional systems of care coordinating hospitals and EMS have reduced the time-to-reperfusion, increased the number of patients undergoing PPCI in timely manner, and may have improved survival of patients with STEMI. Advances in interventional techniques, the development of newer generations of DES, and newer antithrombotic drugs have enhanced the effectiveness of PPCI in patients with STEMI. In addition, PCI is very helpful not only after failed fibrinolysis but may also represent a valuable adjunct to initially successful pharmacological reperfusion in the setting of a pharmacoinvasive therapy. Although the proportion of patients with STEMI treated with PCI has been increasing steadily in recent years, major efforts are required to make this therapy available to all patients within a short time from symptom onset. Additional work is needed to develop new effective adjunct therapies able to promote further myocardial salvage by preventing or attenuating distal embolization, MVO, and reperfusion-related myocardial injury. Intensive experimental and clinical research aiming at myocardial cell regeneration is ongoing and offers new prospects for the improvement of prognosis and quality of life in patients with STEMI.

KEY REFERENCES

12. Keeley EC, Boura JA, Grines CL. Primary angioplasty versus intravenous thrombolytic therapy for acute myocardial infarction: a quantitative review of 23 randomised trials. *Lancet*. 2003;361(9351): 13–20.
24. Schomig A, Mehilli J, Antoniucci D, et al. Beyond 12 hours Reperfusion AlternatiVe Evaluation (BRAVE-2) Trial Investigators. Mechanical reperfusion in patients with acute myocardial infarction presenting more than 12 hours from symptom onset: a randomized controlled trial. *JAMA*. 2005;293(23):2865–2872.
50. Boersma E. Primary Coronary Angioplasty vs. Thrombolysis Group. Does time matter? A pooled analysis of randomized clinical trials comparing primary percutaneous coronary intervention and in-hospital fibrinolysis in acute myocardial infarction patients. *Eur Heart J*. 2006;27(7):779–788.
67. Menees DS, Peterson ED, Wang Y, et al. Door-to-balloon time and mortality among patients undergoing primary PCI. *N Engl J Med*. 2013;369(10):901–909.
70. Terkelsen CJ, Sorensen JT, Maeng M, et al. System delay and mortality among patients with STEMI treated with primary percutaneous coronary intervention. *JAMA*. 2010;304(7):763–771.
85. Jollis JG, Al-Khalidi HR, Roettig ML, et al. Regional systems of care demonstration project: American Heart Association Mission: Lifeline STEMI Systems Accelerator. *Circulation*. 2016;134(5): 365–374.
88. Jollis JG, Al-Khalidi HR, Roettig ML, et al. Impact of regionalization of ST-segment-elevation myocardial infarction care on treatment times and outcomes for emergency medical services transported patients presenting to hospitals with percutaneous coronary intervention: Mission: Lifeline Accelerator-2. *Circulation*. 2018;137:376–387.
95. Hochman JS, Lamas GA, Buller CE, et al. Coronary intervention for persistent occlusion after myocardial infarction. *N Engl J Med*. 2006;355(23):2395–2407.
115. Ellis SG, Tendera M, de Belder MA, et al. Facilitated PCI in patients with ST-elevation myocardial infarction. *N Engl J Med*. 2008;358(21):2205–2217.
121. Cantor WJ, Fitchett D, Borgundvaag B, et al. Routine early angioplasty after fibrinolysis for acute myocardial infarction. *N Engl J Med*. 2009;360(26):2705–2718.
125. Armstrong PW, Gershlick AH, Goldstein P, et al. Fibrinolysis or primary PCI in ST-segment elevation myocardial infarction. *N Engl J Med*. 2013;368(15):1379–1387.

144. Gershlick AH, Stephens-Lloyd A, Hughes S, et al. Rescue angioplasty after failed thrombolytic therapy for acute myocardial infarction. *N Engl J Med*. 2005;353(26):2758–2768.
152. Spaulding C, Henry P, Teiger E, et al. Sirolimus-eluting versus uncoated stents in acute myocardial infarction. *N Engl J Med*. 2006;355(11):1093–1104.
158. De Luca G, Dirksen MT, Spaulding C, et al. Drug-Eluting Stent in Primary Angioplasty (DESERT) Cooperation. Drug-eluting vs bare-metal stents in primary angioplasty: a pooled patient-level meta-analysis of randomized trials. *Arch Intern Med*. 2012;172(8):611–621; discussion 621-2.
203. Jolly SS, Yusuf S, Cairns J, et al. Radial versus femoral access for coronary angiography and intervention in patients with acute coronary syndromes (RIVAL): a randomised, parallel group, multicentre trial. *Lancet*. 2011;377(9775):1409–1420.
216. Wald DS, Morris JK, Wald NJ, et al. Randomized trial of preventive angioplasty in myocardial infarction. *N Engl J Med*. 2013;369(12):1115–1123.
218. Engstrom T, Kelbaek H, Helqvist S, et al. Complete revascularisation versus treatment of the culprit lesion only in patients with ST-segment elevation myocardial infarction and multivessel disease (DANAMI-3-PRIMULTI): an open-label, randomised controlled trial. *Lancet*. 2015;386(9994):665–671.
220. Smits PC, Abdel-Wahab M, Neumann FJ, et al. Fractional flow reserve-guided multivessel angioplasty in myocardial infarction. *N Engl J Med*. 2017;376(13):1234–1244.
224. Stone GW, Webb J, Cox DA, et al. Distal microcirculatory protection during percutaneous coronary intervention in acute ST-segment elevation myocardial infarction: a randomized controlled trial. *JAMA*. 2005;293(9):1063–1072.
230. Fröbert O, Lagerqvist B, Olivecrona GK, et al. Thrombus aspiration during ST-segment elevation myocardial infarction. *N Engl J Med*. 2013;369(17):1587–1597.
232. Jolly SS, Cairns JA, Yusuf S, et al. Randomized trial of primary PCI with or without routine manual thrombectomy. *N Engl J Med*. 2015;372(15):1389–1398.
258. Mehta SR, Tanguay JF, Eikelboom JW, et al. Double-dose versus standard-dose clopidogrel and high-dose versus low-dose aspirin in individuals undergoing percutaneous coronary intervention for acute coronary syndromes (CURRENT-OASIS 7): a randomised factorial trial. *Lancet*. 2010;376(9748):1233–1243.
260. Wiviott SD, Braunwald E, McCabe CH, et al. Prasugrel versus clopidogrel in patients with acute coronary syndromes. *N Engl J Med*. 2007;357(20):2001–2015.
265. Montalescot G, van 't Hof AW, Lapostolle F, et al. Prehospital ticagrelor in ST-segment elevation myocardial infarction. *N Engl J Med*. 2014;371(11):1016–1027.
275. Stone GW, Witzenbichler B, Guagliumi G, et al. Bivalirudin during primary PCI in acute myocardial infarction. *N Engl J Med*. 2008;358(21):2218–2230.
282. Valgimigli M, Frigoli E, Leonardi S, et al. Bivalirudin or unfractionated heparin in acute coronary syndromes. *N Engl J Med*. 2015;373(11):997–1009.
286. Montalescot G, Zeymer U, Silvain J, et al. Intravenous enoxaparin or unfractionated heparin in primary percutaneous coronary intervention for ST-elevation myocardial infarction: the international randomised open-label ATOLL trial. *Lancet*. 2011;378(9792):693–703.
362. Thiele H, Akin I, Sandri M, et al. PCI strategies in patients with acute myocardial infarction and cardiogenic shock. *N Engl J Med*. 2017;377(25):2419–2432.

 Additional references available online at expertconsult.com

中文导读

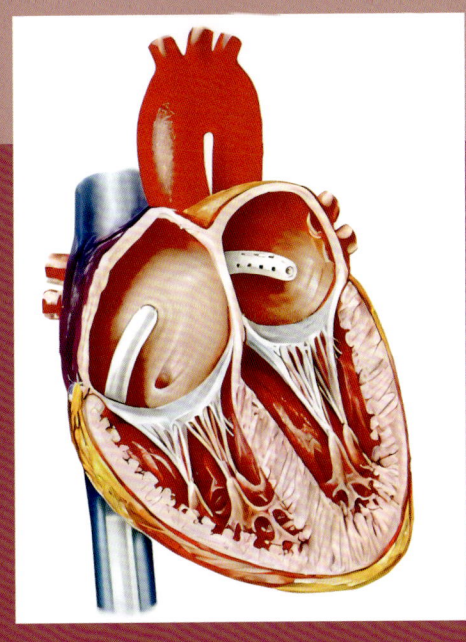

第21章
经皮冠状动脉介入术后的住院治疗、住院时长及出院计划

  经皮冠状动脉介入治疗是目前治疗缺血性心脏病的最常用手段。术后对患者进行长时间的监测，确保手术成功、提前识别并发症的发生是十分必要的。嘱患者卧床休息，遥测监测的同时，需要重点关注其穿刺部位的恢复情况。经皮冠状动脉介入治疗术后，仅建议对存在心肌梗死症状/体征或虽无症状但存在血管造影并发症的患者进行CK-MB或cTn值的检测，其余患者不建议常规检测。术后对血小板功能的检测缺乏临床获益的数据支持。随着诊疗技术、药理学和医疗程序的不断进步和创新，经皮冠状动脉介入治疗的安全性和有效性整体得到明显提高，新的技术显著减少了血管入路并发症和出血的风险。基于这些发展及支付结构的变化，术后患者总体住院时长较以前有明显的缩短。经选择无围术期或血管造影并发症的患者甚至可以在术后当日出院。这种术后当日出院的模式，不仅能提高患者的满意度，同时还可以节省临床医疗开支。但安全的术后当日出院模式，需要充足的术前评估、规范的手术操作及细致的术后管理。对患者出院后的随访计划和健康指导随之也应更加具体，应向患者提供伤口注意事项，以及关于体力活动、术后复查的明确指示。对于术后双联抗血小板的治疗及其他药物治疗方案的调整，也应在出院书面材料中注明。

  本章节较为全面地阐述了介入治疗术后管理、出院计划和指导、心脏生物标记物检测的作用及意义，并详尽介绍了"术后当日出院（一日病房）"这一医疗模式的发展趋势。

苗旭光 崔 松

章节要点

- 经皮冠状动脉介入治疗术后全面的出院管理是术后护理的重要组成部分，包括与患者的直接沟通、对手术或血管并发症的监测，以及通过具体的随访计划来进行出院后的指导。
- 药物调整尤其是经皮冠状动脉介入治疗术后的双联抗血小板治疗方案，对冠心病二级预防和预防晚期并发症而言至关重要。
- 经皮冠状动脉介入治疗术后对心脏生物标记物的检测尚有争议。尽管所有患者经皮冠状动脉介入治疗术后检测生物标记物都合理，但对于有冠状动脉造影并发症或症状、体征提示存在术后心肌缺血的患者，有必要并建议对其进行检测。
- 经皮冠状动脉介入治疗术后，常规进行血小板功能检测毫无作用。
- 由于技术、药物和手术的革新，以及来自于医疗费用支付方对医疗费用的控制压力，经皮冠状动脉介入治疗术后的总住院天数变得越来越短。这导致越来越多的人对术后当天出院模式产生了兴趣。
- 对于手术过程顺利且没有手术并发症的择期经皮冠状动脉介入治疗患者，术后当天出院可能是一个合理的选择。
- 术后当天出院可提高患者满意度，并节省可观的医疗成本，这主要归因于术后监测时间的缩短。

21 Post-Percutaneous Coronary Intervention Hospitalization, Length of Stay, and Discharge Planning

Amit N. Vora, Sunil V. Rao

KEY POINTS

- Comprehensive post-percutaneous coronary intervention (PCI) discharge management is an integral aspect of postprocedure care and includes direct patient communication, monitoring for procedural or vascular complications, and clear discharge instructions with a specific follow-up plan.
- Medication reconciliation, especially regarding dual antiplatelet therapy (DAPT) post-PCI, is critical for aggressive secondary prevention and to prevent late complications.
- Evaluation of cardiac biomarkers post-PCI is controversial. Although it is reasonable to check biomarkers in all patients post-PCI, it is necessary and recommended in patients with procedural angiographic complications or with signs or symptoms suggestive of postprocedure ischemia.
- There is no role for routine measurement of platelet function post-PCI.
- Overall length of stay following PCI has become shorter over time, a change attributable to technological, pharmacological, and procedural innovations but also to payer expectations. This has led to increasing interest in same-day discharge programs.
- Same-day discharge may be a reasonable option for elective PCI patients with no procedural complications and an uneventful postprocedure course.
- Same-day discharge is associated with improved patient satisfaction and considerable cost-savings, primarily attributed to the shorter duration of monitoring postprocedure.

INTRODUCTION

Percutaneous coronary intervention (PCI) is one of the most common procedures in the United States, performed approximately 500,000 times annually,[1] and remains a cornerstone in the management of ischemic heart disease. Historically, a large proportion of PCI procedures were performed during inpatient hospitalization, allowing for a significant amount of time for monitoring postprocedure to ensure procedural success and identify bleeding or vascular complications, as well as for initiating secondary prevention. However, technological, pharmacological, and procedural innovations, as well as payer expectations and cost considerations, have led to a shorter length of stay (LOS) postprocedure and obviated hospital admission. Most nonacute myocardial infarction (MI) PCIs performed in the United States now are performed under an outpatient designation, and this has led to differential risk profiles of PCI patients over time.[2] In this environment, many institutions have developed programs allowing for same-day discharge (SDD) of patients undergoing elective, uncomplicated PCI. As PCI performance measures track not only the proportion of patients discharged on guideline-recommended medical therapies but also post-PCI readmission rates, discharge planning has taken an increasingly important role not only to ensure safe, event-free discharge on appropriate guideline-recommended therapies but also to minimize hospital readmission. This chapter will focus on postprocedural management of patients undergoing PCI, with an emphasis on appropriate discharge planning and instructions, the role of cardiac biomarker testing, and the evolution of successful SDD programs.

POST-PERCUTANEOUS CORONARY INTERVENTION DISCHARGE PLANNING

Discharge planning following PCI should begin prior to the procedure, with an emphasis on gathering information regarding preprocedure activity levels, medication adherence, and patient social support at home. Postprocedure management focuses on: (1) access site management and monitoring for new ischemia and bleeding or vascular complications and (2) appropriate communication, both oral and written, between the provider team and the patient regarding procedural outcome, medication changes, and safety plan in the setting of an adverse event. The Society for Cardiovascular Angiography and Interventions (SCAI) has offered a consensus statement regarding postprocedure best practices following PCI.[3]

Physician-to-Patient Communication

The results of the procedure, including any complications and/or unexpected findings, should be explained clearly to the patient and his or her family. The type of intervention, if any, and the duration of DAPT should also be introduced and reinforced repeatedly by the team of care providers throughout the patient stay.

Access Site Management

Typically, manual compression, a compression device, and/or a vascular closure device (VCD) is used in patients following transfemoral access, whereas a wristband compression device is used most frequently among patients undergoing transradial (TR) access. For patients undergoing transfemoral access and anticoagulated with heparin, the access sheaths can generally be removed once the activated clotting time (ACT) falls below 175 seconds if a closure device is not used. The use of bivalirudin typically does not necessitate checking an ACT unless there is significant renal impairment (i.e., creatinine clearance <30 mL/min or hemodialysis); in that situation, sheaths may be removed once the ACT falls below 180 seconds. In patients without significant renal dysfunction, the femoral arterial sheath can be removed 2 hours after the discontinuation of the bivalirudin infusion if a closure device is not used.

Postprocedure Ambulation

The access site, method of hemostasis, intensity of procedure sedation, and anticoagulation strategy drive recommendations for activity immediately postprocedure. Patients undergoing TR catheterization may ambulate as soon as sedation wanes. For patients undergoing transfemoral catheterization and PCI, strict bed rest is typically recommended for 4 to 8 hours if manual compression is used or 1 to 4 hours if a VCD is used; prior to ambulation, a care provider must ensure that hemostasis is achieved and there is no diminution of downstream peripheral pulses.

Postprocedure Monitoring

Patients are generally monitored in a telemetry setting postprocedure, with monitoring of vital signs every 15 minutes for the first 2 hours by trained nursing personnel. Although most patients go home on the same day within 2 to 6 hours following diagnostic cardiac catheterization, there are varying lengths of monitoring following PCI, which will be discussed in greater detail below. Additionally, the role of laboratory testing post-PCI will be discussed below.

Discharge Physical Examination

Although a full physical examination is generally performed prior to discharge, additional focus should be directed to the patient's access site to ensure adequate hemostasis and perfusion. The access site should be auscultated to ensure no bruit, which may be concerning for a pseudoaneurysm or arteriovenous fistula, each of which requires additional testing to confirm, typically via ultrasound. Distal pulses should be palpated to ensure no decrease in downstream perfusion. Patients should also be able to demonstrate their baseline level of ambulation without difficulty and ensure pain is well controlled prior to consideration of discharge postprocedure.

Discharge Instructions

Patients should be provided with clear instructions regarding physical activity, follow-up, and the need for additional laboratory testing postprocedure. Discharge instructions should also have clear contact information for the recovery unit or the physician in case of complications following discharge. Additionally, discharge instructions should address the following concerns:

Site management: Patients should be advised that there may be minor bruising and/or pain at the access site, which should resolve within 1 month postprocedure. Patients undergoing transfemoral access should not strain or lift anything greater than 5 pounds for 48 hours postprocedure and should apply pressure to the access site when sneezing or coughing. Clear instructions for an action plan for access site complications, including active arterial bleeding, hematoma, erythema or purulence at the access site, or downstream neurologic symptoms such as numbness/tingling or paresthesia, should be provided.

Activity levels: Although important to maintain preprocedure activity levels, most patients are advised to refrain from physical exercise for at least 48 hours postprocedure. Patients undergoing PCI should be enrolled in a cardiac rehabilitation program postprocedure to develop a plan of graded exercise.

Driving and return to work: Most patients are advised to refrain from driving for at least 48 hours, if not 1 week, postprocedure. The decision to return to work is individualized and often is related to job satisfaction, financial stabilities, and/or company policies.[4] Recommendations regarding return to work also depend on the type of work the patient performs, including physical demands, mental stress, and safety considerations.

Sexual activity: Most patients are advised to refrain from sexual activity for 1 week postcardiac catheterization to allow for access site healing. Other recommendations are based on the patient's level of fitness. According to an American Heart Association (AHA) consensus statement,[5] sexual activity is reasonable for patients at low risk for cardiovascular complications or who can exercise for 3 to 5 metabolic equivalents (METs) without symptoms or electrocardiogram (ECG) changes. In previous studies of sudden cardiac death related to sexual activity, most patients who died during intercourse were men (82% to 93%) who participated in extramarital sexual activity (75%), typically with a younger partner, after excessive food and alcohol consumption.[6,7] A recent analysis of 536 patients with incident MI reported that only 3 patients (0.7%) reported sexual activity in the hour prior to the MI and 1.5% in the 3 to 6 hours prior.[8]

Medication Reconciliation

Medication reconciliation is a critical aspect of postprocedure discharge planning and major changes are typically reinforced at multiple instances during the patient stay by trained personnel, which may include physicians, nurses, trainees, or pharmacists. Barring specific contraindications, many patients undergoing PCI will be on dual antiplatelet therapy (DAPT) with aspirin and an additional platelet inhibitor (currently available agents are $P2Y_{12}$ antagonists), a β-blocker, an angiotensin converting enzyme (ACE) inhibitor, and a high-intensity statin.[9-11] Patients should be provided with clear instructions regarding which medications should be stopped, which medications have changed in dosage, and which medications they should begin to take postprocedure. Recommendations for postprocedure DAPT should be clearly stated on the discharge paperwork, and given the critical nature of uninterrupted therapy, a clear plan should be outlined for the patient to obtain the antiplatelet as an outpatient. SCAI has recommended that diabetic patients should withhold their metformin for 48 hours postprocedure. Patients previously on warfarin who have stopped it for the procedure should be restarted on their regimen and have an international normalized ratio (INR) value checked within 1 week postprocedure to ensure a therapeutic range. No consensus guidelines have been provided for the novel oral anticoagulants (NOACs), but they are generally started postprocedure as hemostasis is achieved and do not require close monitoring.

Communication to Referring Physician

An appropriate transition of care from the invasive cardiologist to the primary cardiologist or referring physician is also an integral component of postprocedure care. This communication is typically performed verbally as well as in the form of a procedure note clearly identifying the indications for the procedure, the diagnostic findings, interventions performed, and plan for postprocedure management.

TABLE 21.1 Checklist for Discharge

Physician-to-patient communication
- Operator has spoken to the patient or patient representative and described the procedure and complications or unexpected findings, if any.

Postprocedure monitoring
- No signs of symptoms of new ischemia
- No new abnormalities on telemetry or electrocardiogram
- Patient able to ambulate without difficulty
- Patient able to tolerate food

Access site management
- Hemostasis achieved
- No significant pain/tenderness at site
- No bruit or thrill
- Intact distal pulses

Medication reconciliation
- Plan for dual antiplatelet therapy reviewed
- Other medications reviewed and reconciled

Follow-up
- Follow-up scheduled
- Follow-up labs

Follow-Up

SCAI has recommended that the patient follow up with his or her primary care physician, cardiologist, or midlevel physician extender within 2 to 4 weeks postprocedure, or sooner for patients with procedural complications or comorbidities such as anemia or renal dysfunction requiring more frequent laboratory test monitoring. The purpose of this follow-up visit is to: (a) ensure compliance with the medication regimen, especially with regard to DAPT; (b) reconcile medications to ensure that the medication changes upon discharge have been followed; (c) reinforce aggressive secondary prevention measures, including dietary and exercise habits and smoking cessation; and (d) confirm that the patient has enrolled in a cardiac rehabilitation program.

A sample discharge checklist is provided in Table 21.1.

THE ROLE OF POST-PERCUTANEOUS CORONARY INTERVENTION MONITORING OF CARDIAC BIOMARKERS, PLATELET INHIBITION, AND RENAL FUNCTION

The purpose of checking cardiac biomarkers after a PCI procedure is to assess for evidence of periprocedural myocardial damage. Historically, cardiac biomarkers had been checked serially every 8 to 12 hours postprocedure. However, the routine measurement of cardiac biomarkers post-PCI is controversial because the clinical implications and prognostic significance of an elevated biomarker level in the absence of angiographic complications or signs and symptoms of a new acute MI are unclear. In this setting, ascribing significant importance to biomarker elevation in the absence of clear evidence of adverse clinical outcomes may lead to a longer hospital LOS and may subject the patient to unnecessary evaluation and testing, increasing the potential for iatrogenic complications. As hospital LOS is decreasing, there is increasing tension regarding the role of routine biomarker testing post-PCI.

Traditionally, creatine kinase-muscle/brain (CK-MB) levels were checked routinely post-PCI; now, at some institutions, there has been a transition to cardiac troponin (cTn), a much more sensitive and specific biomarker able to detect even small amounts of myocardial damage. Unsurprisingly, rates of detection of myocardial injury have risen using the more sensitive assay. In one series of 4930 patients undergoing elective PCI, Novack et al. report that only 7.2% of patients had CK-MB levels of ≥3 × upper limit of normal (ULN) but 24.3% had cTn levels ≥3 × ULN.[12] Previous studies have noted an association between elevated biomarkers postprocedure and mortality, but it is unclear whether this is an epiphenomenon, due primarily to the extent of complex coronary disease and not necessarily to the actual procedure.[13] The importance of relatively small biomarker increases is uncertain. In a series of 5850 patients, Jeremias et al. report an association between periprocedural MI and 1-year mortality, but only in patients with CK-MB greater than eight times normal or with a Q-wave MI.[14] Additionally, that study questioned the importance of biomarker elevations postprocedure in the absence of an angiographically evident complication.

In 2007, the first proposed universal definition for myocardial infarction[15] proposed that a peri-PCI MI (type 4a) was defined as a biomarker elevation of ≥3 × the 99th percentile of the upper reference limit (URL) in patients with normal biomarker levels preprocedure. However, the authors clearly note that this designation was by arbitrary convention in the absence of clear data. In the third universal definition for MI,[16] this was further refined to greater than 5 × URL of the cTn and evidence of: (a) prolonged ischemia (chest pain >20 minutes), (b) ischemic ECG changes or pathologic Q-waves, or (c) angiographic evidence of a flow-limiting complication (i.e., loss of side branch, no-reflow, embolization), or (d) imaging evidence of loss of viable myocardium.

In this setting, a consensus statement from SCAI[17] suggests that a clinically relevant MI after coronary revascularization be defined as an MI resulting in a CK-MB elevation of ≥10 × ULN, with a lower threshold of ≥5 × ULN in patients with new pathologic Q-waves post-MI; the ratio of cTn to CK-MB should be 7:1 (i.e., a clinically relevant MI would be ≥70 × ULN using a cTn assay) if a CK-MB assay is unavailable. For patients with elevated baseline CK-MB or cTn levels that are stable or decreasing, the elevation should rise by an absolute increment to those described above. For patients with elevated CK-MB or cTn levels that are increasing, the elevation should rise by an absolute increment, but additionally there should be new ECG or clinical signs concerning for a clinically relevant MI (new heart failure or hypotension). Table 21.2 describes the evolution of the definition of a peri-PCI MI, incorporating the proposed definition of a clinically relevant MI.

The current PCI guidelines recommend measurement of a CK-MB or cTn value for patients with signs or symptoms of MI or in asymptomatic patients with significant persistent angiographic complications such as large side occlusion no-reflow, or thrombosis (class I, level of evidence [LOE] C), but offer only a weak recommendation for routine measurement of cardiac biomarkers in all patients post-PCI (class IIb, LOE C).[10] In the absence of routine testing, a consensus document[17] recommends performing an ECG 1 to 4 hours postprocedure after an uncomplicated PCI; if normal, biomarkers do not need to be checked. In the presence of clinical symptoms, angiographic complications, or ECG changes, CK-MB (or cTn if CK-MB is unavailable) should be measured 8 to 12 hours postprocedure, and, if elevated, every 8 to 12 hours thereafter until they peak.

Platelet Function

Platelet function testing has been used to assess the degree of platelet reactivity; although high levels of platelet reactivity have been associated with adverse outcomes,[18–20] antiplatelet strategies tailored to platelet reactivity have failed to show a benefit. In the Gauging Responsiveness with A VerifyNow assay-Impact on Thrombosis And Safety (GRAVITAS) Trial,[21] 2214 patients with high platelet reactivity were randomized to high- or low-dose clopidogrel; at 6 months, there was no difference in the primary composite end point (2.3% vs. 2.3%, hazard ratio [HR] 1.01; 95% confidence interval [CI] 0.58 to 1.76; $P = .97$). Similarly, in the Assessment by a Double Randomization of a Conventional Antiplatelet Strategy versus a Monitoring-guided Strategy for Drug-Eluting Stent Implantation and of Treatment Interruption versus Continuation One Year after Stenting (ARCTIC) Trial,[22] 2440 patients scheduled for PCI were randomized to a strategy of platelet function testing and dose adjustment in those with elevated platelet reactivity but did not show a reduction in the primary

TABLE 21.2 Changes in the Definition of a Peri-Percutaneous Coronary Intervention Myocardial Infarction As Well As the Proposed Definition of a Clinically Relevant Myocardial Infarction

Biomarker Elevation Pattern	First Definition	Third Definition	Clinically Relevant Myocardial Infarction
Normal biomarkers at baseline	Elevation of biomarkers >3 × 99th percentile URL	Elevation of cTn >5 × 99th percentile URL AND either: (a) evidence of prolonged ischemia; (b) ischemic ST-changes or new Q-waves; (c) angiographic evidence of flow limiting lesion; (d) imaging evidence of loss of viable myocardium	Peak CK-MB (cTn) rises to ≥10 × ULN (≥70 × ULN for cTn) or ≥5 × ULN (≥35 × ULN for cTn) with new pathologic Q-waves in ≥2 contiguous leads or new left bundle branch block (LBBB)
Elevated at baseline but stable	No guidance; continue to measure biomarkers and use features of ECG and imaging	>20% rise of cTn from the most recent preprocedure value	CK-MB (or cTn) rises by absolute increment as those described above from the most recent preprocedure level
Elevated at baseline and not stable or falling	No guidance	No guidance	CK-MB (or cTn) rises by absolute increment as those described above from the most recent preprocedure level + ST-elevation or depression along with signs of clinically relevant MI (new/worsening heart failure, hypotension, etc.)

CK-MB, Creatine kinase-muscle/brain; *cTn*, cardiac troponin; *MI*, myocardial infarction; *ULN*, upper limit of normal; *URL*, upper reference limit.

composite end point in the monitored group (HR 1.13; 95% CI 0.98 to 1.29; P = .10). Given the lack of clinical benefit, routine platelet function testing is not currently recommended.[9,10]

Renal Function

Postprocedure renal injury is common, especially in patients with preexisting renal insufficiency, and may be due to aortic atheroemboli, contrast-induced injury, or a combination of the two. Currently, the only strategies proven to minimize risk include volume expansion and minimization of contrast use. Because creatinine increase is observed 48 to 72 hours post-PCI in those affected, there is limited utility in measuring renal function within the first 24 hours postprocedure. SCAI recommends that patients at increased risk for contrast-induced nephropathy (CIN) should have a serum creatinine value checked about 5 to 7 days postprocedure.[3]

TRENDS IN POSTPROCEDURE LENGTH OF STAY

Over the last decade, there has been a significant push toward shorter LOS for all hospitalizations and most procedures, and PCI has not escaped this general trend. With respect to PCI, the drivers for shorter LOS have focused on procedure-specific technological advances and payer considerations.

Technological, Pharmacological, and Procedural Advances

Over the previous three decades, there have been significant technological, pharmacological, and procedural advances that have fundamentally improved both safety and efficacy of PCI. The initial development of stent technology to supplement balloon angioplasty has markedly reduced rates of acute vessel closure. Iterative improvements in stent technology in materials, polymer coating, and antimitogenic drug delivery have made stents more durable, easier to deliver, and less likely to incite neointimal hyperplasia, further decreasing the need for repeat intervention. Advances in miniaturization and guidewire technology have virtually eliminated femoral and brachial cutdown techniques, as catheters have decreased in size from 9-Fr to 5-Fr. Even more "slender" 4- and 3-Fr guide catheters are available in some countries.[23]

These changes have been paralleled by improvements in pre- and periprocedural pharmacological management. The development of more potent oral antiplatelet agents, such as prasugrel[24] and ticagrelor,[25] as well as strategies for appropriate upstream utilization have led to a more tailored approach to periprocedural antithrombotic strategy, including the use of heparin as monotherapy during PCI.[26] More tailored provisional use of glycoprotein (GP) IIb/IIIa inhibitors rather than routine use has led to decreased bleeding with similar efficacy.[27] The introduction and widespread adoption of the direct thrombin inhibitor bivalirudin has led to further increases in safety with similar efficacy.[28–30]

Additionally, these advances have been coupled with procedural innovations, namely TR PCI, to further improve efficacy and safety. Although first described in 1989 by Campeau and by Otaki in 1992[31,32] and popularized by Kiemeneij and Laarman in 1994,[33,34] the TR technique has historically seen poor uptake by operators in the United States, though that has been changing more recently. Feldman et al. performed an analysis of 2.8 million patients in the American College of Cardiology's (ACC) National Cardiovascular Data Registry (NCDR) CathPCI Registry and noted that TR adoption has increased almost 16-fold, from 1.2% in 2007 to 16.1% in 2012, now accounting for 6.3% of total procedures.[35] The main advantage for TR access appears to be dramatic reductions in vascular access complications and bleeding, as shown in the RIVAL (RadIal Versus femorAL access for coronary intervention) Trial, which randomized 7021 acute coronary syndrome (ACS) patients to either TR (n = 3507 patients) or transfemoral (n = 3514 patients) and demonstrated no difference in the primary composite outcome of death/MI/stroke/noncoronary artery bypass grafting major bleeding at 30 days (3.7% vs. 4.0%, HR 0.92; 95% CI 0.72 to 1.17; P = .50) but reduction in vascular access complications (1.4% vs. 3.7%, HR 0.37; 95% CI 0.27 to 0.52; P < .0001) and ACUITY (Acute Catheterization and Urgent Intervention Triage strategY) major bleeding (1.9% vs. 4.5%, HR 0.43; 95% CI 0.32 to 0.57; P > .0001).[36] Additional patient-centered benefits of TR access include easier hemostasis and earlier ambulation postprocedure. Radial approach has also been associated with lower cost of care and shorter hospital LOS.[37]

The data for VCDs, though popular in the United States, has been mixed. Although randomized clinical trial data has shown limited benefit, a recent NCDR analysis by Marso et al. assessed the effects of different bleeding avoidance strategies and found modestly decreased bleeding with VCDs, bivalirudin, or both compared with manual compression alone.[38] Meta-analyses have been conflicting, with one study showing some benefit (pooled odds ratio [OR] 0.89; 95% CI 0.86 to 0.91)[39] but another showing similar complication rates with VCDs and manual compression.[40]

Payer Expectations

As PCI has become safer and more effective, there have been significant changes in payment structures that additionally have driven shorter LOS and increase in outpatient setting in patients undergoing PCI. In 2007, the InterQual criteria (McKesson Corporation, San Francisco, CA), a set of criteria used by hospitals nationwide to offer guidance on admissions decisions, were modified such that PCI was no longer an inpatient procedure by default. While procedures performed on an urgent or emergent basis (such as for acute MI) were still eligible for inpatient status, this change effectively made PCI predominantly an outpatient procedure.

Nevertheless, given differential reimbursement schedules, there was still a significant incentive to perform PCI and submit for reimbursement at the inpatient level. This was driven by the fact that the Centers for Medicare and Medicaid Services (CMS) reimburse outpatient procedures using the Ambulatory Payment Classification (APC) system and inpatient procedures using the more lucrative Diagnosis Related Group (DRG) framework, making the same procedure eligible for vastly different reimbursement based on admission status. For example, an uncomplicated PCI using a drug-eluting stent (MS-DRG 147) would be reimbursed $11,497 under the inpatient DRG system but only $7763 (APC 0656) under the outpatient APC system, a difference of more than $3700. As hospitals attempted to seek reimbursements for PCI procedures under the inpatient DRG system, CMS instituted the Recovery Audit Contractors (RAC) program as part of the Medicare Modernization Act of 2003 to recover possible overpayments to hospitals, even retrospectively; to date, the program has recovered more than $3.65 billion in 2013 alone. Facing increased scrutiny for inpatient billing of PCI, hospitals now perform the majority of nonacute PCI in the outpatient setting.

In 2013, the inpatient and outpatient designations were further refined as CMS implemented the "two-midnight" rule, stipulating that an acute inpatient admission will require a stay that spans at least two midnights, in effect classifying even more patient encounters as outpatient instead of inpatient. This has led to even further interest in SDD programs.

SAME-DAY DISCHARGE FOLLOWING PERCUTANEOUS CORONARY INTERVENTION
History and Background

The concept of SDD originated two decades ago, as Kiemeneij, one of the pioneers of TR access, *a priori* initiated his patients on warfarin, performed PCI via the TR approach, and discharged them on the same day.[41–43] Despite other early reports of the safety of SDD,[44,45] there has been low adoption of SDD in the United States. In an analysis of the NCDR CathPCI Registry, Rao et al. note that the prevalence of SDD was only 1.25% among the 107,018 elective PCI patients hospitalized for 1 day or less between 2004 and 2008.[16] Of note, although both strategies of SDD and overnight observation are outpatient admissions and discharges, SDD occurs when the patient is discharged home on the same calendar day of the procedure, whereas overnight hospitalization requires at least one midnight of observation prior to discharge.

Safety of Same-Day Discharge

The safety of SDD compared with overnight observation has been demonstrated both in observational studies and randomized trials; however, results have been difficult to compare directly across

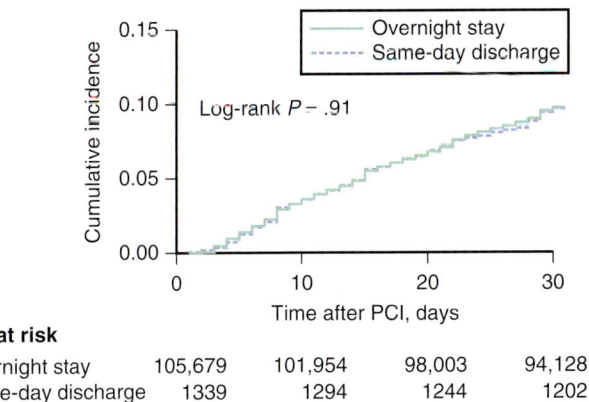

Fig. 21.1 Cumulative incidence of 30-day mortality or rehospitalization between patients undergoing same-day discharge versus overnight hospitalization. *PCI*, Percutaneous coronary intervention. (From Rao SV, Kaltenbach LA, Weintraub WS, et al. Prevalence and outcomes of same-day discharge after elective percutaneous coronary intervention among older patients. *JAMA*. 2011;306[13]:1461–1467.)

studies, given variance in underlying patient population, study setting, and outcomes of interest. The Rao CathPCI analysis noted no significant difference in 30-day death or hospitalization between patients undergoing SDD or overnight hospitalization (Fig. 21.1).[46] Abdelaal et al. performed a meta-analysis of 13 studies (five randomized trials, eight observational experiences) encompassing 111,830 patients and found similar complication rates between SDD and overnight observation in both the randomized (OR 1.20; 95% CI 0.82 to 1.74) and observational (OR 0.67; 95% CI 0.27 to 1.66) cohorts (Fig. 21.2).[47] Another meta-analysis of 37 studies including 12,803 patients found that there was no difference between SDD and overnight observation with regard to death/MI/target-vessel revascularization (OR 0.90; 95% CI 0.43 to 1.87) among randomized patients and a low rate of the composite end point among the observational cohort (1.0%, 95% CI 0.35% to 1.32%), suggesting that SDD is a safe and feasible strategy among patients undergoing elective PCI.[18]

Patient Selection

Patient selection for SDD is controversial. A previous SCAI consensus document released in 2009 suggests that the only patients eligible for an abbreviated observation period prior to discharge are patients with: (a) age less than 70 years; (b) stable angina on presentation with no biomarker elevation; (c) asymptomatic with an abnormal stress test; (d) no significant comorbidities including chronic heart failure, chronic obstructive pulmonary disease, peripheral vascular disease, bleeding predisposition, or contrast allergy; (e) normal renal function, (f) fully loaded on thienopyridine and no GP IIb/IIIa inhibitor use; (g) single-vessel PCI with less than 28 mm stent, no periprocedural complications; and (h) patient and family willingness.[49] However, these criteria were criticized as being too conservative. Gilchrist et al. reported safe SDD in 100 patients undergoing successful elective PCI without complications (defined as no unstable dissection, no major side-branch loss, no prolonged periprocedural ischemia); 85% of these patients would not have met SCAI criteria for SDD, with the main contraindications to discharge being age, distance from hospital, and no pretreatment with thienopyridine or GPIIb/IIIa used.[50] In the setting of multiple studies that documented safe SDD in higher-risk patients, SCAI released a revised consensus document in 2018.[51] The updated consensus recommendations that favor SDD include the following: (a) patient characteristics (clinically stable, baseline functional status, baseline comorbidities); (b) procedural characteristics (successful procedure [including an uncomplicated chronic total occlusion (CTO) attempt], adequate hemostasis, and effective DAPT), and (c) program

SECTION III Coronary Intervention

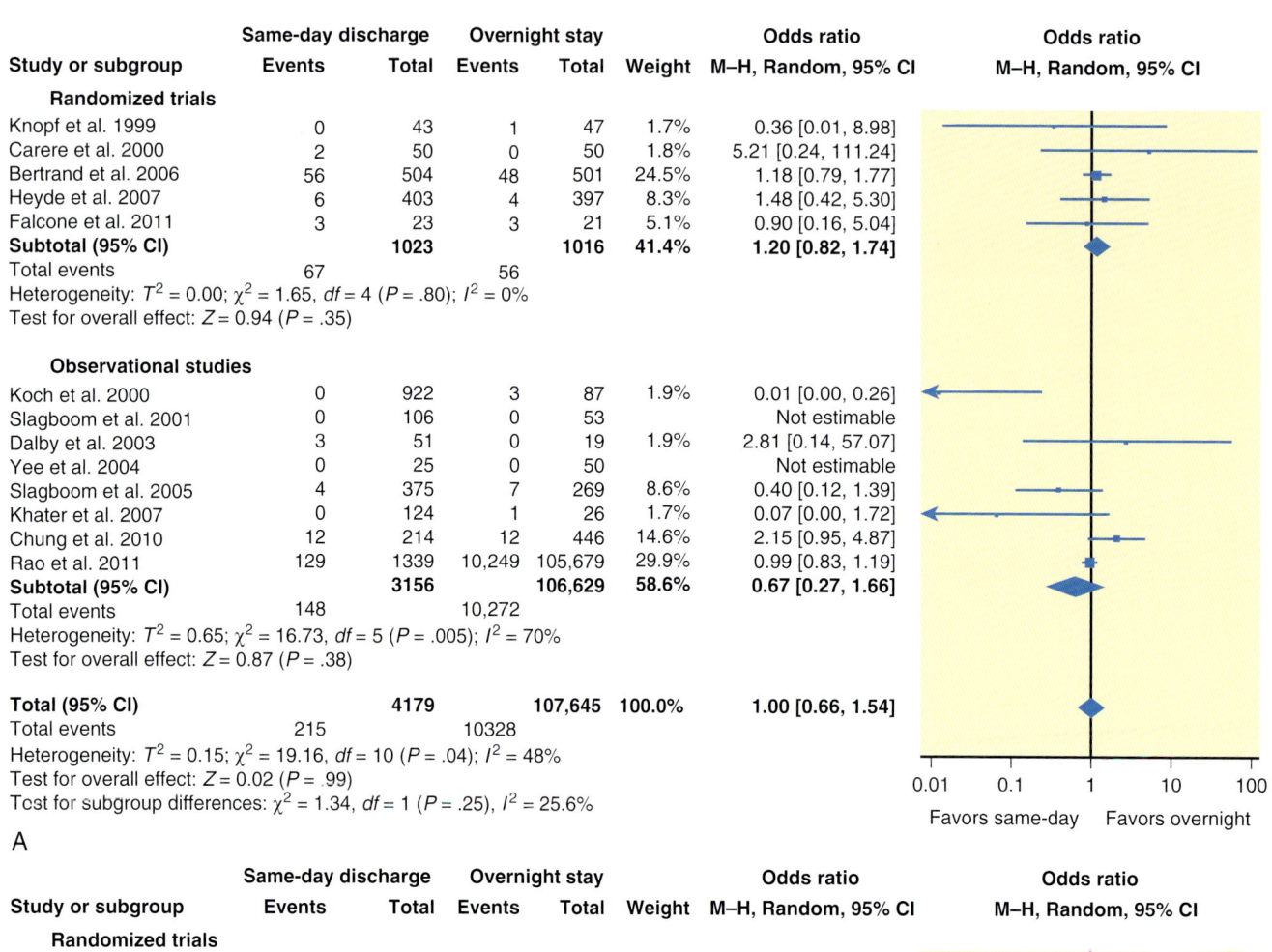

Fig. 21.2 Forest plot of the Incidence of 30-day total complications (A) and 30-day major adverse cardiac events (B). *CI,* Confidence interval; *M–H,* Mantel–Haenszel. (From Abdelaal E, Rao SV, Gilchrist IC, et al. Same-day discharge compared with overnight hospitalization after uncomplicated percutaneous coronary intervention: a systematic review and meta-analysis. *JACC Cardiovasc Interv.* 2013;6[2]:99–112.)

characteristics (appropriate education and social support at home, plan for P2Y$_{12}$ inhibitor, and updated contact information).[50,51] A revised patient flow diagram is shown in Fig. 21.3.

The dominant feature of safe SDD appears to be the absence of periprocedural or angiographic complications and not necessarily underlying patient characteristics. Hodkinson et al. assessed prospective 30-day outcomes among patients undergoing SDD 6 hours post-PCI using criteria that focused on the technical result of the procedure instead of clinical presentation or lesion complexity.[52] Among the 1059 patients selected for SDD, 27.7% presented with an ACS and 40.8% had high-risk lesions as defined by the ACC/AHA definition. Almost all patients (98%) underwent PCI via a TR approach. Among this group, rates of major adverse cardiovascular events (MACEs) at 30 days was 0.85% and rates of subacute stent thrombosis 0.4%; no MACEs were observed within 24 hours postdischarge, suggesting minimal, if any, benefit from prolonged monitoring with regard to preventing short-term readmissions.

Selected Patient Populations

Acute Coronary Syndrome

Although most studies of SDD have excluded patients with ACS, there are a number of studies that have demonstrated low event rates even in these high-risk patients. In the Early Discharge After TR Stenting of the Coronary Arteries (EASY) trial,[53] which randomized 1005 patients to bolus abciximab and SDD (n = 504 patients) or to bolus plus 12-hour abciximab infusion and overnight monitoring (n = 501 patients), 66% of patients presented with unstable angina and 18% to 19% of patients presented with an acute MI; the SDD discharge was noninferior to overnight monitoring at 30-day follow-up. Hodkinson et al. describe a cohort of 1059 SDD patients of whom 293 (27.7%) were ACS patients and describe no MACEs 24 hours postdischarge and a 30-day MACE rate of 0.85%.[52]

Transfemoral Access

Given low rates of radial uptake in the United States, many studies have demonstrated safe SDD among patients undergoing femoral access with or without VCD use. In the Elective PCI in Outpatient Study (EPOS), all 800 patients randomized to SDD or overnight monitoring underwent elective PCI via a transfemoral approach; only 3 cases of access site complications were reported.[54] In a meta-analysis, there was no difference in major bleeding or vascular complications among patients randomized to SDD versus overnight monitoring (OR 0.75; 95% CI 0.19 to 2.98; P = .69).[48] In the CathPCI analysis, more than 96% of SDD cases incorporated femoral access and a VCD was used in 65% of cases.[46] Patel et al. assessed outcomes in 2400 patients undergoing SDD after PCI and describe low rates of bleeding (0.58%), vascular complications (0.04%), and major adverse cardiovascular and cerebrovascular events (MACCEs) (0.96%) at 30 days among low-risk patients overwhelmingly undergoing PCI via a transfemoral technique (99.6%).[55] This was further studied by Antonsen et al. among 1809 low-risk patients undergoing PCI via a femoral approach and undergoing vascular closure using the AngioSeal device.[56] Of note, in this study, stable non–ST-elevation acute coronary syndromes (NSTE-ACS) was not an exclusion criterion for SDD. Among the 355 (19.6%) patients who underwent SDD, 78 (22.0%) presented with unstable angina/non–ST-segment elevation myocardial infarction (UA/NSTEMI); although there were no significant differences in rates of MACCE at 24 hours or 30 days postprocedure (except for one patient who underwent target-lesion revascularization at 4 days), three patients had vascular complications: two were readmitted within 24 hours for access site hematoma and one patient developed a femoral pseudoaneurysm postprocedure, necessitating treatment with thrombin injection.

Elderly

SDD, even among carefully selected elderly patients, appears to be safe as well. Ziakas et al.[57] report that despite high rates of minor access site complications, there were no significant differences in major access site complications, stent thrombosis, or readmission among elderly patients. Ranchord et al. assessed the safety of SDD in 212 patients (13.4% of the study population) ≥75 years of age undergoing elective PCI and found no deaths, similar rates of readmission within 24 hours (<0.7%), and similar rates of MACE (3.3% vs. 3.6%, P = 1.0) in both groups of patients.[58] The analysis

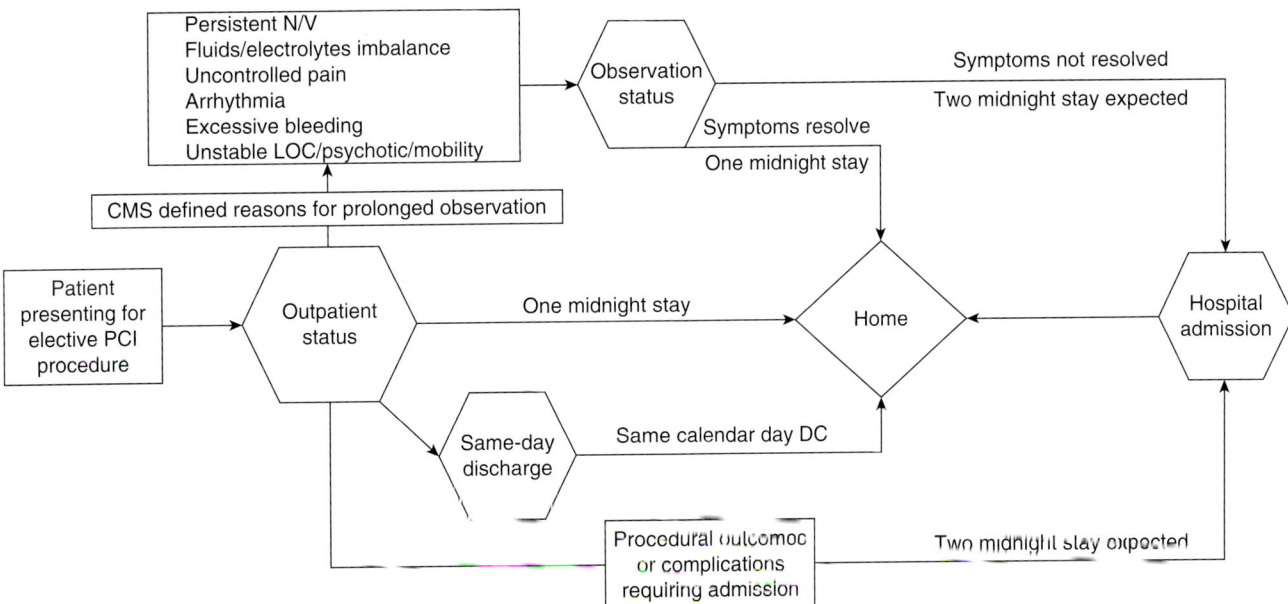

Fig. 21.3 Sample pathway for discharge following percutaneous coronary intervention (PCI). CMS, Centers for Medicare and Medicaid Services; DC, discharge; LOC, level of consciousness; N/V, nausea/vomiting. (From Seto AH, Shroff A, Abu-Fadel M, et al. Length of stay following percutaneous coronary intervention: an expert consensus document update from the society for cardiovascular angiography and interventions. Catheter Cardiovasc Interv. 2018;92[4]:717–731.)

from the CathPCI registry was performed entirely in patients over the age of 65 years and showed similar rates of 30-day death or readmission between SDD and overnight observation.[46]

Patient Satisfaction With Same-Day Discharge

Previous studies[59–61] have shown that many patients prefer SDD to overnight monitoring. Kim et al. recently assessed patient preference with SDD versus overnight observation in a randomized trial of 298 patients undergoing elective PCI and found that perceived readiness for discharge assessed prior to discharge was high and similar between SDD (97.9%) and next-day discharged (96.6%), $P = .69$.[62] At 30-day follow-up, 79% of patients randomized to SDD, compared with 49% of patients randomized to overnight observation, were satisfied with the timing of their discharge. Whereas 9% of the SDD patients preferred to have stayed for longer observation, 37% of the overnight observation patients would have preferred to have been discharged sooner.

Economic Impact of Same-Day Discharge

The economic impact of SDD depends largely on the prevailing admissions and reimbursement criteria. Historically, a low rate of uptake for SDD has been attributed to the fee-for-service model wherein additional services provided during the inpatient hospitalization were fully reimbursed. However, over the last decade, almost all elective PCI cases in the United States are reimbursed at a fixed rate regardless of overall LOS or resource utilization under the outpatient APC system. Given that one hospital day can cost up to $4000,[37] there is an increasingly valuable opportunity to create care pathways that increase value by facilitating SDD among appropriately selected patients by reducing costs associated with unnecessary overnight monitoring and prolonging LOS, if even by hours.

Bundled payment schemes require providers to absorb costs related to postprocedure complications and preventable readmissions. In this context, a SDD system can only be cost-saving if it reduces costs associated with post-PCI monitoring and maintains a low rate of complications.[63]

Providers who have created innovative new care pathways to appropriately select, monitor, and discharge stable, uncomplicated patients have noted significant decreases in resource utilization and increasing bed capacity. Brewster and colleagues describe the creation of an outpatient "radial lounge" for postprocedure monitoring of patients undergoing TR coronary procedures and describe significantly increased rates of SDD after PCI procedures (from 2.3% to 51.2%, $P < .005$) with a concomitant reduction in inpatient bed utilization.[64] An example of a successful radial lounge from Pilsen Hospital, Czech Republic, is shown in Fig. 21.4.

The potential cost savings of SDD compared with standard overnight monitoring was studied by Rinfret et al., in a post hoc analysis of the EASY trial, a randomized, open-label study comparing SDD with abciximab only bolus with overnight monitoring and bolus in addition to a 12-hour infusion of abciximab, found that the SDD strategy was noninferior to the overnight monitoring strategy.[65] The mean post-PCI hospital LOS was 8.9 hours for the SDD patients but 26.5 hours for the overnight monitoring patients. Associated costs were $1117 ± $1554 for SDD patients compared with $2258 ± $1328 for overnight monitoring patients, a cost difference of $1141 that was primarily attributed to hospital costs related to post-PCI ward-related costs, estimated to be $65 per hour in this Canadian study. These savings may be higher in environments where costs are higher. In another study by Amin and colleagues using data from the NCDR CathPCI Registry, SDD occurred in 5.3% of patients (though 23.1% of patients undergoing TR access) that were eligible for SDD. The study authors estimated that the cost difference between TR access and SDD and transfemoral access and non-SDD was $3689 ($13,389 vs. $17,076, $P < .001$).[66]

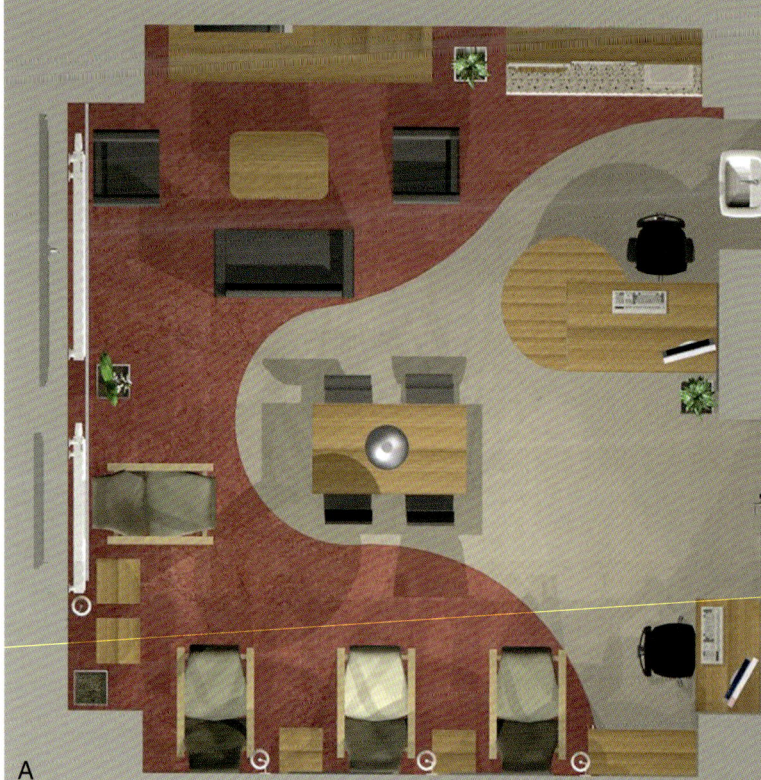
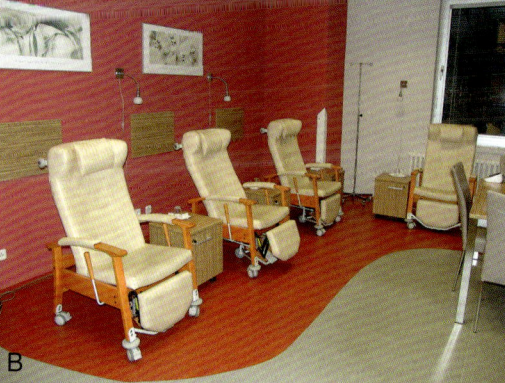
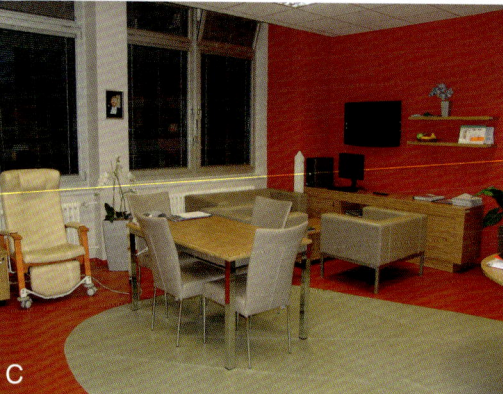

Fig. 21.4 The radial lounge at Pilsen Hospital in Pilsen, Czech Republic, which facilitates same-day discharge. (Photographs courtesy Ivo Bernat, MD.)

Recommendations for Safe Same-Day Discharge

Preprocedure Screening

Preprocedural screening should focus on baseline demographic, clinical, and social factors precluding SDD. Although older patients (>65 to 75 years of age) and patients presenting with ACS have been discharged safely, most programs typically favor overnight management in these groups. Other patient factors warranting overnight management include impaired renal function (glomerular filtration rate <60 mL/min), severe left ventricular dysfunction (<30%), or contrast allergy. Additionally, patients should live close to a medical facility in case of a medical emergency and have adequate social support.

Procedural Characteristics

The sine qua non of SDD is a successful procedure without complications. Most complications manifest within 6 hours of PCI and thus can be readily identified during postprocedure monitoring.[67] Although safely used in the EASY Trial,[53] most operators feel that the use of a postprocedure infusion of GP IIb/IIIa inhibitor warrants overnight monitoring. However, the use of an abbreviated infusion or bolus only (as in the EASY trial) may be suitable for SDD. Other procedural factors that may warrant consideration of overnight monitoring include significant left main disease, use of mechanical circulatory support (intra-aortic balloon pump), or complex PCI (including a bifurcation lesion, multi-vessel intervention, or atherectomy). Angiographic complications such as a significant dissection, side-branch loss, slow or no-reflow phenomenon, and procedural complications such as periprocedural ischemia or ventricular arrhythmias also warrant longer observation. According to the new SCAI consensus document, an unsuccessful uncomplicated CTO attempt may be feasible for SDD.

Postprocedural Monitoring

Patients are typically monitored for 4 to 8 hours postprocedure. Symptoms or signs of ischemia, including chest pain, shortness of breath, hemodynamic instability, or new or worsening ECG changes, should warrant careful management and longer observation. Patients should be able to achieve their preprocedure level of ambulation without significant discomfort prior to discharge as well. Additionally, the access site should be evaluated carefully to ensure appropriate hemostasis and no early signs of distal vascular compromise. The role of checking biomarkers post-PCI is controversial and is discussed elsewhere in this chapter. If the procedure was uncomplicated and there are no signs or symptoms of ischemia, checking cardiac biomarkers prior to SDD is not warranted; however, if there was an angiographic complication or signs of new myocardial dysfunction, a CK-MB or cTn should be checked 8 to 12 hours postprocedure and repeated if newly abnormal; in that situation, SDD is not a feasible strategy. Additionally, prior to discharge, clear instructions, including medication changes and plan for DAPT, activity recommendations, and clear contact information in the event of an adverse event, should be provided. It is advisable to have the patient's family obtain at least a 30-day supply of DAPT prior to discharge. This is most feasible at hospitals that have on-site pharmacies.

After Discharge

SDD patients should be contacted within 24 to 72 hours of discharge to ensure no ischemic or vascular/bleeding complications since returning home. Additionally, compliance with DAPT should be confirmed at this time, as well as plans for routine postprocedure follow-up within 2 to 4 weeks.

A proposed checklist for eligibility of SDD is provided in Table 21.3.

TABLE 21.3 Proposed Checklist for Eligibility for Same-Day Discharge

Preprocedural factors
- No acute decompensated heart failure or shock
- No contrast allergy
- Nonemergent PCI
- Adequate social support
- Lives close to medical facility

Procedural/angiographic factors
- Uncomplicated access
- Lesion details—the lesion is NOT:
  1. Unprotected left main
  2. Atherectomy
- Infusion glycoprotein IIb/IIIa not used (bolus is acceptable)
- No angiographic complication (side branch occlusion, dissection, no-reflow phenomenon)

Postprocedure monitoring
- No signs or symptoms of ischemia
- No biomarker elevation (if checked)
- Patient able to ambulate without difficulty
- Patient able to tolerate oral intake
- Has $P2Y_{12}$ inhibitor on hand prior to discharge

PCI, Percutaneous coronary intervention.

CONCLUSIONS

The importance of appropriate postprocedure management in patients undergoing PCI cannot be understated and has taken on additional meaning as postprocedure LOS has continued to decrease. Clear patient communication, both verbal and written, rigorous medication reconciliation (including a plan for DAPT), and a well-defined plan in case of complications, may minimize adverse outcomes post-PCI. The role of measuring cardiac biomarkers continues to evolve. Although current recommendations strongly support biomarker testing in patients with a procedural complication or evidence of myocardial injury but offer only weak support for routine testing postprocedure, the clinical relevance of small levels of myocardial necrosis continues to be debated as newer and more sensitive assays to detect myocardial injury are available. Finally, as LOS postprocedure continues to shorten, there is a valuable opportunity to design new, innovative care pathways to safely manage patients postprocedure and discharge eligible patients on the same day of their procedure, which, if performed safely and effectively, may lead to increased patient satisfaction as well as cost-savings.

KEY REFERENCES

19. Thygesen K, Alpert JS, Jaffe AS, et al. Third universal definition of myocardial infarction. *J Am Coll Cardiol*. 2012;60(16):1581–1598.
46. Rao SV, Kaltenbach LA, Weintraub WS, et al. Prevalence and outcomes of same-day discharge after elective percutaneous coronary intervention among older patients. *JAMA*. 2011;306(13):1461–1467.
51. Seto AH, Shroff A, Abu-Fadel M, et al. Length of stay following percutaneous coronary intervention: an expert consensus document update from the society for cardiovascular angiography and interventions. *Catheter Cardiovasc Interv*. 2018;92(4):717–731.
63. Gilchrist IC. Same day discharge after elective percutaneous coronary intervention. *Curr Cardiol Rev*. 2014;16(4):470.
66. Amin AP, Patterson M, House JA, et al. Costs associated with access site and same-day discharge among medicare beneficiaries undergoing percutaneous coronary intervention: an evaluation of the current percutaneous coronary intervention care pathways in the United States. *JACC Cardiovasc Interv*. 2017;10(4):342–351.

Additional references available online at expertconsult.com.

中文导读

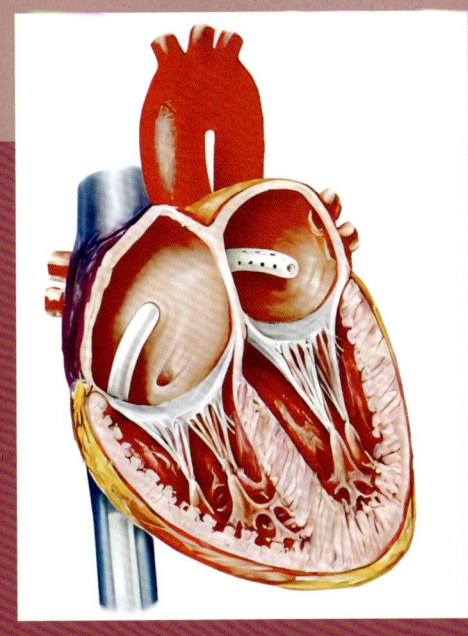

第22章
心源性休克的干预

在药物治疗、护理措施、循环支持设备和更积极的冠状动脉血运重建等方面取得进展的同时，心源性休克的院内死亡率仍处于较高水平。全身动脉低血压和组织低灌注是心源性休克的两大因素。临床大多数急性心肌梗死患者发生心源性休克是由左心室功能障碍引起的，此外室间隔和乳头肌的机械损伤、某些药物的使用都可能会导致心源性休克的发生和发展。急性心肌梗死时因左心室功能障碍引起的心源性休克在临床表现上存在差异，仅有少部分患者能在发病时被明确诊断。梗死后6小时内46.6%的患者出现心源性休克，24小时为74.1%，这提示医师们在心源性休克发展之前进行及时干预的必要性。大部分临床研究表明，早期进行血运重建依然是心源性休克患者预后的最强预测因子。对于心源性休克的患者，早期行右心导管检查可协助快速寻求病因，以及完善后续诊疗计划。一线处理仍是静脉注射正性肌力药物、血管升压药物等，尽可能地维持其血流动力学的稳定，为进一步的检查和干预提供可能。而终末期心力衰竭的患者，行IABP等机械循环支持能带来血流动力学益处。尽早行血运重建可以提高急性心肌梗死后心源性休克患者的短期和长期存活率，血运重建在各个危险分级都有好处。如果在无法立即进行血运重建，且无禁忌证情况下首要方案仍为溶栓治疗。对于严重的三支病变或左主干病变患者，立即行冠状动脉旁路移植术是首选的血运重建方法。本章节对急性心肌梗死患者心源性休克早期血运重建的必要性给予了较为全面的阐述。

苗旭光　崔　松

章节要点

- 心源性休克仍然是急性心肌梗死住院患者的主要死亡原因。
- 大多数急性心肌梗死患者发生心源性休克是由左心室功能障碍引起的。早期恢复梗死相关动脉供血区域的血液灌注，对于预防心源性休克和改善心源性休克预后至关重要。
- SHOCK试验表示，早期、即时的血管重建可明显降低死亡率。
- 心源性休克患者通过经皮冠状动脉介入治疗改善预后的主要预测因素是再灌注时间、血管通畅程度，以及TIMI血流分级增加。
- 大多数心源性休克患者合并多支血管病变。干预非梗死相关动脉的病变可能会带来益处。冠状动脉解剖结构不适合经皮冠状动脉介入治疗的患者应选择外科手术进行血运重建。
- 心源性休克是一种可治愈的疾病状态，在直接经皮冠状动脉介入治疗时代早期有相当大的机会可恢复。早期有创策略可以提高短期和长期生存率，存活的患者通常可以恢复良好的生活质量。

22 Interventions in Cardiogenic Shock

Satya S. Shreenivas, Scott M. Lilly, Howard C. Herrmann

KEY POINTS

- Cardiogenic shock (CS) remains the leading cause of death among patients hospitalized with acute myocardial infarction (AMI).
- Left ventricular (LV) dysfunction accounts for most CS in AMI patients. Early restoration of perfusion to the territory supplied by the infarct-related artery is of paramount importance in preventing CS and changing outcomes once it has developed.
- The Should We Emergently Revascularize Occluded Coronaries for Cardiogenic Shock (SHOCK) trial and registry demonstrated the mortality benefit of early, immediate revascularization compared with medical stabilization.
- Major predictors of improved outcomes with percutaneous coronary intervention (PCI) in CS are time to reperfusion, achievement of vessel patency, and increase in thrombolysis in myocardial infarction (TIMI) flow grade.
- The majority of patients who present with CS have multi-vessel disease. Interventions on noninfarct-related artery (IRA) lesions may be beneficial. Patients with coronary anatomy not deemed suitable for PCI should be surgically revascularized.
- CS is a treatable illness with a reasonable chance of recovery in the primary PCI era. An early invasive approach can increase both short- and long-term survival, and survivors often regain an excellent quality of life.

BACKGROUND

The combination of a systolic blood pressure less than 90 mm Hg, elevated intracardiac filling pressures, and target organ damage due to cardiac dysfunction defines cardiogenic shock (CS).[1] Early case series of CS revealed an in-hospital mortality approaching 80%.[2] Advances in intravenous (IV) drug therapy, systems of care, newer circulatory support devices, and more aggressive attempts at coronary revascularization have all led to an improvement in survival, but CS continues to have an in-hospital mortality approaching 50%. To understand which therapies might benefit patients with CS, it is necessary to review the pathophysiology and examine in detail the trials of drugs, circulatory support devices, and percutaneous coronary intervention (PCI).

PATHOPHYSIOLOGY

CS is a state of end-organ hypoperfusion caused by cardiac failure. Manifestations may include cold extremities, decreased urine output (<30 mL/h), alteration in mental status, or both in the setting of low systemic arterial blood pressure. Hemodynamically, CS is characterized by low cardiac output (CO) and systemic arterial hypotension in the setting of normal or elevated left ventricular (LV) filling pressure.

LV pump failure is the primary insult in most forms of CS. LV dysfunction may reflect new irreversible injury, reversible ischemia, damage from prior infarction, or a combination of these. Ventricular pump failure is caused by both systolic and diastolic dysfunction (Fig. 22.1). *Systolic dysfunction* results in a decreased stroke volume and resultant decreased CO, which clinically presents as a lower blood pressure. The body's response is an attempt to raise the blood pressure by increasing the heart rate and peripheral vasoconstriction, which although temporarily effective, also leads to increased myocardial work. The combination of the decreasing blood pressure, higher heart rate, and increased myocardial work leads to decreased coronary perfusion that is dependent on diastolic blood pressure and the diastolic filling period, which shortens as the heart rate increases. This decreased coronary perfusion leads to further myocardial ischemia. The lower blood pressure also triggers the renin-angiotensin-aldosterone system (RAAS), which results in fluid retention and peripheral vasoconstriction. These two effects, combined with the aforementioned tachycardia, further increase myocardial workload and contributes to worsening myocardial dysfunction. Finally, diastolic dysfunction leads to an increased LV end-diastolic pressure (LVEDP), which causes pulmonary congestion and hypoxia. The elevation in LVEDP and the lower diastolic blood pressure also contribute to lower coronary perfusion pressure. Both the hypoxia and the lower coronary perfusion pressure result in further myocardial ischemia.

Right ventricular (RV) dysfunction may also cause or contribute to CS. RV failure may limit LV filling via a decrease in CO, ventricular interdependence, or both. Additionally, as the intraventricular septum can account for up to 40% of RV function, proximal left anterior descending (LAD) occlusions that result in poor septal branch coronary blood flow can lead to significant RV dysfunction. Shock caused by isolated RV dysfunction carries nearly as high a mortality risk as shock caused by LV failure. Additionally, the benefit of revascularization was similar in the Should We Emergently Revascularize Occluded Coronaries for Cardiogenic Shock (SHOCK) trial and in the registry in patients with primarily RV dysfunction versus primarily LV dysfunction.[3]

Mechanical complications such as ventricular septal rupture and papillary muscle rupture may lead to CS without severe reduction in LV function.[4,5] Ultimately, most patients with CS complicating acute myocardial infarction (AMI) develop shock after presenting at the hospital. In some, medication use contributes to the development of shock. Classes of medications used to treat AMI that have been associated with shock include beta-blockers, angiotensin-converting enzyme (ACE) inhibitors, nitrates, diuretics, and morphine.

CLINICAL PRESENTATION

Whereas severe cardiac dysfunction that might lead to CS has many causes, by far the most common cause of CS in hospitalized inpatients in the United States is coronary artery disease (CAD).[6] The incidence and mortality of patients with CS in the setting of AMI remained unchanged during the 1980s and 1990s despite a progressive decline in the overall mortality of AMI, the development of the coronary care unit and early defibrillation in the

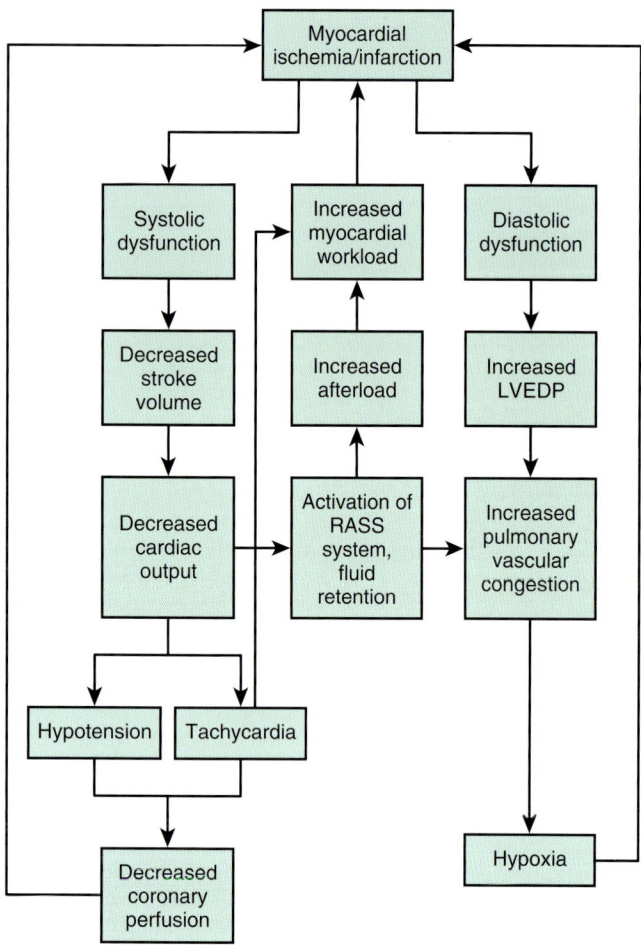

Fig. 22.1 Progression of myocardial infarction to cardiogenic shock. *LVEDP*, Left ventricular end-diastolic pressure; *RASS*, renin-angiotensin-aldosterone system.

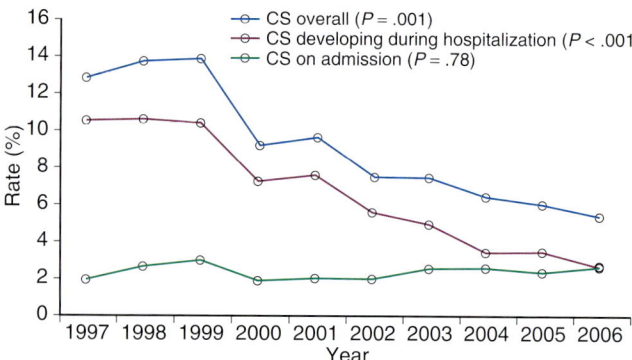

Fig. 22.2 Temporal trends of cardiogenic shock *(CS)* from 1997 to 2006. These demonstrate a reduction in the overall incidence and development of CS during hospitalization in patients presenting with an acute coronary syndrome. (Redrawn from Jeger RV, Radovanovic D, Hunziker PR, et al. AMIS Plus Registry investigators: ten-year trends in the incidence and treatment of cardiogenic shock. *Ann Intern Med.* 2008;149:618–626.)

1970s, the routine use of aspirin and β-blockers in the 1980s, and the introduction of reperfusion therapy with thrombolytics in the early 1990s.[7-10] The mortality associated with an acute coronary syndrome (ACS) and CS started to improve with attempts at percutaneous revascularization (Figs. 22.2 and 22.3).[11,12]

The SHOCK Trial and the SHOCK Registry

The SHOCK trial is the largest randomized trial to compare early, immediate revascularization, accomplished by either PCI or coronary artery bypass grafting (CABG), and initial medical stabilization in the setting of CS complicating AMI, which includes reperfusion therapy with thrombolytics.[13,14] The SHOCK trial and its registry provide insight into the etiology, risk factors, hemodynamic profile, clinical features, timing, and prognosis of CS complicating AMI. Eligible patients had to have an ST-segment elevation myocardial infarction (STEMI) complicated by shock caused by LV failure (mechanical and iatrogenic causes excluded), clinical and hemodynamic confirmation of CS, and shock developing within 36 hours of infarction. Intraaortic balloon pump (IABP) counterpulsation was permitted in both arms. Randomization had to occur within 12 hours of the diagnosis of shock. Patients with severe systemic illness, mechanical complications of myocardial infarction (MI), dilated cardiomyopathy (DCM), and severe valvular heart disease were excluded. A total of 302 patients were randomized in the SHOCK trial; a simultaneous registry prospectively enrolled patients who did *not* fulfill the eligibility criteria for entry into the trial. The SHOCK trial and registry included patients with mechanical complications of AMI, those with shock secondary to medications, those who presented more than 36 hours after infarction or who were not randomized within 12 hours of shock, and patients with shock diagnosed on clinical grounds alone (no hemodynamic confirmation). A total of 1190 patients were enrolled in this prospective, nonrandomized registry.

Etiology

Among all the patients enrolled in the SHOCK trial and registry, 78.5% had predominant LV failure, most often with electrocardiography (ECG) findings consistent with recent anterior MI (58%). Shock complicating inferior MI was less common (34.4%) and was associated with a prior MI in one-third of patients and a mechanical cause of shock in the remainder. Mechanical complications accounted for a minority of causes of CS. Severe mitral regurgitation was found in 6.9% of cases, ventricular septal rupture in 3.4%, RV infarction in 2.8%, and tamponade and rupture in 1.4%. Additionally, a minority of cases were iatrogenic, induced by medications such as β-blockers, calcium channel blockers, ACE inhibitors, diuretics, nitrates, and morphine. Risk factors for the development of CS in the context of AMI included older age, anterior MI, hypertension, diabetes mellitus, multivessel CAD, prior MI or angina, prior diagnosis of heart failure, STEMI, and left bundle branch block (LBBB).

Clinical Manifestations

Variability exists in the clinical manifestations of CS caused by LV failure in the setting of AMI.[15] Although the majority of patients with CS from predominant LV failure have classic findings of peripheral hypoperfusion and pulmonary congestion in the setting of arterial hypotension, approximately 25% of patients manifest hypotension and hypoperfusion in the *absence* of clinical pulmonary congestion. Consequently, the absence of pulmonary congestion on physical evaluation should not be considered a surrogate for low risk; clearly, LV compromise can coexist with a normal initial pulmonary evaluation. CS is diagnosed at presentation in only a minority of patients, but the majority of patients who ultimately develop shock following AMI do so within the first 24 hours. In a report from the SHOCK trial and registry that included CS patients with predominant LV failure, only 9% of the patients were diagnosed at presentation (median delay from MI symptom onset to hospital admission was 1.25 hours).[16] About

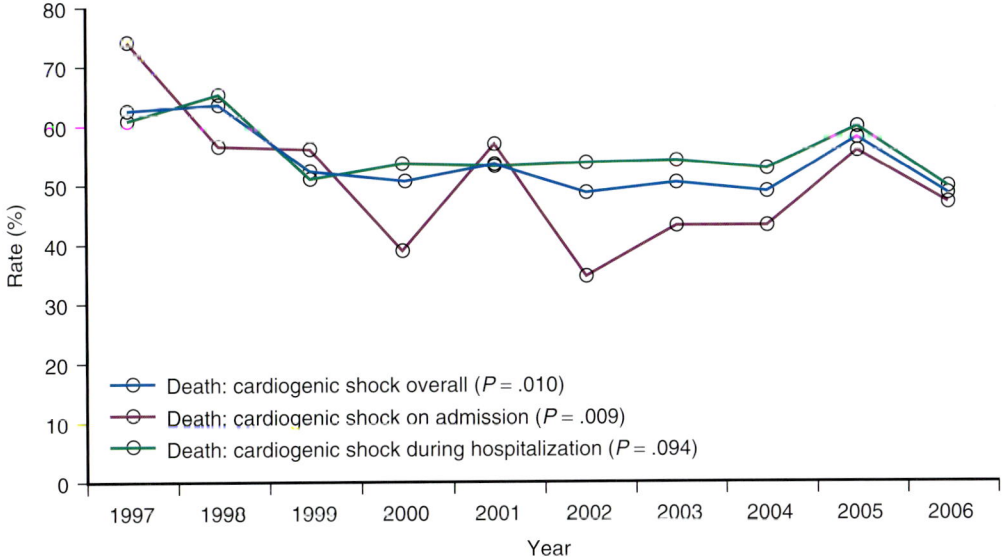

Fig. 22.3 Temporal trends in mortality in patients with an acute coronary syndrome and cardiogenic shock (CS) from 1997 to 2006. The data demonstrate a reduction in the rate of death in CS overall, in patients with CS on admission, and in those developing CS during hospitalization. (Redrawn from Jeger RV, Radovanovic D, Hunziker PR, et al. AMIS Plus Registry investigators: ten-year trends in the incidence and treatment of cardiogenic shock. *Ann Intern Med.* 2008;149:618–626.)

half of the patients (46.6%) who developed CS did so within 6 hours of infarct onset. By 24 hours, 74.1% of the patients who developed CS were diagnosed, and late shock (onset >24 hours) occurred in 25.9% of the study patients. By implication, then, often a therapeutic window exists that could allow for intervention either before CS develops or early in its course. However, the median time from hospital admission to shock onset was only 4.6 hours, which indicates that this window is relatively narrow for many patients. Other studies have shown a higher incidence of late shock. These studies included CS caused by the mechanical complications of MI, which usually manifest later than CS caused by LV failure.[17] Angiographic data from patients enrolled in the SHOCK trial revealed extensive, severe CAD in the majority. Almost two-thirds had three-vessel coronary disease, and 21% had left main CAD. The LAD coronary artery was the culprit vessel in 49% of the cases, and the right coronary artery (RCA) was the problem in 29%.[18] The mortality rates from CS in the modern era (50% to 60%) are far lower than the historic figures of 80% to 90%. However, mortality rates can range from 10% to 80%, depending on demographic, clinical, and hemodynamic factors. Specific factors include age, clinical signs of peripheral hypoperfusion, anoxic brain damage, left ventricular ejection fraction (LVEF), and stroke. Female sex does not appear to be an independent predictor of poor outcome, although hemodynamic data are predictive of short-term mortality but not long-term mortality; however, early revascularization remains the strongest predictor of outcome.

TREATMENT

Role of Right Heart Catheterization

With severe acute heart failure, it is sometimes difficult to accurately predict hemodynamic status or response to medical interventions.[19,20] For this reason, early right heart catheterization with a "leave-in" Swan-Ganz catheter may be considered in patients who are thought to be in CS. Not only does this allow for the quick and accurate diagnosis of a cardiac etiology, it also allows for subsequent tailored medical therapy. The Evaluation Study of Congestive Heart Failure and Pulmonary Artery Catheterization Effectiveness (ESCAPE) trial examined the role of routine right heart catheterization in acute decompensated heart failure patients and did not reveal a mortality difference between patients treated with invasive monitoring compared with those treated without invasive monitoring.[21] However, this study did not enroll all patients at each site who presented with acute decompensated heart failure, and it is possible that physicians may not have enrolled the sickest patients because of the possibility of randomization to no invasive monitoring. This study also confirmed the lack of sensitivity of physical exam findings at predicting the hemodynamic state of the CS patient (Table 22.1).

In addition to helping diagnose the etiology of shock and helping tailor medical interventions, an invasive monitoring approach also allows for prediction of in-hospital outcomes. Both pulmonary capillary wedge pressure (PCWP) and CO were shown to have independent prognostic value in the Global Utilization of Streptokinase and Tissue Plasminogen Activator for Occluded Coronary Arteries (GUSTO-I) trial.[22] Another invasively derived parameter, the *cardiac power output* (CPO: mean arterial pressure [MAP] × CO ÷ 451) has been shown to be a powerful predictor of in-hospital mortality. In the SHOCK trial, CPO was the strongest independent hemodynamic predictor of in-hospital mortality (Fig. 22.4).[23] Based on these results, patients with a CPO of fewer than 0.53 have an in-hospital mortality that approaches 60%. Hemodynamics can help guide medical therapy and can help the clinician make decisions as to which patients might benefit from more aggressive treatment.

Inotropes

One of the first lines of medical treatment in a patient with CS is the initiation of IV inotropes and vasopressors, despite the lack of evidence supporting this practice.[24] Frequently, the use of these medications may help to stabilize the hemodynamics while further investigations and/or interventions can proceed (coronary revascularization, valve surgery, workup for ventricular assist devices, and/or orthotopic heart transplantation).

TABLE 22.1 Sensitivity and Specificity of Physical Exam Findings in Predicting a Pulmonary Capillary Wedge Pressure Greater Than 22 mm Hg

	Sensitivity (%)	Specificity (%)
Elevated jugular venous pressure	67	74
Rales	15	85
Ascites	21	88
Pedal edema	48	69
Orthopnea	40	60
Hepatomegaly	15	92

ESCAPE Investigators. Evaluation study of congestive heart failure and pulmonary artery catheterization effectiveness: the ESCAPE trial. *JAMA*. 2005;294:1625–1633.

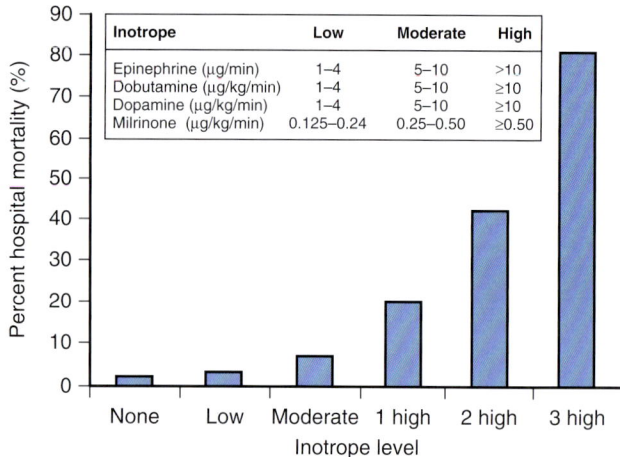

Fig. 22.5 **Mortality based on inotrope requirements.** (Reproduced from Samuels LE, Kaufman MS, Thomas MP, et al. Doses and types of vasopressors and inotropes and increasing mortality. *J Card Surg*. 1999;14:288–293.)

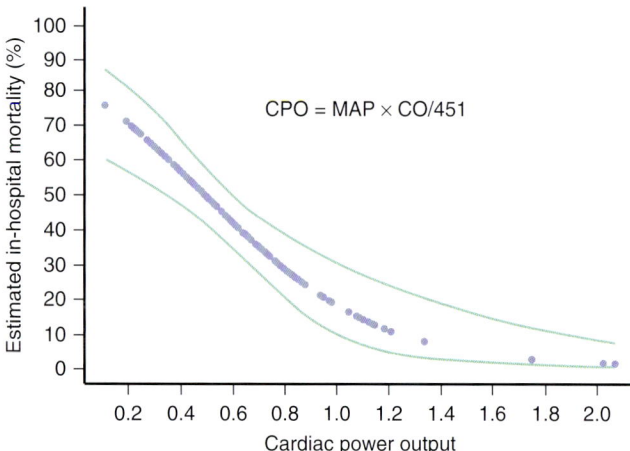

Fig. 22.4 Cardiac power output *(CPO)* and in-hospital mortality. *CO,* Cardiac output; *MAP,* mean arterial pressure. (Reproduced from Fincke R, Hochman JS, Lowe AM, et al. Cardiac power is the strongest hemodynamic correlate of mortality in cardiogenic shock: a report from the SHOCK trial registry. *J Am Coll Cardiol*. 2004;44:340–348.)

Two types of inotropes are currently available, phosphodiesterase inhibitors (milrinone) and catecholamines (dobutamine). Both work by increasing intracellular cyclic adenosine monophosphate (cAMP) but via two different mechanisms: *catecholamines* bind to extracellular adrenergic surface receptors and increase the production of cAMP, whereas *phosphodiesterase inhibitors* block the intracellular degradation of cAMP to adenosine monophosphate (AMP). Despite the widespread use of inotropes, both the Acute Decompensated Heart Failure National Registry (ADHERE) and the Outcomes of a Prospective Trial of Intravenous Milrinone for Exacerbations of Chronic Heart Failure (OPTIME-CHF) study have examined the role of inotropes in severe heart failure and have shown that patients on long-term inotrope therapy have increased mortality.[25,26] These findings have led to a decrease in the use of inotropes routinely, although these medications are still frequently used in rapidly deteriorating CS patients.

When inotropes fail to stabilize the patient, the use of vasopressors such as dopamine, norepinephrine, and/or epinephrine can be used to maintain perfusion pressure, but the use of these medications has also not been proven to improve symptoms or survival. Comparative studies between these vasopressors have yielded mixed results. Prevailing dogma was that the use of dopamine was superior to the use of norepinephrine in patients with CS because of the greater action of dopamine on the β-receptors compared with the peripheral α-receptors.[27] This was thought to promote cardiac contractility and to not appreciably increase peripheral vasoconstriction, and thus afterload, when compared with the greater effect of norepinephrine on the peripheral α-receptors. However, in the Sepsis Occurrence in Acutely Ill Patients II (SOAP II trial), which compared dopamine with norepinephrine in the treatment of shock, the subset of CS patients treated with dopamine had a significantly higher mortality than the patients treated with norepinephrine.[28] These data are clouded by the fact that patients treated with norepinephrine were also more likely to receive concomitant treatment with dobutamine. It is possible that instead of the beneficial effects of one vasopressor over another, the use of a potent inotrope is responsible for the difference in survival.

Whereas there may be a paucity of data on the best use of inotropes and vasopressors in CS, the amount and types of IV drugs has long been shown to have a strong correlation with increased mortality (Fig. 22.5). Once a patient is on more than one inotrope or vasopressor, their in-hospital mortality is greater than 40%.[29] Likewise, trials comparing the use of surgical ventricular assist devices with ideal medical therapy (mostly inotropes and vasopressors) have also shown that medical therapy is inferior to definitive surgical LV-assist device implantation.[30] The use of inotropes and vasopressors should be limited to patients who can be stabilized while a precipitating cause is found and treated. Longer treatment or the use of these medications in end-stage heart failure patients without a reversible cause increases mortality and is inferior to mechanical surgical circulatory support.

Mechanical Support

(See also Chapter 37.)

IABP counterpulsation has long been the mainstay of mechanical therapy for CS. Use of IABP improves coronary and peripheral perfusion and augments LV performance. The use of the IABP in CS was first described by Adrian Kantrowitz and colleagues in 1968,[31] and its use increased in the 1980s and 1990s, when studies on the use of IABP and thrombolysis in AMI revealed increased patency of the infarct-related artery (IRA) and improved thrombolysis in myocardial infarction (TIMI) flow grade.[32,33] Despite the improvement in hemodynamics, no large randomized trial has shown any mortality advantage to the use of the IABP in CS, especially in the current PCI era. A large meta-analysis of several randomized trials and cohort studies on the use of IABP in STEMI complicated by CS showed no survival benefit to the use of the IABP.[34] Because of the conflicting prior data with the use of IABP during the thrombolysis era and the equivocal meta-analysis results, two subsequent large randomized trials of the IABP were conducted. The Intraaortic Balloon Pump in Cardiogenic Shock II (IABP–SHOCK II) trial randomized 595 patients who presented with an acute MI and CS to IABP and early revascularization versus early revascularization alone and revealed that the use of IABP does not decrease 12-month all-cause mortality.[35] In addition to not changing the mortality of patients in CS, the use of IABP in reducing infarct size was also questioned by the Counterpulsation to Reduce Infarct Size Pre-PCI for Acute Myocardial Infarction (CRISP-AMI) trial.[36] This trial randomized patients with STEMI to an IABP prior to PCI versus PCI alone to examine whether the use of the IABP would reduce infarct size, but it revealed no difference between the two groups in LV mass as measured by cardiac magnetic resonance imaging (CMRI). One good outcome in these two trials was that the use of IABP, although of questionable therapeutic benefit, was also not associated with significant side effects or complications. Small randomized trials of the use of IABP versus extracorporeal membrane oxygenation (ECMO) and peripheral LV-assist devices (TandemHeart [CardiacAssist, Pittsburgh, PA] and Impella [Abiomed, Danvers, MA]) have shown that the use of IABP is frequently safer than more invasive modalities and that the use of the IABP confers some hemodynamic benefit.[37] Based on the relative safety profile and the hemodynamic benefits, it is reasonable to use the IABP as part of a stepwise algorithm to treat CS patients who are not responsive to inotropes and to do so prior to the initiation of more invasive mechanical circulatory support.[38] Mechanical circulatory support is currently playing an increasing role in treatment of CS (see Chapter 37).

Reperfusion in Cardiogenic Shock

The only way to prevent CS in the setting of AMI appears to be very early reperfusion therapy. In a randomized trial of early, in-ambulance thrombolysis versus primary PCI (PPCI), the incidence of CS was 0% among patients assigned to prehospital thrombolysis and only 0.5% in the group randomized within 2 hours from symptom onset.[39] However, reperfusion with thrombolytics is inferior to revascularization with PCI in achieving sustained TIMI grade 3 flow in the IRA. The survival benefit of early revascularization in CS, reported in several observational studies, was demonstrated convincingly in the randomized SHOCK trial, which demonstrated lower 6-month and 12-month mortality rates with a strategy of early emergency revascularization compared with initial medical stabilization, which included IABP placement and thrombolytic therapy.[40–42] A 13% absolute increase in 1-year survival was reported in patients assigned to early revascularization (Fig. 22.6).[43] This corresponds to a number needed to treat (NNT) of fewer than eight patients to save one life. Numerous registry studies have confirmed the survival advantage of early revascularization in CS, whether percutaneous or surgical, both in the young and in older adults. Although thrombolytic therapy is less effective, in the absence of contraindications, thrombolytics should be administered when immediate revascularization is not possible. Ideally, such patients should have IABP and should be transferred immediately to a facility that offers revascularization.

Percutaneous Coronary Intervention in Cardiogenic Shock

Multiple trials have demonstrated the superiority of emergency revascularization with PCI compared with fibrinolytics in achieving sustained TIMI grade 3 flow in STEMI, with improvement in mortality rates and preservation of LV function. In the SHOCK trial, PCI was the most frequent mode of revascularization, with

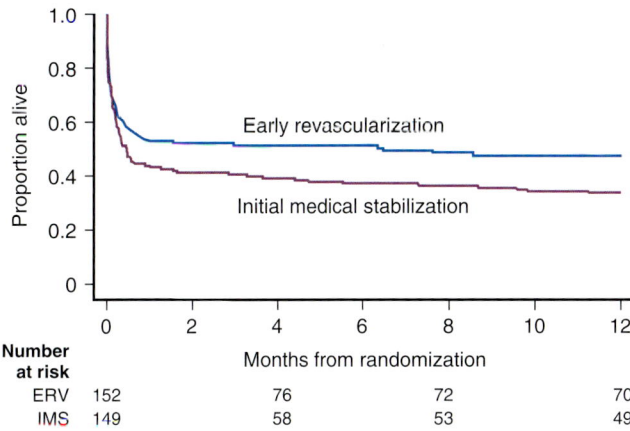

Fig. 22.6 Survival rates among patients undergoing early revascularization *(ERV)* or initial medical stabilization *(IMS)* in the SHOCK trial. Both 6-month and 12-month survival rates were significantly higher in those randomized to early revascularization. (Redrawn from Hochman JS, Sleeper LA, White HD, et al. SHOCK investigators: one-year survival following early revascularization for cardiogenic shock. *JAMA*. 2001;285:190–192.)

84 of 132 patients randomized to immediate revascularization with PCI.[44] Success with PCI—defined as the combination of a residual stenosis less than 50%, a greater than 20% reduction in stenosis, and TIMI grade 2 or 3 flow—was achieved in 76% of patients. Overall survival in the patients selected for PCI was 54% at 30 days and 50% at 1 year. Thirty-day survival was 65% after successful PCI, but it was only 20% if PCI was unsuccessful ($P > .001$). At 1 year, these values were 61% and 15%, respectively ($P > .001$). Post-PCI patency and TIMI grade 3 flow in the IRA was strongly associated with survival, even after adjustment for important clinical and hemodynamic characteristics. No patient who had an occluded IRA (TIMI flow grade 0 or 1) after PCI survived. Among CS patients undergoing PCI, age, time from symptom onset to PCI, and post-PCI flow grade are independent predictors of mortality. Of note, revascularization provided benefit at every level of risk.

In the SHOCK trial, the success rate of PCI was relatively low (76%) and not unexpected, given that most patients had diffuse disease and occluded arteries and were hemodynamically unstable. This study predates the era of widespread stenting and adjunctive antiplatelet therapies in the setting of AMI. The majority of these patients underwent balloon angioplasty. Stents were used in 34% of patients, mainly to salvage a failed balloon PCI; the stents were largely first-generation devices implanted without the benefit of current adjunctive therapies. The culprit-artery stenting rate increased during the study from 0% in 1993 to 10% in 1996 and to 74% by 1998 ($P > .001$). PCI was more often successful in stented patients than in unstented patients (93% vs. 67%, $P < .013$), although 1-year survival was similar (54% vs. 48%, $P < .82$). This discrepancy between the success rate and the mortality rate for PCI is probably a result of bias because most stenting was performed following unsuccessful balloon angioplasty. The use of glycoprotein (GP) IIb/IIIa inhibitors (abciximab) also increased during the study period from 0% in 1993 to over 80% by 1998. Although the use of stents and GP IIb/IIIa inhibitors did not improve the mortality rate in the SHOCK trial, more recent data from multiple registries demonstrated that increased use of routine stenting and GP IIb/IIIa inhibitors were independent predictors of procedural success rates, TIMI grade 3 flow, and mortality in patients undergoing PCI for CS.[45] Although 81% of patients in the SHOCK trial had multivessel disease, most patients with PCI underwent single-vessel procedures

(87%). During the study period, an increase was reported in the frequency of multivessel procedures from 0% to 23% ($P = .018$). One-year survival was 55% after single-vessel PCI but only 20% after a single-stage multivessel procedure. More recent data demonstrated no mortality difference between those undergoing only culprit-vessel PCI and those undergoing multivessel PCI in CS despite a high percentage of use of stenting and GP IIb/IIIa inhibitors.[46] Although PCI of the culprit lesion alone has been advocated in the management of AMI, the prevalence of multivessel disease and the possibility of ischemia far from the infarct zone and of progressive deterioration in LV function may argue for a strategy of more complete revascularization with multivessel PCI or surgery. As in STEMI without shock, earlier revascularization is better in CS. Presentation 0 to 6 hours after symptom onset was associated with lower mortality rates among CS patients undergoing primary PCI in the *Arbeitsgemeinschaft Leitende Kardiologische Krankenhausarzte* (ALKK) registry, in which door-to-angiography times were less than 90 minutes in approximately three-fourths of patients.[45] In the SHOCK trial, long-term mortality rates appeared to increase as time to revascularization increased from 0 to 8 hours. However, a survival benefit was seen as long as revascularization was performed within 48 hours after MI and 18 hours after shock onset. The initial misperception that older patients do not benefit from PCI arose from the interaction between treatment effect and age in the SHOCK trial. The apparent lack of benefit for older adults in the trial was likely caused by imbalances between groups in the baseline ejection fraction. Several studies, including the SHOCK trial and registry, have shown the consistent benefit of revascularization in older patients, which suggests that clinicians are capable of identifying older patients who are most appropriate for revascularization.[47] The American College of Cardiology (ACC)/American Heart Association (AHA) guidelines recommend early revascularization in CS for those younger than 75 years of age (class I) and for suitable candidates over 75 years of age (class IIa).[48] In a certain group of patients, however, additional treatment is futile, particularly when irreversible multiple end-organ failure or anoxic brain damage has occurred.

MULTIVESSEL DISEASE

The optimal revascularization strategy (i.e., percutaneous or surgical revascularization, single or multivessel PCI) for patients with multivessel CAD and CS is not clear. This is of particular importance because multivessel disease is common; 87% of patients in the SHOCK trial had multivessel disease. Both percutaneous and surgical methods of revascularization were permitted in the SHOCK trial. Thirty-seven percent of patients assigned to the early revascularization strategy underwent CABG at a median of 2.7 hours after randomization.[49] Despite a higher prevalence of triple-vessel or left main CAD and diabetes mellitus in patients who underwent CABG compared with those who underwent PCI, survival and quality of life were similar. The coronary anatomy may be most amenable to CABG in some patients. Immediate CABG is the preferred method of revascularization when severe triple-vessel or left main CAD is present and should be performed, as needed, when ventricular septal rupture or severe mitral regurgitation exists. In the SHOCK trial, the rate of multivessel PCI increased over the study period, which perhaps suggests that operators had gained experience with PCI in patients with CS. However, this small subset had a worse adjusted outcome than those who had single-vessel PCI.

Although current ACC/AHA guidelines suggest avoiding PCI in non-IRAs unless the patient is in CS, recent trial data suggest a possible benefit for complete revascularization even in patients who are not in CS. The Preventive Angioplasty in Acute Myocardial Infarction (PRAMI) trial[50] and other trials (see Chapter 21) examined the role of multivessel PCI in both infarct and nonculprit arteries and showed that those patients randomized to the preventative PCI group of more complete revascularization had a significantly reduced risk of adverse cardiovascular events (hazard ratio [HR], 0.35; 95% confidence interval [CI], 0.21 to 0.58; $P < .001$). Although promising, the PRAMI trial was relatively small (465 patients), and follow-up was limited to 23 months because of early discontinuation of the trial. Another criticism of the trial has been that revascularization in the nonculprit lesions occurred without any further testing for ischemia, which is the most commonly used practice. (See Chapter 21 for further review of trials examining multivessel PCI in both CS and non-CS patients.)

Based on the current trial data and the ACC/AHA guidelines, PCI of the IRA is recommended in the case of single-vessel or double-vessel disease or moderate triple-vessel disease and when CABG is not possible for patients with more extensive disease. Staged multivessel PCI may be performed if surgery is not an option, and a single-stage procedure may be considered if the patient remains in shock after PCI of the IRA and if the other vessels have a flow-limiting lesion and supply a large region at risk.

LONG-TERM SURVIVAL AND QUALITY OF LIFE

Long-term survival data from the SHOCK trial revealed persistence of treatment benefit with remarkable 3- and 6-year survival rates in the early revascularization group of 41.4% and 32.8%, respectively, with persistence of treatment benefit (Fig. 22.7).[51] These findings are consistent with the 11-year survival rate of 55% observed in the GUSTO-I trial with 30-day CS survivors.[52] Furthermore, in GUSTO-I, annual mortality rates after 1 year (2% to 4%) were similar for those with shock and those without.

In survivors, quality of life is at least as important as long-term survival. At 2 weeks after discharge, 75.9% of patients assigned to revascularization and 62.5% assigned to medical stabilization in the SHOCK trial were in New York Heart Association (NYHA) functional classes I or II.[53] Among patients who were in NYHA functional class III to IV at 2 weeks, 55% of survivors improved to class I or II by 1 year. Similarly, in a series of patients with CS treated with early revascularization, 80% of survivors were completely asymptomatic at a median of 18 months, and all were in NYHA functional class I or II.[54] Bicycle exercise testing in a subgroup showed age-appropriate exercise capacity in all. Finally, in a series of patients treated with circulatory support, nearly all performed activities of daily living 1 year after the event, and some had even returned to full-time employment.[55]

CONCLUSION

CS is a treatable illness with a reasonable chance for recovery, although the literature has traditionally focused on the very high mortality associated with this diagnosis. It is important to recognize that although patients with CS are at very high risk for early death, great potential exists for salvage. Revascularization is associated with some benefit at every level of risk. An early invasive approach can increase short-term and long-term survival and results in patients regaining an excellent quality of life.

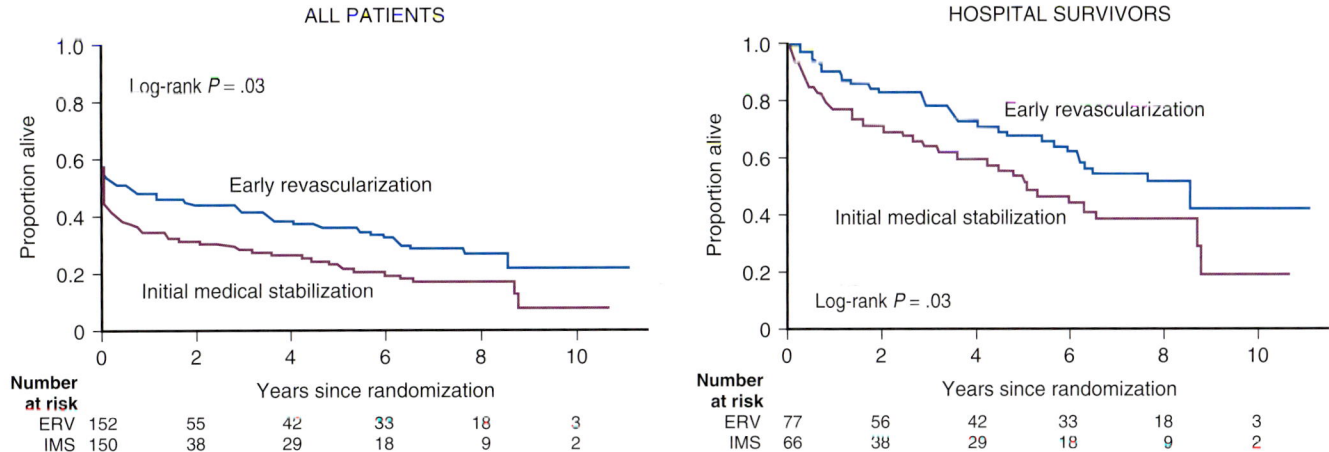

Fig. 22.7 Long-term survival rates by Kaplan-Meier analysis of patients undergoing early revascularization *(ERV)* or initial medical stabilization *(IMS)* in the SHOCK trial. The mortality benefit of immediate revascularization persisted during the 6 years of mean follow-up. (Redrawn from Hochman JS, Sleeper LA, Webb JG, et al. for the SHOCK Investigators. Early revascularization and long-term survival in cardiogenic shock complicating acute myocardial infarction. *JAMA*. 2006;295:2511–2515.)

KEY REFERENCES

1. Hollenberg SM, Davinsky CJ, Parillo JE. Cardiogenic shock. *Ann Intern Med*. 1999;131:47–59.
12. Babaev A, Frederick PD, Pasta DJ, et al. Trends in the management and outcomes of patients with acute myocardial infarction complicated by cardiogenic shock. *JAMA*. 2005;294:448–454.
13. Hochman JS, Sleeper LA, Webb JG, et al. Early revascularization in acute myocardial infarction complicated by cardiogenic shock. SHOCK Investigators. Should We Emergently Revascularize Occluded Coronaries for Cardiogenic Shock. *N Engl J Med*. 1999;341:625–634.
19. Stevenson LW, Perloff JK. The limited reliability of physical signs for estimating hemodynamics in chronic heart failure. *JAMA*. 1989;261:884–888.
21. ESCAPE Investigators and ESCAPE Study Coordinators. Evaluation study of congestive heart failure and pulmonary artery catheterization effectiveness: the ESCAPE trial. *JAMA*. 2005;294:1625–1633.
23. SHOCK Investigators. Cardiac power is the strongest hemodynamic correlate of mortality in cardiogenic shock: a report from the SHOCK trial registry. *J Am Coll Cardiol*. 2004;44:340–348.
25. Abraham WT, Kirkwood KF, Fonarow GC, et al. In-hospital mortality in patients with acute decompensated heart failure requiring intravenous vasoactive medications: an analysis from the Acute Decompensated Heart Failure National Registry (ADHERE). *J Am Coll Cardiol*. 2005;46:57–64.
26. Cuffe MS, Califf RM, Adams KF, et al. Short-term intravenous milrinone for acute exacerbation of chronic heart failure: a randomized controlled trial (OPTIME-CHF). *JAMA*. 2002;287:1578–1580.
28. De Backer D, Biston P, Devriendt J, et al. Comparison of dopamine and norepinephrine in the treatment of shock. *N Engl J Med*. 2010;362:779–789.
29. Samuels LE, Kaufman MS, Thomas MP, et al. Doses and types of vasopressors and inotropes and increasing mortality. *J Card Surg*. 1999;14:288–293.
31. Kantrowitz A, Tjonneland S, Freed PS, et al. Initial clinical experience with intraaortic balloon pumping in cardiogenic shock. *JAMA*. 1968;203:113–118.
35. Thiele H, Zeymer U, Neumann FJ, et al. Intra-aortic balloon counterpulsation in acute myocardial infarction complicated by cardiogenic shock (IABP-SHOCK II): final 12 month results of a randomised, open-label trial. *Lancet*. 2013;382:1638–1645.
38. Shreenivas S, Wilensky R. Percutaneous circulatory support during percutaneous coronary intervention. *Interv Cardiol*. 2012;4:449–460.
50. Wald DS, Morris JK, Wald NJ, et al. Randomized trial of preventive angioplasty in myocardial infarction. *N Engl J Med*. 2012;369:1115–1123.
54. Ammann P, Straumann E, Naegeli B, et al. Long-term results after acute percutaneous transluminal coronary angioplasty in acute myocardial infarction and cardiogenic shock. *Int J Cardiol*. 2002;82:127–131.

Additional references available online at expertconsult.com.

中文导读

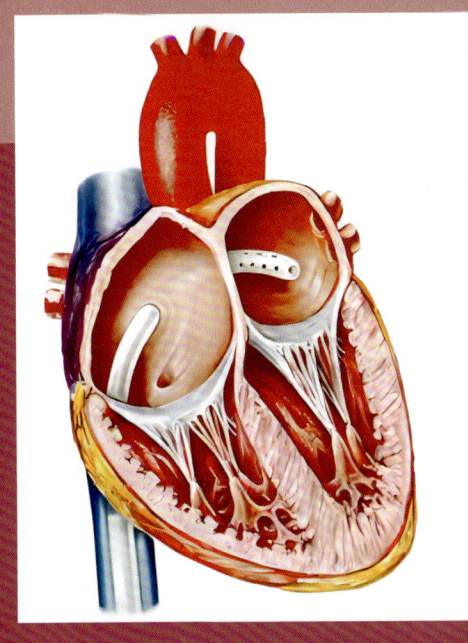

第23章
分叉和边支血管支架置入术

　　冠状动脉分叉病变是指发生在心外膜冠状动脉主要分支处附近的病变。最重要的分类是将分叉病变分为"真性"分叉和"非真性"分叉，前者指主分支和侧分支均存在明显狭窄（>50%直径狭窄），后者则包括涉及分叉的所有其他病变类型。在常规临床实践中，Medina分类法仍然是对冠状动脉分叉病变进行分类的最简单和应用最广泛的方法。

　　尽管有各种治疗手段，药物洗脱支架仍然是治疗分叉病变的常规方法，而在主分支上置入一个支架是最广泛使用的方法。多项比较单支架和双支架治疗冠状动脉分叉病变效果的随机试验结果表明，仅在主分支内置入支架仍是首选策略；在大多数情况下，可行必要性（边支）支架术置入术。现有的随机试验得出的结论是，对于大多数冠状动脉分叉病变患者，常规双支架置入并没有改善血管造影或临床结局。

　　分叉病变不仅在解剖结构上表现出差异性（斑块负荷、斑块位置、分支间的角度、分支的直径、分叉位置），而且在治疗过程中解剖结构的动态变化（斑块/嵴的移位、夹层）也有差异，因此在分叉病变经皮冠状动脉介入治疗中最重要的问题是根据病变的特点选择最合适的策略。本章详细清晰地梳理了常见的单支架和双支架术式的步骤流程和适用的病变解剖结构。合理应用腔内影像学、旋磨术等技术可以有效辅助分叉病变的介入治疗。

何松原　柳景华

章节要点

- 除了开口位于主动脉位置的开口病变外,其他部位的开口病变被视为一种可能的分叉病变。
- 6 F指引导管在大多数情况下是合适的;如果不确定,则应使用7 F或8 F指引导管。
- 不要冒失去分支的风险;如果不确定,一定要用导丝去保护边支。
- 如果导丝进入边支困难,可考虑首先扩张主支。
- 必要性支架置入术并不意味着可接受一个重要分支的不良最终结果。
- 用双支架(主支支架和分支支架)治疗分叉病变是一种可接受的策略。
- 在置入两个支架时,不要忘记高压扩张分支后进行最终对吻扩张。
- 当专门用于分叉病变的药物洗脱支架可用时,许多理念会发生变化,包括双支架策略更灵活用途的出现。
- 最佳抗血小板治疗始终是短期和长期介入治疗成功的关键因素,对于最新进展应做到与时俱进。

23 Bifurcations and Branch Vessel Stenting

Antonio Colombo, Goran Stankovic

KEY POINTS

- Always consider an ostial lesion as a possible bifurcation lesion, except in cases of aortoostial location.
- A 6-Fr guiding catheter is appropriate most of the time; when in doubt, use 7- or 8-Fr.
- Do not risk losing the side branch (SB); when in doubt, always protect it with a wire.
- If there are difficulties wiring the SB, consider dilating the main branch first.
- Provisional stenting does not mean accepting a poor final result for an important SB.
- Treatment of a bifurcation lesion with two stents (main and SBs) is an acceptable approach.
- Do not forget the final kissing inflation preceded by high-pressure inflation on the SB when implanting two stents.
- When dedicated drug-eluting stent (DES) for bifurcation lesions become available, many concepts may change, including the emergence of a more liberal usage of a two-stent strategy.
- Optimal antiplatelet therapy is always a key factor for short- and long-time success: keep yourself updated for new developments.

BIFURCATION LESIONS

A bifurcation coronary lesion is a lesion occurring at, or adjacent to, a significant division of a major epicardial coronary artery. Coronary bifurcation lesions have been the subject of several classifications, with the underlying assumption that each type could be associated with a specific treatment. However, attempts to classify bifurcation lesions[1-6] suffer all the limitations of coronary angiography (different plaque distribution and extent of disease when evaluated by intravascular ultrasound [IVUS]).[7] At the present time, there are six different classifications of bifurcation lesions (Fig. 23.1). The most important distinction to is to divide bifurcation lesions into "true" bifurcations, where the main branch (MB) and the side branch (SB) are both significantly narrowed (>50% diameter stenosis), and "nontrue" bifurcations, which include all the other lesions involving a bifurcation. In routine practice, the "Medina" classification is still the most simplified and widely used approach to classify distribution of atherosclerotic plaque at bifurcation site.[5] The presence of "1" means >50% diameter stenosis and "0" the absence of stenosis, in each of the three bifurcation segments, starting with proximal MB, distal MB, and proximal SB: 1,1,1 when there is a critical stenosis in all three segments and 1,1,0 when only the proximal and distal MB are affected. Many other combinations are possible. A limitation of the Medina classification is that the length of the stenosis involving the SB is not specified and we think that this distinction is a key element to properly plan the treatment.

Despite an array of devices available, stenting utilizing drug-eluting stent (DES) remains the default approach to treat bifurcation lesions, and the implantation of a single stent on the MB is the most widely used approach.

Contemporary Studies

Several major randomized trials comparing one or two stents in the treatment of coronary bifurcations demonstrated that the implantation of a stent only in the MB remains the preferred strategy.

The sirolimus-eluting stent (SES) bifurcation study was the first attempt to provide specific information in this subset of lesions.[8] Eighty-five patients were randomly assigned to either stenting both branches or stenting the MB only with provisional stenting (PS) of the SB. Data were analyzed by actual treatment received, not by intention-to-treat. Crossover rate was very high, 51.2% in the provisional group and 4.7% in the two-stent group. Restenosis at 6 months did not differ significantly between the stent/stent (28.0%) and the stent/percutaneous transluminal coronary angioplasty (18.7%) groups ($P = .53$). During the 6-month follow-up, there was no significant difference between groups in death, myocardial infarction (MI), target-vessel revascularization (TVR), or target-vessel failure (19.0% vs. 13.6%). Therefore, this study demonstrated that compared with historical studies utilizing bare-metal stents,[1,9,10] a clear improvement has been achieved in the treatment of bifurcation lesions when one or two DESs were implanted.

In a second study, Pan and coworkers compared two strategies for the SES treatment of bifurcation lesions in 91 patients with "true" coronary bifurcation lesions.[11] Six-month major adverse cardiac events (MACEs) and restenosis rate of the MB and of the SB were similar in the two study groups.

A third randomized study was the Nordic Bifurcation Study (Nordic), in which 413 patients were randomized to two stents ($n = 206$) or PS ($n = 207$) with SES implantation.[12] The crossover from provisional to stenting two branches was allowed if thrombolysis in myocardial infarction (TIMI) flow following SB dilation was 0 and was only 4.3%. At 6 months, there was no difference between the two groups regarding cardiac death, MI, index lesion MI, TVR, target-lesion revascularization (TLR) and stent thrombosis (ST). At 5-year follow-up, the combined safety and efficacy end point of cardiac death, nonprocedure-related MI, and TVR remained similar and were seen in 15.8% of patients in the PS group, as compared with 21.8% in the two-stent group ($P = .15$).[13]

In a fourth trial, Bifurcations Bad Krozingen (BBK) study, Ferenc et al. compared 202 patients randomly allocated to either provisional T stenting or routine T stenting[14] utilizing SES. Primary end point was percent diameter stenosis of the SB at 9-month angiographic follow-up, and was similar between the two groups ($P = .15$). The overall 1-year incidence of TLR after provisional and routine T stenting was also similar, as well as the primary clinical outcome (composite of death, MI, TLR was 12.9% vs. 11.9%, $P = .83$).

In the CACTUS trial (Coronary Bifurcations: Application of the Crushing Technique Using Sirolimus-Eluting Stents),[15] 350 patients were randomly allocated to either provisional T or crush SES implantation, with mandatory final kissing balloon inflation (FKBI) in both groups. Stent implantation in the SB was allowed by the T stenting technique only when at least 1 of the following conditions was met: residual stenosis ≥50%, dissection of type B or worse, or TIMI flow ≤2. A high proportion of patients (92%) had true bifurcations, and crossover rate in the provisional T group was 31%. The primary angiographic end point was the in-segment restenosis rate, and the primary clinical end point was the 6-month rate of MACEs (cardiac death, MI, or TVR). At 6 months, angiographic restenosis rates were not different between the crush group (4.6% and 13.2% in the MB and SB, respectively) and the PS group (6.7% and 14.7% in the MB and SB, respectively; P = not significant [NS]). The primary clinical outcome (death, MI, revascularization) was also similar in both groups (15.0% provisional vs. 15.8% crush, P = NS).

In the BBC ONE study (British Bifurcation Coronary Study: Old, New, and Evolving Strategies), 500 patients were randomly allocated to either a simple strategy (minimalist provisional T) or a complex strategy (either crush or culotte) using paclitaxel-eluting stents (PESs).[16] In the simple strategy, the MB was stented, followed by optional kissing balloon dilatation/T stent utilizing the following criteria: TIMI flow <3 in the SB, severe ostial pinching of the SB (>90%), threatened SB closure, or SB dissection greater than type A. Only 30% of SB underwent further treatment after MB stenting (27% balloon dilatation and 3% stenting). In the complex strategy, both branches were systematically stented (culotte or crush techniques) with mandatory kissing balloon dilatation. At 9-month clinical follow-up, there was a significant difference between the two groups in terms of death, MI, or revascularization (simple 8.0% vs. complex 15.5%). This difference was largely driven by the higher incidence of MI in the complex group (11.2% vs. 3.6%, P = .001). It is quite surprising to note the very high number of complications that occurred in patients randomized to the complex strategy.

The DKCRUSH-II (Double Kissing Crush Versus Provisional Stenting Technique for Treatment of Coronary Bifurcation Lesions) trial investigated the difference in MACE (cardiac death, MI, or TVR) at 12 months in 370 patients with coronary bifurcation lesions after double kissing crush (DK-crush) or PS techniques.[17] MACE and definite ST rates were similar between the DK (10.3% and 2.2%) and PS groups (17.3% and 0.5%, P = .070 and P = .372, respectively). However, angiographic restenosis rates in the main vessel (MV), and the SB were lower in the DK group (3.8% and 4.9%) than the PS group (9.7% and 22.2%, P = .036 and P < .001, respectively), as well as TVR (6.5% vs. 14.6%, P = .017). At 5 years, MACE tended to occur more frequently in patients treated with a provisional strategy, as opposed to DK-crush (23.8% vs. 15.7%, P = .051).[18] TLR rate was higher in patients with PS versus DK-crush (16.2% vs. 8.6%, P = .027), particularly in patients with anatomically more complex lesions.[18,19]

Most recently, the DKCRUSH-V (Double Kissing Crush Versus Provisional Stenting for Left Main Distal Bifurcation Lesions) randomized trial showed a reduction in a 12-month target lesion failure (TLF) rate with DK-crush versus PS

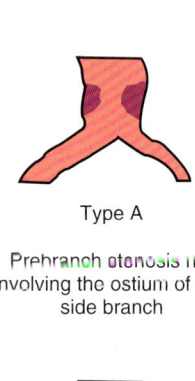

Type A

Prebranch stenosis not involving the ostium of the side branch

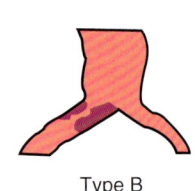

Type B

Postbranch stenosis of the parent vessel not involving the ostium of the side branch

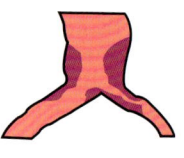

Type I

True bifurcation lesion

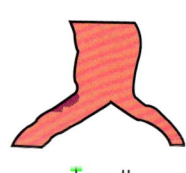

Type II

One-sided asymmetric lesion where only one branch is diseased

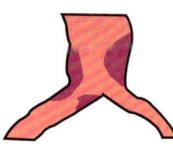

Type C

Stenosis of the parent vessel not involving the ostium of the side branch

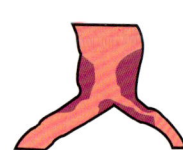

Type D

Stenosis involving the parent vessel and the ostium of the side branch

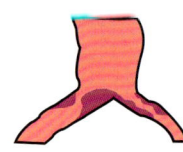

Type III

Branch bifurcation lesion where parent vessel is free of disease and both branches have ostial disease

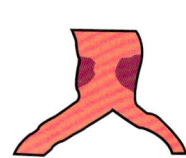

Type IV

Lesion in the parent vessel either before or after the takeoff of a side branch that may or may not have additional ostial disease

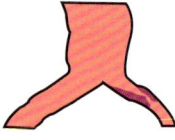

Type E

Stenosis involving the ostium of the side branch only

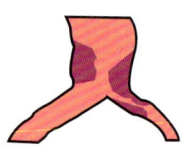

Type F

Stenosis discretely involving the parent vessel and the ostium of the side branch

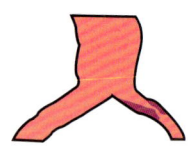

Type V

Single branch point or ostial lesion at a bifurcation

A   B

Fig. 23.1 Various classifications of bifurcations according to plaque distribution: Duke (A), Sanborn (B),

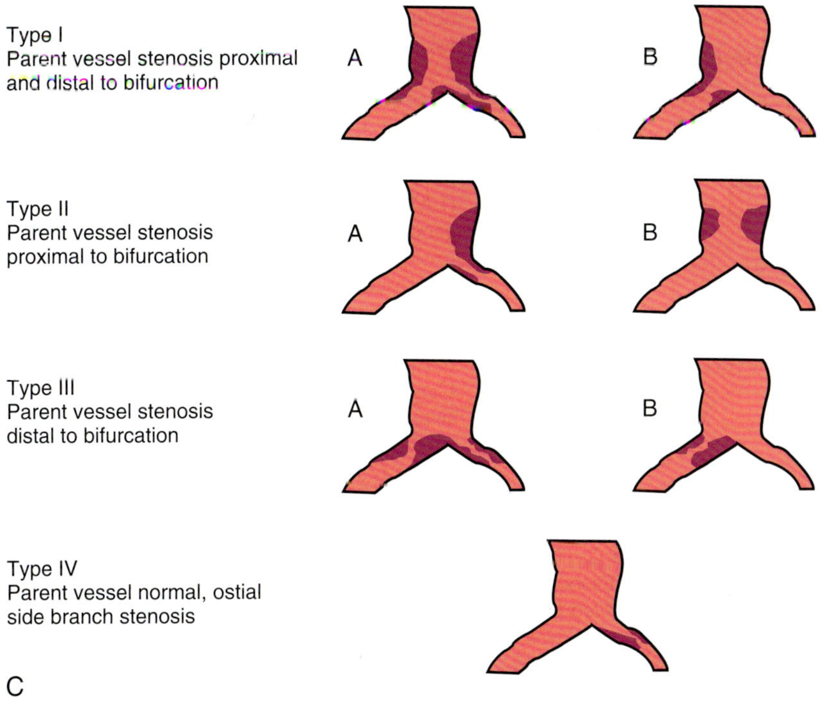

CHAPTER 23 Bifurcations and Branch Vessel Stenting

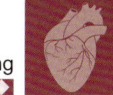

Type I
Parent vessel stenosis proximal and distal to bifurcation

A B

Type II
Parent vessel stenosis proximal to bifurcation

A B

Type III
Parent vessel stenosis distal to bifurcation

A B

Type IV
Parent vessel normal, ostial side branch stenosis

C

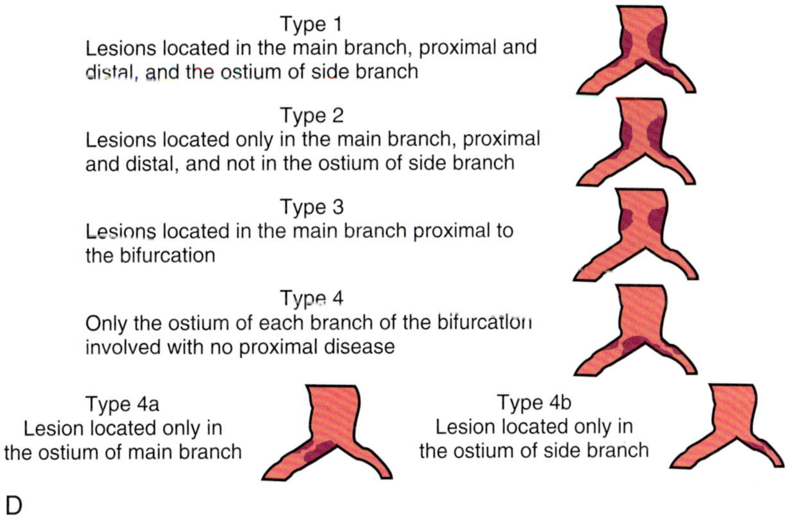

Type 1
Lesions located in the main branch, proximal and distal, and the ostium of side branch

Type 2
Lesions located only in the main branch, proximal and distal, and not in the ostium of side branch

Type 3
Lesions located in the main branch proximal to the bifurcation

Type 4
Only the ostium of each branch of the bifurcation involved with no proximal disease

Type 4a
Lesion located only in the ostium of main branch

Type 4b
Lesion located only in the ostium of side branch

D

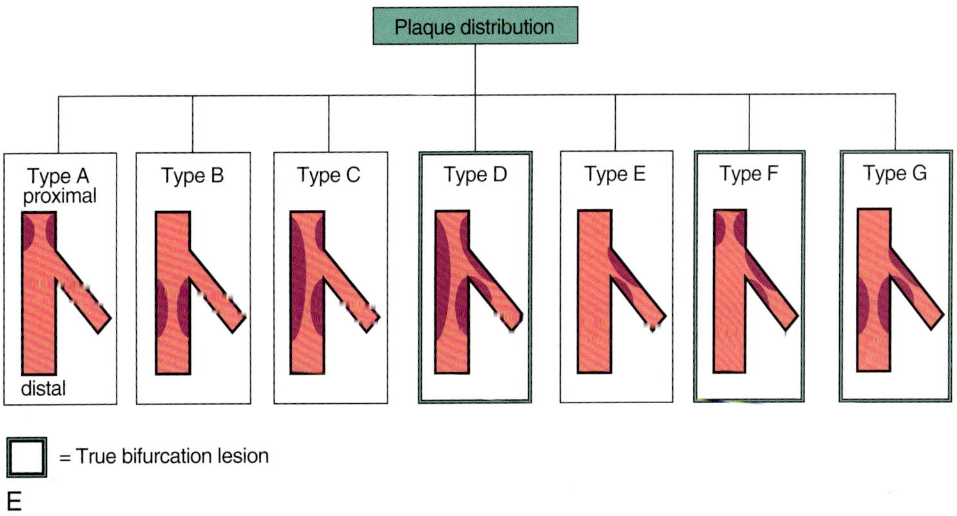

Plaque distribution

| Type A proximal | Type B | Type C | Type D | Type E | Type F | Type G |

distal

☐ = True bifurcation lesion

E

Fig. 23.1—Cont'd Safian (C), Lefevre (D), SYNTAX study (E),

463

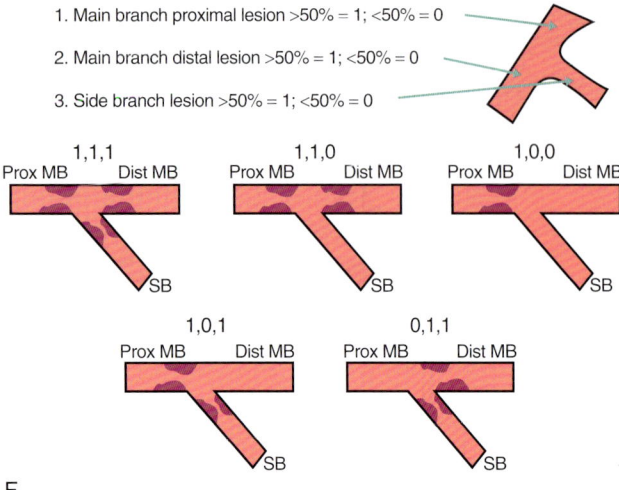

Fig. 23.1—Cont;d Medina (F). *MB*, Main branch; *SB*, side branch. (A, From Popma J, Leon M, Topol EJ. *Atlas of Interventional Cardiology*. Philadelphia: Saunders; 1994; B, From Spokojny AM, Sanborn TM. The bifurcation lesion. In: Ellis SG, Holmes DR, eds. *Strategic Approaches in Coronary Intervention*. Baltimore: Williams and Wilkins; 1996:288; C, From Safian RD. Bifurcation lesions. In: Safian RD, Freed M, eds. *Manual of Interventional Cardiology*. Royal Oak: Physicians' Press; 2001:221–236; D, From Lefevre T, Louvard Y, Morice MC, et al. Stenting of bifurcation lesions: classification, treatments, and results. *Catheter Cardiovasc Interv*. 2000;49:274–283; E, From Sianos G, Morel MA, Kappetein AP, et al. The SYNTAX score: an angiographic tool grading the complexity of coronary artery disease. *EuroIntervention*. 2005;1:219–227; F, From Medina A, Suárez de Lezo J, Pan M. A new classification of coronary bifurcation lesions. *Rev Esp Cardiol*. 2006;59:183.)

(5.0% vs. 10.7%, $P = .02$) in patients with true distal left main (LM) bifurcation lesions.[20] DK-crush was associated with a tendency toward less clinically driven TLR (3.8 vs. 7.9%, $P = .06$), and surprisingly, it also resulted in lower rates of MI (0.4% vs. 2.9%, $P = .03$) and ST (0.4% vs. 3.3%, $P = .02$).

The clinical implication of these trials is that in most cases, provisional rather than elective stenting of the SB should be performed.[21–23] PS appears less expensive and simpler, and can be performed with less contrast and in a shorter procedural time. At the same time, the evidence of comparable results in the two arms does not contradict the choice of crush/culotte stenting in selected cases with complex anatomy or with diffuse disease on the SB. The consensus from available randomized trials was that routine two-vessel stenting did not improve either angiographic or clinical outcomes for most patients with coronary bifurcation lesions, although routine dual vessel stenting did not involve a significant penalty either.[24]

One shortcoming of these trials was that the treatment groups including two stents were heterogeneous, and the techniques used may have resulted in different clinical outcomes.

Clinical outcomes in randomized trials comparing one- versus two-stent strategies in non-LM bifurcations are presented in Fig. 23.2.

To evaluate the impact of specific two-stent technique, the Nordic complex bifurcation stenting study was performed. In this investigation, 424 patients were randomized to either crush or culotte stenting utilizing SES (77% of which were "true" coronary bifurcation lesions).[25] At 6-month clinical follow-up, there was no difference between the two groups in terms of death, post-procedure MI, or revascularization (the primary end point: crush 4.3% vs. culotte 3.7%, $P = .87$). However, there was a trend for a higher incidence of periprocedural MI and significantly higher occurrence of in-stent restenosis in the crush group (crush 10.5% vs. culotte 4.5%, $P = .046$). Clinical outcomes remained similar at 3-year follow-up in the crush and the culotte groups, with MACE rates of 20.6% versus 16.7% ($P = .32$).[26]

The DKCRUSH-III study investigated the difference in MACE rates at 1-year after DK crush and Culotte stenting in 419 patients with unprotected left main coronary artery (LMCA) distal bifurcation lesions.[27] Patients in the Culotte group had higher 1-year MACE rate compared with the DK group (16.3% vs. 6.2%, $P = .001$), which was mainly driven by increased TVR rate (11.0% vs. 4.3%, $P = .016$). In all prespecified subsets, patients with bifurcation angle ≥70 degrees, NERS (New Risk Stratification) score ≥20, and SYNTAX (Synergy between Percutaneous Coronary Intervention with Taxus and Cardiac Surgery) score ≥23, MACE rates at 1 year were consistently lower in the DK group. At 3 years, the occurrence of MACE remains more frequent in the culotte versus DK-crush group (23.7% vs. 8.2%, $P < .001$), mainly driven by a higher rate of TVR (18.8% vs. 5.8%, $P < .001$) and MI (8.2% vs. 3.4%, $P = .037$).[28] Interestingly, the rate of definite ST was 3.4% in patients treated with culotte, whereas no definite ST was documented in the DK-crush group (0.007).

In the BBK II trial, 300 patients with bifurcation lesions requiring SB stenting were randomized to undergo T stenting and small protrusion (TAP) or culotte stenting.[29] Nine-month angiographic follow-up, which was available for 91% of the patients, revealed higher binary restenosis rate after TAP as compared with culotte (17.0% vs. 6.5%, $P = .006$), whereas the 1-year incidence of TLR was 12% in the TAP group and 6% in the culotte group ($P = .069$).[29]

To evaluate the impact of a specific DES type on clinical outcome in patients with bifurcation lesions, Pan et al. enrolled 205 patients in a prospective randomized trial; 103 patients were assigned to SES and 102 patients to PES.[30] All patients were treated by provisional T stenting. Angiographic data and immediate procedural results were similar in both groups. There was no difference in rates of death or MI in-hospital and during follow-up. Primary end point, angiographic restenosis rate, was significantly lower in the SES group (9% vs. 29%, $P = .011$), as well as TLR at 24 months post stenting (4% vs. 13%, $P = .021$). Similar results were obtained in the COBIS (Coronary Bifurcation Stenting) registry, which compared MACEs (MACE defined as cardiac death, MI, or TLR) between SES and PES.[31] At a mean follow-up of 22 months, treatment with SES resulted in a lower incidence of MACE (hazard ratio [HR] 0.53; 95% confidence interval [CI], 0.32 to 0.89; $P < .01$) and TLR (HR; 0.55, 95% CI, 0.31 to 0.97; $P = .02$), but not of cardiac death and cardiac death or MI.

Clinical outcome of newer generation DES in bifurcation lesions was evaluated in several randomized trials. Burzotta et al. randomized 150 consecutive patients with bifurcated lesions undergoing systematic provisional-stenting to SES or everolimus-eluting stent (EES) in the Sirolimus Versus Everolimus-Eluting Stent Randomized Assessment in Bifurcated Lesions and Clinical Significance of Residual Side-Branch Stenosis (SEA-SIDE) study.[32] The primary procedural end point was the occurrence of any trouble in the SB management and was similar between SES and EES (16% vs. 11%, $P = .34$). The primary angiographic end point (post-percutaneous coronary intervention [PCI] three-dimensional quantitative coronary arteriography [QCA]-estimated minimal lumen diameter) showed similar post-PCI results in the MV and better results in the SB with EES than with SES. Clinical outcome at 18 months showed no difference in rates of target bifurcation failure (9.0% in SES vs. 10.7% in EES patients, $P = .57$). SES and EES were also compared in the randomized Cordoba & Las Palmas (CORPAL) study, in which 293 patients with bifurcation lesions were treated utilizing the provisional SB stenting technique.[33] In-hospital outcome and

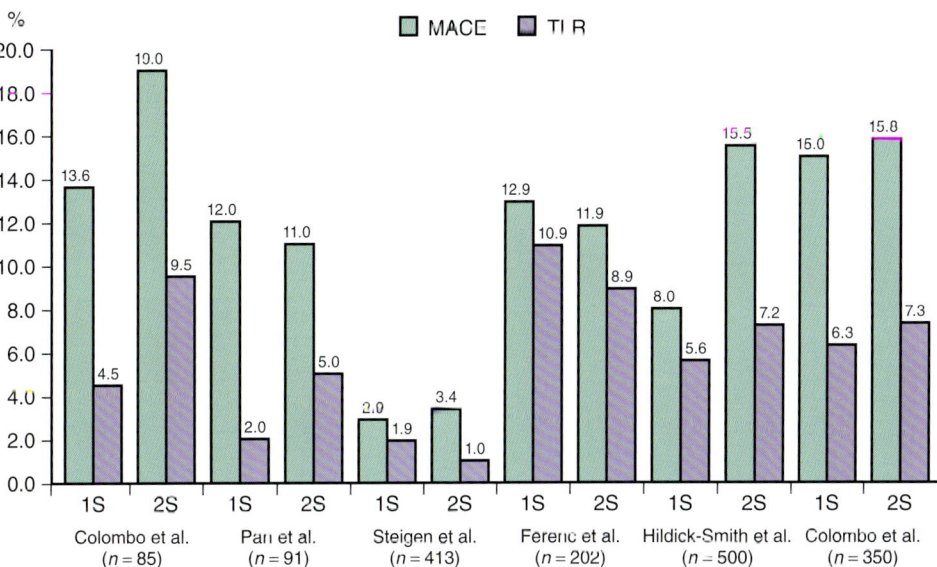

Fig. 23.2 Clinical outcomes in randomized trials comparing one- versus two-stent strategy, utilizing drug-eluting stents. *1S,* Single stent; *2S,* two stents; *MACE,* major adverse cardiac events; *TLR,* target-lesion revascularization. (Data from Colombo A, Moses JW, Morice MC, et al. Randomized study to evaluate sirolimus-eluting stents implanted at coronary bifurcation lesions. *Circulation.* 2004;109:1244–1249; Pan M, de Lezo JS, Medina A, et al. Rapamycin-eluting stents for the treatment of bifurcated coronary lesions: a randomized comparison of a simple versus complex strategy. *Am Heart J.* 2004;148:857–864; Steigen TK, Maeng M, Wiseth R, et al: Randomized study on simple versus complex stenting of coronary artery bifurcation lesions: the Nordic bifurcation study. *Circulation.* 2006;114:1955–1961; Ferenc M, Gick M, Kienzle RP, et al. Randomized trial on routine vs. provisional T stenting in the treatment of de novo coronary bifurcation lesions. *Eur Heart J.* 2008;29:2859–2867; Hildick-Smith D, de Belder AJ, Cooter N, et al. Randomized trial of simple versus complex drug-eluting stenting for bifurcation lesions: the British bifurcation coronary study: old, new, and evolving strategies. *Circulation* 2010;121:1235–1243; and Colombo A, Bramucci E, Sacca S, et al. Randomized study of the crush technique versus provisional side-branch stenting in true coronary bifurcations: the CACTUS [Coronary Bifurcations: Application of the Crushing Technique Using Sirolimus-Eluting Stents] Study. *Circulation.* 2009;119:71–78.)

12-month follow-up MACE was similar between SES and EES (6.2% vs. 6.1%, $P = .84$). A pooled analysis of these two randomized trials (SEA-SIDE and CORPAL) showed similar MACE-free survival at 3 years, while exploratory landmark analysis for late events (occurring after 1 year) showed significantly fewer MACE in the EES group (1.4% vs. 5.4%, $P = .02$).

In a prospective extension of the SEA-SIDE study, the performance of a zotarolimus-eluting stent (ZES) was compared with that obtained using SES and EES (the Z-SEA-SIDE).[34] ZES demonstrated improved performance compared with SES (SB "trouble" rate 4% vs. 16%, $P = .014$) and SB angiographic results, while ZES were similar to EES.

The recent 5-year follow-up study of the LEADERS all-comers randomized trial showed a superior long-term efficacy of a Biolimus A9(TM)–eluting stent (BES) compared with an SES.[35] BES also tended to associate with a lower rate of very late ST between years 1 and 5. The importance of the observed beneficial results of the second-generation DES over the first-generation DES in terms of coronary bifurcation treatment was confirmed by a recent pooled analysis of 3162 patients from the Korean Bifurcation Pooled Cohorts, which suggested comparable results of single- versus double-stenting if second-generation DES were used, contrary to previous reports favoring a single-stent approach if first-generation DES had been used.[36]

Approach to Treatment of Bifurcation Lesions

Bifurcations vary not only in anatomy (plaque burden, location of plaque, angle between branches, diameter of branches, bifurcation site) but also in the dynamic changes in anatomy during treatment (plaque/carina shift, dissection).

Previous pathologic studies demonstrated that atherosclerosis occurs predominantly in low shear-stress regions of bifurcation, but carina (flow divider) involvement by atherosclerosis is extremely unusual. Nakazawa et al. recently demonstrated that in nonstented coronary bifurcations, the lateral wall showed significantly greater intima as well as necrotic core thickness than the flow divider.[37] After stenting, plaque formation and neointimal growth were also significantly less at the flow divider versus the lateral wall. Those observations were also confirmed in vivo by IVUS preintervention evaluation of distal LMCA bifurcations.[38] Oviedo et al. showed that bifurcation disease is usually diffuse and, contrary to angiographic classifications that the carina (flow divider), was spared in all lesions, while the plaque was present predominantly on the opposite side of the flow divider. However, data presented by van der Giessen et al. threw new light on the subject through computed tomography (CT) angiography suggesting that the carina does have some atheroma present in 30% of bifurcations, though the volume of that plaque remains small and was present only if there is significant volume of plaque located at the lateral walls opposite to flow divider (low wall shear stress areas), indicating that atherosclerotic plaque grows circumferentially.[39]

Koo et al. evaluated with IVUS and fractional flow reserve (FFR) the mechanisms of changes in the geometry of the ostium of the SB after the MB stenting, testing the hypothesis that MB stenting may create worsening of an SB ostial lesion as a result of a combination of MB plaque and carina shift.[40] The investigators concluded that the decrease in plaque volume in the proximal MB, with no associated increase in plaque volume in the distal MB, was indirect evidence of plaque shift from the MB to the SB ostium after stent implantation. In addition, the increased luminal volume in the distal MB, with no significant decrease in the plaque volume, was believed to be due to vessel enlargement and provided support to the theory that carina shift is likely to contribute to the degree of luminal narrowing of the SB.

As a result of those investigations, we can conclude that no two bifurcations are identical, and no single strategy exists that can be applied to every bifurcation. Thus the most important issue in bifurcation PCI is selecting the most appropriate strategy for an individual bifurcation and optimizing the performance of this technique.

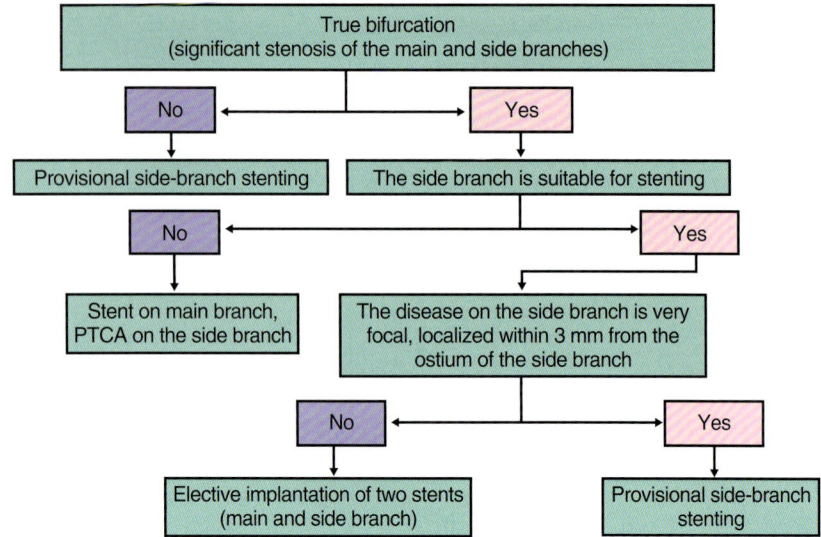

Fig. 23.3 Our proposed algorithm for stenting bifurcation lesions. *PTCA,* Percutaneous transluminal coronary angioplasty.

Guiding Catheter Selection

Most bifurcation lesions can be approached with a 6-Fr guiding catheter because a provisional strategy will be utilized most of the times. The exception is when, due to lesion characteristics, the operator decides from the very beginning to implant two stents (needing a 7- or 8-Fr guiding catheter). When there are doubts regarding the optimal treatment and the operator needs to make a decision following predilatation, we suggest usage of a 7- or 8-Fr guiding catheter.

With currently available very low profile balloons, it is possible to insert two balloons inside a large lumen 6-Fr guiding catheter. If two stents are needed and a 6-Fr guiding catheter is employed, some limitations need to be known. The two stents can only be inserted and deployed sequentially. The standard crush technique and the V or kissing stents technique cannot be performed unless a guiding catheter of 7 or 8 Fr is utilized.

A General Outline When Treating a Bifurcation Lesion

Fig. 23.3 summarizes a proposed approach to bifurcation lesions with an attempt to give directions regarding SB stenting as intention-to-treat only in cases where disease on the SB extends beyond the ostium and the SB has a significant area of distribution.

The most frequently used approach is provisional SB stenting,[23] and it is outlined as follows:

1. Placement of two wires (MB and SB)
2. Predilatation of MB or both branches, when needed[21]
3. Stenting of the MB
4. Stent optimization with proximal optimization technique (POT)
5. Recrossing with a wire into the SB
6. Crossing with a balloon into the SB
7. Performance of FKBI, with moderate pressure (8 atm) in the SB, until the balloon is fully expanded
8. Final POT, if result in the SB is adequate after FKBI[23]
9. Placement of a second stent in the SB when the result is unsatisfactory (>75% residual stenosis, dissection, TIMI flow grade <3 in a SB ≥2.5 mm or FFR <0.80)

An important aspect when stenting bifurcations is the protection of the SB by inserting a wire to be left until the stenting procedure on the MB has been completed, including high-pressure stent deployment or postdilatation. During jailed wire retrieval, attention is paid to avoid any trauma to coronary ostium with the guiding catheter, which tends to be pulled in as jailed wire is removed.

In the provisional technique, wire cross through the distal strut (the "carina strut") following MB stenting is strongly suggested because it creates better SB scaffolding than proximal crossing.[41]

In order to optimize SB access through the carina strut, the POT technique is suggested.[41] Optimization of the stent deployment proximal to the carina by using a short larger-diameter balloon may help access the most distal strut during wire exchange. If the result remains unsatisfactory after MB stenting, SB stenting should be performed with T stenting or TAP-stenting, reverse/internal crush or culotte, followed by kissing balloon inflation.[41] Given the heterogeneity in local resource environment and operators level of experience, both of these variables may need to be taken into account when following the recommended general outlines for treatment of coronary bifurcation lesions.[22,42]

Difficult Side Branch Access

After having attempted different types of wires with variations of curves and other advanced techniques, the operator may be left with the impossibility to advance a wire in the SB. At this point, a few options are available: (1) abort the procedure because the risk of closing the SB is too high, given the size and distribution of the branch (typically an angulated circumflex artery); (2) use a microcatheter in order to navigate a reshaped wire in unfavorable MV anatomies or the SuperCross catheter (Vascular Solutions, Minneapolis, MN) with different preshaped tip curves; (3) perform rotational atherectomy on the MV with the intent to remove the plaque, which prevents entry toward the SB; (4) dilate the MV with a balloon, hoping plaque modification will result in favorable plaque shift and facilitate access toward the SB; (5) use the "reverse wire" technique, creating a unique guidewire tip with two sharp curves (a longer proximal curve to create a loop in the distal MV and an opposite short distal curve to engage the SB ostium during the wire pullback);[21] or (6) use the Venture wire control catheter (Vascular Solutions), a low-profile catheter with a tip that can be deflected up to 90 degrees to facilitate wire orientation and provide excellent backup support (Fig. 23.4).[43] Sometimes the use of a relatively stiff wire can be a solution, due to the better steerability and penetration force. Use of hydrophilic wires can also be considered; however, the risk of subintimal passage is increased when using stiff and/or hydrophilic wires.

Each of these options has its rationale. The specific anatomical condition, the operator's experience, and the clinical scenario may direct the selection of the best strategy.

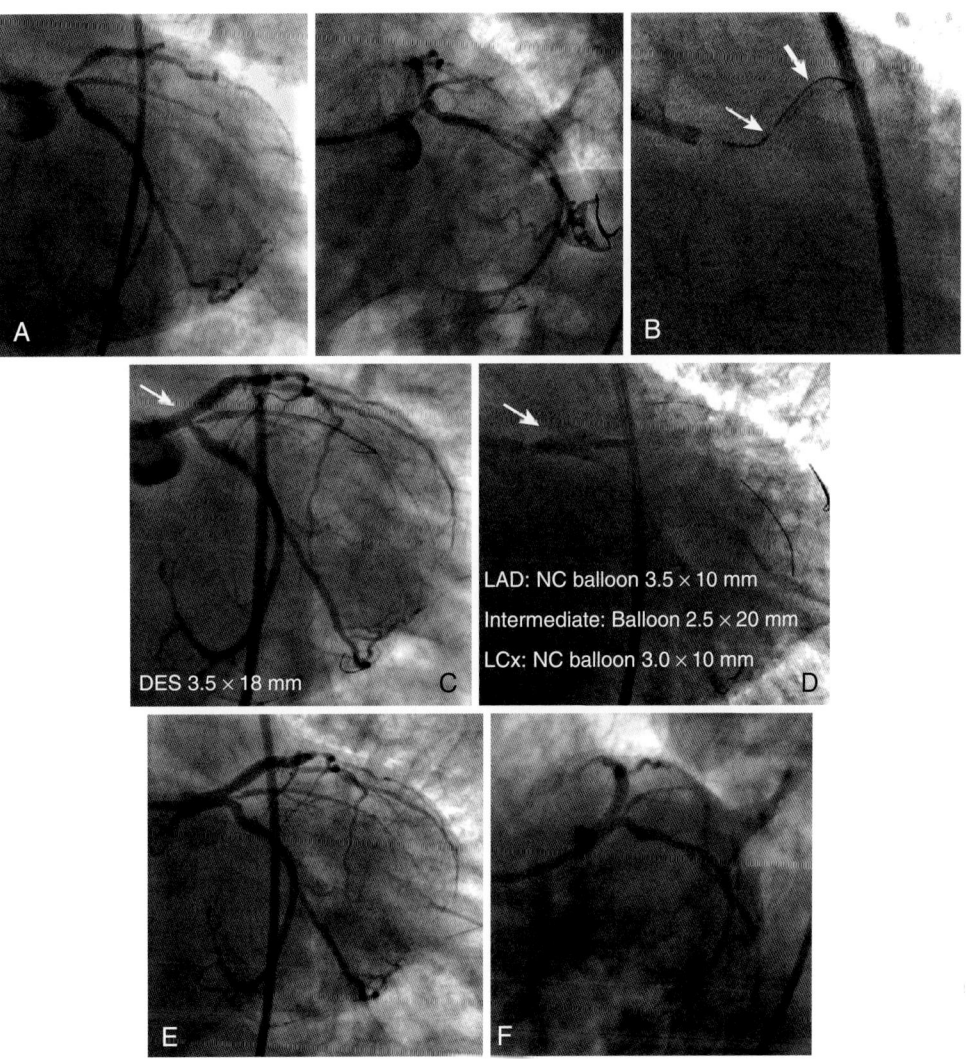

Fig. 23.4 Baseline angiogram presents large eccentric atherosclerotic plaque, which involves the distal part of the left main coronary artery (LMCA) and extends into the ostial segment of the left anterior descending *(LAD)* (A, caudal view; B, spider view). Because of a tight LMCA lesion and unfavorable access to the ostial LAD, a Venture wire control catheter (Vascular Solutions, Minneapolis, MN) *(arrow)* was used to insert a coronary guidewire *(thick arrow)* (C). After that, two guidewires were inserted in intermediate branch and left circumflex *(LCx)*. Following predilatation of the LMCA/ostial LAD lesion, a drug-eluting stent was implanted from the ostium of LMCA toward LAD (D), and final kissing balloon inflation was performed with three balloons, positioned from left main to LAD, intermediate branch and LCx (E). Panel E presents final angiographic result. *DES,* drug-eluting stent; *NC,* noncompliant balloon.

The Role of Final Kissing Balloon Inflation

FKBI is proposed if the SB is dilated through the MB stent struts to correct MB stent distortion and proximal expansion and provide better scaffolding of the SB ostium to facilitate future access to the SB. The long-term clinical benefit of FKBIs (in cases of MV stenting alone) is not proven. Nordic III and CORPAL-KISS studies demonstrated no systematic clinical advantage of routine kissing strategy when a single-stent treatment is used, and retrospective analysis of the COBIS (Coronary Bifurcation Stenting) registry found FKBI may even increase long-term TLR rate in the MV.[11,46] However, angiographic follow-up at 8 months in the NORDIC III study showed lower SB restenosis rate in patients with true bifurcation lesions when FKBI was performed (7.6% vs. 20.0%, P = .024),[44] and a study by Koo et al. found FKBI restores normal FFR in the SB in the majority of patients.[47] A recent randomized study investigated the impact of angiography-guided versus FFR-guided SB treatment, in 320 patients undergoing bifurcation PCI with provisional SB stenting strategy.[48] SB treatment (balloon or stent) tended to be less frequent in the FFR-guided group (56.3% vs. 63.1%, P = .07), and there was no difference in the 1-year rate of MACE or TVR. Several criteria have been proposed to define lesions in which FKBI is required (>75% residual stenosis at the SB, TIMI flow grade <3, or FFR <0.80). Therefore, two appropriate strategies are either to use a pressure wire to interrogate the significance of the SB lesion and treat or not accordingly, or simply to do FKBI on all angiographically significant ostial SB lesions, which reduces the proportion of physiologically significant SB ostial lesions. Of note, Nordic III found no penalty for routine kissing balloon inflations.[44] A sequential MB-SB-MB balloon inflation was proposed as a simpler alternative to FKBI.[49] A recent clinical, optical coherence tomography (OCT) based study confirmed the previously in vitro observed benefits of this technique, which amounts to performing POT, followed by an SB dilatation and a repeated, final POT (rePOT).[50] Although this study confirmed rePOT can be successfully applied in the clinical setting, its impact on patient outcomes needs to be further elucidated.

As a general approach to provisional strategy, we favor the performance of FKBI.

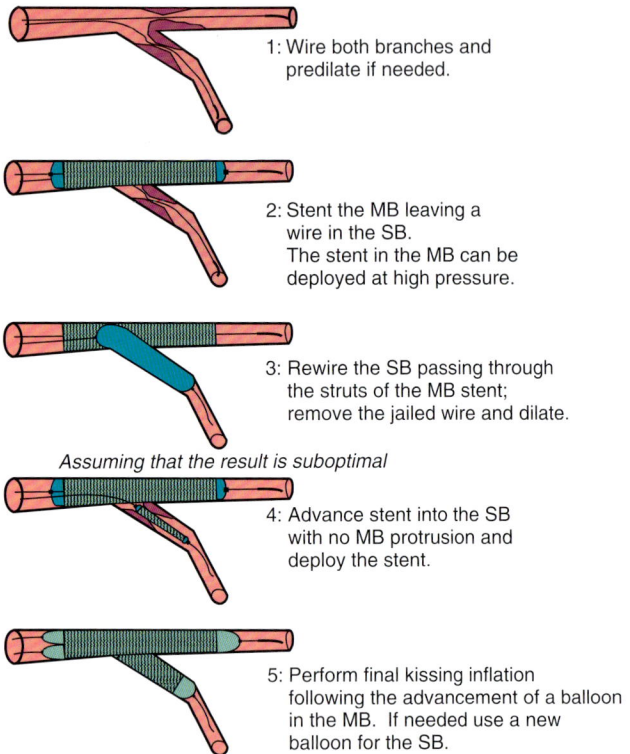

Fig. 23.5 A schematic representation of the T technique. *MB*, Main branch; *SB*, side branch.

A Second Stent in the Side Branch Following Provisional Approach

When we are not satisfied with the result obtained with balloon dilatation of the SB, we implant a second stent using one of the following strategies: T, TAP, culotte, or reverse/internal crush configuration. FFR or new imaging techniques, such as OCT, can be of value in the evaluation of SB result after balloon dilation.

1. **T technique** (Fig. 23.5). This technique is the one most frequently utilized to transition from provisional stenting to stenting the SB.[51,52] The T technique consists in advancing a second stent into the SB (following adequate dilation of the MB stent struts). The stent is positioned at the ostium of the SB trying to minimize any possible gap. A second kissing balloon inflation is also performed. In our view, the T technique is associated with the risk of leaving a small gap between the stent implanted in the MB and the stent implanted in the SB. This gap may be a factor contributing to an uneven distribution of the drug, hence leading to ostial restenosis at the SB.
2. **T stenting and small protrusion (TAP).** The TAP technique is a modification of the T stenting technique and is based on an intentional minimal protrusion of the SB stent within the MB (Fig. 23.6).[53,54] This technique can be described as follows:
    a. A second stent is advanced in the SB in a way to minimally protrude (1 or 2 mm) into the MB.
    b. A balloon is advanced in the MB.
    c. The SB stent is deployed as usual (12 atm or more), and the MB balloon is simultaneously inflated at 12 atm or more.
    d. Both balloons are deflated and removed.

    Despite some concerns about stent protrusion in the MB, in our experience we have been able to perform IVUS in the MB and SB and, when needed, to advance additional stents distally in the MB and in the SB. Three-year clinical follow-up of 95 patients treated with TAP stenting showed a MACE rate of 12.9%, and there were no cases of definite or probable ST.[55]

3. **Reverse/internal crush: crush performed after main branch stenting** (Fig. 23.7).[56,57] The main purpose in performing a reverse crush is to allow an opportunity for provisional SB stenting. This technique was developed with the intent to minimize any possible gap between the MB and SB stents. The reverse crush can be performed utilizing a 6-Fr guiding catheter according to the following steps:
    a. After stenting the MB, a second stent is advanced into the SB and left in position without being deployed.
    b. A balloon sized according to the diameter of the MB, and shorter than the stent already deployed, is advanced in the MB and positioned at the level of the bifurcation, taking care to stay inside the stent previously deployed in the MB.
    c. The stent in the SB is retracted about 3 mm or less into the MB and deployed. The deploying balloon is removed, and an angiogram is obtained to verify the absence of any distal dissection and the need of an additional stent. If such is the case, the wire from the SB is removed and the balloon in the MB is inflated at high pressure (12 atm or more).
    d. The SB struts are recrossed with a wire and a balloon (a 1.5 mm balloon is sometimes needed). The balloon is sized to the SB reference diameter and inflated at high pressure (12 to 20 atm).
    e. The final kissing balloon is performed.

    In our practice, this technique has been completely superseded by the TAP.
4. **The provisional culotte technique.** The culotte technique can be proposed as a provisional SB stenting strategy in Y shape angulated bifurcation lesions, as in the original description,[58] although the first stent can be deployed across the most angulated branch, usually the SB (inverted culotte).[59] This technique can be described as follows:
    a. After MB stenting, a second stent is advanced in the SB protruding into the MB to overlap with the proximal part of the MB stent and expanded following removal of MB wire.
    b. MB is rewired through the stent struts and dilated.
    c. Finally, kissing balloon inflation is performed

The European Bifurcation Club Approach to Bifurcation Stenting

The European Bifurcation Club (EBC) was founded in 2004 in order to devise a common terminology for the description and treatment of bifurcation lesions and to exchange ideas on the clinical, technical, and fundamental aspects of the specific treatment strategies implemented in this setting. A synopsis of these discussions is presented as follows[21–24,41]:

1. The MEDINA classification should be used for bifurcation lesions (1,0) and MADS classification for bifurcation stenting techniques (MADS: Main, Across, Distal, Side, based on the manner in which the first stent has been implanted).
2. Provisional T stenting remains the gold standard technique for most bifurcations.
3. Large SBs with ostial disease extending >5 mm from the carina are likely to require a two-stent strategy.
4. In provisional technique, after wiring both branches, the MB should be predilated when required, while SBs without severe calcification or long significant lesion (>5mm) do not require routine predilatation.
5. The SB wire should be jailed behind the MB stent in true bifurcation lesions.
6. The MB stent is selected according to distal MB diameter and postdilatation, or kissing balloon inflations, are required to optimize the proximal MB stent diameter.
7. The POT technique is carried out after MB stenting by inflating a short balloon just proximal to the carina; POT should be

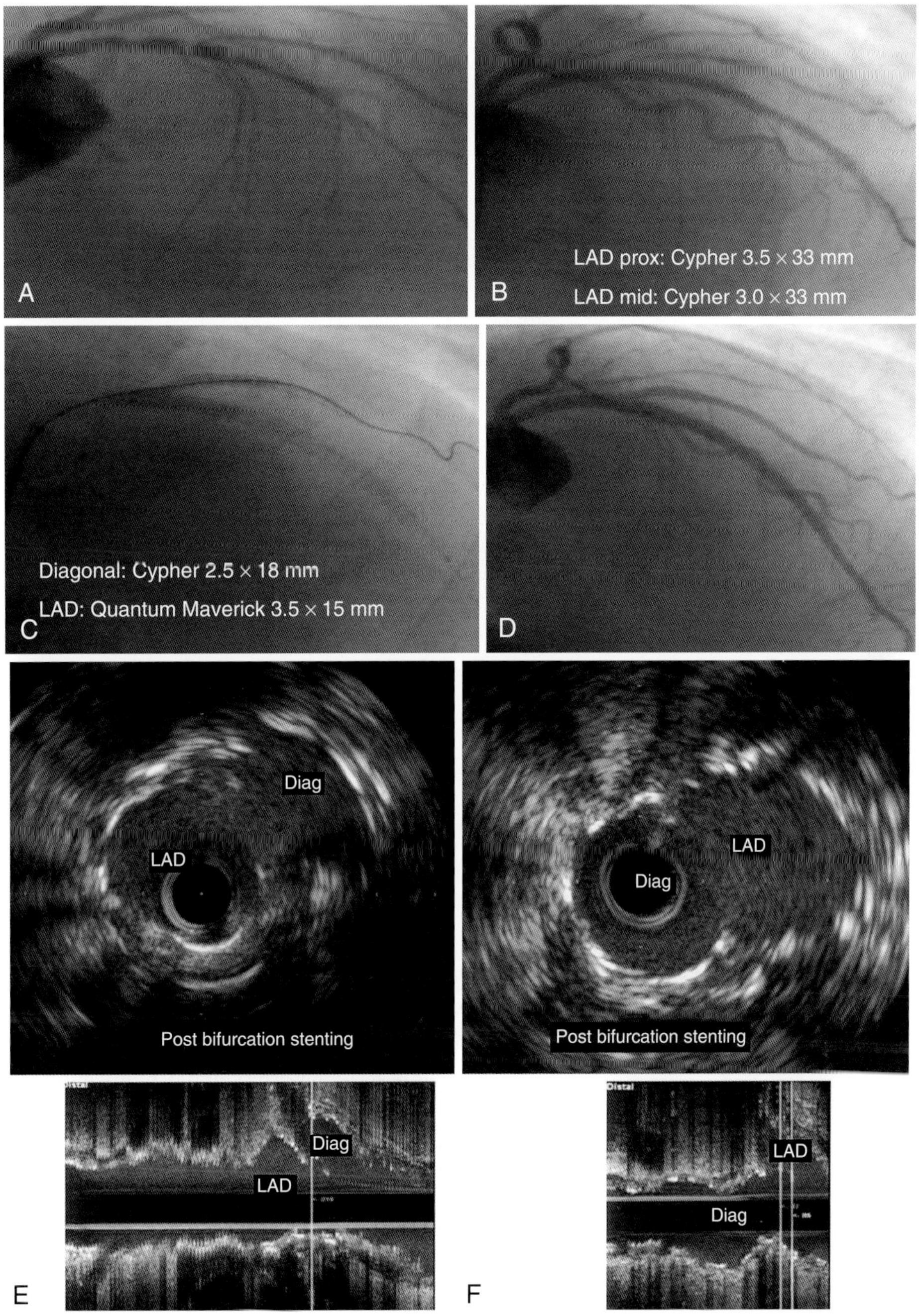

CHAPTER 23 Bifurcations and Branch Vessel Stenting

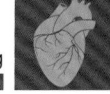

Fig. 23.6 Example of T stenting and small protrusion (TAP) technique. Baseline angiogram presents diffuse disease of the left anterior descending *(LAD)* and ostial/proximal segment of diagonal branch (A). Following stent implantation in proximal and mid segments of the LAD and balloon angioplasty at the diagonal branch, the result appears unsatisfactory (B). A second stent is advanced in the diagonal branch to minimally protrude (1 or 2 mm) into the LAD and balloon is positioned in the LAD. The stent in the diagonal branch is deployed and the balloon in the LAD simultaneously inflated (C). Angiographic view of the final result (D). Transverse and longitudinal views of final intravascular ultrasound in the LAD (E) and the diagonal branch (F) confirm optimal stent position in the diagonal branch, with minimal protrusion in the LAD. *NC,* Noncompliant balloon.

performed before SB rewiring to facilitate access and reduce the risk of accidental abluminal rewiring (wiring behind the MV stent).
8. SB treatment is indicated if the ostium is pinched or the flow is limited after POT.
9. SB wire crosses through the distal strut following MB stenting.
10. Kissing balloon inflation for carina reconstruction is optional in the provisional stenting but mandatory in two-stent techniques.
11. The procedure should be finalized by POT after kissing to correct the proximal MB stent distortion.
12. Intravascular imaging is a valuable supplement in bifurcation treatment and is especially useful in complex lesions due to the limitations of angiography alone.[23]

TWO STENTS AS INTENTION-TO-TREAT

If the operator determines a particular bifurcation will need implantation of two stents—one in the MB and the other in the

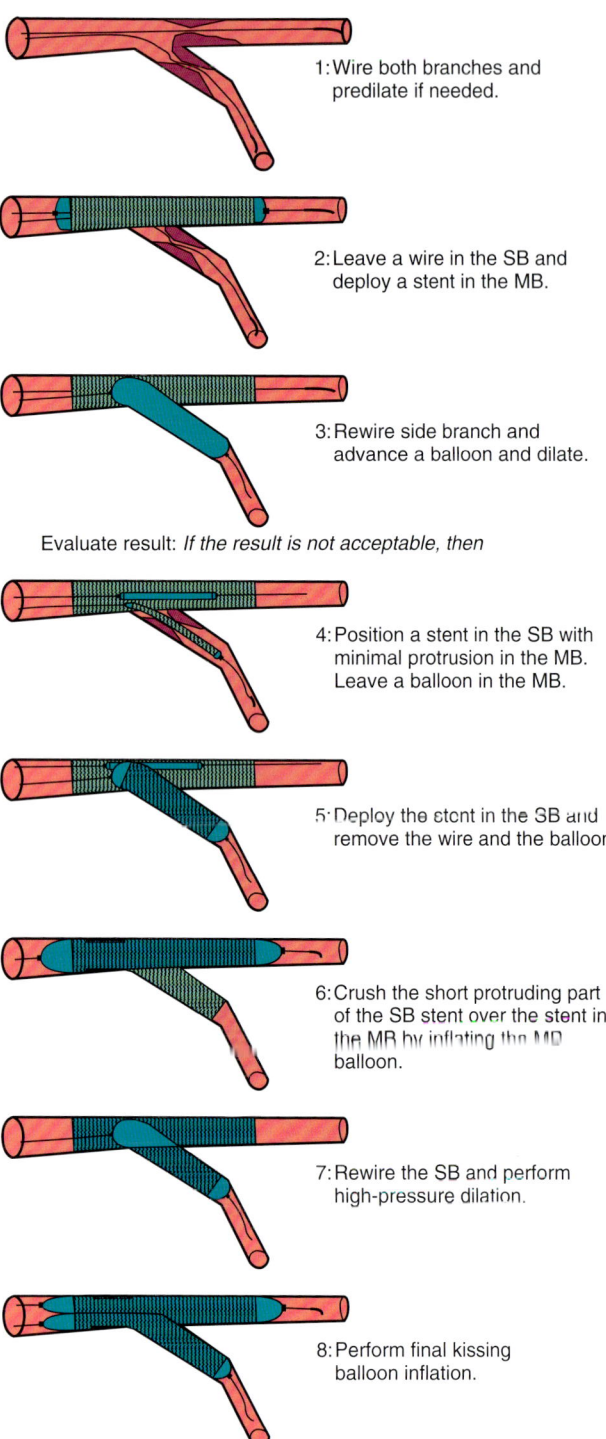

Fig. 23.7 A schematic representation of the reverse/internal crush technique. *MB*, Main branch; *SB*, side branch.

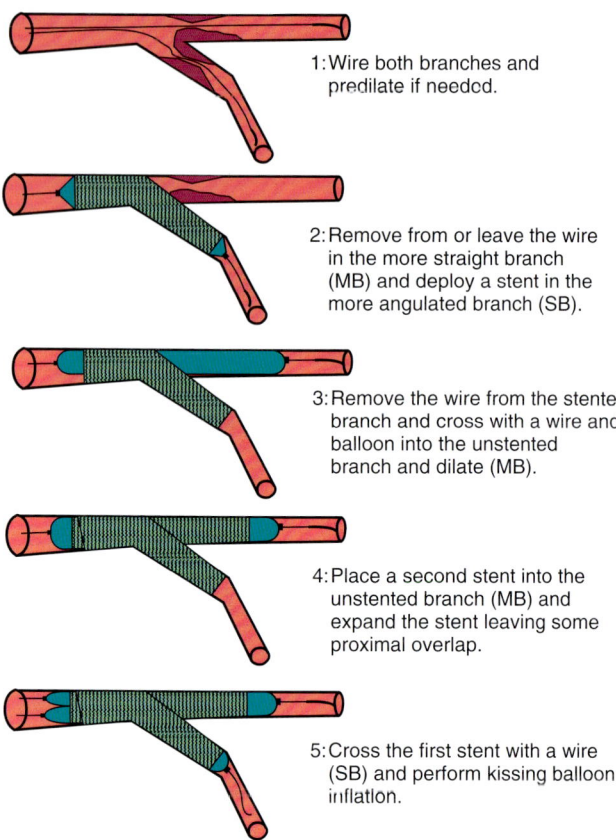

Fig. 23.8 A schematic representation of the culotte technique. *MB*, Main branch; *SB*, side branch.

SB—the techniques we consider suitable in the era of DES are described as follows.

The two-stent approach will be reserved only for selected "true" bifurcations following the evaluation of additional parameters:

A. The size and the territory of distribution of the SB
 The term *SB* is sometimes associated with a misleading connotation. The terminology may convey a vessel of less importance compared to the MB. While this statement may be true in most cases, there are various anatomical conditions in which the SB is as important as the MB, regarding both the size and territory of distribution. An LMCA that bifurcates into left anterior descending (LAD) and left circumflex (LCx), a right coronary artery (RCA) that bifurcates in a posterior descending artery and a number of posterolateral branches, a dominant LCx that bifurcates into a distal circumflex, and a large obtuse marginal branch are all examples in which the SBs are important vessels that may generate a large ischemia if left with a critical narrowing. As outlined in Fig. 23.3, the size of the territory supplied by the SB becomes a valuable element to guide the decision to accept a mediocre result at the SB ostium (following balloon angioplasty) versus the need to have almost 0% residual stenosis following additional SB stenting.

B. The length of the lesion at the ostium of the SB
 While most of the studies found a focal lesion at the ostium of the SB does not prevent a provisional approach, the situation may be different when the stenosis extends for several mm into the SB.

C. The angle between the MB and the SB and the narrowing at the ostium of the SB
 The angle of origin of the SB from the MB can be acute, close to 90 degrees, or obtuse. The narrower the angle between the two branches, the higher the risk of plaque prolapse and compromise of the ostium of the SB.[60] Another element to consider when looking at the angle between the two branches is the difficulty to recross into the SB following stenting of the MB. The severity of the narrowing at the ostium of the SB is another factor influencing placement of two stents. An additional variable to be considered is the result obtained following balloon dilatation of the SB. All these elements mean that the decision to implant a second stent may be made following predilatation of the MB and of the SB.

CHAPTER 23 Bifurcations and Branch Vessel Stenting

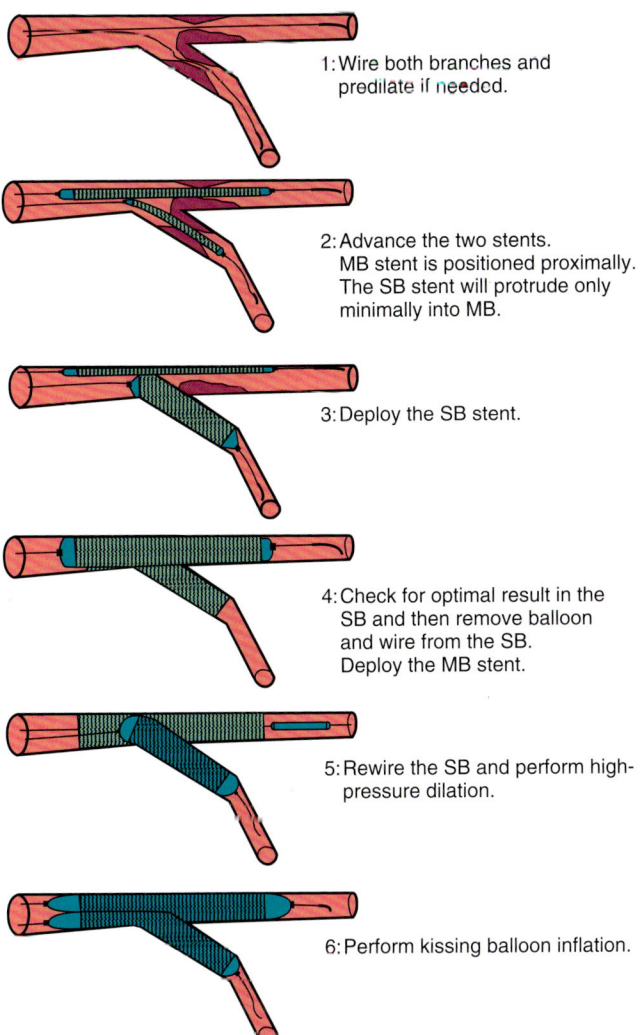

Fig. 23.9 A schematic representation of the mini-crush technique. *MB*, Main branch; *SB*, side branch.

1: Wire both branches and predilate if needed.
2: Advance the two stents. MB stent is positioned proximally. The SB stent will protrude only minimally into MB.
3: Deploy the SB stent.
4: Check for optimal result in the SB and then remove balloon and wire from the SB. Deploy the MB stent.
5: Rewire the SB and perform high-pressure dilation.
6: Perform kissing balloon inflation.

What it is important to know is that if we make the decision to use one stent (in the MB), there is always the possibility of deploying a second stent in the SB if the result is not considered optimal.

TWO-STENT TECHNIQUES

The Culotte Technique

The culotte technique (Fig. 23.8) uses two stents and leads to full coverage of the bifurcation at the expense of an excess of metal covering of the proximal end.[58,59]

The culotte technique is probably the technique that gives the best coverage of the carina. An important caveat to this approach is to dilate the struts toward the SB. Open-cell design stents are recommended for the culotte technique. The Nordic complex bifurcation stenting study compared crush or culotte stenting utilizing SES and demonstrated at 6-month follow-up no difference between the two groups in terms of death, MI, or repeat revascularization, and clinical outcomes remained similar at 3-year follow-up.[25,26]

Technique Description

Step 1: Both branches are predilated.
Step 2: A stent is deployed across the most angulated branch, usually the SB and optimized with POT.
Step 3: The nonstented branch is rewired through the stent struts and dilated.
Step 4: A second stent is advanced and expanded into the non-stented branch, usually the MB and optimized with POT.
Step 5: Finally, kissing balloon inflation and final POT is performed. This technique is suitable for all angles of bifurcations and provides near-perfect coverage of the SB ostium. Disadvantages are that, like the crush, the culotte technique leads to a high concentration of metal with a double-stent layer at the carina and in the proximal part of the bifurcation. Other disadvantages of the technique are that rewiring both branches through the stent struts can be difficult and time-consuming. Performing the POT after each stent implantation may help rewiring.

The Mini-Crush Technique (Side-Branch Stent Crushed by the Main Branch Stent)

The crush technique (Fig. 23.9) originated with the availability of DES.[61] The recent addition of the word "mini" highlights the need to decrease as much as possible the amount of stent overlap between the SB and MB, as described by Galassi et al., compared with modified T stenting, as described by Kobayashi et al.[62,63] Since routine performance of the FKBI was adopted, restenosis at the ostium of the SB appears to be declining.[64]

The main advantage of the crush technique is that immediate patency of both branches is ensured. This objective is notably important when the SB is functionally relevant or difficult to be wired. The main disadvantage is that the performance of the FKBI makes the procedure more laborious, due to the need to recross multiple struts with a wire and a balloon.

The performance of the crush technique requires a 7- or 8-Fr guiding catheter, and the technique commits the operator to implant two stents. Below we will describe a modification of the crush technique that allows provisional SB stenting and permits performing the same or similar approach utilizing a 6-Fr guiding catheter.

An angiographic example of the crush technique is presented in Fig. 23.10.

When the angle between the MB and SB is close to 90 degrees, it is possible to minimize the gap even without crushing the SB stent and utilizing the modified T technique.

Technique Description

Step 1: Both branches are wired and fully dilated. Particular attention is paid to dilate the SB, and we often utilize a 6-mm long cutting balloon if there is evidence that the predilating balloon does not fully expand at the ostium of the SB.
Step 2: The stent for the SB is positioned in the SB, and then the MB stent is advanced.
Step 3: The SB stent is pulled back into the MB for about 2 to 3 mm. This step is verified in at least two projections.
Step 4: The stent in the SB is deployed at least at 12 atm. The balloon is deflated and removed from the guiding catheter. An angiogram is taken to verify that the SB has an appropriate lumen, normal flow, and that no distal dissection or residual lesions are present. If an additional stent is needed in the SB, this is the time to perform the implant. Following this check, the wire is removed from the SB and the stent in the MB is fully deployed at high pressure, usually above 12 atm and optimized with POT. An angiogram is taken following removal of the balloon from the MB.
Step 5: A wire is advanced in the SB aiming to cross through the central or proximal strut.[65] This maneuver may be challenging. In addition to trying with the initial floppy wire (Balance Universal, Abbott Vascular Devices, Redwood City, CA/

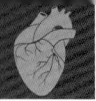

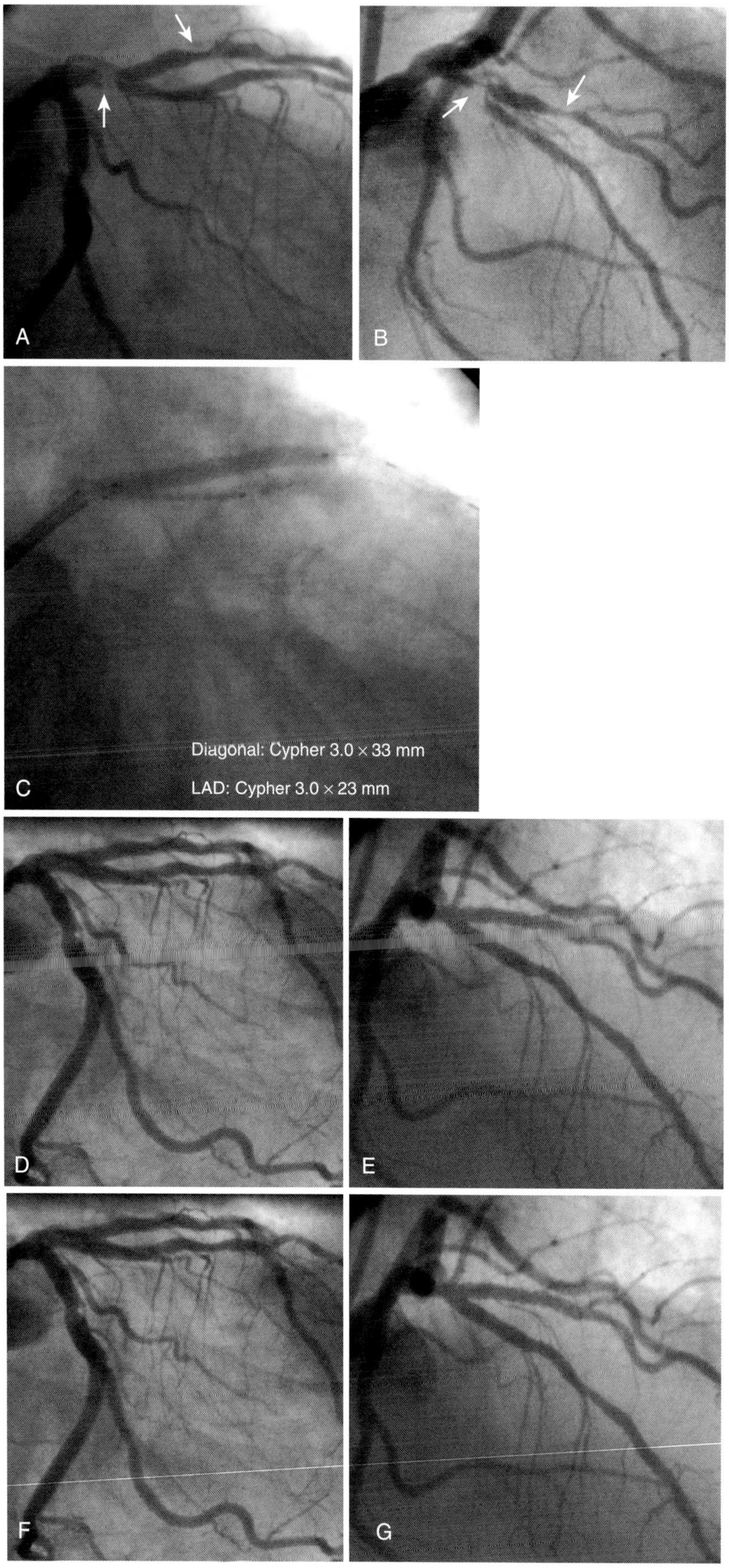

SECTION III Coronary Intervention

Fig. 23.10 Example of crush stenting technique. Baseline angiogram of bifurcation lesion, involving left anterior descending *(LAD)* and a large diagonal branch, is presented in panels A and B. Following lesion predilatation, two stents are positioned with the stent in the LAD placed more proximally than the stent in the diagonal branch (C). Side-branch stent is inflated first (diagonal branch). Note that long stent was chosen for diagonal branch in order to also cover a lesion distal to bifurcation site (A and B, *arrow*). Optimal final result (D and E) was maintained at 10-month angiographic follow-up (F and G).

Guidant, Santa Clara, CA), other choices are Rinato/Prowater (Asahi Intec, Japan/Abbott Vascular Devices), and Pilot 50 and Pilot 150 (Abbott Vascular Devices). We frequently try first to cross through the stent struts into the SB with a 1.5- to 1.25-mm diameter balloon. If this very small balloon cannot cross, we consider repositioning the wire traversing the stent struts in another location. It is important to perform a final dilatation on the stent toward the SB with a balloon appropriately sized to the diameter of this branch and inflated at high pressure (12 atm or more).

Step 6: A second balloon is advanced over the wire which was left in place in the MB, and kissing balloon inflation is performed at 8 atm or more.

Step Crush and Double-Kissing Crush

When there is the need to perform a two-stent technique as intention-to-treat and a 6-Fr guiding catheter is the only available approach (radial approach), the "step crush" or "the modified balloon crush technique" techniques can be used.[66]

The final result is basically similar to that obtained with the standard crush technique, with the only difference that each stent is advanced and deployed separately. The need for a 6-Fr guiding catheter is the main reason to utilize this technique.

The technique named DK-crush and sleeve techniques are other variants of the crush technique, which may optimize stent deployment and apposition.[67,68] In a randomized study, the 12-month rate of TVR using the DK-crush technique was decreased compared with a provisional SB stenting strategy[17] and was recently shown to reduce TLF when compared with provisional SB stenting in patients with distal LM true bifurcation lesions.[20]

Technique Description

Step 1: The same as the standard crush technique.
Step 2: A stent is advanced in the SB protruding a few millimeters into the MB. A balloon is advanced in the MB across the bifurcation.
Step 3: The stent in the SB is deployed, the balloon is removed, an angiogram is performed, and if the result is adequate, the wire is also removed. The MB balloon is then inflated (to crush the protruding SB stent) and removed. Optionally, kissing balloon inflation can be performed at that time (double-kissing crush technique).[17,67]
Step 4: A second stent is advanced in the MB and deployed (usually at 12 atm or more).

The next steps are similar to those of the crush technique and involve recrossing into the SB, SB stent dilatation, and FKBI.

The V and the Simultaneous Kissing Stent Techniques

The V and the simultaneous kissing stent (SKS) techniques (Fig. 23.11) are performed by delivering and implanting two stents together.[69,70] One stent is advanced in the SB; the other one is advanced in the MB. Both stents are pulled back to create a new carina as close as possible to the original one. The main advantage of the V technique is that the operator will never lose access to any of the two branches. In addition, when an FKBI is performed, there is no need to recross any stent. Fig. 23.12 shows an example of V technique performed on LMCA. When the two stents protrude into the MB with the creation of a double barrel and a very proximal carina, the technique is called *SKS*.[70] We prefer the V technique for selected bifurcation lesions where the lesions are distal to the bifurcation (Medina 0,1,1); if there is a proximal stenosis in the MB, we prefer a different approach rather that creating an overlap with the SKS.

Technique Description

Step 1: Both branches are wired and fully predilated. It is important to perform an adequate predilatation in order to allow full stent expansion.
Step 2: The two stents are positioned into the branches with a minimal protrusion of both stents in the main proximal branch. Different operators allow a variable amount of protrusion creating sometimes a rather long (5 mm or more) double barrel in the proximal MB (SKS). Sometimes it is necessary to advance the first stent more distally into the vessel to facilitate the advancement of the second stent. This maneuver is essential when the kissing stent technique is used to stent a trifurcation using three kissing stents (for simultaneous three-stent deployment, a 9-Fr guiding catheter is required). Following accurate stent positioning, it is important to verify their correct placement in two projections before deploying the stents. In our experience, each balloon is first inflated individually at high pressure of 12 atm or more, while other operators inflate the balloons simultaneously.
Step 3: Inflate both balloons simultaneously. The size of the balloon and of the stents is chosen based on the diameter of the vessels to be stented. In the event the reference vessel size proximal to the bifurcation is relatively small and the operator fears the risk that the two balloons inflated simultaneously may be oversized, the kissing inflation is performed at low pressure (4 atm).

Using the V technique, a metallic neocarina is created within the vessel proximal to the bifurcation. Theoretical concerns about the risk of thrombosis due to the new carina have not been confirmed in our and other operators' experience. The types of lesions we consider most suitable for this technique are very proximal lesions, such as bifurcation of a short LMCA free of disease. Ideally, the angle between the two branches should be less than 90 degrees. The V technique is also suitable for other bifurcations, provided the portion of the vessel proximal to the bifurcation is free of disease and there is no need to deploy a stent more proximally. Positioning a stent proximally to the double barrel is problematic, as it will result in a bias toward one of the two branches and will likely leave a gap.

The "Y" and the "Skirt" Techniques

The "Y" technique has a particular historical value because it was the first bifurcation stenting technique demonstrated in a live case course.[71] This technique involves an initial predilatation, followed by stent deployment in each branch. If the results are not adequate, a third stent may also be deployed in the MB.[72] To approximate the proximal stent to the already-deployed stents, it is necessary to modify the stent delivery system by placing one stent over two balloons ("skirt" stenting).[73] This technique is the last resort for treating very demanding bifurcations in which there are needs to maintain uninterrupted wire access to both branches.

Flower Petal Stenting

The technique of "flower petal" stenting involves implanting a stent in the SB with a single strut protruding into the MB; the protruding strut closest to the carina is wired and dilated to create a larger strut or "flower petal"; this protruding petal is then flattened and plastered down over the carina with a series of MB inflations, including a MB stent and kissing balloon inflations, thus ensuring complete ostial coverage and scaffolding.[74] The most challenging part of this technique is wiring a single strut close to the carina, and in the original description, this required IVUS guidance and was not always successful. The technique was modified to allow ex vivo wiring of the proximal strut and subsequent balloon insertion into this strut. This approach needs partial inflation of the proximal segment of the stent, performed

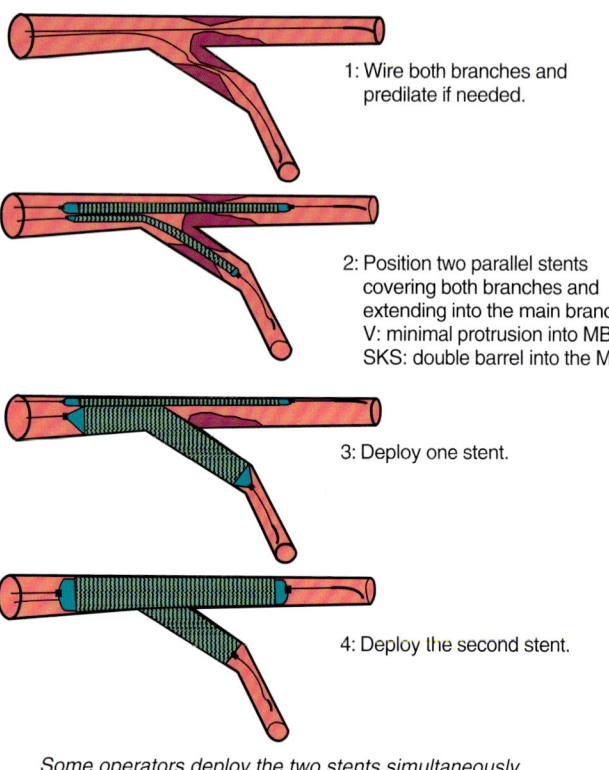

Fig. 23.11 A schematic representation of the V technique. *MB*, Main branch; *SKS*, simultaneous kissing stent.

before stent insertion in the guiding catheter. Although this creates a bulkier dual-wire and balloon system, the technique is suitable for a 6-Fr guide catheter and is mainly applied in bifurcation lesions located in the distal LM.

The most frequently used two-stent techniques are summarized in Table 23.1. While no definitive statement can be made regarding the best strategy to be used, when there is the need to implant two stents in a bifurcation, we present in Fig. 23.13 a schematic approach according to the anatomy of the lesion.

Left Main Bifurcation Stenting

Distinct anatomical features and clinical significance epitomize the approach to percutaneous LM treatment. The 13th Consensus document from the EBC was dedicated to LM stenting.[75]

1. LM anatomy
   Mean LM IVUS-derived reference diameter was estimated to be 5 mm, ranging from 3.5 to 6 mm, with a characteristic plaque distribution involving lateral walls of the LM stem and extending into the LAD and CX.[38] As a consequence, what angiographically may appear as an isolated stenosis at the ostium of LAD or CX is often in fact a continuous atherosclerotic plaque also involving the LM. In addition to the larger mean diameter and characteristic plaque distribution of LM arteries, another defining characteristic of LM anatomy is the fact that the SB (i.e., CX) is frequently clinically relevant, as it supplies >10% of the myocardium in >95% of cases.[75]

2. Indications for LM treatment
   As per current clinical practice guidelines, LM revascularization is indicated in cases of angiographic stenosis >50% and the proof of myocardial ischemia.[76] If there is angiographic ambiguity, accumulated evidence to date suggests IVUS-derived minimal lumen area (MLA) >6 mm^2 and FFR >0.80 are acceptable criteria for deferral of LM treatment (with the limitation that evaluation of a LM stenosis with FFR may be inaccurate if LAD or CX disease is present).[75]

3. Evidence for percutaneous LM treatment
   PCI has been compared with coronary artery bypass grafting (CABG) for treatment of LM disease in six randomized studies.[77-82] The common finding of the early studies appeared to be the noninferiority of PCI to CABG, up to 10-year follow-up, albeit with limitations to the data such as using the first-generation DES and accepting a higher TVR with PCI and being of a small sample size.[77-79,81] The two most recent randomized studies, utilizing contemporary second-generation DES, are the Everolimus-Eluting Stents or Bypass Surgery for Left Main Coronary Artery Disease (EXCEL)[82] and Percutaneous Coronary Angioplasty Versus Coronary Artery Bypass Grafting in Treatment of Unprotected Left Main Stenosis (NOBLE)[80] trials, which included 1905 and 1201 patients with LM disease, respectively. Importantly, in both of those trials, >80% of patients had a distal LM bifurcation stenosis. The EXCEL trial demonstrated noninferiority of PCI with EES to CABG in terms of death, stroke, or MI at 3 years (15.4% vs. 14.7%, P for noninferiority = .02).[82] On the contrary, the NOBLE trial, which utilized a thicker strut stainless steel BES, showed a reduction in the 5-year rate of death, nonprocedural MI, stroke, or any repeat coronary revascularization with CABG compared with PCI (19% vs. 29%, respectively, P = .0066).[80] Due to multiple differences in trial protocols, including the end point definition, most notably of procedural versus nonprocedural MI, and the follow-up length, the EXCEL and NOBLE trials may not be entirely comparable, and the evaluation of the role of PCI for treatment of LM disease in everyday clinical practice is still ongoing. Taken together, the collected evidence seems to suggest the feasibility of percutaneous LM treatment as reflected by mortality rates similar to CABG, albeit with the clinical outcomes of PCI being dependent on the patient's overall coronary artery disease complexity (e.g., higher SYNTAX scores favoring surgical revascularization).[75,83]

4. LM stenting technique
   The 13th EBC consensus document provides an extensive overview of the considerations regarding the technique of LM stenting. In the following, the core messages are presented[75]:
   - The use of one guidewire may be considered in cases of an isolated ostial and/or midshaft LM disease, whereas two guidewires are recommended for all nonostial/midshaft LM PCI.
   - MB preparation (e.g., predilatation, rotational atherectomy) is recommended in the majority of cases prior to LM stenting, whereas SB preparation may be contemplated in case of severe ostial disease, calcified stenosis, and/or difficult SB access.
   - Stent sizing should consider maximum expansion capacities of current DES platforms to accommodate the mean LM diameter of ≈5 mm. If PCI involves distal LM bifurcation, the stent should be sized according to the distal reference diameter (i.e., proximal LAD or CX for most of the cases).
   - Provisional SB stenting is recommended for distal LM disease that does not involve both branches, with implantation of one stent in most cases and the essential role of POT to ensure adequate stent expansion in the LM stem.
   - If both branches of LM bifurcation are stenotic, stepwise provisional strategy is recommended, with the possible extension to a two-stent technique if SB stenting is deemed necessary, most commonly utilizing the T/TAP technique

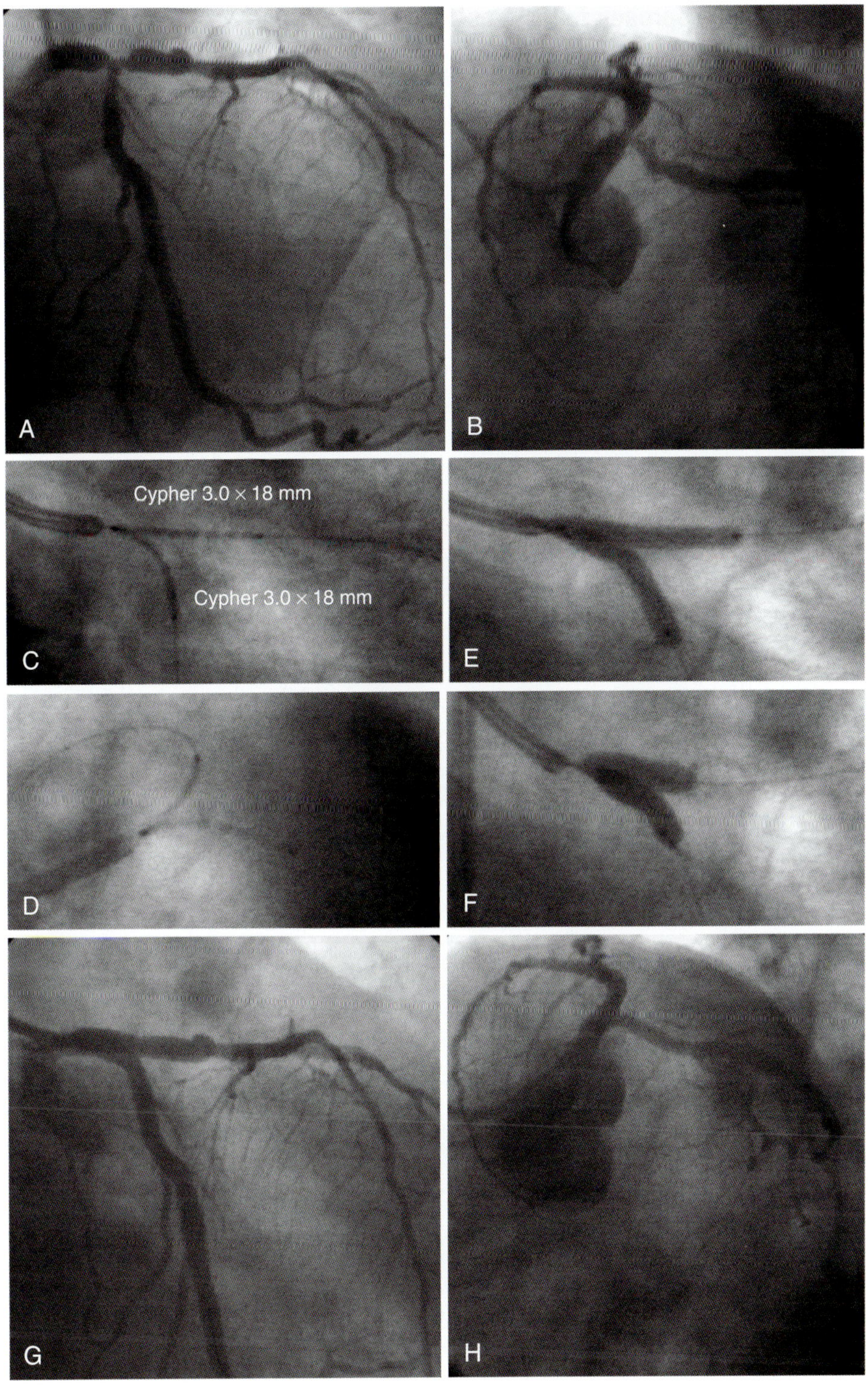

CHAPTER 23 Bifurcations and Branch Vessel Stenting

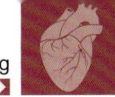

Fig. 23.12 Example of V stenting technique. Baseline angiogram of a left main coronary artery bifurcation lesion, with two large branches, left anterior descending and left circumflex (A and B). The V-stenting was used due to the fact that the disease was mainly at the level of the very distal left main and the angle of the two branches was very favorable for a V-technique. Stent positioning in two projections is shown in panels C and D and stent deployment and postdilatation with the 4-mm balloons is shown in panels E and F. Final result is presented in panels G and H.

in the presence of a wide bifurcation angle or the Culotte technique if the angle is narrower.
- For centers more comfortable with the DK-crush technique, it may be considered a viable alternative, based on the results of a recent randomized DKCRUSH-V trial.[20]
- Regardless of the technique used, high-pressure kissing balloon inflation is considered mandatory if two-stent approach is applied.
- Based on observational evidence indicating clinical benefit of IVUS guidance for LM PCI,[61] the use of intracoronary imaging is encouraged in general, and whenever angiographic ambiguity or unexpected intraprocedural difficulties are encountered, in particular (for more details, see the section on intracoronary imaging).

SECTION III Coronary Intervention

Controversies in the Technical Approach to Isolated Ostial Left Anterior Descending or Circumflex Lesions

1. Approach to ostial LAD lesion
   LM 0,1,0 lesion (ostial LAD) is traditionally considered to be unfavorable for percutaneous intervention because of the technical difficulty and potential risk of serious complications. Two interventional strategies are traditionally used in this lesion subset: precise stent implantation at the LAD ostium level or stenting the LMCA towards LAD. IVUS guidance is encouraged to assess plaque distribution before deciding which technique should be applied in a specific lesion. Precise stenting of LAD ostium is feasible in cases with a large bifurcation angle and IVUS documentation of absence of disease in distal LM. Precise LAD ostial stenting consists of scaffolding the counter-carina, with a mild protrusion of the stent covering the ostium of the circumflex. In this technique, the proximal stent marker should be positioned just proximal to the angiographic carina (the transducer of the IVUS catheter could be filmed when it is positioned at the carina level to have a reference for subsequent stent placement). Disadvantages of precise ostial LAD stenting are as follows: (a) if the device is positioned too proximally, it protrudes into the LMCA, which may compromise an LCx and make repeated intervention difficult; (b) if the ostial LAD lesion is not totally covered by the stent, acute recoil and late restenosis is expected.[41] Therefore, optimal positioning of the stents is critical for the treatment of this lesion. Furthermore, with branch ostial disease, there is frequent involvement of the distal LMCA, and thus the impending danger of incomplete lesion coverage if stenting is not extended to the involved LM. From this perspective, left MB ostial lesion is very similar to bifurcation disease and should be treated in a similar manner. Therefore, many believe ostial disease of LAD and LCx should be treated percutaneously by stenting from the LM into the diseased MB with provisional SB stenting.[41]

2. Approach to isolated SB ostial (0,0,1) bifurcation lesions: lesions at the ostium of a diagonal/obtuse marginal/posterolateral branch
   Ostial SB lesions are particularly important because they have the potential to become the origin of a new lesion on the MB. Isolated SB ostial lesions (0,0,1), although not frequent, are very challenging lesions to treat (especially in narrow, "Y" shape

TABLE 23.1 Main Characteristics of Two-Stent Techniques

	T/TAP	Mini-Crush	Culotte	SKS
Guiding catheter (Fr)	6	7[a]	6	7
Provisional SB stenting	Yes	No	Possible	No
Preserved GW access MB	Yes	Yes	No	Yes
Preserved GW access SB	No	No	No	Yes
Bifurcation angle:				
<70 degrees	Not ideal	Ideal	Suitable	Suitable
>70 degrees	Ideal	Not ideal	Not ideal	Not ideal
MB and SB diameters:				
Similar diameters	Suitable	Suitable	Ideal	Ideal
Discrepancy in diameters	Suitable	Ideal	Not ideal	Not ideal

[a]6 Fr could be used for balloon "Step-Crush" and "Double-Kissing Crush."
GW, Guidewire; *MB*, main branch; *SB*, side branch; *SKS*, simultaneous kissing stent; *TAP*, T and protrusion.

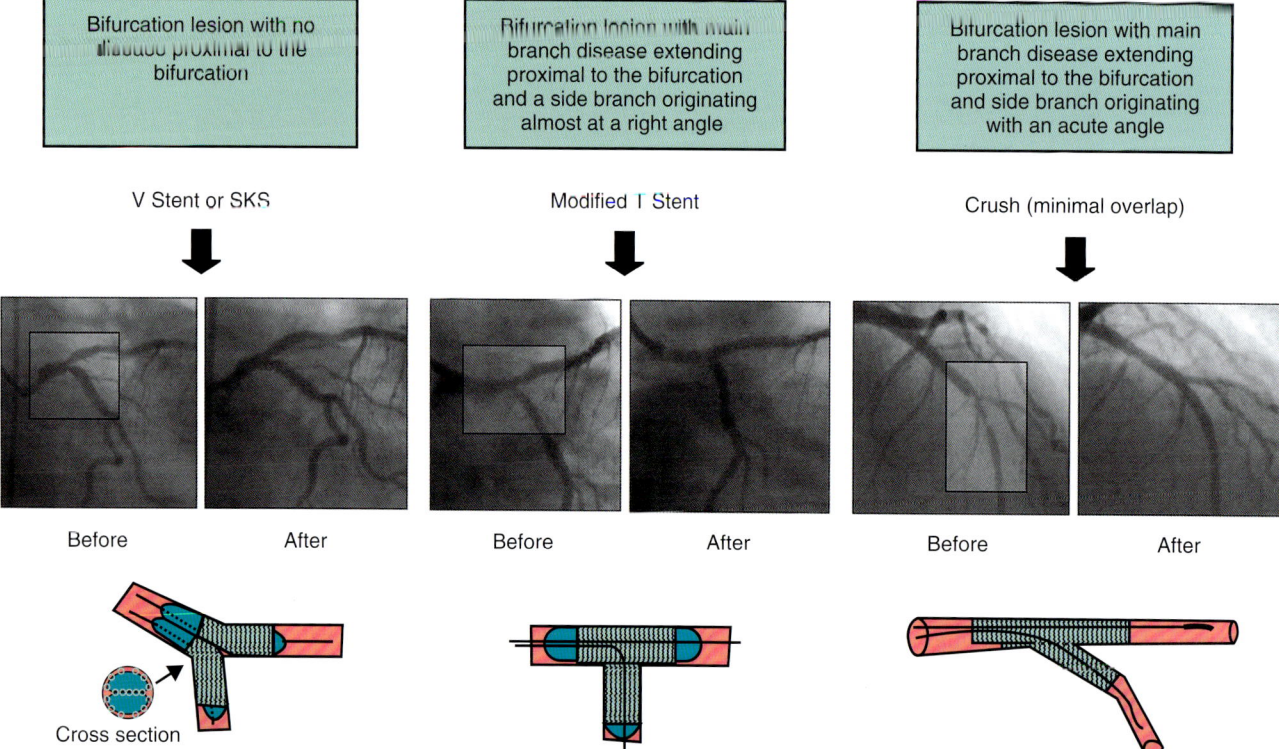

Fig. 23.13 Our proposed approach when implanting two stents on a bifurcation as intention-to-treat. *SKS*, Simultaneous kissing stents.

angulations). Each operator should always remember what we have called the "sad story of the ostial diagonal lesion" and be aware that too aggressive treatment of these lesions may not always be the best approach, leading to trauma to the LAD causing a new stenosis on this vessel. Unfortunately, we cannot propose an easy solution to this conundrum, rather that alerting the operator to this possible risk. Occasionally a simple cutting balloon dilatation at the ostium of a diagonal branch is a minimalistic approach that should be considered.

Brunel et al. have developed an "inverted" technique for the treatment of Medina 0,0,1 lesions, derived from the usual provisional T stenting.[85] The stent is implanted from the proximal MB into the SB, with reopening of the strut through the distal MB and systematic final kissing balloon.

Alternative approaches are use of the single short stent (precise ostial positioning is very difficult and complete ostial coverage is difficult/impossible except for 90-degree bifurcation), shunt technique, or dedicated stents.[41]

One strategy to be considered is to evaluate the functional significance, with FFR, of the lesion located at the SB, and finally we should not dismiss the fact that optimal medical therapy is a reasonable approach.

Dedicated Bifurcation Stents

The conventional approach to bifurcation PCI still has a number of limitations, such as maintaining access to the SB throughout the procedure; MB stent struts jailing the SB ostium, resulting in difficulty in rewiring the SB or passing the balloon/stent into the SB through the stent struts; distortion of the MB stent by SB dilatation; inability to fully cover and scaffold the ostium of the SB; inability of the stent structure to withstand SB balloon dilatation and deformation; and finally, operator skills, and technical experience.[86] Grundeken et al. gives a contemporary overview of the dedicated stents for distal LM stenting.[87] Thus far, the main advantage of most dedicated bifurcation stents is to allow the operator to perform the procedure on a bifurcation lesion without the need to rewire the SB. Dedicated bifurcation stents can be broadly divided into:

1. Stents for provisional SB stenting that facilitate or maintain access to the SB after MB stenting and do not require recrossing of MB stent struts (e.g., Petal, former AST stent, [Boston Scientific, Natick, MA]; Multi-link Frontier/Pathfinder/SBA [Abbott Vascular Devices]; Invatec Twin-Rail [Medtronic/Invatec, Brescia, Italy]; Nile Croco/Pax [Minvasys, Genevilliers, France]; Antares [Trireme Medical, CA]; Y-Med SideKick [Y-Med, San Diego, CA]; Stentys [Stentys SAS, Clichy, France]). These stents allow placement of a second stent on the SB if needed.
2. Stents that usually require another stent implanted in the bifurcation (e.g., Axxess Plus [Devax, Irvine, CA]; Sideguard [Cappella, MA]; Tryton [Tryton Medical, MA]). The Tryton and Sideguard are designed to treat the SB first and require recrossing into the SB after MB stenting for final kissing inflation. The Axxess Plus is the exception, as it is implanted in the proximal MB at the level of the carina and does not require recrossing into the SB, but may require the additional implantation of two further stents in distal MB and SB to completely treat some types of bifurcation lesions.

Most of these bifurcation devices have not yet been compared in a randomized fashion against either a provisional or two-stent strategy using conventional DES, except for the Tryton stent, which is compared with the provisional approach in the randomized Tryton IDE trial.[88]

The TRYTON IDE trial (Randomized Controlled Study to Evaluate the Safety & Effectiveness of the Tryton Side Branch Stent Used with DES in Treatment of de Novo Bifurcation Lesions in the Main Branch & Side Branch in Native Coronaries) did not meet its primary end point of statistical noninferiority in patients who underwent stenting of the MV and SB versus those who underwent stenting of the MV alone with a provisional strategy to stent the SB if necessary (the composite end point of TVF for the provisional arm was 12.8%, and for the Tryton arm was 17.4%, $P = .11$).[88] However, the Tryton Confirmatory Study suggested the safety and efficacy of this dedicated stent in treatment of coronary bifurcations with a large SB.[89]

Dedicated bifurcation stents may potentially overcome limitations of conventional stents in bifurcations (SB protection, multiple layers, distortion, SB access, crossing through side of the stent, gaps in scaffolding). However, although efforts to produce dedicated bifurcation stent delivery systems are strongly encouraged and research fostered, none of the currently available systems can at present challenge the results offered by the provisional T stent strategy in the majority of bifurcation lesions.

BioResorbable Scaffolds

The first clinically tested bioresorbable stents (BRSs) (Absorb BVS, Abbot Vascular) showed increased rates of major cardiovascular events, driven by a higher device thrombosis rate, as compared with contemporary second-generation DES,[90] which led to a global halt of sales announced by the manufacturer on September 14, 2017.

As a new generation of BRSs is being increasingly tested, the recent experimental studies, evaluating the use of the Magmaris magnesium alloy bioresorbable scaffold (Biotronik, Bulach, Switzerland) for treatment of complex bifurcation lesions, reinforced the need for a selective approach at this early stage of the technology development, preferentially in a single stent strategy with an extension to TAP technique if needed.[91]

ROLE OF ADJUNCTIVE PROCEDURES

Intracoronary Imaging

EBC recommends the use of IVUS for most interventions involving the LM, as several pooled analyses indicated the benefit of IVUS-guidance over angiography only when performing LM PCI, especially if treating the distal bifurcation with a two-stent strategy.[92,93] In 2018, the EBC Consensus document on the use of IVUS guidance for the evaluation and treatment of LM disease was published. The following are the most important messages from this document[94]:

- Atherosclerotic plaque is usually of diffuse nature in the LM and often difficult to be adequately assessed by angiography only, as reflected by a study of 38 patients with angiographically normally appearing LM, which, in 10 cases, proved to be diffusely diseased on IVUS.[95]
- Isolated plaque at the ostium of LAD is seen angiographically in only 9% of cases, whereas using advanced imaging, in >90% there is a continuous plaque stretching from proximal LAD into the LM.[38]
- In case of a discrepancy in the measured MLA on IVUS pullback from both LAD and CX, the smallest MLA is the most accurate.
- IVUS-derived data can be used for the following stages of procedure planning:
  - Assessment of the risk of SB compromise—stenosis proximal or distal to the SB, as well as at the SB ostium, together with the eyebrow sign and significant calcium, predispose to adverse shift of the carina toward the SB (i.e., usually in the CX)
  - Determining the adequate stent diameter and length

- Anticipating proximal optimization—reference diameter and length of the segment from carina to the proximal stent edge
- After stent implantation in the MV, IVUS can be used to optimize the final result:
  - Detection of edge stenosis/dissection (geographic miss)
  - Evaluation of stent apposition and expansion in the MV including the LM stem
  - Control of SB rewiring (e.g., abluminal wire position)
  - Evaluation of stent expansion and apposition in the SB, particularly at the level of SB ostium, if the second stent is needed
  - Ruling out longitudinal stent distortion

Rotational Atherectomy

Rotational atherectomy is important to allow optimal stent expansion in lesions with severe superficial calcifications. Even if no data are available regarding the role of this technology with DES, we think it is intuitive to aim for optimal stent expansion and symmetry. In a setting of a very calcific lesion, this goal can only be obtained with adequate lesion preparation.

The main area of discussion is how frequently a calcific lesion should be pretreated with rotational atherectomy and when, conversely, a high-pressure balloon is sufficient. Except for information obtained with IVUS or in circumstances where no balloon will cross the lesion, we cannot provide additional objective guidelines to make a scientific decision. The operator's judgment remains the most frequent tool dictating the choice of rotational atherectomy. Burr size is typically small, with the intent to modify the plaque, minimizing the risk of embolization.

In our experience, SB stent under-deployment due to inadequate preparation remains the most important cause of restenosis at the ostium of the SB.[96]

Cutting and Scoring Balloons

Bifurcation lesions with a fibrotic plaque at the SB ostium are an ideal setting for this device. The REDUCE III (Restenosis Reduction by Cutting Balloon Evaluation) randomized trial evaluated the role of cutting balloon dilatation before stenting versus standard balloon dilatation in a variety of lesions.[97] This trial reported a lower restenosis rate (11.8% vs. 18.8%, $P = .04$) when lesions were predilated with the cutting balloon. The fact that the final postprocedure lumen diameter was larger in the cutting balloon arm and that the late loss was 0.74 mm for both strategies leads us to believe that the main advantage was toward better stent expansion.

As just discussed in the context of rotational atherectomy, it is difficult to demonstrate that a niche device has an advantage in every lesion. For this reason, we suggest the usage of the cutting balloon in selected moderately calcific and fibrotic lesions, especially involving the origin of the SB. As an alternative, the AngioSculpt catheter, which includes nitinol spiral wires that wrap around the balloon catheter, can be used for lesion preparation. As the balloon inflates, the spiral wires score fibrotic or fibro-calcific plaque, stabilizing balloon position (which avoids slippage) and may lower the risk of dissection. The AGILITY trial (Angiosculpt Coronary Bifurcation Study) supported a provisional stent strategy for complex true bifurcation lesions, with deployment of a DES in the MB, after dilatation of the SB with a scoring balloon.[98]

Associated Pharmacological Treatment

When performing bifurcation stenting with one or two stents, we do not usually change our protocol of periprocedural heparin administration (100 U/kg without elective glycoprotein IIb/IIIa inhibitors and 70 U/kg with elective glycoprotein IIb/IIIa inhibitors). Usage of glycoprotein IIb/IIIa inhibitors is reserved to thrombus-containing lesions and in selected patients with acute coronary syndromes.

We pay a lot of attention to preprocedural preparation with thienopyridines, and when in doubt, we administer a 600-mg loading dose of clopidogrel in the catheterization laboratory,[99] or use a loading dose of ticagrelor or Prasugrel.

In our current practice, the duration of combined thienopyridine and aspirin treatment following bifurcation two-stent strategy is usually for a minimum of 6 months and usually extended to 1 year.

CONCLUSIONS

The introduction of DES has made a remarkable improvement in the treatment of bifurcation lesions. However, several randomized DES trial data showed that routine two-vessel stenting does not improve either angiographic or clinical outcomes for most patients with coronary bifurcation lesions. Therefore, provisional SB stenting remains the gold standard technique for most bifurcations. Nevertheless, there are several bifurcation lesions where two stents are required from the outset, and operators should be confident in such settings.

Finally, the introduction of DES, dedicated for different types of bifurcations, may further facilitate the conquest of one of the most challenging areas in Interventional Cardiology.

KEY REFFRENCES

6. Louvard Y, Lefevre T, Morice MC. Bifurcation lesions. In: Eeckhout E, Serruys PW, Wijns W, eds. *Percutaneous Interventional Cardiovascular Medicine: The PCR-EAPCI Textbook*. Spain: Europa; 2012:283–320.
8. Colombo A, Moses JW, Morice MC, et al. Randomized study to evaluate sirolimus-eluting stents implanted at coronary bifurcation lesions. *Circulation*. 2004;109:1244–1249.
12. Steigen TK, Maeng M, Wiseth R, et al. Randomized study on simple versus complex stenting of coronary artery bifurcation lesions: the Nordic bifurcation study. *Circulation*. 2006;114:1955–1961.
15. Colombo A, Bramucci E, Sacca S, et al. Randomized study of the crush technique versus provisional side-branch stenting in true coronary bifurcations: the CACTUS (Coronary Bifurcations: Application of the Crushing Technique Using Sirolimus-Eluting Stents) study. *Circulation*. 2009;119:71–78.
16. Hildick-Smith D, de Belder AJ, Cooter N, et al. Randomized trial of simple versus complex drug-eluting stenting for bifurcation lesions: the British Bifurcation Coronary Study: old, new, and evolving strategies. *Circulation*. 2010;121:1235–1243.
17. Chen SL, Santoso T, Zhang JJ, et al. A randomized clinical study comparing double kissing crush with provisional stenting for treatment of coronary bifurcation lesions: results from the DKCRUSH-II (Double Kissing Crush versus Provisional Stenting Technique for Treatment of Coronary Bifurcation Lesions) trial. *J Am Coll Cardiol*. 2011;57:914–920.
25. Erglis A, Kumsars I, Niemela M, et al. Randomized comparison of coronary bifurcation stenting with the crush versus the culotte technique using sirolimus eluting stents: the Nordic stent technique study. *Circ Cardiovasc Interv*. 2009;2:27–34.
47. Koo BK, Park KW, Kang HJ, et al. Physiological evaluation of the provisional side-branch intervention strategy for bifurcation lesions using fractional flow reserve. *Eur Heart J*. 2008;29:726–732.
51. Carrie D, Karouny E, Chouairi S, Puel J. "T"-shaped stent placement: a technique for the treatment of dissected bifurcation lesions. *Cathet Cardiovasc Diagn*. 1996;37:311–313.
53. Burzotta F, Gwon HC, Hahn JY, et al. Modified T-stenting with intentional protrusion of the side-branch stent within the main vessel stent to ensure ostial coverage and facilitate final kissing balloon: the T-stenting and small protrusion technique (TAP-stenting). Report of bench testing and first clinical Italian-Korean two-centre experience. *Catheter Cardiovasc Interv*. 2007;70:75–82.
58. Chevalier B, Glatt B, Royer T, et al. Placement of coronary stents in bifurcation lesions by the "culotte" technique. *Am J Cardiol*. 1998;82:943–949.

61. Colombo A, Stankovic G, Orlic D, et al. Modified T-stenting technique with crushing for bifurcation lesions: immediate results and 30-day outcome. *Catheter Cardiovasc Interv*. 2003;60:145–151.
63. Kobayashi Y, Colombo A, Akiyama T, et al. Modified "T" stenting: a technique for kissing stents in bifurcational coronary lesion. *Cathet Cardiovasc Diagn*. 1998;43:323–326.
69. Schampaert E, Fort S, Adelman AG, Schwartz L. The V-stent: a novel technique for coronary bifurcation stenting. *Cathet Cardiovasc Diagn*. 1996;39:320–326.
70. Sharma SK. Simultaneous kissing drug-eluting stent technique for percutaneous treatment of bifurcation lesions in large-size vessels. *Catheter Cardiovasc Interv*. 2005;65:10–16.
75. Burzotta F, Lassen JF, Banning AP, et al. Percutaneous coronary intervention in left main coronary artery disease: the 13th consensus document from the European Bifurcation Club. *EuroIntervention*. 2018;14:112–120.

 Additional references available online at expertconsult.com.

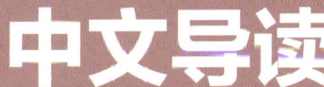

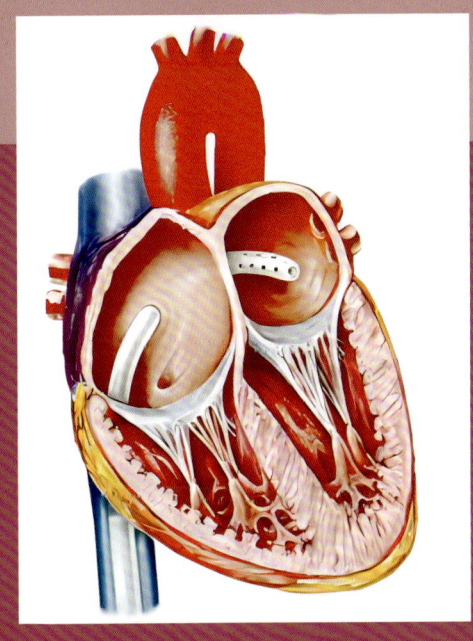

第24章
无保护左主干病变的经皮冠状动脉介入治疗

在所有接受冠状动脉造影的患者中，3%~5%的患者存在冠状动脉左主干病变，在接受搭桥手术的患者中，10%~30%的患者有冠状动脉左主干病变。传统定义中，冠状动脉造影狭窄直径达到50%被认为是冠状动脉左主干显著狭窄的临界值；血流储备分数和血管内超声也可评估冠状动脉左主干狭窄，当FFR<0.80，最小管腔面积<4.5 mm²时，认为冠状动脉左主干存在显著狭窄。冠状动脉左主干病变可根据病变位置分为开口病变、体部病变和分叉病变。冠状动脉左主干开口或体部病变需要在严密的血流动力学监测和精细的指引导管操作下完成。对于冠状动脉左主干分叉病变，往往需要选择必要性单支架技术或双支架技术。必要性单支架技术与双支架技术相比，与较好的结局相关，包括较低的主要不良心血管事件、死亡、心肌梗死、支架内血栓形成和靶血管血运重建风险。因此，在冠状动脉左主干分叉病变的治疗中，首选必要性单支架技术。如果左回旋支供血范围大（左优势型），支架跨开口置入后血流受损风险高（分叉角度小或明显的开口病变），首选双支架技术。这些技术主要分为四大类：T-支架、crush技术、culotte技术、SKS技术。血管内超声可用于冠状动脉左主干病变的介入治疗以优化支架的直径、长度和定位。对于高危患者（左室功能低、冠状动脉重度钙化、血栓病变），术中可应用血流动力学支持（IABP、Impella）以预防可能发生的循环崩溃。冠状动脉左主干病变的最佳血运重建方式仍具有争议，经皮冠状动脉介入治疗具有早期安全性优势，主要缺血事件较少，而冠状动脉旁路移植术具有较好的持久性，包括更低的再次血运重建发生率。因此血运重建方式的选择需要根据患者的病变解剖特点、个人偏好等具体情况综合确定。

何松原　柳景华

章节要点

- 冠状动脉造影在评估左主干病变和指导治疗方面存在局限性。冠状动脉生理学和影像学检查的互补应用有助于改善左主干支架术的预后。
- 左主干开口或体部支架置入术的长期预后良好。
- 在治疗左主干远端分叉时，介入医师应了解每种支架策略的优缺点。无论选择何种经皮冠状动脉介入治疗策略，术后获得足够大的最小支架横截面积对于预防支架内再狭窄和不良临床结果至关重要。
- 经皮冠状动脉介入治疗具有早期安全性优势，而冠状动脉旁路移植术在避免再次血运重建方面具有更大的持久性。
- 左主干病变的最佳血运重建方式的选择应考虑到每个患者的具体情况、患者的偏好，以及经皮冠状动脉介入治疗或冠状动脉旁路移植术的适用性。

24 Percutaneous Coronary Intervention for Unprotected Left Main Coronary Artery Stenosis

Jung-Min Ahn, Duk-Woo Park, Seung-Jung Park

KEY POINTS

- Coronary angiography has limitations in assessing left main coronary artery (LMCA) disease and guiding treatment. The complementary use of coronary physiology and imaging modalities is helpful to improve outcomes following LMCA stenting.
- Long-term prognosis following ostial or shaft LMCA stenting is excellent.
- When treating the distal LMCA bifurcation, the interventionalist should understand the advantage and disadvantage of each stenting strategy. Whatever percutaneous coronary intervention (PCI) strategy is selected, achieving sufficient minimal stent cross-sectional area after LMCA stenting is of paramount importance to prevent in-stent restenosis and adverse clinical outcomes.
- PCI offers early safety advantages, whereas coronary artery bypass grafting (CABG) offers greater durability with respect to freedom from repeat revascularization.
- The optimal choice of revascularization modality for LMCA disease should take into account the specific circumstances of each patient, patient preferences, and suitability of PCI or CABG.

INTRODUCTION

Left main coronary artery (LMCA) disease was first described by James Herrick in 1912 in patients dying of cardiogenic shock after acute myocardial infarction (MI).[1] Clinically significant LMCA disease has been found in 3% to 5% of all patients who undergo coronary angiography and in 10% to 30% of patients who undergo bypass surgery.[2] Owing to the large area of jeopardized myocardium, LMCA disease was associated with high morbidity and mortality, and thus coronary artery bypass grafting (CABG) has been the standard revascularization strategy. However, over several decades, there has been a considerable evolution in the field of percutaneous coronary intervention (PCI). Remarkable advancements in stent devices, technical refinement, and adjunctive medical therapy have led to improved PCI outcomes for unprotected LMCA disease. With a widespread use of drug-eluting stents (DES), PCI for LMCA lesion has become technically more feasible and associated with favorable long-term clinical outcomes. Recently, several clinical trials using first- and second-generation DES found similar survival rates after PCI and CABG.[3–6] Thus unprotected LMCA stenting has become more generalized as primary revascularization strategy.[7]

ANATOMY AND PATHOLOGY

The LMCA arises from the left aortic sinus just below the sinotubular junction of the aortic root. In approximately two-thirds of patients, the LMCA bifurcates into the left anterior descending (LAD) and left circumflex (LCX) arteries; in one-third of patients, the LMCA trifurcates into the LAD, LCX, and ramus intermedius. The LMCA supplies, on average, 75% of the left ventricle. Examination of 100 autopsy cases found that the LMCA had an average length of 10.8 mm (±5.2 mm, range 2 to 23 mm), an average diameter of 4.9 (±0.8) mm, with an average branches angle of 86.7 degrees (±28.8, range 40 to 165 degrees).[8] The anatomic portion of the LMCA stenosis is divided into three anatomic regions: the ostium, midshaft, and distal bifurcation. Histologically, the ostial portion resembles the aorta, being rich in aortic smooth muscle cells and elastic fibers. The distal bifurcation is the part of the LMCA most susceptible to the development of an atherosclerotic lesion because of low shear flow disturbance. Especially in the bifurcation, the lateral wall—that is, the wall opposite the flow divider—is the most frequent site of atherosclerotic plaque accumulation, whereas the flow divider (the bifurcation carina) is usually spared because of high shear stress.[9]

Several etiologies contribute to LMCA stenosis (Table 24.1). The most frequent cause is atherosclerosis. The pathologic plaque composition of LMCA disease varies from the pathologic intimal thickening to thin-cap fibroatheroma with or without plaque rupture.[10] In cases of minimal LMCA disease, the most frequent underlying plaque type is pathologic intimal thickening (64%), followed by fibroatheroma with early or late core (17%). However, most lesions with significant LMCA stenosis, defined as more than 50% narrowing, showed more complex plaques, such as fibroatheromas with late core, thin-cap fibroatheroma, surface ruptures, fissures, and intraplaque hemorrhage. In addition, intravascular ultrasound (IVUS) analysis demonstrates the diffuse nature of LMCA disease that extends from the LMCA to the LAD in 90% of patients and to the LCX in 62% of patients.[11]

Definition of Significant Left Main Coronary Artery Stenosis

Traditionally, an angiographic stenosis diameter of 50% has been considered the cutoff for significant LMCA stenosis. Angiography, however, has limitations in assessing lesion morphology and the true luminal size of the LMCA. In addition, noninvasive testing is often not helpful due to clinical and technical limitations. The intermediate LMCA stenosis can be directly assessed by fractional flow reserve (FFR), with an FFR below 0.80 considered a significant LMCA stenosis. Previous studies found patients with an insignificant FFR can be safely treated medically with comparable outcomes to those undergoing CABG.[12] In case of LMCA with downstream stenoses in the LAD and/or LCX, FFR measured across the LMCA stenosis will be increased leading to underestimation of the lesion significance. However, in vivo study found that unless downstream stenosis is very significant, its impact is clinically negligible.[13]

TABLE 24.1 Causes of Left Main Coronary Artery Stenosis
Atherosclerosis
Nonatherosclerotic causes
Idiopathic causes
• Irradiation
• Takayasu arteritis
• Syphilitic aortitis
• Rheumatoid arthritis
• Aortic valve disease
• Kawasaki disease
• Cardiac surgery or transcatheter aortic valve implantation
• Injury after left main coronary intervention

TABLE 24.2 Favorable or Unfavorable Anatomic Features for Single-Stent Crossover Stenting in the Treatment of Unprotected Left Main Coronary Artery Stenosis	
	Anatomic Features
Favorable	• Insignificant stenosis at the ostial LCX with Medina classification 1,1,0 or 1,0,0 • Diminutive LCX with <2.5 mm in diameter right-dominant coronary system • Wide angle with LAD • No concomitant disease in LCX • Focal disease in LCX
Unfavorable	• Insignificant stenosis at the ostial LCX with Medina classification 1,1,1; 1,0,1; or 0,1,1 • Large size of LCX with ≥2.5 mm in diameter left-dominant coronary system • Narrow angle with LAD • Concomitant disease in LCX • Diffuse disease in LCX

LAD, Left anterior descending coronary artery; *LCX*, left circumflex coronary artery.
From Moussa ID, Colombo A, eds. *Tips and Tricks in Interventional Therapy of Coronary Bifurcation Lesions*. New York: Informa Healthcare; 2010:135.

IVUS is another useful tool to determine the significance of LMCA stenosis. Jasti and colleagues reported that a minimal luminal area (MLA) of 5.9 mm² had the highest sensitivity and specificity (93% and 95%, respectively) for determining a significant LMCA stenosis, compared with FFR as the gold standard.[14] Park and colleagues more recently addressed 112 patients with isolated intermediate LMCA stenosis who underwent preinterventional IVUS and FFR measurements to determine the IVUS MLA criteria that correspond to an FFR below 0.80. They found the IVUS MLA value within the LMCA that best predicted FFR below 0.80 was less than 4.5 mm².[15] In addition, in contrast to non-LMCA stenosis, the positive predictive value of IVUS-measured MLA less than 4.5 mm² is high, at 84%. Thus, if an FFR measurement is not feasible or unreliable, IVUS MLA criteria can be used.

STENTING TECHNIQUES

Ostial and Shaft Lesion

Stenting of LMCA ostial and shaft lesion can be performed safely if meticulous guiding technique and careful hemodynamic monitoring are performed. Coaxial alignment of the guiding catheter is important to minimize ostial injury and to ensure proper positioning of the stent. As long as coaxial alignment is maintained, it is usually easy to advance and position the balloon or stent at the target lesion. Once the balloon or stent is properly positioned, the guiding catheter can be gently retracted 1 to 2 cm into the aorta with gentle forward pressure on the device catheter. The ostial LMCA lesion is dilated and stented with the guide tip positioned in the aortic sinus. The proximal stent edge is positioned very slightly outside the ostium and is expanded against the aortic wall. After deployment of the stent, the stented segment is further dilated with high-pressure balloon inflations an to achieve an optimal stent cross-sectional area. Balloon inflations are brief (<30 seconds) to avoid prolonged global ischemia and ischemia-related complications. Aortoostial coverage may not be mandatory for treatment of disease limited to the shaft of the LMCA.

Bifurcation Lesion

PCI for LM bifurcation is technically demanding and has been associated with a high rate of adverse clinical events, and thus should be restricted to experienced interventionalists who understand the risk/benefit ratio of the percutaneous approaches.

Selection of Left Main Coronary Artery Bifurcation Treatment Strategy

Based on nonrandomized studies and extrapolations of non-LMCA bifurcation trials, the provisional one-stent approach has been considered as a preferred strategy over the elective two-stent technique. However, because of the large myocardium territory supplied by the LCX, there is a possibility of acute circulatory collapse after main vessel stenting. In addition, a provisional one-stent approach for LMCA bifurcation with angiographic significant LCX ostial disease found a higher risk of early target-vessel MI and target-vessel revascularization at 1 year. Therefore, the presence of significant disease in the LCX ostium is regarded as an important factor in choosing a stenting strategy. Table 24.2 summarizes the selection criteria for stenting strategies based on the anatomic features involving the LMCA bifurcation. The provisional one-stent approach is preferred for LM bifurcations with insignificant stenosis at the ostial LCX or a nondominant left coronary system. By contrast, the elective two-stent technique is preferred in patients with significant LCX ostial stenosis with a dominant left coronary system. When there is angiographic ambiguity of LCX ostium, direct imaging of LCX ostium using IVUS may prevent circumflex occlusion or unnecessary complex bifurcation intervention.

Provisional One-Stent Strategy

If the operators choose to use a one-stent approach, there is always the possibility of placing a second stent in the LCX if the result is suboptimal. This strategy is defined as *provisional stenting*. To facilitate rewiring, a wire is placed in the LCX before stenting with the LAD when there is (1) narrowing at the LCX ostium; (2) severe stenosis of the main branch, with a large plaque burden at risk for plaque shifting; (3) a narrow angle of the LCX origination; and (4) deterioration of the LCX ostium after predilation of the main branch.

Patients who develop ischemic symptoms require further side branch intervention. As a bailout procedure for a suboptimal balloon result or significant dissection at the ostial LCX, provisional T-stenting or a reverse crush technique are often used, in which case a final kissing balloon inflation (FKBI) is mandatory. However, FKBI after single-stent crossover in LMCA bifurcation is not routinely performed unless the LCX flow is compromised.[16] FFR-guided decision making for LCX intervention after main vessel stenting is often helpful.[17]

Compared with two-stent techniques, the provisional one-stent approach for distal LMCA bifurcation is associated with more favorable outcomes, including lower risks of major adverse cardiac events, death, MI, stent thrombosis, and target-vessel revascularization.[18] Therefore, the provisional one-stent approach has been preferred in the treatment of LMCA bifurcation stenosis.

TABLE 24.3	Advantages and Disadvantages of Different Two-Stent Techniques	
Mini-Crush	Minimizes multiple layers of struts Good scaffolding at SB ostium Facilitates FKBI Compatible with 6-Fr guider using balloon crushing	Still leaves multiple layers of strut
DK-crush	Good scaffolding at SB ostium Facilitates FKBI Compatible with 6-Fr guider	Complex procedural steps
T-stenting	Good SB scaffolding with angles >70 degrees	Potential gap at SB ostium Protrusion of SB stent into the MB (in the case of TAP)

DK, Double kissing; *FKBI*, final kissing balloon inflation; *MB*, main branch; *SB*, side branch; *TAP*, T-stenting and small protrusion.

Elective Two-Stent Strategy

If the LCX is large (left-dominant system) and at high risk of flow compromise after crossover stenting (narrow angle and significant ostial stenosis), an initial two-stent technique is preferred. These techniques fall mainly into four broad categories: T-stenting, crush stenting and its variants, culotte stenting, and simultaneous kissing stenting. Although better outcomes were reported with the double kissing-crush technique than with the culotte technique in the randomized trial,[19] no consensus has been reached as to which two-stent approach might be better than others. Thus selecting a proper stenting technique should depend on the patient's clinical manifestations, LMCA bifurcation morphology, and the operator's preference. Advantages and disadvantages of different two-stent techniques are summarized in Table 24.3.[20]

Several procedural factors can influence the clinical outcomes of LMCA bifurcation stenting. FKBI should be accompanied in all two-stent techniques to avoid malapposition or underexpansion of stents. The proximal optimization technique is also important because it promotes adequate stent apposition in the left main stem, helps avoid abluminal rewiring, and facilitates rewiring the LCX through a distal stent cell, which is important for complete scaffolding of the LCX ostium.[21] Finally, each segment of the left main should achieve sufficient stent expansion by applying poststent high pressure ballooning, which could be confirmed by final IVUS surveillance. Fig. 24.1 summarizes the integrated use of IVUS and FFR in the treatment of LMCA bifurcation stenosis.[22]

Recently, several dedicated stents for bifurcations have been tested for the treatment of LMCA disease. Theoretically, the advantages offered by these devices may improve clinical outcomes. However, the success of currently available systems depends on the specific bifurcation anatomy. Further studies are needed to define the role of dedicated bifurcation stents in LM disease.[23]

Intravascular Ultrasound Guided Left Main Stenting

IVUS provides more reliable data than angiography on lesion characteristics regarding lumen size, plaque characterization, and disease distribution, which result in optimal stent sizing, length, and positioning. For distal LMCA bifurcation lesions, IVUS helps decide stenting strategy by providing accurate information regarding main-branch and side-branch disease pattern and vascular remodeling. Following PCI, IVUS evaluation ensures optimal stent strut apposition and expansion, guiding subsequent postdilatation to achieve larger stent diameters to maximize clinical benefit. IVUS minimal stent area correlating with lower angiographic restenosis are 5.0 mm² for the LCX ostium, 6.3 mm² for the LAD

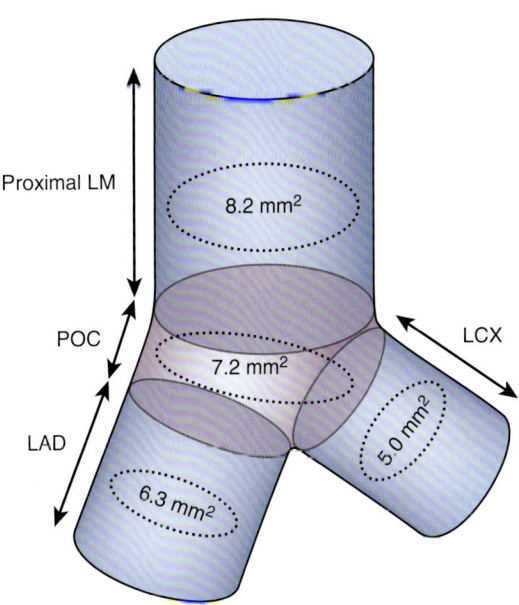

Fig. 24.1 Cutoff values of minimal stent area for the prediction of angiographic in-stent restenosis on a segmental basis. *LAD*, Left anterior descending artery; *LCX*, left circumflex artery; *LM*, left main; *POC*, polygon of confluence.

ostium, 7.2 mm² for the polygon of confluence, and 8.2 mm² for the proximal LMCA (the so-called 5-6-7-8 rule of criteria) (Fig. 24.2).[24] The operator should perform IVUS evaluation after stent implantation and should make an effort to achieve above stent areas using adjunctive high pressure balloon dilations.

Currently, all studies uniformly indicate that IVUS guided LMCA stenting plays a role in improving long-term clinical outcomes, despite the inherent limitations of nonrandomized observational design.[25-27]

Hemodynamic Support and Cardiogenic Shock

Patients with normal left ventricular (LV) function are tolerant of global ischemia during balloon and stent occlusion. Although an intraaortic balloon pump (IABP) is not routinely recommended during the procedure, it should be used to prevent hemodynamic collapse in patients with severely depressed LV function. More advanced support (e.g., Impella; Abiomed, Danvers, MA) may be indicated for high-risk patients, such as those with low left ventricular ejection fraction (LVEF), very calcified stenosis, or thrombus-containing LMCA stenosis.

Despite the remarkable advancement of hemodynamic support, outcomes of cardiogenic shock due to LMCA disease have not much improved. Considering its very high mortality, if possible, more aggressive treatment including heart transplantation or LV assist devices should be considered earlier, unless the patient's hemodynamics respond well to revascularization and/or inotropic agents.

Medical Treatment Versus Revascularization

The natural prognosis of patients with medically treated LMCA disease was very poor: early observational studies found 3-year survival rates of 50%.[28-30] Small controlled trials to compare CABG with medical therapy found that CABG provided a survival benefit in patients with angiographically significant LMCA stenosis. The subsequent meta-analysis of seven randomized trials demonstrated that the 5-year relative risk reduction for mortality provided by CABG over medical therapy was greater for LMCA disease than for three-vessel or one- or two-vessel disease, and the absolute survival benefit time from CABG was 19.3

SECTION III Coronary Intervention

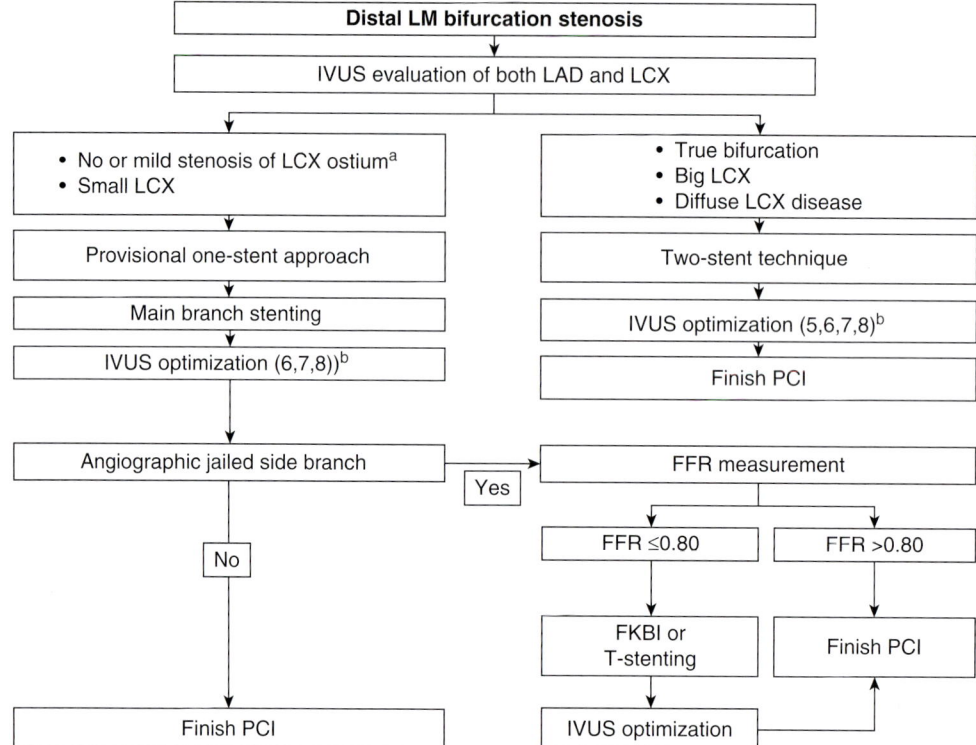

Fig. 24.2 Algorithm for the interventional treatment of distal left main bifurcation lesions. [a]In general, minimal lumen area >4 mm² or plaque burden <50% of the ostium of the left circumflex artery is considered insignificant stenosis. [b]Fig. 24.1. *FKBI*, Final kissing balloon inflation; *IVUS*, intravascular ultrasound; *LAD*, left anterior descending artery; *LCX*, left circumflex artery; *LM*, left main; *PCI*, percutaneous coronary intervention.

months.[31] Since then, CABG has been the treatment of choice in LMCA stenosis. Recently, a Bayesian cross-design and network meta-analysis of 12 studies (four randomized clinical trials and eight observational studies) found that use of PCI for patients with LMCA stenosis is associated with higher 1-year mortality than the medical treatment only.[32]

Percutaneous Coronary Intervention for Unprotected Left Main Coronary Artery

Balloon Angioplasty and Bare-Metal Stenting

Although LMCA stenosis might be considered an attractive target for balloon angioplasty because of its large caliber, short lesion length, and lack of tortuosity, the initial results of balloon angioplasty were not favorable but rather had a high procedural complication rate and early mortality.[33,34] The adoption of metallic stents dramatically overcame the inherent limitations of balloon angioplasty (i.e., acute recoil, abrupt closure, or dissection) and rejuvenated interest in PCI for complex LMCA lesions. In the era of bare-metal stents (BMS), among elective low-risk patients, PCI with stenting showed acceptable in-hospital or midterm outcomes.[35-39] However, excessive risks of restenosis and repeat revascularization hampered the wide expansion of LMCA stenting.

Drug-Eluting Stent Implantation

After a widespread use of DES found a lower risk of angiographic and clinical restenosis, PCI for LMCA disease became more feasible, demonstrating favorable short- and long-term clinical outcomes.[40-43] Several observational studies found promising outcomes for PCI using DESs compared with BMSs.[40,43] In addition, two first-generation DES showed similar clinical performance for the treatment of LMCA stenosis in observational studies[44,45] and a randomized trial.[46] Currently, second- and third-generation DESs have replaced first-generation devices. The Intracoronary Stenting and Angiographic Results: Drug-Eluting Stents for Unprotected Coronary Left Main Lesions 2 (ISAR LEFT MAIN 2) trial found that the zotarolimus-eluting stent and the everolimus-eluting stent for treatment of unprotected LMCA disease provided comparable clinical and angiographic outcomes at 1-year follow-up.[47] In a large pooled analysis (*n* = 2692) of three prospective, clinical-practice registries involving unrestrictive use of DESs for LMCA disease, there were no significant differences in stent-related and patient-related outcomes at 3-year follow-up between different types of newer-generation DES devices.[48] Therefore, patient and lesion selection and optimal technique are more important than the stent platform to determine early and late outcomes in LMCA PCI.

STENT THROMBOSIS AND ANTIPLATELET THERAPY AFTER DRUG-ELUTING STENT IMPLANTATION

Since the introduction of the DES, concerns have been raised regarding the long-term safety of DES use with particular regard to late stent thrombosis and late mortality. However, recent data alleviate some of the concerns about the safety of PCI with DES for the treatment of LMCA disease. The Synergy between Percutaneous Coronary Intervention with Taxus and Cardiac Surgery (SYNTAX) trial found LMCA PCI with DES was associated with a lower risk of stent thrombosis.[49] In addition, reported rates of stent thrombosis in patients who received DES implantation for LMCA disease among several large observational and randomized studies have been lower or, at worst, similar to rates of stent thrombosis compared with patients with other coronary lesions in routine clinical practice.[46-48,50-52] Therefore, prolonged dual-antiplatelet therapy or a more potent regimen may not be necessary for the prevention of stent thrombosis after LMCA stenting.

In-Stent Restenosis After Left Main Coronary Artery Drug-Eluting Stenting

In spite of the good initial and long-term outcomes of PCI for LMCA stenosis, in-stent restenosis (ISR) remains a challenging problem. The rates of angiographic restenosis after LMCA stenting with a DES has been found to vary widely, from 8% to 42%.[53,54] Restenotic lesions, complex stenting with two or more stents in a bifurcation lesion, the total number of stents, and bifurcation lesions were identified as independent predictors of ISR.[53] The LCX ostium was the most common location of the restenosis.[55] Both underexpansion of stents and neointimal hyperplasia were the most important mechanisms of ISR.[56] Real-world registry studies reported that most patients with left main ISR were treated by PCI, and approximately 10% of patients received CABG as an initial treatment strategy.[54] Long-term outcome was favorable regardless of revascularization strategies. In addition, the angiographic surveillance did not affect the patient's long-term outcomes; therefore, routine angiographic follow-up is not recommended after LMCA PCI.[53]

Percutaneous Coronary Intervention Versus Coronary Artery Bypass Graft in Left Main Coronary Artery Stenosis

Registry Data

The Revascularization for Unprotected Left Main Coronary Artery Stenosis: Comparison of Percutaneous Coronary Angioplasty Versus Surgical Revascularization (MAIN-COMPARE) registry included 2240 patients with unprotected LMCA disease who underwent stenting (BMS: $n = 318$, first-generation DES: $n = 784$) or CABG ($n = 1138$) at 12 major cardiac centers. The 5-year follow-up results found that the risk of mortality and composite of death, Q-wave MI, or stroke were similar between the PCI and CABG groups; however, the rate of repeat revascularization was significantly higher in the PCI group.[57] The Drug Eluting Stent for Left Main Coronary Artery (DELTA 1) registry included 1874 patients who underwent LM PCI with mostly first-generation DES and 900 patients who underwent CABG. Similarly, no difference was observed in the occurrence of death, stroke, and MI between PCI and CABG at a median follow-up of 3.5 years. Target-vessel revascularization was higher in the PCI group. For the treatment of LMCA ostial and shaft lesions, PCI showed very favorable clinical outcomes, comparable to CABG.[51] The DELTA 2 registry, which enrolled 3986 patients who underwent LMCA PCI with second-generation DES, compared outcomes with the CABG cohort from the DELTA 1 registry. Compared with the CABG cohort, PCI was associated with a similar rate of death or MI, but stroke was higher in CABG and target-vessel revascularization was higher in PCI.[52]

The large, multinational, all-comers Interventional Research Incorporation Society-Left MAIN Revascularization (IRIS-MAIN) registry evaluated secular trends in patient characteristics, treatment, and outcomes over the last two decades. This registry showed that over time, the proportion of PCI treatment has progressively increased, whereas the opposite trend has been noted for CABG treatment. Notably, risk-adjusted survival, composite outcomes, and repeat revascularization have significantly improved for PCI over time, but remained stable for CABG. As a result, the gap of treatment-effect between PCI and CABG has gradually diminished from the BMS period through the early DES period to the late DES period. Although the outcomes of medical therapy alone were also observed to improve, medical therapy has always been inferior to revascularization strategies in LMCA.[7]

Randomized Trials

The Left Main Coronary Artery Stenting (LE MANS) trial[3] was the first randomized comparison of PCI with stenting (52 patients) and CABG (53 patients) for treatment of LMCA stenosis with or without multivessel coronary artery disease. DES were placed in 35% of PCI patients, and left internal mammary artery (LIMA) grafts were used in 72% of CABG patients. At 1 year, the primary end point of absolute change in LVEF was significantly greater in the PCI group compared with the CABG group, whereas the secondary end points—survival and major adverse cardiac or cerebrovascular events (MACCEs)—were comparable in the two groups.

In the left main subgroup of the SYNTAX trial,[4,58] there were no significant differences in the primary end point of MACCE (37% vs. 31%), death (13% vs. 15%), or MI (8% vs. 5%) between PCI with paclitaxel-eluting stent and CABG of up to 5 years. PCI patients had a lower stroke (2% vs. 4%), but a higher revascularization (27% vs. 16%) compared with CABG patients. Patients with high SYNTAX scores (≥33)—that is, those with increased lesion numbers and complexity—had higher death and revascularization rates in the PCI arm.

The Premier of Randomized Comparison of Bypass Surgery versus Angioplasty Using Sirolimus-Eluting Stent in Patients With Left Main Coronary Artery Disease (PRECOMBAT) trial is a first, LMCA-specified, moderate-sized, randomized controlled trial comparing PCI with sirolimus-eluting stent and CABG.[6,59] At 5 years, the rates of MACCE (18% vs. 14%), death (6% vs. 8%), MI (2% vs. 2%), or stroke (1% vs. 1%) were similar between PCI and CABG. However, target-vessel revascularization occurred more commonly after PCI than after CABG (11% vs. 6%).

The Everolimus-Eluting Stents or Bypass Surgery for Left Main Coronary Artery Disease (EXCEL) trial enrolled 1,905 patients with LMCA disease and low or intermediate anatomical complexity (SYNTAX score ≤32), and PCI was performed with a second-generation everolimus-eluting stent. At 3 years, PCI was noninferior to CABG with respect to the primary composite end point of death, stroke, or MI (15.4% vs. 14.7%). While the primary end point was lower after PCI than after CABG at 30 days (4.9% vs. 7.9%), fewer primary end point events occurred in the CABG group than in the PCI group between 30 days and 3 years. The rates of early MI and major periprocedural adverse events within 30 days were significantly lower with PCI than with CABG (3.9% vs. 6.2% and 8.1% vs. 23.0%, respectively), but ischemia-driven revascularization during follow-up was more frequent after PCI than after CABG (12.6% vs. 7.5%). Overall, these findings suggest PCI offers an early safety advantage and CABG offers greater long-term durability.[60]

The Nordic-Baltic-British left main revascularization study (NOBLE) trial enrolled 1201 patients. PCI was performed with a first-generation DES (11%) or a biolimus-eluting stent (89%). The 5-year rate of the primary end point of MACCE (death, nonprocedural MI, repeat revascularization, or stroke) was significantly higher after PCI compared with CABG (28% vs. 18%). The 5-year rate of nonprocedural MI (6% vs. 2%) and any revascularization (15% vs. 10%) were also higher after PCI. Unexpectedly, at 5-year follow-up, the rate of stroke tended to be higher in PCI patients than in CABG patients (5% vs. 2%). However, the 5-year rate of death was similar between PCI and CABG (36% vs. 32%).[61] Fig. 24.3 depicts the primary end points of these four randomized trial.

Meta-analysis

A metanalysis of six randomized trials found at a median follow-up of 39 months, there were no significant between-group differences in the risk of all-cause mortality, cardiac mortality, MI, or stroke (Fig. 24.4). PCI was associated with higher rates of repeat revascularization compared with CABG in all tertiles of SYNTAX score, and therefore is associated with a greater risk for the long-term composite end point of death, MI, stroke, or repeat revascularization. Based on SYNTAX score category, there were no significant differences in the incidence of all-cause mortality, MI, or stroke. However, the incidence of repeat revascularization was lower in the CABG group regardless of SYNTAX score.[62]

CURRENT STATUS OF LEFT MAIN CORONARY ARTERY PERCUTANEOUS CORONARY INTERVENTION AND SELECTION OF REVASCULARIZATION STRATEGY

As favorable results continue to accrue, recommendations concerning LMCA PCI has been updated. In the current 2014 European Society of Cardiology and American College of Cardiology/

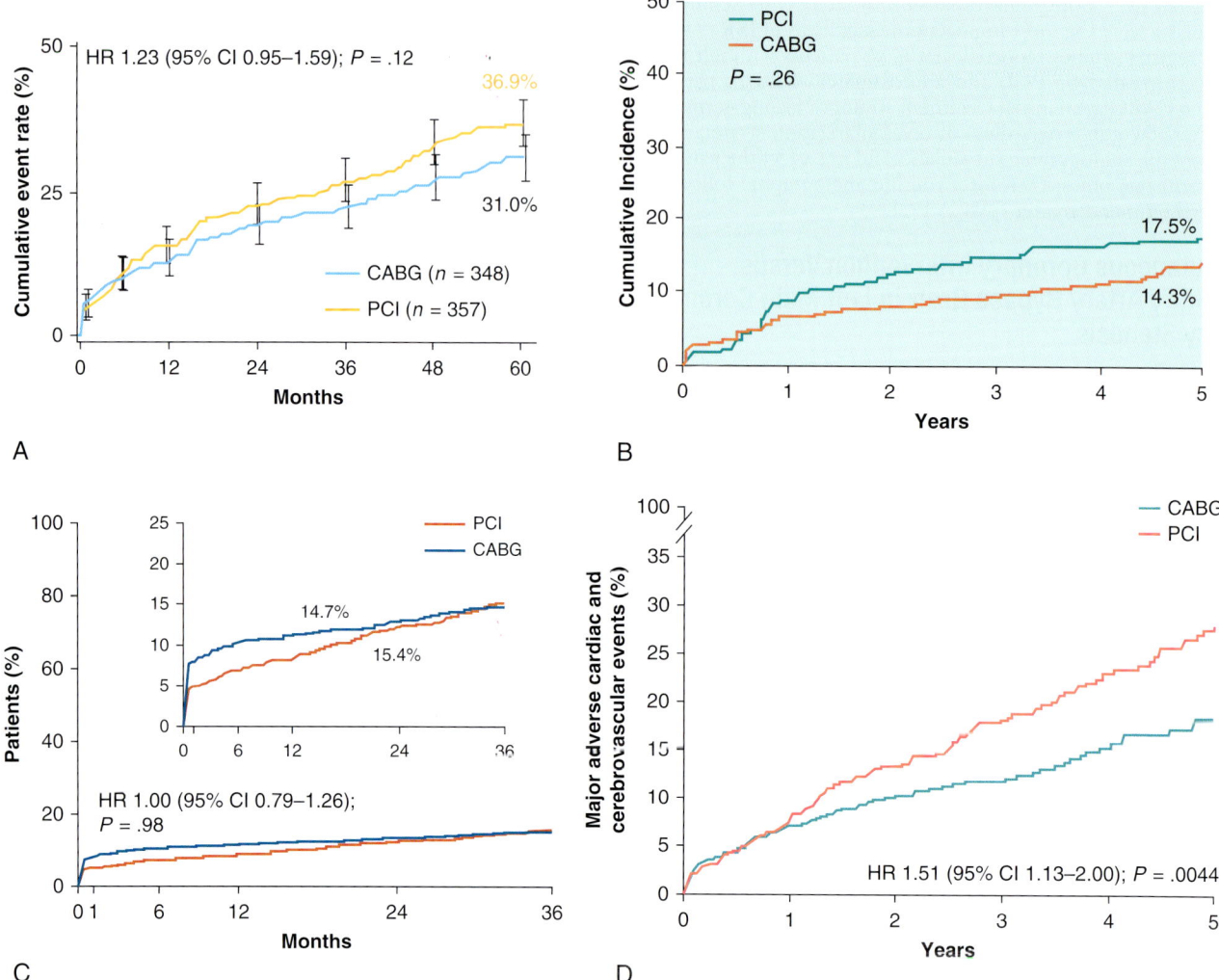

Fig. 24.3 Primary end point of four randomized trials to compare percutaneous coronary intervention *(PCI)* with coronary artery bypass graft *(CABG)*. (A) SYNTAX: all-cause death, myocardial infarction, stroke, and repeat revascularization; (B) PRECOMBAT: all-cause death, myocardial infarction, stroke, and ischemic driven target-vessel revascularization; (C) EXCEL: all-cause death, stroke, or myocardial infarction; and (D) NOBLE: all-cause death, nonprocedural myocardial infarction, stroke, and repeat revascularization. *CI*, Confidence interval; *HR*, hazard ratio.

American Heart Association Guidelines, CABG is a class I, level of evidence B recommendation for LMCA revascularization and PCI is a I B, IIa, or III B based on SYNTAX score tertile.[63,64]

The optimal revascularization strategy, for LMCA disease is still controversial. Some patients prefer CABG surgery, and some patients prefer PCI because PCI offers an early safety advantage with fewer major ischemic events, whereas CABG offers greater durability, including freedom from repeat revascularization. Therefore, the optimal choice of revascularization modality for LMCA disease should take into account the specific circumstances of each patient, individual preferences, and eligibility of PCI or CABG by communication among surgeons, cardiologists, and the patient (Fig. 24.5).[65]

CONCLUSIONS

Over several decades, there has been a remarkable evolution in surgical and percutaneous revascularization for patients with LMCA disease. Current evidence from clinical trials and extensive off-label experience indicates that LMCA PCI shows mortality and morbidity rates comparable to CABG, especially in patients with low and intermediate lesion complexity. This may prompt many interventional cardiologists to choose DES PCI as the preferred treatment option for patients with LMCA disease. An integrated approach that combines more advanced devices with specialized techniques, adjunctive physiologic and imaging support, and adjunctive pharmacologic agents has greatly improved PCI success rates and long-term clinical outcomes for these complex lesions.

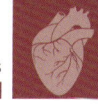

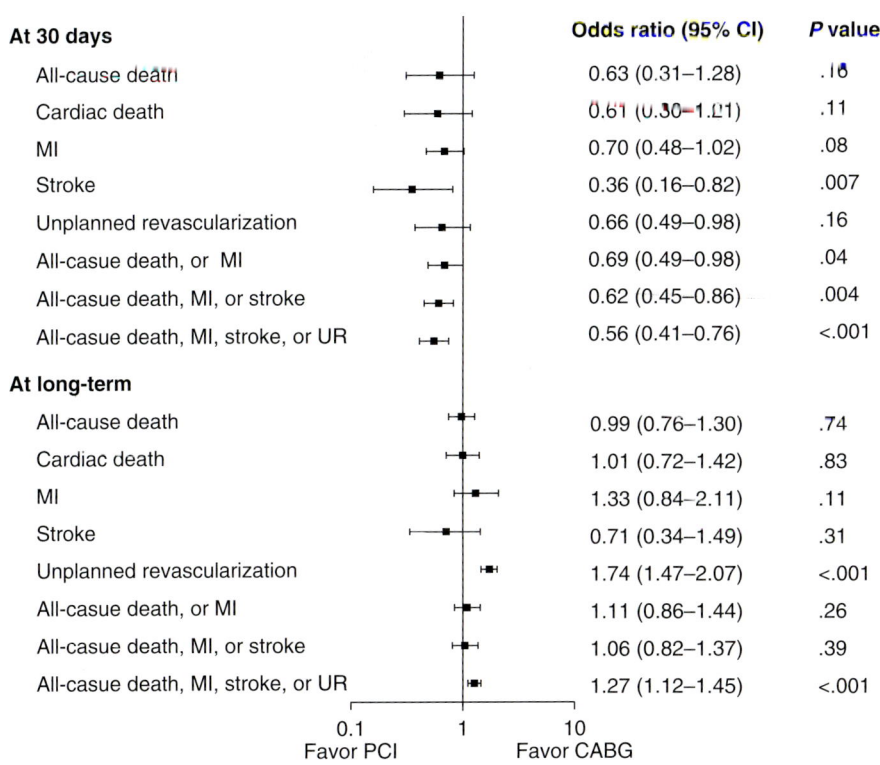

	Odds ratio (95% CI)	P value
At 30 days		
All-cause death	0.63 (0.31–1.28)	.16
Cardiac death	0.61 (0.30–1.21)	.11
MI	0.70 (0.48–1.02)	.08
Stroke	0.36 (0.16–0.82)	.007
Unplanned revascularization	0.66 (0.49–0.98)	.16
All-casue death, or MI	0.69 (0.49–0.98)	.04
All-casue death, MI, or stroke	0.62 (0.45–0.86)	.004
All-casue death, MI, stroke, or UR	0.56 (0.41–0.76)	<.001
At long-term		
All-cause death	0.99 (0.76–1.30)	.74
Cardiac death	1.01 (0.72–1.42)	.83
MI	1.33 (0.84–2.11)	.11
Stroke	0.71 (0.34–1.49)	.31
Unplanned revascularization	1.74 (1.47–2.07)	<.001
All-casue death, or MI	1.11 (0.86–1.44)	.26
All-casue death, MI, or stroke	1.06 (0.82–1.37)	.39
All-casue death, MI, stroke, or UR	1.27 (1.12–1.45)	<.001

0.1 — Favor PCI — 1 — Favor CABG — 10

Fig. 24.4 Meta-analysis of six randomized trials. *CABG*, Coronary artery bypass graft; *CI*, confidence interval; *MI*, myocardial infarction; *PCI*, percutaneous coronary intervention; *UR*, unplanned revascularization.

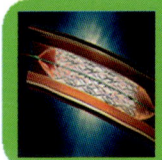

PCI
- Less invasive and early recovery
- Eally safety advantage (less MI, less stroke, or less major periprocedural adverse events)
- Similar mortality

Heart Team Approach

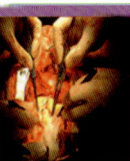

CABG
- Long-term durability
- Less revasculaization
- Lass spontanaous MI
- Similar mortally

⬅ Favor for PCI — **Recommendation** — Favor for CABG ➡

Clinical Factors
- **Urgent revascularization**
- **Serious comorbidity and high surgical risk** (ie., chronic lung disease, advanced age, disability from prior stroke, prior bypass surgery, or poor general performance)

- Clinical equipose

- Low ejection fraction
- Longstanding diabetes
- Need for any concomitant cardiac surgery
- High-bleeding risk unable to comply with DAPT

Anatomical Factors
- Ostial or trunk LM disease
- Isolate LM disease (non-bifurcational or bifurcational)
- LM plus additional one-vessel disease

- LM plus additional two-vessel disease

- **LM plus additional three-vessel disease**
- **Combined complex anatomy not suitable for PCI** (i.e., severe calcification or tortuosity, CTO, multiple/diffuse long lesions, or complex in-stent restenosis)

Each patient's individual circumstances and preferences

Fig. 24.5 Selection of revascularization strategy. *CABG*, Coronary artery bypass graft; *CTO*, chronic total occlusion; *DAPT*, dual antiplatelet therapy; *LM*, left main; *MI*, myocardial infarction; *PCI*, percutaneous coronary intervention.

KEY REFERENCES

6. Park SJ, Kim YH, Park DW, et al. Randomized trial of stents versus bypass surgery for left main coronary artery disease. *N Engl J Med.* 2011;364:1718–1727.
7. Lee PH, Ahn JM, Chang M, et al. Left main coronary artery disease: secular trends in patient characteristics, treatments, and outcomes. *J Am Coll Cardiol.* 2016;68:1233–1246.
14. Jasti V, Ivan E, Yalamanchili V, et al. Correlations between fractional flow reserve and intravascular ultrasound in patients with an ambiguous left main coronary artery stenosis. *Circulation.* 2004;110:2831–2836.
15. Park SJ, Ahn JM, Kang SJ, et al. Intravascular ultrasound-derived minimal lumen area criteria for functionally significant left main coronary artery stenosis. *JACC Cardiovasc Interv.* 2014;7:868–874.
22. Ahn JM, Lee PH, Park SJ. Practical based approach to left main bifurcation stenting. *BMC Cardiovasc Disord.* 2016;16:49.
24. Kang SJ, Ahn JM, Song H, et al. Comprehensive intravascular ultrasound assessment of stent area and its impact on restenosis and adverse cardiac events in 403 patients with unprotected left main disease. *Circ Cardiovasc Interv.* 2011;4:562–569.
48. Lee PH, Kwon O, Ahn JM, et al. Safety and effectiveness of second-generation drug-eluting stents in patients with left main coronary artery disease. *J Am Coll Cardiol.* 2018;71:832–841.
50. Chieffo A, Park SJ, Meliga E, et al. Late and very late stent thrombosis following drug-eluting stent implantation in unprotected left main coronary artery: a multicentre registry. *Eur Heart J.* 2008;29:2108–2115.
60. Stone GW, Sabik JF, Serruys PW, et al. Everolimus-eluting stents or bypass surgery for left main coronary artery disease. *N Engl J Med.* 2016;375:2223–2235.
61. Makikallio T, Holm NR, Lindsay M, et al. Percutaneous coronary angioplasty versus coronary artery bypass grafting in treatment of unprotected left main stenosis (NOBLE): a prospective, randomised, open-label, non-inferiority trial. *Lancet.* 2016;388:2743–2752.

 Additional references available online at expertconsult.com.

中文导读

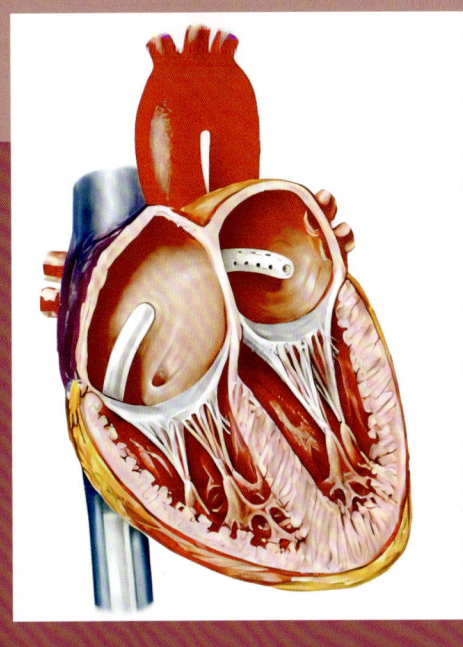

第25章
复杂多支病变

冠状动脉多支血管病变的血运重建治疗是冠心病治疗中复杂且重要的领域。冠状动脉旁路移植术曾是多支血管病变血运重建的唯一选择。近年来，经皮冠状动脉介入治疗的技术进步与器械发展大幅改善了临床结果，尤其是新型药物洗脱支架的出现逐步拓宽了经皮冠状动脉介入治疗在多支血管病变领域的适用范围。如何选择经皮冠状动脉介入治疗与冠状动脉旁路移植术治疗多支血管病变是冠心病学界争论的焦点。一系列大型临床试验结果显示，冠状动脉旁路移植术与经皮冠状动脉介入治疗就临床硬终点而言基本持平，但经皮冠状动脉介入治疗难以撼动冠状动脉旁路移植术对于糖尿病患者的生存优势。冠状动脉旁路移植术天然的高完全血运重建率，以及经皮冠状动脉介入治疗自身存在的再狭窄及多次手术的问题使提高其治疗效果显得十分重要。因此积极使用并联合多种临床手段提升经皮冠状动脉介入治疗效果有着重要意义。SYNTAX系列评分可以简单快速识别高风险患者，冠状动脉功能学评估避免了不必要的支架植入，而腔内影像学是指导支架正确选择与优化经皮冠状动脉介入治疗结果的有力工具。对于部分解剖适宜的患者，联合两种血运重建策略不失为一种良好选择。无论选择何种血运重建方式，需要心脏内外科医师共同决策，综合二级预防措施，优化药物治疗尤其是双联抗血小板策略是多支血管病变治疗的重要基石。

程子超　柳景华

章节要点

- 心血管血运重建旨在缓解未治疗冠心病对预后的负面影响，现已发展为改善多支血管病变患者预后与生活质量的重要策略。
- 经过40年的发展，经皮冠状动脉介入治疗已成为安全且可重复的技术，新器械的出现使复杂病变的经皮冠状动脉介入治疗变得触手可及。
- 近年来，一系列具有里程碑意义的临床试验结果表明，在排除了糖尿病患者以后，经皮冠状动脉介入治疗与冠状动脉旁路移植术治疗多支病变患者的临床硬终点（例如，死亡、心肌梗死）几乎没有差异。
- 在所有的临床试验中，冠状动脉旁路移植术优于经皮冠状动脉介入治疗的最主要原因是经皮冠状动脉介入治疗存在更高的再次血运重建率。
- 采用临床和介入策略，包括危险分层、利用缺血或影像指导介入治疗，可以帮助临床医师合理地选择经皮冠状动脉介入治疗患者，并进一步改善经皮冠状动脉介入治疗手术结果——这将有希望弥补冠状动脉旁路移植术与经皮冠状动脉介入治疗在预后方面所观察到的临床差异。
- 将严格的科学证据转化为临床实践将进一步完善我们在解剖与临床层面对多支血管病变患者进行合适的经皮冠状动脉介入治疗。

25 Complex and Multivessel Percutaneous Coronary Intervention

Sergio Buccheri, Davide Capodanno

KEY POINTS

- Myocardial revascularization, which aims to relieve the negative prognostic impact of coronary artery disease left untreated, has emerged as a strategy to improve prognosis and quality of life in patients with multivessel disease (MVD).
- Over the past four decades, percutaneous coronary intervention (PCI) has evolved into a safe and reproducible procedure that, using an armamentarium of cutting-edge devices, has extended the possibility of noninvasive revascularization in complex anatomical settings.
- Results of the recent landmark clinical trials in patients with MVD have consistently shown a substantial equipoise between PCI and coronary artery bypass grafting (CABG) in terms of hard clinical outcomes (i.e., mortality, myocardial infarction), with the exception of MVD in the context of diabetes mellitus.
- Consistently across trials, differences favoring CABG over PCI were mainly driven by higher rates of repeat revascularization.
- The adoption of clinical and interventional strategies (i.e., risk stratification, use of ischemia- or imaging-guided percutaneous revascularization) to properly guide the selection of PCI candidates, as well as to improve PCI procedural results, will hopefully contribute to filling the observed gap between CABG and PCI outcomes.
- Translating rigorous scientific evidence into clinical practice will further contribute to refining our understanding of proper anatomical and clinical thresholds for the appropriateness of percutaneous revascularization in patients presenting with MVD.

INTRODUCTION

A complex interplay of clinical and anatomical factors lies behind the naive angiographic definition of multivessel coronary artery disease (CAD). Indeed, while multivessel disease (MVD) is scholastically defined as the presence of significant atheromatous disease involving two or three coronary arteries as detected by coronary angiography, a wide spectrum of clinical and anatomical circumstances enters the clinical definition of MVD in the real world. Thoroughly weighting all these factors challenges decision making in daily clinical practice, so that pinpointing the optimal balance between safety and efficacy issues in the selection of a proper revascularization strategy becomes a clinical hurdle.[1] Comprehensively looking at these clinical and angiographic factors in the context of multidisciplinary heart team discussion, as advocated by current guidelines, has emerged as a key factor for improving outcomes after revascularization.[2,3] Also, risk stratification tools have been developed to accurately support decision making between coronary artery bypass grafting (CABG) and percutaneous coronary intervention (PCI).[4,5]

PCI has evolved from a hazardous technique allowing simple balloon angioplasty of isolated proximal coronary lesions to a safe and reproducible procedure that, using an armamentarium of cutting-edge devices, has extended the possibility of noninvasive revascularization in complex anatomical settings.[6] The advent and iteration of stent device technology has been crucial in this process. Newer generation drug-eluting stents (DES) have consistently demonstrated to sizably improve the safety and efficacy outcomes of coronary stenting.[7] As such, nowadays studies looking at plain old balloon angioplasty (POBA) or the use of bare-metal stents (BMS) for PCI in patients with MVD can be considered mainly of historical interest since these procedural strategies are not used any longer as a default approach in modern interventional cardiology practice.[8–18] This chapter will provide a comprehensive overview of the modern strategies to properly select patients, as well as perform and optimize PCI results in patients with MVD based on available evidence from landmark studies in the field.

MULTIVESSEL DISEASE: PREVALENCE AND PROGNOSTIC IMPLICATIONS

Estimating the true unbiased prevalence of MVD is challenging since patients undergoing coronary angiography generally have a clinical indication prompting for invasive cardiac catheterization. Patients with cardiac valve diseases undergoing preoperative coronary angiography represent a cohort where the risk of referral bias for angiography is lowered. In these patients, a small study found that the prevalence of MVD, defined as two or more vessels with clinically significant stenosis or stenosis of the left main (LM) coronary artery, was 21.2%.[19] As expected, the prevalence of MVD is higher, reaching 32.3% for three-vessel disease, in patients undergoing clinically driven angiography as reported in the Swedish Coronary Angiography and Angioplasty Registry.[20] Similarly, data from the CathPCI registry in the United States showed a prevalence of two- and three-vessel disease in patients undergoing coronary angiography for different clinical indications of 29.3% and 16.0%, respectively.[21]

It is intuitive that the higher the burden and extent of CAD the poorer the prognosis and the expected survival. Indeed, a simultaneous presence of CAD in multiple coronary arteries increases the total amount of myocardium at jeopardy and increases the risk of myocardial ischemia.[22] The negative clinical consequences of ischemia, including myocardial infarction (MI), arrhythmias and heart failure, clinically translate into poorer outcomes and survival in the long term. Data on the prognostic impact of MVD left untreated mainly derive from the first randomized clinical trials comparing CABG with optimal medical therapy and no revascularization. A patient-level meta-analysis of these trials showed that patients undergoing revascularization with CABG had significantly lower mortality compared to patients who were managed conservatively both at 5 years (10.2% vs. 15.8%; odds ratio [OR] 0.61; 95% confidence interval [CI] 0.48 to 0.77; P = .0001) and at 10 years (26.4% vs. 30.5%; OR 0.83; 95% CI 0.70 to 0.98; P = .03).[23] The risk of mortality at 5 years was reduced by 68% and 42% in patients with LM and three-vessel disease, respectively. Also, the prognostic benefits of revascularization are demonstrated when looking at the outcomes of patients who are denied surgery due to the presence of distal CAD.[24] Indeed, among these patients, cardiac mortality and MI at 1 year were excessively high, reaching 39.2% and 37.2%, respectively. Patients with three-vessel CAD left untreated had a significant (fourfold) increase in the risk of death (51.6% vs. 20%, P = .039; OR 4.26; 95% CI 1.16 to 15.69). As such, revascularization, which aims to relieve the negative prognostic impact of CAD left untreated, has emerged as a strategy to improve prognosis and quality of life in this scenario and, nowadays, is the cornerstone of treatment in patients with MVD.

REVASCULARIZATION IN PATIENTS WITH MULTIVESSEL DISEASE: STRATEGIES, LANDMARK STUDIES, AND OUTCOMES

While surgical revascularization initially represented the only option for myocardial revascularization, the advent of PCI opened a clinical path to a less-invasive revascularization strategy.[25] A plethora of randomized clinical trials have compared the clinical outcomes following revascularization with CABG or PCI. The initial studies were conducted comparing CABG with POBA or PCI with BMS implantation.[8–18] However, drawbacks of POBA and BMS use (e.g., procedural complications, restenosis, need for repeat revascularization) are well known, especially in patients with MVD. Therefore, studies comparing the outcomes of CABG versus POBA or BMS implantation can nowadays be considered of historical interest since, as reported above, these procedures do not represent a default approach in modern interventional cardiology practice. Results of studies comparing CABG with POBA, or PCI with BMS implantation are summarized in Table 25.1.

The iteration of stent device technology has been crucial to fill the consistent gap in terms of clinical outcomes seen between CABG and PCI using BMS/POBA. Indeed, DES have been consistently demonstrated to sizably improve the safety and efficacy of coronary stenting.[26] DES iteration has proceeded along two main directions: a progressive reduction of stent strut thickness, and the use of antiproliferative drugs eluted from permanent or bioresorbable polymers, to counteract neointimal hyperplasia.

Almost 10 years ago, the Synergy Between Percutaneous Coronary Intervention with Taxus and Cardiac Surgery (SYNTAX) trial was the first of a series of landmark studies assessing the comparative performance of PCI using DES and CABG in patients with MVD.[27]

The SYNTAX Trial

The SYNTAX trial was an all-comer, multicenter, noninferiority randomized clinical trial that enrolled and randomized 1800 patients with three-vessel/LM CAD to undergo CABG or PCI with paclitaxel-eluting stents in a 1:1 ratio.[27] A total of 705 patients had CAD with isolated LM involvement, while three-vessel disease (not including LM) was encountered in 1095 patients. Patients were enrolled only if the local cardiac surgeon and the interventional cardiologist deemed the patient equally eligible to undergo revascularization by CABG or PCI. The primary clinical end point of the study was a composite of major adverse cardiac and cerebrovascular events (MACCE) including death from any cause, stroke, MI, or repeat revascularization at 1 year after randomization. For the first time in a revascularization trial, the evaluation of the anatomical burden and complexity of underlying CAD for each patient was evaluated using the SYNTAX score (SS).[4] The SS is a multiparametric angiographic quantification tool (i.e., 12 questions ranging from anatomy to characteristics of lesions subsets such as bifurcations or chronic total occlusions), which numerically expresses the complexity of CAD in patients undergoing revascularization. A user-friendly online calculator of the score is available at http://www.syntaxscore.com/calculator/start.htm. Patients in the SYNTAX trial were stratified according to the SYNTAX into: low SS group defined as SS ≤22, intermediate SS ranging from 23 to 32, and a high SS when the SS was ≥33. The study was powered to demonstrate noninferiority of PCI as compared to CABG at 1 year using a noninferiority margin of 6.6%.

In the overall study cohort, the 1-year rates of MACCE were significantly higher in the PCI group (17.8% vs. 12.4% for CABG, P = .002) and noninferiority was not met. The difference in the primary end point was largely driven by the higher rates of repeat revascularization in patients treated with PCI (13.5% vs. 5.9%, P < .001). The number needed to treat; that is, the number of CABG procedures needed to prevent one repeat revascularization, was 13.2. There was a significant interaction between the SS and the treatment groups concerning the primary end point (P = .01). Indeed, PCI was comparable to CABG in the lower SS group but had significantly higher rates of MACCE in the intermediate and high SS groups.

In the subgroup of patients with LM disease (36.6% of these patients had three-vessel disease), the rate of MACCE was similar between CABG and PCI groups (13.7% and 15.8%, respectively; P = .44), while in patients having three-vessel disease without LM involvement, MACCE rates were significantly increased in the PCI group compared to the CABG group (19.2% vs. 11.5%, P < .001).

The results of the SYNTAX trial, stratified by the anatomical burden of CAD (LM involvement or MVD without LM disease), were consistent at the intermediate and longest available follow-up (3 and 5 years, respectively).[28,29] In analyses based on SS terciles, PCI had comparable clinical outcomes for patients with LM disease in the low and intermediate SS groups, while in patients with three-vessel disease, PCI and CABG had similar rates of MACCE only in the lowest SS tercile.

The BEST Trial

The Randomized Comparison of Coronary Artery Bypass Surgery and Everolimus-Eluting Stent Implantation in the Treatment of Patients with Multivessel Coronary Artery Disease (BEST) trial compared the outcomes of CABG and PCI with second-generation everolimus-eluting stents in patients with MVD. The study was conducted at 27 centers in East Asia, and a total of 880 patients were randomized to CABG or PCI in a 1:1 ratio.[30] The primary end point of the study was a composite of death, MI, or target-vessel revascularization. Due to slow enrollment, the initial sample size of 1776 patients—required to demonstrate the noninferiority of PCI with respect to CABG at 2 years using a noninferiority margin of 4%—was not achieved. MVD was defined in the study as the presence of two- or three-vessel disease without LM involvement. At 2 years, the primary end point occurred in 11.0% of patients assigned to PCI and in 7.9% of patients randomly assigned to CABG (absolute risk difference, 3.1 percentage points; 95% CI –0.8 to 6.9; P = .32 for noninferiority). During long-term follow-up, the primary end point was more frequently encountered in the PCI group than in the CABG group (15.3% vs. 10.6%; hazard ratio [HR] 1.47; 95% CI, 1.01 to 2.13; P = .04). Consistent with the results of the SYNTAX trial, the difference was mainly driven by significantly higher rates of repeat revascularization in the PCI group. The composite of death, MI, or stroke did not differ between PCI and CABG (11.9% and 9.5%, respectively; P = .26).

TABLE 25.1 Randomized Controlled Trials Comparing Noncontemporary Percutaneous Coronary Intervention Strategies with Coronary Artery Bypass Grafting

Trial	Population	Treatment	Follow-Up	Principal Findings
BARI	Symptomatic patients with MVD ($n = 1,829$)	POBA vs. CABG	10 years	Survival was 71% for PTCA and 73.5% for CABG ($P = .18$). The PTCA group had substantially higher subsequent revascularization rates compared with the CABG group (76.8% vs. 20.3%, $P < .001$)
RITA	1,011 patients (45% single-vessel and 55% multivessel disease)	POBA vs. CABG	6.5 years (median)	Death or nonfatal MI occurred in 17% of the PTCA group and in 16% of the CABG group ($P = .64$). The prevalence of angina and repeat CABG were consistently higher in the PTCA group
GABI	Symptomatic patients with MVD ($n = 8,981$)	POBA vs. CABG	1 year	One year after treatment, 74% of the patients in the CABG group and 71% of those in the PTCA group were free of angina
EAST = Emory Angioplasty versus Surgery	Patients with MVD ($n = 392$)	POBA vs. CABG	3 years	The primary end point of death, MI, or a large ischemic defect was not different, and repeat revascularization was significantly greater in the angioplasty group. Survival was comparable at 8 years
CABRI	Patients with MVD ($n = 1,054$)	POBA vs. CABG	1 year	Patients randomized to PTCA required significantly more reinterventions, took more medications and more frequently had clinically significant angina
ERACI = **Argentine** Randomized Study: Coronary Angioplasty with Stenting versus **Coronary Bypass Surgery** in patients with Multiple-Vessel Disease	Patients with MVD ($n = 127$)	POBA vs. CABG	3 years	Freedom from death, Q-wave MI, angina, and repeat revascularization procedures was significantly greater for the CABG group
ARTS	Patients with MVD ($n = 1,205$)	BMS vs. CABG	5 years	The overall freedom from death, stroke, or MI was not significantly different between the groups. The incidence of repeat revascularization was significantly higher in the stent group
AWESOME = **Angina With Extremely Serious Operative Mortality Evaluation**	Patients with refractory angina and one risk factor for adverse outcome with CABG ($n = 454$)	BMS vs. CABG	3 years	No significant difference in survival was reported, which was 79% and 80% for CABG and PCI, respectively. However, there was a difference in survival free of revascularization: 66% and 44% for CABG and PCI, respectively ($P = .001$)
MASS II = **Medicine, Angioplasty, or Surgery Study II**	611 patients randomly assigned to undergo CABG ($n = 203$), PCI ($n = 205$), or medical therapy ($n = 203$)	MT vs. BMS vs. CABG	10 years	After multivariate Cox analysis at 10-year follow-up, a protective effect of CABG compared with MT = medical therapy (HR 0.43; 95% CI 0.32 to 0.58; $P < .001$) and PCI (HR 0.53; 95% CI 0.39 to 0.72; $P < .001$) was observed for the combined incidence of overall mortality, MI, or refractory angina
SoS = Stent or Surgery	Symptomatic patients with multivessel CAD ($n = 988$)	Stent-assisted PCI vs. CABG	6 years (median)	Higher risk of death with PCI (HR 1.66; 95% CI, 1.08 to 2.55; $P = .022$). The combined incidence of death or Q-wave MI was similar in both groups
ERACI II	450 patients with MVD	BMS vs. CABG	5 years	Similar survival and freedom from nonfatal acute MI was observed between PCI and CABG (92.8% vs. 88.4% and 97.3% vs. 94%, respectively, $P = .16$)

ARTS, Arterial Revascularization Therapies Studies; *AWESOME*, Angina With Extremely Serious Operative Mortality Evaluation; *BARI*, Bypass Angioplasty Revascularization Investigation; *BMS*, bare-metal stents; *CABG*, coronary artery bypass grafting; *CABRI*, Coronary Angioplasty versus Bypass Revascularisation Investigation; *CAD*, coronary artery disease; *CI*, confidence interval; *EAST*, Emory Angioplasty versus Surgery; *ERACHI*, Argentine Randomized Study: Coronary Angioplasty with Stenting versus Coronary Bypass Surgery in patients with Multiple-Vessel Disease; *GABI*, German Angioplasty Bypass Surgery Investigation; *HR*, hazard ratio; *MASS II*, Medicine, Angioplasty, or Surgery Study II; *MI*, myocardial infarction; *MT*, medical therapy; *MVD*, multivessel disease; *PCI*, percutaneous coronary intervention; *POBA*, plain old balloon angioplasty; *PTCA*, percutaneous transluminal coronary angioplasty; *RITA*, randomized intervention treatment of angina; *SoS*, Stent or Surgery.

The FREEDOM Trial

The Future Revascularization Evaluation in Patients with Diabetes Mellitus: Optimal Management of Multivessel Disease (FREEDOM) trial explored the comparative performance of CABG and PCI in diabetic patients with MVD.[31] MVD was defined as the presence of a stenosis of more than 70% by angiography in two or more major epicardial vessels involving at least two separate coronary-artery territories and without LM involvement. Sirolimus- or paclitaxel-eluting stents were the types most frequently used in the study. The primary outcome of the trial was a composite of all-cause death, nonfatal MI, and nonfatal stroke. A total of 1900 patients with a mean SS of 26.2 ± 8.6 were randomized in the study. The median follow-up time was 3.8 years (interquartile range, 2.5 to 4.9). The rate of the primary end point was significantly lower in the CABG group as compared to the PCI group ($P = .005$ by the log-rank test). The divergence of the curves started to become more evident at 2 years. At 5 years, the event rates were 26.6% and 18.7%

in the PCI and CABG groups, respectively (absolute difference of 7.9 percentage points, 95% CI, 3.3 to 12.5; number of CABG procedures needed to prevent one event = 12.7). Importantly, all-cause death was significantly increased in patients who underwent PCI (P = .049). The results were consistent in the subgroup of patients with two-or three-vessel disease (P for interaction = .75).

Clinical Outcomes From Meta-Analyses and Large Registries

By pooling the results of multiple and homogeneous clinical trials, meta-analyses may offer more robust and powered evidence about comparative clinical outcomes between different treatment strategies. Previous meta-analyses conducted by merging study-level results have highlighted the risk of increased mortality after revascularization with PCI compared to CABG.[32] However, study-level meta-analyses suffers the important limitation of the lack of subgroup characterization, based on important clinical characteristics, where pooled results may significantly differ. Patient-level meta-analyses may overcome these limitations. Indeed, a patient-level meta-analysis of 11 trials, which included individual data from 11,518 subjects undergoing revascularization with CABG or PCI, still found a survival benefit with CABG over PCI in patients with MVD (11.5% and 8.9% after PCI and CABG, respectively; HR 1.28; 95% CI 1.09 to 1.49; P = .0019) but differences in survival between CABG and PCI were mainly driven by the presence of diabetes. Indeed, in patients without diabetes, no differences between CABG and PCI were evident (8.7% and 8.0% after PCI and CABG, respectively; HR 1.08; 95% CI 0.86 to 1.36; P = .49).[33]

Unfortunately, the generalizability of randomized controlled trials (RCTs) and related meta-analyses is often hampered by too stringent selection criteria and nonconsecutive enrollment. Real-world registries may overcome these limitations, and their results are particularly useful to complement and corroborate RCT findings in the real world. Initial result from large registries of patients with MVD, which compared CABG and PCI outcomes, such as the ACCF-STS Database Collaboration on the Comparative Effectiveness of Revascularization Strategies (ASCERT) and Coronary Revascularization Demonstrating Outcomes Study in Kyoto (CREDO-Kyoto) PCI/CABG cohort-2 registries, raised concerns about a survival benefit with CABG over PCI and highlighted significant differences for other hard clinical outcomes favoring CABG (i.e., MI).[34,35] These results were confirmed even after extensive statistical adjustment. However, in these registries, first-generation DES were mainly employed, and findings about mortality were concerned by the presence of residual confounding.[36] Recently, a large and more contemporary analysis from the Cardiac Surgery Reporting System (CSRS) and Percutaneous Coronary Intervention Reporting System (PCIRS) registries of the New York State Department of Health looked at the comparative clinical outcomes of patients with MVD undergoing revascularization with CABG or PCI with everolimus-eluting stents.[37] More than 18,000 patients were compared in propensity score-matched analyses (1:1 matching ratio) in the study. At a mean follow-up of about 3 years, PCI was associated with a similar mortality (HR 1.04; 95% CI, 0.93 to 1.17; P = .50) but a higher risk of MI (HR 1.51; 95% CI, 1.29 to 1.77; P < .001) and repeat revascularization (HR 2.35; 95% CI, 2.14 to 2.58; P < .001). Interestingly, the stroke risk was significantly lower with PCI (HR 0.62; 95% CI, 0.50 to 0.76; P < .001) and the difference in the adjusted risk for MI between CABG and PCI was not evident in patients achieving complete revascularization (P for interaction = .02).

Meaningful Message for Clinical Practice

In aggregate, results of the landmark clinical trials comparing CABG and PCI in patients with MVD showed a substantial equipoise between CABG and PCI in terms of hard clinical outcomes (i.e., mortality, MI). Consistently across the studies, the differences favoring CABG were mainly driven by higher rates of repeat revascularization with PCI. Indeed, despite the advent of modern DES technology, which has significantly lowered the rate of in-stent restenosis with respect to BMS and POBA, CABG continues to portend lower rates of repeat revascularization in the long term. However, trials showed that differences in restenosis might become attenuated when the complexity of CAD is low. However, the paradigm of similarities in hard clinical outcomes between CABG and PCI may not hold true in diabetic patients, where a survival advantage of CABG has been clearly depicted.

Shared decision making has become increasingly important when making a choice between CABG or PCI for multivessel disease. The stakeholders for shared decision making include the heart team as well as the patient and family. When communicating differences in CABG versus PCI outcomes, it can be useful to consider the number of CABG procedures required to prevent one event if PCI was selected instead. For example, as described above, in the SYNTAX trial the primary end point difference was largely driven by higher rates of repeat revascularization in patients treated with PCI (13.5% vs. 5.9%, P < .001). The absolute difference of 7.6 means that the number needed to treat with CABG to prevent one repeat revascularization was 13.2. This can be a useful data point when the heart team communicates options to individual patients. Another perspective on the same data is to add "*freedom from* repeat revascularization" to the "repeat revascularization" data. Informing a patient that repeat procedures were needed in 13.5% of PCI patients, compared to only 5.9% of CABG patients (a relative 56% reduction), provides a very different message compared to communicating that freedom from revascularization was improved from 86.5% with PCI to 94.1% with CABG (a much smaller, relative 9% improvement).

STRATEGIES TO IMPROVE OUTCOMES AFTER PERCUTANEOUS CORONARY INTERVENTION FOR MULTIVESSEL DISEASE

As reported above, DES have substantially lowered the rate of repeat revascularization by reducing neointimal hyperplasia and late lumen loss compared to BMS. However, the persisting gap in outcomes between CABG and PCI has fostered the quest for additional clinical and interventional strategies to support the proper selection of PCI candidates, and to improve PCI procedural results. In this context, different strategies have proven their value, including the use of fractional flow reserve (FFR) and intravascular imaging, and the iteration of naive anatomical classification of CAD toward a combined anatomical and clinical approach for risk stratification.

Fractional Flow Reserve and the FAME Trial

Identification of ischemia-provoking lesions, beyond angiographic stenosis severity, has been the object of extensive research in patients with MVD. Since stenting itself is associated with a sizeable rate of stent-related adverse events (stent thrombosis, restenosis), avoiding unnecessary stenting is key to improving clinical outcomes in the long term. FFR, a technique that evaluates the trans-stenotic pressure gradient after achieving maximal hyperemia, has emerged as a simple, robust, and reproducible tool to assess the functional relevance of coronary lesions.[38] An FFR value below 0.80 identifies ischemia-provoking lesions with an accuracy of more than 90%.[39]

In the FFR versus Angiography for Multivessel Evaluation (FAME) trial, a total of 1005 patients with MVD were randomized to PCI guided by angiography alone or by angiography and FFR.[40] MVD was defined in the study as the presence of stenoses of at least 50% by angiography in two of the three major epicardial coronary arteries. Patients with LM disease were excluded. The primary end point of the study was a composite of death, MI, and any repeat revascularization at 1 year.

The mean SS in the study population was 14.5 and significantly more stents per patient were implanted in patients undergoing PCI guided by angiography alone (2.7 ± 1.2 vs. 1.9 ± 1.3, $P < .001$). At 1 year, the rate of the primary end point was significantly lower in patients in the FFR-guided PCI group compared to patients randomized to angiography guidance alone (13.2% vs. 18.3%, $P = .02$, respectively). Significance for the primary end point was driven by a trend toward a reduction in the rate of MI and repeat revascularization, while all-cause death did not differ across the groups. Rates of angina were comparable between the two groups. The ongoing FAME 3 trial (NCT 02100722) will explore whether PCI, guided by FFR measurements with the use of the newer generation zotarolimus-eluting stent, is noninferior with respect to CABG for the combined end point of death, MI, stroke, and repeat revascularization at 1 year in patients with three-vessel disease without LM involvement.

Refining the SYNTAX Score

As already advocated by the 2014 European guidelines,[41] the SS is a central tool to inform the therapeutic decision making between CABG and PCI in daily clinical practice. In patients with MVD, an SS value >22 contraindicates revascularization by PCI (class III/level of evidence B), while in patients with LM disease, the cutoff value contraindicating PCI is 32.

The concept behind the SS is robust and straightforward. Indeed, using a single number, the SS allows a simple and meaningful quantification of CAD complexity, and allows the discriminating presence of simple or diffuse CAD burden. However, the anatomical SS has a series of intrinsic limitations.[42] Calculating the SS is time-consuming, and unintended errors during the rating process are possible (in particular when rating the characteristics of bifurcations and chronic total occlusions). All these factors lead to a significant amount of variability when the SS is calculated by different operators (inter-observer variability). As an example, in the EXCEL trial, approximately one-third of patients had discordant core-lab and site-reported SS values and some patients not meeting the inclusion criterion of an SS threshold value below 32 were included in the trial due to erroneous calculations.[43] Importantly, the lack of refinement by clinical variables into a merely anatomical evaluation tool lowers the predictive ability of the score in complex clinical settings. To overcome these limitations, a series of refinements of the SS have been recently proposed and some of these have been progressively permeating clinical practice.[44] The conceptual groundwork for iteration of the anatomical SS has followed different directions, namely: integration of the anatomical score with clinical variables (i.e., global risk classification, SS II),[5,45] quantification of the functional relevance of CAD (functional SS),[46] and assessment of the prognostic relevance of CAD left untreated (residual SS, residual functional SS).[47,48]

SYNTAX II Score

The SYNTAX II score has been developed as a prognostic tool for individualizing the decision making between PCI and CABG.[5] Clinical variables with significant interaction (i.e., opposite direction of the treatment effect) between PCI and CABG with respect to mortality at 4 years entered the SYNTAX II score. The final score includes eight predictors: (1) anatomical SS, (2) age, (3) creatinine clearance, (4) left ventricular ejection fraction, (5) the presence of unprotected LM CAD, (6) peripheral vascular disease, (7) female sex, and (8) chronic obstructive pulmonary disease. The SYNTAX II score was externally validated in the multicenter DELTA registry and outperformed the anatomical SS alone in terms of discrimination (discrimination of the SYNTAX II score above 0.70 in the derivation and validation cohort). In a pooled analysis of patients enrolled in the Premier of Randomized Comparison of Bypass Surgery versus Angioplasty Using Sirolimus-Eluting Stent in Patients with Left Main Coronary Artery Disease (PRECOMBAT) and BEST trials,[49] the SYNTAX II score demonstrated good calibration and discrimination in patients with and without diabetes (C-statistic of 0.68 and 0.67, respectively). These results further support the external validity of the SYNTAX II score in patients with either MVD and/or LM involvement.

Residual and Coronary Artery Bypass Grafting SYNTAX Score

The detrimental prognostic impact of CAD left untreated has been well characterized in the literature and has been previously mentioned in this chapter. The residual SS (i.e., the SS of lesions which were not addressed by revascularization), may objectively quantify the extent of incomplete revascularization and has demonstrated interesting prognostic performance in patients undergoing revascularization.[47] In the PCI cohort of the SYNTAX trial, a residual SYNTAX score (rSS) >8 was associated with increased risk of mortality at 5 years, which peaked up to 35% compared to patients with residual rSS values below 8.

Similarly, in patients treated with surgery, the CABG SS is calculated by deducting points from the baseline anatomical SS, which are weighted using the Leaman score and depend on the relative importance of the diseased coronary artery segments that have a functional bypass graft anastomosed distally.[50] The CABG SS has had limited penetration into clinical practice.

Functional SYNTAX Score

The functional SYNTAX score (fSS) integrates FFR evaluation with the anatomical SS.[46] The fSS is defined as the SS of only ischemia-provoking lesions (FFR values below 0.80). In the FAME trial, the fSS demonstrated a better predictive accuracy for major adverse cardiac events compared to the anatomical SS (C-statistic for the functional SS of 0.677 vs. 0.630 for the anatomical SS, $P = .02$). Interestingly, a recent study has demonstrated significant improvements in risk discrimination when the rSS and fSS are integrated and combined into the residual-functional SS.[48]

Intravascular Imaging to Guide and Optimize Percutaneous Coronary Intervention Procedures

As reported above, the proper selection of lesions to be treated with PCI is a critical step to avoid unnecessary stenting and to improve long-term clinical outcomes. Besides proper lesion selection, optimization of stent implantation is also crucial to pursue the goal of improving long-term outcomes after PCI. The use of intravascular imaging may be instrumental to achieve this target.

Currently, there is an emerging belief regarding the sizable prognostic benefits of intravascular imaging use in daily clinical practice.[51] In complex anatomical settings, the use of intravascular imaging has emerged as a powerful tool to guide proper stent selection and to optimize PCI results. Indeed, relying on angiography only in complex anatomies can be potentially misleading, and can increase the likelihood of stent failure in the long term. Angiography has several drawbacks, including poor ability to characterize plaque anatomy and burden, limited precision when assessing vessel dimensions, and low sensitivity in the evaluation of results after stent implantation (the presence of dissection at stent edges, malapposition, geographical missing of the lesion to cover). Intravascular imaging techniques, including intravascular ultrasound (IVUS) and optical coherence tomography (OCT), are useful aids made available to PCI operators in order to optimize PCI results.[52] IVUS is characterized by lower spatial resolution compared to OCT and allows for an accurate characterization of the entire vessel anatomy (i.e., vessel diameter and lesion length). On the contrary, the higher spatial resolution and lower tissue penetration of OCT is particularly useful when looking at intimal and subintimal abnormalities either before stenting (i.e., dissection, plaque erosion or rupture, presence of thrombus), or after stenting (plaque protrusion, presence of dissection at the stent edges, stent malapposition). Several trials have investigated and consistently demonstrated the incremental prognostic benefits conveyed by intravascular imaging techniques used during complex PCI procedures. Moreover, imaging guidance during complex interventions (i.e., LM or chronic total occlusion PCI) has become accepted as a relevant quality metric in PCI practice. To date, only a limited number of trials has compared the head-to-head performance of IVUS and OCT. Among 450 patients enrolled in the OCT compared with IVUS and with angiography to guide coronary stent implantation (ILUMIEN III) trial, OCT-guided PCI using a predefined strategy (e.g., based on measurements at the external elastic lamina) for stent selection and procedural optimization resulted in similar minimum stent area as compared to IVUS and angiography guidance.[53] Also, the Optical Frequency Domain Imaging vs. Intravascular Ultrasound in Percutaneous Coronary Intervention (OPINION) trial showed that IVUS and OCT guidance yield similar clinical outcomes at 1 year for the composite end point of cardiac death, target-vessel–related MI, and ischemia-driven target-vessel revascularization.[54] As such, the selection of a specific intravascular imaging technique in contemporary PCI practice mainly depends on operators' preference and experience. The ongoing Intravascular Imaging- Versus Angiography-Guided Percutaneous Coronary Intervention for Complex CAD (RENOVATE) trial (NCT03381872) and the planned ILUMIEN IV studies will shed definitive light about the prognostic benefits of intravascular imaging use in patients with complex coronary anatomy undergoing percutaneous revascularization.

Secondary Prevention: An Important Clinical Goal After Revascularization

The rate of recurrent thrombotic events in patients with MVD is noteworthy.[55,56] Among possible thrombotic events, stent thrombosis remains a feared complication after stenting, and is associated with relevant mortality.[57] Despite the reduced rate of stent thrombosis observed with DES compared to BMS, the cumulative number of events at long-term follow-up is not negligible.[58,59] The pharmacologic cornerstone for preventing stent thrombosis is dual antiplatelet therapy (DAPT). Beyond stent thrombosis, DAPT may exert its protective effects against thrombosis over a ruptured/ulcerated plaque in other vascular territories.[60] The optimal duration of DAPT, defined as the combination of aspirin and a $P2Y_{12}$ inhibitor, has been investigated in several clinical trials.[61,62] Prolonging DAPT duration has been advocated as a strategy to reduce the rate of stent thrombosis and recurrent ischemic events. The emerging concept from trials is that tailoring proper DAPT duration on patients' clinical characteristics (i.e., clinical presentation as acute coronary syndrome or stable angina) and anatomical factors (complexity of the PCI procedure) should be preferred over an indiscriminate approach.[63,64] Indeed, DAPT prolongation is associated with an increased risk of bleeding, which may sizably impact on mortality.[65] Therefore, an individualized approach, informed by modern risk stratification tools,[66,67] has emerged as a key factor to identify the optimal balance between thrombotic and bleeding risks.

Also importantly, the presence of MVD CAD should be viewed as merely the local manifestation of atherosclerosis. Atherosclerosis is a multifactorial, progressive pan-vascular disease, which, over time, continues to put the heart, as well as other target organs at jeopardy for ischemia (i.e., brain with ischemic stroke, peripheral limb circulation with critical limb ischemia).[68] Targeting all factors contributing to the progression of atherosclerosis according to well-established secondary preventive measures is of paramount importance to reduce the burden of recurrent events.[69] Physicians have a central role in spreading the concepts of and recommending a healthier lifestyle to delay, and possibly counteract, the several factors that contribute to the progression of atherosclerotic disease. These include smoking cessation and moderate physical activity, proper care of metabolic risk factors prompting atherosclerosis progression (i.e., diabetes and dyslipidemia), and a careful assessment of blood pressure values over time. Guideline recommendations in patients with CAD have reported in detail the desired targets and goals for both primary and secondary prevention measures.[69–71] Regrettably, a meta-analysis of five contemporary trials comparing myocardial revascularization using PCI or CABG found that the adherence to guideline-directed medical therapy in patients with CAD is low and further decreases over time.[72] Indeed, the rate of use of any antiplatelet agent plus β-blocker plus statin was 67% at 1 year and decreased to 53% at 5 years in patients enrolled in contemporary clinical trials of myocardial revascularization. These percentages were even lower when an angiotensin-converting enzyme inhibitor/angiotensin receptor blocker was considered as part of the guideline-recommended medical therapy.

Combining Different Strategies to Improve Percutaneous Coronary Intervention Outcomes of Multivessel Disease: The SYNTAX II Study

The SYNTAX II study sought to investigate whether PCI performed according to a modern strategy (SYNTAX II strategy) in patients with MVD may contribute to improve clinical outcomes and reduce the gap in clinical outcomes compared with surgery.[73] The SYNTAX II strategy is shown in Fig. 25.1. SYNTAX II was an all-comers, European multicenter, and single-arm study, which included patients with de novo three-vessel disease (LM disease not included). Patients were deemed eligible for inclusion in the study if they had an SS II value (site-reported) predicting equipoise between CABG and PCI for 4-year mortality. In addition, all patients were evaluated in the context of the heart team and were asked to volunteer in the study only if "equivalent anatomical revascularization" could have been obtained with either CABG or PCI. PCI was conducted in the study according to modern state-of-the-art technical practice, namely: use of FFR/instantaneous wave-free ratio to select ischemia-provoking lesions, the use of intravascular imaging to select and optimize stent implantation, the use of a newer generation everolimus-eluting DES with bioabsorbable polymer, a recommendation for revascularization of chronic total occlusions by dedicated operators, as well as guideline-directed medical therapy. The primary end point was a MACCE at 1-year follow-up, defined as the composite of all-cause death, stroke, any MI, or any revascularization.

A total of 454 patients underwent PCI in SYNTAX II. Patients were compared to historical cohorts of patients (treated with PCI and CABG) derived from the SYNTAX trial based on predicted equipoise in 4-year mortality using SS II. At 1 year, patients undergoing PCI according to the SYNTAX-II strategy had lower rates of MACCE compared to the historical SYNTAX cohort (10.6% vs. 17.4% in SYNTAX II vs. SYNTAX-I PCI cohort; HR 0.58; 95% CI 0.39 to 0.85; $P = .006$). The difference in MACCE was driven by a significant reduction in the incidence of MI (HR 0.27; 95% CI 0.11 to 0.70; $P = .007$) and repeat revascularization (HR 0.57; 95% CI 0.37 to 0.9; $P = .015$). Results were consistent when patients in the SYNTAX II study were compared

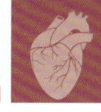

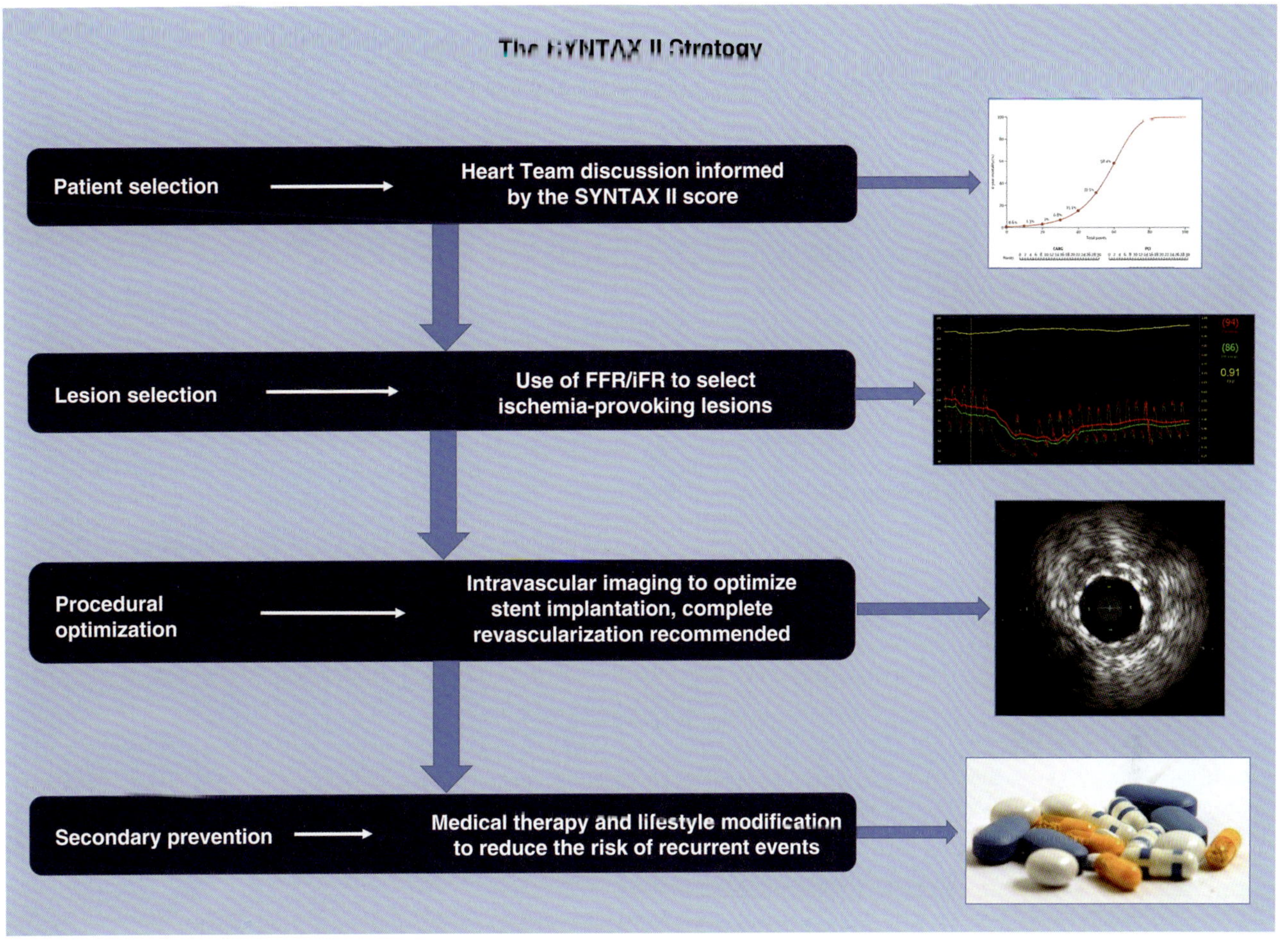

Fig. 25.1 The SYNTAX II strategy. *FFR*, Fractional flow reserve; *iFR*, instantaneous wave-free ratio; *IVUS*, intravascular ultrasound; *PCI*, percutaneous coronary intervention.

to patients who underwent surgery in the SYNTAX trial (HR for MACCE at 1 year 0.91; 95% CI 0.59 to 1.14; P = .684). In aggregate, the findings from the SYNTAX II trial emphasize the prognostic benefits conveyed by performing PCI according to the highest standards of modern clinical and technical practice (i.e., heart team careful evaluation of patients, physiology-guided revascularization, optimization of stent implantation with intravascular imaging, and optimization of medical therapy after the procedure). Long-term results of the SYNTAX-II study and a randomized trial looking at the comparative outcomes of PCI performed in keeping with the SYNTAX II strategy and a cohort of patients undergoing CABG are awaited.

Meaningful Message for Clinical Practice

Clinical and technical iteration of PCI practice has been demonstrated to positively impact on clinical outcomes after revascularization. Importantly, selecting the right patient and lesion subset using a modern approach, which introduces significant refinements to support clinical and technical decision making, may provide the opportunity to fill current gaps in clinical outcomes between PCI and CABG. As such, adhering to this modern strategy may offer the highest standards of quality to patients undergoing percutaneous revascularization. Large and prospective confirmative studies are awaited to corroborate these results and to prompt a wider adoption of a combined clinical and technical selection approach in daily clinical practice.

MANAGING MULTIVESSEL DISEASE IN PATIENTS WITH STEMI

Restoration of blood flow to the myocardium in order to relieve the negative consequences of prolonged ischemia is the cornerstone of the interventional management of patients presenting with ST-elevation myocardial infarction (STEMI).[74] Often, the presence of bystander lesions beyond the culprit increases the complexity of therapeutic management. Indeed, the presence of additional nonculprit lesions is frequently encountered in STEMI, and is reported in up to 40% of cases.[75] Consistent with stable CAD, the increasing burden of CAD in STEMI patients is associated with worse prognosis compared to the treatment of isolated culprit lesions, especially with respect to subsequent risk of recurrent MI events.[76] Therefore, fixing all lesions beyond the culprit at the time of the index procedure or before discharging the patient home may seem an intuitive strategy in light of the prognostic benefits demonstrated for complete revascularization. However, findings from multiple observational studies have challenged this paradigm, leading to an initial contraindication in clinical guidelines for the revascularization of nonculprit lesions during primary PCI, except in patients presenting with cardiogenic shock.[77–79] Recently, a series of large RCTs (listed in Table 25.2) have consistently demonstrated that achieving complete revascularization of nonculprit lesions, either during the index or in a staged procedure, may reduce the risk of major cardiac adverse events.[80–84] These trials often differed with respect to the timing of when complete revascularization was

TABLE 25.2 Principal Randomized Clinical Trials in STEMI Patients With Multivessel Disease

Studies	Sample Size	Definition of MVD	Timing of CR and Severe Stenosis Definition	Primary End Point	Follow-Up	Main Findings
PRAMI	465	One or more coronary arteries other than the infarct artery	Immediate (lesions >50%)	Composite of cardiac death, nonfatal MI and refractory angina	23 months	Early stopped, primary end point significantly reduced with CR = complete revascularization. CR associated with lower risk of nonfatal MI and refractory angina.
CvLPRIT	296	One additional noninfarct-related epicardial artery with at least one angiographically significant lesion	Preferably immediate or in-hospital staged (>70% diameter stenosis in one plane or >50% in 2 planes)	Composite of all-cause mortality, recurrent MI, heart failure, repeat revascularization	12 months	Primary end point significantly reduced with CR. Nonsignificant reduction in all primary end point components.
DANAMI-3-PRIMULTI	627	Nonculprit vessels with angiographic stenosis >50%	In-hospital staged (FFR<0.80 or lesion >90%, artery diameter >2 mm)	Composite of all-cause mortality, nonfatal MI, ischemia driven revascularization of non-IRA = infarct-related artery lesions	12 months	Primary end point significantly reduced with CR. Significant reduction in repeat revascularization with CR.
PRAGUE 13	214	One or more stenoses of non-IRA coronary artery (arteries)	Staged PCI between 3rd and 40th day after pPCI = primary PCI (≥70% stenosis and diameter artery ≥2.5 mm)	Composite of all-cause mortality, nonfatal MI and stroke	38 months	Primary end point did not differ between groups.
COMPARE-ACUTE	885	Noninfarct-related coronary arteries of at least 2.0 mm in diameter with stenosis of 50% or more	FFR-guided revascularization (FFR, ≤0.80) performed generally during the same intervention; possible delays at the operator's discretion	Composite of death from any cause, nonfatal MI, revascularization, and cerebrovascular events	12 months	Primary end point significantly reduced with CR. Significant reduction in the rate of repeat revascularization.

COMPARE-ACUTE, Comparison Between FFR-Guided Revascularization Versus Conventional Strategy in Acute STEMI Patients With Multivessel Disease; *CR*, complete revascularization; *CvLPRIT*, ; *DANAMI-3-PRIMULTI*, complete revascularisation versus treatment of the culprit lesion only in patients with ST-segment elevation myocardial infarction and multivessel disease; *FFR*, fractional flow reserve; *IRA*, infarct-related artery; *MI*, myocardial infarction; *MVD*, multivessel disease; *PCI*, percutaneous coronary intervention; *pPCI*, primary PCI; *PRAGUE 13*, Multivessel Disease Diagnosed at the Time of PPCI for STEMI: Complete Revascularization Versus Conservative Strategy; *STEMI*, ST-elevation myocardial infarction.

achieved (i.e., immediate, in-hospital, or post-discharge staged) and the modality to guide revascularization (i.e., based on angiography or FFR). Remarkably, the prognostic benefits in these studies was mainly driven by a reduction in the need for repeat revascularization (a soft end point). An updated comprehensive study-level meta-analysis, including nine trials of complete versus culprit-only revascularization in 2663 STEMI patients, found a significantly lowered risk for long-term cardiovascular mortality, long-term revascularization, and long-term nonfatal MI in patients undergoing complete revascularization.[85] However, the overall methodologic quality of current studies is quite low and the total amount of information is not conclusive. Consistently, newly released European guidelines for the management of STEMI patients have given a class IIa/level of evidence A (i.e., should be considered) for revascularization of nonculprit lesions, either at the time of the index procedure or in a staged in-hospital procedure.[74] Ongoing and larger studies with sufficient statistical power to detect differences in hard clinical end point, such as mortality and MI, will provide more definitive evidence on this topic (i.e., FULL REVASC [NCT02862119], COMPLETE [NCT01740479]).

CONCLUSIONS

Over the past four decades, the role of PCI as an alternative technique for achieving myocardial revascularization in complex disease and MVD has progressively emerged. Currently, PCI represents a valid alternative to CABG in selected anatomical and clinical contexts. The iteration of materials and stent technology alongside a better awareness of proper pre- and intraprocedural planning strategies (from proper patient selection to ischemia- or imaging-guided functional revascularization) have contributed to reducing the gap in clinical outcomes compared to CABG. Translating rigorous scientific evidence into clinical practice has been key to achieving this goal and, certainly, will further contribute to refining our understanding of proper anatomical and clinical thresholds for the appropriateness of percutaneous revascularization in patients presenting with MVD.

KEY REFERENCES

4. Sianos G, Morel M-A, Kappetein AP, et al. The SYNTAX score: an angiographic tool grading the complexity of coronary artery disease. *EuroIntervention*. 2005;1(2):219–227.
5. Farooq V, van Klaveren D, Steyerberg EW, et al. Anatomical and clinical characteristics to guide decision making between coronary artery bypass surgery and percutaneous coronary intervention for individual patients: development and validation of SYNTAX score II. *Lancet*. 2013;381(9867):639–650. https://doi.org/10.1016/S0140-6736(13)60108-7.
6. Serruys PW, Rutherford JD. the birth, and evolution, of percutaneous coronary interventions: a conversation with Patrick Serruys, MD, PhD. *Circulation*. 2016;134(2):97–100. https://doi.org/0.1161/CIRCULATIONAHA.116.023681.
7. Stefanini G, Byrne R, Windecker S, et al. State of the art: coronary artery stents—past, present and future. *EuroIntervention*. 2017;13(6):706–716. https://doi.org/10.4244/EIJ-D-17-00557.

23. Yusuf S, Zucker D, Passamani E, et al. Effect of coronary artery bypass graft surgery on survival: overview of 10-year results from randomised trials by the Coronary Artery Bypass Graft Surgery Trialists Collaboration. *Lancet*. 1994;344(8922):563–570. https://doi.org/10.1016/S0140-6736(94)91963-1.

27. Serruys PW, Morice M-C, Kappetein AP, et al. Percutaneous coronary intervention versus coronary-artery bypass grafting for severe coronary artery disease. *N Engl J Med*. 2009;360(10):961–972. https://doi.org/10.1056/NEJMoa0804626.

28. Kappetein AP, Feldman TE, Mack MJ, et al. Comparison of coronary bypass surgery with drug-eluting stenting for the treatment of left main and/or three-vessel disease: 3-year follow-up of the SYNTAX trial. *Eur Heart J*. 2011;32(17):2125–2134. https://doi.org/10.1093/eurheartj/ehr213.

29. Mohr FW, Morice M-C, Kappetein AP, et al. Coronary artery bypass graft surgery versus percutaneous coronary intervention in patients with three-vessel disease and left main coronary disease: 5-year follow-up of the randomised, clinical SYNTAX trial. *Lancet*. 2013;381(9867):629–638. https://doi.org/10.1016/S0140-6736(13)60141-5.

31. Farkouh ME, Domanski M, Sleeper LA, et al. Strategies for multivessel revascularization in patients with diabetes. *N Engl J Med*. 2012;367(25):2375–2384. https://doi.org/10.1056/NEJMoa1211585.

33. Head SJ, Milojevic M, Daemen J, et al. Mortality after coronary artery bypass grafting versus percutaneous coronary intervention with stenting for coronary artery disease: a pooled analysis of individual patient data. *Lancet*. 2018;391(10124):939–948. https://doi.org/10.1016/S0140-6736(18)30423-9.

37. Bangalore S, Guo Y, Samadashvili Z, et al. Everolimus-eluting stents or bypass surgery for multivessel coronary disease. *N Engl J Med*. 2015;372(13):1213–1222. https://doi.org/10.1056/NEJMoa1412168.

39. Pijls NHJ, de Bruyne B, Peels K, et al. Measurement of fractional flow reserve to assess the functional severity of coronary-artery stenoses. *N Engl J Med*. 1996;334(26):1703–1708. https://doi.org/10.1056/NEJM199606273342604.

60. Capodanno D, Alberts M, Angiolillo DJ. Antithrombotic therapy for secondary prevention of atherothrombotic events in cerebrovascular disease. *Nat Rev Cardiol*. 2016;13(10):609–622. https://doi.org/10.1038/nrcardio.2016.111.

62. Gargiulo G, Valgimigli M, Capodanno D, et al. State of the art: Duration of dual antiplatelet therapy after percutaneous coronary intervention and coronary stent implantation—past, present and future perspectives. *EuroIntervention*. 2017;13(6):717–733. https://doi.org/10.4244/EIJ-D-17-00468.

66. Costa F, van Klaveren D, James S, et al. Derivation and validation of the predicting bleeding complications in patients undergoing stent implantation and subsequent dual antiplatelet therapy (PRECISE-DAPT) score: A pooled analysis of individual-patient datasets from clinical trials. *Lancet*. 2017;389(10073):1025–1034. https://doi.org/10.1016/S0140-6736(17)30397-5.

67. Yeh RW, Secemsky EA, Kereiakes DJ, et al. Development and validation of a prediction rule for benefit and harm of dual antiplatelet therapy beyond 1 year after percutaneous coronary intervention. *JAMA*. 2016;315(16):1735. https://doi.org/10.1001/jama.2016.3775.

73. Escaned J, Collet C, Ryan N, et al. Clinical outcomes of state-of-the-art percutaneous coronary revascularization in patients with de novo three vessel disease: 1-year results of the SYNTAX II study. *Eur Heart J*. 2017;38(42):3124–3134. https://doi.org/10.1093/eurheartj/ehx512.

 Additional references available online at expertconsult.com.

中文导读

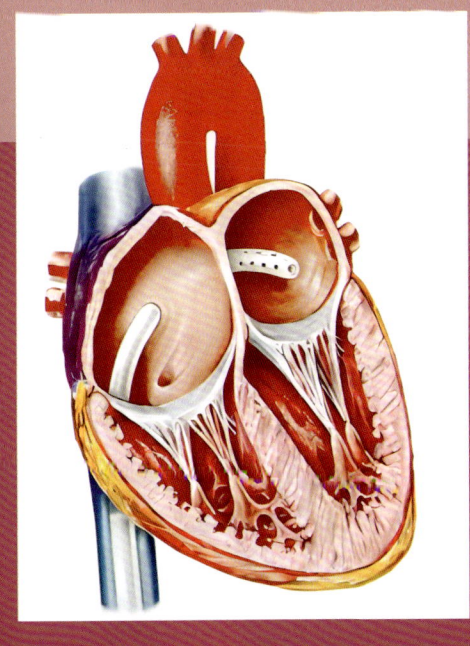

第26章
慢性完全闭塞病变的介入治疗

慢性完全闭塞病变是介入心脏病学中最复杂的领域之一。以往较低的手术成功率与较高的并发症发生率限制了慢性完全闭塞病变介入治疗的开展。近年来，这一领域的技术取得了重大进展，一些中心及术者可以安全高效地对慢性完全闭塞病变进行介入治疗。尽管观察性研究得出了十分积极的结果，但由于不同中心及术者水平的广泛差异，以及相关随机对照试验证据的缺乏，慢性完全闭塞病变的介入治疗仍然难以大规模普及。如何提升慢性完全闭塞病变介入治疗的成功率，降低其并发症的发生率应作为术者的共同目标。遵循Hybrid流程图，使用评分系统及充分的术前准备有助于决胜千里。熟悉先进的器械与各类技术方可稳操胜券。慢性完全闭塞病变介入治疗以建立远端位于血管真腔内的正向导丝轨道为技术目标，因此正向导丝升级是最为常用的基本技术。逆向技术操作复杂，并发症较多，但有力地提升了手术成功率。得益于理念与器械的发展，正、逆向导丝内膜下再入技术解决了以往导丝进入内膜下而被迫结束的一系列复杂慢性完全闭塞病变，其中CrossBoss导管及Stingray球囊的出现使正向内膜下再入技术变得更为安全、可控且高效。未来，随着技术的进一步发展，以及新证据的出现，慢性完全闭塞病变介入治疗的适应证将逐步拓宽。

程子越　柳景华

章节要点

- 慢性完全闭塞病变在冠状动脉疾病患者中极为常见，这种病变是冠心病患者未能接受经皮冠状动脉介入治疗的常见原因。
- 观察性研究结果表明，成功的慢性完全闭塞病变介入治疗可以改善缺血症状，提高射血分数和临床生存率。但随机对照试验的证据极为有限，这些研究也存在诸多不足。
- 临床上，慢性完全闭塞病变可以近似视为血流储备分数≤0.8的狭窄病变。
- 慢性完全闭塞病变介入治疗的成功率已得到大幅提高，有经验术者的成功率可接近90%。
- 慢性完全闭塞病变介入治疗的并发症发生率明显高于非慢性完全闭塞病变介入治疗。某些特殊并发症与逆向技术有关。
- Hybrid策略联合慢性完全闭塞病变专用导丝及器械已极大程度提高了慢性完全闭塞病变介入治疗的可重复性与成功率。

26 Intervention for Coronary Chronic Total Occlusions

Ravi S. Hira, William L. Lombardi

KEY POINTS

- Chronic total occlusion (CTO) is a common feature in patients with coronary artery disease (CAD) and is a frequent reason for not proceeding with percutaneous coronary intervention (PCI).
- Observational data suggests that ischemic reduction from successful CTO PCI improves symptoms, ejection fraction (EF), and long-term clinical survival compared with failure of CTO PCI. Available randomized trial data are limited and have several limitations.
- Clinically, a CTO imitates a lesion with a fractional flow reserve (FFR) of 0.8 or less.
- The success rate of CTO PCI has dramatically improved, approaching 90% among experienced operators.
- Complications are higher with CTO PCI compared with non-CTO PCI; some unique complications are related to retrograde techniques.
- The hybrid approach in conjunction with CTO-specific guidewires and devices has provided a dramatic improvement in reproducibility and success with CTO PCI.

CHRONIC TOTAL CORONARY OCCLUSION

Chronic total coronary occlusions (CTOs), along with major bifurcations (including the left main coronary artery) and long lesions, constitute a disease type that remains a major technical challenge for interventional cardiologists individually, and represents a significant limitation for interventional cardiology as a field. Percutaneous coronary intervention (PCI) is still predicated upon a steerable guidewire spanning the target lesion and acting as a rail over which therapies are delivered and as a "safety line" in case of target-vessel complications. The essential challenge of CTO PCI lies in the initial traversing of the lesion with a guidewire. Length of the occlusion, as well as presence of calcification and suture line fibrosis after graft failure, further increase the complexity of CTO PCI.

In the past few years, important advancements have been made in techniques that safely and more predictably overcome this essential challenge.[1] Dissemination of these techniques along with increasing risk profiles that make patients poor candidates for cardiac surgery has led to an accelerated adoption of CTO PCI into mainstream interventional practice. Most major PCI programs now have, or are planning for, specialized competence in contemporary CTO procedures. An understanding of the field has become essential knowledge for all interventionalists and arguably for any cardiologist who advises patients regarding revascularization options. This chapter strives to provide that understanding.

DEFINITION

A CTO is most often defined as a coronary occlusion known to be present for 3 or more months or a newly documented occlusion not attributable to a similarly recent ischemic event. The term *occlusion* is most accurately reserved for a stenosis within which there is neither a continuous visible lumen nor any visible antegrade flow that cannot be accounted for by collaterals (Thrombolysis in Myocardial Infarction [TIMI] grade 0).[2] Lesions with trace antegrade lumenal flow (TIMI grade 1) are referred to as *functional* or *subtotal* occlusions. Lesions with a residual lumen but without antegrade flow because of competing collateral flow are referred to as *pseudo-occlusions*. Functional and pseudo-occlusions overlap in practice and may be difficult to distinguish from a true CTO unless imaged with dual-catheter angiography or probed with a guidewire. Finally, spontaneously recanalized CTOs are sometimes identified, wherein a long, tortuous microchannel exists within the presumed architecture of a previous occlusion.

Detection of coronary occlusions remains the domain of catheter-based angiography. Current coronary computed tomography (CT) angiography has limited spatial resolution and does not capture the temporal information required to determine flow rate or directionality. As such, it cannot readily be used to distinguish a CTO from a functional or pseudo-occlusion or even reliably from a high-grade stenosis with preserved flow.

PREVALENCE

Reports that describe the prevalence of CTOs vary widely depending on the cohort studied. Moreover, unless developed specifically for the study of CTOs, angiographic and interventional databases generally do not contain data fields that reliably distinguish subacute from chronic occlusions, true occlusions from subtotal or pseudo-occlusions, or potentially bypassed from nonbypassed occlusions. Thus the literature reveals an inconsistency of methods for determining the true prevalence of CTOs in the population.

A retrospective study from a large U.S. Veterans Administration (VA) center extracted patients with at least one 70% stenosis (by visual estimate), no prior coronary artery bypass grafting (CABG), and no myocardial infarction (MI) within 3 months from 8004 consecutive patients undergoing cardiac catheterization between 1990 and 2000.[3] Within the derived cohort of 3087 patients, 52% (1612) had a CTO.

In a prospective study, Fefer and colleagues[4] reported data on more than 14,000 patients undergoing nonemergent angiography at three tertiary Canadian centers in 2008 and 2009. They found nonacute coronary occlusions present in 14.7%. After excluding patients with prior CABG, as well as those without significant CAD, they reported that 18.4% of the remaining 7680 patients had at least one nonacute occlusion.

A prospectively collected population-based Swedish registry[5] of nonacute general angiography and PCI found a similar CTO prevalence of 16% in over 91,000 patients with significant coronary artery disease (CAD). Like the Canadian registry, this prevalence was calculated after exclusion of those with prior CABG. An unexpected finding was a decline in CTO prevalence over the 8-year period examined, from 17.2% in 2005 to 15.1% in 2012.

PATHOLOGY

The histopathology of CTOs is an evolving area that has grown from necropsy and ex vivo tissue analyses to include the use of intravascular micro–computed tomography (MCT), micro–magnetic resonance imaging (MMRI), and intravascular ultrasound (IVUS). Studies characterizing the histology of CTOs have led to further insights regarding procedural success and failure.

Postnecropsy samples of CTOs consistently demonstrate preservation of vessel architecture; a multilayered structure in which the intima and neointima (including atherosclerotic plaque) is distinguishable from the muscularis and adventitia. Importantly, the external elastic lamina remains intact. This preservation of architecture is a fundamental feature enabling percutaneous recanalization (Fig. 26.1). Early necropsy studies to examine human CTOs have shown that angiographic characteristics, such as proximal cap morphology, correlate with histology. Tapered-tip occlusions contain areas of luminal recanalization with microchannels and loosely packed fibrous tissue. Such occlusions also tend to be shorter.[6] Conversely, lesions with a blunt cap are typically composed of densely packed fibrous material and fibrocalcific intimal plaque and tend to be longer.[7]

Studies in mice, porcine, and rabbit femoral arterial occlusion models have provided experimental insights into the development of CTOs. Recent thrombotic occlusions display an inflammatory infiltrate dominated by neutrophils and mononuclear cells that penetrate the occlusive thrombus. The density of this infiltrate peaks at 2 weeks after occlusion and declines thereafter. Proteoglycan-enriched extracellular matrix replaces thrombus; deposition occurs early, between weeks 2 and 6 after occlusion. It is concentrated at the proximal and distal ends of the lesion. Over time, these areas are replaced by densely packed collagen.[8] Negative remodeling of the surrounding vessel and variable decay of the internal elastic lamina accompany this process.[7,8] These experimental observations may in part explain the clinical paradigm of mechanically resistant proximal and distal caps.

Human and animal necropsy studies and advanced imaging studies have confirmed the frequent presence of recanalization microvascular channels (*microchannels*) within chronically occluded segments. Microchannels in human CTOs were first described by Katsuragawa et al.,[6] wherein small vascular channels ranging from 160 to 230 μm in diameter were noted at both proximal and distal lesion segments. This observation led to speculation that microchannels might consistently provide a through-and-through route for fine guidewires to track. Subsequent human and experimental pathologic studies suggested these microchannels are more typically configured as corkscrews or sharply angulated channels that become fragmented and discontinuous as occlusions age and typically do not traverse the full length of an occlusion.[7-9] Thus, while microchannels are unlikely to provide a continuous channel for guidewire passage, especially in longer CTO segments, they may still render a "path of low resistance" through the CTO segment tissue.

CLINICAL PROFILE AND PRESENTATION

When compared with a cohort of CAD patients without CTO, patients with CTO display important differences in baseline characteristics that point toward more advanced atherosclerosis. Patients are on average 1 to 2 years older, more likely to be male, and more likely to have diabetes and hypertension. Multivessel CAD is more commonly present, as is peripheral arterial disease and cerebrovascular disease.

A twofold excess in history of prior MI was observed among CTO patients in both Canadian[4] and Swedish[5] registries (40% vs. 23% and 37% vs. 17%, respectively, $P < .01$ in both). However, the relationship between a CTO, the presence and extent of infarction in the subtended territory, and the degree of left ventricular (LV) dysfunction attributable to the CTO is not well established. Half of the patients in the Canadian registry had a left ventricular ejection fraction (LVEF) less than 50%, but significant Q-waves were present in only 32% of right coronary arteries (RCAs), 13% of left anterior descending (LAD) coronary arteries, and 26% of left circumflex (LCX) artery occlusions. In the VA registry,[3] chronic CAD patients with CTO had a significantly lower LVEF than those without a CTO (LVEF 53% vs. 60%, $P < .0001$) but also had significantly more multivessel CAD (66% vs. 42%, $P < .0001$).

Despite the long-term presence of a CTO, an acute coronary syndrome (ACS) arising in other coronary segments is a common trigger for cardiac catheterization that leads to CTO detection. ACS immediately preceded CTO detection in 46% of the Canadian cohort and 40% of the Swedish cohort. Conversely, in a prospective single-center registry[10] of nearly 3300 consecutive primary PCI procedures for ST-elevation MI (STEMI) the prevalence of a preexisting CTO was 12.8%. Patients with a CTO detected at primary PCI had significantly worse prognosis than patients with single-vessel CAD (infarct vessel only) or those with multivessel CAD without a CTO.

INDICATIONS FOR REVASCULARIZATION

Published indications for CTO revascularization largely mirror the indications for revascularization in otherwise obstructive nonocclusive stable CAD. In this regard, the primary indication for CTO PCI in the setting of single-vessel CAD is the relief of ischemic symptoms that persist despite antiischemic medical therapy. However, the frequency with which PCI is offered to patients with a CTO (but otherwise limited CAD not warranting CABG) is much lower than for obstructive nonocclusive CAD in practice and moreover varies widely among physicians and PCI centers.

Multicenter U.S. registries[11,12] of patients treated in the 1990s indicate that only 8% to 15% of patients with a CTO at angiography underwent PCI. The subsequent prospective VA registry[3] found that the presence of a CTO at angiography was an independent predictor of a physician recommending CABG or medical therapy as opposed to PCI. In the Canadian CTO registry[4] that enrolled patients in 2008 and 2009, PCI was undertaken in only 10%. Importantly, there is wide practice variation, with as few as 1% and as many as 16% of patients with CTOs treated with PCI ($P < .001$), despite similar rates of CABG at all centers (22% to 28%, P = not significant [NS]). The low and variable use of PCI for CTO likely reflects many factors, among them a wide variation in technical expertise of operators and lack of evidence of benefit of CTO PCI on hard outcomes such as death and MI.

Neither American nor European guidelines distinguish between CTOs and obstructive nonocclusive lesions with respect to the threshold for undertaking revascularization, whether by PCI or CABG. The European guidelines[13] consider CTO PCI a complex procedure that demands experienced operators at centers with specialized CTO equipment and access to circulatory support and cardiac surgery. Ad hoc CTO PCI (coincident with diagnostic catheterization) is discouraged. The American College of Cardiology (ACC)/American Hospital Association (AHA)/Society for Cardiovascular Angiography and Interventions (SCAI) guidelines[14] state that "(CTO PCI) in patients with

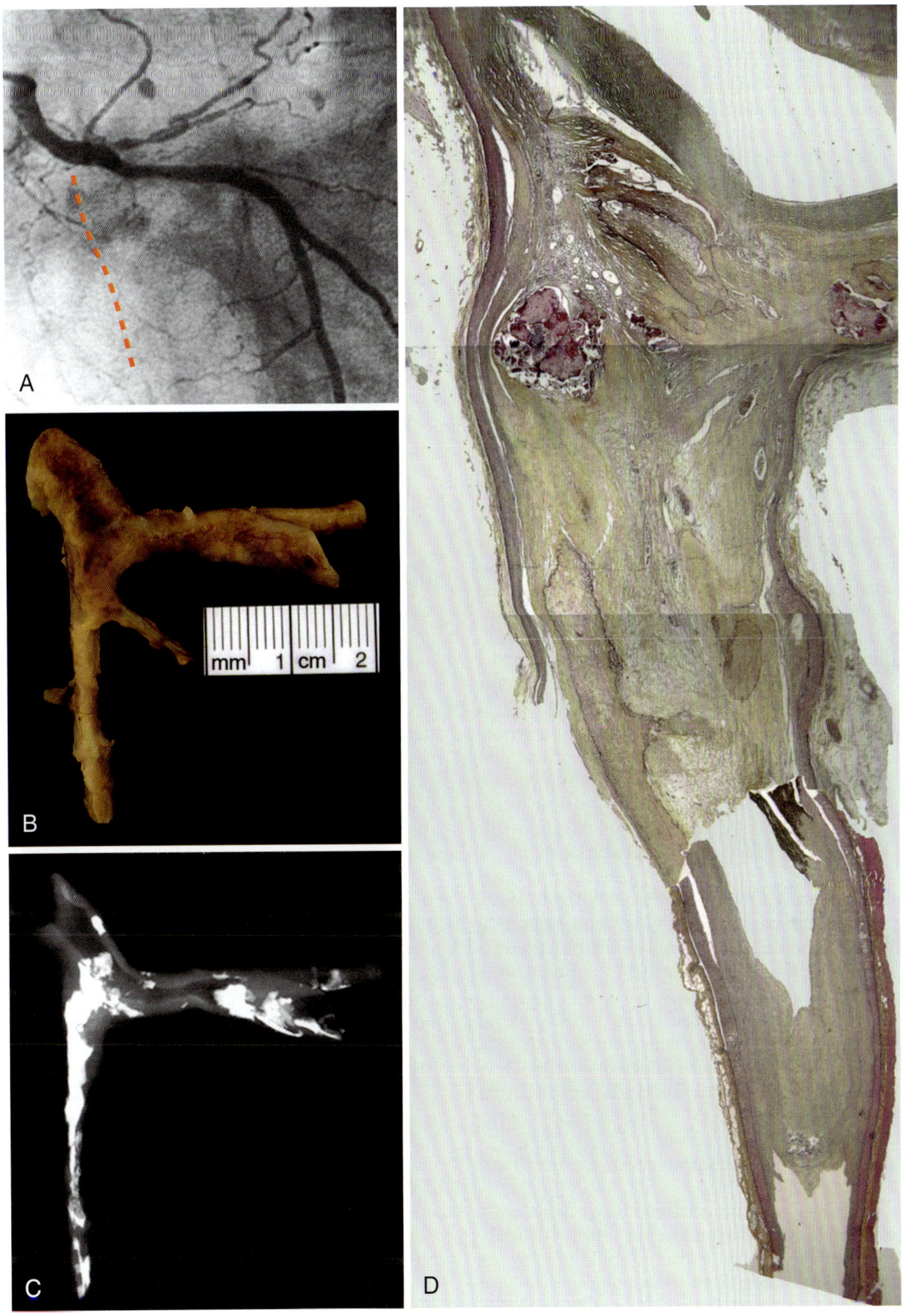

CHAPTER 26 Intervention for Coronary Chronic Total Occlusions

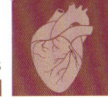

Fig. 26.1 Postmortem example of a chronically occluded atherosclerotic left anterior descending (LAD) coronary artery. (A) Ante mortem angiography (left anterior oblique cranial projection) of left coronary demonstrates a flush occlusion of the LAD with small bridge collaterals arising from the left main. The *dotted line* represents the approximate course of the occluded vessel. (B) Postmortem, the left main, proximal circumflex, and proximal LAD arteries have been dissected en bloc; apart from negative remodeling, few external cues are present to suggest that the LAD lumen is occluded. (C) Postmortem radiograph of the specimen emphasizes the extent of dystrophic calcium typical in a chronic occlusion; (D) longitudinal histopathology confirms preservation of vessel architecture, including a multilayered structure in which the intima and neointima (and extensive atherosclerotic plaque) is distinguishable from the muscularis and adventitia. Importantly, the external elastic lamina remains intact (apparent breaches are due to fixation artifact). The preservation of gross vessel architecture is the pathologic feature that most enables contemporary techniques for percutaneous recanalization.

appropriate clinical indications and suitable anatomy is reasonable when performed by operators with appropriate expertise" (class IIa, level of evidence B).

The updated 2017 Appropriate Use Criteria for Coronary Revascularization in Patients With Stable Ischemic Heart Disease[15] from the American Societies no longer distinguish between appropriate indications for CTO PCI and PCI of obstructive nonocclusive lesions. Asymptomatic patients are classified as "inappropriate" in many scenarios, but may be appropriate in the setting of high risk findings on noninvasive testing, including severe LV dysfunction. Given these recommendations, we advise caution in pursuing CTO PCI in asymptomatic patients, with careful review for these special indications.

ISCHEMIA AND LEFT VENTRICLE FUNCTION

The burden of ischemia in a territory subtended by a CTO is presumably determined by the left ventricular mass supplied by the occluded segment, the degree of infarction in that zone, the degree of collateralization, and the severity of coronary obstruction, if any, in vessels that supply those collaterals. Because the intracoronary pressure beyond an occlusion is inherently low, the myocardium subtended may be especially vulnerable to subendocardial ischemia that is exacerbated by elevation of end-diastolic pressure. No systematic study has been done to quantify the degree of ischemia in an unselected cohort of patients with CTO. However, in a study of 569 consecutive patients with multivessel disease undergoing myocardial scintigraphy after incomplete revascularization by PCI, 126 had at least one residual CTO. Of these, 64 patients (50.8%) had a severely abnormal scan (with summed stress score >8). There was a linear relationship between the global summed stress score and the summed stress score of the territory subtended by the CTO. At a median follow-up period of 44 months, summed stress score was incrementally and significantly associated with hard (cardiac death and MI) and soft (unstable angina and repeat PCI procedures) end points.[16]

The Clinical Outcomes Utilizing Revascularization and Aggressive Drug Evaluation (COURAGE)[17] trial failed to show a difference in death or MI in patients with CAD who had stable angina and myocardial ischemia randomized to an initial strategy of PCI versus medical therapy. While CTO patients were excluded from the study, angina was improved in the PCI group. There was also significant crossover in the medical therapy arm, with 32.6% of patients undergoing revascularization with PCI or CABG at 4.6 years. A substudy[18] that evaluated serial nuclear imaging at baseline and 1-year postrandomization revealed that PCI with optimal medical therapy (OMT) led to greater ischemia reductions compared with OMT alone (33% vs. 19%; P = .0004), especially patients with moderate to severe pretreatment ischemia (78% vs. 52%; P = .007).

The International Study of Comparative Health Effectiveness with Medical and Invasive Approaches Study (ISCHEMIA) trial[19] is currently underway, and randomizing patients with moderate to severe ischemia to revascularization and OMT versus OMT alone may contribute to our understanding of ischemia-guided revascularization including patients with CTOs.

The relationship between CTO, ischemia, regional and global LV dysfunction, and post-PCI LV recovery is complex and incompletely characterized. Patients undergoing primary PCI for STEMI who are also found to have a CTO in a noninfarct-related vessel are significantly more likely to have moderate or severe LV impairment (28% vs. 17%, P < .01) and are more than twice as likely to suffer progressive LV impairment at follow-up (39% vs. 17%, P < .01) compared with patients who do not have a CTO.[10]

The available reports exploring the relationship between CTO revascularization and LV function do not include medically treated comparators. With this important limitation, patients with regional LV dysfunction in whom the abnormal wall segment is subtended by the CTO commonly demonstrate regional LV improvement after CTO PCI.[20] Improvement in global LVEF following CTO PCI is less easily demonstrated, in part because more than half of CTO patients have normal baseline ejection fraction (EF). In the Total Occlusion Study of Canada (TOSCA),[21] 244 patients had paired baseline and 6-month core laboratory evaluated LV angiograms, and 106 of these (43%) had an impaired EF at baseline (EF <60%, mean 46% ± 9%). EF did not change at follow-up among those with normal baseline EF but rose 3.8% (± 8.4%) in the cohort with impaired baseline EF (P < .001). The direction and magnitude of these EF changes are consistent with those observed in smaller series.[20,22]

Further, in patients with akinetic segments or significant LV dysfunction and remodeling, myocardial viability should be considered prior to CTO PCI. Multiple studies have linked viability to improvement in regional function following PCI.[22–25] While its use is controversial in the face of two negative trials,[26,27] they are limited by significant crossover and lack of adherence to viability results.

COLLATERAL CIRCULATION

Viability of myocardium distal to a CTO is dependent upon collateral circulation. Present in humans from birth, both ischemia and flow-mediated shear stress stimulate collateral development.[28–30] Collateral flow has been characterized functionally by both angiographic and hemodynamic criteria. Rentrop et al.[31] described four collateral grades: (0) no visible filling of any collateral channels, (1) filling of side branches of the occluded artery, (2) partial filling of the recipient main vessel, and (3) complete filling of the epicardial vessel. Although this classification was originally described during acute balloon occlusion of the receiving vessel, it is now used to classify collateral circulation in CTO studies. The presence of angiographically visible collaterals conveys positive prognostic information. A recent meta-analysis[32] of 12 studies to examine the association between visible collaterals in acute, subacute, and chronic coronary disease involving 6529 patients found that those with high collateralization had lower risk of death during follow-up (relative risk [RR] for all coronary occlusions 0.64; 95% confidence interval [CI] 0.45 to 0.91; P = .012; RR for chronic occlusions 0.59; 95% CI 0.39 to 0.89; P = .012).

Hemodynamic quantitation of collateral function most commonly uses the *collateral pressure index* (CPI), defined as mean pressure of collateral circulation (P_w) divided by mean aortic pressure (P_a), each with central venous pressure (CVP) subtracted ($[P_w - CVP]/[P_a - CVP]$).[33] Both wedge and direct measurements of collateral pressure have been described. CPI values >0.3 are considered adequate to prevent ischemia at rest but have not been rigorously validated. Threshold CPI values that correspond to provocable ischemia are uncertain, as are the thresholds for pressure-derived fractional flow reserve (FFR) and instantaneous flow reserve (IFR) measured distal to occlusions. In the case of FFR and IFR, threshold values established in nonocclusive lesions may apply. A single-center prospective study of 107 patients undergoing CTO PCI measured CPI (with direct rather than wedge collateral pressure), distal bed postadenosine FFR, and doppler-based collateral flow velocity reserve (CFVI). Whereas CPI at rest was above 0.3 in 78% of patients, only one patient demonstrated an FFR value above 0.75 (the conventional ischemic threshold), and more than one-third of patients had evidence of inducible coronary steal by CFVI.[34]

PREPARATION FOR CHRONIC TOTAL OCCLUSION PERCUTANEOUS CORONARY INTERVENTION

The femoral or radial approach can be used for CTO PCI with emphasis on dual angiography to visualize collateral flow and length of the occlusion. The guiding principle of access selection is that operators should use access routes that they are comfortable with. The relative merits of potentially larger sheath/guide sizes (femoral) can be weighed against the reduction in vascular complications and improved patient comfort (radial).[35,36] When femoral access is used, long (45 cm) sheaths can overcome iliac tortuosity and increase guide catheter support. Guiding catheter size is usually limited to 6 Fr (occasionally 7 Fr) from the radial approach. Good passive support with coaxial alignment is crucial, especially in complex CTO procedures. Although the choice of the guiding catheter shape is generally dictated by personal experience, it is important for operators to seek a guide with optimal backup support at the onset of the procedure, rather than accepting one with merely satisfactory support. The radial operator should be familiar with active guide manipulation to augment the support, and all operators should be versed in balloon anchoring and mother-and-child guide extension techniques to improve support when needed.[37]

When the distal vessel is filled by ipsilateral collaterals, flow may be impaired after wire and catheter advancement, resulting in a collateral or preferential collateral shift to the retrograde collaterals during the procedure. Therefore, to achieve the best diagnostic angiography (i.e., to fill the entire collateral bed), contralateral injection should be performed at the start of the procedure if any visible contralateral collaterals are present. Operators from the EuroCTO Club have used contralateral injection in 62% of their cases,[38] whereas dual injection was used in 78% of cases in a more recent North American series.[39] Dual-injection collateral analysis is best performed using low magnification, so that the entire coronary tree is visualized without panning. Careful study of the collaterals not only provides important information in choosing the most appropriate collateral, but will also alert the operator to the risk of ischemia and hemodynamic or electrical instability if the wired collateral becomes occluded. Three typical collateral pathways are demonstrated in Figs. 26.2–26.4. A careful and detailed review of the angiogram is critical for creating primary and alternative CTO treatment strategies to optimize the efficacy, efficiency, and safety of the procedure.[1]

Anticoagulation during CTO PCI is best achieved with unfractionated heparin (UFH) because it allows for titration of the anticoagulant effect (an activated clotting time [ACT] of >350 seconds is recommended by many operators during retrograde CTO PCI to minimize the risk of donor vessel and guide thrombosis).[40] Bivalirudin requires ongoing flow and exposure to blood to maintain its pharmacotherapeutic effect and therefore has the potential for higher guide catheter thrombotic rates. As with all PCI, preloading with a $P2Y_{12}$ adenosine diphosphate (ADP) receptor inhibitor and aspirin is important to reduce the risk of acute stent thrombosis and periprocedural MI.

Scoring Systems to Stratify Difficulty of Chronic Total Occlusion Percutaneous Coronary Intervention

Predicting the difficulty of CTO crossing with a guidewire is important for case selection and procedural planning. The Multicentre CTO Registry of Japan (J-CTO) score was developed to determine likelihood of successful wire crossing within 30 minutes. It involves assigning one point to each of five variables: (1) previously failed lesion, (2) blunt type of entry, (3) presence of calcification within the CTO segment, (4) bending >45 degrees within the CTO segment, and (5) occlusion length ≥20 mm. Patients are classified into four difficulty groups: *easy* (J-CTO score of 0), *intermediate* (a score of 1), *difficult* (a score of 2), and *very difficult* (a score of ≥3). The J-CTO score correlated well with the probability of successful guidewire crossing within 30 minutes (87.7%, 67.1%, 42.4%, and 10.0%, respectively)[41] and was recently validated in an independent single-center Canadian

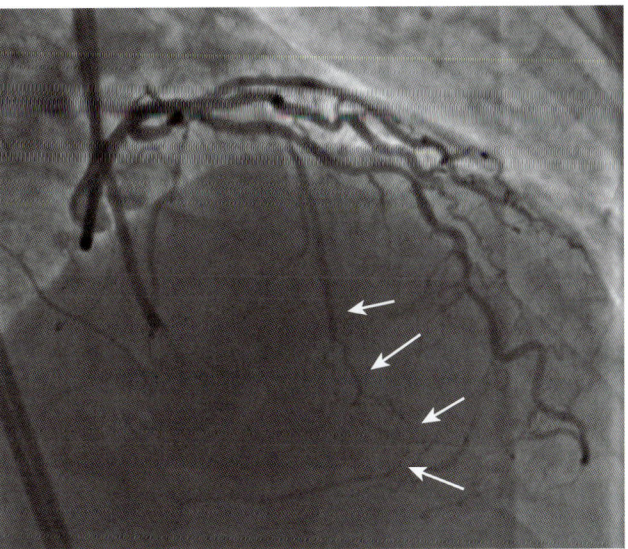

Fig. 26.2 Typical fine, moderately tortuous transseptal collateral *(arrows)* connecting the left anterior descending (LAD) coronary artery to the right posterior descending artery. Transseptals are the most commonly used collaterals for retrograde chronic total occlusion techniques and can serve to access an occluded dominant right coronary artery or dominant left circumflex artery from the LAD, or in the opposite direction, to access an occluded LAD from a dominant right or left circumflex artery. Another transseptal collateral is visible arising from the distal LAD. Because transseptal collaterals are generally contained within septal myocardium, their rupture rarely poses a hazard with respect to tamponade.

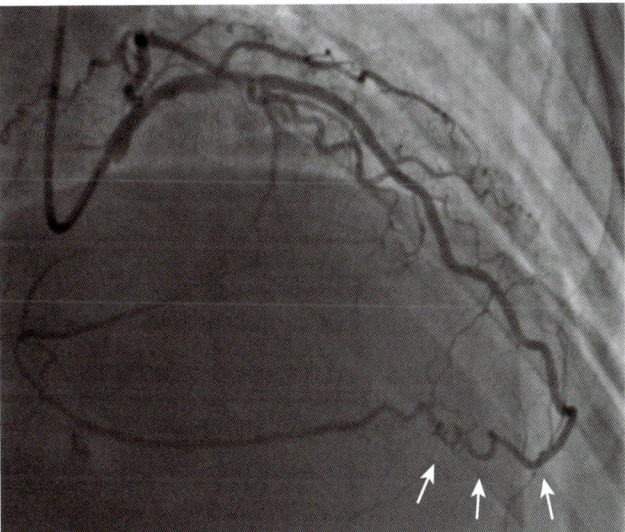

Fig. 26.3 A large, dominant, tortuous, transapical epicardial collateral *(arrows)* supplies the right posterior descending artery from the distal left anterior descending artery. This collateral is likely to become kinked when instrumented with a guidewire or microcatheter, resulting in loss of visualization of the distal target and creating the potential for acute intraprocedural ischemia. Collaterals of this configuration are rarely helpful as conduits for retrograde access.

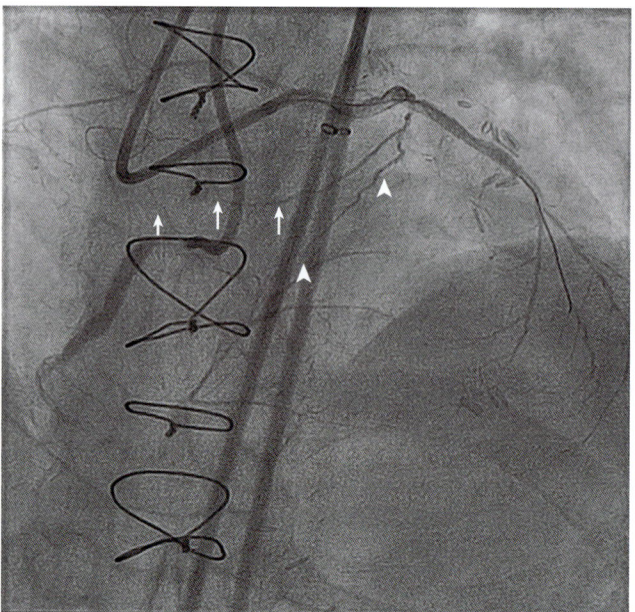

Fig. 26.4 Two typical atrioventricular groove epicardial collaterals from the circumflex artery to the right posterolateral branch; *arrows* indicate a straight connection, and *arrowheads* show a tortuous connection.

cohort.[42] Recent reports using a hybrid-based CTO algorithm have shown that the J-CTO score predicts an increasing need for retrograde procedures to obtain success (Fig. 26.5).[43]

The Prospective Global Registry for the Study of Chronic Total Occlusion Intervention (PROGRESS CTO) Score[44] is another novel scoring system to predict technical success of CTO PCI performed using the hybrid approach that is described as follows. It involves assigning one point to each of four variables: (1) proximal cap ambiguity, (2) absence of interventional collaterals, (3) moderate-severe tortuosity with 2 bends >70 degrees or 1 bend >90 degrees, and (4) circumflex CTO.

These tools provide a guide for anticipating procedure time, contrast, and radiation exposure[42] with reasonable prediction of successful PCI.

APPROACHES AND TECHNIQUES

Antegrade Approach

Antegrade Wire Escalation

Antegrade guidewire-based recanalization of CTOs has been and remains the most common approach worldwide.[45–47] In general, an over-the-wire catheter is delivered to the proximal cap on a workhorse wire, and then CTO-specific techniques and wire shaping are applied. The approach of gradually escalating wire stiffness to achieve crossing has become more nuanced and

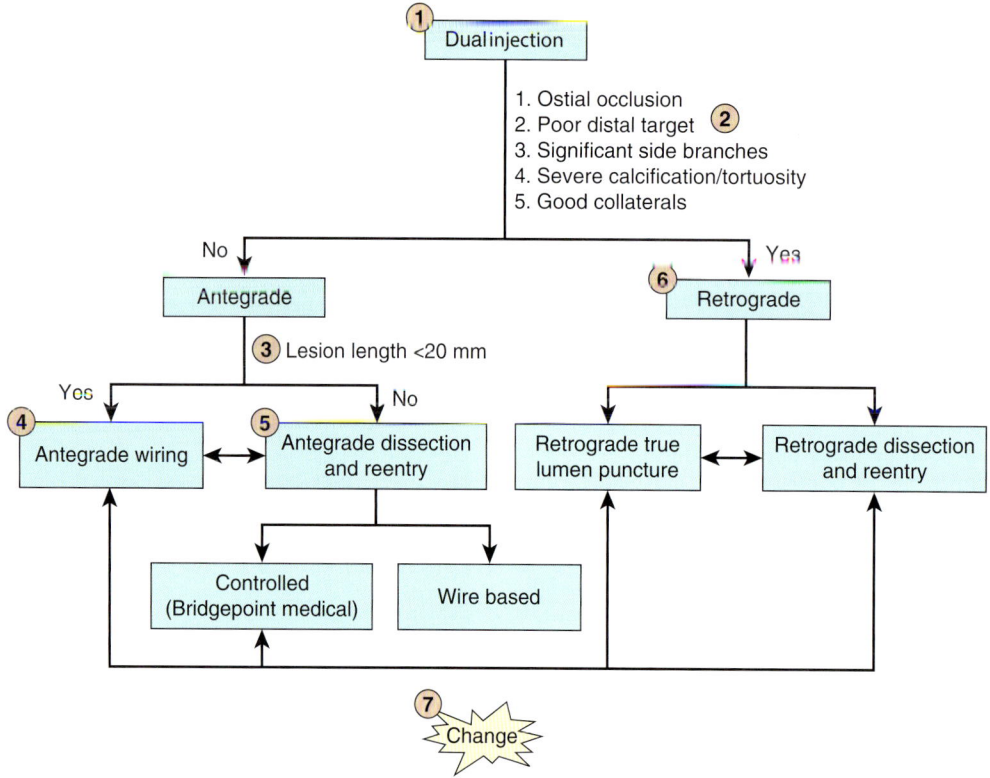

Fig. 26.5 The hybrid approach to chronic total occlusion (CTO) percutaneous coronary intervention (PCI) uses sentinel features of the coronary anatomy to guide the initial approach to CTO recanalization. Antegrade approaches are favored by a clearly identified nonostial occlusion inlet (proximal cap), a large and well-visualized target segment beyond the distal cap, absence of severe calcification or tortuosity, and absence of an important side branch adjacent to the distal cap that might be excluded during dilation and stenting of a subintimal tract. Retrograde approaches are favored when suitable collaterals or bypass grafts exist through which delivery of PCI equipment to the distal cap appears feasible, particularly when the anatomy does not favor an antegrade approach. An important feature of hybrid CTO procedures is the operator's predisposition to timely changes of strategy when progress toward the goal of recanalization stalls.

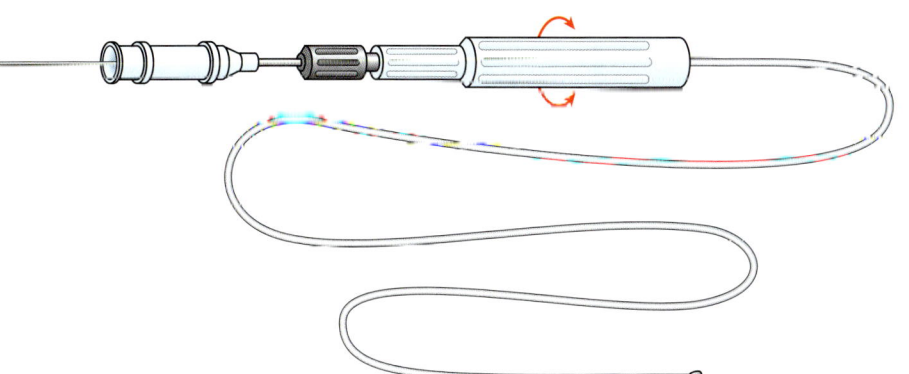

Fig. 26.6 The CrossBoss catheter is used to make a controlled dissection from the proximal cap to the point of planned reentry with the Stingray balloon. This catheter uses blunt dissection to avoid perforation. Unlike wire-based blunt dissection ("knuckle" wires), the CrossBoss was designed to create a small channel that avoids subintimal hematoma and consequent compression of the reentry zone.

flexible. Modern step-up/step-down techniques start with soft, tapered, polymer/hydrophilic wires but step up promptly to stiff, spring-coil tapered wires to overcome any hard, calcified, or fibrotic segments of the occlusion and then step back down to soft, polymer/hydrophilic wires to continue tracking along the occluded segment and complete the crossing of the CTO.[1,48] A rapidly expanding range of CTO guidewires demands that the CTO specialist has an organized approach to wire choice that keeps pace with evolving global experience and new guidewire designs.[49]

Balloons or catheters should never be advanced over a wire unless it is certain that the wire is in the architecture of the vessel (within the boundary of the external elastic lamina) because small diameter wire perforations that occur within the occluded segment are usually benign but can become catastrophic if larger equipment is advanced outside the vessel, thereby enlarging the size of the perforation. Moreover, once they access the distal true lumen, the relatively stiff CTO-crossing wires should be exchanged for safer workhorse wires to avoid distal plaque disruption/dissection, and in particular to prevent inadvertent distal perforation of small vessels, causing delayed tamponade.[50]

Antegrade Dissection/Reentry

The primary mode of failure when recanalizing a chronically occluded vessel using wire-based techniques is failure of the wire to enter the distal true lumen and to instead reside within plaque or within the subintimal plane. Reentering the true lumen from these positions can be extremely challenging with wire-based techniques alone. Recent technologies such as the CrossBoss catheter, Stingray balloon, and Stingray reentry guidewire (Boston Scientific, Natick, MA) have addressed this limitation and have provided a much more reproducible and systematic method for successfully gaining reentry into the coronary lumen. The CrossBoss catheter is a metal-braided, over-the-wire support catheter with a 1-mm rounded distal tip that can be used to support standard guidewire manipulation or can be advanced using rapid rotation. This can be done with or without the wire leading in order to perform blunt dissection in the subintimal space while controlling the amount of subintimal hematoma till the targeted reentry zone is reached (Fig. 26.6). The catheter could potentially cross into the distal true lumen in approximately 40% of lesions or enter into a side branch, which is important to recognize to avoid perforation. Once the CrossBoss catheter or standard wire is in the subintimal position next to the targeted reentry zone, coronary reentry can be systematically achieved with Stingray coronary reentry technologies (Boston Scientific). The Stingray balloon is a flat, 1-mm thick, over-the-wire balloon catheter with three exit ports (one distal and two 180-degree diametrically opposed side ports). When the balloon is inflated, it effectively wraps the artery with one of the two exit ports, directed toward the lumen and the other toward the adventitia. Using fluoroscopy and collateral angiography, operators can select the lumen port with the dedicated Stingray reentry wire or other stiff, tapered wires to puncture into the distal true lumen and achieve control by either advancing the stiff wire into the distal vessel (stick-and-go technique) or switching for a soft, tapered, polymer/hydrophilic wire (stick-and-swap technique) (Fig. 26.7).

Occasionally, subintimal wire manipulation can cause significant subintimal hematoma that can compress the distal true lumen and can thus require decompression through aspiration. The Stingray balloon or other microcatheters can be used for this purpose with a subintimal transcatheter withdrawal (STRAW) technique. These technologies have been highly successful and have had low complication rates, even in early experiences and refractory cases.[50,51]

The CrossBoss First trial[52] was a multicenter randomized controlled trial of initially attempting CTO crossing using the CrossBoss catheter or using antegrade wire escalation (AWE) in patients planned for a primary antegrade approach. Patients were excluded if they had ostial CTO lesions (within 5 mm of vessel ostium) or if the operator planned to use a primary retrograde approach for CTO crossing. Technical and procedural success, crossing time, and incidence of major adverse cardiovascular events were similar between the two groups. On subgroup analysis, CrossBoss was associated with shorter crossing time than wire escalation in CTOs due to in-stent restenosis (median time 41 [interquartile range (IQR): 23 to 58] vs. 66 [IQR: 32 to 111] minutes; $P = .047$).

Other antegrade techniques used to reenter the true lumen from the subintimal space are less precise and controlled. These include IVUS guided reentry, parallel wire technique, subintimal tracking and reentry, and limited antegrade subintimal tracking.

Retrograde Approach

In 2005, Katoh and colleagues pioneered the modern era of retrograde CTO recanalization by introducing new techniques such as targeted septal or epicardial collateral crossing, retrograde lesion crossing, and management of the subintimal space through the use of balloon dilation for connecting antegrade and retrograde channels.[53] Currently, retrograde procedures account for 15% to 34% of specialist CTO PCI procedures recorded in dedicated European and U.S. registries.[38,54–57] These methods require access to the vessel distal to the CTO from a collateral or occasionally a bypass graft vessel with successful placement of a support catheter into the distal target vessel.[58]

Retrograde Wire Escalation

The term *retrograde wire crossing* refers to successful lesion crossing in the retrograde direction from true lumen in the distal vessel

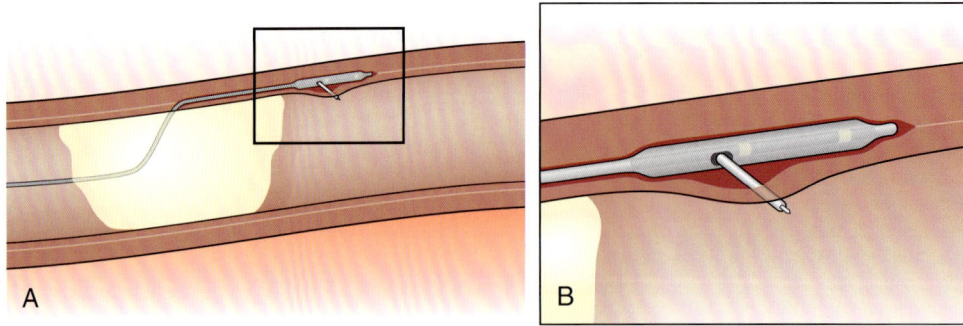

Fig. 26.7 The Stingray dedicated antegrade dissection and reentry system. After establishing an antegrade subintimal tract using a CrossBoss (A) or other low-profile catheter or small angioplasty balloon, the Stingray balloon (B) is delivered and inflated in a position adjacent to the preferred segment for reentry. The flat profile of the Stingray balloon leads to its self-orientation circumferentially within the arterial wall such that one of the exit ports inevitably faces the arterial lumen. This port can then be selected using the dedicated steerable Stingray guidewire, designed to facilitate puncture back into the true lumen.

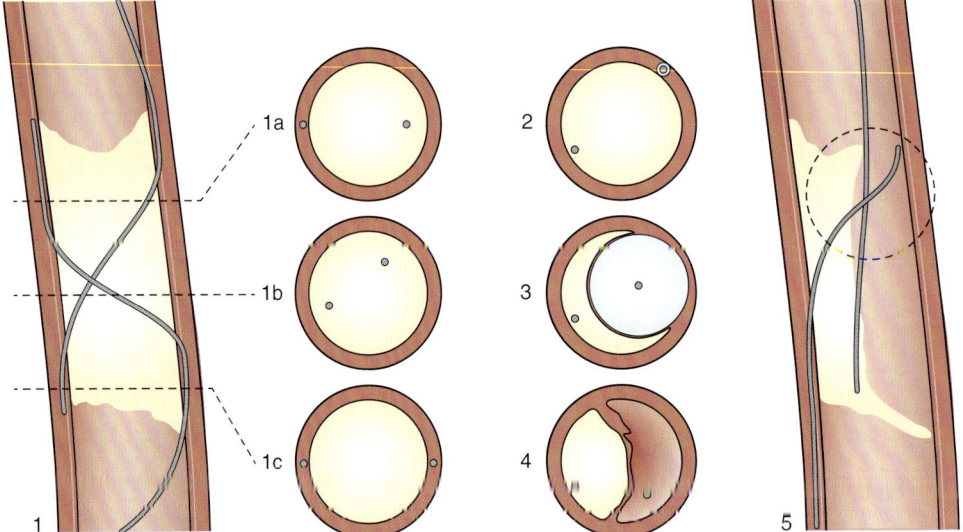

Fig. 26.8 Controlled antegrade-retrograde tracking (CART). Through directed penetration or knuckling, antegrade and retrograde guidewires are brought into overlap within the occluded segment *[1]*; wires may be on opposite sides of the internal elastic lamina (one subintimal, the other within the occluded true lumen *[1a]*; both within the occluded true lumen *[1b]*; or both in a subintimal plane *[1c]*). Regardless, a balloon is advanced over one of the wires *[2]*; it is inflated and deflated *[3]*; and it is then withdrawn, leaving behind iatrogenic dissection that often includes breaches of the internal elastic lamina within the occluded segment *[4]* that allow the retrograde wire to be moved into a plane common with the antegrade wire and then advanced into the patent proximal true lumen *[5]* and ultimately externalized. CART was originally described with the balloon positioned on the retrograde wire; the term reverse CART refers to the now common practice of positioning the balloon on the antegrade wire.

to true lumen in the proximal vessel; it is successful in less than 30% of retrograde procedures.[40] The standard approach after successful retrograde wire manipulation includes placing the retrograde wire and then the microcatheter into the antegrade guide catheter and then exchanging those for a long wire to be externalized from the antegrade guide.[59] The externalized wire—such as the R350 (Vascular Solutions, Minneapolis, MN), RG3 (Asahi Intecc, Nagoya, Japan), or ViperWire Advance (CSI, St. Paul, MN)—is then used as the interventional platform to complete the PCI procedure.[60] It is important for the portion of the retrograde guidewire that is traversing fine collaterals to remain covered by a microcatheter to protect the collateral vessel from laceration and perforation. Equally important is careful attention to retrograde guide movement to prevent guide-induced donor vessel injury.

Retrograde Dissection and Reentry Techniques

Controlled antegrade and retrograde subintimal tracking (CART; Fig. 26.8) with intentional dissection followed by reentry has become the dominant retrograde technique for successful crossing of CTOs. The principle of this technique is to create a limited subintimal dissection space at the CTO segment that is connected with the proximal and distal true lumen, thereby facilitating antegrade or retrograde wire crossing. The current evolution of this technique, termed *reverse CART*, uses retrograde delivery of a microcatheter within the CTO segment either with traditional wire or knuckle-wire techniques. An antegrade wire is then advanced distal to the retrograde equipment, followed by dilation of the occlusion segment with a balloon delivered over the antegrade wire. This tears (dissects) together the two spaces occupied by antegrade and retrograde equipment to create a single, common subintimal space that is in continuity with the lumen. The retrograde wire can then be advanced into the proximal vessel true lumen.

Ultrasound observations suggest this maneuver is easiest when both the antegrade and retrograde guidewires are on the same side of the internal elastic lamina, either both within the subintimal space or both within the original true lumen. The most common reason for failure of this technique is use of undersized balloons, a problem overcome with experience and use of IVUS for optimal balloon sizing and positioning.[61] After the retrograde wire is advanced into the antegrade guide, externalization of the retrograde wire is performed as described previously. The use of an antegrade mother-child guide extension catheter positioned immediately proximal to the reverse-CART segment can expedite retrograde wire capture and externalization.

STRUCTURED ALGORITHMS FOR CHRONIC TOTAL OCCLUSION PERCUTANEOUS CORONARY INTERVENTION

Hybrid Algorithm

Contemporary antegrade, retrograde, and dissection and reentry techniques are complementary and necessary for the full spectrum of CTO PCI. Exploring sequential CTO crossing options can increase success, shorten procedure times, and reduce radiation exposure. The CTO expert operator needs broad skill sets, versatility, and flexibility to accommodate the wide range of anatomic scenarios that will be present in patients with CTOs and a strong indication for revascularization. Although significant variability exists between operators with respect to procedural approach and skill, the "hybrid method" for CTO PCI is an effort to standardize initial and provisional technique selection based on patient anatomy (see Fig. 26.6).[1] The implementation of the hybrid method requires skill-set development in all techniques—optimal wire manipulation, dissection/reentry, and retrograde techniques. The development and adoption of only one or two of these skill sets will ultimately limit the options available to the operator and, therefore, the likelihood of successful revascularization in all patients with an appropriate indication.

Asia-Pacific Algorithm

The Asia-Pacific CTO club proposed a new algorithm[62] that allows for differing skill sets and equipment availability. Similar to the hybrid algorithm, it recommends a systematic approach to determine whether the primary strategy should be antegrade or retrograde. However, unlike the hybrid algorithm, occlusion length alone does not determine the choice of either a wire escalation strategy or a dissection reentry strategy. Rather, a combination of factors, including ambiguity of the vessel course, severe calcification, tortuosity, length, and previous failure, are used to determine this. It includes the use of IVUS–guided puncture to overcome proximal cap ambiguity, the parallel wire technique, IVUS-guided wiring, and limited subintimal tracking and reentry as options in the algorithm.

CLINICAL OUTCOMES

It is logical to believe that revascularization of severely ischemic viable territories, such as those subtended by a CTO, would provide clinical benefit. Yet the scientific evidence to support this remains variable. The CTO population is inherently difficult to study, given heterogenous anatomy, complexity, and varying operator skill level leading to significant selection bias. In the absence of prospective randomized data, retrospective reports have focused on procedural, in-hospital, and long-term cardiovascular outcomes between patients with CTO PCI success versus failure. Recent randomized controlled trials have been reported, though they suffer from several limitations.

Observational Data

The first retrospective report examined approximately 2000 patients undergoing CTO PCI at a single center over a 20-year period. Ten-year Kaplan-Meier analyses showed CTO PCI success to be associated with an absolute survival advantage of 8.5% when compared with failure (73.5% vs. 65.0%). In a multivariable model, CTO success remained an independent predictor of long-term survival.[63] In population-based analysis from the British Columbia Cardiac Registries, PCI success among approximately 1400 CTO PCI procedures was associated with a 9% absolute survival advantage at 6-year follow-up (adjusted HR 0.44; 95% CI 0.30 to 0.64; $P < .0001$), with a nearly 20% absolute reduction in early and late coronary bypass.[64] The U.K. National Institute for Cardiovascular Outcomes Research examined the data from nearly 15,000 patients who underwent elective PCI between 2005 and 2009 to target one or more CTOs. After adjustment for recorded baseline characteristics, PCI success was significantly associated with lower all-cause mortality at mean follow-up of 2.7 years (HR 0.71; 95% CI 0.62 to 0.82; $P < .001$; Fig. 26.9).[65]

In the National Cardiovascular Data Registry CathPCI database, success rate of CTO PCI was only 59% compared with 96% in non-CTO PCI, with twice the incidence of major adverse cardiac events (MACE) at 1.6% versus 0.8%.[66] Procedural success of CTO PCI improved over the study period from 2009 to 2013, and was related to operator volume. The Canadian multicenter registry reported a procedural success rate of 70% in CTO PCI,[4] while the European RECHARGE registry reported an overall success rate of 74% using the hybrid algorithm.[43]

Procedural MACE in CTO PCI with experienced providers has previously been reported at 1.8%.[67] Coronary perforation and MI were the most common adverse events in a meta-analysis of more than 18,000 patients undergoing CTO PCI.[68] Coronary perforation leading to tamponade, emergency CABG, and death were reported at <1%, each with tamponade occurring more frequently in retrograde cases.[66,68,69]

In a meta-analysis of six CTO studies that reported symptoms using various methodologies and follow-up, PCI success was associated with a much higher likelihood of freedom from residual or recurrent angina ($n = 1601$, HR 2.2; 95% CI 1.5 to 3.3; $P = .0001$).[70] Use of early and late coronary bypass surgery was also decreased after successful CTO PCI, concordant with both the effectiveness and durability of symptom relief attributable to these procedures.[64,70]

In the largest contemporary dataset of CTO PCI from the PROGRESS CTO registry,[71] outcomes of CTO PCI using the hybrid algorithm were examined in 3055 patients at 20 centers in the United States, Europe, and Russia. The overall technical success rate was 87%, and the rate of in-hospital major complications was 3.0%. The final successful crossing strategy was AWE in 52.0%, retrograde in 27.1%, and antegrade dissection reentry (ADR) in 20.9%, with >1 crossing strategy required in 40.9%. Median contrast volume was 270 mL (IQR: 200 to 360 mL), air kerma radiation dose was 2.9 Gy (IQR: 1.7 to 4.7 Gy), and procedure time was 123 min (IQR: 81 to 188 min).

In a prospective study from the FlowCardia's Approach to Chronic Total Occlusion Recanalization (FACTOR) trial,[72] the benefit of CTO PCI on health status was evaluated. Successful CTO PCI was independently associated with improvements in

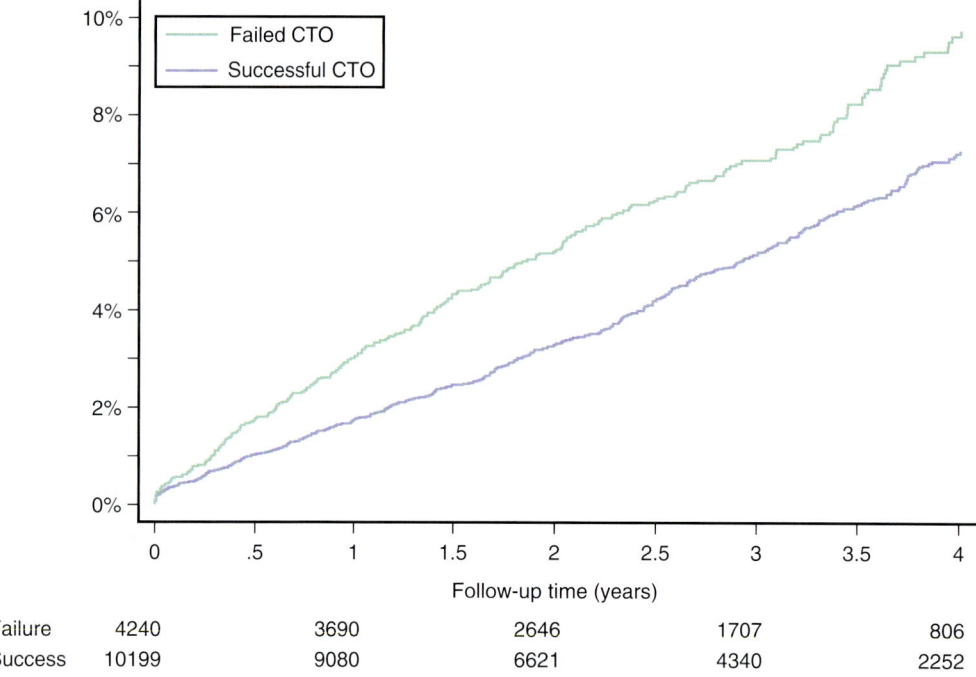

Fig. 26.9 Kaplan-Meier curve showing differences in mortality between those with failed versus successful percutaneous coronary intervention (PCI) procedures targeting a chronic total occlusion *(CTO)*. Successful intervention was associated with a significant decrease in mortality (hazard ratio 0.71; 95% confidence interval 0.62 to 0.82; $P < .001$). Data drawn from nearly 15,000 patients enrolled in a population-based U.K. PCI registry. (From British Cardiovascular Intervention Society; National Institute for Cardiovascular Outcomes Research; et al. Long-term follow-up of elective chronic total coronary occlusion angioplasty: analysis from the U.K. Central Cardiac Audit Database. *J Am Coll Cardiol.* 2014;64:235–243.)

angina frequency, physical limitations, and enhanced quality of life at 1 month follow-up as assessed by the Seattle Angina Questionnaire (SAQ).

The short duration of follow-up, lack of adjudicated, and patient reported outcomes in the observational studies provided led to the development of the OPEN CTO registry. This is an adjudicated, prospective cohort of more than 1000 consecutive CTO patients who underwent PCI at 14 high-volume centers in the United States with 30-day, 6-month, and 1-year patient follow up. Success rates have been reported at 86% with 0.9% in-hospital and 1.3% 1 month mortality. Perforations requiring treatment occurred in 4.8%.[73] This registry includes post-CABG, as well as inoperable patients.

Randomized Controlled Trials

There have been three randomized trials evaluating CTO PCI versus OMT.

The Evaluating Xience and Left Ventricular Function in Percutaneous Coronary Intervention on Occlusions After ST-Elevation Myocardial Infarction (EXPLORE) trial[74] evaluated 304 patients from 14 centers in Canada and Europe with STEMI and concurrent CTO in a noninfarct-related artery. Shortly after, primary PCI patients were randomized to CTO PCI or conservative treatment without CTO PCI. There was no significant difference between groups in the primary outcomes of LVEF and LV end diastolic volume on cardiac magnetic resonance imaging or MACE after 4 months. However, subgroup analysis revealed that patients with CTO located in the LAD coronary artery who were randomized to the CTO PCI strategy had significantly higher LVEF compared with patients without CTO PCI (47.2 ± 12.3% vs. 40.4 ± 11.9%; $P = .02$).

The DECISION-CTO trial[75] from Korea planned to enroll 1284 patients but was stopped early because of slow enrollment, after randomizing 834 patients with coronary CTOs to CTO PCI with OMT alone versus OMT alone. CTO PCI was performed with a high success rate (91%). Concurrent nonocclusive lesions were revascularized following randomization in many patients in both groups (77% and 79% for the OMT and CTO PCI groups, respectively). Nearly 20% of the OMT group crossed over to CTO PCI. At 3 years, the primary end point of death, MI, stroke, or repeated revascularization occurred in 19.6% of the OMT versus 20.6% of the CTO PCI group, suggesting noninferiority of OMT. Measures of quality of life (QoL; SAQ) were similar between study groups. The trial suffered from important design and execution limitations, hindering interpretation of its results, and limiting their applicability to daily clinical practice. These limitations include the following: (1) high prevalence of non-CTO lesions that were treated after enrollment in both study groups without knowledge of the presence of ischemia or symptoms after non-CTO lesion revascularization; (2) high rates of crossover from OMT to CTO PCI; (3) mild baseline symptoms; (4) hard clinical primary end points including death and MI rather than symptom improvement which would be the expected benefit of CTO PCI; (5) noninferiority design as opposed to superiority in order for CTO PCI to replace the less invasive OMT; and (6) low power.

In contrast to DECISION-CTO, the EuroCTO trial[76] was the first randomized controlled trial of CTO PCI to look at QoL outcomes. Werner et al. initially planned to enroll 1200 patients, but because of slow enrollment, only 407 patients were randomized 2:1 to CTO PCI versus OMT (aspirin, statin, angiotensin-converting enzyme inhibitor where tolerated, plus at least two antianginal agents at maximum tolerated dose). The primary efficacy end point was health status at 12 and 36 months. Patients with non-CTO lesions were enrolled only after such lesions were successfully revascularized and if patients continued to experience anginal symptoms. The study showed significant improvement in angina frequency with CTO PCI over OMT ($P = .009$) as well as greater improvements in Canadian Cardiovascular Society angina scores with PCI over OMT ($P < .001$). Improvements in physical limitation, QoL, angina stability, and treatment satisfaction were numerically higher in the PCI-treated patients. Major adverse cardiovascular and cerebrovascular events at 12 months was similar between the PCI and OMT arms (5.2% vs. 6.7%; $P = .52$).

It is important to recognize the challenges of conducting randomized controlled trials in patients randomized to CTO PCI versus OMT—they will need to evaluate symptomatic improvement as the primary outcome as opposed to hard clinical end points but will likely include less symptomatic patients at baseline. However, the most symptomatic patients are likely the ones to derive the most benefit from CTO PCI. Therefore, the effect of CTO PCI is likely to be underestimated.

CONCLUSION

With the development of a multitude of new techniques and devices for CTO PCI, we are now able to successfully revascularize the vast majority of patients with an appropriate indication. Training of new operators has led to further growth and adoption of CTO PCI. As operators and programs acquire these skills, it is imperative that the culture of scientific investigation and collaboration continues in order to improve procedural success, minimize care variability, and ensure that all patients receive appropriate therapy.

KEY REFERENCES

1. Brilakis ES, Grantham JA, Rinfret S, et al. A percutaneous treatment algorithm for crossing coronary chronic total occlusions. *JACC Cardiovasc Interv*. 2012;5:376–379.
3. Christofferson RD, Lehmann KG, Martin GV, et al. Effect of chronic total coronary occlusion on treatment strategy. *Am J Cardiol*. 2005;95:1088–1091.
4. Fefer P, Knudtson ML, Cheema AN, et al. Current perspectives on coronary chronic total occlusions: the Canadian Multicenter Chronic Total Occlusions Registry. *J Am Coll Cardiol*. 2012;59:991–997.
34. Werner GS, Surber R, Ferrari M, et al. The functional reserve of collaterals supplying long-term chronic total coronary occlusions in patients without prior myocardial infarction. *Eur Heart J*. 2006;27(20):2406–2412.
40. Brilakis ES, Grantham JA, Thompson CA, et al. The retrograde approach to coronary artery chronic total occlusions: a practical approach. *Catheter Cardiovasc Interv*. 2012;79:3–19.
41. Morino Y, Abe M, Morimoto T, et al. Predicting successful guidewire crossing through chronic total occlusion of native coronary lesions within 30 minutes: the J CTO (Multicenter CTO Registry in Japan) score as a difficulty grading and time assessment tool. *JACC Cardiovasc Interv*. 2011;4:213–221.
43. Maeremans J, Walsh S, Knaapen P, et al. The Hybrid Algorithm for Treating Chronic Total Occlusions in Europe: The RECHARGE Registry. *J Am Coll Cardiol*. 2016;68:1958–1970.
44. Christopoulos G, Kandzari DE, Yeh RW, et al. Development and Validation of a Novel Scoring System for Predicting Technical Success of Chronic Total Occlusion Percutaneous Coronary Interventions: The PROGRESS CTO (Prospective Global Registry for the Study of Chronic Total Occlusion Intervention) Score. *JACC Cardiovasc Interv*. 2016;9(1):1–9.
48. Brilakis ES, Karmpaliotis D, Patel V, et al. Complications of chronic total occlusion angioplasty. *Intervent Cardiol Clin*. 2012;1:373–389.
50. Whitlow PL, Burke MN, Lombardi WL, et al. Use of a novel crossing and re-entry system in coronary chronic total occlusions that have failed standard crossing techniques: results of the FAST-CTOs (Facilitated Antegrade Steering Technique in Chronic Total Occlusions) trial. *JACC Cardiovasc Interv*. 2012;5:393–401.
53. Surmely JF, Tsuchikane E, Katoh O, et al. New concept for CTO recanalization using controlled antegrade and retrograde subintimal tracking: the CART technique. *J Invasive Cardiol*. 2006;18:334–338.
54. Thompson CA, Jayne JE, Robb JF, et al. Retrograde techniques and the impact of operator volume on percutaneous intervention for coronary chronic total occlusions an early U.S. experience. *JACC Cardiovasc Interv*. 2009;2:834–842.
65. British Cardiovascular Intervention Society, National Institute for Cardiovascular Outcomes Research. Long-term follow-up of elective chronic total coronary occlusion angioplasty: analysis from the U.K. Central Cardiac Audit Database. *J Am Coll Cardiol*. 2014;64(3):235–243.
66. Brilakis ES, Banerjee S, Karmpaliotis D, et al. Procedural outcomes of chronic total occlusion percutaneous coronary intervention: a report from the NCDR (National Cardiovascular Data Registry). *JACC Cardiovasc Interv*. 2015;8:245–253.
73. Sapontis J, Salisbury AC, Yeh RW, et al. Early procedural and health status outcomes after chronic total occlusion angioplasty: a report from the OPEN-CTO registry (Outcomes, Patient Health Status, and Efficiency in Chronic Total Occlusion Hybrid Procedures). *JACC Cardiovasc Interv*. 2017;10(15):1523–1534.
74. Henriques JP, Hoebers LP, Råmunddal T, et al. Percutaneous intervention for concurrent chronic total occlusions in patients with STEMI: the EXPLORE trial. *J Am Coll Cardiol*. 2016;68(15):1622–1632.
75. Park S. *Drug-Eluting Stent Implantation Versus Optimal Medical Treatment in Patients with Chronic Total Occlusion (DECISION-CTO)*. Washington, DC: American College of Cardiology's 66th Annual Scientific Session & Expo; 2017.
76. Werner GS, Martin-Yuste V, Hildick-Smith D, et al. A randomized multicentre trial to compare revascularization with optimal medical therapy for the treatment of chronic total coronary occlusions. *Eur Heart J*. 2018;39(26):2484–2493. https://doi.org/10.1093/eurheartj/ehy220.

Additional references available online at expertconsult.com.

中文导读

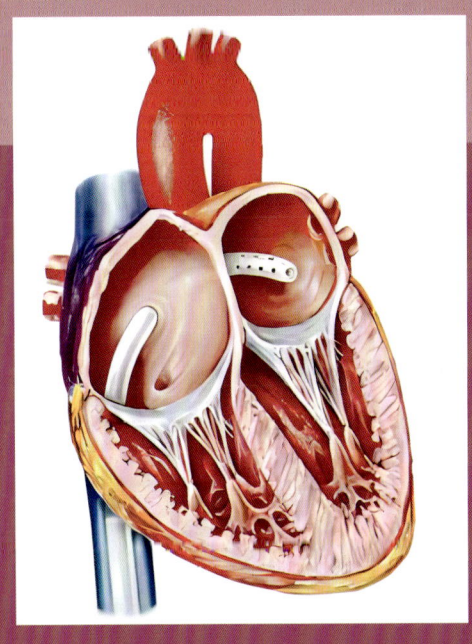

第27章
桥血管介入治疗

  冠状动脉旁路移植术是一种常见的外科治疗冠状动脉粥样硬化性心脏病的手术，其长期预后依赖于桥血管移植物的寿命。通过使用动脉移植物、非体外循环手术和微创外科技术、抗血小板及调脂药物治疗，桥血管移植物寿命及冠状动脉旁路移植术预后已得到明显改善。然而，桥血管失败仍然是心血管医师无法回避的技术难题，而介入治疗可能是大多数冠状动脉旁路移植术患者桥血管失败唯一的血运重建方案。

  本章节概括了冠状动脉旁路移植术后不同时期桥血管失败发生的机制、临床表现及手术策略。搭桥术后早期缺血（＜30天）通常是桥血管闭塞或狭窄所致，此时通常可对桥血管行经皮冠状动脉介入治疗。冠状动脉旁路移植术后数年出现不稳定型心绞痛或ST段抬高型心肌梗死最常见的原因是大隐静脉桥血管病变，在这种情况下，尽可能选择自体冠状动脉血管行经皮冠状动脉介入治疗术。本章节还重点总结了桥血管尤其是大隐静脉桥血管进行经皮冠状动脉介入治疗的相关技术技巧、器械选择及并发症处理。然而，静脉桥血管病变与冠状动脉自身血管病变在病理生理学机制、手术策略及支架置入后临床结局并不完全相同，尚需更多研究证据指导临床决策，改善这类患者的临床结局。

申学谦　柳景华

章节要点

- 搭桥术后早期缺血（<30天）通常是因为桥血管闭塞或狭窄所致，此时经皮冠状动脉介入治疗通常是可行的策略。

- 冠状动脉旁路移植术后数年出现不稳定型心绞痛或ST段抬高心肌梗死多数是由于大隐静脉桥血管病变所致。在这种情况下，应尽可能优先选择冠状动脉自身血管行经皮冠状动脉介入治疗术。

- 血栓保护装置可以降低SVG PCI术中因斑块栓塞所致的心肌梗死风险，推荐用于大多数冠状动脉旁路移植术后多年才出现的大隐静脉桥血管原位病变。

- 如果患者存在多个大隐静脉桥血管病变或闭塞、左心室功能降低且有可用的动脉桥来源，建议优先选择再次行冠状动脉旁路移植术。如果与前降支吻合的左乳内动脉桥血管通畅，则选择经皮冠状动脉介入治疗术。

- 尽管药物洗脱支架在大隐静脉桥血管中的有效性不如冠状动脉自身血管，但药物洗脱支架可降低冠状动脉自身血管的再狭窄，因此它已经成为许多术者在处理大隐静脉桥血管时的默认策略。5个关于药物洗脱支架和裸金属支架应用于大隐静脉桥血管的随机试验得出了相互矛盾的结果。

27 Bypass Graft Intervention

John S. Douglas Jr.

KEY POINTS

- Early postoperative ischemia (<30 days) is frequently due to graft occlusion or stenosis, and percutaneous coronary intervention (PCI) is often feasible.
- Unstable angina or ST–segment–elevation myocardial infarction (STEMI) years after coronary artery bypass grafting (CABG) is most often due to a saphenous vein graft (SVG) lesion; in such cases, native vessel PCI is preferred whenever possible.
- Embolic protection reduces the risk of atheroembolic myocardial infarction during SVG PCI and should be used in the treatment of most de novo SVG lesions that occur years after CABG.
- Multiple diseased or occluded SVGs, reduced left ventricular (LV) function, and available arterial conduits favor repeat CABG; a patent left internal mammary artery (LIMA) to the left anterior descending (LAD) coronary artery favors PCI.
- Drug-eluting stents (DESs) reduce restenosis in native coronary arteries and have become the default strategy in SVGs for many operators in spite of reduced efficacy in SVGs compared with native vessels. Five randomized trials of DESs and bare-metal stents (BMSs) in SVGs yielded conflicting results.

THE SCOPE OF THE PROBLEM

Coronary artery bypass grafting (CABG) is a commonly performed surgical procedure whose efficacy has been enhanced by the use of arterial grafts, off-bypass procedures, and minimally invasive surgical techniques. In addition, attempts have been made to improve graft longevity with antiplatelet agents and lipid-lowering therapy. In spite of these efforts, the temporary nature of the palliative effect of CABG remains a significant health care problem. Severe myocardial ischemic syndromes occur in 3% to 5% of patients immediately after surgery; thereafter, recurrent ischemic symptoms appear in 4% to 8% of post-CABG patients annually. Saphenous vein graft (SVG) attrition, the most common cause, is up to 40% during the first year; 1% to 2% of grafts occlude annually 1 to 5 years after surgery, and 5% occlude each year over the next 5 years. At 10 years, one half of all SVGs are occluded, and half of the patent SVGs are diseased.

In experience at Emory University Hospital and the Cleveland Clinic, reoperation was required in about 3% of patients by 5 years, 15% by 10 years, and 30% by 15 years. For reoperation, even in the most experienced centers, the risk of in-hospital death and nonfatal Q-wave myocardial infarction (MI) is triple that of the initial operation. In the state of New York, in-hospital mortality was 4.1% for initial operations but 11%, 25%, and 39% for first, second, and third reoperations, respectively.[1] In addition to being more risky, reoperative surgery was associated with less complete anginal relief and reduced graft patency, probably attributable to more advanced disease and poorer graft conduits. These factors have promoted a conservative approach to reoperation and have favored the use of percutaneous coronary intervention (PCI).[2–5] In addition, many symptomatic patients who are candidates for percutaneous methods would not be considered for reoperation because of a limited amount of myocardial ischemia, risk to patent grafts, lack of suitable conduits, poor left ventricular (LV) function, advanced age, or coexisting medical problems. Recently published data from the Society of Thoracic Surgery (STS) national database showed that among patients aged 65 years and older who survived following an initial CABG operation, rates of repeat revascularization at 1, 5, 10, and 18 years were 2%, 8%, 16%, and 25%, respectively, and that the mode of revascularization was mostly PCI (93%).[6] Factors associated with a higher rate of repeat revascularization included female sex, diabetes, prior PCI, dialysis, and incomplete revascularization. In the past decade at Emory, approximately 10% of the patients who underwent PCI had had a prior CABG, and bypass graft intervention was the most common indication. It is in this difficult group of patients, those who require bypass graft intervention, that decision making is particularly critical owing to the increased up-front risk and reduced long-term benefit of such intervention.

INDICATIONS FOR INTERVENTION

Patients who experience recurrent ischemia after coronary bypass surgery have diverse anatomic problems; therefore selection for PCI must be based on careful analysis of the projected outcomes of competing strategies. The status of the left anterior descending (LAD) and its graft significantly influences revascularization choices because of its impact on long-term outcome and the lack of survival benefit of reoperative surgery to treat non–LAD-related ischemia.[6,7] Factors that favor surgical revascularization include multiple-vessel involvement, severe vein graft disease, poor LV function, total occlusions of native coronary arteries, and the availability of arterial conduits.[8] Because the choice among percutaneous methods and the relative effectiveness of each are often influenced by the time elapsed since surgery, indications are considered relative to this factor.

Early Postoperative Period

The performance of routine intraoperative angiography at the conclusion of CABG at one center and four recent trials in which routine angiography was performed at 12 months to assess graft patency have provided sobering insights regarding contemporary CABG.[9–13] Among 366 consecutive patients who underwent intraoperative completion angiography, Zhao and colleagues[9] found that 12% of bypass grafts had defects important enough to require intervention (open surgical revision, 3.4%; open-chest PCI, 6%; and minor adjustment, 2.8%). In a randomized trial in over 100 high-volume U.S. centers that included over 3000 patients in whom modern surgical techniques and medications were utilized, graft failure at 1 year occurred in 41.6% of SVGs with a single distal anastomosis and 50.6% with multiple distal anastomoses.[10] In the PRAGUE-4 (randomized comparison between off-pump and on-pump surgery) trial, angiographic follow-up at 1 year revealed that 40% of SVGs and 9% of left internal mammary artery (LIMA) grafts were occluded.[11] In the Veterans Affairs Randomized On/Off Bypass (ROOBY) study, 23% of SVGs and 11% of LIMA grafts performed off-pump failed at 1 year.[12] In the DACABG trial conducted in 2014 to 2015, patients undergoing elective CABG and treated with aspirin postoperatively experienced a 24% rate of SVG failure.[13] Graft failure was associated with death, new MI, or repeat revascularization in 26% of patients.[10] Recurrent ischemia within days of surgery is usually related to acute vein graft thrombosis due to endothelial damage during harvesting and initial exposure to arterial pressure. However, stenosis may exist at proximal or distal anastomoses (Fig. 27.1); a bypass graft may be kinked; the wrong vessel may have been bypassed; or the revascularization may have been rendered incomplete as a result of diffuse disease, stenoses distal to graft insertion, or inaccessible intramyocardial position of a recipient artery. To determine the cause of severe early postoperative myocardial ischemia and define therapeutic options, coronary arteriography has been carried out within a few hours of surgery in 3% to 4% of patients in some centers,[14–16] and this strategy is recommended. PCI in patients with early ischemia after CABG is a class I indication in the American College of Cardiology(ACC)/American Heart Association (AHA)/Society for Cardiovascular Angiography and Interventions (SCAI) PCI guidelines and the European guidelines on revascularization.[17,18] Although 44 of 145 patients (30%) catheterized because of ischemia early after surgery had no apparent cause for ischemia, many patients had correctable problems; 30 patients had emergency reoperation and 44 underwent PCI.[14–16] In a recent report, emergency coronary angiography was performed in 118 of 5427 CABG patients, of whom 57% had graft failure and 60% underwent repeat revascularization.[19] In seven patients, focal stenosis was present in a venous or arterial graft distal anastomosis, and balloon dilation across suture lines was safe in these patients. However, in our experience (Fig. 27.2) and in that of others, extreme care is warranted within a few hours after surgery to ensure an intracoronary position of the steerable guidewire, indicating that the guidewire has not penetrated a suture line. In addition, balloon sizing should be conservative; we are aware of unreported cases of suture-line disruption and severe hemorrhagic complications. It is noteworthy that European guidelines advise against PCI of a graft anastomosis early after CABG because of this risk of perforation.[18] Immediate access to a covered stent is essential, should suture line perforation occur. Mild to moderate imperfections at the anastomosis observed in the early postoperative period should not be dilated because they frequently disappear on subsequent angiography, suggesting the presence of edema.[20] Some have attributed these observations to the self-reparative ability of the LIMA.[21] If a thrombosed graft is discovered, PCI of the native coronary artery is recommended, but mechanical thrombectomy can be attempted—or a return to the operating room may be considered—if the jeopardized vessel is of significant importance. Use of thrombolytic agents or glycoprotein (GP) IIb/IIIa inhibitors in the early postoperative period carries substantial risk of bleeding. Patients at increased risk for early postoperative ischemia include those undergoing minimally invasive and "off-bypass" techniques and those who receive non-internal mammary arterial grafts.

When ischemia recurs 1 to 12 months after surgery, perianastomotic stenoses are among the most common problems (Fig. 27.3). Stenotic lesions of the distal anastomosis of saphenous vein or arterial grafts can be successfully dilated with balloon angioplasty at this time with little morbidity and good long-term patency in 80% to 90% of patients without stent implantation.[3,22] Among 34 patients with distal anastomosis lesions reported from our early experience, 25 (74%) presented within 1

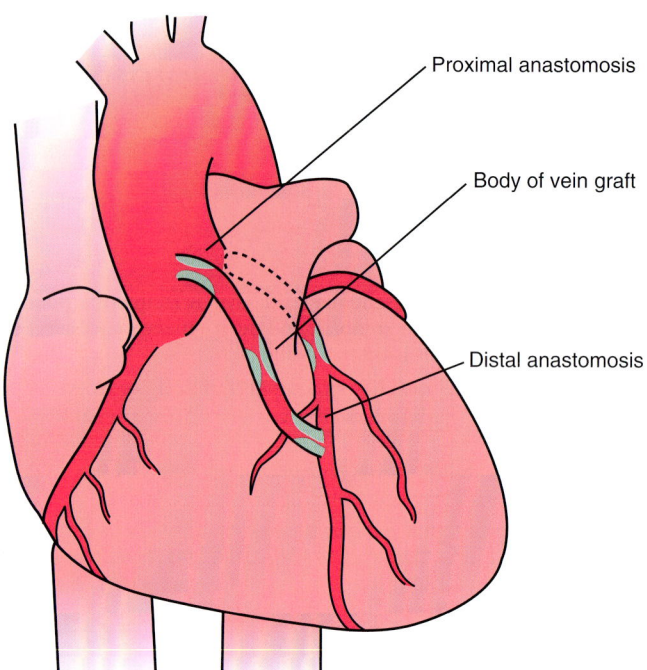

Fig. 27.1 Sites of saphenous vein graft stenoses. All lesions between the proximal and distal anastomoses are considered midgraft lesions.

year of CABG.[3] Thirty-two were successfully dilated, and three of four restenosis lesions redilated. A total of 30 of 32 patients were asymptomatic at 10 months. Stenoses, or in some cases total occlusions, of the middle or distal portions of the internal mammary artery (IMA) or radial artery grafts may be dilated successfully (Fig. 27.4), especially when the presence of a short occlusion can be documented. Stenotic lesions of mid-SVGs that occur within a year of surgery are usually the result of intimal hyperplasia; these lesions can be dilated with balloon angioplasty and/or stented with little risk of distal embolization, but recurrence has been noted in about 50% of cases in our experience, and periprocedural graft perforation has been observed. Stents, directional coronary atherectomy, and excimer laser angioplasty have all been tried for the treatment of proximal anastomotic lesions that occur within a year of surgery with excellent initial results but significant rates of restenosis. Data are sparse regarding the use of drug-eluting stents (DESs) at this site.

One to Three Years After Surgery

Patients with recurrent ischemia 1 to 3 years after surgery frequently have new stenoses in graft conduits and native coronary arteries that are amenable to percutaneous intervention. Whenever possible, native coronary lesions are targeted. The ACC/AHA/SCAI PCI guidelines consider focal ischemia–producing graft lesions in patients 1 to 3 years after CABG with preserved LV function to be a class IIa indication ("conflicting evidence, weight of evidence/opinion in favor of usefulness").[17]

More Than Three Years After Surgery

Beginning about 3 years after implantation, atherosclerotic lesions appear in vein grafts with increasing frequency. Unstable ischemic syndromes are common, and aggressive invasive evaluation and therapy are indicated. In about 70% of post-CABG patients who present with an acute coronary syndrome (ACS), the culprit lesion is located in an SVG.[23] Atherosclerotic plaques in vein grafts contain foam cells, cholesterol crystals, blood elements, and necrotic debris, with less fibrocollagenous tissue and

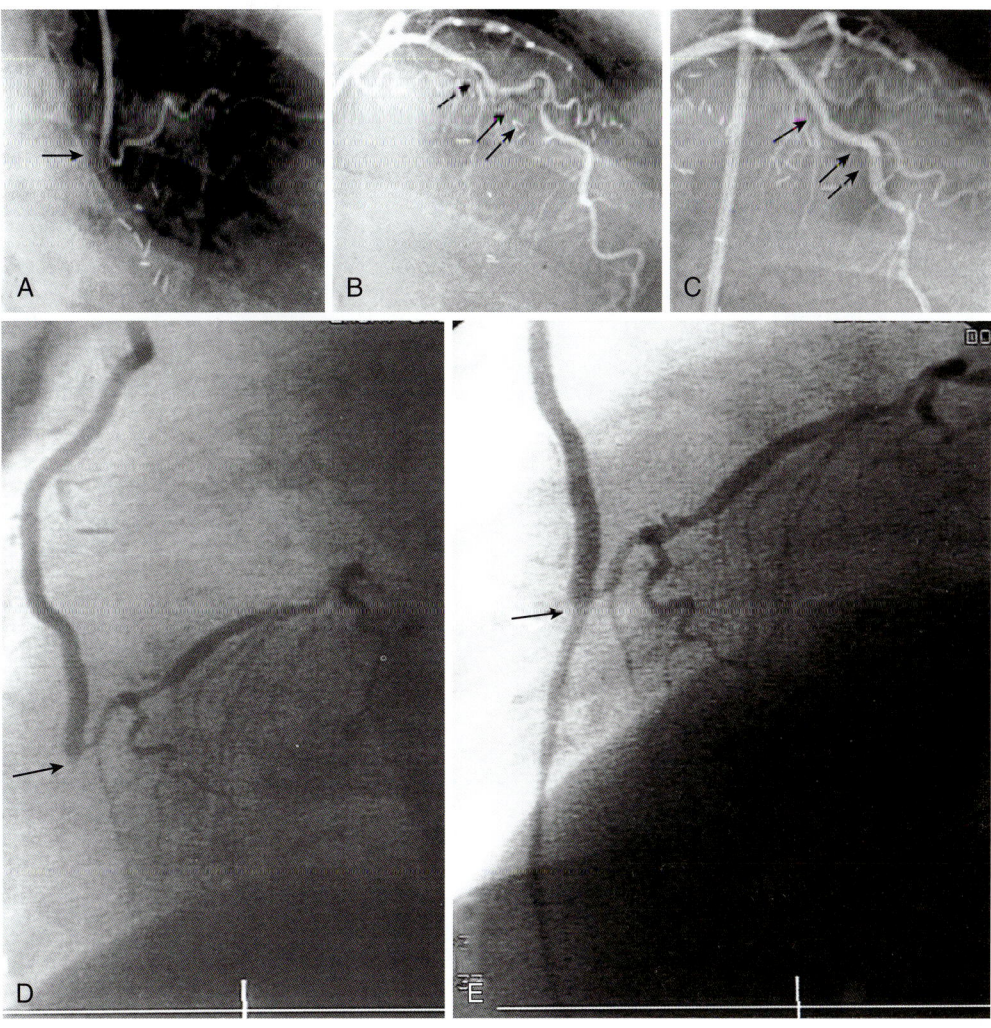

Fig. 27.2 Two cases of failure of minimally invasive coronary artery bypass graft treated with percutaneous catheter-based intervention. *Case 1:* A 78-year-old woman underwent left internal mammary artery (LIMA) to left anterior descending (LAD) coronary artery surgery through a left fourth intercostal incision without cardiopulmonary bypass because of refractory angina and a long stenosis of a tortuous LAD. Angina at rest recurred within a few hours after surgery, and angiography on the second postoperative day revealed occlusion of the LIMA graft about 4 cm from its insertion into the LAD (A, *arrow*). The LAD was tortuous, with multiple, severe stenoses (B, *arrows*); left ventricular function was normal. Angioplasty and stent implantation in the native vessel yielded an excellent angiographic result (C, *arrows*) and favorable short-term follow-up. *Case 2:* Because of disabling angina and a long proximal LAD stenosis, a 60-year-old man underwent minimally invasive LIMA to LAD. About 2 hours after surgery, an electrocardiogram showed anterior ST-segment elevation, and emergency coronary arteriography revealed occlusion of the distal LAD at the graft insertion (D, left lateral view, *arrow*). Balloon angioplasty through the LIMA graft was successful (E, *arrow*), and the patient remained asymptomatic at 6-month follow-up.

calcification than are present in native coronary arteries (Fig. 27.5). Consequently, the plaques in older vein grafts may be softer and more friable, as well as being larger than those observed in native coronary arteries, and they frequently have thin fibrous caps and associated thrombus formation (Fig. 27.6). Recently published optical coherence tomography (OCT) studies of older SVGs in patients with stable angina surprisingly documented the presence of thrombus in most patients[24] and in patients with ACSs revealed the enormous complexity of SVG lesions (Fig. 27.7).[25] Atheroembolism related to graft intervention may have catastrophic consequences. Consequently, bulky vein graft lesions (those with a large potential atheroma mass) should be avoided if possible. Improved initial outcome has been reported with stent placement compared with balloon dilation in SVGs. However, long-term results in SVGs have been disappointing. Data on long-term outcomes with DESs in SVGs are limited (see Drug-Eluting Stents in Vein Grafts section), and the role of percutaneous techniques in totally occluded SVGs is controversial.

Acute ST-Segment Elevation Myocardial Infarction

After coronary bypass surgery, approximately 3% of patients experience ST-segment elevation myocardial infarction (STEMI) annually. Because these patients were excluded from early reperfusion trials, therapy has been based on clinical experience and remains controversial. In a majority of patients, the culprit vessel has been found to be a vein graft, and considerable lesion-associated thrombus was a common accompaniment (see Fig. 27.6). Intravenous thrombolytic therapy is relatively ineffective in SVGs.[26] Most investigators currently favor emergency coronary arteriography

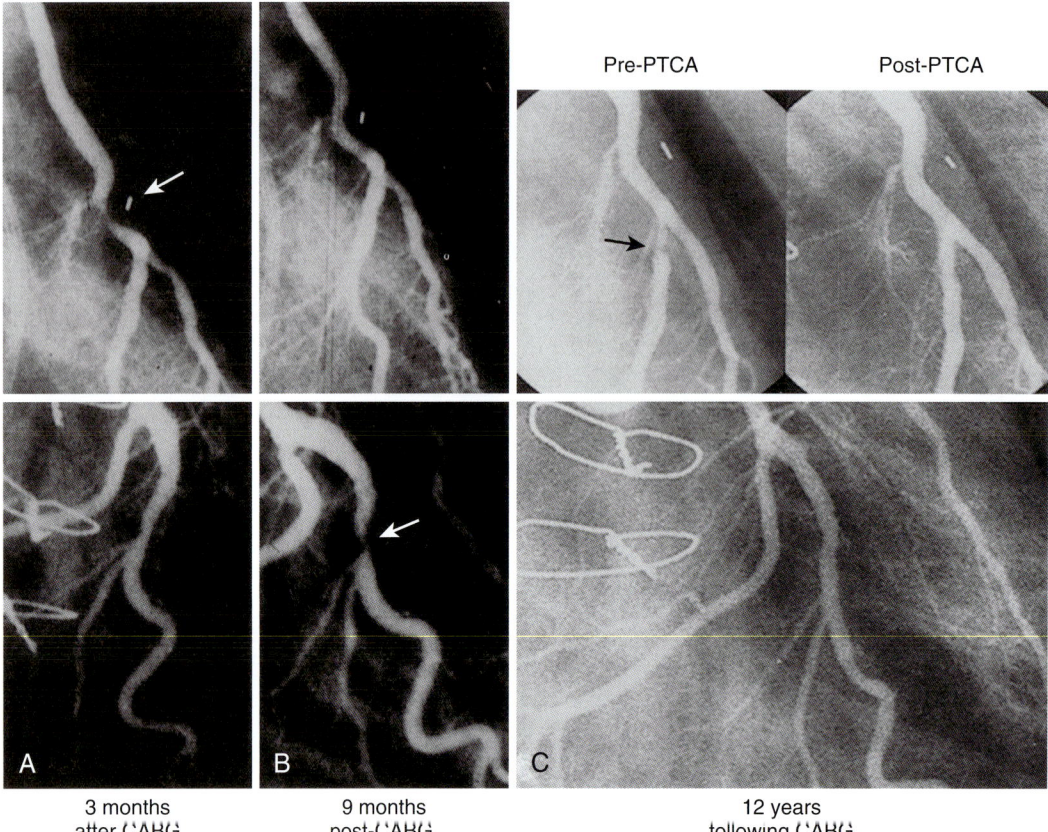

Fig. 27.3 A 37-year-old woman had placement of saphenous vein grafts (SVGs) to the left anterior descending (LAD) and posterior descending coronary arteries. Unstable angina recurred 3 months later, and high-grade stenosis was present at the junction of the SVG to the LAD (A, *top: arrow*). The circumflex coronary artery had minimal disease (A, *bottom*). The SVG to the posterior descending coronary artery was patent, and balloon angioplasty of the distal anastomosis was successful. Disabling angina recurred 9 months following coronary artery bypass grafting *(CABG)*. Coronary arteriography (B, *top*) showed a widely patent distal anastomosis but high-grade stenosis of the circumflex coronary artery (B, *bottom: arrow*) that was unresponsive to nitroglycerin. Balloon angioplasty of the circumflex stenosis was successful (residual stenosis 0%). Twelve years following CABG, angina recurred and recatheterization showed high-grade stenosis of the mid-LAD just beyond the takeoff of a large diagonal (C, *top left: arrow*); the vein graft to the posterior descending coronary artery was occluded. Previous percutaneous transluminal coronary angioplasty *(PTCA)* sites at the distal anastomosis of the vein graft to the LAD and the circumflex artery (C, *bottom*) were widely patent. Balloon angioplasty of the mid-LAD was successful. The patient remained asymptomatic for 4.5 years, when a new thrombotic stenosis in the midportion of the SVG to the LAD led to replacement of this graft with a left internal mammary artery graft. All prior PTCA sites were patent, and surgical benefit was extended over 16 years with three percutaneous procedures.

and the option of more specific intervention, including thrombectomy and mechanical recanalization. Among approximately 1000 patients with STEMI and a history of prior CABG reported from the National Cardiovascular Data Registry (NCDR), post-CABG patients were older, had more lesion complexity, and had lower likelihood of a door-to-balloon time ≤90 minutes (76%).[27] This delay to treatment warrants a "call to action" in the post-CABG patient with STEMI.[28] Among almost 80,000 patients undergoing primary PCI in England and Wales between 2007 and 2012, 2658 had prior CABG,[29] and these patients had more comorbidities and higher mortality at 30 days and 1 year. The culprit vessel was a bypass graft in 56% and native coronary artery in 44%. Recent reports indicate that both acute and long-term results of PCI in SVGs for treatment of STEMI are inferior to those of native vessel PCI for STEMI. In a study of 2240 consecutive patients with STEMI, Brodie and colleagues[30] observed that patients who underwent SVG PCI were sicker (had poorer LV function, more three-vessel disease, and prior MI) than patients who underwent native vessel PCI. Patients with SVG occlusion had lower rates of thrombolysis in myocardial infarction (TIMI) grade 3 blood flow, higher in-hospital mortality (21% vs. 8%, $P = .0004$), and worse 10-year survival (49% vs. 76%, $P < .0001$). SVG patency was 64% at 1 year. In the Mayo Clinic STEMI experience, treatment of an SVG was independently associated with adverse cardiac events.[31] In a report of 192 post-CABG patients with acute MI, 30-day mortality with SVG PCI was significantly higher than that with native vessel PCI (14.3% vs. 8.4%, $P = .03$).[32] The ACC/AHA Task Force Report on Early Management of Acute Myocardial Infarction classified PCI for vein graft recanalization as a class IIa intervention: "acceptable, of uncertain efficacy and may be controversial; weight of evidence in favor of usefulness/efficacy."[33]

TECHNICAL STRATEGY

The postoperative patient offers unique challenges to the PCI operator. The selection of a guide catheter to achieve coaxial alignment and provide adequate back-up support is often the key to success. Fig. 27.8 illustrates the shapes of guide catheters commonly

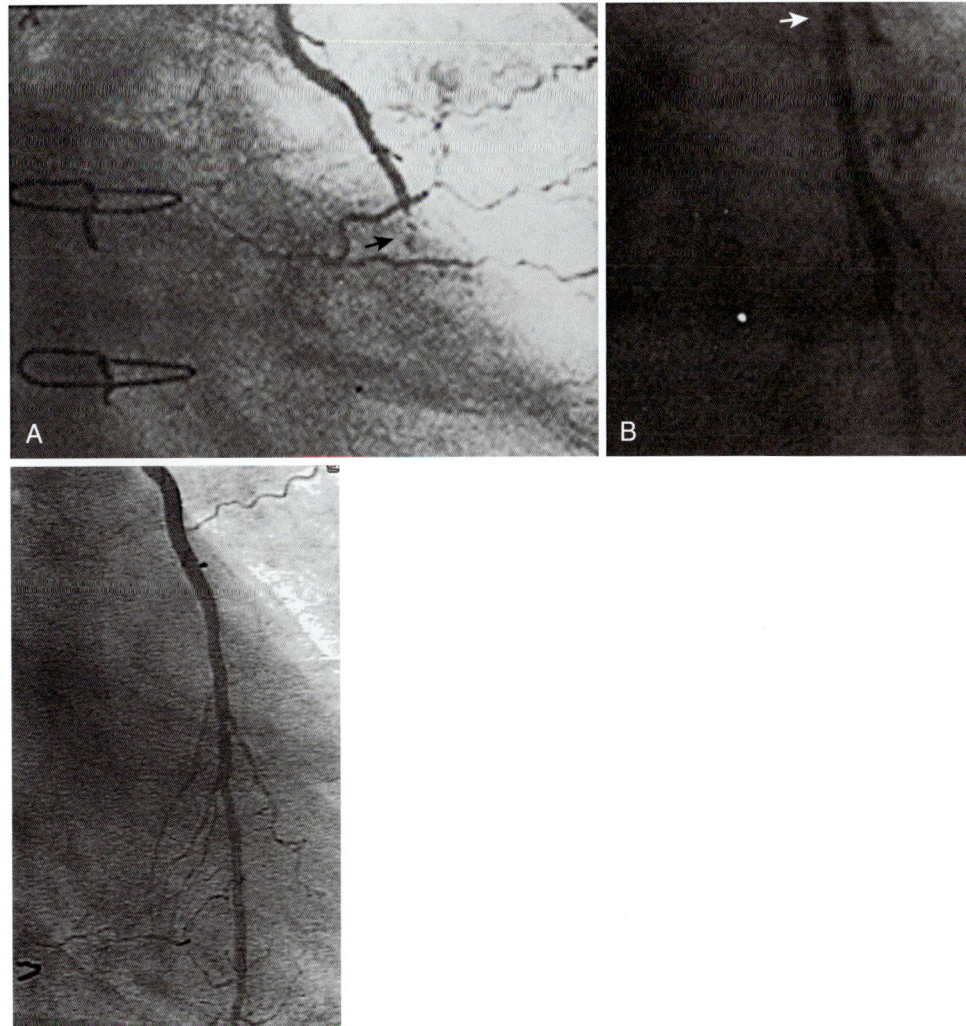

Fig. 27.4 A 52-year-old man experienced recurrence of angina 5 months after a triple coronary bypass. Coronary arteriography revealed total occlusion of the left internal mammary artery (LIMA) 1 to 2 cm proximal to insertion into the left anterior descending (LAD) coronary artery (A, *arrow*), severe stenosis of a large diagonal, and patent grafts to the obtuse marginal and right coronary arteries. The LIMA was recanalized by use of an 8-Fr internal mammary artery guide catheter for good backup, progression to a relatively stiff guidewire to punch across the total occlusion, and a 2-mm over-the-wire balloon (result after percutaneous transluminal coronary angioplasty: B, *arrow*). The diagonal was successfully dilated. The patient presented again 5 years later with recurrent angina and was found to have an occluded saphenous vein graft to the obtuse marginal artery; the native obtuse marginal artery was successfully dilated. The LIMA-to-LAD anastomosis was widely patent (C), as was the diagonal, 5 years after recanalization.

used for vein graft interventions; 7-Fr catheters are favored for many vein graft procedures (for optimal visualization, to facilitate stenting, and to accommodate large balloons, stents, and embolic protection devices [EPDs] and large covered stents needed to treat bypass graft perforations). Although some have recommended routine use of slightly oversized balloons and stents for vein graft procedures, it is prudent to size balloons and stents no larger than the normal reference segment. This is especially true in older vein grafts, in which vein graft rupture has been reported with moderate oversizing. In addition, Iakovau and colleagues[31] reported no benefit of oversizing with respect to target-vessel revascularization (31% vs. 26%, $P = .3$), and MI was increased (29% vs. 17%, $P < .05$). Notably, Hong and colleagues[35] have reported favorable outcomes using slightly undersized stents in SVGs. In general, most experienced operators stent from "normal to normal." When vein grafts that encircle the heart are encountered, or in the case of IMA grafts to far distal locations, balloon catheters with extra-long (145-cm) shafts or shorter guide catheters (80 to 90 cm) may be needed, or the guide catheter can be shortened and a flared, short sheath one size smaller can be used to close the cut end of the catheter. Embolic protection strategies, a class I indication in PCI guidelines for de novo SVG lesions, have been shown to reduce atheroembolic MI (as discussed later) and should be considered in PCI of de novo SVG lesions.

RESULTS OF INTERVENTION

Percutaneous Coronary Intervention Versus Reoperation

At Emory University over a fourteen year period, a total of 2613 post-bypass patients underwent catheter-based myocardial

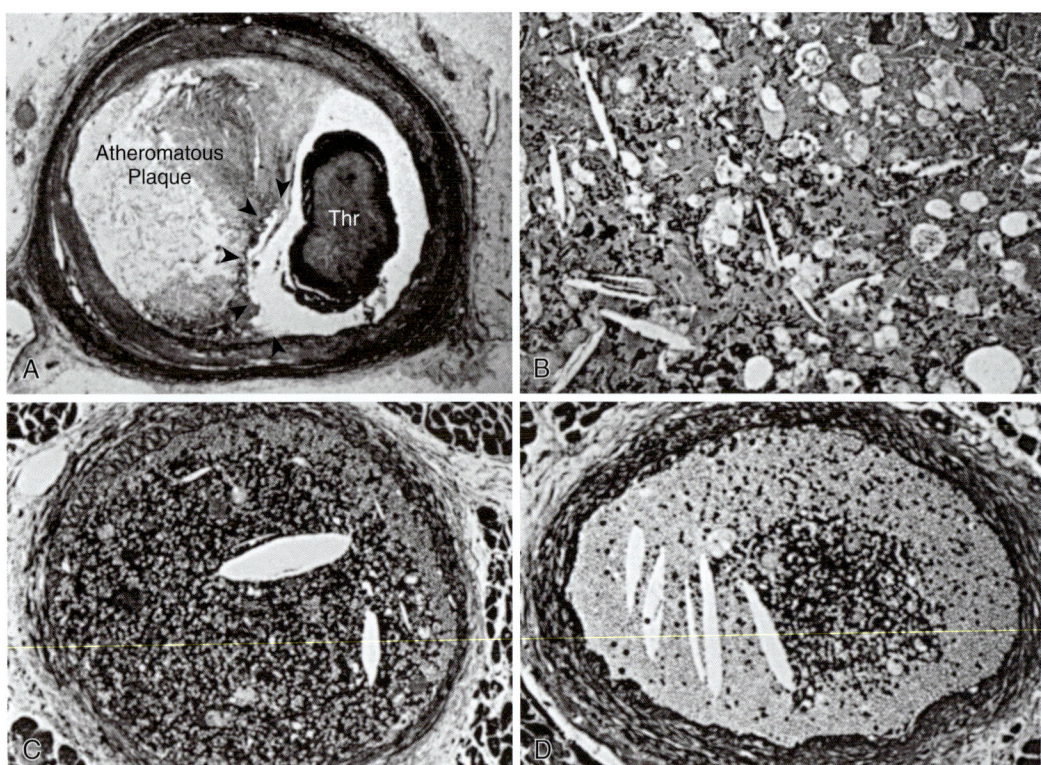

Fig. 27.5 Vein graft. (A) Low-power photomicrograph shows rupture *(arrowheads)* of atheromatous plaque caused by balloon angioplasty and secondary thrombosis *(Thr)*. Sections taken at adjacent sites were involved by such extensive disruption that luminal boundaries were obliterated. (B) High-power photomicrograph demonstrates the nature of the plaque, with foam cells, cholesterol clefts, blood elements, and necrotic debris. (C and D) Intramural coronary artery branches. Atheromatous emboli obstruct vessels in anterolateral (C) and inferoseptal (D) walls of left ventricle (compare with B). (From Saber RS, Edwards WD, Holmes DR Jr, et al. Balloon angioplasty of aortocoronary saphenous vein bypass grafts: a histopathologic study of six grafts from five patients, with emphasis on restenosis and embolic complications. *J Am Coll Cardiol.* 1988;12:1501–1509.)

revascularization.[36] Compared with 1561 patients treated with reoperative surgery, in-hospital outcomes were more favorable for mortality (1.1% vs. 6.9%; $P < .001$), Q-wave infarction (1.4% vs. 5.4%; $P < .001$), stroke (0% vs. 2.8%; $P = .27$), length of stay (3.0 vs. 10.5 days; $P < .001$), and cost ($8500 vs. $24,200; $P < .01$); in-hospital CABG was required in 2.9% of PCI patients. Ten-year survival was better in the angioplasty group. By 5 years, approximately 50% of the PCI patients required either repeated PCI or CABG, and survival was better in patients who underwent native vessel, compared with graft, interventions. In 2191 post-CABG patients who underwent multivessel revascularization at the Cleveland Clinic between 1995 and 2000, a total of 1487 had reoperation and 704 had PCI.[8] Initial outcomes were more favorable with PCI for completeness of revascularization, 30-day mortality, periprocedural Q-wave infarction, and stroke. At 5 years, unadjusted survival was 79% for CABG and 75% for PCI ($P = .008$). The only randomized comparison of PCI and CABG in post-bypass patients was reported by Morrison and colleagues,[37] who randomized 143 patients (67 to PCI and 75 to CABG). At 3 years, survival was approximately 75% in both groups, comparable to the 5-year survival in the Cleveland Clinic study; no significant advantage of one procedure over the other was apparent. An Emory University experience with 1712 diabetic patients who required repeat revascularization (1123 with PCI, 589 with reoperation) indicated relatively poor long-term outcomes. Survival at 5 years with PCI and reoperation was about 60%.[38] Data from the STS registry shows an increasing use of PCI as the revascularization strategy of choice as the patient's age increases.[7]

Vein Graft Intervention

Although the benefit of PCI for native vessel stenoses has been firmly established and enhanced with DESs, graft conduit lesion interventions have been more controversial. Guideline statements[17,18] and appropriate use criteria[39] encourage the use of PCI in early graft failure but are less supportive of PCI in vein grafts in place for more than 3 years because of the risk of embolic MI and poor durability. Vein graft intervention is a class IIa indication for patients with severe symptoms, good LV function, and patent arterial grafts, and for patients who are poor candidates for reoperation. Appropriate use criteria indicated that SVG PCI was appropriate in patients with stable class III or IV symptoms or intermediate to high risk findings on non invasive testing.[40] Criteria for determining whether a vein graft stenosis is "significant" are similar to those for native vessel lesions, but the use of fractional flow reserve (FFR) has not been well studied in this setting. Because progression of atherosclerosis in SVGs exceeds that in native coronary arteries, some operators have been more aggressive in SVGs. Ellis and colleagues[41] noted that patients with moderate, untreated stenoses in SVGs had a much higher late cardiac event rate than patients without (45% vs. 2%). However, Rodes-Cabau and associates reported in a randomized comparison of PCI and medical therapy that PCI of intermediate nonobstructive SVG lesions did not reduce cardiac events at 3-year follow-up.[42] Therefore, PCI of moderate nonobstructive stenosis in SVGs is not supported.

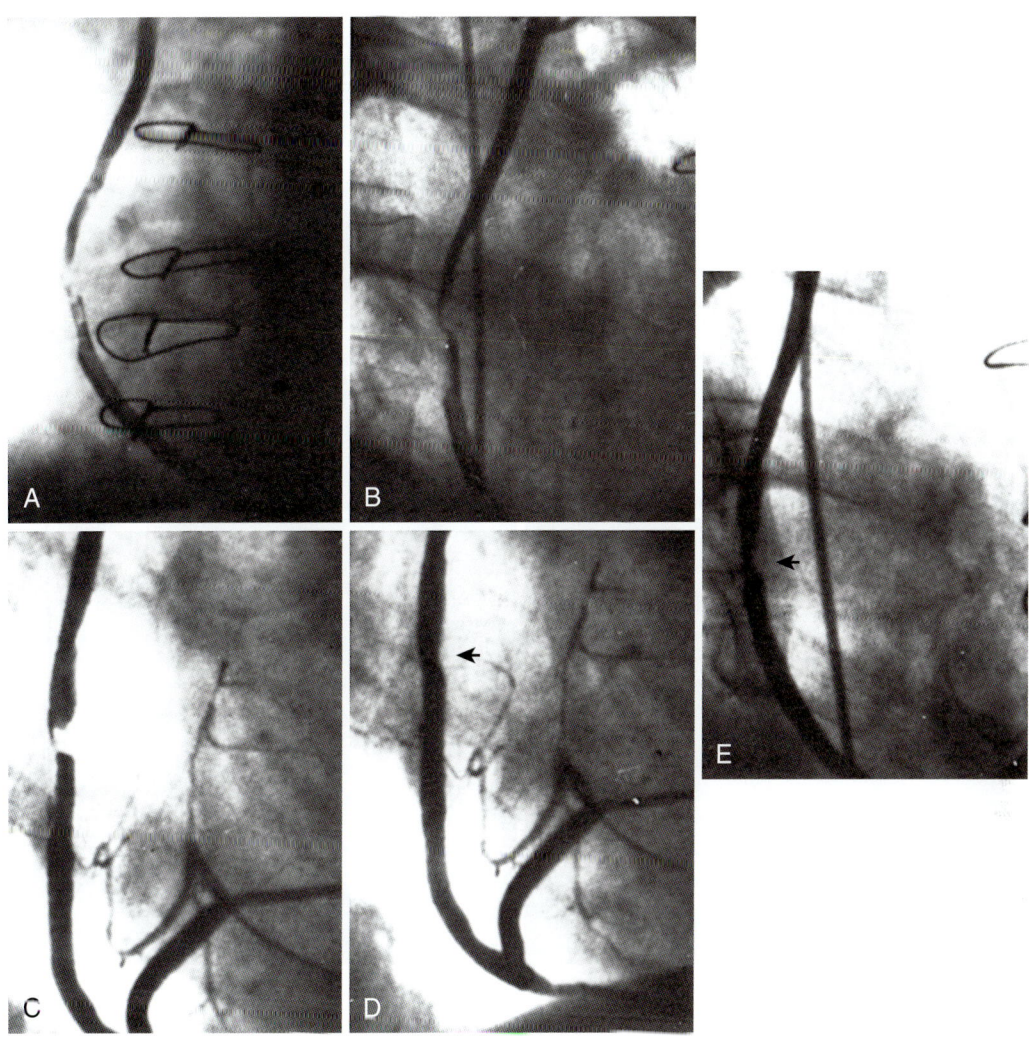

Fig. 27.6 A 59-year-old man developed recurrent rest pain 10 years after coronary bypass surgery. (A) Coronary arteriography revealed high-grade stenosis with thrombus and poor flow in a sequential saphenous vein graft (SVG) to the posterior descending and circumflex coronary arteries. No narrowing was present in the left anterior descending coronary artery, diagonal, and large anterior marginal systems. The inferior left ventricular wall was moderately hypokinetic. (B) After infusion of thrombolytic agent into the graft for approximately 1 hour, flow improved and thrombus was diminished. The patient was maintained on intravenous heparin for several days. (C) Coronary arteriography then showed that an eccentric, high-grade focal stenosis was present in the proximal SVG to the right coronary artery without thrombus. (D) After placement of a 4.0-mm stent *(arrow)*, the patient became asymptomatic. (E) Recatheterization 6 months later revealed excellent patency of the SVG with mild narrowing of approximately 40% at the stent site *(arrow)*. At last follow-up, the patient remained asymptomatic. The availability of thrombectomy and embolic protection make a more direct approach with thrombectomy appealing in some patients with extensive SVG thrombus.

Bare-Metal Stents Versus Balloon Angioplasty in Vein Grafts

In the first report of balloon angioplasty in SVGs, Grüntzig noted a higher than expected restenosis rate,[2] and subsequent experiences confirmed this finding.[3,4] Initial success rates of balloon angioplasty were higher in relatively ideal SVG lesions that were discrete and free of thrombus, but non–Q-wave MI occurred in 13% of 599 consecutive patients at Emory. Restenosis occurred in 68% of proximal lesions, 61% of midvein graft lesions, and 45% of distal lesions. These relatively poor results of balloon angioplasty in SVGs prompted use of bare-metal stents (BMSs). BMS implantation in native vessels had been shown to improve initial results by opposing elastic recoil achieving a larger lumen, to stabilize dissections avoiding need for emergency CABG and to reduce restenosis. However, the benefits associated with BMS in SVGs proved to be modest, as demonstrated in the Saphenous Vein De Novo (SAVED) trial, the seminal study that compared balloon angioplasty and BMS in SVGs.[43] A total of 220 patients with new SVG lesions and angina pectoris or objective evidence of myocardial ischemia were randomly assigned to implantation of Palmaz-Schatz BMS or standard balloon angioplasty. Patients with lesion length greater than two stents, MI within 7 days, or evidence of intragraft thrombus were excluded. Stented patients received warfarin anticoagulation. Patients assigned to stenting had a higher rate of procedural efficacy, defined as a reduction of stenosis to less than 50% of the vessel diameter with the assigned therapy, than did those assigned to angioplasty (Fig. 27.9), but they experienced more hemorrhagic complications resulting from warfarin anticoagulation. In-hospital complications were otherwise similar in the two groups, although a trend was observed toward fewer non–Q-wave infarctions in the

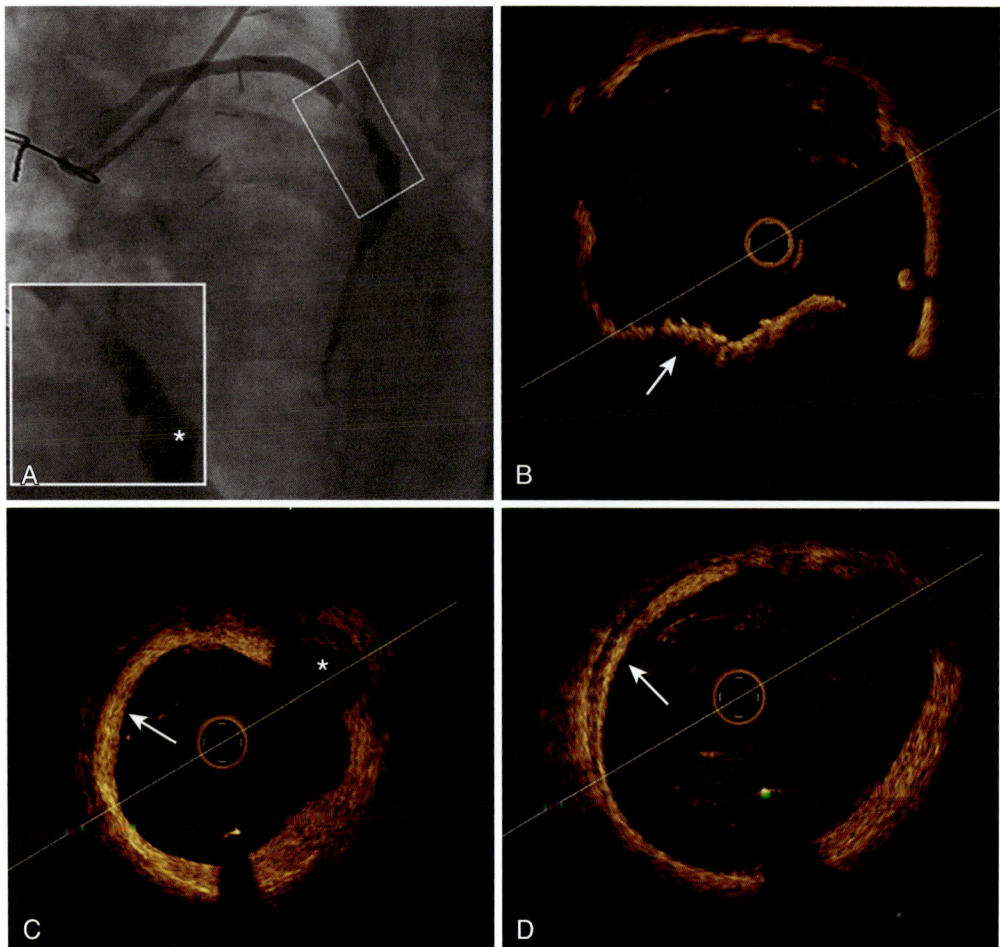

Fig. 27.7 Angiography and optical coherence tomography (OCT) of a saphenous vein graft (SVG) lesion in a patient with non–ST-segment elevation myocardial infarction. (A) Angiography of an SVG to left anterior descending coronary artery with severe narrowing and thrombus (white box). Plaque ulceration with a flap is shown in the magnification ( ). (B) OCT at the site of the lesion reveals red thrombus (arrow). (C) Intimal rupture with a large cavity underneath (*) is also apparent. In (C) and (D), arrows point to a signal-rich layer, under which a signal-free layer is evident that separates the former from the SVG wall. In all OCT frames, fibrofatty composition of the intima is evident. (From Davlouros, P, Damelou A, Karantolis V, et al. Evaluation of culprit saphenous vein graft lesions with optical coherence tomography in patients with acute coronary syndromes. J Am Coll Cardiol Intcrv. 2011,4:683–693.)

stent group. Whether stents have a significant effect in reducing particulate matter embolization is not certain, but it is a possible explanation for this trend. Restenosis occurred in 37% of the stented patients and in 46% of the angioplasty group ($P = .24$). The outcome in the SAVED trial with respect to freedom from death, MI, repeated bypass surgery, or revascularization was better in the stent group (73% vs. 58%; $P = .03$). The lack of a significant difference in restenosis rates in the treatment groups was due to the greater late lumen loss in the stent group and the small sample size.

Drug-Eluting Stents in Vein Grafts

Although BMSs improve the initial and intermediate-term outcomes of SVG PCI, the impact is modest owing to restenosis and disease progression. A number of published reports of the use of DESs in SVGs have shown conflicting results, leading some to question their use for this indication.[44] Five randomized comparisons of DESs with BMSs in SVGs have been reported involving a total of 1535 patients.[45–52] Two reported benefits, one harm, and two equal outcomes. Vermeersch and coworkers[45] implanted sirolimus-eluting stents (SESs) in 38 patients and BMSs in 37. At 6 months, patients who received SESs had less restenosis (14% vs. 33%, $P = .03$) and target-lesion revascularization (TLR; 5% vs. 22%, $P = .047$) but similar rates of death and MI. At a median follow-up of 32 months, "late catch-up" had occurred, and target-vessel revascularization (TVR) rates were comparable. Eleven deaths had occurred after DES, and none after BMS ($P = .001$).[46] A second randomized trial compared the outcomes of 41 patients treated with paclitaxel-eluting stents (PESs) with 39 treated with BMSs. Angiographic restenosis at 1 year occurred in 57% of BMS-treated SVGs and in 11% of PES-treated SVGs ($P < .0001$), and TLR was significantly less common with a PES at 1.5 years (5% vs. 28%, $P = .003$).[48] At 35 months, the target-vessel failure rate remained less in DES treated patients.[48]

The third randomized comparison of DES and BMS use in SVGs, the Is Drug-Eluting–Stenting Associated with Improved Results in Coronary Artery Bypass Grafts (ISAR-CABG) study, is the first powered for clinical end points.[49] In this superiority trial, 610 patients were randomly assigned to receive a BMS or one of three DESs. The primary end point—the combined incidence of death, MI, and TLR—was reduced significantly at one year by

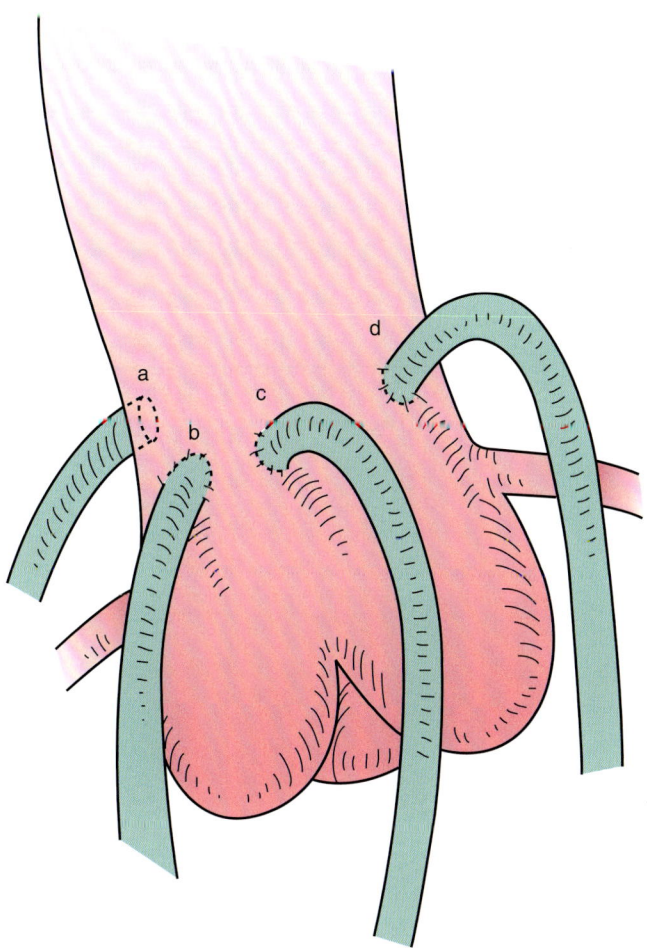

Fig. 27.8 Selection of guide catheters in vein graft angioplasty: *a*, Multipurpose shape; *b*, multipurpose, right Judkins; *c*, hockey stick, left Amplatz, right Judkins; *d*, hockey stick, left Amplatz. Obtaining adequate backup becomes more difficult in positions c and d.

DES use (15% vs. 22%, P = .02), as was TLR (7% vs. 13%, P = .01). No differences were observed in death, MI, or stent thrombosis at 1 year. Seventy-two percent of patients underwent routine follow-up angiography at a median of 6.7 months, and less restenosis (15% vs. 29%, P < .0001) and graft occlusion (6% vs. 12%, P = .008) were noted in DES-treated patients. At 5 years, the primary end point (death, MI or TLR) advantage of DES was lost (55% in DES; 54% in BMS group; P = .89) (Table 27.1).[50] At 5 years, TLR occurred in 33% of the DES group and 26% of the BMS group (P = .27) (Fig. 27.10A). Landmark analysis (see Fig. 27.10B) showed lower TLR rates in the DES group at 1 year but higher rates between 1 and 5 years.

The fourth randomized comparison of DES versus BMS in SVGs, known as BASKET-SAVAGE, was presented at the 2016 European Society of Cardiology.[51] A total of 173 patients with SVG disease were randomized to BMS (n = 84) or paclitaxel-eluting stents (DES, n = 89). The patients had a median age of 72 years and had received their SVGs a median of 13 years earlier. The primary end point (12 month major adverse cardiovascular event [MACE]) occurred significantly less often in the DES-treated group (2% vs. 18%, P < .001), driven largely by less TVR (0% vs. 12%, P < 0.001) and less MI (2% vs. 12%, P = .025). In a subgroup of patients followed up to 3 years, MACE was lower with DES-treatment (12% vs. 30%, P = .001), and the safety profile was similar.

The fifth randomized trial, the Drug-Eluting Stents Versus Bare Metal Stents in Saphenous Vein Graft Angioplasty (DIVA), is a blinded comparison of DES (89% second-generation DES) versus BMS in 25 Veterans Administration Hospitals.[52,53] Patients, mostly men, treated about 13 years after CABG, had similar characteristics, angiographic finding, and procedural techniques, including embolic protection in 69%. There was a significantly higher rate of periprocedural MI in the BMS group (8% vs. 3%, P = 0.016). There was no routine angiographic follow-up, which differs from some of the earlier randomized trials such as ISAR-CABG, where angiographic follow-up was encouraged and performed in 72% of patients. The primary end point, a 12-month composite of cardiac death, target-vessel MI, and TVR, was similar in DES and BMS treated patients (17% vs. 19%, P = .67), as were multiple secondary end points at 12 months (Fig. 27.11). Antiplatelet therapy was similar out to 36 months. Target-vessel failure during long-term follow-up (median 2.7 years) was similar with DES and BMS (see Fig. 27.11F).

The three randomized trials that focused on SVG patency suggested better results with DES, whereas the largest randomized trials, DIVA and ISAR-CABG, assessed important long-term clinical outcomes (death, MI, TLR, and TVR) and reported similar long-term outcomes. Because SVGs placed to arteries with noncritical lesions are more likely to fail and commonly without a clinical event, there is not a clear relationship between graft failure and clinical events. Although two-thirds of patients in ISAR-CABG received early-generation DES, which are no longer in clinical use, 89% of patients in DIVA received second-generation DES. The observation of late catch-up in adverse clinical events and restenosis is not a new phenomenon, as late lumen creep out to 2 to 4 years has been described following DES implantation, whereas neointimal formation peaks about 6 months after BMS implantation. The difference in coronary arterial and saphenous vein substrates may account for the more prominent late loss of benefit with DES implantation in SVGs. The similar and relatively poor long-term results in DIVA and ISAR-CABG emphasize the need to perform PCI on native vessels rather than SVGs whenever possible and call into question the use of more costly DES in SVGs.

Embolic Protection

Recently attention has refocused on the importance of periprocedural elevations of troponin, which indicate myocardial necrosis most often as a result of atheroembolism. Even when mostly straightforward, single-lesion, single-stent SVG PCI procedures were carried out prior to the availability of embolic protection, significant creatine kinase (CK) elevations were noted in 20% of patients (see Fig. 27.5). The rate of MI and procedural risk were shown to increase with lesion complexity, length, and estimated plaque volume.[54] In more than 3000 patients who underwent SVG stenting, CK-MB elevation was the most powerful predictor of late mortality.[55] The key role played by atheroembolization and confirmation of effective protective strategies were the products of several observational and randomized studies.[56–58] The GuardWire system (Medtronics, Minneapolis, MN [no longer available]) utilized a hollow 0.014-inch wire incorporating a compliant, inflatable distal occlusion balloon. During inflation of the distally placed balloon, flow in the graft was interrupted; the stent was then implanted, followed by aspiration of the graft using a special monorail catheter and deflation of the balloon to restore flow. The effectiveness of this strategy in a broad range of patients was confirmed in the Saphenous Vein Graft Angioplasty Free of Emboli Randomized (SAFER) trial,[56] in which 801 patients were randomly assigned to stent implantation with or without use of the GuardWire distal protection device. This study is the only randomized controlled trial of embolic protection versus no protection. Thirty-day MACEs were reduced by 42% with use of embolic protection (16.5% to 9.6%, P = .004), primarily because of the lower rates of MI. This system, frequently applicable even

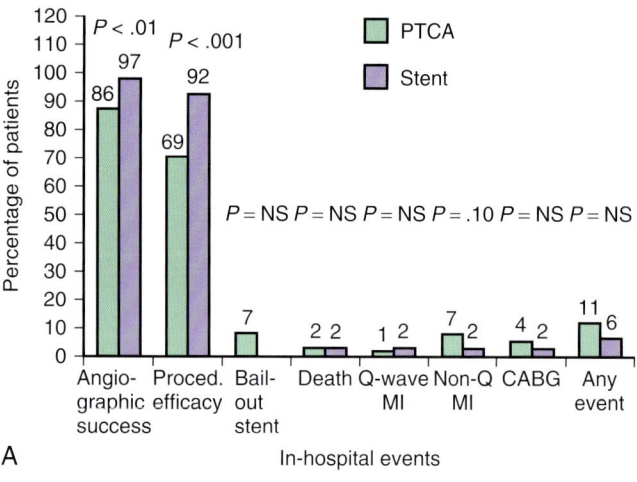
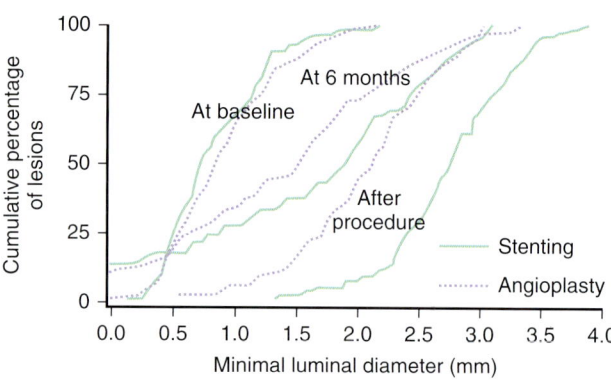
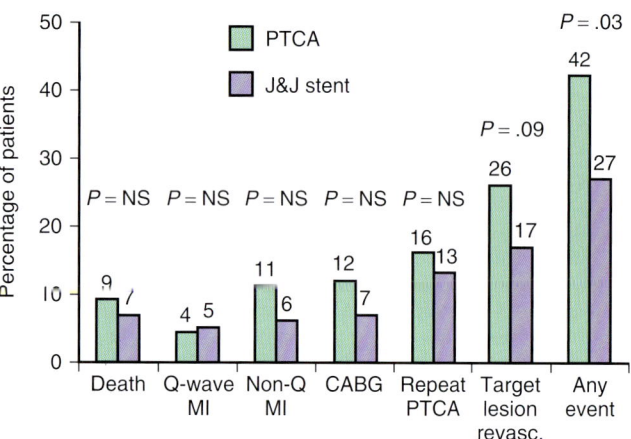

Fig. 27.9 Results from the Saphenous Vein De Novo trial, a randomized comparison of bare-metal stenting and standard balloon angioplasty. (A) Stents were associated with a higher procedural success rate, whereas other in-hospital events were similar. (B) The minimal luminal diameter at 6 months was larger in the stent group (1.73 vs. 1.49 mm; $P = .01$). (C) Late cardiac events were significantly more common in patients in the percutaneous transluminal coronary angioplasty *(PTCA)* group. *CABG,* Coronary artery bypass grafting; *J&J,* Johnson and Johnson; *MI,* myocardial infarction; *NS,* non significant; *revasc.,* revascularization. (From Savage MP, Douglas JS Jr, Fischman DL, et al.; for the Saphenous Vein De Novo Trial Investigators. Stent placement compared with balloon angioplasty for obstructed coronary bypass grafts. *N Engl J Med.* 1997;337:740–747.)

TABLE 27.1 Clinical Results at 5 Years in ISAR-CABG

	DES	BMS	*P* Value
N	303	307	
Cardiac death	18%	20%	.7
MI	8%	10%	.37
Stent thrombosis	2%	0.4%	.14
TLR	33%	25%	.27
TVR	40%	33%	.57
Death, MI, TLR	55%	54%	.89

BMS, Bare-metal stent; *DES,* drug-eluting stent; *ISAR-CABG,* Is Drug-Eluting–Stenting Associated with Improved Results in Coronary Artery Bypass Grafts; *MI,* myocardial infarction; *TLR,* target-lesion revascularization; *TVR,* target-vessel revascularization.
From Colleran R, Kufner S, Mehilli J, et al. Efficacy over time with drug-eluting stents in saphenous vein graft lesion. *J Am Coll Cardiol.* 2018;71:1973–1982.

in the presence of severe stenosis owing to its relatively low profile, captured small particles and soluble vasoactive agents such as endothelin, serotonin, and a variety of coagulation components that have been shown to be liberated during SVG PCI.[57] Analysis of the benefit of embolic protection in relation to lesion length in SAFER showed that even with lesions less than 10 mm in length, a 77% reduction in 30-day MACEs was experienced (2.2% vs. 8.1%). The use of this system increased costs at 30 days by less than $650 per patient, with a cost-effectiveness ratio of $3700 per year of life, making it highly cost-effective. Disadvantages of this form of embolic protection include the need to completely occlude the target SVG during stent deployment and aspiration (not always well tolerated), a requirement for a relatively long "parking" segment distal to the lesion, inability to protect side branches, the complexity of the system and added procedural time, cost, and potential for complications.

A variety of filters have been applied to SVG interventions, and filters have become the only form of embolic protection currently available (Fig. 27.12). In a 651-patient randomized multicenter trial, the FilterWire (Boston Scientific, Natick, MA) was compared with the GuardWire. The 30-day MACE rate, the primary end point,

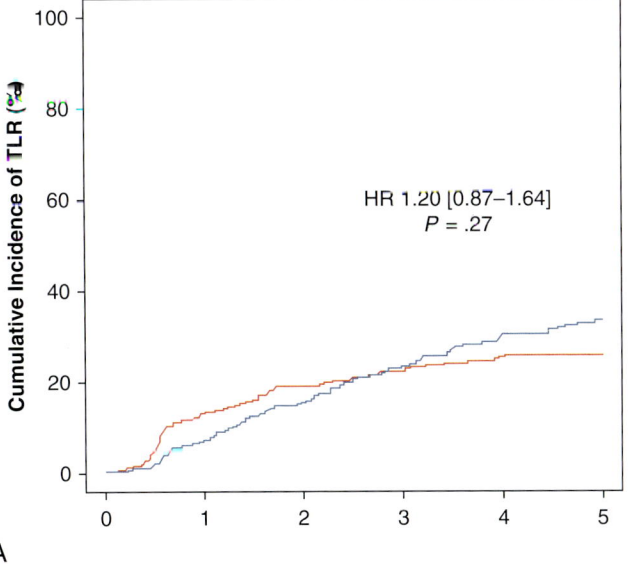

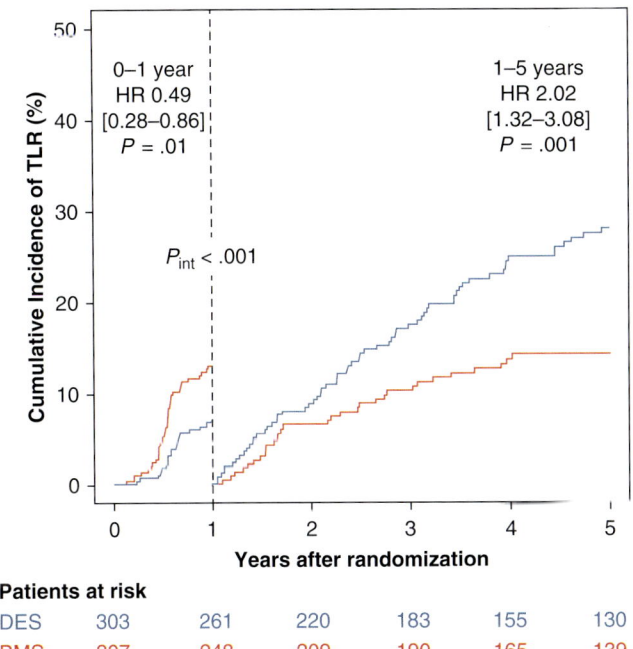

Fig. 27.10 Kaplan-Meier curves of target-lesion revascularization *(TLR)* from ISAR-CABG. (A) Kaplan-Meier curves showing cumulative incidence of TLR at 5 years. (B) Kaplan-Meier curves with landmark analysis showing cumulative incidence of TLR at 1 year and between 1 and 5 years. *BMS,* Bare-metal stent; *DES,* drug-eluting stent; *HR,* hazard ratio; *ISAR-CABG,* Is Drug-Eluting–Stenting Associated with Improved Results in Coronary Artery Bypass Grafts; *HZ,* Hazard ratio. (From Colleran R, Kufner S, Mehilli J, et al. Efficacy over time with drug-eluting stents in saphenous vein graft lesions. *J Am Coll Cardiol.* 2018;71:1973–1982.)

was similar—9.9% with the FilterWire compared with 11.6% with the GuardWire—and no difference was seen in rates of death or MI.[38] Some of the advantages of filters include ease of use, avoidance of ischemia because of preserved coronary flow, and good visualization of the site to be stented. Disadvantages include the need to cross the lesion with a somewhat bulky filter, which may require predilation and could cause embolization; these sequelae have been shown to increase the occurrence of Q-wave MI. In addition, some material may not be captured, including particles smaller than the 100-micron pore size and soluble agents. The former may not be relevant based on studies reporting that filtering was just as efficient as balloon occlusion in particle capture, despite pore sizes larger than the majority of embolic particles. Other problems with filters include the long distal parking segment required and the potential for overwhelming the filter, resulting in diminished antegrade flow that mimics the no-reflow phenomenon. Should this occur, the optimal strategy is to aspirate the stagnant dye column—which may contain suspended debris—followed by filter removal and replacement if more interventional work is needed. Unfortunately, a proximal protection device, applicable in patients with an inadequate "landing zone" beyond the lesion, is no longer available. When proximal protection was compared with either the FilterWire or GuardWire in a randomized trial, the rate of MACEs was comparable (9.2% vs. 10%, *P* = nonsignificant).[59] A number of filters are currently available that appear to be equally effective.

Expanding on the work of Liu and colleagues,[54] in an analysis of SVG stenting in 3958 patients from six studies, angiographic variables were found to be potent predictors of 30-day MACEs.[55] SVG degeneration score and large estimated plaque volume were the most potent predictors; thrombus, advanced patient age, and active tobacco use also contributed. When the occurrence of MACEs was analyzed relative to degeneration score or plaque volume, the use of embolic protection had similar relative treatment benefit across all categories of risk. The almost halving of MACE associated with embolic protection across all risk strata strongly supports its routine use in all PCIs of old SVGs. This contrasts sharply with the observation that embolic protection was used in only 22% of almost 20,000 patients who underwent SVG PCI in the NCDR in spite of a class I indication for the use of embolic protection in SVGs in the PCI guidelines statements.[60] Analysis of 49,325 senior patients showed a similar frequency of use of embolic protection (21.2%) and that EPD use was more common in high-risk subgroups (acute coronary syndrome, de novo lesions, and midgraft lesions).[61] The more frequent use of EPDs in high-risk patients helps explain the similar outcomes of EPD-treated patients and those without embolic protection in observational studies.[62] It is of interest that in the important ISAR-CABG study, in which 610 patients underwent SVG stenting, embolic protection was used in a minority of patients (<5%) and the 30-day MACE rate was low (4%).[49] The very selective use of embolic protection with favorable outcomes suggests that patient selection and current management strategies and more effective pharmacotherapy may all be contributing. The fact that 40% of patients in the control arm of SAFER underwent postdilation with a mean balloon size of 4.2 mm (mean reference vessel diameter of the entire group was 3.4 mm) may be one example of a change in technique that has occurred. Currently, most operators avoid postdilation of stents in SVGs and would certainly avoid use of a balloon larger than the reference vessel diameter. Clinical scenarios in which embolic protection may be expected to have little impact include lesions with very little plaque volume, in-stent restenosis lesions in which neointimal hyperplasia is the predominant pathology, and lesions that occur less than 3 years after CABG. In patients judged to have a high probability of atheroembolization, direct stenting, slight stent undersizing, use of longer stents, and use of embolic protection (filters) are potential strategies to mitigate this risk. The use of filters during stent implantation in ostial SVG lesions has been associated with serious complications due to difficulty in filter retrieval (see Chapter 29 for more information on embolic protection).[63]

Adjunctive Pharmacotherapy

Accepted adjunctive therapy during PCI of native vessels and SVGs includes antithrombotic measures—aspirin, antithrombin,

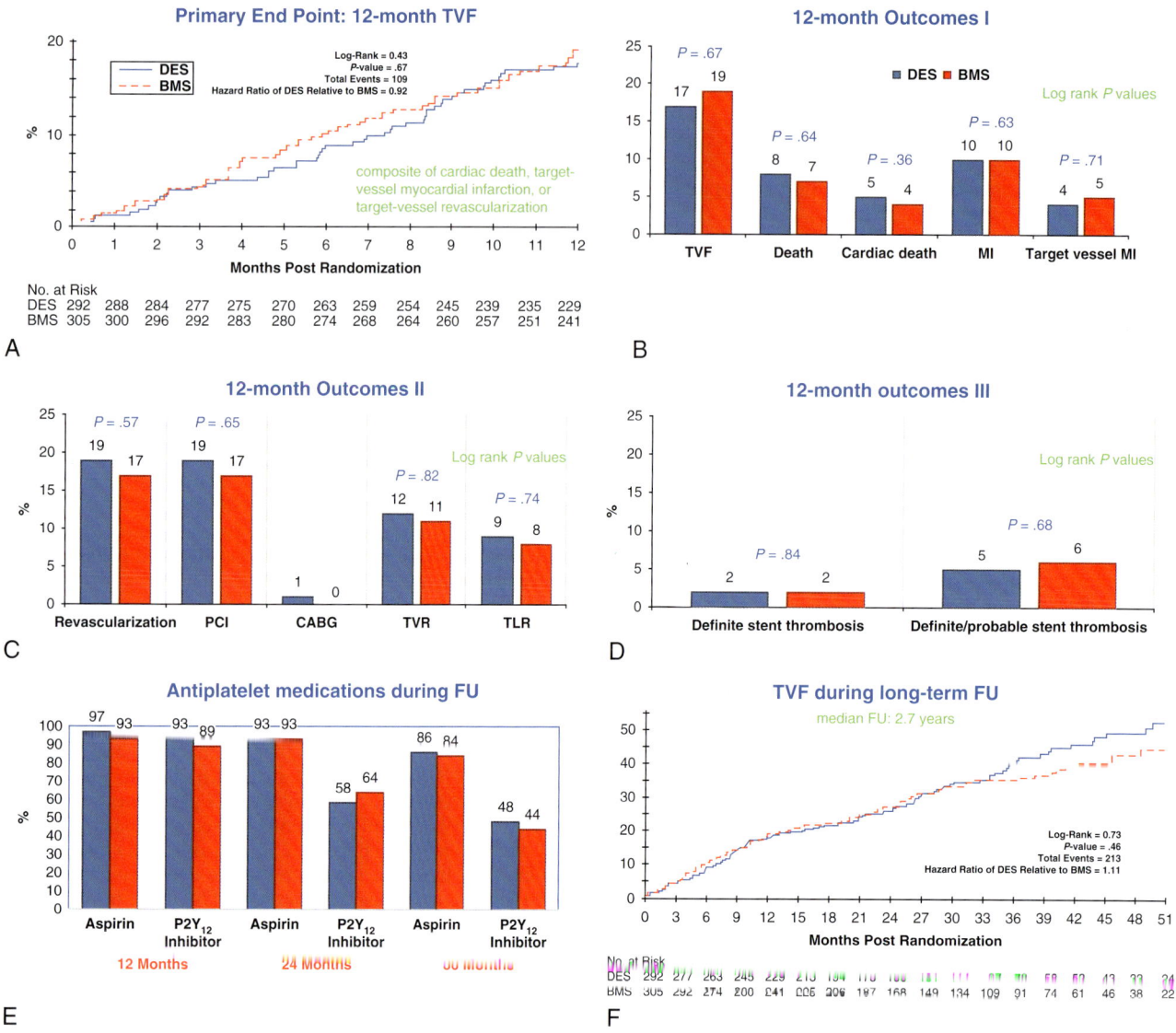

Fig. 27.11 Comparison of outcomes following drug-eluting stents *(DESs)* versus bare-metal stents *(BMSs)* implantation in saphenous vein graft (SVG) in the randomized Drug-Eluting Stents Versus Bare Metal Stents in Saphenous Vein Graft Angioplasty trial. *CABG,* Coronary artery bypass grafting; *FU,* follow-up; *MI,* myocardial infarction; *PCI,* percutaneous coronary intervention; *TLR,* target-lesion revascularization; *TVF,* target-vessel failure; *TVR,* target-vessel revascularization. (From Brilakis ES. Drug-eluting stents vs bare metal stents in saphenous vein graft angioplasty (DIVA) presented on behalf of the DIVA Trial Investigators and the Veterans Affairs Cooperative Studies Program #571 Study Group at the European Society of Cardiology Congress; August 26, 2017; Barcelona, Spain.)

other antiplatelet agents—and vascular dilators as needed for the prevention and treatment of slow or no reflow. Unfractionated heparin was used in the vast majority of SVG studies reported. Among the 403 SVG patients in the first and second Randomized Evaluation in PCI Linking Angiomax to Reduced Clinical Events (REPLACE) trials randomized to heparin or bivalirudin, logistic regression analysis revealed no difference in the combined end point—death, MI, urgent revascularization, or major bleeding—but less minor bleeding was observed with bivalirudin.[64] A somewhat increased risk of perforation with SVGs makes the use of bivalirudin, which is not reversible, less appealing in this group of patients; however, bivalirudin may be the best choice in certain patients with high bleeding risk. Optimal dosing and duration of dual-antiplatelet therapy (DAPT) following SVG PCI have not been well studied. Most operators recommend a bolus of 600 mg of clopidogrel prior to SVG PCI, followed by a dose of 75 mg daily for at least a year. A recently published cohort study of 411 post-SVG PCI patients who were event free at the time of clopidogrel cessation revealed a clustering of death or MI within 90 days. The cumulative 5-year event rate was lowest in patients treated with clopidogrel for more than 2 years ($P < .001$), which supports long-term DAPT following SVG PCI.[65]

The relatively large embolic burden encountered in SVG procedures provides some explanation of the failure of GP IIb/IIIa platelet receptor inhibitors to prevent periprocedural MI in these patients.[66–68] When data from five large trials—Evaluation of 7E3 for the Prevention of Ischemic Complications (EPIC), Evaluation of Percutaneous Transluminal Coronary Angioplasty to Improve Long-Term Outcome with Abciximab GP IIb/IIIa Blockade (EPILOG), Evaluation of Platelet IIb/IIIa Inhibitor for Stenting (EPISTENT), Integrilin to Minimize Platelet Aggregation and Coronary Thrombosis (IMPACT II), and Platelet

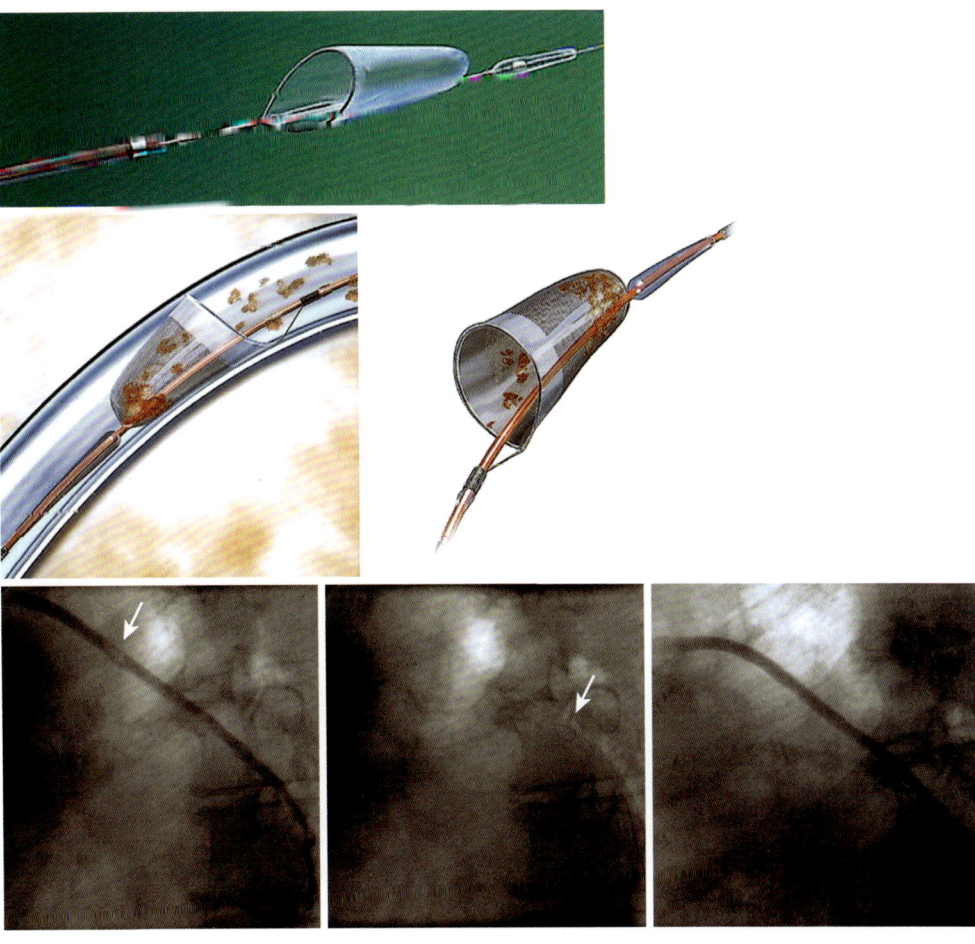

Fig. 27.12 The FilterWire. *Top panel:* The polyurethane nonocclusive filter with 110-μm pore size mounted on a nitinol loop fixed to a guidewire. *Middle, left panel:* The filter is deployed distal to the lesion and the nitinol is expanded to the size of the vessel (3.0 to 5.5 mm). *Middle, right panel:* Filter is removed with a large embolic load. *Bottom, left panel:* Thrombus (arrow) containing saphenous vein graft lesion. *Bottom, middle panel:* Deployed filter (arrow). *Bottom, right panel:* Excellent result after stenting. (From Gorog DA, Foale RA, Malik I, et al. Distal myocardial protection during percutaneous coronary intervention. When and where? *J Am Coll Cardiol.* 2005;46:1434–1445.)

Glycoprotein IIb/IIIa in Unstable Angina: Receptor Suppression Using Integrilin Therapy (PURSUIT)—with a total of more than 600 SVG PCI patients and data from the Cleveland Clinic registry were analyzed, there was no apparent benefit from GP IIb/IIIa inhibitors.[67] In spite of the class III recommendation in the 2011 PCI guidelines for the use of GP IIb/IIIa inhibitors in SVG PCI, selective use in certain patients with significant thrombus burden may be indicated.[68] The use of microvascular dilators to treat no or slow reflow following PCI, or their use prophylactically before the procedure, has not been well studied but is an important strategy in SVG PCI (see the discussion of the no-reflow phenomenon in the section that follows).

Restenosis Lesions in Saphenous Vein Grafts

The management of patients with restenosis of SVG stent sites is a topic of considerable interest and a significant clinical problem. As is true in native coronary intervention, treatment of in-stent restenotic lesions in SVGs is safer than treatment of de novo SVG lesions primarily because of reductions in slow or no reflow and periprocedural MI and reductions in dissection. In-stent restenosis lesions are a subset in which embolic protection can often be omitted because the pathology is mostly neointimal hyperplasia. In a double-blind randomized trial that included 120 patients with in-stent restenosis who received gamma radiation with Iridium-192 or placebo, Waksman[69] reported significantly lower restenosis in the irradiated group at 6 months compared with the control group and noted a 79% reduction in the need for repeat intervention. However, intracoronary brachytherapy is not currently available in most centers, and DESs have become the default strategy in spite of a paucity of data to support this application.

Total Occlusion of Saphenous Vein Grafts

Considering the relatively poor results of PCI in SVGs with focal stenoses, it is not surprising that complete occlusion with attendant large clot burden is hugely problematic. In the setting of STEMI and newly formed thrombus, results are suboptimal (as discussed previously); and as acuity wanes, thrombus resistance heightens, making percutaneous revascularization extremely challenging. In the subacute setting, thrombectomy (aspiration or rheolytic) with or without balloon angioplasty plus a strategy to dissolve thrombus (local or systemic GP IIb/IIIa or lytic agents, prolonged anticoagulation) achieved reasonable initial success in small cohort studies. Delaying stent implantation for days or weeks until the thrombus burden had largely resolved was the principal strategy in some reports,[70–73] and use of embolic protection and undersized stents was noted to avoid the consequences of embolization.[74] Although intervention in chronic total SVG occlusion received a class III recommendation in the 2011 PCI guidelines,[68] successful PCI was recently reported in about 70% of almost 100 patients, with 1- to 3-year cardiac mortality of 4.2%, MI in 14%, and TVR in about 30%.[73] Considering the narrow risk-benefit relationship, most experienced PCI operators do not attempt PCI in chronic total SVG occlusion.[72]

Internal Mammary Artery Grafts

Favorable results have been reported with balloon dilation of IMA graft stenoses. Lesions at the anastomoses of arterial grafts with the native coronary artery behave much like distal anastomotic lesions of SVGs. They usually occur within a few months of surgery and often respond to low-pressure balloon inflations.

Successful dilation and stenting of ostial or extremely proximal IMA graft lesions is infrequently required. In a report of PCI of 32 IMA graft lesions, 12 were in the midportion of the artery and 20 were at the anastomosis.[75] Gruberg and colleagues[76] reported outcomes of 174 patients with LIMA PCI (63% had lesions at the anastomosis) with 97% procedural success and TLR of 7% at 1 year. Success was achieved in over 90% of approximately 1000 patients in over 20 reports in the literature. Complications were infrequent, the most common being IMA dissection and spasm. No very large series or long-term data are available regarding stenting in IMA grafts or PCI in gastroepiploic or radial artery grafts.

COMPLICATIONS

Improved techniques, and especially stents, have made PCI safer, but complications still occur. Fortunately, the need for emergency surgery for failed PCI has plummeted from the 3.5% reported for 1263 post-CABG patients in the 1980s to less than 1%.[77] The most common complications are atheroembolic MI, bleeding, no reflow, and graft perforation. Embolic MI is minimized by avoidance of bulky SVG, lesions, by performing native vessel PCI, using embolic protection in SVGs when possible, using direct stenting and slight stent undersizing, and avoiding postdilation of stents in SVGs. In every case, the interventionalist is balancing risks and benefits: for instance, significant undersizing of a stent could lead to stent thrombosis or undesirable interactions between the stent and other equipment, such as intravascular ultrasound catheters or filters, which can become "entangled" by the unopposed stent edge. Bleeding is a major issue in elderly post-CABG patients and in women, and it is reduced by avoidance of GP IIb/IIIa inhibitors, use of radial access, and selective use of bivalirudin. Graft perforation and no-reflow phenomenon are discussed in the following sections.

Perforation

Coronary artery perforation is a potential complication of all coronary interventions. It has been attributed to vessel wall penetration with guidewires, inflation of a balloon in a subintimal location, overexpansion of a coronary artery or graft, atheroablative techniques, and stent implantation. SVG perforation is a rare but greatly feared complication. Prolonged balloon inflation and reversal of anticoagulation are effective in stabilizing most patients. However, in spite of the absence of pericardium and the scarring present after bypass surgery, vessel perforation may result in extensive hemorrhage, vessel occlusion, and cardiac tamponade or atrial compression, necessitating emergency surgery. Covered stents have had an increasing role in the treatment of perforation. In one report of 35 perforations, a polytetrafluoroethylene (PTFE)–covered stent was successful in sealing 100%.[78] Because of their large diameter, SVGs are favorable conduits for use of this strategy for sealing perforations. Although the use of oversized balloons has been advocated for vein graft dilations, older vein grafts may rupture with only modest oversizing. Because of this potential risk, it seems wise to size balloons and stents to the normal adjacent vessel or slightly smaller, and to plan ahead by having a covered stent of proper size available and by using a guide catheter capable of delivering the device.

No-Reflow Phenomenon

The cause of slow or no reflow following SVG PCI is multifactoral and includes vasospasm and embolization of atheromatous debris and thrombus. The importance of microvascular spasm is suggested by the observation that vasoconstrictors are released during SVG stent procedures, by the relief in no-reflow phenomenon when a calcium channel blocker is administered before SVG PCI, by the apparent treatment effect of small vessel dilators (calcium channel blockers, adenosine, nitroprusside), and by the lack of benefit of nitroglycerin.[79–83] When no reflow occurs or is expected, intracoronary administration of these agents is frequently effective. It is noteworthy that one study reported that aspiration of the stagnant dye column retrieving plaque gruel, and probably soluble vasoconstrictors liberated during SVG PCI,[81] was more effective than calcium channel–blocking agents in relieving no reflow. The important role of atheroembolism is apparent from the studies of embolic protection and pathology (see Fig. 27.5).[56–58]

THE FUTURE OF BYPASS GRAFT INTERVENTION

Thorny issues related to bypass graft intervention occupy both ends of the temporal spectrum. Intraoperative angiography has identified significant bypass graft problems, the treatment of which may enhance graft patency, improve clinical outcomes, and reduce the need for subsequent ischemia-driven repeat revascularization However, moderate anastomotic imperfections noted early after surgery have been shown to disappear subsequently (suggesting edema). It is not clear whether the information gained by routine intraoperative angiography is worth the added cost. Late-term SVG PCI is encumbered by atheroembolic MI and a high number of subsequent cardiac events due to restenosis and progressive vein graft disease. However, embolic protection strategies documented to be beneficial across the entire range of risk strata are markedly underutilized, and recent studies question the value of routinely employing embolic protection in SVG PCI. Are DESs sufficiently effective in SVGs to warrant the increased cost associated with their use? Is one DES more effective than others? The data are not compelling. And finally, can disease progression in nontarget sites be forestalled? Will the use of "plaque sealing" of moderate SVG lesions by DES implantation, which appeared promising in a pilot trial, be tested in the multicenter study required to corroborate these findings? In the future of bypass graft intervention, questions will outnumber answers.

KEY REFERENCES

2. Grüntzig AR, Senning A, Siegenthaler WE. Nonoperative dilatation of coronary-artery stenosis: percutaneous transluminal coronary angioplasty. *N Engl J Med.* 1979;301:61–68.
3. Douglas Jr JS, Gruentzig AR, King 3rd SB, et al. Percutaneous transluminal coronary angioplasty in patients with prior coronary bypass surgery. *J Am Coll Cardiol.* 1983;2:745–754.
4. Douglas Jr JS, King 3rd SB, Roubin GS. Percutaneous transluminal coronary angioplasty in patients with prior coronary artery bypass grafting. *J Thorac Cardiovasc Surg.* 1987;93:272–275.
8. Brener SJ, Lytle BW, Casserly IP, et al. Predictors of revascularization method and long-term outcome of percutaneous coronary intervention or repeat coronary bypass surgery in patients with multivessel coronary disease and previous coronary bypass surgery. *Eur Heart J.* 2006;27:413–418.
9. Zhoa DX, Leacche M, Balaguer JM, et al. Routine intraoperative completion angiography after coronary artery bypass grafting and 1-stop hybrid revascularization: results from a fully integrated hybrid catheterization laboratory/operating room. *J Am Coll Cardiol.* 2009;53:232–241.
25. Davlouros P, Damelou A, Karantalis V, et al. Evaluation of culprit saphenous vein graft lesions with optical coherence tomography in patients with acute coronary syndromes. *JACC Cardiovasc Interv.* 2011;4:683–693.
43. Savage MP, Douglas Jr JS, Fischman DL, et al., for the Saphenous Vein De Novo Trial Investigators. Stent placement compared with balloon angioplasty for obstructed bypass grafts. *N Engl J Med.* 1997;337:740–747.
49. Mehili J, Pache J, Abdel-Wahab M, et al. Drug-eluting versus bare-metal stents in saphenous vein graft lesions (ISAR-CABG): a randomized controlled superiority trial. *Lancet.* 2011;378:1071–1078.

50. Colleran R, Kufner S, Mehilli J, et al. Efficacy over time with drug-eluting stents in saphenous vein graft lesions. *J Am Coll Cardiol*. 2018;71:1973–1982.
53. Brilakis ES. Drug-eluting stents vs. bare metal stents in saphenous vein graft angioplasty (DIVA) presented on behalf of the DIVA Trial Investigators and the Veterans Affairs. Barcelona, Spain: Cooperative Studies Program #571 Study Group at the European Society of Cardiology Congress; 2017.
56. Baim DS, Wahr D, George B, et al. Randomized trial of a distal embolic protection device during percutaneous intervention of saphenous vein aorto-coronary bypass grafts. *Circulation*. 2002;105:512–590.
68. Levine GN, Bates ER, Blankenship JC, et al. 2011 ACCF/AHA/SCAI guideline for percutaneous coronary intervention. A report of the American College of Cardiology Foundation/American Heart Association Task Force on Practice Guidelines and the Society for Cardiovascular Angiography and Interventions. *J Am Coll Cardiol*. 2011;58:e44–e122.
83. Fischell TA, Subraya RG, Ashraf K, et al. "Pharmacologic" distal protection using prophylactic, intragraft nicardipine to prevent no-reflow and non-Q-wave myocardial infarction during elective saphenous vein graft intervention. *J Invasive Cardiol*. 2007;19:58–62.

Additional references available online at expertconsult.com.

中文导读

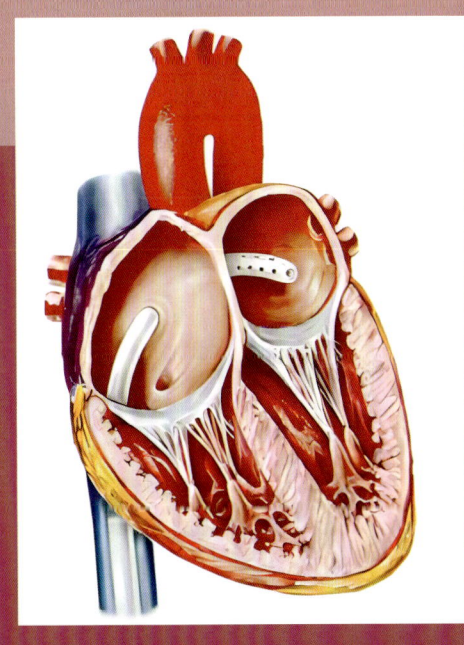

第28章
富含血栓病变

  由于冠状动脉疾病是全球导致死亡和发病的主要原因，含血栓病变的病理生理学和治疗具有极其重要的临床意义。血栓在急性和慢性缺血性冠状动脉综合征的病理生理学中都扮演着重要角色。在冠状动脉造影和介入治疗过程中发现含血栓的病变都提示手术变得复杂。这些病变表现为活跃、不稳定和复杂的血管动脉粥样硬化状态，通常需要特殊且迅速地处理。

  本章回顾了急性冠状动脉综合征病理生理学中的与血栓相关的最新概念，描述了血栓的结构及主要成分，包括纤维蛋白、血小板、红细胞和血管活性物质；并说明了其既是复杂介入的原因，又是其结果；描述了用于血栓识别、专用药物治疗和血栓清除策略；介绍了主要的血栓清除技术：手动抽吸、机械装置和栓塞保护系统；提出了一系列具有挑战性的含血栓病变及其相应的治疗方案。

  与上一版相比，本章节引用了与血栓的物理特征和生物学特征有关的新研究和独特发现。这一发展伴随着对含血栓病变的新认识，特别是关于胆固醇在动脉粥样硬化血栓病变的病理生理学中的存在作用。血栓对冠状动脉介入治疗的即时结果、短期和长期结果，以及主要和抢救的成本有重大影响。药物治疗和机械血栓切除装置可以单独使用或联合使用。尽管学者对含血栓病变的认识日益增加，但最佳治疗仍存在争议，且仍需进一步研究。

申学谦　柳景华

章节要点

- 从病理生理学而言，血栓在急性冠状动脉综合征、慢性缺血性冠状动脉综合征中都扮演着重要角色。
- 血栓是不稳定的动脉粥样硬化斑块的一个标志。
- 斑块破裂、斑块侵蚀和钙化结节是导致冠状动脉血栓形成的主要组织病理学基础。
- 动脉粥样硬化斑块的坏死核心及脂质含量，特别是坏死核内部胆固醇结晶的形态变化和动态变化，可影响血栓形成。
- 血栓的主要成分是纤维蛋白、血小板、红细胞和血管活性物质。
- 理解血栓的结构及成分、准确评估血栓负荷，对于制定适当的血运重建策略至关重要。
- 提高对血栓的诊断能力并加以分类可提高血栓病变治疗的有效性。
- 血栓对经皮冠状动脉介入治疗有着深远的影响，既可作为复杂介入治疗的原因，也可以是介入治疗所带来的后果。
- 尽管处理富含血栓病变，可直接参考ACC/AHA急性冠状动脉综合征治疗指南，但制定一套精确的经皮冠状动脉介入治疗流程治疗血栓病变仍然是一项具有挑战性的任务，这是因为冠状动脉血栓的复杂特征、局部潜在的动脉粥样硬化斑块，以及患者血管解剖特征并不完全相同。
- 当代血栓移除技术包括手动抽吸、电动机械装置和栓塞保护系统。
- 血栓专用技术应用经验存在很大差异。因此，目前对含血栓病变的治疗策略还存在很大分歧。
- 在急性冠状动脉综合征和其他血栓性心血管疾病中，为了确保血栓病变介入治疗的结局能得到进一步改善，开发新型药物和新技术就显得至关重要。

28 The Thrombus-Containing Lesion

On Topaz

KEY POINTS

- Thrombus plays a major role in the pathophysiology of acute and chronic ischemic coronary syndromes.
- Thrombus is a marker of active, unstable atherosclerotic plaques.
- Plaque rupture, plaque erosion, and calcified nodules are prominent histopathologic components causing coronary thrombosis.
- The necrotic core of the atherosclerotic plaque and its lipid content, especially the morphologic changes and dynamic movement of embedded cholesterol crystals, affect thrombus formation.
- The main constituents of thrombus are fibrin, platelets, red blood cells and vasoactive compounds.
- Understanding the architecture and structural components of the thrombus and proper burden assessment are essential for tailoring appropriate revascularization strategies.
- Enhanced capabilities of thrombus-defining diagnostic modalities and incorporation of thrombus classifications can increase the effectiveness of treatment.
- Thrombus has a profound impact on percutaneous coronary intervention (PCI), acting as a cause and a sequala of complicated interventions.
- Useful American College of Cardiology/American Heart Association guidelines for the management of patients with acute coronary syndromes are readily available, yet developing precise PCI algorithms for the management of thrombus-containing lesions remains a challenging task owing to the complex characteristics of the coronary thrombus, the presence of underlying atherosclerotic plaque, and the anatomic characteristics of the host vessels.
- The main contemporary technologies for thrombus removal are manual aspiration, power-sourced mechanical devices, and embolic protection systems.
- Experience with thrombus-dedicated technologies differs widely; therefore current treatment approaches to thrombus-containing lesions diverge considerably.
- The development of new pharmaceuticals and technologies is critical to ensure further improvement in the outcomes of interventions for thrombus-containing lesions in acute coronary syndromes and other thrombotic cardiovascular conditions.

INTRODUCTION

Thrombus and thrombotic lesions occupy the daily agenda of interventional cardiologists all over the world.[1] Accordingly, since coronary artery disease is the leading global cause of mortality and morbidity, the pathophysiology and management of thrombus-containing lesions are of paramount clinical importance. Based on the reports of the American Heart Association (AHA), the overall prevalence of myocardial infarction in the United States is at 7.6 million and that of stroke at 6.8 million.[2] The incidence and pathologic interrelationship between coronary plaque and associated thrombosis are displayed in Table 28.1.

The identification of thrombus-containing lesions during coronary angiography and intervention is ominous. These lesions represent active, unstable, and complex vascular atherosclerotic conditions that require specific and often expeditious management. Although significant progress has been made in the field as percutaneous coronary intervention (PCI) increasingly targets complex lesions with a remarkable high success rate,[3] thrombus-containing lesions continue to serve as markers of PCI-associated major adverse coronary events (MACEs), larger myocardial damage, stent thrombosis, increased rates of in-hospital complications, 6-month recurrent myocardial infarction (MI), and death.[4–9] Overall, there is a persistent impression that thrombus-containing lesions remain a considerable challenge to the performance of safe and efficacious revascularizations.[10,11] Consequently thrombus should be seen as a dual biovascular factor that, on the one hand, participates in the pathophysiology of coronary syndromes[12] and, on the other, serves as an initiator of PCI-related complications.[13,14]

Since the publication of the previous (seventh) edition of the *Textbook of Interventional Cardiology* in 2014, new research and unique discoveries pertaining to the physical characteristics and biologic features of thrombus have emerged.[15,16] This development has been accompanied by new insights into the understanding of thrombus-containing lesions, especially regarding the presence and the cardinal role of cholesterol in the pathophysiology of atherothrombotic lesions.[17] Accordingly, this chapter reviews updated concepts related to thrombus involvement in the pathophysiology of acute coronary syndromes (ACSs), describes the structural architecture of thrombus, and delineates its impact on interventions and outcomes. Specific imaging modalities for thrombus identification, dedicated pharmacotherapy, and thrombus removal strategies are delineated. A series of challenging thrombus-containing lesions and their corresponding management options are presented.

PROCESSES OF THROMBUS FORMATION: HISTOPATHOLOGY AND TYPES

Understanding the processes of thrombus formation in an atherosclerotic plaque and familiarity with the unique structural components of thrombus and their physical characteristics is crucial for the lesion-centered revascularization of atherosclerotic lesions and vessels.[18] Thrombotic lesions are formed when the fibrous cap of an atherosclerotic plaque develops structural defects.[19] Significant morphologic changes in the plaque become manifest by rupture, erosion, or fissure. Such weakening of the plaque's integrity exposes its necrotic core, an event that enables the movement of plaque material into the arterial lumen. The seminal research of Abela

TABLE 28.1 Coronary Thrombosis: Incidence and Etiology

Until 2000	Main Causes	
1. Plaque rupture	See footnote[a]	
2. Plaque fissure	See footnote[b]	
After 2000	**Main Causes**	
Autopsy-Based[c]	*OCT*-Based[d]	
1. Plaque rupture	65%	44%
2. Plaque erosion	30%	31%
3. Calcified nodule	5%	8%

[a]Stary HC, Chandler AB, Dinsmore RE, et al. A definition of advanced types of atherosclerotic lesions and a histological classification of atherosclerosis. A report from the Committee on Vascular Lesions of the Council on Arteriosclerosis, American Heart Association. *Circulation*. 1995:92:1355–1374.
[b]Davies MJ, Thomas AC. Plaque fissuring—the cause of acute myocardial infarction, sudden ischemic death and crescendo angina. *Br Heart J*. 1985;53:363–373.
[c]Yahagi K, Davis HR, Arbustini E, et al. Sex differences in coronary artery disease: pathological observations. *Atherosclerosis*. 2015;239:260–267
[d]Jia H, Abtahian F, Aguirre AD, et al. In vivo diagnosis of plaque erosion and calcified nodule in patients with acute coronary syndrome by intravascular optical coherence tomography. *J Am Coll Cardiol*. 2013;62:1748–1758.
OCT, Optical coherence tomography.

and colleagues has demonstrated the critical role played by cholesterol deposits within the plaque.[20] They elegantly demonstrated that cholesterol crystals within the plaque exhibit unique physical properties including dynamic movement that leads to perforation of the tunica intima, which in turn triggers further disruption (Fig. 28.1). These researchers clearly identified the cholesterol crystals as independent predictors of thrombus formation and subsequent adverse coronary and cerebrovascular clinical events.[20] The ensuing contact of exposed, disrupted, and highly thrombogenic subendothelial matrix and plaque with circulating platelets and white blood cells activates the coagulation cascade. The resultant platelet adhesion and aggregation leads to thrombus formation (Fig. 28.2). Furthermore, released tissue factor from the arterial injury directly activates the extrinsic coagulation cascade and promotes fibrin formation. Activated platelets release powerful promoters of vasoconstriction and aggregation, including serotonin, adenosine diphosphate, thromboxane A2, oxygen-derived free radicals, endothelin, and platelet activating factor.[21] Importantly, plaque rupture should be distinguished from plaque fissures. Plaque rupture is usually surrounded by an apparent luminal thrombus, whereas plaque fissure, in most instances, involves intraluminal thrombus composed of fibrin and platelets with interspersed erythrocytes. The thrombus related to fissure is most commonly small.[22] The delicate vessels within the plaque (i.e., the vasa vasorum) are a major cause of intraplaque hemorrhage. The mechanism behind this phenomenon is the disruption of microvessels lined by discontinuous endothelium without supporting pericytes.[23,24] Moreover, plaque erosion is generally associated with negative remodeling, whereas plaque

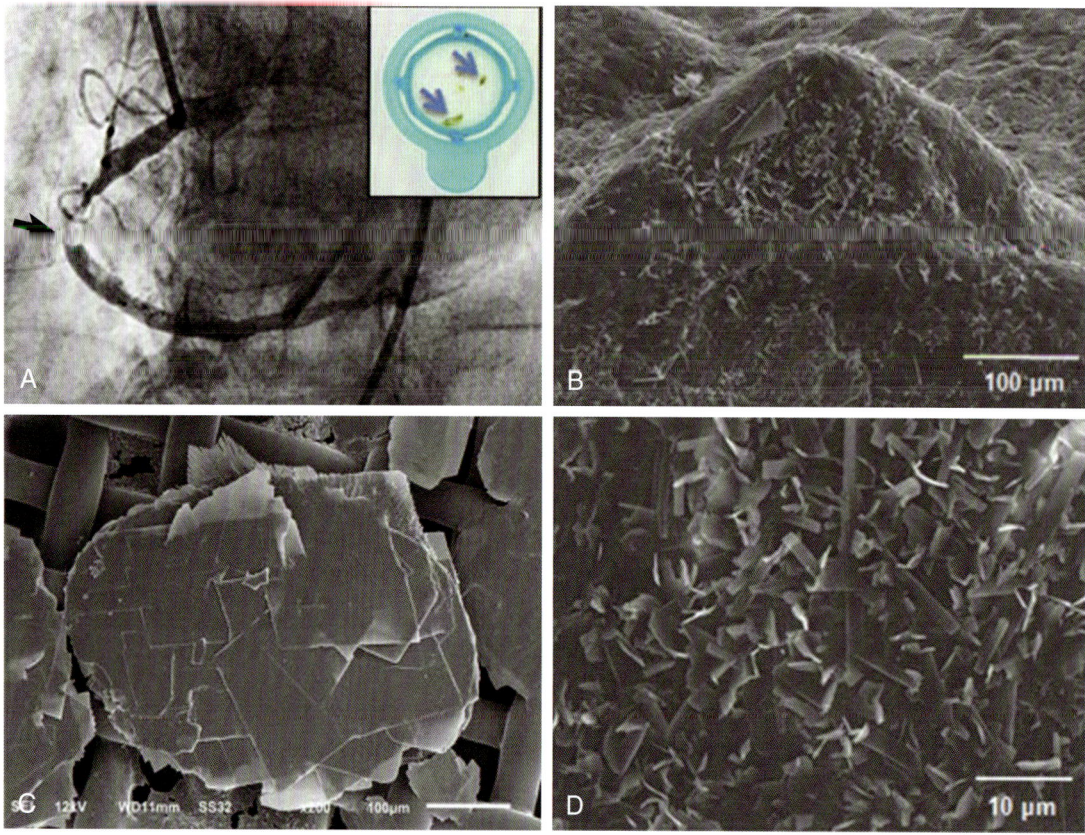

FIG. 28.1 Cholesterol crystals obtained from aspiration of an infarct-related coronary artery during acute myocardial infarction. (A) The right coronary artery exhibits angiographic filling defect *(black arrow)*. The insert demonstrates aspirate collected in a cup *(arrows)*. (B) A heap of aspirated materials with extensive cholesterol crystals embedded in debris. (C) Scanning electron microscope imaging of a large cholesterol crystal cluster (0.187 mm²) composed of many layers of merged individual plate crystals. (D) Dense aggregate of needle shaped cholesterol crystals. (From Lamichhane M, Salehi N, Ahmadjee A, et al. Pathology of arterial thrombosis: characteristics and thrombus types. In: Topaz O, ed. *Cardiovascular Thrombus: From Pathology and Clinical Presentations to Imaging, Pharmacotherapy and Interventions*. Philadelphia: Elsevier; 2018:15–30.)

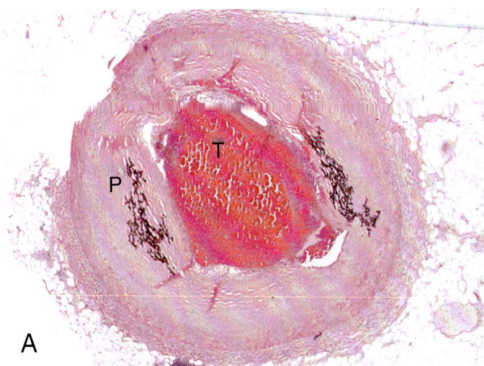
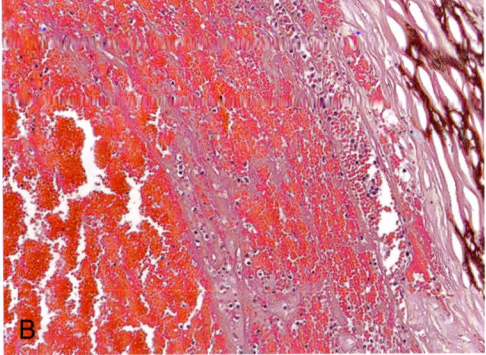

FIG. 28.2 High-power view of the right coronary artery. (A) Layering of acute thrombus *(T)*. (B) Red blood cells alternate between layers of fibrin (hematoxylin and eosin, 20×). *P*, Plaque. (Courtesy Shannon Mackey-Bojack MD, Jesse E. Edwards Registry of Cardiovascular Disease Collection, Nasseff Heart Center, United Hospitals, University of Minnesota School of Medicine, St. Paul, MN.)

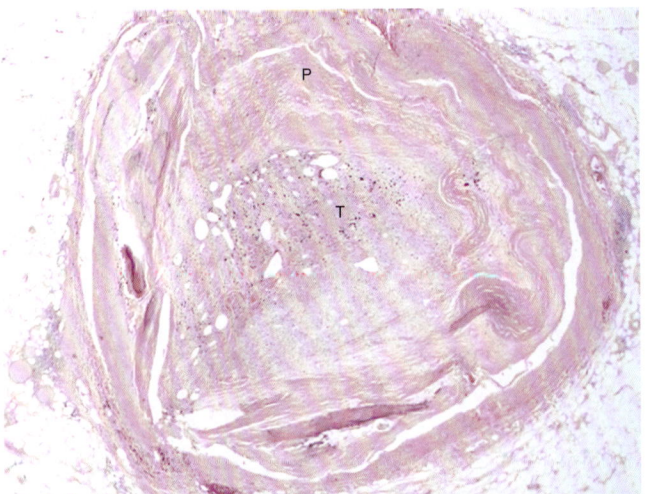
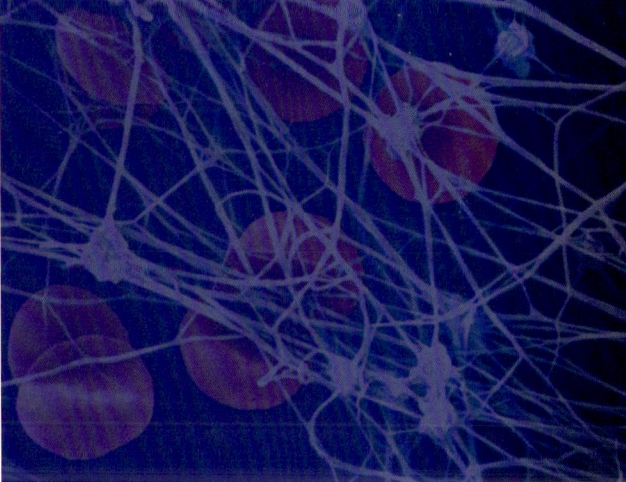

FIG. 28.3 Cross section of right coronary artery occluded by calcified, complicated atherosclerotic plaque *(P)* and organized thrombus *(T)* (hematoxylin and eosin, magnification 2×). (Courtesy Shannon Mackey-Bojack, MD, Jesse E. Edwards Registry of Cardiovascular Disease Collection, Nasseff Heart Center, United Hospitals, University of Minnesota School of Medicine, St. Paul, MN.)

FIG. 28.4 Scanning electron microscopy of a thrombus. Note the crisscrossing thick and thin fibrin fibers, which provide a scaffolding system for the thrombus. Platelets and red blood cells are attached to the fibrin net. (Courtesy Marc Carr Jr, MD, PhD, and Hemodyne Inc., Richmond, VA.)

rupture is associated with positive remodeling.[25] Also, erosions are frequently the cause of distal microembolization and resultant microvascular obstruction as compared with lesions constituting plaque rupture (71% vs. 42% respectively).[26] At the site of rupture or erosion, the thrombus is predominantly made up of aggregated platelets, whereas a propagated thrombus is red and consists of fibrin and red cells.[24] As the thrombus accumulates to form a critical obstacle (Fig. 28.3), impaired flow dynamics along and distal to the thrombotic lesion develop, frequently accompanied by vasoconstriction and resultant clinical ischemic coronary events.[27] During PCI, thrombus frequently exhibits structural variability as it adheres either loosely or sometimes quite firmly to the underlying plaque and the vessel's wall. Consequently and unpredictably, it exhibits either marked friability or unyielding rigidity in response to the mechanical forces generated by balloon and stent deployment. These contradictory physical properties stem from the cumulative effects of an assortment of the intra thrombus components.

THROMBUS ARCHITECTURE AND RELATED CHARACTERISTICS

Structurally, the thrombus is held by a scaffolding or platform made of fibrin fibers.[28,29] Two distinct types of branching fibers are organized in a three-dimensional (3D) network within the thrombus. Dense, thin fibers resist deforming mechanical forces and are poorly dissolved by thrombolytic agents. Thick fibers, on the other hand, are susceptible to the effects of external mechanical forces and are readily dissolved by thrombolytic therapy.[30] Recent discoveries have illuminated the major role that the clot's structure and function play in the pathogenesis of atherosclerosis, serving as novel risk factors for arterial and venous thrombosis and thromboembolism.[28] Platelets, red blood cells, vasoconstrictors, and procoagulant compounds are anchored to the matrix of the crisscrossing fibers within the clot (Fig. 28.4). Platelet dynamics also play a crucial role in the pathogenesis of atherosclerotic ischemic conditions.[31] Abnormalities in platelet function can persist and predict clinical events following PCI.[32] In patients presenting with ACS, the clot-adhering platelets typically effect a significant increase in the clot's contractile force, leading to increased platelet aggregation and causing the entire thrombus to exhibit a greater elastic modulus.[33] The platelets sustain and amplify the coagulant response at the plaque site and release procoagulant platelet-derived microparticles.[34]

Various biochemical processes and interactions between activated platelets, red blood cells, fibrinogen, vasoconstrictors, atherosclerotic material and the vessel's wall all have a substantial impact on the fibrin network. These constituents

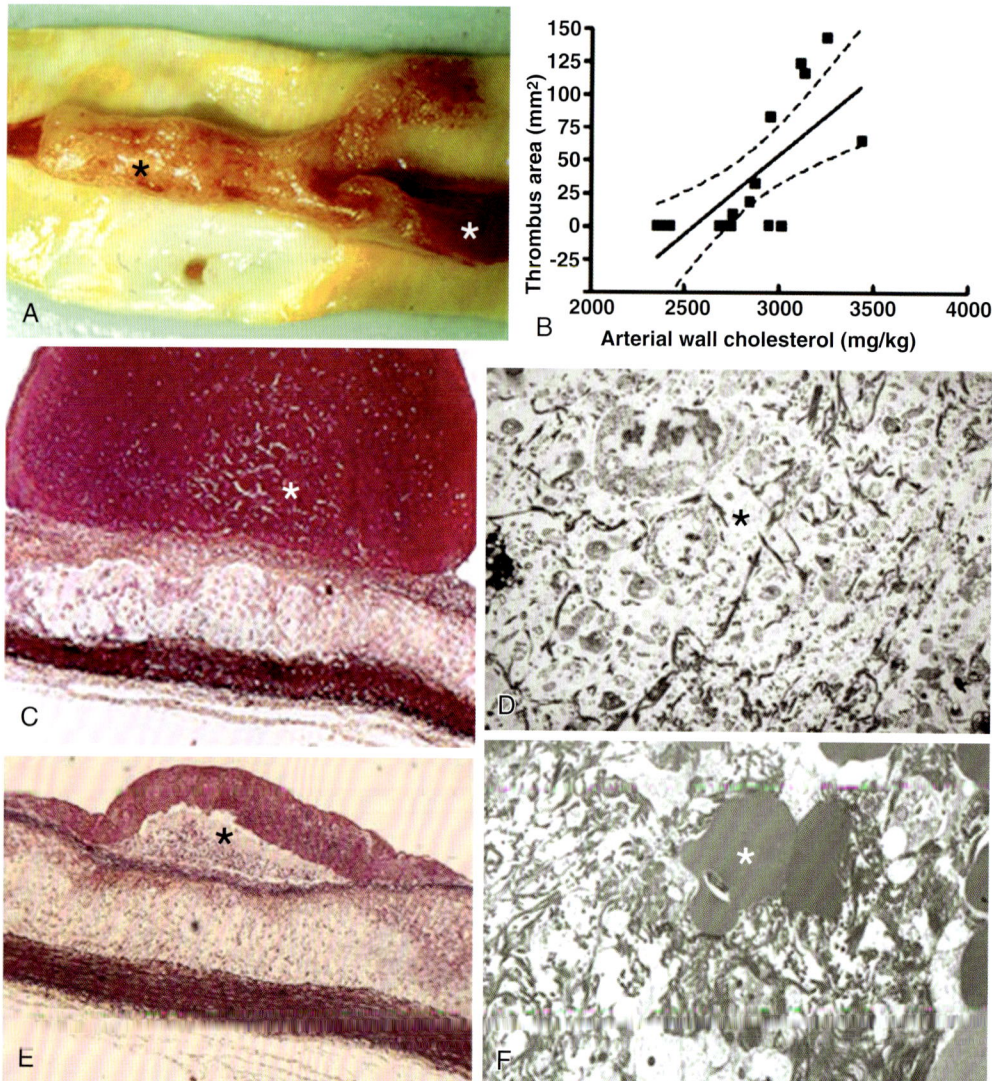

FIG. 28.5 Gross view of a predominantly white thrombus, as often seen in the atherosclerotic model of plaque disruption and thrombosis. (A) Gross view of a predominantly white thrombus. (B) Correlation between thrombus surface area and cholesterol content in an atherosclerotic arterial wall ($r = .71$, $P < .002$). (C) Light micrograph of a white thrombus overlying a plaque on the intimal surface of the aorta (Movat pentachrome stain, platelets stain red, magnification ×160). (D) Transmission electron micrograph of a white thrombus demonstrating a high platelets concentration with fibrin and few red blood cells (magnification = 3.4 × 2.5). (E) Light micrograph of a red thrombus overlying a plaque located on the intimal surface of the aorta (Movat pentachrome stain, magnification ×180). This demonstrates a dense surface thrombus layer with a loose inner core. (F) Transmission electron micrograph of red thrombus with loosely packed fibrin and many interspersed red blood cells (magnification ×2.5).(*) (From Lamichhane M, Salehi N, Ahmadjee A, et al. Pathology of arterial thrombosis: characteristics and thrombus types. In: Topaz O, ed. *Cardiovascular Thrombus: From Pathology and Clinical Presentations to Imaging, Pharmacotherapy and Interventions.* Philadelphia: Elsevier; 2018:15–30.)

account for the thrombus's level of activity, stability or instability, and for the overall "aggressiveness" of the thrombus as encountered during intervention. The presence and ratio of the previously mentioned components lead to the formation of distinct types of thrombi, each with unique rheolytic and mechanical properties. The two most prominent are the red and white thrombi. They can be detected by angioscopy[35] and their angiographic characteristics correlate with the histology of extracted thrombi.[36] The red thrombus has a dense surface and a loose inner core. Transmission or scanning electron microscopy demonstrates loosely packed fibrin and many interspersed red blood cells. The white thrombus consists of a dense structure lacking loose inner spaces, yet it contains a high concentration of platelets with fibrin and only few red blood cells (Fig. 28.5).[37] Based on histopathologic analysis of aspirated thrombotic contents, erythrocyte-rich (red) thrombus is found in about 35% of patients, mainly in those presenting with a low thrombosis in myocardial infarction (TIMI) flow. The platelet-rich (white) thrombus is identified in 65% of cases, especially in the early course of acute myocardial infarction (AMI).[38] Indeed, Silvan and colleagues found that the platelet and fibrin contents of the occlusive thrombi in acute ST-elevation myocardial infarction (STEMI) evolve rapidly; here ischemic time was found to have a high impact on the composition of thrombi, resulting in a positive correlation with intracoronary thrombotic fibrin content ($r = .38$, $P = .01$) and a negative correlation with platelet content

($r = -.34$, $P = .02$). Even within a population of patients treated with aggressive antithrombotic regimens, ischemic time was a key determinant of thrombus composition.[39] Sebben and colleagues analyzed the influence of the histopathologic features of coronary thrombi on the clinical outcomes in patients with STEMI. Among 331 patients who underwent thrombus aspiration, they identified a group of 199 whose aspirate was available for analysis. Recent thrombus was identified in 116 patients (58%) and old thrombus in 83 patients (42%). Recent thrombi had greater infiltration of red blood cells than old thrombi ($P = .02$), but there were no statistically significant differences between other clinical, angiographic, laboratory, or histopathologic features or medications in both group of patients. The clinical outcomes were similar in both groups.[40]

In many patients the occlusive thrombus is a mixture of red and white clot and the frequent resistance encountered in attempts to extract the thrombus suggests that certain clots contain layers upon layers of one thrombus type interspersed with the other.[41,42] Calcified nodules are an important albeit the least frequent cause of coronary thrombosis (5% prevalence). These lesions reside in highly calcified, tortuous arteries; they are characterized by a disrupted luminal surface and many calcified nodules with overlying thrombus and no necrotic core or only a minimal one.[4,43] From the perspective of the clinical management of coronary artery disease, the presence of major risk factors—such as smoking, male gender, and hypercholesterolemia—in patients with ACSs is known to influence plaque morphology adversely and is associated with a higher frequency of thrombus. Once the thrombus has formed, the size of the culprit lesion correlates with larger infarcts and worse left ventricular function. The size of the thrombus also relates to PCI-induced distal embolization. This was demonstrated in a pathologic analysis of aspirated embolized debris where the larger the thrombus at a culprit lesion was, the larger were the dimensions of the debris collected inside a filter.[44] In turn, the dimensions of the debris predicted arteriolar occlusion. A list of factors contributing the formation of high-grade thrombus in atherosclerotic lesions is given in Table 28.2.

DETECTION OF THROMBUS-CONTAINING LESIONS

Various invasive imaging modalities are available for the diagnosis of intracoronary thrombus. Numerous studies have demonstrated the poor sensitivity of angiography, although its specificity approaches 100% when multiple angiographic views are obtained for verification and strict definitions. Nevertheless, angiography remains the practical gold standard for the recognition of thrombus, demonstrating the classical findings of reduced contrast density, staining, haziness, irregular lesion contour, "filling defect," or a smooth convex meniscus at the site of a total thrombotic occlusion. When thrombus is suspected but not apparent angiographically, the optical coherence tomography (OCT) imaging modality[45,46] is the tool of choice (Fig. 28.6). Because of its user-friendly application and remarkable imaging quality, this technology has rapidly gained recognition and popularity among interventionalists.[47,48] Recently Negishi et al. demonstrated the usefulness of OCT in the evaluation of thrombi to determine whether a distal protection device should be applied in the setting of STEMI. Investigating the unique no-reflow phenomenon that affects filter protection devices, they found, through OCT analysis, that the length of the plaque's lipid pool plus the length of the thrombus served as an independent predictor of the filter protection no-reflow phenomenon.[49] Thrombus also appears to be involved in the long-term processes that determine plaque repair in the presence of an ACS. Souteyrand and colleagues used OCT to decipher the mechanisms of plaque complications causing ACS.[50] They discovered that in the months following a successfully dissolved acute thrombosis, OCT revealed that the cavities of ruptured fibrous cap plaques persist and are bordered by a smooth neointima, whereas intact fibrous cap plaques exhibited partial incorporation of the deepest layers of thrombus within the plaque. Other technologies for the detection of thrombi, which today are less commonly used, include intravascular coronary ultrasound[51,52] (Fig. 28.7) and, in some centers, percutaneous angioscopy.[53]

THE GRADING AND CLASSIFICATION OF THROMBI

Angiography remains the most practical imaging modality for the identification and quantification of intracoronary and peripheral arterial thrombi during the diagnostic and intervention portions of cardiac and vascular catheterization. The classification systems for thrombi and related scoring systems are useful for the quantification and qualification of the thrombus burden.[54] Then these classifications provide a clinical/angiographic correlation that affects management decisions prior to, during, and after intervention.

The widely used TIMI grading classification was published in 1985 by the TIMI study investigators.[55] This pioneering scale was based on the recognition that the yield of thrombolytic therapy for evolving AMI was defined by the varying sizes and load of angiographically evident intracoronary thrombi. Relying on visual assessment of angiographic views demonstrating the thrombus size as compared with the diameter of the host vessel, this classification defined thrombus as follows: grade 0 means the absence of angiographic characteristics indicating thrombus; grade 1—determined by reduced contrast density, haziness, irregular lesion contour, or a smooth convex meniscus at the site of total occlusion—is suggestive but not diagnostic of thrombus; grade 2 means that thrombus is definitely present, its greatest dimension being half the

TABLE 28.2 Factors Contributing to the Formation of a High-Grade Thrombus

MYOCARDIAL INFARCTION–RELATED
1. Absence of preinfarction angina
2. Late presentation (>12 h) after onset of acute myocardial infarction
3. Recent Q-wave myocardial infarction with continuous chest pain and ischemia
4. Cardiogenic shock

LESION-RELATED
1. Acute plaque rupture; complex morphology and proximal culprit lesion

VESSEL-RELATED
1. Slow or stagnant antegrade coronary or SVG flow
2. Large anatomic size increasing thrombus formation; accumulation in native coronary vessels and SVGs
3. Morphology: ectasia, aneurysm, old SVG
4. Failed thrombolysis

PERCUTANEOUS CORONARY INTERVENTION-RELATED
1. Triggering of the plaque and accompanying thrombus with guidewire, balloon, or stent: formation of the angry clot phenomenon
2. Inadequate anticoagulation during intervention
3. Poor stent apposition to the vessel's wall
4. Lack of/premature or abrupt cessation of thienopyridines
5. Hypercoagulopathy
6. Heparin-induced thrombocytopenia and thrombosis (HITT)
7. Vasculitis
8. Increased white blood cells
9. Hyperglycemia
10. Methamphetamines
11. Cocaine
12. Sports performance enhancing agents

SVG, Saphenous vein graft.

SECTION III Coronary Intervention

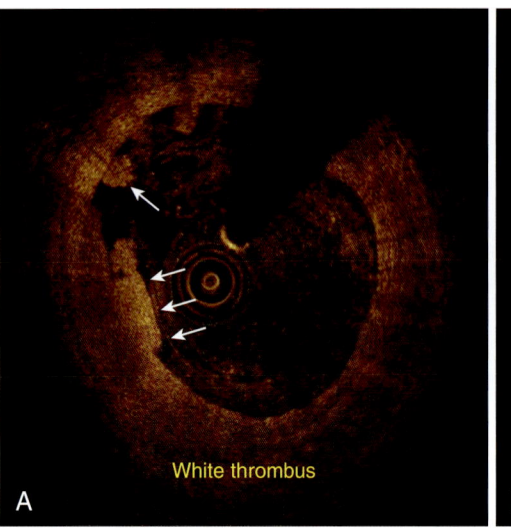
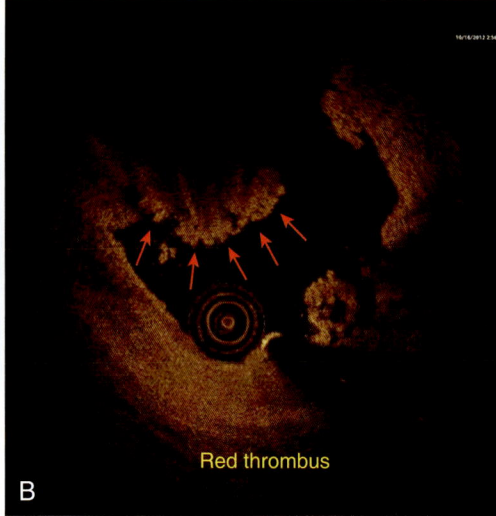

FIG. 28.6 Optical coherence tomography demonstrates white thrombus (A, *arrows*) and red thrombus (B, *arrows*). (Courtesy Peter O'Kane, MD, Cardiac Intervention Unit, Department of Cardiology, Dorset Heart Center, Royal Bournemouth Hospital, Bournemouth, UK.)

FIG. 28.7 Utilization of coronary intravascular ultrasound (IVUS) for thrombus detection. A 65-year-old diabetic smoker, noncompliant with medications, had a history of coronary artery disease including previous stenting and developed an acute coronary syndrome. Intracoronary thrombus *(red arrow)* in the middle segment of the left anterior descending artery was identified with a 45-MHz Revolution IVUS catheter (Volcano, San Diego, CA). The thrombus was aspirated with a Priority One aspiration catheter. The culprit plaque received a Synergy drug-eluting stent, and the clinical results were adequate.

TABLE 28.3 The Thrombolysis in Myocardial Infarction Angiographic Thrombus Classification

	Definition[a]
Grade 0	No angiographic characteristics of thrombus
Grade 1	Possible angiographic features of thrombus include decreased density of contrast, haziness, irregular lesion contour, or a smooth convex meniscus at the site of total occlusion suggestive but not diagnostic of thrombus
Grade 2	Definite thrombus present in multiple angiographic views: markedly irregular lesion contour with a significant filling defect. The thrombus's greatest dimension is half of the vessel's diameter
Grade 3	Definite thrombus in multiple views with its greatest dimension ranging from one-half to two vessel diameters
Grade 4	Definite large thrombus with greatest dimension larger than two vessel diameters
Grade 5	Complete thrombotic occlusion of the vessel: a convex margin that stains with contrast and persists for several cardiac cycles

[a]Gibson CM, de Lemos JA, Murphy SA, et al. Combination therapy with abciximab reduces angiographically evident thrombus in acute myocardial infarction—a TIMI 14 sub-study. *Circulation.* 2001;103:2550–2554.

vessel's diameter; grade 3 also means that thrombus is present, its greatest dimension being between half the vessel's diameter and less than two vessel diameters; grade 4 indicates the presence of thrombus with its largest dimension being more than twice the vessel's diameter; and grade 5 indicates that the vessel is completely occluded. Table 28.3 details the parameters of the classic TIMI thrombus grading scale.

Specific angiographic images representing the classic TIMI thrombus grading scale are demonstrated in Fig. 28.8.

Although this classification is user friendly and universally accepted, the accuracy of both the score's lowest level (i.e., grade 0) and the highest level (i.e., grade 5) is considerably suboptimal. With its hallmark characteristic of TIMI 0 flow, the ischemia or infarct-related vessel containing a thrombus grade 5 is totally occluded. Consequently the actual ratio between the volume of the underlying plaque and the associated thrombotic volume is unknown, yet the assumption of the TIMI score is that this grade represents the greatest thrombotic burden. Therefore interventionalists from the Thoraxcenter, Rotterdam, in the Netherlands,[7] introduced an important step of restratification for the evaluation and management of grade 5 thrombus as detailed in Table 28.4.

The first step of this process involves the advancement of a PCI guidewire or a 1.5-mm balloon aimed at crossing the occlusive thrombus (Fig. 28.9). This intervention is expected to

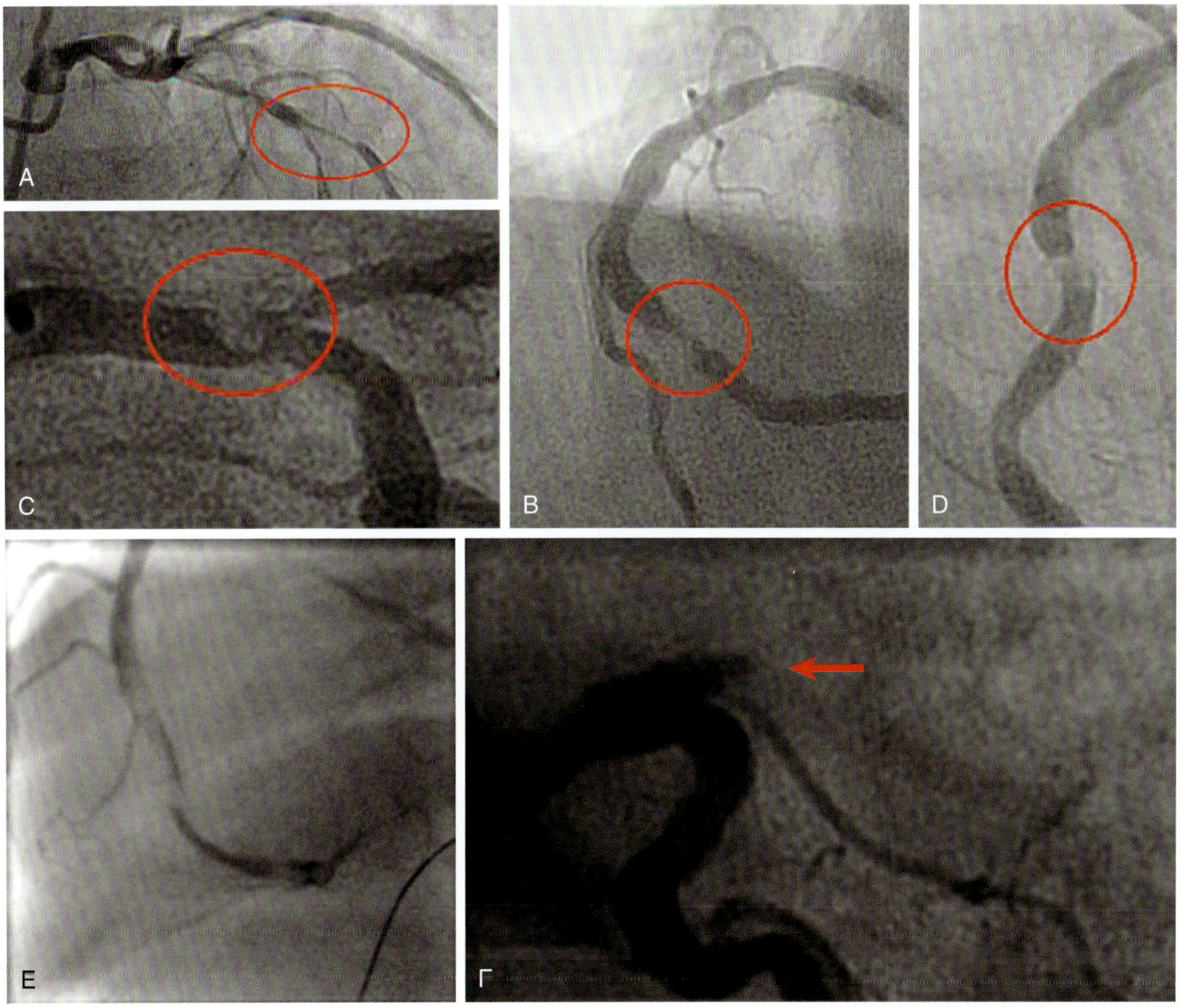

CHAPTER 28 The Thrombus-Containing Lesion

FIG. 28.8 Grades of thrombus as defined by the classic thrombolysis in myocardial infarction (TIMI) thrombus grading. (A) Grade 0: No thrombus present. The marked plaque *(red circle)* exhibits smooth and clear borders without haziness located in the middle segment of the left anterior descending artery. (B) Grade 1: Suspected thrombus in the plaque occupying the middle-distal right coronary artery *(red circle)*. (C) Grade 2: Eccentric plaque and associated thrombus located in the distal left main coronary artery *(red circle)*. (D) Grade 3: Thrombus in the middle segment of the right coronary artery *(red circle)*. (E) Grade 4: Represented by heavy layers of thrombus almost completely obstructing distal flow. (F) Grade 5: Total thrombotic occlusion of the proximal left anterior descending artery in a patient with an acute anterior wall myocardial infarction *(red arrow)*. (From Topaz O, Topaz A. Thrombus classifications: critical tools for diagnostic and interventional cardiovascular procedures. In: Topaz O, ed. *Cardiovascular Thrombus: From Pathology and Clinical Presentations to Imaging, Pharmacotherapy and Interventions*. Philadelphia: Elsevier; 2018:175–187.)

TABLE 28.4 Thrombus Grade 5: The Reclassification Process[a]

Intervention aimed at crossing the thrombotic occlusion in order to restore antegrade flow. Once a measure of flow has been gained, the size of the exposed underlying thrombus is stratified as follows:

Small thrombus—grades 1–3

Large thrombus—grade 4

[a]Sianos G, Papafaklis MI, Daemen J, et al. Angiographic stent thrombosis after routine use of drug-eluting stents in ST-segment elevation myocardial infarction: the importance of thrombus burden. *J Am Coll Cardiol*. 2007;50:572–583.

recanalize the thrombus and restore antegrade flow. Accordingly a newly exposed thrombus scored as grade 1, 2, or 3 is a relatively *small* thrombus; one scored as grade 4 is a relatively *large* thrombus. Therefore additional revascularization devices can be applied. From a practical stand point, a stratified small residual thrombus can be successfully managed with an aspiration catheter and adjunctive stenting. Adjunctive pharmacotherapy can be chosen as well. For postrecanalization removal of a large thrombus, especially when resistance is encountered during initial aspiration, utilization of a power-based mechanical thrombectomy device may be required.[41] Among the useful devices for this task are rheolytic thrombectomy,[56,57] excimer laser,[58,59] and the X-Sizer thrombectomy device.[60,61] When stenting is required in the presence of a large thrombotic load, the choice of a dedicated thrombus-capturing stent is a valid management option.[62,63]

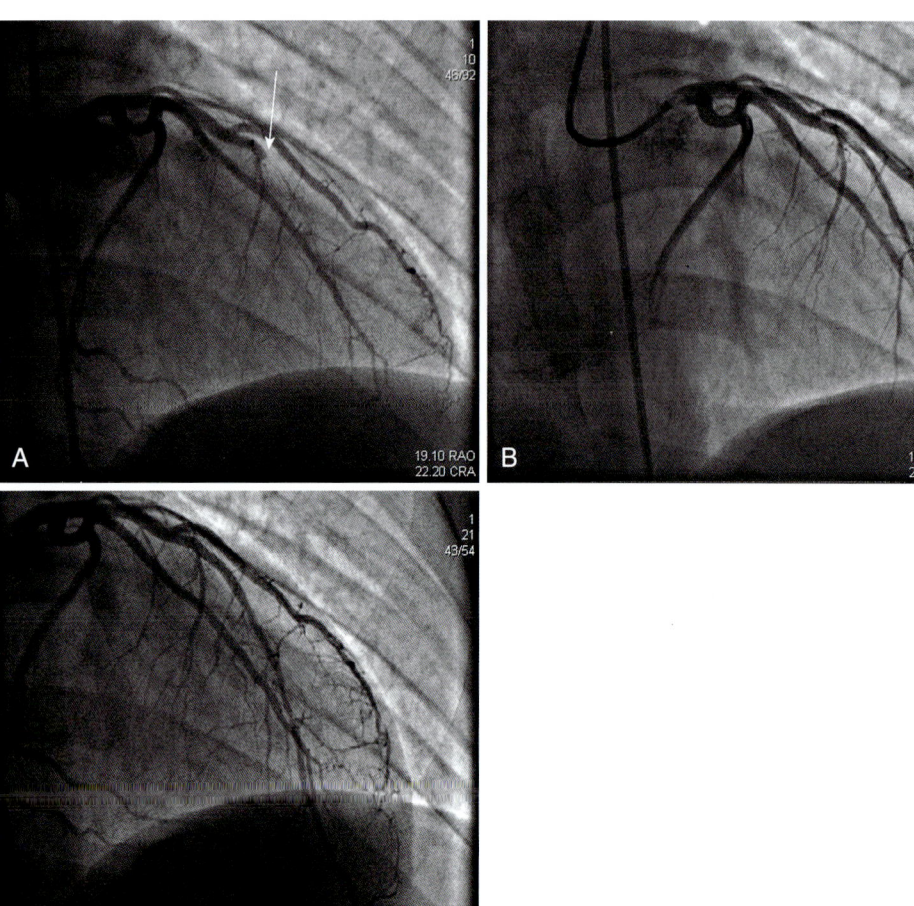

FIG. 28.9 **Grade 5 thrombus.** (A) Intervention-based reclassification of grade 5 with a guidewire traversing the occlusive left anterior descending coronary artery thrombus *(arrow)*. (B) Guidewire restratification of the thrombus to a small residual burden at the site of the underlying plaque. (C) Restratification enabled a revascularization strategy based on treatment with standard balloon intervention and stenting.

The usefulness of this reclassification extends beyond its application in all patients with AMI and ischemic coronary disease who exhibit TIMI 0 antegrade flow due to grade 5 thrombus. However, growing experience with dedicated thrombus removal strategies reveals that the Thoraxcenter's restratification method calls for a modification to correct the inherent erroneous a priori assumption that *every* grade 5 thrombus can be restratified. In reality, all grade 5 thrombi are not alike, and they certainly exhibit varying responses to the process of restratification. Recognizing these facts, we have recently introduced a new modification to the restratified TIMI score for grade 5 thrombi based on the identification of three distinct types of thrombi (i.e., A, B, and C).[64]

The angiographic features of the new modification are presented in Table 28.5 and illustrated in Fig. 28.10.

Another innovative classification was introduced by Aleong and colleagues. It relies on the combined analysis of edge detection and video-densitometry-based quantitative coronary angiography for the enhancement of quantitative thrombus assessment. Their experience with this method indicates that it quantifies the thrombotic volume accurately.[66] A different, practical classification by Niccoli is presented in Table 28.6.

Altogether, while the usefulness and merits of the contemporary angiography-based classifications of thrombus scores are highly valuable, some limitations must be recognized. First, reliance on the visual interpretation of angiography implies an inherent observer bias that can decrease accuracy. Indeed, underestimation of presence and size of thrombus occurs when angiographic assessments are compared with more accurate imaging methods such as OCT, coronary ultrasound, and angioscopy. Moreover, the current classifications fall short of differentiating between types of thrombus (i.e., white vs. red) and do not define the thrombotic content within chronic total occlusions. Third, thrombus classifications neither describe nor take into account the underlying morphology and severity of the accompanying atherosclerotic plaque. This is of a concern especially when heavily calcified lesions may also contain thrombus. Nevertheless, it should be recognized that angiography remains the most user friendly and least expensive imaging modality currently available for thrombus-related management decisions during PCI. As such, angiographic thrombus classifications continue to serve as highly relevant clinical tools. In that regard, it is intriguing to realize that the Syntax scoring system[67,68]—which is a useful scoring system serving as a differentiator for the outcome of patients undergoing PCI for three-vessel and unprotected left main coronary disease—gives only one point for the presence of thrombus without any further classification.[69]

TARGETED THROMBUS REVASCULARIZATION STRATEGIES

The indications for targeted thrombus revascularization are displayed in Table 28.7.

For patients with a suspected or small thrombus (corresponding to TIMI grades 1 to 2), the aspiration catheter is considered

TABLE 28.5 A New Modification of the Thrombus Grade 5 Restratification Process: Identification of Three Distinct Thrombus Types[a]

Type A: Guidewire successfully crosses and recanalizes the occlusive thrombus with partial or complete restoration of forward flow.
Type B: Guidewire crosses the occlusive thrombus and is positioned distally but fails to restore any forward flow.
Type C: Guidewire fails to cross the occlusive thrombus and TIMI 0 flow remains.
Grade 5 type A: This type of occlusive thrombus permits a guidewire or a small balloon to cross; as a result, at least partial restoration of antegrade flow is achieved.
Grade 5 type B: Represents a thrombus that initially permits guidewire recanalization and a small balloon inflation, yet *restoration of antegrade flow* cannot be achieved and TIMI 0 flow remains. The interventionalist can then choose to apply a larger balloon or a mechanical thrombectomy tool. If this succeeds, the target is regraded as a type A. Otherwise this thrombus remains as a grade 5 type B.
Grade 5 type C: Represents a thrombus that totally resists crossing by the guidewire. Consequently there is no change in the shape and size of the targeted thrombotic occlusion and TIMI 0 flow remains. Such a scenario suggests that practically, the combined morphology of the underlying atherosclerotic plaque and the large thrombus burden constitute an impenetrable chronic total occlusion. Another practical thrombus grading classification was published by Nicoli and colleagues.[65] It is delineated in Table 28.6.

[a]Topaz O, Topaz A. Thrombus classifications: critical tools for diagnostic and interventional cardiovascular procedures. In: Topaz O, ed. *Cardiovascular Thrombus: From Pathology and Clinical Presentations to Imaging, Pharmacotherapy and Interventions*. Philadelphia: Elsevier; 2018:175–187.

TIMI, Thrombolysis in myocardial infarction.

---

to be the tool of choice. However, management of a significant (TIMI grade 3) or heavy thrombus burden (TIMI grades 4 to 5) is challenging due to the common occurrence of friable thrombotic material dislodged by the balloon and stent.[70] Embolization of fragmented thrombotic particles obstructs flow within the distal arterial segments, side branches, and myocardial microvessels. Overall, in patients with ACS who undergo standard PCI, distal embolization occurs in the range of 6% to 15% for all lesion types and is associated with up to a sevenfold increase in the rate of periprocedural MI. In most instances resultant severe ischemia, microinfarctions, an inflammatory response, and contractile dysfunction reduce coronary reserve, causing deleterious effects on recovery and salvage.[71] Moreover, the optimal myocardial blush score of grade 3 is gained in only 28% to 35% of PCI patients who had a final TIMI 3 epicardial flow,[72,73] thus attesting to the limited yield of standard PCI in thrombus-containing lesions. This condition is classically termed the "illusion of reperfusion,"[74] which succinctly presents the marked discrepancy between primary PCI-gained TIMI 3 flow versus the disappointing suboptimal degree of subsequent myocardial salvage. The main cause is the prevalent intracoronary thrombus and related distal embolization, microvessel obstruction, no reflow, and myocardial necrosis.[73,75] Clearly patients who develop procedure-related no reflow tend to sustain larger infarct sizes, significantly worse left ventricular function, and a greater risk of adverse cardiac events and death. A recent Australian study by Mazhar and colleagues identified the phenomenon in a series of 189 patients in whom multivariate analysis identified thrombus scores ≥4, symptom-to-balloon time ≥360 minutes, and age above 60 years as independent predictors of no reflow.[76] Similarly, a recent Chinese study determined the factors related to the no-reflow phenomenon in 203 patients with STEMI who underwent direct PCI, finding five risk factors including high thrombus burden.[77] Indeed, cumulative evidence shows that these complications are especially pronounced among patients who undergo primary PCI for AMI.[6,7,78] The Thrombus Aspiration during Percutaneous coronary intervention in Acute myocardial infarction Study (TAPAS) project studied the sequelae of angiographically visible distal embolization in 883 STEMI PCI patients on triple antiplatelet therapy.[6] The aspirated thrombus was larger in patients with evidence of angiographic embolization versus those without ($P = .002$), and it more often contained erythrocytes (50% vs. 15.7%, $P < .001$, respectively). Those who sustained angiographically evident embolization had significantly worse outcomes than patients without, as indicated by a lower myocardial blush grade, impaired ST-segment resolution and a higher level of myocardial enzyme leakage. As compared with the revascularization of thrombus-free lesions, embolization significantly increased the need for emergency bypass surgery and the procedure-related death rate.[79] At 1-year follow-up, reinfarction occurred in 8.9% of the TAPAS patients versus only 3.0% in patients without embolization ($P = .018$). Thus the thrombus's effect on the development of adverse coronary events and suboptimal outcomes should be taken into consideration and dealt with promptly before, during, and after PCI.[80–82] The overall impact of thrombus on PCI is presented in Table 28.8.

The principles governing the mechanisms of action and interaction with targeted thrombus that involve specific thrombus treatment strategies are described in Table 28.9.

PHARMACOTHERAPY

The mainstay pharmacologic therapies for the management of thrombus-containing lesions include aspirin, heparin, 2b/3a platelet receptor antagonists, thienopyridines (clopidogrel, prasugrel, ticlopidine), and direct thrombin inhibitors.[83] The benefit of a decreased thrombotic burden can be achieved even before an intervention, thus improving the PCI results and reducing the risk of distal thrombotic embolization. Specifically, chronic aspirin therapy has been shown to decrease the burden of thrombus before stent deployment[84]; heparin reduces fibrin formation and platelet contractile forces, and the 2b/3a receptor antagonists markedly reduce platelet aggregation and aggregate size while also increasing the access of thrombolytic agents to platelet-rich clots.[83,85,86] Nevertheless these pharmaceutical agents are less effective in an already formed active unstable thrombus,[7] especially in the presence of a high thrombus grade. For example, significant limitations of pharmacologic therapy are apparent in the PCI to old saphenous vein grafts (SVGs) containing a large thrombus burden.[87] Suboptimal PCI results in these thrombotic grafts are manifested by inadequate ST resolution at 60 minutes, limited prevention of distal embolization, and an insufficient degree of revascularization. Thus in ACSs with lesions containing a significant clot burden, improved PCI outcomes require a mechanical removal strategy.[88]

MECHANICAL THROMBUS REMOVAL

Adjunctive Thrombectomy

Contemporary mechanical thrombus removal or dissolution devices can be categorized into four main types according to their activation mode: (1) manual aspiration catheters, (2) embolic protection, (3) power-sourced thrombectomy, and (4) ultrasound-induced sonication.

Overall, thrombus removal devices are user friendly owing to their relatively small size and convenient rapid delivery. Their efficiency contributes to the reduction of procedure-related radiation exposure. A different classification defines thrombus extraction devices as "simple" (i.e., aspiration based) or "complex" (i.e., mechanically based).[89] This categorization is supported by a meta-analysis of 17 randomized trials on thrombus removal versus standard PCI comprising 3909 patients[90] which found that thrombus removal was associated with a significantly greater likelihood of TIMI 3 flow, grade 3 myocardial

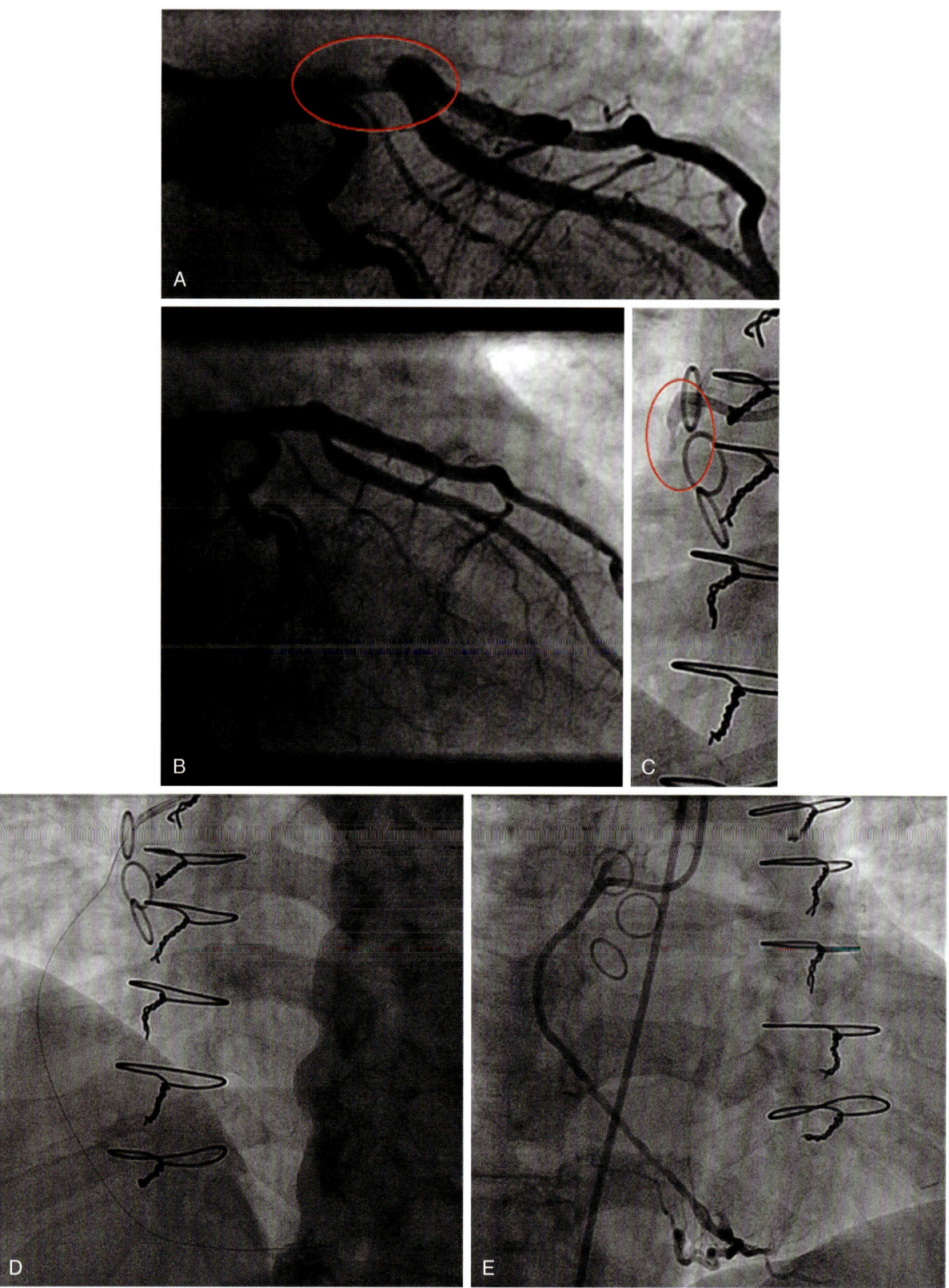

FIG. 28.10 (A) The new modification of the Thoraxcenter grade 5 thrombus. Restratification of the grade 5: with a guidewire and a small balloon, the thrombus was transformed to grade 2 *(red circle)*. Thus the initial thrombus corresponds to thrombus grade 5 type A. (B) Final percutaneous coronary interventions results after stenting of the target lesion, demonstrating marked patency of the vessel and no residual thrombus (final grade 0). (C) Thrombus grade 5 in the ostium-proximal portion of an old saphenous vein bypass graft in a patient with unstable angina and ischemia of the inferior lateral wall *(red circle)*. (D) Grade 5 stratification enabled in guidewire to cross the total thrombotic occlusion and be positioned distally, but antegrade flow was not restored. This corresponds to grade 5 type B. (E) Final angiography after application of excimer laser and stenting over the guidewire reveals adequate patency of the old graft with no residual thrombus. (From Topaz O, Topaz A. Thrombus classifications: critical tools for diagnostic and interventional cardiovascular procedures. In: Topaz O, ed. *Cardiovascular Thrombus: From Pathology and Clinical Presentations to Imaging, Pharmacotherapy and Interventions.* Philadelphia: Elsevier; 2018:175–187.)

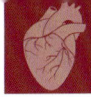

CHAPTER 28 The Thrombus-Containing Lesion

TABLE 28.6 Thrombus Grading: A Two-Grade Scale[a]

A *low* thrombus grade corresponds to TIMI thrombus grades 1–3.
A *high* thrombus grade corresponds to TIMI thrombus grades 4 and 5.

[a]Niccoli G, Spaziani C, Marino M, et al. Effect of chronic aspirin therapy on angiographic thrombotic burden in patients admitted for a first ST-elevation myocardial infarction. *Am J Cardiol.* 2010;105:587–591.
Due to the frequent difficulty of precisely differentiating between TIMI thrombus grade 1 and TIMI thrombus grade 3, this bilevel classification incorporates only two grades of angiographic thrombus: a *low* grade corresponding to TIMI thrombus grades 1–3 and a *high* grade representing TIMI thrombus grades 4 and 5. It is noteworthy that, similar to the traditional TIMI classification, this bilevel categorization is useful in the assessment of thrombus burden in old saphenous vein bypass grafts. Nevertheless, this classification is less useful when the underlying thrombus is angiographically assessed as of an "*intermediate*" size (i.e., between a "*small*" and a "*large*" load).
TIMI, Thrombolysis in myocardial infarction.

TABLE 28.7 Indications for a Targeted Thrombus Revascularization Strategy

CLINICAL

Stable and unstable angina, acute coronary syndromes: ST-elevation myocardial infarction and non–ST-elevation myocardial infarction when the clinical condition is associated with a need to
1. significantly decrease the thrombus burden in atherosclerotic lesions
2. remove thrombus acting as a barrier to antegrade flow
3. reduce the threat of thrombotic embolization
4. reduce the risk of no reflow

PATHOLOGIC

1. Atherosclerotic thrombotic plaques
2. Stent thrombosis
3. Intracoronary thrombus secondary to hypercoagulability or to the formation of an angry clot
4. Thrombus emboli lodged in a coronary artery or saphenous vein graft

TABLE 28.8 Impact of Thrombus on Percutaneous Coronary Interventions

- Thrombus risks clinical outcome during and post intervention
- Thrombus negates and adversely effects crossing of the target lesion and related vessel
- Thrombus specifically Increases intervention related risk of distal embolization and subsequent no-reflow phenomenon; creation of acute thrombotic occlusion; periprocedural myocardial infarction; emergency bypass surgery and death
- Thrombus is a strong predictor of major adverse coronary events; early and late stent thrombosis; in-hospital complications; risk of 6-month recurrent myocardial infarction and death
- Thrombus management may prolong procedures and increase their cost
- Thrombus embedded in chronic thrombotic occlusion can provide microvascular channels that in some cases may be helpful in crossing the lesion

TABLE 28.9 Thrombus Treatment Strategies: Mechanisms of Action

Pharmacotherapy: dissolution and suppression
Displacement: guidewire, balloon, covered stent
Removal: aspiration catheters
Capture: dedicated stent platforms
Extraction: rheolytic thrombectomy, X-Sizer
Maceration: Thrombocat
Vaporization: laser
Ultrasonication: intracoronary ultrasound

blush, and ST-segment resolution. The investigators concluded that thrombus removal devices appear to improve markers of myocardial perfusion in patients undergoing primary PCI with no difference in overall 30-day mortality but an increased likelihood of stroke. The clinical benefits of thrombectomy appeared to be influenced by the device type, with a trend toward survival benefit with manual aspiration catheters and worsening outcomes with mechanical devices. Nevertheless, in view of the great variability in thrombus content and size among patients with ACSs, interventionalists can choose the proper device in association with the morphologic characteristics of the targeted thrombus while achieving excellent results with either of these tools. This last point was reemphasized by a large Dutch study of 812 consecutive patients who were treated with drug-eluting stents for STEMI. Examining the effect of the underlying thrombus's size on procedural outcome, the researchers demonstrated a direct proportional effect on the initial and final thrombotic burden on mortality and the role the thrombus's size as an independent predictor of postprocedural MACEs and stent thrombosis.[7] Importantly, the role played by mechanical thrombectomy devices in the management of unresolved large thrombotic burdens during PCI should be recognized, as the existence of such a thrombus clearly increases the rate of MACEs and stent thrombosis (Fig. 28.11). The previously mentioned TAPAS study found that thrombus aspiration is applicable in a large majority of patients with STEMI, affording better reperfusion and clinical outcomes than PCI without a mechanical thrombus removal strategy.[91] These findings confirm previous observations from smaller trials and give credence to the notion that manual aspiration protects the microcirculation during primary PCI. However, whether these findings are attributable to an immediate reduction in thrombus burden, facilitation of direct stenting, or a combination of these two mechanisms remains unclear.[92] The benefits and limitations of mechanical thrombectomy devices are described in Table 28.10.

Embolic Protection

These tools are used to prevent the propagation of atheromatous or thrombotic debris downstream. They fall into three categories: filter-based, proximal occlusion, and distal flow occlusion devices.[60,93] The use of embolic protection devices does not require any special preparation of the patient other than the standard anticoagulation therapy for percutaneous intervention. These devices are user friendly; however, a clear limitation relates to the need for crossing the very same clot that required protection in the first place and the need for a distal landing zone of adequate length. Overall, embolic protection devices are useful adjuncts in primary PCI for ACS and have been shown to effectively reduce the rate of periprocedural infarction.[94] The embolic protection devices have a class I indication for SVG interventions due to the prevalence of thrombus-containing lesions.[95,96] However, studying the value of distal protection during rescue PCI, the Enhanced Myocardial Efficacy and Removal by Aspiration of Liberated Debris (EMERALD) investigators found that patients with AMI undergoing rescue PCI compared with primary PCI have similar myocardial perfusion, infarct size, and clinical outcomes, concluding that distal protection apparently does not offer any detectable benefit in this patient population.[97] In fact, there is concern that the routine use of filter protection for PCI of STEMI may increase the incidence of stent thrombosis, and

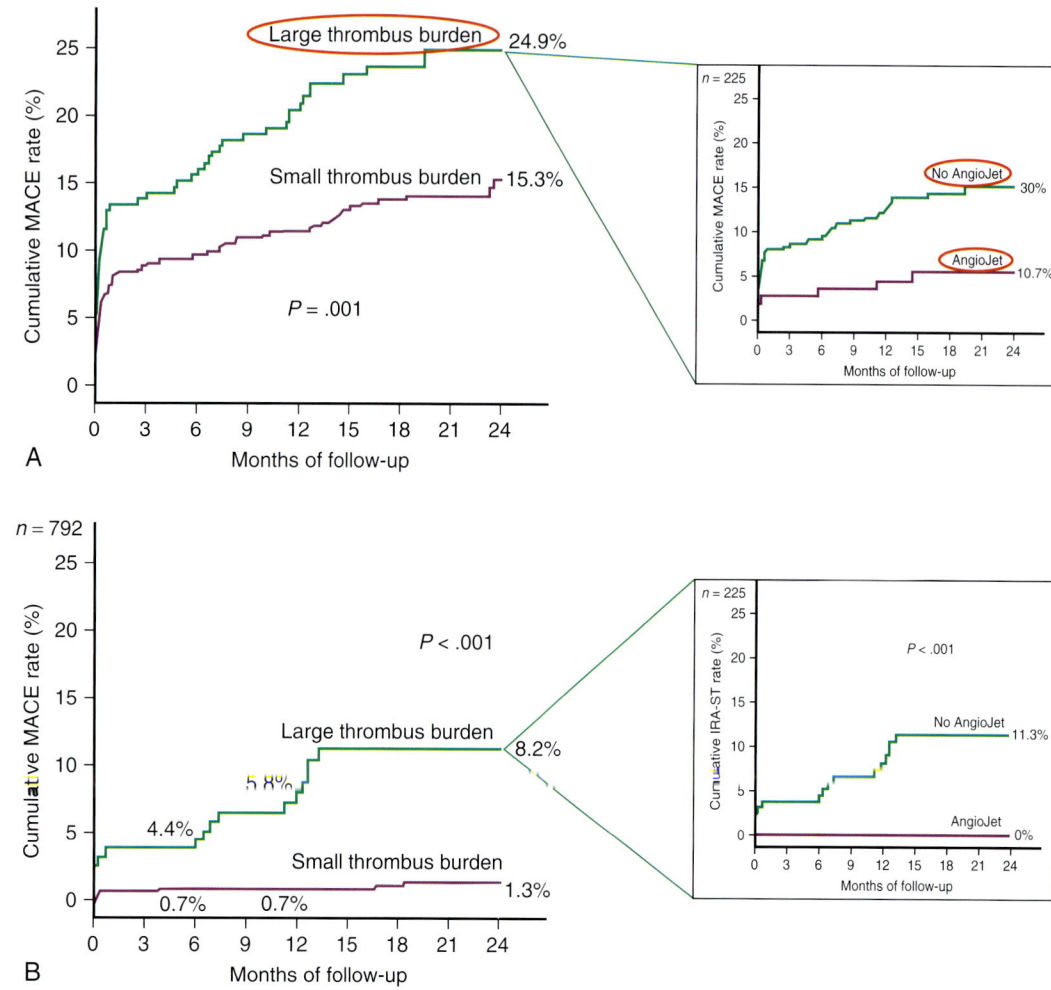

FIG. 28.11 (A) A large unresolved thrombus increases major adverse cardiac events (*MACEs*). (B) A large unresolved thrombus increases stent thrombosis. (Adapted from Sianos G, Papataklis MI, Daemen J, et al. Angiographic stent thrombosis after routine use of drug-eluting stents in ST-segment elevation myocardial infarction: the importance of thrombus burden. *J Am Coll Cardiol.* 2007;50:572–583.)

TABLE 28.10 Usefulness of Mechanical Thrombectomy Devices

Advantages
1. Decreasing "door-to-thrombus clearance" time
2. Efficient thrombus extraction through direct contact
3. Removal of the thrombus based prothrombotic coagulants and promoters of vasoconstriction and platelet aggregation
4. Combined activity with selective infusion of vasodilators, platelet aggregation inhibitors, and thrombolytic agents
5. Restoration of antegrade flow, improved myocardial blush score, and lowering of cTFC
6. Enabling accurate assessment of the underlying plaque morphology and stenosis
7. Facilitating stenting
8. Reducing distal embolization and no-reflow phenomena
9. Improving post-MI rate 6 months and 1-year MACE and survival rates

Limitations
1. May prolong percutaneous coronary intervention duration
2. Higher dependency on operator's technique
3. Can cause distal embolization due to device manipulations
4. Do not completely eliminate the risk of "no reflow"
5. May not achieve complete thrombus removal
6. Do not reduce the need for adjunct stenting
7. Increased cost

cTFC, Corrected thrombolysis in myocardial infarction frame count; *MACE*, major adverse cardiac event; *MI*, myocardial infarction.

the clinically driven target-lesion and -vessel revascularization.[98] In general, a selective rather than routine strategy of device utilization should be applied and limited to those patients at highest risk for clinically relevant embolization.[99]

Aspiration Catheters: Manual thrombus aspiration offers a safe, straightforward approach for the rapid reduction of thrombotic burden, prevention of thrombotic embolization, preservation of microvascular integrity, and reduction of infarct size.[93,100] This technology is by far the most widely utilized in current practice in patients with thrombotic lesions. Several prospective trials have demonstrated an increased myocardial blush grade of 2 to 3 and adequate ST-segment resolution of more than 70% in a substantial number of patients who received this treatment.[93,101] In addition, manual thrombus aspiration improves the perfusion of myocardial tissue as well as left functional ventricular recovery and modeling.[102] In a study similar to the Randomized Evaluation of the effect of Mechanical reduction of distal Embolization by thrombus aspiration in primary and rescue Angioplasty (REMEDIA) trial, investigators observed a significant decrease in the elevation of procedure-related cardiac enzymes in comparison with patients who did not receive aspiration, as well as only 3% of no reflow versus 15%, respectively. Follow up over 6 months demonstrates a significantly decreased occurrence of left ventricular dilation in comparison with patients who underwent standard PCI.[103] Meta-analysis of randomized studies of aspiration catheters shows a significant benefit in reduced mortality compared with standard PCI alone (2.7% vs. 4.4%, P = .05, respectively).[104] It should be noted that several studies failed to find advantage to the routine use of aspiration catheters in *all* STEMI patients, observing that it does not increase myocardial salvage and, in fact, may increase the final infarct size.[105] Similarly, a cautionary observation was offered by the multicenter, prospective, randomized, controlled open-label Thrombus Aspiration in ST-Elevation Myocardial Infarction in Scandinavia (TASTE) study,[106] a STEMI registry that compared manual thrombus aspiration followed by PCI to standard PCI. The investigators reported no reduction in all-cause 30-day mortality among the study's 7224 patients (2.8% in the aspiration catheter group vs. 3.0% in the PCI only group). However, the inclusion criteria could have led to selection bias and the relatively low statistical power of analysis in this study met with considerable criticism. Certain limitations of aspiration catheters should be recognized, such as the difficult delivery along tortuous vessels, reduced capability to aspirate at the distal coronary segments, and the risk of dissection/perforation in cases where the guidewire was not located within the true lumen.[107] The low, negative aspiration pressure and small evacuation holes also limit yield in the presence of a large thrombotic volume. Commonly, the application of aspiration catheters results in inadequate clot extraction, leaving at least 30% to 50% residual volume.[108] The risk of catheter-induced distal embolization, especially during a hurried maneuver, and the need to pass both antegrade and retrograde while crossing a large thrombus should be taken into account in using aspiration catheters. At present it is also unclear whether any one aspiration catheter provides a significant advantage over others. Notably, even the sequential use of thrombus aspiration catheters and distal protection filters can result in inadequate thrombus removal.[104,108,109]

Since thrombus aspiration is most frequently used for STEMI, a valid question regards the role of aspiration thrombectomy in patients with non–ST-elevation myocardial infarction (NSTEMI). The Thrombus Aspiration in ThrOmbus containing culprit lesions in Non-ST-Elevation Myocardial Infarction (TATORT) NSTEMI study, a prospective controlled multicenter randomized trial, compared adjunctive thrombus removal with aspiration with conventional PCI in patients with thrombus-containing lesions. The trial randomized 460 patients in a 1:1 fashion to aspiration thrombectomy and standard PCI.[110] The primary end point was the extent of microvascular obstruction as defined by cardiac magnetic resonance within 4 days of randomization. Clinical end points—including death, myocardial reinfarction, target-vessel revascularization, and new congestive heart failure—were analyzed at 6 months. Microvascular obstruction was not different between the aspiration thrombectomy and the standard PCI groups (1.7% left ventricle [LV] vs. 1.6% LV, respectively, P = .65). Similarly, no significant differences were observed in infarct size, myocardial salvage index, or angiographic parameters such as blush grade or TIMI flow grade. Clinical follow-up at 6 months also found no differences (P = .85) in the combined clinical end point between the aspiration catheters and the standard PCI approach. Accordingly the investigators concluded that aspiration thrombectomy in patients with NSTEMI undergoing early PCI in thrombus-containing lesions does not reduce the extent of no reflow in comparison with standard PCI without thrombectomy.

Power-Sourced Thrombectomy

The mainstay representatives of this group include the rheolytic thrombectomy, excimer laser, and the X-Sizer devices. The question of whether power based-mechanical thrombectomy offers any advantage over aspiration catheters is pertinent to practical management. However, only a limited number of prospective studies with direct comparisons between these two modalities have been conducted. Parodi and colleagues prospectively studied 80 AMI patients and compared rheolytic thrombectomy with manual aspiration catheters.[111] OCT was used to detect postremoval residual thrombus. Interestingly, all but one patient had residual thrombus after both rheolytic thrombectomy and aspiration. The number of OCT quadrants containing thrombus in the manual aspiration arm was higher than that in the rheolytic group, but the difference did not reach statistical significance. Large residual thrombus was more frequently identified in the manual aspiration (P = .039) and all markers of reperfusion were better with rheolytic thrombectomy. At 6 months, the percentage of poorly positioned stent struts in the manual aspiration group was higher than that in the rheolytic thrombectomy group (2.7% ± 4.5% and 0.81% ± 1.6%, respectively; P = .02). The investigators concluded that although both technologies can result in incomplete removal of thrombus, rheolytic thrombectomy offers more effective thrombus removal and improved myocardial reperfusion.

Overall there is a strong clinical impression that the larger the target thrombus, the higher the extraction yield of a power-based mechanical thrombectomy device.[112–114] A meta-analysis of 24 randomized trials comparing thrombus removal strategies in 4927 STEMI patients lends support to the benefits of mechanical thrombectomy, but only when used in patients with high thrombus burdens.[115] Intriguingly, many hold the opinion that a comparison between manual aspiration and power-based mechanical thrombectomy should be considered unethical in patients with lesions containing large thrombus burdens as they should be treated specifically with mechanical power-based thrombectomy devices.[116]

The AngioJet rheolytic thrombectomy (AngioJet, Boston Scientific, Boston, MA) device is approved by the U.S. Food and Drug Administration (FDA) for thrombus-containing lesions in coronary and peripheral interventions. The principle of activation is the creation of saline jets inside the catheter traveling backward at high speed, creating a zone of negative pressure (the Venturi effect). Side windows along the catheter's tip optimize fluid flow, drawing thrombus into the catheter for fragmentation and removal. Proper thrombectomy technique incorporates slow advancement of the catheter. Temporary pacing should be considered in patients with thrombus in a large target vessel or in cases with limited myocardial reserve. The device's success and safety in the management of large thrombus burdens in STEMI patients and resultant improvement in effective myocardial perfusion as compared with standard PCI has been well documented.[117–120] The Thoraxcenter interventional group elegantly demonstrated that rheolytic thrombectomy in STEMI patients is a significant independent predictor of reduced risk for stent thrombosis and MACEs, specifically when applied for the removal of large thrombus burdens.[5] In the Florence Appraisal of Rheolytic Atherectomy (FAST) study, the AngioJet was used in 116 AMI patients with extensive thrombus load, leading to significant perfusion improvement as compared with a control group with similar thrombotic burdens who received standard PCI.[121] The in-hospital rate of MACEs for the AngioJet was relatively low at 8%. Nevertheless, this device together with the entire concept of thrombus extraction sustained a major setback in 2006 when negative results from the AngioJet Rheolytic Thrombectomy In Patients Undergoing Primary Angioplasty for Acute Myocardial Infarction (AIMI) multicenter study were published.[122] In retrospect, this study was poorly designed: thrombus was not a criterion for enrollment, and operators were required first to passively advance the device to the distal target vessel and then perform retrograde thrombectomy. The prospective multicenter JetStent study addressed questions raised by and about the AIMI study, comparing the effect of rheolytic thrombectomy with direct stenting on myocardial reperfusion, infarct size, and clinical outcomes in STEMI.[123] The study exclusively focused on AMI patients with angiographically visible thrombus, using only slow single-pass antegrade technique and a narrower temporal definition of early ST-segment resolution (more than 50% within 30 minutes). Overall, 501 STEMI patients with visible thrombus (grades 1 to 4) or with a totally occluded infarct-related vessel (thrombus grade 5, which underwent restratification) were enrolled. At baseline both groups had a thrombus grade

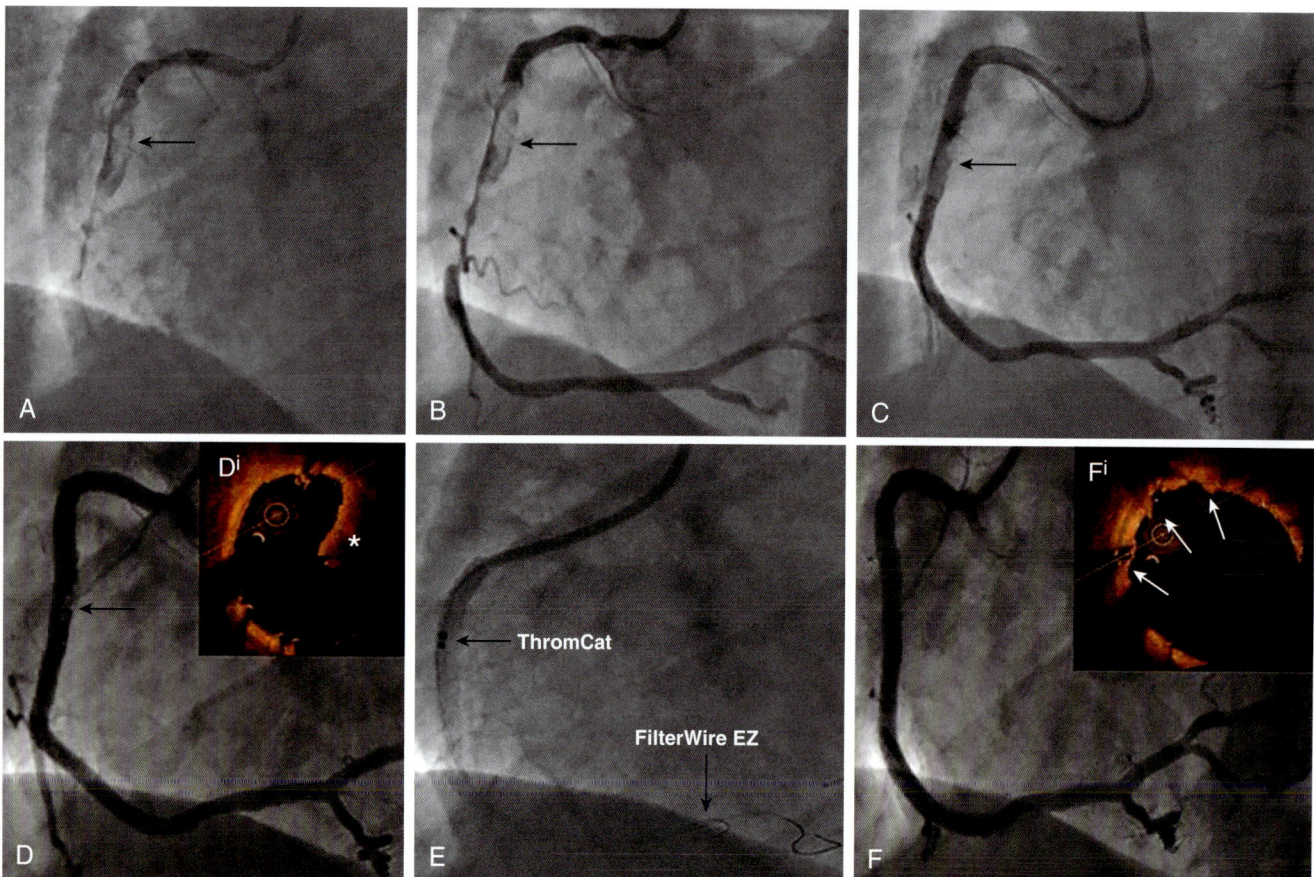

FIG. 28.12 Application of the ThromCat device, which uses a high-speed rotational helix to macerate and extract thrombus. This thrombectomy tool can be synergistically applied with a filter protection device and with other thrombectomy devices, such as laser. (A) Occluded dominant right coronary artery with a massive intracoronary thrombus *(arrow)*. (B) Establishment of TIMI 2 flow following excimer laser thrombectomy. (C) Angiographic results after treatment with laser and throm. (D₁) the treated site as demonstrated by optical coherence tomography technique, the *asterisk* indicates residual thrombosis. (E) The residual thrombus was cleared by application of the ThromCat device. (F¹) Final view of treated site *(arrows)* as observed through optical coherence tomography. (From Rawlins J, Sambu N, O'Kane P. Strategies for the management of massive intra-coronary thrombus in acute myocardial infarction. *Heart.* 2013;99:510.)

of 3 to 5 (in 99% of the patients) and TIMI 0 flow (in 83% of the patients). A platelet receptor antagonist was used in 97% and 98%, respectively. A 93% procedural success rate was achieved in both groups. The results demonstrate improved myocardial reperfusion with rheolytic thrombectomy as determined by higher rates of early ST-segment resolution (86% vs. 79%, respectively, $P = .04$). A significant difference in MACEs was observed between the groups at 1 and 6 months: 3.1% AngioJet versus 6.9% direct stenting ($P = .05$), and 12% versus 21% ($P = .01$), respectively. No difference was found between the two strategies regarding myocardial blush score and corrected TIMI frame count. Multivariate regression analysis showed that randomization to rheolytic thrombectomy was a predictor of ST-segment resolution (odds ratio 1.7, 95 % confidence interval [CI] 1.03–2.8; $P < .039$) and 6-month MACEs rate (hazard ratio 0.5, 95% CI 0.31–0.82; $P = .06$). Another mechanical thrombectomy device, the Thrombcat (Spectranetics, Colorado Springs, CO) catheter, is also used for the treatment of heavy thrombus burden, as demonstrated in Fig. 28.12.

Lasers are useful debulking devices for the treatment of lesions deemed unsuitable for standard PCI[124,125] and specifically for the revascularization of thrombus-containing lesions.[126] These devices create a smooth coronary lumen after debulking, which in turn facilitates stent deployment and improved long-term results.[127] The FDA-approved pulsed-wave ultraviolet wavelength excimer laser (Spectranetics, Philips, Colorado Springs, CO) interacts favorably with several components of the occluding thrombus. Laser-generated acoustic shock waves can dissolve fibrin fibers[128] and suppress platelet aggregation.[129] This laser has been successfully applied in patients with ACSs including AMI,[129–131] as depicted in Fig. 28.13. The thrombus dissolution capability of this laser was studied in the Cohort of Acute Revascularization in Myocardial Infarction with Excimer laser (CARMEL) multicenter study,[113] which enrolled 151 "real world" AMI patients with continuous chest pain and ischemia caused by either STEMI or non-STEMI, including late presentation, cardiogenic shock (13%), failed thrombolytic therapy (11%), or contraindications for this therapy (17%). The target vessel was a coronary artery in 79% and a venous bypass graft in 21%. Using independent core laboratories, the quantitative and statistical analyses demonstrated that despite the presence of compromised baseline hemodynamics and a heavy thrombotic burden in 65% of the patients, the laser had 95% device success, 97% angiographic success, and 91% procedural success. The laser increased the baseline TIMI 0 flow of 1.2 ± 1.1 to 2.8 ± 0.5 with a poststenting final TIMI flow of 3.0 ± 0.2 ($P < .001$ vs. baseline). Distal embolization occurred in only 2%, no reflow in 3%, device-induced small dissection in 4%, and a small perforation in 0.6%. Total MACEs were relatively low at 13%. The most significant finding was that the maximal removal effect was directly proportional to the baseline thrombotic burden (i.e., the larger

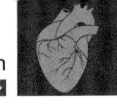

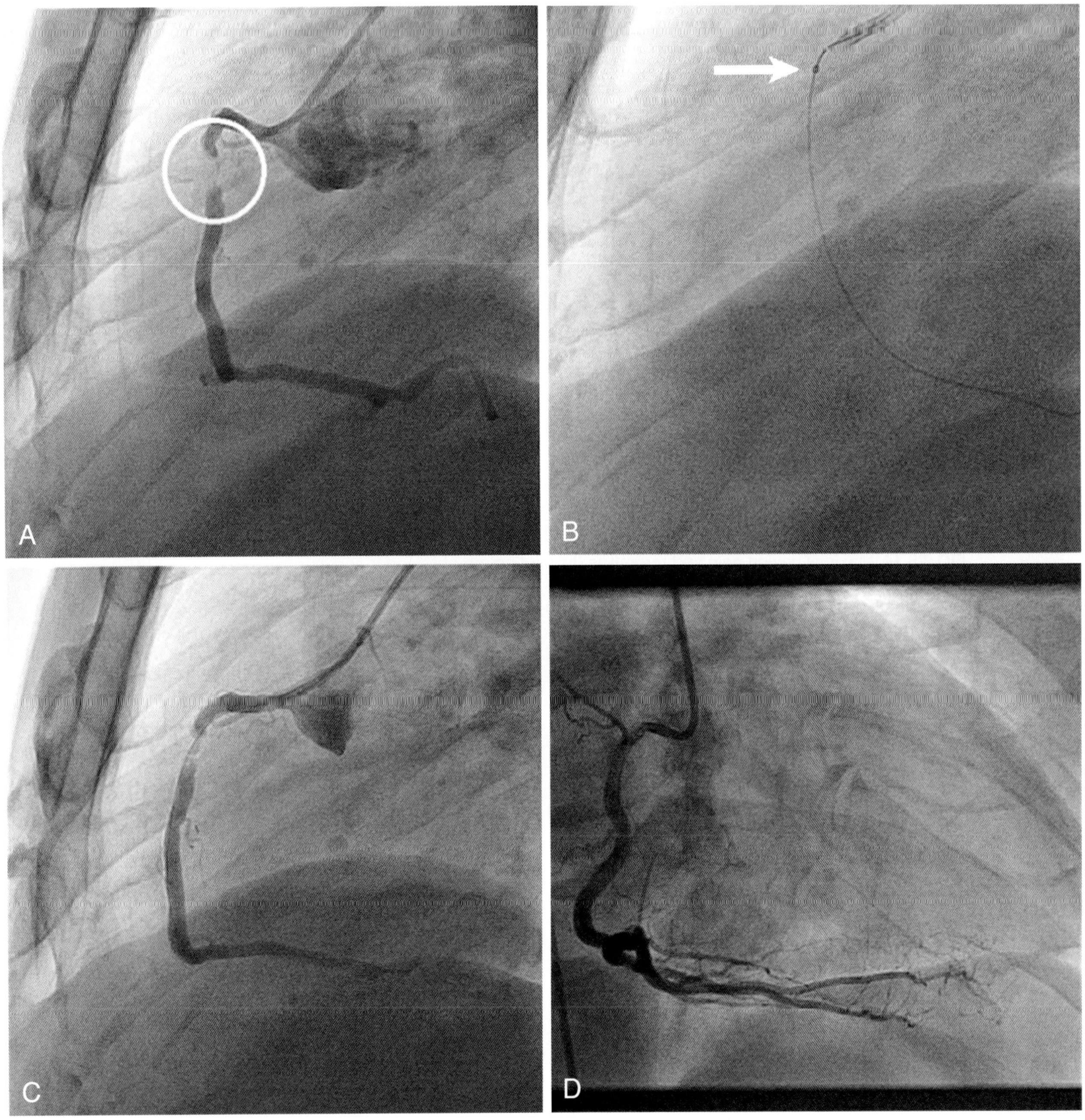

FIG. 28.13 Excimer laser in acute inferolateral myocardial infarction. (A) The circle surrounds ruptured plaque and thrombosis of the proximal right coronary artery. (B) The tip of the arrow points to the excimer laser catheter as it debulks the target plaque while crossing it. (C) An angiogram demonstrating plaque and thrombus removal. Residual plaque and thrombus were managed with adjunct stenting. (D) Final angiogram depicting complete patency of the infarct-related vessel. Marked clinical improvement was observed. (From Topaz O, Topaz A. Power-sourced mechanical thrombectomy in the management of thrombus-containing atherosclerotic lesions. In: Topaz O, ed. *Cardiovascular Thrombus: From Pathology and Clinical Presentations to Imaging, Pharmacotherapy and Interventions.* Philadelphia: Elsevier; 2018:261–283.)

the initial thrombotic burden at the target lesion, the higher the absorption of the laser and the more effective and higher the gain for the laser application). Importantly, thrombus was not identified as a predictor of PCI failure. Thus this study provided the first quantitative evidence of the considerable benefit associated with utilization of a dedicated mechanical thrombectomy device in thrombus-removal and, in particular, in AMI, as presented in Fig. 28.14. Subsequent subgroup analysis recognized a specific gain for the laser among patients (mainly those presenting late for treatment) who exhibited a heavy thrombotic burden and unstable hemodynamic parameters.[132] Ultrasound-induced thrombus dissolution can be used as an adjunctive therapy intended to increase the efficacy of thrombolytic therapy.[52,133]

As for thrombus focused sonication therapy, two distinct approaches rely on an invasive catheter delivering sonication directly to the targeted thrombus or on an external device delivering transcutaneous therapeutic ultrasound energy.[134] Additional studies will be needed to investigate the efficacy and safety issues

	QCA per TIMI Thrombus				
GRADE	0	1	2	3	4
	No thrombus	Small thrombus	Medium thrombus	Large thrombus	Extensive thrombus
Patients (n)	11	14	28	45	63
MLD: Baseline (mm)	.87 ± .69	.72 ± .43	.65 ± .45	.59 ± .49	.37 ± .49
Post laser	1.74 ± .46	1.48 ± .49	1.51 ± .51	1.50 ± .41	1.62 ± .62
Laser acute gain	.90 ± .63	.76 ± .52*	.84 ± .60	.94 ± .48	1.21 ± .72*
Final	2.97 ± .60	2.54 ± .55	2.47 ± .62	2.62 ± .55	2.76 ± .62
%DS: Baseline	74% ± 21%	76% ± 16%	77% ± 16%	82% ± 16%	89% ± 15%
Post laser	47% ± 13%	51% ± 11%	52% ± 15%	51% ± 13%	53% ± 17%
Laser acute reduction	27% ± 18%	25% ± 15%	25% ± 19%	31% ± 16%	36% ± 20%
Final	16% ± 17%	15% ± 13%	22% ± 14%	16% ± 17%	22% ± 16%

*$P = .03$

FIG. 28.14 Maximal device gain and thrombus dissolution are obtained in the extensive thrombus group. *DS,* Diameter of stenosis; *MLD,* minimal luminal diameter; *QCA,* quantitative coronary angiography; *TIMI,* thrombolysis in myocardial infarction. (Adapted from Topaz O, Ebersole D, Das T. Excimer laser angioplasty in acute myocardial infarction [the CARMEL multicenter study]. *Am J Cardiol.* 2004;93:694–701.)

of the external delivery system in order to examine whether it provides improved enhancement of pharmacologic thrombolytic agents and superior thrombus dissolution in comparison with the invasive intracoronary delivery method and other approaches.

The X-Sizer thrombectomy system (eV3, Plymouth, MN) enjoyed popularity in the United States; however, today it is used mainly in Europe.[135] This technology is built with a helical cutter enclosed in a protective housing attached to a dual-bore catheter shaft containing a guidewire and vacuum/extraction lumens. Activation of the handheld controller simultaneously rotates the helical cutter (2100 rpm), which entraps and macerates soft atherosclerotic plaque and thrombus for transfer to a vacuum collection bottle. The device operates 1.5-, 2.0-, and 2.3-mm-diameter cutters and is compatible with 0.014 inch guidewires. Napodano and colleagues demonstrated in 92 AMI patients that direct PCI with X-Sizer thrombectomy followed by stenting significantly improved myocardial reperfusion as assessed by myocardial blush score and ST-segment resolution.[135] The large, prospective X-Sizer for Thrombectomy in Acute Myocardial Infarction (X-AMINE) multicenter study that followed demonstrated an 87% device success rate and 95% adequate thrombus removal from the targeted lesions.[136]

Combined Pharmacothrombectomy

This reperfusion strategy targets lesions and vessels laden with a very heavy thrombotic burden accompanied by slow antegrade flow. Combining power-sourced mechanical thrombectomy with selective intracoronary injection of thrombolytic agents, it offers the benefit of direct contact with the underlying clot and adequate removal of large thrombus associated with a decreased risk of systemic lytic effect.[137,138]

STENTS FOR TARGETED THROMBUS CAPTURE

Direct stenting during PCI of thrombus-containing lesions with either bare-metal or drug-eluting stents is a commonly used strategy.[139] Nonetheless, despite the popularity and perceived success

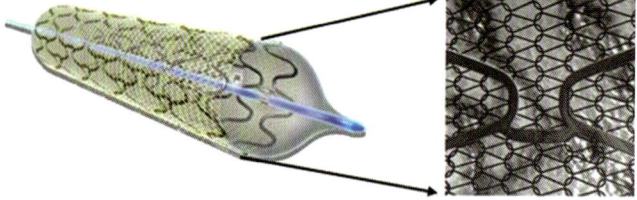

FIG. 28.15 MGuard thrombus-capturing stent system. (InspireMD, Tel Aviv, Israel.)

of direct stenting, distal embolization and no flow do occur, mainly due to the mobilization of fragmented clot.[118,140] As for thrombus-dedicated stent technology, two concepts are noted—thrombus capture and thrombus exclusion, both aiming to prevent thrombotic distal embolization and consequently to improve the microcirculation. The MGuard stent (Inspire-MD, Tel-Aviv, Israel) offers a trapping stent-based mechanism for the dedicated management of intracoronary thrombus and reduction of embolization.[62] This platform is made of a stainless steel bare-metal stent covered with an ultrathin 150 by 180 μm flexible mesh net fabricated by circular knitting (Fig. 28.15). During stent deployment, the net stretches and slides over the expanding stent struts, creating custom-designed pores parallel to the vessel wall. Once deployed, the MGuard stent seals the thrombus and associated plaque and captures[141] potential embolic debris between the fiber net and the arterial wall (Figs. 28.16 and 28.17). Early experience with this stent included 100 STEMI patients who enrolled in a prospective multicenter study, all with angiographic evidence of thrombus in the infarct-related artery. The stent achieved 90% myocardial blush grade 3 and 90% complete (>70%) ST-segment resolution.[142] The investigators concluded that the MGuard stent offers a safe and feasible option for PCI in STEMI patients, providing a very high perfusion grade and significant electrocardiographic improvement. Romaguera and associates specifically studied the usefulness of this stent in 56 STEMI patients with a residual high thrombotic burden (angiographic TIMI grade 4 or 5)

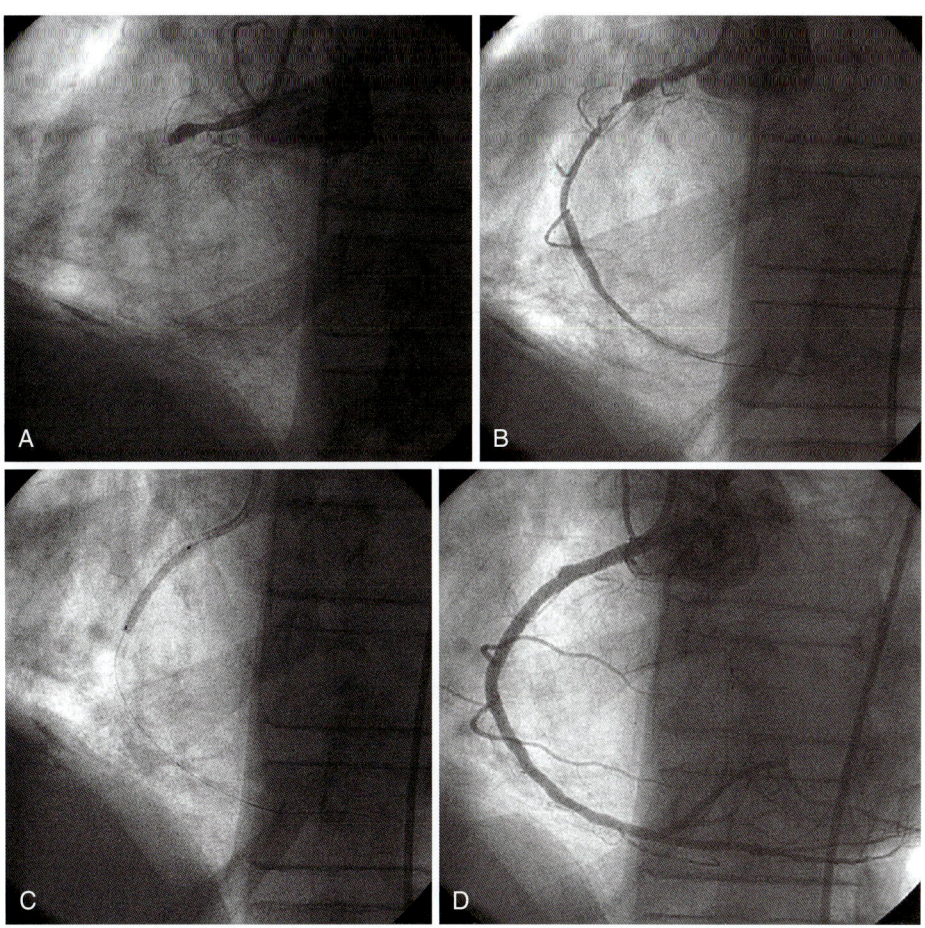

FIG. 28.16 An 81-year-old patient with inferior ST-elevation myocardial infarction. (A) Grade 5 thrombus occludes the right coronary artery (RCA). (B) After aspiration and balloon dilation, antegrade flow was restored but grade 2 thrombus is present. (C) Deployment of a 3.0/24-mm MGuard thrombus-capturing stent. (D) Final results demonstrate complete patency of the RCA with thrombolysis in myocardial infarction (TIMI) grade 3 blush. The ST-segment resolved. (Courtesy Ran Kornowski MD, Rabin Medical Center, Israel.)

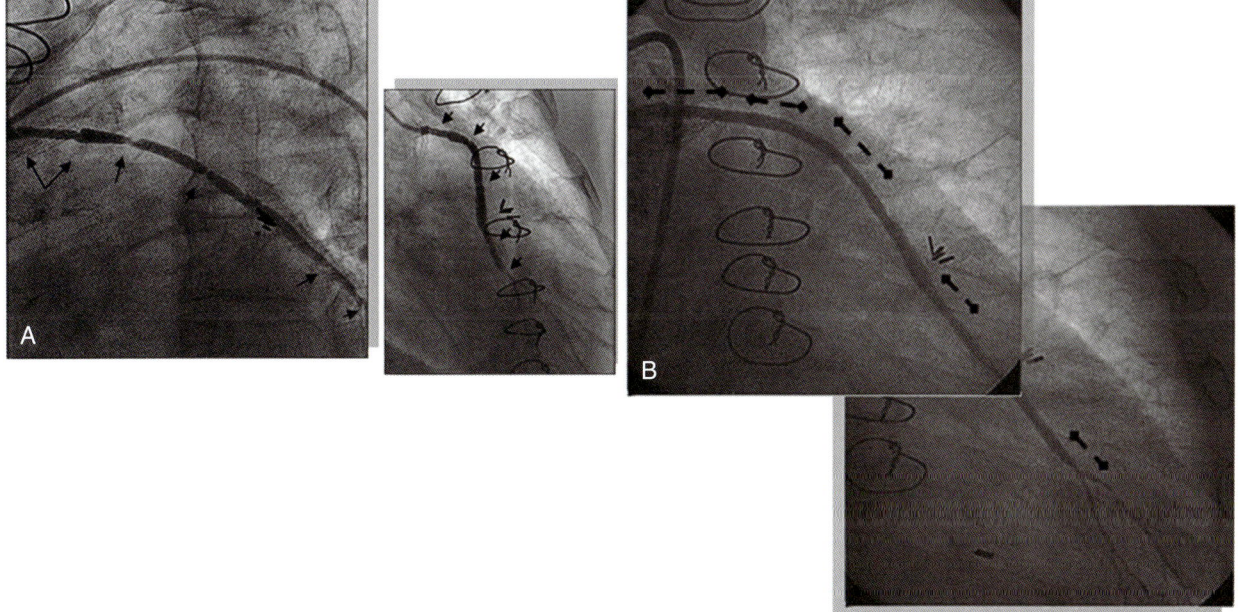

FIG. 28.17 Thrombus capturing in an ischemic patient with a degenerated saphenous vein graft to the obtuse marginal branch. (A) Five consecutive lesions *(arrows)* along the graft. (B) Treatment with four consecutive MGuard stents (3.5 × 24 mm, 3.5 × 15 mm, 3.25 × 12 mm, and 2.75 × 12 mm) and a bare-metal stent distally. A protection device was not used. (Courtesy Ran Kornowski, MD, Rabin Medical Center, Israel.)

persisting despite aggressive manual aspiration.[137] Following MGuard stent implantation, more than 85% of the patients had thrombus grade 0 and a final TIMI 3 flow was gained in 82%; there was a normal myocardial blush in 55% and complete ST-segment resolution in 59%. Occlusion of a side branch occurred in two cases (3.5%), embolization in five cases (8.9%) and transient no reflow in four cases (7.1%). The MACEs at 9-month follow up were 3.6%, including one definite stent thrombosis and one target-vessel revascularization. Accordingly the investigators concluded that this stent may be useful for preventing distal embolization in STEMI patients who remain with high thrombotic burdens after manual aspiration.

A different approach to thrombus eradication with stents involving the concept of thrombus exclusion/displacement was studied by Gunn and colleagues, who inserted a novel pericardium-covered stent graft to treat massive thrombus in the setting of ACS. The Aneugraft stent graft (ITGI Medical, Or-Akiva, Israel) consists of a conventional balloon-expandable 316L stainless steel stent that is sutured externally, at either end, with a single layer of blemish-free equine pericardium 105 μm thick. The initial experience with 10 lesions demonstrated immediate elimination of the large thrombus-related angiographic filling defect and restoration or maintenance of TIMI grade 3 blood flow. In one patient who could take only aspirin, the stent thrombosed.[143] It appears that this unique stent technology may be considered for select patients who have failed established thrombus removal technologies.[144]

SPECIFIC THROMBOTIC LESIONS: LOCATION, EFFECTS, AND MANAGEMENT OPTIONS
The Hostile Clot

The terms *hostile thrombus* or *angry clot* describe a very unique pathologic vascular phenomenon with distinctive angiographic features and worrisome clinical sequalae. This is recognized during PCI and peripheral endovascular interventions alike. Its hallmark is a sudden, rapid, and aggressive large-volume accumulation accompanied by angiographic and clinical instability. Such a thrombus can grow to a very significant size from a sudden, "natural" plaque rupture, as demonstrated in Fig. 28.18, or it may be caused by mechanical provocation during PCI. Such a provocation can be triggered by a guidewire and/or other equipment crossing an atherosclerotic thrombotic plaque, as demonstrated in Fig. 28.19. In most instances, the angry thrombus phenomenon occurs in lesions that are already considered to be thrombus-containing plaques.[37] Nevertheless they can also be formed in clean plaques (i.e., those with a TIMI thrombus grade 0). Such an aggressive thrombus can be formed at any stage of the coronary (or peripheral) intervention, and once recognized, it serves as an ominous marker for imminent complications. Moreover, the angry thrombus can even develop abruptly upon completion of a seemingly routine, uncomplicated balloon inflation or stent deployment. In the vast majority of instances identification of an angry thrombus is accompanied by rapidly developing deleterious clinical effects. Once an angry thrombus has been formed, it rapidly aggregates at the target lesion and beyond, frequently expanding distally and even proximally into the treated vessel with devastating effect on the ischemic myocardium.[145]

Application of a thrombus classification method can assist in both the recognition and the timely management of this abnormal vascular structure, since the angry thrombus can expeditiously and aggressively expand to reach TIMI thrombus grade 4 to 5. Consequently acute vessel closure can ensue, as well as thrombus fragmentation, distal embolization, and occlusion of smaller arteries. The hostile thrombus commonly causes severe ischemia, dangerous arrhythmias, and conduction abnormalities due to the cessation of antegrade flow, distal embolization, and a marked decrease in myocardial perfusion. This process frequently leads to AMI accompanied by severe hemodynamic instability. From a technical viewpoint, the angiographic identification of such rapid increase in the thrombotic load should be followed by expeditious clot removal. Noteworthy, the angry thrombus commonly resists treatment with standard pharmacotherapy, balloon angioplasty, or aspiration catheters and standard stenting.[37] Specifically, in many cases an aggressive angry thrombus does not readily respond to aspiration catheters, thus requiring the application of motorized mechanical thrombectomy and administration of enhanced pharmacotherapy in order restore antegrade flow and distal perfusion for myocardial salvage.[88,146]

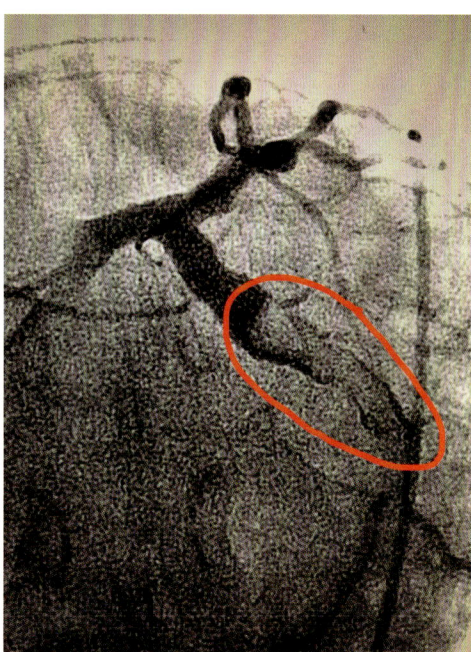

FIG. 28.18 The formation of a "natural" hostile, megasize thrombus *(red elliptic)* following plaque rupture in a patient with an acute coronary syndrome. (Courtesy Kristine Owen, MD, FACC, Director, Cardiac Catheterization Laboratory, Charles George VAMC, Asheville, NC.)

Stent Thrombosis

Early, late, and very late stent thromboses are considered major adverse clinical developments that have a significant impact on clinical outcomes (Fig. 28.20).[147,148] Stent thrombosis is often multifactorial,[148] where a major cause is the presence of residual thrombus after PCI that either accumulates gradually over time or rapidly aggregates to form a subtotal or fully occlusive thrombus. Stent thrombosis can be marked by serious complications such as nonfatal and fatal AMI[149,150] and hemodynamic instability. Expedient management is a key to a favorable outcome, especially for patients who present with STEMI.[151,152] Primary PCI, including additional stenting with or without thrombectomy, is effective in restoring vessel patency, but reocclusion and restenosis are frequent.[153] The often raised practical question as to which device is best for the management of stent thrombosis can be addressed in consideration with the burden of the targeted thrombus burden and related clinical picture.[153,154] Although a small to medium thrombotic volume in a stable patient can be managed with combination therapy consisting of pharmacologic agents and aspiration catheters, a large thrombotic burden, especially in the presence of hemodynamic instability and ongoing ischemia, calls for enhanced removal by a power-based mechanical thrombectomy device.[153,155] Nevertheless, even successful

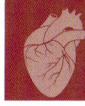

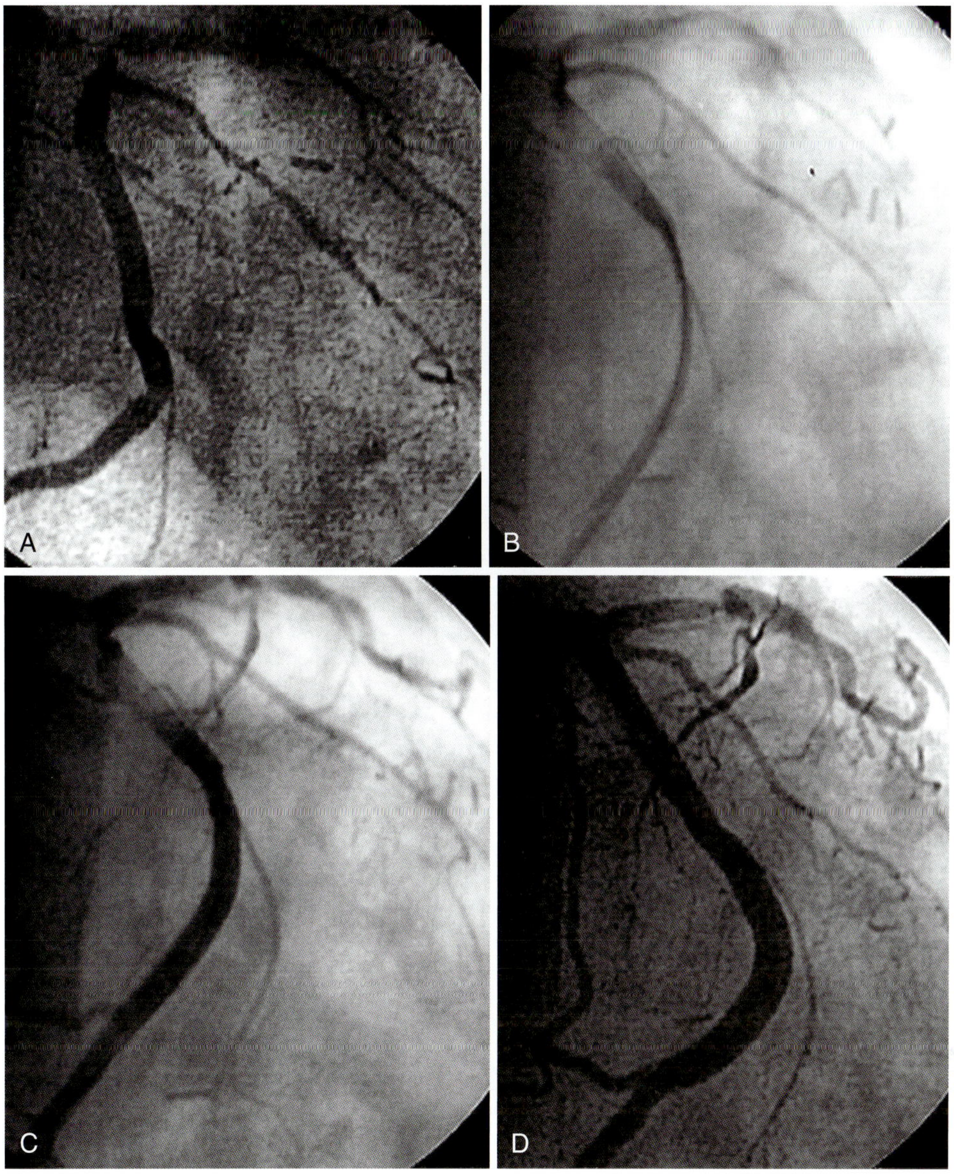

FIG. 28.19 The so-called angry clot phenomenon: a patient after coronary artery bypass grafting who presented with unstable angina, severe ischemia, and hemodynamic compromise. A left internal mammary artery graft to a diffusely diseased left anterior descending artery was patent. (A) The left main exhibits critical stenosis with grade 2 thrombus. (B) Percutaneous coronary intervention of the left main lesion: the patient received a IIb/IIIa platelet receptor antagonist, heparin, aspirin, and clopidogrel. However, as soon as the guidewire crossed the left main stenosis and was positioned at the distal circumflex artery, rapid and aggressive thrombus accumulation occurred along the entire vessel and resulted in marked narrowing and slow flow. Increased chest pain, ischemia, and hypotension ensued, requiring immediate thrombus dissolution. This was achieved with a 0.9-mm rapid exchange X-80 excimer laser catheter (Spectranetics, Colorado Springs, CO), which was activated at maximal flow (80 mJ/mm²/80 Hz). (C) Angiography after laser debulking and thrombolysis demonstrated restoration of flow, with reversal of the clot accumulation and mild residual clot remaining at the proximal vessel. (D) Final results after stenting of the left main were accompanied by a clinical recovery.

PCI for stent thrombosis can be associated with a larger infarct and poorer outcome than in patients with de novo lesions and STEMI.

LEFT MAIN CORONARY LESIONS

Atherosclerotic lesions of the left main coronary artery comprise unique morphologic features.[81,156] Thrombus-containing lesions in the left main coronary artery are an ominous angiographic finding (Fig. 28.21) as they are among the most challenging targets for PCI. The performance of percutaneous revascularization for left main disease continues to generates great global interest,[157,158] recognizing that the thrombus stands to have a major impact on clinical and procedure-related risks, complications, and outcome. Acute thrombosis of an underlying left main plaque has potentially grave consequences; in cases of acute total occlusion,[159] the only realistic option for lifesaving revascularization is emergency PCI (Fig. 28.22). Prasad and colleagues reported a 28-patient series with unprotected thrombotic left main lesions who underwent standard PCI.[160] Only a modest angiographic success rate of 83%

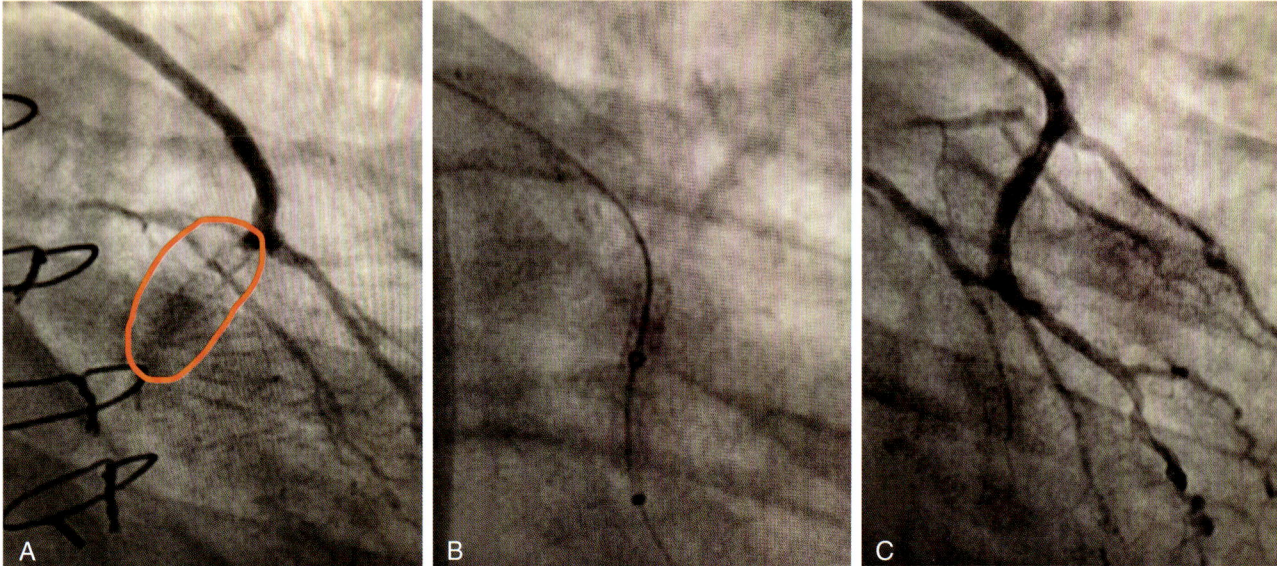

FIG. 28.20 Stent thrombosis and rheolytic thrombectomy application. (A) Magnified angiographic view demonstrating total thrombotic occlusion of a stent *(red ellipse)* in a saphenous vein graft to an obtuse marginal branch. Three weeks after stopping dual antiplatelet therapy the patient presented with an acute coronary syndrome accompanied by congestive heart failure and a compromised hemodynamic condition. (B) AngioJet rheolytic thrombectomy was performed along the entire length of the thrombosed stent while a large volume thrombus was retrieved, resulting in an immediate hemodynamic improvement and resolution of the ischemia. (C) Final results of the stent revascularization. Minimal residual thrombus was noted and treated with a IIb/IIIa platelet receptor antagonist for 12 hours. Complete clinical recovery ensued.

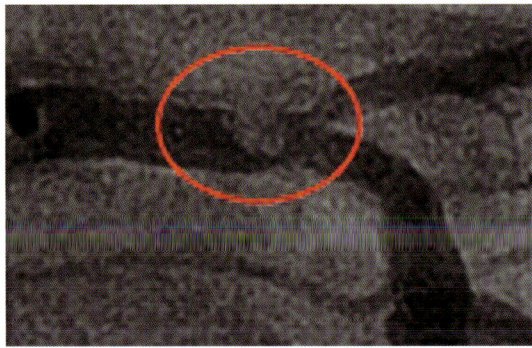

FIG. 28.21 Marked thrombosis *(red circle)* accompanying an atherosclerotic lesion of the left main coronary artery with protrusion onto the left anterior descending artery. (From Topaz O, Topaz A. Thrombus classifications: critical tools for diagnostic and interventional cardiovascular procedures. In: Topaz O, ed. *Cardiovascular Thrombus: From Pathology and Clinical Presentations to Imaging, Pharmacotherapy and Interventions.* Philadelphia: Elsevier; 2018:175–187.)

(comprising 24 patients) was achieved, accompanied by a cumulative in-hospital mortality of 36%. These outcomes raise valid concern that thrombus-containing stenoses may not be treated by a dedicated thrombus removal approach. For such a high-risk interventional scenario and in order to reduce the risk of distal embolization, our experience points to a need to first focus on the thrombus removal strategy, preferably with a mechanical thrombectomy device. The merits of this approach are expeditious clot clearance leading to proper exposure and tailored treatment of the underlying atherosclerotic plaque. This in turn, facilitates stent delivery and deployment with a high subsequent success rate.[161] For select symptomatic patients with chronic thrombotic occlusion (CTO) of the left main coronary artery,[160] PCI can be a viable management option utilizing either antegrade or retrograde recanalization through one of the angiographically distinct collateral channels that connect the right coronary artery to the left coronary vessels.[156]

MULTIVESSEL CORONARY THROMBOSIS

This presumably rare condition is most probably angiographically underrecognized due to the prevalent focus on identification of the one infarct-related artery and the inherent pressure surrounding expeditious STEMI management. Multivessel thrombotic lesions in ACS patients pose crucial management challenges. These patients frequently present with severe hemodynamic compromise. The multivessel thrombosis can affect coronary arteries and old bypass grafts alike (Fig. 28.13). The pathophysiologic process accounting for this scenario begins when plaque ruptures and acute thrombosis of a single artery leads to the development of cardiogenic shock. This, in turn, further decreases coronary perfusion pressure; consequently multivessel thrombi involving other significant lesions are formed.[162] Another etiology accounting for multivessel coronary thrombosis involves a left chamber cardiac tumor with dislodgement and embolization of thrombotic material and subsequent occlusion of multiple coronary vessels.[163] The optimal treatment approach to multivessel coronary thrombosis is unknown, varying considerably from PCI to urgent bypass surgery. In instances whereby the most critical culprit thrombotic lesion can be identified with certainty, selective treatment with an aspiration catheter, aggressive pharmacotherapy, and subsequent stenting can be beneficial. However, in a case of PCI failure or in patients with continuous global ischemia due to thrombus-laden lesions in the other coronary arteries (especially during hemodynamic deterioration), urgent coronary bypass surgery is the preferred management option.

MULTIPLE THROMBI IN A SINGLE VESSEL

The initial angiogram in patients with ACS can show several thrombotic occlusions appearing simultaneously (Fig. 28.24). These thrombi may be mobile or rigid, and they may differ in morphology, size, and mobility. The etiology in most instances relates to progression of the atherosclerotic process; however, this unusual occurrence may sometimes represent hypercoagulation, the angry-clot phenomenon, or breakup of the original thrombus

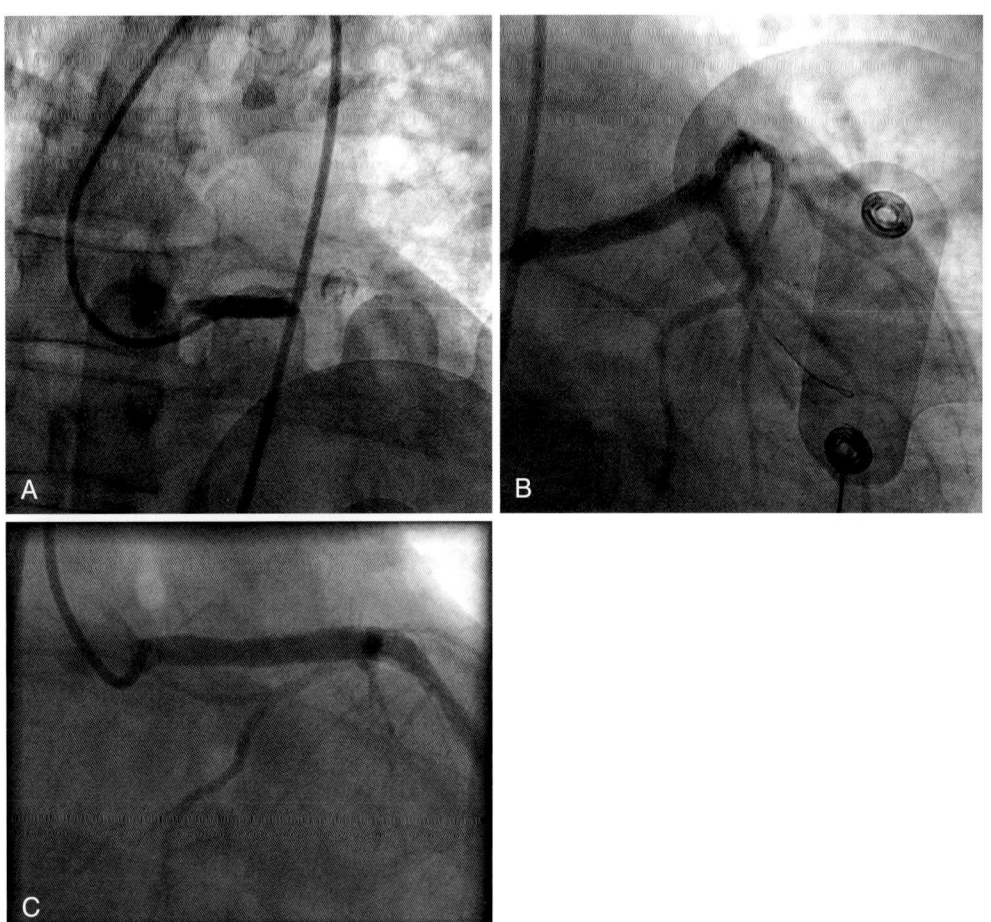

FIG. 28.22 Acute left main thrombosis. This 48-year-old patient suddenly collapsed in a public place. Following cardiopulmonary resuscitation, an anterior wall ST-elevation myocardial infarction was diagnosed. A stormy course during transfer to the medical center included repeated episodes of intense chest pain, hypotension, increased ischemia, and ventricular tachycardia, which culminated in full arrest upon entry to the cardiac catheterization suite. At 45 minutes, full code was required, including intubation, defibrillation ×17, amiodarone, and epinephrine prior to relative stabilization and catheterization. (A) Total occlusion of the left main artery. (B) A 0.014-inch ATW guidewire (Cordis/Johnson & Johnson, Bridgewater, NJ) recanalized the occlusion, followed by Export aspiration catheterization, which extracted clot. (C) The target left main lesion was dilated and successfully stented with a 5.0/16-mm Liberté stent (Boston Medical, Natick, MA), yielding a diameter of 5.7 mm. Thrombolysis in myocardial infarction grade 3 flow was restored; however, refractory arrhythmias ensued that required additional cardiopulmonary resuscitation, antiarrhythmics, defibrillation ×24, and the insertion of an intraaortic balloon pump. Following stabilization, the patient received therapeutic hypothermia for 2 days. Cardiac catheterization was repeated and intravascular ultrasound on day 7 demonstrated in patency of the stent and adequate coronary flow. The patient was discharged without angina or congestive heart failure with a left ventricular ejection fraction of 30%, anterolateral hypokinesis, and no neurologic deficit. (Courtesy William R. Hathaway, MD, and William D. Kuehl, MD, Mission Memorial Heart Center, Asheville, NC.)

into separate particles. In consideration of PCI, in most instances the use of thrombin inhibitors or platelet receptor antagonists in synergy with a powered mechanical thrombectomy device can yield adequate removal of thrombus. A filter protection device can be applied as well, provided that it does not interrupt the occluding thrombi during the initial placement manipulations.

CHRONIC THROMBOTIC OCCLUSION

Thrombus usually resides in the main body of the CTO. In a majority of CTO cases, the presence of thrombus in this diseased segment plays a critical role.[164] Conceivably the thrombus can provide a more promising "crossing medium" than that offered by the rigid calcium deposits and the resistive fibrotic tissue. Technically, CTO is seen as a challenging target for revascularization[165] owing to the presence of fibrotic tissue, calcifications, and atherosclerotic material. The latter, indeed, frequently comprises a formidable obstacle that diverts or deflects the tip of the guidewire, causing it to buckle away or even perforate the vessel's wall. Importantly, these lesions frequently contain layers of organized thrombus of various ages. Microchannels commonly recanalize the organized thrombus within the CTO (Fig. 28.25), enabling the propagation, albeit limited, of antegrade flow distal to the plaque.[166] Accordingly, although the angiographic hallmark of a CTO points to a 100% stenosis, the histopathologic domain and the clinical realm suggest that about half of these lesions are actually less than 100% occluded.[165] PCI in such cases could specifically aim at crossing the CTO through the microchannels, followed by removal of the obstructive plaque.[167] The same approach can be taken in instances of revascularization of CTOs within old saphenous bypass vein grafts. From a technical viewpoint, proper selection of the guiding catheter and subsequent

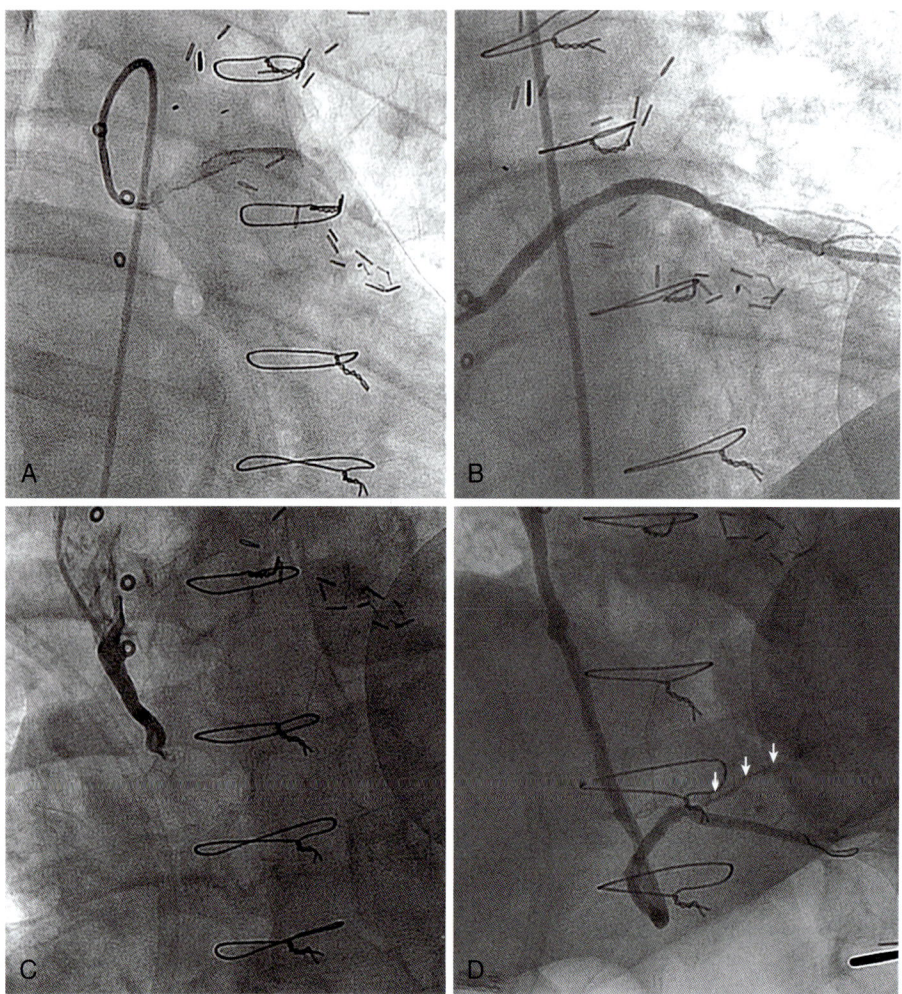

FIG. 28.23 Simultaneous multivessel thrombosis in the bypass grafts of a patient with anterior and inferior non–ST-elevation myocardial infarction. (A) Grade 4 thrombus burden in the saphenous vein graft (SVG) to the left anterior descending coronary artery. (B) Final revascularization results after aspiration catheter and stenting. (C) Grade 5 thrombotic occlusion of the SVG to the posterior descending artery. (D) Final revascularization results after aspiration catheter and stenting. (Courtesy William B. Abernethy III, MD, Asheville Cardiology Associates, Mission Memorial Hospital Heart Center, Asheville, NC.)

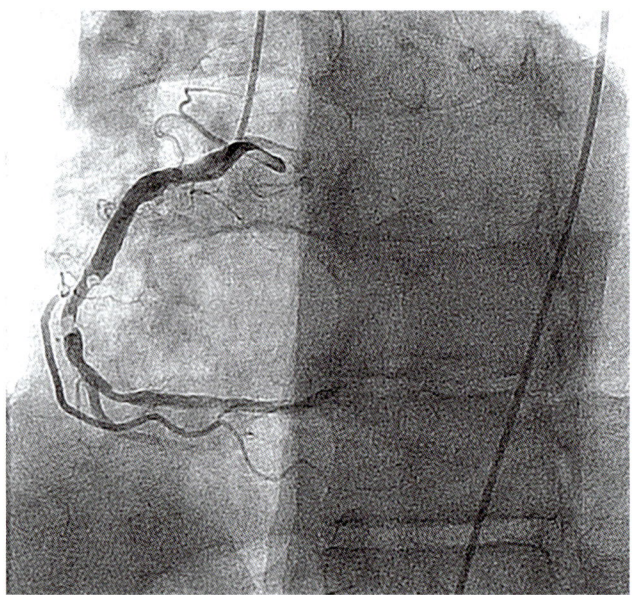

FIG. 28.24 Multiple thrombi with varying morphology presenting in a patient with acute coronary syndrome and severe inferolateral ischemia.

careful maneuvering of dedicated guidewires either via the antegrade or retrograde recanalization approach[168] are prerequisites to successful revascularization of the CTO. However, efforts to cross a CTO can be hampered by the triggering of uncontrolled thrombosis, whereby an underlying thrombus is provoked, culminating in the rapid accumulation of a large thrombus. Such an unwarranted development can threaten the entire PCI procedure and its outcome. Thus, ways of decreasing the burden of the embedded occlusive thrombus should be considered. This usually calls for the application of a mechanical removal device. Once most or all of the thrombotic content has been extracted, balloon dilatation and stenting are facilitated. In fact, evidence from the National Heart, Lung and Blood Institute registry corroborates the benefit of focusing on the thrombotic component of CTO during targeted PCI. Multivariate regression analysis has demonstrated that the presence of thrombus is a strong predictor of success in CTO revascularization (adjusted odds ratio 0.31, 95% CI 0.15– 0.61; P = .0008). This intriguing finding attests to the fact that thrombus removal clears the way for subsequent successful dilatation and precise stent delivery and deployment.[169] In the absence of bleeding complications, select intracoronary injection of low-dose thrombolytic therapy can also be administered until the completion of thrombus removal and subsequent stenting.

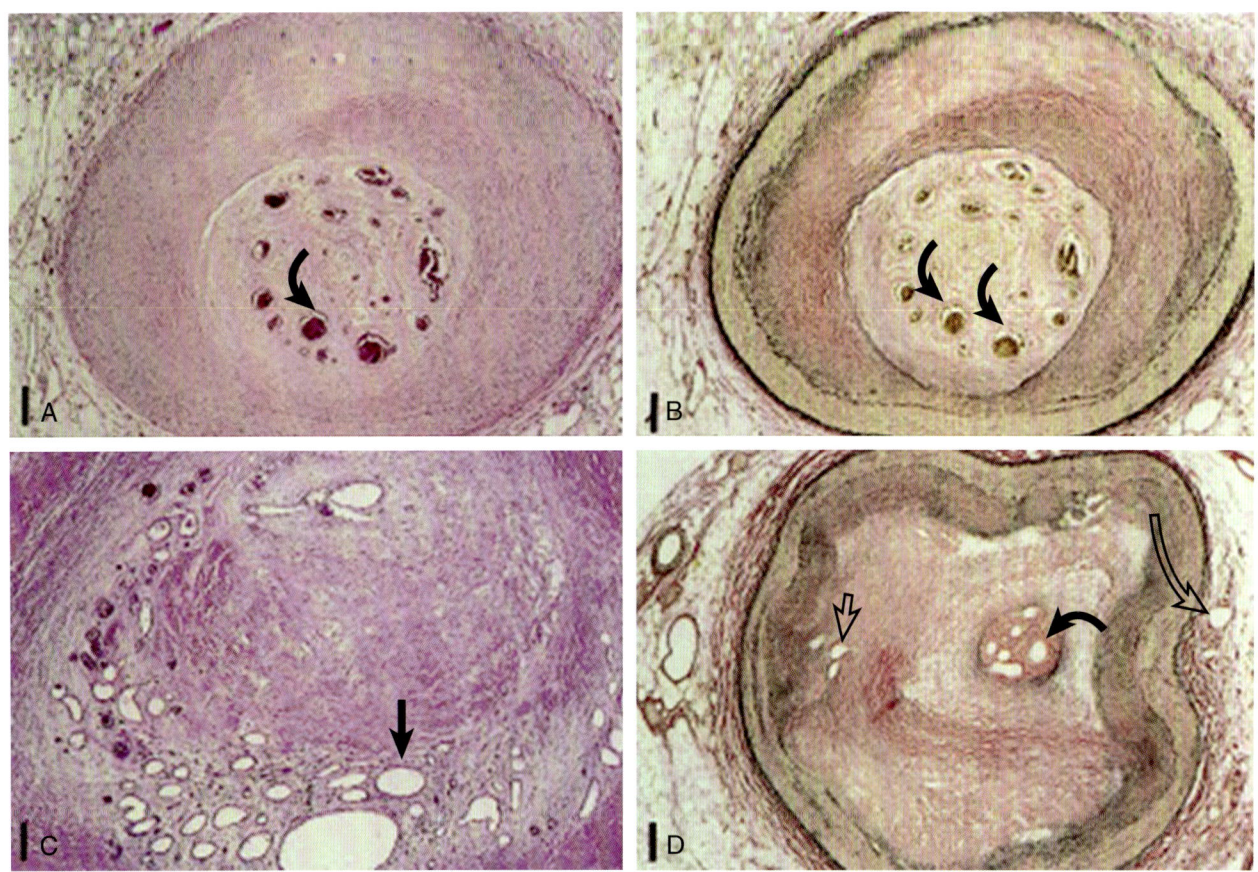

FIG. 28.25 Histopathology of chronic total occlusions. (A and B) Low-power views (hematoxylin-eosin and Lawson elastic van Gieson stains) showing recanalization of a chronic total occlusion by large central neovascular channels (NCs) *(arrows)*. Scale bar indicates 385 μm. (C) High-power view (hematoxylin-eosin stain) demonstrating extensive small, medium, and large intimal plaque (IP) NCs *(arrows)*. Scale bar indicates 167 μm. (D) Low-power view (elastic van Gieson stain) demonstrating central lumen, IP and adventitial NC formation (*solid*, *open* and *curved open arrows*, respectively). Scale bar indicates 500 μm. (From Strivatsa SS, Edwards WD, Boos CM, et al. Histologic correlates of angiographic chronic total coronary artery occlusions. *J Am Coll Cardiol.* 1997;29:955–963; Topaz O. *Cardiovascular Thrombus: From Pathology and Clinical Presentations to Imaging, Pharmacotherapy and Interventions.* Elsevier; 2018:311–320.)

For the removal process of atherosclerotic and thrombotic content within CTOs, multiple dedicated and innovative technologies are available. These include standard, coated, and fortified cutting balloons; balloon-mounted radiofrequency combined with thermal energy; acoustic ultrasound energy catheters; vibrational energy; magnetic navigation; blunt microdissection catheters; and collagenase infusion. Two of the most useful debulking and thrombus removal tools are rheolytic atherectomy (AngioJet, Boston Scientific, Boston, MA) and excimer laser (Spectranetics, Philips, Colorado Springs, CO) (Fig. 28.26). Both of these technologies utilize direct thrombus engagement for the removal of its constituents. Most procedures of PCI or endovascular peripheral interventions for CTOs include a final step of stenting. The preferable stent for this task is the drug-eluting type. In select patients with markedly long coronary CTOs, the intervention may require implantation of a "full metal jacket" (i.e., final stents 60 mm or longer without gap) in order to provide complete lesion coverage.[170]

SAPHENOUS VEIN GRAFT

Thrombus formation is among the most critical elements accountable for the development of degenerative venous graft disease.[171]

The classic pathologic features of thrombus in old SVGs are shown in Fig. 28.27. This relentless disease accounts for the failure of vein grafts following coronary artery bypass surgery. Consequently, at 10 years after surgery, the patency rate of old vein grafts is only 40% to 50%.[172] Distinct pathologic processes tend to develop in these vascular bypass conduits at different times.[173] Therefore thrombosis is the leading cause of early graft failure whereas atherosclerotic degeneration and neointimal hyperplasia are predominant at the midterm stage. Then thrombus plays a significant role in the pathogenesis of late venous graft disease, especially in association with the rupture of atherosclerotic plaques.[174] Fig. 28.28 demonstrates thrombosis and corresponding management in an old SVG. In general, thrombus superimposition is found in as many as 80% of old SVGs.[175] During the last two decades, percutaneous vein graft intervention has been established as the preferred treatment strategy for patients with degenerative vein grafts who experience angina pectoris, ischemia, and MI[176] as demonstrated in Fig. 28.29. Accordingly, the incorporation of dedicated thrombus-removal strategies for the treatment of SVGs—including pharmacotherapy, distal protection filters, aspiration catheters, power-based mechanical thrombectomy,[146,171] and implantation of standard as well as unique thrombus capturing/displacing stents[177]—have all contributed to a steady improvement in SVG PCI-related adverse angiographic

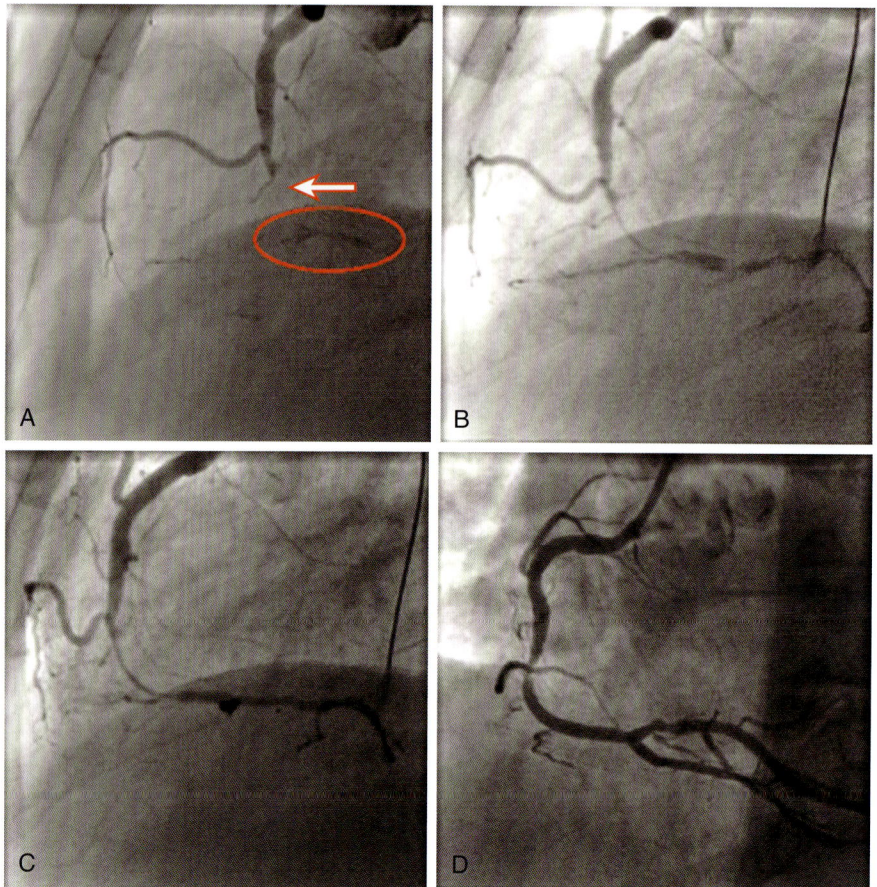

FIG. 28.26 Percutaneous coronary interventions in a patient with a chronic total occlusion who presented with exertion-related angina pectoris and shortness of breath. (A) Diagnostic angiogram in the lateral view demonstrates a chronic total occlusion in the middle segment of the right coronary artery. The proximal cap of the chronic total occlusion is marked by an *arrow*. The intraplaque middle segment of the occlusion contains a long linear thrombus *(red circle)*. (B) Angiographic results following successful crossing of the chronic total occlusion with a guidewire and activation of a 0.9-mm excimer laser catheter along the entire length of the occlusion. A recanalization channel was created with resultant restoration of antegrade flow. (C) Angiographic results following additional removal of thrombus burden by application of a 2.0-mm X-Sizer catheter. (D) Final angiographic results after adjunctive stenting of the chronic total occlusion site. The target vessel is completely patent with excellent distal flow. Clinically, the patient improved with no further angina pectoris and shortness of breath. (From Topaz A, Topaz O. The role and impact of thrombus in formation and revascularization of chronic total occlusions. In: Topaz O, ed. *Cardiovascular Thrombus: From Pathology and Clinical Presentations to Imaging, Pharmacotherapy and Interventions*. Elsevier; 2018:311–328.)

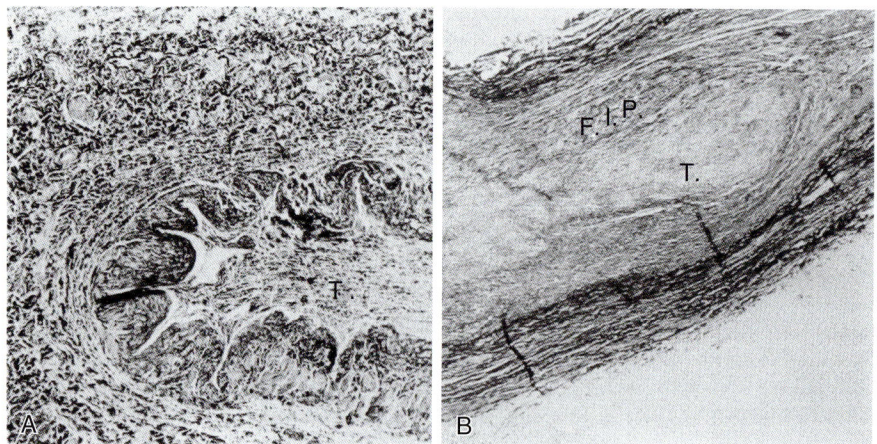

FIG. 28.27 Exhibition of thrombus in diseased saphenous vein grafts (SVGs). (A) SVG graft in place for 7 months. The lumen is occluded by an organized thrombus *(T)*. (Elastic tissue stain, ×57.) (B) SVG graft in place for 3 ½ months. Longitudinal section of SVG. The intima shows fibrous proliferation *(F.I.P.)*. In addition, luminal occlusion results from a superimposed organized thrombus *(T)*. (Elastic tissue stain, ×25.) (From the landmark article by Vlodaver Z, Edwards JE. Pathologic changes in aortic-coronary arterial saphenous vein grafts. *Circulation*. 1971;44:719–728, fig. 3. With permission.)

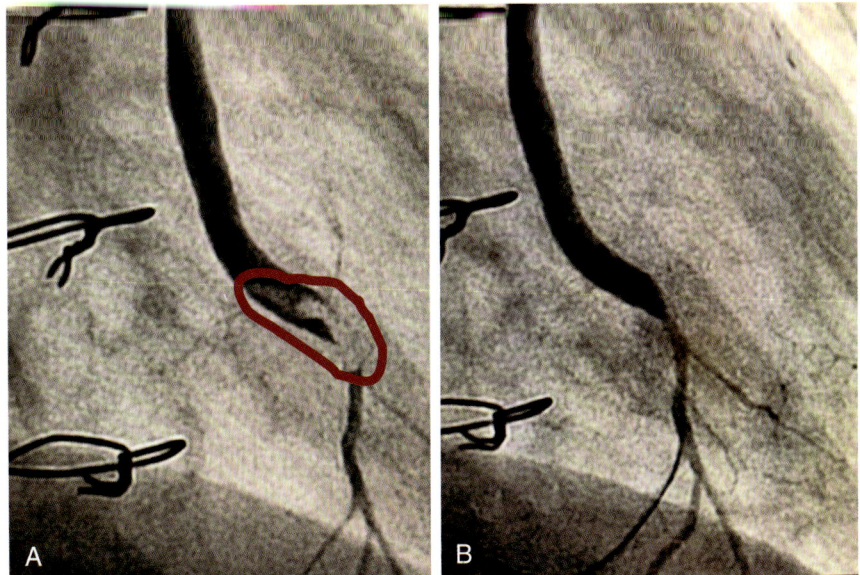

FIG. 28.28 Thrombosis and thrombus management in an old saphenous vein graft. A 70-year-old patient with a history of severe coronary artery disease after coronary artery bypass grafting 5 years earlier. Known atherosclerotic aorta and chronic atrial fibrillation on triple anticoagulation/antiplatelet therapy presented with severe chest pain and ischemia with evidence of a large non–ST-elevation myocardial infarction. The international normalization ratio (INR) was therapeutic and the ventricular rate under control. (A) Magnified angiographic view demonstrating a large thrombus burden *(red elliptic)* lodged at the distal anastomosis of the SVG to the obtuse marginal branch. Thrombolysis In myocardial infarction 1 (TIMI 1) compromised antegrade flow was present. (B) Several runs with an aspiration catheter retrieved yellow-beige granular atherosclerotic material. Antegrade flow markedly improved and the chest pain and ischemia disappeared. No underlying atherosclerotic plaque was identified at the site of the cleared occlusion. Therefore, while recognizing a graft-recipient "mismatch," adjunctive stenting was not performed. Subsequent pathologic examination demonstrated abundant deposits of calcium associated with scattered cholesterol clefts, foreign body giant cells, histiocytes, chronic inflammatory cells and small amounts of organizing thrombotic material that was eosinophilic, suggesting platelet deposition. Thus, this flow-limiting thrombus originated from the atherosclerotic ascending aorta. (Courtesy David H. Serfas, MD, FACC, Interventional Cardiology, Asheville Cardiology Associates, Mission Memorial Hospital, Asheville, NC.)

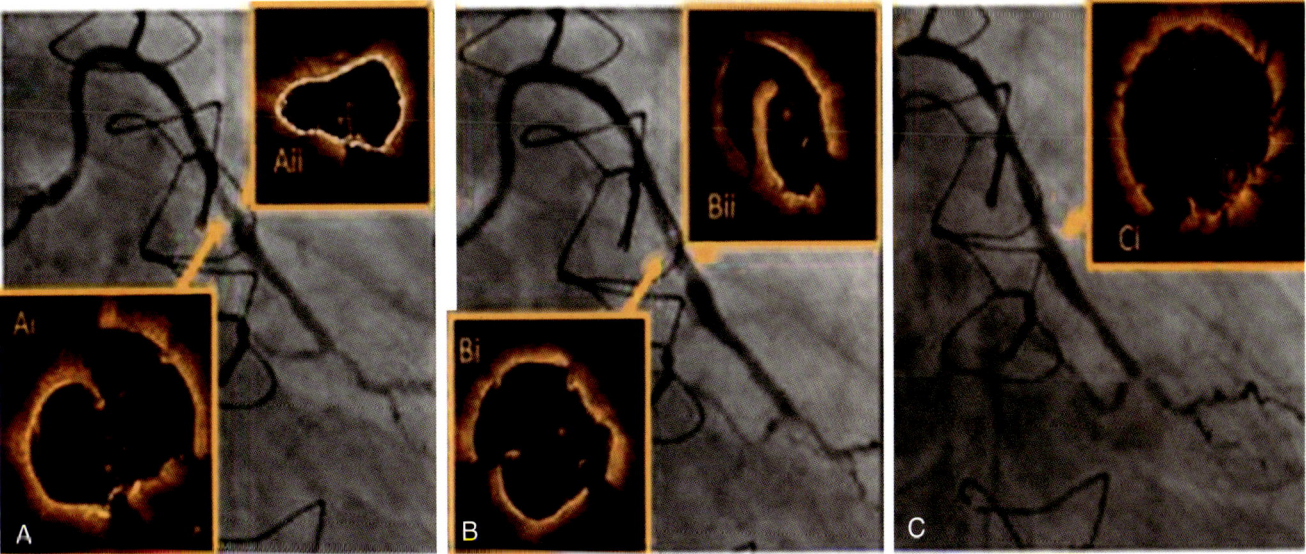

FIG. 28.29 (A) A severe lesion in the middle portion of a diffusely diseased saphenous vein graft (SVG) to the obtuse marginal from a patient presenting with an acute coronary syndrome. Upon optical coherence tomography (OCT) interrogation, a dissection flap is evident (Ai) proximal to a severe stenosis, with a minimal luminal area of 3.38 cm (Aii). The imaging suggested atheromatous plaque rupture within the SVG. Excimer laser revascularization was undertaken, on this occasion without a distal protection device. Analysis of the OCT image after laser application demonstrates a significant reduction in the burden of atheromatous plaque. (Bi) Extension of the atheromatous dissection is clearly shown, although it is not clearly seen angiographically. The case was completed with deployment of a single drug-eluting stent with excellent angiographic and OCT results (C). (Courtesy Dr. Peter O'Kane FRSC, FACC, Dorset Heart Centre, The Royal Bournemouth Hospital, Bournemouth, Dorset, UK.)

and clinical outcomes.[178] Although both bare-metal and drug-eluting stents are the most common devices applied in the management of thrombotic vein grafts, growing evidence demonstrates that the drug-eluting stents achieve better results.[179,180]

In consideration with the risk of poststenting thrombosis in treated vein grafts, it appears that a more potent and longer-lasting antiplatelet therapy may be required as compared with the treatment of native coronary arteries.[171] Nevertheless, owing to the prevalence of thrombus in old SVGs, interventions continue to be associated with a higher risk of distal embolization, the no-reflow phenomenon, myocardial tissue injury, and a considerably higher risk of 2-year major adverse ischemic events as compared with interventions in native coronary arteries.[180]

SUMMARY

Thrombus has a major impact on the performance, results, short- and long-term outcome, and cost of primary and rescue coronary interventions. Treatment can be successful with dedicated tools that incorporate any of the following mechanisms: displacement, extraction, dissolution, maceration and vaporization. Pharmacotherapy and mechanical thrombectomy devices can be used either separately or in combination. Despite the growing understanding of thrombus-containing lesions, the optimal management is still a study in progress and at times a controversial one.

KEY REFERENCES

1. Ligthart J, Ren C, Evelyn Regar E, et al. Encounters with thrombus and thrombosis in a major academic center: cases as "Pictures at an Exhibition." In: Topaz O, ed. *Cardiovascular Thrombus: From Pathology and Clinical Presentations to Imaging, Pharmacotherapy and Interventions*. Philadelphia: Elsevier; 2018:321–336 [chapter 22].
7. Sianos G, Papafaklis MI, Daemen J, et al. Angiographic stent thrombosis after routine use of drug eluting stents in ST-segment elevation myocardial infarction. The importance of thrombus burden. *J Am Coll Cardiol*. 2007;50:572–583.
10. Topaz O. Revascularization of thrombus laden lesions in AMI-the burden on the interventionalist. *J Invas Cardiol*. 2007;19:324–325.
11. Topaz O. Thrombectomy during primary PCI for STEMI-call of the thrombus. *Cath Cardiovasc Interv*. 2012;80:1181–1182 [Editorial].
13. Karacsonyi J, Henry T, Ungi I, et al. The impact of thrombus as a cause and as a result of complicated percutaneous coronary intervention. In: Topaz O, ed. *Cardiovascular Thrombus: From Pathology and Clinical Presentations to Imaging, Pharmacotherapy and Interventions*. Philadelphia: Elsevier; 2018:203–216 [chapter 14].
14. Napodano M, Landi A. Impact of thrombus burden on myocardial damage in the setting of primary percutaneous coronary intervention. In: Topaz O, ed. *Cardiovascular Thrombus: From Pathology and Clinical Presentations to Imaging, Pharmacotherapy and Interventions*. Philadelphia: Elsevier; 2018:189–201 [chapter 13].
15. Vilahur G, Ben-Aicha S, Badimon L. Animal models of thrombosis. In: Topaz O, ed. *Cardiovascular Thrombus: From Pathology and Clinical Presentations to Imaging, Pharmacotherapy and Interventions*. Philadelphia: Elsevier; 2018:87–97 [chapter 6].
16. Leiderman K, Bannish BE, Kelley MA, et al. Mathematical models of thrombus formation and fibrinolysis. In: Topaz O, ed. *Cardiovascular Thrombus: From Pathology and Clinical Presentations to Imaging, Pharmacotherapy and Interventions*. Philadelphia: Elsevier; 2018:67–86 [chapter 5].
17. Lamichhane M, Salehi N, Ahmadjee A, et al. Pathology of arterial thrombosis: characteristics and thrombus types. In: Topaz O, ed. *Cardiovascular Thrombus: From Pathology and Clinical Presentations to Imaging, Pharmacotherapy and Interventions*. Philadelphia: Elsevier; 2018:15–30.
28. Baker SR, Ariens RAS. Fibrin clot structure and function: a novel risk factor for arterial and venous thrombosis and thromboembolism. In: Topaz O, ed. *Cardiovascular Thrombus: From Pathology and Clinical Presentations to Imaging, Pharmacotherapy and Interventions*. Philadelphia: Elsevier; 2018:31–49 [chapter 3].
31. Layne K, Passacquale G, Ferro A. The role of platelets in the pathophysiology of atherosclerosis and its complications. In: Topaz O, ed. *Cardiovascular Thrombus: From Pathology and Clinical Presentations to Imaging, Pharmacotherapy and Interventions*. Philadelphia: Elsevier; 2018:51–65 [chapter 4].
38. Vlaar PJ, Svilaas T, Vogelzang M, et al. A Comparison of 2 thrombus aspiration devices with histopathological analysis of retrieved material in patients presenting with ST-segment elevation myocardial infarction. *JACC Cardiovasc Interv*. 2008;1. 265–226.
41. Topaz O. On the hostile massive thrombus and the means to eradicate it. *Cath Cardiovasc Interv*. 2005;65:280–281 [Editorial].
51. Rawlins J, Shah N, O'Kane P. Adjunct interventional techniques for the treatment of intra-coronary thrombus. *Heart*. 2013;99:216–222.
54. Topaz O, Topaz A, Owen K. Thrombus grading for coronary interventions: The role of contemporary classifications. *Interv Cardiol*. 2011;3:705–712.
58. Dahm JB, Ebersole D, Das T, et al. Prevention of distal embolization and no-reflow in patients with acute myocardial infarction and total occlusion in the infarct-related vessels. *Cath Cardiovasc Interv*. 2005;64:67–74.
126. Polkampally PR, Topaz A, Topaz O. Lasers in cardiology and cardiothoracic surgery. In: Nouri K, ed. *Lasers in Dermatology and Medicine*. New York: Springer; 2011:573–580.
127. Rawlins J, Talwar S, Green M, et al. Optical coherence tomography following percutaneous coronary intervention with excimer laser coronary atherectomy. *Cardiovasc Revasc Med*. 2014;15:29–34.
132. Topaz O, Ebersole D, Dahm JB, et al. Excimer laser in myocardial infarction: a comparison between STEMI patients with established Q-wave versus patients with non-STEMI [non-Q]. *Lasers Med Sci*. 2008;23:1–10.
155. Parodi G, Memisha G, Bellandi B, et al. Effectiveness of primary percutaneous coronary interventions for stent thrombosis. *Am J Cardiol*. 2009;103:913–916.

Additional references available online at expertconsult.com.

中文导读

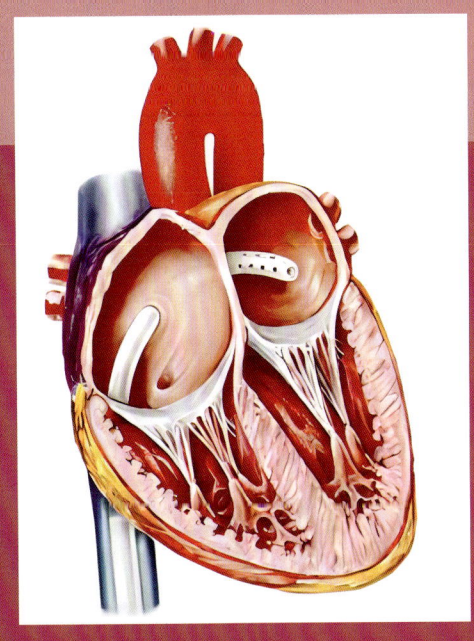

第29章
经皮冠状动脉介入治疗的并发症

　　尽管过去40年里经皮冠状动脉介入治疗术的并发症已明显下降，但并发症会直接影响介入治疗所带来的临床获益，这值得临床医师关注。本章节介绍了急性闭塞、冠状动脉穿孔、器械脱载、紧急冠状动脉旁路移植术、心肌梗死、无复流等常见并发症，详细分析相关机制，并给予防治指导。

　　急性闭塞病因以冠状动脉夹层及损伤最为常见，分为5大类，治疗目标是稳定血流动力学及减轻心肌缺血。急性闭塞也可由血栓导致，如确有血栓形成，充分抗凝极为重要。冠状动脉破裂主要由导丝挫伤及血管破裂导致，可根据病变严重程度分为3级，对应不同治疗方式及预后。冠状动脉破裂的治疗核心是封闭穿孔部位、维持血流动力学稳定、酌情心包穿刺及适时停用抗凝药物。医源性升主动脉夹层偶有发生，绝大多数患者可保守治疗。经皮冠状动脉介入治疗相关器械血栓是一个灾难性的并发症，本章节提到处理多种置入物血栓的方法。围术期心肌梗死亦有发生，需留意患者心肌酶及肌钙蛋白变化，针对该并发症预防，抗血小板药物效果确切，远端栓塞装置有待探索。无复流机制较为复杂，在一定程度上可通过预处理及后处理降低发生率。对比剂过敏很常见但一般较轻，必要时可通过类固醇、肾上腺素等药物治疗以改善症状。出血是较为常见的并发症，相关治疗策略包括选择合适的患者、个性化药物应用、通路管理及使用桡动脉通路。

　　预防是并发症治疗的最佳策略，而及时识别并正确处理是并发症治疗的关键，这也是一位成熟术者必须具备的能力。通过本章节介绍，将有助于提高介入心脏病医师处理经皮冠状动脉介入治疗相关并发症的能力和经验。

赵天禄　柳景华

章节要点

- 尽管大多数并发症可以避免，但如果发生，快速诊断及正确处置对于减少诸如心肌梗死或死亡等不良事件十分重要。
- 急性闭塞及术中支架血栓形成或急性支架内血栓是导致心肌梗死及死亡的严重并发症。这类患者需要快速恢复血流灌注、选择最优药物治疗、谨慎评估、确定病因并加以治疗。
- 冠状动脉穿孔主要由导丝、过度扩张、旋磨装置导致。应用球囊封堵穿孔部位并停用抗凝药物极为重要。如果穿孔持续存在，关于植入PTFE覆膜支架或进行急诊心脏手术的必要性尚存争议。
- 涉及内膜下扩张的现代慢性完全闭塞病变介入治疗技术会增加并发症发生率。例如，心肌内血肿、主动脉开口部夹层、侧支循环丢失等并发症过去罕见，但对于慢性完全闭塞病变介入治疗就显得更为多见。
- 支架脱载栓塞是一种并不常见的并发症。如果可能，需保留导丝在支架结构中心通过。支架取出涉及一系列技术，包括远端球囊扩张、抓捕及导丝缠绕。必要时可将脱载支架在原位（非计划部位）释放。
- 正接受经皮冠状动脉介入治疗的患者需转运紧急心脏外科手术，其死亡率和并发症发生率很高。这是由于患者正处于心肌梗死状态，经皮冠状动脉介入治疗术所采取的强效抗凝治疗所致。
- 围术期心肌梗死与并发症发生率及死亡率密切相关。预防围术期心肌梗死发生的策略除了包括药物优化治疗，还包括合理使用诸如远端保护伞等辅助器械。
- 远端微循环血管床受阻可导致冠状动脉血流受损，从而引起最终的冠状动脉无复流。尽管无复流有时可通过血管扩张剂逆转，但预防仍然是最佳策略。
- 大多数空气栓塞是医源性的，可以通过细致的导管管理加以预防。
- 对比剂过敏很少发生且有时难以诊断。为了稳定过敏患者血流动力学情况，类固醇激素治疗必不可少，有时也需要肾上腺素。
- 出血与住院期间及术后30天内死亡率升高密切相关。避免出血的策略包括优化患者选择、药物治疗及血管入路选择与管理。

29 Complications of Percutaneous Coronary Intervention

Marvin H. Eng, Jeffrey W. Moses, Paul S. Teirstein

Good judgment comes from experience and experience comes from bad judgment.
—Unknown

KEY POINTS

- Although most complications are avoidable, when they occur, rapid recognition and corrective response are necessary to mitigate adverse consequences such as myocardial infarctions or death.
- Abrupt closure and intraprocedural stent thrombosis/acute stent thrombosis (<24 hours) are serious complications that can result in myocardial infarctions and death. Treating them requires rapid steps to restore perfusion, optimization of pharmacology, and careful evaluation to identify and treat the cause.
- Coronary perforations are generally caused by guidewires, overdilation, and atheroablative devices. Sealing the perforation with balloon occlusion is imperative, followed by halting anticoagulation. Should it be necessary, either implantation of a polytetrafluoroethylene (PTFE)-stent graft or referral to emergent cardiac surgery remains an option if the perforation persists.
- Contemporary chronic total occlusion percutaneous coronary intervention (PCI) techniques involving subintimal dilation are associated with increased complication rates. Complications that were formally rare, such as intramyocardial hematoma, aortoostial dissection, and side branch loss, are surfacing more frequently at busy chronic total occlusion programs.
- Stents embolization is an infrequent complication. If possible, retain wire access through the center of the stent. Retrieval involves an array of techniques, including distal balloon inflation, snaring, and wire wrapping. Deployment of an embolized stent in an unintended location may be necessary.
- Emergent referral of patients undergoing PCI for cardiac surgery is associated with significant morbidity and mortality due to ongoing myocardial infarction and the powerful anticoagulants used during PCI.
- Periprocedural myocardial infarction is associated with increased morbidity and mortality. Strategies to avoid periprocedural myocardial infarction include pharmacologic optimization and appropriate use of adjunctive devices such as distal protection filters.
- Coronary no-reflow results when the distal microcirculatory bed is overwhelmed resulting in impaired coronary flow. Although sometimes reversible with vasodilators, prevention remains the best strategy.
- Air embolism is almost always iatrogenic and preventable through meticulous catheter management.
- Radiocontrast hypersensitivity occurs rarely and is sometimes difficult to recognize. Treatment with steroids and sometimes epinephrine may be necessary to stabilize the patient's hemodynamics.
- Bleeding is associated with significant in-hospital and 30-day mortality. Strategies to avoid bleeding include optimization of patient selection, pharmacology, and access site selection and management.

INTRODUCTION

Over the past 40 years, complications of percutaneous coronary intervention (PCI) have decreased dramatically. The contemporary procedural risk of death, myocardial infarction (MI), or urgent referral for bypass surgery is 1.54% to 1.67%, 1.5%, and 0.2%, respectively.[1-3] The lower complication rate is partially responsible for a growing trend towards same-day discharge following PCI.[4] Nevertheless, prompt recognition of complications and a calm and effective response are essential components of success as a PCI operator. This chapter will explore the most common procedural complications.

ABRUPT CLOSURE

Incidence

The term abrupt closure dates back to the prestent era, referring to cessation of coronary flow often related to dissection or thrombosis. In contemporary interventional practice, vessel closure is a relatively rare event that may be related to inadequate pharmacology, residual thrombus, stent edge-dissection, or inability to contain a major coronary dissection. The incidence of abrupt closure (often called "acute closure") during PCI has steadily decreased from 3% in the balloon angioplasty era to 0.3% in the current era (Fig. 29.1). The trend in decreasing acute closure rates corresponds to the increased utilization of stents and effective antithrombotics, including glycoprotein IIb/IIIa inhibitors, dual antiplatelet therapy, and direct thrombin inhibitors. The decrease in abrupt closure resulted in a decrease in emergent coronary artery bypass grafting (CABG) and reduced periprocedural PCI mortality from 1.4% in 1985–1986 (as observed from the National Heart, Lung and Blood Institute [NHLBI] Dynamic Registry), to an in-hospital mortality rate of 0.13%–0.16% and 1.54%–1.67% for elective and all PCI, respectively, as a result of the most recent iterative improvements in technology and quality.[5]

Mechanisms

The most common mechanism of acute closure is dissection and injury to the media (Fig. 29.2; Table 29.1).[6] Intramural hematoma can develop, along with intimal flaps, causing mechanical obstruction.

With mechanical obstruction and the exposure of subintimal tissue, thrombus formation is often initiated. Vasoconstriction further complicates this milieu but is rarely a major mechanism of closure.[7]

Although the predominate causes of acute closure in the prestent era were dissection (28%), thrombus (20%), or both (7%), the cause is indeterminate in almost 50% of patients.[8,9] Patient factors predictive of abrupt closure include unstable angina, multivessel disease, and female gender.[10,11] When examining the angiographic risk factors of dissection-mediated acute closure, proximal tortuosity was the strongest predictor followed by American College of Cardiology (ACC) lesion grade C (Table 29.2), longer lesion length, and de novo stenosis. Similarly, risks for thrombotic closure include presence of preexisting thrombus, degenerated vein grafts, and recent MI.[11] Air embolism and no-reflow phenomenon are also part of the differential diagnosis of abrupt closure (discussed elsewhere).

As techniques in interventional cardiology have evolved to include intentional dissection and reentry for recanalization of chronic total occlusions (CTOs), the breadth of complications from dissections have changed. Formerly, there were concerns only of abrupt closure for untreated dissections; however, now that extensive dissections are created with the ultimate goal of successful recanalization and stenting along its entire length, the implications of dissections differ. The range of complications currently include abrupt closure of unstented dissections should the operators be unable to stent the length of the exposed subintima, propagation of subintimal hematomas that unintentionally extend the dissection, and stenting of the subintimal space unintentionally closing side branches resulting in ischemia or infarction.

Prognostic Significance

Most data regarding outcomes of patients experiencing abrupt closure are derived from the prestent era. In studies from the balloon angioplasty era, 6% of patients died, 36% suffered nonfatal MI, and 30% were referred for emergency CABG.[8]

Treatment

Abrupt closure results in acute ischemia that may be manifested by dramatic electrocardiogram (ECG) changes, hypotension, hypertension, chest pain, ventricular arrhythmias, and/or bradycardia.

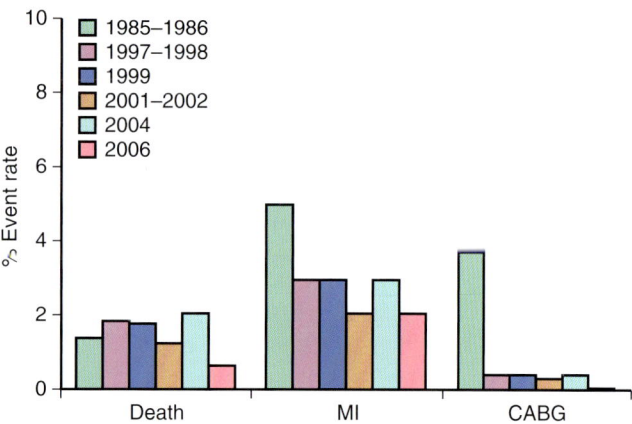

Fig. 29.1 Improvements in percutaneous coronary intervention outcomes through its evolution from the balloon angioplasty to the drug-eluting stent era are reflected in the National Heart, Lung and Blood Institute Dynamic Registry. *CABG,* Coronary artery bypass grafting; *MI,* myocardial infarction. (From Venkitachalam L, Kip KE, Selzer F, et al. Twenty-year evolution of percutaneous coronary intervention and its impact on clinical outcomes: a report from the National Heart, Lung, and Blood Institute-Sponsored, Multicenter 1985–1986 PTCA and 1997–2006 Dynamic Registries. *Circ Cardiovasc Interv.* 2009;2:6–13.)

TABLE 29.1 Classification of Coronary Dissection

Type	Description	Acute Closure (%)
A	Minor radiolucencies within lumen during angiography without dye persistence	0–2
B	Parallel tracks or double lumen separated by radiolucent area during angiography without dye persistence	2–4
C	Extraluminal cap with dye persistence	10
D	Spiral luminal filling defects	30
E	New persistent filling defects	9
F	Non-E types that lead to impaired flow or total occlusion	69

Permission obtained by author from Klein LW. Coronary complications of percutaneous coronary intervention: a practical approach to the management of abrupt closure. *Catheter Cardiovasc Interv.* 2005;64:395–401.

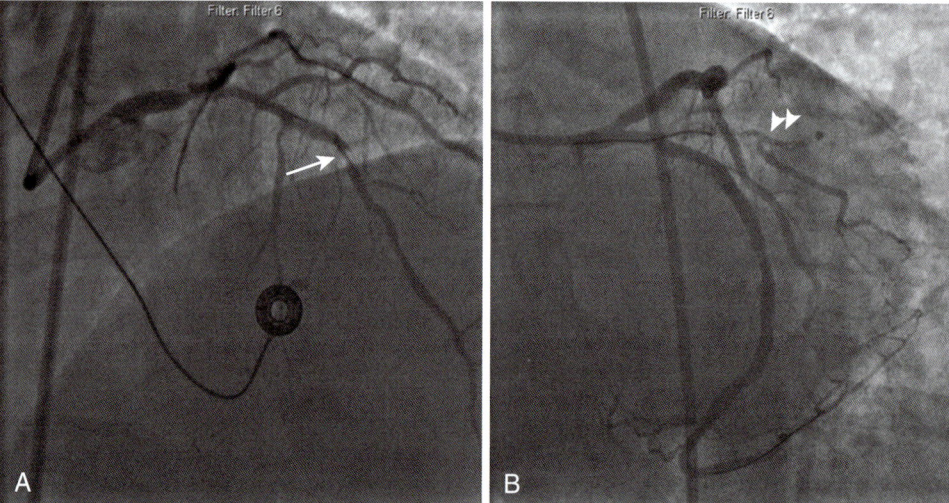

Fig. 29.2 Coronary dissection. (A) Nonflow limiting dissection in the left anterior descending artery *(arrow).* (B) Flow-limiting spiral dissection of the obtuse marginal branch with incomplete distal filling *(arrowheads).*

CHAPTER 29 Complications of Percutaneous Coronary Intervention

TABLE 29.2 American College of Cardiology/American Heart Association Lesion Classification System

TYPE A
- Discrete (<10 mm length)
- Concentric
- Readily accessible
- Nonangulated segment, <45 degrees
- Smooth contour
- Little or no calcification
- Less than totally occlusive
- Not ostial in location
- No major side branch involvement
- Absence of thrombus

TYPE B
- Tubular (10–20 mm length)
- Eccentric
- Moderate tortuosity of proximal segment
- Moderately angulated segment, >45 degrees, <90 degrees
- Irregular contour
- Moderate to heavy calcification
- Total occlusions <3 months old
- Ostial in location
- Bifurcation lesions requiring double guidewires
- Some thrombus present

TYPE C
- Diffuse (>2 cm length)
- Excessive tortuosity of proximal segment
- Extremely angulated segments >90 degrees
- Totally occlusion >3 months old
- Inability to protect major side branches
- Degenerated vein grafts with friable lesions

B1, One adverse characteristic; B2, ≥2 adverse characteristics.

The first priorities are to stabilize hemodynamics and relieve ischemia. Vasopressors, inotropes, intraaortic balloon pump (IABP), or ventricular assist device insertion should be considered for hemodynamic instability. Extreme vagal reactions may also cause bradycardia or hypotension and should be treated with atropine, intravenous (IV) fluid boluses, and vasopressors if necessary. Immediate recognition and treatment of electrical instability with antiarrhythmic medications and cardioversion are imperative.[7]

Expeditious efforts to restore antegrade flow such as repeat angioplasty must be quickly attempted. Urgent stenting is usually required to stabilize dissections. Glycoprotein IIb/IIIa or IV $P2Y_{12}$ inhibitors can be helpful if thrombus is responsible for the acute closure. Prospective use of abciximab was compared with placebo in both balloon angioplasty and stenting cohorts in the Evaluation of Platelet IIb/IIIa inhibitor for Stenting (EPISTENT) trial and demonstrated that abciximab decreased rates of abrupt closure and side branch loss.[12] However, the utility of glycoprotein IIb/IIIa inhibitors as a bailout is controversial because the available data are more supportive of upstream use during PCI.[12,13]

In the case of persistent acute closure, one should consider the use of intravascular ultrasound (IVUS) to better define pathology, such as the presence and extent of dissections. Multiple stents may be required to restore patency and stabilize a dissection. If the IVUS findings are suspicious for thrombus, aspiration thrombectomy may be valuable and the addition of a glycoprotein IIb/IIIa inhibitor should be considered. Intracoronary thrombolytic delivery has been used for rescue of abrupt closure but is associated with significant morbidity and not recommended.[10] When wiring dissections, it is important to confirm selection of the true lumen prior to stenting or otherwise suffer the result of false-lumen stenting and loss of myocardial perfusion. In the process of troubleshooting the dilemma of true versus false-lumen location, IVUS can help to distinguish the two without potentially pressurizing the subintimal space with selective injections (Fig. 29.3).

Factors affecting the inflow and outflow should be investigated. The use of multiple angiographic views, IVUS, and selective distal injections may better delineate the anatomy. Guide catheter dissections may cause poor in-flow and can easily be overlooked. Pressure dampening, ventricularization, ECG changes, or severe ischemic pain may indicate an ostial guide catheter dissection. Distal wire dissections that occlude outflow may require stenting or prolonged balloon inflation.

In the prestent, balloon angioplasty era, approximately 40% of cases with acute closure ultimately achieved procedural success.[10] The predominant treatment was repeat balloon dilation with prolonged inflation facilitated by autoperfusion balloon catheters. Historically, the use of stents as a bail-out device for abrupt or impending closure dramatically decreased the need for emergent CABG.[14] Although no randomized trial has been performed, the dramatic decrease in urgent and emergent CABG, from 3% to 0.7% in the NHLBI Dynamic Registry was clearly associated with the use of stents and more effective anticoagulation, primarily glycoprotein IIb/IIIa inhibitors and $P2Y_{12}$ inhibitors.[5]

Patients with a successful outcome following treatment of abrupt closure require close monitoring in an intensive care setting. If needed, intraaortic balloon counterpulsation or left ventricular (LV) assist devices should be considered until the patient is stable. Serial cardiac enzyme assessments, ECGs, and echocardiography to assess the extent of myocardial damage are also recommended (see Fig. 29.4 for acute vessel closure management algorithm).

Unsuccessful Outcome

If recanalization is unsuccessful, the interventionalist is faced with the choice of referral for emergent coronary bypass surgery or medical management. Medical management is essentially acceptance that the patient will sustain an MI. The quantity of myocardium subtended by the closed vessel, versus the likelihood of a successful surgical result and risks of undergoing emergent surgery, is the most important factor when deciding between surgical or medical management of abrupt closure. Care must be taken to distinguish "refractory closure" from "no-reflow" because CABG is ineffective in the latter. Certainly the degree of supportive therapy may include use of devices to treat cardiogenic shock and utilization of percutaneous ventricular assist devices ranging from axial flow catheters (Impella, Abiomed, Danvers, MA) or extracorporeal support either in the form of TandemHeart (LivaNova, London, U.K.) or extracorporeal membrane oxygenation (ECMO).

Stent Thrombosis

Intraprocedural and acute stent thrombosis both comprise a form of contemporary abrupt closure. Stents serve to improve patency after dilating stenotic lesions and stabilize dissections, but metal is inherently thrombogenic, and early experience with stents showed thrombosis rates as high as 8% to 16% if implanted for rescuing abrupt closure.[15,16] The early stent thrombosis (<30 days) rate for elective PCI in stable coronary artery disease (CAD) patients is 0.3% to 0.5%, but stenting for acute coronary syndromes demonstrated early stent thrombosis rates as high as 3.4% and 1.4% for ST-elevation MI (STEMI) and non-STEMI (NSTEMI), respectively, indicating the presence of a thrombogenic milieu.[17–20] Intraprocedural stent thrombosis (IPST) and acute stent thrombosis are rare events, occurring 0.8% to 1.2% and 0.1% to 0.9% of cases, respectively.[21–24] For purposes of this chapter, we will focus on intraprocedural and acute stent thrombosis (<24 hours from implantation).

Factors leading to stent thrombosis include a combination of patient comorbidities, suboptimal pharmacology, and procedural

567

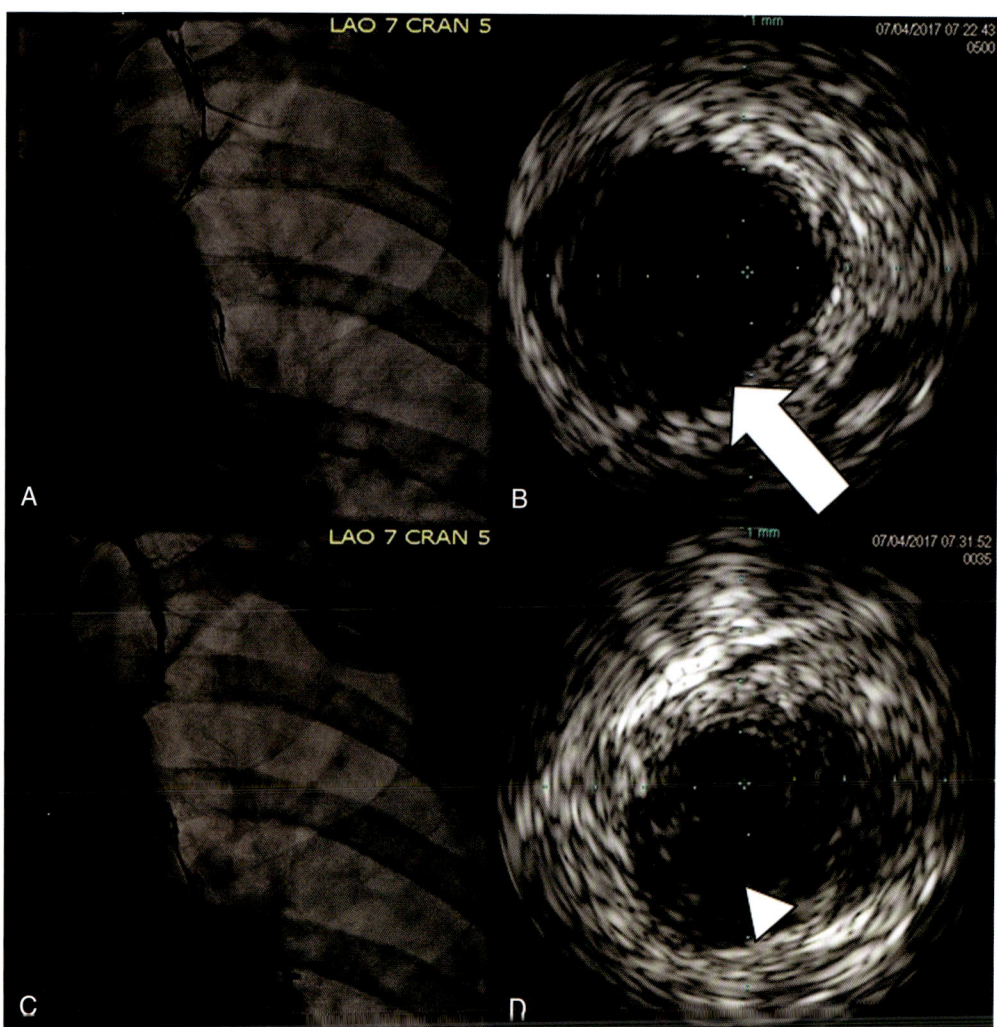

Fig. 29.3 Intravascular ultrasound (IVUS) Interrogation for troubleshooting true- versus false-lumen wire location. (A) Left internal mammary artery hydraulic dissection and attempt to wire the true lumen. (B) Questioning the wire location, IVUS demonstrates a lumen that is compressed by subintimal hematoma *(arrow)*. This lumen appears to have a media and the fact that the wire cannot be easily advanced corroborates false lumen location. (C) The wire was withdrawn and redirected, this time finding the true lumen, confirmed by IVUS. (D) IVUS confirmed true lumen location, and this time the false lumen is observed *(arrowhead)*. This time the wire can be advanced easily.

variables related to stent implantation, plaque disruption, and vessel injury. Multivariate analysis from the Cangrelor versus Standard Therapy to Achieve Optimal Management of Platelet Inhibition-PHOENIX (CHAMPION-PHOENIX) study identified NSTEMI and STEMI at presentation (NSTEMI odds ratio [OR] 1.87, $P = .04$; STEMI OR 2.07, $P = .004$), angiographic thrombus prior to PCI (OR 1.79, $P = .01$), and total stent length (OR 1.03 per mm, $P < .0001$) as independent predictors of IPST.[22] Post hoc inspection of the Acute Catheterization and Urgent Intervention Triage Strategy (ACUITY) trial revealed insulin-dependent diabetes (OR 3.48), renal insufficiency (OR 2.09), Duke jeopardy score (OR 1.15), final stent minimal luminal diameter (OR 0.32), preprocedural thienopyridine administration (OR 0.30), baseline hemoglobin (OR 1.28), and extent of CAD (OR 1.01) as independent factors associated with early stent thrombosis.[17] In an IVUS substudy of stent thrombosis from the Harmonizing Outcomes with Revascularization and Stents in Acute Myocardial Infarction (HORIZONS-AMI) trial, small cross-sectional area (<5 mm^2), stent malapposition, plaque protrusion, edge dissection, and residual stenosis played significant roles in predicting early stent thrombosis.[25] All cases of stent thrombosis had at least one abnormality, and 50% of patients had two or more IVUS abnormalities.[25] Ex vivo histologic analysis of fatal stent thrombosis cases corroborated plaque prolapse and incomplete apposition as contributors of stent thrombosis; however, medial tears were found in 27% of analyzed segments, suggesting that deep vessel wall injuries play a significant role in stent thrombosis.[26] Finally, complex PCI, particularly stenting using the crush technique, carries a higher rate of IPST of 0.5% to 1.3%.[27]

Mortality of stent thrombosis ranges from 26% to 45% overall when looking at all-comers.[28] Those who present with STEMI are found to have less successful reperfusion compared with their STEMI counterparts who do not have stent thrombosis (stent thrombosis 80.4% vs. nonstent thrombosis 96.9%, $P < .0001$).[29] Along with less successful reperfusion, those with STEMI in the context of stent thrombosis have greater rates of in-hospital mortality (stent thrombosis–STEMI 17.4% vs. nonstent thrombosis–STEMI 7.1%, $P = .03$) and composite major adverse cardiovascular and cerebrovascular event (MACCE) (stent thrombosis–STEMI 25.6% vs. nonstent thrombosis–STEMI 9.2%, $P = .003$).[29] Similarly IPST has a 30-day mortality rate of 10.1% and carries an adjusted OR of 12.3 of death compared with non-IPST cases. In addition, IPST predicts a higher rate of 30-day post-PCI stent thrombosis (5.6%, adjusted OR 7.6).[22]

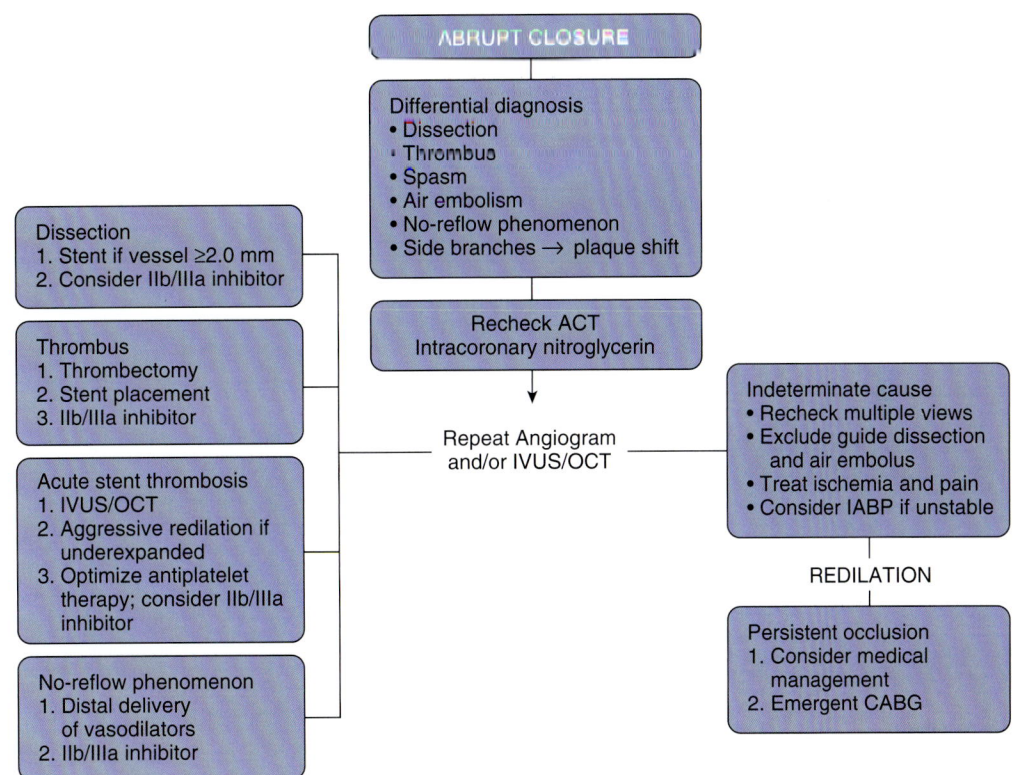

Fig. 29.4 Suggested algorithm for management of abrupt closure. *ACT*, Activated clotting time; *CABG*, coronary artery bypass grafting; *IABP*, Intraaortic balloon pump; *IVUS*, intravascular ultrasound; *OCT*, optical coherence tomography. (Adapted from Klein LW. Coronary complications of percutaneous coronary intervention: a practical approach to the management of abrupt closure. *Catheter Cardiovasc Interv.* 2005;64:395–401.)

Avoiding stent thrombosis requires operators to be meticulous about anticoagulation and stent implantation. A fundamental axiom is confirming adequate outflow prior to stent implantation. Placing a stent in an artery with no-reflow due to microvascular obstruction or a vessel with poor distal runoff is risky and may increase the likelihood of stent thrombosis. In the highest thrombotic risk acute coronary syndrome, STEMI, it appears that preprocedure pharmacology may be efficacious for reducing stent thrombosis. Preprocedure prasugrel did not seem to impact stent thrombosis and was associated with excessive bleeding complications; however, pre-hospital ticagrelor decreased definite stent thrombosis (OR 0.26, 95% confidence interval [CI] 0.07 to 0.91).[30,31] Cangrelor utilization was associated with a 35% decrease in intraprocedural stent thrombosis (OR 0.65, CI 0.42 to 0.99, *P* = .04) in the CHAMPION-PHOENIX study, further emphasizing the important role of platelet blockade in stent thrombosis.[22] Routine use of intravascular imaging has been shown to be important in left main stenting, and summated evidence from a recent meta-analysis shows a significant decrease in stent thrombosis when using IVUS and optical coherence tomography (OCT) with an OR of 0.42 (95% CI 0.2 to 0.72) and 0.39 (95% CI 0.1 to 1.20), respectively.[32,33] When using IVUS, reductions in cardiovascular death, MI, and target-lesion revascularization were observed.[33]

When confronted with acute or IPST, one must be very prompt at restoring perfusion to minimize myocardial damage and the approach to treatment should include both pharmacologic and mechanical optimization. Certainly, if intracoronary thrombus develops, prompt aspiration thrombectomy or angioplasty should be performed immediately to restore patency. Therapeutic anticoagulation should be confirmed and more potent antiplatelet therapy considered, as both IV cangrelor and glycoprotein inhibition were both associated with less IPST.[22,34]

Bailout glycoprotein inhibitor, loading with either prasugrel or ticagrelor, or switching to cangrelor to rapidly reach maximal steady state platelet inhibition may be helpful if not already using these medications. If there is suspicion the patient could have heparin-induced thrombocytopenia (HITT), switching to a direct-thrombin inhibitor such as bivalirudin should be considered. Intravascular imaging with either IVUS or OCT should be used to determine stent apposition, expansion, and presence of edge dissections. Optimization of stent deployment with appropriate postdilation and treatment of edge dissections with additional stents will be imperative to prevent repeat stent thrombosis.[35] Additional stent implantation should be done judiciously because each millimeter of stent increases the probability of IPST.[22]

CORONARY PERFORATION

Incidence

Coronary perforation is a serious complication with an incidence ranging from 0.19% to 3.0% of cases (Table 29.3). Lesions associated with perforation are more complex in nature. ACC type B or C, calcified lesions, or CTOs are more likely to sustain perforation (see Table 29.3).[36,37] Women and the elderly are at greater risk of perforation.[8] Since the introduction of CTO PCI, two multicenter registries have described a perforation rate of 0.33% to 0.34% of all cases and a prospective multicenter U.S. registry describes a 4.1% rate of perforations in a 5-year history of CTO cases.[38–40]

Mechanism

There are two basic mechanisms of perforation: guidewire penetration and vessel rupture. Vessel rupture is usually caused by

TABLE 29.3 Incidence and Outcome of Coronary Perforation Across Reported Studies

Author	Number of Procedures	Perforation Incidence (%)	Tamponade (%)	CABG (%)	MI (%)	Death (%)
Aljuni et al.[44] (1988–1992)	8932	0.4	17	37	26	9
Dippel et al.[41] (1995–1999)	6214	0.58	22	22	NA	11
Ellis et al.[165] (1990–1991)	12,900	0.4	24	24	16	5
Fasseas et al.[37] (1990–1991)	16,298	0.58	11.6	10.5	12.6	7.5
Gruberg et al.[42] (1990–1999)	30,746	0.27	31	39	34	10
Gunning et al.[43] (1995–2001)	6245	0.8	46	15	NA	12
Javaid et al.[166] (1996–2005)	38,559	0.19	19	35	NA	17
Kiernan et al.[36] (2000–2008)	14,281	0.48	18	3	7.4	5.9
Shimony et al.[45] (2001–2008)	9568	0.59	15.8	7	NA	7
Stankovic et al.[167] (1993–2001)	5728	1.5	12	13	18	8
Ramana et al.[168] (2001–2004)	4886	0.5	4	20	32	8
Witzke et al.[169] (1995–2003)	12,658	0.3	18	5	5	2.6

CABG, Coronary artery bypass grafting; *MI*, myocardial infarction; *NA*, not available.

balloon or stent mismatch with oversizing of the dilatation catheter. Occasionally, an appropriate-sized balloon or stent will result in perforation due to extensive dissection, lack of vessel wall integrity, or subintimal wire placement. Early balloon angioplasty studies found increasing the balloon:artery ratio greater than 1.2:1 increased perforation risk.[8] Use of atherectomy devices such as excimer laser or rotational atherectomy increases perforation risk as well.[41] Recanalization of CTOs has become a common setting for perforation, sometimes due to small guidewire perforations; however, the increasingly aggressive maneuvers of high-pressure dilations and use of atheteroablative devices in the subintimal space have led to more frequent perforations.[36,38,40]

Ellis graded perforations (Table 29.4) by separating them into three classes of severity ranging from small endovascular leaks into the adventia (grade I) to frank extravasation into the pericardial space (grade III). Grade I perforations are frequently caused by guidewires but atheroablative devices and stents can cause small endovascular leaks. Occasionally, guidewires can cause very large distal perforations; therefore extreme vigilance should be maintained, particularly when using stiff and hydrophilic guidewires into distal tortuous vessels. Grade II and grade III perforations are usually caused by high-pressure balloon inflations, oversized balloon catheters, stents, the use of atheroablative devices, or aggressive interventions in the subintimal space (Fig. 29.5).

Prognosis

Perforation severity predicts prognosis. Grade III perforations can quickly result in cardiac tamponade, rapid hemodynamic collapse, MI, and/or death (Table 29.5).[8,36,37,41–45] Either immediate covered stent implantation or referral for emergency CABG is often indicated. With the dissemination of subintimal techniques for CTO PCI, perforation is associated with a 7.1% rate of death and 25.9% rate of major adverse cardiac events (MACEs).[40] A legacy effect has been reported with a 1.6 odds for death at 12 months in perforation survivors of CTO PCI.[46]

Diagnosis

Given the dire consequences of coronary perforation, the interventionalist must be especially attuned to recognizing this complication early. Patients may experience hypotension, severe chest pain, dizziness, or nausea disproportional to symptoms typically associated with balloon inflation. There may be persistent ST segment changes after balloon deflation. Vasovagal reactions may also accompany perforations along with severe bradycardia and hypotension.[47] Awareness and vigilance post-PCI is vital because cardiac tamponade as late as 24 hours post-PCI has been reported.[8,48] Perforations have been associated with a cardiac tamponade rate of 14.1% to 14.2% in two separate registries and 10% in the subset of CTO-PCI in post-CABG patients. Late tamponade risk can be minimized with careful "final" angiograms visualizing all instrumented vessels and their branches.

Management

Grade I perforations can generally be treated with reversal of anticoagulation and/or prolonged balloon inflation at/or proximal to the perforated vessel segment. Guidewire perforations are often best treated by balloon occlusion but have been treated with delivery of occlusive coils, fat, or beads. Occasionally, grade I perforations can resolve without an intervention but small endovascular leaks may persist and require the use of a covered stent or referral to emergent CABG. Grade III perforations are catastrophic and more likely require urgent pericardiocentesis, deployment of a polytetrafluoroethylene (PTFE)-covered stent, and/or referral for emergent surgery.[47]

TABLE 29.4 Ellis Classification of Coronary Perforations

Classification	Description	Possible Clinical Sequelae
I	Focal extraluminal crater without extravasation limited to media or adventitia	Usually benign, may rarely cause delayed cardiac tamponade
II	Pericardial or myocardial blush without contrast in pericardium; limited extravasation producing patch of blushing or staining within the myocardium or pericardium	
III	Persistent extravasation with streaming or jet of contrast	High risk, increased morbidity and mortality
IIIA	Directed toward pericardium	High risk of acute cardiac tamponade
IIIB	Directed toward myocardium (e.g., ventricular cavity)	More benign course; possible fistula formation

Permission obtained by author from Klein LW. Coronary artery perforation during interventional procedures. *Catheter Cardiovasc Interv*. 2006;68:713–717.

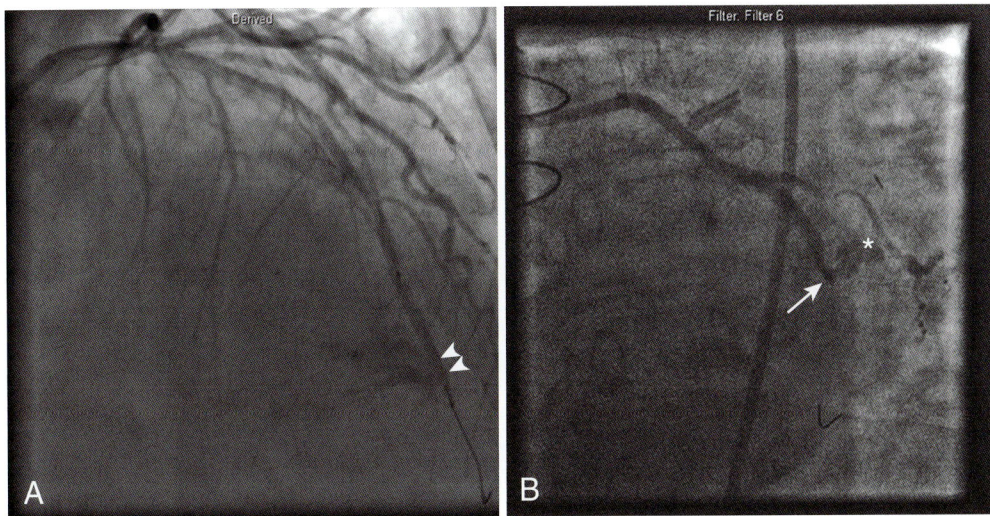

Fig. 29.5 Coronary perforations. (A) Distal perforation in the left anterior descending artery leading to extravasation *(arrowheads)* while treating a severe plaque. (B) Perforation in a midobtuse marginal branch *(arrow)* due to rotational atherectomy with extravasation into the pericardium *(*)*. (Adapted from Klein LW. Coronary complications of percutaneous coronary intervention: a practical approach to the management of abrupt closure. *Catheter Cardiovasc Interv*. 2005;64:395–401.)

TABLE 29.5 Coronary Stent Embolization Is Associated With Significant Major Adverse Cardiac Events

	Incidence (%)	n	Death (%)	MI (%)	CABG (%)
Brilakis et al.[62]	0.32	38	3	11	5
Bolte et al.[68]	1.7	387	6.2	3.9	17
Cantor et al.[170]	8.3	108	2.8	5	16
Eggebrecht et al.[171]	0.9	20	15	NA	15

CABG, Coronary artery bypass grafting; *MI*, myocardial infarction; *n*, number of procedures; *NA*, not available.

Once a perforation occurs, the first step is to remain calm and advance a balloon from the guide catheter across the perforation without losing guidewire position. If the perforation results from a guidewire, then balloon inflation proximal to the perforation is indicated. This highlights an essential interventional cardiology fundamental: balloons should remain in the guide or within the lesion following any inflation until angiography confirms there is no perforation. When perforation is recognized, balloon expansion to a pressure sufficient to occlude flow (usually 2 to 4 atm) is the first and urgent step. Once the vessel is occluded, the patient's hemodynamics may normalize; however, aggressive treatment with IV fluids, atropine, vasopressors, and perhaps IABP insertion may be required.

When treating perforations, anticoagulation should be stopped after all of the interventional devices have been removed from the artery. If heparin was used as the anticoagulant, reversal with protamine is usually indicated. However, operators should be cautious to ensure that a bloody effusion is not present because, once the blood in the pericardium coagulates, it may not be possible to evacuate it from pericardium without a pericardial window. Glycoprotein IIb/IIIa inhibitors must also be stopped, and abciximab can be reversed with an infusion of platelets. The effects of tirofiban and eptifibatide cannot be reversed with platelet infusions, but both have a shorter half-life compared to abciximab. Although IIb/IIIa inhibitors can increase bleeding complications, they have not been demonstrated to increase the incidence or severity of perforations.[41] Direct thrombin inhibitors such as bivalirudin are sometimes used for procedural anticoagulation, and its effects cannot be reversed with protamine, although bivalirudin has not been associated with an increased hazard in death or life-threatening complications for high-risk PCI.[49] Infusion of fresh frozen plasma may be the only means to reverse anticoagulation with bivalirudin; however, this requires a time delay to thaw the blood products.[50]

The presence of coronary perforation should trigger urgent echocardiography. If a large pericardial effusion is present and associated with tamponade physiology, emergent pericardiocentesis is indicated. Should echocardiography not be available, the diagnosis of tamponade can be made on clinical grounds; use of right heart catheterization or fluoroscopy of the heart borders may be helpful.

A major advance in the treatment of coronary perforation is the development of PTFE-covered stents. Prior to the advent of PTFE stents, the presence of a grade III perforation often required emergency CABG and carried significant mortality.[48] The currently available PTFE stent (Jostent Graftmaster, Abbott Vascular, Santa Clara, CA) is a PTFE graft layered between two bare-metal stents that can exclude perforations. Available outside of the United States, the PK Papyrus (Biotronik, Lake Owego, OR) has a delivery profile of 1.19 mm and increased flexibility to improve deliverability, but there are scant clinical data regarding its use.[51] The initial experience using PTFE grafts was reported in a small case series, demonstrating a decrease in cardiac tamponade and emergency coronary bypass surgery.[52] PTFE-covered stents are bulky, and delivery into tortuous vessels can be challenging. A separate guide catheter for the PTFE-covered stent delivery is recommended because most guide catheters cannot accommodate both an angioplasty balloon and PTFE-stent graft simultaneously (Fig. 29.6). Therefore a two-guide technique has been developed, wherein contralateral access is established and a separate guide catheter is used to deliver the stent. A wire from the second guide catheter is advanced down the coronary vessel and the angioplasty balloon momentarily deflated to allow guidewire passage. The PTFE-stent is then quickly advanced across the perforation and deployed after the removal of the angioplasty balloon. The two-guide catheter technique has been documented to decrease adverse event rates and offers the operator the luxury of more time to position the stent.[53] Side-branch vessels near the perforation site may be excluded by the PTFE-covered stent, which may result in a periprocedure MI.[52] IVUS should be routinely be used to verify adequate covered stent expansion because deploying this dual stent layer may require aggressive (≥18 atm) post dilation. Occasionally, collateral filling may cause persistent extravasation despite exclusion of the perforation with a stent graft and surgical management or occlusion of the supplying collateral may be required. Keep in mind that

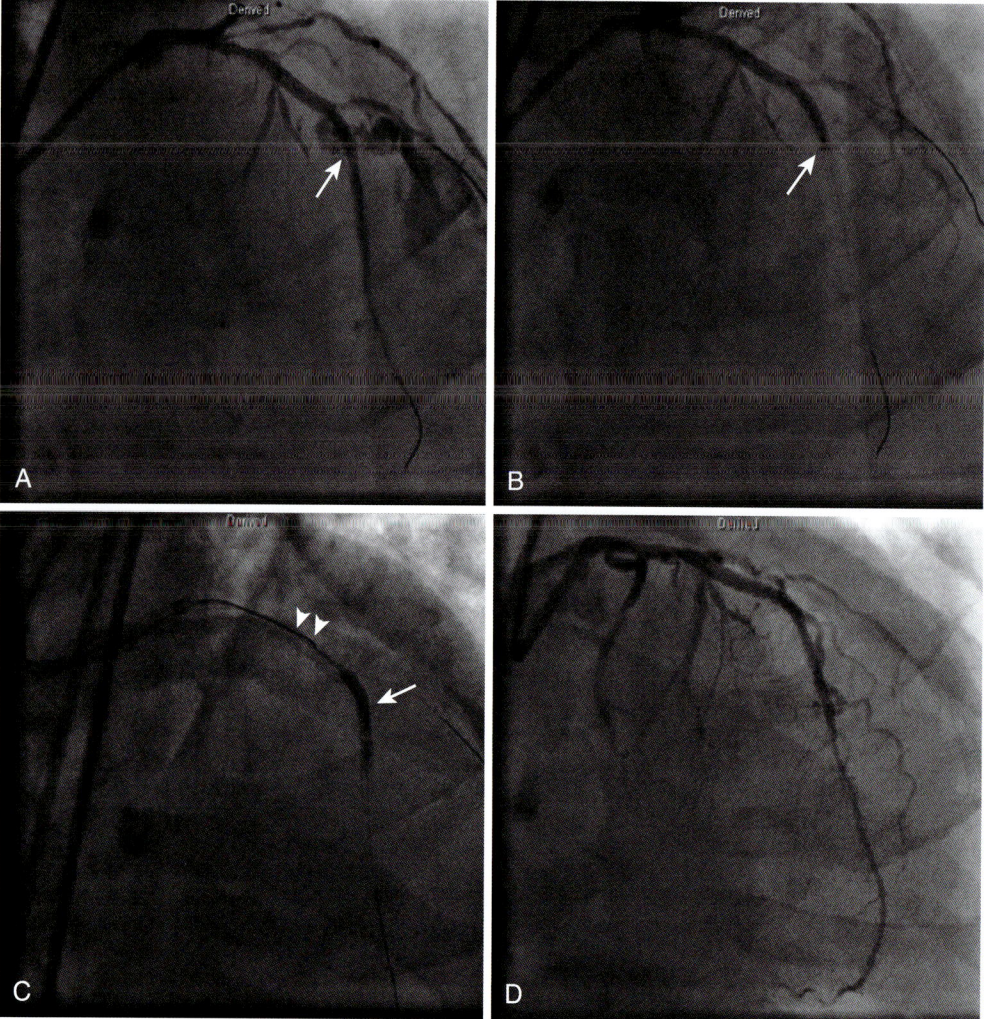

Fig. 29.6 Successful exclusion of a coronary perforation with a polytetrafluoroethylene-covered stent graft. (A) An Ellis class III perforation at the mid-left anterior descending artery (LAD) with streaming into the pericardial space *(arrow)*. (B) Balloon tamponade of the perforation. (C) Dual guide technique is shown as the original coronary wire is withdrawn *(arrowheads)* while a JoStent *(arrow)* (Abbott Vascular, Santa Rosa, CA) covered stent graft is deployed in the mid-LAD to exclude the perforation. (D) Final angiogram demonstrating no extravasation post stent graft deployment.

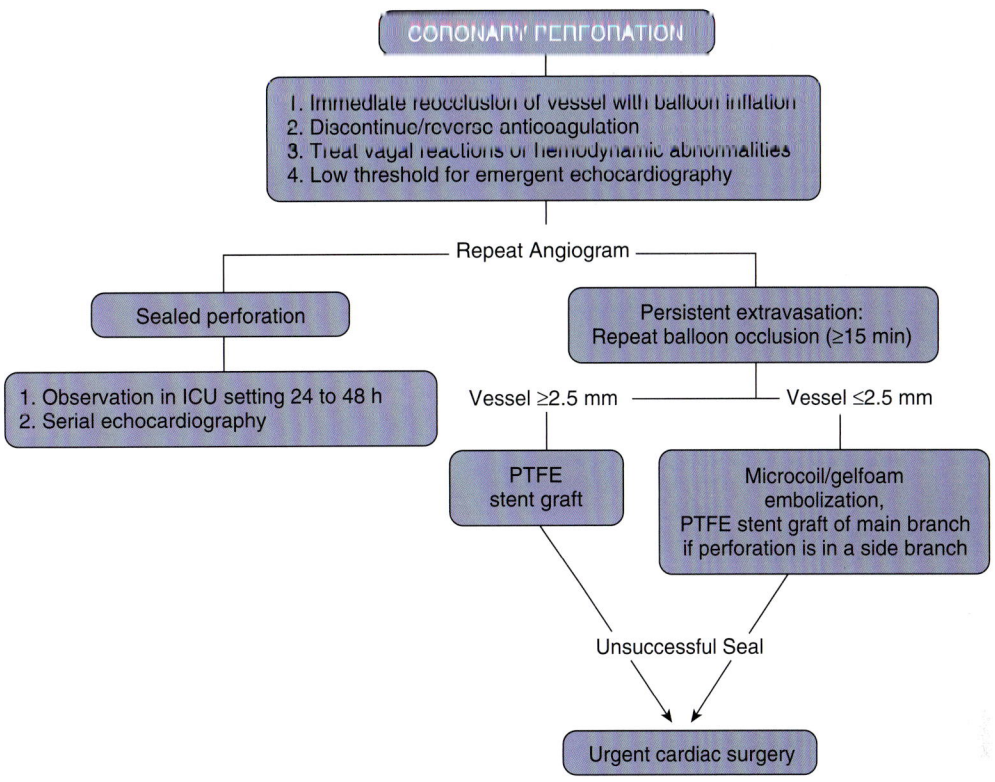

Fig. 29.7 Suggested algorithm for management of coronary perforation. *ICU,* Intensive care unit; *PTFE,* polytetrafluoroethylene. (From Klein LW. Coronary artery perforation during interventional procedures. *Catheter Cardiovasc Interv.* 2006;68:713–717.)

PTFE-covered stents are associated with high rates of restenosis and a 22% 1-year MACE rate.[54]

Perforations in small vessels can be addressed with either additional prolonged balloon inflations or the injection of thrombin, polyvinyl alcohol, Gelfoam, collagen, or the embolization of microcoils or beads (see Fig. 29.7 for suggested strategy for the management of coronary perforation).[55,56]

With more aggressive subintimal recanalization techniques used for CTO PCI, a variation of perforation, formation of myocardial hematomas, has arisen. During aggressive wiring while performing retrograde dissection and reentry via septal collaterals, a perforation can occur and the resultant breach can cause a hematoma to form in the ventricular septum, disrupting the myocardial architecture causing hypokinesis or akinesis.[57] Similarly, a subintimal breach can cause the bleeding to track towards the myocardium instead of the pericardium, disrupting myocardial contractility or compressing certain chambers.[58–60] Understanding the extent of the hematoma and taking corrective action is difficult to assess in the midst of the PCI, but the effects are most apparent with the development of cardiogenic shock. Special attention should be paid to the location of the possible hematoma and the implicated ventricle because significant depression of myocardial function may call for the use of left, right, or both ventricular assist devices. For the time being, the treatment is supportive and waiting for the hematoma to resolve.

Iatrogenic Ascending Aortic Dissection

As PCI has become more aggressive in the CTO era, more and more complications have arisen from either aggressive guiding catheter use, wire trauma, or subintimal dissection near the coronary ostium resulting in aortic dissection (Fig. 29.8). The rate of aortic dissection in a European multicenter registry was 0.06% and typically caused by catheter trauma. The majority of cases were due to guiding catheters of the Judkins and Amplatz variety, and 90.5% of catheters were 6-Fr. Sealing the breach as the site of coronary ostium with a stent stabilizes the dissection. None of the patients suffering from the iatrogenic dissection suffered late complications with a follow-up period of 51 months, indicating that the great majority of these dissections can be treated conservatively.[61]

EMBOLIZATION OF PERCUTANEOUS CORONARY INTERVENTION EQUIPMENT

Incidence

Embolization of equipment such as coronary stents and guidewire fragments is a potentially catastrophic complication of PCI. Stents are the most common device embolized, with an incidence ranging from 3% for first generation, hand-crimped stents to a much lower 0.32% rate for current manufacturer-mounted stent delivery systems.[62,63] More recently the incidence of lost angioplasty equipment fragments was found to be 0.38% among 2238 consecutive cases, indicating a relatively rare phenomenon.[64] Equipment embolized ranged from guidewires, broken catheters, stents, and a coronary filter. Extreme tortuosity, angulation, and calcification increase the risk of stent embolization due to dislodgement from delivery balloons. For this reason, stents are more frequently lost in the right coronary artery and circumflex artery and less commonly in the left anterior descending artery.[62,65]

The incidence of retained coronary angioplasty equipment components is reported to be 0.2% in a single center series of 5400 consecutive cases.[66] A recent case series focused on guidewire entrapment identified that 31 cases in the literature were predominantly associated with CTO PCI (13.5%) and jailed wire technique in bifurcations (29%).[67] Other factors contributing to

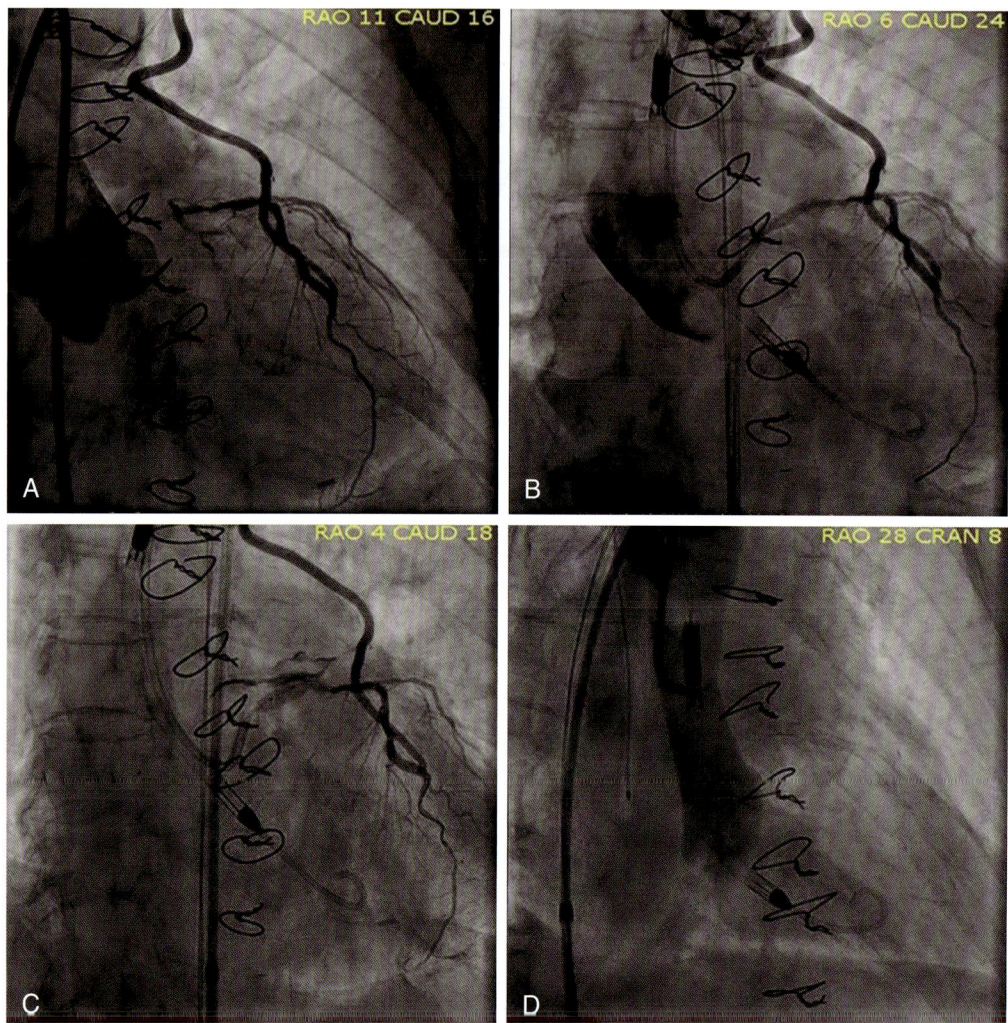

Fig. 29.8 Iatrogenic aortic dissection from ostial left main trauma. (A) Occluded left main targeted for antegrade and retrograde dissection reentry. (B) Retrograde wire reentry into the aorta but staining of the aortic root is present representing intimal dissection of aortic root. Note the Impella insertion to manage hemodynamic instability. (C) Greater than one channel was open and prolonged balloon tamponade was attempted to stabilize the dissection. (D) Aortography demonstrating intimal flap extending past the mid ascending aorta.

the fracture and embolization of guidewires include significant tortuosity, calcified vessels, and in-stent restenosis lesions. Excessive force when withdrawing or torqueing wires >180 degrees may eventually fracture the tip of the wire.

Prognosis

Embolization of coronary stents is associated with worse prognosis and an increased risk of adverse cardiac events (see Table 29.5).[62,65,68] Successful retrieval is associated with good prognosis; however, unsuccessful management or retrieval results in high rates of periprocedural MI, emergent referral to CABG, and death.[68] Peripheral embolization of stents is rarely associated with significant clinical sequelae. In one noninvasive assessment of 20 patients with peripheral stent embolization, there were no peripheral vascular complications over a mean duration of 5 years.[65]

The adverse consequences of retained wire fragments ranged from MI, stent thrombosis, perforation with tamponade, and occasionally death. However, these adverse consequences occur in a minority of cases. In one study, 23 of 31 such cases suffered no adverse immediate consequences.[67]

Treatment

There are numerous approaches to the removal of embolized stents. If possible, maintain guidewire position through the center of the stent. This will facilitate retrieval using one of many commercially available snares (Fig. 29.9). Placing a small (5 mm) snare over the angioplasty guidewire through the stent and carefully tracking it to the stent may enable removal, but operators should be warned that if sufficiently trapped, the stent may elongate. Another option is to advance a small diameter balloon through the unexpanded stent, inflate the balloon, and attempt to drag the stent back into the guide catheter. A third approach is to pass a second wire alongside the embolized stent, attempting to enter one of the struts and then attach a single torquing device to both wires used to twist the wires together followed by withdrawal of the wire wrapped stent from the artery. A fourth approach is to deploy the embolized stent in its unintended location. Retrieval devices such as biliary forceps or bioptomes can easily damage the arterial wall and should be avoided or handled with great care. Deploying a new stent alongside the embolized stent such that the dislodged stent is embedded into the arterial wall is a reasonable option should retrieval be difficult, but this

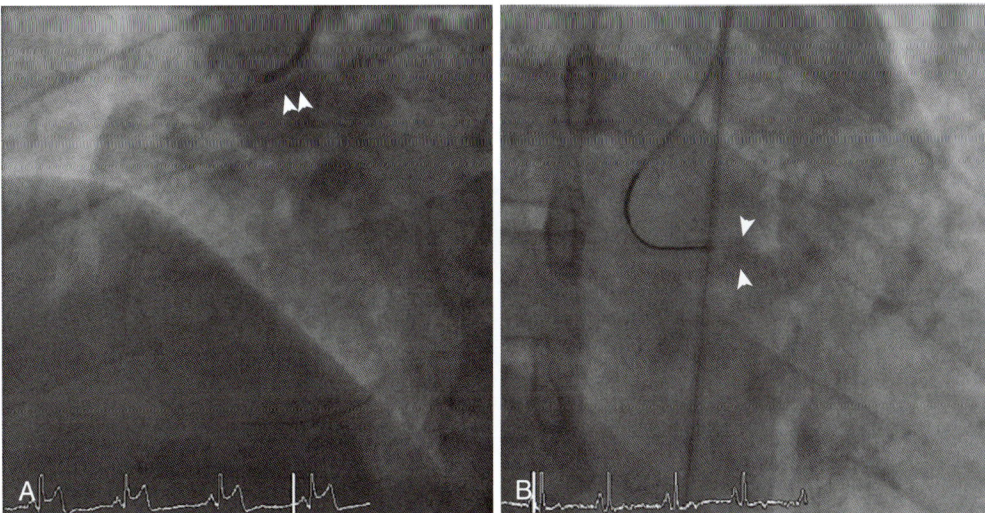

Fig. 29.9 Snaring of an embolized coronary stent at the right coronary ostium. (A) A coronary stent *(arrowheads)* was stripped from the balloon and is located at the right coronary ostium. (B) Using a gooseneck snare, the stent *(arrowheads)* is retrieved and retracted into the guide.

TABLE 29.6 Unadjusted Rates of Major Adverse Clinical Event Following Emergent Coronary Artery Bypass Grafting for Failed Percutaneous Coronary Intervention in Contemporary Retrospective Single-Center Registries

	Time Period	Incidence (%)	n	Death (%)	MI (%)	Stroke (%)
Seshadri et al.[71]	1992–2000	0.6	113	15	12	53
Roy et al.[72]	1994–2008	0.4	90	7.8	5.7	10
Yang et al.[70]	1995–2003	0.5	77	13	NA	NA

MI, Myocardial infarction; *n,* number of procedures; *NA,* not available.

technique may be associated with an elevated risk of periprocedural MI, death, and referral to CABG.[68]

Treatment of retained angioplasty wire bears similarities to treating embolized stents with some exceptions. Some fragments can be manage conservatively; review of embolized guidewires from 1980 to 2012 revealed 14.9% of cases were managed conservatively.[69] In this series, the most commonly used percutaneous technique was snaring of the fragment followed by deep guide catheter intubation and angioplasty balloon inflation to trap the guidewire fragment in the guiding catheter. Advancing coronary wires alongside the embolized fragment and twisting them together to entangle the fragment is another option. It should be kept in mind that all of these rescue maneuvers carry risks of extensive coronary dissection, rupture, or abrupt closure. The option of covering the embolized guidewire with a coronary stent is a theoretical solution, the conditions leading to guidewire fracture but must be overcome. Surgical extraction of the guidewire is an option but unplanned, emergent cardiac surgery is associated with significant mortality and morbidity, as explained next.

EMERGENCY CORONARY BYPASS SURGERY

Incidence

The incidence of emergency CABG has steadily decreased from the balloon angioplasty era of 1.5% to 2.9% to 0.14% to 0.41% in the stent era (Table 29.6).[70–72] Recent data from The NHLBI Dynamic Registry describe an incidence of 0.7% for early CABG 30 days or less from PCI.[5] Patient characteristics associated with emergent CABG included cardiogenic shock, acute MI, multivessel disease, and a prior history of MI. Procedural variables distinguishing patients referred for emergent CABG include ACC type C lesions, placement of an IABP, dissection, perforation, and abrupt closure. Analysis from one single center study found that most patients referred for CABG had at least one or two high-risk characteristics and those with four high-risk factors had a 9.3% incidence of emergent CABG.[72]

Prognosis

Emergent CABG following PCI is associated with significant morbidity and mortality, with a death rate ranging between 7.8% and 15.4% among three single center studies.[73] Q wave MIs, stroke, and/or renal insufficiency commonly complicate emergent CABG procedures.[70] Q wave MI accounts for most of the patient deaths, followed by cardiac arrhythmias, suggesting that delay in perfusion while transitioning to surgery is the most common mechanism of demise.[70] Therefore it is advisable to attempt all possible solutions expeditiously and, if success from PCI does not appear likely, request emergency CABG sooner rather than later and strongly consider intraaortic counterpulsation, LV support device insertion, and/or aggressive pharmacologic support to maintain perfusion pressure en route to surgery.

Myocardial Infarction

Incidence

Periprocedural myonecrosis during PCI is common, occurring with a 0% to 47% incidence based on reported series.[74] The definition of MI varies between studies with respect to biomarker assay, threshold values, frequency of blood specimen sampling, and use of ECG data among studies resulting in wide ranges of reported incidence.[75] Whether myonecrosis is directly responsible for late adverse outcomes or is simply a symptom of disease severity is debated. However, the prognostic significance of higher

TABLE 29.7 Incidence and Implication of Periprocedure Myocardial Infarction From Major Studies

Authors	n	Cardiac Marker Cutoff Level	Incidence (%)	Follow-Up Implication
Abdelmeguid et al.[172]	4484	CK 1–2 × ULN	5.8	Death (RR 1.27)
Abdelmeguid et al.[173]	4664	CK 2–5 × ULN	2.6	Death (RR 2.19)
Kong et al.[174]	2812	CK 5 × ULN CK 1–1.5 × ULN CK 1.5–3 × ULN CK >3 × ULN	1.3 2.3 3.8 2.9	Death (RR 1.05)
Ghazzal et al.[175]	15,637	CK 1–2 × ULN CK 2–3 × ULN CK >3 × ULN	4.6 1.1 1.6	Death (OR 1.84)
Tardiff et al.[176]	1616	CK-MB >1 × ULN	18.0	Death/MI/Revasc. 6-month end point 1–3 × ULN 32.4% 3–5 × ULN 37.9% 5–10 × ULN 35.3% >10 × ULN 43.6%
Waksman et al.[177]	3265	CK-MB >2 × ULN, ST/T changes or CP	4.7	Death 7.8%
Simoons et al.[178]	5025	CK-MB 1–3 × ULN	13.2	Death (log enzyme ratio OR 1.82)
Roe et al.[179]	2384	CK-MB >3 × ULN CK-MB 1–3 × ULN CK-MB 3–5 × ULN CK-MB 5–10 × ULN CK-MB >10 × ULN	6.6 21.3 6.0 7.1 9.5	Death (OR 1.06)
Mehran et al.[79]	2256	CK-MB >4 ng/mL	25.8	NR
Stone et al.[180]	7147	CK-MB >4 ng/mL	14	Death (adjusted OR 8.00)
Dangas et al.[181]	4085	CK-MB >4 ng/mL	36.9	Death (OR 1.5)
Ajani et al.[182]	1326	CK-MB >4 ng/mL	45	Death/MI/TVR (OR 1.57)
Brener et al.[183]	3478	CK-MB >8.8 ng/mL	24	Death (OR 1.89)
Ellis et al.[184]	8409	CK-MB >8.8 ng/mL	17.2	Death
Brener et al.[185]	3573	CK-MB >8.8 ng/mL	38	Death (HR 1.1)
Hong et al.[186]	1693	CK-MB 4–20 ng/mL CK-MB >20 ng/mL	32.1 15.2	Death (OR 5.5)
Natarajan et al.[187]	1128	cTnI 1–4 × ULN cTnI >5 × ULN	7.6 9.1	NR
Nallamothu et al.[188]	1157	cTnI 1–<3 × ULN cTnI 3–<5 × ULN cTnI 5–<8 × ULN cTnI ≥8 × ULN	16 4.8 2 6.5	Death cTnI 5–<8 × ULN OR 3.4 cTnI ≥ 8 × ULN OR 2.7
Fuchs et al.[189]	1129	cTnI 1–3 × ULN cTnI >3 × ULN	15 15.5	Death/MI/TVR cTnI >3 × ULN 6.4%
Cavallini et al.[190]	3494	cTnI >0.15 ng/dL CK-MB >5 ng/mL	44.2 16.0	Death (OR 1.9)

CK-MB, Creatine kinase myoglobin; *cTnI*, cardiac troponin-I; *CP*, chest pain; *HR*, hazard ratio; *MI*, myocardial infarction; *NR*, not recorded; *OR*, odds ratio; *RR*, relative risk; *TVR*, target-vessel revascularization; *ULN*, upper limit of normal.
Permission obtained by author from Herrmann J. Peri-procedural myocardial injury: 2005 update. *Eur Heart J.* 2005;26:2493–2519.

biomarker values is reproducible across many studies (Table 29.7). Currently the accepted universal definition for a periprocedural MI is peak creatine kinase myoglobin (CK-MB) ≥10 times the local laboratory upper limit of normal (ULN), or ≥5 times ULN with new pathologic Q waves in two contiguous leads (Table 29.8).[76] Contemporary series published after instituting the new definition of periprocedural MI ranges from 4.3% to 7.1%.[77,78]

Mechanism

Obvious causes of periprocedural MI include side-branch occlusion, distal macroembolizaton, no-reflow, abrupt occlusion, prolonged balloon inflations, and hypotension (Table 29.9). A recent meta-analysis reveals that 57.3% of periprocedural MIs were due to side-branch occlusion, but it should be noted that 21.3% of cases were not associated with a known etiology. Distal microembolization occurs frequently, and the extent of myonecrosis has been shown to be proportional to the plaque burden and degree of calcification.[79] Microvascular embolization is reflected by worsening myocardial perfusion grade, and impaired perfusion grade is directly proportional to a larger infarct size by magnetic resonance imaging (MRI).[80] Doppler coronary flow studies give further credence to importance of distal embolization and microvascular obstruction as the cause of most post-PCI biomarker elevation, which is further supported by delayed enhancement MRI studies.[81,82]

TABLE 29.8 Definition of Clinically Relevant Myocardial Infarction After Both Percutaneous Coronary Interventions and Coronary Artery Bypass Grafting Procedures

1.	In patients with normal baseline CK-MB	The peak CK-MB measured within 48 h of the procedure rises to ≥10 times the local laboratory ULN, or to ≥5 times ULN with new pathologic Q-waves in ≥2 contiguous leads or new persistent LBBB, OR in the absence of CK-MB measurements and a normal baseline cTn, a cTn (I or T) level measured within 48 h of the PCI rises to ≥70 times the local laboratory ULN, or ≥35 times ULN with new pathologic Q-waves in ≥2 contiguous leads or new persistent LBBB.
2.	In patients with elevated baseline CK-MB (or cTn) in whom the biomarker levels are stable or falling	The CK-MB (or cTn) rises by an absolute increment equal to those levels recommended above from the most recent preprocedure level.
3.	In patients with elevated CK-MB (or cTn) in whom the biomarker levels have not been shown to be stable or falling	The CK-MB (or cTn) rises by an absolute increment equal to those levels recommended above plus new ST segment elevation or depression plus signs consistent with a clinically relevant MI, such as new onset or worsening heart failure or sustained hypotension.

CK-MB, Creatine kinase myoglobin; *cTn*, cardiac troponin; *LBBB*, left bundle branch block; *MI*, myocardial infarction; *PCI*, percutaneous coronary intervention; *ULN*, Upper limit of normal.
Permission obtained by author from Moussa ID, Klein LW, Shah B, et al. Consideration of a new definition of clinically relevant myocardial infarction after coronary revascularization: an expert consensus document from the Society for Cardiovascular Angiography and Interventions (SCAI). *J Am Coll Cardiol*. 2013;62:1563–1570.

TABLE 29.9 Mechanisms of Periprocedural Myonecrosis

PROCEDURE-RELATED COMPLICATIONS
- Side-branch occlusion
- Flow-limiting dissection
- Abrupt closure
- Macroscopic embolization
- No-reflow
- Microscopic embolization

LESION-SPECIFIC CHARACTERISTICS
- Large thrombus burden
- Plaque volume
- Plaque vulnerability

PATIENT-SPECIFIC CHARACTERISTICS
- Arterial inflammation
- Aspirin resistance
- Genetic predisposition

Permission obtained by author from Bhatt DL, Topol EJ. Periprocedural cardiac enzyme elevation predicts adverse outcomes. *Circulation*. 2005;112:906–922.

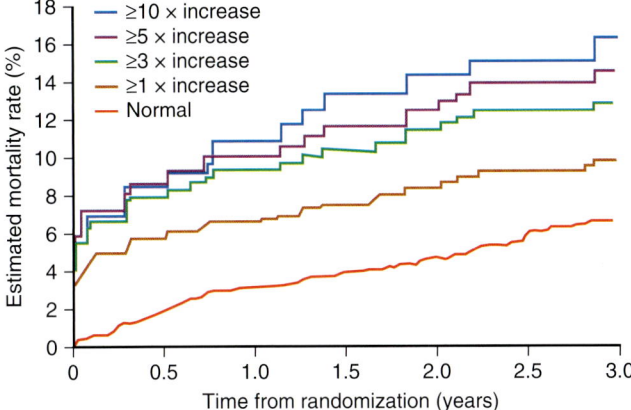

Fig. 29.10 Mortality for patients with 1-fold to 10-fold increases in periprocedural creatinine kinase elevation. The *P* values for comparisons are ≥1 time, *P* = .02; ≥3 times, *P* < .001; ≥5 times, *P* < .001; and ≥10 times, *P* < .001. (From Topol EJ, Ferguson JJ, Weisman HF, et al. Long-term protection from myocardial ischemic events in a randomized trial of brief integrin beta₃ blockade with percutaneous coronary intervention. EPIC Investigator Group. Evaluation of Platelet IIb/IIIa Inhibition for Prevention of Ischemic Complication. *JAMA* 1997;278:479–484).

Of note, when optimizing stent expansion, greater cross-sectional areas were linked to higher CK-MB elevation postprocedure, suggesting that aggressive stent expansion increases the risk of plaque disruption and subsequent distal embolization.[83] Advancing and implanting bulkier devices such as stents has been associated with larger periprocedural MI.[12] Improvement in adjunctive pharmacology during PCI such as glycoprotein IIb/IIIa inhibitors and IV P2Y$_{12}$ inhibitors significantly decreased MI rate following PCI, presumably by mitigating no-reflow and inhibiting platelet adhesion.[84,85]

The use of mechanical atherectomy devices are more likely to result in periprocedural MI. As coronary lesions are debulked, plaque is "pulverized" and sent downstream into the intracoronary vascular bed. Although most embolized particles are small and pass harmlessly through the coronary microcirculation, atherectomy is associated with somewhat increased periprocedural MI and no-reflow phenomenon when compared with balloon angioplasty.[86]

Prognosis

Periprocedural enzyme elevation measured as CK-MB and troponin elevation is directly related to adverse events, including death and Q wave MI (QWMI) (see Table 29.9; Fig. 29.10).[87,88] This has been observed in multicenter trials, as well as in meta-analysis of multiple acute coronary syndrome and stable coronary disease trials.[89] Large scale side-branch loss from subintimal dissection or stenting of the false lumen can cause larger infarctions associated with worse long-term outcomes.[90]

Prevention—Pharmacotherapy

Periprocedural myocardial necrosis appears to be part of "collateral damage" to undertaking PCI, but multiple pharmacologic and device developments have emerged to attenuate the incidence of this complication. Pharmacologic advances such as glycoprotein IIb/IIIa inhibitors, P2Y$_{12}$ receptor inhibitors, and statins decrease periprocedural MI. The use of distal embolic protection during vein graft interventions has been shown to significantly reduce periprocedural MI.

Glycoprotein IIb/IIIa inhibitors target the common final receptor for platelet cross-linking and thrombus formation. Abciximab, a murine monoclonal antibody specific for platelet IIb/IIIa receptors, causes an 80% blockade of platelet function[91] and was the first agent to demonstrate a reduction in periprocedural MI (8.6% vs. 5.2%, *P* = .013) when using balloon angioplasty or atherectomy to

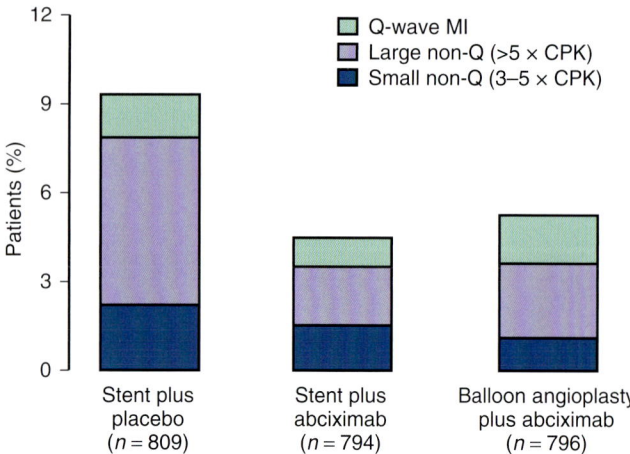

Fig. 29.11 Incidence and type of myocardial infarction for each treatment group. *CPK,* Creatinine phosphokinase; *MI,* myocardial infarction. (From the EPISTENT Investigators. Randomised placebo-controlled and balloon-angioplasty-controlled trial to assess safety of coronary stenting with use of platelet glycoprotein-IIb/IIIa blockade. Lancet. 1998;352:87–92.)

perform PCI.[92] These results were consistently reproduced while implanting stents in subsequent trials such as Evaluation of Platelet IIb/IIIa Inhibitor for Stenting (EPISTENT), Evaluation in PTCA to Improve Long-Term Outcome with Abciximab GP IIb/IIIa Blockade (EPILOG), and the c7E3 FAB antiplatelet therapy in unstable refractory angina (CAPTURE) trial, each with greater than 50% reductions in periprocedural MI compared with PCI with heparin and aspirin alone (Fig. 29.11).[12,85,93] Similar reductions of periprocedural MI were observed with synthetic small molecule glycoprotein IIb/IIIa inhibitors such as eptifibatide and tirofiban. A 40% reduction of MI was seen at 48 hours (5.4% vs. 9.0%, $P = .0015$) in the Enhanced Suppression of the Platelet IIb/IIIa Receptor with Integrilin Therapy (ESPRIT) trial, and most of the clinical benefit of eptifibatide in the Platelet Glycoprotein IIb/IIIa in Unstable Angina: Receptor Suppression Using Integrilin Therapy (PURSUIT) trial were attributed to reductions in periprocedural MI.[94,95] Tirofiban was observed to reduce periprocedural MI when administered in a high-dose fashion in the Additive Value of Tirofiban Administered With the High-Dose Bolus in the Prevention of Ischemic Complications During High-Risk Coronary Angioplasty (ADVANCE) trial.[96]

Adequate platelet inhibition appears to be the key to success with respect to preventing periprocedural MI by not only blocking IIb/IIIa receptors but also inhibiting $P2Y_{12}$-mediated platelet activation. This was first observed with pretreatment using ticlopidine and then clopidogrel in the PCI subset of the Clopidogrel in Unstable Angina to Prevent Recurrent Events (CURE) trial where a 44% reduction in MI was seen at 30 days.[97,98] Preprocedural loading with 300 mg of clopidogrel was found to reduce the primary end point of MI, death, and target-vessel revascularization (TVR) by 38% if given at least 6 hours prior to PCI.[99,100] High-loading dose (600 mg) of clopidogrel caused a 50% reduction in periprocedural MI, likely due to achieving therapeutic inhibition of platelets more rapidly.[101] As expected, resistance to either aspirin or clopidogrel increases the hazard of periprocedural MI.[102] Tailoring anticoagulation strategies by adding eptifibatide to patients without optimal clopidogrel response may reduce periprocedural MI.[103] More powerful $P2Y_{12}$ inhibitors should theoretically decrease periprocedural MI in elective PCI; however, only cangrelor in the CHAMPION-PHOENIX study has been associated with decreased periprocedural MI, whereas most studies investigating either ticagrelor or prasugrel have been in the context of pharmacodynamic or acute coronary syndrome studies.[104]

In addition to optimizing antiplatelet therapy prior to PCI, pretreatment with statins appears to prevent myocardial injury in patients both undergoing elective and emergent PCI.[105,106] Loading patients with atorvastatin 40 mg for 1 week prior to PCI caused a 72% reduction in periprocedural MI (3% vs. 18%, $P = .025$) during elective PCI in the Atorvastatin for Reduction of Myocardial Damage during Angioplasty (ARMYDA) study.[105] The mechanism of myonecrosis attenuation may be related to the decrease in expression of Vascular cell adhesion protein 1 (VCAM-1) and Intercellular adhesion molecule 1 (ICAM-1) post PCI.[107] Even when patients are already receiving chronic statin therapy, reloading with high doses of statins provided added reduction of periprocedural MI.[108]

Because many periprocedural MIs are caused by distal embolization, use of embolic protection devices have been investigated in several settings; however, the benefits have been observed only in saphenous vein graft interventions. In the Saphenous Vein Graft Angioplasty Free Of Emboli Randomized trial (SAFER) trial, a total of 801 patients undergoing elective saphenous vein graft PCI were randomized to distal protection using the Guardwire (Medtronic Vascular, Santa Rosa, CA), resulting in a 41% reduction in periprocedural MI compared with those without embolic protection devices.[109] Proximal protection and aspiration using the PROXIS (St. Jude Medical, MN) produced comparable rates of periprocedural MI, and its use was found to be noninferior to distal embolic protections devices when used in saphenous vein graft interventions.[110] Unfortunately, the PROXIS device is no longer manufactured.

The benefits of distal embolic protection have not been reproduced in native coronary vessels. The Enhanced Myocardial Efficacy and Recovery by Aspiration of Liberated Debris (EMERALD) trial randomized 501 patients to receiving either distal embolic protection using the Guardwire Plus distal protection device (Medtronic Vascular) combined with aspiration thrombectomy or usual care for STEMI.[111] Despite the use of the Guardwire Plus and aspiration thrombectomy, no differences were observed with respect to death, MI, or infarction size. Lack of efficacy in the setting of STEMI was attributed to the delay in reperfusion seen in the treatment group using distal embolic protection devices. Similarly, use of Filterwire EX (Boston Scientific, Natick, MA) distal protection during acute coronary syndromes did confer any decrease of infarct size or reduction of MACE in the Protection Devices in PCI Treatment of MI for Salvage of Endangered Myocardium (PROMISE) study.[112]

Periprocedural MI remains a common complication that predicts future adverse outcomes. Judicious revascularization, optimization of pharmacologic therapy, and use of embolic protection devices when appropriate may reduce its incidence.

CORONARY NO-REFLOW

Incidence and Diagnosis

Coronary no-reflow is the inability to perfuse myocardium after opening of a previously occluded or stenosed epicardial coronary artery.[113] No-reflow is suspected to result from a combination of endothelial damage, platelet and fibrin embolization, vasospasm, and tissue edema that overwhelms the coronary microcirculation. Reperfusion-related injury is hypothesized to contribute to no-reflow via infiltration of the microcirculation with neutrophils and platelets. The incidence of no-reflow ranges from 0.6% to 2% and is more frequently observed when using stents, atherectomy, and performing PCI in saphenous vein grafts.[114,115] Risk factors for no-reflow include the angiographic presence of thrombus, cardiogenic shock, increased reperfusion time, hyperglycemia, and leukocytosis.[116–118] Diagnosis of no-reflow is made angiographically by assessing flow usually using the thrombolysis in myocardial infarction (TIMI) grading system (Table 29.10); however, there are other systems of measuring microcirculatory myocardial perfusion

TABLE 29.10 Thrombolysis in Myocardial Infarction Grading System for Describing Coronary Flow

TIMI Grade	Angiographic Characteristics
0	No antegrade flow beyond the point of occlusion.
I	Contrast material is able to pass through the area of obstruction but fails to opacify the distal coronary bed.
II	Contrast is able to penetrate the area of obstruction and fills the distal coronary bed; however, it is perceptibly slower than other coronary vessels unaffected by the coronary obstruction.
III	Antegrade flow into distal coronary bed of the obstructed artery is as prompt as the flow in an uninvolved coronary vessel.

TIMI, Thrombolysis in myocardial infarction.

TABLE 29.11 Prevention of No-Reflow

- Use of distal protection devices when treating saphenous vein graft lesions.
- When performing rotational atherectomy, routine use of nitroglycerin, verapamil, and heparin in combination with the flush solution.
- Consider pretreatment with a IIb/IIIa inhibitor during percutaneous coronary intervention in patients with acute coronary syndromes.
- Minimize balloon inflation and consider direct stenting in patients with bulky atheroma or saphenous vein grafts.
- Pretreatment with verapamil or adenosine.
- Aspiration thrombectomy for thrombus-laden lesions.

such as myocardial blush score, TIMI frame count, and contrast echocardiography.

Prevention

To some degree, no-reflow can be minimized or prevented during coronary intervention with diligent pharmacologic and mechanical pretreatment and posttreatment (Table 29.11). Pretreatment with intracoronary calcium channel blockers is a helpful adjunct for treatment of saphenous vein grafts.[119] Use of distal protection devices in the context of saphenous vein graft PCI decreased the rate of no-reflow to 4.8% compared with 9.7% when performing PCI without distal protection in the SAFER trial.[109] Rates of no-reflow increase with the use of rotational atherectomy, likely due to the embolization of pulverized plaque into the microcirculation. In one small study, the use of preemptive intracoronary adenosine, and nitroglycerin during rotational atherectomy decreased the rate of no-reflow from 11.4% to 1.4%.[119,120] Recent evidence from a small study showed a 10-minute intragraft infusion of adenosine at 200 μg/min decreases no-reflow in elective vein-graft interventions.[121] Administration of abciximab prior to PCI for STEMI increased the proportion of patients with TIMI III flow both pre- and post-PCI in the Abciximab before Direct Angioplasty and Stenting in MI Regarding Acute and Long-Term Follow-up (ADMIRAL) trial.[122] This increase in TIMI III flow translated into higher patient left ventricular ejection fraction (LVEF) and decreased the composite end point of death, TVR, and reinfarction among patients receiving abciximab. More recently, use of intracoronary abciximab to improve reperfusion during STEMI did not cause an increased rate of TIMI III (intracoronary abciximab 91.3% vs. no intracoronary abciximab 91.5%, $P = .94$) or myocardial blush grade 3 (intracoronary abciximab 80.7% vs. no intracoronary abciximab 82.1%, $P = .71$).[123]

Another tool in preventing no-reflow and optimizing perfusion in the setting of STEMI is aspiration thrombectomy. The Thrombus Aspiration during PCI in Acute Myocardial Infarction Study (TAPAS) trial was a prospective trial randomizing 1071 patients to either routine aspiration thrombectomy prior to coronary stenting versus usual care.[121] Aspiration thrombectomy improved markers of reperfusion such as myocardial blush score and ST segment resolution, but outcomes with respect to death, reinfarction, TVR, and composite MACEs were not found to be different at 30 days. Rates of MACEs correlated with the degree of perfusion as measured by myocardial blush score and ST segment resolution (Fig. 29.12). At 1 year, routine aspiration thrombectomy reduced the rate of cardiac death to 3.4% compared with 6.7% when performing routine primary PCI for reperfusion therapy.[125] Benefits of adjunctive thrombectomy during STEMI were reproduced in both meta-analysis and in a pooled patient analysis of 11 randomized clinical trials for both 30-day and 1-year MACCEs, respectively.[126,127] However, the most recent prospective evaluations of aspiration thrombectomy, Thrombus Aspiration during ST-Segment Elevation Myocardial Infarction (TASTE) and Intracoronary Abciximab Infusion and Aspiration Thrombectomy in Patients Undergoing PCI for Anterior STEMI (INFUSE-AMI), did not recapitulate the benefit seen with aspiration thrombectomy in the TAPAS trial.[123,128] No differences in TIMI III flow (aspiration 92.6% vs. no aspiration 90.1%, $P = .36$), myocardial blush grade 3 (aspiration 83.4% vs. no aspiration 79.3%, $P = .26$), and infarct size (aspiration 17% vs. no aspiration 17.3%, $P = .51$) were observed in INFUSE-AMI.[123] Similarly, TASTE observed no differences with respect to hard clinical end points, because the 30-day all-cause mortality did not change with aspiration (aspiration 2.8% vs. no aspiration 3.0% $P = .63$). Finally, the largest prospective trial (Trial of Routine Aspiration Thrombectomy with PCI versus PCI Alone in Patients with STEMI [TOTAL]) examining the efficacy of aspiration thrombectomy in STEMI demonstrated again no difference in the primary end point of death, recurrent MI, cardiogenic shock, or New York Heart Association class IV heart failure at 1 year with thrombus aspiration after randomizing 10,064 patients.[129]

Treatment

First-line treatment for no-reflow primarily consists of delivery of vasodilators, especially adenosine, calcium channel blockers, and/or nitroprusside into the coronary microcirculation (Table 29.12). Should the dye column stop at midvessel, distal contrast injections through balloons or microcatheters should be performed to exclude dissection. Injection of vasodilators through an infusion catheter close to the distal bed may improve microcirculation drug delivery. Which vasodilator to use has been a subject of controversy; thus far the agent with a slight edge in evidence may be adenosine. One open-label, prospective randomized study comparing large dose adenosine (120-μg bolus followed by a 2-minute infusion of 1 mg/min) showed improved ST resolution compared with both placebo and nitroprusside.[130] One-year follow-up showed less left ventricular (LV) remodeling in the adenosine group compared with placebo; however, differences in LV remodeling and MACE rates between adenosine and nitroprusside were not statistically significant.[131] There is no role for referral for emergent coronary bypass surgery or thrombolytic therapy. If the stenosis is widely patent by angiography or IVUS, additional coronary stenting is not helpful. Cases with cardiogenic shock may require intraaortic balloon counterpulsation or LV support devices to maintain adequate systemic perfusion pressure.

Prognosis

No-reflow is associated with larger infarction size, reduced LVEF, and death.[132–134] Retrospective analysis in patients with no-reflow undergoing primary PCI have an in-hospital and 6-month mortality increase of 6-fold and 10-fold, respectively. The adjusted odds for death at 6 months was 5.4 times higher in patients with no-reflow.[134]

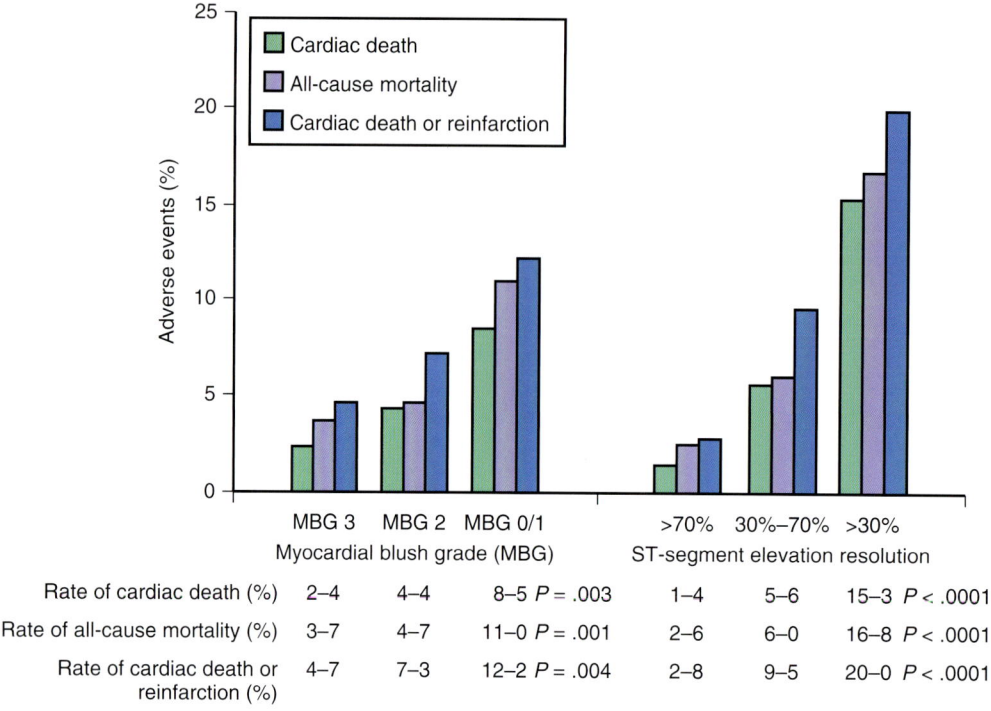

Fig. 29.12 Cardiac death, all-cause mortality, and the combined end point of cardiac death and nonfatal reinfarction are inversely proportional to myocardial blush score and degree of ST segment resolution, proving that outcomes are directly related to the quality of perfusion. (From Vlaar PJ, Svilaas T, van der Horst IC, et al. Cardiac death and reinfarction after 1 year in the Thrombus Aspiration during Percutaneous coronary intervention in Acute myocardial infarction Study [TAPAS]: a 1-year follow-up study. *Lancet.* 2008;371:1915–1920.)

TABLE 29.12 Society for Cardiovascular Angiography and Interventions Suggested Management of No-Reflow

FIRST-LINE MANAGEMENT
Adenosine (10–20 μg bolus)
Verapamil (100–200 μg bolus or 100 μg/min up to 1000 μg total with temporary pacer on standby)
Nitroprusside (50–200 μg bolus, up to 1000 μg total dose)

EVIDENCE LESS STRONG
Rapid, moderately forceful injection of saline or blood (to unplug microvasculature)
Cardizem (0.5–2.5 mg over 1 min up to 5 mg)
Papaverine (10–20 μg)
Nicardipine (200 μg)
Nicorandil (2 μM)
Epinephrine (50–200 μg)

NEVER SHOWN TO BE EFFECTIVE
Intracoronary nitroglycerin
Coronary artery bypass grafting (contraindicated)
Stent placement (if site of original stenosis is widely patent)
Thrombolytics (e.g., urokinase, tissue-type plasminogen activator)

Permission obtained by author from Klein LW, Kern MJ, Berger P, et al. Society of cardiac angiography and interventions: suggested management of the no-reflow phenomenon in the cardiac catheterization laboratory. *Catheter Cardiovasc Interv*. 2003;60:194–201.

Air Embolism

Incidence

Injection of air into the coronary artery is potentially fatal, possibly resulting in "air lock" causing abrupt occlusion of the vessel, possible cardiac arrest, and MI. Almost always iatrogenic, the incidence of this complication is approximately 0.1% to 0.3%.[135] Air embolism usually results from the inadequate aspiration of catheters or the entrainment of air during equipment exchanges. Occasionally, rupture of an inadequately prepared coronary balloon or introduction of air through an intracardiac defect can allow paradoxical embolism into the coronary circulation.

Diagnosis

The degree of danger associated with air embolism is proportional to the amount of air that enters the coronary circulation. Once air is embolized, air lock can prevent perfusion of the distal coronary bed (Fig. 29.13). Air embolism may manifest as chest pain, hypotension, transient ECG changes consistent with myocardial ischemia, arrhythmias (bradycardia, heart block, ventricular tachycardia, and ventricular fibrillation), and even cardiac arrest. The diagnosis of air embolism is made angiographically, and the bolus generally divides into smaller bubbles causing slow flow phenomenon in epicardial vessels.[135]

Treatment

Resolution of air embolism can be accomplished faster by ventilating with 100% oxygen (Table 29.13). Increasing the mean arterial pressure will assist in forcing air bubbles into the coronary microcirculation and overcoming the air lock. Forceful injection of saline or contrast can also assist in dissipating the air. Balloons can be used to pulverize large bubbles. Thrombectomy catheters can be used to aspirate bubbles from the epicardial vessel. While waiting for an air embolus to resolve, the patient will often become profoundly hypotensive and complain of chest discomfort. Expedient treatment of hypotension with systemic vasopressors such as norepinephrine or phenylephrine can be life saving. Intraaortic balloon counter pulsation may also be useful. Of course the most efficacious means of dealing with air embolism is prevention by meticulous aspiration and flushing of catheters between equipment exchanges.[136]

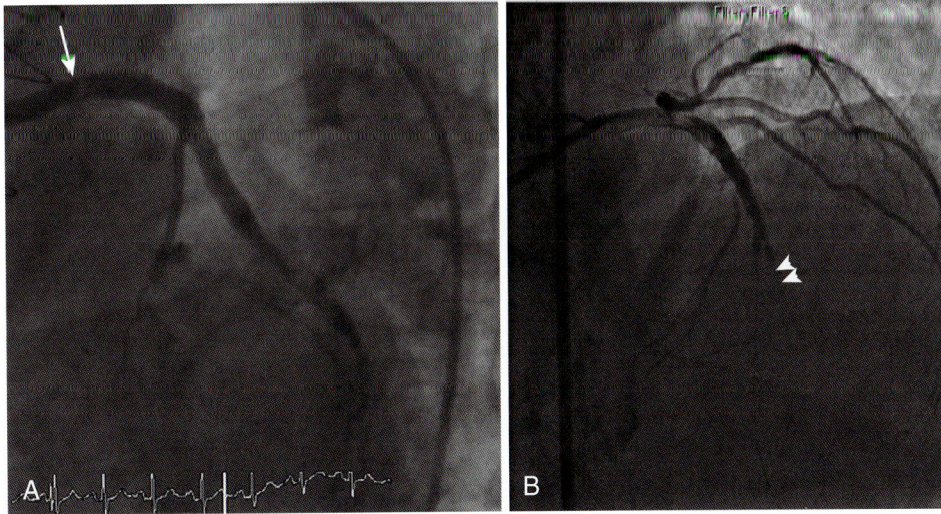

Fig. 29.13 Air embolism. (A) Air embolism *(arrow)* from inadequate flushing of a distal protection filter. (B) "Airlock" created by a large air embolus causing cessation of flow in the left anterior descending artery *(arrowheads)*.

TABLE 29.13 Treatment of Air Embolism

- Ventilate with 100% oxygen
- Aggressive treatment with intravenous fluids, atropine, or vasopressors for hemodynamic support
- Consider intraaortic balloon pump counterpulsation for hemodynamic support
- Dissipate the "airlock" with wires or balloon catheters
- Consider catheter aspiration or air embolus
- Treat no-reflow phenomenon with standard vasodilators (adenosine, verapamil, nitroprusside)

TABLE 29.14 Commonly Used Pretreatment Regimen for Contrast Allergy

- Prednisone 50 mg orally 13, 7, and 1 h prior to procedure or hydrocortisone 100 mg intravenous 1 h prior to procedure
- Cimetidine 300 mg orally 1 h prior
- Diphenhydramine 50 mg orally 1 h prior
- Montelukast 10 mg orally 1 h prior
- Nonionic low or isoosmolar contrast agent

RADIOCONTRAST HYPERSENSITIVITY

Incidence and Prognosis

Allergy to contrast medium is a common but rarely serious complication in the cardiac catheterization laboratory. Since the advent of low-osmolar nonionic agents, contrast intolerance has significantly declined. The risk of allergy to contrast agents is estimated to be 4% to 12% and 1% to 3% for ionic and nonionic contrast agents, respectively.[137] The reported incidence of severe contrast reactions is 0.23%, with a mortality of one per 55,000 cases.[138] Reactions from contrast media include minor events such as nausea, vomiting, and localized uticaria with pruritus and moderate reactions characterized by laryngeal or facial edema and mild bronchospasm. Severe reactions are true emergencies and manifest as respiratory or cardiac arrest and shock. Occasionally, contrast allergy may manifest solely as persistent hypotension during a cardiac procedure. Approximately 2% to 5% of patients may develop delayed reactions characterized by rash 1 hour to 1 week after contrast exposure.[139] Patients may experience pruritus, maculopapular rash, uticaria, angioedema, and/or fever. Often, identification of the agent responsible for the allergy may be confounded due to concomitant delivery of antibiotics or treatment with antithrombotic agents, such as clopidogrel.

Prevention and Treatment

Prophylactic measures can decrease the incidence and severity but do not entirely eliminate the risk of contrast reactions. Pretreatment of patients with contrast allergy usually consists of corticosteroids and antihistamines (Table 29.14). Mild reactions may be treated with a similar regiment; however, moderate reactions such as laryngeal edema, bronchospasm, or hypotension require immediate administration of intramuscular (IM) epinephrine 0.1 to 0.3 mL (1:1000 dilution) or IV epinephrine 1 mg (1:10,000 dilution) to prevent progressive symptoms.[140] Severe bronchospasm, laryngeal edema, or cardiac arrest is treated with IV epinephrine diluted 1:10,000 at a dose of 1 to 3 mL (Table 29.15). Overdose of IV epinephrine may manifest as tachycardia, tremor, pallor, and hypertensive emergency. Preexisting β-blocker therapy may blunt the response of epinephrine and increase the risk of a severe reaction. Supplemental oxygen, endotracheal intubation, aggressive fluid resuscitation, administration of corticosteroids, and use of an epinephrine drip may be required to stabilize the patient. Such patients should be monitored in the intensive care unit until the reaction subsides.[141]

BLEEDING

Bleeding rates vary depending on the definitions used, but it is a relatively common complication, with major bleeding occurring in 1.7% of all-comers when analyzing patients from 2004 to 2011 in the CathPCI Registry.[142] Focused analysis of acute coronary syndrome trials showed that TIMI minor/major bleeding occurs in approximately 2.3% of patients in a pooled registry of acute coronary syndrome studies, and 4.1% patients with STEMI suffered TIMI major bleeding in the HORIZONS trial.[143,144] Given the multiple definitions of bleeding in the literature, a universal definition of bleeding was formed by the Bleeding Academic Research Consortium (BARC) and subsequently validated (Table 29.16).[145,146] Predictors of bleeding from multiple analyses included advanced age, female gender, severe renal impairment, glycoprotein inhibitor use, larger sheath size, peak activated clotting time, simultaneous right heart catheterization, low-molecular-weight heparin use, elevated white cell count, procedure duration, and heparin use post procedure.[147–150]

Bleeding adversely impacts prognosis; the presence of bleeding was associated with an in-hospital mortality of 5.58% versus 0.57% (P < .001) of nonbleeding patients.[142] Patient comorbidities compound the risk of mortality from bleeding events, because death rates are directly proportional to the risk of bleeding. Patients high-risk for bleeding with a subsequent bleeding event had a 6.54% higher rate of death relative to those low-risk for bleeding (P < .001).[142] Nonaccess-site bleeding further increases the hazard of death and elevates the in-hospital mortality rate to 8.25%.[142] Mortality is proportional to bleeding severity. No significant difference in mortality was observed between TIMI minor and no-bleeding in acute coronary syndromes, but a fivefold increase in mortality is seen when bleeding is severe.[143] The mortality increase for major bleeding is greatest in the first 30 days; after 30 days, the mortality hazards drop from a 5-fold to 1.5-fold increase in death compared to no bleeding.[143] Similarly, early hazard towards MI (adjusted hazard ratio [HR] 4.44) and stroke (adjusted HR 6.46) was most prominent in the first 30 days following bleeding.[143] Retroperitoneal bleeding, a particularly devastating event with an in-hospital mortality of 6.4%, is fortunately rare (0.4%).[151] Increased early mortality associated with bleeding may originate from the requirement to discontinue antiplatelet therapy, the increased metabolic stress of having poor oxygen delivery due to anemia, possible hypotension, and possibly the role of blood transfusion, which is independently associated with both a fourfold and threefold increase of death and MI, respectively, even after adjusting for covariates and nadir hemoglobin concentration.[152] Recent data show blood transfusions compound the risk of acute kidney injury nearly fivefold in acute coronary syndromes.[153]

Strategies to mitigate bleeding include appropriate patient selection, tailored pharmacology, access site management, and use of radial access. Avoiding inappropriate revascularization candidates using prospective risk calculators is valuable, because the in-hospital mortality number needed to harm (NNH) for a bleeding event in high-risk patients and those with nonaccess-site bleeding were NNH = 21 and NNH = 16, respectively.[154,155] Appropriate pharmacology selection and drug dosing remain problematic, and as many as 22.3% of patients with chronic renal failure are given contraindicated medications.[156] When analyzing cohorts at high risk for bleeding using vascular closure device (VCD) only, bivalirudin only, and combined use of VCD + bivalirudin, the combined approach was associated with the lowest rate of periprocedural bleeding (VCD 4.6% vs. bivalirudin 3.8% vs. VCD + bivalirudin 2.3%, P < .001).[157] Femoral access using ultrasound guidance may help to mitigate some bleeding complications

TABLE 29.15 Treatment of Anaphylactoid Reactions to Contrast Media

MILD
Nausea, vomiting, and localized urticaria with pruritus, self-limiting
- Observation

MODERATE
Laryngeal or facial edema and mild bronchospasm
- Epinephrine:
  - 1:1000 dilution at 0.1–0.3 mL IM
  - 1:10,000 dilution at 1–3 mL IV
- Diphenhydramine 25–50 mg IV

SEVERE
Respiratory or cardiac arrest and anaphylactoid shock
- Advanced cardiac life support resuscitation (airway, breathing, circulation)
- Epinephrine drip at 10–20 μg/min up to 30 min after symptom resolution
- Aggressive IV fluids

IM, Intramuscular; *IV*, intravenous.
Permission obtained by author from Nayak KR, White AA, Cavendish JJ, et al. Anaphylactoid reactions to radiocontrast agents: prevention and treatment in the cardiac catheterization laboratory. *J Invas Cardiol.* 2009;21:548–551.

TABLE 29.16 Bleeding Academic Research Consortium Definitions of Bleeding.

Type 0: no bleeding
Type 1: bleeding that is not actionable and does not cause the patient to seek unscheduled performance of studies, hospitalization, or treatment by a healthcare professional; may include episodes leading to self-discontinuation of medical therapy by the patient without consulting a healthcare professional
Type 2: any overt, actionable sign of hemorrhage (e.g., more bleeding than would be expected for a clinical circumstance, including bleeding found by imaging alone) that does not fit the criteria for type 3, 4, or 5 but does meet at least one of the following criteria: (1) requiring nonsurgical, medical intervention by a healthcare profession, (2) leading to hospitalization or increased level of care, or (3) prompting evaluation

Type 3:
    Type 3a:
        Overt bleeding + hemoglobin drop of 3 to <5 g/dL (provided hemoglobin drop is related to bleed)
        Any transfusion <with overt bleeding
    Type 3b:
        Cardiac tamponade
        Bleeding requiring surgical intervention for control (excluding dental/nasal/skin/hemorrhoid)
        Bleeding requiring vasoactive agents
    Type 3c:
        Intracranial hemorrhage (does not include microbleeds or hemorrhage transformation, does include intraspinal)
        Subcategories confirmed by autopsy or imaging or lumbar puncture
        Intraocular bleed compromising vision

Type 4: Coronary artery bypass grafting–related bleeding Perioperative intracranial bleeding within 48 h Reoperation after closure of sternotomy for the purpose of controlling bleeding Transfusion of ≥5 U whole blood or packed red blood cells within a 48-h period Chest tube output ≥2 L within a 24-h period

Type 5: fatal bleeding
    Type 5a: Probable fatal bleeding; no autopsy or imaging confirmation but clinically suspicious
    Type 5b: Definite fatal bleeding; overt bleeding or autopsy or imaging confirmation

because it decreases the number of puncture attempts and subsequent vascular complications, but micropuncture technique does not appear to significantly impact vascular complications or bleeding.[158,159] Finally, radial access resulted in a 50% decrease in access-site related major bleeding, and the benefits of radial access are magnified in acute coronary syndromes, particularly STEMI in which radial puncture decreased access-related bleeding 60% in the Radial Versus Femoral Randomized Investigation in ST-Elevation Acute Coronary Syndrome (RIFLE-STACS) trial.[160,161] However, given the 6.1% to 10.0% rate of crossover from radial to femoral access, strategies for mitigating femoral access bleeding remain valuable.[160–162] A prospective superiority trial, Minimizing Adverse Haemorrhagic Events by Transradial Access Site and Systemic Implementation of Angiox (MATRIX), randomized patients with ST and non-ST acute coronary syndromes to either radial or femoral access and found radial access to have lower rates of MACEs through a reduction in bleeding and all-cause mortality.[163] In the National Cardiovascular Data Registry, patients experiencing bleeding less frequently used radial access (5.0% vs. 11.2%, $P < .001$), bivalirudin (43.8% vs. 59.4%), and VCD (32.9% vs. 42.4%, $P < .001$) than those without bleeding, suggesting that bleeding avoidance strategies are important.[164]

CONCLUSION

Avoidance, recognition, and management of procedural complications is central to maintaining competence as an interventional cardiologist. Although the specific complications described in this chapter represent some of the most important and common mishaps, this is not an exhaustive listing. Complications can never be completely avoided. No matter how experienced the interventionalist, complications will teach humility and be a source of continuing education throughout one's career.

KEY REFERENCES

22. Genereux P, Stone GW, Harrington RA, et al. Impact of intraprocedural stent thrombosis during percutaneous coronary intervention: insights from the CHAMPION PHOENIX Trial (Clinical Trial Comparing Cangrelor to Clopidogrel Standard of Care Therapy in Subjects Who Require Percutaneous Coronary Intervention). *J Am Coll Cardiol*. 2014;63:619–629.
24. Dangas GD, Caixeta A, Mehran R, et al. Frequency and predictors of stent thrombosis after percutaneous coronary intervention in acute myocardial infarction. *Circulation*. 2011;123:1745–1756.
28. Iakovou I, Schmidt T, Bonizzoni E, et al. Incidence, predictors, and outcome of thrombosis after successful implantation of drug-eluting stents. *JAMA*. 2005;293:2126–2130.
38. Kinnaird T, Kwok CS, Kontopantelis E, et al. Incidence, Determinants, and outcomes of coronary perforation during percutaneous coronary intervention in the United Kingdom between 2006 and 2013: an analysis of 527 121 cases from the British Cardiovascular Intervention Society Database. *Circ Cardiovasc Interv*. 2016;9(8).
61. Núñez-Gil IJ, Bautista D, Cerrato E, et al. Incidence, management, and immediate- and long-term outcomes after iatrogenic aortic dissection during diagnostic or interventional coronary procedures. *Circulation*. 2015;131:2114–2119.
62. Brilakis ES, Best PJM, Elesber AA, et al. Incidence, retrieval methods, and outcomes of stent loss during percutaneous coronary intervention. *Catheter Cardiovasc Interv*. 2005;65:333–340.
70. Yang EH, Gumina RJ, Lennon RJ, et al. Emergency coronary artery bypass surgery for percutaneous coronary interventions: changes in the incidence, clinical characteristics, and indications from 1979 to 2003. *J Am Coll Cardiol*. 2005;46:2004–2009.
76. Moussa ID, Klein LW, Shah B, et al. Consideration of a new definition of clinically relevant myocardial infarction after coronary revascularization: an expert consensus document from the Society for Cardiovascular Angiography and Interventions (SCAI). *J Am Coll Cardiol*. 2013;62:1563–1570.
129. Jolly SS, Cairns JA, Yusuf S, et al. Outcomes after thrombus aspiration for ST elevation myocardial infarction: 1-year follow-up of the prospective randomised TOTAL trial. *Lancet*. 2016;387:127–135.
143. Eikelboom JW, Mehta SR, Anand SS, et al. Adverse impact of bleeding on prognosis in patients with acute coronary syndromes. *Circulation*. 2006;114:774–782.
163. Valgimigli M, Gagnor A, Calabró P, et al. Radial versus femoral access in patients with acute coronary syndromes undergoing invasive management: a randomised multicentre trial. *Lancet*. 2015;385:2465–2476.

Additional references available online at expertconsult.com.

中文导读

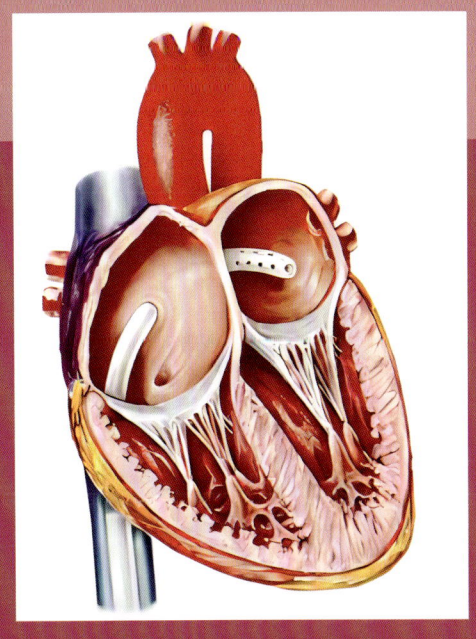

第30章
围术期心肌梗死及栓塞保护装置

  围术期心肌梗死是经皮冠状动脉介入治疗手术常见的一种并发症，程度轻重不一。近年来发生围术期并发症的患者预后趋于改善，但由于检测技术的改良，围术期心肌梗死发生率逐年上升。本章全方位介绍围术期心肌梗死的相关诊疗规范，并着重介绍血栓保护装置。

  本章先以围术期心肌梗死相关定义作为切入点，从心肌酶及肌钙蛋白两方面定义围术期心肌梗死。然后阐述了围术期心肌梗死相关机制，介绍了围术期心肌梗死与远端血栓、血小板激活之间的关系，并且尝试将这些机制与定义相联系。在此之后，作者尝试从患者特点及病变节段特点分析，结合手术其他并发症及器材使用情况，综合阐述围术期心肌梗死相关危险因素。在详尽的介绍后，作者开始阐述预防及治疗围术期心肌梗死的方法。这部分包括抗凝药物、降脂药物及非药物方案。常用的抗凝药物有注射用GPⅡb/Ⅲa血小板抑制剂、直接凝血酶抑制剂及$P2Y_{12}$受体阻滞剂。他汀类药物具有抗炎作用，可能有助于降低围术期心肌梗死发生率。非药物治疗方案部分囊括了直接支架置入、缺血预适应、血栓保护装置、血栓抽吸等内容。本章将栓塞保护装置分为远端过滤装置、远端阻塞装置和近端阻塞装置，并做了相应介绍。最后作者将经皮冠状动脉介入治疗与血栓保护装置联系起来，介绍二者合用的优势，并尝试拓展到颈动脉介入手术及瓣膜介入手术，总结了该技术未来可能的应用领域，体现了该技术的无限潜力。

赵天禄　柳景华

章节要点

- 围手术期心肌梗死仍然是经皮冠状动脉介入治疗的常见并发症。
- 2012版第三通用定义文件将与经皮冠状动脉介入治疗相关的心肌梗死定义如下：如果基线肌钙蛋白正常，术后肌钙蛋白超过正常上限99%的5倍即可诊断；如果基线肌钙蛋白升高，但基线水平稳定或逐渐下降，术后肌钙蛋白升高超过基线值20%可诊断。
- 预防围手术期心肌梗死的策略包括药物治疗和机械治疗。
- 在干预围术期心肌梗死卓有成效的药物有强化抗血小板药物及他汀类降脂药物。
- 机械治疗方法包括在大隐静脉介入治疗、颈动脉支架、经导管主动脉瓣置换术时使用栓塞保护装置。
- 在经导管主动脉瓣置换术期间常规使用脑栓塞保护装置仍存在争议，但部分研究证据表明该策略有益。

30 Periprocedural Myocardial Infarction and Embolism-Protection Devices

Adrian W. Messerli, Khaled M. Ziada, Debabrata Mukherjee

KEY POINTS

- Periprocedural myocardial necrosis remains a common complication of percutaneous coronary intervention (PCI).
- The 2012 Third Universal Definition document defines a myocardial infarction (MI) associated with PCI as elevation of troponin values above five times the 99th percentile of upper reference limit (URL) in patients with normal baseline values or a rise of troponin values above 20% if the baseline values are elevated and are stable or falling.
- Strategies to prevent periprocedural MI (PMI) include pharmacologic and mechanical approaches.
- The primary pharmacologic interventions that have achieved significant success in preventing PMI include aggressive antiplatelet and statin therapy.
- Mechanical approaches include the use of embolic protection devices (EPDs) in the setting of saphenous vein graft (SVG) intervention, carotid stenting, and transcatheter aortic valve replacement (TAVR).
- The use of routine cerebral embolic protection during TAVR remains controversial, with some evidence to suggest benefit.

PERIPROCEDURAL MYOCARDIAL INFARCTION

- The contemporary definition of periprocedural myocardial infarction (PMI) is based on the rise and fall of biomarkers—such as total creatine kinase (CK), creatine kinase MB (CK-MB), and troponin—after percutaneous coronary intervention (PCI) in addition to clinical, electrocardiography (ECG), and imaging evidence of myonecrosis.
- The incidence of PMI varies according to the type of assayed biomarker (CK-MB, troponin I [Tn I], or troponin T [Tn T]) and the preset threshold for diagnosis.
- Larger PMIs are infrequent and usually follow angiographically documented complications, such as side-branch closure or no-reflow phenomenon, but smaller and more common PMIs often follow apparently uncomplicated procedures.
- The primary underlying mechanisms of PMI are side-branch occlusions and distal embolization into the downstream microcirculation of the PCI-related vessel, with platelet aggregation/activation playing a significant role in subsequent myonecrosis.
- Risk factors for development of PMI include acute presentation, heightened systemic inflammation, and advanced coronary and/or noncoronary atherosclerotic disease. Atheroablation devices (directional or rotational) are associated with higher rates of PMI, followed by stents and then balloon angioplasty.
- PMI is associated with increased late mortality, and the association is more robust when the CK-MB or troponin levels exceed five times the upper limit of normal (ULN).
- Potent antiplatelet therapies (intravenous [IV] glycoprotein [GP] IIb/IIIa inhibitors, and/or oral thienopyridine inhibitors) decrease the incidence of PMI, especially in high-risk procedures.
- Pretreatment with statins reduces the incidence of PMI because of their antiinflammatory effects.

EMBOLISM PROTECTION DEVICES

- Embolism protection devices (EPDs) include distal occlusive balloons, filter devices, and proximal flow occlusion/reversal systems; all aim to prevent embolized debris produced at the angioplasty site from reaching the distal microvascular bed.
- Clinical trials have demonstrated that using an EPD during vein graft PCI leads to a significant reduction in PMI. However, newer data suggests they may not be uniformly beneficial, particularly for certain lesion subsets.
- Several randomized trials failed to show any benefit of an EPD in the setting of PCI for acute myocardial infarction (MI), thus highlighting the complexity of the mechanisms of myonecrosis and injury in those settings.
- Good evidence suggests that EPDs reduce cerebral embolism during carotid stenting, but no prospective randomized trials based on clinical end points have been undertaken to confirm that benefit.
- Comparison of carotid stenting with the use of embolic protection with carotid endarterectomy demonstrates similar outcomes in patients with asymptomatic disease.
- The exact role of EPDs during transcatheter aortic valve replacement (TAVR) is yet to be defined. The relationship between imaging evidence for cerebral embolism, or volume of embolic particulate debris captured in devices, with clinical stroke and cognitive decline remains unclear.
- Given the explosive growth of TAVR, keen interest persists in the development and application of new cerebro-protective devices.

Periprocedural myocardial necrosis remains the most common complication of PCI. Such myonecrosis can range from a clinically silent minor elevation of cardiac enzymes to a major MI with short- and/or long-term consequences. With advances in pharmacologic therapies and in interventional technology, the incidence of early major adverse cardiac events (MACEs)—such as large MI and death—has fallen to less than 3%, even in complex multivessel PCI.[1,2] The reduced incidence of these complications can be attributed in large part to the role of coronary stents in treatment of abrupt closure and the aggressive antiplatelet therapies more commonly utilized over the last three decades. This improvement in outcomes is remarkable considering the ever-increasing number and complexity of patients and lesions treated with PCI today compared with 20 to 30 years ago. However, the frequency with which any periprocedural myonecrosis is detected has increased, primarily because of the development and widespread adoption of sensitive biomarkers of myocardial damage. As such, the exact definition and clinical significance of the periprocedural release of cardiac markers are topics for active debate, both in real-world practice and in clinical trial settings.

DEFINITION

The definition of *periprocedural myocardial infarction* (PMI) is continuing to evolve with changing and improving biomarker assays and a better understanding of the prognostic significance of these events. Currently, commonly used definitions for the diagnosis of PMI are based on one of two documents: the Third Universal Definition of Myocardial Infarctions[3] and the definition proposed by the Society of Cardiac Angiography and Interventions (SCAI) expert consensus document.[4]

Both definitions are based on identifying the rise and fall of cardiac biomarkers following PCI in addition to corroborating clinical, ECG, imaging, and/or angiographic evidence of myonecrosis. They differ in the various thresholds considered enough to make the diagnosis and in how they indicate a clinically relevant change in prognosis. It is important to note that both definitions of PMI are complicated by earlier referral of acute coronary syndrome (ACS) and MI patients to the catheterization laboratory. Importantly, the prognostic implication of elevated biomarkers after PCI cannot be known unless the baseline level is taken into account. In patients with elevated biomarker levels at baseline, prognosis is more directly linked to the baseline or initial injury than to the postprocedural level. In fact, biomarker elevation before PCI is the most important determinant of long-term mortality. In those situations, detection of abnormal levels of cardiac markers after PCI may not necessarily be related to the procedure but are simply a reflection of the ongoing myonecrosis caused by the thrombotic event that led to the clinical presentation. In ACS patients, biomarker levels may rise after a normal initial sample, which commonly coincides with the time when angiography and PCI are performed.[5] For these reasons, both definitions include specific criteria to extend the definition of PMI to those who were referred to PCI in the setting of ACS or ST-elevation myocardial infarction (STEMI).

The Third Universal Definition of Myocardial Infarction: Definition of Periprocedural Myocardial Infarction

The 2012 Third Universal Definition document[3] proposed the following updated definition for PMI: an MI associated with PCI is arbitrarily defined by elevation of troponin values greater than five times the 99th percentile (upper reference limit [URL]) in patients with normal baseline values (≤99th percentile URL) or a rise of troponin values greater than 20% if the baseline values are elevated and are stable or falling. The required enzymatic criteria should be associated with (1) symptoms consistent with myocardial ischemia; (2) new ischemic ECG changes or new left bundle branch block (LBBB); (3) angiographic loss of patency of a major coronary artery or a side branch, a persistent slow- or no-flow state, or embolization; or (4) imaging demonstration of new loss of viable myocardium or new regional wall motion abnormality. PCI-related MI (type 4) is distinguished from spontaneous MI (type 1), secondary MI (type 2), and MI associated with sudden death (type 3) or coronary artery bypass grafting (CABG; type 5). A documented stent thrombosis is recognized as a type 4b MI, whereas an MI associated with restenosis greater than 50% is type 4c (Table 30.1).

When a troponin value is elevated but less than or equal to five times the 99th percentile URL after PCI, and the troponin value was normal before the PCI, or when the troponin value is

TABLE 30.1 Categories of Myocardial Infarction Related to Percutaneous Coronary Intervention as Defined in the Third Universal Definition of Myocardial Infarction 2012

Category	Description/Definition
Type 4a: MI related to PCI	MI associated with PCI is arbitrarily defined by elevation of cardiac troponin values greater than five times the 99th percentile URL in patients with normal baseline values or a rise of cardiac troponin values >20% if the baseline values are elevated and are stable or falling. *In addition, one of the following features needs to be present:* 1. Symptoms suggestive of myocardial ischemia 2. New ischemic electrocardiographic changes or new left bundle branch block 3. Angiographic loss of patency of a major coronary artery or a side branch or persistent slow-flow or no-flow or embolization 4. Imaging demonstration of new loss of viable myocardium or new regional wall motion abnormality
Type 4b: MI related to stent thrombosis	MI associated with stent thrombosis is detected by coronary angiography or autopsy in the setting of myocardial ischemia and with a rise and/or fall of cardiac biomarker values with at least one value above the 99th percentile URL.
Type 4c: MI related to restenosis	MI with evidence of 50% or more stenosis at coronary angiography or a complex lesion associated with a rise and/or fall of troponin values above the 99th percentile URL and no other significant obstructive CAD of greater severity following (1) initially successful stent deployment or (2) initially successful PTCA (diameter stenosis <50% at the end of the procedure).

CAD, Coronary artery disease; *MI,* myocardial infarction; *PCI,* percutaneous coronary intervention; *PTCA,* percutaneous transluminal coronary angioplasty; *URL,* upper reference limit.
From Thygesen K, Alpert JS, Jaffe AS, et al. Third universal definition of myocardial infarction. *J Am Coll Cardiol.* 2012;60:1581–1598.

more than the 99th percentile URL in the absence of ischemic, angiographic, or imaging findings, the task force suggested that the term *myocardial injury* should be used.

Notably, the universal definition states that troponin is the preferred biomarker, the prognostic significance of which is less well validated than CK-MB in the setting of post-PCI myonecrosis. A large body of literature has demonstrated that post-PCI CK and CK-MB elevations have serious adverse prognostic implications, even in absence of pathologic Q-waves.[6–9] Three meta-analyses to examine the prognostic impact of periprocedural elevated CK-MB have confirmed a proportionate increase in early and late mortality with rising values.[10–12] The use of abnormal troponin assays to diagnose type 4a MI is supported by some datasets, although supporting evidence is not as wide ranging as has been demonstrated on the basis of abnormal CK-MB. Troponin is a particularly sensitive biomarker used ubiquitously for risk stratification in patients with ACS, but its widespread adoption has by itself increased the incidence of spontaneous MI and PMIs by 40% to 50%. In contrast to its predictive value in type 1 MI (ACS), existing data on peri- or post-PCI troponin elevation do not establish a clear association with an adverse prognosis. To make the definition more clinically relevant, the biomarker threshold for PMI was raised from greater than three times the 99th percentile URL in the earlier version of the Universal Definition document[13] to greater than five times the 99th percentile URL in the most recent one.[3] Nonetheless, the more recently recommended threshold remains arbitrary, and critics argue that any diagnosis of PMI should be associated with meaningful, well-defined prognostic significance.

The Society of Cardiac Angiography and Interventions Expert Consensus Proposed Definition of Periprocedural Myocardial Infarction

To address the limitations of the universal definition of PMI discussed above, an expert consensus group from the SCAI[4] proposed an alternate definition of *clinically relevant* MI after PCI, defined as "an event associated with a worsened prognosis." To this end, the document recommended that CK-MB be the preferred biomarker to assess clinically relevant PMI, defined as a CK-MB 10 or more times the ULN. A lower threshold (≥5 × ULN) may be accepted in the patient in whom new pathologic Q-waves in two or more contiguous leads (or new, persistent LBBB) develop after PCI, although further study is required to validate this threshold. If CK-MB assays are not available, the consensus document suggests a troponin level of 70 or more times the ULN to diagnose a type 4a MI. The authors selected this high troponin threshold so that the prognostic implication would be comparable to that associated with a CK-MB elevation of 10 or more times the ULN.

The following recommendations were made to diagnose post-PCI MI in ACS patients in whom the baseline level has not returned to normal: (1) in patients with elevated troponin (or CK-MB) in whom the biomarker levels are stable or falling, a new CK-MB elevation by an absolute increment of 10 or more times the ULN (or ≥70 × ULN for troponin) from the previous nadir level should be evident; (2) in patients with elevated troponin (or CK-MB) in whom the biomarker levels have *not* been shown to be stable or falling, there should be a further rise in CK-MB or troponin beyond the most recently measured value by an absolute increment of 10 or more times the ULN in CK-MB or 70 or more times the ULN in troponin plus new ST-segment elevation or depression plus signs consistent with a clinically relevant MI, such as new-onset or worsening heart failure or sustained hypotension.

Enzyme Elevation and Imaging Evidence of Myonecrosis

Although substantial debate surrounds the clinical significance of minor biomarker elevation after PCI, there is solid imaging evidence that biomarker release following PCI corresponds to irreversible myocardial injury, both qualitatively and quantitatively.

One study had 48 patients undergo cardiac magnetic resonance imaging (CMRI) before and after PCI to detect newly developed late gadolinium enhancement (LGE) as evidence of procedure-related myonecrosis.[14] Findings were correlated with serum troponin levels recorded 24 hours after the index PCI. Troponin elevation above the ULN was noted in 37% (14 patients), all with evidence of LGE in the target vessel territory. A linear correlation was also apparent between the troponin level at 24 hours after PCI and the mass (in grams) of newly hyperenhanced myocardium, both on the early post-PCI scan and on delayed 8-month scans, thus confirming the correlation between periprocedural biomarker release and irreversible myocardial damage (Fig. 30.1).[14]

In addition to confirming the irreversible nature of the myocardial injury, the location of MR hyperenhancement in relation to the PCI target segment may give insight into the pathophysiologic mechanism underlying PMI. When the hyperenhancement is visualized in proximity of the treated segment, side-branch occlusion (SBO) is the more likely explanation. However, in cases in which the myocardial injury/damage is downstream from the

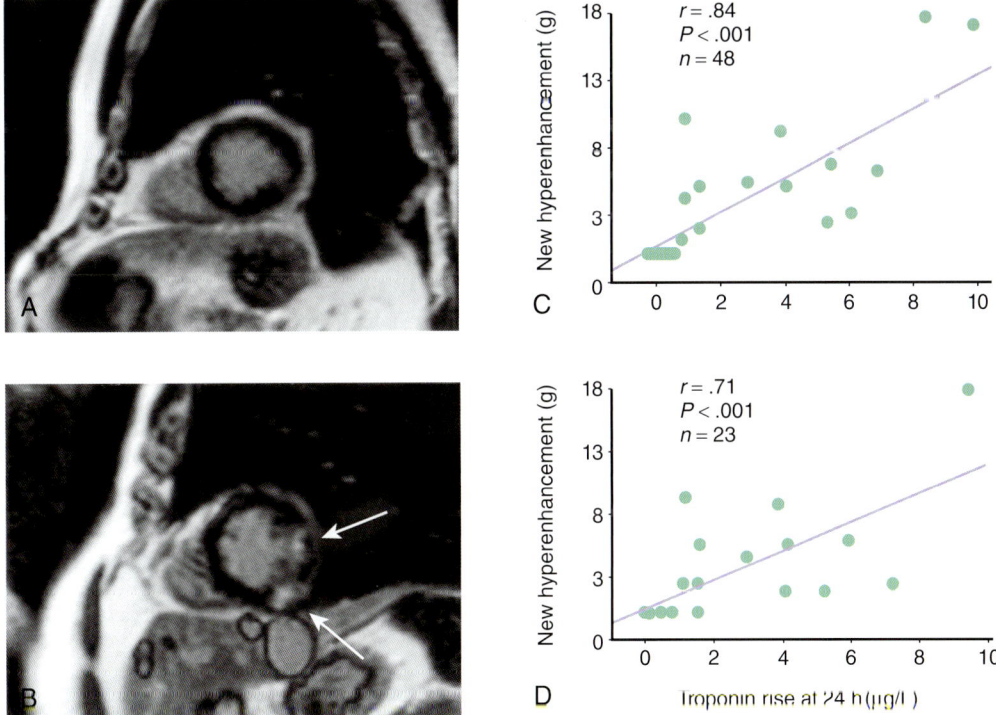

Fig. 30.1 (A) Apical ventricular short-axis image in a patient showing no hyperenhancement before left circumflex/obtuse marginal bifurcation percutaneous coronary intervention (PCI). (B) Image demonstrates two regions of new hyperenhancement in the distribution of the obtuse marginal branch artery after PCI *(arrows)*. Correlation between 24-hour post-PCI troponin I value versus mass of new myocardial hyperenhancement both early (C) and late (D) after PCI. (From Selvanayagam JB, Porto I, Channon K, et al. Troponin elevation after percutaneous coronary intervention directly represents the extent of irreversible myocardial injury: insights from cardiovascular magnetic resonance imaging. *Circulation*. 2005;111:1027–1032.)

treated segment, PMI can be best explained by distal microembolization and adverse platelet and inflammatory reactions in the microcirculation.[15,16]

INCIDENCE

As with its definition, the reported incidence of PMI has varied widely from one published report to another (Table 30.2). This variation can be attributed to several factors, but the predominant predictors are the choice of biomarker assayed and the threshold value used to diagnose PMI.

In a randomized trial of PCI and CABG for triple-vessel disease, 75% of PCI and 100% of CABG patients had biomarker level elevation despite successful revascularization. Use of ultrasensitive troponin resulted in nearly all such patients reaching criteria for a type 4a MI, whereas only about 15% were classified as such using CK-MB.[17] In other studies composed of less complex patients, an appreciable elevation of cardiac troponin above the ULN following PCI was still noted in about 40% to 50%.[18] In one meta-analysis of 15 studies that included more than 7500 patients with normal baseline troponin levels, troponin elevation occurred in 29% of the procedures.[19] When applying the older universal definition of PMI (any troponin elevation >3 × URL), the incidence of PMI is 14.5%. In a patient series that excluded patients with initially positive markers, the average incidence of PMI using CK-MB, troponin T, and troponin I greater than the ULN was 23%, 23%, and 27%, respectively.[16]

When the incidence of PMI is reported for a consecutive series of patients undergoing PCI (irrespective of their clinical condition after the procedure), it is invariably higher than in other series, in which biomarkers are assayed only in patients who developed certain symptoms or signs of ischemia. This is the result of detection of a fairly larger proportion of clinically silent events, with small-magnitude biomarker release.[7] The American College of Cardiology (ACC)/American Heart Association (AHA) PCI guidelines update published in 2011 recommended that for those patients who have signs or symptoms suggestive of MI during or after PCI, or for asymptomatic patients with significant persistent angiographic complications, e.g., large SBO, flow-limiting dissection, no-reflow phenomenon, or coronary thrombosis, CK-MB and/or troponin should be measured (class I recommendation). A class IIb recommendation is proposed for routine measurement of cardiac biomarkers in all patients after PCI.[2] Using a lower biomarker cutoff value to define PMI increases its epidemiologic incidence.[12,20] Other important factors that contribute to the heterogeneity of the conclusions of the various published series include the widely disparate baseline and procedural characteristics in the studied populations, inclusion or exclusion of patients with antecedent MI, and the timing of blood sampling.[5,16]

UNDERLYING PATHOPHYSIOLOGIC MECHANISMS

According to the distribution of hyperenhancement indicative of acute injury, MR myocardial imaging in patients who develop biomarker release after PCI reveals two different types of PMI. In the more commonly seen *distal type* of PMI, hyperenhancement is in the distal distribution downstream from the treated segment. In the *proximal type* of PMI, the injury is primarily detected adjacent to the treated segment.[15,21] Proximal PMI is usually linked to flow impairment in a side branch arising from the treated segment, whereas the more commonly seen distal PMI results from microvascular obstruction in the distribution of the artery subjected to PCI.

Distal Embolization and Periprocedural Myocardial Infarction

Although distal embolization associated with endothelial injury has been recognized for years, the importance of this phenomenon in relation to PCI was not fully appreciated until the last decade.[22] Significant distal embolization can cause no-reflow phenomenon after PCI in large part as a result of microvascular dysfunction, because evidence of myocardial ischemia and reduced antegrade coronary flow are present in the absence of an occlusive epicardial stenosis or side-branch compromise. In a report of patients undergoing PCI for non-STEMI (NSTEMI), those with a postprocedural troponin I elevation were significantly more likely to have reduced tissue-level perfusion than those without a troponin I elevation. Platelet aggregates have been identified in the distal microcirculation and in atherosclerotic debris retrieved from arteries downstream from the site of angioplasty using filter devices (Fig. 30.2).

Clinically, intravascular ultrasound (IVUS) studies provided further insight into the relationship between embolization of plaque material and PMI. Prati and coworkers[23] examined the relationship between change in plaque volume before and after stenting and the degree of CK-MB release in 54 patients. In patients with unstable angina, the reduction in plaque volume was more significant; more importantly, however, such reduction significantly correlated with CK-MB release even after adjusting for

TABLE 30.2 Incidence of Periprocedural Myocardial Infarction in Selected Large Patient Series

Reference	n	Type of PCI	Biomarker Definition of PMI	Incidence of PMI (%)
Harrington et al.[6]	1012	PTCA DCA	CK-MB × 2 ULN	3.8 10.3
Abdelmeguid et al.[7]	4664	PTCA, DCA	CK 2–5 × ULN	2.6
Ellis et al.[8]	8409	PCI	CK-MB >8.8	17.2
Ghazzal et al.[9]	15,637	PCI	CK 1–2 × ULN CK >3 × ULN	4.6 1.6
Simoons et al.[10]	5025	PTCA	CK-MB 1–3 × ULN	13.2
Ioannidis et al.[11]				
Roe et al.[12]	2384	PCI	CK-MB 1–3 × ULN CK-MB 3–5 × ULN CK-MB 5–10 × ULN CK-MB >10 × ULN	21.3 6.0 7.1 9.5
Stone et al.[64]	7147	PTCA Stent Ablation Ablation + stent	CK-MB >4	25.1 34.4 37.8 48.8
Natarajan et al.[180]	1128	PCI	Tn I >0.5	16.8
Nallamothu et al.[20]	1157	PCI	Tn I 1–3 × ULN Tn I 3–5 × ULN Tn I 5–8 × ULN Tn I ≥ 8 × ULN	16.0 4.6 2.0 6.5
Cavallini et al.[18]	3494	PCI	Tn I >0.15 CK-MB >5	44.2 16.0
Testa et al.[19]	7578	PCI	Tn >99% URL Tn >3 × URL	28.7 14.5

CK-MB, Creatine kinase MB; *DCA*, directional coronary atherectomy; *PCI*, percutaneous coronary intervention; *PMI*, periprocedural myocardial infarction; *PTCA*, percutaneous transluminal coronary angioplasty; *Tn*, troponin; *TnI*, trpononin I; *ULN*, upper limit of normal; *URL*, upper reference limit.

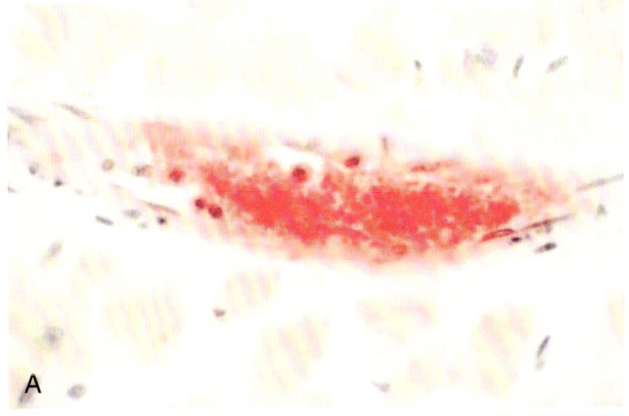

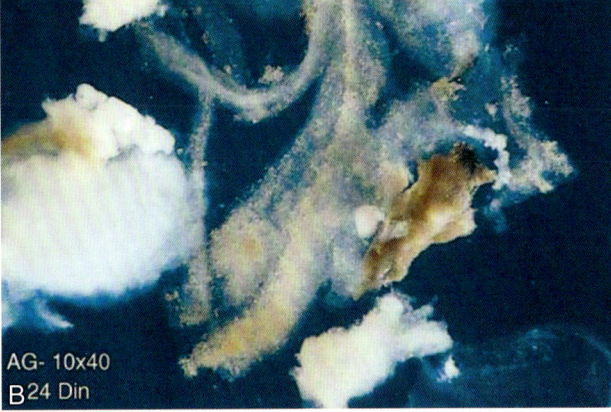

Fig. 30.2 (A) Histologic specimen of intramyocardial microvessel filled with platelets; the specimen stained positive for platelet glycoprotein IIb/IIIa from a patient who suffered sudden cardiac death. (B) Atherosclerotic particulate embolic material retrieved from percutaneous coronary revascularization with an Angioguard guidewire filter. (From Topol EJ, Yadav JS. Recognition of the importance of embolization in atherosclerotic vascular disease. *Circulation*. 2000;101:570–580.)

other variables that influence PMI. A more recent and sophisticated analysis of 62 patients undergoing complex PCI by Porto and colleagues[24] demonstrated a significant association between the change in target lesion plaque area by IVUS and the mass of myonecrosis assessed by hyperenhancement on MR imaging after PCI. The authors also correlated impaired microvascular flow (thrombolysis in myocardial infarction [TIMI] perfusion grade 0 or 1) with MR evidence of hyperenhancement downstream from the treated segment, hence suggesting that particulate matter from the atherosclerotic plaque disrupted by angioplasty drifts downstream and leads to microvascular obstruction and myonecrosis. With the higher resolution of frequency domain optical coherence tomography (OCT), correlations were made between the morphologic features of plaque and subsequent risk of PMI. In a study of 50 patients undergoing single vessel stenting and OCT imaging before and after PCI, a thin-cap fibroatheroma (TCFA) pre-PCI was defined as a lipid-rich plaque (two or more quadrants of lipid core) with a fibrous cap ≤65 μm. TCFA was more frequently seen in those who developed type 4a MI (76% vs. 41%, $P = .017$). The association was statistically significant and independent of other variables that predicted the development of type 4a MI.[24]

Platelet Activation

Platelet activation plays a critical role in the development and perpetuation of coronary microvascular obstruction following PCI. By definition, the interventional devices used to treat an epicardial stenosis will result in a break in the endothelial surface and a release of debris into the coronary bloodstream. The exposed intraplaque contents stimulate platelet activation and aggregation at the site of the PCI and probably also in the downstream microvasculature. Thus, the platelet aggregates that plug the microcirculation not only cause mechanical obstruction but also lead to detrimental biochemical responses due to their interaction with the injured endothelium, the neutrophils, and more platelets. The release of vasoactive substances such as serotonin and endothelin-1 from the activated platelets and the injured endothelium lead to intense microvascular vasoconstriction, which accentuates the ischemic injury and resultant myonecrosis.[16,22] The odds of developing PMI, in a cohort of 151 patients presenting for nonurgent PCI, increased threefold if they were found to be aspirin resistant before the procedure.[25]

Periprocedural ST-Segment–Elevation Myocardial Infarction

A PCI-related infarction presenting with ST-segment elevation is caused by acute and total occlusion of a relatively sizable epicardial coronary branch. This is most commonly the result of abrupt closure of a branch or acute stent thrombosis. On occasion, embolization of large thrombus or atheroma may occlude the distal vessel and cause STEMI; such embolization is more common in degenerated saphenous vein graft (SVG) interventions than in native vessel interventions.

RISK FACTORS PREDISPOSING TO PERIPROCEDURAL MYOCARDIAL INFARCTION

Clinical trials to examine the role of newer interventional devices, GP IIb/IIIa inhibitors, and/or newer anticoagulants—as well as large PCI registries—have provided significant insight into the incidence and significance of PMI. Based on these studies, certain subsets of patients have been identified to be at higher risk of PMI. These subsets can be identified based on clinical, lesion-related, procedural, or device-related variables.

Clinical Characteristics

The risk of PMI is significantly increased in patients with evidence of more severe atherosclerotic disease. Multivessel and/or more diffuse coronary artery disease (CAD) is associated with an approximately 50% increase in the relative risk of developing PMI.[9,12,26] IVUS evidence of increased plaque burden is also a risk factor for development of PMI,[21,23] which may explain why diabetics are at a higher risk.[27] Notably, evidence of advanced noncardiac atherosclerotic disease has been associated with an even higher relative risk of PMI.[26] Other patient risk factors such as advanced age and preexisting renal dysfunction are probably indicative of more advanced atherosclerotic disease.

The clinical presentation at the time of PCI may also play a role in determining the risk of PMI and other adverse events during and after the procedure. Patients with ACS are more likely to develop PMI.[12] However, studies to examine the incidence of PMI in this patient population have been limited by methodologic difficulties. First, it is more complex to define PMI when patients present with elevated markers before PCI; therefore, most of the studies on this topic excluded these patients from the analysis. Second, even if patients with elevated markers are excluded, it is conceivable that those with negative markers who were referred to PCI within minutes to hours of presentation may have been having a spontaneous infarction that was only appreciated after the PCI.[12,16]

A heightened systemic inflammatory state before PCI is also a major predictor of adverse outcomes, which include PMI. Most

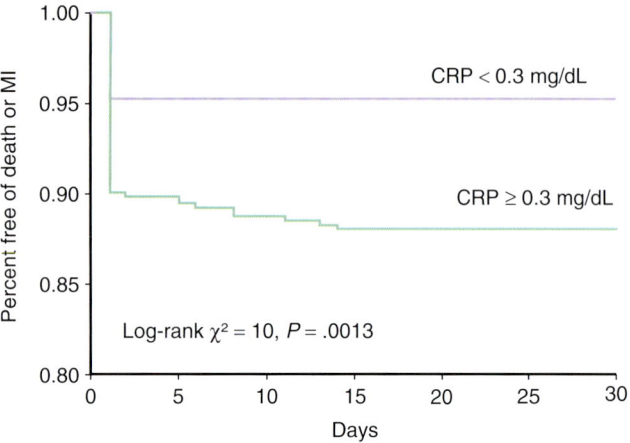

Fig. 30.3 Kaplan–Meier survival curves for 30-day death or myocardial infarction *(MI)* stratified by baseline C-reactive protein *(CRP)*. The majority of the events and the separation of the curves occur within the first 1 to 2 days; that is, the difference is primarily driven by the incidence of periprocedural myocardial infarction. (From Chew DP, Bhatt DL, Robbins MA, et al. Incremental prognostic value of elevated baseline C-reactive protein among established markers of risk in percutaneous coronary intervention. *Circulation.* 2001;104:992–997.)

of the evidence in support of this hypothesis has been based on correlations between pre-PCI C-reactive protein (CRP) levels and evidence of PMI. A small study of 85 patients with stable angina undergoing PCI demonstrated that PMI, defined by an elevated troponin level, is significantly more frequent in patients with elevated CRP (46% of those with elevated CRP, but only 18% of those with a normal CRP, developed the complication).[28] Chew and colleagues[29] examined the relationship between preprocedural CRP and the adverse events (death and MI) in the first 30 days following PCI in a larger series of 727 consecutive patients. The highest quartile of CRP was predictive of worse outcome (odds ratio [OR], 3.68; 95% confidence interval [CI] 1.5 to 9.0) and that association persisted even after adjusting for other variables that influence outcome. The event-free survival curves separated within 24 hours and were primarily driven by a reduction in MI, suggesting that patients with elevated CRP are more susceptible to development of PMI (Fig. 30.3).

Lesion-Related Risk Factors

SVG lesions are notorious for the risk of development of PMI, probably as a result of the increased incidence of both macro- and microembolization with subsequent slow flow and no-reflow phenomenon. In the absence of an EPD, the risk of PMI (defined as CK-MB >3 × ULN) in the contemporary era can be as high 13.7%. This rate almost doubles if the threshold cutoff value to define PMI is any increase in CK-MB.[30] The introduction of EPDs in the last few years has reduced the risk of PMI in those patients.[30–32]

Several lesion characteristics are traditionally associated with a higher risk of PMI, primarily features suggestive of lesion instability such as eccentricity, irregular contour, or visible thrombosis. Complex lesions (ACC/AHA type C) usually contain one or more of those features and are thus associated with a significantly increased risk of PMI.[7,33] In a small study, the value of the Synergy Between Percutaneous Coronary Intervention With Taxus and Cardiac Surgery (SYNTAX) score in predicting PMI was assessed and compared with other lesion-scoring systems. This particular angiographic scoring system expressed lesion severity and complexity, which can be estimates of disease severity. Not surprisingly, increasing SYNTAX scores were associated with increased risk of PMI. Using receiver operator curve (ROC) analysis, a score of 17 or higher predicted PMI with a sensitivity of 75% and a specificity of 70%.[34]

Lesions that involve the ostium of a major side branch are usually among the more complex lesion types and are more prone to result in PMI because of the higher risk of side-branch closure. Other lesion characteristics that confer a higher risk of PMI include those features that suggest a higher plaque burden such as multiplicity of lesions, long lesions, and diffusely diseased arteries. Lesions with a larger necrotic core, as identified by IVUS and virtual histology (IVUS-VH) imaging, may confer a higher risk of PMI; this is because the necrotic core components include fragile tissues such as foam cells, organized intramural hemorrhage, and cholesterol crystals that may embolize and potentiate thrombosis.[35] In this study, embolization of small particles liberated during stenting was detected as high-intensity transient signals (HITS) with a Doppler guidewire (Fig. 30.4). Tanaka and associates[36] utilized OCT to image the culprit plaques in NSTEMI patients undergoing PCI. Plaques with thinner caps (<70 μm) and larger lipid cores (>90-degree arc of the vessel circumference) were more highly associated with periprocedural no-reflow phenomenon.

Procedural Complications and Risk of Periprocedural Myocardial Infarction

SBO, flow-limiting dissections, and transient abrupt closure have been the most recognizable procedural complications that result in relatively large PMIs.[7,9,34,37] However, these complications are rare, and most detected PMIs follow routine procedures with no obvious angiographic complications.[16,22] With universal availability of stents and their routine use, abrupt closure has become quite rare—fewer than 1% of cases in contemporary PCI.[22] The effectiveness of stenting and the availability of potent antiplatelet therapies are probably the primary mechanisms by which large (Q-wave) PMIs and need for emergent coronary surgery have been reduced by almost 50%.[38,39] Abrupt closure and no-reflow phenomenon have not been found to affect outcome when treated promptly, with no subsequent PMIs.[37]

SBO has been, and remains, the most common angiographically recognizable procedural complication to result in PMI.[7,9] Unlike abrupt closure, the incidence of SBO has not decreased with routine use of coronary stenting. In fact, with increasing stent use, SBO has become the most likely cause of acute occlusion during PCI.[40] SBO has been reported in 13% to 19% of cases in which a stent was placed across a major side branch (>1 mm), and most occur after post-stent high-pressure dilation. Side branches that arise from within native coronary artery lesions are at a fivefold to tenfold higher risk for occlusion. Other predictors include branch ostial disease, branch artery size, and balloon/artery ratio. Proposed mechanisms for SBO include plaque shift (the so-called snowplow effect), branch artery ostial dissection or spasm, and/or thrombus formation.[41] A major SBO can be associated with large (possibly Q-wave) infarctions, but even smaller SBOs have been associated with evidence of small areas of MR hyperenhancement, diagnostic of small areas of PMI. The distribution of hyperenhancement in these cases is different from that seen with distal embolization downstream of the target lesion for PCI. With SBO, hyperenhancement is adjacent, rather than distal to, the location of the PCI. The likelihood of development of new hyperenhancement increases 16-fold when SBO can be angiographically recognized.[21]

Some intriguing observations have been made regarding SBO and PMI in the era of PCI for complex lesions using drug-eluting stents. In the Randomized Trial Evaluating Slow-Release Formulation TAXUS Paclitaxel-Eluting Coronary Stents to Treat De Novo Coronary Lesions (TAXUS V) trial, which randomized 1172 patients to receive a paclitaxel-eluting or a bare-metal

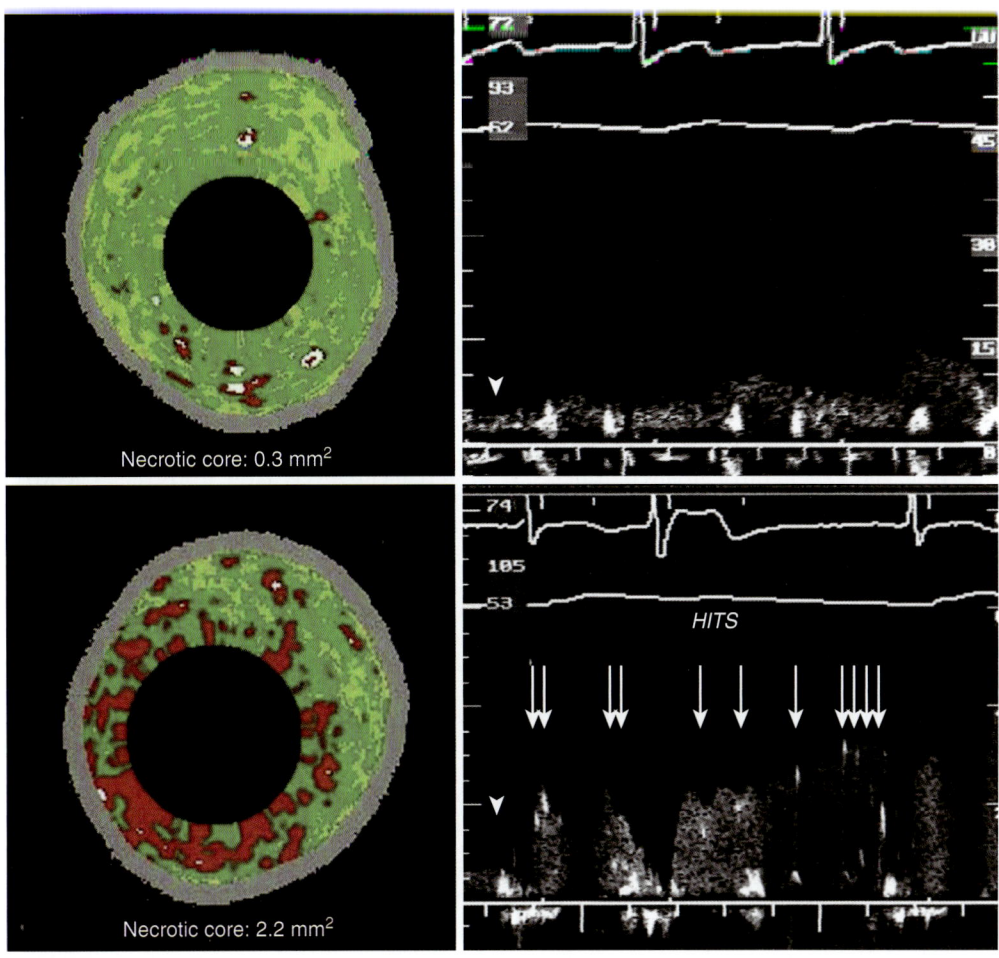

Fig. 30.4 Plaques with a larger necrotic core, as identified by intravascular ultrasound and virtual histology imaging, are more likely to cause distal embolization. The largely fibrotic plaque with minimal necrotic core *(top left)* results in minimal high-intensity transient signals *(HITS; top right)* detected by a Doppler wire placed distal to the lesion during stenting. Conversely, stenting of a plaque with a larger necrotic core *(bottom left)* results in significantly more HITS. (From Kawamoto T, Okura H, Koyama Y, et al. The relationship between coronary plaque characteristics and small embolic particles during coronary stent implantation. *J Am Coll Cardiol.* 2007;50:1635–1640.)

stent, complex lesion subsets (>35% type C) were treated in both groups, and more than 30% of patients received more than one stent. In the subgroup of patients who received multiple stents, the incidence of 30-day MI was significantly higher with paclitaxel-eluting stents (8.3% vs. 3.3%, $P = .047$). Core laboratory angiographic analysis of this patient subset revealed a significantly higher incidence of side-branch compromise or occlusion with paclitaxel-eluting stents than with bare-metal stents (42.6% vs. 30.6%, $P = .03$), resulting in a higher incidence of less than TIMI grade 3 flow in the paclitaxel-eluting stent group. Why paclitaxel-eluting stents are associated with more side-branch compromise and subsequent PMI remains unclear. Possible explanations include the increasing thickness of the stent struts caused by the drug-eluting polymer, increased platelet deposition, and/or paclitaxel-induced spasm.[42] A comparison of paclitaxel- and everolimus-eluting stents demonstrates the importance of the strut and polymer thickness. A post hoc analysis of the Clinical Evaluation of the Investigational Device XIENCE V Everolimus-Eluting Coronary Stent System in the Treatment of Subjects With de Novo Native Coronary Artery Lesions (SPIRIT III) randomized trial[43] compared the incidence of PMI in 113 patients who received the thinner strut and polymer everolimus-eluting stent to 63 patients who received the paclitaxel-eluting stent, in whom a small side branch was "jailed" by the deployed stent. PMI was defined as any increase in CK-MB above the ULN and was much lower in the everolimus-eluting stent group (9.0% vs. 29.7%, $P = .01$).

Risk of Periprocedural Myocardial Infarction by Interventional Device

Some of the earliest investigations to spark interest in PMI and its significance were in the context of comparing newer interventional devices to standard balloon angioplasty. Data from the Coronary Angioplasty Versus Excisional Atherectomy Trial (CAVEAT-I) demonstrated that directional coronary atherectomy (DCA) was associated with more abrupt closure, evidence of PMI, and subsequently a higher rate of clinical adverse events compared with balloon angioplasty.[6,44] These findings were confirmed in the Balloon Versus Optimal Atherectomy Trial (BOAT), in which a more refined technique of DCA failed to demonstrate its superiority to percutaneous transluminal coronary angioplasty (PTCA). However, the incidence of PMI was still significantly higher with DCA than with PTCA (16% vs. 6%).[45] DCA is associated with more distal embolization, particularly in SVG interventions.[46] There is also evidence of a higher degree of platelet activation with DCA,[47] with its subsequent mechanical obstruction and thrombotic and inflammatory responses in the downstream microcirculation. Similarly, owing to its mechanism of action, rotational atherectomy is associated with more platelet activation and more distal embolization of plaque debris than balloon angioplasty.[48]

Although the routine use of coronary stents has dramatically reduced the incidence of most PCI complications—such as abrupt closure, flow-limiting dissections, need for emergent bypass surgery, and restenosis—stenting increases the incidence of PMI compared with balloon angioplasty, with a relative risk increase of about 20%.[16,22,49] In patients who underwent PCI of the left anterior descending coronary artery (LAD) and were randomly assigned to balloon angioplasty or stenting, evidence was found of a higher degree of platelet and neutrophil surface activation after stenting.[50] High-pressure inflations aiming to over-expand stents and reduce restenosis can actually lead to higher CK-MB levels. In a study of approximately 1000 patients undergoing IVUS-guided stenting, the incidence of PMI (defined as CK-MB $3 \times$ ULN) was 16%, 18%, and 25% in three groups of patients, in whom the final stent/reference lumen area was less than 70%, 70% to 100%, and greater than 100%, respectively.[51] Increasing stent length was also associated with increased biomarker release in a smaller study of patients who underwent elective PCI.[52]

PROGNOSTIC IMPLICATIONS OF PERIPROCEDURAL MYOCARDIAL INFARCTION

Although much controversy surrounds the definition and prevalence of PMI with everyday PCI, there is no dispute that significant PMI is associated with an increased mortality risk. Controversy still exists about the pathophysiologic mechanisms that underlie this association and also the definition and size of PMI that would confer such increased risk. However, convincing evidence suggests that any PMI is associated with some degree of increased risk of death, particularly with longer follow-up durations.

The pioneering work of Abdelmeguid and coworkers[7] demonstrated that CK and CK-MB elevation after PCI (primarily balloon angioplasty and DCA in this report) are associated with an approximate 30% relative increase in 3-year mortality. Three-year follow-up of the Evaluation of Abciximab 7E3 for the Prevention of Ischemic Complications (EPIC) trial patients, who underwent angioplasty and DCA as well, revealed an incremental long-term risk of death with increasing degrees of PMI. Among the 2001 patients enrolled in the trial, the mortality risk increased from 7.3% in those with no CK elevation to 13.1% when CK was greater than three times the ULN and again to 16.5% with CK greater than 10 times the ULN.[53] In the EPISTENT trial, in which stenting was routinely used in two-thirds of the patients, the 1-year mortality doubled between patients with minimal to no PMI (CK-MB $>1 \times$ ULN) to those with CK-MB greater than three to 10 times the ULN (1.5% vs. 3.4%).[54] Subsequently, similar conclusions were made by examining outcomes of patients enrolled in PCI clinical trials and large-scale single-center patient registries (see Table 30.2).[6,8,9,12,54,55]

The threshold above which a PMI is considered prognostically significant has been a subject of some debate. It has been traditional to consider a PMI when the CK-MB exceeds three times the ULN, although the recent PCI guidelines suggest CK-MB greater than five times the ULN should be the threshold for defining a PMI.[56] In the large series of Ghazzal and colleagues,[9] minor elevation of total CK ($<3 \times$ ULN) did not confer a statistically significant increase in risk of late mortality. Brener and coworkers[57] suggested that only massive CK-MB release ($>10 \times$ ULN) predicts an increased risk of death over a 3-year period. However, strong evidence shows that smaller CK-MB elevations are associated with increasing risk of death. Abdelmeguid and colleagues[7] examined that question specifically and concluded that any increase in CK-MB above normal limits confers some degree of risk. In a later meta-analysis, any increase in CK-MB, even less than three times the ULN, was associated with a statistically significant increase in the risk of death (OR 1.5). Patients with a CK-MB level three to five times the ULN and those with levels more than five times the ULN had an even higher relative risk of dying over the 3-year follow-up.[11] Similarly, in the large meta-analysis by Roe and colleagues,[12] the increased mortality risk was associated with increasing CK-MB expressed as a continuous variable—that is, with no specific thresholds above or below which the risk changes (Fig. 30.5). A more recent analysis of 5268 patients undergoing elective PCI, using both troponin T and CK-MB postprocedure levels, demonstrated an association of the elevated biomarker levels with 3-month mortality. The optimal thresholds that predicted mortality in this analysis were troponin T greater than 25 times the ULN and CK-MB greater than five times the ULN.[58]

Frequently, very large PMIs (i.e., CK-MB levels >8 to $10 \times$ ULN) are associated with significant complications or an unsuccessful procedural result. The association between PMI and mortality has been attributed to the impact of an unsuccessful procedure on mortality and not to an independent effect. In a study of approximately 6000 patients, the incidence of PMI was three times more frequent when the procedure was unsuccessful, and the size of the infarction was also significantly larger. After adjusting for the success of the procedure—defined as residual stenosis of less than 50%, achievement of TIMI grade 3 flow, absence of significant residual dissection, no need for urgent revascularization, and no stent thrombosis within 24 hours—the presence or absence of PMI was not statistically related to 1-year mortality.[59] However, the study only examined 1-year mortality, and in many investigations that have examined PMI, the effect on mortality was observed with longer-term follow-up. In addition, the initial studies by Abdelmeguid and colleagues[7,33] that established a relationship between PMI and death have excluded unsuccessful procedural results from their analyses. In the recent CK-MB and PCI study[18] to examine the significance of post-PCI troponin elevation, unsuccessful procedures doubled the odds of 2-year mortality; yet the effect of post-PCI CK-MB levels remained a strong and significant predictor of mortality.

The association between mortality and PMI defined by elevated serum troponin levels has been studied, although less extensively. The updated PCI guidelines propose that a PMI becomes clinically significant if the troponin level exceeds five times the ULN. In a study of 1157 patients (>77% receiving stents), 1-year mortality risk increased only in the group of patients with troponin I levels eight or more times the ULN (≥ 16 ng/mL).[20] However, in a large multicenter prospective study of almost 3500 patients that addressed the significance of post-PCI troponin levels, a statistically significant association was found between troponin I elevation and 2-year mortality. As expected, the incidence of troponin I elevation after PCI was significantly higher than that of CK-MB, indicating the higher sensitivity of troponin I in detecting myonecrosis. Yet this high sensitivity appears to reduce the ability of troponin elevation to predict prognosis.[18] As for troponin T, a threshold of greater than 25 times the ULN appears similar to a CK-MB threshold of five times the ULN in predicting 90-day mortality.[58]

A contemporary analysis on the prognostic significance of PMI in patients from the Acute Catheterization and Urgent Intervention Triage Strategy (ACUITY) trial suggests that PMI is a marker of baseline risk, atherosclerosis burden, and procedural complexity but in most cases does not appear to have independent prognostic significance. In this analysis of the 1-year follow-up of the ACUITY patients, development of a spontaneous MI was significantly associated with mortality, whereas a postprocedural MI was not.[60]

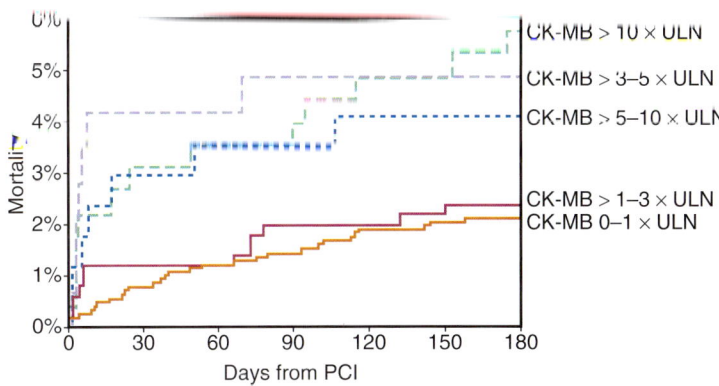

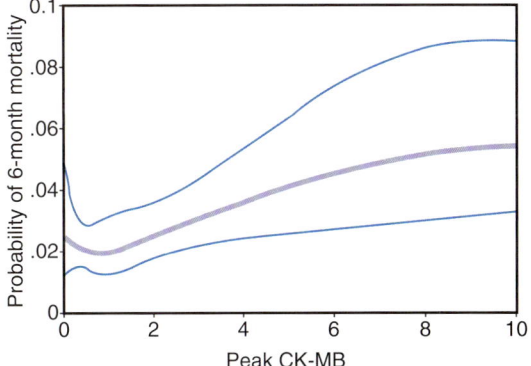

Fig. 30.5 *Top:* Kaplan–Meier curves for 6-month unadjusted mortality after percutaneous coronary intervention *(PCI)* for increments of post-PCI creatine kinase MB *(CK-MB)*. *Bottom:* Continuous unadjusted relationship between peak CK-MB (expressed as times the upper limit of normal [× *ULN*]) and 6 months mortality. The thin–or blue–lines represent the 95% confidence intervals. (From Roe MT, Mahaffey KW, Kilaru R, et al. Creatine kinase-MB elevation after percutaneous coronary intervention predicts adverse outcomes in patients with acute coronary syndromes. *Eur Heart J.* 2004;25:313–321.)

PREVENTION AND MANAGEMENT OF PERIPROCEDURAL MYOCARDIAL INFARCTION

In the majority of cases of PMI, the event is clinically silent and the diagnosis is made based on routine collection of cardiac biomarkers after PCI. Therefore, little can be done to treat the event by any specific measures different from those that should be used with any patient undergoing PCI—that is, effective β-blockade, antiplatelet therapy, lipid lowering, and aggressive risk-factor control. During the procedure, recognition of a side-branch closure usually prompts an attempt at restoration of flow in that branch by balloon angioplasty and stenting if necessary. If distal embolization of thrombus is seen to impair distal flow, aspiration thrombectomy and/or intracoronary (IC) fibrinolytic therapy may improve flow. Embolization of atheromatous debris is not likely to respond to pharmacologic agents.[61] IC injection of vasodilators such as nitroglycerin, calcium channel blockers, nitroprusside, or adenosine can also improve flow by relieving arteriolar spasm and recruiting a larger microvascular bed. Whereas these maneuvers can improve epicardial flow, it is not clear whether they will impact the size or the prognostic significance of the PMI.[62,63] After the procedure, and in the event of a relatively large PMI (e.g., CK-MB ≥5 × ULN), an additional day of telemetry monitoring and more adequate β-blockade (with a target heart rate of about 60 beats/min) may be indicated.

Given the adverse prognostic implications, it is significantly more important to develop strategies to prevent, rather than treat, PMI. Successful strategies to prevent PMI include pharmacologic and nonpharmacologic approaches. The primary pharmacologic interventions that have achieved significant success include aggressive antiplatelet therapy (primarily IV GP IIb/IIIa inhibitors and oral thienopyridine inhibitors) and statin therapy. Nonpharmacologic approaches include the use of EPDs in the setting of SVG intervention. Collectively, these therapies are integrated to prevent or at least reduce distal embolization and to protect the myocardium.

Intravenous Glycoprotein IIb/IIIa Platelet Inhibitors

Periprocedural utilization of GP IIb/IIIa platelet inhibitors provides immediate and near-complete inhibition of platelet aggregation. The IV administration of the appropriate doses and the targeting of the final common receptor for the aggregation process (the GP IIb/IIIa receptor) ensure both an extremely high bioavailability and a very predictable and complete response. Abciximab, the prototype of this class of antiplatelet agents, has been shown in multiple clinical trials to reduce the incidence of post-PCI myonecrosis. In the seminal trials (EPIC, Evaluation in PTCA to Improve Long-Term Outcome With Abciximab GP IIb/IIIa Blockade [EPILOG], and EPISTENT), the cutoff for defining PMI was CK-MB levels three times the ULN. The relative risk reduction in MI at 30 days ranged between 40% and 60%, with the curves separating as early as the first day, thus indicating a significant reduction in PMI.[32,64] In EPISTENT, administration of abciximab significantly reduced the risk of a larger PMI (CK-MB >5 × ULN) irrespective of the device used, stent or balloon angioplasty (Fig. 30.6).[54] In the c7E3 FAB Antiplatelet Therapy in Unstable Refractory Angina (CAPTURE) trial,[65] refractory unstable angina patients were randomized to receive abciximab or placebo many hours before and during PCI. In this trial, the incidence of MI in the hours before undergoing PCI was reduced significantly in the abciximab arm. Additionally, the incidence of PMI was reduced by more than 50% in the abciximab arm (2.6% vs. 5.5%, *P* = .009). With rotational atherectomy, which consistently results in distal microembolization, abciximab bolus and infusion demonstrated a significant advantage over anticoagulation alone in reducing postprocedural CK and CK-MB rise.[48]

Similar effects have been demonstrated with the synthetic small-molecule GP IIb/IIIa inhibitors, eptifibatide and tirofiban. The impact of eptifibatide on PMI was significantly better when the dosing regimen was adjusted from one bolus in the Platelet Glycoprotein IIb/IIIa in Unstable Angina: Receptor Suppression Using Integrilin Therapy (PURSUIT) PCI trial[66] to the

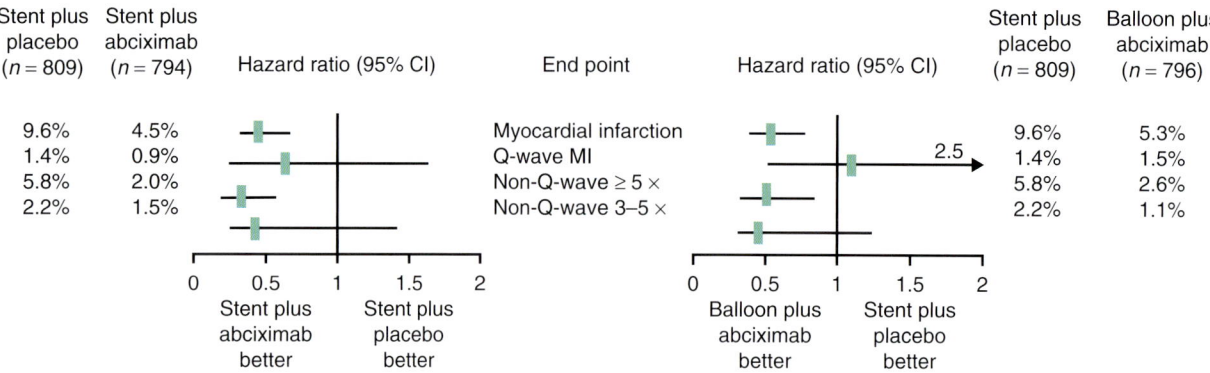

Fig. 30.6 Kaplan–Meier estimates and hazard ratios (95% confidence interval [CI]) for myocardial infarction in the EPISTENT trial. (From The EPISTENT Investigators. Randomized placebo-controlled and balloon-angioplasty-controlled trial to assess safety of coronary stenting with use of platelet glycoprotein-IIb/IIIa blockade. Lancet. 1998;352:87–92.)

double-bolus regimen followed in the Enhanced Suppression of the Platelet IIb/IIIa Receptor with Integrilin Therapy (ESPRIT) trial.[67] This emphasizes the importance of the near-complete inhibition required if an impact on distal embolization is to be expected. In the PURSUIT trial, the incidence of PMI was reduced by 25%, whereas the reduction with the double-bolus regimen was 40%. In both trials, PMI was defined as CK-MB greater than three times the ULN, and the incidence of PMI in the placebo group was very similar in both trials—about 9%. Similarly, in the Randomized Efficacy Study of Tirofiban for Outcomes and Restenosis (RESTORE) trial,[68] which examined the role of tirofiban in patients with ACSs, a small but significant reduction was seen in PMI at the 48-hour mark. However, no statistically significant difference was seen in the incidence of the primary end point (30-day death, MI, or revascularization for recurrent ischemia and use of stents for threatened or abrupt closure) between tirofiban and placebo. With the higher-dose tirofiban bolus, a small study of 202 high-risk patients undergoing PCI demonstrated that PMI defined by troponin rise decreased by about 34% and average CK-MB level (expressed in absolute units) was reduced by more than 50%.[69]

Direct Thrombin Inhibitors (Bivalirudin)

Although it has been clearly established that intensive platelet inhibition does result in reduced PMI, concern has been raised about excess bleeding risk caused by such strategies. Recent focus on bleeding complications demonstrates a significant adverse prognostic implication to periprocedural bleeding on outcome, with convincing evidence of increased 1-year mortality in patients who suffer an early bleeding complication.[70] This recognition has encouraged the use of the direct thrombin inhibitor bivalirudin as the primary anticoagulant during PCI over the last several years. Large trials to compare bivalirudin with a combination of heparin and GP IIb/IIIa inhibitors demonstrated noninferiority of bivalirudin in reducing PMI and its clear superiority in reducing bleeding complications. It thus seems to strike a reasonable balance between reducing PMI and other ischemic complications without paying a price in the form of excess bleeding. In the Randomized Evaluation in PCI Linking Angiomax to Reduced Clinical Events (REPLACE-2) trial, which examined the role of bivalirudin in low-risk PCI patients, the incidence of PMI was slightly higher, but not statistically significant, in the bivalirudin arm: 7.0% compared with 6.2% in the control arm of heparin and GP IIb/IIIa inhibitors.[71] In another large randomized trial of over 4500 low-risk PCI patients (those with stable clinical presentations), bivalirudin therapy was compared with unfractionated heparin, and both groups were preloaded with oral aspirin and clopidogrel.

Neither anticoagulant strategy was superior in reducing ischemic complications (PMI 5.6% with bivalirudin vs. 4.8% with heparin), but bleeding complications were reduced in the bivalirudin arm (3.1% vs. 4.6%, $P = .008$).[72]

In the ACUITY trial, approximately 14,000 ACS patients treated with an early invasive strategy were randomized to one of three antithrombotic regimens: heparin plus a GP IIb/IIIa inhibitor; bivalirudin plus a GP IIb/IIIa inhibitor; or bivalirudin alone. Comparing those who received heparin and GP IIb/IIIa inhibitors to those who received bivalirudin alone, no difference was found in ischemic events, but bleeding complications were reduced by almost 50% at 30 days (5.7% vs. 3.0%, $P < .001$ for noninferiority, $P < .001$ for superiority of bivalirudin).[73]

In a prespecified analysis, the outcomes of 7789 ACUITY patients who underwent PCI were analyzed according to the anticoagulation regimen they received. The results mirrored those of the main trial: no difference was found in PMI or other ischemic events, but a statistically significant reduction in bleeding complications was noted, leading to improved net clinical benefit in favor of bivalirudin alone. A post hoc analysis of this subset demonstrated an important interaction between clopidogrel pretreatment and the choice of anticoagulant strategy. Of the 7789 PCI patients, 129 did not receive any clopidogrel, and 3493 received clopidogrel before angiography, 1572 at the time of PCI, and 814 after PCI. Patients who received clopidogrel before angiography or within 30 minutes of PCI had similar ischemic complications, whether they were randomized to bivalirudin or heparin and GP IIb/IIIa inhibitors. However, when clopidogrel was not given, or when it was given more than 30 minutes after PCI, those randomized to bivalirudin experienced a higher incidence of ischemic events, mostly in the form of PMI (14.1% vs. 8.5%; risk ratio [RR] 1.7; 95% CI 1.05 to 2.63).[74] This interaction between timing of clopidogrel therapy and bivalirudin use emphasizes the need for an effective antiplatelet therapy when direct thrombin inhibitors are used during PCI.

$P2Y_{12}$ Platelet Inhibitors

The proven benefit of IIb/IIIa platelet inhibitors in reducing PMI further supports the central role of platelet aggregation/activation in the pathophysiology of PMI. This is also further emphasized by the very high incidence of PMI and other adverse cardiac events in patients with aspirin resistance. Thus, dual-antiplatelet therapy (DAPT) at the time of PCI has been advocated. The timing and dosing of these agents seems to have a significant impact on PMI and other post-PCI adverse events. Steinhubl and colleagues[75] reported a significant reduction in the incidence of PMI with pre-PCI administration of ticlopidine.

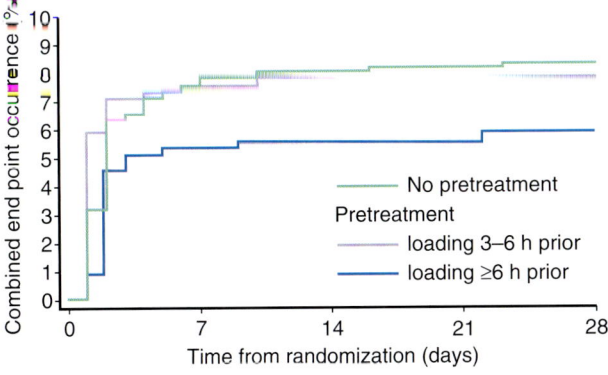

Fig. 30.7 The 28-day combined end point (death, myocardial infarction, urgent revascularization) in the Clopidogrel for Reduction of Events During Observation trial, stratified by use and timing of clopidogrel loading dose. The curves separate within 48 hours, primarily because of differences in incidence of periprocedural myocardial infarction. (From Steinhubl SR, Berger PB, Mann JT 3rd, et al. Early and sustained dual oral antiplatelet therapy following percutaneous coronary intervention: a randomized controlled trial. *JAMA*. 2002;288:2411–2420.)

The longer the duration of therapy, the lower the incidence; and among patients pretreated with ticlopidine, the odds ratio for development of PMI was 0.18 when the duration of pretreatment was 3 or more days. Subsequently, the questions of dosing and duration of pretreatment with another thienopyridine inhibitor, clopidogrel, were addressed in the Clopidogrel for Reduction of Events During Observation (CREDO) trial. The study randomized patients undergoing elective PCI to receive a 300-mg clopidogrel loading dose or placebo 3 to 24 hours before PCI. All patients were taking aspirin, and most of them did undergo PCI. A second randomization to 28 days versus 9 months of DAPT was performed for those in the clopidogrel arm. The results demonstrated a reduction in 30-day major adverse events (primarily early MIs) only in patients who received the loading dose 6 or more hours before PCI (Fig. 30.7).[76] The timing of the loading dose significantly impacted the beneficial effect of thienopyridine on PCI outcomes. In the Clopidogrel in Unstable Angina to Prevent Recurrent Events (CURE) trial, 30% of patients underwent PCI at the discretion of the treating cardiologists. This PCI subgroup included 2658 patients with NSTEMI from non-U.S. centers where the time between admission for ACS and PCI averaged 10 days. In this setting, the 30-day incidence of MI was reduced by more than 50% in patients who received clopidogrel (2.9% vs. 6.2%), suggesting that a longer duration of pretreatment, particularly in high-risk patients, is associated with better protection against procedure-related MI.[77]

Several groups have demonstrated that a higher loading dose (600 mg) of clopidogrel can achieve two important goals: it can reach higher levels of platelet inhibition and can achieve that target within 2 hours of oral administration.[78] The improved efficacy of the higher loading dose is at least partly attributed to the fact that about one-third of patients do not adequately respond to the inhibitory effect of the 300 mg dose.[78] The Antiplatelet Therapy for Reduction of Myocardial Damage During Angioplasty (ARMYDA-2) trial established the superiority of the 600-mg loading dose of clopidogrel in reducing PMI and improving 30-day outcomes. This study enrolled 255 patients undergoing PCI and randomized them to 300 versus 600-mg loading doses of clopidogrel 4 to 8 hours before PCI. The primary end point of death, MI, or urgent revascularization at 30 days was reduced by 66% in the high-loading-dose arm (4% vs. 12%, $P = .04$). The benefit was almost entirely due to the marked reduction in PMI—a reduction of approximately 50% in a multivariate model adjusting for all variables that influence the incidence of PMI (OR 0.48; 95% CI 0.15 to 0.97; $P = .044$).[79] It remains controversial whether a higher loading dose of clopidogrel (900 mg) can lead to further improvement in PMI and other ischemic complications.[80,81]

The main criticism of the routine clopidogrel preloading strategy in patients undergoing coronary angiography is that a fraction of the patients will be referred to bypass surgery; these patients will have an increased risk of bleeding unless their bypass surgery is postponed for at least 5 days. Thus the Antiplatelet therapy for Reduction of MYocardial Damage during Angioplasty (ARMYDA)-5 PRELOAD trial tested the strategy of high-dose clopidogrel loading in the catheterization laboratory against high-dose preloading that was previously established. In this trial, 409 patients were randomized to receive a 600-mg preloading dose 4 to 8 hours before PCI or a 600-mg loading dose in the catheterization laboratory after obtaining diagnostic angiograms. The study revealed no difference in incidence of PMI between the two strategies (8.8% in laboratory vs. 9.3% preload groups, $P = .99$).[82] Point-of-care testing demonstrated that platelet reactivity remained high during the PCI and for the 2 hours that followed in patients treated in the catheterization laboratory, which is not consistent with the previously established association between better platelet inhibition and reduced incidence of PMI. The study was also criticized for the small sample size, which makes it underpowered to detect a difference between the groups.[83]

As the evidence for the effective platelet inhibition caused by clopidogrel mounted, questions arose regarding the need for the more expensive IV GP IIb/IIIa inhibitors in PCI. In sequential investigations, the Intracoronary Stenting and Antithrombotic Regimen Rapid Early Action for Coronary Treatment (ISAR-REACT) trials, the interaction between clopidogrel loading and abciximab infusion for peri-PCI platelet inhibition was examined in low-risk and then in higher-risk patient populations. In ISAR-REACT 1, more than 1000 stable patients were randomized to receive clopidogrel loading plus placebo versus clopidogrel loading plus abciximab bolus and infusion. At 30 days, no statistically significant difference was found between the two groups in the incidence of MI or death.[84] However, the very low incidence of adverse events in the placebo group diminished the statistical power of the study to detect differences between the groups. In the following study, ISAR-REACT 2, more than 2000 patients with non–ST-segment–elevation ACSs were enrolled. All patients received clopidogrel pretreatment, and half of them were randomized to abciximab bolus plus infusion. Unlike ISAR-REACT 1, a significant reduction was seen in the 30-day composite end point in favor of abciximab. This included more than a 20% reduction in infarctions, most of which were PMIs (8.1% vs. 10.5%). Based on the results of those two investigations, it seems that a more complete degree of platelet inhibition is needed in patients at higher risk of PMI and procedural complications. In addition to the more complete platelet inhibition ensured by the use of abciximab, its cross reactivity with $\alpha V\beta 3$ (vitronectin) and $\alpha M\beta 2$ (Mac-1) receptors may provide potent antiinflammatory effects. This appears to be associated with a significant reduction in the degree of rise of inflammatory markers such as CRP, interleukin 6, and tumor necrosis factor alpha (TNF-α) in the 1 to 2 days following PCI, an effect that may contribute to the reduction in PMI seen with abciximab use during PCI.[85]

The association of more effective platelet inhibition and improved outcomes in patients with ACS treated invasively has been further supported by results of clinical trials comparing prasugrel and ticagrelor to clopidogrel. Although the incidence of PMI was not directly reported, both agents were associated with a statistically significant lower incidence of ischemic events in the early phase after PCI, which are typically driven by periprocedural events.[86–88]

Cangrelor is a direct-acting and reversible intravenous $P2Y_{12}$ receptor antagonist. Cangrelor achieves almost complete and immediate inhibition of ADP-induced platelet aggregation when administered as a bolus. The plasma half-life is approximately 3 to 5 minutes, and platelet function is restored within an hour after cessation of infusion. The use of cangrelor in patients undergoing PCI was studied in two phase III trials, the Cangrelor versus Standard Therapy to Achieve Optimal Management of Platelet Inhibition (CHAMPION) PCI and CHAMPION PLATFORM studies.[89,90] Cangrelor was not associated with a significant reduction in the primary efficacy end point in either of these trials but was associated with reductions in secondary end points, including the rate of stent thrombosis, with no excess in severe bleeding. The prospective, double-blind, active-controlled clinical trial Cangrelor versus standard therapy to achieve optimal Management of Platelet InhibitiON (CHAMPION PHOENIX)[91] was designed to evaluate prospectively whether cangrelor does indeed reduce ischemic complications of PCI. The modified intention-to-treat population comprised 10,942 patients, approximately 44% of whom presented with an ACS. Compared with those who received clopidogrel immediately before or after PCI, cangrelor—administered as an IV bolus and an infusion for 2 hours or for the duration of the procedure, whichever was longer—significantly reduced the rate of periprocedural complications of PCI, including stent thrombosis. A reduction in the rate of acute PMI accounted for most of the benefit. Importantly, the incidence of major bleeding or need for transfusion were not significantly different between the groups.[91] A pooled analysis of all three randomized trials of cangrelor demonstrated a significant reduction in MACEs (mostly PMI) by 19% and stent thrombosis by 41% at 48 hours after PCI.[92]

Impact of Statin Therapy

The inflammatory response of distal embolization and platelet aggregate interaction with leukocytes contributes to the degree of myonecrosis that is frequently seen after PCI. The observations made in PCI registries demonstrated a reduction in PMI in patients who were receiving statins at the time of their PCI.[93] Proposed mechanisms that can explain this finding include an antiinflammatory effect and the ability of statins to enhance nitric oxide production.[94] In an analysis of 803 patients undergoing rotational atherectomy, the incidence of any myonecrosis was reduced by statin therapy from 52% to 24%, and the incidence of PMI (CK-MB ≥3 × ULN) was reduced from 22% to 7.5%.[95] These observations were eventually confirmed in two prospective randomized trials. In both trials, statin therapy was started several days before scheduled PCI in the active therapy arm. In one report on 451 patients, statin therapy was not restricted to any specific agents. Median post-PCI troponin level was 0.13 ng/mL in the statin group and 0.21 ng/mL in the control group (P = .03). Similarly, the incidence of troponin I more than five times the ULN was significantly reduced with statin therapy (23.5% vs. 32% in the control group, P = .04).[96] In the similarly designed Atorvastatin for Reduction of Myocardial Damage During Angioplasty (ARMYDA) trial, a smaller number of stable angina patients were randomized to receive atorvastatin versus placebo. A greater than 50% reduction was reported in incidence of PMI, as measured by CK-MB, troponin I, or myoglobin in the atorvastatin group.[97] In ARMYDA-2, an incremental benefit of statin and high-dose loading clopidogrel was found that led to a more impressive 80% reduction in PMI.[79]

A subgroup analysis of the ARMYDA trial confirms the antiinflammatory role of statins in reducing myonecrosis after PCI. In 138 patients, serum levels of adhesion molecules—intracellular adhesion molecule (ICAM), vascular cell adhesion molecule (VCAM), and e-selectin—were similar in patients in the atorvastatin group and the placebo group before PCI. Yet after PCI, the rise in ICAM and e-selectin were significantly attenuated with atorvastatin therapy. This attenuated rise in adhesion molecules paralleled the protective effect against myonecrosis, providing some evidence that the antiinflammatory effect of statins contributes to their observed protective effect against myonecrosis and early mortality, which cannot be attributed to its HMG-CoA reductase inhibitory effect.[98]

The impact of high-dose statin therapy can be demonstrated within days, confirming the existence of mechanisms of action other than lipid lowering. The Novel Approaches for Preventing or Limiting Events (Naples II) trial[99] recently reported that a single, high (80 mg) loading dose (within 24 hours) of atorvastatin reduces the incidence of PMI in elective PCI. The incidence of PMI was 9.5% in the atorvastatin group and 15.8% in the control group (OR 0.56; 95% CI 0.35 to 0.89; P = .014).

Because most patients undergoing PCI are already on statins, the question of pretreatments seemed irrelevant. However, pleiotropic and antiinflammatory effects of statins seem to diminish with time. The Atorvastatin for Reduction of Myocardial Damage During Angioplasty–Acute Coronary Syndromes (ARMYDA-RECAPTURE) clinical trial[100] randomized more than 380 patients undergoing PCI to an intensive "reloading" of atorvastatin (80 mg 12 hours before and 40 mg immediately before PCI) and a standard therapy group (standard daily dose of atorvastatin). All patients were pretreated with clopidogrel and aspirin. At 30 days, a significant reduction was observed in the composite end point in favor of atorvastatin reloading. The incidence of any postprocedure elevation in CK-MB and troponin was significantly lower in the reloading group (13% vs. 24%, P = .017, and 37% vs. 49%, P = .021, respectively). Similar to observations made with abciximab, the benefit of intensive atorvastatin therapy was restricted to patients who presented with ACS, probably because of the higher underlying risk of PMI. A meta-analysis of 14 randomized controlled trials including at total of 3146 patients with stable angina and NSTEMI noted that statin loading before PCI was associated with a 56% relative reduction in PMI (OR 0.44; 95% CI 0.35 to 0.56; P < .00001). The reduction in PMI was statistically significant regardless of the clinical presentation (Fig. 30.8).[101]

Nonpharmacologic Approaches

Few mechanical options to prevent PMI are currently available. Direct stenting (without balloon predilation) was proposed to reduce plaque trauma and distal embolization. A small randomized study compared direct stenting to conventional predilation followed by stent deployment and demonstrated a significant reduction in PMI.[102] In a retrospective analysis that involved 311 stable angina patients, Nageh and associates[103] noted that direct stenting reduced postprocedural troponin I levels when compared with patients in whom predilation was used. Subsequent larger trials did not confirm any concrete advantages of this approach in reducing myonecrosis or any other adverse events.[104]

As mentioned previously, bifurcation stenosis interventions are particularly vulnerable for PMI, primarily as a result of SBO. Trials to evaluate a two-stent strategy versus a one-stent or provisional stent strategy (a one-stent strategy that allows the positioning of a second stent if required) have observed that PMI is more frequent with the two-stent strategy.[105]

The concept of ischemic preconditioning (ICP) and its role in myocyte protection is an intriguing one. Transient and repeated episodes of ischemia followed by reperfusion of the myocardium or any other muscle mass in the body can provide some protection against myocardial damage when a prolonged episode of ischemia ensues by limiting reperfusion injury. This concept has been shown to limit infarct size in patients undergoing bypass surgery.[106] In the Cardiac Remote Ischemic Preconditioning in Coronary Stenting (CRISP Stent)[107] study, 242 stable angina

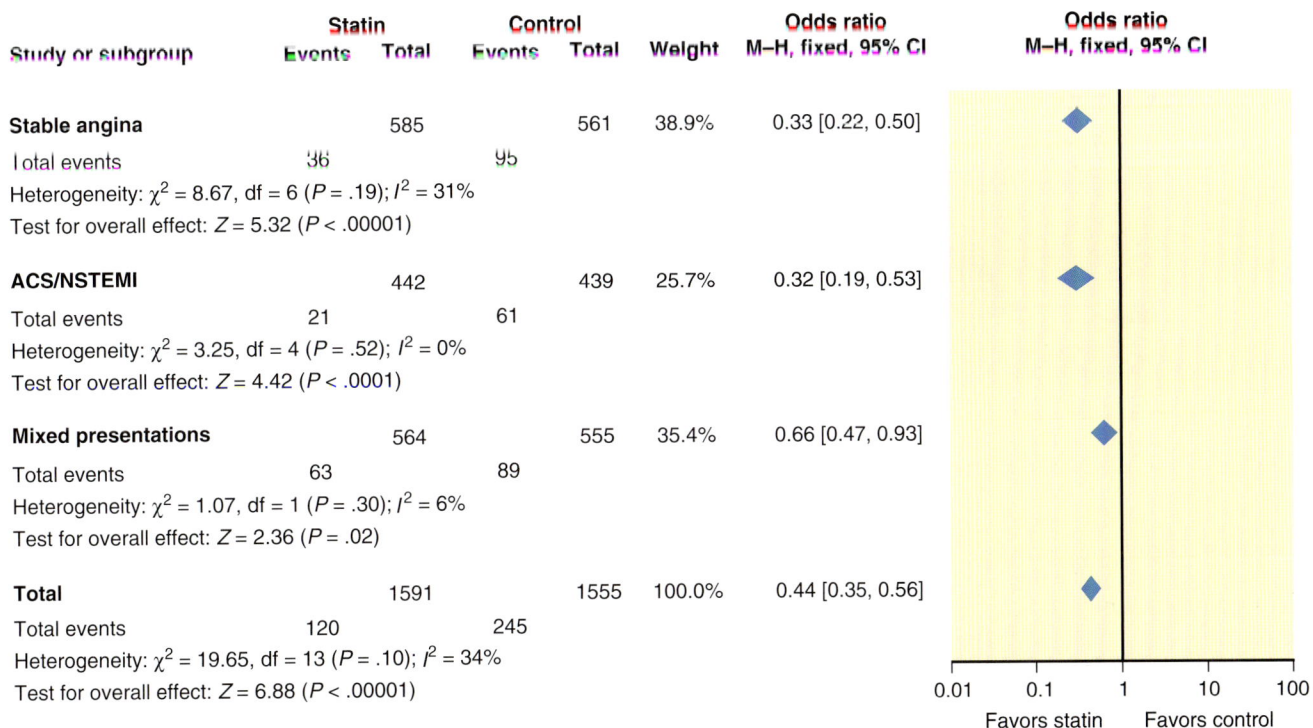

Fig. 30.8 **Impact of statin therapy on periprocedural myocardial infarction.** Odds ratios of periprocedural myocardial infarction in patients loaded with a statin before percutaneous coronary intervention (PCI) are compared with patients treated with statin therapy only after PCI. The figure depicts the results for the overall meta-analysis and the results for the trials that enrolled patients with stable angina, acute coronary syndrome (ACS), and a mixed population of patients. CI, Confidence interval; df, degrees of freedom; I^2, a measure of heterogeneity; M–H, Mantel–Haenszel method; NSTEMI, non–ST-elevation myocardial infarction; Z, Z score. (From Benjo AM, El-Hayek GE, Messerli F, et al. High-dose statin loading prior to percutaneous coronary intervention decreases cardiovascular events: a meta-analysis of randomized controlled trials. *Catheter Cardiovasc Interv.* 2015;85:53–60.)

patients undergoing elective PCI were randomized to receive remote IPC (induced by three 5-minute inflations of a blood pressure cuff to 200 mm Hg around the upper arm, followed by 5-minute intervals of reperfusion) or a control (an uninflated cuff around the arm) before arrival in the catheterization laboratory. The primary outcome was troponin I level at 24 hours after PCI. The median troponin I level at 24 hours after PCI was lower in the remote IPC group compared with the control group (0.06 vs. 0.16 ng/mL; $P = .040$). After PCI, 42% of patients who underwent remote IPC had a normal troponin level, compared with 24% of the control group ($P = .01$). The mechanisms of protection induced by remote ICP are multifactorial; evidence shows an early opening of mitochondrial potassium channels[108] and a later antiinflammatory effect mediated by modified gene expression.[109]

Only two devices have suggested benefit on periprocedural infarct size: embolic protection in the setting of SVG intervention and aspiration thrombectomy in the setting of STEMI. EPDs have some advantage in reducing the incidence of PMI in SVG PCI; these devices are discussed in detail in the following section. Manual thrombectomy with aspiration of the occluding thrombus has been shown to reduce embolization, no-reflow phenomenon, infarct size, and mortality during primary PCI for acute STEMI.[110] Whether that can be considered under the category of PMI remains unclear. Further evidence in support of manual aspiration thrombectomy comes from a 2013 meta-analysis that incorporated 18 trials ($n = 3936$) to compare aspiration thrombectomy/PCI to PCI alone in STEMI patients. Risks of all-cause mortality (the primary end point) and MACE—a composite of death, MI, and target-vessel revascularization—were significantly lower with aspiration thrombectomy (RR 0.71 [95% CI 0.51 to 0.99] and 0.76 [95% CI 0.63 to 0.92]). However, these results were refuted by a larger multicenter, prospective, randomized trial on a very similar patient population in the Thrombus Aspiration in ST-Elevation Myocardial Infarction in Scandinavia (TASTE) trial.[111] This trial randomly assigned 7244 STEMI patients to either manual thrombus aspiration followed by PCI or PCI alone. The primary end point of death from any cause at 30 days was similar in both groups (2.8% vs. 3.0%, respectively; HR 0.61; 95% CI 0.34 to 1.07).

CONCLUSIONS

PMI is not uncommon after PCI. The reported incidence varies according to the biomarker used and the threshold for diagnosis. SBO and/or distal embolization of atherosclerotic debris and platelet aggregates are the most common mechanisms underlying PMI. Overall data suggest that PMI is associated with late mortality, although a cause-effect relationship has been debated. The larger the PMI, the more robust is the association with future mortality and major adverse outcomes. Use of coronary stents has dramatically reduced incidence of abrupt vessel closure, which was a major cause of large PMI in the early balloon angioplasty experience. Potent platelet inhibitor therapy (IV or oral), statins (as antiinflammatory agents), and EPDs (in SVG PCI) had the most success in reducing the incidence of PMI. Cardiac biomarkers should be serially assayed in patients who have signs or symptoms suggestive of MI during or after PCI or in asymptomatic

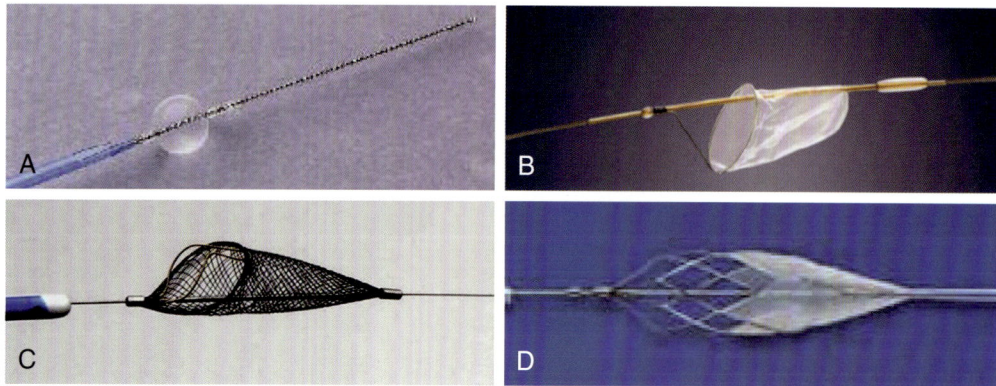

Fig. 30.9 Examples of distal embolic protection devices. (A) The PercuSurge GuardWire, from Medtronic, is the only balloon occlusive distal device. The FilterWire, from Boston Scientific (B); the Spider, from Covidien (C), and the Accunet, from Abbott Vascular (D) are all examples of distal filter devices.

patients with significant persistent angiographic complications (e.g., large SBO, flow-limiting dissection, no-reflow phenomenon, or coronary thrombosis).

EMBOLIC PROTECTION DEVICES

With the wider acceptance of the significance of distal embolization during PCI, efforts to reduce the incidence and impact of this phenomenon have been underway. As discussed earlier, effective antiplatelet therapy with GP IIb/IIIa inhibitors and $P2Y_{12}$ inhibitors significantly reduces procedure-related myonecrosis. Despite routine use of these pharmacologic agents, a small PMI is not uncommon even after uncomplicated procedures. This is of particular concern in the setting of SVG interventions, which have a high propensity for distal embolization, no-reflow phenomenon, and PMI. Lesions with high thrombus burden are another subgroup of procedures with a higher risk of distal embolization with any interventional device. The prototype of such procedures is PCI in the setting of acute MI. Over the last few years, several innovative designs for EPDs have been developed to improve outcomes in these subsets of patients, as well as in those in other clinical settings.

The three basic designs of EPD are (1) distal filters, (2) distal occlusion balloons, and (3) proximal occlusion devices (Fig. 30.9; see also Fig. 30.14 later). Table 30.3 summarizes the differences between the various concepts for EPDs.

Distal Filter Devices

Distal filter devices consist of a filter bag or basket attached to the terminal portion of an angioplasty guidewire. The Angioguard filter wire (Cordis, Hialeah, FL) and the FilterWire (Boston Scientific, Natick, MA) are the prototypes of the filter devices. Generally, these devices consist of a 0.014-inch wire that has a filter basket near its distal end (see Fig. 30.9). Beyond the filter protrudes a short portion of guidewire that can be shaped. The currently used version has pores that are approximately 100 μm in diameter. The smallest nominal filter basket size is currently 3.5 mm, which would be used for vessels larger than 3.0 mm but not more than 3.5 mm; the largest basket size is 8 mm. As a general principle, the filter should be oversized by about 0.5 to 1.0 mm compared with the vessel reference diameter. Once the wire crosses the lesion and the filter basket is in a relatively disease-free portion of the artery, the sheath is retracted and the basket is released to deploy in the artery. It should be positioned about 2.5 to 3 cm distal to the lesion. The sheath is removed over the wire, which then serves as a standard angioplasty wire. During the intervention, blood flow through the pores of the filter is preserved, and the deployed filter does not affect injecting contrast for visualization. When the interventional procedure is complete, a retrieval sheath is advanced over the wire and is used to collapse the filter basket securely. The retrieval sheath and the collapsed filter trapping the embolic debris inside it are then removed as one unit.

The Spider (Covidien, Plymouth, MN), the Accunet (Abbott Vascular, Santa Clara, CA), and the Interceptor Plus Coronary Filter (Medtronic Vascular, Minneapolis, MN) are additional examples of devices that work similarly. The chief advantage of this type of device is the ability to maintain antegrade perfusion throughout the procedure; the chief disadvantage is the inability to capture smaller microparticulate debris and vasoactive mediators.

Distal Occlusion Devices

The PercuSurge GuardWire System (6 Fr; Medtronic), the prototype of the balloon occlusion devices, consists of a 0.014-inch hollow hydrotube with an occlusion balloon toward the distal end and a 2.5-cm steerable tip beyond the balloon (see Fig. 30.9A). The wire is used to cross the lesion, and the balloon is positioned distal to the lesion in a relatively disease-free segment. The balloon is inflated at a low atmospheric pressure to create a seal; the occlusion diameter ranges from 3 to 6 mm. Angioplasty, stenting, and postdilation are all performed as necessary over the hydrotube. The aspiration catheter is then advanced over the wire, and any dislodged debris is removed with a slow distal-to-proximal pullback. The balloon is deflated, the GuardWire is withdrawn, and angiography is performed to confirm distal flow. Provided the balloon is inflated at low pressure, the risk of restenosis is not increased. Although this is the first EPD approved by the Food and Drug Administration (FDA) in the United States, this device is no longer available for commercial use.

A theoretic advantage of distal occlusion includes capture of unlimited debris (regardless of size) and aspiration of inflammatory vasomediators released with angioplasty. However, crossing the lesion with the device may potentiate embolism, and some debris may be shunted into side branches during aspiration of the target artery. In addition, antegrade flow is aborted with inflation of the occlusion balloon, allowing for distal ischemia.

Proximal Occlusion Devices

The Proxis Embolic Protection System (Abbott/St. Jude Medical, Minneapolis, MN) was the best example of a proximal occlusion device in SVG interventions, but it is no longer available for use in the United States. The system contains an

TABLE 30.3 Characteristics of Different Concepts in Embolic Protection Devices

	Distal Filter	Distal Balloon Occlusion	Proximal Occlusion
Antegrade perfusion	Uninterrupted	Temporarily interrupted[a]	Temporarily interrupted[a]
Visualization of the distal vessel	Unhindered	Not possible during inflation	Possible via the inner sheath
Efficacy of emboli protection	May allow passage of emboli smaller than the pore size (100 μm)[b]	Once inflated, traps all emboli	All particles can be aspirated
Vasoactive substances	Pass unimpeded	Can be aspirated completely	Can be aspirated completely
Crossing profile	0.040 to 0.050 inch	0.026 to 0.033 inch	No crossing, deployed proximal to the lesion
Embolization during device positioning	Likely to occur	Less likely to occur	None because device does not cross the lesion
Retrieval profile	Occasionally difficult if filter is full of debris	Not a problem after balloon deflation	Not a problem; device is proximal to the lesion
Flexibility of guidewire use	None because the filter is attached to wire	None because the balloon is attached to wire	Excellent; device can be used with any wire
Effect of distal disease on device	May not be feasible if no disease-free segment is present	May not be feasible if no disease-free segment is present	Device is proximal, distal disease irrelevant

[a]Transient ischemia can occur while the embolism protection system is being used unless adequate retrograde collaterals are present.
[b]In reality, the filter can trap particles smaller than its pore size due to clumping of particles. Numerous trials have demonstrated no clinically significant differences between distal balloon occlusion and distal filter concepts.

inner working sheath about 6 Fr in diameter, which is advanced through a 7- or 8-Fr guiding catheter. An inflatable balloon is attached to the end and to the external surface of the inner sheath. Inflation of this balloon in the target artery proximal to the lesion provides a seal that prevents antegrade flow through the target artery. After the system is in place, the intervention can be performed through the inner working sheath using the wire, balloon, and stent of choice. Small contrast injections for visualization are feasible. At the end of the procedure, the interventional devices are removed, and the stagnant blood in the target artery is aspirated via the working sheath. The final step is to deflate the balloon and remove the working sheath, leaving the guiding catheter in the artery after aspiration of debris and vasoactive substances.

Similar devices are now available for use in carotid stenting procedures. These include the Mo.Ma Ultra Cerebral Protection Device (Medtronic Vascular, Minneapolis, MN) and the Gore Flow Reversal System (W.L. Gore and Associates, Flagstaff, AZ). Both devices contain an inflatable balloon around the main guiding catheter that occludes the common carotid artery during internal carotid angioplasty. They also have a secondary extension balloon that is inflated in the external carotid artery to isolate flow from collaterals that may propel atherothrombotic debris toward the cerebral circulation. After inflation of both common and external carotid balloons, the internal carotid artery is crossed with the angioplasty wire of choice. Balloon dilation and stenting are performed in the usual manner with no internal carotid flow permitted. After stenting and postdilation are complete, the blood and debris trapped distal to the common carotid occlusion balloon are then aspirated manually in the case of the Mo.Ma device. With the Gore Flow Reversal System, the guiding catheter contains an additional channel connected to flow-reversal tubing attached to the femoral vein. As the distal common carotid and internal carotid arteries are isolated by inflation of both balloons, the static blood that includes the debris from the treated lesion is continuously drained by the flow-reversal channel and tubing connected to the lower-pressure femoral vein. The tubing is fitted with a filtering chamber to prevent the atherothrombotic debris from reaching the femoral vein. The Gore Flow Reversal System is no longer commercially available for sale in the United States.

SAPHENOUS VEIN GRAFT PERCUTANEOUS CORONARY INTERVENTION

Traditionally, vein graft PCI is considered a high-risk procedure because of the increased risk of distal macroembolization and microembolization with subsequent slow flow or no reflow and PMI. Degenerated vein grafts contain more diffuse, friable, lipid-rich, concentric plaques than native coronary arteries, which makes them particularly prone to distal embolization.[61,112] Of note, one of the most potent interventions to reduce the risk of PMI in native coronary PCI—namely, GP IIb/IIIa inhibitors—appears to be ineffective in the setting of vein graft PCI. A pooled analysis of several GP IIb/IIIa inhibitor trials, as well as large registry data, demonstrated that addition of IV GP IIb/IIIa inhibitors to standard anticoagulation regimens was not associated with any significant reduction in ischemic complications, including PMI, in patients undergoing vein graft PCI.[113,114]

Several small studies tested the efficacy of EPDs (particularly, the PercuSurge GuardWire) and demonstrated that particulate matter can be aspirated in the majority of cases with an associated reduction in the incidence and magnitude of CK-MB elevation expected with such procedures.[115] Based on these findings, 801 patients from 47 centers were randomized to undergo vein graft PCI with GuardWire protection versus no EPD in the SVG Angioplasty Free of Emboli Randomized (SAFER) trial.[30] The primary end point was death, Q-wave MI, non–Q-wave MI (CK-MB >3 × ULN), emergent bypass surgery, or target-vessel revascularization within 30 days. Almost 40% of patients had angiography that revealed thrombus. Technical success was achieved with the device in 90.1% of the cases. The primary end point was significantly reduced with use of the PercuSurge GuardWire (from 16.5% to 9.6%, $P = .004$), primarily driven by the approximate 50% reduction in non–Q-wave MI, from 13.7% to 7.4% (Fig. 30.10). A number of important secondary end points were also favorably influenced; most important, no-reflow phenomenon was reduced dramatically (9.0% vs. 3.0%; $P = .02$).[30] Moreover, a cost-effectiveness analysis of the SAFER trial demonstrated that the reduction in ischemic complications leads to a shorter hospital stay and reduction in early costs, thus compensating for most of the added expense of the EPD. The projected improved survival on the basis of reduced early complications—namely, reduced

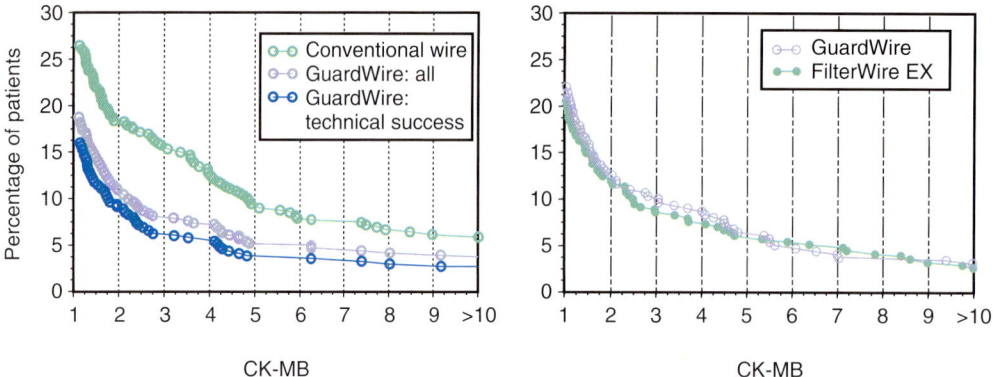

Fig. 30.10 Impact of embolic protection devices on periprocedural myocardial infarction in vein graft percutaneous coronary intervention. *Left:* From the SAFER trial, cumulative distribution-function curve of peak cardiac enzyme values after assignment to placebo or GuardWire and the per-protocol subgroup with technically successful GuardWire use. Creatine kinase MB *(CK-MB)* is represented as multiples of the upper limit of normal. The incidence of periprocedural myocardial infarction of any size is significantly lower with GuardWire use. *Right:* From the FilterWire EX Randomized Evaluation, a similar plot for patients randomized to distal protection with the FilterWire EX versus the GuardWire, showing noninferiority of the FilterWire. (From Baim DS, Wahr D, George B, et al. Randomized trial of a distal embolic protection device during percutaneous intervention of saphenous vein aorto-coronary bypass grafts. *Circulation.* 2002;105:1285–1290; and Stone GW, Rogers C, Hermiller J, et al. Randomized comparison of distal protection with a filter-based catheter and a balloon occlusion and aspiration system during percutaneous intervention of diseased saphenous vein aorto-coronary bypass grafts. *Circulation.* 2003;108:548–553.)

PMI—was calculated to cost less than $4000 per year of life saved, which makes the use of EPD in vein graft PCI a very cost-effective strategy.[116]

This significant improvement in outcome with the use of the GuardWire occlusion device ushered in a new era in which EPD use has become the standard of care with vein graft PCI. Thus, the randomized controlled trials leading to FDA approval of other EPDs for use in vein graft PCI were designed as noninferiority trials, with the GuardWire used in the "active" control arm. In a controlled trial, 651 patients undergoing vein graft PCI were randomized to receive the FilterWire EX versus the GuardWire. Use of GP IIb/IIIa inhibitors was left to the discretion of the operators. The primary end point was a composite similar to that used in the SAFER trial. At 30 days, no difference was seen in the incidence of any MI, with a trend toward a reduction in the primary end point in the FilterWire arm (9.9% vs. 11.6%, P = .53 for superiority, P = .0008 for noninferiority; see Fig. 30.10).[32] Currently, the FilterWire is the most commonly used EPD in SVG PCI.

A more complex study design was used to demonstrate noninferiority of the Proxis system. A total of 639 target vein grafts in 594 patients were prospectively randomized to a test group (use proximal protection when possible, distal protection when not) or a control group (use distal protection when possible). The 30-day composite end point was similar to that used in the SAFER trial. The study demonstrated noninferiority of proximal protection when the analysis was performed by intention to treat or by actual device use.[117]

Noninferiority trials were similarly designed to test the efficacy of other devices. In those trials, the 30-day primary end point was reached in 8% to 11% of patients, achieving the preset standard for noninferiority in comparison to the GuardWire or FilterWire in all studies.[118,119]

The use of EPDs during SVG intervention is a class 1 recommendation per the ACC/AHA/SCAI guidelines.[2] Unfortunately, adoption of EPD use for SVG interventions in the United States has been sluggish. There are numerous reasons to explain the modest use of EPD devices. First, they can be cumbersome to position and deploy, and their use may be limited by technical and anatomic challenges (graft size, inadequate landing zone, distal lesion, and vessel tortuosity). Second, EPD use increases the technical complexity, time, and costs of the procedure. Third, deployment of an EPD carries some risk of procedural complications. Fourth, there is skepticism that the benefits of EPD apply to all SVG lesions (for instance, focal plaques, in-stent restenosis, or proximal or distal fibrotic anastomosis).

Recently published data challenges the effectiveness of EPD in improving outcomes and calls into question the relevance of existing randomized data in contemporary practice.

Brennan et al.[120] interrogated the National Cardiovascular Data Registry (NCDR) CathPCI Registry to retrospectively analyze and compare 49,325 patients with SVG lesions treated with and without EPD between 2005 and 2009. Their results corroborate the previously reported underuse of EPD in the United States at only 21%, when one-third of the centers did not use EPD at all and only 5.6% used EPD in >50% of SVG PCI. The majority of these patients presented with ACS and had longer lesions with higher plaque burden and degenerative score—patients who should derive benefit from use of an EPD. However, EPD use was not associated with reduced adverse events after 3 years of follow-up. In fact, there was an increased adjusted risk of no-reflow, dissection and perforation, and PMI in short-term follow-up with the use of EPD. The study suffered from selection bias, and lack of information on plaque morphology and volume, vein graft degenerative score, and procedural technique specifics.

Based on this information, operators may elect to reserve the use of EPDs for SVG lesions presumed to be associated with the highest risk of embolism. In a pooled analysis of 3958 patients included in five randomized trials and one registry, a prediction model was developed to estimate the risk of major adverse events after SVG PCI. Angiographic scoring of the severity of degeneration, volume of plaque, and presence of thrombus were among the strongest predictors of adverse events. However, the value of EPD use in reducing PMI (by ~40%) was demonstrated across all categories of angiographically estimated risk.[121] These findings suggest a clear need for continuing education and training of interventional operators on the potential value of these devices and for intensifying efforts to develop more affordable and easy-to-use devices (Fig. 30.11).

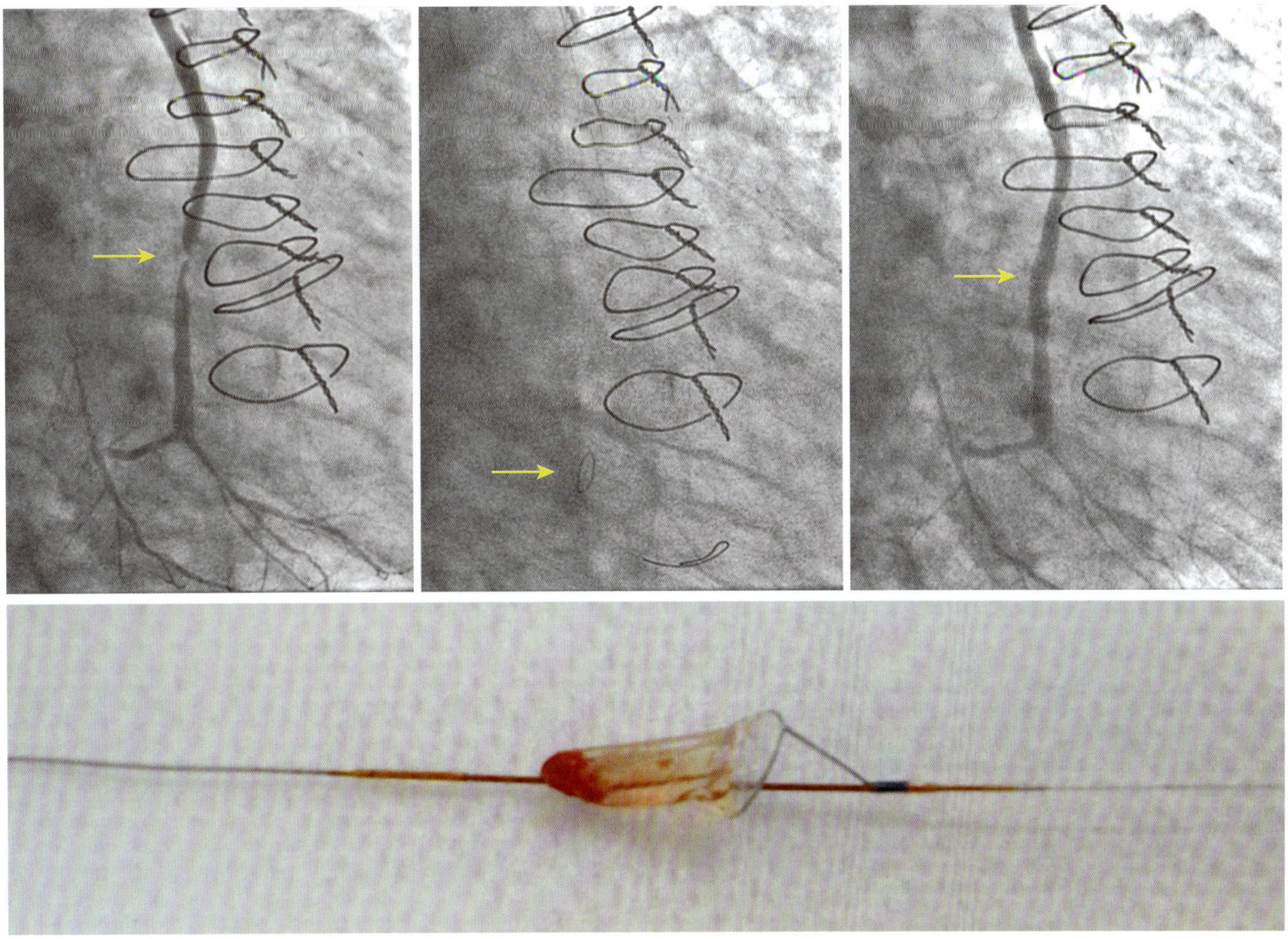

Fig. 30.11 Use of the FilterWire in contemporary saphenous vein graft percutaneous coronary intervention. Angiograms of a saphenous vein graft (SVG) to an obtuse marginal branch in a patient presenting with non–ST-segment–elevation myocardial infarction. *Left:* A subtotal lesion is noted in the body of the SVG *(arrow)*. *Middle:* The lesion is crossed with a FilterWire EZ, which is then deployed in the distal graft, as noted by the radioopaque nitinol ring at the base of the filter basket *(arrow)*. The radioopaque spring coil tip is folded in the native vessel beyond the anastomosis. *Right:* The final angiogram after stent deployment and removal of the FilterWire with no residual stenosis within the stented segment *(arrow)* and good runoff into the distal obtuse marginal branch. *Bottom:* The FilterWire contains macroscopic evidence of thrombotic material and fatty debris from the degenerated lesion. (From Foley JD, Ziada KM. Embolic protection devices for saphenous vein graft percutaneous coronary interventions. Interv Cardiol Clin. 2013;2[2]:259–271.)

Percutaneous Coronary Intervention for Acute Myocardial Infarction

The concept of EPD use in primary PCI is both attractive and intuitive. These are the prototypical thrombotic lesions with a very high likelihood of distal embolization. The success of EPD in vein graft PCI led to clinical trials to examine the feasibility of the concept. In a small study, use of the PercuSurge GuardWire during primary stenting of infarct-related artery resulted in improved flow and subsequently improved ventricular function when compared with procedures performed without EPD use.[121]

However, the larger randomized trials did not confirm the initial favorable impression regarding EPD use in primary PCI. The Enhanced Myocardial Efficacy and Removal by Aspiration of Liberated Debris (EMERALD) trial[123] was an international, multicenter, prospective, randomized trial that enrolled 501 patients with STEMI undergoing primary or rescue PCI. Patients were randomized to PCI with the PercuSurge GuardWire distal protection device versus PCI without an EPD. Among 252 patients assigned to the GuardWire, debris was retrieved in 73%. Disappointingly, no difference was found between the two groups in any of the primary or secondary end points (ST resolution in 63% vs. 62%; infarct size 12% vs. 9.5%; *P* = nonsignificant [NS] for both). The Protection Devices in PCI Treatment of MI for Salvage of Endangered Myocardium (PROMISE) trial tested the efficacy of the FilterWire in the setting of PCI for acute MI. This study included patients with NSTEMI and used different surrogate end points: coronary flow velocity measured by an intravascular Doppler wire and the size of the infarction measured by hyperenhancement on MRI scans 3 days after the procedure. Similar to the results of the EMERALD trial, FilterWire protection provided no additional benefit.[124] Other trials to examine filter-based EPD in the setting of primary angioplasty have not demonstrated any clinical benefit to this approach.[125]

Use of proximal protection combined with thrombus aspiration was examined in the Proximal Embolic Protection in Acute Myocardial Infarction and Resolution of ST-Elevation (PREPARE) trial. In this prospective randomized trial, 284 patients were randomized to primary PCI with the Proxis system versus primary PCI alone after angiography. The primary end point was the occurrence of complete (≥70%) ST-segment resolution at 60 minutes. The results demonstrated an earlier resolution of the ST segment in the proximal protection arm, but no difference was found between the groups in the primary end point, infarct size by MR, or clinical adverse outcomes.[126,127]

Several potential explanations exist for the disappointing results of EPD use in primary angioplasty. Using EPD may delay restoration of epicardial flow, and the devices may cause further embolization while crossing the lesion, thus negating any favorable effects of subsequent protection. The incomplete aspiration of liberated debris or leaking of vasoactive substances released from the ruptured plaques may lead to further downstream damage at the time of EPD removal. Embolization into side branches may play a role, particularly in cases with acute thrombotic occlusion, leading to initial TIMI flow grade 0 and absence of visualization of the distal artery at the time of EPD positioning. Notably, these results also indicate a relative underestimation of the degree of existing damage and the role of reperfusion injury in determining the final infarct size after primary PCI.[128]

High-Risk Native Plaques

Certain native coronary plaque phenotypes may be particularly susceptible to distal embolization and resultant PMI after PCI, specifically lipid-rich fibroatheromas. Recently, case reports and registries have suggested that plaque characterization by invasive imaging by IVUS, OCT, and near-infrared spectroscopy (NIRS) may help select emboli-prone lesions. Brilakis et al.[129] reported that use of a filter-based EPD before PCI of high-risk plaques, identified by NIRS, may protect from PMI. The CANARY (Coronary Assessment by Near-infrared of Atherosclerotic Rupture-prone Yellow) Study was the first prospective, multicenter investigation, and it sought to determine whether pre-PCI plaque characterization using NIRS could identify lipid-rich plaques at risk of PMI. In addition, the study was designed to evaluate the feasibility of using a distal EPD as a means to prevent heart attacks triggered by the embolization of plaque during PCI. Eighty-five patients were enrolled at nine U.S. sites. The authors noted that use of NIRS did help identify lipid-rich lesions with an increased risk of PMI, presumably due to distal embolization during PCI. However, the use of a filter EPD did not protect against PMI. So while preinterventional intravascular imaging with NIRS is able to identify lesions at increased risk of PMI, the routine use of filter EPD during PCI of such lesions cannot be recommended.

Carotid Stenting

Although the clinical implications of embolization were first elucidated for coronary interventions, the paradigm is applicable and relevant in angioplasty procedures in other arterial beds. Interventional procedures in the carotid and renal arteries are two areas where embolization may be particularly significant; embolization appears to occur more frequently after carotid stenting than after carotid endarterectomy (CEA). Using transcranial Doppler (TCD) monitoring, microscopic embolization occurs at least eight times more frequently with carotid angioplasty and stenting than with CEA.[130] Indeed, the vast majority of patients who undergo carotid stenting have TCD evidence of microembolization (Fig. 30.12). Similar to embolization related to coronary interventions, it appears that evidence of systemic inflammatory response can lead to more embolization. In a small study of 43 patients who underwent carotid stenting with TCD monitoring of the ipsilateral middle cerebral artery, a positive correlation was found between TCD-identified microembolism and preprocedural leukocyte count (a marker of systemic inflammation). This correlation remained significant even after adjusting for age, sex, comorbidities, medical therapy, and use of an EPD.[131]

Potentially, even small embolic particles are poorly tolerated by the cerebral microcirculation.[132] In an ex vivo model of carotid angioplasty, particles generated from human carotid plaques were injected into the cerebral circulation of rats. Of interest, stenting produced almost twice as much embolization as balloon angioplasty in this model; passage of the guidewire also produced embolization, although only about a quarter as many emboli were produced than with balloon angioplasty. Particles smaller than 200 μm in size did not cause cerebral ischemia during the first 3 days after the procedure, whereas particles of 200 to 500 μm did cause neuronal death. However, at 7 days, injury was detected by fragments of both sizes. Thus if smaller sizes of emboli are relevant in humans, an occlusion device may be better than a filter device. Although filters can be designed with smaller pore sizes, the disadvantage is that this can increase the risk of thrombosis by the filter itself and can decrease distal flow.

Thus, several EPDs were designed for use in conjunction with carotid angioplasty and stenting in the hope of reducing the incidence of procedure-related strokes. The earlier and more extensive experience thus far is with distal filter devices (balloon occlusion and filter types). More recently, proximal occlusion devices have become available, and early experience has shown significant promise that these devices might be associated with further reduction in stroke rates.

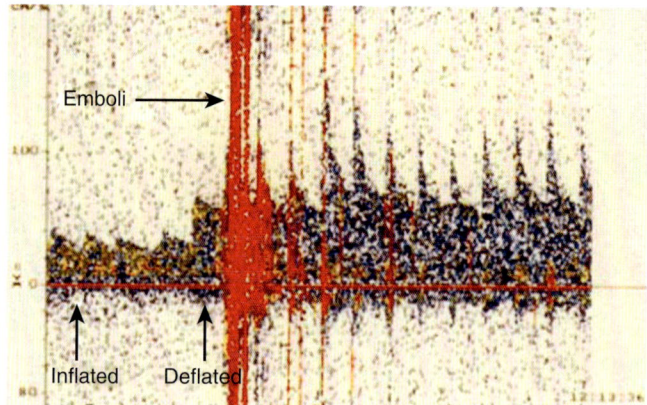

Fig. 30.12 Transcranial Doppler monitoring of middle cerebral artery flow during elective carotid artery stenting. The high-intensity transients observed at the time of balloon deflation represent a surge of microemboli from the extracranial site of angioplasty to the intracranial circulation. (From Topol EJ, Yadav JS. Recognition of the importance of embolization in atherosclerotic vascular disease. *Circulation*. 2000;101:570–580.)

Distal Embolism Protection Devices in Carotid Stenting

Reimers and colleagues[133] reported their initial experience with three different filter designs (Angioguard, NeuroShield [MedNova, Galway, Ireland], and FilterWire) in 84 patients undergoing carotid stenting. Macroscopic debris was collected in 53% of filters, and histologic analysis of the debris revealed lipid-rich macrophages, fibrin, and cholesterol clefts. The early experience with the balloon-occlusion variety of EPD (PercuSurge GuardWire) was reported in a series of 75 patients. In this series, macroscopic debris was collected from all patients (100%), and histologic analysis was very similar to particles obtained from filter devices.[134]

In addition to retrieval of macroscopic and microscopic debris, additional evidence suggests that the use of EPD during carotid stenting effectively reduces embolism to the cerebral microcirculation. These data have been gleaned from studies using MR diffusion-weighted imaging (DWI), the most sensitive imaging modality for detection of early cerebral ischemia.[135,136] Comparison of DWI scans before and after carotid stenting reveals that use of an EPD significantly reduces both the incidence and number of new lesions identified on the postprocedure scan. Most new lesions were small (<10 mm) and

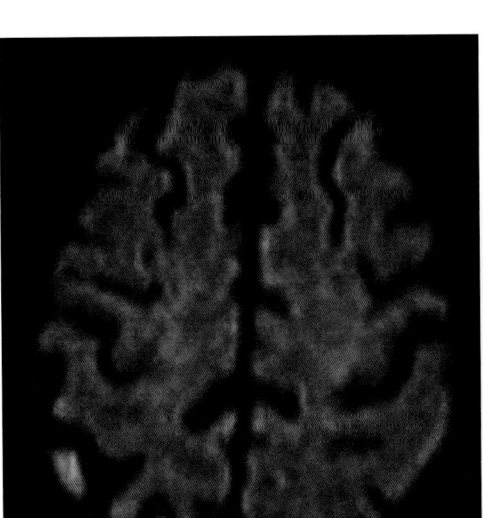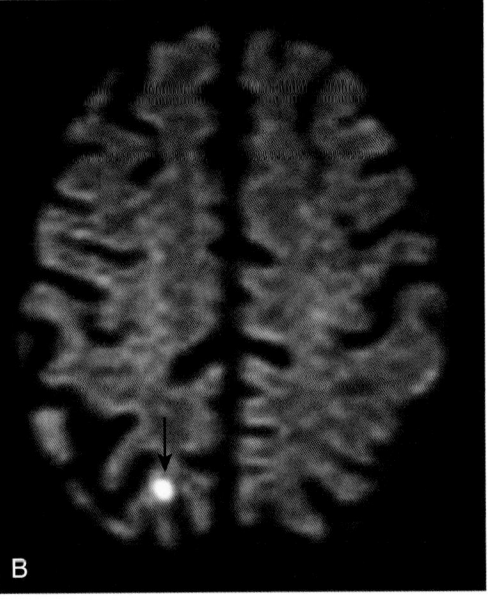

Fig. 30.13 Axial diffusion-weighted imaging of the brain. (A), Preprocedure. (B), Postprocedure. Despite carotid stenting with an embolic protection device in place, an ipsilateral hyperintense lesion *(arrow)* related to silent cerebral embolism is appreciable at the cortical-subcortical junction of the right parietal lobe. (From Cosottini M, Michelassi MC, Puglioli M, et al. Silent cerebral ischemia detected with diffusion-weighted imaging in patients treated with protected and unprotected carotid artery stenting. *Stroke.* 2005;36:2389–2393.)

asymptomatic (Fig. 30.13). In a study of 206 patients, no difference was reported in the incidence of stroke between patients who did and did not receive EPD protection, but the number of DWI-visualized new lesions was significantly higher in patients who did develop a stroke.[136]

Although no randomized trial has been done to compare outcomes of carotid stenting with and without EPD protection, evidence from large multicenter registries demonstrates that EPD use has resulted in a significant reduction in neurologic adverse events. In a systematic review of published reports, Kastrup and coworkers[137] compared outcomes of 2357 patients undergoing carotid stenting without an EPD with outcomes of 839 patients in whom stenting was performed with an EPD in place. A significant reduction was seen in 30-day death/stroke rate with EPD use (1.8% vs. 5.5%, $P < .001$). Both minor and major strokes were significantly reduced in patients who received EPDs (minor stroke 0.5% vs. 3.7%, $P < .001$; major stroke 0.3% vs. 1.1%, $P < .05$). The larger Global Carotid Artery Stent Registry surveys the major interventional centers worldwide and collects self-reported data on technical details and outcomes. In the most recent update, 6753 patients had undergone stenting without EPD protection, and 4221 patients did receive EPD protection. The 30-day incidence of stroke and procedure-related death was reduced by more than 50%, from 5.3% to 2.2%. Despite EPD use, symptomatic patients remained at higher risk for developing stroke or procedure-related death compared with the asymptomatic subgroup (2.7% vs. 1.75%).[138]

Few randomized trials have compared contemporary carotid artery stenting with CEA. The Stenting and Angioplasty with Protection in Patients at High Risk for Endarterectomy (SAPPHIRE) trial randomized patients to either endarterectomy or carotid stenting with the Angioguard filter device. Both symptomatic and asymptomatic patients were included if they had a coexisting condition that placed them at a higher risk of complications during a CEA. The primary composite end point was death, stroke, or MI at 30 days plus death due to neurologic causes or ipsilateral stroke between day 31 and 1 year. Because of slowing recruitment, the trial was terminated after randomizing 334 patients. In this high-risk population, the primary composite end point was reduced in the stent group compared with the surgical group (12.2% vs. 20.1%, $P = .004$ for noninferiority, $P = .053$ for superiority). At 30 days, the incidence of stroke was 3.6% and 3.1% in the stent and CEA arms, respectively. This reduction in primary end point was driven primarily by a reduction in MI in the stent arm rather than by differences in cerebral events.[139]

To gain FDA approval, several manufacturers of EPDs and stents initiated a number of large patient registries to demonstrate safety and efficacy of their novel devices. Most of these enrolled patients at high risk of complications, similar to the SAPPHIRE design. The low incidence of death or stroke compared with historic adverse event rates in CEA resulted in the eventual FDA approval of many of these devices.[140,141]

Two European-based randomized trials attempted to demonstrate noninferiority of carotid stenting compared with CEA, the Stent-Supported Percutaneous Angioplasty of the Carotid Artery Versus Endarterectomy (SPACE) trial and the Endarterectomy Versus Angioplasty in Patients with Symptomatic Severe Carotid Stenosis (EVA-3S). Both studies included patients with symptomatic carotid stenosis and attempted to demonstrate the noninferiority of stenting.[142,143] The endpoints were relatively similar: death or stroke at 30 days. Both studies did not emphasize EPD use; only 25% of patients in SPACE had EPDs. In EVA-3S, EPD use was mandated only after evidence of excess stroke in the first 80 patients.[144] Both studies failed to demonstrate noninferiority, and excess stroke (mostly minor) was evident in the stenting arm.

The two larger randomized trials to compare carotid stenting with endarterectomy, the International Carotid Stenting Study (ICSS) and the Carotid Endarterectomy Versus Stenting Trial (CREST), have been completed. ICSS enrolled 1713 symptomatic patients, emphasized EPD use (80%), and had a primary end point of fatal or disabling stroke at 3 years. At 120 days, the investigators reported an excess of minor strokes in the stenting arm (7.6% vs. 4.1% in the endarterectomy group) and an excess of laryngeal nerve palsy in the endarterectomy arm.[145] Alternatively, CREST randomized 2502 patients with both symptomatic and asymptomatic disease, making it the largest study to date to address this question. The primary composite end point was periprocedural stroke, death, or infarction plus ipsilateral stroke within 4 years. All stenting procedures included EPD use. At 30 days, the stroke rate was 4.1% for stenting and 2.3% for endarterectomy, and the rate of major stroke was less than 1% in both groups. The study showed no difference between the groups in the composite end point and no difference between symptomatic and asymptomatic patients. An excess of minor strokes occurred with stenting, balanced by an excess of MIs in the endarterectomy group.[146]

Based on the totality of evidence, several factors can be seen to have a significant impact on outcomes of carotid stenting: symptomatic status, EPD use, and operator experience. In the two trials that mandated use of an EPD and restricted enrollment to experienced operators (SAPPHIRE and CREST), there is more evidence of equipoise between stenting and endarterectomy. Of note, both studies included asymptomatic patients, who are considered to be at lower risk for events. On the other hand, trials that did not mandate EPD use on a large scale and/or that included interventional operators with minimal or no experience (SPACE, EVA-3S, and ICSS) had a higher event rate with stenting, albeit these trials focused on symptomatic patients.

Proximal Embolism Protection Devices in Carotid Stenting

The single-center experience using the Mo.Ma Ultra Proximal Cerebral Protection Device (Fig. 30.14) generated significant promise in this approach. In a series of 1300 patients who underwent carotid stenting using this device, the incidence of all strokes was 0.84%, with a surprisingly low 1.38% incidence of death and stroke at 30 days.[147] The Proximal Protection With the Mo.Ma Device During Carotid Stenting (ARMOUR) prospective registry was intended to provide U.S. data for FDA approval. Among 225 pivotal patients, primarily asymptomatic, device success exceeded 98%. The 30-day incidence of stroke was 0.9% and the combined death and stroke rate was 2.7%, emphasizing both the safety and efficacy of the device.[148] A similar prospective single-arm study examined the outcome of carotid stenting using the Gore Flow Reversal System in 245 pivotal high-surgical-risk patients. The primary end point was a major adverse event—stroke, death, MI, or transient ischemic attack—within 30 days of stenting. The adverse event rate was compared with an objective performance criterion derived from studies that included carotid stenting with embolic protection. At 30 days, the composite end point was reached in 11 patients (4.5%), which statistically was significantly better than the objective criterion ($P = .002$). The stroke and death rate was 2.9%, and no patient had a major ischemic stroke.[149]

A subsequent meta-analysis of 2397 patients from six independent databases of the two proximal occlusion devices examined the incidence and predictors of 30-day major adverse clinical events including stroke, MI, and death using random effects models. The incidence rates were 1.71% for stroke, 0.02% for MI, and 0.40% for death. The composite primary end point at 30 days was 2.25%. Age and diabetic status were the only significant independent risk predictors; however, total stroke rates remained below 2.6% in all subgroups, including symptomatic octogenarians. The authors concluded that carotid stenting with proximal occlusion devices yields a very low incidence of adverse events at 30 days.[150]

The improved outcomes noted with proximal protection devices in carotid stenting raise the question of whether another large randomized trial to compare stenting with endarterectomy is warranted. This may be of particular importance because the stroke risk of procedures performed with these devices was not affected by symptomatic status and old age, the two important predictors of adverse outcome with stenting in the CREST trial.

Cerebral Embolic Protection Device Use During Transcatheter Aortic Valve Replacement

As the use of TAVR is rapidly expanding to more patient subsets, concern regarding periprocedural strokes becomes more relevant. In earlier trials,[151] TAVR was associated with a significant (~5%) rate of stroke, mostly in the first 48 hours postprocedure. With evolution of the valves and the procedure, the stroke rates may have decreased. A recent large meta-analysis[152] demonstrated a weighted risk of 2.4%, which represents a significant decrease compared to the early experience. On the other hand, the recent Placement of Aortic Transcatheter Valves II (PARTNER-II) trial conducted in intermediate-risk patients still noted a major stroke rate of 3.2%.[153]

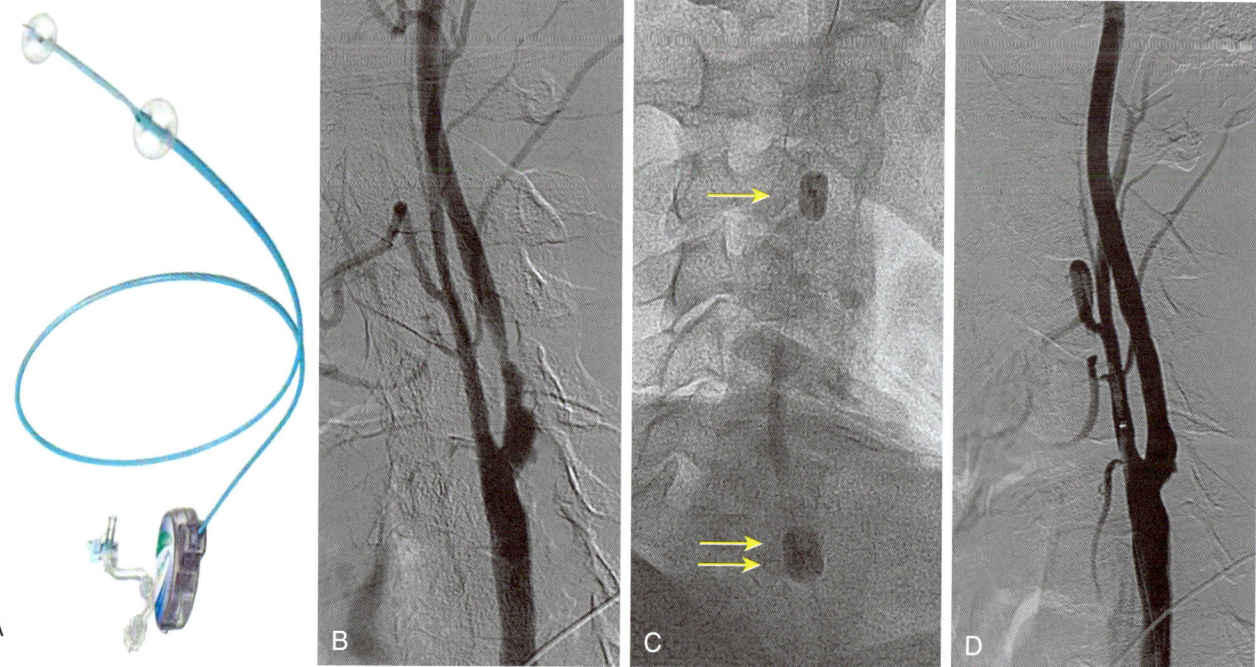

Fig. 30.14 Example of carotid stenting using Medtronic's Mo.Ma proximal protection system. This embolic protection device is based on preventing antegrade flow and potential retrograde flow through the internal carotid artery during carotid angioplasty by use of common carotid and external carotid occlusive balloons. (A) The catheter with its two occlusive balloons. (B) The lesion in the left internal carotid artery is severe. (C) The external carotid balloon (yellow arrow) and the common carotid balloon (double arrows) are inflated to occlude flow. Contrast stain is seen indicating absence of antegrade flow. After stenting and dilation, debris in the isolated segment is aspirated before occlusive balloons are deflated. (D) Final angiographic result.

Importantly, clinically evident stroke only accounts for a minority of cerebral insults from embolic events. According to diffusion weighted magnetic resonance (DW-MRI) imaging studies,[152] silent cerebral embolism (CE) following TAVR occurs in >75% of cases, regardless of the specific device deployed or vascular access used.[152] The long-term clinical consequences of silent CE are not well understood. The mere presence of particulate emboli to the brain does not predictably correlate with manifest clinical compromise or cognitive dysfunction; in fact, most are silent and transient. But while most are inconsequential, associations with neurocognitive decline, future stroke, and/or frank dementia have been reported.[154,155]

Several recent studies have observed that the occurrence of silent ischemic embolism was not associated with a measurable post-TAVR neurocognitive impairment.[156,157] Ghanem et al.[158] reported that 91% of patients realized preserved cognitive function 2 years after TAVI. Even so, the potential benefit of neuroprotection should not be ignored as TAVR widens its scope to include younger and lower-risk patients wherein preventing CE might prevent longer-term neurocognitive impairment.

Various definitions of stroke, central nervous system infarction, and silent CE have been proposed,[159,160] confounding interpretation of clinical research trials and registries. However, given the relatively low rate of clinical neurological events at short-term follow-up and the high frequency of new CE lesions after TAVR, total new lesion volume on DW-MRI has been used as a surrogate end point for TAVR-related neurological damage and as the primary end point in studies evaluating the efficacy of cerebral embolic protection (CEP) devices.

History of cerebrovascular disease and prior stroke are clinical risk factors for new periprocedural stroke. In addition, manipulating large-caliber catheters through an atherosclerotic and calcified aortic arch incurs embolic risk, as does the positioning of stiff wires across the diseased valve, balloon inflation, and valve deployment.[161] Other procedural risk factors include postdilation, multiple device repositioning, and smaller annulus size.

One strategy to attenuate the risk of CE, although not exclusive, is the use of CEP devices. These can work as filters capturing debris or deflectors redirecting emboli away from the cerebral circulation. Embolic deflectors are usually deployed in the aortic arch to deflect debris away from the great vessels into the descending aorta, whereas current filter-based systems are deployed in the brachiocephalic trunk and left common carotid artery to capture debris en route to the brain.[162] Currently the only FDA-approved CEP device for TAVR is the Sentinel dual filter system (Claret Medical Inc., Santa Rosa, CA). Delivered via a right radial artery approach, this EPD consists of a 6F-compatible catheter with deployable proximal and distal filters; the proximal embolic filter is delivered to the brachiocephalic artery, and a distal embolic filter is delivered to the left common carotid artery prior to beginning the TAVR procedure (Fig. 30.15).[163]

The Claret Embolic Protection and TAVI (CLEAN TAVI) study[164] randomized 100 patients receiving a CoreValve to Sentinel embolic protection or versus no protection. All patients had a baseline brain DW-MRI before and postprocedure at 2, 7, and 30 days. Patients randomized to Sentinel protection had significantly fewer ischemic lesions and a smaller total lesion volume on days 2 and 7 post-TAVR. The control arm had more neurological changes, especially ataxia. The MRI Investigation in TAVR with Claret (MISTRAL-C) study[165] enrolled 65 patients undergoing TAVR with either balloon-expandable or self-expanding transcatheter valves. Patients with Sentinel protection had numerically fewer new lesions, smaller total brain lesion volume, and better preserved neurocognitive performance. However, this study suffered from a 40% dropout rate for the follow-up brain MRI study, so it was ultimately underpowered for its primary neurologic end point.

The SENTINEL (Cerebral Protection in Transcatheter Aortic Valve Replacement) Trial[163] is the largest multicenter TAVR trial to date to evaluate CEP using the Sentinel filter-based device. The study enrolled 363 patients from 19 centers undergoing TAVR to a safety arm (Sentinel device, n = 123), an active arm (brain imaging before and after procedure with Sentinel device use, n = 121), and a control arm (brain imaging before and after procedure with no CEP device use, n = 119). Patients in the randomized imaging arms underwent DW-MRI scanning of the brain before and 2 to 7 days after the TAVR procedure. Four types of transcatheter valves were used in the trial. Embolic debris were captured in 99% of Sentinel filters used. The rate of major adverse cardiac and cerebrovascular events (MACCE) at 30 days, the primary safety end point, was 7.3% in the two Sentinel arms combined and 9.9% in the control arm ($P = .41$). The primary efficacy end point, median total *new* lesion volume, was 102.8 mm^3 for CEP vs. 178.0 mm^3 in controls ($P = .33$). This reduction did not achieve statistical significance, although it is important to note that the study was not powered for clinical end points. However, when adjusting for preexisting lesion volume and type of valve in a post hoc analysis, Sentinel protection did significantly reduce new lesion volume, and demonstrated a correlation between lesion volume and neurocognitive decline.

In another recent study, Seeger et al.[166] enrolled 802 consecutive patients at a single center, and using propensity scoring, matched 280 patients undergoing TAVR with Sentinel CEP with 280 patients in the control group. The device was successfully positioned in 91.8% of patients. Debris was retrieved in 85.1% of

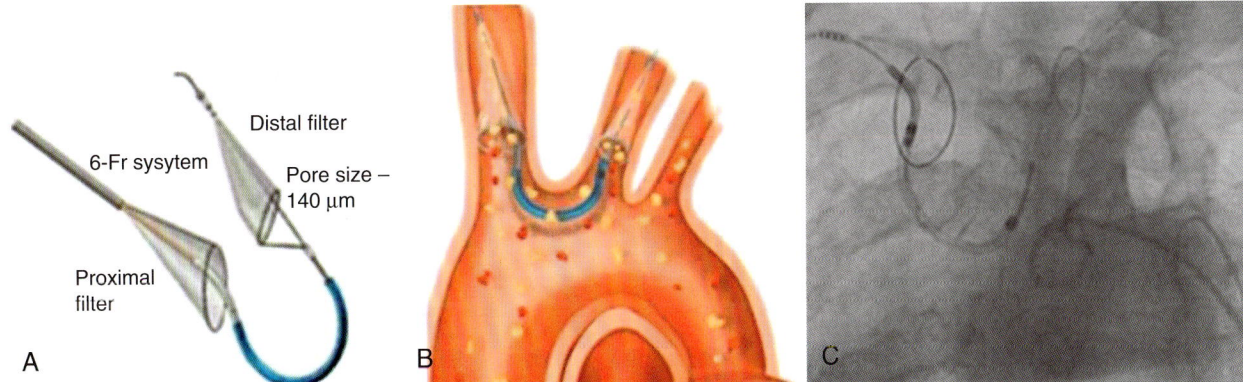

Fig. 30.15 The sentinel dual-filter embolism protection device. (A) The device with its dual filters. The pore size of the filter is 140 μm. (B) The proximal filter is placed in the brachiocephalic artery and the distal filter in the left carotid artery. (C) A fluoroscopic image of the device. (From Kapadia SR, Kodali S, Makkar R, et al. Protection against cerebral embolism during transcatheter aortic valve replacement. *J Am College Cardiol.* 2017;69[4]:367–377.)

the protection devices upon removal. One-week cerebrovascular accident rates were 1.4% in the CEP cohort versus 4.6% in the unprotected cohort. Patients with the device had a 2.1% incidence of all-cause death or stroke, compared to 6.8% in the control group. This translates into one stroke or death being prevented for every 21 TAVR procedures with Sentinel device protection.

Debris captured in embolic protection devices is surprisingly varied; isolated thrombus is rare (about 20%). The majority consists of fibrin and calcification particulates, and aortic or valve connective tissue. Size of captured particulate debris varies throughout the different studies, with the majority of CE measuring <500 μm, but on rare occasion ranging to several centimeters in maximum diameter.[167] The number and diversity of captured debris is significantly more frequent compared with other interventional procedures using filter devices (e.g., carotid stenting).[168] To that end, traditional periprocedural anticoagulation regimens favored in PCI may be of marginal benefit in prevention of TAVR-resultant CE.[169]

The Embrella Embolic Deflector (Edwards Lifesciences Ltd.) and the TriGuard (Keystone Heart Ltd.) are deflecting devices that are deployed in the aortic arch to partially or completely cover the ostia of the brachiocephalic trunk and the left carotid and subclavian arteries (Fig. 30.16)[170] (www.keystoneheart.com/us/, accessed April 30, 2018). The data gathered from trials on the neuroprotective benefit of these CEPs has provided mixed results. The Prospective Randomised Outcome Study in Patients Undergoing TAVI to Examine Cerebral Ischemia and Bleeding Complications (PRO-TAVI-C) trial[171] was a pilot study of the Embrella device. According to MRI data, Embrella placement resulted in an increased new cerebral lesion burden, without discernable improvement on neurological event rates or neurocognitive function. Further, a transcranial Doppler sub-analysis noted more high-intensity signals as surrogate for debris embolization while placing the device.[172]

Efficacy and safety of the TriGuard device was tested in the SMT Embolic Deflection CE Mark Trial (DEFLECT I) study.[173] Total cerebral vessel coverage was obtained in 80% of cases, but device instability was noted in one-third of the cases. TriGuard use resulted in numerically lower total lesion volume detected by DW-MRI compared to historical data of TAVR patients without protection. DEFLECT-III was a randomized controlled trial[174] testing a second-generation TriGuard (with a smaller pore size of 130 μm, compared to 250 μm on the first generation). Patients were randomized to TriGuard protection versus no protection, and underwent DW-MRI 4 days posttranscatheter aortic valve implantation. Complete cerebral vessel coverage was successfully obtained in nearly 90% of cases. New neurological deficit (defined by National Institutes of Health Stroke Scale) was noted in only 3% of TriGuard-protected patients compared to 15% of unprotected patients. In addition, neurocognitive decline, both at discharge and 30-day follow-up, was more common in unprotected patients. Total lesion volume measured by DW-MRI was lower in TriGuard-protected patients, particularly in those patients receiving the SAPIEN 3 valve. The Cerebral Protection to Reduce Cerebral Emboli Lesions After Transcatheter Aortic Valve Implantation (REFLECT) study is currently enrolling and should provide further insights about Triguard device. The study will randomize TAVR patients 2:1 into TriGuard protection versus no protection and assess total volume of cerebral lesions on postprocedure DW-MRI.

In aggregate, the data in support of routine CEP device use are still not uniformly compelling. Importantly, individual EPD trials have been mostly underpowered for their primary end points. One meta-analysis[175] on the Sentinel CEP suggests that its use may be associated with smaller volume of ischemic lesions, yet CEP use may not necessarily lead to reductions in the number of new single, multiple, and total number of lesions and may even be associated with a numerically increased risk of HITS in certain studies. The investigators reported no significant differences were found with respect to hard end points, such as clinically evident stroke or mortality, between patients undergoing TAVR either with or without CEP (Fig. 30.17).

Another meta-analysis[176] included five studies that, overall, enrolled 625 patients (376 had been randomized to undergo TAVR with CEP and 249 to undergo unprotected TAVR). The primary clinical end point was the risk of stroke or death at the longest follow-up point available according to the intention-to-treat principle. The use of CEP had a lower risk of death or stroke on relative and absolute terms (6.4% vs. 10.8% for without embolic protection; $P = .04$), representing a 4% absolute reduction in the risk of stroke or death with a number needed to treat of 22.

It is important to remember that only approximately one-half of strokes occur during the TAVR procedure. The other 50% of strokes occur within the ensuing 2 months, and are likely due to greater thrombogenicity from unendothelialized stent struts, arterial wall injury, and new flow turbulence. Moreover, new onset of atrial fibrillation after TAVR has been reported in up

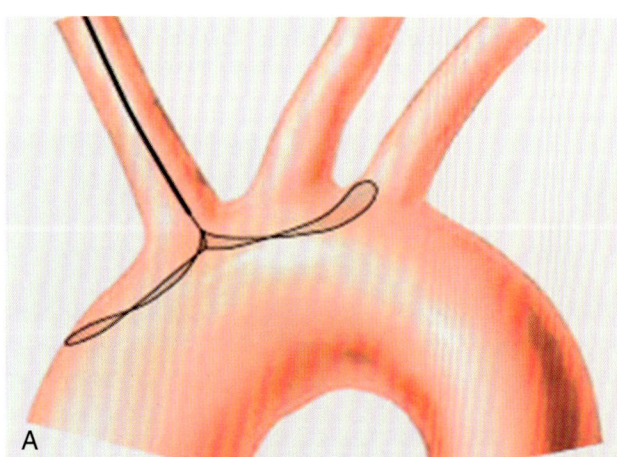 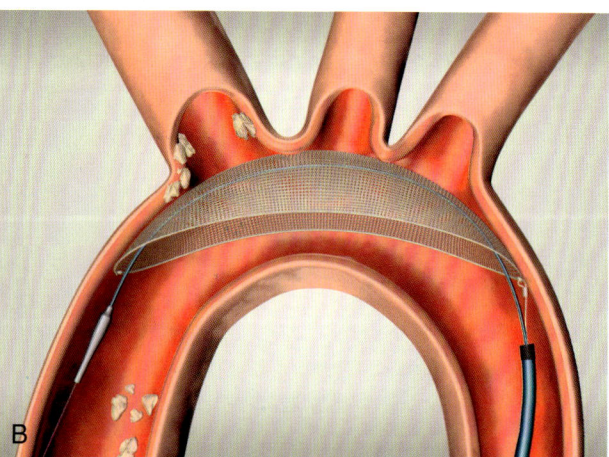

Fig. 30.16 Embolism deflector devices. (A) The Embrella Embolic Deflector System, delivered via right radial access, consisting of two petals placed in the aortic arch to cover the brachiocephalic trunk and the left carotid artery. (B) The TriGuard transcatheter aortic valve replacement cerebral embolic protection system, composed of a single-wire nitinol frame and mesh filter (pore size 130 μm) and delivered via a 9-Fr femoral sheath into the aortic arch to cover all three great arteries. (A, From Samim M, Agostoni P, Hendrikse J, et al. Embrella embolic deflection device for cerebral protection during transcatheter aortic valve replacement. *J Thoracic Cardiovasc Surg.* 2015;149[3]:799–805.e2; and B, TriGUARD 3 illustration courtesy Keystone Heart, 2019.)

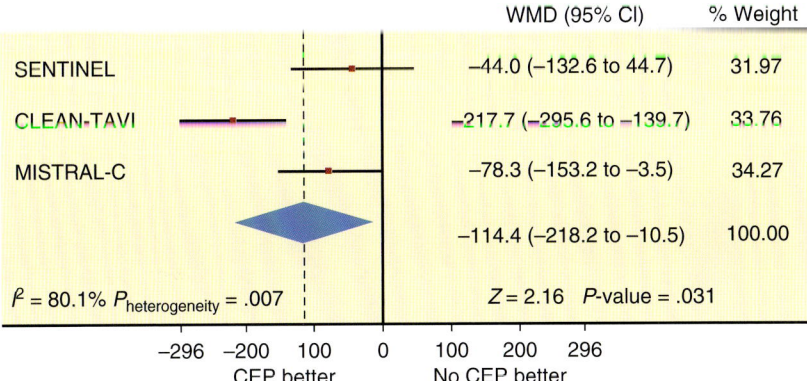

Fig. 30.17 Meta-Analysis of Randomized Controlled Trials Investigating Filter (Claret Medical, Santa Rosa, CA) Cerebral Protection Filters. Forest plot shows results for new total lesion volume in patients undergoing transcatheter aortic valve replacement with versus without cerebral embolic protection *(CEP)* filters. The weighted mean difference *(WMD)* among groups equals −114.4 mm^3 (95% confidence interval *[CI]*: −218.2 mm^3 to −10.5 mm^3), thus confirming a significant reduction in the analyzed end point (*P* value of .031). (From Latib A, Pagnesi M. Cerebral embolic protection during transcatheter aortic valve replacement: a disconnect between logic and data? *J Am Coll Cardiol.* 2017;69:378–380.)

to 30% of patients.[177] Counterintuitively, DAPT and not systemic anticoagulation is widely prescribed after TAVR, likely as a holdover from PCI recommendations. The potential merits of modern systemic anticoagulation after TAVR is currently being tested in the ongoing ATLANTIS (Anti-Thrombotic Strategy After Trans-Aortic Valve Implantation for Aortic Stenosis) (apixaban 5 mg × 2 vs. DAPT or vitamin K antagonist) and GALILEO (Global Study Comparing a rivAroxaban-based Antithrombotic Strategy to an antiPLatelet-based Strategy After Transcatheter aortIc vaLve rEplacement to Optimize Clinical Outcomes) (rivaroxaban + acetylsalicylic acid vs. DAPT) trials.

Since silent cerebral lesions occur in almost all patients and CEP use has consistently been shown to reduce such lesions,[161] the central question is whether CEP devices should be used in all TAVRs. For the most part, CEP device use appears to be feasible and safe, but inconsistent clinical benefit and increased cost have likely prevented more uniform adoption. Future trials will seek to identify particularly vulnerable populations, and need to consider uniform definitions of cerebral insult. In all likelihood, and for widespread acceptance, proof of benefit will need to extend beyond just reduction in silent embolic lesion, but rather in the form of reduced acute clinical neurologic events.

CONCLUSIONS

EPDs have gained widespread acceptance in the interventional cardiology and vascular community over the last decade. Solid evidence shows that they are safe to use and effective in reducing distal embolism during interventional procedures. Clinical outcomes have been excellent in vein graft PCI, and EPD protection is now considered the standard of care. For various reasons, results of EPD use in the setting of primary and rescue PCI have been disappointing, and at this point in time, there does not seem to be a future for those devices in acute MI intervention. However, solid evidence shows that carotid stenting with EPD protection is associated with reduced risk of stroke. Carotid stenting with proximal EPD protection seems to be even more protective against risk of stroke, although randomized comparative trials are lacking. With more innovation in EPD design, and as the ongoing clinical trials are completed, the potential exists for future application of EPDs in other settings of coronary and peripheral interventions.

KEY REFERENCES

2. Levine GN, Bates ER, Blankenship JC, et al. 2011 ACCF/AHA/SCAI Guideline for Percutaneous Coronary Intervention: a report of the American College of Cardiology Foundation/American Heart Association Task Force on Practice Guidelines and the Society for Cardiovascular Angiography and Interventions. *Circulation.* 2011;124(23):e574–e651.
4. Moussa ID, Klein LW, Shah B, et al. Consideration of a new definition of clinically relevant myocardial infarction after coronary revascularization: an expert consensus document from the Society for Cardiovascular Angiography and Interventions (SCAI). *J Am Coll Cardiol.* 2013;62(17):1563–1570.
7. Abdelmeguid AE, Topol EJ, Whitlow PL, et al. Significance of mild transient release of creatine kinase-MB fraction after percutaneous coronary interventions. *Circulation.* 1996;94(7):1528–1536.
11. Ioannidis JP, Karvouni E, Katritsis DG. Mortality risk conferred by small elevations of creatine kinase-MB isoenzyme after percutaneous coronary intervention. *J Am Coll Cardiol.* 2003;42(8):1406–1411.
13. Thygesen K, Alpert JS, White HD. Universal definition of myocardial infarction. *J Am CollCardiol.* 2007;50(22):2173–2195.
31. Naidu SS, Turco MA, Mauri L, et al. Contemporary incidence and predictors of major adverse cardiac events after saphenous vein graft intervention with embolic protection (an AMEthyst trial substudy). *J Am Coll Cardiol.* 2010;105(8):1060–1064.
32. Stone GW, Rogers C, Hermiller J, et al. Randomized comparison of distal protection with a filter-based catheter and a balloon occlusion and aspiration system during percutaneous intervention of diseased saphenous vein aorto-coronary bypass grafts. *Circulation.* 2003;108(5):548–553.
72. Kastrati A, Neumann FJ, Mehilli J, et al. Bivalirudin versus unfractionated heparin during percutaneous coronary intervention. *N Engl J Med.* 2008;359(7):688–696.
90. Bhatt DL, Lincoff AM, Gibson CM, et al. Intravenous platelet blockade with cangrelor during PCI. *N Engl J Med.* 2009;361(24):2330–2341.
110. Svilaas T, Vlaar PJ, van der Horst IC, et al. Thrombus aspiration during primary percutaneous coronary intervention. *N Engl J Med.* 2008;358(6):557–567.
122. Stone GW, Webb J, Cox DA, et al. Distal microcirculatory protection during percutaneous coronary intervention in acute ST-segment elevation myocardial infarction: a randomized controlled trial. *JAMA.* 2005;293(9):1063–1072.
142. Mas JL, Chatellier G, Beyssen B, et al. Endarterectomy versus stenting in patients with symptomatic severe carotid stenosis. *N Engl J Med.* 2006;355(16):1660–1671.
145. Brott TG, Hobson 2nd RW, Howard G, et al. Stenting versus endarterectomy for treatment of carotid-artery stenosis. *N Engl J Med.* 2010;363(1):11–23.
163. Haussig S, Mangner N, Dwyer MG, et al. Effect of a cerebral protection device on brain lesions following transcatheter aortic valve implantation in patients with severe aortic stenosis: the CLEAN-TAVI randomized clinical trial. *JAMA.* 2016;316(6):592–601.
168. Van Belle E, Hengstenberg C, Lefevre T, et al. Cerebral embolism during transcatheter aortic valve replacement: the BRAVO-3 MRI study. *J Am Coll Cardiol.* 2016;68(6):589–599.
174. Latib A, Pagnesi M. Cerebral embolic protection during transcatheter aortic valve replacement: a disconnect between logic and data? *J Am Coll Cardiol.* 2017;69(4):378–380.

 Additional references available online at expertconsult.com.

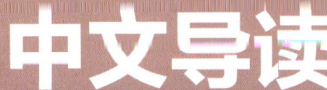

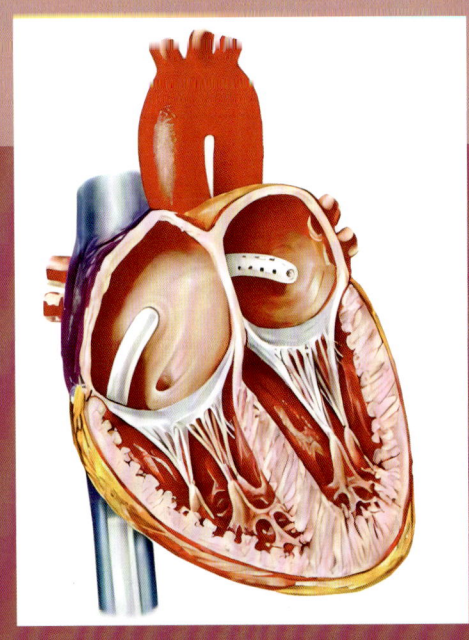

第31章
血管入路管理与血管闭合装置

近年来,介入心脏病学成功进一步扩大了其在各种血管和非血管领域治疗心血管疾病的使用领域。在这种背景下,血管入路的适当选择及正确管理,对于患者的安全至关重要。选择合适的入路通常是手术成功的关键。除了常用的股动脉逆行穿刺外,还可根据手术需要选择股动脉顺向穿刺入路、肱动脉入路、桡动脉入路、腘动脉入路或经心尖左心室穿刺。

血管入路相关并发症包括血肿、闭塞、栓塞、夹层、假性动脉瘤、动静脉瘘、神经损伤和血管感染等。这些入路并发症会增加患者痛苦,延长患者住院时间,并增加相关手术费用。更为重要的是,其还与围术期非心脏事件、术后1年非致死性心肌梗死或死亡密切相关。因此,加强动脉入路选择和管理就成为介入心脏病学的首要任务。本章总结了股动脉穿刺、动脉闭合装置的使用和并发症处理的相关知识。

陈文杰　柳景华

章节要点

- 穿刺部位的并发症仍然是心血管介入治疗后最常见的不良事件，可延长患者住院时间，并增加相关手术费用。
- 选择合适的入路部位往往是成功完成冠状动脉、外周血管或结构性心脏病介入治疗的关键问题。入路选择取决于靶血管或结构性心脏病介入治疗、术者技术和患者意愿。
- 超声引导下股总动脉穿刺术安全有效，可减少相关并发症的发生。
- 几种股动脉闭合装置与徒手和机械压迫相比，可以提供同等甚至更好的患者结局和满意度。
- 最常用的股动脉闭合装置可提供两种经皮止血机制：使用缝线或钉子关闭股动脉穿刺点，或使用可吸收塞子临时性封堵动脉穿刺处。
- 在使用闭合装置时，术者应谨慎选择股动脉的插管位置。
- 血管闭合装置使患者能够早期行走，从而改善了患者的舒适度，它的使用也减轻了医务人员的负担，潜在地降低了腹股沟并发症的发生率。

31 Access Management and Closure Devices

Fernando Cura, Marcelo Abud

KEY POINTS

- Access-site complications continue to be the most common adverse events after cardiovascular interventions, extending the patient's hospital stay and increasing the associated procedural costs.
- Selection of the appropriate access site is frequently a key issue for the successful completion of coronary, peripheral vascular, or structural procedures. Selection depends on the target vessel or structural intervention, the operator's skills, and the patient's preferences.
- The ultrasound-guided common femoral artery puncture is safe and effective to reduce associated complications.
- Several femoral access closure technologies are on the interventional field that offer equivalent or even better patient outcomes and satisfaction compared with manual and mechanical compression.
- The most commonly used femoral closure devices provide two types of mechanisms for percutaneously controlling bleeding: deploying sutures or staples to close the femoral puncture site or using resorbable plugs to temporarily seal the arteriotomy.
- When using closure devices, the operator should be careful in choosing the site of cannulation of the femoral artery.
- Vascular closure devices have improved patient comfort by enabling early ambulation, and their use has decreased the burden on the medical staff with a potential reduction in groin complication rates.

INTRODUCTION

In recent years, interventional cardiology has succeeded in further expanding its field of action for the treatment of cardiovascular diseases in a variety of vascular and nonvascular territories. In this context, the appropriate selection of vascular access, as well as its proper management, are fundamental for patient's safety.

Percutaneous coronary interventions (PCI) have usually been performed by the femoral approach; however, to reduce complications and increase patient comfort, radial access is increasingly used and is becoming the preferred access site by many interventionalists.[1] Moreover, the use of radial approach has demonstrated a reduction not only in major bleeding events but also in hospital stay when compared to femoral access using manual compression for hemostasis.[1-4] Despite this, femoral access is still the preferred access in multiple settings, as in the case of complex PCI (e.g., chronic total occlusions or left main trunk interventions).[5,6]

Furthermore, femoral access is especially necessary in interventions that require large-bore access. In this sense, the transfemoral approach is the commonly used access for transcatheter aortic valve replacement and for mechanical circulatory support (intraaortic balloon pump, Impella [Abiomed, Danvers, MA], or venoarterial extracorporeal membrane oxygenation).

In general, the most common noncardiac catheterization adverse event is related to the vascular access site.[7,8] Vascular complications are also associated with an increased risk of nonfatal myocardial infarction or death in the year following the procedure, in particular when accompanied by significant bleeding.[9] Additionally, major access-site complications increase medical costs and the length of hospital stay, and delay social reinsertion. Moreover, there is an increasing proportion of patients undergoing therapeutic interventions and being discharged the same day.[10] Therefore, enhancing the safety of arterial access and hemostasis has become a priority in the catheterization laboratory.

The aggressive level of anticoagulation used during therapeutic procedures requires the achievement of safe and reliable hemostasis of the access site. The use of manual or mechanical compression was until recently the only way to control bleeding by allowing clot formation at the arteriotomy site. The appearance and clinical use of vascular closure devices (VCDs) for rapid hemostasis after femoral access started more than 25 years ago. Since then, these devices have improved patient comfort by enabling early ambulation, and their use has decreased the burden on the medical staff.[11]

The use of passive femoral devices (pads impregnated with procoagulant material, and mechanical compression devices that replace manual compression) has not resulted in a reduction in groin complication rates. With the development of more refined devices, such as active femoral closure devices (including sutured-based, collagen-based, or patches), observational data has demonstrated a reduction of bleeding and vascular complication rates compared to manual compression.[12] However, these effects were not always evident in randomized studies.[13] The introduction of newer femoral closure devices, a better patient selection, as well as the development of a learning curve has probably improved the safety of this intervention.[14]

This chapter summarizes the concepts of femoral access puncture, the use of arterial closure devices, and postprocedural management.

PLANNING ACCESS

The selection of an appropriate access site is frequently a key issue for the successful completion of coronary, peripheral vascular, or structural procedures. Proficiency with all available vascular puncture techniques is a basic requirement for the interventionalist. The selection of a vascular access site is related to the interventional target, sheath diameter, access to target lesion length, atheromatosis burden of the route, and patient clinical characteristics.

It is important to review clinical reports and perform a high-quality preprocedural vascular assessment of all peripheral pulses, presence of bruits, blood pressure difference between arms, and other pertinent findings, such as skin color, trophic changes, ulcerations, or the presence of intermittent claudication. This important decision deserves full analysis of the target vessel for treatment, consideration of the patient's preference, and assessment of the interventionalist's skills. Some aspects of the vascular access are crucial to the safety and success of the procedure.

The retrograde femoral access and radial access are the two preferred approaches for coronary interventions. Ulnar and brachial accesses are seldom utilized. There are several techniques for endovascular peripheral therapies according to the target treatment vessel: crossover femoral approach for contralateral iliofemoral treatment; antegrade femoral puncture for ipsilateral treatment of below-the-knee arteries; femoral retrograde access for aortic, carotid, iliac, and renal vessels; local puncture for dialysis access treatment; and direct retrograde access from below-the-knee arteries. Moreover, the common femoral artery (CFA) is the preferred access for percutaneous aortic artery and aortic valve interventions.[15,16]

RETROGRADE PUNCTURE TECHNIQUE FOR THE FEMORAL ARTERY

The CFA is the preferred site for percutaneous arterial cannulation because it is large, accessible, and easily compressible. However, strict adherence to meticulous technique is necessary to avoid vascular complications, in particular when larger sheaths are being used.

The reduction in the sheath size was presumed to result in fewer access complications, but there was not a clear association with a decrement in the bleeding rate. Retrograde femoral access can be considered the standard technique for coronary, renal, iliac, and crossover for contralateral femoral interventions (Fig. 31.1). Endovascular repair of abdominal and thoracic aortic aneurysms has become the standard of care for anatomically appropriate patients. All the devices developed to date are deployed through relatively large (12- to 24-Fr) sheaths.

Transcatheter aortic valve implantation is the treatment of choice for patients with aortic valve stenosis and moderate to high surgical risk and its indication is rapidly expanding toward lower-risk patients. The fully transfemoral percutaneous approach with VCDs is considered the standard of care, as well as a fundamental component of the minimalistic approach.[16] The use of larger sheaths for these interventions requires a meticulous puncture technique in the anterior wall of the CFA.

Patient Preparation

Any vascular puncture should be performed under sterile technique. The groin is shaved in the area that spans approximately 10 cm around the specified puncture site, preferably using electric clippers with a single-use sterile razor. A variety of antimicrobial agents are available, but povidone-iodine solutions and chlorhexidine-based preparations are most commonly used.[17] There is evidence that chlorhexidine-based solutions are more effective and cause less irritation than povidone-iodine ones.[18]

Since the vascular access is generally the only painful part of the procedure, generous local anesthesia with approximately 20 mL of 1% to 2% lidocaine is needed, as well as adequate pressure and rhythm monitoring to identify any possible vagal reaction. First, create an intradermal wheal with 3 to 4 mL of lidocaine at the desired level of entry. The remaining lidocaine will be used to infiltrate the deeper planes covering the anticipated path of the needle to the artery.

Anatomical Considerations

The CFA originates as a continuation of the external iliac artery immediately after the take-off of the inferior epigastric artery and after crossing the inguinal ligament, which represents an important anatomical landmark. When drawing an imaginary line between the anterior superior iliac supine and the pubis tubercle, it is near or at the midpoint of the line. Then, the CFA descends almost vertically down and ends at the hiatus of the adductor muscle, where it branches into the superficial femoral artery and the profunda femoral artery (Fig. 31.2).

One important aspect is to puncture only the anterior wall of the femoral artery with open-bore needles, which have the advantage of demonstrating blood return immediately (Fig. 31.3).

Based on angiographic evaluation, the mean luminal diameter of the CFA is 6.9 ± 1.4 mm and its mean length is 43.3 ± 16.2 mm. This is theoretically large enough to comfortably accommodate the typical range of femoral sheath sizes for most diagnostic and interventional procedures. Note that diabetics, women, and patients with small body surface area have disproportionately smaller CFA.[19]

Choice of Puncture Site

In order to avoid complications, the operator should be careful in choosing the site of cannulation at the level of the CFA (see Fig. 31.2). Puncture sites not located at the appropriate level are responsible for the majority of vascular access complications.[20] Cannulation of the artery too low increases the chance of entering the superficial femoral artery rather than the CFA. This entry site may predispose to dissection, arterial occlusion, pseudoaneurysm, bleeding, and arteriovenous fistula formation.[21] Entering the artery above the inguinal ligament may lead to problems in compressing the artery against the inguinal ligament, increasing the risk of hematoma formation and favoring retroperitoneal hemorrhage. It was reported that puncture performed above the inferior epigastric artery was associated with retroperitoneal bleeds.[22,23]

The *safest zone* to puncture is located from 1 to 2 cm below the inguinal ligament (1 to 2 cm below the line traced from the anterosuperior iliac spine to the pubic tubercle) and above the femoral bifurcation (see Fig. 31.2). There are different ways to ascertain this location: palpatory method, fluoroscopic evaluation, and ultrasound-guided puncture. In a multinational survey, 60% of operators used the classic palpation technique, while fluoroscopic evaluation and ultrasound-guided puncture are used by only 11% and 2% of operators, respectively (60%).[24]

Traditional Palpatory Method

This method is based on the identification of landmarks to identify the inguinal ligament and hence the position of the CFA distal to it: *inguinal crease, the point of maximal pulsation, and bony landmarks.*

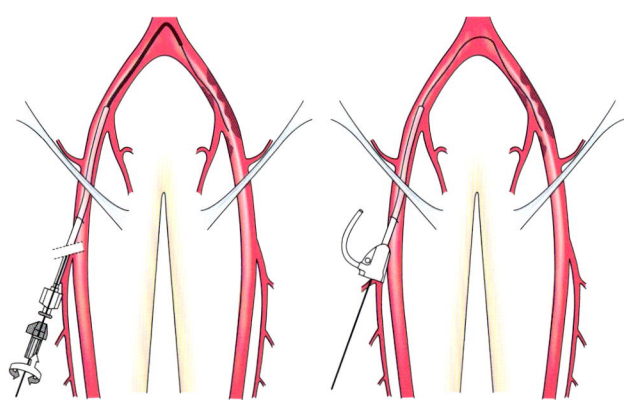

Fig. 31.1 Retrograde femoral access for a contralateral approach.

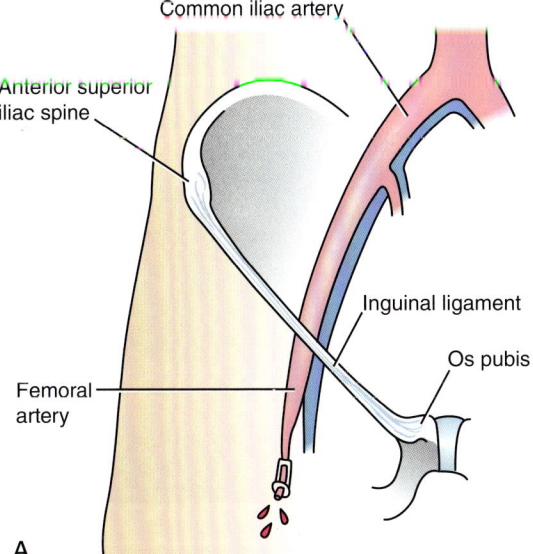

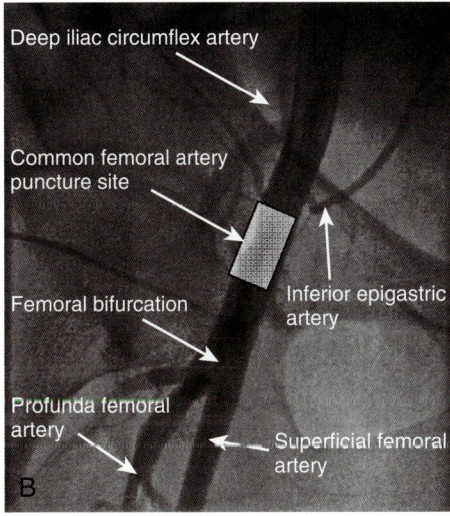

Fig. 31.2 Accessing the femoral artery. (A) An imaginary line between the superior anterior crest and the pubis is constructed; this line usually corresponds to the location of the inguinal ligament. The needle should enter approximately 1 cm below the imaginary line while advancing at a 30- to 45-degree angle. (B) An excellent method for localizing the puncture site is to use fluoroscopy of the femoral head. The needle point should be over the lower inner quadrant (see also Video 31.1).

The puncture at or just below the *inguinal crease* has been extensively used as a landmark based on the belief that it was closely related to the inguinal ligament, but there is a lot of evidence against that concept. First, the distance between both is highly variable, ranging from 0 to 11 cm with an average of 6.5 ± 1.9 cm. In addition, a significant variation between the inguinal crease and the femoral bifurcation has been reported.[25,26] The point of maximal pulsation is more reliable than the inguinal crease to localize the CFA since it has been reported that it is projected over the CFA in 92.7% of limbs.[26] Finally, bony landmarks are based on the midpoint of a line between the anterior superior iliac spine and the pubic symphysis,[20] in particular a point located 2.5 cm distally to this line. It is important to note that the surface landmarks could be altered in many conditions, such as obesity, prior hematoma, scarring, and low blood pressure, making this traditional method very unreliable.

Fluoroscopic Visualization Method

The CFA correlates well to the area that is at the mid-third of the femoral head in the majority of cases.[27,28] Accessing the CFA using fluoroscopy compared to traditional anatomic landmark guidance has improved the arterial puncture site.[10] To note, femoral artery bifurcation is below the inferior border of the femoral head in 65% to 80% of cases, lies on the medial third of the femoral head in 92% of patients, and only 8% have the arterial completely medial to the femoral head.[26,29,30]

Ultrasound-Guided Femoral Access

Ultrasound guidance has emerged as an alternative method to identify the puncture site. In the last decade, it has become the standard of care outside the cardiac catheterization laboratory for vascular access, especially for central venous catheterization with guideline recommendations endorsing its use.[31] Multiple randomized trials and meta-analysis have demonstrated a reduction in complications rates, number of attempts, and time to access. However, few operators use ultrasound routinely for vascular access in the cardiac catheterization laboratory.[24]

Ultrasound allows for direct visualization of the CFA and the identification of the origin of the inferior epigastric artery superiorly and the femoral bifurcation inferiorly. Furthermore, applying some pressure with a transducer allows for the differentiation between the femoral artery and the femoral vein (Fig. 31.4).

Several studies have examined the usefulness of ultrasound-guided femoral access. The largest study addressing this issue was FAUST (Femoral Arterial Access With Ultrasound Trial).[30] It was a prospective, multicenter trial that randomized 1004 patients

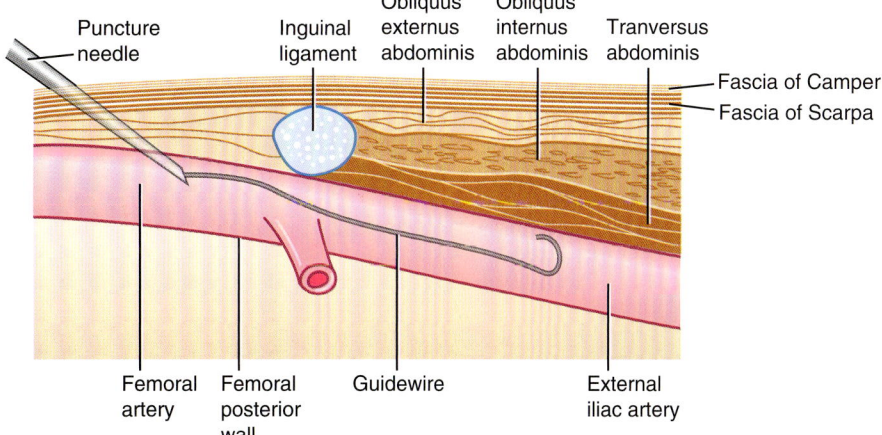

Fig. 31.3 The femoral artery must be entered using a large-bore needle with backflow of blood. As soon as the needle passes into the vessel through the anterior wall, flow is brisk and pulsatile. The guidewire is advanced and prevents occult bleeding through the posterior wall.

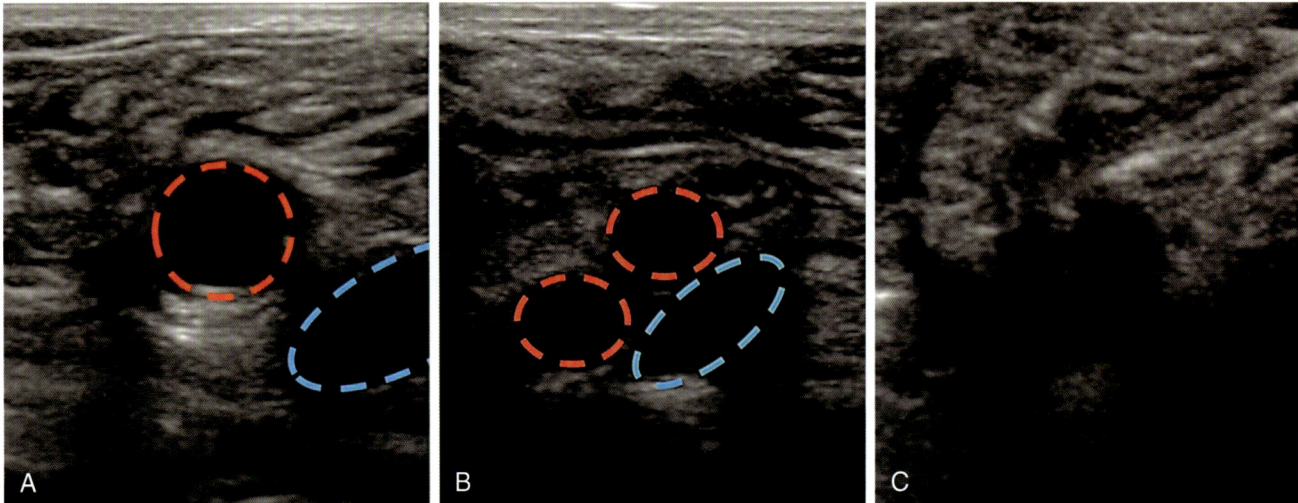

Fig. 31.4 (A) Ultrasound visualization of common femoral artery *(red circle)* and its relationship with femoral vein *(blue semicircle)*. (B) Ultrasound visualization of femoral artery bifurcation into superficial and profunda *(red circles)* and its relationship with femoral vein *(blue circle)*. (C) Ultrasound visualization of needle tip entering at the anterior wall of the common femoral artery.

undergoing retrograde femoral approach to either fluoroscopic or ultrasound guidance. The primary end point was successful CFA cannulation. Secondary end points were time to sheath insertion, number of forward needle advancements, first pass success, accidental venipunctures, and vascular access complications at 30 days. Regarding the primary outcome, ultrasound guidance did not reach higher rates of CFA cannulation (86.4% vs. 83.3%, P .17). However, in patients with high femoral bifurcations, ultrasound-guided access was more likely to puncture at the level of the CFA (82.6% vs. 69.8%, P .01). With regard to secondary outcomes, ultrasound-guided puncture significantly improved first-pass success rate (83% vs. 46%, P .0001), and reduced the number of attempts (1.3 vs. 3.0, P .0001), venipuncture (2.4% vs. 15.8%, P .0001), and median time to access (136 s vs. 148 s, P .003). Moreover, vascular complications were less frequent in this group (1.4% vs. 3.4% P .04), a result driven by a significant reduction in groin hematomas >5 cm (0.6% vs. 2.2%, P .03).

A meta-analysis and systematic review with a total of 1551 subjects (782 in the ultra-sound–guided group and 769 in the palpation group)[32] compared both femoral access techniques demonstrating that ultra-sound–guided femoral access was associated with 60% reduction in bleeding events, a 76% reduction in the number of puncture attempts, an 80% reduction in venipunctures, and similar rates of catheter insertion outside of the CFA boundaries (Table 31.1).

Micropuncture

Standard access via the CFA is obtained with an 18-gauge needle and a 0.035- or 0.038-inch J-tip wire. In an effort to reduce local trauma to the artery and surrounding tissues, a 21-gauge needle system (Micropuncture Access Set, Cook Medical) has been introduced for femoral access to reduce arteriotomy access by 56% compared with the 18-gauge needle.

However, there are few studies that investigated the role of the micropuncture system for a reduction in access-site related complications and at present there is no clear evidence to sustain the routine use of micropuncture needles.[33] An observational study showed a significantly higher frequency of retroperitoneal hemorrhage in the micropuncture group (0.7% vs. 0.18%; P = .04).[34] Therefore, the 0.018-inch wire advancement should be performed under fluoroscopy guidance in order to prevent inadvertent wiring of side branches.

TABLE 31.1 Risk of Adverse Events of Ultra-Sound–Guided Femoral Puncture Versus Fluoroscopic Guidance

Outcomes	US-guided	Control	OR (95% CI)
Bleeding events	11/782	26/769	0.41 (0.20–0.83)
≥1 puncture attempt	144/728	357/721	0.24 (0.19–0.31)
Venipunctures	23/621	105/621	0.18 (0.11–0.29)
Puncture outside of the CFA	76/558	87/549	0.84 (0.60–1.17)

Summary of outcomes evaluated in the meta-analysis conducted by Marquis-Gravel et al, demonstrating the safety and efficacy of the ultra-sound–guided femoral puncture technique vs. fluoroscopic guidance.
CFA, Common femoral artery; *CI*, confidence interval; *OR*, odds ratio; *US*, ultra-sound.

ANTEGRADE PUNCTURE TECHNIQUE FOR THE FEMORAL ARTERY

The antegrade puncture technique provides more direct access to many lesions in the femoropopliteal segment and the infraglenoidal arteries. It allows reduction of the volume of contrast and provides stronger support for superficial femoral artery chronic occlusions. However, antegrade puncture is technically more challenging. Although a high puncture of the CFA is required to have enough space for navigation of the guidewire into the superficial femoral artery, suprainguinal puncture should be avoided because of the higher risk for retroperitoneal bleeding (Fig. 31.5). Ultrasound-guided puncture helps to identify the femoral bifurcation anatomy.

PUNCTURE TECHNIQUE FOR THE BRACHIAL ARTERY

Brachial access is an alternative technique that can be used for coronary, renal, and lower limb interventions. However, the radial access is usually preferred because of a higher rate of brachial access-site complications compared to femoral access, such as artery occlusion or hematoma (odds ratio [OR] 2.41; confidence interval [CI] 2.15 to 2.69; $P < .001$).[14] Puncture of the brachial artery should be performed in its distal part above the antecubital fossa, where the artery is relatively superficial. At this level, after sheath removal, the artery can be compressed against the humerus to obtain hemostasis (Fig. 31.6). Direct puncture of the axillary artery, which has been performed in the past, has largely been abandoned.

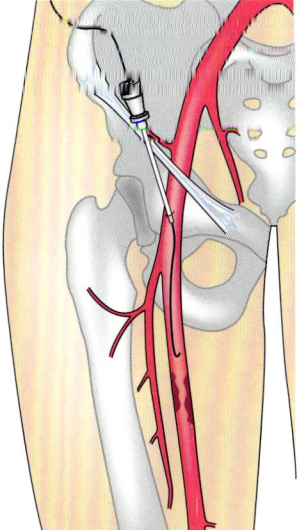

Fig. 31.5 Anterograde puncture technique for the femoral artery.

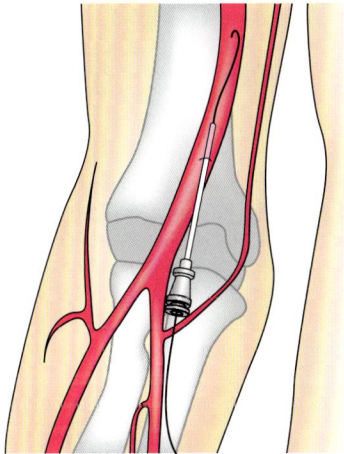

Fig. 31.6 Puncture technique for the brachial artery.

PUNCTURE TECHNIQUE FOR THE POPLITEAL ARTERY

Transpopliteal retrograde access becomes useful when the superficial femoral artery cannot be crossed using other antegrade techniques. Patients are placed in a prone position. The puncture is performed with the assistance of roadmap fluoroscopy after the injection of contrast from an ipsilateral femoral catheter or guided with ultrasound (Fig. 31.7). Particular attention should be paid to achieving complete hemostasis after intervention by careful manual compression. The incidence of access-site complications is potentially higher with transpopliteal access than with conventional techniques.[35]

TRANSAPICAL LEFT VENTRICULAR PUNCTURE

Percutaneous interventions are becoming increasingly complex, but in some instances the target lesion may be difficult to reach using conventional transvenous or transarterial access.

Transapical left ventricular puncture gives direct access to the left ventricle and although frequently used in the past for diagnostic reasons, has largely been abandoned. Nevertheless, there are multiple clinical circumstances where direct transapical access is required for interventional indications including access to the left ventricle for inaccessible percutaneous mitral paravalvular leak

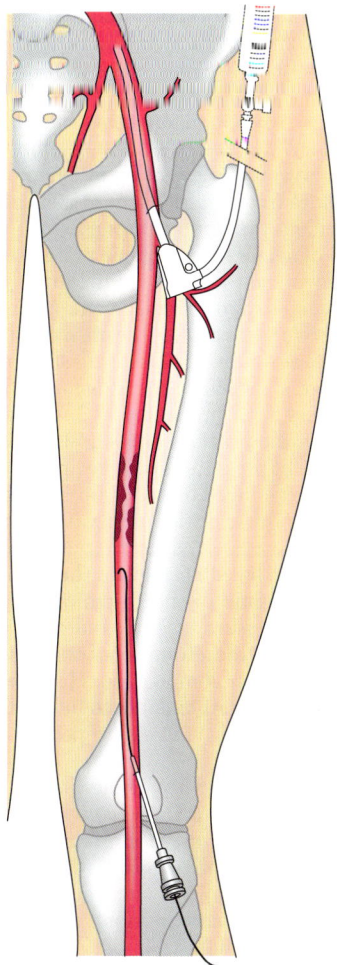

Fig. 31.7 Puncture technique for the popliteal artery.

repair, percutaneous aortic valve implantation, and the promising field of percutaneous mitral valve implantation.[36,37]

Percutaneous transthoracic puncture is appealing for an interventional cardiologist, but can be complicated with lung puncture resulting in pneumothorax or hemothorax due to damage of the internal mammary and subcostal arteries, or persistent leak after sheath withdrawal. Damage to the coronary artery can be avoided by doing selective coronary angiography before puncture. However, most of these complications can be diminished by puncturing "under direct vision" after a mini thoracotomy. Computed tomography (CT) scanning is useful to guide the access site either for direct puncture or to perform the mini thoracotomy.[38]

HEMOSTATIC METHODS AFTER PERCUTANEOUS CARDIOVASCULAR PROCEDURES

Proper technique is essential for achieving successful femoral artery hemostasis without complications. Methods used to achieve hemostasis after percutaneous procedures include manual compression, mechanical compression, vascular plugs, percutaneous vascular suturing or staples, and topical hemostasis accelerators.

Manual and Mechanical Compression

Digital compression should be considered the gold standard for compressive methods. Performed properly, it can prevent bleeding and maintain distal perfusion. This procedure may be performed by a physician, nurse, or technician who has received formal training.

Before sheath removal, it is important to assess distal pulses and the access site for signs of any existing complication. It is also necessary to wait until heparin has increased the activated clotting time (ACT) to less than 160 to 180 seconds.[11] The use of protamine to reverse heparin remains controversial after coronary interventions. The incidence of adverse reactions to protamine is relatively low; however, some of them could be life-threatening. These are more frequent in insulin-dependent diabetics and patients with previous protamine exposure.[39]

The duration of manual compression and the time of immobilization are proportional to the size of the introducer sheath and the level of anticoagulation. Although the manual compression technique is effective with smaller sheath sizes, it becomes more challenging and hazardous with increasing sheath sizes. The recommended compression time is 10 minutes of "firm" pressure, 2 to 5 minutes of "less firm" pressure, and 2 minutes of light pressure while applying the pressure dressing. If bleeding continues, another 15 minutes of pressure should be applied.

Risk factors for prolonged bleeding include severe atherosclerosis at the puncture site and a loss of elasticity without adequate approximation of the vessel edges after removing the sheath. Other risk factors for bleeding include the sheath size, anticoagulation level at the time of sheath removal, aortic regurgitation, elevated blood pressure, obesity, and older age. The use of manual compression has the advantage of continuous observation and modulation of vascular compression. However, it has the disadvantage of requiring a staff member to be available, prolonged immobilization, and bedrest, increasing patient discomfort and length of hospital stay.

To avoid this, there are a variety of mechanical devices to apply similar local pressure. Their main benefit is to provide a hands-free hemostasis and improve operator productivity, and outcomes are as good or even better than manual compression. A meta-analysis conducted by Jones and McCutcheon included two studies that compared mechanical compression versus manual compression. Mechanical compression was more effective for preventing hematoma formation but the prevalence of bleeding did not differ significantly between the different methods of compression.[40]

However, a subanalysis of the CathPCI Registry found that mechanical compression devices have shown significantly higher odds of "bleeding or vascular complications" than manual compression (OR 1.15; CI 1.10 to 1.20; $P < .001$).[14]

The CompressAR (Advanced Vascular Dynamics, Vancouver, WA) is a mechanical compression-assist device developed to enhance comfort for patients and practitioners. It includes a handle and a detachable sterile and disposable disk. There are seven styles of CompressAR discs to choose from in varying shapes and sizes. Practitioners apply external pressure using the system in much the same way that they would apply manual pressure (Fig. 31.8). This device is associated with a 63% increased risk of serious femoral vascular complications when compared with manual compression and with shorter compression time.[41]

The FemoStop (Abbott) is a pneumatic pressure device that uses a clear plastic compression bag that molds to skin contours (Fig. 31.9). The FemoStop is composed of a plastic arch, inflatable transparent dome, connection tubing, a stopcock, an elastic or adjustable belt, and a handheld manometer. It is held in place by straps passing around the hip. The amount of applied pressure may be modulated and observed with sphygmomanometer gauge. It allows visualization of the puncture site. The FemoStop is frequently indicated for compression to repair pseudoaneurysms and it achieves hemostasis more quickly when compared with manual compression.[42]

Femoral Closure Devices

Among endovascular interventions, bleeding and vascular complications are the most common noncardiac, procedure-related

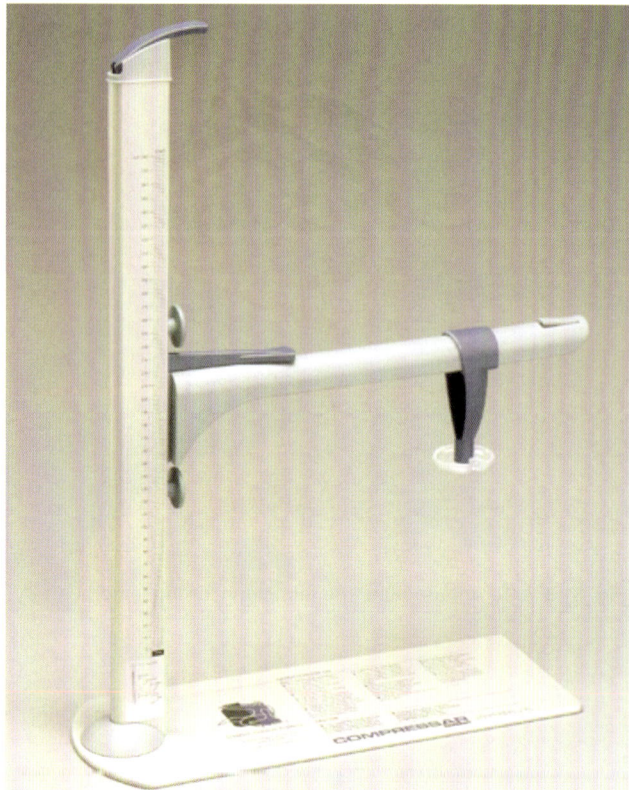

Fig. 31.8 Compass compression-assist device is placed over the femoral sheath before pulling it. Then, more comfortable manual pressure is applied. (Photo courtesy Advanced Vascular Dynamics, Vancouver, WA.)

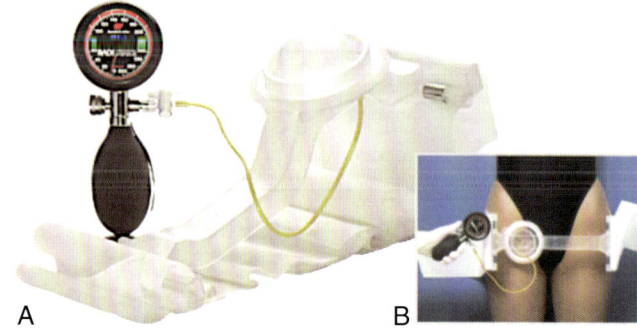

Fig. 31.9 (A) The FemoStop pressure system with sphygmomanometer. (B) The belt should be aligned with the puncture site equally across both hips.

adverse outcomes, occurring in 1.72% of procedures whether or not a vascular closure device is utilized.[9] It is well known that they are associated with increased morbidity and mortality, longer hospitalization, and a higher cost of care.[12] VCDs have emerged as an alternative to traditional manual or mechanical compression with important benefits not only in hemostasis and ambulation but also in patient satisfaction and quality of life.[43]

Numerous randomized control trials (RCTs) have compared the use of VCD versus manual compression or surgical cutdown. Regarding patient satisfaction and quality of life, some studies addressed this issue as a secondary outcome. The Continued Access Protocol (CAP) trial compared the Angio-Seal VIP (Terumo, Leuven, Belgium) with Perclose ProGlide (Abbott Vascular Devices, Redwood City, CA) and manual compression

TABLE 31.2 Risk of Adverse Events After Cardiac Catheterizations by Hemostasis Device

Complication	Type of Hemostasis Strategy								
	Manual (%)	Mechanical (%)	Angio-Seal (%)	PerClose (%)	BCW (%)	StarClose (%)	Mynx (%)	Patches (%)	Total (%)
Entry-site bleed	0.95	1.10	0.61	0.62	0.70	0.80	0.71	0.82	0.82
Retroperitoneal bleed	0.26	0.26	0.38	0.22	0.11	0.36	0.39	0.18	0.29
Occlusion	0.04	0.03	0.04	0.05	0.00	0.03	0.02	0.03	0.04
Embolization	0.05	0.04	0.04	0.03	0.00	0.02	0.02	0.04	0.04
Dissection	0.25	0.45	0.19	0.15	0.15	0.14	0.09	0.29	0.24
Pseudoaneurysm	0.59	0.63	0.19	0.12	0.40	0.14	0.37	0.51	0.41
Arteriovenous fistula	0.08	0.09	0.03	0.03	0.07	0.02	0.01	0.07	0.06
All bleeding	1.18	1.32	0.95	0.80	0.80	1.12	1.07	0.98	1.08
All vascular	0.97	1.20	0.47	0.35	0.60	0.35	0.49	0.92	0.76
Bleeding or vascular	1.99	2.34	1.36	1.10	1.27	1.42	1.48	1.77	1.72

BCW, Boomerang Closure Wire.
From Tavris DR, Wang Y, Jacobs S, et al. Bleeding and vascular complications at the femoral access site following percutaneous coronary intervention (PCI): an evaluation of hemostasis strategies. *J Invasive Cardiol*. 2012;24:328–334.

following PCI.[44] The discomfort was evaluated with a scale of 1 to 4 (most pain). There was significantly greater patient satisfaction with VCD in regard to pain, mainly driven by the use of Angio-Seal VIP (there was an important trend toward less pain with Perclose ProGlide). The Percutaneous Endovascular Aneurysm Repair (PEVAR) trial was a multicenter RCT conducted to assess the safety and effectiveness of Perclose ProGlide and Prostar XL (Abbott) versus standard surgical cutdown in patients undergoing endovascular aortic aneurysm repair. Quality of life was assessed before and after the procedure by the Medical Outcomes Study short form SF-36.[45] One month after the procedure there were greater changes in the mean scores in Perclose ProGlide (+9) and Prostar XL (+6) versus cutdown (0). Compared with cutdown, prescribed analgesics for groin pain were significantly lower in Prostar XL (12% vs 34%; P .039) and trended lower in Perclose ProGlide (18% vs 34%; P .241). A systematic review conducted by Cox et al. has confirmed these results.[46]

Regarding the efficacy of VCD to reduce vascular complications, there are numerous registries and RCT with mixed results. First, the operator experience plays an important role. Tavris et al. performed a trend analysis in which VCD were associated with decreasing bleeding and vascular complication rates over time.[14] Along the same lines, Jiang et al. performed a network meta-analysis of 40 studies in 2015.[47] The overall population was divided according to trials that were run before or after 2005. They observed a significant reduction in the risk for major access site complications with the use of VCD when analyzing trials after 2005 but no differences among trials conducted before 2005. Moreover, in the entire population, VCD were associated with a lower risk for hematomas (relative risk [RR] 0.80; 95% CI 0.71 to 0.90).

A large observational registry from the National Cardiovascular Data Registry (NCDR) showed evidence that VCD are associated with safety profiles that are significantly different from manual compression.[14] In a multivariate analysis involving only PCIs with femoral access sites, the majority of VCDs performed better than manual compression to achieve hemostasis with lower bleeding and vascular complications (Table 31.2).

One of the largest randomized trials conducted to evaluate the role of VCD for the achievement of hemostasis in patients undergoing transfemoral catheterization was the Instrumental Sealing of Arterial Puncture Site—CLOSURE Device versus Manual Compression (ISAR-CLOSURE).[13] It included 4524 patients undergoing diagnostic coronary angiography with a 6-Fr sheath who were randomized to intravascular VCD, extravascular VCD, or manual compression. The primary end point (incidence of vascular access site complications, i.e., the composite of hematoma at least 5 cm in size, pseudoaneurysm, arteriovenous fistula, access site–related major bleeding, acute ipsilateral leg ischemia, need for vascular surgical or interventional treatment, or local infection at 30 days after randomization) was observed in 6.9% of patients assigned to VCD and 7.9% assigned to manual compression ($P < .001$ for noninferiority). Closure-device failure occurred less frequently with intravascular VCD (FemoSeal) than with extravascular VCD (Exoseal) (5.3% vs. 12.2%; $P < .001$). VCD use compared with manual compression resulted in shorter time to hemostasis (median 1 minute vs. 10 minutes; $P < .001$).

An RCT conducted by Hermanides et al. compared the Angio-Seal versus manual compression in 627 patients undergoing PCI.[48] The primary end point was the in-hospital incidence of severe hematoma >5 cm at the puncture site or groin bleeding resulting in prolonged hospital stay, transfusion and/or surgical intervention at the puncture site, arteriovenous fistula formation, and/or any surgical intervention at the puncture site. Although they found similar rates of complications (Angio-Seal 2.6% vs. manual compression 4.5%, P .195), in the predefined subgroup of patients with a history of hypertension the combined primary end point was significantly reduced after use of the closure device (Angio-Seal 0.8% vs. manual compression 7.2%; $P = .008$).

In the aforementioned CAP Trial,[44] there was no significant difference in major vascular complications (retroperitoneal bleeding, pseudoaneurysm, thrombosis, arteriovenous fistula) between groups.

In the Ensure's Vascular Closure Device Speeds Hemostasis (ECLIPSE) trial, 401 patients undergoing PCI were randomized in a 2:1 fashion to Exoseal versus manual compression.[49] The primary efficacy end points were time to hemostasis and time to ambulation, whereas the primary safety end points were periprocedural and 30-day incidence of arterial access-related complications. Both time to hemostasis (4.4 ± 11.6 minutes vs. 20.1 ± 22.5 minutes, $P < .0001$) and time to ambulation (2.5 ± 5 hours vs. 6.2 ± 13.3 hours, P .003) were significantly shorter with the use of Exoseal. Interestingly, there were no major adverse events reported in both groups.

Numerous studies have reported that VCDs are safe and effective to allow immediate mobilization after the procedure. The RISE Clinical Trial evaluated the safety and efficacy of the StarClose in patients undergoing diagnostic coronary or peripheral catheterizations.[50] Immediate hemostasis was achieved in 91.2% of patients and time to ambulation was 8.29 ± 10.75 minutes. There were no deaths or major vascular complications (i.e., vascular repair or the need for repair, new ipsilateral lower extremity ischemia documented by patient symptoms, physical exam and/or decreased or absent blood flow on lower extremity angiogram, access site-related bleeding requiring transfusion, and/or any access site-related surgery). An RCT by Hvelplund et al. compared immediate versus delayed (4 hours) mobilization in patients treated with Angio-Seal.[51] There were no differences in all vascular complications (18.8% vs. 16%, P .53) nor major vascular complications (4.1% vs. 5.1%, P .69) between groups. In the SCOAST study, Angio-Seal and StarClose were compared in the setting of immediate mobilization.[52] There was no significant bruising in either group at either 30 or 60 minutes postprocedure. At 1 week, there was significantly more bruising in the Angio-Seal group than the StarClose group (63.1 vs. 38.5 cm^2, P = .02). Patient satisfaction and pain perception were not significantly different between the groups.

A meta-analysis of 31 RCTs conducted by Biancari et al. included 7528 patients who were randomized to VCDs or manual/mechanical compression after diagnostic angiography and/or therapeutic interventions.[53] Most of these studies excluded patients at high risk of puncture-site complications. In terms of groin hematoma, bleeding, pseudoaneurysm, and blood transfusion there were no differences between groups. However, lower limb ischemia and other ischemic complications (0.3% vs. 0%, P .07), the need of surgery for vascular complications (0.7% vs. 0.4%, P .10), and the incidence of groin infection was significantly more frequent with VCDs (0.6% vs. 0.2%, P .02).

All closure devices have been reported to be safe in patients receiving glycoprotein (GP) IIb/IIIa inhibitors.[54,55] However, some reports have raised concerns about an increased risk of bleeding complications with the use of VCD compared with manual compression in this setting (in combination with anticoagulation drugs, oral antiplatelets, and GP IIb/IIIa inhibitors).[14] A sub-analysis of the Harmonizing Outcomes With Revascularization and Stents in Acute Myocardial Infarction (HORIZONS-AMI) trial evaluated the relationship of VCD use to bleeding and ischemic events in patients undergoing primary PCI for ST-segment elevation myocardial infarction.[55] The primary outcome was the net adverse clinical events (NACE), defined as the composite of major bleeding unrelated to coronary artery bypass graft (CABG) surgery and major adverse cardiac events (comprised of death, reinfarction, ischemia-driven target-vessel revascularization, and stroke) at 30 days and 1 year. At 30 days, patients in the VCD group had significantly less NACE driven by a lower rate of non–CABG-related major bleeding. These results were maintained regardless of the anticoagulant treatment.

Studies comparing the benefits and cost-effectiveness of closure devices and manual compression found that the use of closure devices is not only safe but also cost saving.[56,57] Although the use of VCD has a cost implication, it allows a reduction in hospitalization time, leading to significant cost savings due to decreased personnel and infrastructural demands.

Based on their mechanism of action, VCD can be divided into *passive devices* and *active closure devices*.

Passive Devices

Passive devices are impregnated with procoagulant material which is deposited in the arteriotomy site at the same time of mechanical compression. The use of this type of VCD has demonstrated a marginal reduction in the time to hemostasis compared with manual compression, but it did not translate into a reduction in the overall bedrest time and there was no reduction in the risk for access-site complications.[58,59] Conversely, Tavris et al. found that bleeding and vascular complications were reduced by 30% with hemostasis pads.[14] According to the paucity of data and the development of newer devices, hemostasis pads are considered as tools to aid manual compression to obtain hemostasis.

Active Devices

Active devices involve a wide variety of devices with different mechanism of action: compression discs that are removed after hemostasis is achieved, and those that use plugs, sutures, or clips that are either absorbed or remain in place to close the arteriotomy. The safety and efficacy of these devices is dependent on arteriotomy in the safe zone, the dimension of the CFA, and the artery being free from atherosclerosis at puncture site.

Plug-Based Sealing Devices

Collagen is considered one of the most thrombogenic components of the vascular wall. It attracts and binds platelets. Collagen also plays an important role in healing wounds by carrying growth factors and by providing a matrix for cellular proliferation. Because it is highly compatible and easily manufactured in many different forms, collagen is an ideal component for hemostasis products. Collagen can be used alone to plug the vessel wall or tissue tract, or it can be combined with thrombin or gelfoam. Thrombin converts fibrinogen to fibrin, accelerating and strengthening clot formation. Moreover, other substances rather than collagen can be used as sealants.

The *Angio-Seal* (Terumo)[60] mechanically closes the site by sandwiching the arteriotomy site between a bioabsorbable polymer anchor inside the vessel and an extravascular collagen sponge covering the arterial surface within the skin tract (Fig. 31.10). It consists of four components within a delivery device: anchor, collagen plug, connecting suture, and a tamper. All three components deployed into the patient are completely resorbable. The small plug contains only about 15 mg of collagen, and the anchor is made from polyglycolic and polylactic acids which dissolve within 60 to 90 days. Before Angio-Seal deployment, the access site should be assessed by injecting contrast through the sheath under fluoroscopy. If the introducer enters the femoral artery above the inguinal ligament, at the bifurcation, at a branch vessel, or at an atherosclerotic vessel, there is an increased risk of device failure or embolization, and an alternative method for hemostasis should be used. Proper technique must be followed to avoid bleeding complications, anchor embolization, thrombosis, and infection.

A large number of randomized and observational trials supports the use of Angio-Seal in diagnostic and interventional procedures with high success rates (more than 90%).[44,61]

It was reported that an 8-Fr Angio-Seal was safe and efficient to close 9-Fr femoral artery puncture sites, even under recombinant tissue plasminogen activator.[62]

The ExoSeal (Cordis Corporation, Miami Lakes, FL) consists of a feltlike plug made of polyglycolic acid (PGA) that completely dissolves into carbon dioxide and water over about 3 months. It can be used following diagnostic angiography or interventional procedures and is anchored in place on top of the puncture in the femoral artery, after the catheter is removed. The device uses an indicator nitinol wire to locate the arterial anterior wall to ensure extravascular plug placement. The wire is removed before the plug is delivered. Because none of the plug is inserted into the artery itself, it does not interfere with blood flow.[63,64]

It showed high success rates (>90%),[65] similar to other passive and active devices[66] and it was associated with significantly lower pain levels and discomfort when compared to manual compression.[67]

The Mynx (Cardinal Health, Inc., Dublin, OH) uses an extravascular, bio-inert sealant to provide immediate hemostasis of the puncture site.[68,69] The device met the challenge of simultaneously sealing the puncture hole in the artery and in the tissue track by generating a thrombus. It incorporates a unique,

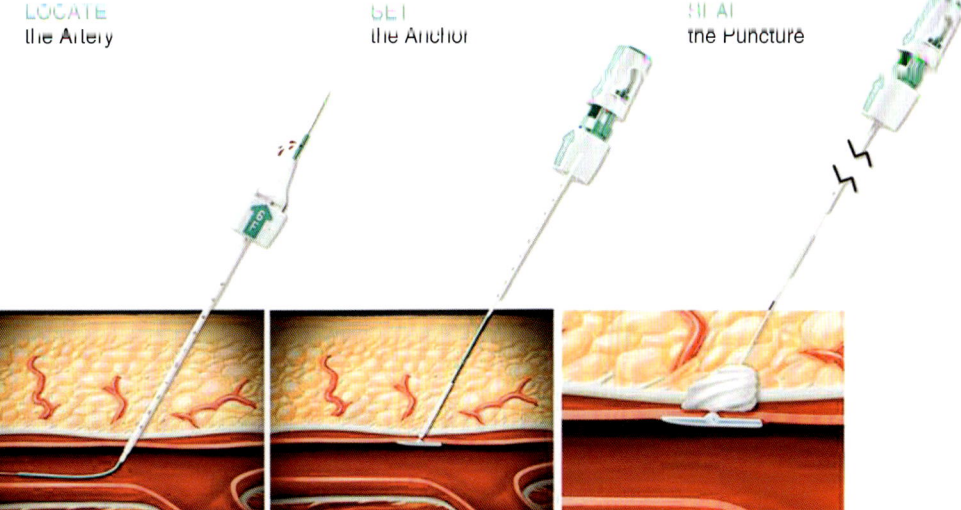

Fig. 31.10 Angio-Seal hemostasis system. The anchor is deployed, and retraction of the system secures the anchor against the anterior vessel wall. The collagen plug is deployed outside of the artery, and the suture is cut at the skin line, leaving the subcutaneous vascular closure components hidden. (Image courtesy St. Jude Medical, St. Paul, MN.)

low-profile, balloon-positioning catheter in combination with a biologic, procoagulant compound.[68] In a registry-based analysis, the Mynx device performed similarly to Perclose and Angio-Seal (Fig. 31.11).[70]

The Vascade Vascular Closure System (Cardiva Medical, Sunnyvale, CA) is a new-generation extravascular technology that consists of a bioresorbable thrombogenic collagen patch. The device is compatible with 5-, 6-, or 7-Fr introducer sheaths and consists of an expandable nitinol disk that locates the vessel wall and provides temporary hemostasis and a retractable/lockable sleeve that houses a bovine-derived collagen patch. At the completion of the procedure, the Vascade device is inserted through the existing introducer sheath, the disk is deployed in the lumen of the artery, the sheath is removed over the device, and the disc is brought against the vessel wall to achieve temporary hemostasis.[71]

Suture-Based Closure Devices

The percutaneous suture-mediated closure device is a method to achieve arteriotomy hemostasis in a safe and timely manner. Several studies have shown the efficacy of percutaneous suture-mediated closure devices in decreasing time to hemostasis and time to ambulation without increasing the rate of access-site complications. However, experience suggests that the devices may result in infrequent but challenging vascular complications of the groin, such as retroperitoneal hemorrhage, arterial thromboses, infections, dissections, and large pseudoaneurysms. Proper training and operator skills are necessary for the successful use of these suture-based closure devices. The use of standard aseptic techniques in all cases, along with a single dose of prophylactic intravenous antibiotics during placement of the percutaneous suture-mediated closure device in high-risk patients, appears to prevent infectious complications.

The Perclose ProGlide (Abbott Vascular Devices) was the first suture-based closure device in the market, and it is based solely on sutures. The main advantage of Perclose ProGlide compared with other closure devices is that no material is left at the puncture site, except for the sutures. Needles are used to guide the sutures through the vessel wall. The Prostar (Abbott) device uses four needles and two sutures while the ProGlide devices use two needles and one suture. They can be used with 6- to 10-Fr sheaths. Perclose consists of several components, including an automatic knot-pushing tool, and the suture-containing device itself. This tool consists of a sheath connected to a handle by a guide that is introduced into the vessel by means of the 0.035-inch guidewire after the angioplasty sheath has been removed.

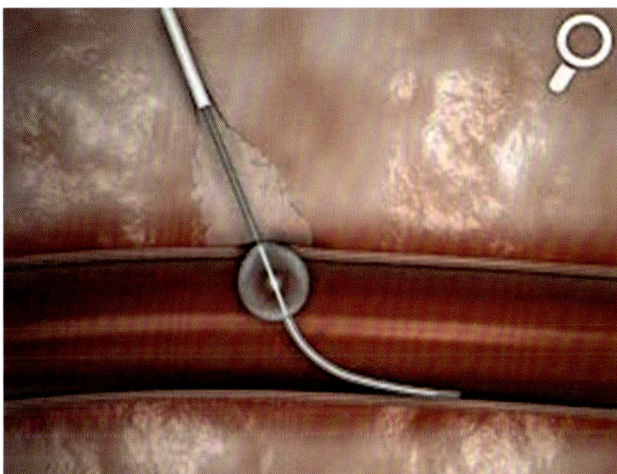

Fig. 31.11 The Mynx hemostatic device uses a low-profile, balloon-positioning catheter in combination with a biologic, procoagulant-containing bovine collagen and thrombin solution.

When the intravascular position has been achieved, the device is secured by pulling the lever and releasing the anchor. Using the needle plunger, needles are inserted through the vessel wall and grip the sutures. The needles are then retracted until they are outside of the skin with the sutures. Each of the two suture ends can be retrieved and pulled down to the surface of the artery with the help of a knot pusher. This improved device has shortened the time of deployment and improved handling. After it is apparent that hemostasis will be achieved, the guidewire is removed with further sequential tightening of the suture pairs.

In the contemporary era of interventional cardiology that requires large-bore sheaths for structural heart procedures and advanced mechanical circulatory support devices, this devices uses the "preclosing technique."[72] This technique allows the operator for the "off-label" use of the Prostar or two ProGlide devices to achieve hemostasis for larger sheaths. After accessing the CFA with a 6- to 10-Fr sheath, a Prostar suture-mediated closure device is deployed without tying it. As an alternative, two sequential and perpendicular ProGlides can be implanted. After the intervention is finalized, the preloaded sutures are tied over the large sheath while it is removed. The modified "preclosure" technique is a feasible alternative for hemostasis after using larger sheaths (12- to 18-Fr) to avoid the open surgical cutdown and diminish the need for general anesthesia.[45] Observational data and one randomized trial suggest that a percutaneous approach to transcatheter aortic valve replacement or Endograft using VCD with preclosure offers similar vascular outcomes to surgical cutdown for arterial access.[73,74]

The StarClose SE (Abbott Vascular Devices, Redwood City, CA) is a clip-based femoral closure device (Fig. 31.12).[75] The clips are made of nitinol alloy that are deployed through the existing procedural sheath. The extravascular approach closes by apposing the tissue at and above the arteriotomy site, leaving nothing in the arterial lumen. The artery may be accessed again shortly after hemostasis has been achieved.

Although relatively high success rates have been reported with the use of the device (≈88%),[76–78] the information is contradictory.[79]

Electrical-Based Sealing Pads

The use of noninvasive closure devices for interventional procedures has rapidly increased in the past few years.[80] The patch technologies are a new form of biologically active, superficially applied therapies that accelerate local hemostasis at the puncture site.[81] One of the substances used in these pads is chitosan, derived from the deacetylation of chitin. Chitin is obtained from the shells of lobsters, crab, and shrimp. Chitin has a slightly positive charge, and chitosan has a strong positive charge, but erythrocytes and platelets are negatively charged. Because of their positive charges, chitin and chitosan attract negatively charged platelets and red blood cells to the applied area. Other hemostatic pads are impregnated with chemicals such as bovine thrombin or potato starch. These agents, combined with effective manual compression, may result in a shorter time to hemostasis and a stronger blood clot at the puncture site. These devices are effectively used for adjunctive closure devices or as hemostatic accelerators for manual compression of the access site. The simple application and the low cost make this system attractive. The reliability of these devices, however, still needs to be evaluated in a larger number of patients.

Chito-Seal Topical Hemostasis Pad (Abbott Vascular Devices, Redwood City, CA) is intended for use in the management of bleeding wounds such as vascular access sites. The pad is coated with chitosan gel, which is a powerful hemostatic agent twice as chemically active as chitin. The Clo-Sur P.A.D. (Scion Cardio-Vascular, Miami, FL) is a pad consisting of hydrophilic, naturally occurring biopolymer polyprolate acetate. It also activates electrical interference between erythrocytes and the pad, leading to red blood cell agglutination and clot formation. The SyvekPatch (Marine Polymer Technologies, Danvers, MA), an external device used to control bleeding from vascular access sites, consists of a poly-N-acetyl glucosamine polymer, which is isolated from a microalga. The mechanism of action involves clot formation and local vasoconstriction as part of its hemostatic effect. Neptune Pad, BIOTRONIK's noninvasive hemostasis device, is made of calcium alginate derived from seaweed with antimicrobial and wound-healing properties.

ACCESS-SITE COMPLICATIONS

Local bleeding or vascular complications at the site of catheter insertion constitute the most common adverse events after cardiovascular interventions. Access-site complications can extend the patient's length of hospitalization and increase the associated procedural costs.

Access-site bleeding complication is defined as blood loss at the site of arterial or venous access, or due to perforation of an artery or vein requiring transfusion, prolonging the hospital stay, or causing a drop in hemoglobin of >3.0 g/dL. Bleeding attributable to the vascular site could be retroperitoneal, a local hematoma (defined as >10 cm with femoral access, >2 cm with radial access, or >5 cm with brachial access), or external at the entry site. However, vascular complication includes the presence of any

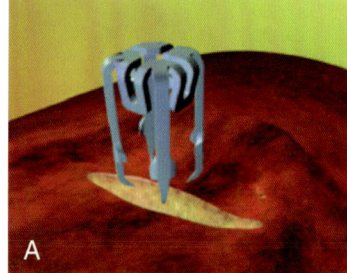
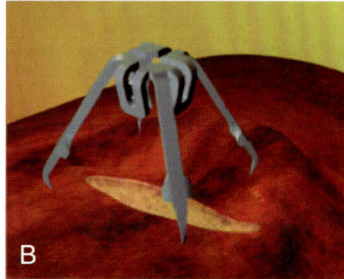
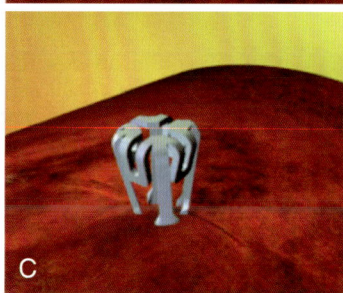
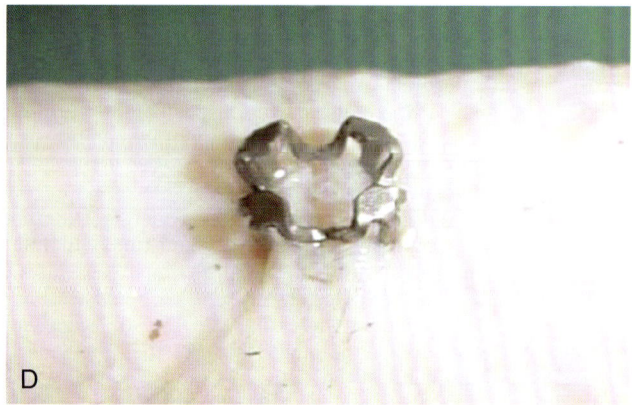

Fig. 31.12 Expanding staple-based closure device. (A) Staple tracks are small and deployed through a sterile delivery system, reducing the chance of touch contamination. (B) The device expands wide above the arteriotomy to close the arteriotomy. (C) It purses the arteriotomy closed to promote healing, does not remodel the vessel, and has no intraluminal components to impede flow. (D) The staple gathers the full thickness of the vessel media and adventitia for a secure mechanical closure. (Photograph courtesy Medtronic, Minneapolis, MN.)

one of the following vascular complications: occlusion (defined as total obstruction of the artery by thrombus or dissection), embolization, dissection, pseudoaneurysm (defined as the occurrence of a disruption and dilation of the arterial wall without identification of the arterial wall layers at the site of the catheter entry), or arteriovenous fistula. Other rare complications are neural damage and vascular infection.

Patient characteristics associated with an increased risk of bleeding or vascular complications include age, female gender, body mass index, renal failure, peripheral vascular disease, hypertension, congestive heart failure, acute myocardial infarction, recent angioplasty, use of intraaortic balloon pump during the procedure, emergency procedure, and use of IIb/IIIa inhibitors, thrombolytics, low-molecular-weight heparin, or unfractionated heparin during the procedure.[14]

The American College of Cardiology-National Cardiovascular Data Registry (ACC-NCDR) reported an overall in-hospital serious adverse event rate related to vascular access of 1.72% among 1,819,611 percutaneous coronary intervention procedures performed via femoral access site at 1089 American sites that submitted data to the CathPCI Registry from 2005 through 2009.

Before vascular closure device placement, a femoral artery angiogram through the sheath should be obtained to assess the puncture site, vessel diameter, and presence and severity of atherosclerosis. It can help to identify patients at higher risk for groin complications. Some femoral closure devices should be avoided when the artery diameter is less than 5 mm and in cases of higher or lower femoral punctures.

Bleeding complications occur more frequently while obtaining access and positioning sheaths or early after removal when local pressure is not properly achieved. Several comorbid conditions have been associated with groin complications.

Hematoma

Hematoma is considered a significant complication when it has a diameter of more than 10 cm. The incidence of local hematoma varies from 1% to 5%, and most hematomas require only observation and no further intervention. Occasionally, hematoma-mediated femoral nerve compression accompanying limb weakness may occur. It resolves spontaneously within 2 to 3 weeks.

Retroperitoneal Hemorrhage

Retroperitoneal hemorrhage remains an infrequent but occasionally devastating consequence of percutaneous cardiovascular intervention. The incidence of retroperitoneal hemorrhage is 0.29%; 73% of these patients require blood transfusions, and 10% die during hospitalization.[33] Retroperitoneal hemorrhage is independently associated with "high femoral artery stick" when femoral artery sheaths are placed superior to the inferior epigastric artery, with female gender, with the use of an Angio-Seal device, with the use of a GP IIb/IIIa inhibitor, with a presentation of acute myocardial infarction, and inversely with the patient's weight.[23] Other studies have confirmed three factors to be predictive for retroperitoneal hemorrhage (female gender, low body weight, and high femoral puncture), whereas the use of GP IIb/IIIa, sheath size, and the use of a closure device did not correlate with bleeding complications.[82] Bleeding complications should be considered when a patient has a new onset of hypotension, flank pain, or decreased hematocrit level. Strict adherence to meticulous vascular access technique, the judicious use of closure devices, and appropriate and rapid management when this complication is suspected should lessen the occasionally serious consequences related to this problem.

A major cause of retroperitoneal bleeding is a puncture above the inguinal ligament. When the posterior arterial wall is punctured, blood can spread into the retroperitoneal space. The location of the inferior epigastric artery may be helpful in judging the location of the puncture with regard to the inguinal ligament. The inferior border of this vessel defines the border of the inguinal ligament and represents a marker by which femoral punctures can be assessed for possible risk of retroperitoneal bleeding. The inferior epigastric artery arises from the distal external iliac artery just before it crosses under the inguinal ligament to enter the thigh and become the femoral artery. It typically originates opposite the deep iliac circumflex branch and bears a direct relation to the inferior extent of the peritoneal transversalis fascia. When the entry site of the sheath is superior to the origin of

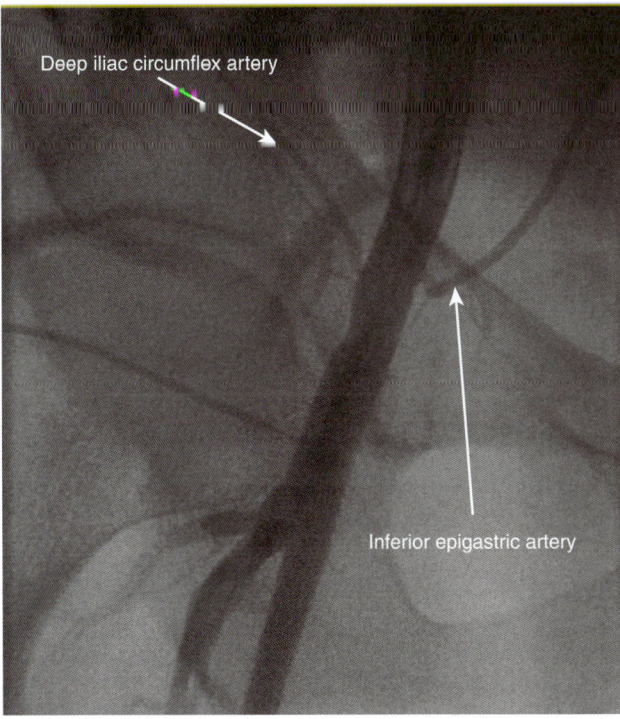

Fig. 31.13 Angiogram through the sheath to assess the femoral artery and puncture location. The right anterior oblique, 30-degree projection of a typical femoral artery access site shows the inferior epigastric entry in relation to its surrounding anatomy. The inferior epigastric artery arises from the distal external iliac artery just before it crosses under the inguinal ligament; the inferior border of this vessel defines the border of the inguinal ligament.

the inferior epigastric artery, the sheath passes through various layers of the anterior abdominal wall, including superficial fascia and muscles, before entering the artery (Fig. 31.13). The collagen plug–based closure devices may not reach the wall of the artery in some cases. Therefore, the operator should be careful in choosing the site of cannulation of the femoral artery. Fluoroscopy can be used to ascertain the relative location of the femoral head and pelvic brim in that endeavor (see Fig. 31.2B). The retroperitoneal space appears to be able to sequester large amounts of blood. Volume and blood product support and correction of thrombin and platelet inhibition are central to management when this complication is suspected. Although CT or other forms of imaging are occasionally useful in diagnosing retroperitoneal hemorrhage, this modality is usually not required, and it may delay treatment. Peripheral vascular surgery or endovascular treatment is appropriate if blood product transfusion does not result in hemodynamic stabilization or if there is clinically significant organ or nerve compression.

Pseudoaneurysm

The incidence of iatrogenic femoral pseudoaneurysm after percutaneous procedures is around 0.4%. A pseudoaneurysm is a hematoma that remains in continuity with the artery, allowing flow in and out of the hematoma. It can be differentiated from a simple hematoma by the presence of a bruit and a palpable pulsatile mass. Pseudoaneurysms are normally detected by ultrasound (Fig. 31.14). Older age, obesity, female gender, larger sheath size, peripheral vascular disease, a low arterial puncture site below the common femoral bifurcation, and the level of anticoagulation are associated with this complication. A pseudoaneurysm larger than 3 cm in diameter usually is treated by mechanical compression, thrombin

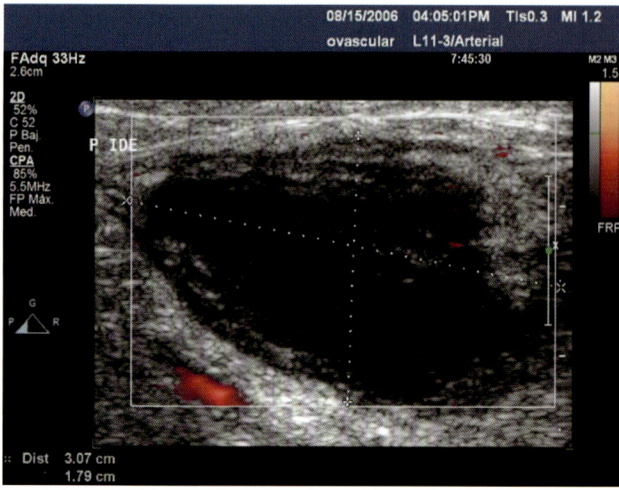

Fig. 31.14 Pseudoaneurysm arising from the common femoral artery is assessed by duplex ultrasound.

injection, or surgery. Smaller pseudoaneurysms can be followed by serial ultrasound. Ultrasound-guided manual or mechanical compression is often used to convert the pseudoaneurysm to a thrombosed hematoma by compressing the neck connecting it to the artery. Ultrasound-guided, low-dose thrombin injection appears to be more effective in reducing the need for surgical repair, is better tolerated by the patient, and requires a shorter hospital stay.[83]

Arteriovenous Fistula

Arteriovenous fistula is defined as an abnormal connection between an artery and vein. This may be caused by trauma, improper removal of adjacent arterial and venous sheaths, or inadvertent puncture of a vein while accessing an artery. It is an uncommon and low-risk groin complication that is suspected by the detection of a continuous bruit at the access site, and it is diagnosed by ultrasound. In cases of arterial insufficiency, the fistula can be treated with ultrasound-guided compression, endovascular stenting, or surgical repair.

Vessel Occlusion

Vessel occlusion associated with manual compression may occur because of excessive occlusive pressure during the compression process. Patients with diabetes, female patients, or those with peripheral vascular disease have arteries with reduced lumen diameters and may be more susceptible to this complication. Vessel occlusion is characterized by a sudden onset of pain and possible paresthesia. The affected limb is cyanotic, is cool, and has diminished or absent pulses. Treatment methods for vessel occlusion include administration of heparin or lytic agents or an endovascular or surgical thrombectomy procedure.

Access-Site Infections

Although relatively uncommon, vascular closure device–related infection is an emerging and serious phenomenon with a high morbidity rate. It requires aggressive medical and surgical intervention to achieve cure.[84] Access-site infections manifest with high fever, femoral abscess, septic thrombosis, and mycotic aneurysm. The predominant source of pathogens is the endogenous flora of the patient's skin. Attention to skin preparation is part of the infection prevention strategy. Diabetes mellitus and obesity are the most common associated comorbidities. Infectious groin complications are significantly increased with suture-based closure devices. Surgical removal of the percutaneous closure device

and debridement to normal arterial wall are recommended for all patients with suspected femoral endarteritis. Before inserting a closure device, it is recommended to again prepare the skin insertion site and remove any pooled blood before beginning the arterial closure, especially in the case of a prolonged procedure. If compromise of sterile technique is suspected, the operator should consider a change of gloves before beginning the arterial closure and a change of towels around the skin insertion site, especially if the drape has become saturated with blood. Some interventionalists routinely administer one or more doses of intravenous antibiotics when using a vascular closure device. Although some differences may exist regarding local complications with the use of femoral closure systems, neither device has been shown to reduce major local complications.

CONCLUSIONS AND FUTURE TRENDS

Access-site complications continue to be the most common adverse events after cardiovascular interventions extending patient's length of hospitalization and increasing the associated procedural costs.

Several femoral access closure technologies are on the interventional field offering equivalent or even better patient outcomes compared with manual compression. There has been a consistent improvement of the safety profile of VCDs over time. The ease of use is continuing to improve, patients are being more carefully selected, and operators are gaining more experience with them. Sealing and suturing closure devices have been shown to shorten hemostasis time, reduce the discomfort of manual or mechanical compression, and allow earlier ambulation after cardiovascular procedures compared with conventional compression techniques. The patch technologies are a new form of biologically active, superficially applied therapies that have found acceptance in many practices. Ultimately, the further expansion of femoral closure devices will depend on which device provides a simple approach with reliable hemostasis at a cost that can justify their incorporation into routine practice. There is still a special need for dedicated femoral closure devices for larger arteriotomies for aortic endovascular repair and aortic valve replacement.

KEY REFERENCES

1. Jolly SS, Amlani S, Hamon M, et al. Radial versus femoral access for coronary angiography or intervention and the impact on major bleeding and ischemic events: a systematic review and meta-analysis of randomized trials. *Am Heart J*. 2009;157:132–140.
4. Romagnoli E, Biondi-Zoccai G, Sciahbasi A, et al. Radial versus femoral randomized investigation in ST-segment elevation acute coronary syndrome: the RIFLE-STEACS (Radial Versus Femoral Randomized Investigation in ST-Elevation Acute Coronary Syndrome) study. *J Am Coll Cardiol*. 2012;60:2481–2489.
13. Schulz-Schüpke S, Helde S, Gewalt S, et al. Comparison of vascular closure devices vs manual compression after femoral artery puncture: the ISAR-CLOSURE randomized clinical trial. *JAMA*. 2014;312(19):1981–1987.
14. Tavris DR, Wang Y, Jacobs S, et al. Bleeding and vascular complications at the femoral access site following percutaneous coronary intervention (PCI): an evaluation of hemostasis strategies. *J Invasive Cardiol*. 2012;24:328–334.
23. Ellis SG, Bhatt D, Kapadia S, et al. Correlates and outcomes of retroperitoneal hemorrhage complicating percutaneous coronary intervention. *Catheter Cardiovasc Interv*. 2006;67:541–545.
24. Damluji AA, Nelson DW, Valgimigli M, et al. Transfemoral approach for coronary angiography and intervention: a collaboration of international cardiovascular societies. *JACC Cardiovasc Interv*. 2017;10(22):2269–2279.
27. Abu-Fadel MS, Sparling JM, Zacharias SJ, et al. Fluoroscopy vs. traditional guided femoral arterial access and the use of closure devices: a randomized controlled trial. *Catheter Cardiovasc Interv*. 2009;74:533–539.

30. Seto AH, Abu-Fadel MS, Sparling JM, et al. Real-time ultrasound guidance facilitates femoral arterial access and reduces vascular complications: FAUST (Femoral Arterial Access With Ultrasound Trial). *JACC Cardiovasc Interv*. 2010;3(7):751–758.
32. Marquis-Gravel G, Tremblay-Gravel M, Levesque J, et al. Ultrasound guidance versus anatomical landmark approach for femoral artery access in coronary angiography: a randomized controlled trial and a meta-analysis. *J Interv Cardiol*. 2018;31(4):496–503. https://doi.org/10.1111/joic.12492.
33. Ambrose JA, Lardizabal J, Mouanoutoua M, et al. Femoral micropuncture or routine introducer study (FEMORIS). *Cardiology*. 2014;129(1):39–43.
44. Martin JL, Pratsos A, Magargee E, et al. A randomized trial comparing compression, Perclose Proglide and Angio-Seal VIP for arterial closure following percutaneous coronary intervention: the CAP trial. *Catheter Cardiovasc Interv*. 2008;71(1):1–5.
46. Cox T, Blair L, Huntington C, et al. Systematic review of randomized controlled trials comparing manual compression to vascular closure devices for diagnostic and therapeutic arterial procedures. *Surg Technol Int*. 2015;27:32–44.
51. Hvelplund A, Jeger R, Osterwalder R, et al. The Angio-Seal™ femoral closure device allows immediate ambulation after coronary angiography and percutaneous coronary intervention. *EuroIntervention*. 2011;7(2):234–241.
52. Veasey RA, Large JK, Silberbauer J, et al. A randomised controlled trial comparing StarClose and AngioSeal vascular closure devices in a district general hospital—the SCOAST study. *Int J Clin Pract*. 2008;62(6):912–918.
53. Biancari F, D'Andrea V, Di Marco C, et al. Meta-analysis of randomized trials on the efficacy of vascular closure devices after diagnostic angiography and angioplasty. *Am Heart J*. 2010;159(4):518–531.
63. Pieper CC, Wilhelm KE, Schild HH, et al. Feasibility of vascular access closure in arteries other than the common femoral artery using the ExoSeal vascular closure device. *Cardiovasc Interv Radiol*. 2014;37(5):1352–1357.
67. Pieper CC, Thomas D, Nadal J, et al. Patient satisfaction after femoral arterial access site closure using the ExoSeal(®) vascular closure device compared to manual compression: a prospective intra-individual comparative study. *Cardiovasc Intervent Radiol*. 2016;39(1):21–27.

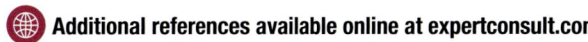

Additional references available online at expertconsult.com.

中文导读

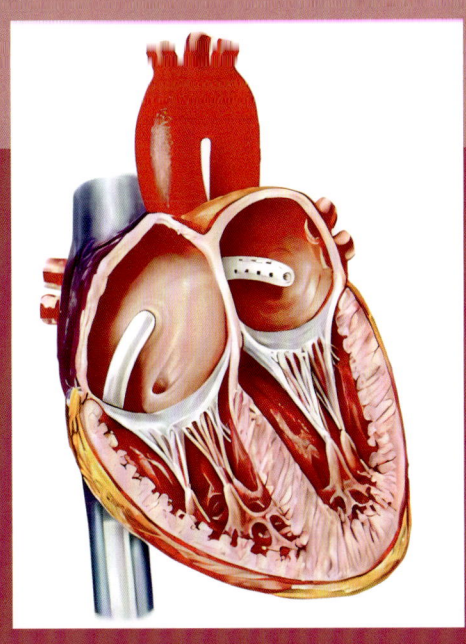

第32章
经桡动脉途径的心血管诊疗

  桡动脉和尺动脉通常是肱动脉的末端分支，多起源于肘部以下。它沿着前臂外缘到达手腕，通过掌浅弓和掌深弓与尺动脉的分支相连。在手腕前的远端3~5 cm处，非常表浅。桡神经在此改变方向，使得与刺穿相关的神经损伤几乎不可能发生。桡动脉周围没有大静脉，也降低了动静脉瘘的风险。由于这样的解剖结构，经桡动脉入路进行诊断性血管造影和经皮冠状动脉介入治疗具有更高的可靠性和安全性。

  经股动脉入路曾经是冠状动脉造影和经皮冠状动脉介入治疗最常用的方式。为了降低经皮冠状动脉介入治疗相关血栓并发症，围术期抗栓治疗方案就显得必不可少，然而，这也同时增加了股动脉通路—部位相关的出血并发症。因此，在过去20年里越来越多术者开始选择经桡动脉入路进行心脏介入诊疗手术。本章介绍了经桡动脉入路的使用、禁忌证、并发症等相关知识。在"现实世界"中，只要手术操作和器械能为≤7 F指引导管所兼容，均可采用经桡动脉入路。因此，经桡动脉入路是冠状动脉介入治疗的一个重要且安全的血管入路。

陈文杰   柳景华

章节要点

- 经皮冠状动脉介入治疗后入路部位和非入路部位出血并发症与包括死亡在内的不良预后相关。
- 诊断性血管造影术和经皮冠状动脉介入治疗采用经桡动脉入路，几乎不会发生穿刺部位大出血，而且便于患者早期活动，并增加随后的临床净获益。
- 在经过最初较短的学习曲线之后，经桡动脉入路与经股动脉入路的手术成功率基本接近。
- 在任何临床情况下，所有能与5 F、6 F或7 F指引导管相兼容的手术和器械均可采用经桡动脉入路。
- 当急性冠状动脉综合征行经皮冠状动脉介入治疗时，经桡动脉入路可降低包括死亡在内的主要不良心血管事件的发生率。

32 Transradial Access for Cardiovascular Catheterization and Intervention

Farzin Beygui, Olivier F. Bertrand, Gilles Montalescot

KEY POINTS

- Access-site and nonaccess-site bleeding complications after percutaneous coronary intervention (PCI) are associated with poor outcome, including mortality.
- A transradial approach (TRA) for diagnostic angiography and PCI is associated with virtually no major access-site bleeding, early ambulation, and subsequent increase of net clinical benefit.
- After an initial short learning curve, the procedural success rates of TRA become similar to those of the transfemoral approach.
- TRA can be used in any clinical condition for all procedures and devices compatible with 5-, 6-, or 7-Fr guiding catheters.
- A TRA is associated with a reduction of major adverse cardiovascular event rates including mortality in the setting of PCI for acute coronary syndromes.

INTRODUCTION

Although both diagnostic coronary angiography and percutaneous coronary intervention (PCI) are still most commonly performed via transfemoral access in a large number of catheterization laboratories in the United States, the transradial access is now the default approach in Europe and Asia, accounting for more than 80% of PCI procedures. The development of highly potent antithrombotic regimens associated not only with a major reduction in thrombotic complications of PCI, but also with an increase in femoral access-site–related bleeding complications, has led to the development of the transradial approach (TRA) for PCI during the past two decades. While TRA adoption in the United States has been relatively slow, recent reports document a steady increase, now encompassing 30% to 40% of PCI.[1] Similarly, primary PCI is more and more frequently performed with TRA, as shown in the international randomized Acute ST-elevation myocardial infarction (STEMI) Treated With Primary Angioplasty and Intravenous Enoxaparin or unfractionated heparin (UFH) to Lower Ischemic and Bleeding Events at Short- and Long-Term Follow-Up (ATOLL) study, in which 66% of procedures used the radial artery.[2] The growing interest in TRA is also apparent in the medical literature, as more than 1500 publications concerning the subject have been reported within the past 5 years.

RATIONALE FOR TRANSRADIAL APPROACH TO PERCUTANEOUS CORONARY INTERVENTION

Anatomic Considerations

The radial artery, as well as the ulnar artery, is usually a terminal branch of the brachial artery, originating below the elbow. In some cases, the radial artery originates from the upper brachial artery or even directly from the axillary artery. It follows the external margin of the forearm to reach the wrist, where it divides (most of the time) into two branches, joining branches of the ulnar artery through superficial and deep palmar arches. The palmar arches also may be irrigated by branches of the common interosseous artery, a high-originating branch of the ulnar artery. Quite superficial all along, the radial artery is covered by the brachioradialis muscle proximally. It becomes very superficial and accessible in its 3- to 5-cm distal portion before the wrist, considered the puncture site. Moreover, the satellite radial nerve changes direction at this final portion, making puncture-related nerve injury almost impossible. The absence of major veins around the radial artery also reduces the risk of arteriovenous fistula. Because of such anatomy, TRA for diagnostic angiography and PCI appears to be very safe. Very recently, some radial operators have described the use of the distal radial artery, which is accessed at the "snuffbox" dorsal level of the hand at the junction of the intersection of the thumb and first finger.[3] Although early results seem promising especially for left distal TRA in postcoronary artery bypass grafting (CABG) patients, few data have been reported on safety and benefits compared to standard TRA.

FEASIBILITY AND SECURITY

Following the initial study in 1989,[4] the feasibility and safety of TRA for coronary diagnostic or interventional procedures have been widely demonstrated by studies in the 1990s and early 2000s showing rates of successful PCI ranging from 90% to 100%.

As with any technique, TRA requires a learning curve, which has been ascribed to be less than 100 cases.[5,6] Beyond that curve, experience leads to higher rates of procedural success and lower x-ray exposure. A recent meta-analysis demonstrated that, although they are associated with a statistically significantly higher operator x-ray exposure, the difference between transradial and transfemoral approaches becomes less significant with operators' experience.[7] The importance of the learning curve was also highlighted by the American National Cardiovascular Data Registry (NCDR), based on a study population of 54,561 patients. It showed that, on the one hand, as the operators' transradial intervention volume increases, more high-risk patients are treated, whereas on the other hand, fluoroscopy time, contrast volume, and bleeding risk are reduced. The threshold to overcome the learning curve is still debated but is around 30 to 50 cases.[8]

Both operator and patient x-ray exposures may be reduced by simple methods such as reducing the fluoroscopy rate from 15 to 7.5 frames per second, using leaded shields and patient support (e.g., starsystem), as well as maintaining the longest distance between x-ray source and operators. The recently developed robotic-assisted PCI solutions—Corindus, Robocath—may, in the future, dramatically reduce the operators' x-ray exposure regardless of the vascular approach.

Overall the feasibility of a TRA for diagnostic or interventional coronary procedures is high (>90%), especially in experienced centers (>95%). In a series of 1119 consecutive South Korean patients, the mean radial artery diameter measured by ultrasound was 2.6 (±0.41) mm in men and 2.43 (±0.38) mm in women.[9] In another series of 250 Japanese patients, the radial artery diameter was larger than 7- and 8-Fr catheters in 71.5% and 44.9% of male patients, respectively, and 40.3% and 24% of female patients, respectively.[10] Although such data may not be totally generalized to all other populations, it underlies the fact that the TRA could potentially be used in a vast majority of patients with 5-, 6-, and even 7-Fr catheters. In some patients with sufficiently large artery diameter, 8-Fr catheters may also be used if needed. Yet it must be remembered that catheter–radial artery diameter mismatch is associated with a higher risk of radial artery occlusion.

TRA has been used for different types of procedures with various devices and methods such as intravascular ultrasound (IVUS)–guided stenting, coronary brachytherapy, distal protection, embolectomy, rotational atherectomy, bifurcated stents, and so on. However, this approach is still incompatible with the intraaortic balloon pump (IABP) and all other devices or procedures needing 8-Fr or greater access. It is interesting to note that TRA is now becoming more popular for peripheral interventions too.

The use of sheathless guiding catheters with smaller outer diameters—6.5- and 7.5-Fr catheters, equivalent to 5- and 6-Fr introducer diameters, respectively—has been reported to be feasible and safe.[11] Although their use remains somewhat limited, such catheters may allow more complex procedures, such as simultaneous "kissing" stenting, in patients with small radial arteries.

More recently, the 5- to 7-Fr thin-walled slender sheaths with outer diameters smaller than standard sheaths have been developed. The 6-Fr slender was compared to a 5-Fr standard sheath in a multicenter study reporting no significant difference between the two groups in terms of radial artery occlusion rates. However, the noninferiority for the slender sheath was not demonstrated because of the very low event rates.[12] If confirmed by further studies, such technology may allow the use of larger devices in small radial arteries.

TRA may be somewhat limited in patients who have previously undergone CABG. A recently published small ($n = 128$) monocentric randomized study in this setting (58% diagnostic angiography alone) reported higher crossover rates, contrast volume, procedure time, and patient and operator exposure in the global group associated with a left transradial compared with a transfemoral approach. Nevertheless, as acknowledged by authors (most of them trained femoralists), with the first operator being always a trainee, the study may have been biased for the radiation exposure and contrast volume parameters. Furthermore, in the subgroup of patients who underwent PCI, procedural success was similar between the two groups.[13] In patients with a left mammary graft, it is usually easier to cannulate the ostium selectively by using a left radial approach. However, selective catheterization of left or right internal thoracic bypasses is often possible via the contralateral approach, such as by using a Judkins left or other dedicated catheter. In patients with bilateral left internal thoracic bypasses, technical difficulties can be overcome easily by a bilateral radial access.

In a recent publication from a high radial volume center with a radial-first strategy, based on a consecutive series of more than 1600 patients, a transfemoral approach was directly used in 2.7% of patients, and in another 1.8%, it was used after a failed attempt at a TRA.[14] Female sex, previous CABG, and cardiogenic shock were independent predictors of TRA failure.

TRANSRADIAL VERSUS TRANSFEMORAL APPROACH FOR PERCUTANEOUS CORONARY INTERVENTION

The transfemoral approach represents an easily accessible superficial arterial access point, through which large catheters delivering all types of devices could be introduced. Compared with the transfemoral approach, TRA is associated with fewer vascular complications, more comfort for patients, and the possibility of rapid ambulation, lower procedure cost, and reduced hospital stay and cost. Several randomized trials comparing advantages and disadvantages of each method are summarized in Table 32.1.

The first landmark international randomized trial comparing the transradial and transfemoral approaches was the Radial Versus Femoral Access for Coronary Intervention (RIVAL) trial,[15] which included 7021 acute coronary syndrome (ACS) patients randomly assigned to each of the approaches for angiography and/or PCI. Indications for angiography were ST-elevation myocardial infarction (STEMI) in 27.2% and 28.5%, and non-STEMI (NSTEMI) in 28.5% and 25.8% in transradial and transfemoral groups, respectively. Angiography was performed in 99.8% and PCI was performed in approximately 66% of patients in both groups. PCI success rates were comparable between the two groups (95.4% vs. 95.2%), with higher access-site crossover rates in the transradial group (7.6% vs. 2%, $P < .0001$). The rates of the primary end point—the composite of death, myocardial infarction (MI), stroke, or non-CABG bleeding at 30 days—were comparable between the transradial and transfemoral groups (3.7% and 4%) as were each of the individual components. However, the secondary end point of major vascular complications occurred more often in the transfemoral group (1.4% vs. 3.7%, $P < .0001$). Moreover, all post hoc exploratory outcomes including major bleeding, the composite of death or MI or major bleeding and the composite of major non-CABG bleeding and vascular complications were met more often in the transfemoral group.

Although RIVAL failed to show a significant difference between the two groups regarding the primary end point used in the protocol, two major findings in the subgroup analysis should be underlined: first, in the STEMI subgroup of the study, the TRA was associated not only with a significant reduction of the primary end point, but also a reduction in mortality; second, the primary end point was also significantly reduced by the TRA in the centers with the highest radial PCI volume (hazard ratio [HR] 0.49; 95% confidence interval [CI] 0.28 to 0.87), which highlights the importance of the learning curve and operator experience for the TRA. The results of the RIVAL trial in the setting of ACS were more recently confirmed in the Minimizing Adverse Haemorrhagic Events by TRansradial Access Site and Systemic Implementation of angioX (MATRIX Access) trial, which randomly assigned 8404 ACS patients with or without ST-segment elevation, to radial or femoral access for angiography and PCI. The study showed a reduction of major adverse cardiovascular events, (relative risk [RR] 0.85; $P = .03$), net adverse clinical events (NACEs) (RR 0.83; $P = .009$), major bleeding unrelated to coronary artery bypass surgery (RR 0.67; $P = .013$) and all-cause mortality (RR 0.72; $P = .045$).[16] The results were consistent among all patient subgroups, including the ACS presentation type, with the exception of a significant interaction, supporting the highest benefit in high radial volume centers. A meta-analysis of studies comparing transradial versus transfemoral approach in the setting of ACS incorporated in the latter publication confirmed the significant benefit of TRA in reducing rates of death, major cardiovascular events, and major non-CABG bleeding.

The overall advantages of TRA also have been underscored by three meta-analyses showing an initial higher procedural success rate for the transfemoral approach, but a clear trend toward equalization of procedural success rates between the two approaches through the years, and significant advantages of TRA in terms of bleeding complications, mainly through a dramatic reduction of entry-site complications as well as composite end points of cardiovascular events, including mortality.[17–19]

Such advantages make the TRA the access of choice for same-day PCI, which has been reported to be highly feasible, safe, and cost effective in such indication.[20] Several centers in Europe and the United States are now introducing the concept of "radial lounges" to accommodate patients before and after catheterization in an environment similar to an "airport lounge."

TABLE 32.1 Randomized Trials Comparing Transradial and Transfemoral Approaches for Percutaneous Coronary Intervention

Study/Author	Type of Procedure	N	Technical Success (%)		Access-Site Complication (%)		Other End points
			TR	TF	TR	TF	
MATRIX[59]	Diagnostic ± PCI for ACS	8404 6721	100 92.7	99.9 92.8	0.1	0.4	Significant superiority of TR approach in terms of the death/MI/stroke, net clinical benefit, all-cause mortality, BARC 1, 2 and 3 bleeding
RIVAL trial[15]	Diagnostic and/or PCI for ACS	7021	92.4	98	1.4	3.7	Comparable rates of the primary end point—death, MI, stroke, and major bleeding at 30 days—significantly higher rates of femoral access-site complications
OCTOPLUS[22]	PCI in pts. >80 years	371	89	91	1.6	6.6	Trend to longer TR procedure duration
RADIAL-AMI[27]	Primary or rescue PCI	50	99.6	100	0.4	0.4	Similar fluoroscopy time and contrast media quantity
STEMI-RADIAL trial[32]	Primary PCI	707	96	97	0.3	0.8	Significant superiority of the TR approach for net adverse clinical events, bleeding, and duration of ICU stay
RIFLE-STEACS trial[33]	Primary or rescue PCI	1001	94	99	2.6	6.8	Significant superiority of TR approach for the 30-day primary end point of net adverse clinical events, death, bleeding, and duration of hospital stay
Mann et al.[60]	Stenting TR vs. TF with PerClose	218			0	3.4	TR reduced length of procedure, hospital stay, and total cost. PerClose: Inadequate in 18%, failure of hemostasis in 10%
Louvard et al.[61]	Diagnostic ± ad hoc PCI in ~43%	210	100	100	2	6	TR reduced length of stay, total cost, and was patient preferred, but it increased x-ray exposure length
Saito et al.[62]	Primary stenting	149	96	97	0	3	Comparable in-hospital MACE rates
Slagboom et al.[63]	Outpatient PCI	644	96	97	0	6	Similar rates of major bleeding, higher rates of same-day discharge, and lower rates of minor bleeding with TRA
Brasselet et al.[64]	Primary PCI with abciximab	114	91.6	96.5	3.5	19.3	Similar rates of bleeding, transfusion, and MACE; higher fluoroscopy time and earlier ambulation with TRA
Li et al.[65]	Primary PCI	370	98.4	98.9	2	7	Similar procedure times
Achenbach et al.[66]	PCI in patients aged >75	307	91	100	1.3	9	Higher examination time with TR but similar fluoroscopy time, number of catheters, and amount of contrast media
RADIAMI[67]	Primary PCI	100	94	98	2	12	Similar procedure times, clinical event rates, and bleeding rates
RADIAMI II[68]	Primary PCI, femoral access closure device	109	96	98	0	3	Longer door-to-balloon time in transradial approach, similar clinical adverse event and bleeding rates, successful closure of femoral access 93%

ACS, Acute coronary syndrome; *BARC,* Bleeding Academic Research Consortium; *ICU,* intensive care unit; *MACE,* major acute coronary events; *MATRIX,* Minimizing Adverse Haemorrhagic Events by TRansradial Access Site and Systemic Implementation of angioX; *MI,* myocardial infarction; *OCTOPLUS,* comparison of transradial and transfemoral approaches for coronary angiography and angioplasty in octogenarians; *PCI,* percutaneous coronary intervention; *pts.,* patients; *RADIAL-AMI,* Radial vs. femoral access for emergent PCI with adjunct glycoprotein IIb/IIIa inhibition in acute MI; *RADIAMI,* RADIal vs. femoral approach for PCI in patients with Acute MI; *RIVAL,* Radial Vs femorAL access for coronary intervention; *RIFLE-STEACS,* Radial Versus Femoral Randomized Investigation in ST-Elevation Acute Coronary Syndrome; *STEMI-RADIAL,* Trial Comparing Radial and Femoral Approach in Primary PCI; *TF,* transfemoral; *TR,* transradial; *TRA,* transradial approach.

The TRA is also of particular interest in patients at high risk for bleeding (older adults, women, patients with renal failure, the obese, or patients on multiple antithrombotic agents, especially glycoprotein [GP] IIb/IIIa inhibitors). The TRA has been reported to be associated with fewer vascular complications in obese patients (multivariate odds ratio [OR] 0.12; 95% CI 0.02 to 0.94; P = .043) in a retrospective series of 5234 diagnostic or interventional (56.6%) procedures,[21] as well as in older adults (1.6% vs. 6.5%, P = .03).[22] Other patients with obvious advantages for a radial, rather than a femoral, approach are patients with severe and/or proximal peripheral artery disease (PAD), patients with bilateral aortofemoral bypass grafts, those with aortic aneurysms, and patients with a prior history of femoral complication after catheterization. Unfortunately, data from NCDR registry illustrated the so-called "radial paradox" in which higher bleeding-risk patients are, in fact, less likely to undergo TRA in U.S. centers.[23]

TRA has been associated with reduced risks of acute kidney injury compared to the transfemoral approach concordantly demonstrated in different patient cohorts.[24,25] Such findings may be related to the reduced atheroembolic potential of the transradial access. Yet, further data from randomized comparison are required to better establish the mechanism of TRA impact and the magnitude of benefit for TRA compared to standard femoral access.

Finally, when considering all-comer PCI registries such as the RIVIERA registry,[26] which prospectively included 7962 unselected patients or the Canadian MORTAL registry of 38,872 procedures, the TRA appears to be independently associated to reduced rates of bleeding, death, or MI, at 30-day and 1-year mortality.[26,27]

The 2007–12 report of the NCDR (n = 2,820,874 procedures) comparing transradial and transfemoral approaches confirmed the prior findings with overall higher success rates (94.7% vs. 93.8%, adjusted OR 1.13, P < .001) and fewer vascular (0.16% vs. 0.45%, adjusted OR 0.51, P < .001) and bleeding complications (2.67% vs. 6.08%, adjusted OR 0.39, P < .001) with the TRA.[28]

TRANSRADIAL APPROACH IN ST-ELEVATION MYOCARDIAL INFARCTION

TRA is of particular interest in the setting of primary PCI for STEMI (Tables 32.1 and 32.2) performed by experienced operators in patients treated by aggressive antithrombotic regimens, in which life-threatening access-site bleeding complications and the subsequent major cardiovascular events may be avoided by such an approach. In this setting, growing evidence suggests that TRA is associated with overall similar door-to-balloon times, lower rates of vascular complication and bleeding in the presence of triple antithrombotic therapy,[27,29,30] and even reduced 30-day mortality compared with a femoral approach.[31] As mentioned above, in the STEMI subgroup of the RIVAL trial,[15] TRA was associated not only with a significant reduction of the primary end point (HR 0.6; 95% CI 0.38 to 0.94), but also with mortality (HR 0.39; 95% CI 0.20 to 0.76).

Two studies in the specific setting of PCI for STEMI confirmed overall the superiority of the transradial versus the transfemoral approach in terms of NACEs, combining bleeding, and thrombotic events.[32,33] Moreover, the Radial Versus Femoral Randomized Investigation in ST-Elevation Acute Coronary Syndrome (RIFLE-STEACS) trial reported a highly significant reduction of 30-day mortality and bleeding associated with a TRA (5.2% vs. 9.2%, P = .02, and 7.8% vs. 12.2%, P = .03).[33] Although the benefit of the TRA in terms of mortality were not specifically demonstrated in the MATRIX trial, the recently published comparison of STEMI versus non-ST ACS patients included in the trial showed that the results were consistent between groups of ACS patients based on the type of presentation.[34] Table 32.2 summarizes the results of the TRA versus transfemoral studies in the setting of STEMI.

A recent meta-analysis of 16 randomized trials, confirmed the latter data showing significant and consistent reductions in all-cause mortality (RR 0.68; 95% CI 0.54 to 0.85), major adverse cardiac events (RR, 0.80; 95% CI 0.68 to 0.94), and major bleeding (RR 0.56; 95% CI 0.42 to 0.74) by the transradial compared with the transfemoral approach.[35] It should be remembered that the exact mechanisms on how TRA might directly impact on survival benefit in primary PCI compared to femoral approach remains largely unknown and are likely multifactorial.

Finally, although based on observational studies, the feasibility and the benefit of the TRA seem to be preserved even in the setting of cardiogenic shock complicating STEMI.[36]

Considering such compelling data, the latest European Society of Cardiology (ESC) guidelines for the management of STEMI recommended a transradial over a transfemoral approach in the setting of primary PCI (level of recommendation Ia). Upcoming

TABLE 32.2 Recent Randomized Trials Comparing Transradial and Femoral Approaches in ST-Elevation Myocardial Infarction

30-Day End point	Transradial		Transfemoral		OR/RR (95% CI) Radial vs. Femoral Approach	P
	N/Total	%	N/Total	%		
Death						
RIVAL	12/955	2.7	32/1003	3.2	0.39 (0.20–0.76)	.026
RIFLE-STEACS[a]	26/500	5.2	46/501	9.2	—	.020
STEMI-RADIAL	8/348	2.3	11/359	3.1	—	.64
MATRIX[34]	48/2001	2.4	55/2009	2.7	0.87 (0.59–1.29)	.5
Death/MI/Stroke						
RIVAL	26/955	2.7	46/1003	4.6	0.59 (0.36–0.95)	.032
RIFLE-STEACS[b]	36/500	7.2	57/501	11.4	—	.029
STEMI-RADIAL	12/348	3.5	15/359	4.2	—	.7
MATRIX	121/2001	6.1	126/2009	6.3	0.96 (0.75–1.24)	.8
Major Bleeding						
RIVAL	8/955	0.8	9/1003	0.9	0.92 (0.0.36–2.39)	.87
RIFLE-STEACS	39/500	7.8	61/501	12.2	—	.026
STEMI-RADIAL	5/348	1.4	26/359	7.2	—	.0001
MATRIX	28/2001	1.5	50/2009	2.6	0.56 (0.35–0.89)	.01
Access-Site Crossover						
RIVAL	51/955	5.3	16/1003	1.6	3.32 (1.89–5.82)	<.0001
RIFLE-STEACS	47/500	9.4	14/501	2.8	—	—
STEMI-RADIAL	13/348	3.7	2/359	0.6	—	.003
MATRIX	144/2001	2.2	32/2009	1.6	—	<.0001

[a]Cardiac death.
[b]Death/myocardial infarction/target-lesion revascularization/stroke.
CI, Confidence interval; *MATRIX*, Minimizing Adverse Haemorrhagic Events by TRansradial Access Site and Systemic Implementation of angioX; *MI*, myocardial infarction; *OR*, odds ratio; *RIVAL*, Radial Vs femorAL access for coronary intervention; *RIFLE-STEACS*, Radial Versus Femoral Randomized Investigation in ST-Elevation Acute Coronary Syndrome; *RR*, relative risk; *STEMI-RADIAL*, Trial Comparing Radial and Femoral Approach in Primary PCI.

statements from U.S. scientific societies will also recommend higher use of TRA in catheterization laboratories.

TRANSRADIAL VERSUS TRANSBRACHIAL APPROACHES

Two of the previous randomized trials also had a transbrachial approach subgroup of patients. The Radial Versus Femoral Access for Coronary Angiography of Intervention and the Impact on Major Bleeding and Ischemic Events (ACCESS) study[37] reported comparable procedural success rates, equipment consumption, and procedural and fluoroscopy time among the three approaches for PCI. Nevertheless, the transbrachial approach was associated with higher rates of vascular complications compared with the TRA (2% vs. 0%, P = .035). The Brachial, Radial, or Femoral Approach for Elective Palmaz-Schatz Stent Implantation (BRAFE) stent study compared transradial and transfemoral approaches with a transbrachial cutdown approach, reporting no local vascular complication with the latter.[38] Such a brachial approach is not commonly used anymore (outside Japan) and still bears a higher risk of vascular complications. The brachial access does not need a cutdown and can be done with a classic percutaneous approach, but it is usually preferred when neither femoral nor radial approaches are possible.

TRANSRADIAL VERSUS TRANSULNAR APPROACH

The ulnar artery is usually less superficial than the radial artery, and both its puncture and compression may be technically more difficult. The Transulnar Versus Transradial Artery Approach for Coronary Angioplasty (PCVI-CUBA) study randomized 413 patients with a normal direct or reverse Allen test to undergo coronary angiography followed, or not, by PCI[39] through a transradial versus a transulnar approach. The two methods were associated with similar access success (96% vs. 93%), PCI success (96% vs. 95%), and asymptomatic access-site artery occlusion (5% vs. 6%) rates. A more recent noninferiority-designed randomized trial comparing the two approaches showed somewhat more conflicting results.[40] In this study, the transulnar approach was associated with more attempts before successful access (three vs. one, P < .001), longer procedural time, higher contrast volume, and much higher rates of crossover (32.3% vs. 5.9%, P = .004). Although the composite primary end point of crossover and major adverse cardiovascular and vascular events at 60 days was inconclusive, the transulnar approach appears to be only an alternative to transradial access for PCI and not a first-line strategy. Indeed, it remains technically more challenging; and with the ulnar nerve being closer to the ulnar artery, nerve injury remains an issue during puncture attempts and the hemostasis phase.

COST-EFFECTIVENESS

Systematic and concordant evidence suggests that because of a shorter length of hospital stay, possibility of same-day out, reduced nursing workload, reduced rates of complications, and absence of need for closure devices, the TRA is associated with significant cost reductions in both diagnostic angiography and PCI settings.

PRACTICAL CONSIDERATIONS FOR A TRANSRADIAL APPROACH

Contraindications to the Transradial Approach

The relative contraindications to a TRA are the presence of forearm arteriovenous fistula or a proven absence of collateral ulnar circulation (e.g., known occlusion of the ulnar artery). The TRA should be considered with precaution and after assessing the balance between other access-site complications and the risk of radial access in end-stage renal disease patients with the potential need for forearm arteriovenous fistula, and in patients with small or heavily calcified radial arteries. Ultimately, there are no absolute contraindications for TRA or transulnar catheterization, but it remains an important duty for the interventional cardiologist to explain to patients the risks-benefits of using the wrist access versus the standard femoral approach.

Assessment of Ulnopalmar Arterial Arches

The assessment of collateral ulnar circulation has traditionally been recommended prior to the TRA to PCI. The early postprocedure occlusion of the radial artery could occur in 0% to 19% of patients depending on the clinical or ultrasound assessment of the radial artery patency, the type of procedure (diagnostic or interventional), whether anticoagulation was used, the duration and the technique of arterial compression after the procedure, and the size of the introducers and catheters. In 40% to 60% of cases, the pulse could be redetected within hours to weeks after the occlusion, which remained asymptomatic in virtually all patients. Nevertheless, the description of incomplete palmar arches and very rare cases of transient or definitive hand or finger ischemia have been reported, theoretically justifying the evaluation of the ulnopalmar arch prior to the radial puncture. However, most reported cases of distal ischemia have been associated with distal emboli and normal Allen testing prior to catheterization. Although the assessment of the collateral ulnar circulation is of theoretical interest, the low specificity of the Allen test and the absence of symptomatic ischemic complications in the abundant literature have made this recommendation obsolete in many experienced radial centers.

The Allen Test

A simple clinical way of testing the adequacy of the collateral ulnar circulation is the modified Allen test (Fig. 32.1A and B). The test consists of the simultaneous compression of radial and ulnar arteries, followed by several flexion–extension movements of the fingers, leading to uncoloring of the palm. The ulnar compression is then ceased. The recoloration time of the palm after the end of the ulnar artery compression defines the Allen test: normal is less than 5 seconds, intermediate is 5 to 10 seconds, and abnormal is 10 seconds or more. The reverse Allen test, comprising all steps with the exception of a transient radial—instead of ulnar—compression, could be used in the case of a transulnar approach.

A potentially more accurate method for the evaluation of the ulnopalmar arch may be the plethysmooxymetric test (see Fig. 32.1C and D, and Video 32.1). The radial artery is compressed after the detector is positioned on the thumb. The persistent damping of the plethysmographic curve and a decrease of the blood oxygen saturation indicate inadequate ulnar collateral circulation. Barbeau and colleagues[41] compared such a method with the Allen test in 1010 consecutive patients. The study showed that 6.3% of patients would be excluded based on the Allen test, but only 1.5% had an abnormal plethysmooxymetric test.

In clinical practice, the use of the Allen test is highly variable from one center or operator to another. In centers where the test is systematically performed, the TRA is usually attempted in normal or intermediate patient groups. The issue is highly controversial because on one hand, many operators do not test the collateral circulation, and on the other, in most clinical trials, the abnormality of the test is an exclusion criterion.

One recent study demonstrated reduced blood flow and increased capillary lactate levels in the thumb following 30 minutes of occlusive compression of the radial artery in patients with an abnormal Allen test compared with those with a normal test,[42]

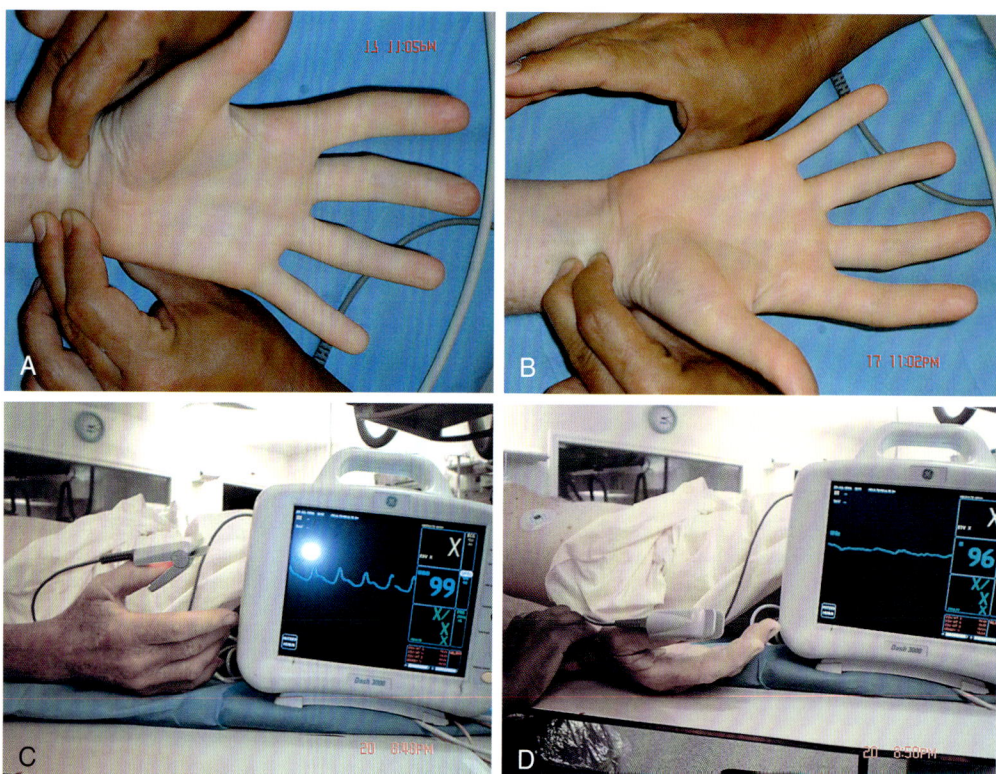

Fig. 32.1 Ulnopalmar arch assessment. (A) Allen test: compression of both radial and ulnar arteries. (B) Allen test: homogeneous recoloration of the palm after ulnar artery compression is released in a patient with normal palmar arch. (C) Plethysmooxymetric test: before radial artery compression. (D) Plethysmooxymetric test: dumping of the plethysmographic curve and decrease of oxygen saturation of the thumb after radial compression in a patient with incomplete palmar arch.

which suggests potential ischemic complications in patients with an abnormal test. A more recent trial in 203 patients undergoing a TRA with a normal, intermediate, or abnormal Allen test did not confirm the previous findings on increased lactate levels.[43] Moreover, the latter study—based on plethysmographic frame counts—demonstrated an enhancement of the ulnar flow only in patients with an abnormal Allen test after radial artery occlusion. Hence the prognostic relevance of the Allen test remains controversial, and its relation to the safety of the procedure has never been shown. A few cases of severe hand ischemia have been reported but never in relation to an abnormal Allen test.

Because of the rare occurrence of radial artery occlusion and the exceptionally symptomatic character of such a complication, the prognostic value of neither of the previous tests has been demonstrated, and many operators use the TRA without prior evaluation of the ulnopalmar arch. Today, many believe the abnormal Allen test should not deter patients to undergo TRA diagnostic angiography and/or PCI. Conversely, the plethysmographic curve performed prior to the procedure might help to verify that radial artery remains patent during radial artery compression until hemostasis is completed.

Right Versus Left Transradial Approach
The left radial access may have some advantages over the right TRA. Such reported advantages include more comfort and less hypothetic risk in case of hand ischemia for the right-handed majority of patients, easier coronary cannulation using standard Judkins catheters, less guidewire usage, lower rates of unusual artery branching or vessel tortuosity needing less catheter manipulation, shorter procedure and fluoroscopy times, and selective opacification of the left internal thoracic artery bypass grafts.

In a randomized trial that compared 232 left and 205 right transradial diagnostic procedures, the left approach was associated with shorter duration of catheter manipulation and shorter procedure and fluoroscopy times, as well as lower rates of guidewire usage, suggesting increased procedural efficacy.[44] A meta-analysis that involved 22 randomized trials and included more than 10,000 patients confirmed the lower fluoroscopy time and contrast volume with the left, compared with the right, TRA.[45]

Nevertheless, the right TRA is clearly more ergonomic for the majority of operators, and the differences between the two approaches may not be of clinical relevance. The choice of the side remains mainly a matter of operator preference—the right radial approach being the default side in 90% of cases. Recently, to avoid the patient pronation of the left wrist, a distal approach TRA from the "snuffbox" has been proposed and seems particularly attractive in overweight post-CABG patients.

As mentioned before, previous bi-internal thoracic artery CABG is a specific situation in which a double left and right radial approach for diagnostic angiography could be used, allowing direct access to internal thoracic arteries' ostia for further intervention through the grafts.

Patient Preparation, Arterial Puncture, and Sheath Insertion

Explanations and premedication should be given to patients based on local practice (Video 32.2). Because excessive anxiety may favor radial artery spasm, premedication may be used prior to radial artery puncture (see below). When possible, local anesthesia of the puncture site with an anesthetic cream 30 to 60 minutes prior to the puncture may improve patient comfort and can reduce the risk of radial artery spasm and cannulation failure.

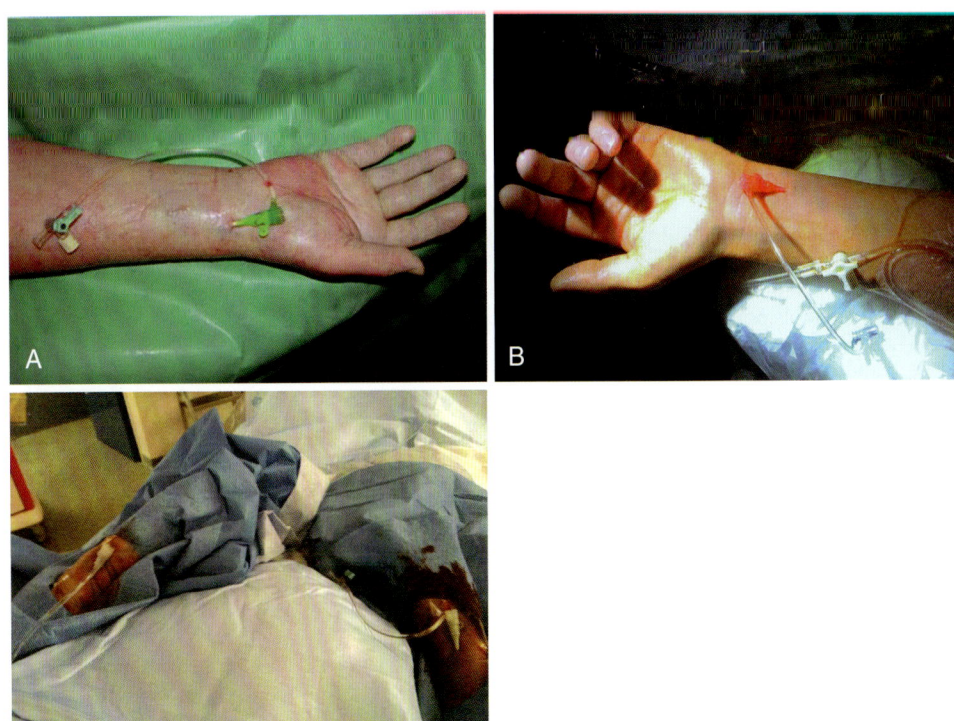

Fig. 32.2 (A) Right transradial approach. (B) Left ulnar sheath approach. (C) Bilateral radial approach for selective catheterization of both internal thoracic arteries.

Some operators also recommend local vasodilation by apposition of a nitrate patch or paste on the puncture site. To be effective, it seems that the treatment must be administered at least 1 hour prior to radial puncture. An alternative technique is to mix nitroglycerin (100 μg in 1 mL) and lidocaine (1 mL of 1% solution) and to administer 0.5 to 1 mL subcutaneously prior to the initial radial artery puncture. In case of spasm, tiny radial artery, or multiple repeat procedures, an interesting technique is to use the sphygmomanometer inflated for 5 to 10 minutes around the arm to induce a reactive and transient hyperemic state in the forearm arterial system and induce maximal vasodilation of the radial artery. The forearm should be shaved if necessary and aseptically prepared. Usually the groin is also prepared in case of radial access failure or if greater than 7-Fr material is needed. The arm and wrist rest on an armrest, and a roll of gauze can be inserted under the wrist to make the puncture easier.

Prior to puncture, a small dose of subcutaneous lidocaine 1% or 2% solution (0.5 to 2 mL) is injected at the puncture site. The radial artery might be accessed either by direct (anterior) puncture or using a through-and-through technique. Although access is somewhat faster with the through-and-through technique, the choice remains a matter of operator preference because there are no differences in the rate of complications. The artery is punctured either with a short 18- to 19-gauge entry needle (anterior) or a 20-gauge venous-type catheter entry needle, usually with a 30-degree angle to the horizontal plane. The needle is advanced until blood appears and stops. The inner needle is then retrieved in case of venous-type needle use. The needle or the catheter is then retrieved until a pulsatile blood flow appears. A 0.025-inch straight, preferably hydrophilic coated guidewire is introduced through the needle or the catheter, which is then removed. A 70-mm long arterial hydrophilic sheath is then introduced on the wire eventually after a very small superficial skin incision. Fig. 32.2 shows single right radial, left ulnar, and bilateral radial sheaths in place. The use of hydrophilic coated sheaths (Fig. 32.3) and the smallest sheath size—4 Fr for diagnostic and 5 Fr for PCI, with further upsizing if needed to 6, 7, or even 8 Fr—are recommended because they are associated with less radial artery

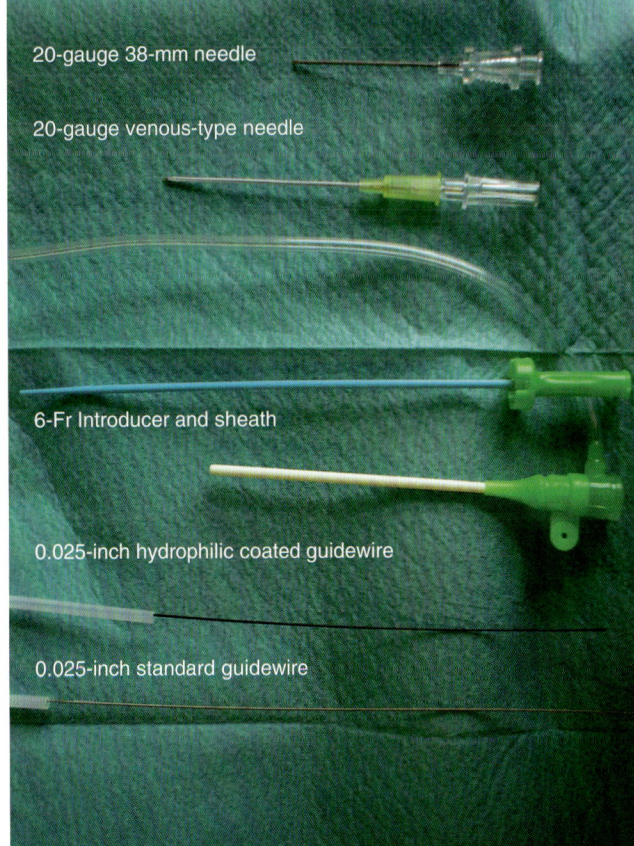

Fig. 32.3 Transradial approach kit (Terumo Medical, Somerset, NJ).

occlusion and spasm and less extraction force at removal. The use of long sheaths (23 cm), initially recommended, has now been largely abandoned. The use of recently developed thin-walled slender sheaths with outer diameters smaller than standard sheaths is of interest in patients with small radial arteries.

Prevention of Radial Artery Spasm

An intraarterial spasmolytic drug or drug cocktail is injected through the sheath after its introduction. Different cocktails have been evaluated based on various treatments—nitroglycerin, nitroprusside, molsidomine, phentolamine, diltiazem, or verapamil—alone or in combination.

In a randomized trial that included 406 patients, the rates of clinical and/or angiographic radial artery spasm were significantly reduced by the intraarterial injection of nitroglycerin 100 µg with or without combination therapy with verapamil 1.25 mg (3.8% and 4.4%, respectively) compared with placebo (20.4%).[46] However, the effect of nitrates depends on the dose used, and a high dose is recommended when used alone. In another randomized trial that included 1219 patients, the combination of verapamil 2.5 mg and molsidomine 1 mg was associated with less radial spasm (4.9%) compared with verapamil 2.5 or 5 mg (8.3% and 7.9%) or molsidomine 1 mg (13.3%) alone and placebo (22.2%).[47] In another randomized trial, verapamil 2.5 mg alone was more effective in the prevention of radial artery spasm compared with the α-blocker phentolamine 2.5 mg (spasm rates were 13.8% vs. 23.2%, respectively).[48]

The intraarterial injection of verapamil, nitroglycerin, or a combination of the two seems to be associated with the lowest spasm rates and could be recommended in all patients after the introduction of the sheath in the radial artery. Patients should be warned that they might experience cold and/or heat lasting a few seconds in the forearm and arm after the intraarterial injection.

A randomized trial of 2013 patients compared an association of intravenous (IV) opioid/benzodiazepine with no treatment during the preparation of the access site in patients undergoing elective transradial PCI. In this study, patients received intraarterial glyceryl trinitrate (GTN) and verapamil, and guiding catheters smaller than 7 Fr were used. The authors found a significant reduction of angiography-confirmed radial artery spasm (2.6% vs. 8.3%, OR 0.29; $P < .001$) with significant reductions of access-site crossover rates and patient discomfort.[49] The general use of such a strategy may nevertheless increase the complexity of a routine procedure performed on an outpatient basis.

Anticoagulation

Because of the potential risk of radial artery occlusion, and for the full control of local bleeding complications, all patients not already on anticoagulation therapy undergo full-dose anticoagulation after the arterial sheath is placed in the radial artery prior to both diagnostic and interventional procedures. Although the role and the type of anticoagulation for TRA have not been adequately assessed by randomized trials, several prospective registries have reported a significant reduction of the rates of radial artery occlusion associated with full anticoagulation. Overall, full anticoagulation is recommended in all patients undergoing transradial procedures, and different regimens should be considered based on validated guidelines and local practice: fixed-dose, weight-adjusted, or activated clotting time (ACT)-adjusted unfractionated heparin; weight-adjusted low-molecular-weight heparin; bivalirudin; and so on. Anticoagulants may be injected through the arterial sheath or through venous access because the route has not been associated with the risk of radial artery occlusion.

Glycoprotein IIb/IIIa Inhibitors and Fibrinolytics

Because of the extremely low vascular site complication rates, TRA to PCI is clearly the method of choice in the setting of PCI with highly active antithrombotic regimens and early or rescue PCI after thrombolysis.

Although the use of IIb/IIIa inhibitors has decreased due to the advent of the more recent rapidly and highly active P2Y12 inhibitors, their use in STEMI or bail-out situations is still relatively common. In a series of mostly ACS patients undergoing PCI with abciximab through transradial ($n = 83$) or transfemoral access ($n = 67$), the 30-day rate of major acute coronary events was similar between the two approaches, but bleeding complications occurred in 0% of the former versus 7.4% of the latter ($P = .04$).[50]

A small, randomized pilot trial comparing transradial and transfemoral approaches for urgent PCI in 50 patients after thrombolysis (in 66% of patients) and/or GP IIb/IIIa inhibitor therapy (94%) reported comparable results in terms of procedural success (only one failure in the transradial group) and vascular complication rates (one pseudoaneurysm in each group) but slightly longer average local anesthesia–to–first balloon time in the transradial group (32 vs. 26 min, $P = .04$).[27] In the noninferiority, randomized Early Discharge After Transradial Stenting of Coronary Arteries (EASY) study, which compared transradial PCI either with same-day discharge and abciximab bolus or hospitalization and abciximab infusion in 1005 patients (66% with unstable angina), the 30-day composite end point of death, MI, urgent revascularization, major bleeding, repeat hospitalization, access-site complications, and severe thrombocytopenia were comparable. The overall rates of access-site complication (4.8% vs. 4.2%), major bleeding (0.8% vs. 0.2%), and transfusion were impressively low.[51]

A post hoc analysis of the ATOLL randomized trial limited to the population receiving GP IIb/IIIa inhibition in the setting of primary PCI for STEMI also found that such drugs were used more safely and with lower rates of major bleeding with a TRA compared with other access sites (4% vs. 9%, $P = .03$).[52]

Finally, in the setting of fibrinolysis a recent propensity score analysis of the CathPCI registry including 9494 patients demonstrated a significant reduction of bleeding complications in case of rescue PCI in association with the transradial versus the transfemoral approach (OR 0.67; 95% CI 0.52 to 0.87; $P < .003$). In another analysis of post thrombolysis rescue PCI with adjuvant GP IIb/IIIa inhibitor therapy in 111 patients, 47 had a TRA, showed lower rates of access-site bleeding (0% vs. 9%, $P = .04$) and transfusion (4% vs. 19%, $P = .02$) with the transradial access. The fluoroscopy time, contrast media volume, and time to first balloon inflation were comparable between the two approaches.[53]

Despite the absence of adequately sized randomized trials in the specific setting of transradial PCI with GP IIb/IIIa inhibitors or after thrombolysis, the extremely low access-site–related bleeding complications associated with such an approach firmly suggests its use in patients receiving highly active antithrombotic therapy.

Guiding Catheters

The guidewire used for the TRA is usually a standard 0.032- to 0.035-inch guidewire. In case of anatomic difficulties, such as radial or subclavian loops, a hydrophilic coated guidewire could be used. The progression of the guidewire should be done under fluoroscopic control, especially with hydrophilic coated guidewires. The catheter exchange can be done using a long, 260- to 300-cm exchange guidewire or with a nonhydrophilic wire placed in the aortic root using a flush syringe to inject over the wire. The syringe and the catheter are retrieved during the flush injection, under fluoroscopic control (Video 32.3). Such exchange methods are extremely useful in case of difficult access.

The cannulation of the coronary arteries via a left or right TRA can be done using standard Judkins right and left catheters in the majority of patients. The cannulation of both right and left coronary ostia is very similar between the left radial and transfemoral approaches, and all standard catheters can be used through such access. In a series of 412 consecutive left transradial diagnostic procedures, only 5.5% of left main and 3% of right coronary ostia needed to be cannulated by catheters other than standard left or right Judkins catheters.[54]

For the right TRA, both left and right Judkins catheters usually end up in the right coronary or noncoronary sinuses. The Judkins right catheters are to be manipulated similarly as through transfemoral access, intubating the right coronary ostia after a slight clockwise rotation. For the cannulation of the left main coronary ostium, an initial clockwise rotation is needed, eventually followed first by a gentle pull or push and then a slight anticlockwise rotation.

In most high-volume centers, the guiding catheters used are the long-tip extra back-up 3.5 to 4 for left coronary and Judkins right 4 for right coronary PCI. Several other guiding catheters have been used for transradial PCI, such as the Amplatz left 2, Champ, or a multipurpose catheter, used for both left and right TRAs. Finally, specific transradial guiding catheters have been developed, although a majority of operators use standard guiding catheters. A list of guiding catheters used for the TRA is given in Table 32.3.

The diameter of the guiding catheters is also to be considered because 6-Fr guide catheters are more often associated with spasm and radial artery occlusion than 5-Fr catheters. The limitations of the 5-Fr compared with the 6-Fr catheter are less strong backup due to higher flexibility of the catheters and incompatibility with some devices (rotational atherectomy, thrombectomy, and distal protection devices; >4 mm coronary stents) or procedures (kissing stent or balloon for bifurcation lesions). Special attention also should be paid to the possibility of bubble formation as a result of the Venturi effect when balloons or devices are rapidly removed from a 5-Fr catheter. On the other hand, deep but cautious arterial intubation can be performed with 5-Fr catheters when needed; for example, for crossing calcified coronary curves.

The recent developments of 5- to 7-Fr guideline extension catheters (GuideLiner, Guidezilla, Guidion) represent a major advance in the situations were coronary artery intubation is difficult and the support is insufficient (Videos 32.4–32.6). The extensions can be advanced over the PCI guidewire and deeply intubate the coronary artery either on the guidewire alone or on a small sized PCI balloon, and allow stent delivery (only with ≥6-Fr extensions) with adequate support.

Difficult Anatomy

The arterial circulation of the upper limbs is subject to frequent variation among patients. During the initial phase of the learning curve, the failure of the TRA is usually the result of puncture failure, whereas for experienced operators, the failure is related to difficult radial artery anatomy. A series of 1191 consecutive cases reported anomalous upper branching of the radial artery in 3.2%, a high origin of the radial artery in 2.4%, and radial or brachial artery tortuosity in 4.2% (arteries were S- and Ω-shaped in 31% each).

In another series of 2211 consecutive patients, the authors reported a 98.9% success rate, and 22.8% of patients had anatomic variations that included tortuosity (3.8%), stenosis (1.7%), hypoplasia (7.7%), abnormal origin of the radial artery (8.3%), and retroesophageal (lusoria) subclavian artery (0.45%).[55] Notably, rates of success in this experienced radial center were high in all anatomic variations (83% to 96.7%) except the lusoria subclavian artery (60% success rate), which should be considered as a relative contraindication to the TRA (Fig. 32.4, Videos 32.4

TABLE 32.3 Guiding Catheters Used for Transradial Percutaneous Coronary Intervention

Guiding Catheter (Curves)	Left Coronary	Right Coronary	Bypass Grafts
STANDARD CATHETERS			
Judkins left (3.5 or 4)	+	– (+3.5 curve)	–
Judkins right (4)	–	++++	Left/right IMA
Amplatz left (2)	++	+	Left SVG
Amplatz right	–	+	–
Extra back-up (3.0 or 3.5)	++++	–	–
Multipurpose	+	+	Right SVG
Internal mammary	–	–	Left/right IMA
LCB/RCB	–	–/+	Left/right SVG
Ikari left	+	+	
BRAND NAME CATHETERS			
Kimny (Boston Scientific)	+	+	–
MUTA L/R (Boston Scientific)	+	+	–
Radial curve (Boston Scientific)	+	+	–
Fajadet L/R (Cordis)	+	+	–
Mann IM (Boston Scientific)	–	–	Left or right IMA
Barbeau L/R (Cordis)	+	+	–
Brachial type K (Terumo Medical)	+	+	–
Tiger II (Terumo Medical)	+	+	–

IMA, Internal mammary artery; *LCB,* left coronary bypass; *RCB,* right coronary bypass; *SVG,* saphenous vein graft.

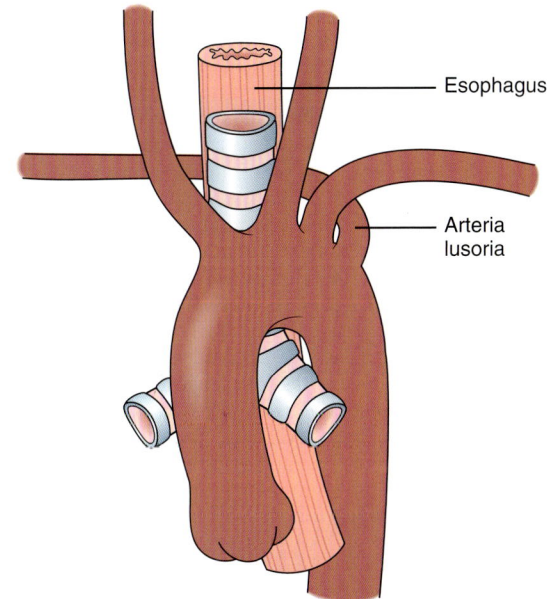

Fig. 32.4 Schematic representation of retroesophageal subclavian artery (arteria lusoria).

and 32.5). The most common anatomic variations and difficulties are listed in Table 32.4, and some examples are shown in Figs. 32.5, 32.6, 32.7, 32.8 and in Videos 32.7–32.10.

Repeat Transradial Procedures

Because of the risk of postprocedure radial artery occlusion—although such complication is rare and usually asymptomatic—repeated procedures may be questioned. The reported rates of access failure through the same radial artery range from 3% for the second attempt up to 50% for a fifth attempt. Such data should be considered with caution because the number of patients with multiple procedures was very low in the previous study. In a series of consecutive 480 patients with more than two repeat radial access procedures, the same radial artery could be used up to 10 times, but each repeat attempt was associated with a 5% failure rate due to chronic radial artery occlusion.[56]

Finally, pathology examinations of radial arteries used for coronary artery bypass graft, as well as optical coherence tomography (OCT), have provided evidence of acute and chronic injuries, such as intimal and medial tears and dissection, intimal thickening, and stenosis (Fig. 32.9), especially in those with repeat transradial interventions.[57] Such findings have led some to recommend a transfemoral approach in patients at a low risk of femoral access-site complication and a high risk of repeated procedures, such as those with complex, multivessel lesions with a high restenosis risk or heart transplant recipients undergoing systematic annual angiography. However, this does not appear to be a concern at high-volume radial centers. The use of 4-Fr diagnostic and 5-Fr guiding catheters, adequate anticoagulation regimens, and less intense and shorter radial compression after the procedure is associated with lower rates of radial artery occlusion and allows multiple procedures in the majority of patients.

Complications

The transradial access is associated with very low major access-site–related complications. The two most common complications are radial artery spasm (Fig. 32.10; Videos 32.11–32.13), often related to painful procedures or excessive catheter manipulations, and asymptomatic, often reversible radial artery occlusion (Video 32.14) that may occur in 3.8% to 22% and 0% to 19% of patients, respectively. Female sex, diabetes, small body surface area, low body mass index, short stature, smoking history, small diameter of the radial artery, number of catheters used, and catheter size (6 vs. 5 Fr) have been related to radial artery spasm. Reported predictors of radial artery occlusion are small radial artery diameter, low difference between radial artery and sheath diameters, diabetes, low-dose or no anticoagulation, and repeated procedures using the same access site. Predicting the risk of radial artery spasm may be possible before puncture by the ultrasound assessment of the arterial diameter and the flow-mediated artery dilation. Nevertheless, the clinical usefulness of such a strategy remains hypothetic. A list of reported transradial access–related complications is provided in Table 32.5. More recently, the concept of patent hemostasis has emerged as a nonpharmacologic method of ensuring lower risks of radial artery occlusion. Indeed, it seems that occlusive and prolonged hemostasis is a strong predictor of radial artery occlusion. An interesting method to maximize the success of "patent-hemostasis" is to apply dual (i.e., radial and ulnar graded) compression of radial and ulnar arteries until hemostasis is completed.[58]

Conclusions

Bleeding complications after PCI have been associated with higher rates of hard clinical events, including mortality. The

TABLE 32.4 Anatomic Abnormalities

Anatomic Difficulties	Solution
Forearm	
Lateral position of the radial artery on the wrist	Change puncture site or access site
Hypoplastic radial artery	Change access site
Radial artery remnants	Guidewire progression under angiographic control
Radial artery loops	Hydrophilic coated guidewires under angiographic control, 0.014-inch angioplasty guidewires; change access site in case of calcified, "unloopable" loops
Arm	
Brachial artery remnants High origin of the radial artery	Guidewire progression under angiographic control
Brachial artery loops	Hydrophilic coated guidewires under angiographic control, 0.014-inch angioplasty guidewires; change access site in case of calcified, "unloopable" loops
Shoulder-Thorax	
Axillary or subclavian artery loops Arteria lusoria (retroesophageal right subclavian artery)	Hydrophilic coated guidewires under angiographic control, deep inspiration change access site in case of calcified, "unloopable" loops
Brachiocephalic arterial trunk abnormalities Posterior origin Bicarotidian trunks Thoracic aortic rotations	Guidewire progression under angiographic control, deep inspiration Guidewire progression under angiographic control, deep inspiration, catheters adapted to aortic angulation

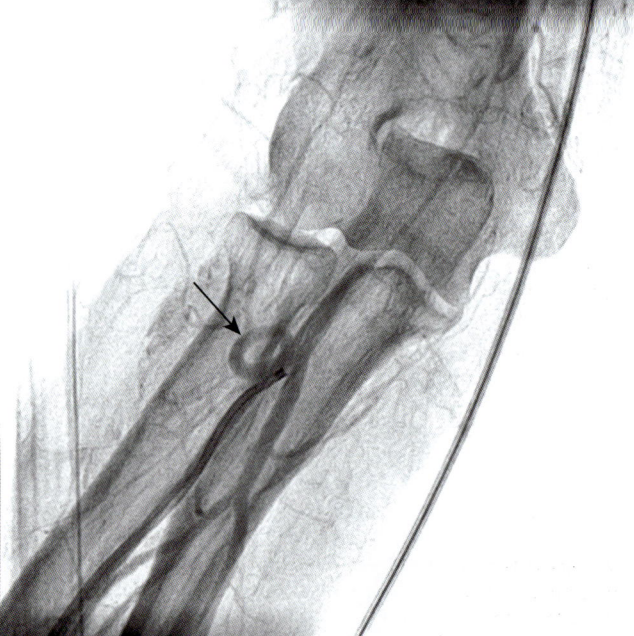

Fig. 32.5 Radial artery omega-shaped complete loop *(arrow)*.

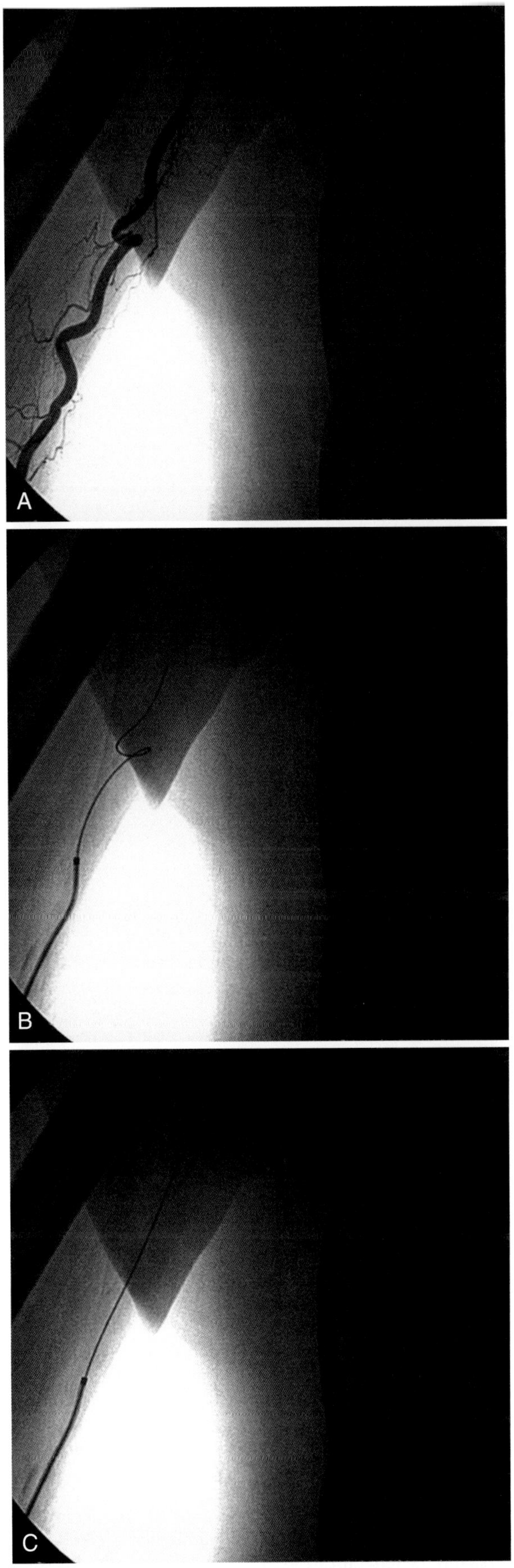

Fig. 32.6 Brachial artery loop. (A) Before wiring. (B) During wiring. (C) Artery unlooped by a hydrophilic coated guidewire.

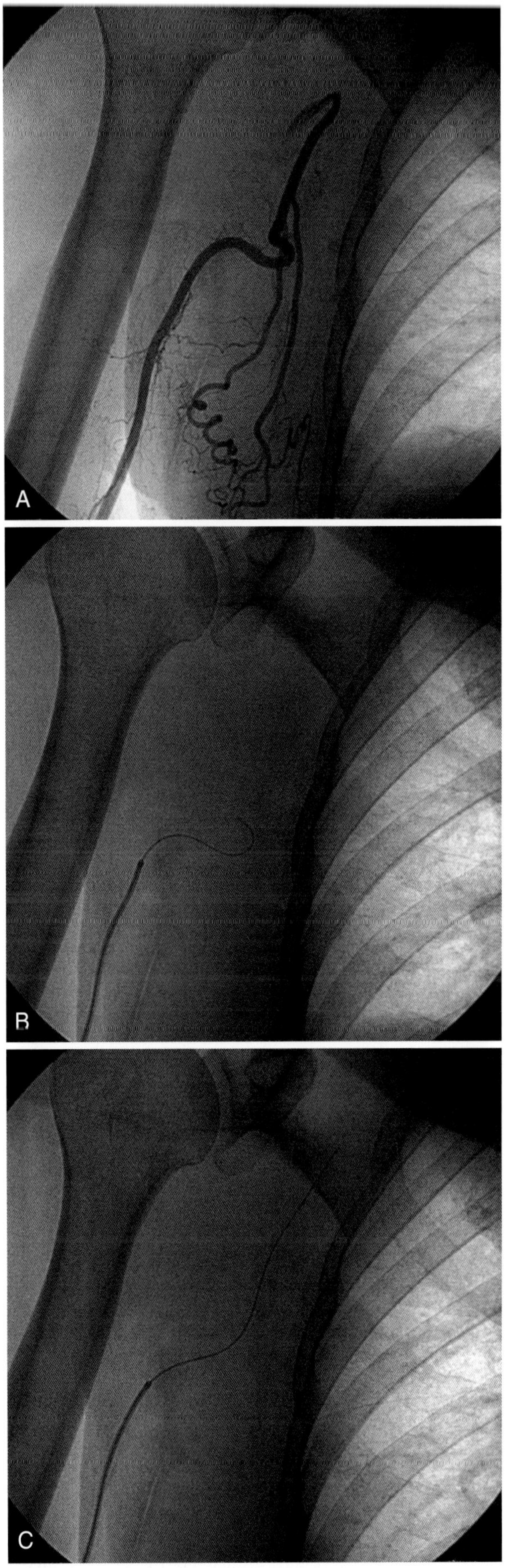

Fig. 32.7 High brachial artery loop. (A) Before wiring. (B) During wiring. (C) Artery unlooped by a hydrophilic coated guidewire.

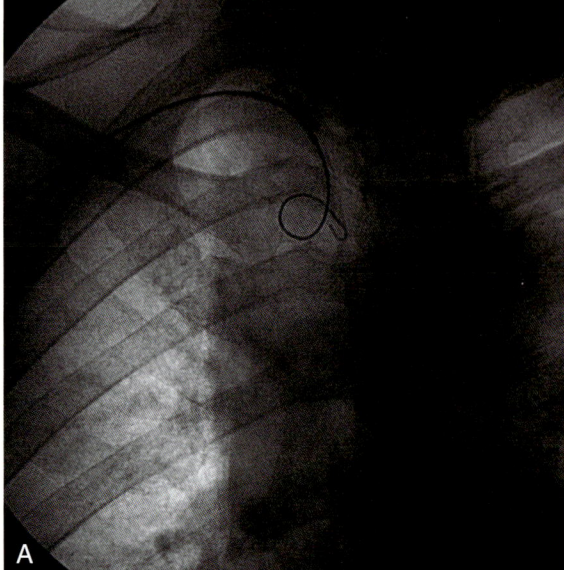

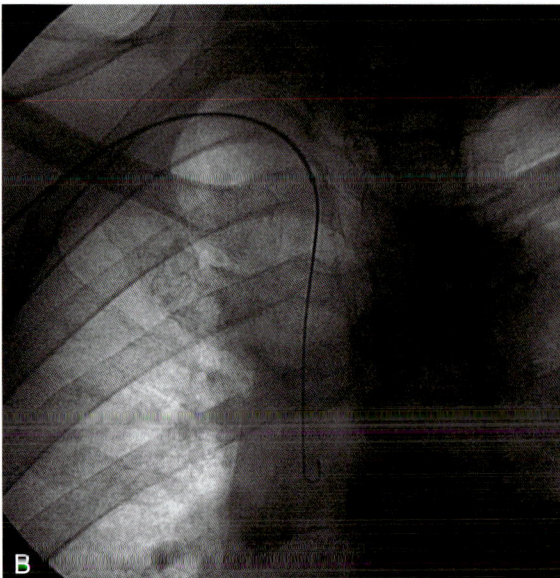

Fig. 32.8 Subclavian loop. (A) Before wiring. (B) Artery unlooped by a standard preshaped guidewire.

TRA is associated with a dramatic risk reduction for entry-site complication, compared with the transfemoral approach, and appears to be the easiest, safest, and most cost-effective way to control bleeding complications and to improve clinical outcome, including survival, after PCI. Growing evidence in large observational studies and randomized trials shows significant reduction in major cardiovascular events and even mortality with the TRA to PCI in the settings of ACS in general and STEMI in particular, as recently demonstrated in the randomized MATRIX, RIVAL, and RIFLE-STEACS trials. TRA is associated with easy entry-point hemostasis, more comfort for patients, quick postprocedure ambulation, and the possibility of outpatient procedures.

The only theoretic contraindication to the TRA is the inadequate ulnar collateral circulation detected by the increasingly controversial Allen test, although most operators proceed without such a test because of its unknown value in predicting postprocedure complications. Initially appearing to be a more difficult access site, compared with the femoral artery, after a short learning curve and with knowledge of potential anatomic difficulties and ways to overcome such difficulties, the procedural

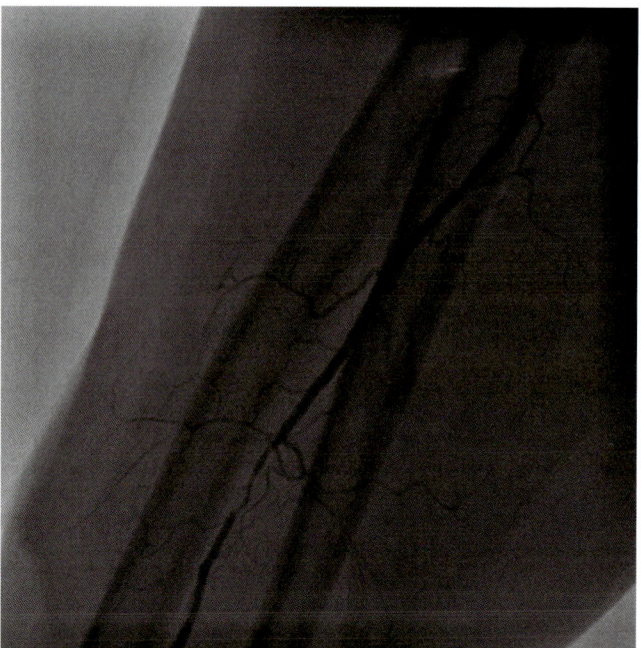

Fig. 32.9 Radial artery stenosis (visualized after transulnar opacification).

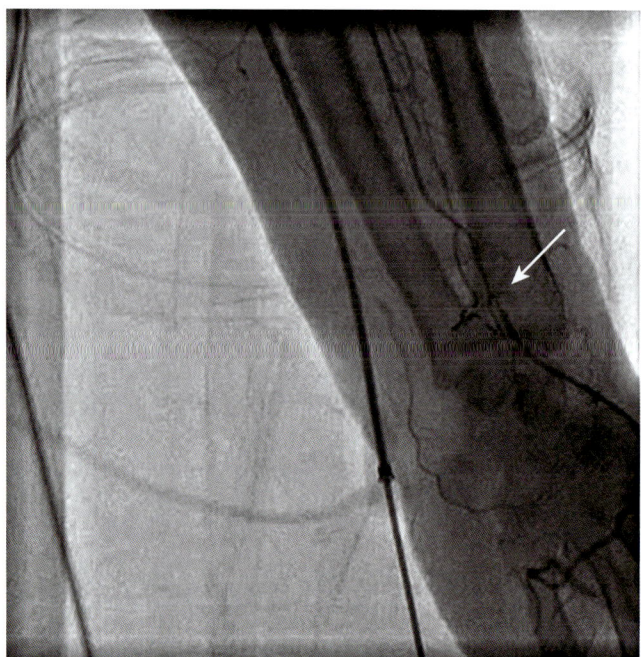

Fig. 32.10 Radial artery spasm *(arrow)*.

success rates of the TRA become virtually identical to those of the transfemoral approach, without the access-site complications. There still is a need for more adequately sized randomized trials, as well as academic educational programs to promote a TRA among interventionalists, in order to develop this obviously superior technique.

The TRA—initially considered as an alternative to transfemoral access—is already the preferred method for PCI in many centers, and its generalization as the first-line method is likely to be just a matter of time.

TABLE 32.5 Transradial Approach–Related Reported Complications

Complications	Frequency	Prevention	Solution
Asymptomatic loss of radial pulse (reversible in ~50% of cases)	0%–9%	Spasmolytic cocktail, 5-Fr catheters	—
Radial artery spasm	4%–23%	Lidocaine cream prior to puncture; anxiolytic preparation; avoid excessive catheter manipulation and change; preventive spasmolytic cocktail; hydrophilic coated sheath guidewires and catheters	Spasmolytic cocktail General sedation
Radial artery extraction (refractory spasm)	Exceptional	Avoid excessive force to remove catheter or sheath	Spasmolytic cocktail General sedation
Radial artery false aneurysm	Exceptional	—	Local compression Surgery
Arteriovenous fistula	Exceptional	Avoid perforation	Local compression Surgery
Symptomatic finger and/or hand ischemia	Exceptional	Avoid radial puncture if Allen test is inadequate; 5-Fr catheters; adequate antithrombotic cocktails; spasmolytic cocktails	Anticoagulation Surgery
Bleeding at the puncture site	0%–2%	—	Local compression
Forearm hematoma and compartment syndrome	Exceptional	Control progression of guidewire; long arterial sheath to stop the bleeding in case of perforation; covered stent in case of uncontrollable perforation	Surgery Leeches
Vascular injury/dissection (radial, brachial, subclavian, carotid arteries)	Exceptional	Control progression of guidewire, especially hydrophilic coated wires	Anticoagulation Stent Surgery

KEY REFERENCES

1. Badri M, Shapiro T, Wang Y, et al. Adoption of the transradial approach for percutaneous coronary intervention and rates of vascular complications following transfemoral procedures: insights from NCDR. *Catheter Cardiovasc Interv*. 2018;92:835–841. https://doi.org/10.1002/ccd.27490.
4. Campeau L. Percutaneous radial artery approach for coronary angiography. *Cathet Cardiovasc Diagn*. 1989;16(1):3–7.
5. Rao SV, Tremmel JA, Gilchrist IC, et al. Best practices for transradial angiography and intervention: a consensus statement from the society for cardiovascular angiography and intervention's transradial working group. *Catheter Cardiovasc Interv*. 2014;83(2):228–236. https://doi.org/10.1002/ccd.25209.
15. Jolly SS, Yusuf S, Cairns J, et al. Radial versus femoral access for coronary angiography and intervention in patients with acute coronary syndromes (RIVAL): a randomised, parallel group, multicenter trial. *Lancet*. 2011;377(9775):1409–1420. https://doi.org/10.1016/S0140-6736(11)60404-2.
16. Valgimigli M, Gagnor A, Calabró P, et al. Radial versus femoral access in patients with acute coronary syndromes undergoing invasive management: a randomised multicentre trial. *Lancet*. 2015;385(9986):2465–2476. https://doi.org/10.1016/S0140-6736(15)60292-6.
17. Agostoni P, Biondi-Zoccai GGL, de Benedictis ML, et al. Radial versus femoral approach for percutaneous coronary diagnostic and interventional procedures; systematic overview and meta-analysis of randomized trials. *J Am Coll Cardiol*. 2004;44(2):349–356. https://doi.org/10.1016/j.jacc.2004.04.034.
19. Bertrand OF, Bélisle P, Joyal D, et al. Comparison of transradial and femoral approaches for percutaneous coronary interventions: a systematic review and hierarchical Bayesian meta-analysis. *Am Heart J*. 2012;163(4):632–648. https://doi.org/10.1016/j.ahj.2012.01.015.
23. Rao SV, Ou F-S, Wang TY, et al. Trends in the prevalence and outcomes of radial and femoral approaches to percutaneous coronary intervention: a report from the National Cardiovascular Data Registry. *JACC Cardiovasc Interv*. 2008;1(4):379–386. https://doi.org/10.1016/j.jcin.2008.05.007.
34. Vranckx P, Frigoli E, Rothenbühler M, et al. Radial versus femoral access in patients with acute coronary syndromes with or without ST-segment elevation. *Eur Heart J*. 2017;38(14):1069–1080. https://doi.org/10.1093/eurheartj/ehx048.
43. Valgimigli M, Campo G, Penzo C, et al. Transradial coronary catheterization and intervention across the whole spectrum of Allen test results. *J Am Coll Cardiol*. 2014;63(18):1833–1841. https://doi.org/10.1016/j.jacc.2013.12.043.
51. Bertrand OF, De Larochellière R, Rodés-Cabau J, et al. A randomized study comparing same-day home discharge and abciximab bolus only to overnight hospitalization and abciximab bolus and infusion after transradial coronary stent implantation. *Circulation*. 2006;114(24):2636–2643. https://doi.org/10.1161/CIRCULATIONAHA.106.638627.

Additional references available online at expertconsult.com

中文导读

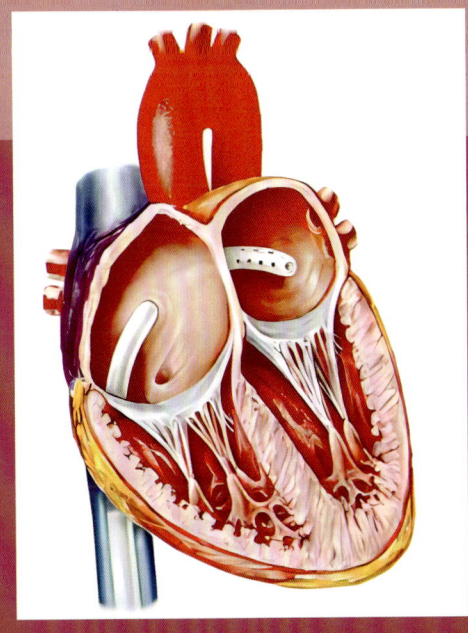

第33章
心脏外科医师及心脏团队的作用

在过去很长一段时间里，心脏介入治疗需要有丰富经验的心脏外科团队随时待命，以便在发生危急情况时立即提供外科支持。然而，伴随研究的深入、经验的积累、技术的发展和器械的更新，需要外科干预的介入并发症已经变得相当罕见。尽管如此，当前的指南仍然建议择期经皮冠状动脉介入治疗应当在具有心脏外科支持能力的中心开展。事实上，心脏外科和心脏介入并不孤立，近年来兴起的杂交手术恰恰反映了紧密的学科交叉，例如，经导管治疗结构性心脏病、经皮冠状动脉介入治疗与冠状动脉旁路移植术的联合开展等，将两大学科紧密结合在一起，促成了心脏介入与心脏外科的共同进步。在此过程中，"心脏团队"的概念被进一步强调，心脏团队的设立使得外科与介入优势互补，在面对复杂病变时能够从容应对。优秀的心脏团队能为患者制定更为合理的治疗策略，降低手术风险，紧密的协作更有助于推动技术创新，因此，提倡将心脏团队模式作为所有心脏中心的标准配置。就目前而言，将心脏外科与介入心脏病学进行技术整合仍然有很长的路要走，学科交叉与默契合作不仅需要制定详细的处置流程、组织跨学科的理论学习和技术培训，还需要建立杂交手术室，以及能满足介入与外科要求的设备，并需要多个部门的协调配合。本章节对外科医师的应急待命职责、心血管杂交手术、心脏团队等几大方面进行了系统的阐述，描述了外科在当前心脏介入治疗中的重要角色，列举了学科交叉的技术突破，并对今后的学科发展进行了展望。

张宇超　柳景华

章节要点

- 心脏外科医师在导管室中扮演的传统角色是介入心脏病学医师的后援支持。然而，随着介入治疗的发展和经验积累，以及医疗器械与技术的更新，这种后援支持作用正在失去其存在的必要。

- 新型微创杂交手术建立在传统外科开放手术的基础上，给出了一条从概念到临床实践的明确路径。这条路径需要外科医师、介入医师、医疗器械制造商，以及美国食品药品监督管理局等监管机构之间的合作。

- 外科医师和心脏病学专家面对面交流的心脏团队模式，应作为所有心脏中心处理复杂冠状动脉病变和结构性心脏病的标准模式。

- 由于未来介入心脏病学和心脏外科需要外科医师和心脏病学医师的密切合作，因此有必要建立一条将外科及心脏病学培训项目的基本原则和技能结合起来的临床培训路径。

33 Role of the Cardiac Surgeon and the Heart Team

Kazuhiro Hisamoto, Danielle N. Sin, Mathew R. Williams

KEY POINTS

- The role of the cardiac surgeon in the catheterization laboratory has traditionally been surgical backup for the interventional cardiologist. Such service is losing necessity as the development and mastery of new interventional procedures progress and correlate with the advancement of medical device technology.
- New minimally invasive interventional procedures are founded upon the historical open surgical approach and take a defined pathway from conception to clinical acceptance. This pathway requires collaboration among surgeons, interventionalists, medical device manufacturers, and regulatory bodies such as the U.S. Food and Drug Administration.
- The heart team model, with face-to-face communication between surgeon and cardiologist, should be considered the standard of care in all cardiac centers for approaching complex coronary lesions and structural heart defects.
- Because the future of interventional cardiology and cardiac surgery will require close collaboration between surgeons and cardiologists, a clinical training pathway that incorporates certain fundamental principles and skills from both surgery and cardiology training programs will be necessary.

INTRODUCTION

The role of the cardiac surgeon is first to do surgery with respect to invasive techniques involving structures of the heart. In regard to interventional cardiologists and in the catheterization (cath) lab, the cardiac surgeon can be broadly described in three categories. The first and most historical undertaking is providing backup for the interventional cardiologist in case of an untoward complication or surgical emergency. This role has lost relevancy with the advent and subsequent mastery of new procedures. Formal surgical standby for routine percutaneous coronary intervention (PCI), in which a surgeon is preemptively notified and available, is no longer required or routine because complications that require surgical intervention have become quite uncommon, reaching 0.56%,[1] in established PCI centers. However, current published guidelines for elective PCI still recommend the availability of an experienced surgical team that can be activated quickly in the event of an emergency in the cath lab.[2,3]

The second role is a hybrid between a surgeon and an interventionalist. The hybrid cardiac surgeon takes an active role in interventional procedures and, in some cases, has formal cross-training in interventional cardiology. Hybrid cardiac surgeons serve an important function in today's more complex cardiac interventional procedures such as transcatheter aortic valve replacement (TAVR), percutaneous mitral valvuloplasty, perivalvular leak intervention, percutaneous mitral valve repair, transcatheter mitral valve replacement (TMVR), and combined coronary artery bypass grafting (CABG)/PCI or valve/PCI procedures. With the heart team model becoming widely adopted, hybrid surgeons will help to shape the cath lab of the future. As complex surgical procedures are combined with a catheter-based approach, there is a need for skill sets from both a surgeon and interventionalist simultaneously at the interventional table.

Lastly, the cardiac surgeon serves as an innovation consultant. The cardiovascular surgeon's intraoperative experience and technical development are deeply rooted in the surgical correction of structural heart disease. From years of performing open-heart procedures, cardiac surgeons gain mastery and develop unique perspectives on the three-dimensional (3D) anatomy of the heart and great vessels. The cardiac surgeon continues to contribute valuable insight to the development and refinement of new techniques and procedures, which will ultimately become the standard of care for the cardiovascular interventionalist of tomorrow.

This chapter explores the roles and close collaboration between cardiac surgeons and interventional cardiologists. As the two fields merge, respective knowledge is combined for innovation to advance science of complex cardiovascular diseases and to create unique plans for patients from a repertoire of therapeutic options that reduce risk and provide better outcomes.

ROLE OF THE SURGEON ON SURGICAL STANDBY

During the early years of percutaneous transluminal coronary angioplasty (PTCA) and PCI, surgeons were, by necessity, to remain in house on surgical standby for urgent consultations and surgical emergencies that resulted from early interventional procedures. Fraught with technical pitfalls and clinical unknowns, early complications in the cath lab required an emergent trip to the operating room (OR), often with a patient in extreme cardiogenic shock.[4-7] These PCI complications are life threatening, with hemodynamic instability and associated prolonged periods of ischemia. As a result, indications for emergency CABG after failed PCI have become well established. The most common indications include abrupt vessel closure, dissection, incomplete revascularization, coronary perforation, and unsuccessful dilation or PCI, in addition to other miscellaneous clinical scenarios.[8,9] Such emergencies require the availability of a cardiac surgery team experienced in emergency aortocoronary operations and on-site cardiac surgical backup to provide all aspects of readily available cardiac surgical support.

As angiography, PTCA, and surgical techniques improved and medical equipment became more advanced, surgeons were no longer required to remain in such close proximity to the cath lab.[10,11] This was particularly true after introduction of the Gianturco–Roubin stent and its rapid adoption as a "bailout" device by the interventional cardiology community.[12,13] Almost uniformly, and for decades, active PCI centers have enjoyed a steady reduction in the percentage of cases that require emergency CABG after failed PCI (Fig. 33.1).[1,14] However, despite near universal trends that demonstrate decreased morbidity and mortality from PCI, the consequences of complications remain

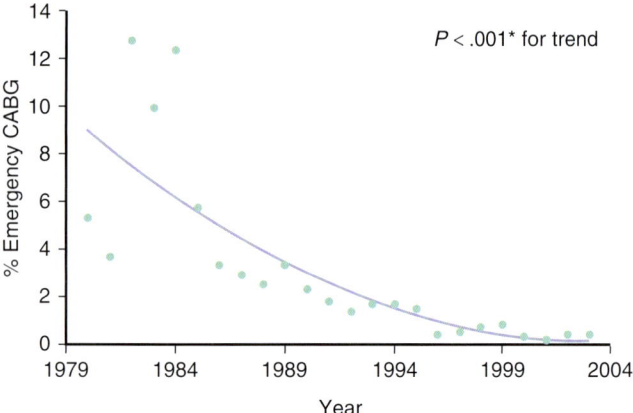

Fig. 33.1 Percentage of patients who required emergency coronary artery bypass grafting *(CABG)* after percutaneous coronary intervention from 1979 to 2003 (n = 23,087). The Armitage test for trend is indicated by an *asterisk*. (From Yang EH, Gumina RJ, Lennon RJ, et al. Emergency coronary artery bypass for percutaneous interventions: changes in the incidence, clinical characteristics, and indications from 1979 to 2003. *J Am Coll Cardiol.* 2005;46:2004–2009.)

TABLE 33.1 Coronary Artery Bypass Grafting and Mortality Rates Following Percutaneous Coronary Intervention at Hospitals Without and With On-Site Coronary Artery Bypass Grafting Surgery

	Patients (%)				
Outcomes	Without On-Site CABG	With On-Site CABG	Unadjusted *P* Value	Adjusted OR (95% CI)[a]	Adjusted *P* Value
ALL PCIs					
No. of patients	8168	617,686		621,530[b]	
Mortality	492 (6)	20,393 (3.3)	<.001	1.29 (1.14–1.47)	<.001
CABG	160 (2)	8321 (1.4)	<.001	1.05 (0.87–1.27)	.59
PRIMARY/RESCUE PCI					
No. of patients	1795	34,537		36,235[b]	
Mortality	202 (11.3)	4209 (12.2)	0.24	0.93 (0.80–1.08)	.34
CABG	82 (4.6)	1772 (5.1)	0.29	0.95 (0.73–1.22)	.67
NONPRIMARY/RESCUE PCI					
No. of patients	6373	583,149		585,295[b]	
Mortality	290 (4.6)	16,184 (2.8)	<.001	1.38 (1.14–1.67)	.001
CABG	78 (1.2)	6549 (1.1)	.45	0.92 (0.73–1.17)	.52

[a]Adjusted for age, gender, race, year, Charlson comorbidity score, primary diagnosis of acute myocardial infarction, acuity, multivessel PCI, and stent use.
[b]Adjusted models excluded 4324 patients (0.7%) missing on patient covariates; 45 (4 among primary/rescue PCI) among patients without on-site CABG and 4279 (93 among primary/rescue PCI) among patients with on-site CABG.
CABG, Coronary artery bypass grafting; *CI*, confidence interval; *OR*, odds ratio; *PCI*, percutaneous coronary intervention.
Data from Wennberg DE, Lucas FL, Siewers AE, et al. Outcomes of percutaneous coronary interventions performed at centers without and with on-site coronary artery bypass graft surgery. *JAMA.* 2004;292:1961–1968.

potentially catastrophic. Thus it is still common practice and is recommended by the American College of Cardiology (ACC)/American Heart Association (AHA)/Society of Cardiovascular and Angiography and Interventions (SCAI) practice guidelines that the majority of elective PCI be performed at centers with an active open heart surgery program and that certain interventional decisions be discussed with a cardiac surgeon before proceeding with PCI.[2,3]

In the event of emergent need for aortocoronary bypass, outcomes have been shown to be better in centers with an open heart surgery program (Table 33.1).[7,14] According to current guidelines, on-site surgical backup for elective PCI at centers that have acceptable annual volume of at least 75 procedures or more should provide emergency hemodynamic support and expeditious revascularization to manage complications that cannot be addressed in the cath lab.[15]

The ACC/AHA/SCAI 2014 Expert Consensus Document provides recommendations for PCI without on-site surgery that are a composite of recommendations that include requirements for both facilities and personnel.[3] The issues of cardiac surgical backup and the level of committed resources needed are frequently revisited, and most centers use the first-available OR model to remain efficient and maximize resources. Some centers rely on off-site surgical backup, but this is the exception rather than the rule because such practice exposes the patient to a finite but potentially fatal risk and is deemed unnecessary in most areas. Recommendations for primary PCI for ST-elevation myocardial infarction (STEMI) without on-site cardiac surgery require: (1) a highly experienced physician and catheterization team, (2) a proven plan for rapid transport to a nearby hospital with appropriate support and resources, and (3) that it be executed in a timely fashion.[15] The apparent success of centers that perform PCI without on-site cardiac surgery programs depends on operator experience and volume and can also be attributed to fairly strict patient selection and criteria defined by Wharton et al.[16]

It should be noted that, in low-volume centers (<200 PCIs per year), adverse event estimates lose stability and may therefore be unreliable.[2] The 2013 PCI competency document identified a signal that suggested that these low-volume centers were associated with worse outcomes. Thus laboratories that perform fewer than 200 procedures annually and that are not serving isolated or underserved populations should be questioned. Multiple low-volume and partial-service PCI centers within a geographic area diffuse the PCI expertise, increase costs for the overall health care system, and have not been shown to improve access. If the transfer time is 30 minutes or less, it is reasonable to assume that transfer to the nearest PCI center will provide reperfusion as rapidly as if it were available at the first hospital. For this reason, development of PCI facilities within a 30-minute emergency transfer time to an established facility is strongly discouraged.[3]

TRANSCATHETER AND HYBRID CARDIOVASCULAR PROCEDURES

Many procedures that were historically performed by surgeons as open surgeries are currently routinely performed percutaneously or with a cutdown in the cath lab or interventional suite such as hybrid OR by interventionalists of various disciplines, including cardiovascular surgeons, cardiologists, vascular surgeons, and interventional radiologists. These procedures are growing in number and variety and include pacemaker insertion, mechanical ablation of atrial fibrillation (Maze procedure), closure of patent foramen ovale, and repair of atrial septal defect, in addition to endovascular alternatives to open carotid endarterectomy, repair and resection of abdominal and thoracic aortic aneurysms, and peripheral artery bypass. The most recent surgical procedures performed with a small cutdown or percutaneous interventional approach include TAVR, TMVR, and mitral valvuloplasty or clipping. Although not as prevalent as vascular surgeons performing many of their traditionally open surgeries percutaneously in the interventional suite (i.e., endovascular abdominal aneurysm repair [EVAR]), analogous procedures such as thoracic endovascular aortic repair (TEVAR) are performed more and more in the hybrid OR by cardiac surgeons. In addition, a few hybrid cardiac surgeons have acquired formal coronary angiography and PCI training and possess skills sufficient for hospital privileging.

TRANSCATHETER AORTIC VALVE REPLACEMENT

Rapid development and miniaturization of valve-deployment technology have led to the rapid adoption of *transfemoral transcatheter aortic valve replacement* (TF-TAVR), and, since its commercial development in 2011, TF-TAVR has put itself into the domain of the interventional cardiologist. However, cardiac surgeons are required to be part of the transcatheter heart team that performs these procedures.[17]

In contrast to TF-TAVR and inherent to the design of the procedures, transapical TAVR (TA-TAVR) and transaortic TAVR (TAo-TAVR) can be performed only in a hybrid OR with a trained cardiac surgeon who can gain exposure to and manage surgical control of the ascending aorta and left ventricle (LV). These approaches require the ready availability of the cardiopulmonary bypass machine, an experienced perfusionist, and the surgeon's direction to coordinate these pieces.

In the TA-TAVR procedure, a small left anterolateral thoracotomy is made over the point of maximal impulse (PMI) on the anterolateral chest wall to gain control of the apex of the LV (Fig. 33.2A). This allows the surgeon to place a circular series of pledgeted sutures in the myocardium before the apical puncture and to place a transmyocardial guidewire using the Seldinger technique (see Fig. 33.2B). Once control of the LV apex is attained and guidewire placement across the aortic valve is confirmed, a long sheath is placed and a balloon aortic valvuloplasty (BAV) is performed. Following the BAV, the balloon-expandable transcatheter heart valve (THV) bioprosthesis is deployed in the aortic position under rapid ventricular pacing (see Fig. 33.2C and D). The integrity and position of the newly placed THV is confirmed intraoperatively by both aortography and transesophageal echocardiography (TEE) before the chest is closed by the surgeon.

In the TAo-TAVR procedure, a partial J sternotomy or a right anterior mini thoracotomy (Fig. 33.3)[18] is used for gaining access to the ascending aorta. Appropriate preoperative planning entails careful evaluation of the position of the ascending aorta in the chest with respect to the sternum, using a computed tomography (CT) scan (Fig. 33.4).[18] A partial J sternotomy suffices in most TAo cases; however, with unusual anatomy in which 50% of the aorta lies to the right of the outer table of the sternum, a second intercostal approach may provide better access. Once the aorta has been surgically exposed, a site is selected that is at least the minimum distance requirement from the annulus for proper THV deployment (Fig. 33.5).[18] This site should be free of excessive calcium and in a location that will allow sufficient sheath depth for proper THV deployment. The sheath must be placed in a straight line to the annulus after properly identifying the "TAo zone" along the upper outer quadrant of the aorta (Fig. 33.6). Two purse-string sutures large enough to accommodate the THV sheath are placed, and heparin is administered. Using the Seldinger technique, the aortic lumen is entered and the native valve is crossed, exchanging a stiff, preshaped wire into the LV using a multipurpose catheter and standard exchange

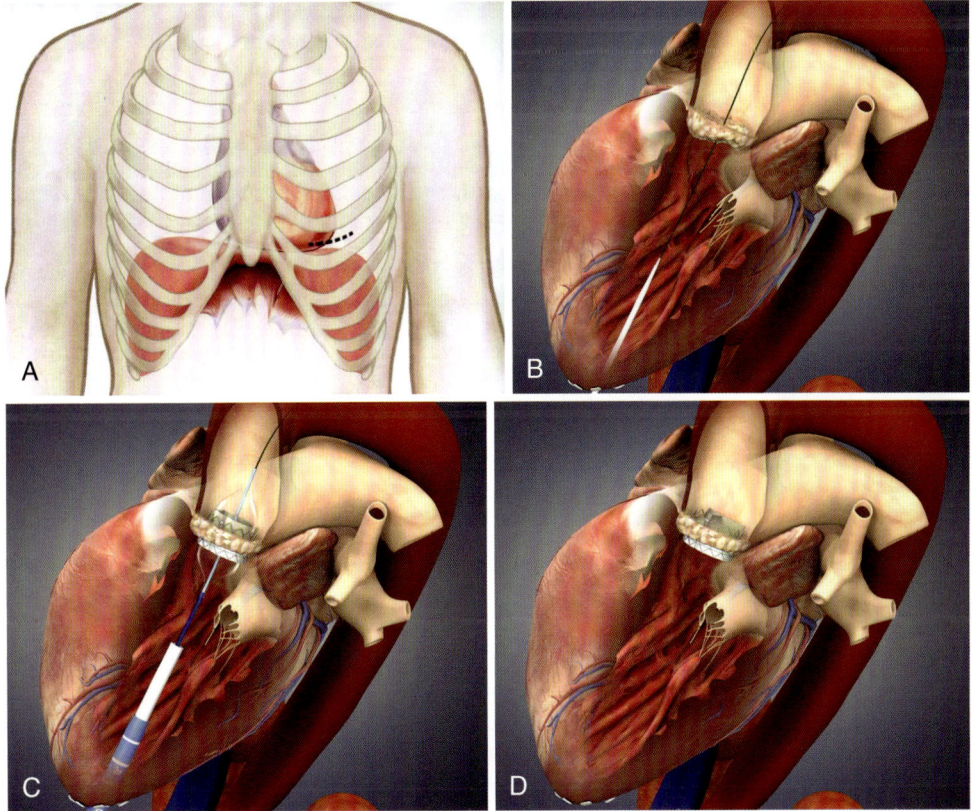

Fig. 33.2 Transapical transcatheter aortic valve insertion (TA-TAVR). (A) Keyhole left anterolateral thoracotomy for apical access. (B) Seldinger technique used for wire insertion and dilation of transmural myocardial tract before balloon aortic valvuloplasty. (C) Balloon expansion of percutaneous aortic valve. (D) Well-seated percutaneous bioprosthesis in the aortic position.

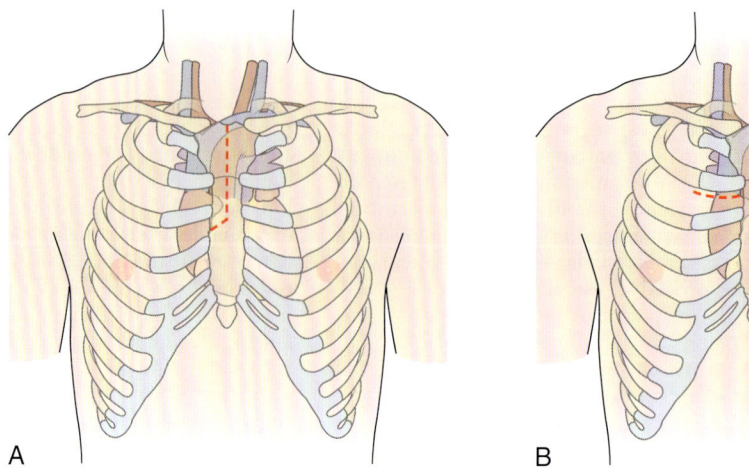

Fig. 33.3 Transaortic (TAo) approach. (A) Access ascending aorta, J sternotomy to second or third right intercostal space. (B) Anterior right mini thoracotomy, second intercostal space. Used if partial J sternotomy is not possible because of previous surgery or unusual anatomy.

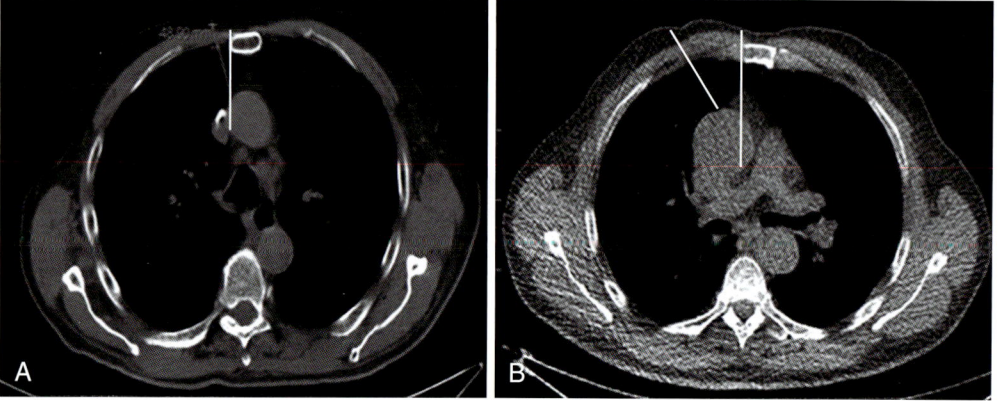

Fig. 33.4 Transaortic access-site selection. Computed tomography (CT) scan is used to screen for transaortic (Tao) approach. (A) CT slice at the upper end of the aorta at the level of the second intercostal (IC) space demonstrates a left-sided aortic arch (*white line* from outer table of sternum perpendicularly down the aorta). (B) CT slice of right-sided aorta present when 50% of the aorta lies to the right of a line drawn from the outer table of the sternum. The second IC approach can be used in this case.

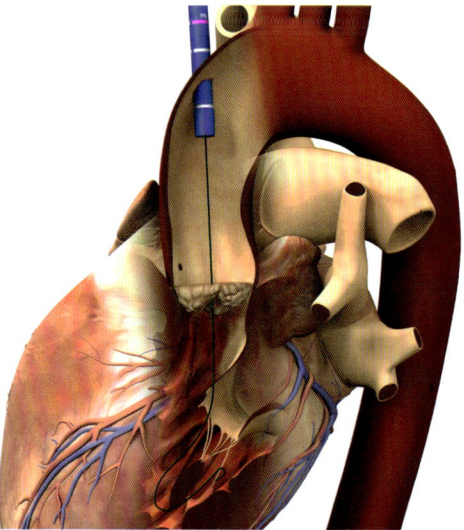

Fig. 33.5 Transaortic access-site selection. Access site is selected that is at least the minimum distance required from the annulus for proper transcatheter heart valve deployment. The access site should be free of calcium and should allow the sheath to be placed in a straight line perpendicular to the annulus.

techniques. The large THV sheath is then positioned above the native valve over the stiff wire for deployment of the THV, which is performed under fluoroscopy with rapid pacing similar to other THV approaches. Once the THV has been deployed and postdeployment echocardiography assessment is complete, the sheath is removed and the purse-string sutures are secured. The chest is then closed in standard surgical fashion.

Recently, the subclavian or axillary TAVR approach (SCA-TAVR) has become a popular technique. The multiinstitutional CoreValve clinical trial showed major morbidity and mortality rates of SCA-TAVR are equivalent to TF-TAVR.[19] In the SCA-TAVR procedure, the fibers of the pectoralis major are split retracted through a 3- to 5-cm incision in the deltopectoral groove. The pectoralis minor can be retracted or divided to expose the subclavian artery, which is then controlled with vessel loops. It is very important to avoid injury to the brachial plexus, which is located immediately superior to the subclavian artery. Direct Seldinger technique or 10-mm Dacron graft anastomosed to the artery can be used. There are two important considerations when using the subclavian artery. The subclavian artery of either side may be used, but the use of the right subclavian artery becomes technically difficult for device positioning if the aortic valve annulus is more than 30 degrees off the horizontal plane. In addition, if a patent internal mammary artery (IMA) graft is present, sheath obstruction or artery injury may limit flow during

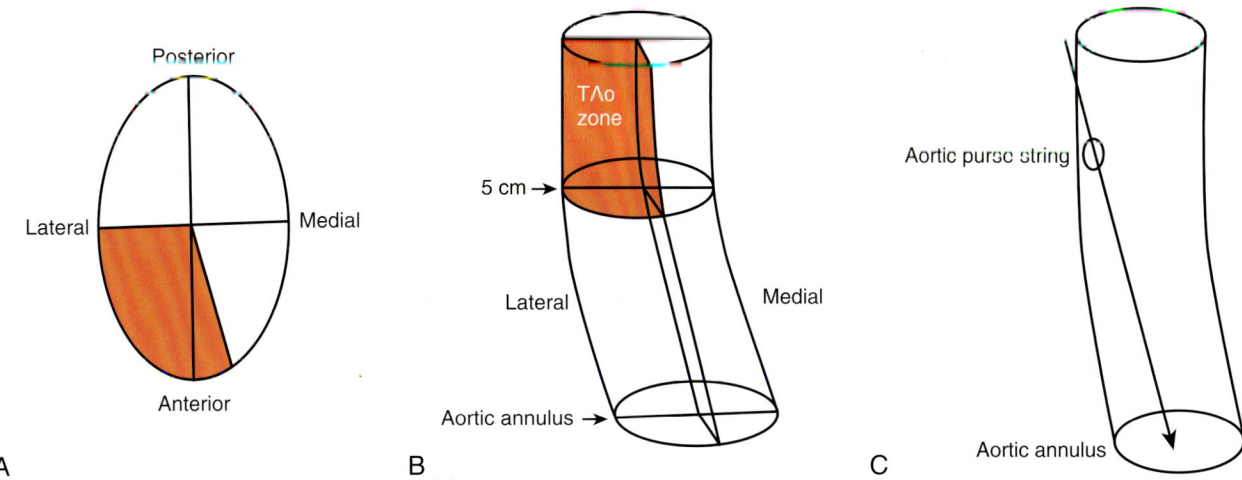

Fig. 33.6 (A and B) The transaortic *(TAo)* zone for cannulation of the aorta along the upper outer quadrant. (C) This will allow for a direct line of approach perpendicular to the aortic valve. (From Bapat V, Attia R. Transaortic transcatheter aortic valve implantation: step-by-step guide. *Semin Thorac Cardiovasc Surg.* 2012;24:206–11.)

or after device placement, causing ischemic complications. Alternative access techniques such as transcarotid access or transcaval access are used for select patients at some institutions. TF-TAVR remains the least invasive TAVR procedure. The heart team approach is critical in assessing the optimal access site for individual patients, particularly in those with poor options for access.

It is with procedures such as the TAVR, which will ultimately be combined with PCI in the same setting, that the new cardiac interventionalist will come of age. For the increasingly frail, aging population in the United States, an attractive alternative to current open heart surgery will be to have well-trained hybrid cardiac surgeons who can perform minimally invasive surgical and interventional procedures expeditiously in one setting, thus eliminating the need for multiple costly hospital visits and repeated exposures to anesthesia.

Percutaneous Mitral Valve Repair

As TAVR has become an established technique, device manufacturers and investigational cardiologists have set their sights on the mitral valve. Due to complex anatomy and a wide variety of associated pathologies that place patients at high risk, a percutaneous approach to mitral valve disease is a greater challenge than that of aortic valve stenosis. MitraClip (Abbot Vascular Structural Heart, Menlo Park, CA), which is the only U.S. Food and Drug Administration (FDA)-approved commercially available percutaneous mitral valve repair platform, is designed for edge-to-edge plication of the mitral leaflets. This technique is based on the surgical edge-to-edge repair "Alfieri stitch."[20] During the MitraClip procedure, access is obtained from a femoral vein followed by transseptal puncture to access the left atrium from the right atrium. Unlike many cardiac interventional procedures, implantation is guided by transesophageal ultrasound more often than fluoroscopy and 3D echocardiographic images are used to confirm orientation of the MitraClip (Fig. 33.7). A deep understanding of mitral valve anatomy is essential for this procedure. Cardiac surgeons who routinely analyze mitral valve anatomy in the OR have an advantage in positioning the MitraClip, which is the key portion of the procedure. Collaboration among interventional cardiologists, echo cardiologists, and cardiac surgeons is critical for a successful procedure.

Transcatheter Mitral Valve Replacement

Currently, the MitraClip system is the most well-studied transcatheter approach for mitral valve repair. However, the randomized, controlled Endovascular Valve Edge-to-Edge Repair Study II (EVEREST2) showed that the MitraClip was significantly less effective at reducing mitral regurgitation than surgical mitral valve repair.[21] Although there is no available TMVR device commercially approved in the United States, TMVR should theoretically provide a more complete and reproducible MR reduction than transcatheter mitral repair such as the MitraClip. Specific challenges facing the development of TMVR devices include more complex 3D anatomy, asymmetric shape, less calcification, and higher risk of left ventricular outflow tract (LVOT) obstruction in TMVR compared with TAVR. Although a fully percutaneous transfemoral venous approach would be the least invasive approach for TMVR, challenges exist regarding the delivery of a high-profile device system through the atrial septum. Most TMVR systems currently under clinical evaluation have a transapical delivery system. Preprocedural multimodal imaging, including ECG-gated cardiac CT scans, provide an abundance of important information regarding mitral valve anatomy and assessment of chest wall access sites.

Transcatheter mitral valve-in-valve implantation is a promising therapy for the patients with severe comorbidities who have had a previous mitral valve replacement. Recent studies have suggested successful feasibility of this approach.[22–24] Transvenous transseptal balloon-expandable THV implantation for failed mitral bioprosthesis is associated with a high procedural success rate of 97%, 95% 30-day survival, 86% 1-year survival, and durable prosthesis function at 1 year of follow-up.[25] However, treatment of patients with failed annuloplasty rings and severe mitral annular calcification (MAC) was associated with significant rates of LVOT obstruction. In particular, patients with MAC had higher 30-day mortality (17%), complication rates including valve migration, LVOT obstruction, and paravalvular leaks.[25] Treating mitral valve disease in patients with severe MAC is still a significant challenge for experienced interventional cardiologists using a transcatheter approach and experienced cardiac surgeons using an open surgical approach. Direct vision through an atriotomy using a balloon-expandable THV may prevent the complications associated with MAC (Fig. 33.8).[26,27] Hybrid cardiac surgeons who have both interventional and surgical skill sets have an advantage in adapting to novel hybrid techniques.

Endovascular Aortic Repair

The development of endovascular aortic repair has allowed a minimally invasive approach for treatment of thoracic and abdominal aortic pathologies. TEVAR has become the first-line therapy in many descending aortic pathologies. Recent systemic

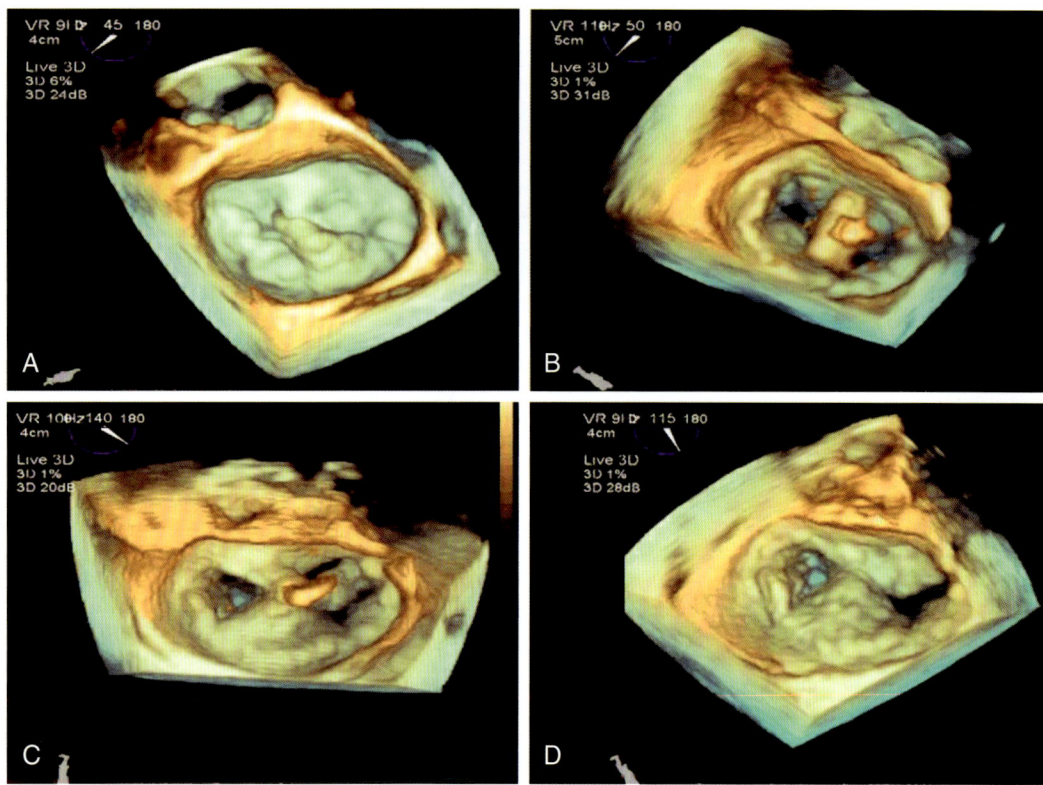

Fig. 33.7 (A) P2 flail. (B) Clip positioning. (C) Leaflets grabbed; clip still attached to delivery catheter. (D) Clip released; no more flail segment is seen.

review showed that TEVAR was associated with lower mortality and lower complication rate without an increased reintervention rate compared with open surgical repair.[28]

TEVARs may also be considered for ascending aortic arch pathologies in high-risk patients. A hybrid aortic arch repair has been described using an open vascular bypass procedure performed to secure a proximal landing zone with concomitant antegrade endovascular stent graft placement in the aortic arch (Fig. 33.9).[29] For aortic dissection, TEVAR is an option for treating type B aortic dissections in the setting of contained rupture and/or malperfusion.[30] A recent study revealed TEVAR in patients with stable type B aortic dissection may improve survival and delay disease progression compared with traditional medical management.[31] TEVAR may also be used in the setting of traumatic aortic transection. Although long-term data are not available, endovascular aortic repair has been associated with significantly lower perioperative morbidity and mortality compared with an open surgical repair.[32]

For most patients and aortic pathologies, open surgical repair remains the gold standard and provides excellent and durable result. However, the role of TEVAR is expected to continue rapidly expanding. Cardiac and aortic surgeons need to acquire these endovascular skills and collaborate with interventional cardiologists, vascular surgeons, and peripheral interventionalists to offer the full spectrum of therapeutic options for complex aortic pathologies. This collaboration will help us to deliver appropriate therapy for patients on an individualized basis.

Hybrid Coronary Revascularization

Hybrid procedures that have gained the most acceptance include hybrid coronary revascularization (HCR), hybrid valve surgery with PTCA or PCI, and hybrid procedures for atrial fibrillation. In addition, some centers have also undertaken hybrid therapies for coronary artery disease associated with carotid artery disease and aortic arch pathology. In centers with busy hybrid programs, HCR most often refers to minimally invasive direct coronary artery bypass (MIDCAB), in which the anastomosis of the left internal mammary artery (LIMA) to the left anterior descending artery (LAD) is the focus of the surgical portion of the operation and is combined with PCI with drug-eluting stents (DESs) to the non-LAD targets.[33–35] This approach accepts the notion that the surgical LIMA-to-LAD anastomosis is the most durable form of revascularization currently available but also recognizes that the patency rates of traditional saphenous vein grafts (SVGs) are less than robust, and their ability to remain open in the long term is greatly inferior to the LIMA approach.[36,37]

In the era of the modern DES, the SVG as a conduit for CABG must become suspect. Whereas excellent data exist that demonstrate 10- to 20-year patency for the LIMA-to-LAD anastomosis, similar data on SVG patency are quite discouraging; thus the DES is currently an attractive alternative.[36,37]

An alternative to the use of an SVG conduit in CABG is the use of multiple arterial grafts. A recent meta-analysis study showed the use of multiple arterial grafts including right internal mammary artery (RIMA) graft may improve survival.[38] However, some surgeons may be reluctant to perform bilateral internal mammary artery (BIMA) grafting due to concerns of an increased risk of mediastinitis, particularly in patients with uncontrolled diabetes mellitus, obesity, and chronic obstructive pulmonary disease. Although current Society of Thoracic Surgeons guidelines recommend the use of multiple arterial grafts when possible, only approximately 7% of CABG operations are performed with more than one arterial graft in the United States.[39]

The LIMA-to-LAD portion of the HCR procedure can be performed in a variety of ways, including totally endoscopic atraumatic CABG, robotically assisted CABG, or CABG performed through a keyhole incision. In these approaches, the

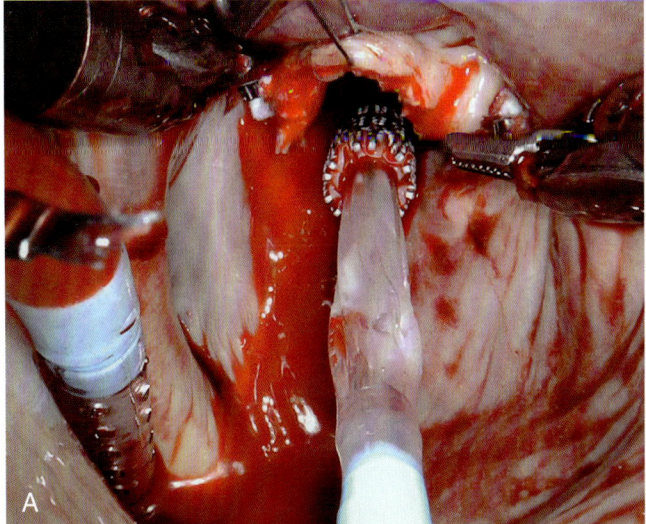

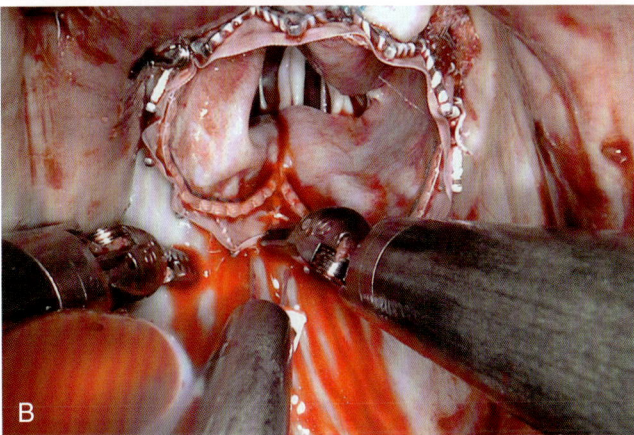

Fig. 33.8 (A) Robotic transcatheter mitral valve replacement via direct atrial approach. Positioning of the Sapien valve prior to deployment. Traction stitch at top image in the center of the residual anterior leaflet. (B) Postdeployment of the Sapien valve, securing the final anchoring stitch.

LIMA is taken down either endoscopically or robotically, and a LIMA-LAD anastomosis is either performed by hand or with robotic assistance on an arrested or beating heart. The design and techniques for these procedures are still evolving but are being brought to the forefront of mainstream cardiovascular medicine.

Postoperative survival and LIMA patency rates in patients who had HCR were excellent (98.7% to 100% and 96% to 100%, respectively) (Table 33.2).[40] Intermediate-term rates of MACCEs in the HCR group were low across the series.[40] In the only randomized prospective study to date, Gasior et al. conducted a feasibility study comparing HCR with conventional CABG.[41] Although this study has fundamental limitations as a small single-center trial lacking power analysis for either primary or secondary end points, it demonstrated that major adverse cardiovascular and cerebrovascular events (MACCEs) (89.8% HCR vs. 92.2% conventional CABG) and LAD graft patency rates (94% vs. 93%) were no different between groups at 1 year. A multicenter, observational study compared the HCR outcomes with multivessel PCI in patients with low Synergy Between PCI with Taxus and Cardiac Surgery (SYNTAX) scores.[42] This study revealed the risk-adjusted MACCE rates were similar between groups through 12-month follow-up. A large prospective randomized trial of HCR versus multivessel PCI has been funded by the National Heart, Lung and Blood Institute and started the enrollment in 2017 (NCT03089398).

The hybrid alternative to the traditional CABG or valve operation has become a reality.[43–47] Following the same premise that the LIMA-LAD is the most durable method of surgical coronary revascularization (with SVG being a distant contender), valve surgery with PCI using DES to non-LAD targets, such as the RCA and the circumflex, is currently a viable option. This is especially true in the case of frail older adults who have already undergone cardiac surgery. This approach allows the surgeon to perform minimally invasive valve surgery using only a mini thoracotomy or partial sternotomy to replace or repair the valve, thus minimizing overall morbidity. The non-LAD coronary revascularization portion of the procedure can be done with PCI with a DES either in the same setting or during a second-stage procedure. The results of published series of hybrid valve surgery or PCI are summarized in Table 33.3.[43–47] More investigation needs to take place, but the benefits derived from the current hybrid approach for treating valvular disease seem quite apparent at this initial stage.

HYBRID CARDIAC SURGEON

With time, many elective open heart surgical procedures will become less prevalent. However, complications and challenging scenarios such as hostile chest entry and difficult intravascular access to vital structures will remain. Because of this, a need for surgeons who are facile with open heart surgical techniques and who can proceed expeditiously will persist, especially for the patient presenting in extremis. As a result, the future cardiovascular surgeon will likely need to become more of a cardiovascular interventionalist than currently envisioned. Related fields such as vascular surgery have shown that additional formal endovascular training can and must be integrated into fellowship programs to achieve excellence. Today's vascular surgical community is comfortable in the interventional suite performing complex vascular interventions that combine percutaneous, endovascular, and cutdown approaches to achieve the desired clinical result. Cardiovascular surgery must follow suit to maintain excellence and safety in treating the growing aging, more complex patient population.

Surgeons have continued to perform open heart surgeries while keeping their eyes on more minimally invasive approaches. Femoral cannulation allows major operations to be performed through "mini sternotomies" or via keyhole thoracotomy incisions with very fine surgical instruments. Miniature jaws and extended hand pieces that facilitate even the most delicate maneuvers required for complex minimally invasive surgical procedures, such as mitral valve reconstruction, are currently available. Recent development of robotic technologies allows surgeons to perform totally endoscopic cardiac surgery in patients with complicated mitral valve disease. Despite these strides toward less invasive techniques, some patients remain better served without the trauma of any surgery, in particular surgery that involves cardiopulmonary bypass.

Advancing in parallel to their surgical colleagues, interventional cardiologists for decades have been performing all their cath lab procedures through the percutaneous approach. They have been extremely successful in traversing the peripheral vasculature to perform a spectrum of cardiovascular procedures ranging from very delicate coronary interventions for coronary artery disease to stenting of larger proximal and distal vessels for peripheral vascular disease and to currently replacing the aortic and mitral valves via the femoral vessels. With both disciplines working from opposite directions—the surgeon from open to minimally invasive and the interventional cardiologist from straightforward PTCA to transcatheter valve therapies—it has now become clear that the two disciplines are

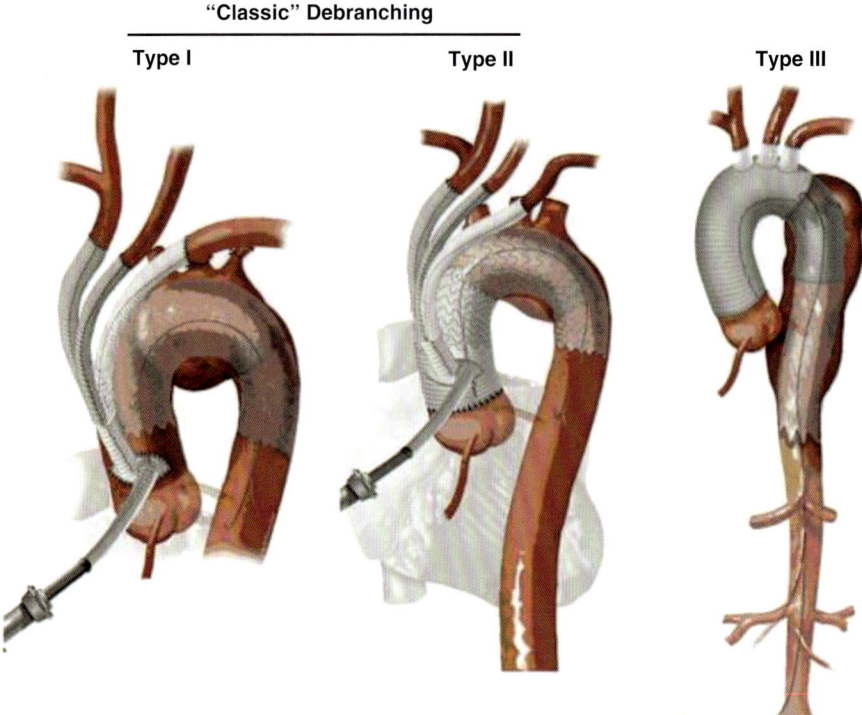

Fig. 33.9 Debranching procedure using thoracic endovascular aortic repair. Type 1: good proximal and good distal landing zone. Type 2: good distal but poor proximal landing zone. Type 3: poor proximal and poor distal landing zone. (From Milewski RK, Szeto WY, Pochettino A, et al. Have hybrid procedures replaced open aortic arch reconstruction in high-risk patients? A comparative study of elective open arch debranching with endovascular stent graft placement and conventional elective open total and distal aortic arch reconstruction. *J Thorac Cardiovasc Surg*. 2010;140[3]:590–597, Copyright © 2010 The American Association for Thoracic Surgery.)

TABLE 33.2 Results of Recent Hybrid Coronary Revascularization Series

Authors, Publication Year	Surgical Technique	n	Survival (%)	LIMA Patency (%)	MACCE (%)	Hospital LOS (days)	Conversion Rate (%)
Hu et al., 2011	MIDCAB	104	100	100	1 (18 months)	8.2	1
Bonatti et al., 2012	TECAB	140	100	97.3	20 (5 years)	6	9.7
Repossini et al., 2013	MIDCAB	166	98.8	100	17 (5 years)	6.5	2.4
Adams et al., 2014	Robotic	96	100	94	21 (5 years)	4	2.1
Bonaros et al., 2014	TECAB	180	100	NR	20 (5 years)	6	2.2
Gasior et al., 2014	MIDCAB	98	100	99	10.2 (1 years)	8.8	6
Halkos et al., 2014	Robotic	300	98.7	97.6	NR	5	2
Modrau et al., 2015	MIDCAB	100	100	95	20 (5 years)		

LIMA, Left internal mammary artery; *LOS*, length of stay; *MACCE*, major adverse cardiac and cerebrovascular events; *MIDCAB*, minimally invasive direct coronary artery bypass; *NR*, not reported; *TECAB*, totally endoscopic coronary artery bypass.
Data from Kayatta MO, Halkos ME. Reviewing hybrid coronary revascularization: challenges, controversies and opportunities. *Expert Rev Cardiovas Ther.* 2016;14(7):821–830.

poised to intersect and converge, overlapping in an unprecedented manner. It is only through close collaboration and open recognition of each other's unique, yet complementary skill set that the field of cardiovascular medicine can advance and new therapies manifest.

Hybrid Suite

Hybrid operating rooms function as a space for the integration of procedures performed both by the cardiothoracic surgeon and the interventional cardiologist. An existing cath lab or existing OR can both be fitted appropriately to accommodate the correct equipment for endovascular interventions and structural heart procedures. Imaging tools such as an image intensifier (I-I) for high-quality fluoroscopy, ultrasound, and angiography should be present for visualizing, planning, and performing minimally invasive procedures such as PCI or TAVR. However, the hybrid room must be amenable to a conversion to major surgical interventions, such as an open chest approach (in the event of an emergency), aortocoronary bypass, and open valve procedures. Appropriate materials that may not be necessary in an interventional procedure but needed in a surgical case must be present at all times. In addition, space and storage are also required for a perfusion team and equipment (Fig. 33.10).

To create an effective and functional hybrid suite, it is imperative to consider input from all those who will be potentially working in the room. The personnel, including the surgical, catheterization, anesthesia, echo, and radiologic teams, should discuss information such as equipment and placement of said equipment and staff. Plans for preparing and draping the patient in advance to accommodate both the surgeon and interventional cardiologist should be discussed because this

TABLE 33.3 Results of Hybrid Valve Surgery or Percutaneous Coronary Intervention

Author, Publication Year	n	Age (Years)[a]	ACS (%)	CHF (%)	Reop. (%)	MIS (%)	Operative Mortality (%)
PTCA ± PCI AND MVR, AVR, OR BOTH							
Byrne et al., 2005	26	72 (53–91)	92	N/A	42	30.8	3.8
Santana et al., 2014	202	76.5 (68–82)	N/A	21.6	15.3	100	3.6
George et al., 2015	26 (primary 12, reop 14)	81 (54–98), 78.5 (63–87)	N/A	66.7, 100	53.8	16.7, 7.1	0
PCI AND AVR							
Brinster et al., 2006	18	75 (56–89)	N/A	N/A	27.8	100	5.6
PCI AND MVR							
Umakanthan et al., 2009	32	69 (44–85)	15	43	38	100	3

[a]Data presented as median (range).
ACS, Acute coronary syndrome; AVR, aortic valve replacement; CHF, congestive heart failure; MIS, minimally invasive surgery; MVR, mitral valve replacement; n, number of patients; N/A, not available; PCI, percutaneous coronary intervention; PTCA, percutaneous transluminal coronary angioplasty; Reop., reoperative procedure.
Data from Leacche M, Umakanthan R, Zhao DX, et al. Surgical update: hybrid procedures, do they have a role? Circ Cardiovasc Interv. 2010;3:511–518; and Santana O, Singla S, Mihos C, et al. Outcomes of a combined approach of percutaneous coronary revascularization and cardiac valve surgery. Innovations. 2017;12:4–8.

often requires stocking a combination of standard prep packs from both the catheterization lab and OR. Planning new or updating standard operating procedures and operations manual is also critical.

Room architectural structure is also an important consideration because proper ceiling height is needed to allow screens and monitors to retract reasonably. Space and pathways should be adequate for staff and equipment to be moved, added, or removed based on the procedure. Connectivity of all imaging and monitoring equipment should be ensured and readily visible to all members of the operating staff and those in the control room. A body of literature discusses the proper methodology and construction of hybrid suites based on the extensive trial-and-error experiences of some of the earliest and most experienced hybrid centers.[48–50]

Cardiac Surgeon in Innovation

Alongside their colleagues in cardiology, radiology, and other disciplines, cardiac surgeons have led pioneering efforts for invasive procedures and technical innovations. The input of the surgeon has always been highly regarded for advice on the anatomic aspects and physiologic practicality of proposed invasive cardiac procedures. Once deemed surgically feasible, new clinical techniques are developed and adopted by the medical community, often with a less invasive approach. New interventional procedures are largely based on open surgical approaches, first converted to minimally invasive procedures by surgeons and later translated to percutaneous techniques by interventionalists. Continual refinement of interventional tools and equipment requires close collaboration among surgeons and interventionalists to continually provide state-of-the art care to cardiovascular patients

For example, in 1929 Werner Forssmann, a surgical trainee at the time, passed a urinary catheter through the vein in his own arm to his heart and subsequently irradiated himself. After successfully demonstrating the catheter to be in the right atrium, Forssmann was credited with performing the first cardiac catheterization—a procedure currently routine for the interventional cardiologist.[51,52] In 1953 Sven-Ivar Seldinger, who trained briefly as a surgeon before becoming a radiologist, developed a percutaneous approach for the introduction of vascular catheters for both right and left heart catheterization.[53] His technique is currently the most common percutaneous

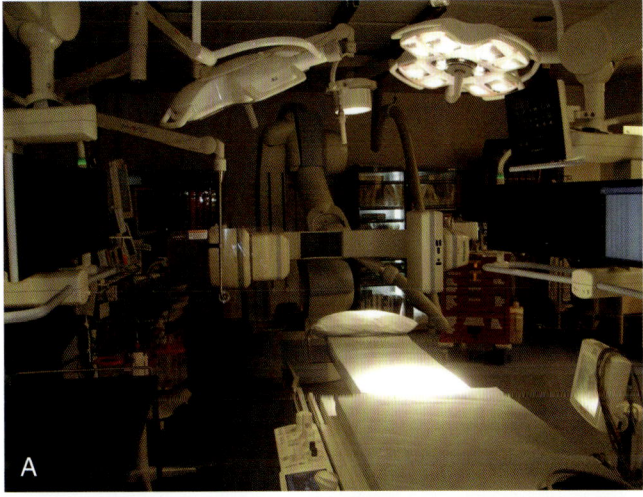
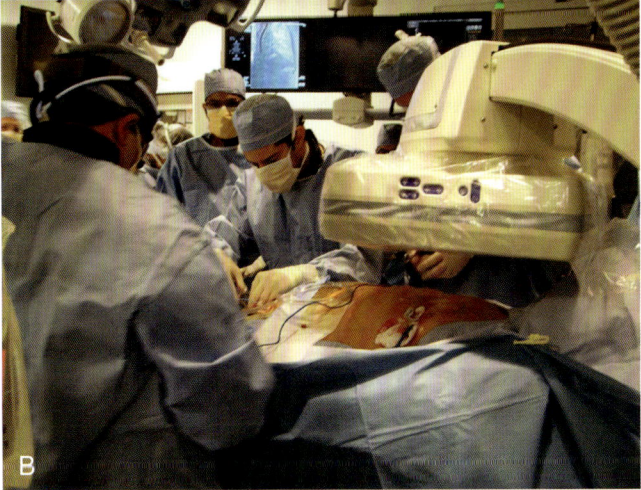

Fig. 33.10 Hybrid suite. (A) Hybrid interventional suite. (B) Transapical transcatheter aortic valve implantation (intraoperative photo). Note the cardiac surgeon in the foreground in proximity to the left mini thoracotomy used to access and control the left ventricular apex. Interventional cardiologists prepare the groin for instrumentation on the far side of the operating table.

approach used for gaining access to the vascular tree. Andreas Grüntzig and, along with his surgical colleague Richard Myler, in 1977 inflated the first catheter-guided balloon in a coronary artery during a coronary bypass operation.[54] Grüntzig's novel procedure eventually became known as *percutaneous transluminal coronary angioplasty* (PTCA) and set the stage for modern interventional cardiology and PCI.

These, among other events and milestones, illustrate that surgeons have remained steadfast throughout history. This stays constant today as the cardiac surgeon transcends disciplines and roles to allow for new ideas and creativity that pave the way for revolutionary changes. As new procedures alter the current standard of care and are adopted into practice, it is critical for the cardiac surgeon's role and knowledge be expanded to the entire heart team.

Training for Future Hybrid Cardiac Surgeon/Interventionalist

The discipline of cardiac surgery remains too complex for practicing interventional cardiologists to cross-train without completing a lengthy formal residency in surgery. However, focused and well-thought-out surgical rotations integrated throughout medical residency training and cardiology fellowship could prepare an interventionalist to perform more complex and minimally invasive techniques in conjunction with surgical colleagues. However, it is important to note that as the integument is violated in an increasingly invasive manner, the risk and magnitude of major complications escalates rapidly, and there is no substitute for the complete mastery of grounded surgical principles and technique. Likewise, presuming that much of the discipline of interventional cardiology can be mastered in short courses that claim to impart interventional "wire skills" is of equal misconception and fraught with great hazard. The true mastery of such a specialized discipline requires intense study through a formal interventional cardiovascular fellowship, which is currently almost exclusively available through the traditional cardiology pathway.

The American Board of Thoracic Surgery recently published new minimum annual case number requirement of 5 cases as primary operator and 10 cases as assistant for TAVR endovascular skills training and 5 cases for interventional wire-based procedures such as left heart catheterization, PCI, TEVAR, and MitraClip.[55] Cardiothoracic surgery training programs have been preparing for the expansion of novel percutaneous technology by making efforts to provide educational endovascular opportunities to trainees. However, a recent study showed a significant number of trainees reported feeling uncomfortable performing key steps of TAVRs (52%) and TEVARs (49%).[55] Ideally, competency in endovascular techniques should be acquired during residency. Realistically, specialized and dedicated cross-training for at least 6 months to 1 year is probably required to become a true hybrid cardiac surgeon. As of now, structural heart disease fellowship programs are available at select institutions administered jointly by the departments of surgery and medicine and require fellows to function clinically in both cardiac surgery and cardiology. According to the website of the SCAI Foundation (www.SCAI.org), 34 U.S.-based structural heart fellowship programs are currently available. Most programs are 1 year in length and impart excellent experience in all aspects of general interventional cardiology including diagnostic angiography, PCI, TAVR, endovascular graft techniques, and hybrid cardiac surgery procedures. Some programs are providing high-level exposure to emerging technology and basic to advanced interventional training opportunities for surgeons who do not have a background of interventional cardiology training.

KEY REFERENCES

14. Wennberg DE, Lucas FL, Siewers AE, et al. Outcomes of percutaneous coronary interventions performed at centers without and with onsite coronary artery bypass graft surgery. *JAMA*. 2004;292:1961–1968.
17. Leon MB, Smith CR, Mack M, et al. Transcatheter aortic-valve implantation for aortic stenosis in patients who cannot undergo surgery. *N Engl J Med*. 2010;363:1597–1607.
21. Feldman T, Kar S, Elmariah S, et al. Randomized Comparison of percutaneous repair and surgery for mitral regurgitation: 5-year results of everest II. *J Am Coll Cardiol*. 2015;66:2844–2854.
25. Eleid MF, Whisenant BK, Cabalka AK, et al. Early outcomes of percutaneous transvenous transseptal transcatheter valve implantation in failed bioprosthetic mitral valves, ring annuloplasty, and severe mitral annular calcification. *JACC Cardiovasc Interv*. 2017;10:1932–1942.
29. Bavaria J, Milewski RK, Baker J, et al. A Classic hybrid evolving approach to distal arch aneurysms: toward the zone zero solution. *J Thorac Cardiovasc Surg*. 2010;140:S77–S80.
36. Alexander JH, Hafley G, Harrington RA, et al. Efficacy and safety of edifoligide, an E2F transcription factor decoy, for prevention of vein graft failure following coronary artery bypass graft surgery: PREVENT IV: a randomized controlled trial. *JAMA*. 2005;294:2446–2454.
41. Gasior M, Zembala MO, Tajstra M, et al. Hybrid revascularization for multivessel coronary artery disease. *J Am Coll Cardiol Intv*. 2014;7:1277–1283.
42. Puskas JD, Halkos ME, DeRose JJ, et al. Hybrid coronary revascularization for the treatment of multivessel coronary artery disease: a multicenter observational study. *J Am Coll Cardiol*. 2016;68:356–365.
55. Vardas PN, Stefanescu Schmidt AC, Lou X, et al. Current status of endovascular training for cardiothoracic surgery residents in the United States. *Ann Thorac Surg*. 2017;104:1748–1754.

 Additional references available online at expertconsult.com.

中文导读

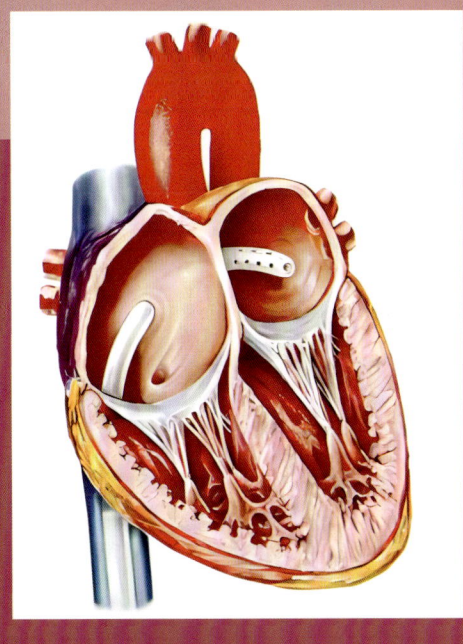

第34章
再狭窄

再狭窄是血管受损后出现的一种病理反应，内皮细胞与血小板活化、炎症反应、平滑肌细胞增殖等因素均与再狭窄有关，可能有多条通路共同参与了再狭窄的发生。经历了普通球囊和裸金属支架时代，药物洗脱支架置入术已成为当代临床实践中冠状动脉粥样硬化性心脏病介入治疗的主要手段。正是因为细胞增殖和生长因子信号在再狭窄病变中扮演了核心角色，因此形成了药物洗脱支架表面附着抗增殖药物的药理学基础。不幸的是，尽管支架不断革新，支架内再狭窄仍然是困扰术者的一类临床结局，也成为术者不得不面对的一类棘手的病变类型。得益于冠状动脉腔内影像学的应用，术者能够对再狭窄病变进行更细致的参数测量与病理评估，以期窥探再狭窄的机械性或生物性成因，为进一步干预寻找合适的解决方案。随着研究的深入，学者们尝试通过改进支架设计、抗增殖药物涂层、聚合物及洗脱系统以期减少再狭窄，但仍未能完全避免其发生。治疗再狭窄有多种策略可供选择，如药物洗脱支架置入、应用药物涂层球囊、血管内近距离放射治疗、准分子激光销蚀术或旋磨术等斑块修饰手段。对于再狭窄最好的策略是避免其发生，一旦再狭窄发生，尝试应用腔内影像学评估既往失败因素、评价再狭窄机制，有助于临床分型并指导进一步治疗。本章节汇总了当代循证医学证据，梳理了再狭窄机制、临床特征、分型、预测因素，阐述了当代预防再狭窄的举措和治疗再狭窄的策略。

张宇超　柳景华

章节要点

- 再狭窄是血管对损伤的一种病理反应，是由于血管的负性重塑和血管平滑肌细胞的新生增殖而导致的血管节段狭窄。
- 支架内再狭窄的临床和血管造影预测因素包括糖尿病、非吸烟状态、女性、急性冠状动脉综合征、既往经皮冠状动脉介入治疗、大隐静脉桥血管病变、小血管、长病变、解剖特征复杂、开口病变和慢性完全闭塞病变。
- 手术结束时所获得的管腔大小是一个重要且可控的再狭窄预测因子。
- 细胞增殖和生长因子信号是再狭窄病变的核心理论，现已成为当代药物洗脱支架的技术基础。
- 药物洗脱支架的使用极大地减少了造影再狭窄及临床再狭窄的发生率，但对于再狭窄病变、糖尿病、旁路移植物疾病和分叉病变疗效不佳。
- 在使用新一代药物洗脱支架的当代临床试验中，不良事件由靶病变失败和冠状动脉疾病原位病变进展所驱动，具有相似的预测因子。

34 Restenosis

David A. Zidar, Marco A. Costa, Daniel I. Simon

KEY POINTS

- Restenosis is a pathologic response to injury that leads to narrowing of the vessel segment as a result of negative vascular remodeling and neointimal proliferation of vascular smooth muscle cells.
- Clinical and angiographic predictors of stent restenosis include diabetes, nonsmoking status, female sex, acute coronary syndrome, previous percutaneous coronary intervention (PCI), saphenous vein graft disease, small vessel diameter, long lesions, high angiographic complexity, ostial location, and chronic total occlusions.
- The lumen size achieved at the end of the procedure is an important modifiable predictor of restenosis.
- The central roles of cellular proliferation and growth factor signaling within the restenotic lesion provide the basis for contemporary drug-eluting stent (DES) technology.
- DES use has drastically reduced angiographic and clinical restenosis across broad lesion and patient subsets, but those with restenotic lesions, diabetes mellitus, bypass graft disease, and bifurcations continue to be problematic.
- In contemporary trials using newer-generation DESs, adverse events are driven as much by progression of coronary artery disease (CAD) in untreated sites (de novo disease) as by target-lesion failure, with similar predictors.

Nature does nothing without purpose or uselessly.
Aristoteles (384–322 BC)

INTRODUCTION

Restenosis, the arterial wall healing response to mechanical injury, has plagued cardiologists since the introduction of balloon angioplasty by Gruntzig and collaborators.[1] This chapter will describe our current understanding of the mechanisms, clinical features, impact, and treatment of restenosis in contemporary percutaneous coronary intervention (PCI).

ARTERIAL INJURY AND MECHANISMS OF RESTENOSIS

Normal Versus Pathologic Response to Arterial Injury

The initial consequences of balloon angioplasty or coronary stenting are de-endothelialization, mechanical disruption of atherosclerotic plaque, often with dissection into the tunica media and occasionally adventitia, and stretch of the entire artery.[2] Endothelial injury, platelet aggregation, inflammatory cell infiltration, release of growth factors, medial smooth muscle cell (SMC) modulation and proliferation, proteoglycan deposition, and extracellular matrix remodeling are the major milestones in the temporal sequence of the response to this trauma. In the majority of patients, the healing response includes both stabilization of the SMC structures and reendothelialization of the artery without significant reduction in vessel diameter. In contrast, restenosis is a pathophysiologic response to injury, which leads to narrowing of the vessel segment, due to negative vascular remodeling and/or neointimal proliferation (Fig. 34.1).[3] Neointimal hyperplasia (NIH) ultimately is a result of inappropriate migration and proliferation of vascular SMC, and is driven by multiple factors (Fig. 34.2). Bare-metal stents (BMS) were developed to mitigate elastic recoil and negative remodeling, but they remain prone to NIH. Drug-eluting stents (DES) were developed to prevent NIH, and these devices (especially first-generation DES) can be accompanied by delayed reendothelialization, which has been associated with stent thrombosis. Thus, the durability of coronary interventions largely depends on a healthy healing response to arterial injury. While a great deal is known about the general response to injury, what remains less clear are the particular mechanisms that differentiate an optimal "healthy" injury pattern leading to reendothelialization without NIH from a pathologic one resulting in either NIH or incomplete reendothelialization.

Endothelial Cell and Platelet Activation

In animal models, denuding the endothelium is sufficient for the development of NIH. Several mechanisms appear to directly link endothelial activation to restenosis. First, nitric oxide-mediated responses to flow and shear stress provide a protective response. Therefore, the loss of a functional endothelium likely contributes to pathological healing.[4] Second, endothelial injury leads to the production of cytokines such as platelet derived growth factor (PDGF) and transforming growth factor β (TGF β) which can induce migration and proliferation of vascular smooth muscle cell (VSMC).[5] Endothelial response to injury also promotes platelet adhesion. Platelet activation and deposition has been shown to occur almost immediately after endothelial injury in vivo,[6,7] and results in the platelet production of cytokines and growth factors including PDGF. Elevated platelet reactivity measured at the time of PCI has been associated with increased restenosis rates after balloon angioplasty.[8]

Inflammation

The central role that inflammatory pathways play in the pathophysiology of restenosis is also generally well accepted.[9] After a layer of platelets and fibrin are deposited at the injured site, adhesion molecules such as P-selectin on platelets attach to circulating leukocytes via receptors such as P-selectin glycoprotein ligand (PSGL-1) to promote leukocyte rolling along the injured surface. Leukocytes then bind tightly to platelets through the interaction of leukocyte Mac-1 with platelet glycoprotein (GP) Ibα and through leukocyte integrin cross linking with fibrinogen which is bound to the platelet GP IIb/IIIa receptor. Migration of leukocytes occurs across the platelet-fibrin layer as these cells diapedese through tissue, driven by chemical gradients of chemokines released from SMCs and resident macrophages.

The precise cellular and molecular mechanisms of inflammation following arterial injury are dependent on the specific type of injury (i.e., atherogenic vs. balloon mechanical vs. stent). For example, experimental stent deployment in animal arteries causes sustained elevation of monocyte chemotactic protein-1 (MCP-1) postinjury (~14 days) compared to balloon-injured arteries (<24 hours).[10] Antibody-mediated blockade of C-C chemokine receptor 2 (CCR2), a primary leukocyte receptor for MCP-1, markedly diminished neointimal thickening after stent-induced, but not balloon-induced, injury in nonhuman primates.[11]

Inflammatory responses to the stent itself have also been proposed. Innate immune responses, which have a predominance of monocyte/macrophage infiltrates, have been described. Antigen-specific adaptive immune hypersensitivity responses typified by infiltration of T-cells and B-cells in conjunction with eosinophils may also play a role in restenosis (reviewed by Byrne et al.[12]). The corrosion of stent material, leading to the activation of thrombospondin-1-dependent inflammatory pathways may also play a role in the restenotic processes following stenting.[13]

Investigators have pursued antirestenosis strategies using systemic antiinflammatory therapies, including liposome-encapsulated bisphosphonates,[14] prednisone,[15] anti-CD18 or anti-CCR2 blockade,[11] and peroxisome proliferator-activated receptor (PPAR-γ) activator rosiglitazone. Experimental observations support a causal

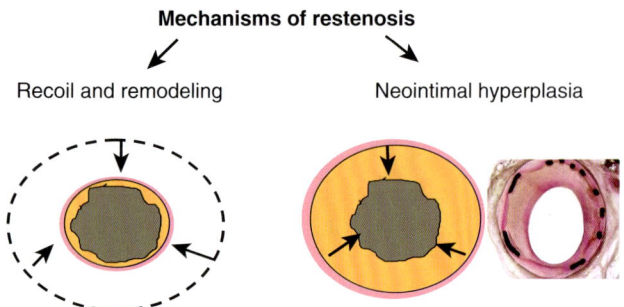

Fig. 34.1 Illustration of the two main mechanisms of restenosis. Negative vessel remodeling and elastic recoil are mainly observed after balloon angioplasty, while in-stent restenosis is mainly associated with intimal hyperplasia (in-stent restenosis histology, *right panel*).

A Diseased artery before stent
Atherosclerotic plaque with resident macrophages

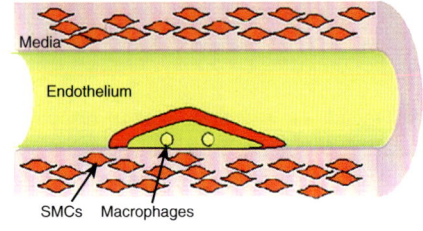

B Immediate after stent
Endothelial denudation, platelet/fibrinogen deposition

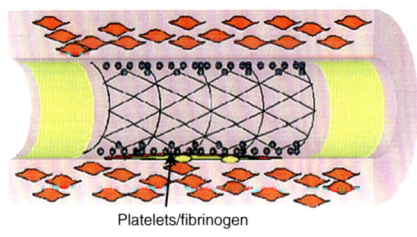

C Leukocyte recruitment
Cytokine release

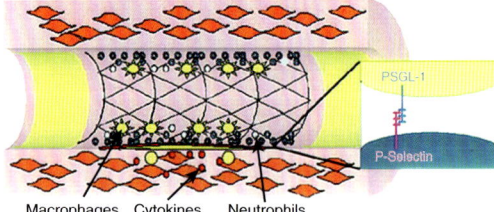

D Leukocyte infiltration
SMC proliferation/migration

E Neointimal growth
Continued SMC proliferation and macrophage recruitment

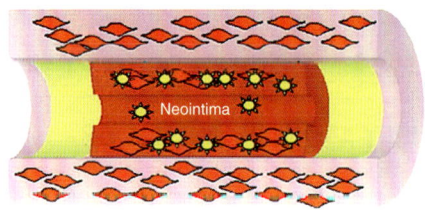

F Restenotic lesion
More ECM rich over time

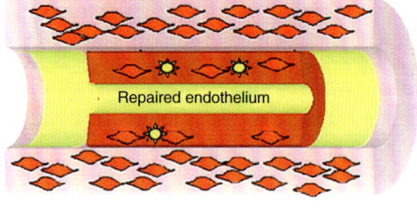

Fig. 34.2 Schematic of the integrated cascade of restenosis. (A) Atherosclerotic vessel before intervention. (B) Immediate result of stent placement with endothelial denudation and platelet/fibrinogen deposition. (C and D) Leukocyte recruitment, infiltration, and smooth muscle cell *(SMC)* proliferation and migration in the days after injury. (E) Neointimal thickening in the weeks after injury, with continued SMC proliferation and monocyte recruitment. (F) Long-term (weeks to months) change from a predominantly cellular to a less cellular and more extracellular matrix-rich plaque. (Reprinted with permission from Frederick GP, Welt FGP, Rogers C. Inflammation and restenosis in the stent era. *Arterioscler Thromb Vasc Biol.* 2002;22:1769–1776. *ECM,* Extracellular matrix; *FGF,* fibroblast growth factor; *GP,* glycoprotein; *IGF,* insulin-like growth factor; *IL,* interleukin; *MCP-1,* monocyte chemotactic protein-1; *PDGF,* platelet derived growth factor; *PSGL-1,* P-selectin glycoprotein ligand-1; *SMC,* smooth muscle cells; *TGF-β,* transforming growth factor-β; *VEGF,* vascular endothelial growth factor.)

relationship between inflammation and experimental restenosis. Antibody mediated blockade[16,17] or selective absence of Mac-1[18] diminished leukocyte accumulation and limited neointimal thickening after experimental angioplasty or stent implantation. Corticosteroids have been shown to reduce the influx of mononuclear cells, to inhibit monocyte and macrophage function, and to influence SMC proliferation.[19] However, clinical trials with systemic corticosteroids to prevent restenosis have shown disappointing results.[20]

Smooth Muscle Cell Proliferation

The SMC is vital to the healing process after arterial injury[21] due to its ability to migrate, proliferate, and synthesize extracellular matrix (ECM) upon stimulation.[22] Growth factors released from platelets, leukocytes, and SMC stimulate a granulation or cellular proliferation phase. SMCs from the media and adventitia migrate into the intima layer. Aided by fracture of the internal elastic membrane, these cells migrate into the intima, where they shift from a contractile to the synthetic phenotype. SMCs may proliferate from 24 hours to 2 to 3 months after vascular injury, returning to a contractile phenotype after this period. The PDGF is a potent promoter of this SMC migration.[23] Adventitial myofibroblasts (an α-actin staining cell) also proliferate and migrate into the neointimal[24] and appear to play an important role in supplying the intima layer with proliferative cellular elements for new lesion formation. Assessment of cellular proliferation status in atherectomy suggests that cells of the monocyte/macrophage lineage also proliferate within human in-stent restenotic tissue.[25]

While cellular division is essential for the subsequent development of restenosis, so too is the synthesis of various collagen subtypes and proteoglycans.[26] Over a longer period of time, the artery enters a phase of remodeling involving ECM protein degradation and resynthesis. Accompanying this phase is a shift to less cellular elements and greater production of ECM. This ECM actually constitutes the major component of the restenotic lesion; NIH has been shown to be predominately a low cellular tissue.[27]

Cell Cycle Regulation and the Rationale for Drug-Eluting Stent Development

The central role of cellular proliferation and growth factor signaling within the restenotic lesion provided the basis for antirestenosis pharmacological strategies targeting cell cycle division early after stent implantation. The clinical success targeting cellular division pathways illustrate the central role these pathways play in the formation of NIH.

In the absence of injury, SMCs are quiescent and exhibit very low levels of proliferative activity. However, during restenosis, SMCs that migrate to the intima progress through the G1/S transition of the cell cycle.[28] The different phases of the cell cycle of eukaryotic cells are regulated by a series of protein complexes composed of cyclins (D, E, A, B), cyclin-dependent kinases (CDKs; CDK4, CDK2, p34^{cdc2}) and their cyclin-dependent kinase inhibitors (CKIs; p27^{Kip1}, p70, p16^{INK4}). The function of CKIs is regulated by changes in their concentration as well as in their localization in the cell.[29] SMC p27^{Kip1} is downregulated after arterial injury when cell proliferation increases. p21^{Cip1} is not observed in normal arteries, but is upregulated along with p27^{Kip1} in later phases of arterial healing response and is associated with a significant decline in cell proliferation and an increase in procollagen and TGF-β synthesis.[29] These findings suggest that p27^{Kip1} and p21^{Cip1} are endogenous regulators of G1 transit in vascular SMC and inhibit cell proliferation after arterial injury. p27^{Kip1} and p21^{Cip1} bind and alter the activities of cyclin D–, cyclin E–, and cyclin A–dependent kinases (CDK2) in quiescent cells, leading to failure of G_1/S transition and cell cycle arrest.[30,31] Overexpression of p27^{Kip1} results in cell cycle arrest in the G1 phase. Conversely, inhibition of p27^{Kip1} increases the number of cells in S phase.[32]

The level of p27^{Kip1} is also regulated by constituents of the ECM. Mature collagen (polymerized type 1 collagen) suppresses p70^{S6k} and has been shown to increase the levels of p27^{Kip1}, while monomeric collagen, which is present during degradation of ECM in the synthesis phase of restenosis, downregulates p27^{Kip1}.[33] Consistent with its regulatory role in SMC proliferation and the pathobiology of restenosis, polymorphisms in P27^{kip1} that enhance the production of this cell cycle inhibitor are associated with reduced SMC proliferation and decreased risk of restenosis following PCI.[34]

Sirolimus and Its Analogues

Sirolimus (Rapamycin) was initially discovered in 1975 as an antifungal produced by *Streptomyces hygroscopicus* isolated from an Easter Island soil sample.[35] Sirolimus binds the ubiquitously expressed FK506-binding protein 12 (FBP12) protein and blocks activation of the serine/threonine kinase named mammalian target of rapamycin (mTOR).[36] Blockade of mTOR in this manner leads to inhibitory effects on cell-cycle kinases including p27, cyclins, and pRb phosphorylation resulting in cell cycle arrest at G1/S phase (Fig. 34.3).[37] In cellular models and animal experiments, sirolimus inhibits VSMC migration and proliferation[38] and has important antiinflammatory effects.[39,40]

Newer generation DES have employed sirolimus analogues with only minor pharmacokinetic differences. For example, the chemical structure of zotarolimus differs from sirolimus at the carbon 40 position in which a tetrazole substitution is made in place of the hydroxyl group of sirolimus. This modification does not affect FKBP12 binding, nor in vitro T cell and VSMC effects. However, it does lead to more lipophilicity and a shorter half-life compared to sirolimus.[41] Everolimus is another sirolimus analogue with a 2-hydroxyethyl substitution at position 40. It results in decreased in vitro potency but similar in vivo efficacy in immunosuppression and transplant models.[42,43]

Paclitaxel

Paclitaxel (Taxol) was discovered from the bark of the pacific yew tree and was noted to have potent antiproliferative properties. Its mechanism of action is achieved through the induction of tubulin polymerization, which leads to cell cycle arrest and cyostasis at G_0 (see Fig. 34.3). Systemically administered paclitaxel had favorable effects in preclinical models of restenosis.[44] In addition to blocking VSMC migration and proliferation, paclitaxel has also been shown to inhibit neutrophil function,[45] endothelial cell migration, angiogenesis, and allogenic T-cell responses.[46] Paradoxically, the effect of paclitaxel on macrophages is stimulatory in a manner similar to lipopolysaccharide.[47,48]

ANGIOGRAPHIC AND CLINICAL FEATURES OF RESTENOSIS

Definitions–Angiographic Restenosis

Angiographically detected obstruction of 50% diameter stenosis (DS) or more at the site of a previously treated coronary segment has been historically defined as restenosis.[49] This cutoff point was based on early physiological experimental studies, which demonstrated that when the arterial lumen diameter is reduced to 50% or less, coronary flow reserve becomes impeded.[50] For purposes of scientific studies, many definitions of angiographic restenosis have been used, although the classical binary definition based on percentage DS is the most widely accepted. Unfortunately, percent DS does not depict the degree of deterioration in lumen diameter and does not convey a measure of the vessel response to injury.[51,52]

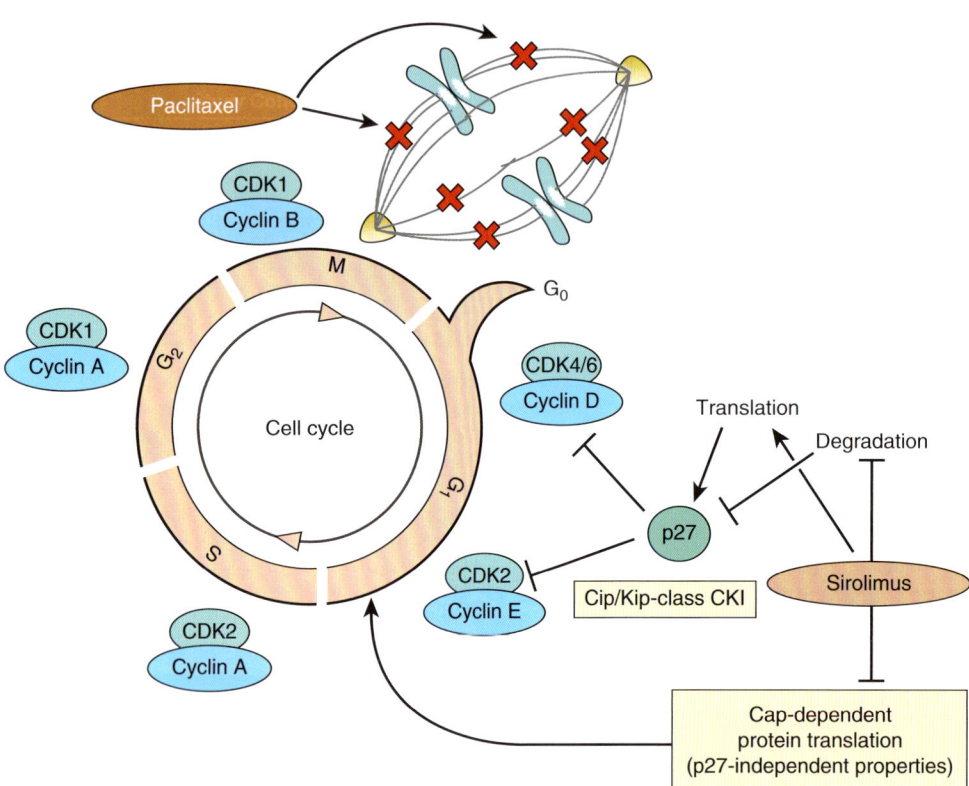

Fig. 34.3 Schematic representation of vascular smooth muscle cell cycle regulation and the mechanism of sirolimus and paclitaxel. *CDK,* Cyclin-dependent kinase; *CKI,* cyclin-dependent kinase inhibitor.

In view of these considerations, clinical restenosis studies have been adopting a more comprehensive approach in reporting findings from both perspectives (categorical and continuous), to determine whether the agent under investigation had a restraining or inhibitory effect, and whether the ultimate clinical/angiographic outcome has been improved by the use of any new therapy. However, the more subtle facets of potent antiproliferative devices, such as DES, challenge the validity of conventional angiographic parameters[53-55]; also, advanced imaging techniques, such as intravascular ultrasound (IVUS)[56] and optical coherence tomography (OCT),[57,58] have greatly improved the ability to visualize restenosis and to make quantitative assessments of strut coverage, neointimal thickness, neointimal volume, and minimal lumen diameter (MLD).

Late loss (LL) is a continuous angiographic measure of lumen deterioration. LL is conventionally calculated by subtracting the MLD value at follow-up from the immediate postprocedural MLD. These computations are made irrespective of the locations of MLD measurements. LL has traditionally served as a major outcome measure in BMS trials and continues to play a similar role in the era of DES.[59,60] It represents a surrogate marker of NIH when measurements are performed within stented segments, because stents abolish the remodeling component of the restenotic process.[51,61] However, conventional LL measurements may be methodologically flawed, because of changes in the location of MLD between postprocedure and follow-up measurements.[55,62] As a result, LL frequently derives from measurements performed in different (unmatched) locations in the target segment. Sites with higher degrees of lumen deterioration and neointimal proliferation may be overlooked, potentially leading to inaccurate conclusions regarding the antiproliferative efficacy of a given device.

Angiographic restenosis parameters have been reported in two ways: in-lesion and in-stent analyses (Fig. 34.4). "In-lesion" LL analysis encompasses the stented segment and 5 mm distally and proximally in an attempt to depict edge restenosis. Furthermore, in-lesion LL is affected by vascular remodeling or vessel spasm, and may not be a valid surrogate for intimal hyperplasia or for determining antiproliferative device efficacy.

Clinical and research assessment of restenosis has been markedly improved by IVUS and OCT, which enable high fidelity measurement of restenotic area, neointimal volume, and MLD, in addition to enabling three-dimensional rendering of restenotic segments. OCT is a particularly useful technology for the evaluation of stent healing and restenosis because current generation commercially available OCT systems produce high-resolution *in vivo* images of coronary arteries and deploy stents with 10 to 15 μm resolution compared to the 150 to 200 μm resolution of IVUS. Although limited in its ability to image deep into the blood vessel wall beyond 1 to 3 mm, OCT increases the diagnostic accuracy of near-luminal structures. Thin fibrous caps associated with plaque rupture, strut coverage, and high resolution assessment of the neointima can be visualized and quantified (reviewed by Bezerra et al.[58]) (Fig. 34.5). In clinical trials, OCT outperformed IVUS for the detection of small degrees of NIH[63] and was more sensitive in detecting stent malapposition, tissue protrusion, and edge dissections.[64,65] In addition, OCT-based single stent-strut-level analysis provides clear assessment of stent-strut coverage and apposition,[66] which are important clinical parameters that have been linked to DES-induced delayed arterial healing and the risk of stent thrombosis.[67,68]

Clinical Restenosis

Although angiography and intravascular imaging have been widely used as the initial guiding tool for the diagnosis and management of restenosis, such anatomic assessments—especially when moderate in-stent restenosis (ISR) is detected—may correlate poorly with clinical and functional assessments. Restenosis may cause no symptoms in up to 50% of patients, even when silent ischemia is demonstrable.[69] Exercise electrocardiographic testing may be of limited value to detect "silent"

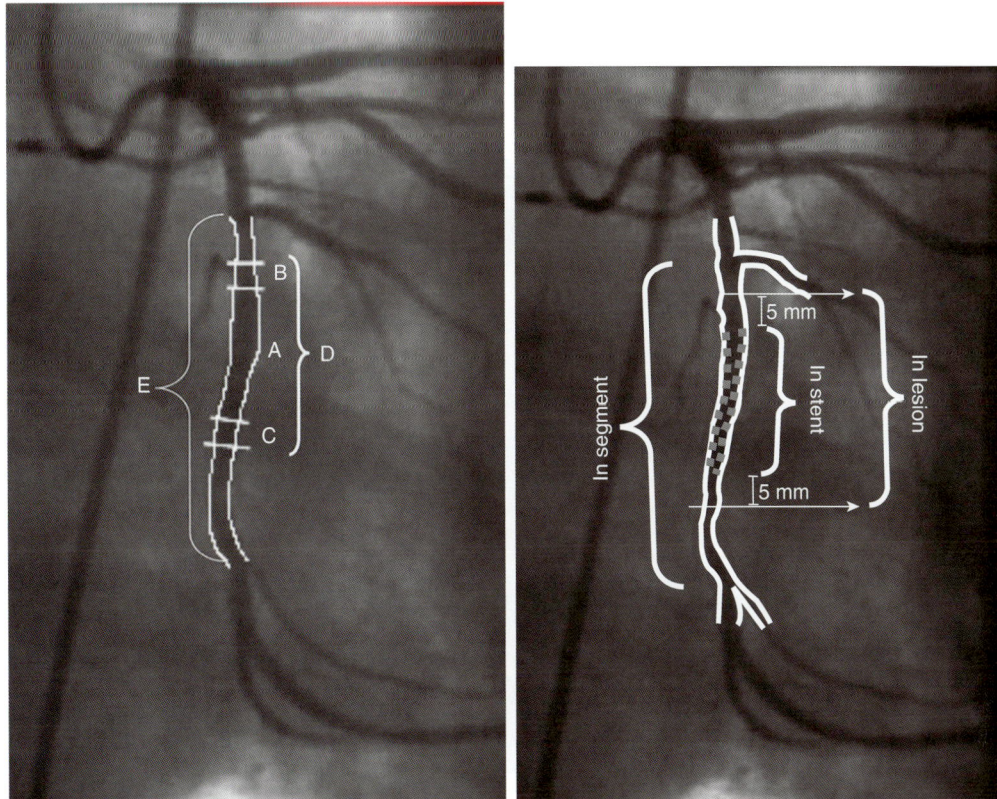

Fig. 34.4 Coronary angiography and model illustrating a segmental approach to analyze and report the effects of drug-eluting stents on coronary arteries. (Reprinted with permission from Sousa JE, Serruys PW, Costa MA. New frontiers in cardiology: drug-eluting stents: Part II. *Circulation*. 2003;107[18]:2383–2389.)

restenotic lesions[70] and computer-aided tomography angiography (CTA) detection of restenosis can be unreliable because of stent metal radiographic artifacts.[71,72] Other noninvasive tests, such as thallium scintigraphy, plus cardiac and stress echocardiography, have been used to improve the sensitivity and specificity of noninvasive assessment of restenosis.[73] Ischemia, even when quantified invasively via fractional flow reserve, has a low correlation with angiographic measurements.[74] On the other end of the clinical spectrum, restenosis may present itself in the form of an acute coronary syndrome (ACS) in up to one-third of patients, which challenges the notion that restenosis is benign.[75,76] Restenosis is of particular concern following left main PCI because of the potential risk of sudden cardiac death associated with early "silent" restenosis.

Target-lesion revascularization (TLR) is defined as any repeat percutaneous intervention of the treated coronary segment or bypass surgery of the target vessel. Target-vessel revascularization (TVR) expands the definition of TLR to include repeat percutaneous intervention of the target vessel, irrespective of the location of the stenosis within the treated segment. Target-lesion failure (TLF) is typically defined as a composite of ischemia driven TLR, myocardial infarction (MI) related to the target vessel, and death related to the target vessel.[51,77]

In clinical practice, older studies suggest patients with nonfunctional angiographic restenosis may experience a benign course,[78] and the so-called oculostenotic reflex leads to a higher rate of repeat revascularization with no clear clinical benefit at 12 months after the initial intervention.[79] If repeat angiography shows moderate ISR without clear clinical evidence of ischemia, invasive assessment of distal flow velocity or pressure can be used to enable a physiologic-based decision making regarding the need for reintervention.[80–82]

Incidence of Restenosis

The incidence of LL and binary restenosis in key stent clinical trials are described in the table 34.2.[60,83–94] One should consider differences in time of the follow-up assessment, the percentage of patients with angiographic follow-up data, and the patient population when interpreting clinical trial restenosis data.

Patterns of Restenosis

The extent and distribution of in-stent restenosis after BMS can be characterized based upon the distribution of angiographic NIH.[95] Focal restenosis (Pattern 1) is defined as less than 10 mm in length. Diffuse ISR (Pattern 2) involves a length greater than 10 mm. Proliferative ISR is greater than 10 mm in length and extends outside the stent (Pattern 3). ISR that leads to chronic total occlusion constitutes pattern 4. After Palmaz-Schatz stent implantation, of those who experienced ISR, focal restenosis occurred most frequently (42%), diffuse ISR was seen in 21%, proliferative ISR in 30%, and total occlusion in 7%.[95,96] Restenosis after bifurcation PCI frequently occurs focally at the ostium of the side branch.[97] The pattern of restenosis also influences the durability of repeat PCI. For instance, Mehran et al showed that, TLR rates in the pre DES era for BMS restenosis ranged from 19.1% for focal lesions, compared to 50% for proliferative lesions, and 83.4% for total occlusions.[98]

In general, technique-related failures (geographic miss, stent fracture, edge dissections) may account for a proportion of focal

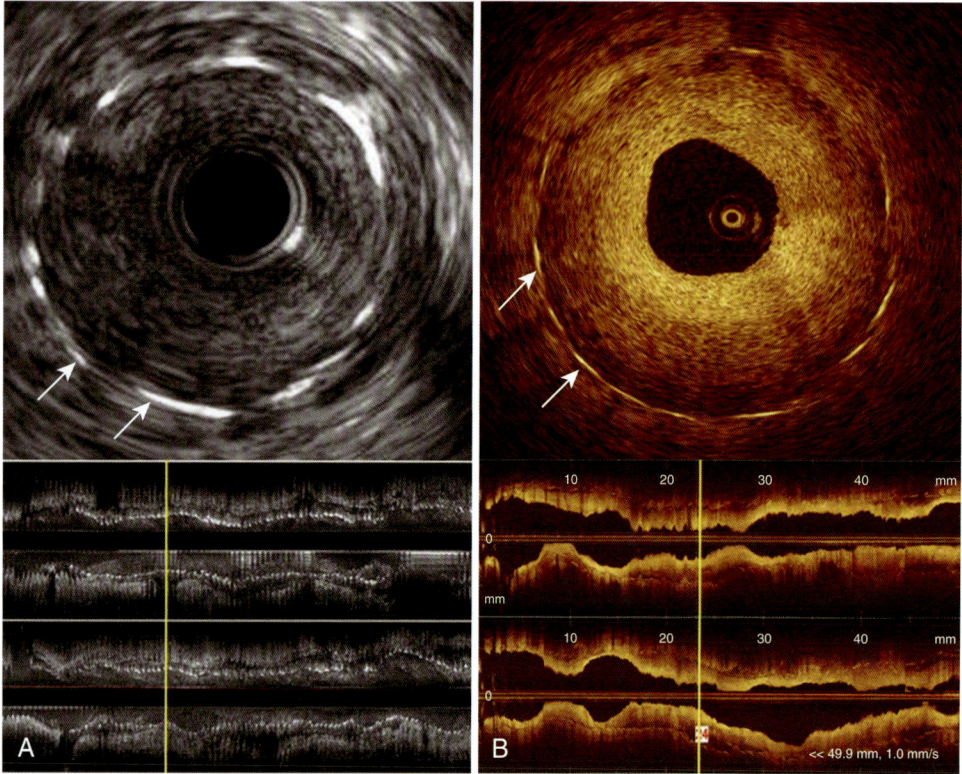

Fig. 34.5 Intravascular ultrasound (IVUS) and optical coherence tomography (OCT) imaging of bare-metal stent restenosis: 6 months after implantation in a human coronary artery, a 3.0 × 32 mm Taxus Liberte stent was evaluated by IVUS with the Boston Scientific Atlantis IVUS Catheter (A) or by OCT with the Light Lab-M3 OCT catheter (B). Stent struts *(white arrows)* are clearly visible in the cross-sectional images *(top panels)*. The higher resolution OCT system enables markedly better visualization and quantification of neointimal tissue compared to IVUS in both cross sectional *(top panels)* and longitudinal representations *(bottom panels)*. In addition, compared to IVUS (0.097-inch), the smaller profile of the OCT imaging catheter (0.016-inch") enables visualization and quantification of neointimal stenosis in areas of critical narrowing where the neointimal tissue completely contacts the IVUS catheter.

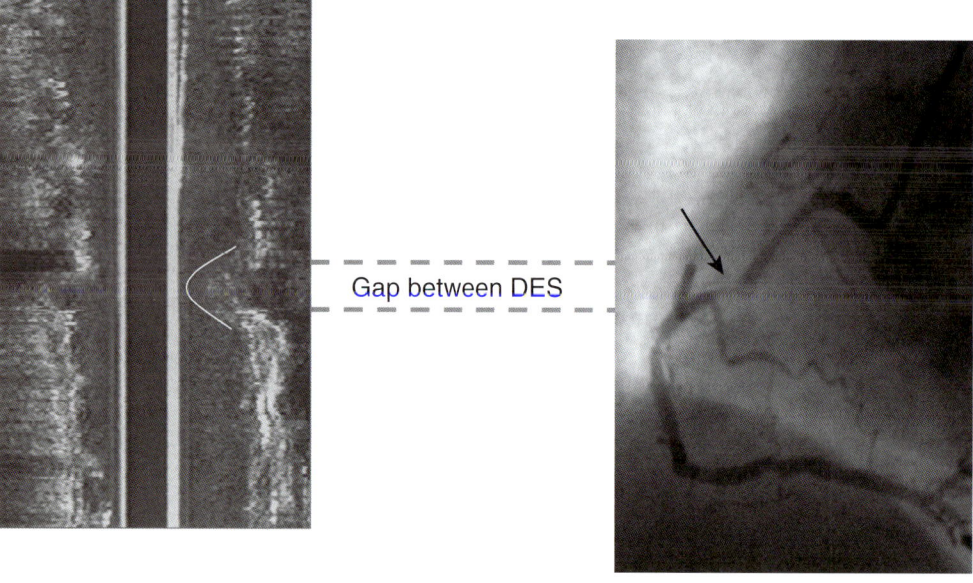

Fig. 34.6 Longitudinal intravascular ultrasound image showing a focal intimal hyperplasia formation (delineated) in a gap between two sirolimus-eluting stents. Note the lack of intimal hyperplasia within the stents. Right panel shows the corresponding focal angiographic restenosis *(black arrow)*. Mechanical and procedural related factors are key determinants of restenosis after drug-eluting stents. *DES*, Drug-eluting stent.

ISR and are observed at the stent edges or gaps between stents in noncomplex cases (Fig. 34.6). On the other hand, complex biological factors may be more likely to contribute to diffuse patterns of in-stent restenosis, which is seen in more challenging clinical scenarios such as patients with bypass graft disease or diabetes mellitus. These distinctions also have clinical relevance since a diffuse pattern of ISR predicts worse long-term outcomes after repeat PCI.[98–100]

Important differences exist when comparing in-stent restenosis after DES compared to BMS. NIH, in response to BMS, tends to occur within the first 9 months.[101] In contrast, restenosis after DES is delayed, and neointimal tissue can continue to accrue out to at least 5 years. Intravascular imaging often shows a heterogenous appearance to the NIH within DES, compared to a smooth homogenous pattern typically observed after BMS (Fig. 34.7). Comparative studies also suggest DES NIH is relatively hypocellular and proteoglycan rich, compared to BMS where there is an abundance of SMCs.[102] Pathologic studies also show that the accumulation of lipid laden foamy macrophages, so called neoatherosclerosis,[103] is frequently found within the neointima and can be accompanied by a necrotic core and thin layer fibroatheroma. Neoatherosclerosis has been reported to occur earlier after DES than after BMS,[104] but is also highly prevalent in BMS,[103] especially in the setting of very late stent thrombosis. Moreover, the characteristics of DES restenosis may vary

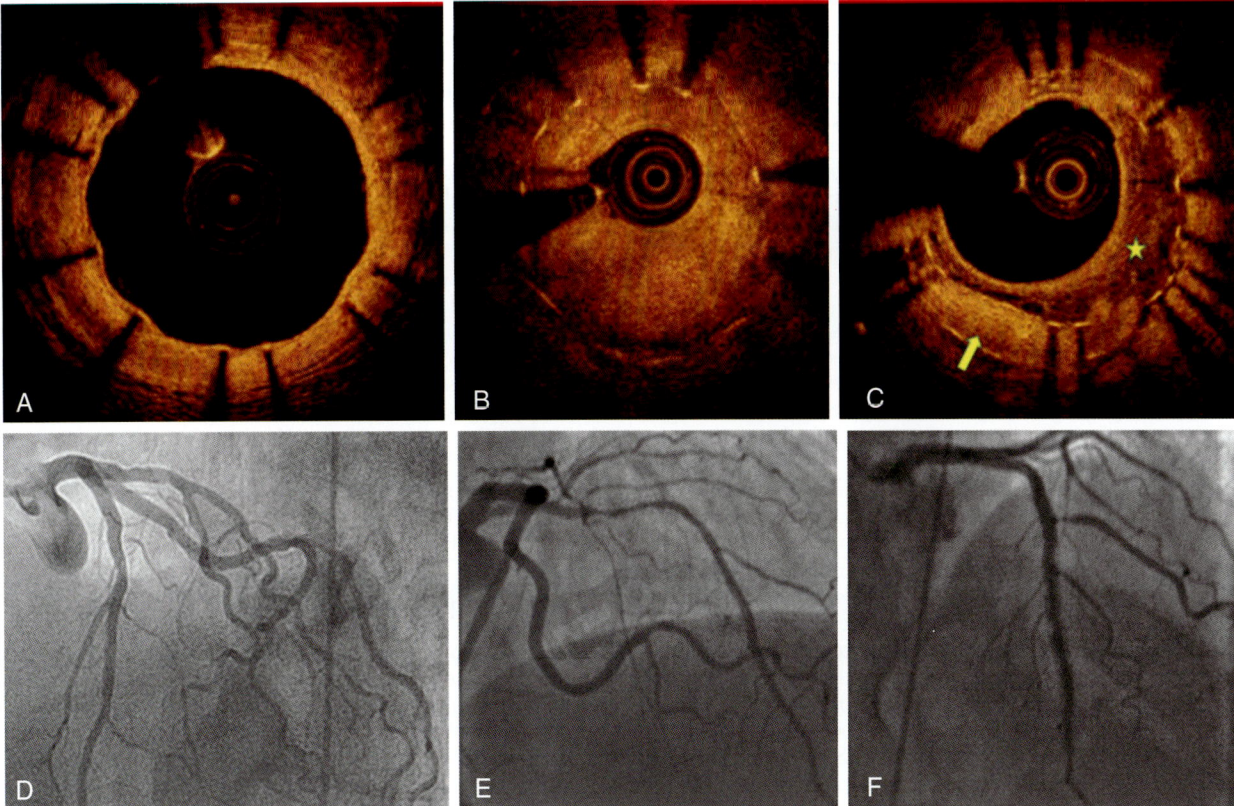

Fig. 34.7 Variable neointimal patterns as revealed by optical coherence tomography (OCT). An OCT cross-sectional image of an everolimus-eluting stent shows complete strut coverage without evidence of in-stent restenosis (ISR) at 9 months follow-up (A). ISR with a typical homogeneous fibrotic neointima is typically observed after bare-metal stent (BMS), and can also be observed after drug-eluting stent (DES), as seen in this example, 6 years after sirolimus-eluting stent implantation (B). Atypical patterns of ISR can also been seen after DES (C). This is an example of a heterogeneous, low-intensity neointima within an everolimus-eluting stent *(star)*, 1 year after implantation to treat ISR of a sirolimus-eluting stent *(arrow)* implanted 4 years earlier. Note the differences in the intensity of the neointima observed in response to the first and second percutaneous coronary intervention. Corresponding angiograms for the vessel depicted by OCT are shown (D, E, and F, respectively). (From Elmore JB, Mehanna E1, Parikh SA, et al. Restenosis of the coronary arteries: past, present, future directions. *Interv Cardiol Clin.* 2016:5(3);281–293.)

depending on the device. For example, restenosis after sirolimus-eluting stents (SES) were mostly (>90%) focal and often located at the stent edges,[105,106] while diffuse intimal proliferation or total occlusion accounted for approximately half of the restenosis cases after first-generation polymer-coated paclitaxel-eluting stents.[107]

Predictors of Restenosis

Previous studies have identified clinical and procedural factors associated with a higher risk of restenosis (Table 34.1). Diabetes mellitus has consistently been demonstrated to be an important clinical risk factor for restenosis whether it be after balloon angioplasty, BMS, or DES implantation.[108] Anatomical features associated with an increased likelihood of restenosis includes saphenous vein graft disease and small vessel diameter, long lesions, and chronic total occlusions.[109–113] Angiographic and intravascular imaging studies have extensively demonstrated that the principal determinant of restenosis is the lumen size achieved at the end of the procedure.[114,115] While DES has drastically reduced angiographic and clinical restenosis across broad lesion and patient subsets, certain anatomical and clinical scenarios—such as patients with diabetes mellitus, restenotic lesions after brachytherapy or DES,[116] bypass graft disease,[117] and bifurcations—continue to be problematic.[90,118]

TABLE 34.1 Clinical and Angiographic Predictors of Bare-Metal Stent Restenosis

Diabetes mellitus
Nonsmoking status
Female gender
Acute coronary syndrome
Previous percutaneous coronary intervention
Small-vessel diameter
Lesion length >20 mm
Multiple stents
ACC/AHA type C lesion
Ostial location

ACC, American College of Cardiology; *AHA,* American Heart Association.

The potent antiproliferative effects of DES have also exposed the importance of procedural factors as major causes of target-vessel failure (TVF). Since NIH is uncommon within the DES early after implant, the role of iatrogenic factors may be more pronounced in the current era. For example, the S.T.L.L.R (prospective evaluation of the impact of Stent deployment Techniques on clinical outcomes of patients treated with the cypheR stent) trial was a large scale study (*n* = 1567, 43 participating institutions) prospectively investigating the SES deployment technique and its relationship to clinical outcomes in the modern PCI era. This study reported a high incidence of geographical miss as defined by the mismatching of lesion and injury vascular targets with subsequent SES treatment deployment sites, and highlights the importance of procedural-related factors on clinical restenosis. Other mechanical-related failures, which may trigger restenosis, include stent under-expansion[119] and strut fracture[120]—both of which are associated with higher rates of TLR.

Stent under-expansion appears to predispose to restenosis after DES implantation. For example, in a cohort 76 patients undergoing IVUS for DES restenosis, 42% had stent under-expansion, which is a problem particularly important for longer stents where under-expansion may be more difficult to recognize without intravascular imaging.[121]

In the DES era, the predictors and mechanisms related to stent failure, especially when delayed, are poorly understood. Stent-induced or polymer-induced inflammation has also been identified as a possible contributor to first-generation DES restenosis and stent thrombosis. Polymer-induced inflammation might be especially operant in cases where there is late DES failure (restenosis >6 months after implantation) or late stent thrombosis (>12 months after implantation) occurring long after DES antiproliferative drugs have been eluted from the polymer.[13,122,123]

Altered vasomotor function with DES has been shown in arterial segments adjacent to the stented sites in DES compared to BMS treated arteries.[124,125] Even 6 months following the implantation of DES, intracoronary acetylcholine injection[126] or hand grip exercise provocation[127] induce abnormal vasoconstrictive responses in artery segments distal to DES.[128] The clinical relevance of vasomotor dysfunction has not been established, although one study demonstrated that impaired endothelial function was related to in-stent restenosis compared with matched controls.[129] DES-associated abnormalities in endothelial function could be related to delayed vascular repair, or the DES drug itself, but the drugs are completely eluted within months after implantation.[130–133] Vasomotor dysfunction may be less problematic in newer DES designs, including everolimus-eluting stents and bioresorbable scaffolds.[134–139]

PREVENTION OF RESTENOSIS—DRUG-ELUTING STENT EVOLUTION AND REDESIGNS

Scaffold Design

Preclinical studies suggest that restenotic responses may be affected by biomechanical conditions (architecture, material composition, and strut thickness) related to the stent, independent of vessel injury.[140,141] Early generation BMS and DES were mounted on stainless steel platforms with relatively large strut sizes. For instance, the Cypher stent utilized 316L stainless steel, and a strut thickness of 140 μm. The first generation Taxus was also manufactured with 316L stainless steel and had a strut thickness of 132 μm. While stainless steel has an extensive safety track record and excellent radial strength, the bulky design of these stainless-steel stents limited deliverability to distal, calcified, or tortuous segments. The development of cobalt chromium and platinum alloys for BMS and DES platforms led to substantial reductions in strut thickness with preserved radial strength.[142]

Randomized trials support the notion that stent characteristics, particularly strut size, affects the risk of restenosis.[143,144] The Intracoronary Stenting and Angiographic Results-Strut Thickness Effect on Restenosis Outcome (ISAR-STEREO) trial showed that a thin strut (50 μm) RX multilink design resulted in marked reduction in binary restenosis and TVR (12.3% vs. 21.9%) compared to the thick strut (140 μm) BX velocity.[145] Contemporary BMS and newer-generation DES have taken advantage of these advances in stent scaffold design and this may account, in part, for improved outcomes associated with newer DES compared to their first-generation counterparts. Platinium chromium alloys may offer greater radial strength, conformability, trackability, and radiopacity[145] compared to cobalt chromium in bench testing, and appear to be noninferior to cobalt chromium stents in vivo.[142]

Bioresorbable stents are also under development to function as a temporary stent structure that biodegrades once the need for redial strength and mechanical support is gone. The best studied device of this type—the Absorb Bioresorbable Vascular Scaffold (BVS, Abbott Laboratories, Abbott Park, IL)—is comprised of a backbone of poly-L-lactide, which has a strut thickness of 150 um, but degrades to water and carbon dioxide within 3 years.[146] Based upon 1 year results from the ABSORB III trial,[147] the first BVS was approved by the U.S. Food and Drug Administration (FDA) in 2016. However, due to increased rates of adverse events between years 1 and 3,[148] this device was subject to a class 1 device recall by the FDA and pulled from the worldwide market in 2017. Other bioresorbable stent platforms remain under development, including designs with lower strut thickness and greater distensibility.[146]

Drug Elution

As detailed above, BMS restenosis is typically caused by unregulated VSMC proliferation leading to NIH. As such, several antiproliferative agents were studied in early preclinical models of restenosis. Sirolimus and paclitaxel each disrupt cellular proliferation through inhibition of G1/S phase and M phase, respectively (see Fig. 34.1). These agents proved efficacious in animal models and could be delivered locally.[149–151] These two agents then resulted in striking reductions in LL and angiographic restenosis during first-in-human testing,[152,153] culminating in the SIRIUS (Sirolimus-Eluting Stent in De-Novo Native Coronary Lesions) and TAXUS (evaluating safety and feasibility of the TAXUS NIRx stent system compared with bare NIR stents [control] for treatment of coronary lesions) trials confirming the impressive efficacy of the Cypher and Taxus stents, respectively, against restenosis. These first-generation devices provided unambiguous proof that local drug delivery to disrupt the cell cycle could prevent restenosis, thus ushering in a new era of interventional cardiology.

Newer-generation DES use derivatives of sirolimus, which are engineered to have only minimal pharmacokinetic differences and similar biologic effects. Both the Endeavor and Resolute stents use zotarolimus. The chemical structure of zotarolimus differs from sirolimus at the carbon 40 position in which a tetrazole substitution is made in place of the hydroxyl group of sirolimus. This modification leads to more lipophilicity and a shorter half-life, but does not substantially alter VSMC effects compared to sirolimus.[41] The in vivo potency of zotarolimus was fourfold less than sirolimus when studied in assays of immunosuppression in rats.[41] In a porcine model of restenosis, zotarolimus-eluting stents led to effective inhibition of NIH compared to stents containing polymer only.[41] Everolimus is also a sirolimus analogue with a 2-hydroxyethyl substitution at position 40. This compound has decreased in vitro potency, but has similar in vivo efficacy in immunosuppression and transplant models.[42,43]

Polymer and Elution Kinetics

Early preclinical studies with DES showed that the prevention of restenosis requires an extended period of drug delivery.[154,155] Thus, various polymers and elution systems have now been developed not only to attach the drug to the stent during processing, sterilization, and storage, but also to allow controlled drug delivery upon stent implantation. The polymer design used in the Cypher DES consisted of three layers. The steel struts were coated with a primer layer of Parylene C. Sirolimus was contained in a middle layer of 67% polyethylene-co-vinyl acetate

(PEVA) and 33% poly(n-butyl methacrylate) (PBMA) dissolved in the organic solvent Tetrahydrofuran (THF). This system leads to controlled elution of sirolimus over 30 to 60 days.[156]

The Taxus stent had a polymer composed of poly(styrene-b-isobutylene-b-styrene) (SIBS, Translute). Preclinical testing of the kinetics of paclitaxel elution from SIBS show that the drug is eluted as an initial burst of drug release via dissolution within the first 48 hours, followed by slow release over 10 days through diffusion from the polymer.[157] Complete drug elution from SIBS extends out to 90 days.

The Xience V/Promus stent was designed to capitalize on the biocompatibility of fluorinated surfaces. Several reports suggest that fluoropassive coatings offer improved long-term biocompatibility.[158] The stent is first coated with a primer layer consisting of PBMA. The polymer is a single-phase layer of 7.8 μm consisting of an 83%/17% mixture of the semi-crystalline poly(vinylidene fluoride-co-hexafluoropropylene) and everolimus. The elution of everolimus occurs over the course of 4 months, with 25% released within the first day and an additional 50% over the first month.[159] In a rabbit model, the Xience V stent design resulted in improved endothelialization compared to first-generation DES.[160] The Promus Element DES uses the same fluoropolymer/everolimus combination on a platinum chromium platform.

The polymer used in the Endeavor (Medtronic, Minneapolis, MN) stent system was designed to provide more rapid drug elution. The polymer is based on the biomimicry of phosphorylcholine (PC), a phospholipid found on red blood cells, to optimize the biocompatibility of the surface coating. Four PC-based monomers are cross-linked to achieve adequate adhesion and durability.[161] Biocompatibility testing in porcine coronary arteries show no differences in endothelialization or inflammatory changes after PC-coated stent implantation compared to uncoated stents.[162-164] Ninety-eight percent of zotarolimus elutes from the Endeavor DES within 14 days.[165]

In contrast to the Endeavor system, the Resolute stent utilizes the BioLinx polymer, which provides extended drug elution. This formulation of three copolymers consists of a hydrophilic C19 polymer, polyvinylpyrrolidone (PVP), and a hydrophobic C10 polymer, combined in a ratio of 63%/10%/27%. The stent is covered with a primer coat of Parylene C and then zotarolimus is added in a drug/polymer ratio of 35%:65%. Due in part to its hydrophilic surface, the BioLinx appears to be relatively inert in vitro.[166] Eighty-five percent of zotarolimus elutes from the Resolute DES within 60 days and the remainder elutes by 180 days.[167]

The Synergy (Boston Scientific, Marlborough, MA) DES uses a bioabsorbable polymer attached to the abluminal surface of stent, leaving the luminal surface polymer free. This stent employs a thinner (74 μm) strut platinum chromium platform, which delivers everolimus via a polymer comprised of poly(D,L-lactide-co-glycolide) (PLGA) on the abluminal stent surface only. This stent system leads to complete drug elution as well as polymer reabsorption by 4 months.[168]

Clinical Outcomes With Newer Generation Drug-Eluting Stent

Trials of newer-generation DES have shown both improved efficacy in terms of TLR and improved safety with reduced stent thrombosis rates compared to first-generation DES designs (Table 34.2). For instance, the SPIRIT IV trial compared the Xience V everolimus eluting stent (X-EES) to the first-generation paclitaxel-eluting stent (PES) in 3687 patients with stable coronary artery disease (CAD).[169] TLF rates at 1 year were significantly lower with X-EES (4.2% vs. 6.8%; relative risk [RR] = 0.62, 95% confidence interval [CI] 0.46 to 0.82). Individual end points of MI (1.9% vs. 3.1%, P = .02) and stent thrombosis (0.17% vs. 0.85%, P = .004) also favored X-EES over PES at 1 year. The results held at 2 years, and EES was still associated with superior outcomes[170] for TLF (6.9% vs. 9.9%, P = .003) and MI (2.5% vs. 3.9%, P = .02). Stent thrombosis rates at 2 years were still considerably lower for the newer-generation stent (0.4% vs. 1.2%, P = .008). The COMPARE trial tested X-EES versus PES in a broader population of 1800 patients (60% had ACS and 25% had ST-elevation myocardial infarction [STEMI]) and involved more complex lesions (45% had type C lesions, with an average of 1.4 lesions per patient).[171] The primary end point, a composite of all-cause mortality, MI, and TVR at 12 months, was lower with X-EES (6% vs. 9%, P = .02), TLR was also reduced with X-EES (2% vs. 5%, P = .0002), as was definite and probable stent thrombosis (0.7% vs. 3%, P = .002). The advantages for X-EES held up after 2 years for the primary end point (9.0% vs. 13.7%, P = .0016) and definite/probable stent thrombosis (0.9% vs. 3.9%, P < .0001).[172] Rates of very late stent thrombosis between years 1 and 2 were also low with the X-EES (0.3% vs. 1.5%, P = .02) despite the fact that only 13% of this relatively high-risk population continued dual antiplatelet therapy beyond 1 year. Five-year outcomes from the SPIRIT III trial showed continued superiority of X-EES over PES for TLF (12.7% vs. 19.0%, P = .008) as well as reduced all-cause death (5.9% vs. 10.1%, P = .02).[173]

The Resolute All Comers trial compared the Resolute Zotorolimus-eluting stent (R-ZES) system to X-EES in 2292 patients, (over 50% presented with ACS); it was powered for clinical events with a noninferiority design.[174] Rates of TLF were similar for both stents (8.2% for R-ZES vs. 8.3%, P < .001 for noninferiority). In-stent late lumen loss was not statistically different between the two stents (0.27 ± 0.43 mm for R-ZES vs. 0.19 ± 0.40 for X-EES, P = .08). Rates of definite, probable, or possible stent thrombosis were similar for both stents (2.3% vs. 1.5% X-EES, P = .17). These findings were confirmed in the TWENTE trial, a second head-to-head comparison of R-ZES with X-EES designed to test these two stent designs across broad patient populations, including those with ACS and higher risk "off-label" lesion subsets.[175] Patients treated with R-ZES had a TVF rate of 8.2% compared to 8.1% in patients treated with X-EES (difference 0.1%, CI–2.8% to 3.0%, P = .001 for noninferiority). Definite-or-probable stent thrombosis rates were similar for both stents (0.9% and 1.2% for X-EES, P = .59).

Whereas trials of first-generation DES versus BMS convincingly demonstrated that local cell cycle inhibition could lead to a dramatic reduction in restenosis rates, the trials of newer generation DES versus first-generation DES establish that very late stent thrombosis risk is not a "necessary evil" of DES. Newer-generation DES achieved additional reductions in restenosis while also lowering stent thrombosis rates, which suggests that a better balance between reendothelialization and NIH prevention was possible. In fact, contemporary DES now have very late stent thrombosis rates similar to BMS.[176]

Predictors of restenosis after newer generation DES appear similar to first-generation DES[118,177] and include diabetes mellitus, previous PCI, angiographic complexity, vein graft disease, ostial lesions, and prior restenosis.[178] It is also notable that predictors of DES restenosis, including angiographic complexity, also predict the future need for revascularization at de novo sites.[178] This suggests that in the current era, mechanisms that drive the progression of de novo atherosclerosis may overlap with, and be as important as, those that drive stent failure.

TREATMENT OF RESTENOSIS

After Percutaneous Transluminal Coronary Angioplasty

Repeat PCI for restenosis stemming from balloon angioplasty (alone), as the index procedure, has a relatively favorable prognosis. Treatment with BMS in this setting has been associated

TABLE 34.2 Summary of Pivotal Restenosis Trial Data

Study (n)	Randomized	Drug/Agent	Device Type	In-Stent Late Loss (Time of f-up)	In-Lesion Restenosis (Time of f-up)
BMS vs. PTCA STRESS (n = 410)	Yes	None	Palmaz-Schatz Balloon angioplasty	0.74-mm (6-month)[a] 0.38-mm (6-month)[a]	31.6% (6-month) 42.1% (6-month)
BENESTENT (n = 520)	Yes	None	Palmaz-Schatz Balloon angioplasty	0.65-mm (6-month)[a] 0.32-mm (6-month)[a]	22% (6-month) 42% (6-month)
MUSIC (n = 161)	No	None	Palmaz-Schatz	0.77-mm (6-month)	8.3% (6-month)
1st-Gen DES **RAVEL** (n = 238)	Yes	Sirolimus	BX Velocity BX Velocity	−0.01-mm (6-month) 0.8-mm (6-month)	0% (6-month) 26.6% (6-month)
SIRIUS (n = 1058)	Yes	Sirolimus None	BX Velocity BX Velocity	0.17-mm (8-month) 1.00 mm (8 month)	8.9% (9-month) 36.3% (9-month)
TAXUS IV (n = 1314)	Yes	Paclitaxel None	Express 2 Express 2	0.39-mm (9-month) 0.92-mm (9-month)	7.9% (9-month) 26.6% (9-month)
REALITY (n = 1386)	Yes	Sirolimus Paclitaxel	BX Velocity Express 2	0.09-mm (8-month) 0.31-mm (8-month)	9.6% (8-month) 11.1% (8-month)
SIRTAX (n = 1012)	Yes	Sirolimus Paclitaxel	BX Velocity Express 2	0.13-mm (9-month) 0.25-mm (9-month)	6.7% (9month) 11.9% (9-month)
Newer Gen DES **ENDEAVOR II** (n = 1197)	Yes	Zotarolimus None	Driver Driver	0.61-mm (9-month) 1.03-mm (9-month)	13.2% (9-month) 35% (9-month)
SPIRIT III (n = 1002)	Yes 2:1	Everolimus Paclitaxel	Vision Express 2	0.16-mm (8-month) 0.30-mm (8-month)	2.3% (8-month) 5.7% (8-month)
PLATINUM QCA (n = 100)	No	Everolimus	Element	0.20-mm (9-month)	1.1% (9-month)[b]
RESOLUTE FIM (n = 139)	No	Zotarolimus	Driver	0.22-mm (9-month)	2.1% (9-month)[b]
Diabetes Trials **DIABETES-I** (n = 160)	Yes	Sirolimus None	BX Velocity BX Velocity	0.08 (9-month) 0.66-mm (9-month)	7.7% (9-month) 33% (9-month)
DIABETES-II (n = 80)	No	Paclitaxel	Express 2	0.42-mm (9-month)	7.6% (9-month)
ISAR-DIABETES (n = 250)	Yes Yes	Sirolimus Paclitaxel	BX Velocity Express 2	0.19-mm (6-month) 0.49-mm (6-month)	6.9% (6-month) 16.5% (6-month)

[a]These measurements reflect "In-lesion" late loss instead of "In-stent."
[b]These measurements reflect "In-segment" restenosis instead of "In-lesion."
BMS, Bare-metal stent; *DES*, drug-eluting stent; *f-up*, follow-up; *PTCA*, percutaneous transluminal coronary angioplasty.

with an 18% rate of repeat restenosis, which compares favorably with restenosis rates for de novo lesions.[179] Therefore, restenosis after balloon angioplasty should typically be treated with stenting when technically feasible, given the randomized data that shows improved angiographic and clinical results compared to repeat balloon angioplasty alone.[179]

After Bare-Metal Stents

Prior to the DES era, the treatment of BMS restenosis was associated with high rates of repeat TLR.[180] Several studies compared the use of balloon angioplasty (alone) with repeat BMS placement.[181,182] For instance, the Restenosis Intra-Stent: Balloon Angioplasty Versus Elective Stent Implantation (RIBS-I) trial (n = 450) showed that patients with BMS restenosis had TVR rates of 24.3% and 19.6% after balloon angioplasty versus BMS, respectively, at 12 months.[180]

Intracoronary radiation has also been extensively studied in the setting of BMS restenosis.[183-185] For instance, the Washington Radiation for In-Stent Stenosis Trial (WRIST) study showed brachytherapy results in improved early TVR rates (26% vs. 68%), but higher rates of TLR between 6 months and 5 years (21.5% vs. 6.1%).[186] Brachytherapy is also associated with very late stent thrombosis,[185] which is probably due to delayed endothelial healing.[187]

The introduction of DES has significantly improved the treatment of BMS restenosis. First-generation DES have been shown to be superior to balloon angioplasty as well as brachytherapy for the treatment of BMS restenosis.[188-191] Observational trials of contemporary DES designs suggest these newer devices also lead to durable results with low restenosis and major adverse cardiovascular events (MACE) rates (10% to 15% at 9 to 12 months).[192,193] Thus, BMS restenosis is often best treated by restenting with DES.

Angioplasty with a drug-coated balloon (DCB) has been shown to be superior to plain balloon angioplasty in those with BMS restenosis. For instance, Scheller et al. showed that patients with BMS ISR randomized to DCB had lower rates of restenosis and MACE (31% vs. 4%, P = .01) compared to those who had angioplasty with an uncoated balloon.[194] A paclitaxel DCB had similar results to restenting with a paclitaxel DES.[195] The RIBS V study randomized patients with BMS ISR to the newer-generation EES versus DCB. The EES was associated with superior angiographic results, but the DCB led to similarly low rates of TVR and MACE at 1 year.[196]

After Drug-Eluting Stents

Patients who develop DES restenosis should be viewed as a population for recurrent events regardless of the strategy used for repeat PCI. For instance, among 392 patients with first-generation DES ISR, the MACE rates after a median of 3 years were 32.8%.[197] The rate of treatment failure for DES restenosis depends on the pattern of restenosis, with the highest repeat restenosis rates observed in patients with diffuse patterns.[100,197,198]

Similar to BMS ISR, various interventional approaches have been compared for DES ISR. For instance, in patients (n = 96) with focal (<10 mm) ISR from a first-generation DES, repeat PCI using an SES led to improved angiographic results at 9 months, and similar TVR rates compared to cutting balloon angioplasty (0.0% vs. 6.3%, P > .05) at 12 months.[199] The Intracoronary Stenting and

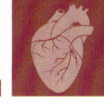

Angiographic Results: Drug Eluting Stents for In-Stent Restenosis 2 (ISAR-DESIRE 2) trial compared repeat stenting with SES or PES in patients with SES restenosis.[200] These two first-generation DES were equally effective at treating DES restenosis, however, 1 year MACE rates were relatively high (≈20%) in both groups. Intravascular brachytherapy has also been studied for DES ISR as an alternative to repeat PCI with DES.[201] DCB use leads to improved rates of TVR compared to balloon angioplasty[202,203] and may be similar to repeat stenting with a first-generation DES.[204]

Whether DCB is superior to newer-generation DES is less clear based upon observational studies.[205,206] A network analysis comparing the multitude of available interventional strategies for DES ISR suggests that repeat PCI with a newer-generation DES is associated with the lowest rates of recurrent TVR.[207] However, as these patients represent a heterogeneous group, personalized approaches to their treatment are advisable until more definitive studies are available.

Role of Intravascular Imaging

Intravascular imaging may provide information as to the mechanism of stent failure, and may guide the intervention. It is particularly important to exclude stent under-expansion, especially when restenting is planned. Defining the bulk of NIH may also guide debulking strategies. Stent fracture, geographic miss, and other potential etiologies or restenosis may be defined via intravascular imaging. Thus the use of IVUS or OCT should be considered to define the mechanism ISR. If mechanical failures are encountered and the stenosis is discrete, properly sized balloon angioplasty may suffice. If the disease is mostly outside the stent, that is, edge restenosis, or there is substantial NIH burden, another DES may be needed.

Debulking and Other Plaque Modifying Modalities

Numerous debulking/plaque modifying devices have been used for lesion modification at the time of repeat intervention for ISR. Laser atherectomy relies on high-intensity light, heat, and shock waves for the ablation of tissue, and may facilitate greater expansion upon stent delivery. Rotational atherectomy utilizes a diamond-tipped burr, rotating at high speeds, to mechanically debulk the lesion. The cutting balloon, with its three to four blades on the outer surface, makes cuts along the endothelium upon expansion and purportedly improves the dilatability of the intended segment. The AngioSculpt scoring balloon has nitinol struts that encircle the balloon to facilitate complete expansion of ISR tissue. Each of these devices has been shown to result in greater luminal diameter, but this has not consistently resulted in demonstrable improvements in clinical event rates in the pre-DES era.[208–210] Additional study is needed to determine the efficacy and optimal manner of debulking in the current DES era.

SUMMARY

Restenosis is a major limitation to PCI and limits the durability of PCI. The development of first-generation and newer-generation DES has drastically reduced, but not eradicated, restenosis. As a result of this in combination with improved deliverability of these newer designs, PCI is a feasible treatment option in the great majority of patients with CAD. Given the increased utilization of PCI, restenosis remains a significant problem requiring individualized treatment strategies.

Our experiences from Gruentzig to the present have consistently highlighted that coronary atherosclerosis is a formidable adversary; thus this generation of devices, no matter how much improved, are unlikely to be the last. The current challenge is to improve the efficacy of PCI by developing new strategies that treat complex obstructive atherosclerosis, prevent restenosis, and restore arterial healing. It is notable that the same predictors of restenosis after BMS are relevant even after newer-generation DES, predicting both failure at the stented segment as well as progression elsewhere. Thus, despite the gains achieved in improving the durability of PCI procedural success, a greater understanding of the basic biologic mechanisms that promote healthy arterial healing and durable resistance to de novo and recurrent atherosclerosis are still needed.

KEY REFERENCES

1. Gruntzig AR, Senning A, Siegenthaler WE. Nonoperative dilatation of coronary-artery stenosis: percutaneous transluminal coronary angioplasty. *N Engl J Med*. 1979;301:61–68.
67. Finn AV, Kolodgie FD, Harnek J, et al. Differential response of delayed healing and persistent inflammation at sites of overlapping sirolimus- or paclitaxel-eluting stents. *Circulation*. 2005;112:270–278.
76. Rathore S, Kinoshita Y, Terashima M, et al. A comparison of clinical presentations, angiographic patterns and outcomes of in-stent restenosis between bare metal stents and drug eluting stents. *EuroIntervention*. 2010;5:841–846.
83. Serruys PW, de Jaegere P, Kiemeneij F, et al. A comparison of balloon-expandable-stent implantation with balloon angioplasty in patients with coronary artery disease. Benestent Study Group. *N Engl J Med*. 1994;331:489–495.
84. Fischman DL, Leon MB, Baim DS, et al. A randomized comparison of coronary-stent placement and balloon angioplasty in the treatment of coronary artery disease. Stent Restenosis Study Investigators. *N Engl J Med*. 1994;331:496–501.
86. Moses JW, Leon MB, Popma JJ, et al. Sirolimus-eluting stents versus standard stents in patients with stenosis in a native coronary artery. *N Engl J Med*. 2003;349:1315–1323.
87. Stone GW, Ellis SG, Cox DA, et al. A polymer-based, paclitaxel-eluting stent in patients with coronary artery disease. *N Engl J Med*. 2004;350:221–231.
94. Stone GW, Midei M, Newman W, et al. Comparison of an everolimus-eluting stent and a paclitaxel-eluting stent in patients with coronary artery disease: a randomized trial. *JAMA*. 2008;299:1903–1913.
95. Mehran R, Dangas G, Abizaid AS, et al. Angiographic patterns of in-stent restenosis: classification and implications for long-term outcome. *Circulation*. 1999;100:1872–1878.
98. Bossi I, Klersy C, Black AJ, et al. In-stent restenosis: long-term outcome and predictors of subsequent target lesion revascularization after repeat balloon angioplasty. *J Am Coll Cardiol*. 2000;35:1569–1576.
147. Ellis SG, Kereiakes DJ, Metzger DC, et al. Everolimus-eluting bioresorbable scaffolds for coronary artery disease. *N Engl J Med*. 2015;373:1905–1915.
148. Kereiakes DJ, Ellis SG, Metzger C, et al. 3-Year Clinical outcomes with everolimus-eluting bioresorbable coronary scaffolds: the ABSORB III trial. *J Am Coll Cardiol*. 2017;70:2852–2862.
170. Stone GW, Rizvi A, Sudhir K, et al. Randomized comparison of everolimus- and paclitaxel-eluting stents: 2-year follow-up from the SPIRIT (Clinical Evaluation of the XIENCE V Everolimus Eluting Coronary Stent System) IV trial. *J Am Coll Cardiol*. 2011;58:19–25.
171. Kedhi E, Joesoef KS, McFadden E, et al. Second-generation everolimus-eluting and paclitaxel-eluting stents in real-life practice (COMPARE): a randomised trial. *Lancet*. 2010;375:201–209.
175. von Birgelen C, Basalus MWZ, Tandjung K, et al. A randomized controlled trial in second-generation zotarolimus-eluting resolute stents versus everolimus-eluting Xience V stents in real-world patients: the TWENTE trial. *J Am Coll Cardiol*. 2012;59:1350–1361.
178. Taniwaki M, Stefanini GG, Silber S, et al. 4-Year clinical outcomes and predictors of repeat revascularization in patients treated with new-generation drug-eluting stents: a report from the RESOLUTE All-Comers trial (A Randomized Comparison of a Zotarolimus-Eluting Stent With an Everolimus-Eluting Stent for Percutaneous Coronary Intervention). *J Am Coll Cardiol*. 2014;63:1617–1625.
187. Costa MA, Sabaté M, van der Giessen WJ, et al. Late coronary occlusion after intracoronary brachytherapy. *Circulation*. 1999;100:789–792.
191. Kastrati A, Mehilli J, von Beckerath N, et al. Sirolimus-eluting stent or paclitaxel-eluting stent vs balloon angioplasty for prevention of recurrences in patients with coronary in-stent restenosis: a randomized controlled trial. *JAMA*. 2005;293:165–171.

 Additional references available online at expertconsult.com.

中文导读

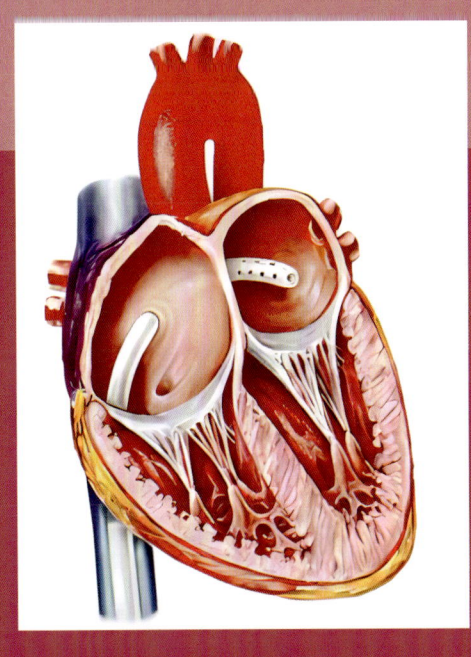

第35章
辅助器械：切割球囊、激光、冠状动脉斑块旋切术

在过去的30年里，已经开发了几种消融或切割动脉粥样斑块的器械，以优化经皮冠状动脉介入治疗的急性结果，提供手术成功率，并减少再狭窄。尽管每种器械使用不同的机制来修饰动脉粥样硬化斑块，但目标都是为了获得比球囊经皮腔内冠状动脉成形术更大的管腔、更高的成功率和更低的再狭窄率。

经过数十项临床试验后发现，常规使用斑块修饰并没有产生比单独经皮腔内冠状动脉成形术更好的临床结果，建议无须常规进行斑块销蚀。但是，在某些情况下，这可能是获得程序性和临床成功的唯一手段。本章节根据临床研究结果，阐明了对于高度钙化或无法扩张的高阻力病变，在支架植入之前进行斑块修饰或销蚀是至关重要的预处理步骤。

陈思源　范　谦

章节要点

- 旋磨和轨道旋磨术有助于在无法扩张、坚硬的或严重钙化的病变部位进行支架置入。
- 切割或刻痕球囊与传统球囊滑动相比不易滑动,可用于治疗再狭窄或开口部病变。
- 通过热机械机制,激光血管成形术可用来预处理坚硬或无法扩张的病变,便于支架置入。
- 动脉粥样斑块销蚀装置并不能减少再狭窄。
- 动脉粥样斑块销蚀装置会增加冠状动脉穿孔的风险。
- 病变修饰技术的安全应用需要丰富的经验。

35 Role of Adjunct Devices: Atherectomy, Cutting Balloon, and Laser

John A. Bittl

KEY POINTS

- Rotational and orbital atherectomy facilitate stent implantation in undilatable, rigid, or heavily calcified lesions.
- Cutting or scoring balloons slip less often than conventional balloons and may be useful for treating restenotic or ostial lesions.
- Laser angioplasty uses a thermomechanical mechanism to prepare rigid or undilatable lesions for stent implantation.
- Atheroablative devices do not reduce restenosis.
- Atheroablative devices increase the risk of coronary perforation.
- The safe use of lesion-modifying approaches requires advanced technical skills.

INTRODUCTION

Several devices that ablate or section atheromatous plaque have been developed during the past 30 years to optimize the acute results of percutaneous coronary intervention (PCI) and reduce restenosis. After dozens of clinical trials found that the routine use of plaque modification did not produce better clinical outcomes than percutaneous transluminal coronary angioplasty (PTCA) alone,[1] clinical practice guidelines recommended against the routine use of ablative approaches during PCI.[2] However, in selected circumstances, atheroablative approaches may be the only means of achieving procedural and clinical success.[3] This chapter analyzes the results of clinical trials and illustrates the complementary but crucial role that atheroablative devices fill in current practice in the preparation of rigid, highly calcified or undilatable lesions for stent implantation.

HISTORICAL BACKGROUND

Before the modern era of coronary stenting, the search for treatments to overcome the shortcomings of PTCA was based on experimental findings that suggested that the healing response of treated coronary arteries was directly proportional to the degree of imposed injury.[4] This was supported by angiographic analyses that suggested that late restenosis was directly proportional to the acute gain achieved during treatment with different treatments.[5] Based on research that suggested that plaque excision could improve clinical outcomes and lower the rate of restenosis after PCI, directional coronary atherectomy (DCA) entered clinical trials in 1987. Excimer laser coronary angioplasty (ELCA) and percutaneous transluminal rotational atherectomy (PTRA) appeared in 1988. Holmium laser angioplasty (HLA) premiered in 1990, cutting balloon angioplasty (CBA) debuted in 1991, and the newest ablative device, orbital atherectomy (OA), entered investigation in 2008.

Although each device used a different mechanism for modifying atheromatous plaque, the common goal was to obtain larger lumens, higher success rates, and lower restenosis rates than could be achieved with balloon PTCA alone. When evidence from randomized trials (Table 35.1)[1,6–32] seemed to refute the ablation hypothesis, coronary stenting (see Chapter 15) rapidly replaced atheroablative therapies. Clinical practice guidelines currently specify that no atheroablative device should be used routinely during PCI,[2] but the guidelines add the provision that rotational atherectomy is reasonable for fibrotic or heavily calcified lesions that might not be crossed by a balloon catheter or adequately dilated with high-pressure balloons before stent implantation (class IIa).[2] Cutting and scoring balloons may be considered to reduce slippage and trauma during PCI for in-stent restenosis (ISR) or ostial lesions in side branches (class IIb).[2] Laser angioplasty might be considered for fibrotic or moderately calcified lesions that cannot be crossed or dilated with high-pressure balloons before stent implantation (class IIb).[2] Because treatments that ablate or section atheromatous plaque continue to be used in many interventional programs, each approach is reviewed in the following sections.

PERCUTANEOUS TRANSLUMINAL ROTATIONAL ATHERECTOMY

Mechanism of Action

PTRA removes tissue and reduces lesion rigidity by attacking calcified atherosclerotic plaque like a dental drill, which bores into enamel but leaves pulp unharmed. Based on the theory of differential cutting, rotary ablation pulverizes rigid atherosclerotic plaque, which is not able to deflect, and yet preserves the integrity of the flexible artery wall. The hard plaque is abraded into small particles that average 5 µm in diameter and are taken up by the reticuloendothelial system.

Equipment

The Rotablator system (SciMed/Boston Scientific, Natick, MA) contains: (1) a preconnected burr with an advancing device that houses an air turbine and drive shaft; (2) a console that regulates an air supply and monitors the rotation of the burr; and (3) a DynaGlide foot pedal to activate the device. The burr has an abrasive tip that is welded to a long flexible drive shaft covered by a plastic sheath, and it tracks over a central coaxial RotaWire (0.009-inch diameter, 3.3-m length) that has a flexible radiopaque platinum distal part (20 mm-length) that does not rotate during abrasion. The wire and the burr can be advanced independently.

The elliptical nickel-coated brass burr has 2000 to 3000 microscopic diamond crystals on its leading face (Fig. 35.1). The diamond crystals are 20 µm in size, with only 5 µm protruding from the nickel coating, and the trailing edge of the burr is smooth. Burrs are available in various diameters that range from 1.25 to 2.50 mm in 0.25-mm increments.

TABLE 35.1 Randomized Trials Comparing Atheroablative or Thrombectomy Devices

Acronym	Definition	Primary End Point[a]	Patients (n)	Year[b]	Indications	Comparison
AMIGO[6]	Atherectomy Before Multi-Link Improves Luminal Gain and Clinical Outcomes	Binary restenosis	753	2002	Native vessel	DCA vs. PTCA
AMRO[7]	Amsterdam Rotterdam Randomized Trial	6-month MACE	308	1993	Native vessel	ELCA vs. PTCA
ARTIST[8]	Angioplasty/Rotational Atherectomy for Treatment of Diffuse In-Stent Restenosis Trial	6-month MACE	298	2002	ISR in native vessel	PTRA vs. PTCA
BETACUT[10]	Beta Radiation Assisted by Cutting Balloon Angioplasty for In-Stent Restenosis	Binary restenosis	100	2002	ISR in native vessel	CBA vs. PTCA before BT
BOAT[11]	Balloon/Optimal Atherectomy Trial	Binary restenosis	989	1995	Native vessel	DCA vs. PTCA
CAPAS[12]	Cutting Balloon Atherotomy Versus Plain Old Balloon Angioplasty Study	Binary restenosis	232	1997	Native vessel	CBA vs. PTCA
CARAT[13]	Coronary Angioplasty and Rotablator Atherectomy Trial	Postprocedure diameter stenosis	222	2000	Native vessel	PTRA vs. PTRA
CAVEAT-I[14]	Coronary Angioplasty Versus Excisional Atherectomy Trial I	Binary restenosis	1012	1992	Native vessel	DCA vs. PTCA
CAVEAT-II[15]	Coronary Angioplasty Versus Excisional Atherectomy Trial II	Binary restenosis	305	1993	SVG	DCA vs. PTCA
CBASS[18]	Cutting Balloon for Small-Size Vessels[c]	Binary restenosis	99	1999	Native vessels <2.6 mm	CBA vs. PTCA
CCAT[16]	Canadian Coronary Atherectomy Trial	Binary restenosis	274	1992	LAD	DCA vs. PTCA
COBRA[17]	Comparison of Balloon Angioplasty/Rotational Atherectomy	Binary restenosis	502	1996	Native vessel	PTRA vs. PTCA
CUBA[18]	Cutting Balloon Versus Conventional Balloon Angioplasty Trial[c]	Binary restenosis	306	1997	Native vessel	CBA vs. PTCA
DART[19]	Dilation/Ablation Revascularization Trial	Binary restenosis	446	1998	Small vessel	PTRA vs. PTCA
ERBAC[21]	Excimer Rotablator Balloon Angioplasty Comparison	Procedural success	454	1996	Native vessel	ELCA vs. PTCA
ERBAC[21]	Excimer Rotablator Balloon Angioplasty Comparison	Procedural success	453	1996	Native vessel	PTRA vs. PTCA
GRT[23]	Global Randomized Trial	Binary restenosis	1238	1997	Native vessel	CBA vs. PTCA
LAVA[26]	Laser Angioplasty/Coronary Angioplasty	6-month MACE	215	1997	Native vessel	HLA vs. PTCA
REDUCE 1[1]	Restenosis Reduction by Cutting Balloon Evaluation 1[c]	Binary restenosis	802	2001	Native vessel	CBA vs. PTCA
REDUCE 2[18]	Restenosis Reduction by Cutting Balloon Evaluation 2[c]	Binary restenosis	492	2002	ISR	CBA vs. PTCA
REDUCE 3[27]	Restenosis Reduction by Cutting Balloon Evaluation 3	Binary restenosis	521	2003	Stenting	CBA vs. PTCA
RESCUT[28]	Restenosis Cutting Balloon Evaluation	Binary restenosis	428	2002	ISR	CBA vs. PTCA
ROSTER[29]	Rotational Atherectomy Versus Balloon Angioplasty for Diffuse In-Stent Restenosis	Target-lesion revascularization	200	2001	ISR	PTRA vs. PTCA

TABLE 35.1 Randomized Trials Comparing Atheroablative or Thrombectomy Devices—cont'd

Acronym	Definition	Primary End Point[a]	Patients (n)	Year[b]	Indications	Comparison
ROTAXUS[32]	Rotational Atherectomy Prior to Taxus Stent Treatment for Complex Native Coronary Artery Disease	In-stent late lumen loss	120	2013	Native vessel calcified lesions	PTRA vs. PTCA
SPORT[1]	Stenting Post Rotational Atherectomy Trial[c]	30-day MACE	735	1999	Native vessel calcified lesions	PTRA vs. PTCA
STRATAS[30]	Study to Determine Rotablator System and Transluminal Angioplasty Strategy	Acute success	497	2000	Native vessel	PTRA vs. PTRA

[a]If the primary end point was not stated or if multiple primary end points were listed, the end point used in power calculations for sample size estimation was used.
[b]Year that patient recruitment was completed. Otherwise, the year the study was reported or published.
[c]Unpublished, with data approved by investigators where cited.[1]
BT, Brachytherapy; *CBA*, cutting balloon atherotomy; *DCA*, directional coronary atherectomy; *ELCA*, excimer laser coronary angioplasty; *HLA*, holmium laser angioplasty; *ISR*, in-stent restenosis; *LAD*, proximal segment of the left anterior descending artery; *MACE*, major adverse cardiac event (death, myocardial infarction, or revascularization); *PTCA*, percutaneous transluminal coronary angioplasty; *PTRA*, percutaneous transluminal rotational atherectomy; *SVG*, saphenous vein graft.

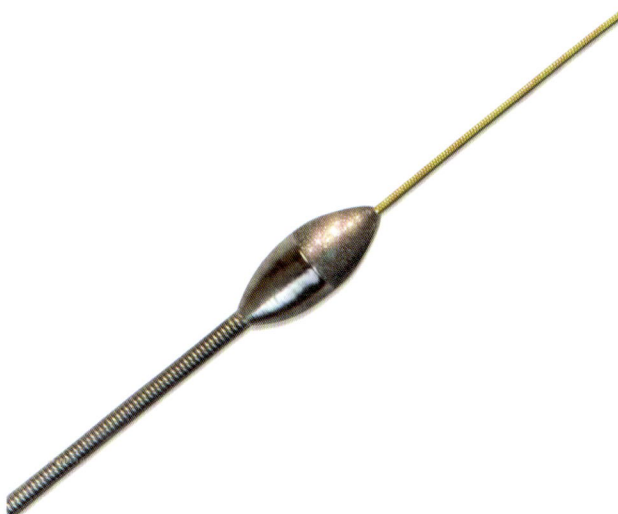

Fig. 35.1 Rotablator burr. (Courtesy Boston Scientific, Natick, MA.)

During use, a rotaflush solution containing a lubricant, verapamil 5 mg, 5000 units of heparin, and 1000 μg of nitroglycerin per 500 mL saline irrigates the catheter sheath to lubricate and cool the rotating parts. In recent years, many centers omit all but the lubricant to avoid hypotension. The number of revolutions per minute (rpm) is measured by a fiberoptic light probe and is displayed on a control panel. The advancer has preset delimiters for retraction and advancement. The wireClip Torquer and guidewires are critical components of the system. RotaGlide lubricant may be useful for crossing resistant lesions.

Procedure

All patients are pretreated with aspirin and an anticoagulant. The size of the guide catheter depends on the size of the burr. A 6-Fr Runway Guide (Boston Scientific) with a 0.070-inch inner lumen accommodates a 1.25-mm burr, allowing conversion to PTRA if an undilatable or uncrossable lesion is encountered during PTCA, even during transradial PCI with low-profile 5/6-Fr sheaths.

Rotary ablation is preceded by placing the RotaWire across the lesion and parking the unfolded wire tip in a straight segment of the distal vessel, not in a side branch. Many practitioners initially place their workhorse wire into the distal vessel and use a microcatheter to replace it with the RotaWire. During rotablation, protection of side branches is unnecessary because a "snow plow" effect is rare. When treating large coronary arteries, particularly the right coronary artery, many cardiologists insert a prophylactic temporary pacemaker because of the possibility of bradyarrhythmias. Before advancing the burr into the guide catheter, the rotational speed of the burr is checked outside the body at the Y-adaptor with flush running. An outside-body speed of 155,000 rpm translates to an unimpeded speed of 140,000 rpm within the coronary artery. A recent study has suggested no difference in clinical or angiographic outcomes at speeds of 140,000 or 190,000.[33]

The burr and drive shaft are manually advanced over the guidewire to a proximal segment of the target vessel. Before rotablation, a three-point checklist is completed to prevent abrupt burr advancement and vessel dissection: (1) the advancer knob is loosened and moved back and forth approximately 5 mm to unload stored tension on the drive cable; (2) the Y-adaptor is loosened to unload stored tension in the Rotablator sheath; and (3) the DynaGlide mode is activated at lower rotational speeds to unload any residual tension within the system and then switched off to allow the burr to advance into the vessel at ablative speeds. The burr is moved into the target lesion with a pecking motion that maintains a high speed of rotation. Decelerations of greater than 5000 rpm are avoided to reduce the risk of vessel trauma, heat formation, and large particle generation. Ablation runs are limited to 15 to 20 seconds each. If the lesion cannot be crossed after five attempts, downsizing of the burr may be required. After successful crossing, several polishing runs complete lesion preparation for stent delivery. Occasionally, an initial smaller burr is exchanged for a larger diameter burr for more complete ablation prior to stent implantation, although the benefit of this approach has not been demonstrated (see later).

Clinical Results

Several trials have defined the optimal use of PTRA. The Study to Determine Rotablator and Transluminal Angioplasty Strategy (STRATAS) trial[30] compared an aggressive debulking strategy (burr/artery ratio of 0.7 to 0.9 followed by balloon inflation of less than 1 atm or no inflation) with a moderate debulking strategy (burr/artery ratio of less than 0.7 followed by conventional balloon angioplasty). The clinical success was similar, but the aggressive strategy caused more myocardial infarctions (11% vs. 7%) and a higher rate of restenosis (58% vs. 52%). The Coronary

Angioplasty and Rotablator Atherectomy Trial (CARAT)[13] compared a large-burr strategy (burr/artery ratio >0.7) with a small-burr strategy (burr/artery ratio <0.7). The large-burr strategy achieved similar immediate lumen enlargement and rate of target-vessel revascularization (TVR) as the small-burr strategy but caused more angiographic complications (12.7% vs. 5.2%, $P < .05$). Taken together, these two trials are the basis for recommending a single burr for each procedure, selecting a burr/artery ratio of 0.5 to 0.6, and avoiding burr over-sizing.

In a series of multicenter randomized trials,[1,8,17,19,21,32] rates of major adverse cardiac events (MACEs) at 30 days and rates of angiographic restenosis were higher after PTRA than after balloon PTCA alone (Fig. 35.2).

Lesion Selection

Because PTRA confers a slightly increased risk, it should be used selectively.[3] Most practitioners find that they must maintain expertise with PTRA because undilatable lesions are encountered regularly. Approximately 1% to 3% of lesions that can be crossed with a guidewire are uncrossable with balloon catheters or are undilatable at pressures higher than 20 atm. Rotational atherectomy successfully improves the compliance of most rigid lesions, allowing balloon dilation and stent implantation to be completed successfully (Fig. 35.3). For long calcified lesions, small burrs are recommended to alter the compliance of the vessel to allow balloon angioplasty and spot stenting of the segments with dissection (Fig. 35.4).

Certain precautions need emphasis. Angulated lesions in bends of more than 60 degrees are a relative contraindication to the use of PTRA, and lesions in a bend greater than 90 degrees are an absolute contraindication because dissection or perforation may occur. When PTRA is performed in nonangulated lesions, the rotating burr should never be advanced to the point of contact with the spring tip of the RotaWire. The rotating burr should not be allowed to remain in one location within the artery; a gentle retraction and readvancement motion is needed to avoid dissection or welding. The rotating burr should not be advanced within the guide catheter. Rotational atherectomy should be avoided in dissected segments after balloon angioplasty, in lesions with visible thrombus, and in degenerated saphenous vein grafts (SVGs). Hemodynamic support with either balloon pumping or Impella (see Chapter 22) may be needed for patients with ischemic cardiomyopathy and borderline hemodynamics that might deteriorate in the presence of microembolization.

ORBITAL ATHERECTOMY

Mechanism of Action

Although OA shares common features with PTRA, it uses a different mechanism based on the principle of elliptical burr movement, in which rotational speed determines the effective burr size.[3] The OA device uses an eccentrically mounted, diamond-coated crown (Fig. 35.5) that orbits over an atherectomy wire at speeds of 80,000 to 120,000 rpm.[33] Repeated passes of the crown across a calcified lesion "sands" away rigid plaque but allows elastic tissue to flex away from the crown. The orbital diameter of the crown expands radially via centrifugal force. The elliptical orbit may allow blood to flow around the crown during treatment, theoretically dispersing heat more efficiently and generating smaller particles than PTRA.[33]

Equipment

The Diamondback 360° OA System (Cardiovascular Systems, St. Paul, MN) works on a 0.012-inch, 325-cm ViperWire. The system is composed of a handheld device and an atherectomy controller.

Procedure

Some technical aspects of the OA procedure (Fig. 35.6) are like the techniques used during PTRA, but some differences are highlighted here. OA is performed with a 1.25-mm diamond-encrusted crown. The crown is eccentrically mounted on the atherectomy catheter which allows an orbital motion as the device spins at 80,000 or 120,000 rpm. The crown's orbit will grow as time in lesion and rpm speed increases, which eliminates the need for larger-diameter devices for varying vessel sizes. The diamond-encrusted sanding surface will ablate hard material while deflecting away from softer healthy tissue. OA requires the use of the ViperWire guidewire, a unique 0.012-inch, 330-cm tapered wire that provides support while allowing for orbital movement for the spinning crown. Also required is a specially designed pumping mechanism that can be mounted on a standard IV pole. The pump is designed to push a lubricant, called Viperglide, along with saline through the device which allows the spinning catheter to run smoothly during operation. The leading tip of the atherectomy device is never advanced within 5 mm of the distal opaque portion of the ViperWire, and ablation runs are limited to 30 seconds each. A single OA crown was used in 80% of patients enrolled in clinical trials.[34]

Lesion Selection

OA is recommended for severely calcified coronary lesions, defined in the pivotal clinical trial (see later) as severe calcification detected fluoroscopically in both sides of the arterial wall for at least 15 mm when viewed longitudinally or the presence of at least a 270-degree arc of calcium viewed in cross section using intravascular ultrasound (IVUS).[35]

Clinical Results

In the Safety and Feasibility of OA for the Treatment of Calcified Coronary Lesions (ORBIT I) study,[34] a registry of 50 patients with severely calcified lesions treated with OA followed by stent placement, procedural success was achieved in 47 patients (94%), and MACEs were reported in 2 patients (4%). Angiographic complications included dissections in six patients (12%) and a coronary perforation in one patient (2%).

In the Pivotal Trial to Evaluate the Safety and Efficacy of the OA System in Treating De Novo, Severely Calcified Coronary Lesions (ORBIT II),[35] a registry of 443 patients with severely calcified coronary lesions treated at 49 U.S. sites, the primary safety end point of freedom from 30-day MACE was achieved in 89.6% of patients. Stent delivery was successful in 97.7% of cases, with less than 50% diameter stenosis (DS) achieved in 98.6% of subjects. Low rates of in-hospital Q wave myocardial infarction (0.7%), cardiac death (0.2%), and TVR (0.7%) were reported. Angiographic complications included severe dissections in 15 patients (3.4%) and perforations in 8 patients (1.8%).

The role of OA vis-à-vis PTRA for the treatment of patients with severe calcified coronary lesions will likely depend on several factors, including local expertise and the relative cost of the two devices.

DIRECTIONAL CORONARY ATHERECTOMY

After approval of a DCA device by the U.S. Food and Drug Administration (FDA) in 1990 using registry data, several randomized trials comparing DCA with PTCA with and without stenting failed to demonstrate a clinical benefit of DCA

CHAPTER 35 Role of Adjunct Devices: Atherectomy, Cutting Balloon, and Laser

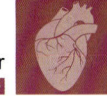

	Rotational atherectomy (PTRA)		PTCA		Favors PTRA	Favors PTCA
30-Day mortality	n	%	n	%		
ARTIST[8]	0/152	(0.0)	1/146	(0.7)		
COBRA[17]	1/252	(0.4)	4/250	(1.6)		
DART[19]	1/227	(0.4)	0/219	(0.0)		
ERBAC[21]	2/231	(0.9)	2/222	(0.9)		
ROTAXUS[32]	2/120	(1.7)	0/120	(0.0)		
Total (OR 0.8 [0.3–2.5])	6/982	(0.6)	7/957	(0.7)		
30-Day MI						
ARTIST[8]	7/152	(4.6)	2/146	(1.4)		
COBRA[17]	10/252	(4.0)	5/250	(2.0)		
DART[19]	5/227	(2.2)	3/219	(1.4)		
ERBAC[21]	8/231	(3.5)	8/222	(3.6)		
Total (OR 1.6 [0.9–3.0])	30/862	(3.5)	18/837	(2.2)		
30-Day MACE						
ARTIST[8]	13/152	(8.6)	7/146	(4.8)		
COBRA[17]	25/252	(9.9)	19/250	(7.6)		
DART[19]	12/227	(5.3)	5/219	(2.3)		
ERBAC[21]	7/231	(3.0)	6/222	(2.7)		
ROTAXUS[32]	5/120	(4.2)	5/120	(4.2)		
SPORT[1]	9/360	(2.5)	5/375	(1.3)		
Total (OR 1.5 [1.1–2.2])	71/1342	(5.3)	47/1332	(3.5)		
Angiographic restenosis						
ARTIST[8]	80/124	(64.5)	62/121	(51.2)		
COBRA[17]	80/163	(49.1)	87/170	(51.2)		
DART[19]	55/108	(50.9)	56/111	(50.5)		
ERBAC[21]	86/145	(59.3)	51/109	(46.8)		
ROTAXUS[32]	15/124	(12.1)	17/123	(13.8)		
SPORT[1]	82/269	(30.5)	73/263	(27.8)		
Total (OR 1.2 [1.0–1.5])	398/932	(42.7)	346/906	(38.2)		
Cumulative revascularization						
ARTIST[8]	60/152	(39.5)	46/146	(31.5)		
COBRA[17]	54/252	(21.4)	60/250	(24.0)		
DART[19]	64/227	(28.2)	61/219	(27.9)		
ERBAC[21]	90/205	(43.9)	64/191	(33.5)		
ROSTER[29]	28/100	(28.0)	40/100	(40.0)		
SPORT[1]	53/360	(14.7)	61/375	(16.3)		
Total (OR 1.0 [0.9–1.2])	349/1296	(26.9)	333/1281	(26.0)		
Cumulative MACE						
ARTIST[8]	31/152	(20.4)	13/146	(8.9)		
COBRA[17]	75/210	(35.7)	75/213	(35.2)		
DART[19]	59/227	(26.0)	54/219	(24.7)		
ERBAC[21]	94/205	(45.9)	70/191	(36.6)		
ROSTER[29]	40/100	(40.0)	53/100	(53.0)		
SPORT[1]	63/360	(17.5)	51/375	(13.6)		
Total (OR 1.2 [1.0–1.4])	362/1254	(28.9)	316/1244	(25.4)		

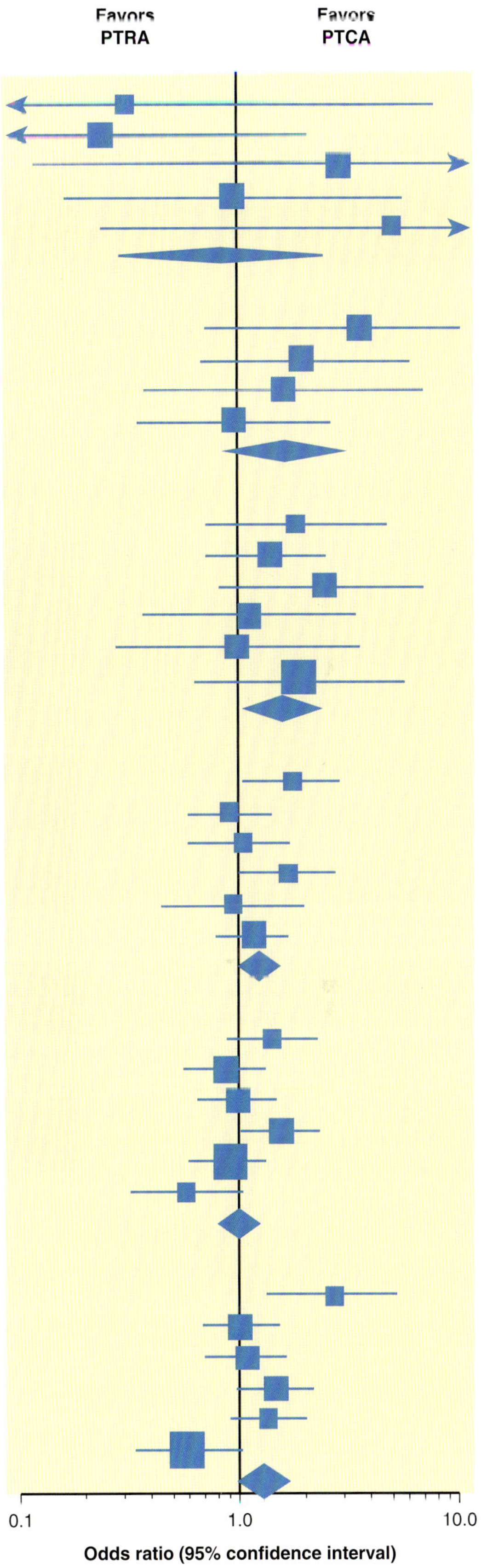

Odds ratio (95% confidence interval)

Fig. 35.2 Systematic overview of randomized trials of percutaneous transluminal rotational atherectomy (PTRA) versus percutaneous transluminal coronary angioplasty (PTCA). Pooled odds ratios (ORs) and 95% confidence intervals are presented, and trial abbreviations are given in Table 35.1. MACE, Major adverse cardiovascular event; MI, myocardial infarction. (Updated and reprinted from Bittl JA, Chew DP, Topol EJ, et al. Meta-analysis of randomized trials of percutaneous transluminal coronary angioplasty versus atherectomy, cutting balloon atherotomy, or laser angioplasty. J Am Coll Cardiol. 2004;43:936–942.)

(Fig. 35.7). At the current time, no DCA devices are marketed in the United States for coronary indications, but renewed interest is emerging.[36]

CUTTING BALLOON ANGIOPLASTY

CBA, or atherotomy, is a variation of conventional PTCA. In CBA, three or four sharp metal microtomes mounted on a noncompliant balloon incise and score coronary atheroma during balloon inflation.

Mechanism of Action

The aim of cutting balloon atherotomy is to reduce the appearance of uncontrolled longitudinal tears in the vessel wall induced during conventional balloon dilation. Compared with conventional PTCA, CBA makes controlled microincisions in the atheromatous plaque at lower pressures. Small mechanistic studies have confirmed that lesions can be dilated at lower pressure with cutting balloons than with conventional balloons.[22]

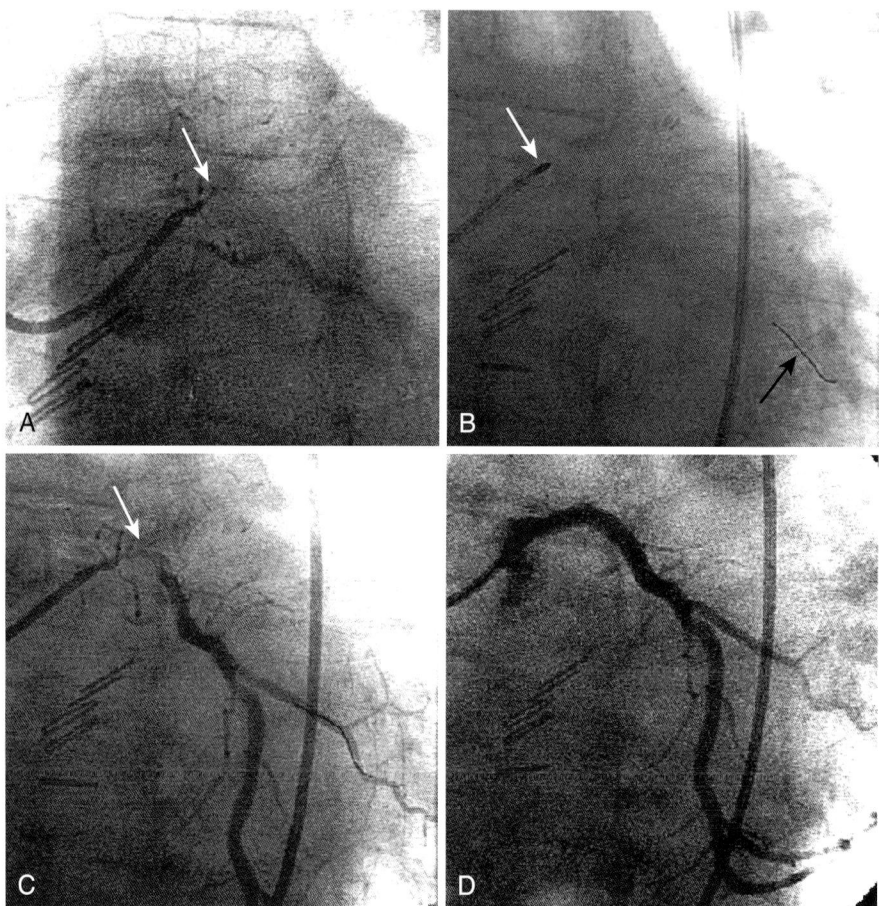

Fig. 35.3 Rotational atherectomy for uncrossable left main stenosis. (A) The left main occlusion jeopardized a large, unbypassed left circumflex coronary artery; it could be crossed with a guidewire but not with a balloon catheter *(arrow)*. (B) After placement of a RotaWire with tip positioned distally *(black arrow)*, a 1.25-mm burr was advanced through the left main occlusion *(white arrow)*. (C) The residual stenosis *(arrow)* was successfully treated with a sirolimus-eluting stent and was dilated to 4 mm. (D) The final result.

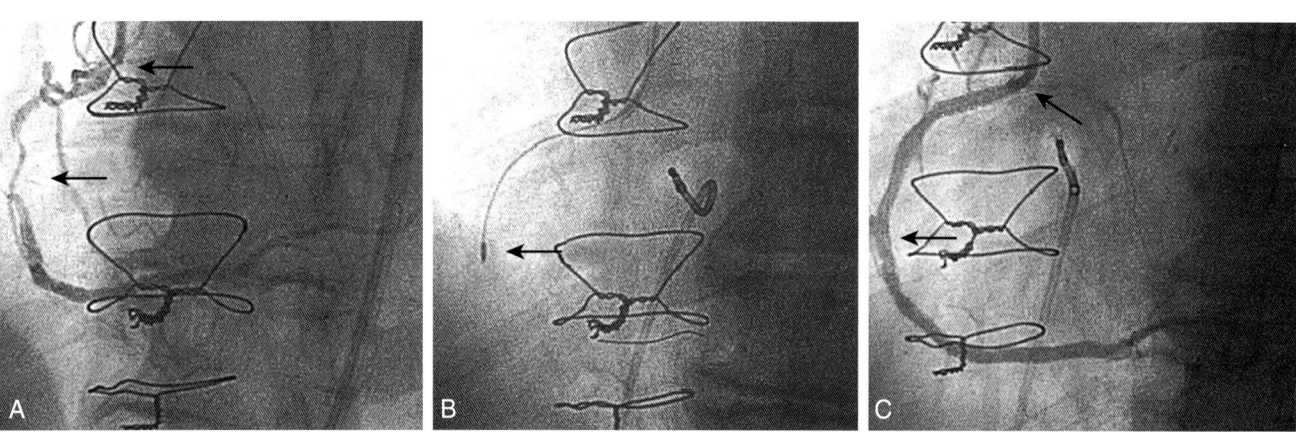

Fig. 35.4 Rotational atherectomy for uncrossable lesions in the right coronary artery. Proximal and midportion stenoses (A, *arrows*) could not be crossed with low-profile balloon catheters but were successfully treated with a 1.25-mm burr (B, *arrow*), leaving dissections that were successfully treated with stents (C, *arrows*).

Equipment

The Cutting Balloon Ultra-2 (Boston Scientific) is a monorail device, whereas the Flextome Cutting Balloon (Boston Scientific) has two configurations (Fig. 35.8). The Flextome device contains a flex point every 5 mm along the length of the atherotomes for greater flexibility and deliverability. It is available in over-the-wire and monorail configurations. Cutting balloons are available in balloon lengths of 6, 10, and 15 mm. The cutting blades, or atherotomes, are mounted longitudinally along the balloon surface. The atherotomes are not directly affixed to the balloon but rather are bonded to a pad mounted on the balloon. The double bond allows flexibility but ensures that atherotomes remain firmly fixed in place. The number of atherotomes depends on balloon diameter. Three atherotomes are on 2.0- and 3.25-mm balloons, and four are on 3.5- and 4.0-mm balloons.

Technique

The guidewires, catheters, and techniques used for CBA are like the equipment traditionally used for PTCA. However, the cutting balloons are less compliant and may not track as well as conventional balloon catheters. During CBA, the risk of blade fracture or retention is reduced by slowly inflating and deflating the balloon and by avoiding balloon pressures at or above rated burst pressures.

Clinical Results

Several small trials, all enrolling fewer than 200 patients, compared CBA with PTCA and reported that CBA reduced restenosis by 41% to 69% (Fig. 35.9).[12,18,22,24,25] However, other small studies that compared CBA with PTRA[31] or balloon PTCA[10] as pretreatment before brachytherapy for ISR found no difference in restenosis, and several large trials that compared CBA with PTCA generally found no difference in restenosis (see Fig. 35.9). The Global Randomized Trial (GRT)[23] randomized 1238 patients and reported no difference in angiographic restenosis between CBA and balloon PTCA (31.4% vs. 30.4%). The Restenosis Cutting Balloon Evaluation Trial (RESCUT)[28] enrolled 428 patients with ISR and reported no difference in restenosis between CBA and balloon PTCA (29.8% vs. 31.4%). The Restenosis Reduction by Cutting Balloon Evaluation (REDUCE 1) study[1] enrolled 802 patients and reported slightly higher restenosis rates with CBA than with PTCA (32.7% vs. 25.5%). The REDUCE 2 study[18] enrolled 416 patients and also observed a trend toward higher restenosis rates after CBA than after PTCA (52.1% vs. 44.2%). The REDUCE 3 study[27] randomized 453 patients undergoing coronary stenting and reported lower restenosis rates after the use of CBA than after PTCA (11.8% vs. 19.6%).

Lesion Selection

Many interventional cardiologists consider using CBA for ostial lesions or for ISR because cutting balloons appear to slip less often than conventional balloons.[23,27,28]

Complications

The risk of coronary perforation (Fig. 35.10) is slightly higher after the use of CBA than after conventional PTCA, as reported in the GRT (0.8% vs. 0.0%).[23]

SCORING BALLOON ANGIOPLASTY

The AngioSculpt scoring balloon catheter (AngioScore, Spectranetics, Colorado Springs, CO) is an alternative to the cutting balloon. The scoring balloon contains a flexible nitinol scoring ribbon with three rectangular spiral struts to incise the atheromatous plaque at pressures up to 18 atm.[37] The system, which has a low crossing profile (2.7 Fr), is promoted as a more flexible alternative to the cutting balloon. A small randomized trial of 252 patients with restenosis within drug-eluting stents

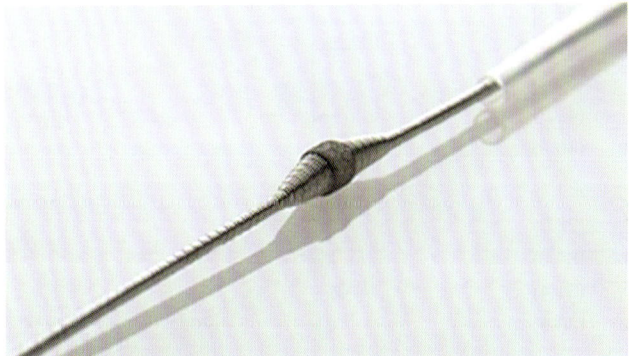

Fig. 35.5 Orbital atherectomy crown. (Courtesy Cardiovascular Systems, St. Paul, MN.)

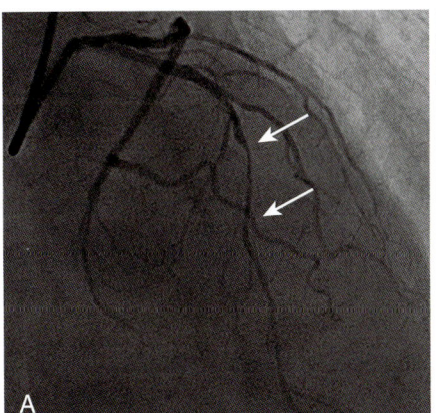
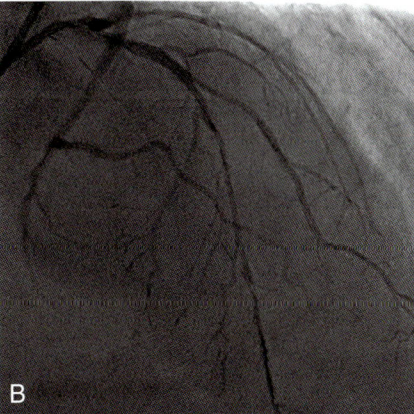
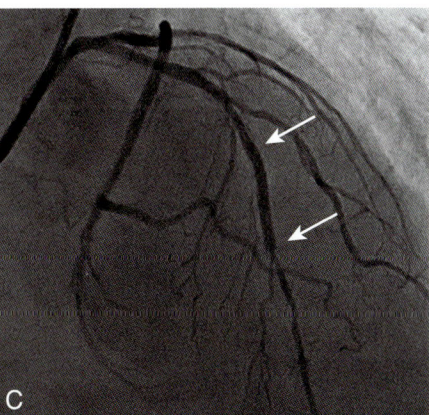

Fig. 35.6 Orbital atherectomy of left anterior descending (LAD) artery. A heavily calcified lesion in the midportion of the LAD artery (A, *arrows*) is treated with a 1.25-mm orbital atherectomy crown (B) and a drug-eluting stent (C, *arrows*).

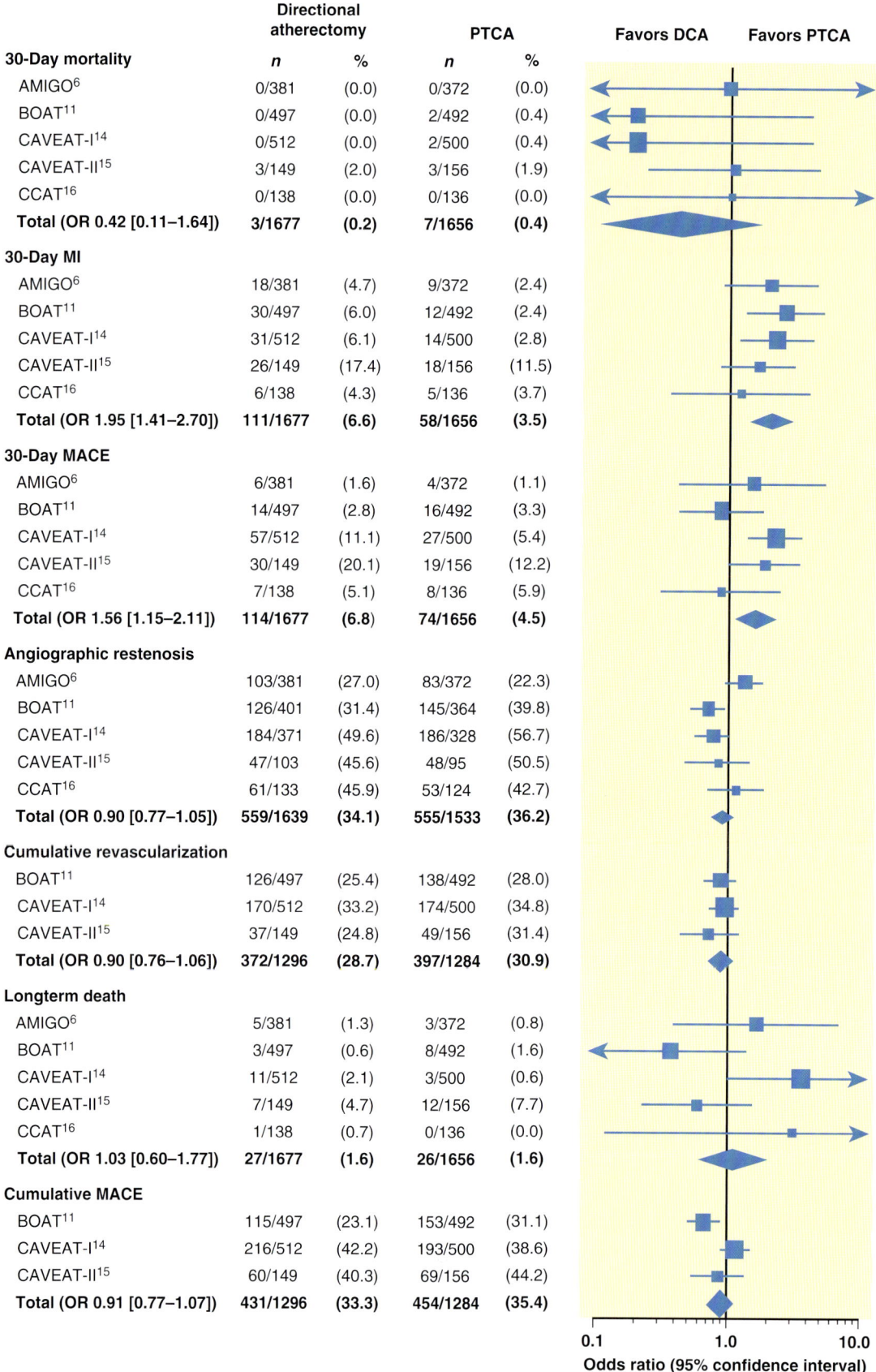

Fig. 35.7 Systematic overview of randomized trials of directional coronary atherectomy *(DCA)* versus percutaneous transluminal coronary angioplasty *(PTCA)*. Pooled odds ratios *(ORs)* and 95% confidence intervals are presented. Trial abbreviations are given in Table 35.1. *MACE,* Major adverse cardiovascular event; *MI,* myocardial infarction. (Updated and reprinted from Bittl JA, Chew DP, Topol EJ, et al. Meta-analysis of randomized trials of percutaneous transluminal coronary angioplasty versus atherectomy, cutting balloon atherotomy, or laser angioplasty. *J Am Coll Cardiol* 2004;43:936–942.)

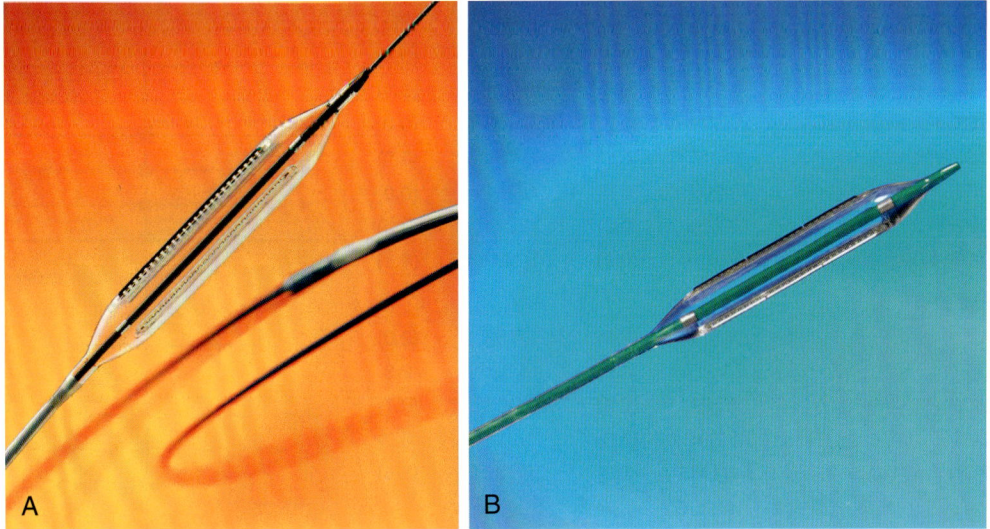

Fig. 35.8 The Cutting Balloon Ultra 2 (A) is a monorail device, and the Flextome Cutting Balloon (B) is an over-the-wire catheter. (Courtesy Boston Scientific, Natick, MA.)

suggested that use of the scoring balloon compared with standard therapy resulted in lower in-segment DS at follow-up (35% ± 17% vs. 40% ± 21%) but no difference in clinical outcomes.[38]

LASER ANGIOPLASTY

The use of lasers has broad appeal. Most people assume that medical lasers vaporize tissue through the mechanism of photochemical dissociation, but the predominant mechanism of all medical lasers involves a thermomechanical process. In the case of the excimer laser, protein and nucleic acid chromophores absorb laser light at 308 nm and transfer heat to water. Intracellular water vaporizes and generates bubbles twice the diameter of the laser catheter (Fig. 35.11). The explosive increase in volume lyses cells and generates stress waves up to tens of kilobars within the irradiated tissue.[39] The resulting barotrauma can be exploited to prepare rigid and undilatable lesions for stent implantation.

Technique

The size of laser catheters used for angioplasty should be no more than two-thirds the reference diameter of the target vessel. For severe stenoses, the smallest laser catheters are recommended to increase the likelihood of successful crossing. The elimination of blood and contrast from the coronary artery during ELCA reduces collateral damage and dissection.[40] This is achieved by flushing all lines with saline and by injecting saline through the guide catheter at a rate of 2 to 3 mL per second during laser activation (Fig. 35.12). However, if lesions are found to be undilatable or uncrossable, using ELCA in a blood field without saline flush will enhance the thermomechanical effects and may increase successful crossing.[39,41,42]

Clinical Results

Several randomized studies have compared pulsed wave lasers with other treatment modalities,[7,21,26] but none have shown a benefit over conventional PTCA (Fig. 35.13).

Lesion Selection

Although ELCA has been approved for seven lesion types—(1) long lesions, (2) moderately calcified lesions, (3) ISR before brachytherapy, (4) SVG lesions, (5) ostial lesions, (6) total occlusions, and (7) undilatable lesions—some interventional cardiologists reserve its use for nondilatable lesions (Fig. 35.14).[2]

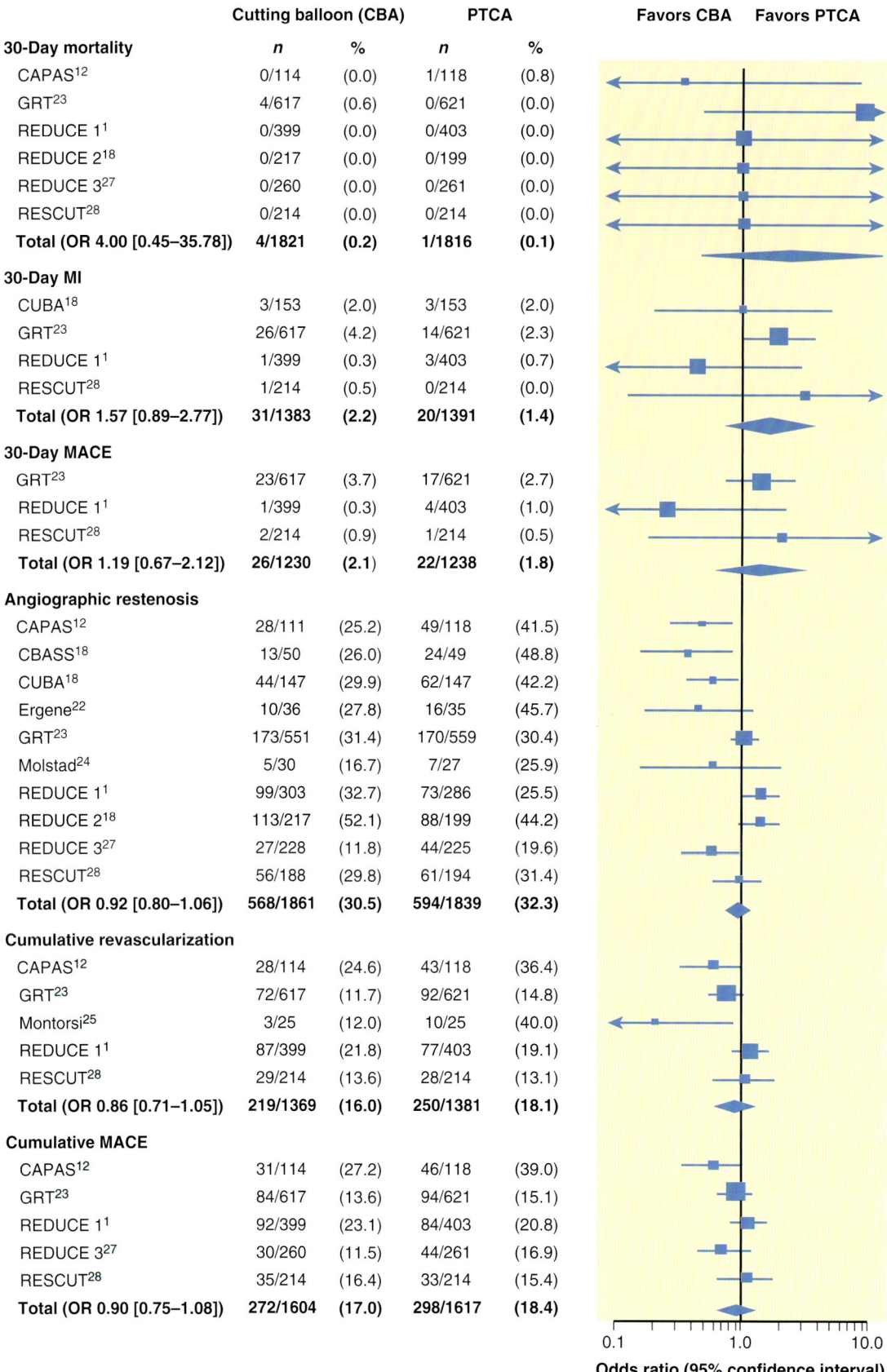

Fig. 35.9 Systematic overview of randomized trials of cutting balloon angioplasty *(CBA)* versus percutaneous transluminal coronary angioplasty *(PTCA)*. Pooled odds ratios *(ORs)* and 95% confidence intervals are presented. Trial abbreviations are given in Table 35.1. *MACE,* Major adverse cardiovascular event; *MI,* myocardial infarction. (Updated and reprinted from Bittl JA, Chew DP, Topol EJ, et al. Meta-analysis of randomized trials of percutaneous transluminal coronary angioplasty versus atherectomy, cutting balloon atherotomy, or laser angioplasty. *J Am Coll Cardiol.* 2004;43:936–942.)

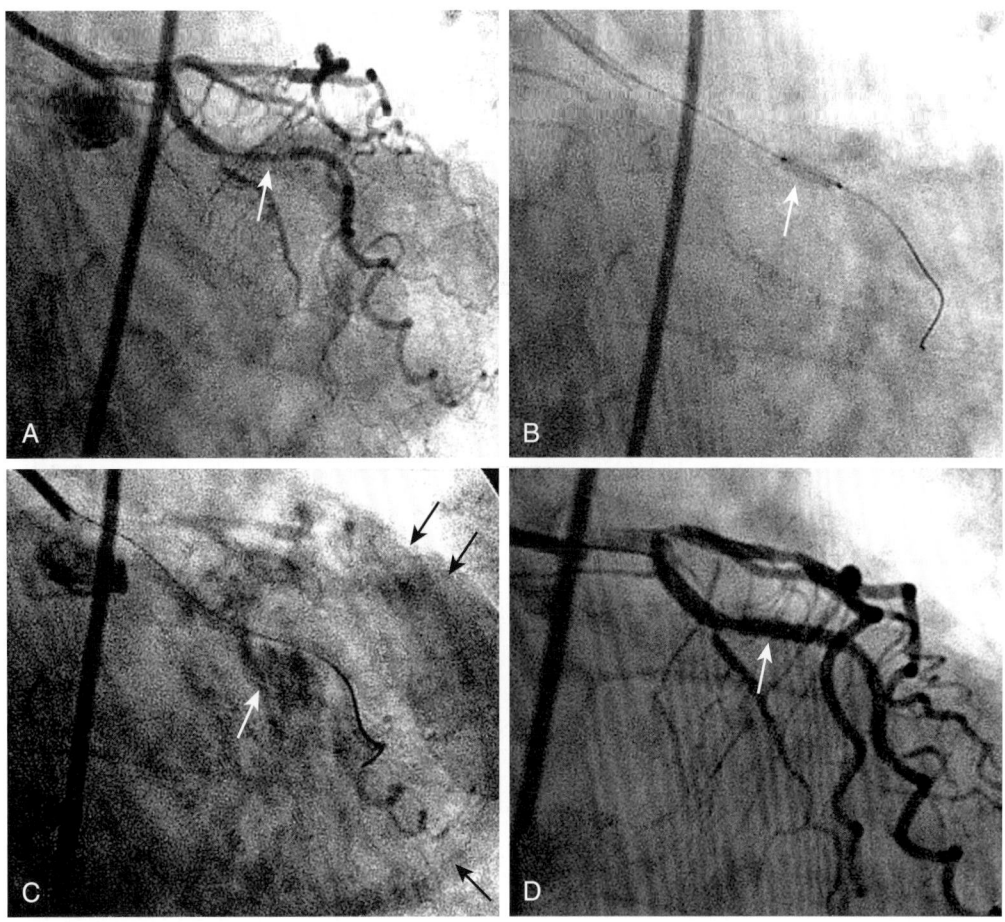

Fig. 35.10 Perforation after cutting balloon angioplasty. The first marginal branch had been treated previously with a 3.0-mm bare-metal stent and showed moderate restenosis 7 months later (A, *arrow*), causing angina. A 3.0-mm cutting balloon was positioned within the stented segment (B, *arrow*), but inflation was complicated by free perforation (C, *white arrow*), circumferential hemopericardium (C, *black arrows*), and cardiac tamponade. The patient was rapidly stabilized with pericardiocentesis and placement of a polytetrafluoroethylene-covered stent to seal the coronary perforation (D, *arrow*).

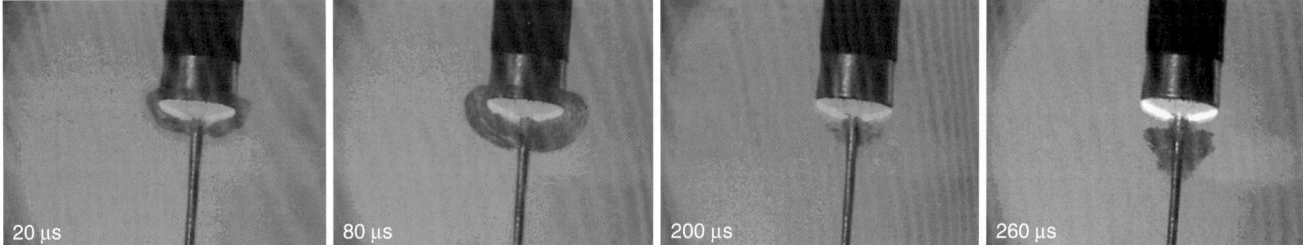

Fig. 35.11 Laser-tissue interaction. Excimer laser light penetrates approximately 100 μm deep into tissue and rapidly converts cellular water into steam, causing a vapor bubble to rapidly expand and implode at the catheter tip.

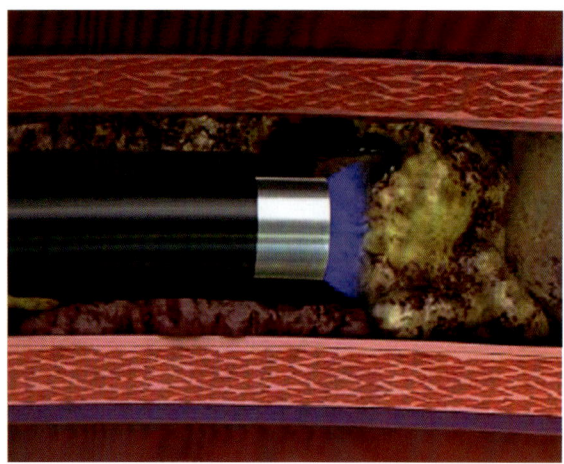

Fig. 35.12 Schematic rendition of excimer laser angioplasty procedure. (Courtesy Spectranetics, Colorado Springs, CO.)

	Laser angioplasty		PTCA		
30-Day mortality	n	%	n	%	
AMRO[7]	0/151	(0.0)	0/157	(0.0)	
ERBAC[21]	2/232	(0.9)	2/222	(0.9)	
LAVA[26]	2/117	(1.7)	0/98	(0.0)	
Total (OR 1.9 [0.3–10.5])	4/500	(0.8)	2/477	(0.4)	
30-Day MI					
AMRO[7]	5/151	(3.3)	5/157	(3.2)	
ERBAC[21]	9/232	(3.9)	8/222	(3.6)	
LAVA[26]	5/117	(4.3)	0/98	(0.0)	
Total (OR 1.4 [0.7–2.9])	19/500	(3.8)	13/477	(2.7)	
30-Day MACE					
AMRO[7]	9/151	(6.0)	6/157	(3.8)	
ERBAC[21]	10/232	(4.3)	6/222	(2.7)	
LAVA[26]	12/117	(10.3)	4/98	(4.1)	
Total (OR 1.9 [1.0–3.5])	31/500	(6.2)	16/477	(3.4)	
Angiographic restenosis					
AMRO[7]	64/124	(51.6)	52/126	(41.3)	
ERBAC[21]	82/143	(57.3)	51/109	(46.8)	
Total (OR 1.5 [1.1–2.2])	146/267	(54.7)	103/235	(43.8)	
Cumulative revascularization					
AMRO[7]	48/151	(31.8)	46/157	(29.3)	
ERBAC[21]	100/211	(47.4)	64/191	(33.5)	
Total (OR 1.5 [1.1–2.0])	148/362	(40.9)	110/348	(31.6)	
Cumulative MACE					
AMRO[7]	50/151	(33.1)	47/157	(29.9)	
ERBAC[21]	101/211	(47.9)	70/191	(36.6)	
LAVA[26]	41/117	(35.0)	33/98	(33.7)	
Total (OR 1.3 [1.0–1.7])	192/479	(40.1)	150/446	(33.6)	

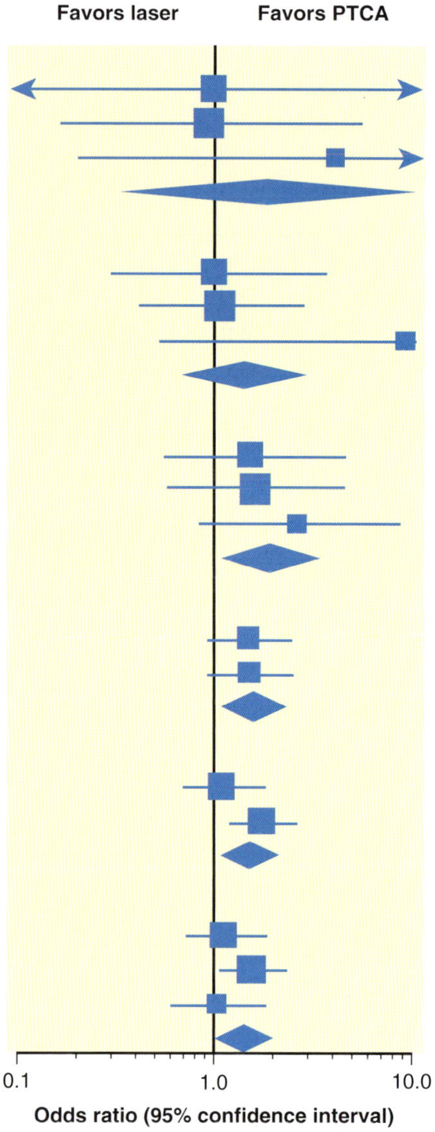

Odds ratio (95% confidence interval)

Fig. 35.13 Systematic overview of randomized trials of laser angioplasty versus percutaneous transluminal coronary angioplasty *(PTCA)*. Pooled odds ratios *(ORs)* and 95% confidence intervals are presented, and trial abbreviations are given in Table 35.1. *MACE,* Major adverse cardiovascular event; *MI,* myocardial infarction. (Updated and reprinted from Bittl JA, Chew DP, Topol EJ, et al. Meta-analysis of randomized trials of percutaneous transluminal coronary angioplasty versus atherectomy, cutting balloon atherotomy, or laser angioplasty. *J Am Coll Cardiol.* 2004;43:936–942.)

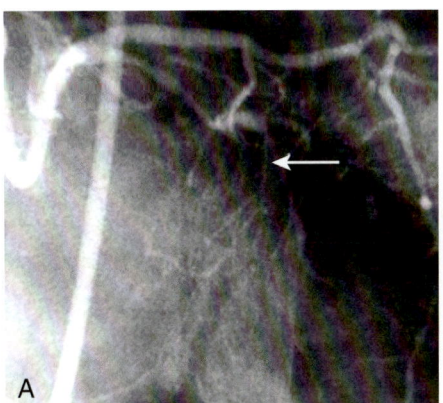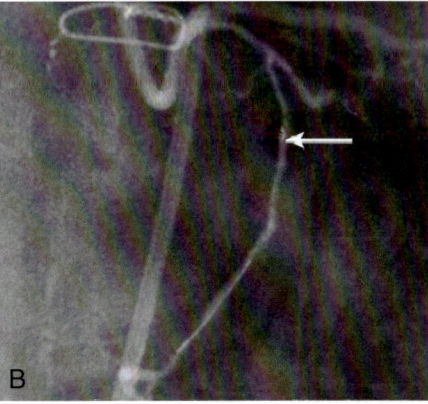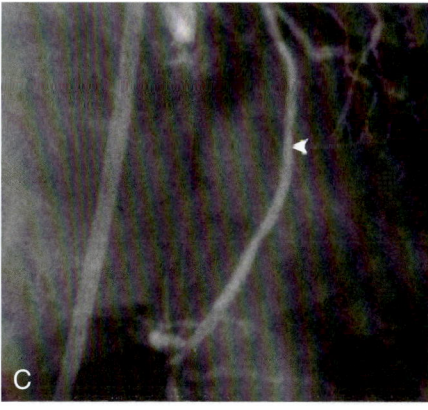

Fig. 35.14 Long undilatable lesion treated with excimer laser angioplasty. The occluded left circumflex coronary artery (A, *arrow*) was crossed with a guidewire and treated with a 1.4-mm excimer laser catheter (B, *arrow*) followed by PTCA (C, *arrow*). *PTCA,* Percutaneous transluminal coronary angioplasty.

KEY REFERENCES

1. Bittl JA, Chew DP, Topol EJ, et al. Meta-analysis of randomized trials of percutaneous transluminal coronary angioplasty versus atherectomy, cutting balloon atherotomy, or laser angioplasty. *J Am Coll Cardiol.* 2004;43:936–942.
2. Levine GN, Bates ER, Blankenship JC, et al. 2011 ACCF/AHA/SCAI guidelines for percutaneous coronary intervention: a report of the American College of Cardiology Foundation/American Heart Association task force on practice guidelines and the Society for Cardiovascular Angiography and Interventions. *J Am Coll Cardiol.* 2011;58:e44–e122. plus Data Supplements 123–124.
11. Baim DS, Cutlip DE, Sharma SK, et al. Final results of the Balloon vs Optimal Atherectomy Trial. *Circulation.* 1998;97:322–331.
13. Safian RD, Feldman T, Muller DW, et al. Coronary angioplasty and Rotablator atherectomy trial (CARAT): immediate and late results of a prospective multicenter randomized trial. *Catheter Cardiovasc Interv.* 2001;53:213–220.
21. Reifert N, Vandormael M, Krajcar M, et al. Randomized comparison of angioplasty of complex coronary lesions at a single center: Excimer Laser, Rotatational Atherectomy, and Balloon Angioplasty Comparison (ERBAC) study. *Circulation.* 1997;96:91–98.
23. Mauri L, Bonan R, Weiner BH, et al. Cutting balloon angioplasty for the prevention of restenosis: results of the Cutting Balloon Global Randomized Trial. *Am J Cardiol.* 2002;90:1079–1083.
30. Whitlow PL, Bass TA, Kipperman RM, et al. Results of the Study to Determine Rotablator and Transluminal Angioplasty Strategy (STRATAS). *Am J Cardiol.* 2001;87:699–705.
32. Abdel-Wahab M, Richardt G, Joachim Büttner H, et al. High-speed rotational atherectomy before paclitaxel-eluting stent implantation in complex calcified coronary lesions: the randomized ROTAXUS (Rotational Atherectomy Prior to Taxus Stent Treatment for Complex Native Coronary Artery Disease) trial. *JACC Cardiovasc Interv.* 2013;6:10–19.
40. Deckelbaum LI, Natarajan MK, Bittl JA, et al. Effect of intracoronary saline on dissection during excimer laser coronary angioplasty: a randomized trial. *J Am Coll Cardiol.* 1995;26:1264–1269.

Additional references available online at expertconsult.com.

中文导读

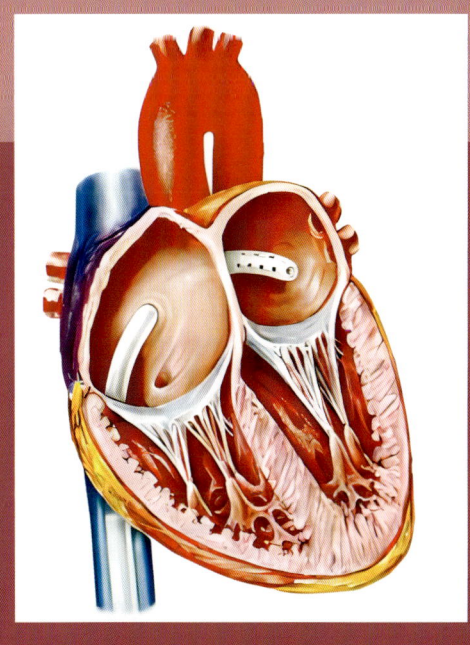

第36章
支持性经皮介入治疗

　　本章节介绍了各种循环支持器械的工作原理、适应证及循证医学证据。随着技术发展和老龄化社会的到来，越来越多的患者可能正在接受高危的经皮冠状动脉介入治疗，包括高龄患者、左主干病变、多支血管病变和严重心功能不全的患者。在许多情况下，外科搭桥手术并不是一个可行或令人满意的选择，因为其复苏时间较长，这使得经皮冠状动脉介入治疗成为改善心功能和减少缺血症状的唯一可能的办法。但这类特殊患者不仅是外科搭桥手术的高危患者，亦是经皮冠状动脉介入治疗的高危患者，在围术期容易发生循环崩溃。因此，术者必须准确识别风险，并考虑对手术并发症和住院死亡率高风险的患者预防性使用血流动力学支持。此外，在急性心肌梗死合并心源性休克的情况下接受经皮冠状动脉介入治疗的患者是使用血流动力学支持装置的特别高危人群，现有证据支持在最初的医疗尝试稳定后使用血流动力学支持装置。

陈思源　范　谦

章节要点

- 选择性高危患者的临床特征包括高龄、有心肌梗死病史、低射血分数、充血性心力衰竭、近期血流动力学不稳定、肾功能不全和外周血管疾病。

- 选择性患者的高危冠状动脉造影特征包括左主干病变、残留唯一血管通畅、多支血管病变、复杂病变（钙化、曲折、分叉）、术前血流TIMI分级降低，以及血栓性病变。

- 应根据特定患者围术期临床失代偿的风险状况对选择性高危患者使用循环支持装置做出决定。ACCF/AHA临床指南将高危经皮冠状动脉介入治疗中的血流动力学设备作为Ⅱb类推荐，将急性心肌梗死合并心源性休克应用IABP或替代循环支持装置分别作为Ⅱa类推荐和Ⅱb类推荐。表现为急性心肌梗死和冠状动脉综合征的患者代表了在经皮冠状动脉介入治疗前可能需要急性血流动力学稳定的患者中的一个独特的亚群。器械的选择取决于所需支持程度、是否是单一心室或双心室受到影响、患者是否存在低氧、技术专长相关实际问题、启动支持所需的时间和设备的可用性。

- IABP支持提供高达0.5 L/min的心排血量；其在择期高风险经皮冠状动脉介入治疗中的益处得到了大量稳定心律患者的经验数据的支持，但是最近公布的随机数据和Meta分析质疑其益处。IABP在随机数据中也没有显示出对出现心源性休克患者的好处，促使欧洲指南将其降级为Ⅲ级推荐。

- 心肺支持可以完全支持循环（双室支持）和氧合，无论心律如何，经验丰富的医师可以快速启动；然而，其会导致血管和进入部位并发症的高发生率，并且在单独使用时不会卸载左心室。

- TandemHeart设备可间接减轻左心室负荷，提供中间水平的循环支持，流量高达3.5 L/min，且使用时间可以很长。但它的应用受限于复杂插入技术，且支持证据相对较少。

- Impella设备可直接减轻左心室负荷，提供高达2.5 L/min、3.5~4.0 L/min（Impella CP）或5.0 L/min（Impella 5.0）的循环支持，使用时间很长。由于更容易的插管技术和在高危经皮冠状动脉介入治疗中相对可靠的观察和随机化的试验数据，它得到了更广泛的应用。

- 基于大量观察和随机数据，Impella设备已获得美国食品药品监督管理局的批准，用于高风险的经皮冠状动脉介入治疗和心源性休克。Impella RP右侧支持装置最近已可用于治疗右侧衰竭，无论是单独使用还是与左室辅助装置结合使用，都可用于治疗双室衰竭。

- 针对高危经皮冠状动脉介入治疗队列，报告了精心设计的IABP及无支持的随机对照试验和IABP与Impella 2.5[Impella 2.5与IABP在接受高风险经皮冠状动脉介入治疗患者中的血流动力学支持的前瞻性随机临床试验（PROTECT Ⅱ）]的随机对照试验，但两项试验都没有达到主要终点的优势。PROTECT Ⅱ的次要终点提示对重复血管重建和再住院有好处。然而，接受支持的经皮冠状动脉介入治疗的患者在功能状态和射血分数方面有明显的改善，这表明无论使用何种设备进行支持，高危经皮冠状动脉介入治疗都是有益的。对于合并心源性休克的急性心肌梗死（ST段抬高型心肌梗死）患者，在直接经皮冠状动脉介入治疗之前早期减轻左心室负荷的随机试验目前正处于研究阶段。

36 Supported Percutaneous Intervention

Srihari S. Naidu, Madhur A. Roberts, Howard C. Herrmann

KEY POINTS

- Clinical characteristics of the elective high-risk patient include older age, history of myocardial infarction (MI), low ejection fraction, congestive heart failure (CHF), recent hemodynamic instability, renal insufficiency, and peripheral vascular disease.
- High-risk angiographic characteristics for the elective patient include left main coronary artery (LMCA) disease, last patent conduit, multivessel coronary artery disease, complex lesions (calcified, tortuous, bifurcation), decreased preprocedure thrombolysis in myocardial infarction (TIMI) flow, and thrombotic lesions.
- The decision to use a circulatory support device for the elective high-risk patient should be made within the context of the risk profile of the specific patient for periprocedural clinical decompensation. American College of Cardiology Foundation (ACCF)/American Heart Association (AHA) clinical guidelines support hemodynamic devices in high-risk percutaneous coronary intervention (PCI) as a class IIb recommendation and for acute myocardial infarction (AMI) complicated with cardiogenic shock (CS) as a class IIa for intraaortic balloon pump (IABP) and class IIb for alternative circulatory support devices. Patients presenting with AMI and CS represent a unique subset of patients who may require acute hemodynamic stabilization prior to primary PCI. Choice of device is guided by the degree of support necessary, whether one or both ventricles are affected, and whether the patient is hypoxemic, as well as practical issues related to technical expertise, time necessary to initiate support, and availability of devices.
- IABP support provides up to 0.5 L/min of cardiac output; its benefit in elective high-risk PCI is supported by a large amount of experiential data in patients with stable cardiac rhythm, although recently presented randomized data and meta-analyses question its benefit. The IABP has also not shown benefit in randomized data for patients presenting in CS, prompting a reduction to class III in the European guidelines.
- Cardiopulmonary support (CPS) can completely support the circulation (biventricular support) and oxygenation irrespective of cardiac rhythm and can be instituted quickly by experienced practitioners; however, it leads to high rates of vascular and access-site complications and does not unload the left ventricle (LV) when used in isolation.
- The TandemHeart device (Cardiac Assist, Pittsburgh, PA) indirectly unloads the LV, provides an intermediate level of support that reaches flows of up to 3.5 L/min, and can be used for an extended period, but it is limited by the complex insertion technique and is supported by relatively meager clinical data.
- The Impella device (Abiomed, Danvers, MA) directly unloads the LV, can provide up to 2.5 L/min (Impella 2.5), 3.5 to 4.0 L/min (Impella CP), or 5.0 L/min (Impella 5.0) of circulatory support, and it can also be used for an extended period. It has gained more widespread use because of the easier insertion technique and relatively robust observational and randomized trial data for high-risk PCI.
- Impella devices have gained U.S. Food and Drug Administration (FDA) approval for high-risk PCI and cardiogenic shock, based on a large body of observational and randomized data. The Impella RP right-sided support device has recently become available for right-sided failure either in isolation or, when combined with LV support devices, for biventricular failure.
- Well-designed randomized controlled trials (RCTs) of the IABP versus no support (the Balloon Pump-Assisted Coronary Intervention Study [BCIS-1]) and the IABP versus Impella 2.5 (A Prospective Randomized Clinical Trial of Hemodynamic Support With Impella 2.5 Versus IABP in Patients Undergoing High-Risk Percutaneous Coronary Intervention [PROTECT II]) have been reported for the high-risk PCI cohort, but neither trial met its primary end point for superiority. Secondary end points in PROTECT II suggest benefits in repeat revascularization and rehospitalization. However, patients with supported PCI evidenced improvements in functional status and ejection fraction, suggesting that high-risk PCI is beneficial regardless of device used for support.

Randomized trials of early unloading of the LV prior to primary PCI in acute myocardial infarction (ST-elevation MI) with CS are currently underway.

INTRODUCTION AND RATIONALE: IDENTIFYING THE HIGH-RISK PATIENT

Complications of balloon angioplasty that threaten coronary blood flow, termed *acute and threatened occlusions*, usually require urgent surgical intervention and are the main causes of procedure-related morbidity and mortality. Before the advent of stents as a bail-out treatment for impending vessel closure, this complication occurred in approximately 6% of balloon angioplasty procedures. Patients who required emergent surgery in this setting had a 50% likelihood of suffering myocardial infarction (MI), and mortality rates were as high as 10%.[1] In these early studies, patient characteristics that included compromised ventricular function, left main coronary artery (LMCA) disease, multivessel disease, and older age were identified as risk factors for balloon angioplasty–related mortality.[2,3] With the development of coronary stents and advanced pharmacotherapy to seal dissections and improve blood flow in thrombotic lesions, respectively, the need for urgent surgery was reduced with a concomitant reduction in percutaneous coronary intervention (PCI)-related morbidity and mortality.[4]

In the current era, studies have demonstrated that the need for urgent surgery after PCI has been reduced to less than 1%, with a marked reduction in procedure-related mortality.[5] In one comparison of patients treated in 1997 and 1998 with those treated in 1985 and 1986, the rate of in-hospital deaths, MI, and coronary artery bypass grafting (CABG) fell from 7.9% to 4.9%, despite the treatment of more complex lesions and stent use in only 71% of patients.[6] Most of the differences between these periods were accounted for by the reduction in the need for emergent CABG from 3.7% to 0.4%.[6] Nonetheless, morbidity and mortality among patients who required emergent CABG remained high.[5] Moreover, the increased confidence afforded by stents and improved operator techniques and experience have prompted interventions on more complex lesions and in patients with more severe cardiac and noncardiac diseases. In particular, results of the Synergy Between Percutaneous Coronary Intervention With Taxus and Cardiac Surgery (SYNTAX) trial confirm reasonable outcomes in select patients with LMCA disease or multivessel coronary disease, and completed and ongoing trials of high-risk PCI with cardiac assist device placement indicate that extremely high-risk patient populations are, indeed, being increasingly considered for PCI.[7,8] American College of Cardiology Foundation (ACCF)/American Heart Association (AHA) clinical guidelines have kept pace and currently support percutaneous unprotected left main stenting in appropriate high-risk surgical patients as a class IIa and IIb indication.[9] The more recent American College of Cardiology (ACC)/AHA/ Society for Cardiovascular Angiography and Interventions (SCAI) 2017 appropriate use document also considers left main stenting appropriate in a subset of patients, depending on the location of the stenosis, disease burden in other territories, and use of antianginal therapy.[10] Given the large amount of the myocardium in jeopardy in these subsets, as well as the baseline comorbidities frequently present (including reduced ventricular reserve), the potential for severe clinical decompensation in such patients is a real concern. It has therefore become essential to precisely identify the predictors of risk and to consider the use of hemodynamic support for patients at high risk for procedural complications and in-hospital mortality.

A number of variables have been defined that contribute to increased procedural risk in PCI. These can be patient related, be lesion related and depend on clinical presentation. Patient-related variables include age, symptoms of heart failure, impaired left ventricular function, prior cardiovascular disease (CVD) such as prior MI, other known coronary artery disease (CAD) (multivessel or left main disease), peripheral arterial disease (PAD), diabetes mellitus, and chronic kidney disease.[11-18] Lesion-related variables incorporate left main stenosis, bifurcation disease, saphenous vein grafts, last patent vessel, heavily calcified lesions, ostial lesions, and chronic total occlusions.[19-23] Clinical acuity of presentation also confers a high risk.[24]

Although a number of investigators have used commonsense definitions to classify patients at high risk, two studies systematically developed risk models.[19,25-27] In the *Mayo Clinic model*, clinical and angiographic variables were used to predict in-hospital complications after PCI.[26] The variables were age, shock, renal insufficiency, urgent procedures, heart failure, thrombus, and LMCA or multivessel disease. A score based on these factors predicted the risk of complications and identified a "highest risk" group with an event rate that exceeded 25%.[26] In a similar study of 46,000 procedures in the mandatory New York State Hospital PCI reporting system, investigators included nine factors in a risk score: (1) ejection fraction (EF), (2) previous MI, (3) gender, (4) age, (5) hemodynamic state, (6) PAD, (7) congestive heart failure (CHF), (8) renal failure, and (9) LMCA disease. Using this *New York State Hospital model*, a graded risk score for in-hospital mortality was derived and validated. Approximately 2% of all patients had a greater than 5% risk for in-hospital death, and approximately 4% of patients had a greater than 3% risk.[27] Other studies have confirmed these risk factors for PCI-related complications,[3,11,28] but neither model may accurately represent the higher-risk patient populations undergoing intervention in the current era.

More recently, CathPCI registry data were used to develop "full," "precatheterization," and "bedside risk prediction" mortality models.[24] The precatheterization model consisted of age, body mass index (BMI), CVD, PAD, chronic lung disease, prior PCI, glomerular filtration rate (GFR), EF, cardiogenic shock (CS), acuity of PCI, New York Heart Association (NYHA) class symptoms within past 2 weeks, and cardiac arrest within 24 hours. The CathPCI registry risk prediction score performed well, and the study also showed that clinical acuity remains the strongest predictor of PCI procedural mortality.[24] In addition to these clinical risk factors, angiographic factors of lesion complexity—thrombus, calcification, and bifurcations—have been shown to be associated with more dissections, distal embolization, and side-branch occlusions, resulting in a threefold increase for in-hospital death.[29]

Several patient characteristics deserve separate discussion. Although female sex was initially associated with complications in early studies of balloon angioplasty, more recent studies have failed to demonstrate an important effect on outcome.[26,27,30,31] When compared with CABG, PCI has increased rates of mortality in patients with diabetes. However, when looking at the subset of patients undergoing PCI with and without diabetes, patients with diabetes have more complex lesion characteristics and risk factors but no increase in in-hospital mortality after multivariable adjustment.[32]

More recently, baseline left ventricle (LV) dysfunction and the extent of the myocardium in jeopardy during the procedure have reemerged as perhaps the strongest clinical risk factors for intraprocedural decompensation and in-hospital mortality. Accordingly, recent studies on high-risk PCI have used the combination of severe ventricular dysfunction (represented by EF <30% to 35%) and either LMCA disease, last patent conduit, or multivessel disease as high-risk PCI inclusion criteria.[20] Thus it is clear that despite major advances in the technical and procedural performance of modern PCI, clinical and angiographic predictors of significant morbidity and mortality can be identified (Table 36.1). Moreover, it appears likely that increasing numbers of patients will be undergoing high-risk PCI, including the very old and those with LMCA disease, multivessel disease, and significant ventricular dysfunction. In many cases, bypass surgery is not a viable or palatable option, with prolonged recovery, leaving PCI as the only remaining possible mechanism to improve ventricular function and reduce ischemic symptoms.

Finally, patients undergoing PCI in the setting of acute myocardial infarction (AMI) with CS represent an especially high-risk group in whom hemodynamic support devices have been used, and national guidelines currently support their use after initial attempts at medical stabilization.[9] Lately, there has been emphasis on the timing of hemodynamic support devices in AMI complicated by CS. The concept of door-to-support time has been developed and seems to have significant effect on outcomes in preclinical studies. As the hemodynamic instability in CS progresses, the reduced cardiac output and elevated filling pressures lead to decreased systemic perfusion, lactic acidosis, multiorgan ischemia, hepatic and venous congestion, and multiorgan failure.[33] This trail of events subsequently transitions CS from a potentially reversible hemodynamic problem to a more complex hemometabolic problem. Initiating mechanical circulatory support (MCS) early (i.e., prior to PCI or pharmacotherapy for hemodynamic support) may theoretically lead to improved survival. A retrospective study from the continuous ventricular assist device (cVAD) Registry found that early implantation of Impella (Abiomed, Danvers, MA) before PCI and before requiring inotropes/vasopressors was associated with increased survival. Furthermore, they demonstrated that with increasing time from shock onset to MCS, the survival

TABLE 36.1 Predictors of Risk During Percutaneous Coronary Intervention

Factor	References
CLINICAL AND PATIENT RELATED	
Older age	3, 27, 26, 75, 13, 14
Cardiogenic shock	6, 27, 26, 75
Recent myocardial infarction	6, 27, 26, 75
Congestive heart failure	26-28, 75
Prior coronary artery bypass grafting/revascularization	111
Peripheral vascular disease	27, 75
Chronic renal insufficiency	26, 27, 75
Diabetes Mellitus	15, 17, 18
Acuity of cardiogenic shock	24
ANGIOGRAPHIC	
Left main coronary artery/multivessel disease	27, 26, 75, 113, 118, 15, 16, 21, 22
Complex lesions (bifurcation, calcification, total occlusion)	29
Saphenous vein graft	23
Decreased thrombolysis in myocardial infarction (TIMI) flow	114
Left ventricular dysfunction	6, 27, 28, 11, 75, 12
Thrombus	26, 29

decreased (66%, 37%, and 26% when MCS was initiated <1.25 hours, 1.25 to 4.25 hours, and after 4.25 hours, respectively; $P = .017$).[34] A smaller subset of patients from the cVAD Registry who underwent unprotected left main PCI as a culprit lesion in patients with MI complicated by CS was then looked at. The number of patients was small ($n = 36$); however, the data showed that patients who received Impella prior to PCI had better early survival as compared with the ones who received the Impella after the PCI.[35] Similar results were also noted in the USPella Registry that showed significantly higher in-hospital survival (63% higher) when Impella was initiated prior to revascularization.[36] This concept will be further evaluated in an ongoing randomized clinical trial: Door to Unloading With Impella CP System in AMI trial.

Together, these data provide the rationale and impetus for the increased use of hemodynamic support during complex or high-risk PCI in various clinical settings in the current era, including CS. The remainder of this chapter will discuss the approach to such patients, historical and current data, the devices currently available to provide support, and the results that may be achieved by using them.

APPROACH TO THE PATIENT

Mechanical circulatory support at the time of PCI has historically been instituted in one of two settings: *electively* for presumed high-risk intervention and *emergently* for periprocedural hemodynamic instability. The latter may occur during a planned elective PCI or occur on presentation, such as with AMI and CS. However, specific indications remain unclear because of limitations in performing large-scale randomized trials and evaluating specific devices in individual patient subsets, especially for the latter indication. Nevertheless, a review of existing literature and ongoing clinical trials provides a framework for both patient and device selection when evaluating patients for elective or emergent support.

Electively placed mechanical support is aimed at improving procedural success by minimizing myocardial ischemia and maintaining hemodynamic stability, thereby reducing clinical decompensation and resultant mortality in high-risk preselected patient subsets, as discussed in the previous section. In this setting, prophylactic insertion of the intraaortic balloon pump (IABP) or the Impella ventricular assist device (VAD) appears to have the most robust observational data for improving procedural success with a minimal increase in complications.[20,37-44] Despite encouraging registry data, however, a randomized controlled trial (RCT) failed to show clinical benefit to routine prophylactic IABP insertion in patients undergoing high-risk PCI.[45] The more powerful Impella device was subsequently studied in patients deemed to need hemodynamic support for high-risk PCI. Whereas the device was successful in providing superior hemodynamic support, in comparison to routine IABP use (based on magnitude of drop in cardiac power output [CPO] during the case), no difference was reported in major adverse events at 30 days.[46] However, secondary end points in each of these trials were hypothesis generating, in that procedural complications and long-term mortality were improved with routine IABP use in the Balloon Pump-Assisted Coronary Intervention Study (BCIS-1) trial, and repeat revascularization, total length of stay, and 90-day major adverse events were improved with Impella, especially in patients who did not undergo rotational atherectomy.[46,47]

The use of mechanical circulatory support in the emergent setting for patients with documented hemodynamic instability or CS is more familiar to interventional cardiologists. Instability may be present before PCI (as in acute MI with compromised ventricular function) or may develop as a consequence of procedural complications such as coronary dissection, poor coronary reflow, or thromboembolism. A common underlying finding in most of these patients is ventricular dysfunction. Although there is paucity of RCT data in this arena, a pooled meta-analysis of IABP use in patients with acute ST-elevation myocardial infarction (STEMI) found no benefit to IABP use in conjunction with primary angioplasty, but some benefit was seen in those receiving thrombolytic therapy.[48] The more recent Intraaortic Balloon Pump in Cardiogenic Shock II (IABP-SHOCK II)[49] trial similarly found no benefit to routine IABP use in patients presenting with CS, prompting a downgrading of the European guidelines to class III.[50] Available percutaneous ventricular assist devices (pVADs) appear to improve hemodynamic parameters in patients with acute clinical decompensation, but only registry data are available to suggest improved outcome.[36] As a result, determining whether and which device to use in specific settings remains controversial and is primarily guided by experience and expert consensus, with the field as a whole shifting toward more powerful support earlier in the course of clinical deterioration.

Device selection is based on several factors; these include ease and rapidity of institution, level of invasiveness and complications, physician familiarity, requisite technical expertise, level of anticipated circulatory support, available supportive clinical trial data, and, in the case of the Impella device, Food and Drug Administration (FDA) approval for both high-risk PCI and CS. An IABP is the least invasive and most familiar device and may be instituted rapidly, but it also provides the least support, averaging 0.5 L/min augmentation in cardiac output.[51] It may be left in place for several days and has a low vascular complication rate.[52] Conversely, full cardiopulmonary support (CPS) is significantly more invasive, and it requires timely surgical and perfusionist collaboration for institution and removal, but it can produce greater improvement in cardiac output, approximating normal physiology. However, CPS cannot be maintained indefinitely because hematologic and pulmonary complications increase as bypass time approaches 6 hours and, in the absence of concomitant LV venting or unloading, its deleterious effect on myocardial oxygen consumption remains a concern.[52] pVADs, such as the TandemHeart or the Impella 2.5 or

CP, provide an intermediate level of support that approaches 2.5 to 4 L/min; in addition, these devices can be placed emergently in the catheterization laboratory (cath lab) without surgical backup, which has prompted their increased use recently. Unlike the Impella, the TandemHeart requires transseptal puncture to deliver the inflow cannula into the left atrium, and it requires a somewhat larger arterial cannula. Thus only patients with a larger femoral arterial diameter are able to accommodate device placement, which can be performed only by those skilled in the transseptal technique. Consequently, compared with the Impella device, cath lab utilization rate of the TandemHeart appears to have stabilized or decreased in recent years. In both devices, the cannulae are larger than with an IABP and may result in significant vascular morbidity. However, unlike full CPS, the use of a pVAD has been successful for intermediate lengths of time (up to 14 days). Relatively smaller cannulae, as with the Impella, are likely to reduce femoral complications.

Historically, elective high-risk PCI has been performed safely with either provisional or prophylactic IABP support. However, as described earlier, RCT data have suggested that routine prophylactic IABP support may offer little meaningful benefit in these patients over the short term.[45] pVAD has been shown to have superior hemodynamic parameters (e.g., mean arterial pressures) as compared with IABP.[53] In those select patients who appear to require additional circulatory support, as defined by the inclusion criteria of completed and ongoing randomized trials, a pVAD may be considered, with the caveats that the inherent increase in delay and invasiveness (particularly access-site complications) may partially offset the benefit and that definitively supportive RCTs remain absent.[46] However, some observational and retrospective data do suggest significant reduction in mortality with pVADs when compared with IABPs in patients undergoing PCI.[54] For patients who develop severe hemodynamic instability, CS, or frank arrest during PCI, bail-out use of the IABP appears beneficial and is certainly the most familiar and rapid strategy; however, the support provided may be insufficient.[49] Cath labs experienced in rapid pVAD placement may opt for these larger, more powerful devices as either an initial or rapidly escalating strategy. Developing data on hemodynamic parameters that might predict meaningful recovery, such as CPO (measured in Watts), would at least theoretically support their use.[55] Although full CPS may be considered in cath labs equipped and staffed for timely initiation, its clinical use had been relegated to anecdotal experience over the past decade until more compact CPS units were recently developed. Consequently, there has been a rise in their utilization in some cath labs. Nevertheless, in emergent settings, pVADs appear most promising and consequently have become increasingly prominent, but they require specialized technical expertise for optimal patient selection, device placement, and postprocedural management. Although two pVADs currently exist, the TandemHeart and the Impella devices, the vast majority of the data and clinical experience have centered around the Impella device, based on the large amount of observational data and subsequent FDA approvals.

DESCRIPTION OF DEVICES AND AVAILABLE CLINICAL DATA

Intraaortic Balloon Pump

The IABP was first used clinically in CS by Kantrowitz in 1968.[56] As its application expanded to include refractory angina, severe hemodynamic compromise, and postcardiotomy pump failure and with the advent of percutaneous insertion, the IABP was one of the first hemodynamic devices used to support high-risk PCIs.[56-58]

The IABP catheter is a double-lumen 7.5- to 8.0-Fr catheter that has a polyethylene balloon attached to its distal end. One central lumen is used for guidewire placement and pressure transduction. Second lumen is attached to the pump that inflates the balloon with helium gas. Helium is a low-viscosity gas that facilitates rapid transfer in and out of the balloon, and it absorbs very rapidly in blood in the case of balloon rupture. The rapid filling of the balloon in early diastole augments diastolic pressure and thereby leads to increased coronary perfusion pressure, whereas deflation of the balloon at end diastole reduces effective aortic volume and decreases aortic systolic pressure, which leads to lower LV afterload. The net effect is a decrease in myocardial oxygen requirements from lower systolic wall tension and an increase in coronary perfusion pressure, which improves the myocardial supply/demand balance. Cardiac output increases because of the improved myocardial contractility as a result of the increased coronary blood flow and the reduced afterload.[59-61]

Insertion Technique

Evaluation of the iliac and femoral arteries is recommended to exclude significant arterial disease. Access in the common femoral artery is obtained via the Seldinger technique. The balloon can be inserted through an 8- or a 9-Fr sheath or directly in a sheathless fashion. Before insertion, all the air in the balloon should be evacuated with a large syringe attached to the one-way valve to maintain the lowest possible profile during insertion. The balloon catheter is advanced under fluoroscopic guidance over a stiff 0.021-inch guidewire until the radiopaque tip marker reaches a level just distal to the left subclavian artery. After removal of the guidewire, the central lumen is flushed and connected to a pressure transducer. The balloon is then connected to the console, the system is purged with helium, and counterpulsation is started. Proper placement and inflation of the balloon should be done fluoroscopically, and the timing of inflation and deflation should be optimized by either the surface electrocardiogram (ECG) or the transduced pressure tracing to achieve optimal hemodynamic support. Newer IABP algorithms and software upgrades allow for autoinflation and more precise timing. Vascular complications such as thromboembolism and stroke should be kept in mind while considering the use of IABP. Severe peripheral vascular disease or aortoiliac disease increases the risk of vascular complications.[62]

Clinical Trials

Much of the observational data on the use of IABPs and other circulatory support devices during high-risk PCI come from the prestent era of coronary interventions. Voudris and colleagues[39] found that support with IABP use during elective high-risk angioplasty is both safe and feasible. During a 13-month period (in 1987 and 1988), 27 patients considered high risk because of decreased LV function or multivessel disease underwent angioplasty with IABP support. Primary success, according to contemporary ACC guidelines, was achieved in all 27 patients. No major cardiac events occurred during hospitalization, and only one IABP-related vascular complication was reported. After a mean follow-up period of 13 months, two deaths, one cardiac transplantation, and six cases of symptom-driven target-vessel revascularization (TVR, 22% rate of recurrent angina) were reported, and the TVR was also successfully performed with IABP support.[39]

Similar outcomes were reported by Kahn and associates[38] in a group of 28 high-risk patients during the same period. The most common high-risk feature in this cohort of patients was severe LV dysfunction, but some patients had critical stenosis in the LMCA or a single remaining coronary artery. Procedural success was 96% (90 of 94 lesions were successfully dilated). Eleven patients had intraprocedural hypotension, although the augmented diastolic pressure was maintained over 90 mm Hg in all cases, and angioplasty was completed in all patients. Vascular complications associated with the IABP occurred in 11% of the patients. In another series[40] of 21 patients with similar high-risk features, 90% of lesions attempted were successfully dilated without hemodynamic compromise; device-related complications (hematoma) occurred in 10% of the cases, and procedure-related complications occurred in 14%.

The beneficial effects of IABP support were also shown in high-risk coronary rotational atherectomy.[63] In a retrospective analysis, 28 patients scheduled to undergo rotational atherectomy were placed on IABP support before the coronary intervention. This group was compared with 131 patients with high-risk coronary lesions who did *not* have an IABP placed a priori. The group that received a planned IABP comprised patients who were older and had more LV dysfunction and a higher incidence of multivessel disease. Although systolic hypotension occurred in 11% of the patients in the study group, diastolic pressure augmentation provided by the IABP allowed successful completion of the procedure in all patients. Hypotension that necessitated IABP placement occurred in 7% of the patients in the comparison group. Slow flow occurred at a similar rate in both groups; however, 27% of the patients in the comparison group who experienced slow flow developed a non-Q wave MI, compared with none in the study group. No differences were reported in the rate of transfusion requirements or vascular complications.[63]

In a more recent study by Brodie and colleagues,[2] IABP was shown to reduce periprocedural events in a group that consisted of 213 patients who presented with acute MI and received an IABP. In contrast to the earlier studies discussed, the majority of patients in this group were treated with stents, and approximately a third were treated with abciximab, reflecting the then-contemporary treatments. Whereas the indication for the IABP in most cases was CS, 80 patients were hemodynamically stable but were considered high risk because of LV dysfunction. In this group, the use of IABP support led to a decreased incidence of prolonged hypotension, cardiac arrest, and ventricular fibrillation; however, the difference was not statistically significant because of the low number of patients in this group. IABP use was associated with an increased risk of major bleeding and higher transfusion rates.

Although IABP use during high-risk coronary interventions had been shown, at least in registry and case series data, to be effective in supporting the circulation, the increased rates of vascular and hemorrhagic complications associated with its use demanded careful patient selection.[2,38,39,41,63] For this reason, a strategy of provisional IABP support was compared with prophylactic placement of IABP in high risk interventions in a retrospective, nonrandomized study.[64] Sixty-one patients who received elective IABP were compared with 72 patients in whom support was initiated only when clinically necessary. The patients in the elective IABP group were slightly older, but other high-risk features were similar, including severity of LV dysfunction (EF <30%) and rates of multivessel disease and unstable angina. Rates of stent and glycoprotein inhibitor use were similar between the two groups. The rates of slow flow were similar in both groups, but hemodynamic deterioration occurred only in patients (15%) in the provisional IABP group, and all received urgent IABP support. Rates of vascular complications were low in this study, with only two patients in the provisional IABP group developing groin hematomas. No cases of major bleeding were reported. Although not statistically significant, three deaths occurred in the provisional IABP group in patients who required urgent placement of an IABP compared with one death in the elective group.[64] Similarly, in a study of 48 patients undergoing primary PCI for AMI complicated by CS, IABP placement prior to PCI resulted in reduced major adverse cardiac events (MACEs), including mortality, than postprocedure placement.[65]

More contemporary observational data have been less supportive. In particular, evaluation of collected data from the National Cardiovascular Data Registry (NCDR) found no difference in overall mortality with use of the IABP for high-risk PCI, and wide national variation was apparent in its use for this purpose.[66] Furthermore, a meta-analysis of IABP use in AMI found no benefit to IABP use in this setting and found a higher incidence of stroke.[48] A summary of the published observational trials that used IABP during high-risk PCI is shown in Table 36.2.

Routine prophylactic use of IABP in high-risk PCI or CS has recently come into question, however, following the results of two large randomized trials.[45,49] Patients undergoing high-risk PCI, defined as severe LV systolic dysfunction (left ventricular ejection fraction [LVEF] <30%) and extensive CAD were randomized in the BCIS-1 trial to either routine IABP or no planned IABP prior to PCI.[45] No difference was reported in the primary end point of major adverse cardiac and cerebrovascular events (MACCEs) at 28 days despite a marked

TABLE 36.2 Intraaortic Balloon Pump Observational Trials

First Author	Year	Procedure	Number of Patients	Revasc. Success Rate (%)	Device-Related Complication Rate (%)	In-Hospital Mortality Rate
Anwar[37]	1990	PTCA	97	85.6	2	1
Kahn[38]	1990	PTCA	28	96	11	7.1
Voudris[39]	1990	PTCA	27	100	3.7	0
Kreidieh[40]	1992	PTCA	21	90	9.5	0
O'Murchu[63]	1995	Atherectomy/PTCA	28	100	7.1	0
Kaul[82]	1995	PTCA	20	95	0	5
Schreiber[83]	1998	PTCA	91	87	27	8.7
Brodie[2]	1999	PTCA/Stent[a]	108[b]	89.8	8[c]	37[d]
Briguori[64]	2003	PTCA/Stent	61	94	0	8
Abdol-Wahab[65]	2010	Stent	48 (26 pre-PCI, 22 post-PCI)	100	NR	19% vs. 59%
Curtis[66]	2012	Stent	18,990	NR	4.8%–5.1%	4.9%

[a]Stents were used in the last 3 years of the study.
[b]Includes patients with shock or congestive heart failure; the number of patients undergoing high-risk PCI was not defined.
[c]Includes patients who received an intraaortic balloon pump after PTCA.
[d]Thirty-day mortality that includes patients with cardiogenic shock.
NR, Not reported; *PCI*, percutaneous coronary intervention; *PTCA*, percutaneous transluminal coronary angioplasty; *Revasc.*, revascularization.

reduction in procedural complications. In addition, bleeding and access-site complications trended higher with routine IABP use. Mortality was no different at 6 months but was significantly reduced at long-term follow-up of 51 months, a finding that can be deemed only hypothesis generating because the trial was not powered to reveal a mortality difference.[47]

In the setting of AMI complicated by CS, the IABP remains the most commonly used support device. Despite its widespread use, the data for its support in AMI complicated by CS are unsatisfactory. The IABP-SHOCK II trial randomized 600 patients to routine IABP versus no IABP.[49] All patients were expected to undergo early revascularization. By 30 days, no difference in mortality or any secondary end points was noted, and rates of bleeding, sepsis, and stroke were similar.[49] These findings highlight the importance of RCT data and appropriate selection and timing of clinical end points to fully elucidate the proper role of any cardiac assist device in high-risk PCI. Accordingly, the IABP was given a class III indication (no benefit) in the most recent European guidelines.[50] A summary of the randomized trials in high-risk PCI, including the BCIS-1 and IABP-SHOCK II trials, is shown in Table 36.3.

Percutaneous Cardiopulmonary Support (CPS, ECMO)

The introduction in 1985 of the portable Bard CardioPulmonary Bypass Support system (CR Bard, Murray Hill, NJ) expanded the application of percutaneous CPS.[67] Although the most common application for temporary circulatory support is for patients who cannot be weaned from cardiopulmonary bypass after cardiac surgery, CPS has also been implemented in the cath lab either emergently as a bridge to cardiac surgery or prophylactically to support high-risk coronary interventions. Full CPS incorporates a heat exchanger, an adjustable blood reservoir, a pump, and an oxygenator and can temporarily substitute for the entire circulation and oxygenation, irrespective of cardiac rhythm. Because blood comes in contact with various biomaterials in the perfusion circuit, activation of blood proteins and cells leads to morbidity that limits the length of time it can be maintained. Other more simplified strategies use only a blood pump and extracorporeal membrane oxygenation (ECMO).

CPS unloads the right ventricle but does not unload the left.[67] Pulmonary and systolic aortic pressures have been shown to decrease, whereas diastolic and mean systemic arterial pressures remain unchanged.[67,68] In normal functioning hearts, the reduction in preload and a small increase in afterload produced by the arterial inflow reduces wall stress and produces smaller end-diastolic LV volumes because the LV is able to eject the blood it receives. However, in dilated and poorly contracting hearts, especially after cardiac arrest, the increase in afterload may impair LV emptying, and another means of assisting emptying of the ventricle (e.g., IABP or Impella) may be necessary to avoid further deterioration of heart function. Another very simple approach is to provide an external cardiac compression approximately every minute while the patient is on CPS. Studies have also shown that CPS does not increase coronary perfusion in the setting of an occlusion, so bypass surgery should be considered if circulation cannot be restored percutaneously. For these reasons, CPS may, at least in theory, be a poor choice for patients undergoing high-risk PCI, in whom unloading the LV and maintaining antegrade coronary blood flow are primary concerns.

Insertion Technique

Before arterial cannulation, angiography of the iliofemoral arteries is performed to exclude significant arterial disease. Care should be taken to access the artery below the inguinal ligament in the common femoral artery. Invasive monitoring with a pulmonary artery catheter is recommended during support. Once venous access and arterial access are obtained with a flexible 0.038-inch guidewire and an 8-Fr dilator, anticoagulation is started with an antithrombin agent. The flexible wire is replaced with a stiff 0.038-inch guidewire, and both the vein and the artery are progressively dilated with 12- and 14-Fr dilators. Finally, 18-Fr cannulae are placed, with the inflow at the level of the right atrium and the outflow at the level of the aortic bifurcation. The cannulae are then clamped before being connected to the primed perfusion circuit. Priming of the circuit should be performed by a perfusionist while access is being obtained. After carefully de-airing the system, the cannulae are connected to the perfusion circuit; support is started at 2 L/min and then progressively advanced by 0.5-L/min increments as needed.[68]

After successful coronary intervention or hemodynamic support for CS, CPS is weaned quickly in those who can tolerate it, usually over 15 minutes, by gradually reducing the flow rate. Volume is infused to increase the LV filling pressure to at least 8 to 10 mm Hg or to prebypass levels, whichever is less. If necessary, inotropic agents may be used to facilitate the weaning of support. An intraaortic balloon or Impella device can also be used if weaning causes difficulties for the patient. The Bard

TABLE 36.3 Major Randomized Controlled Trials of Hemodynamic Support Devices

Study (Year)	Comparator Groups	Outcomes
BCIS-1[45,47] (2010)	IABP vs. no IABP in high-risk PCI	• 28-day MACCEs (primary end point) 15.2% vs. 16.0%, P = NS • NS difference 6-month mortality but significant by 1 year • Routine IABP reduced procedural complication rate
IABP-SHOCK II[49] (2012)	IABP vs. no IABP in cardiogenic shock complicating acute myocardial infarction	• 30-day all-cause mortality (primary end point) 39.7% vs. 41.3%, P = NS • NS difference in any secondary end points, including complications and length of stay
ISAR-SHOCK[53] (2008)	Impella 2.5 vs. IABP in cardiogenic shock caused by AMI	• Cardiac index after 30 minutes of support was significantly increased in patients with the Impella (Impella: ΔCI = 0.49 ± 0.46 L/min/m^2; IABP: ΔCI = 0.11 ± 0.31 L/min/m^2; P = 0.02). • 30-day mortality was 46% in both groups.
PROTECT II[46] (2012)	Impella 2.5 vs. IABP in high-risk PCI	• 30-day MAEs (primary end point) 35.1% vs. 40.1%, P = NS • 90-day per protocol definition MAE reduced with Impella • Impella provided statistically significant superiority in cardiac power output
IMPRESS in Severe Shock[112] (2017)	Impella 2.5 vs. IABP in AMI with CS	• 30-day mortality were similar (46% and 50%, P = 0.92) • 6-month mortality were also similar (50%) in both groups

AMI, Acute myocardial infarction; *CS,* cardiogenic shock; *IABP,* intraaortic balloon pumping; *MACCEs,* major adverse cardiovascular and cerebrovascular and events; *MAE,* major adverse event; *NS,* not significant; *PCI,* percutaneous coronary intervention.

percutaneous CPS system is a portable, battery-operated system that consists of a centrifugal pump (Bio-Medicus; Medtronic, Minneapolis, MN), a heat exchanger, and a membrane oxygenator. Venous inflow is achieved by active suction—not by gravity, as in the classic cardiopulmonary bypass system—which makes it essential that patients be well hydrated. To prevent air embolism, central venous access should be avoided while the pump is operating. Another portable CPS device, Cardiohelp (Maquet Cardiovascular, Rancho Dominguez, CA), is also available. Percutaneous CPS can only be performed for 6 hours. After that, platelet aggregation, hemolysis, and increased capillary permeability with plasma loss become major complications. However, longer durations of support out to several days are increasingly commonplace. Given the large sheath sizes, vascular complications are a major concern, often requiring antegrade perfusion via a second arterial cannulation in the affected limb. Venting of the LV will help to improve cardiac recover and can also avoid risks of stroke due to LV thrombus. Other methods for prolonged support, such as bilateral axillary arterial access, may further reduce vascular complications.

Clinical Trials

Early reports on small numbers of patients showed that using CPS for high-risk angioplasty was feasible, even though it had high rates of femoral access-site complications.[69-71] The national registry of elective supported angioplasty reported data on 801 patients who underwent elective angioplasty with CPS in 25 centers from 1988 to 1992. The suggested inclusion clinical criteria were (1) the presence of severe or unstable angina; (2) at least one likely dilatable coronary artery stenosis; and (3) LVEF less than 25% or a target vessel that supplies more than half of the viable myocardium or both.[72] Although the initial angioplasty success rate was high in this registry, the rates of device-related complications were also high. The strategy was thus changed to one of standby support for these high-risk interventions. Prophylactic support was implemented in 73% of the patients, and the last 27% registered had standby support. The overall primary success rate was 93%, and the success rate in the group that had standby support was 91%.[73] The rates of vascular complications (15% vs. 6.1%) and transfusions (31% vs. 14%) decreased with the change in strategy from prophylactic support to standby support. The mortality rate (6.3% vs. 6% in the prophylactic and standby groups, respectively) and the rate of emergent bypass surgery (2.5% vs. 3.2%) did not change, however, which reflects the high-risk profile of the patients in the registry. Only 16 of 217 patients (7.4%) in the standby strategy group required emergency initiation of bypass support. Of these 16 patients, 75% had successful angioplasty without any need for bypass surgery, which suggested that standby support reduced the need for emergency bypass surgery. The only group of patients who demonstrated a clear benefit to using prophylactic support was the group with an LVEF of 20% or less. In these patients, those treated with prophylactic placement of CPS before coronary intervention had a lower mortality compared with those who had CPS on standby (7% vs. 18%, $P < .05$). A separate analysis was done of the 42 patients in the registry with 60% or more LMCA stenosis who underwent balloon angioplasty, and the results were compared with those for high-risk patients who had another vessel dilated.[74] The hospital mortality was 14.3% in patients who had angioplasty of the LMCA (prior to the stent era), notably higher than the 4.6% hospital mortality in patients who did not have significant LMCA disease and had angioplasty of another vessel ($P < .001$).[74]

In the present era, additional support with CPS did not improve the outcome of percutaneous intervention in LMCA disease. As the insertion technique evolved from requiring surgical cutdown to a percutaneous approach, as described by Shawl and colleagues,[75] the experience with CPS continued to grow in the cath lab; this group reported one of the largest series of supported angioplasty from 1988 to 1991.[75-77] Among the first 51 patients, 94% had three-vessel disease, 70% had an LVEF of 35% or less, and the majority had been turned down for bypass surgery.[75] All the patients tolerated the coronary intervention, and the mean coronary stenosis improved from 89% to 21%. The hospital mortality was 6%, which compared well with the 6.9% mortality in patients undergoing CABG with an LVEF of 35% or less at that time.[78] The most frequent complication was bleeding that required transfusion, which occurred in 40% of the patients. Other complications included pseudoaneurysm (8%), hematoma (2%), and femoral nerve weakness (8%). With improvement in the cannula removal technique, the requirement for transfusion decreased in later patients to 4% and eliminated the occurrence of femoral nerve injury.[76] CPS showed promising short- and long-term results in patients at particularly high risk (mean LVEF ≤ 19.5% ± 3.5%, 54% with dilation of the single remaining patent artery, 17% with dilation of an unprotected LMCA).[77] Angiographic success was achieved in 98.7% of the arteries attempted in 105 patients. Despite the occurrence of asystole in five patients (4.8%) and of electromechanical dissociation in 40 (38.1%) with balloon inflation, no procedural deaths were reported, and all patients were weaned off CPS after the angioplasty. The hospital mortality was 4.7%. After a mean follow-up of 24 (± 13) months, 97% of patients were in Canadian Cardiovascular Society (CCS) functional class I or II, compared with only 3% before the intervention ($P < .001$).[77]

Because of the high rate of complications, attention was turned to using CPS on a standby basis. Two retrospective analyses showed that the incidence of hemodynamic collapse that required support during angioplasty was less than 1%.[71,79] Subsequently, the National Registry of Elective Cardiopulmonary Support compared the usefulness of prophylactic percutaneous CPS with standby percutaneous CPS in patients undergoing high-risk angioplasty.[80] Mortality rates were similar: 6.4% in the prophylactic group and 6.1% in the standby group. The rates of procedural success were also similar in the two groups. However, morbidity was significantly higher in the prophylactic CPS group: 42% of patients had femoral access-site complications that necessitated blood transfusions compared with only 11.7% of patients in the standby group. Of 180 patients in the standby group, only 13 (7.2%) suffered irreversible hemodynamic collapse, and emergency CPS was initiated in less than 5 minutes in 12 of these 13 patients. The patients who did benefit from prophylactic CPS were those with an EF of 20% or less, and mortality was lower with support initiated before angioplasty (4.8% vs. 18.8%, $P < .05$).[80]

A more recent European study evaluated the usefulness of CPS during the stent era.[81] The report included two groups of patients: group I comprised 68 patients undergoing elective high-risk coronary intervention, and group II consisted of 24 patients who presented with acute MI and CS. In the elective group, primary success was achieved in 66 patients (97%), with complete revascularization obtained in 44% of the group. Four patients (5.9%) developed femoral artery complications, and one patient (1.5%) died before discharge. After 28 (± 19) months of follow-up, MACEs occurred in 30% of patients and included 7 deaths (10.3%). Compared with the previous literature on angioplasty supported by CPS, this study demonstrated that CPS could be used effectively during coronary stenting and also showed an improvement in the rate of complications.

Two studies compared CPS and IABP for high-risk coronary interventions. One prospective trial randomized patients to either CPS or IABP support during PCI that was considered high risk because of the presence of unstable angina with poor LV function in a target vessel supplying more than half of the remaining viable myocardium.[82] Between June 1991 and November 1993, 40 patients were randomized. All patients had a history of a prior

MI, the majority had three-vessel disease, and the mean EF in both groups was lower than 25%. All patients were treated with angioplasty using balloon inflations lasting longer than 2 minutes. Patients in both groups tolerated balloon inflations lasting 2 to 3 minutes without hemodynamic decompensation. Primary success was achieved in 19 of 20 patients in both groups with similar angiographic results. No vascular or hemorrhagic complications were reported in the IABP group, whereas two patients assigned to CPS developed vascular complications that required surgical repair, and five other patients required blood transfusions.[82] One death occurred in each group, thought to be caused by acute vessel closure after discontinuation of support. The study authors concluded that both IABP and CPS were effective in supporting high-risk coronary interventions in the presrent era, but IABP had lower rates of complications.

Schreiber and colleagues[83] reported retrospective observational data to compare outcomes in a larger group of patients who had undergone high-risk PCI with hemodynamic support. Over a 4-year period, 149 patients who had high-risk PCI underwent prophylactic placement of either an IABP ($n = 91$) or CPS ($n = 58$). Patients who presented with acute MI, unstable angina, and stable angina were included if they were hemodynamically stable before the procedure. Patients were considered high risk if they had poor ventricular function, had a culprit vessel supplying the majority of the myocardium, or required multivessel PCI. Patients who received CPS were more likely to be male (91% vs. 73%, $P < .01$) and more likely to have a history of chronic angina (91% vs. 69%, $P = .003$), CHF (59% vs. 35%, $P = .008$), and a lower mean EF ($26\% \pm 13\%$ vs. $32\% \pm 14\%$, $P < .01$). Multivessel PCI was performed more often in the CPS group (40% vs. 20%, $P < .01$). Despite the higher severity of their disease, angioplasty was successful more often in the CPS group compared with the IABP group (99% vs. 87% of lesions, $P = .005$). MACEs—which included MI, stroke, need for CABG, and death—occurred at similar rates in both groups, although the rate of CABG trended higher in the IABP group without reaching statistical significance (1.7% vs. 6.5%, $P = .33$). Of note, the rate of death was high in both groups (12% in the CPS group, 8.7% in the IABP group, $P = .71$).[83] As in the study by Kaul and colleagues,[82] access-site complications and transfusions occurred more frequently in the CPS group. The higher angioplasty success rate in the CPS group is likely explained by the longer duration of balloon inflation tolerated by this group. This difference would likely not exist with the use of stents. More recent case series in the stent era have generally supported the feasibility of temporary cardiopulmonary support for high-risk PCI with high procedural success but at the continued cost of vascular complications.[84,85]

Accordingly, use of CPS for high-risk PCI has decreased with the advent of minimally invasive pVADs and is virtually nonexistent currently for this elective high-risk PCI indication. The studies that describe CPS in high-risk PCI are summarized in Table 36.4. Complications of prolonged use of CPS and ECMO include bleeding, infection, thrombocytopenia, and compromised perfusion to the lower extremity. The complexity of therapy and the requirements for a surgeon and a bedside perfusionist are the drawbacks to this therapy. Nonetheless, the high level of support may be the only option for some patients who experience full cardiopulmonary collapse that requires intervention, especially when both respiratory and circulatory support are required.

Percutaneous Left Ventricular Assist Devices
Left Atrial–Femoral Artery Bypass

The left atrial–femoral artery bypass strategy, first described in 1962 by Dennis,[86–88] was initially used in patients who could not be weaned from cardiopulmonary bypass after surgery. More recently, a dedicated system with a compact centrifugal pump, the TandemHeart pVAD, was developed to allow relatively rapid percutaneous institution of left atrial–femoral artery bypass (Fig. 36.1).[61] The pump cycles oxygenated blood from the left atrium (via a transseptally placed cannula) to the femoral artery without the need for an external oxygenator or a heat exchanger.

TABLE 36.4 Percutaneous Cardiopulmonary Support Observational Trials

First Author	Year	Procedure	n	Revasc. Success Rate (%)	Device-Related Complication Rate (%)	Transfusion Rate (%)	In-Hospital Mortality Rate(%)	Bypass Time (Minutes)
Vogel[119]	1988	PTCA	9	100	11	100	11.0	NR
Shawl[75]	1989	PTCA	511[a]	100	14	38	5.8	37
Shawl[76]	1990	PTCA	121[b]	NR	9.9	29.7	NR	37[c]
Teirstein[80]	1993	PTCA	389[d]	88.7	12.6	39	6.4	NR
Sivananthan[70]	1994	PTCA	13	83	83	100	7.7	92.8 ± 46
Kaul[82]	1995	PTCA	20	95	10	25	5	NR
Vogel[73]	1995	PTCA	801[e]	93	15[f]	31[f]	6.9	NR
Shawl[77]	1995	PTCA	107	98	4.7	1.9	4.7	46 ± 30
Schreiber[83]	1998	PTCA	58	99	50	60	12	60 ± 45
de Lezo[120]	2002	PTCA	68[g]	97	6	NR	1.5	NR
Vainer[84]	2007	Stent	15	93	13	53	27[h]	NR
Bagai[85]	2011	Stent	20	100	NR	NR	28.2%	NR

[a]Includes 20 patients with left ventricular ejection fraction of 25% of less, which are included in the 1996 report.
[b]A total of 121 patients were reported, 101 of which underwent elective coronary interventions.
[c]Time reported for the elective interventions.
[d]Number of patients with prophylactic percutaneous cardiopulmonary support (CPS) device placement.
[e]27% of patients were treated with a standby strategy.
[f]Complication and transfusion rates were reported for the group with percutaneous CPS devices placed prophylactically.
[g]A total of 92 patients were reported, 68 of whom had elective procedures.
[h]Death rate at 15 months and in-hospital mortality were not reported.
NR, Not reported; PTCA, percutaneous transluminal angioplasty; Revasc., revascularization.

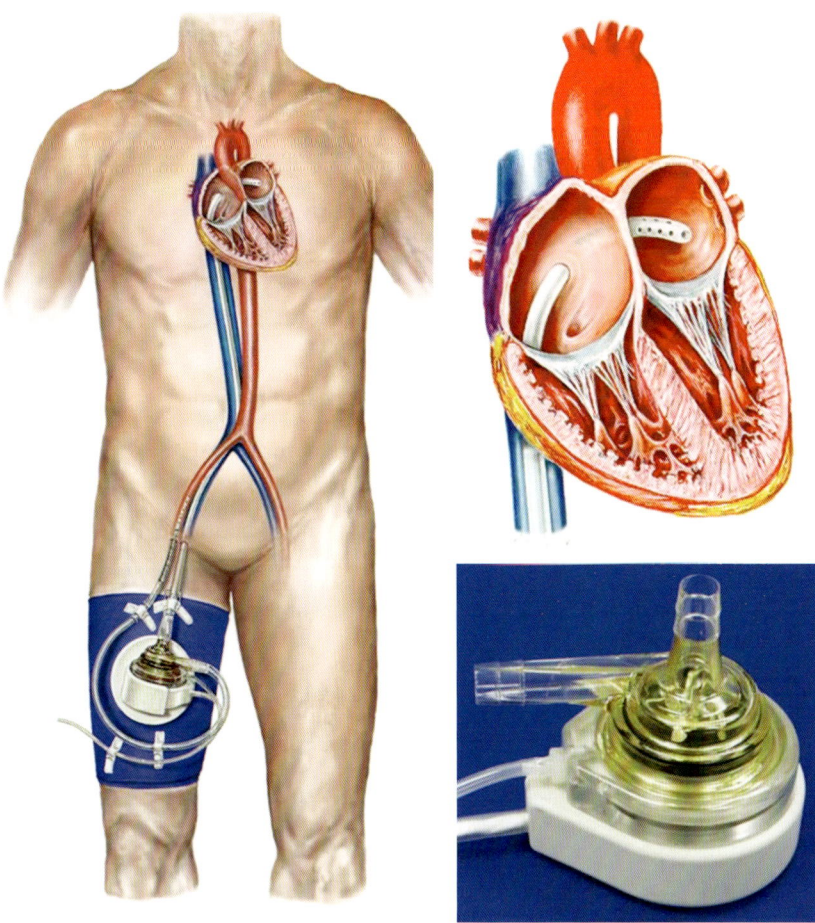

Fig. 36.1 The TandemHeart percutaneous left ventricular assist device. The inflow cannula to the centrifugal pump is inserted transseptally to the left atrium, and the outflow is inserted in the femoral artery.

The left atrial–femoral artery bypass system indirectly unloads the LV and decreases cardiac filling pressures, cardiac workload, and myocardial oxygen demand.[89,90] Similar to CPS, however, patients with CS as a result of severe LV dysfunction may paradoxically exhibit a rise in myocardial oxygen demand due to an increase in afterload. Such cases may require additional LV unloading maneuvers, such as IABP or Impella placement. Predominant right ventricular failure and left atrial thrombus are contraindications to the use of a transseptal left ventricular assist device (LVAD). In the setting of right ventricular failure, a concomitant right ventricular assist device (RVAD) is usually necessary to maintain left atrial volume. This may be achieved through use of a second device positioned from the right atrium to the pulmonary artery, or through a dedicated Impella right-sided device, discussed later. Although aortic regurgitation is not a contraindication, the experience with the use of TandemHeart in this condition is limited.[91] Like other devices, vascular complications may occur with the TandemHeart owing to the large arterial sheath diameter, and patients must be monitored for this complication.

Insertion Technique

After angiography of the distal aorta and iliac vessels to exclude significant arterial occlusive disease, access in the femoral vein is obtained. After a transseptal puncture is performed, the interatrial septum is dilated in two stages with 14- and 21-Fr dilators, and the 22-Fr inflow cannula is advanced to the left atrium under fluoroscopic and echocardiographic guidance.[90,92] The outflow 15- to 17-Fr cannula (chosen based on the caliber of arterial vessels and desired flow rate) is then inserted by using the Seldinger technique over a stiff guidewire, and it is advanced to the common iliac artery. The cannulae are de-aired and connected to the pump.

The TandemHeart pVAD is a continuous-flow centrifugal pump that operates at 7500 rpm and provides up to 5.0 L/min of blood flow. The pump contains a single moving part, an impeller suspended by a magnetic force on a thin lubricating film of fluid.[93] A continuous infusion of heparinized saline solution provides this hydrodynamic bearing for the pump, as well as local anticoagulation and cooling of the motor. Full systemic anticoagulation with heparin is required. The TandemHeart has FDA approval to provide extracorporeal circulatory support for up to 6 hours and a Conformité Européene (CE) mark for use up to 30 days.

Clinical Trials

A small prospective feasibility study evaluated the hemodynamic effects of the TandemHeart pVAD in short-term stabilization of patients with CS.[90] The device was safely implanted in 18 patients, with a mean duration of support of 4 (± 3) days. Hemodynamic indices, including pulmonary capillary wedge pressure (PCWP), pulmonary arterial pressure (PAP), cardiac output, and systemic blood pressure showed a significant improvement on TandemHeart pVAD support. During support, hemolysis was negligible, bleeding that required transfusion occurred in five patients, and two with PAD required surgical placement of an antegrade perfusion cannula to relieve limb ischemia.

To date, mostly case reports and small series on the experience with the left atrial–femoral artery bypass system remain to support high-risk coronary interventions[89,92–96] (see Case Study 1); two small randomized trials have been undertaken, but no trials have been completed and no ongoing large randomized trials are underway. In early series, the device was shown to be easily implanted by interventionalists experienced in transseptal puncture and to provide circulatory support to allow high-risk coronary interventions to be done successfully in a controlled fashion (Table 36.5). Three case series were recently published.[97–99] In one, between 2000 and 2006, 23 patients with a mean age of 59 years underwent high-risk PCI using the TandemHeart device. Implantation was successful in all patients, and PCI was successful in 21 patients (91.3%). Hemodynamic parameters improved, including PCWP and systemic arterial pressure. Five patients died with the device in place, primarily from preexisting CS. Mild to moderate access-site bleeding was reported in 27% of patients. In the second series, 37 patients received the device for high-risk PCI or CS. The mean age was 73 years, and 97% were in NYHA class III CHF or CS. Technical PCI success was reported in all patients, but 82% required blood transfusion after the procedure. Overall, however, 71% of patients in this extremely high-risk group survived to discharge. In the third study, from the Mayo Clinic, 54 patients were supported with the TandemHeart for high-risk PCI that included left main and multivessel stent placement in 64% of patients. Hemodynamics improved during support, including cardiac output and LV filling pressure; procedural success was high at 97%, and 6-month survival was 87%, but vascular complications occurred in 13%.[99]

Two small randomized trials have compared the TandemHeart with IABP in patients with CS.[100,101] Although benefit was seen in terms of hemodynamic parameters, a small meta-analysis that combined both studies did not suggest an effect on survival with use of the device.[102] Because of the transseptal puncture required, the TandemHeart pVAD may ultimately be best suited for elective initiation of hemodynamic support because insertion times tend to be longer compared with IABP and other pVAD devices (Impella). In addition, because it can provide up to 5.0 L/min of flow, the TandemHeart pVAD may be useful for high-risk PCI in the setting of CS, particularly when more potent Impella (CP or 5.0) or CPS devices are unavailable. Nonetheless, the current landscape has shown a decline in use of TandemHeart in favor of

CASE STUDY 1

An 80-year-old man with severe chronic obstructive pulmonary disease (COPD), chronic renal insufficiency, and carotid artery disease presented with unstable angina. Echocardiography revealed severe LV dysfunction (LVEF 10%), anterior wall akinesis, and moderate mitral regurgitation. Positron emission tomography (PET) showed lateral wall ischemia and high anterolateral viability. Cardiac catheterization revealed 95% distal LMCA disease involving the ostia of both the left anterior descending (LAD) and left circumflex (LCx) arteries (Fig. 36.2) and also revealed a 50% stenosis in the mid right coronary artery. The patient was thought to be at high risk for surgical revascularization; thus hemodynamically supported LMCA intervention with the TandemHeart pVAD was undertaken. After transseptal placement of a 21-Fr inflow cannula in the left atrium and placement of a 15-Fr outflow cannula in the right common iliac artery, left atrial–distal aorta bypass was achieved with a nonpulsatile flow rate of 3 L/min. Bifurcation stenting of the LAD and LCx arteries was performed with two sirolimus-eluting stents deployed simultaneously using the "kissing" technique (Figs. 36.3 and 36.4). The decrease in aortic pulse pressure was significant because of diminished stroke volume, but the mean perfusion pressure was maintained, and the patient remained hemodynamically stable without angina or arrhythmia (Fig. 36.5). The patient was discharged 2 days after the procedure and remained angina-free at 1-month follow-up.[103]

TABLE 36.5 Left Atrial–Femoral Artery Bypass Observational Trials

First Author	Year	n	Insertion Time (min)	Revasc. Success Rate (%)	Mean Support Duration	In-Hospital Mortality (n)	Other Complications
Glassman[96a]	1993	13	b	100	43 ± 17 minutes	0	• Transfusion in 1 of 13 patients • Small left-to-right shunts in 2 of 13 patients
Lemos[92]	2003	7[c]	31 to 69	92.3	55 ± 96 hours	1	• Bleeding in 4 of 7 patients • Hypothermia in 2 of 7 patients
Aragon[89]	2005	8	b	100	d	1	• Acute renal failure requiring dialysis in 1 of 8 patients
Kar[95]	2006	5	b	100	107 minutes[e]	1	• Blood transfusions in all patients • Groin hematomas in 2 of 5 patients
Al-Husami[121]	2008	6	36.5	100	b	1	• No vascular complications (all devices removed in the OR) • In 1 of 6, possible TIAs/seizure
Vranckx[97]	2008	23	35	91.3	31 ± 49.8 hours	5	• Bleeding in 27% • Hypothermia in 6 of 23 patients
Vranckx[122]	2009	9	27	100	93 minutes	0	• Vascular complications 44.4%
Thomas[98]	2010	37	b	100	b	11	• 82% transfusion rate
Alli[99]	2012	54	+	97	+	10[f]	• 13% major vascular complication rate

[a]The device used in this series was not the TandemHeart percutaneous ventricular assist device (pVAD).
[b]Not reported.
[c]Five patients were hemodynamically stable prior to insertion of the pVAD.
[d]Not reported, but all patients had the pVAD removed in the catheterization laboratory at the end of the coronary intervention. The mean procedure time was 169 ± 21 min.
[e]Excludes duration of support for one patient who required support for an additional 48 hours because of persistent poor left ventricular function.
[f]30-day mortality.
OR, Operating room; Revasc., revascularization; TIA, transient ischemic attack.

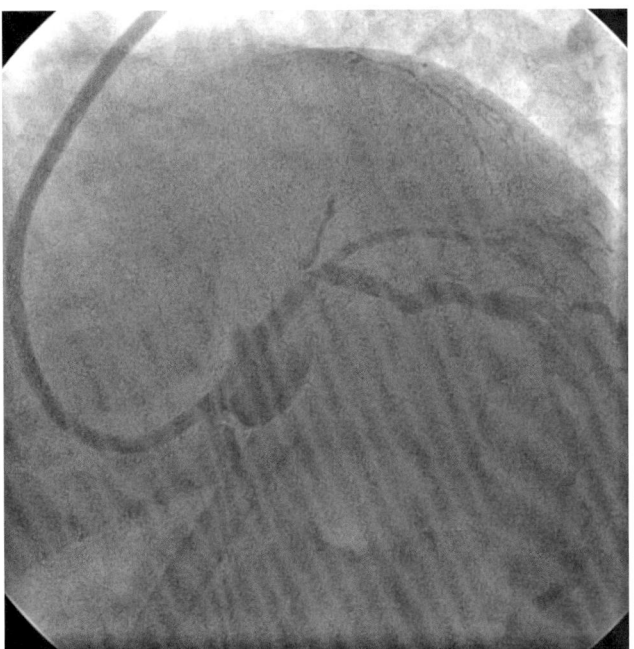

Fig. 36.2 Baseline angiography showing distal left main coronary artery stenosis and subtotal occlusion of the proximal left anterior descending artery.

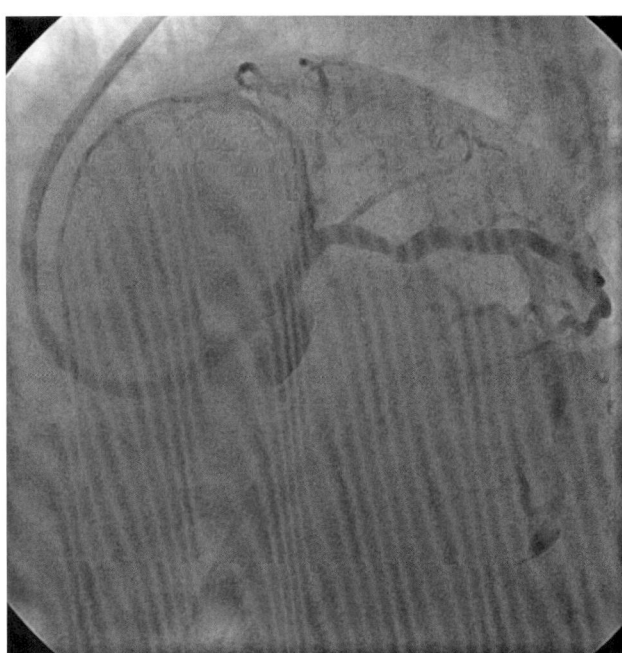

Fig. 36.4 Final angiography showing reconstruction of the distal left main coronary artery, proximal left anterior descending artery, and left circumflex coronary artery.

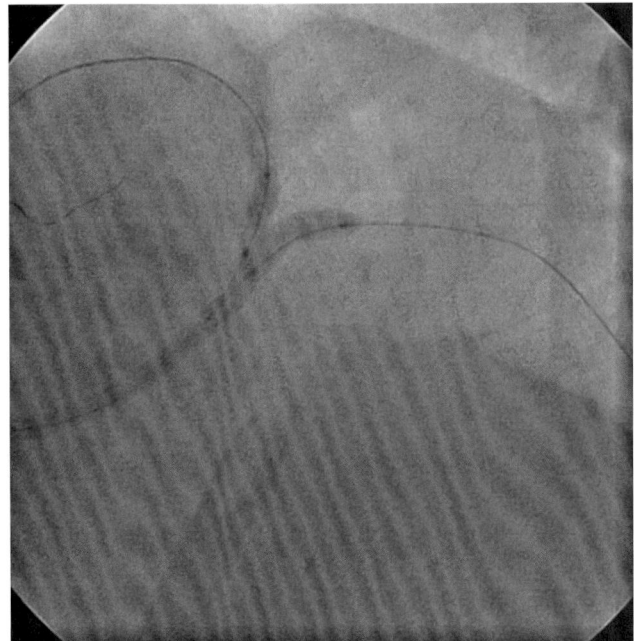

Fig. 36.3 Percutaneous coronary intervention using two sirolimus-eluting stents in a "kissing" technique.

Impella for high risk elective PCI and either Impella or CPO/ECMO for CS, depending on magnitude of support required.

TRANSVALVULAR LEFT VENTRICULAR ASSIST DEVICES

In 1988 Wampler and colleagues[104] described a new catheter-mounted transvalvular LVAD, which was initially placed surgically via the femoral artery. Development of a smaller (13-/14-Fr) system allowed percutaneous insertion of the device. Two investigational devices, the Impella (Abiomed Inc.) and the Hemopump (Medtronic), have been tested clinically, although only the Impella is currently available for clinical use. The Impella 2.5 is a microaxial rotary blood pump that unloads the LV by expelling blood from the LV to the aorta (Fig. 36.6). The device can deliver an output of up to 2.5 L/min. The Impella device has been shown to directly unload the LV by decreasing the end-diastolic pressure, decreasing the end-diastolic and end-systolic volumes, and increasing the combined (device plus native heart) cardiac output, simultaneously improving coronary blood flow.[61,105,106] Notably, because the device withdraws blood from the LV during all phases of the cardiac cycle, including during isovolumic contraction and relaxation, theoretic benefits extend beyond comparable flow rates of other, indirect unloading devices (i.e., the TandemHeart and IABP). The LV unloading with Impella reduces end-diastolic wall stress, improves diastolic compliance, increases aortic and intracoronary pressure and coronary flow velocity reserve, and stimulates a decrease in coronary microvascular resistance.[107,108] Larger Impella CP devices (delivering 3.5 to 4.0 L/min) and 5.0 devices with greater hemodynamic benefits are also available, but the 5.0 device typically requires surgical cutdown for placement. As with the other devices, vascular complications increase with the catheter size and duration of support.

Insertion Techniques

Before the procedure, an echocardiogram should be performed to exclude the presence of an LV thrombus or critical aortic stenosis. Angiography of the distal aorta and iliac vessels should also be performed before insertion of the femoral sheath. The Impella 2.5 percutaneous device has a maximal outer diameter of 12 Fr, whereas the Impella CP has a maximal outer diameter of 13 Fr. Often the vascular access site is "preclosed" with a suture-based closure device for high-risk PCI indication because

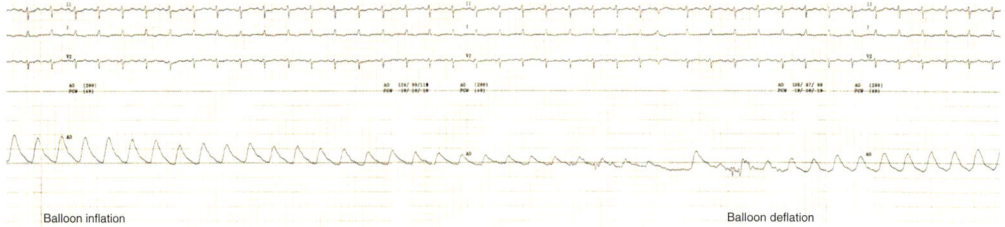

Fig. 36.5 Aortic pressure tracing during balloon inflation shows a significant decrease in pulse pressure caused by diminished stroke volume with preserved mean perfusion pressure via the TandemHeart bypass circuit.

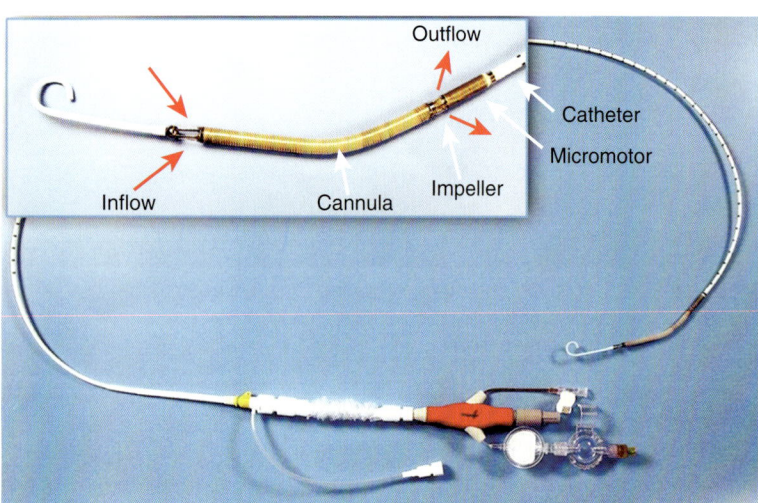

Fig. 36.6 Impella Recover LP 2.5 device. (Adapted from Valgimigli M, Steendijk P, Sianos G, et al. Left ventricular unloading and concomitant total cardiac output increase by the use of percutaneous Impella Recover LP 2.5 assist device during high-risk coronary intervention. *Catheter Cardiovasc Interv.* 2005;65[2]:263–267.)

the device is usually weaned and explanted postprocedure. For CS, where the device may stay in place longer, manual compression is used for eventual catheter removal. After inserting an appropriately sized (usually 14 Fr) sheath in the femoral artery, an exchange length (300 cm) 0.014-inch guidewire is delivered to the LV with an end-hole angiographic catheter (Judkins Right 4 [JR4], Multipurpose A [MPA], etc.). The device is then advanced over the wire and is positioned across the aortic valve under fluoroscopic guidance. The pigtail conformation helps to maintain a stable positioning within the LV and prevents adherence to the endocardium. Recently, a wireless insertion technique has also been described.

Proper placement is critical to ensure unimpeded outflow of blood and catheter stability, and recent device modifications have improved on both of these aspects. The proximal part of the catheter connects to a portable mobile console that provides power and allows control of the pump.[106] The Impella 2.5 device is mounted on a 9-Fr pigtail catheter (see Fig. 36.6), which sits in the LV cavity. The device provides flows of up to 2.5 L/min at its maximal rotational speed of 50,000 rpm and can be safely left in place for up to 5 days.[105] The Impella CP can provide up to 4.0 L/min of flow, whereas the 5.0 provides up to 5 L/min of flow with similar implantation durations. A heparinized 20% dextrose solution continuously lubricates the pump. For prolonged support, peripheral heparin infusion to an activated clotting time (ACT) of 160 to 180 seconds is required.

For high-risk PCI, the Impella 2.5 and CP are FDA approved for 6 hours, whereas in CS, Impella 2.5, and CP have FDA approval for short-term use of 4 days, and 6 days for Impella 5.0. Contraindications to the use of Impella include severe aortic stenosis, mechanical aortic valve, presence of LV thrombus, and greater than moderate aortic regurgitation.

Clinical Trials

Initial case studies evaluating the Impella 2.5 device in high-risk PCI suggested safety, feasibility, and minimal complications, with one report suggesting no significant benefit.[109] This was followed by A Prospective Feasibility Trial Investigating the Use of the Impella 2.5 System in Patients Undergoing High-Risk Percutaneous Coronary Intervention (PROTECT I),[20] the primary safety and feasibility study of 20 patients in the United States. Enrolling patients with LMCA or sole remaining conduit and severe LV dysfunction, the device was technically successful in all cases with a low complication rate. Several smaller registries have reported on use of the Impella 2.5 device in high-risk PCI, but the largest published series are the multicenter Europella Registry and the USpella Registry.[42,51,110,111] Case Study 2 represents an example of high-risk PCI using Impella 2.5 support.

The baseline characteristics of the 144 patients in the Euro-Pella Registry suggested that these patients were indeed at high risk: 70% had an LVEF less than 30%, 36% had recent MI, 42% had prior surgical revascularization, 76% had previous MI, 20% had prior stroke, 26% had chronic lung disease, and 62% had diabetes. In addition, 55% had more than three target lesions, 52.8% had LMCA disease, 17.4% had intervention on a last remaining patent vessel, and 43.1% had refused CABG. The logistic EuroSCORE was 15 (± 12.2), which further indicated the high-risk nature of this population. Despite this, overall mortality was 5.5% at 30 days. Another 5.5% required blood transfusion, and 0.7% required surgery for bleeding. No MI or need for emergent CABG was noted. Stroke occurred in 0.7% and vascular complications occurred in 4%.[42]

More recently, the results of the multicenter USPella Registry described outcomes in 251 patients using the Impella 2.5 device for a variety of real-world indications, including 178 for high-risk PCI.[111] Of these, 63% were in NYHA class III or IV heart failure, and 62% had an LVEF less than 30% before intervention. In addition, 56% of patients did not qualify for CABG because of excessive comorbidities. Results showed a 90% success rate and an 8% rate of 30-day MACEs. Survival was 96% at 30 days, 91% at 6 months, and 88% at 1 year. In addition, only 30% of patients remained in NYHA class III or IV heart failure, consistent with an absolute increase in mean EF from 31% to 37%. This latter improvement resulted in a 29% reduction in the anticipated need for implantable cardioverter defibrillators (ICDs) because the percentage of patients with an EF less than 30% was reduced from 62% to 44%.[36,111] Thus in real-world observational practice, Impella use appeared safe, feasible, and efficacious in improving signs and symptoms of heart failure and ventricular dysfunction. In the subset of patients who presented with AMI and CS, Impella also appeared to be safe and feasible; in addition, preprocedure placement of the Impella 2.5 appeared to improve survival compared with postprocedure placement, suggesting that early unloading may impact myocardial salvage and resultant long-term outcomes.[36]

Although Impella seems to have better hemodynamic properties as compared with IABP, the effect on long-term hard outcomes is undetermined. There remains a paucity of large RCTs in this arena. The ISAR-SHOCK (Efficacy Study of LV Assist Device to Treat Patients With Cardiogenic Shock) trial was a small study ($n = 25$) that demonstrated significant improvement in cardiac index 30 minutes after Impella was placed as compared with IABP.[53] However, no mortality benefit was shown between the two devices. A prospective, randomized trial (Percutaneous Mechanical Circulatory Support Versus Intra-Aortic Balloon Pump in Cardiogenic Shock After Acute Myocardial Infarction [IMPRESS] trial) also failed to show any mortality benefit at 30 days between the Impella and IABP group.[112] Of note, this study also had a small sample size consisting of 48 patients.

The multicenter PROTECT II superiority trial randomized patients with similar inclusion criteria to PROTECT I to prophylactic IABP or Impella 2.5 support for elective high-risk PCI.[46] To date, PROTECT II is the largest RCT of high-risk PCI ever performed. Although the trial was terminated early for futility, 452 patients were ultimately randomized to IABP or Impella 2.5 for elective high-risk PCI. In general, enrolling a sicker patient population than the BCIS-1 trial, the primary end point, a composite of 11 end points at 30 days by intention-to-treat analysis, was no different between groups. However, the primary end point trended favoring Impella in the per-protocol population of patients who received the device per the inclusion and exclusion criteria (34.3% Impella vs. 42.2% IABP, $P = .092$). By 90 days, a prespecified secondary end point, the differences were magnified in the intention-to-treat population (40.6% Impella vs. 49.3% IABP, $P = .066$) and reached statistical significance in the per-protocol population (40.0% Impella vs. 51.0% IABP, $P = .023$).[46] Tables 36.3 and 36.6 provide a summary of these trials. These data, together with observational data, prompted FDA approval in high-risk PCI.

The other transvalvular assist device, the Hemopump system, also expels blood from the LV to the aorta by using a rotating turbine that imparts both rotational and longitudinal velocities to the blood. This device has been shown to increase cardiac output and reduce mean PAP in clinical trials.[113–115] However, the Hemopump was not shown to significantly affect coronary blood flow velocities before or after angioplasty.[114] Small feasibility

CASE STUDY 2

A 71–year-old man presented with accelerating angina over 1 month. A stress echo was performed but was terminated at 3 minutes because of chest pain and diffuse ST-segment depressions. EF was 30%. The patient's metoprolol was increased, and he was scheduled for cardiac catheterization. Patient history included hypertension, distant MI (treated medically), and significant vascular disease that included emergent repair of both an ascending aortic dissection and an abdominal aortic aneurysm, 10 and 3 years prior, respectively. The patient's coronary anatomy was not assessed at these times because of the emergent nature of his surgeries. At cardiac catheterization, he was found to have distal left main bifurcation disease and moderate to severe systolic dysfunction, with an estimated EF of 25% (Video 36.1). Because of his prior operations, severe vascular disease, and COPD, he was felt to be a poor candidate for surgical revascularization. IABP placement was also relatively contraindicated because of the risk of repeated balloon-induced vascular trauma. Impella 2.5 supported high-risk PCI and was therefore considered. A right heart catheterization was performed to assess and maintain filling pressures, and the Impella device was inserted and placed across the aortic valve (Video 36.2). The LAD and LCx arteries were wired, and simultaneous kissing stents were placed in the left main and daughter vessels (Video 36.3). During inflation, the patient remained hemodynamically stable with minimal decrease in systolic pressure (and pulse pressure) but with maintenance of diastolic pressure. After postdilation, the final angiographic result is seen in Video 36.4. Hemodynamics were reassessed, and the patient was weaned off the device over 15 minutes. The device was then removed. Preclose technique sutures were subsequently tied down with achievement of hemostasis. At 6 months, the EF improved to 35%, and the patient did not require implantable defibrillator placement. His angina was relieved after the procedure, and he was maintained on ischemic cardiomyopathy medications.[103]

TABLE 36.6 Transvalvular Left Ventricular Assist Device Observational Trials

First Author	Year	n	Revasc. Success Rate	MACEs	Hemolysis	Support Duration (hour)
Dens[a,110]	2006	23	100%	17%	22%	2.1 ± 1.6
Valgimigli[109]	2006	10	100%	30%[b]	60%	2.4 ± 1.5
Henriques[51]	2006	19	100%	5%	[d]	2.0[c]
Burzotta[118]	2008	10	100%	0%	[d]	[d]
Dixon[20]	2009	20	100%	20%	10%	1.7 ± 0.6
Sjauw[42]	2009	144	100%	12.5%	<1%	1.45 ± 0.8
Maini[111]	2010	175	99%	8%	0%	1.0

[a]Revascularization (Revasc.) strategy included percutaneous coronary intervention (PCI) and off-pump coronary artery bypass.
[b]Four of 10 patients also received a transfusion.
[c]Maximum support time reported.
[d]reported.
MACE, Major adverse cardiac events.

trials have shown the Hemopump to be safe in supporting high-risk interventions.[113-115] However, to date, the Hemopump is not available clinically. A third device, the HeartMate PHP (St. Jude Medical) is not currently approved within the United States. This device is 14 Fr but can expand to 24 Fr, potentially offering higher flow rates. Clinical data and experience with this device are limited.

Guidelines on Use of Hemodynamic Support Devices in High-Risk Percutaneous Coronary Intervention, Including Cardiogenic Shock

With the increasing dataset in recent years regarding percutaneous support devices, both observational and randomized, national guidelines have modified their recommendations in both high-risk PCI and CS subsets.[9] Accordingly, use of an appropriate percutaneous hemodynamic support device is currently categorized as "may be reasonable" as an adjunct to high-risk PCI in carefully selected patients (class IIb recommendation).[9] Ideal patients include predominantly those with the inclusion criteria specified within the BCIS-1 and PROTECT II trials, including left main and last patent conduit or multivessel disease in the setting of markedly reduced EF. Therefore the IABP and Impella appear particularly suited for this indication, with Impella favored due to the specific FDA indication. A class IIa (for IABP) and class IIb (for alternative circulatory support device) recommendation is given to the use of cardiac support devices for patients with STEMI and persistent CS despite successful revascularization.[116] Potent devices that include the TandemHeart, Impella CP or 5.0, or a CPS seem particularly suited for this indication; choice varies based on local experience, extent of support required, and device-specific complication rates. Impella has several advantages, both practical and hemodynamic, as well as an FDA indication for CS. Currently, guidelines continue to support device placement after successful revascularization for patients who present with CS in the setting of AMI; whether earlier unloading prior to PCI will prove beneficial remains to be seen and is the subject of ongoing investigation. For those patients in refractory CS, especially with biventricular failure and/or impaired oxygenation, CPS/ECMO is the primary support strategy, whereas biventricular support can be accomplished by separate percutaneous LVAD and RVAD support.

CONCLUSIONS

With the development of stents and technical improvements in coronary wires, guiding catheters, and balloons, the rates of abrupt closure and hemodynamic collapse during percutaneous interventions have decreased. The improved technology has also allowed for higher-risk procedures, which would have been referred for bypass surgery in the early days of coronary angioplasty. Moreover, recent clinical trials have suggested that PCI may be a reasonable option in some patients with LMCA or multivessel coronary disease, many of whom are very old or have concomitant ventricular dysfunction, and recent PCI guidelines currently allow LMCA stenting in appropriate candidates.[9] Furthermore, patients with AMI and CS remain an extremely high-risk PCI population. As a result, the field of high-risk PCI has evolved to include the use of cardiac assist devices to minimize periprocedural risk and improve short-term and long-term ventricular function and survival in both these clinical scenarios.

Although formal guidelines on the use of circulatory support devices during high-risk PCI are just now becoming available, much decision making continues to be left to the clinician. The

TABLE 36.7 Comparison of Circulatory Support Modalities

	Insertion Technique	Major Complications	Effect on Circulation	Length of Support	Advantages	Limitations	Contraindications
IABP	Percutaneous or surgical	• Limb ischemia • Stroke	Augments CO by up to 0.5 L/min	Days to weeks	• More prolonged support duration • Indirectly unloads the LV	• Requires stable rhythm • Lowest level of hemodynamic support	• Moderate to severe AI • Aortic disease • Uncontrolled sepsis • Coagulopathy • PAD
CPS	Percutaneous or surgical	• Bleeding, hemolysis • Stroke • Embolus	Provides complete circulatory support	Up to 6 hours	• Independent of rhythm • Allows controlled transfer to the OR • Full support	• Limited duration of support • Requires perfusionist • Does not unload the LV	• Moderate to severe AI • PAD • Coagulopathy
LA-FA pVAD	Percutaneous or surgical	• Pericardial tamponade • Aortic puncture • Limb ischemia	Augments CO by up to 5.0 L/min (TandemHeart)	Up to 14 days	• Prolonged support duration • Partial LV support • Indirectly unloads the LV	• Large arterial cannulae • Requires transseptal puncture • LV unloading may be limited in marked LV dysfunction	• PAD • RV failure • LA thrombus • Profound coagulopathies and bleeding diathesis
LV-AO pVAD	Percutaneous or surgical	Limb ischemia	Augments CO by up to 2.5 L/min (2.5 device), 3.5 to 4.0 L/min (CP device) or 5.0 L/min (5.0 device)	Up to 14 days	• Prolonged support duration • Partial LV support • Markedly unloads the LV • Ease of use	Relatively large arterial cannula	• LV thrombus • VSD • Aortic stenosis • Mechanical Aortic valve • RV failure • Severe PAD

AI, Aortic insufficiency; *CO*, cardiac output; *CP*, cardiac power; *CPS*, cardiopulmonary support; *IABP*, intraaortic balloon pump; *LA*, left atrium; *LA-FA*, left atrium to femoral artery; *LV*, left ventricle; *LV-AO*, left ventricle–aorta; *OR*, operating room; *PAD*, peripheral arterial disease; *pVAD*, percutaneous ventricular assist device; *RV*, right ventricle; *VSD*, ventricular septal defect.

decision to implement these devices, for example, is often at the discretion of the individual interventionalist and is based on the cumulative experience of completed and ongoing clinical trials. A thorough understanding of the high-risk clinical characteristics discussed in this chapter and the procedural and angiographic factors that portend a high risk of decompensation and mortality is the first step in the proper use of support devices. The choice of these devices should be based on the level of support provided by each device compared with the level of support necessary for the given clinical situation, the level of complexity of device insertion and maintenance of support, specific device-related risks, benefits and contraindications, local experience, and a working knowledge of the increasing evidence that supports their clinical use (Table 36.7). A multisociety consensus statement—2015 SCAI/ACC/HFSA/STS Clinical Expert Consensus Statement on the Use of Percutaneous Mechanical Circulatory Support Devices in Cardiovascular Care[117]—on the use of these devices in cardiovascular practice has been published and provides more in-depth information on the different clinical settings that may benefit from mechanical circulatory support and the guidance on device choice in different settings. It is expected that these recommendations and formal guidelines will evolve over time, based on incremental data and experience and the availability of new devices.

KEY REFERENCES

9. Levine GN, Bates ER, Blankenship JC, et al. 2011 ACCF/AHA/SCAI Guidelines for Percutaneous Coronary Intervention: a report of the American College of Cardiology Foundation/American Heart Association Task Force on Practice Guidelines and the Society for Cardiovascular Angiography and Interventions. *J Am Coll Cardiol.* 2011;58(24):e44–e122.
45. Perera D, Stables R, Thomas M, et al. Elective intra-aortic balloon counterpulsation during high risk percutaneous coronary intervention: a randomized controlled trial. *JAMA.* 2010;304(8):867–874.
46. O'Neill WW, Kleiman NS, Moses J, et al. A prospective randomized clinical trial of hemodynamic support with Impella 2.5 versus intra-aortic balloon pump in patients undergoing high-risk percutaneous coronary intervention: the PROTECT II study. *Circulation.* 2012;126(4):1717–1727.
47. Perera D, Stables R, Clayton T, et al. Long-term mortality data from the balloon pump-assisted coronary intervention study (BCIS-1): a randomized, controlled trial of elective balloon counterpulsation during high-risk percutaneous coronary intervention. *Circulation.* 2013;127(2):207–212.
49. Thiele H, Zeymer U, Neumann FJ, et al. Intraaortic balloon support for myocardial infarction with cardiogenic shock. *N Engl J Med.* 2012;367(14):1287–1296.
50. Roffi M, Patrono C, Collet JP, et al. 2015 ESC guidelines for the management of acute coronary syndromes in patients presenting without persistent ST-segment elevation: task force for the management of acute coronary syndromes in patients presenting without persistent ST-segment elevation of the European Society of Cardiology (ESC). *Eur Heart J.* 2016;37:267–315.
53. Seyfarth M, Sibbing D, Bauer I, et al. A randomized clinical trial to evaluate the safety and efficacy of a percutaneous left ventricular assist device versus intra-aortic balloon pumping for treatment of cardiogenic shock caused by myocardial infarction. *J Am Coll Cardiol.* 2008;52(19):1584–1588.
112. Ouweneel DM, Eriksen E, Sjauw KD, et al. Percutaneous mechanical circulatory support versus intra-aortic balloon pump in cardiogenic shock after acute myocardial infarction. *J Am Coll Cardiol.* 2017;69(3):278–287.
116. O'Gara PT, Kushner FG, Ascheim DD, et al. 2013 ACCF/AHA guideline for the management of ST-elevation myocardial infarction: a report of the American College of Cardiology Foundation/American Heart Association task force on practice guidelines. *J Am Coll Cardiol.* 2013;61(4):e78–e140.
117. Rihal CS, Naidu SS, Givertz MM, et al. 2015 SCAI/ACC/HFSA/STS clinical expert consensus statement on the use of percutaneous mechanical circulatory support devices in cardiovascular care (Endorsed by the American Heart Association, the Cardiological Society of India, and Sociedad Latino Americana de Cardiologia Intervencion; Affirmation of Value by the Canadian Association of Interventional Cardiology-Association Canadienne de Cardiologie D'intervention). *J Am Coll Cardiol.* 2015;65(19):e7–e26.

 Additional references available online at expertconsult.com.

中文导读

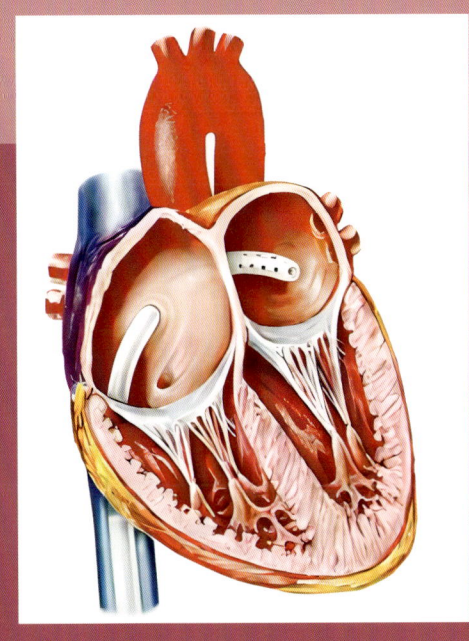

第37章
区域性急性缺血性心脏病救治中心

　　直接经皮冠状动脉介入治疗能快速恢复冠状动脉血流，减少心肌坏死范围，并降低ST段抬高型心肌梗死患者的死亡率，已成为ST段抬高型心肌梗死的首选血运重建方式。然而，由于医疗资源、地理环境等因素存在明显的地区差异，针对急性冠状动脉综合征患者，特别是心源性休克和院外心搏骤停患者，如何因地制宜开展高效的医疗救治就变得极为复杂。因此，美国就提出了发展急性冠状动脉综合征、心源性休克和院外心搏骤停的区域性救治中心理念。

　　本章节从区域性救治体系的相关组成、网络化合作机制到为了持续改进救治质量的质控机制，全面地介绍了美国关于急性冠状动脉综合征和心源性休克的区域性救治中心和区域性救治体系。"他山之石可以攻玉"，鉴于我国在医疗资源上的地区差异可能较美国更为严重，因此美国"区域性救治体系"的理念值得我们加以借鉴，建立一个符合我国国情的高效救治体系必不可少。

李长江　彭红玉

章节要点

- 目前针对ST段抬高型心肌梗死患者处置的临床实践指南均推荐，"所有社区都应建立和保持一个ST段抬高型心肌梗死处置的区域性体系，涵盖急救医疗服务和医院医疗行为的评估和持续质量改进"（Ⅰ类推荐，证据等级B）。

- 在无法提供高级心血管治疗的社区和郊区医院与可提供这些治疗的医院之间建立"有意义的网络化联系"，这是急性冠状动脉综合征患者接受"区域性"救治的含义。其中"网络化"的定义包括从成为同一医院系统的附属机构到共享通用患者诊疗方案，以及跟踪、报告和审核诊疗遵循临床实践指南的依从性、核心措施和临床结局。

- 对于医师和医院/设施而言，心血管手术（冠状动脉搭桥手术、冠状动脉成形术和支架置入术）的每年数量与最佳临床结果[包括急性冠状动脉综合征和（或）心源性休克患者的生存率]之间存在直接关系。对于那些年手术量高的医师和医院，手术的临床结果更好。

- 急性ST段抬高型心肌梗死的院前阶段至关重要。首次医疗接触时急救医疗服务在现场提供12导联心电图，而现场心电图的表现和传输已被证明可显著减少ST段抬高型心肌梗死治疗开始的时间延迟并降低死亡率。为了进一步减少治疗的时间延迟，须持续评估策略包括通过急救医疗服务院前启动导管室、绕过急诊科将ST段抬高型心肌梗死患者直接转运至导管室。

- ST段抬高型心肌梗死救治系统应由多个必需环节组成，其中包括患者治疗重点、提高手术效率、适当的系统激励机制（绩效薪酬）、特定的结果和过程指标，以及持续质量改进的质控机制。

- 由于急救医疗服务和医院资源、地理环境、人口密度及运输距离存在明显的地区差异，在美国没有一种单一"体系模式"在救治急性冠状动脉综合征和心源性休克方面具有可行性。而"区域救治系统示范计划"通过协作式救治，近来已被证实可改善患者临床结局，其具体目标包括：①选择性地在美国大都市地区加快实施ST段抬高型心肌梗死救治系统；②推动实施更有效的ST段抬高型心肌梗死救治；③改善临床结果。该计划近来已被证实通过合作式的救治可改善临床结局。也有类似项目正在进行以进一步加强心源性休克的合作救治。

- 完全冠状动脉血运重建可以改善急性冠状动脉综合征患者的短期和长期预后。鉴于冠状动脉疾病的复杂性日益增加，救助区域化使得医院开展复杂冠状动脉治疗的机会增加，这也让存在复杂冠状动脉病变的患者能更多地得到完全性血运重建。

37 Regional Centers of Excellence for the Care of Patients With Acute Ischemic Heart Disease

Robert F. Riley, Timothy D. Henry, Dean J. Kereiakes

KEY POINTS

- Current clinical practice guidelines for the care of patients who present with ST-segment elevation myocardial infarction (STEMI) provide a class I recommendation that "all communities should create and maintain a regional system of STEMI care that includes assessment and continuous quality improvement of emergency medical services (EMS) and hospital-based activities" (class I, level of evidence B).

- "Regional" care for patients with acute coronary syndromes implies "meaningful networking associations" between community and rural hospitals that do not provide tertiary cardiovascular services and a tertiary cardiovascular service provider. The definition of *networking* ranges from being a merged affiliate (same hospital system) to sharing common patient care protocols, as well as tracking, reporting, and auditing clinical practice guideline compliance, core measures, and clinical outcomes.

- For both physician operators and hospitals/facilities, a direct relationship exists between annual volume of cardiovascular procedures—coronary bypass surgery, coronary angioplasty, and stenting—and optimal clinical outcomes, including survival for both patients presenting with acute coronary syndrome (ACS) and/or cardiogenic shock. Those doctors and hospitals performing the highest annual volumes of procedures have the best outcomes.

- The prehospital phase of acute STEMI is critically important. The performance and transmission of a 12-lead electrocardiogram by EMS providers in the field at the point of first medical contact has been demonstrated to significantly reduce time delays to initiation of STEMI treatment and to reduce mortality. Strategies continue to be evaluated to further reduce time delay to treatment, and these include prehospital catheterization laboratory (cath lab) activation by EMS and emergency department bypass with direct transport of STEMI patients to the catheterization laboratory.

- A system for STEMI care should comprise multiple integral components that include a patient care focus, enhanced operational efficiency, appropriate system incentives (pay for performance/value), specific outcome and process measures, and mechanisms for quality review with continuous quality improvement.

- Because of marked regional variation in EMS and hospital resources, geography, population density, and transport distances, no single "system model" for ACS and cardiogenic shock care is likely to be either practical or achievable in the United States. With specific goals to (1) accelerate the implementation of STEMI care systems in selected U.S. metropolitan areas, (2) facilitate more effective delivery of STEMI care, and (3) improve clinical outcomes, the regional systems of care demonstration project—Mission: Lifeline STEMI Accelerator—has recently shown an improvement in outcomes through coordination of care. Similar projects are underway to further coordinate care for cardiogenic shock.

- Complete coronary revascularization has shown to improve both short- and long-term outcomes in patients with ACS. Given the increasing complexity of coronary artery disease, regionalization will also enable more complete revascularization in this patient group with increased access to complex coronary therapeutics.

INTODUCTION

The rapid restoration of normal coronary blood flow via pharmacologic and/or mechanical recanalization of an occluded coronary artery limits the extent of myocardial necrosis and reduces mortality of patients who present with ST-elevation myocardial infarction (STEMI).[1] Furthermore, primary percutaneous coronary intervention (PPCI) has demonstrated more frequent, complete, and durable coronary reperfusion in both randomized controlled trials (RCTs) and observational studies when compared to thrombolysis with medical therapy alone and is the preferred revascularization modality for treating STEMI by current guidelines if PPCI can be provided in a prompt, expert manner. In light of this, current American College of Cardiology Foundation (ACCF)/American Heart Association (AHA) guidelines recommend emergency medical services (EMS) transport directly to a percutaneous coronary intervention (PCI)-capable hospital for PPCI as the recommended strategy for STEMI patients, with an ideal first medical contact to PCI device-time system goal of 90 minutes or less (class I, level of evidence B).[1] Mounting data also supports the idea of complete coronary revascularization in patients with acute coronary syndromes (ACS).[2–6] However, a concerted, integrated approach to caring for patients with ACS, particularly those in cardiogenic shock and out-of-hospital cardiac arrest (OHCA), has been complicated by the diversity and extent of resources required for comprehensive treatment and by the various settings (urban, suburban, rural) in which care is delivered. Data from national registries have demonstrated a failure to achieve recommended system goals, particularly among STEMI patients who presented to hospitals without PCI capability and required interhospital transfer for PPCI.[7] The creation of specialized care centers for other medical emergencies, such as trauma and acute stroke, has been shown to improve clinical outcomes; therefore the concept of developing regional centers of excellence for the care of ACS (including STEMI), cardiogenic shock, and OHCA has become the focus of a collaborative initiative of the AHA and the ACCF as well as individual states.[7–11]

The term *regional* implies meaningful networking associations between all prehospital and hospital-based constituents that enable rapid recognition and timely care delivery in an integrated fashion.[7,12] These initiatives have been in part prompted by studies that demonstrate shortfalls in the achievement of quality-ensured, guideline-compliant care in addition to disparities in treatment on the basis of age, sex, race, geographic location, or time of STEMI presentation.[7] Similarly, hospitals with a higher proportion of transfer-in non–ST-elevation myocardial infarction (NSTEMI) patients tend to provide higher overall quality of care with lower overall in-hospital mortality, though the proportion of NSTEMI patients transferred into revascularization-capable hospitals varies significantly as shown in the CRUSADE (Can Rapid Risk Stratification of Unstable Angina Patients Suppress Adverse Outcomes With Early Implementation of the ACC/AHA Guidelines) National Quality Improvement Initiative.[13]

Through focus on system process components, multiple national initiatives such as Get With The Guidelines (GWTG), the Guidelines Applied to Practice (GAP) project, the National Registry of Myocardial Infarction (NRMI), the CRUSADE registry, and the D2B (door-to-balloon) Alliance have demonstrated a positive impact as reflected by increased clinical practice guideline (CPG) adherence for early (≤24 hours) and predischarge medical therapies and a reduction in D2B and door-to-needle (D2N) times, as well as door-in–door-out (DIDO) times, for STEMI patients who require interhospital transfer.[14] Nevertheless, broader and more region-specific system-based initiatives such as Mission: Lifeline continue to be vital in reducing total ischemic time—that is, time from chest pain symptom onset to coronary recanalization—which is the principal determinant of outcome.[12] Any delay in reperfusion (i.e., prolongation of total ischemic time) is associated with higher short-term (in-hospital, 30-day) and late (1-year) mortality in a continuous, nonlinear fashion (Fig. 37.1).[15–18] Because only a minority of U.S. hospitals are capable of performing PCI, the provision of prompt, expert PCI as the preferred reperfusion modality for the majority of ACS patients is a formidable challenge that will ultimately require regional integration of resources.[7] Not surprisingly, a very similar relationship can be seen between clinical volume and outcomes with cardiogenic shock, given that it is a complex acute condition that requires a multidisciplinary treatment team to provide procedural, surgical, and medical care. A study from the Nationwide Inpatient Sample illustrated this direct relationship between adjusted in-hospital mortality and hospital volume. The adjusted hazard ratio (HR) for mortality in the lowest quartile (<27 cases of cardiogenic shock treated per year) was 1.27 (1.15, 1.40) compared to the highest quartile (≥107 cases of cardiogenic shock treated per year).[19] Therefore, establishing systems of care with higher-volume hospitals utilized as regional hubs integrated with clearly defined protocols for management of cardiogenic shock for all ACSs including STEMI and OHCA has the potential to improve patient outcomes.[9]

THE CASE FOR REGIONALIZED CARE

Based in part on experience with trauma and stroke care in the United States, several basic tenets form the foundation of the premise behind regionalized systems for ACS, cardiogenic shock, and OHCA, including observations that (1) annual procedural volumes are directly related to clinical outcomes, (2) medical resources are limited, and (3) regionalization facilitates CPG adherence, quality, and outcomes monitoring, along with access to advanced technology and expertise.

A direct relationship has been demonstrated between both hospital facility and physician operator annual procedural volumes and optimal clinical outcomes following either elective or primary PCI and coronary artery bypass graft (CABG) surgery.[20–25] Physicians and hospitals with the highest procedure volumes have lower risk-adjusted in-hospital mortality to the extent that the relative benefit of PPCI versus fibrinolysis for the treatment of STEMI may be lost when PPCI is performed in a low-volume institution.[20] Similarly, risk-adjusted hospital mortality was increased (HR 1.20; 95% confidence interval [CI] 1.08 to 1.33) among centers that perform in the lowest tertile of annual PPCI volumes (<36 procedures/year) when compared with those in the highest tertile (>60 procedures/year).[25] A pooled analysis of multiple studies that included over one million PCI procedures confirmed the relationship between lower annual hospital PCI volumes (≤200 cases) with an increase in in-hospital mortality and need for emergent CABG surgery following PCI.[26] These specific data on annual institutional volume and outcome have been acknowledged by both the ACCF/AHA/Society for Cardiovascular Angiography and Interventions (SCAI) 2013 Update of the Clinical Competence Statement on Coronary Artery Interventional Procedures and the SCAI/ACC/AHA 2014 Expert Consensus Document regarding PCI without on-site surgical backup as follows: "It is important to note that a signal exists suggesting that an institutional volume threshold [below] 200 PCI/year appears to be consistently associated with worse outcomes across various studies." The Clinical Competence Statement then continues, "Accordingly, the writing committee recommends that an institution without on-site surgery with a volume fewer than 200 PCI annually, unless in a region underserved because of geography, should strongly consider whether or not it should continue to offer this service."[27,28]

A similar PCI volume–outcome (in-hospital mortality) relationship has been demonstrated for physician operators by the New York statewide database for PPCI and by the National Cardiovascular Data Registry (NCDR) for both elective and acute PCI (Fig. 37.2).[24,29] In-hospital mortality was increased for elective PCI (HR 1.27; 95% CI 1.11 to 1.45) and acute PCI (HR 1.10; 95% CI 1.00 to 1.21) among physician operators who performed fewer than 75 PCIs per year (vs. ≥75 PCIs/year). Similar results were reproduced recently from the NCDR in 2017, showing that the median annual number of procedures performed per operator was 59, with 44% of operators performing <50 PCI procedures per year. This study showed that low-volume operators more frequently performed emergent PPCI procedures and practiced at hospitals with lower annual PCI volumes. This is important because 26% of all centers that report to the NCDR performed fewer than 200 PCIs per year, and 38% performed fewer than 36 PCIs per year.[25,30] The adjusted risk of in-hospital mortality was

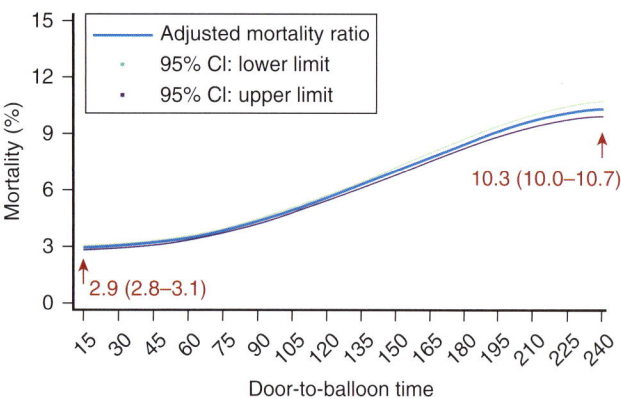

Fig. 37.1 Impact of door-to-balloon time on mortality from the NCDR CathPCI registry from 2005 to 2006. *ACC,* American College of Cardiology; *CI,* confidence interval; *NCDR,* National Cardiovascular Data Registry; *PCI,* percutaneous coronary intervention. (From Rathore SS, Curtis JP, Chen J, et al; National Cardiovascular Data Registry. Association of door-to-balloon time and mortality in patients admitted to hospital with ST elevation myocardial infarction: national cohort study. *BMJ.* 2009;338:b1807.)

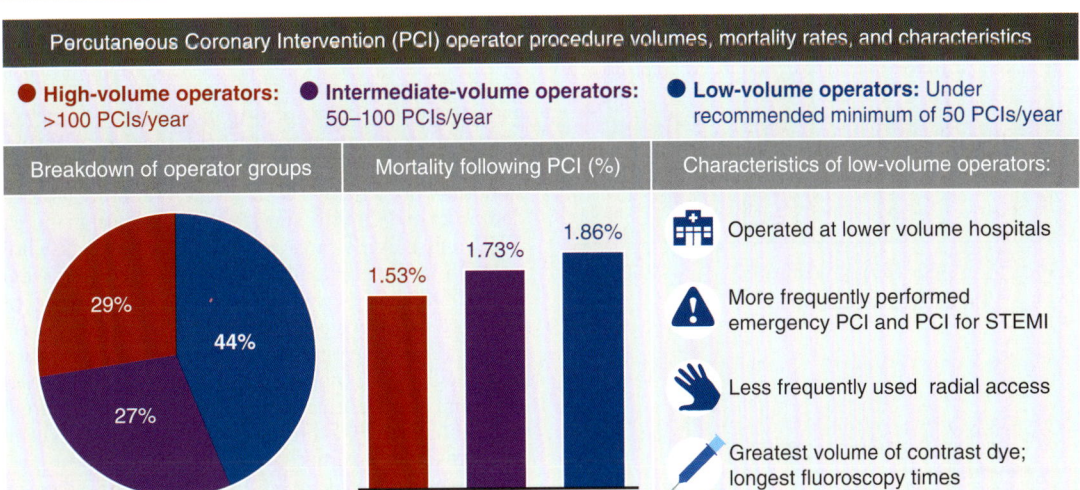

Fig. 37.2 Primary percutaneous coronary intervention (PPCI) annual volume was shown to be inversely related to in-hospital mortality among 86,044 ST-segment elevation myocardial infarction patients reported by 738 participating American College of Cardiology/National Cardiovascular Data Registry hospitals from 2006 through 2009 following multivariate adjustment. Hazard for in-hospital death was increased (1.20; 95% confidence interval 1.08 to 1.33; P = .001) in low-volume (≤36 PCI/year) versus high-volume (>60 PCI/year) centers. STEMI, ST-segment elevation myocardial infarction. (Reproduced from Fanaroff AC, Zakroysky P, Dai D, et al. Outcomes of PCI in relation to procedural characteristics and operator volumes in the United States. *J Am Coll Cardiol*. 2017;69:2913–2924.)

higher for PCI procedures performed by low- and intermediate-volume operators compared with those performed by high-volume operators (see Fig. 37.2).

Despite these data showing a direct correlation between operator volume and outcomes, both the 2013 Clinical Competency Statement and the 2014 Expert Consensus Document allow for lower annual PCI volumes (≥50 total PCI and ≥ 11 PPCI/year) for credentialing.[27,28] Considering the declining number of PCI procedures performed annually in the United States, the increasing complexity of coronary artery disease (CAD), and the need for medical cost reduction while maintaining or increasing quality, a more reasonable approach might be to promote regionalization, with fewer institutions providing PCI, allowing operators to maintain higher annual volume and thus optimize care delivery.[31]

Furthermore, the case for regionalization extends beyond the care delivered in the cath lab. Each of the process of care metrics for ACS patients as measured by ACC/AHA guideline adherence has been linked to both in-hospital and late (6- to 12-month) survival following presentation of ACS.[32] An analysis of hospital composite guideline adherence quartiles demonstrated an inverse relationship between the adherence to guideline-compliant care and the risk-adjusted in-hospital mortality rate.[33] For every 10% increase in guideline adherence, a 10% relative reduction in in-hospital mortality was observed.[33] This observation supports the central hypothesis that better adherence with evidence-based care practices throughout the scope of patient care for patients with ACS will result in better outcomes.[34] Additionally, lower-volume small community hospitals may be less likely to allocate the capital resources and personnel required to adequately track, collate, and report clinical outcomes or process measures (i.e., guideline compliance). Indeed, in a survey commissioned by the AHA, only slightly more than half of the hospitals queried were systematically tracking STEMI treatment times (D2N or D2B times) or rates of infection, readmission, stroke, recurrent myocardial infarction (MI), or mortality following either PCI or CABG.[7] This observation is made more meaningful by the fact that multiple national initiatives—such as GWTG, the Cardiac Hospitalization Atherosclerosis Management Program (CHAMP), the GAP project, the NRMI, and the CRUSADE Acute Coronary Treatment and Intervention Outcomes Network (ACTION) registry—have recently placed emphasis on system quality through systematic measurement of both care processes and clinical outcomes.[14]

The D2B Alliance was initiated in November of 2006 and has resulted in increased use of recommended strategies for process improvement and a greater number of patients being treated within guideline recommendations.[35] Despite documented process improvement as reflected by progressive reduction in D2B times, concurrent improvement in mortality following PPCI appears to have plateaued, and focus has now turned toward total ischemic time as the principal determinant of outcomes.[36] Because the relationship between total ischemic time and the extent of myocardial necrosis is nonlinear (Fig. 37.3), even optimally short D2B times may have little impact on the degree of myocardial salvage or survival in patients who present to the hospital late following infarct symptom onset.[16,17,37] Furthermore, because of a lack of integrated systems for STEMI care, patients who require transfer from non–PCI-capable facilities for PPCI continue to experience long door-to-door-to-balloon (D2D2B) times, as well as total ischemic times, with consequent poorer clinical outcomes.[38] This trend is also seen for patients presenting with NSTEMI who require transfer for definitive revascularization compared to those presenting to hospitals with on-site access to the full spectrum of resources required to care for this group.[13,39] Multiple factors including worse clinical outcomes, decreased ability to track and report clinical metrics, inability to adequately manage patients with complications of ACS, including cardiogenic shock and OHCA, and incomplete longitudinal care continue to provide strong evidence for the regionalization of care for patients with ACS.

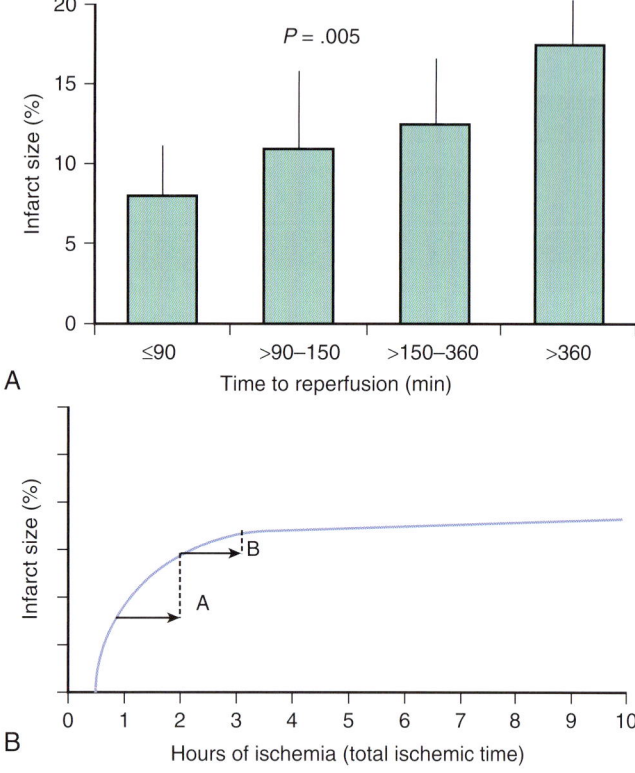

Fig. 37.3 (A) Relationship between chest pain symptom onset to balloon inflation (time to perfusion/total ischemic time) and infarct size as determined by gadolinium-enhanced cardiovascular magnetic resonance imaging. (B) Relationship between a 1-hour door-to-balloon (D2B) time percutaneous coronary intervention (PCI) delay and infarct size as a function of total ischemic time. Infarct size may be variably influenced by a similar D2B time (1 hour) depending on the length of the time delay to PCI-hospital presentation (A vs. B). (A, From Francone M, Bucciarelli Ducci C, Carbone I, et al. Impact of primary coronary angioplasty delay on myocardial salvage, infarct size, and microvascular damage in patients with ST-segment elevation myocardial infarction: insight from cardiovascular magnetic resonance. *J Am Coll Cardiol*. 2009;54:2145–2153; B, From Garcia-Dorado D, Garcia del Blanco B. Door-to-balloon time and mortality. *N Engl J Med*. 2014;370:179.)

PERCUTANEOUS CORONARY INTERVENTION CENTERS WITHOUT ON-SITE CARDIAC SURGERY

There continues to be a trend toward proliferation of "PCI centers" that lack on-site cardiac surgical facilities for the performance of PCI. Elective PCI at hospitals without surgery on site (no-SOS sites) has been evaluated in two large-scale randomized trials.[40,41] The Cardiovascular Patient Outcomes Research Team Elective Angioplasty Study (C-PORT E) screened 99,479 patients with both acute and elective PCI indications (excluding PPCI for STEMI), consented 75,674 subjects for trial participation, and randomized 18,867 subjects on a 3:1 basis to have PCI either at a no-SOS or an SOS facility, respectively.[40] Approximately 75% of consented subjects were excluded from randomization in large part because of clinical and/or angiographic risk. The hypothesis of C-PORT E was that PCI performed at no-SOS facilities would be noninferior with respect to the primary end points (death at 6 weeks and major adverse cardiovascular events [MACE] at 9 months) when compared with PCI at SOS facilities, though this was an interesting end point given that PCI has never been demonstrated to reduce mortality in stable ischemic heart disease patients when compared with medical therapy alone. As such, the absence of a difference in mortality between randomly assigned treatment groups (both PCI) was predictable. Nevertheless, despite the inherent low-risk characteristics of the randomized cohort, PCI failure was increased on both a per-patient ($P < .01$) and per-lesion ($P = .04$) basis when performed at the no-SOS facilities (Fig. 37.4A). In addition, a significant ($P < .01$) increase in target-vessel revascularization (TVR, the need for additional procedures performed on the intervened-upon artery) and a trend ($P = .09$) toward an increased frequency of MACE was observed by intention-to-treat (ITT) analysis through 9 months follow-up (see Fig. 37.4). Furthermore, a per-protocol analysis of subjects who actually received the randomly assigned treatment demonstrated highly statistically significant increases in both TVR and MACE rates among those subjects who had PCI at no-SOS facilities. Finally, PCI was more costly when performed at no-SOS centers, driven largely by the relative cost increment observed in lower-volume (<200 PCI/year) centers.

The PCI Outcomes in Community Versus Tertiary Settings (MASS-COMM) trial randomly assigned 3691 patients with both acute and elective indications for PCI (excluding PPCI for STEMI) on a 3:1 basis to PCI at no-SOS ($n = 2774$) or SOS centers ($n = 917$), respectively.[41] No differences in MACE or repeat revascularization was observed by type of PCI site at either 30 days or 12 months. Wide variability was apparent in outcomes among participating hospitals as reflected by absolute differences between sites of 14% and 17% in MACE rates at 30 days and 12 months, respectively. This interhospital variation in treatment effect was most marked among no-SOS centers and raises concern with regard to the credibility of pooling such widely discrepant outcomes data. In addition, although an annual operator PCI volume requirement of 75 or more procedures per year is stated in the MASS-COMM study methods section, minimum annual operator volumes of fewer than 30 PCIs per year were recorded during 4 of the 6 years of the study.[41] Finally, the PCI success rates achieved in MASS-COMM are concerning on both a per-patient and a per-lesion basis. In an adjudicated angiographic review cohort, the per-patient PCI success rates were 81.3% and 74.7% in non-SOS and SOS centers, respectively.[41] The MASS-COMM authors did not report a cost economic analysis for this trial as was performed in C-PORT E.

The impact of C-PORT E and MASS-COMM has been the proliferation of low-volume PCI programs, particularly those with no SOS, which perform PPCI for STEMI, despite the exclusion of these patients from both of these trials. Indeed, 49% of centers that currently report to the NCDR perform 400 or fewer PCIs per year, and 25% perform 200 or fewer PCIs per year. Of note, about 90% of no-SOS centers perform 400 or fewer PCIs per year, and 83% of the centers that perform 200 or fewer PCIs per year are no-SOS centers.[30] Furthermore, the impact of no-SOS centers in geographic proximity to SOS centers on SOS-center PCI volume has been a point of concern. Indeed, during the 6-year duration of the MASS-COMM study, a 40% reduction in SOS-center operator annual PCI volume was observed (vs. a 9% reduction in participating no-SOS centers).[41] Clearly, the growth in the number of PCI centers has exceeded by almost threefold the growth in the U.S. population and has occurred despite a concomitant significant decline in STEMI volumes.[42] In fact, despite a 44% increase in PCI capacity (521 new PCI programs) in the United States between 2000 and 2006, only a 1% increase in PCI access was achieved when a ground transport time to PCI of 60 minutes or less is used to define *access*.[43] This systematic reduplication of PCI services at an estimated cost of several billion dollars appears to be driven by market share competition and not the desire to strategically improve access to PPCI.[44] Indeed, it has been estimated that about 80% of new PCI programs have opened within a 12-mile radius of an existing SOS PCI center.[44]

Additionally, in a study that included data from the Nationwide Inpatient Sample of over 6.9 million patients who received PCI in the United States between 2003 and 2012, 5.7% of the procedures were performed at centers without on-site cardiac

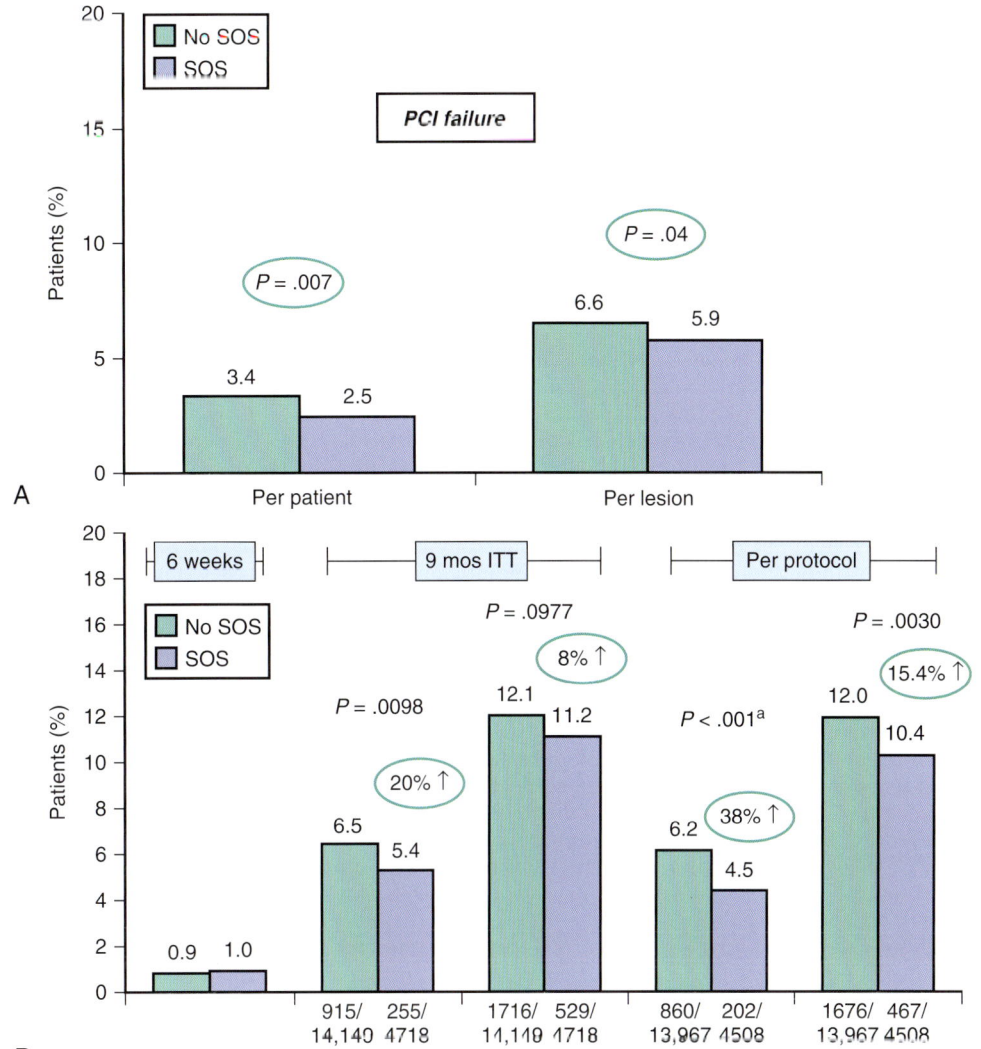

Fig. 37.4 Analysis in the cardiovascular patient outcomes research team elective angioplasty study trial. (A) Per-patient and per-lesion percutaneous coronary intervention (PCI) failure rates by randomly assigned site for PCI. (B) Outcomes by PCI site, intention to treat (ITT), and actual treatment received (per protocol). MACE, Major adverse cardiovascular event; SOS, surgery on site; TVR, target-vessel revascularization. [a]Chi-squared analysis. (Adapted from Aversano T, Lemmon CC, Liu L; for the Atlantic CPORT Investigators. Outcomes of PCI at hospitals with or without on-site cardiac surgery. N Engl J Med. 2012;366:1792–1802.)

surgery capabilities, and the overall proportion of PCIs performed at these centers increased with time (1.8% in 2003 to 12.7% in 2013; $P < .01$). Notably, elective PCI tended to be performed mostly at hospitals with CABG availability (38.2% vs. 24.1%) during that time. The authors found that the unadjusted in-hospital mortality was lower for patients treated at PCI centers with on-site surgery (odds ratio [OR] 0.74; 95% CI 0.72 to 0.75), but the difference disappeared after adjustment for demographics, risk factors, hospital characteristics, and procedural indication (OR 1.01; 95% CI 0.98 to 1.03). In subgroup analyses however, in-hospital mortality was lower for patients undergoing PCI at centers with surgical backup for those ≤75 years old (OR 0.94, $P < .01$), diabetics (OR 0.94, $P < .01$), and those with prior CABG (OR 0.83, $P < .01$). Notably, annual PCI volume was ≤200 cases in almost two-thirds of the off-site surgery centers, while 81% of the on-site surgery center cases were at hospitals with annual PCI volumes >400.[45] In an analysis of 625,854 Medicare patients undergoing PCI, in-hospital and 30-day mortality was increased in those centers without on-site cardiac surgery with the greatest hazard observed in hospitals that performed the lowest number of PCI procedures (≤50).[46] Even in the context of a completely integrated community hospital–tertiary hospital system, the performance of PPCI without on-site cardiac surgery was associated with a trend toward increased hospital mortality when compared with PPCI performed at the tertiary center.[47] Although single-center studies have reported excellent outcomes in patients undergoing PPCI at hospitals without on-site cardiac surgery, the one randomized trial that compared fibrinolysis to primary PCI at hospitals without surgery on site (C-PORT PPCI) was flawed by an inadequate sample size, relatively high rates of stroke and recurrent MI observed in the fibrinolytic treatment arm, and a large portion of subjects (31%) enrolled at a single center.[48,49] As recently as 2017, large registry data have shown a similar risk for mortality following both PPCI and elective PCI performed at hospitals with, versus those without, cardiac surgical facilities.[41,50]

With these concerns in mind, the writing group of the 2014 SCAI/ACCF/AHA Expert Consensus Document Update on PCI without on-site surgical backup states "the development of PCI facilities within a 30-minute emergency transfer time to an established facility is strongly discouraged."[28] Additionally, the current ACCF/AHA guidelines for the performance of PCI designate a class IIb (procedure/treatment may be considered, usefulness/efficacy is less well established) level of evidence B indication for elective PCI and a class IIa (it is reasonable to perform the procedure) level of evidence B for primary PCI in no-SOS hospitals; they also note the need for appropriate planning for program development to be accomplished at all no-SOS facilities and the importance of using rigorous clinical/angiographic criteria for proper patient selection for elective PCI.[1,51] These recommendations underpin the growing concern that these types of facilities may be providing suboptimal care, particularly for patients presenting with ACS.

BENEFITS OF CATHETER-BASED THERAPY FOR ACUTE CORONARY SYNDROMES
ST-Elevation Myocardial Infarction

The relative advantage of PCI versus fibrinolytic therapy depends on several factors. First, because primary PCI entails an obligate time delay for implementation in the catheterization laboratory compared with fibrinolysis administration in the emergency department (ED), the relative advantage of PCI depends on the relative time delay to definitive treatment (balloon inflation). Pooled analyses of multiple RCTs suggest that the survival advantage in favor of PCI is inversely proportional to the relative time delay for PCI implementation and may be lost if the PCI-related time delay (D2B time minus DTN time) exceeds 60 to 110 minutes.[52–54] Differences between these analyses may be explained by differences in patient risk profiles. Indeed, a survival advantage in favor of PCI is evident only when the risk of death to 30 days following fibrinolytic therapy exceeds about 4%.[55] Longer relative time delays may still be associated with a PCI survival advantage in those patients at highest risk for death following fibrinolysis.[56] The PCI-related time delay associated with mortality equipoise compared with fibrinolysis is influenced significantly by patient-related variables that include age and infarct location regardless of patient-related time delays (less than vs. more than 120 minutes) to presentation.[53] Thus accurate risk assessment should be part of any STEMI treatment triage algorithm.

As noted previously, the relative survival advantage of PCI versus fibrinolysis is also dependent on the case volume experience of both the interventional cardiologist and the facility. In general, optimal outcomes have been correlated with higher procedural volumes on the part of both the facility and operator. Transport of the STEMI patient to a center capable of performing PCI yields superior clinical outcomes compared with on-site (community hospital) fibrinolytic therapy when the D2D2B time is less than 120 minutes.[57]

Despite significant improvement in D2B treatment times for patients who present to PCI-capable facilities, STEMI patients who present first to a non-PCI facility and are subsequently transported to a PCI facility often incur prolonged time delays to definitive treatment.[58,59] Indeed, initial presentation to a non-PCI center has been identified as a major determinant of prolonged time delay to PCI treatment due to the lack of a well-defined integrated system with protocol-driven algorithms for care and dedicated transport facilities.[60] Data from NMRI demonstrated that D2D2B times for patients who required transport for PCI were a median of 180 minutes, and only 15% received PCI within 120 minutes from initial hospital presentation.[58] Not surprisingly, although both the diagnosis of STEMI and in-hospital mortality rates associated with STEMI have declined over the past 8 to 15 years, mortality rates remain consistently higher for those STEMI patients who require transfer for PCI, compared with those who do not, and likely reflect the incremental, protracted delay to treatment.[59,61,62] This outcome and performance gap exists despite the availability of technology that allows EMS personnel to transmit a prehospital 12-lead electrocardiogram (ECG) and makes the diagnosis of STEMI evident at the point of first medical contact. The integration of EMS and incorporation of the prehospital phase for ACS evaluation and diagnosis are integral components of any regionalized system for STEMI care. Earlier STEMI diagnosis via a transmitted prehospital 12-lead ECG facilitates expedited in-hospital STEMI treatment.[63–65] Hospitals that demonstrate the shortest D2B times incorporate prehospital STEMI diagnosis (transmitted ECG) with a multidisciplinary team approach in which either the emergency physician or specially trained EMS providers activate the cardiac cath lab prior to cardiology consultation.[66] Indeed, the facilitation of in-hospital PCI treatment for STEMI patients with a transmitted prehospital ECG has resulted in significant reductions in D2B times and has also shown improvement in in-hospital and 30-day survival.[67–70] The consistent, significant relationships that have been demonstrated between earlier STEMI diagnosis, more rapid treatment, and improved outcomes has prompted a consensus recommendation for the implementation of prehospital 12-lead ECG systems by all EMS providers.[71] Multiple reports from established STEMI systems of care that use EMS integration with prehospital 12-lead ECG diagnosis of STEMI and prehospital ambulance triage to the nearest PCI-capable facility (bypassing non–PCI-capable facilities) have demonstrated reduced time delays to treatment, reduced infarct size, and improved survival among triaged patients compared with those who require subsequent interhospital transfer for PCI.[72–76] Indeed, prehospital ECG capability, specialized EMS training, and integration have spawned a new paradigm for prehospital diagnosis and triage of STEMI patients (Fig. 37.5).[77]

Nevertheless, the rapid transport of patients with STEMI to the nearest PCI-capable facility for care may be limited by several factors. First, only a minority (≤5%) of EMS-transported patients with chest pain actually have STEMI. Second, only a minority (<50%) of EMS systems have 12-lead ECG capabilities. Third, a precedent mandate exists for transport of patients with suspected STEMI to the nearest facility, even when fibrinolysis may be contraindicated and/or that facility does not provide primary PCI. Fourth, evolution toward a more integrated process of prehospital care is complicated by the fact that 329 different EMS regions exist in the United States with more than 993 hospital-based EMS systems.[7,78] Remarkably, hospital-based EMS systems represent only 6.5% of all EMS providers with the remainder comprised of private, third-party systems (48.6%) and fire station–based systems (44.9%).[7] Although the transport time to a specialized PCI center may appear long, it can be more than counterbalanced by an integrated EMS system that incorporates prenotification. A doubling of the recommended transport time has been proposed for suspected STEMI patients who are transported to a "center of excellence," where the target D2B time is 60 minutes or less.[28,79] Such efficiency of process can be achieved only through an integrated system for STEMI care that incorporates the prehospital ECG for earlier diagnosis; expedited triage; and readily available, rehearsed transport systems. A "network" approach with earlier activation of transport systems between the referral and PCI centers has achieved sustainable first D2B times of 90 minutes or less for STEMI patients who required interhospital transfer for PCI.[80,81] Finally, a more uniform evolution toward integration in the process of STEMI care has been impeded by diverging incentives, the lack of coordinated objectives, and ostensibly competing strategies. For example, in many regions, particularly those without state-regulated certificate of need requirements, a proliferation of new cath labs for the provision of primary PCI in no-SOS centers has occurred, as previously noted.[42,44] Conversely, other regions—including Minneapolis, Los Angeles, Boston, and the state of North Carolina—have developed integrated EMS systems with a focus on prehospital diagnosis and triage to an established center of excellence proficient in both primary and elective PCI. These competing strategies—one focused on building more small PCI centers, the other on more efficient and effective utilization of existing PCI centers through prehospital-EMS integration—have drawn support from the divergent financial incentives present among various stakeholders in the process of care. Only recently have sophisticated modeling techniques been utilized to compare the relative efficacy and/or cost of these "build more" versus "use more effectively" strategies for PCI facilities as they specifically pertain to the care of STEMI patients.[82] Of note, the strategy focused on EMS integration, prehospital diagnosis, and triage with more effective utilization of existing PCI facilities was found to be more effective and less costly than the strategy of creating new PCI facilities (Fig. 37.6).[82] The coordination of strategies and the integration of essential prehospital and hospital

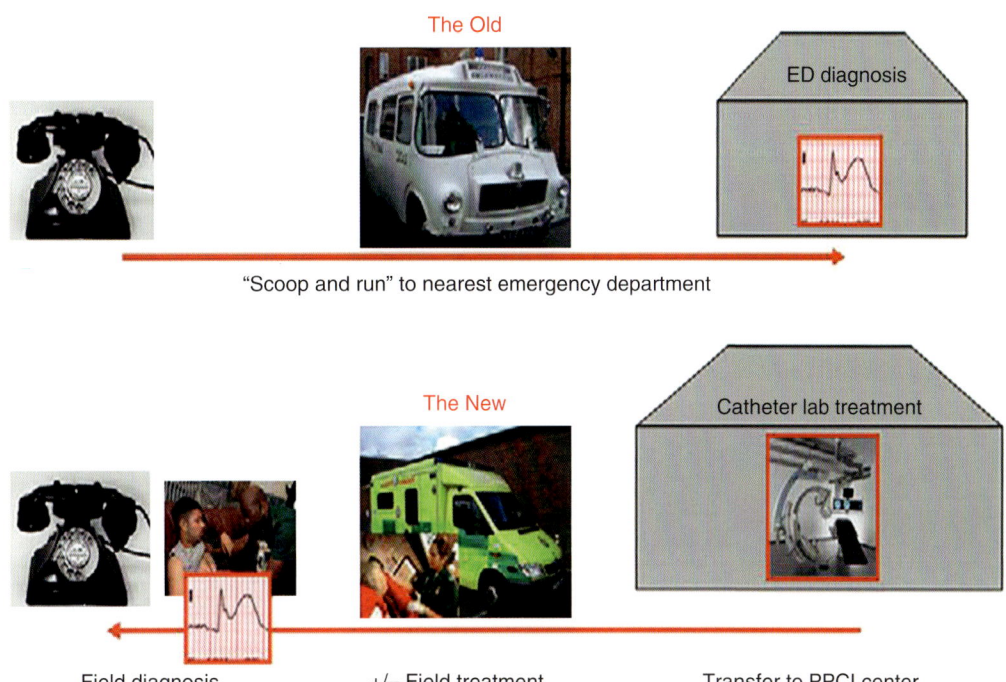

Fig. 37.5 Evolving paradigms in prehospital diagnosis, triage, and treatment of ST-elevation myocardial infarction (STEMI). Prehospital diagnosis (with or without field treatment) and triage to a primary percutaneous coronary intervention *(PPCI)* center ("the new") has reduced total time delays to STEMI treatment. *ED*, Emergency department. (From Dalby M, Whitbread M. The role of the emergency services in the optimization of primary angioplasty: experience from London and the Heart Attack Team. *EuroIntervention*. 2013;9:517–523.)

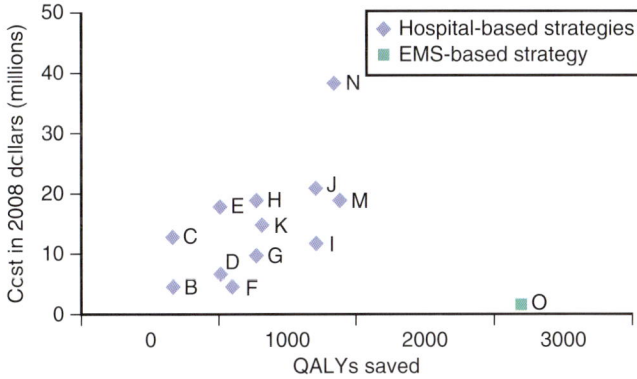

Fig. 37.6 Comparative effectiveness of ST-segment elevation myocardial infarction regionalization strategies. Hospital-based (expansion of percutaneous coronary intervention [PCI]-capable facilities) versus emergency medical services *(EMS)*-based (regionalization with EMS integration for existing PCI facilities) demonstrates that the EMS-based strategy is less costly and more effective. *QALY*, Quality adjust life-year. (From Concannon TW, Kent DM, Normand SL, et al. Comparative effectiveness of ST-segment-elevation myocardial infarction regionalization strategies. *Circ Cardiovasc Qual Outcomes*. 2010;3:506–513.)

resources for ACS care on the state level has been the focus of the national Mission: Lifeline initiative of the AHA in conjunction with the ACC.

New data has also shown the importance of complete coronary revascularization for patients presenting with STEMI. In 2013, the randomized trial of Preventive Angioplasty in Myocardial Infarction (PRAMI) evaluated treatment of culprit-only versus culprit plus significant obstructive nonculprit coronary lesions in patients presenting with STEMI. They enrolled 465 patients from 2008 to 2013 at five centers throughout the United Kingdom (U.K.). Subjects were randomly assigned to either preventive PCI (234 patients) or culprit-lesion-only PCI (231 patients). The primary outcome was a composite of death from cardiac causes, nonfatal MI, or refractory angina. During a mean follow-up of 23 months, the primary outcome occurred in 21 patients assigned to preventive PCI and in 53 patients assigned to no preventive PCI (infarct-artery-only PCI), which translated into a HR of 0.35 (95% CI 0.21 to 0.58), significantly favoring preventative PCI. Analysis of the three individual components of the primary outcome showed a HR of 0.34 (95% CI 0.11 to 1.08) for death from cardiac causes, 0.32 (95% CI 0.13 to 0.75) for nonfatal MI, and 0.35 (95% CI 0.18 to 0.69) for refractory angina, all favoring preventative PCI. The authors concluded that for patients with STEMI and multivessel CAD, in addition to culprit artery PCI, preventive PCI in nonculprit coronary arteries with severe stenoses significantly reduced the risk of MACE, as compared with PCI limited to the culprit artery alone.[2] In 2015, the randomized trial of complete versus lesion-only revascularization in patients undergoing PPCI for STEMI and multivessel disease (CvLPRIT trial) compared complete revascularization at index admission with treatment of the infarct-related artery (IRA) only. A total of 296 patients in 7 U.K. centers were randomized to either in-hospital complete revascularization ($n = 150$) or IRA-only revascularization ($n = 146$). Complete revascularization was performed either at the time of PPCI or before hospital discharge. The primary end point was a composite of all-cause death, recurrent MI, heart failure, and ischemia-driven revascularization within 12 months. As shown in Fig. 37.7, the primary end point occurred in 10.0% of the complete revascularization group versus 21.2% in the IRA-only revascularization group (HR 0.45; 95% CI 0.24 to 0.84), though the trial was not powered to show a difference in any of the individual components of MACE.[3] Additionally, the Fractional Flow Reserve–Guided Multivessel Angioplasty in Myocardial Infarction (Compare Acute) trial published in 2017 tested a similar hypothesis of

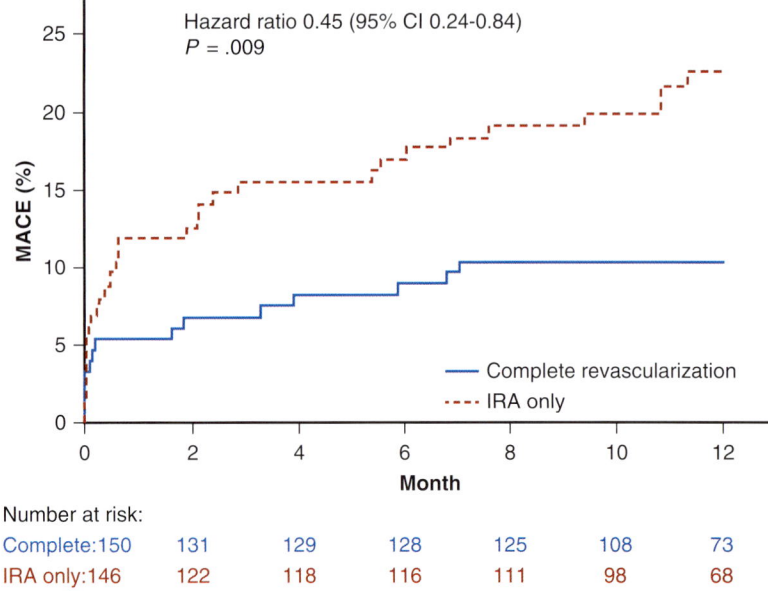

Fig. 37.7 Analysis from the CvLPRIT trial showing decreased major adverse cardiovascular events (MACE) following complete coronary revascularization compared to culprit-only percutaneous coronary intervention during ST-elevation myocardial infarction. *CI,* Confidence interval; *IRA,* infarct-related artery. (From Gershlick AH, Khan JN, Kelly DJ, et al. Randomized trial of complete versus lesion-only revascularization in patients undergoing primary percutaneous coronary intervention for STEMI and multivessel disease: the CvLPRIT trial. *J Am Coll Cardiol.* 2015;65:963–972.)

culprit-only versus culprit plus fractional flow reserve (FFR)-guided complete revascularization in STEMI patients. A total of 885 patients with STEMI and multivessel disease who had undergone primary PCI of an infarct-related coronary artery were randomized in a 1:2 ratio to undergo complete revascularization of non infarct-related coronary arteries guided by FFR (295 patients) or to forgo revascularization of non infarct-related coronary arteries (590 patients). The primary end point was a composite of death from any cause, nonfatal MI, revascularization, and cerebrovascular events at 12 months. The primary outcome occurred in 23 patients in the complete-revascularization group and in 121 patients in the infarct-artery-only group who did not receive complete revascularization (HR 0.35; 95% CI 0.22 to 0.55), favoring FFR-guided complete revascularization in this group. On breakdown of the individual components of the primary end point, only repeat revascularization was significant (HR 0.32; 95% CI 0.20 to 0.54).[4] This trial was based on prior studies showing the validity of FFR values for nonculprit lesions during ACS, including STEMI.[83] The cumulative evidence of these trials heavily favors a strategy of complete coronary revascularization in patients presenting with STEMI and is reflected in the 2015 ACC/AHA/SCAI guidelines for the treatment of STEMI. These guidelines reflect a change in the recommendation for treating noninfarct coronary lesions, either at the time of culprit lesion PCI or in a staged fashion which was modified from a previous class III ("harm") recommendation to a class IIB recommendation.[84] Similarly, the 2016 Appropriate Use Criteria (AUC) from the ACC/American Association for Thoracic Surgery/AHA/American Society of Echocardiography/American Society of Nuclear Cardiology/SCAI/Society of Cardiovascular Computed Tomography/Society of Thoracic Surgeons gave the recommendation of "A" appropriate for revascularizing nonculprit lesions in patients presenting with STEMI.[85]

The only caveat to this strategy may be in patients presenting with STEMI and concurrent cardiogenic shock. For the last several decades, several retrospective analyses of randomized trials provided evidence that the only therapy found to improve survival in patients with cardiogenic shock was complete coronary revascularization.[86] However, both a recent meta-analysis and a recent large-scale randomized trial of culprit-only versus complete revascularization in patients presenting in cardiogenic shock (CUPRIT-SHOCK trial) have shown increased mortality in patients undergoing complete revascularization during the index culprit PCI procedure.[87,88] Therefore, staging nonculprit lesions in this group may improve outcomes in this high-risk patient group, though this remains an area of ongoing investigation.

The timing of when to perform nonculprit PCI in patients presenting with STEMI remains controversial. Hannan et al. performed a retrospective analysis of STEMI patients in New York who underwent complete revascularization, either during the index hospitalization versus within 60 days of the hospitalization, and found no significant difference in MACE between these groups.[89] This contrasts with the Single-Staged Compared With Multi-Staged PCI in Multivessel NSTEMI Patients (SMILE Trial) that evaluated the timing of complete revascularization in patients with multivessel CAD presenting with NSTEMI which found that primary end point (major adverse cardiovascular and cerebrovascular events [MACCEs]) were significantly lower in the single procedure PCI group (n = 36 [13.63%] vs. the staged-procedure prior to discharge group (n = 61 [23.19%]) with a HR of 0.549 (95% CI 0.36 to 0.83). While these populations differ in pathophysiology (STEMI vs. NSTEMI), the optimal timing for complete coronary revascularization in the acute setting remains to be determined.

NON–ST-SEGMENT ELEVATION ACUTE CORONARY SYNDROMES

In the context of therapeutic innovation in catheter-based technology and adjunctive pharmacotherapy, the cumulative weight of data from RCTs supports the use of an early invasive (angiography followed by revascularization if feasible) versus conservative (medical therapy with angiography for spontaneous or provoked ischemia) strategy in the treatment of NSTEMI, though the relative benefit of invasive versus conservative treatment is directly proportional to patient risk profile as reflected by the Thrombolysis in Myocardial Infarction (TIMI) study, the Platelet Glycoprotein IIb/IIIa in Unstable Angina: Receptor Suppression Using Integrilin Therapy (PURSUIT) trial, and the Global Registry of Acute Coronary Events (GRACE) risk-stratification schemes.[90]

In addition, the magnitude of benefit attributable to the invasive treatment strategy appears to be inversely correlated with the duration of time delay from presentation to revascularization and directly correlated with both the relative extent of revascularization in the active treatment versus the control/conservative groups and the duration of clinical follow-up.[91–96] Data suggest that earlier revascularization (≤24 hours after presentation) provides greater benefit as reflected by a reduction in the occurrence of cardiovascular death, MI, or stroke than later (≥36 hours) revascularization, particularly in those NSTEMI patients at highest risk.[97]

Similarly, pooled patient-level data from the Fast Revascularization During Instability in Coronary Disease (FRISC II), Invasive Versus Conservative Treatment in Unstable Coronary Syndromes (ICTUS), and Randomized Intervention Treatment of Angina 3 (RITA-3) randomized trials show durable long-term (5-year) relative clinical benefit for the invasive treatment strategy.[96] The major source of controversy no longer surrounds the choice of treatment strategy (invasive vs. conservative) but rather the fact that although the benefit of an early invasive strategy is proportional to patient risk, the propensity to receive such treatment is greatest in patients at lower risk.[97–100] This treatment-risk paradox may be due to physician misconceptions regarding benefit-harm tradeoffs, concerns about treatment complications, or public reporting, and has been observed in relationship to the performance of angiography and/or PCI and in the use of platelet inhibitor therapies.[101]

Additionally, the benefits of transporting patients from a non-PCI facility to one capable of performing PCI for NSTEMI has been shown to be inversely proportional to patient risk strata.[102] The importance of the treatment-risk paradox is further magnified by the observation that compliance with the current ACC/AHA CPG recommendations, including early angiography, is inversely correlated with in-hospital mortality for ACS.[33] Furthermore, evidence-based therapies—which includes antiplatelet agents, β-blockers, lipid-lowering agents, and angiotensin-converting-enzyme inhibitors—initiated before hospital discharge are associated with an incremental survival advantage in follow-up. The fact that performance measures such as CPG compliance relate process of care to mortality presents an opportunity to define strategies that enhance current CPG compliance and utilization, further emphasizing a need for regionalization models of care with triage to centers of excellence.

Finally, data continues to support complete coronary revascularization in patients presenting with NSTEMI. Shishehbor et al. performed a retrospective analysis of patients presenting with unstable angina or NSTEMI and multivessel CAD at the Cleveland Clinic from 01/1995 to 06/2005 and compared the incidence of a composite end point including death, MI requiring hospitalization (excluding periprocedural MI), or any target or nontarget-vessel revascularization (PCI or CABG) to a mean follow-up of 2.3 years between those who had culprit lesion only PCI versus those who underwent complete coronary revascularization. Complete revascularization was associated with a lower composite end point following adjustment for baseline and angiographic characteristics (HR 0.80; 95% CI 0.64 to 0.99) as well as in propensity matched analysis (HR 0.67; 95% CI 0.51 to 0.88) and was primarily driven by a lower rate of repeat revascularization.[6] Additionally, Rosner et al. performed a retrospective analysis of the Acute Catheterization and Urgent Intervention Triage Strategy (ACUITY) trial to evaluate rates of MACE at 1-year follow-up for those patients who underwent complete versus incomplete (residual lesion ≥70% in any vessel ≥2 mm in size) revascularization and found that incomplete coronary revascularization was strongly associated with 1-year MI, ischemia-driven unplanned revascularization, and MACEs (Fig. 37.8).[5] Based on these studies, among others, the most recent 2014 ACC/AHA guidelines for the treatment of NSTEMI give a class IIB recommendation for a strategy of multivessel PCI, in contrast to culprit-lesion-only PCI, for the treatment of patients presenting with NSTEMI.[103]

Models of Regional Systems of Care

Given the substantial amount of data supporting the regionalization of care for patients with ACS, significant efforts have been made to regionalize the provision of PPCI therapy for STEMI in major U.S. metropolitan areas such as Minneapolis, Minnesota and Charlotte, North Carolina.[80,104,105] Through partnership with community hospitals in standardized protocol-driven algorithms for care and designated transport systems—along with enhanced multidisciplinary communication among EMS personnel, ED physicians, and interventional cardiologists—the Minneapolis Heart Institute at Abbott Northwestern Hospital and the Sanger Heart and Vascular Institute at Carolinas Medical Center have both demonstrated the ability to promptly access and treat STEMI patients who originate from up to 200 miles from the PCI center.[80,105] By focusing on collaboration and integration of resources, community hospitals initiate adjunctive pharmacotherapies in patients who present with STEMI and emergently transport them to the interventional team waiting at the central PCI center. These data demonstrate that regional systems in the United States can achieve results at least similar to those of smaller European centers with organized transfer systems. Indeed, D2D2B times for transfer-in patients with STEMI were 90 minutes or less in 56% and 120 minutes or less in greater than 90% of patients, respectively, using an integrated regional system approach. Similar results have been duplicated in other regional STEMI systems.[69,106–109]

A statewide approach is also being used in North Carolina, known as *Reperfusion of Acute Myocardial Infarction in North Carolina Emergency Departments* (RACE). This initiative uses standardized protocols and integrated systems for the treatment and timely transfer of patients with STEMI in five regions in North Carolina. The RACE program demonstrated a significant improvement in time to treatment at both PCI and non-PCI hospitals and resulted in increased timely access to PCI on a statewide level.[110,111] The success of these regional programs resulted in a new class I recommendation in the ACC/AHA STEMI guidelines that "each community should develop a STEMI system of care."[1,112]

The limitations of the prior nonintegrated, nonregionalized process for STEMI care in the United States was reflected by the absence of improvement in prolonged times to treatment despite widespread dissemination of benchmark goals for therapy (door-to–fibrinolytic infusion times of 30 minutes or less or a D2B time of 90 minutes or less) in the form of CPGs.[113] With marked regional variation in both EMS and hospital resources along with geography, population density, and transport facility distances, no single "system model" for STEMI care is likely to be either practical or achievable in the United States.[114,115] In addition to larger regional and statewide initiatives for STEMI care process integration, a number of smaller local and community STEMI systems have been developed. In a survey of 381 separate systems across 47 states, 202 involved a single PCI hospital, 150 included two to five PCI hospitals, and 29 included more than five PCI-capable hospitals.[114] Marked intersystem variability in the processes of STEMI care was observed. With specific goals to accelerate the implementation of STEMI care systems in selected U.S. metropolitan areas, to facilitate more effective delivery of STEMI care, and to improve clinical outcomes following STEMI, the regional systems of care demonstration project Mission: Lifeline STEMI Accelerator was created as a national outcomes research study initiated by the Duke Clinical Research Institute (DCRI) in collaboration with the AHA.[12] Participating regions were selected through a competitive application process. A total of 17 regions were selected to participate, and variability was wide in the number of PCI hospitals (3 to 33), non-PCI hospitals (3 to 30), and EMS agencies (1 to 500) in each region. Regional meetings of stakeholders were held that included cardiologists and emergency medicine physicians from both PCI-capable and non-PCI hospitals, EMS directors, senior hospital administrators, and regional AHA and Department of Health representatives. Region-specific data were examined, and specific

STEMI case examples focused on prehospital ECG early STEMI identification and transmission and overread; "single call" cath lab activation and interhospital transfer protocols and resources were reviewed. All participating centers entered patient-level data in the ACTION–GWTG registry. ACTION–GWTG is a comprehensive acute MI database jointly owned and managed by the ACC and AHA that permits assessment of both individual hospital and regional performance with inclusion of prehospital, ED, cath lab, and in-hospital management and outcome data.[116] Multiple system performance and outcome measures are analyzed by region and among regions with a focus on first medical contact to device activation (reperfusion) times in addition to in-hospital mortality, bleeding, stroke, congestive heart failure, and cardiogenic shock. The central goal of the Mission Lifeline Accelerator project is to facilitate and expedite implementation of STEMI care systems in 17 selected metropolitan regions with the aim to improve utilization and timeliness of reperfusion therapy to improve clinical outcomes in STEMI.[12] An early report from this initiative by Jollis et al. in 2016 demonstrated that the establishment of leadership teams, coordinated protocols, and systematic, regular feedback for 484 hospitals and 1253 EMS agencies in 16 regions across the United States led to a significant increase in the proportion of patients meeting guideline goals of first medical contact–to–device time, both for those directly presenting via EMS (50% to 55%; $P < .01$) as well as transferred patients (44% to 48%; $P < .01$).[117]

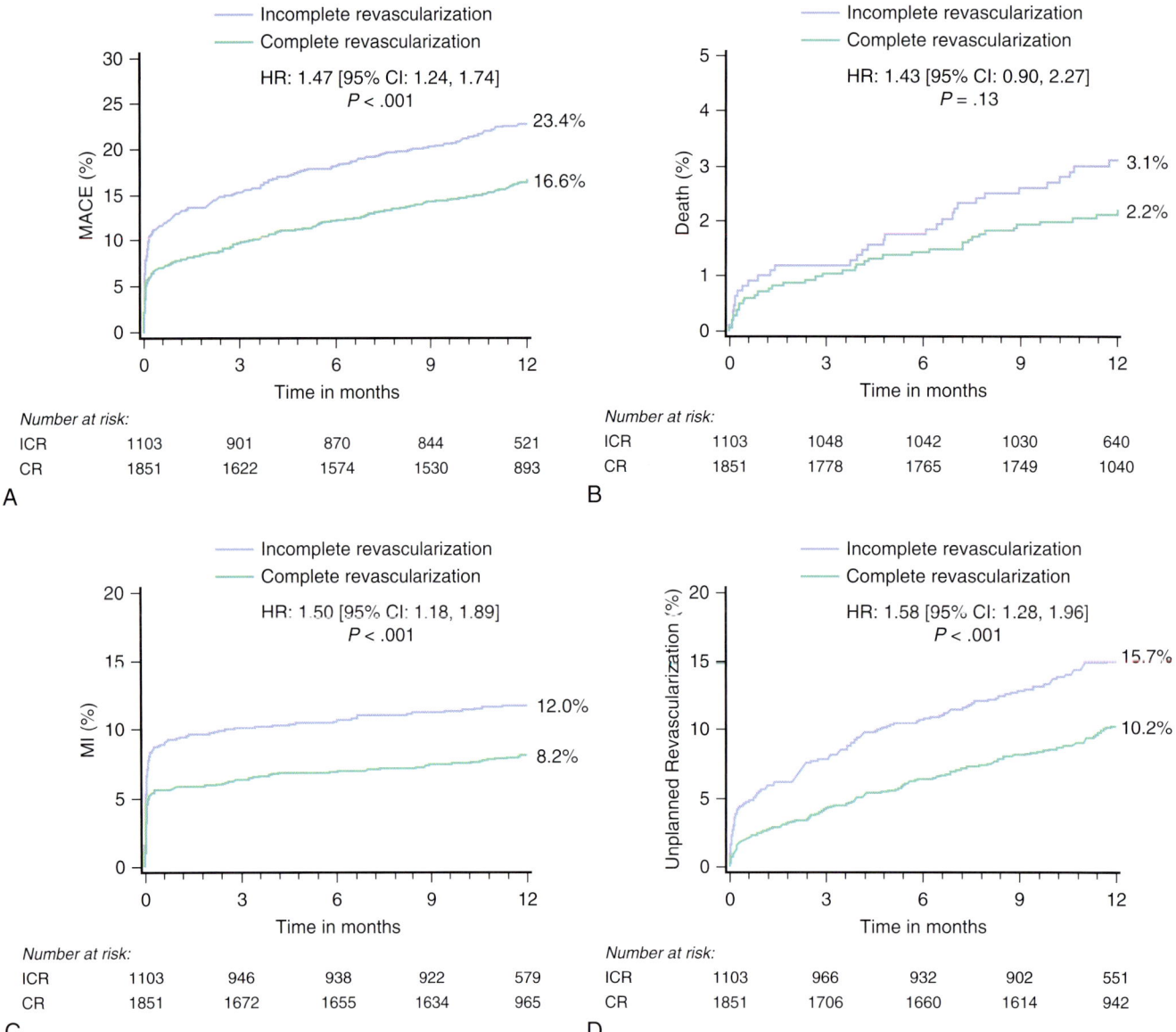

Fig. 37.8 Comparison of outcomes between incomplete *(ICR)* and complete revascularization *(CR)* in patients presenting with non–ST-elevation myocardial infarction from the acute catheterization and urgent intervention triage strategy trial. Complete revascularization was associated with reductions in the composite end point of major adverse cardiovascular events *(MACE)* (A), as well as the individual end points of death (B), myocardial infarction *(MI)* (C) and unplanned revascularization (D). *CI,* Confidence interval; *HR,* hazard ratio. (From Rosner GF, Kirtane AJ, Genereux P, et al. Impact of the presence and extend of incomplete angiographic revascularization after percutaneous coronary intervention in acute coronary syndromes: the Acute Catheterization and Urgent Intervention Triage Strategy (ACUITY) trial. *Circulation.* 2012;125:2613–2620.)

REGIONALIZATION OF CARE FOR CARDIOGENIC SHOCK

Given the significant clinical association between ACS and cardiogenic shock, similar variability can be seen for care delivery to patients with cardiogenic shock and, therefore, the same argument can be made for regionalization of the care for this patient group. The most recent Scientific Statement from the AHA regarding the contemporary management of cardiogenic shock advocates for the development of regionalized systems of care.[9] Despite advances in reperfusion therapy and mechanical circulatory support that have been associated with improvements in survival, significant regional disparities in evidence-based care have been reported, and in-hospital mortality remains high (27% to 51%).[118,119] Regionalized systems of care coupled with specific treatment algorithms have improved survival in high-acuity time-sensitive conditions such as acute myocardial infarction, out-of-hospital cardiac arrest, and trauma. Applying a similar framework to cardiogenic shock management may lead to improvements in survival and, although no consensus exists regarding structure, systems of care are emerging within existing regional cardiovascular emergency care networks (Fig. 37.9).

One of the earliest regional care systems for cardiogenic shock was implemented in New York in the 1990s for the management of refractory postcardiotomy shock requiring temporary mechanical support as bridge to transplantation or recovery. The program consisted of a network of spoke hospitals located within a 250-mile radius of a hub institution. Implementation of this network was associated with a 66% survival rate, compared with the 25% historical survival rate.[120] The concept of a "traveling shock team" within a regional hub-and-spoke model was further developed in the cardiac-RESCUE study, where investigators created a network of 22 tertiary and 53 community hospitals that transferred patients with cardiogenic shock to three designated centers using a mobile extracorporeal membrane oxygenation team, consisting of a surgeon, a perfusionist, and a nurse. Stabilized patients were subsequently transferred to the hub institution.[121] Similar teams have been successfully implemented at the Mayo Clinic Arizona and Columbia University Medical Center in the U.S.[122,123] These studies demonstrated the feasibility of mobile shock teams that can be used to successfully facilitate early support and treatment of patients with cardiogenic shock within a hub-and-spoke model. Characteristics of hub centers for care of patients with cardiogenic shock have been proposed by the AHA Scientific Statement (Table 37.1).[9]

LIMITED MEDICAL RESOURCES

The current trend for proliferation of small "heart centers" under the premise of patient convenience is counter to the well-established link between higher procedural volumes and better clinical outcomes, and it taxes critically limited resource pools, including those of specialized nurses and subspecialty-trained physician providers.[124] One strategy for dealing with the mismatch between the consensus evidence in favor of an interventional (catheter-based) approach to the treatment of ACS along with the resources required to care for patients with cardiogenic shock and the ability to deliver such care is to construct regionalized systems for ACS care and to have medical centers extend care coordination beyond the traditional boundaries of a hospital.[8,14,79] A *system* is defined as an integrated group of entities within a region that coordinate the provision of diagnostic and treatment services. A *STEMI care system* or a *cardiogenic shock care system* includes EMS providers, referral (non–PCI-capable) hospitals, PCI-capable hospitals, and others.[7,12] Participants share protocols and have predefined action plans based on regional consensus of how best to provide optimal patient care that complies with contemporary professional society guidelines.

The proliferation of small "heart" programs focused on PCI with duplication of services further taxes limited resource pools

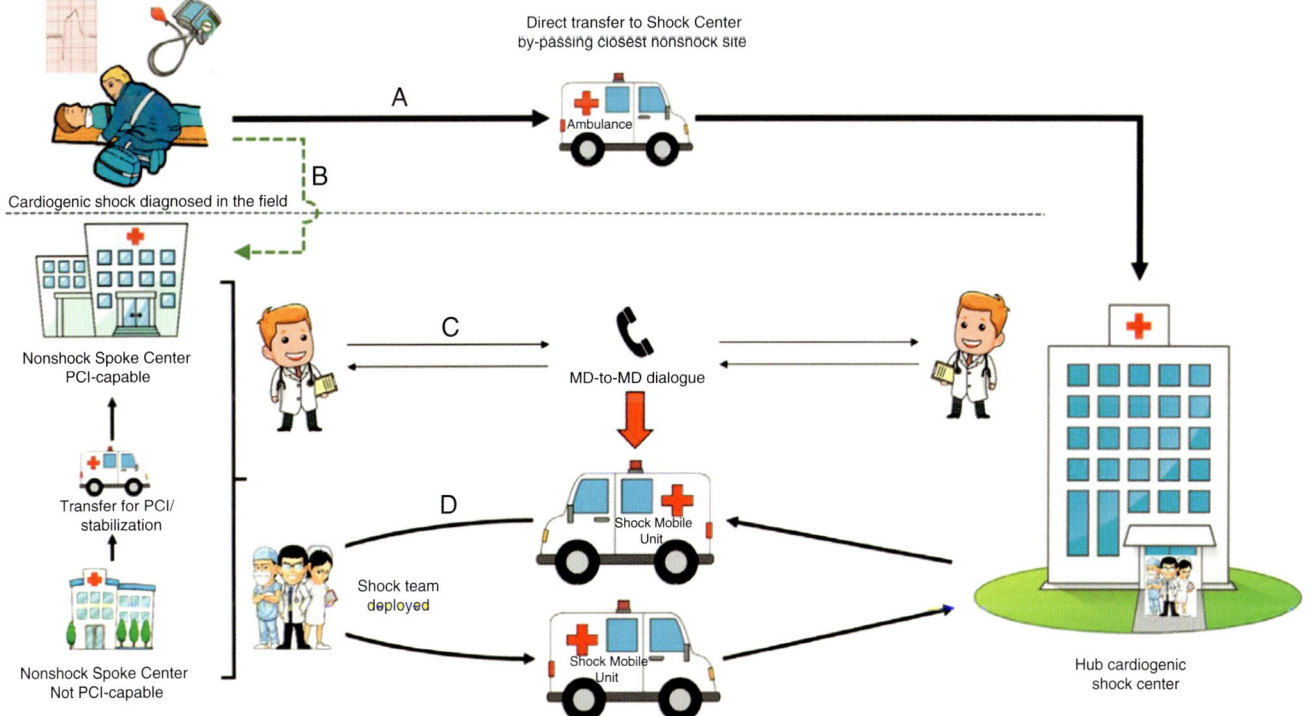

Fig. 37.9 Example of a proposed regional system of care for cardiogenic shock. *MD*, Medical doctor; *PCI*, percutaneous coronary intervention. (Reprinted with permission. *Circulation*. 2017;136:e232–e268 ©2017 American Heart Association, Inc.)

TABLE 37.1 Proposed Requirements for a "Hub" Care Center for Cardiogenic Shock

Critical Care Unit	Medical and Technological Capabilities	On-site Medical Consultants	Professional Consultants	Academic Characteristics
CICU or ICU	24-h/7-day Primary PCI	Cardiology: interventionalists, echocardiographers, advanced HF/transplantation specialists Electrophysiology	Pharmacy	CS research or participation in national registries
		Palliative care		
		Neurology		
24-h/7-day In-house unit coverage by MD, PA, NP, or resident	Cardiac surgery	Cardiologist-intensivists or intensive care	Social work	Quality improvement and auditing
1:1 Nurse-to-patient ratio	IABP	Cardiac surgery	Respiratory therapist	Trainee education
Vasoactive infusions	Percutaneous VAD	Nephrology	Physical therapy	
Mechanical ventilation	Implantable VAD	Palliative care	Occupational therapy	
Invasive cardiac and hemodynamic monitoring	ECMO: mobile ECMO team and eCPR capabilities		Dietician	
CRRT	Echocardiography		Pharmacy	
Temporary transvenous pacing			Social work	

CICU, Cardiac intensive care unit; *CRRT*, continuous renal replacement therapy; *CS*, cardiac sciences; *ECMO*, extracorporeal membrane oxygenation; *eCPR*, extracorporeal cardiopulmonary resuscitation; *HF*, heart failure; *IPPB*, intraaortic balloon pump; *ICU*, intensive care unit; *MD*, medical doctor; *NP*, nurse practitioner; *PA*, physician assistant; *PCI*, percutaneous coronary intervention; *VAD*, ventricular assist device.
Source: American Heart Association, Inc.

and appears unnecessary in the context that the majority (>80%) of the adult U.S. population lives within a 60-minute ground transport commute to an existing PCI center.[43] In fact, the proliferation/expansion of PCI-capable hospitals in the United States has been largely confined to urban and suburban regions and has had very limited impact on an increase in access to PCI for STEMI patients.[125] Indeed, it appears that most metropolitan regions in the United States would be better served from a cost-effectiveness perspective to adopt the strategy of EMS integration with existing PCI-capable facilities rather than to build additional PCI centers in geographic proximity.[82] A recent analysis suggests that statewide legislated mandates for hospital transport of STEMI patients successfully expedites guideline compliant STEMI care without an increase in PCI-providing centers.[62] Thus, mandated modification of EMS process significantly reduced total ischemic time to PPCI without change in existing PCI capacity.[126]

Future Care of ST-Elevation Myocardial Infarction Patients

At present, the lack of a coordinated system of care denies many patients the benefit of timely PPCI. A coordinated system for the provision of PCI could prevent an estimated six to eight MACCEs per 100 STEMI patients treated and might thus affect 35,000 patients yearly.[7,78] However, the current scheme for cardiovascular reimbursement could penalize community hospitals without cardiac cath labs when patients are transferred or admitted directly to a regional center.[7] An adjustment to the reimbursement strategy, possibly to include regional networks of partnering community and tertiary care centers, must be addressed. Non–PCI-capable hospitals could be incentivized to risk stratify and transfer patients presenting with STEMI, cardiogenic shock, and/or OHCA based on risk as well as transport time and distance. Such contractually defined networks could provide similar quality-ensured and monitored, protocol-driven algorithms for care with predefined systems for prompt patient transport. Confounding issues such as case mix index could be defined by the system rather than by the individual hospital.

Credentialing and criteria for development of a center of excellence for STEMI, cardiogenic shock, and OHCA care should include the established ability to provide prehospital diagnosis of STEMI with a transmitted 12-lead ECG via integration with local and regional EMS providers and generally accepted protocols for diagnosis, treatment, and triage.[7,78] To be successful, a system for care should comprise multiple integral components that include a patient care focus, enhanced operational efficiency, appropriate system incentives (pay for performance, pay for value), specific outcome and process measures, and mechanisms for quality review with continuous quality improvement. Professional societies and organizations are in the process of developing the credentialing criteria for these centers. State and/or local government agencies could be charged with the oversight of legitimacy for regional STEMI, cardiogenic shock, and OHCA networks, and CPG adherence and monitoring could be performed by established systems rather than by individual hospitals and centers. Treatment, outcome, and performance data acquisition and analysis will be standardized with appropriate and timely feedback to participating systems and centers. Individual states have been charged with development of regional coordinators to provide oversight, monitoring, and support for participating systems and centers. We support the development and credentialing for the designation in a manner similar to established stroke and trauma center designations. Suggested criteria are listed in Table 37.2.

The process for development of systems of care for STEMI patients has already been initiated by the AHA and is the subject of ongoing stakeholder meetings. The AHA has issued a call to action to improve the implementation and timeliness of infarct reperfusion with PPCI that carefully considers the ideal system from the perspective of each constituent, which includes the patient, physician, EMS provider, non-PCI capable hospital, PCI-capable center, and payer. Given the importance of time to treatment for STEMI patients, the ideal system of care will likely be different for various geographic locales (urban/suburban vs. rural) and will consider the risk of MI in the individual patient. Recommendations should be forthcoming for additional research and requisite changes in policy to support the construct and implementation of systems that will improve quality care and outcomes for STEMI patients. In a similar fashion, the AHA has also established initial criterion for caring for patients with cardiogenic shock that includes developing regional care networks. Patients with these critical illnesses will be better served through further collaborative efforts to deliver optimal care.

TABLE 37.2 Criteria for Acute Cardiovascular Care Centers

CRITERIA FOR A LEVEL 1 ACUTE CARDIOVASCULAR EMERGENCY CENTER
1. 24-h cardiac catheterization laboratory available
2. 24-h cardiovascular surgery availability
3. Comprehensive interventional cardiology and cardiovascular surgery services
4. More than 200 PCI patients/year (>36 STEMI) per hospital
5. More than 75 PCI patients/year per interventional cardiologist
6. EMS integration with prehospital 12-lead ECG transmission
7. Standardized protocols at referral and receiving hospitals
8. Transfer agreements in place/transportation system available
9. Education and training programs for transport, referral, and receiving hospital personnel
10. Quality assurance program
11. Comprehensive care for cardiogenic shock including advanced hemodynamic support (i.e., ECMO, LVAD, Impella, and/or TandemHeart)
12. Comprehensive care for out-of-hospital cardiac arrest (i.e., hypothermia, Lucas device, etc.)
13. Comprehensive care for acute aortic dissection and abdominal aortic aneurysm

CRITERIA FOR A LEVEL 2 ACUTE CARDIOVASCULAR EMERGENCY CENTER
Same as in 1 through 10 above with transfer agreements/protocols in place with a level 1 center for cardiogenic shock, out-of-hospital cardiac arrest, and aortic disease

CRITERIA FOR A LEVEL 3 ACUTE CARDIOVASCULAR EMERGENCY CENTER
Same as for level 2 but without 24-h surgical availability and with transfer agreements/protocols in place with level 1 and/or 2 centers

CRITERIA FOR A LEVEL 4 ACUTE CARDIOVASCULAR EMERGENCY CENTER
No PCI or surgical availability but with transfer agreements/protocols in place with level 1, 2, and 3 centers

ECG, Electrocardiography; *ECMO,* extracorporeal membrane oxygenation; *EMS,* emergency medical services; *LVAD,* left ventricular assist device; *PCI,* percutaneous coronary intervention; *STEMI,* ST-elevation myocardial infarction.
Modified from Henry TD, Atkins JM, Cunningham MS, et al. ST-segment elevation myocardial infarction: recommendations on triage of patients to heart attack centers—is it time for a national policy for the treatment of ST-segment elevation myocardial infarction? *J Am Coll Cardiol.* 2006;47:1339–1345.

In conclusion, an abundance of data supports the regionalization of care for patients with ACS and cardiogenic shock. Centers of excellence provide higher levels of guideline-based care, both in the catheterization laboratory and throughout the care continuum. Limited medical resources and care delivery gaps should prompt a refocus on developing pathways to optimize care delivery for ACS/shock, particularly as the complexity of CAD increases and the importance of a HEART team approach to these increasingly complex patients becomes more mainstream.

KEY REFERENCES

7. Jacobs AK, Antman EM, Ellrodt G, et al. American Heart Association's Acute Myocardial Infarction Advisory Working Group. Recommendation to develop strategies to increase the number of ST-segment-elevation myocardial infarction patients with timely access to primary percutaneous coronary intervention. *Circulation.* 2006;113:2152–2163.
8. Topol EJ, Kereiakes DJ. Regionalization of care for acute ischemic heart disease: a call for specialized centers. *Circulation.* 2003;107:1463–1466.
9. van Diepen S, Katz JN, Albert NM, et al. American Heart Association Council on Clinical Cardiology; Council on Cardiovascular and Stroke Nursing; Council on Quality of Care and Outcomes Research; Mission: Lifeline. Contemporary management of cardiogenic shock: a scientific statement from the American Heart Association. *Circulation.* 2017;136:e232–e268.
17. Garcia-Dorado D, Garcia del Blanco B. Door-to-balloon time and mortality. *N Engl J Med.* 2014;370:179.
24. Srinivas VS, Hailpern SM, Koss E, et al. Effect of physician volume on the relationship between hospital volume and mortality during primary angioplasty. *J Am Coll Cardiol.* 2009;53:574–579.
25. Kontos MC, Wang Y, Chaudhry SI, et al. NCDR. Lower hospital volume is associated with higher in-hospital mortality in patients undergoing primary percutaneous coronary intervention for ST-segment-elevation myocardial infarction: a report from the NCDR. *Circ Cardiovasc Qual Outcomes.* 2013;6:659–667.
28. Dehmer GJ, Blankenship JC, Cilingiroglu M, et al. Society for Cardiovascular Angiography and Interventions; American College of Cardiology; American Heart Association. SCAI/ACC/AHA expert consensus document: 2014 update on percutaneous coronary intervention without on-site surgical backup. *Catheter Cardiovasc Interv.* 2014;84:169–187.
36. Menees DS, Peterson ED, Wang Y, et al. Door-to-balloon time and mortality among patients undergoing primary PCI. *N Engl J Med.* 2013;369:901–909.
40. Aversano T, Lemmon CC, Liu L. For the Atlantic C-PORT Investigators. Outcomes of PCI at hospitals with or without on-site cardiac surgery. *N Engl J Med.* 2012;366:1792–1802.
41. Jacobs AK, Normand SL, Mauri L. PCI at hospitals with or without on-site cardiac surgery. *N Engl J Med.* 2013;369:392–393.
42. Langabeer JR, Henry TD, Kereiakes DJ, et al. Growth in percutaneous coronary intervention capacity relative to population and disease prevalence. *J Am Heart Assoc.* 2013;2:e000370.
43. Nallamothu BK, Bates ER, Wang Y, et al. Driving times and distances to hospitals with percutaneous coronary intervention in the United States: implications for prehospital triage of patients with ST-elevation myocardial infarction. *Circulation.* 2006;113:1189–1195.
44. Concannon TW, Nelson J, Kent DM, et al. Evidence of systematic duplication by new percutaneous coronary intervention programs. *Circ Cardiovasc Qual Outcomes.* 2013;6:400–408.
64. Diercks DB, Kontos MC, Chen AY, et al. Utilization and impact of pre-hospital electrocardiograms for patients with acute ST-segment elevation myocardial infarction: data from the NCDR (National Cardiovascular Data Registry) ACTION (Acute Coronary Treatment and Intervention Outcomes Network) Registry. *J Am Coll Cardiol.* 2009;53:161–166.
71. Garvey JL, MacLeod BA, Sopko G, et al. National Heart Attack Alert Program (NHAAP) Coordinating Committee; National Heart, Lung, and Blood Institute (NHLBI); National Institutes of Health. Pre-hospital 12-lead electrocardiography programs: a call for implementation by emergency medical services systems providing advanced life support—National Heart Attack Alert Program (NHAAP) Coordinating Committee; National Heart, Lung, and Blood Institute (NHLBI); National Institutes of Health. *J Am Coll Cardiol.* 2006;47:485–491.
72. Dieker HJ, Liem SS, El Aidi H, et al. Pre-hospital triage for primary angioplasty: direct referral to the intervention center versus interhospital transport. *JACC Cardiovasc Interv.* 2010;3:705–711.
78. Jacobs AK, Antman EM, Faxon DP, et al. Development of systems of care for ST-elevation myocardial infarction patients: executive summary. *Circulation.* 2007;116:217–230.
82. Concannon TW, Kent DM, Normand SL, et al. Comparative effectiveness of ST–segment-elevation myocardial infarction regionalization strategies. *Circ Cardiovasc Qual Outcomes.* 2010;3:506–513.

84. Levine GN, Bates ER, Blankenship JC, et al. 2015 ACC/AHA/SCAI focused update on primary percutaneous coronary intervention for patients with ST-elevation myocardial infarction: an update of the 2011 ACCF/AHA/SCAI guideline for percutaneous coronary intervention and the 2013 ACCF/AHA guideline for the management of ST-elevation myocardial infarction. *J Am Coll Cardiol*. 2016;67:1235–1250.
94. Bavry AA, Kumbhani DJ, Rassi AN, et al. Benefit of early invasive therapy in acute coronary syndromes: a meta-analysis of contemporary randomized clinical trials. *J Am Coll Cardiol*. 2006;48:1319–1325.
96. Fox KA, Clayton TC, Damman P, FIR Collaboration, et al. Long-term outcome of a routine versus selective invasive strategy in patients with non–ST-segment elevation acute coronary syndrome a meta-analysis of individual patient data. *J Am Coll Cardiol*. 2010;55:2435–2445.
101. McCabe JM, Joynt KE, Welt FG, et al. Impact of public reporting and outlier status identification on percutaneous coronary intervention case selection in Massachusetts. *JACC Cardiovasc Interv*. 2013;6:625–630.
103. Amsterdam EA, Wenger NK, Brindis RG, et al. 2014 AHA/ACC guideline for the management of patients with non–ST-elevation acute coronary syndromes: a report of the American College of Cardiology/American Heart Association Task Force on Practice Guidelines. *J Am Coll Cardiol*. 2014;64:e139–228.
105. Henry TD, Sharkey SW, Burke MN, et al. A regional system to provide timely access to percutaneous coronary intervention for ST-elevation myocardial infarction. *Circulation*. 2007;116:721–728.
111. Jollis JG, Al-Khalidi HR, Monk L, et al. Regional Approach to Cardiovascular Emergencies (RACE) Investigators. Expansion of a regional ST-segment-elevation myocardial infarction system to an entire state. *Circulation*. 2012;126:189–195.
114. Jollis JG, Granger CB, Henry TD, et al. Systems of care for ST-segment-elevation myocardial infarction: a report From the American Heart Association's Mission: Lifeline. *Circ Cardiovasc Qual Outcomes*. 2012;5:423–428.
117. Jollis JG, Al-Khalidi HR, Roettig ML, et al. Mission: Lifeline STEMI Systems Accelerator Project. Regional systems of care demonstration project: American Heart Association Mission: Lifeline STEMI Systems Accelerator. *Circulation*. 2016;134:365–374.

Additional references available online at expertconsult.com.

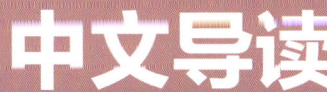

中文导读

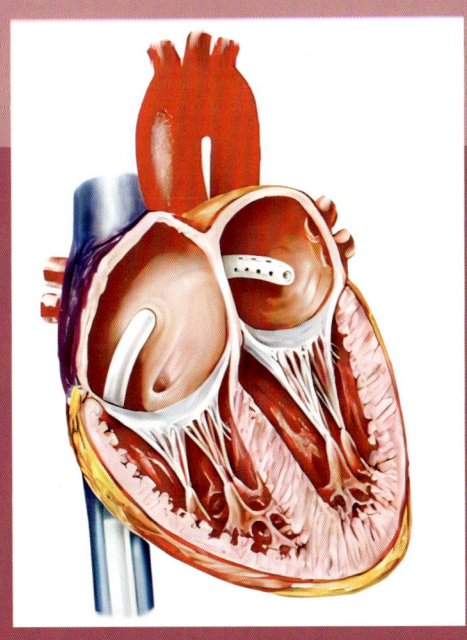

第38章
冠状动脉微血管疾病的诊断与治疗

　　冠状动脉循环包括微循环和心外膜冠状动脉，其中与冠状动脉微循环相关的疾病即为冠状动脉微血管疾病，它在有心血管危险因素的患者中普遍存在，并且与不良事件风险增加相关。研究表明，冠状动脉微血管疾病患者也存在大血管动脉粥样硬化，包括阻塞性和非阻塞性。如果患者的心绞痛症状、无创应激试验和冠状动脉造影之间存在不一致时，必须系统地评估冠状动脉微血管疾病是否是心源性胸痛的生理学合理原因。

　　本章主要作为评估有症状非阻塞性冠状动脉疾病患者的概述。从涉及病史和物理、实验室和潜在无创成像的初始检查开始，下一步是根据冠状动脉造影、生理学手段（如血流储备分数、瞬时无波型比率）和影像学评估（如冠状动脉CT血管造影、CT-FFR、血管内超声、光学相干断层成像等）排除阻塞性冠心病。一旦梗阻性冠心病被消除，需要对冠状动脉微循环的侵入性进行评估，该评估将通过适当的方案和设备以标准的方式进行。这是通过冠状动脉内腺苷、乙酰胆碱和硝酸甘油来实现的，以获得CFRne、CFRe，并评估心外膜血管痉挛和平滑肌功能。医师应及时准确地报告这些结果，并提供详细的解释。通过这些简单的策略，可以安全有效地评估和医师护理冠状动脉微血管疾病患者。冠状动脉微血管疾病患者的治疗应以功能性血管造影的结果为指导，大多数在策略上应侧重基本预防原则，如减肥、合理饮食、运动等。对于有功能性血管造影异常的患者，治疗应以心外膜异常、微血管异常、血管扩张剂异常和非血管扩张剂异常的机制和部位为指导。最后，应考虑建立一个专门的胸痛诊所，以规范评估胸痛的流程，建立持续和长期治疗症状的最佳实践，并为这些患者提供持续的随访。

林小龙　范　谦

章节要点

- 血管生理学基于以下基本方程：CO（流量）＝压差（ΔP）÷阻力（R）。因此，冠状动脉血流在很大程度上是由心肌氧合的供求不匹配驱动的，需要增加心肌基质的输送。
- 冠状动脉微循环是心肌灌注的主要调节器，在很大程度上取决于血管张力对内皮衍生因子如一氧化氮的反应。
- 基线时，心肌几乎处于循环中的最大吸氧量。因此，心肌耗氧量的任何增加都高度依赖于冠状动脉血流的增加。
- 冠状动脉血流储备是冠状动脉生理学中的一个重要概念，因为它代表了正常循环能力，以增加冠状动脉血流应对心肌需求和压力的增加。
- 冠状动脉血流储备可以通过多普勒血流图进行有创性评估，该图可以捕捉腺苷输注后红细胞速度的变化；然后可以得到多普勒速度与静止速度的比值。
- 冠状动脉血流储备异常提示需对可能主要损害心肌微循环的潜在疾病进行检查。

38 Diagnosis and Treatment of Coronary Microvascular Disease

Amir Lerman, R. Jay Widmer

KEY POINTS

- Vascular physiology is grounded in the following basic equation: CO (flow) equals the pressure difference (ΔP) divided by the resistance (R). Resultantly, coronary blood flow (CBF) is largely driven by supply/demand mismatches in myocardial oxygenation, requiring increased delivery of substrate to the myocardium.
- The coronary microcirculation is the primary regulator of myocardial perfusion and is largely dependent on vessel tone in response to endothelial-derived factors such as nitric oxide (NO).
- At baseline, the myocardium is almost at maximal oxygen extraction from the circulation. Thus any increase in myocardial oxygen consumption is highly dependent on an increase in CBF.
- Coronary flow reserve (CFR) is an important concept in coronary physiology as it represents the normal circulatory ability to increase CBF in response to increased demands and stressors on the myocardium.
- CFR can be assessed invasively using a Doppler flow wire that captures changes in red cell velocity after the infusion of adenosine; thereafter a ratio of the Doppler velocity to the resting velocity can be obtained.
- Abnormal CFR should prompt a workup for underlying diseases that might primarily impair the microcirculation of the myocardium.

INTRODUCTION

Conventional angiography visually and subjectively assesses only approximately 5% to 10% of coronary arteriolar anatomy.[1] The remaining 90% to 95% of the coronary vasculature requires a detailed and systematic approach to successfully evaluate patients with typical symptoms of cardiac angina without obvious obstructive coronary artery disease (CAD). In the visible conduits, an atherosclerotic lesion greater than 70% has traditionally been treated with revascularization—surgical or percutaneous—for the resolution of symptoms.[2] In cases where there is discordance between the patient's anginal symptoms, noninvasive stress testing, and the coronary luminogram, one must methodically evaluate for coronary microvascular dysfunction (CMD) as a physiologically plausible cause of cardiac chest pain. This chapter aims to inform the reader of the basics of coronary arterial physiology with special attention to the coronary microcirculation, which should be of benefit to the practicing interventional cardiologist.

Epidemiology of Coronary Microvascular Dysfunction

Current estimates state that anywhere from 40% to 60% of patients undergoing coronary angiography for compelling symptoms or positive noninvasive testing have nonobstructive CAD (NOCAD).[3,4] Moreover, the majority of patients who have been referred for coronary angiography were found to have microvascular dysfunction.[5–7] These diagnostic and treatment dilemmas are typically overlooked because percutaneous intervention cannot address the pathophysiologic process. The evaluation of coronary epicardial and microvascular disease on top of traditional risk models like the Framingham score can correctly reclassify cardiovascular risk in nearly one-fourth of patients.[8] That these patients deserve particular attention and further evaluation is underscored by their increased morbidity, mortality, low quality of life, and high medical expenses.[8–10]

Initial Workup of Coronary Microvascular Dysfunction

The initial workup of NOCAD should include a good history and physical examination. Some clues in the history—although not absolutely indicative of microvascular disease—could include conventional risk factors (e.g., sex, smoking, hypertension, hyperlipidemia, autoimmune or inflammatory diseases such as hypothyroidism, and Reynaud disease).[5] Other important information to be obtained in the history should include chronic and acute medications and toxin ingestion. Agents documented to cause coronary vasospasm are listed in Table 38.1.

Specifically in women, a history of polycystic ovaries and toxemia of pregnancy, and in men the presence of endothelial dysfunction outside of the coronary vasculature, can be associated with CMD. Physical examination is less revealing in CMD. Laboratory abnormalities are typically nonspecific; however, abnormal thyroid function, uric acid levels, markers of inflammation such as lipoprotein PA_2 ($LpPA_2$) and C-reactive protein (CRP), white blood cell counts, and even brain natriuretic peptides can be seen in these patients. Other noninvasive imaging such as coronary computed tomography (CT) can often rule out obstructive CAD; however there is no functional testing component to assess the endothelium or microcirculation. Therefore the utilization of coronary CT may not provide appropriate information on microvascular function.

If clinically compelled by a history of typical cardiac angina, an abnormal noninvasive stress test, or even elevated cardiac biomarkers, cardiac catheterization is performed in these patients, generally revealing no obvious obstructive coronary lesion. One must make sure that obstructive coronary disease is ruled out by thoroughly inspecting the results of angiography to determine whether causative "flush" coronary occlusions or other coronary anomalies may have been missed. In several instances, the presence of coronary vasospasm can be documented; one should use intracoronary nitroglycerin to reduce vascular tone, as this can cause typical angina without obstructive CAD. Furthermore, lesions thought to be nonobstructive

TABLE 38.1 Medications, Drugs, and Toxins Known to Induce Sudden, Severe Coronary Artery Spasm

Tobacco smoking	Butane
Khat	Alcohol
Cocaine	Ecstasy/lysergic acid diethylamide
Methamphetamines	Triptans/sumatriptans
Marijuana	Chemotherapy (5-flououracil, capecitabine)

in orthogonal views should be carefully evaluated with physiologic means such as fractional flow reserve (FFR) or instantaneous flow reserve (iFR) to make sure that no hemodynamically significant lesion is present. Established metrics for nonobstructive disease in patients with 40% to 70% luminal stenosis include an FFR value above 0.80,[11] or iFR above 0.89.[12,13] Imaging with intravascular ultrasound (IVUS) or optical coherence tomography (OCT) can also be of importance to investigate potentially unstable/vulnerable plaques that may be smoldering culprit lesions. OCT is also of great importance in patients with chest pain and CMD to rule out spontaneous coronary artery dissection (SCAD), as treatment pathways will certainly diverge based on the underlying diagnosis. Evidence of moderate CAD and conditions such as anemia, tachycardia, sepsis, and so on can cause a type 2 myocardial infarction and should prompt a review looking for the underlying cause of the myocardial supply/demand mismatch, amelioration of the inciting cause, and potential adjustment of secondary prevention medications such as chronotropic, vasodilator, or antiplatelet agents in treating these patients.

Indications for further invasive testing beyond coronary angiography include a discrepancy between the degree of epicardial disease as detected by the coronary angiogram and the patient's symptoms and/or the results of the noninvasive stress test. Angina or "chest pain syndrome" can include typical and atypical features, such as exertional dyspnea; chest, neck, and shoulder discomfort; or similar symptoms with certain triggers such as physical activity, anxiety, social situations, or emotional prompts.[14] These patients could also have inconclusive or likely abnormal noninvasive testing such as exercise electrocardiography (ECG), stress imaging, CT, or magnetic resonance imaging (MRI). Stress testing often reproduces symptoms, but there could be some other abnormal component such as poor exertional effort, cardiac output limitation on VO_2 testing, abnormal anaerobic thresholds, abnormal O_2 pulse rise, a sudden increase in heart rate upon reaching anaerobic threshold, or other anginal symptoms.[15] In many cases, noninvasive stress testing can reproduce symptoms in these patients; however, there may be a discrepancy between noninvasive stress testing and both the epicardial and microvascular abnormalities found via invasive angiography.[16]

Noninvasive Imaging—Computed Tomography Angiography and Fractional Flow Reserve

CT has recently become an emerging diagnostic modality for assessing obstructive coronary disease in low-risk patients. Coronary CT can detect obstructive CAD, and these findings have correlated with overall cardiac outcomes.[17] There are, however, inherent limitations regarding lower sensitivity in women, poor specificity in the setting of coronary calcium, and exposure to radiation and contrast dye. CT-FFR has now developed into a means by which to assess the physiologic significance of obstructive CAD with an improvement in diagnostic accuracy of 36% compared with coronary CT alone (A Randomised Controlled Trial to Compare Routine Pressure Wire Assessment With Conventional Angiography in the Management of Patients With Coronary Artery Disease [RIPCORD])[18] as well as improved sensitivity and specificity (area under the curve increased to .92) in the Diagnosis of Ischemia-Causing Stenoses Obtained Via Noninvasive Fractional Flow Reserve (DISCOVER-FLOW) trial.[19] CT-FFR values below .80 nearly doubled the probability of revascularization (2.9 to 4.3, $P = .03$) compared to those above .80 without any change in cardiovascular outcomes in the PROspective Multicenter Imaging Study for Evaluation of Chest Pain (PROMISE) trial [20] with the caveat that only one-third of the patients had diagnostic CT-FFR images. Finally, in results from the Prospective LongitudinAl Trial of FFRct: Outcome and Resource IMpacts (PLATFORM) trial, CT-FFR demonstrated improved specificity in which patients were sent to the catheterization lab without a difference in clinical outcomes.[21] These imaging modalities are certainly promising in the realm of assessing obstructive CAD; however, they have not been tested or validated in assessing the microcirculation—only in excluding obstructive CAD. Further invasive assessments in the catheterization laboratory are likely still necessary should coronary CT be unrevealing.

Physiologic Basis of Functional Coronary Assessment

The primary role of epicardial coronary vessels is conductance, while the microcirculation matches blood supply to myocardial oxygen requirements (mostly though modulation of arteriolar tone) and makes possible the interchange of oxygen, nutrients, and metabolites between myocytes and blood in the capillary network. The mechanism for ischemia generation in epicardial vessels is the impairment of conductance caused by inward plaque growth during atherogenesis, intraluminal obstruction caused by thrombus, and/or coronary spasm. Conversely, CMD results mostly from inadequate coronary arteriolar autoregulation and, less frequently, from structural remodeling of arterioles of the capillary bed, intraluminal plugging, or microvascular edema/hemorrhage impairing the conductance of the microvasculature (Fig. 38.1).

The invasive assessment of vascular function has been historically described[5,10,22-26] and should be divided based on the mechanism of reduction in coronary flow reserve (CFR) to determine if the abnormalities in the CFR are nonendothelial-dependent (CFRne) or endothelial-dependent (CFRe). These invasive measures recorded in the cardiac catheterization lab can be performed with very high fidelity and safety, including intracoronary vascular reactivity testing.[28,29] Assessing the ability of the microvasculature to meet myocardial demand, CFR is one measure of the ability of the coronary circulation to augment blood flow with stress measured as a ratio of maximal coronary blood flow (CBF) (usually drug-induced) and baseline physiological blood flow.

Protocol for Functional Coronary Artery Assessment

Approach

In patients without obstructive CAD as determined by imaging and physiologic assessment wherein further invasive assessment of the microcirculation is indicated, one must carefully plan the procedure, including the equipment used (Fig. 38.2), vessels studied, and order of microvascular assessments. Traditionally these investigations are performed from a femoral approach. This is considered best for two main reasons. First, to avoid the need for vasodilators routinely administered during radial access, and, second, to accommodate the guiding and infusion catheters plus the wire required to perform the test. Ideally all vasoactive drugs should be withheld prior to testing. This is particularly important with regard to nitrates and calcium channel blockers. Other vasoactive substances, such as nicotine and caffeine, should be withheld for 12 hours prior to testing. Furthermore, operators experienced in performing and interpreting these tests should be consulted in the study of these patients so that technical success is maximized in addition to arriving at a proper diagnosis.

Unless otherwise indicated by regional abnormalities on a noninvasive stress testing, the left anterior descending (LAD) artery is the vessel of choice for these studies. This vessel subtends the most myocardium, is typically very approachable with the equipment

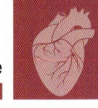

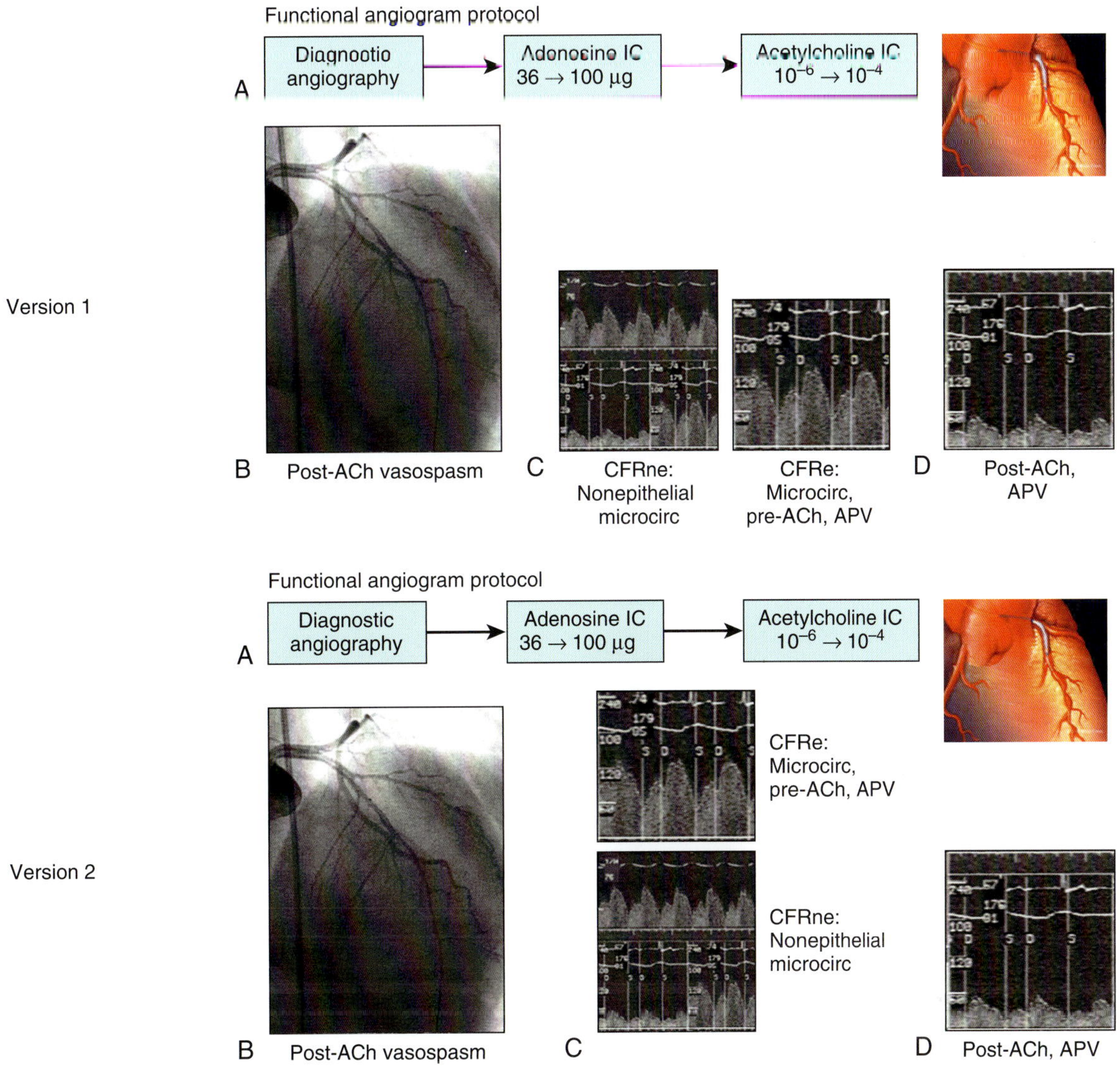

Fig. 38.1 Typical functional angiograms demonstrating changes in coronary flow reserve (CFR) in an endothelial-dependent *(CFRe)* and non–endothelial-dependent *(CFRne)* manner. The protocol, initiated with diagnostic angiography (A) and moving on to adenosine and acetylcholine *(ACh)* infusion, is depicted on top. The angiogram (far left) shows an example of vasoconstriction after the administration of ACh. (B) CFRne is assessed using blood-flow-velocity profiles *(APV,* average peak velocity) at rest and after adenosine infusion (bottom middle). Assessment of CFRe is depicted on the far right (C) with a normal pre-ACh reading consisting of a predominant diastolic component on the top. The lower right panel (D) shows a marked reduction in APV after the infusion of ACh, indicative of poor microvascular recruitment of blood flow as seen in patients with microvascular disease. *IC,* Intracoronary.

due to its large caliber, and can easily be assessed in terms of Doppler velocities and diameter quantifications. The left circumflex or right coronary arteries can be studied if inferior or lateral changes are seen on the noninvasive test or if transient ischemic mitral regurgitation secondary to posterior/lateral ischemia is in question. If these arteries are to be studied, changes in the selection of a guiding catheter may have to be made, in addition to reductions in dosing of provocative medications.

Some patients who have previously undergone stent implantation for obstructive CAD can have further angina symptoms without the reemergence of obstructive CAD or restenosis. There are data that show abnormal coronary reactivity in vessel segments distal to the stented segment.[30-33] Assessing coronary reactivity mainly distal to the stent and pertaining to the microcirculation can be important in evaluating chest pain in these patients. The protocols described below can be conducted distal to previously placed stents using careful wiring of these vessels to avoid trapping the wire beneath a stent strut or deforming the stent.

Equipment

A 7-Fr guide is predominantly used. This is typically an extra backup (EBU/XB) or Judkins left shape depending on the anatomy (Figs. 38.3 and 38.4). Recently the ability to utilize a 7.5-Fr sheathless guide or 7-Fr radial sheaths and guides has allowed these procedures to be performed using the radial approach. One caveat to this approach is the potential for radial artery spasm requiring intraarterial vasodilators such as nitroglycerin and verapamil, which may influence the results of the catheterization and velocity measurements, thereby interfering with an accurate assessment of the microvasculature. To avoid catheter or wire thrombosis, intravenous heparin should be administered at a standard dose (60 to 80 IU heparin/kg body weight) to ensure an activated clotting time (ACT) greater than 250 seconds. An additional safety measure is having a syringe for intraarterial nitroglycerin readily available should coronary spasm unexpectedly occur.

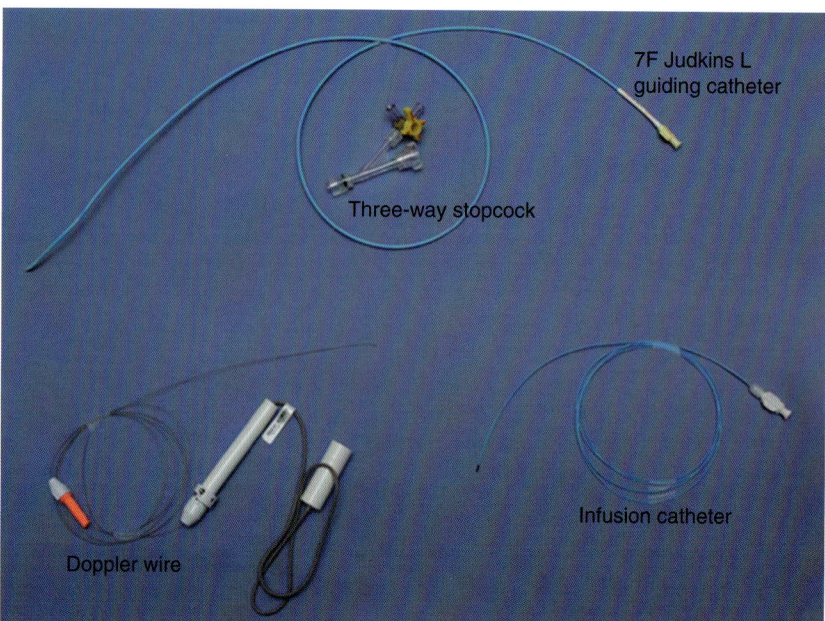

Fig. 38.2 Equipment used in functional angiography, including a guide catheter and three-way stopcock *(top)*, 3-Fr infusion catheter *(bottom right)*, and Doppler wire *(bottom left)*.

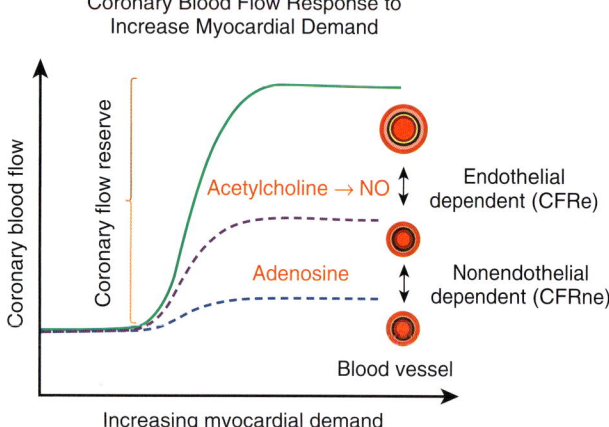

Fig. 38.3 Increasing myocardial demand leads to an increase in coronary blood flow (CBF). The ratio of CBF above baseline is referred to as coronary flow reserve (CFR) and comprises a nonendothelial component *(CFRne)* and an endothelial-dependent component *(CFRe)*. *NO*, Nitric oxide.

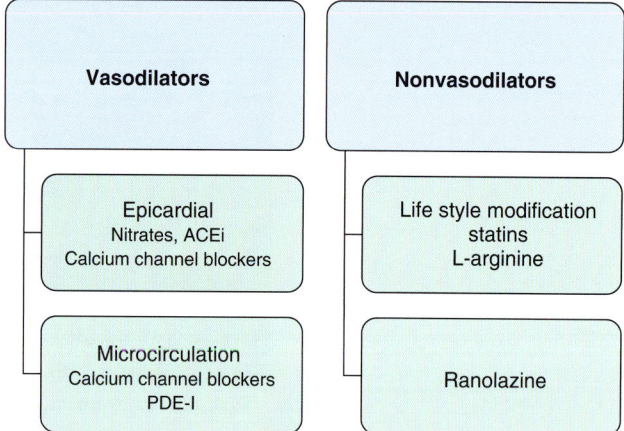

Fig. 38.4 Vasodilator and nonvasodilator strategies to improve anginal symptoms arising from either the epicardial vessels or microvasculature. *ACEi*, Angiotensin converting enzyme inhibitors; *PDE-1*, phosphodiesterase 1.

Once the 7-Fr guide has been positioned within the ostium of the left main coronary artery, the Doppler wire and infusion catheter are positioned. The infusion catheter should be positioned at the proximal to middle portion of the vessel (if the vessel is large enough to accommodate it without creating ischemia) to ensure adequate drug delivery to the distal portion of the artery with plenty of upstream vessel not directly affected by the drug infusion to test upstream flow-mediated vasodilation. Once the vessel has been successfully instrumented with the infusion catheter, one can carefully position the 0.014-inch Doppler velocity wire through the infusion catheter into the vessel being studied. Once testing is ready to begin, the guide and infusion catheter should both be properly flushed with heparinized saline and equalized. The system should not be pretreated with intracoronary nitroglycerin as this will alter blood flow independent of the endothelium or microcirculation with the smooth muscle–directed vasodilation.

An alternative to an infusion catheter placed in the coronary artery is to advance the flow wire into the LAD without the use of an infusion catheter and to infuse drug directly through the guide. While it is overall safe to perform, there is a risk of left main or proximal LAD dissection with this method, and the possibility of vasospasm throughout the left-sided coronary arteries without placement of workable coronary wires in the distal vessels.

Endothelial-Independent Microvascular Blood Flow

It is recommended to begin by obtaining CFRne once the Doppler wire and infusion catheter are both in place. The administration of intracoronary adenosine (up to 72 µg) allows for the measurement of maximal coronary endothelial independent vasodilation (intravenous adenosine would be inexact to test coronary microcirculation). This hyperemic average peak velocity (APV) is compared with the resting APV and a CFRne ratio is obtained (see Fig. 38.1). This should be repeated two to three times until a stable maximal APV is obtained.

Endothelial-Dependent Microvascular Blood Flow

Once the assessment of the nonendothelial-dependent microcirculation has been ascertained via adenosine administration and the CFRne obtained, the next step in the workup of patients with CMD is assessing the endothelial-dependent epicardial diameter and microcirculation, CFRe (based on changes of APV). This is performed with the intracoronary administration of the endothelium-dependent vasodilator acetylcholine (ACh). This will assess the endothelial-dependent vasodilatory properties of the epicardial, as well as the coronary, microvasculature. Two measurements are needed to calculate CFRe—the APV and the coronary artery luminal diameter.

Following stable positioning of the infusion catheter and with the Doppler wire in place, graded infusion of ACh should be initiated with increasing doses of ACh (10^{-6} M → 10^{-4} M, or equivalently, ACh 0.001 mmol → 0.1 mmol) for up to 3 minutes at 1 mL/min via an infusion pump. The infusion should be quickly stopped should symptoms or complications occur. During the infusion, concomitant measurement of epicardial diameter via any angiographic imaging software and APV will allow calculation of CBF. The purpose of this testing is twofold: (1) assessment of coronary epicardial vasoreactivity and (2) assessment of the ability of the endothelium of the coronary microcirculation to appropriately increase CBF. This particular protocol involves the measurement of coronary epicardial diameter at three sites along the artery: 5 mm proximal and 5 mm distal to the infusion catheter for CBF calculations (usually mid-LAD), and at the distal LAD, as well as measurement of APV after 3 minutes of each ACh infusion. Hemodynamic data as well as patient symptoms should be assessed at baseline, at the end of each 3-minute period of infusion, and after the administration of 100 to 200 μg of intracoronary nitroglycerin. Some operators will choose to administer ACh, then nitroglycerin, and finish with adenosine to obtain CFRne with the thought being to remove epicardial vessel tone with nitroglycerin prior to adenosine. Both protocols have been used and reported with comparable results.

Alternative Measurement of Coronary Blood Flow
The Kety method involves inserting a catheter in the coronary sinus and assuming N_2O concentrations. Typically there is an injection of 250 mL/min (3% to 5% CO). Another thermodilution-like method involves using radioactive nuclides (thallium, sestamibi), which measure active myocardium, or others (technetium-PYP), which detect infarcted tissue. 133-Xe washout in combination with angiography can be used to detect bulk volume over time, which is tantamount to CBF.[34]

A similar method but based on slightly different physical properties by which to test coronary microcirculatory function deals with thermodilution and index of microcirculatory resistance. This technique is similar to pharmacological and pressure-based techniques but instead uses intracoronary temperature measurements to approximate flow.[9] This has been shown to be independent of epicardial vascular function; it is reproducible and has even been evaluated in patients with ST-elevation myocardial infarction, providing important prognostic information regarding ventricular function at 3 months.[35,36] Despite reasonable prediction of events and outcomes following percutaneous intervention,[37,38] there are no guideline-based recommendations for its regular utilization in the catheterization laboratory.

Medications
Medications such as ACh and methylergometrine, a synthetic analog of ergonovine, are used in the catheterization lab to test the potential of the coronary arteries for vasospasm—providing an explanation for angina in a patient chest pain and NOCAD. directly. Normally functioning endothelium should invoke smooth muscle relaxation in response to ACh administration; however, dysfunctional endothelium will paradoxically constrict and potentially spasm. Intracoronary nitrates should be immediately available when these tests are being performed to reverse any spasm that may occur.

Methylergometrine, or methergine, is a potent nonendothelial-dependent alpha-adrenergic, dopaminergic, and serotonergic agonist that can also be used to produce coronary vasoconstriction in patients prone to coronary vasospasm. Accordingly this agent has largely fallen out of favor in testing for coronary spasm, as the risk and danger of irreversible and fatal spasm during testing outweighs the benefit of making the diagnosis. ACh has an advantage as it has a known mechanism of action with a shorter duration of action, in addition to having been extensively studied in the clinical testing of endothelial function.

Adenosine

Intracoronary adenosine administration in the catheterization laboratory serves to replicate the stressor of increased myocardial oxygen demand. As adenosine is released in response to low oxygen tension, this should induce microvascular vasodilation, which induces a potential space with the recruitment of volume of blood vessels and the decreased distal pressures create a driving force for increased CBF. The subsequent augmentation of flow—not directly dependent on the release of nitric oxide (NO) from the endothelium—correlates to the velocity reading (i.e., the APV).

In order to assess CBF, we recommend administering escalating doses of adenosine through the infusion catheter microvascular bolus administration of 36 to 72 μg.[16] Measurement should not be made until a plateau response of maximal APV is reached. If CFR is thought to be submaximal, then a further administration up to 100 μg can be given. If the testing is in the right coronary artery (RCA) (only if the RCA is the suspected culprit), 24 to 72 μg of intracoronary adenosine is recommended. If there is a clinical need to administer adenosine intravenously in order to measure FFR, one might also consider CFR testing as well as testing with ACh afterward to ensure normal endothelial function.

Acetylcholine

Under normal physiologic conditions, ACh stimulates the production and release of NO from the endothelium, which results in vasodilation and increased CBF. In patients with epicardial or microvascular endothelial dysfunction, the bioavailability of endothelial NO is reduced, and its direct action on smooth muscle cells causes vasoconstriction (called paradoxical vasoconstriction).

ACh should be infused through either the infusion catheter (see earlier) or the guide (must be prepared by careful bolusing). As mentioned previously, the doses of ACh are (in increasing fashion) 10^{-6} M (0.001 mmol), 10^{-5} M (0.01 mmol), and 10^{-4} M (0.1 mmol) for endothelial function testing. The infusion rate for each dose should be 1 mL/min for 3 minutes. One should obtain an angiogram and APV at the end of 3 minutes of infusion.

Nitroglycerin

At the completion of these tests, intracoronary nitroglycerin (an endothelium-independent epicardial vessel dilator) should be administered at a dose of 100 to 200 μg.[39] This dose will depend on systemic blood pressure; however, it has been noted that intracoronary nitroglycerin up to 200 μg has little effect on systemic blood pressure and should not affect the microcirculation. The response to intracoronary nitroglycerin is a qualitative measure of epicardial smooth muscle function manifested by an increased vessel diameter after administration. There is no appreciable direct effect of nitroglycerin on the microcirculation.[39] APV should usually decline appropriately with increased arterial diameter to maintain CBF.

Procedural Safety
Though not without risk, these additional invasive measures recorded in the cardiac catheterization lab, including the use of

TABLE 38.2 Recommended Diagnostic Parameters to Assess Endothelial-Dependent and Nonendothelial-Dependent Coronary Circulation

Medication	Nonendothelial-Dependent Function (CFRne)	Epicardial Endothelial Function	Microcirculatory Endothelial Function (CFRe)
Adenosine (microcirculation)	% change in CFR >2.5	—	—
Acetylcholine (epicardial and microcirculation)	—	% change in coronary artery diameter >20%	% change in CBF >50%
NTG (epicardial)	% change in coronary diameter, >20%	—	—

CBF, Coronary blood flow; *CFR*, coronary flow reserve; *CFRe*, endothelial-dependent CFR; *CFRne*, nonendothelium-dependent CFR; *NTG*, nitroglycerin.

intracoronary vascular reactivity testing[28,29] and IVUS,[40] can be performed with very high fidelity and safety. Aside from the usual risks of invasive coronary angiography,[41,42] there have been only rare reports of coronary artery dissection with instrumentation of the artery with the infusion catheter or wire and even more rare reports of pathological vasospasm.[5,8,28] With careful attention to safety and detail following a steady learning curve, these potential complications can be avoided or quickly reversed to avert serious patient harm.

INTERPRETATION OF THE TEST RESULTS

To assess the coronary circulation with ACh administration, we propose the following parameters for the diagnosis of epicardial versus microvascular dysfunction. Often the diagnosis of epicardial spasm—or acute and sudden vessel constriction—can be made without specific calculations and with the combination of angiographic appearance of vasoconstriction and symptoms with ACh administration. Coronary diameter can be measured with any standard catheterization laboratory imaging software and should be measured proximal to the infusion catheter, 5 mm distal to the site of ACh administration, and in the distal LAD. CBF can be calculated from measurements of coronary flow velocity and coronary cross-sectional area with the modified hydraulic equation CBF = 0.5 × velocity × area. Using the metrics obtained during testing, CBF = 0.5 × APV × (radius^2 × Π).[43] Coronary radius (diameter/2) and CBF obtained at the site and distal to the site of ACh administration assesses the direct endothelial response to ACh, whereas the diameter and CBF proximally assesses the ability of the vessel to respond to increases in blood flow. This should also include vasodilation and increase in CBF. An increase in coronary diameter of greater than 20% and/or an increase in flow of greater than 50% are considered normal (Table 38.2).[a]

Suggested Therapies

The therapy of patients with CMD should be guided by the outcomes and the results of the functional angiogram. There are no large randomized clinical trials aimed at addressing therapeutic options for these patients. Furthermore, many of the trials focus either on symptom relief or improvement in physiological CBF. Few results, however, are overtly positive. Therefore most of the treatment strategies for CMD should focus on basic prevention principles such as weight loss, proper diet,[45] and exercise.[46] In patients with an abnormal functional angiogram, the treatment should be guided by the mechanism and site of the abnormality—epicardial versus microvascular and vasodilator versus nonvasodilator therapies (see Fig. 38.4). Finally, consideration should be given to the establishment of a dedicated chest pain clinic so as to formalize procedures and protocols for the evaluation of chest pain, establish best practices for ongoing and long-term treatment of symptoms, and provide consistent follow-up for these patients.

---

[a]References 5, 10, 22, 23, 25, 32, 44.

Treatment—Nonvasodilators

Lifestyle Modification—Diet and Exercise

Some of the most intuitive evidence toward managing symptoms and recurrent events revolves around lifestyle modification[45] including the Mediterranean diet,[47] weight loss,[48] exercise,[49] and foods such as dark chocolate,[50] nuts,[51] olive oil,[52] plant-based foods,[53] and green tea,[54] and moderate alcohol consumption. Furthermore, an abbreviated version (8 weeks) of cardiac rehabilitation focusing on exercise prescription has been found to reduce symptoms in women with CMD.[55] Finally, larger meta-analytic data, despite bias secondary to inability to blind patients as well as marked heterogeneity, have demonstrated a reduction in chest pain symptoms up to 9 months following the initiation of psychological interventions, including therapy.[56]

Statins

Intuitively, the antihyperlipidemic, antiinflammatory, and pleiotropic effects of statins would seem to make them an attractive therapeutic tactic in combating microvascular disease.[57] Unfortunately the majority of our data regarding the reported efficacy of statins improving microvascular function are based on animal and human models of microvascular disease caused by diabetes. Certainly there will be some mechanistic crossover, as there are data supporting the use of statin therapy for CMD. Furthermore, one should be careful that SCAD is not the primary pathology, as case series data show a potential harm in treating SCAD patients with statins.[58]

In patients with CMD, small randomized controlled trials (RCTs) have indicated an improvement in exercise times as well as macrovascular arterial vasoreactivity after 3 to 6 months of statin use.[59–61] Nonrandomized data show a 50% improvement in invasively measured CBF in response to ACh in six patients treated for 6 months with pravastatin.[62] Although no randomized long-term data exist regarding symptom management or CBF,[57] cross-sectional data from patients with nonobstructive CAD and hyperlipidemia appropriately treated with statins demonstrate positive remodeling and improved vasoreactivity to adenosine.[63]

Treatment—Epicardial Vasodilators

Nitrates

Long-acting oral nitrates have little benefit unless preload reduction is beneficial or there is epicardial smooth muscle–dependent spasm present on cardiac catheterization, as these agents have little beneficial effect on the microcirculation. This was shown in a small comparator RCT with nitrates, amlodipine, and atenolol where there was no benefit in terms of symptoms with oral isosorbide mononitrate.[64] Similarly, no improvement in exercise performance or CBF assessed by echocardiography was found after short-term administration of isosorbide dinitrate.[65] Nevertheless, use of oral or transdermal nitroglycerin can result in symptom relief particularly for patients with clinical and physiologic evidence of epicardial vasospasm.

Angiotensin Converting Enzyme Inhibitors

ACE inhibitors are a mainstay in treating obstructive CAD in patients after myocardial infarction or with reduced left ventricular function.[66,67] The potential beneficial impact on the coronary microcirculation through enhanced vasodilatory pathways, reduced oxidative stress, and improvement in NO bioavailability, creates the potential to offer therapeutic benefit for those with CMD. Small RCTs show a benefit on exercise capacity/symptoms,[61,68,69] as well as angina frequency[68] using both ramipril and quinapril. Furthermore, data from the Women's Ischemia Syndrome Evaluation (WISE) study indicate that quinapril can be effectively used to improve symptoms in CMD patients in conjunction with an improvement in CFR.[70] Improvements in CBF could be related to improved NO bioavailability and activity.[71]

β-Blockers

β-Blocker properties include reducing myocardial oxygen consumption through reductions in heart rate and preload/afterload, which make them useful in obstructive CAD and theoretically in CMD. There is also the converse theory that β-blockers could cause unopposed alpha vasoconstriction; however, this has never been seen clinically. Small trials have demonstrated benefit of atenolol (100 mg daily) in patients with symptomatic CMD in terms of angina attacks and diastolic echocardiographic parameters, but it had minimal effect on symptoms during exercise.[72] Exercise benefits were also not seen with other β-blockers, including 4 weeks of acebutolol therapy (400 mg daily)[73] or propranolol (160 mg daily) for 2 weeks.[74] Only nebivolol has been shown to improve CFR as a one-time dose in patients with obstructive CAD and low CFR at baseline.[75] Another small RCT of nebivolol versus atenolol demonstrated no significant differences in CFR or endothelial dysfunction between the two cohorts at 1 year.[76] Moreover, fatigue was a substantial side effect of such high doses of beta blockade in all of these small RCTs.

Treatment—Microvascular Vasodilators
Calcium channel antagonists

Most practitioners find success in reducing symptoms with calcium channel blockade.[77] Small crossover RCTs have demonstrated symptomatic benefit using dihydropyridine calcium channel blockers.[68,78] There are, however, some conflicting data regarding the dihydropyridine calcium channel blocker amlodipine[65]; this could be secondary to an unpredictable reflex sympathetic activation seen with peripheral vasodilation in some patients.[79] Nondihydropyridine calcium channel antagonists have variable effects, as some studies show a benefit on symptoms related to vasospasm[78] and others show no benefit over placebo using verapamil.[80] Initial work showed little effect of acute intravenous diltiazem on CBF.[81] However, more recent data with larger patient samples and longer follow-up using low-dose (90 mg twice daily) diltiazem showed marked improvements in CBF assessed by CFR and angina symptoms.[82]

L-Arginine

L-arginine, a precursor of NO, may ameliorate chest pain in patients with macrovascular or microvascular disturbances mostly secondary to endothelial dysfunction.[83] Oral L-arginine supplementation improves peripheral endothelial function in hyperlipidemic men,[84] and along these lines some data from small trials do demonstrate that large doses of L-arginine for 6 months significantly improve coronary endothelial function and anginal symptoms.[85,86] Furthermore, acute infusions of L-arginine show an improvement in CBF in the catheterization laboratory.[87] For most patients, the large dosage of L-arginine makes compliance difficult as patients start with 3 g daily in divided doses working up to 9 g daily. Potential drawbacks of this therapy include the large dose required and potential for gastrointestinal or pulmonary side effects.

Treatment—Microvascular Nonvasodilators
Ranolazine

Ranolazine, an inhibitor of the late inward sodium currents that reduces cytosolic calcium levels, thus enhancing ventricular relaxation, has shown promise in improving CMD symptoms. Others have shown ranolazine to alter fatty acid metabolism or reduce heart rate and blood pressure. Therefore it could also improve myocardial perfusion, thus theoretically reducing angina triggers.[88] To those points, initial pilot data in small (15 to 20 patients) RCTs utilizing 375 to 1000 mg of ranolazine twice daily for 4 weeks showed symptomatic benefit in patients with CMD.[89,90] Furthermore, 8 weeks of ranolazine therapy has shown an improvement in CFR as assessed by echocardiography.[91] Unfortunately, randomized data recently published from the Treatment With Ranolazine in Microvascular Coronary Dysfunction (MCD): Impact on Angina Myocardial Ischemia (RWISE) study showed that 128 CMD patients (96% female) randomized to 2 weeks of ranolazine versus placebo experienced no improvement in their angina symptoms as assessed by the Seattle Angina Questionnaire, quality of life, or cardiac MRI perfusion.[92]

Enhanced Extracorporeal Counterpulsation

In an attempt to restore the balance between myocardial oxygen supply/demand and improve coronary perfusion pressure, external counterpulsation delivered by pneumatic cuffs applied to the lower extremities, or enhanced extracorporeal counterpulsation (EECP), has found limited use in refractory angina secondary to severe CAD.[93] Additionally, there appears to be benefit of EECP on vascular endothelium in patients with refractory angina secondary to CAD.[94] Geographic sparsity, cost, extensive treatment duration, and lack of large-scale benefit seen in dedicated CMD trials make EECP a less common treatment strategy in CMD.

CONCLUSIONS

This chapter should serve as an overview for evaluating patients with symptomatic NO CAD. Beginning with the initial workup involving history and physical, laboratory, and potentially noninvasive imaging, the next step is the exclusion of obstructive CAD based on coronary angiographic, physiologic, and imaging assessment. Once obstructive CAD has been eliminated, the coronary microcirculation is evaluated in a standard way with appropriate protocols and equipment. This is accomplished with the administration of intracoronary adenosine, ACh, and nitroglycerin to obtain CFRne, CFRe, and to evaluate epicardial vasospasm and smooth muscle function. These results should be promptly and correctly reported and a detailed interpretation provided. With these simple strategies, one can safely and effectively evaluate and care for patients with CMD.

KEY REFERENCES

2. Gould K, Lipscomb K, Hamilton GW. Physiologic basis for assessing critical coronary stenosis. Instantaneous flow response and regional distribution during coronary hyperemia as measures of coronary flow reserve. *Am J Cardiol*. 1974;33:87–94.
5. Sara J, Widmer RJ, Matsuzawa Y, et al. Prevalence of coronary microvascular dysfunction among patients with chest pain and nonobstructive coronary artery disease. *JACC Cardiovasc Interv*. 2015;8:1445–1553.
8. Reriani M, Sara JD, Flammer AJ, et al. Coronary endothelial function testing provides superior discrimination compared with standard clinical risk scoring in prediction of cardiovascular events. *Coron Artery Dis*. 2016;27:213–220.

10. Suwaidi J, Hamasaki S, Higano ST, et al. Long-term follow-up of patients with mild coronary artery disease and endothelial dysfunction. *Circulation*. 2000;101:948–954.
14. Shaw L, Bairey Merz CN, Pepine CJ, et al. Insights from the NHLBI-Sponsored Women's Ischemia Syndrome Evaluation (WISE) Study: Part I: gender differences in traditional and novel risk factors, symptom evaluation, and gender-optimized diagnostic strategies. *J Am Coll Cardiol*. 2006;47:S4–S20.
16. Cassar A, Chareonthaitawee P, Rihal CS, et al. Lack of correlation between noninvasive stress tests and invasive coronary vasomotor dysfunction in patients with nonobstructive coronary artery disease. *Circ Cardiovasc Interv*. 2009;2:237–244.
22. Borlaug B, Olson TP, Lam CS, et al. Global cardiovascular reserve dysfunction in heart failure with preserved ejection fraction. *J Am Coll Cardiol*. 2010;56:845–854.
27. Yoshino S, Cassar A, Matsuo Y, et al. Fractional flow reserve with dobutamine challenge and coronary microvascular endothelial dysfunction in symptomatic myocardial bridging. *Circ J*. 2014;78:685–692.
28. Wei J, Mehta PK, Johnson BD, et al. Safety of coronary reactivity testing in women with no obstructive coronary artery disease: results from the NHLBI-sponsored Women's Ischemia Syndrome Evaluation (WISE) Study. *JACC Cardiovascular interventions*. 2012;5:646–653.
29. Ong P, Athanasiadis A, Borgulya G, et al. Clinical usefulness, angiographic characteristics, and safety evaluation of intracoronary acetylcholine provocation testing among 921 consecutive white patients with unobstructed coronary arteries. *Circulation*. 2014;129:1723–1730.
38. McGeoch R, Watkins S, Berry C, et al. The index of microcirculatory resistance measured acutely predicts the extent and severity of myocardial infarction in patients with ST-segment elevation myocardial infarction. *JACC Cardiovasc Interv*. 2010;3:715–722.
40. Khuddus M, Pepine CJ, Handberg EM, et al. An intravascular ultrasound analysis in women experiencing chest pain in the absence of obstructive coronary artery disease: a substudy from the National Heart, Lung and Blood Institute-Sponsored Women's Ischemia Syndrome Evaluation (WISE). *J Interv Cardiol*. 2010;23:511–519.
43. Doucette J, Corl PD, Payne HM, et al. Validation of a Doppler guide wire for intravascular measurement of coronary artery flow velocity. *Circulation*. 1992;85:1899–1911.
44. Herrmann J, Higano ST, Lenon RJ, et al. Myocardial bridging is associated with alteration in coronary vasoreactivity. *Eur Heart J*. 2004;25:2134–2142.
47. Klonizakis M, Alkhatib A, Middleton G, et al. Mediterranean diet- and exercise-induced improvement in age-dependent vascular activity. *Clin Sci (Lond)*. 2013;124:579–587.
85. Lerman A, Burnett Jr JC, Higano ST, et al. Long-term L-arginine supplementation improves small-vessel coronary endothelial function in humans. *Circulation*. 1998;97:2123–2128.
92. Bairey Merz C, Handberg EM, Shufelt CL, et al. A randomized, placebo-controlled trial of late Na current inhibition (ranolazine) in coronary microvascular dysfunction (CMD): impact on angina and myocardial perfusion reserve. *Eur Heart J*. 2016;37:1504–1513.

Additional references available online at expertconsult.com.

SECTION IV

第四部分

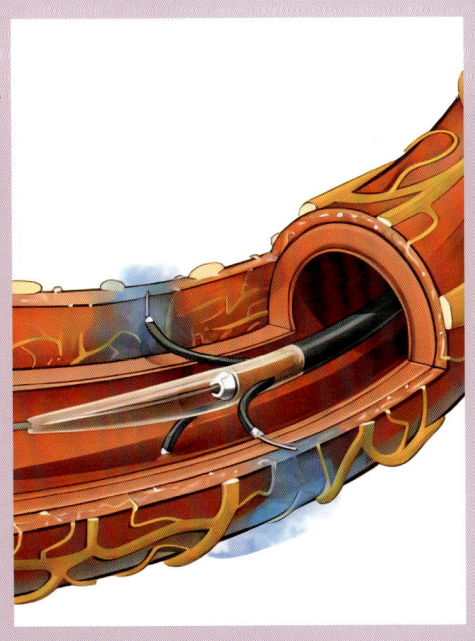

Peripheral Vascular Interventions

外周血管介入治疗

中文导读

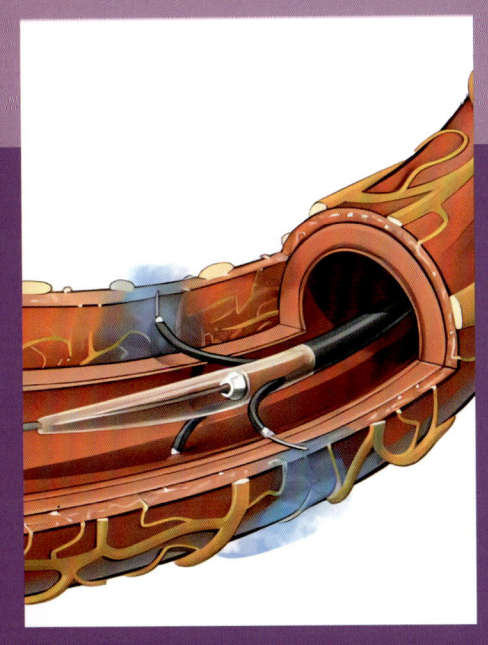

第39章
下肢血管介入

下肢血管疾病是一种较为常见的血管疾病，其发病率高达3%～10%，并随年龄增长，发病率呈上升趋势，在年龄大于70岁的患者中发病率高达10%～15%。下肢血管疾病的主要临床表现为间歇性跛行、缺血性静息痛、坏疽等。然而超过半数的患者并无明显的临床症状，可通过踝肱比来确定疾病的严重程度。上述患者均应进行血管评估。下肢动脉系统解剖复杂，分支血管较多，病变类型复杂，尤其是闭塞性病变严重影响患者生活质量甚至威胁患者生命。

本章详细介绍了下肢血管解剖特点、下肢血管疾病的诊断及评价方法，并针对常见的近端下肢动脉疾病，以及膝下动脉疾病、急性下肢缺血、血栓性血管炎、动脉瘤、动脉粥样硬化症等，详细介绍了介入治疗指征和方法，以及外科手术的治疗要点。

牛冠男　张洪亮

章节要点

- 存在行走障碍、跛行、缺血性静息痛及不易愈合的溃疡的患者应接受血管检查以评估是否存在下肢外周动脉疾病的风险。
- 尽管近年来在无创评估下肢外周动脉疾病方面取得了进展，但血管造影仍然是诊断的"金标准"。下肢血管造影可提供动脉解剖的详细信息，对拟行下肢血运重建的患者，推荐直接进行血管造影以评估下肢外周动脉疾病。
- 髂动脉闭塞患者发病年龄相对较小，与腹股沟以远的下肢疾病相比，对其生产力和生活方式影响较大。
- 下肢动脉经皮介入治疗后极佳的中期至长期通畅率使其成为适合病变的患者手术之外的一种有吸引力的替代方法。血管内介入是TASC A型和B型髂动脉及股腘动脉病变的首选血管重建技术。
- 支架置入术是治疗髂总动脉及髂外动脉狭窄或闭塞病变的有效方法。
- 髂动脉狭窄的血管内介入治疗的技术和临床成功率超过90%，其中长期通畅率与外科手术血管重建相当。因此，介入治疗成为大多数髂动脉狭窄的首选治疗方法。
- 手术仍然是治疗股总和股深近端闭塞性下肢血管疾病的首选策略。
- 经皮介入治疗长期通畅度略低，但其创伤较小，且与外科手术相比其死亡率及并发症发生率较低。
- 如果介入治疗失败，可以再次尝试，但反复进行有难度的外科手术在技术上更具挑战性。
- 在解剖结构合适的病变患者中，优先选择血管内介入治疗作为首选治疗方案。

SECTION IV Peripheral Vascular Interventions

39 Lower Extremity Interventions

Debabrata Mukherjee

KEY POINTS

- Individuals at risk for lower extremity peripheral artery disease (PAD) should undergo a vascular review of symptoms to assess walking impairment, claudication, ischemic rest pain, and the presence of nonhealing wounds.
- Despite recent advances in noninvasive evaluation of lower extremity PAD, contrast angiography remains the gold standard for definitive evaluation. Contrast angiography provides detailed information about arterial anatomy and is recommended for evaluation of patients with lower extremity PAD when revascularization is contemplated.
- Occlusive disease of the iliac arteries appears to occur in relatively young patients and may have a greater impact on productivity and lifestyle compared with infrainguinal lower extremity disease.
- The excellent intermediate- to long-term patency rates following percutaneous intervention of the lower extremity arteries has led to its emergence as an attractive alternative to surgery in patients with suitable lesions. Endovascular intervention is recommended as the preferred revascularization technique for TransAtlantic Inter-Society Consensus (TASC) type A and B iliac and femoropopliteal artery (FPA) lesions.
- Stenting is effective as primary therapy for common iliac and external iliac artery stenosis and occlusions.
- Technical and clinical success rates of endovascular interventions for iliac artery stenosis exceed 90% with a fairly comparable intermediate- and long-term patency to that of surgical revascularization, making them the initial therapy of choice for most iliac stenoses.
- Although controversial, surgery remains the preferred strategy for patients with common femoral and proximal profunda femoris obstructive PAD.
- Lower durability of percutaneous intervention may be offset by the less invasive nature of endovascular interventions and resultant decreased morbidity and mortality compared with vascular surgery.
- Interventions can be repeatedly done if they fail, but repeat surgery is technically more challenging and may be limited by availability of conduit.
- In patients with anatomically appropriate lesions, most practitioners use endovascular interventions preferentially as the initial therapy of choice.

EPIDEMIOLOGY AND NATURAL HISTORY

Peripheral arterial disease of the lower extremity is a common health problem.[1] Epidemiologic studies have mostly used intermittent claudication (IC) as a symptomatic marker of the disease and an abnormal ankle-brachial index (ABI) to define the burden of asymptomatic peripheral artery disease (PAD).[2] The prevalence of the disease is dependent on the age of the population studied and the underlying atherosclerotic risk profile of the cohort. It is estimated that the overall disease prevalence is in the range of 3% to 10%, increasing to about 15% to 20% in persons older than 70 years. More than half of all patients with lower extremity PAD may be asymptomatic.[3-9]

History that includes standardized questionnaires, such as the Rose Claudication Questionnaire used in the Framingham Heart Study, and physical examination may grossly underestimate the true burden of lower extremity PAD.[4] Criqui and colleagues[10] evaluated the prevalence of lower extremity PAD in a population of 613 men and women in Southern California using four different modalities: the Rose Questionnaire, pulse examination, ABI, and pulse wave velocity. The detection rate of PAD with ABI and pulse-wave velocity was two to seven times higher than the detection rate of the Rose Questionnaire. Of interest, clinical examination of the pulse overestimated the prevalence of PAD by twofold.

To optimally manage patients with lower extremity PAD, whether symptomatic or asymptomatic, it is important to understand the global vascular disease burden, the natural history of the disease process, its impact on the patient's lifestyle, and the risk factors for an individual patient. Such knowledge is key to reducing the mortality and morbidity of the individual patient.

VASCULAR ANATOMY OF THE LOWER EXTREMITY

The abdominal aorta bifurcates at the level of the fourth lumbar vertebra into two branches, the right and the left common iliac arteries, which further divide into the *external iliac artery*, which normally follows the same axis of the common iliac artery, and the *internal iliac arteries*, which take a posteromedial track in relation to the common iliac artery. In addition to its terminal branches, the common iliac artery gives branches to the surrounding tissues, peritoneum, psoas muscle, ureter, and nerves. Occasionally, the common iliac artery provides accessory renal arteries to a normal or ectopic kidney. Fig. 39.1 depicts the arterial circulation of the lower extremity.

The external iliac arteries are larger than the internal iliac arteries. They descend along the medial border of the psoas major muscle and enter the thigh posterior to the inguinal ligament to become the common femoral arteries. The inferior epigastric artery arises medially from the distal external iliac artery and ascends behind the rectus abdominis muscle. This vessel is a useful landmark in predicting higher bleeding risk in arterial punctures proximal to its origin.[11] The external iliac artery gives off other branches—namely, the deep circumflex, cremasteric, and several muscular and cutaneous branches—before it continues as the common femoral artery (CFA). Together the common iliac and the external iliac arteries contribute to the inflow of the lower extremity.

The CFA starts as a continuation of the external iliac artery, giving multiple branches to surrounding tissues, such as the pudendal arteries and the superficial circumflex artery; then it becomes the superficial femoral artery (SFA) after giving rise to the deep femoral artery (DFA) roughly 3.5 cm distal to the inguinal ligament. The DFA arises laterally and posteriorly from the CFA, whereas the SFA continues its pathway to end as the popliteal artery when it passes through the abductor canal. The DFA gives off perforating branches, usually three—the lateral and medial circumflex arteries and muscular branches—and the end of the DFA is the fourth perforating branch. The popliteal artery continues through the abductor's canal, and after giving muscular, cutaneous, genicular, and sural branches, it terminates into the anterior tibial artery and the tibioperoneal trunk. The CFA, SFA, DFA, and the popliteal artery comprise the outflow of the lower extremity.

The anterior tibial artery runs between the two heads of the tibialis posterior muscle and then through the upper part of the interosseous membrane to the front of the leg medial to the head of the fibula. It descends down to the ankle and then continues to the dorsum of the foot, where it becomes the dorsalis pedis artery. The posterior tibial artery arises from the popliteal artery distal to the origin of the anterior tibial artery as the tibioperoneal trunk. After giving rise to the peroneal artery, the tibioperoneal trunk continues as the posterior tibial artery behind the leg and passes behind the medial malleolus to end by giving rise to the arteries of the foot, namely the calcaneal, which anastomoses with the calcaneal and malleolar branches of the peroneal

and medial and lateral planter arteries. The anterior tibial artery, posterior tibial artery, and the peroneal artery are considered the runoff vessels.

DIAGNOSIS OF LOWER EXTREMITY PERIPHERAL ARTERIAL DISEASE

History and Physical Examination

Patients with lower extremity PAD may be asymptomatic (disease is detected during physical examination or screening tests), or they may present with IC, rest pain, nonhealing ulcers, or intractable foot infections. In light of the limitations of clinical assessment in defining patients with asymptomatic PAD, additional assessment of patients with risk factors for atherosclerosis may be required in identifying patients with asymptomatic advanced PAD. Symptomatic patients can be classified based on the severity of ischemia based on either the Fontaine or Rutherford categories (Table 39.1).

Ankle-Brachial Index

The ABI is a ratio of the blood pressure in the dorsalis pedis or the posterior tibial artery, whichever is higher, to the blood pressure in the brachial arteries. ABI measurement is one of the most cost-effective methods for assessing PAD of the lower extremity, and it typically is done with a handheld Doppler ultrasound device. This is a noninvasive, fairly reproducible, and inexpensive test. The resting ABI should be used to establish the lower extremity PAD diagnosis in patients with *suspected* lower extremity PAD, defined as individuals with one or more of the following: exertional leg symptoms, nonhealing wounds, age 65 and older, or 50 years and older with a history of smoking or diabetes.[12] The ABI should also be measured in both legs in all new patients with PAD of any severity to confirm the diagnosis of lower extremity PAD and establish a baseline.[11] ABI results should be uniformly reported: *noncompressible* values are defined as greater than 1.40, *normal* values are 1.00 to 1.40, *borderline* is 0.91 to 0.99, and *abnormal* is 0.90 or less. The most widely accepted definition of lower extremity PAD is a resting ABI of less than 0.9, which is usually associated with 50% or greater angiographic arterial stenosis with a reported sensitivity

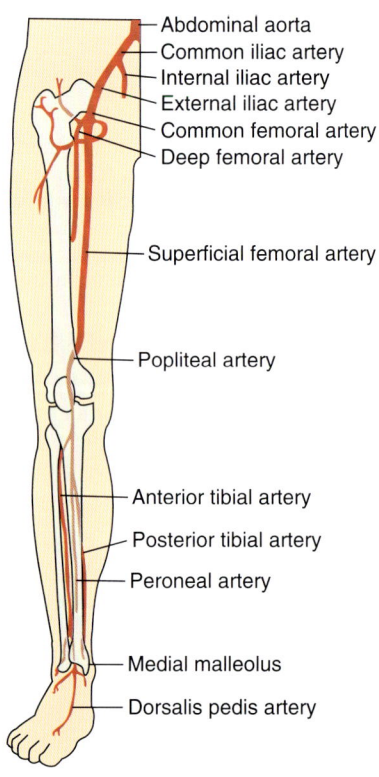

Fig. 39.1 Arterial tree of the lower extremity.

TABLE 39.1 Classification of Lower Extremity Peripheral Artery Disease by the Fontaine Stages and Rutherford Categories

Fontaine		Rutherford		
Stage	Clinical	Grade	Category	Clinical
I	Asymptomatic	0	0	Asymptomatic
IIa	Mild claudication	I	1	Mild claudication
IIb	Moderate to severe claudication	I	2	Moderate claudication
		I	3	Severe claudication
III	Ischemic rest pain	II	4	Ischemic rest pain
		III	5	Minor tissue loss
IV	Ulceration or gangrene	IV	6	Ulceration or gangrene

From Dormandy JA, Rutherford RB. Management of peripheral arterial disease (PAD). TASC Working Group. Trans-Atlantic Inter-Society Consensus (TASC). *J Vasc Surg.* 2000;31:S1–S296.

of 95% and close to 100% specificity.[7] A resting ABI of 0.4 to 0.9 is suggestive of mild to moderate PAD, and a resting ABI below 0.4 is suggestive of severe PAD (Table 39.2). Resting ABI measurement can be artifactually high in the setting of tibial artery calcification usually seen in diabetics. The toe-brachial index (TBI) should be used to establish a diagnosis in patients in whom lower extremity PAD is clinically suspected but in whom the ABI test is not reliable because of noncompressible vessels (usually patients with long-standing diabetes or advanced age). A TBI below 0.7 is considered abnormal.

TABLE 39.2 Grading Lower Extremity Peripheral Arterial Disease by Ankle-Brachial Index[a]

	Supine Resting ABI	Postexercise ABI
Normal	>1.0	>1.0
Mild	0.8–0.9	>0.4
Moderate	0.4–0.8	>0.2
Severe	<0.4	<0.2

[a]Postexercise ABI is measured following treadmill exercise at 1–2 mph, 10% to 12% grade, for 5 min or is symptom limited.
ABI, Ankle-brachial index.
From Mukherjee D, Yadav JS. Update on peripheral vascular diseases: from smoking cessation to stenting. *Cleveland Clinic J Med.* 2001;68(8):723–733; table 2.

The use of exercise ABI may be helpful in equivocal cases. For this, the patient walks on the treadmill at a constant speed of 1 to 2 miles per hour and at a 10% to 12% incline for 5 minutes, or the exercise can be done with active pedal plantar flexion. A decrease of at least 15 mm Hg in the ankle systolic pressure following the exercise challenge is considered an abnormal test. Patients with no significant PAD are expected to have an increase or no change in their ankle systolic pressure. Exercise treadmill tests may also be performed in individuals with claudication who are to undergo exercise training (lower extremity PAD rehabilitation), so as to determine functional capacity, assess nonvascular exercise limitations, and demonstrate the safety of exercise.

Pulse Volume Recording

Plethysmography is used to detect volumetric changes in the lower extremity blood flow and is performed with pressure cuffs inflated to 60 to 65 mm Hg at various segments of the lower extremity. A normal tracing will have a rapid systolic upstroke and downstroke with a prominent dicrotic notch. This pattern changes as PAD develops and progresses, with a noted attenuation and widening of the arterial waveform. Ultimately, the waveform becomes flat (nonpulsatile) in patients with advanced PAD (Fig. 39.2). Pulse volume recordings are reasonable to establish the initial lower extremity PAD diagnosis, assess localization and severity, and follow the status of lower extremity revascularization procedures.

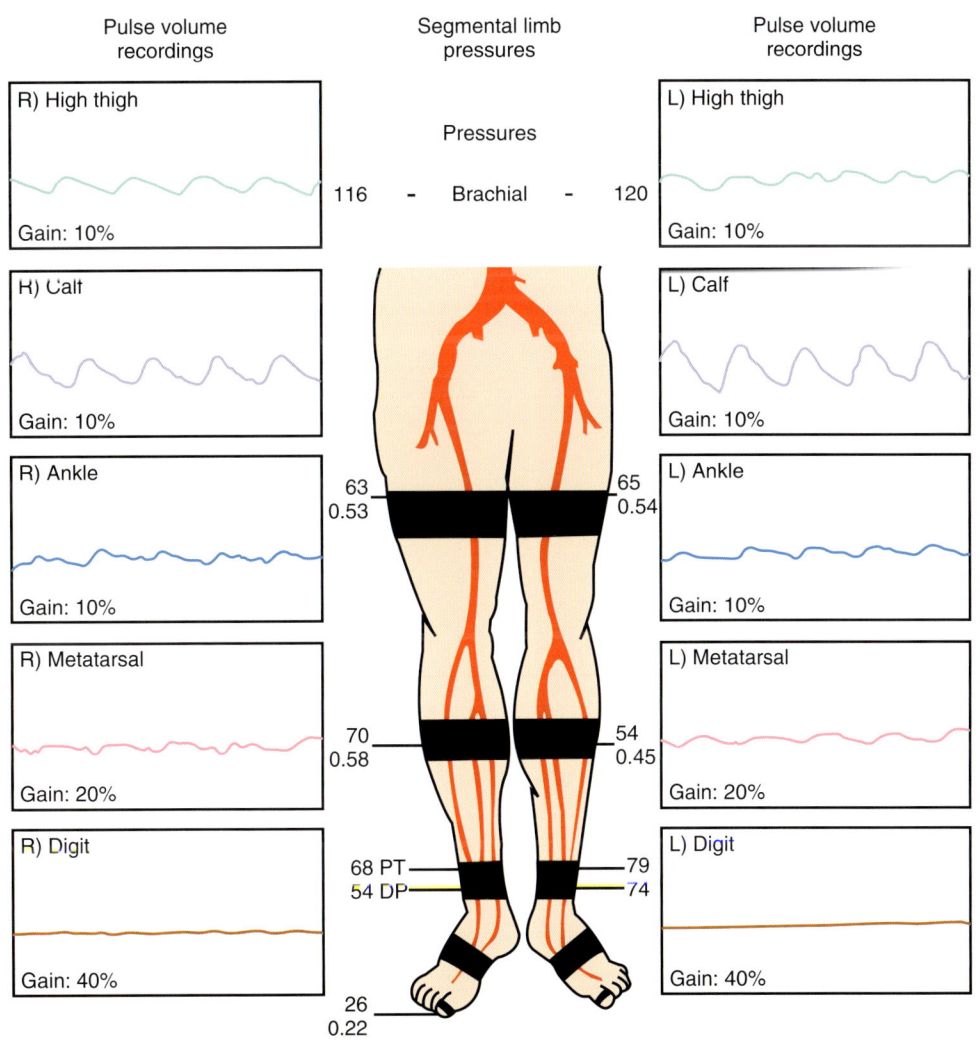

Fig. 39.2 **Segmental limb pressures and pulse volume recordings (PVRs) demonstrating aortoiliac disease.** The PVR waveforms in the thigh segment are dampened, and the segmental pressures in the thigh are decreased when compared with the brachial pressures. *DP,* Dorsalis pedis; *L,* left; *PT,* posterior tibial; *R,* right. (From Rajagopalan S, Mukherjee D, Mohler E, eds. *Manual of Vascular Diseases.* Philadelphia: Lippincott Williams & Wilkins; 2004:17.)

Segmental Blood Pressure

For this test, a series of blood pressure cuffs are placed at the level of the thigh (one or two cuffs), calf, ankle, foot, and the big toe. These cuffs are then inflated sequentially to about 20 mm Hg above the systolic pressure in that segment. The cuff pressure is then released slowly, and a continuous-wave Doppler probe is used to obtain the pressure at each segment. A decrease between two consecutive levels of 30 mm Hg or more indicates the presence of a stenosis in the segment proximal to the blood pressure cuff. Also, the presence of a 20- to 30-mm Hg difference in the pressure at one limb, when compared with the contralateral limb at the same level, is suggestive of significant PAD proximal to the cuff in that limb.

Duplex Ultrasonography

Duplex ultrasound uses a 5- to 7.5-MHz transducer to assess and characterize suprainguinal and infrainguinal PAD with a high sensitivity and specificity (over 90%). Doppler velocities are obtained (60-degree Doppler angle) to complement two-dimensional ultrasonography. Traditionally, arteries are classified into five categories based on the degree of stenosis: category 1 is considered normal, 2 indicates stenosis of 1% to 19%, 3 is stenosis of 20% to 49%, 4 indicates 50% to 99% stenosis, and 5 signifies total occlusion. Duplex ultrasonography may be useful to operators in planning access to a lesion that is amenable to endovascular therapy. It is also very helpful in identifying iatrogenic traumatic lesions and pseudoaneurysms. Direct ultrasound-guided compression or thrombin injection to repair femoral artery pseudoaneurysms is widely used in treating such lesions without the need for surgical procedures. One important limitation of Duplex ultrasonography is that it may overestimate residual stenosis following interventions, which limits its usefulness as a follow-up tool in this setting. Duplex ultrasound is recommended for routine surveillance after femoral-popliteal or femoral-tibial-pedal bypass with a venous conduit. Minimum surveillance intervals are approximately 3, 6, and 12 months and then yearly after graft placement.[11,12]

Computed Tomography Angiography

The use of spiral computed tomography angiography (CTA) in assessing lower extremity PAD has 93% sensitivity and 96% specificity in detecting greater than 50% stenosis with high accuracy when compared with digital subtraction angiography (DSA). A systematic review and meta-analysis[13] suggested that CTA is highly accurate for assessment of PAD in detecting stenosis of the aortoiliac and femoral arteries. However, diagnostic accuracy of CTA in below-knee vessels is poor and contrast angiography should be considered where below-knee disease needs to be accurately identified.[14] CTA correctly identified hemodynamically significant lesions and also accurately distinguished between greater than 50% stenoses and occlusions. Ninety-four percent of occlusions and 87% of nonoccluded segments with more than 50% stenosis detected by contrast angiography were correctly identified by CTA.[13] The accuracy of CTA may potentially be even higher than reported in this study because all studies used contrast angiography as the reference standard but did not report whether biplanar views were used routinely. Because CTA reconstructions allow three-dimensional (3-D) assessment, significant disease may be detected by CTA but may not be recognized by angiography, which may lead to the underestimation of specificity. CTA has advantages over magnetic resonance angiography (MRA) in patients with pacemakers and defibrillators and in those with metal clips, stents, or prosthesis (no significant artifact is seen in CTA as opposed to MRA), and it is significantly faster to perform than MRA. However, CTA requires the use of iodinated contrast, and it entails exposure to ionizing radiation. Dose-saving algorithms are very effective in reducing radiation exposure and should be used whenever possible.[15]

Magnetic Resonance Angiography

The use of gadolinium-enhanced magnetic resonance angiography (GEMRA; Fig. 39.3) in the assessment of lower extremity PAD has been compared with standard catheter angiography, with a reported sensitivity and specificity for detecting stenosis greater than 50% of about 90% and 100%, respectively. Most contemporary studies report an agreement of 91% to 97% between MRA and catheter angiography. GEMRA is superior to duplex ultrasound in detecting greater than 50% stenotic lesions (sensitivity of 98% vs. 88% and specificity of 96% vs. 95%).[7]

Limitations of this technology include the tendency to overestimate the severity of stenosis and the fact that metal clips

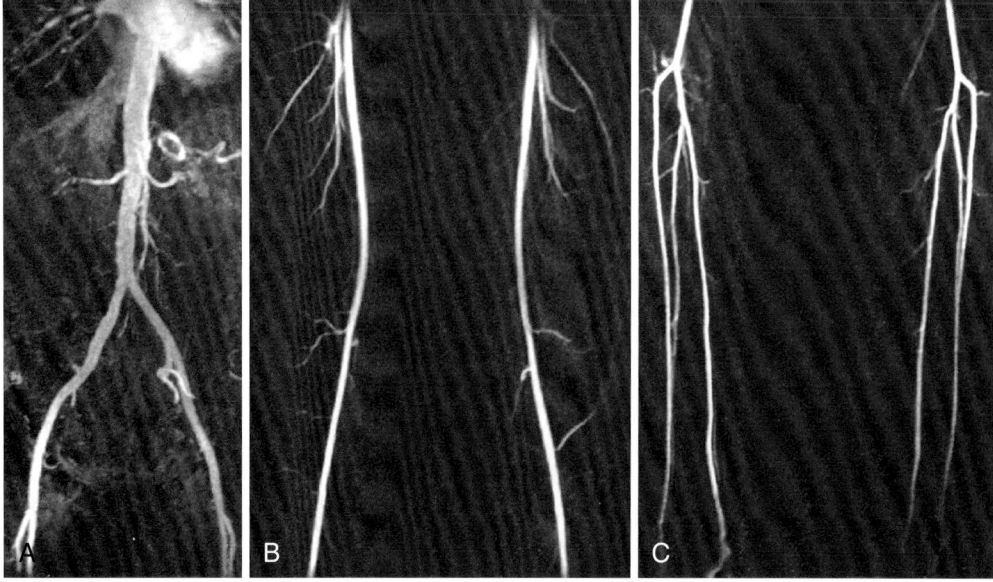

Fig. 39.3 Maximal intensity projection images of a normal lower extremity runoff three-dimensional contrast-enhanced magnetic resonance angiography. (A) Aortoiliac region; (B) superior femoral artery and profunda femoris; and (C) three-vessel below the knee runoff with anterior tibial, peroneal and posterior tibial arteries. (From Rajagopalan S, Mukherjee D, Mohler E, eds. *Manual of Vascular Diseases*. Philadelphia: Lippincott Williams & Wilkins; 2004:65.)

may give the impression of total occlusion, and metal stents can obscure vascular flow as well. In addition to these limitations, certain subsets of patients may not be able to be studied with MRA, such as those with pacemakers and defibrillators and those with certain types of cerebral aneurysm clips.[7] The principle role of MRA is in the initial evaluation for PAD, especially in patients with inflow disease, using "bolus chase" 3-D imaging, in which a single bolus of contrast is followed to the foot.

Contrast Angiography

Despite recent advances in noninvasive evaluation of lower extremity PAD, contrast angiography remains the gold standard. Traditionally, a pelvic/abdominal aortogram in the anteroposterior projection is done using a straight pigtail catheter (5 or 6 Fr) placed at the level of the L1-L2 vertebrae. Approximately 10 to 15 mL of isoosmolar contrast is injected at a rate of 15 mL/s with DSA technology. This allows an excellent view of the distal aorta, the origin of the common iliac arteries, and the external iliac and common femoral arteries. Angulated views (left anterior oblique [LAO] of 30 degrees) can then be used to visualize the iliac and femoral bifurcations without overlap. Next, the pigtail catheter is placed above the aortic bifurcation (L3 to L4) and DSA with bolus chase, 8 mL/s for 10 seconds, is used to assess the outflow and distal runoff. Selective injections and sheath injections can then be used to further define the territory of interest as needed. The use of "road map" technology can be used subsequently to help operators in their intervention and placement of balloons and stents. Contrast angiography remains the most readily used and widely available imaging technique in patients with PAD of the lower extremity when revascularization is contemplated. The use of noninvasive technologies, such as MRA or CTA, may be used prior to contrast angiography to help identify the potential culprit lesion and plan the best approach (access point, catheter selection, etc.) to study such a lesion invasively.[7] Contrast angiography may be associated with vascular access complications (bleeding, infections, pseudoaneurysms, and vascular disruption), atheroembolism, contrast nephropathy, and contrast-induced anaphylactoid reactions. These complications, although rare, should be considered in the decision-making process with regard to the assessment of PAD.

Overall, contrast angiography provides detailed information about arterial anatomy and is recommended for evaluation of patients with lower extremity PAD when revascularization is contemplated. When conducting a diagnostic lower extremity arteriogram in which the significance of an obstructive lesion is ambiguous, transstenotic pressure gradients and supplementary angulated views should be considered.[12]

INTERVENTIONS

Percutaneous or surgical interventions are indicated for severe lifestyle-limiting symptoms, to reduce tissue breakdown in the context of critical limb ischemia (CLI), or for salvage in the context of acute limb ischemia (ALI). In general, endovascular procedures are indicated for individuals with a vocational or lifestyle-limiting disability due to IC when clinical features suggest a reasonable likelihood of symptomatic improvement with endovascular intervention and (1) the response to exercise or pharmacologic therapy has been inadequate or (2) the risk-benefit ratio is a very favorable (e.g., focal aortoiliac occlusive disease). The Society of Vascular Surgery (SVS) recommends objective performance goals to assess efficacy of interventions in a patient-centric manner to include major adverse cardiovascular events (MACE), 30-day major adverse limb events (MALE), 30-day amputation rate, amputation-free survival, and freedom from MALE,[16] and can objectively assess efficacy of interventions on hard outcomes.

Iliac Artery Intervention for Inflow Disease

Indications

The indications for iliac artery (or aortoiliac) percutaneous intervention include (1) symptom relief in patients with IC who failed medical therapy; (2) management of CLI (rest pain, ulceration, or gangrene) prior to a planned distal lower extremity bypass surgery to restore or to preserve the inflow to the lower extremity; (3) in preparation for other invasive procedures, such as the placement of an intraaortic balloon pump (IABP); and (4) for treatment of flow-limiting dissection following invasive catheterization-based procedures.

Revascularization Options

Occlusive disease confined to the iliac arteries appears to occur in relatively young patients and may therefore have a greater impact on productivity and lifestyle. For instance, the mean age of the cohort in the Dutch Iliac Stent Trial was approximately 59 years.[17] These patients, over 90% of whom were smokers, were otherwise healthy compared with those with infrainguinal disease or more diffuse PAD. In general, any type of revascularization for this subset of patients can offer satisfactory long-term results. Historically, aortobifemoral bypass surgery has been the gold standard for PAD that involves the iliac arteries, because this procedure is associated with excellent long-term patency rates (85% to 90% at 5 years, 75% to 80% at 10 years, and 60% at 20 years); however, it may be associated with an intraoperative mortality of roughly 1% to 3% and a major complication rate of 5% to 10%. This, combined with the excellent intermediate- to long-term patency rates following percutaneous intervention, has led to the emergence of percutaneous revascularization as an attractive alternative to surgery in patients with suitable lesions for such intervention. In a Swedish randomized controlled trial (RCT)[18] in which 37% of randomized patients had iliac artery stenosis, equivalence in outcomes was evident between percutaneous transluminal angioplasty (PTA) and surgery. In the iliac disease subgroup, the patency rate at 1 year was 90% in the PTA arm versus 94% in the surgical arm. Table 39.3 summarizes the recommendation of the Trans-Atlantic Inter-Society Consensus (TASC) working group for the revascularization strategy of iliac lesions. The TASC group classifies peripheral arterial lesions into Type A, B, C, or D according to anatomic distribution, number and nature of lesions (stenosis, occlusion), and according to the overall success rates of treating the lesion percutaneously or surgically.[19]

Techniques

Access and Recanalization Techniques
In patients with a unilateral stenotic iliac lesion that does not involve the CFA, ipsilateral access through the CFA with retrograde PTA is usually preferred because it provides direct access to the diseased segment and provides a coaxial alignment of the equipment (Fig. 39.4). Contralateral access with the use of a crossover sheath is reserved for patients with disease that involves the ipsilateral CFA (Fig. 39.5) when the surgeon plans to intervene on more distal lesions in the same limb or when jeopardizing flow to the affected limb by placement of the sheath in the ipsilateral CFA is a concern. Various crossover sheaths are available; the ArrowFlex sheath (Arrow International, Reading, PA) is more flexible and can be helpful in crossing over acute aortic bifurcation angles, but it provides less support than the Flexor Ansel, Raabe, and Balkin sheaths (Cook Medical, Bloomington, IN); these provide more support but are less compliant. If the iliac artery is occluded, both approaches may be needed. For aortic bifurcation lesions, a bilateral retrograde approach is used; the placement of kissing balloons—and, subsequently, kissing stents—is the optimal approach in this setting.

SECTION IV Peripheral Vascular Interventions

TABLE 39.3 The Recommendation of the Trans-Atlantic Inter-Society Consensus Working Group for the Revascularization Strategy of Aortoiliac Femoropopliteal Lesions

	Iliac Disease	Femoral Lesions
TASC A	Single, <3 cm of CIA or EIA (unilateral/bilateral)	Single, ≤3 cm in length, does not involve the SFA or popliteal artery
TASC B	1. Single, 3–10 cm, not extending into the CFA 2. Two stenoses <5 cm long in the CIA and/or EIA, does not extend to the CFA 3. Unilateral CIA occlusion	1. Single stenoses or occlusion 3–5 cm long, does not involve the distal popliteal artery 2. Heavily calcified, ≤3 cm, or multiple stenoses or occlusions each <3 cm 3. Single or multiple lesions in the absence of continuous tibial runoff
TASC C	1. Bilateral 5- to 10-cm stenosis of the CIA and/or EIA, does not extend to CFA 2. Unilateral EIA occlusion or stenosis, does not extend into the CFA 3. Bilateral CIA occlusion	1. Single stenosis/occlusion >5 cm 2. Multiple stenoses or occlusions 3–5 cm, with or without heavy calcification
TASC D	1. >10-cm lesions or diffuse, multiple, unilateral stenoses that involve the CIA, EIA, and CFA 2. Unilateral occlusion that involves both the CIA and EIA 3. Bilateral EIA occlusions 4. Diffuse disease that involves the aorta and both iliac arteries or lesions in a patient that require aortic or iliac surgery (AAA)	Complete CFA or SFA occlusions

An endovascular procedure is the treatment of choice for type A, and surgery is the procedure of choice for type D. At present, endovascular treatment is more commonly used in type B lesions, and surgical treatment is more commonly used in type C lesions. Evidence is insufficient to make firm recommendations, particularly in cases with type B and C lesions.

AAA, Abdominal aortic aneurysm; *CFA*, common femoral artery; *CIA*, common iliac artery; *EIA*, external iliac artery; *SFA*, superficial femoral artery.
From Dormandy JA, Rutherford RB. Management of peripheral arterial disease (PAD). TASC Working Group. Trans-Atlantic Inter-Society Consensus (TASC). *J Vasc Surg.* 2000;31:S1–S296; and Norgren L, Hiatt WR, Dormandy JA, et al. Inter-Society Consensus for the Management of Peripheral Arterial Disease (TASC II). *J Vasc Surg.* 2007;45(suppl S):S5.

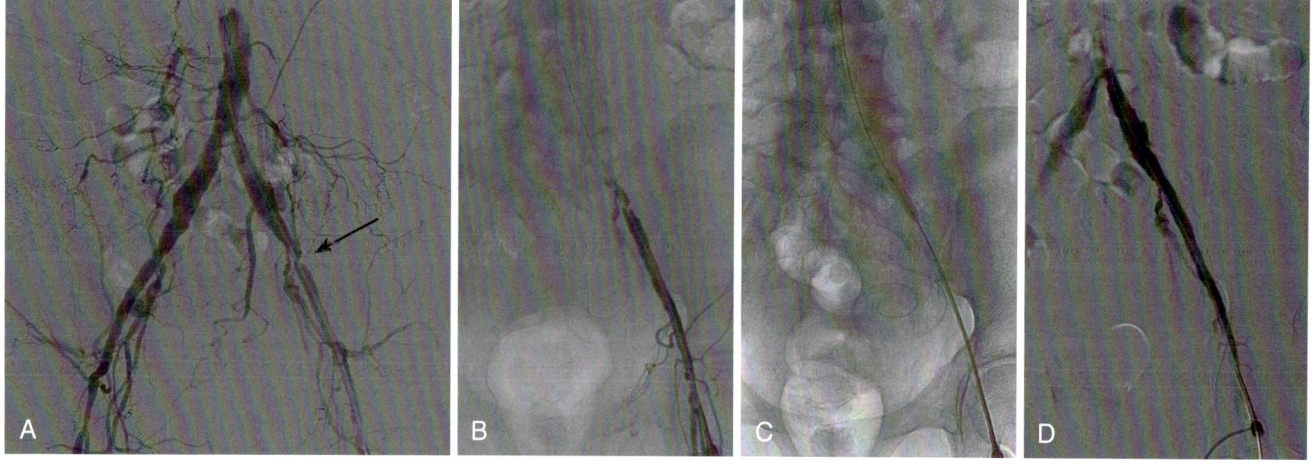

Fig. 39.4 **Left external iliac artery intervention.** (A) Abdominal aortogram with runoffs where the lesion is noted (*arrow*). (B) Using an ipsilateral approach, the lesion is crossed with a guidewire. (C) Angioplasty is done. (D) Successful final result with resolution of the obstructive lesion and no flow-limiting dissection or significant elastic recoil.

In lesions distal to the aortic bifurcation (in the body of the common iliac artery or the external iliac artery), PTA is attempted, and if satisfactory results are achieved (<5 mm Hg residual gradient and <30% residual stenosis with no flow-limiting dissection), stenting may not be indicated. However, ostial lesions of the common iliac arteries (i.e., aortoiliac bifurcation lesions) are preferably stented with kissing stents. In general, 0.035-inch guidewires are used in PTA and in stenting of the iliac arteries, but 0.018- or 0.014-inch guidewires may be used as well. In nonocclusive lesions, a regular nonhydrophilic guidewire can be used; however, if crossing such lesions is difficult, the use of a hydrophilic wire is indicated.

Stent Choice

Both balloon- and self-expandable stents can be used in aortoiliac disease. The balloon-expandable stent is advantageous in the context of an aortic bifurcation lesion, in which kissing stents are usually placed. It is also superior to self-expandable stents when precision in stent placement is needed. The self-expanding stent provides the flexibility in flexion points, which reduces the risk of stent deformity and fracture, and is ideal in the setting of common iliac lesions that do not involve the ostium and those in the external iliac artery. Self-expanding stents were generally favored for the external iliac artery because they reduce the perforation risk.

Clinical Data

In the management of patients with IC secondary to iliofemoral disease, percutaneous revascularization (specifically PTA without stenting) has been compared with conservative management (specifically with exercise training, smoking cessation counseling,

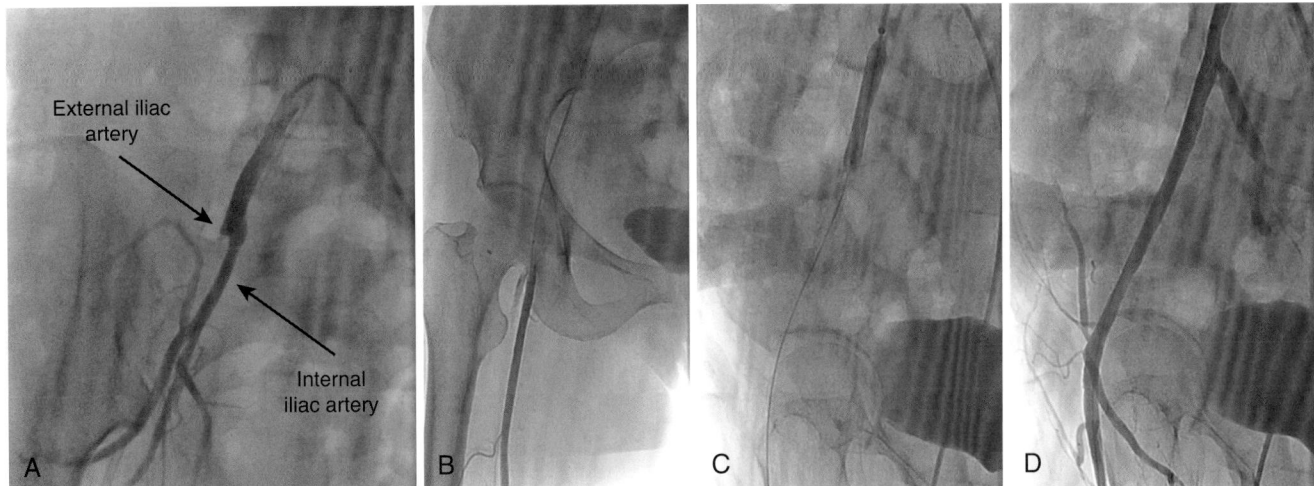

Fig. 39.5 Ostial external iliac artery occlusion. (A) The lesion is approached from a contralateral access point utilizing a crossover sheath. (B) The lesion is crossed with a hydrophilic guidewire, a balloon is placed at the level of the noted distal external iliac artery lesion, and angioplasty is done. (C) The first stent is deployed and a second, more proximal stent is placed. (D) Final result after stent placement.

and antiplatelet therapy with aspirin). The results revealed two important findings: First, PTA can effectively alleviate patients' symptoms, improve treadmill distance, and improve ABI during a short-term follow-up period, although these benefits are mostly lost by 2 years. Second, although PTA improves perfusion to the feet, which may confer protection—particularly for populations at higher risk for limb loss, such as diabetics—supervised exercise improves functional outcome and at the same time enhances global conditioning. These two strategies should therefore be considered complementary to each other because they address different but interrelated issues.[20–22]

Overall, for iliofemoral lesions, the clinical results of percutaneous revascularization are generally comparable to those of surgical bypass or reconstruction. A Swedish trial[23] randomized patients with threatened limb loss (40% with rest pain or gangrene) or claudication who did not improve with exercise training (60%) to either PTA or surgical revascularization. The study population had a mean age of 70 years, a 26% prevalence of diabetes, and an average symptom duration of 18 months. No differences were found between the PTA or surgery treatment groups with regard to 1-year primary and secondary patency rates, which were 61% and approximately 72%, respectively. The complication rates were not statistically different between treatment groups, although most of the adverse events involved patients who presented with rest pain or gangrene, which highlights the impact of baseline limb status on subsequent outcomes. Adverse events included a 1-year death rate of about 10% and a reocclusion rate of 5% (both treatment groups), a major amputation rate of 5.7% versus 16%, and a hematoma rate of 7.5% versus 4.1% (PTA vs. surgery, respectively). The infection and embolization rates were 8.2% each and were seen only in the surgical group, not with PTA. These findings were corroborated by the Veterans Administration (VA) cooperative study,[24] which randomized 255 male patients with iliac or femoropopliteal disease and claudication or rest pain. To be eligible, patients had to be suitable for either PTA or surgery, which may have resulted in a case mix with less diffuse disease compared with the typical vascular surgery population. The average age was 61.5 years, 29% had diabetes, 20% had a history of myocardial infarction (MI), more than 25% had previous surgery or PTA for PAD, and 99% were current or previous smokers (~48 pack-years each). Three study-related deaths occurred, all in the surgery group (*n* = 126). Of the 129 patients randomized to PTA, 20 procedural failures (15.5%) were reported but no deaths; also noted were an inability to cross the lesion with a wire in 7.8%, inability to dilate the lesion in 2.3%, thrombosis within 24 hours in 3.9%, and no hemodynamic improvement after PTA in 1.6%. No stents were available for this trial. Seventeen of the patients who failed PTA subsequently underwent successful surgical revascularization. At a median follow-up of 2 years, no statistically significant difference was found between the PTA and surgery groups with regard to death and major amputations. This pattern of equivalent outcome held true at 4 years follow-up. However, the 2-year target-limb repeat revascularization rate was higher after PTA compared with surgery.[22] In a review of the available literature from 1989 through 1997, Bosch and Hunink[25] reported a higher technical success with stenting with no difference in complication rates and 30-day mortality rates in their meta-analysis of six studies that included 2116 patients with IC secondary to aortoiliac disease. The severity-adjusted primary patency rates were 65% with PTA versus 77% with stenting for stenotic lesions and 54% for PTA versus 61% with stenting for occlusions.

A strategy of primary stenting, as opposed to provisional stenting, is generally recommended for aortoostial lesions. Although an equivalent outcome between primary versus provisional stenting was reported in the Dutch Iliac Stent Trial,[26] only 57% of patients randomized to PTA did *not* require stenting. In comparison, a strategy of routine implantation of the same stent (a Palmaz balloon-expandable stent) gave results that were superior to PTA in an RCT of 185 patients by Richter and colleagues.[27] The authors reported a 4-year patency rate of 94% in the stent arm versus 69% with PTA. Cumulative clinical success, defined as improvement of clinical stage of one level or more, was 89% for stenting and 67% for PTA, respectively. Major periprocedural complications were noted in four patients in the stent group as opposed to three in the PTA group (3.7% overall). These findings were confirmed in the meta-analysis by Bosch and Hunink[25] because stenting offered superior technical success rates and long-term patency compared with PTA in occluded arteries. The outcome of two different self-expanding stents, the stainless steel Wallstent (Boston Scientific, Natick, MA) and the nitinol S.M.A.R.T. stent (Cordis Endovascular, Warren, NJ), for the treatment of iliac artery lesions was compared in a multicenter prospective randomized trial.[28] The acute procedural success was higher with the S.M.A.R.T. stent (98.2%, vs. 87.5% with the Wallstent; *P* = .002). At 1 year, the patency rate was similar for both stents (91.1% with the Wallstent and 94.7% with the S.M.A.R.T. stent) with similar complication rates (5.9% vs. 5.9%, respectively; P = nonsignificant [NS]).

Overall, the technical and clinical success rates of endovascular interventions for iliac artery stenosis exceeds 90% and approaches almost 100% in focal iliac lesions, with a fairly comparable intermediate- and long-term patency to that of surgical revascularization. Factors that negatively affect the long-term patency for either modality are the quality of the distal runoff vessels, the severity of ischemia, and the length of the diseased segment.[29,30] Female sex has also been associated with decreased patency following external iliac stents.[31] Technical success is commonly defined as less than 30% residual stenosis (*anatomic success*), a postintervention mean translesion gradient of 5 mm Hg or less and an increase in the ABI of more than 0.1, or a decrease in symptoms by one category (*hemodynamic success*). Another criterion that has been suggested is an improvement of at least one category of symptoms (*clinical success*).[32] At this time, stenting is an effective primary therapy for common iliac artery and external iliac artery stenoses and occlusions.

Complications and Their Management

Complications rates are generally low in aortoiliac interventions. These include access-site complications (such as groin hematoma, retroperitoneal bleeding, pseudoaneurysm, and arteriovenous fistula [AVF] formation), thrombosis at the intervention site, arterial rupture, and distal embolization. These complications happen at a rate of less than 5% to 6% in most series.[33] Death, contrast-induced nephropathy, MI, and cerebrovascular accident (CVA) occur at a rate of less than 0.5%. The need for urgent vascular repair is reported to be around 2%. With regard to serious complications, rupture—particularly of the external iliac artery—seems to be reported more frequently with the iliac arteries than with percutaneous interventions in other lower extremity arteries.[33,34]

When to Refer to Surgery

Surgery is usually reserved for patients with diffuse disease or those with long total occlusions. It is also the appropriate approach in those with associated infrarenal aortic aneurysms. Table 39.3 summarizes the recommendations of the TASC working group for the appropriate revascularization strategy of iliac lesions.

Femoropopliteal Intervention for Outflow Disease

Common Femoral Artery

Although controversial, many clinicians believe CFA revascularization should be done surgically. Concerns about elastic recoil and dissection following PTA and concerns about mechanical compression of stents and acute stent thrombosis have limited endovascular intervention to this territory. PTA has been used in cases of severe fibrotic lesions following previous surgery.

The SFA and the proximal popliteal artery are the most common anatomic sites of stenosis and occlusion in patients with IC. It is estimated that slightly more than a quarter of diseased SFAs progress over a 3-year period, and 17% may go on to occlusion. Predictors of progression are continued smoking, worsening symptoms, and the presence of an already occluded contralateral SFA.[35] For patients who have disease confined to the SFA, a supervised exercise program might offer a functional outcome that is equivalent or even superior to percutaneous revascularization. This could be due to preserved iliac inflow and the DFA, which is a common and important source of collaterals for patients with SFA stenoses or occlusion. Surgery remains the gold standard when therapy is indicated, and primary femoropopliteal graft patency rates of about 80% at 5 years have been documented.[35] Continued improvements in technology include metal alloys with shape memory and superelastic properties and stents coated with antiproliferative agents, and these are helping to surmount the problem of poor long-term durability, which is currently the main limitation of endovascular techniques. Femoropopliteal angioplasty can be considered for discrete single lesions less than 10 cm, less than 5 cm for calcified stenosis, or less than 3 cm for multiple lesions, so long as the SFA origin or distal popliteal artery is not involved. Endovascular treatment of longer SFA lesions is more controversial. Factors that have been found to adversely impact long-term patency are CLI (gangrene or rest pain), multiple stenoses or diffuse disease, and poor distal runoff.[36,37]

Indications

The low morbidity and mortality of endovascular intervention makes this the strategy of choice in patients with suitable lesions (see Table 39.3). It is an appropriate option in the management of symptomatic patients with (1) femoropopliteal lesions less than 10 cm in length (unilateral or bilateral), (2) multiple stenoses or occlusions less than 5 cm (not involving the trifurcation), (3) a single stenosis less than 15 cm (not involving the trifurcation), and (4) prior to surgery in patients with no continuous tibial runoffs in order to improve inflow for surgical bypass.

Techniques

Common Femoral Artery

Access is usually obtained via the contralateral femoral artery (with a crossover sheath) or via the brachial artery. Lesions that involve the bifurcation of the CFA represent a challenging problem, and sometimes kissing balloons are needed to achieve desirable angiographic outcome.

Stents have historically not been recommended; however, the use of self-expanding nitinol stents is gaining popularity among some interventionalists. Stents are routinely used in salvage situations, and the flexible self expanding stent is the appropriate choice in this vessel. Stenting, however, poses many concerns because stent compression or fracture can occur and may render future surgical repair more complicated. It is important to point out that although restenosis rates are high in the CFA (>50%), restenosis may be associated with less limiting symptoms in patients who needed the PTA for persistent or critical symptoms.

Deep Femoral Artery

Revascularization of the DFA may be needed in the setting of total occlusion of the SFA, or of a femoropopliteal bypass graft, because the DFA plays an important role as a source of collaterals to the lower extremity. Surgery is the preferred strategy in this vessel; however, PTA may be tried in the setting of severe limb-threatening ischemia when surgery is contraindicated or if the disease involves the distal portion of the descending branch of the DFA, which is less accessible for surgeons.

Access via the contralateral femoral artery (with a crossover sheath) or from the brachial artery can be used. Interventions are usually done in the context of limb-threatening ischemia; thus it is important to emphasize that a rather conservative approach with regard to balloon sizing is best in this setting, especially with no data available regarding the placement of stents in the DFA. Stents are used provisionally in the context of flow-limiting dissections or severe residual lesions.

Superficial Femoral Artery

Four approaches are possible to access the SFA, through (1) a contralateral femoral artery (with a crossover sheath), (2) an ipsilateral antegrade common femoral approach, (3) a retrograde popliteal approach, or (4) a brachial artery approach. By accessing the contralateral CFA and then using a curved catheter—such as an internal mammary (IM), Judkins right, Cobra, or Simmons catheter—to engage the ostium of the common iliac artery of the diseased limb, a long, kink-resistant sheath (e.g., Balkin, Raabe, ArrowFlex) is placed. The contralateral approach is more popular because it provides excellent support and helps access other segments (iliac or infrainguinal vessels) on the same limb; however, the antegrade CFA access—which is relatively more challenging than the retrograde approach—is still widely used. An antegrade brachial approach might be the only viable option in patients with bilateral iliofemoral disease. The popliteal approach is the least used because it is associated with a higher risk of complications associated with the smaller size of the popliteal artery and the nearby vital structures that may be injured and because it is uncomfortable for the patient. In general, a familiarity with all the different approaches is necessary because the underlying anatomy of each patient will determine what would be a feasible vascular access point. Fig. 39.6 shows an example of an SFA intervention.

Stent Choice

Stenting as the primary approach for femoropopliteal lesions is typically not indicated. Stents and other adjunctive techniques, such as lasers, cutting balloons, atherectomy devices, and thermal devices, can be useful in the femoral, popliteal, and tibial arteries as salvage therapy for a suboptimal or failed result from balloon dilation (e.g., persistent translesional gradient, residual diameter stenosis >50%, or flow-limiting dissection).[38] If stenting is indicated, self-expanding nitinol stents are generally used in SFA lesions in light of the high risk of stent compression and fracture. One small randomized study of 104 patients suggested that treatment of SFA disease by primary implantation of a self-expanding nitinol stent yielded results superior to those with the currently recommended approach of balloon angioplasty with optional secondary stenting at 6 to 12 months.[39] Another study in 73 patients confirmed that primary stenting with a self-expanding nitinol stent for treatment of intermediate-length SFA disease resulted in morphologically and clinically superior midterm results compared with balloon angioplasty with optional secondary stenting.[40] However, in a meta-analysis of 934 patients, Mwipatayi and colleagues[41] concluded that stent placement in femoropopliteal occlusive disease does not increase the patency rate when compared with PTA alone at 1 year.

The use of sirolimus-eluting S.M.A.R.T. stents for SFA occlusion was evaluated in the Sirolimus-Eluting Versus Bare Nitinol Stent for Obstructive Superficial Femoral Artery Disease (SIROCCO II)[42] study and did not show any significant differences in clinical outcome compared with bare-metal stents (BMSs). At 24 months, the restenosis rate in the sirolimus group was slightly higher than in the BMS group (22.9% vs. 21.1%, $P > .05$). Stent fractures, defined as one or more broken struts, were detected by the independent angiographic and radiographic core laboratory in eight patients in the BMS group and nine in the sirolimus stent group.[42] The Zilver PTX paclitaxel-eluting stent (PES) (Cook Medical)—a polymer-free, paclitaxel-coated, nitinol drug-eluting stent (DES)—was also evaluated in several clinical studies.[43,44] Dake and colleagues[44] compared the 12-month safety and effectiveness of the Zilver PTX with PTA and provisional BMS placement in patients with femoropopliteal PAD. Compared with the PTA group, the primary DES group exhibited superior 12-month event-free survival (90.4% vs. 82.6%, $P = .004$) and primary patency (83.1% vs. 32.8%, $P < .001$). Overall, femoropopliteal PAD treatment with the PES was associated with superior 12-month outcomes compared with PTA and provisional BMS placement. Longer term follow-up of this cohort at 2 years demonstrated that outcomes with the PES support its sustained safety and effectiveness in patients with femoropopliteal artery (FPA) disease, including the long-term superiority of the DES to PTA and to provisional BMS placement.[44] Based on outcome data, the Zilver PTX is the first and only DES approved by the U.S. Food and Drug Administration (FDA) for SFA lesions. Recently, 5-Year Results of the Zilver PTX Randomized Trial were reported, which suggests that the Zilver PTX DES provided sustained safety and clinical durability in comparison with standard endovascular treatments.[45] Despite the benefit of Zilver PTX over PTA and Zilver BMS noted in this trial, the superiority of Zilver PTX over other contemporary newer nitinol BMS has not been established.[46]

The IntraCoil (Sulzer IntraTherapeutics, St. Paul, MN) self-expanding peripheral stent, the LifeStent FlexStar (Bard, Murray Hill, NJ) peripheral vascular stent, the Complete SE (Medtronic Vascular, Santa Rosa, CA) vascular stent system, the Supera (Abbott Vascular, Abbott Park, IL) peripheral stent, the Viabahn (W.L. Gore, Flagstaff, AZ) endoprosthesis, and the EverFlex (Covidien, Mansfield, MA) self-expanding stent are examples of some FDA-approved BMSs used in the femoral and peripheral arteries.

Specific Techniques: Laser, Atherectomy, SilverHawk

Although anecdotal experiences and reported case series have suggested some benefits, the use of directional atherectomy and laser angioplasty has not been shown to offer any clear advantage

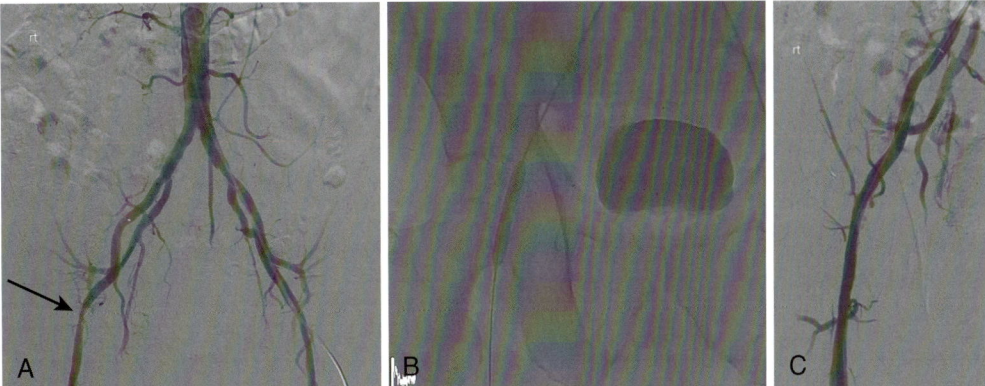

Fig. 39.6 Right superficial femoral artery (SFA) intervention. (A) Abdominal aortogram reveals the right SFA lesion *(arrow)*. (B) The lesion is crossed and angioplasty is done using a contralateral access point. (C) Successful percutaneous transluminal angioplasty (PTA) result with no significant residual lesion or flow-limiting dissection.

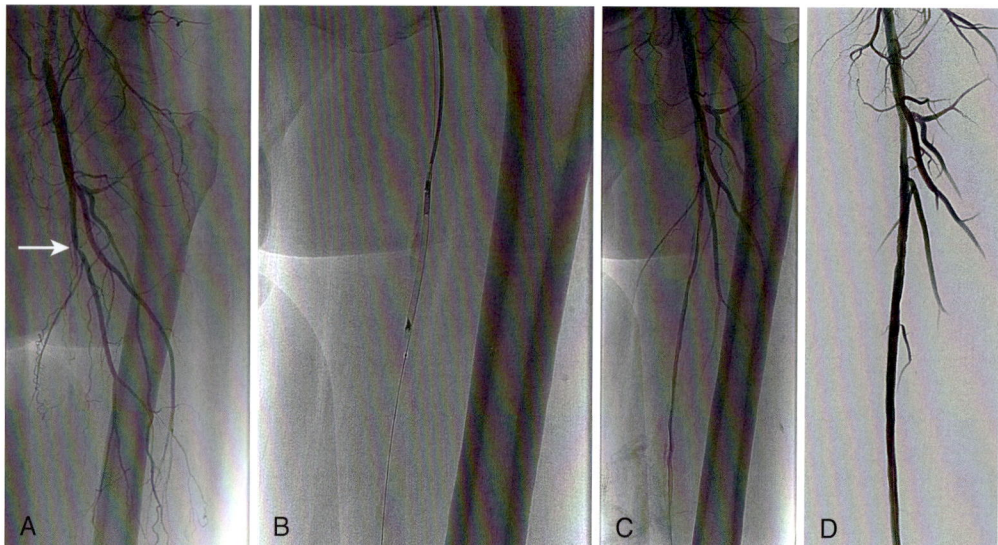

Fig. 39.7 Superficial femoral artery (SFA) ostial bifurcation lesion. (A) Angiogram revealed the right SFA ostial occlusion *(arrow)*. (B) The lesion is crossed and atherectomy is done using a contralateral access point. (C) Percutaneous transluminal angioplasty (PTA) result with significant residual lesion. (D) Stenting is performed with no residual stenosis, and normal flow is noted in the deep femoral artery.

over PTA in femoropopliteal PAD.[47,48] A prospective database of 275 patients suggested that the SilverHawk device (Fox Hollow Technologies, Redwood City, CA) was an effective endovascular therapy for peripheral arterial intervention with a low mortality, low complication rate, low amputation rate, and rare need for conversion to surgical bypass.[49] Atherectomy devices may be particularly useful for ostial SFA bifurcation lesions (Fig. 39.7) and calcified lesions.

Clinical Data

RCTs in patients with IC and FPA disease that compared medical therapy with PTA consistently revealed that PTA offers early symptomatic relief at 3 to 6 months compared with medical therapy, and outcomes were similar at 2 years.[48,50] Clinical acute success rates of PTA of FPA disease in the contemporary era exceeds 95%.[38] Contemporary endovascular approaches that include stenting offer acute technical success rates of up to 99%, and short- to medium-term patency rates are superior to PTA alone.[39] The mid- to long-term data of endovascular interventions in patients with IC or CLI and FPA disease are summarized in Tables 39.4 and 39.5.

The advantage of placing a sent in the SFA is that it limits elastic recoil, scaffolds flow-limiting dissection, and provides a higher acute technical support; however, these advantages are counterbalanced by a stent-induced enhanced endothelial hyperplasic response that can result in in-stent restenosis (ISR) and negate the noted advantages of stenting on long-term follow-up. Restenosis following endovascular interventions depends on the severity of the disease (total occlusion vs. patent vessel with a high-grade lesion), the status of the distal runoffs, and the length of the lesion. Whether different stent material and/or drug elution with antiproliferative agents would result in improved outcomes will remain to be seen in future investigations.

Restenosis remains a limiting factor in achieving optimal intermediate to long-term patency. The use of brachytherapy in treating ISR resulted in a 50% reduction in the restenosis rate with no noted increased risk of late thrombosis. The use of sirolimus-eluting stents was not associated with superior

TABLE 39.4 Estimated Pooled Primary Patency Rates Following Balloon Dilation and Stent Implantation in Patients With Intermittent Claudication Secondary to Femoropopliteal Stenoses

Lesion Type and Year After Treatment		Balloon Dilation		Stent Implantation	
		Patency (%)[a]	Range (%)	Patency (%)[a]	Range (%)
Stenosis	0	100 (1.0)	98–100	100 (1.2)	99–100
	1	77 (1.7)	78–80	75 (2.2)	73–79
	2	66 (2.0)	63–71	67 (2.4)	65–71
	3	61 (2.2)	55–68	66 (2.7)	64–70
	4	57 (2.5)	54–63	NA	NA
	5	55 (2.8)	52–62	NA	NA
Occlusion	0	88 (2.9)	81–94	99 (2.3)	92–100
	1	65 (3.0)	55–71	73 (2.8)	69–75
	2	54 (3.1)	45–61	66 (3.0)	61–68
	3	48 (3.3)	40–55	64 (3.2)	59–67
	4	44 (3.5)	36–53	NA	NA
	5	42 (3.7)	33–51	NA	NA

Note: Ranges are derived from sensitivity analyses.
[a]Numbers in parentheses represent the standard error.
NA, Not available.
From Muradin GS, Bosch JL, Stijnen T, et al. Balloon dilation and stent implantation for treatment of femoropopliteal arterial disease: meta-analysis. *Radiology*. 2001;221(1):137–145.

results when compared with BMSs.[42] However, the Zilver PTX, a DES that elutes paclitaxel, showed sustained safety and effectiveness in patients with FPA disease and has been approved by the FDA for use in the SFA.[45] Nitinol, an alloy of nickel and titanium, is flexible and more likely to recover from being crushed when compared with stainless steel. A small single-center clinical trial compared the use of a self-expanding nitinol stent versus PTA with optional stenting (32% in this arm received stents) in symptomatic SFA disease (i.e., severe IC or CLI). In this trial, the use of stents was associated with lower rates of angiographic restenosis at 6 months (24% vs. 43%, *P* = .05) and improved treadmill time at 6 to 12 months. This study is limited by its small size and short-term follow-up.[40] Fig. 39.8 lists the overall success and patency rates of PTA (with and without stenting) versus surgery in all claudicants.

Drug-eluting balloons (DEBs) have shown efficacy in patients undergoing intervention for FPA disease. In the Local Taxan with Short Time Contact for Reduction of Restenosis in Distal Arteries (THUNDER) trial,[51] investigators randomly allocated patients undergoing FPA intervention to a paclitaxel-iopromide DEB or standard balloon angioplasty and found a significant reduction in the primary end point of late lumen loss with the DEB strategy (0.4 ± 1.2 mm vs. 1.7 ± 1.8 mm; $P < .001$). Positive results were also observed in the randomized Femoral Paclitaxel (FemPac) trial, in which late lumen loss was significantly lower with a paclitaxel-iopromide DEB compared with balloon angioplasty (0.5 ± 1.1 vs. 1.0 ± 1.1 mm; $P = .031$).[52] The Lutonix Paclitaxel-Coated Balloon for the Prevention of Femoropopliteal Restenosis Trial (LEVANT I) sought to evaluate the safety and efficacy of the Lutonix DEB, which is coated with 2 μg/mm² paclitaxel and a polysorbate-sorbitol carrier for treatment of FPA lesions.[53] At 6 months, late lumen loss was 58% lower for the Lutonix DCB group (0.46 ± 1.13 mm) than for the control group (1.09 ± 1.07 mm; $P = .016$).[53] Similarly effectiveness data were seen with a paclitaxel-urea DEB (IN.PACT Pacific; Medtronic Vascular).[54] Another recent study compared a paclitaxel-eluting balloon (PEB) with conventional PTA, followed by systematic implantation of a self-expanding nitinol BMS in patients at risk for restenosis.[55] A total of 104 patients (110 FPA lesions in 110 limbs) were randomly assigned to either a PEB plus a BMS or regular balloon angioplasty plus a BMS. The primary end point was 12-month binary restenosis, and secondary end points were freedom from target-lesion revascularization (TLR) and major amputation. Post hoc subanalyses were performed for the comparison of long (≥100 mm) versus short lesions and true lumen versus a subintimal approach. The study found that predilation with DEB angioplasty prior to BMS implantation, compared with a regular balloon plus BMS in complex FPA lesions, reduces restenosis and TLR at 12-month follow-up.[55] The FDA approved Bard's Lutonix 035 DEB in October 2014 and Medtronic's IN.PACT Admiral DEB in January 2015. Two separate meta-analyses of the available data from 11 randomized trials showed a significant improvement in clinical and angiographic outcomes with DEBs.[56,57]

TABLE 39.5 Estimated Pooled Primary Patency Rates Following Balloon Dilation and Stent Implantation in Patients With Critical Limb Ischemia Secondary to Femoropopliteal Stenoses

Lesion Type and Year After Treatment		Balloon Dilation		Stent Implantation	
		Patency (%)[a]	Range (%)	Patency (%)[a]	Range (%)
Stenosis	0	83 (3.7)	69–88	100 (3.3)	94–100
	1	60 (4.0)	46–63	74 (3.8)	68–80
	2	49 (4.0)	35–54	66 (3.9)	59–72
	3	43 (4.1)	30–51	65 (4.1)	58–71
	4	40 (4.3)	26–46	NA	NA
	5	38 (4.5)	24–44	NA	NA
Occlusion	0	70 (3.5)	62–75	98 (3.2)	94–100
	1	47 (3.5)	40–51	73 (3.6)	68–75
	2	36 (3.6)	28–41	65 (3.7)	60–68
	3	30 (3.7)	20–37	63 (3.9)	58–68
	4	27 (3.9)	16–34	NA	NA
	5	25 (4.1)	13–32	NA	NA

Note: Ranges are derived from sensitivity analyses.
[a]Number in parentheses is the standard error.
NA, Not available.
From Muradin GS, Bosch JL, Stijnen T, et al. Balloon dilation and stent implantation for treatment of femoropopliteal arterial disease: meta-analysis. *Radiology*. 2001;221(1):137–145.

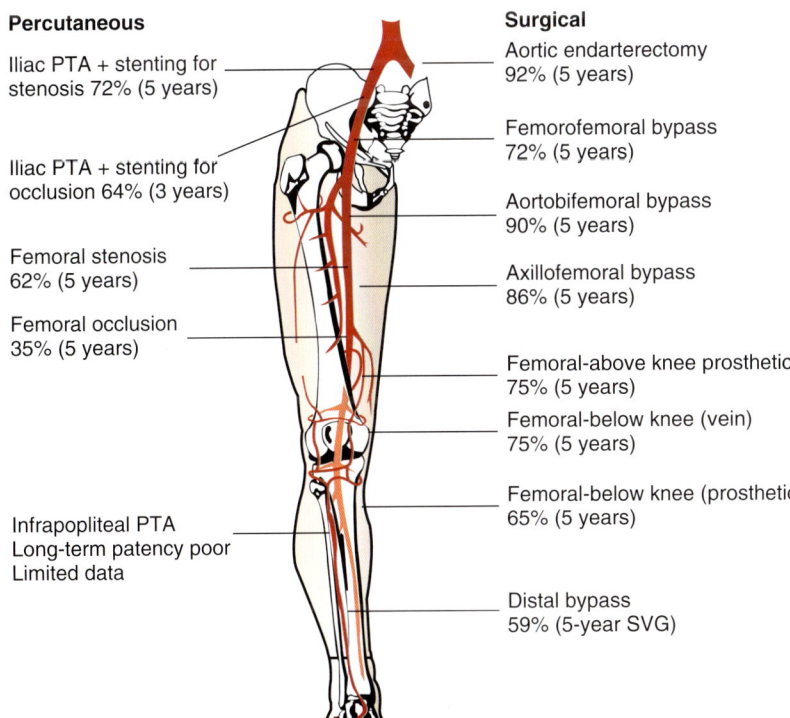

Fig. 39.8 Patency rates for percutaneous and bypass procedures in intermittent claudication. *PTA*, Percutaneous transluminal angioplasty; *SVG*, saphenous vein graft. (Data adapted from the TransAtlantic Inter-Society Consensus [TASC] recommendation.)

RCTs that compare PTA with surgery in the management of infrainguinal PAD are limited. This is partly because the choice of the revascularization modality will depend on how extensive the disease is in the individual patient, surgery being the most likely route of action in the setting of extensive long lesions and in those with CLI. In a multicenter RCT of 263 men, Wolf and associates[22] reported three operative deaths in the surgical arm ($n = 126$) and none in the PTA arm ($n = 129$). No difference in survival was noted, although a trend was seen in favor of the PTA arm. Although patients in both arms had sustained improvement in both hemodynamics and quality of life, the success rate was higher in the surgical arm, and more limb salvage was reported than in the PTA arm. No differences were reported in clinical outcome on median follow up of 4 years. In a small randomized trial, a 1-year patency rate of 43% in the PTA arm ($n = 30$) versus 82% in the surgical arm ($n = 24$) was reported.[58]

Complications and Their Management

Dissection, perforation, and distal embolization are the complications encountered in femoropopliteal interventions. Although the use of stenting is discouraged as a primary strategy, its use as a bailout strategy in the context of flow-limiting dissections and perforations has been well established. The appropriate use of anticoagulation and antiplatelet therapy safeguard against acute and subacute thrombosis and may limit the incidence and the consequences of distal embolization.

When to Refer to Surgery

Although somewhat controversial, surgery remains the preferred strategy for patients with common femoral and proximal DFA obstructive PAD. It is also the preferred strategy for patients with a heavily calcified or completely occluded CFA, femoropopliteal calcified stenosis, occlusions more than 15 cm in length, total occlusions (TOs) of the SFA that are more than 20 cm, and TOs of the popliteal artery or of the proximal trifurcation.[19] It is important to point out that a strategy of initial PTA in lieu of surgery in selected patients is also reasonable.[23]

Infrapopliteal (Runoff) Disease

Indications

Despite the fact that the first reported cases of endovascular interventions in the management of infrapopliteal PAD was in 1964 by Dotter and Judkins, endovascular therapy has had a limited role in the management of infrapopliteal PAD. In patients with IC secondary to infrapopliteal PAD, medical therapy is the most appropriate initial strategy.[2] Tibioperoneal angioplasty is limited by recurrence and also by the need for skilled operators, because the need for emergency surgical bailout is associated with considerable risk that cannot be justified in patients with stable IC, especially when medical management is known to produce similar outcomes with limited risk.[2] However, in carefully selected patients, and in the hands of experienced operators, an acute success rate of 95% (98% for stenosis, 86% for chronic TO) with less than 1% significant complication rates can be achieved.[19,59,60] The role of angioplasty in patients with CLI is more promising and justified because its results are comparable, if not superior, to infrapopliteal/tibial bypass surgery.[59] Endovascular techniques can thus be used as a primary therapy or as an adjunctive therapy to bypass surgery to improve inflow in a diseased segment or to improve the outflow. Up to a quarter of patients with CLI have lesions isolated to arteries below the knee, and these occur mostly in patients with diabetes and other comorbid conditions. Historically, the main concerns with regard to endovascular interventions of the infrapopliteal vessels were the long-term patency, complications, and technical failure of such interventions. With improved equipment, appropriate patient selection, and meticulous technical approach, acute success rates of over 90% and 5-year limb salvage rates of close to 90% are now possible on a more consistent basis, particularly in the context of a comprehensive strategy that includes medical, endovascular, and surgical modalities, as well as lesion surveillance long term.[60]

Techniques

Access and Recanalization Techniques and Devices
Antegrade ipsilateral femoral access is usually used for infrapopliteal interventions. The advantages of such access include a straight-line approach to the lesion and that it allows a shorter length of catheter or balloon shaft, more torque control, and a better mechanical advantage and "pushability" for occlusions or lesions that are difficult to cross. This approach requires experience to minimize complications at the access site. If combined below- and above-knee PTA is necessary, angioplasty of the tibioperoneal arteries initially might lower the risk of peripheral embolization. In the Uppsala series, 6 of the initial 40 procedures had embolization that required either transcatheter embolectomy or local streptokinase infusion. After altering their practice so that distal angioplasty was performed prior to more proximal lower limb angioplasty, no embolization was seen in the subsequent 54 procedures.

Because occlusion of these end arteries jeopardizes the feet and leaves no surgical bailout options, the characteristics of reported successful series must be carefully considered. In Dorros and colleagues' series,[59] tibioperoneal lesions had to be less than 10 cm in length, and distal vessels were visualized. Occlusions were less successfully opened than stenoses (73% vs. 98%), and a residual stenosis of up to 50% was acceptable for these relatively small vessels. Complete multivessel revascularization may not be necessary, especially when a significant improvement in ABI is already documented. If angioplasty results in straight-line flow to the foot, clinical success rates of up to 80% at 24 months have been reported; conversely, the lack of straight-line flow portends failure within 11 months. Vasospasm usually abates with intra-arterial nitroglycerin or verapamil.

Stent Choice

Stents are not recommended in the management of infrapopliteal disease; however, stent placement may be used as a bailout in the context of flow-limiting dissections. The Percutaneous Transluminal Angioplasty and Drug-Eluting Stents for Infrapopliteal Lesions in Critical Limb Ischemia (PADI) trial[61] was a prospective, multicenter, randomized, controlled, double-arm study to investigate the safety and efficacy of primary PES implantation versus PTA in infrapopliteal lesions in CLI. The 5-year rates of amputation- and event-free survival (survival free from major amputation or reintervention) were significantly higher in the DES arm compared with PTA—BMS (31.8% vs. 20.4%, $P = .043$; and 26.2% vs. 15.3%, $P = 0.041$, respectively), but survival rates were comparable.

Specific Techniques

Zeller and colleagues[62] reported that below-knee native vessel lesions with a diameter of at least 2 mm can be treated with the SilverHawk catheter with a high success rate and a low complication rate. Orbital atherectomy was tested as a unique approach to infrapopliteal disease and provided predictable and safe lumen enlargement.[63] The real-world multicenter study CONFIRM prospectively followed 728 consecutive patients, in 57 institutions, treated with orbital atherectomy.[64] The study showed that orbital atherectomy effectively reduced the degree of stenosis with the use of adjunctive low-pressure balloon angioplasty.[65] Overall, atherectomy devices can reduce the burden of soft atheromatous or calcific plaque, change vessel compliance, leading to a decrease in the need for bail-out stenting, but have not shown improvement in hard end points.

Clinical Data

Despite advances in modern aggressive revascularization techniques, the mortality and morbidity rates for this cohort of patients have remained substantial, with 30-day mortality rates of around 4% to 10%, a 6% to 14% amputation rate, and 90-day graft failure rates of close to 5%.[66] The 5-year patency rate for femoral below-knee bypass is about 75% (vein graft) to 60% (prosthetic grafts), whereas for distal bypass, it is about 50%.[4] An important contributor to these poor outcomes is the substantial disease burden in this cohort of patients, who have a preponderance of coronary artery disease (CAD), diabetes mellitus, and baseline tissue loss (foot ulcer, gangrene, or nonhealing wound).[4]

No RCTs have compared strategies for the treatment of below-knee arterial occlusive disease. Dorros and colleagues[67] reported the largest prospective series of infrapopliteal angioplasty on 284 limbs with CLI (Fontaine stages III and IV) in 235 patients between 1983 and 1996. The mean age was 67 years, 69% were males, half had diabetes, more than a quarter had previous MI, a third had prior coronary artery bypass surgery, and 39% had prior peripheral vascular surgery. The overall acute technical success rate was 100% for inflow lesions and 92% for infrapopliteal lesions. The success rate was 98% for stenoses but only 73% for occlusions. Complications were infrequent: 0.7% in-hospital all-cause mortality, 0.7% emergency vascular surgery, 9% in-hospital major amputation, and 0.4%, or one case each, of compartment syndrome, major infection, and transfusion were reported. A series ($n = 60$) reported by Söder and associates[60] involved an older (mean age, 72 year) and sicker cohort: more than 75% had diabetes, almost 25% had baseline renal insufficiency, 90% presented with minor (81%) or major (9.7%) tissue loss, and the majority were not eligible for distal bypass surgery (no runoff in 70 limbs, single-vessel runoff in two limbs). This group reported a primary angiographic success rate of 84% (102 of 121) for stenosis and 61% (41 of 67) for occlusions with corresponding restenosis rates of 32% and 52% at follow-up angiography performed at a mean of 10 months after primary PTA. The rate of major complications was 2.8% (access-site pseudoaneurysms in two patients). The primary clinical success was 63% (45 of 72). A 48% cumulative primary patency rate, a 56% secondary patency rate, and an 80% cumulative limb-salvage rate were reported at 18 months. Factors that independently correlated with continued lesion patency up to 12 months were angiographic improvement to the site of most severe ischemia (6-month primary patency of 68% vs. 16%; $P = .001$) and absence of renal insufficiency (patency of 63% vs. 24%; $P = .06%$). Clinical success, defined as relief of claudication or avoidance of major amputation, was achieved in only 45 of 72 limbs (63%) acutely, but this is comparable to results from surgical series. No patient in this series had a subsequent surgical bypass operation for the limbs, largely because of poor distal targets or pedal arteries.

Local delivery of paclitaxel via DEBs had shown promising results in the infrapopliteal area, with a reduction in 3-month binary restenosis compared with historic controls treated with PTA.[68] Subsequently, several randomized trials examined the efficacy of DEBs in infrapopliteal disease. In the Drug-Eluting Balloon Evaluation for Lower Limb MUltilevel TreatMent (DEBELLUM) trial, 50 consecutive patients with 122 lesions in the femoral–popliteal and/or infrapopliteal arteries were randomized to DEBs or standard PTA.[69] Late lumen loss was lower in the DEB group (0.5 ± 1.4 vs. 1.6 ± 1.7 mm, $P < .01$), and target lesion revascularization was necessary in 6.1% of the DEB group versus 23.6% of the standard PTA group ($P = .02$). The Drug-eluting balloon in peripheral intervention for below the knee angioplasty evaluation (DEBATE-BTK) trial examined a paclitaxel DEB for the reduction of restenosis in diabetic patients with CLI.[70] DEB compared with PTA strikingly reduce 1-year restenosis, target lesion revascularization, and target vessel occlusion in the treatment of below-the-knee lesions in diabetic patients with CLI. The Infrapopliteal Drug-Eluting Angioplasty versus Stenting (IDEAS) trial randomized 50 patients to infrapopliteal DEB angioplasty (25 arteries in 25 limbs) or primary DES placement (30 arteries in 27 limbs).[71] Compared with DEB in long infrapopliteal lesions, DES were associated with significantly lower residual immediate postprocedure stenosis and significantly reduced restenosis at 6 months.[71] Even though RCTs have demonstrated technical superiority of DEBs over standard PTA, there are still concerns that need to be addressed prior to their widespread use as primary treatment for patients with infrapopliteal PAD. One of the main issues is the lack of a significant difference in hard end points such as major amputation or mortality rates between DEBs and standard PTA.

Current guidelines espouse the angiosome concept for infrapopliteal CLI, which entails establishing direct blood flow to the infrapopliteal artery directly responsible for perfusing the region of the leg or foot with the nonhealing wound.[2]

When to Refer to Surgery

In the management of infrapopliteal disease, bypass surgery has been associated with disappointing results. Just as with PTA, the patency rate of bypass grafting remains inferior to that of bypass grafting in more proximal PAD as shown in Fig. 39.7. Success in achieving limb salvage with minimal periprocedual complication is dependent on the status of distal circulation and on the overall risk profile of the patient. Amputation—primary, when no antecedent attempt is made on revascularization, or secondary, following failure of revascularization—may be necessary in patients with CLI complicated by intractable infections or uncontrollable rest pain.

ACUTE LIMB ISCHEMIA

Acute limb ischemia (ALI) is defined as a sudden or rapidly developing loss of limb perfusion that results in the development or worsening of symptoms and signs of limb ischemia with an eminent threat to limb viability. ALI may be the first manifestation of PAD in previously asymptomatic patients.[7] More commonly, patients with IC will experience progression in their disease with development of rest pain, ischemic ulcers, and eventually gangrene. Although it may be gradual, this progression is usually the result of recurrent acute ischemic events. Two mechanisms are implicated in ALI: embolism and in situ thrombosis. Differentiation based on history and clinical examination alone may be clinically impossible in 10% to 15% of cases. Although little information is available on the incidence of ALI in the general population, it is estimated to be 14 per 100,000 and is the indication for 10% to 16% of all vascular procedures performed. Patients with embolic ALI are more likely to die than those with thrombosis, usually secondary to underlying cardiac disease, whereas patients with thrombotic ALI are more likely to lose their limbs when compared with those who have embolic ALI.

The natural history of ALI has remained largely unchanged despite the advances in the surgical, endovascular, and pharmacologic therapies. Patients who present with ALI continue to have a particularly poor short-term outlook both in terms of loss of the leg and mortality, with 30-day amputation rates of between 10% and 30% and a mortality rate of 15%. The fact that overall mortality rates after intervention for acute ischemia have not improved dramatically over the past 20 years reflects the severity of the underlying atherosclerotic burden in these high-risk patients.[2]

An embolic event complicates atrial fibrillation, MI with left ventricular thrombus, or peripheral pseudoaneurysm. Thrombosis in situ is usually encountered in patients with PAD and tenuous collateral circulation, or it may be seen in patients with prior bypass surgery with an acute thrombosis of the graft. Also of importance are other mechanisms of ALI such as septic or cardiac tumor emboli; trauma, such as popliteal artery disruption; and dissection of large vessels with distal progression, such as aortic dissection with iliac artery occlusion. Table 39.6 shows a recommended classification of ALI, which is useful in estimating the impact for the individual patient and in determining the prognosis of the limb at presentation.[72]

Management Strategies of Acute Limb Ischemia

In approaching patients with suspected ALI, history and physical examination should be focused on establishing the underlying mechanism of the ALI to categorize the patient based on the underlying leg symptoms and signs, in addition to the Doppler assessment of the peripheral pulses. Once the diagnosis of ALI is made, the objective should be to prevent thrombus propagation and worsening ischemia. Thus anticoagulation with heparin, if not contraindicated, is the first step in management. Restoration of the flow as soon as possible is the next step (for viable limbs in Fontaine class I and II), using either pharmacologic or endovascular versus open catheter thromboembolectomy. If the patient has a true late nonviable limb (class III), amputation is the only option because revascularization of such limbs is of no benefit but rather is associated with a high risk of mortality. Table 39.7 gives the recommended medications and doses of thrombolytic therapy. In general, patients with clear embolic etiology and a discernible location of obstruction by physical exam are taken to surgery for open embolectomy. If there is no clear embolic etiology, an arteriogram should be performed and the decision is made, based on the findings, regarding endovascular versus surgical interventions.

Interventional Treatment

Pharmacologic Thrombolysis

Although systemic thrombolysis has no role in the management of ALI, catheter-directed thrombolytic therapy is effective in the management of patients with class I and IIa ischemia. This approach is clearly less invasive, has less morbidity and mortality when compared with open surgery, and may reduce the risk of reperfusion injury. The choice of lytic therapy will depend on the location, anatomy, and patient comorbidities. Contraindication to thrombolysis should be observed.

Percutaneous Aspiration Thrombectomy

Percutaneous aspiration thrombectomy (PAT) is an alternative nonsurgical modality to treat ALI that uses large-lumen catheters and suction with a 50-mL syringe to remove embolus or thrombus from native vessels, bypass grafts, and runoff vessels. PAT devices such as the Amplatz Clot Buster (BARD-Microvena, White Bear Lake, MN) and the Straub Rotarex System (Straub Medical, Wangs, Switzerland) have been used with fibrinolysis to reduce the time and dose of the fibrinolytic agent or as a stand-alone procedure.

Percutaneous Mechanical Thrombectomy

The concept of creating a "hydrodynamic recirculation vortex" that would dissolve a thrombus and remove its fragments is the underlying thought behind most percutaneous mechanical thrombectomy (PMT) devices, such as AngioJet (Possis Medical, Minneapolis, MN), Hydrolyser (Cordis, Warren, NJ), Penumbra's Indigo Mechanical Thrombectomy System (Alameda, CA) and Oasis (Boston Scientific/Medi-tech, Natick, MA) thrombectomy systems. The efficacy of PMT depends on the age of the thrombus because fresh thrombi can be efficiently removed, unlike old, organized thrombi.

Surgery

The indications for surgery include patients with clear embolic etiology, where an open embolectomy can be performed, and patients with CLI (classes IIb and III). Surgery is associated with the risk of infection, hemorrhage, and periprocedural cardiovascular adverse events.

Critical Leg Ischemia

Critical leg (or limb) ischemia (CLI) is characterized by persistent rest pain with or without ongoing tissue loss, ischemic ulceration,

TABLE 39.6 Classification of Acute Limb Ischemia

		Neuromuscular	
Category	Description	Findings	Doppler
I	Viable	No sensory or muscle weakness	Audible arterial and venous
IIa	Threatened (marginally)	Minimal	Often inaudible arterial, audible venous
IIb	Threatened (immediately)	Mild to moderate, associated with pain	Usually inaudible arterial, audible venous
III	Irreversible	Profound deficit	No signals

From Weaver FA, Comerota AJ, Youngblood M, et al. Surgical revascularization versus thrombolysis for nonembolic lower extremity native artery occlusions: results of a prospective randomized trial. The STILE Investigators. Surgery versus thrombolysis for ischemia of the lower extremity. J Vasc Surg. 1996;24(4):513–521, discussion 521–523.

TABLE 39.7 Recommended Doses of Antiplatelet, Antithrombotic, and Thrombolytic Medications for Management of Acute Limb Ischemia

Medication	Route	Dosage	Laboratory
Aspirin	PO/PR	81–325 mg	None
Clopidogrel	PO	300–600 mg loading dose; 75 mg maintenance dose	None
Heparin	IV	60 U/kg bolus then 12 U/kg/h	aPTT, plts, Hct
Vorapaxar[b]	PO	2.08 mg daily	None
Mannitol	IV	12.5–25 g	Creatinine
Plasminogen activator	IA	Depends on agent[a]	Hct, fibrinogen, FSP
Urokinase	IA	80,000–200,000 U/h tapered infusion	Hct, fibrinogen, FSP

[a]Depends on thrombolytic (retaplase 0.25–1.0 U/h; alteplase 0.2–1.0 mg/h; tenecteplase 0.25–0.5 mg/h).
[b]Do not use in patients with a history of stroke, TIA, or ICH.
aPTT, Activated partial thromboplastin; FSP, fibrin split products; Hct, hematocrit; IA, intraarterial; ICH, intracranial hemorrhage; IV, intravenous; plts, platelet count; PO, per os (orally); PR, per rectum (rectally).
From Rajagopalan S, Mukherjee D, Mohler E, eds. Manual of Vascular Diseases. Philadelphia: Lippincott Wilkins & Williams; 2004:92.

or gangrene. The term *critical limb ischemia* is traditionally used to describe patients with ischemic symptoms of more than 2 weeks duration. Patients with CLI usually have ankle systolic pressure below 40 mm Hg, toe systolic pressure below 30 mm Hg, reduced transcutaneous oxygen concentration ($TCPO_2$) of less than 50 mm Hg, or combinations of these.

In general, the underlying etiology is almost exclusively atherosclerosis, and frequently it is a multivessel and multisegment disease. Smoking and diabetes are the most potent risk factors and are associated with higher rates of amputation. The prognosis in patients with CLI is poor secondary to comorbid conditions: mortality rates approach 10% per year, and amputation rates of 25% to 45% at 1 year.[7]

Interventional Treatment and Surgery

Management of CLI depends on the patient's *risk profile* (expected operative mortality, underlying renal function, and the risk of contrast nephropathy, etc.) and *anatomic profile* (multisegment, multivessel, the number of runoffs, the suitability of the disease to PTA vs. surgery, etc.). Fig. 39.9 outlines a general approach to the management of CLI.

Periprocedural Antithrombotic Therapy

PTA and stenting are usually conducted with weight-based heparinization to achieve an activated clotting time of 200 to 250 seconds. A front load of aspirin (325 mg) and clopidogrel (300 to 600 mg) at least 12 hours prior to intervention is widely used. The use of glycoprotein IIb/IIIa may be useful in the context of diabetes or evidence of angiographic thrombus or ulceration and in patients with poor runoff (one vessel or none) to prevent distal embolization. After PTA and stenting, life-long aspirin therapy is recommended in light of the high cardiovascular event rate in patients with advanced PAD. Most clinicians prescribe adjunctive clopidogrel for 1 to 12 months after a lower extremity percutaneous intervention.

Post Peripheral Bypass Surgery Patient

Various types of vascular bypass grafts are used in the management of lower extremity PAD. A detailed discussion of this subject is beyond the scope of this chapter; however, interventionalists are likely to encounter graft-related complications, the most serious of which is ALI secondary to graft thrombosis.

In general, acute thrombosis of bypass grafts is secondary to technical problems and usually presents in the early postoperative period and requires an urgent intervention. In this setting, patients should be anticoagulated and then evaluated for balloon catheter thrombectomy. Mature graft thrombosis occurs at a rate of 10% at 5 years and rarely presents with ALI. Such patients are managed with thrombolytic therapy to clear the thrombus burden, and then the underlying etiology should be addressed either through an endovascular approach or by open surgery.[73]

MISCELLANEOUS CONDITIONS

Buerger Disease (Thromboangiitis)

Buerger disease is a nonatherosclerotic inflammatory vasculitis of the small and medium-sized arteries, veins, and nerves. It can affect upper and lower extremities and occurs most commonly in young male smokers. The etiology is uncertain, although a clear and strong association exists with smoking and tobacco use. The mainstay of therapy is smoking cessation, and in fact without

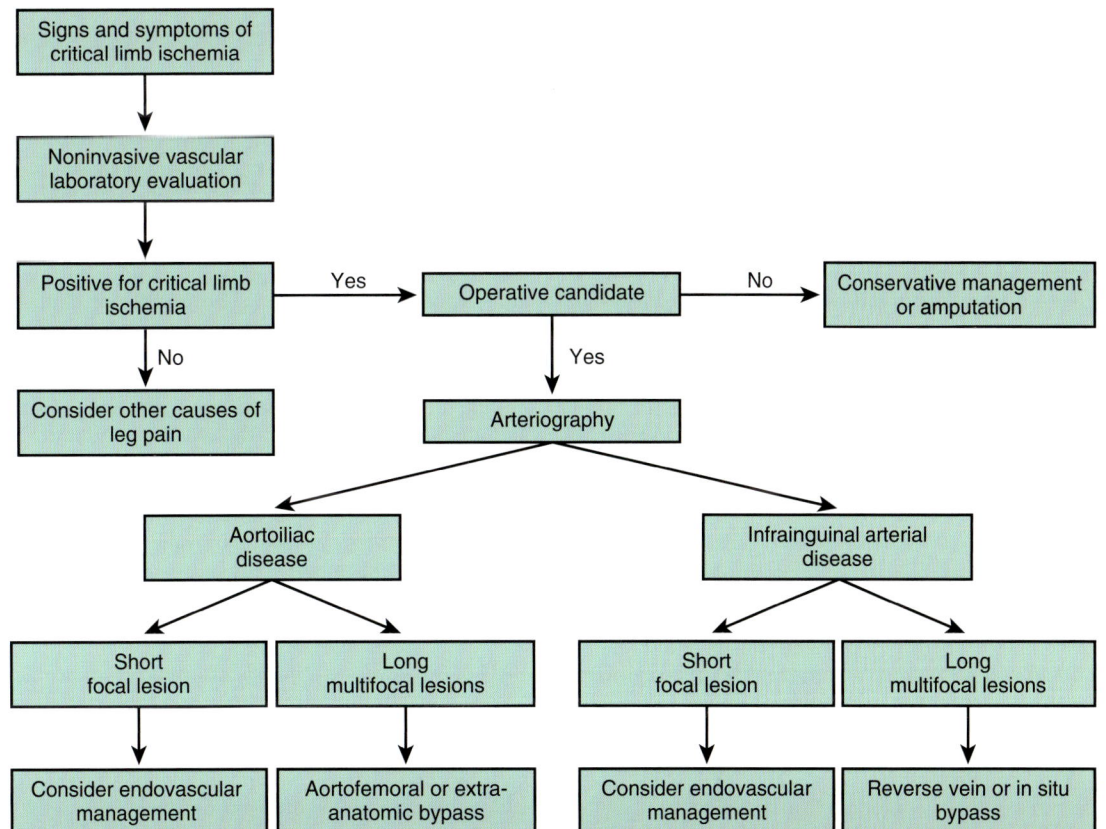

Fig. 39.9 Treatment algorithm for patients with critical limb ischemia. (From Rajagopalan S, Mukherjee D, Mohler E, eds. *Manual of Vascular Diseases*. Philadelphia: Lippincott Williams & Wilkins; 2004:92.)

complete cessation of smoking and tobacco use, the prognosis for limb salvage is dismal.[74] Medical therapy with antiplatelets, immunosuppressants (cyclophosphamide), and analgesics has been used.

Surgical revascularization of the lower extremity in the context of Buerger disease has a limited role in light of the diffuse nature of the disease and its tendency to involve distal small vessels before progressing proximally. Bypass surgery, when feasible, should be done with an autologous vein and veins not affected by the disease process. Percutaneous intervention has no clear role in the management of patients with Buerger disease.

Peripheral Aneurysm

The most common cause of peripheral aneurysm formation is atherosclerosis. Other predisposing factors include hypertension, inflammatory and infectious processes, trauma, connective tissue diseases, and familial tendencies. Whereas most aneurysms are asymptomatic, they can become the source of distal embolization, they can become infected, they may compress surrounding tissues, or they may rupture. Aneurysms of the lower extremity have particular complications depending on their location.

Iliac artery aneurysms are associated with atheroembolism, obstructive uropathies, iliac vein obstruction, and perineal or groin pain. The use of MRA or multidetector contrast computed tomography (CT) is the preferred strategy for diagnosis. Traditionally speaking, surgical resection is indicated if the aneurysm is symptomatic or is more than 3 cm in diameter. Endovascular treatment using a variety of options available today, such as coil embolization or stent-graft placement, may be an alternative to surgery. Early experience indicates that endovascular treatment is safe and effective in the hands of skilled operators; however, large long-term follow-up studies are needed to determine whether this approach is a practical alternative to open surgery.[75]

Femoral artery aneurysm is associated with atheroembolism and venous obstruction. It can be diagnosed with ultrasound and is managed surgically if symptomatic. Case series of endovascular interventions have been reported, but the data are limited, and larger studies with long-term follow-up are needed to help identify the role of this approach in the setting of femoral artery aneurysm.[76]

Popliteal artery aneurysm is associated with thrombosis, atheroembolism, venous obstruction, popliteal neuropathy, and infection. It can be bilateral in 50% of patients. Ultrasound can be used to make the diagnosis, although contrast angiography is generally needed prior to surgery to assess the proximal and distal circulation (Fig. 39.10). Once diagnosed, popliteal artery aneurysm should be resected to prevent its potentially devastating thromboembolic complications. Endovascular repair of popliteal artery aneurysms is a new technique that has emerged as an alternative to open surgical bypass. The evidence to support its use is limited, but early results have been promising and have shown high rates of initial treatment success.[77]

Atheroembolism

Atheroembolism refers to the occlusion of arteries secondary to the detachment and embolization of atheromatous debris, which includes cholesterol crystals, platelets, fibrin, and calcium. Atheroemboli can originate from any atherosclerotic segment, although typically they originate from aortic atheromas and from aneurysms of the large and medium-sized arteries. They tend to occlude small end arteries and arterioles such as those of the kidneys, retina, brain, and extremities.

Clinical features of this disorder are usually reflective of acute ischemic complications and depend on the affected organ. Atheroembolic events in the lower extremity would result in painful cyanotic toes (blue toe syndrome) and are associated with

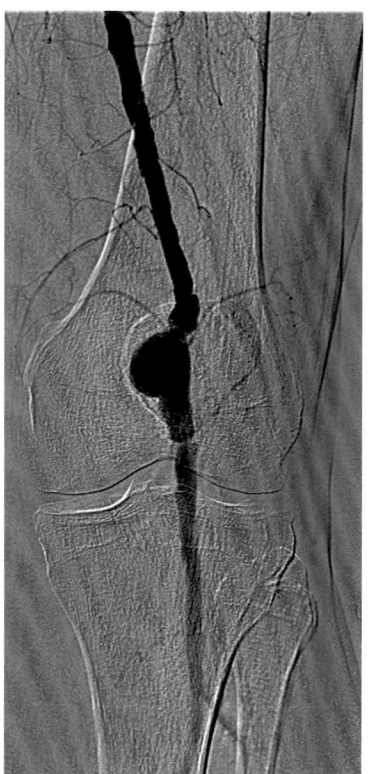

Fig. 39.10 Digital subtraction angiography of left popliteal artery showing aneurysm.

digital and foot ulcerations in addition to multiorgan dysfunction, depending on the extent of the embolic burden. Levido reticularis is common in patients with atheroembolism and is encountered in up to 50% of patients. It is important to point out that distal pulses will remain intact, unlike with CLI and ALI secondary to thromboembolism, in which pulses are usually abnormal because atheroemboli occlude smaller, more distal vessels. The differential diagnosis includes many conditions such as vasculitis and prothrombotic conditions, such as antiphospholipid syndrome and heparin-induced thrombocytopenia.

Affected patients may have an elevated erythrocyte sedimentation rate, thrombocytopenia, eosinophilia, eosinophiluria, and hypocomplementemia. The finding of cholesterol crystals in small arteries is a pathognomonic sign when found in skin or muscle biopsies. Transesophageal echocardiography, CT scan, and MRA can be used to visualize the aorta (searching for shaggy, mobile atheromas), and assessment of aneurysms by ultrasound and angiography is part of the workup to identify the source of the emboli if possible.

If the source cannot be identified, no definitive therapy exists, but antiplatelet therapy with aspirin has been advocated. If the source is identified, surgical removal or endovascular isolation of the source of the emboli is the only definitive therapy.[78]

CONCLUSIONS AND FUTURE DIRECTIONS

PAD of the lower extremity is a serious health problem associated with significant morbidity, and it is a reflection of advanced atherosclerosis that often affects other vascular trees. Although the management of patients with IC is based on an integrated exercise program and pharmacologic modification of the associated risk factors, percutaneous interventions have emerged as an effective alternative to surgical revascularization in patients who remain symptomatic or those who progress to CLI. Advances in technology will likely continue to optimize the role of percutaneous interventions in the management of PAD, and whereas such interventions are already very effective in the management of IC caused by iliofemoral disease, room for improvement remains in the use of such interventions in the management of infrapopliteal disease and of ALI and CLI. The use of DEB therapy for de novo PAD has been quite effective.[79] Future studies need to define the optimal antiplatelet therapy (drug or drugs and dosage) for prevention of cardiovascular and limb-related events in patients with PAD, and compare efficacy and cost effectiveness of the different endovascular technologies for treatment of claudication and CLI, including drug-coated balloons and DESs. Such studies should include patient-centered end points, such as functional parameters, time to wound healing, and quality of life in addition to standard patency-focused outcomes. Finally, optimal management of the patient with peripheral arterial disease should involve a multidisciplinary team consisting of the patient's primary care physician, cardiologist, vascular interventionalist and a vascular surgeon, to decide on the best strategy for the individual patient.

KEY REFERENCES

2. Gerhard-Herman MD, Gornik HL, Barrett C, et al. 2016 AHA/ACC guideline on the management of patients with lower extremity peripheral artery disease: a Report of the American College of Cardiology/American Heart Association Task Force on Clinical Practice Guidelines. *Circulation*. 2017;135(12):e726–e779.
12. Anderson JL, Halperin JL, Albert NM, et al. Management of patients with peripheral artery disease (compilation of 2005 and 2011 ACCF/AHA guideline recommendations): a report of the American College of Cardiology Foundation/American Heart Association Task Force on Practice Guidelines. *Circulation*. 2013;127(13):1425–1443.
14. Lim JC, Ranatunga D, Owen A, et al. Multidetector (64+) computed tomography angiography of the lower limb in symptomatic peripheral arterial disease: assessment of image quality and accuracy in a tertiary care setting. *J Comput Assist Tomogr*. 2017;41(2):327–333.
16. Stoner MC, Calligaro KD, Chaer RA, et al. Reporting standards of the Society for Vascular Surgery for endovascular treatment of chronic lower extremity peripheral artery disease. *J Vasc Surg*. 2016;64(1):e1–e21.
19. Norgren L, Hiatt WR, Dormandy JA, et al. Inter-Society Consensus for the Management of Peripheral Arterial Disease (TASC II). *J Vasc Surg*. 2007;45(suppl S):S5–S67.
45. Dake MD, Ansel GM, Jaff MR, et al. Durable clinical effectiveness with paclitaxel-eluting stents in the femoropopliteal artery: 5-year results of the Zilver PTX randomized trial. *Circulation*. 2016;133(15):1472–1483.
51. Tepe G, Zeller T, Albrecht T, et al. Local delivery of paclitaxel to inhibit restenosis during angioplasty of the leg. *N Engl J Med*. 358(7):689–699.
53. Scheinert D, Duda S, Zeller T, et al. The LEVANT I (Lutonix paclitaxel-coated balloon for the prevention of femoropopliteal restenosis) trial for femoropopliteal revascularization: first-in-human randomized trial of low-dose drug-coated balloon versus uncoated balloon angioplasty. *JACC. Cardiovasc Interv*. 2014;7(1):10–19.
56. Kayssi A, Al-Atassi T, Oreopoulos G, et al. Drug-eluting balloon angioplasty versus uncoated balloon angioplasty for peripheral arterial disease of the lower limbs. *Cochrane Database Syst Rev*. 2016;8:CD011319.
61. Spreen MI, Martens JM, Knippenberg B, et al. Long-term follow-up of the PADI trial: percutaneous transluminal angioplasty versus drug-eluting stents for infrapopliteal lesions in critical limb ischemia. *J Am Heart Assoc*. 2017;6(4):e004877.
65. Das T, Mustapha J, Indes J, et al. Technique optimization of orbital atherectomy in calcified peripheral lesions of the lower extremities: the CONFIRM series, a prospective multicenter registry. *Catheter Cardiovasc Interv*. 2014;83(1):115–122.
71. Siablis D, Kitrou PM, Spiliopoulos S, et al. Paclitaxel-coated balloon angioplasty versus drug-eluting stenting for the treatment of infrapopliteal long-segment arterial occlusive disease: the IDEAS randomized controlled trial. *JACC Cardiovasc Interv*. 2014;7(9):1048–1056.
77. Ronchey S, Pecoraro F, Alberti V, et al. Popliteal artery aneurysm repair in the endovascular era: fourteen-years single center experience. *Medicine (Baltimore)*. 2015;94(30):e1130.
79. Schneider PA, Laird JR, Tepe G, et al. Treatment effect of drug-coated balloons is durable to 3 years in the femoropopliteal arteries long-term results of the IN.PACT SFA Randomized Trial. *Circulation: Cardiovasc Interv*. 2018;11:e005891. https://doi.org/10.1161/CIRCINTERVENTIONS.117.005891.

 Additional references available online at expertconsult.com.

中文导读

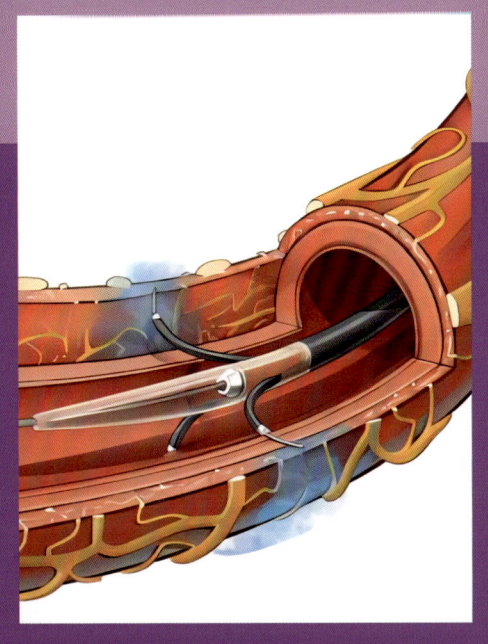

第40章
上肢和主动脉弓

　　心脏病学在血管医学领域的持续发展是一个自然的延伸，因为动脉粥样硬化是一个不仅仅与冠状动脉系统相关的系统性过程，冠状动脉、颈动脉和肱动脉等外周血管的动脉粥样硬化程度之间存在高度的相关性。大多数冠状动脉疾病的管理概念、保守治疗和经皮介入治疗技术可借鉴到外周血管疾病的治疗中。本章节讨论涉及上肢（如腋动脉和肱动脉）和近主动脉弓血管（如锁骨下动脉）的外周血管的解剖学、流行病学、危险因素、诊断和治疗。由于症状的相似性，例如，血管病变、动脉瘤或夹闭综合征、栓塞现象、药物和化学物质暴露等情况可能使诊断复杂化。因此，涉及上肢和主动脉弓血管的疾病往往需要具备广泛的知识面，掌握全面的病史和通过系统的体格检查来准确诊断与鉴别诊断。有20%～30%的人群存在上肢及主动脉弓的解剖变异，临床意义取决于其异常情况。由于介入治疗成功率高、再狭窄率低、通畅率高、成本低、恢复时间快，经皮血运重建已取代外科手术成为治疗动脉粥样硬化性头臂动脉或锁骨下动脉狭窄的一线治疗方法。在对上肢大血管疾病进行经皮介入治疗之前，应充分评估分支血管与病变的关系，以及病变的开口受累情况。由于栓塞大脑前循环的可能性，经皮介入治疗头臂动脉比锁骨下动脉血运重建更为复杂。上肢动脉和主动脉弓血管疾病的管理需要识别患者手术指征及时机，并了解动脉瘤疾病的管理。

周　政　张洪亮

章节要点

- 一个血管床的动脉疾病往往是其他血管床疾病的先兆。
- 涉及上肢、主动脉弓及分支血管的疾病较为复杂,需要全面地了解病史、详细的体格检查,并具备丰富的知识面才能更好地进行鉴别诊断。
- 对于疑似动脉血管疾病的患者,应测量双上肢血压;如果疑似大动脉炎,应测量四肢血压。
- 上肢及主动脉弓血管的解剖变异发生率为20%~30%,有无病理学意义取决于其具体异常表现。
- 合并上肢血管疾病的体格检查需包含评估是否存在胸廓出口综合征的可能。
- 在对上肢大血管疾病进行经皮介入治疗前,应充分评估分支血管与病变的关系及开口受累情况。
- 由于栓塞大脑前循环的可能性,经皮介入头臂动脉比锁骨下动脉血运重建更为复杂。
- 经皮介入治疗因其成功率高、再狭窄率低、通畅率高、成本低、恢复时间快已成为治疗动脉粥样硬化性头臂动脉或锁骨下动脉狭窄的一线疗法。
- 上肢和主动脉弓血管疾病的诊治需要掌握手术时机,并了解动脉瘤疾病的管理。

40 Upper Extremities and Aortic Arch

Kimberly S. Delcour, Ivan P. Casserly, Robert S. Dieter

KEY POINTS

- Arterial disease in one vascular bed is a harbinger of disease in other vascular beds.
- The differential diagnosis of diseases involving the upper extremity (UE) and aortic arch branch vessels is vast and requires extensive knowledge and a thorough history and physical examination.
- In patients with suspected arterial disease, blood pressure should be measured in both UEs, and if Takayasu arteritis is suspected, blood pressure should be measured in all four extremities.
- Anatomic variation in the UE vessels and aortic arch occurs in 20% to 30% of the population, and the pathologic significance depends on the anomaly.
- The physical examination of a patient with UE disease is incomplete in the absence of performing diagnostic maneuvers to evaluate for thoracic outlet syndrome (TOS).
- Before performing percutaneous intervention for UE large vessel disease, the relationship of branch vessels to the lesion and ostial involvement of the lesion should be thoroughly evaluated.
- Percutaneous intervention in the brachiocephalic artery is more complicated than revascularization of the subclavian artery due to the potential for embolization to the anterior cerebral circulation.
- Percutaneous revascularization has become first-line therapy instead of surgery for treating atherosclerotic brachiocephalic or subclavian stenosis because of the high technical success rates, the low restenosis and high patency rates, and lower cost with quicker recovery times.
- Management of UE arterial and aortic arch vascular disease requires discernment of when to refer patients to surgery and an understanding of the management of aneurysmal disease.

INTRODUCTION

From the inception of the subspecialty of interventional cardiology, to the Centers for Medicare and Medicaid Services (CMS) physician specialty designation for interventional cardiology, the scope of interventional cardiology has continued to expand. The discipline has grown beyond percutaneous management of coronary artery disease to include therapy for valvular and structural heart disease and endovascular treatment of aortic aneurysm, venous disease, and peripheral arterial disease (PAD), including management of vascular disease in the upper extremity (UE) and proximal arch vessels.

The continued evolution of cardiology in the field of vascular medicine has been a natural extension because atherosclerosis is a systemic process that is not isolated to the coronary vasculature, and a high degree of correlation exists between the extent of atherosclerosis in the coronary, carotid, and brachial arteries.[1] Coronary disease is associated with an increased risk of PAD, and among those with PAD, the risk of coronary and cerebrovascular ischemic events with significant morbidity and mortality is extremely high.[2-6] Most of the management concepts and techniques for coronary arterial disease are transferable to the treatment of PAD when a conservative medical strategy or percutaneous therapy is employed.

General and interventional cardiologists care for patients with coexistent coronary and peripheral vascular disease and those with significant risk factors for the development of arterial vascular disease. These clinicians must have a thorough understanding of PAD, including the application of screening tools and management strategies.

This chapter discusses the anatomy, epidemiology, risk factors, diagnosis, and treatment of PAD involving the UE (i.e., axillary and brachial arteries) and proximal arch vessel (i.e., subclavian artery). It excludes carotid arterial disease evaluation and management, which are discussed in Chapter 46.

EPIDEMIOLOGY AND RISK FACTORS FOR PERIPHERAL ARTERIAL DISEASE

Considering an age-adjusted prevalence of about 12%, PAD is estimated to affect at least 8 to 12 million individuals in the United States.[2,7] Advancing age is strongly associated with the increased prevalence of PAD, and approximately 20% of U.S. adults older than 70 years have PAD.[6,8]

PAD has been reported to affect males and females equally, but studies have demonstrated a greater predilection for PAD among blacks versus nonHispanic whites (38% vs. 25% of men), and the ethnic propensity is independent of traditional risk factors for cardiovascular disease such as hypertension, hyperlipidemia, diabetes, kidney disease, and tobacco use.[6-9] An estimated 25% to 40% of patients seen in the general cardiology clinic have PAD,[2,3,5] and up to 50% of patients with PAD may be asymptomatic, illustrating the need for careful evaluation of patients of advancing age and those with risk factors for cardiovascular and peripheral vascular disease.[6]

Unlike PAD involving the lower extremities, atherosclerosis is estimated to account for only about 5% of cases of UE ischemia. Obstruction of the brachiocephalic (innominate) or subclavian (inflow) arteries accounts for most cases due to the propensity for atherosclerosis at those sites, with a fourfold higher occurrence on the left than the right.[10,11] However, not all UE ischemia is related to inflow obstruction. Because of the relatively uncommon occurrence of atherosclerosis distal to the inflow arteries, numerous causes of UE arterial disease involving the large or medium-sized arteries (proximal to the wrist) or small arteries (distal to the wrist) must be considered. Conditions such as vasculopathies, aneurysm or entrapment syndromes, embolic phenomena, medications, and chemical exposures can complicate the diagnosis due to the similarity of symptoms. Additional testing beyond the comprehensive history and physical examination may be required to elucidate the cause.[12] Table 40.1 provides the differential diseases, exposures, and other conditions that should be considered.[12,13]

VASCULAR ANATOMY OF THE UPPER EXTREMITY AND AORTIC ARCH

Normal Anatomy

The normal branching pattern of vessels coming off the aortic arch in approximately 70% of the population[14] includes the initial

TABLE 40.1 Differential Diagnosis of Upper Extremity Vessel Obstructive Disease

Vessel Size	Site, Disease State, and Substance	Symptoms and Physical Examination Findings	Symmetry and Acuity
MEDIUM TO LARGE			
Atherosclerosis	Brachiocephalic artery Subclavian artery Axillary artery	Arm claudication Hand or finger pain Bruit, pulse deficit	Typically unilateral Chronic and progressive
Aneurysm	Thoracic outlet syndrome Trauma, crutch syndrome Vasculitis Fibromuscular dysplasia	Pulsatile mass in the supraclavicular fossa, hoarseness, dyspnea, transient ischemic attack (subclavian artery)	Unilateral Chronic and progressive
Thromboembolism	Heart Aortic arch Proximal great vessels	Varies (e.g., ischemia, pallor) according to cause Skin ulcers Osler nodes Janeway lesions	Unilateral, can be bilateral Typically acute
Entrapment	Trauma Thoracic outlet syndrome Neoplasm	Pain, especially with movement or certain positions	Unilateral Chronic and progressive unless it is an acute injury
Vasculitis or arteritis	Giant cell (temporal) arteritis Kawasaki disease Takayasu arteritis Radiation-induced arteritis	Constitutional symptoms (e.g., fever, weight loss, fatigue, arthralgias, myalgias), rash, bruit, pulse deficit	Unilateral or bilateral
Vasospasm	Nicotine Cocaine Methamphetamine	Digital pallor Cyanosis	Unilateral or bilateral Acute on chronic
SMALL			
Hematologic disorders	Cryoglobulinemia (types I, II, III) Myeloproliferative syndrome Multiple myeloma Leukemia Primary macroglobulinemia	Constitutional symptoms	Unilateral or bilateral, typically bilateral Progressively worsening
Hypercoagulable states	Antiphospholipid syndrome Antithrombin III, protein C, or protein S deficiency Heparin-induced thrombocytopenia	Variable, typically mimicking thromboembolic disease	Unilateral or bilateral, typically bilateral Progressively worsening
Rheumatologic disorders (vasculitis)	Rheumatoid arthritis Systemic lupus erythematosus Scleroderma, CREST syndrome, mixed connective tissue disease Henoch-Schönlein purpura	Constitutional symptoms, dysphagia, nail pitting, prominent nailbed capillary loops, skin lesions (e.g., erythema nodosum, petechial rash, pyoderma gangrenosum, palpable purpura), sclerodactyly, telangiectasias	Unilateral or bilateral, typically bilateral Progressively worsening
Infectious diseases	Hepatitis C *Mycoplasma* pneumonia	Variable, typically mimicking thromboembolic disease	Unilateral or bilateral, typically bilateral Progressively worsening
Embolic and thrombotic diseases	Buerger disease Atheromatous disease Aneurysms Atrial fibrillation Atrial myxomas Left ventricular thrombus ASD/PFO Endocarditis or valvular disease	Varies according to cause Skin ulcers Osler nodes Janeway lesions	Bilateral Acute
Vasospasm	Raynaud phenomenon Medications or illicit substances	Finger pain, fixed cyanosis, ulcers, gangrene	Typically bilateral Acute, chronic, or acute on chronic
Exposures	Vinyl chloride	Digital pallor Cyanosis	Unilateral or bilateral Chronic and progressive

ASD/PFO, Atrial septal defect or patent foramen ovale; *CREST*, calcinosis cutis, Raynaud phenomenon, esophageal dysfunction, sclerodactyly, telangiectasia. Data from Rajagopalan S, Mukherjee D, Mohler E. *Manual of Vascular Diseases*. Philadelphia: Lippincott Williams & Wilkins; 2005:216; and Stone JH. Immune complex-mediated small vessel vasculitis. In: Firestein GS, Budd RC, Gabriel SE, et al, eds. *Kelley's Textbook of Rheumatology*. 9th ed. Philadelphia: Saunders; 2012.

branch, the right brachiocephalic artery, the left common carotid artery, and the left subclavian artery. Variations from the typical branching pattern are discussed in the next section.

The right brachiocephalic artery (innominate) divides into the right subclavian and the right common carotid artery behind the right sternoclavicular joint. The right subclavian artery then becomes the axillary artery at the lateral border of the first rib. The brachial artery, a continuation of the axillary artery, begins at the lateral border of the teres major muscle and terminates at the neck of the radius as it divides into the radial and ulnar arteries. The radial artery continues in the hand as the deep palmar arch, whereas the ulnar artery continues in the hand as the superficial

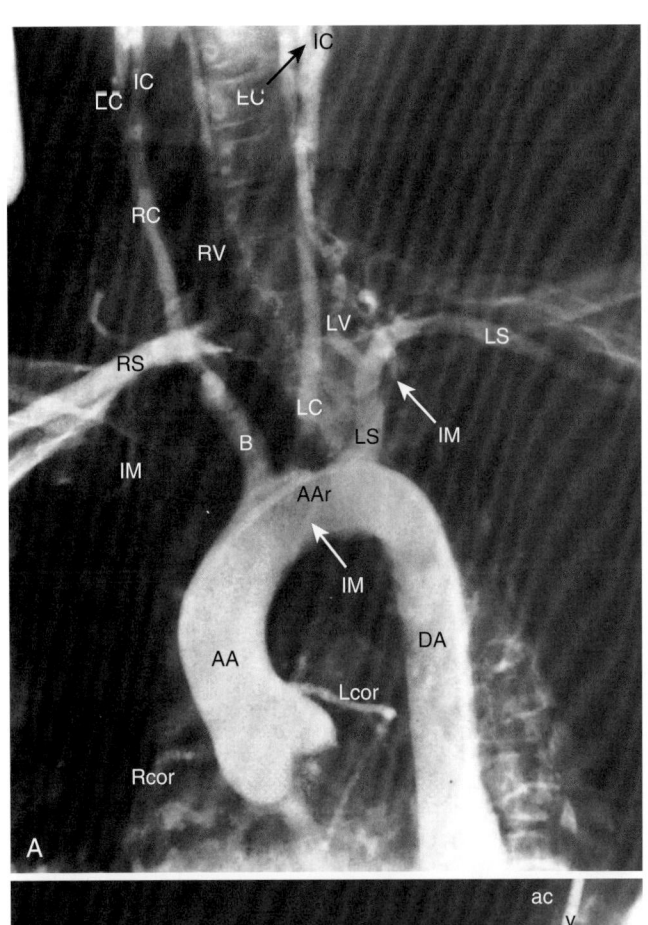
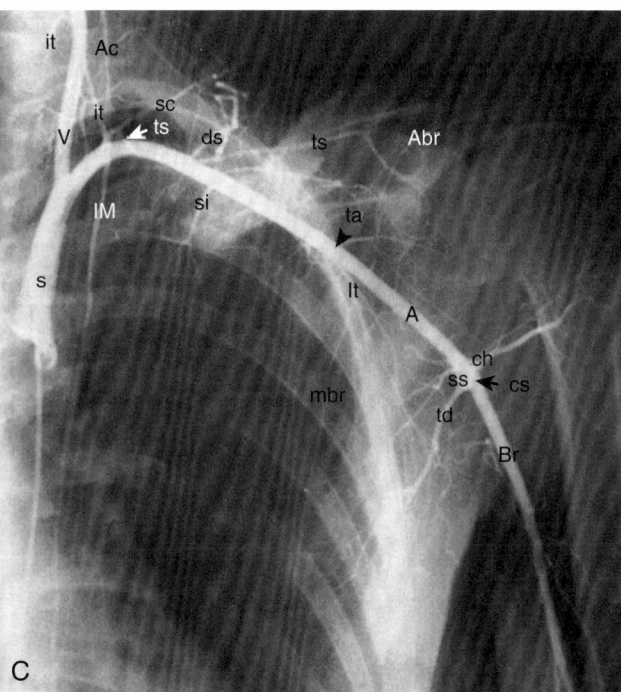
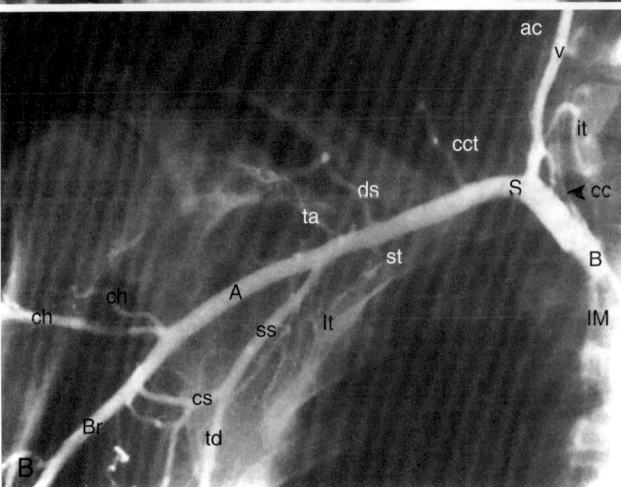

Fig. 40.1 Normal anatomy. (A) Left anterior oblique arch aortogram. (B) Right subclavian arteriogram. (C) Left subclavian arteriogram. *A*, Artery; *AA*, ascending aorta; *AAr*, aortic arch; *B*, brachiocephalic artery; *DA*, ductus arteriosus; *EC*, external carotid artery; *IC*, internal carotid artery; *IM*, internal mammary; *LC*, left carotid; *Lcor*, left coronary artery; *LS*, left subclavian artery; *LV*, left ventricle; *RC*, right carotid; *Rcor*, right coronary artery; *RS*, right subclavian artery; *RV*, right ventricle; *ta*, truncus arteriosus; *V*, vein. (From Kadir S. *Atlas of Normal and Variant Angiographic Anatomy.* Philadelphia: WB Saunders; 1991.)

palmar arch, which gives rises to the digital arteries.[15] The left subclavian artery, the third branch off the aorta after the innominate and the left common carotid, has a branching pattern in the left UE that is analogous to the right. Fig. 40.1 demonstrates normal anatomy angiographically.

Smaller vessels provide extensive collateral circuits in the shoulder, elbow, and palm regions and are protective in allowing perfusion to the UE despite significant obstruction. UE large vessel disease is typically asymptomatic until the collateral support is insufficient or exhausted. Despite having protective collateral circuits, the UE remains vulnerable to ischemia if the obstruction occurs proximally because the UE is supplied by only one artery from the aorta.

Anatomic Variants

The anomalous circulation in the UE and aortic arch primarily results from alterations in embryologic development (Fig. 40.2).

SECTION IV Peripheral Vascular Interventions

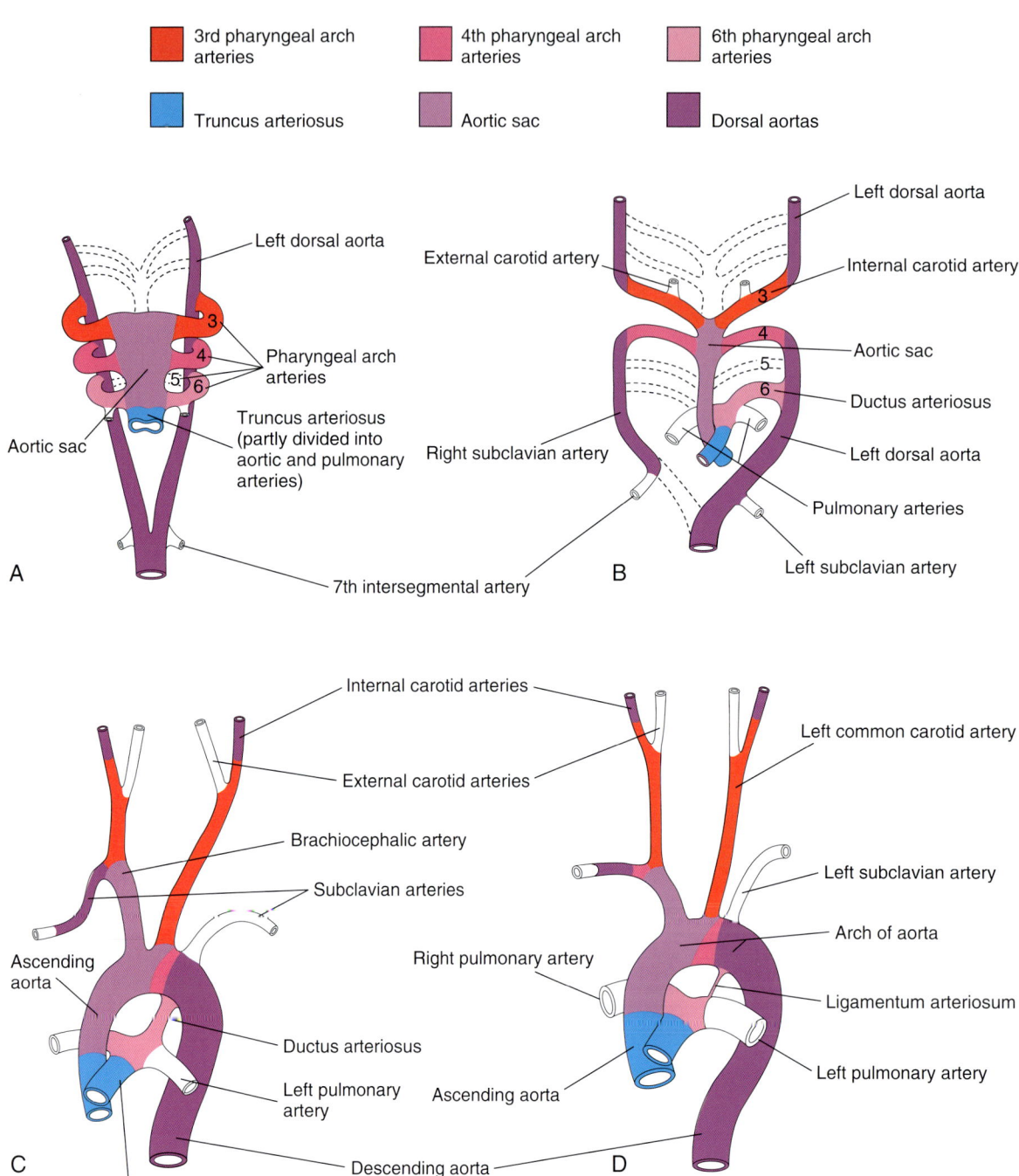

Fig. 40.2 Embryologic transformation of the aorta to a normal adult pattern. The vessels that are not colored are not derived from these structures. (A) Pharyngeal arch arteries at 6 weeks; by this stage, the first two pairs of arteries have largely disappeared. (B) Pharyngeal arch arteries at 7 weeks; the parts of the dorsal aortae and pharyngeal arch arteries that normally disappear are indicated with *broken lines*. (C) Arterial arrangement at 8 weeks. (D) Sketch of the arterial vessels of a 6-month-old neonate. Note that the ascending aorta and pulmonary arteries are considerably smaller in C than in D. This represents the relative flow through these vessels at the different stages of development. Observe the large size of the ductus arteriosus (DA) in C and that it is essentially a direct continuation of the pulmonary trunk. The DA normally becomes closed within the first few days after birth. Eventually the DA becomes the ligamentum arteriosum, as shown in D. (From Moore K, Persaud TVN. The cardiovascular system. In: Moore K, Persaud TVN, eds. *Before We Are Born: Essentials of Embryology and Birth Defects*. 6th ed. Philadelphia: WB Saunders; 2003:264.)

TABLE 40.2 Arterial Variants and Collateral Pathways of the Upper Extremity and Aortic Arch

Anatomic Variants	Prevalence (%)	Pathologic Significance	Physical Examination Clues
Bovine arch: common origin of brachiocephalic and left common carotid arteries	22	None	No specific findings
Origin of left common carotid from the brachiocephalic (middle to upper)	8–10	None	No specific findings
Origin of left vertebral artery from the aorta	4–6	None	No specific findings
Origin of right subclavian from left aortic arch, distal to left subclavian (arteria lusoria)	2	Compression due to esophageal ring, prone to rupture and aneurysm (Kommerell diverticulum)	Dysphagia
Common origin of carotids	<1	None	No specific findings
Origin of radial artery from brachial or axillary artery	15–20	None	No specific findings
Origin of ulnar artery from brachial or axillary artery	2–3	None	No specific findings
Collateral Obstruction Site	**Donor Artery**	**Pathologic Significance**	**Physical Examination Clues**
Proximal subclavian or innominate obstruction	Vertebral, other neck, abdominal, or pelvic	Subclavian steal syndrome	Weak or absent pulse Decreased blood pressure Arm weakness or pain
Distal subclavian or axillary	Subscapular, intercostals, lateral thoracic	None, unless collateral supply insufficient, then ischemia	No specific findings
Brachial artery	Profunda brachialis, radial, ulnar	None, unless collateral supply insufficient, then ischemia	No specific findings

Data from Rajagopalan S, Mukerjee D, Mohler E. *Manual of Vascular Diseases*. Philadelphia: Lippincott Williams & Wilkins; 2005:39–43, 215; Kadir S. *Atlas of Normal and Variant Angiographic Anatomy*. Philadelphia: WB Saunders; 1991:xi, 529; Kaufman JA, Lee MJ. *Vascular and Interventional Radiology: The Requisites*. 2nd ed. Philadelphia: Elsevier; 2014 [chapter 6]; and Pellerito JS, Polak JF. *Introduction to Vascular Ultrasonography*. 6th ed. Philadelphia: Saunders; 2012 [chapter 13].

Although an exhaustive review of embryologic development is beyond the scope of this chapter, the resultant aortic arch and proximal branching vessel variants are the consequence of aberrant formation, including persistence or abnormal regression, of the endocardial tube, the ventral and dorsal aortae, and the six paired branchial arch arteries or the intersegmental arteries.

Table 40.2 lists some of the more commonly encountered variants, their frequencies in the population, associated pathologic significance, and diagnostic physical examination findings.[12,14,16,17] The more common arterial variants in the forearm and collateral pathways that may form in the presence of main arterial obstruction are included. Figs. 40.3-40.5 show examples of variant anatomy.

DIAGNOSTIC EVALUATION AND DISEASE CLASSIFICATION

History and Physical Examination

As with many other facets of medicine, the importance of a thorough history and physical examination in patients with suspected PAD cannot be overstated. Although they are often not sufficient to elucidate the diagnosis because of the broad differential, they should nonetheless be complete so as to narrow the focus and avoid extraneous testing or referrals.

Because of the broad differential for UE ischemia, the history and review of systems should be comprehensive and should include detailed descriptions of the symptoms, comorbidities, exposures (e.g., chemicals, vibratory tools, radiation), trauma, and a complete medication history including prescription drugs, illicit drugs, and tobacco use. Keys to narrowing the differential diagnosis include consideration of the previously described elements, the acuity of onset and time course (intermittent versus constant), exacerbating and alleviating factors, symmetry or asymmetry of symptoms, and physical examination findings (see Table 40.1).

Unilateral symptoms suggest a more localized process (e.g., entrapment, stenotic lesion), whereas bilateral symptoms are more characteristic of a systemic disease process. The acuity or time course can be confusing because an acute onset of symptoms may be a manifestation of a chronic process with an acute exacerbation or simply an acute condition. In arterial ischemia, signs of acute or chronic arterial insufficiency can be distinct and aid in diagnosis (Table 40.3).[18]

In vasospastic disease, the intermittent or constant nature of the symptoms helps differentiate primary (nonobstructive) Raynaud disease from the secondary (obstructive) form. Primary Raynaud disease is typically intermittent, and the vasospastic symptoms resolve completely between bouts, whereas in secondary Raynaud disease, symptoms are persistent but may wax and wane in intensity. Normal vasomotor function must be differentiated from abnormal vasospastic disease. Normal physiologic arterial vasoconstriction of the cutaneous circulation in the hands and fingers occurs in response to stimuli such as cold exposure. During normal physiologic vasoconstriction, blood flow is continuous, whereas with vasospastic disease (i.e., Raynaud disease), there is cessation of blood flow.[12]

Blood pressure should be manually measured in both arms because a systolic gradient of greater than 15 to 20 mm Hg suggests a significant stenosis, with a gradient of 20 mm Hg or more having a specificity of 94%.[19] A systolic gradient of more than 10 mm Hg may indicate hemodynamic significance and justify further investigation.[11] If Takayasu (giant cell) arteritis is suspected, blood pressure should be measured in all four extremities to evaluate the differential pressure between the upper and lower extremities.

Palpation should begin in the supraclavicular fossa because a pulsatile mass suggests a subclavian artery aneurysm, and distal

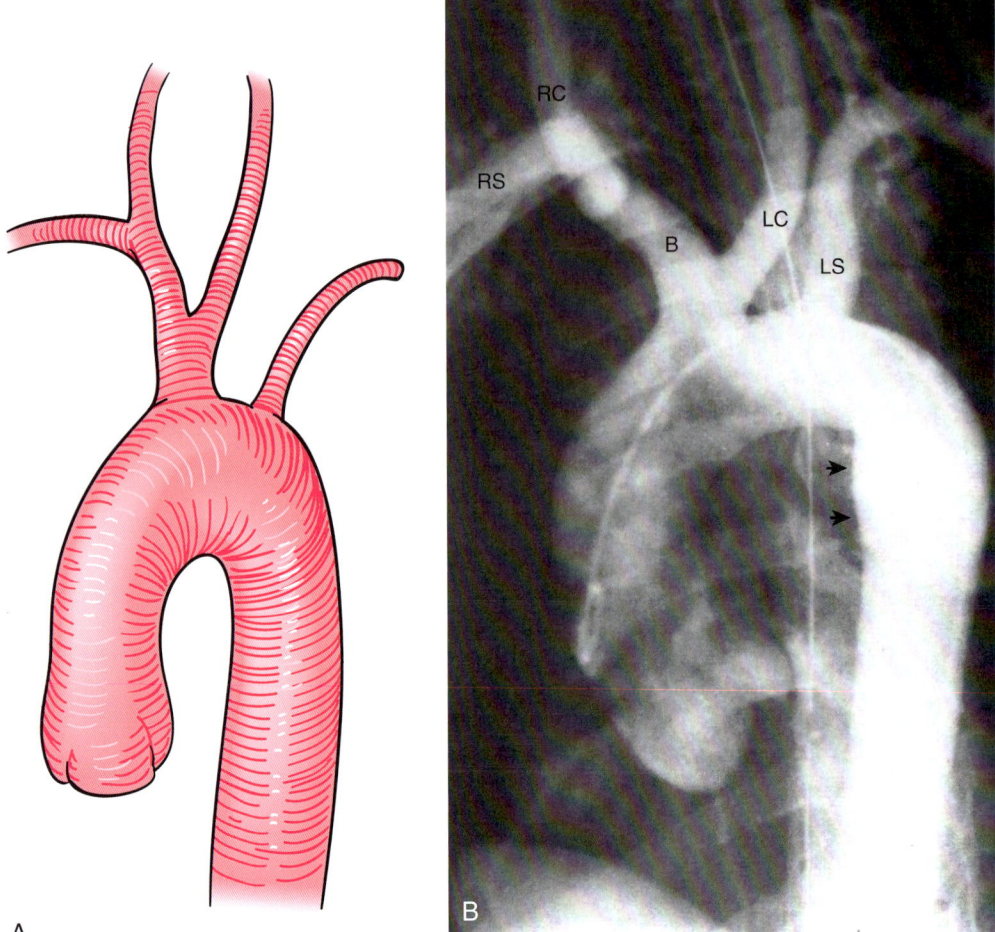

Fig. 40.3 Common origin of left common carotid and brachiocephalic arteries (i.e., bovine arch). (A) Schematic drawing. (B) Left anterior oblique arch aortogram of a bovine arch. *B*, Brachiocephalic artery; *LC*, left carotid; *LS*, left subclavian artery; *RC*, right carotid; *RS*, right subclavian artery. (From Kadir S. *Atlas of Normal and Variant Angiographic Anatomy*. Philadelphia: WB Saunders; 1991.)

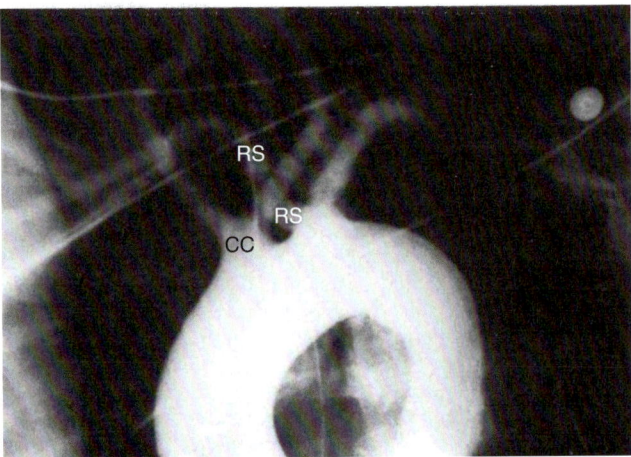

Fig. 40.4 Aberrant right subclavian *(RS)* artery and a common carotid *(CC)* trunk. (From Kadir S. *Atlas of Normal and Variant Angiographic Anatomy*. Philadelphia: WB Saunders; 1991.)

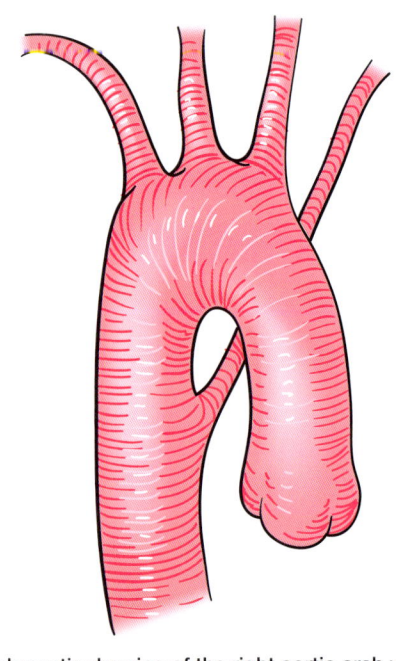

Fig. 40.5 Schematic drawing of the right aortic arch with aberrant left subclavian artery. (From Kadir S. *Atlas of Normal and Variant Angiographic Anatomy*. Philadelphia: WB Saunders; 1991.)

TABLE 40.3 Signs of Arterial Ischemia	
Course	Signs
Acute	Pulselessness
	Palor
	Poikilotherima
	Pain
	Paresthesias
Chronic	Muscle atrophy
	Skin bronzing
	Focal hair loss
	Digital gangrene
Acute or chronic	Nonhealing ulcer

Data from Johnston, SL, Dieter RS. Upper extremities and aortic arch. In: Topol EJ, Teirstein PS, eds. *Textbook of Interventional Cardiology*. 6th ed. Philadelphia: Saunders; 2012 [chapter 38].

subclavian artery aneurysms are typically caused by compression over a cervical rib (i.e., thoracic outlet syndrome [TOS]). Tenderness in the supraclavicular fossa and along the scalene muscles also suggests TOS. The brachial, radial, and ulnar arteries should be palpated because pulse deficits, especially radial or brachial, in a younger and otherwise previously healthy patient suggest Takayasu arteritis, whereas a unilateral pulse deficit in an older adult patient with comorbidities of cardiovascular disease typically represents atherosclerotic disease.

The supraclavicular fossa should be auscultated for the presence of a bruit or murmur. A bruit suggests subclavian artery stenosis, whereas a continuous murmur suggests an arteriovenous fistula.[12] The skin should be inspected for ulcers (e.g., atherosclerosis, embolism, vasculitis, Buerger disease), rashes, petechiae, purpura (e.g., vasculitis, rheumatologic illnesses), and cyanosis (e.g., vasospasm, drug or chemical exposure). The nails should be examined for pitting and nail bed capillary loops or splinter hemorrhages, which suggest vasculitis or endocarditis, respectively.

Capillary refill (normal <5 seconds) should be evaluated bilaterally, and special techniques such as the Allen maneuver, the Halstead maneuver, or the Adson test can be performed if TOS is suspected. However, because the Adson sign (i.e., loss of the radial pulse in the arm) elicited by the test can be positive in asymptomatic patients, it should not be used as an independent indicator but considered in conjunction with other objective findings.[20] If subclavian steal syndrome is suspected, the Dieter test, in which a blood pressure cuff is inflated and then rapidly deflated (on the limb with subclavian stenosis) to induce hyperemia, vertebral flow reversal, and provocation of posterior cerebral symptoms, can clinically establish the diagnosis.[21]

Laboratory Testing

Initial laboratory tests in the evaluation of UE ischemia include a complete blood cell count (CBC), comprehensive metabolic panel (CMP), lipid panel, erythrocyte sedimentation rate (ESR), C-reactive protein (CRP), activated partial thromboplastin time (aPPT), and prothrombin time (PT) or international normalized ratio (INR). Some authorities also recommend tests for rheumatoid factor (RF) and antinuclear antibodies (ANAs).

Based on the initial differential diagnosis, additional testing may be needed. For example, if an embolic phenomenon, an idiopathic thrombosis, or a hypercoagulable state is suspected, tests for factor V Leiden mutation, protein C and protein S deficiencies, antithrombin III deficiency, and prothrombin 20210A polymorphism may be useful. If an infectious cause is suspected, a hepatitis panel, rapid plasma reagin (RPR) test, and blood cultures may be needed. Similarly, if a rheumatologic disorder is likely, tests for antiphospholipid antibodies and lupus anticoagulant may be helpful in addition to tests for RF and ANA. Because the laboratory workup can be time-consuming and expensive, a comprehensive history and physical examination are essential for guiding the investigation and selecting patients who require a more extensive evaluation.[22]

Vascular Laboratory Testing

Various noninvasive and invasive vascular diagnostic tests and imaging studies may be used in assessing the cause and severity of disease. Measuring segmental limb pressures in the arm, analogous to testing performed for lower extremity arterial disease, can identify the level of obstruction and the severity of disease. A difference in blood pressures between the left and right sides of 10 mm Hg or more is considered abnormal, a pressure gradient between adjacent segments in the same limb of more than 20 mm Hg indicates significant obstructive disease, and a gradient of more than 30 mm Hg suggests an occlusion.[10] Similar to the ankle-brachial index in the lower extremity, a wrist-brachial index (WBI) or a finger-brachial index (FBI) of less than 0.85 or 0.70, respectively, is considered to be abnormal and indicates arterial insufficiency. Other diagnostic tools are listed in Table 40.4, along with the benefits and limitations of each study.[8,10,11,17]

Catheter-Based Angiography

Before performing selective angiography of the brachiocephalic or subclavian arteries, an aortic arch angiogram using a soft, multi-sidehole catheter (e.g., pigtail catheter) and 30 to 40 mL of contrast material delivered by autoinjection (e.g., 15 to 20 mL/s delivered over 2 seconds, 0.3 to 0.5 seconds rate of rise, 900 psi) in a 30- to 40-degree left anterior oblique (LAO) projection using digital subtraction angiography (DSA) should be performed.[10,12,23] Based on improved tolerance, lower tonicity, and fewer side effects, the recommended contrast medium is iodixanol, an isoosmolar, nonionic agent.[10,24,25] Access is typically obtained from the common femoral artery (CFA) for catheter-based diagnostic angiography and for percutaneous intervention for stenosis, whereas radial and more commonly ipsilateral brachial artery access in combination with CFA access is used for treating occlusions. Indications for UE diagnostic angiography are given in Table 40.5.[10-12]

For selective engagement and angiography of the brachiocephalic and left subclavian arteries, various catheters can be used with hand-injected contrast of 5 to 10 mL on DSA. Commonly, the Judkins right 4 (JR4) catheter is selected, but alternatives include the internal mammary artery (IMA) and multipurpose (MP-A) catheter or specialty shaped catheters such as the Vitek (VTK), Simmons 1 or 2 (SIMS), or Headhunter-1 (H-1). Catheter selection should be guided by the arch aortogram, with the initial catheter choice matching the level of difficulty of the arch type. For example, a JR4 is appropriate for a type 1 arch, whereas a VTK or H-1 is recommended for type 2, and the SIMS is used for a type 3 arch.[10,12] Care should be taken when engaging, disengaging, or manipulating catheters to avoid vascular trauma or excessive scraping of the aorta (i.e., to minimize the risk of stroke).

After selective engagement, orthogonal oblique projections are recommended for proper delineation and reduction in overlap. The right anterior oblique (RAO) view is recommended for the brachiocephalic bifurcation, origin of the right subclavian artery, and origins of the left vertebral artery and IMA from the left subclavian artery. The LAO view is recommended for improved visualization of the right vertebral artery and IMA.[10,16] Patient positioning is neutral (i.e., anatomic position), but abduction and external rotation may be needed for the evaluation when TOS is suspected of causing vascular compression.

For axillary and brachial artery angiography, the diagnostic catheter should be placed in the distal subclavian artery.

TABLE 40.4 Vascular Diagnostic Testing

Test	Benefit	Limitations
WBI/FBI	Simple, economical, noninvasive	Inaccurate in heavily calcified, noncompressible vessels
Segmental limb pressures	Establishes presence, severity, and anatomic location of disease Useful for surveillance after revascularization	Inaccurate in heavily calcified, noncompressible vessels
Finger pulse volume recording with plethysmography	Differentiates normal from diseased limbs or obstructive from vasospastic disease Useful for surveillance after revascularization	Accuracy decreases with multilevel disease, less accurate in identifying level of disease, can be abnormal in low cardiac output states
Duplex ultrasound	Simple, economical, noninvasive High sensitivity and specificity (>90%) Color flow and spectral analysis used to identify flow reversal, turbulence at aneurysms or other arterial lesions, and stenosis vs. occlusion in low-flow states Useful for surveillance after revascularization	Highly operator dependent Diagnostic accuracy limited with dense calcification Difficult to image left proximal subclavian and other segments of the subclavian arteries under the clavicle
CTA	High-resolution definition of anatomy Allows visualization in multiple planes Used to determine candidacy for endovascular procedures	Radiation and contrast exposure Limited use in patients with contrast allergy or severe renal disease Acoustic shadowing artifact with pacemakers
Magnetic resonance angiography	Excellent anatomic resolution Lack of exposure to radiation Provides associated soft tissue definition, including vascular wall inflammation, cysts, aneurysms	Cannot be used if metal present (e.g., AICD, pacemaker) Time consuming, costly, requires prolonged breath holding Prone to artifacts (coil dropout and venous susceptibility) Gadolinium limits use in CKD stage 4 or 5
Catheter-based angiography	Allows direct visualization of vessels Allows for assessment of pressure gradients Allows structural and functional assessment with IVUS and FFR	Invasive Contrast and radiation exposure

AICD, Automatic implantable cardioverter defibrillator; *CTA*, computed tomography angiography; *CKD*, chronic kidney disease; *FFR*, fractional flow reserve; *FBI*, finger-brachial index; *IVUS*, intravascular ultrasound; *WBI*, wrist-brachial index.
Data from Olin JW, Sealove BA. Peripheral artery disease: current insights into the disease and its diagnosis and management. *Mayo Clin Proc*. 2010;85(7):678–692; Casserly IP, Sachar R, Yadav JS. *Practical Peripheral Vascular Intervention*. 2nd ed. Philadelphia: Lippincott Williams & Wilkins; 2011 [chapters 2, 3, and 24]; Ochoa VM, Yeghiazarians Y. Subclavian artery stenosis: a review for the vascular medicine practitioner. *Vasc Med*. 2010;16(1):29–34; and Pellerito JS, Polak JF. *Introduction to Vascular Ultrasonography*. 6th ed. Philadelphia: Saunders; 2012 [chapter 13].

TABLE 40.5 Indications for Aortic Arch and Upper Extremity Diagnostic Angiography

Screening before planned coronary artery bypass grafting with internal mammary artery grafting in the following patients
- Bilateral arm blood pressure differential > 10 mm Hg
- History of radiation therapy for the neck or chest
- History of vasculitis or known peripheral arterial disease, especially angiographic aortic arch or iliofemoral disease, even if asymptomatic

Evaluation of acute symptoms
- Cyanosis
- Acute limb ischemia
- Blue digit syndrome

After blunt or penetrating trauma with signs of vascular injury

Evaluation of symptomatic arm claudication

Evaluation for unilateral upper extremity embolization when a proximal arterial embolic source is suspected (e.g., vascular thoracic outlet syndrome)

Evaluation of suspected steal syndrome
- Subclavian steal syndrome (i.e., vertebrobasilar insufficiency)
- Coronary steal syndrome (i.e., angina from internal mammary graft insufficiency)

Data from Casserly IP, Sachar R, Yadav JS. *Practical Peripheral Vascular Intervention*. 2nd ed. Philadelphia: Lippincott Williams & Wilkins; 2011 [chapters 2, 3, and 24]; Ochoa VM, Yeghiazarians Y. Subclavian artery stenosis: a review for the vascular medicine practitioner. *Vasc Med*. 2010;16(1):29–34; and Rajagopalan S, Mukerjee D, Mohler E. *Manual of Vascular Diseases*. Philadelphia: Lippincott Williams & Wilkins; 2005;215:39–43.

The anteroposterior projection, with the patient in the neutral position, is used to visualize the distal subclavian, axillary, and brachial arteries, although slight arm abduction may enhance visualization.[10,16]

TREATMENT

Management of UE disease ranges from medical management to percutaneous intervention or surgical treatment. Modification of risk factors and medical therapy for atherosclerotic disease are considered the standard of care for all patients, regardless of the degree of disease. When intervention is indicated, percutaneous management is favored over the surgical approach because of improved efficacy and patency rates with angioplasty and stenting in the modern era (Fig. 40.6) and the desire to avoid factors of surgery associated with increased morbidity and mortality, such as increased cost, general anesthesia, and longer hospitalization and recovery times.[11,12,26]

Before initiating a brachiocephalic or subclavian intervention, the diagnostic images should be studied to determine the proximity of the lesion to the vertebral, carotid, and internal mammary arteries, and the vessel takeoff from the aortic arch (left subclavian) or the brachiocephalic (right subclavian).

Access for percutaneous angioplasty and stenting (PTAS) is typically obtained from the CFA for intervention in stenosis, whereas ipsilateral brachial (less commonly, radial) artery access in combination with CFA access is used for treating occlusions, provided there is a lack of severe aortoiliac disease. If CFA access is prohibited by severe aortoiliac disease, brachial access is recommended for the treatment of stenosis and occlusive disease.[10]

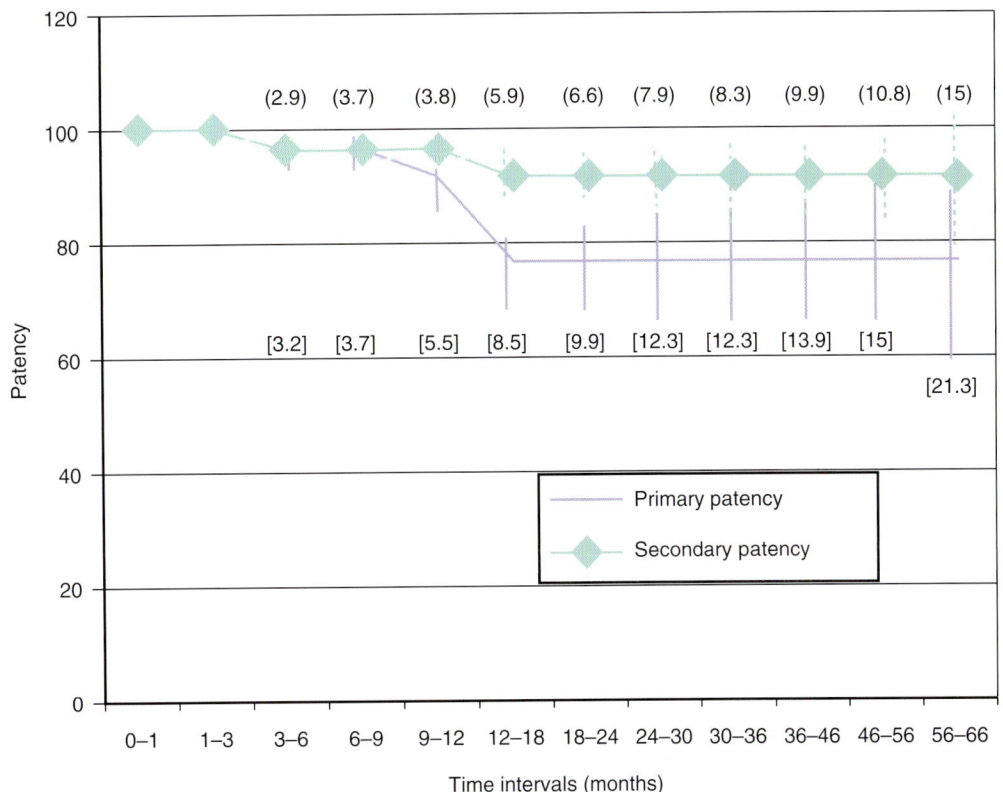

Fig. 40.6 Long-term patency of innominate and subclavian artery stenting. (From Brountzos EN, Petersen B, Binkert C, et al. Primary stenting of subclavian and innominate artery occlusive disease: a single center's experience. *Cardiovasc Intervent Radiol.* 2004;27:616–623.)

TABLE 40.6 Complications of Percutaneous Angioplasty and Stenting of the Upper Extremity or Proximal Arch Vessels

Vascular complications, including dissection, perforation, intrathoracic hemorrhage
Embolization, including thrombotic and atheroembolic material
Cerebrovascular accident or transient ischemic attack
Restenosis
Vascular access complications (e.g., hematoma, thrombosis, pseudoaneurysm, especially with brachial artery access)
Stent migration, malposition, dislodgement, or embolization

All endovascular operators should be aware of the complexities and potential complications of PTAS involving the UE or proximal arch vessels (Table 40.6) and appreciate that intervention in the innominate artery is more complex than subclavian intervention because of the potential for embolization to the anterior cerebral circulation through the right common carotid artery.[10–12] With that knowledge, the use of an embolic protection device should be considered. Similarly, balloon angioplasty as a stand-alone therapy is rarely performed now because of the excellent, durable results obtained with the combination of balloon angioplasty and stenting.

A long sheath- or guide-based system can be used. The sheath or guide is parked proximal to the lesion, taking care to avoid atheroembolization, and the PTAS is carried out with an undersized balloon for predilation to avoid the risk of dissection (i.e., approximately 70% of the estimated vessel diameter). Balloon-expandable stents, which offer more accurate stent placement, are typically used for stenosis proximal to the vertebral artery. Self-expanding stents, which offer more flexibility and less deformability, are typically used to treat stenosis distal to the vertebral artery, where less placement accuracy is required but where flexion points related to the subclavian to axillary transition exist.

Because of the risk of dissection or rupture, conservative stent sizing is recommended. Typically, 6 to 8 mm is used for the subclavian and 8 to 10 mm is used for the innominate artery.[10,12]

After stenting, lifelong aspirin and at least 4 weeks of clopidogrel are recommended with suggested follow-up intervals of 1 month, 6 months, 12 months, and then annually.[26] Bilateral cuff pressures should be taken at each visit, along with eliciting recurrent symptoms by the history and physical examination. Symptom recurrence or a more than 10 mm Hg change in the arm cuff pressure differential should be evaluated with duplex ultrasonography because early detection and intervention are important for maintaining patency.[10,26]

SPECIAL CONSIDERATIONS

The causes of large vessel disease of the UE are relatively limited and typically are categorized as embolic, aneurysmal, vasculopathic (including vasculitis and atherosclerosis), and entrapment syndromes. The following sections discuss common disease processes of the UE vessels that require specific knowledge and attention when suggested by the history or physical examination findings during evaluation.

Thoracic Outlet Syndrome

TOS is a term used to describe an array of symptoms that result from compression of the neurovascular structures passing through the scalene triangle (i.e., subclavian artery, subclavian vein, and brachial plexus), which has an anterior and posterior boundary of the anterior and middle scalene muscles, respectively, and a base of the cervical or first rib.[27] Compression may also occur at the

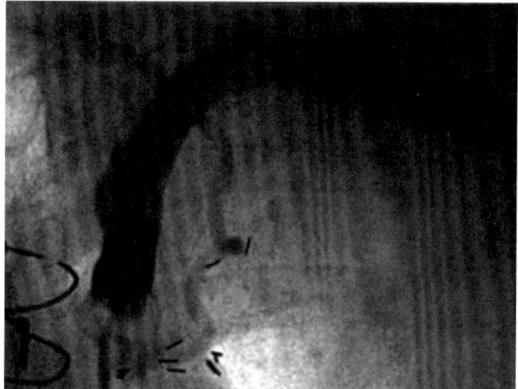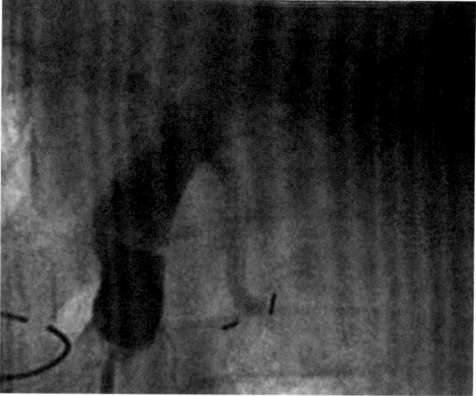

Fig. 40.7 Dynamic left subclavian artery obstruction (i.e., Dieter sign) and exacerbation of a proximal subclavian artery kink with expiration. The subclavian arteriograms were obtained during inspiration *(left)* and expiration *(right)*. (From Dieter RS, Morshedi-Meibodi A, Ahmed MH, et al. Description of a new angiographic sign: dynamic left artery obstruction. *Vasc Dis Manage.* 2006;3:298–299.)

costoclavicular space (i.e., costoclavicular space syndrome), which is bounded by the clavicle, first rib, costoclavicular ligament, and middle scalene muscle, or under the pectoralis minor and coracoid process (i.e., pectoralis minor space).[28]

Classification of symptoms is typically based on whether the brachial plexus (i.e., neurogenic TOS), the subclavian artery (i.e., arterial TOS), or rarely, the subclavian vein (i.e., venous TOS) accounts for the primary site of compression. Neurogenic TOS accounts for 90% to 95% of cases and is more common in women. Vascular TOS (arterial and venous), which accounts for the most serious morbidity associated with this condition due to a tendency for aneurysm formation, occurs in 5% to 10% of patients. Arterial TOS is equally distributed among males and female patients, whereas venous TOS tends to occur two times more often in men than women. Most patients with TOS tend to be 20 to 40 years of age and have a history of repetitive motion of the UE, especially overhead movements, or neck trauma, with whiplash being the most common cause.

Symptoms of arterial TOS include claudication, pallor, coolness, digital ischemia, and pain in the hand and are typically caused by aneurysm-induced emboli or embolization from thrombus formation distal to a subclavian stenosis. Arm heaviness, swelling of the arm, cyanosis, and paresthesias of the fingers or hand are symptoms suggesting venous TOS.[29] Arm swelling is an important discriminator because it is typically absent in neurogenic or arterial TOS. As previously described, various provocative maneuvers can be used to elicit symptoms, although all suffer from low specificity. When vascular TOS is suspected, further evaluation, including duplex ultrasound, magnetic resonance imaging (MRI), and angiography (arteriography or venography), may be useful.[10,18] Angiography should be performed initially in the neutral position and then repeated in the provocative position.

Treatment of vascular TOS is reserved for patients who are symptomatic or have evidence of embolization. Surgical intervention is considered for decompression in the setting of an acute vascular syndrome, whereas endovascular management using catheter-directed thrombolytics or embolectomy can be used if necessary in the setting of acute embolization.[10,12,29] However, other than thrombolysis, surgical decompression is considered mandatory for first-line, definitive therapy. Endovascular therapy is reserved for second-line treatment.

Subclavian Steal Syndrome

In the setting of a significant brachiocephalic or subclavian stenosis or obstruction, blood flow from the vertebrobasilar or posterior cerebral circulation can be redirected in a retrograde fashion along the ipsilateral vertebral artery toward the arm, causing symptoms of ischemia such as dizziness, unsteadiness, vertigo, ataxia, nystagmus, diplopia, or other visual changes. The condition, called *subclavian steal syndrome* (SSS), is somewhat controversial, and some argue that patients remain asymptomatic in the absence of concurrent cerebrovascular lesions such as contralateral carotid artery stenosis, contralateral vertebral artery stenosis, or hypoplastic posterior communicating arteries. In patients with those vascular lesions, there is inadequate blood flow to the posterior or vertebrobasilar circulation, resulting in ischemic symptoms, especially during vigorous arm activity.[12,30] Transient obstruction in the proximal subclavian (Fig. 40.7) with respiration (i.e., Dieter sign) has been reported.[21]

Only an estimated 2.5% of patients are symptomatic, with 80% of them having concurrently contralateral carotid or vertebral artery stenosis. SSS has a threefold higher incidence in left subclavian artery stenosis compared with brachiocephalic artery lesions and is twice as likely to occur in 40- to 60-year-old men compared with women.[31] Further evaluation of symptomatic patients is indicated, and the recommended initial study is duplex ultrasonography of the carotid and vertebral arteries. Based on the results of the noninvasive studies, angiography of the aortic arch and the brachiocephalic, subclavian, carotid, and vertebral arteries may be warranted to confirm the diagnosis and for anatomic definition before intervention.

Intervention is indicated only for symptomatic patients. A fresh thrombus is the primary contraindication to brachiocephalic (subclavian) PTAS in this setting. In a study of 252 patients that compared endovascular treatment with extrathoracic bypass surgery, Song and colleagues found that endovascular treatment was safe and effective and had patency rates comparable to those of surgery in the short and medium terms, whereas surgery provided a more durable result in the long term.[32]

Coronary Steal Syndrome

Similar to SSS, *coronary steal syndrome* (CSS) is a phenomenon in which coronary ischemia results from coronary blood flowing retrograde through the IMA away from the heart to supply the arm with a proximal stenosis in the subclavian artery. CSS has become increasingly recognized over the past 2 decades because of the increased use of the IMA as a conduit in 75% to 90% of coronary arterial bypass graft operations.[33] Similar to SSS, catheter-based intervention is considered first-line therapy for symptomatic patients, and surgery for CSS is similar to that for SSS.[34,35]

CONCLUSIONS

Diagnosis and management of UE vascular disease is similar to that for lower extremity disease, with important differences in the differential diagnoses for UE disease, unique catheter-based interventional challenges based on the UE and aortic arch anatomy and important branch vessels, and the potential for rare but serious complications. Because of the high technical success rate, low restenosis or high patency rates, and minimal complications with careful catheter manipulation and conservative balloon and stent choices, percutaneous catheter-based intervention of symptomatic subclavian artery atherosclerotic disease remains the first-line therapy in the absence of acute thrombus.

Understanding when to refer patients to surgery is also important. Further reading regarding aneurysmal disease is recommended for practitioners managing UE or aortic arch vascular disease.

Acknowledgments

We offer special thanks to Samuel L. Johnston for his contributions to this chapter in previous editions.

KEY REFERENCES

1. Sorensen KE, Kristensen IB, Calermajer DS. Atherosclerosis in the human brachial artery. *J Am Coll Cardiol*. 1997;29(2):318–322.
5. Dieter RS, Morshedi-Meibodi A, Ahmed MH, et al. Lower extremity peripheral arterial disease in hospitalized patients with coronary artery disease. *Vasc Med*. 2003;8(4):233–236.
13. Stone JH. Immune complex-mediated small vessel vasculitis. In: Firestein GS, Budd RC, Gabriel SE, et al., eds. *Kelley's Textbook of Rheumatology*. 9th ed. Philadelphia: Saunders; 2012.
19. English JA, Carell ES, Guidera SA, et al. Angiographic prevalence and clinical predictors of left subclavian stenosis in patients undergoing diagnostic cardiac catheterization. *Catheter Cardiovasc Interv*. 2001;54(1):8–11.
21. Dieter RS. The Dieter test. *Expert Rev Cardiovasc Ther*. 2009;7(3):221.
29. Sanders RJ, Hammond SL, Rao NM. Diagnosis of thoracic outlet syndrome. *J Vasc Surg*. 2007;46(3):601–604.

Additional references available online at expertconsult.com.

中文导读

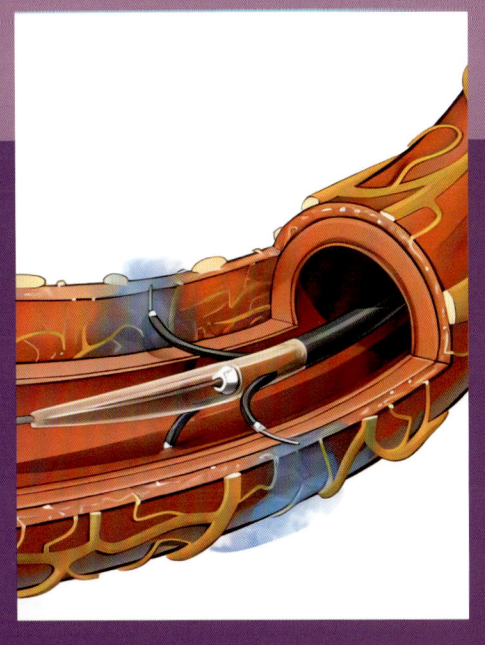

第41章
慢性肠系膜缺血：诊断和治疗

　　慢性肠系膜缺血是肠道血管供血异常时最常见的病因。尽管如此，慢性肠系膜缺血却是一种十分罕见的疾病。其中，动脉粥样硬化是慢性肠系膜缺血的最常见病因。此外，纤维肌性发育不良、Buerger病和主动脉夹层等疾病也可导致慢性肠系膜缺血。动脉粥样硬化性血管狭窄常常可累及肠系膜动脉及其主要分支（如腹腔干、肠系膜上动脉和肠系膜下动脉）。因此，当罹患动脉粥样硬化性疾病的患者行主动脉造影时，常常可发现肠系膜动脉及其分支的开口处狭窄。然而，这些患者却很少出现肠系膜缺血的症状。这是因为内脏血管床之间存在丰富的侧支循环连接。由于症状性肠系膜缺血在临床上较为罕见，因此容易漏诊和误诊，导致延误病情。慢性肠系膜缺血的典型临床表现是餐后腹痛伴体重减轻。相比之下，功能性肠病的患者虽然也会有餐后腹痛，但很少会出现体重减轻。一般情况下，两个或多个肠系膜分支血管存在显著狭窄，才会引发慢性肠系膜缺血的典型症状。当疑诊慢性肠系膜缺血时，可优选CT血管成像技术作为筛查手段。当前，支架植入是慢性肠系膜缺血的初始治疗策略。尽管术后影像学检查的再狭窄率较高，但临床症状复发率较低。因此，通过无创性检查进行密切随访十分重要。

张而立　张洪亮

章节要点

- 动脉粥样硬化性血管狭窄常常可累及肠系膜动脉及其主要分支（如腹腔干、肠系膜上动脉和肠系膜下动脉），但却很少引起肠系膜缺血的症状。这是因为内脏血管床之间存在丰富的侧支循环连接。
- 慢性肠系膜缺血的典型临床表现是餐后腹痛伴体重减轻。相比之下，功能性肠病的患者虽然也会有餐后腹痛，但很少会出现体重减轻。
- 慢性肠系膜缺血的疑诊患者，经常会同时具有其他动脉粥样硬化性疾病的临床表现，例如，冠状动脉粥样硬化性心脏病、缺血性脑卒中、肾血管狭窄性疾病或下肢动脉粥样硬化性疾病。
- 一般情况下，两个或多个肠系膜分支血管存在显著狭窄，才会引发慢性肠系膜缺血的典型症状。单个肠系膜血管狭窄很少引发症状，可在腹部外科手术影响内脏血管侧支循环时发生。
- 当疑诊慢性肠系膜缺血时，可优选CT血管成像技术作为筛查手段。目前，支架植入已基本替代外科开腹手术，成为慢性肠系膜缺血的初始治疗策略。
- 术后造影随访提示支架再狭窄的发生率约为40%，但临床症状的复发率仅为20%。因此，通过无创性检查进行密切随访是十分重要的。

41 Chronic Mesenteric Ischemia: Diagnosis and Intervention

Christopher J. White

KEY POINTS

- Atherosclerotic stenoses commonly involve the major mesenteric arteries (celiac, superior mesenteric, and inferior mesenteric) but rarely cause symptomatic mesenteric ischemia because of the excellent collateral circulation that interconnects the visceral vascular beds.
- The classic presentation is postprandial abdominal pain with weight loss. Patients with functional bowel complaints rarely have significant weight loss.
- Patients with suspected chronic mesenteric ischemia (CMI) commonly have atherosclerosis involving other vascular territories such as coronary artery disease, stroke, renovascular disease, or lower extremity atherosclerotic disease.
- Symptomatic mesenteric ischemia usually results from significant stenosis affecting two or more vessels. Single-vessel disease of the mesenteric circulation is a rare cause of symptomatic mesenteric ischemia but may occur after an abdominal surgery that interrupts the collateral circulation.
- Noninvasive testing with computed tomographic angiography is the preferred screening test in patients with suspected CMI.
- An endovascular-first strategy with stents has largely replaced open surgery as the initial treatment for this disease.
- Angiographic restenosis after stenting approaches 40%, but the clinical recurrence rate appears to be about 1 in 5 patients, so careful clinical and noninvasive follow-up is warranted.

BACKGROUND

Although the most common vascular disorder involving the intestines is ischemia, the clinical syndrome of chronic mesenteric ischemia (CMI), or chronic intestinal ischemia, is very unusual. Other etiologies associated with this uncommon syndrome include fibromuscular dysplasia, Buerger disease, and aortic dissection, but atherosclerosis is by the far the most frequent cause. Atherosclerotic disease of the aorta with associated aortoostial stenosis of the visceral vessels is a relatively common angiographic finding but an infrequent clinical problem.

In a population-based prevalence study of mesenteric artery stenosis, 553 healthy Medicare beneficiaries were screened with abdominal ultrasound for evidence of mesenteric disease.[1] In 17.5% of the total cohort, there was significant narrowing of a mesenteric vessel (>50% diameter stenosis), and more than 97% of these cases represented isolated celiac artery narrowing. There was no correlation with age, race, gender, or body mass index and the presence of mesenteric artery stenosis. Only 1.3% of the patients had involvement of more than one mesenteric vessel.

Another natural history study reported on a group of 980 asymptomatic patients with mesenteric ischemia who were monitored clinically.[2] Only three patients eventually developed symptoms, each with three mesenteric vessels severely affected. The most likely explanation for the infrequent occurrence of CMI in clinical practice is the redundancy of the visceral circulation, which has multiple interconnections between the superior mesenteric artery (SMA) and the inferior mesenteric artery (IMA).

CLINICAL PRESENTATION

Women are much more commonly affected (70%) than men. The classic presentation of this disease is postprandial abdominal discomfort with significant weight loss (Fig. 41.1). The abdominal discomfort associated with eating leads these patients to avoid food, causing them to lose weight. Patients with CMI typically avoid food and demonstrate significant weight loss. However, patients with ischemic gastropathy may have atypical presenting symptoms, such as vomiting, diarrhea, constipation, ischemic colitis, or lower gastrointestinal bleeding. Most patients have evidence of atherosclerosis in other vascular beds and may have experienced prior myocardial infarction, stroke, or claudication.[3]

Patients with atypical symptoms can be very difficult to diagnose, but a high degree of suspicion for CMI in those with other manifestations of atherosclerosis and unexplained weight loss is appropriate. Often the diagnosis is delayed in patients who are being evaluated for a possible malignancy as an explanation for their weight loss. Patients with functional bowel complaints rarely experience significant weight loss, which helps to differentiate them from CMI patients. Evidence of significant obstruction of two or more of the mesenteric vessels is often found when classic symptoms and endoscopy suggest bowel ischemia, although single-vessel disease, usually of the SMA, has been described, particularly if collateral connections have been disrupted by prior abdominal surgery.

DIAGNOSIS

The diagnosis of CMI is a clinical one, based on symptoms and consistent anatomic findings. If there is high clinical suspicion of CMI, patients should undergo Doppler ultrasound (duplex) imaging or noninvasive angiography with computed tomographic angiography (CTA) and magnetic resonance angiography (MRA) to confirm their anatomy, although for imaging resolution CTA is preferred.[3]

Visualization of the mesenteric vessels with duplex ultrasound is technically challenging and requires a skilled and dedicated sonographer. The reported accuracy for duplex imaging in identifying significant stenoses of the celiac artery and SMA approaches 90%, with the caveat that ultrasound velocities will be

SECTION IV Peripheral Vascular Interventions

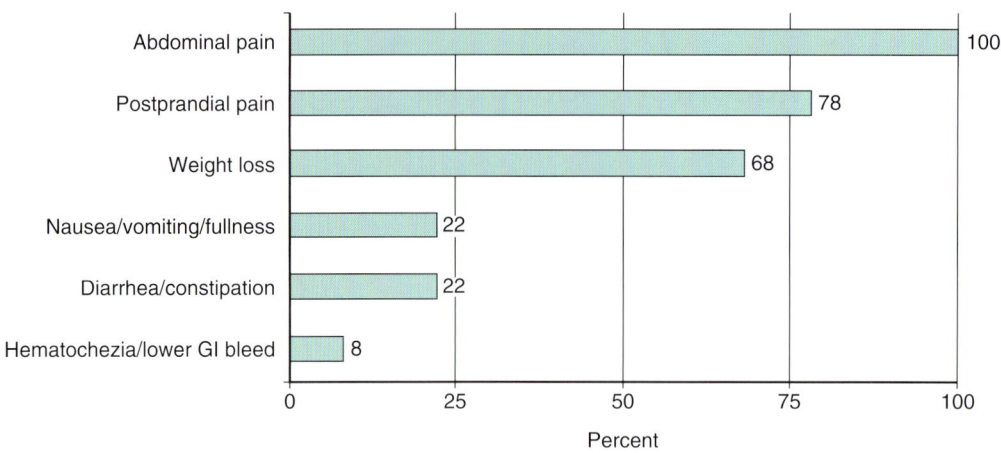

Fig. 41.1 Initial clinical presentation of patients with chronic mesenteric ischemia. *GI,* Gastrointestinal. (From Silva JA, White CJ, Collins TJ, et al. Endovascular therapy for chronic mesenteric ischemia. *J Am Coll Cardiol.* 2006;47:944–950.)

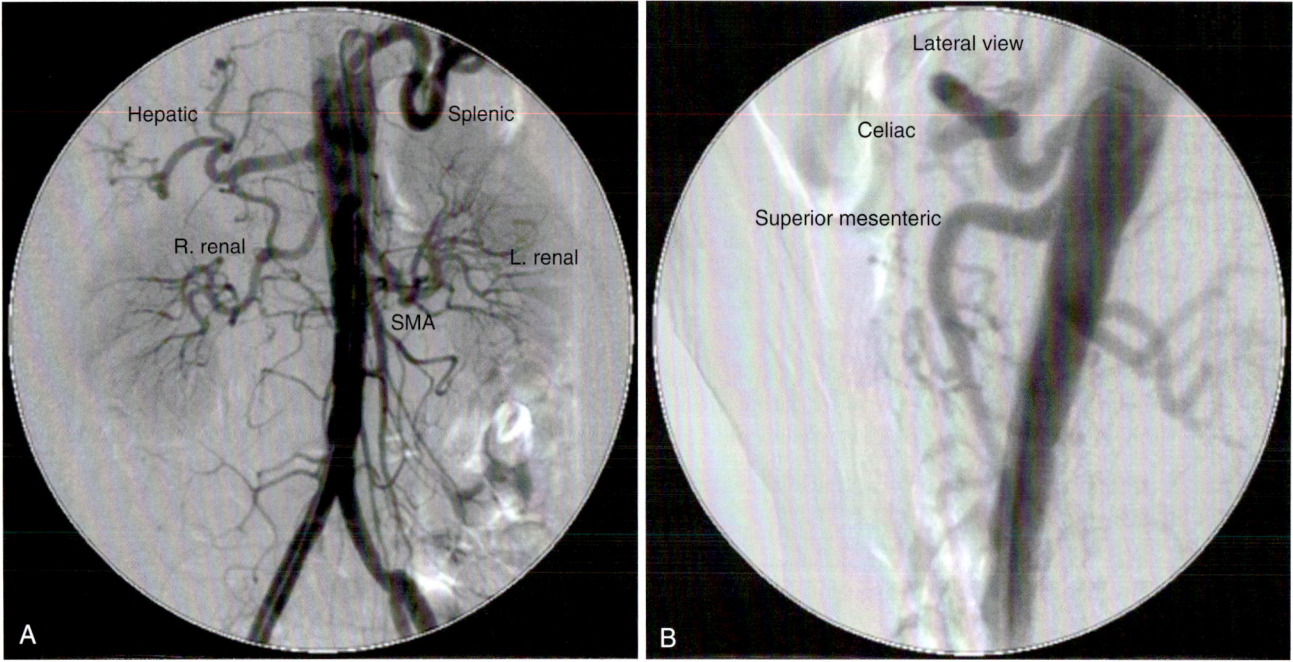

Fig. 41.2 (A) An abdominal aortogram (anteroposterior view) shows the branches of the celiac artery (hepatic and splenic), the right *(R.)* and left *(L.)* renal arteries, and the superior mesenteric artery *(SMA)*. (B) An abdominal aortogram (lateral view) shows the origins of the celiac and superior mesenteric arteries.

higher in stented arteries than native arteries, making the diagnosis of in-stent restenosis more difficult.[4,5] With the relatively common application of CTA and MRA imaging for abdominal pathology, it is now possible to make the "anatomic" diagnosis without performing an invasive procedure.[6]

Invasive digital subtraction angiography is useful for diagnosis but requires a lateral aortogram to visualize the ostia of the mesenteric vessels (Fig. 41.2). Occasionally an enlarged collateral vessel connecting a branch of the IMA with the SMA (arc of Riolan) is seen on the anteroposterior aortogram; it is an indication of proximal mesenteric artery disease. When critical stenoses (≥70%) in multiple vessels are found in symptomatic patients, revascularization is appropriate. However, in patients with borderline lesions or questionable symptoms, there is no stress test to confirm mesenteric ischemia.

TREATMENT

Revascularization has traditionally been performed via open surgery with either endarterectomy or bypass grafting. However, this patient group has a high incidence of underlying coronary artery disease, and the perioperative surgical mortality rate ranges from 3.5% to 15% (Table 41.1),[7–23] with the highest incidence of complications occurring in patients older than 70 years of age.[24,25]

Atherosclerotic aortoostial obstructions of the visceral vessels are similar to those of the renal arteries, and the technical considerations for percutaneous transluminal angioplasty (PTA) with stent placement are similar to those for renal artery intervention (Fig. 41.3). As with renal interventions, stent placement offers a superior late patency compared with PTA alone.[26] The endovascular approach circumvents the need for general anesthesia

TABLE 41.1 Surgical Outcomes for Chronic Mesenteric Ischemia

Author	Year	No. Patients	No. Vessels	Technical Success (%)	30-Day Mortality (%)	Symptom Relief (%)	Restenosis (%)
Kieny et al.[7]	1990	60	69	100	3.5	NA	25
Cormier et al.[8]	1991	32	90	100	9	NA	9
Cunningham et al.[9]	1991	74	194	100	12	86	NA
McAfee et al.[10]	1992	58	119	100	10	90	10
Calderon et al.[11]	1992	20	36	100	0	100	0
Christensen et al.[12]	1994	90	109	100	13	NA	NA
Gentile et al.[13]	1994	26	29	100	10	89	11
Johnston et al.[14]	1995	21	43	100	0	NA	16
Moawad and Gewertz[15]	1997	24	38	100	4	78	23
Mateo et al.[16]	1999	85	130	100	8	87	24
Sivamurthy et al.[17]	2006	41	59	100	15	68	17
Atkins et al.[18]	2007	49	88	100	4	88	20

NA, Not applicable.

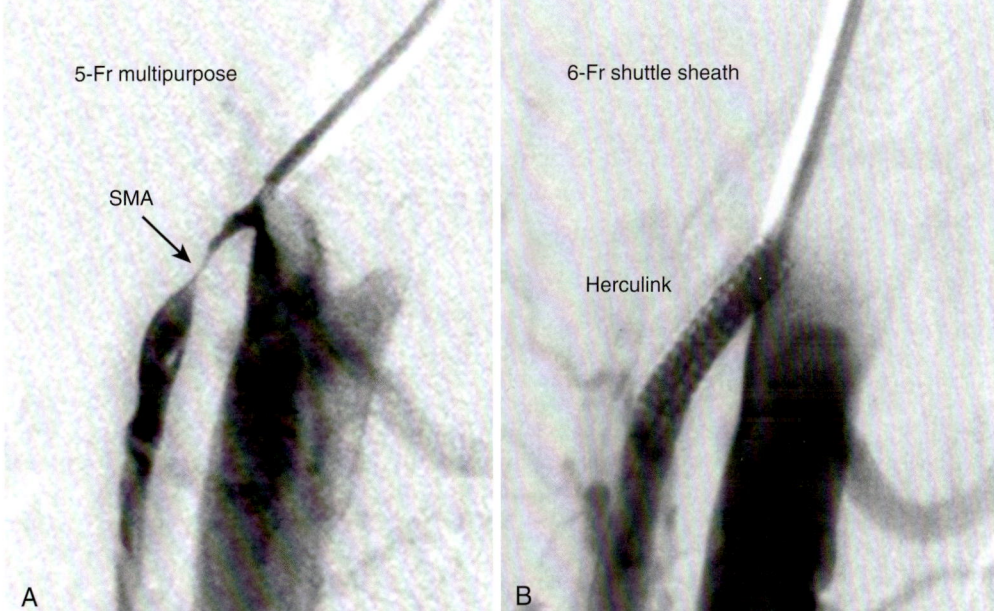

Fig. 41.3 (A) Baseline angiogram with brachial artery access showing tight stenosis in the proximal superior mesenteric artery *(SMA)*. (B) Final angiogram after deployment of a balloon-expandable stent.

and the morbidity associated with open surgery; it is believed to result in lower rates of acute mortality and morbidity (Table 41.2).[18,26–40]

Because of the relative infrequency of this disease, there are no randomized trials comparing surgery to endovascular treatment for CMI. The early 20-year (1977–97) Cleveland Clinic experience in 85 patients who had CMI treated with surgery demonstrated an 8% perioperative mortality rate, and one-third of the patients had a major complication of surgery.[16] Advanced age, hypertension, coronary artery disease, and disease in other vascular beds correlated with surgical complications. At late follow-up, 23% (n = 18) had objective evidence of restenosis, 21% (n = 16) had recurrent CMI symptoms, and 12% (n = 9) underwent target-vessel revascularization. The 5-year survival rate after surgery was 64% (95% confidence interval [CI] 53% to 75%), and the 3-year symptom-free survival rate was 81% (95% CI 72% to 90%).

The Mayo Clinic experience in 229 consecutive CMI patients demonstrated a propensity for higher-risk patients with more comorbidities to be referred for angioplasty with stenting, whereas lower-risk patients tended to have open repair.[23] The researchers found that despite their lower-risk status, the surgical patients had greater morbidity and longer hospitalization compared with the endovascular group. They noted a higher restenosis rate for endovascular therapy (EVT), but there was no difference in secondary patency between surgical and stented patients.

In a series of 59 patients and 79 vessels with CMI treated with balloon expandable stents at the Ochsner Clinic, the technical success rate was 96%, and symptom relief was achieved in 88% of patients.[36] There was one perioperative death (1.7%) and two access site complications. At a mean follow-up of 38 ± 15 months, 17% of the patients had recurrence of their symptoms but none had developed acute mesenteric ischemia. All patients with recurrent symptoms underwent successful retreatment without

TABLE 41.2 Percutaneous Outcomes for Chronic Mesenteric Ischemia

Author	Year	No. Patients	No. Vessels	Technical Success (%)	30-Day Mortality (%)	Symptom Relief (%)	Restenosis (%)
Matsumoto et al.[27]	1995	19	20	79	0	52	NA
Hallisey et al.[28]	1995	16	25	84	6	75	25
Allen et al.[29]	1996	19	24	95	5	79	NA
Maspes et al.[30]	1997	23	41	90	0	75	12
Nyman et al.[31]	1998	5	6	100	0	80	60
Sheeran et al.[32]	1999	12	13	92	8	75	16
Kasirajan et al.[33]	2001	28	32	100	11	66	27
AbuRahma et al.[34]	2003	22	24	95	0	67	30
Sharafuddin et al.[35]	2003	25	26	96	4	85	8
Landis et al.[26]	2005	29	33	97	6.9	90	16.3
Sivamurthy et al.[17]	2006	21	29	95.3	16	27	32
Silva et al.[36]	2006	59	79	96	1.7	83	29
Atkins et al.[18]	2007	31	42	97	3	84	20
Oderich et al.[37]	2013	42	42	98	0	98	12
Guo et al.[38]	2017	32	35	96.9	0	90.7	26.9

NA, Not applicable.

complication. The in-stent restenosis rate at 14 ± 5 months—with 90% of the vessels imaged with CTA, invasive angiography, or duplex ultrasound—was 29% (see Table 41.2). The target-vessel revascularization rate was 17%. The 5-year cumulative rates of freedom from death, symptom recurrence, or both were 72%, 79%, and 57%, respectively.

To compare surgery with EVT, the administrative database of the National Inpatient Sample (NIS) was used to retrospectively examine 4150 patients treated for CMI between 2007 and 2014.[41] In this propensity-matched cohort, major adverse cardiovascular and cerebrovascular events (MACCEs) and composite in-hospital complications occurred significantly less often after EVT than after surgery (8.6% vs. 15.9%; $P < .001$; and 15.3% vs. 20.3%; $P < .006$, respectively). EVT was also associated with lower median hospital costs ($20,807.00 vs. $31,137.00; $P < .001$, respectively) and shorter length of stay (5 vs. 10 days, respectively; $P < .001$) compared with open surgery.

A recent meta-analysis of eight CMI studies compared EVT with surgery and demonstrated that there was no difference in 30-day mortality or 3-year cumulative survival rate; compared with surgery, EVT resulted in a significantly lower rate of in-hospital complications ($P = .002$), whereas the recurrence rate within 3 years after revascularization was significantly greater for EVT ($P < .00001$).[42] A comparative effectiveness and cost-effectiveness comparison analysis of EVT versus surgery demonstrated that EVT was the preferred treatment for CMI patients despite more reinterventions.[43]

Complications of EVT can lead to serious consequences. In a series of 156 patients reported from the Mayo Clinic, serious complications—including branch perforation, distal embolization, vessel dissection, and stent embolization—occurred in 7%.[44] The use of antiplatelet therapy reduced the risk of embolization, and smaller platform equipment (0.014- vs. 0.035-inch) reduced the risk of complications.[44]

The Achilles' heel of EVT has been restenosis. Recently a nonrandomized 225-patient CMI case series suggested a possible advantage for balloon-expandable covered stents compared with bare-metal stents.[37] A significant reduction in restenosis was seen in both de novo lesions and restenosis lesions. No increased risk of stent thrombosis was observed. The disadvantage of the balloon-expandable covered stents is the requirement for a larger, 0.035-inch stent platform rather than the smaller, safer, 0.014-inch stent platform. These encouraging data need confirmation in controlled trials; also the benefits of drug-eluting balloons and stents—which have improved patency in other vascular beds—need to be explored.

CONCLUSION

The infrequent occurrence of CMI has made randomized controlled trials comparing treatment outcomes very difficult to perform. Current evidence suggests that compared with surgery, EVT is a cost-effective choice for patients with CMI. The current treatment recommendation is that patients who are candidates for either surgery or percutaneous therapy should receive percutaneous therapy with stent placement.

KEY REFERENCES
3. Clair DG, Beach JM. Mesenteric ischemia. *N Engl J Med*. 2016;374:959–968.
4. AbuRahma AF, Stone PA, Srivastava M, et al. Mesenteric/celiac duplex ultrasound interpretation criteria revisited. *J Vasc Surg*. 2012;55:428–436.
5. AbuRahma AF, Scott Dean L. Duplex ultrasound interpretation criteria for inferior mesenteric arteries. *Vascular*. 2012;20:145–149.
23. Oderich GS, Bower TC, Sullivan TM, et al. Open versus endovascular revascularization for chronic mesenteric ischemia: risk-stratified outcomes. *J Vasc Surg*. 2009;49:1472–1479.e3.
41. Lima FV, Kolte D, Kennedy KF, et al. Endovascular versus surgical revascularization for chronic mesenteric ischemia: insights from the national inpatient sample database. *JACC Cardiovasc Interv*. 2017;10:2440–2447.
42. Cai W, Li X, Shu C, et al. Comparison of clinical outcomes of endovascular versus open revascularization for chronic mesenteric ischemia: a meta-analysis. *Ann Vasc Surg*. 2015;29:934–940.
43. Hogendoorn W, Hunink MG, Schlosser FJ, et al. A comparison of open and endovascular revascularization for chronic mesenteric ischemia in a clinical decision model. *J Vasc Surg*. 2014;60:715–725.

 Additional references available online at expertconsult.com.

中文导读

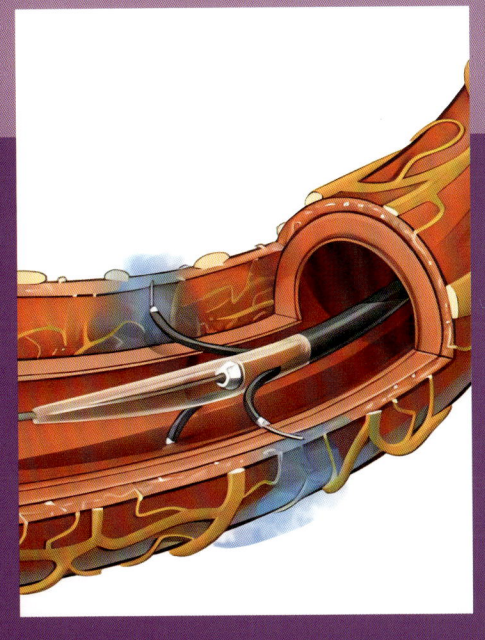

第42章
肾动脉狭窄

　　在65岁以上人群中，肾动脉狭窄患病率为6.8%。在冠心病和高血压患者中，超过19%的患者罹患肾动脉狭窄；在外周动脉疾病患者中，超过14%的患者罹患肾动脉狭窄。90%的肾动脉狭窄由动脉粥样硬化引起，除此之外，纤维肌发育不良是第二常见的病因。目前对于肾动脉狭窄的主要无创性检查有双功能超声、CTA和MRA。尽管目前在动脉粥样硬化性肾动脉狭窄患者中使用肾动脉支架改善血压和肾功能的有效性尚存在争议，但对于接受强化药物治疗的严重肾动脉狭窄且合并难治性高血压及肾功能下降的患者，以及严重肾动脉狭窄合并反复急性肺水肿且无其他诱因的患者，仍可从肾动脉支架植入术中获益。多项前瞻性、对照临床试验已证实经皮去肾交感神经术治疗重度难治性高血压的安全性和有效性。目前正在开发多种去肾交感神经的新技术，包括射频、超声波和局部给药。

　　本章节重点详细介绍肾脏缺血的有创评估、肾动脉造影术、肾动脉支架植入术的详细操作流程及防止动脉粥样硬化栓塞的远端保护装置，以及支架内再狭窄的处理和肾动脉支架植入术的并发症。

张而立　张洪亮

章节要点

- 肾动脉狭窄是由一组异质性疾病引起的，其病因、临床表现、病程、治疗和结局各不相同。动脉粥样硬化性肾动脉硬化和纤维肌发育不良是肾动脉狭窄的最常见原因。

- 动脉粥样硬化进行性发展的患者可能有慢性缺血性肾病的症状和体征，导致肾血管性高血压和肾功能不全。然而，肾动脉狭窄、高血压和肾功能不全之间的因果关系很难证明。

- 当在高容量、有经验的血管实验室进行非侵入性检查时，双功能多普勒超声检查是一种极好的诊断工具和理想的检测手段。超声的特异性和敏感性与CTA、MRA具有竞争力，且超声的成本较低。

- 肾动脉造影仍然是诊断动脉粥样硬化性肾动脉硬化的"金标准"，它允许对肾周腹主动脉进行全面定义，并对肾动脉及其分支血管的直径和轮廓进行评估。然而，动脉粥样硬化严重程度的血管造影评估（直径狭窄百分比）可能不足以确定动脉粥样硬化性肾动脉硬化和高血压或肾功能障碍之间的因果关系。

- CORAL研究表明，在肾动脉狭窄合并收缩期高血压或慢性肾脏疾病患者的综合多因素药物治疗的基础上，肾动脉支架植入并不能带来预防临床事件的显著获益。

- 公认的肾动脉血运重建适应证包括严重的、难治性高血压，复发性肺水肿，以及在最佳药物治疗下仍有进展的肾功能不全。然而，这些建议基于有限的临床试验证据支持。

- 使用新发布的大直径冠状动脉药物洗脱支架进行经皮血管重建，是具有适当临床适应证的肾动脉血管重建的新的优势选择（指征外，未经批准）。辅助性的肾脏血管内技术（远端保护装置）和药物（GPⅡb/Ⅲa抑制剂）的临床有效性和安全性还没有在强有力的临床试验中得到证实。

- 经皮肾交感神经射频消融术是安全的，但其疗效尚未在随机、盲法、假手术对照的研究中得到证实。

42 Renal Artery Stenosis

Waleed Alharbi, Nilesh J. Goswami, Jeffrey A. Goldstein

KEY POINTS

- Renal artery stenosis (RAS) is caused by a heterogeneous group of diseases with various causes, clinical manifestations, courses, treatments, and outcomes. Atherosclerotic renal artery sclerosis and fibromuscular dysplasia are the most common causes of renal artery sclerosis.
- Patients in whom atherosclerosis is progressive may have signs and symptoms of chronic ischemic renal disease, resulting in renovascular hypertension and renal dysfunction. However, the causal relationship between RAS, hypertension, and renal dysfunction is difficult to prove.
- Duplex Doppler ultrasonography, when performed noninvasively in a high-volume, experienced vascular laboratory, is an excellent diagnostic tool and ideal for surveillance. The specificity and sensitivity of ultrasound are competitive with computed tomography angiography and magnetic resonance angiography, but ultrasound has a lower cost.
- Renal arteriography remains the "gold standard" for the diagnosis of atherosclerotic renal artery sclerosis, allowing full definition of the perirenal abdominal aorta and assessment of the diameter and contour of the renal artery and its branch vessels. However, angiographic evaluation of the severity of atherosclerosis (i.e., percent diameter stenosis) alone may be inadequate in establishing the cause and effect between atherosclerotic renal artery sclerosis and hypertension or renal dysfunction.
- The Cardiovascular Outcomes in Renal Atherosclerotic Lesions (CORAL) study demonstrated that renal artery stenting does not confer a significant benefit for the prevention of clinical events when added to comprehensive, multifactorial medical therapy in people with RAS and hypertension or kidney disease.
- Accepted consensus indications for renal artery revascularization include severe, refractory hypertension; recurrent pulmonary edema; and progressive renal insufficiency despite optimal medical therapy. However, these recommendations are based on limited supporting clinical trial evidence.
- Percutaneous revascularization with newly released large diameter coronary drug-eluting stents represents a new advantageous option (off label) for renal artery revascularization with appropriate clinical indications. The clinical effectiveness and safety of adjunctive renal endovascular technologies (i.e., distal protection devices) and medications (i.e., glycoprotein IIb/IIIa inhibitors) have not been established in robust clinical trials.
- Percutaneous radiofrequency renal sympathetic denervation is safe, but its efficacy has not been demonstrated in a randomized, blinded, sham-controlled study.

INTRODUCTION

Atherosclerotic renal artery stenosis (ARAS) is associated with chronic renal ischemia and increased cardiovascular morbidity and mortality. The primary aim of renal revascularization therapies is to improve blood pressure control, salvage renal function, and reduce cardiovascular risk. Although technical advances in the endovascular treatment of ARAS have improved dramatically in the past decade, allowing patients with more extensive ARAS to be considered for revascularization, the indications for treating these patients remain controversial and highlight the major divergence in practice among physicians regarding the appropriate treatment for patients with ARAS.[1] Small and large prospective, randomized clinical trials from Europe have failed to demonstrate the clinical benefit of renal revascularization in reducing cardiovascular events or poor renal outcomes compared with medical therapy alone.[2-4] Determining the essential role of renal revascularization and appropriate patient selection has become the central issue among physicians. Consensus regarding the technical aspects of renal stent revascularization has reached a general level of acceptance among interventionists.

The emergence of percutaneous renal sympathetic denervation as a safe and effective technology in the treatment of drug-resistant hypertensive patients has highlighted the important role of the sympathetic nervous system in hypertension.[5] Ongoing large clinical trials in the treatment of hypertension and renal insufficiency in these patient populations, with and without ARAS, will ensure that renal interventional therapies for hypertension control will remain an exciting area of clinical research.

EPIDEMIOLOGY AND NATURAL HISTORY

ARAS is the most common secondary cause of hypertension. Left untreated, it may progress to renal dysfunction. The prevalence of end-stage renal disease in the United States is 372,407 patients per year, with approximately 100,000 new cases diagnosed each year[6]; 2.1% of these new cases are attributed to ARAS.[7] ARAS is reported in 0.5% to 5%[8] of all hypertensive patients and 45% of patients with severe or malignant hypertension.[9]

The prevalence of ARAS increases with age, especially in patients with diabetes, hypertension, coronary artery disease (CAD), or aortoiliac occlusive disease.[10] A population-based study reported a prevalence of renal artery stenosis (RAS) (>60% stenosis) to be 6.8% among patients older than age 65.[11]

In a Mayo Clinic series, more than 19% of patients with CAD and hypertension were found to have greater than 50% stenosis of the renal arteries.[12] In another series, more than 14% of patients with peripheral artery disease (PAD) were found to have significant angiographic stenosis of the renal arteries.[13] The risk factors for the development of ARAS are similar to those of CAD. Similarly, stroke and PAD are highly prevalent among patients with end-stage renal disease on hemodialysis. ARAS is progressive in 36% to 71% of patients with this condition, and 39% of patients with greater than 75% ARAS progress to complete occlusion within the 3-year follow-up.[14] In a prospective study of 84 patients with at least one abnormal renal artery, progression of RAS occurred at a rate of approximately 20% per year.[15]

Unfortunately, it is difficult to identify the subset of patients who will progress to renal failure.

Although 90% of renal artery lesions are atherosclerotic, the remaining 10% result from other causes. Fibromuscular dysplasia (FMD), the second most common cause of RAS, results in fibrous thickening of the intima, media, or adventitia of the arterial wall. FMD is more common among women between the ages of 15 and 50 years and is recognized by its beaded appearance on angiography.[16] Less common causes include trauma, dissection, external compression by a tumor or mass, thromboemboli, renal artery aneurysms, neurofibromatosis, vasculitis, retroperitoneal fibrosis, and radiation-induced stenosis.[17]

PATHOPHYSIOLOGY OF RENOVASCULAR HYPERTENSION AND ISCHEMIC NEPHROPATHY

The renal vasculature is richly innervated by sympathetic afferent and efferent nerve fibers that control renovascular resistance and the resultant increase in renin release.[18] Efferent renal nerve activity is controlled by several inputs, such as aortic and carotid baroreflexes[19] and cardiac stretch receptors.[20] Renal nerves often receive greater sympathetic activation than others, especially in the setting of essential hypertension.[21] This disproportionate increase in renal sympathetic activity results in increased renovascular resistance and increased plasma renin activity, and it promotes the retention of sodium and water.[22] The afferent renal nerves contribute to the pathogenesis of renovascular hypertension by increasing activation of the sympathetic nervous system.[18]

In unilateral ARAS, decreased blood flow through the affected kidney results in increased production of renin, which cleaves angiotensin to produce angiotensin I, which is converted to angiotensin II. Angiotensin II is a direct vasoconstrictor that stimulates aldosterone secretion and results in sodium reabsorption. The retained salt and water are then excreted by the unaffected kidney, producing a renin-dependent hypertensive state. In bilateral ARAS or ARAS in a solitary functioning kidney without the ability to sense an elevated blood pressure, pressure natriuresis does not occur, resulting in volume expansion and suppression of renin activity. These patients become highly dependent on angiotensin II for glomerular filtration. Angiotensin II maintains the efferent arteriolar tone of the glomeruli. When angiotensin-converting enzyme inhibitors (ACEIs) or angiotensin receptor blockers (ARBs) are administered, the efferent arteriolar tone is no longer maintained, and glomerular filtration is decreased, resulting in renal insufficiency. Sodium restriction and diuresis convert bilateral RAS to a renin-mediated form of hypertension.[23]

DIAGNOSTIC TESTS AND IMAGING

Duplex ultrasound, computed tomography angiography (CTA), and magnetic resonance angiography (MRA) are contemporary noninvasive imaging modalities used to diagnose RAS. Other tests can be used to assess the potential physiologic effect of RAS.

Ultrasonography

Duplex ultrasonography is a useful noninvasive test to screen for RAS, with sensitivity between 75% and 98% and specificity between 87% and 100%.[24] Its sensitivity in identifying accessory renal arteries is 67% (Fig. 42.1). Duplex ultrasonography can produce images of the renal arteries, assess blood flow velocity and pressure waveforms, and measure kidney size without contrast or radiation exposure (Figs. 42.2 and 42.3). Estimation of renal artery percent diameter stenosis is based on the renal artery velocity and the ratio of renal artery to aortic velocity (Table 42.1), and antihypertensive medications do not interfere with duplex imaging. It can also provide information regarding renal parenchymal disease, tumors, and calculi. It is less expensive than CTA or MRA, can be used for renal artery stenting surveillance, and can be easily performed at the patient's bedside. Unfortunately, early studies of this technology reported a 10% to 20% rate of failure due to operator inexperience, patient obesity, or bowel gas.[24] The test may be time consuming when done by inexperienced technologists.

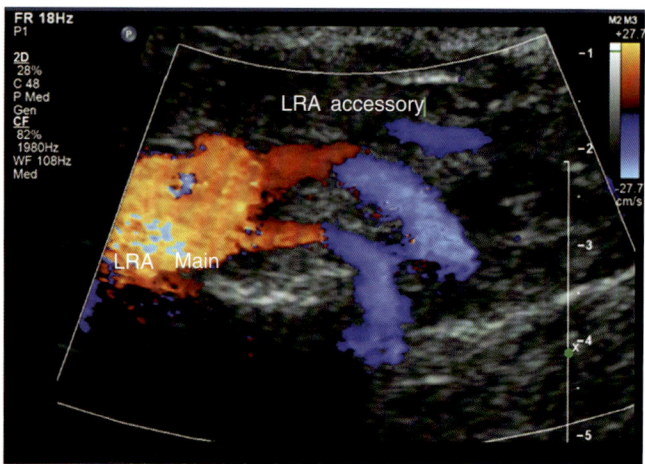

Fig. 42.1 Main and accessory left renal arteries *(LRA)* as defined on duplex ultrasound.

The renal resistive index (RI) is a commonly used measure of resistance to arterial flow within the renal vascular bed. It is calculated during duplex ultrasonography (see Fig. 42.3).

Peak Systolic Renal Parenchymal Velocity

An elevated RI is considered to be an indicator of nephrosclerosis and intrinsic kidney disease. Radermacher and colleagues used an RI greater than 0.8 as the sole screening tool to identify a patient subset that may have a less than optimal response of blood pressure control and improved renal function with renal artery stent revascularization.[25] However, these findings were refuted by other studies suggesting improved renal function and blood pressure control after successful renal artery stenting.[26,27] RI should not be considered the sole parameter in deciding whether a patient will have a clinically favorable response to percutaneous renal revascularization.

Magnetic Resonance Angiography and Computed Tomography Angiography

MRA and CTA, both excellent noninvasive techniques to evaluate patients for possible renal pathology, are widely available. If duplex ultrasonography is nondiagnostic, these modalities can be used to confirm the findings of duplex ultrasound and used for patients whose anatomy is unfavorable for invasive angiography. However, CTA does require the use of iodinated contrast. Both CTA and MRI can provide additional visualization of the aorta, accessory renal arteries, and renal parenchymal anatomy.

MRA requires no contrast but cannot be used in patients with ferromagnetic devices or those who are claustrophobic. Stented vessels cannot be adequately evaluated by MRA. Grobner and Marckmann and colleagues postulated that the gadolinium used in MRA was causative in the development of nephrogenic fibrosing dermopathy.[28,29] Since then, the use of MRA has been restricted to patients with a serum creatinine level less than 1.5 to 2.0 mg/dL. The sensitivity and specificity of MRA are 62% and 84%, respectively.[30] The drawbacks of CTA include large contrast load and nephrotoxicity, along with the radiation exposure. The sensitivity and specificity of CTA are 64% and 92%, respectively.[30] CTA can also be used for stent surveillance if duplex ultrasonography is nondiagnostic (Fig. 42.4).

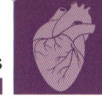

CHAPTER 42 Renal Artery Stenosis

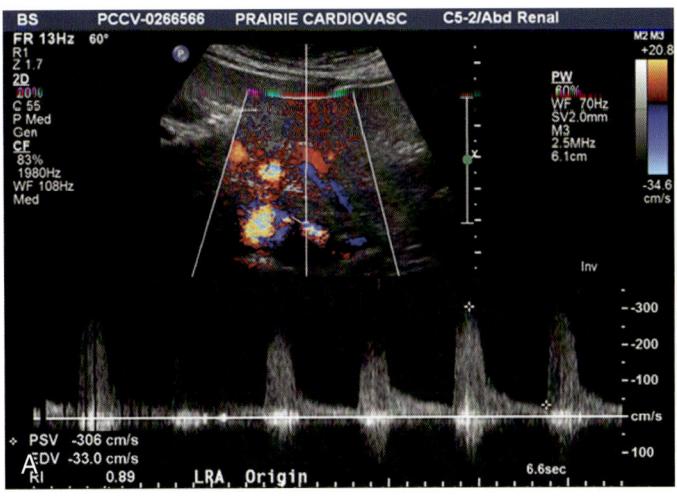
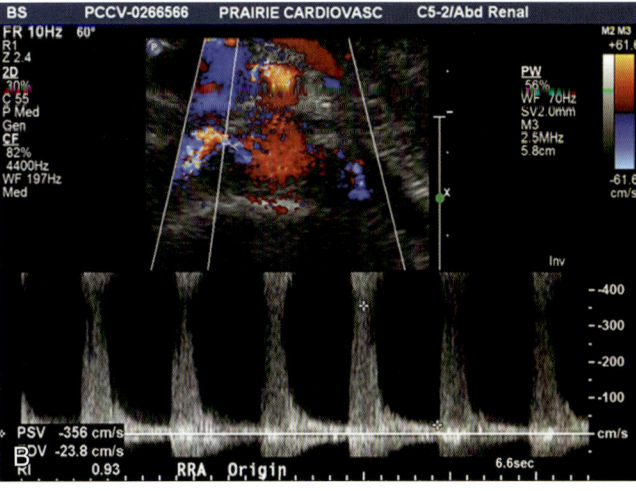

Fig. 42.2 (A and B) Bilateral renal artery stenosis of 60% to 99% on duplex ultrasonography in a 69-year-old woman.

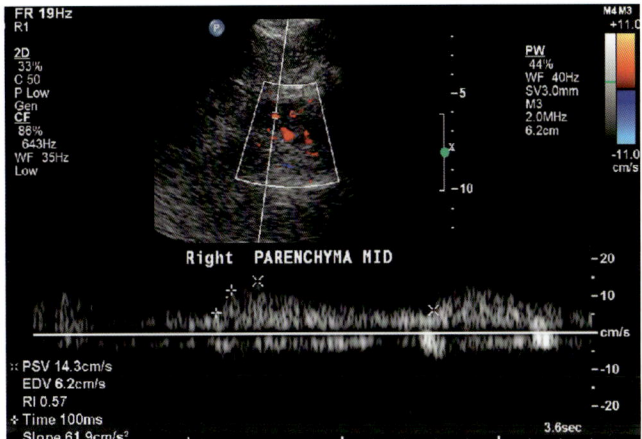

Fig. 42.3 Resistive index *(RI)* and prolonged acceleration time (≥100 ms) in a patient with 60% to 99% renal artery stenosis.

TABLE 42.1 American College of Cardiology/American Heart Association Peripheral Arterial Guidelines for the Management of Renal Artery Stenosis

Degree of Stenosis (%)	Duplex Criteria
0–59	RAR <3.5 and renal artery PSV <200 cm/s
60–99	RAR ≥3.5 or renal artery PSV >200 cm/s (and flow turbulence)
Occluded	Absence of arterial flow and low-amplitude signal

PSV, Peak systolic velocity; *RAR*, renal-aortic ratio.

FUNCTIONAL ASSESSMENT OF RENAL ARTERY STENOSIS

Brain natriuretic peptide (BNP) is secreted by ventricular myocytes in response to increased myofibril stretch. Its production is also stimulated by angiotensin II, which is elevated in patients with RAS, and by hypertension. BNP antagonizes plasma renin activity and promotes diuresis and sodium excretion. Silva and colleagues studied the role of BNP levels in patients with RAS and hypertension.[31] In this small study, baseline BNP was elevated in patients with severe ARAS. A significant blood pressure response to renal stenting was seen in patients with elevated baseline BNP levels. The test may be useful in identifying patients with renovascular hypertension who would be likely to respond to stent revascularization; however, larger confirmatory studies are required to prove this.

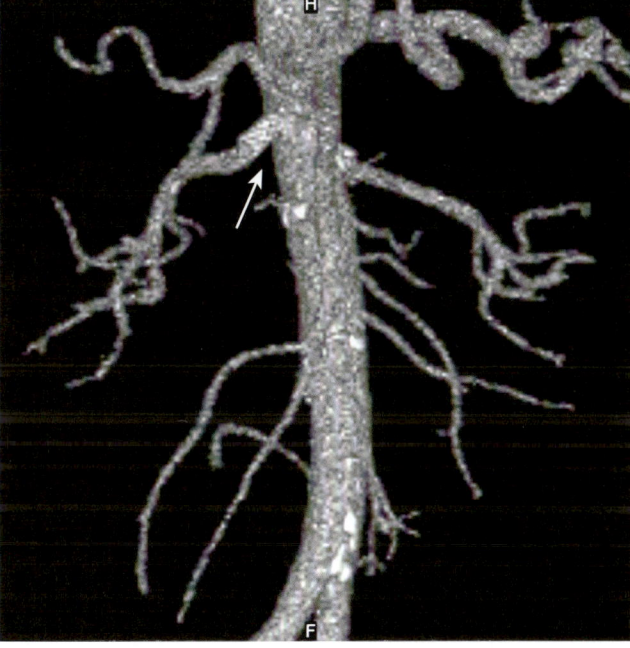

Fig. 42.4 Computed tomography angiography images after right renal artery stenting demonstrates patency *(arrow)*.

Radionuclide imaging has been historically used to diagnose unilateral RAS. With this technique, a detector gamma camera is used to assess baseline renal flow by injecting a radionuclide tracer (Technetium-99m diethylenetriaminepentaacetic acid [DTPA]). Repeat scans are performed after administering the ACEI captopril, which decreases renal function on the ipsilateral side of RAS, whereas the uptake of the unaffected side is normal or increased. The reported sensitivity and specificity are 90% and 93%, respectively.[32,33] The wide availability of duplex ultrasound, CTA, and MRA has resulted in the near elimination of this test to diagnose RAS. It is occasionally used for cortical functional assessment of the ipsilateral and contralateral kidney in the setting of renal atrophy and RAS or for cortical functional assessment of a horseshoe kidney with RAS.

Plasma renin activity or plasma renin assay (PRA) has also been used as a screening test for renovascular hypertension. Plasma renin levels have a low specificity in the diagnosis of RAS, but the concomitant use of an ACEI improves the specificity of PRA levels. PRA is measured at baseline and 1 hour after oral administration of 50 mg of captopril. Unfortunately, the sensitivity ranges widely, between 34% and 100%, and the specificity varies from 80% to 90%.[34,35] In patients with bilateral or unilateral RAS in a solitary kidney, the sensitivity and specificity is this assay is much lower because the resultant volume overload suppresses PRA levels.

Assessment of renal vein renin level is another test for diagnosing renovascular hypertension. It is performed using a catheter to compare the renin levels of both kidneys. Although it may identify blood pressure responders to endovascular intervention or surgery, it has fallen out of favor because of the invasive nature of the test. Measurement of plasma renin and renal vein renin activity is seldom needed in contemporary diagnosis and management of RAS because of the availability of noninvasive imaging modalities.

Identification of At-Risk Patients and Indications for Renal Artery Revascularization

ARAS should be suspected in patients with resistant hypertension or progressive renal insufficiency who have CAD or PAD. Specific clinical clues are listed in Table 42.2. Preprocedural identification of the patient with poorly controlled hypertension who is likely to benefit from renal stent revascularization is challenging. The recommendations of the American College of Cardiology/American Heart Association (ACC/AHA) for the management of PAD, including revascularization in RAS, are as listed in Table 42.3.[36] Appropriate indications for renal revascularization include unilateral RAS, bilateral RAS, or RAS involving a solitary functioning kidney in patients in whom blood pressure cannot be adequately controlled with maximal tolerable doses of at least three antihypertensive medications of different classes or if side effects of the antihypertensive medication prohibit sufficient control.[37]

In patients with unilateral RAS with normal renal function and well-controlled hypertension, revascularization may not be required. Instead, close follow-up for potential loss of pharmacologic control and accelerating hypertension or a potential decline in renal function may suffice. In these instances, a renal duplex ultrasound should be considered.

Patients who have undergone successful stent revascularization are often prescribed antiplatelet and statin therapies. The routine use of clopidogrel (Plavix) in combination with aspirin after successful stent revascularization has not been adequately evaluated, but most investigators use this combination in light of other indications (i.e., drug-eluting coronary stent implantation). Statins (3-hydroxy-3-methyl-glutaryl-coenzyme A reductase inhibitors) are frequently given to patients with ARAS; these agents may slow the progression of renal atherosclerosis

TABLE 42.2 Clinical Clues Suggesting Renal Artery Stenosis

Hypertension beginning before age 30 or after age 55
Acute elevation of plasma creatinine levels or azotemia after initiation of ACEI or ARB
Patients with hypertension and asymmetric kidney size
Moderate to severe hypertension in patients with diffuse atherosclerosis
Recurrent congestive heart failure or flash pulmonary edema in a patient with hypertension
Malignant hypertension
Resistant hypertension
Epigastric bruit

ACEI, Angiotensin-converting enzyme inhibitor; *ARB,* angiotensin receptor blocker.

after renal revascularization and in some instances induce plaque regression.[38] Cheung and coworkers found a reduction of ARAS progression from 30% to 6% in patients without and with statins, respectively.[38] They also found 12 of 79 patients exhibited signs of disease regression.[38] Statins should therefore be considered for all patients with established dyslipidemia and ARAS.

CORAL Study

The Cardiovascular Outcomes in Renal Atherosclerotic Lesions (CORAL) study was an open-label, randomized, international, multicenter, controlled clinical trial, sponsored by the National Heart, Lung, and Blood Institute (NHLBI) of the National Institutes of Health (NIH).[39] The study compared medical therapy alone with medical therapy plus renal artery stenting in patients with atherosclerotic RAS and elevated blood pressure or chronic kidney disease, or both. Patients with severe ARAS (>60% angiographic stenosis) with a systolic blood pressure of 155 mm Hg or higher although on two or more antihypertensive medications were eligible for enrollment in the trial. Although 5322 patients were screened, only 947 were randomized.

The primary end point was death from cardiovascular or renal causes, myocardial infarction, stroke, hospitalization for congestive heart failure, progressive renal insufficiency, or need for kidney replacement. Although the stent group had a modest but statistically significant lowering of systolic blood pressure (2.3 mm Hg, $P = .03$), this did not translate into a lowering of clinical events. Over a median follow-up time of 43 months, there was not a significant difference between the two treatment groups in the occurrence of the primary end point or any of its individual components or all-cause mortality. The study concluded that renal artery stenting did not confer a significant benefit with respect to the prevention of clinical events when added to comprehensive, multifactorial medical therapy in people with RAS and hypertension or kidney disease.

There have been criticisms of the study. Patients with RAS of 60% or more could be enrolled in the study, and the mean degree of stenosis in the trial was 68%. There is debate about the severity of stenosis necessary to justify intervention. The study authors reported that in patients with more than 80% stenosis, as measured by the investigators, no clear benefit was seen. Although a significant proportion of subjects in the CORAL study subgroup

TABLE 42.3 Duplex Ultrasound Criteria for a Diagnosis of Renal Artery Stenosis

Indication	Classification of Recommendation	Level of Evidence
Asymptomatic bilateral or unilateral RAS in a solitary kidney	IIb	C
Accelerated hypertension	IIa	B
Resistant hypertension	IIa	B
Hypertension and unexplained unilateral small kidney	IIa	B
Hypertension with intolerance to antihypertensive medications	IIa	B
Progressive kidney disease and bilateral RAS or RAS in a solitary kidney	IIa	B
Chronic renal insufficiency and unilateral RAS	IIb	C
Recurrent, unexplained CHF or sudden and unexplained pulmonary edema	I	B

CHF, Congestive heart failure; *RAS,* renal artery stenosis.

had high-grade stenosis, severe hypertension at entry, and significant translesional systolic pressure gradients, there was no positive treatment effect of stenting observed in these subgroups.[40] The trial took almost 5 years to complete enrollment. Some patients who were eligible were not enrolled because of the preference of their physicians, who might have been convinced of the clinical benefit of the RAS. In a recent updated systemic review of seven randomized clinical trials in ARAS patients, five of seven randomized controlled trials did not show significant differences between renal stenting and medical therapy in blood pressure control, kidney function, mortality, or pulmonary edema.[41]

Despite the negative results of the studies, there are still situations in which patients can benefit from renal artery stenting. Patients with severe RAS and refractory hypertension or declining renal function despite intensive medical therapy may benefit from renal artery stenting. Renal artery stenting should be considered for patients with severe RAS and recurrent acute pulmonary edema without an alternative cause. These indications are broadly consistent with the consensus statement from the Society for Cardiovascular Angiography and Interventions (SCAI).[42]

Clinical Follow-Up

Patients must be monitored closely after renal artery intervention for recurrent or worsening hypertension or renal dysfunction. Although no medical society has offered guidelines, surveillance duplex ultrasonography should be considered every 6 months after the placement of a renal artery stent (Figs. 42.5 and 42.6). Four duplex ultrasound criteria have been reported for the diagnosis of in-stent restenosis (ISR) (Table 42.4). If ISR is identified in a patient with stable renal function and well-controlled hypertension, the original indication for renal artery intervention should be reviewed and close clinical monitoring should continue.

RENAL ENDOVASCULAR INTERVENTIONS

Invasive Assessment of Renal Ischemia

The first renal artery balloon angioplasty was reported by Andreas Grüntzig in Zurich, Switzerland, in 1977.[43] The initial endovascular strategies consisted of balloon angioplasty alone and were associated with relatively poor acute procedural success and poor patency rates. These outcomes were the direct result of heavy renal aortoostial plaque burden and calcification with resultant vessel recoil and/or dissections. However, with the introduction of balloon-expandable metal stents, many of the mechanical limitations of primary balloon angioplasty were overcome, with resultant acute procedural success rates as high as 98% and 9-month duplex Doppler binary restenosis rates of approximately 20% to 25%.[44]

Over the subsequent decade, the tools used for percutaneous renal artery intervention evolved rapidly, from hand-crimped stents on 5- or 6-Fr balloons designed on 0.035-inch wire systems to low-profile, 6-Fr, guiding catheter–compatible, premounted stent-balloon combinations on 0.014- to 0.018-inch wire systems designed specifically for renal interventions. Despite technical improvements, the enthusiasm for percutaneous renal artery stent revascularization has waxed and waned, in part because of the lack of clinical evidence supporting the effectiveness of renal stenting in ARAS patients to improve blood pressure and renal function.[2,4,45–47]

Although the limitations of the trials (i.e., visual estimate of ARAS degree of stenosis, significant crossover to the intervention therapy, lack of standardized methods of blood pressure and microcirculation assessment, and the definition of clinical success) have been well enumerated, patients in these studies were ll

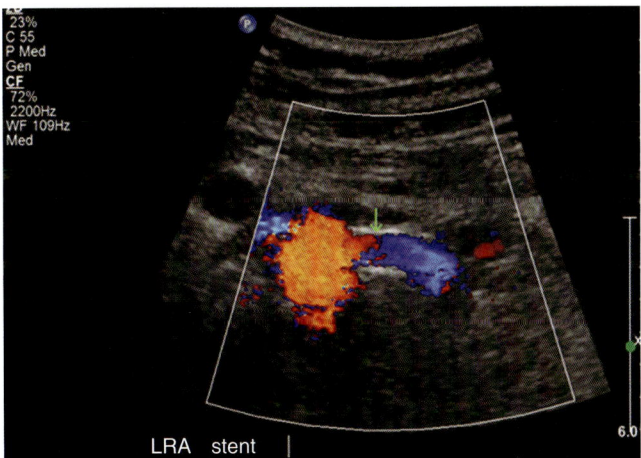

Fig. 42.5 Follow-up renal artery duplex ultrasonography demonstrates a patent stent *(arrow)*. *LRA,* Left renal artery.

TABLE 42.4 Ultrasound Criteria for the Diagnosis of In-Stent Restenosis

Percent In-Stent Restenosis (%)	Criteria
>60	PSV >200 cm/s or RAR >3.5[39]
>60	PSV >225 cm/s or RAR >3.5[75]
>70	PSV >395 cm/s or RAR >5.1[76]
>60	PSV >280 cm/s or RAR >4.5[77] (PTRAS after fenestrated and branched endovascular repair)

PSV, Peak systolic velocity; *PTRAS,* percutaneous transluminal renal artery stenting; *RAR,* renal-aortic ratio.

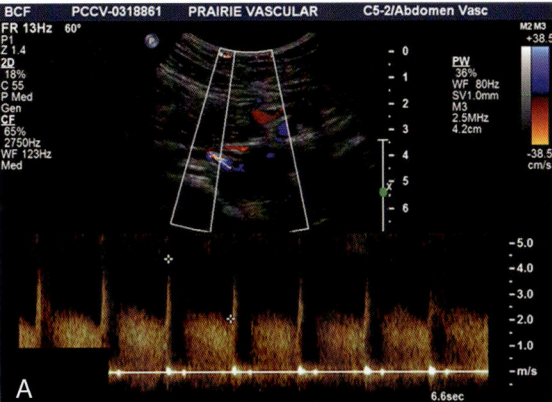
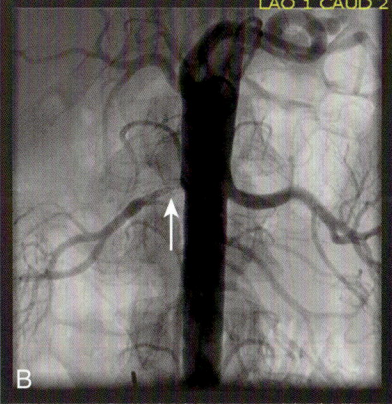

Fig. 42.6 (A) In-stent restenosis is demonstrated by duplex ultrasound with very high peak systolic (440 cm/s) and end-diastolic (206 cm/s) velocities. (B) Right renal artery in-stent restenosis *(arrow)* is confirmed by contrast angiography.

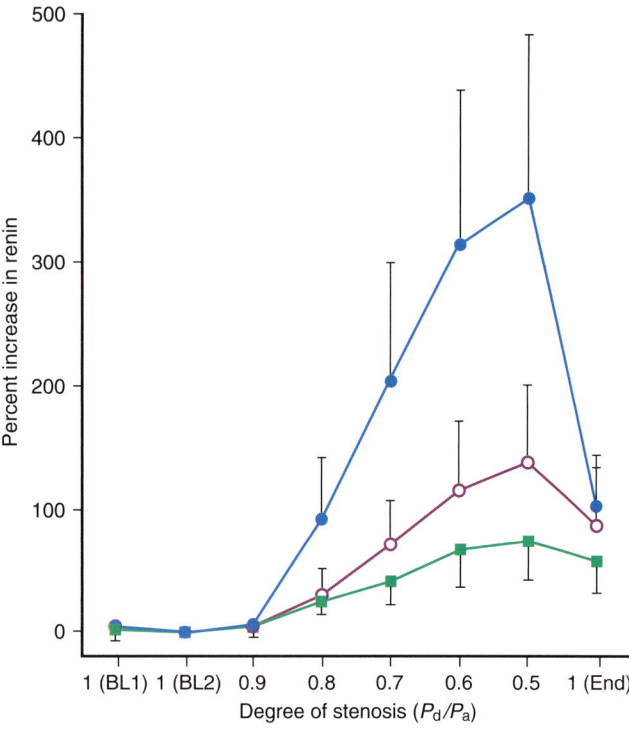

Fig. 42.7 Effects of a balloon-induced, unilateral, controlled, graded stenosis, expressed as the ratio of distal pressure (P_d) corrected for aortic pressure (P_a). (Modified from De Bruyne B, Manoharan G, Pijils M, et al. Assessment of renal artery stenosis severity by pressure gradient measurements. *J Am Coll Cardiol.* 2006;48:1851–1855.)

selected on the basis of angiographic lesion severity. Use of this inclusion criterion reflects the commonly held belief that angiographic lesion severity is proportional to renal ischemia and that stent revascularization will result in clinical benefit. However, this paradigm has been challenged by several investigators,[48,49] underscoring the fact that although quantitative angiography improves the accuracy of assessment compared with visual estimation, it does not improve the accuracy of diagnosing renal ischemia. ARAS angiographic severity may often be overestimated compared with other modalities that may reflect the presence of renal ischemia.[50]

Among the other invasive modalities that can be used to assess ischemia is renal fractional flow reserve (FFR).[51] However, the evidence for outcome improvement using intrarenal functional assessment of RAS severity is insufficient due to heterogeneity in methodology and subjects' characteristics.[52] FFR seems to be able to discriminate responders from nonresponders to renal revascularization using intrarenal infusion of hyperemic agents such as dopamine or fenoldopam. A series of reports by Belgian investigators emphasized the importance of the invasive physiologic assessment of ARAS lesions in preparation for renal revascularization in a well-selected group of patients. De Bruyne and colleagues demonstrated that the magnitude of the renal artery occlusion was proportional to the activation of the renin-angiotensin system and required at least a 10% gradient (Fig. 42.7). Follow-up work by Mangiacapra and coworkers suggested that similar invasive translesional pressure gradient assessment after a bolus administration of intraarterial dopamine might further improve the patient selection for renal stenting. In this small study ($n = 53$), a dopamine-induced mean pressure gradient of 20 mm Hg or more before revascularization was the sole independent predictor of blood pressure improvement at the 3-month follow-up. However, the investigators described an 18% nonresponder rate despite a dopamine-induced gradient of 20 mm Hg or more,

underscoring the heterogeneity of the potential pathophysiologic mechanisms responsible for hypertension in this patient cohort.[1]

Renal Contrast Angiography

Abdominal aortography should be performed before renal stenting. It assists in identifying the renal ostia, extent of ostial disease, accessory renal arteries, degree of perirenal aortic calcification, angulation of the renal artery takeoff from the aorta, and degree of aneurysmal enlargement of the abdominal aorta. If indicated, subsequent selective renal angiography can be performed with a series of 4-, 5-, or 6-Fr diagnostic catheters. Typical catheter configurations include internal mammary, renal double curve, Sos, and Cobra catheters. Left anterior oblique–angled views often assist in the identification of the right and left renal ostia.[53]

Renal Artery Stenting

All patients should be pretreated with aspirin therapy; the efficacy of adjunctive use of clopidogrel, although widely practiced, has not been adequately studied in renal stent patients. After sheath insertion, the patient should be fully anticoagulated with unfractionated heparin to obtain an activated coagulation time of at least 250 seconds. In most cases, arterial access is acquired in a retrograde approach from either common femoral artery. However, in patients with severe bilateral aortoiliac disease or tortuosity or a sharply downward-angulated renal artery, an antegrade radial or brachial approach may be considered.

In most cases, renal artery revascularization is performed using a 6-Fr guiding catheter. The guiding catheter should reflect the angle at which the renal artery arises off the aorta, location of the stenosis, anatomy of the perirenal aorta, and operator preference. The most commonly used guides are the internal mammary artery, renal standard curve, renal double curve, or hockey stick. The multipurpose guide is well suited for a brachial or radial approach. For the common femoral arterial approach, a sheath 35-cm long is preferable because it minimizes guide catheter manipulation in a potentially heavily diseased perirenal aorta and can facilitate guiding catheter exchanges over smaller diagnostic catheters if required.

The goal of renal artery intervention is to achieve an optimal angiographic and hemodynamic result with minimal manipulation of the renal artery and to minimize potential atheroembolization and dissection of the renal artery or aortic wall. The no-touch technique can be used in an attempt to minimize distal atheroembolization (Fig. 42.8). To use this technique, a 35-cm sheath is placed below the renal artery and a hand injection of contrast is performed to locate the renal ostium (see Fig. 42.8A). A 0.035-inch, J-tip guidewire is advanced in the abdominal aorta superior to the renal arteries. Over this wire, the guide catheter is advanced in proximity to the renal artery. The 0.035-inch wire is then retracted to the soft portion of the wire so that the guide catheter begins to assume its shape and approach the ostium of the renal artery. The J-shaped portion of the wire is left outside to guide against the aortic wall (see Fig. 42.8B).

The ostium of the guiding catheter is gently rotated and aligned with the renal ostium, with the J wire preventing guiding catheter intubation into the renal artery. From this position, a 0.014-inch wire is directed through the guide and into the distal renal artery (see Fig. 42.8C). The 0.035-inch J wire is then removed, and the guide catheter is allowed to gently engage the ostium of the renal artery (see Fig. 42.8D).

Another method for safely engaging the renal ostium is the exchange technique (Fig. 42.9). A 35-cm sheath is placed below the renal artery, and a hand injection of contrast is used to locate the renal ostium. A 4-Fr, soft-tipped diagnostic catheter is used to gently locate and engage the renal ostium (see Fig. 42.9B). Use of a small, soft catheter minimizes the possibility

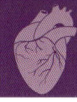

CHAPTER 42 Renal Artery Stenosis

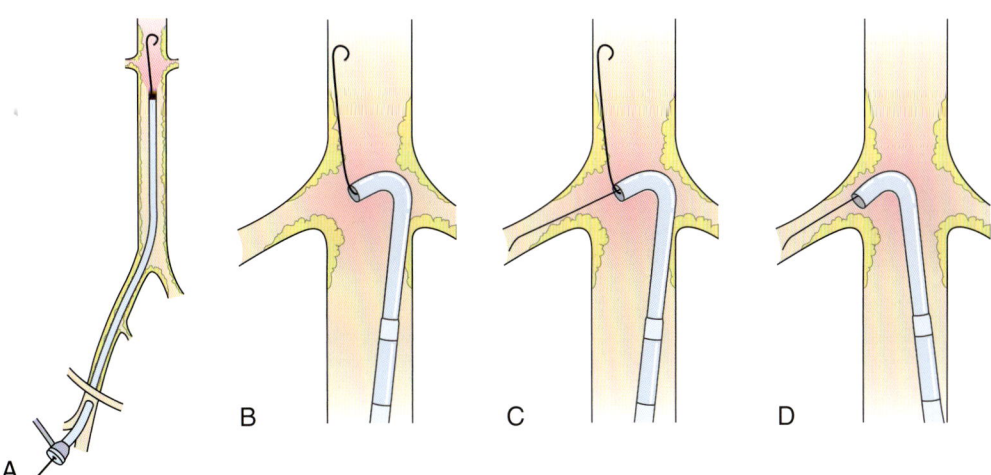

Fig. 42.8 No-touch technique: guiding the catheter. (A) A 35-cm sheath inserted over 0.035-inch guidewire. (B) Guide catheter is positioned near renal artery ostium with soft portion of 0.035-inch wire out to protect the ostium. (C) A 0.014-inch wire is advanced into the renal artery. (D) A 0.035-inch guidewire is removed.

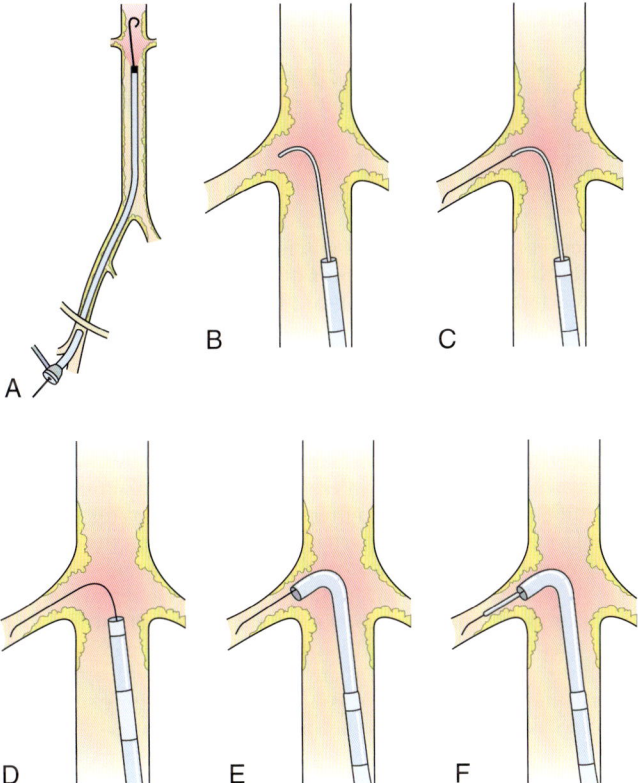

Fig. 42.9 Exchange technique. (A) A 35-cm sheath inserted over 0.035-inch guidewire. (B) Renal artery engaged with a 5-Fr diagnostic catheter. (C) A 0.014-inch wire inserted into the renal artery through the diagnostic catheter. (D) Diagnostic catheter removed. (E) Guide inserted over the 0.014-inch guidewire. (F) Interventional equipment can be inserted.

Another commonly used method for engaging the renal artery involves a dilator/guide system (Veripath Peripheral Guiding Catheter, Abbott Vascular Devices, Mountain View, CA). With this technique, the renal artery is wired with a 0.014-inch wire through the softer selective diagnostic catheter. With the 0.014-inch wire in the renal artery, the diagnostic catheter is removed, and the renal dilator/guide system is back-loaded onto the 0.014-inch wire. The dilator provides a smooth transition across the lesion and is gently withdrawn, allowing the guiding catheter to advance to the renal ostium; however, dottering of the renal lesion occurs with this technique, and the possibility of atheroembolization is a concern. The average diameter of a normal renal artery is approximately 5.0 to 6.0 mm, which depends on the presence of accessory renal arteries and poststenotic dilation.

Predilation of the renal lesion is highly recommended and should be performed with a balloon diameter slightly smaller than that of the renal reference vessel. Inflation is performed to full expansion of the balloon. Flank pain should be closely monitored because it indicates stretching of the adventitia. If detected, higher-pressure inflations should be avoided because further dilation could result in perforation. Most atherosclerotic renal artery lesions demonstrate significant recoil after balloon angioplasty and therefore require stent placement. Balloon-expandable stents should be positioned such that 1 to 2 mm of the stent protrudes into the aorta to ensure proper coverage of the arterial ostium. It is often necessary to place the stent in two views to ensure proper placement.

Historically, one challenge for the use of drug-eluting stents in the renal arteries is sizing, where the largest-diameter coronary artery drug-eluting stent is 4.0 mm, and overdilation of an undersized stent may reduce its radial strength. Currently, the introduction of 4.5- and 5.0-mm coronary (off-label) Drug-eluting stent Resolute Onyx sizes from Medtronic (Medtronic, Minneapolis, MN) resolved the stent sizing issue of renal arteries. Use of the Ostial Pro Stent positioning system (Ostial Solutions, Kalamazoo, MI) can assist in proper stent placement and adequate coverage of the ostium of the renal artery (Fig. 42.10). It is a disposable device compatible with 6-, 7-, and 8-Fr systems. It has opaque gold-plated feet that are used to identify the ostium and assist in placement of the stent to confirm coverage of the ostium.

After correct placement, the stent should be deployed with the proper pressure to achieve a 1:1 ratio with the diameter of the reference vessel. After stent deployment to nominal balloon pressures, the deflated balloon is reduced to within the stent confines, with the proximal aspect of the balloon protruding into the aorta.

of atheroembolization or dissection, which could be caused by a larger, stiffer guide. Once engaged, a 0.014- or 0.018-inch guidewire is passed through the diagnostic catheter and into the main renal artery (see Fig. 42.9C). The diagnostic catheter is then removed (see Fig. 42.9D), leaving the guidewire in place. A 6- or 7-Fr guide is placed over the guidewire, maintaining the 35-cm sheath below the renal artery and facilitating placement of the guide (see Fig. 42.9E). The renal predilation balloon can then be safely passed into the renal artery (see Fig. 42.9F).

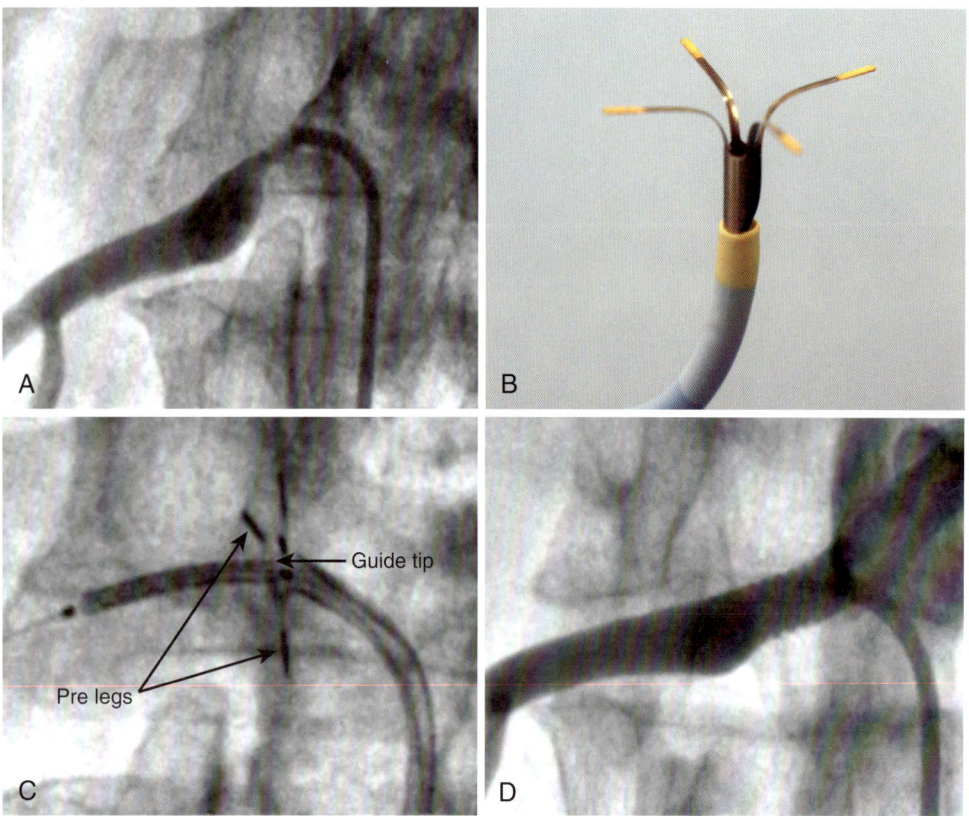

Fig. 42.10 (A) High-grade renal lesion is identified using a 5-Fr diagnostic catheter. (B) Ostial Pro Stent (Ostial Solutions, Kalamazoo, MI) demonstrates four gold-plated feet in the deployed position through a 6-Fr guide catheter. (C) The deployed radiopaque feet are deployed against the aortic wall. These markers are aligned with the proximal balloon marker before stent deployment. (D) After stent placement, the angiogram demonstrates excellent renal stent deployment at the aortorenal ostium.

The balloon is then taken to high pressures for the postdilation step. For this maneuver, as the balloon is being deflated, the guide can be advanced forward to reengage the renal artery. The deflating balloon is used as a dilator to less traumatically advance the guide back into proper position if necessary. A completion angiogram should be done to assess proper coverage of the renal ostium by the stent, the main renal artery, and its branches for signs of dissection or spasm and the renal parenchymal blush to exclude evidence of atheroembolization. Although there are no data to establish the routine use of aspirin and clopidogrel after stenting, most operators continue the use of these agents for at least 30 days. The illustrative case in Video 42.1 shows step by step technique for renal artery stenting.

Distal Protection Devices to Prevent Atheroembolization

Despite successful renal artery revascularization, renal function may deteriorate in 8% to 32% of patients.[53] Although this decline in renal function may reflect the continued effects of underlying disease processes (e.g., diabetes, hypertension) or reperfusion injury, atheroembolization may also be a potential cause. During a simulated renal stent procedure, Hiramoto and coworkers demonstrated that angioplasty and stenting of ex vivo aortorenal atheroma specimens can produce thousands of atheroemboli particles.[54] Intuitively, distal protection devices may provide beneficial results in selected patients by preventing distal atheroembolization, but limited clinical studies have proven inconclusive. Although several study authors[55–57] have suggested an improvement in renal function or its stabilization associated with the use of distal protection devices, they are designed primarily for use in carotid artery stent procedures and coronary artery bypass grafts. Which patient cohort may potentially benefit from the use of these devices has not been clearly established.

Insight into the potential mechanism of atheroembolic decline in renal function was provided by Cooper and colleagues.[58] This study randomized 100 patients in a 2 × 2 factorial design to distal protection (filter type) versus no distal protection and the glycoprotein IIb/IIIa platelet receptor inhibitor abciximab or placebo. Renal artery stenting with distal protection or abciximab alone was associated with a decline in estimated glomerular filtration rate (GFR) at 30 days. However, the combination of distal protection and abciximab use was not associated with a decline in GFR. Abciximab use also was associated with lower incidence of platelet-rich emboli in the filter device.

The use of distal protection in the renal arteries is not without risk; occlusive devices (e.g., PercuSurge) can predispose to renal ischemia, and filter devices not specifically designed for the renal vasculature may cause renal artery spasm. Moreover, the distal filter wire may cause dissection of the distal renal vessel. These filters are associated with various filter efficiencies and may not trap all of the atheromatous debris generated by the renal intervention. Use of the filters is limited to renal arteries with sufficient "landing zones," excluding their use in patients with early renal artery bifurcations. They are associated with a learning curve, and inexperience may prolong the procedure and increase contrast use. Filter retrieval also may be problematic because the recapture catheter can become entrapped within the newly deployed stent.

Management of In-Stent Restenosis

Duplex Doppler–defined restenosis rates after successful stenting depend on a variety of anatomic and patient-related factors. Smaller-diameter vessels (<4 mm) can have restenosis rates as high as 40%, whereas larger vessels (>6 cm) usually have restenosis rates of less than 10%.[58] A history of tobacco use, diabetes, and time to restenosis evaluation also appear to be associated with higher restenosis rates.[59]

Although the endovascular options for ISR treatment are many—including repeat balloon angioplasty, repeat stenting deployment (i.e., bare-metal or drug-eluting stent), drug-coated balloon, or placement of a covered stent (iCAST, Atrium Medical,

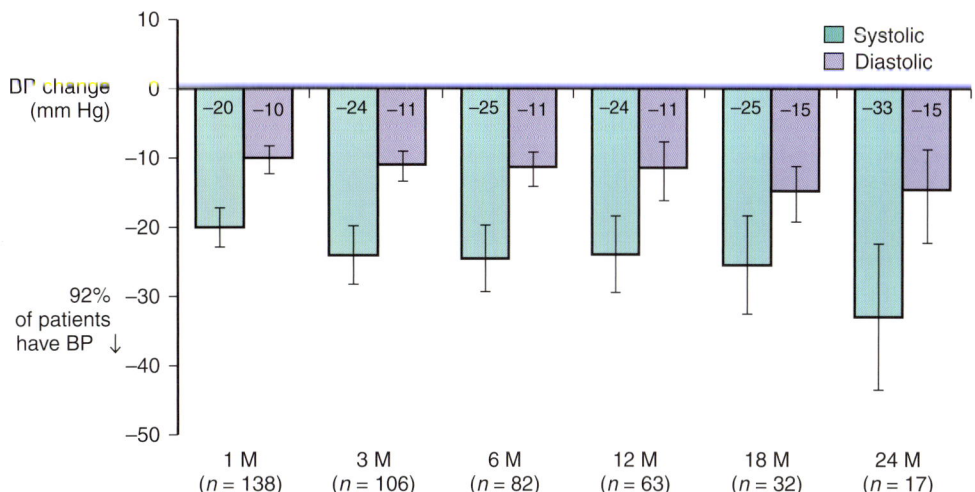

Fig. 42.11 Sustained improvement in blood pressure *(BP)* response during a 2-year follow-up.

Hudson, NH)—there are few data to suggest the superiority of any one modality.[60] Because of the recoil in the vessel, balloon angioplasty for ISR usually does not provide a durable result. Placement of more metal into the vessel often results in recurrent restenosis.[61] Brachytherapy,[62] atherectomy, cryoplasty,[63] and laser debulking[64] techniques have been described.[62]

Although the efficacy of drug-eluting stents in the coronary vasculature is well established, their use in renal revascularization is less clear. The Palmaz Genesis Peripheral Stainless Steel Balloon Expandable Stent in Renal Artery Treatment (GREAT) trial was a randomized evaluation of bare-metal stents versus drug-eluting stents in 105 patients with ARAS. At 6 months, no significant difference in stent patency between the two treatment arms was discerned (6.7% vs. 14.6%, $P = .30$). At 1 year, target-lesion revascularization rates were 11.5% for bare-metal stents and 1.9% for drug-eluting stents (i.e., sirolimus-eluting balloon expandable stent versus bare-metal low-profile stent for renal artery treatment[65]). Although the rate of adverse events was lower in the treatment group, statistical significance was not demonstrated in this small patient cohort.

Renal stenting has been compared with balloon angioplasty for the treatment of ISR in a retrospective study of 101 patients with renal artery ISR, which found patients treated with repeat stent placement were 6.89 times more likely to lose patency after treatment than patients with balloon angioplasty ($P < .01$).[66] Drug-eluting stents also have been compared with brachytherapy for the treatment of renal ISR. At 3 years, there were lower rates of major adverse clinical events and target-lesion revascularization with drug-eluting stents, but they did not reach statistical significance.[67]

Another option for treatment of ISR is placement of a balloon-expandable covered stent (iCast). In theory, this strategy could reduce the risk of neointimal proliferation through the stent struts. Use of this stent has been reported in the renal and iliac beds for treatment of restenosis.[68] Drug-eluting balloons may eventually play a role in this space as well but are clearly an off-label indication at this point.

Complications

Most complications associated with percutaneous renal artery revascularization are related to arterial access. They include groin hematomas, retroperitoneal hemorrhage, pseudoaneurysm, arteriovenous fistula, and infection. These complications should be treated as usual and are discussed in other sections of this textbook. Serious complications may arise due to atheroembolization to the kidneys, bowel, or lower extremities, resulting in renal failure, ischemic bowel, or digital ischemia, respectively.

Renal artery dissection can usually be treated with stent placement. Distal wire perforation may resolve spontaneously with reversal of anticoagulation or may require coil embolization. Renal artery perforation may respond to prolonged balloon inflation with reversal of anticoagulation or may require the placement of a stent graft.

Percutaneous Renal Sympathetic Denervation to Treat Resistant Hypertension

The kidney plays an essential role in the regulation of blood pressure through sodium, volume, and renin modulation and renal sympathetic neuronal activation. Renal sympathetic drive, which contributes to the development and perpetuation of hypertension and sympathetic outflow to the kidney, is activated in patients with essential hypertension. Studies indicate that the renal nerves contribute to the development and maintenance of hypertension and all hypertensive processes. Efferent sympathetic outflow stimulates renin release, increases tubular sodium reabsorption, and reduces renal blood flow. Afferent signals from the kidney modulate central sympathetic outflow and directly contribute to neurogenic hypertension.

Early studies in nonselective surgical sympathectomy have demonstrated effective control of severe hypertension. Catheter-based technologies enable selective denervation of the human kidney with radiofrequency energy (Medtronic, Minneapolis, MN) delivered to the renal artery lumen, ablating the renal nerves located in the adventitia of the renal arteries. Krum and colleagues, in a first study of this approach in humans, demonstrated successful renal denervation with resultant reduction of sympathetic activity, renin release, and central sympathetic outflow.[5] This feasibility trial demonstrated that percutaneous sympathetic renal denervation was safe and effective in reducing blood pressure in patients with severe resistant hypertension.

A subsequent case report suggested that renal denervation was also associated with a decrease in norepinephrine level spill-over and in muscle sympathetic activity.[69] Two-year follow-up of this patient cohort demonstrated a substantial reduction in blood pressure, averaging 33 mm Hg, which persisted without significant adverse events (Fig. 42.11).[70] The Renal sympathetic denervation in patients with treatment-resistant hypertension (SYMPLICITY HTN-2) trial extended these original observations.

The SYMPLICITY HTN-2 trial[71] was a multicenter, prospective, randomized, crossover trial of patients with baseline systolic hypertension of 160 mm Hg or higher despite taking three or more antihypertensive medications. The trial randomized 106 patients in a 1:1 ratio to undergo renal denervation or previous drug treatment alone with a primary end point of blood pressure control assessed at 6 months. Six-month office-based blood pressure assessment demonstrated a mean reduction of 31/12 mm Hg below the pretreatment baseline values in the renal denervation cohort. The blood pressure values in the control group were unchanged, whereas 84% of the patients who underwent renal denervation had a reduction of systolic blood pressure of at least 10 mm Hg. There were no serious procedure- or device-related complications or adverse events in the renal denervation group. The trials demonstrated that catheter-based renal denervation could be safely used to substantially reduce blood pressure in patients with resistant hypertension.

In an effort to gain approval from the U.S. Food and Drug Administration, the SYMPLICITY HTN-3 trial was performed at 88 sites in the United States. This study was a prospective, single-blinded, randomized, sham-controlled study evaluating patients with refractory hypertension.[72] Patients with refractory hypertension were randomized in a 2:1 fashion to renal denervation or sham procedure. After almost 2 years, the study enrolled 535 patients. Of the 1441 patients assessed for inclusion in this trial, only 37.1% (535) were randomized. The primary end point was the change in office systolic blood pressure at 6 months. The mean reduction in office systolic blood pressure was 14.13 ± 23.93 mm Hg in the renal denervation group compared with 11.74 ± 25.94 mm Hg in the sham group. This resulted in an absolute difference of 2.39 mm Hg, which was importantly *not* statistically significant (P = .26). The difference was even less when ambulatory systolic blood pressures were compared. The renal denervation group had a lower ambulatory systolic blood pressure, but the difference was only 1.96 mm Hg. The prespecified superiority margin for systolic blood pressure reduction was determined to be 5 mm Hg.

These results did not meet this end point for superiority. The safety end point showed no concerns, and there was no change in GFRs for patients receiving renal denervation therapy. The results were in conflict with prior nonblinded, nonsham studies and took most observers by surprise. There were many differences between SYMPLICITY HTN-3 and prior studies. Most important, this was a sham-controlled trial. In this study, the sham group had almost a 12-mm Hg reduction in systolic blood pressure.

Similar impressive placebo effects have been seen in prior clinical trials with a sham arm. In the Direct Myocardial Revascularization In Regeneration of Endomyocardial Channels Trial (DIRECT),[73] percutaneous myocardial laser revascularization was randomized to treatment or to sham arms and evaluated the effect on angina. Remarkably, significant improvement in angina as measured by Canadian Cardiovascular Society class was seen for all treatment groups at 6 months: 2.0 ± 1.2, 1.9 ± 1.3, and 2.2 ± 1.2, in high-dose, low-dose, and placebo groups, respectively (P = .413).

SYMPLICITY HTN-3 was the first blinded and sham-controlled study to evaluate renal denervation for the treatment of hypertension. Based on its results, any subsequent studies will likely be required to include a sham arm. The size of the study was also different from the preliminary studies. It was the largest randomized study of renal denervation, and the larger sample size in the study might have influenced results based on the theory of regression to the mean: the more data points obtained, the more accurate the result. Randomization also tends to eliminate selection bias. Both factors likely played a role in the neutral result obtained.

Results of the trial could also have been affected by the population studied. In the renal denervation arm, 25% of the patients treated were African American. This subgroup showed a decreased or no response to therapy compared with non-African Americans.

Efficacy of the denervation is difficult to assess objectively. There were many new, inexperienced operators performing these procedures in this trial. Many of the operators performed fewer than five procedures. The equipment used also was the newer-generation catheter and control unit. Despite the presence of error messages, the treatments were counted as completed. The efficacy of the procedure may be in question.

A combination of the described factors may have played a role in the negative results seen in SYMPLICITY HTN-3. Alternatively, the technology may not be clinically efficacious. However, in a small blinded trial the Catheter-based renal denervation in patients with uncontrolled hypertension in the absence of antihypertensive medications (SPYRAL HTN-OFF MED) of 80 patients without resistant hypertension (24-hour systolic pressure 140 to 170 mm Hg on no antihypertensive medications), catheter-based renal denervation reduced ambulatory blood pressure by 5/4 mm Hg compared with a sham procedure.[74] Although this trial provides proof of principle, establishing the benefit of catheter-based renal denervation on no antihypertensive medications will require a large blinded trial of patients with resistant hypertension.

Various new technologies are being developed to achieve renal denervation. They include radiofrequency energy, ultrasound, and locally delivered drugs. The application of current and evolving technologies needs to be evaluated in the United States and be required to compare its results to that of a sham group. These new trials will ultimately determine the fate of this strategy for the treatment of hypertension and other medical conditions.

Acknowledgments

We recognize Drs. Rocha-Singh, Mishkel, and Kolluri for their contribution to the prior edition of this chapter.

KEY REFERENCES

4. Bax L, Woittiez A, Kouwenberg H, et al. Stent placement in patients with atherosclerotic renal artery stenosis and impaired renal function: a randomized trial. *Ann Intern Med.* 2009;150:840–848.
5. Krum H, Schlaich M, Whitbourn R, et al. Catheter-based renal sympathetic denervation for resistant hypertension: a multicentre safety and proof-of-principle cohort study. *Lancet.* 2009;373:1275–1281.
9. Mann SJ, Pickering TG. Detection of renovascular hypertension. State of the art. 1992. *Ann Intern Med.* 1992;117(10):845–853.
12. Rihal CS, Textor SC, Breen JF, et al. Incidental renal artery stenosis among a prospective cohort of hypertensive patients undergoing coronary angiography. *Mayo Clin Proc.* 2002;77(4):309–316.
25. Radermacher J, Chavan A, Bleck J, et al. Use of Doppler ultrasonography to predict the outcome of therapy for renal-artery stenosis. *N Engl J Med.* 2001;344(6):410–417.
26. Zeller T, Frank U, Muller C, et al. Predictors of improved renal function after percutaneous stent-supported angioplasty of severe atherosclerotic ostial renal artery stenosis. *Circulation.* 2003;108(18):2244–2249.
39. Cooper CJ, Murphy TP, Cutlip DE, et al. Stenting and medical therapy for atherosclerotic renal-artery stenosis. *N Engl J Med.* 2014;370(1):13–22.
40. Murphy TP, Cooper CJ, Matsumoto AH, et al. Renal Artery stent outcomes: effect of baseline blood pressure, stenosis severity, and translesion pressure gradient. *J Am Coll Cardiol.* 2015;66(22):2487–2494.
41. Raman G, Adam GP, Halladay CW, et al. Comparative effectiveness of management strategies for renal artery stenosis: an updated systematic review. *Ann Intern Med.* 2016;165(9):635–649.
44. Gruntzig A, Vetter W, Meier B, et al. Treatment of renovascular hypertension with percutaneous transluminal dilatation of a renal artery stenosis. *Lancet.* 1978;15:801–802.
48. Van Jaarsveld BC, Krijnen P, Pieterman H, et al. For the Dutch Renal Artery Stenosis Intervention Cooperative Study Group. The effect of balloon angioplasty on hypertension in atherosclerotic renal-artery stenosis. *N Engl J Med.* 2000;342:1007–1014.
49. De Bruyne B, Manoharan G, Pijls M, et al. Assessment of renal artery stenosis severity by pressure gradient measurements. *J Am Coll Cardiol.* 2006;48(48):1851–1855.
52. van Brussel PM, van de Hoef TP, de Winter RJ, et al. Hemodynamic measurements for the selection of patients with renal artery stenosis. A systematic review. *JACC Cardiovasc Interv.* 2017;10(10):973–985.
63. Chrysant GS, Goldstein JA, Casserly IP, et al. Endovascular brachytherapy for treatment of bilateral renal artery in-stent restenosis. *Catheter Cardiovasc Interv.* 2003;59(2):251–254.

68. Holmes D, Teirstein P, Satler L, et al. 3-year follow-up of the SISR (Sirolimus-Eluting Stents Versus Vascular Brachytherapy for In-Stent Restenosis) trial. *JACC Cardiovasc Interv.* 2008;1(4):439–448.
72. Bhatt DL, Kandzari DE, O'Neill WW, et al. for the SYMPLICITY HTN-3 Investigators. A controlled trial of renal denervation for resistant hypertension. *N Engl J Med.* 2014;370.1393–1401.
73. Leon MB, Kornowski R, Downey WE, et al. A blinded, randomized, placebo-controlled trial of percutaneous laser myocardial revascularization to improve angina symptoms in patients with severe coronary disease. *J Am Coll Cardiol.* 2005;46.1812–1819.

Additional references available online at expertconsult.com.

中文导读

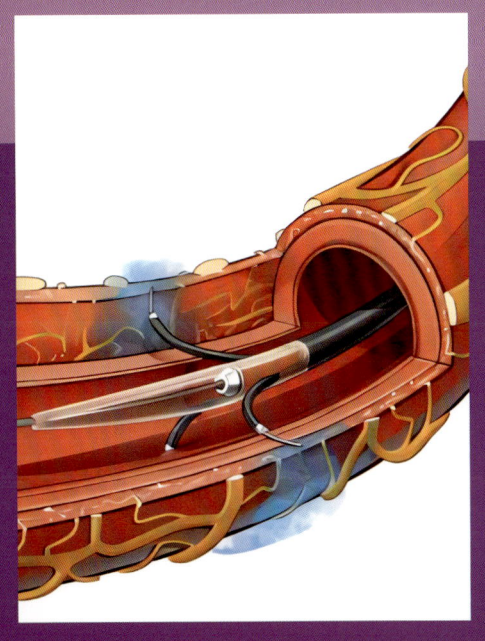

第43章
难治性高血压的器械治疗

  60岁以上人群高血压患病率高达60%～75%，51%的脑卒中和45%的缺血性心脏病可归因于高血压，高血压的发病机制极其复杂，神经内分泌调节在其中发挥了重要作用，交感神经调节和血管顺应性改造是目前比较常用的高血压器械治疗手段。自主神经系统在维持水钠潴留、血管张力方面发挥重要作用，肾交感神经在其中起主导作用。肾交感神经调节被证明可以降低血压，目前最常用的技术手段是肾动脉交感神经消融术。多个临床试验探究了肾动脉交感神经消融术治疗难治性高血压的效果，大多数临床试验获得阳性结果。肾动脉交感神经消融术的严重并发症发生率较低，主要有血管痉挛、严重疼痛、肾动脉夹层、肾动脉狭窄和血管入路并发症。应用超声、化学试剂、放射线等手段进行交感神经消融也在探索当中。目前需要研发更精准的工具来识别适合进行交感神经消融的人群和进行消融部位定位。颈动脉窦在血压调节中也发挥重要作用，目前多种手段包括颈动脉窦切除、植入式压力感受器激动治疗、压力感受器机械调节都被用来尝试治疗难治性高血压。针对单纯收缩性高血压、脉压差增大的患者，其高血压主要机制是由于动脉顺应性变差，肾动脉交感神经消融术难以取得满意效果，通过制造动静脉瘘来降低血管阻力成为此类人群可行的治疗手段。程序性高血压控制是高血压治疗的新理念，它通过植入双腔起搏器，程序性调控起搏方式来调节血压。高血压器械治疗目前蓬勃发展，但基于器械治疗高血压的临床试验存在众多问题，如血压监测方式与基线药物治疗、器械治疗洗脱期、主要终点事件、假手术与否，这些临床试验参数的变化对试验结果与解读非常重要。而不同器械治疗的适用人群选择也是需要关注的热点问题。

孟　真　张洪亮

章节要点

- 未控制的高血压是目前广泛影响公共卫生并造成严重经济后果的重大健康问题。
- 新的治疗手段通过针对神经内分泌调节和血管顺应性的机械改造来治疗高血压。
- 减少肾脏神经交感信号输出的治疗手段取得了一些有效的临床数据,但仍在试验阶段。
- 一系列的技术手段可以通过阻断肾脏神经来调节肾交感张力,最常用的手段是射频消融。

43 Device Therapy for Resistant Hypertension

Marat Fudim, Marvin H. Eng, Paul A. Sobotka

KEY POINTS

- Uncontrolled hypertension presents a significant health care problem with far-reaching public health and economic consequences.
- Novel therapies target neurohumoral modulation and mechanical alteration of vascular compliance to treat hypertension.
- Reduction of the sympathetic nervous output from the renal nerves has some supporting clinical data but remains experimental at the time of this publication.
- A variety of technologies can be used to modulate renal sympathetic tone through destruction of renal nerves with the most common being radiofrequency ablation.

DEFINITION AND EPIDEMIOLOGY

Hypertension (HTN) is estimated to be present in 77.9 million adults and 60% to 75% of patients older than 60 years.[1] Globally, 51% of stroke and 45% of ischemic heart disease are attributable to HTN.[2] HTN-related stroke, cardiac disease, and renal failure are preventable with adequate lowering of blood pressure (BP), which may be achieved across several modalities.[3,4]

Surveys suggest that in the United States, nearly 50% of identified and treated hypertensive patients have systolic blood pressure (SBP) >140 mm Hg, and 13% (26% of the uncontrolled) have systolic BPs of >160 mm Hg.[5] Despite the wide availability of effective drugs for BP control, as much as 51% of patients have low adherence, in turn resulting in 38% increased rate of cardiovascular (CV) morbidity relative to those compliant with medications.[6] Even in clinical trial settings, only 57% of patients elect to persist and adhere to medication recommendations after 2 years, signaling the futility of relying on patient compliance for chronic HTN management.[7] Furthermore, a subset of patients who choose to be compliant with complex multidrug formulations, remain above target pressures, and are designated resistant hypertensive patients. Despite compliance with medications, patients with BP above clinical targets continue to have excess CV mortality, stroke, myocardial infarction, and onset of renal insufficiency.[4,8,9] Treatment strategies to complement pharmacotherapy to reduce BP would address a large unmet clinical need and potentially reduce the CV morbidity of uncontrolled HTN among patients either nonadherent or resistant to HTN pharmacotherapy.

The pathophysiology of HTN is multifactorial with neurohumoral activation making a significant contribution to its genesis (Fig. 43.1). Secondary pathologies such as arteriosclerosis and loss of vascular compliance further accelerate disease progression. Consequently, a treatment approach addressing the separate components of the pathophysiology resulted in the emergence of several separate and perhaps complimentary device driven strategies: sympathetic nervous modulation to decrease downstream maladaptive events in vascular tone and sodium balance or mechanical alteration of the systemic vascular resistance using an arterial-venous anastomosis to change vascular compliance.

NEURO MODIFICATION: TARGETING THE SYMPATHETIC NERVOUS SYSTEM AND HYPERTENSION

Renal Denervation: Science and Clinical Application

Maintenance of body fluid composition, volume, and vascular tone is a complex integrated process regulated by the autonomic nervous system that is heavily renal driven.[10] The sympathetic nervous system (SNS) acquires signals reflecting changes in renal hydrostatic pressure and chemistry and processes information in the central SNS, and efferent signals from the central nervous system adjust renal contribution to vascular tone and volume homeostasis. Afferents nerve endings from the kidney vasculature and parenchyma relay information to the ipsilateral cell bodies in the dorsal root ganglia to the posterior gray column, and finally the brain stem and mid-brain integrate afferent signals from multiple end-organ sensors and baroreceptors (Fig. 43.2).[10] Efferent fibers from the central nervous system extend to the sympathetic preganglionic neurons in the intermediolateral cell column. At approximately T10 to T12 and L1 to L2, splanchnic nerves connect via prevertebral ganglia (e.g., celiac and mesenteric) to postganglionic neurons and communicate to the kidneys bilaterally.[10] In addition, the renal nervous system may reflexively autoregulate without central nervous system output.[11]

Efferent and afferent nerves function in a reflex loop where afferent signals from the kidney to the central nervous system regulate the efferent sympathetic nerve output back to the kidney. Renal afferent nerves are complex and diverse because they represent a heterogeneous population of fibers including myelinated and nonmyelinated fibers.[12,13] Two main physiologic types of renal afferents are responsible for signaling information to the central nervous system, mechanosensitive and chemosensitive receptors. Mechanosensitive receptors transmit hydrostatic data from the renal arteries, veins, and pelvis. Renal ischemia, ionic composition, adenosine, osmolar concentration, oxidative stress, and chemicals (i.e., bradykinin) activate renal chemoreceptors.[10] Functionally, the renal afferent fibers can be divided in (1) pressor, (2) renorenal, and (3) depressor types.[14,15] This means that some fibers contribute to the elevation of the sympathetic tone (sympathostimulant), whereas others reduce the sympathetic tone (sympatholytic). This is supported by increasing preclinical and clinical evidence suggesting that endovascular electrical mapping with stimulation of renal arteries can result in a differential response including an elevation in BP,[16–19] no effect,[20] and in some instances a reduction in BP.[21] Several investigators have suggested a specific anatomic distribution of the functional fibers, with preferentially sympathostimulatory fibers in the proximal renal artery[19] and sympathoinhibitory fibers more distal in the renal hilum.[14]

The efferent arm of the reflex loop innervates renal tubules, the juxtaglomerular apparatus, and renal vasculature. Increased renal sympathetic efferent activity stimulates the β1 receptor of the juxtaglomerular apparatus to release renin.[22,23] Alpha-1B subtype receptor stimulation increases sodium resorption.[23,24]

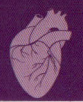

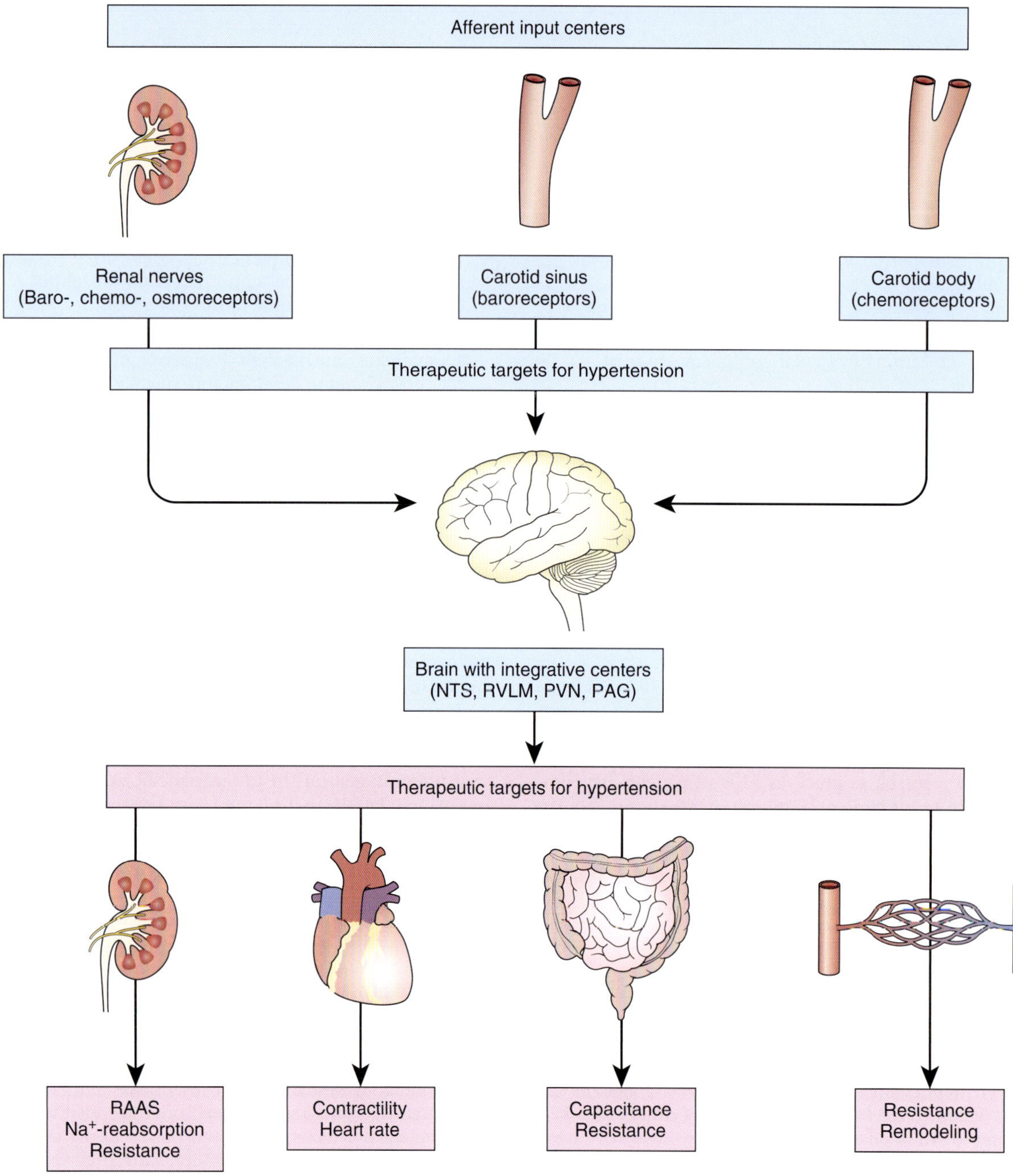

SECTION IV Peripheral Vascular Interventions

Fig. 43.1 Some of the key neurohumoral contributors to hypertension and the effected target organs. *NTS*, Solitary nucleus; *PAG*, periaqueductal gray; *PVN*, paraventricular nucleus of the hypothalamus; *RAAS*, renin angiotensin aldosterone system; *RVLM*, rostral ventrolateral medulla.

Alpha-1A stimulation vasoconstricts renal arterioles, decreasing renal blood flow.[23,25] Graded response of low- or high-frequency signals from the central nervous system modify renal activity. Coincidentally, the efferents are colocated with the afferents in the renal adventitia, providing the anatomic feasibility for percutaneous ablation technology (Fig. 43.3).[26]

Data Supporting Renal Denervation
Preclinical Research

Of the vast preclinical research on renal sympathetic innervation in HTN, a few studies merit mention. Electrical stimulation of feline and canine renal afferents increases vasoconstriction-mediated BPs rises.[27] Interruption of afferent fibers via dorsal rhizotomy in a rodent nephrectomy model of chronic renal failure model causes a decrease in norepinephrine (NE) turnover, attenuates HTN, and improves renal function confirming the renal contribution to BP regulation.[28] Surgical renal denervation (RDN) across several HTN models consistently lowers BP[29,30] and improves natriuresis.[31]

Surgical Denervation for Hypertension Control

Prior to the development of antihypertensive pharmacotherapy, surgical thoracolumbar splanchnectomy served as a therapeutic option for reducing BP.[32,33] A large, prospective, observational study where 1266 and 467 patients undergoing splanchnectomy

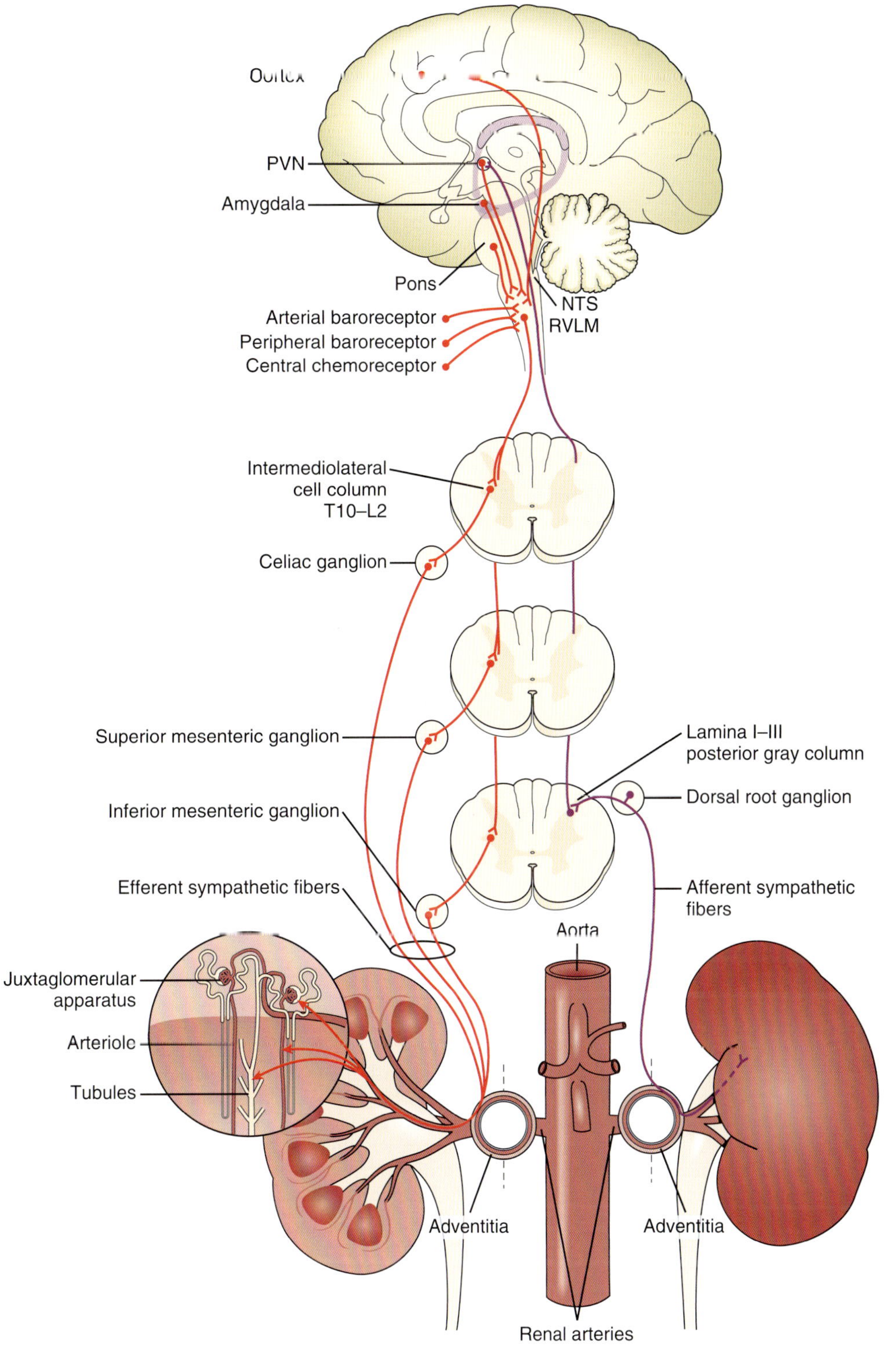

Fig. 43.2 Anatomy of the sympathetic autonomic nervous system and renal innervation. *NTS*, Solitary nucleus; *PVN*, paraventricular nucleus of the hypothalamus; *RVLM*, rostral ventrolateral medulla. (From Bertog SC, Sobotka PA, Sievert H. Renal denervation for hypertension. *JACC Cardiovasc Interv*. 2012;5[3]:249–258.)

and medical therapy, respectively, showed durable BP lowering in conjunction with improved 5-year survival (surgical 81% vs. medical 46%).[34] In addition, symptomatic relief for headaches and precordial pain, reduction in cardiac size, and renal function improvement were observed[33,35,36] at the cost of significant operative mortality (5%).[34] Subsequent studies in nephrectomized patients observed postsurgical reductions in resting sympathetic tone corresponding to substantial lowering of BP, reinforcing the pathophysiological evidence for modulating renal sympathetic output as a treatment for HTN.[37,38]

RENAL ARTERY DENERVATION

Sympathetic modulation for treatment of HTN was rediscovered, and various methodologies have been explored to ablate renal nerves. Given a lack of techniques to screen for different functional afferent renal fiber types, the initial development targeted an undifferentiated global renal denervation. The most developed technology is endovascular radiofrequency (RF) ablation. Initial devices use unipolar or bipolar RF ablation in repeated spiral patterns in energy levels, attempting to achieve

SECTION IV Peripheral Vascular Interventions

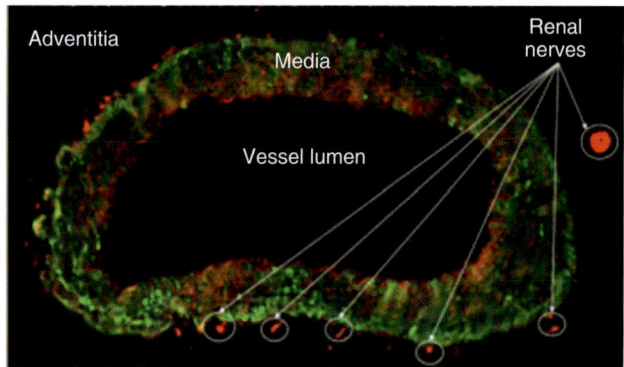

Fig. 43.3 Cross-sectional histology revealing the adventitial location of renal nerves. (From Sobotka PA, Mahfoud F, Schlaich MP, et al. Sympatho-renal axis in chronic disease. *Clin Res Cardiol*. 2011;100[12]:1049–1057.)

sufficient depth to reach the adventitia and disrupt nerve traffic. Delivery of pharmacoablative agents or transmission of focused ultrasonic energy to ablate renal nerves are investigational at the time this chapter is authored.

Radiofrequency Ablation-SYMPLICITY Catheter and Clinical Evidence

SYMPLICITY Catheter system (Ardian LLC/Medronic, Minneapolis, MN) is a 6-Fr RF catheter that directs energy (8 W) to the endoluminal surface to ablate renal nerves located in the adventitia. This single electrode catheter requires a manual 360-degree rotation to accomplish a circumferential ablation. The SYMPLICITY I and II studies were performed with multiple independent ablations using a unipolar RF system, and the catheter underwent iteration from a fixed arch to a physician enabled bend for the SYMPLICITY HTN-3 study (FLEX catheter). This later catheter iteration enabled physicians to both alter the pressure of the ablation lead on the artery wall, and also the angle of attack of the lead—both of which appear to be determinates of depth of RF injury.

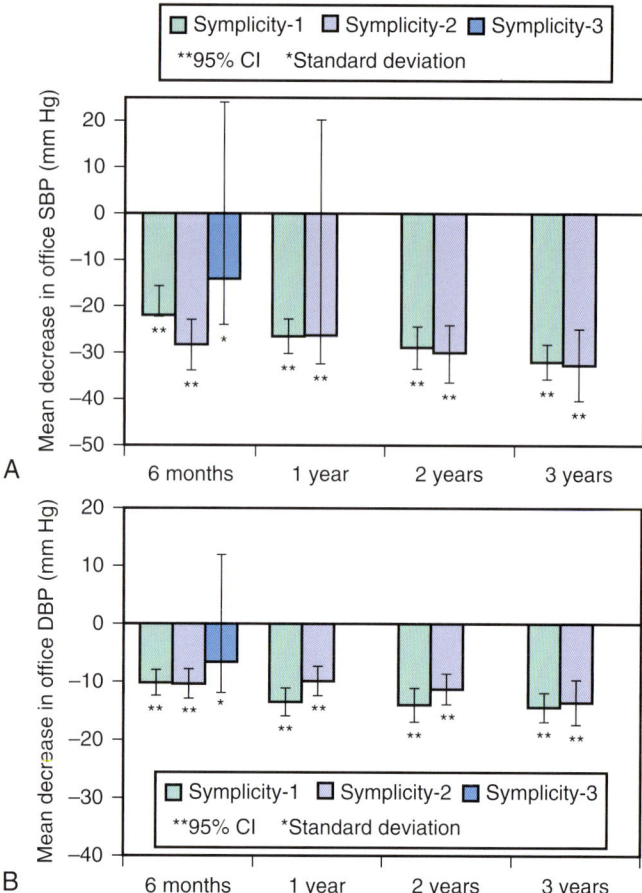

Fig. 43.4 Blood pressure lowering among treatment and control groups across all three SYMPLICITY trials through long-term follow-up. (A) Mean decrease in office systolic blood pressure *(SBP)* through 3 years of follow-up in SYMPLICITY HTN-1/2 and 6 months in SYMPLICITY HTN-3. (B) Mean decrease in office diastolic blood pressure *(DBP)* of SYMPLICITY HTN 1/2 and 6 months in SYMPLICITY HTN-3. *CI,* Confidence interval.

Efficacy

SYMPLICITY HTN-1 is a proof-of-concept, first-in-human trial testing the safety and efficacy of RF ablation for HTN therapy. Here, 45 treatment-resistant patients were followed prospectively following bilateral renal nerve RF ablation. Despite treatment with a mean of 4.7 antihypertensive drugs, mean baseline office BP of 177/101 mm Hg decreased to −27/17 mm Hg by 12 months post ablation (Fig. 43.4). Of the 45 patients, noradrenaline turnover was assessed in 10 patients and found to decrease 47% (95% confidence interval [CI] 28% to 65%), confirming a relationship between renal nerve ablation, reduction of sympathetic tone, and BP lowering.[39]

SYMPLICITY HTN-2 randomized 106 drug-resistant hypertensive patients to either medical therapy or RF ablation in conjunction with medical therapy. Mirroring SYMPLICITY HTN-1, patients took an average of 5.2 to 5.3 medications, and mean office BP readings were 178/97 to 98 mm Hg for both RF and medical therapy cohorts. Post-RF ablation, office BP measurements decreased by a mean −32/−12 mm Hg at 6 months, whereas the medical therapy group saw no changes (+1/0 mm Hg) ($P < .0001$) (see Fig. 43.4).[40]

Long-term follow-up at 3 years observed a durable reduction of −32/14 mm Hg ($n = 88$) and −33/14 mm Hg ($n = 40$) in patients from SYMPLICITY 1 and 2, respectively (see Fig. 43.4).[41,42]

SYMPLICITY HTN-3 is a U.S.-based prospective, blinded, randomized, sham-controlled premarket approval trial for Medtronic's SYMPLICITY FLEX ablation catheter.[43] Entry criteria included a stable medication regiment of three or more drugs prescribed at fully tolerated doses, including a diuretic, with an office systolic BP of 160 mm Hg or greater. The trial randomized 530 patients to achieve 95% statistical power for detecting a mean difference of 15 ± 25 mm Hg in office SBP between treatment and control cohorts. Although the trial did confirm safety in the RDN cohort, no significant difference in BP between the treatment and control arms were seen (6 months office SBP RDN −14.13 ± 23.93 mm Hg vs. control −11.74 ± 25.94 mm Hg, $P = .26$), resulting in a negative study (see Fig. 43.4).

This trial, although elegant in design, had unique trial elements that may have contributed to the negative findings of SYMPLICITY HTN-3. In the 6 weeks prior to enrollment and postrandomization, approximately 20% and 40% of patients, respectively, were subject to medication changes. Thiazide diuretics and aldosterone antagonists require up to 6 to 8 weeks to reach maximal BP-lowering effects, suggesting that the BP baselines may not have been stable for some patients enrolled.[44–46] Previously, RDN had been tested on predominantly white people of European decent, but 26% of the enrollment in SYMPLICITY HTN-3 were African-American (AA). Notably, medical therapy was more effective at lowering BP in AA patients (RDN −15.5 mm Hg vs. sham −17.8 mm Hg, $P = .641$) compared with their non-AA

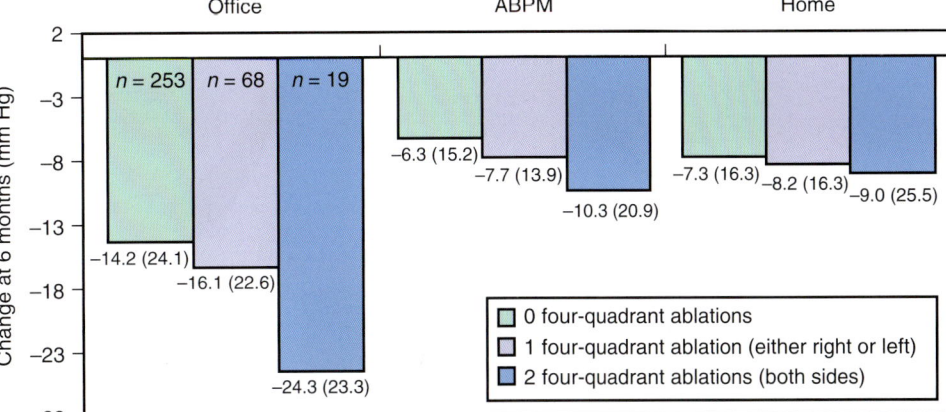

Fig. 43.5 Blood pressure changes according to completeness of ablation with respect to circumferential location in either none, one, or both renal arteries. *ABPM,* Ambulatory blood pressure monitoring. (Kandzari DE, Bhatt DL, Brar S, et al. Predictors of blood pressure response in the SYMPLCITY HTN-3 trial. *Eur Heart J.* 2015;36:219–227.)

counterparts (RDN −15.2 mm Hg vs. −8.6 mm Hg, $P = .012$), suggesting that pharmacogenomic variances related to race may play a role in HTN management.[46] Finally, procedural variability may have played a significant role in the lack of efficacy. Approximately 74% of patients received ablation in less than four quadrants of any renal artery, whereas approximately 6% patients had ablation of all four quadrants of the renal artery circumference bilaterally. Those with less than four quadrant ablation demonstrated decreases in office and ambulatory BP of −14.2 and −6.3 mm Hg, respectively, whereas those with four-quadrant bilateral RDN were found to have −24.3 and −10.3 mm Hg decreases in office and ambulatory BP, respectively (Fig. 43.5).[47,48] Insufficient training at trial onset and use of a newer iteration of the ablation catheter (FLEX catheter) may have contributed to differences in efficacy seen between SYMPLICITY HTN-2 and -3.

The neutral SYMPLCITY HTN-3 trial was followed by the randomized, controlled, Renal Denervation for Hypertension (DENERHTN) trial, sponsored by the French government.[49] This trial randomized 106 patients with resistant HTN to either RDN or a control group. The main difference to previous studies was the implementation of a standardized stepped-care antihypertensive treatment in both arms. In this trial, the RDN met its primary efficacy end point and showed superiority of RDN in combination with optimized pharmacotherapy when compared with pharmacotherapy alone (baseline-adjusted difference of −5.9 mm Hg [−11.3 to −0.5; $P = .0329$]).

The subsequent SPYRAL OFF-MED and ON-MED trials were developed to address some of the trial, operator, and device-related problems outlined previously. SPYRAL OFF-MED was a multicenter, international, single-blind, randomized, sham-controlled, proof of-concept trial.[50] Compared with the SYMPLICITY HTN-3, three major distinctions were introduced in the patient population, catheter technology used, and concomitant treatment. SPYRAL-OFF excluded patients with isolated systolic HTN because this phenotype has an attenuated response to RDN,[51] and used a modified multielectrode catheter with a revised ablation technique of distally focused treatment allowing a more circumferential and random ablation site selection and theoretically more complete renal denervation of both afferent and efferent fibers.[47] The new Simplicity Spyral (Medtronic Minneapolis, MN) is a multielectrode 4-Fr catheter delivered via a 0.014-inch guidewire in a rapid-exchange fashion (Fig. 43.6). The first-in-human trial results in 29 patients presented at Transcatheter Therapeutics (TCT) 2013 showed a −16 ± 21/7 ± 12 mm Hg reduction in office BP.[52] Patients had to be off medication; therefore resistant hypertensive individuals were not included. Adherence to the study protocol and especially the lack of antihypertensive medication intake at follow-up was confirmed by toxicologic analyses, allowing a proper intention to treat and per protocol analysis.[53]

SPYRAL OFF-MED randomized 80 patients to either RDN or sham-RDN. At 3 months' follow-up the mean difference between the groups favored RDN for change in both 24-hour and office BP from baseline: 24-hour SBP −5.0 mm Hg (95% CI −9.9 to −0.2; $P = .0414$), 24-hour diastolic blood pressure (DBP) −4.4 mm Hg (−7.2 to −1.6; $P = .0024$), office SBP −7.7 mm Hg (−14.0 to −1.5; $P = .0155$), and office DBP −4.9 mm Hg (−8.5 to −1.4; $P = .0077$) (Fig. 43.7). Given the unique and rigorous design of this study, these results provide the most robust biologic proof of principle for the effect of RDN on BP in humans. Extended follow-up and the results for the SPYRAL ON-MED trial are expected to be released soon. At the time this chapter was authored, RDN remains experimental in the United States, and the proper selection of patients, optimal device design, and demonstration of technical success remain ill-defined.

The SYMPLICITY Global Registry will plan to enroll 5000 patients and assess both safety and efficacy of RDN. Twelve-month data for 846 patients showed a mean reduction of −12.7 mm Hg office SBP.[54]

Complications and Management of Radiofrequency Ablation in Renal Denervation

The rate of serious complications documented with RDN is low, and the most frequently reported complications are: vasospasm, severe pain, renal artery dissection, renal artery stenosis, and vascular access complications. Vasospasm is mild and may be preempted with calcium channel blockers or nitrates.[55] Adventitial depth of ablation stimulates pain fibers that may trigger strong vagal reactions. Renal artery dissection resulting from catheter manipulation was reported in SYMPLICITY-1, and those attempting ablation should be trained in renal artery stenting.[56] Endovascular complications and bleeding are the most frequently reported complication, and careful, fundamentally sound vascular access remains paramount.[56-58]

Additional Radiofrequency Devices

Efforts to provide more consistent ablation, improve ease of use, and shorten procedure times have resulted in the development of alternate RF devices attempting to improve on the single lead, unipolar RF first-generation device. Later iterations apply multilead unipolar RF to deliver predictable circumferential denervation over a shorter duration, bipolar RF energy with greater precision. An updated list of ongoing clinical trials in the space of RDN can be found in the most recent European clinical consensus conference for device-based therapies for HTN.[53]

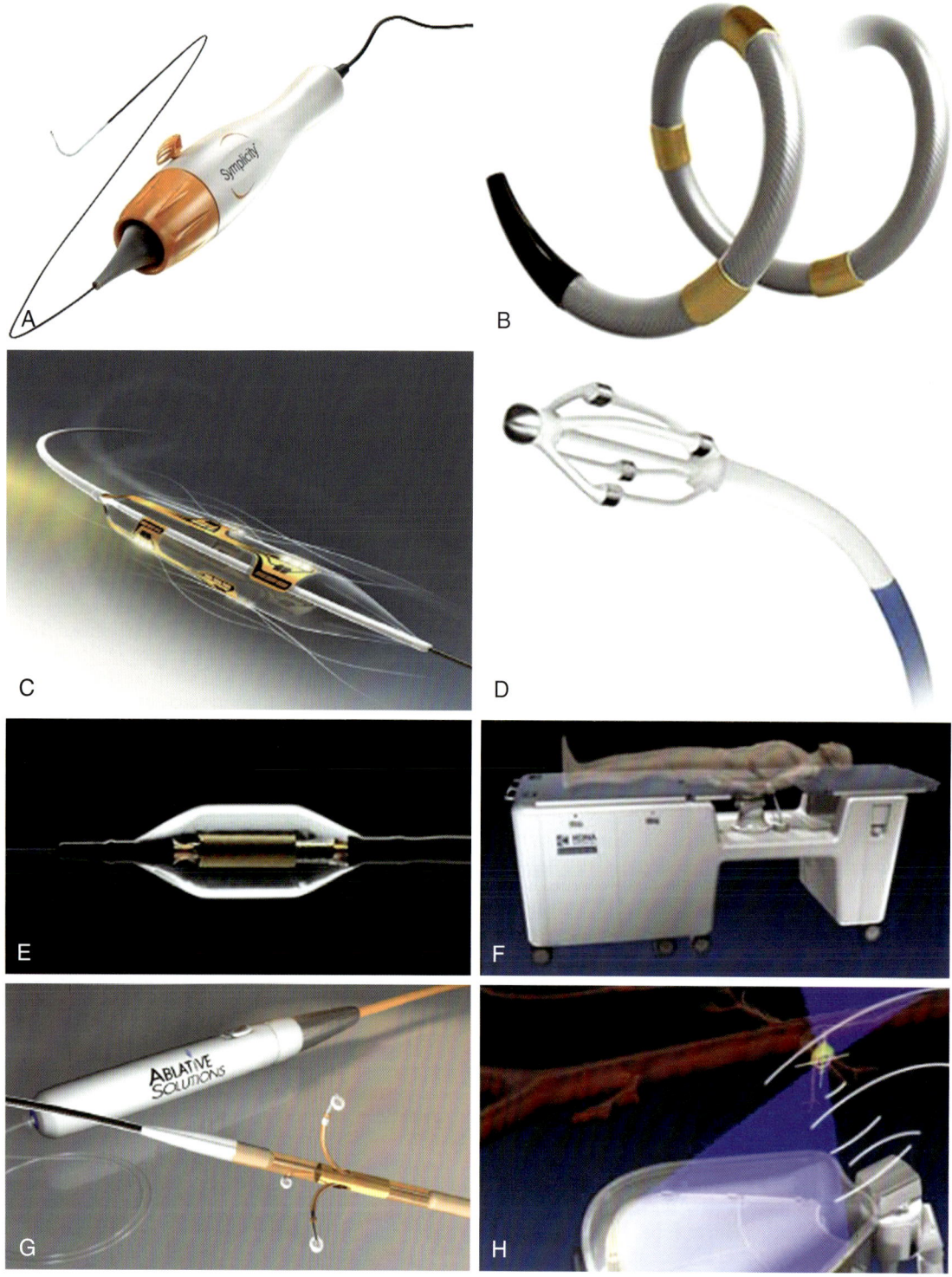

Fig. 43.6 A nonexhaustive representation of ablation catheters and technologies currently applied for renal denervation. RF energy: (A) SYMPLICITY Flex, (B) SYMPLICITY Spyral, (C) Vessix (Boston Scientific), and (D) EnligHTN (St. Jude). Ultrasound: (E) intravascular by ReCor Medical's Paradise catheter, (F and H) extravascular by Kona. (G) Perivascular chemical ablation by Ablative Solutions' Peregrine catheter. (Images courtesy the respective manufacturers.)

Multielectrode Radiofrequency Ablation

The EnligHTN Renal Denervation System (St. Jude Medical, St. Paul, MN) has a basketlike catheter design that causes contact with the endoluminal surface in a predictable pattern (see Fig. 43.6). The Ablation-induced Renal Sympathetic Denervation Trial (ARSENAL) enrolled 44 patients, recapitulating the inclusion/exclusion criteria and primary efficacy end point (office BP) from SYMPLICITY HTN-1. At 6 months, BP reduction of −26/−10 mm Hg was sustained out to 18 months (−24/−10 mm Hg).[58,59] The design of the EnligHTNed IDE trial in resistant hypertensive patients is being finalized in discussion with the U.S. Food and Drug Administration (FDA). The trial is randomized, double-blinded, and sham-controlled. Participants will

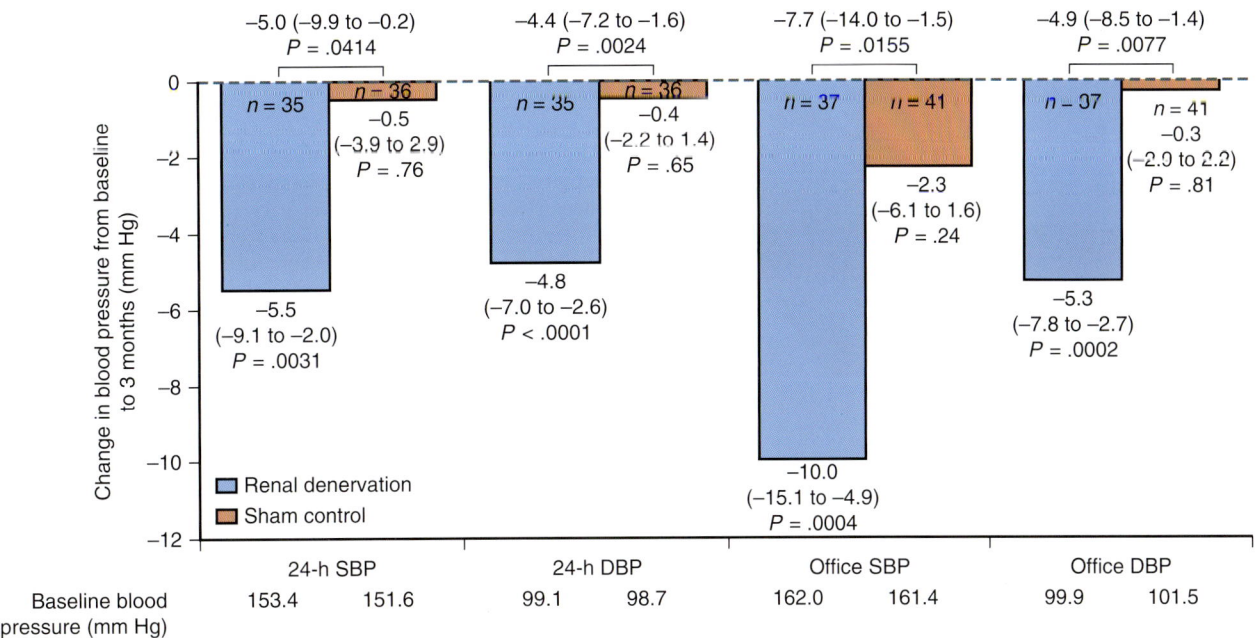

Fig. 43.7 Changes at 3 months in office and ambulatory systolic blood pressure *(SBP)* and diastolic blood pressure *(DBP)* for renal denervation and sham control groups. The 95% confidence intervals and unadjusted *P* values are shown. (From Townsend RR, Mahfoud F, Kandzari DE, et al. Catheter-based renal denervation in patients with uncontrolled hypertension in the absence of antihypertensive medications (SPYRAL HTN-OFF MED): a randomised, sham-controlled, proof-of-concept trial. *Lancet.* 2017;390:2160–2170.)

discontinue their current antihypertensive drugs and switch to standardized single-pill triple therapy to be maintained at least 12 months after randomization. The primary efficacy end point is reduction in 24-hour SBP at 6 months compared with baseline.

The Vessix V2 Catheter (Boston Scientific, Natick, MA) is another RF system consisting of an over-the-wire balloon catheter mounted with bipolar RF electrodes (see Fig. 43.6). Combined results from the REDUCE-HTN first-in-human and postmarketing studies of the Vessix renal denervation system showed a mean reduction in office BP of −25/−10 mm Hg at 6 months (*n* = 139).[60] The REDUCE HTN: REINFORCE (NCT02392351) study was initiated to test the performance of the balloon-based bipolar Vessix system over a 2-month period comparing the effects with those from a sham procedure of percutaneous renal angiography on mean reduction in daytime ambulatory SBP. The Reduce-HTN trial has been terminated due to poor enrolment and statistical futility.

Ultrasonic

Ultrasound energy consists of high-frequency sound waves which can penetrate surrounding fluids and generate frictional heating in tissues resulting in a rise in temperature that induces renal nerve injury.[61] This technology would permit ablation without contact with the endoluminal surface of the renal arteries. The resultant denervation is nonselective and theoretically results in total renal afferent and efferent nerve denervation. Long-term potential of reinnervation following ultrasonic denervation has not been reported.

The PARADISE Ultrasonic (ReCor Medical, Menlo Park, CA) is a balloon catheter that causes renal artery ablation using ultrasound directed energy. Its first-in-human study of 20 patients (Renal denervation by ultraSound Transcatheter Emission [REALISE] trial) with resistant HTN showed a reduction in BP of −32/−16 mm Hg over 3 months, but no follow-up data have been released since 2012 (see Fig. 43.6).[62] The new Study of the Recor Medical Paradise System in Clinical Hypertension (RADIANCE-HTN) trial (NCT02649426) will compare the ReCor Medical Paradise ultrasound system to a sham procedure, with the primary end point change in average daytime ambulatory SBP from baseline to 2 months postprocedure in two separate on- (TRIO) and off-medication (SOLO) cohorts of patients with uncontrolled HTN.[63] In the TRIO cohort, participants with resistant HTN will discontinue their current antihypertensive drugs and switch to standardized single-pill triple therapy. Furthermore, the Renal Denervation on Quality of 24-hr BP Control by Ultrasound In Resistant Hypertension (REQUIRE) trial (NCT02918305, *n* = 140) is designed to evaluate resistant HTN patients on standard of care medication in Japan and South Korea.

The TIVUS system (therapeutic intravascular ultrasound system) from Cardiosonic, Ltd, Tel Aviv, Israel, completed enrolling its first-in-human trial in the winter of 2013.[64] The follow-up TIVUS II study is recruiting 25 patients (NCT01835535) targeting three groups of patients: 1) severe resistant HTN, 2) moderate resistant HTN, and 3) failed prior RF therapy.

Externally delivered ultrasound energy ablating renal nerves Kona Medical Inc. (Bellevue, Washington) reported a −29/−12 mm Hg 6 month (*n* = 24) and −19.4/6.5 mm Hg (*n* = 17) for the Sham Controlled Study of Renal Denervation for Subjects With Uncontrolled Hypertension (WAVE) I and WAVE II studies, respectively.[65] WAVE-IV (NCT02029885) was a sham-controlled, double-blind study with the noninvasive ultrasound-based Kona Medical Surround Sound System for bilateral RDN. This trial used change in office SBP from screening to 6 months postrandomization as the primary efficacy end point. The trial was stopped for futility on 19 July 2016 because it had by this time point not demonstrated any differences between the groups in either office BP or 24-hour ambulatory blood pressure (ABP). There had been no safety concerns.

Tissue-Directed Pharmacological Ablation

The failure of the RF approach in the SYMPLICITY HTN-3 trial raised the possibility that "point-by-point" ablation with a limited number of focal burns may result in ineffective global RDN. Even under ideal conditions, with perfect "circumferential" energy delivery, RF (thermal) injury is likely to miss >50% of the renal sympathetic nerves due to a lack of depth energy penetration.[66] Moreover, individual applications of RF energy may fail to successfully cause complete circumferential denervation or

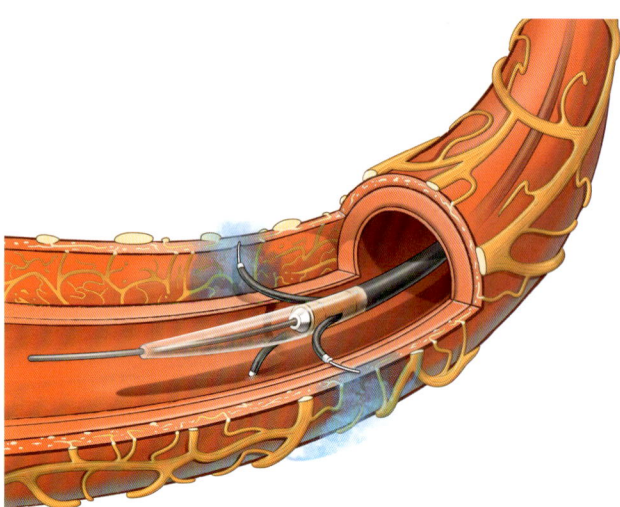

Fig. 43.8 A three-needle delivery device (Peregrine) for injection of dehydrated ethanol into the adventitial and periadventitial space.
(© Justin A. Klein, CMI, 2013. All Rights Reserved.)

fail to successfully target key nerve trunks. It may be possible to achieve more complete denervation using a specialized drug delivery catheter to perform "chemical" RDN, with ethanol (EtOH), a well-characterized and predictable neurolytic agent. A novel microneedle-based drug delivery catheter (Peregrine, Ablative Solutions, Inc. Menlo Park, CA) has obtained FDA clearance to cause predictable periarterial adventitial deep and circumferential renal sympathetic denervation, with minimal injury to the normal structures (intima and media) of the renal arterial wall (Fig. 43.8). In preclinical and clinical testing, microdoses of EtOH were delivered locally to the adventitial and periadventitial space of the renal artery (PeriVascular Renal Denervation; PVRD), with evidence of rapid and nearly complete sympathetic denervation, as assessed by renal parenchymal NE, and histopathologic evaluation.[67,68] Furthermore, studies support a potential benefit compared with RF-based RDN techniques, indicating a more complete ablation of nerves and reduction of nerve function.[69] This device, although cleared by the FDA to cause periarterial denervation on the basis of renal nerve studies, is not specifically approved for RDN, and clinical trials for this specific indication are anticipated across multiple clinical applications, including HTN, heart failure, and sympathetically mediated tachyarrhythmias. Guanethidine is another agent considered for injection because it is already approved by the FDA for treatment of moderate to severe HTN.[64]

β-Radiation of the Renal Artery

Prior research using radiation therapy in atrial fibrillation noted histological evidence of nerve fibrosis.[70] Vascular brachytherapy is a well-developed treatment for coronary restenosis and investigators postulated that it may have potential for inducing nerve damage in the renal vasculature in lieu of using RF ablation. Preclinical experiments in swine showed 50% nerve damage with doses of 50 Gy. No damage was seen to adjacent tissues.[71]

QUANTIFYING PROCEDURAL TECHNICAL SUCCESS, TITRATING ABLATIVE THERAPY, AND TARGETING IDEAL PATIENTS FOR RDN

The failure of the SYMPLICITY HTN-3 to demonstrate a significant benefit associated with RDN and the only mild improvement in BP seen in DENERHTN[49] and SPYRAL OFF-MED trial[50] may represent technical failure of the device or physician to cause significant RDN, unselective of sympatholytic and sympatho-stimulant fibers, or selection of a population whose renal nerve contribution to HTN is negligible. Both suggest the importance of tools to assist in patient selection and verification of successful denervation. In the past, measurement of renal noradrenaline spillover or assessment of muscle sympathetic nerve activity (MSNA) quantified sympathetic activity and confirmed successful denervation during early experience of RDN.[39,72,73] However, not only is renal noradrenaline spillover technically challenging, but it gives no insight into renal afferent nerve activity. Likewise, few centers have the technical expertise to perform MSNA measurements, and it likely is not acceptable to patients for repeated testing. Importantly, a reduction in sympathetic tone is not automatically reflected by a reduction of BP.[74] This can probably be explained by the complexity of pathophysiology and the variable role that SNA can play in it. Ineffective reduction in BP following RDN ranges from 10% to 50%.[39,75] Comparably, changes in left ventricular hypertrophy following RDN were observed to be independent from BP improvement.[76] This indicates that BP may not necessarily be the best surrogate marker of technical success in RDN.

The recurrent observation of lack of BP reduction or BP elevations after RDN have raised concern for the detrimental effects of unselective global RDN potentially targeting renal afferent fibers that exert a sympatholytic function on the autonomic nervous system.[50,77] Conceptually, the ideal site for RDN should raise arterial BP when stimulated. Sites in the renal artery that are without biologic effect or reduce BP when stimulated are potentially perilous to denervate and should be avoided. The development of an appropriate tool to document the renal nerve contribution to elevated BP and technical success of RDN may be in the near future. Preliminary work using simple or more advanced electroanatomic mapping systems has been applied to renal arteries to demonstrate the presence or absence of sympatho-stimulation or sympatholytic fibers.[16–21] The introduction of dedicated diagnostic and ablation systems (Jie Wang: Mapping sympathetic nerve distribution for renal ablation and catheters for same. U.S. Patent 8702619, published on December 15, 2011 and issued on April 22, 2014) could enable proper patient selection through screening for candidates whose BP is renal nerve activity dependent and allow targeting of optimal ablation sites with documentation of technical success through the loss of systemic BP and heart rate changes following RDN. The Sympathetic Mapping/Ablation of Renal Nerves Trial (SMART) using the SyMapCath I catheter and SYMPIONEER S1 Stimulator/Generator is currently ongoing (NCT02761811).

The pathophysiology of multiple chronic diseases such as diabetes, arrhythmias, obstructive sleep apnea, heart failure, and chronic renal insufficiency are strongly attributed to SNS and modulation of sympathetic tone may have additional salutary effects beyond lowering BP.[78–81] Thus a clinically meaningful and reproducible metric of systemic sympathetic state ultimately may be required to select ideal candidates for RDN and document technical success of the intervention as alternative therapeutic targets such as diastolic heart failure or glucose intolerance may become future indications.

ALTERNATIVE APPROACHES TO SYMPATHETIC MODULATION

Carotid Body and Sinus

Given the role of excessive sympathetic tone in the pathogenesis of HTN and several chronic disease states, there is a long history of investigating sources of sympathetic tone, including the carotid body (CB) and sinus. Located in at the bifurcation of common carotid artery, the CB is a 1.5- to 7.0-mm ovoid bilateral organ innervated by the nerve fibers of the glossopharyngeal, vagal, and sympathetic nerve of the adjacent superior cervical ganglion. The CB is the body's primary peripheral chemoreceptor, sensing changes in oxygen saturation, carbon dioxide tension, acidosis, glycemia, and hypoperfusion.[82] CB stimulation signals to the solitary nucleus in the rostral ventrolateral medulla oblongata to elevate sympathetic tone, increasing BP and minute ventilation.[83] The carotid sinus is an outpouching of the internal carotid artery, housing mechanoreceptors that detect BP changes and maintains arterial tone by modulating parasympathetic and sympathetic signaling. Chemoreflex and baroreflex controls are intertwined; heightened chemoreflex can cause sympathoactivation and inhibition of the baroreflex function.[84]

Preclinical research shows that the CB chemoreceptor plays a significant role in HTN.[85,86] Surgical CB denervation in both young and adult spontaneous hypertensive rats (SHRs) both prevented the onset of HTN and reduced systolic arterial pressures by approximately 20 mm Hg through the decrease of sympathetic vasomotor tone.[86] Hypertensive and normal human male MSNA were measured at baseline and following the inactivation of the chemoreceptor by administrating 100% oxygen.[87] Following chemoreceptor inactivation, hypertensive patients demonstrated a significant decrease in MSNA, whereas normal healthy patients showed no changes in sympathetic activity, confirming that chemoreceptor sympathetic input contributes to HTN. Prior experience in surgical CB excision showed an approximately 20 mm Hg decrease in SBP in 29 hypertensive asthmatic patients.[88] In the first study of CB resection in resistant HTN patients ($n = 15$), the unilateral resection did not result in significant change in either office or ambulatory BP up to 12 months. However, patients with drop in MSNA did experience a significant BP reduction as well.[89] Preliminary data from a trial of unilateral endovascular ablation of the CB for patients with resistant HTN ($n = 10$) indicated a reduction in the 24-hour BP by an average of $9 \pm 9/4 \pm 6$ mm Hg at 1 month postprocedure.[90] The effect on BP continued to be observed at 6 months, with BP reduction of $10 \pm 15/4 \pm 7$ mm Hg compared with baseline BP. Follow-up for all the patients up to 12 months is underway (Cibiem, Los Altos, CA) (NCT 02099851). The current iteration of the device enables a transvenous approach, ultrasonic imaging of the CB, and selective CB denervation without intraarterial and carotid manipulations. Clinical trials at the time of this publication are underway.

Modulation of BP through manipulation of the carotid sinus is an old concept recently revived. Arterial baroreceptors rapidly reset in response to BP fluctuations and increase the firing of baroreceptor afferents with elevated BP. However, with chronically elevated BP, adjustment of baroreceptor response diminishes and the threshold for activation changes. Therefore baroreceptors become less sensitive to change in the context of chronic HTN.[82] Experiments exploring the role of the carotid sinus elucidated the role of electrical impulse stimulation to chronically regulate BP.[91] Researchers attempted to leverage this knowledge into a device therapy for HTN, but limitations in the technology of the 1960s failed to create an appropriate stimulator for patients. Technological limitations in conjunction with emergence of pharmacotherapy caused baroreceptor stimulation to disappear from the therapeutic armamentarium. Recognition of populations resistant to pharmacotherapy stimulated renewed interest in baroreceptor pacing, culminating in the clinical development of mature pacing systems for HTN management. The Rheos baroreceptor pacing system (CvRX, Minneapolis, MN) was tested in the randomized, double-blind, parallel-design Rheos Pivotal trial in patients with resistant HTN.[92] All patients underwent implantations, but baroreceptor activation therapy (BAT) implementation was randomized for the first 6 months. There was no difference in first degree of acute response (BAT 54% vs. no-BAT 46% responders, $P = .97$) and the second-degree end point of mean BP decrease just missed statistical significance (BAT 16 ± 29 vs no-BAT 9 ± 29 mm Hg, $P = .08$).[92] Evaluation of the second-generation device Barostim *neo* (Fig. 43.9) was done in a prospective, open-label fashion in 30 patients in Canada and Europe. Six months postimplantation, BAT reduced mean BP 26 ± 4.4 mm Hg, $P \leq .001$).[93] With respect to safety, the Rheos trial showed 74.8% event-free procedural safety which improved to 90% in the Barostim *neo* trial. A publication by Heusser et al.[94] demonstrated that 12 of 18 patients experienced stimulation-related side effects after implantation of the neo System, so that stimulation intensity had to be reduced. However, chronically tolerable levels resulted in less-pronounced BP reductions compared with bilateral stimulation.[94] A pivotal trial seeking FDA approval for the device is still underway (NCT01679132). Furthermore, the ESTIM-rHTN trial (Economic Evaluation of Baroreceptor Stimulation for the Treatment of Resistant Hypertension), funded by the French Ministry of Health and CvRX, which aims to study BAT in patients with resistant HTN and renal impairment (estimated glomerular filtration rate, 30 mL/min/1.73 m² or higher; NCT02364310), is currently recruiting.

In addition to electrical baroreceptor stimulation, mechanical modulation of the same receptors as an antihypertensive is being explored. Likely an extrapolation from hypotensive responses observed postcarotid stenting, Controlling and Lowering Blood Pressure With The MOBIUSHD™ (CALM-FIM_EUR), was the first major prospective study ($n = 30$) to investigate the BP-lowering effects of an implantable device in the carotid sinus that influences autonomic output via carotid sinus mechanoreceptors, the MobiusHD device (Vascular Dynamics, Mountain View, CA) (Fig. 43.10). The mean baseline 24-hour ambulatory BP of 166/100 mm Hg (17/14) was reduced by 21/12 mm Hg (14 to 29/7 to 16) at 6 months ($P < .0001$ for SBP and DBP). Five serious adverse events had occurred in four patients (13%) at 6 months: hypotension ($n = 2$), worsening HTN ($n = 1$), intermittent claudication ($n = 1$), and wound infection ($n = 1$).

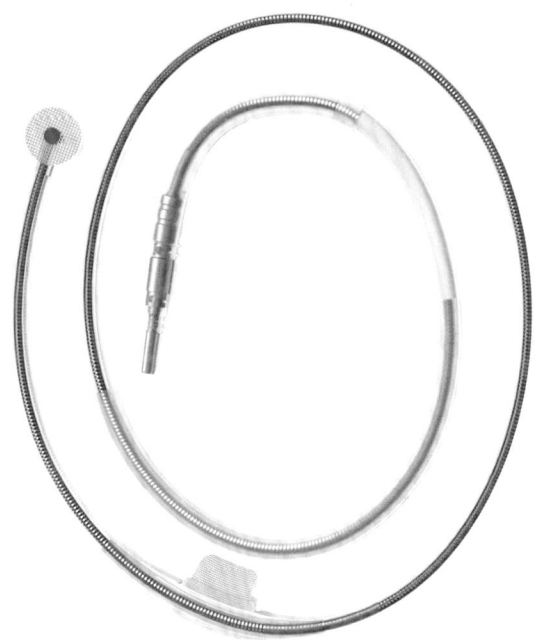

Fig. 43.9 Second-generation Barostim *neo* lead. (Image provided by CvRX.)

Mechanical Solutions

Studies have demonstrated that the isolated systolic HTN phenotype predicts a less pronounced response than combined HTN to therapy targeting neurologic and humoral interventions such as RDN,[51] suggesting that, in patients with widened pulse pressures (isolated systolic HTN), underlying structural changes such as aortic stiffness and pressure wave reflection are important factors.[95,96]

ARTERIOVENOUS ANASTOMOSIS FOR THE REDUCTION OF VASCULAR RESISTANCE AND INCREASE OF COMPLIANCE FOR HYPERTENSION MANAGEMENT

While investigating the implantation of a percutaneous arterial venous fistula (AVF) (ROX Medical Inc., San Clement, CA) intended for treating dyspnea in chronic obstructive pulmonary disease (COPD) patients, investigators noticed an instantaneous significant lowering of BP in hypertensive patients.[97] This observation spurred interest in using small central AVF to treat chronic HTN. Similar to observations in new fistula implantation in chronic renal failure patients, the mechanism is thought to be due to adding a fixed volume, central arterial-venous anastomosis reducing BP by adding a low resistance and high compliance venous attachment to the central arterial tree.[98] With addition of a low-capacitance circuit, total systemic vascular resistance and the effective arterial volume decrease.[97] Another possible salutary effect may be improvement of compliance of the arterial tree and reduction of the pulse wave. Multiple analyses consistently demonstrate the association of reduced arterial compliance and increase pulse wave velocity with adverse CV outcomes.[99] The absence of increases in heart rate following BP reduction imply an additional mechanism of action being suppression of the baroreflex by activation of the cardiopulmonary mechanoreceptors. This mechanism explains the absence of acute and chronic compensations and implies that the mechanism of action combines mechanical reduction of central arterial strain with suppression of the baroreflex.[100]

The ROX AV-Fistula device (ROX Medical Inc., San Clemente, CA), is a nitinol clip that creates a 4-mm fixed diameter, common iliac arterial-venous fistula. To implant the ROX Coupler, the venous and arterial wall is punctured from the venous side, and a balloon-expandable nitinol clip is deployed (Fig. 43.11). Real-time invasive hemodynamic assessment allows immediate verification of technical success, and little pain is experienced during the creation of the anastomosis. An immediate and significant reduction of BP accompanies the opening of the anastomosis. Long-term patency of the device can easily be confirmed with bedside noninvasive techniques, and its effects may be reversed with application of a covered arterial stent. Complications seen in its use in COPD patients, using a larger-diameter anastomosis, include episodes of right heart failure, edema formation, venous stenosis, and the usual femoral access complications.[101,102] In the open-label, multicenter ROX CONTROL HTN study, 83 patients (mean age: 58 to 59 years, mean office and ambulatory SBP 175 and 157 mm Hg in the ROX coupler group and 171 and 156 mm Hg in the control group, respectively) were randomized to treatment with the ROX coupler ($n = 44$) or normal care ($n = 39$).[103] Although at 6-month follow-up there was no significant systolic office or systolic ambulatory BP reduction in the group receiving standard care (by 3.7 mm Hg, $P = .31$ and .5 mm Hg, $P = .86$, respectively), there was a pronounced reduction in the group treated with the ROX coupler (by 27 mm Hg, $P < .0001$ and 14 mm Hg, $P < .0001$, respectively). Results at 1 year have

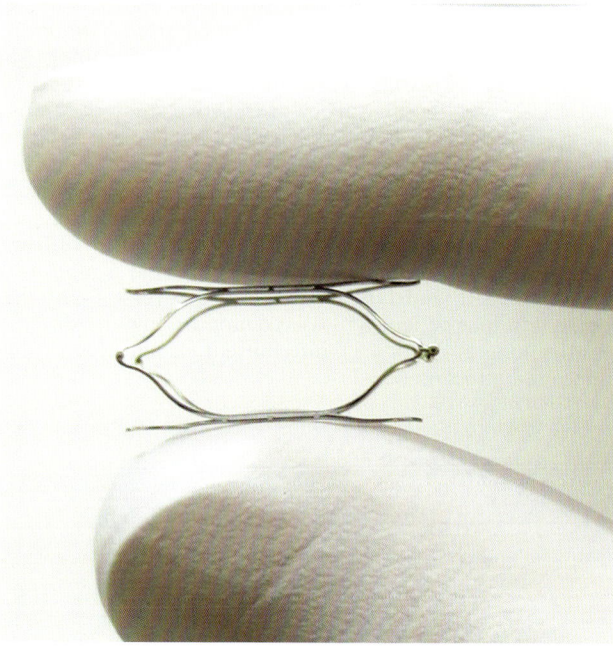

Fig. 43.10 Mobius-HD carotid stent. (Image provided by Vascular Dynamics.)

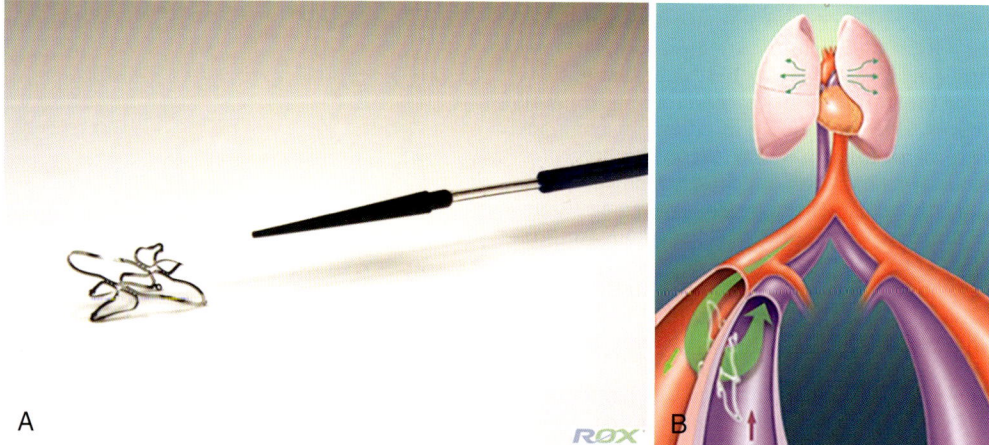

Fig. 43.11 The ROX Coupler (A) is a 4-mm nitinol clip that is designed to cause a fistula between the iliac vein and artery (B). (Courtesy ROX Medical, San Clemente, CA.)

demonstrated stable reduction of both office and ambulatory BP, with no loss of clinical effect and the identification of no additional adverse events.[104] The 1-year ABP reduction was 12.4 ± 14.4 mm Hg (n = 9).

In a post hoc analysis, the observed reduction in BP occurred both in patients with isolated systolic HTN and combined HTN, and the magnitude was similar.[105] This differs from the effect of renal denervation that is less pronounced in patients with isolated HTN.[51,106] The encouraging results have led to the setting up of an ongoing 1:1 randomized, sham (arterial puncture)-controlled multicenter U.S. trial with an estimated range of enrolment of 250 to 500 (adaptive end point) patients with uncontrolled HTN and anticipated completion in 2019 (NCT02895386). The trial will enroll patients with isolated systolic and combined HTN. Primary end point will be the change in mean ambulatory SBP at 6 months compared with baseline. Furthermore, a global registry is recruiting patients for continued safety and efficacy assessment (NCT01885390).

PACEMAKER-MEDIATED PROGRAMMABLE HYPERTENSION CONTROL THERAPY

Programmable Hypertension Control (PHC) therapy tests a new concept of HTN control put forward by Backbeat Medical. PHC therapy is an algorithm embedded in a standard dual-chamber pacemaker with regular transvenous leads and implant procedure. The algorithm delivers a sequence of alternating shorter and longer atrioventricular (AV) intervals pacing. The algorithm reduces BP by reducing ventricular filling and modulating the baroreflex responses, preventing activation of the autonomic nervous system. The main mechanism of BP reduction is by short AV delay pacing, which reduces left ventricular (LV) filling and thus reduces LV pressure (Starling mechanism). Reduction in ventricular filling immediately reduces BP.[107] In the first-in-human study, following a run-in period, PHC therapy reduced office BP by 16 ± 15 mm Hg and 24–hour ambulatory SBP decreased by an additional 10 ± 13 mm Hg (both P < .01) at 3 months.[108] A long-term safety and efficacy study has been initiated (NCT02837445).

REGULATORY TRIAL EXECUTION

With the advent of device-based interventional therapies for HTN in the mid-2000s, a large number of clinical trials were initiated and completed in a short time frame. Although HTN was never an easy disease to study, due to inherent differences in the disease population and various pitfalls in the selection and assessment of end points, the introduction of device-based therapies has uncovered several new obstacles to be considered.

1. Role of drug monitoring to demonstrate adherence and persistence with baseline drug therapy: In device-based therapies, it is imperative to reduce variation in adherence or persistence to oral antihypertensive treatment through the trial and limit lifestyle modification measures that might be a consequence of trial enrollment. Modern technologies such as mass spectrometry have made it easier to measure drug adherence using either blood or urine samples,[109] and these methods have been used to assess adherence as a factor in resistant HTN before and after RDN.[110,111] However, measuring drug metabolites by itself is a trial intervention and creates mischief when generalizing the results of the trials to clinical practice.
2. Run-in phase prior to device therapy: A run-in phase with repeated BP assessments (office and ABP measurements) has become integral to clinical device trials in HTN to reduce bias introduced by regression to the mean.[112] When studying treatments for the resistant populations, therapeutic regimens should be consistent between the groups. For trials in drug-treated populations, a standardized, stepped titration scheme used in trials with antihypertensive drugs, such as the he LIFE study[113] or the DENERHTN trial,[49] is highly preferable to reduce heterogeneity and ensure that all patients receive appropriate CV protection. Unfortunately, to date no established and validated tool exists to adjust BP changes after an intervention, if dose or drug regimen has been changed.
3. Timing of primary end points: Traditional importance in drug trials of 12 and 24 weeks for device trials requires reexamination. Although cumulative evidence indicates that early onset of antihypertensive effect improves CV outcomes, the time to BP control remains long. The objective of HTN management cannot be simply to achieve and maintain the goal BP, but to do so quickly to improve short-term and long-term CV outcomes. Although no randomized controlled data are available regarding the urgency to treat HTN, a number of clinical trials and retrospective reviews support the hypothesis that rapid BP reduction is safe and the time needed to attain target BP influences the outcome of both standard and high-risk populations.[114–116] Prompt BP control reduced the risk of CV events, and delays of 1 month to 2 years in starting antihypertensive therapy increased the risk of certain CV end points, particularly stroke. Certain high-risk populations require even more rapid and aggressive BP-lowering therapies. Upcoming therapies such as the ROX, Cibiem, and Mobius trials hold the promise of significant and rapid BP reduction, which may render sham efforts ineffective because treatments may result in such immediate and obvious changes in pressures that patients become aware of their randomization and equipoise of treating physicians is embarrassed.
4. Sham, where it is needed and where not: The RDN experience has reinvigorated the debate about the need for sham trials. The recently reported SPYRAL trial shows no change in the control population's BP as a result of sham, the first definitive demonstration of the lack of sham effect in a prospective randomized trial of HTN with an end point duration of >3 months, and raising theoretical concerns about the justification for sham in objective measures trials. A majority of upcoming device HTN trials, nonetheless, now have a sham-control arm, and it has become a common belief that a sham-control group is a prerequisite for a successful proof-of-concept trial of device-based therapies in HTN. However, the use of a sham procedure is associated with certain degree of complexity, including the ethics of performing a procedure conferring an immediate risk of adverse event in those trials recruiting especially untreated patients with grade I to II HTN who are at low immediate CV and cerebrovascular risk. These could be instances where sham adds complexity and risk and expense without added benefit to our understanding of the studied therapy. A blinding index can be used to assess the efficacy of blinding in clinical device trials.[117] The index can be used for any blinded group, not only study subjects and researchers. An assessment of appropriate blinding is particularly important in randomized controlled device trials where proper blinding can be highly challenging. Furthermore, the ability to create and sustain sham groups is in doubt when the treatment effect is large and immediate.

MATCHING PATIENTS WITH DEVICES—PATIENT SELECTION

Patients in whom HTN is not related to renal sympathetic hyperactivity, and therefore denervation for the purpose of reducing BP is futile and ought to be spared needless procedures. For example, those whose HTN is related to loss of aortic elasticity may be unresponsive to RDN and may be more ideal for HTN strategies targeting mechanical underlying causes. Similarly, there may exist populations of hypertensive patients for whom medications will compound risk of adverse events without effecting substantial

BP changes. Transitioning from the era of drug escalations and limiting devices to drug failures will occur with the development of diagnostic devices that identify when neurohormonal intervention will be futile or identification of patients who are uniquely ideal for mechanical interventions. Currently, patient age, pulse pressure (isolated systolic HTN), and pulse wave velocity are crude predictors of futility of neurologic and humoral interventions.

KEY REFERENCES

18. Chinushi M, Izumi D, Iijima K, et al. Blood pressure and autonomic responses to electrical stimulation of the renal arterial nerves before and after ablation of the renal artery. *Hypertension*. 2013;61:450–456.
26. Sobotka PA, Mahfoud F, Schlaich MP, et al. Sympatho-renal axis in chronic disease. *Clin Res Cardiol*. 2011;100:1049–1057.
39. Krum H, Schlaich M, Whitbourn R, et al. Catheter-based renal sympathetic denervation for resistant hypertension: a multicentre safety and proof-of-principle cohort study. *Lancet*. 2009;373:1275–1281.
40. Symplicity HTN-2 Investigators, Esler MD, Krum H, et al. Renal sympathetic denervation in patients with treatment-resistant hypertension (the Symplicity HTN-2 trial): a randomised controlled trial. *Lancet*. 2010;376:1903–1909.
41. Krum H, Schlaich MP, Böhm M, et al. Percutaneous renal denervation in patients with treatment-resistant hypertension: final 3-year report of the Symplicity HTN-1 study. *Lancet*. 2013;383(9917):622–629.
48. Kandzari DE, Bhatt DL, Brar S, et al. Predictors of blood pressure response in the SYMPLICITY HTN-3 trial. *Eur Heart J*. 2015;36:219–227.
49. Azizi M, Sapoval M, Gosse P, et al. Optimum and stepped care standardised antihypertensive treatment with or without renal denervation for resistant hypertension (DENERHTN): a multicentre, open-label, randomised controlled trial. *Lancet*. 2015;385:1957–1965.
50. Townsend RR, Mahfoud F, Kandzari DE, et al. Catheter-based renal denervation in patients with uncontrolled hypertension in the absence of antihypertensive medications (SPYRAL HTN-OFF MED): a randomised, sham-controlled, proof-of-concept trial. *Lancet*. 2017;390:2160–2170.
51. Mahfoud F, Bakris G, Bhatt DL, et al. Reduced blood pressure-lowering effect of catheter-based renal denervation in patients with isolated systolic hypertension: data from SYMPLICITY HTN-3 and the Global SYMPLICITY Registry. *Eur Heart J*. 2017;38:93–100.
53. Mahfoud F, Schmieder RE, Azizi M, et al. Proceedings from the 2nd European Clinical Consensus Conference for device-based therapies for hypertension: state of the art and considerations for the future. *Eur Heart J*. 2017;38:3272–3281.
63. Mauri L, Kario K, Basile J, et al. A multinational clinical approach to assessing the effectiveness of catheter-based ultrasound renal denervation: the RADIANCE-HTN and REQUIRE clinical study designs. *Am Heart J*. 2018;195:115–129.
104. Lobo MD, Sobotka PA, Stanton A, et al. Central arteriovenous anastomosis for the treatment of patients with uncontrolled hypertension (the ROX CONTROL HTN study): a randomised controlled trial. *Lancet*. 2015;385:1634–1641.
113. Pocock SJ, Bakris G, Bhatt DL, et al. Regression to the Mean in SYMPLICITY HTN-3: Implications for Design and Reporting of Future Trials. *J Am Coll Cardiol*. 2016;68:2016–2025.

 Additional references available online at expertconsult.com.

中文导读

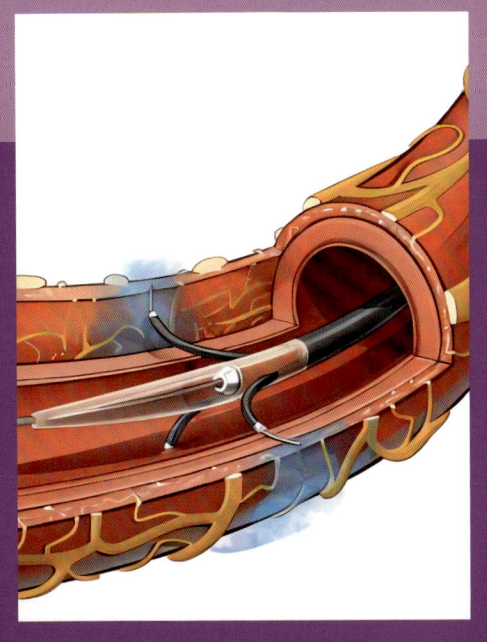

第44章
主动脉（胸腹）介入治疗

　　主动脉（胸腹）疾病包括主动脉夹层、胸主动脉瘤和腹主动脉瘤三部分，本章节将依次讲述疾病的发病率、临床分型、治疗指征和治疗策略，以及最常见并发症——内漏的处理。

　　急性主动脉夹层是一种罕见但危及生命的疾病，分为Stanford分型和DeBakey分型，前兆包括壁内血肿、穿透性主动脉溃疡和局部内膜撕裂，最主要的并发症在于主动脉重要侧支灌注不良。治疗策略主要是封闭近端破口以引导血流进入真腔，降低假腔压力，并诱导假腔内血栓形成，继而血管壁纤维化，从而实现主动脉壁重塑。主动脉覆膜支架主要用于重建受压真腔，从头颈动脉到主动脉主要分支，并增加主动脉远端血流。大多覆膜支架采用不锈钢、镍钛合金或非磁性合金制成金属骨架。对B型主动脉夹层而言，经皮主动脉覆膜支架植入术比传统外科手术更安全且效果更好。

　　胸腹主动脉瘤主要见于老年人，发病率逐年增加，其病理机制在于瘤样主动脉壁变弱，最终导致破裂出血而危及生命。开放性修复通常用于低风险患者，而腔内覆膜支架植入修复是一种可代替传统外科且微创的治疗方法。胸主动脉瘤修复评估考虑患者的总体风险状况、动脉瘤迅速扩大的证据、直径≥5.5 cm和症状，并且腔内修复适用性主要基于患者的临床和解剖特征。主动脉弓杂交手术也是一种选择。对于腹主动脉瘤而言，术前评估患者整体风险和瘤体解剖特征至关重要，腔内修复手术成功率和长期结果取决于近端和远端覆膜支架的固定和密封。胸腹主动脉瘤覆膜支架植入术后并发症包括植入物感染、脑卒中和截瘫等，最常见的并发症是内漏，内漏治疗包括经导管弹簧圈或胶水栓塞、球囊血管成形术、腔内覆膜支架植入术和开放性外科修复术。

陈　阳　张洪亮

章节要点

- 急性主动脉夹层是一种罕见、具有潜在灾难的疾病，发病率约为3.5例/100万人/年，美国每年至少发生8000例。
- 主动脉覆膜支架主要用于重建受压真腔，从头颈动脉到主动脉主要分支，并增加主动脉远端血流。封闭近端破口以引导血流进入真腔，降低假腔压力，并诱导假腔内血栓形成，继而血管壁纤维化，从而实现主动脉壁重塑。
- 经皮主动脉覆膜支架植入术治疗B型主动脉夹层比传统外科手术更安全且效果更好。
- 对于胸主动脉瘤修复，腔内覆膜支架植入术是一种可代替传统外科手术、有希望且微创的治疗方法。大多数器械采用不锈钢、镍钛合金或非磁性合金制成金属骨架。
- 胸主动脉瘤修复评估考虑患者的总体风险状况、动脉瘤迅速扩大的证据、直径≥5.5 cm和症状，腔内修复适用性主要基于患者的临床和解剖特征。
- 内漏是胸主动脉瘤覆膜支架植入术后最常见的并发症。治疗内漏的方案包括经导管弹簧圈或胶水栓塞、球囊血管成形术、腔内覆膜支架植入术和开放性外科修复术。
- 腹主动脉瘤腔内修复手术成功率和长期结果取决于近端和远端覆膜支架的固定和密封。

44 Aortic Vascular Interventions (Thoracic and Abdominal)

Christoph A. Nienaber, Ibrahim Akin

KEY POINTS

- Acute aortic dissection is an uncommon but potentially catastrophic illness that occurs with an incidence of approximately 3.5 per 1 million person-years, with at least 8000 cases occurring annually in the United States.
- Aortic stent grafts are primarily used to reconstruct the compressed true lumen cranial to major aortic branches and to increase distal aortic flow. Proximal communications are sealed to direct flow into the true lumen, depressurize the false lumen, and induce thrombosis in the false lumen, with fibrotic transformation and subsequent remodeling of the aortic wall.
- Percutaneous stent graft placement in the dissected aorta is safer and produces better results than surgery for type B dissections.
- Use of endovascular stent grafts for repair of thoracic aortic aneurysms is a promising and less invasive therapeutic alternative to conventional surgical treatment.
- Most devices use a metal skeleton made of stainless steel, nitinol, or Elgiloy.
- Evaluation for repair of a thoracic aortic aneurysm considers the patient's overall risk profile, evidence of rapid enlargement of the aneurysm, diameter equal to or greater than 5.5 cm, and symptoms. Suitability for endovascular repair is based on clinical and anatomic considerations.
- Endoleaks are the most prevalent complications after stent graft treatment of thoracic aortic aneurysms. Treatment options include transcatheter coil or glue embolization, balloon angioplasty, placement of endovascular graft extensions, and open repair.
- Procedural success and long-term outcome of endovascular repair of abdominal aortic aneurysms depend on proximal and distal fixation and sealing.

AORTIC DISSECTION

Acute aortic dissection is an uncommon but potentially catastrophic illness. It occurs with an incidence of approximately 3.5 per 100,000 person-years, and at least 8000 cases occur each year in the United States.[1,2] About 0.5% of patients with chest or back pain have an aortic dissection.[3] Two-thirds of patients are male, with an average age at presentation of approximately 65 years. A history of systemic hypertension, found in up to 72% of patients, is by far the most common risk factor.[1,2]

Acute aortic dissection is diagnosed within 2 weeks of onset of symptoms, which is the high-mortality period. Patients surviving 2 weeks are considered to have subacute disease, and chronic aortic dissection is diagnosed after 8 weeks. Aortic dissections are further classified according to their anatomic location using the Stanford and DeBakey classifications. The fundamental distinction is whether the dissection is proximal (i.e., involving the aortic root or ascending aorta) or distal (i.e., beyond the left subclavian artery) (Fig. 44.1).

Important precursors of typical aortic dissection include intramural hematoma (IMH), penetrating aortic ulcers (PAU), and localized intimal tears that are variants of a wall-dissecting process. Chronic hypertension affects arterial wall composition, causing intimal thickening, fibrosis, and calcification and extracellular fatty acid deposition. The extracellular matrix also undergoes accelerated degradation, apoptosis, and elastolysis with hyalinization of collagen. Both mechanisms may eventually lead to intimal disruption. Adventitial fibrosis may obstruct nutrient vessels feeding the arterial wall and the small intramural vasa vasorum. Both result in necrosis of smooth muscle cells and fibrosis of elastic structures, rendering the vessel wall vulnerable to pulsatile forces and creating a substrate for aneurysms and dissections.[1,2]

In addition to chronic hypertension, smoking, dyslipidemia, and use of crack cocaine are risk factors. Rarely, inflammatory diseases destroy the media layers and cause weakening, expansion, and dissection of the aortic wall. Iatrogenic aortic dissection may be associated with invasive retrograde catheter interventions or occur during or after valve or aortic surgery.[1,2]

Men are affected twice as often as women by acute aortic dissection, with 60% of cases classified as proximal (type A) and 40% as distal (type B) according to the Stanford classification.[1,2] Historical data for untreated aortic dissection of the ascending aorta show a mortality rate of 1% to 2% per hour within the first 24 hours, resulting in a mortality rate of up to 50% to 74% during the acute phase.[1,2] Uncomplicated acute type B dissection is less frequently lethal, with survival rates for medically treated patients of 89% at 1 month, 84% at 1 year, and up to 80% within 5 years.[1,2] Survival may be significantly improved by the timely institution of appropriate therapy. Prompt clinical recognition and definitive diagnostic testing are essential in the management of aortic dissection.

Conventional treatment of Stanford type A (DeBakey types I and II) dissection (see Fig. 44.1) consists of surgical reconstruction of the ascending aorta with complete or partial resection of the dissected aortic segment. In type A dissections, interventional endovascular strategies have no clinical application except to relieve critical malperfusion before surgery of the ascending aorta. This is done by distal endovascular interventions in cases of thoracoabdominal extension of a proximal dissection (DeBakey type I) with distal ischemic complications. In Stanford type B dissections, stent graft placement aims to remodel the thoracic descending aorta, typically by sealing one or multiple proximal entry tears with a Dacron-covered stent, initiating thrombosis of the false lumen.[4–7]

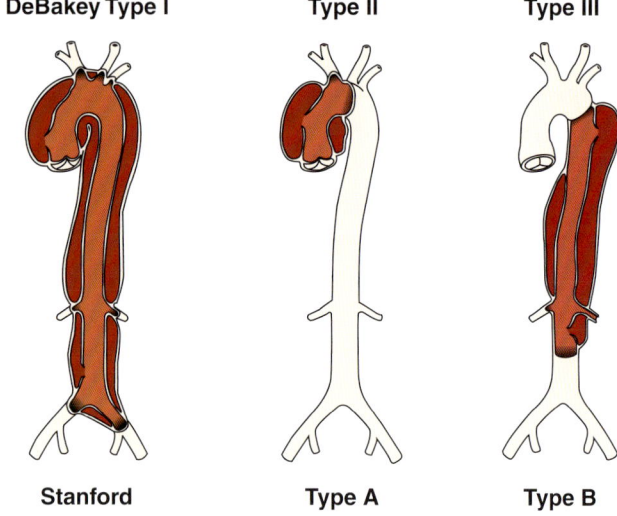

Fig. 44.1 Common classifications of thoracic aortic dissection.

DeBakey
- Type I — Originates in the ascending aorta, propagates at least to the aortic arch and often beyond it distally
- Type II — Originates in and is confined to the ascending aorta
- Type III — Originates in the descending aorta and extends distally down the aorta or, rarely, retrograde into the aortic arch and ascending aorta

Stanford
- Type A — All dissections involving the ascending aorta, regardless of the site of origin
- Type B — All dissections not involving the ascending aorta

Reconstruction of a collapsed true lumen may reestablish side branch flow (Fig. 44.2). Various scenarios of malperfusion syndrome are amenable to endovascular management, including static or dynamic collapse (i.e., intima invagination) of the aortic true lumen (i.e., pseudocoarctation) (Fig. 44.3), static or dynamic occlusion of one or more vital side branches, and an enlarging false aneurysm due to a patent proximal entry tear. Although peripheral pulse deficits often can be reversed with surgical repair of the dissected thoracic aorta, patients with signs of mesenteric or renal ischemia do not fare well. Mortality rates for patients with renal ischemia are between 50% and 70% and may be as high as 87% in cases with mesenteric ischemia.[8–10]

Surgical mortality rates for patients with acute peripheral vascular ischemic complications are similar to those for patients with mesenteric ischemia, and the in-hospital mortality rate may reach 89%.[11–14] Operative mortality rates for surgical fenestration are between 21% and 61%, which has encouraged percutaneous interventional management by endovascular balloon fenestration of a dissecting aortic membrane to treat mesenteric ischemia, a concept often discussed as a niche indication in complicated cases of malperfusion.[13–15]

Management of Stanford type B (DeBakey type III) dissection with the use of endovascular stent grafts has evolved slowly in anticipation of an unknown risk of paraplegia from spinal artery occlusion, as seen in up to 18% of cases after open surgery.[14,15] After technical improvements, a large series of patients has been successfully treated in various specialized centers by endovascular stent grafts placed to cover entry tears in the descending aorta and in the aortic arch. Studies have demonstrated that closure of proximal entry tears is essential to reconstruct the aortic wall and reduce the total aortic diameter. Entry tear closure promotes depressurization of the false lumen, thrombus formation in the false lumen (Fig. 44.4), and remodeling of the entire aorta.[5,6,15] In the near future, combined surgical and interventional procedures are likely to be developed for proximal dissections.[16–18]

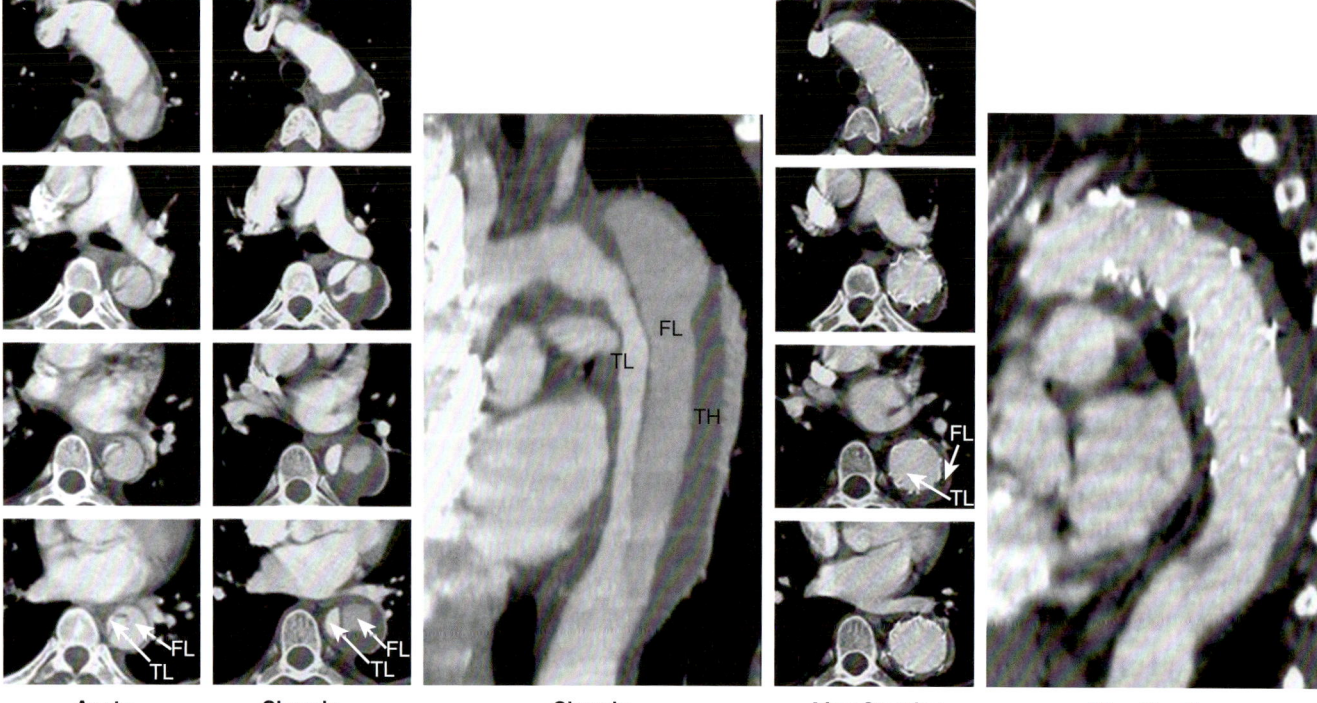

Fig. 44.2 Type B aortic dissection in a 48-year-old man. Notice the dynamic obstruction of the true lumen *(TL)* in the acute phase. After stent graft placement across the proximal thoracic entry, the entire true lumen of the thoracic aorta is reconstructed over time, with complete healing of the dissected aortic wall and shrinking of the completely thrombosed *(TH)* false lumen *(FL)*.

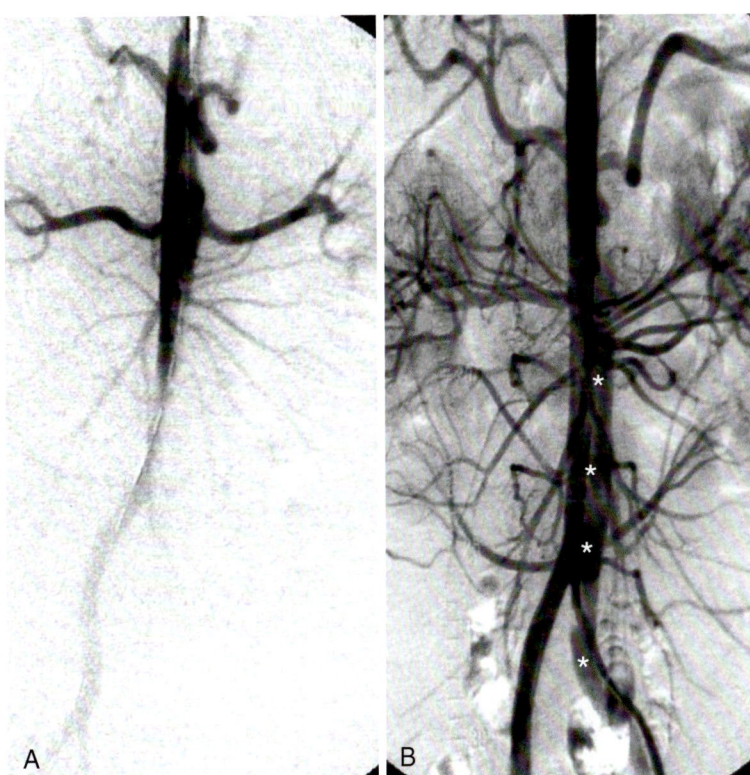

Fig. 44.3 Digital subtraction angiography of a thoracoabdominal type B dissection. (A) Dynamic obstruction of the true lumen distal to the renal arteries causes malperfusion of the mesentery and both lower extremities. (B) At follow-up 3 months after stent graft placement in the proximal descending aorta, the true lumen has widened as a consequence of aortic remodeling, and the patient is asymptomatic. However, the false lumen *(stars)* in the abdominal aorta is not completely thrombosed.

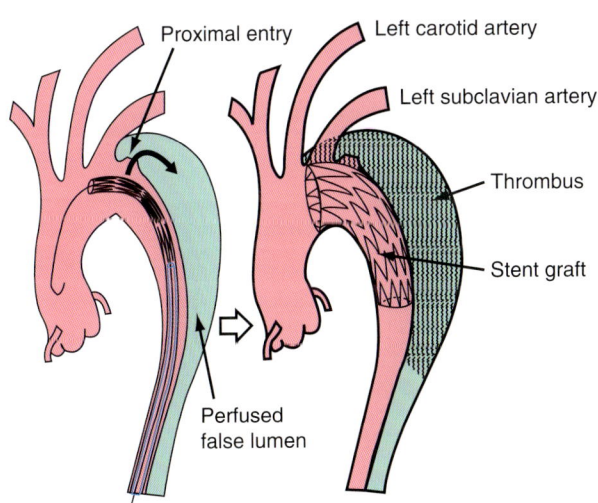

Fig. 44.4 Interventional reconstruction of the dissected aorta with sealing of the proximal entries, depressurization of the false lumen, and initiation of the false lumen thrombosis.

Indications for Endovascular Aortic Interventions

Significant perioperative morbidity and mortality in cases of acute, complicated type B dissection have prompted alternative therapeutic concepts. Thoracic endovascular aortic repair (TEVAR), even though it is an off-label indication for dissection, has been approved by the U.S. Food and Drug Administration (FDA) for aneurysmal disease of the aorta. The natural course of aortic dissection is determined by two elements: early complications and late events. In the acute phase, TEVAR has abrogated impending rupture and relieved static and dynamic malperfusion. A later benefit appears to be false lumen thrombosis, mitigating the risk of aneurysmal dilation and subsequent rupture.

The role of interventional management of static or dynamic obstruction of aortic branch arteries in complicated and complex distal dissection was settled in 2010, when static obstruction of a branch was overcome by placing endovascular stents in the ostium of a compromised side branch. Dynamic obstruction may benefit from stents in the aortic true lumen, sometimes combined with side branch stenting and preferentially without additional balloon fenestration because fenestration does not improve stress and tension on the thin aortic wall.[19]

Sometimes, bare-metal stents deployed from the true lumen into side branches can buttress the flap in a stable position.[20] In rare cases, fenestration helps to create a reentry tear for the dead-end false lumen back into the true lumen, with the aim of preventing thrombosis of the false lumen and compromise of branches fed exclusively from the false lumen; however, this concept lacks clinical proof of benefit. Conversely, fenestration increases the long-term risk of aortic rupture because a large reentry tear promotes flow in the false lumen, which promotes aneurysmal expansion. There is also a risk of peripheral embolism from a patent but partly thrombosed false lumen.[20,21]

The most effective method to avoid an enlarging false lumen is sealing of proximal entry tears with a customized stent graft (Fig. 44.5). Absence of a distal reentry tear is desirable for optimal results but is not a prerequisite. Compression of the true aortic lumen cranial to the main abdominal branches with distal malperfusion (i.e., pseudocoarctation) is usually corrected by stent grafts that expand the compressed true lumen and improve distal aortic blood flow.[5,6,13,15] Depressurization and shrinking of the false lumen is the most beneficial result to be gained, ideally followed by complete thrombosis of the false lumen and remodeling of the entire dissected aorta (see Fig. 44.2).[17]

Like previously accepted indications for open surgical repair in complicated type B dissections, factors such as intractable pain with descending dissection, rapidly expanding false lumen diameter, extraaortic blood collection as a sign of imminent rupture, and distal malperfusion syndrome are accepted indications for emergent stent graft placement.[17,18,20–22] Even late-onset

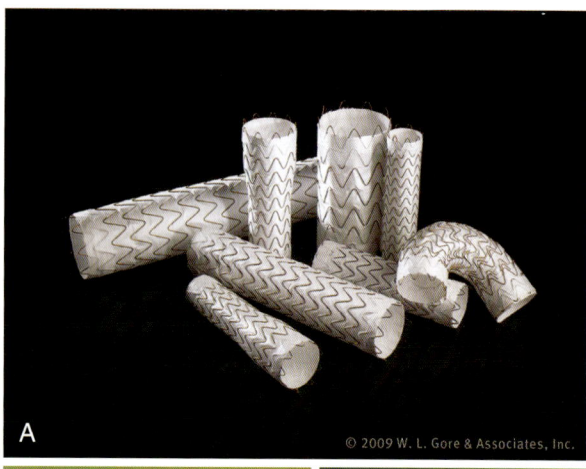
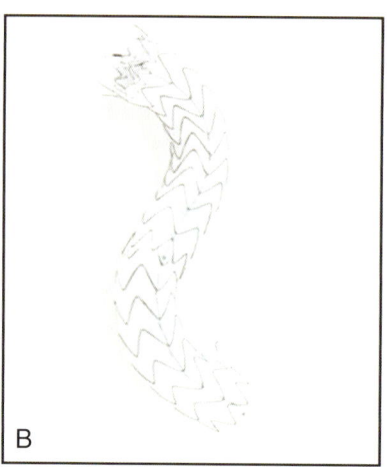
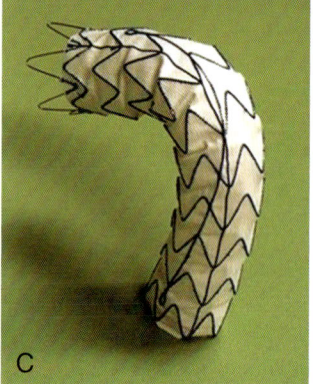
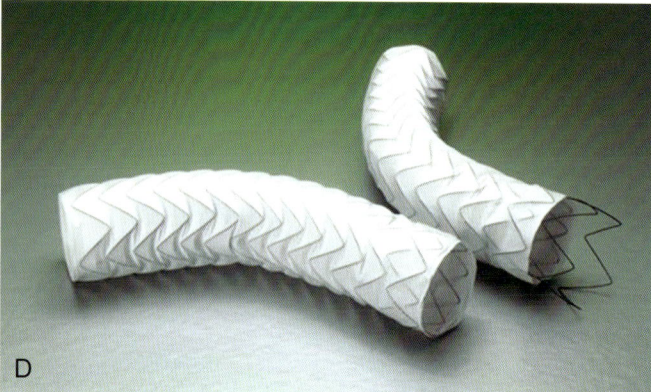

Fig. 44.5 A selection of thoracic stent grafts from American manufacturers that are available in Europe: (A) TAG. (B) Valiant. (C) Relay stent-graft. (D) EndoFit. (A, Gore, Flagstaff, AZ. B, Medtronic AVE, Santa Rosa, CA. C, Duke Vascular, Inc., Santa Cruz, CA. D, Bolton Medical, Sunrise, FL.)

complications such as malperfusion of vital aortic side branches are likely to justify endovascular stent grafting of an occlusive lamella to improve distal true lumen flow as a first option. Surgery is employed only after an unsuccessful attempt because surgical repair has failed to prove superior to interventional treatment even in uncomplicated cases. In complicated cases, endoluminal treatment has replaced open surgery in advanced aortic centers.[4–6,20–23] Even in some cases of retrogradely extended type A dissections, TEVAR is feasible as a primary approach to seal the entry or as a secondary step after open repair of the ascending aorta.[17] Open surgery may include an "elephant trunk" or transposition of arch vessels to provide optimal landing zones for endovascular completion in a hybrid approach.[24,25] Treatment options are summarized in Table 44.1.

Stable Acute Type B Aortic Dissection

Patients with suspected acute aortic dissection should be admitted to intensive care and subjected to immediate diagnostic evaluation. Reduction of systolic blood pressure to 100 to 120 mm Hg with an eye on renal function and pain relief is an initial priority and is usually achieved by morphine sulfate and intravenous β-blocking agents with or without vasodilating drugs such as sodium nitroprusside or angiotensin-converting enzyme inhibitors (Table 44.2).

The heart rate should be kept low; a heart rate below 60 beats per minute significantly decreases secondary adverse events (e.g., aortic expansion, recurrent aortic dissection, aortic rupture, need for aortic surgery) in type B aortic dissections compared with a conventional rate of more than 60 beats per minute.[26] After stable blood pressure and symptom relief are obtained, a patient with an uncomplicated type B aortic dissection can be discharged (usually within 14 days) on oral drugs. Clinical and imaging follow-up are advised at 3 and 6 months and annually thereafter.

TABLE 44.1 Therapeutic Strategies for Aortic Dissection

SURGERY
Type A aortic dissection
Acute type B dissection complicated by the following:
  Retrograde extension into the ascending aorta
  Dissection in fibrillinopathies (e.g., Marfan syndrome, Ehlers–Danlos syndrome)
  Rupture or impending rupture (historically classic indication)
  Progression with compromise of vital organs

MEDICAL THERAPY
Uncomplicated type B dissection
Stable, isolated arch dissection
Uncomplicated chronic type B dissection

INTERVENTIONAL THERAPY
Unstable acute or chronic type B dissection
Malperfusion
Rapid expansion (>1 cm/year)
Critical diameter (≥5.5 cm)
Refractory pain
Type B dissection with retrograde extension into the ascending aorta
Hybrid procedure for extended type A aortic dissection

Of 384 patients with type B dissections from the International Registry of Aortic Dissection (IRAD), 73% were managed medically with an in-hospital mortality rate of 10%.[1,27] Short-term survival rates were 91% at 1 month and 89% at 1 year. The reported long-term survival rate with medical therapy varies between 60% and 80% at 4 to 5 years and is about 40% to 45% at 10 years.[1,27] Potential beneficial effects of early stenting is proved in the ADSORB trial (Acute Uncomplicated Aortic Dissection Type B: Evaluation of Stent Graft Placement or Best Medical Treatment Alone).[28] Of 61 patients being randomized in best

TABLE 44.2	Initial Medical Treatment for Aortic Dissection		
Drug	Mechanism	Dose	Cautions and Contraindications
Esmolol	Cardioselective β_1-blocker	Load: 500 µg/kg IV Drip: 50 µg/kg/min IV Increase by increments of 50 µg/min	Asthma or bronchospasm Bradycardia Second- or third-degree AV block Cocaine or methamphetamine abuse
Labetalol	Nonselective $\beta_{1,2}$-blocker Selective α_1-blocker	Load: 20 mg IV Drip: 2 mg/min IV	Asthma or bronchospasm Bradycardia Second- or third-degree AV block Cocaine or methamphetamine abuse
Enalaprilat	ACE inhibitor	0.625–1.25 mg IV q6h Maximum dose: 5 mg q6h	Angioedema Pregnancy Renal artery stenosis Severe renal insufficiency
Nitroprusside	Direct arterial vasodilator	Begin at 0.3 µg/kg/min IV Maximum dose: 10 µg/kg/min	May cause reflex tachycardia Cyanide/thiocyanate toxicity, especially in renal or hepatic insufficiency
Nitroglycerin	Vascular smooth muscle relaxation	5–200 µg/min IV	Decreases preload; contraindicated in tamponade or other preload-dependent states Concomitant use of sildenafil or similar agents

ACE, Angiotensin-converting enzyme; *AV*, atrioventricular; *IV*, intravenous; *q*, every.

medical therapy group (n = 31) and best medical therapy group in addition to aortic stent graft placement (n = 30), the latter group had a significantly lower rate of primary end point, which was a combination of incomplete/no false lumen thrombosis, aortic dilatation, or aortic rupture at 1 year (P < .001).

Unstable Acute Type B Aortic Dissection

About 30% to 42% of acute type B aortic dissections are complicated, as evidenced by hemodynamic instability or peripheral vascular ischemia, and they have an unpredictable outcome.[27] Acute lower limb and visceral ischemia has been reported in 30% to 50%, and malperfusion syndrome occurs frequently with extended dissections, with mortality between 50% and 85% if untreated.[29] However, operative mortality rates for patients with acute aortic dissection complicated by renal ischemia are about 50% and can be as high as 88% for those with mesenteric malperfusion.[30] Of 571 patients with acute type B aortic dissection in the IRAD, 390 were treated medically. In the 125 complicated cases, 59 patients underwent standard open surgery, and 66 were subjected to TEVAR. The in-hospital mortality rate was significantly lower with TEVAR than after open surgery (10.2% vs. 33.9%, P = .002) (Fig. 44.6).[31]

The provisional extension to induce complete attachment (PETTICOAT) technique pushes the idea of endothoracic reconstruction further by extending the stent graft scaffold distally with open-cell bare-metal stents until distal malperfusion is corrected.[32] Using this technique, aortic fenestration maneuvers and branch vessel revascularization with side branch stents usually are not needed and have almost become obsolete.

A meta-analysis of outcomes for 942 patients from 29 studies found an in-hospital mortality rate of 9% and reintervention rate of 10.4%.[33] Emergency surgical conversion or periprocedural stroke was rare (0.6% and 3.1%, respectively), and the survival rate was 88% at mean follow-up of 20 months. A second meta-analysis of outcomes for 1304 patients subjected to TEVAR for complicated acute type B aortic dissection found a technical success rate of 99% and a 30-day mortality rate of 2.6%.[34] At late follow-up, false lumen thrombosis was documented in 92.9% of patients, and surgical conversion was required in 0.8%, with endovascular reintervention performed in 1.6%. Retrograde extension into the ascending aorta and neurologic complications were reported in 0.4% and 0.6%, respectively.[34] Further results are listed in Table 44.3 and elsewhere.[31,35–51]

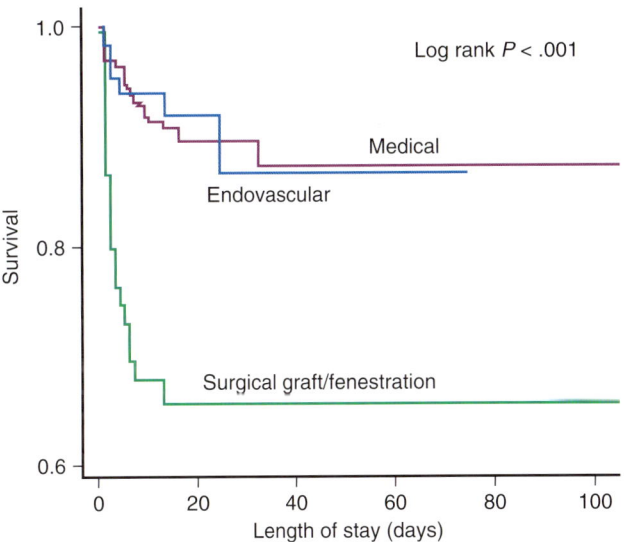

Fig. 44.6 Comparison of medical, surgical, and endovascular treatment of complicated type B aortic dissection. (From Fattori R, Tsai TT, Myrmel T, et al. Complicated acute type B dissection: is surgery still the best option? A report from the International Registry of Acute Aortic Dissection. *JACC Cardiovasc Interv.* 2008;1[4]:395–402.)

In patients deemed unsuitable candidates for conventional open surgical repair, 1- and 5-year survival rates were 74% and 31% with TEVAR compared with 93% and 78% (P < .001) survival rates for patients considered candidates for conventional open repair.[35] A comparison between endovascular treatment of complicated type B aortic dissection and medical therapy of uncomplicated type B dissection in 56 patients with a follow-up of 18.1 ± 16.9 months found similar outcomes in both groups but a better midterm fate of the descending thoracic aorta in the stent graft group and no associated paraplegia. There were no differences in the 5-year survival rates (86.3% for both groups).[36]

Chronic Type B Aortic Dissection

Evolution of an acute dissection to a chronic dissection involves progressive thickening of the intimal flap due to fibrosis. More

TABLE 44.3 Results of Endovascular Stent Graft Implantation in Various Clinical Conditions

Study	Year	n	Technical Success (%)	Paraplegia (%)	Mortality (%)	Follow-Up (Months)
ACUTE COMPLICATED TYPE B DISSECTION						
Bortone et al.[23]	2004	43	100	0	7	21
Xu et al.[40]	2006	63	95	0	10.6	48
Verhoye et al.[41]	2008	16	100	0	27	36
Fattori et al.[31]	2008	66	100	3.4	10.6	1
Szeto et al.[42]	2008	35	97.1	2.8	2.8	18
Khoynezhad et al.[111]	2009	28	90	NA	18 (1 year) 22 (5 years)	36
Alves et al.[112]	2009	106	99	1.8	18 (acute AD) 7 (chronic AD)	35.9
Parsa et al.[113]	2010	55	100	2	37 (overall) 6 (aorta related)	14.4
Shu et al.[43]	2011	45	100	NA	4.4 (1 year)	13
Ehrlich et al.[44]	2013	29	100	10	21 (1 year) 39 (5 years)	53
Wiedemann et al.[45]	2014	110	100	4.5	15 (1 year) 27 (5 years)	60
Massmann et al.[46]	2014	14	93	0	0	30
Bavaria et al.[172]	2015	50	100	NA	15 (1 year)	12
CHRONIC TYPE B DISSECTION						
Nienaber et al.[5]	1999	12	100	0	0	12
Kato et al.[173]	2001	15	100	0	0	24
Eggebrecht et al.[47]	2005	28	100	0	13.6	12
Jing et al.[59]	2008	35	100	0	7.6	48
Nienaber et al.[52]	2009	72	95.7	2.8	11.1 (overall) 5.6 (aorta related)	24
Kang et al.[174]	2011	76	100	0	15.7	34
Nienaber[50]	2013	72	100	2.8	11.3 (overall) 6.9 (aorta)	60
Andersen[51]	2014	75	100	0	14 (1 year) 35 (5 years)	34
Lu et al.[175]	2015	51	100	0	1.9 (3.5)	44
Conway et al.[176]	2017	125	98.4	NA	2.4 (in-hospital)	8

AD, Aortic dissection; *NA*, not applicable.

intimal tears are reported in chronic type B aortic dissection than acute dissection. The growth rate of the chronically dissected distal aorta is estimated to be between 0.10 and 0.74 cm in diameter per year, depending on the initial aortic diameter and state of hypertension.[1,25]

Unfortunately, the long-term outcome after medical therapy alone is suboptimal, with a reported 50% mortality rate at 5 years and delayed expansion of the false lumen in 20% to 50% of patients at 4 years.[1,25] Expansion of the false lumen, for which an initial diameter beyond 4 cm and persistent perfusion of the false lumen are predictors, predisposes patients to aortic rupture or retrograde migration of the dissection toward the ascending aorta.[1,25] TEVAR should be considered when the aortic diameter exceeds 5.5 mm or when there is persistent thoracic pain or uncontrolled hypertension and rapid growth of the dissecting aneurysm (>1 cm/year).

Our group prospectively evaluated elective TEVAR in 12 patients with chronic type B dissection and compared the results with 12 matched surgical controls. Proximal entry closure and complete thrombosis of the false lumen at 3 months were achieved in all patients. Stent graft treatment resulted in no morbidity or mortality, whereas surgical treatment resulted in four deaths (33%, $P = .04$) and five adverse events (42%, $P = .04$).[5] These results were confirmed by similar observations (see Table 44.3).

Whether prophylactic use of TEVAR in patients with chronic type B aortic dissections is superior to medical treatment alone was evaluated in the prospective, randomized, controlled Investigation of Stent Grafts in Aortic Dissection (INSTEAD) trial.[52] A total of 140 patients in stable clinical condition at least 2 weeks after the index dissection were randomly subjected to elective stent graft placement in addition to optimal medical therapy ($n = 72$) or to optimal medical therapy alone ($n = 68$). There was no difference in the all-cause death rate and a 2-year cumulative survival rate of 95.5% ± 2.5% with optimal medical therapy versus 88.9% ± 3.7% with TEVAR ($P = .15$) (Fig. 44.7). Moreover, the aorta-related death rate was not different (2.9% vs. 5.6%, $P = .68$), and the risk for the combined end point of aorta-related death and progression was similar ($P = .65$). Aortic remodeling (with true lumen recovery and thoracic false lumen thrombosis) occurred in 91.3% of patients with TEVAR and in 19.4% of those who received medical treatment ($P < .001$), which suggests ongoing aortic remodeling.

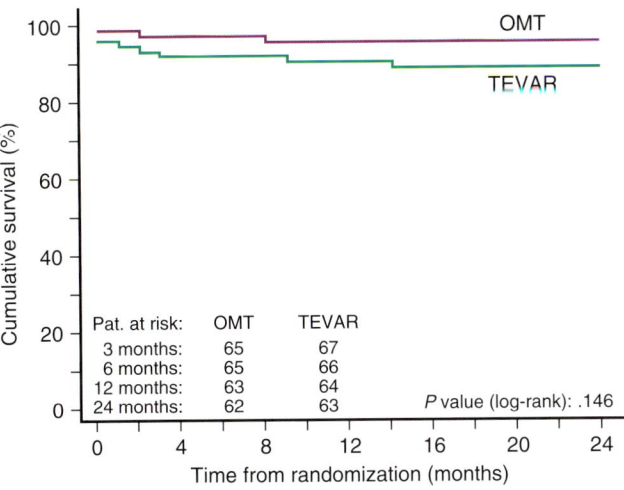

Fig. 44.7 Cumulative survival of patients with chronic type B aortic dissection within 24 months after randomization. *OMT*, Optimal medical therapy; *TEVAR*, thoracic endovascular aortic repair. (From Nienaber CA, Rousseau H, Eggebrecht H, et al. Randomized comparison of strategies for type B aortic dissection: the Investigation of STEnt grafts in Aortic Dissection (INSTEAD) trial. *Circulation*. 2009;120:2519–2528.)

The 5-year follow up, which was evaluated in the INSTEAD-XL trial, revealed an all-cause mortality rate of 11.1% for TEVAR versus 19.3% for medical therapy ($P = .13$), whereas the aorta-specific mortality rate was 6.9% versus 19.3 ($P = .04$), with a progression rate of 27.0% versus 46.1% ($P = .04$). Landmark analysis suggested a benefit of TEVAR for all-cause mortality (0% vs. 16.9%, $P = .0003$), aorta-specific mortality (0% vs. 16.9%, $P = .0005$), and progression (4.1% vs. 28.1%, $P = .004$) between 2 and 5 years.[51]

Aortic Stent Graft Placement

Aortic stent grafts are primarily used to reconstruct the compressed true lumen cranial to major aortic branches and to increase distal aortic flow. Proximal communications are sealed to direct flow into the true lumen, depressurize the false lumen, and induce thrombosis in the false lumen, with fibrotic transformation and subsequent remodeling of the aortic wall. Stent graft placement across the origin of the celiac, superior mesenteric, and renal arteries may lead to fatal organ failure.

Important descriptive features of the thoracic aorta are derived from multislice computed tomography (CT), including the shape and size of the aortic pathology (i.e., diameter, length, and shape) and the condition of the aortic wall (e.g., atheroma, calcification, thrombus), and data are used for three-dimensional reconstruction. Although there is no standard convention for the measurement of vessel diameters, many operators measure the inner wall of the vessel (i.e., endothelial trailing edge) because it can ensure some degree of oversizing that is considered desirable for endograft placement. Contrast angiography does not provide reliable measurements.

In addition to the initial obligatory diagnostic CT angiography or magnetic resonance angiography (MRA), transesophageal echocardiography (TEE) and intravascular ultrasound may be performed to obtain additional valuable information. For instance, flow-sensitive MRA sequences or contrast-enhanced TEE views show the communication sites between true and false lumens and provide insights into the dynamic flow pattern in the false lumen before stent graft placement. Access vessels must also be evaluated for size and tortuosity because the stent graft delivery systems are quite large (up to 24 Fr) and can cause significant trauma to the femoral access site and iliac arteries.

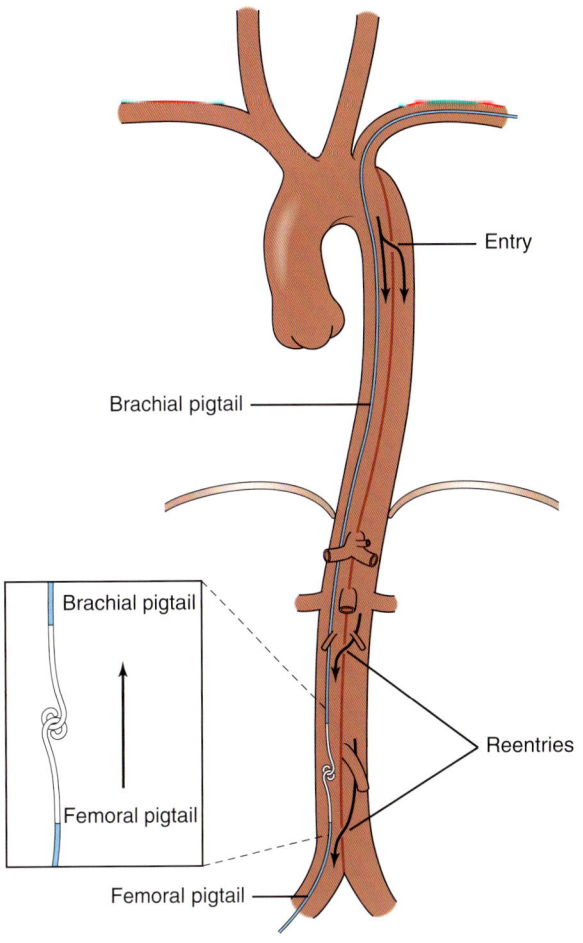

Fig. 44.8 In complex cases with multiple reentries in the abdominal aorta, the embracement technique using two pigtail catheters ensures navigation of the guidewire in the true lumen before stent graft placement.

Features that are unfavorable for thoracic stent graft use include severe aortic angulation or tortuosity, friable atheroma or thrombus lining the aortic wall, and aortic pathology involving the ascending aorta. The vicinity of relevant side branches, usually the left subclavian artery (LSA) or left common carotid artery, is critical when planning to place a stent graft for type B dissection. Appropriate periinterventional image reconstruction of the aortic arch pathology enhances the result in individual cases.

The procedure is best performed in the catheterization and imaging laboratory using digital angiography and general anesthesia. The femoral artery is the most popular access site and can usually accommodate a 24-Fr stent graft system. In the Seldinger technique, a 260-cm stiff wire is placed over a pigtail catheter that is navigated with a soft wire in the true lumen under both fluoroscopic and transesophageal ultrasound guidance. In complex cases with multiple reentries in the abdominal aorta, the embracement technique, which uses two pigtail catheters, is useful (Fig. 44.8).

A pigtail catheter that has been installed in the true aortic lumen through the left brachial artery picks up the femoral pigtail catheter in the true lumen of the abdominal aorta and pulls it up into the aortic arch. This procedure ensures definite positioning of the stiff guidewire in the true lumen, which is essential for correct deployment of the stent graft. The stent is carefully advanced over the stiff wire, and the launching of the stent graft is performed with systolic blood pressure lowered to 50 to 60 mm Hg by infusion of sodium nitroprusside or by rapid right ventricular pacing to prevent dislodgement.[53,54] After deployment, short inflation of a latex balloon can improve apposition of the stent struts to the aortic wall, although only if proximal sealing of thoracic communications is incomplete.

Paraplegia may occur after the use of multiple stent grafts, but this appears to be a rare phenomenon, especially when the stented segment does not exceed 16 cm long. Both Doppler ultrasound and contrast fluoroscopy are instrumental for documenting the immediate result or initiating adjunctive maneuvers. The navigation of wires and instruments is easier for thoracic aortic aneurysms (TAAs) or ulcers, but dual imaging using ultrasound and fluoroscopy simultaneously is equally important.

A frequent anatomic consideration is the short distance between the origin of the LSA and the primary tear in type B dissections. Coverage of the ostium to the LSA must sometimes be accepted to perform endovascular aortic repair in the aortic pathology adjacent to the artery. According to observational evidence, prophylactic surgical maneuvers are not imperative or always required for safety reasons but may be relegated to an elective measure after an endovascular aortic intervention if intolerable signs or symptoms of ischemia occur.[55] However, before intentional LSA occlusion, careful attention must be paid to potential supraaortic variants (e.g., aberrant subclavian artery, nonintact vertebrobasilar system, dominant left vertebral artery) that originate directly from the aortic arch and other pathologies recognized during preinterventional vascular staging.

Retrograde Type A Thoracic Aortic Dissection

TEVAR is associated with complications. New and unexpected complications such as endoleak, graft migration, device separation, and retrograde type A thoracic aortic dissection (rATAD) have emerged. A European multicenter registry of 4750 procedures estimated the incidence of rATAD at 1.33%, with 25% being asymptomatic cases.[56] One single center reported a 2.5% rate of rATAD (n = 11); three of the patients had Marfan syndrome.[57] Of interest, rATAD developed intraoperatively in two patients, occurring 2 hours after the procedure in one patient, at 1 week in one patient, and in seven patients a month after TEVAR; eight of these cases were converted to open surgery, and two received medical treatment.[57]

Open surgery is the treatment of choice for potentially fatal complications, but the procedure-related mortality rate after rATAD surgery is between 20% and 57%.[56,57] The mechanisms of rATAD after TEVAR are unclear, but observations suggest that rATAD may have several causes, such as oversize ballooning, procedure- or device-related factors, unfavorable aortic dissection anatomy, and natural progression of initial aortic dissection. Among possible TEVAR-related factors, injury from proximal bare spring with outward pointing radial force was suspected. Lack of conformability of stent grafts when passively bent at the aortic arch may cause traumatic strain to the wall and create a tear. Balloon dilation after TEVAR can cause injury to the inner layers and retrograde extension. Additional balloon dilation was performed in 11 cases (23%) of rATAD in one series.[56] Oversizing of the stent graft by more than 20% in relation to the landing zone diameter was considered a risk factor for rATAD.

Genuine fragility of the aortic wall may predispose to rATAD and be a sign of natural disease progression. Newly developed type A dissections were observed in four of 180 and in five of 66 patients under medical treatment for acute type B dissection.[48,58]

Timing and Application of Endovascular Repair

The optimal timing for endovascular intervention in type B dissections remains controversial. Bortone and colleagues favor an early intervention within 2 weeks of the initial diagnosis; stent graft placement was successful in all patients referred for intervention within the first 2 weeks.[23] A high rate of reverse remodeling is likely when the patient is treated early after development of the dissection flap. With the passage of time, the dissection flap becomes more fibrosed, thickened, and matured, and it is less amenable to TEVAR.

Shimono and coworkers reported that complete obliteration and resolution of the false lumen after endovascular stent graft treatment was more frequently achieved in cases of acute aortic dissection than those of chronic aortic dissection (70% vs. 38.5%).[49] Conversely, others have observed higher mortality rates for patients with acute type B aortic dissection.[47,59] Morphologic change of the initially fragile dissecting membrane to a more fibrotic and seemingly stable membrane in the chronic phase are critical for endovascular repair, suggesting that TEVAR is safer after a minimum of 4 weeks after the onset of aortic dissection but before the chronic stage.[60] The more stable clinical status of patients in the chronic phase of aortic dissection may be an important determinant of better survival after TEVAR.

Because of the lack of prospective, randomized data comparing immediate and delayed intervention in various clinical and anatomic conditions, no general recommendation has been issued about the timing of endovascular treatment. However, observational evidence may favor an early intervention during the window of aortic plasticity when justified by a low complication rate.

Endovascular stent grafting has emerged as an alternative therapy to the open surgical repair of aortic dissection. Although patients at high surgical risk can benefit from the endovascular technology, the exact role of stent grafting awaits definition as long-term data and experience continue to accumulate and as devices and techniques evolve. Instead of replacing conventional surgical treatment completely, endovascular repair will likely play a complementary role and offer a less invasive option. The limitations of both approaches are distinct. What is considered high risk for surgery is defined by clinical parameters in terms of comorbidities, but contraindications to endovascular stent grafting are defined by anatomic constraints. Both strategies will continue to coexist and may merge to generate hybrid procedures.

DESCENDING THORACIC AORTIC ANEURYSM
Endovascular Repair by Stent Grafts

TAAs, which were classified by Crawford and Safi (Fig. 44.9), occur predominantly in the elderly and have been increasing in incidence as the population ages and diagnostic capabilities advance.[61] With an incidence of 6 to 10 per 100,000 person-years, TAAs are less common than abdominal aortic aneurysms (AAAs) but remain life-threatening.[61-63] In several series, the ascending aorta was involved in 51%, the aortic arch in 11%, and the descending thoracic aorta in 38% of TAA cases. One-fourth of the patients had concomitant infrarenal aneurysmal aortic disease, and up to 13% had multiple aneurysms, whereas the risk of having a TAA when AAA was diagnosed was between 3.5% and 12%.[63]

The pathogenesis of aortic aneurysms has not been fully established, but it is thought to be multifactorial and include atherosclerosis, increased tissue protease activity, antiprotease deficiency, and genetic collagen defects such as Marfan syndrome and Ehlers–Danlos syndrome. Up to 20% of patients with an aneurysm have a first-degree relative with the same disorder.[64]

Weakening of the aortic wall can also be induced by inflammation resulting from microbiologic diseases or multisystem inflammation disorders. Aortitis induced by syphilis and *Staphylococcus aureus* infection is well known. Kawasaki syndrome is characterized by more circumscriptive wall thickening and aneurysm formation, whereas syphilis can induce diffuse wall thickening and aneurysm formation of the ascending aorta. Behçet disease, like other forms of vasculitis, may lead to local aneurysm formation and perforation rather than dissection. Thoracic and abdominal aneurysm may develop in giant cell arteritis.

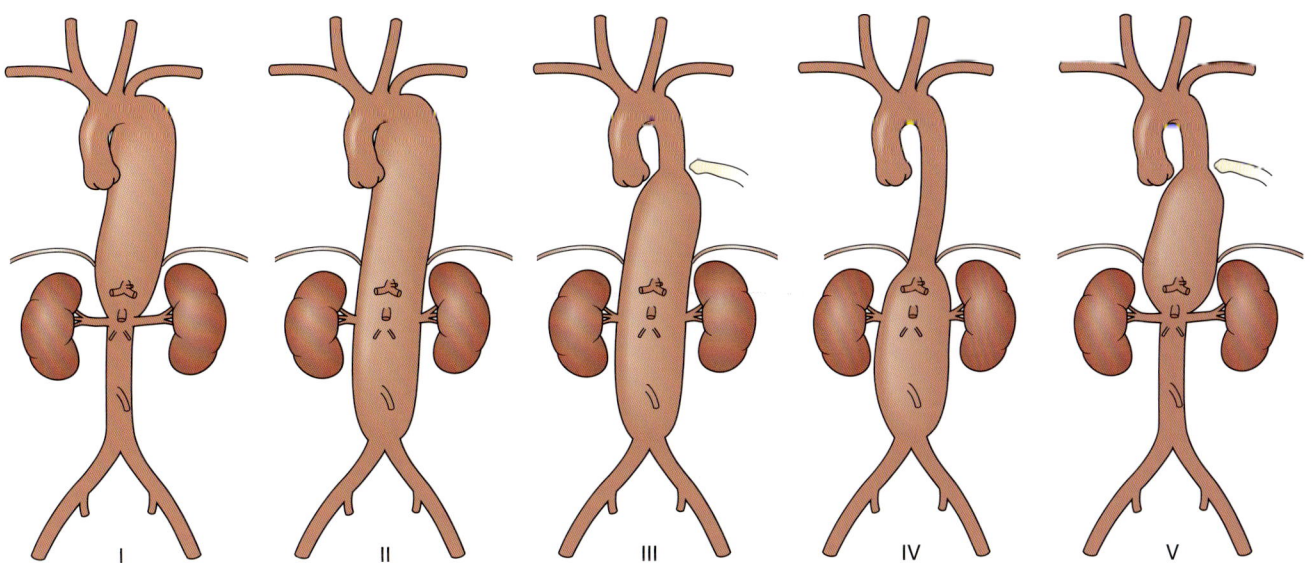

Fig. 44.9 Classification of thoracoabdominal aortic aneurysms.

The use of cocaine and amphetamines can lead to aortic wall thinning and aneurysm formation. In aortic stenosis, poststenotic aneurysm formation can occur, which may be enhanced after aortic valve prosthesis implantation. An important cause of aneurysm formation is related to trauma, particularly high-speed deceleration trauma involving the aortic isthmus in 95%. About 15% to 20% of deaths are related to aortic trauma in these patients.

The natural history of TAAs is one of progressive expansion and weakening of the aortic wall, leading to eventual rupture.[65–67] Initial aneurysmal size can also be an important predictor of aneurysm growth. A study of 721 patients found that TAA size had a profound impact on the risk of rupture, with an annual rate of 2% for aneurysms less than 5 cm, 3% for aneurysms 5 to 5.9 cm, and 7% for aneurysms larger than 6 cm in diameter. The risk appears to rise abruptly as thoracic aneurysms reach a size of 6 cm.[68] Nondimensional variables with an impact on the expansion rate and risk of rupture should also be evaluated. In a multivariate regression analysis, the Mount Sinai group identified older age, pain (even uncharacteristic pain), and a history of chronic obstructive pulmonary disease as independent risk factors for TAA rupture.[69]

With an associated mortality rate of 94%, TAA rupture is usually a fatal event.[62,70] Olsson and colleagues found that 22% of the patients in their survey with ruptured aortic aneurysms and dissection did not reach the hospital alive and that the diagnosis was made at autopsy.[71] The 5-year survival rate of unoperated TAA patients approximates 13%, whereas 70% to 79% of those who undergo elective surgical intervention are alive at 5 years.[72–74]

A novel predictor for TAA rupture, the aortic size index, may be useful for predicting increasing rates of rupture, dissection, or death. Individual body surface area is used for the aortic size index (aortic diameter/m^2), enabling improved selection of individual patients for surgical repair. An aortic size index of 2.75 cm/m^2 or less represents a low risk of rupture (≈4% per year), 2.75 to 4.24 cm/m^2 correlates with a moderate risk (≈8% per year), and greater than 4.25 cm/m^2 indicates a high risk (≈20% per year), underlining the importance of aortic size for predicting complications.[75] The risk of rupture should be assessed for all patients who are suitable candidates for surgical treatment.

The use of endovascular stent grafts for the repair of TAAs is emerging as a promising, less invasive therapeutic alternative to conventional surgical treatment. Endovascular treatment of aortic aneurysms is achieved by transluminal placement of one or more stent graft devices across the longitudinal extent of the lesion. The prosthesis bridges the aneurysmal sac to exclude it from high-pressure aortic blood flow, allowing sac thrombosis around the endograft and possible remodeling of the aortic wall (Fig. 44.10).

Endovascular aortic repair techniques were initially applied in cases of AAA, and efforts to adapt this technology for TAAs are ongoing. As is the case for AAAs, a less invasive approach to TAA repair is highly desirable because the patient population tends to be elderly and harbors multiple comorbidities.[67,74,76] Continued development of endovascular therapy for thoracic aneurysms is likely to provide greater benefits in terms of patient outcomes than those observed with AAAs. Conventional surgical treatment of TAA is physiologically more demanding and carries a greater operative risk. It mandates open thoracotomy, aortic cross-clamping, resection of the aneurysm, and replacement with a prosthetic graft; this often requires cardiopulmonary bypass.[77] For the aortic arch, surgical intervention is most likely the best method, and it is frequently combined with stent graft implantation to seal the distal aortic arch to the descending aorta.

Special systems have been designed so that implantation can be performed using an antegrade strategy.[74–77] For thoracic descending or thoracic-abdominal aortic aneurysms, the surgical strategy has been developed over the last 15 years to prevent ischemic complications. The operation requires permissive hypothermia (32°C to 34°C nasopharyngeal value), moderate heparinization (1 mg/kg), renal artery perfusion with 4°C crystalloid solution, aggressive reattachment of segmental arteries (especially between T8 and L1), sequential aortic clamping and cerebrospinal fluid drainage, left heart bypass during proximal anastomosis, and selective perfusion of celiac and superior mesenteric arteries during intercostal, visceral, and renal anastomosis.[74–77]

Despite advances in operative technique, intraoperative monitoring, and postoperative care, the mortality and morbidity rates for surgery remain substantial and less favorable than outcomes for open AAA repair. The mortality rate for TAA surgical repair ranges from 5% to 20% in elective cases and up to 50% in emergent situations.[74,78–82]

Major complications associated with surgical TAA treatment include renal and pulmonary failure, visceral and cardiac ischemia, stroke, and paraplegia. Paraplegia is a particularly devastating complication that is almost unique to the surgical treatment of TAAs, occurring in 5% to 25% of cases, compared with less than 1% for AAAs.[72,74,81–84] For these reasons, significant numbers of TAA patients are not candidates for open repair and have been without a treatment option until recently.

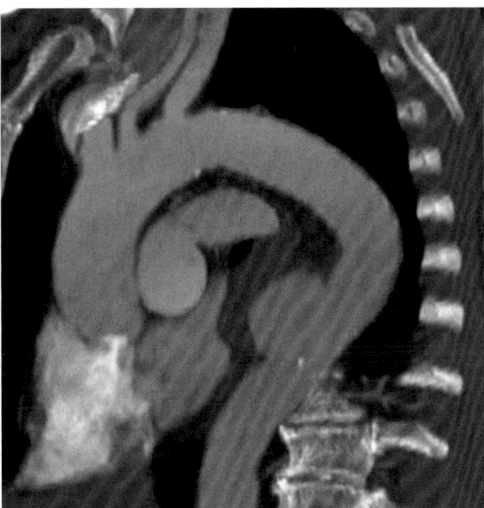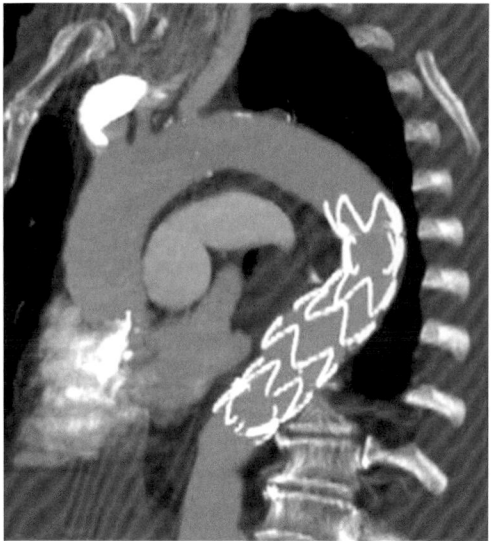

Fig. 44.10 Computed tomography angiography shows a circumscribed aneurysm of the descending thoracic aorta in a middle-aged man selected for endografting *(left)*. One-year follow-up after successful endovascular exclusion of the aneurysm by stent graft placement demonstrates marked shrinkage of the periprosthetic aneurysm and optimal wall apposition of the stent graft *(right)*.

Endovascular aneurysm repair of the thoracic aorta currently focuses on the descending portion. This aortic segment provides a substrate more amenable for endovascular stent graft repair due to avoidance of the great vessels proximally and major visceral branches and aortic bifurcation distally. Despite these anatomic advantages and the ability to draw from early experiences with endovascular AAA repair, the development of stent grafting in the thoracic aorta has progressed more slowly than that involving its infrarenal counterpart.

The thoracic aorta poses several challenges that have impeded simple adaptation of the endovascular devices and techniques developed for the abdominal aorta.[85] First, the hemodynamic forces of the thoracic aorta are significantly more aggressive and place greater mechanical demands on thoracic endografts. The potential for device migration, kinking, and late structural failure are important concerns. Second, greater flexibility is required of thoracic devices to conform to the natural curvature of the proximal descending aorta and to lesions with tortuous morphology. Third, because larger devices are necessary to accommodate the diameter of the thoracic aorta, arterial access is more problematic. More TAA patients than AAA patients are women, and access vessels tend to be smaller in women. Fourth, as with conventional open TAA repair, paraplegia remains a potential complication of the endovascular approach despite the absence of aortic cross-clamping.[86,87] Fifth, TAAs often extend beyond the boundaries of the descending thoracic aorta and involve more proximal or distal aorta than desired. Management of the LSA in particular has gained considerable attention.[88–90] With these challenges in mind, significant progress has been achieved since the first stent graft was deployed for TAA exclusion in 1992.[55,86,91]

Technical Aspects of Endovascular Repair

Early clinical experience with stent grafting of the thoracic aorta was based on the use of first-generation, homemade devices that were rigid and required large delivery systems (24- to 27-Fr).[91,92] Since then, several commercial manufacturers of abdominal endografts have created derivatives for the thoracic aorta with dramatic improvements over homemade devices. The endoprostheses are composed of a stent (nitinol or stainless steel) covered with fabric (i.e., polyester or polytetrafluoroethylene [PTFE]).

Evaluation for repair of a TAA considers the patient's overall risk profile, evidence of rapid enlargement of the aneurysm, a diameter of 5.5 cm or greater, and symptoms. The suitability of the patient for endovascular repair is based on clinical and anatomic considerations. Preprocedural imaging with spiral CT or magnetic resonance imaging (MRI) is essential to characterize the lesion and access route. Measurements from imaging data are used to select the appropriate diameter and length of a device. The aneurysm's location is determined in relation to the LSA and celiac axis.

Successful TAA exclusion requires normal segments of native aorta at both ends of the lesion (i.e., landing zone or neck) of at least 15 to 25 mm to ensure adequate contact between the endoprosthesis and the aortic wall and formation of a tight circumferential seal. Landing zones that are markedly angled or conical or that contain thrombus can result in poor fixation. Devices are oversized by 10% in diameter to provide sufficient radial force for adequate fixation. The vascular access route for device introduction and delivery to the pathologic target must be of sufficient size and suitable morphology. The preferred and most common site (41% to 58%) of vascular access is the common femoral artery. Less frequently, access to the iliac artery (9% to 44%) through an extraperitoneal approach is required.[92,93] Severe stenosis and tortuosity of the abdominal and thoracic aorta distal to the target are also contraindications for endovascular repair.

Despite these criteria, treatment failures can occur. However, the specific contributing factors and frequencies are unknown, particularly over the long term. Follow-up surveillance with serial CT scans at 1, 6, and 12 months and annually thereafter is recommended to monitor changes in aneurysm morphology, identify device failures, and detect endoleaks.

Hybrid Procedures for Aortic Arch Pathologies

The aortic arch morphology is challenging because of angulation and the proximity of the supraaortic branches that need to be preserved. Traditionally, open arch reconstruction using hypothermic cardiac arrest, extracorporeal circulation, and selective cerebral perfusion has been demonstrated to effectively manage aortic arch pathologies. However, this standard procedure for any arch pathology carries a significant mortality rate (2% to 9%) and risk of paraplegia and cerebral stroke in 4% to 13% of cases.[94,95] Open repair is therefore often reserved for low-risk patients.

Hybrid arch procedures are a combination of debranching bypass (i.e., supraaortic vessel transposition) to establish cerebral perfusion and subsequent thoracic endografting to provide patient-centered solutions for complex aortic arch lesions. Hybrid arch procedures are performed without hypothermic circulatory arrest and extracorporeal circulation. These procedures could expand the treatment group to older patients with severe comorbidities and to those requiring repeat surgery who are currently ineligible for open surgical intervention. The key to

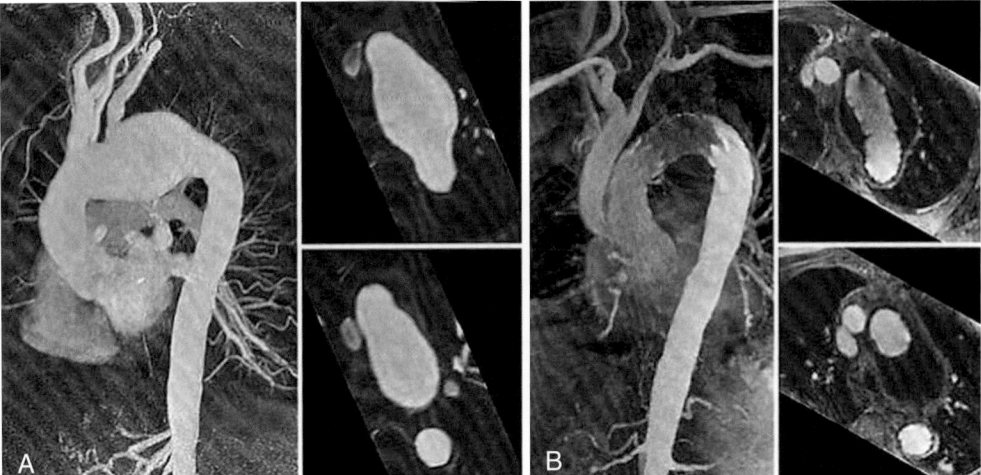

Fig. 44.11 Contrast-enhanced magnetic resonance angiography of the aorta in a case of an aortic aneurysm. (A) Aneurysm of the aortic arch involves the supra-aortic branches. (B) Postinterventional surgical result after a hybrid procedure with debranching of the supraaortic vessels and stent graft implantation in the aortic arch.

success is the quality of the unimpaired suitable ascending aorta as a donor site for the debranching bypass and proximal landing zone for the endografts (Fig. 44.11).

Clinical Experience

The literature on thoracic stent grafting consists mostly of small to medium-sized case series with short- to medium-term follow-up (Table 44.4). Nevertheless, these studies illustrate a consensus pattern of outcomes when viewed in the aggregate. Overall, successful device deployment is achieved in 85% to 100% of cases, and the periprocedural mortality rate ranges from 0% to 14%, falling within or below elective surgery mortality rates of 5% to 20%.[85,92–110] Outcomes have improved over time with accumulated technical expertise, the use of commercially manufactured devices, and improved patient selection criteria.

The published collective experiences of the European Collaborators on Stent-Graft Techniques for Abdominal Aortic Aneurysm Repair (EUROSTAR) and United Kingdom Thoracic Endograft registries ($n = 249$) demonstrate successful deployment in 87% of cases, a 30-day mortality rate of 5% for elective cases, and paraplegia and endoleak rates of 4% each.[110] The FDA phase II trial data from exclusive deployment of the Gore TAG endograft in 142 patients with TAA revealed similar results: technical success in 98%, a 30-day mortality rate of 1.5%, paraplegia in 3.5%, and endoleak in 8.8%.[109] These results cannot be directly compared with the outcomes of contemporary surgical studies. Most patients with TAA repaired by the endovascular approach in these studies were older and sicker, having been deemed high-risk patients or not suitable for open surgical repair. For example, according to the American Society of Anesthesiologists (ASA) physical status classification, which predicts procedural risk (i.e., low risk, 1 to 2; intermediate risk, 3; high risk, 4 to 5; organ donor, 6), 52% of patients in the combined EUROSTAR and United Kingdom registries were preoperatively classified as ASA 3 or higher.[110]

True comparisons between conventional therapy and the endovascular alternative can be made only after the completion of prospective, randomized, controlled trials. Although these trials are being conducted, a few studies have compared endovascular treatment with anatomically similar open surgery historical controls. As part of the phase II Gore Excluder study, 19 TAA patients who were candidates for open repair received stent graft therapy and were compared with a nonrandomized cohort of 10 patients who had undergone open repair before the availability of thoracic stent grafts.[101] All aneurysms met the same inclusion and exclusion criteria for anatomic involvement. The 1-year survival rate was 89.5% for the endovascular group and 70% for the operative group. As expected, mean hospital stay (6.2 vs. 16.3 days) and length of intervention (155 vs. 256 minutes) were significantly less for those treated endovascularly. In a similar study, Ehrlich and colleagues found a decreased 30-day mortality rate (10% vs. 31%), mean hospital stay (6 vs. 10 days), and mean intervention time (150 vs. 325 minutes) with endovascular repair; the paraplegia rate was also decreased (0% vs. 12%).[96]

Complications and Outcomes

The thoracic aorta has unique anatomic features and a distinctive biomechanical and hemodynamic environment, which explain some of the rare late complications specific to devices used in this location. The descending thoracic aorta, unlike the abdominal aorta, is relatively mobile in the chest and is subject to a complex and vigorous three-dimensional motion. Fixation points are the aortic root, origins of major branches, and a long, mobile aortic segment extending from the LSA to the celiac artery. The thoracic aorta elongates, angulates, and enlarges between these points, and aneurysms may develop.

The mechanical forces exert a complex pattern of dynamic circumferential, radial, and axial forces on thoracic stent grafts, resulting in a stress field significantly different from that exerted on abdominal stent grafts. Development of aneurysms of the dissected aorta after stent graft treatment is an infrequent event. False-lumen thrombosis due to thoracic endografting is essential to prevent late aortic expansion, and close clinical and imaging follow-up are essential to monitor anatomic changes over time.

An unresolved problem, even after successful thoracic stent graft placement, is the fate of the distal aortic segment. In the case of large reentry points, the thoracic-abdominal segment of the false lumen has a tendency to remain patent and remodel completely, setting the stage for late complications such as aneurysmal enlargement at the proximal or distal end of the stent graft. Other complications include perforations of the fragile aortic intima by the ends of the metallic stent, especially in the early phase of acute aortic dissection, and injuries caused by stiff guidewires and devices manipulation, setting the stage for aneurysmal evolution. The risk of these complications seems to be reduced by introducing the more flexible and soft-tip delivery systems with the aid of minimally traumatic thoracic guidewires specifically designed for the interventions. The duration of an endovascular procedure may also correlate with complications such as stroke or bleeding, both of which may be reduced by experienced operators requiring less than 30 minutes to complete a case.

TABLE 44.4 Summary Data on Studies of Endovascular Repair of Thoracic Aortic Aneurysm

Study	n	Mean Follow-Up (Months)	Devices	Technical Success	30-Day Mortality (%)	Long-Term Survival (%)	Paraplegia (%)	Endoleak (%)
Dake et al.[92]	103	22	Homemade	83% complete thrombosis	9	73 (actuarial 2 year)	3	24
Ehrlich et al.[96]	10	NA	Talent	80% complete thrombosis	10	NA	0	20
Cartes-Zumelzu et al.[97]	32	16	Excluder, Talent	90.6%	9.4	90.6 (32 months)	3.1	15.4
Grabenwoger et al.[98]	21	NA	Talent, Prograft	100%	9.5	NA	0	14.3
Greenberg et al.[99]	25	15.4	Homemade	NA	20 (12.5 for elective, 33 for emergent)	NA	12	12
Temudom et al.[100]	14	5.5	Homemade, Vanguard, Excluder	78.6%	14.3	NA	7.1	14.3
Najibi et al.[101]	24	12	Excluder, Talent	94.7%	5.3	89.5 (1 year)	0	0
Heijmen et al.[102]	28	21	Talent, AneuRx, Excluder	96.4%	0	96.4 (mean, 21 months)	0	28.6
Schoder et al.[103]	28	22.7	Excluder	100%, 89.3% complete exclusion	0	96.1 (1 year), 80.2 (3 years)	0	0 25
Marin et al.[104]	94	15.4	Excluder, Talent	85.1%	NA	NA	NA	24
Lepore et al.[105]	21	12	Excluder, Talent	100%	9.5	76.2 (1 year)	4.8	19
Sunder-Plassman et al.[106]	45	21	Corvita, Stenford, Vanguard, AneuRx, Talent, Excluder	NA	6.7	NA	2.2	22.2
Ouriel et al.[85]	31	6	Excluder, Talent, Other commercial	NA	12.9	81.6 (1 year)	6.5	32.3
Bergeron et al.[107]	33	24	Excluder, Talent	NA	9.1	75.8 (mean 24 months)	0	0
Czerny et al.[108]	54	38	Excluder, Talent	94.4%	9.3	63 (3 years event free)	0	27.8
Makaroun et al.[109]	142	29.6	TAG	97.9%	1.5	75 (2 years freedom from death)	3.5	8.8
Leurs et al.[110]	249	1–60	Excluder, Talent, Zenith, EndoFit	87%	10.4 (5.3 for elective, 27.9 for emergent)	80.3 (1 year)	4	4.2
Greenberg et al.[114]	100	14	Zenith	NA	NA	83 (1 year)	1	6
Wheatley et al.[115]	156	21.5	Gore	98.7%	3.8	76.6 (1 year)	0.6	11.5
Bavaria et al.[169]	140	24	Gore	98%	2.1	NA	2.9	10
Fairman et al.[170]	195	12	Talent	99.5%	2.1	83.9 (1 year, all cause); 96.9 (1 year, aneurysm related)	1.5 (paraplegia); 3.6 (stroke)	NA
Hughes et al.[171]	79	23	Zenith, Gore, Talent	98.7%	5.1	77 (55 months, overall); 86 (aorta specific)	1.3 (paraplegia); 2.5 (stroke)	2.5
Foley et al.[116]	195	60	Talent	100%	NA	43.9	NA	5.7 (type I, III)
Fossaceca et al.[117]	53	25.6	NA	100%	7.5	39	3.8	22.6
Matsumura et al.[118]	16	60	Zenith	100%	NA	37	NA	5.7
Nathan et al., 2015[177]	47	35	NA	NA	4.3	89 (50 months)	6.4	NA
Farber et al., 2017[178]	1333	60	Bolton Relay	97	5.3	91.3 (60 months, aneurysm related)	2.6	4.5

NA, Not applicable.

Patency of the abdominal aortic false lumen may be related to persistent communications between the true lumen and false lumen. Treatment of these communications at the level of distal thoracic and abdominal aorta can obliterate the false lumen and reduce the aortic diameter, but in practice, closure is difficult to achieve because of the proximity or involvement of the visceral branches. Another source of late complications is distention of the aorta beyond the portion covered by the stent graft due to the mechanical weakness of the dissected aortic walls. Prevention of these complications can be partially achieved during the primary procedure by ensuring adequate landing zones proximal and distal to the stent graft and by closure of large fenestrations along the length of the false lumen.

Prosthetic graft infection is a rare complication. The diagnosis requires imaging, hematologic, and clinical studies. The findings of air in the aneurysm sac or excessive soft tissue accumulation and progressive enlargement of the aneurysm sac point to a stent infection. Similarly, in the setting of suspicious imaging results, raised levels of systemic inflammation markers may be informative, as are the clinical symptoms of an infection. In most cases, positron emission tomography (PET) radionuclide studies are helpful.

Treatment of thoracic endograft infection depends on the diagnostic certainty, pathogenesis of the organism, extent of infection, and the presenting features and medical comorbidities of the patient. The spectrum of management strategies includes conservative treatment with targeted antibiotics delivered peripherally or by direct puncture and instillation into the perigraft space, insertion of another stent graft inside the infected graft, and excision of the infected stent graft with debridement of the surrounding tissue and in situ or extraanatomic vascular reconstruction.

Treatment of aortic graft infection remains problematic. In the absence of management algorithms that can define treatment in particular conditions based on patient presentation and degree of infection, decisions must be tailored to each patient and weigh the risks of the available options. A decision must be made about whether treatment is intended to be curative or palliative. Curative treatment that requires an aggressive approach with open surgery and that is associated with a relatively high mortality rate may be justified. In cases of palliation, placement of an endovascular graft (graft-in-graft approach) to prevent life-threatening bleeding or fistulation may be considered. Patients with complex graft disease should always be treated in experienced centers that have the required treatment modalities at their disposal.

With avoidance of aortic cross-clamping and prolonged iatrogenic hypotension, endovascular TAA repair was expected to result in lower incidences of paraplegia compared with conventional treatment. The initial concern after stent graft placement was the risk of spinal cord ischemia due to the frequent need to cover multiple intercostal arteries and the artery of Adamkiewicz, usually the only prominent intersegmental branch from the aorta at the lower thoracic or upper lumbar level. Paraplegia rates have ranged from 0% to 5% in endovascular studies,[85,92–110] compared with 5% to 25% for open repair cases.[72,74,79–82] Although low, these rates remain significant, especially because it is impossible to reimplant intercostal arteries in this setting. Some evidence suggests that the occurrence of paraplegia is associated with concomitant or prior surgical AAA repair and increased exclusion length due to the absence of lumbar and hypogastric collateral circulation.[99–119] Adjunctive measures to further reduce spinal cord ischemic complication rates in endovascular TAA repair are being investigated.[120]

Endoleaks are the most prevalent complications after TAA stent graft treatment. However, their observed frequency is substantially less than that reported for AAA endograft repair,[121] and the distribution of endoleak types is also different. TAA endoleaks occur more commonly at the proximal or distal attachment site (type I endoleak), whereas most AAA endoleaks are type II.[122] Type I endoleaks are more serious and require expeditious intervention because they represent direct communications between the aneurysm sac and aortic blood flow.[123]

Treatment options for endoleaks include transcatheter coil or glue embolization, balloon angioplasty, placement of endovascular graft extensions, and open repair.[124,125] Although current anatomic criteria limit thoracic stent graft exclusion to lesions located at least 15 to 25 mm away from the origin of the LSA and celiac trunk, it is common for descending TAAs to be located within the proximal or distal neck length necessary for adequate fixation. At the proximal end, the landing zone can be extended by prophylactic transposition of the LSA to the left carotid artery or by bypass graft placement.[86] Alternatively, the uncovered proximal portion of the Talent endograft can be placed across the LSA origin to achieve fixation without blocking flow. However, case reports of inadvertent coverage of the LSA origin found no resulting complications,[126] and subsequent studies determined that these maneuvers may not be necessary as long as there is no obstruction of the right vertebral or carotid artery and the left internal mammary artery is not used as a coronary bypass conduit.[88–90] Complications such as left arm ischemia have been rare, possibly due to collateral blood supply through retrograde left vertebral flow. Most centers intentionally cover the LSA origin if necessary and reserve secondary revascularization procedures for treatment of related symptoms if they develop.[55,86]

For more proximal TAAs involving the aortic arch, branched and fenestrated stent grafts are being developed to accommodate perfusion through the great vessels.[127,128] Although feasibility has been demonstrated, it is already apparent that the required implantation techniques would be highly complex and would demand considerable technical expertise. Some centers have been investigating techniques to create fenestrations intraoperatively after device deployment and coverage of critical branches.[129]

In contrast, there are no easy management strategies to deal with a short distal neck. In this setting, fenestrated and branched grafts have been used in isolated cases, but the overall experience is limited. Intentional coverage of the celiac artery is not recommended given the risk of hepatic and visceral ischemia. Although a normal superior mesenteric artery may provide collateral flow, no methods exist to predetermine whether the collateral supply would be sufficient. Moreover, the celiac trunk may serve as a prominent source of retrograde endoleak if the artery is covered without adjunctive transcatheter occlusion.

In distal aneurysms that involve the descending thoracic and the abdominal aorta, combined open AAA repair and endovascular TAA exclusion is a novel treatment approach under investigation. Stent grafts are also being used to treat patients with diffuse aneurysmal disease involving the entire thoracic aorta. In these patients, the traditional surgical treatment is a two-stage procedure called the *elephant trunk technique*.[130] In the first stage, the ascending aorta and aortic arch are repaired by a median sternotomy, and an extra-long graft is used for reconstruction, which leaves the excess portion of the graft, the elephant trunk, dangling within the lumen of the remaining diseased aorta. In the second stage, the lesion in the descending aorta is repaired by a left thoracotomy, and the graft replacement is connected to the elephant trunk proximally. To bypass the need for thoracotomy, a few centers have successfully deployed thoracic stent grafts into the elephant trunk extension, replacing the second stage of the traditional elephant trunk procedure.[131]

Following closely on the heels of early clinical experiences with stent grafting for TAA repair, experimental application of the less invasive approach has been extended to a growing number of other pathologies of the thoracic aorta. They include aortic dissection,[5] traumatic aortic injury,[132] penetrating atherosclerotic ulcer,[133] and aortic rupture.[62]

ABDOMINAL AORTIC ANEURYSM

Therapeutic Strategies

Aneurysm of the abdominal aorta represents a potentially life-threatening scenario affecting an increasingly important segment of the aging patient population. With improved overall health care, many patients reach an advanced age despite severe cardiovascular, hypertensive, and pulmonary comorbidities, providing time for an AAA to enlarge to a critical diameter and qualify for open surgical or endovascular treatment.

Although surgical resection and interposition of an abdominal aortic prosthesis (i.e., Dacron or Gore-Tex) have long been considered standard treatment, despite a well-known perioperative mortality risk, endovascular strategies have evolved over the past decade and have become an accepted standard of care for patients considered too sick or too old for open surgery. Advanced technology, ease of use, and the temptation of a fully percutaneous procedure have attracted a new breed of endovascular surgeons propelled by the prospect of avoiding surgical risk and inducing reconstructive remodeling of the aneurysmatic aorta through depressurization and complete exclusion of the aneurysmal sac.

After deployment, the stent graft bridges the region of the aneurysm, excluding it from the circulation while allowing aortic blood flow to continue distally through the prosthetic stent graft lumen. Between 30% and 60% of AAAs are anatomically suitable for endovascular repair. When repair is undertaken, the rate of successful stent graft implantation has ranged from 78% to 94%.

A major technical difficulty associated with the stent graft technique that has yet to be overcome is endoleaks. They occur in 10% to 20% of cases[134] and are seen angiographically as persistent contrast flow into the aneurysmal sac due to failure to completely exclude the aneurysm from the aortic circulation. If left untreated, endoleaks can leave the patient at risk for aneurysmal expansion or rupture. In a follow-up study of outcomes at 12 months or longer for more than 1000 stent graft recipients, the EUROSTAR investigators reported that almost 10% of patients per year required secondary interventions, suggesting that there should be caution in the broad application of endovascular aneurysmal repair (EVAR).[135]

Physicians have embraced EVAR as the method of choice to treat AAAs in high-risk patients. EVAR has great appeal for this older population because it leads to faster recovery with fewer systemic complications than open repair.[136-141] Parodi and colleagues[142] reported the first endovascular repair of an AAA in a human in 1991; they used a graft fashioned from prosthetic vascular grafts and expandable stents. More than 20,000 EVARs take place each year in the United States, representing 36% of all AAA repairs. More than 12% of procedures in Europe involve EVAR, and the expected annual growth rate is 15% (Medtronic Marketing Department, personal communication, 2006). EVAR is the method of choice for high-risk older patients because of its minimal incisions, shorter operating time, and reduced blood loss.

Indications for Treatment

Most asymptomatic AAAs are discovered serendipitously, often on imaging examinations for other complaints. Increasing evidence indicates that there is value to screening patients for AAA, and it is likely that screening will be approved in the near future.[143]

After the diagnosis of AAA is made, two critical questions need to be answered: when to intervene and how to intervene. The availability of EVAR has made these decisions somewhat more complex while adding a significant treatment option. Studies have questioned whether aneurysms smaller than 5 cm in diameter should be treated.[144] However, the clinical recommendation remains to offer treatment for aneurysms between 5 and 5.5 cm in diameter, depending on the results of clinical trials.[145] An exception to this guideline is that intervention should be offered despite the size of the aneurysm if symptoms develop or the aneurysm increases in size by 1 cm/year.[146] If the patient is a woman with smaller native vessels, the relative size that represents aneurysmal disease may be less than the conventional 5- to 5.5-cm range.

Patient selection has emerged as the most important factor for successful EVAR. Assessment begins with consideration of the body habitus and gender of the patient; small body size and female gender have been associated with a higher risk of procedure abortion.[147,148] The comorbidities of the patient must be assessed, with careful attention to cardiac, pulmonary, and renal conditions. Risk stratification analysis indicates that survival for those at low to minimal risk is excellent over 10 years. Those at highest risk succumb to cardiac disease or cancer, and survival is poorest for those patients.[149] EVAR has shown a reduction in 30-day mortality relative to that achieved with open repair (1.2% vs. 4.6%). Risk stratification determines survival in general and shows that both open surgery and EVAR decrease the risk of death from AAA rupture.[150]

The characteristics of the aneurysm must be matched to the most suitable device; this has a direct impact on outcomes and the complication profile of the procedure. The aneurysm is evaluated from a three-dimensional reconstruction CT scan or aortography with a calibrated catheter. At least four important features must be assessed before a patient's eligibility for EVAR can be determined, and this analysis leads to a list of contraindications (Table 44.5).[151] Experienced interventionists can deal with some of these challenges, but morphologic features of the aneurysm and access vessels may preclude EVAR.

The key features of endovascular repair of AAAs that determine procedural success and long-term outcomes are proximal and distal fixation and sealing. Most devices have a metal skeleton made of stainless steel, nitinol, or Elgiloy. Attachment is facilitated by the use of hooks or radial force. After the graft is inserted through the sheath, it can be deployed by a self-expanding mechanism or by balloon expansion. Some grafts attach superior to the renal arteries (i.e., suprarenal attachment), but most devices require at least 15 mm of proximal neck to achieve fixation and sealing in the infrarenal position. The grafts require different delivery system sizes (i.e., profiles). Low-profile devices permit access through smaller arteries.

Most complications associated with EVAR are minor and can be watched carefully or treated easily with additional interventional procedures. Some complications occur during or soon after the procedure, whereas others may be noticed only during graft surveillance.[152] A study by Ohki and colleagues[153] analyzed complication and death rates within 30 days after EVAR and reported them to be 17.6% and 8.5%, respectively. This remains an active and important area of EVAR research, and standards have been developed to facilitate reporting of endovascular abdominal aortic repair complications.[154]

TABLE 44.5 Evaluation for Endovascular Aneurysm Repair

Computed tomography assessment for EVAR eligibility
Proximal neck: diameter, length, angle, and presence or absence of thrombus
Distal landing zone: diameter and length
Iliac arteries: aneurysms and occlusive disease
Access arteries: diameter, occlusive disease
Contraindications for EVAR
Short proximal neck
Thrombus in proximal landing zone
Conical proximal neck
Greater than 120-degree angulation of the proximal neck
Critical inferior mesenteric artery
Significant iliac occlusive disease
Tortuosity of iliac vessels

EVAR, Endovascular aneurysm repair.

Endoleaks can have substantial clinical significance because they carry an increased risk of symptoms or aneurysmal rupture. The term *endoleak* describes the continuation of blood flow into the extragraft portion of the aneurysm; this flow increases the size of the aneurysmal sac.[155] Endoleaks occur in the acute setting during graft implantation or during the postoperative surveillance period. Most procedural endoleaks disappear without intervention. Endoleaks are graft related or nongraft related, and a classification system has been developed (Table 44.6).[156] Type I endoleaks occur when the attachment is not complete proximally or distally; blood can flow into the aneurysmal sac, and it is not completely occluded by endograft attachment to the arterial wall. Type II endoleaks result from continued backflow from aortic branches, such as the inferior mesenteric artery and lumbar arteries. Flow occurs retrograde into the aneurysmal sac around the endograft. Type III endoleaks are caused by defects in the endograft structure that lead to leakage of blood flow from inside the endograft to the aneurysmal sac. Type IV endoleaks occur early after endograft placement and resolve when the fabric's porosity is decreased by clotted blood.

Because endovascular repair uses a relatively new technology, graft surveillance for complications such as endoleaks is essential. Endoleaks are diagnosed by a variety of techniques: arteriography, pressure monitoring during or after the procedure, CT scanning, and duplex Doppler scanning. CT is the preferred method of detecting endoleaks. An analysis of 2463 patients from the EUROSTAR registry revealed that 171 had an endoleak by the time of their 1-month postoperative evaluation and 317 developed an endoleak at a later date.[157] Of these, 7.8% had a type II endoleak, and 12% had a type I, type III, or combination leak.

Endoleaks are treated by coil embolization, placement of stent graft cuffs and extensions, laparoscopic ligation of inferior mesenteric and lumbar arteries, open surgical repair, and repeat EVAR procedures. Type I and III endoleaks require fairly urgent intervention because blood flow and sac pressure will continue to increase and lead to rupture. Type IV endoleaks usually resolve on their own. The management of type II endoleaks is more controversial because some of them thrombose on their own, whereas others lead to sac enlargement.

Endograft surveillance is important to document normal and abnormal morphologic changes in the repair and in the involved vessels. This process is vital for the detection of endoleaks, increased aneurysm diameter, and device migration.[158] The recommended surveillance routine includes a CT scan at 1, 6, and 12 months and annually thereafter. If an endoleak is detected, scanning frequency increases to every 6 months until resolution of the endoleak is confirmed.

The use of EVAR technology has led to a greater understanding of the basic science of aneurysmal disease. For example, Curci and Thompson[159] have been studying the relationship between the secretion of matrix metalloproteinases (MMPs) and AAAs. They have measured increased levels in the aneurysmal wall compared with the normal arterial wall.

Randomized Trial Data and Analysis

The EVAR Study Group has provided important revelations from randomized studies on the treatment of the moving target called AAA in the context of increasing age of patients, continuously refined technology, and improving operator skills. Whereas treatment of large AAAs with EVAR reduced the 30-day mortality rate to 1.7%, compared with 4.7% with open repair ($P < .009$) on an intention-to-treat basis, the investigators were prudent to judge the early benefits only as a license to continue evaluation of EVAR by the use of longer follow-up.[160,161] However, no differences were seen in total mortality or aneurysm-related mortality in the long-term follow-up.[162]

In the Dutch Randomized Endovascular Aneurysm Repair (DREAM) study, 6 years after randomization, endovascular and open repair of AAAs resulted in similar rates of survival (68.9% vs. 69.9%, $P = .97$).[163] Scores for measures of quality of life and sexual functioning favored EVAR only in the early postoperative period but equalized after 6 months compared with open repair, in parallel with a need for continued reinterventions with EVAR. A closer look, however, revealed that many late complications after successful EVAR had low prognostic impact, such as endoleak type II requiring reintervention in only 17 of 79 cases. Severe complications such as graft rupture ($n = 9$), graft migration ($n = 12$), endoleak type I ($n = 27$), and graft thrombosis ($n = 12$), which required reintervention in 35 of 60 cases, were likely to be attributed to technical or procedural problems with the stent graft or unsuitable anatomy, underscoring the inherently immature nature of an emerging technology. Moreover, at least six different brands of endovascular devices were used by surgeons with different levels of experience.

Endovascular repair of AAAs was associated with a significantly lower rate of aneurysm-related mortality than no repair in patients who were ineligible for open repair (adjusted hazard ratio [HR] = 0.53; 95% confidence interval [CI] 0.32 to 0.89; $P = .02$). The 30-day operative mortality was 7.3% in the endovascular repair group. The overall rate of aneurysmal rupture in the no-intervention group was 12.4 (95% CI 9.6 to 16.2) per 100 person-years. This advantage did not result in any benefit in terms of total mortality (adjusted HR = 0.99; 95% CI 0.78 to 1.27; $P = .97$). A total of 48% of patients who survived endovascular repair had graft-related complications, and 27% required reintervention within the first 6 years. During 8 years of follow-up, endovascular repair was considerably more expensive than no repair (cost difference, £9826 [U.S. $14,867]; 95% CI 7638 to 12,013 [11,556 to 18,176]).[164,165]

The data presented by the EVAR trialists (30-day and midterm outcomes in EVAR 1 and data from EVAR 2 for patients unfit for open surgery) are sobering, but they also are provocative and revealing.[166,167] In accordance with the DREAM studies,[161,163,168,169] EVAR 1 showed significant early survival benefit after 30 days with endovascular repair due to reduced periinterventional risk, corroborating previous observational evidence.[37,38,170] Careful analysis of randomized data has provided highly valuable information.

Health status comprising age, comorbidities, and prognostic confounders was the most important denominator of individual prognosis, followed by, to a lesser degree, the nonsurgical nature of EVAR (which can be performed percutaneously with local anesthesia). Assessment of the general state of health of older and sicker patients and serious attempts at improvement should precede EVAR. Examples are cardiopulmonary workup, potentially including percutaneous coronary intervention, and respiratory improvement as integral parts of strategic planning. For some

TABLE 44.6 Classification of Endoleaks

Type I: Attachment-site leaks
   Proximal end of endograft
   Distal end of endograft
   Iliac occluder (plug)

Type II: Branch leaks (without attachment-site connection)
   Simple or to-and-fro (from only one patent branch)
   Complex or flow-through (with two or more patent branches)

Type III: Graft defect
   Junctional leak or modular disconnect
   Fabric disruption (midgraft hole)
   Minor (≤2 mm, such as suture holes)
   Major (≥2 mm)

Type IV: Graft wall (fabric) porosity (30 days after graft placement)

conditions, it appears justified to reject EVAR when conservative care is more appropriate.

The nature of complications requiring reinterventions after EVAR is often related to technical shortcomings with current-generation devices or to unsuitable anatomy. Physicians and the industry must recognize those limitations and develop better devices and improved selection algorithms for treatment with EVAR.

Although the endovascular community should always embrace the *primum non nocere* principle and avoid well-intended but harmful treatment, it should also appreciate the evolving nature of the problem. Some patients considered unfit for surgery do improve and find themselves in a lower-risk category and fit for surgery or EVAR. EVAR technology and interventional skills improve with time and training, and the short-term differential advantage over open surgery is likely to increase.

Elderly patients may express a personal preference for a less traumatic procedure such as EVAR performed by an expert despite the lack of a clear-cut midterm advantage and accept surveillance and interventions during follow-up. The higher costs of follow-up imaging needed with EVAR may be dramatically reduced with a smarter surveillance strategy based on clinical and ultrasound interrogation instead of serial CT or MRI.

Although EVAR may not improve the AAA prognosis compared with classic surgery at midterm, resulting in a current draw after an early advantage, EVAR is here to stay. Better staging and selection of patients, constantly improving technology,[37] and the expertise of centers of excellence for aortic diseases can enhance matching patients with therapeutic options, including EVAR or conservative treatment. It is still wise to use clinical judgment and to offer a holistic approach with intelligent use of prognosticating tools and interdisciplinary cooperation, especially for the growing segment of older patients with multiple comorbidities.

Whether the results of the EVAR trials and the Cautious voice of Jonathan Michaels[39] will halt the trend of increasing use of EVAR instead of open surgery remains to be seen. It is certain, however, that the randomized data from EVAR 1 and EVAR 2 will refocus the debate on natural history and patient selection for a forward-moving technology.

KEY REFERENCES

1. Hagan PG, Nienaber CA, Isselbacher EM, et al. The International Registry of Aortic Dissection (IRAD). *JAMA*. 2000;283:897–903.
2. Erbel R, Aboyans V, Boileau C, et al. 2014 ESC Guidelines on the diagnosis and treatment of aortic disease: document covering acute and chronic aortic disease of the thoracic and abdominal aorta of the adult. The Task Force for the diagnosis and treatment of aortic diseases of the European Society of Cardiology (ESC). *Eur Heart J*. 2014;35:2873–2926.
5. Nienaber CA, Fattori R, Lund G, et al. Nonsurgical reconstruction of thoracic aortic dissection by stent graft placement. *N Engl J Med*. 1999;340:1539–1545.
25. Svensson LG, Kouchoukos NF, Miller DC, et al. Expert consensus document on the treatment of descending thoracic aortic disease using endovascular stent grafts. *Ann Thorac Surg*. 2008;85:S1–S41.
27. Tsai TT, Fattori R, Trimarchi S, et al. Long-term survival in patients with type B acute aortic dissection: insight from the International Registry of Acute Aortic Dissection. *Circulation*. 2006;114:2226–2231.
31. Fattori R, Tsai TT, Myrmel T, et al. Complicated acute type B dissection: is surgery still the best option? *JACC Cardiovasc Interv*. 2008;1:395–402.
32. Nienaber CA, Kische S, Zeller T, et al. Provisional extension to induce complete attachment after stent graft placement in type B aortic dissection: the PETTICOAT concept. *J Endovasc Ther*. 2006;13:738–746.
47. Eggebrecht H, Herold U, Kuhnt O, et al. Endovascular stent graft treatment of aortic dissection: determinants of postinterventional outcome. *Eur Heart J*. 2005;26:489–497.
50. Nienaber CA, Kische S, Rousseau H, et al. Endovascular repair of type B aortic dissection: long-term results of the randomized investigation of stent grafts in aortic dissection trial. *Circ Cardiovasc Interv*. 2013;6:407–416.
52. Nienaber CA, Rousseau H, Eggebrecht H, et al. Randomized comparison of strategies for type B aortic dissection: the Investigation of STEnt grafts in Aortic Dissection (INSTEAD) trial. *Circulation*. 2009;120:2519–2528.
54. Koschyk DH, Nienaber CA, Knap M, et al. How to guide stent graft implantation in type B aortic dissection? Comparison of angiography, transesophageal echocardiography, and intravascular ultrasound. *Circulation*. 2005;112(suppl I):I-260–I-264.
56. Eggebrecht H, Thompson M, Rousseau H, et al. European Registry on Endovascular Aortic Repair Complications. Retrograde ascending aortic dissection during or after thoracic aortic stent graft placement: insight from the European registry on endovascular aortic repair complications. *Circulation*. 2009;120(suppl 11):S276–S281.
66. Crawford ES, DeNatale RW. Thoracoabdominal aortic aneurysm: observations regarding the natural course of the disease. *J Vasc Surg*. 1986;3:578–582.
110. Leurs LJ, Bell R, Degrieck Y, et al. Endovascular treatment of thoracic aortic diseases: combined experience from the EUROSTAR and United Kingdom Thoracic Endograft registries. *J Vasc Surg*. 2004;40:670–679.
142. Parodi JC, Palmaz JC, Barone HD. Transfemoral intraluminal graft implantation for abdominal aortic aneurysms. *Ann Vasc Surg*. 1991;5:491–497.
162. Greenhalgh RM, Brown LC, Powel JT, et al. for The United Kingdom EVAR Trial Investigators. Endovascular versus open repair of abdominal aortic aneurysm. *N Engl J Med*. 2010;362:1863–1871.
163. DeBruin JL, Baas AF, Buth J, for the DREAM Study Group, et al. Long-term outcome of open or endovascular repair of abdominal aortic aneurysm. *N Engl J Med*. 2010;362:1881–1889.

Additional references available online at expertconsult.com.

中文导读

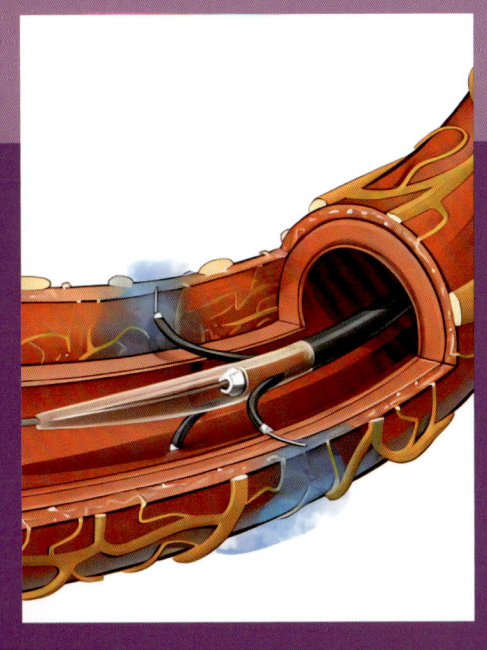

第45章
静脉介入

　　静脉疾病是外周血管疾病的重要组成部分，近年来静脉病变的发病率逐年上升，影响到多达1/4的人口。外周静脉疾病若得不到及时治疗，将会出现外周组织肿胀、色素沉着及溃疡等；而若重要器官的静脉系统发生病变，可能会严重影响器官功能甚至危及生命。外科手术是静脉疾病的经典治疗手段，但在外科治疗过程中出现的疗效不确切、手术创伤较大等问题日益引起业界的关注。近年来，随着冠状动脉介入的蓬勃发展，冠状动脉介入相关的技术逐步在静脉系统展开应用，使得以往许多棘手的疾病都可以通过静脉腔内介入技术得到治疗。介入微创手术因其疗效显著、并发症低、术后恢复迅速，已经成为未来静脉治疗发展的大趋势。在本章节中，作者从静脉系统的解剖特点与病理生理机制切入，由浅入深阐述了中心静脉狭窄、上下肢深静脉血栓的诊断、药物和导管治疗，以及下腔静脉过滤器的插入和取回。整个章节全面细致、贴合临床实际操作，为有志于从事静脉介入领域的医师搭建了一条高效学习的快车道。

孟　真　张洪亮

章节要点

- 静脉疾病——包括急性（深静脉血栓、肺栓塞）和慢性（血栓形成后综合征、溃疡、静脉曲张）疾病，在全世界范围内广泛流行，影响到多达1/4的人口。
- 浅静脉疾病可以有明显的症状，但通常很容易用微创消融技术治疗。
- 上腔静脉综合征表现为面部、手臂和上胸部的严重充血和水肿，并可能导致呼吸困难、认知功能障碍和头痛症状。病因常与恶性肿瘤、导管留置和起搏器导线有关。
- Paget-Schroetter综合征表现为剧烈运动后上肢自发性深静脉血栓形成，部位通常在患者的优势臂。重复性的高强度运动导致血管内膜的微创伤，进一步引发凝血级联的激活。
- 与导管留置或起搏器导线无关的上肢深静脉血栓应促使进一步检查血管压迫综合征。
- 多普勒超声检查因其具有易获取、便携、可重复性好和成本低廉等优势，通常是诊断深静脉血栓（上肢或下肢）的首选检查方法。然而，多普勒超声对中心静脉狭窄的诊断效能有限。
- 在未经治疗的近端深静脉血栓中，临床肺动脉栓塞的发病率很高，并且与高死亡率有关。经过规范治疗，肺动脉栓塞的发病率可下降到5%，死亡率可低于1%。
- 目前越来越多的证据表明下腔静脉完全闭塞是静脉系统疾病的主要来源。使用静脉内介入技术进行髂—腔静脉重建具有较好的长期通畅性。
- 可回收的下腔静脉过滤器是治疗有抗凝禁忌证或复发性肺动脉栓塞患者的重要辅助工具，同时对治疗"自由漂浮"的髂静脉血栓患者或心肺功能受损的患者也有获益。
- 经皮机械血栓切除术是导管溶栓治疗的重要辅助技术，可缩短静脉闭塞时间，缩短住院时间，减少出血风险，并节省总体费用。

45 Venous Intervention

Michael A. Jolly, Mitchell J. Silver

KEY POINTS

- Venous disease, both acute (deep vein thrombosis [DVT], pulmonary embolism [PE]) and chronic (postthrombotic syndrome, ulcers, varicose veins), is widely prevalent, affecting up to a quarter of the population.
- Superficial vein disease can be highly symptomatic but often easily treated with minimally invasive ablative techniques.
- The superior vena cava (SVC) syndrome manifests as severe congestion and edema of the face, arms, and upper thorax, and may progress to dyspnea, cognitive dysfunction, and headache. It is commonly associated with malignancy, indwelling catheters, or pacemaker leads.
- Patients with Paget-Schroetter syndrome (PSS) develop spontaneous DVT of the upper extremity, usually in the dominant arm, after strenuous physical activity. Heavy repetitive exertion causes microtrauma to the vessel intima and leads to activation of the coagulation cascade.
- Upper extremity DVT not associated with indwelling catheters or pacemaker leads should prompt further workup for a vascular compression syndrome.
- Duplex ultrasonography is generally the initial test of choice for the diagnosis of DVT (in upper or lower extremities) due to its widespread availability, portability, reproducibility, and cost. However, it has a limited role for central venous stenosis.
- Clinical PE has a high prevalence in untreated proximal DVT and is associated with a high mortality rates. Under treatment, the incidence of PE decrease to 5%, and the mortality to less than 1%.
- Complete inferior vena cava occlusion is becoming increasingly recognized as a major source of venous morbidity. Iliocaval reconstruction using modern endovenous techniques has excellent long-term patency.
- Retrievable inferior vena cava filters are important adjuncts in the care of patients with contraindications to anticoagulation or recurrent PE. They can also be beneficial in the treatment of patients with "free-floating" iliac vein thrombus, or in patients with compromised cardiopulmonary reserve.
- Percutaneous mechanical thrombectomy is an important adjunct to catheter-directed thrombolysis and may result in a shorter time to vein patency, shorter length of hospitalization, reduction in hemorrhagic risk, and overall cost savings.

INTRODUCTION

As interventional cardiologists have expanded their skill set from coronary interventions to the endovascular management of peripheral arterial disease, venous intervention has also gradually become a common part of the "global cardiovascular interventionalist's" repertoire. In fact, as more and more interventional cardiologists recognize the high prevalence, morbidity, and mortality associated with venous disease in their patient populations, more have become interested in the management of venous disorders. These include both the medical and catheter-based treatment of central venous stenosis, upper and lower extremity deep venous thrombosis (LEDVT), and the insertion and retrieval of inferior vena cava (IVC) filters, to name a few.

THE VENOUS SYSTEM: BASIC HISTOLOGY AND PHYSIOLOGY

Veins are larger in caliber and more numerous then arteries. Arteries of the extremities run in the deep compartments, protected from superficial injury. Veins, on the other hand, course in both the deep and superficial spaces. In addition, the venous system has a much greater volume capacity than the arterial system, with thinner and less elastic walls. Most anatomists distinguish three layers in the walls of veins: tunica intima, tunica media, and tunica adventitia. While the distinctions between the layers are subtle, in general the venous internal elastic membrane is poorly defined, and the tunica media is much less developed compared to that of arteries.

Similar to the arterial system, veins are commonly categorized into three major groups: large size veins, medium size veins, and venules and small size veins. Only medium and large size veins will be discussed in this chapter; for a complete review of venous embryology and anatomy, please refer to an anatomic text book.

Medium size veins range between 2 and 9 mm in diameter. These include veins from extremities distal to the axillary or inguinal crease, and cutaneous veins. The intima consists of endothelium, basal lamina, and reticular fibers. The media consists of a very thin layer of circular smooth muscle and few collagen fibers. The adventitia, the thickest of all the layers, consists of both collagen and elastic fibers.

The large size veins consist of veins central to the axillary or inguinal crease, superior vena cava (SVC), IVC, renal veins, hepatic veins, and azygos veins. The intima is similar to the medium size veins. Interestingly, a tunica media is lacking in most of the large veins, with the exception of the gravid uterus and pulmonary veins. A thick adventitia makes up the greater part of the thickness of the wall. This layer is rich in elastic fibers and longitudinally oriented collagen. The IVC is exceptional in that its adventitia contains scattered longitudinal bundles of smooth muscle. Large size veins, similar to large arteries, get their nutrient blood supply from very small penetrating vessels called vasa vasorum.

Vein Valves

Valve leaflets are a thin fold of the intima, with a thin layer of collagen and a network of elastic fibers that extend toward the intima of the vessel wall. Anatomically, valves are generally bicuspid in structure and are more numerous in the veins of the lower extremity, where the force of gravity is greatest. In general, small and large size veins have no valves. The wall of the vessel becomes thinner and slightly expanded just above the attachment of each valve cusp, creating a cavity called the *valve sinus*. When competent, the valves are forced shut by the weight of the column of blood above and the manner in which this column interacts with the valve sinus. This interaction causes valvule coaptation, preventing venous reflux (Fig. 45.1).

Only medium size veins have valves, as their predominant function is to ensure the antegrade flow of blood. This includes flow both peripheral to central and superficial to deep, with unidirectional valves preventing retrograde flow of blood away from the heart

Physiology

The venous system has a large capacity, accounting for approximately two-thirds of the systemic blood volume. Veins, because of their unique vascular structure, can undergo a large change in volume with minimal change in transmural pressure. This characteristic is called *venous capacitance*.

Because of their low elastic tissue content and collagen dense adventitia, veins are actually stiffer than arteries when compared at the same distending pressure. A person standing at rest has significantly elevated venous pressures at the level of the feet and calves, accumulating a large volume of blood in the lower extremities. The calf muscles augment venous return by working as a hydraulic pump. During walking or exercise, calf muscle contraction pushes the accumulated blood toward the heart, decreasing the venous pressures close to zero. The venous pressure remains low even during calf muscle relaxation. At this time, the unidirectional venous valves prevent backflow of blood, but allow antegrade flow towards the heart. It is imperative that the venous valves are competent for the calf pump system to work efficiently. A normal pump system reduces venous pressures and volume in the exercising muscle, increases venous return, and improves arterial perfusion.

Varicose Veins

Incompetent valves in the saphenous system permit reflux of blood from the central veins to the peripheral veins. The superficial veins dilate once the volume of retrograde flow exceeds their capacity; this ultimately leads to poor coaptation and venous valve incompetence. This valve incompetence can occur in the deep and superficial systems, creating a standing column of blood with a constant increase in pressure. The transmission of an elevated venous pressure into the superficial system leads to the characteristic clinical sequalae known as varicose veins.

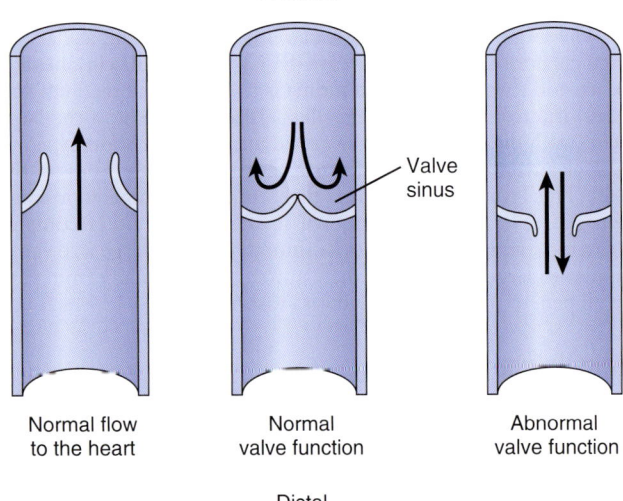

Fig. 45.1 Venous valves with schematic representation of normal and abnormal function.

Chronic Venous Disease

Chronic venous insufficiency is a significant problem in the United States, affecting as much as 25 to 40 million people. Venous valve incompetence is central to the underlying venous hypertension that appears to underlie most or all signs of chronic venous disease. Chronic venous disease afflicts a younger segment of the population, and the morbidity of edema, leg pain, and ulceration may result in lifestyle alterations, loss of work, and frequent hospitalizations. The prevalence of venous ulcerations is not restricted to the elderly, but certainly increases with age.[1] It has been estimated that venous ulcers have had a major negative economic impact, with the loss of approximately 2 million working days, and incur treatment costs of approximately $3 billion dollars per year in the United States.[2] The chief clinical manifestations of chronic venous disease are aching, leg pain, heaviness, a sensation of swelling, itching, cramping, and restless legs. Chronic venous disease can be graded according to the descriptive clinical, etiologic, anatomical, and pathophysiological (CEAP) classification, which provides an orderly framework for communication and decision making (Table 45.1).[3] The pathophysiology of chronic venous disease in regard to its clinical expression has been well described, involving venous valve incompetence,

TABLE 45.1 Revised CEAP Classification of Chronic Venous Disorders

CLINICAL CLASSIFICATION	
C_0	No visible or palpable signs of venous disease
C_1	Telangiectasias, reticular veins, malleolar flares
C_2	Varicose veins
C_3	Edema without skin changes
C_4	Skin changes ascribed to venous disease (e.g., pigmentation, venous eczema, lipodermatosclerosis)
C_{4a}	Pigmentation or eczema
C_{4b}	Lipodermatosclerosis or atrophie blanche
C_5	Skin changes as defined above with healed ulceration
C_6	Skin changes as defined above with active ulceration
S	Symptomatic, including ache, pain, tightness, skin irritation, heaviness, and muscle cramps, and other complaints attributable to venous dysfunction
A	Asymptomatic
ETIOLOGIC CLASSIFICATION	
Ec	Congenital
Ep	Primary
Es	Secondary (postthrombotic)
En	No venous cause identified
ANATOMIC CLASSIFICATION	
As	Superficial veins
Ap	Perforator veins
Ad	Deep veins
An	No venous location identified
PATHOPHYSIOLOGIC CLASSIFICATION	
Pr	Reflux
Po	Obstruction
Pr,o	Reflux and obstruction
Pn	No venous pathophysiology identifiable

CEAP, Clinical, etiologic, anatomical, and pathophysiological. Adapted from Eklöf B, Rutherford R, Bergan J, et al. Revision of the CEAP classification for chronic venous disorders: consensus statement. *J Vasc Surg*. 2004;40:1248–1252.

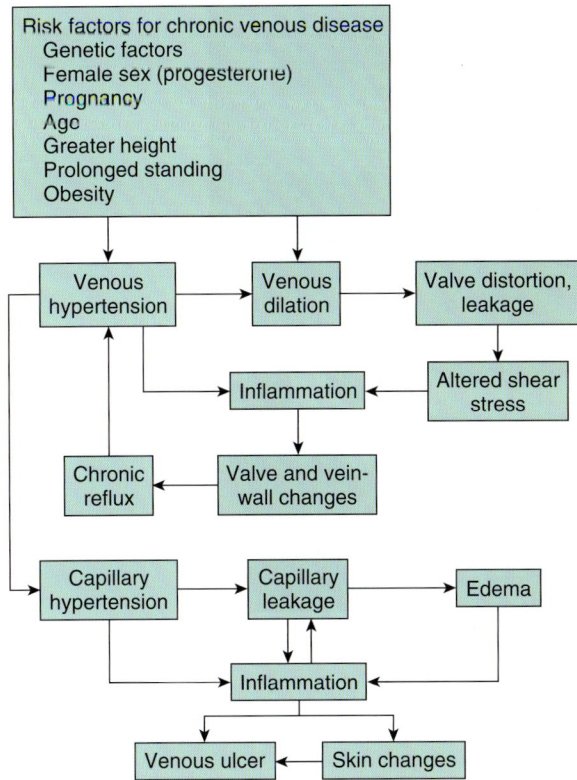

Fig. 45.2 Venous hypertension as the hypothetical cause of the clinical manifestations of chronic venous disease, emphasizing the importance of inflammation.

structural changes in the vein wall (manifest as hypertrophy), and the role of elevated venous pressure and shear stress.[4] There has been new progress made in understanding the pathophysiology of the skin changes of chronic venous disease. These studies have emerged to validate that chronic inflammation has a key role in the skin changes of chronic venous disease. Support for the role of chronic inflammation in chronic venous disease has come to be known as the microvascular leukocyte-trapping hypothesis, where elegant studies have shown elevated numbers of macrophages, T lymphocytes, and mast cells in skin biopsy specimens from lower limbs affected by chronic venous disease.[5] The chronic inflammatory state in patients with chronic venous disease is related to the skin changes that are typical of the condition.[4] Increased expression and activity of metalloproteinase (MMP, especially MMP2) has been reported in lipodermatosclerosis,[6] venous leg ulcers,[7] and wound fluid from nonhealing ulcers.[8]

The treatment of chronic venous disease has evolved considerably over the past few years and is aimed at preventing venous hypertension, venous reflux, and chronic inflammation (Fig. 45.2). Compression stockings remain the initial therapy for controlling venous hypertension, and are often the initial treatment before undertaking an interventional procedure such as endovenous laser ablation (EVLA). Endovenous ablation procedures utilizing laser energy or radio frequency are now available to treat venous reflux, and are becoming a common part of the armamentarium used to combat chronic venous disease. As such, this has become an area of interest of those "vascular minded" interventional cardiologists.

Superficial Vein Ablation

EVLA is a percutaneous technique that uses laser energy to ablate incompetent superficial veins. The axial veins are the primary target for this therapy and include the great saphenous vein (GSV), small saphenous vein (SSV), and accessory saphenous veins (ASVs).

The other alternative approaches to the treatment of chronic venous disease include radiofrequency energy, liquid and foam sclerotherapy, and open surgical management. A review of these other modalities is beyond the scope of this chapter and, as such, we will focus on EVLA.

The indications for EVLA are the same as other vein ablation therapies, including radiofrequency ablation, sclerotherapy, and open surgical stripping. The use of open surgical vein stripping for symptomatic varicose veins has become less as these other percutaneous options have evolved.

Venous ablation is indicated in patients with symptoms and signs of venous disease that persist in spite of a trial of medical management. This constellation of symptoms and clinical findings would include chronic leg pain and achiness, recurrent stasis cellulitis, venous stasis ulcers, and preulcerative skin changes. From a physiologic standpoint, documenting reflux in the target vein (i.e., retrograde flow >0.5 seconds) is essential before entertaining EVLA (Fig. 45.3). In addition, the patient's symptoms should directly relate to the incompetent veins being treated.

Absolute contraindications for EVLA would include patients with acute deep vein thrombosis (DVT) and pregnancy, due to the risk of developing a new DVT.[9] We prefer to wait a minimum of 6 weeks after delivery in pregnant patients before performing EVLA.

Relative contraindications to EVLA for a given vein segment include

- Chronic or recurrent phlebitis in the target vein, since formation of synechiae in the vein can prevent passage of the laser sheath. This decision should be based on duplex ultrasound screening.
- Passage of the device may not be possible in severely tortuous venous segments.
- Due to the concern of skin burns, the target vein should ideally be at least 1 cm deep to the skin dermis after the tumescent anesthesia is applied.
- Aneurysms of the GSV are at a greater risk of procedural failure. In general, an aneurysmal vein segment of greater than 2.5 cm is not ideal for EVLA.

As patients may present with "mixed" arterial and venous disease, patients with lower extremity venous ulcers should be evaluated for peripheral arterial disease. These patients should at a minimum have a lower extremity ankle/brachial index (ABI) measurement to ensure the adequacy of the arterial circulation. If the patient is found to have peripheral arterial disease, especially if the ABI is 0.7 or less, the arterial disease should be addressed prior to treating the venous disease.

PREOPERATIVE EVALUATION AND PREPARATION

The preoperative evaluation should include a comprehensive history and physical exam, and obtaining noninvasive vascular laboratory studies. A venous duplex ultrasound of the affected lower extremity should evaluate the deep veins, GSV, ASVs, if present, and SSV for patency, as well as the presence of reflux (see Fig. 45.3). Ideally, a "treatment roadmap" should be drawn out for every patient that illustrates the target vein, important perforators that may require foam sclerotherapy, and anatomic details such as vein tortuosity that may influence the procedural approach (Fig. 45.4).

Medications

Aspirin, antiplatelet agents, and nonsteroidal antiinflammatory drugs (NSAIDs) are sometimes discontinued to limit postoperative bruising. The decision to withhold these medications must

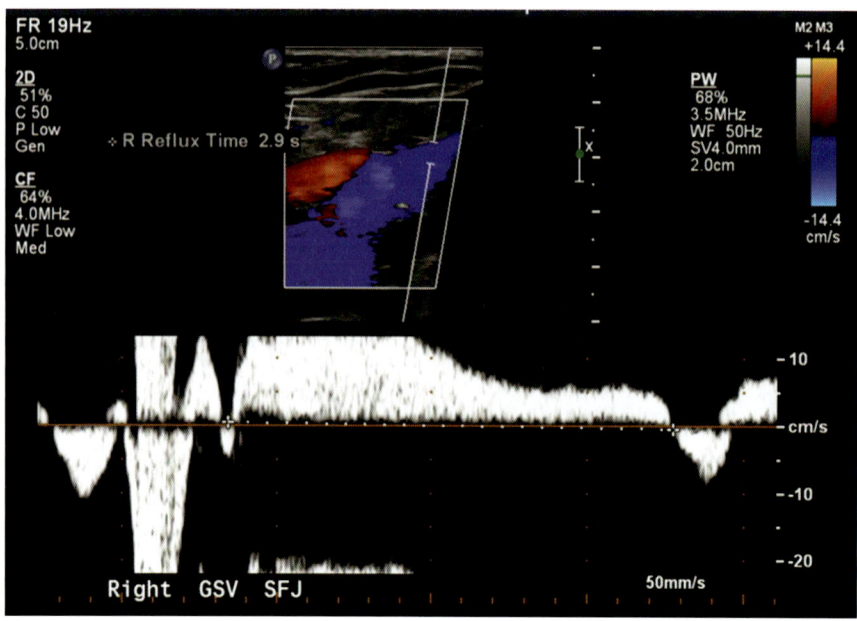

Fig. 45.3 Duplex ultrasound of the right saphenofemoral junction demonstrating significant venous reflux.

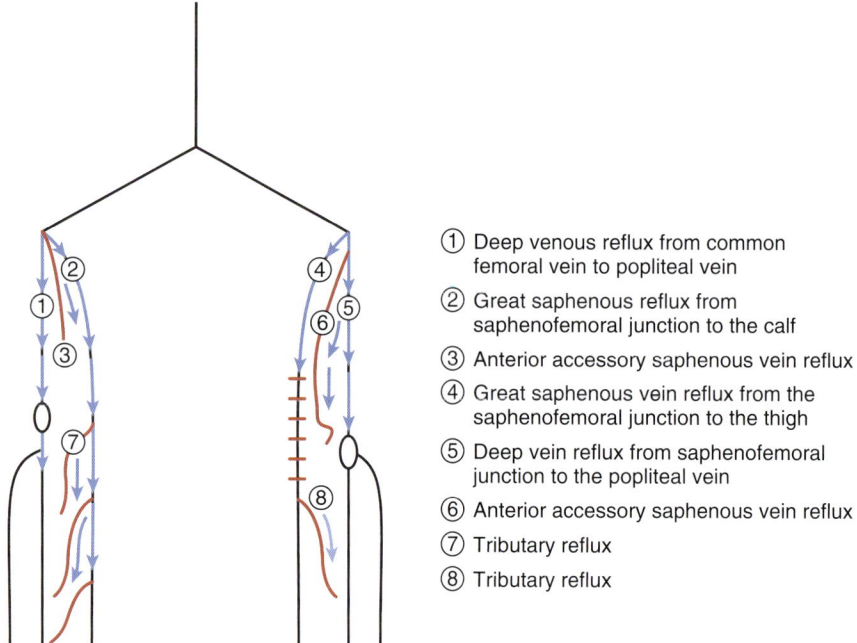

Fig. 45.4 Representative example of a preprocedure venous anatomy diagram used to simplify understanding of location and extent of superficial venous reflux in a given patient. The use of this type of tool can be incredibly useful in planning and executing a successful ablation.

be made on a case-by-case assessment of risk/benefit in individual patients.

For patients who are on full dose anticoagulation, cessation of anticoagulation is **not** necessary prior to EVLA. Perioperative anticoagulation with low molecular weight heparin or warfarin does not appear to affect the success of EVLA.[10–13]

If cessation is selected, warfarin may be temporarily discontinued or bridging anticoagulation initiated with heparin or low-molecular-weight heparin. If the patient is on a direct oral anticoagulant (DOAC), and cessation is felt to be clinically indicated for EVLA, the DOAC can be withheld for 24 hours before EVLA.

Prophylactic Antibiotics

Antibiotic prophylaxis is generally not needed prior to EVLA. However, when EVLA is combined with vein excision, antibiotics should be administered to decrease the risk of surgical site infection.[14]

Deep Vein Thrombosis Prophylaxis

EVLA is a brief outpatient procedure with an overall low risk of DVT. DVT prophylaxis is needed only for high-risk patients.

Planning Supplemental Procedures

Considerations for adjunctive procedures should be based on the preprocedure history and physical, and the venous duplex "treatment roadmap" done prior to EVLA. The adjunctive procedures may include percutaneous phlebectomy and/or foam sclerotherapy at the same time as EVLA, or in a staged fashion.

Compression Stockings

Patients are typically prescribed knee high/thigh high compression stockings (20 to 30 mm Hg), which they should obtain prior to the day of the scheduled procedure. However, the type of compression prescribed and the length of time in compression may vary widely, and is ultimately up to the treating physician.[15]

Schedule Duplex Appointment

A prescheduled appointment should be made for follow-up duplex examination 2 to 3 days after EVLA to assess for DVT.

Vein Mapping/Marking

On the day of the procedure, the veins to be ablated can be marked (i.e., marked with indelible ink) with duplex ultrasound to aid in the administration of tumescent anesthesia, but it is generally not necessary. This may be useful when first getting started using EVLA.

PROCEDURE

EVLA can be performed in a clinic or office or other outpatient surgery setting with oral diazepam and local anesthesia with or without supplemental venous procedures.[16] The dose and type of oral sedative should be made on a case-by-case basis, based on the patient's comorbid medical conditions. If moderate sedation is used, a nurse should be dedicated to monitoring the patient's level of consciousness, heart rate, blood pressure, and oxygen saturation. Local tumescent anesthesia is always required, even if the patient undergoes general anesthesia in an operating room. It is beyond the scope of this chapter to provide specific instructions on how to perform EVLA. There are numerous textbooks now available on both the techniques and technology of EVLA.[17]

Perform Supplemental Procedures

Following successful closure of the target veins, the extremity is evaluated for any significant residual varicose veins, which can be managed with phlebectomy or sclerotherapy, depending on their size or operator preference.

FOLLOW-UP CARE

Pain Management

EVLA is generally well tolerated and controlled with over-the-counter pain medications (e.g., acetaminophen). In one study, 85% of patients complained of no or minimal pain.[18] Moderate to severe pain is experienced in 4% to 9% of patients.[19,20] Extensive concurrent vein excision may require stronger analgesics (e.g., codeine). Pain gradually resolves with time and is improved by wearing compression stockings.

NSAIDs can be added in patients who develop a significant phlebitic reaction. An ice pack can also be applied to the affected areas for comfort.

Compression Stockings

The type of compression and the length worn following EVLA vary widely in the literature.[21] A number of trials have addressed this issue and have randomized patients to wearing compression stockings for 1 to 2 weeks versus 0 to 2 days following EVLA.[22-24] Most of these trials[22-24] have found diminished edema, pain, and use of pain medication for the first 1 to 2 weeks in patients who wore compression stockings longer. There was no difference in time to return to work, vein closure rates, or DVT.

Postoperative Duplex Ultrasound

All patients should undergo duplex ultrasound within 2 to 3 days following the procedure to rule out DVT.[19,25] The main purpose of the postoperative duplex study is to carefully evaluate the proximal extent of the ablated vein for thrombus and to determine whether any thrombus extends into the deep veins. Thrombus extending from the saphenous vein into the proximal deep vein cephalad to the level of the ablation can lead to DVT, although this is uncommon.[19] This process has been termed endovenous heat-induced thrombus (EHIT). If the initial ultrasound demonstrates no thrombus in the deep vein, repeat ultrasound is not required unless the patient develops new symptoms. Thrombus within the deep vein is treated accordingly.

CENTRAL VENOUS STENOSIS—SUPERIOR VENA CAVA SYNDROME

SVC syndrome is a serious disorder resulting from impeded venous return from the upper body caused by obstruction of the SVC. The symptoms include severe congestion and edema of the face (facial plethora), arms, and upper thorax, and may progress to dyspnea, headache, and ultimately cognitive dysfunction. A clinical classification system has been used by several clinicians, which helps the classify symptom severity (Table 45.2). The SVC syndrome is usually caused by obstruction, extrinsic or intrinsic, of the SVC, although bilateral obstruction of both brachiocephalic venous segments can also result in a similar clinical syndrome. Extrinsic compression caused by mediastinal malignancy or lymphadenopathy is the most common cause of true

TABLE 45.2 Clinical Scoring System for Central Venous Stenosis

Signs and Symptoms	Grade
Neurologic Symptoms	
Stupor, coma, blackout	4
Blurry vision, headache, dizziness, amnesia	3
Changes in mentation	2
Uneasiness	1
Laryngotracheal or Thoracic Symptoms	
Orthopnea, laryngeal edema	3
Stridor, hoarseness, dysphagia, shortness of breath	2
Cough, pleural effusion	1
Nasal and Facial Signs or Symptoms	
Lip edema, nasal stiffness, epistaxis, rhinorrhea	2
Facial swelling	1
Venous Dilation	
Neck vein or arm vein distension, upper extremity swelling or upper body plethora	1

Modified from Kish K, Sonomura T, Mitsuzane K, et al. Self expandable metallic stent therapy for superior vena cava syndrome: clinical observations. *Radiology*. 1993;189:531–535.

SVC syndrome.[26] The syndrome can also result from extension of central venous DVT to the SVC, usually in the presence of bilateral subclavian vein stenosis. Other etiologies include thrombosis caused by underlying stenosis from long-term indwelling central venous catheters or other transvenous instruments (discussed later), or benign compressive or constrictive conditions of the mediastinum, such as adenopathy from earlier histoplasmosis, fibrosing mediastinitis, previous irradiation, tuberculosis, and histiocytosis.[27-31]

Diagnosis of Superior Vena Cava Syndrome

The clinical presentation of SVC syndrome is relatively consistent and can be verified with multiple diagnostic modalities. Computed tomography (CT) is helpful for the initial workup of SVC syndrome and often gives enough information to proceed directly to an endovascular procedure.[32] An upper extremity venogram will reveal multiple collaterals if the obstruction has been long standing, but with acute SVC obstruction there are often surprisingly few collaterals. In most cases, the venogram will demonstrate the level of involvement, but it can still overestimate the length of involvement of the innominate veins and even the SVC because of the high resistance to flow. Magnetic resonance imaging (MRI) is helpful for the evaluation of SVC syndrome, and procedure planning can be based solely on MRI findings.[33] MRI shows excellent, detailed anatomical information regarding the extent of occlusion and collateral flow. Ultrasound, on the other hand, is not accurate in pinpointing the location of the central obstruction, especially when the obstruction is more proximal than the subclavian veins due to poor acoustic penetration. However, the Doppler signal will raise a suspicion of obstruction because of the flattened character of the waveform as a result of loss of venous pulsatility and respiratory phasicity. Ultrasound with Doppler can, however, be a useful tool for follow-up after endovascular repair. Obstructive changes in the waveform will raise suspicion of recurrent narrowing or occlusion of the recanalized vessel.

Technique

Endovascular therapy has emerged to be first-line treatment for central vein stenosis.[34] It is important to have a plan of approach before attempting SVC recanalization or stent placement. Taking into account the patient's clinical presentation and preprocedure noninvasive imaging is essential to a successful outcome.

Many operators have used femoral vein access, but others have used jugular, subclavian,[35] and arm vein or even transhepatic venous approaches for stent delivery.[36] One may use any combination of these approaches, but it is always paramount to have a guidewire "through and through," especially when stenosis are severe and difficult to pass.[37] A guidewire externalized from two separate access points allows for better overall support and control during stent delivery and deployment. This is particularly important in regard to preventing stent migration into the right side of the heart or pulmonary artery when the stenosis is near the SVC and right atrial junction. The stent is more likely to stay on the wire and can be more safely manipulated, removed, or moved to a different location. Initially accessing the SVC from the anterograde direction such as the right internal jugular vein or upper extremity veins has several benefits. First, manipulation is easier because of the limited space in the internal jugular vein compared with the right atrium, which one has to work through when coming from a femoral vein access. Second, the distance from the access site to the obstruction is shorter, often making it easier to cross chronic total occlusions. Finally, accessing from the anterograde direction allows for good contrast visualization during injections. Other upper extremity access points, such as the brachial or basilic veins, are also viable options, especially in patients with short or obese necks. The entire venous intervention can be performed from this access, including thrombolysis, angioplasty, and stent placement in most cases.[38] Hemostasis is not usually problematic; placing a pressure dressing for 20 minutes or holding pressure for 5 to 10 minutes is usually successful. If double-barrel stenting is required to treat the SVC, bilateral upper extremity access is ideal, with the stents each traversing the brachiocephalic veins.

Stent Selection

Early reports of SVC stenting described the use of Gianturco stents (now, the Cook-Z stent; Cook Medical, Bloomington, IN). This was the first self-expanding stent in wide use and had diameters that were acceptable. Although few complications have been reported, large sheath introducers (14- to 16-Fr) are required for this stent, and it is now used only in cases where inflow vessels must be covered because of the large spaces between the stent's interstices. Similarly, the Palmaz stent (now, the Palmaz Genesis stent; Cordis Corporation, Miami, FL) was once commonly used for treatment of SVC syndrome but is now rarely used in this anatomic location. This stent is balloon-expandable and has a higher radial force than self-expanding stents. However, when extra radial force is needed, it can be used either primarily or secondarily within a deployed self-expanding stent that cannot sustain the radial force of SVC recoil. In today's era of endovascular therapy, self-expanding stent delivery systems are now mostly used for SVC stenting (Fig. 45.5).[29,30] Modern self-expanding stent delivery systems are easily deployed and come on a 6- to 7-Fr delivery platform. The Wallstent (Boston Scientific Corporation, Natick, MA) was one of the earlier versions of a self-expanding stent, and is still widely used for venous interventions, including SVC stenting. Its main shortcoming is foreshortening that can occur on delivery or postdilatation, which makes precise placement challenging. More modern generations of self-expanding nitinol stents, a shape memory superelastic alloy that offers greater flexibility and vessel adaptability, are being developed and used specifically for venous indications (as discussed later). For the SVC, a 12- to 16-mm stent diameter is usually adequate; however, the use of intravascular ultrasound (IVUS) can be an extremely useful adjunct to both the diagnosis and treatment of SVC syndrome, as with most venous interventions.[39]

Complications

In a group of 59 patients with malignant disease, Lanciego reported six reocclusions, all of which were treated successfully with re-stenting in combination with thrombolysis.[40] One of the patients in this series had stent migration to the right atrium, which was successfully treated.

Hemopericardium has been reported by several operators in the literature. This complication most commonly occurs during the procedure itself or immediately after stent placement,[41] but delayed bleeding into the pericardium has also been described.[42,43] The pericardial reflection can extend very high in the mediastinum, and the position is unpredictable. In this regard, it is advisable to place stents high in the SVC without compromising clinical results. If there is a high index of suspicion for hemopericardium, an echocardiogram or right heart catherization should be done immediately.

Central Venous Stenosis—Inferior Vena Cava

Anatomy and Symptoms

The IVC is the major venous structure responsible for returning deoxygenated blood from the lower extremities, abdomen, and pelvic organs. It is a retroperitoneal structure that typical lies just right and anterior of the spinal column, flanked by the abdominal aorta that sits alongside it and leftward. It forms as a confluence of the right and left common iliac veins at L5 and is fed by several other important confluences as it courses to the right atrium, including the gonadal veins, lumbar veins, renal veins, and hepatic veins. As with most venous anatomy, when stenosis or occlusion occurs, various other venous plexi or anatomic routes are recruited to accommodate venous return from the lower extremities. These may include collateralization of the azygous-hemiazygos system, lumbar-lateral sacral venous plexus, epidural venous plexus, and extensive abdominal wall superficial venous collaterals.[44] Symptoms of total occlusion of the IVC or iliocaval segments is often varied and may range from completely asymptomatic to severe with chronic lower extremity edema or active venous leg ulcers. These clinical manifestations are closely related to etiology. For example, acute IVC thrombosis, such as from IVC filter thrombosis, typically presents with pain and lower extremity swelling, whereas more chronic presentations may be more subtle and mirror symptoms typically seen with chronic superficial venous disease (Table 45.3).

Causes of Inferior Vena Cava Occlusion

The etiology of IVC occlusion is generally subdivided between nonthrombotic causes, acute thrombotic causes, or chronic postthrombotic causes. Nonthrombotic etiologies include extrinsic compression from malignant tumors or nonmalignant masses (uterine fibroids, large infrarenal abdominal aortic aneurysms), anatomical compressive syndromes such as May-Thurner syndrome, and IVC atresia or agenesis. Acute IVC thrombosis can occur as a result of any of the aforementioned nonthrombotic causes but is also commonly seen with preexisting IVC filters. Chronic postthrombotic IVC occlusion occurs following acute thrombosis and includes all of the typical sequalae of the postthrombotic state including venous injury, contraction, and fibrosis.

Diagnosis

The diagnosis of IVC occlusion is typically suggested by the constellation of historical factors and exam findings described previously. Clinically, patients may present with varied symptoms, but generally lower extremity edema is present or has been previously significant (see Table 45.3). In addition, it may be suggested by routine venous duplex ultrasonography when deep venous reflux is noted in the external iliac, common femoral, or proximal femoral veins. As with SVC occlusions, the Doppler waveform, when insonated more peripheral to the occlusion, may show a blunted waveform and lack the pulsatility or respiratory phasicity typically expected. Standard CT is useful in showing advanced chronic IVC occlusion, even without contrast, because the IVC will appear unusually retracted and small. When CT venography is appropriately performed, the contrast will opacify the extensive venous collateralization often seen in addition to demonstrating

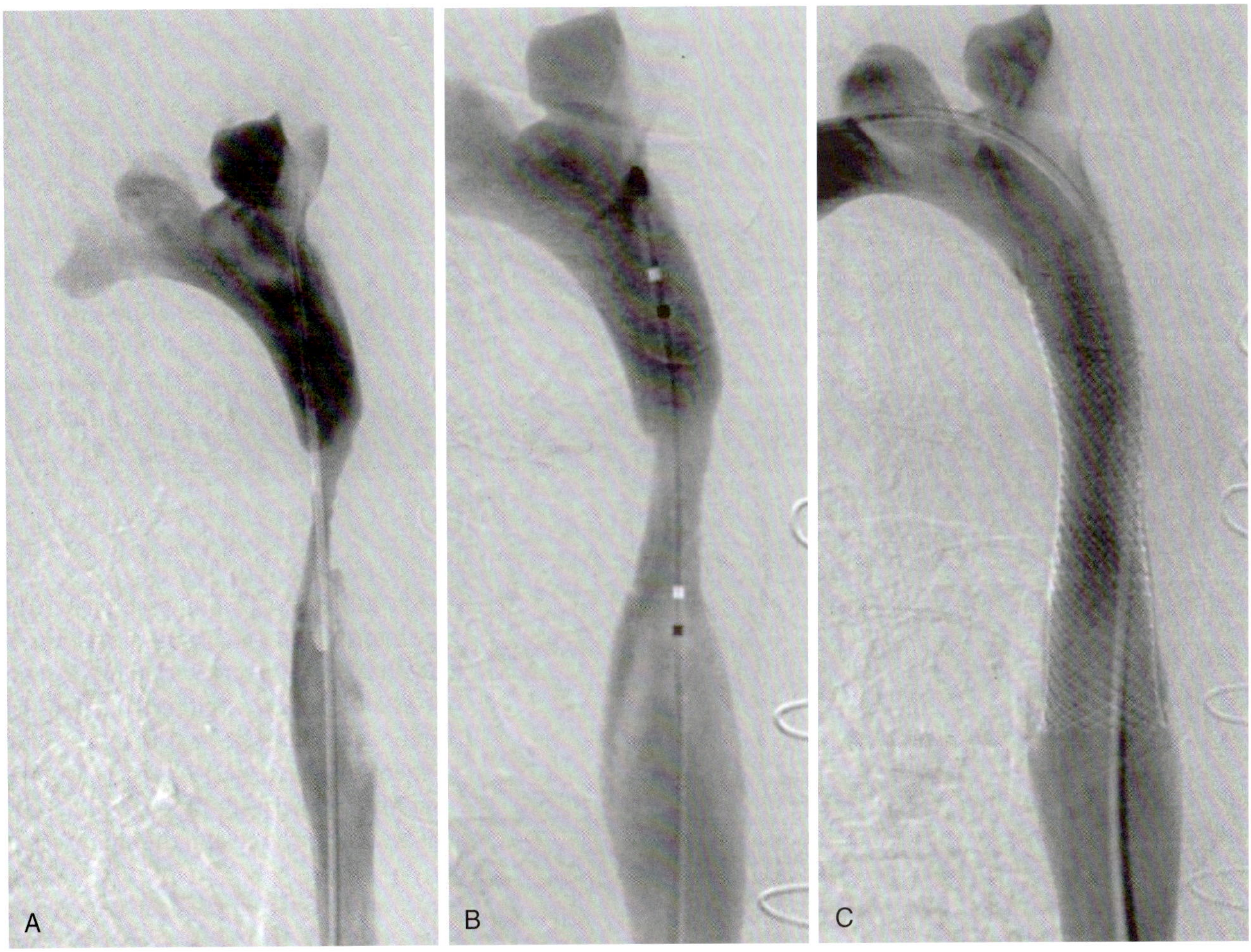

Fig. 45.5 (A) Venogram of significant superior vena cava (SVC) stenosis. (B) Venogram of SVC after 12-mm diameter balloon was used for angioplasty. (C) Venogram after 14-mm WALLSTENT (Boston Scientific Corporation, Natick, MA).

the level of occlusion and any associated extrinsic compressive processes. Magnetic resonance venography (MRV) is also exceptionally good and demonstrates high-resolution images of the venous vasculature associated with iliocaval obstruction. Invasive venography remains important in the diagnosis and treatment of IVC occlusion, but we typically reserve this for use in endovenous recanalization or in conjunction with IVUS when it is necessary to rule out extrinsic compressive diseases such as May-Thurner.

Treatment/Technique

Revascularization of the chronically occluded IVC or iliac veins can be achieved using modern endovascular techniques with high rates of success (Fig. 45.6). Until recently, the majority of the required equipment has been adapted from arterial procedures and include hydrophilic guidewires, standard angioplasty balloons, IVUS, and large, braided, closed-cell stents, such as the Wallstent (Boston Scientific, Minneapolis, MN). In Europe and more recently in the United States, nitinol stents have been developed specifically for use in venous applications. These stents hope to address the unique properties desirable in venous stenting including large diameters, ease of delivery, long lengths, high overall strength, and resistance to external compression.

Several caveats regarding venous revascularization make it unique when compared with arterial revascularization. Unlike the iliac arteries or aorta, which both have a generous smooth muscle media layer making them cylindrical, the IVC and iliac veins are thin-walled vessels designed for low-pressure, high volume blood flow. This makes predicting overall vessel diameter extremely challenging using standard contrast venography, since they often assume a more oval geometry with sometime extremely varying diameters based on volume status and venous loading conditions. In addition, when stenting the iliocaval segments, considerable attention must be paid to the quality of the venous inflow and outflow. The spot-stenting techniques utilized in arterial revascularization do not adapt well on the venous side, where typical caval reconstruction requires complete vessel coverage by stents. Finally, stenting across the inguinal ligament and into the common femoral vein is very frequently required in order to maintain adequate inflow or continuity. While this is considered a relatively taboo technique on the arterial side, extension of stents into the common femoral vein is associated with excellent long-term patency and no significant difference when compared with stents that terminate above the inguinal ligament.[45]

Most complex iliocaval reconstructions are done in the supine position and under general anesthesia due to discomfort with large balloon inflations and procedural time. Vascular access is typically done under ultrasound guidance, with placement of sheaths in the proximal femoral vein. This allows enough "running room" for stenting of the common femoral vein, if necessary. Jugular access may also be required in order to attempt wiring from both the antegrade and retrograde directions. In general, 0.035-inch hydrophilic guidewires are used with support catheters to cross chronic total occlusions. Care is taken to avoid subintimal wiring and to avoid following collateral pathways, many of which can be extremely large and may closely parallel the occluded segments. Once the lesion is crossed with a guidewire, balloon angioplasty and stenting can then be completed in standard fashion. The iliofemoral confluence is typically stented in a "kissing" fashion into a previously placed IVC stent. Stent sizing decisions for veins are generally made on the basis of what the normal diameter *should* be, rather than attempting to match the stents to adjacent venous segments.

When completed successfully, endovenous iliocaval reconstruction plays an extremely important role in the management

TABLE 45.3 Clinical Features of Iliocaval Obstruction

Asymptomatic
Edema
Venous Claudication
Recurrent DVTs
Varicose veins
Venous leg ulcers
Abdominal wall varicosities
Testicular varicoceles
Ovarian vein reflux, chronic pelvic pain
Dyspnea/syncope (from restricted cardiac preload)

DVT, Deep vein thrombosis.

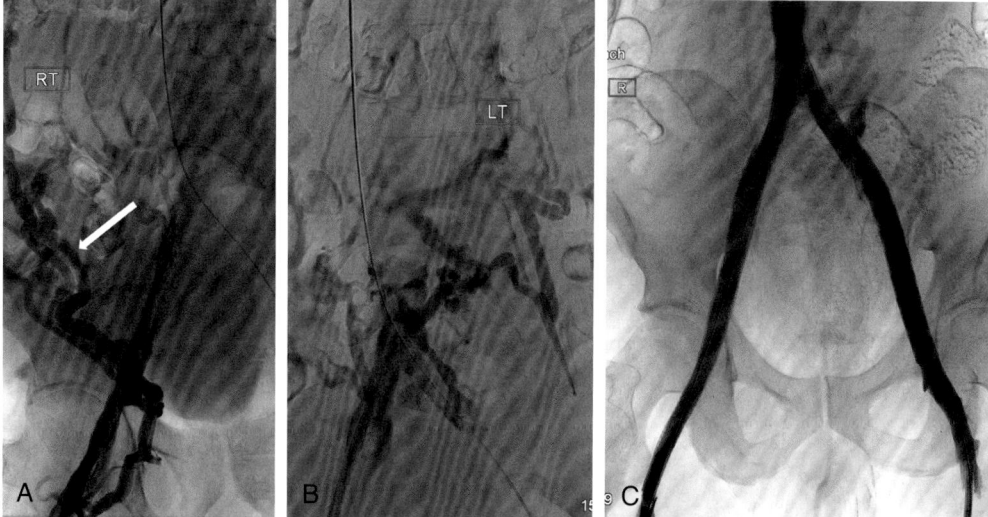

Fig. 45.6 (A) Venogram from the right common femoral vein. Note the extensive, mature, abdominal wall collaterals *(arrow)* that develop to shunt venous return around the occluded inferior vena cava. (B) Venogram from the iliac vein confluence. There are multiple lumbar venous collaterals noted. (C) Final venography following endovenous iliocaval reconstruction demonstrating return of anatomic venous flow.

of this highly symptomatic patient population. Relief of pain is achieved in nearly 90% of these patients, reduction in edema in up to 80%, and up to 70% to 80% healing of venous leg ulcers is typically enjoyed. Technical success is more than 90% in experienced centers, and the rate of major complication is less than 1%. Patency, when measured up to 5 years, is generally in the 80% to 90% range for nonthrombotic etiologies and 74% to 89% for postthrombotic causes.[46]

DEEP VENOUS THROMBOSIS—UPPER EXTREMITY

Upper extremity deep vein thrombosis (UEDVT) is an increasingly important clinical condition with potential consequences of significant morbidity and mortality. Subclinical pulmonary embolism (PE) may be present in 33% of patients with an UEDVT, but symptomatic pulmonary embolization is detected in only 4% to 9% of such patients.[47,48] The venous pathway of the upper limb is less likely to develop a DVT compared with the lower limb because of the relatively high blood flow rate, gravitational effects, and lack of stasis.

Historically named after James Paget and Leopold von Schroetter, Paget-Schroetter syndrome (PSS) remains a leading cause of primary UEDVT. Also known as *effort thrombosis* or *thoracic outlet syndrome* (TOS), PSS was often regarded as a benign condition. As available case reports and literature grew in the 1990s, UEDVT was increasingly regarded as a more common and less benign disease with potential for increased PE, postthrombotic syndrome (PTS), and mortality.[49–51] This change in view regarding UEDVT is reflected by a higher degree of clinical awareness, more sensitive and ubiquitous noninvasive diagnostic techniques, and more effective contemporary treatments.[52–54]

Primary UEDVT remains a rare disorder (1 to 2/100,000 persons/year)[55,56] and generally refers to effort thrombosis (PSS), venous TOS, or idiopathic UEDVT. Patients with effort thrombosis develop spontaneous UEDVT, usually in their dominant arm, after repetitive strenuous activities such as rowing, wrestling, weight lifting, or baseball pitching, but they are otherwise young and healthy.[57] The heavy exertion causes microtrauma to the vessels' intima, leading to activation of the coagulation cascade. Significant thrombosis may occur with repeated insults to the vein wall, especially if mechanical compression of the vessel is also present.[58]

TOS refers to compression of the neurovascular bundle (brachial plexus, subclavian artery, subclavian vein) as it exits the thoracic inlet (Fig. 45.7).[59,60] Although this disorder may initially cause intermittent positional extrinsic vein compression, repeated trauma to the vessel can result in dense perivascular fibrous scar tissue formation that will persistently compress the vein.[59] Compression of the subclavian vein typically develops in young athletes with hypertrophied muscles who do heavy lifting or frequently abduct their arms. Cervical ribs, long transverse processes of the cervical spine, musculofascial bands, and clavicular or first rib anomalies are sometimes found in these patients. Therefore, plain films of the cervical spine and chest should be obtained in all patients undergoing evaluation for TOS.[59] Presenting signs and symptoms of UEDVT can be found in Table 45.4.

Secondary UEDVT is associated with both exogenous and endogenous risk factors and usually develops in older, ill patients, with a slight preference for females.[61] Among exogenous risk factors, the positioning of central venous lines, malignancy, previous or actual episodes of LEDVT, treatment with oral contraceptives, and trauma appear to have the highest impact on the development of UEDVT. Patients with indwelling central venous catheters constitute a particularly high risk population, especially when undergoing chemotherapy, invasive hemodynamic monitoring, chronic parenteral nutrition, hemodialysis, or transvenous pacing, with a more than 60% prevalence of either symptomatic or asymptomatic UEDVT.[62–64] In fact, ipsilateral catheter related UEDVT may account for up to 70% of all secondary UEDVT cases.[61] Malignancy, either overt or undiagnosed, is also frequently associated with UEDVT (more than 30% of cases).[56,65] In fact, the discovery of an otherwise unexplained UEDVT in the older population should prompt a malignancy workup, as some data indicate that occult malignancy, especially lung cancer and lymphomas, may be discovered during follow-up in up to 24% of patients with UEDVT, mostly during the first week of hospital admission.[66]

A history of previous episodes or an ongoing DVT of the lower extremities is associated with UEDVT in up to 18% of cases.[61] In an ultrasound surveillance study, nearly 30% of high risk trauma patients develop UEDVT during the course of hospitalization that may be asymptomatic in up to 30% of the cases.[67] Treatment with oral contraceptives may also represent a significant risk factor in females (up to 14%), although these data are conflicting.[68] Infrequently, UEDVT arises in carriers of peripheral venous catheters, generally from a superficial phlebitis spreading to the deep venous system,[64] or is associated with intravenous drug abuse, especially of cocaine.[69]

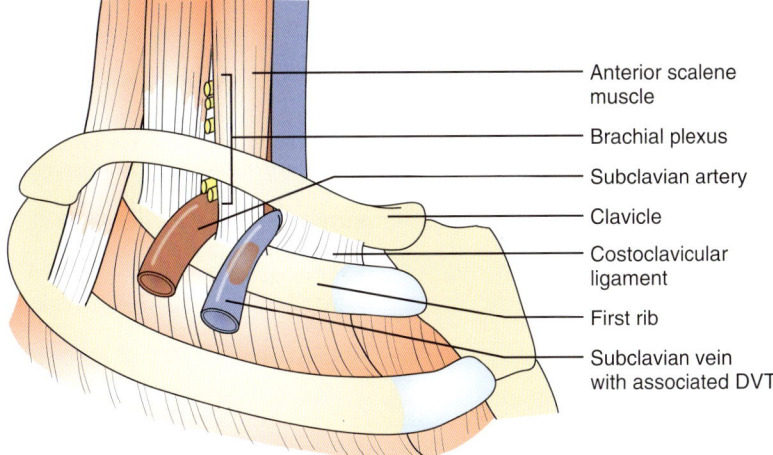

Fig. 45.7 Illustration of the thoracic outlet anatomy. Note the relationship of the subclavian vein to the surrounding structures; the anterior scalene muscle posteriorly, the first rib inferiorly, the clavicle superiorly, and the costoclavicular ligament anteriorly.[60] In this example, the costoclavicular ligament is abnormal and constricting venous flow. *DVT,* Deep vein thrombosis. (Modified from Urschel HC, Patel AN. Surgery remains the most effective treatment for Paget-Schroetter syndrome: 50 years' experience. *Ann Thorac Surg.* 2008;86[1]:254–260, Fig. 2.)

The prevalence of hypercoagulable states in patients with UEDVT is uncertain because observational studies report varying results; however, the best available data estimates rates as high as 24%.[56,70] Furthermore, screening for coagulation disorders is controversial and has never been shown to be cost effective.[71] The yield of these tests is highest for patients with idiopathic UEDVT, a family history of DVT, a history of recurrent, unexplained pregnancy loss, or a personal history of a prior DVT. Finally, the increasing use of device therapy in the cardiac patient has undoubtedly led to an increased prevalence of UEDVT and other venous obstructive complications. Unlike catheter-associated complications, which may be transient and treatable with removal of the device, cardiac pacemaker or defibrillator leads are generally permanent. Moreover, it is now common to have two or even three leads traversing the subclavian vein and repeat procedures for device upgrades or lead revisions are frequent. In some studies, the incidence of angiographic venous lesions following pacemaker implantation near 64%, with UEDVT as high as 23%.[72,73] Fortunately, the majority of these UEDVTs are asymptomatic. Advanced age (≥65), left ventricular ejection fraction ≤0.40, and atrial fibrillation have all been associated with increased risk for subclavian vein obstruction following pacemaker implantation.[72,74,75]

Diagnostic Testing

Historically, the gold standard for the diagnosis of UEDVT, which involves direct imaging of the whole deep venous system of the arm, is contrast venography. In contemporary practice, however, contrast venography has a limited initial role due to its invasive nature, inconvenience for patients, technical difficulty in performing and interpretation, and possible contrast dye-related complications. Instead, there are several noninvasive imaging modalities that are widely available that serve as alternatives to contrast venography; these are highlighted as follows.

Duplex Ultrasonography

Duplex ultrasound has largely replaced invasive venography for the initial diagnosis of deep venous thrombosis. Its most advantageous features include no requirement for nephrotoxic contrast agents, its noninvasive nature, and the absence of ionizing radiation. In addition, it is widely available, portable, inexpensive, and can readily be performed at the bedside. Duplex ultrasonography has a high sensitivity and specificity for peripheral (jugular, distal subclavian, axillary) UEDVT.[76] Acoustic shadowing from the clavicle, however, limits visualization of a segment of subclavian vein and may result in a false-negative study.[77] Some technical recommendations regarding the use of duplex ultrasonography for the diagnosis of UEDVT would include utilizing a combination of real-time compression grayscale ultrasonography, color Doppler, and flow measurements using duplex technique with a 7.5-MHz linear-array probe.

In considering the diagnosis of UEDVT utilizing duplex ultrasonography, the definition of thrombosis is critical. It is widely accepted that noncompressibility of a venous segment with or without visible thrombus constitutes thrombosis. There is a building body of evidence regarding the use of isolated flow abnormalities as predictors of venous thrombosis. Due to acoustic shadowing from the clavicle, these flow abnormalities can be crucial clues to underlying thrombosis that is otherwise not well-visualized in the venous segments beyond the clavicle.[77] These flow abnormalities seen on duplex ultrasound are only suggestive of thrombosis, and contrast venography may be necessary if there is a high clinical index of suspicion for UEDVT. No studies have specifically addressed interobserver and intraobserver variability, but it is widely accepted in clinical practice that duplex ultrasonography is operator-dependent and that some patients may be more difficult to investigate, especially those with extensive edema or morbid obesity.

Magnetic Resonance Imaging

MRV is an accurate, noninvasive method for detecting thrombus in the central chest veins, such as the SVC and brachiocephalic veins. MRV provides a complete evaluation of central collaterals, central veins, and blood-flow patterns. The correlation with traditional contrast venography is very good; therefore, MRV is a valuable imaging modality for the diagnosis of UEDVT when contrast venography is contraindicated or impossible. However, the increased use of pacemakers and internal defibrillators, the longer time required for image acquisition, and claustrophobia are potential drawbacks to MRV. Once considered a preferred alternative to contrast dye-based techniques such as contrast venography or CT venography for patients with renal disease, the recognition of nephrogenic systemic fibrosis and its association with gadolinium has also impacted the widespread adoption of MRV.[78,79]

Computed Tomography Venography

Already a mature technology, CT continues to evolve with the use of multidetector CT equipment where coronal and sagittal slice reformation and 3D reconstruction are possible. Even more, the ability for rapid image acquisition gated to the cardiac cycle provides for high-resolution imaging without motion artifact. As such, this imaging modality will likely play a greater role in the management of patients with UEDVT going forward. One major advantage of CT venography is the ability to assess for the presence of pulmonary emboli and other anatomic abnormalities, which may underlie a patient's upper extremity complaints (such as malignancy). Limitations to this technology include the need for contrast, the use of ionizing radiation, and overall cost.

Treatment Options

The optimal approach for the treatment of UEDVT remains unknown, but in general there are two overarching goals: first, to prevent thrombus propagation, and second, to restore normal venous anatomy. Arresting further thrombus formation reduces

TABLE 45.4 Signs and Symptoms of Deep Venous Thrombosis of the Upper Extremity[a]

	Symptoms	Signs
Axillary or subclavian vein thrombosis	Vague shoulder or neck discomfort Arm or hand edema	Supraclavicular fullness Palpable cord Arm or hand edema Extremity cyanosis Diluted cutaneous veins Jugular venous distention Unable to access central venous catheter
Thoracic outlet syndrome	Pain radiating to arm/forearm Hand weakness	Brachial plexus tenderness Arm or hand atrophy Positive Adson[b] or Wright[c] maneuver

[a]These are nonspecific and may be recognized with provocative maneuvers.
[b]Adson maneuver: The examiner extends the patient's arm on the affected side while the patient extends the neck and rotates the head toward the same side. The test is positive if there is weakening of the radial pulse with deep inspiration and suggests compression of the subclavian artery.
[c]Wright maneuver: The patient's shoulder is abducted and the humerus externally rotated. The test is positive if symptoms are reproduced and there is weakening of the radial pulse.

the risk of secondary events such as pulmonary embolization or disease recurrence. Restoration of normal venous anatomy is achieved typically by recanalization of existing thrombus and is important in the prevention of PTS. It is quite likely that henceforth more patients with UEDVT will be approached with a multimodal effort. These treatment options will include either individually or in combination anticoagulant therapy, thrombolytic therapy, endovascular intervention, and/or vascular surgery.

Anticoagulation

Anticoagulation represents the mainstay of therapy for UEDVT. Anticoagulation helps maintain patency of venous collaterals and reduces thrombus propagation, even in the absence of complete thrombus resolution.[80] Unfortunately, anticoagulation alone rarely achieves vessel recanalization, thus leading to permanent obstruction of the upper extremity veins. Collateral veins typically develop, but these are generally not accessible for placement of intravenous lines and usually inadequate for the normal efflux of venous blood from the arm. Typically, standard anticoagulation includes unfractionated heparin or low molecular weight heparin for 5 to 7 days, as a "bridge" to oral warfarin. Warfarin is typically continued for a minimum of 3 months, with a goal international normalized ratio of 2.0 to 3.0. A longer duration of warfarin anticoagulation may be indicated if some form of coagulation abnormality is detected or if an underlying mechanical etiology is not definitively treated. Alternatives to warfarin in contemporary practice include the use of the DOACs such as dabigatran, rivaroxaban, and apixaban in the treatment of DVT.[81]

Thrombolytic Therapy

Because many patients with UEDVT are young, active, and healthy, thrombolytic therapy rather than conservative anticoagulation should be strongly considered on a case-by-case basis. Certainly, a young healthy patient with UEDVT may have significant long-term morbidity if treated with only anticoagulation.[82] In this regard, thrombolysis restores venous patency early, minimizes damage to the endothelium, and reduces the risk of long-term complications, especially the development of PTS, with its disabling chronic aching and swelling of the arm and hand. The obvious disadvantage of thrombolytic therapy is greater risk of a bleeding complication.

The ideal candidate for thrombolytic therapy for UEDVT would be an otherwise healthy young patient with a primary UEDVT or those patients with an indwelling central venous catheter, where it is essential to maintain patency for central venous access.

Results from a large series of patients with UEDVT who were treated with catheter-directed thrombolysis (CDT) showed that treatment restored venous drainage, with subsequent low frequency of mild postthrombotic syndrome at follow-up.[83] No intracerebral bleeding, clinical PE, or death occurred during treatment follow-up.[83] Thrombolysis has the best chance of success if used within 4 to 6 weeks of the symptom onset, as older, organized thrombus is more resistant to thrombolysis. When performing CDT, the catheter should be placed directly within the entire length of visible thrombus; otherwise the potential for collateral circulation to divert drug distribution away from the thrombus may lead to an unsuccessful procedure.

There are no randomized, prospective controlled clinical trials comparing different thrombolytic agents for treating UEDVT. At our tertiary referral center, catheter-directed alteplase (tPA) or tenecteplase (TNK) are administered at 0.25 to 0.5 U/h for 8 hours.[84] Clinical examination and serial venography are used to assess response to treatment. We often utilize a percutaneous mechanical thrombectomy (PMT) device in combination with thrombolytic therapy. This adjunctive catheter-based thrombectomy technique has the benefit of thrombus extraction prior to thrombolytic therapy, which often initiates some blood flow, thereby improving drug distribution and reducing dose and duration of thrombolytic therapy.[85] A complete description of PMT devices can be found in the section that discusses the management of LEDVT.

Interventional Therapy

Catheter-based mechanical thrombectomy is an important adjunct to thrombolytic therapy, as stated previously. Theoretically advantageous, the ability to perform instant thrombus removal and thereby restore some anterograde flow through the DVT allows for better overall drug distribution and delivery. Moreover, the ability to deliver thrombolytic agents directly into the clot instead of systemically reduces both the dose and treatment time.[86]

Adjunctive percutaneous transluminal angioplasty (PTA) or, rarely, stenting of the subclavian vein has utility, especially for catheter-related stenosis, when there is a hemodynamically significant pressure gradient following successful thrombolytic therapy.[87] Fig. 45.8 demonstrates CDT of an acute right UEDVT in a patient with classic effort thrombosis. The routine practice of stenting the subclavian vein location should be avoided, when possible, due to the high rates of restenosis. The treatment of subclavian vein stenosis resulting from transvenous permanent pacemaker or internal cardiac defibrillator leads is becoming increasingly common. While they can sometimes present as UEDVT or even SVC syndrome,[88] such patients more often are discovered during the elective upgrade of the cardiac device or during the addition or revision of leads. In such instances, the predominant role of interventional therapy is to assist with lead delivery through what is often a chronically occluded or near-occluded vein comprised of dense, scar-like adhesions. In this scenario, the use of balloon angioplasty to facilitate sheath insertion across the stenosis is usually adequate to provide a path through which the electrophysiologist can work.

Surgical Therapy

Subclavian vein compression in patients with primary UEDVT represents an important cause of recurrent thrombosis and long-term morbidity.[89] As such, after successful treatment of an acute UEDVT, it is paramount that some form of imaging be undertaken to evaluate for the presence of vein compression. Following successful thrombolysis, venography in the neutral and shoulder abducted position can help demonstrate vein compression. Recent surgical series recommend surgical correction of extrinsic vein compression,[89] which typically requires resection of part of the first rib or clavicle. Lysis of adhesions around the subclavian vein may also be required if anatomic anomalies have caused chronic, repeated trauma to the subclavian vein. Today, surgical thrombectomy is rarely required due to advancements in pharmacologic and catheter-based therapies. However, in symptomatic patients who are refractory to other therapies, surgical thrombectomy can restore venous patency.

Treatment of UEDVT is aimed at preservation of venous anatomy, prevention of potentially fatal PE, and to decrease the risk of PTS. Treatment is dependent on the cause, duration of thrombosis, and clinical circumstances. For the majority of patients with UEDVT, anticoagulation for 3 to 6 months of oral anticoagulation is usually sufficient, especially for reversible conditions such as catheter-associated UEDVT. However, there is a tendency to be more aggressive with thrombolytic therapy and catheter-based thrombectomy in individual cases, especially in younger patients who are at risk of chronic venous insufficiency or in an effort to minimize long-term morbidity and optimize functionality. A structured physical therapy program aimed

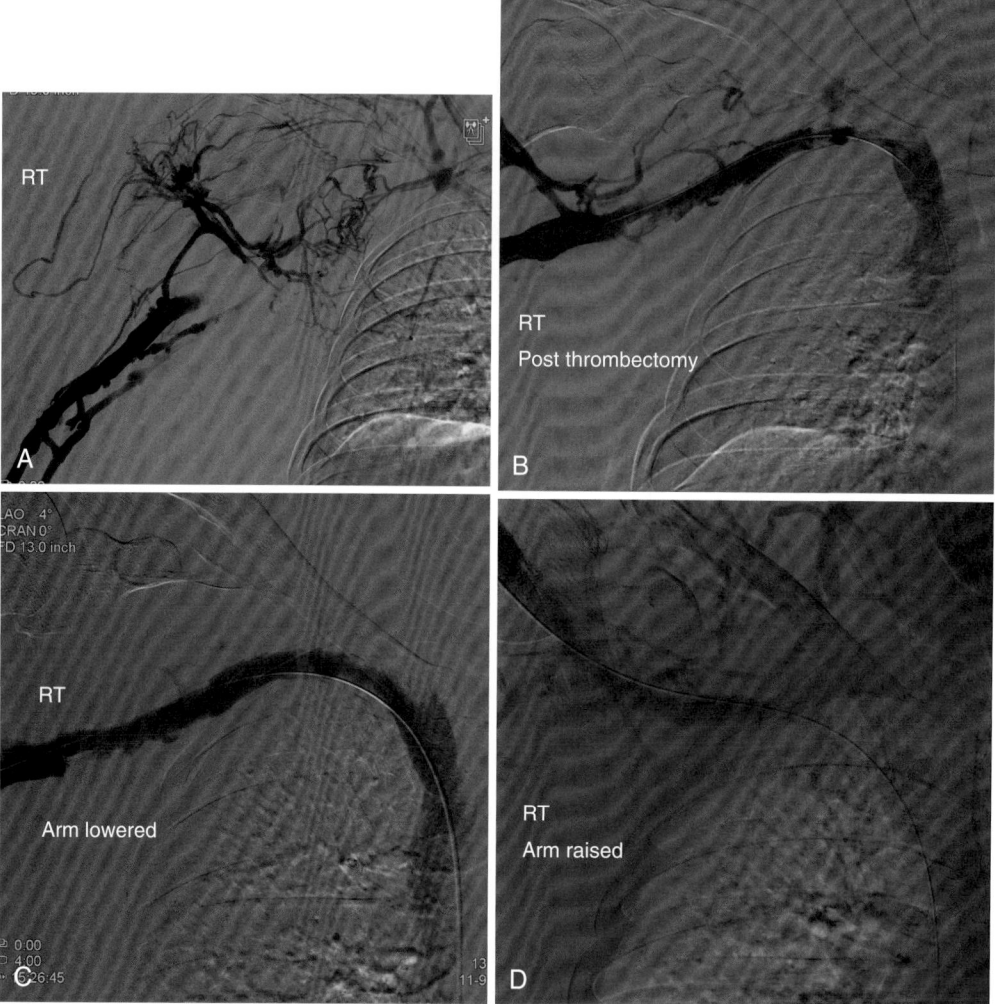

Fig. 45.8 (A) Right upper extremity venogram of a 42-year-old right-handed painter with acute right subclavian vein deep venous thrombosis. (B) Venogram in same patient after successful "on-the-table" catheter-directed thrombolysis and rheolytic thrombectomy. Provocative maneuvers show excellent flow with the arm in a neutral position after treatment (C), but provoked outlet obstruction with the arm in the raised and externally rotated position (D), as evidenced by cessation of venous flow despite successful treatment. *RT*, Right.

at loosening the muscles compressing the subclavian vein and weight loss, if indicated, are other important adjuncts to complete therapy.

DEEP VENOUS THROMBOSIS—LOWER EXTREMITY

DVT is a process that can affect any of the deep veins of the body, but is most frequently discovered in the deep veins of the lower extremity. Venous thrombus formation is initiated by intravascular clotting and is increased in the presence of several risk factors. These risk factors were postulated more than 100 years ago by Virchow and are summarized by his classic triad of coagulation abnormalities, endothelial damage, and stasis. The main contributing risk factors for DVT of the lower extremities included advanced age, prolonged bed rest, and major surgery—particularly large abdominal operations and orthopedic procedures. Other commonly described risk factors include previous DVT, malignancy, trauma, varicose veins, chronic venous insufficiency, high estrogen states (i.e., pregnancy and the postpartum period, estrogen-containing contraceptive devices or pills), and hypercoagulable states, either primary or secondary. May-Thurner syndrome is a rarely diagnosed condition in which patients develop iliofemoral DVT due to an anatomical variant in which the right common iliac artery overlies and compresses the left common iliac vein against the lumbar spine (Fig. 45.9). This variant has been shown to be present in more than 20% of the population; however, it is rarely considered in the differential diagnosis of DVT, particularly in patients with other risk factors. The major complications of LEDVT include PE and PTS, and therefore the treatment paradigms are aimed largely at the prevention of both. The incidence of venous thromboembolism (VTE) in the general population may reach 1.92/1000 person-years. Even more interesting, nearly half of all cases are idiopathic. For those patients with first episode of VTE, the 28-day mortality may reach 11% and as high as 25% in the cancer-associated subgroups.[90] Clinical PE occurs in 26% to 67% of the cases of untreated proximal DVT and is associated with a mortality rate of 11% to 23% if untreated. Under treatment, the incidence of PE decreases to 5% and the mortality to less than 1%.

PTS, however, is a cause of increased morbidity and disability as well. Up to two-thirds of patients with iliofemoral DVT develop edema and pain, with 5% developing venous ulcers despite adequate anticoagulation.[82] Early diagnosis and treatment of DVT is essential to prevent mortality and morbidity from PE and PTS.

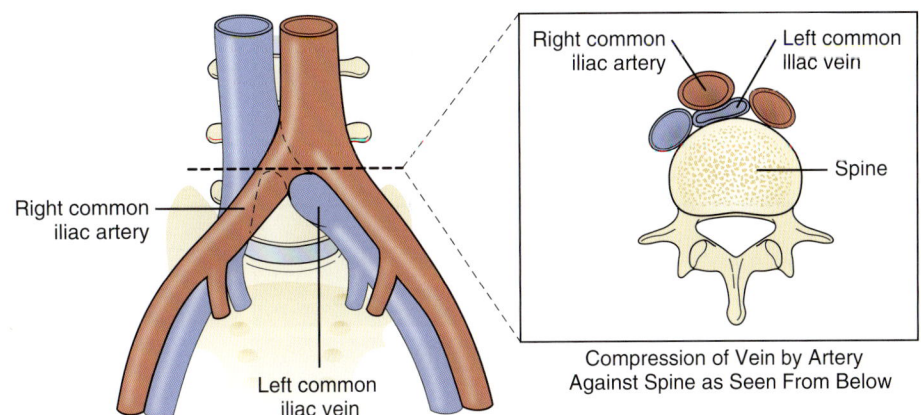

Fig. 45.9 Typical May-Thurner anatomy demonstrated by extrinsic compression of the left common iliac vein between the lumbar vertebrae and the overriding right common iliac artery.

Diagnosis of Acute Deep Venous Thrombosis of the Lower Extremity

Venous Duplex Ultrasound

The clinical diagnosis of LEDVT is notoriously inaccurate, with the classic signs and symptoms of DVT being as common in patients without DVT as they are in those with confirmed DVT. Objective confirmation of clinically suspected DVT is therefore required. Despite its many limitations, contrast venography has historically been considered the "gold standard" for the diagnosis of acute DVT. It is invasive, not easily reproducible, impossible to perform or interpret in 9% to 14% of patients, fails to visualize all venous segments in 10% to 30% of studies, and may be associated with interobserver disagreements in 4% to 10% of studies. Not surprisingly, contrast venography has been replaced by venous duplex ultrasound as the most widely used diagnostic test for acute DVT. In comparison with contrast venography, duplex ultrasound has the advantages of being widely available, noninvasive, portable, inexpensive, and easily repeatable. A complete ultrasound evaluation of the lower extremities includes an assessment of venous compressibility, intraluminal echogenic signals, venous flow characteristics, and luminal color filling. Venous incompressibility, or failure to completely coapt the venous walls with gentle probe compression, is the most widely used diagnostic criteria for acute DVT.[91] Normal flow in the proximal veins should be spontaneous and vary with respiration, increasing during expiration and decreasing during inspiration. Adjunctive grayscale imaging may allow for more subtle characterization of the thrombus, including the degree of intraluminal echogenicity, surrounding tissue edema, and amount of venous dilation—all of which may assist the provider in determining the age of the DVT.

Other noninvasive imaging techniques for the diagnosis of LEDVT include MRV and CT venography. These modalities are comparable to conventional contrast venography, but are subject to the multitude of limitations described previously.

Intravascular Ultrasound

IVUS has emerged as a precise 360-degree imaging modality used in the diagnostic, therapeutic, and posttherapy surveillance of DVT. IVUS helps provide information about defects within the lumen, degree of stenosis, and structures that may be immediately adjacent to veins (Fig. 45.10). As with other ultrasound studies, image artifacts are important to recognize and understand in order to appropriately interpret imaging results.[92] A study utilizing CT venography in patients who presented with acute iliofemoral DVT is best to illustrate why IVUS should be utilized when performing IVC or iliac vein intervention.[93] Chung found that approximately two-thirds of patients with iliofemoral DVT have an anatomic abnormality of their iliac vein in addition to a large thrombus burden. These anatomic abnormalities may include extrinsic compression or vascular webs/strictures. Importantly, standard venography has a very low sensitivity (about 45%) of diagnosing these anatomic abnormalities, and therefore IVUS should be considered the standard of care when performing IVC or iliac vein intervention.[93]

Diagnostic Testing and Clinical Risk Stratification

D-dimer, which is formed as a by-product in the degradation of crosslinked fibrin by plasmin, reflects thrombus formation and has been proposed as an alternative or adjunct to initial diagnostic testing. Although D-dimer is sensitive for the diagnosis of DVT, D-dimer measurements are nonspecific, and elevated levels may be associated with preeclampsia, malignancy, infection, trauma, age, or recent surgery. The high sensitivity of D-dimer measurements and its favorable negative predictive value makes it advantageous in the exclusion of DVT when used in the correct patient population and typically in conjunction with other predictive models[94]; however, the low specificity and positive predictive value necessitate confirmatory noninvasive testing for positive results. A combined strategy using an assessment of clinical probability, D-dimer testing, and venous duplex ultrasound may hold the greatest diagnostic promise. This approach relies on observations that its negative predictive value approaches 100% in outpatients with a low pretest clinical probability for DVT.[95]

Goals of Therapy

As our understanding of the pathophysiology of VTE has evolved, coupled with the constant refinement of endovascular devices and thrombotic therapy, so too have our overall goals of care. There are four general treatment strategies for patients with LEDVT: (1) diminishing the severity and duration of lower extremity symptoms, (2) preventing PE, (3) minimizing the risk of recurrent venous thrombosis, and (4) preventing the PTS. To successfully achieve these goals, usually a comprehensive treatment approach using multiple modalities is employed. This may be as simple as a brief duration of anticoagulation, compression stockings, and avoidance of prolonged immobility in some patients. In others, it may include an extensive biological workup for inherited thrombophilia, some form of catheter-based interventional therapy, and IVC filter placement.

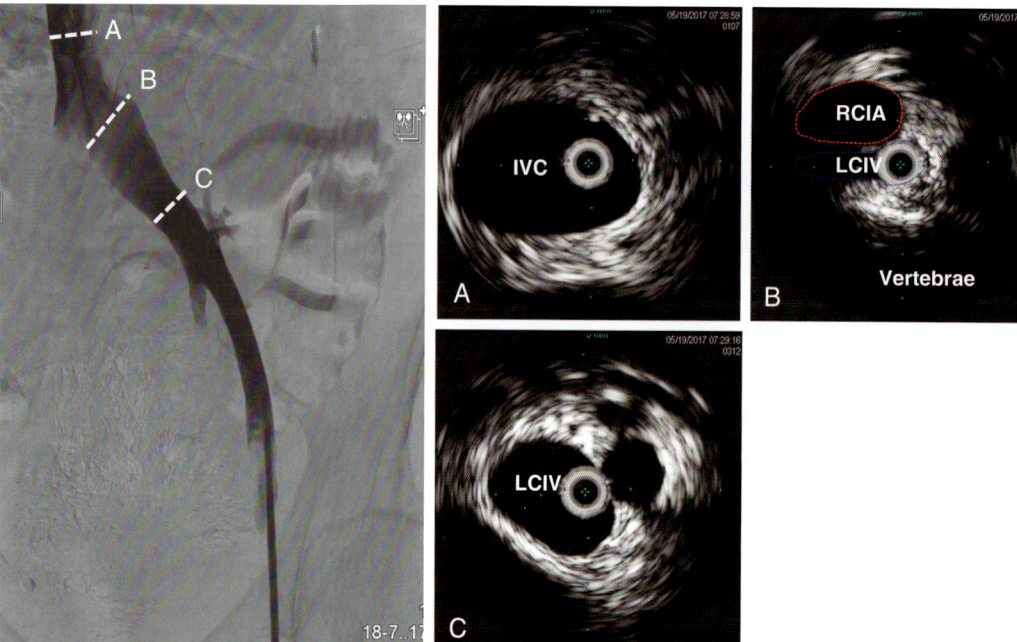

Fig. 45.10 Intravascular ultrasound (IVUS) images taken at corresponding levels depicted on the venogram of the left iliac veins and IVC. The inferior vena cava *(IVC)* has normal dimensions (A), but severe extrinsic compression of the left common iliac vein *(outlined by dashed blue line)* by the right common iliac artery *(outlined by dashed red lines,* B) is seen, followed by return to normal left common iliac vein dimensions (C). *LCIV,* left common iliac vein; *RCIA,* right common iliac artery.

TABLE 45.5 Direct Oral Anticoagulant Pharmacokinetics

Key Points	Rivaroxaban	Apixaban	Edoxaban	Dabigatran
Target	Factor Xa	Factor Xa	Factor Xa	Factor IIa
T½	7–11 h	12 h	6–11 h single doses; 9–10 h multiple doses	12–17 h
Clearance	30% Renal 60% Liver	25% Renal 75% Liver	33% Renal 60% Liver	80% Renal
Metabolism CYP 450	CYP3A4 CYP2J2	CYP3A4	No	No
P-GP	Yes	Yes	Yes	Yes
P-GP	Yes	Yes	Yes	Yes

Detailed monographs and practice guidelines regarding the medical management of LEDVT are numerous and readily available.[96] There is uniform agreement that adequate initial anticoagulant therapy is required to arrest further thrombus propagation and PE. Intravenous unfractionated heparin remains in widespread use but is gradually being replaced by low-molecular-weight heparin as the anticoagulant of choice for the initial treatment of LEDVT. Both agents are relatively safe and effective when used in this context, with low-molecular-weight heparin suitable for outpatient therapy because of improved bioavailability and more predictable anticoagulant response. Serious potential complications of heparin therapy, such as heparin-induced thrombocytopenia and osteoporosis, seem less common with low-molecular-weight heparin. The introduction of the DOACs have simplified the outpatient management of LEDVT. This is due to their favorable pharmacokinetics (Table 45.5), and efficacy and safety data compared with vitamin K antagonists (Tables 45.6 and 45.7). Although medical therapy with anticoagulation is the mainstay of the initial management of LEDVT, many patients, particularly with large proximal iliofemoral DVTs, have persistent leg edema, pain, and difficulty ambulating. Even worse, some patients progress to develop phlegmasia cerulea dolens, a rare condition marked by severe venous hypertension, cyanosis, venous gangrene, compartment syndrome, and eventually limb loss or circulatory collapse. These morbid symptoms arise from venous hypertension caused by outflow obstruction, and the latter demands a treatment strategy more aggressive than simple anticoagulation. Indeed, anticoagulation alone is associated with thrombus regression in only 50% of patients,[97] a fact that severely limits anticoagulation monotherapy, particularly in patients with very proximal DVTs. Fortunately the modern evolution of endovascular techniques (including CDT, mechanical thrombectomy, and stenting) has significantly increased the number of viable treatment options for LEDVT.[98,99] The details of endovascular venous intervention—which are targeted to restore venous patency, preserve valvular function, and minimize the risk of late postthrombotic complications—are discussed as follows.

Catheter-Directed Thrombolysis

In the early 1990s, Semba and Dake first reported the feasibility of CDT for iliofemoral vein thrombosis as an alternative to systemic anticoagulation, systemic thrombolysis, or surgical venous thrombectomy.[100] CDT, or the delivery of thrombolytic agents directly into the thrombus offers significant advantages over systemic therapy, which may fail to reach and penetrate an occluded

TABLE 46.6 Monotherapy Summary

Study	Recurrent VTE		Major Bleeding	
EINSTEIN DVT				
Rivaroxaban	2.1%	Noninferior	0.8%	Noninferior
Standard Rx	3.0%		1.2%	
EINSTEIN PE				
Rivaroxaban[a]	2.1%	Noninferior	1.1%	HR = 0.49 P = .003
Standard Rx	1.8%		2.2%	
AMPLIFY				
Apixaban[b]	2.3%	Noninferior	0.6%	RR 0.31 $P \leq .001$
Standard Rx	2.7%		1.8%	

[a]Major Bleeding (HR = 0.49; 95% CI 0.31–0.79; P = .003).
[b]Major Bleeding (RR, 0.31; 95% CI 0.17–0.55; $P \leq .001$).
CI, Confidence interval; *DVT*, deep vein thrombosis; *HR*, hazard ratio; *PE*, pulmonary embolism; *RR*, relative risk; *VTE*, venous thromboembolism.
EINSTEIN Investigators, Bauersachs R, Berkowitz SD, et al. Oral rivaroxaban for symptomatic venous thromboembolism. *N Engl J Med.* 2010;363:2499–2510; EINSTEIN–PE Investigators, Büller HR, Prins MH, et al. Oral rivaroxaban for the treatment of symptomatic pulmonary embolism. *N Engl J Med.* 2012;366:1287–1297; Agnelli G, Buller HR, Cohen A, et al. Oral apixaban for the treatment of acute venous thromboembolism. *N Engl J Med.* 2013;369:799–808.

TABLE 45.7 Lead In Therapy Venous Thromboembolism

Study	Recurrent VTE		Major Bleeding	
RE-COVER				
Dabigatran	2.4%	Noninferior	1.8%	HR = 0.84
Standard Rx	2.1%		1.9%	
HOKUSAI VTE				
Edoxaban	3.2%	Noninferior	1.4%	HR = 0.82
Standard Rx	3.5%		1.6%	

Subgroup Analysis N-terminal pro-brain natriuretic peptide.
Edoxaban 3.3% HR 0.52; 95% CI 0.28 to 0.98.
Standard 6.2%.
CI, Confidence interval; *HR*, hazard ratio; *VTE*, venous thromboembolism.
Schulman S, Kearon C, Kakkar AK, et al. Dabigatran versus warfarin in the treatment of acute venous thromboembolism. *N Engl J Med.* 2009;361:2342–2352.
The Hokusai-VTE Investigators, Büller HR, Décousus H, et al. Edoxaban versus warfarin for the treatment of symptomatic venous thromboembolism. *N Engl J Med.* 2013;369:1406–1415.

TABLE 45.8 Single-Center Case Studies Supporting Catheter-Directed Thrombolysis for Deep Venous Thrombosis[a]

Author	n	Agent	Outcome	Hemorrhage, %
Molina et al.	12	UK	95% lysis	0%
Comerota et al.	7	UK	71% lysis	0%
Semba and Dake	27	UK	92% lysis	0%
Bjarnason et al.	87	UK	86% lysis	6.9% major/14.9% minor
Patel et al.	10	UK	100% lysis	0%
Ouriel et al.	11	r-PA	73% lysis	0%
Castenada et al.	25	r-PA	92% lysis	4%
Chang et al.	10	t-PA	90% lysis	0%
Horne et al.	10	t-PA	90% lysis	30% minor
Razavi et al.	36	TNK	83%	2.7% major 8.3% minor

[a]Series evaluating catheter-directed thrombolysis for deep venous thrombosis.
N, Number of patients; *R-PA*, reteplase; *TNK*, tenecteplase; *t-PA*, alteplase; *UK*, urokinase.

venous segment. Because thrombolytic agents activate plasminogen within the thrombus, the local delivery of the drug directly into the thrombus enhances its overall effectiveness. By focusing the delivery of higher concentrations of the drug, lysis rates can be improved, the duration of treatment reduced, and complications associated with the exposure of the patient to systemic thrombolytic therapy potentially minimized. Furthermore, with enhanced removal of obstructive thrombus, it is believed that venous valvular function will remain preserved, and consequently, the incidence of PTS will be reduced. In addition, successful CDT facilitates detection and correction of any underlying venous obstructive lesions with balloon angioplasty and/or stent placement. Currently there are no thrombolytic agents that are approved for CDT by the U.S. Food and Drug Administration (FDA). The use of thrombolytic agents in CDT for venous thrombosis constitutes an "off-label" use. While there are multiple thrombolytic agents available in the United States for use in CDT, the majority of reported contemporary use involve alteplase and tenecteplase. Although the various agents have unique properties that might theoretically confer an advantage of one over another, there remains no peer-reviewed consensus on a superior agent for CDT for venous thrombosis. The literature on CDT for venous thrombosis has a paucity of prospective randomized comparative trials. Therefore, the choice of thrombolytic agent is generally individualized to the physician's discretion. The largest published experience with CDT has come from the National Venous Thrombolysis Registry,[100] which included 287 patients treated with urokinase and followed up for 1 year. Overall, 71% of the patients were treated for iliofemoral DVT. Complete dissolution of thrombus was achieved in 31% of cases, and partial thrombus dissolution was reported in an additional 52%. Primary patency at 1 year was 60%. Preservation of valvular competence was demonstrated in 72% of patients with complete thrombolysis. Table 45.8 reviews the available clinical experience for CDT for the treatment of DVT.

The location of the LEDVT and the patient's symptoms determine the access technique. For most cases of iliofemoral DVT, the ipsilateral popliteal vein is favored if the clinical situation allows. With the patient prone on the angiographic table, the popliteal vein should be accessed under ultrasound guidance, typically with a small-gauge micropuncture echogenic needle, with care to avoid inadvertent puncture of the popliteal artery, especially since the popliteal vein is often thrombosed. The ipsilateral posterior tibial vein may also be accessed, a technique that confers the advantage of maintaining the patient in a supine position and treatment of the popliteal thrombosis. Following popliteal vein cannulation, a short sheath is then introduced, through which all subsequent catheters can be exchanged. Next, a baseline venogram is obtained through the venous sheath using standard Digital subtraction angiography imaging techniques. Then, a combination of 0.035-inch straight and curved hydrophilic guidewires are typically used to easily cross the occluded venous segment. Following wire and then catheter traversal of the occluded venous segment, venography is then repeated to confirm the intraluminal position of the catheter. At this point, modern techniques generally favor moving directly to mechanical thrombectomy (described as follows), followed by the insertion of a multisidehole infusion catheter for dedicated, prolonged administration of thrombolytics if necessary. When positioning an infusion catheter for the direct delivery of thrombolytic agents, it is essential to position the delivery system directly across the thrombus in order to maximize plasminogen activation at the site of obstruction. Fig. 45.11 illustrates the endovascular management of an acute left common

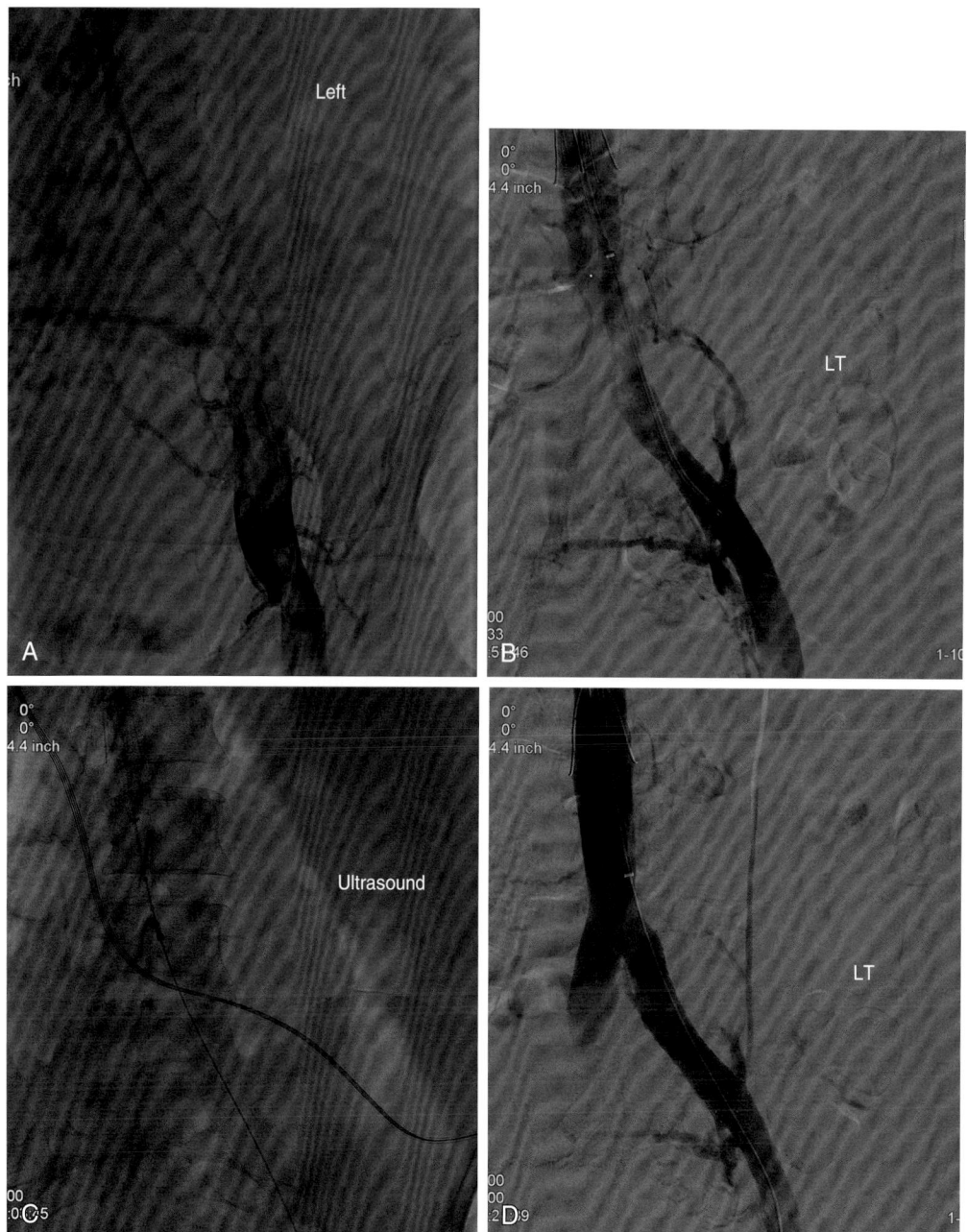

Fig. 45.11 (A) Extensive thrombotic occlusion of left common and external iliac veins with some extension into the common femoral veins. Note the severely dilated iliac veins. (B) Following pharmacomechanical thrombolysis utilizing rheolytic thrombectomy and thrombolysis. (C) Intravascular ultrasound to confirm extrinsic compression of the left common iliac vein and to assist with stent sizing. (D) Final venogram of left common and external iliac vein status poststenting. *LT,* Left.

iliac DVT. Patients are then closely monitored in an interventional recovery unit during thrombolytic infusion. It is common, particularly with an extensive thrombus burden, for the duration of therapy to exceed 24 hours. Follow-up venography should be performed every 8 to 12 hours to assess and/or reposition the infusion catheter as necessary. Weighing the risk versus benefit of thrombolytic therapy, the infusion should ideally be continued until complete lysis is achieved.

In patients in whom venous patency has been restored and there is no underlying stenotic/occlusive lesion, thrombolysis is discontinued and anticoagulation is initiated. The presence of venous stenosis as the cause of acute iliofemoral DVT should generally be ruled out formally with IVUS following thrombolysis. Hemodynamically significant lesions that are uncovered in the iliac veins should be considered for endovascular stenting; however, many operators delay stenting for several months to allow for the hypercoagulable acute phase to pass. IVC filter placement during CDT for LEDVTs are commonly used according to their standard indications and to prevent iatrogenic PE if extensive mechanical thrombectomy is to be utilized. Their routine use during CDT has always been controversial because of the low incidence of complications observed when thrombolysis is performed without filter protection. Acknowledging this controversy, we have generally been using retrievable IVC filters during CDT for LEDVTs, especially in patients in whom the venogram defines a true "free-floating" iliac vein thrombus or in patients

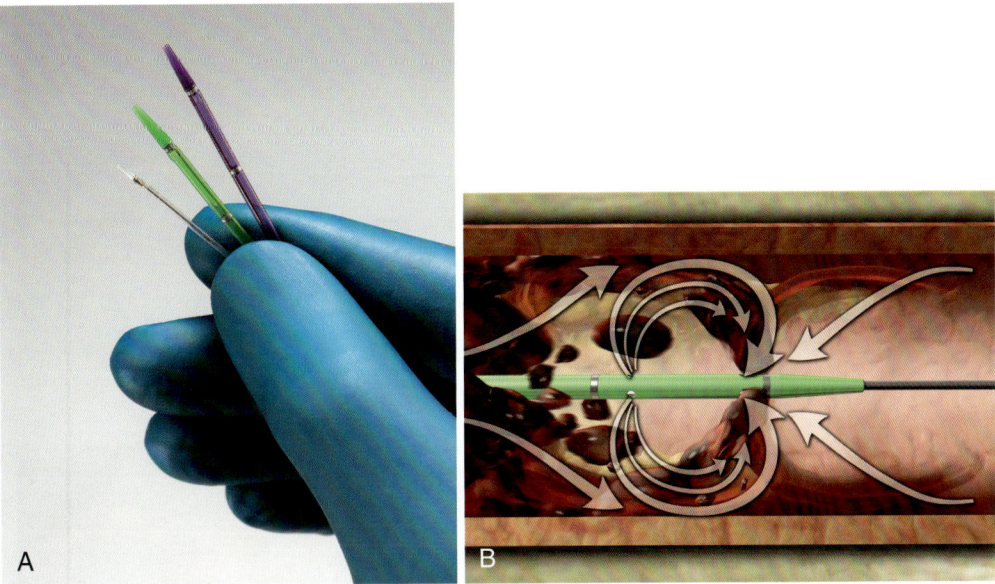

Fig. 45.12 (A) The AngioJet System (Boston Scientific, Marlborough, MA) comes in multiple sizes and emits high-velocity saline jets that are directed backward from the tip of the device to outflow channels in a coaxial fashion. (B) This generates a vacuum force that draws the thrombus into the catheter by the Venturi effect. (Image courtesy Boston Scientific. © 2014 Boston Scientific Corporation or its affiliates. All rights reserved.)

with a documented pulmonary embolus and limited cardiopulmonary reserve.

Percutaneous Mechanical Thrombectomy

Several drawbacks to CDT as a monotherapy for LEDVT include the time necessary for thrombolysis, the need for intensive care monitoring, associated hemorrhagic risks, cost, and lack of prospective, randomized clinical trials. With these issues in mind, PMT is conceptually attractive because such a technique may obviate or reduce the time required for thrombolytic drug administration. In turn, this may result in a shorter time to vein patency, shorter length of stay, reduction in hemorrhagic risk, and overall cost savings. From a mechanistic standpoint, PMT devices can be categorized as rotational, hydrodynamic, or ultrasound-facilitated. *Pharmacomechanical thrombectomy* is a term used to describe the treatment of thrombosis using both thrombolytic drugs and mechanical thrombectomy during the same procedure. Some PMT devices have the unique capability of being able to deliver thrombolytics directly into the thrombus, whereas others may be used only as an adjuvant prior to the use of a standard multisidehole infusion catheter. Rotational thrombectomy devices employ a high-speed rotating basket or impeller to pulverize or fragment thrombus. Preclinical evaluation of these devices have focused on clot removal and assessment of potential valve injury. In one such study, the Arrow-Trerotola (Arrow) percutaneous thrombectomy device did not cause physiologically significant damage to valves 7 mm or larger in diameter.[101] Hydrodynamic, or "rheolytic," recirculation devices have become a common treatment modality for LEDVT. The AngioJet system (Boston Scientific, Minneapolis, MN) is the prototypical device in this category, which works based on the Venturi effect. Rapidly flowing saline jets are directed backward from the tip of the device to outflow channels in a coaxial fashion, which, in turn, generates a vacuum force that draws thrombus into the catheter (Fig. 45.12). Newer iterations of this device also include the ability to spray thrombolytic agents directly into areas of thrombus using the Power Pulse technology, making it a simple device for pharmacomechanical thrombectomy (Fig. 45.13). In addition, a new 8-Fr catheter (Zelante, Boston Scientific, Minneapolis, MN) with a venous only indication offers four times the thrombectomy power over the 6-Fr system. Using Power Pulse, the operator delivers the thrombolytic agent after a standard thrombectomy run and then allows the drug to dwell, typically for 30 minutes. Following the dwell period, a final "cleanup" run is performed, again using the standard thrombectomy settings. The Zelante catheter in our experience offers an "on the table" result two-thirds of the time, alleviating the need for a prolonged thrombolytic infusion with its associated costs and risks. Two contemporary series utilizing pharmacomechanical thrombectomy and the Power Pulse technique both report high technical success rates with acceptable safety and long-term improved functional outcomes.[102,103]

In an effort to improve thrombolytic penetration and enhance thrombus disruption, an ultrasound based infusion system, the EkoSonic Endovascular System (BTG International, London, U.K.), was developed. The EkoSonic catheter combines high frequency, low power ultrasound with simultaneous CDT to accelerate clot dissolution. The exposure of nonfragmenting ultrasound to clot has no thrombolytic effect on its own. However, the combination of directed ultrasound with local thrombolytic infusion accelerates the thrombolytic process.[104] Mechanistically, it is thought that the ultrasound waves work by loosening the fibrin matrix, increasing clot permeability, and ultimately driving the thrombolytic agent deep into the thrombus for better drug distribution. In addition, the ultrasound energy is atraumatic with regard to the venous valves, a property theoretically important in the prevention of PTS. The EkoSonic catheter system consists of a 5.2-Fr, multilumen drug delivery catheter with one central lumen and three separate infusion ports (Fig. 45.14). Each catheter has a matched ultrasound core wire that is placed in the central lumen that delivers the ultrasound energy evenly along the entire infusion pathway. After the catheter is positioned in the thrombus, an infusion of thrombolytic agent is started, along with saline to serve as a coolant. Ultrasound energy is then started and delivered simultaneously with the thrombolytic agent infusion. In a multicenter series of 53 patients, ultrasound-accelerated thrombolysis was shown to be a safe and efficacious treatment for DVT with a high incidence of complete thrombolysis and a reduction in bleeding rates.[105] However, the Ultrasound-enhanced Thrombolysis Versus Standard Catheter Directed Thrombolysis for Ilio-femoral Deep Vein Thrombosis (BERNUTIFUL) Trial, which compared

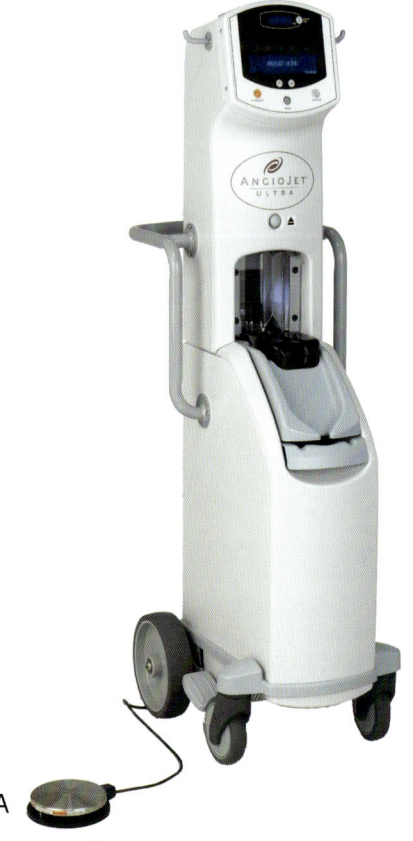
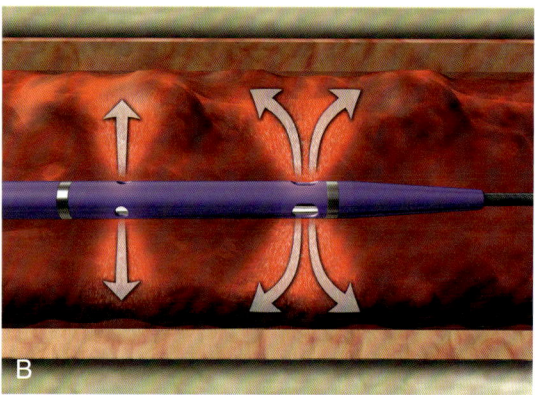

Fig. 45.13 (A) AngioJet Thrombectomy System (Boston Scientific, Marlborough, MA) with a simplified set-up process. (B) It also has the ability to directly spray thrombolytics onto the clot using the Power Pulse spray feature. (Image courtesy Boston Scientific. © 2014 Boston Scientific or its affiliates. All rights reserved.)

EKOS ultrasound assisted thrombolysis versus standard CDT, did not show any benefit of ultrasound assisted thrombolysis in thrombus resolution.[106] This device has recently gained FDA approval for the use in the pulmonary arteries in the treatment of PE.[107]

A catheter based thrombectomy system, the Indigo Mechanical Thrombectomy catheter (Penumbra Inc., Alameda, CA), can be used to remove emboli and thrombi from the venous system (Fig. 45.15). It is indicated for use on its own when thrombolytic therapy and surgery may be contraindicated, as well as in conjunction with thrombolysis to shorten lengthy infusions and costly intensive care unit stays. These features are driven by the Indigo System's Pump Max and proprietary separator, which maximize aspiration power and efficiency. These two technologies ensure continuous aspiration throughout the system without clogging the catheter's tip. This percutaneous system is available in four diameter options (CAT3, CAT5, CAT6, and CAT8), ranging from 3.4- to 8-Fr and lengths ranging from 85 to 150 cm.

Finally, another catheter-based thrombectomy system, the ClotTriever by Inari Medical (Irvine, CA), offers another option to patients with acute iliofemoral DVT. The advantages of the ClotTriever system would include the ability to capture and remove large thrombus volumes, mechanically core clot from the vein wall, treat in a single session, and potentially reduce or eliminate the need for thrombolytics. The system includes the ClotTriever sheath (Fig. 45.16) that is 13 Fr. and the ClotTriever catheter (Fig. 45.17) that includes the "Coring Element" with the collection bag that can contour to effectively treat vessels as small as 6 mm and as large as 16 mm.

These exciting combination strategies continue to be developed and investigated, and with further follow-up and study will be better defined for their use in the evolving treatment paradigms for DVT.

The Research Gap in Deep Vein Thrombosis Intervention

The Catheter-Directed Thrombolysis for Deep Vein Thrombosis (CaVevT) study was a multicenter, open-label, randomized trial examining the use of CDT versus standard anticoagulation in patients with a first-time iliofemoral DVT. The primary end point was the incidence of PTS at 24 months. The final result was a 14% absolute risk reduction in PTS, favoring CDT over standard anticoagulation at 2-year follow-up.[108] At 5-year follow-up, the absolute risk reduction increased to 28%, and the number needed to treat decreased from seven to four.[109] More recently, the results of the National Institutes of Health-sponsored Acute Venous Thrombosis: Thrombus Removal with Adjunctive Catheter-Directed Thrombolysis (ATTRACT) trial were published following a nearly 5-year enrollment period.[110] The ATTRACT trial was a multicenter, randomized, open-label clinical trial that randomized patients with acute proximal DVT to receive interventional therapy and standard therapy versus standard therapy alone. The primary end point was the development of PTS at 2 years. The ATTRACT trial found that among patients with acute proximal DVT, interventional therapy did not prevent PTS, but did increase major bleeding. The study was clearly underpowered to draw any conclusions on the population of patients with iliofemoral DVT, but intervention did reduce PTS severity scores with a trend of benefit toward the iliofemoral DVT group. There has been considerable criticism on the ATTRACT trial design and the lack of follow-up imaging to adequately address the open vein hypothesis. Only a subgroup of patients in ATTRACT had imaging at 1 year to assess vein patency (20%); therefore, any firm correlation of an "open vein" to the rate of PTS is limited. In addition, current interventional techniques have progressed since the completion of the ATTRACT trial,

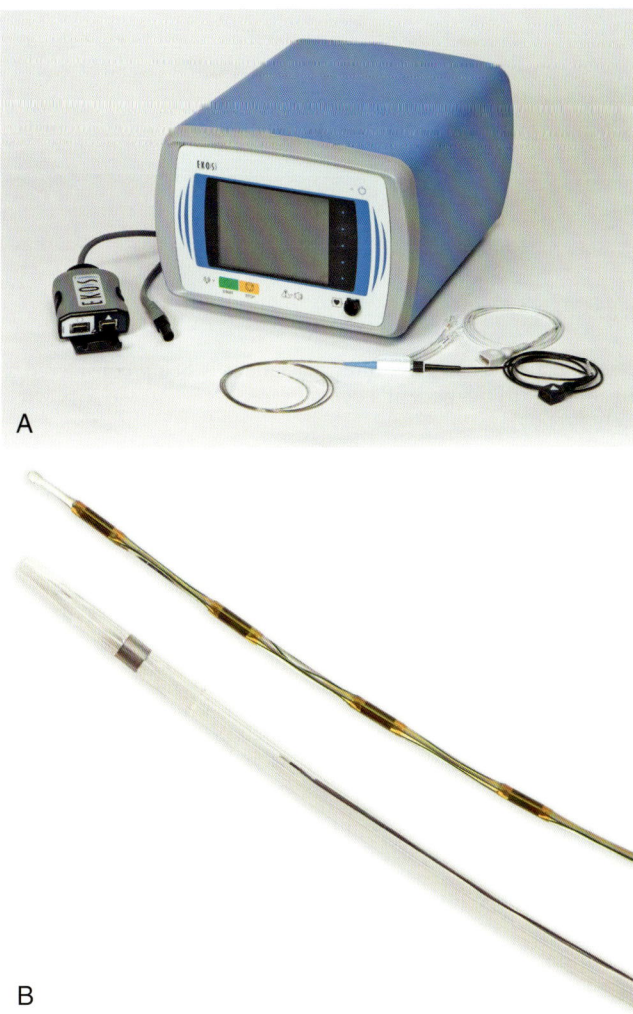

Fig. 45.14 (A) The EkoSonic Endovascular System (EKOS Corporation, Bothell, WA) has an ultrasound-generating console with simplified set-up. (B) The catheter is placed directly into the thrombus, where microtransducers transmit high-frequency, low-power sound waves.

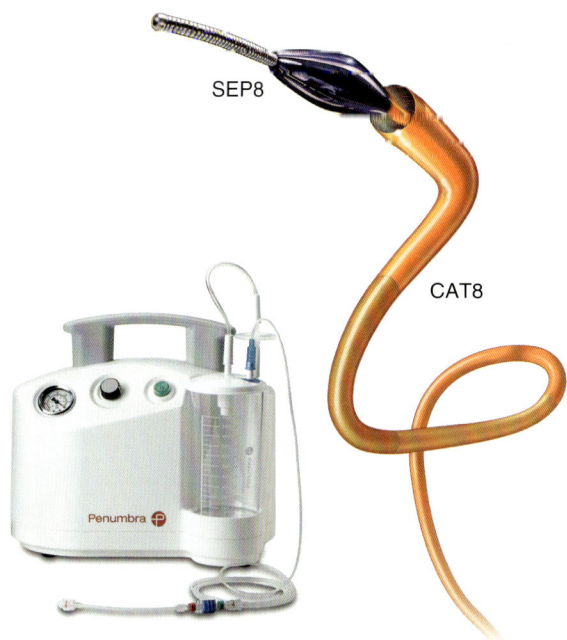

Fig. 45.15 Penumbra Indigo Continuous Aspiration Mechanical Thrombectomy, 8 Fr (CAT 8) catheter and pump. (Courtesy Penumbra, Inc., Alameda, CA.)

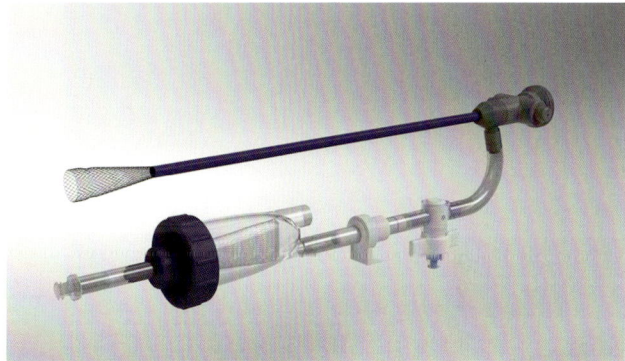

Fig. 45.16 ClotTriever sheath, 13 Fr. (Courtesy Inari Medical, Inc., Irvine, CA.)

including improved thrombectomy devices and utilization of IVUS to determine the need for adjunctive venous stenting. The limitations of standard venography that was utilized in the ATTRACT trial have been reviewed above. Therefore, further research must be done using modern-day interventional techniques in a population of iliofemoral DVT patients before the results of the ATTRACT trial may impact current practice patterns.

Inferior Vena Cava Filters

The primary indications for IVC filter placement include absolute contraindications to anticoagulation or recurrent thromboembolism while receiving therapeutic doses of anticoagulation for LEDVT. IVC filters can also be placed in the setting of massive or submassive PE when it is believed that any further pulmonary emboli may be lethal due to a compromised cardiopulmonary reserve. Although effective in reducing the risk of further pulmonary embolization, IVC filters do not afford protection from further DVT. In fact, IVC filters may result in an increased risk of secondary DVT. In a study by Decousus, in high-risk patients with proximal DVT, the initial beneficial effect of IVC filters for the prevention of pulmonary embolus was counterbalanced by an excess of recurrent DVT (20.8%) versus standard anticoagulation (11.6%), without any difference in mortality.[111]

Today, IVC filters are designed as permanent or optionally retrievable (Fig. 45.18). Optionally retrievable filters are approved for permanent placement but are designed to facilitate retrieval once the risk of further PE or contraindication to anticoagulation has passed. Currently, there are 11 permanent or optionally retrievable IVC filters with FDA approval in the United States. Percutaneous transjugular or transfemoral insertion is most commonly utilized. Smaller delivery sheaths and lower device profiles have also facilitated access via the brachial vein or popliteal vein. The choice of filter depends on the IVC size and required duration of insertion prior to safely starting anticoagulation. The popularity of IVC filters has increased dramatically over the last decade due to expanding indications for insertion—particularly primary prevention and the increasing utilization of retrievable filters. Manufacturer recommended retrieval times vary by product, with some filters having on-label retrieval times for up to 1 year following implantation. A recent FDA mandate (August 2010) recommends that implanting physicians and clinicians responsible for the ongoing care of patients with retrievable IVC filters consider removing the filter as soon as protection from PE is no longer needed. Complications of IVC filters generally fall

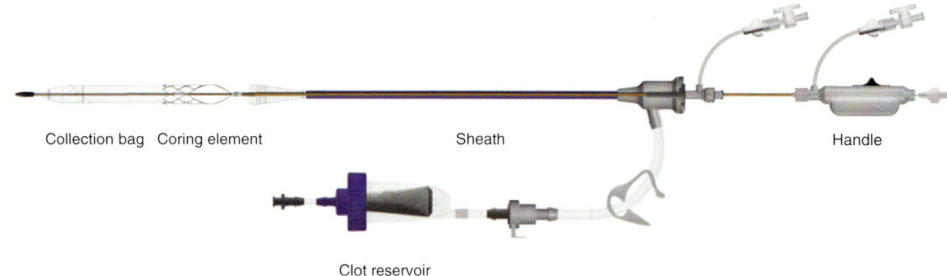

Fig. 45.17 Clottriever thrombectomy catheter. (Courtesy Inari Medical, Inc., Irvine, CA.)

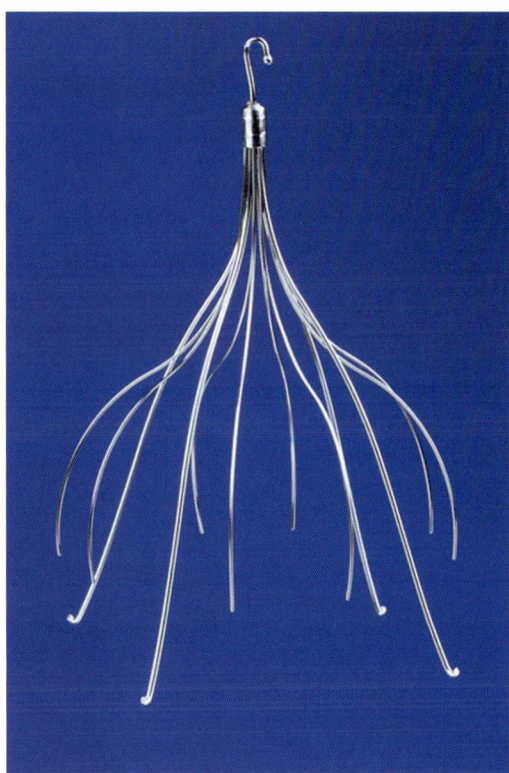

Fig. 45.18 Cook Celect retrievable inferior vena cava (IVC) filter, which has nitinol construction, is used in IVCs up to 30 mm in diameter and is delivered via a 7-Fr delivery sheath. (Courtesy Cook Medical, Bloomington, IN.)

into three separate categories: procedure-related, device-related, and thrombosis-related. Procedure-related complications include primarily insertion site complications, whereas device-related complications include malpositioning, tilting, failure of complete deployment, migration, fracture, and IVC perforation. These device-related complications affect the efficacy of the filter in secondary PE prevention. Thrombotic complications include PTS, recurrent DVT, and IVC thrombosis. The seriousness of these complications highlights the importance of appropriate case selection when IVC filter placement is being considered as an adjuvant to the patient's overall care.

KEY REFERENCES

1. Moffatt CJ, Franks PJ, Doherty DC, et al. Prevalence of leg ulceration in a London population. *QJM*. 2004;97:431–437. https://doi.org/10.1093/qjmed/hch075.
4. Bergan JJ, Schmid-Schonbein GW, Smith PDC, et al. Chronic venous disease. *N Engl J Med*. 2006;355:488–498.
20. Desmyttère J, Grard C, Wassmer B, et al. Endovenous 980-nm laser treatment of saphenous veins in a series of 500 patients. *J Vasc Surg*. 2007;46(6):1242–1247. https://doi.org/10.1016/j.jvs.2007.08.028.
33. Hartnell GG, Hughes LA, Finn JP, et al. Magnetic resonance angiography of the central chest veins. A new gold standard? *Chest*. 1995;107:1053–1057. https://doi.org/10.1378/chest.107.4.1053.
34. Rizvi AZ, Kalra M, Bjarnason H, et al. Benign superior vena cava syndrome: stenting is now the first line of treatment. *J Vasc Surg*. 2008;47:372–380. https://doi.org/10.1016/j.jvs.2007.09.071.
44. Carvalho DZ, Hughes JD, Liebo GB, et al. Venous congestive myelopathy due to chronic inferior vena cava thrombosis treated with endovascular stenting: case report and review of the literature. *J Vasc Interv Neurol*. 2015;8(1):49–53.
46. Raju S. Treatment of iliac-caval outflow obstruction. *Semin Vasc Surg*. 2015;28(1):47–53. https://doi.org/10.1053/j.semvascsurg.2015.07.001.
91. Lensing AW, Prandoni P, Brandjes D, et al. Detection of deep-vein thrombosis by real-time B-mode ultrasonography. *N Engl J Med*. 1989;320(6):342–345. https://doi.org/10.1056/NEJM198902093200602.
93. Chung JW, Yoon CJ, Jung SI, et al. Acute iliofemoral deep vein thrombosis: evaluation of underlying anatomic abnormalities by spiral CT venography. *J Vasc Interv Radiol*. 2004;15(3):249–256.
94. Wells PS, Anderson DR, Rodger M, et al. Evaluation of D-dimer in the diagnosis of suspected deep-vein thrombosis. *N Engl J Med*. 2003;349(13):1227–1235. https://doi.org/10.1056/NEJMoa023153.
107. Kucher N, Boekstegers P, Müller OJ, et al. Randomized, controlled trial of ultrasound-assisted catheter-directed thrombolysis for acute intermediate-risk pulmonary embolism. *Circulation*. 2014;129:479–486. https://doi.org/10.1161/CIRCULATIONAHA.113.005544.
110. Vedantham S, Goldhaber SZ, Julian JA, et al. Pharmacomechanical catheter-directed thrombolysis for deep-vein thrombosis. *N Engl J Med*. 2017;377(23):2240–2252. https://doi.org/10.1056/NEJMoa1615066.

 Additional references available online at expertconsult.com.

中文导读

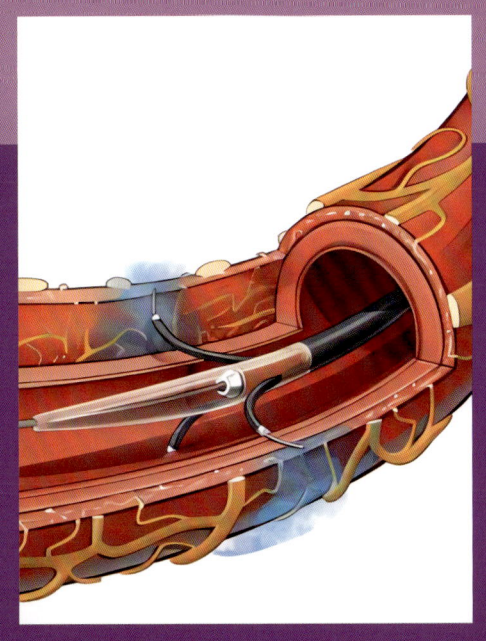

第46章
颈动脉及脑血管介入

　　缺血性脑卒中是成年人主要的致残病因，20%的脑卒中是颅内外动脉硬化狭窄造成的，本章概述了颈动脉分叉部、椎动脉近段及颅内动脉病变的介入治疗。

　　颈动脉分叉狭窄是最常见的颅外动脉病变部位，分叉病变和脑卒中关系明确，狭窄严重程度及病变症状稳定性是主要决定因素，介入再血管化治疗能明显减少脑卒中及近期和长期风险。本章详述了颈动脉介入治疗的流程，包括术前评估，围手术期准备，手术通道的建立，远端栓塞保护装置的应用，球囊预扩张及后扩张的必要和风险，支架的类型及合理选择等。对术后的并发症处理也很精细，包括术中、术后血流动力学障碍、高灌注综合征、心脏并发症、长期支架再狭窄等。通过大量的临床数据，针对不同风险等级的颈动脉狭窄患者，真实世界研究展示介入手术治疗风险及获益。

　　椎动脉近段病变以开口病变为主，目前介入干预是主要治疗手段，针对椎动脉介入手术操作要点进行详解，并汇总了椎动脉血管内治疗的临床研究结果。

　　颅内大动脉病变也是脑卒中的主要病因，本部分阐述了颅内大动脉的概念、病理及自然病史，以及相关的内外科治疗研究证据。尤其基于近些年急性脑卒中颅内动脉介入治疗的基础，阐述了今后颅内动脉介入治疗的方向。

　　通过本章节的介绍，有助于临床医师详细了解头颈部动脉病变的介入治疗，根据不同的病变特点选择合适的支架种类和再血管化治疗方式。

王彬成　张洪亮

章节要点

- 颈动脉动脉硬化行介入治疗进展迅速。基于潜在神经系统并发症风险,许多介入手术研究重在全面评估介入手术相较药物治疗的临床获益。
- 颈动脉分叉疾病和颅内动脉粥样硬化占所有缺血性卒中病因的15%~20%,是中风预防的重要靶标。
- 颈动脉分叉病变介入治疗是在栓塞保护系统辅助下的自膨支架植入,能更好地降低远端栓塞风险。对于高危颈动脉病变患者,该技术和颈动脉内膜剥脱等效。对于普通风险患者是否行颈动脉介入治疗,RCT研究结果尚无明确定论。
- 10%的后循环卒中是由于椎动脉近端病变导致的。这个部位的手术操作简单,安全性高,但未证实优于单纯药物治疗。
- 颅内动脉介入治疗进展迅速,是急性脑卒中的重要治疗手段。
- 通过提高手术技术、改进材料工艺、更精确地患者筛选,以及随机对照试验的开展,脑卒中血管介入治疗的作用会逐步显现出来。

46 Carotid and Cerebrovascular Intervention

R. Kevin Rogers, Joshua Seinfeld, Ivan P. Casserly

KEY POINTS

- Carotid intervention for the treatment of atherosclerotic disease has evolved considerably. The potential for serious neurologic complications during such procedures places a premium on careful studies documenting the overall clinical efficacy of intervention compared with medical therapy.
- Carotid bifurcation disease and intracranial atherosclerosis account for 15% to 20% of all ischemic strokes and represent an important target for stroke prevention.
- Contemporary carotid bifurcation intervention involves the use of self-expanding stents with embolic protection systems to reduce the risk of distal embolization. The technique has proven to be equivalent to carotid endarterectomy in high-risk patients. There remains debate on the interpretation of randomized trial data for carotid stenting and on Medicare reimbursement in normal-risk patients.
- Proximal vertebral artery disease may account for up to 10% of posterior circulation ischemic events. Intervention at this site is straightforward and safe but has not proven to be superior to medical therapy alone.
- Intracranial intervention is evolving to be an important therapy for acute stroke at qualified institutions.
- Further refinements in technique, technology, and patient selection, together with dedicated randomized controlled trials, will allow cerebrovascular intervention to realize its true potential in patients with stroke.

INTRODUCTION

Stroke is the leading cause of adult disability and the third leading cause of death in North America, Europe, South America, and Asia. Most strokes (80% to 85%) are ischemic in etiology. In the United States, atherosclerotic disease affecting the extracranial and intracranial arterial circulation accounts for approximately 20% of ischemic strokes (Fig. 46.1) and thus is an important target for stroke prevention.[1] Carotid intervention has evolved largely for the treatment of atherosclerotic disease with the goal of stroke prevention. Based on dramatic technological advances and increased operator expertise, these procedures can currently be performed with a high rate of technical success. However, because of the potential for serious neurologic complications from endovascular intervention in the cerebrovascular circulation, clear documentation of the safety of these procedures and their overall clinical efficacy is of paramount importance. These considerations have raised the bar for cerebrovascular intervention compared with other peripheral vascular procedures.

In the field of cerebrovascular intervention, carotid bifurcation intervention is unique in that the natural history of carotid artery bifurcation disease has been well defined and large randomized trials have previously documented the clinical effectiveness of surgical revascularization for this disease. There is already a large evidence base supporting carotid intervention in specific patient subgroups, and several randomized trials are ongoing in the remaining patient populations. With more than 140,000 carotid endarterectomy (CEA) procedures performed each year in the United States, and more than 280,000 worldwide, the potential impact of percutaneous revascularization has captured the interest of endovascular specialists who are keen to offer an alternative to surgery.

In contrast, endovascular intervention in the cerebrovascular circulation outside of the carotid bifurcation has been hampered by two important considerations: the natural history of noncarotid bifurcation cerebrovascular disease is less well defined, and there is a notable absence of randomized data documenting the benefit of revascularization compared with medical therapy alone. However, despite these obstacles, dramatic advances in the technical aspects of these interventions have been made, and there is an increased recognition of the need for well-designed clinical studies that address these deficiencies. What is often underappreciated is that noncarotid bifurcation cerebrovascular disease is responsible for at least the same number of ischemic strokes as carotid bifurcation disease and represents an equally important target for stroke prevention.

This chapter summarizes the current status of carotid bifurcation intervention and the most frequently performed noncarotid bifurcation cervical cerebrovascular interventions, notably of the proximal vertebral artery (VA). The emerging role of intracranial intervention in acute stroke management is also introduced.

CAROTID BIFURCATION INTERVENTION

Carotid Bifurcation Atherosclerosis and Stroke

The carotid bifurcation has a remarkable predilection for the development of atherosclerosis, which is typically located at the origin of the internal carotid artery (ICA) (Fig. 46.2). This plaque is similar to that found at other sites throughout the arterial system in that it contains a dense cap of connective tissue with embedded smooth muscle cells and an underlying core of lipid and necrotic debris.[2] Histologic studies of plaque from the carotid bifurcation of symptomatic and asymptomatic individuals have revealed features associated with the development of symptoms that are similar to those associated with plaque vulnerability in the coronary circulation: reduced amounts of collagen, increased inflammation, thinning of the fibrous cap, and increased cholesterol in the necrotic core.[2,3] Based on our current understanding, these processes result in plaque fissuring or rupture at the carotid bifurcation, causing either occlusive or nonocclusive thrombus formation. The dominant mechanism of stroke is believed to result from distal thromboembolism to the anterior cerebral circulation. However, a number of considerations, such as the size and composition of the embolus, the presence of contralateral disease, the anatomy of the circle of Willis, and the activity of fibrinolytic pathways, may attenuate or accentuate the clinical consequence of the pathologic event. Consequently, the same pathologic event may result in a reversible neurologic deficit (i.e., transient ischemic attack [TIA]), an irreversible neurologic deficit (i.e., stroke), or no symptoms at all.

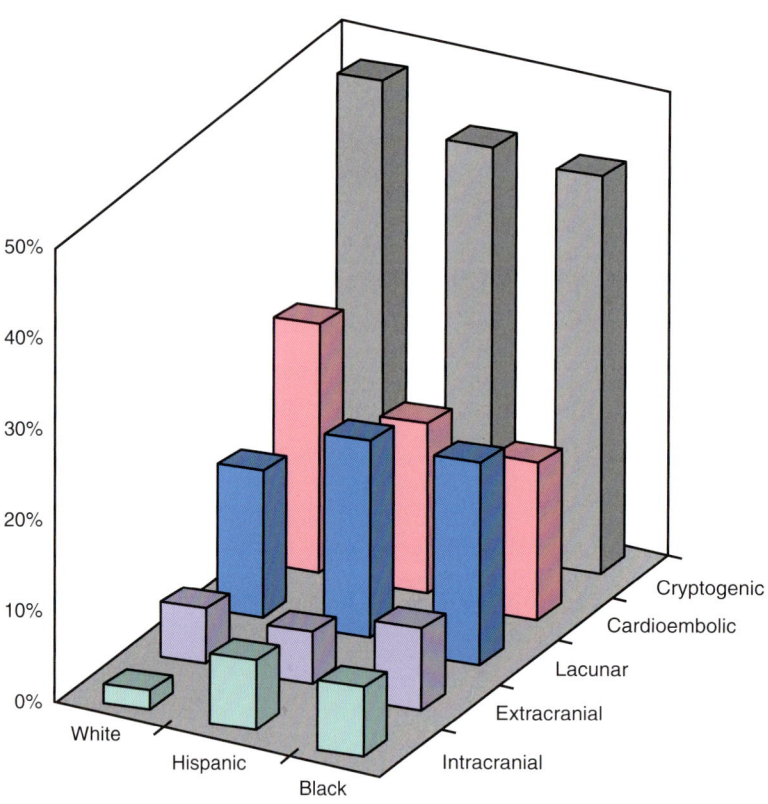

Fig. 46.1 Proportion of ischemic stroke subtypes according to race in the Northern Manhattan Study. (Adapted from White H, Boden-Albala B, Wang C, et al. Ischemic stroke subtype incidence among whites, blacks, and Hispanics: the Northern Manhattan Study. *Circulation*. 2005;111[10]:1327–1331.)

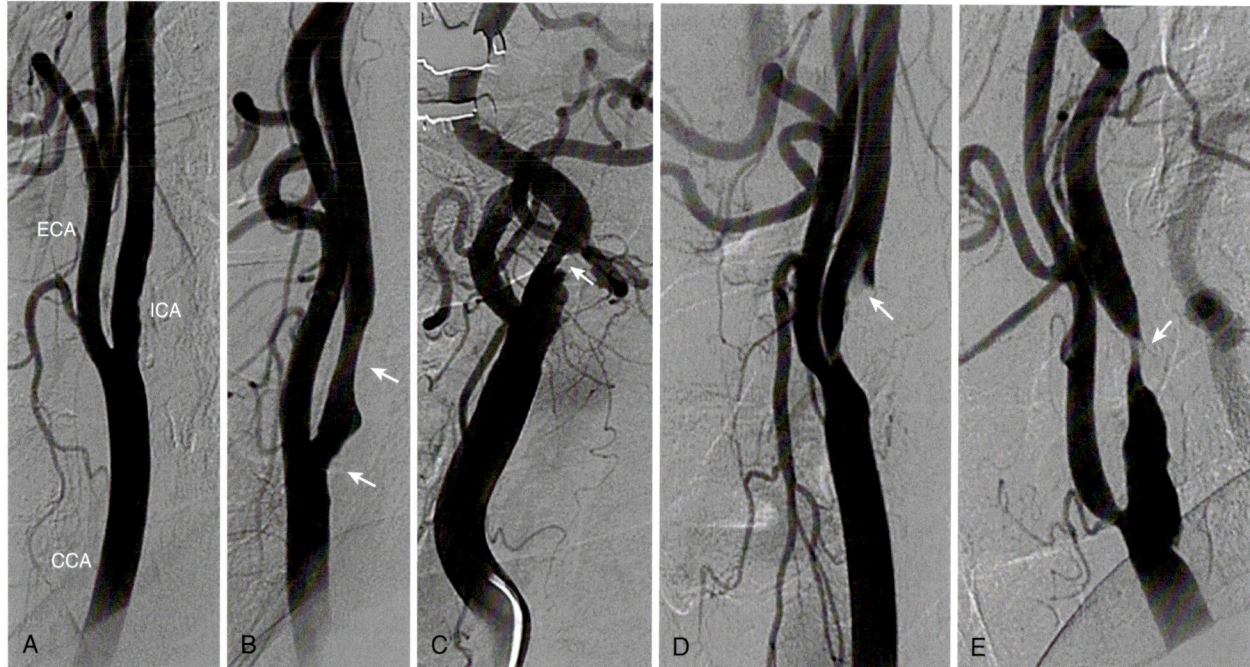

Fig. 46.2 Angiographic images from the carotid bifurcation show the spectrum of atherosclerotic disease at this site. (A) Minimal disease at the origin of the internal carotid artery *(ICA)*. (B) Mild stenosis extending from the distal common carotid artery *(CCA)* into the proximal ICA. (C) Moderate eccentric stenosis in the proximal portion of the ICA. (D) A thrombotic lesion in the proximal portion of the ICA in a patient with recent stroke. (E) High-grade stenosis in the proximal portion of the ICA. Notice that atherosclerotic plaque tends to accumulate in the posterior aspect of the ICA. *Arrows* indicate location of plaque. *ECA*, External carotid artery.

Natural History of Carotid Artery Bifurcation Disease

In clinical practice, two dominant factors are used to determine the risk of ischemic complications from a lesion of the carotid artery bifurcation: the symptomatic status of the lesion and the severity of stenosis. Although many of these data are derived from the medical arms of the large randomized CEA trials performed between the late 1980s and early 2000s, these considerations continue to be used as the major criteria for choosing patients for endovascular procedures and for enrolling subjects in carotid endovascular trials.

Symptomatic lesions of the carotid bifurcation are associated with a high risk of recurrent ischemic stroke. In the North American Symptomatic Carotid Endarterectomy Trial (NASCET), the risk of any ipsilateral stroke at 2-year follow-up in medically treated patients with symptomatic stenoses of 70% to 99% was 26%.[4] Among patients with symptomatic stenoses of 50% to 69%, the 5-year risk of any ipsilateral stroke was 22.2%.[5] There is a close temporal relationship between these recurrent strokes and the index event, with a steep exponential decline in risk within the first months, followed by a more gradual decline and ultimate normalization of risk at 2 to 3 years (Fig. 46.3).

By contrast, asymptomatic lesions of the carotid bifurcation are associated with a much lower risk of ischemic stroke. Over a 5-year period after an asymptomatic carotid stenosis was diagnosed (more than 60% by ultrasound), the risk of any stroke among medically treated patients in the Asymptomatic Carotid Surgery Trial (ACST) was 11%.[6] Not surprisingly, the risk of stroke was constant over the duration of the study. The implication from these findings is that carotid revascularization should be performed as expediently as possible after a neurologic event

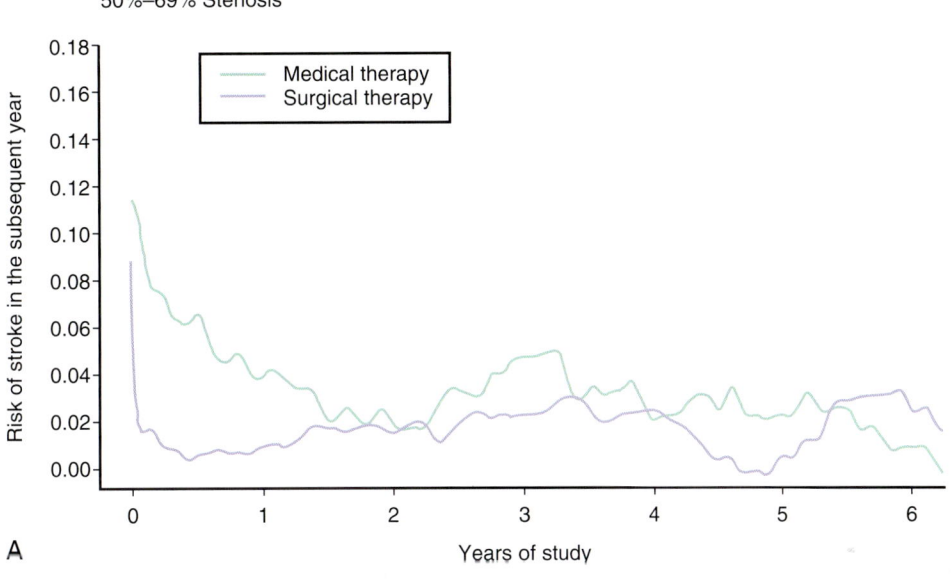

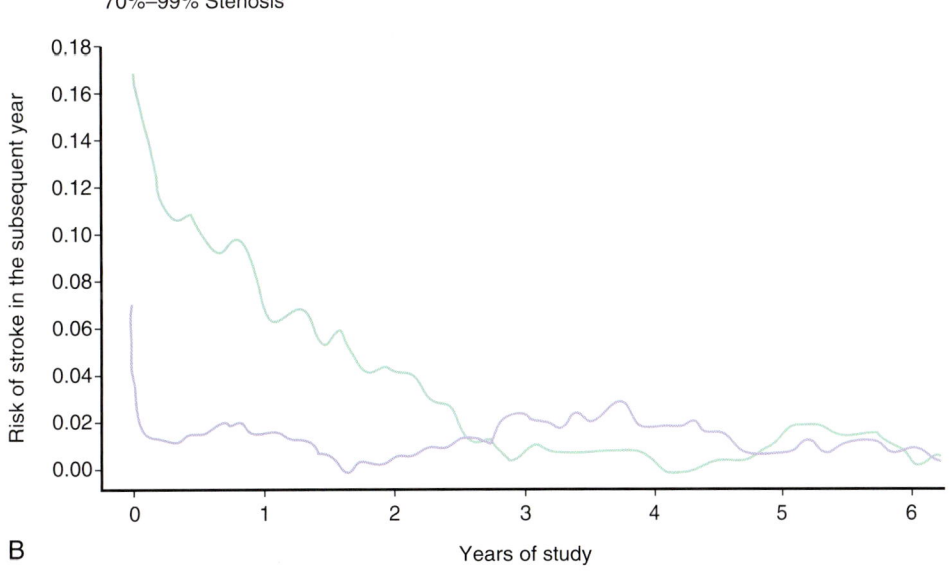

Fig. 46.3 Change in risk of ipsilateral stroke over time in medically treated *(green line)* and surgically treated *(purple line)* patients with symptomatic stenosis of 50% to 69% (A) or 70% to 99% (B) in the NASCET trial (North American Symptomatic Carotid Endarterectomy Trial). (Adapted from Barnett HJ, Taylor DW, Eliasziw M, et al. Benefit of carotid endarterectomy in patients with symptomatic moderate or severe stenosis. North American Symptomatic Carotid Endarterectomy Trial Collaborators. *N Engl J Med.* 1998;339[20]:1415–1425.)

caused by a culprit symptomatic stenosis, whereas intervention for an asymptomatic lesion may be approached in a more elective fashion.[7]

Among symptomatic patients, a close relationship between the severity of stenosis as assessed by careful angiographic methods and subsequent risk of ipsilateral stroke has been demonstrated.[8] The relationship is nonlinear, with a steep increase in risk associated with the tightest degree of stenosis (Fig. 46.4). However, for symptomatic patients with "near-occlusion" of the ICA—defined as a stenosis causing obstruction to flow sufficient to result in a decrease in the ICA diameter beyond the lesion (Fig. 46.5)—there are data to suggest that the risk of recurrent stroke is reduced compared with patients with severe stenosis without features of near-occlusion.[9] One potential explanation for this finding is the reduced likelihood of distal cerebral embolization caused by diminished flow distal to a critical stenosis. Among asymptomatic patients, the association between stenosis severity and risk of subsequent stroke has been inconsistent.[6,10] This finding likely underscores the heterogeneous nature of carotid plaque histology in asymptomatic patients and suggests that assessments of plaque vulnerability may be a more potent predictor of recurrent events than severity of stenosis in this patient group.

Currently there are more sophisticated models to predict the risk of stroke in patients with carotid disease, particularly for symptomatic patients.[11,12] In addition to stenosis severity, these models incorporate variables such as age, sex, nature of the presenting symptomatic event, time since the index event, plaque surface morphology, and transcranial Doppler findings to provide a more individualized estimate of risk. However, these models have yet to be incorporated into patient selection criteria in randomized trials to more fully establish their clinical relevance.

Benefit of Carotid Revascularization

The benefit of carotid revascularization in patients with carotid artery disease has been documented in several randomized controlled trials (RCTs) comparing medical therapy with surgical revascularization (i.e., CEA). These data are extremely important in any discussion of endovascular therapy for carotid bifurcation disease because they form the cornerstone justifying revascularization in certain subsets of patients. In a pooled analysis of data from the three major RCTs in symptomatic patients, CEA compared with medical therapy reduced the end point of stroke or operative death at 5 years in patients with carotid stenoses of 50% or greater, as assessed by carotid angiography using the NASCET criteria (Fig. 46.6).[13] This benefit was more pronounced in patients with stenoses of 70% to 99% (absolute risk reduction [ARR] 15.3%; 95% confidence interval [CI] 9.8% to 20.7%) than in those with stenoses of 50% to 69% (ARR 7.8%; 95% CI 3.1% to 12.5%). In addition, the crossover of the event-free curves occurred very early in the patient cohort with 70% to 99% stenoses (1 to 2 months) compared with the patient cohort with 50% to 69% stenosis (1 year). The incidence of perioperative stroke and/or death in these studies was uniformly less than 6%; the benefits derived from CEA are predicated on the maintenance of similar procedural outcomes. No significant benefit was observed in patients with near-occlusion of the carotid artery (ARR 0.1%; 95% CI –10.3 to 10.2), likely related to the lower risk of recurrent stroke with medical therapy in this group. These studies were performed in the late 1980s and early to mid-1990s; therefore the only stipulated medical therapy in the nonsurgical arm was aspirin. Contemporary medical therapy would likely attenuate the observed benefit associated with CEA. However, given the magnitude of the observed benefit associated with CEA in symptomatic patients, investigators have been reluctant to repeat randomized studies using contemporary medical therapy alone as a treatment arm.

Compared with medical therapy, CEA has also been shown to significantly reduce the incidence of stroke or operative death at 5-year follow-up in asymptomatic patients with carotid stenoses of 60% or greater, as assessed by carotid ultrasound (11.8% vs. 6.4%; ARR 5.4%; 95% CI 3% to 7.8%).[6] It is important to

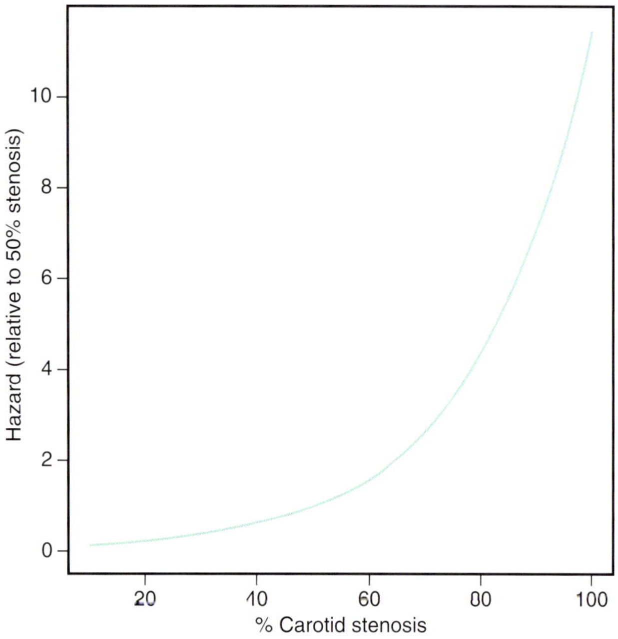

Fig. 46.4 Hazard of ipsilateral ischemic stroke within 3 years after index transient ischemic attack or stroke as a function of the percent of carotid stenosis, determined with the use of biplane angiographic views. (Adapted from Cuffe RL, Rothwell PM. Effect of nonoptimal imaging on the relationship between the measured degree of symptomatic carotid stenosis and risk of ischemic stroke. *Stroke.* 2006;37:1785–1791.)

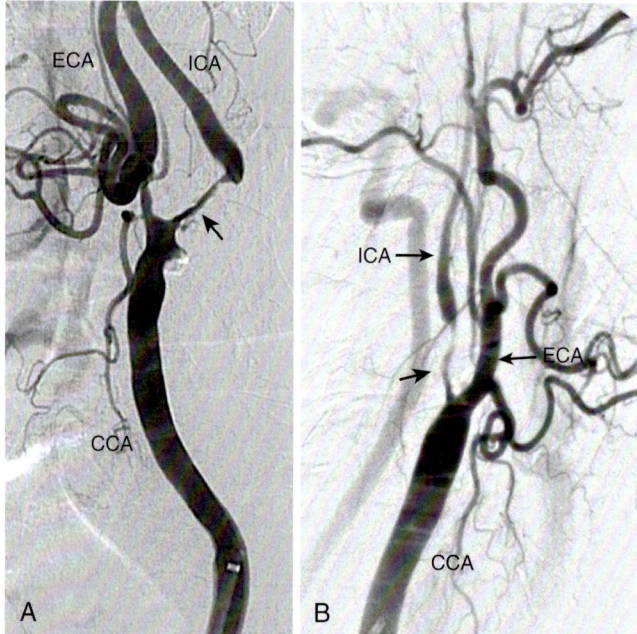

Fig. 46.5 Angiographic appearance of "near-occlusion" of the internal carotid artery *(ICA)*. (A) Reduction in diameter of the ICA compared with the external carotid artery *(ECA)* reflects a mild form of near-occlusion of ICA *(arrow)*. (B) Major collapse of the ICA beyond critical stenosis *(arrow)* reflects a severe form of near-occlusion of the ICA and is often referred to as a string sign. *CCA,* Common carotid artery.

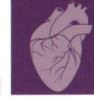

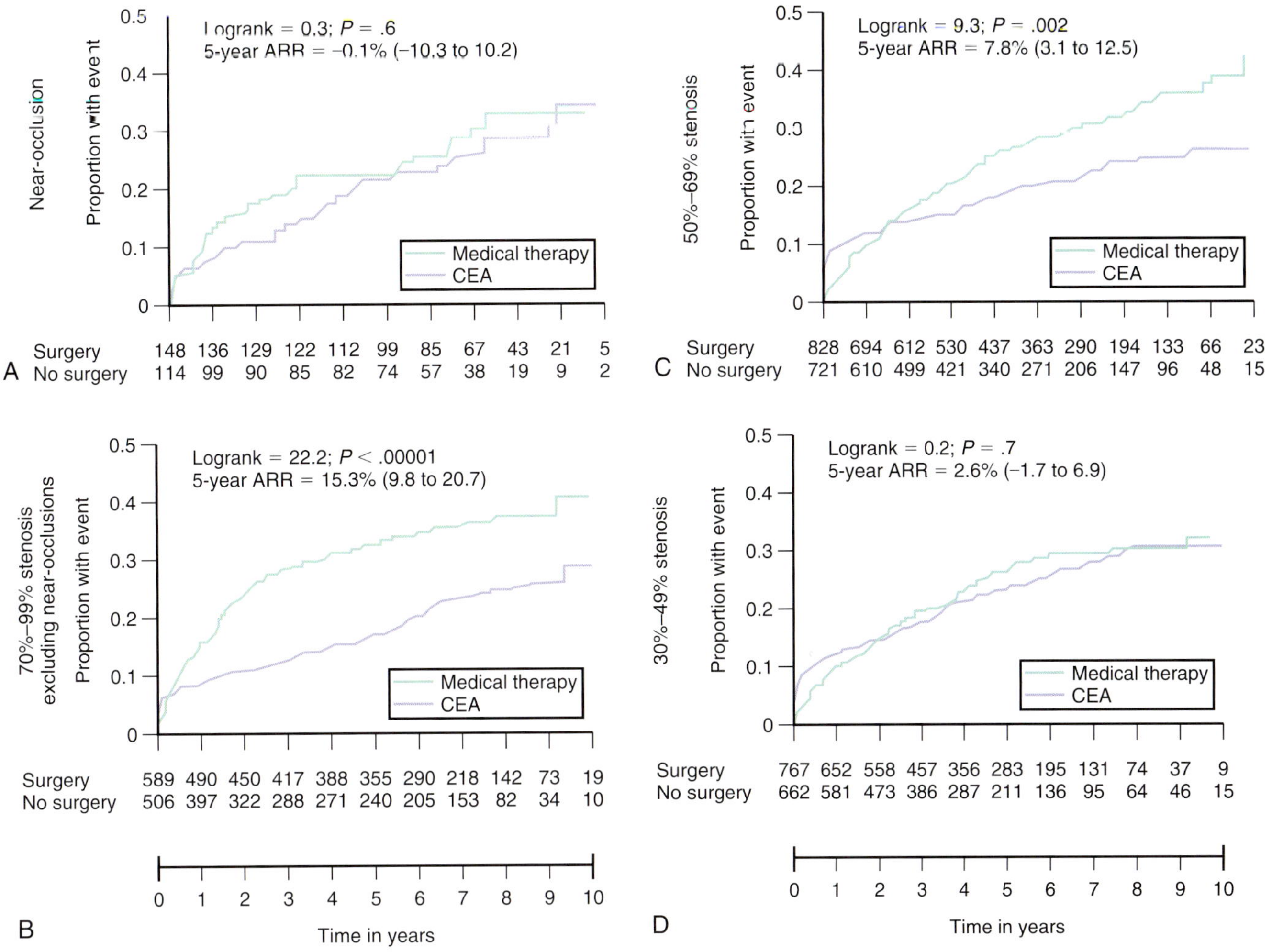

Fig. 46.6 Risk of any stroke or operative death in medically treated *(green line)* and surgically treated *(purple line)* symptomatic patients with varying degrees of carotid artery stenosis. (A) Near-occlusion. (B) 70% to 99%. (C) 50% to 69%. (D) 30% to 49%. *ARR*, Absolute risk reduction; *CEA*, carotid endarterectomy. (Adapted from Rothwell PM, Eliasziw M, Gutnikov SA, et al. Analysis of pooled data from the randomised controlled trials of endarterectomy for symptomatic carotid stenosis. *Lancet*. 2003;361:107–116.)

emphasize that in this asymptomatic population, the early hazard associated with revascularization persists up to 2 years from the time of CEA. If the life expectancy of the patient is less than 5 years, then significant benefit should not be anticipated. In addition, participation in these trials involving patients with asymptomatic carotid stenoses required documentation of a perioperative stroke and death rate of less than 3% at the investigation site, and the generalization of these findings is predicated on reproducing similar procedural outcomes.

Percutaneous Carotid Revascularization

Initial animal experimentation with percutaneous carotid revascularization began in the late 1970s and was followed by the first clinical reports of carotid angioplasty in the early 1980s. The first rigorous clinical testing of percutaneous carotid revascularization began in the mid-1990s. Although these studies demonstrated feasibility, two subsequent pivotal developments allowed percutaneous carotid revascularization to emerge as a viable alternative to CEA in the treatment of carotid disease: the ability to provide protection from distal embolization at the time of intervention, using a variety of embolic protection devices (EPDs), and the use of self-expanding stents. Carotid artery stenting (CAS) using self-expanding stents in combination with embolic protection represents the contemporary approach to carotid revascularization.

Carotid Artery Stenting: The Procedure

Preprocedural Assessment

Before any CAS procedure is undertaken, clinical assessment of the patient and anatomic assessment of the aortic arch and carotid/cerebral vasculature are essential.[14] Advanced age (>80 years) has been associated with significantly worse outcomes with CAS and should be carefully considered for the appropriateness of intervention.[15,16] Decreased cerebral reserve, manifested by the presence of dementia or cognitive impairment, and a history of prior strokes or lacunar infarcts increase the likelihood that distal embolization will be clinically manifested and are relative contraindications for the procedure.[17] Anatomic assessments usually can be made based on noninvasive studies, notably computed tomography (CT) angiography and magnetic resonance (MR) angiography. CT angiography offers higher spatial resolution and superior visualization of the aortic arch compared with MR angiography, and it allows an assessment of the degree of calcification of the aortic arch and carotid bifurcation lesion that is

TABLE 46.1 Anatomic Assessments Recommended Before Carotid Artery Stenting and Their Impacts on Interventional Planning

Angiographic Assessment	Impact on Interventional Procedure
ARCH ANATOMY	
Type I, II, or III arch	Predict difficulty of percutaneous approach and influence strategy for delivery of guide or sheath to CCA
Anomalies of origin of great vessels	
Tortuosity of proximal portion of great vessels	
LESION CHARACTERISTICS	
Precise location of lesion, with definition of proximal and distal extent of lesion	Influence planned location for stent placement and stent length
Lesion length	Influence strategy for delivery of guide or sheath to distal CCA
Complex lesion ulceration	Influence choice of stent length
Severity of stenosis	Predict difficulty of crossing lesion with filter device or wire
Severity of lesion calcification	Predict need for predilation of lesion before filter delivery
Diameter of vessel(s) proximal and distal to lesion	Influence choice of stent diameter
ICA DISTAL TO LESION	
Assess cervical portion of ICA for presence of disease and tortuosity	Influence choice of landing zone for filter or proximal occlusion EPD
Diameter of cervical ICA	Increased tortuosity favors use of guide to provide support for delivery of filter
	Influence choice of diameter of filter-type or proximal occlusion EPD
PATENCY OF EXTERNAL CAROTID ARTERY	
	Influences strategy for delivery of guide or sheath to distal CCA

CCA, Common carotid artery; *EPD,* embolic protection device; *ICA,* internal carotid artery.

not possible with MR angiography. Table 46.1 lists the anatomic features that should be reviewed and highlights the importance of each. Overall, these anatomic features allow the operator to more accurately determine the procedural risk and facilitate the planning of appropriate technique for procedural success.

Baseline Angiography

In most circumstances, CAS procedures are performed with the use of femoral artery access. Although the extent of baseline angiography varies depending on the preprocedural noninvasive assessment, high-quality angiography of the carotid bifurcation, the ipsilateral ICA, and intracranial anterior circulation is essential. We administer a heparin bolus of 25 mg/kg before any diagnostic cerebrovascular procedure in an effort to minimize the risk of thrombotic complications. A variety of catheter types are used to perform angiography, depending on the personal preference of the operator and the anatomy of the aortic arch and great vessels. For patients with uncomplicated anatomy (i.e., type I aortic arch, no tortuosity of the great vessels), a Bernstein catheter functions well. For more complicated anatomies (e.g., type II or III arch, tortuosity of the great vessels, bovine origin of the left common carotid artery [CCA]), a Vitek or Simmons catheter is usually required.

Interventional Technique

The technique for CAS placement follows a number of well-defined steps. Before CAS placement, all patients should receive aspirin. In addition, it is our practice to administer clopidogrel before the procedure. During the procedure, anticoagulation using unfractionated heparin to achieve an activated clotting time (ACT) of 275 to 300 seconds is standard.[18] For patients with a contraindication to heparin, a direct thrombin inhibitor such as bivalirudin has been shown to be safe.[19] In a cohort of 3555 patients from the Carotid Artery Revascularization and Endarterectomy (CARE) registry, bivalirudin was associated with less need for transfusion (0.9% vs. 1.5%; $P = .01$) and no difference in myocardial infarction (MI), stroke, and death at 30 days, compared with unfractionated heparin in a propensity score analysis.[20] Most operators perform the procedure without the administration of sedatives, which enhances the ability to screen for any neurologic change during the procedure.

Delivery of Sheath or Guide to the Common Carotid Artery

To deliver the range of contemporary equipment required for CAS, a 6-Fr sheath or 8-Fr guide must be placed in the distal CCA. In patients with difficult aortic arch anatomy, bovine origin of the left CCA, occlusion of the external carotid artery (ECA), distal CCA lesions, or significant tortuosity of the great vessels, this can be one of the most technically challenging parts of the procedure. This portion of the procedure is "unprotected" in that there is no distal EPD to protect against distal embolization, so the safety of this step is heavily operator dependent.

The standard procedure for delivery of a 6-Fr sheath in the CCA is as follows. The CCA of interest is engaged with a diagnostic catheter. A stiff-angled Glidewire is advanced into the ECA, and the diagnostic catheter is advanced over it. The Glidewire is exchanged for a superstiff Amplatz or SupraCore wire, and then the diagnostic catheter is removed. The 6-Fr sheath and its dilator are delivered over the stiff wire to the distal CCA, after which the dilator is removed.

Although this standard approach is sufficient for approximately 70% of cases, a number of variations to the technique may be necessary, depending on the specific anatomic features of the individual patient. Much of the learning curve in CAS involves achieving experience with these variations and learning how to predict which variation is appropriate for an individual patient's anatomy. One of the pivotal dogmas in CAS is that guidewires and catheters should never be placed across the carotid lesion to deliver the sheath or guide to the CCA. It is preferable to refer the patient for CEA than to persist in risky attempts to deliver the guide or sheath.

Delivery of Embolic Protection Device

The use of EPDs is currently considered the standard of care during CAS. Compelling observational data support this recommendation. Several studies have demonstrated that distal embolization is ubiquitous during CAS,[21,22] and observational series have shown a significant association between decreased periprocedural rates of stroke and death and the use of EPDs.[16,23] Over the past decade, three different device systems that provide protection from distal embolization at the time of carotid intervention have been developed.[24,25] In clinical practice, the most popular and most user friendly of these systems is the filter-type EPD (Table 46.2). These systems allow continued antegrade flow during carotid intervention—an important consideration for patients with compromised collateral flow to the ipsilateral carotid territory (e.g., patients with contralateral carotid artery disease or occlusion).

Because filter-type EPDs have been used in most contemporary CAS registries and RCTs, more data exist to support their use in carotid intervention compared with other EPDs. Based on the submission of these data to the U.S. Food and Drug Administration (FDA), multiple filter-type EPDs have received FDA approval, including Accunet, EmboShield, Spider, Angioguard, FilterWire, and FiberNet devices (Fig. 46.7; see Table 46.2).

TABLE 46.2 Filter-Type Embolic Protection Devices Used During Carotid Intervention

Filter	Manufacturer	Diameter (mm)	Pore Size (μm)
Interceptor	Medtronic	4.5, 5.5, 6.5	100
FilterWire EZ	Boston Scientific	3.5–5.5	80
Angioguard XPAngioguard RX	Cordis	4, 5, 6, 7, 8	100
EmboShield NAV	Abbott Laboratories	2.5–4.8, 4–7	140
Spider	ev3	3, 4, 5, 6, 7	50–200
Accunet OTW Accunet RX	Abbott Laboratories	4.5, 5.5, 6.5, 7.5	120
FiberNet	Medtronic	3.5–5, 5–6, 6–7	40

OTW, Over the wire; *RX*, monorail.

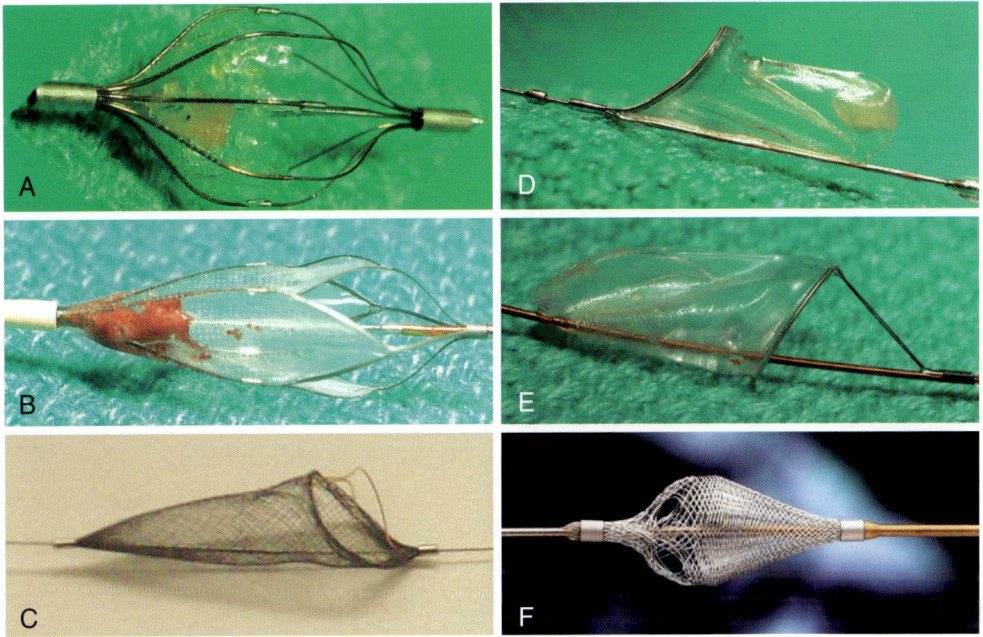

Fig. 46.7 Examples of filter-type embolic protection devices used during carotid intervention. (A) Angioguard XP (Cordis, Warren, NJ). (B) Accunet (Abbott Vascular, Abbott Park, IL). (C) Spider (ev3, Plymouth, MN). (D) FilterWire EX (Boston Scientific, Natick, MA). (E) FilterWire FZ (Boston Scientific). (F) Interceptor (Medtronic, Minneapolis, MN). (From Casserly IP, Sachar R, Yadav JS. *Manual of Peripheral Vascular Intervention*. Philadelphia, PA: Lippincott Williams & Wilkins; 2005.)

Although there is some variation in the individual design of these devices, they typically contain a polyurethane membrane with pores of fixed size (ranging from 80 to 140 μm in different devices), supported by a nitinol frame. The Spider and Interceptor EPDs are unique in that the filter pores are formed by a nitinol mesh. Each filter is integrated with a 0.014-inch guidewire with a 3- to 4-cm shapeable floppy tip. With the exception of the EmboShield and Spider devices, the filter is fixed to the wire.

The technique for delivery of a filter-type EPD varies according to the design of the system. In systems such as the Accunet, FilterWire EZ, or Angioguard, the filter is delivered in a collapsed form across the carotid lesion on the attached guidewire. With the EmboShield system, a unique 0.014-inch wire (BareWire) is used to cross the lesion first; the filter is then delivered in a collapsed form over this wire and deployed over the distal portion of the wire. The Spider system allows the lesion to be crossed using any 0.014-inch wire followed by a 2.9-Fr delivery catheter. It allows delivery of the Spider filter, which is integrated with a dedicated 0.014-inch wire that allows a small range of independent motion of the wire and filter. Predilation of the carotid lesion before delivery of the filter-type EPD is required in fewer than 1% to 2% of cases. If it is required, a small-caliber coronary balloon (i.e., 2.0-mm diameter) that minimizes the risk of distal embolization should be used. Regardless of the filter-type EPD that is used, the filter should ideally be deployed in a straight and nondiseased portion of the cervical ICA, which is typically in the distal cervical portion of the vessel. The presence of tortuosity or disease in the cervical portion of the ICA may necessitate an alternative placement, but there must be at least 3 to 4 cm of distance between the proximal margin of the filter and the distal margin of the ICA lesion to allow subsequent delivery of interventional equipment. These filter-type systems have replaced distal occlusion balloon EPDs, which were the first type of EPD used during a carotid intervention (c.1998).[26]

The most recent group of EPDs developed for carotid intervention are the proximal occlusion devices (e.g., the Parodi Antiembolism System from Gore Medical, Flagstaff, AZ, and the MO.MA System from Medtronic). These systems attempt to protect the brain from distal embolization by eliminating antegrade flow in the ICA during the procedure, essentially generating an

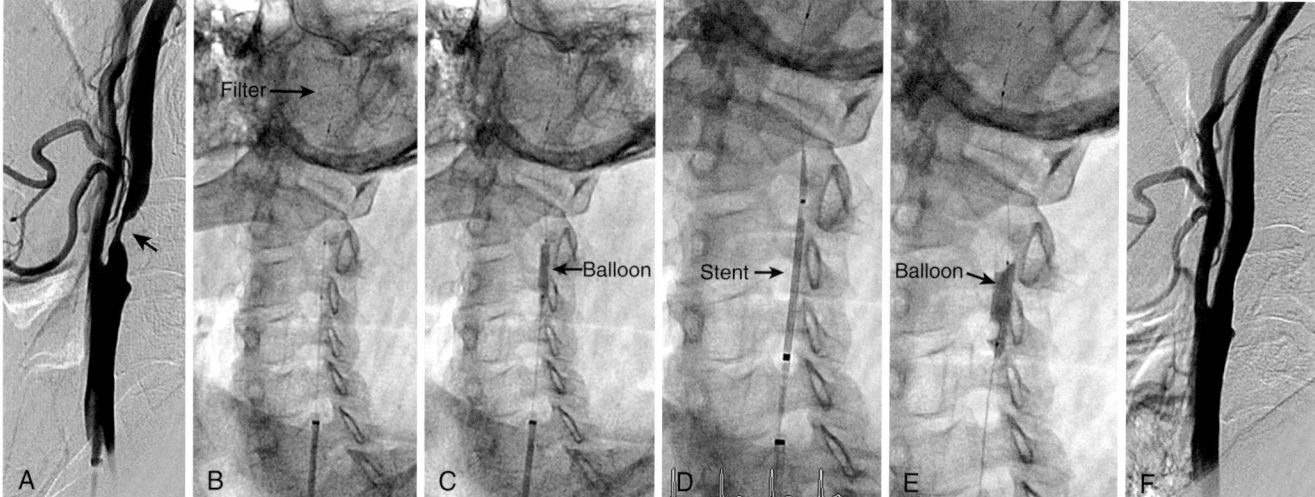

Fig. 46.8 Angiographic images from a carotid artery stent procedure. (A) Baseline angiographic image shows severe internal carotid artery stenosis *(arrow)*. (B) Placement of filter-type embolic protection device (5.5-mm-diameter Accunet filter, Abbott Vascular, Abbott Park, IL). (C) Predilation (4.0- by 20-mm Maverick balloon, Boston Scientific, Natick, MA). (D) Placement of tapered 6- to 8-mm-diameter by 30-mm-long self-expanding nitinol stent (Acculink, Abbott Vascular). (E) Postdilation with 5.0- by 20-mm Aviator balloon (Cordis, Warren, NJ). (F) Final angiographic appearance after removal of filter.

endovascular clamp.[27] Compliant balloons are inflated in the distal CCA and ECA, interrupting antegrade carotid flow and theoretically eliminating the risk of distal embolization from debris liberated during angioplasty and stenting. The success of such systems is predicated on adequate collateral circulation from the circle of Willis to maintain cerebral perfusion. With the Parodi device (not currently available in the United States), retrograde flow is generated in the ICA by connecting the lumen of the catheter, whose tip is in the CCA and distal to the occlusive balloon, to a catheter in the femoral vein. Blood flows down its pressure gradient from the CCA, through the blood return system, and to the femoral vein. In contrast, the MO.MA device simply creates a static column of blood in the ICA without continuous flow reversal, and removal of this unfiltered column of blood is achieved by aspiration with a syringe. Proximal EPDs appear to be particularly useful for cases in which tortuosity or disease distal to the carotid bifurcation lesion precludes the use of filter-type or distal balloon-occlusion EPDs.

Data with proximal EPDs are more limited than those for distal EPDs, but they are emerging. The Proximal Flow Blockage Cerebral Protection During Carotid Stenting (PRIAMUS) study,[28] an initial large registry using a proximal balloon-occlusion system, enrolled 416 "real-world" patients with carotid disease and reported a high rate of technical success (~99%) and acceptable clinical outcomes (4.5% incidence of in-hospital stroke, death, or MI). Two prospective registries using the MO.MA system have also been reported. In the Proximal Protection with the MO.MA Device During Carotid Stenting (ARMOUR) study, 262 high-risk patients undergoing CAS with embolic protection were enrolled, with a reported 30-day rate of stroke, death, or MI of 2.7%.[29] In a larger, single-center registry of 1300 patients who underwent CAS with embolic protection from the MO.MA device, the 30-day rate of stroke or death was a remarkable 1.4%, and the procedural success rate was 99.7%.[30] Finally, in a meta-analysis of four studies including 2397 patients (mix of normal and high surgical risk and symptomatic and asymptomatic status) undergoing CAS, the 30-day stroke rate was an impressive 1.7%.[31] A small randomized trial examining the incidence of diffusion-weighted MR imaging defects also showed that there was clearly less distal embolization with proximal EPDs compared with distal EPDs,[17,32] but a significant effect on clinical outcome has yet to be demonstrated. Although these results are encouraging, a direct comparison of proximal versus distal embolic protection in a randomized trial with hard clinical outcomes is needed.

Angioplasty and Stenting

Fig. 46.8 shows angiographic images from a carotid artery stent procedure.

Predilation

After placement of the EPD system, the lesion is usually predilated to facilitate stent delivery. Low-profile coronary balloons with diameters of 3.0 to 4.0 mm are used. Attempts to deliver the stent without predilation have been associated with a greater amount of atheroembolism, likely related to increased trauma to the lesion with forcible passage of the stent across a tight stenosis.[17]

Stent Selection and Placement

As in other vascular territories, the ability to stent carotid lesions has allowed operators to achieve a predictable angiographic result, deal with procedural complications such as dissection and abrupt vessel closure, and improve long-term patency by eliminating vessel recoil. Initial attempts at carotid stenting using relatively inflexible stainless steel balloon-expandable stents (e.g., Palmaz stent, Cordis, Warren, NJ) were associated with acute technical success. However, their use was abandoned owing to the subsequent development of stent crushing, likely related to compression of the superficially located carotid stent from neck movements.[33] This complication led to the development and use of flexible self-expanding stents that could conform to the tortuous anatomy of the carotid bifurcation and changes in vessel shape associated with neck movements (Table 46.3). The functional properties of these stents are defined by their metal composition and design.[34] Nitinol, a nickel-titanium alloy, is the most widely used material for carotid self-expanding stents; because of its large elastic range, it confers an ability to withstand significant

TABLE 46.3 Self-Expanding Carotid Artery Stents

Stent	Manufacturer	Metal Composition	Design	Tapered Version Available	FDA-Approved
Carotid WALLSTENT	Boston Scientific, Natick, MA	Cobalt chromium	Closed-cell	No	Yes
Exponent	Medtronic, Minneapolis, MN	Nitinol	Open-cell	No	Yes
Precise	Cordis, Warren, NJ	Nitinol	Open-cell	No	Yes
Protégé	ev3, Plymouth, MN	Nitinol	Open-cell	No	Yes
AccuLink	Abbott, Abbott Park, IL	Nitinol	Open-cell	Yes	Yes
X-Act	Abbott, Abbott Park, IL	Nitinol	Closed-cell	Yes	Yes
Zilver	Cook, Bloomington, IN	Nitinol	Open-cell	No	No
Cristallo Ideale	Invatec, Roncadelle, Italy	Nitinol	Hybrid	Yes	No

FDA, U.S. Food and Drug Administration.

deformations. A variety of nitinol stents with either a closed- or an open-cell design is available. The closed-cell design offers superior scaffolding at the cost of reduced flexibility.

Carotid stents come in a variety of sizes that match the typical diameter of the ICA and CCA (5 to 10 mm), and they are typically 20 to 40 mm long. The nominal diameter of the stent used should be 1 to 2 mm larger than the diameter of the largest treated vessel (usually the CCA). Stent lengths are chosen to provide complete lesion coverage. Initially, all carotid stents were cylindrical. However, tapered stents that conform to the size mismatch between the ICA and the CCA and facilitate treatment across the carotid bifurcation are currently commonly used. The tapered stents used are usually 6 to 8 mm or 7 to 9 mm in diameter and either 30 or 40 mm long. The cylindrical stents used are usually 8 mm in diameter and of similar length (i.e., 30 to 40 mm). For most cases, any of the available carotid stents will achieve similar technical success and clinical outcomes. In the remaining cases (~25%), assuming that all stents are available to the operator, the choice of stent should be individualized and is largely influenced by arterial anatomy and lesion morphology.[35] For example, stents with the greatest degree of flexibility—that is, open-cell-design nitinol stents with large open-cell areas and highly flexible interconnecting bridges (e.g., Precise stent, Cordis; Zilver stent, Cook, Bloomington, IN)—may be optimal for treating lesions in tortuous locations. Calcified lesions should be treated with stents that have a high radial force and a moderate outward expansive force, such as nitinol stents with a closed-cell design (e.g., Xact stent, Abbott). Finally, lesions with the greatest risk for distal embolism should be treated with stents that provide greater vessel scaffolding (closed-cell nitinol or cobalt alloy stents; e.g., WALLSTENT, Xact).

Postdilation

Postdilation of the self-expanding stent is typically performed with the use of a 4.5- to 5.5-mm diameter noncompliant balloon (e.g., Aviator, Cordis; Sterling, Boston Scientific). There is general agreement that postdilation is associated with the greatest propensity for plaque embolization; therefore experienced operators advocate a conservative approach to postdilation balloon sizing. A residual stenosis of less than 20% is usually accepted.

After predilation, stent deployment, and postdilation, contrast angiography is performed to assess the angiographic result and detect any potential complications. When filter-type EPDs are being used, this practice allows the detection of "slow flow," which is an important finding that requires special management.[36] Slow flow is manifested by delayed antegrade flow in the ICA and may vary from complete cessation of antegrade flow to mild delay of ICA flow compared with the ECA (Fig. 46.9). Most likely, this phenomenon is caused by excessive distal embolization of plaque elements that occlude the filter pores, compromising

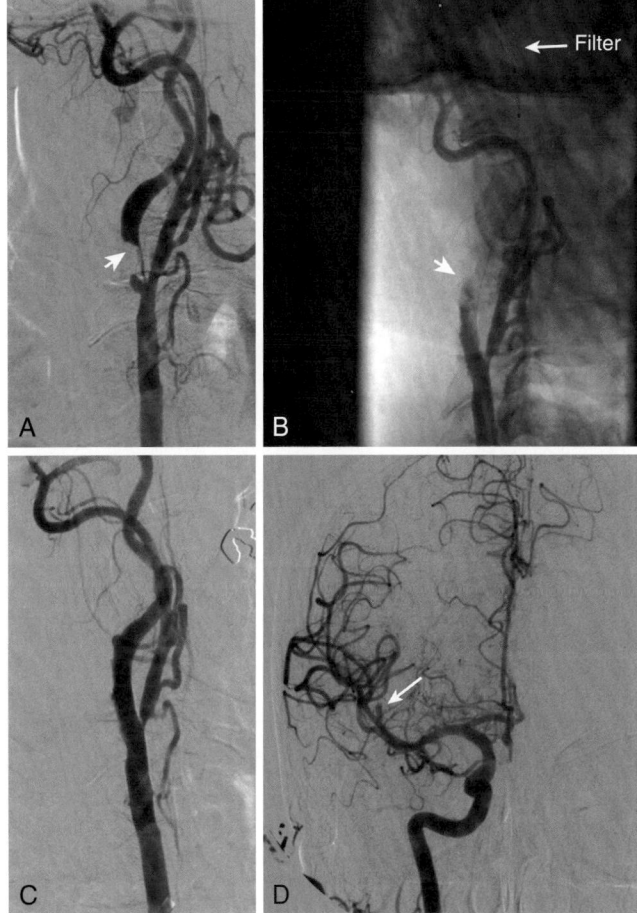

Fig. 46.9 Angiographic appearance and complication of slow flow during carotid intervention. (A) Baseline angiogram shows critical bulky stenosis at the origin of the right internal carotid artery (ICA) (arrow) in a symptomatic patient. (B) Angiographic appearance after poststent dilation shows cessation of flow in the ICA (arrow). Notice the complete filling of the external carotid artery. (C) Angiographic appearance after aspiration of the column of blood proximal to the filter and subsequent retrieval of the filter. (D) Angiogram of the middle cerebral artery after retrieval of the filter shows occlusion of one of its branches (arrow).

antegrade flow through the filter (Fig. 46.10). The phenomenon can occur in up to 8% to 10% of cases[14,36] and is most commonly observed after postdilation of the stent (75% of cases) or after stent deployment (25% of cases). Predictors of this event include treatment of symptomatic lesions, increased patient age, and increased stent diameter.[14] In patients with slow flow, the column of blood proximal to the filter has not been appropriately cleared of debris embolized from the treatment site by the filter EPD. In an effort to prevent distal embolization of this debris at the time of filter retrieval, use of an Export catheter to aspirate 40 to 60 mL of blood from the column of blood proximal to the filter before retrieval of the filter EPD is recommended. If slow flow is observed after stent deployment, poststent dilation is discouraged because it will probably exacerbate the degree of embolization from the treatment site.

Removal of the Embolic Protection Device and Final Angiography

Removal of filter-type EPD devices is achieved by advancing a retrieval sheath over the interventional wire and collapsing the filter. The collapsed filter is then withdrawn carefully across the stent and removed. Most retrieval sheaths are available in a straight or angled shape to allow them to be advanced past the stent. Rarely, the patient may have to turn his or her head or external compression may have to be applied to the carotid to facilitate this maneuver. Final angiography at the treatment site, the EPD landing zone, and the ipsilateral anterior cerebral circulation is performed to assess the procedural outcome and detect any procedural complication (e.g., distal embolization, spasm at the filter site).

Postprocedural Care and Follow-Up

At most centers, patients are admitted overnight to a step-down telemetry floor and typically discharged the next day. Neurologic and hemodynamic monitoring are the most important components of care. All patients should receive lifelong aspirin therapy unless contraindicated, and clopidogrel is recommended for a minimum of 4 weeks after the procedure. Patients are seen at 1 month and 12 months after the procedure for clinical assessment and a carotid ultrasound study to screen for in-stent stenosis. Thereafter, yearly carotid ultrasound examination is recommended.[37]

COMPLICATIONS OF CAROTID INTERVENTION

Stroke

Stroke is the most important complication of CAS. Regardless of whether the patient is deemed to be at high or normal risk for CEA, the risk of periprocedural stroke is most strongly related to the patient's symptomatic status.[30] In studies of high-risk patients, most were asymptomatic. The 30-day incidence of stroke after CAS in multiple observational studies of high-risk patients has ranged from 2.3% to 6.9%,[29,36,38-43] with a majority of high-risk registry studies in recent years reporting stroke rates of 2.3% to 4.4%.[29,36,38,40,41,43] These rates are comparable to the 30-day stroke rate of 3.1% that was observed in the sole randomized trial of high-risk patients.[44] Approximately 80% of these reported strokes were ipsilateral to the treatment site; of these, 25% to 33% were classified as major strokes (i.e., persistence of neurologic deficit beyond 30 days based on a National Institutes of Health [NIH] Stroke Scale score >3). The 30-day rate of stroke in the four contemporary trials of normal-risk, symptomatic patients ranged from 5% to 9% (Table 46.4).[45-48] A lower 30-day stroke rate of 2.5% was also reported in an asymptomatic subgroup from one trial of normal-risk patients.[45]

Although it has been poorly documented in most studies, our experience is that the majority of strokes occur at the time of the CAS procedure. This impression is corroborated by data from the Carotid and Vertebral Artery Transluminal Angioplasty Study (CAVATAS), in which 16 of 22 ischemic strokes

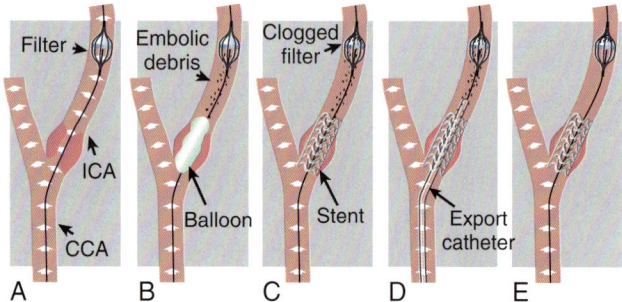

Fig. 46.10 Schematic diagram of proposed mechanism of slow flow and rationale for aspiration. (A) Carotid bifurcation lesion with filter placed distally. (B and C) Balloon angioplasty and stenting result in embolization of debris from atherosclerotic plaque toward the filter, causing occlusion of filter pores and accumulation of debris in the column of blood proximal to the filter. (D and E) Aspiration proximal to the filter removes debris from the column of blood without affecting the debris causing occlusion of the filter. *CCA*, Common carotid artery; *ICA*, internal carotid artery. (From Casserly IP, Abou-Chebl A, Fathi R. Slow-flow phenomenon during carotid artery intervention with embolic protection devices: predictors and clinical outcome. *J Am Coll Cardiol.* 2005;46[8]:1466–1472.)

TABLE 46.4 Thirty-Day Outcomes From Randomized Trials of Carotid Artery Stenting and Carotid Endarterectomy in Normal-Risk Patients

Trial	Stroke (%)			Myocardial Infarction (%)			Death (%)		
	CAS	CEA	P Value	CAS	CEA	P Value	CAS	CEA	P Value
CREST									
Total	4.1	2.3	.01	1.1	2.3	.03	0.7	0.3	.18
Symptomatic	5.5	3.2	.04	1.0	2.3	.08	3	0	NR
Asymptomatic	2.5	1.4	.15	1.2	2.2	.2	0	0	NA
ICSS	7.0	3.3	<.01	0.4	0.5	NR	1.3	0.5	.07
EVA-3S	8.8	2.7	<.01	0.4	0.8	.62	0.8	1.2	.68
SPACE	7.5	6.2	NS	NR	NR	NR	0.7	0.9	NS
ACT 1	2.8	1.4	.23	0.5	0.9	.41	0.1	0.3	.43

ACT, Asymptomatic Carotid Trial; *CAS,* carotid artery stenting; *CEA,* carotid endarterectomy; *CREST,* Carotid Revascularization Endarterectomy Versus Stenting Trial; *EVA-3S,* Endarterectomy Versus Angioplasty in Patients with Symptomatic Severe Carotid Stenosis; *ICCS,* International Carotid Stenting Study; *NA,* not applicable; *NR,* not reported; *NS,* not statistically significant but specific *P* values not reported; *SPACE,* Stent-Supported Percutaneous Angioplasty of the Carotid Artery Versus Endarterectomy trial.

in the 30-day period after carotid intervention occurred within the first 24 hours after the procedure.[49] Beyond 30 days, the risk of ipsilateral stroke with CAS is extremely low. In the Stenting and Angioplasty With Protection in Patients at High Risk for Endarterectomy (SAPPHIRE) trial, there were only two additional strokes (both minor) in the period between 30 days and 1 year after CAS among 167 patients, emphasizing the long-term safety of the procedure.[44] Most procedure-related strokes (>80%) are ischemic in nature, with the dominant mechanism being distal embolization of plaque due to manipulation of catheters and wires in the aortic arch and CCA and embolization of plaque elements associated with angioplasty and stent placement at the treatment site. Hemorrhagic strokes accounted for 15% to 20% of all strokes in larger high-risk stent registries.[42,43] The timing of these strokes is slightly later than that of ischemic strokes, and the dominant mechanism is probably related to cerebral hyperperfusion after CAS.

Neurologic deficits during the CAS procedure should be assumed to be ischemic in nature, and immediate cerebral angiography should be performed. A normal angiogram is associated with an excellent clinical outcome, and no further treatment should be instituted. In contrast, occlusion of a large artery (≥2 to 2.5 mm diameter) is associated with a poor neurologic outcome, and attempted recanalization using a combination of mechanical (i.e., angioplasty) and pharmacologic (i.e., thrombolytics, glycoprotein IIb/IIIa inhibitors) therapies by qualified interventionalists with experience in intracranial intervention are reasonable.[50] However, even in skilled hands, the outcome of such rescue maneuvers is unpredictable because conventional therapies have largely been designed to treat thrombus and the occlusive emboli in the setting of CAS are composed of atheromatous debris.

Hemodynamic Depression

Baroreceptors located in the adventitia of the carotid sinus form part of the rapidly acting pressure control mechanism of the body and are activated by increases in blood pressure. Signals from these receptors are transmitted through the glossopharyngeal nerve (cranial nerve IX) toward the vasomotor center in the medulla, which in turn activates the vagus nerve (cranial nerve X) and reticulospinal tract, resulting in peripheral vasodilation, bradycardia, and decreased cardiac contractility (Fig. 46.11). Transient pressure from angioplasty and more prolonged pressure from self-expanding stents activates these baroreceptors, causing the hypotension and bradycardia that is frequently associated with CAS. In general, these hemodynamic effects are seen immediately at the time of intervention; in some patients, they persist into the postprocedural period for 24 to 48 hours.[51–53] It is uncommon for significant effects to be seen beyond 48 to 72 hours, because the baroreceptors gradually adapt to the pressure from the self-expanding stent.

In a retrospective analysis of 500 consecutive CAS cases from a single center, the frequency of procedural hemodynamic depression—defined as a systolic blood pressure less than 90 mm Hg or bradycardia of less than 60 beats/min—was 42%, with persistent hemodynamic depression after the procedure in 17% of cases.[53] Not surprisingly, the location of the lesion at the carotid bulb was a predictor of the event. Prior endarterectomy was associated with a reduced incidence of hemodynamic depression, most likely because of denervation of the carotid sinus.

The management of hemodynamic depression is usually straightforward. Prophylactic measures include withholding antihypertensive medications on the morning of the procedure and ensuring adequate hydration with intravenous (IV) fluids before and during the procedure. Some operators routinely administer atropine (0.25 to 0.5 mg IV) before the angioplasty and stenting portion of the procedure, whereas others restrict its use to patients who have critical aortic stenosis or critical coronary artery disease or who demonstrate an exaggerated hemodynamic response to angioplasty or stent deployment. In the presence of severe asymptomatic (i.e., systolic blood pressure <75 mm Hg) or any symptomatic hemodynamic depression, the use of IV vasopressors (e.g., phenylephrine, dopamine, epinephrine) is indicated. For less severe asymptomatic hemodynamic depression, oral pseudoephedrine (40 to 60 mg every 4 to 6 hours) may be used in an effort to avoid IV vasopressors. For patients with persistent postprocedural hemodynamic depression, it is important to withhold routine antihypertensive medications and to carefully titrate these medications as the patient's blood pressure returns to baseline. Providing the patient with an automated blood pressure cuff and ensuring daily contact between the patient and the health care provider is advisable to optimize this management after hospital discharge.

Hyperperfusion Syndrome

Cerebral hyperperfusion syndrome is a rare but potentially life threatening complication of carotid and vertebral revascularization procedures that improve flow to a chronically ischemic cerebral territory.[54] The syndrome is thought to be caused by significant increases in cerebral blood flow (>100% of baseline) after revascularization,[55] which in combination with impaired cerebral autoregulation results in transudation of fluid into the brain's interstitium and cerebral edema (Fig. 46.12). Although hypertension is often present in these patients, it is not a universal finding. Clinically, patients typically complain of a throbbing headache that is ipsilateral to the revascularization site, although the headache may be diffuse. Associated symptoms include nausea, vomiting, confusion, and visual disturbances. In the most severe cases, patients develop focal neurologic deficits and seizures.

The feared complication of the hyperperfusion syndrome is intracerebral or subarachnoid hemorrhage, which is associated with a high mortality rate (40% to 60%) and severe morbidity among survivors. In 12 observational studies published since 2003 reporting rates of hyperperfusion syndrome after carotid stenting, the incidence of hyperperfusion syndrome was 1.3% (73 of 5431 cases).[56–59] There is some variation in the timing of the syndrome, but most cases manifested within 24 hours after the procedure, and cases beyond 2 to 4 days were rare. Based on data in patients undergoing carotid revascularization with CEA, an increased risk of the syndrome likely persists up to 28 days after CAS. The rate of hemorrhagic complications of the syndrome after CAS appears to be high, with 25% to 60% of cases being complicated by intraparenchymal or subarachnoid hemorrhage.[60–62]

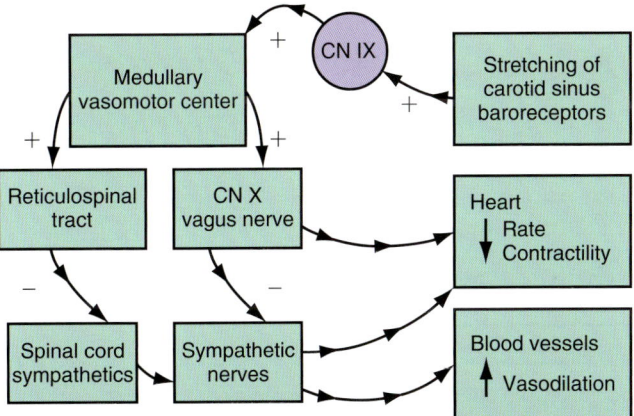

Fig. 46.11 Diagrammatic representation of the effect of activation of mechanoreceptors in the carotid sinus during carotid intervention. *CN,* Cranial nerve.

The low event rates for hyperfusion syndrome in these reports preclude multivariate analyses of predictors of the syndrome after CAS. Several risk factors have been reported in the CEA literature, and these probably also apply in patients undergoing CAS. They include preexisting hypertension, postprocedural hypertension, contralateral carotid occlusion, critical ipsilateral carotid stenosis, and incomplete circle of Willis.[60] These risk factors permit the identification of patients who are at high risk for cerebral hyperperfusion after CAS. However, aggressive control of blood pressure after CAS is recommended in all patients to prevent it. One study reported an incidence of hyperperfusion syndrome of 3 (0.5%) among a cohort of 570 patients with the implementation of an aggressive blood pressure-lowering algorithm after carotid stenting.[63]

The cornerstones of management of hyperperfusion syndrome are prompt diagnosis and emergent institution of therapy. The diagnosis is initially a clinical one, based on the patient's symptoms. Although confirmatory studies are helpful, the clinical diagnosis of hyperperfusion syndrome mandates immediate medical therapy. Because blood flow is pressure dependent in patients with cerebral hyperperfusion syndrome, the major focus of therapy is a reduction in systemic arterial pressure.[60] Several antihypertensive agents are contraindicated because they are associated with increased cerebral blood flow, including glycerol trinitrate, nitroprusside, calcium channel antagonists, and angiotensin-converting enzyme inhibitors. Recommended agents include β-blockers, labetalol (mixed α- and β-adrenergic antagonist), and clonidine (central $α_2$-adrenergic antagonist), which have favorable effects on cerebral blood flow and cerebral perfusion pressure in this clinical situation. Patients should be cared for in an intensive care setting that facilitates meticulous control of systemic arterial pressure. After institution of treatment, imaging studies (i.e., CT and MR imaging) are helpful to screen for hemorrhagic complications and assess for the presence of cerebral edema. In addition, transcranial Doppler ultrasonography documenting a significant increase in flow velocity (>150% to 300% compared with baseline) in the ipsilateral middle cerebral artery is useful in confirming the diagnosis.

Adverse Cardiac Events

MI has not been included in the outcome analysis of all RCTs of normal-risk patients. However, the importance of MI as a component of the primary composite end point is underscored by the increased risk of death among patients who suffer MI in the perioperative period after vascular surgery (Fig. 46.13).[64,65] For this reason, the incidence of MI, as determined by preprocedural and postprocedural electrocardiograms and serial measurements of creatine kinase (CK) and CK-MB fraction, has been included in the end point of most high-risk CAS registries and trials. In this patient cohort, the 30-day incidence of MI has been in the range of 0% to 2.4%.[29,36,38–44] More than 80% of these MIs were non-Q wave in type. When CAS was compared with CEA in high-risk patients in the SAPPHIRE trial, there appeared to be a significant and consistent reduction in MI with CAS (2.4% versus 6.1%; $P = .04$).[44] The risk of MI among normal-risk patients undergoing CAS is likely to be lower, a contention supported by data from the Carotid Revascularization Endarterectomy versus Stenting Trial (CREST), which reported 30-day MI rates of 1.1% in the CAS arm and 2.3% in the CEA group ($P = .03$) (see Table 46.4).[66]

Restenosis

In-stent restenosis (ISR) is an important late complication of CAS. Because of its acceptable sensitivity, safety, and accessibility, duplex ultrasound screening for carotid ISR[67] has largely been used for frequency estimates. Based on this method, the incidence of severe ISR (≥80%) is 3% to 4% at approximately 18 months of follow-up.[68,69] The rate of ISR at 2 years in a randomized trial of CAS and CEA was higher (11.1%) when a lower cutoff value (i.e., ≥70%) was used to define it.[70] However, for

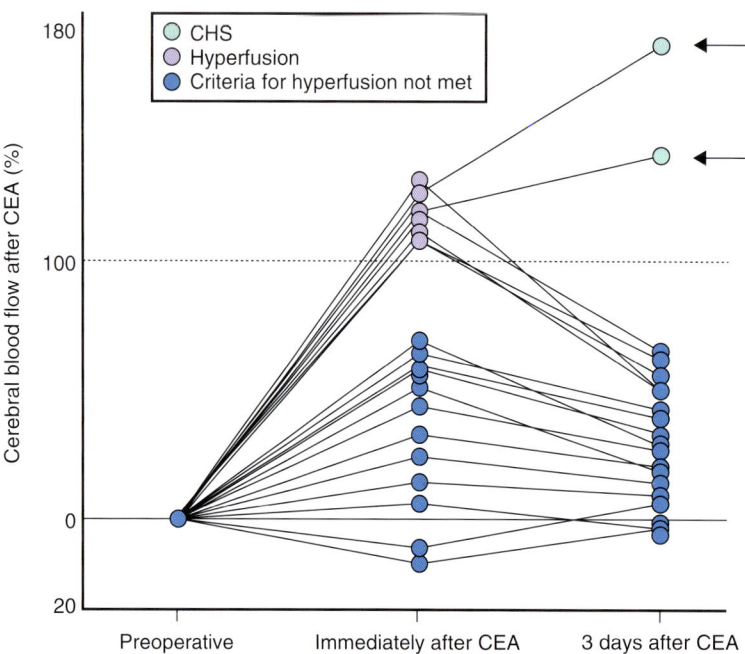

Fig. 46.12 Graph showing the increase in cerebral blood flow (CBF) after carotid endarterectomy. Increase in CBF >100% from baseline defines the patient group with cerebral hyperperfusion *(purple circles)*. Within this group, two patients *(arrows)* developed clinical signs and symptoms consistent with cerebral hyperperfusion syndrome *(CHS)*. *CEA,* Carotid endarterectomy. (From van Mook WN, Rennenberg RJ, Schurink GW, et al. Cerebral hyperperfusion syndrome. *Lancet.* 2005;4:877–888.)

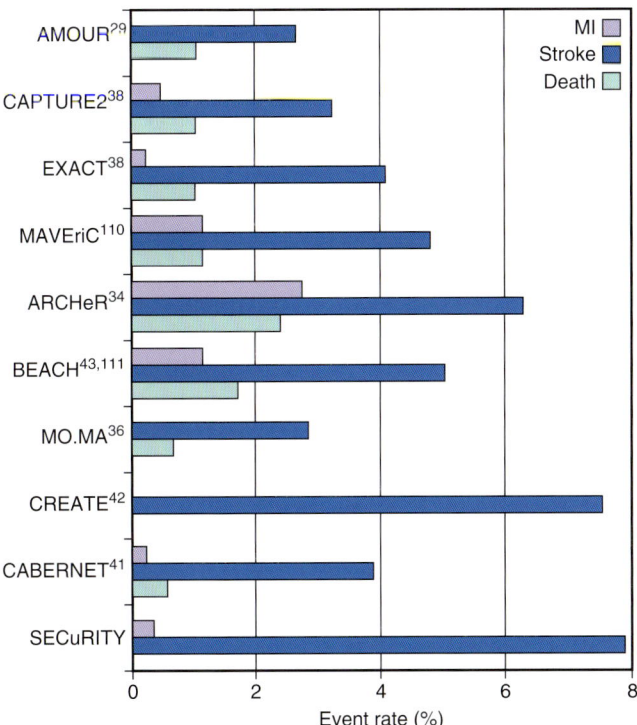

Fig. 46.13 Incidence of death, stroke, and myocardial infarction *(MI)* at 30 days in high-risk carotid artery stent registries. The registries are ordered, with the most recently published at the top and the earliest published at the bottom. From references[29,36,38,39,41–43,110,111].

TABLE 46.5 Criteria Used to Define a High-Risk Population in Studies of Carotid Artery Stenting

CLINICAL CRITERIA
Age >75–80 years
Congestive heart failure (class III/IV)
Known severe left ventricular dysfunction (LVEF <30%–35%)
Planned CABG or heart valve surgery
Recent MI (>24 h and <4–6 weeks)
Unstable angina (CCS class III/IV)
Severe pulmonary disease[a]
Contralateral cranial nerve injury

ANATOMIC CRITERIA
Previous CEA with recurrent stenosis
Surgically inaccessible lesion
High cervical lesion (at or above C2)
Below the clavicle
Contralateral carotid occlusion
Radiation therapy to neck
Prior radical neck surgery
Severe tandem lesions
Spinal immobility of the neck

[a]Defined as need for home oxygen, partial pressure of oxygen (Po_2) <60 mm Hg on room air, forced expiratory volume in 1 s (FEV_1) <30%–50% of predicted.
CABG, Coronary artery bypass surgery; *CCS,* Canadian Cardiovascular Society; *CEA,* carotid endarterectomy; *LVEF,* left ventricular ejection fraction; *MI,* myocardial infarction.

less-severe degrees of ISR, conventional ultrasound criteria for determination of the degree of stenosis in a nonstented carotid artery may overestimate stenosis after CAS because of alterations in the compliance of the stented artery.[71] Nonetheless, data suggest that ISR is associated with low rates of clinical events. In two large series, only 1 of 12 patients with severe ISR (>80%) was symptomatic,[68,69] and only 2 of 54 patients with ISR greater than 70% were symptomatic.[70] In addition, the rate of clinically driven target-vessel revascularization was only 2.4% at 3 years in a randomized trial of high-risk patients.[41]

A serial intravenous ultrasound (IVUS) study demonstrated that the immediate postprocedural minimal carotid stent area is negatively correlated with the percentage of restenotic area at follow-up.[72] Before this study, it was thought that such a relationship would not exist owing to the large caliber of the carotid artery. This finding emphasizes the need to balance the short-term procedural risk of distal embolization and stroke from aggressive poststent dilation against the long-term risk of ISR. As in the case of restenosis after CEA, the clinical benefits of revascularization for ISR after CAS have not been demonstrated. Both of these pathologies appear to be associated with a relatively benign clinical outcome,[72] suggesting that a conservative approach is appropriate. Repeat revascularization is usually limited to patients with severe ISR and may be influenced by other considerations, such as the presence of contralateral disease or occlusion. A variety of interventional techniques have been reported for treatment of carotid ISR, including angioplasty, cutting-balloon angioplasty, repeat stenting, and brachytherapy, with recurrence rates ranging from 0% to 50%.[68,69,73,74]

CAROTID ARTERY STENTING—CLINICAL DATA

Although the benefits of CEA compared with medical therapy have been clearly demonstrated in RCTs, these trials systematically excluded patients with certain baseline comorbidities or high-risk anatomic features (Table 46.5). Subsequent "real-world" assessments of clinical outcomes with CEA have suggested that the conclusions of these trials might not be broadly applicable in clinical practice. For example, Wennberg and colleagues[75] analyzed outcomes in 113,000 Medicare patients undergoing CEA between 1992 and 1993 and reported mortality rates at least three times greater than those reported in prior RCTs. A single-center CEA registry of more than 3000 patients demonstrated that comorbidities such as severe coronary artery disease, chronic obstructive pulmonary disease, and renal insufficiency were associated with a 7.4% incidence of perioperative death, stroke, or MI, compared with 2.9% in a low-risk cohort of patients without these comorbidities.[76] Based on such data, initial attempts to demonstrate equipoise between contemporary percutaneous carotid revascularization and CEA focused on a high-risk patient cohort as the study population of interest. Accepting that carotid revascularization has not been proven in RCTs to be more efficacious than medical therapy in this study population, surgical CEA has been widely used by vascular surgeons on the basis that a beneficial effect in high-risk patients could be extrapolated from trial data in normal-risk study populations.

Carotid Artery Stenting in High-Risk Patients

Among high-risk patients, outcomes of CAS using contemporary techniques have been reported in the form of case series, industry-sponsored registries, and a single RCT. In general, studies of high-risk patients have grouped symptomatic and asymptomatic patients together, with most patients (~75%) being asymptomatic. The enrollment criteria have relied heavily on data from prior RCTs in normal-risk patients—symptomatic patients with 50% or greater carotid stenosis and asymptomatic patients with 70% to 80% carotid stenosis being eligible for inclusion. Case series were particularly helpful in the early stages of the development of CAS but generally have suffered from a lack of stringent oversight. A large number of multicenter, industry-sponsored registries with stricter oversight have been performed (Table 46.6, see Fig. 46.13).

TABLE 46.6 "High-Risk" Registries of Carotid Artery Stenting With Embolic Protection

Study	Sponsor	Sample Size	Stent	Embolic Protection Device	Status
SAPPHIRE (CAS registry)	Cordis	409	Precise	Angioguard	3-year outcomes published
ARCHeR 2, 3	Guidant	ARCHeR 2—278 ARCHeR 3—145	Acculink (OTW & RX)	Accunet	2-year outcomes published
SECuRITY	Abbott Vascular Devices	320	MedNova Xact	MedNova NeuroShield/EmboShield	1-year outcomes presented
BEACH	Boston Scientific	480	WALLSTENT	FilterWire EX and EZ	1-year outcomes published
CABERNET	EndoTex	380	NexStent	FilterWire EX	3-year outcomes published
MAVErIC International	Medtronic	51	Exponent	Interceptor	1-year outcomes published
MAVErIC II	Medtronic	Phase I—99 Phase II—399	Exponent	GuardWire	1-year outcomes published
PASCAL	Medtronic	115	Exponent	Any CE mark–approved device	30-day outcomes presented
CREATE	ev3	400	Protégé	Spider	30-day outcomes published
MO.MA[a]	Invatec	157	Any carotid stent	MO.MA	30-day outcomes published
CAPTURE2	Abbott	4175	Acculink	Accunet	30-day outcomes published
EXACT	Abbott	2145	Xact	EmboShield	30-day outcomes published
ARMOUR	Invatec	262	Any carotid stent	MO.MA	30-day outcomes published

[a]Seventy-five percent of patients were considered high risk.
ARCHeR, Acculink for Revascularization of Carotids in High-Risk Patients; *BEACH,* The Boston Scientific EPI: A Carotid Stenting Trial for High-Risk Surgical Patients; *CABERNET,* Carotid Artery Revascularization Using the Boston Scientific EPI FilteRwire EX/EZ and the EndoTex NexStent; *CAPTURE2,* Carotid RX ACCULINK/RX ACCUNET Post-Approval Trial to Uncover Unanticipated or Rare Events; *CAS,* carotid artery stent; *CREATE,* the Carotid Revascularization With ev3 Arterial Technology Evolution trial; *EXACT,* EmboShield and Xact Post Approval Carotid Stent Trial; *MAVErIC,* Evaluation of the Medtronic AVE Self-Expanding Carotid Stent System With Distal Protection in the Treatment of Carotid Stenosis; *MO.MA,* a prospective multicenter clinical registry for carotid stenting with a new neuro-protection device based on endovascular clamping; *OTW,* over-the-wire; *PASCAL,* Performance and Safety of the Medtronic AVE Self-Expandable Stent in Treatment of Carotid Artery Lesions; *Rx,* Monorail; *SAPPHIRE,* Stenting and Angioplasty With Protection in Patients at High Risk for Endarterectomy; *SECuRITY,* a registry study to evaluate the NeuroShield bare wire cerebral protection system and Xact stent in patients at high risk for carotid endarterterectomy.

The largest of these registries are the EmboShield and Xact Post Approval Carotid Stent Trial (EXACT; *n* = 2145) and the Carotid RX ACCULINK/RX ACCUNET Post-Approval Trial to Uncover Unanticipated or Rare Events study (CAPTURE2; *n* = 4175). In both of these studies, there was independent adjudication of neurologic outcomes. At 30 days, the rate of death was 0.9% in both trials; the rate of stroke was 3.6% in EXACT and 2.8% in CAPTURE2.[38] These event rates are somewhat lower than what was reported in smaller, earlier published registries of carotid stenting with distal EPDs, in which the study populations ranged from approximately 200 to 500 participants and the stroke rates were 3.4% to 6.9% (see Table 46.6 and Fig. 46.13).[38,41–43] This temporal trend suggests that increased operator experience has played a role in reducing adverse outcomes.

Emerging data on the use of proximal EPDs also suggest that these devices may be associated with reduced rates of stroke. In a European multicenter registry of 157 high-risk patients treated with CAS and proximal embolic protection with MO.MA, the 30-day rate of stroke was 2.5%. Similarly, in another multicenter registry of 263 subjects treated with CAS and MO.MA, the stroke rate was 2.3% (see Table 46.6 and Fig. 46.13).[29,36] The SAPPHIRE trial is the sole randomized trial comparing CEA with CAS in high-risk patients.[44] Enrollment in this study differed from the multicenter industry-sponsored registries in one important respect: the carotid lesion had to be deemed amenable to revascularization by both surgical and percutaneous methods. As a result, the overall risk of the cohort in the randomized portion of this trial was likely somewhat less than in registry-type studies.

Given its randomized design, the SAPPHIRE trial has provided the most robust data supporting the role of CAS with filter-type EPDs compared with CEA in high-risk patients. At 30-day and 1-year follow-up, there was a trend toward a reduction in the incidence of death in the CAS group, a significant reduction in the incidence of MI in the CAS arm, but no significant difference in stoke rate (Table 46.7). Target-lesion revascularization (0.7% vs. 4.6%; P = .04) and cranial nerve palsies (0% vs. 5.3%; P = .003) were also significantly reduced in the CAS arm. At 3-year follow-up in this RCT, event rates were comparable between CAS and CEA patients: death occurred in 19% of patients in the CEA arm and 21% of patients in the CAS arm (P = .68), and stroke occurred in 9% of patients in each arm. Overall, these data support the conclusion that CAS with embolic protection is not inferior to CEA in high-risk patients and provides equivalent long-term protection from stroke events.[74]

Carotid Artery Stenting in Normal-Risk Patients

Carotid intervention remains investigational in normal-risk patients. In contrast to high-risk CAS trials, studies in normal-risk patients have typically included symptomatic and asymptomatic patients seen in isolation, according to the clearly established differences in their natural history based on symptomatic status. In addition, most major normal-risk studies have had a randomized design and in general have compared CAS with CEA. A total of six randomized trials of carotid intervention in normal-risk patients have been completed (Table 46.8; see Table 46.4).

The CAVATAS trial was the first of these and included a largely symptomatic patient cohort with carotid disease.[49] However, because this study enrolled patients between 1992 and 1997, the endovascular arm largely used a strategy of angioplasty alone—EPDs were not available, and carotid stents became available only toward the end of the trial. Despite the lack of a

TABLE 46.7 Outcomes in the SAPPHIRE Trial (Based on Intention-to-Treat Analysis)

	Randomized Trial	
	CAS (%)	CEA (%)
30-DAY OUTCOMES		
Death	0.6	2.0
Stroke	3.1	3.3
MI	1.9	6.6
Death/stroke/MI	4.4	9.9
1-YEAR OUTCOMES		
Death	7.4	13.5
Stroke	6.2	7.9
MI	3.0	7.5
30-day death/stroke/MI plus death and ipsilateral stroke between 31 days and 1 year	12.2	20.1
3-YEAR OUTCOMES		
Death	18.6	21.0
Stroke	9.0	9.0
MI	5.4	8.4
30-day death/stroke/MI plus death and ipsilateral stroke between 1 and 3 years	24.6	26.9

CAS, Carotid artery stenting; *CEA*, carotid endarterectomy; *MI*, myocardial infarction; *SAPPHIRE*, Stenting and Angioplasty with Protection in Patients at High Risk for Endarterectomy.

contemporary CAS technique, the 30-day incidence of death or disabling stroke was identical in each arm (6%; *P* = not significant). Not surprisingly, the low rate of stent use was associated with a high rate of restenosis in the endovascular arm. Given the absence of EPD and carotid stent use in this trial, the relevance of the CAVATAS data to contemporary practice is limited.

The Stent-Protected Percutaneous Angioplasty of the Carotid Versus Endarterectomy (SPACE) trial and the Endarterectomy Versus Angioplasty in patients With Symptomatic Severe Carotid Stenosis (EVA-3S) trial were the first two RCTs comparing contemporary CAS technique (i.e., EPD and carotid stent use) with CEA.[46,77] Both were performed in Europe, and the 30-day and long-term (2- to 4-year) outcomes have been published. In the EVA-3S trial, the 30-day incidence of stroke or death was 9.6% in the CAS arm versus 3.9% in the CEA arm (*P* = .01).[46] The SPACE trial reported the incidence of ipsilateral stroke and death at 30 days in the CAS arm as 6.8% versus 6.3% in the CEA arm.[77] Based on predefined statistical rules to prove the equivalence of CAS versus CEA, the SPACE investigators concluded that CAS failed to demonstrate equivalence. Because enrollment would have had to be doubled to provide enough power to prove equivalence, they stopped further patient recruitment into the trial.

For proponents of CAS, these results were disappointing and certainly raised concern regarding the safety of CAS in this patient subset. However, the results of both of these studies need to be interpreted in the context of several factors that challenge the validity of the findings. Neither study had a roll-in phase to ensure that operators were completely familiar with the equipment for CAS and to audit their clinical outcomes. This limitation was compounded by the fact that the threshold carotid interventional experience required for operators in both of these studies was suboptimal. For example, in the EVA-3S trial, an operator who had performed only five prior CAS procedures was eligible to treat randomized patients. Similarly, in the SPACE trial, eligible operators for the CAS arm need not have ever performed carotid stenting; rather, eligibility was set by a threshold of having performed 25 successful angioplasty procedures in any vascular bed. There were additional issues with regard to the interventional technique used in these studies. Despite the availability of EPDs, the EVA-3S study did not initially mandate their use. Only after an interim analysis demonstrated an increased incidence of stroke among patients in whom EPDs were not used was the protocol amended to mandate their use. In the SPACE trial, the use of EPDs was left to the discretion of the operator, and they were ultimately used in only 27% of all patients. Predilation before stenting was performed in only 17% of patients in the EVA-3S trial, which is a definite deviation from accepted CAS technique in the United States. In a further deviation from accepted U.S. practice, 15% of patients in EVA-3S were not administered dual antiplatelet therapy after carotid stent placement. In summary, the data provided by the EVA-3S and SPACE trials did not support equivalence of CAS versus CEA in symptomatic patients at normal risk for CEA, but deficiencies in trial design and execution are believed by proponents of CAS to explain the signal of harm associated with CAS in these trials.

The remaining three RCTs of CAS versus CEA in normal-risk symptomatic patients were the International Carotid Stenting Study (ICSS), the CREST trial, and the Asymptomatic Carotid Trial (ACT1).[46,66,78,79] More than 1700 patients from Europe, Australia, New Zealand, and Canada were enrolled in the ICSS. Unfortunately, this study did not have a roll-in phase, and the minimum training requirement for CAS operators was set at 50 total stenting procedures, of which only 10 had to be in the carotid territory. In addition, the use of EPDs was not mandated; they appear to have been used in approximately 80% of cases. Considerable controversy has been generated by the finding that there was an increased incidence of new ischemic lesions on diffusion-weighted MR imaging in patients treated at centers in which EPDs were used versus centers in which EPDs were not used. It is unclear whether this finding represents real harm due to EPD use or whether operators were inexperienced with their use. Accepting these limitations, the major finding of ICSS was that the incidence of stroke at 30 days was significantly lower with CEA than with CAS (3.9% vs. 7.6%). This difference was driven largely by an excess of nondisabling strokes in the CAS group. At 120-days follow-up, the rates of death and stroke were significantly lower with CEA than with CAS (0.8% vs. 2.3%, and 4.1% vs. 7.7%, respectively). There was an extremely low rate of MI in both arms (0.4% for CAS and 0.5% for CEA).[78]

The CREST trial was a U.S.-based trial sponsored by the NIH that enrolled more than 2500 patients. Unlike other RCTs in normal-risk populations, both symptomatic (53%) and asymptomatic patients were included, a decision that was driven by initial problems with patient recruitment. In contrast to other trials of normal-risk patients, there was a stringent lead-in phase to ensure that operators were familiar with the single carotid stent and filter system used in the study and to audit clinical outcomes before approval for recruitment of patients into the randomized portion of the trial. The primary end point of the trial (periprocedural death, stroke, or MI plus ipsilateral stroke up to 4 years after carotid revascularization) occurred in 7.2% of the CAS group compared with 6.8% of the CEA group (*P* = .51). There was an increased incidence of stroke at 30 days in the CAS group (4.1% vs. 2.3%; *P* = .01), driven by an increased incidence of minor rather than major stroke. There was a lower rate of periprocedural MI in the CAS group (1.1% vs. 2.3%; *P* = .03), and, not surprisingly, cranial nerve palsies were more frequent in the CEA group (4.8% vs. 0.3%; *P* < .01).[66] Proponents of CAS are likely to promote CREST as an example of a well-designed and executed U.S.-based trial in which stroke rates with CAS were lower than in earlier, non–U.S.-based trials with recognized limitations.

Finally, ACT1 was a multicenter, randomized trial of CEA versus CAS in patients at standard risk for CEA.[79] The intention was to enroll 1658 subjects, but the trial was stopped early

TABLE 46.8 "Normal-Risk" Carotid Artery Stent Trials

Trial	Planned Sample Size	Sites of Enrollment	Funding	Clinical Enrollment Criteria	Lesion Enrollment Criteria	Endovascular Strategy	Primary End Points	Status of Trial
ICSS (CAVATAS-2)	1500	Europe Australia Canada	Stroke Association Sanofi Synthelabo European Commission	TIA/stroke within 12 months	>50% by NASCET method or noninvasive equivalent	CAS + EPD	30-day death/stroke/MI 3-year death/disabling stroke	120-day outcomes published
EVA-3S	900	France	National Research Organization	TIA/stroke within 4 months	>60% by NASCET or noninvasive equivalent	CAS + EPD	30-day death/stroke 30-day death/stroke + ipsilateral stroke at 2–4 years	4-year outcomes published
SPACE	1900	Germany Austria Switzerland	Federal Ministry of Education and Research German Research Foundation Industry Funding	TIA/stroke within 6 months	>50% by NASCET or 70% by Doppler	CAS ± EPD	30-day death/ipsilateral stroke	2-year outcomes published
CREST	2500	North America Europe	National Institute of Neurological Disorders and Stroke—NIH Guidant Corporation	Symptomatic Asymptomatic	>50% by NASCET >70% by ultrasound >60% by NASCET >70% by ultrasound	CAS + EPD	30-day death/stroke/MI Ipsilateral stroke after 30 days	30-day outcomes published
ACT I	1540	North America	Abbott Vascular	Asymptomatic		CAS + EPD	Stroke/death/MI within 30 days + ipsilateral stroke at 30–365 days	April 2005
TACIT	3700	North America Europe	NIH, Pharma, Device Industry	Asymptomatic	>60% by ultrasound	CAS + EPD	Stroke/death at 3–5-year follow-up	Held due to lack of funding
SPACE2	3523	Germany Austria Switzerland	Federal Ministry of Education and Research German Research Foundation Industry Funding	Asymptomatic	>50% by ultrasound	CAS + EPD	30-day stroke/death Ipsilateral stroke at 5 years	5-year results published

ACT I, Asymptomatic Carotid Stenosis, Stenting Versus Endarterectomy Trial; *CAS*, carotid artery stenting; *CAVATAS*, Carotid and Vertebral Artery Transluminal Angioplasty Study; *CREST*, Carotid Revascularization Endarterectomy Versus Stent Trial; *EPD*, embolic protection device; *EVA-3S*, Endarterectomy Versus Angioplasty in Patients With Symptomatic Severe Carotid Stenosis; *ICCS*, International Carotid Stenting Study; *MI*, myocardial infarction; *NASCET*, North American Symptomatic Carotid Endarterectomy Trial; *NIH*, National Institutes of Health; *SPACE*, Stent-Supported Percutaneous Angioplasty of the Carotid Artery Versus Endarterectomy Trial; *TACIT*, Transatlantic Asymptomatic Carotid Intervention Trial; *TIA*, transient ischemic attack.

due to enrollment challenges, with follow-up in 1453 patients. There was no difference in the primary outcome (freedom from death, stroke, and MI at 30 days and ipsilateral stroke at 1 year) between the CAS and CEA (event rate 3.8% vs. 3.4%, $P = .01$ for noninferiority). Although debate is likely to continue, CREST and ACT1 appear to have restored confidence among the interventional community that CAS will ultimately become a viable option for normal-risk symptomatic (and asymptomatic) patients.

In summary, results from trials of CEA versus CAS in normal-risk symptomatic patients are mixed. The optimal method of carotid revascularization may depend on patient age, operator experience, and patient preference regarding the risks of periprocedural MI (higher with CEA), periprocedural stroke (higher with CAS, particularly if operators are inexperienced), and cranial nerve palsy (higher with CEA). Regarding asymptomatic patients at normal risk for CEA, results from CREST 2 are eagerly awaited. CREST 2 is a randomized trial comparing CEA, CAS, and optimal medical therapy in symptomatic and asymptomatic patients with carotid artery disease.

CAROTID ARTERY STENTING—FUTURE PERSPECTIVE

Realizing the potential of CAS will require further refinements in interventional tools and technique. Perhaps more dramatic may be a reevaluation of the current paradigm for choosing patients for carotid revascularization. We need to move beyond using symptomatic status and percent carotid stenosis as the sole determinants of need for revascularization. Combining more sophisticated prediction models that incorporate multiple clinical variables with advanced imaging studies of carotid plaque (e.g., tissue characterization with MR imaging or ultrasound) that allow a more accurate estimation of an individual's risk of recurrent neurologic events is necessary. In addition, considering the individual's estimated procedural risk (for either CEA or CAS), based on clinical and anatomic assessments, will allow physicians to make a more valid judgment regarding the risk-benefit ratio for the individual patient (Fig. 46.14).

Furthermore, the current culture of viewing CAS and CEA as competitive strategies for carotid revascularization is counterproductive and reminiscent of the debate on percutaneous coronary intervention versus coronary artery bypass surgery. Instead, these strategies should be viewed as complementary. In fact, there have been advancements in a hybrid carotid stenting technique with the ENROUTE carotid stenting and flow reversal system (Silk Road Medical Inc., Sunnyvale, CA). In this transcarotid stenting technique, a 2- to 4-cm incision for common carotid exposure is performed under local or general anesthesia. A 10-Fr sheath is placed in the CCA and connected to a venous return sheath in the femoral vein, creating flow reversal in the carotid for embolic protection. The stenting procedure is then performed. In a single-arm prospective study of 141 patients (symptomatic and

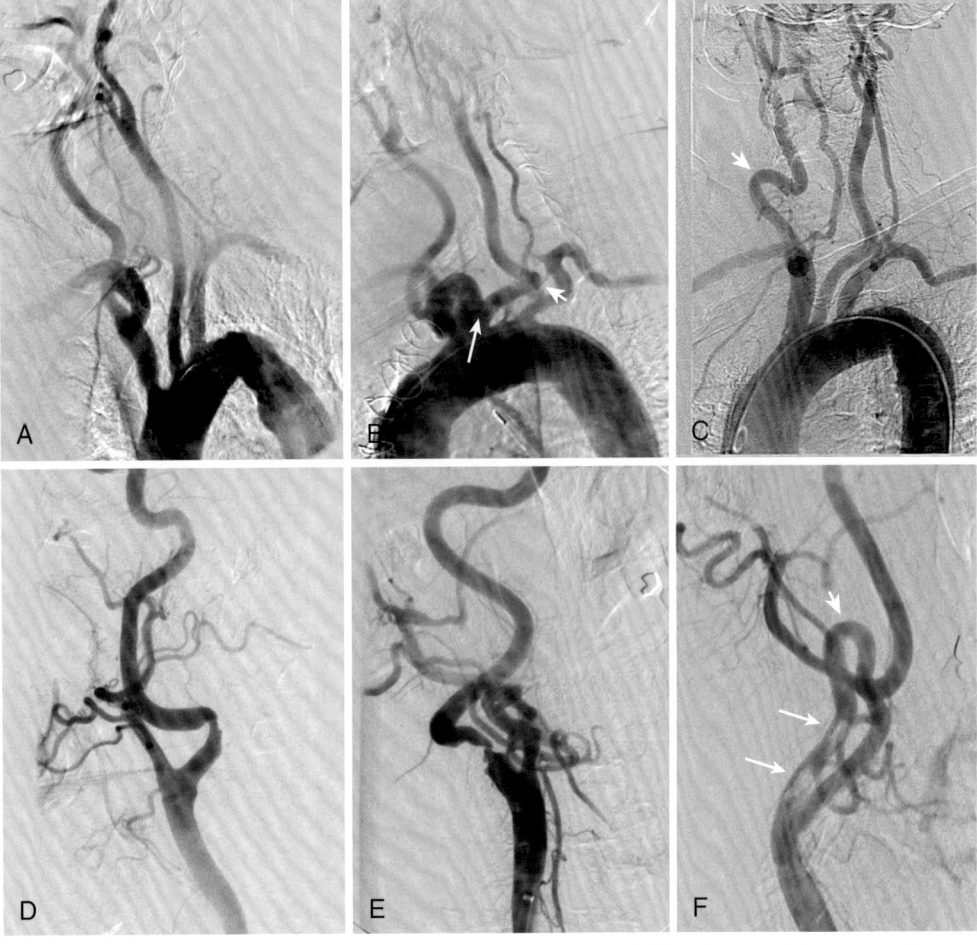

Fig. 46.14 Examples of anatomic variations that increase procedural risk during carotid artery stenting. (A) Type III aortic arch. (B) Bovine origin of the left common carotid artery (CCA) *(long arrow)* and severe tortuosity in the left CCA *(short arrow)*. (C) Severe tortuosity in the right CCA *(arrow)*. (D) Marked angulation in the internal carotid artery (ICA) at the site of stenosis. (E) Tandem areas of angulation distal to stenosis of the ICA. (F) Dense circumferential calcification at lesion site *(long arrows)* and severe tortuosity distal to the ICA stenosis *(short arrow)*.

asymptomatic) at high risk for CEA, the rate of stroke, MI, or death at 30 days was 5%.[80]

In summary, the mode of revascularization that is most likely to achieve the safest procedural outcome for an individual patient should be chosen. Close examination of outcomes from CAS versus CEA trials should help to elucidate those variables that favor one mode of revascularization over the other.

PROXIMAL VERTEBRAL ARTERY INTERVENTION

Atherosclerotic disease of the VA is most commonly located at the origin and proximal V1 extracranial segment of the vessel. Typically, disease at this location represents extension of plaque from the subclavian artery into the proximal VA. In a large prospective New England registry of patients with symptomatic ischemia of the posterior circulation, proximal VA disease was deemed the primary mechanism of stroke in 9%, underscoring the importance of atherosclerotic disease at this site.[81,82] The mechanism of stroke was attributed predominantly to either hemodynamic compromise or artery-to-artery embolism (i.e., VA to distal posterior circulation).

Contemporary surgical revascularization of proximal VA disease typically involves transposition of the VA to the ipsilateral CCA or ICA. Other surgical options include VA endarterectomy and vein patch angioplasty.[82] Although some centers have reported excellent procedural and long-term results,[83] these surgical techniques have currently been almost completely replaced by endovascular therapies. However, lack of RCT data demonstrating a benefit of revascularization over medical therapy alone in patients with proximal VA disease makes clinical decision making problematic. Moreover, there is almost a complete absence of data regarding the natural history of asymptomatic patients with proximal VA disease and a relative paucity of data regarding the natural history in symptomatic patients. Given these uncertainties, most operators restrict endovascular revascularization to symptomatic patients, especially those for whom medical therapy has failed. Intervention in asymptomatic patients should be strictly limited to those deemed at high risk based on the appearance of the lesion, the presence of poor collateral flow from the carotid circulation, and the existence of contralateral VA disease.

Technique

Most proximal VA interventions are performed using femoral artery access, but the ipsilateral brachial artery may also be used, particularly if the VA origin has a retroflexed takeoff from the subclavian artery (Fig. 46.15).[84] Radial access has also been described as a feasible alternative.[85] An appropriately sized sheath or guiding catheter is delivered to the proximal subclavian artery, and the lesion is crossed using a soft-tipped 0.014-inch coronary wire. This wire is advanced to the distal V2 segment of the VA to provide support for device delivery. Predilation with a coronary balloon is routinely performed to facilitate stent delivery. Stenting with a balloon-expandable stent is recommended to provide radial strength and reduce restenosis. For smaller-sized VAs (i.e., diameter <3.75 mm), we typically use a coronary stainless steel drug-eluting or bare-metal stent. For larger-sized VAs (>4 mm diameter), stainless steel or cobalt-chromium peripheral balloon-expandable stents may be used. There is a lack of consensus regarding the need for EPDs during proximal VA intervention. If the V2 segment of the vessel is sufficiently large to accommodate current-generation filter-type EPDs (i.e., ≥4 mm) and the ostial lesion has a high-risk appearance (e.g., ulceration), the use of such devices is recommended.

Endovascular Outcomes

Data regarding the endovascular treatment of proximal VA disease are largely derived from a number of single-institution case series treating a symptomatic patient population.[84] With the use of contemporary stenting techniques, procedural success approaches 100% and periprocedural neurologic complications are rare (Table 46.9). The high restenosis rates associated with angioplasty alone have been significantly improved with stenting, with most series reporting ISR in 3% to 10% of patients. As expected, lesion length has been identified as an independent predictor of ISR, and this may have implications for the selection of drug-eluting rather than bare-metal stents for longer lesions.[86] Long-term follow-up shows a late stroke rate of less than 1%, reinforcing the overall safety of the procedure.

Coward and colleagues reported an analysis of a small subset of patients from the CAVATAS trial with proximal VA disease

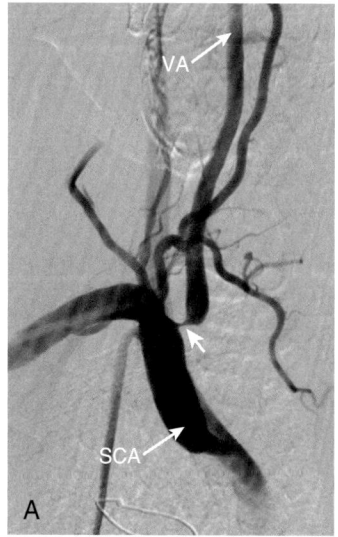 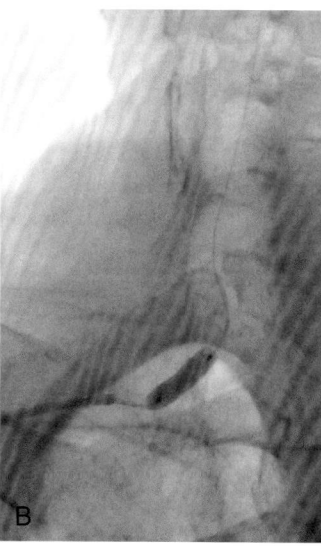 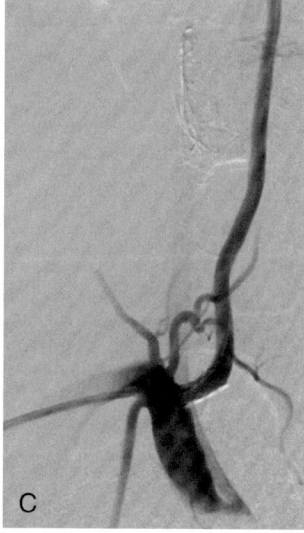

Fig. 46.15 Vertebral artery intervention. (A) Right subclavian artery *(SCA)* angiography shows severe stenosis *(arrow)* at the origin of right vertebral artery *(VA)*. Because of the takeoff angle of the right VA, it was decided to approach the lesion from the right brachial artery. (B) Inflation of a 5.0- by 12-mm Palmaz Blue balloon-expandable cobalt-chromium stent (Cordis, Warren, NJ) at the ostium of the right VA. (C) Final angiographic appearance.

TABLE 46.9 Clinical Outcomes in Selected Series of Proximal Vertebral Artery Stenting

Study	n	Technical Success (%)	Procedural Complications	Improvement in Symptoms	Mean Follow-Up (Months)	Late Stroke	Restenosis
Mukherjee et al.[112]	12	100	None	12/12	6.4	0	1/12
Malek et al.[113]	13	100	1 TIA	11/13	20.7	0	N/A
Jenkins et al.[114]	32	100	1 TIA	31/32	10.6	0	1/32
Chastain et al.[115]	50	98	None	48/50	25	1	5/50
Qureshi et al.[116]	12	92[a]	None	N/R	1	0	N/R
Ogilvy et al.[117]	50	100	None	41/43	21	0	11/36
Jenkins et al.[82]	105[b]	100	1 TIA, 1 dissection	95/105	29	5	14/105[c]
Parkhutik et al.[118]	29	100	1 stroke	N/A	32	1	1/29

[a]Technical success defined as successful deployment of distal protection device and final residual stenosis of <30%.
[b]Ninety-seven cases involved proximal vertebral artery.
[c]Target-vessel revascularization.
N/A, Not available; *TIA*, transient ischemic attack.

(mean stenosis, approximately 75%).[87] From a cohort of 16 patients, 8 patients received endovascular therapy (angioplasty in 6, stenting in 2), and 8 patients received medical therapy. There were two procedure-related posterior circulation TIAs in the endovascular therapy group and no neurologic events in the medically treated group. Although this trial subgroup involved a small number of patients and does not reflect contemporary endovascular techniques, it does reinforce the need for dedicated trials of endovascular revascularization versus medical therapy in patients with proximal VA disease to help define the benefit, if any, of endovascular revascularization in this patient cohort.

INTRACRANIAL INTERVENTION

Intracranial large-vessel atherosclerosis is estimated to account for 5% to 10% of all ischemic strokes in the United States. In Asian, Hispanic, and black populations, the incidence of intracranial atherosclerosis is significantly greater and accounts for a greater proportion of all ischemic strokes.[1,88] As in the extracranial circulation, atherosclerosis of the intracranial circulation has a predilection for specific anatomic sites. In the anterior cerebral circulation, these include the petrous, cavernous, and supraclinoid (Fig. 46.16) portions of the ICA and the main trunk of the middle cerebral artery (MCA); in the posterior cerebral circulation, the distal VA (Fig. 46.17), vertebrobasilar junction, and midportion of the basilar artery are most commonly affected.

Intracranial atherosclerosis can cause ischemic stroke by a variety of mechanisms, including hypoperfusion, thrombotic occlusion at the site of disease, distal embolization from the site of disease, and occlusion of small penetrating arteries due to plaque extension. In identifying those patients most likely to benefit from revascularization therapy, it is important to develop an understanding of the likely mechanism of stroke in each patient based on clinical evaluation, noninvasive imaging, and contrast angiography.

The natural history of asymptomatic intracranial atherosclerosis is largely unknown, but limited data suggest a benign course.[89] By contrast, the Warfarin-Aspirin Symptomatic Intracranial Disease (WASID) trial provided a reasonable estimate of the high risk of recurrent events in patients with a recent TIA or stroke due to angiographically verified 50% to 99% stenosis of a major intracranial vessel.[90] In this cohort, the 1-year risk of an ischemic stroke in the distribution of the diseased intracranial artery in medically treated patients was approximately 12%. Additional retrospective studies have suggested a variety of clinical and angiographic variables to further risk-stratify patients with symptomatic intracranial atherosclerosis, including recurrent symptoms despite medical therapy,[91] lesion location (e.g., vertebral and ICA lesions proximal to major points of collateral supply have a lower risk than lesions involving the basilar artery or MCA), and severity of stenosis.[92]

Surgical revascularization of intracranial ICA and MCA disease was first performed in 1967 and subsequently tested in a large RCT of almost 1400 patients, which was reported in 1985.[93] Patients were randomly assigned to surgical revascularization (by anastomosis of branches of the ECA to the cortical branches of the MCA) or to medical therapy with aspirin (325 mg four times daily). Surgical therapy was associated with a 14% increase in the relative risk of nonfatal and fatal stroke. This therapy was revisited with the Carotid Occlusion Surgery Study (COSS) randomized trial, the results of which were reported in 2011. In this trial, 195 patients were randomized, 97 to bypass surgery and 98 to medical management. Despite excellent bypass patency, 98% at the 1-month postoperative visit, there was no significant difference in 2-year stroke risk between cohorts and the 30-day stroke rate was 14.4% for the surgical arm of the study versus 2% for the medically managed patients. Given the lack of evidence supporting the routine use of surgical bypass to reduce future stroke risk in the setting of intracranial occlusions, attempts at percutaneous revascularization of intracranial disease were made in the 1980s. The initial experience was similarly disappointing, with limited technical success and prohibitively high complication rates. However, by the mid-1990s, a variety of technological advances, borrowed from the coronary intervention field, and improved operator expertise resulted in a renewed enthusiasm for the technique. Technological advances included the availability of 0.014-inch wires that could negotiate the tortuous intracranial anatomy and low-profile, flexible balloon dilation catheters.

As in other vascular territories, stents were used to address some of the shortcomings associated with angioplasty of intracranial vessels (i.e., vessel recoil, abrupt vessel closure, and restenosis). However, the tortuosity of the intracranial circulation presented a significantly greater challenge for stent delivery than that encountered in the coronary circulation, so it was not until the availability of third- and fourth-generation coronary stents with improved flexibility and lower crossing profiles that stenting of intracranial disease became more widespread. Currently, a number of stents designed specifically for use in intracranial intervention, most notably the nitinol self-expanding Wingspan Stent (Boston Scientific), the balloon-expandable stainless steel Apollo stent (MicroPort Medical, Shanghai, China), and the balloon-expandable Pharos device (Micrus Endovascular, Sunnyvale, CA) have been developed and tested in prospective studies.[94,95]

Although stenting offers an effective treatment for arterial dissection and vessel recoil and improves restenosis rates, the use of stents in intracranial vessels raises a number of unique concerns.

SECTION IV Peripheral Vascular Interventions

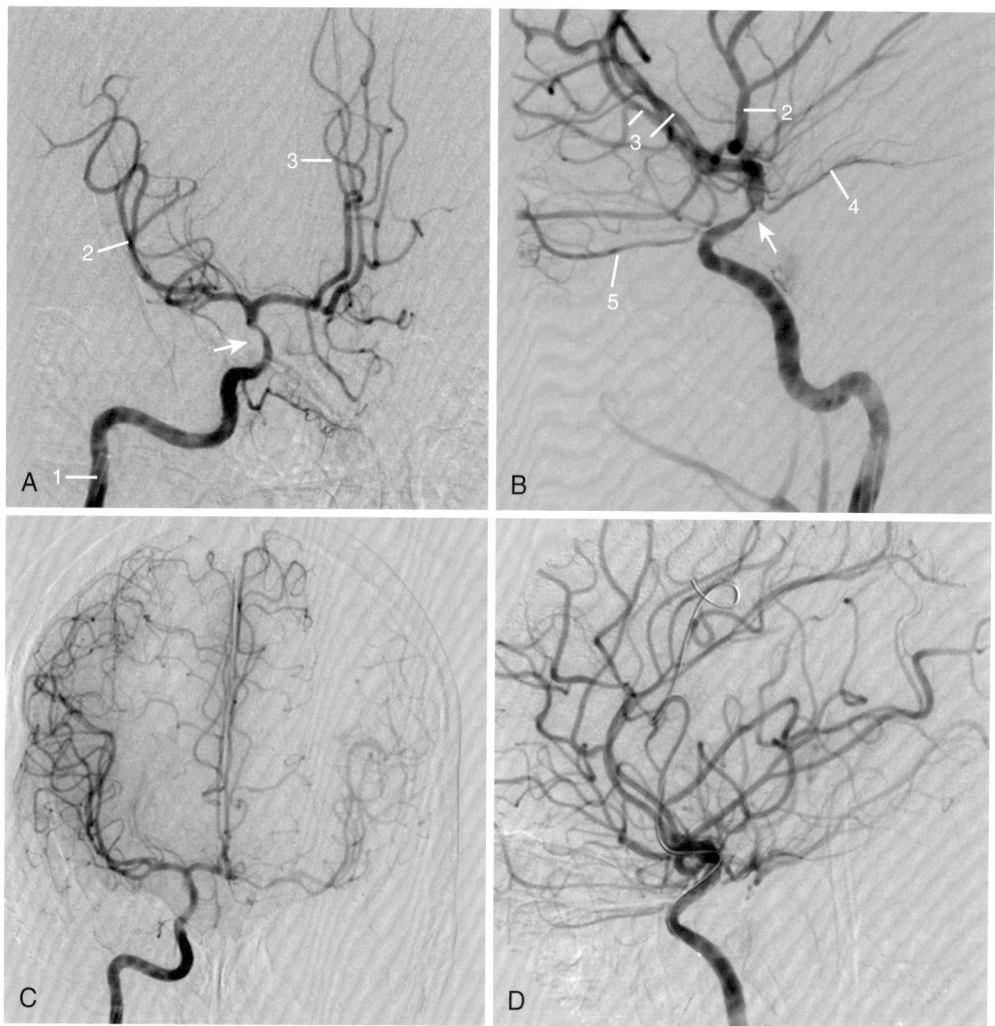

Fig. 46.16 Intracranial intervention. (A and B) Baseline cerebral angiography in posteroanterior (PA) cranial and lateral projections, respectively, show severe stenosis in the supraclinoid portion of the internal carotid artery *(arrows)*. (C and D) Cerebral angiography in PA cranial and lateral projections, respectively, after placement of 3.0- by 8-mm balloon-expandable Multilink Vision stent (Guidant Corporation, Indianapolis, IN). *1*, Internal carotid artery; *2*, middle cerebral artery; *3*, anterior cerebral artery; *4*, anterior choroidal branch; *5*, ophthalmic branch.

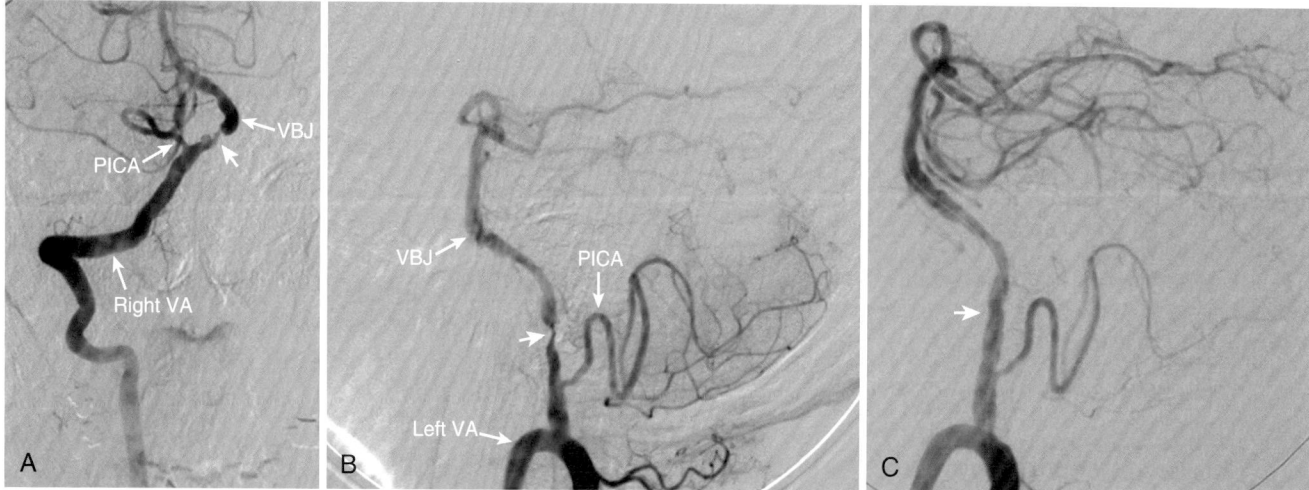

Fig. 46.17 Intracranial intervention. (A and B) Baseline angiography of right vertebral artery *(VA)* demonstrates severe stenosis *(arrows)* in intracranial portion of vessel between the origin of the posterior inferior cerebellar artery *(PICA)* and the vertebrobasilar junction *(VBJ)*. (C) Vertebral artery angiography after placement *(arrow)* of 3.0- by 12-mm Multilink Vision stent (Abbott Vascular, Abbott Park, IL).

Intracranial arteries are particularly fragile because of the sparse adventitia and elastic layers of the media and hence are prone to perforation. Depending on the lesion location, such perforations result in either subarachnoid or intraparenchymal hemorrhages, which are associated with high morbidity and mortality.[96] Given this consideration, intracranial stents are typically undersized and inflated to lower pressures (4 to 8 atm). However, several studies of stenting in the coronary circulation have shown that the use of stents that are appropriately sized to the reference vessel diameter and inflated to high pressures (14 to 16 atm) is required for optimal stent deployment and apposition of stent struts to the vessel wall. The latter considerations are believed to minimize the risk of stent thrombosis and to reduce the rate of restenosis.

As described, potentially serious consequences are associated with the current practice of intracranial stenting. Moreover, stenting is associated with significantly more plaque shifting than angioplasty alone. Although the occlusion of small side branches in the coronary circulation is usually a benign event, compromise of critical side branches from intracranial vessels (e.g., lenticulostriate branches of the MCA and perforating branches of the basilar artery) can have severe neurologic consequences.[97] Finally, significant complications (e.g., stent dislodgement, vessel dissection, distal embolization of plaque) may occur with attempts to deliver stents through the technically challenging vascular terrain of the intracranial circulation.

Technique

Intracranial intervention is almost universally performed with the use of femoral arterial access. Most operators use general anesthesia, in contrast to other cerebrovascular interventions, but conscious sedation has been shown to be a viable alternative.[98] Preprocedural antiplatelet and procedural anticoagulation regimens mirror those practiced during carotid bifurcation intervention. The first task during anterior or posterior circulation intracranial intervention is the delivery of a guide or sheath to the internal carotid or VA, respectively. Sheaths are most commonly used (e.g., Shuttle sheath, Cook), although the inner luminal diameter of a 6-Fr sheath is adequate for delivery of standard interventional equipment required for angioplasty and stent deployment in the intracranial circulation. Numerous intermediate catheters of varying diameters and lengths can be used to address tortuous anatomy requiring additional support. Having achieved this platform, a variety of 0.010- to 0.014-inch wires (e.g., Synchro, Boston Scientific) may be used to cross the intracranial lesion. To provide sufficient support for device delivery, the wire is usually advanced to the second- or third-order branches of the middle or posterior cerebral artery for anterior or posterior circulation interventions, respectively.

Angioplasty is performed with the use of coronary balloons (e.g., Maverick, Boston Scientific), and the angioplasty technique is modified to minimize the risk of vessel perforation. These modifications include using balloon diameters that are 70% to 80% of the vessel diameter and performing slow, prolonged inflation of the balloon to less than nominal pressures (4 to 8 atm), followed by slow deflation. In addition, the minimal balloon length required to treat the lesion is chosen to minimize the risk of compromising flow in side or perforating branches. Although some operators adopt a strategy of "provisional" stenting (i.e., stenting only if the angioplasty result is suboptimal), an increasing number practice primary stenting (stent placement regardless of the initial angioplasty result). Currently, the most popular stents used for intracranial intervention are the recent generation of cobalt-chromium balloon-expandable coronary stents (e.g., Multilink Vision, Abbott; Driver, Medtronic), which have superior deliverability compared with stainless steel coronary stents. Balloon-expandable stents are sized 0.5 mm smaller than the estimated vessel diameter and are inflated to moderate pressures (6 to 8 atm). The minimal stent length is used to attenuate the risk of plaque shift into critical side or perforating branches. Final angiography of the lesion site and distal cerebral circulation is performed, and patients recover in a neurointensive care setting.

Clinical Outcomes

The initial data regarding intracranial intervention were derived mostly from retrospective observational case series at a small number of institutions with highly experienced operators; as such, they had significant limitations in applicability to broad clinical settings. Case series from the late 1990s and early 2000s reported the experience with intracranial angioplasty. However, the availability of balloon-expandable coronary stents appears to have improved the technical success rate to greater than 90% without a significant increase in periprocedural complications. A systematic review of 31 studies, many of which were early case series, reported results from 1177 intracranial stenting procedures. The median rate of technical success was 96% (interquartile range, 90% to 100%), whereas the median rate of stroke and death was 7.7% (interquartile range, 4.4% to 14.3%).[99] A number of multicenter prospective studies of intracranial stenting for symptomatic atherosclerotic lesions have been performed in the past decade.[100–104] Each of these studies reported procedural success rates of 90% or better, and four of the five studies reported procedural success of 95% or better.

Early complications rates have ranged from 2% to 7% for ischemic stroke, 1% to 3% for intracerebral hemorrhage, and 0% to 5% for death (Table 46.10). The evidence for long-term complication rates (e.g., restenosis) are less robust because there are fewer data, varying definitions of restenosis, and differing

TABLE 46.10 Multicenter Prospective Observational Studies of Intracranial Stenting

Study	Year	n	Lesions	Lesion Location		Technical Success (%)	Follow-Up	Adverse Outcomes		
				Anterior	Posterior			Ischemic Stroke	Intracerebral Hemorrhage	Death
SSYLVIA	2004	61[a]	61	20	23	95	30 days	3 (5%)	1 (2%)	0
WINGSPAN[100]	2007	45	45	23	22	100	30 days	1 (2%)	1 (2%)	0
Fiorella et al.[119]	2007	78	82	54	28	99	Periprocedural	4 (5%)	1 (1%)	4[b] (5%)
Zaidat et al.[104]	2008	129	129	76	53	97	30 days	6 (5%)	3 (2%)	4[c] (3%)
INTRASTENT[d]	2010	372	388	223	165	90	Periprocedural	28 (7%)	12 (3%)	8 (2%)

[a]Forty-three lesions were intracranial.
[b]Deaths were due to the four ischemic strokes.
[c]Three deaths were due to either ischemic or hemorrhagic strokes.
[d]One-hundred and forty-nine patients were enrolled prospectively. A study center could enter consecutive patients retrospectively if done completely (n = 239).
 SSYLVIA, Stenting of Symptomatic Atherosclerotic Lesions in the Vertebral or Intracranial Arteries.

strategies for patient surveillance. Nonetheless, in the Stenting of Symptomatic Atherosclerotic Lesions in the Vertebral or Intracranial Arteries (SSYLVIA) trial, between 30 days and 1 year of follow-up, there were two strokes, giving a cumulative 1-year stroke incidence of 14%. Repeat angiography at 6 months documented a restenosis rate of 32% in the intracranial cohort. In the overall group (intracranial and extracranial procedures), 39% of patients with restenosis were symptomatic (i.e., with TIAs or strokes).[101] In contrast to the SSYLVIA study, all patients in the Wingspan study with restenosis were asymptomatic. In this latter registry, the restenosis rate (>50% by angiography) at 6 months was 7.5%, and the incidence of ipsilateral stroke or death was 7.0%.[100] These prospective studies underscore the technical success of intracranial procedures, mirroring the rates reported in other observational series. However, the 6-month and 1-year rates of death and stroke in prospective cohort studies appear to be greater than in retrospective longitudinal studies, highlighting potential publication bias in the latter type of study design. Indeed, the 14% rate of stroke at 1 year in the SSYLVIA study is remarkably similar to the 1-year risk of stroke reported in the WASID trial in medically treated patients.[90,101]

The Stenting and Aggressive Medical Management for Preventing Recurrent Stroke (SAMMPRIS) trial compared intracranial stenting with the Wingspan system plus optimal medical therapy versus optimal medical therapy alone in patients with symptomatic, severe intracranial arterial stenosis.[105] The primary end point was stroke or death at 30 days. The trial was stopped early after results from the first 451 of a planned 764 enrolled patients were obtained because of higher event rates in the intervention arm. At 30 days, stroke and death had occurred in 14.7% of the stenting and medical therapy group, compared with only 5.8% of the medical therapy alone group ($P = .002$). The disparity in outcome rates was driven primarily by intraprocedural complications, indicating that technical advances could potentially improve outcomes for intracranial intervention. Nonetheless, results from SAMMPRIS have dampened enthusiasm for endovascular therapy for obstructive intracranial arterial disease.

In contrast, intracranial intervention for acute stroke is showing great promise for improving outcomes in this devastating disease. Multiple trials of endovascular therapy compared with standard care in acute stroke are currently showing marked improvements in functional outcomes (Table 46.11).[2,106–109] Although these relatively small trials differ in several design features, a few common signals are emerging: (1) outcomes strongly favor a timely percutaneous approach by skilled operators in the early treatment of acute stroke patients as compared with systemic fibrinolysis alone, (2) advanced imaging assessment of the amount of at-risk but viable cerebrum is important for patient selection, and (3) the use of retrievable stents are prevalent in this evidence base as the endovascular treatment of choice. This new paradigm of stroke management has tremendous implications on system-wide efforts at delivering acute stroke care and on training programs to ensure there are a sufficient volume of skilled interventionalists.

TABLE 46.11 Randomized Trials of Endovascular Therapy Versus Standard Treatment in Patients With Acute Stroke, Large Vessel Occlusion, and Viable Brain

Trial	n	Setting	Endovascular Therapy	Timing after Stroke Onset (h)	Systemic Fibrinolytic Use in Trial	Primary Outcome	Results
ESCAPE	316	Worldwide	Available thrombectomy devices Retrievable stents recommended	<12	75%	mRA scale at 90 days	Percent with mRA 0–2: 53.0%, vs. 29.3%, $P < .001$ favoring intervention
EXTEND 1A	70	Australia	Retrievable stent	<4.5	100%	Reperfusion at 24 h and early neurologic improvement (≥8-point reduction on the NIHSS or an mRA score of 0 or 1 at day 3)	Percent with mRA 0–2: 71% vs. 40%; $P = .01$ favoring intervention
MR CLEAN	500	The Netherlands	Intra-arterial fibrinolytic and/or mechanical thrombectomy (81% retrievable stents)	<6 h of anterior stroke onset	89%	Modified Rankin scale at 90 days	Percent with mRA 0–2: 32.6% vs. 19.1% $P < .01$ favoring intervention
REVASCAT	206	Spain	Retrievable stent	<8 h of anterior stroke onset	73%	Severity of disability at 90 days, according to the distribution of scores on the modified Rankin scale	Percent with mRA 0–2: 43.7% vs. 28.2%; $P < .05$ favoring intervention
THRACE	414	France	Available thrombectomy devices	<4–5 h	100%	Proportion of patients achieving functional independence at 3 months, defined by a score of 0–2 on the modified Rankin scale	Percent with mRA 0–2: 42% vs. 53% $P = .028$ favoring intervention

ESCAPE, Endovascular treatment for Small Core and Anterior circulation Proximal occlusion with Emphasis on minimizing computed tomography to recanalization times; *EXTEND 1A*, Extending the Time for Thrombolysis in Emergency Neurological Deficits—Intra-Arterial trial; *MR CLEAN*, Multicenter Randomized CLinical trial of Endovascular treatment for Acute ischemic stroke in the Netherlands; *mRA*, modified Rankin; *n*, number of participants in study; *NIHSS*, National Institutes of Health Stroke Scale; *REVASCAT*, Randomized Trial of Revascularization with Solitaire FR Device versus Best Medical Therapy in the Treatment of Acute Stroke Due to Anterior Circulation Large Vessel Occlusion Presenting within Eight Hours of Symptom Onset; *THRACE*, THRombectomie des Art.res CErebrales.

CONCLUSIONS

Cerebrovascular intervention has evolved dramatically over the past decade. It is clear that these procedures are feasible and—when performed by experienced endovascular specialists using contemporary interventional equipment and techniques—are safe. The challenge for the future is to advance understanding of the natural history of cerebrovascular atherosclerosis, more accurately predict those patients who will develop recurrent events, and refine the patient populations in whom endovascular revascularization provides meaningful clinical benefit.

KEY REFERENCES

29. Ansel GM, Hopkins LN, Jaff MR, et al. Safety and effectiveness of the INVATEC MO.MA(R) proximal cerebral protection device during carotid artery stenting: results from the ARMOUR pivotal trial. *Catheter Cardiovasc Interv.* 2010;76(1):1–8.
30. Stabile E, Salemme L, Sorropago G, et al. Proximal endovascular occlusion for carotid artery stenting: results from a prospective registry of 1,300 patients. *J Am Coll Cardiol.* 2010;55(16):1661–1667.
31. Bersin RM, Stabile E, Ansel GM, et al. A meta-analysis of proximal occlusion device outcomes in carotid artery stenting. *Catheter Cardiovasc Interv.* 2012;80(7):1072–1078.
37. Bates ER, Babb JD, Casey Jr DE, et al. ACCF/SCAI/SVMB/SIR/ASITN 2007 clinical expert consensus document on carotid stenting: a report of the American College of Cardiology Foundation Task Force on clinical expert consensus documents (ACCF/SCAI/SVMB/SIR/ASITN clinical expert consensus document committee on carotid stenting). *J Am Coll Cardiol.* 2007;49(1):126–170.
38. Gray WA, Chaturvedi S, Verta P. Thirty-day outcomes for carotid artery stenting in 6320 patients from 2 prospective, multicenter, high-surgical-risk registries. *Circ Cardiovasc Interv.* 2009;2(3):159–166.
44. Yadav JS, Wholey MH, Kuntz RE, et al. Protected carotid-artery stenting versus endarterectomy in high-risk patients. *N Engl J Med.* 2004;351(15):1493–1501.
45. Brott TG. The Randomized Carotid Revascularization Endarterectomy vs Stenting Trial (CREST): primary results. In: *Program and Abstracts of the 2010 International Stroke Conference.* 2010.
66. Brott TG, Hobson 2nd RW, Howard G, et al. Stenting versus endarterectomy for treatment of carotid-artery stenosis. *N Engl J Med.* 2010;363(1):11–23.
79. Rosenfield K, Matsumura JS, Chaturvedi S, et al. Randomized trial of stent versus surgery for asymptomatic carotid stenosis. *N Engl J Med.* 2016;374(11):1011–1020.
80. Kwolek CJ, Jaff MR, Leal JI, et al. Results of the ROADSTER multicenter trial of transcarotid stenting with dynamic flow reversal. *J Vasc Surg.* 2015;62(5):1227–1234.
106. Goyal M, Demchuk AM, Menon BK, et al. Randomized assessment of rapid endovascular treatment of ischemic stroke. *N Engl J Med.* 2015;372(11):1019–1030.
107. Campbell BC, Mitchell PJ, Kleinig TJ, et al. Endovascular therapy for ischemic stroke. *N Engl J Med.* 2015;372(24):2365–2366.
108. Berkhemer OA, Fransen PS, Beumer D, et al. A randomized trial of intraarterial treatment for acute ischemic stroke. *N Engl J Med.* 2015;372(1):11–20.

 Additional references available online at expertconsult.com.

中文导读

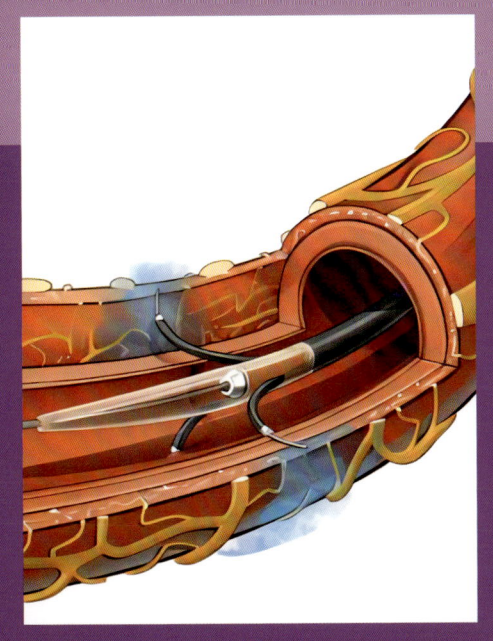

第47章
卒中中心与介入心脏病学

　　脑卒中是致死和致残的主要原因，80%以上的脑卒中是缺血性的。急性脑卒中的早期快速评估，尤其是CT或MRI等影像学评估，有助于快速明确病因、启动治疗，以降低死亡率和致残率。缺血性脑卒中的治疗原则是尽快实现再灌注，最主要的治疗策略为静脉注射组织型纤溶酶原激活剂（Ⅳ tPA），其他还包括动脉内溶栓、机械血栓切除术及球囊血管成形术等。神经保护的药物和设备仍有待进一步研发。卒中中心的建设有助于缩短救助时间、提高对卒中患者的初步评估和护理能力、提高卒中治疗的成功率。急性脑卒中和急性心肌梗死的治疗有相似之处，然而，不同于介入心脏病专家队伍的全天候介入治疗，缺乏能够提供随时救治能力的神经介入医师是目前的主要短板。回顾性研究发现，神经血管专家和心血管专家进行的血管内卒中治疗手术均有良好的临床结局，其结果没有显著差异。介入心脏病专家加入卒中团队，解决人力短缺的问题，对于帮助迎接按需快速再灌注治疗的挑战具有重要作用。

　　本章节重点介绍了急性脑卒中的影像学评估，血压、血糖、发热等生理指标的管理，再灌注策略，以及卒中中心的建设。另外还强调了介入心脏病学在卒中项目中的重要作用，建议可以将介入心脏病学专家纳入卒中队伍，共同建设卒中团队。

李秋忆　张洪亮

章节要点

- 卒中的三大类型是出血性、血栓性和栓塞性（即从动脉到动脉和从心腔到动脉）。
- 与冠状动脉病变不同，颈动脉斑块最常见于动脉粥样硬化而不是血栓闭塞引起症状。
- 脑梗死的大小取决于再灌注发生所需的时间、作为侧支来源的Willis环的通畅性，以及周围缺血半暗带的活力。
- 唯一被批准的急性缺血性卒中的治疗方法是在发病后3~4.5小时无禁忌证的情况下进行静脉溶栓。
- 卒中静脉溶栓治疗并发颅内出血的风险增加，与卒中的范围、治疗时间（＞3小时）、患者年龄（＞85岁）和未控制的高血压直接相关。
- 最近完成的涉及缺血性卒中的随机对照试验证实，在大血管闭塞的患者中，无论是否使用静脉组织型纤溶酶原激活剂（Ⅳ tPA），机械取栓均优于单独使用Ⅳ tPA，可获得更高的再通率、更好的临床结果和相似的并发症发生率。
- 由卒中团队中的介入心脏病专家提供的血管内卒中治疗的结果，不劣于由神经血管专家提供的治疗结果。

47 Stroke Centers and Interventional Cardiology

Christopher J. White

KEY POINTS

- The three broad categories of stroke are hemorrhagic, thrombotic, and embolic (i.e., artery to artery and chamber to artery).
- Carotid plaque, unlike coronary lesions, most often causes symptoms due to atheroembolization rather than thrombotic occlusion.
- The size of a brain infarction is determined by the time it takes for reperfusion to occur, the patency of the circle of Willis as a collateral source, and the viability of the surrounding penumbra of ischemic tissue.
- The only approved treatment for acute ischemic stroke is intravenous thrombolysis within 3 to 4.5 hours of onset and without contraindications.
- The risk of intracranial hemorrhage complicating intravenous thrombolytic therapy for stroke is increased in direct relation to the size of the stroke, time to treatment (>3 hours), patient age (>85 years), and uncontrolled hypertension.
- Recently completed randomized controlled trials involving ischemic stroke have established that mechanical thrombectomy in patients with large-vessel occlusions with or without intravenous tissue-type plasminogen activator (IV tPA) is preferred over IV tPA alone, yielding higher recanalization rates, higher rates of favorable clinical outcomes, and similar complication rates.
- Outcomes of endovascular stroke therapy given by interventional cardiologists on a stroke team are not inferior to the outcomes of therapy given by neurovascular specialists.

INTRODUCTION

Stroke affects approximately 70,000 Americans each year, resulting in almost 150,000 deaths.[1] Stroke is the third leading cause of death in the United States, after heart disease and cancer. It is the number one cause of disability and the number one reason for rehabilitation. There are more than 3 million stroke survivors in the United States, and one-third of them are young adults with long-term disabilities.[2]

The causes of stroke include hemorrhage, thrombus, and embolus. Embolic strokes may extend artery to artery or from a heart chamber (left atrium or ventricle) to an artery, particularly in patients with atrial fibrillation. A major tenet of the treatment of ischemic stroke is that *time is brain*.

The extent of ischemic brain injury is determined by the time from the onset of symptoms to reperfusion; the collateral circulation, including an intact circle of Willis; and the penumbra of viability surrounding the infarcted brain tissue. The penumbra is the region of brain surrounding the infarct area where the blood supply is significantly reduced but energy metabolism is maintained due to collateral flow. The viability of this area depends on the severity and duration of ischemia. If blood flow is rapidly restored, some ischemic brain tissue can be saved. For ischemic and hemorrhagic strokes, there are opportunities to minimize injury early after the onset of the stroke. This puts a premium on the rapid assessment of patients with stroke (Table 47.1).[3]

The goals of treatment include preventing or limiting the mortality and morbidity of the acute event and preventing recurrent events. More than 80% of strokes are ischemic.[4] Ischemic stroke therapy, designed to achieve reperfusion as quickly as possible and to minimize further damage, consists of intravenous thrombolysis with or without catheter-based reperfusion therapy, which can include intra arterial thrombolysis, mechanical thrombectomy, or balloon angioplasty with or without stent placement.[3]

Rapid initiation of intravenous tissue-type plasminogen activator (IV tPA) with a door-to-needle time of less than 60 minutes is important for a good outcome. However, the American Heart Association's Get With the Guidelines–Stroke national registry has reported that fewer than one in three stroke patients are treated within less than 60 minutes of arrival at the hospital.[5] Although a national heart attack quality initiative has enabled interventional cardiologists to achieve dramatic reductions in door-to-balloon times,[6] acute stroke therapy languishes without a mandate to provide early reperfusion. Currently there is no goal for time to reperfusion or door-to-treatment time in the United States, and it is not the standard of care for stroke therapy as it is for heart attacks.[7] Unfortunately, owing to a variety of issues—including time to presentation, availability of stroke programs, and a lack of national focus on time to treatment—the majority of patients with ischemic stroke in the United States do not receive reperfusion therapy.[8–10]

NEW IMAGING STRATEGIES

The American Heart Association/American Stroke Association (AHA/ASA) has a class I recommendation to perform noncontrast computed tomography (CT) or magnetic resonance imaging (MRI) for patients who are evaluated within 3 hours of stroke symptom onset so as to exclude intracranial bleeding.[2] Imaging is the cornerstone for triaging candidates for stroke therapy. The purpose of the baseline CT is to detect conditions that make the patient ineligible for thrombolysis, such as subdural, subarachnoid, or parenchymal intracranial hemorrhage (ICH). CT may also detect mass lesions or hemorrhagic infarctions.

Brain imaging in the setting of an acute stroke has four major goals. First, ICH must be excluded. The patient with ICH has a neurosurgical emergency, and the neurosurgeon must be involved immediately. Second, CT and MRI can be used to identify intravascular thrombus noninvasively. Data regarding the geographic distribution and size of the thrombus burden can assist in deciding between IV tPA and endovascular mechanical thrombectomy. Third, the ratio of the volume of viable to nonviable brain (penumbra) predicts the patient's potential for recovery.

Multimodal CT includes unenhanced CT, CT angiography (CTA), and CT perfusion. Noncontrast CT can identify ICH and detect early signs of acute ischemic stroke. CTA can identify

TABLE 47.1 The Seven Ds of Stroke Care
• Detection
• Dispatch
• Delivery
• Door-to-treatment time
• Data
• Decision
• Drug and device administration

the occlusion site, detect arterial dissection, and grade collateral blood flow, whereas CT perfusion can differentiate between tissue at risk (the so-called penumbra) and irreversibly damaged brain tissue.

THE MANAGEMENT OF PHYSIOLOGIC VARIABLES

A cornerstone of managing acute stroke is reducing the risk of recurrent events and minimizing the disability due to the established stroke. Acute therapy involves the management of physiologic variables, reperfusion of ischemic tissue, and reduction of the risk of ICH. The patient's level of consciousness, airway status, and oxygenation must be determined immediately. An electrocardiogram is needed to rule out a concomitant myocardial infarction.

Hypertension

Most patients with stroke have arterial hypertension, which is associated with a poorer outcome, but lower blood pressure may decrease perfusion to the ischemic penumbra, extending the size of the infarction. Hypertensive patients who are eligible for treatment with IV tPA should have their blood pressure carefully lowered so that their systolic blood pressure is <185 mm Hg and their diastolic blood pressure is <110 mm Hg before fibrinolytic therapy is initiated. If medications are given to lower blood pressure, the clinician should be sure that the blood pressure is stabilized at the lower level before beginning treatment with IV tPA and that it is maintained below 180/105 mm Hg for at least the first 24 hours after intravenous IV tPA treatment.[2]

In patients with markedly elevated blood pressure who do not receive fibrinolysis, a reasonable goal is to lower blood pressure by 15% during the first 24 hours after the onset of stroke. The level of blood pressure that would mandate such treatment is not known, but consensus exists that medications should be withheld unless the systolic blood pressure is >220 mm Hg or the diastolic blood pressure is >120 mm Hg. Restarting antihypertensive medications is reasonable after the first 24 hours for patients who have preexisting hypertension and are neurologically stable unless a specific contraindication to restarting treatment is known. Patients who have malignant hypertension or other medical indications for the aggressive treatment of blood pressure should be treated accordingly.[2]

Hypoglycemia

Severe hypoglycemia may mimic a stroke and can be detected by a finger-stick glucose determination. Immediate reversal is warranted with intravenous or oral glucose solutions, or both.

Hyperglycemia

Elevated blood glucose levels are associated with worse outcomes for patients with acute stroke. This may be related to increased lactate production, which increases infarct size, reduces the effectiveness of thrombolytic therapy, and may increase the risk of hemorrhagic transformation of infarcted brain tissue. Hyperglycemia can increase the extent of infarction in cerebral ischemia, and a blood glucose level above 200 should be controlled to as close to the normal range as possible, using insulin if necessary.

Fever

Fever is associated with poorer stroke outcomes, possibly because of a detrimental effect on brain metabolism, increased free radical production, or deterioration of the blood-brain barrier function. If bacterial endocarditis is suspected, samples for blood cultures should be drawn and an echocardiogram should be obtained before interventional management. Current recommendations are to use antipyretics to maintain normothermia.

REPERFUSION STRATEGIES

Intravenous Thrombolysis

IV tPA is the only therapy for acute ischemic stroke approved by the U.S. Food and Drug Administration (FDA) (Tables 47.2 and 47.3). The original time limit of 3 hours from the onset of stroke has been extended to 4.5 hours in selected cases.[11] IV tPA was shown to be an effective therapy for stroke in a meta-analysis of 2775 patients treated within 6 hours of onset.[12] Patients treated within 90 minutes of onset had an almost threefold increase in good outcomes—a rate that dropped to a 1.6-fold increase if they were treated between 91 and 180 minutes. For those treated between 180 and 270 minutes,

TABLE 47.2 Eligibility for Thrombolysis for Stroke
Indication: ischemic stroke within 3 h of onset of symptoms
Clinical contraindications
• History of intracranial hemorrhage (ICH)
• Systolic blood pressure >185 mm Hg, diastolic blood pressure >110 mm Hg
• Rapid improvement in neurologic status
• Mild neurologic impairment
• Symptoms of subarachnoid bleeding
• Stroke or head trauma within the last 3 months
• Gastrointestinal or genitourinary hemorrhage within 3 weeks
• Major surgery within 3 weeks
• Recent heart attack
• Seizure with stroke
• Taking oral anticoagulants
• Received heparin within 48 h
Radiologic contraindications
• Evidence of ICH
Laboratory contraindications
• International normalized ratio >1.7
• Platelet count <100,000
• Elevated activated partial thromboplastin time
• Blood glucose <50 mg/dL

TABLE 47.3 Treatment of Ischemic Stroke

Intravenous Thrombolysis	Mechanical Thrombectomy
≤4.5 h from onset of symptoms	≤6 h from onset of symptoms
Widely available	ASPECTS score >6
Restricted population	Large-vessel occlusion
• No bleed on head CT scan	Disabling stroke (NIHSS ≥5)
• SBP <185 mm Hg	• MCA occlusion
• DBP <110 mm Hg	• Speech impairment
• Low bleeding risk	• Vision impairment

ASPECTS, Alberta Stroke Program Early Computed Tomography Score; *CT*, computed tomography; *DBP*, diastolic blood pressure; *MCA*, middle cerebral artery; *NIHSS*, National Institutes of Health Stroke Scale; *SBP*, systolic blood pressure.

the odds ratio for benefit was 1.4 times greater than for placebo. The risk of ICH was greater for the thrombolysis group (5.9%) compared with the placebo group (1.1%).

IV tPA has limited effectiveness in recanalizing proximal stroke-related arteries with a large clot burden. Recanalization rates range from less than 10% for internal carotid artery occlusions to approximately 50% for middle cerebral artery distal branch occlusions.[13,14]

The risk-to-benefit ratio for IV tPA in ischemic stroke is narrow. About 11% more patients benefit at 3 months from intravenous lysis, whereas 6.4% develop ICH. Unfortunately, only a minority of eligible patients with acute ischemic stroke receive reperfusion treatment in the United States.[15] Seven stroke patients must be treated with intravenous lysis to achieve an excellent outcome and avoid one stroke death or disability. For every 100 stroke patients treated with intravenous thrombolysis within 3 hours, 32 have a better outcome despite the 3 who suffer significant ICH. At 1 year after treatment, those treated with intravenous lysis have a 30% increased likelihood of minimal or no disability compared with placebo, but there were no differences in the rates of mortality and recurrent strokes.[16] The risk of hemorrhage is increased for older adult patients and those with larger strokes, diabetes mellitus, a history of stroke, or thrombocytopenia.

Intra arterial Thrombolysis

Intra arterial thrombolysis involves the selective placement of a catheter into the cerebral vessels. The benefit of catheter-based intracranial therapy is the ability to use smaller doses of lytic agents and to employ mechanical clot disruption and extraction with guidewires, balloons, and thrombectomy devices.

The effectiveness of intra arterial thrombolysis has been established in several trials. The Prolyse in Acute Cerebral Thromboembolism II (PROACT II) trial randomized patients admitted within 6 hours with stroke and angiographically documented occlusion of the middle cerebral artery to 9 mg of intra arterial prourokinase plus unfractionated heparin or to unfractionated heparin alone.[17] Successful reperfusion was achieved in 66% of the intra arterial prourokinase group compared with only 18% of the control group ($P < .001$). Forty percent of the prourokinase group had slight or no neurologic disability (modified Rankin Scale score of ≤2) at 90 days compared with only 25% of the control group ($P = .04$).

There were more symptomatic cases of ICH in the thrombolysis group compared with controls (11% vs. 3%, $P = .03$). The number needed to treat to make one patient independent was seven. This trial extended the efficacy for stroke treatment to 6 hours from onset of symptoms, but only 2% of all screened patients were enrolled. Contraindications to catheter-directed thrombolysis include recent brain surgery, unknown time of onset of the deficit, uncontrolled hypertension, and CT evidence of hemorrhage or tumor.

Mechanical Thrombectomy

Between December 2014 and April 2015, five randomized controlled trials provided compelling evidence that mechanical thrombectomy improves outcomes after acute ischemic stroke (Tables 47.4 and 47.5). Endovascular treatment significantly improved clinical outcome in patients with proximal intracranial occlusion of the anterior circulation compared with IV tPA, indicating that the preferred treatment of these patients is no longer IV tPA but endovascular revascularization (Figs. 47.1–47.5).[18–22]

The major differences between these new positive trials and past negative trials was (1) the use of CTA to select patients with proximal intracranial occlusion; (2) the selection of patients with more viable brain tissue (penumbra); and (3) the use of new, more flexible and user-friendly thrombectomy devices. The percentage of patients achieving a favorable clinical outcome with mechanical thrombectomy varied between 33% and 71%. There was a consistent favorable clinical outcome (defined as a modified Rankin Score [mRS] of 0 to 2 at 90 days) across all studies. In the trials in which penumbral imaging with CT perfusion was used, the advantage for mechanical thrombectomy was even more pronounced. Importantly, mechanical thrombectomy with or without intravenous thrombolysis was consistently effective overall and among important prespecified patient subgroups of sex, age, stroke severity, and time of presentation.

TABLE 47.4 Randomized Trials of Mechanical Thrombectomy With IV tPA vs. IV tPA

Trial	Number of Patients (MT/IV tPA)	Inclusion Criteria	Exclusion Criteria	Primary End Point	Devices Used
MR CLEAN[18]	500 (233/267)	Age ≥18 NIHSS >2 6 h from onset		mRS at 90 days	Retrievable stents in 81% IAT in 10%
EXTEND-IA[19]	70 (35/35)	Age ≥18 IV t-PA within 4.5 h Penumbral imaging with CT or MRI	Groin puncture after 6 h from onset	NIHSS improvement Reperfusion at 24 h	Retrievable stents
ESCAPE[20]	315 (165/150)	Age ≥18 NIHSS >2 12 h from onset Groin puncture within 60 min of baseline CT	ASPECTS score ≤5 Poor collaterals on CTA Large infarct core	mRS at 90 days	Retrievable stents in 86%
SWIFT PRIME[21]	196 (98/98)	Age 18–80 NIHSS ≥8 to <30 IV tPA within 4.5 h	extracranial cervical carotid occlusion	mRS at 90 days	Retrievable stents
REVASCAT[22]	206 (103/103)	Age 18–85 NIHSS >6 8 h from onset	ASPECTS score <7	mRS at 90 days	Retrievable stents

ASPECTS, Alberta Stroke Program Early Computed Tomography Score; *CT*, computed tomography; *CTA*, computed tomographic angiography; *ESCAPE*, Endovascular Treatment for Small Core and Anterior Circulation Proximal Occlusion with Emphasis on Minimizing CT to Recanalization Times; *EXTEND-IA*, Extending the Time for Thrombolysis in Emergency Neurological Deficits–IntraArterial; *IAT*, intra arterial thrombolysis; *IV tPA*, intravenous tissue-type plasminogen activator; *MR CLEAN*, Multicenter Randomized Clinical Trial of Endovascular Treatment for Acute Ischemic Stroke in the Netherlands; *MRI*, magnetic resonance imaging; *mRS*, modified Rankin scale; *MT*, mechanical thrombectomy; *NIHSS*, National Institutes of Health Stroke Scale; *SWIFT PRIME*, Solitaire with the Intention for Thrombectomy as Primary Endovascular Treatment; *REVASCAT*, Randomized Trial of Revascularization with Solitaire FR Device versus Best Medical Therapy in the Treatment of Acute Stroke Due to Anterior Circulation Large Vessel Occlusion Presenting within 8 Hours of Symptom Onset.

TABLE 47.5 Results of Randomized Trials of Mechanical Thrombectomy With IV tPA vs. IV tPA

	Patients (n)	mRS 0–2 MT (%)	mRS 0–2 IV tPA (%)	sICH MT (%)	sICH IV tPA (%)	Mortality MT (%)	Mortality IV tPA (%)
MR CLEAN[18]	500	33[a]	19	7.7	6.4	21	22
EXTEND-IA[19]	70	71[b]	40	0	6	9	20
ESCAPE[20]	315	53[a]	29	3.6	2.7	10	19[c]
SWIFT PRIME[21]	196	60[a]	36	0	3	9	12
REVASCAT[22]	206	44[a]	28	1.9	1.9	18	16

[a]$P < .001$.
[b]$P = .01$.
[c]$P = .04$.

ESCAPE, Endovascular Treatment for Small Core and Anterior Circulation Proximal Occlusion with Emphasis on Minimizing CT to Recanalization Times; *EXTEND-IA*, Extending the Time for Thrombolysis in Emergency Neurological Deficits -Intra-Arterial; *IV tPA*, Intravenous tissue-type plasminogen activator; *MR CLEAN*, Multicenter Randomized Clinical Trial of Endovascular Treatment for Acute Ischemic Stroke in the Netherlands; *mRS*, modified Rankin scale; *MT*, mechanical thrombectomy; *sICH*, symptomatic intracranial hemorrhage; *SWIFT PRIME*, Solitaire with the Intention for Thrombectomy as Primary Endovascular Treatment; *REVASCAT*, Randomized Trial of Revascularization with Solitaire FR Device versus Best Medical Therapy in the Treatment of Acute Stroke Due to Anterior Circulation Large Vessel Occlusion Presenting within 8 Hours of Symptom Onset.

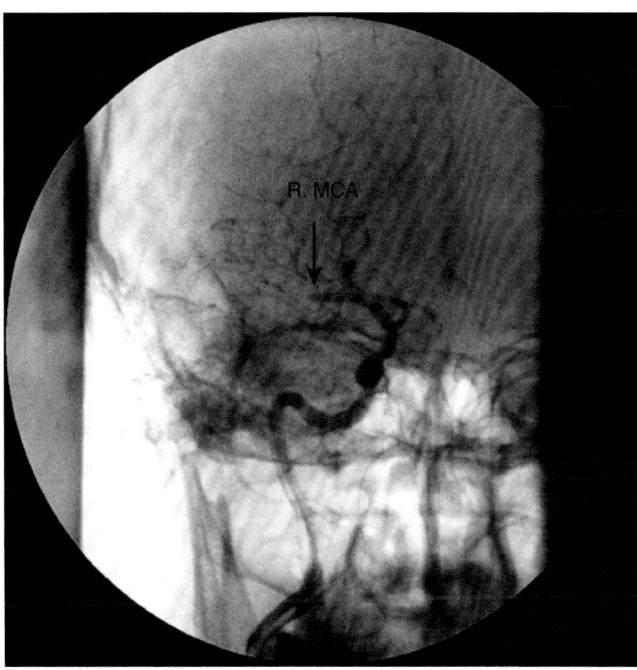

Fig. 47.1 A patient with atrial fibrillation who had an acute occlusion of the right middle cerebral artery *(R. MCA)*.

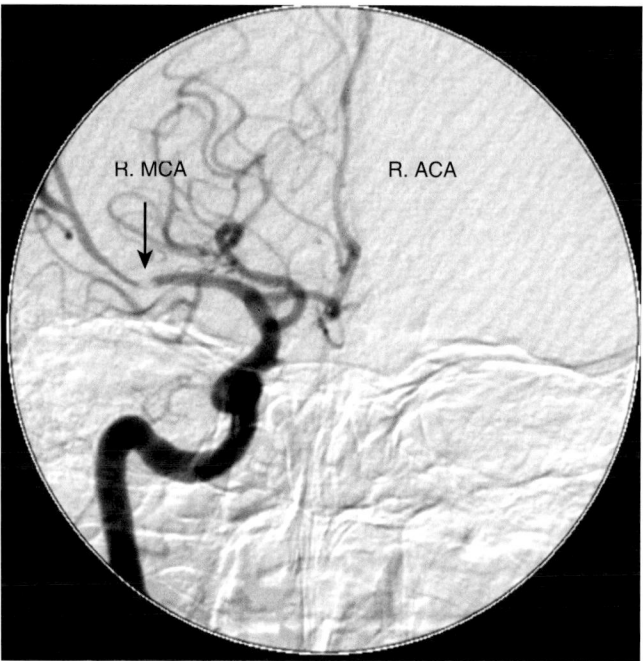

Fig. 47.2 Intracranial administration of 2 mg of recombinant tissue-type plasminogen activator produced partial recanalization *(arrow)* of the right middle cerebral artery *(R. MCA)*. *R. ACA*, Right anterior cerebral artery.

The use of mechanical thrombectomy added no additional risk of ICH over standard management with IV tPA. The risk for ICH in both the interventional and control arms ranged from 0% to 7%. The fact that mechanical thrombectomy in all trials carried no higher bleeding risk compared with IV tPA demonstrates that thrombectomy is safe and that any bleeding risk is caused mainly by thrombolysis. Although mechanical thrombectomy is associated with higher costs, it also resulted in improved patient outcomes. From the cost-effectiveness studies, mechanical thrombectomy seems to be good value for money when a threshold of $50,000 per quality-adjusted life year gained is adopted.[23]

Neuroprotection

Although many drugs and devices are under investigation to prolong the life of the penumbra, maintain the blood-brain barrier, and reduce hemorrhage and reperfusion injury, none has been proven effective in humans. The latest AHA/ASA Guidelines for the Early Management of Adults With Ischemic Stroke, published in 2007, conclude that "no intervention with putative neuroprotective actions has been established as effective in improving outcomes after stroke, and therefore none currently can be recommended," assigning neuroprotection a class III (do not do) recommendation in the guidelines.[2,24]

Despite this pessimism, there has been enthusiasm for therapeutic hypothermia as an emerging therapy for stroke. Hypothermia provides neuroprotection by decreasing cellular metabolism, limiting cytotoxicity, reducing the formation of free radicals, and preventing breakdown of the blood-brain barrier. Mechanisms of cooling include invasive central venous catheters and surface methods. Many data support the neuroprotective effects of hypothermia in animal models, but the utility of induced hypothermia in the treatment of patients with ischemic stroke is not well established and further trials are needed. A more recent meta-analysis showed that the latest

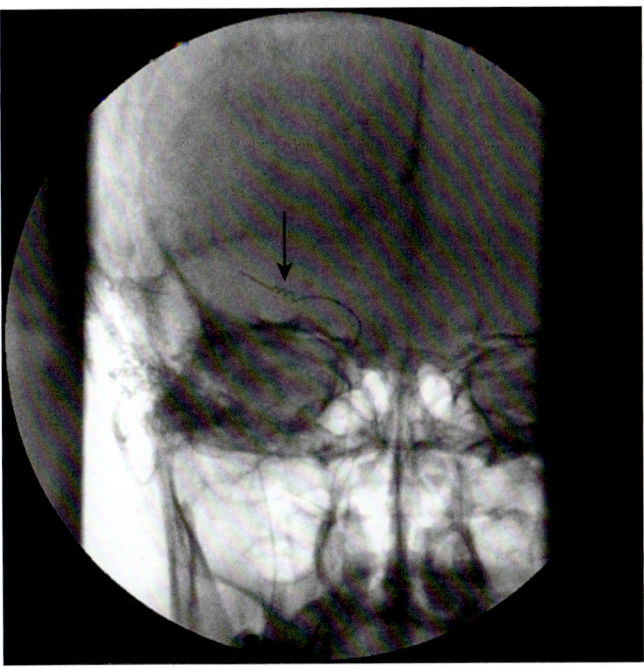

Fig. 47.3 Placement of the MERCI thrombectomy catheter *(arrow)* in the right middle cerebral artery.

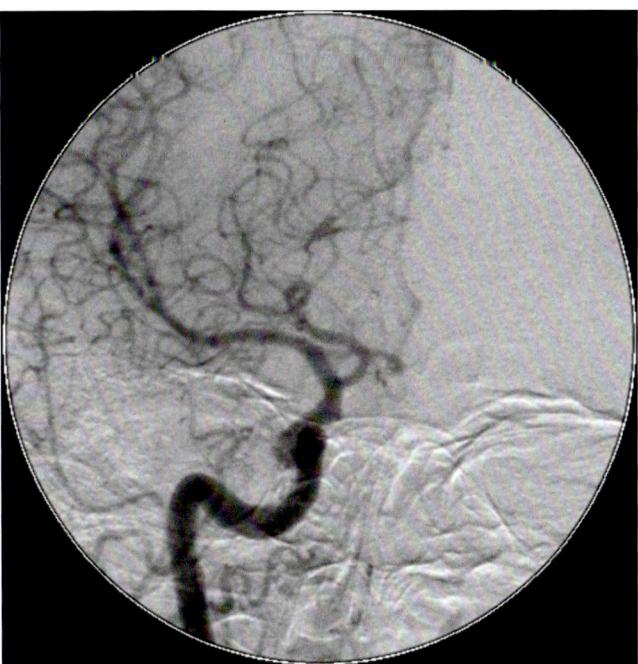

Fig. 47.5 Result after recanalization of the right middle cerebral artery.

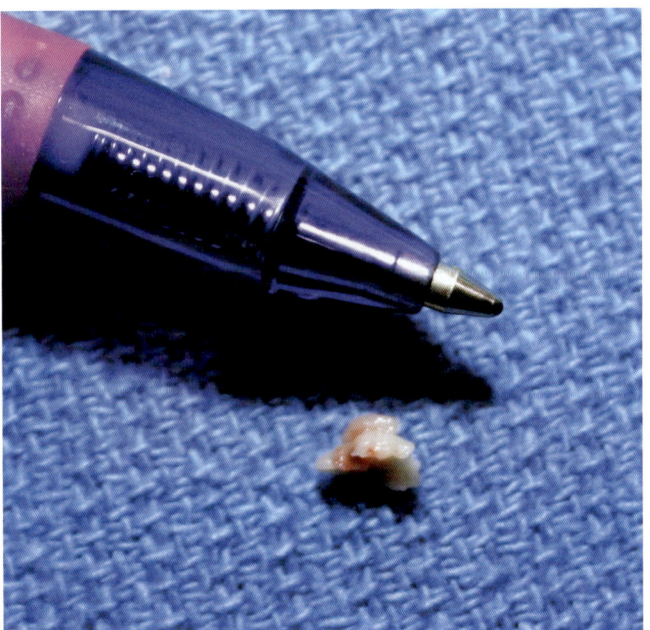

Fig. 47.4 **Retrieval of fibrous clot with the MERCI device.** The imprint from the left atrial appendage can be seen.

preclinical data are of higher quality than previous reports, and the data continue to support consideration of therapeutic hypothermia for cerebral ischemia in larger clinical trials of acute ischemic stroke.[25]

STROKE CENTERS

Stroke centers are a key component of building a successful stroke program. The concept of stroke centers was outlined by the Brain Attack Coalition (BAC) in 2000.[26] Stroke centers are modeled after streamlined trauma care and the treatment of acute myocardial infarction in that they require the most rapid possible identification and triage of patients in order to provide the most timely treatment.

This systems-based approach requires community-wide coordination and planning. It includes empowering ambulances to bypass hospitals and bring stroke patients to facilities with specialized treatment capabilities. Certified primary stroke centers provide basic acute stroke care, including the initial assessment and treatment of stroke patients by stroke teams, stroke units, and 24-hour access to CT scans. Comprehensive stroke centers are intended for complicated or high-risk stroke patients and offer specialized stroke personnel, including specialized neurologic intensive care units; advanced neuroimaging capabilities; on-demand neurosurgical and endovascular interventional capabilities; and the infrastructure to support these activities.[27]

The comprehensive stroke center has an endovascular specialist and neurosurgeon available at all times for consultation and immediate procedural support, including aneurysm clipping, placement of a ventriculostomy device or intracranial pressure transducer, and percutaneous catheter-based therapy for stroke. Dedicated stroke units enable close monitoring of stroke patients by providers who are accustomed to treating stroke patients and familiar with their unique needs. Part of the infrastructure includes rigorous data collection and outcomes assessment to advance the field of stroke care. Community education regarding stroke risk factors and recognition and ambulance bypass systems are crucial components in building successful stroke treatment centers.

THE ROLE OF CARDIOLOGY IN A STROKE PROGRAM

There are similarities in the treatment of acute stroke and acute myocardial infarction. Both emphasize achieving early reperfusion, which is driven by early patient recognition of symptoms, early hospital admission, and early initiation of treatment. However, there are also significant differences. For example, stroke thrombi usually have an embolic origin, making them

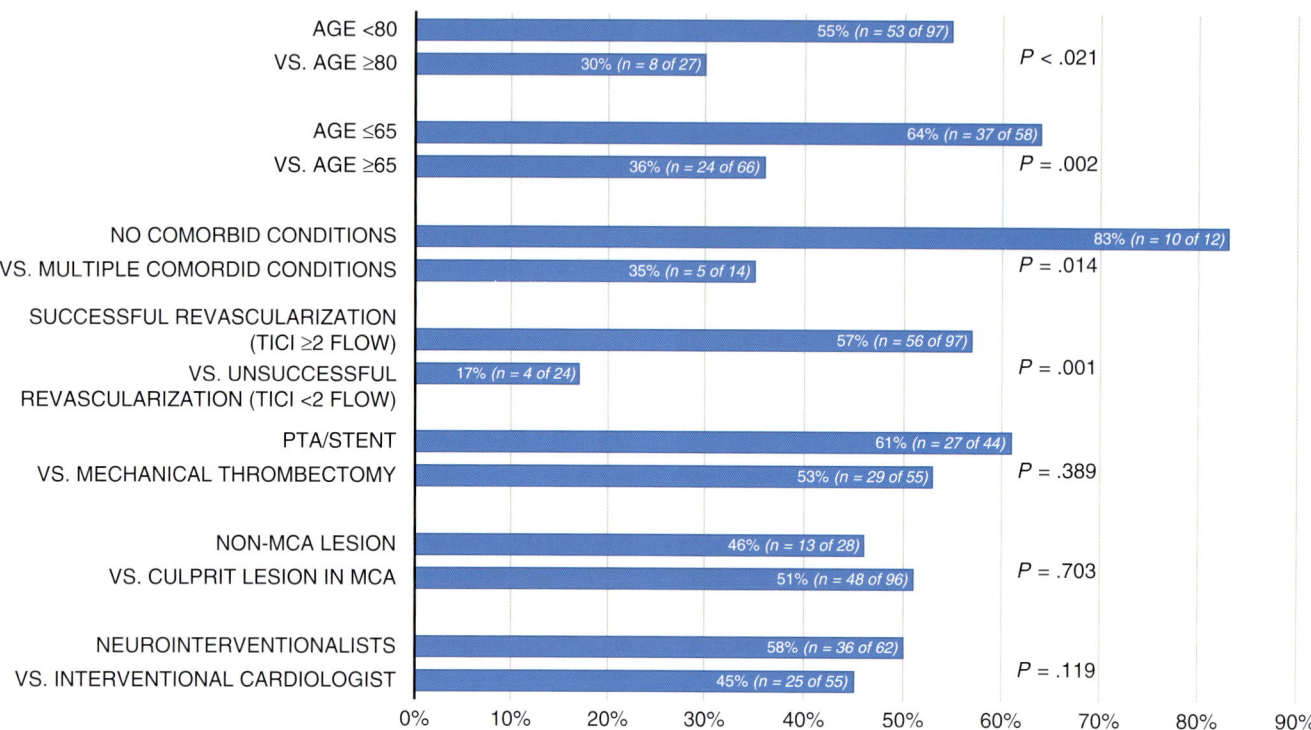

Fig. 47.6 Primary outcome data with clinical variables are listed on the left y axis. Bar graphs are those with good clinical outcome (mRS ≤2), presented as a percentage of those observed within that specific group of patients. P values are listed for each comparison. *MCA,* middle cerebral artery; *PTA,* percutaneous transluminal angioplasty; *TICI,* thrombolysis in cerebral infarction. (Reprinted with permission from Htyte N, Parto P, Ragbir S, et al. Predictors of outcomes following catheter-based therapy for acute stroke. *Catheter Cardiovasc Interv.* 2015;85:1043–1050, fig. 1.)

older, more organized, and more resistant to lysis. The volume of clot is larger in stroke patients, and the tortuosity of cerebral vessels can make clot-busting therapy more difficult than the treatment of acute myocardial infarction.

My colleagues and I have reported our experience with a multidisciplinary team that included interventional cardiologists and provided emergent endovascular therapy for patients with acute ischemic stroke who were ineligible for intravenous thrombolysis.[28,29] A stroke neurologist in consultation with the interventional cardiologist and neuroradiologist is initially called to assess the patient and determine the need for intervention. We considered stroke patients eligible for intervention if they were less than 8 hours from symptom onset. No specific cutoff or lower limit was used for their National Institutes of Health Stroke Scale (NIHSS) score to exclude patients from intervention. Instead, patients were eligible if they had a serious deficit, even if the corresponding NIHSS score was comparatively low (e.g., monocular blindness).

In reviewing the most recent 124 consecutive stroke patients treated with catheter-based therapy, we found that successful revascularization led to good neurologic outcomes for selected patients. Medical comorbidities and higher age (>65 years) contributed to poor outcomes for stroke patients despite successful recanalization. We compared procedures performed by neurovascular specialists versus cardiovascular specialists and found no differences in outcomes (Figs. 47.6 and 47.7).[30]

The most important problem facing stroke therapy is a lack of on-demand interventional therapy for most patients who are not candidates for lysis. Unlike the national standard of care for heart attacks, for which an army of interventional cardiologists have been mobilized behind a national effort to minimize door-to-balloon time for early reperfusion, endovascular therapy for stroke is uncommon because of the scarcity of neurointerventional physicians to provide this service around the clock in most communities.[9] Relatively few neuroradiologists are available to provide coverage at all times in every hospital that accepts stroke patients for treatment. One way to expand this service would be to take advantage of the army of specialists available from interventional cardiology.[31,32]

Interventional cardiologists are currently providing around-the-clock interventional treatment for acute myocardial infarction. With training and the formation of a multidisciplinary stroke treatment group including neurology, radiology, and surgical specialties, the treatment capabilities that are so badly needed in many communities could be extended. Many interventional cardiologists are currently performing carotid stent placement and intracerebral angiography. It is a reasonable and achievable step to enable competent carotid interventionalists who have cerebral angiography experience to perform acute stroke intervention (Table 47.6).

Interventional cardiologists are poised to join the stroke team to aid in the significant manpower shortage in treating acute stroke. As skilled angiographers, experienced interventionalists, and productive members of a multidisciplinary team, they can meet the challenge of providing on-demand rapid reperfusion therapy for this devastating disease.[33]

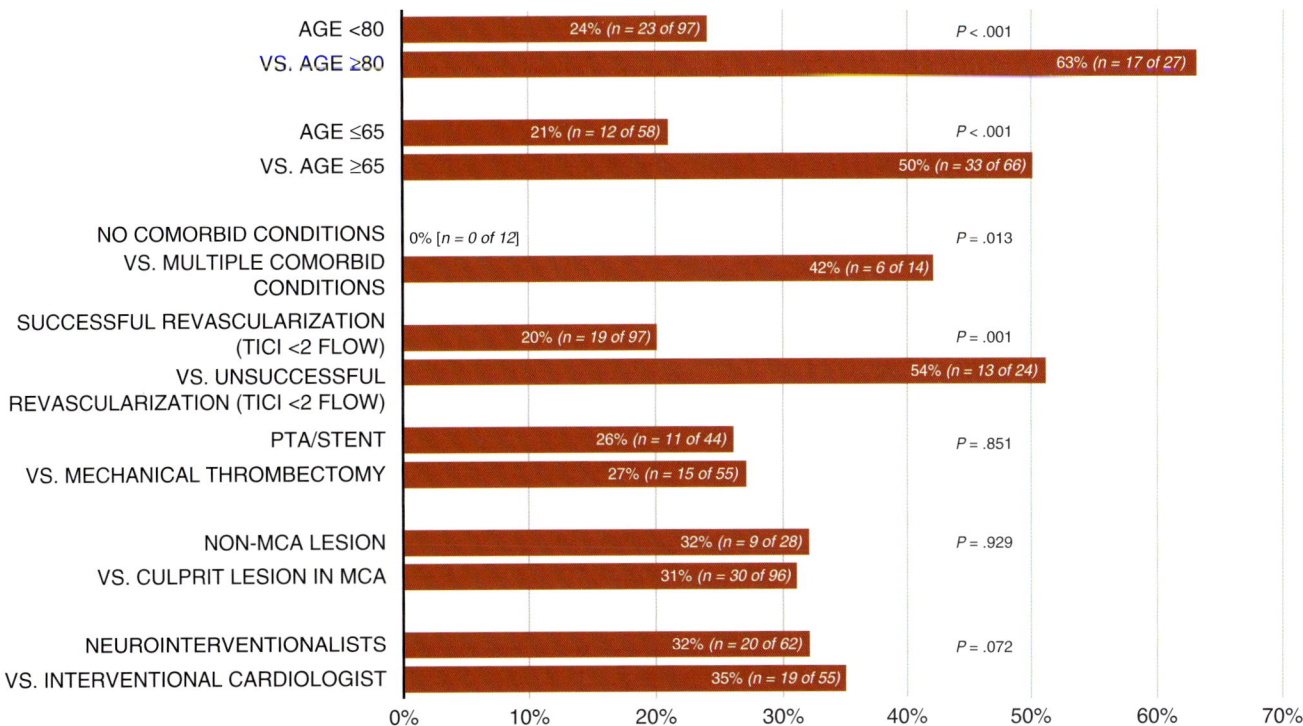

Fig. 47.7 This bar graph shows 30-day mortality data looking at the same variables from primary outcome data in this study. Clinical variables are listed on left y axis. Bar graphs are those with 30-day mortality presented as a percentage of those observed within that specific group of patients. P values are listed for each comparison. (Reprinted with permission from Htyte N, Parto P, Ragbir S, et al. Predictors of outcomes following catheter-based therapy for acute stroke. *Catheter Cardiovasc Interv.* 2015;85:1043–1050, fig. 2.)

TABLE 47.6 Strengths and Weaknesses of Cardiologists on the Stroke Intervention Team

STRENGTHS

Excellent catheter skills

Experience with carotid stent placement and cerebral angiography

Management of atherosclerotic risk factors for stroke

Rapid response 24/7 to assist and relieve interventional neuroradiology

Management of coexisting cardiac disease (e.g., atrial fibrillation)

Weaknesses

Limited knowledge of

   Cerebral anatomy

   Computed tomography and magnetic resonance imaging interpretation

   Localization of deficit

   National Institutes of Health Stroke Scale and neurologic examination

   Management of stroke complications (e.g., intracranial hemorrhage)

KEY REFERENCES

9. Suzuki S, Saver JL, Scott P, et al. Access to intra-arterial therapies for acute ischemic stroke: an analysis of the US population. *AJNR Am J Neuroradiol.* 2004;25:1802–1806.
10. Clott HJ, Rabinstein A, Lanzino G, et al. Intra-arterial stroke therapy: an assessment of demand and available work force. *AJNR Am J Neuroradiol.* 2009;30:453–458.
12. Hacke W, Donnan G, Fieschi C, et al. Association of outcome with early stroke treatment: pooled analysis of ATLANTIS, ECASS, and NINDS rt-PA stroke trials. *Lancet.* 2004;363:768–774.
18. Berkhemer OA, Fransen PS, Beumer D, et al. A randomized trial of intraarterial treatment for acute ischemic stroke. *N Engl J Med.* 2015;372:11–20.
19. Campbell BC, Mitchell PJ, Kleinig TJ, et al. Endovascular therapy for ischemic stroke with perfusion-imaging selection. *N Engl J Med.* 2015;372:1009–1018.
20. Goyal M, Demchuk AM, Menon BK, et al. Randomized assessment of rapid endovascular treatment of ischemic stroke. *N Engl J Med.* 2015;372:1019–1030.
21. Saver JL, Goyal M, Bonafe A, et al. Stent-retriever thrombectomy after intravenous t-PA vs. t-PA alone in stroke. *N Engl J Med.* 2015;372:2285–2295.
22. Jovin TG, Chamorro A, Cobo E, et al. Thrombectomy within 8 hours after symptom onset in ischemic stroke. *N Engl J Med.* 2015;372:2296–2306.
30. Htyte N, Parto P, Ragbir S, et al. Predictors of outcomes following catheter-based therapy for acute stroke. *Catheter Cardiovasc Interv.* 2015;85:1043–1050.
33. Hopkins LN, Holmes Jr DR. Public health urgency created by the success of mechanical thrombectomy studies in stroke. *Circulation.* 2017;135:1188–1190.

Additional references available online at expertconsult.com.

SECTION V
第五部分

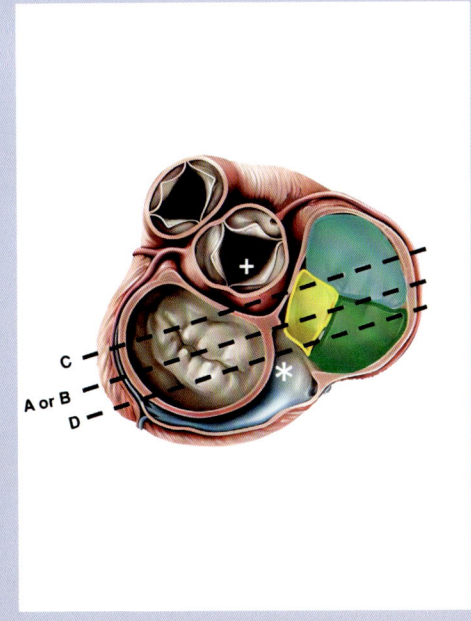

Structural Interventions
结构性心脏病介入治疗

中文导读

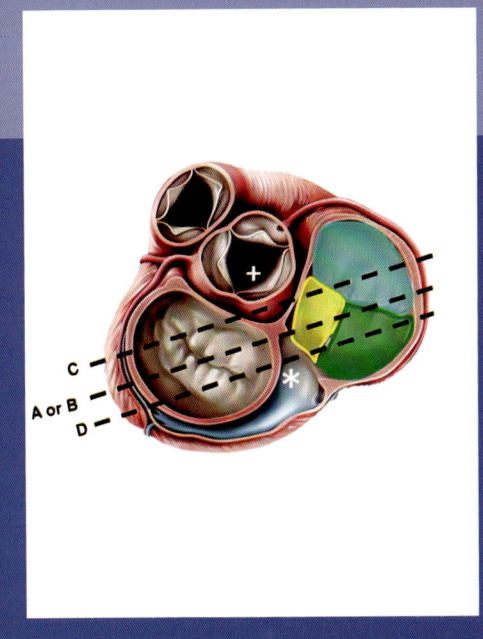

第48章
心腔内介入手术的影像学评估

　　随着介入影像学技术的日益成熟，结构性心脏病介入手术的开展取得了重大的突破。多模态影像学成像是结构性心脏病医师的另一双"眼睛"。目前众多影像学评估被用于结构性心脏病的手术干预，如超声心动图技术、CT、荧光透视技术及心脏MRI。本章详细阐述了在介入手术操作中常规使用的影像学技术。

　　围绕影像学评估这一主题，本章节对现有成像技术做了概括性介绍，包括经胸超声心动图技术、经食道超声心动图技术、荧光透视技术（左心房造影技术，左心室造影技术，主动脉造影技术，右心室造影技术，肺血管造影技术）和CT。此外，本章重点介绍了常见疾病和术式的影像学评估，如房间隔穿刺、卵圆孔未闭、继发性房间隔缺损、左心耳封堵、经皮二尖瓣修复、主动脉瓣/肺动脉瓣修复、经皮主动脉瓣/二尖瓣置换、机械瓣与生物瓣和瓣周漏封堵术。影像学成像的选择是基于手术干预类型、团队经验、术者的熟悉程度、操作能力及医疗财政的支出。随着结构性心脏病手术的日益复杂，CT、MRI和混合成像技术的快速发展和支付能力的提升，高质量的实时多模态成像正成为介入手术的必要环节。

李子昂　张洪亮

章节要点

- 开展结构性心脏病手术需要多模态影像学技术的辅助,包括荧光透视检查和超声心动图检查,以及CT和心脏MRI。
- 多模态影像学技术的功能是相互补充的。在手术过程中,荧光透视技术可以实时成像,超声心动图技术可以探查瓣膜结构。
- 荧光透视技术可以将三维解剖学结构转换为二维平面结构。因此,需要多次投影来准确定位三维空间中的解剖学结构。
- 超声心动图对手术指导至关重要,可实现瓣膜结构可视化,以及对手术器械的引导。
- 超声心动图技术通常用于指导间隔手术(卵圆孔未闭和房间隔缺损闭合)、左心耳封堵术和二尖瓣介入术,也常规应用于经导管瓣膜置入术和瓣周漏封堵术。
- CT提供了三维空间解剖结构,这对手术计划的制定和手术器材的选择至关重要,可能会引领介入手术影像技术的变革。
- 荧光透视检查、CT和超声心动图检查等影像学辅助技术的应用对于结构性心脏病的手术开展至关重要。

SECTION V Structural Interventions

48 Imaging for Intracardiac Interventions

Nyal Borges, Serge C. Harb, Samir R. Kapadia

KEY POINTS

- Structural heart disease interventions rely on multimodality imaging, including fluoroscopy and echocardiography (intracardiac, transthoracic, or transesophageal) during the procedure, and computed tomography and cardiac magnetic resonance for procedural planning.
- These modalities are complimentary. During the procedure, fluoroscopy allows real-time imaging of radio opaque devices, while intraprocedural ultrasound is ideal for soft tissue visualization including valvular structures.
- Fluoroscopy projects three-dimensional anatomy in two dimensions. Therefore, multiple projections (commonly biplane imaging) are needed to precisely locate devices and structures in three-dimensional space.
- Three-dimensional and biplane echocardiography are critical for procedural guidance, allowing optimal visualization of valvular structures, and catheter and device guidance.
- Ultrasound-based imaging using intracardiac (ICE) or transesophageal echocardiography (TEE) are typically used to guide septal interventions (trans-septal puncture, patent foramen ovale, and atrial septal defect closures), left atrial appendage closure, and mitral valve interventions. They are also routinely used during transcatheter valve implantations and for paravalvular leak closure.
- Computed tomography provides three-dimensional data that is important for candidate selection, procedural planning, and device sizing. The advent of has the potential to revolutionize procedural imaging.
- Integration of fluoroscopic, computed tomographic, and echocardiographic images in the catheterization laboratory is critical for the success of structural heart interventions.

FLUOROSCOPY AND ANGIOGRAPHY

Left-Sided Structures

Left Atrial Angiogram

Left atrial (LA) angiogram is rarely performed by direct injection, but the LA is frequently seen on the levophase of the right-sided angiogram or ventriculogram. Direct injection in the left atrial appendage (LAA) is performed to evaluate the anatomy prior to percutaneous closer (Fig. 48.1). Typically the right anterior oblique (RAO) cranial view shows the LAA opening in the medial-lateral diameter, and RAO caudal view delineates the superior-inferior opening diameter (see Fig. 48.1). These views are also important to study the shape of the LAA for percutaneous closure planning, as certain shapes are more amenable to percutaneous closure.[1]

Left Ventriculogram

The left ventricle is typically divided into inflow and outflow segments.[2] The inflow consists of the mitral valve apparatus, and the outflow portion includes the apex, left ventricular outflow tract (LVOT), and the aortic valve, as seen in Fig. 48.2. The angle between the inflow and outflow tract is around 30 degrees in young patients and increases with "unfolding of aorta." Since the interventricular septum maintains its position while the aorta is transposed anteriorly and more horizontally, there can be "bulging" of the septum.

Left ventriculogram is typically performed in the RAO projection 30 degrees; however, different views should be considered, depending on the purpose of the procedure. The RAO projection delineates the separation of atria from ventricles. Various structures seen on the RAO projection are delineated in Fig. 48.2. Anterior and inferior walls as well as the apex are seen without overlap in this view. The lateral wall and septum are overlapped, and their motion is perpendicular to the x-ray beam. Anterior and posterior mitral valve leaflets are seen from the side in a longitudinal plane, along with the inflow portion of the ventricle. This relationship is critical to recognize when performing mitral valve intervention when devices have to be advanced coaxially in the inflow (e.g., Inoue balloon or MitraClip). In this view, the anterior and posterior leaflets of the mitral valve are foreshortened. The anterolateral and posteromedial commissures are superiorly and inferiorly positioned, as shown in Fig. 48.2. The aortic valve and the coronary sinuses can be appreciated in this view. The right coronary sinus and the noncoronary sinus are located on the right and left side of the aortic root. The left coronary sinus is located between the right and the noncoronary sinus. In this view, the ostia of the right and left main coronary arteries appear close to one another, and this view is useful for anterior-posterior (AP) localization of either coronary artery within the aortic root.

The anatomical structures seen in the left anterior oblique (LAO) view are outlined in Fig. 48.3. The LAO projection delineates the interventricular groove and separates the right ventricle from the left ventricle. In order to align the mitral inflow to the apex of the ventricle, some caudal angulation can be added to the LAO projection. This allows one to see the left ventricle in end-on projection, where papillary muscles as well as anterior and posterior leaflets can be clearly identified. Note that the inflow and outflow of the ventricle are typically well separated in this view. The left and the right coronary sinuses and coronary ostia are separated clearly, and the noncoronary sinus is overlapped with the right coronary cusp (RCC; albeit located lower in the aortic root).

Unconventional views allow better delineation of certain parts of the left ventricle. The LAO cranial projection is typically better to assess LVOT. The purpose of this projection is to see the anterior leaflet of mitral valve in a longitudinal view when it does not overlap with the interventricular septum. It is also the view of choice to see the interventricular septum in the muscular portion for assessment of ventricular septal defect (VSD). The LAO caudal projection allows one to see the mitral valve end-on, and can place the anterolateral and posteromedial commissures in the context of the bifurcation of left main into the left anterior descending artery and left circumflex artery, respectively.

SECTION V Structural Interventions

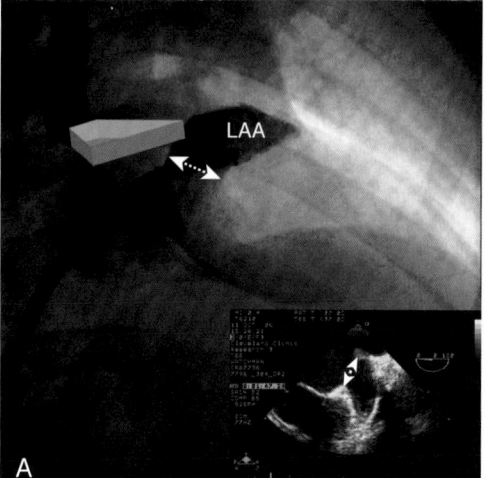
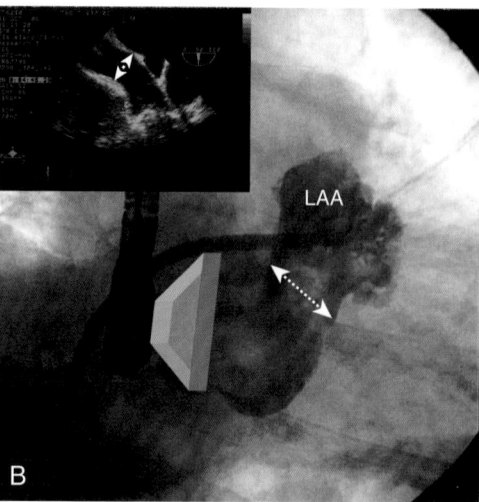

Fig. 48.1 (A) Shows right anterior oblique (RAO) cranial view of left atrial appendage *(LAA)* injection. The "width" of the LAA opening is shown *(dotted arrows)*, which is also depicted by horizontal view in transesophageal echocardiography (TEE) *(inset)*. (B) Shows RAO caudal view of the LAA in the same subject, showing the "height" of the opening *(dotted arrows)*, which corresponds to a vertical view by TEE *(inset)*.

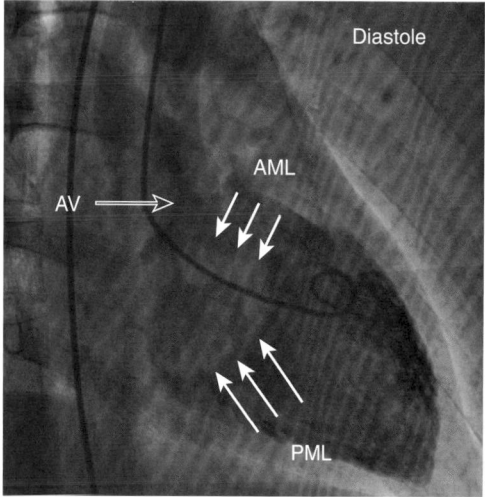
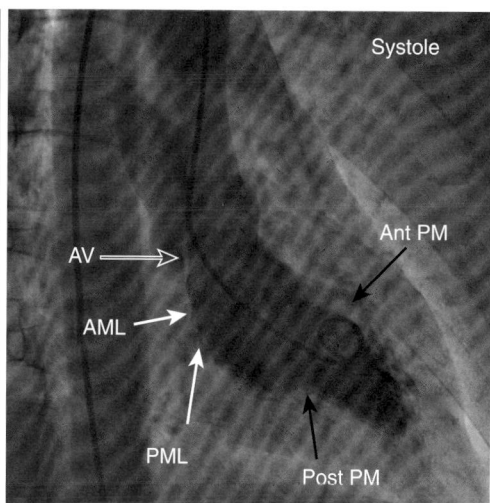

Fig. 48.2 Right anterior oblique 30-degree view of the left ventricle in diastole and systole. The aortic valve *(open arrow)*, mitral valve *(solid white arrows)*, and the papillary muscles *(solid black arrows)* are shown. In diastole, mitral valve is open and there is clearance of contrast as the blood enters the left ventricle from left atrium. Anterior and posterior leaflets are seen separate in diastole *(left panel)*. In systole, the mitral valve is closed and the aortic valve is open *(right panel)*. In this view, anterior, apex, and the inferior walls can be assessed. *AML*, Anterior mitral leaflet; *Ant PM*, anterolateral papillary muscle; *AV*, aortic valve; *PML*, posterior mitral leaflet; *Post PM*, posterolateral papillary muscle.

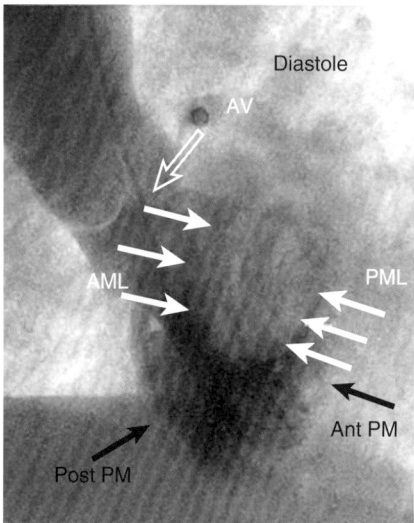
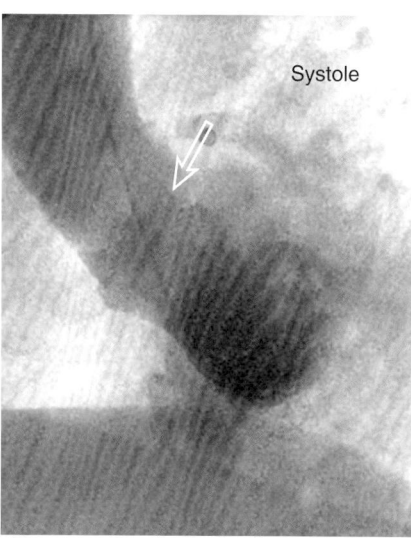

Fig. 48.3 Left anterior oblique 60-degree view of the left ventricle in diastole and systole. The aortic valve *(open arrow)*, mitral valve *(solid white arrows)*, and the papillary muscles *(solid black arrows)* are shown. In diastole, the mitral valve is open and there is clearance of contrast as the blood without contrast enters the left ventricle from left atrium. Anterior and posterior leaflets are seen separate in diastole *(left panel)*. In this view, lateral and the septal walls can be assessed. *AML*, Anterior mitral leaflet; *Ant PM*, anterolateral papillary muscle; *AV*, aortic valve; *PML*, posterior mitral leaflet; *Post PM*, posterolateral papillary muscle.

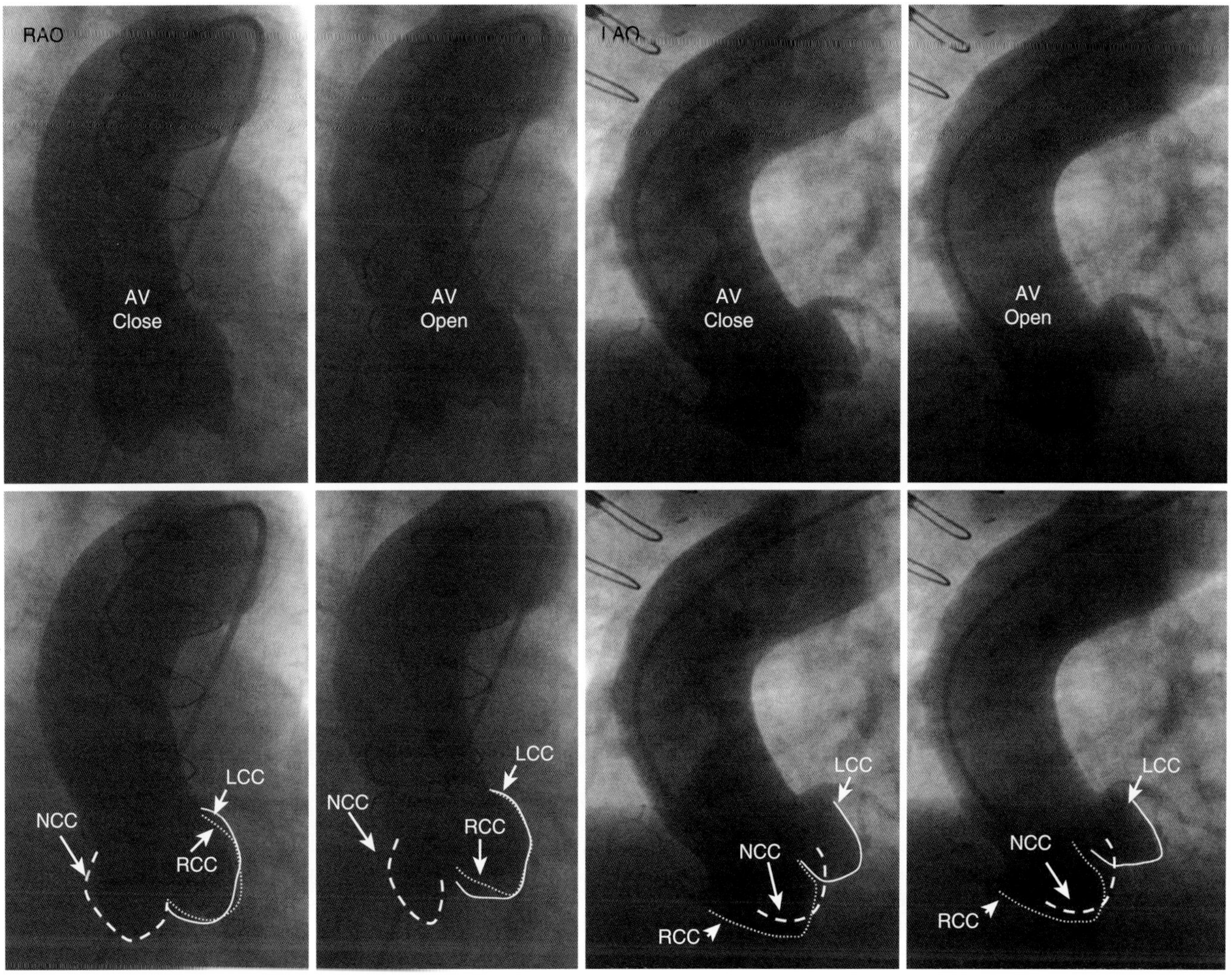

Fig. 48.4 Shallow right anterior oblique *(RAO)* and left anterior oblique *(LAO)* aortograms in a subject with aortic stenosis and restricted leaflet motion are shown. Different structures are delineated by *dashed lines* and *arrows* in the bottom panel. For each view, the aortic valve in the closed and open position is shown. Note the overlap of the left and right coronary cusps in the RAO projection and the right and noncoronary cusps in the LAO projection. *AV*, Aortic valve; *LCC*, left coronary cusp; *NCC*, noncoronary cusp; *RCC*, right coronary cusp.

Aortogram

Ascending aortogram is used to examine the aortic valve and root and can be of diagnostic utility with aortic aneurysms, aortic valve insufficiency, and rarely aortic dissection. Aortogram is performed in the RAO (30 degrees) and LAO (40 degrees) projections. Rapid injection (20 mL/s for 2 to 3 seconds) using an assist device and proper catheter positioning allows for the assessment of different aortic cusps. Aortogram is usually performed with a multi-side-hole pigtail catheter positioned just 2 to 3 cm above the sinus of Valsalva (Fig. 48.4). The grading of aortic regurgitation can be made by comparing the degree of opacification of the left ventricle to the aorta two cardiac cycles after contrast injection, as well as evaluating for delayed contrast clearance within the ventricle. Rapid, dense opacification of the ventricle to a greater density than the aorta and delayed contrast clearance indicate significant severe aortic insufficiency. It is critical to assess the aortogram in both the LAO and RAO projections because opacification in the LAO projection is exaggerated due to left ventricle (LV) foreshortening. Information regarding the severity of aortic regurgitation from aortography should be correlated with hemodynamic tracings of LV end systolic pressure, rate of rise of LV diastolic pressures, and the LV end diastolic pressure value itself to increase diagnostic accuracy.[3]

Right Sided Structures

Right atrial angiogram is typically performed to look at the interatrial septum (IAS). A pigtail catheter, Berman angiographic catheter, or National Institutes of Health (NIH) catheter with rapid injection rate is used. Various anatomical relationships are important to recognize on fluoroscopy, including relation of noncoronary cusp (NCC) to IAS for transseptal puncture, superior vena cava (SVC) for intracardiac echocardiography (ICE) imaging, and anterior leaflet of the mitral valve for antegrade interventions. These relationships are well demonstrated in a anteroposterior (AP) view on right atrial angiogram (Fig. 48.5). This procedure can be used to guide transseptal puncture, patent foreman ovale (PFO), and atrial septal defect (ASD) closures.

Right Ventriculogram

Right ventricle is usually heavily trabeculated with the inflow and outflow tract at the right angles to each other. Most typically, right ventriculogram is performed in AP and lateral projection with the catheter positioned in midcavity to prevent ventricular ectopy. A pigtail catheter, Berman angiographic catheter, or NIH

SECTION V Structural Interventions

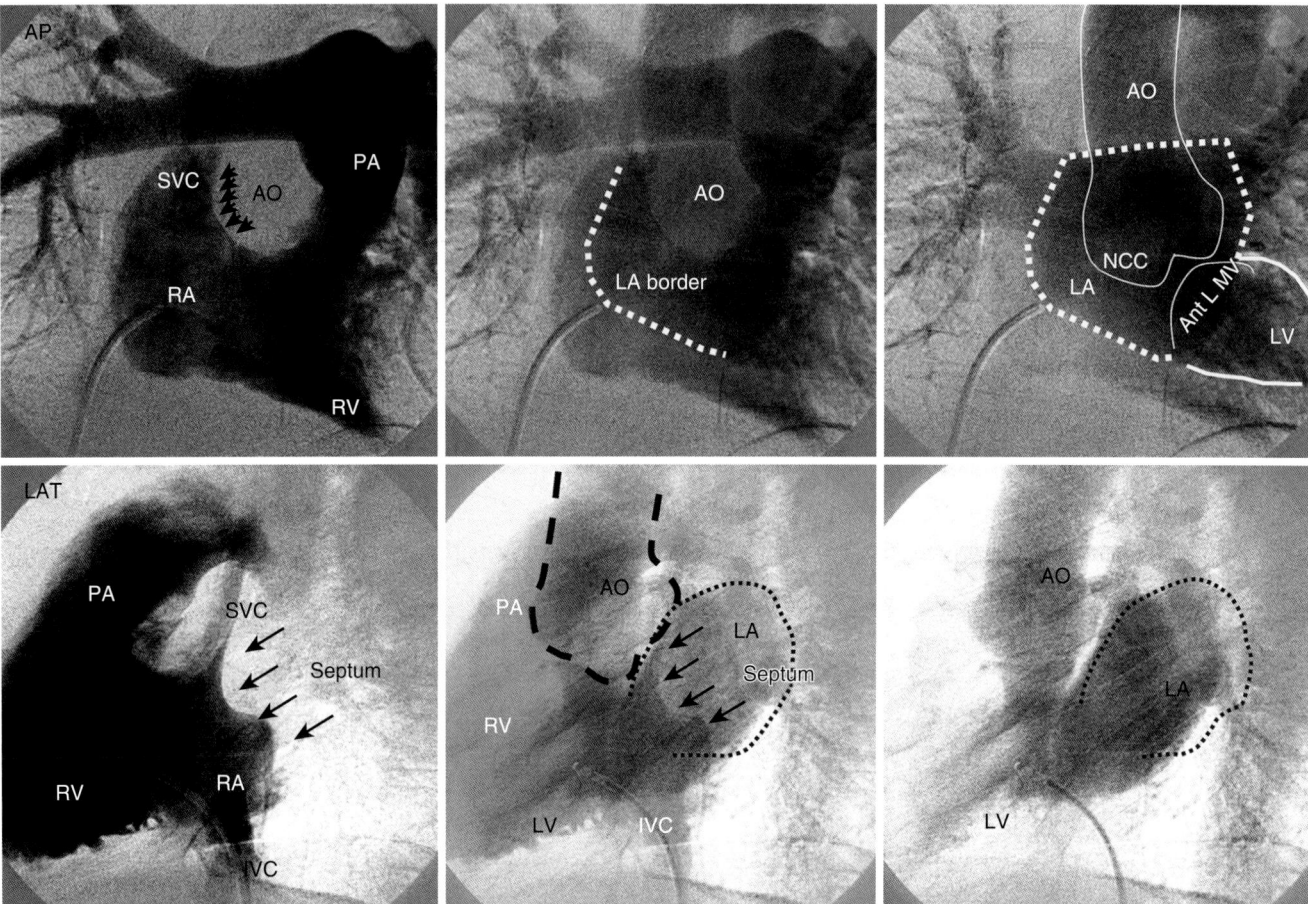

Fig. 48.5 Anteroposterior *(AP; top panel)* and lateral *(LAT; bottom panel)* view of a right atrial angiogram is shown. Dextro phase *(left panel)*, levo phase *(right panel)*, and two phases superimposed on each other *(middle panel)* are presented. *antL MV*, Anterior leaflet of the mitral valve; *AO*, aorta; *IVC*, inferior vena cava; *LA*, left atrium; *LV*, left ventricle; *NCC*, noncoronary cusp; *PA*, pulmonary artery, *RA*, right atrium, *RV*, right ventricle, *SVC*, superior vena cava.

catheter can be used to perform a right ventriculogram. Rate of injection (>25 mL/s) and the volume of contrast (60 mL) administered has to be higher in order to delineate the components of the right ventricular cavity. Right ventriculogram can be used to assess the tricuspid valve, right ventricular outflow tract, pulmonary valve, pulmonary arteries, pulmonary veins, and left atrium (see Fig. 48.5).

Pulmonary Angiogram

Pulmonary angiography is the gold standard technique for diagnosing pulmonary embolism.[4] In addition, it is used to assess a variety of other conditions, such as pulmonary valve stenosis, pulmonary artery stenosis, anomalous pulmonary venous return, and pulmonary arteriovenous malformation. Frequently, pulmonary artery angiogram is performed in the AP and lateral views to visualize the LA and assess pulmonary vein drainage prior to ASD closure (Fig. 48.6). Most commonly, multi-side-hole pigtail or NIH catheters are used with high injection rates of 40 mL/s to visualize pulmonary veins. The dextro and levo phases of the injections are shown in Fig. 48.7.

TRANSESOPHAGEAL ECHOCARDIOGRAPHY

Transesophageal echocardiography (TEE) is heavily relied upon in structural interventions, including transcatheter valve repair and replacement, particularly with the advent of new techniques to intervene on the mitral and tricuspid valves, defect closures, including paravalvular leaks (PVLs); PFO, ASD, and VSD closures; and LAA occlusion devices.[5] In our experience, most patients in the catheterization laboratory can tolerate TEE placement in the supine position without endotracheal intubation. Judicious use of short-acting sedatives such as midazolam and good suction of the posterior pharynx are critical for patient comfort.

The TEE probe contains a 3- to 7.5-MHz ultrasound transducer at its tip and can be advanced to the esophagus or stomach for proper visualization of cardiac structures.[6] The tip of the probe can be anteflexed, retroflexed, or moved side to side as needed to optimize visualization of cardiac structures. The currently available TEE transducers allow for multiplane and three-dimensional imaging. The common positions for the TEE transducer are the upper and mid esophagus, and transgastric positions. Standard views include 0, 45, 60, 90, and 120 degrees, with the understanding that these angles provide rough references and need to be adapted to patient's anatomy.

The 0-degree transgastric view shows the mitral valve in short axis (Fig. 48.8). At the 45-degree midesophageal view, the aortic valve, right ventricular outflow tract, right atrium, IAS, and the left atrium can be seen (Fig. 48.9). The 60-degree midesophageal level is called the *commissural view*, since it allows visualization of both mitral valve commissures in addition to the LV and left atrium (see Fig. 48.9).

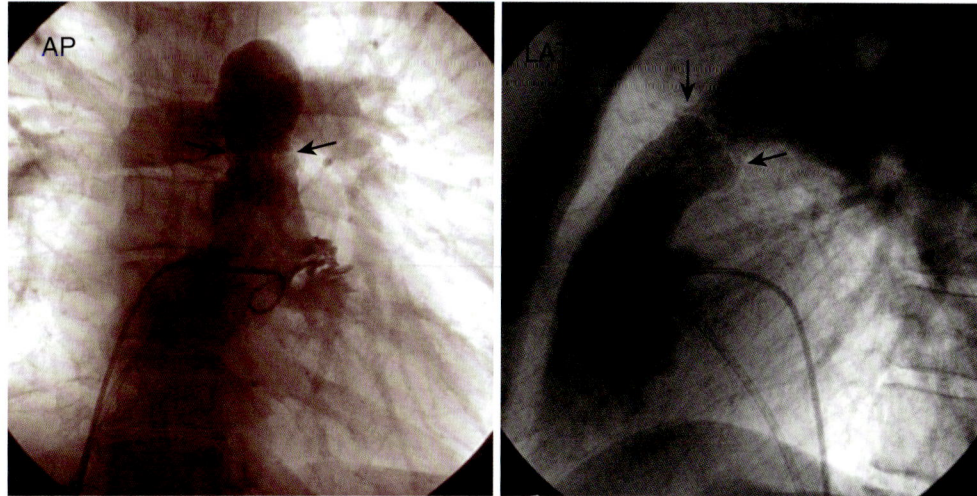

Fig. 48.6 Anteroposterior *(AP)* and lateral *(LAT)* view of the right ventricle with the pigtail catheter in the right ventricular outflow tract is shown. Note doming of the pulmonic valve as shown by the *black arrows*.

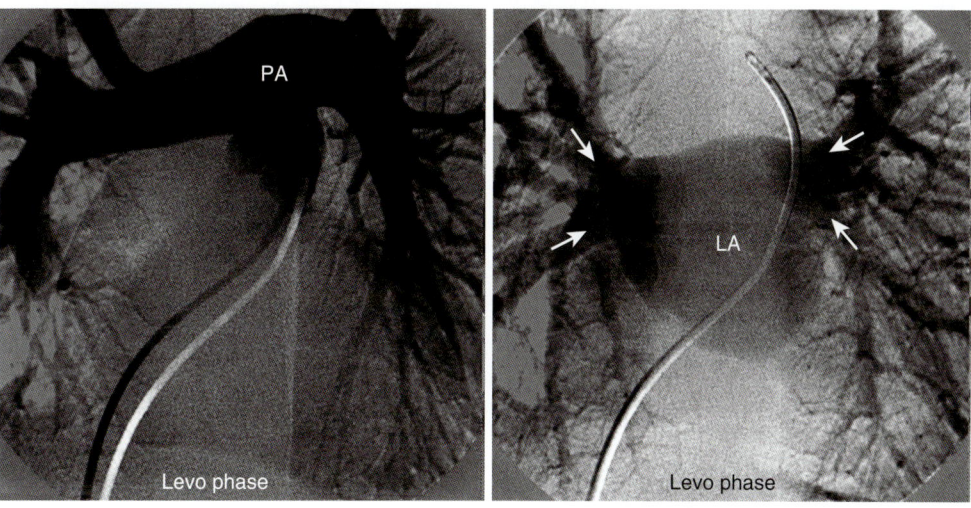

Fig. 48.7 Normal pulmonary angiogram is shown in the anteroposterior view. Large volume of dye (40 mL/s) is rapidly injected using a National Institute of Health catheter. Left panel shows the pulmonary artery trunk and the left and right pulmonary arteries and their branches. Right panel shows opacification of the left atrium in the levo phase. Digital subtraction is used to visualize the pulmonary veins *(solid white arrows)*. *LA*, Left atrium; *PA*, pulmonary artery.

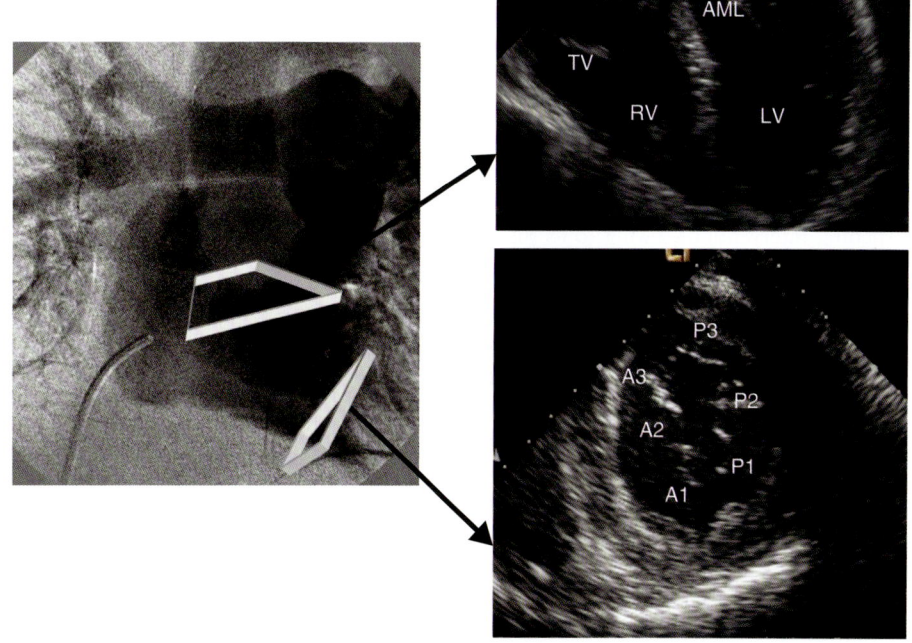

Fig. 48.8 Transesophageal echocardiography shows "0-degree" (horizontal) midesophageal and transgastric views *(right panels)*. The left panel shows the heart in anteroposterior view (refer to Fig. 48.4 for orientation). The upper right panel is the four-chamber view, and the lower right panel is a short-axis view of the mitral valve with the corresponding leaflet segments. The posterior leaflet is divided into P1 to P3 and the anterior leaflet into A1 to A3 from lateral to medial. *AML*, Anterior mitral leaflet; *LA*, left atrium; *LV*, left ventricle; *PML*, posterior mitral leaflet; *RA*, right atrium; *RV*, right ventricle; *TV*, tricuspid valve.

SECTION V Structural Interventions

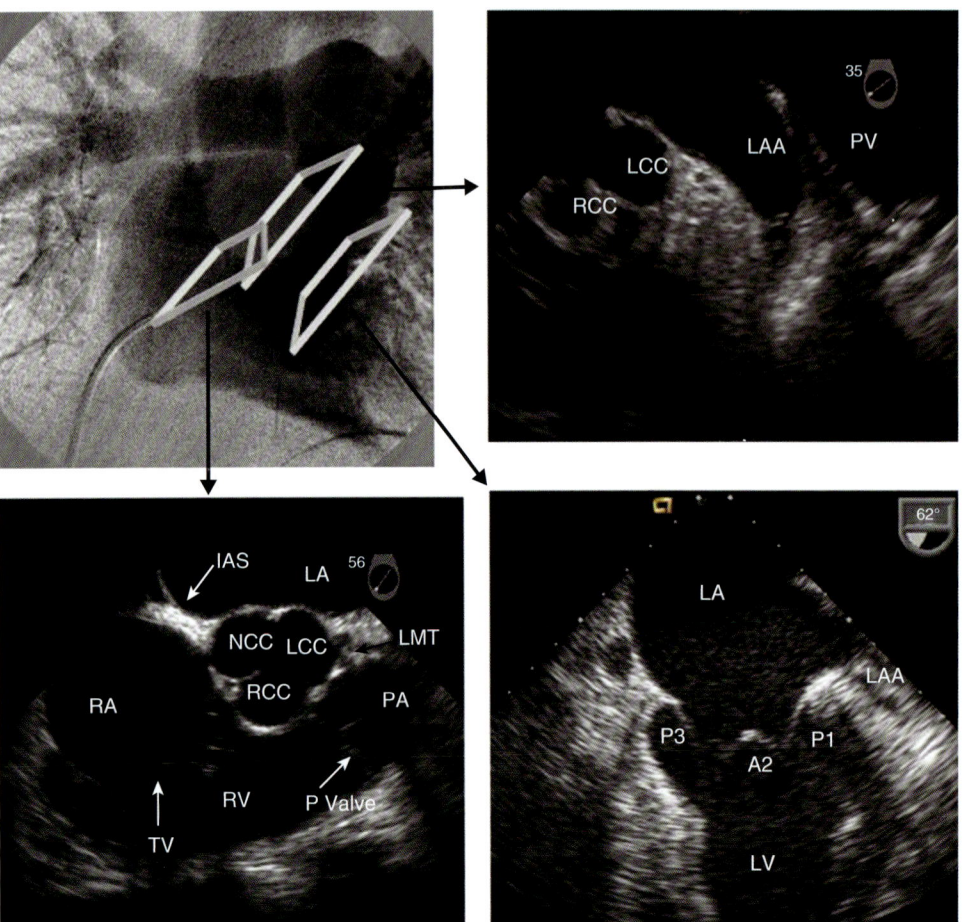

Fig. 48.9 Transesophageal echocardiography "40- to 60-degree" views in the upper to midesophagus with probe turned to the left *(right upper panel)*, upper to midesophageal junction with probe directed anteriorly *(left lower panel)*, and midesophageal commisural view *(right lower panel)*. Left panel shows the heart in anteroposterior view (refer to Fig. 48.4 for orientation). *IAS*, Interatrial septum; *LA*, left atrium; *LAA*, left atrial appendage; *LCC*, left coronary cusp; *LMT*, left main trunk; *LV*, left ventricle; *NCC*, noncoronary cusp; *PA*, pulmonary artery; *PV*, pulmonic vein; *RA*, right atrium; *RCC*, right coronary cusp; *RV*, right ventricle; *TV*, tricuspid valve.

At the 90-degree midesophageal view, the anterior and inferior LV walls, LAA, mitral valve, and coronary sinus can be visualized (Fig. 48.10). Rightward rotation with slight elevation brings in the bicaval view, where the SVC, right atrium, inferior vena cava, IAS, and left atrium can be seen (see Fig. 48.10). Leftward rotation allows the LAA to be examined for the presence of thrombus.

The 120-degree midesophageal (long-axis view) shows the left ventricle, left atrium, aortic valve, LVOT, mitral valve, and ascending aorta (Fig. 48.11). In this view, the anterior and posterior mitral leaflets are visualized. Therefore, combining the commissural and long views (via biplane imaging) allows simultaneous visualization of the anterior and posterior leaflets and the commissures, allowing precise localization of the defect and proper guidance of device deployment.

Three-dimensional TEE technology has become standard in structural interventions, owing to its superior representation of the anatomy and spatial relationships. With the introduction of the new pyramidal ultrasound beam probes, 3D images can be created in real time. The primary advantage of 3D TEE is the ability to provide real-time intraprocedural guidance and confirmation of optimal catheter and device positioning. Three-dimensional TEE can be extremely helpful in mitral valve interventions. The mitral valve surgeon's view allows visualization of both leaflets with all six scallops and both commissures in one view, which is of paramount importance in transcatheter valve repair and replacement, allowing optimal device positioning. In PVL closures, 3D TEE is essential for clear delineation of the defect location and size and to assess for any residual. This technique is also superior for device sizing and to verify optimal sealing of the LAA in LAA occlusion procedures. Three-dimensional imaging also allows simultaneous visualization of all tricuspid valve leaflets, which is very helpful in transcatheter tricuspid therapies. It is also a valuable tool for transseptal punctures and in defect (PFO, ASD, and VSD) closures.

INTRACARDIAC ECHOCARDIOGRAPHY

ICE provides excellent images of the intracardiac structures without the associated patient discomfort and airway issues that are inherent to other modalities, such as TEE.[7] In addition, in certain situations, ICE can produce a clearer, well-defined image compared to TEE. These include assessments of the posterior part of the IAS, where the TEE probe is too close to the area of interest, the pulmonary valve due to its anterior position, the aortic arch for dissection due to air shadowing from the bronchus, and in some cases, the mechanical aortic valve because of shadowing. ICE is less optimal for evaluating mitral regurgitation (MR), LAA, and LV wall motion (e.g., contrast distribution for alcohol ablation).

The two main ICE transducers systems are the mechanical/rotational and phased-array systems. The mechanical transducers typically operate at 9 MHz or higher, and produce a circular scan path perpendicular to the catheter. Mechanical catheters are imaging catheters without color or Doppler capabilities and are less useful than the phased-array systems, which allow complete evaluation that is comparable to TEE. In our catheterization laboratory, we exclusively use phased-array systems to guide structural heart disease interventions. The phased-array systems use 64 piezoelectric elements with frequencies of 5.5, 7.5, 8.5, and 10 MHz to produce a single sector scan that is perpendicular to the long axis of the catheter. The probe is available as an 8-Fr or 11-Fr catheter with

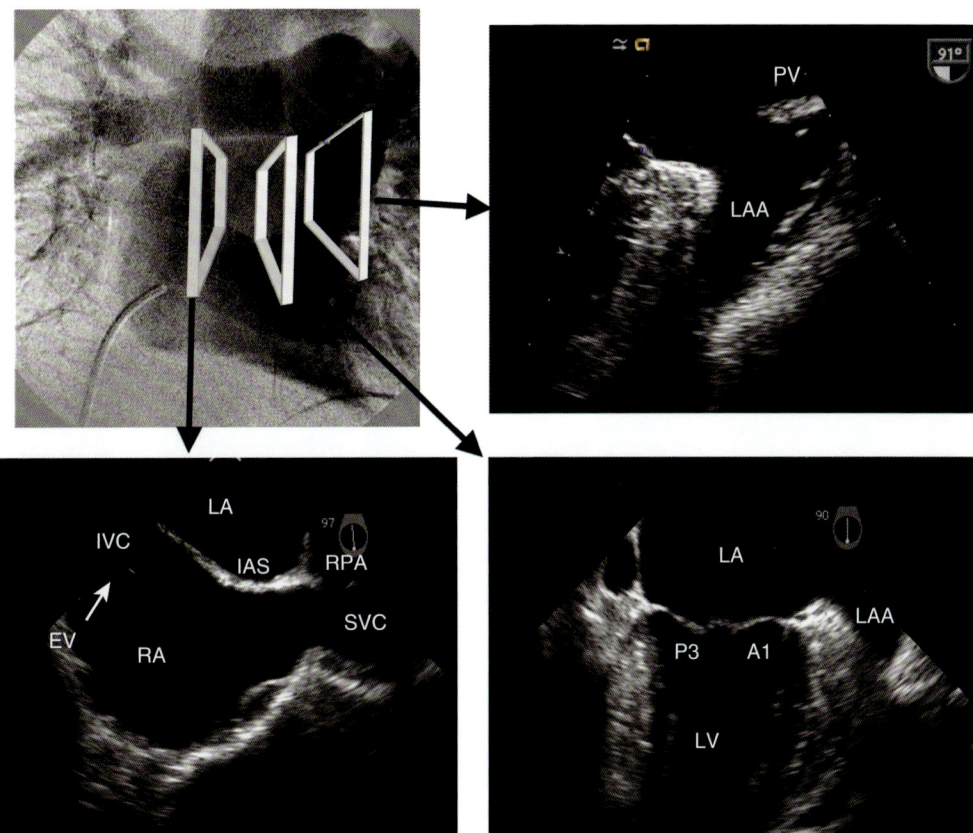

Fig. 48.10 Transesophageal echocardiography shows "90-degree" midesophageal view of the left atrial appendage *(upper right panel)*, bicaval *(lower left panel)*, and the two-chamber *(lower right panel)* views as the probe is directed from left to right. Left panel shows the heart in anteroposterior view (refer to Fig. 48.4 for orientation). *EV*, Eustachian valve; *IAS*, interatrial septum; *IVC*, inferior vena cava; *LA*, left atrium; *LAA*, left atrial appendage; *LV*, left ventricle; *PV*, pulmonic vein; *RA*, right atrium; *RPA*, right pulmonary artery; *RV*, right ventricle; *SVC*, superior vena cava.

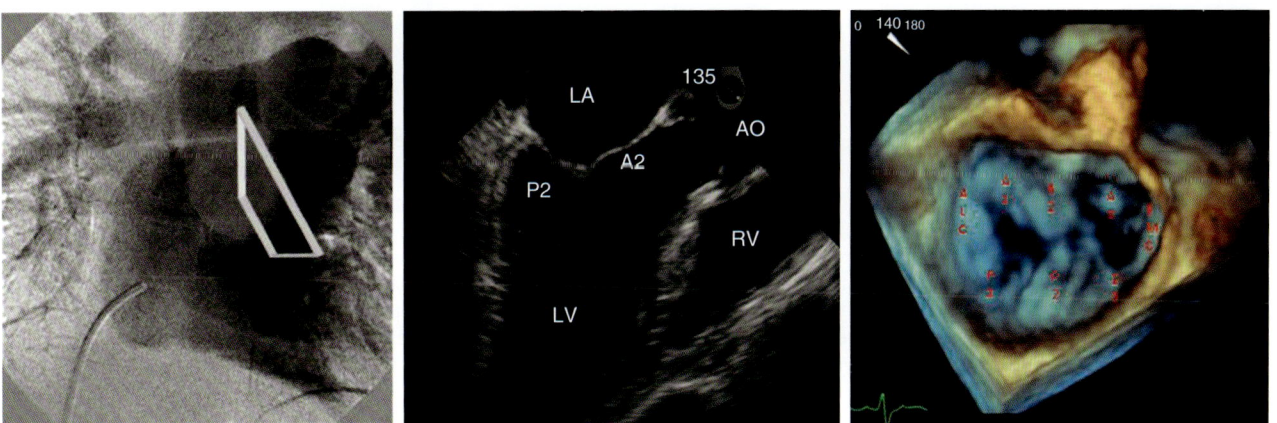

Fig. 48.11 Transesophageal echocardiography shows "130-degree" midesophageal long-axis view of the ascending aorta *(middle panel)*. Left panel shows the heart in anteroposterior view (refer to Fig. 48.4 for orientation). P2 and A2 refer to the posterior and anterior middle scallops of mitral leaflets. Right panel shows the mitral valve with 3D TEE. *A*, Anterior leaflet; *ALC*, anterolateral commissure; *AO*, aorta; *LA*, left atrium; *LV*, left ventricle; *P*, posterior leaflet; *PMC*, posteromedial commissure; *RV*, right ventricle; *TEE*, transesophageal echocardiography.

"monoplane" imaging. Each device has two handles, which allows the operator to move the probe tip in the AP and lateral directions. Maximum tissue penetration with ICE is around 10 to 12 cm.

ICE is currently being used for assessment of IAS, pulmonary veins, crista terminalis, the Eustachian valve, the tricuspid annulus, coronary sinus ostium, the aortic valve, the ascending aorta, the aortic arch, and for the assessment of the mitral valve in some cases. In general, there are three standard views; however, modification of these views by clocking or counter-clocking may be necessary. One can typically start from the SVC and pull the probe back caudally for visualization of different structures. The initial view is from the SVC when the transducer is in the neutral position (Fig. 48.12). Subsequent counterclockwise rotation will rotate the transducer anteriorly where the ascending aorta, the aortic valve, part of pulmonary trunk, and tricuspid valve can be seen (see Fig. 48.12). Clockwise rotation from this neutral position will rotate the transducer posteriorly, where IAS, right pulmonary artery, and descending aorta may be seen (see Fig. 48.12). The next view is typically obtained from the right atrium at the level of tricuspid valve (see Fig. 48.12). This view shows the tricuspid valve and the ascending aorta. Further clockwise rotation delineates part of the IAS. In order to see the entire IAS,

SECTION V Structural Interventions

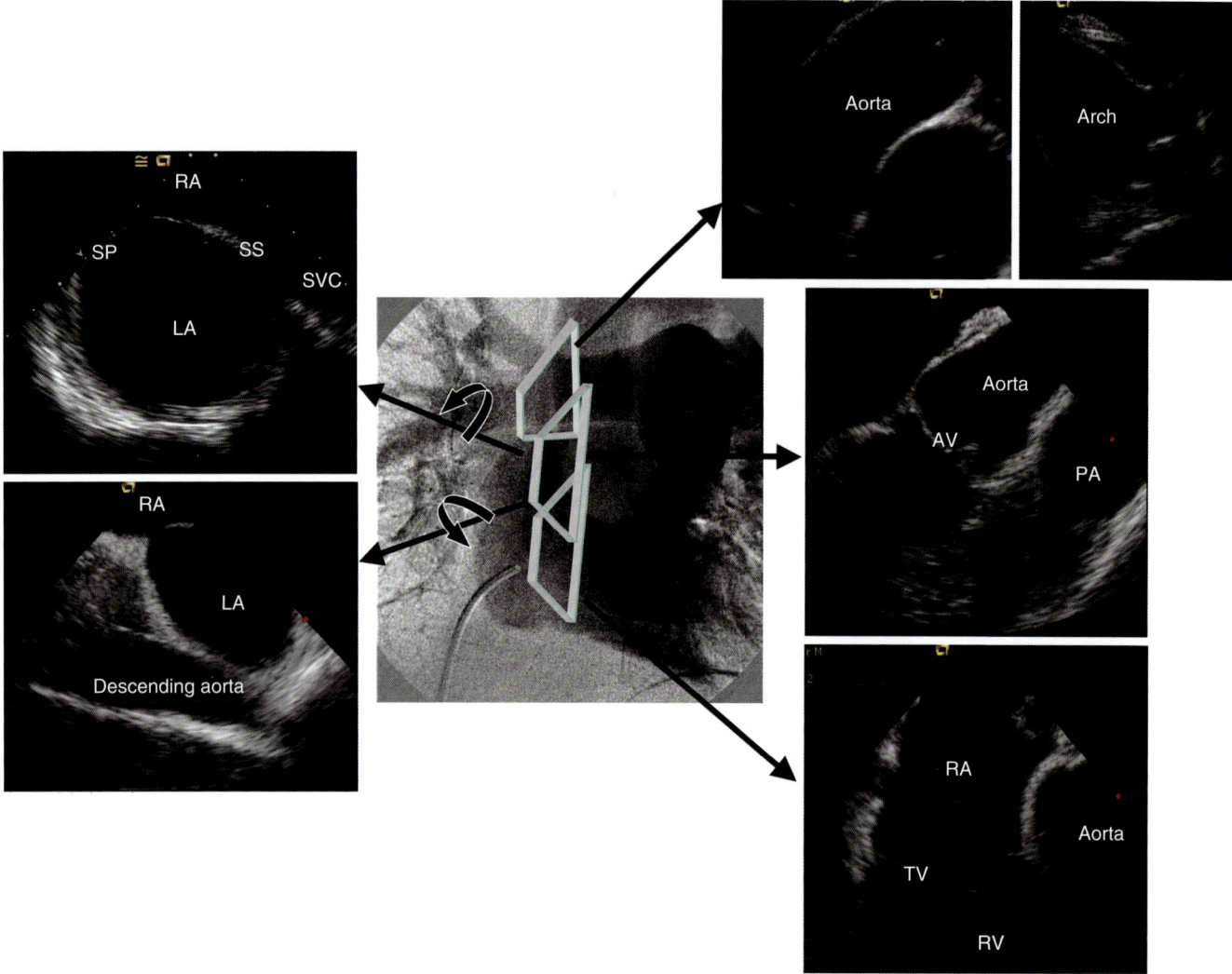

Fig. 48.12 The basic views obtained by intracardic echocardiography in the neutral position *(right panel)* and with progressive clockwise rotation *(left panel)*. The corresponding planes are shown on the fluoroscopy *(center panel)*. Refer to Fig. 48.4 for orientation of fluoroscopic image. In the neutral position from superior vena cava *(top panel)*, mid right atrium *(right middle panel)*, and at the level of tricuspid valve *(right bottom panel)*, the above structures can be seen. The panel on the left is obtained by turning the probe clockwise from the mid right atrium to visualize the entire interatrial septum from anterior to posterior aspect. *AV*, Aortic valve; *LA*, left atrium; *PA*, pulmonary artery; *RA*, right atrium; *RV*, right ventricle; *SP*, septum primum; *SS*, septum secundum; *SVC*, superior vena cava; *TV*, tricuspid valve.

posterior flexion is applied to the probe. This will allow enough depth so the entire IAS can be visualized (Fig. 48.13). The third standard view (anterior horizontal view) is obtained by flexing the probe in the mid right atrium with some clockwise rotation (Fig. 48.14). This generates a short-axis view of the aortic valve and produces a better visualization of the anteroposterior section of the septum. Further clockwise rotation will demonstrate the mitral valve and its apparatus. It is possible to see the aortic valve in cross section by rotating the probe clockwise and posteriorly; however, this view is less reproducible compared to the anterior horizontal view described previously (see Fig. 48.12). Occasionally, the mitral valve can be visualized from the coronary sinus, the right ventricle, or the superior aspect of the right atrium.

COMPUTED TOMOGRAPHY AND "FUSION" FLUOROSCOPY

Computed tomography (CT) has long been used to assess anatomic structures during the planning of surgical cardiac interventions and has also been adopted as a core imaging modality for the planning of transcatheter-based procedures. The high spatial resolution of CT allows detailed assessments of the valvular structures to determine anatomic candidacy for certain procedures. In general, the utility of CT-based imaging for structural interventions lies in its use for anatomic evaluation, quantitative assessment, procedure guidance/planning, and postprocedure monitoring. For example, gated cardiac CT is vital to assess the aortic valve leaflet length vis-à-vis coronary ostial height to determine risk of coronary obstruction in transcatheter aortic valve replacement and also provides a reliable assessment of the aortic annulus area for valve size determination. CT imaging is useful in nonvalvular procedures as well, such as LAA occlusion, as the LAA length, shape, and ostial dimension can all be obtained with ease and are critical to device choice and sizing to obtain a successful result. Integration of CT information is also accurate, safe, and reproducible for determining the optimal co-planar view for valve deployment.[8] While this technology does not reduce overall radiation exposure for the majority of patients, in certain patients with complex aortic rotation/angulation, contrast, and radiation exposure can certainly be reduced with preplanning using CT.

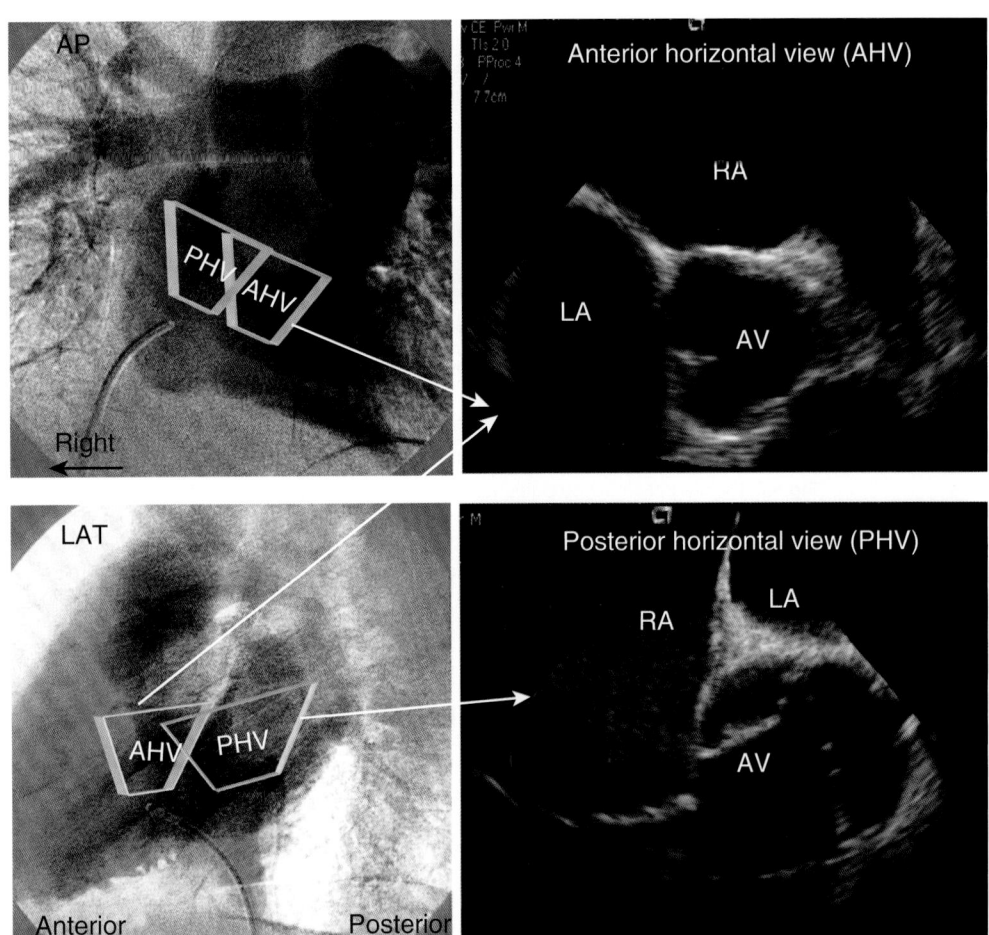

Fig. 48.13 Intracardic echocardiography in the anterior and posterior horizontal views *(right panel)*. The corresponding planes are shown in the anteroposterior *(AP; left upper panel)* and lateral view *(left lower panel)* on fluoroscopy (see text for detail). *AV*, Aortic valve; *LA*, left atrium; *LAT*, lateral view; *RA*, right atrium.

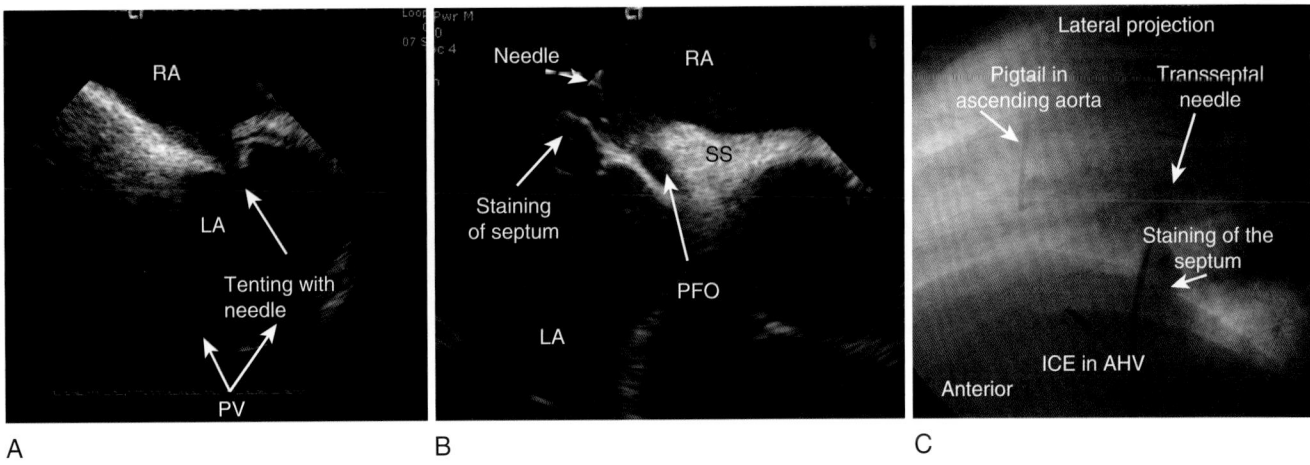

Fig. 48.14 Intracardiac echocardiography *(ICE)* shows a good location of puncture demonstrated by needle tenting opposite to the pulmonary veins (A). Panels (B) and (C) show a transseptal puncture in a patient patent foreman ovale with a long tunnel. (B) Shows the needle with stained septum. Note the puncture site is close to the end of septum secundum *(SS)*. (C) Shows the position of ICE probe and septal staining in the lateral projection for the same patient shown in panel B. Note that ascending aorta is anterior while the Brockenbrough needle is pointing posteriorly (C). *AHV*, Anterior horizontal view; *LA*, left atrium; *PFO*, patent foramen ovale; *PV*, pulmonary vein; *RA*, right atrium.

CT with fluoroscopy "fusion" imaging is an emerging technology that could potentially result in significant reductions in fluoroscopy time, esophageal intubation time for TEE, and total procedural time, and provide more detailed catheter guidance than fluoroscopy alone. Preprocedural multidetector computed tomography (MDCT) imaging is obtained, and areas of interest are marked on this image data set to be used as a reference. The Syngo DynaCT (Siemens Healthcare, Forcheim, Germany) is acquired intraprocedurally via the C-arm during a breath hold, and the C-arm CT is then "matched" to the preprocedural MDCT using an automatic software algorithm. One limitation of this software is the limited spatial resolution of the C-arm CT due to breath

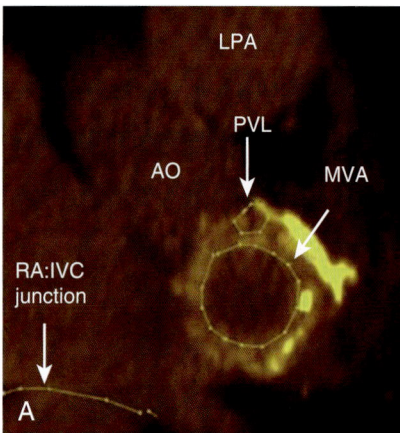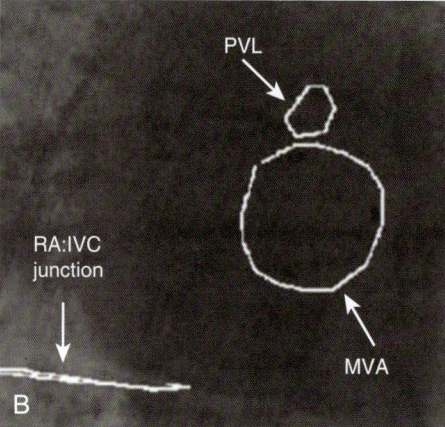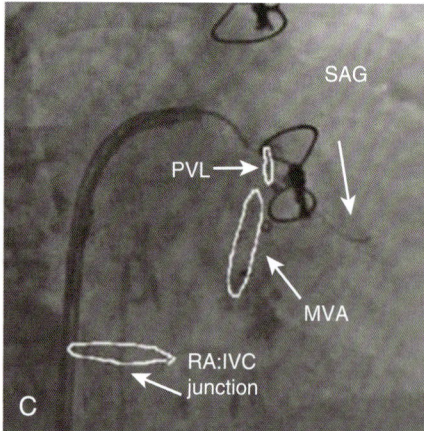

Fig. 48.15 Integration of computed tomography (CT) and real-time fluoroscopy. (A) Areas of interest are marked on the preprocedural CT (LAO projection). (B) CT markings are overlaid onto the real-time fluoroscopic image in the catheter laboratory (LAO). (C) Markings facilitate crossing of the leak (RAO projection). *AO,* Aorta; *IVC,* inferior vena cava; *LAO,* left anterior oblique; *LPA,* left pulmonary artery; *MVA,* mitral valve annulus; *PVL,* paravalvular leak; *RA,* right atrium; *RAO,* right anterior oblique; *SAG,* stiff-angled Glide wire.

motion artifact, which is greater than what is observed with more rapid MDCT imaging. Therefore, manual calibration is required to ensure perfect "matching" and can be achieved by moving the C-arm to align cardiac structures with the MDCT image. Once the data sets have been registered, the MDCT markings can be overlaid on live fluoroscopy, as seen in Fig. 48.15.[9] These markings allow for the navigation of catheters with increased accuracy and confidence in complex interventions. In transcatheter aortic valve implantation (TAVI), C-arm CT can be utilized to confirm important anatomic considerations, such as native leaflet length, coronary ostial height, and aorta-left ventricular outflow angulation, prior to valve deployment to ensure procedural success. It can also be utilized during PVL closure to limit the amount of time required to cross the leak, which can often be time-consuming using fluoroscopic and echocardiographic guidance alone. With further advances in real time C-arm CT, it is highly likely that this technology will be routinely used in all structural cardiac interventions.

Fusion of fluoroscopic images with 3D TEE has also gained increasing popularity over the last decade.[10,11] Patented fusion software such as EchoNavigator (Phillips Medical Systems, Netherlands) have received U.S. Food and Drug Administration (FDA) approval for live 3D TEE guidance as an overlay on fluoroscopy. Co-registration of the TEE probe and fluoroscopy is achieved by altering the C-arm and table positioning to permit the TEE probe to be visible on fluoroscopy. Once co-registration is complete, the TEE or C-arm can be moved without loss of imaging fusion. The EchoNavigator software can be used to mark anatomic targets, such as PVL sites, and this marking can then be overlaid on fluoroscopy for catheter guidance. Since its introduction, this software has been utilized successfully in various structural interventions and, with increasing adoption among interventionalists, is likely to become integral in structural interventions.[12,13]

Specific Procedural Uses for Intracardiac Imaging
Transseptal Puncture

Transseptal puncture has become an integral part of many intracardiac procedures, including percutaneous mitral valvuloplasty, mitral valve repair, LAA closure, some cases of PFO closure, and atrial fibrillation ablation.[14] The goal is to cross the IAS through the fossa ovalis, a 2-cm in diameter area that is bound superiorly by septum secundum, called the *limbus*. It is located posterior and inferior to aortic root in the mid portion of IAS. The procedure is performed using the Brockenbrough needle (USCI, Billerica, MA), which is introduced through an 8-Fr Mullins sheath and dilator combination. Procedure is performed primarily by fluoroscopic guidance with ultrasound imaging (ICE or TEE guidance) as an important supplement. Fluoroscopically, the most important landmarks are position of the aorta (determined by placing a catheter in aortic root), and margins of right and left atrium. This can be determined by right atrial angiogram in the AP and lateral projections (see Fig. 48.4). The needle is withdrawn caudally in the AP projection from SVC; three medial drops are identified, which correspond to SVC-right atrial junction, noncoronary sinus of aorta, and limbus of the fossa ovalis. Needle position is then checked in lateral projection to ensure posterior direction in relation to the aorta (see Fig. 48.14). The needle is advanced to the LA with close monitoring of pressure through the needle to ensure that there is no drop in pressure as the needle traverses the IAS. Staining of the septum can be very helpful if there is any doubt regarding the location of the puncture site (see Fig. 48.14).

TEE can also help determine the appropriate location of the puncture site. The vertical distance from the mitral valve and aorta can be determined by four-chamber and bicaval views, respectively (Fig. 48.16). TEE also helps rule out thrombus in the left atrium or the LAA appendage, and monitor pericardium for presence of effusion. The puncture site must be identified through recognition of tenting, as it indicates the precise location of the needle tip (see Fig. 48.16).

Three-dimensional TEE can also be used to guide safe transseptal puncture. The IAS is typically visualized in the bicaval view which shows the superoinferior extent of the IAS, including the fossa ovalis and both the superior and inferior vena cava. This orientation is important, as a more inferior puncture is required to reach the LAA while a more superior puncture is typically needed for mitral valve interventions. A biplane image at this level shows the anteroposterior extent of the IAS, allowing a better appreciation of the anterior and posterior adjacent structures, specifically the aortic valve, which is critical to localize as the operator needs to position his transseptal puncture posteriorly away from it. Another alternative would be a 3D acquisition at the level of the IAS that includes all adjacent structures. Appropriate manipulation of such image allows visualization of the septum and adjacent structures from both the right-atrial and left-atrial perspective.

ICE is commonly used to guide this procedure and can identify the anteroposterior and superoinferior boundaries of the IAS. The ICE catheter is introduced in the right atrium and then steered to the right with posterior flexion, and this gives rise to the posterior horizontal view. In this view, the superior and inferior cavo-atrial junction is delineated, the aortic rim is well seen,

CHAPTER 48 Imaging for Intracardiac Interventions

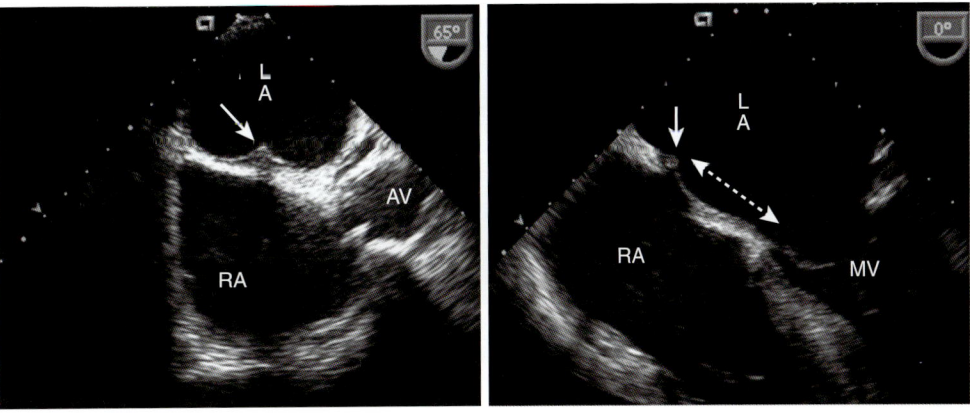

Fig. 48.16 Transesophageal echocardiography shows "65-degree" (midesophagus) and "0-degree" (four-chamber) location of the puncture site. The distance between the puncture site and the aortic (left panel) and the mitral valve (right panel) can be determined on these views. Presence of tenting (white arrow) confirms the location and position of the needle. *AV*, Aortic valve; *LA*, left atrium; *MV*, mitral valve; *RA*, right atrium.

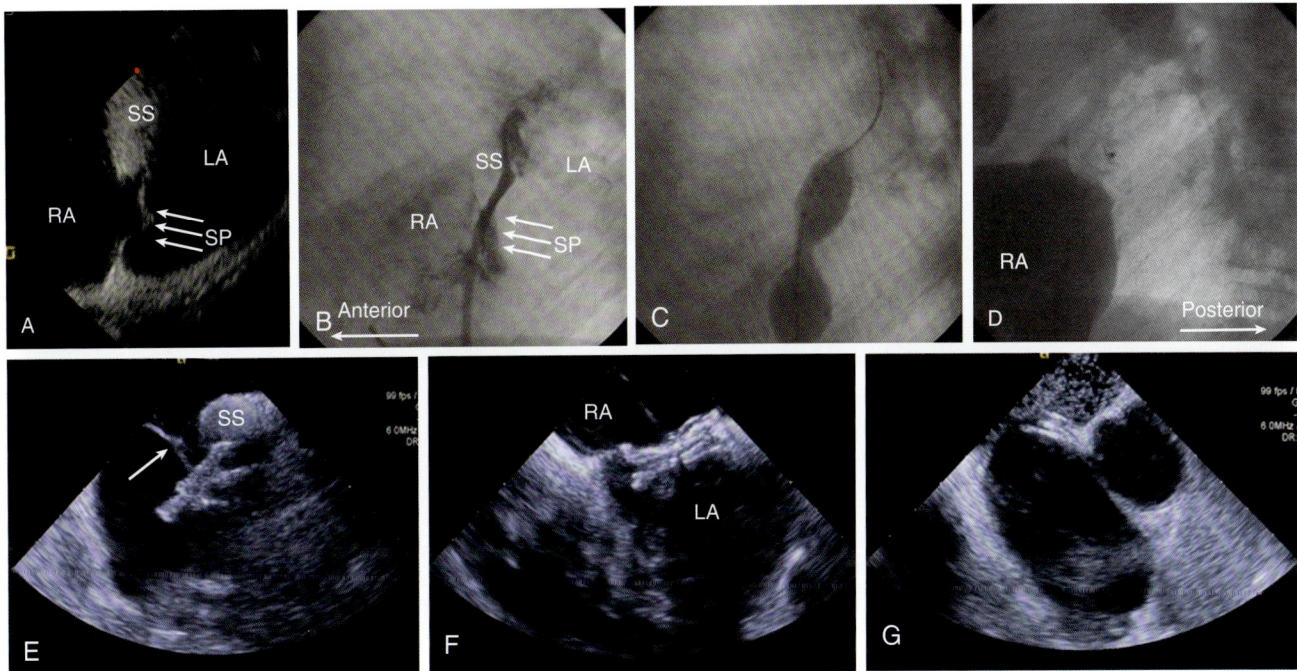

Fig. 48.17 (A) Shows patent foreman ovale (PFO) with septum primum (SP) and septum secundum (SS) on intracardiac echocardiography. The image is rotated to match the fluoroscopic image (B). SP is flimsy (atrial septal aneurysm). Lateral view on fluoroscopy shows a patent PFO (B), "feeling" of PFO with sizing balloon (C), and proper positioning of the device with a right atrial angiogram prior to detachment (D). PFO occluder device in the left atrium via trans-septal access (E). PFO occluder device is positioned across the PFO optimally (F). Bubble study showing lack of right to left shunting after device deployment (G). *LA*, Left atrium; *RA*, right atrium.

and the right upper pulmonary vein is seen. While keeping the catheter in this orientation, the whole system is then rotated in a clockwise fashion and placed below the aortic valve. This denotes the anterior horizontal view and localizes the short axis of the IAS and delineates the posterior extent of the IAS (see Fig. 48.14A). The appropriate site can also be confirmed in the anterior horizontal view (Fig. 48.17).[15]

Patent Foramen Ovale

The details of this procedure are covered in the separate chapter. Briefly, under normal embryologic development, the IAS is composed of the septum primum and septum secundum, which are two independent crescent-shaped membranes. In utero, the mobile septum primum allows right to left shunting, permitting delivery of oxygenated blood to the fetal systemic circulation. At birth, there is a rise in LA pressure that drives the fusion of the septum primum and secundum. In approximately 15% to 20% of individuals, this fusion does not occur, resulting in a patent foramen ovale and occasionally permitting right to left shunting, depending on transseptal pressure gradients

Fluoroscopy and ICE are used in conjunction for percutaneous PFO closure. The most common views are the shallow LAO (10 degrees), cranial (10 degrees), or lateral view (60 degrees LAO), which allows better appreciation of the PFO orientation. Typically, a Gudel-Lubin catheter is used to cross the PFO, and while the catheter is being pulled back, contrast injection is used to visualize the PFO on fluoroscopy (see Fig. 48.17B). This allows visualization of the length of the tunnel (overlap between septum primum and secundum) and the thickness of septum secundum. Additionally, balloon inflation in the PFO not only helps determine the size of the PFO but also helps delineate the shape and size of the tunnel and allows one to "feel" the quality of the tissue around the PFO (see Fig. 48.17C). Deployment of the device is

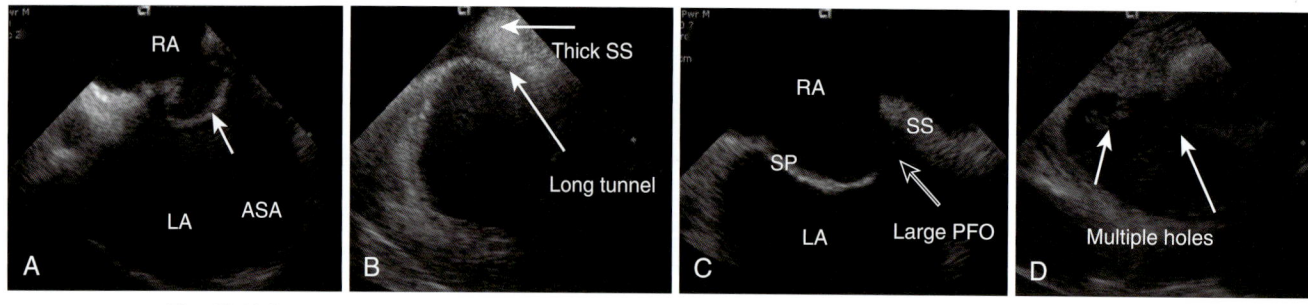

Fig. 48.18 Intracardiac echocardiography shows presence of atrial septal aneurysm (A), the overlap of septum primum and septum secundum showing the "tunnel" (B), the thickness of septum secundum (B), size of patent foreman ovale *(PFO)* (C), and the presence of additional openings (D). *ASA,* Atrial septal aneurysm; *LA,* left atrium; *RA,* right atrium; *SP,* septum primum; *SS,* septum secundum.

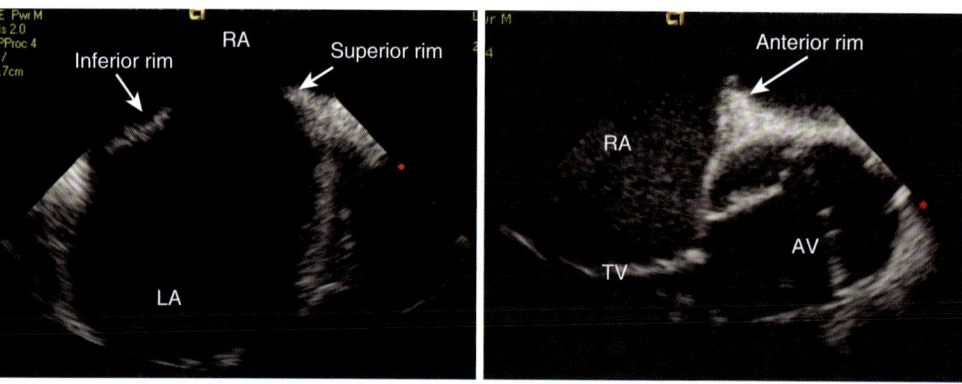

Fig. 48.19 Intracardiac echocardiography shows the inferior and superior rim of secundum atrial septal defect *(left panel)*. Note the presence of small anterior rim *(right panel)*. *AV,* Aortic valve; *LA,* left atrium; *RA,* right atrium; *TV,* tricuspid valve.

usually done in the shallow LAO cranial view (10 to 10 degrees), which allows perpendicular visualization of the IAS. Lastly, injection of the contrast under fluoroscopy from the guide catheter prior to release confirms good apposition (see Fig. 48.17D).

ICE is commonly used to first assess the IAS in the longitudinal plane from top to bottom in the anterior and the posterior direction. This is done by turning the probe in the clockwise and counterclockwise directions at various heights in the right atrium (see Fig. 48.12). Next the probe is flexed anteriorly, and the ultrasound beam is directed superiorly and posteriorly in order to visualize the anteroposterior length of the IAS (see Fig. 48.13). ICE should be carefully performed with the following points in consideration: (a) presence or absence of atrial septal aneurysm (Fig. 48.18A), (b) the relationship of septum primum to septum secundum to determine the length of the "tunnel" (see Fig. 48.18B), (c) thickness of septum secundum (see Fig. 48.18B), (d) size of PFO (see Fig. 48.18C), (e) presence of additional foramina (see Fig. 48.18D), (f) degree of interatrial shunting, and (g) presence of a prominent Chiari network. ICE can be used to confirm that the wire has crossed the PFO when multiple foramina are present. Similarly, ICE can be very useful when transseptal puncture for a tunneled PFO is necessary (see Fig. 48.17). Typically the puncture has to be made fairly anterior near the PFO to adequately cover PFO with the device. Device deployment is typically performed under ICE and fluoroscopy guidance. Once the operator is satisfied, the device is released and a bubble study is performed to detect the presence of any residual right to left shunting.

In our institution, almost all PFOs are closed using fluoroscopy and ICE guidance. TEE is associated with greater patient discomfort and requires an additional operator. Two views are most helpful when using TEE; the first is the (30 to 40 degrees) midesophageal short-axis view of the aortic valve and the IAS, the second is the (90 to 100 degrees) midesophageal bicaval view, which shows the inferior and SVC, the right atrium, and the IAS. However, subtle changes in these views and angles may be necessary for better visualization, owing to variations in anatomy among individual patients. At present, only the Amplatzer PFO occluder (St. Jude Medical, Inc., Abbott Park, IL) is FDA approved for PFO indication, with the HELEX/Cardioform septal occluder (Gore and Associates, Newark, DE) also commercially available with premarket approval (both shown in Fig. 48.17).

Secundum Atrial Septal Defect

Secundum ASD results from underdeveloped septum secundum, resulting in a true opening in the IAS. The key elements in the assessment of ASD with echocardiography for percutaneous closure include (a) identifying the location of the defect in the septum secundum (superior, inferior, anterior, or posterior), (b) size of the defect, (c) identification of multiple defects, and (d) adequacy of rims (Fig. 48.19). Pulmonary angiogram is the most helpful modality to identify anomalous venous drainage in the catheterization laboratory (see Fig. 48.5).

ICE is the preferred imaging method for this procedure.[16] In general, the two views described herein for PFO are adequate for visualizing ASD and its structural detail. Individualization of views should be considered, as the ASD occurs in many different sizes and shapes. Obliteration of color flow with balloon inflation allows proper sizing without oversizing, as commonly happens when only the waist of the balloon is used with fluoroscopy (Fig. 48.20). Device deployment is guided by ICE, and proper gripping can be tested with "push and pull." Impingement of surrounding structures (e.g., mitral valve, SVC, roof the LA, aorta, and coronary sinus) should be carefully assessed prior to releasing the device. Right atrial angiogram with end-on view of the device allows clear visualization of the device margins and its relation to LA walls and aorta (Fig. 48.21).

Left Atrial Appendage Occlusion

The LAA is derived from the embryonic left atrium and is a blind pouch located on the anterior surface of the heart and has

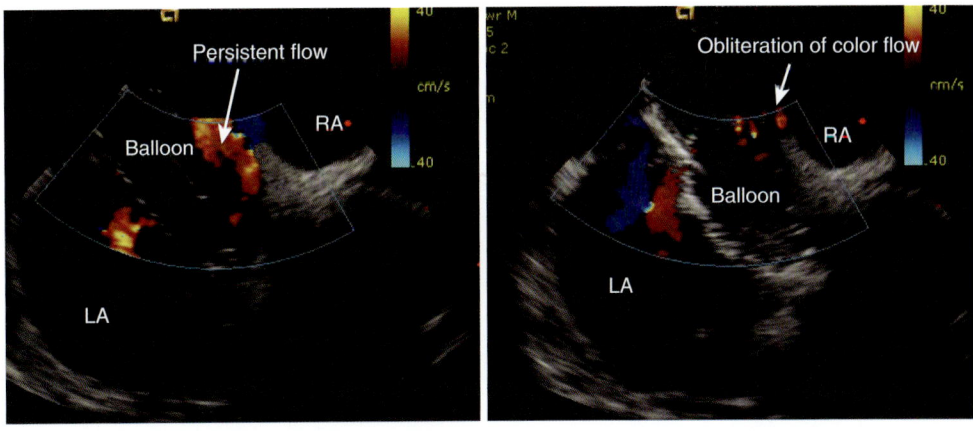

Fig. 48.20 Intracardiac echocardiography shows the process of atrial septal defect (ASD) sizing. Balloon is inflated with color interrogation of the ASD. Initially there is presence of persistent flow around ASD balloon *(left panel)*. Balloon is inflated further to barely obliterate flow across ASD and size is measured. This allows choosing the proper size of ASD closure device without oversizing. *LA*, Left atrium; *RA*, right atrium.

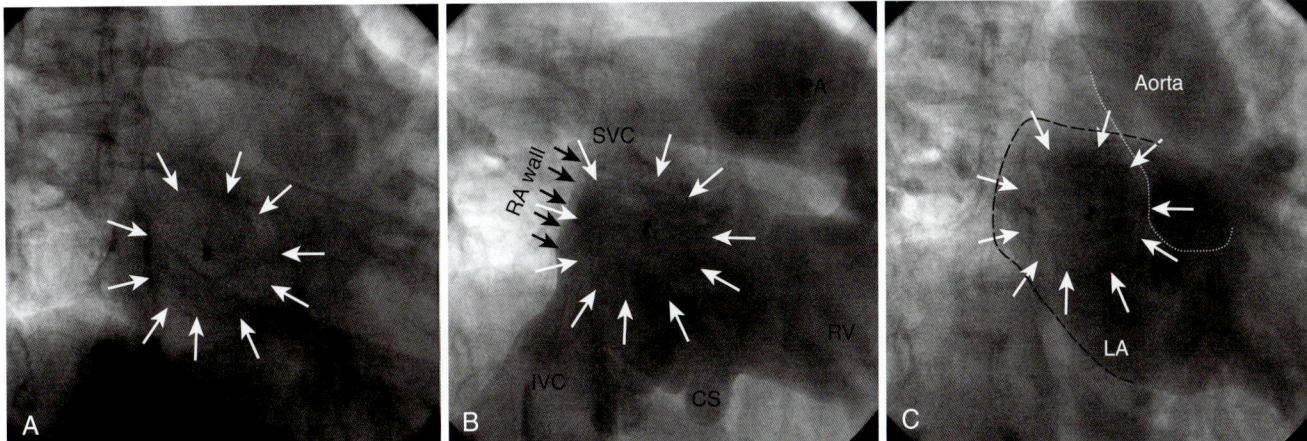

Fig. 48.21 Right anterior oblique caudal view of a right atrial angiogram shows atrial septal defect device "end on" (A) with surrounding structures in the dextro (B) and levo (C) phase of contrast injection. Note the relation of the device with right atrial walls, left atrial walls, and the aorta. *White arrows* show the margin of the left atrial device disk. *Black arrows* point to the right atrial wall. Aortic silhouette is traced with *dashed white line*. Left atrial border is shown by the *dashed black line*. *CS*, Coronary sinus; *IVC*, inferior vena cava; *LA*, left atrium; *PA*, pulmonary artery; *RA*, right atrium; *RV*, right ventricle; *SVC*, superior vena cava.

several anatomical variations.[17] The ostium of the LAA is ellipsoid in shape, and the ostium enlarges progressively with severity of atrial fibrillation.[1] The pectinate muscles within the LAA must be delineated, as they can be misidentified as thrombus. The use of real-time 3D TEE can help distinguish between pectinate muscles and thrombi.[18] The combination of TEE and CT imaging is effective in assessing LA and LAA anatomy. TEE can assess functional and anatomical features that increase the risk for thrombogenicity.

Computed tomographic imaging can assess the morphology and provide anatomical information to guide LAA closure. Specifically, it can delineate the 3D orientation of the LAA relative to the pulmonary artery, the number and shapes of lobes, and the general orientation of the appendage.[19] The morphological appearance of the LAA has been divided into four distinct categories based on CT analysis: (1) wind sock (long, dominant lobe), (2) cauliflower (short length with complex internal structure), (3) chicken wing (one prominent end in the LAA), and (4) cactus (dominant central lobe with secondary lobes).[20]

Several important anatomic considerations can be obtained from cardiac MDCT imaging and should be evaluated in the planning stages of LAA occlusion procedures to ensure optimal results and minimize the risk of complications. Optimal sizing of the LAA ostium can be easily obtained, along with the distance from ostium to the first bend in the LAA, as well as the angulation of the LAA to the plane of the ostium. The anatomic relationship and proximity of the left superior pulmonary vein, which is typically located superior and slightly posterior to the LAA and the mitral valve annulus (located inferiorly), can be clearly visualized as well. Furthermore, approximate distances between the IAS and LAA ostium can be established to minimize risk of LAA perforation with wires or catheters.[21,22]

Once transseptal assess is obtained and the delivery sheath is placed in the LAA, a pigtail catheter is placed in the LAA, and LAA images are obtained. The best working view is a RAO 30-degree caudal, which correlates with the TEE image at 135 degrees. A simple RAO view correlates with the TEE image at 45 to 90 degrees, whereas the cranial RAO correlates with the TEE image at 0 degrees. Once the device is deployed, a TEE is used to interrogate adequate sealing of all the LAA lobes.

Mitral Valvuloplasty

Proper guidance with imaging can make percutaneous mitral valvuloplasty (PMV) safer and more effective, especially in developed countries where patients are older and valves are less optimal for balloon valvuloplasty.[23]

TEE is most helpful in guiding PMV (Fig. 48.22). It helps (1) with guidance for transseptal puncture, (2) to rule out clots in LAA prior to the procedure, (3) with determining the degree and the mechanism of MR with each balloon inflation, and (4) in documenting the size of the defect in the IAS as a result of transseptal puncture after removal of the balloon. We prefer to use TEE in the cardiac catheterization laboratory for this procedure.[24] This

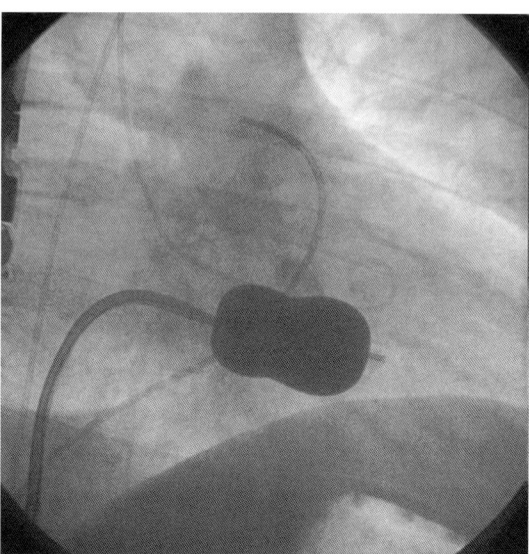
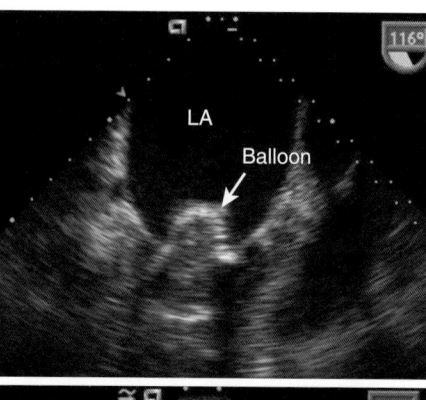
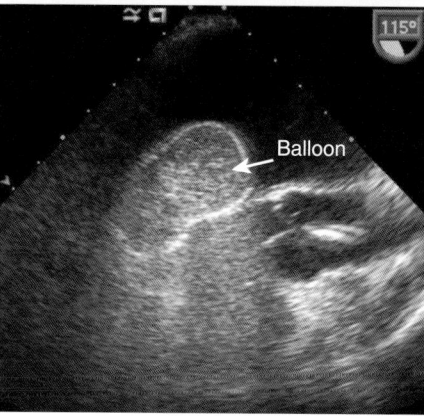

Fig. 48.22 Mitral valvuloplasty using the Inoue balloon in the right anterior oblique projection under fluoroscopy *(left panel)*. Upper and lower right panels show a stepwise balloon inflation in the 110- to 120-degree long-axis view under transesophageal echocardiography guidance. *LA*, Left atrium.

can be safely accomplished in supine position without endotracheal intubation if proper sedation and suctioning of the posterior pharynx is performed. Careful interrogation of the mitral valve with TEE in the midesophageal as well as transgastric views is helpful for determining the mechanism and severity of MR. Currently, ICE is not very helpful for mitral valve interrogation and assessment.

Fluoroscopy is also an important component of this procedure. Left ventricular angiogram can assess the severity of MR; however, an adequate volume of dye should be injected to visualize opacification in typically dilated left atria. Fluoroscopy in the RAO projection is helpful to ensure coaxial entry of balloon through the mitral valve without entanglement in the chordae. Partial inflation of the Inoue balloon and advancement of balloon to the cardiac apex in this projection prior to engagement and inflation within the MV can also help in confirming that the balloon is free from chordal apparatus.

Aortic Valvuloplasty

Fluoroscopy plays a significant role in visualizing the aortic valve and its orifice. Using fluoroscopy in the LAO and RAO projections can help determine which leaflet has the most motion (see Fig. 48.7). Typically, an AL-1 catheter should be pointed under the moving leaflet to cross the valve with a straight wire. If RCC is moving, this motion is best appreciated in RAO projection. If LCC or NCC has the most motion, then the LAO projection is helpful. The LAO view is the safest view to cross the aortic valve to prevent inadvertent entry into coronary ostia with a straight wire.

This procedure is done with fluoroscopy only.[25,26] Hemodynamic measurements are important to guide the aggressiveness of balloon valvuloplasty. In the event of complications, TEE or ICE can help determine the exact cause (e.g., severity and mechanism of aortic insufficiency).

Pulmonary Valvuloplasty

Pulmonary valve stenosis is a common congenital abnormality. Many of these patients undergo pulmonary valvuloplasty in adulthood. Cineangiography, transthoracic echocardiography (TTE), TEE, and ICE are helpful modalities used for this procedure.[27] Pulmonary artery angiogram in AP and lateral views is helpful in order to visualize the pulmonary annulus size and preexisting pulmonary insufficiency (Fig. 48.23). Occasionally, right ventriculography in the same views may be performed to assess the right ventricular outflow tract (Fig. 48.24). Severe subpulmonary hypertrophy may be associated with significant dynamic right ventricular outflow tract obstruction post pulmonary valvuloplasty.

Both TTE and TEE can be helpful in assessing pulmonary valve annular size. ICE provides useful assessment of pulmonary insufficiency, allows for measurement of the annulus, and can be placed in the right ventricular outflow tract for assessment of the pulmonary valve (see Fig. 48.24).

Percutaneous Mitral Valve Repair

A mitral valve apparatus consists of the annulus, leaflets, chordae, and the papillary muscles. The mitral annulus is saddle shaped, with the highest points being the left and right trigones and lateral commissure. There is some suggestion that the shape of the annulus changes when the LA and LV dilate. The posterior leaflet is larger in length but covers one-third of the circumference of the annulus, while the shorter anterior leaflet covers two-thirds of the annulus.[28] Unlike any other interventional procedures, the use of real-time echocardiographic imaging guidance is critical, and clear communication is needed between the interventionalist and the imaging specialist. It is recommended that an imaging protocol consisting of predetermined views for each step be created. An ideal puncture site in the IAS should be in the superior and posterior aspect of the IAS, to achieve a height of

3.5 to 4.0 cm above the mitral valve coaptation plane. The clip is then ideally positioned in the center of the regurgitant jet, with the clip arm aligned perpendicular to the commissural line. The midesophageal long-axis view is used to guide the anteroposterior positioning, and the commissural view guides the medial-lateral position. The addition of 3D TEE in addition to 2D TEE provides superior guidance of the MitraClip procedure. The 3D images of the mitral valve from both the LA and ventricular side provide better navigation, accurate alignment of the clip at the middle scallops of the mitral valve, and visualization of the clip arms perpendicular to the commissural line (Fig. 48.25). In addition, TEE imaging is useful for assessment of residual MR with each attempt at treatment. The most common views include the midesophageal short-axis view (typically for transseptal puncture and to guide catheter manipulation), midesophageal commissural or "two-chamber" view, a midesophageal long-axis view ("LVOT"; multiplane angle of approximately 120 to 150 degrees), and a transgastric short-axis view (multiplane angle 0 to 30 degrees) at the mitral valve level. For coronary sinus–related procedures, fluoroscopy and TEE are helpful for proper positioning of the device and evaluating the effectiveness of the intervention. Angiography helps determine left circumflex and coronary sinus relationships. CT can help patient selection by defining the relationship between coronary sinus, mitral annulus, and left circumflex coronary artery.

Percutaneous Aortic Valve Replacement

Percutaneous aortic valve replacement is currently approved for intermediate-risk, high-risk, and inoperable patients with aortic stenosis.[29] There are multiple different approaches that are being investigated with balloon expandable, self-expanding stented, or unstented valves. Accurate positioning of the valve is critical for both balloon expandable and self-expanding valves; therefore, proper imaging in the catheterization laboratory is of paramount importance.

In the planning stages for percutaneous aortic valve replacement, CT is invaluable and provides critical information related to candidacy for transfemoral approach, including calcification, size and tortuosity of the iliac, and femoral vasculature. 4D Cardiac CT can be used to visualize the aortic valve apparatus and determine the extent of pathologic changes, including calcification, and also to verify their relation with coronary ostia to assess the risk of coronary obstruction (Fig. 48.26).

Intraprocedurally, fluoroscopy is used to accurately define the aortic valve plane (see Fig. 48.7). Fluoroscopy with minimal contrast injection at times can determine appropriate angles so that the aortic valve plane is seen without any overlap of the sinuses (Fig. 48.27). Typically LAO cranial and RAO caudal views are used. It is also important to note which leaflets and commissures are calcified and/or restricted. Accurate definition of leaflet morphology, especially length, may help identify patients where compromise of coronary ostia is likely at the time of valve deployment. Injection of dye at the time of balloon valvuloplasty may also help predict this relationship. The ascending aortic slope (horizontal versus vertical in LAO projection) may determine the ease or difficulty in delivering the valve. TEE is also important for valve assessment (calcification, annulus size, and severity), accurate positioning of the valve, and assessing the results of valve replacement (valvular or perivalvular leak and function).

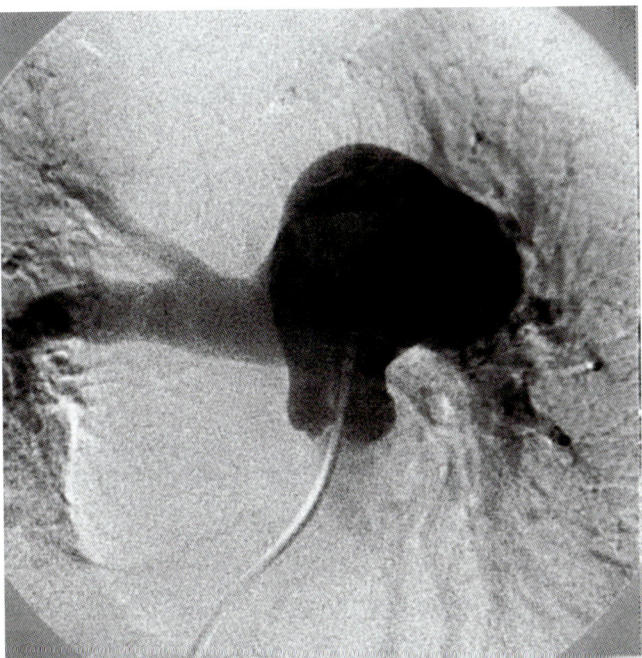

Fig. 48.23 Pulmonary angiogram assesses pulmonic valve using the National Institute of Health catheter. Note the presence of mild pulmonary insufficiency and poststenotic pulmonary artery dilatation. Digital subtraction was used for better visualization.

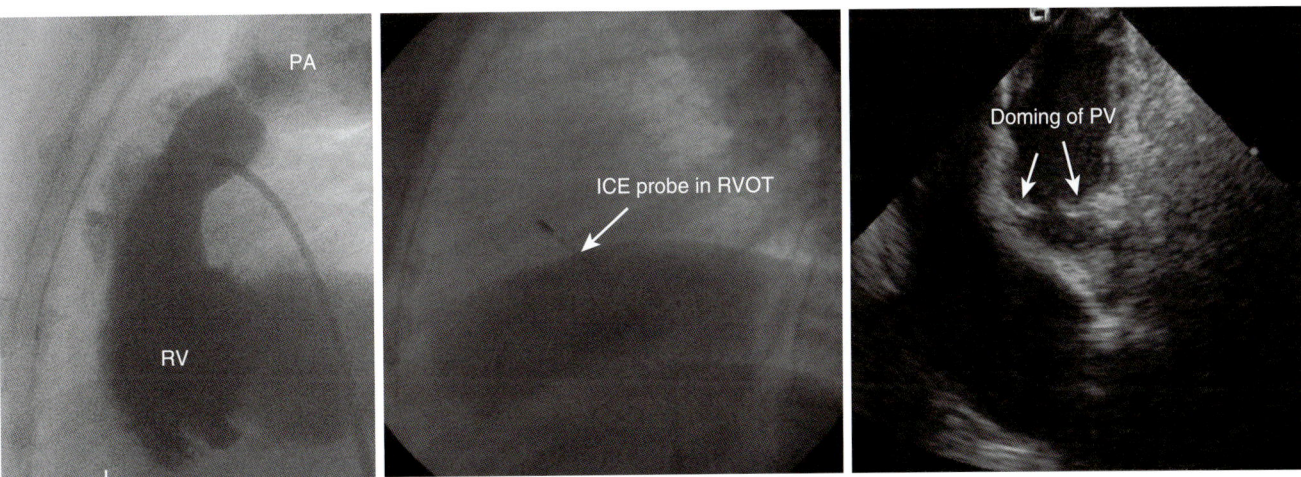

Fig. 48.24 Right ventriculogram showing pulmonary stenosis in the lateral view *(left panel)*. Middle panel shows intracardiac echocardiogram *(ICE)* probe in the right ventricular outflow tract in the lateral view (same projection as the *left panel*). The right panel shows pulmonary valve doming in the corresponding ICE view. *PA,* Pulmonary artery; *PV,* pulmonary valve; *RV,* right ventricle; *RVOT,* right ventricular outflow tract.

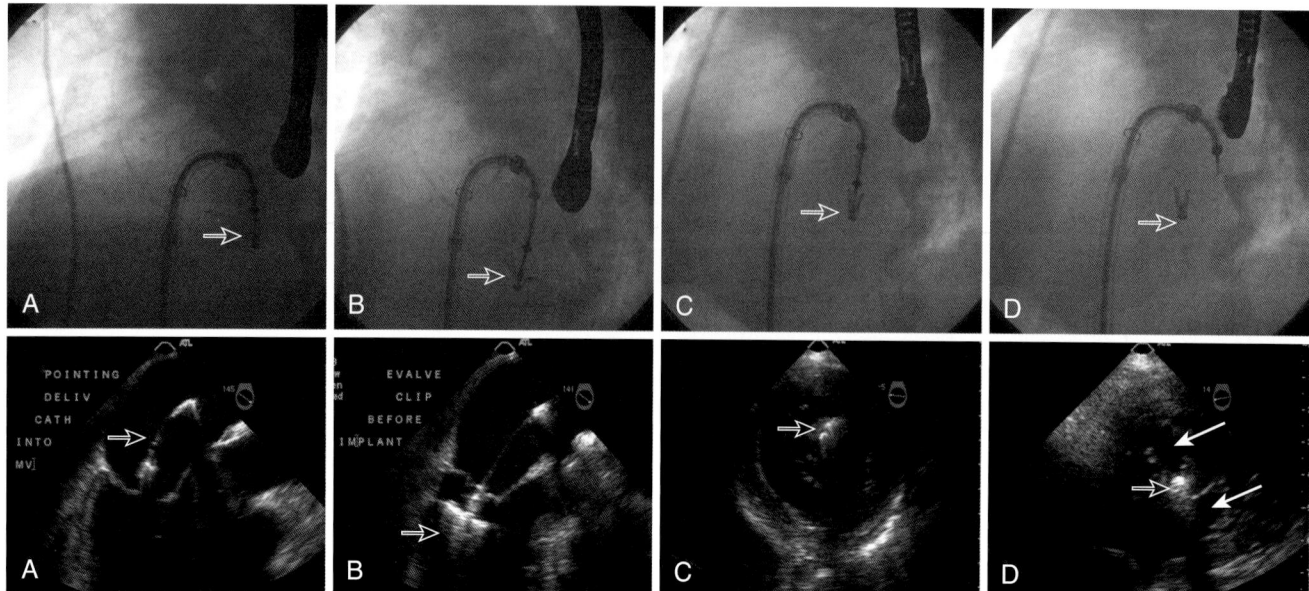

Fig. 48.25 Upper panel shows the MitraClip in the left atrium pointing towards the mitral valve (MV; A), the opening of the clip and advancing across MV (B), grabbing the leaflet tips (C), and releasing the clip (D). Lower panel depicts the transesophageal echocardiography images of the device in left atrium pointing towards the MV (A), the opening of the clip and advancing across MV (B), perpendicular orientation of the clip to the MV coaptation line in transgastric view (C), and final result with double orifice *(two white arrows)* (D).

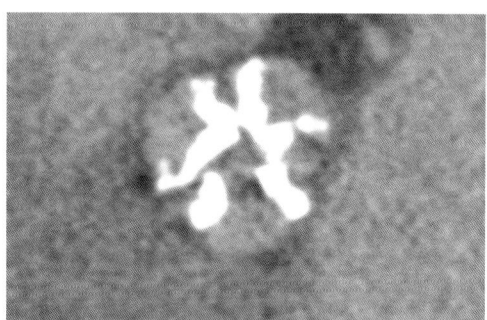 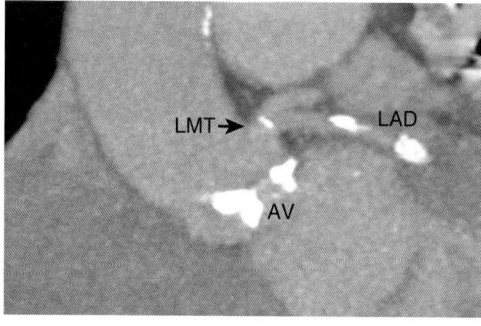

Fig. 48.26 Four-dimensional computed tomography (CT) of the aortic valve in short axis *(left panel)* and longitudinal cuts *(right panel)*. Note significant calcification on the aortic valve and left anterior descending artery. CT can also help determine the distance between aortic valve and left main trunk. *AV,* Aortic valve; *LAD,* left anterior descending; *LMT,* left main trunk.

A straight flush catheter can be used to opacify the NCC selectively to ensure optimal position of the TAVI valve within the LVOT, as shown in Fig. 48.28. For the Edwards Sapien S3 valve, fluoroscopic angulation can be optimized to reveal a light "band" across the collapsed valve stent (as seen in Fig. 48.28), which can also assist in optimal positioning of this valve by ensuring this "band" is level with the NCC. Aortography is used post deployment to confirm final positioning of the valve, as well as to evaluate for potential PVLs. Often, both the native and prosthetic valve leaflets can be visualized by aortography (see Fig. 48.28).

Mechanical Prosthetic Valve Assessment

Occasionally mechanical valves require a full assessment for the presence of dehiscence, vegetations, or obstruction secondary to thrombus or pannus formation. While TTE and TEE can provide valuable information, some limitations persist, including shadowing, pressure recovery phenomena, and difficulty in visualizing the aortic valve secondary to its anterior location.

Fluoroscopy has been used to measure opening and closing angles of mechanical aortic valves. To determine this, fluoroscopy cameras should be positioned so tangential views of the leaflets are obtained (Fig. 48.29). As during the placement of the prosthetic aortic valve the rotational orientation can vary from patient to patient, there is no single view that can correctly visualize this valve. Therefore, we recommend a systematic approach, starting with the 20- to 30-degree RAO caudal view, and gradually increasing this angle toward an LAO cranial projection (see Fig. 48.29). Occasionally ventriculography may be helpful to see the subvalvular pathology, like pannus. In patients with low-profile tilting disks (i.e., Bjork-Shiley, [Pfizer Inc. New York, NY] St. Jude, Medtronic-Hall valve [Medtronic PLC, Minneapolis, MN]), transseptal puncture and pressure measurements with or without ventriculography may be necessary for better assessment of the prosthetic valve. Although prosthetic aortic valve can be crossed with a 0.014-inch pressure wire, the safety of such a procedure is unclear. In situations where both the mitral and the aortic valves have mechanical prostheses, either apical puncture or crossing the aortic or mitral valves with a pressure wire can be considered (see Fig. 48.29) to obtain direct pressure gradients.

Cardiac CT also allows for the assessment of opening and closing angles of the mechanical prosthetic valves. ICE can also be used to assess prosthetic aortic valve function from a hemodynamic perspective. ICE can be utilized to visualize the LVOT below a mechanical aortic valve from the right atrium, but typically has poor image quality of the valve itself due to reflection and shadowing from metallic surfaces.

Paravalvular Leak Closure

Multimodality imaging using TTE and TEE usually provides the initial diagnosis of PVL. Procedural guidance often requires

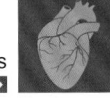

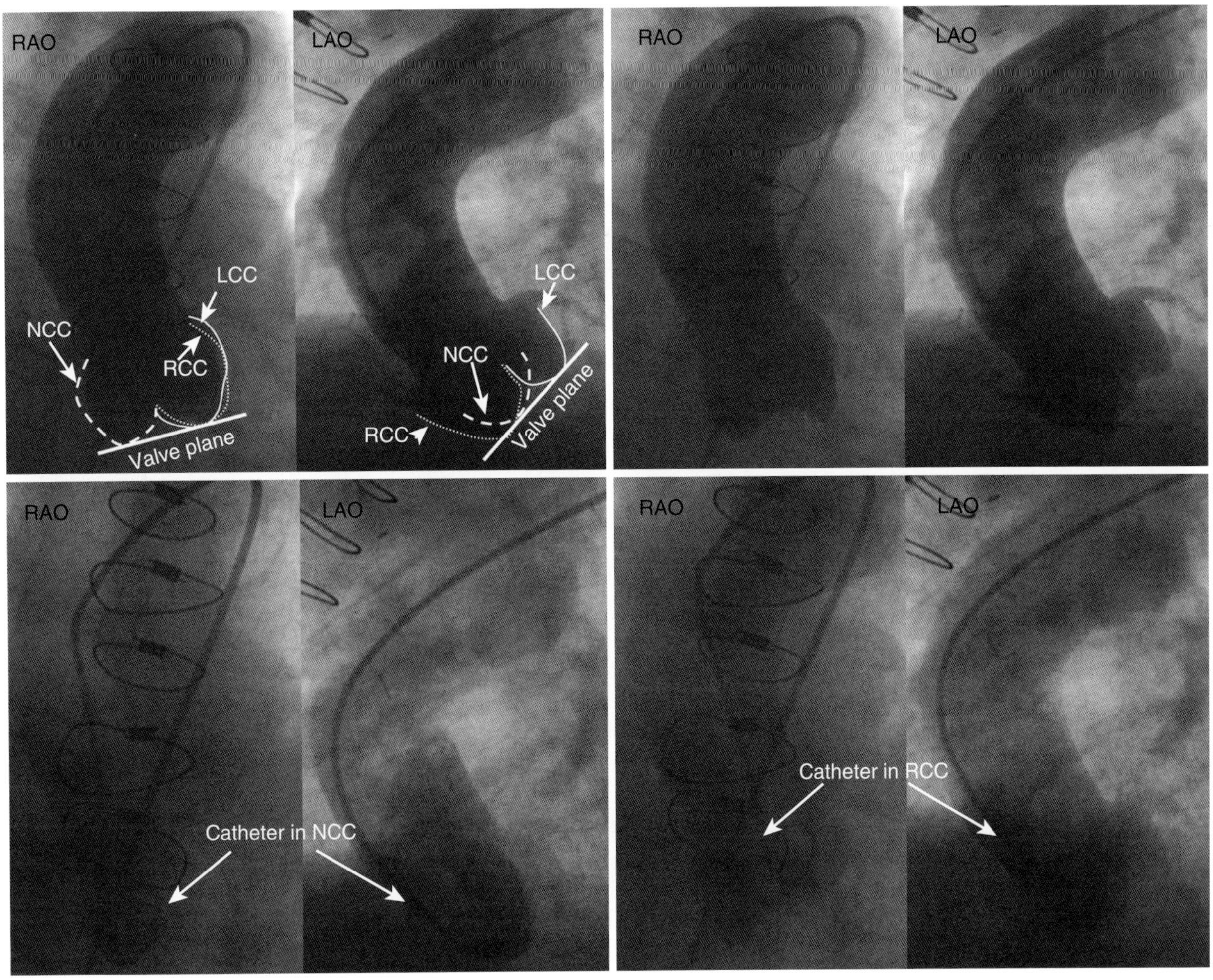

Fig. 48.27 Left anterior oblique *(LAO)* cranial "40/20 degree" and right anterior oblique *(RAO)* caudal "20/20 degree" views of the aortic valve and its plane. The proper angulation of the camera has to be customized in each patient so that the all cusps are superimposed. Note that catheter is in different sinuses in different phases of injection. *LCC*, Left coronary cusp; *NCC*, noncoronary cusp; *RCC*, right coronary cusp.

the aide of 2D and 3D TEE, ICE, fluoroscopy/angiography, and more recently the combination of CT and fluoroscopy. The mitral valve is viewed as a clockface and leak origin defined by the position on the clock (Fig. 48.30) from the LA, or "surgeon's" view. The most common locations for mitral PVL are anteromedial (between 10 and 11 o'clock) and posterolateral (between 5 and 6 o'clock).[30] When using TEE, localizing the PVL requires reconstruction of the virtual clock face with multiple imaging planes. Fig. 48.31C, demonstrates the clock-face orientation of the MV as viewed from the left ventricle, which is also the position of the MV in the typical LAO C-arm angulation. The 90-degree TEE view demonstrates the leak origin (see Fig. 48.31A), which is confirmed by the 134-degree view (see Fig. 48.31B), with both views showing the PVL origin at approximately 11 o'clock. Similarly, the aortic valve can also be referenced as a clockface, as shown in Fig. 48.30. Aortic PVLs are most commonly encountered at the 7 to 11 o'clock position (46%), followed by the 11 to 3 o'clock position (36%).[30,31] An alternative designation is to identify the origin of the PVL with respect to the native cusp location (i.e., RCC, LCC, and NCC). The short-axis view of the aortic valve, either by TTE or TEE, is usually the most helpful in defining the leak with respect to the cusps (Fig. 48.32). When closure of the PVL is attempted, the location of the PVL on TEE and markings are made on a preprocedural noncontrast CT (see Fig. 48.32).

A CT-like image using the catheterization laboratory's C-arm (Syngo DynaCT Cardiac, Siemens Healthcare, Forcheim, Germany) is used to establish the position of the patient on the table, and landmarks are used to register the preprocedural CT to the "rotational" DynaCT. The overlay is then fused with the real-fluoroscopic image to provide a dynamic, integrated record of the location of the PVL in relation to the mitral or aortic valve (see Fig. 48.32). Provision of these stenciled "targets" allows optimal guidance for wires and interventional devices. In addition, we use ICE for puncture of the IAS, as well as initial wire/catheter guidance if the PVL is well seen (Fig. 48.33). In general, we place the TEE probe after crossing the leak with a wire (if possible) to minimize the duration of TEE intubation in patients who are usually under conscious sedation alone (without endotracheal intubation or general anesthesia). In lateral mitral PVL, the ICE catheter situated in the right atrium is inadequate to provide appropriate procedural guidance. In addition to ICE imaging, a TEE image is used for wire/catheter guidance, evaluation of procedural success and the need for additional closure devices due to residual PVL, and assessment of complications, such as valve impingement by the device.

Transcatheter Mitral Valve replacement

Transcatheter mitral valve replacement (TMVR) is an emerging technique that is on the cutting edge of structural transcatheter interventions and holds significant promise for the future. The mitral valve is a dynamic, variable, and complex structure. Mitral valve geometry changes during each cardiac cycle, and loading conditions, volume status, and numerous other factors result

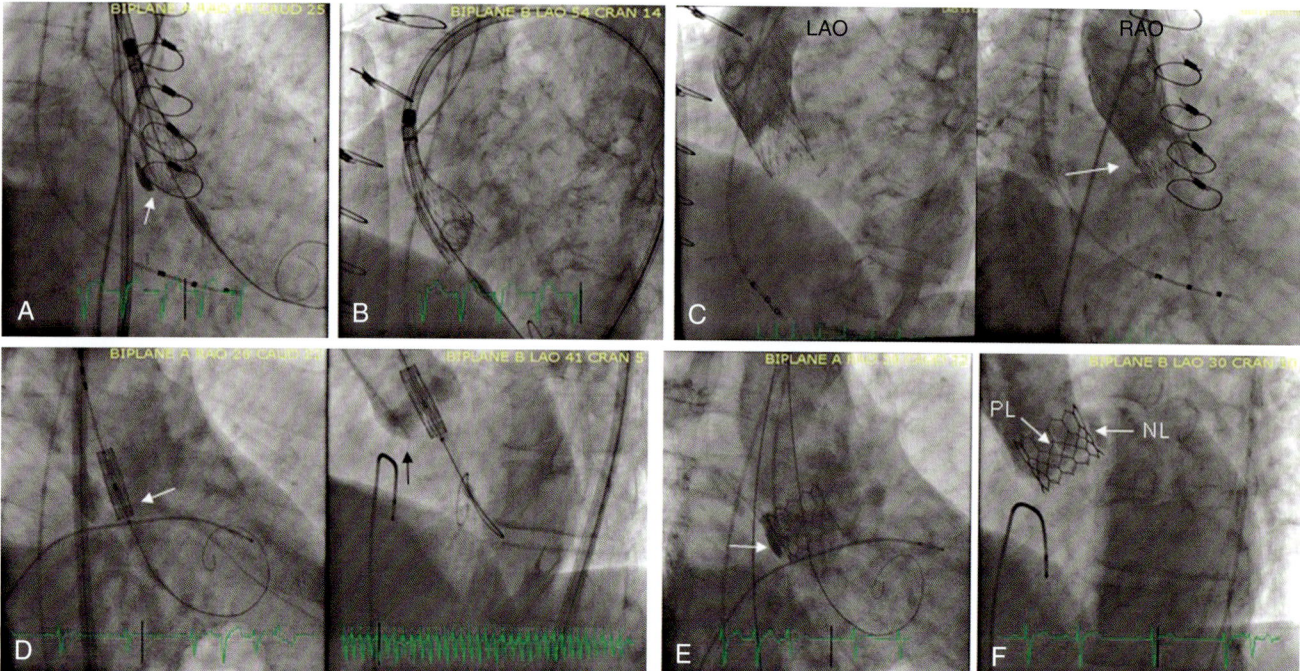

Fig. 48.28 Percutaneous aortic valve replacement. (A) Corevalve positioning in the left ventricular outflow tract. Contrast injection into the noncoronary cusp via a straight flush catheter *(arrow)* is used to delineate the ideal position for valve placement (B). Corevalve being unsheathed (C). Corevalve fully deployed in the aortic root appears clearly supravalvular on aortography with native coronary sinus seen as well *(arrow)* in left anterior oblique *(LAO)* (left) and right anterior oblique *(RAO; right)*. (D) Edwards Sapien S3 valve being positioned in the left ventricular outflow tract—optimization of fluoroscopy to create a straight line *(white arrow)* along the collapsed valve stent and alignment with noncoronary cusp (opacified by injection via straight flush catheter, *black arrow*) facilitates optimal positioning. (E) Fully deployed Edwards Sapien S3 valve with optimal positioning; the noncoronary cusp is opacified *(arrow)*. (F) Final aortogram postdeployment of Edwards Sapien S3 valve showing native leaflet *(NL)*, prosthesis leaflets *(PL)*, and slightly supravalvular deployment of Edwards Sapien S3 valve.

in variations in mitral annulus geometry in the short and long term, highlighting the dynamic nature of mitral valve anatomy. Significant interpatient variability in annular and subvalvular geometry exists, further complicating the standardization of transcatheter mitral interventions. Mitral valve interventions have inherently lower margins for error than equivalent procedures at the aortic position, owing to the multitude of nearby structures that could be compromised by inappropriate positioning or sizing of devices, including pulmonary veins, LAA, papillary muscles, left ventricular apex and outflow tracts, and the aortic valve. For the provided reasons, preprocedural and intraprocedural imaging is of vital importance to obtaining a successful result without complications.

In regard to preprocedural planning, 4D gated cardiac CT imaging is most commonly used. The determination of mitral annular size is vital to appropriate device selection. The mitral annulus is composed of the anterior horn, which is contiguous with the aortomitral curtain, and posterior horn, which is formed by basal insertion of the posterior mitral leaflet. The medial and lateral trigones form the nadirs, with the medial trigone being contiguous with the interventricular septum. The mitral annulus is a D-shaped structure, with the flat segment of the "D" formed by truncation of the anterior horn at the annular plane, connecting the medial and lateral trigones (Fig. 48.34A). The sizing of the annulus is complex but reproducible, and accurate techniques have been established by Leipsic and colleagues involving manual tracking of the insertion of the posterior leaflet and fibrous anterior continuity (anterior horn) along LV long axis and truncation of the anterior leaflet at the intertrigonal plane, as seen in Fig. 48.34B.[32] The landing zone for TMVR is also carefully evaluated to identify the presence of an LV basal shelf or mitral annular calcification that may affect valve sealing resulting in PVL development. Risk stratification for development of postprocedural LVOT obstruction can also be performed via CT with the presence of steep aortomitral angle (>70 degrees), septal bulge, small LV cavity, small neo LVOT cross-sectional area (<2 cm^2), or elongated anterior MV leaflet conferring increased risk (see Fig. 48.34C).[33] CT is also useful for determining the optimal apical access site (intercostal space), delivery system, and fluoroscopy angulation to permit coaxial deployment of the prosthesis.

Intraprocedural Guidance During TMVR Is Largely Dependent on TEE and Fluoroscopy at Present

Transapical access can be visualized by TEE in the midesophageal two-chamber view. As an example, images of the deployment of a Tendyne valve (Tendyne System, Roseville, MN) have been included in this chapter. Once the guidewire is freely advanced into the LA under TEE and fluoroscopic guidance, the valve delivery system can be advanced across the mitral valve (Fig. 48.35A). The X-plane can be used to center the valve in the AP dimension, while en face 3D TEE can be used to ensure that the delivery system is in the A2 to P2 plane prior to device unsheathing (see Fig. 48.35B). The en face (LA view) 3D TEE view is useful to rotate D-shaped valves so the flat surface is aligned with the aortomitral curtain. Under fluoroscopic and TEE guidance (X-plane or 2D TEE in midesophageal two- or four-chamber view), the valve is unsheathed and appropriate seating is confirmed (see Fig. 48.35C and E). TEE also permits detection of PVLs and baseline transvalvular gradients (see Fig. 48.35D).

CHAPTER 48 Imaging for Intracardiac Interventions

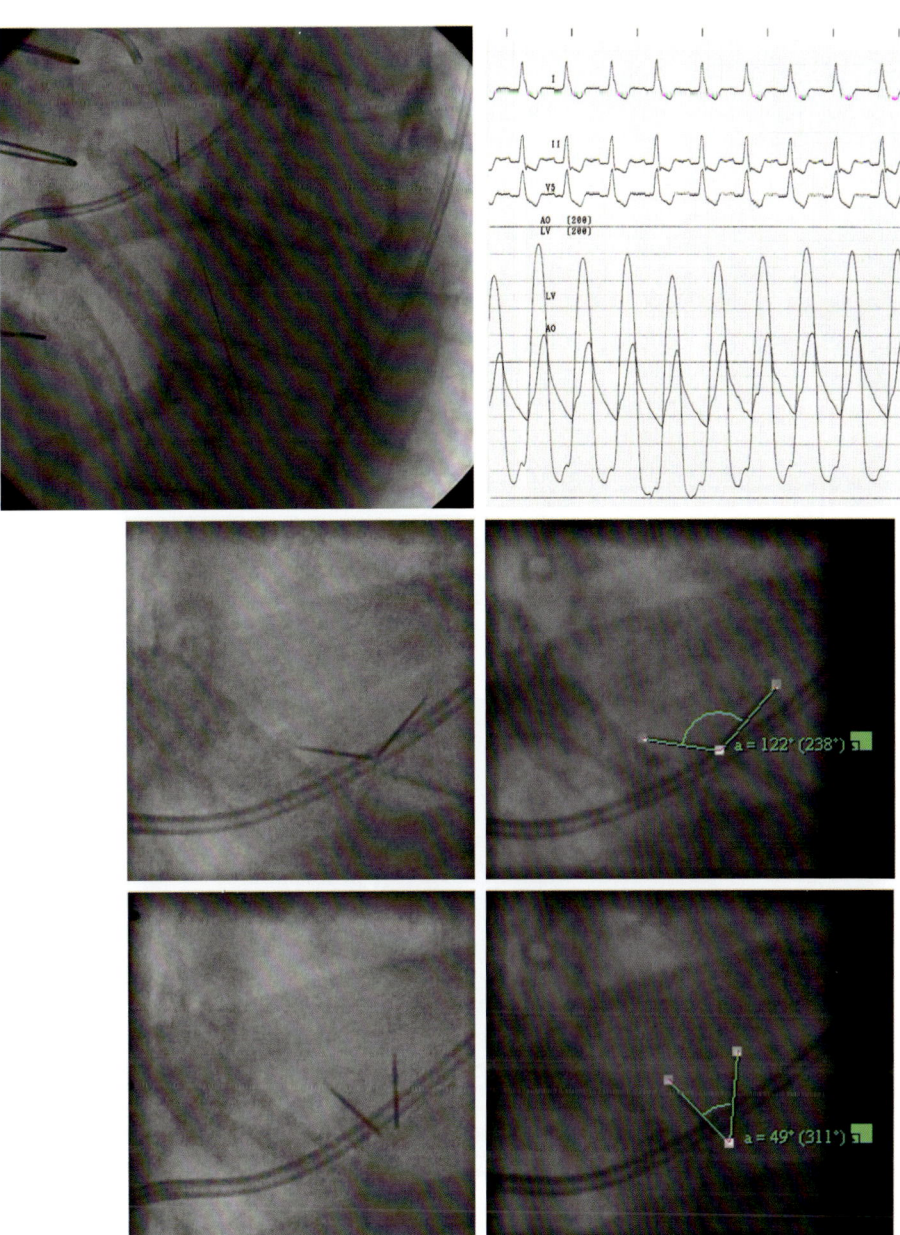

Fig. 48.29 This figure shows prosthetic aortic valve (AV) assessment using fluoroscopy. This valve was crossed with 0.014-inch pressure wire. Hemodynamic tracings show significant gradient across AV. Opening and closing angles are measured in lower panel. Note that valve is imaged so that the leaflets are seen end-on.

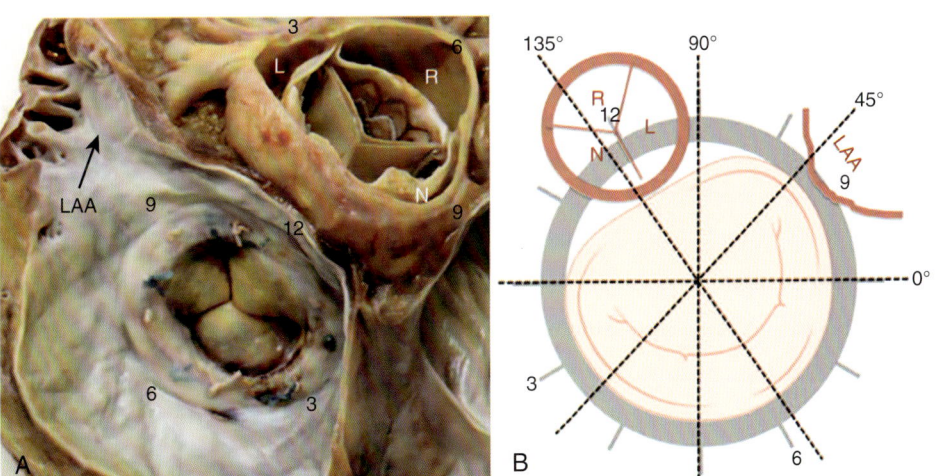

Fig. 48.30 Mitral valve orientation. (A) Clock-face designation of the mitral and aortic valves *(left atrial view)*. (B) Transesophageal echocardiography planes *(dashed lines)* along the mitral valve (viewed from the left ventricle); typical left anterior oblique C-arm angulation. *L*, Left coronary cusp; *LAA*, left atrial appendage; *N*, noncoronary cusp; *R*, right coronary cusp.

897

SECTION V Structural Interventions

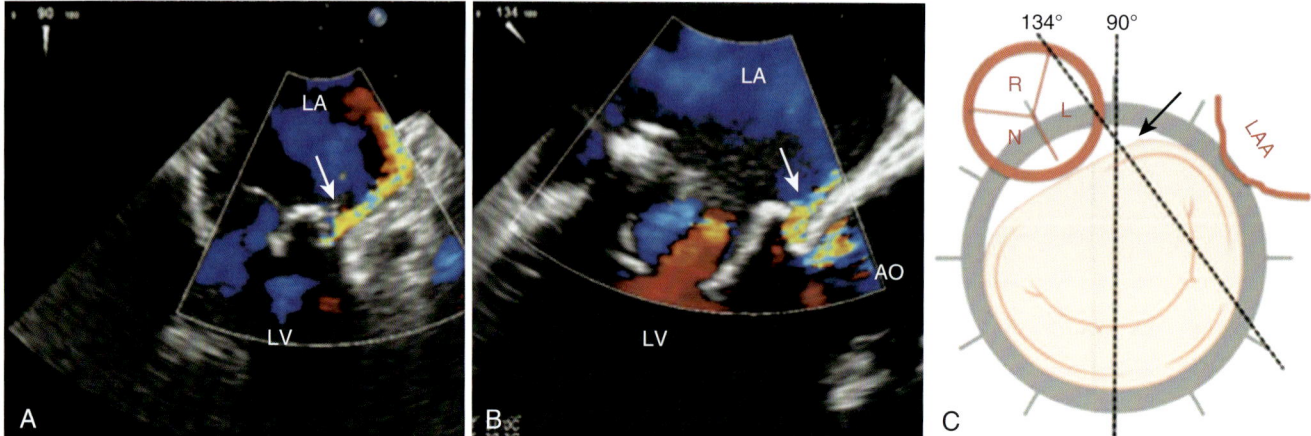

Fig. 48.31 Transesophageal echocardiography (TEE) localization of mitral paravalvular leak. (A) TEE 90-degree view demonstrates leak *(arrow)*. (B) TEE 134-degree view also demonstrates the leak. (C) The two TEE planes interrogating the MV: leak is at the intersection *(arrow)*. *AO*, Aorta; *LA*, left atrium; *LAA*, left atrial appendage; *LV*, left ventricle; *MV*, mitral valve; *TEE*, transesophageal echocardiography.

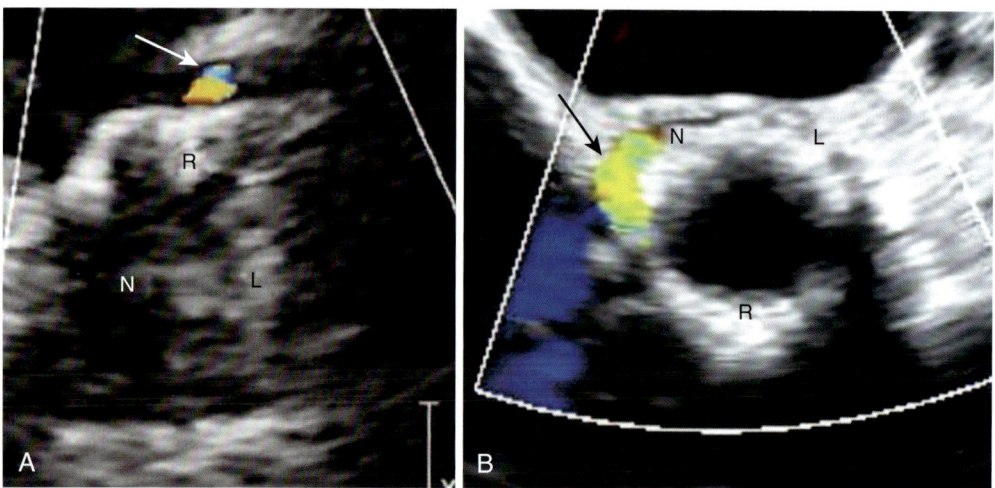

Fig. 48.32 Aortic paravalvular leak localization. (A) Transthoracic echocardiogram in the parasternal short-axis view shows the leak at the native right coronary cusp *(R)*. (B) Transesophageal echocardiogram in the short-axis view (45 degrees) shows the leak at the noncoronary *(N)* cusp. *L*, Native left coronary cusp.

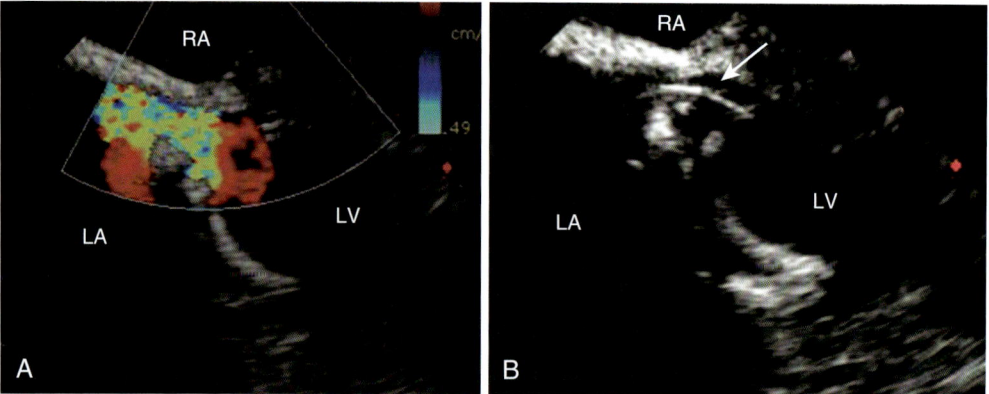

Fig. 48.33 Use of intracardiac echocardiography to guide mitral paravalvular leak closure. (A) Color-flow Doppler demonstration of the leak. (B) Wire across the leak *(arrow)*. *LA*, Left atrium; *LV*, left ventricle; *RA*, right atrium.

898

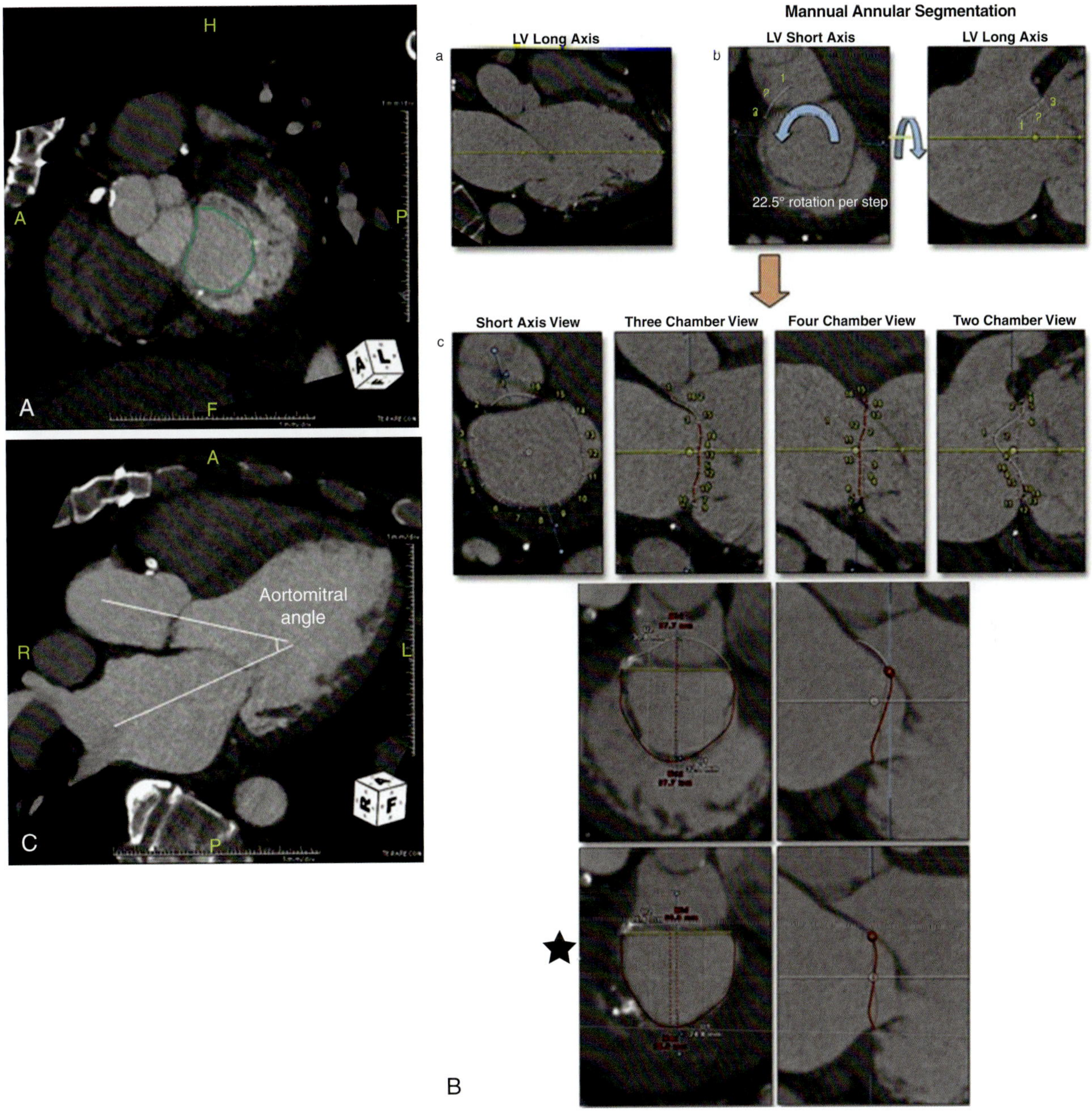

Fig. 48.34 The D-shaped mitral annulus on 4D multidetector computed tomography (CT) imaging outlined in green (A). The measurement of mitral valve annulus by CT using manual plotting of insertion of posterior mitral leaflet and anterior fibrous continuity along left ventricle *(LV)* long axis yields a saddle shaped annulus. Truncation of the annular perimeter in the intertrigonal plane *(yellow line* on starred image) yields a D-shaped annulus (B). Aortomitral angle as assessed by 4D multidetector CT (C). (B, From Blanke P, Dvir D, Cheung A, et al. Mitral annular evaluation with CT in the context of transcatheter mitral valve replacement. *JACC Cardiovasc Imaging.* 2015;8[5]:612–615.)

Transcatheter Tricuspid Valve Repair and Replacement

The tricuspid valve provides unique challenges in regard to catheter-based therapies, owing to its large orifice and annulus and interpatient variability in regard to annulus shape. Tricuspid regurgitation (TR) is the most common form of valve dysfunction, and severe TR is typically associated with right ventricle dilation, resulting in tricuspid annular dilation and eventual restriction of the TV leaflets, creating a self-propagating cycle of worsening valvular incompetence. Currently, multiple technologies are under development for native transcatheter tricuspid valve intervention that focus on one of three pathologic processes: annulus reduction (Mitralign device, Mitralign, Inc. Tewksbury, MA; TriCinch system, 4Tech Cardio Ltd., Galway, Ireland), improvement in leaflet coaptation (Forma device, Edwards Lifesciences, Irvine, CA; MitraClip, Abbott Laboratories, Abbott Park, IL), or reduction in preload by placement of stented valves in the IVC (Sapien valve, Edwards Lifesciences, Irvine, CA). Balloon expandable valves such as the Edwards Sapien S3 valve have deployed within previously placed degenerated tricuspid prostheses or dysfunctional valvuloplasty rings with encouraging outcomes.[34] The GATE tricuspid atrioventricular stent (Navigate Cardiac Structures Inc., Lake Forest, CA) is a valved stent designed for

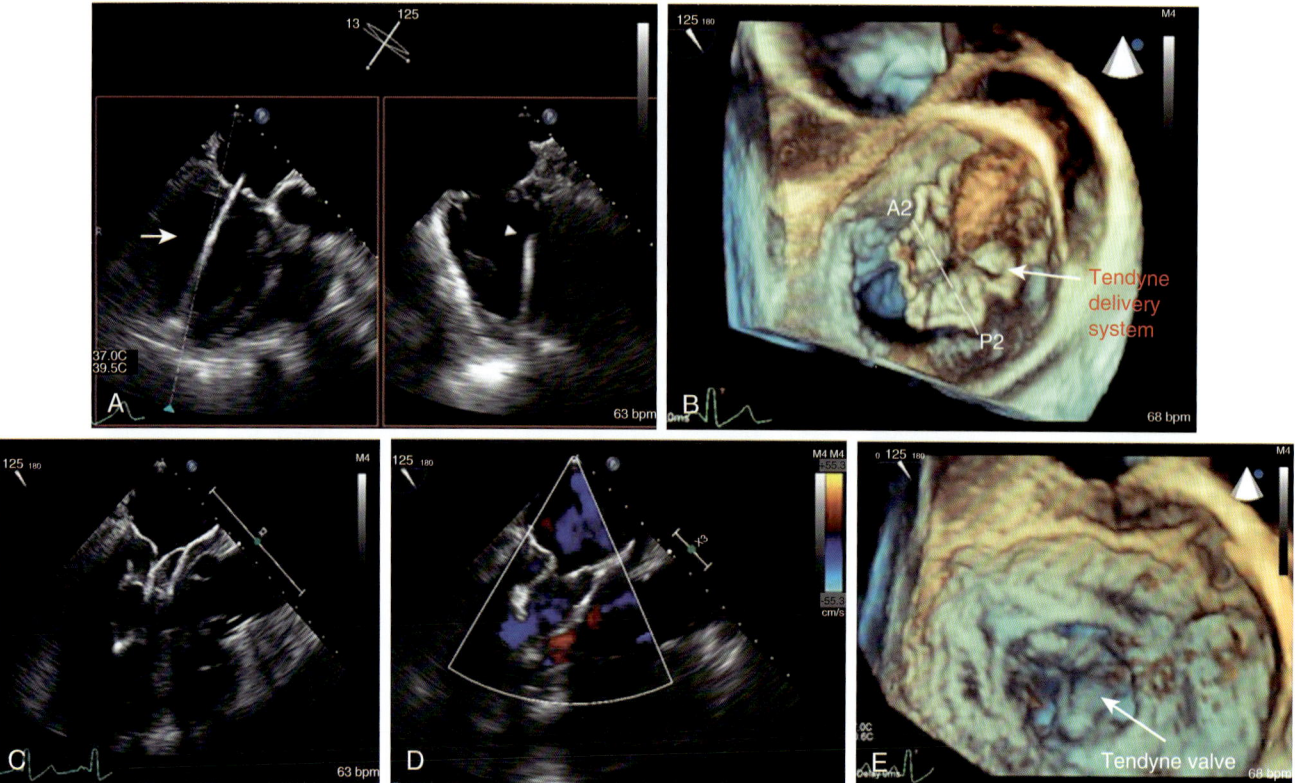

Fig. 48.35 A guidewire *(arrow)* is seen across the mitral valve from apical access (A). Tendyne valve centered between A2 and P2 prior with partially unsheathed valve (B). Deployed valve seen by 2D transesophageal echocardiography (TEE) in long-axis (125-degree) midesophageal view (C). No residual mitral regurgitation or paravalvular leak seen by color-flow Doppler (D). 3D TEE view from left atrial perspective showing well-seated Tendyne valve (E). *A2*, Anterior leaflet, segment 2; *P2*, posterior leaflet, segment 2.

transcatheter tricuspid valve repair and replacement (TTVR) of the native TV via internal jugular (percutaneous) or transatrial (minimally invasive) approach, with first-in-human deployment successfully completed in 2016 in the United States.[35]

Accurate tricuspid annulus sizing is critical to successful transcatheter tricuspid valve replacement and is typically performed using 4D MDCT imaging. Given that transcatheter tricuspid interventions are in the early stages of clinical use, there is no consensus on optimal imaging technique for the tricuspid valve. CT-based imaging is used to size the tricuspid annulus and assess its geometry, evaluate the relationship between the tricuspid annulus and right coronary artery (RCA) to determine risk of RCA impingement with tricuspid annular manipulation, to determine anatomic relationship of the right ventricle apex to the tricuspid annulus for placement of spacer devices, and to assess the inferior vena cava dimensions for placement of transcatheter valves.[36] Intraprocedural imaging for tricuspid valve interventions typically involves the use of ICE, TEE, and fluoroscopy. To illustrate the utility of each modality, the deployment of the GATE atrioventricular valve stent (NaviGate Cardiac Structures Inc., Lake Forest, CA) device is illustrated in Fig. 48.36. TEE can be used intraprocedurally to document baseline TR in midesophageal 0-degree view, which shows the right atrium, TV, and right ventricle clearly (see Fig. 48.36A). The delivery system is advanced across the tricuspid annulus under fluoroscopy and TEE guidance (see Fig. 48.36B). Right coronary artery angiography can be utilized to delineate the atrioventricular groove to further assist in centering the valve between the right atrium and ventricle. Intracardiac echo provides detailed imaging of TV annulus in the low atrial horizontal view (see Fig. 48.12, *bottom right panel*), and this view can be used to ensure adequate positioning and seating of the GATE AVS device (see Fig. 48.36C). Three-dimensional TEE can also be used to visualize the device delivery system across to the TV (see Fig. 48.36D and E). Once the positioning has been optimized, the device is deployed. Postdeployment imaging is obtained with fluoroscopy, ICE, and 2D/3D TEE to confirm proper positioning and color-flow Doppler evaluation is performed to evaluate for paravalvular TR (Fig. 48.37).

SUMMARY

The realm of imaging in intracardiac interventions is a wide topic and not all the procedures are covered in this chapter, but this chapter serves as a framework for understanding the different modalities available and their respective roles during these procedures. Multimodality imaging serves as the starting point for appropriate patient selection, ruling out complications, and postprocedural follow-up. The ideal choice of an imaging modality is based on the type of intervention, local expertise, operator familiarity, training, and financial constraints. With the increasing complexity of structural interventions and rapid advances and increased affordability in CT, MRI, and hybrid imaging technologies with fluoroscopic registration, high-quality real-time multimodality imaging is becoming integral for intraprocedural success and safety.

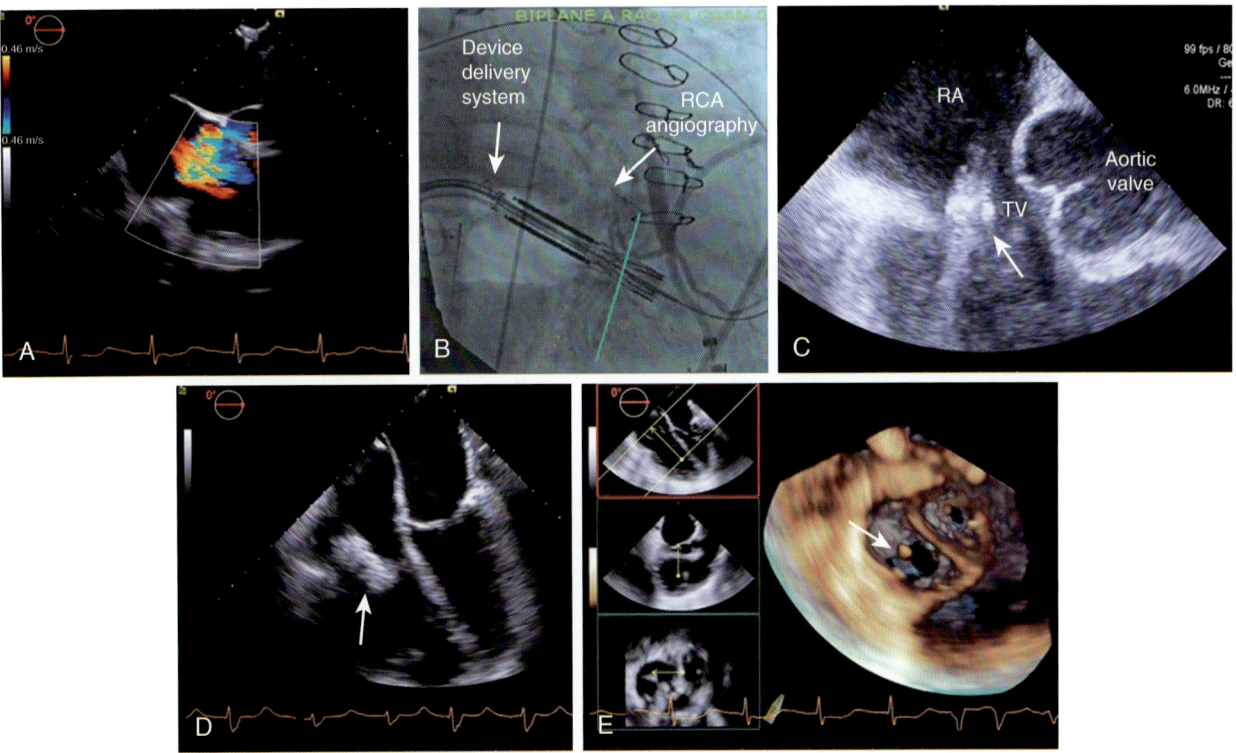

Fig. 48.36 Baseline tricuspid regurgitation evaluation by color-flow Doppler on transesophageal echocardiography (TEE) (A). Advancement of Navigate delivery system across tricuspid valve *(TV)* with fluoroscopy with RCA angiogram and TEE guidance (B). GATE AVS delivery system across TV on intracardiac echocardiography imaging; *arrow* showing device (C). 2D TEE showing device across the tricuspid valve; *arrow* showing device (D). 3D TEE image showing device across the tricuspid valve; *arrow* showing device (E). *green line*, Atrioventricular groove; *AVS*, atrioventricular valve stent; *RA*, Right atrium; *RCA*, right coronary artery.

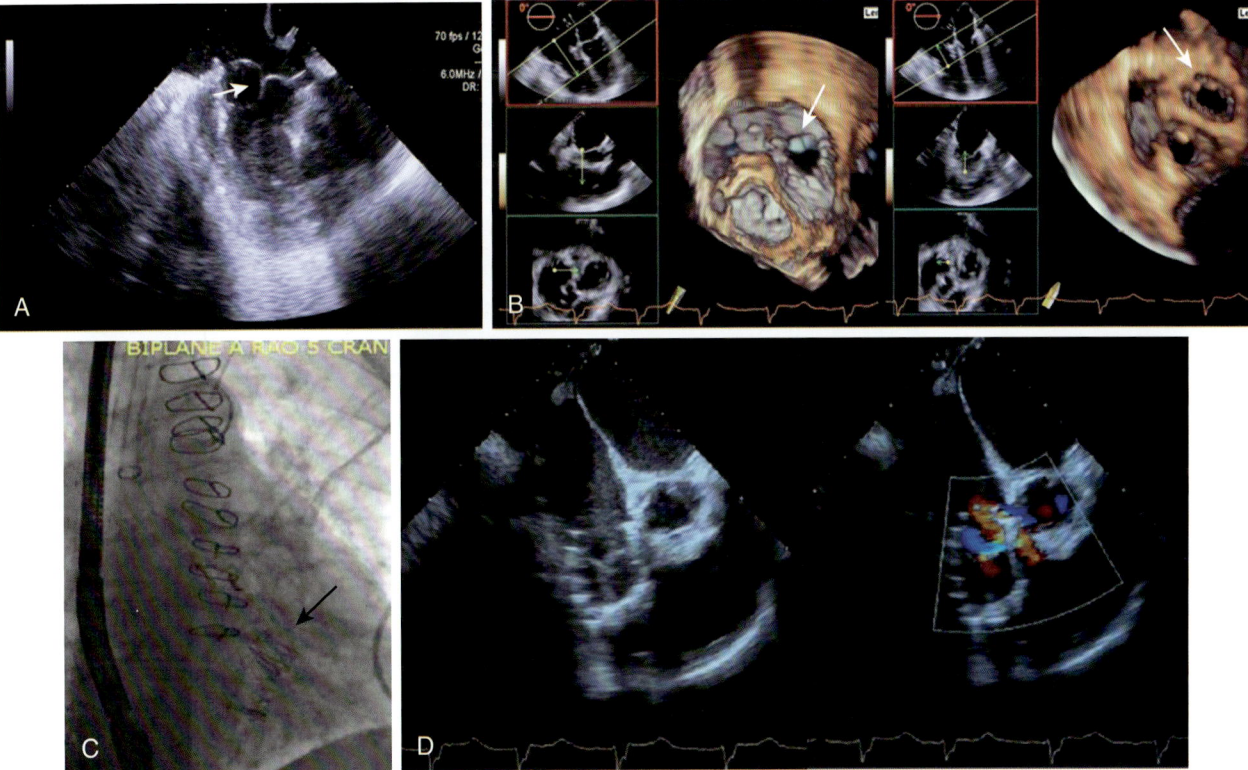

Fig. 48.37 Deployed GATE AVS device seen on intracardiac echocardiography in low atrial view, *arrow* shows device (A). 3D transesophageal echocardiography (TEE) from atrial *(left)* and ventricular view *(right)* showing well seated GATE AVS device, *arrow* shows device (B). Fluoroscopy showing deployed GATE AVS device, *arrow* shows device (C), 2D TEE with color flow showing mild-moderate paravalvular leak (D). *AVS*, Atrioventricular valve stent.

KEY REFERENCES

3. Kapadia SR, Tuzcu EM. Accurate procedural assessment of AR—critical for successful TAVI. *EuroIntervention*. 2016;11(10):1088–1091.
9. Krishnaswamy A, Tuzcu EM, Kapadia SR. Integration of MDCT and fluoroscopy using C-arm computed tomography to guide structural cardiac interventions in the cardiac catheterization laboratory. *Catheter Cardiovasc Interv*. 2015;85(1):139–147.
16. Salomé N, Braga P, Gonçalves M, et al. Transcatheter device occlusion of atrial septal defects and patent foramen ovale under intracardiac echocardiographic guidance. *Rev Port Cardiol*. 2004;23(5):709–717.
19. Nucifora G, Faletra FF, Regoli F, et al. Evaluation of the left atrial appendage with real-time 3-dimensional transesophageal echocardiography: implications for catheter-based left atrial appendage closure. *Circ Cardiovasc Imaging*. 2011;4(5):514–523.
21. Wang Y, Di Biase L, Horton RP, et al. Left atrial appendage studied by computed tomography to help planning for appendage closure device placement. *J Cardiovasc Electrophysiol*. 2010;21(9):973–982.
22. Krishnaswamy A, Patel NS, Ozkan A, et al. Planning left atrial appendage occlusion using cardiac multidetector computed tomography. *Int J Cardiol*. 2012;158(2):313–317.
24. Roberts JW, Lima JA. Role of echocardiography in mitral commissurotomy with the Inoue balloon. *Cathet Cardiovasc Diagn*. 1994;(suppl 2):69–75.
27. Shively BK. Transesophageal echocardiographic (TEE) evaluation of the aortic valve, left ventricular outflow tract, and pulmonic valve. *Cardiol Clin*. 2000;18(4):711–729. http://www.ncbi.nlm.nih.gov/pubmed/11236162.
31. Krishnaswamy A, Kapadia SR, Tuzcu EM. Percutaneous paravalvular leak closure- imaging, techniques and outcomes. *Circ J*. 2013;77(1):19–27.
33. Naoum C, Blanke P, Cavalcante JL, et al. Cardiac computed tomography and magnetic resonance imaging in the evaluation of mitral and tricuspid valve disease: implications for transcatheter interventions. *Circ Cardiovasc Imaging*. 2017;10(3):e005331.
35. Navia JL, Kapadia S, Elgharably H, et al. First-in-Human Implantations of the NaviGate Bioprosthesis in a Severely Dilated Tricuspid Annulus and in a Failed Tricuspid Annuloplasty Ring. *Circ Cardiovasc Interv*. 2017;10(12):e005840.
36. van Rosendael PJ, Kamperidis V, Kong WKF, et al. Computed tomography for planning transcatheter tricuspid valve therapy. *Eur Heart J*. 2016;38(9):ehw499.

Additional references available online at expertconsult.com.

中文导读

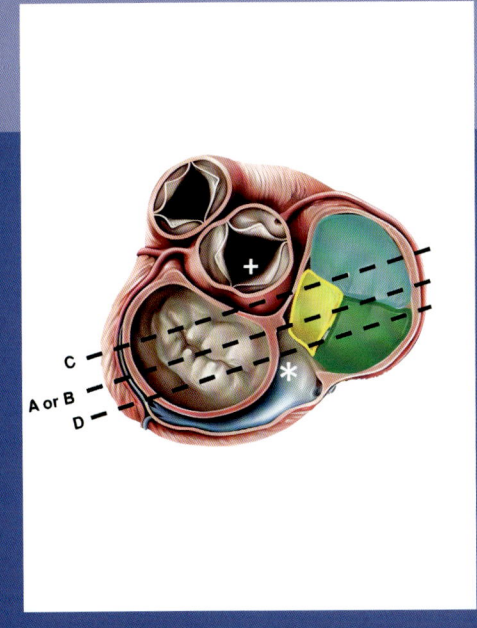

第49章
卵圆孔未闭及房间隔缺损的经皮封堵治疗

　　卵圆孔未闭和房间隔缺损是常见的先天性心脏病类型，二者都会导致左右心房间的分流，但病因并不完全相同。卵圆孔未闭在普通成年人群中检出率为25%左右，其发生率不受性别、种族影响。其被证实与反常性栓塞、不明原因的卒中、偏头痛、减压病，以及直立性低氧血症相关。房间隔缺损患者通常直到儿童期仍无症状，部分患者可能出现反复的心力衰竭，儿童期出现反复的呼吸道感染，容易乏力及活动后气短等。在成年后，持续的房间隔缺损伴随分流量较大时，患者可能出现房性心律失常、肺动脉高压及心力衰竭。介入封堵治疗是临床中治疗卵圆孔未闭和房间隔缺损的常用手段。在卵圆孔未闭中，其被用于减少卒中发生率，但目前关于其效果的数据仍在争议。由于部分房间隔缺损会自行愈合，介入封堵治疗常推荐在患者4~5岁时进行，对于成年患者，封堵的指征包括右心扩大、反常性栓塞，以及直立性低氧血症等。本章节详细介绍了两种疾病的病理生理机制，临床表现，介入封堵治疗的指征，操作详情等，内容夯实。尽管由于解剖的变异，部分患者需要更先进的装置来实现成功的封堵治疗，但总体来说，经皮封堵房间隔缺损或卵圆孔未闭都是非常安全的操作。

丰德京　张洪亮

章节要点

- 卵圆孔未闭和房间隔缺损都会导致左右心房间的分流,但二者的病因并不相同。卵圆孔未闭是由于胚胎时期原发隔和继发隔之间未完全融合导致,而房间隔缺损则是由于房间隔发育过程中部分缺失导致。
- 卵圆孔未闭被证实与反常性栓塞、不明原因的卒中、偏头痛、减压病及直立性低氧血症综合征相关。
- 尽管目前的数据支持卵圆孔未闭封堵治疗以预防复发性缺血性脑血管事件,但仍存在争议。
- 由于部分房间隔缺损会自行愈合,因此,在患者4~5岁时行房间隔缺损封堵治疗是推荐的,但如果成年时期才诊断出房间隔缺损,封堵的指征包括右心扩大、反常性栓塞,以及直立性低氧血症综合征等。
- 尽管由于解剖的变异,部分患者需要更先进的装置来实现成功的封堵治疗,但总体来说,经皮封堵房间隔缺损或卵圆孔未闭都是非常安全的操作。

49 Percutaneous Closure of Patent Foramen Ovale and Atrial Septal Defect

Nishtha Sodhi, Alan Zajarias, David T. Balzer, John M. Lasala

KEY POINTS

- Although patent foramen ovale (PFO) and atrial septal defect (ASD) both involve an abnormal communication across the interatrial septum, their causes are different. PFO results from lack of fusion between the septum primum and the septum secundum, whereas a secundum ASD is caused by the absence of a segment of the atrial septum.
- PFO has been associated with paradoxical embolization, cryptogenic stroke, migraine headache, decompression sickness, and platypnea-orthodeoxia syndrome.
- The role of PFO closure for recurrent ischemic cerebrovascular events is supported with recently published data, but remains controversial.
- Elective closure of ASDs by 4 to 5 years of age is usually recommended, but if undetected until adulthood, indications for closure include right heart enlargement, paradoxical embolism, and platypnea-orthodeoxia syndrome.
- Anatomic variations may require advanced closure techniques for successful closure, but in general, percutaneous closure of a PFO or a secundum ASD is a technically straightforward and safe procedure.

INTRODUCTION

Atrial septal defects (ASDs) are some of the most common congenital cardiac anomalies. The first surgical repair of an ASD occurred in 1952. Nearly 25 years later, in 1976, King and Mills reported the first percutaneous ASD closure in five patients using a double-umbrella device.[1,2] The early successes were followed by use of the Rashkind device and subsequently the Lock Clamshell Occluder in the late 1980s.[3,4] Refinements in percutaneous interventional technology and advances in cardiac imaging techniques have largely swayed contemporary management of ASDs to the cardiac catheterization lab. Patent foramen ovale (PFO), which had been rarely treated surgically, despite its known association with paradoxical embolism, is also now considered for percutaneous closure.

This chapter describes the embryology, pathophysiology, and clinical associations of these anatomic defects, followed by a technical description of the procedure, its indications, complications, and the relevant data.

PATENT FORAMEN OVALE

Embryology

PFO is a remnant of the fetal circulation. By day 18 of gestation, the primordium of the heart becomes evident. At the end of the fourth week, the endocardial cushions fuse to form the right and left atrioventricular canals. The endocardial cushions serve as the primordium of the atrioventricular valves and the inferior wall of the atrium.

At this time, the common atrium undergoes a process of septation. The *septum primum* grows caudally toward the endocardial cushions, closing the interatrial communication (*ostium primum*). As the septum primum reaches its destination, the cells in its superior portion undergo apoptosis and coalesce to form the *ostium secundum*. A muscular *septum secundum* forms to the right of the septum primum and extends to reach the caudal border of the ostium secundum, forming a flaplike valve between both atria (Fig. 49.1 and Video 49.1).[5]

Oxygenated placental blood enters the right atrium from the inferior vena cava (IVC) and is directed toward the interatrial septum (IAS) by the eustachian valve. The low left atrial pressure, the lack of blood flow through the pulmonary veins, and the preferential flow of the IVC to the IAS allow oxygenated blood to cross the foramen ovale and enter the systemic circulation. Blood entering the right atrium from the superior vena cava (SVC) is directed away from the IAS by the *crista interveniens*, preventing the mixture of nonoxygenated blood in this chamber. The right horn of the *sinus venosus* incorporates the SVC and IVC into the right atrium (Video 49.2).

At birth, the pulmonary vascular resistances and the right cardiac pressures fall, and the left atrial pressure increases, forcing the *septum primum* against the *septum secundum* and occluding the valvelike foramen ovale. Complete occlusion occurs in most of the population, but in approximately 25%, the fusion is incomplete, giving rise to a PFO (Video 49.3).[6]

Incidence

The echocardiographic estimate for the incidence of PFO in the adult population is approximately 25%.[6] Autopsy studies revealed probe-patent PFOs of 0.2 to 0.5 cm in 29%.[7] The frequency of PFO decreases with age, but the size of the defect increases with each decade of life.[8] The incidence rate of PFO is equal for both genders and among all ethnic groups; however, PFOs in whites and Hispanics are more prevalent and are associated with a greater degree of shunting.[9] Spontaneous PFO closure may occur during adulthood, although data suggest that PFOs may recanalize over time.[10]

PFO was thought to be an inconsequential finding until 1877, when Cohnheim postulated that a venous thrombosis might paradoxically traverse a foramen ovale and produce a systemic embolism.[11-14] Since then, PFOs have been associated with various disease processes, including cryptogenic stroke, paradoxical embolization, platypnea orthodeoxia syndrome, hypoxemia with

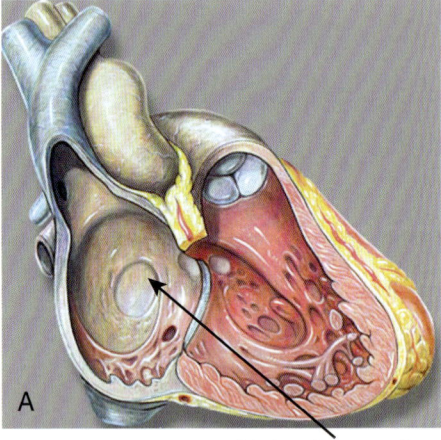

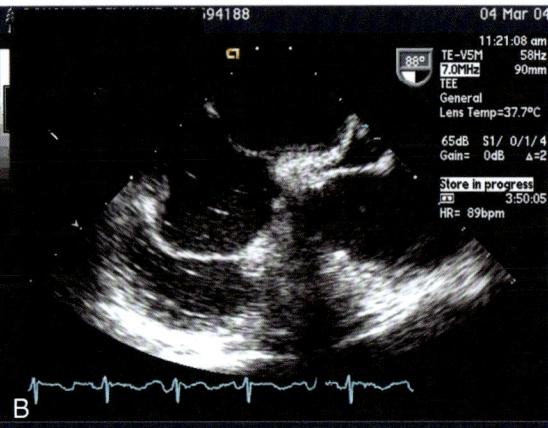

Fig. 49.1 Diagram (A) and sonogram (B) of the interatrial septum depict the limbus of the fossa ovalis and the anatomic location of the patent foramen ovale.

TABLE 49.1 Evaluation of Cryptogenic Stroke

Condition	Diagnostic Test
Cerebrovascular disease	Carotid Doppler, magnetic resonance angiography
Cardiac source of embolism (in specific patient populations as per the updated 2018 AHA/ASA Guidelines)	
Left atrial appendage thrombus	Transesophageal echocardiogram
Left ventricular aneurysm	Transthoracic or transesophageal echocardiogram
Ascending aorta atheroma	Transesophageal echocardiogram
Paroxysmal atrial fibrillation	Holter monitor
Hypercoagulable state	Protein C and S activity Antithrombin III level Lupus anticoagulant Anticardiolipin antibody Factor V Leiden Prothrombin 20210A mutation

AHA, American Heart Association; *ASA*, American Stroke Association.

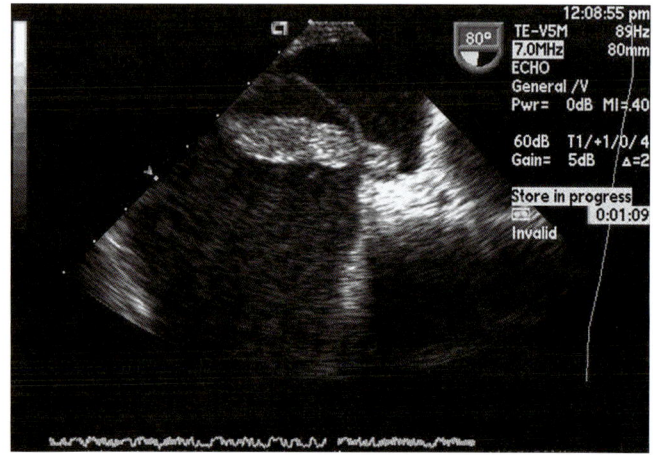

Fig. 49.2 The thrombus in transit from the right atrium through a patent foramen ovale into the left atrium illustrates the concept of paradoxical embolization.

normal pulmonary pressures, decompression sickness (DCS) in scuba divers and high-altitude pilots, and migraine headaches.[15–20]

Cryptogenic Stroke

The cause of cerebrovascular accidents (CVAs) varies among age groups. Atrial fibrillation and small vessel disease contribute to most strokes in patients older than 50 years. Among patients younger than 35 years, the most common causes include nonatherosclerotic arteriopathies, arterial dissection, and thromboembolism.[10] However, in 35% to 40% of patients with CVAs, the causes remain unknown, even after a thorough evaluation. Such CVAs are classified as *cryptogenic* and are largely a diagnosis of exclusion.

Evaluation includes: a hypercoagulable evaluation, heart rhythm evaluation, and carotid doppler (Table 49.1). In the 2018 updated American Heart Association/American Stroke Association (AHA/ASA) guidelines, routine use of echocardiography in all patients presenting with acute ischemic stroke to plan subsequent secondary preventive treatment is deemed not cost-effective and is not recommended (class III; Level of Evidence [LOE] B-NR).[21,22]

The search for the probable causes of cryptogenic strokes has implicated PFOs. In a retrospective case-control study, PFOs were four times more prevalent among young adults who experienced a stroke without an identifiable cause compared with others with known causes.[16] In a prospective trial of 503 patients, Handke and colleagues showed that PFOs were more frequent among patients experiencing cryptogenic strokes irrespective of age (<55 years: 43.9% vs. 14.3%, odds ratio [OR] = 4.70, $P < .001$; >55 years: 28.3% vs. 11.9%, OR = 2.92, $P < .001$).[23] More recently, preoperative PFO was found to be significantly associated with increased risk of perioperative ischemic stroke within 30 days of noncardiac surgery (Ng et al.). Among patients with cryptogenic strokes, patients with PFOs were less likely to have traditional cardiovascular risk factors such as hypertension, hypercholesterolemia, and tobacco use.[24]

Proposed mechanisms for PFO-associated cryptogenic strokes include in situ thrombosis, paradoxical embolization, and predisposition to atrial arrhythmias.[25] Paradoxical embolization (i.e., passage of a venous thrombus into the systemic circulation through a PFO) has been the predominant theory (Fig. 49.2 and Video 49.4). Evidence that supports the role of PFOs in cryptogenic strokes includes case reports of the transit of thrombi across PFOs, cerebral distribution of cryptogenic CVAs that suggests an embolic nature, and the increased frequency of deep venous thrombosis in patients who had cryptogenic CVAs.[26–28]

The Paradoxical Embolism from Large Veins in Ischemic Stroke (PELVIS) trial found an increased frequency of positive magnetic resonance venography testing for pelvic thrombus in patients with PFOs and cryptogenic CVAs compared with patients with known causes (20% vs. 4%, $P < .03$).[29]

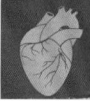

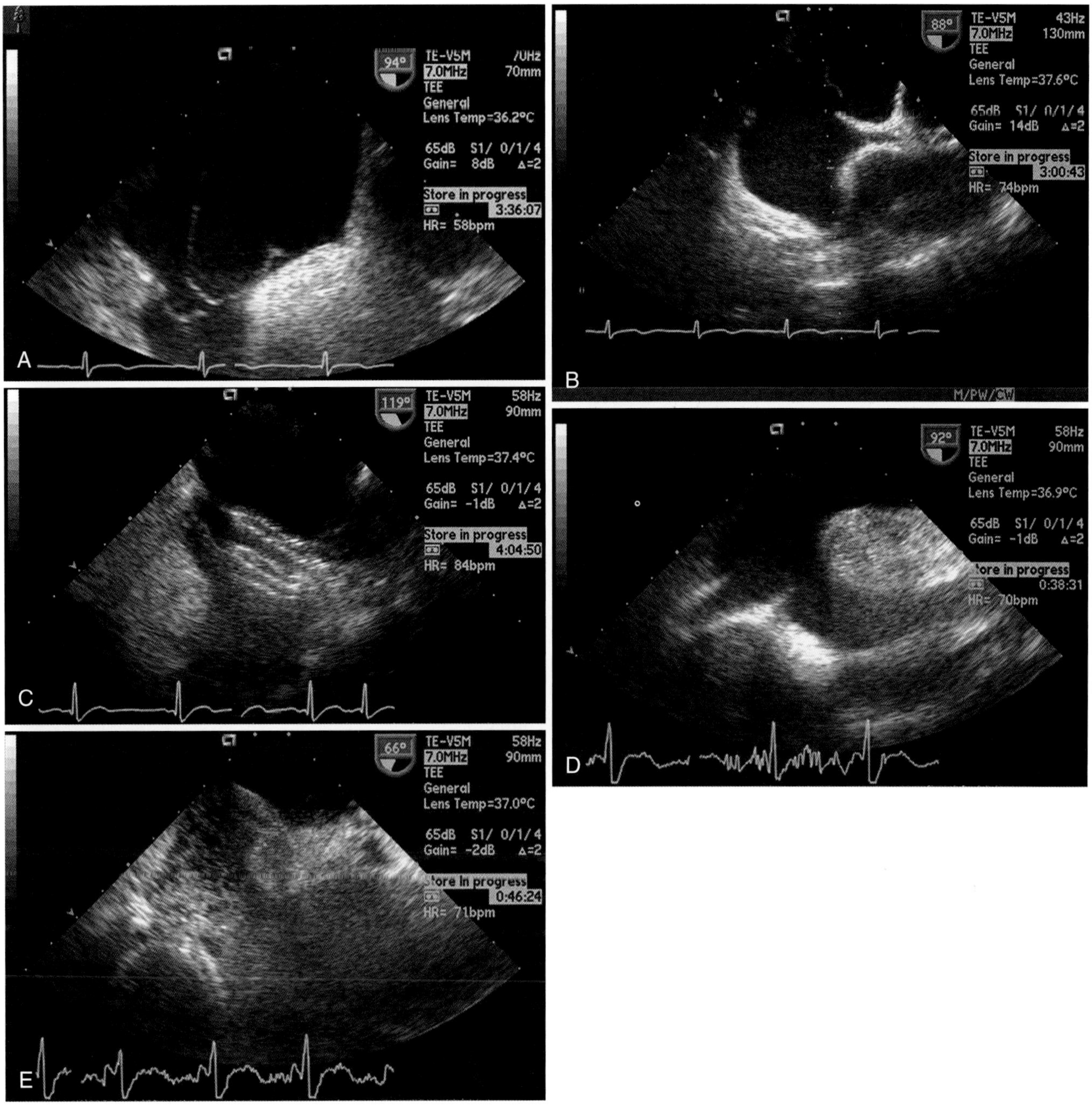

Fig. 49.3 Transesophageal echocardiogram in the bicaval view (90 degrees) identifies right atrial cardiac structures that may increase the degree of right-to-left shunt across a patent foramen ovale (PFO) or may complicate the closure procedure. (A) Prominent eustachian valve. (B) Atrial septal aneurysm. (C) A 25-mm AGA foramen occluder (AGA Medical, Plymouth, MN) successfully captures the septum secundum and primum closing the PFO. (D and E) Lipomatous hypertrophy of the atrial septum also creates a challenge in placing the closure device. Immediately after device deployment, the saline contrast study is mildly positive.

These data underline the causative role of paradoxical embolization in patients who had cryptogenic strokes.

Stroke Recurrence and Risk Identification

The reported recurrence rate of cryptogenic stroke varies from 1.2% to more than 16%, but usually is about 2%.[30,31] Retrospective studies have found the risk of recurrence to be related to PFO size, patency at rest, shunt severity, and the presence of atrial septal aneurysm (ASA).[32–34] A prominent eustachian valve has been associated with increased patency of the foramen ovale and the risk of stroke recurrence because it preferentially directs blood flow to the IAS (Fig. 49.3 and Video 49.5).[35] It has been postulated that a mobile IAS may increase the size of the foramen ovale, facilitating the passage of thrombi. Recurrences of cryptogenic CVAs have been associated with the degree of septal protrusion. Patients with a septum excursion greater than 6.5 mm had a risk of recurrence of 12.3% compared with 4.3% for controls at 3 years.[30] Finally, the combination of ASA and PFO was associated with an increased risk of recurrence in a French PFO/ASA study (hazard ratio [HR] = 4.17; 95% confidence interval [CI] 1.47 to 11.84).[36]

TABLE 49.2 RoPE Score Calculator: An Index to Assess the Statistical Attributability of Cryptogenic Stroke to Patent Foramen Ovale Has Been Developed (ROPE Score)

Characteristic	Points	RoPE score
No history of hypertension	1	
No history of diabetes	1	
No history of stroke or TIA	1	
Nonsmoker	1	
Cortical infarct on imaging	1	
Age, years		
18–29	5	
30–39	4	
40–49	3	
50–59	2	
60–69	1	
≥70	0	
Total score (sum of individual points)		
Maximum score (a patient <30 years with no hypertension, no diabetes, no history of stroke or TIA, nonsmoker, and cortical infarct)		10
Minimum score (a patient ≥70 years with hypertension, diabetes, prior stroke, current smoker, and no cortical infarct)		0

RoPE, Risk of Paradoxical Embolism; *TIA*, transient ischemic attack.

An index to assess the statistical attributability of cryptogenic stroke to PFO has been developed (RoPE Score), with emerging work correlating severity of right to left shunting by contrast transcranial doppler (Table 49.2).

Treatment of Cryptogenic Stroke

Medical Treatment

Medical treatment with aspirin or oral anticoagulants has traditionally been utilized with mixed results on efficacy against recurrent neurologic events. In the French PFO/ASA study, 267 patients who experienced cryptogenic strokes and had PFOs only or PFOs with ASAs were treated with aspirin or with aspirin and warfarin if they had a venous thrombosis.[36] After 4 years of follow-up, there were 12 episodes of recurrent strokes and 9 recurrent transient ischemic attacks (TIAs). All episodes occurred in patients treated with aspirin alone.

The PFO in Cryptogenic Stroke Study (PICSS) was the only prospective, blinded, randomized trial that compared the efficacy of aspirin versus oral anticoagulation in patients with CVAs.[37] It found no statistically significant difference in stroke recurrence between patients with PFOs treated with aspirin and those treated with warfarin (17.9% vs. 9.5%; HR = 0.52; 95% CI 0.16 to 1.67; $P = .28$). Furthermore, the incidence of recurrent stroke in PFO patients with ischemic stroke was high: 14.8% at 2 years.[38]

The 2014 AHA/ASA guidelines state that for patients with an ischemic stroke or TIA and a PFO who are not undergoing anticoagulation therapy, antiplatelet therapy is recommended (class I; LOE B). For patients with an ischemic stroke or TIA and both a PFO and a venous source of embolism, anticoagulation is indicated, depending on stroke characteristics (class I; LOE A). When anticoagulation is contraindicated, an IVC filter is reasonable (class IIa; LOE C). The updated 2018 AHA/ASA guidelines do not suggest superiority of either antiplatelet or anticoagulation management in cryptogenic stroke in PFO patients.

Surgical Treatment

Surgical closure of PFOs in patients who had cryptogenic strokes has been reported. The largest series included 91 consecutive patients with a mean age of 44 years and one prior CVA. Surgery was evaluated with intraoperative transesophageal echocardiography (TEE), and suture or patch closure was employed. Closure was achieved in 98% of cases, and the actuarial freedom from recurrence was 93% at 1 year and 83% at 4 years. The surgical procedure was associated with significant morbidity in 21%.[39] Smaller series reflected similar closure rates and significant morbidity.

Percutaneous Treatment

Despite medical therapy, the stroke recurrence rate in ischemic stroke patients with PFO is estimated at 4.5% within a 4-year period.[38] Thus secondary preventive treatment, such as percutaneous closure, in addition to medical therapy has been a topic of debate.[40–45] Prior to 2017, three multicenter, randomized, controlled trials (RCTs) comparing PFO closure for recurrent cryptogenic stroke with medical therapy (CLOSURE I, PC, and RESPECT) had largely negative results, showing no statistically significant benefit of PFO closure over medical therapy for ischemic stroke recurrence. In addition, there was a significantly higher incidence of atrial fibrillation development in the patients who received the STARFlex closure device (Fig. 49.4), but not the AMPLATZER PFO Occluder, compared with medication.

Based on these three RCTs, the 2014 AHA/ASA guidelines did not recommend PFO closure in cryptogenic stroke (class III, LOE A). However, in the setting of PFO and deep vein thrombosis (DVT), PFO closure by a transcatheter device might be considered, depending on the risk of recurrent DVT (class IIb; LOE C). The American Academy of Neurology discouraged routine PFO closure in cryptogenic stroke patients outside of research trials until July 2016, when an updated statement was issued criticizing its use altogether. However, in September 2017, three trials with positive results were published (Fig. 49.5).

CLOSURE 1 (evaluation of the STARFlex septal closure system in patients with a stroke or TIA due to presumed paroxysmal embolism through the PFO) evaluated PFO closure with the CardioSeal and STARFlex septal occluders (see Fig. 49.4) compared with aspirin or warfarin, or both, in 909 patients 18 to 60 years old with a cryptogenic CVA or TIA during the 6 months before enrollment. Over a 2-year follow-up, the composite end point of CVA or TIA, all-cause death at 30 days, and death from neurologic causes between 31 and 730 days was similar among groups: 5.5% versus 6.8% for closure compared with antiplatelet or anticoagulant therapy (HR = 0.78; 95% CI 0.45 to 1.35; $P = .37$).

The PC trial (Patent Foramen Ovale and Cryptogenic Embolism) compared PFO closure using the Amplatzer PFO occluder with medical therapy (i.e., at least one antiplatelet or anticoagulant drug) in 414 patients aged younger than 60 years with a history of cryptogenic stroke, TIA, or peripheral embolism and documented PFO. The composite end point of death, nonfatal stroke, TIA, or peripheral embolism was similar for the groups (3.4% vs. 5.2%; HR = 0.63; 95% CI 0.24 to 1.62; $P = .34$).

The RESPECT trial (Randomized Evaluation of Recurrent Stroke Comparing PFO Closure to Established Standard of Care Treatment) compared PFO closure using the Amplatzer PFO occluder with antiplatelet or anticoagulation therapy (i.e., aspirin, warfarin, clopidogrel, aspirin plus dipyridamole, or aspirin plus clopidogrel) in 980 patients followed over a mean of 2.6 years. Although the primary end point was negative by intention-to-treat analysis (recurrent CVA for closure: 1.8% vs. 3.4% for antiplatelet/anticoagulant therapy; HR = 0.49; 95% CI 0.22 to 1.11; $P = .08$), three patients randomized to device closure had a stroke before receiving the device. The as-treated cohort analysis showed a positive trend favoring the device closure cohort (1.1% vs. 3.3%; HR = 0.27; 95% CI 0.10 to 0.75; $P = .007$), and the

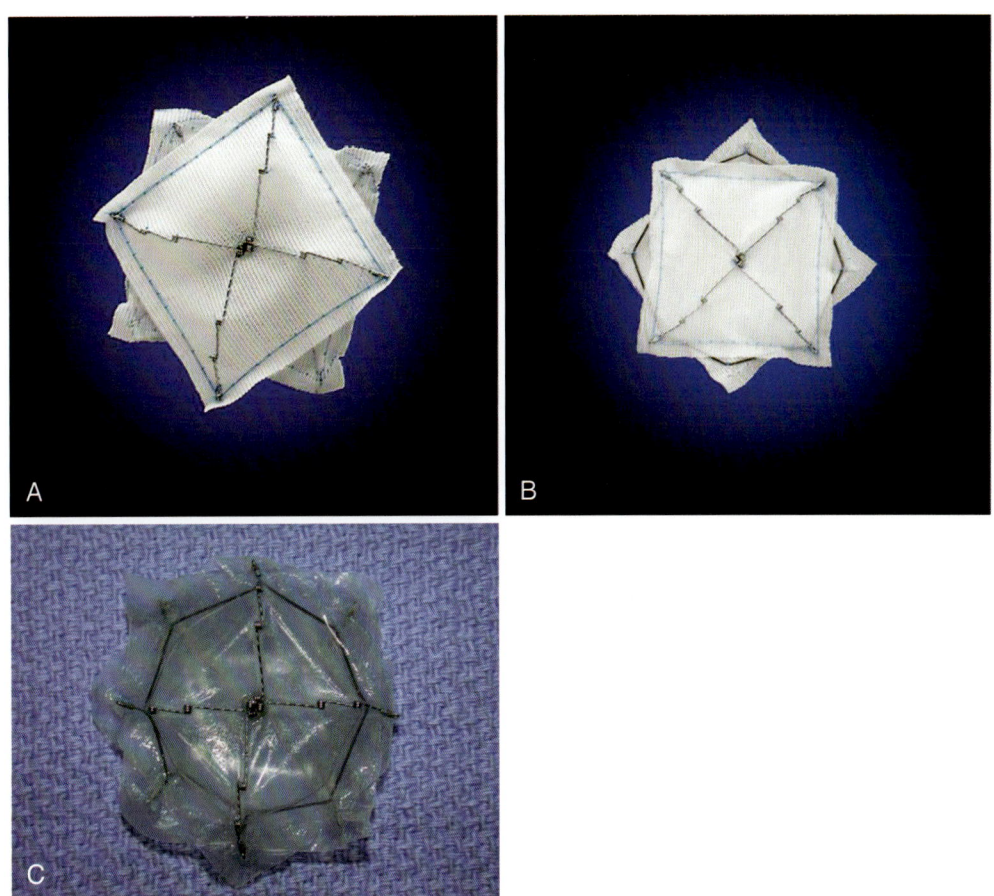

Fig. 49.4 Photographs of the CardioSeal (A), STARFlex (B), and BioSTAR (C) septal occluders. These devices are no longer available. (Courtesy NMT Medical, Boston, MA.)

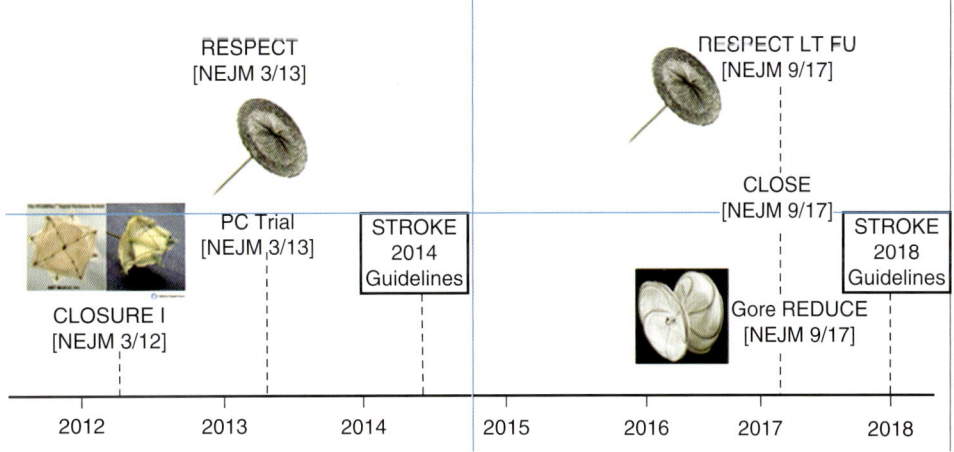

Fig. 49.5 Evolution of clinical trials, device development, and guidelines for transcatheter patent foramen ovale closure. *CLOSURE 1,* Evaluation of the STARFlex Septal Closure System in Patients with a Stroke and/or Transient Ischemic Attack due to Presumed Paradoxical Embolism through a Patent Foramen Ovale; *LT FU,* long-term follow-up; *NEJM;* New England Journal of Medicne; *RESPECT,* Randomized Evaluation of Recurrent Stroke Comparing PFO Closure to Established Current Standard of Care Treatment; *PC trial,* Comparing Percutaneous Closure of Patent Foramen Ovale (PFO) Using the Amplatzer PFO Occluder with Medical Treatment in Patients with Cryptogenic Embolism. (Courtesy Mustafa Husaini MD.)

per-protocol cohort analysis favored transcatheter closure (1.3% vs. 3%; HR = 0.37; 95% CI 0.14 to 0.96; P = .03). The subset analysis favored device closure for PFO with associated ASAs.

The final long-term results of RESPECT showed that after 10 years, in an intention-to-treat analysis, PFO closure with the AMPLATZER PFO Occluder resulted in a 62% relative risk reduction (RRR) for recurrent ischemic stroke compared with medical management (HR 0.38; 95% CI 0.18 to 0.79; 10-year event rates 2.3% vs. 11.1 %; P = .007). The rates of atrial fibrillation, major bleeding, and death from any cause were comparable or lower in the device study arm.[38]

The GORE HELEX Septal Occluder/GORE CARDIO-FORM Septal Occluder for PFO Closure in Stroke Patients (REDUCE) trial[46] demonstrated that through at least 2 years,

PFO closure with the GORE HELEX or GORE CARDIOFORM (both W.L. Gore & Associates) septal occluder plus antiplatelet therapy was superior to antiplatelet treatment alone in reducing the risk of recurrent (77% RRR; HR 0.23; 95% CI 0.09 to 0.62) and new clinical ischemic stroke or in silent brain infarct on MRI (49% RRR; HR 0.51; 95% CI 0.29 to 0.91).[38]

The Patent Foramen Ovale Closure or Anticoagulants Versus Antiplatelet Therapy to Prevent Stroke Recurrence (CLOSE)[47] study was a multicenter randomized superiority trial, comparing transcatheter PFO closure plus antiplatelet therapy to antiplatelet therapy alone for the prevention of recurrent stroke in patients aged 16 to 60 years who had a recent cryptogenic ischemic stroke attributed to PFO with an associated ASA or large right-to-left shunt.[38] Recurrent fatal or nonfatal stroke was significantly reduced in the PFO closure group as compared with the antiplatelet therapy alone group (97% RR; HR 0.03; 95% CI 0.00 to 0.26; $P < .001$).

In both REDUCE and CLOSE, a higher incidence of atrial fibrillation was detected, but this was largely periprocedural and transient. The 2018 American College of Cardiology (ACC)/AHA Guidelines do not clearly support or disprove transcatheter closure, citing potential biases for the recent data.

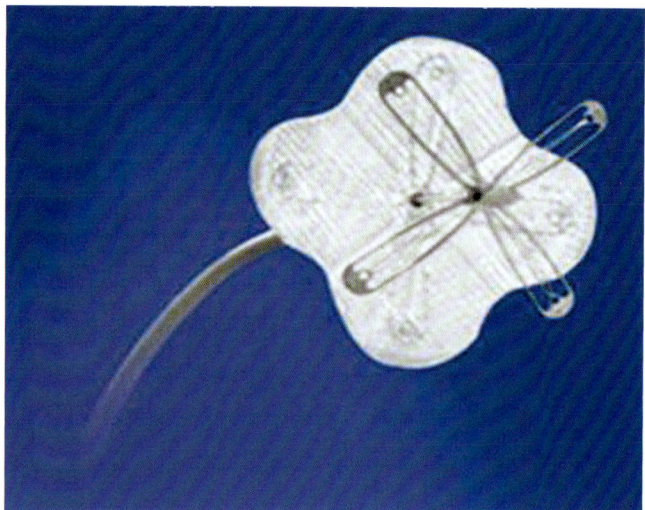

Fig. 49.6 Photograph of the St Jude's patent foramen ovale occluding system. (Courtesy St. Jude's Medical, St. Paul, MN.)

Related Disorders

Migraine Headache

PFO is present in up to 60% of migraine patients, and up to 50% of patients with PFO suffer from migraines. Retrospective analysis of patients who underwent PFO closure for cryptogenic strokes revealed a decrease in the frequency of attacks of migraine with aura in 80% or even complete resolution in 56%.[48,49] Other studies have demonstrated that after a 12-month follow-up, the frequency and intensity of the migraine attacks were significantly decreased in patients who underwent PFO closure.[50] These observational studies, however, are largely masked by three randomized controlled trials that do not suggest PFO closure for migraines is warranted.

The Migraine Intervention with STARFlex Technology (MIST) trial[51] tested the association between PFOs and migraine headaches with aura. It was a multicenter, blinded study that randomized 432 patients with migraine to PFO closure with a STARFlex Septal Repair (NMT Medical, Boston, MA) implant or a sham procedure. The primary end point of cessation of migraines was not met. However, reduction in headache days in at least 50% occurred more frequently in the PFO closure group (42% vs. 23%, $P = .038$).[51] The MIST II trial (evaluated PFO closure to treat migraine with aura; sponsored by NMT Medical, Boston, MA) and the ESCAPE trial (Effect of Septal Closure of Atrial PFO on Events of Migraine with the PFO Occlusion Device [Fig. 49.6]; sponsored by St. Jude Medical Corp., Fullerton, CA) have been discontinued because of slow enrollment. The Percutaneous Closure of Patent Foramen Ovale in Patients with Migraine (PREMIUM) trial (evaluating use of the Amplatzer PFO occluder; sponsored by AGA Medical, Golden Valley, MN) also demonstrated negative results with no difference in responder rate, defined by reduction in migraine attacks.[52] Based on these data, PFO closure for primary prevention of migraines is not recommended.[53–58]

Platypnea-Orthodeoxia Syndrome and Hypoxia

PFO has been associated with the rare platypnea-orthodeoxia syndrome. It is postulated that right-to-left shunting occurs across a patent foramen, particularly in the setting of an ASA.

Platypnea-orthodeoxia syndrome is seen primarily in very old patients and is associated with an event that alters the geometry of intrathoracic organs, such as a pneumonectomy or an enlarged ascending aorta. Extrinsic compression of the right atrium or decreased compliance of the right ventricle may also predispose to shunting at the atrial level in these patients.[59] It is postulated that in patients with an elongated aorta, the heart is shifted laterally so that the IVC drains directly toward the atrial septum, although this is not fully understood. This anatomic shift maintains the PFO open throughout the cardiac cycle and generates the physical findings.[60]

The diagnosis of platypnea-orthodeoxia syndrome is made by using saline contrast echocardiography with the patient in the supine and seated positions.[11] Surgical or percutaneous closure has been done successfully, leading to marked improvement in the patient's symptoms.[61,62] The 2008 ACC/AHA guidelines for the management of adults with congenital heart disease have a class IIa, LOE B indication for reasonable closure of an atrial septal defect, either percutaneously or surgically, in the presence of documented platypnea-orthodeoxia.

Hypoxia related to PFOs may be observed in patients with severe pulmonary hypertension or obstructive sleep apnea.[63] The mechanism involves transient or persistent elevation of the right atrial pressure in relation to the left atrial pressure or redirection of the IVC blood flow toward the IAS. Hypoxia related to right-to-left shunting at the atrial level has been associated with pulmonary arteriovenous malformations, liver disease, amiodarone toxicity, pulmonary emboli[64] with transient pulmonary hypertension, positive-pressure ventilation, hypovolemia, aortic aneurysm, right ventricular infarction, Ebstein anomaly, and carcinoid valve disease.

Making the diagnosis may be challenging because it requires documentation of right-to-left shunting while the patient is hypoxic, and frank improvement occurs after closure. In patients with severe pulmonary hypertension with decreased right ventricular function, the PFO serves as an escape valve, which aids emptying of the right atrium into a lower pressure circuit (i.e., left atrium). In these patients, PFO closure may be fatal.

Decompression Sickness

DCS is caused by nitrogen bubbles that come out of solution in blood as the ambient pressure decreases when a person ascends from a dive. The amount of nitrogen bubbles generated depends on the total time spent in the dive, the speed of ascent, compliance with decompression stops, and individual factors such as cardiac output. The nitrogen bubbles usually stay in the venous circulation and make it to the lungs, where they are rapidly diffused. In a person with a PFO, the nitrogen bubbles may enter the systemic circulation and travel superiorly toward the brain, occluding a small arterial branch.[65-67]

DCS in patients with PFOs is associated with early onset of cerebral or vestibular symptoms, which occurs within 30 minutes after a dive, even after the person has performed all the appropriate rest stops.[68] Accordingly, professional divers or military personnel may undergo screening for PFO with a bubble contrast transthoracic echocardiography (TTE) or TEE study.[38] The presence of a PFO is considered a contraindication to diving. PFO closure is not recommended in this scenario. Recreational scuba divers may choose to undergo screening for the presence of a PFO at their own discretion.[38]

Diagnosis of Patent Foramen Ovale

Echocardiography plays an important role in the diagnosis of abnormalities of the atrial septum. Traditionally, TEE has been considered the gold standard to diagnose a PFO. The advantage of TEE is that it can identify all portions of the IAS, enabling the diagnosis of all subtypes of ASDs, fenestrated atrial septum, and PFOs. TEE also allows detailed identification of lipomatous hypertrophy of the septum, ASAs, a prominent eustachian valve, or a long PFO tunnel that may alter a planned closing procedure (Video 49.6; see Fig. 49.3).

TEE can identify other potential sources of embolization (e.g., left atrial appendage thrombus, cardiac tumors, aortic atheroma). An ASA is defined as a redundancy of the atrial septum with excursion greater than 10 mm into either of the atria and a 15-mm base. The degree and direction of the interatrial shunt depend on the net pressure difference between the atria. The interatrial shunt direction changes with the phase of respiration and the cardiac cycle. It can be documented by color Doppler interrogation of the IAS (Fig. 49.7). Color interrogation along the fossa ovalis may cause erroneous identification of a PFO because of color cross-contamination when lowering the Nyquist limit.

TEE's diagnostic sensitivity is significantly lower than that of a saline contrast study; the addition of saline contrast improves TEE's diagnostic sensitivity.[69] The injection of saline contrast through the femoral vein is superior for the diagnosis of PFOs by TEE and for the appropriate sizing of ASDs.[70] Appropriate provocative measures that transiently increase the right atrial pressure (i.e., Valsalva maneuver) may be difficult to perform during a TEE because of the patient's sedation, relative hypovolemia from a fasting state, and the inability to close the glottis against the echo probe (Figs. 49.8 and Figs. 49.9 and Videos 49.7–49.9).

Fundamental imaging TTE has been considered inferior for the diagnosis of PFOs. However, the advent of second harmonic imaging has improved the sensitivity of TTE to 90%.[71] An easier and more effective performance of a provocative maneuver (e.g., no sedation, euvolemia, complete glottic closure) during TTE may improve the image quality and is associated with a higher sensitivity than that of TEE for the diagnosis of PFOs.[72]

Closure Devices for Patent Foramen Ovale

Amplatzer Patent Foramen Ovale Occluder

The Amplatzer patent foramen ovale occlude (APO) is a self-expanding, double-disk device made from 0.005-inch nitinol wire (i.e., nickel-titanium alloy), with a polyester fabric sewn into both disks (Fig. 49.10). The device has radiopaque marker bands and comes in 18 mm, 25 mm, and 35 mm sizes, and is recapturable and repositionable.

Device size represents the right atrial disk diameter. The right atrial disk stabilizes the device, preventing embolization from right to left. The thin stem allows various degrees of disk mobility that permit the PFO occluder to seat appropriately in

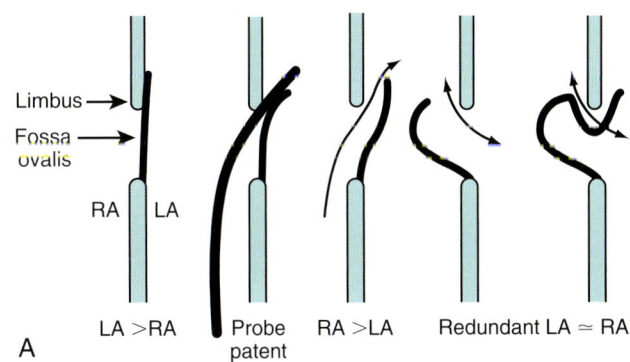

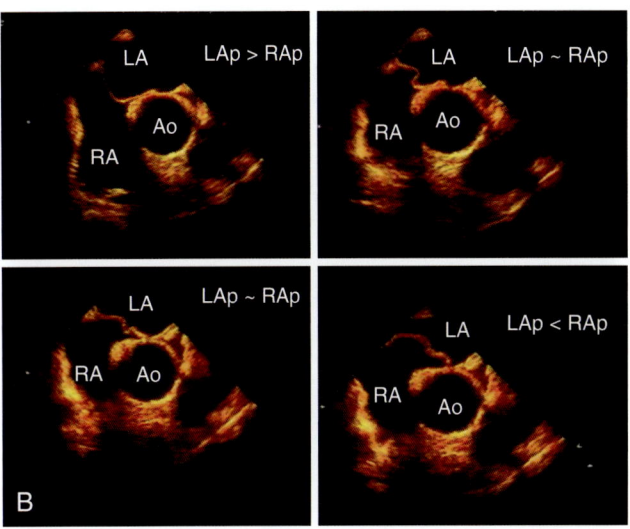

Fig. 49.7 (A) Association of interatrial septal anatomy and direction of interatrial shunt. (B) Transesophageal echocardiograms depict interatrial septal mobility related to left and right atrial pressures. *Ao*, Aorta; *LA*, left atrium; *LAp*, left atrial pressure; *RA*, right atrium; *RAp*, right atrial pressure. (Modified from Amplatz K, Moller II. *Radiology of Congenital Heart Disease*. St. Louis: Mosby; 1993.)

a long tunnel or around a hypertrophied septum. The left atrial disk dimensions are designed to decrease interference with pulmonary venous drainage or with the mitral valve and to minimize the thrombogenic material in the systemic circulation.

Device sizing depends upon the measurement from the foramen ovale to the SVC and from the foramen ovale to the aorta. The right disk radius should not exceed the shortest distance obtained, unless there is an ASA in which case a larger occlude should be utilized to cover the aneurysm (Table 49.3). The 25-mm device is used in most cases. The APO has the advantage of being self-expanding, has a simple deployment, and is placed through a small venous sheath (8 Fr for 18 mm and 25 m sizes and 9 Fr for the 35-mm size). It is fully retractable until it is released. In October 2016, the U.S. Food and Drug Administration (FDA) approved the APO occluder for reduction of recurrent ischemic stroke risk in patients who had a cryptogenic stroke presumed secondary to a paradoxical embolism, as determined by a neurologist and cardiologist.[73]

Closure of Patent Foramen Ovale

Indications

Based on the initial three RCTs, the 2014 AHA/ASA guidelines did not recommend PFO closure in cryptogenic stroke (class III, LOE A). The American Academy of Neurology discouraged

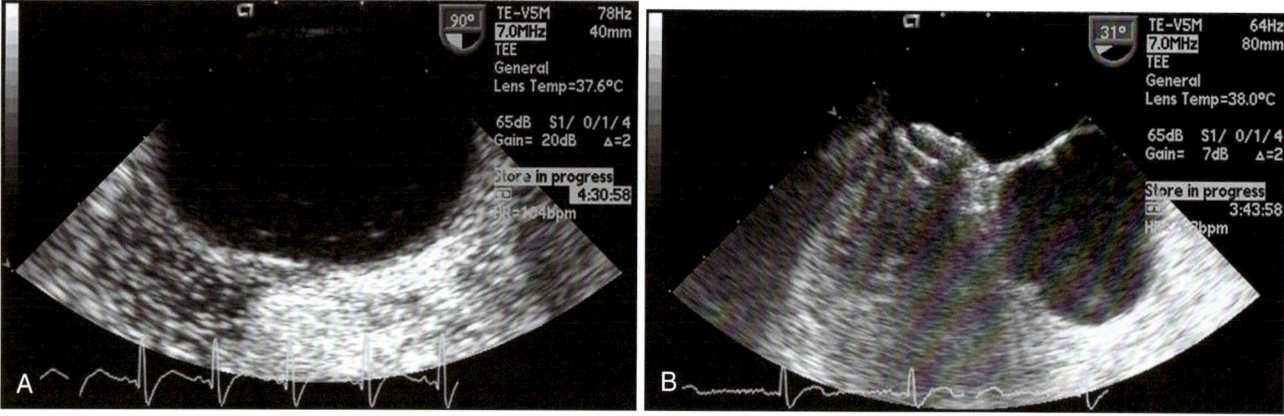

Fig. 49.8 Transesophageal echocardiogram before (A) and after (B) placement of a 25-mm AGA foramen occluder (AGA Medical, Plymouth, MN). Saline contrast is present in the left atrium before device placement. After device placement, the saline contrast study is negative.

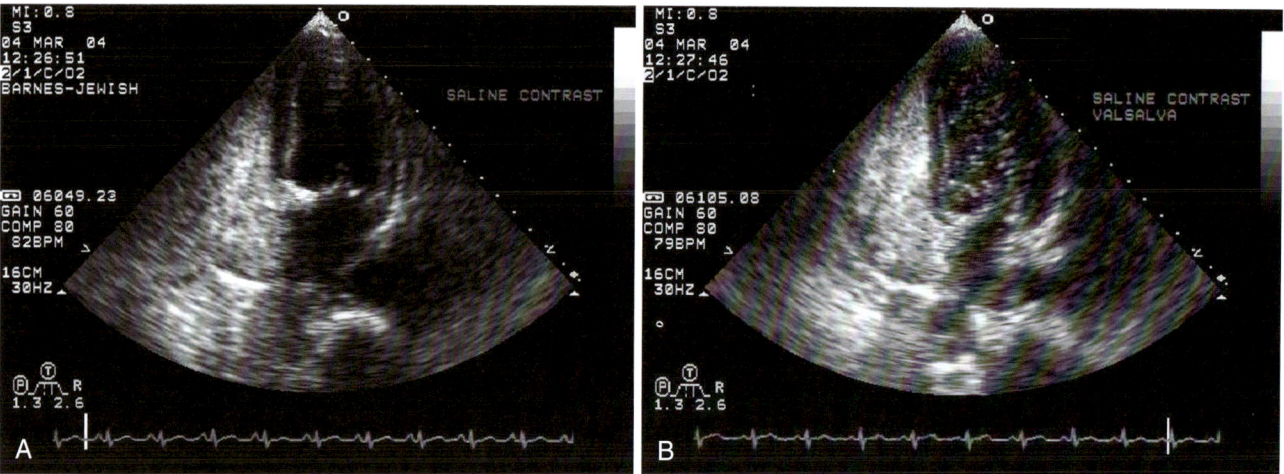

Fig. 49.9 Transthoracic echocardiogram with a saline contrast study at rest (A) and during a Valsalva maneuver (B). Transient increase in the right atrial pressure during the release phase of the Valsalva maneuver demonstrates a large right-to-left shunt at the atrial level due to a patent foramen ovale.

Fig. 49.10 Frontal view of the AGA Amplatzer PFO occluder. (Courtesy AGA Medical, Golden Valley, MN.)

TABLE 49.3 Selection Criteria for AGA Medical Patent Foramen Ovale Occluders and Delivery Systems

Distance From Defect to Superior Vena Cava or Aorta	Suggested Device Size	Delivery Sheath Size
>17.5 mm	35 mm	9 Fr
12.5–17.4 mm	25 mm	8 Fr
9–12.4 mm	18 mm	8 Fr
<9 mm	None	

routine PFO closure in cryptogenic stroke patients outside of research trials until July 2016, when an updated statement was issued criticizing its use altogether. However, in September 2017, three trials with positive results were published which may change future practice patterns.

Preprocedure Considerations

The diagnosis should be confirmed before arrival at the catheterization laboratory. Percutaneous closure of secundum ASDs or

CHAPTER 49 Percutaneous Closure of Patent Foramen Ovale and Atrial Septal Defect

PFO is performed under ultrasound (TEE or intracardiac echocardiography [ICE]) and fluoroscopic guidance. The procedure begins with an explanation of the risks and benefits of the procedure, and with patient consent to treatment.

Adequate hydration decreases the risk of an air embolism. To decrease the risk of prosthetic infection, procedures are postponed until indolent infections (e.g., urinary tract infections, upper respiratory infections) are cleared. Patients are given intravenous antibiotics (i.e., cefazolin, vancomycin, or clindamycin) in transit to the catheterization laboratory. Indwelling urinary catheters are not recommended to avoid transient bacteremia or a nidus for infection.

Venous Access

Femoral venous access provides a favorable angle of entry and is obtained with a 7-Fr to 8-Fr short sheath. Generous soft tissue predilation is advised in preparation for a larger sheath exchange. A second venous sheath (8 or 10 Fr) is placed for ICE. If the contralateral vein is punctured, a 25-cm sheath is preferred for ease of ICE catheter manipulation.

An accessory venous variant should be suspected if resistance is met, which should lead to cessation of sheath advancement and to wire and catheter repositioning toward the larger venous channel (Fig. 49.11). Hepatic vein access (Fig. 49.12) may be used for infrahepatic venous interruption as an alternative to a jugular approach.

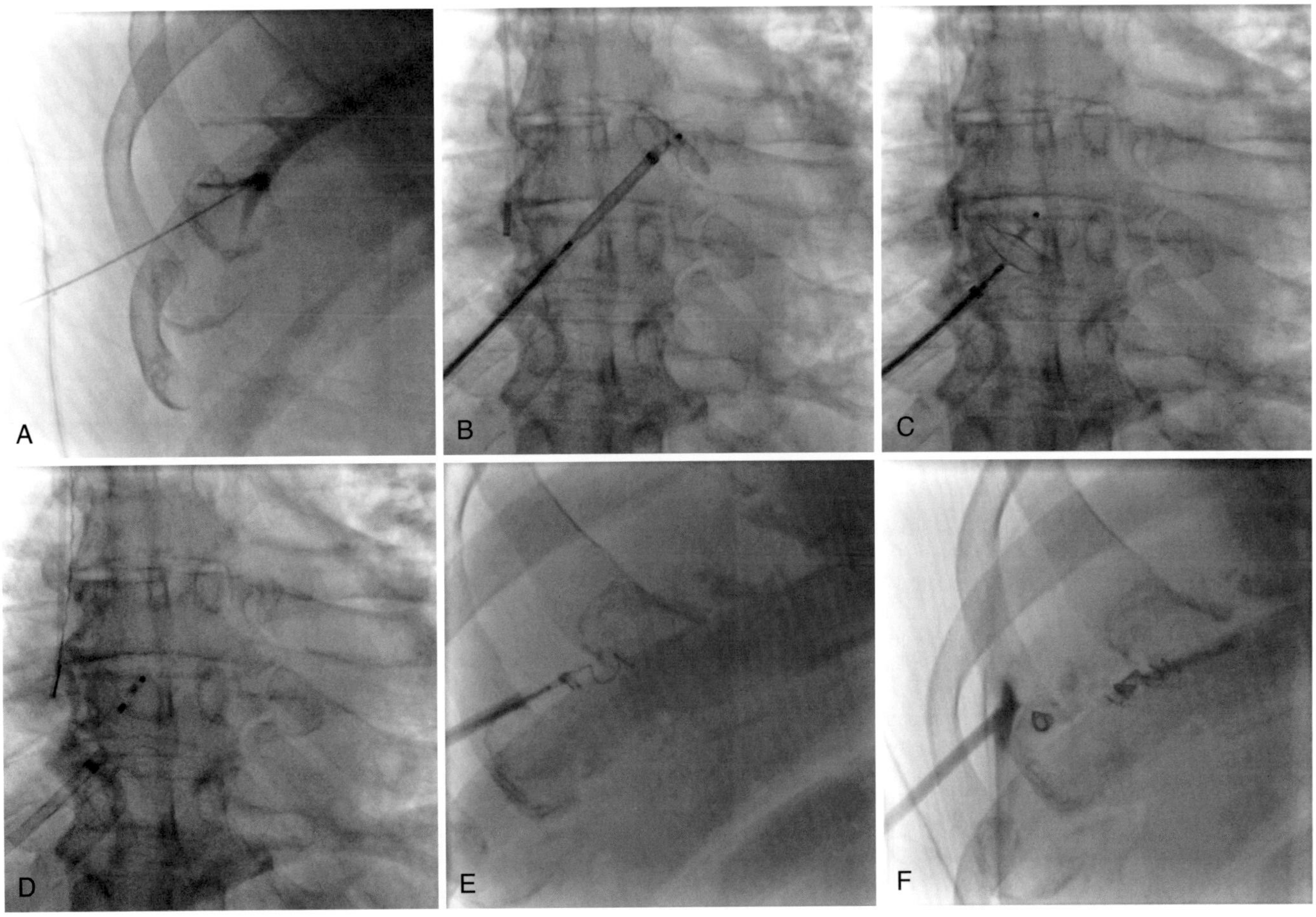

Fig. 49.11 Venogram demonstrates accessory venous drainage into the left common iliac vein. Finding an aberrant wire course or resistance during sheath advancement should prompt a search for variations.

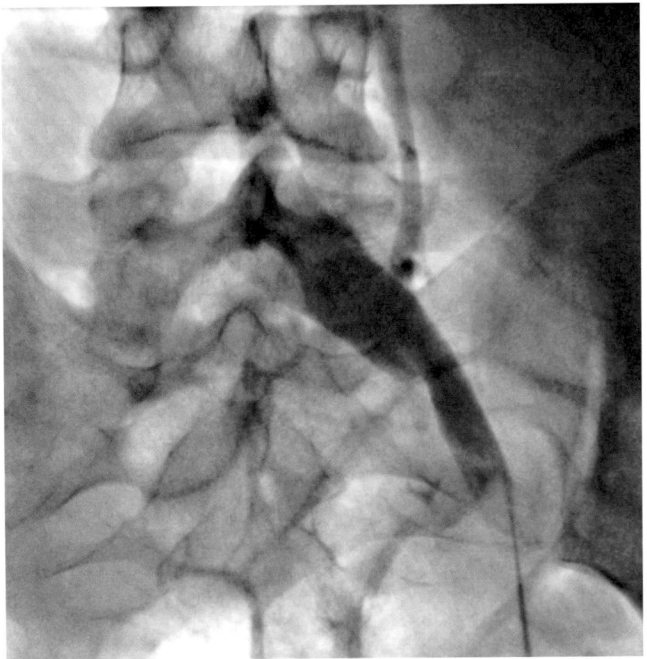

Fig. 49.12 Cine images. (A) Hepatic vein access is obtained. (B–D) Amplatzer multifenestrated cribriform septal occluder components are serially deployed. Coils are then deployed at the hepatic venous entry site (E) and near the liver capsule (F) to ensure hemostasis.

Crossing the Interatrial Septum

An end-hole multipurpose catheter (MPA) is advanced over a stiff 0.035-inch or 0.038-inch, 1.5-mm-long, J-tipped guidewire (Amplatzer wire). On arrival to the junction of the right atrium and IVC, the wire is advanced toward the IAS at the level of the aortic valve. The catheter may be advanced or rotated medially to direct the wire across the PFO.

If the guidewire does not cross easily, a Judkins right coronary catheter may be used instead. If the wire still cannot be threaded through the PFO, a hydrophilic-coated wire (Glidewire, Terumo Medical Corporation, Tokyo, Japan) may be used to negotiate through the tunnel. If the crossing cannot be achieved after a significant amount of time or effort, it is important to confirm or refute the diagnosis of a PFO by repeating a bubble study from the femoral vein (see Video 49.7). For an extant PFO, intracardiac shunting occurs within the first five beats; the presence of late bubble passage into the left atrium implies an intrapulmonary shunt. If significant passage of contrast is seen, septal puncture and closing the opening of the PFO with a device instead of inserting the device through the tunnel itself may be considered.

After entry into the left atrium, the guidewire is advanced to the left upper pulmonary vein, extending beyond the left main stem bronchus. Passage of the guidewire should occur without resistance. The wire tip should be kept in the pulmonary vein to avoid perforation of the left atrium or stimulation of a cough reflex. Placing the guidewire in the left atrial appendage is not recommended because it may lead to perforation. Incorrect localization of the wire is visualized as the wire coiling within the cardiac silhouette or detected as premature atrial depolarizations.

Anticoagulation

After passage across the foramen ovale, systemic anticoagulation is done with heparin to yield an activated clotting time of 200 seconds or greater. Heparin is administered. Aspirin (325 mg) should be administered before the procedure and clopidogrel after the procedure.

Measurement for Device Selection

Echocardiographic measurements are made to aid in device selection (see Table 49.3). Some operators prefer to measure the PFO diameter with a sizing balloon to select the appropriate device, or identify a long PFO tunnel. Balloon inflation must be done carefully to avoid tearing of the septum primum. With the use of the Amplatzer APO occluder, more than 95% of cases are done with a 25-mm or 30-mm device. The use of a sizing balloon is controversial with this device.

Delivery Sheath Insertion and Device Preparation

After the device is selected, the short sheath is removed and replaced with a long delivery sheath. The sheath is advanced until the dilator has crossed the IAS. The dilator is then separated, and the sheath is advanced slowly into the middle left atrium. The dilator and the guidewire are removed, and the sheath is connected to the manifold while ensuring that air bubbles are cleared meticulously. The occluder devices are loaded according to the manufacturers' instructions. The device usually is attached to its delivery cable and retracted into the delivery catheter. Special care must be exercised to meticulously flush the delivery catheter and device to remove all air bubbles from the system. The delivery catheter is then introduced into the delivery sheath.

Device Positioning and Release

The device is pushed through the delivery sheath under fluoroscopy. If air bubbles are seen, the device is removed and prepared again while the sheath is allowed to bleed back. After the device reaches the tip of the delivery sheath, the sheath is withdrawn slowly until the entire left atrial disk is exposed. Echocardiographic confirmation of left disk deployment is required to ensure that the left atrial disk is not in the PFO tunnel (see Video 49.9). Traction is then applied on the device and the delivery sheath to ensure that the left atrial disk abuts the atrial septum.

After the left disk is in place, the delivery sheath is withdrawn until the right atrial disk is expanded. As this is confirmed by fluoroscopy and echocardiography, the device is wiggled back and forth to ensure appropriate seating. Echocardiographic evaluation of pulmonary veins and the mitral valve is performed to avoid device obstruction by these structures. It is normal to see color flow across the center but not around the newly placed and anticoagulated Amplatzer PFO occluder device, particularly those positioned in patients with ASAs.

If no obstruction exists and the device appears stable, in appropriate position, and fully expanded, release can be done according to the manufacturer's recommendations. It is important to retract the delivery cable back into the delivery sheath to avoid cardiac perforation. After the device is released, its conformation changes slightly as a result of released tension. Rotation of up to 45 degrees is not unusual. A saline contrast study is performed to assess shunt severity. Shunting may be absent or significantly decreased after the device is released. Results of the bubble study become progressively negative as the device reaches its normal conformation and becomes endothelialized (Videos 49.10 through 49.12).

Postprocedure Care

A postprocedure chest radiograph is obtained to confirm device position, and a TTE with bubble study is done to quantify any residual shunting or development of pericardial effusion. Patients are prescribed 75 mg of clopidogrel daily for 1 to 3 months and daily 81 mg aspirin for 6 months and generally discharged same day (unless closure of large/fenestrated defects which may require overnight monitoring). For patients with histories of CVAs or TIAs, aspirin therapy may be continued indefinitely. Standard precautionary measures against subacute bacterial endocarditis should be followed for 6 months.

Special Considerations

Transseptal Puncture

Transseptal puncture is rarely required to close a PFO. It is favored in two instances: when the PFO tunnel is long and passage with a guidewire or delivery sheath is unsuccessful, and when the inferior border of an appropriately measured device interferes with the mitral valve. A SafeSept transseptal guidewire (Pressure Products Medical Supplies, Inc., Santa Barbara, CA), Bovie cauterizer attached to the transeptal needle, or laser or radiofrequency energy may be used for cases with a redundant septum to enhance puncture safety.

Prominent Chiari Network and Redundant Eustachian Valve

Herniation of the Chiari network or a redundant eustachian valve should be sought before device release. These structures can be deflected using a steerable radiofrequency ablation catheter.

Multiple Shunts

For an ASD associated with a PFO, a single cribriform septal occluder may be used to minimize the shunt. If there is persistent shunting, a second device may be placed as long as there is no interaction with the mitral valve or pulmonary veins (Fig. 49.13).

Atrial Septal Aneurysms

Closure of an ASA with a PFO usually does not require a larger device. Closure of these PFOs is successful with a standard

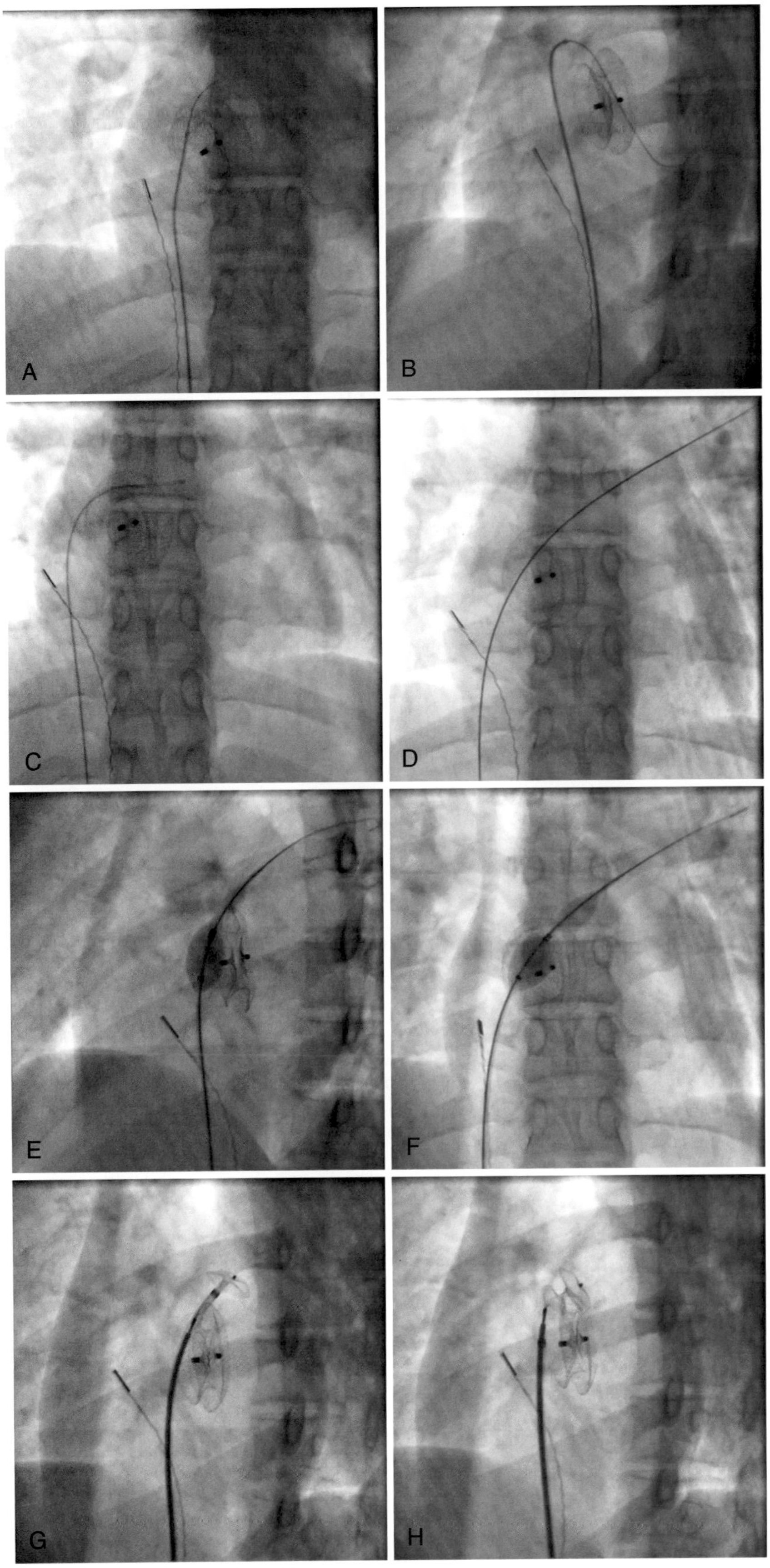

CHAPTER 49 Percutaneous Closure of Patent Foramen Ovale and Atrial Septal Defect

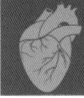

Fig. 49.13 Cine images of a symptomatic patient with a residual shunt after closure of an atrial septal defect. (A and B) A multipurpose catheter and guidewire are used to cross the defect. (C) The catheter is then advanced into the left atrium. (D) The wire is exchanged for an Amplatz Extra Stiff guidewire positioned in the left upper pulmonary vein. (E and F) The "stop flow" diameter and residual defect contour are obtained with the use of a sizing balloon. (G and H) A second device is deployed.

technique at 6 months (see Fig. 49.3).[74] It is imperative to capture the septum secundum with the device to ensure a stable position, closure, and prevent device embolization or slippage.

Lipomatous Hypertrophy of the Atrial Septum

When closing a PFO in patients with lipomatous hypertrophy of the atrial septum, the device needs to straddle the septum secundum. Under fluoroscopy, a properly seated device produces the Pacman sign, in which cranial halves of the left and right atrial disks look like open jaws biting into the septum secundum. This position ensures device stability and PFO closure. The off-label use of an ASD or ventricular septal defect (VSD) occluder may be required for hypertrophy greater than 2 cm.

Complications

Percutaneous closure of PFOs is a safe procedure. Procedural complications occur in 4% to 7% of patients but are usually mild.[75-77] A short procedural learning curve and significant device modifications have transformed PFO closure into an effective and safe procedure. Periprocedural complications include air embolism, device migration, pericardial effusion and tamponade, device erosion, vascular complications, and atrial arrhythmias. Complications occurring after discharge include endocarditis, device fracture and erosion, and device thrombosis.

Procedure-Related Complications

Air embolus is a potentially devastating complication, but it can be easily recognized and avoided. Air embolus is caused by air entering the delivery sheath as the dilator is removed or during its preparation. It may also be associated with incomplete flushing of the device when introducing it to the delivery catheter or delivery sheath.

Adequate hydration before starting the procedure minimizes negative pressure swings and decreases the chances of air entry into the equipment. Maintaining catheters below atrial level at all times is key. Gentle flushing during slow dilator and wire withdrawal can offset the negative pressure void created by their retrieval. Preemptive use of positive-pressure ventilation in patients with airway or pulmonary disease helps minimize dangerous wide intrathoracic pressure swings during sedation.

Air bubbles in the delivery catheter can be easily recognized as the device is being pushed through the delivery sheath if done under fluoroscopy. Inferior leads should be monitored; air embolism can manifest as sudden onset of hypotension, heart block, ventricular tachycardia, inferior ST-segment elevation (because the right coronary artery is anterior), and transient neurologic decline. If air is seen within the delivery sheath, it is important to remove the device slowly to reduce the ensuing vacuum and let the delivery sheath bleed back. If the air bubble has entered the circulation, hypotension or ensuing arrhythmias should be treated with the standard advanced cardiac life support (ACLS) protocol. Supplemental oxygen may aid in bubble resolution. The placement of patients in the Trendelenburg position may decrease the risk of cerebral embolization. Direct aspiration of the right coronary artery may be warranted if an airlock exits. If warranted, transfer to a hyperbaric chamber may be considered.

Device-Related Complications

Device migration is characterized by the loss of the correct position of the device (Fig. 49.14). It may be related to incomplete device exit from the tunnel or placement of a smaller device in a large PFO or in an unrecognized ASD. If migration occurs, devices may be removed percutaneously with a snare. If this cannot be done, surgical removal is recommended.

Device arm fracture was mostly seen with the use of the earlier-generation PFO-Star closure device. However, it is now rarely encountered.

Device erosion rarely can occur in closures of large ASDs that lack an appropriate aortic rim of tissue.

Device thrombosis has been seen in patients with concomitant hypercoagulable states who undergo PFO closure and generally requires surgical removal.

Transient arrhythmias may occur. In both REDUCE and CLOSE, a higher incidence of atrial fibrillation was detected, but this was largely periprocedural and transient.

Endocarditis may complicate PFO closure. Bacterial device infection or colonization may prove catastrophic. Strict sterile technique should be followed throughout the procedure, and antibiotic prophylaxis for subacute bacterial endocarditis should be continued for 6 months. Surgical excision is warranted if endocarditis occurs.

ATRIAL SEPTAL DEFECT

Among the various congenital cardiac anomalies encountered in the adult population, ASD is one of the most common. It is easily treated and has an excellent long-term prognosis. Less than a decade ago, surgical repair was considered the standard of care and provided durable long-term results. Since the FDA approved a device for percutaneous ASD closure in December 2001, there has been a dramatic shift toward catheter-based closure of ASDs, which provides durable results paralleling surgical techniques, with remarkably less morbidity and extremely short recovery time and hospitalization. Patients and physicians alike prefer the less invasive percutaneous approach, although no studies have directly compared the surgical and percutaneous techniques for efficacy and safety.

The preceding section provided an in-depth discussion on the PFO with regard to its embryology, physiology, clinical pathophysiology, diagnosis, and catheter-based management. Because there is a considerable overlap between the PFO and ASD, the following discussion highlights salient characteristics that are specific to ASD.

Embryology

Unlike a PFO, an ASD occurs when a portion of the IAS is absent. Incomplete caudal growth of the septum secundum or excessive resorption of the septum primum gives rise to a *secundum ASD*. If the septum primum fails to reach the endocardial cushions, a primum ASD occurs with its associated abnormalities (e.g., cleft mitral valve, inlet VSD). A sinus venosus ASD occurs when there is abnormal resorption of atrial septal tissue adjacent to the caval-atrial junction. An unroofed coronary sinus or the absence of atrial tissue adjacent to the site of coronary sinus drainage into the right atrium results in a coronary sinus ASD (Table 49.4 and Fig. 49.15).[78]

Anatomic and Morphologic Considerations

The secundum defect is located at the center of the atrial septum, involving the fossa ovalis. This is a true tissue defect compared with a PFO. This is the only type of ASD that is amenable to transcatheter closure techniques. To permit percutaneous closure, there should be adequate tissue margins of the defect for securing the closure device to the tissue. Lack of an adequate tissue margin predisposes to device prolapse or potential embolization. Large defects also predispose the device to encroaching on the adjacent aortic root and the mitral valve, which can result in major complications.

A thorough assessment of the atrial septum using echocardiography is a prerequisite for optimal closure. The choice of imaging depends on the operator's experience and preferences. Sinus venosus–type defects are located in the perimeter of the atrial septum near the entry of the SVC. This defect prevents the

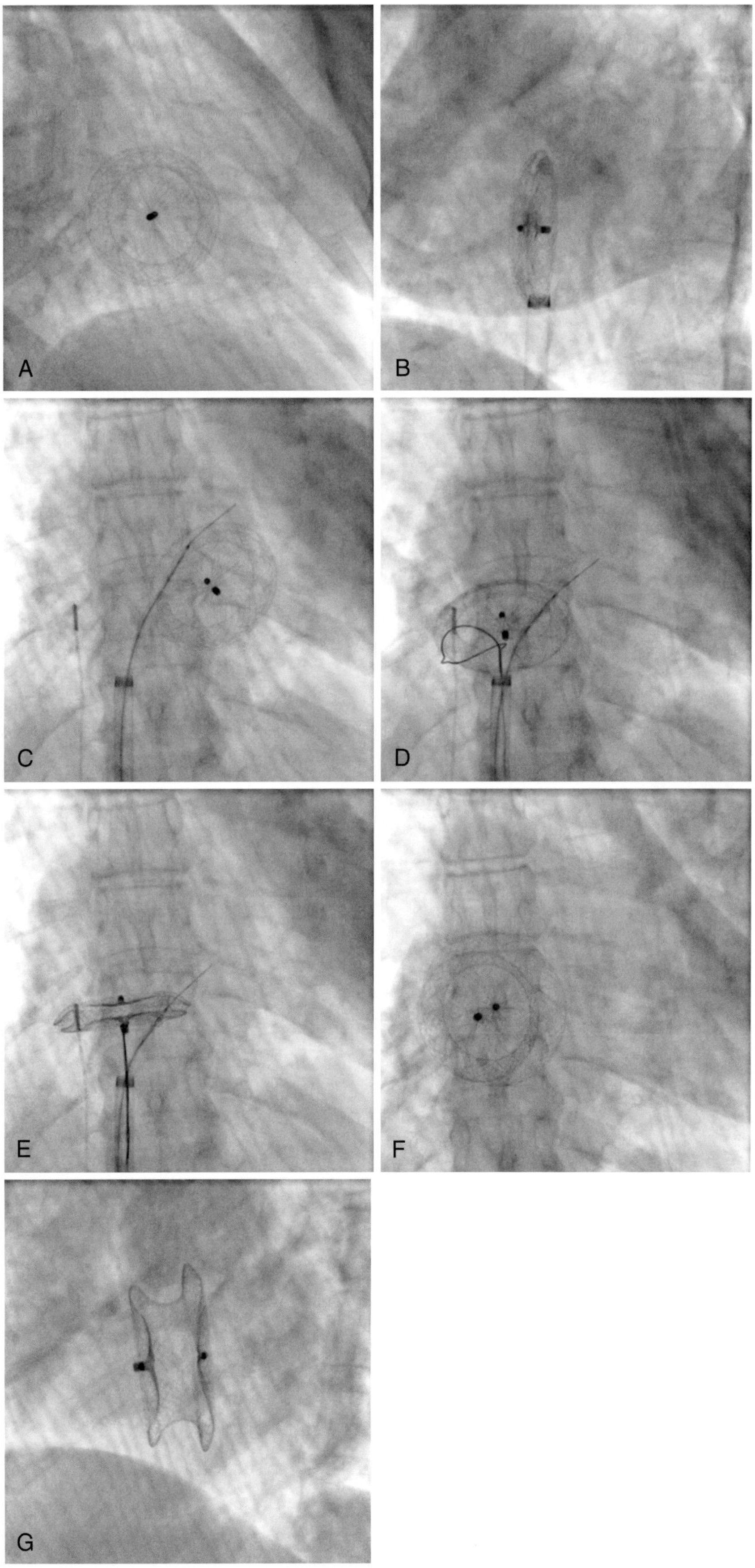

Fig. 49.14 Cine images of device migration noticed after development of ventricular ectopy after closure of a large atrial septal defect. (A and B) A 32-mm Amplatzer septal occluder (AGA Medical, Plymouth, MN) migrated into the right ventricular cavity. (C) An internal mammary artery guide catheter directs a Cook retrieval forceps (Cook Medical, Bloomington, IN) to hold the device position. (D) After device migration to the right atrium, the Cook retrieval forceps holds the device position, and a 25-mm Gooseneck Snare is used to lasso the detachment pin. (E) The device is externalized with a large sheath. (F and G) A new 34-mm Amplatzer septal occluder device is then successfully deployed across the atrial septal defect.

TABLE 49.4 Atrial Septal Defect and Patent Foramen Ovale Characteristics

Feature	Patent Foramen Ovale	Atrial Septal Defect
Embryology	Failure of the septum primum and the septum secundum to fuse completely Pathway or channel between tissue flaps	Failure of the septum primum or the septum secundum, or both, to develop normally Tissue defect
Direction of shunt	RA pressure greater than LA pressure; shunts right to left LA pressure greater than RA pressure; may stay closed or shunt left to right Shunt is dynamic and bidirectional Shunt direction depends on RA-to-LA pressure difference, RVEDP-to-LVEDP difference, phase of respiration, and volume status	Usually RA pressure equal to LA pressure but shunts left to right because the RV is more compliant Shunt reverses with Eisenmenger physiology Shunt is dynamic and bidirectional Shunt direction depends on RA-to-LA pressure difference, RVEDP-to-LVEDP difference, phase of respiration, and volume status

ASD, Atrial septal defect; *LA*, left atrium; *LVEDP*, left ventricular end-diastolic pressure; *PFO*, patent foramen ovale; *RA*, right atrium; *RV*, right ventricle; *RVEDP*, right ventricular end-diastolic pressure.

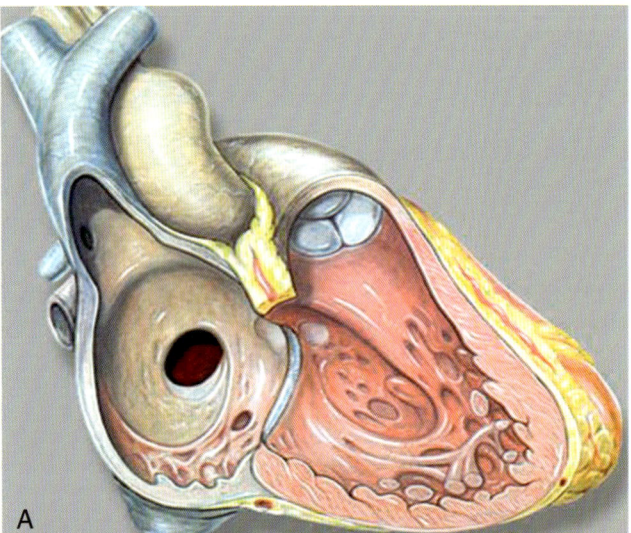
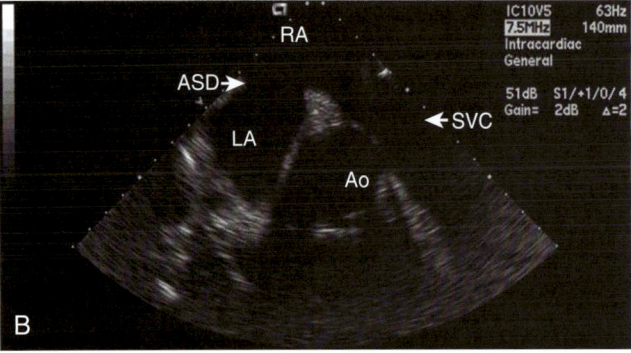
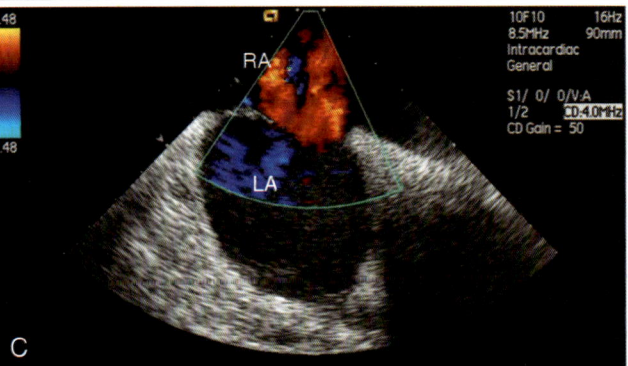

Fig. 49.15 (A) Diagram of a secundum atrial septal defect *(ASD)*. (B) ASD as seen on an intracardiac echocardiogram. (C) Color Doppler interrogation identifies a left-to-right shunt. *Ao,* Aorta; *LA,* left atrium; *RA,* right atrium; *SVC,* superior vena cava. (Modified from Patrick J. Lynch, Director, ITS Web Services Department, Yale University, New Haven, CT.)

normal separation of pulmonary veins from the right lung, the SVC, and the right atrium, and the result is anomalous drainage of one or more pulmonary veins.[79] Typically, defects located close to the IVC are rare and are called *caval defects.* They can be associated with anomalous pulmonary venous drainage. Ostium primum ASDs, also known as *endocardial cushion defects or atrioventricular canal defects,* may be accompanied by VSDs and a cleft mitral valve. With the exception of secundum defects, the management of other types of ASDs requires surgical repair and is not detailed here.

Clinical Presentation

Patients with ASDs usually remain asymptomatic during childhood. Typically, the pulmonary outflow murmur or a fixed split of the second heart sound detected during routine physical examination prompts further evaluation, which results in the diagnosis. Some patients may experience recurrent heart failure, have a predilection for recurrent respiratory infection during childhood, and have easy fatigability and exertional dyspnea.[80] In adults, a long-standing ASD with significant shunting may manifest with atrial arrhythmias, pulmonary arterial hypertension, and heart failure.

Hemodynamics

The direction and magnitude of the shunt across an ASD depend on the size of the defect, right and left atrial pressures, right and left ventricular compliance and end-diastolic pressures, vascular resistance in the pulmonary and systemic circuits, the phase of respiration, intrathoracic pressure, and intravascular volume status.[81] In most patients with moderate- to large-sized ASDs, both atria are in open communication, and the mean atrial pressure is equal. The shunt is directed left to right because compliance of the right atrium and right ventricle is higher than that of the left atrium and left ventricle. In those with very small ASDs without equalization of atrial pressures, the gradient across the atria also plays a role in the direction of the shunt.

A close review of the Doppler performed across the defect shows that the flow occurs during the entire cardiac cycle. Left-to-right shunting occurs mostly during late systole and early diastole, but atrial contraction also provides additional flow augmentation. The shunt results in diastolic overloading of the right ventricle and increased pulmonary blood flow. Depending on the size of the defect, pulmonary blood flow may be as high as five times the systemic flow. In those with long-standing and untreated ASDs, pulmonary hypertension may ensue, which can result in reversal of the shunt's direction, depending on the status of the right ventricle. Even in an uncomplicated ASD, a transient and small right-to-left shunt occurs during the early phase of ventricular systole and is further accentuated by respiration that decreases intrathoracic pressure. This is the rationale behind performing a saline contrast study during echocardiography for the detection of ASDs (Video 49.13).

Diagnosis

Physical examination findings usually initiate the evaluation for suspected ASDs. This includes a hyperdynamic precordium, a fixed split of the second heart sound without respiratory variation, a loud pulmonic component of the second heart sound, and a pulmonary outflow tract murmur. Primum-type defects may have associated tricuspid and mitral regurgitation murmurs. The electrocardiogram further supports the clinical findings. Right-axis deviation, right ventricular hypertrophy, rSR′, and rsR′ pattern in the right precordial leads with normal QRS duration are common electrocardiographic findings in ostium secundum defects. An inverted P wave in lead III is seen in sinus venosus defects, whereas left-axis deviation may denote an ostium primum defect. Lengthening of the PR interval due to atrial enlargement and conduction delay can be seen in all three types of ASD.[82] Chest radiographic findings include right atrial and ventricular enlargement, prominent pulmonary artery, and increased pulmonary vascular markings.

Echocardiography

Echocardiography has replaced cardiac catheterization techniques for the diagnosis of ASDs.[83,84] Even shunt fraction can be reliably calculated using an echocardiogram. A TTE with a saline contrast study should be done first. The defect may be visualized directly by TTE imaging, particularly from a subcostal view of the IAS, but a TEE can provide much better anatomic characterization of the septum and the adjoining structures.[85,86]

Typical echocardiographic findings include right atrial and right ventricular enlargement, increased pulmonary artery pressure, and Doppler demonstrating continuous flow across the atrial septum.[87] Three-dimensional echocardiography with image reconstruction has been used to plan closure procedural details. ICE can also be used, but its use is mostly restricted to providing imaging guidance for percutaneous closure (Video 49.14).

Cardiac Catheterization

In current clinical practice, cardiac catheterization primarily for diagnostic purposes is uncommon, but it is used when there is a discrepancy between the clinical and echocardiographic findings. Invasive hemodynamic assessment is performed during a planned percutaneous closure. A defect in the atrial septum is usually obvious when the guidewire or the catheter crosses the midline (i.e., atrial septum) into the left atrium. The site at which the catheter crosses provides diagnostic clues about the defects. In secundum defects, the site of crossing is midseptal, whereas in sinus venosus and primum defects, the catheter crosses the IAS at a high level and a low level, respectively. Angiograms can further demonstrate shunting and other associated anomalies (see Video 49.8).[88] In the past, an injection in the right upper pulmonary vein was recommended, but this is rarely performed in current clinical practice.

We recommend a pulmonary arteriogram in a straight pulmonary artery projection to rule out associated partial anomalous pulmonary venous return (PAPVR). A right heart catheterization with measurement of oxygen saturations in the innominate vein, the SVC, the right atrium, the right ventricle, and pulmonary arteries is also important to assess the magnitude of the shunt and rule out associated problems such as pulmonary hypertension and PAPVR. It is also important to measure left atrial pressure or left ventricular pressure, or both, especially in older adults (discussed later).

Closure of Atrial Septal Defect

Indications

Unrepaired ASDs that result in right heart volume overload can lead to progressive exertional dyspnea and exercise intolerance, atrial arrhythmias, and pulmonary hypertension. Calculation of

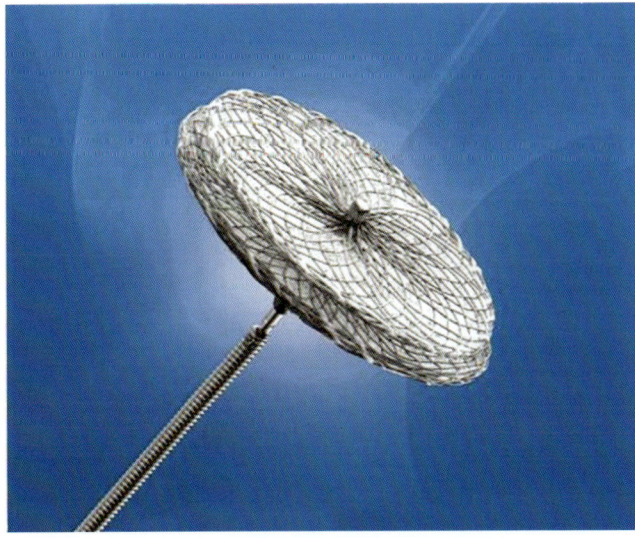

Fig. 49.16 Photograph of the AGA cribriform septal occluder. (Courtesy AGA Medical, Golden Valley, MN.)

the pulmonary to systemic flow ratio (Qp/Qs) estimates shunt direction and magnitude, which is related to defect size and interventricular pressure and compliance differences. Over time, long-standing right-sided volume overload may alter Qp/Qs. A small Qp/Qs in the setting of right atrial or right ventricular overload should not preclude closure.

Right chamber enlargement as documented by echocardiography is accepted as an indication for percutaneous ASD closure. Other indications, including platypnea-orthodeoxia syndrome, paradoxical embolus, DCS, and migraine headaches, are controversial (as discussed earlier).

Devices for Percutaneous Closure

Percutaneous closure of ASD has proved to be reliable, safe, and effective as indicated by the available data, but choosing defects with appropriate anatomic characteristics is critical for successful closure. Currently, the Amplatzer Septal Occluder, the Amplatzer multifenestrated septal occluder Cribiform device, and the Gore Cardioform are the only FDA-approved devices (Fig. 49.16).

Amplatzer Septal Occluder and Amplatzer Multifenestrated Septal Occluder Cribiform

The Amplatzer septal occluder (ASO) is a self-expandable, double-disk device made from nitinol wire mesh (Fig. 49.17). The two disks are linked together by a connecting waist, which corresponds to the balloon size of the ASD. To increase its closing ability, the disks and the waist are filled with Dacron polyester fabric. The polyester fabric is securely sewn to each disk by a polyester thread. The device is available in various sizes ranging from 4 to 38 mm (4 to 20 mm at 1-mm increments, 22 to 38 mm at 2-mm increments), and the size refers to the diameter of the waist. Device selection is based on the stretched diameter of the defect (i.e., a 10-mm stretched defect requires a 10-mm device).

The pivotal study reported technical success rates of 95.7%.[89] Technical success was defined as successful deployment of a device. The 12-month closure success rate was 98.5%, with closure success defined as a shunt of less than 2 mm in patients in whom a device was successfully placed. Patient selection and optimal imaging are key to success.

Multiple ASDs in a patient may be closed with more than one device (Fig. 49.18). A cribiform device that is approved for closure of multifenestrated ASDs is available in four diameters: 18, 25, 30, and 35 mm. Modifications to the basic technique may be needed to close very large ASDs; they are discussed separately.

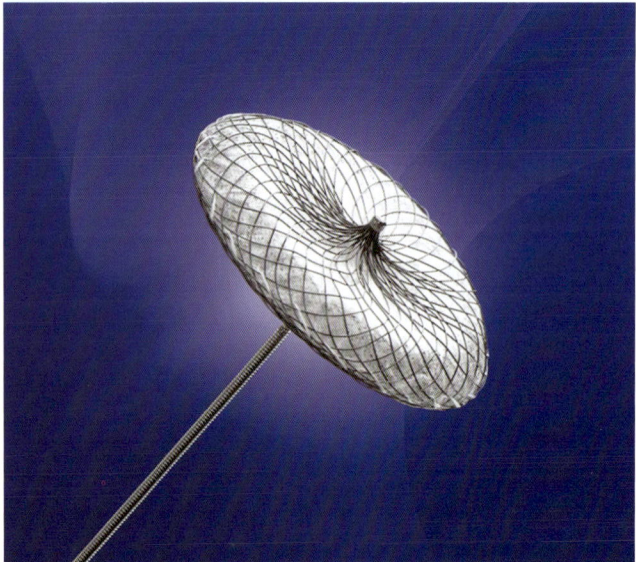

Fig. 49.17 Amplatzer septal occluder. (Courtesy AGA Medical, Golden Valley, MN.)

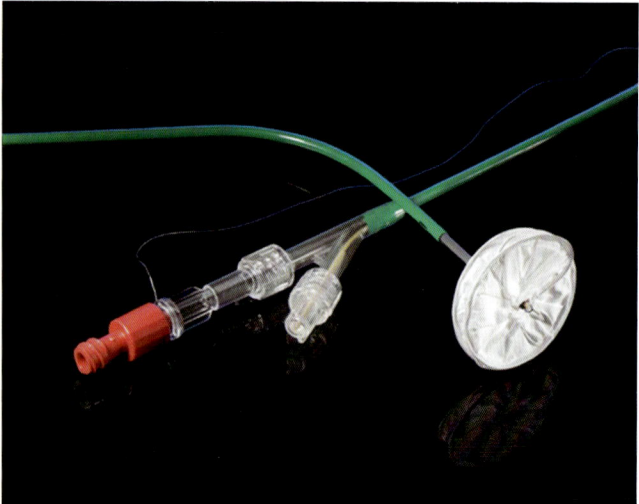

Fig. 49.19 Gore Helex septal occluder and delivery system. (Courtesy W.L. Gore & Associates, Newark, DE.)

TABLE 49.5 GORE CARDIOFORM Septal Occluder Device Sizing

Labeled Occluder Diameter (mm)	Maximum Recommended Defect Size Measured With Stop Flow Balloon Sizing (mm)
15	8.5
20	11
25	14
30	17

From Kent DM, Ruthazer R, Weimar C, et al. An index to identify stroke-related vs incidental patent foramen ovale in cryptogenic stroke. *Neurology*. 2013;81:619–625.

is not self-centering, a ratio of the device to balloon-stretched defect of at least 1.75:1 is required to prevent residual shunting or device embolization.

In the pivotal study with 50 patients, 97.9% patients met procedural success, defined as technical success with completely occluded defect or residual shunt ≤2 mm at the completion of the implant procedure. No 30-day or 6-month serious adverse events of device events were reported.

Theoretical advantages for the Cardioform occluder compared with the ASO are that it is a lower-profile device, has less nitinol and therefore less nickel exposure (of particular consideration in those patients with a nickel allergy), and may have a lower risk of erosions. Primary disadvantage is the inability to close defects larger than 17 mm in diameter. Currently, the device is also being used in an off-label fashion for PFO closure, but will likely meet full approval shortly.

Procedural Details

Aspirin therapy is started days before the procedure. Antibiotics are given within 30 minutes of achieving access. Patients should be adequately anticoagulated with unfractionated heparin during the entire procedure and the activated clotting time maintained above 250 seconds before device placement.

Typically, femoral venous access is used, and the size of the sheath is based on the size and type of the device and delivery sheath system chosen. TEE or ICE is used for imaging guidance during the procedure. If ICE is used, a second venous sheath is required during the procedure.

We recommend performing a right heart catheterization with every ASD closure. This includes measurements of

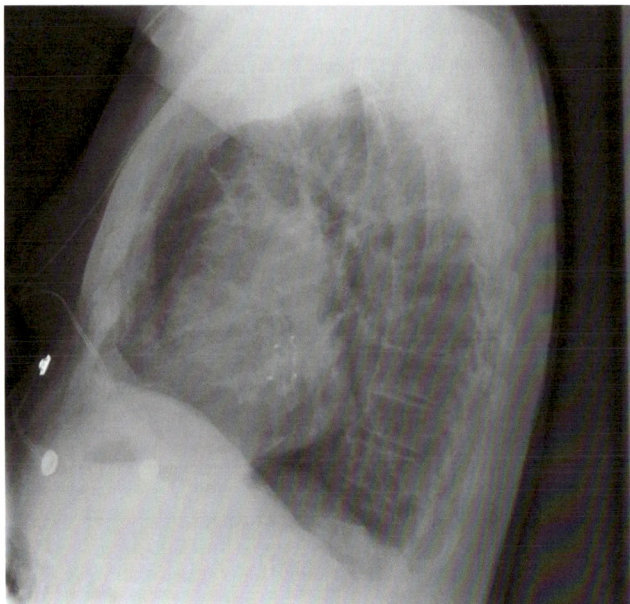

Fig. 49.18 Chest radiograph obtained after deployment of two AGA septal occluders.

The reported advantages of the Amplatzer device include ease of use, delivery with smaller-diameter catheters, and the facility to retrieve and reposition it before complete deployment. The device design also permits it to self-center across the defect.

Gore Cardioform Occluder

The Gore Cardioform septal occluder consists of a device and special delivery system (Fig. 49.19). The device is a nonself-centering, double-disk device that consists of a nitinol wire frame covered by an expanded polytetrafluoroethylene (ePTFE) membrane. The ePTFE membrane is treated with a hydrophilic coating to facilitate echocardiographic imaging during device implantation.

The device is approved for closure of ASDs less than 17 mm in diameter. The device is available in 15 mm, 20 mm, 25 mm, and 30 mm open disk diameter sizes (Table 49.5). Because the device

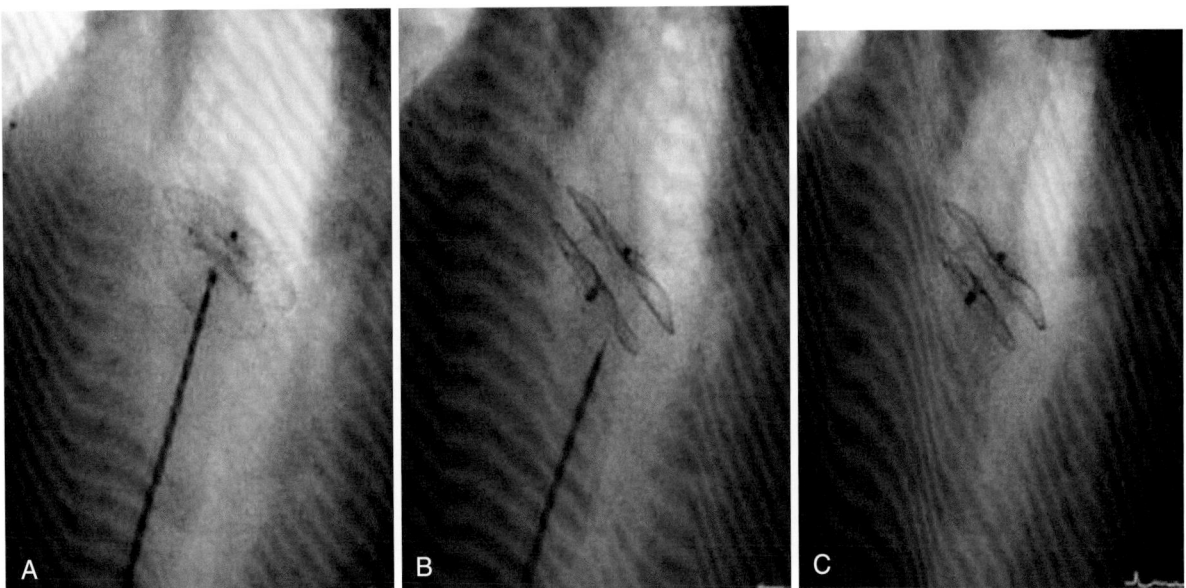

Fig. 49.20 Deployment of an AGA septal occluder (AGA Medical, Plymouth, MN). (A) Once in place, the device is wiggled to ensure stability. (B) After stability is confirmed, the device is released by rotating the delivery cable. (C) After it is released, the cable is withdrawn into the delivery sheath to avoid trauma.

oxygen saturations and pressures in the innominate vein, SVC, right atrium, and pulmonary arteries, as well as performance of pulmonary arteriography. This information is important to assess PAPVR and pulmonary hypertension. If PAPVR is documented in the setting of a secundum ASD, it is important to decide how much of the total lung parenchyma is draining anomalously. If a single segmental vein is anomalous in the setting of a moderate-sized or larger ASD, device closure of the ASD is still indicated, and the anomalous vein can be left in situ. It is also important to measure left atrial pressure or left ventricular end-diastolic pressure, or both, especially in older adults because left ventricular diastolic dysfunction can complicate transcatheter ASD closure and precipitate left heart failure due to an inability of the left ventricle to adjust to the increased preload.

After the right heart catheterization has been completed, a 0.035-inch J-tipped guidewire guided through a 6-Fr MPA is the best tool to cross the defect. The wire is positioned in the left upper pulmonary vein. After crossing the defect, the ASD diameter is measured with a balloon specifically designed for sizing atrial communications, such as the Amplatzer (AGA Medical, Plymouth, MN) or the NuMed (NuMed, Inc., Hopkinton, NY) sizing balloon.

Under fluoroscopic and echocardiographic guidance, the balloon catheter is placed across the defect and gently inflated with diluted contrast until the left-to-right shunt ceases, as observed with echocardiography. The maximum achieved occlusive diameter is measured at the balloon waist. This is the stop-flow diameter. It is critical not to overinflate the balloon because this can lead to selection of an inappropriately large device and increase the risk of erosion. The diameter of the balloon is measured fluoroscopically and with echocardiography, and the measurements should be in close agreement (<1 mm difference).

If an ASO is chosen, the sizing balloon is removed, and the appropriately sized sheath for delivery is advanced into the right atrium. The dilator is removed, and the sheath is de-aired and then advanced over the wire into the left atrium. Alternatively, the sheath and the dilator can be advanced over the guidewire into the left upper pulmonary vein, and the wire and the dilator can then be removed. It is important to de-air the sheath completely if the latter approach is taken because an air embolus can otherwise result.

The device is loaded and advanced into the delivery sheath under fluoroscopic and echocardiographic guidance (Fig. 49.20; also see Videos 49.10 through 49.12). Meticulous attention must be paid to avoid suction of air into the system, which occurs particularly when using large-caliber delivery sheaths.

If the Cardioform occluder is chosen, its size needs to be at least 1.75 times the stop-flow diameter of the defect. The device can be delivered in two ways: by removing the sizing balloon and guidewire and advancing the chosen device and delivery system through a 10-Fr sheath across the defect under echocardiographic guidance or by removing the sizing balloon and leaving the guidewire in place and then sliding the guidewire through the tip of the catheter. The catheter is then advanced across the defect and into the left atrium, at which point the guidewire is removed.

Complications

The Amplatzer pivotal trial described a major adverse cardiac event (MACE) rate of 1.6% (7 of 442 patients). This included two arrhythmias requiring treatment, three device embolizations with surgical removal, one embolization with percutaneous removal, and one delivery system failure. This compares with a MACE rate of 5.2% (8 of 154) in the surgical control group in this study. Minor adverse cardiac events occurred in 6.1% of patients (27 of 442), compared with a rate of 18.8% (29 of 154) in the surgical group.

Erosions associated with the use of the ASO are the most common life-threatening complication. They are reported to occur with a frequency of approximately 1 to 3 per 1000 implants (0.1% to 0.3%).

Amin and colleagues described erosions associated with the use of the ASO and, based on a panel of physicians, developed recommendations to avoid this complication.[90] They recommended using the stop-flow method of balloon sizing. They also recommended only a gentle to-and-fro motion on the device after it is implanted. Patients at high risk for erosions were thought to be those needing an ASO greater than 1.5 times the unstretched diameter of the defect and those with deficient superior or aortic

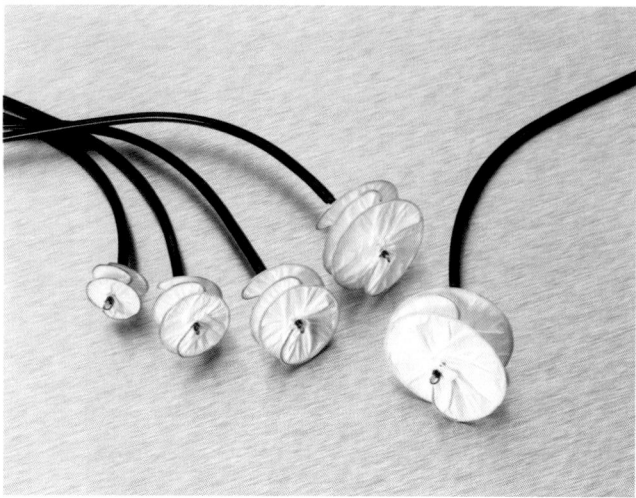

Fig. 49.21 Photograph of the Helex septal occluder. (Courtesy W.L. Gore & Associates, Newark, DE.)

rims. It was also thought that devices that were deformed at the level of the aortic root (splayed around the aorta) were at higher risk of erosion.

The FDA convened an advisory panel on May 24, 2012, to address the erosion issue, and the current instructions for use of the ASO state, "absence of the anterior superior (aortic) rim and device oversizing may be related to causation of erosion due to increased likelihood of device-tissue contact in the dynamic anatomic area of highest risk for erosion."[91] The instructions for use and the FDA recommend clinical follow-up with a cardiologist and an echocardiogram at implantation, 1 day after the procedure, before discharge, and at 1 week, 6 months, and 12 months after implantation. Annual cardiology follow-up is recommended thereafter (without the specific recommendation for an echocardiogram).

The new Cardioform device was designed to address many of the issues with the older Helex device (Fig. 49.21), and like the Amplatzer devices has a safe profile. Embolization is a rare phenomenon that can happen with any of the devices, and operators must be familiar with retrieval techniques (see Fig. 49.14).

Device embolization can occur to the right heart, the left heart, or the aorta. Most device embolizations occur at the time of or shortly after implantation, although late embolization has been reported. Percutaneous device retrieval is possible in a significant number of cases. The device should initially be stabilized with a bioptome or a gooseneck snare so that it does not cause hemodynamic compromise. This may require a second venous line from an inferior or superior approach; one site of access is used to hold the device, and the second is used to snare and subsequently retrieve the device. A long, relatively stiff sheath can be advanced adjacent to the device. The tip of the sheath can be beveled by cutting it at a 30- to 45-degree angle. This facilitates pulling the device into the sheath. The right atrial microscrew can then be snared using a gooseneck snare delivered through a 6-Fr cut pigtail catheter or other angled guiding catheter delivered through the retrieval sheath. The pigtail can be cut such that the distal end assumes a 90-degree angle in relation to the shaft of the catheter. This allows turning of the snare so that it may be steered to the microscrew.

After the microscrew is snared, the device is pulled back into the sheath. This may require rotation of the delivery sheath, the snare, or traction placed on the device from the bioptome to allow the microscrew to enter the beveled portion of the sheath. After the microscrew enters the sheath, the entire device may be withdrawn. A fully deployed device should not be pulled across

the mitral or tricuspid valves because of the risk of valve damage. Instead, the long delivery sheath should be placed next to the device for retrieval if the device lies within the ventricle. Devices that embolize to the atria may be snared and pulled into the IVC. Traction using a bioptome from above may then be applied to the superior portion of the device to facilitate entry into the retrieval sheath. Devices may also be retrieved from the pulmonary artery or aorta using modifications of this technique. If the device cannot be percutaneously removed, surgical removal is necessary.

Special Considerations

Closure of Large Atrial Septal Defects

Closure of large ASDs (30 to 36 mm) or those with deficient rims (<5 mm) can be difficult. Because the Cardioform device cannot be used to close large ASDs, the focus of this discussion is on techniques that have been described for use with the ASO.

In patients with a deficient SVC (superior or anterosuperior rims [retroaortic]), it is very easy for the left atrial disk to prolapse through the defect on initial deployment. This can also occur with deficient posteroinferior rims. If multiple rims are deficient, the likelihood of successful closure decreases further. The operator's familiarity with advanced techniques of deployment greatly improves the chances of procedural success, and it is imperative that the implanter become comfortable with several of these techniques.

In right upper pulmonary vein deployment, the delivery sheath is positioned with the tip in the right upper pulmonary vein.[92] The left atrial disk is partially deployed in the os of the right upper pulmonary vein or near the roof of the left atrium, and the remainder of the device is then rapidly deployed by pulling down on the delivery sheath while fixing the delivery cable. After the device is fully exposed, the cable can be pushed forward to reorient the device if necessary. Unsheathing of the device in this technique must be performed rapidly to be successful (Video 49.15).

In the left upper pulmonary vein (LUPV) deployment, the delivery sheath is placed in the LUPV, and the left atrial disk is deployed.[93] The left atrial disk is held in place in the LUPV and assumes an oblong shape. The remainder of the device is unsheathed by retracting the delivery sheath over the cable. Tension on the cable is then released, allowing the right atrial disk to reconfigure against the septum. This results in the left atrial disk being released from the LUPV and orienting correctly against the atrial septum. The unsheathing maneuver and the release of tension on the delivery cable must be performed sequentially and rapidly for the procedure to be successful. Proper deployment of the left atrial disk in the LUPV is paramount; if the left atrial disk is deployed too far into the LUPV, it will not be released from the vein. Conversely, if the left atrial disk is not deployed far enough in the LUPV, it will be released prematurely, and the technique will not be successful. The left bronchus is a useful fluoroscopic landmark for the ostium of the LUPV and should be used as a guide for placement.

Alternative sheath uses are described subsequently. The Hausdorf sheath (Cook, Bloomington, IN) has a double curve at the distal end, which facilitates appropriate alignment of the left atrial disk against the septum. This sheath is available in 10-, 11-, and 12-Fr sizes. Its use is particularly helpful in patients with deficient superior or anterosuperior rims.

A Mullins sheath may also be used. It has more of a curve compared with the standard 45-degree TorqVue delivery sheath and may help align the left atrial disk appropriately. Kutty and colleagues described the use of a Mullins sheath.[94] The sheath is modified by cutting off the distal curved portion of the sheath parallel to the shaft. This results in what they called a *straight sidehole sheath*.[94] The very sharp distal end of the modified sheath is then cut off to reduce the risk of perforation. This modification

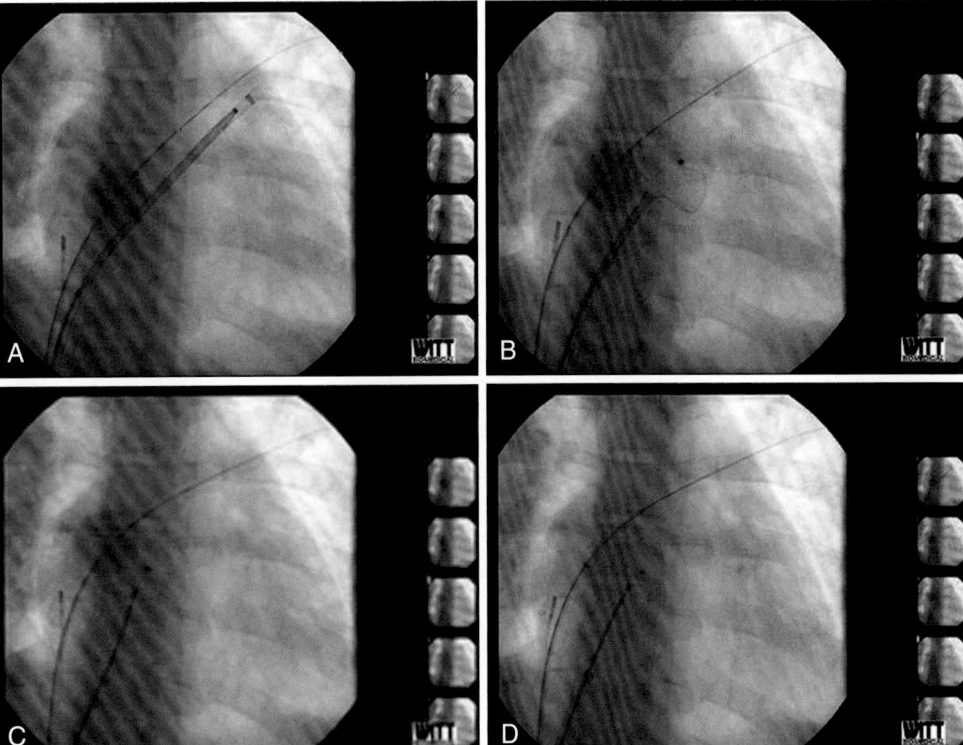

Fig. 49.22 Steps in balloon-assisted technique. (A) Inflation of an occlusion balloon against the right atrial side of the atrial septum with the Amplatzer delivery sheath in place. (B) Deployment of the left atrial disk using an occlusion balloon as a buttress to prevent prolapse of the disk. (C) Deployment of the right atrial disk with the occlusion balloon still in place. (D) Deflation of the occlusion balloon and reconfiguration of the Amplatzer device without prolapse of disk (see Video 49.14, and 49.16 through 49.18).

of the Mullins sheath results in the device exiting the tip of the delivery sheath at an angle that makes deployment of the left atrial disk parallel to the septum much easier.

For the balloon-assisted technique (Fig. 49.22 and Videos 49.16 through 49.18; see Video 49.14), Dalvi and associates[95] reported a technique that uses a balloon as a buttress to prevent prolapse of the left atrial disk through the ASD during deployment. This technique is easy to learn and quite successful in our experience. To perform this procedure, a second venous line is inserted. The ASD is crossed in a standard fashion, and the defect is sized using the stop-flow technique. The appropriate device and delivery sheath are chosen and placed in the left atrium in the standard fashion. Through the second venous sheath, a catheter is placed in the LUPV, and a 0.035-inch guidewire is placed. The sizing balloon or a Meditech occlusion balloon can be placed over the guidewire. The balloon is inflated in the right atrium and placed against the right side of the atrial septum. The left atrial disk of the device is then deployed and pulled against the left side of the septum. The balloon helps prevent prolapse of the device at this time. The remainder of the device is deployed while the balloon remains in place against the septum. After the entire device is deployed, the sizing balloon is deflated.

TEE or ICE is used to assess the results. If the device has been correctly placed, the deflated balloon and guidewire are removed from across the septum. One disadvantage of this technique is that a second or third (if ICE is used) venous access is required.

Several other techniques have been described to assist in closure of large ASDs or those with deficient rims. They include the use of the dilator as a buttress similar to that described for the balloon-assisted technique, use of a right coronary guiding catheter, and use of a deflectable electrophysiology sheath.[95,96]

Multifenestrated Atrial Septal Defects

Fenestrations are frequently encountered with secundum ASDs. These additional defects are often found along the posteroinferior portion of the atrial septum. In many situations, closure of the primary defect within the fossa ovalis is enough to provide closure of the secondary defects. If the secondary fenestrated portion of the septum is fairly remote (>7 mm) from the primary defect, closure using multiple devices may be required (discussed later). If the fossa ovalis has multiple fenestrations, use of a nonself-centering device such as the Cardioform device or the Amplatzer cribriform device is appropriate.

The procedural details for closure of fenestrated ASDs are different from those for a standard secundum ASD in that the defect is *not* balloon sized. Instead, the distance from the central-most defect to the furthest reaches of the outer-most defect is measured under TEE or ICE guidance. It is important to measure this in multiple views and to use the largest diameter measured to choose a device. This measured dimension represents the radius of the device to be chosen. The device must have a diameter at least twice the measured radius to ensure that all the holes are covered with device material.

After the device is chosen, the central-most defect is crossed under ultrasound guidance. The operator must ensure that the central defect is crossed and not one of the satellite lesions. This may be difficult, especially in the setting of a septal aneurysm. A variety of catheters may be used for this purpose, but we have found that a multipurpose or Judkins right coronary catheter is often successful. Because the fenestrations are often small, the use of a non–J-tipped wire such as a Wholey wire or Terumo wire is necessary. The wire within the catheter makes identification of the catheter on ultrasound easier. As the catheter or wire crosses a very thin, floppy septum, the tissue is often moved out of plane on the echocardiogram, and it is important to look in several views to decide whether the appropriate hole has been crossed.

After the correct hole has been crossed, the guidewire is placed in the LUPV. If the Amplatzer cribriform device is chosen, the appropriate delivery sheath is advanced across the septum, and the device is deployed as previously described. If a Cardioform device is chosen, the sheath should be advanced over the guidewire as mentioned in the procedural section earlier. After the Cardioform sheath is across the defect, the guidewire is removed and the device deployed in the standard fashion. A full TEE or

ICE study should be repeated after device deployment to make certain that all the defects have been covered with the device.

Multiple Atrial Septal Defects

Multiple ASDs have been reported to occur in up to 7.3% of cases.[97] They can often be treated with a single device. If the secondary defect is not covered appropriately by a single device, deployment of a second device is necessary if the secondary defect is thought to be hemodynamically significant. Use of a second device may be anticipated if an Amplatzer septal occluder is chosen to close the primary defect and if the distance between the edges of the primary and secondary defects is 7 mm or more.

Several techniques have been used to close multiple defects, including simultaneous defect sizing and device deployment and sequential sizing and closure. We think either approach is acceptable. We typically perform sequential defect sizing and closure, in which one of the defects is crossed, sized, and then closed with an appropriate device. This is followed by crossing the secondary defect, sizing it, and closing it.

It does not matter which defect is addressed first. The relationship of the two devices to each other is likewise not critical. On some occasions, the larger device can sandwich the smaller device; at other times, the disks are intercalated. Either approach is acceptable. Smaller defects are often at the posteroinferior portion of the septum, and after they are closed, the two devices may orient themselves at almost 90 degrees to each other. This is to be expected because the atrial septum is a three-dimensional structure. On rare occasions, more than two devices are necessary to close additional defects. Meticulous attention to echocardiographic images is required to make certain that there is enough room in the left atrium to accommodate additional devices without impinging on adjacent structures.

Atrial Septal Defect Closure and Pulmonary Hypertension

Pulmonary hypertension occurs anywhere from 6% to 50% of adults with ASDs[98–103] and is an important consideration prior to deciding on ASD closure. A higher baseline pulmonary artery systolic pressure (PASP), younger age, and smaller body size have been found to be independent factors associated with a reduction in PASP after transcatheter ASD closure.[100]

ASD closure is recommended in patients with any level of pulmonary hypertension and a left-to-right shunt. Those with a bidirectional shunt and systemic desaturation (aortic saturation <92%) should undergo pulmonary vasodilator testing with test occlusion of the ASD. If the response is favorable, percutaneous ASD closure may be performed. A favorable response is defined as a fall in the mean pulmonary arterial pressures with oxygen and test occlusion, with no decrease in the cardiac output and no increase in the right atrial pressure. If the response is unfavorable, the patient should be started on pulmonary vasodilator therapy, and cardiac catheterization should be repeated after several months to reassess the hemodynamics. If there has been a favorable change, the ASD may be closed at that time with a fenestrated device designed for such cases (Fig. 49.23).

Diastolic Left Ventricular Dysfunction and Atrial Septal Defect Closure

An increasing number of patients older than 60 years are being referred for transcatheter closure of ASDs. Up to 25% of these patients may have left ventricular restrictive physiology.[104] Closure of the ASD in this situation may result in an acute increase in left atrial pressure and precipitation of pulmonary edema and left heart failure.[105] Anticipation of this complication is important, and proper evaluation of the patient before ASD closure is necessary.

We recommend a protocol similar to that described by Schubert and colleagues, in which patients have their left atrial pressure assessed with and without balloon occlusion.[104] If the

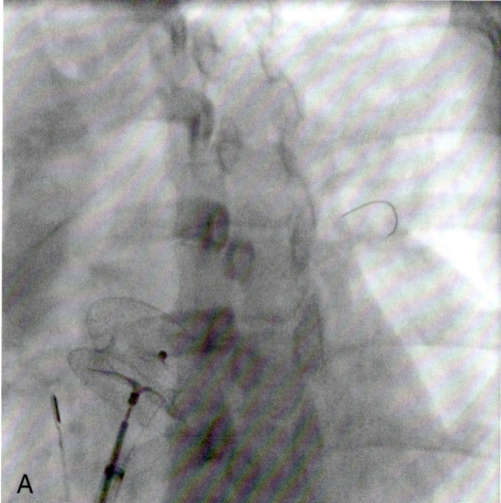
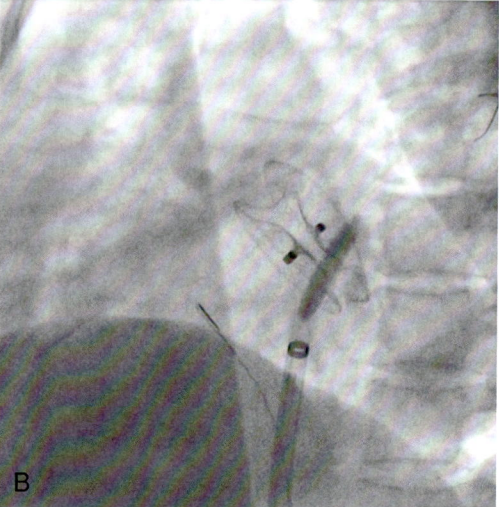
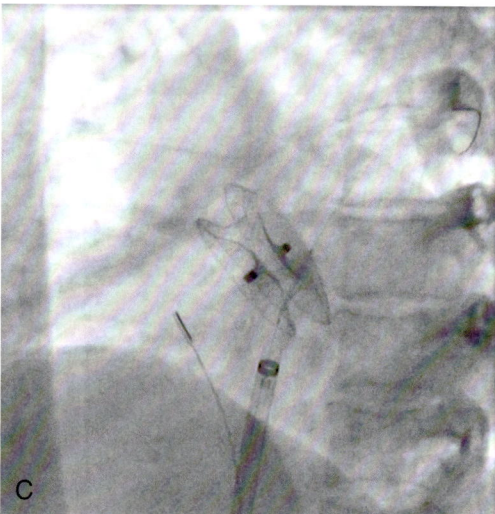

Fig. 49.23 Cine images show the deployment of a fenestrated device for atrial septal defect closure in a patient with a bidirectional shunt and severe pulmonary hypertension responsive to pulmonary vasodilator therapy. After ex vivo creation of the fenestration, the fenestration is crossed with the use of an extra support wire before device loading. (A) After it is deployed, the device is observed in a stable position. The extra support coronary wire tip is kept in the left upper pulmonary vein for support. (B) After measurements, a coronary balloon is advanced over the wire and used to expand the fenestration. (C) A bare-metal stent is then deployed across the fenestration.

left atrial pressure increases significantly (>10 mm Hg) with test occlusion, the patient should undergo medical conditioning with diuretics and a drug such as milrinone or nesiritide. A Swan-Ganz catheter can be placed in these patients to monitor wedge pressures. After 48 to 72 hours of medical therapy, the patient can then undergo a repeat catheterization, and if the left atrial pressure does not increase by more than 10 mm Hg, the ASD can be closed and the patient weaned from the medications over the next 48 hours. Diuretics are usually necessary on discharge.

CONCLUSIONS

Transcatheter PFO closure for recurrent ischemic strokes is more supported with emerging data, but remains controversial. Transcatheter secundum ASD closure is standard therapy for not only simple secundum ASDs, but also large, multiple, or multi-fenestrated defects and for complex patients, such as those with pulmonary hypertension and restrictive left ventricular physiology.

KEY REFERENCES

8. Wu LA, Malouf JF, Dearani JA, et al. Patent foramen ovale in cryptogenic stroke. Current understanding and management options. *Arch Intern Med.* 2004;164:950–956.
38. Atianzar K, Casterella P, Zhang M, Sharma R, Gafoor S. Update on the management of patent foramen ovale in 2017: indication for closure and literature review. *USC.* Fall 2017;11(2) https://www.uscjournal.com/articles/update-management-patent-foramen-ovale-2017-indication-closure-and-literature-review.
43. Furlan AJ, Reisman M, Massaro J, et al. Closure or medical therapy for cryptogenic stroke with patent foramen ovale. *N Engl J Med.* 2012;366:991–999.
44. Riaz IB, Dhoble A, Mizyed A, et al. Transcatheter patent foramen ovale closure versus medical therapy for cryptogenic stroke: a meta-analysis of randomized clinical trials. *BMC Cardiovasc Disord.* 2013;13:116.
46. NCT00738894 trial. *Gore Helex Septal Occluder for Patent Foramen Ovale Closure in Stroke Patients* (Gore REDUCE). http://www.clinicaltrials.gov/ct2/show/NCT00738894?term=NCT&rank=1. Accessed January 20, 2014.
47. NCT00562289 trial. *Patent Foramen Ovale Closure or Anticoagulants Versus Antiplatelet Therapy to Prevent Stroke Recurrence* (CLOSE). http://www.clinicaltrials.gov/ct2/show/NCT00562289?term=PFO+AND+stroke&rank=4.
73. Melikian N, MacCarthy PA. The spectrum of PFO closure Devices. *Cardiac Interventions Today.* 2017.
74. Zajarias A, Thanigaraj S, Lasala J. Predictors and clinical outcomes of residual shunt in patients undergoing percutaneous transcatheter closure of patent foramen ovale. *J Invasive Cardiol.* 2006;18:533–537.

Additional references available online at expertconsult.com

中文导读

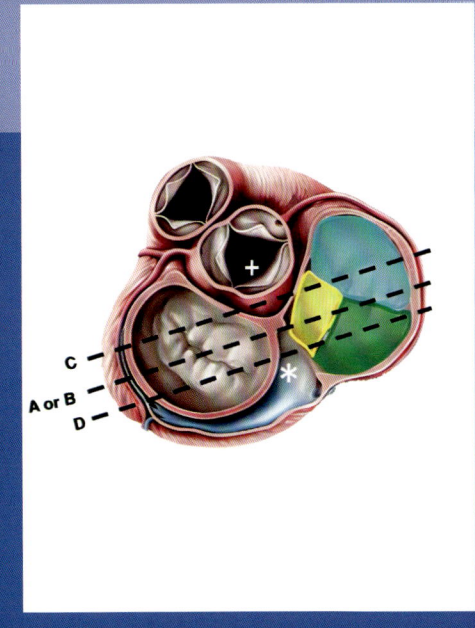

第50章
左心耳封堵与卒中：防止心源性卒中的局部器械治疗

　　心房颤动是卒中和系统性栓塞的重要危险因素。随着全球人口的老龄化，心房颤动的患病率正在大幅增加。虽然口服抗凝药可以降低血栓栓塞的风险，但随之而来的高出血风险限制了其广泛应用。研究证实左心耳是心房颤动患者血栓栓塞的主要来源，并将其描述为"人类最致命的附属器官"。窦性心律下左心耳的舒缩可使出入的血流增加，但心房颤动时左心耳的收缩功能障碍，容易导致局部血液淤滞及血栓形成。因此，针对存在抗凝禁忌和高风险的患者群体，有学者提出了将左心耳隔离于全身循环之外的局部封堵治疗，为这类患者的心源性卒中预防提供了抗凝以外的替代方案。截至目前已有包括Watchman、Amplatzer Cardiac Plug等在内的多种经导管左心耳封堵器械应用于临床。

　　鉴于此，本章总结了心房颤动患者的风险评估，描述了左心耳封堵的作用机制，综述了获得CE认证或美国食品药品监督管理局许可的左心耳封堵器械及其安全性和有效性数据，并对如何选择适合的患者进行左心耳封堵治疗提供了系统的评估方法，包括患者的血栓栓塞风险、长期口服抗凝药物的出血风险、器械植入的手术风险、药物治疗的不依从性，以及患者的偏好等。

张　斌　张洪亮

章节要点

- 心房颤动可以引起中风和系统性栓塞，导致高致残率及死亡率。
- 左心耳是心房颤动中血栓的主要来源，因此也是减少中风的一个介入治疗目标。
- 在高风险患者的外科心脏手术过程中，尽管通常会同时进行左心耳切除或者隔离，但经常发生切除不充分或术后残余，与后续的血栓和栓塞事件有关。
- 针对外科左心耳封堵有效性，不同观察性研究之间存在矛盾的结果。
- 两项随机临床试验比较了Watchman LAA封堵器与华法林在符合口服抗凝条件的患者中的效果，结果显示用该装置封堵是一种可接受的长期华法林替代方案，可预防心血管死亡、中风和系统性栓塞。
- Amplatzer Cardiac Plug和第二代Amulet使用与Watchman不同的机制来封堵LAA。小规模的观察性研究表明Amplatzer与Watchman没有明显差异。
- 对心房颤动患者的评估包括使用有效的风险方案评估血栓栓塞和出血风险，应基于个人的合并症情况，如CHA2DS2-VASc和HAS-BLED评分。
- 适当选择经导管LAA封堵的患者需要综合评估：包括患者的血栓栓塞风险、长期口服抗凝药物的出血风险、器械植入的手术风险、药物治疗的不依从性及患者的偏好等。

50 Left Atrial Appendage Closure and Stroke: Local Device Therapy for Cardiocmbolic Stroke Protection

Matthew J. Price, Miguel Valderrábano

KEY POINTS

- Atrial fibrillation (AF) is associated with substantial morbidity and mortality due to stroke and systemic embolism.
- The left atrial appendage (LAA) appears to be the primary source of thromboembolism in AF and therefore is a target for mechanical therapies for stroke reduction.
- Although concomitant LAA excision or exclusion is commonly performed during cardiac surgery in high-risk patients, insufficient resection or postoperative residual leaks occur frequently and may be associated with thrombus and embolic events.
- Observational studies have provided conflicting results regarding the efficacy of surgical LAA closure for stroke reduction.
- Two randomized clinical trials that compared the Watchman LAA occluder with warfarin in oral anticoagulation–eligible patients have shown that closure with the device is an acceptable alternative to long-term warfarin in some patients for the prevention of cardiovascular death, stroke, and systemic embolism.
- The Amplatzer Cardiac Plug and the second-generation Amulet occlude the LAA using a mechanism different from that of the Watchman. Several small-scale, observational case series suggest that outcomes for the Amplatzer devices are similar to those for the Watchman device.
- Evaluation of the patient with AF incorporates an assessment of thromboembolic and bleeding risk using well-validated risk schemes, such as the CHA_2DS_2-VASc and HAS-BLED scores, which are based on individual comorbidity profiles.
- Appropriate patient selection for transcatheter LAA closure requires the assessment of the individual's risk of thromboembolism, long-term bleeding risk on oral anticoagulation, short-term procedural risk of device implantation, medication noncompliance, and patient preference.

INTRODUCTION

Atrial fibrillation (AF) is associated with a significant risk of stroke and systemic embolism. The worldwide prevalence of this arrhythmia is increasing substantially as the global population ages. Although long-term treatment with oral anticoagulation (OAC) reduces thromboembolic risk, it is associated with an ongoing bleeding hazard and other limitations that deter its use.

The left atrial appendage (LAA) appears to be the dominant source of thromboembolism in patients with AF and has been described as "our most lethal human attachment."[1] LAA contraction during sinus rhythm leads to vigorous blood flow in and out the appendage cavity, but LAA contractile dysfunction during AF can predispose to local stasis, thrombosis, and systemic embolization. Local therapies that exclude the LAA from the systemic circulation offer a mechanical alternative to OAC for cardioembolic stroke protection in these patients, and several devices for transcatheter LAA closure have been developed.

This chapter summarizes the approaches to risk assessment for AF patients, describes the mechanistic basis for LAA closure, reviews the devices with the Conformité Européenne (CE) mark or U.S. Food and Drug Administration (FDA) clearance and their safety and efficacy data sets, and provides a framework for selecting the appropriate patient for device therapy.

ATRIAL FIBRILLATION AND STROKE

AF is the most common arrhythmia in the United States and is associated with significant morbidity and mortality.[2] AF results in up to a fivefold increased risk of stroke,[3,4] a twofold increased risk of dementia,[5–7] a threefold increased risk of heart failure,[4] and a 40% to 90% increased risk of overall mortality.[8] The overall global burden of AF, its incidence, its prevalence, and its associated mortality have progressively increased over the past two decades,[9] and the prevalence of AF in the United States is expected to rise to between 5.6 and 12 million cases in 2050.[10]

Risk factors for AF include advancing age, male sex, diabetes mellitus, obesity, hypertension, and European ancestry. The cumulative risk of AF by 80 years of age in the Atherosclerosis Risk in Communities (ARIC) study was 21% among white men, 17% among white women, and 11% among African Americans.[11]

In addition to symptoms such as fatigue, palpitations, and shortness of breath, AF is associated with substantial morbidity, primarily due to stroke and thromboembolism. Paroxysmal, persistent, or permanent forms of AF increase stroke risk to a similar degree.[12] Subclinical AF of more than 6 minutes' duration has been associated with an increased risk of ischemic stroke or systemic embolism.[13]

The relative contribution of AF to stroke is particularly large among the elderly. AF accounted for approximately 24% of strokes in those 80 to 89 years of age in the Framingham Heart Study.[14] AF-related ischemic strokes are more likely to be fatal than non-AF strokes, and among survivors, AF-related strokes are greater in severity and recur more frequently.[15]

ASSESSMENT OF THROMBOEMBOLIC AND BLEEDING RISK

An individualized assessment of thromboembolic risk is a critical part of the therapeutic decision-making process. The $CHADS_2$ and CHA_2DS_2VASc scores are well-validated schemes for the risk stratification of ischemic stroke and systemic thromboembolism. Based on the individual comorbidities defined in Table 50.1, the scores are used to estimate the yearly risk of thromboembolic events and identify patients with AF who may derive clinical benefit from OAC (Table 50.2).[16,17] The CHA_2DS_2VASc

TABLE 50.1 The CHADS$_2$ and CHA$_2$DS$_2$VASc Scoring for Thromboembolic Risk in Atrial Fibrillation

Characteristic	Points
CHADS$_2$	
C: congestive heart failure	1
H: hypertension	1
A: age ≥75 years	1
D: diabetes mellitus	1
S$_2$: prior stroke, transient ischemic attack, or thromboembolism	2
Maximum score	6
CHA$_2$DS$_2$VASc	
C: congestive heart failure	1
H: hypertension	1
A$_2$: age ≥75 years	2
D: diabetes mellitus	1
S$_2$: prior stroke, transient ischemic attack, or thromboembolism	2
V: vascular disease (i.e., prior MI, PAD, or aortic plaque)	1
A: age 65–74 years	1
Sc: sex category (e.g., female)	1
Maximum score	9

MI, Myocardial infarction; *PAD*, peripheral arterial disease.
Modified from January CT, Wann LS, Alpert JS, et al. 2014 AHA/ACC/HRS guidelines for the management of patients with atrial fibrillation: a report of the American College of Cardiology/American Heart Association Task Force on Practice Guidelines and the Heart Rhythm Society. *J Am Coll Cardiol*. 2014;64:e1–e76.

TABLE 50.2 Yearly Risk of Stroke Based on CHADS$_2$ and CHA$_2$DS$_2$VASc Scores

Score	Adjusted Yearly Stroke Rate (%)
CHADS$_2$	
0	1.9
1	2.8
2	4.0
3	5.9
4	8.5
5	12.5
6	18.2
CHA$_2$DS$_2$VASc	
0	0
1	1.3
2	2.2
3	3.2
4	4.0
5	6.7
6	9.8
7	9.6
8	6.7
9	15.2

Modified from January CT, Wann LS, Alpert JS, et al. 2014 AHA/ACC/HRS guidelines for the management of patients with atrial fibrillation: a report of the American College of Cardiology/American Heart Association Task Force on Practice Guidelines and the Heart Rhythm Society. *J Am Coll Cardiol*. 2014;64:e1–e76.

TABLE 50.3 HAS-BLED Bleeding Risk Score for Hemorrhage Risk in Patients With Atrial Fibrillation

Characteristic	Points
H: hypertension (uncontrolled systolic blood pressure >160 mm Hg)	1
A: abnormal liver or renal function[a]	1 each, maximum 2
S: prior stroke	1
B: bleeding history or disposition (e.g., anemia)	1
L: labile INR (i.e., time in therapeutic range <60%)	1
E: elderly age (>65 years)	1
D: drugs promoting bleeding or excess alcohol consumption (>7 units/week)	1 each, maximum 2
Maximum score	9

[a]Abnormal liver function was defined as cirrhosis or biochemical evidence of significant hepatic derangement; abnormal renal function was defined as serum creatinine >200 μmol/L (2.26 mg/dL).
INR, International normalized ratio.
Modified from Pisters R, Lane DA, Nieuwlaat R, et al. A novel user-friendly score (HAS-BLED) to assess 1-year risk of major bleeding in patients with atrial fibrillation: the Euro Heart Survey. *Chest* 2010;138:1093–1100.

score refines the CHADS$_2$ score by providing greater weight for elderly age (A$_2$) and incorporating the sex category (Sc) and vascular disease (VA). The CHA$_2$DS$_2$VASc score can better identify patients who are at low risk (i.e., CHA$_2$DS$_2$VASc score = 0) and those who may not require OAC.[17] The CHA$_2$DS$_2$VASc score can also identify those at risk for stroke despite anticoagulation.[18]

The 2014 American Heart Association (AHA), American College of Cardiology (ACC), and Heart Rhythm Society (HRS) guidelines for the management of patients with AF recommend calculation of the CHA$_2$DS$_2$VASc score to assess stroke risk (class I, level B evidence) and the use of oral anticoagulants in patients with a CHA$_2$DS$_2$VASc score of 2 or greater (class I, level A evidence).[19] The European Society of Cardiology (ESC) guidelines also recommend OAC in patients with a CHA$_2$DS$_2$VASc score of 2 or greater (class I, level A evidence) and state that OAC should be considered in patients with a CHA$_2$DS$_2$VASc score of 1 (class IIa, level A evidence).[20]

The decision to treat a particular patient with OAC is often influenced by a real or perceived risk of bleeding. Several bleeding risk stratification schemes have been proposed. The HAS-BLED score, as defined in Table 50.3, provides better predictive capacity for bleeding events in OAC-treated patients compared with other scores and highlights risk factors that can be actively managed to reduce the bleeding risk.[21–23] The 2016 update of the ESC guidelines for the management of AF recommend that the HAS-BLED score should be used to assess bleeding risk. In that system, a score of 3 or higher indicates high risk, and some caution and regular review is needed after the initiation of antithrombotic therapy (class IIa, level A evidence). The guidelines further recommend that the HAS-BLED score be used to identify modifiable bleeding risks that need to be addressed, but they do not recommend that it be used on its own to exclude patients from OAC therapy (class IIa, level B evidence).[20]

The 2014 AHA/ACC/HRS guidelines make no formal recommendations regarding bleeding risk scores. However, it observes that a HAS-BLED score of 3 or higher indicates a high risk of bleeding that requires closer observation of a patient for adverse events, closer monitoring of international normalized ratios (INRs), and differential dose selections of oral anticoagulants or aspirin.[19]

TABLE 50.4 Bleeding Outcomes in Randomized Trials of Nonvitamin K Antagonist Oral Anticoagulants Compared With Warfarin in Patients With Atrial Fibrillation

Study	Study Drug	Major Bleeding[a] (% Events/100 pt-yr)				GI Bleeding (% Events/100 pt-yr)			
		Interv.	Warf.	HR (95% CI)	P Value	Interv.	Warf.	HR (95% CI)	P Value
RE-LY[26]	Dabigatran[b]	3.11%	3.36%	0.93 (0.81–1.07)	.31	1.51%	1.02%	1.50 (1.19–1.89)	< .001
ARISTOTLE[27]	Apixaban	2.13%	3.09%	0.69 (0.60–0.80)	< .001	0.76%	0.86%	0.89 (0.70–1.15)	.37
ROCKET-AF[28]	Rivaroxaban	3.60%	3.4%	1.04 (0.90–1.20)	.58	3.15%	2.16%	NR	< .001
ENGAGE-AF[29]	Edoxaban[b]	2.75%	3.43%	0.80 (0.71–0.91)	< .001	1.51%	1.23%	1.23 (1.02–1.50)	.03

[a]Definitions of major bleeding: *RE-LY*, clinically overt bleeding with decrease in hemoglobin of ≥2 g/dL, transfusion of ≥2 U of packed red blood cells (PRBCs), or symptomatic bleeding in a critical area or organ; *ARISTOTLE* and *ENGAGE-AF*, clinically overt bleeding with a decrease in hemoglobin of ≥2 g/dL or transfusion of ≥2 U of PRBCs, occurring at a critical site or resulting in death; *ROCKET-AF*, fatal outcome, involvement of a critical anatomic site, decrease in hemoglobin of ≥2 g/dL, transfusion of ≥2 U of PRBCs, or permanent disability.
[b]Event rates are listed for dabigatran (150 mg bid) and edoxaban (60 mg daily) dosages.
CI, Confidence interval; *GI*, gastrointestinal; *HR*, hazard ratio; *Interv.*, intervention; *NR*, not reported; *pt-yr*, patient-years; *Warf.*, warfarin.

ORAL ANTICOAGULATION FOR STROKE PREVENTION

Oral anticoagulants reduce the risk of thromboembolism in patients with nonvalvular AF. Warfarin, a vitamin K antagonist, reduces the risk of ischemic stroke by approximately two-thirds.[24] Successful therapy with warfarin, however, is challenging. Warfarin has a narrow therapeutic window. The pharmacokinetics and pharmacodynamics of warfarin vary considerably because they are influenced by genetics, diet, and numerous drug-drug interactions.[25] Regular laboratory monitoring and dose adjustment are required, and maintenance of anticoagulation in the therapeutic range can be difficult. Patients enrolled in clinical trials were in the therapeutic range 55% to 65% of the time.[26–29]

The nonvitamin K antagonist oral anticoagulants (NOACs) are noninferior or superior to warfarin for the prevention of stroke and systemic embolism, and they are more convenient because they do not require ongoing monitoring.[26–29] The efficacy of the NOACs compared with warfarin is driven primarily by reductions in hemorrhagic stroke; rates of ischemic strokes are similar or only modestly reduced. The NOACs are associated with a similar or lower rate of major hemorrhage than warfarin, with the exception of gastrointestinal bleeding, which is greater with all NOACs except apixaban, for which the risk of gastrointestinal bleeding is similar (Table 50.3).[26–29]

Oral anticoagulants are underused despite their proven efficacy in reducing stroke and systemic embolism.[30–32] In the 2009 U.S. National Health and Wellness Survey, 36% of AF patients at high risk for thromboembolism were not being treated with an oral anticoagulant.[33] In a large study of commercially insured patients with AF, 47% were not receiving an oral anticoagulant despite being at moderate to high risk for stroke.[34] OAC prescription prevalence did not exceed 50% among AF patients with CHA$_2$DS$_2$-VASc ≥3 in the more than 429,000 patients enrolled in the ACC/National Cardiovascular Data Registry (NCDR) PIN-NACLE (Practice Innovation and Clinical Excellence) registry between 2009 and 2012.[35] The prevalence of OAC use in high-risk patients was only modestly improved with the introduction of NOACs in 2014.[36] Indeed, patients with highest risk of stroke tend to be associated with lower rates of OAC prescription.

Patient characteristics associated with lower use of OAC include advancing age, perceived barriers to compliance, dementia, falls, hepatic or renal impairment, drug and alcohol abuse, gastrointestinal bleeding, and intracranial hemorrhage.[37] In the Outcomes Registry for Better Informed Treatment of Atrial Fibrillation (ORBIT) study, patient refusal or preference, fall risk, and frailty were the factors associated with the lowest use of OAC among patients at high risk for stroke.[38]

Therapeutic challenges with the NOACs include cost, lack of widely available antidotes (with the exception of dabigatran), side effects, and the need for long-term compliance. The overall

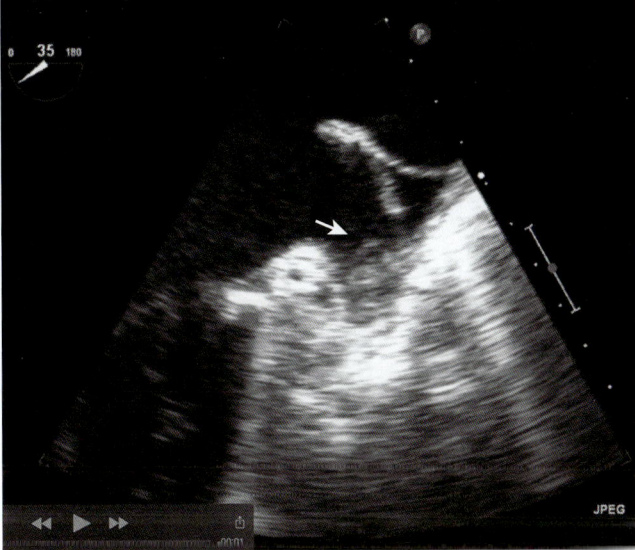

Fig. 50.1 A left atrial appendage thrombus *(arrow)* in a patient with atrial fibrillation is identified by transesophageal echocardiography.

bleeding hazard with the NOACs (see Table 50.4) must be evaluated in the context of a therapy that needs to be administered for years. The safety and efficacy of NOACs for patients at higher risk for bleeding has not been defined because patients with prior bleeding events or those thought to be at high risk for bleeding were excluded or not well represented in the pivotal randomized trials.[26–29,39]

LEFT ATRIAL APPENDAGE CLOSURE

Rationale

The LAA is a multilobed, trabeculated, broad-shaped structure with a narrow neck. During AF, there is decreased LAA contractility and function, leading to dilation and remodeling and causing the appendage to function as a static pouch, predisposing patients to blood stagnation and thrombosis (Fig. 50.1).[40] Anatomic characteristics of the LAA, such as neck diameter, depth,[41] extent of trabeculations,[42] and cauliflower-type morphology,[43,44] have been associated with AF stroke risk (Fig. 50.2).

The LAA was the source of more than 90% of thrombi in cases of stroke in which the thrombus could be identified.[45] These data lend support to the hypothesis that elimination of the LAA may offer a preventive strategy for AF-related stroke.

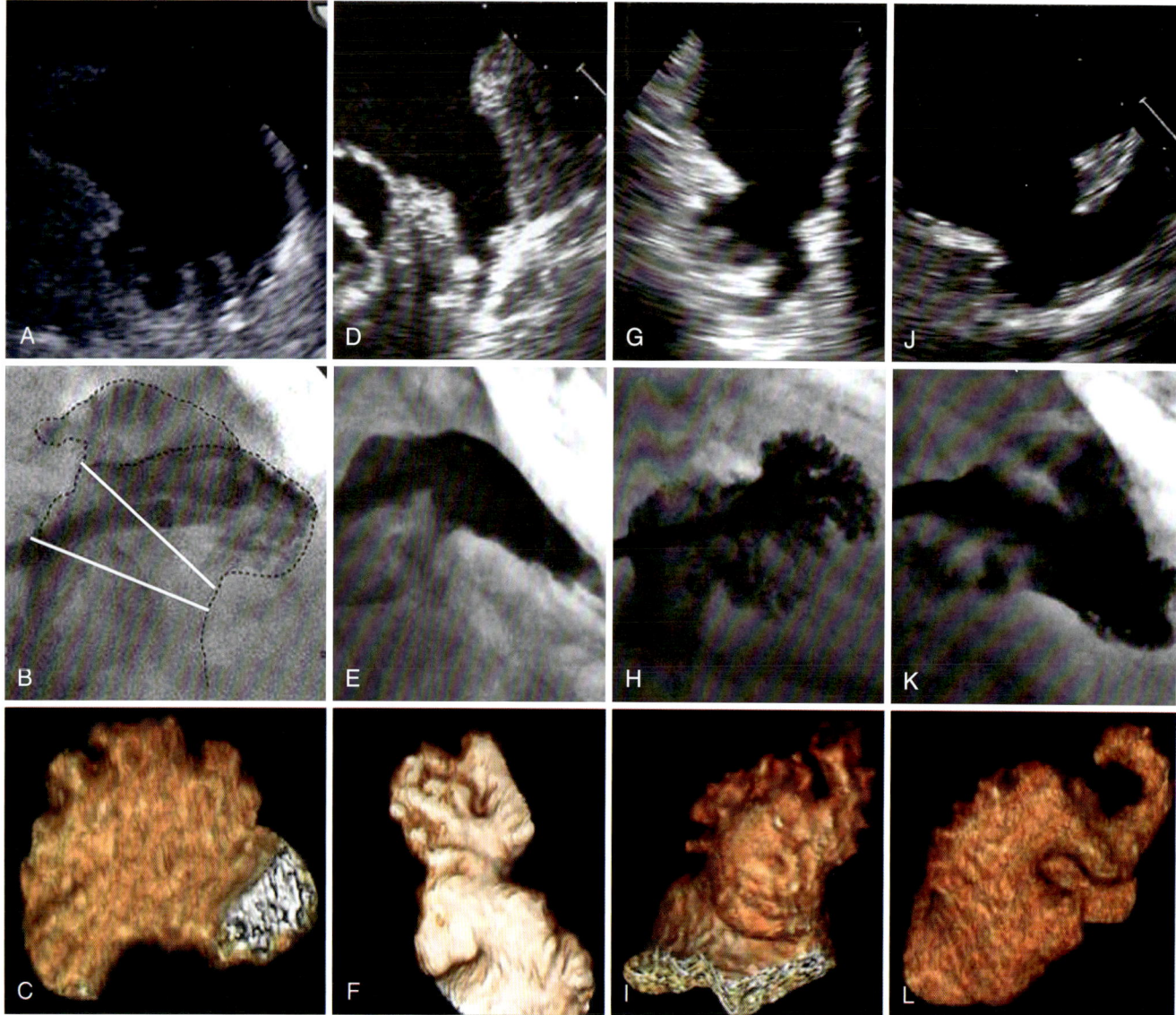

Fig. 50.2 The four morphologic classifications of the left atrial appendage are shown by transesophageal echocardiography *(top)*, cine-angiography *(middle)*, and three-dimensional computed tomography *(bottom)*. (A–C), Cauliflower morphology. (D–F), Windsock morphology. (G–I), Cactus morphology. (J–L), Chicken wing morphology. (Modified from Beigel R, Wunderlich NC, Ho SY, et al. The left atrial appendage: anatomy, function, and noninvasive evaluation. *JACC Cardiovasc Imaging.* 2014;7:1251–1265.)

Surgical Approaches

More than 60 years ago, Madden suggested that surgical resection of the LAA in patients with AF could prevent recurrent arterial emboli,[46] and concomitant exclusion or removal of the LAA during cardiac surgery in high-risk AF patients has become commonplace. The heterogeneity of surgical techniques that are used and the lack of randomized data make it particularly challenging to assess whether this approach is effective in reducing the risk of thromboembolism in the absence of long-term OAC.

The two general approaches to surgical LAA closure are exclusion and excision. Exclusion can be performed with running or mattress sutures, with or without felt pledgets, from the endocardial or epicardial surface or with a stapler (Fig. 50.3). Excision can be performed by stapled excision or removal and oversewing.[47] However, postoperative residual leaks and insufficient resection occur frequently and can be associated with thrombus and neurologic events.[48,49] Incomplete or insufficient closure is more common with suture or staple exclusion than with excision.[47–50]

The results of observational studies that have examined the association between surgical LAA closure and stroke reduction are conflicting (Table 50.5).[47,50] The Left Atrial Appendage Occlusion Study III (LAAOS III) is recruiting participants and will randomly assign approximately 4500 patients with AF undergoing cardiac surgery to concomitant surgical LAA excision or exclusion or to conventional medical therapy (clinicalTrials.gov identifier NCT01561651). The primary end point is the first occurrence of stroke or systemic arterial embolism over a mean follow-up period of 4 years.[51] The results of this trial (scheduled to be completed in 2020) will help define the efficacy of surgical approaches to stroke prevention.

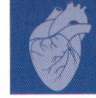

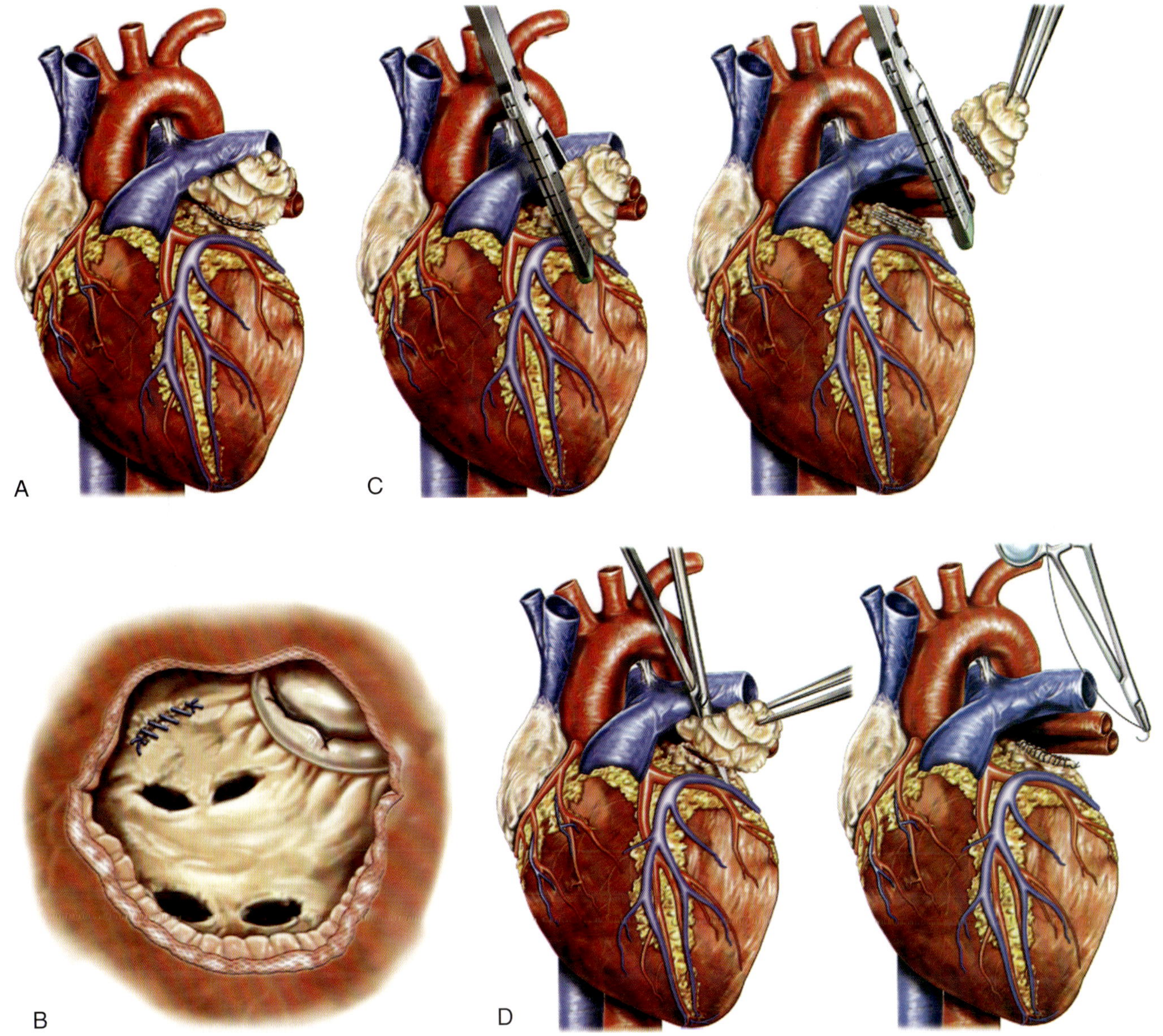

Fig. 50.3 Surgical techniques used to close the left atrial appendage (LAA). (A) Epicardial suture exclusion. (B) Endocardial suture exclusion. (C) Stapled excision, with the stapler positioned across the base of the LAA *(left)* and the LAA removed with an intact stump *(right)*. Thrombotic complications may occur if the residual stump is too large. (D) Removal of the LAA by scissors or electrocautery *(left)*, followed by two-layer suture closure of the LAA stump flush with the heart surface *(right)*. (Modified from Chatterjee S, Alexander JC, Pearson PJ, et al. Left atrial appendage occlusion: lessons learned from surgical and transcatheter experiences. *Ann Thorac Surg.* 2011;92:2283–2292.)

Transcatheter Approaches

Percutaneous Left Atrial Appendage Transcatheter Occlusion System

The Percutaneous Left Atrial Appendage Transcatheter Occlusion (PLAATO) system (ev3, Plymouth, MN) was the first percutaneous device to be prospectively evaluated for the purpose of LAA closure.[59] The device consisted of a self-expanding nitinol cage covered with an occlusive expanded polytetrafluoroethylene (ePTFE) membrane, with small anchors along the struts and passing through the membrane to help anchor the device in the LAA (Fig. 50.4). The device was delivered through a 14-Fr delivery sheath guided by transesophageal echocardiography (TEE) and fluoroscopy.

Device feasibility and long-term outcomes were evaluated in a prospective, nonrandomized, multicenter study of 64 AF patients in North America who were at high risk for thromboembolism (CHADS$_2$ score ≥2) but who were not candidates for warfarin.[60] Patients were treated after the procedure with indefinite aspirin and 4 to 6 weeks of clopidogrel. Anatomic closure at the time of the procedure (i.e., residual flow area ≤3 mm wide) was achieved in 98% of cases, and safety outcomes were excellent (i.e., only one major device-related adverse event within 1 month of the procedure). At the 5-year follow-up, the observed rate of stroke or transient ischemic attack was 3.8% per year, compared with an expected rate of 6.6% based on the CHADS$_2$ score of the study population.

The European prospective, multicenter, observational experience provided further insight into device feasibility and clinical

TABLE 50.5 Comparisons of Surgical Left Atrial Appendage Closure Techniques

Study	Country	No. Studied	Closure Method	Closure Success Rate (%)[a]	Effect of LAA Closure on Stroke Prevention
Johnson et al.[1]	United States	437	Excision	100	Positive
Katz et al.[48]	United States	50	Endocardial suture	64	None
Garcia-Fernandez et al.[52]	Spain	205	Endocardial suture	90	Positive
Bando et al.[53]	Japan	812	Endocardial suture	Not measured	Negative
Blackshear et al.[54]	United States	15	Thoracoscopic epicardial purse-string	93[b]	Positive
Pennec et al.[55]	France	30	Endocardial Excision	70–80 100	Negative Positive
Schneider et al.[56]	Germany	6	Endocardial suture	17	Negative
Healey et al.[57]	Canada	77	Epicardial suture Stapler	45 72	Positive
Kanderian et al.[49]	United States	137	Excision Suture exclusion Stapler	73 (20% stapler) 23 0	Positive trend
Bakhtiary et al.[58]	Germany	259	Clamp and epicardial suture	100[b]	Positive

[a]Assessed by transesophageal echocardiography.
[b]Remnant size not measured.
LAA, Left atrial appendage.
Adapted from Chatterjee S, Alexander JC, Pearson PJ, et al. Left atrial appendage occlusion: lessons learned from surgical and transcatheter experiences. Ann Thorac Surg. 2011;92:2283–2292.

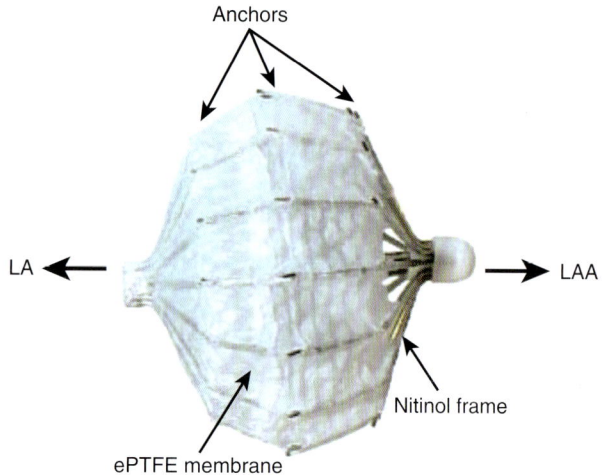

Fig. 50.4 The Percutaneous Left Atrial Appendage Transcatheter Occlusion device was the first to be prospectively evaluated in patients with atrial fibrillation. It consists of a self-expanding nitinol cage covered with an occlusive expanded polytetrafluoroethylene (ePTFE) membrane, with small anchors along the struts and passing through the membrane to help anchor the device in the appendage. LA, Left atrium; LAA, left atrial appendage. (From Sievert H, Lesh MD, Trepels T, et al. Percutaneous left atrial appendage transcatheter occlusion to prevent stroke in high-risk patients with atrial fibrillation: early clinical experience. Circulation. 2002;105:1887–1889.)

efficacy over a relatively short-term clinical follow-up. In this registry, a total of 180 high-risk AF patients were treated with the PLAATO device.[61] LAA occlusion was successful in 90%. The major periprocedural complication was cardiac tamponade, which occurred in 3.3% of cases. At 129 patient-years of follow-up, the observed incidence of stroke was 2.3% per year, compared with the expected 6.6%.[61] The device was not evaluated beyond these studies due to financial considerations. However, the PLAATO experience serves as proof of the principle for transcatheter occlusion of the LAA for stroke prevention.

Watchman Occluder

Device Characteristics

The Watchman LAA closure device (Boston Scientific, Natick, MA) is parachute shaped and consists of a nitinol frame and a polyethylene terephthalate (PET) fabric membrane cap that faces the body of the left atrium (Fig. 50.5). Small tines that project toward the left atrium line the circumference of the distal portion of the device and help anchor the device in the LAA trabeculae. The device is connected to a delivery cable by a threaded insert in the proximal cap.

Device size corresponds to the diameter of the device measured at the proximal shoulders, which is its widest portion. The five sizes range from 21 to 33 mm, in 3-mm increments. The manufacturer recommends oversizing the device by 8% to 20%, although some operators have advocated more aggressive oversizing.[62] The Watchman device is used to occlude LAAs between approximately 17 and 30 mm in diameter, as long as there is sufficient depth to accommodate the device, whose length is approximately equal to its fully expanded diameter. The device can be partially recaptured and redeployed before release from the delivery cable if the implant location is too deep, or it can be fully recaptured and removed if it is deployed too proximally or a different device size is required. This device is CE marked for sale within the European Economic Area and is approved for use in the United States. The FDA indications for use, and the Center for Medicare and Medicaid Services (CMS) coverage decision, are shown in Box 50.1 and 50.2, respectively.

Implantation Procedure

Device selection is determined by LAA size, which is derived from a combination of TEE and fluoroscopic measurements (Fig. 50.6). Cardiac computed tomography (CT) can also be used for preprocedural planning,[63] but the presence of LAA thrombus should be excluded by TEE at the time of the procedure itself. A 14-Fr double- or single-curved access sheath is introduced into the left atrium through a transseptal puncture in the inferoposterior aspect of the interatrial septum. The 14-Fr access sheath is carefully placed deep within the LAA and often telescoped over a diagnostic pigtail catheter to prevent laceration or perforation of the thin-walled, friable LAA.

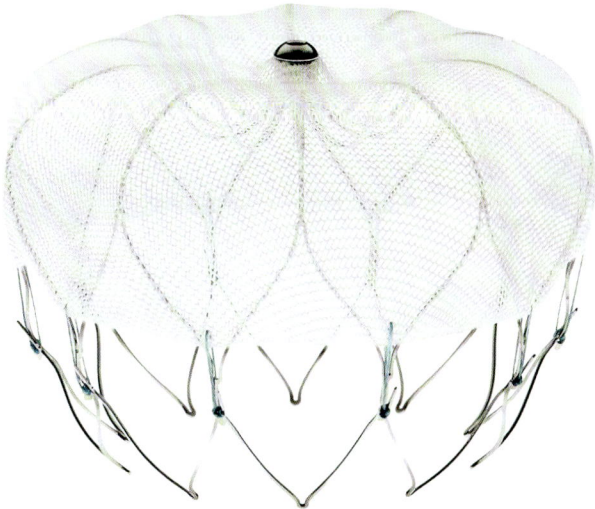

Fig. 50.5 The Watchman device is composed of a self-expanding nitinol frame with a polyethylene terephthalate fabric cap. Distal tines secure the device in the left atrial appendage trabeculae. The device length is approximately equal to its diameter. The device is fully retrievable before release from the delivery cable.

BOX 50.1 Food and Drug Administration Indication for Use for the Watchman Left Atrial Appendage Occluder

The WATCHMAN is indicated to reduce the risk of thromboembolism from the left atrial appendage in patients with nonvalvular atrial fibrillation who:

- Are at an increased risk of for stroke and systemic embolism based on $CHADS_2$ or CHA_2DS_2VASc scores and are recommended for OAC
- Are deemed by their physicians to be suitable for warfarin
- Have an appropriate rationale to seek a nonpharmacologic alternative to warfarin, taking into account the safety and effectiveness of the device compared to warfarin

Specific factors may include one or more of the following:

- A history of major bleeding while taking therapeutic anticoagulation therapy
- The patient's prior experience with OAC (if applicable),
- A medical condition, occupation, or lifestyle placing the patient at high risk of major bleeding secondary to trauma

OAC, Oral anticoagulation.
From https://www.accessdata.fda.gov/scripts/cdrh/cfdocs/cfpma/pma.cfm?id=P130013. Accessed April 12, 2018.

The device, which is provided preloaded in a delivery system and attached to a delivery cable, is advanced to the tip of the access sheath, after which the sheath is withdrawn and the device deployed. Device implantation is guided by a combination of TEE and fluoroscopy, and TEE imaging plays a critical role in assessing the adequacy of device deployment (Figs. 50.7 and 50.8). The device is then released by counterclockwise rotation of the delivery cable if the appropriate TEE and fluoroscopic measurements are met. Recently, interventionalists have proposed using intraprocedural intracardiac echocardiography (ICE) to guide the Watchman LAA closure procedure, with an aim to simplify the procedural logistics, as this would avoid the use of TEE, which in turn generally requires general anesthesia.[64,65]

BOX 50.2 Summary of Centers for Medicare and Medicaid Services National Coverage Decision for Left Atrial Appendage Closure

1. The device must have received FDA approval
2. The patient must have:
   - A $CHADS_2$ score ≥2 or a CHA_2DS_2VASc score ≥3
   - A formal shared-decision making interaction with an independent physician using an evidence based tool on OAC in patients with AF prior to LAA closure
   - A suitability for short-term warfarin but deemed unable to take long-term oral anticoagulation
3. The patient is enrolled in, and the hospital must participate in, a prospective, national, audited registry (i.e., the American College of Cardiology NCDR LAAO registry)
4. The operator has performed ≥25 interventional cardiac procedures that involve transseptal puncture through an intact septum

FDA, Food and Drug Administration; *LAA*, left atrial appendage; *LAAO*, left atrial appendage occlusion; *NCDR*, National Cardiovascular Data Registry.

Clinical Data

Clinical outcomes for the Watchman device have been evaluated in several studies (Table 50.6). Safety and clinical efficacy have been evaluated in two Bayesian, randomized clinical trials that tested whether LAA occlusion was noninferior to warfarin therapy for the primary efficacy end point of stroke, systemic embolism, and cardiovascular or unexplained death in AF patients who were eligible for long-term OAC. The trials had different study sizes, entry criteria, and follow-up durations.

The Watchman Left Atrial Appendage System for Embolic Protection in Patients with Atrial Fibrillation (PROTECT-AF) trial randomly assigned 707 AF patients with a $CHADS_2$ score of 1 or greater who were eligible for long-term OAC to Watchman LAA closure or warfarin in a 2:1 ratio.[66] The Prospective Randomized Evaluation of the Watchman Left Atrial Appendage Closure Device in Patients with Atrial Fibrillation Versus Long-Term Warfarin Therapy (PREVAIL) trial randomly assigned 407 AF patients with a $CHADS_2$ score of 2 or greater to Watchman LAA closure or warfarin in a 2:1 ratio. In these trials, patients who received the Watchman device were continued on warfarin therapy for approximately 6 weeks after the procedure, at which time they were transitioned to dual antiplatelet therapy (DAPT) with aspirin and clopidogrel for 6 months, followed by indefinite aspirin monotherapy if LAA sealing was confirmed by TEE (Fig. 50.9).

PROTECT-AF

In the PROTECT-AF trial, Watchman LAA closure was noninferior and superior to warfarin for the primary efficacy end point at a mean follow-up of 3.8 ± 1.7 years (2625 patient-years; rate ratio = 0.60; 95% credible interval [CrI] 0.41 to 1.05; posterior probability of noninferiority >99.9%, posterior probability for superiority = 96%; Fig. 50.10). LAA closure was also superior to warfarin therapy when the results were analyzed using traditional, frequentist statistical methods (hazard ratio [HR] 0.61; 95% confidence interval [CI] 0.38 to 0.97; $P = .04$). The clinical efficacy of LAA closure was maintained after the completion of the protocol-mandated postprocedural adjunctive pharmacotherapy in the device group (i.e., warfarin and DAPT; HR 0.32; 95% CI 0.17 to 0.63; $P < .001$). Safety events were initially greater in the device group and driven by procedural complications, although by the end of follow-up, the overall rate of safety events in both arms were similar due to bleeding events in the warfarin group (see Fig. 50.10).

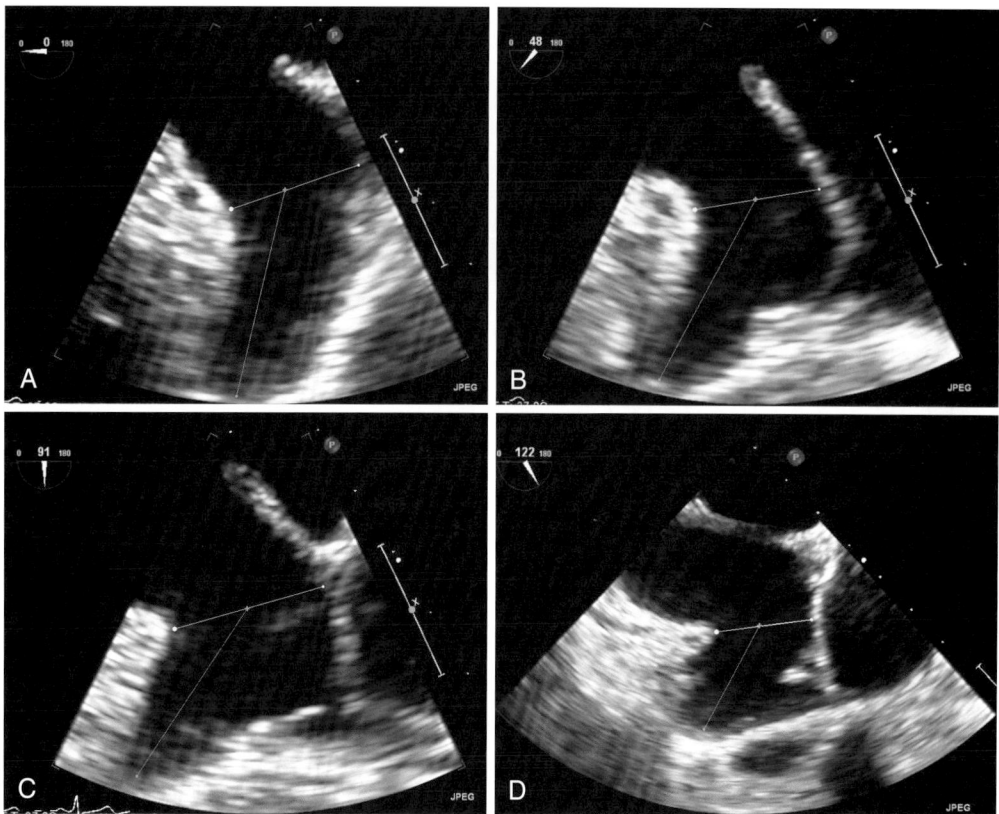

Fig. 50.6 Preprocedural transesophageal echocardiographic assessment of the left atrial appendage (LAA) before Watchman occluder implantation. The diameter and depth of the LAA is measured at 0, 45, 90, and 135 degrees (A, B, C, and D, respectively). The diameter of the LAA is defined as the distance from a point just distal to the left circumflex artery (i.e., mitral valve annulus) to roughly 1 to 2 cm from the tip of the ridge of the left upper pulmonary vein. Alternatively, the LAA ostium can be measured by drawing a line from the mitral valve annulus across to the ridge of the left upper pulmonary vein perpendicular to the planned axis of the delivery sheath. The initially selected device size is often modified after the delivery sheath is introduced into the LAA because this may clarify the maximal implantation depth. (Copyright © MedReviews, LLC. Reprinted with permission of MedReviews, LLC. Price MJ. Left atrial appendage occlusion with the WATCH-MAN™ for stroke prevention in atrial fibrillation. *Rev Cardiovasc Med*. 2014;15[2]:142–151. *Reviews in Cardiovascular Medicine* is a copyrighted publication of MedReviews, LLC. All rights reserved.)

The rates of ischemic stroke did not differ between groups in the PROTECT-AF trial, although the rate of fatal and disabling stroke was lower in the device group (rate ratio = 0.37; 95% CrI 0.15 to 1.00; Fig. 50.11). Cardiovascular and all-cause mortality were also reduced with LAA closure (HR 0.40; 95% CI 0.21 to 0.75; P = .005 and HR 0.66; 95% CI 0.45 to 0.98; P = .04, respectively). Peri-device flow on follow-up TEE was a common finding (41% and 32% of patients at 6 weeks and 1 year after the procedure, respectively). It was mostly less than 3 mm in diameter and did not appear to be associated with thromboembolic events.[67] Quality-of-life measurements were significantly improved for the patients randomly assigned to the device compared with those on warfarin.[68]

The final 5-year follow-up of PROTECT-AF is in line with these findings.[69] At a mean follow-up of 2717 patient-years, the primary efficacy end point was significantly reduced with Watchman LAA closure compared with warfarin (2.66 events per 100 patient-years vs. 3.66 events per 100 patient-years, P = .04), as was cardiovascular mortality (2.32 events per 100-patient-years vs. 1.03 events per 100 patient-years, P = .009).

PREVAIL

The aim of the smaller PREVAIL trial was to confirm procedural safety, particularly among newer operators, and to further explore clinical efficacy of LAA closure compared with warfarin.[70] Operators without prior Watchman experience implanted the device in approximately 40% of the enrolled patients. Three coprimary end points were examined: procedural safety, primary clinical efficacy (i.e., composite of stroke, systemic embolism, and cardiovascular or unexplained death), and late clinical efficacy (i.e., ischemic stroke and systemic embolism occurring >7 days after the procedure).

The Watchman met the performance goal for procedural and device safety prespecified by the sponsor and the FDA, with safety events occurring in 2.2% of patients. Implantation by new operators was not associated with reduced rates of implant success or an increased risk of major adverse events, indicating that the training program implemented during the trial mitigated any substantial learning curve with the device. The rate of procedural complications, including stroke and serious pericardial effusions, were significantly reduced in the PREVAIL trial compared with PROTECT-AF and were consistent with that of the prospective continued access registry that followed the PROTECT-AF trial (Table 50.7).[71]

At a mean follow-up of 11.8 ± 5.8 months, the primary efficacy end point of stroke, systemic embolism, or cardiovascular death was similar between study arms, but LAA closure did not achieve noninferiority due to wide 95% credible intervals (device event rate of 0.064 vs. warfarin event rate of 0.064; rate

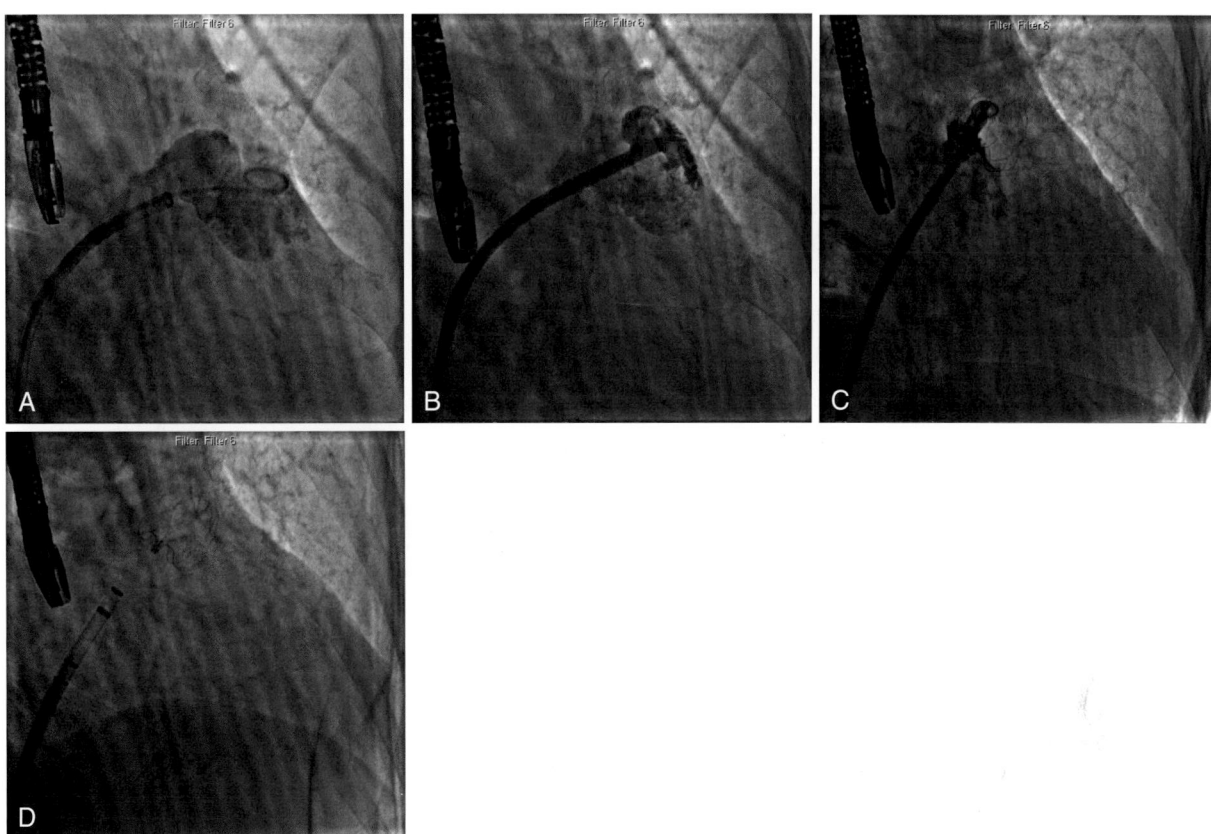

Fig. 50.7 Watchman left atrial appendage closure. (A) Left atrial appendage (LAA) angiography is performed in the right anterior oblique caudal projection through a 6-Fr diagnostic pigtail catheter that has been advanced through a dedicated 14-Fr access sheath. (B) The access sheath is advanced deeply into the LAA over the pigtail catheter while applying counterclockwise rotation to orient the sheath coaxially with the LAA ostium. (C) Left atrial angiography after device deployment demonstrates successful LAA closure. Contrast can enter the LAA through the perforated cap of the device, which endothelializes in the weeks after implantation. (D) Fluoroscopy of the device after release from the delivery cable. (Modified from Price MJ, Holmes DR. Mechanical closure devices for atrial fibrillation. *Trends Cardiovasc Med.* 2014;24:225-231.)

TABLE 50.6 Studies of Left Atrial Appendage Occlusion With the Watchman Device for Stroke Prevention in Nonvalvular Atrial Fibrillation

	PROTECT AF	CAP	PREVAIL	CAP2	ASAP	Ewolution	Post-Approval Registry
Design	Noninferiority versus warfarin, 2:1 randomization	Prospective Observational	Noninferiority versus warfarin, 2:1 randomization	Prospective Observational	Prospective Observational	Prospective Observational	Prospective Observational
Population	n = 463 OAC eligible	n = 566 OAC eligible	n = 269 OAC eligible	n = 578 OAC eligible	n = 150 OAC ineligible 4 European centers	n = 1025 73% OAC ineligible 47 centers in Europe, Russia, Middle East	n = 3822
CHA_2DS_2VASc	3.2	3.9	4.0	4.5	4.4	4.5	4.0
Postimplantation therapy	Warfarin × 45 days DAPT × 5 months ASA lifelong	Warfarin × 45 days DAPT × 5 months ASA lifelong	Warfarin × 45 days DAPT × 5 months ASA lifelong	Warfarin × 45 days DAPT × 5 months ASA lifelong	DAPT × 6 months ASA lifelong	Operator discretion: 60% DAPT 15% warfarin 11% NOAC + ASA lifelong	Operator discretion

ASA, Aspirin; *ASAP,* ASA Plavix Feasibility Study with Watchman Left Atrial Appendage Closure Technology; *CAP,* Continuing Access to PROTECT-AF; *CAP2,* Continued Access to PREVAIL; *DAPT* dual antiplatelet therapy, *NOAC;* nonvitamin K antagonist oral anticoagulant; *OAC,* oral anticoagulation; *PREVAIL,* Prospective Randomized Evaluation of the Watchman LAA Closure Device in Patients With Atrial Fibrillation Versus Long-Term Warfarin Therapy; *PROTECT-AF,* Watchman Left Atrial Appendage System for Embolic Protection in Patients With Atrial Fibrillation.

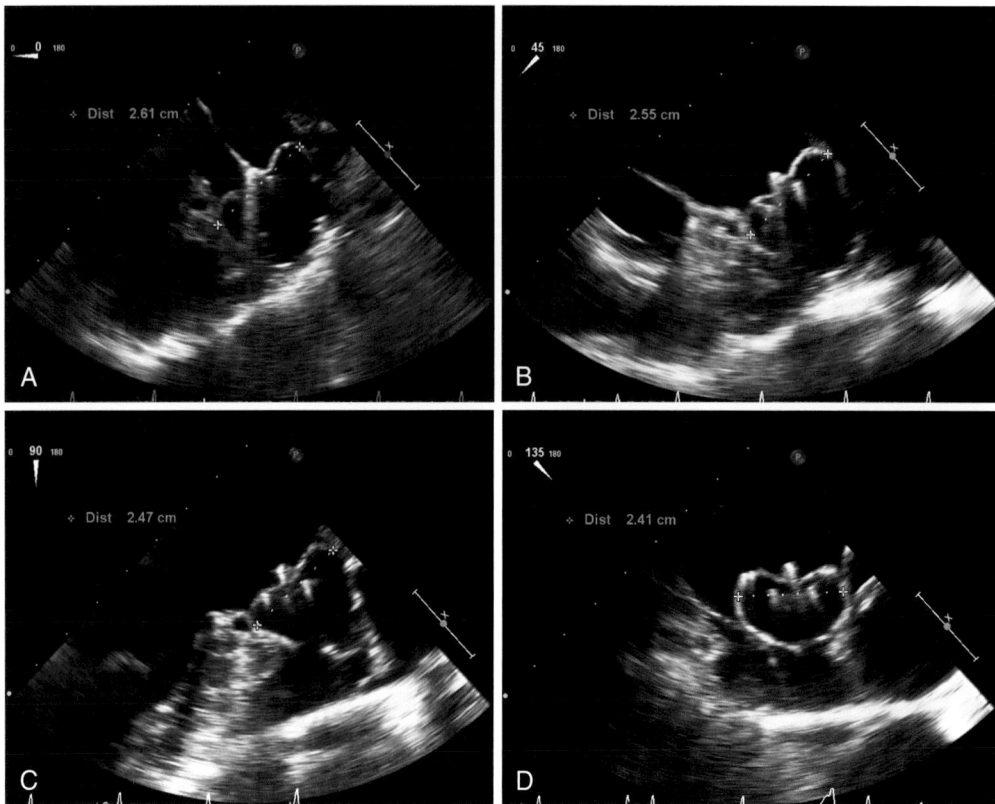

Fig. 50.8 Transesophageal echocardiographic *(TEE)* assessment of Watchman occluder implantation. After deployment of a Watchman 30-mm left atrial appendage *(LAA)* occluder, the device is assessed at 0, 45, 90, and 135 degrees (A, B, C, and D, respectively). Compression is determined by measuring the distance across the shoulders of the device. The device is released if compression and position are adequate, the LAA is shown to be sealed by color Doppler and left atrial angiography, and the device is well anchored according to a tug test. In this case, the device is approximately 13% to 20% compressed and is well positioned, no color flow is seen around the device into the LAA, and the LAA moved with the device as a unit when the delivery cable was tugged gently. The device was therefore released from the cable with successful LAA occlusion. According to the protocol in research studies, the patient was treated with warfarin and aspirin for 6 weeks, when repeat TEE confirmed LAA closure without thrombus, and the warfarin was then discontinued. The patient was treated with aspirin and clopidogrel for 5 more months and then was continued on aspirin monotherapy. (Copyright © MedReviews, LLC. Reprinted with permission of MedReviews, LLC. Price MJ. Left atrial appendage occlusion with the WATCHMAN™ for stroke prevention in atrial fibrillation. *Rev Cardiovasc Med.* 2014;15[2]:142–151. *Reviews in Cardiovascular Medicine* is a copyrighted publication of MedReviews, LLC. All rights reserved.)

ratio = 1.07; 95% CrI 0.57 to 1.89; rate ratio for noninferiority criterion: upper bound of 95% CrI <1.75, posterior probability for noninferiority = 93.0%). The rate of ischemic stroke or systemic embolism was noninferior to Watchman LAA closure. The final, longer-term outcomes of the PREVAIL trial have also been reported. At a mean of follow-up of 47.9 ± 19.4 months (1626 patient-years), Watchman LAA closure was still not noninferior to warfarin for the primary efficacy end point of stroke, systemic embolism, or cardiovascular death (rate ratio = 1.33; 95% CI 0.78 to 2.13; posterior probability for noninferiority = 88.4%), and achieved noninferiority for the end point of ischemic stroke or systemic embolism (posterior probability of noninferiority = 97.5%).

The clinical efficacy findings in the PREVAIL trial should be interpreted in the context of a much lower than expected rate of stroke and systemic embolism in the warfarin control group despite the baseline high-risk characteristics of the enrolled population.[70]

Meta-Analysis of Protect-AF and Prevail

A meta-analysis of pooled, patient-level data from long-term follow-up of PROTECT-AF (total follow-up, 2717 years) and the PREVAIL (total follow-up, 1626 years) further assessed the outcomes of LAA closure with the Watchman compared with warfarin in AF patients suitable for long-term warfarin (Table 50.8).[69] The rate of the primary efficacy end point (cardiovascular/unexplained death, stroke, or systemic embolism) was similar between device closure and warfarin therapy (HR 0.82; 95% CI 0.58 to 1.17; P = .27), as was the rate of all-cause stroke and systemic embolism (HR 0.96; 95% CI 0.60 to 1.54; P = .87). The rate of cardiovascular or unexplained death and the rate of all-cause mortality was both significantly lower with device therapy (HR 0.59; 95% CI 0.37 to 0.94; P = .027 and HR 0.73; 95% CI 0.54 to 0.98; P = 0.035). Hemorrhagic stroke was significantly and substantially reduced by device closure (HR 0.20; 95% CI 0.07 to 0.56; P = .0022). The rate of ischemic stroke and systemic embolism more than 7 days postprocedure (i.e., not related to the procedure) was numerically higher in the device group, although the difference did not reach statistical significance (HR 1.40; 95% CI 0.76 to 2.58; P =.24). Significantly fewer disabling strokes occurred with device closure compared with warfarin (HR 0.41; 95% CI 0.19 to 0.90; P = .027). There were no significant interactions between various sub-groups and the treatment effect of LAA closure.

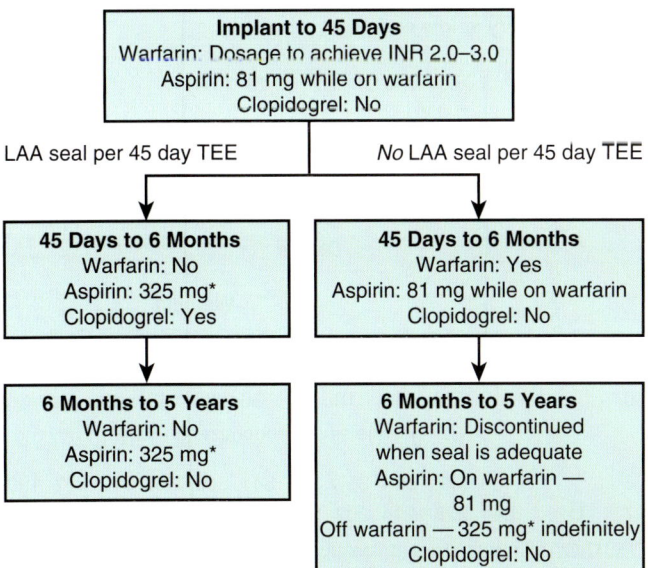

Fig. 50.9 Anticoagulant and antiplatelet management strategy for patients receiving device therapy in the PROTECT-AF and PREVAIL randomized clinical trials of the Watchman left atrial appendage *(LAA)* occluder. After device implantation, patients were treated with a combination of warfarin and aspirin for approximately 6 weeks, at which time transesophageal echocardiography *(TEE)* was performed. If the LAA was sealed (i.e., residual leak <5 mm wide without evidence of thrombus), warfarin was discontinued, and the patient was treated with aspirin and clopidogrel until 6 months after the procedure, at which time the clopidogrel was discontinued and the patient continued on aspirin monotherapy. In the PROTECT-AF trial, patients could also receive clopidogrel at study entry if clinically indicated. *Asterisk*, Recommended dosage; *INR*, international normalized ratio; *PREVAIL*, Prospective Randomized Evaluation of the Watchman Left Atrial Appendage Closure Device in Patients with Atrial Fibrillation Versus Long-Term Warfarin Therapy; *PROTECT-AF*, Watchman Left Atrial Appendage System for Embolic Protection in Patients with Atrial Fibrillation. (Modified from Holmes DR Jr, Kar S, Price MJ, et al. Prospective randomized evaluation of the Watchman Left Atrial Appendage Closure device in patients with atrial fibrillation versus long-term warfarin therapy: the PREVAIL trial. *J Am Coll Cardiol.* 2014;64:1–12.)

In another pooled analysis of PROTECT-AF and PREVAIL, Watchman LAA closure significantly reduced major bleeding compared with continued warfarin therapy once the 6-month period of postprocedure pharmacotherapy was completed (1.0 events vs. 3.5 events per 100 patient-years; RR 0.28; 95% CI 0.16 to 0.49; P < .001).[72] This benefit was driven by reductions in gastrointestinal bleeding and intracranial hemorrhage (Table 50.9 and Fig. 50.12). Although reductions in major bleeding were observed across all subgroups studies, LAA closure had particular benefit among patients who were elderly, female, and at low baseline bleeding risk (Table 50.10).

Watchman LAA closure in OAC-contraindicated patients. Although the PROTECT-AF and PREVAIL trials studied LAA closure in an OAC-eligible population, stroke prevention strategies are particularly challenging in patients who cannot tolerate anticoagulation or in whom anticoagulation is contraindicated. The ASA Plavix Feasibility Study With Watchman Left Atrial Appendage Closure Technology (ASAP) trial was a prospective, multicenter, nonrandomized study that examined the clinical efficacy of Watchman LAA closure in 150 AF patients who were ineligible for warfarin therapy.[18] After implantation, patients were treated with clopidogrel for 6 months and with aspirin indefinitely. The rate of stroke or systemic embolism was 2.3% per year at a mean follow-up of 14.4 ± 8.6 months, which was significantly less than the expected rate of 7.3% per year based on a hypothetical patient population with similar $CHADS_2$ treated with aspirin alone. At a median follow-up of 55.4 months, the annual rate of ischemic stroke or systemic embolism was 1.8% (95% CI 0.9% to 3.3%), approximately 75% lower than the expected rate.[73] Further data are required to robustly define the early safety of the Watchman device with postprocedural DAPT rather than a brief course of OAC. The prospective, multicenter ASAP-TOO (Assessment of the WATCHMAN Device in Patients Unsuitable for Oral Anticoagulation) trial will enroll approximately 900 AF patients who are deemed unsuitable for OAC and randomize them to either medical therapy (single or no antiplatelet therapy per operator discretion) or Watchman LAA closure followed by a modified postimplant drug regimen of DAPT that does not include OAC.[74]

Amplatzer Cardiac Plug and Amulet

Device Characteristics and Procedural Approach
The Amplatzer Cardiac Plug (ACP, St. Jude Medical, Minneapolis, MN) consists of a self-expanding nitinol mesh that forms a distal lobe and proximal disk, each with a sewn polyester patch, and they are connected by a short, central waist. The distal lobe has hooks around its circumference that anchors the device in the LAA, and the proximal disk covers the mouth of the LAA from within the left atrium, akin to a baby pacifier (Fig. 50.13).[75]

The mechanism of LAA occlusion is different from that of the Watchman, which occludes the LAA by filling the appendage itself. Device sizing is based on the maximal diameter of the distal lobe's landing zone. The second-generation ACP, the Amulet, has a slightly longer distal lobe, more stabilizing hooks, a longer central waist, and a larger-diameter proximal disk with a recessed threaded insert (Fig. 50.14).[76] These modifications improve device stability, position, residual leak, and the incidence of device-associated thrombi.[77]

For the ACP or Amulet, the landing zone is measured approximately 12 to 15 mm from the LAA orifice.[78] The device is delivered through a 12- to 14-Fr double-curved sheath that is introduced into the LAA from the right femoral vein through a transseptal puncture. The ACP and Amulet have the CE mark but are not approved for use in the United States.

Clinical Data
The safety and clinical efficacy of the ACP and Amulet devices for stroke prevention in AF have been examined in several nonrandomized, retrospective and prospective, observational studies, many of which were single-center experiences (Table 50.11). Most studies evaluated the device in patients with intolerance or contraindications to OAC, and patients were usually treated with a limited course of antiplatelet therapy after device implantation.

Several tentative conclusions can be gleaned from the reported experience with the ACP and the Amulet. The rates of successful LAA closure are excellent. The most frequent procedural complication appears to be pericardial effusion, occurring at rates similar to those seen in the randomized Watchman experience, and clinical efficacy appears acceptable, with the important caveat that the data set is substantially limited by the study designs.

Several randomized trials of the Amulet device are either planned or ongoing. The STROKECLOSE trial (Prevention of Stroke by Left Atrial Appendage Closure in Atrial Fibrillation Patients After Intracerebral Hemorrhage; clinicaltrials.gov identifier, NCT02830152) will randomly assign 750 AF patients with prior intracranial hemorrhage in a 2:1 fashion to Amulet LAA occlusion or medical therapy. The primary end point is the composite of any stroke, major bleeding, and death at 2 years. The Amulet LAA Occluder trial (clinicaltrials.gov identifier,

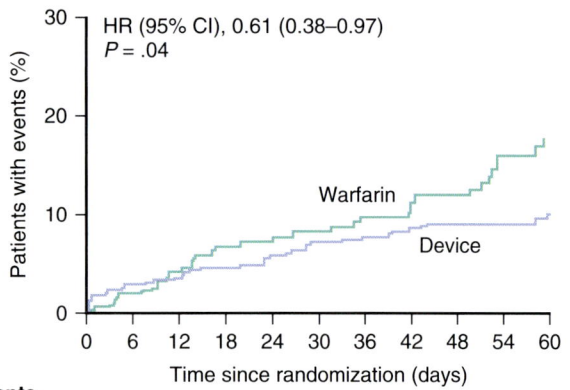
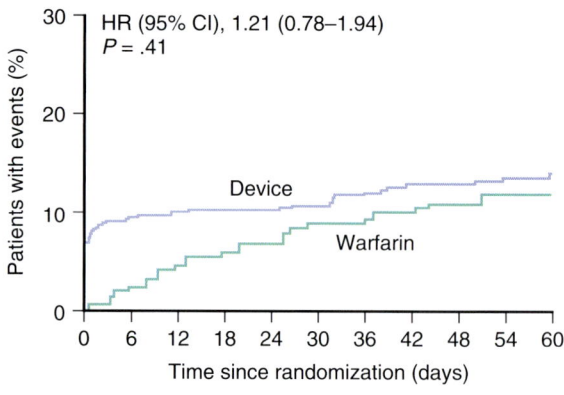

Fig. 50.10 Long-term clinical and safety outcomes in the PROTECT-AF randomized clinical trial of the Watchman left atrial appendage (LAA) closure compared with warfarin therapy. (A) Primary efficacy outcome of cardiovascular death, stroke, or systemic embolism. At a mean of 3.8 years (2621 patient-years) of follow-up, transcatheter LAA occlusion with the Watchman met prespecified criteria for noninferiority and superiority compared with warfarin. (B) The primary safety outcome was a composite of major bleeding events and procedure-related complications. Although an early hazard was apparent in the periprocedural period with device therapy, the overall rate of safety events was similar in both groups, primarily due to ongoing bleeding events in the warfarin group. *PROTECT-AF*, Watchman Left Atrial Appendage System for Embolic Protection in Patients with Atrial Fibrillation. (Modified from Reddy VY, Sievert H, Halperin J, et al. Percutaneous left atrial appendage closure vs warfarin for atrial fibrillation: a randomized clinical trial. *JAMA*. 2012;312:1988–1998.)

NCT02879448) is a prospective, randomized, noninferiority trial of the Amulet versus the Watchman LAA occluder in approximately 1600 AF patients at high thromboembolic risk who are deemed suitable for short-term warfarin but not good candidates for long-term OAC. Patients randomly assigned to the Amulet device will be treated with either DAPT or OAC (according to operator preference), while patients assigned to the Watchman will be treated with the on-label regimen of warfarin and aspirin followed by DAPT. Three primary outcomes will be measured: device closure at 45 days, safety (the composite of procedure related complications, all-cause death, or major bleeding) at 1-year, and efficacy (stroke or systemic embolism) at 18 months.

Transcatheter Left Atrial Appendage Ligation With the Lariat Device

Device Characteristics and Procedural Approach

The Lariat (SentreHeart, Redwood City, CA) is 510(k) cleared by the FDA (i.e., safety and effectiveness information in the premarketing notification has been reviewed) for the approximation of soft tissue. It enables percutaneous delivery of a pretied surgical suture to ligate the LAA.[89] This is accomplished through a combined subxyphoid (i.e., transpericardial) and transseptal approach (Fig. 50.15).

Anatomic eligibility for the procedure is determined by cardiac CT. Appendages with a diameter greater than 40 mm, lobes behind the pulmonary artery, or a posterior orientation should be avoided. A larger, second-generation device will allow closure of appendages as large as 45 mm in diameter. The procedure cannot be performed in patients with prior cardiac surgery because it requires an intact pericardium. The procedure should also be avoided in patients with prior pericarditis because pericardial adhesions can prevent manipulation in the pericardial space and hinder procedural success.

A 14-Fr, slightly curved, and soft-tipped sheath is introduced into the anterior pericardial space using an epidural or micropuncture needle under fluoroscopic guidance. After pericardial access is established, an 8.5-Fr, transseptal sheath is introduced into the left atrium from the right femoral vein using the standard technique; an inferoposterior location in the interatrial septum is preferred. A magnet-tipped guidewire is advanced through the transseptal sheath into the anterior aspect of the LAA, and a complementary magnet-tipped guidewire advanced through the pericardial sheath and connected with the magnet-tipped wire in the LAA, forming a rail over which the Lariat snare is delivered.

The Lariat snare is advanced through the pericardial sheath and over the LAA and then closed at the LAA ostium using TEE and fluoroscopic guidance. The snare contains a preloaded and tied surgical suture. The operator releases the suture with a proximal actuator and then tightens the pretied knot using a suture-tensioning device, after which the snare is removed and the suture cut using a suture cutter. The pericardial sheath is exchanged for a drain, which is left in place for at least 4 to 6 hours.

Clinical Outcomes

The data set for the safety and efficacy of LAA closure with the Lariat has been limited to a few small, observational studies.[90,91] The studies suggest that the major complications associated with the procedure are significant pericardial effusions and postprocedural pericarditis. Results are insufficient to determine the clinical efficacy of the device for stroke prevention.

Bartus and colleagues conducted a single-center, nonrandomized study that enrolled 92 patients who had adequate anatomy for Lariat ligation according to CT imaging.[90] The procedure was aborted in three patients (3.2%) due to unexpected pericardial adhesions. Successful closure, defined as a residual leak of less than 1 mm in diameter, was achieved in 96% of cases. Procedural complications, all of which were significant pericardial effusions, occurred in three patients (3.2%), and pericarditis occurred in two patients (2.2%). At the 1-year follow-up assessment, slightly more than one-half of the patients remained on warfarin therapy. There was no evidence of late leaks on follow-up TEE, and there were no thromboembolic events.

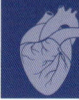

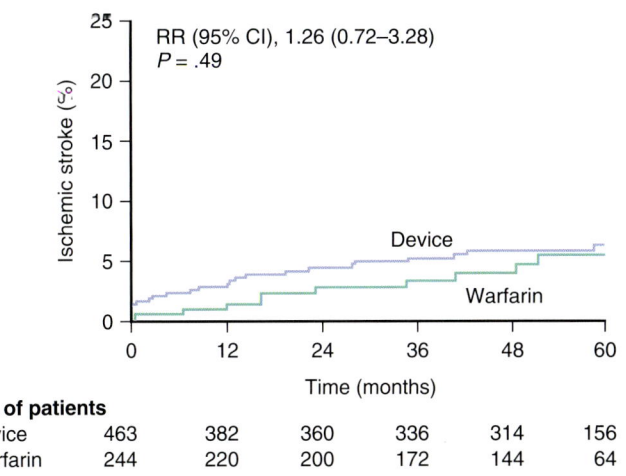
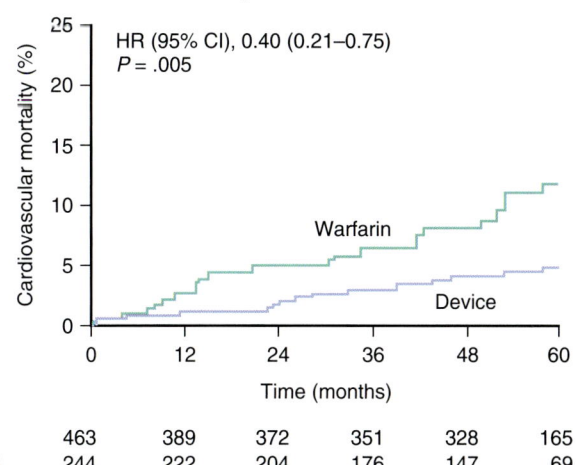
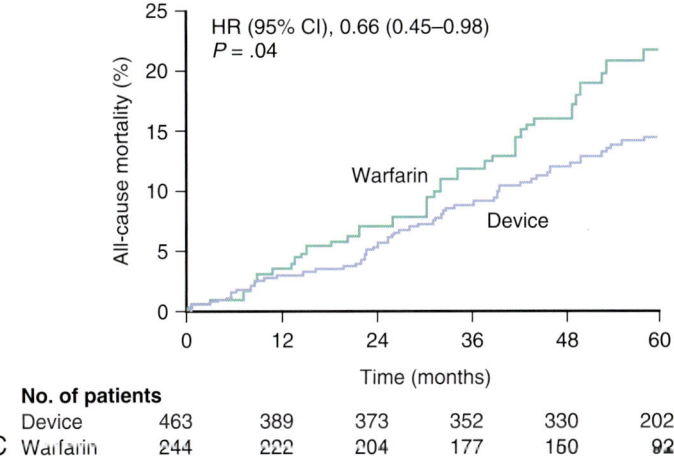

Fig. 50.11 Ischemic stroke and mortality outcomes in the PROTECT-AF randomized clinical trial of Watchman left atrial appendage (LAA) closure compared with warfarin therapy. Ischemic stroke (A), cardiovascular mortality (B), and all-cause mortality (C) at a mean of 3.8 years (2621 patient-years) of follow-up. Compared with warfarin, transcatheter LAA occlusion resulted in a similar rate of ischemic stroke, and it significantly reduced the rates of cardiovascular and all-cause mortality. *PROTECT-AF,* Watchman Left Atrial Appendage System for Embolic Protection in Patients with Atrial Fibrillation. (Modified from Reddy VY, Sievert H, Halperin J, et al. Percutaneous left atrial appendage closure vs warfarin for atrial fibrillation: a randomized clinical trial. *JAMA.* 2012;312:1988–1998.)

TABLE 50.7 Safety Outcomes in Randomized Trials and Continued Access Registries of Left Atrial Appendage Occlusion With the Watchman Device Compared With Warfarin in Patients With Nonvalvular Atrial Fibrillation

	Study			
Outcome	PROTECT-AF (n = 463)	CAP (n = 566)	PREVAIL (n = 269)	P Value
Any complication within 7 days of procedure	8.7%	4.2%	4.5%	.004
Procedure-related stroke	1.1%	0%	0.7%	.02
Pericardial effusion requiring surgery	1.6%	0.2%	0.4%	.03
Pericardial effusion requiring pericardiocentesis	2.4%	1.2%	1.5%	.32
Device embolization	0.4%	0.2%	0.7%	.37

CAP, Continued Access to PROTECT-AF; *PREVAIL,* Prospective Randomized Evaluation of the Watchman Left Atrial Appendage Closure Device In Patients with Atrial Fibrillation Versus Long-Term Warfarin Therapy; *PROTECT-AF,* Watchman Left Atrial Appendage System for Embolic Protection in Patients with Atrial Fibrillation.
Modified from Holmes DR Jr, Kar S, Price MJ, et al. Prospective randomized evaluation of the Watchman Left Atrial Appendage Closure device in patients with atrial fibrillation versus long-term warfarin therapy: the PREVAIL trial. *J Am Coll Cardiol.* 2014;64:1–12.

In a single-center study of 21 patients undergoing Lariat ligation, successful closure was achieved in 20 patients, complicated by a significant pericardial effusion in two patients (10%) and pericarditis in three patients (15%).[91] There were no thromboembolic events over 352 ± 143 days of follow-up.

A multicenter, retrospective study examined the early safety and efficacy of LAA closure with the Lariat device in 154 patients undergoing the procedure in the United States.[92] Enrolled patients were at high risk of thromboembolic and bleeding, with mean CHA_2DS_2VASc score of 4.1 ± 1.6 and a mean HAS-BLED score of 3.2 ± 1.2. Device success (i.e., suture deployment and a less than 5 mm leak by postprocedure TEE) was 94%. Similar to the Bartus experience,[90] 3% of cases were aborted due to unanticipated pericardial adhesions. Procedure-related major bleeding (i.e., Bleeding Academic Research Consortium type 3 bleeding or greater) occurred in 9.1%, and significant pericardial effusion occurred in 10.4% of patients. The incidence of pericarditis was not investigated. Among the 63 patients with immediate closure and TEE follow-up, 3 patients had LAA stump thrombus (4.8%) and 13 (20%) had residual leaks, approximately one-third of which were 5 mm or greater in diameter.

Another multicenter, observational study of 41 patients reported relatively frequent safety events after Lariat LAA ligation.[93] Pericardial effusions that required pericardiocentesis occurred in eight patients (20%), LAA perforation occurred in four patients (9%), and late LAA leaks seen on follow-up imaging occurred in 24%.[93]

The consequences of residual leaks after the Lariat procedure are unknown, although incomplete surgical LAA ligation has been associated with subsequent thrombus formation and clinical events.[49] In addition, even in incomplete ligation cases, the residual LAA tissue seems to undergo significant remodeling and atrophy.[94] Residual leaks after the Lariat procedure can be treated successfully with percutaneous approaches.[95–97]

LAA ligation can have an antiarrhythmic effect in selected patients because the LAA can be a source of AF. The Lariat procedure appears to isolate LAA electrical activity,[98] and in an observational study, the AF burden in patients with known

TABLE 50.8 Safety and Efficacy of Watchman Left Atrial Appendage Closure Compared With Long-Term Warfarin Therapy at 5 Years According to a Patient-Level Meta-analysis of the PROTECT-AF and PREVAIL Clinical Trials

	Device Group (n = 732)		Control Group (n = 382)		Hazard Ratio (95% Confidence Intervals)	P-Value
	No. of Events	Rate (per 100 pt-yrs)	No. of Events	Rate (per 100 pt-yrs)		
2:1 Randomization						
Efficacy: Stroke/SE/CV death	79/2856.0	2.8%	50/1472.8	3.4%	0.82 (0.58–1.17)	.27
All stroke or SE	49/2849.4	1.7%	27/1472.9	1.8%	0.96 (0.60–1.54)	.87
Ischemic stroke or SE	45/28550.2	1.6%	14/1479.1	0.95%	1.71 (0.94–3.11)	.08
Hemorrhagic stroke	5/2954.8	0.17%	13/1499.0	0.87%	0.20 (0.07–0.56)	.0022
Ischemic stroke or SE >7 days	37/2862.1	1.3%	14/1479.1	0.95%	1.40 (0.76–2.59)	.28
Disabling stroke	11/2944.5	0.37%	14/1493.8	0.94%	0.41 (0.19–0.90)	.027
Nondisabling stroke	30/2884.5	1.0%	9/1490.0	0.60%	1.79 (0.85–3.77)	.13
CV/unexplained death	39/2960.5	1.3%	33/1505.2	2.2%	0.59 (0.37–0.94)	.027
All-cause death	106/2961.6	3.6%	73/1505.2	4.9%	0.73 (0.54–0.98)	.035
Major bleeding, all	85/2748.4	3.1%	50/1414.7	3.5%	0.91 (0.64–1.29)	.60
Major bleeding, non–procedure-related	48/2853.6	1.7%	51/1411.3	3.6%	0.48 (0.32–0.71)	.0003

CV, Cardiovascular; *SE,* systemic embolism. Adapted from Reddy VY, Doshi SK, Kar S, et al. 5-Year outcomes after left atrial appendage closure: from the PREVAIL and PROTECT AF trials. *J Am Coll Cardiol.* 2017;70:2964–2975.

TABLE 50.9 Types and Frequencies of Major Bleeding Events in the Pooled PROTECT-AF and PREVAIL Trials That Occurred After the Period of Postimplant Pharmacotherapy (Oral Anticoagulation and Dual Antiplatelet Therapy) in the Device Group (>6 Months Postrandomization)

Bleeding Event	LAA Closure n = 732	Warfarin n = 382	P Value
Gastrointestinal bleeding, n (%)	10 (1.4%)	21 (5.5%)	< .001
Epistaxis, n (%)	1 (0.1%)	1 (0.3%)	1.0
Hematuria, n (%)	0 (0)	2 (0.5%)	.12
Hemorrhagic stroke, n (%)	2 (0.3%)	7 (1.8%)	.01
Cranial bleed, n (%)	3 (0.4%)	1 (0.3%)	1.0
Anemia requiring transfusion, n (%)	2 (0.3%)	1 (0.3%)	1.0
Major bleed requiring transfusion, n (%)	1 (0.1%)	1 (0.3%)	1.0
Other bleeding, n (%)	0 (0)	1 (0.3%)	.35

Patients were randomly assigned to LAA closure or warfarin therapy in a 2:1 fashion.
LAA, Left atrial appendage.
Adapted from Price MJ, Reddy VY, Valderrabano M, et al. Bleeding outcomes after left arial appendage closure compared with long-term warfarin: a pooled, patient-level analysis of the WATCHMAN randomized trial experience. *JACC Cardiovasc Interv.* 2015;8:1925–1932.

AF triggers in the LAA was significantly reduced at 12 months after the Lariat procedure compared with baseline AF activity.[99] Based on this finding, LAA ligation is being studied as an adjunct to catheter ablation of AF in the aMAZE trial (LAA Ligation Adjunctive to PVI for Persistent or Longstanding Persistent Atrial Fibrillation; clinicaltrials.gov Identifier: NCT02513797). This prospective, multicenter, randomized controlled study will evaluate the safety and effectiveness of the Lariat procedure to percutaneously isolate and ligate the LAA from the left atrium as an adjunct to planned pulmonary vein isolation (PVI) catheter ablation in the treatment of subjects with symptomatic persistent or longstanding persistent AF. The primary end point is the freedom from episodes of AF >30 seconds in duration at 12 months post index PVI, measured by 24-hour monitoring. Secondary end points include freedom from other atrial arrhythmias as well as stroke and systemic embolism. However, this clinical trial is not powered to adequately define the role of Lariat LAA ligation for thromboembolic risk reduction in patients with AF.

The Lariat appears to provide high rates of immediate anatomic closure of the LAA, although procedural morbidity is not uncommon. Bleeding events and pericardial effusions drive procedural complications. Several questions regarding the Lariat remain unanswered, including whether safety events can be reduced with increased operator experience, what amount or type of postprocedure medical therapy is required (i.e., brief duration of antiplatelet or anticoagulation therapy), what are the rates and clinical consequences of late residual leaks, and whether the Lariat is effective in reducing thromboembolic events in the absence of long-term oral anticoagulant therapy.

WaveCrest Occluder

Device Characteristics and Procedural Approach

The WaveCrest LAA occlusion system (Coherex Medical, Salt Lake City, UT) has CE mark, and initiation of a pivotal trial in the United States is planned. The occluder consists of a self-expanding nitinol cage with a proximal ePTFE cap (Fig. 50.16). A foam skirt is incorporated through the distal portion of the occluder cap, which could potentially enhance LAA sealing. The system separates the act of LAA occlusion from device anchoring.

When the device is implanted, the occluder is positioned to occlude the LAA, and a set of anchors or tines are then deployed in a separate step to anchor the device in the LAA. Potential advantages of this device include less traumatic deployment and more flexibility in closing the LAA irrespective of its depth. To date, there are no peer-reviewed publications validating the safety and efficacy of LAA closure with the WaveCrest. The WaveCrest2 (WAveCrest vs. Watchman TranssEptal LAA Closure to REduce AF-Mediated STroke-2) study is a randomized clinical trial that will enroll approximately 1250 patients and compare the rates of procedural complications, death, bleeding, and stroke or systemic embolism in patients undergoing WaveCrest versus the Watchman implant (clinicaltrials.gov Identifier: NCT03302494).

PATIENT SELECTION

Appropriate patient selection for transcatheter LAA closure incorporates a particular individual's risk of thromboembolism, long-term bleeding risk on OAC, and the short-term procedural risk of device implantation. Other factors include patient compliance, personal preference, and relative or absolute contraindications to chronic OAC. Thromboembolic risk can be assessed using the $CHADS_2$ and CHA_2DS_2-VASc scores (see Tables 50.1 and 50.2), and bleeding risk can be assessed using schemes such as HAS-BLED (see Table 50.3).

Not all strokes can be prevented by LAA-targeted strategies, and OAC can reduce the risk of stroke in AF patients independent of its role in preventing LAA thrombus. For example, as many as 25% of strokes in AF patients are linked to intrinsic

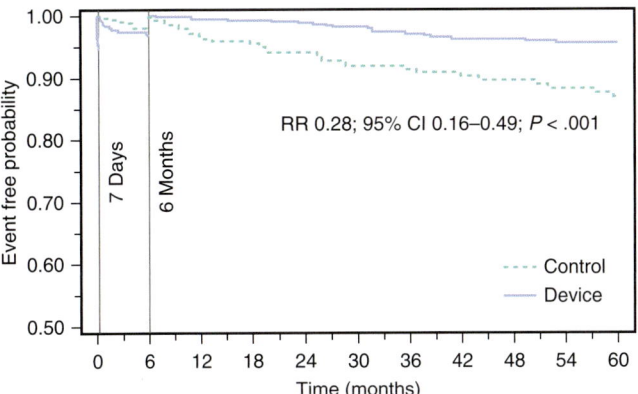

Fig. 50.12 Freedom from first major bleed in a pooled, patient level analysis of the PROTECT-AF and PREVAIL trials. Freedom from major bleeding is divided into three intervals: from randomization to day 7, representing the periprocedural period for patients randomly assigned to LAA closure; from 8 days to 6 months postrandomization, during which device-treated patients received warfarin and aspirin followed by dual antiplatelet therapy; and beyond 6 months, when device-treated patients were eligible to receive aspirin alone. (Adapted from Price MJ, Reddy VY, Valderrabano M, et al. Bleeding outcomes after left atrial appendage closure compared with long-term Warfarin: A pooled, patient-level analysis of the WATCHMAN randomized trial experience. *JACC Cardiovasc Interv.* 2015;8:1925–1932.)

TABLE 50.10 Major Bleeds Beyond 6 Months Postrandomization According to Subgroup in the PROTECT-AF and PREVAIL Randomized Clinical Trials

Subgroup	n (LAA Closure)	n (Warfarin)	Hazard Ratio	P Value	P Interaction
Age ≤75 years	1.4% (6/436)	7.8% (17/217)	0.17 [95% CI: 0.147–0.196]	<.001	.005
Age >75 years	4.4% (13/296)	10.9% (18/165)	0.43 [95% CI: 0.264–0.701]	.001	
CHA_2DS_2-VASc ≤4	1.8% (10/551)	8.5% (22/258)	0.21 [95% CI: 0.138–0.321]	<.001	.28
CHA_2DS_2-VASc >4	5.1% (9/178)	10.7% (13/121)	0.47 [95% CI: 0.161–1.378]	.17	
Modified HAS-BLED <3	1.4% (8/561)	7.9% (23/291)	0.17 [95% CI: 0.173–0.174]	<.001	.001
Modified HAS-BLED ≥3	6.4% (11/171)	13.2% (12/91)	0.55 [95% CI: 0.282–1.070]	.078	
No history of TIA/stroke	2.3% (13/570)	8.9% (26/292)	0.26 [95% CI: 0.216–0.305]	<.001	.67
History of TIA/stroke	3.7% (6/162)	10.0% (9/90)	0.35 [95% CI: 0.102–1.225]	.10	
Female	1.8% (4/224)	12.0% (13/108)	0.17 [95% CI: 0.074–0.369]	<.001	.02
Male	3.0% (15/508)	8.0% (22/274)	0.35 [95% CI: 0.320–0.393]	<.001	

LAA, Left atrial appendage; *TIA*, transient ischemic attack.

SECTION V Structural Interventions

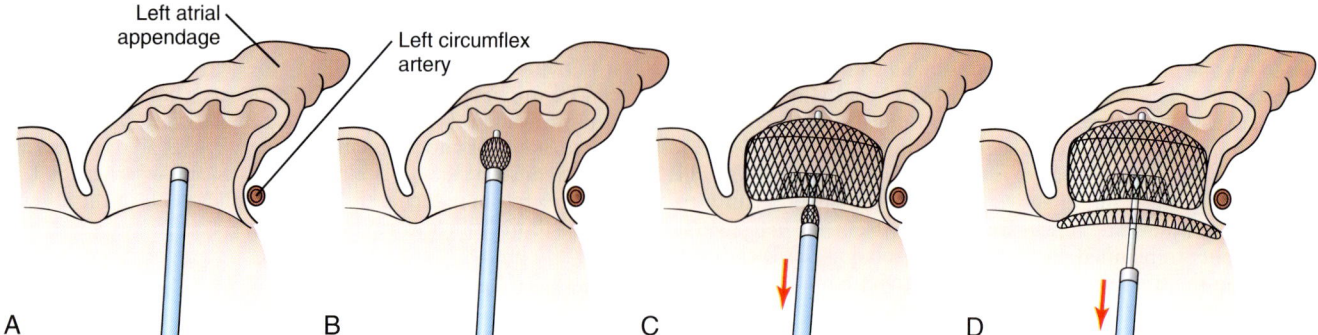

Fig. 50.13 Amplatzer Cardiac Plug device deployment. (A) Initial sheath position. (B) Adjustment of the sheath position with a portion of the distal lobe extruded from the sheath to form a safe, ball-like tip. (C) Device deployment by withdrawal of the sheath over the device delivery cable. (D) Final device position, with the distal lobe acting as an anchor in the left atrial appendage (LAA) and the proximal disk forming an occlusive lid over the mouth of the LAA. (Modified from Meerkin D, Butnaru A, Dratva D, et al. Early safety of the Amplatzer Cardiac Plug for left atrial appendage occlusion. *Int J Cardiol.* 2013;168:3920–3925.)

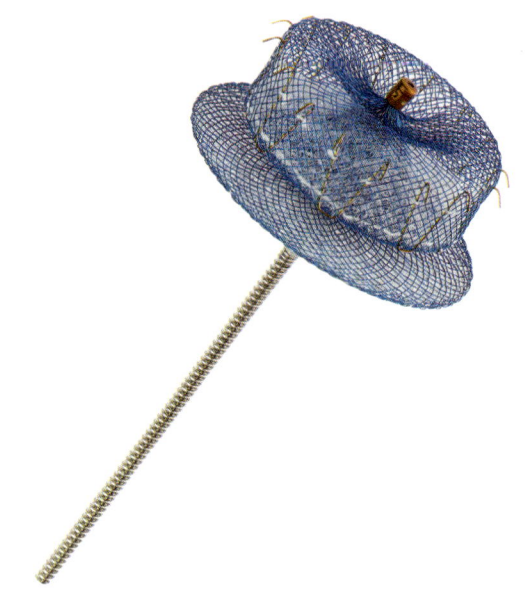

Fig. 50.14 The Amulet left atrial appendage occluder consists of a self-expanding nitinol mesh that forms a distal lobe and proximal disk, each with a sewn-in polyester patch. The distal lobe and proximal disk are connected by a short, central waist. The distal lobe has hooks around its circumference that anchor the device in the left atrial appendage (LAA), and the proximal disk covers the mouth of the LAA from within the left atrium. (Courtesy St. Jude Medical, Minneapolis, MN. AMPLATZER, Amulet, and St. Jude Medical are trademarks of the St. Jude Medical, Inc. or its related companies. Reprinted with permission of St. Jude Medical, © 2015. All rights reserved.)

cerebrovascular disease.[100] The mechanistic connections between the LAA and many risk factors that predict stroke in AF, including several components of the CHA_2DS_2VASc score, have not been fully elucidated. AF also is associated with platelet activation and a hypercoagulable state.[101] For these reasons, LAA closure should not be considered a panacea for stroke prevention in the AF patient who is not an optimal candidate for OAC.

Society recommendations for LAA occlusion are listed in Table 50.12. In brief, the AHA/ACC/HRS guidelines state that surgical excision of the LAA during concomitant cardiac surgery may be considered, but its efficacy is uncertain (class IIb, level C evidence).[19] The ESC guidelines state that surgical excision may be considered during concomitant cardiac surgery (class IIb, level C evidence) and that transcatheter LAA closure may be considered in patients with a high stroke risk and contraindications to long-term OAC (class IIb, level B evidence).[20]

CONCLUSIONS

AF is associated with increased risk of stroke and systemic embolism, and its prevalence is growing significantly due to aging of the global population. Although chronic anticoagulation with vitamin K antagonists and the NOACs reduce the risk of stroke, they are substantially underused, in large part because of therapeutic challenges such as long-term bleeding risk.

The LAA appears to be the primary source of thromboembolism in AF, and it is therefore an attractive target for mechanical approaches to stroke prevention in this patient population. Several devices have been developed to percutaneously occlude or ligate the LAA. Robust safety and efficacy data are limited for most devices. The totality of the clinical trial data suggests that the Watchman LAA occluder is an acceptable alternative to warfarin therapy in many patients. Studies of larger cohorts are needed to determine the safety and clinical efficacy of the other devices beyond their ability to provide immediate anatomic LAA closure. Patient selection for LAA closure must consider the risk of procedural complications, baseline thromboembolic risk, the risk and suitability of OAC, and patient preference.

TABLE 50.11 Studies of Left Atrial Appendage Occlusion Using the First- and Second-Generation Amplatzer Cardiac Plug

Study	Study Design	n	Patient Population	Duration of Follow-Up	Postprocedure Medical Regimen	Safety Outcomes (%)[b]	Efficacy Outcomes (%)
Park et al.[75]	Retrospective, multicenter, observational	143	NR	24 h	NA	PRCs: 7.0 SPE: 3.5 DE: 1.4 Stroke: 2.1	NA
Uena et al.[79]	Prospective, multicenter, observational	52	OAC ineligible	20 ± 5 months	ASA/clopidogrel for 1–6 months, then ASA monotherapy	PRCs: 5.8 SPE: 0 DE: 1.9% Stroke: 0	CV death: 1.9% Stroke: 1.9%
Meerkin et al.[80]	Retrospective, single operator, observational	100	OAC ineligible	In-hospital	NA	PRCs: 1.0% SPE: 1.0% DE: 0 Stroke: 0	NA
Lam et al.[81]	Prospective, two-center, observational	20	OAC ineligible	12.7 ± 3.1 months	ASA/clopidogrel for 1 month	PRCs: 10 SPE: 0 DE: 0 Stroke: 0	Stroke: 0
Chun et al.[82]	Prospective, single-center, observational	40	OAC ineligible	1 year	ASA/clopidogrel for 6 weeks (76%)	PRC: 5% SPE: 2.5 DE: 2.5 (late) Stroke: 0	Death: 5 Stroke: 0
Guérios et al.[83]	Single-center, observational	86	OAC ineligible	25.9 pt-yr	ASA/clopidogrel for 1 month, then ASA for 3–4 months	PRCs: 5.6 SPE: 2.2 DE: 1.1 Stroke: 2.3	Death: 3.5 Stroke: 0
Danna et al.[84]	Single-center, observational	37	OAC ineligible	1 year	ASA/clopidogrel for 1 month, then ASA for at least for 5 months	PRCs: NR SPE: 2.7 DE: 5.9 Stroke: 0	Death: 5 Stroke: 2.9
Horstmann et al.[85]	Single-center, observational	20	OAC ineligible (prior ICH)	13.6 ± 8.2 months	ASA and clopidogrel for 3 months, then ASA monotherapy	PRCs: 0 SPE: 0 DE: 0 Stroke: 0	Stroke: 0
Santoro et al.[86]	Retrospective, multicenter, observational	134	OAC unsuitable	680 ± 351 days 238 pt-yr	ASA and clopidogrel for 1–3 months, then ASA monotherapy	PRCs: 2.2 SPE: 2.2 DE: 0 Stroke: 0	Stroke 0.8 TE: 2.5
Wiebe et al.[87]	Single-center, observational	60	OAC unsuitable	1.8 year	ASA and clopidogrel for 3 months, then ASA monotherapy	PRCs: 11.7 SPE: 1.6 DE: 3.3 Stroke: 0	Death: 4.8 Stroke: 0
Freixa et al.[88a]	Single-center, observational	25	OAC ineligible or stroke with labile INR	1–3 months	NR	PRCs: 0 SPE: 0 DE: 0 Stroke: 0	Stroke: 0
Lam et al.[77a]	Single-center, observational	17	OAC unsuitable	90 days	ASA and clopidogrel for 3 months, then ASA monotherapy	PRCs: 5.8 SPE: 5.8 DE: 0 Stroke: 0	Stroke: 0
Landmesser et al.[102]	Multi-center, observational	1088	OAC unsuitable or ineligible	90 days	None (2%), SAPT (23%), DAPT (54%), OAC ± SAPT (19%)	PRCs: 3.2 SPE: 1.2 DE: 0.1 Stroke: 0.2	Ischemic stroke, SE, CV Death: 1.4

[a]Case series using the second-generation Amulet device.
[b]Definitions of procedure-related complications and significant pericardial effusion varied across studies.
ASA, Aspirin; CV, cardiovascular; DAPT, dual antiplatelet therapy; DE, device embolization; ICH, intracranial hemorrhage; INR, international normalized ratio; NA, not applicable; NR, not reported; OAC, oral anticoagulation; PRC, procedure-related complication; pt-yr, patient-years; SAPT, single antiplatelet therapy; SE, systemic embolism; SPE, significant pericardial effusion; TE, thromboembolism.

SECTION V Structural Interventions

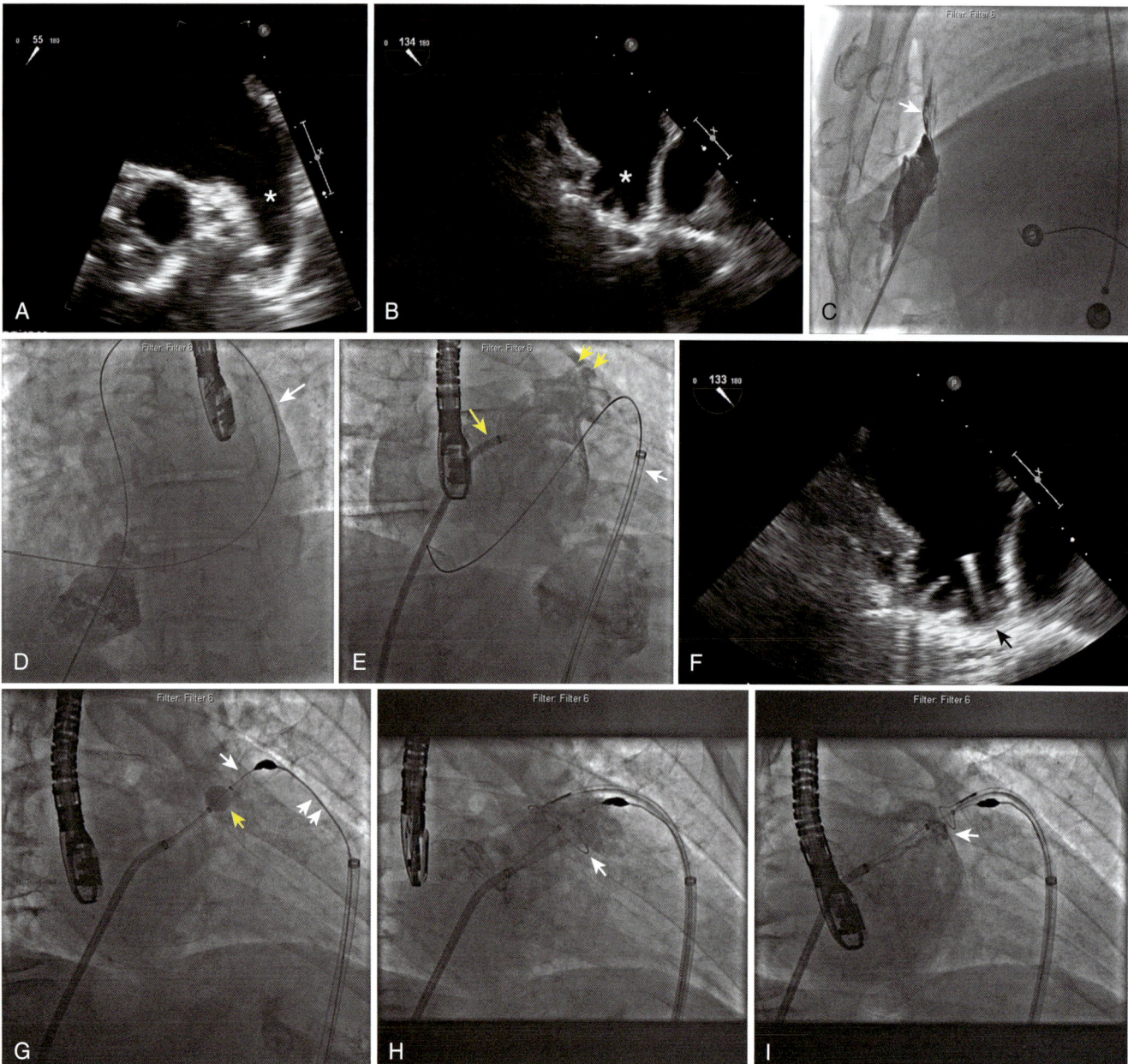

Fig. 50.15 Transcatheter ligation of the left atrial appendage (LAA) with the Lariat. (A) Baseline transesophageal echocardiography (TEE) of the LAA *(asterisk)* at approximately 45 degrees. (B) Baseline TEE of the LAA *(asterisk)* at approximately 135 degrees. (C) Dry pericardial access is obtained by carefully advancing a 17-gauge, 150-mm Tuohy (Pajunk) needle just below the xyphoid process and directed slightly laterally using fluoroscopy in the 90-degree lateral position. Dilute contrast can be injected through the needle lumen to confirm the position, identify tenting of the parietal pericardium, and visualize contrast filling the pericardial space *(arrow)*. A micropuncture needle can also be used. (D) A 0.035-inch wire is advanced through the needle into the pericardium. In the shallow left anterior oblique projection, the wire should lie along the lateral border of the heart *(arrow)*, confirming the pericardial location. (E) A soft-tipped, slightly curved 14-Fr sheath is advanced over the wire into the pericardium *(white arrow)*, and an 8.5-Fr transseptal sheath *(yellow arrow)* is advanced into the left atrium using the standard technique. Left atrial angiography demonstrates the left atrial appendage *(double yellow arrows)*. (F) The magnet-tipped endocardial wire is advanced through the transseptal sheath into the anterior lobe of the LAA and confirmed by TEE *(arrow)*. (G) The magnet-tipped epicardial wire *(double arrows)* is advanced through the pericardial sheath and connected, preferably end to end, with the epicardial wire *(single white arrow)*. The over-the-wire balloon catheter is advanced, and the compliant balloon is inflated with dilute contrast *(yellow arrow)* to coregister the location of mouth of the LAA on fluoroscopy with TEE. (H) The Lariat snare *(arrow)* is introduced into the pericardium over the epicardial wire and then opened and advanced over the LAA. (I) The Lariat snare is closed over the LAA, and the operator delivers a pretied surgical knot by means of an actuator at the proximal end of the device. Left atrial angiography through the transseptal sheath confirms LAA closure *(arrow)*.

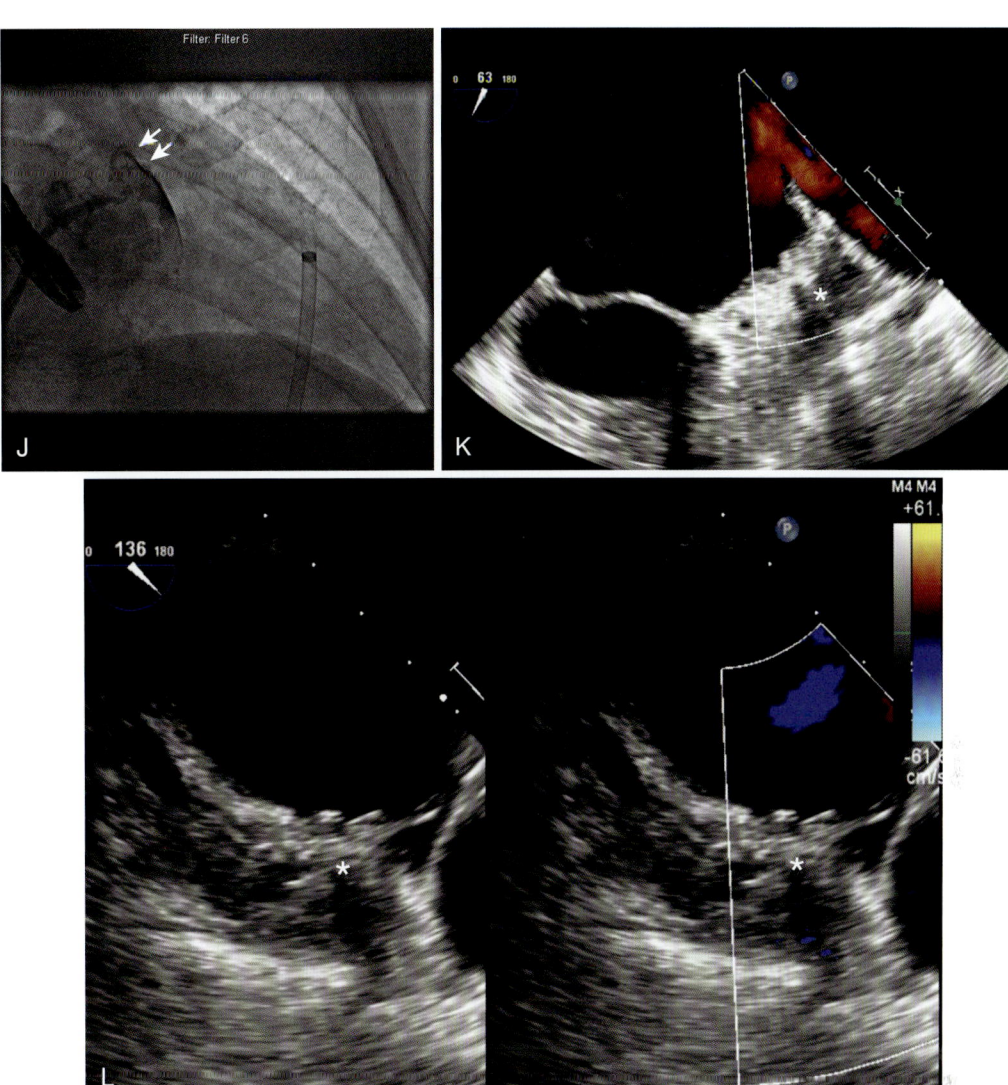

Fig. 50.15, cont'd (J) The suture is tightened with a tensioning device, the Lariat snare and wires are removed, and the suture is cut with a specialized cutter. LAA angiogram demonstrates complete ligation of the LAA without residual leak *(double arrows)*. (K) TEE with color Doppler of the LAA at 60 degrees after Lariat ligation shows complete closure without residual flow. An asterisk indicates the remnant LAA. (L) TEE with color Doppler of the LAA at 135 degrees after Lariat ligation shows complete closure without residual flow. An asterisk indicates the remnant LAA.

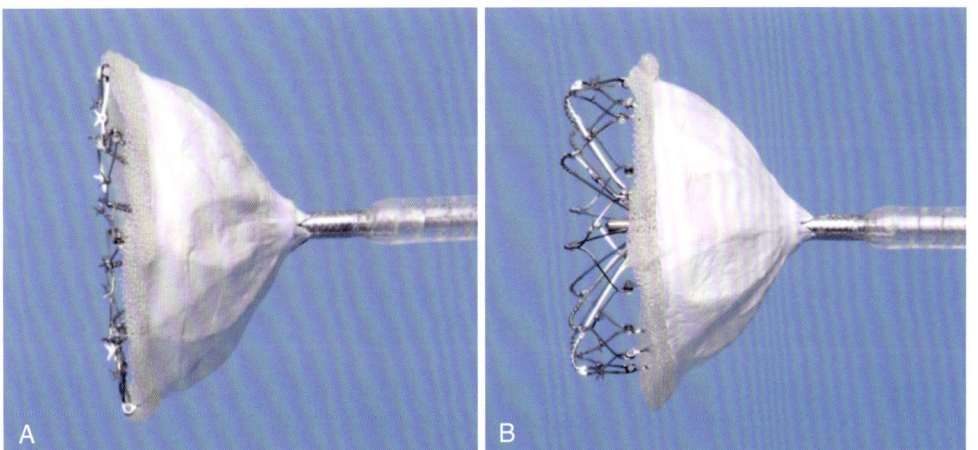

Fig. 50.16 The WaveCrest left atrial appendage (LAA) occlusion system. (A) The occluder has an expanded polytetrafluoroethylene cap and tines in the withdrawn position. (B) The occluder has tines rolled forward to anchor the device in the LAA. The tines can be withdrawn if required for device repositioning or recapture. (Courtesy Coherex Medical, Salt Lake City, UT.)

TABLE 50.12 Recommendations for Left Atrial Appendage Closure

Society Guidelines	Classification	Level of Evidence	Recommendation
American Heart Association/American College of Cardiology/Heart Rhythm Society 2014 guidelines for management of patients with atrial fibrillation[19]	IIb	C	Surgical excision of the left atrial appendage may be considered in patients undergoing cardiac surgery.
European Society of Cardiology 2012 guidelines for management of atrial fibrillation[20]	IIb	C	Surgical excision of the left atrial appendage may be considered in patients undergoing open heart surgery.
	IIb	B	Interventional, percutaneous left atrial appendage closure may be considered in patients with a high stroke risk and contraindications for long-term oral anticoagulation.

KEY REFERENCES

17. Lip GY, Nieuwlaat R, Pisters R, et al. Refining clinical risk stratification for predicting stroke and thromboembolism in atrial fibrillation using a novel risk factor-based approach: the Euro Heart Survey on atrial fibrillation. *Chest*. 2010;137:263–272.
18. Lip GY, Frison L, Halperin JL, Lane DA. Identifying patients at high risk for stroke despite anticoagulation: a comparison of contemporary stroke risk stratification schemes in an anticoagulated atrial fibrillation cohort. *Stroke*. 2010;41:2731–2738.
19. January CT, Wann LS, Alpert JS, et al. 2014 AHA/ACC/HRS guideline for the management of patients with atrial fibrillation: a report of the American College of Cardiology/American Heart Association Task Force on Practice Guidelines and the Heart Rhythm Society. *J Am Coll Cardiol*. 2014;64:e1–e76.
21. Pisters R, Lane DA, Nieuwlaat R, et al. A novel user-friendly score (HAS-BLED) to assess 1-year risk of major bleeding in patients with atrial fibrillation: the Euro Heart Survey. *Chest*. 2010;138:1093–1100.
22. Lip GY, Frison L, Halperin JL, Lane DA. Comparative validation of a novel risk score for predicting bleeding risk in anticoagulated patients with atrial fibrillation: the HAS-BLED (Hypertension, Abnormal Renal/Liver Function, Stroke, Bleeding History or Predisposition, Labile INR, Elderly, Drugs/Alcohol Concomitantly) score. *J Am Coll Cardiol*. 2011;57:173–180.
40. Beigel R, Wunderlich NC, Ho SY, et al. The left atrial appendage: anatomy, function, and noninvasive evaluation. *JACC Cardiovasc Imaging*. 2014;7:1251–1265.
63. Wang DD, Eng M, Kupsky D, et al. Application of 3-dimensional computed tomographic image guidance to watchman implantation and impact on early operator learning curve: single-center experience. *JACC Cardiovasc Interv*. 2016;9(22):2329–2340.
66. Reddy VY, Sievert H, Halperin J, et al. Percutaneous left atrial appendage closure vs warfarin for atrial fibrillation: a randomized clinical trial. *JAMA*. 2012;312:1988–1998.
69. Reddy VY, Doshi SK, Kar S, et al. 5-Year outcomes after left atrial appendage closure: from the PREVAIL and PROTECT AF trials. *J Am Coll Cardiol*. 2017;70(24):2964–2975.
72. Price MJ, Reddy VY, Valderrabano M, et al. Bleeding outcomes after left atrial appendage closure compared with long-term Warfarin: a pooled, patient-level analysis of the WATCHMAN randomized trial experience. *JACC Cardiovasc Interv*. 2015;8:1925–1932.
73. Sharma D, Reddy VY, Sandri M, et al. Left atrial appendage closure in patients with contraindications to oral anticoagulation. *J Am Coll Cardiol*. 2016;67(18):2190–2192.
74. Holmes DR, Reddy VY, Buchbinder M, et al. The assessment of the watchman device in patients unsuitable for oral anticoagulation (ASAP-TOO) trial. *Am Heart J*. 2017;189:68–74.
78. Saw J, Lempereur M. Percutaneous left atrial appendage closure: procedural techniques and outcomes. *JACC Cardiovasc Interv*. 2014;7:1205–1220.
92. Price MJ, Gibson DN, Yakubov SJ, et al. Early safety and efficacy of percutaneous left atrial appendage suture ligation: results from the U.S. Transcatheter LAA Ligation Consortium. *J Am Coll Cardiol*. 2014;64:565–572.
94. Kreidieh B, Rojas F, Schurmann P, et al. Left atrial appendage remodeling after lariat left atrial appendage ligation. *Circ Arrhythm Electrophysiol*. 2015;8(6):1351–1358.
95. Mosley 2nd WJ, Smith MR, Price MJ. Percutaneous management of late leak after lariat transcatheter ligation of the left atrial appendage in patients with atrial fibrillation at high risk for stroke. *Catheter Cardiovasc Interv*. 2014;83:664–669.

Additional references available online at expertconsult.com.

中文导读

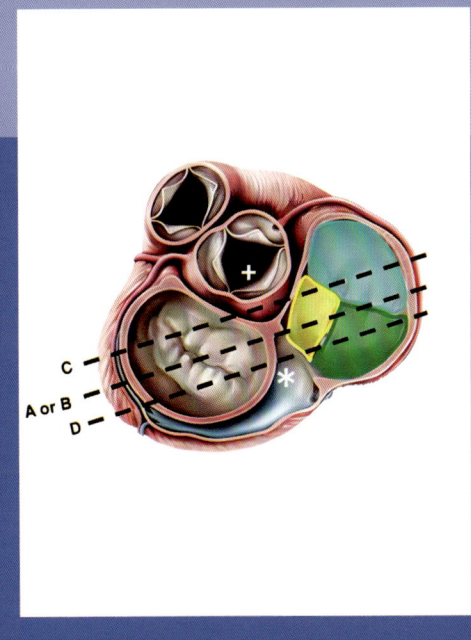

第51章
二尖瓣成形术

经皮二尖瓣连合部切开术是二尖瓣狭窄患者的重要治疗方法。其原理是将融合的联合部打开，与外科连合切开术相同。本章主要介绍了经皮二尖瓣连合切开术的技术路线、监测方法、即刻和长期结果、患者选择及适应证。

目前，使用Inoue球囊经静脉或经间隔入路占主导地位，Inoue球囊技术的有效性、安全性和适用性使其成为经皮二尖瓣连合部切开术的参考点。Inoue技术在超声心动图指导下使用逐步扩张技术，手术结束的标准是瓣膜面积足够大或二尖瓣反流程度增加。超声心动图是重要的监测方式，可提供关于瓣膜面积、压力梯度、反流和连合部开度的基本信息；此外，也可用于检测早期并发症，如心包出血和严重二尖瓣反流。

经皮二尖瓣连合部切开术可提供良好的即时和长期临床结果。瓣膜功能的改善会立即降低左心房压力，改善泵功能。经皮二尖瓣连合部切开术最初成功后，存活率很高，二尖瓣反流程度在随访期保持稳定或略有下降，栓塞发生率低。关于术后长期结局，经皮二尖瓣连合部切开术后最常见的事件是二尖瓣再狭窄。多项研究将外科连合切开术与经皮二尖瓣连合部切开术进行对比，结果显示在解剖特征良好的患者中，经皮二尖瓣连合部切开术在术后7年的短期和中期随访中，至少可与外科手术相当。

患者的选择基于解剖和其他预后预测因素。技术经验对于手术的安全性和患者的选择至关重要。经皮二尖瓣连合部切开术是具有良好特征患者的首选治疗方法，其他患者的决策必须个性化制定。经皮二尖瓣连合部切开术和瓣膜置换术应被视为互补技术，而不是对立的。

王 璨　张洪亮

章节要点

- Inoue球囊技术的有效性、安全性和适用性使之成为经皮二尖瓣连合部切开术的技术参考点。
- 技术经验对于手术安全和患者选择至关重要。
- 经皮二尖瓣连合部切开术即时和长期临床结果良好，由经验丰富的团队执行时风险较低。
- 患者选择基于解剖学特征和其他预后预测因子。
- 经皮二尖瓣连合部切开术是具有良好特征患者的首选治疗方法。
- 其他患者的治疗必须进行个体化决策，经皮二尖瓣连合部切开术和瓣膜置换应被视为互补技术。

51 Mitral Valvuloplasty

Alec Vahanian, Dominique Himbert, Eric Brochet, Bernard Iung

KEY POINTS

- The efficacy, safety, and applicability of the Inoue balloon technique make it the point of reference for percutaneous mitral commissurotomy (PMC).
- Technical experience is essential for the safety of the procedure and the selection of patients.
- PMC provides good immediate and long-term clinical results and carries a low risk when performed by experienced teams.
- Patient selection is based on anatomy and other predictors of outcome.
- PMC is the treatment of choice for patients with favorable characteristics.
- The decision must be individualized for other patients, and PMC and valve replacement should be considered complementary techniques.

INTRODUCTION

Until the first publication by Inoue and coworkers describing percutaneous mitral commissurotomy (PMC) in 1984, open chest surgery was the only treatment for patients with mitral stenosis.[1] Since then, many patients with a wide range of clinical conditions have been treated, enabling efficacy and risk to be assessed.

DEVICES AND TECHNIQUES

Acting in the same way as surgical commissurotomy, PMC opens the fused commissures (Fig. 51.1). PMC is of little or no help in cases of restricted valvular mobility caused by valve fibrosis or severe subvalvular disease, or in cases of degenerative calcified mitral annulus (Video 51.1).[2] The techniques and devices used for PMC have varied over time. Currently, the transvenous or transseptal approach using the Inoue balloon is largely predominant.

Transseptal Approach

The transvenous, or antegrade, approach is performed through the femoral vein. Transseptal catheterization is the crucial first step of the procedure, usually performed under fluoroscopic guidance and continuous pressure monitoring. Echocardiography is not used systematically during transseptal catheterization, but it can enhance its safety, especially for less experienced operators and when technical difficulties are encountered (e.g., severe anatomic distortion). Intracardiac echocardiography may be used without additional operators or general anesthesia, although the price of the device seriously limits its use.[3]

In experienced centers, the whole procedure can be performed using a single venous approach and noninvasive monitoring, which reduces the risk of vascular complications, discomfort, and cost. The retrograde transatrial approach has been abandoned due to its complexity.

Inoue Technique

The Inoue technique was the first to be described, and extensive experience has been acquired by many groups worldwide. The Inoue balloon, composed of nylon and rubber micromesh, is self-positioning and pressure extensible. It is large (24 to 30 mm in maximal diameter) and has a low profile (4.5 mm balloon diameter). The balloon has three distinct parts, each with a specific elasticity, enabling the parts to be inflated sequentially. This sequence allows fast, stable positioning across the valve. Each of the four balloon sizes (i.e., 24, 26, 28, and 30 mm) is pressure dependent, and its diameter can be varied by up to 4 mm, as required by circumstances.

After transseptal catheterization, a stiff guidewire is introduced into the left atrium. The femoral entry site and the atrial septum are dilated with a rigid dilator (14 Fr), and the balloon is introduced into the left atrium. Inoue recommended the use of a stepwise dilation technique under echocardiographic guidance. Balloon size is chosen according to patient's height and then inflated sequentially. First, the distal portion is inflated with 1 or 2 mL of diluted contrast; it acts as a floating balloon catheter when crossing the mitral valve. Second, the distal part is further inflated, and the balloon is pulled back into the mitral orifice. Inflation next occurs at the level of the proximal part and then in the central portion, with the disappearance of the central waist at full inflation (Fig. 51.2). The first inflation is performed 4 mm below the maximal balloon size, and the balloon size is increased in 1-mm increments. The balloon is then deflated and withdrawn into the left atrium. If mitral regurgitation (assessed by color Doppler echocardiography) has not increased by more than one grade and the valve area is less than 1 cm^2/m^2 of body surface area, the balloon is advanced again across the valve, and PMC is repeated with a balloon diameter increased by 1 mm.[1] The criterion for ending the procedure is an adequate valve area or an increase in the degree of mitral regurgitation.

Other Techniques

The double-balloon technique has been described extensively and long-term results are comparable to those of the Inoue balloon.[4,5] The multitrack system, which is a refinement of the double-balloon technique, and the metallic commissurotome have a limited use.

MONITORING THE PROCEDURE AND EVALUATING RESULTS

Echocardiography provides essential information on valve area, gradient, regurgitation, and commissural opening when using the stepwise Inoue technique. Echocardiography enables detection of early complications such as pericardial hemorrhage and severe mitral regurgitation.

Monitoring the Procedure

Planimetry using two-dimensional echocardiography is the reference method. Color Doppler assessment is preferred for

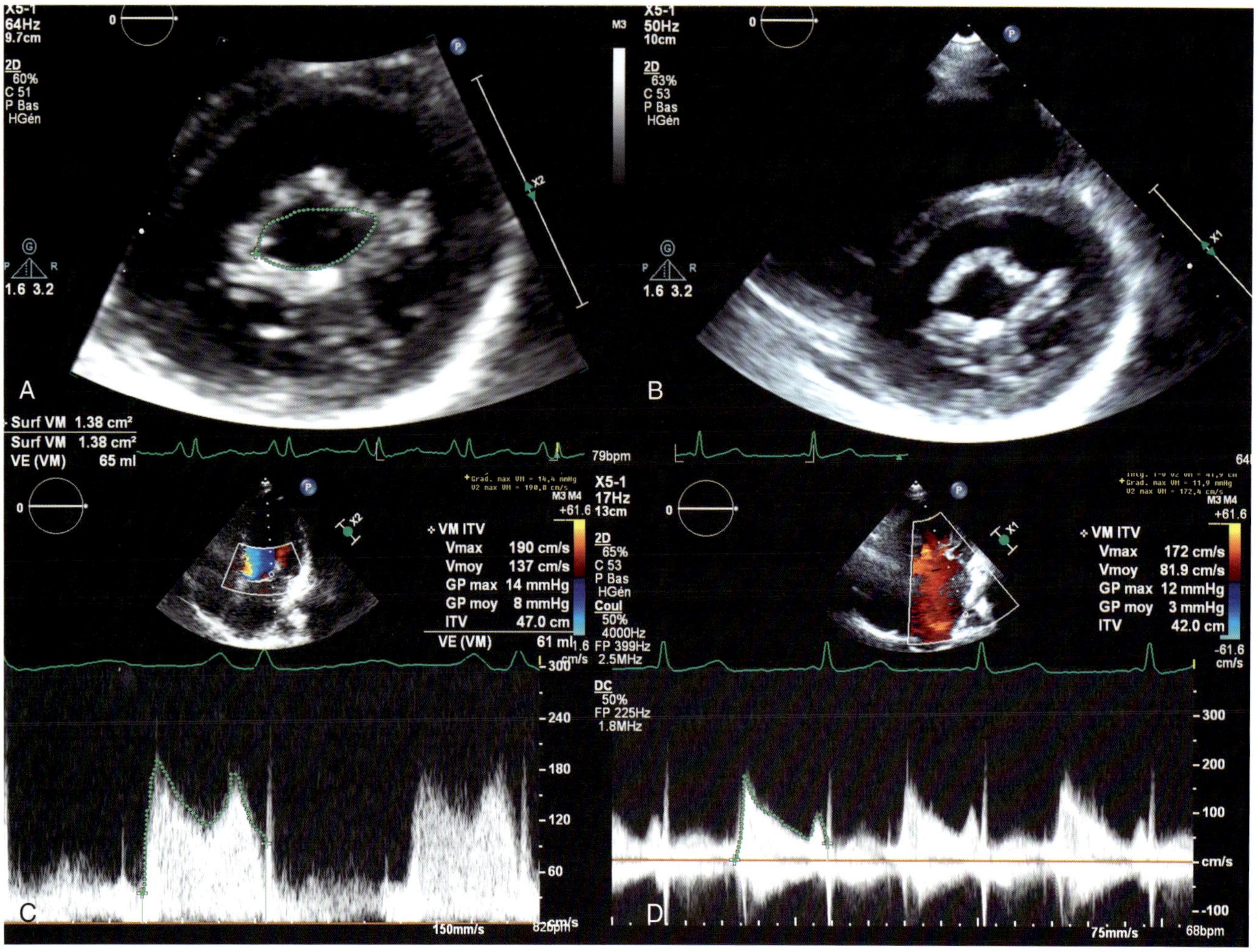

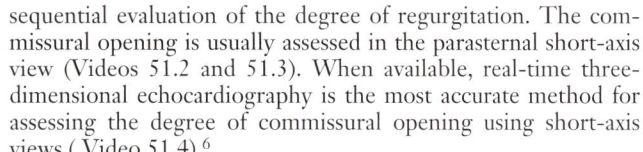

Fig. 51.1 Echocardiographic assessment of a good result of percutaneous mitral commissurotomy (PMC). (A) Parasternal short-axis view before PMC. Severe mitral stenosis with fusion of both commissures and valve area 1.38 cm². (B) Parasternal short-axis view after PMC. Complete opening of both commissures and valve area 2.0 cm². (C) Mean mitral gradient (Doppler) 8 mm Hg before PMC. (D) Mean mitral gradient (Doppler) 3 mm Hg after PMC.

sequential evaluation of the degree of regurgitation. The commissural opening is usually assessed in the parasternal short-axis view (Videos 51.2 and 51.3). When available, real-time three-dimensional echocardiography is the most accurate method for assessing the degree of commissural opening using short-axis views (Video 51.4).[6]

An integrative assessment using the following criteria has been proposed for the desired end point of the procedure: mitral valve area >1 cm²/m² of the body surface area; complete opening of at least one commissure; or appearance or increment of regurgitation > grade 1. The strategy must be tailored to individual circumstances. After the procedure, the most accurate evaluation of the valve area is achieved by echocardiography. Color Doppler flow is used to assess the degree of regurgitation and interatrial shunting.

Immediate Results

Failures

The failure rate for PMC ranges from 1% to 17%.[4,7–10] Failure is often caused by an inability to puncture the atrial septum or position the balloon correctly across the valve. Most failures occur early in the operator's experience.

Hemodynamics

PMC usually provides an increase of approximately 100% in the valve area (Table 51.1).[4,5,9,11–20] Improvement in valve function immediately decreases left atrial pressure (Fig. 51.3) and slightly increases the cardiac index. Pulmonary arterial pressure and pulmonary vascular resistance gradually decrease.[21] Rest and exercise pulmonary arterial pressure are also determined by atrioventricular compliance.[22]

PMC has a beneficial effect on exercise capacity.[23] PMC improves the pump function of the left atrium and the left atrial appendage and decreases left atrial stiffness. It also decreases the intensity of spontaneous echocardiographic contrast in the left atrium.[24]

Complications

Large series have enabled assessment of the risks of the technique.[4,7–10,25] The procedural mortality rate ranged from 0% to 3% and depends mainly on patient condition.

The incidence of hemopericardium is between 0.5% and 12%. Pericardial hemorrhage may be related to transseptal catheterization or to apex perforation by guidewires or the balloon and has become unusual with the Inoue technique. If hypotension occurs

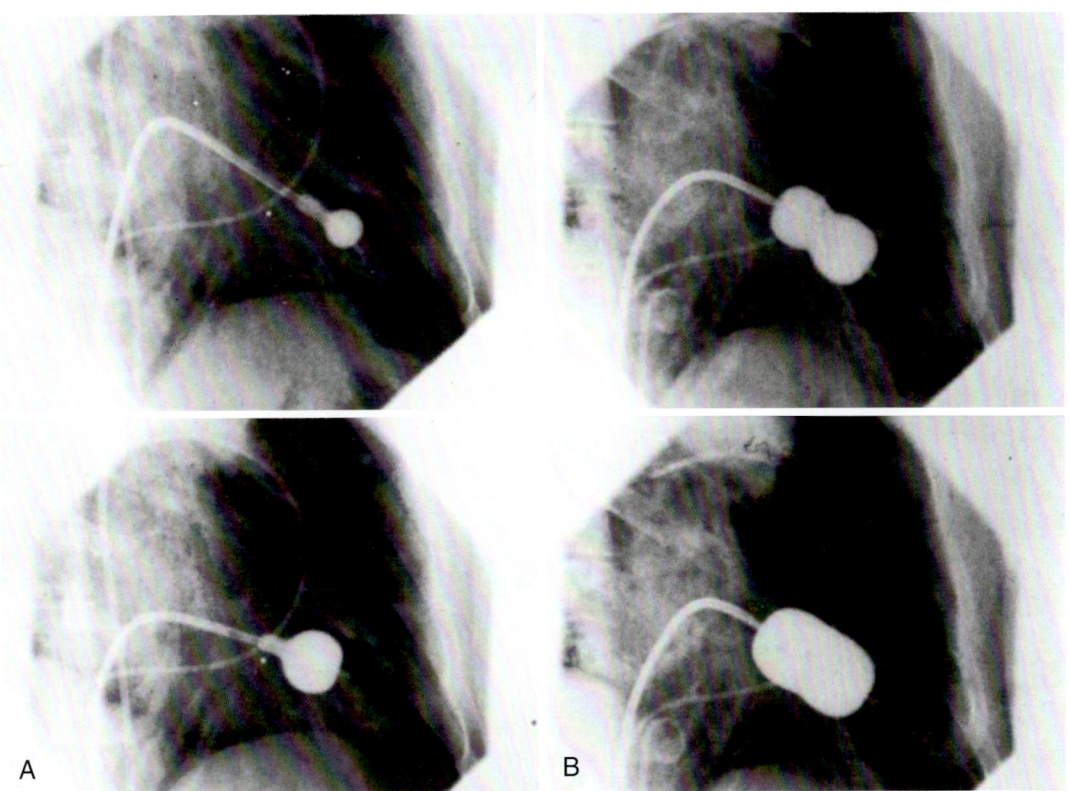

Fig. 53.2 Inoue's percutaneous mitral commissurotomy technique. (A) Inflation of the distal portion of the balloon, which is then pulled back and anchored at the mitral valve. (B) Subsequent inflation of the proximal and middle portions of the balloon. At full inflation, the waist of the balloon in its midportion has disappeared.

TABLE 51.1 Late Results After Balloon Mitral Commissurotomy (Series With Follow-Up ≥5 Years)

	n =	Age (Years)	Mitral Valve Area		Maximum Follow-Up (Years)	Event-Free Survival (%) at Maximum Follow-Up
			Before PMC	After PMC		
Lee et al.[5]	302	41	0.9	1.9	24	52 at 20 years[a]
Bouleti et al.[11]	1024	49	1.1	1.9	20	30[b]
Tomai et al.[c12]	482	55	1.0	1.9	20	36[a]
Fawzy et al.[c13]	547	32	0.9	2.0	19	28[b]
Palacios et al.[4]	879	55	0.9	1.9	12	33[b]
Ben Farhat et al.[9]	654	34	1.0	2.1	10	72[b]
Stefanadis et al.[14]	441	44	1.0	2.1	9	75[b]
Song et al.[15]	402	44	1.0	1.9	9	90[a]
Meneveau et al.[16]	532	54	1.0	1.7	7.5	52[b]
Hernandez et al.[17]	561	53	1.0	1.8	7	69[b]
Wang et al.[18]	310	53	1.1	1.7	6	80
Orrange et al.[19]	132	44	1.0	1.9	7	65[a]
Cohen et al.[20]	146	59	1.0	2.1	5	51[a]

[a]Survival without intervention.
[b]Survival without intervention and in New York Heart Association class I or II.
[c]Patients with good immediate results.
PMC, Percutaneous mitral commissurotomy.

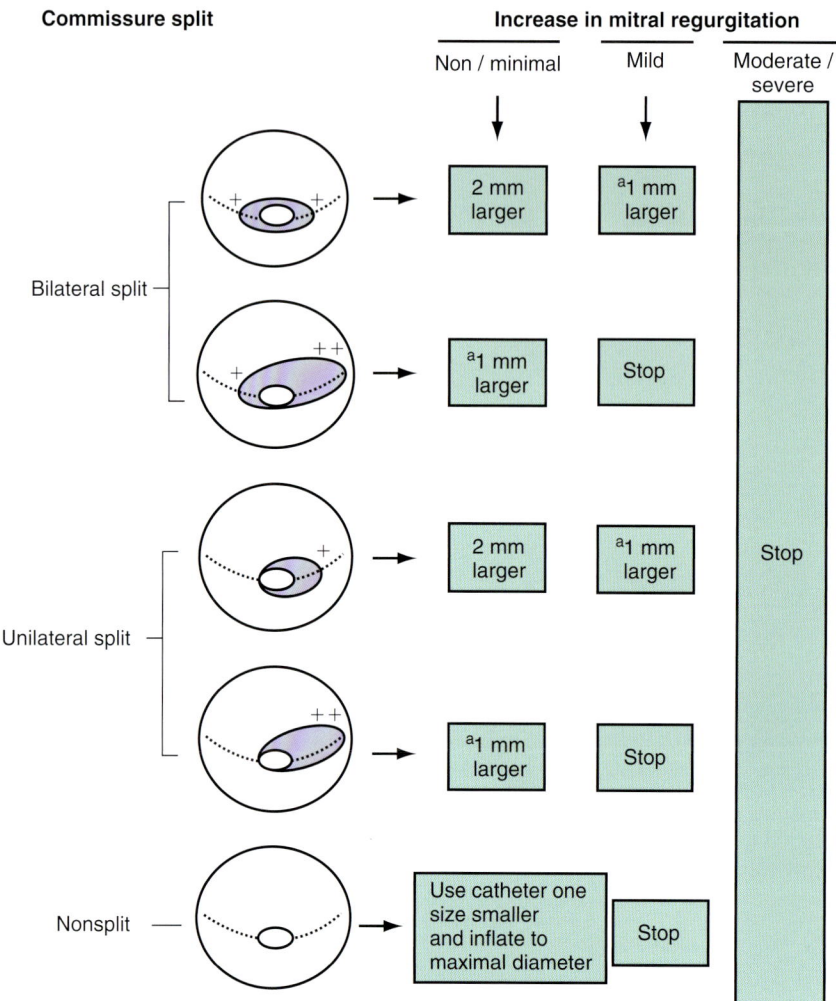

Fig. 51.3 Hemodynamic changes after percutaneous mitral commissurotomy.

^{a}Stop in cases of severely diseased valve or age older than 65 years.

during PMC, hemopericardium must be suspected and echocardiography immediately performed, followed by pericardiocentesis in the catheter laboratory and secondary transfer for cardiac surgery.

Embolism occurs in 0.5% to 5% of cases. It can be caused by gas immediately after balloon rupture, by fibrinothrombotic material, or occasionally, by calcium accumulation.

Severe mitral regurgitation is uncommon, between 2% and 19%, was approximately 5% in large series, and remains largely unpredictable for a given patient.[26,27] It often is related to noncommissural leaflet tearing.[28] In these cases, one or both commissures are too tightly fused to be split. It may also be caused by excessive commissural splitting or rarely by rupture of a papillary muscle. Development of severe regurgitation depends more on the distribution of morphologic changes than on their severity. Severe mitral regurgitation may be well tolerated; more often it is not, and open chest surgery must be scheduled. In most cases, valve replacement is necessary and is more closely related to the extent of valve disease than to the tear itself.

Atrial septal defects are frequent after PMC but generally lead to small shunts which often disappear during follow-up without clinical consequences.

Urgent surgery (within 24 hours) is seldom needed, mainly because of massive hemopericardium or severe and poorly tolerated mitral regurgitation.[28]

Predictors of Immediate Results

Good immediate results are defined in most series by a final valve area ≥1.5 cm^2 with mitral regurgitation grade ≤2/4. Predictive factors of poor immediate results are older age, prior surgical commissurotomy, high functional class, small mitral valve area, atrial fibrillation (AF), high pulmonary artery pressure, severe tricuspid regurgitation, and procedural factors such as balloon size.[4,29–31] Multivariate models have been developed to predict immediate results of PMC.[29,30]

Long-Term Results

Long-term follow-up has been reported in large series of PMC (see Table 51.1, Fig. 51.4).[4,5,9,11–20] In our series, which included 1024 patients, the 20-year survival rate was 73% ± 2%; the survival rate without any reintervention was 34% ± 2%.[11] When analyzing survival without surgery only, this figure increases to between 46% ± 2% and 57% ± 3% for patients younger than 50 years. Good functional results, defined as survival with no cardiovascular death or intervention, were reported for 30% ± 6% of patients with New York Heart Association (NYHA) class I or II disease.[11]

Prediction of long-term results is based on clinical variables such as age, valve anatomy, factors related to the evolutionary stage of the disease (i.e., higher NYHA class before valvuloplasty), prior commissurotomy, severe tricuspid regurgitation, AF, high pulmonary vascular resistance, results of the procedure in terms

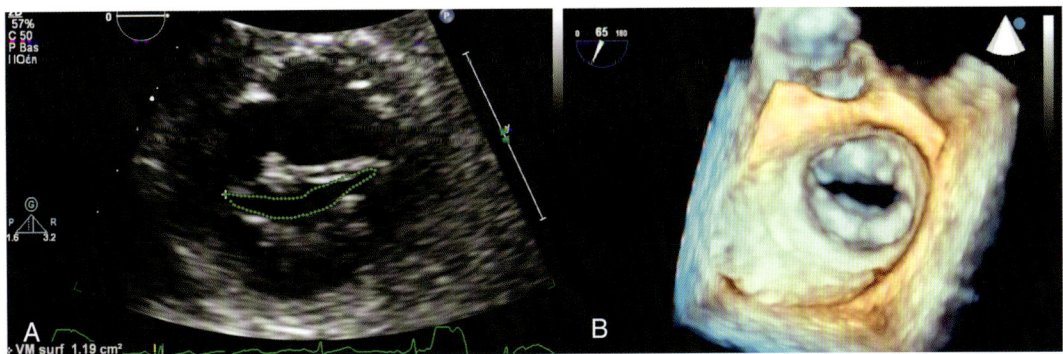

Fig. 51.4 Mitral restenosis 27 years after percutaneous mitral commissurotomy with persistent opening of both commissures. (A) Parasternal short-axis view. (B) Three-dimensional transesophageal echocardiography, view from the left atrium.

of final gradient, valve area and quality of commissural opening, and existence of mitral regurgitation.[4,5,9,11–20] A score combining these variables may be useful for patient selection and is relevant to follow-up.[11] Patients who have favorable immediate results but who are at high risk for further events must be carefully monitored to detect deterioration and institute timely intervention.

If PMC is initially successful, survival rates are excellent and the most frequent event is mitral intervention due to restenosis. After successful PMC, the incidence of restenosis, defined as a valve area <1.5 cm^2 with a loss >50% of the initial gain, is usually between 2% and 40% at 3 to 10 years.[15,17,18,32–34] Age, mitral valve area after PMC, and anatomy are predictors of restenosis.

Repeat PMC can be performed for restenosis if it is due to commissural refusion.[35–39] Using these criteria, repeat valvuloplasty may be performed in up to one-fourth of cases of late reintervention, allowing surgery to be postponed for a substantial number of patients. In a series comprising 85 repeat PMCs, the 10-year rate of cardiovascular survival without surgery was 60% and 50% for survival without intervention.[38]

If the immediate results are unsatisfactory, surgical treatment is usually necessary in the following months.[11,12] In cases of an insufficient initial opening, delayed surgery is usually performed. Valve replacement is necessary in almost all cases.

The degree of mitral regurgitation remains stable or slightly decreases during follow-up.

The low incidence of embolism during follow-up, the decrease in intensity of spontaneous echocardiographic contrast, and the improved left atrial function after PMC suggest a beneficial effect on left atrial blood stasis, and a lower risk of thromboembolism may be expected.[40]

There is no direct evidence that PMC reduces the incidence of AF.[41] It is recommended that electric cardioversion be performed early after successful PMC if the AF is of recent onset and in the absence of severe enlargement of the left atrium. Paroxysmal or persistent AF is an indication for lifelong anticoagulant therapy regardless of the degree of stenosis. Vitamin K blockers should be used due to the lack of data with direct oral anticoagulants.[42,43]

Several studies have compared surgical commissurotomy with PMC, mostly in patients with favorable characteristics.[44] They have shown that valvuloplasty is at least comparable with surgical commissurotomy with regard to short-term and midterm follow-up up to 7 years. There is no randomized comparison of PMC and surgical commissurotomy in patients with less favorable anatomy, and the results of observational series are somewhat contradictory.[36,45]

SELECTION OF PATIENTS

Patient Evaluation

Evaluation of the patient must take into account symptoms, stenosis severity, contraindications to PMC, and the risks involved in surgery as a function of the underlying cardiac and noncardiac status. Because of the small but definite risk inherent in the technique, the indications for intervention are limited to truly symptomatic patients with severe mitral stenosis.

PMC can be proposed for patients who are declared to be asymptomatic but who have pulmonary hypertension, increased thromboembolic risk, or in young women who wish to be pregnant. The American Heart Association/American College of Cardiology (AHA/ACC) guidelines suggest that PMC is reasonable in cases with very severe mitral stenosis (valve area <1 cm^2).[42] Under these conditions, PMC should be performed only by experienced interventionalists when the anatomy is favorable. Contraindications to transseptal catheterization include mainly suspected left atrial thrombosis, severe hemorrhagic disorder, and severe cardiothoracic deformity.

PMC is the only solution when surgery is contraindicated and is favored in patients for whom cardiac surgery poses a high risk, as in the following situations.

In cases of *severe pulmonary hypertension*,[21] PMC may produce a decrease in pulmonary pressures and therefore reduce the operative risk.

For *critically ill patients*, valvuloplasty may be the sole treatment available when there is an absolute contraindication to surgery, or it may be used as a bridge to surgery in other cases.

For *older patients*, valvuloplasty results in a moderate but significant improvement in valve function at an acceptable risk, although subsequent functional deterioration is common.[32,46] PMC can be attempted first according to valve anatomy or performed as a palliative procedure.

During pregnancy, surgery under cardiopulmonary bypass carries a substantial risk of fetal mortality and morbidity.[47] From a technical point of view, the procedure may be challenging and should be performed only by experienced operators. The procedure is effective and allows for normal delivery in most cases. PMC is safe for the fetus, provided that shield protection is provided and the procedure is performed after the 20th week.

For patients with a previous surgical commissurotomy, reoperation is associated with a higher risk of morbidity and mortality and requires valve replacement in most cases. PMC is feasible in this setting, although the procedure may be technically difficult. PMC enables valve replacement to be postponed with a low-risk procedure in selected patients. Echocardiographic examination must be conducted with care to exclude patients in whom restenosis is mainly caused by valve rigidity without significant commissural refusion (Fig. 51.5, Videos 51.5 and 51.6). In patients who have undergone mitral ring annuloplasty for correction of mitral regurgitation, PMC can be proposed if there is commissural fusion. Otherwise, surgical or transcatheter valve implantation (i.e., valve in a ring) can be performed after discussion with the heart team.

Assessment of Valve Anatomy

The assessment of anatomy has several aims when establishing indications and prognosis. Anatomic contraindications to the technique must be excluded. Left atrial thrombosis must be excluded by systematic transesophageal echocardiography (TEE) a few days before the procedure.[48] PMC may be considered only if TEE shows that the thrombus disappeared after 2 to 6 months of vitamin K antagonist therapy.[49]

Another contraindication is moderate mitral regurgitation. PMC can, however, be carried out in selected patients with grade 2 mitral regurgitation if other anatomical conditions are favorable. In cases of combined mitral stenosis and severe aortic disease, surgery is indicated in the absence of contraindications. However, the coexistence of moderate aortic valve disease and severe mitral stenosis is another situation for which PMC is preferable so that the inevitable later surgical treatment of both valves can be postponed.

Combined severe tricuspid stenosis and tricuspid regurgitation with clinical signs of heart failure is an indication for surgery on both valves. Tricuspid regurgitation is not a contraindication to the procedure if there is no marked enlargement of right cardiac chambers.

When mitral valve area is >1.5 cm^2, the risks probably outweigh the benefits, indicating medical treatment only. However, PMC may be considered in selected patients with large body surface area and symptoms and no other cause, even more so if exercise testing is positive.[42,43]

Echocardiographic assessment allows the classification of patients into anatomic groups with a view to predicting the results. Most widely used scores have a prognostic value on immediate and late results but should be analyzed in conjunction with other patient characteristics.[31,50] More recently, a score including a quantitative approach of leaflet motion and commissural area seems to have an improved prognostic value, but validation remains limited so far (Table 51.2).[34]

EXPERIENCE OF THE MEDICAL AND SURGICAL TEAMS

The incidence of technical failures and complications and the quality of results are related to the operator's experience.[25,29,51] Because of the low prevalence of mitral stenosis in developed countries, PMC should be performed in a limited number of expert centers with regards to patient selection and the procedure.[52]

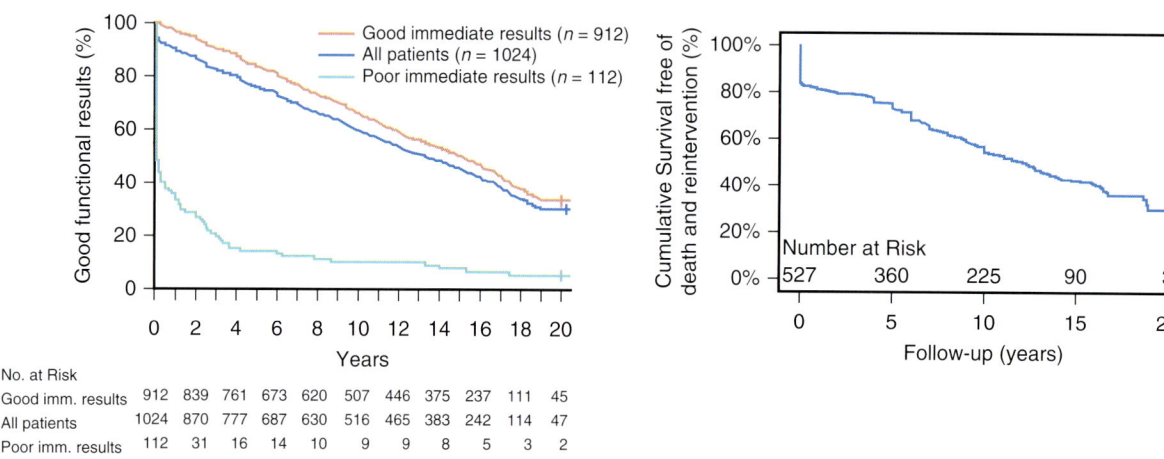

Fig. 51.5 **Long-term results of percutaneous mitral commissurotomy.** (A) Good functional results (cardiovascular survival without intervention and in New York Heart Association functional class I or II) in 1024 patients. (B) Freedom from death or reintervention in 527 patients. (A, Modified from Bouleti C, Iung B, Laouénan C, et al. Late results of percutaneous mitral commissurotomy up to 20 years: development and validation of a risk score predicting late functional results from a series of 912 patients. *Circulation.* 2012;125[17]:2119–2127; B, Modified from Tomai F, Gaspardone A, Versaci F, et al. Twenty year follow-up after successful percutaneous balloon mitral valvuloplasty in a large contemporary series of patients with mitral stenosis. *Int J Cardiol.* 2014;177[3]:881–885.)

TABLE 51.2 Score Using Quantitative Echocardiographic Assessment for the Prediction of Immediate Outcome After BMC

Variable	Prevalence n (%)	Odds Ratio (95% Confidence Interval)	P	Points for Score
Mitral valve area ≤1 cm^2	73 (36)	2.73 (1.32–5.66)	.007	2
Maximum leaflet displacement ≤12 mm	71 (35)	3.40 (1.65–6.99)	.001	3
Commissural area ratio ≥1.25	75 (37)	3.10 (1.51–6.38)	.002	3
Subvalvular involvement[a]	37 (18)	3.23 (1.35–7.71)	.008	3

[a]Absent vs. mild or extensive thickening
Three risk groups are defined according to the score:
- Low risk (17% suboptimal results): score 0–3
- Intermediate risk (56% suboptimal results): score 5
- High risk (74% suboptimal results): score 6–11

Modified from Nunes MCP, Tan TC, Elmariah S, et al. The echo score revisited: impact of incorporating commissural morphology and leaflet displacement to the prediction of outcome for patients undergoing percutaneous mitral valvuloplasty. *Circulation.* 2014;129(8);886–895.

INDICATIONS FOR PERCUTANEOUS MITRAL COMMISSUROTOMY

Selection of a candidate for PMC must be based on clinical and anatomic variables. Anatomy is a simple, practical way to select patients for PMC, even though it should not be the sole criterion (Fig. 51.6).[42,43]

The indication for PMC is clear when surgery is contraindicated and in ideal candidates such as young adults with good anatomy. In these patients, PMC can be considered at an early stage in patients with severe mitral stenosis and few or no symptoms.[53] If restenosis occurs, repeat PMC is often feasible to further defer surgery.

Indications are more debated for other patients, especially those with unfavorable anatomy, who are more common in Western countries and who represent a growing proportion of candidates to PMC.[54] Despite less satisfying results, PMC can be considered as an initial treatment for selected candidates, reserving surgery for cases of failure or late deterioration.[43] Unfortunately, data on these patients from randomized studies are not available, and a comparison of the results of PMC with those of surgical series is difficult because of differences in the patients involved and because the surgical alternative is valve replacement in most cases. Valve replacement is a radical treatment when valve anatomy is impaired, but is associated with higher operative mortality and prosthesis-related complications, which are of particular importance in young patients.

Current opinion is that open surgery can be considered the treatment of choice for patients with bicommissural or heavy calcification. Conversely, data suggest that balloon valvuloplasty can be attempted as a first approach in patients with somewhat unfavorable anatomy, especially if their clinical status argues in favor of it. The following cases fall into this category: extensive lesions of the subvalvular apparatus; mild or moderate calcification, for which the 15-year event-free survival rates are 35% ± 4% and 24% ± 6%, respectively[55]; and unicommissural calcification, for which successful PMC can be achieved in 73% of patients.[56]

In these cases, open chest surgery should be considered reasonably early if the results are unsatisfactory or there is secondary deterioration.

FUTURE PROSPECTS

PMC is a proof of concept in the field of percutaneous structural intervention. It reproduces an effective surgical procedure, with a less invasive approach, and its long-term efficacy has been demonstrated.

The diffusion of PMC is still needed in developing countries, where rheumatic mitral stenosis remains frequent, but with an underuse of PMC because of economic constraints. In developed countries, the problems are different because most candidates are older and have somewhat less favorable anatomy. Careful evaluation of results in this population is still needed to clearly define the indications for PMC and valve replacement.

Evaluation and treatment can be improved through better imaging, including three-dimensional echocardiography and

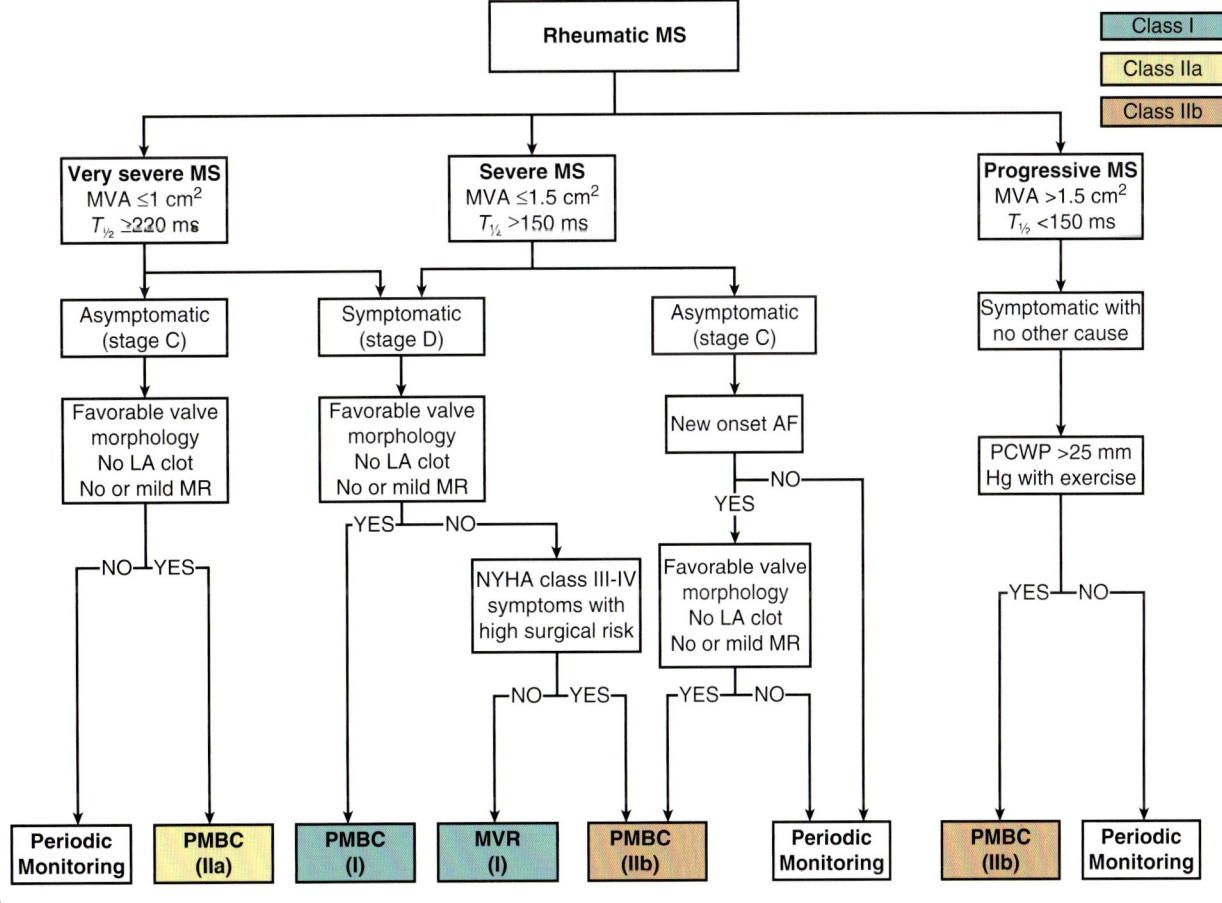

Fig. 51.6 Guidelines on indications for intervention in mitral regurgitation. (A) Indications for intervention for rheumatic mitral stenosis according to the 2014 American College of Cardiology/American Heart Association (ACC/AHA) guidelines for the management of valvular heart disease.

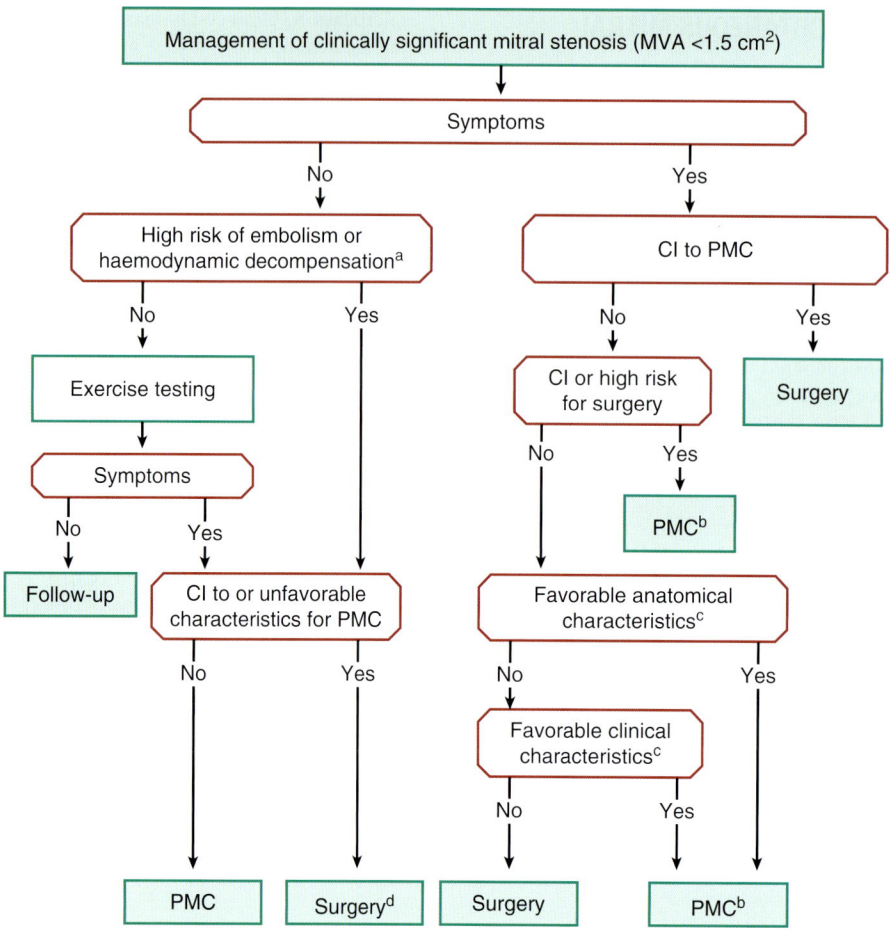

Fig. 51.6, cont'd (B) Management of clinically significant mitral stenosis according to the 2017 ESC/EACTS guidelines for the management of valvular heart disease. [a]High thromboembolic risk: history of systemic embolism, dense spontaneous contrast in the left atrium, new-onset atrial fibrillation. High risk of hemodynamic decompensation: systolic pulmonary pressure >50 mm Hg at rest, need for major noncardiac surgery, desire for pregnancy. [b]Surgical commissurotomy may be considered by experienced surgical teams or in patients with contraindications to PMC. [c]Unfavorable characteristics for PMC can be defined by the presence of several of the following characteristics. Clinical characteristics: old age, history of commissurotomy, New York Heart Association class IV, permanent atrial fibrillation, severe pulmonary hypertension. Anatomical characteristics: echocardiographic score >8, Cormier score 3 (calcification of mitral valve of any extent as assessed by fluoroscopy), very small mitral valve area, severe tricuspid regurgitation. [d]Surgery if symptoms occur for a low level of exercise and operative risk is low. *AF*, Atrial fibrillation; *CI*, Contra-indication; *LA*, left atrial; *MR*, mitral regurgitation; *MS*, mitral stenosis; *MVA*, mitral valve area; *MVR*, mitral valve surgery (repair or replacement); *NYHA*, New York Heart Association; *PCWP*, pulmonary capillary wedge pressure; *PMBC*, percutaneous mitral balloon commissurotomy; *PMC*, percutaneous mitral commissurotomy; $T^{1/2}$, pressure half-time. (A, Modified from Nishimura RA, Otto CM, Bonow RO, et al. 2014 AHA/ACC guideline for the management of patients with valvular heart disease: a report of the American College of Cardiology/American Heart Association Task Force on Practice Guidelines. *J Am Coll Cardiol.* 2014; 63[22]:e57–e185; B, Modified from Baumgartner H, Falk V, Bax JJ, et al. 2017 ESC/EACTS guidelines for the management of valvular heart disease: The Task Force for the Management of Valvular Heart Disease of the European Society of Cardiology (ESC) and the European Association for Cardio-Thoracic Surgery (EACTS). *Eur Heart J.* 2017;38[36]:2739–2791.)

multimodality imaging, in particular computed tomography to quantitate calcification. Further improvement may be achieved by combining PMC with other interventional procedures such as closure of the left atrial appendage, ablation of the pulmonary veins, and in the distant future, percutaneous mitral valve implantation in cases of contraindication and failure or deterioration after PMC. When treating mitral stenosis, we think that PMC and valve replacement must be considered complementary, not opposing, techniques. Each is applicable at the appropriate stage of the disease.

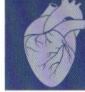

KEY REFERENCES

11. Bouleti C, Iung B, Laouenan C, et al. late results of percutaneous mitral commissurotomy up to 20 years: development and validation of a risk score predicting late functional results from a series of 912 patients. *Circulation*. 2012;125(17):2119–2127.
12. Tomai F, Gaspardone A, Versaci F, et al. Twenty year follow-up after successful percutaneous balloon mitral valvuloplasty in a large contemporary series of patients with mitral stenosis. *Int J Cardiol*. 2014;177(3):881–885.
17. Hernandez R, Banuelos C, Alfonso F, et al. Long-term clinical and echocardiographic follow-up after percutaneous mitral valvuloplasty with the Inoue balloon. *Circulation*. 1999;99(12):1580–1586.
25. Complications and mortality of percutaneous balloon mitral commissurotomy. A report from the National Heart, Lung, and Blood Institute Balloon Valvuloplasty Registry. *Circulation*. 1992;85(6):2014–2024.
29. Iung B, Cormier B, Ducimetiere P, et al. Immediate results of percutaneous mitral commissurotomy. A predictive model on a series of 1514 patients. *Circulation*. 1996;94(9):2124–2130.
30. Cruz-Gonzalez I, Sanchez-Ledesma M, Sanchez PL, et al. Predicting success and long-term outcomes of percutaneous mitral valvuloplasty: a multifactorial score. *Am J Med*. 2009;122(6):581e511–e589.
31. Nunes M, Nascimento B, Lodi-Junqueira L, et al. Update on percutaneous mitral commissurotomy. *Heart*. 2016;102(7):500–507.
34. Nunes MC, Tan TC, Elmariah S, et al. The echo score revisited: impact of incorporating commissural morphology and leaflet displacement to the prediction of outcome for patients undergoing percutaneous mitral valvuloplasty. *Circulation*. 2014;129(8):886–895.
38. Bouleti C, Iung B, Himbert D, et al. Reinterventions after percutaneous mitral commissurotomy during long-term follow-up, up to 20 years: the role of repeat percutaneous mitral commissurotomy. *Eur Heart J*. 2013;34(25):1923–1930.
42. Nishimura RA, Otto CM, Bonow RO, et al. 2014 AHA/ACC guideline for the management of patients with valvular heart disease: a report of the American College of Cardiology/American Heart Association task force on practice guidelines. *J Am Coll Cardiol*. 2014;63(22):e57–e185.
43. Baumgartner H, Falk V, Bax JJ, et al. 2017 ESC/EACTS guidelines for the management of valvular heart disease: the task force for the management of valvular heart disease of the European Society of Cardiology (ESC) and the European Association for Cardio-Thoracic Surgery (EACTS). *Eur Heart J*. 2017;38(36):2739–2791.
44. Ben Farhat M, Ayari M, Maatouk F, et al. Percutaneous balloon versus surgical closed and open mitral commissurotomy: seven-year follow-up results of a randomized trial. *Circulation*. 1998;97(3):245–250.
50. Wunderlich NC, Beigel R, Siegel RJ. Management of mitral stenosis using 2D and 3D echo-Doppler imaging. *JACC Cardiovasc Imaging*. 2013;6(11):1191–1205.
51. Badheka AO, Shah N, Ghatak A, et al. Balloon mitral valvuloplasty in the United States: a 13-year perspective. *Am J Med*. 2014;127(11):1126e1–1126e12.

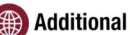 **Additional references available online at. expertconsult.com.**

中文导读

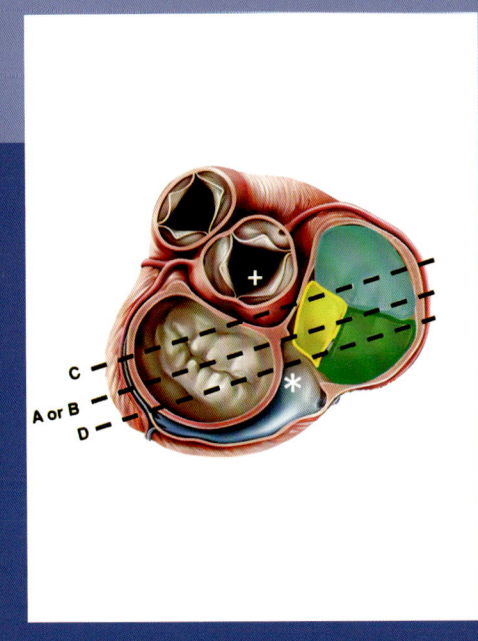

第52章
经皮二尖瓣修复和置换

  慢性二尖瓣反流给公众健康带来了巨大负担。如果不进行治疗，慢性二尖瓣反流会导致左心房和左心室扩大、心房颤动、肺动脉高压、左心室收缩功能障碍和心力衰竭。药物治疗仅可部分缓解二尖瓣反流症状，因此，二尖瓣修复术或二尖瓣置换术的外科手术仍然是慢性二尖瓣反流的主要治疗方法。然而，由于心脏内直视手术的创伤性，以及经常出现的并发症，高达50%的严重二尖瓣反流患者可能不接受外科手术治疗。并且，外科手术在功能性二尖瓣反流患者中的作用亦未得到证实。因此，经皮介入技术有望改变慢性二尖瓣反流的治疗模式。与心脏直视手术相比，经皮二尖瓣修复术具有创伤小和恢复时间短的优势。目前经皮介入技术的原理主要基于4种外科修复技术。虽然很多二尖瓣治疗器械处于临床前和临床评估的早期阶段，但经皮二尖瓣介入技术获得了巨大的关注和可喜的成绩。本章节对二尖瓣反流的病理生理、影像学评估到各种治疗方法均进行了阐述，并强调需要仔细选择适合介入治疗的二尖瓣反流患者及适合的介入治疗器械。相信通过这一章节的学习可对读者理解和掌握经皮二尖瓣修复技术有非常大的收获。

赵振燕   张洪亮

章节要点

- 二尖瓣反流是一个很重要的问题,随着充血性心力衰竭患者数量的增加,二尖瓣反流患者的数量也在不断增加。
- 正在进行的各种临床前和临床经皮二尖瓣修复方法的研究都显示出良好的应用前景。这些方法主要基于已有的外科手术策略,包括缘对缘修复、直接和间接瓣环成形术,以及腱索重建技术。
- 近年来,新器械的早期试验给经导管二尖瓣置换术带来了可喜的结果。
- 对于许多患者来说,通过瓣中瓣技术将经导管主动脉瓣瓣膜植入退化的二尖瓣环或外科生物瓣膜,是一种安全有效的策略。
- 由于瓣膜栓塞和左心室流出道梗阻,在退化的二尖瓣环中置入经导管主动脉瓣瓣膜(环中瓣)的风险高于瓣中瓣手术。
- 根据二尖瓣反流的解剖和功能特点,不同的经皮介入技术具有各自特定的优势。为每个患者选择合适的技术将最终决定这些新兴技术是否成功。
- 在导管室内外整合已有的成像方法对于经皮修复技术的安全性和有效性至关重要。新兴成像设备的发展很可能在未来的经皮介入技术中发挥作用。

52 Percutaneous Mitral Valve Repair and Replacement

Amar Krishnaswamy, Samir R. Kapadia

KEY POINTS

- Mitral regurgitation (MR) is a significant problem, and the number of patients with MR is growing together with increased numbers of patients with congestive heart failure.
- Various percutaneous approaches to mitral valve repair are under preclinical and clinical investigation and show promise. These approaches are predominantly based on established surgical strategies and include edge-to-edge repair, direct and indirect annuloplasty methods, and chamber remodeling strategies.
- In recent years, transcatheter mitral valve replacement techniques have gained a foothold with promising results from early trials of new devices.
- Replacement of degenerated surgical bioprosthetic valves using the valve-in-valve (ViV) approach of placing a transcatheter aortic valve prosthetic within a degenerated mitral ring or valve is a safe and effective strategy for many patients.
- Placement of a transcatheter aortic valve prosthetic in a patient with a degenerated mitral valve ring (valve-in-ring) carries greater risk than the ViV procedure due to valve embolization and left ventricular outflow tract obstruction
- Different percutaneous techniques provide specific advantages, depending on the anatomic and functional characteristics of MR. Selection of the appropriate technique or techniques for each patient will ultimately determine the success of these emerging technologies.
- Integration of established imaging modalities both in and out of the catheterization laboratory is critical for the safety and efficacy of percutaneous repair technologies. The development of emerging imaging modalities will likely play a role in the future of percutaneous technologies.

INTRODUCTION

Chronic mitral regurgitation (MR) poses a significant public health burden, with more than 3 million people in the United States alone suffering from moderate or severe MR.[1] Left untreated, chronic MR results in heart failure symptoms, left ventricular (LV) cavity dilatation and systolic dysfunction, enlargement of the left atrium (LA), atrial fibrillation, and pulmonary hypertension. Medical therapy may provide some relief from symptoms and is necessary to treat ischemic heart disease and heart failure in patients with MR complicating these underlying disease states. However, there has been no proven benefit of these treatments in MR itself.[2] Therefore, surgical correction with mitral valve repair (MVRe) or replacement remains the mainstay of therapy for chronic MR. However, because of the invasive nature of open-heart surgery and the frequent presence of comorbidities in this group, up to 50% of patients with severe MR may not be offered surgery.[3] This is especially true for older patients and those with impaired LV function.[4] Further, the role of surgery in patients with functional MR (FMR) remains unproven.

As a result, percutaneous technology is poised to significantly alter the treatment paradigm for chronic MR. Percutaneous MVRe offers the potential benefits of decreased morbidity, improved recovery time, and shorter hospital stay compared with open-heart surgery. Current percutaneous options are loosely based on surgical repair techniques, with four primary methods to accomplish a reduction in MR: (1) edge-to-edge (E2E) leaflet repair, (2) indirect annuloplasty via the coronary sinus, (3) direct annuloplasty, and (4) septal-lateral (SL) annular cinching. Percutaneous MVRe has gained significant traction over the past few years, with a number of devices in pre- and clinical stages demonstrating early feasibility. However, despite these early successes, no device has yet achieved commercial approval. Overall, the field is very exciting, with promising initial studies highlighting the need for a better understanding of patient selection for appropriate management of MR.

MITRAL VALVE DISEASE

Mitral Valve Anatomy

The mitral valve (MV) complex is composed of the mitral annulus, anterior and posterior leaflets, chordae tendineae, and papillary muscles.[5] The mitral annulus is the elliptical area of attachment of the MV to the base of the LA (Fig. 52.1). The posterior leaflet has three lobes or "scallops": the lateral (P1), central (P2), and medial scallops (P3). The anterior leaflet scallops are named A1, A2, and A3, respectively, corresponding to the posterior scallops. The anatomic position of the valve is such that the two leaflets meet at the anterolateral and posteromedial commissures. Chordae connect both the leaflets and the anterolateral and posteromedial papillary muscles. The primary chordae connect to the free edge of the leaflet; the secondary chordae ("strut" chords) are thicker and connect to the rough zone of the leaflet; and the tertiary chordae are short and connect the basal zone of the leaflet to the ventricular free wall.

Etiology and Mechanism of Mitral Regurgitation

Anatomic or functional abnormalities of any of the structures in the MV apparatus may lead to MR.[6,7] The disease process leading to MR may be primary MV disease, secondary regurgitation resulting from another cardiac disease, or MV involvement in a systemic inflammatory disease (Table 52.1). Various terminologies are used to characterize the mechanisms of MR. The morphologic description, proposed by Carpentier, classifies the mechanism of regurgitation according to leaflet pathophysiology (Fig. 52.2).[8] Type I regurgitation occurs in the presence of

SECTION V Structural Interventions

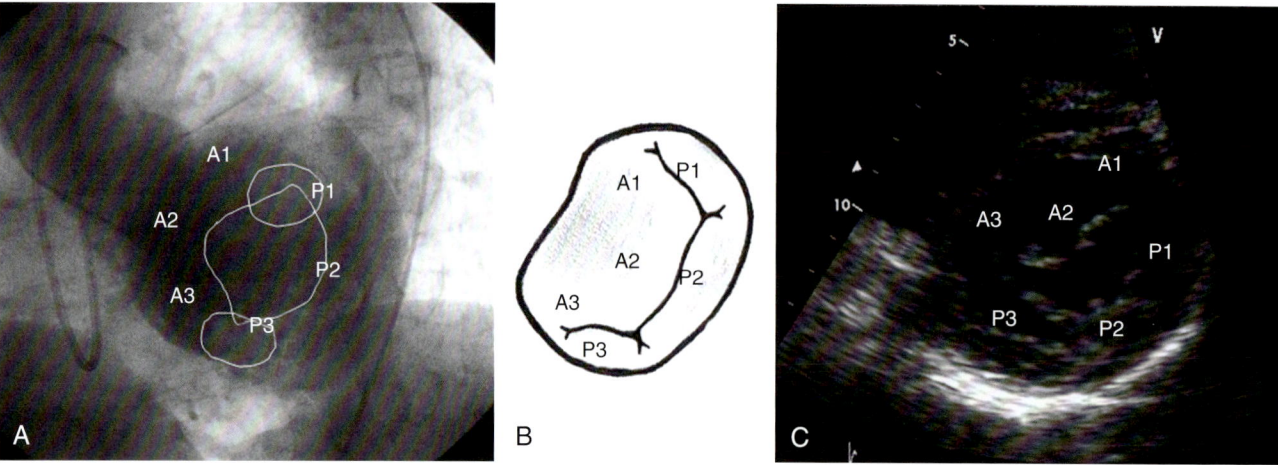

Fig. 52.1 Mitral valve anatomy. (A) Left ventriculogram in the left anterior oblique projection shows the mitral valve in short axis, with labeled leaflet segments. (B) A schematic diagram of the mitral valve in short axis. (C) A transthoracic echocardiographic image of the mitral valve in the parasternal short-axis projection. *A1*, *A2*, and *A3*, Lateral, central, and medial scallops of the anterior leaflet; *P1*, *P2*, and *P3*, lateral, central, and medial scallops of the posterior leaflet.

TABLE 52.1 Causes of Chronic Mitral Regurgitation
Primary mitral valve disorder
Degenerative valve disease
Myxomatous degeneration
Fibroelastic deficiency
Rheumatic valve disease
Infective endocarditis
Chordal rupture
Idiopathic causes
Traumatic causes
Congenital lesions
Cleft anterior mitral leaflet or fenestration
Parachute mitral valve abnormality
Prosthetic valve disorder
Paravalvular regurgitation
Prosthetic valve degeneration
Prosthetic valve endocarditis
Secondary mitral valve disorder (cardiac cause)
Ischemic mitral regurgitation (coronary artery disease)
Papillary muscle dysfunction or rupture
Mitral valve annular dilatation
Global or regional ventricular dysfunction
Left ventricular dilatation
Dilated (nonischemic) cardiomyopathy
Hypertrophic cardiomyopathy
Systemic or inflammatory disease
Systemic lupus erythematosus
Amyloidosis
Connective tissue disorder
Rheumatoid arthritis

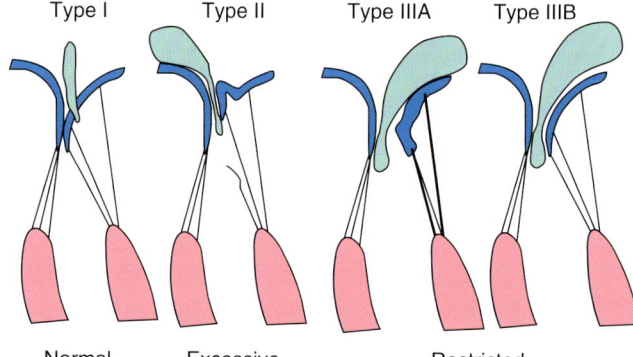

Fig. 52.2 Carpentier classification of mitral regurgitation according to function leaflet mobility. Type I exhibits normal leaflet mobility, as with endocarditis. Type II exhibits excessive leaflet mobility, as in degenerative disease or mitral valve prolapse. Type IIIA exhibits restricted leaflet motion caused by chordal and leaflet thickening due to rheumatic heart disease. Type IIIB exhibits restricted leaflet motion caused by ventricular wall motion abnormality resulting from dilated or ischemic cardiomyopathy.

normal leaflet motion and is usually caused by annular dilatation or leaflet perforation. Type II is caused by leaflet prolapse, which is commonly the result of degenerative (myxomatous) disease, chordal elongation or rupture, or papillary muscle elongation or rupture. Type III is caused by restricted leaflet motion, which may arise from posterior wall motion abnormality or papillary muscle dysfunction due to ischemic cardiac disease. The restricted leaflet motion may also be caused by commissural fusion, leaflet or chordal thickening from rheumatic heart disease, or both. This simplification has usefulness in terms of both the surgical approach and the percutaneous approach, because the goal of therapy is to restore normal leaflet function but not necessarily normal valve anatomy.

Another common method of categorizing MR is based on the etiology and mechanism of the MR. This classification is commonly used in the literature to study the clinical outcomes of patients (Table 52.2). In this classification scheme, MR is loosely categorized on the basis of an abnormal or normal MV as degenerative or rheumatic disease (*primary MR*) and functional or ischemic disease (*secondary MR*), respectively. However, the terms *functional MR*, *ischemic MR*, and *secondary MR* are often used interchangeably and may represent many different mechanisms and morphologic variants.

Degenerative disease includes Barlow disease (myxomatous degeneration) and fibroelastic deficiency, both of which can result in MV leaflet prolapse and degenerative MR (DMR). Fibroelastic deficiency is the most common etiology (approximately 70%) among patients undergoing surgical MVRe in the United States. MR in rheumatic disease is a result of leaflet deformity caused by severe thickening and calcification of the leaflets and subvalvular apparatus and apical leaflet doming resulting in malcoaptation. Although this is a common cause of mitral disease worldwide, it is less frequently encountered in the United States.

TABLE 52.2 Carpentier's Morphologic Classification with Mechanisms of Mitral Regurgitation

TYPE I: NORMAL LEAFLET MOTION
Annular dilatation
Dilated cardiomyopathy—"functional MR"[a]
Leaflet perforation
Annular calcification

TYPE II: LEAFLET PROLAPSED
Chordal rupture or flail leaflet
Chordal elongation—"degenerative MR"
Papillary muscle elongation
Papillary muscle rupture

TYPE III: RESTRICTED LEAFLET MOTION
IIIA: Fibrosis of the subvalvular apparatus—"rheumatic MR"
IIIB: Regional left ventricular remodeling or wall motion abnormality—"ischemic MR"

[a]The term "functional MR" is sometimes used to describe both ischemic and nonischemic MR because they share the characteristics of left ventricular geometric remodeling and annular dilatation with normal leaflet morphology.
MR, Mitral regurgitation.

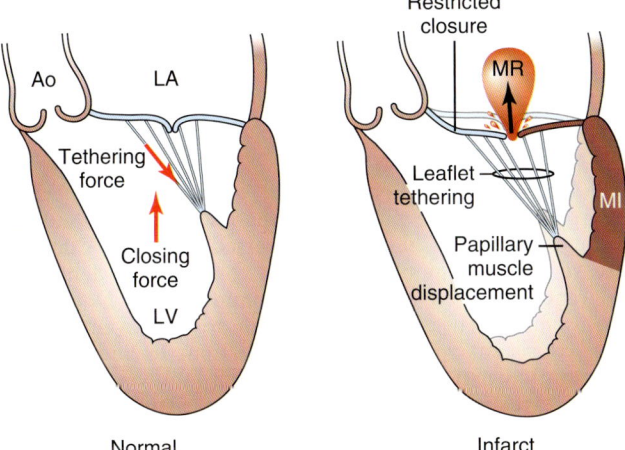

Fig. 52.3 *Left panel*, Balance of forces acting on mitral leaflets in systole. *Right panel*, Infarction causes LV cavity dilatation and papillary muscle displacement, which together result in annular dilatation, leaflet tethering, and restricted leaflet motion. Both factors contribute to functional mitral regurgitation *(MR)*. Dark shading indicates inferobasal myocardial infarction *(MI)*; light shading indicates normal baseline. *Ao*, Aorta; *LA*, left atrium; *LV*, left ventricle. (Modified from Liel-Cohen N, Guerrero JL, Otsuji Y, et al. Design of a new surgical approach for ventricular remodeling to relieve ischemic mitral regurgitation: insights from three-dimensional echocardiography. *Circulation*. 2000;101:2756–2763.)

FMR occurs in the setting of LV dysfunction and is seen in patients with coronary artery disease (ischemic MR) or with dilated cardiomyopathy from other causes. Ischemic MR results from decreased closing force and increased tethering force on the leaflets.[9] Various factors can lessen the closing force, including diminished left ventricular ejection fraction (LVEF), LV dyssynchrony, and decreased annular contraction; similarly, many factors can increase the tethering force, including papillary muscle displacement, LV remodeling, and annular dilatation.[10–13] It is becoming increasingly clear that significant interaction among ventricular, valvular, and annular factors is involved in the generation, perpetuation, and progression of so-called functional MR (Fig. 52.3). More recently, investigators have demonstrated the incidence of typical FMR due to annular dilation but with normal LVEF that results instead from progressive LA enlargement.[14]

Natural History

The natural history of chronic MR depends on the degree of regurgitation, the cause of the underlying disorder, and the degree of LV dysfunction.[15-17] Available data on the natural history of the disease are limited by small sample size, selection bias, inconsistent measures of MR severity, and the inclusion of disparate etiologies of regurgitation. However, it appears that many patients with chronic MR remain asymptomatic for many years.[18] Among patients with mild MR, there is an inconsistent rate of progression to severe MR that appears to be independent of medical treatment.[19] When chronic severe MR is present, approximately 5% to 10% of patients per year develop significant symptoms, clinical indication for surgery, death, or all of these.[18,20]

Whether there is a small risk of sudden cardiac death in patients with severe asymptomatic MR remains controversial, and the data are not compelling enough to subject patients to intervention for this reason alone in the absence of other indications for MVRe.[20] The importance of symptoms in regard to long-term prognosis is demonstrated by the high mortality rate reported for patients with New York Heart Association (NYHA) class III or IV symptoms, even in degenerative MV disease. LVEF is also an important independent predictor of outcome in patients with FMR.[17]

Patients with degenerative MV disease have a favorable long-term prognosis whether they are treated conservatively or, when indicated, surgically. However, patients with degenerative MV disease and coronary disease are fundamentally different from those with degenerative disease alone; the former have a worse prognosis that is dominated by the contribution of coronary disease.[16] Conversely, in the absence of degenerative disease, the presence and degree of MR after myocardial infarction is an independent predictor of mortality, emphasizing the need for accurate quantification; further studies are needed to investigate whether treatment of MR in these patients modifies outcomes.[21,22]

Imaging: Echocardiography

Echocardiography is the dominant modality for imaging the MV and for the assessment of MR severity. Two-dimensional transthoracic echocardiography (TTE) is useful to evaluate the valvular anatomy, to determine the structure and function of the LV, and to assess the origin and degree of regurgitation. Therefore, TTE provides an understanding of MR severity as well as an insight into the primary or secondary nature of the disease. Furthermore, the anatomic assessment of the MV and the LV also allows determination of whether surgical or percutaneous MVRe may be feasible or whether valve replacement will be necessary. Longitudinal data collected by serial echocardiography may be used to determine the timing of intervention and to follow up the results. If transthoracic images are not adequate, transesophageal echocardiography (TEE) provides an excellent assessment of MV anatomy and severity of regurgitation. This can be particularly useful to determine whether valve repair is feasible.

Evaluation of the severity of valvular regurgitation with echocardiography relies heavily on Doppler methods, including color, pulsed-wave, and continuous-wave Doppler. The American Society of Echocardiography has determined the qualitative and quantitative echocardiographic parameters that are useful in grading MR (Table 52.3).[23] The assessment of severity should rely on the integration of both quantitative

TABLE 52.3 Qualitative and Quantitative Parameters Useful in Grading Mitral Regurgitation Severity

	Mild	Moderate	Severe
STRUCTURAL PARAMETERS			
LA size	Normal	Normal or dilated	Usually dilated
LV size	Normal	Normal or dilated	Usually dilated
Mitral leaflets or support apparatus	Normal or abnormal	Normal or abnormal	Abnormal/flail leaflet/ruptured papillary muscle
DOPPLER PARAMETERS			
Color flow jet area	Small, central jet (usually <4 cm^2 or <20% of LA area)	Variable	Large central jet (usually >10 cm^2 or >40% of LA area) or variable size wall-impinging jet swirling in LA
Mitral inflow—PW	A wave dominant	Variable	E wave dominant
Jet density—CW	Incomplete or faint	Dense	Dense
Jet contour—CW	Parabolic	Usually parabolic	Early peaking—triangular
Pulmonary vein flow	Systolic dominance	Systolic blunting	Systolic flow reversal
QUANTITATIVE PARAMETERS			
Vena contracta width (cm)	<0.3	0.3–0.69	≥0.7
Regurgitant volume (mL/beat)	<30	30–59	≥60
Regurgitant fraction (%)	<30	30–49	≥50
EROA (cm^2)	<0.20	0.20–0.39	≥0.40

CW, Continuous wave; *EROA*, effective regurgitant orifice area; *LA*, left atrium; *LV*, left ventricle; *PW*, pulse wave.
Data from Zoghbi WA, Enriquez-Sarano M, Foster E, et al. Recommendations for evaluation of the severity of native valvular regurgitation with two-dimensional and Doppler echocardiography. *J Am Soc Echocardiogr.* 2003;16(7):777–802.

and qualitative measures obtained by Doppler techniques.[24] In addition, structural findings such as a flail leaflet or an enlarged LA can add useful information with regard to regurgitation severity.

Color Doppler provides a number of qualitative and quantitative means to determine MR severity. A proximal flow convergence on color Doppler is present in severe regurgitation. The proximal isovelocity surface area (PISA) of this flow convergence can be used to accurately quantitate the effective regurgitant orifice area (EROA).[25] The width of the regurgitant jet at or just downstream from the regurgitant orifice is known as the *vena contracta* and is slightly smaller than the anatomic regurgitant orifice.[26] This distinction is particularly relevant in some patients with FMR, in which the regurgitant orifice has a slit-like rather than an oval shape. The area of the MR jet occupying the LA can provide a rapid semiquantitative assessment of regurgitation severity. However, this is influenced by instrument factors (e.g., gain) and by jet orientation (e.g., a central jet may appear more severe than an equally large jet that adheres to the atrial wall). In addition, the color jet area is influenced by the driving pressure across the valve and can be enhanced by elevated blood pressure. Color Doppler imaging is also important in the parasternal short-axis view to determine the origin of the MR jet because percutaneous approaches (especially the MitraClip) are more effective in centrally originating jets than in medial or lateral ones.

Regurgitant volume can be assessed with the use of continuous-wave Doppler data. Regurgitant volume is calculated by applying the continuity equation (conservation of mass), in which left-sided regurgitation volume is calculated as the difference between Doppler-derived flows across the aortic and mitral valves.[27] The stroke volume equals the cross-sectional area of the valve annulus, multiplied by the velocity-time integral of flow across the annulus. The regurgitant volume at the MV is calculated as the difference between stroke volumes across the MV and the aortic valve. This can also be expressed as a regurgitant fraction.

Pulsed-wave Doppler is useful to assess the effect of regurgitation on the pulmonary venous flow. A pulmonary venous flow that is blunted or reversed in systole can indicate severe regurgitation.[28,29] The contour and density of the regurgitant envelope on continuous-wave Doppler is also useful: a dense, early-peaking, or triangular envelope is most consistent with severe regurgitation. In addition, the mitral inflow pattern is typically E-wave dominant (>1.2 m/s) in severe regurgitation, reflecting increased flow across the valve.

Alternative Imaging Modalities

Although historically echocardiography has been the dominant imaging modality in the assessment of MR, cardiac computed tomography (CT), cardiac magnetic resonance imaging (MRI), and three-dimensional (3-D) echocardiography are beginning to play more important roles.[24,30–32] Coronary sinus devices that indirectly alter annular geometry are under development, so the relationship of the coronary sinus to the mitral annulus is becoming increasingly important (Fig. 52.4). In addition, the coronary sinus and left circumflex arteries are close to each other and overlap in more than 90% of patients, creating the potential for cinching devices to hinder coronary blood flow.[33] Cardiac CT has the potential to provide significant anatomic details in the screening of patients and procedural planning.

With cardiac MRI, it is possible to obtain significant structural information regarding the geometry of the LV, mitral annulus, and leaflets, as well as quantitative regurgitant volumes.[32] It is likely that regurgitant volumes calculated with the use of cardiac MRI are more accurate and more operator or reader independent compared with those derived from TTE. However, limited experience with this modality currently limits its usefulness for research purposes.

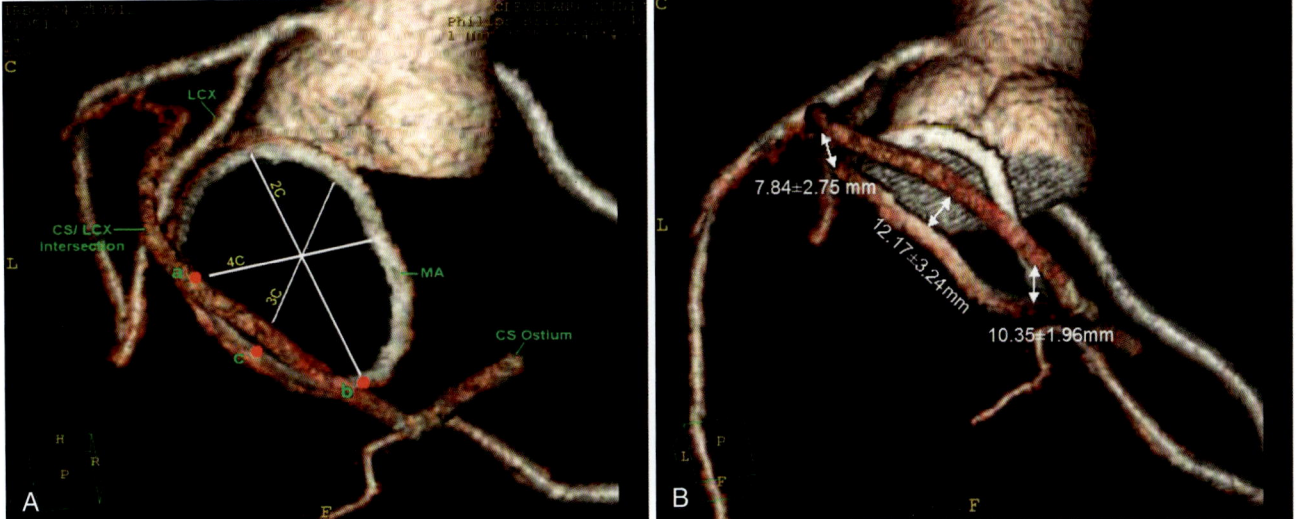

Fig. 52.4 Computed tomographic images of the relationships among the mitral annulus (MA), the coronary sinus (CS), and the left circumflex (LCX) coronary artery. (A) The CS travels along the posterior MA and crosses over the LCX artery. (B) The distance between the MA and the CS varies depending on the location along the annulus.

3-D echocardiography provides a more in-depth understanding of the anatomy of the MV apparatus and the changes of MR. Because the position of the MV apparatus in the LV can be disrupted in all directions, 3-D echocardiography is more likely to define the exact mechanism of MR in ischemic disease and to detect multiple jets of MR that may affect the treatment approach.[34] Furthermore, the ability to acquire real-time 3-D images with color flow allows the team to gauge safety and efficacy during both percutaneous and traditional surgical repairs.

SURGICAL MITRAL VALVE REPAIR

The American College of Cardiology and American Heart Association (ACC/AHA) guidelines provide a framework for patient selection and timing of MV surgery.[35] Any patient with acute severe MR should undergo valve surgery. Valve surgery is also recommended for patients with chronic severe MR in the presence of symptoms and for patients without symptoms in the presence of LV systolic dysfunction or LV cavity dilatation (end-systolic dimension >40 mm). Valve surgery results in the preservation of LV function and improved survival.[36,37]

The onset of atrial fibrillation or the development of significant pulmonary hypertension (pulmonary artery systolic pressure >50 mm Hg at rest or >60 mm Hg with exercise) in an asymptomatic patient with normal LV size and systolic function is a reasonable indication for surgery. Management of asymptomatic patients with severe MR and normal LV size and function remains controversial, but surgery is considered reasonable at centers where repair is likely (>95% chance) and has a low operative risk (<1%); this is provided a class IIa recommendation in the most recent ACC/AHA Guidelines.[35,38,39]

MVRe is the preferred method for surgical management of MR to restore normal leaflet function and annular size.[35] When compared with MV replacement, the major advantages of MVRe are improved survival, preservation of LV function, freedom from anticoagulation, and fewer complications.[40,41] Despite the advantages of MVRe, this technique appears to be underutilized: fewer than 50% of the patients undergoing MV surgery currently receive a repair procedure, even though about 90% are suitable.[42,43]

Surgical Approach

MV surgery can be performed via median sternotomy, a minimally invasive approach that uses partial upper sternotomy or small right thoracotomy, or it can be performed robotically through multiple "ports." Median sternotomy is required if concomitant coronary artery bypass is undertaken. Cardioplegic arrest and cardiopulmonary bypass are necessary regardless of the type of chest wall incision, although typically less than 1 hour is required for a valve repair.[8] Techniques of repair address the annulus (annuloplasty with or without a rigid or flexible ring, decalcification, débridement), the leaflets (triangular or quadrangular resection, sliding annuloplasty, patch enlargement, decalcification, E2E repair), the chordae (resection or elongation of chords), the myocardium itself (e.g., remodeling through the Dor procedure, plication of scar, pericardial cushions, transventricular slings), the papillary muscles (realignment), or some combination of all these.

Isolated Annuloplasty

Isolated mitral annuloplasty is usually reserved for patients with FMR. Available annuloplasty techniques include suture alone, suture with buttressing material, and prosthetic annuloplasty devices. The choice of annuloplasty technique is surgeon and patient specific. A prosthetic annuloplasty band or ring is placed to correct annular dilatation, increase leaflet coaptation by reducing the anteroposterior dimension of the annulus, and prevent future annular dilatation.

Annuloplasty for FMR results in significant improvement in NYHA class, decreased hospital admissions for heart failure, and modest survival rates of 71% to 82% at 2 years and 58% at 5 years. Although favorable changes in LV size, shape, and function have been demonstrated after successful MVRe, a propensity analysis failed to demonstrate any mortality benefit compared with

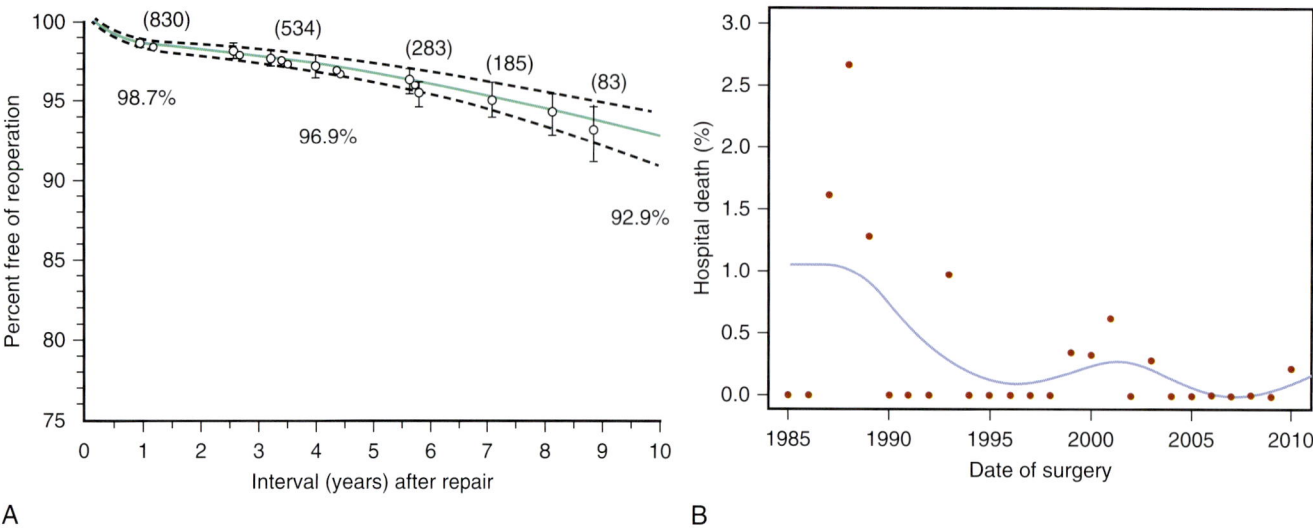

Fig. 52.5 Results of surgical mitral valve repair at Cleveland Clinic. (A) 10-year freedom from reoperation and (B) Trends in hospital mortality 1985–2010. (A, From Gillinov AM, Cosgrove DM, Blackstone EH, et al. Durability of mitral valve repair for degenerative disease. *J Thorac Cardiovasc Surg.* 1998;116:734–743; B, From Yazdchi F, Koch CG, Mihaljevic T, et al. Increasing disadvantage of "watchful waiting" for repairing degenerative mitral valve disease. *Ann Thorac Surg.* 2015;99:1992–2000.)

matched patients not undergoing valve surgery.[39,44] The recurrence rate of FMR after isolated annuloplasty is disappointing (28% at 1 year) and, along with the usually comorbid conditions of this patient population, remains a limitation to widespread use of the procedure.[45]

Annuloplasty With Leaflet Repair

The combination of annuloplasty and leaflet repair, referred to as *Carpentier's techniques*, is most frequently performed for degenerative MV disease. Among the surgical methods of mitral leaflet repair, correction of posterior leaflet or bileaflet prolapse is the most common. Posterior leaflet prolapse occurs in most cases of degenerative MV disease and is the primary cause of regurgitation in approximately 50% of patients. Prolapse results from chordal elongation or rupture and affects the central P2 segment most frequently. This type of problem is most often corrected by posterior leaflet quadrangular resection and plication of the valve annulus,[8] usually accompanied by the placement of a prosthetic annuloplasty ring except in cases of severe calcification of the annulus.

Anterior leaflet prolapse, although less common than posterior leaflet prolapse, is a more challenging problem and has been commonly treated with initial valve replacement due to poor results of repair in this group and greater parity with replacement outcomes.[46] However, when appropriate, several methods have been developed to treat anterior leaflet prolapse with leaflet repair. The most common are chordal transfer, artificial chordae creation, and the Alfieri E2E repair. Chordal transfer is performed by resection of a segment of the posterior leaflet, which is then transferred and sewn to the prolapsing segment of the anterior leaflet. A quadrangular repair of the anterior leaflet completes this procedure. Another method of anterior leaflet repair involves the creation of artificial chordae from Gore-Tex sutures. These artificial chordae are attached to the prolapsing leaflet and the papillary muscle by pledgeted sutures.

The long-term results for mortality, recurrent MR, and reoperation with MVRe in experienced centers are outstanding, are far superior than those for MV replacement, and the mortality rate is similar to that of the general population (86% to 93% survival at 5 years).[47-50] At clinical centers of excellence, such as The Cleveland Clinic, MVRe provides durable results with a 10-year freedom-from-reoperation rate of 93% (Fig. 52.5A) and contemporary rates of in-hospital mortality of well under 0.1% (see Fig. 52.5B).[47,51]

Isolated Leaflet Repair with Edge-to-Edge Technique

Dr. Ottavio Alfieri (Milan, Italy) pioneered a creative repair known as the double-orifice, or E2E, technique. This procedure was initially developed for anterior leaflet prolapse: the free edges of the anterior and the posterior leaflets are sewn together in an attempt to increase leaflet contact and coaptation and reduce regurgitation.[52] This technique also works for repair of posterior leaflet and bileaflet prolapse.[53] The resulting double-orifice MV usually does not cause stenosis, even when combined with an annuloplasty ring.

The first report of this technique was published in 1998.[52] A larger series, published in 2001, consisted of 260 patients who underwent E2E repair, 81% of whom had DMR, and 80% of whom also had an annuloplasty ring placed.[54] There was a low rate of in-hospital mortality (0.7%), and overall survival was good (94% at 5 years), with 95% freedom from reoperation (Fig. 52.6). Most patients (>80%) were NYHA class I or II. A subsequent report comparing patients who did with patients who did not receive concomitant annuloplasty demonstrated worse freedom from significant MR and a higher rate of reoperation in those with isolated E2E repair.[55]

Following Dr. Alfieri's lead, the technique was adopted into practice at many prominent institutions performing MVRe, although usually as a specialized technique and not as a primary method. The introduction of percutaneous E2E repair has fueled interest in the surgical outcomes of this procedure, leading to the publication of a number of single-center case series.[53,54,56-59] The procedure has been applied to both DMR and ischemic MR with favorable results. Although the surgical double-orifice MVRe has been shown to be effective as a treatment for structural or functional MV disease, the surgical literature is limited by a lack of data on isolated E2E repair.[60]

A series of patients with up to 18 years (mean 9.2 years) of follow-up after surgical E2E repair was recently published by Dr. Alfieri's group.[61] Of the 61 patients, 36 did not have concomitant annuloplasty due to heavy annular calcification or limited annular

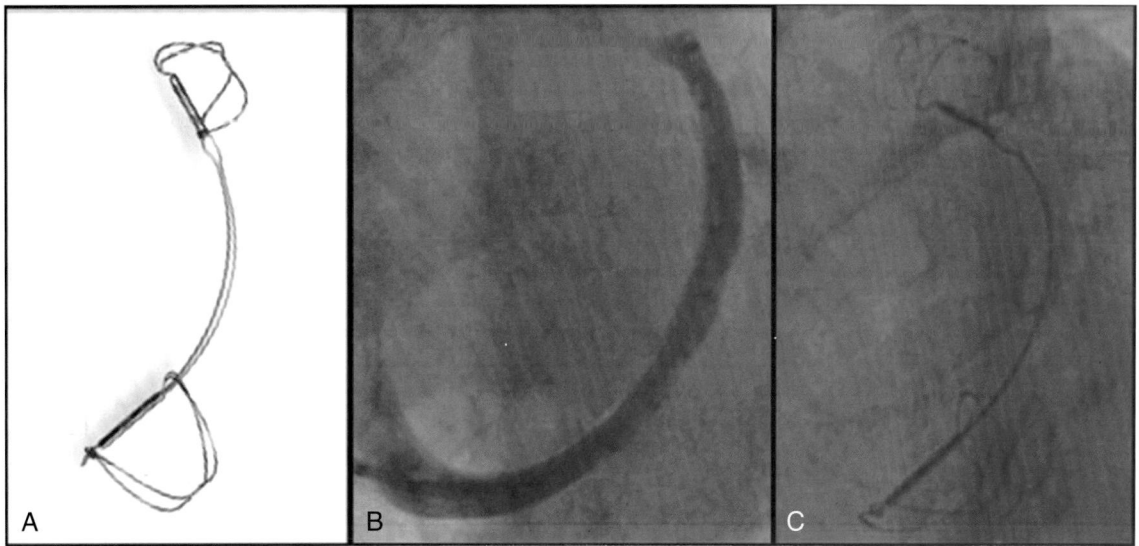

Fig. 52.6 Carillon indirect mitral annuloplasty system. (A) Device with proximal and distal anchors and tensioning band; (B) coronary sinus venography; (C) device in place. (Adapted from Lipiecki J, Siminiak T, Sievert H, et al. Coronary sinus-based percutaneous annuloplasty as treatment for functional mitral regurgitation: the TITAN II trial. *Open Heart*. 2016;3[2]:e000411.)

dilatation. The average age was 64 years, the average LVEF was 60%, and the indications for surgery were bileaflet prolapse/flail (46%), anterior prolapse/flail (18%), and posterior prolapse/flail (36%). Survival at 12 years was 51%, and freedom from reoperation was only 58%. Of these 36 patients, 55% had 3+ or greater MR, and residual MR greater than 1+ at hospital discharge was a significant predictor of severe MR at follow-up (hazard ratio 3.8; 95% confidence interval 1.7 to 8.2; P = .001). Although this was a small series, these results question the long-term benefit of isolated E2E repair in a group of relatively young patients with DMR and may be relevant to the discussion of percutaneous E2E repair in young and otherwise healthy patients.

Percutaneous Mitral Valve Repair

The aim of percutaneous strategies for MVRe is to provide relief from severe MR in patients who would otherwise not be candidates for surgical correction or in those who prefer a less invasive approach without the need for cardiopulmonary bypass. The latter is a more difficult proposition, especially in patients with primary (degenerative) MR, given the historical success and safety of surgical MVRe in treating this problem as detailed previously.

There are currently five major approaches to percutaneous repair. The best-studied approach is the E2E repair, based loosely on the surgical repair championed by Dr. Alfieri. The second approach uses the proximity of the coronary sinus to the mitral annulus to accomplish favorable changes in annular geometry, bringing the posterior leaflet toward the anterior leaflet and thereby improving coaptation. In the third approach, LV reshaping, which accomplishes a reduction in septal-to-lateral diameter and improves leaflet coaptation, can reduce MR. In the fourth approach, called the transventricular (direct) approach, mitral annuloplasty is performed by various methods. Another novel approach involves the implantation of artificial chordae. Finally, recent preclinical and clinical work in transcatheter MV replacement has produced interesting results (Table 52.4).

Edge-to-Edge (Double-Orifice) Leaflet Repair with the MitraClip System

The MitraClip system (Evalve, Menlo Park, CA) is the best-studied of the options for percutaneous MVRe, and results of a randomized trial of its use were reported in 2010.[62] The device uses a 24-Fr steerable delivery guide catheter and a transseptal approach to place a V-shaped clip (MitraClip) on the mitral leaflets, effectively achieving a double-orifice repair similar to the Alfieri stitch (Fig. 52.7).[63] The clip is introduced via the guiding catheter into the LA. The arms of the clip are rotated until they are perpendicular to the line of coaptation of the valve leaflets, most easily accomplished via 3-D TEE guidance. The open clip is advanced into the LV and retracted to grasp the middle scallops of the anterior and posterior valve leaflets in the gripper arms. Positioning is confirmed with TEE, and the clip is locked into position. If needed, the clip can be reopened, detached from the leaflets, and withdrawn into the LA, and the process can be repeated until a satisfactory functional double orifice is created. Care should be taken, especially when manipulating the device near the commissures, not to enter the ventricular cavity too deeply in order to avoid chordal entanglement. When the positioning is considered adequate, the clip is released and remains attached to the MV leaflets. Eventually, fibrosis and scarring occur in the bridging segment, similar to that seen with surgical E2E repair.[64]

MitraClip for Degenerative Mitral Regurgitation

Initial results from 27 patients in the phase I prospective, multicenter safety and feasibility trial called EVEREST I (Endovascular Valve Edge-to-Edge Repair Study I) were published in 2005.[65] The clip was successfully deployed initially in 24 patients (89%), and 3 patients went on to successful surgical repair[6] or replacement.[5]

The pivotal EVEREST II trial randomized 279 patients in a 2:1 fashion, assigning 184 to the MitraClip group and 95 to surgery.[66] Of these subjects, 73% had DMR. One primary end point was a safety end point (major adverse events such as death, stroke, myocardial infarction, reoperation, and transfusion), which was designed to show superiority of the endovascular strategy. At 30 days, the primary safety end point was experienced by 9.6% of the percutaneous group and 57% of the surgical (control) group, although much of this difference was accounted for by the need for transfusion of more than 2 units of blood in the surgical group (53.2%, compared with 8.8% in the percutaneous group). Also notable, however, was the lack of death, major stroke, urgent/

TABLE 52.4 Percutaneous or Minimally Invasive Mitral Valve Repair Devices Under Development

Device	Development Phase	Ongoing Trial and Stage
EDGE-TO-EDGE LEAFLET REPAIR		
MitraClip (Abbott Vascular, Minneapolis, MN)	FDA approval for DMR 2013 FDA approval for FMR 2019 CE Mark approval	No major trials ongoing
INDIRECT ANNULOPLASTY		
CARILLON Mitral Contour System (Cardiac Dimensions, Kirkland, WA)	CE Mark Approval Phase II trials published	*Phase III Trial:* Carillon Pivotal: enrolling (Device vs. Sham + OMT)
DIRECT ANNULOPLASTY		
Mitralign (Mitralign, Salem, NH)	CE Mark Approval	N/A
Cardioband (Edwards Lifesciences, Irvine, CA)	CE Mark Approval Phase II trial published	*Phase III Trial:* ACTIVE: enrolling (Device vs. OMT)
CARDIAC CHAMBER REMODELING		
Accucinch Percutaneous Ventricular Repair System (Ancora Heart, Santa Clara, CA)	First-in-human implants	*Phase II Trial:* Planning underway
ARTO Septal Sinus Shortening System (MVRx Inc, Belmont, CA)	First-in-human implants	N/A
ARTIFICIAL CHORDAE INSERTION		
NeoChord DS1000 (Neochord, Minneapolis, MN)	CE Mark Approval Phase II trial published	N/A
Harpoon MVRS (Edwards Lifesciences, Irvine, CA)	Phase II trial published	
TRANSCATHETER MITRAL VALVE REPLACEMENT		
Tiara (Neovasc, Inc., Richmond, Ontario)	First-in-human implants	N/A
Intrepid (Medtronic Inc., Minneapolis, MN)	Phase II trial published	*Phase III Trial:* APPOLO: enrolling (TMVR vs. SMVR)
Tendyne (Abbott Vascular Santa Clara, CA)	Phase II trial published	*Expanded Phase II Trial:* Expanded Clinical Study of the Tendyne System: enrolling (TMVR registry alone)
CardiAQ (Edwards Lifesciences, Irvine, CA)	First-in-human implants	*Phase II Trial:* CardiAQ Early Feasibility Trial: enrolling (TMVR registry alone)
LivaNova Caisson (LivaNova, Maple Grove, MN)	First-in-human implants	*Phase II Trial:* PRELUDE: enrolling (TMVR registry alone)
SAPIEN M3 (Edwards Lifesciences, Irvine, CA)	First-in-human implants	N/A

ACTIVE, Annular ReduCtion for Transcatheter Treatment of Insufficient Mitral ValvE; *APPOLO,* Transcatheter Mitral Valve Replacement With the Medtronic Intrepid TMVR System in Patients With Severe Symptomatic Mitral Regurgitation; *CE, Conformite Europeenne; COAPT,* Cardiovascular Outcomes Assessment of the MitraClip Percutaneous Therapy for Heart Failure Patients With Functional Mitral Regurgitation; *DMR,* degenerative mitral regurgitation; *FDA,* U.S. Food and Drug Administration; *FMR,* functional mitral regurgitation; *PRELUDE,* Caisson Transcatheter Mitral Valve Replacement (TMVR) System Early Feasibility Study; *SMVR,* surgical mitral valve replacement; *TMVR,* transcatheter mitral valve replacement.

emergent surgery, or MV reoperation in any of the 136 MitraClip patients who achieved acute procedural success.

The second primary end point was for efficacy and was designed to show noninferiority to cardiac surgery with respect to a composite end point of freedom from surgery for valve dysfunction, death, or MR 2+ or worse. Analysis of clinical effectiveness showed the MitraClip to be noninferior to surgery (72.4% vs. 87.8%, with a prespecified margin for noninferiority of 31%). At 4 years' follow-up, Mauri and colleagues demonstrated similar survival (mortality rate, 17.4% vs. 17.8%) and functional improvement, although patients receiving the clip had a much higher need for MV surgery (24.8% vs. 5.5%).[67] The presence of MR of 3+ or 4+ (18.8% vs. 3.0%) was greater with MitraClip at 1 year, although there was no significant difference in worsening MR or need for MV intervention between years 1 and 4. Subgroup analysis demonstrated that patients with FMR may derive greater benefit from the MitraClip (see later discussion).

Given the excellent results of MVRe in patients with DMR who had acceptable surgical risk, interest turned to the use of the MitraClip for those patients at prohibitive surgical risk. The published experience consists of 127 patients in EVEREST II and the high-risk Real-World Expanded Multi-Center Study of the MitraClip System (REALISM) continued access registry.[68] The mean age of the group was 82 years; 48% had prior cardiac surgery; and 86% had NYHA III or IV symptoms. Despite a predicted 30-day mortality rate of 13.2% based on mean Society of Thoracic Surgeons (STS) score, the observed mortality rate was only 6.3%. Mortality at 1 year was 23.6% and was correlated to the degree of residual MR at the time of index hospital discharge. Of the surviving patients, 87% were in NYHA class II or II at 1 year, and 85% had 2+ or less MR.

Given the encouraging safety and efficacy of the MitraClip in extreme surgical risk patients, the U.S. Food and Drug Administration (FDA) in 2013 approved the device for use in patients with DMR who are considered to be at prohibitive risk for surgery. Unfortunately, the group did not approve its use for FMR patients given the predominance of DMR patients enrolled in the U.S.-based clinical trials, despite the fact that the majority of worldwide MitraClip use has been in FMR patients.[69]

The ACC/STS/Transcatheter Valve Therapies registry recently published the initial outcomes of commercial MitraClip implantation in the U.S. among 564 patients with a median STS-predicted risk of

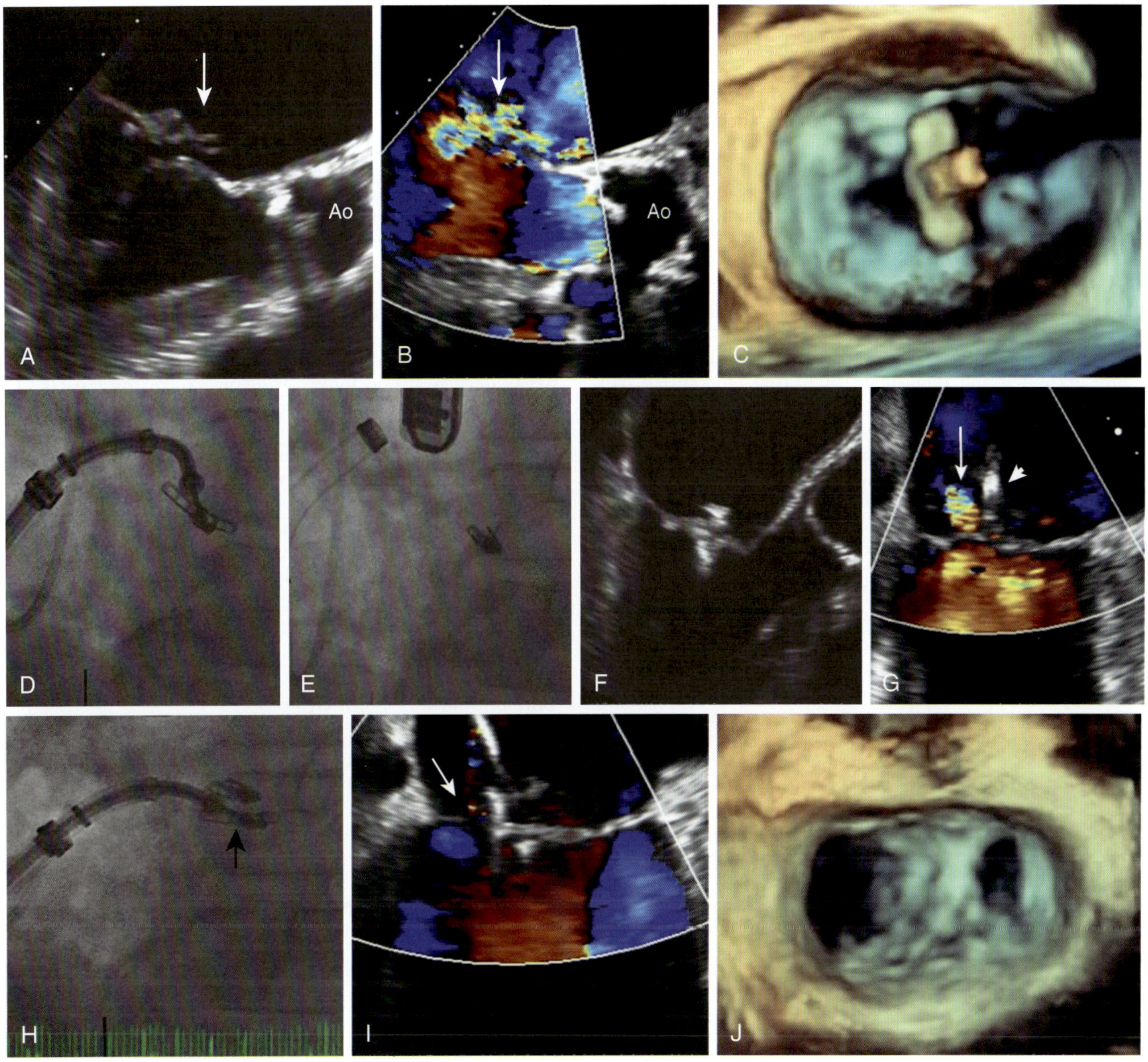

Fig. 52.7 MitraClip repair of posterior leaflet flail. (A) P2 flail *(arrow)* with (B) anteriorly directed mitral regurgitation (MR) *(arrow)*; (C) 3-D transesophageal echocardiography shows the clip in the left atrium perpendicular to the coaptation line; fluoroscopic projections of the clip (D) open in the left ventricle and (E) closed on the valve; (F) clip grasping the mitral valve (MV); (G) moderate residual MR *(arrow)* just medial to the clip *(arrowhead)*; (H) second clip *(arrow)* placed just medial to the first; (I) trivial residual MR *(arrow)*; (J) double-orifice MV after two clips placed. *Ao,* Aorta.

mortality (PROM) of 7.9%.[70] Most patients had either DMR alone (85.5%) or combination DMR/FMR (5.1%), and only a few (9.2%) had FMR, consistent with the U.S. FDA labeled indication. Approximately 97% of patients had successful device implantation, and 93% of patients had ≤2+ MR at discharge. Procedure-related complications were rare, with cardiac perforation seen in 0.7%, stroke in 1.1%, need for open-heart surgery in 0.7%, and single-leaflet device attachment in 1.1%. In this highly comorbid group of patients, in-hospital mortality was relatively low at 2.3%. The report is encouraging with regard to the commercial roll-out of the device as a demonstration of the overall safety and efficacy of the MitraClip device.

MitraClip for Functional Mitral Regurgitation

As mentioned previously, surgery in patients with FMR is generally high risk, has poor durability, and is associated with worse overall survival than in patients with DMR.[71,72] As a result, the major professional societies, including the ACC/AHA, the European Society of Cardiology (ESC), and the International Society for Heart and Lung Transplantation (ISHLT) provide a class IIb indication for MV surgery in patients with FMR. A percutaneous strategy to improve MR and quality of life in these patients would be an important advance and use of the MitraClip for this indication has produced encouraging results.

Among 149 patients with FMR included in the high-risk surgical cohort of EVEREST II and the continued access registry, 63% had prior cardiac surgery and 87% had NYHA class III or IV symptoms.[73] Despite their high-risk profile, these patients demonstrated a low (4.7%) mortality rate at 30 days. At 1 year, 82% had 2+ or less MR, and patients demonstrated significant reduction in LV volumes. The ACCESS-EU trial (A Two-Phase Observational Study of the MitraClip System in Europe) involved 567 high-risk patients, including 393 patients (69%) with FMR; the average Logistic EuroSCORE (predicted mortality according to a logistic regression equation) was 23.[69] Of the patients with FMR, 66% had an LVEF of less than 40%. Despite the high-risk profile, the mortality rate was only 2.8% at 30 days and 17% at 1 year. At 1 year, 78.6% of the FMR patients had 2+ or less MR, and 71% of the entire group had NYHA class I or II symptoms.

The belief that FMR patients fare relatively better with MitraClip than with surgical repair (as opposed to patients with DMR who are able to undergo surgery) is reflected in the enrollment of the contemporary high-risk patient trials and worldwide commercial use. Whereas FMR patients constituted only 26% of the EVEREST I trial, they made up 71% of the EVEREST II/REALISM high-risk cohort and 77% of the ACCESS-EU registry. Furthermore, 67% of the European commercial MitraClip experience has been in patients with FMR.

The landmark Cardiovascular Outcomes Assessment of the MitraClip Percutaneous Therapy for Heart Failure Patients With Functional Mitral Regurgitation (COAPT) trial was recently presented and published.[74] The trial randomized 614 patients with ≥3+ FMR at high or extreme surgical risk to either guideline-directed medical therapy (GDMT) alone (312 patients) or MitraClip plus GDMT (302 patients). Notably, all patients' GDMT regimen was optimized by a heart failure specialist prior to enrollment. Crucial exclusion criteria included LVEF <20% or LV cavity dilation >7.0 cm, significant right-ventricular dysfunction, other significant heart valve disease, and oxygen-dependent lung disease. Important baseline characteristics included an average age of 72 years and STS-PROM 8.2%, LVEF 31%, and 61% of patients with ischemic and 39% of patients with nonischemic cardiomyopathy. The primary safety end point of freedom from all device-related complications at 12 months was achieved in almost 97% of patients, demonstrating excellent safety of the procedure in a highly comorbid group of patients (and similar to that seen in the DMR population). The primary effectiveness end point of annualized rate (up to 24 months) of hospitalizations for heart failure was reduced from 68% in the control group to 36% in the device group ($P < .001$). At 12 months, 95% of patients had ≤2+ MR. Impressively, and not previously seen in any FMR correction trial, there was a 38% relative-risk reduction in all-cause mortality at 2 years with the MitraClip (29.1 vs. 46.1%, $P < .001$). To put these findings in perspective, the number needed to treat to prevent one hospitalization was three patients, and to prevent one death was six. Overall, COAPT is an important step forward in demonstrating the safety and efficacy of this treatment strategy for appropriately selected FMR patients. While this indication for MitraClip is not currently approved by the U.S. FDA, there is tremendous hope that the trial will provide the impetus for such an extension.

It bears mention that in the month prior to presentation of the COAPT results, the Percutaneous Repair with the MitraClip Device for Severe Functional/Secondary Mitral Regurgitation (MITRA-FR) was presented and published.[75] The trial randomized 304 patients with FMR in a 1:1 fashion to medical therapy or MitraClip. At 1 year, there was no difference in death or hospitalization between the two strategies. There are a number of explanations for this difference in comparison to COAPT with regard to trial methodology, procedural results, and follow-up. In MITRA-FR, patients were included with ≥2+ FMR, while COAPT included only ≥3+ regurgitation. Further, COAPT excluded patients with very severe LV dilation (>7.0 cm), though this was not an exclusion to MITRA-FR. Medical therapy at trial enrollment was highly standardized in COAPT with few changes during follow-up, which was not the case in MITRA-FR. Patients available for echocardiography follow-up at 12 months in the MITRA-FR trial was limited, and of those available, 17% had ≥3+ and 50% had ≥2+ FMR (in comparison to 5% and 31% of patients in COAPT, respectively). Finally, with regard to the mortality benefit seen in COAPT, this was noted only beyond 1-year follow-up (there was no difference at 1 year); as such, the 1-year follow-up presented in MITRA-FR (along with half the sample size) may be limited to discern a treatment benefit.

ANNULOPLASTY-BASED MITRAL VALVE REPAIR

Annuloplasty is an integral part of MVRe in most surgical approaches to improving MV leaflet coaptation and reducing MR, and it usually achieves a reduction in mitral annulus diameter of 25% or more. The coronary sinus covers about 50% of the mitral annulus perimeter and 80% of the posterior intertrigonal distance.[76] Indirect annuloplasty uses the anatomic proximity of the coronary sinus to the mitral annulus to modulate annular size and shape. However, there are several challenges to exploiting this relationship. The proximity and location of the coronary sinus to the annulus is variable (see Fig. 52.4).[77] Furthermore, the left circumflex artery crosses between the myocardium and the coronary sinus in almost 50% of patients, increasing the risk of arterial compromise.[76,77] Due to marginal results and financial difficulties, most of the indirect annuloplasty devices are no longer available except the CARILLON Mitral Contour System developed by Cardiac Dimensions (Kirkland, WA). Other approaches include direct annuloplasty, radiofrequency or ultrasound energy delivery to shrink the annulus, and "cinching" devices to remodel the annulus. These are all in various phases of development and clinic use. Proper definition of the anatomic relationships with various imaging techniques, including cardiac CT, angiography, and echocardiography, may be helpful in matching the appropriate approach to the anatomy.

Indirect Annuloplasty
Carillon Mitral Contour System

The CARILLON Mitral Contour System is a fixed-length, double-anchor device (see Fig. 52.6) that is advanced through a catheter and positioned in the coronary sinus. After the device is deployed and locked into position, tension is applied to the anchors of the device, resulting in tissue plication that reduces the MV annular diameter and MR. The procedure is performed percutaneously with internal jugular vein access followed by distal coronary sinus cannulation with a 9-Fr catheter. A measuring catheter is used to determine the optimal positioning of the distal anchor in the coronary sinus. The nitinol annuloplasty device is advanced down the catheter to the target position in the coronary sinus. The distal anchor of the device is deployed by passive expansion and is locked into the fully expanded position by use of the delivery catheter. Tension is placed on the delivery system, bringing the proximal anchor toward the coronary sinus ostium. The amount of tension can be manipulated as needed to optimize reduction in annular dimension (approximately 25%) and reduction in MR, which is verified by real-time echocardiography. If the device position is considered to be optimal, the proximal anchor is deployed and locked into position in a similar fashion. If there is a concern about safety or efficacy, the device can be recaptured by advancing the delivery catheter over the device to collapse the anchors, and the apparatus can be adjusted or removed as necessary.

Clinical feasibility was first evaluated in the prospective, nonrandomized CARILLON Mitral Annuloplasty Device European Union Study (AMADEUS) trial using the next-generation CARILLON XE device in 48 patients with FMR and LV systolic dysfunction.[78] The device was successfully implanted in 30 patients. At the 6-month follow-up, there was a durable and significant decrease in mitral annulus diameter (from 4.2 to 3.78 cm [10%]), MR (average reduction, 23%), and NYHA class (from 2.9 to 1.8), as well as improvement in the quality-of-life score and 6-minute walk test (6MWT) (from 307 to 403 meters). Of the remaining 18 patients, five did not receive implantation because of coronary sinus-related complications ($n = 3$) or fluoroscopic equipment failure ($n = 2$), and 13 patients had retrieval of the device after implantation because of inadequate MR reduction or coronary compromise. With respect to safety, six patients (13%) experienced a total of seven complications within 30 days of the procedure: one patient died of multiorgan failure, three experienced myocardial infarction (none requiring percutaneous coronary intervention), and three experienced coronary sinus dissection or perforation. The complications were clustered early in the experience and resulted in changes to the implantation procedure; improvement in safety was observed later in the study. On the basis of this early work, the CARILLON system was granted the CE mark of approval for use in Europe.

Improvements to the device were evaluated in the follow-up Tighten the Annulus Now (TITAN) study, which enrolled a total of 53 patients. The 36 patients in whom implantation was successful were compared with the 17 patients in whom the device was retrieved. Patients were relatively young (mean age, 62 years) with a mean LVEF of 28% and NYHA class III symptoms. Mortality was 1.9% at 30 days and 22.6% at 12 months, without a substantial difference between those who did and did not receive an implant. There was an average 50% reduction in regurgitant volume in the implanted patients, compared with a relatively stable volume in nonimplanted patients. LV systolic and diastolic volumes were significantly decreased in the implanted patients, whereas those nonimplanted demonstrated increase in volumes. Reduction in NYHA class from III to II was sustained in the implanted group out to 2 years.[79]

In the follow-up TITAN II trial, 36 patients with average age 70 years and average LVEF 34% were enrolled to the newest generation CARILLON mXE2 device (which was modified based on device fractures in TITAN). Of these, 30 had successful implantation, with the other 6 patients having uncomplicated device retrieval due to coronary compromise. The one implanted patient who died (2.8%) within 30 days died at day 17 during treatment for acute cholecystitis (and without evidence of arrhythmia on defibrillator interrogation). Results were effective and durable, with 1-year improvement in 6MWT from 284 to 381 meters and 75% of patients with 2+ MR. There was no change in the 15% reduction achieved in mitral annular dimension seen acutely over 1 year (see Fig. 52.6).

The most recent data regarding the CARILLON system is eagerly anticipated from the randomized REDUCE-FMR trial that completed enrollment in June 2017. The 120 patients had LV systolic dysfunction and significant FMR and were randomized in a 3:1 fashion to device versus medical management alone. Similarly, the CARILLON trial beginning enrollment in the United States and Europe will be the largest and pivotal randomized trial with plans to enroll 400 patients at 50 centers in a 2:1 fashion (ClinicalTrials.Gov NCT03142152). The study design is unique, as even those patients randomized to medicines alone will still undergo a sham procedure as control.

Direct Annuloplasty

Mitralign Direct Annuloplasty System

Based on the concept of direct suture annuloplasty, the Mitralign Direct Annuloplasty System (Mitralign, Tewksbury, MA) uses a device composed of three metal anchors connected by standard suture material. The anchors are placed in the mitral annulus, and the suture is cinched to perform the annuloplasty. The device is placed via retrograde ventricular access with the use of a unique translation catheter with a two-pronged "bi-dent" design for device delivery. The initial design used a magnetic guiding catheter placed in the coronary sinus, but in the most recent iteration, the anchors are placed from the ventricular side using standard imaging techniques. The two anchors are positioned below the valve at the level of each posterior leaflet scallop and then deployed directly through the mitral annulus; they

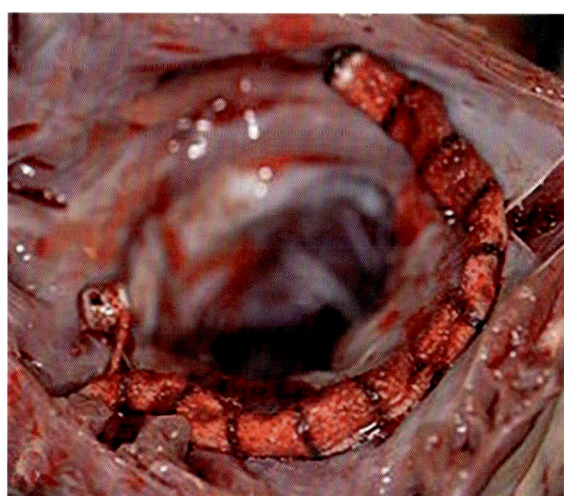

Fig. 52.8 Cardioband direct annuloplasty system (Edwards Lifesciences, Irvine, CA) in place in the posterior mitral annulus. (Modified from Taramasso M, Maisano F. Transcatheter mitral valve repair: transcatheter mitral valve annuloplasty. *EuroIntervention.* 2014;10:U129–U135.)

remain connected by suture material. The suture is then cinched, directly plicating the annulus and emulating the results of a surgical, suture-based annuloplasty.

Successful implantation in one patient in South America and two patients in Europe was reported in 2008 as part of the pilot clinical study. Nickenig and colleagues recently presented the largest experience using the Mitralign system.[80] In the feasibility study of 71 patients, 50 (70%) had implantation of at least one pledget. Thirty-day follow-up data were presented for 45 patients (63% of the initial intention to treat [ITT] cohort) and 6-month clinical follow-up was presented for 30 patients (42% of ITT). In this limited group of patients with follow-up, there were significant reductions in LV systolic and diastolic volumes out to 6 months. Among the treated patients, there was a reduction of 1.3 MR grades (on average) among 50% of the patients. Functionally, 23/30 patients had NYHA I-II symptoms at 6 months (in comparison to 14/30 patients at baseline) and 6MWT was increased by almost 60 m. The device has obtained CE Mark, and another iteration of the device has been applied to the tricuspid valve as the "Trialign" device.

Edwards Cardioband Annuloplasty System

The Edwards Cardioband Annuloplasty System, purchased from Valtech Cardio (Or-Yehuda, Israel) is implanted via a transseptal route. The device consists of a Dacron band that is implanted from trigone to trigone using multiple anchors (Fig. 52.8). The length of the band is then shortened under echocardiography guidance to provide optimal leaflet coaptation. Initial results of the procedure in 24 patients with FMR are encouraging.[81] There was an average 20% reduction in annular dimension, and 85% of patients had 1+ or less MR at hospital discharge. At 6 months, 88% had NYHA I or II symptoms, and 88% had MR 2+ or less.

The Edwards Cardioband Mitral CE Mark Trial has completed enrollment, and while results have not yet been published, they were recently presented.[82] Of 62 patients in the ITT group, 1 was implanted with compassionate use and 1 was not implanted due to patient instability. Of the 60 patients treated per-protocol, ≤2+ MR was seen in 91% at 30 days and 94% at 12 months. This reduction in MR was accomplished with a substantial reduction in SL diameter from 37 to 26 mm. Importantly, there was a sustained clinical benefit seen at 12 months with improvement in 6MWT from 308 to 372 feet and improvement in NYHA class from III or IV at baseline in >80% to class I or II in 79% at 12 months. With regard to adverse events, there were 16 among 9 patients and included death (2), pericardial effusion (2), stroke (1), cardiac surgery (1), and MR recurrence due to partial anchor detachment (2) among others.

The Annular Reduction for Transcatheter Treatment of Insufficient Mitral Valve (ACTIVE) trial is a prospective, randomized trial currently enrolling patients with FMR to either device or medical therapy alone. Importantly, the co-primary end point will include a hierarchical comparison of heart failure hospitalizations and functional capacity in addition to mortality.

Cardiac Chamber Remodeling Devices

FMR caused by dilatated cardiomyopathy and ischemic MR caused by geometric alterations affect not only the mitral annulus but also the LA and the LV and their relationships to the annulus. One potential limitation of the typical ring annuloplasty is that it does not address these alterations in paravalvular geometry. Devices have therefore been engineered with this consideration in mind. However, financial hardship has led to abandonment of the Coapsys device, and the PS3 and BACE devices have been demonstrated only in limited use. They are included here for historical reference.

AccuCinch Percutaneous Ventricular Repair System

The AccuCinch Percutaneous Ventricular Repair system (Ancora Heart, Santa Clara, CA) provides a catheter-based, retrograde transventricular approach to place anchors in the myocardium approximately 10 to 20 mm apical to the MV. The aim is to reduce the LV radius and thereby reduce MV tenting and resultant FMR. A total of 49 patients have been implanted, and most recently results were reported of 18 patients implanted in Europe and the United States during 2016 to 2017 using the latest device iteration.[83] The patients had an average LVEF of 28% with an average left ventricular internal diameters (LVIDs) of 5.5 cm and 94% had 3 or 4+ MR. A total of 16 patients had successful device implantation, 1 patient suffered fatal cardiac arrest prior to deployment, and 1 patient could not be implanted due to anatomic constraints and was discharged home uneventfully. Thirty-day safety was reasonable; in addition to the one death during the procedure, one patient died at day 10 due to renal failure, one died at day 14 due to pneumonia, and two patients experienced access-site complications. Granular data on clinical and echocardiographic outcomes is not available. The Safety and Performance Evaluation of the AccuCinch Ventriculoplasty System for Functional Mitral Regurgitation Due to Dilated Ischemic or Non-Ischemic Cardiomyopathy Trial, an international nonrandomized trial of the device, is anticipated but not yet enrolling at the time of this writing (ClinicalTrials.Gov NCT03183895).

ARTO Septal Sinus Shortening System

The ARTO System (MVRx Inc, Belmont, CA), previously known as the Percutaneous Septal Sinus Shortening (PS3) system (Ample Medical, Foster City, CA) differs from the Coapsys system in that it creates a transatrial bridge rather than a transventricular bridge. This device uses the coronary sinus and a septal closure device to place a cord across the atrium, create tension on the annulus, and remodel the mitral annulus and the LA. SL annular cinching occurs because of traction applied between the interatrial septum and the coronary sinus at the level of the P2 mitral segment.

Palacios and colleagues published the first human use of the PS3 in two patients with FMR. Both patients received implants before planned open-heart surgery (at which time the device was removed). The results were encouraging, with a reduction in MR grade from 2 to 1 in one patient and from 3 to 1 in the other. There was a substantial reduction in mitral annulus diameter (31% in one patient and 29% in the other), comparable to that achieved with surgical annuloplasty and greater than that achieved by other percutaneous coronary sinus-based indirect annuloplasty devices.

The Mitral Valve Repair Clinical Trial (MAVERIC) was published in 2015 and involved 11 patients with an average LVEF of 38% and were all treated at a single center. Postprocedure, 10 patients had 2+ or less MR and 1 patient had 3+ MR; at 30 days, 2 patients had 3+ MR. There were no adverse events within 3 days (death, stroke, etc.), although 1 patient was found to have cardiac tamponade after day 3 and 1 patient required mitral valve surgery at day 65 after asymptomatic T-bar dislodgement was noted at day 35. Further clinical investigation at international centers is underway.

Coapsys and iCoapsys

The Coapsys (Myocor, Maple Grove, MN) annuloplasty system involves the surgical placement of pericardial implants off pump. These implants are placed on the epicardial surface of the heart, with a tethering subvalvular cord that crosses the ventricle internally. This cord is then cinched to decrease the mitral annulus diameter and eliminate MR. Advantages of the Coapsys system include the ability to treat FMR off pump, which allows the combination of off-pump bypass and MVRe. Conceptually, the device provides a more comprehensive mechanism of action by preserving normal valve dynamics and addressing the mitral annulus as well as the subvalvular space and abnormal LV geometry.

In the initial clinical feasibility trial, the device was successfully implanted in 34 patients with FMR at the time of bypass surgery. Data on the first 11 patients completing 1-year follow-up confirmed the durability of MR decrease (grade, from 2.9 to 1.1; jet area, from 7.4 cm^2 to 3.0 cm^2) and NYHA class improvement (from 2.5 to 1.2) at 12 months.[69] A U.S. randomized trial (Randomized Evaluation of a Surgical Treatment for Off-Pump Repair of the Mitral Valve [RESTORE-MV]) enrolled patients with coronary artery disease and ischemic MR, comparing traditional open-heart coronary artery bypass grafting (CABG) with MVRe to CABG with Coapsys device placement. Intraoperative results from this trial were reported for the first 19 patients receiving the implant and showed a reduction in MR grade, from 2.7 ± 0.8 to 0.4 ± 0.7, after implantation ($P < .0001$).[76] Because of funding issues, the trial was prematurely terminated after randomization of 165 patients (77 treated with MVRe and 87 with Coapsys); the results of this trial have not yet been published.

A percutaneous version of the system, the iCoapsys, is implanted through a pericardial access sheath. The ingeniously designed device was tried in two patients, but the Valvular and Ventricular Improvement Via iCoapsys Delivery (VIVID) trial of clinical feasibility was prematurely discontinued because of financial constraints.[77]

Basal Annuloplasty of the Cardia Externally

The Basal Annuloplasty of the Cardia Externally (BACE) device (Mardil, Plymouth, MN) is a silicone band that is slipped around the base of the heart and positioned at the atrioventricular groove to "cinch" the annular and subvalvular LV and provide improved MV coaptation.[84] The device is sutured to the myocardium, and chambers in the band are filled with saline to provide the appropriate level of LV support. A report of the first 11 patients treated at four centers in India was recently published.[85] Patients were 56 years of age on average and had a mean LVEF of 31%. All patients were planned for CABG and had at least moderate FMR.

The degree of MR was reduced to trivial or less in all patients, with a durable result on 3-month echocardiography. The device was placed without issue in all patients, though 1 patient returned to the operating room due to bleeding unrelated to the BACE device, and 1 patient died ultimately of complications related to lower extremity ischemia after balloon pump placement which was performed 12 hours postoperatively. Further trials of the device are not currently ongoing.

Artificial Chord Implantation

NeoChord DS1000 System

The NeoChord DS1000 system (NeoChord, Minneapolis, MN) allows transapical implantation of chordae on a beating heart without the need for cardiopulmonary bypass. The Transapical Artificial Chordae Tendineae (TACT) trial was a prospective study in 30 patients at seven centers.[86] Patients on average were 64 years of age with an LVEF of 59%, and all had severe MR due to isolated posterior leaflet prolapse. Six patients underwent conversion to standard MVRe: four suffered early chord dehiscence and two did not demonstrate acute procedure success and required standard MVRe. Acute procedural success was defined as reduction of MR to 2+ or less and was achieved in 26 patients (86.7%); four patients did not have NeoChords placed and underwent standard MVRe. One patient died as a result of sepsis. At 30-day follow-up, 17 (58.6%) of 29 patients continued with 2+ or less MR. Although these results are not as good as those of traditional MVRe, the less invasive nature of this procedure demonstrates an interesting option for these patients. The device received CE Mark approval in 2012, and more than 500 patients have been implanted thus far.

Harpoon Mitral Valve Repair System

The Harpoon Mitral Valve Repair System (MVRS) (Edwards Lifesciences, Irvine, CA) allows implantation of expanded polytetrafluoroethylene (ePTFE) cords on the beating heart via a small left thoracotomy and into the free leaflet edge of the prolapsing segment of the MV. Once the length of the cord is adjusted (using TEE guidance), the cord is secured to the epicardial surface using a pledget. The TRACER (mitral transapical neochordal echo-guided repair) trial was recently published and included 30 patients with normal LVEF and posterior leaflet prolapse; patients with anterior leaflet pathology or FMR were excluded.[87] Two patients were converted to conventional cardiac surgery during the case, and 1 patient had surgery at day 27 due to endocarditis. There was no perioperative mortality or stroke. At the end of the procedure, 86% of patients had none/trace MR and 14% had mild MR. At 6 months, only 54% had none/trace MR, 31% had mild MR, 8% had moderate MR, and 8% had severe MR. While the authors comment that the procedure took less than half the time of conventional MV repair, and that outside of large centers MV repair is not as frequent or effective, it is difficult to ignore the mid-term MR recurrence in comparison to other DMR-specific procedures such as conventional surgical MVRe and MitraClip.

TRANSCATHETER MITRAL VALVE IMPLANTATION

Whereas transcatheter aortic valve implantation has made significant progress, and thousands of successful implantations have been performed, transcatheter mitral valve implantation is currently in its infancy. Challenges to transcatheter mitral valve replacement (TMVR) include the lack of a rigid/calcified annulus (unlike the diseased aortic annulus), an irregular and saddle-shaped annulus that is dynamic during the cardiac cycle, as well as the larger size of the MV annulus that requires larger devices and therefore larger sheaths. Many of these challenges, such as sheath/device size and resultant catheter manipulation in the left atrium, present even greater difficulty for implantation via the transfemoral/septal route than the apical route. Nevertheless, a number of valves are in preclinical or early clinical use and data have been published or presented at major meetings.

Transcatheter Mitral Valve Devices

Tendyne Valve

The Tendyne valve (Tendyne Holdings, LLC; subsidiary of Abbott Vascular, Roseville, MN) is a transapically delivered self-expanding prosthesis that consists of porcine pericardial leaflets (Fig. 52.9). As a unique design feature, the valve is secured in place via a tether that is attached to a "pad" on the epicardial surface (via the transapical puncture). Early results (30 days) of the feasibility trial were published in 2017 and consisted of 30 patients (28 with successful implantation, 93.3%) with an average age of 75 years, average STS-PROM 7.3%, and average LVEF 47% (though almost 50% of patients with an LVEF 30% to 50%).[88] Almost all patients had either FMR (80%) or mixed FMR/DMR (10%). Of the two patients who were not successfully implanted, one was removed due to significant LV outflow tract (LVOT) obstruction and one was removed due to a lack of coaxiality from the LV apical puncture to the MV annulus that did not allow proper valve seating. Of the 28 implants, all patients had grade 0 residual MR except for one patient who had mild paravalvular MR due to valve malpositioning that was not recognized until after full release and apical access site closure. Other important 30-day results included one mortality (at day 13 due to pneumonia), no strokes, and no need for cardiac surgery. One-year results were presented and show continued durability of MR reduction (one patient with grade 1 MR), functional capacity change (95% with NYHA class I or II symptoms), and improvement in Kansas City Cardiomyopathy Questionnaire (KCCQ) score.[89]

The most recent data was presented for 90 patients implanted at 24 sites worldwide. The device was successfully placed in 87 patients (97%) with no procedural deaths and 30-day mortality of 5.5%.[90] One patient suffered a stroke within 30 days and no patients underwent cardiac surgery. Of the 57 patients with echocardiography data available at 1 month, 56 had no MR and 1 had mild MR.

Medtronic Intrepid Valve

The Intrepid TMVR system (Medtronic Inc., Redwood City, CA) is also a self-expanding, transapically delivered prosthetic that consists of a Nitinol frame and a trileaflet bovine pericardial valve. The recently published feasibility trial consisted of 50 patients with an average age of 73 years, average LVEF of 43%, and most had either FMR (72%) or combination MR (12%).[91] One patient did not have valve implantation due to excessive apical site bleeding, though implantation was successful in 48 of the remaining 49 patients (98%). There were seven deaths within 30 days (14%), three due to apical-site bleeding, one due to device malpositioning, and three due to refractory heart failure. A total of five patients (10%) underwent early reoperation due to apical site bleeding and two patients suffered a stroke (4%). At a median of 173 days, 74% of patients had no MR and 26% had mild MR, and 79% had NYHA class I or II symptoms. The Transcatheter Mitral Valve Replacement With the Medtronic Intrepid TMVR System in Patients With Severe Symptomatic Mitral Regurgitation (APOLLO, ClinicalTrials.Gov NCT03242642) is currently ongoing with plans to enroll 1380 patients in a 1:1 fashion to Intrepid TMVR versus conventional surgery.

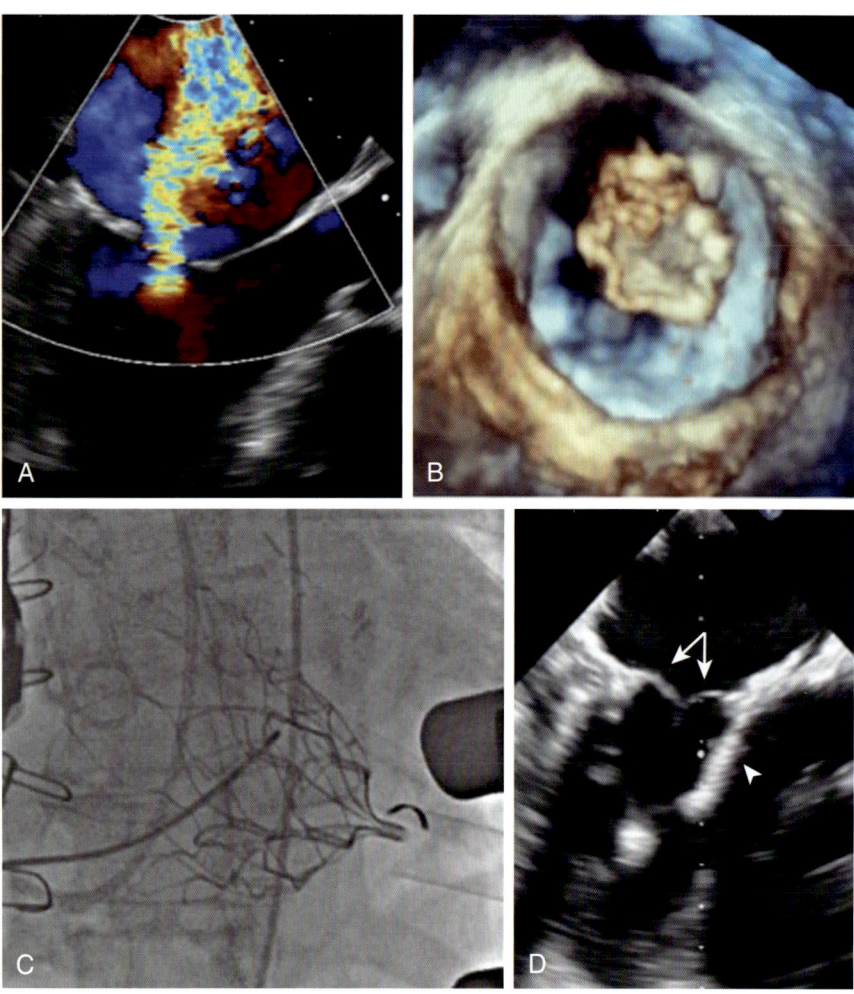

Fig. 52.9 Tendyne transcatheter mitral valve replacement (Abbott Vascular, Santa Clara, CA) to treat functional mitral regurgitation (FMR). (A) Transesophageal echocardiography (TEE) demonstrates severe FMR; (B) 3-D TEE demonstrates initial unsheathing of the valve in the left atrium; (C) fluoroscopy of the valve fully unsheathed; (D) final TEE demonstrates the valve frame (arrowhead) and leaflets (arrows).

Edwards CardiAQ

First developed as an apically or femorally delivered self-expanding valve, the ongoing CardiAQ-Edwards TMVR Early Feasibility Study (ClinicalTrials.Gov NCT02718001) using the most recent device iteration is focused on transfemoral delivery alone. The initial compassionate use experience included 13 patients, 12 of whom had a successful procedure.[92] Unfortunately, there was a 54% 30-day mortality, demonstrating the highly comorbid nature of the patients and thereby providing little insight more than early procedural experience. More recently, a cursory presentation of results demonstrated an 8% 30-day mortality among 26 patients who received the device, showing the substantial improvements that have been achieved with operator experience and device modifications.[93]

Edwards SAPIEN M3

Limited but encouraging experience was recently presented using the transfemoral SAPIEN M3 system (Edwards Lifesciences, Irvine, CA) that consists of a "dock" that is first delivered to the subvalvular apparatus followed by delivery of the valve that shares the tissue and frame of the SAPIEN-3 transcatheter aortic valve prosthesis.[94] The first 10 patients were treated at five centers and had an average age of 74 years and LVEF of 38%. There was no procedural death and there was one procedural stroke. Of the 10 patients, 8 had none or trace residual MR at 30 days, 1 had mild MR, and 1 (the first patient treated) had severe MR at 30 days that was subsequently treated with paravalvular leak closure (and reduced the MR to 2+).

LivaNova Caisson Transcatheter Mitral Valve Replacement

The LivaNova Caisson valve (LivaNova, Maple Grove, MN) is a unique, transfemorally delivered device that consists of two separate structures. First, an "anchor" is delivered to the MV annulus to hold back the native leaflets and provide a foundation for the second step of valve implantation. Recently, the results of 15 patients implanted were presented.[95] Among the group, 57% had FMR and 24% had mixed disease. Procedural success was achieved in 12 patients (80%), and none of these patients had moderate MR. Thirty-day mortality was experienced by 2 of the 12 patients (17%) and the longest valve follow-up was seen at 480 days. The PRELUDE (Caisson TMVR System Early Feasibility Study) study of the Caisson valve is currently recruiting (ClinicalTrials.Gov NCT02768402).

Tiara Valve

The Tiara valve (Neovasc, Richmond, Ontario, Canada) is a transapically implanted, self-expanding valve constructed of a metal alloy frame and bovine pericardial leaflets. It is implanted via a transapical approach. Initial animal studies demonstrated successful implantation in 29 of 36 swine without any migration or embolization.[96] Subsequent implantation was performed in seven cows that were monitored for 150 days. Six of these animals had mild or moderate paravalvular leak over the

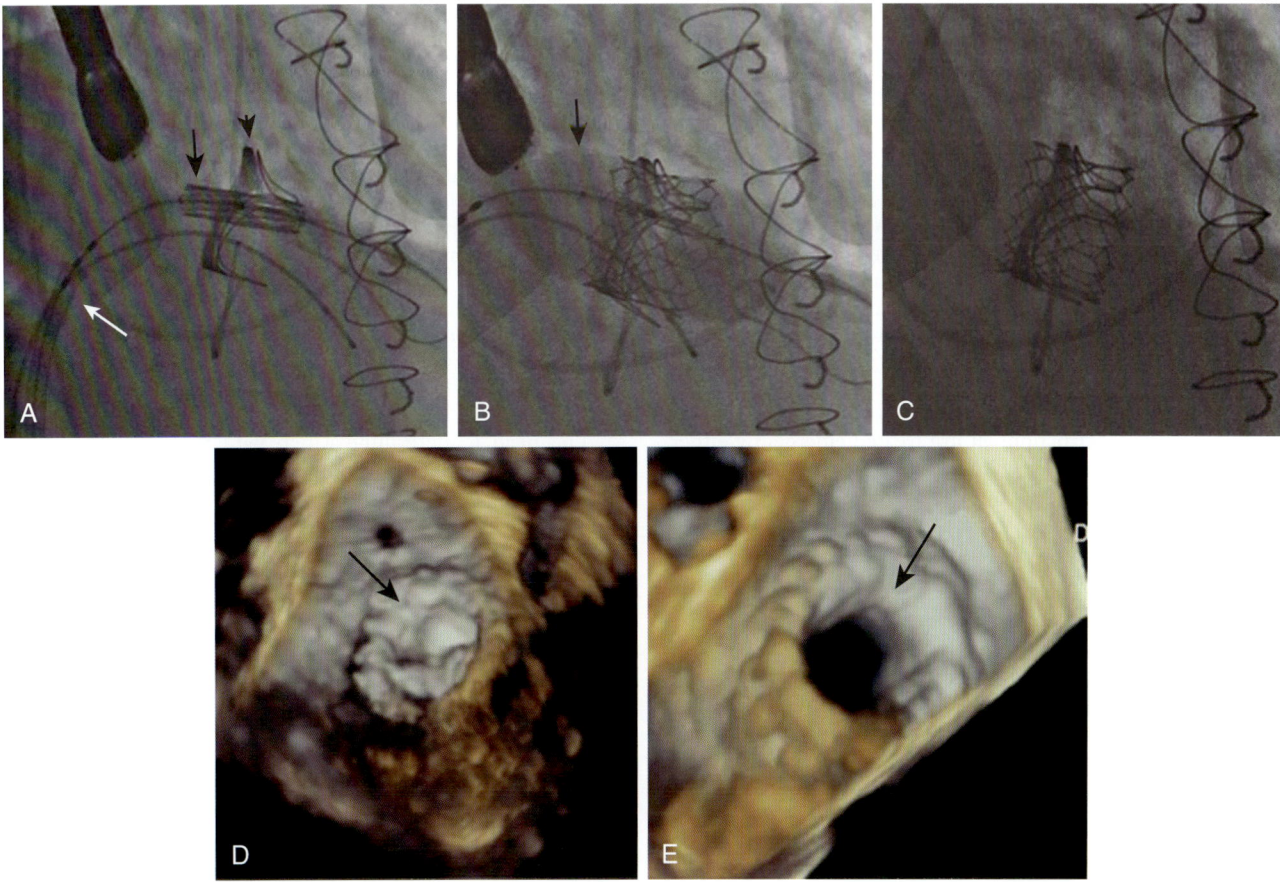

Fig. 52.10 Transfemoral mitral valve-in-valve replacement for a degenerated surgical prosthetic. (A) Catheter via femoral vein *(white arrow)* and crossing the interatrial septum with unexpanded valve in place *(black arrow)* within the mitral prosthesis *(arrowhead)*; (B) balloon inflation of the transcatheter aortic valve replacement prosthesis *(black arrow)*; (C) fully expanded valve in place; (D) 3-D transesophageal echocardiographic view from the left atrium of the stenosed mitral valve *(arrow)*; (E) mitral valve open *(arrow)* after valve-in-valve placement. (From Krishnaswamy A, Mick S, Navia J, et al. Transcatheter mitral valve replacement: a new frontier in interventional cardiology. *Cleve Clin J Med*. 2016;83:S10–S17.)

follow-up period, perhaps due to size mismatch in the setting of only one available prosthesis size. Two patients underwent implantation in early 2014; both were not candidates for surgery because of their severe FMR with an LVEF of 20% to 30%. The procedures were performed without complication. One patient had trivial paravalvular leak and a well-functioning valve but died 69 days later due to progressive cardiac and renal failure. The other patient had no paravalvular leak at follow-up and was alive at 5 months with NYHA class II symptoms.

Surgical Bioprosthetic Valve or Valve Ring Failure

With an aging population and limited durability of surgical mitral valve bioprostheses, there has been substantial interest in catheter-based valve-in-valve (ViV) and valve-in-ring (ViR) implantation to avoid reoperation in a group of patients who are often elderly and comorbid. Clinical experience has included transapical, transfemoral, and direct atrial approaches to implantation of a number of different TAVR prosthetics, though the largest experience has been using the SAPIEN series of valves (Fig. 52.10).[97]

While somewhat dated, the Valve-in-Valve International Data (VIVID) registry provides the largest single published experience of mitral ViV and ViR and included 349 patients who underwent ViV placement and 88 patients who underwent ViR procedures. On average, the patients were 74 years of age with a mean STS score of 12.9% among both groups.[98] Reflecting the fact that the registry was an early experience, most patients had transapical implantation. The procedures were performed with a low rate of stroke (2.9% for ViV, 1.1% for ViR), though the rate of moderate or greater residual MR was significantly higher in patients undergoing ViR procedures (14.8% vs. 2.6%, $P < .001$). Importantly, the risk of LVOT obstruction was substantially higher in the ViR group (8% vs. 2.6%), and highlights the significance of understanding the orientation of the MV prosthesis to the LVOT and the concept of the "neo LVOT."[99] There was a trend toward worse 30-day mortality in the ViR group (11.4% vs. 7.7%, $P = .15$), and small surgical mitral valves (≤25 mm) were associated with higher postprocedural gradients.

In the contemporary era, operators are shifting toward transfemoral/transseptal delivery, given the less invasive nature of this approach and the ability to perform the procedure under conscious sedation (see Fig. 52.10). In a recent series of transfemoral procedures (33 ViV and 9 ViR), there were 31 successful implantations in the ViV group with 2 intraprocedural deaths due to LV perforation. Of the 9 ViR patients, 2 had acute embolization of the valve and were converted to open surgery. Among the seven successfully implanted patients, two developed significant LVOT obstruction; one was treated with surgical resection of the anterior MV leaflet and the other was medically managed.

Degenerative Mitral Stenosis

While outside the scope of this chapter, the use of TAVR prosthetic placement in native mitral annular calcium (MAC) of patients with severe degenerative mitral stenosis (MS) bears mention. As these patients often have no hope for surgery given the high-risk nature of the operation, usually in the setting of concomitant severe pulmonary hypertension, catheter-based alternatives are being actively pursued. The TMVR in MAC global registry consisted of 64 patients with an average age of 73 years and mean STS score of 14%. The transapical route was chosen in 45%, direct atrial in 14%, and transseptal in 41%. Technical success was achieved in 72%, with conversion to open-heart surgery in 6% due to valve embolization (2), LVOT obstruction (1), or LV perforation (1). A second valve was necessary in 17% of procedures. Of note, six patients (9.3%) experienced hemodynamically significant LVOT obstruction; all five treated emergently either surgically or percutaneously, and the one who was stable enough to treat subsequently with alcohol septal ablation, survived. At 30 days, mortality was 29.7%, with 12.5% due to cardiac causes and 17.2% due to noncardiac causes. In a more granular analysis of patients from the registry presented, of 104 patients divided into roughly equal 1/3 groups, in comparison to the first third, the last third of patients enjoyed greater technical success (80% vs. 62.5%), better 30-day survival (85% vs. 68.5%), and no conversion to open surgery (0% vs. 12.5%).[100] These improved outcomes likely reflect improved patient selection with regard to comorbidities and LVOT anatomy along with lessons learned from shared experience. While TMVR in MAC is not commercially approved, multiple registries are currently underway to study outcomes for this group of patients without a good alternative.

Patient Selection

Indications for percutaneous intervention for MR remain similar to those for surgical intervention.[34] Although there has been some interest in lowering the threshold for the severity of MR for percutaneous therapies, with the contention that these treatments are less invasive and safer, there are no data to implement such liberalization. The major excitement in the field is derived from the ability to provide options for patients with higher surgical risk who are symptomatic with severe MR and who do not have any other options. The surgical risk assessment should take into consideration not just the estimated mortality but also the morbidity and the risk of compromising quality of life. With this in mind, the most common target for these therapies, at least initially, are older patients (irrespective of the etiology of MR) with poor LV function and patients with severe FMR, as identified in the Euro Survey, who are not undergoing surgical intervention. It is difficult to justify the use of these techniques in young patients with degenerative MV disease who are otherwise appropriate candidates for surgical MVRe. However, the fact that some of these therapies usually do not impair future surgical options is encouraging.

In many ways, percutaneous MV therapies fit the mold of "personalized medicine," which has been cast in the world of pharmacotherapy. Identifying the mechanisms of MR and then defining the anatomy to predict whether a certain device will work is critical to the clinical application of these procedures. A clear understanding of the specific pathology causing MR is necessary to determine whether a percutaneous E2E repair is required or whether annular dilatation needs to be addressed with a direct or indirect annuloplasty device. A comprehensive understanding of imaging technologies and parameters is key to success. Currently, in the United States, only the MitraClip is available as a commercial device, and only for patients with DMR. With the availability of some of these devices in Europe under the CE mark of approval, clinical data are accumulating to shed more light on the proper selection of patients.

FUTURE DIRECTIONS

Percutaneous MV repair and replacement is an exciting new field with many devices at early stages of preclinical and clinical evaluation. Most strategies are based on principles learned from surgical MVRe techniques. The most advanced technique is the E2E repair, although interesting data are accumulating for a variety of the direct and indirect annuloplasty techniques and transcatheter MV replacement. It is unclear whether percutaneous devices need to eliminate all the MR to be effective. If a percutaneous repair can achieve a significant and durable reduction of MR, albeit not complete elimination, it may still remain a worthy procedure if it prevents clinical events. Indeed, some upcoming trials are either looking at quality of life outcomes and heart failure hospitalization as a primary or co-primary end point.

The need to determine which patients should be targeted in clinical trials is still present.[101] Trials may have to address specific populations and progressively expand the role of these therapies to lower-risk surgical populations. Surgical techniques are beginning to be tailored to the specific valve anatomy, but the percutaneous techniques, in their investigational stages, continue to be limited to one type of device per patient. It seems likely that the future of percutaneous repair will be a combination of techniques to address the complexity of MR in most patients. However, this poses significant limitations to the device development process with current regulations, and the use of multiple devices in the same patient is unlikely at the present time in the United States.

Percutaneous devices are becoming more specifically tailored to the etiology of MR and the anatomy of the individual patient; thus, the proper imaging and patient selection criteria for each device will have to be learned by interventionalists. Improvements both in imaging techniques and in the interpretation of these techniques with regard to percutaneous repair and replacement will be necessary in preprocedural planning, in assessing intraprocedural efficacy and complications, and in postprocedural follow-up.

KEY REFERENCES

22. Mihaljevic T, Lam BK, Rajeswaran J, et al. Impact of mitral valve annuloplasty combined with revascularization in patients with functional ischemic mitral regurgitation. *J Am Coll Cardiol*. 2007;49(22):2191–2201.
35. Nishimura RA, Otto CM, Bonow RO, et al. 2017 AHA/ACC Focused Update of the 2014 AHA/ACC Guideline for the management of patients with valvular heart disease: a report of the American College of Cardiology/American Heart Association Task Force on Clinical Practice Guidelines. *J Am Coll Cardiol*. 2017;70(2):252–289.
48. Mohty D, Orszulak TA, Schaff HV, et al. Very long-term survival and durability of mitral valve repair for mitral valve prolapse. *Circulation*. 2001;104(12 suppl 1):I1–I7.
67. Mauri L, Foster E, Glower DD, et al. Four-year results of a randomized controlled trial of percutaneous repair versus surgery for mitral regurgitation. *J Am Coll Cardiol*. 2013;62(4):317–328.
68. Lim DS, Reynolds MR, Feldman T, et al. Improved functional status and quality of life in prohibitive surgical risk patients with degenerative mitral regurgitation after transcatheter mitral valve repair. *J Am Coll Cardiol*. 2014;64:182–192.
74. Stone GW, Lindenfeld J, Abraham WT, et al. Transcatheter mitral-valve repair in patients with heart failure. *N Engl J Med*. 2018;379(24):2307–2318.

 Additional references available online at expertconsult.com.

中文导读

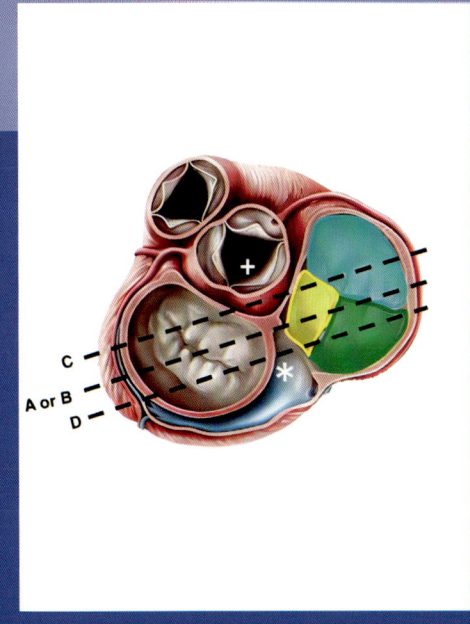

第53章
球囊扩张式瓣膜经导管主动脉瓣置换术

  本章回顾经皮球囊扩张主动脉瓣成形术时代的技术、适应证和结局，综述球囊扩张式瓣膜经导管主动脉瓣植入术的进展，详尽描述了操作技术要点，回顾接受该治疗患者的短期和中期随访结果，并总结了球囊扩张式瓣膜经导管主动脉瓣植入术目前的临床进展及应用情况。在欧洲常用的缩写是TAVI（经导管主动脉瓣植入术），而在美国通常用TAVR，用"置换"代替"植入"。

  有症状的主动脉瓣狭窄预后较差。最早外科主动脉瓣置换术是唯一有效的治疗方式，围术期死亡率为4%。由于高龄、并发症多等原因，有1/3的患者无法进行手术。单纯经皮球囊扩张主动脉瓣成形术后再狭窄率高，中远期预后不佳。经皮球囊扩张主动脉瓣成形术可作为经导管主动脉瓣植入术和外科主动脉瓣置换术禁忌证患者的姑息性治疗和换瓣术前的过渡治疗，也可以改善需要行紧急非心脏手术的危重AS的血流动力学。

  随着更好的设备、新的方法和植入策略的发展，经导管主动脉瓣植入术变得更加简单和安全。针对经导管主动脉瓣植入术的更准确的评分系统正在创建和研究中。作者详细介绍了球囊扩张式瓣膜的特点、经导管主动脉瓣植入术不同入路及手术操作过程；回顾了相关临床研究充分显示其安全性和有效性；并对经导管主动脉瓣植入术围术期卒中、传导阻滞、肾功能不全、瓣周漏、瓣膜血栓、血管并发症、主动脉夹层破裂，以及冠状动脉阻塞等并发症进行详细介绍。建议对于外科主动脉瓣置换术和经导管主动脉瓣植入术后均需要定期超声检查，并确定瓣膜毁损诊断标准。目前经导管主动脉瓣植入术对于年龄更低和低危患者效果尚不清楚，期待更多关于经导管主动脉瓣植入术应用长期持久性的研究。

李　喆　张洪亮

章节要点

- 经皮球囊扩张主动脉瓣成形术可用于缓解重度主动脉瓣狭窄患者的症状，在获益不确定时可作为明确治疗策略前的桥接方式。
- 经导管主动脉瓣置换术为外科手术并发症风险高或极其严重主动脉狭窄患者提供了生存和改善症状的机会，是此类患者治疗的一种选择。
- 对于解剖结构合适的外科手术脑卒中风险患者，经导管主动脉瓣置换术提供了一种非劣效的治疗选择。
- 正在进行的研究将明确经导管主动脉瓣置换术在主动脉瓣二瓣化畸形患者或低风险患者中的作用。
- 多学科团队评估合适的患者、导管输送系统的进步，以及多入路的可选择性，降低了经导管主动脉瓣置换术血管并发症和瓣周漏的发生率。
- 瓣中瓣技术仍然是生物瓣毁损高危患者的合理治疗选择。

53 Balloon-Expandable Transcatheter Aortic Valve Replacement Systems

Alain G. Cribier, Helene Eltchaninoff, Alan Zajarias

KEY POINTS

- Balloon aortic valvuloplasty is used to palliate the symptoms of severe aortic stenosis and as a bridge to more definitive therapy when benefit is uncertain.
- Transcatheter aortic valve replacement (TAVR) provides a survival and symptomatic advantage for patients with severe aortic stenosis who are at high or extreme risk for surgical complications, and it is the treatment of choice for this patient population.
- TAVR provides a noninferior treatment option to surgical aortic valve replacement in intermediate-risk patients with appropriate anatomy.
- Ongoing studies will define the role of TAVR in the patients with bicuspid aortic valve or those who are of low risk.
- Appropriate patient selection by a multidisciplinary team, advances in catheter delivery systems, and the availability of alternative access routes have improved the rates of vascular complications and paravalvular aortic insufficiency.
- Placement of a transcatheter prosthetic (valve-in-valve) remains a reasonable treatment option for high-risk patients with degenerated bioprostheses.

DISCLOSURES

Dr. Cribier is a consultant for Edwards LifeSciences.
Dr. Zajarias is a consultant for Edwards LifeSciences.

INTRODUCTION

Aortic stenosis (AS) remains the most common form of adult acquired valvular heart disease in developed countries, increasing in prevalence with age.[1] As noted earlier by Ross and Braunwald,[2] the natural history of symptomatic AS carries a poor prognosis. Medically treated patients with symptomatic AS have a 1- and 5-year survival of 60% and 32%, respectively.[3] Surgical aortic valve replacement (SAVR) has been for decades the only effective treatment for symptomatic severe AS that alleviates symptoms and improves survival. In the ideal candidate, SAVR has an estimated operative mortality of 4%.[4] However, the operative mortality and incidence of postoperative complications increase with age, and becomes significantly higher when surgery is done urgently and when preexistent comorbidities such as coronary artery disease, poor left ventricular function, renal insufficiency, pulmonary disease, and diabetes are present.[5,6] These factors are considered one of the main reasons for which one-third of patients with valve disease are not referred for surgery.[7]

Prior to the introduction of balloon aortic valvuloplasty (BAV) by our group in 1986,[8] SAVR was the only recommended therapy for patients with symptomatic severe AS but was declined if patients were thought to be "too old" or "high risk."[9] The concept of "old age" has continued to be redefined and has resulted in a moving target for comparison as these techniques have been evolving and the population has been aging. Age is no longer considered a surgical contraindication, and very old patients (octogenarians and nonagenarians) were offered the option if they did not have significant physical or psychological comorbidities.[10–12] The percentage of patients 90 years of age and older undergoing heart surgery has doubled from 1994 to 2001.[11] Patients with poor left ventricular function were also more aggressively managed surgically.[13–15] However, in Europe and the United States a large number of patients with severe AS who were not offered valve replacement remained.[16,17]

In the 1990s the early enthusiasm for BAV in adult patients as a possible alternative to SAVR disappeared following the recognition of the problem of restenosis. The procedure appeared to provide only temporary benefit in symptoms and, at best, a modest survival benefit with a relatively high complication rate.[18,19] The role of BAV in adults remained controversial as reflected in the updated American College of Cardiology (ACC) guidelines.[20] In spite of being determined to be too sick for surgery, BAV was not offered to them in most centers because of its perceived limitations.[16] Interest for learning this technique resurged with the development of transcatheter aortic valve implantation (TAVI) because balloon predilatation of the aortic valve is integrated in the procedure. Furthermore, BAV remains currently indicated as a palliative procedure in patients with contraindications to both TAVI and SAVR and can also be used as a bridge to those procedures in subsets of patients.

Developing TAVI has been for our group a fascinating 20-year odyssey with a happy ending. TAVI emerged in 2002 to profoundly alter the landscape of cardiovascular medicine.[21] Note that TAVI is the common abbreviation used in Europe, whereas in the United States TAVR is commonly used with "replacement" substituting for "implantation." This new "disruptive" technology is among the important "medical breakthroughs" to date. It evoked skepticism and criticism in the beginning, but thanks to innumerable clinical trials and evidence-based investigations, it is currently widely accepted by the medical community and its acceptance has continued to grow. In the past decade, TAVI has been performed in more than 100,000 patients around the world, and its use keeps growing by 40% annually. The field of TAVI is rapidly evolving, with major refinements in technology, procedural techniques, patient selection, and biomedical engineering. With the development of better devices, new approaches, and new implantation strategies, TAVI has become much simpler and safer. Although the indications were initially limited to elderly AS patients with multiple comorbidities, they are currently appropriately expanding to include a broader population of patients with lower surgical risk, degenerated surgical bioprosthesis, and even patients with other valvular diseases such as pure aortic or even mitral insufficiency. Most of our knowledge is founded on the extensive experience acquired with two devices, the balloon-expandable Edwards prosthesis and the self-expanding Medtronic CoreValve prosthesis, which, outside of the United States, have been implanted in equal numbers. U.S. Food and Drug Administration (FDA) approval for nonsurgical patients and high-risk patients was

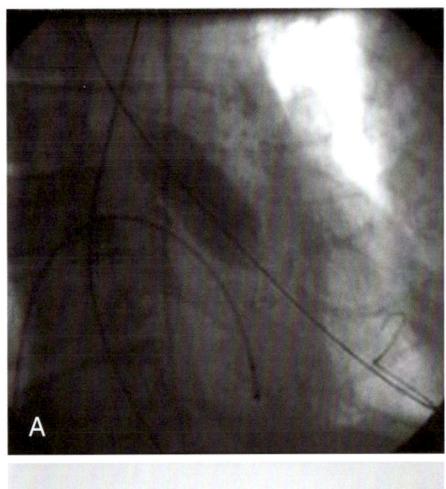
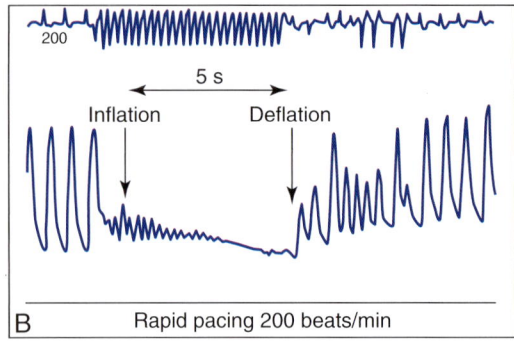
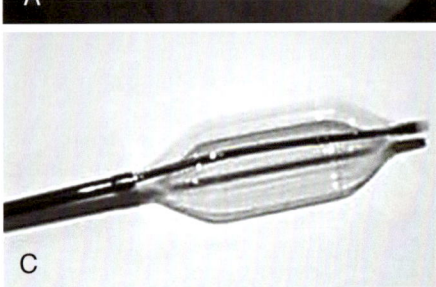
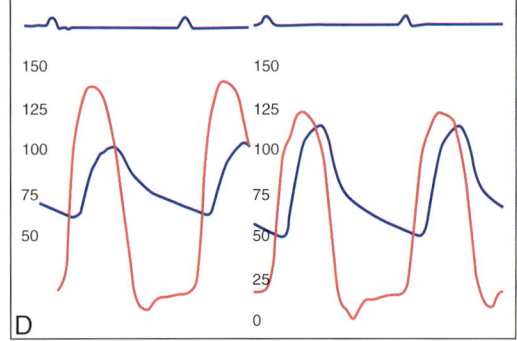

Fig. 53.1 Balloon aortic valvuloplasty (A) is performed under rapid ventricular pacing (B), which decreases the effective cardiac output by inducing ventricular tachycardia. The balloon catheter (C) must be sized to the aortic annulus to avoid severe aortic insufficiency. Doubling of the valve area or decreasing the transvalvular gradient by greater than 50% (D) is considered a successful procedure.

obtained for the Edwards device based on the results of the U.S. Pivotal Placement of Aortic Transcatheter Valve (PARTNER) trial[22,23] and, for the CoreValve device, after the results of the U.S. CoreValve Pivotal trials.[24,25] Indications of TAVI were specified in the European and U.S. Guidelines in 2012, 2014, and 2017 respectively.[20,26–28] Briefly, TAVI can be performed in patients with severe AS without surgical option and as an alternative to surgery in high-risk patients, intermediate-risk patients, and patients with degenerated surgical bioprosthesis in whom TAVI is favored by the heart team based on the individual risk profile and anatomic suitability. The objectives of this chapter are

1. To review the techniques, indications, and results of BAV in the era of TAVI
2. To review the development of balloon-expandable TAVI for calcific AS in adults, describe the implantation technique, review the short-term and midterm follow-up of patients who have received this therapy, and provide insight into the future advances and clinical applications.

BALLOON AORTIC VALVULOPLASTY

Since our first reported cases,[8] we have published our continuing experience which currently exceeds 1500 cases.[29–36] Like others,[18,19] we could obtain immediate improvement in symptoms, hemodynamics, and left ventricular function but had disappointing midterm and long term results. In our hands, BAV remains a valuable palliative procedure for frail patients who are extremely old, often with compromised clinical status due to concomitant coronary artery disease and other extracardiac comorbidities. Most of our patients have been turned down by the surgeons, and BAV is attempted as a "bridge to TAVI or surgical valve replacement" in approximately 50% of the cases. The technique currently used allows us to obtain improved hemodynamic results and reduced complications in this high-risk subset of patients.[36]

The goal of the procedure is to achieve a 100% increase in aortic valve area which is a determinant of prognosis,[18] and in some reported series, the increase in aortic valve area postprocedure was very modest.[37–39] The results of BAV are limited by the pathology involved in the disease. Degenerative AS is its most common etiology[40–42] and appears to be associated to a chronic inflammatory process.[43] Unlike rheumatic mitral stenosis, commissural fusion is not the predominant feature in the majority of elderly patients with calcific AS,[44] and the primary mechanism of the balloon action is fracture of the nodular calcium deposits, thereby improving leaflet mobility during left ventricular contraction.[45] Early restenosis occurring within hours or days is due to early recoil and could be related to the pathology of the valve components, or inappropriate balloon diameter (due to size or insufficient inflation).[32,46] When restenosis occurs after several months, the process may be multifactorial, including the original degenerative process and an altered healing process with fibrosis and ossification.[47,48] When patients develop recurrent symptoms, BAV can be repeated, usually after an interval of 12 to 24 months, and the dilations can be done serially.[34–36,49,50] In many cases the patient may be "bridged" to AVR or TAVI.[20] Despite its limitations, BAV has the interest of providing an often-marked symptomatic relief for selected elderly patients with no other option.[18–20,37] In the vast majority of cases, BAV is done using the retrograde approach, whereas in limited cases with poor femoral access it can be performed via the antegrade approach. For both approaches, we typically perform the baseline hemodynamic study to confirm the presence of severe AS at the same setting as the planned BAV intervention.

RETROGRADE APPROACH: EQUIPMENT AND PROCEDURAL STEPS

Using our current technique, the procedure is usually performed in less than 1 hour, with few complications (Fig. 53.1). Technical "pearls" that we have learned are helpful to make the procedure fast and safer in this critically ill, fragile, elderly patient population. For patient preparation, we use mild sedation with intravenous (IV) midazolam, and local anesthesia. Unfractionated heparin is given IV (3000 to 5000 IU) at the start of the procedure.

Cardiac Catheterization and Rapid Ventricular Pacing

Femoral arterial and venous access is obtained with 8-Fr sheaths. Coronary angiography is obtained, and if indicated, coronary intervention is performed in the same setting but usually after the BAV is completed. Right heart catheterization is performed using a Swan-Ganz thermodilution catheter. If the patient is being considered for TAVI, ascending aortic angiography is obtained, followed by abdominal aortic, iliac, and femoral angiography. When using the appropriate technique, the stenotic aortic valve can be crossed within a few minutes in most cases. An Amplatz left coronary catheter 2 (AL-2) is commonly used for this task. A straight tip, fixed core, 0.035-inch guidewire is positioned at the tip of the catheter. In the 40-degree left anterior oblique projection, the catheter tip is positioned at the rim of the valve. The catheter is slowly pulled back while maintaining firm clockwise rotation, to direct the catheter tip toward the center of the valve plane. The guidewire is carefully moved in and out of the catheter tip over a short distance, sequentially mapping the valve surface and exploring for the valve orifice. Once the wire crosses the valve, the catheter is advanced over the wire in the RAO view and positioned in the middle of the left ventricle (LV). The transvalvular gradient is obtained using the sidearm of the femoral sheath or through a dual-lumen catheter to record aortic pressure. Cardiac output can then be measured and the aortic valve area calculated using the Gorlin formula.[51] An extra-stiff Amplatz 0.035-inch, 270-cm length guidewire (Cook, Bjaeverskov, Denmark) is used to perform all catheter exchanges and to assist in stabilizing the valvuloplasty balloon during inflation, deflation, and withdrawal. Prior to inserting the wire, a large pigtail-shaped curve is formed at the distal end of the wire using a dull instrument to prevent ventricular perforation and decrease ectopy. A 6-Fr temporary bipolar pacing lead is positioned in the right ventricle posterior wall and connected to a pulse generator capable of pacing at up to 220 beats per minute (bpm). Pacing and sensing parameters are determined, and then the blood pressure response to pacing at 200 to 220 bpm is evaluated. The rapid ventricular pacing (RVP) causes a precipitous fall of blood pressure to at least 50 mm Hg to be effective. If this is not achieved at a rate of 200 bpm, then the response is checked again at 220 bpm. If 2:1 conduction block is seen, then the rate will need to be reduced to 180 bpm or the lead position modified. The pacer is set on demand mode at 80 bpm, serving as a backup in the event that a vagal episode or interruption of atrioventricular conduction occurs resulting in bradycardia or asystole in response to balloon inflations.

Balloon Preparation and Balloon Aortic Valvuloplasty

The diagnostic catheter is removed from the LV over the extra-stiff wire while carefully maintaining the looped flexible segment of wire in the LV cavity. The 8-Fr sheath is replaced by a 10-Fr sheath over the extra-stiff wire. In our center, all procedures are performed using a 10-Fr sheath (Cook, Bjaeverskov, Denmark). The evolution of the technique has seen a reduction in the profile of the devices, reducing local complications at the femoral artery puncture site; this was previously the most common complication reported.[52] At the end of the procedure, hemostasis is obtained by using an 8-Fr Angioseal device (Angioseal Vascular Closure Device, St. Jude Medical, Zaventem, Belgium). The majority of our experience was obtained with specifically designed balloon catheters for BAV, the double-sized Cribier-Letac catheters. When the production of those catheters was discontinued, we chose the Z-Med II balloon catheter (Numed Inc., Hopkinton, NY), compatible with a 12- or 14-Fr sheath. Currently we use the lower-profile Cristal balloons (Balt Extrusion, Montmorency, France) which are compatible with a 10-Fr sheath. The 20- and 23-mm diameter balloons are 45 mm in length, and the 25-mm diameter balloon is 50 mm in length. In general, we start with a 23-mm balloon. A 20-mm balloon is used if the valve is densely calcified or the aortic annulus is small (<19 mm by echo). In up to 25% of the cases, the 25-mm diameter balloon size can be used if the aortic annulus diameter is larger than 24 mm. Other catheters have recently become available, such as the TRUE balloon (Bard, New Providence, NJ) or the V8 (Intervalve, Inc, Minnetonka, MN) that minimize balloon migration and facilitate valve expansion. The Trueflow balloon (Bard, NJ) can be used without the need of rapid pacing in patients with a precarious hemodynamic condition. A short extension tubing with a three-way stopcock attached is connected to a handheld 30-mL Luer-Lok syringe filled with diluted contrast. The contrast is diluted 15%:85% contrast to saline to reduce viscosity and facilitate the inflation/deflation cycles. After flushing the distal lumen, the balloon is partially inflated and then completely deflated one or more times to completely purge it of air bubbles. The balloon catheter is advanced across the aortic valve, centering the valve between the two markers. Before using RVP, it was always challenging to maintain the balloon in optimal position during balloon inflation. There must be clear communication between the operators manipulating the balloon catheter and the pacing device. RVP is turned on, and balloon inflation is started quickly and with enough pressure to rapidly inflate the balloon as soon as the blood pressure falls. RVP is continued for a few seconds after the balloon reaches maximal inflation. The balloon is rapidly deflated, the pacer is turned off, and the balloon is withdrawn from the valve. This step requires coordination of the two operators to quickly allow restoration of antegrade flow while maintaining safe wire position in the LV. Rapid balloon deflation and restoration of blood flow is important to minimize the time of hypotension and hypoperfusion. Time must be allowed for the heart rate and blood pressure to return to preinflation values before deciding to inflate the balloon again. Because the pressure gradient cannot be measured through the current generation of balloon catheters, it is important to assess the effects of the balloon dilation and the hemodynamic consequences by observing the waveform of the aortic pressure tracing, as well as the heart rate response, rhythm, and blood pressure recovery. A sudden change in waveform with loss of the dicrotic notch or falling diastolic blood pressure could indicate the presence of severe aortic regurgitation. An improvement in the pressure slope is suggestive of a successful procedure. If the balloon does not appear to be fully expanded or there is no hemodynamic improvement, then repeat inflations are usually carried out before remeasuring the transaortic gradient. The residual gradient is obtained by simultaneous measurement of the pressure in the LV and aorta. If there is a significant gradient, the next larger size balloon may be chosen, and the sequence is repeated. A pullback gradient is also obtained after the final balloon inflation. For the final results, the pacemaker is removed, the cardiac output measured, and the final aortic valve area is calculated. An optimal result is considered to be doubling of the valve area or decreasing the gradient by 50% compared with the baseline value. Supravalvular angiography to determine the presence and/or severity of aortic regurgitation may be performed. If contrast cannot be used, assessment of the presence of aortic insufficiency (AI) and its severity may be performed by transthoracic echocardiography (TTE).

Immediate Management After Balloon Aortic Valvuloplasty

Manual compression is used for hemostasis at the venous entry site. Arterial hemostasis is achieved with the closure device as specified earlier. If a technical failure occurs, a pneumatic pressure device is used (FemoStop II Plus, Radi Medical Systems AB, Uppsala, Sweden). When the case is uncomplicated, the patient is usually discharged within 2 days. However, when BAV is performed in patients with severely impaired LV function or when rescuing a patient from cardiogenic shock, hemodynamic monitoring with inotropic support is usually required in the intensive care unit (ICU). Vagal reactions are the most common cause of hypotension associated with BAV. There must be a low threshold for ruling out the occurrence of pericardial tamponade or retroperitoneal bleed when evaluating the hypotensive patient after BAV.

ANTEGRADE TRANSSEPTAL APPROACH

Patient preparation is similar to the one described for the retrograde approach. Transseptal catheterization is performed via the right femoral vein, using the left lateral view. The puncture is made in the mid third of a virtual line connecting the aortic calcification and the posterior border of the heart. When entry into the left atrium is confirmed, heparin, 5000 IU, is administered intravenously. The Mullins sheath is then used to direct a 7-Fr Swan-Ganz catheter which has an inner lumen compatible with a 0.035-inch guidewire (Edwards LifeSciences, Irvine, CA) across the mitral valve into the LV under fluoroscopic guidance in the 40-degree right anterior oblique (RAO) projection. The transaortic gradient is determined with the Swan-Ganz catheter in the LV and the pigtail catheter in the aorta. The aortic valve area is calculated using the Gorlin formula. For crossing the aortic valve, the Mullins sheath is advanced approximately 2 cm beyond the mitral valve. The balloon of the Swan-Ganz catheter is inflated and directed into the LV outflow approaching the native aortic valve. A 0.035-inch straight wire may facilitate crossing the aortic valve with the balloon deflated, as the catheter is pushed over the wire into the ascending aorta. The wire is removed, and the balloon is reinflated. The catheter is advanced into the descending aorta and positioned at the level of the distal aortic bifurcation with an Amplatz 0.035-inch, 360-cm long extra-stiff guidewire (Cook, Bjaeverskov, Denmark). The balloon is deflated, and the Swan-Ganz is catheter removed. The 8-Fr venous sheath is replaced with a 10-Fr sheath for the subsequent balloon dilations using the Cristal balloon catheter (12 or 14 Fr if NuMed balloons are used). The atrial septum is then dilated with an 8-mm diameter balloon septostomy catheter through the 10-Fr sheath. The same balloon catheters are used as for the retrograde approach. Dilation of the aortic valve is done preferentially with the 23-mm diameter balloon, which is advanced through the 10-Fr sheath and positioned across the aortic valve while the loop in the LV is maintained carefully. BAV is then performed as described previously using RVP. TTE can assess the residual gradient. When two to three inflations using the largest selected balloon size are completed, the balloon catheter is removed. A 6-Fr pigtail catheter is advanced over the extra-stiff wire and positioned over the arch so that the wire can be removed shielded by the catheter, avoiding injury to the aorta or mitral valve. The final gradient is obtained with the pigtail catheter in the LV and another catheter in the aorta. Supraaortic angiograms may be obtained. Hemostasis is obtained with manual compression of the femoral artery and vein after sheath removal. Bed rest is recommended for 24 hours. ICU observation with inotropic support and prolonged hemodynamic monitoring is rarely required, only for hemodynamically unstable patients, typically those presenting in cardiogenic shock.

Results Using Contemporary Balloon Aortic Valvuloplasty Techniques

Over the past 20 years, the results of BAV have been reported in innumerable series and multicenter registries[53-57] showing clashing results depending on various experiences and techniques used. Our most recent series[36] including 323 consecutive patients with severe AS who underwent BAV (with the exception of patients undergoing percutaneous heart valve implantation) between January 2005 and December 2008 has been reported.[35,36] In this group of patients, the average age was 80.5 ± 10 years, 42% were women, and the mean logistic EuroSCORE (European System for Cardiac Operative Risk Evaluation) was 28.7 ± 12.5. New York Heart Association (NYHA) functional class III or IV was observed in 82% of patients, and the procedure was done emergently for patients in cardiogenic shock in 15% of cases. BAV was done using the retrograde approach in 100% of cases. Procedural success was achieved in 80.8% of the procedures. In-hospital mortality rate was 2.5%. Discharge from the hospital was at 5.6 ± 3 days. Over a mean follow-up of 20.7 ± 20.0 months, 26.3% of patients were bridged to SAVR or TAVI and 8.7% had repeat BAV. The other patients were left with medical treatment alone. Patients bridged to SAVR had the most favorable outcomes. Patients bridged to TAVR had better outcomes compared with those treated by single BAV. Finally, our study confirmed that survival was poor in patients treated by a single BAV (56% mortality at 1 year). In our series, the frequency of clinically apparent neurologic events was less than 2%. This compares favorably with the reported incidence of cerebrovascular events in a series of retrograde catheterizations of the aortic valve without intervention.[57] Minimizing the duration of RVP and balloon inflation are important technical issues, and maintaining optimal heart rate and blood pressure during the procedure are crucial. Improvements in the procedure such as RVP and vascular closure devices, as well as continued experience, have resulted in decreased complications despite an increasingly aged and sicker population of patients (Table 53.1).

CURRENT PERSPECTIVES OF BALLOON AORTIC VALVULOPLASTY

The updated ACC/American Heart Association (AHA) guidelines for the management of patients with valvular heart disease continue to regard the role of BAV as controversial.[20] There are no

TABLE 53.1 Comparisons of Complication Rates in the Rouen Series and in the Mansfield Registry

Complications	Mansfield Scientific Aortic Valvuloplasty Registry 1986–1988 (n = 492)	Rouen Series 2002–2005 (n = 141)
Procedural death	2 (4.9%)	3 (2.1%)
Postprocedural death (<7 days)	12 (2.6%)	3 (2.1%)
Cerebral embolic events	11 (2.2%)	2 (1.4%)
Transient ischemic attacks	5 (1.1%)	0 (0%)
Ventricular perforation with tamponade	11 (2.2%)	0 (0%)
Severe aortic insufficiency	5 (1.1%)	2 (1.4%)
Vascular complications (surgical repair)	27 (5.5%)	0 (0%)
Nonfatal arrhythmias	5 (1.1%)	5 (3.5%)
Other: myocardial infarction, sepsis, renal failure	8 (1.6%)	1 (1%)

class I or IIa recommendations for BAV. The class IIb indications for adult patients with severe AS are for patients who are at high risk for SAVR because they are hemodynamically unstable and who would be candidates for "a bridge to surgery" or as a palliative procedure because they have a serious comorbid condition which would preclude SAVR. Other potential indications for BAV are:

1. For the management of patients who present with critical symptomatic AS in need for emergent noncardiac surgery. The hemodynamic improvement of BAV is immediate and may decrease the risk of general anesthesia. In these situations, the BAV should be reserved only for those patients with severe AS and who have the potential for hemodynamic compromise.
2. To determine the contributing role of AS to dyspnea in patients with concomitant severe lung disease to gauge the potential improvement and risks to undergo AVR or TAVI.
3. To assess the myocardial contractile reserve in patients with low gradient/low ejection fraction in whom associated cardiomyopathy is questionable. The patients with no demonstrated contractile reserve can have a perioperative mortality as high as 62%.[58] The indication of AVR or TAVI in those patients can be clarified 2 to 3 weeks after BAV if marked improvement of the left ventricular ejection fraction occurs.

In 2018, BAV continues to have a role in the management of AS, particularly as a palliative modality for our increasing elderly population for whom the risk of valvular intervention is too high or not appropriate.[34,35,50,59,60] Interventional cardiologists and surgeons should become familiar with this technique, particularly if they are interested in TAVI, because it plays a crucial role for patient selection and valve implantation.

TRANSCATHETER AORTIC VALVE IMPLANTATION WITH THE EDWARDS BALLOON-EXPANDABLE PROSTHESIS

Background and Development of Transcatheter Aortic Valve Implantation

Percutaneous catheter-based systems for the treatment of patients with valvular disease have been an exciting area for research since the mid-1960s. The initial animal investigations were performed by Davies in 1965,[61] followed by Moulopoulos in 1971,[62] Phillips in 1976,[63] and Matsubara in 1992.[64] These investigators reported various catheter-based systems for temporary relief of AI, but no further human application was possible due to unsolved major limitations. A new era of investigations started with the development of endovascular stents, raising the concept of balloon-expandable valvular prosthesis. In 1992, Andersen et al.[65] reported their work in a porcine model in which they evaluated a transluminal stented heart valve. Here again, despite encouraging experimental results, there was no development of human application. Subsequently in 2000, Bonhoeffer and coworkers, using a valve from a bovine jugular vein mounted within an expandable stent, reported the feasibility of delivering such a device inside the native pulmonary valve of lambs[66] and thereafter were able to perform the first successful human percutaneous replacement of a pulmonary valve in a right ventricle to pulmonary artery prosthetic conduit with valve dysfunction.[67] Our team in Rouen has been working since the early 1990s on the development of a catheter-based treatment for nonsurgical patients with severe calcific AS that could overcome the high restenosis rate seen after BAV. Early cadaver work in 1994 provided early information on the ability to deploy a Palmaz stent in the aortic position and contributed to appropriate stent dimensions. In 1999, under the auspices of Percutaneous Valve Technologies (PVT; Fort Lee, NJ, USA), an original catheter valve was developed and tested in the sheep model.[68] In vitro testing confirmed the valve hemodynamic profile and durability. An original animal model of chronic aortic regurgitation which allows for the long-term evaluation of the catheter valve in the systemic circulation was developed for in vivo testing.[69] The first TAVI in a human was performed by our group in April 2002[21] followed by an initial series of human implantations for compassionate use that were serially reported.[70–74] Following the acquisition of PVT by Edwards LifeSciences (Irvine, CA) in 2003, further modifications of the Cribier-Edwards device were achieved with the development of the Edwards SAPIEN Heart Valve that preceded multi-center clinical trials and the pivotal randomized PARTNER study in the United States.[22,23] The first series of patients with severe AS treated with the self-expanding CoreValve Revalving System (Medtronic Inc, Minneapolis, MN) was reported by Grube et al. afterwards.[75] Since the first implantation of this device in 2004, several technological improvements were obtained and the efficacy of the CoreValve demonstrated in multiple registries and in the U.S. CoreValve Pivotal trials.[24,25] Over the past years, Edwards Lifescience and Medtronic have been developing new models of transcatheter valves and delivery systems, leading to a clear-cut improvement of the results with decreased rate of complications, whereas a number of other models of transcatheter valves were launched by several companies, some of them being already approved in Europe.

This section will provide a review of the patient selection, procedural techniques, results, and future strategies with balloon-expandable valves.

Risk Stratification

According to the guidelines, TAVI is currently being offered to patients who are at high risk or intermediate risk due to their age or comorbidities. Surgical risk is most commonly estimated by the Society of Thoracic Surgeons Predicted Risk of Mortality (STS-PROM) and the EuroSCORE. The EuroSCORE II has been validated in patients undergoing valvular surgery.[76] Previous versions of the EuroSCORE had shown to overestimate surgical mortality in high-risk patients, and as a result the logistic EuroSCORE II was developed.[76–78] The STS-PROM score is derived from the STS database, a voluntary registry of practice outcomes, and estimates the risk of mortality, morbidity, renal failure, and length of stay after valvular and nonvalvular cardiac surgery.[79,80] This score has been shown to underestimate the true mortality rate after cardiac surgery, but it more closely reflects the operative and 30-day mortality for the highest-risk patients having aortic valve replacement.[81]

The STS-PROM and the EuroSCORE provide an objective way to quantify risk. Although thorough, these risk scores do not include certain characteristics that would complicate surgery and increase the operative mortality such as: previous mediastinal irradiation, chest wall deformity, presence of a severe calcification in the thoracic aorta (porcelain aorta), history of mediastinitis, liver cirrhosis, previous bypass graft preventing safe reentry to the chest, or patient's frailty. In addition, the algorithms were calculated from patients who underwent surgery, thus limiting their applicability to patients who were not considered surgical candidates. Clinical judgment and the patient's level of independent function are subjective parameters that influence outcomes after cardiac surgery but are difficult to measure. A dedicated in-hospital mortality calculator for patients undergoing TAVR has been created with improved accuracy.[82] More accurate risk calculators that will more precisely estimate the risk of patients selected for TAVI are currently being investigated.

Patient Selection for Transcatheter Aortic Valve Implantation

Over the past decade, heart valve teams have transitioned from being able to perform TAVI to become more proficient in

TABLE 53.2 Patient Characteristics Associated with Poor Prognosis After Transcatheter Aortic Valve Implantation

Chronic kidney disease (>stage 3)
    Severe lung disease
    Oxygen dependence
    Slow 5-minute walk
Frailty
Low body mass index
Low mean aortic gradient
Abnormal Mini-Mental Status Examination
Limited 6-minute walk test distance
Nontechnical reasons for inoperability
Moderate/severe tricuspid regurgitation

TABLE 53.3 Outer sheaths diameters and minimal internal vessel diameters required with the three generations of Edwards balloon expandable valve

Valve	Valve Size (mm)	Sheath OD (mm)	Minimum Vessel Diameter (mm)
SAPIEN 3	20	6	5
SAPIEN	23	8.4	7.0
SAPIEN XT	23	6.7	6.0
SAPIEN 3	23	6	5.5
SAPIEN	26	9.2	8.0
SAPIEN XT	26	7.2	6.5
SAPIEN 3	26	6	5.5
SAPIEN XT	29	8.0	7.0
SAPIEN 3	29	6.7	6.0

OD, Outer diameter.

performing TAVI while minimizing complications and obtaining perfect outcomes. Not every high-risk patient with symptomatic severe AS needs to be treated with TAVI. Special emphasis should be placed on performing this procedure in patients who will benefit consistently from this procedure. Certain patient characteristics have been associated with poor prognosis after TAVI. Of inoperable patients, those who were inoperable for technical reasons had a better prognosis that those who were considered inoperable for medical reasons.[83] Preprocedural risk assessment is performed using the EuroSCORE or the STS score as described previously. Patients are usually classified as high risk for surgery when the logistic EuroSCORE and the STS score are greater than 20% and 8%, respectively. However, further expansion of TAVI to intermediate-risk patients has been recently validated by the FDA and appears in the European and U.S. recommendations after the positive results of two randomized studies with the Edwards SAPIEN XT valve[84] (PARTNER 2 trial with a STS Score between 3% and 8%) and the Medtronic CoreValve[85] (SURTAVI trial, with a STS Score between 3% and 15%). These studies showed comparable benefit of TAVI and SAVR on the primary end point of death and disabling stroke at 2 years.

Patient frailty, which has been shown to have a significant impact on clinical outcome after SAVR and TAVI,[86] has become another inclusion criterion. Severe lung disease, oxygen dependence, low body mass index (BMI), worsening renal function, and low transvalvular gradients are also factors associated with poor prognosis.[87–89] Until a dedicated TAVR risk score is created, patient selection should be based on objective evidence associated with elevated surgical mortality and a multidisciplinary approach. The indication of TAVI and the benefit/risk profile must be discussed in detail by a multidisciplinary team (heart valve team) of primary cardiologists, interventional cardiologists, cardiac surgeons, echocardiographers, radiologists, anesthesiologists, and geriatricians. Inclusion requires patients to have severe symptomatic AS, be considered high risk for surgical complications, have a greater than 1-year survival from their comorbidities, and likely benefit from valve replacement (Table 53.2).

Meticulous preprocedure planning with multimodality imaging assessment must be obtained for each patient to determine the feasibility and safety of TAVI and select the best approach. Current prosthesis can be placed via a transfemoral (TF), transapical, transaortic, axillary, transcaval, or carotid approach.[7,8,22,23] The minimum femoral artery diameters according to the different generation of Edwards valves are shown in Table 53.3.

Cardiac Catheterization and Angiographies

Right and left catheterization will determine the presence of pulmonary hypertension and concomitant coronary artery disease which may need to be treated prior to valve implantation. Aortic angiography notes the correct angulation of the image intensifier during valve positioning and determines potential complicating factors in the aortic arch that may interfere with the procedure. Iliofemoral angiography is regularly performed as a first evaluation of vessels diameters, calcification, and tortuosity.

Echocardiography

TTE and/or transesophageal echocardiography (TEE) will assess the anatomy of the aortic valve (trileaflet or bicuspid valve), the severity of AS, the degree and distribution of valvular calcification, the annulus diameter that has been for many years the only way for selecting the appropriate prosthesis size, the left ventricular function, the pulmonary pressures, and concomitant valvular diseases. Cross-sectional three-dimensional TEE can be usefully added to this baseline evaluation.[90]

Computed Tomography

Computed tomography (CT) with three-dimensional reconstruction is invaluable to assess the valvular (calcium distribution, leaflet length) and aortic root anatomy (diameters, angulation, calcification, sinus of Valsalva), the distance coronary ostia/annulus (to assess the risk of coronary occlusion during TAVI), and the aortobifemoral anatomy. CT is currently considered the best tool to accurately evaluate the dimensions of the ovoid-shaped aortic annulus (diameters, circumference, and area) and select the appropriate prosthesis size to prevent valve embolization and paravalvular regurgitation (too small device) or annulus rupture (too large device). This information will be adapted to the model of prosthesis used (Fig. 53.2).

CT has a key role for evaluating the peripheral arteries and preventing complication of the TF approach using large introducers and delivery systems. The prosthesis may be delivered by various approaches, the TF approach being considered the default approach by most teams because it is less invasive than alternative routes. Recent decrease in sheath size allows the TF approach to be used in more than 80% of cases, whereas it was limited to 50% of cases with the first-generation devices. Selection depends on tortuosity, calcification, and internal diameter of the femoral, external iliac, and common iliac arteries. The presence of abdominal aortic aneurysms or history of their repair would favor the use of alternative approaches. Vascular complications have been

Sapien XT Valve Sizing Chart

	23 mm	26 mm	29 mm
Annulus diameter (mm)	18–22	21–25	24–27
Annulus area (mm^2)	332–395	425–506	528–660
Expanded length (mm)	14	17	19

Sapien 3 Valve Sizing Chart

	20 mm	23 mm	26 mm	29 mm
Annulus diameter (mm)	16–19	18–22	21–25	24–28
Annulus area (mm^2)	273–345	338–430	430–546	540–680
Expanded height (mm)	15.5	18	20	22.5

Fig. 53.2 Annular sizing chart for determining the valve size using the SAPIEN XT and SAPIEN 3 devices.

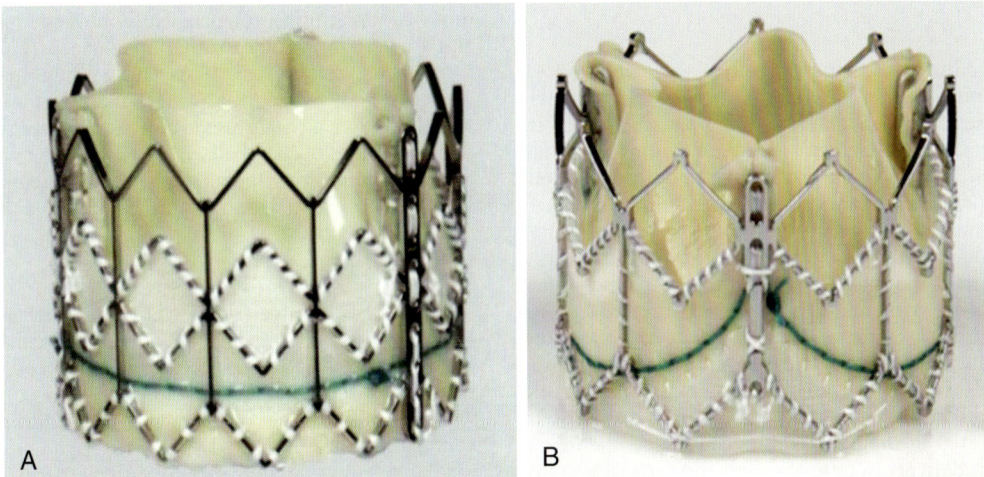

Fig. 53.3 (A) The Edward SAPIEN valve is a trileaflet bovine pericardial valve mounted on a balloon-expandable stainless steel stent. (B) The second-generation SAPIEN XT valve has a new bovine pericardial leaflet design and is mounted on a cobalt chromium stent, reducing its profile.

associated with significant mortality and may be prevented with appropriate screening.[91,92] Safety should not be sacrificed if other approaches than the TF approach are available and patients are considered good candidates. If chronic renal insufficiency precludes the use of a fully contrasted study, then intraarterial administration of a small contrast bolus[93] or a noncontrasted CT may provide appropriate images for the necessary measurements.

EDWARDS TRANSCATHETER AORTIC VALVES

Edwards SAPIEN Valve

The Edwards SAPIEN prosthesis is the first generation of balloon-expandable valve developed by Edwards Lifescience in 2005 (Edwards LifeSciences, Irvine, CA), after the acquisition of PVT. This device is a modified version of the percutaneous valve used in the first-in-human implantations and subsequent feasibility studies performed between 2002 and 2005 by our group,[21,70–72] then by other investigators.[73,74] This model of valve has been used in all feasibility studies in Europe and Canada, later on in the U.S. PARTNER trial, and in many Outside United States (OUS) registries, including the SOURCE (Edwards SAPIEN Aortic Bioprosthesis European Outcome Registry) registry. This model of balloon expandable was the first one approved in the United States. The device consists of a bioprosthetic valve, a balloon catheter on which it is mounted, and a crimping tool.

The Edwards SAPIEN prosthesis is a trileaflet bioprosthesis made of bovine pericardium that is mounted in a balloon-expandable stainless steel stent (Fig. 53.3A). It has been pretreated to decrease calcification and functional deterioration. The stent has a fabric cuff placed in the ventricular side that covers one-half of the frame, limiting stent expansion and decreasing perivalvular insufficiency. Due to the lack of a sowing ring, the valve is oversized to the aortic annulus to ensure postdeployment stability and is available in several sizes selected based on the CT measurement of aortic annular dimensions In benchtop testing, its durability is greater than 10 years. The SAPIEN valve provides a larger effective orifice area and lower hemodynamic profile than corresponding surgically implanted valves but has a higher incidence of perivalvular insufficiency.[94] The valve is mounted on a custom-made balloon with balloon diameters that correspond to the prosthesis size and ends in a

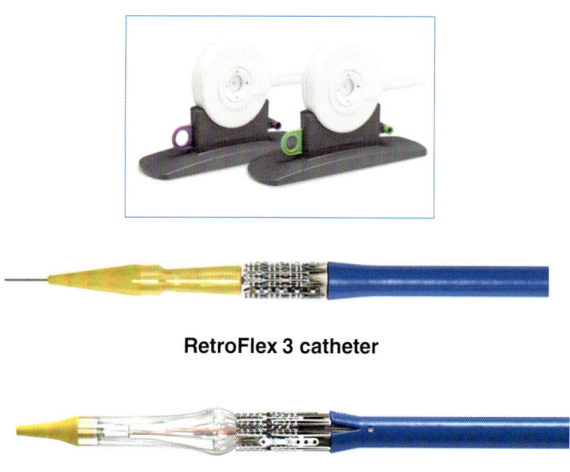

RetroFlex 3 catheter

NovaFlex catheter

Fig. 53.4 From top to bottom: (1) The original crimping device (two sizes adapted to the 23- and 26-mm SAPIEN valves). (2) The RetroFlex 3 delivery system (SAPIEN valve). (3) The NovaFlex delivery system (SAPIEN XT valve). (Courtesy Edwards LifeScience.)

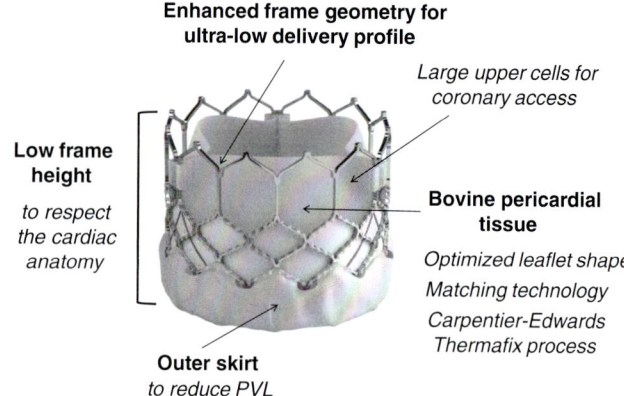

Fig. 53.5 The SAPIEN 3 Transcatheter Heart Valve: Distinguishing Features. *PVL,* Paravalvular leak. (Courtesy Edwards LifeScience.)

nose cone that facilitates crossing the native valve (Fig. 53.4). An original crimping tool is used to manually and symmetrically compress the overall diameter of the prosthesis from its expanded size to its minimal delivery profile. A cylindrical gauge is used to confirm the collapsed profile of the delivery system to ensure that it will move smoothly through the introducer sheath. A measuring ring is used to calibrate the balloon inflation to its desired size and to determine the amount of saline/contrast mixture in the syringe necessary for the proper inflation at the time of deployment. The Retroflex catheter (see Fig. 53.4), an innovation to facilitate the passage of the mounted valve across the aortic arch from the retrograde approach, was initially evaluated by Webb.[74] This catheter has a deflectable tip that changes direction when activated by the rotation of an actuator incorporated in the handle. The catheter is then used to direct the valve delivery system through the arterial system, around the aortic arch, and across the aortic valve providing a less traumatic passage. The Retroflex catheter assists in centering and supporting the valve as it crosses the calcified and stenotic native valve. This system also provides precise positioning at the aortic annulus. The SAPIEN valve and deflecting guiding catheter are introduced through a hydrophilic coated sheath that extends into the abdominal aorta to decrease vascular complications.

SAPIEN XT Valve

A new generation device, Edwards SAPIEN XT (see Fig. 53.3B), is a modified and improved version of the SAPIEN prosthesis, commercialized in Europe since 2009 and approved in the United States in June 2014. It consists of a cobalt chromium, balloon-expandable stent with an integrated, trileaflet bovine tissue valve with a polyethylene terephthalate (PET) fabric cuff. Its design renders it highly resistant to compression postimplantation. The valve's physical properties are similar to surgical bioprosthesis with three sections of bovine pericardium, manufactured with the ThermaFix anticalcification process. The TF kit includes the NovaFlex delivery system (see Fig. 53.4), which consists of a deflectable balloon catheter, with a distal nose cone and a handle consisting of a flexing wheel, a flex indicator, and an alignment wheel used to mount the crimped valve on the balloon after being advanced into the abdominal aorta; a single-use crimper; a 35-cm hydrophilic coated introducer (expandable e-sheath) of 16-, 18-, or 20-Fr for the 23-, 26-, and 29-mm valve sizes, respectively; a 16-, 18-, 20-, or 22-Fr polyethylene iliofemoral arterial dilator (40 cm in length); a dedicated 20-, 23-, or 25-mm valvuloplasty balloon for the 23-, 26-, and 29-mm valve sizes, respectively, (40 mm balloon length), for predilatation of the native aortic valve; and two Atrion balloon inflation devices. The transapical (or transaortic) kit includes: the Ascendra 2 transapical delivery catheter (22 Fr) optimized for a single-hand operation; the Ascendra sheath (24 Fr); a single-use crimper; a 20-mm Ascendra custom-designed valvuloplasty balloon catheter, and two Atrion inflation devices. Dimensions and adequate requirements for the SAPIEN XT and SAPIEN 3 are shown in Table 53.3 and Fig. 53.2.

SAPIEN 3 Valve

The SAPIEN 3 valve (Fig. 53.5) is the latest generation of balloon-expandable valve developed by Edwards Lifesciences. It has been approved and commercialized in several European countries and in the United States and has replaced the SAPIEN XT valve in all countries. This device is a modified and improved version of the SAPIEN XT. It consists of a trileaflet bovine pericardial tissue valve with optimize shape for hemodynamics and durability, mounted into a cobalt chromium frame with enhanced geometry for ultra-low delivery profile. Four sizes are available: 20, 23, 26, and 29 mm. A PET outer skirt has been designed to minimize paravalvular leaks. The Edwards Commander Delivery System for the TF approach (Fig. 53.6) offers a dual articulation for coaxiality. This device can be used in ultralow profile introducer e-sheaths of 14 Fr for the 20-, 23-, and 26-mm valve sizes and 16 Fr for the 29-mm valve size. The Edwards Certitude Delivery System (18 Fr) with articulation features has been designed for the transapical approach. Distinguished features, dimensions, and adequate requirements for the SAPIEN 3 as compared with the other Edwards devices are shown in Figs. 53.2, 53.5 and Table 53.3.

Transfemoral Valve Implantation

Room Requirements

TF TAVI can be performed in the cardiac catheterization laboratory or in the hybrid operating room. The room must be equipped with a fixed fluoroscopy unit that provides high image quality and the ability to store reference images for roadmapping. The room needs to be large enough to allow all operators to work comfortably and the circulators to move freely. A cardiopulmonary bypass machine should be accessible if complications arise. Equipment to treat vascular or coronary complications should be stocked in the room and available on demand.

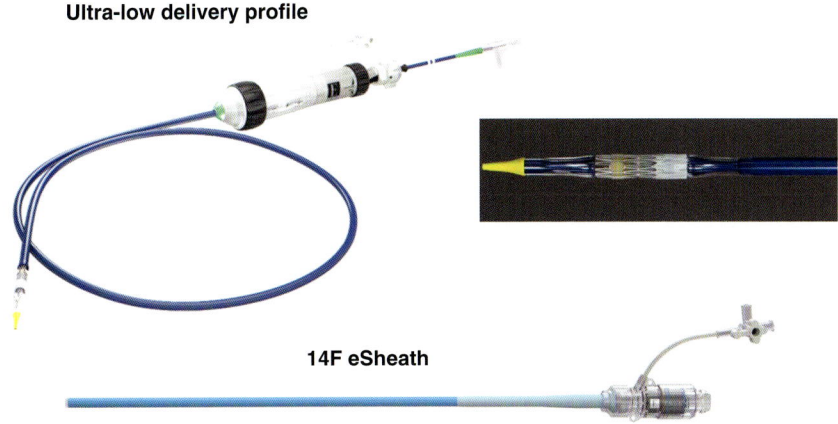

Fig. 53.6 The Commander ultra-low-profile delivery system for transfemoral approach with SAPIEN 3 and the 14-F eSheath arterial introducer. (Courtesy Edwards LifeScience.)

Anesthesia
The procedure can be done under general anesthesia[4] or conscious sedation.[5] General anesthesia is preferred if a TEE is performed simultaneously during the procedure. If not, conscious sedation and local anesthesia do provide enough relief during the procedure and are increasingly accepted since the launch of smaller size devices (SAPIEN XT and SAPIEN 3).[95,96] Continuous invasive hemodynamic monitoring should be used throughout the procedure. Vasopressor support should be used judiciously as vasoconstrictors may interfere with the insertion and removal of the arterial sheath and predispose to vascular complications.

Infection and Antithrombotic Prophylaxis
To decrease the risk of prosthetic infection, activities to reduce infections are followed. Patients are given IV antibiotics (vancomycin or cefazolin) on call to the procedure room and are continued for 48 hours. Aspirin (160 to 325 mg) and clopidogrel (300 mg) are administered at least 24 hours prior to the procedure. After the procedure, clopidogrel 75 mg daily is continued for 1 month and daily aspirin (75 mg) indefinitely.

Venous and Arterial Access
Femoral arterial access is obtained for aortic angiography with a 5- to 6-Fr pigtail catheter and a venous sheath is inserted for RVP. The contralateral artery is cannulated percutaneously or by surgical cutdown. If accessed percutaneously, it can be preclosed with suture-mediated devices. With the new-generation Edwards SAPIEN XT and SAPIEN 3 devices, preclosing with a single 10-Fr Prostar device or with two Proglide devices (Abbott Vascular, Lake Buff, IL) is regularly performed.[97] If a surgical cutdown is performed, the common femoral artery should not be completely dissected in the posterior aspect because sheath insertion is easier when the vessel is partially anchored.

Aortic Angiography
Ascending aortic angiography is performed in a projection that places all aortic cusps in line and perpendicular to the image intensifier. Ideally the best projection is previously determined to minimize the radiation and contrast exposure using CT scan. It can also be facilitated by the use of online three-dimensional reconstruction systems.

Temporary Pacemaker Placement
A ventricular stimulation lead such as the 6-Fr Soloist lead (Medtronic, Minneapolis, MN) is placed in the right ventricle. After testing for appropriate capture, a RVP test is performed at a rate of 180 to 220 bpm as detailed in the BAV section.

Delivery Sheath Insertion
With the guidewire in the aorta, the previously inserted 8-Fr sheath is removed. Serial dilation of the femoral and iliac arteries can be performed with arterial dilators of increasing size to allow sheath delivery. The delivery sheath is then inserted and positioned in the descending aorta

Crossing the Aortic Valve
Once the patient is anticoagulated with heparin (100 IU/kg), the native aortic valve is crossed as described earlier in the BAV section using an Amplatz AL-2 catheter and a straight guidewire. The previously shaped extra-stiff Amplatz 0.035-inch, 270-cm length guidewire (Cook, Bjaeverskov, Denmark) is then exchanged through the AL-2 and the catheter is withdrawn while maintaining the distal wire position in the LV. A pigtail catheter is advanced, and the valve gradient is then obtained. Preshaped guidewires like the Safari (Boston Scientific, Maple Grove, MN) or the Confida (Medtronic, Minneapolis, MN) have been specifically designed for TAVR to minimize LV trauma and perforation.

Balloon Aortic Valvuloplasty
BAV is performed under RVP prior to TAVI with the same technique described previously. A 20-, 23-, or 25-mm Retroflex balloon (Edwards LifeSciences, Irvine, CA) is used for placement of a 23-, 26-, or 29-mm prosthesis, respectively. The valve prosthesis should be ready to be inserted prior to the completion of the BAV on the possibility that severe AI and hemodynamic instability develops. Using the pigtail catheter placed in the ascending aorta above the native aortic valve, contrast administration at the time of full balloon inflation is regularly performed to assess the risk of coronary obstruction by displacement of the native valve leaflet over the left main ostium and to confirm the optimal valve sizing (Fig. 53.7A). In patients with favorable anatomy and valve characteristics, predilatation with a valvuloplasty may not be required. Using a valvuloplasty is beneficial in patients with high transvalvular gradients and very stenosed aortic valves to facilitate device manipulations and positioning.

Valve Insertion and Deployment
The prosthesis and delivery system are then inserted in the sheath over the extra-stiff wire. Once the delivery system reaches the aortic arch, the delivery catheter (RetroFlex for the SAPIEN XT or Commander for the SAPIEN 3) is activated, allowing the safe passage of the delivery system across the aortic arch. The system is then advanced until it reaches the ascending aorta. In the predetermined reference projection, the valve is positioned in the aortic position. After confirmation of the appropriate location

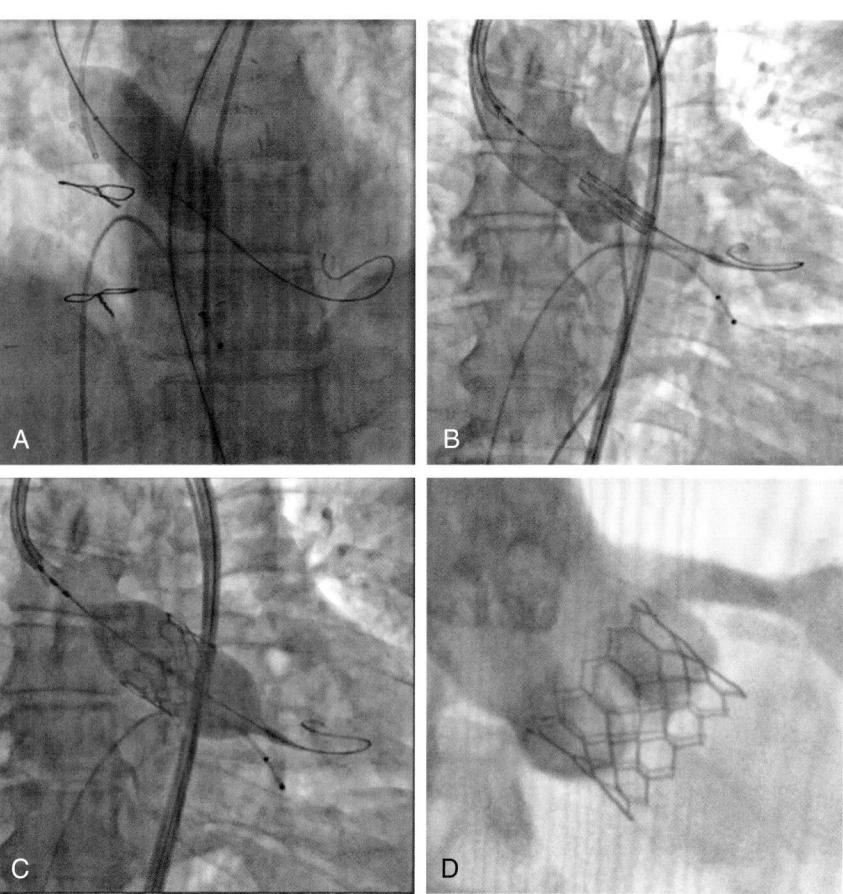

Fig. 53.7 **Transfemoral transcatheter aortic valve implantation.** (A) Balloon aortic valvuloplasty with simultaneous aortography. (B) Correct valve positioning confirmed by angiography. (C) Valve deployment under rapid ventricular pacing. (D) Valve in place after delivery and aortic angiography to confirm valve position, lack of aortic insufficiency, and unrestricted flow through native coronary arteries.

with angiography (and TEE if available) (see Fig. 53.7B), the valve is deployed under RVP (see Fig. 53.7C) after the confirmation that the systemic blood pressure has reached and maintained its nadir. Balloon inflation is held 3 to 5 seconds before deflation, and then RVP is stopped to avoid traction on the prosthesis while the balloon catheter is being withdrawn. The RVP run generally does not last longer than 15 seconds. The delivery system is straightened and withdrawn. The transvalvular gradient can be measured and paravalvular leaks evaluated by angiography (see Fig. 53.7D) and echocardiography.

Sheath Removal and Arteriotomy Closure
The sheath is withdrawn with careful monitoring of the blood pressure and simultaneous contrast administration through a catheter placed at the level of the iliac bifurcation or into the iliac artery. A precipitous drop in the blood pressure or extravasation of contrast media indicates a vascular rupture. This complication should be treated appropriately and expeditiously using covered stent or surgical repair. Immediate tamponade of the ruptured vessel with the large sheath and/or closure of the iliac artery or abdominal aorta with a large size balloon can be urgently performed before arterial repair. The arteriotomy site is then closed surgically or percutaneously with the previously placed preclosure device.[97]

TRANSAPICAL APPROACH

The procedural steps of valve deployment are relatively similar to the TF route and, as such, only the differences will be illustrated (Fig. 53.8).[98–102] Femoral arterial and venous accesses are obtained for aortic root angiography and RVP as previously described. RVP can also be obtained with an epicardial lead. A small left lateral thoracotomy is performed. The planes are dissected until the LV apex is visualized. A purse-string suture is placed in a muscular segment of the apicolateral wall. Once the patient is anticoagulated and the activated clotting time is therapeutic, a direct puncture of the LV is performed and a 7- or 8-Fr sheath is inserted into the LV. A 0.035-inch J-tipped wire is then advanced through the valve into the descending aorta while guided with a Judkins right (JR) curve catheter. The wire must be free of the papillary muscles or mitral chordal structures to avoid complications with the insertion of the delivery sheath. Once in the descending aorta, the wire is exchanged for an extra-stiff wire, the Amplatz 0.035-inch, 270-cm length guidewire (Cook, Bjaeverskov, Denmark), and the JR catheter is removed. The sheath is exchanged for the large delivery sheath that is inserted 3 to 4 cm into the LV cavity. Under RVP, a BAV is performed with a 20-mm Retroflex balloon. The Certitude delivery system (Edwards LifeSciences, Irvine, CA) is advanced into the sheath and deaired. The valve/catheter ensemble is advanced into the aortic position maintaining the balloon marker in the annular plane. After confirmation of the appropriate position by TEE and angiography, RVP and a patient breathhold is begun. The valve is deployed as the blood pressure is at its nadir and the balloon is deflated and withdrawn. Once the degree of AI is assessed and the valve position in confirmed by TEE, the ventricular sheath can be removed. If the valve needs to be postdilated, then this procedure follows. If no further intervention is needed, then the delivery sheath is removed,[99] the puncture site repaired, and the anticoagulation reversed. The thoracotomy is closed over a drain.

Direct Transaortic Approach

The retrograde direct transaortic approach is an interesting alternative to the transapical approach for patients in whom

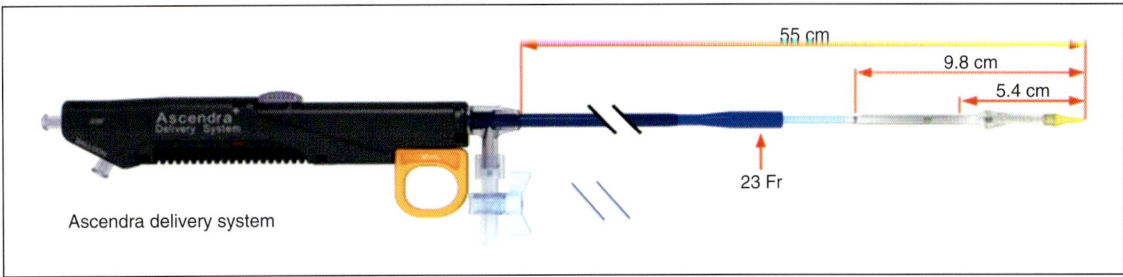

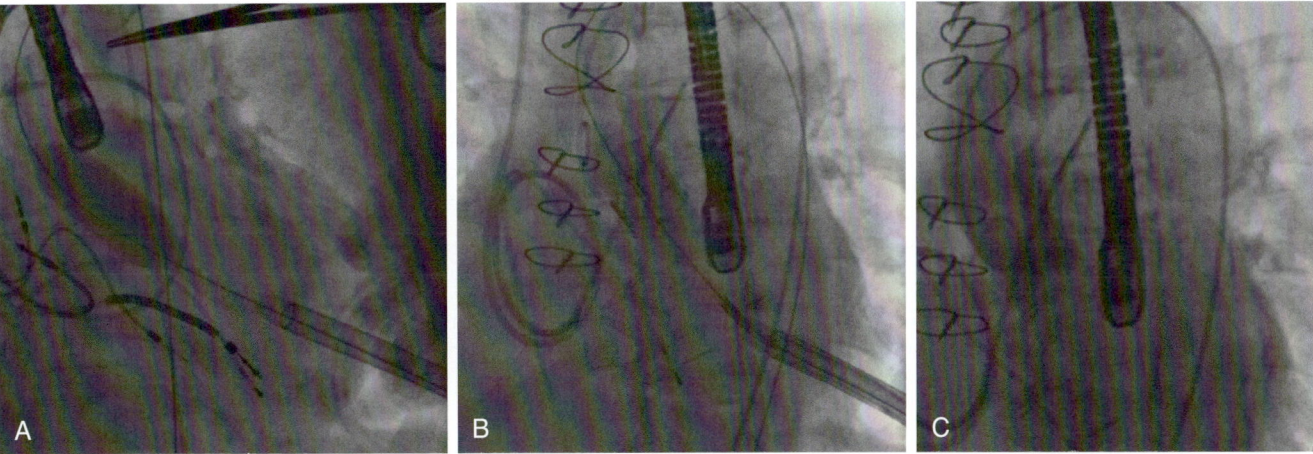

Fig. 53.8 The Ascendra delivery system for transapical delivery of the SAPIEN valve. (A) Balloon valvuloplasty performed under rapid pacing. The delivery sheath is inserted through the apex of the left ventricle after lateral thoracotomy. (B) Valve deployment under rapid ventricular pacing. (C) Aortic angiography post valve implantation confirms the absence of aortic insufficiency

vascular access through the femoral artery cannot be considered.[3] It involves a 5-cm incision in the chest either via ministernotomy or mini-thoracotomy. CT scans are crucial to determine the anatomy and calcification of the aorta, to confirm a minimal distance of 5 cm between the insertion site and the annulus, and to select the best puncture site optimizing the coaxial alignment with the native valve. The advantage of this approach over the transapical route is to avoid any trauma to the LV.

Axillary Approach

Sheath insertion into the left axillary artery is an alternative for patients with poor femoral access. A surgical cutdown or percutaneous approach can be performed following standard technique. A 25-cm sheath that allows access into the aortic arch is preferred after the puncture is performed. Access to the LV follows as previously noted. Once the guidewire is placed safely at the LV apex, the Certitude introducer sheath and system are advanced and the valve is delivered. Dimensions, calcifications, and tortuosity of the subclavian artery may limit the use of this approach.

Transcaval Approach

For patients with poor access arterial access, the transcaval approach has been described. Femoral venous access is obtained and followed by the creation of a puncture from the inferior vena cava to the descending aorta. Once access is obtained in the aorta, the delivery sheath is inserted and the valve is deployed following the traditional steps. At the time of sheath removal, a closure device is deployed which occludes the aortic caval communication.

CLINICAL RESULTS

Historical Results

The initial report of a successful percutaneous implantation of an aortic bioprosthesis in a patient with severe symptomatic AS who presented in cardiogenic shock in April 2002 was greeted with enthusiasm.[21] From 2003 to 2004, single-center registries to document the feasibility of the procedure, on a compassionate basis, were started under the names of Initial Registry of Endovascular Implantation of Valves in Europe (I-REVIVE) and Registry of Endovascular Critical Aortic Stenosis Treatment (RECAST).[70] These registries used a 23-mm bioprosthesis made of equine pericardium mounted on a stainless steel, balloon-expandable stent, and valve placement was primarily done via the antegrade (transseptal) approach. Procedural success was achieved in 75%. Aortic valve area increased consistently from 0.6 cm^2 to 1.6 cm^2 and was accompanied by a fall in mean transvalvular gradient (37 to 9 mm Hg) and an increase in left ventricular ejection fraction (LVEF) (45% ± 18% to 53% ± 14%). The 30-day mortality rate was 23% and the 30-day major adverse cardiovascular and cerebrovascular event (MACCE) rate was 26%.[70] Patient survival was 63% by 6 months and was limited by the severity of patients' comorbidities. Moderate to severe perivalvular AI, seen in 63%, and valve embolization were procedural limitations due to the availability of a single valve size. Due to venous distensibility, sheath insertion was not limited by vessel size, tortuosity, or the presence of peripheral vascular disease. Valve placement was simple as the device crossed the smooth aspect of the aortic valve. However, the technique was challenging due to the need of a transseptal puncture, the navigation of the catheter/valve ensemble across the mitral and aortic valve, and the guidewire interaction with the mitral valve and subvalvular apparatus, contributing to poorly tolerated acute mitral insufficiency. The sum of all these problems limited the diffusion of this approach, prompted technical improvements in the delivery system, and promoted the resurgence of the retrograde approach.

Significant technical and prosthetic modifications followed to solve the previously encountered limitations. To reduce the degree of perivalvular regurgitation, valves were oversized in relation to the aortic annulus, and a second prosthesis size, 26 mm, became available. The perimeter and area of the aortic annulus, at the level of aortic leaflet insertion, were identified for appropriate valve sizing. In addition, the necessary landmarks for valve positioning were recognized, decreasing the risk of valve embolization. Catheters with a manually activated deflectable tip facilitated the valve delivery through the retrograde approach. Modifications in the delivery sheath also reduced vascular complications. Sheath length was increased to deliver the catheter/valve ensemble directly in the descending aorta, decreasing the risk of vascular injury.[100] Minimal arterial diameter, vessel tortuosity, and vessel calcification were still the major limiting factors. Multicenter registries from the United States (Registry Evaluation of Vital Information for VADs in Ambulatory Life [Revival] II), European Union (REVIVE II), and Canada (Canadian Special Access) continued to evaluate procedural safety and efficacy. New valve modifications were added to improve long-term function which included: use of bovine pericardium, elongation of the skirt to decrease perivalvular insufficiency, and the addition of an anticalcification treatment, culminating in the prosthesis that is currently used. The series of retrograde implantation published by Webb and colleagues showed initial procedural success of 78%, which increased to 96% after the first 25 cases, reflecting an important learning curve.[9] Observed 30-day mortality was 12%, and the expected 30-day mortality was 28%. At median follow-up, there was no evidence of valve deterioration, migration, restenosis, or valvular insufficiency. Moderate perivalvular leaks were seen in three cases at 1 month. Perivalvular AI was mild, clinically inconsequential, and stable during follow-up in the majority of the patients. This information led to the approval and valve commercialization in Europe in the Fall of 2007.

The initial experience of the transapical approach in the animal model could be extrapolated to early human experience with promising results.[99,100] The first published data, from Lichtenstein,[100] consisted of seven high-risk patients with AS. Valve implantation was successful in all of them, and there were no procedural deaths. Transvalvular gradient and aortic valve area improvement was seen in all patients, and the results were consistent with those found after retrograde implantation. Observed 30-day mortality was lower than the expected mortality (14% vs. 35%).[98–104] Published multicenter experience using this innovative approach has been growing. Walther et al.[105] reported on 93.2% successful implantations with a conversion rate to traditional AVR of 6.8%. Trace to mild AI was seen in 23 patients. The 30-day mortality was 13.6%, and the predicted operative mortality was 26.8%. Use of extracorporeal circulatory support was frequent (47%) during the initial procedures; however, after familiarization of the technique, the utilization dropped. A U.S.-based feasibility study noted successful valve placement in 90% of the cases accompanied by persistent improvement in symptoms, valve area, mean gradient, AI, and quality of life (QOL). Patient survival was 81.8% at 1 month, 71.7% at 3 months, and 58.7% at 6 months. MACCEs were seen in 65% and included a 5% incidence of stroke, 2.5% need for emergent cardiac surgery, and 17.5% myocardial infarction rate.

Results of Recent Series (Table 53.4)

Over the past 10 years, the Edwards SAPIEN valve and updated devices have been evaluated in a number of national and international registries[106–110] and, in one evidence-based trial, the U.S. PARTNER pivotal trial.[22,23] A second randomized study, the PARTNER 2 trial, using the SAPIEN XT, with results of the main series are summarized as follows.

Canadian Edwards Registry

The Canadian registry of the Edwards SAPIEN valve from 2005 to 2009 in six centers also had very encouraging results.[107] There were 339 high-risk patients (STS 9.8 ± 6.4%) enrolled with 49.6% TF and 50.4% transapical cases. The procedural success was 93.3%, with a 30-day mortality of 10.4%. Mortality was 22% at a mean follow-up of 8 months, with periprocedural sepsis, need for hemodynamic support, chronic kidney disease, and chronic obstructive pulmonary disease as independent predictors of late mortality regardless of the approach. Patients with porcelain aorta and frailty had acute outcomes similar to the overall cohort and patients with porcelain aorta had as good or better survival at 1-year follow-up.

PARTNER European Registry

The majority of short-term and midterm TAVI data have come from European and Canadian registries. The PARTNER European Registry,[111] whose results were published in 2010, is one of three major registries of OUS experience using the Edwards SAPIEN valve. Its primary safety end point was freedom from death from the index procedure to 30 days and 6 months. The primary efficacy end point was hemodynamic status of the valve, QOL, and NYHA improvement at 12 months after implantation. Mean patient age was 82 years, and 84% and 85% of the TF and transapical group had NYHA class III and IV heart failure, respectively. The EuroSCORE was 26 and 34 for the TF and transapical groups, respectively. Not surprisingly, the transapical cohort had greater comorbidities. After valve implantation, the mean aortic gradient fell to 10 mm Hg and aortic valve area rose to 1.6 cm². These values remained the same at 6-month and 1-year follow-up. Mean LVEF, reasonably well preserved at 53% preimplantation, was unchanged. Patients who survived to 1-year follow-up had a dramatic improvement of NYHA class (60% class I to II). To support this, QOL scores improved at 1 year by 23 points. At 18-month follow-up, patients in the TF group had a 71% survival rate, whereas those in the transapical group had a 44% survival. It must be emphasized that comparisons between the TF and transapical groups are not appropriate due to the major differences in comorbidities between the two groups and especially the presence of peripheral vascular disease (a marker of more severe atherosclerotic disease and hence poorer outcomes) in the transapical group.

SOURCE and SOURCE XT Registries

The Source Registry,[112] which included 1123 consecutive patients who underwent TF and transapical TAVI in 32 centers across Europe, was created for postmarketing surveillance. Each center was able to provide 100% of their consecutive patients' data for analysis. Twenty-two of the 32 enrolling centers had no prior experience with the SAPIEN valve and underwent structured training and proctoring. Mean logistic EuroSCORE was 25.7% (TF, $n = 463$) and 29.1% (transapical, $n = 575$). Overall procedural success was 93.8%, with a 30-day mortality of 6.3% and 10.3% with the TF and transapical approach, respectively. At 30 days, functional improvement was dramatic (NYHA class I/II at baseline 19% vs. 86% at 30 days, $P < .001$), and mean survival at 224 days was 74%. The symptomatic improvement persists during follow-up. Mean transaortic gradient decreased from 46.1 ± 6.7 mm Hg to 11.2 ± 4.9 mm Hg at 1 year. The

TABLE 53.4 Baseline and Follow-up Characteristics of Patients Undergoing Transcatheter Aortic Valve Implantation with the Edwards SAPIEN and SAPIEN XT Valve

Study	Patients	Age (Years)	Logistic EuroSCORE (%)	STS Score (%)	Procedural Success (%)	AVA Pre (cm²)	AVA Post (cm²)	Mean Gradient Pre (mm Hg)	Mean Gradient Post (mm Hg)	NYHA III/IV Pre (%)	NYHA III/IV 1 Year (%)	LVEF Pre (%)	LVEF Post (%)	Survival 1 year (%)
Canada[107]	339	81 ± 8	NR	9.8	93.3%	0.63 ± .17	1.55 ± .41	46 ± 17	10 ± 4	90.9	NR	55 ± 14	NR	76
Source TF[106]	463	81.7	25.8	NR	95.2	0.59	1.7	53.5	3.95	76	21.6	NR	NR	81.1
Source TA[106]	575	80.7	29.1	NR	92.7	0.59	1.7	53.5	3.95	77	31	NR	NR	72.1
Partner Cohort B[22]	358	83.1 ± 8	26.4 ± 17.2	11.6 ± 6	96.6	0.6 ± .2	1.5 ± 0.5	44.5 ± 15.7	11 ± 6.9	92	16.7	53.9	57.2	69.3
Partner Cohort A[23]	699	83.6	29.3 ± 16	11.8 ± 3.3	90.2	0.7 ± .2	1.59 ± .4	42.7 ± 14	10.2 ± 4	93	12	52.5 ± 13	56 ± 10	75.8
PARTNER EU (TF)[111]	61	82.3	25.7 ± 11	11.3 ± 6	96.4	0.6 ± 2	1.5 ± .5	48.9 ± 19	12.7 ± 4	82	10.4	52.9 ± 17	56.3 ± 13	79.7
PARTNER EU (TA)[111]	69	81.9 ± 5	33.8 ± 14	11.8 ± 6	95.4	0.6 ± .2	1.6 ± .5	46.6 ± 18	11.5 ± 3	85.5	14.7	52.8 ± 14	55.2 ± 8	50.7
FRANCE (TF)[114]	95	83.2 ± 7	25.6 ± 11	17.4 ± 11	92.6	0.66 ± .1	1.74 ± .4	45 ± 16	10.7 ± 5	70	NR	47 ± 14	55.1 ± 12	NR
FRANCE (TA)[114]	71	82.1 ± 7	26.8 ± 11	18.4 ± 12	92.6	0.68 ± .1	1.74 ± .4	48 ± 16	10.7 ± 5	53	NR	53 ± 12	55.1 ± 12	NR
SAPIEN XT SOURCE XT[112]	2166	81.4 ± 6	20.5 ± 12	8.4	NR	0.7	1.8	47.6	10.8	76.9	12.3	NR	NR	NR
FRANCE 2[116]	2107	82.9 ± 7	22.2 ± 14	15.6 ± 12	96.9	0.7 ± .2	NR	48.6 ± 16	NR	75.5	10.5	53.8 ± 14	NR	76
PARTNER 2[84]	284	84 ± 8.7	NR	10.3 ± 5	96.3	0.6 ± .2	1.6	45.2 ± 14	10	96.8	12	52 ± 13	NR	77.5

AVA, Aortic valve area; LVEF, left ventricular ejection fraction; NR, not reported; NYHA, New York Heart Association classification; STS, Society of Thoracic Surgeons; TA, transapical; TF, transfemoral.

majority of patient mortality and hospital readmission was not valve related. In addition, perivalvular AI remained constant in follow-up and there was no structural deterioration of the valve. Results from the transapical SOURCE registry confirm a similar procedural success (92.7%), with conversion to open AVR in 3.5%. Although vascular injury was less common in the transapical group, when present it was associated with a higher mortality rate. Thirty-day and 1-year mortality rate in the transapical group was higher when compared with the TF group; however, this is likely due to a selection bias. Patients who undergo transapical are generally older, have higher degree of comorbidities, and have a higher EuroSCORE.

Following the SOURCE registry, the SOURCE XT registry (December 2010 to May 2011)[112] included 2189 patients with XT valve in 94 European centers from 17 countries. This registry, which was aimed at monitoring a new technology introduced into the European market, evaluated the results at 30 days and annually to 5 years of the SAPIEN XT valve and NovaFlex delivery system using various approaches (TF 62.7%, transapical 33.3%, other 3.7%). Complications were assessed according to the Valve Academic Research Consortium (VARC) 2.[112] The preliminary results were presented by M. Thomas at the 2012 Transcatheter Therapeutics Meeting. STS score was lower than in the SOURCE registry (8.4% vs. 12.7%). At 30 days, all-cause mortality and cardiac mortality (6.3% and 2.6%, respectively) and stroke rate (2.2%) were significantly lower than in the SOURCE registry ($P < .0001$). Major vascular complications had decreased from 27.5% to 10.1% ($P < .0003$) and major bleeding from 19.3% to 10.6% ($P < .01$).

FRANCE 2 and FRANCE Transcatheter Aortic Valve Implantation Registries

Following the results released in 2009 of the first French TAVI registry,[113] a total of 4201 consecutive patients were enrolled from January 2010 to October 2011 at 34 centers in France in the FRANCE 2 Registry.[113–115] In November, patients in this registry had similar baseline demographics to the European PARTNER Registry, but they received either the Edwards SAPIEN XT valve (67%) or the Medtronic CoreValve (33%). The TF approach was used in 75%, and overall procedural success was 96.9%. Mortality rate at 30 days and 1 year were 9.7% and 24%, respectively. Major stroke, major bleeding, and major vascular complications occurred in 2.3%, 4.5%, and 4.7%, respectively. The only significant difference between the two valves was the rate of new pacemaker implantation: Edwards 11.5%, CoreValve 24.2% ($P < .001$). On multivariate analysis, the only independent predictors of 1-year mortality were increased risk on the logistic EuroSCORE, NYHA functional class III or IV, the use of a transapical approach, and periprosthetic regurgitation grade of 2 or more (on a scale of 0 to 4). At 1 year, 89.5% of surviving patients were in NYHA functional class I or II. The results at 3 years (mean 3.8 years) have been recently reported.[116] The 3-year all-cause mortality was 42%. On multivariate analysis, predictors of mortality were male sex, low BMI, atrial fibrillation, dialysis, NYHA functional class III or IV, higher logistic EuroSCORE, transapical or subclavian approach, need for permanent pacemaker, and paravalvular aortic regurgitation grade of 2 or more. Mean gradient, valve area, and residual aortic regurgitation were stable during follow-up.

In France, a nationwide registry (FRANCE-TAVI registry)[117] was designed to assess nationwide performance trends and clinical outcomes of TAVI during a 6-year period. A total of 12,804 patients treated in 48 centers since 2013 were included in the analysis. Medium age of the population was 84.6 years (males: 49.7%). Mean EuroSCORE was 15%, lower than in the previous national registries. TF TAVI was performed in 80%, whereas periprocedure TEE decreased from 60.7% to 32.7% and general anesthesia from 68.7% to 51.7%. The rate of device success was 96.8%. Thirty-day mortality rate decreased to 4.4% compared with 5.4% in FRANCE 2 registry. Stroke and life-threatening complications remained low and stable over time, whereas rate of pacemaker implantation slightly increased from 12.6% to 17.5%.

PARTNER US Multicenter Pivotal Trial

The U.S. and Canadian multicenter randomized trial PARTNER US[22,23] led to FDA approval of the SAPIEN valve. The primary end point of the PARTNER US multicenter randomized pivotal trial was death from any cause at 1 year. The study design is shown in Fig. 53.9. Between 2007 and March 2009, it included patients from 25 centers with severe symptomatic AS who were poor surgical candidates and had two treatment arms. An arm powered for noninferiority analysis randomized 699 patients with an elevated surgical risk (STS score >10%) to traditional AVR or TAVI (transapical or TF); a second arm powered for superiority analysis randomized 358 patients with severe AS who were deemed inoperable to optimal medical treatment (including BAV) or TAVI. The results of the inoperable arm were first reported.[22] All-cause mortality (30.7% vs. 50.7%, $P < .001$), cardiovascular mortality (19.6% vs. 41.9%, $P < .001$), repeat hospitalization (22.3% vs. 44.1%, $P < .001$), and the composite end point of death or repeat hospitalization (42.5% vs.71.6%, $P < .001$) were seen less frequently in patients randomized to TAVI. In follow-up, there was no evidence degeneration of the valvular prosthesis or restenosis up to 2 years.[118] Heart failure symptoms were less severe in patients treated with TAVI. Patients treated with TAVI had a higher incidence of major vascular complications (16.2% vs 1.1%, $P < .001$), major bleeding (22.3% vs. 11.2%, $P < .001$), and of major strokes (5.0% vs.1.1%, $P = .06$). In patients with severe AS who are not suitable for AVR, TAVI should be the new standard of care.

The results of the high-risk operative cohort were reported 1 year later.[23] All-cause mortality at 30 days was slightly lower with TAVI (3.4% vs. 6.5%, $P = .07$) but was similar at 1- (24.2% vs. 26.8%), 2- (33.9% vs. 35%), and 3-year (44.2% vs. 44.8%) follow-up.[3,8] Although the rates of all neurologic events were higher after TAVI at 30 days and 1 year (5.5% vs. 2.4% and 8.3% vs. 4.3%, $P < .05$), rates of major strokes were not significantly different between TAVI and SAVR at 30 days (3.8% vs. 2.1%, $P = .2$) or at 1 year (5.1% vs. 2.4%, $P = .07$). There were other important differences in periprocedural risks between the two groups, with more major vascular complications at 30 days after TAVI (11.0% vs. 3.2%, $P < .001$), and more major bleeding (19.5% vs. 9.3%, $P < .001$) and new-onset atrial fibrillation (16.0% vs. 8.6%, $P = .006$) after SAVR. Marked improvement of symptoms was similar after TAVI and SAVR and was sustained at 3 years in both the groups.[119] From these results, TAVI emerged as a viable alternative to SAVR in high risk patients, the choice being guided by the decision of the interdisciplinary heart team.

PARTNER 2 Trial

The aim of the PARTNER II trial is to compare the safety and effectiveness of the SAPIEN XT with the NovaFlex delivery system versus the Edwards SAPIEN valve in a randomized controlled trial, using rigorous trial methodologies including the VARC 2 definitions[84] for clinical outcome. The study design is shown on Fig. 53.10. It had two independently randomized populations: (1) the inoperable cohort, which randomized patients to SAPIEN XT vs. SAPIEN via a TF approach, and (2) the moderate risk cohort, which randomized patients to AVR vs. TAVR with the SAPIEN XT and included the transapical, transaortic, or TF approach. In addition to these populations, there were other nonrandomized, nested registries for the inoperable population: (1) inoperable small vessel, (2) inoperable transapical, (3) valve-in-valve (ViV), (4) transaortic, (5) 29-mm SAPIEN XT TF, (6) 29-mm SAPIEN XT TA, and (7) 20-mm SAPIEN 3. The primary end point of

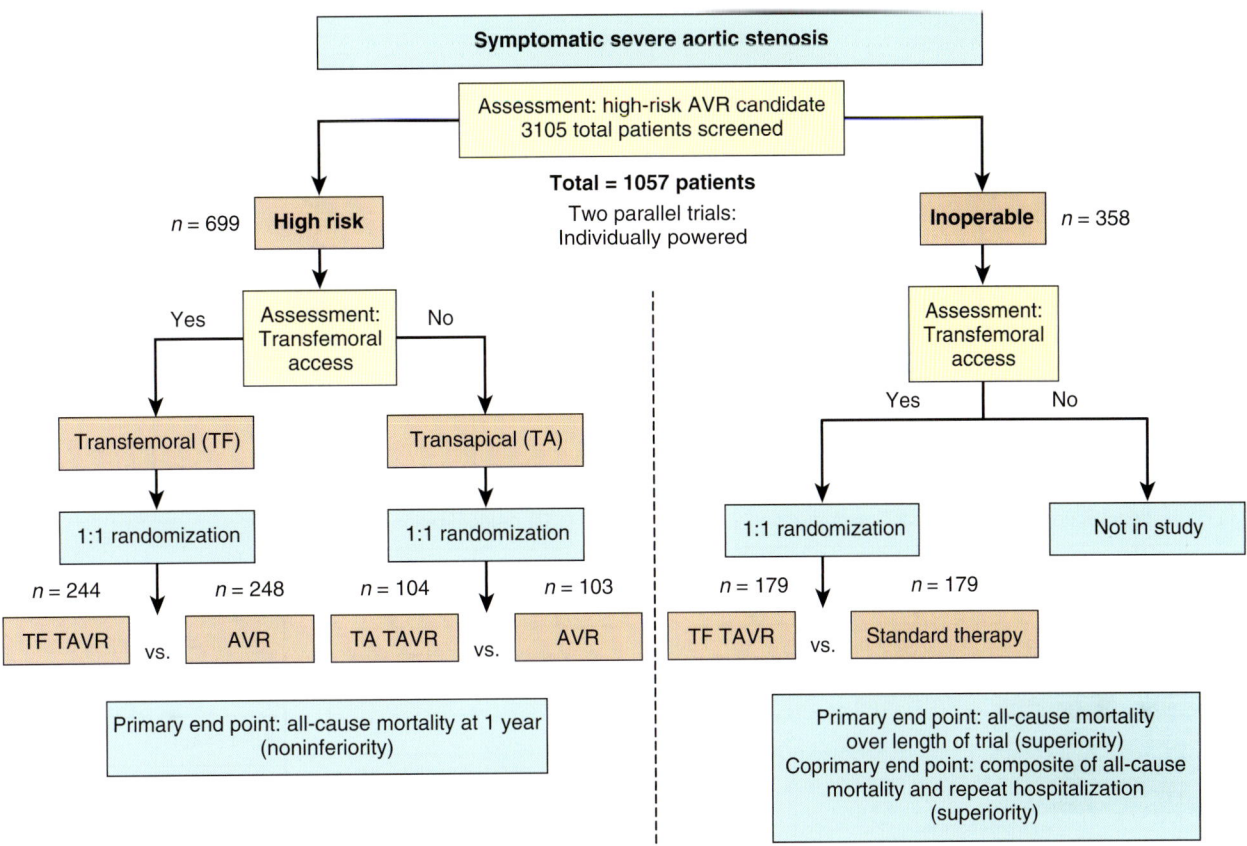

Fig. 53.9 The PARTNER trial is a multicenter randomized trial that evaluated the SAPIEN valve in the inoperable and high-risk operable population of patients with severe symptomatic aortic stenosis. *AVR*, Aortic valve replacement; *TAVR*, transcatheter aortic valve replacement.

the inoperable cohort was composite end point of death, disabling stroke, and repeat hospitalization. In the inoperable/high-risk arm, there was no significant difference in the incidence of the components of the composite end point or in the combined end point (P = .6) at 30 days or 1 year, whereas major vascular events were more common with the SAPIEN system (15.5% vs. 9.6%, P = .04), reaching the noninferiority threshold.[120] Valve performance was similar. The 29-mm prosthesis had a similar performance in the nonrandomized registries.[121,122] The intermediate-risk cohort was composed of patients with an STS score greater than 4% and randomized patients to TAVR vs. AVR. Its primary end point is the nonhierarchical incidence of stroke or death at 2 years. The event rate of all cause death or disabling stroke was 19.3% in the TAVR group and 21% in the surgery group (P = .001 for noninferiority). In the TF cohort, TAVI TF was associated with a lower rate of death or disabling stroke (hazard ration [HR] 0.79; 95% confidence interval [CI] 0.62 to 1; P = .05). TAVR resulted in a larger aortic valve area and a lower rate of acute kidney injury and new-onset atrial fibrillation, whereas surgery resulted in less paravalvular regurgitation and fewer vascular complications.[84]

The SAPIEN 3 valve was evaluated in the high-risk and intermediate-risk population within the PARTNER 2 trial. A single-arm nonrandomized registry included 583 high-risk and inoperable patients in 29 U.S. sites and used a historical control for comparison. With a mean age of 82.7 ± 8.1 years and a median STS score of 8.4%, 1-year survival was 85.6% for all patients. All and disabling stroke occurred in 1.4% and 0.9% at 30 days and 4.3% and 2.4% at 1 year.[123] These results led to the FDA approval of the SAPIEN 3 valve for high-risk and inoperable patients with severe symptomatic AS.

Using historical controls enrolled in the PARTNER 2 intermediate-risk randomized trial as a comparator, the SAPIEN 3 valve was in intermediate-risk patients with similar characteristics in the PARTNER SAPIEN 3 intermediate-risk registry[124]; 1077 patients with severe symptomatic AS who were at intermediate risk for surgical mortality were included. The primary end point was the composite of death from any cause, all strokes, and incidence of moderate or severe aortic regurgitation. At 1-year follow-up, the all-cause mortality and stroke rates were 7.4% and 2%, respectively, in the TAVR group. The primary composite end point was both noninferior (P < .0001) and superior (P < .0001) to surgical valve replacement. These results resulted in the FDA approval of the SAPIEN 3 prosthesis in the intermediate-risk patient group.

PARTNER 3

The PARTNER 3 trial will evaluate low-risk patients with severe symptomatic AS randomized to surgical valve replacement versus TAVI. Enrollment has completed and is in a follow-up phase. The study includes a CT substudy for patients in the surgical or TAVI arm. A continued access registry will be set up for participating centers until the result are available.

Transcatheter Valve Therapy Registry

The STS/ACC Transcatheter Valve Therapy (TVT) Registry was established in the United States as a tool for postmarket surveillance of catheter prostheses and to determine the quality of outcomes in individual centers. Enrollment in the registry is mandatory for any implanting U.S. site. With more than

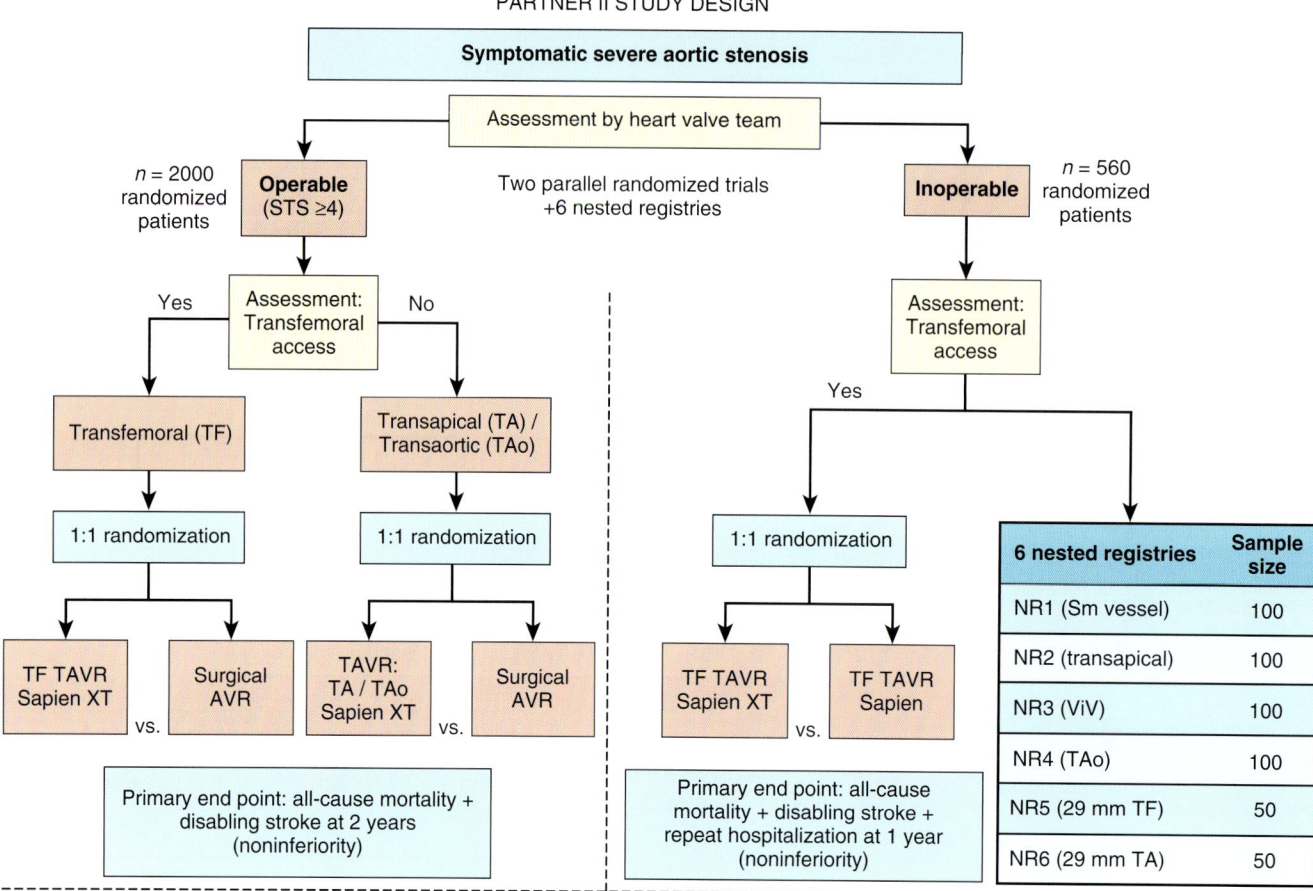

Fig. 53.10 The PARTNER 2 trial (b) evaluated the SAPIEN XT valve and is composed of an inoperable population randomized to SAPIEN XT vs. SAPIEN with multiple nonrandomized nested registries *(NR)* and of an operable intermediate-risk population randomized to transcatheter aortic valve implantation with SAPIEN XT or surgical aortic valve replacement. *AVR*, Aortic valve replacement; *STS*, Society of Thoracic Surgeons; *TAVR*, transcatheter aortic valve replacement; *ViV*, valve-in-valve.

55,000 patients enrolled and followed for up to 1 year, the data have been used to create risk assessment specific for TAVR and benchmark national outcomes. In its latest analysis, the expected 30-day operative mortality (STS-PROM) has decreased from 7% to 6% over 3 years, reflecting a change in the indication for the procedure. In addition, the observed in-hospital (5.7% to 2.9%) and 1-year mortality (25.8% to 21.6%) has decreased from the same time period.[125] Further analysis also suggested sites with larger TAVR volumes were associated with lower in-hospital risk-adjusted outcomes including mortality ($P < .02$), vascular complications ($P < .003$), and bleeding ($P < .001$).[126]

TAVI can be used for the treatment of bioprosthetic valve dysfunction. Originally evaluated in the PARTNER ViV registry, high-risk and inoperable patients presenting with bioprosthetic valve dysfunction were treated with the SAPIEN valve. With significant procedural success and a low 30-day mortality,[127] the SAPIEN and SAPIEN XT valves were approved for this indication. Valve type and build, internal dimensions, and radiographic characteristics define the TAVI size and position. The TAVI prosthesis is placed so that in the expanded position, the ventricular side of the TAVI is at the level of sowing ring. Patients undergoing ViV procedures are at risk for coronary obstruction. Preprocedural planning with CT assessment is critical to avoid coronary obstruction. A virtual ring to coronary distance of greater than 4 mm and large sinus of Valsalva are useful characteristics in avoiding coronary obstruction in patients whose coronary arteries are below or at the level of the valve posts. Survival is dependent on the nature of valve dysfunction, and AI is associated with better survival than AS.[128] A smaller bioprosthetic valve is associated with a higher postprocedural gradient and a higher likelihood of patient prosthetic mismatch. The impact of patient prosthetic mismatch in patients undergoing ViV procedures needs to be assessed. Bioprosthetic valve dysfunction can be treated with the SAPIEN 3 valve in the aortic, mitral, tricuspid, and pulmonary position.

Complications After Balloon-Expandable Transcatheter Aortic Valve Replacement (Table 53.5)

Stroke

The general incidence of clinically significant stroke is 2.5% to 4.2%,[99,100,103,105,116] and it seriously affects survival and QOL.[23] Stroke etiology is obviously multifactorial, as shown by the occurrence of cardiovascular events either during, shortly after, or even far from the TAVI procedure.[129] Strokes occur in 87% of patients within 24 hours post-TAVI. It was originally postulated that the rate of cerebrovascular accident was going to be lower in the transapical approach because the aortic arch was not manipulated; however, the incidence appears to be similar. Recent studies suggest a higher incidence of subclinical perfusion abnormalities documented by magnetic resonance imaging (MRI).[130] Cerebral embolization can occur during the passage of the valve across the aortic arch, while trying to traverse the aortic valve to gain access into the LV, during

TABLE 53.5 Procedural Characteristics and Complications of Patients Undergoing Transcatheter Aortic Valve Implantation with the Edwards SAPIEN, SAPIEN XT, and SAPIEN 3 Valve

Study	Procedural Mortality (%)	30-Day Mortality (%)	Valve-in-Valve (%)	Conversion to Open AVR (%)	AI ≥ 2± (%)	Major CVA/TIA (%)	Major Vascular Complications (%)	MI (%)	Acute Kidney Injury (%)	Pacemaker (%)	Major Bleeding (%)
Canada TF[107]	1.8	9.5	2.4	1.2	6	0.6	13.1	0.6	1.8	3.6	NR
Canada TA[107]	1.7	11.3	2.8	2.3	6	0.6	13	1.7	3.4	6.2	NR
Source TA[106]	NR	10.3	3.3	3.5	2.3	2.6	2.4	0.6	7.1	7	9.9
SourceTF[106]	NR	6.3	0.6	1.7	1.5	2.4	10.6	0.6	1.3	7	8.9
SOURCE XT[112]	NR	4.0			5.5						
PARTNER Cohort B[22]	1.1	5.0	1.7	0	12	5/0	16.2	0	1.1	3.4	16.8
PARTNER Cohort A[23]	0.9	3.4	2	2.6	12.2	5.6	11	0	1.2	3.8	9.3
PARTNER EU TF[111]	1.6	8.2	NR	1.6	5	3.3	7.2	3.3	NR	1.8	NR
PARTNER EU TA[111]	1.4	18.8	1.4	3	5	1.5	NR	6	2	3.8	NR
FRANCE TF[114]	NR	8.4	NR	NR	9	4.2	6.3	2	1	5.3	NR
FRANCE TA[114]	NR	16.9	NR	NR	9	1.4	5.6	0	2.8	5.6	NR
FRANCE 2 TF[116]	2.9	8.5	1.4	0.4%	13.9	1.9	2.7	NR	NR	11.5	2
FRANCE 2 TA[116]	4.1	13.9	2.9	0.7	9	4.4	1.9	NR	NR	13.6	3.4
PARTNER 2A[84]	0.9	3.9	12.3	0.001	0.001	5.5	7.9	1.2	1.3	8.5	NR
SAPIEN 3 HIGH RISK[123]	NR	2.5	14.4	0	0.001	2.6	NR	NR	NR	16.8	NR
SAPIEN 3 Intermediate[126]	NR	1.1	7.4	NR	1.7	2.7	NR	1.5	0.5	10.2	6.1

AI, Aortic insufficiency; *AVR*, Aortic valve replacement; *CVA*, cerebrovascular accident; *MI*, myocardial infarction; *NR*, not reported; *TA*, transapical; *TF*, transfemoral; *TIA*, transient ischemic attack

BAV, and valve implantation. The use of cerebral embolic protection devices during TAVI is currently being evaluated. The Sentinel Trial documented safety of the Claret device (Claret Medical, Santa Rosa, CA) but failed to find a statistically significant difference in neurocognitive function or brain MRI new lesion volume.[131] The patients who are at highest risk of stroke or who would benefit the most from embolic protection are yet to be identified.

Heart Block

Conduction abnormalities are commonly seen in the patients undergoing TAVI due to the proximity of the aortic annulus with the left bundle branch and the atrioventricular node. The incidence of conduction abnormalities in patients undergoing TAVI with the SAPIEN prosthesis is relatively low and not significantly different than after SAVR. In the PARTNER trial, incidence of complete heart block requiring a pacemaker (PPM) was 4.7% (cohort B) and 5.7 % (cohort A), 9% (SAPIEN 3 intermediate risk), left bundle branch block 12%, first-degree aortic valve block 15%. The presence of a preexisting right bundle branch block, calcification in the noncoronary cusp, and the degree of oversizing the prosthesis in relation to the left ventricular outflow tract are predisposing factors to pacemaker dependency.[132,133] Conduction defects are transient when related to trauma to the conduction tissue; however, if there is myocyte necrosis in the interventricular septum, then new atrioventricular block will likely develop. With the CoreValve revalving system, the insertion depth into the LV cavity is associated with more frequent complete heart block.[134]

Renal Dysfunction

Acute kidney injury post-TAVI is not uncommon and has an incidence of 12% to 28% and may progress to the need for renal replacement therapy in 1.4%. The presence of hypertension (odds ratio [OR] = 4.66), chronic obstructive pulmonary disease (OR = 2.64), and transfusion requirement (OR = 3.47) are important risk factors for its development. The presence of acute kidney injury is associated with mortality (28% vs. 7%).[122,123] When compared with surgery, acute kidney injury (9.2% vs. 25%) and need for dialysis (2.5% vs. 8.7%) are less common in patients undergoing TAVI. Patients who develop advanced stages of acute kidney injury postprocedure are associated with mortality.[135]

Severe Aortic Insufficiency

Severe AI is a rare event. According to its etiology, it may be categorized as valvular or perivalvular. Valvular (central) is most commonly caused by the guidewire and disappears once the wire is removed. It is rarely caused by prosthetic malfunction or when the native leaflets interfere with prosthetic function. This is treated with placement of a new valve inside the previously placed valve. Perivalvular insufficiency results in an incomplete coverage of the annulus by the stent frame or a malposition of the prosthesis (too aortic or too ventricular). It is a serious concern because more than mild AI has been shown to be associated with impaired midterm outcome.[84] All effort must be done to prevent paravalvular AI by rigorous assessment of the annulus shape and dimension by CT scan. Paravalvular is due to: (1) inappropriate sizing, (2) malposition, or (3) stent underexpansion. Valve postdilatation may be performed cautiously by adding 1 or 2 mL to the same balloon catheter, which must be centered within the valve. Because the stent has a skirt that does not allow further expansion, postdilatation with a larger balloon may cause flaring of the aortic portion of the stent, changing the conformation of the ventricular portion that may worsen the AI. The incidence of paravalvular AI continues to decrease as new valve sizes become available, valves are sized appropriately, and modifications to the valve skirt are adopted as confirmed by the 1.5% rate of paravalvular AI at 1 year with the SAPIEN 3 prosthesis.[123] As newer-generation valves continue to appear, it is likely that this consequence will be further reduced.

Valve Embolization

Valve embolization is generally due to malposition, undersizing the prosthesis, or inappropriate capture during RVP. Valvular embolization to the LV cavity uniformly requires urgent thoracotomy for removal of the prosthesis and replacement of the aortic valve. If aortic embolization occurs, it is imperative not to remove the guidewire from across the prosthetic valve until it is anchored in the distal aorta, because this prevents it from turning. A balloon catheter is placed in the proximal end of the valve and the valve is then pulled until it can be deployed or fully expanded distal to the left subclavian artery. After the embolized valve is fixed, a new valve can be placed in the aortic position while correcting the original cause of the complication. If the guidewire is removed prior to fixing the valve in place, the valve may become inverted, not allowing the passage of blood through it. Unless the valve can be opened with a stent or surgically, this complication is often fatal. Aortic angiography is recommended after valve manipulation because it can cause aortic dissection.

Vascular Complications

Vascular complications occur in 6.6% of cases. They more commonly occur in the TF approach (8% vs. 3.6%)[103] but are more likely to be fatal in the transapical approach. Vascular complications include small dissection, vascular perforation, and vessel avulsion. Prevention is preferred, hence the importance of vascular screening and the determination of the appropriate luminal diameter and absence of luminal calcification. Although previously associated with higher mortality, with increasing experience, vascular complications are easy to prepare for, thus decreasing their mortality. They may arise from difficult sheath insertion or prolonged sheath time, as the adluminal surface adheres to the endothelium. They are easily recognized by sudden onset of hypotension. Aortic occlusion balloons should be accessible to minimize bleeding while stabilizing the patient. With the availability of expandable sheaths, catheter modifications that allow the passage through a smaller arteriotomy site, the availability of alternative access routes, and the multidisciplinary approach for device implant, the frequency of vascular complications will continue to fall as noted in the PARTNER 2 and SAPIEN 3 registries.[84,123]

Aortic Root Dissection and Annular Rupture

Aortic root dissections may occur if the native valve is not appropriately predilated and the passage of the prosthesis is vigorous or after attempts to capture an embolized valve. Aortic annular tear is seen in patients with a heavily calcified aortic root and can be avoided by limiting the degree of prosthesis oversizing. These rare complications require urgent conversion to surgery and are often fatal.

Coronary Obstruction

The SAPIEN prosthesis in placed in the subcoronary position and should not interfere with the coronary ostia or future attempts of percutaneous revascularization.[136] Coronary obstruction occurs in 0.6% of cases and is seen in patients with effacement of the sinotubular junction, which causes the coronary ostia to migrate.[100] Determination of the distance of the ostia to the aortic annulus by CT angiography is routinely performed during patient screening. Coronary obstruction may be inconsequential if patients have functioning coronary artery bypass grafts. If occlusion occurs, emergency revascularization can be performed.

BALLOON-EXPANDABLE TRANSCATHETER AORTIC VALVE IMPLANTATION

The issue of long-term durability of TAVI valves compared with surgical bioprosthesis has become an important issue with the expansion of TAVI to lower-risk/younger patients. With the balloon-expandable valves, the randomized PARTNER I trial has reported reassuring data at 5 years[137] with no cases of structural valve deterioration in both groups. In the literature, the rate of structural valve deterioration (SVD) after SAVR remains clearly underestimated because it is commonly assessed by the need of reintervention. Standardizing the definition of SVD on echocardiographic assessment was thus mandatory. In Europe a statement from the European Society of Cardiology/European Association for Cardio-Thoracic Surgery has been published,[138] followed by a consensus statement from the Valve In Valve International Data group.[139] Based on annual echocardiography post–balloon-expandable TAVI, in 2018 Eltchaninoff et al. first reported on the Rouen series on durability beyond 5 years[140] from the first-in-human in 2002 to 2012. Using the European criteria, only two patients (0.58%) had reintervention and only 9 patients (3.2%) had moderate SVD. In the series of Deusch et al.[141] with 300 patients and using the same European criteria, the rate of SVD at 7 years was 14.9%. Other studies on long-term durability of transcatheter valves are ongoing. Even though limited by the poor survival of compassionate or high-risk patients in all series, there is no alarm so far on long-term durability of the transcatheter valves. However, how these data will translate in a younger and lower-risk population remains unknown so far.

CONCLUSIONS

TAVI has revolutionized the way we treat patients with severe AS and bioprosthetic valve dysfunction. As patients of all surgical risk profiles are treated with TAVR, it is likely that instead of focusing on surgical risk, consideration for TAVR will be based primarily on anatomic risk. The long-term impact of conduction abnormalities and paravalvular insufficiency will help to guide patient candidacy for current TAVI technologies and future improvement in the TAVI prostheses. Due to its versatility, configuration, and ease of use, the SAPIEN family of valves will continue to be used routinely. Expanding indications to the low-risk, asymptomatic, and heart failure population will be evaluated in ongoing clinical trials. The future of TAVI continues to be written.

KEY REFERENCES

22. Leon MB, Smith CR, Mack M, et al. Transcatheter aortic-valve implantation for aortic stenosis in patients who cannot undergo surgery. *N Engl J Med.* 2010;363:1597–1607.
23. Smith CR, Leon MB, Mack MJ, et al. Transcatheter versus surgical aortic-valve replacement in high-risk patients. *N Engl J Med.* 2011;364:2187–2198.
34. Eltchaninoff H, Durand E, Borz B, et al. Balloon aortic valvuloplasty in the era of transcatheter aortic valve replacement: acute and long-term outcomes. *Am Heart J.* 2014;167:235–240.

68. Cribier A, Eltchaninoff H, Tron C, et al. Early experience with percutaneous transcatheter implantation of heart valve prosthesis for the treatment of end-stage inoperable patients with calcific aortic stenosis. *J Am Coll Cardiol*. 2004;43:698–703.
70. Cribier A, Eltchaninoff H, Tron C, et al. Treatment of calcific aortic stenosis with the percutaneous heart valve: mid-term follow-up from the initial feasibility studies: the French experience. *J Am Coll Cardiol*. 2006;47:1214–1223.
74. Webb JG, Chandavimol M, Thompson CR, et al. Percutaneous aortic valve implantation retrograde from the femoral artery. *Circulation*. 2006;113:842–850.
84. Leon MB, Smith CR, Mack MJ, et al. Transcatheter or surgical aortic-valve replacement in intermediate-risk patients. *N Engl J Med*. 2016;374:1609–1620.
100. Webb JG, Pasupati S, Humphries K, et al. Percutaneous transarterial aortic valve replacement in selected high-risk patients with aortic stenosis. *Circulation*. 2007;116:755–763.
112. Schymik G, Lefevre Y, Bartorelli AL, et al. European experience with the second-generation Edwards SAPIEN XT transcatheter heart valve in patients with severe aortic stenosis: 1-year outcomes from the SOURCE XT Registry. *JACC Cardiovasc Interv*. 2015;8(5):657–669.
116. Gilard M, Eltchaninoff H, Iung B, et al. Registry of transcatheter aortic-valve implantation in high-risk patients. *N Engl J Med*. 2012;366:1705–1715.
117. Gilard M, Eltchaninoff H, Donzeau-Gouge P, et al. Late outcomes of transcatheter aortic valve replacement in high-risk patients. The FRANCE-2 Registry. *J Am Coll Cardiol*. 2016;68(15):1637–1647.
120. Kodali SK, Williams MR, Smith CR, et al. Two-year outcomes after transcatheter or surgical aortic-valve replacement. *N Engl J Med*. 2012;366:1686–1695.
121. Webb JG, Doshi D, Mack M, et al. A randomized evaluation of the Sapien XT transcatheter heart valve system in patients with aortic stenosis who are not surgical candidates. *J Am Coll Cardiol Intv*. 2015;8:1797–1806.
123. Herrmann H, Thourani V, Kodali SK, et al. One year clinical outcomes with Sapien 3 transcatheter aortic valve replacement in high risk and inoperable patients with severe aortic stenosis. *Circulation*. 2016;134:130–140.
124. Thourani V, Kodali S, Makkar R, et al. Transcatheter aortic valve replacement versus surgical valve replacement in intermediate risk patients: a propensity score analysis. *Lancet*. 2016;387:2218–2225.
126. Carroll JD, Vemulapalli S, Dai D, et al. Procedural experience for transcatheter aortic valve replacement and relation to outcomes. *J Am Coll Cardiol*. 2017;70:29–41.
127. Webb JG, Mack M, White J, et al. Transcatheter aortic valve implantation within degenerated aortic surgical bioprostheses. Partner 2 valve in valve registry. *J Am Coll Cardiol*. 2017;69:2253–2262.
128. Dvir D, Webb JG, Bleiziffer S, et al. Transcatheter aortic valve implantation in failed surgical bioprosthetic valves. *JAMA*. 2014;312:162–170.
131. Kapadia S, Kodali S, Makkar S, et al. Protection against cerebral embolism during transcatheter aortic valve replacement. *J Am Coll Cardiol*. 2017;69:367–377.
133. Nazif TM, Williams MR, Hahn RT, et al. Clinical implications of new-onset left bundle branch block after transcatheter aortic valve replacement: analysis of the PARTNER experience. *Eur Heart J*. 2014;35:1599–1607.
137. Mack MJ, Leon MB, Smith CR, et al. 5-Year outcomes of transcatheter aortic valve replacement or surgical valve replacement for high surgical risk patients with aortic stenosis. *Lancet*. 2015;385:2477–2484.
138. Copodamo D, Petronio AS, Prendergast B, et al. Standardized definitions of structural deterioration and valve failure in assessing long-term durability of transcatheter and surgical aortic bioprosthetic valves: a consensus statement from the European Association of Percutaneous Cardiovascular Interventions (EAPCI) endorsed by the European Society of Cardiology (ESC) and the European Association for Cardio-Thoracic Surgery (EACTS). *Eur Cardiothorac Surg*. 2017;52:408–417.
140. Eltchaninoff H, Durand E, Avinee G, et al. Assessment of structural valve deterioration of transcatheter aortic bioprosthetic valves using the new European consensus definition. pii: EIJ-D-18-00358. https://doi.org/10.4244/EIJ-D-18-00358. [Epub ahead of print].

 Additional references available online at expertconsult.com.

中文导读

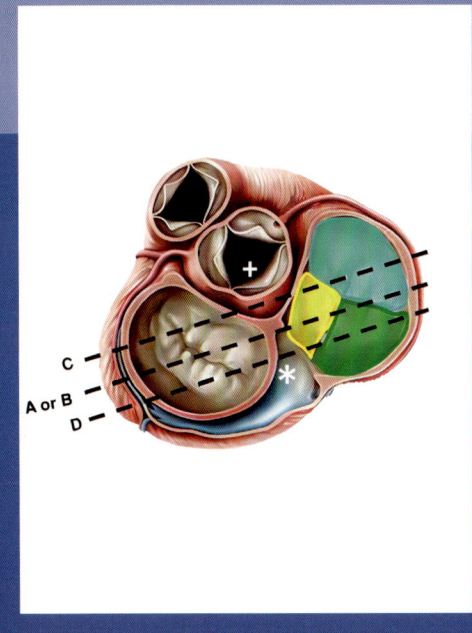

第54章
自膨胀式瓣膜经导管主动脉瓣置换术

经导管主动脉瓣置换术目前已成为主动脉瓣重度狭窄患者治疗的重要选择。在美国，经导管主动脉瓣置换术治疗的患者数量已经超过了外科开胸换瓣手术。最常应用的自膨胀瓣膜包括Core Valve家族经典的Core Valve瓣膜、Evolut-R、Evolut-34 mm、Evolut-PRO等。环上瓣的设计使得自膨胀瓣膜可以获得更低的跨瓣压差，部分可回收的功能可以为瓣膜更好的定位。CT影像学评估是自膨胀瓣膜术前评估选择适宜瓣膜避免并发症的关键工具。与外科手术相比，经导管主动脉瓣置换术新发房颤、出血、急性肾损伤和卒中发生率更低，早期恢复好，生活质量高，但残余主动脉瓣反流和起搏器植入比例高。与球囊扩张瓣膜相比，外科生物瓣毁损应用自膨胀瓣膜因其环上瓣设计，可以提供更小的压差。在终末期肾病、低压差、低心排血量综合征、主动脉瓣反流、二瓣化畸形等特殊患者中，随着新一代器械开发，经导管主动脉瓣置换术也得到了不错的结果。

本章主要从上述方面介绍Core Valve家族和自膨胀经导管主动脉瓣置换术瓣膜的设计特点；通过一系列临床研究结果介绍了夯实自膨胀瓣膜的治疗价值，描述了自膨胀经导管主动脉瓣置换术瓣膜相关的并发症，并展望了未来几年将在美国应用的新型自膨胀生物瓣。

张　倩　张洪亮

章节要点

- 随着大量随机研究证据的积累，经导管主动脉瓣置换术已经成为外科手术风险增加的主动脉瓣狭窄患者的重要治疗方式。在美国，经导管主动脉瓣置换术治疗的患者数量已经超过了外科开胸换瓣手术。

- 最常应用的自膨胀瓣膜包括Core Valve家族的经典Core Valve瓣膜、Evolut-R、Evolut-34 mm、Evolut-PRO等，环上瓣的设计使得自膨胀瓣膜可以获得更低的跨瓣压差，部分可回收的功能可以为瓣膜更好的定位。

- CT影像学评估是自膨胀式瓣膜评估的重要工具，可以通过瓣环周长测量来进行偏大瓣膜选择。可以评估主动脉窦宽度和冠脉高度评估来进行放置安全评估。这些技术可以减少置入后的主动脉瓣残余反流。

- 与外科手术相比，经导管主动脉瓣置换术后房颤、出血、急性肾损伤和部分临床研究中卒中发生率更低，但是残余主动脉瓣反流及术后起搏器植入发生率高。而且经导管主动脉瓣置换术功能恢复更早，生活质量更高。

- 随着自膨胀瓣膜的鞘直径越来越小，直接主动脉入路、锁骨下动脉、颈动脉或经腔静脉入路目前已经很少使用，这些入路仅应用于股动脉入路受限的患者。

- 外科瓣膜毁损应用自膨胀型瓣膜，因为环上瓣设计，任何尺寸外科生物瓣毁损患者自膨胀瓣膜应用后与球囊扩张瓣膜相比压差更低。但外科生物瓣毁损人群应注意避免冠状动脉阻塞。

- 其他自膨胀瓣膜经导管主动脉瓣置换术的指征包括终末期肾病、低压差低输出主动脉瓣狭窄、原发性主动脉瓣反流和主动脉瓣二瓣化相关疾病。新一代经导管主动脉瓣置换术对这些种类的患者处理前景充满希望。

- 自膨胀瓣膜相关并发症正在下降，尤其是随着低风险患者的应用。传导阻滞发生率虽然目前设计器械中有所下降，但仍然在一些患者中是主要问题。

- 新的镍钛非磁性合金经导管主动脉瓣置换术器械，如Acurate Neo、Lotus Edge和Portico在美国很快会进入临床应用。

54 Self-Expanding Transcatheter Aortic Valve Replacement

Mark K. Tuttle, Nima Nasiri, Jeffrey J. Popma

KEY POINTS

- Transcatheter aortic valve replacement (TAVR) has become the default therapy for patients with aortic stenosis who, based on an expanding randomized evidence base, are at increased risk for surgery. TAVR procedures have now surpassed the number of surgical aortic valve replacements in the United States.
- The most frequently used self-expanding bioprostheses—the CoreValve family of CoreValve Classic, Evolut-R, Evolut-34 mm, and Evolut-PRO—have specific design features of annular conformability; supra-annular valve location, resulting in lower gradients; and partial retrievability, allowing for optimal positioning of the bioprosthesis.
- Computed tomographic imaging is an essential tool for self-expanding TAVR, allowing for oversizing relative to the perimeter-based annular dimensions as well as determining the safety of implantation with the assessment of sinus of Valsalva widths and coronary heights. These techniques have enabled a reduction in the rate of residual aortic valve regurgitation after implantation.
- Compared with surgery, TAVR has lower rates of atrial fibrillation, bleeding complications, acute kidney injury, and stroke reduction in some series, but it also means higher rates of residual aortic regurgitation and pacemaker use. TAVR is associated with improved early functional recovery and quality of life.
- Owing to the reduction in sheath size required for self-expanding TAVR, alternative access methods using direct aortic, subclavian, carotid, or transcaval approaches are rarely needed but can provide options for patients with limited iliofemoral access.
- The use of self-expanding TAVR for failed surgical valves is particularly beneficial given the supra-annular design, which allows lower gradients than balloon-expandable TAVR for any given size of surgical valve. Care must be taken to avoid coronary occlusion in this setting.
- Other indications for self-expanding TAVR include end-stage renal disease; low-gradient, low-output aortic stenosis; primary aortic regurgitation; and bicuspid aortic valve disease. TAVR appears promising in this subset of patients with the next generation of devices.
- Complications associated with self-expanding TAVR are decreasing, particularly when lower-risk patients are treated. Conduction disturbances, although lower with contemporary designs, remain problematic for some patients.
- Additional Nitinol-based TAVR devices—such at the Acurate Neo, Lotus Edge, and Portico—will soon be available for patients in the United States.

INTRODUCTION

It has been less that a decade since the initial commercial introduction of transcatheter aortic valve replacement (TAVR) in the United States for patients with symptomatic aortic stenosis who are deemed unsuitable for surgery. Since the advent of percutaneous coronary intervention in 1977, no transcatheter therapy has transformed the management of patients with cardiovascular disease as profoundly as has TAVR. Based on an ever-increasing portfolio of well-designed and executed clinical studies demonstrating the value of TAVR over surgery, practice guidelines now support the use of TAVR for patients deemed at extreme or high risk for surgery (class I) by a multidisciplinary heart team as well as for patients deemed at intermediate risk for surgery (class IIa).[1,2] Most recently, randomized trials of TAVR in patients at low risk for surgery now support this indication as well (NR1, NR2), and practice guidelines are expected to reflect this in their next iteration; their results will likely facilitate further paradigmatic shifts for physicians and patients who seek to determine the most appropriate method of aortic valve replacement.

Two general concepts of TAVR prostheses have been developed: the first facilitates transcatheter valve deployment by means of balloon expansion, using a plastically deformable metal frame; the second facilitates valve deployment using self-expanding or mechanically expanded Nitinol prostheses that provide constant outward force to secure the prosthesis without migration. Although both techniques have led to outstanding results and can be used safely in the majority of patients with severe aortic stenosis, there are differences between the two methods that may render one more appropriate than the other on the basis of clinical and anatomic parameters.

The purposes of this chapter are as follows: (1) to review the design of the CoreValve family of self-expanding TAVR devices; (2) to discuss the clinical results from the expansive array of clinical studies establishing the value of self-expanding TAVR devices; (3) to review the complications associated with self-expanding TAVR devices; and (4) to catalog the additional self-expanding bioprostheses that will be available for commercial use in the United States over the next several years.

COREVALVE AND EVOLUT-R/EVOLUT-PRO SELF-EXPANDING TRANSCATHETER AORTIC VALVE REPLACEMENT

CoreValve "Classic"

Multiple iterations of the CoreValve transcatheter heart valve have been developed over the past decade to improve the performance of the self-expanding prosthesis. The first-generation CoreValve comprised a 25-Fr delivery catheter that housed a self-expanding Nitinol frame supporting a bovine pericardial valve. The second-generation 21-Fr delivery catheter used lower-profile porcine pericardial tissue and scalloped the inflow portion

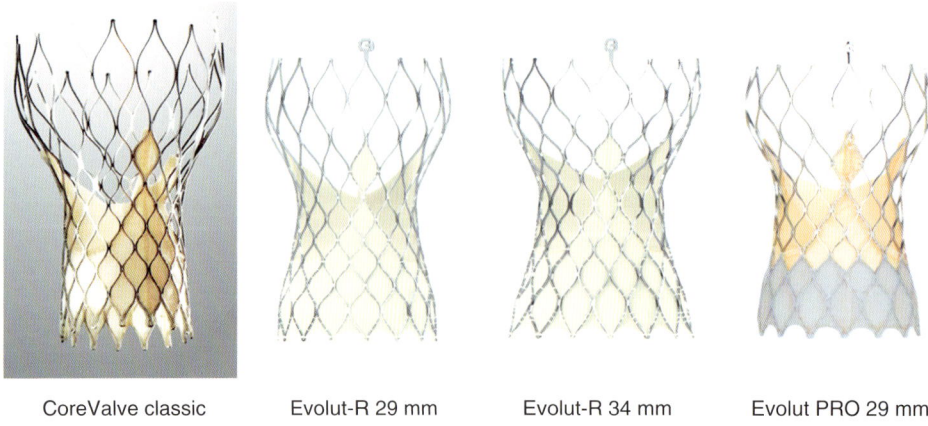

CoreValve classic   Evolut-R 29 mm   Evolut-R 34 mm   Evolut PRO 29 mm

Fig. 54.1 The CoreValve family of self-expanding bioprosthetic designs. (Courtesy Medtronic, 2019.)

of the valve in order to provide better flow hemodynamics. The third-generation 18-Fr CoreValve transcatheter aortic valve achieved its lower profile by cutting the skirt and leaflet into six independent sections and sewing them onto the Nitinol frame. This valve design was approved by the Conformiteé Européenne (CE Mark) in March 2007 and by the U.S. Food and Drug Administration (FDA) for extreme-risk patients in January 2014; it was approved for high-risk patients in April 2014.

The basic design concepts of the CoreValve Classic transcatheter heart valve have been retained over successive generations. They include (1) a self-expanding Nitinol support frame with cells configured in a diamond cell design that anchors a trileaflet supra-annular porcine pericardial tissue valve (Fig. 54.1); (2) an 18-Fr Accutrek delivery catheter that has evolved into a low-profile 14- to 16-Fr Enveo In Line sheath; and (3) a disposable loading system. The CoreValve Classic was available in the following sizes: 23 mm (annular diameter 18 to 20 mm), 26 mm (aortic annular diameter 20 to 23 mm), 29 mm (annular diameter 24 to 26 mm), and 31 mm (annular diameter 26 to 29 mm).[3] The Nitinol frame has three levels of radial and hoop strength. The inflow portion exerts a high radial expansive force to secure the frame within the aortic annulus. The strength of this portion of the frame prevents annular recoil; allows the frame to partially conform to the noncircular shape of the aortic annulus, thus preventing frame migration; and minimizes the occurrence of paravalvular leaks. The "constrained" center portion of the frame has a high hoop strength, which resists size and shape deformation; this is critical, as this portion of the frame contains the supra-annular valve leaflets. The frame is concave at this location to avoid blocking the coronary ostium with the native valve and allows coronary cannulation after the implantation. The outflow portion of the frame exerts low radial forces and serves to orient the frame to the aorta parallel to flow through the valve. Porcine pericardium was selected due to its lower profile (compared with bovine pericardium) and its documented durability. The three leaflet elements are constructed with long commissures, similar to a "suspension bridge." These distribute the aortic pressure load more uniformly to the valve leaflets and the commissural posts. An angled take-off of the posts further reduces stress and optimizes leaflet motion. The ability to maintain functionality in a nonround shape at the inflow is a critical feature of the self-expanding CoreValve system, as the constrained portion of the frame supporting the valve remains in a circular configuration.

Evolut-R, Evolut 34 mm, and Evolut-PRO Self-Expanding Design

To further improve on the CoreValve Classic design, the fourth-generation Evolut-R self-expanding bioprosthesis includes a 14-Fr equivalent EnVeo R Deliver Catheter System, a modified Nitinol design at the annulus that optimizes radial expansive force, a longer porcine pericardial sealing skirt, and a Nitinol delivery catheter capsule that allows resheathing and recapture during deployment (see Fig. 54.1).[4] The partially recapturable Evolut 34 mm allows treatment of annular diameters from 26 to 30 mm and is deliverable with a 16-Fr compatible Enveo delivery system (Fig. 54.2). Finally, the Evolut-PRO leverages the same frame and skirt design as the Evolut-R but adds a thin pericardial wrap around the outside of the frame that decrease the degree of residual aortic regurgitation by increasing the surface area contact by 80% (Fig. 54.3).[5] The Evolut-PRO is delivered with a 16-Fr equivalent EnVeo Delivery catheter.[5]

Anatomic Considerations

Multidetector computed tomographic angiography (CTA) is now the gold standard for transcatheter valve selection and is used to determine annular size and iliofemoral (IF) dimensions prior to the selection of the Evolut-R and Evolut-PRO for TAVR. End-systolic perimeter measurements of the basal annular place should be used for valve size selection to reduce the degree of paravalvular regurgitation after TAVR (Fig. 54.4). In an analysis of patients enrolled in the CoreValve Clinical Trials and Continued Access Registries using the CoreValve Classic, higher device/artery ratios (DARs) were associated with lower rates of moderate or severe paravalvular aortic regurgitation (DAR ≤10%, 17.6%; DAR 10% to 15%, 9.9%; DAR 15% to 20%, 6.3%; and DAR >20%, 4.9%; $P < .001$).[6] Importantly, there was no increase in complications associated with valve oversizing.[6] The preprocedural CTA also permits measurement of the sinus of Valsalva (SOV) diameters and coronary heights prior to the procedure. In general, in order to prevent coronary occlusion during deployment, the average SOV width for the 23-mm Evolut-R or Evolut-PRO should be 25 mm or larger, the average SOV width for the 26-mm Evolut-R or Evolut-PRO should be 27 mm or larger, the average SOV width for the 29-mm Evolut-R or Evolut-PRO should be 29 mm or larger, and the average SOV width for the Evolut 34-mm should be 31 mm or larger. Coronary heights less than 10 mm above the aortic annulus should be approached with caution in order to avoid coronary occlusion from the Evolut skirt (14 to 15 mm in height) during deployment; lower valve implantation is sometimes required in this setting. Aortoventricular angles greater than 70 degrees should be avoided with the CoreValve device.[7]

PROCEDURE DESCRIPTION

In most circumstances patient are pretreated with aspirin and clopidogrel (for those undergoing IF access only), although the incremental benefit of dual antiplatelet therapy (DAPT) has not

CHAPTER 54 Self-Expanding Transcatheter Aortic Valve Replacement

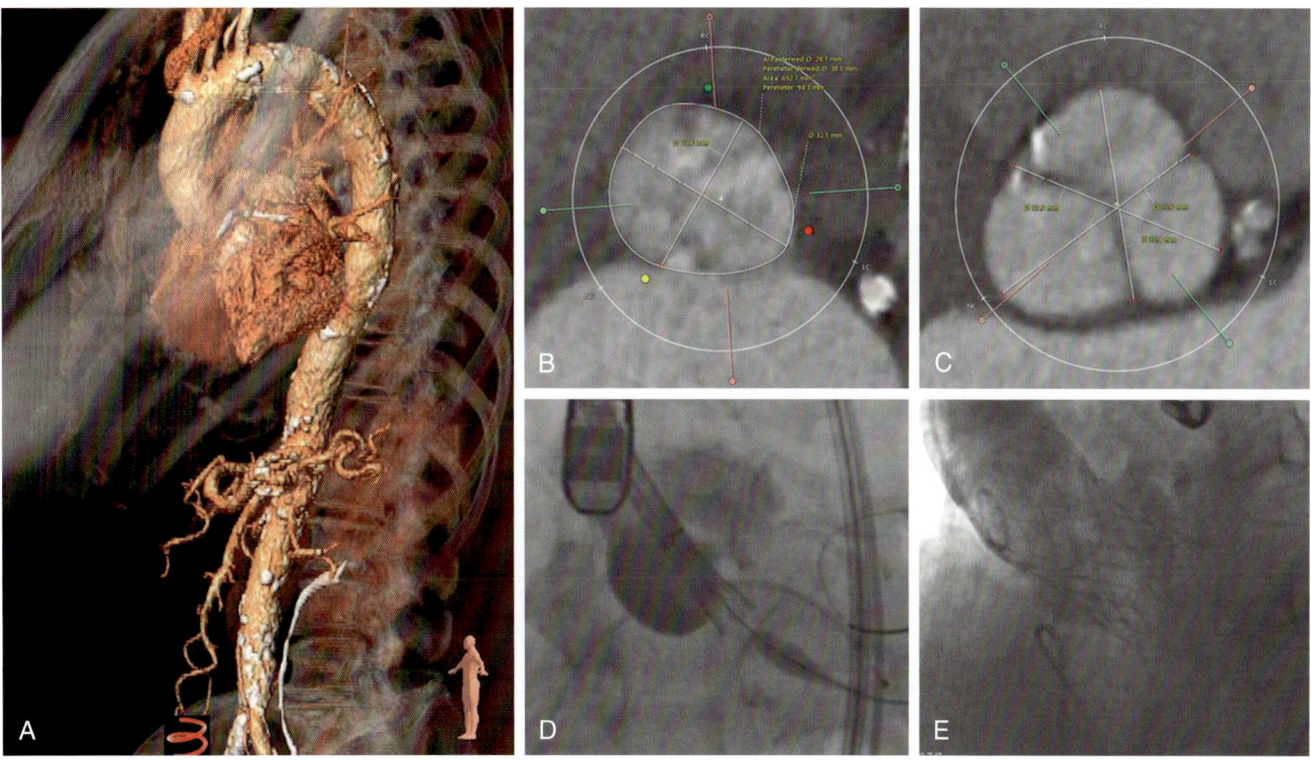

Fig. 54.2 Evolut-R 34 mm deployment for a large aortic annulus. Volume rendering of the ascending and descending aortic and proximal iliac arteries demonstrates a favorable aortic arch for the Evolut-R 34 mm (A). The annular perimeter was 94.3 mm and the perimeter-derived diameter was 30 mm, which is the upper limit for the Evolut-R 34 mm (B). The sinus of Valsalva width is more than 35 mm (C). With the use of a Lunderquist wire, the Evolut-R 34 mm begins deployment 3 mm below the noncoronary sinus (D). The final aortogram demonstrates a 2- to 4-mm implantation depth and mild aortic regurgitation (E).

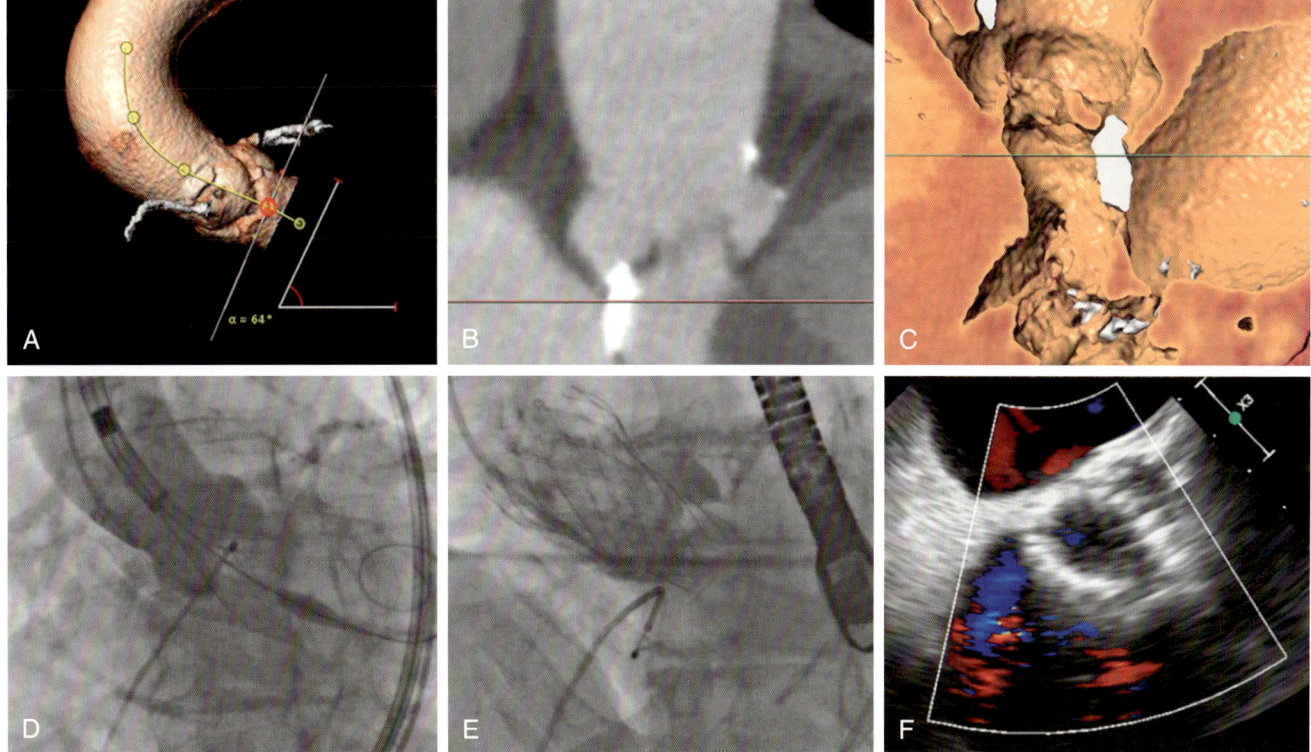

Fig. 54.3 Evolut PRO 29 mm deployment in a patient with extensive left ventricular outflow tract (LVOT) calcium. The aortoventricular angle is favorable for Evolut-PRO Implantation (A). There is extensive LVOT calcium *(white)* (B) that is also visualized with volume rendering (C). The 29-mm Evolut PRO is deployed at 6-mm depth to the noncoronary sinus (D). After deployment, there is no residual aortic regurgitation (E) and no paravalvular regurgitation by transesophageal echocardiography (F).

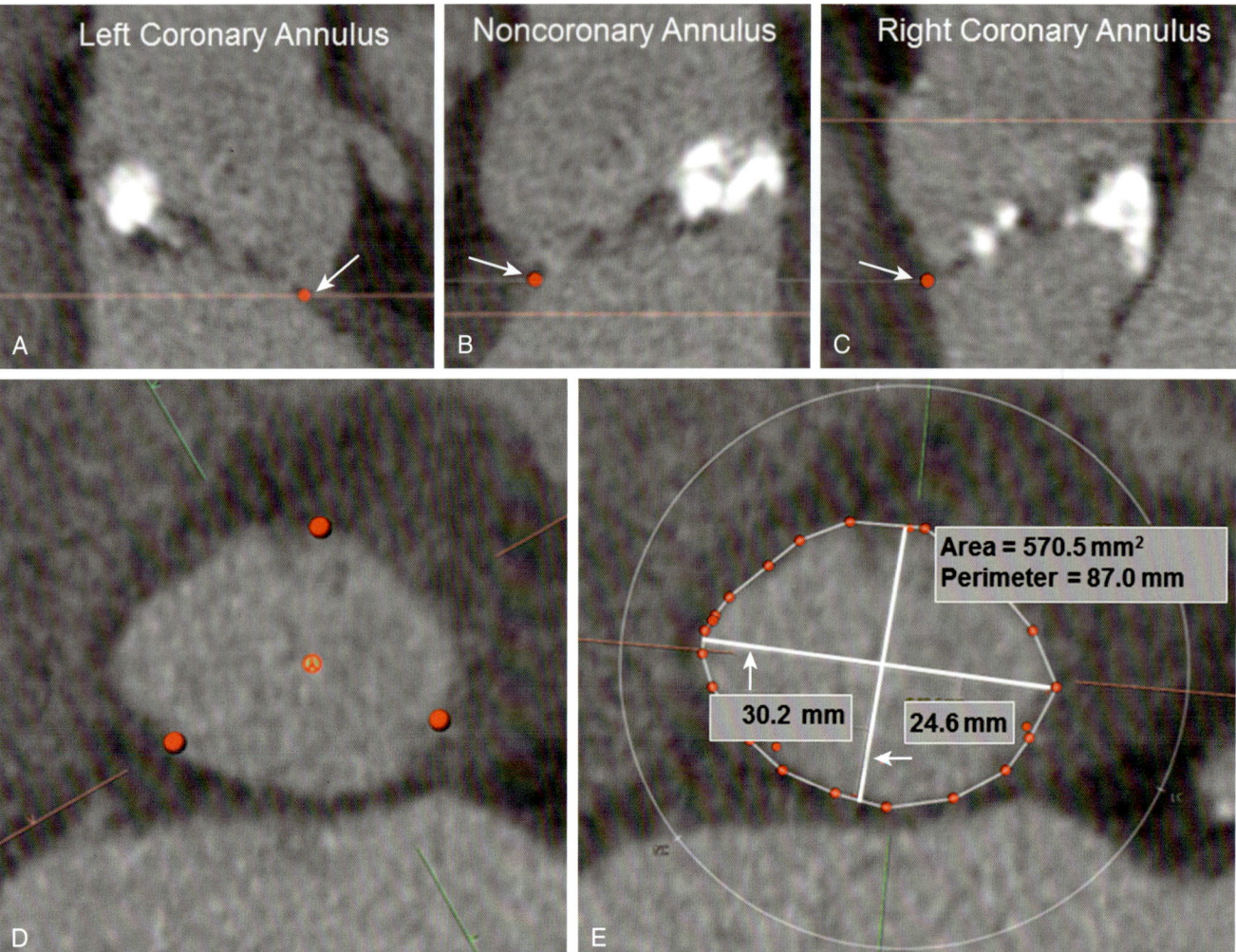

Fig. 54.4 Computed tomographic imaging of the aortic annulus. This is a critical step as measurement of the annulus enables identification of the inferior aspects of the left coronary sinus (A), noncoronary sinus (B), and right coronary sinus (C) as indicated by the red dots. From these points, an annular plane is created that represent the junction of the aorta and the left ventricular outflow tract (D). The long axis and the diameter perpendicular to the long axis are measured and a perimeter area is identified. In the setting of eccentricity of the annulus, the perimeter-determined measures provide more accurate estimates for self-expanding bioprosthesis sizing than area-determined measurements (E).

been demonstrated. Depending on the patient's clinical status and institutional preferences, either general anesthesia or conscious sedation can be used. A temporary 5-Fr pacing wire is positioned within the right ventricle for "fast" or "rapid" pacing during the procedure; in some cases, the TAVR wire has been used for direct left ventricular pacing. Arterial access is then obtained on the side contralateral to the planned 14- to 16-Fr sheath for the EvolutR (14-Fr), Evolut-R 34 mm, or Evolut-PRO (16-Fr) TAVR. Both angiographically guided and ultrasound-guided methods have been used for arterial puncture. Once access has been obtained, anticoagulation is administered to achieve an activated clotting time (ACT) equal to or greater than 250 seconds.

A 5- or 6-Fr pigtail catheter is advanced to the ascending aorta and its distal tip positioned in the noncoronary sinus; a long sheath may be use to stabilize the injection catheter. The gantry position is optimized to allow visualization of all three coronary sinuses in the same plane. An angiographic catheter is then advanced over a standard J-tip guidewire through the primary access sheath and advanced to the ascending aorta. The J-tip guidewire is exchanged for a 0.035-inch straight-tip guidewire, which is used to cross the aortic valve. Once the guidewire is across the aortic valve, the catheter is advanced into the ventricle and hemodynamics are obtained. A 0.035-inch preshaped guidewire (e.g., Confida or Safari preshaped wire) is advanced through the angiographic catheter and positioned in the apex of the left ventricle. Balloon valvuloplasty may then be performed using a balloon sized to the minor axis of the CTA and fast ventricular pacing at 180 beats/min, particularly in the presence of severe valvular calcification (Fig. 54.5).[8–11] Most commonly now, predilation is not performed and the Evolut-R or Evolut-PRO is advanced directly across the annulus.

The Evolut-R or Evolut-PRO is then advanced over the 0.035-inch guidewire and positioned across the native valve. Aortography is used to identify the inferiormost aspect of the valvular plane in the noncoronary sinus. The Evolut bioprosthesis is then positioned with the inflow portion within the aortic annulus (approximately 2 to 4 mm below the annulus). The 0.035-inch wire is used to stabilize the CoreValve along the greater curvature of the aorta, but excessive pressure on the wire in the left ventricular apex should be avoided. As the slow Evolut-R or Evolut-PRO deployment begins, "fast" pacing at 110 to 120 beats/min may be used to lower the intraventricular pressure and stabilize deployment. As the inflow aspect of the device begins to flare outward, aortography is performed sequentially and final positioning is obtained. Once the Evolut frame has been deployed, aortography is performed to assess the degree of

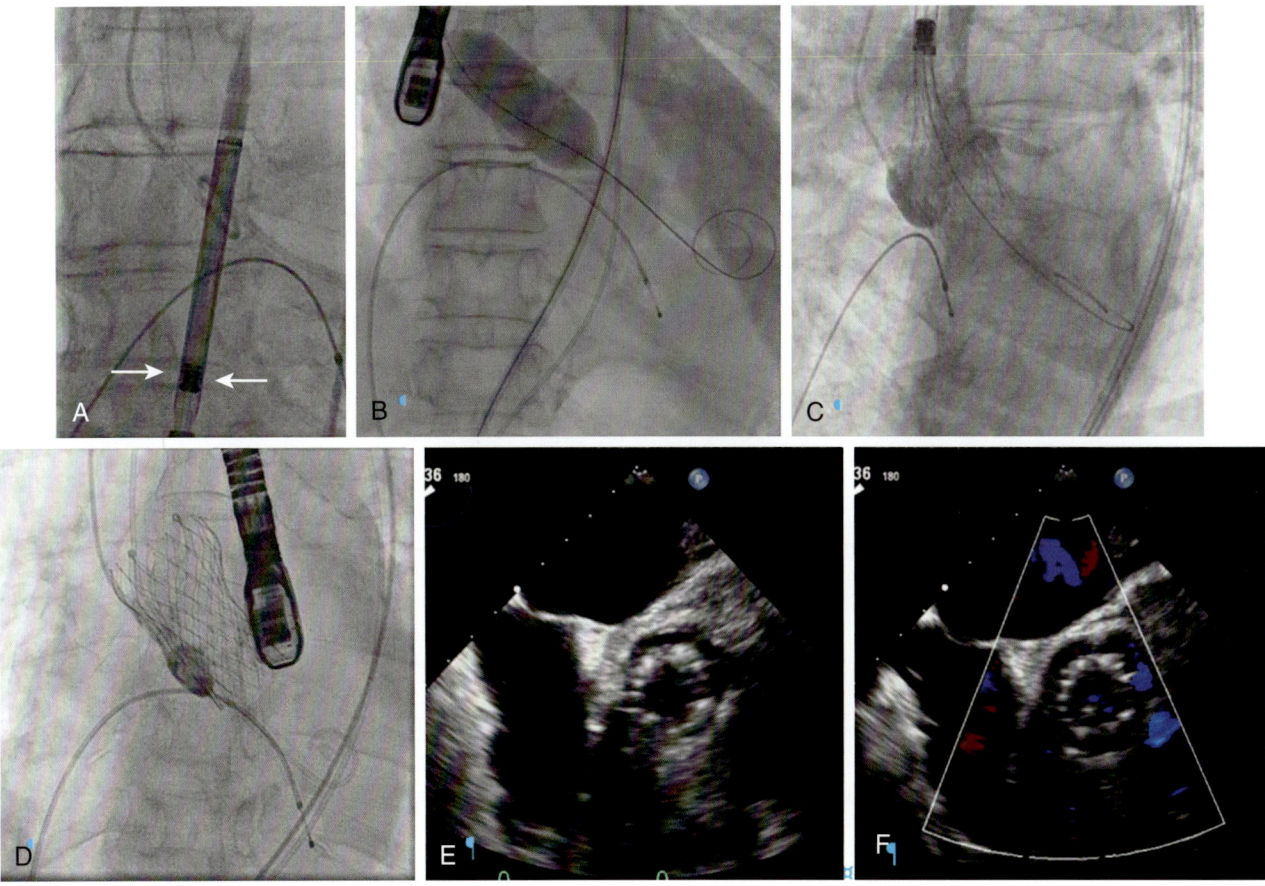

Fig. 54.5 Predilation due to valve calcification prior to self-expanding transcatheter aortic valve replacement. Transfemoral transcatheter aortic valve replacement using a self-expanding prosthesis. (A) Fluoroscopy (extracorporeal) of the valve to make sure that it is loaded correctly with both paddles *(arrows)* in position. (B) Predilation of the annulus can be beneficial in case of a particularly heavily calcified annulus. (C) Partially deployed valve, still attached to the delivery system. At this point the valve can be repositioned or recaptured if adjustments are needed. (D) Final angiographic result. (E) Two-dimensional transesophageal echocardiography after deployment and with (F) color Doppler demonstrating no valvular or paravalvular regurgitation.

residual stenosis within the frame and the degree of aortic regurgitation. Hemodynamics may now be assessed to ensure adequate separation of the left ventricular and aortic diastolic contours. Transesophageal or transthoracic echocardiography is performed to assess the degree of aortic regurgitation. Concordance of the angiographic, hemodynamics, and echocardiography are critical for the determination of the need for balloon postdilatation, which can be performed to expand the frame using the mean diameter of the annulus (Fig. 54.6).[12-17] After a satisfactory result has been achieved, the vascular sheath is removed and percutaneous or open closure is performed. In the event of conduction disturbances during the procedure, patient should be observed with temporary pacemaker placement in a cardiovascular intensive care unit (ICU) for for 24 to 48 hours and monitored for conduction system disturbance. The patient may be discharge 24 to 48 hours after the procedure.

COREVALVE CLINICAL STUDIES BASED ON SURGICAL RISK

Selection of patients suitable for CoreValve TAVR is best facilitated using a multidisciplinary team (MDT) that includes cardiac surgeons, interventional cardiologists, imaging specialists, and geriatricians.[18] The MDT generally reviews the clinical, anatomic, and vascular information for the individual patient and determines his or her suitability for CoreValve TAVR based on estimated surgical risk, which may include convention risk criteria (e.g., Society for Thoracic Surgery Predicted Risk of Mortality [STS PROM]) supplemented by the nontraditional risk factors of severe comorbidities, frailties, and disabilities).

CoreValve Extreme Risk Clinical Study

Extreme-risk patients are those who have an expected mortality or irreversible comorbidities equal to or greater than 50% at 30 days with surgery. The CoreValve Extreme Risk Study was a prospective, multicenter, nonrandomized investigation that recruited 506 patients, of whom 489 underwent attempted treatment with the CoreValve transcatheter heart valve.[19] The rate of all-cause mortality or major stroke at 12 months was 26.0% (versus 43.0% with the objective performance goal; $P < .0001$). Individual 30-day and 12-month events included all-cause mortality (8.4% and 24.3%, respectively) and major stroke (2.3% and 4.3%, respectively) (Table 54.1).[19] Procedural events at 30 days included life-threatening/disabling bleeding (12.7%), major vascular complications (8.2%), and need for permanent pacemaker placement (21.6%).[19] The frequency of moderate or severe paravalvular aortic regurgitation appeared to improve from 30 days to 1 year due to further expansion of the self-expanding prosthesis over time.[19,20] The rates of 2-year all-cause mortality,

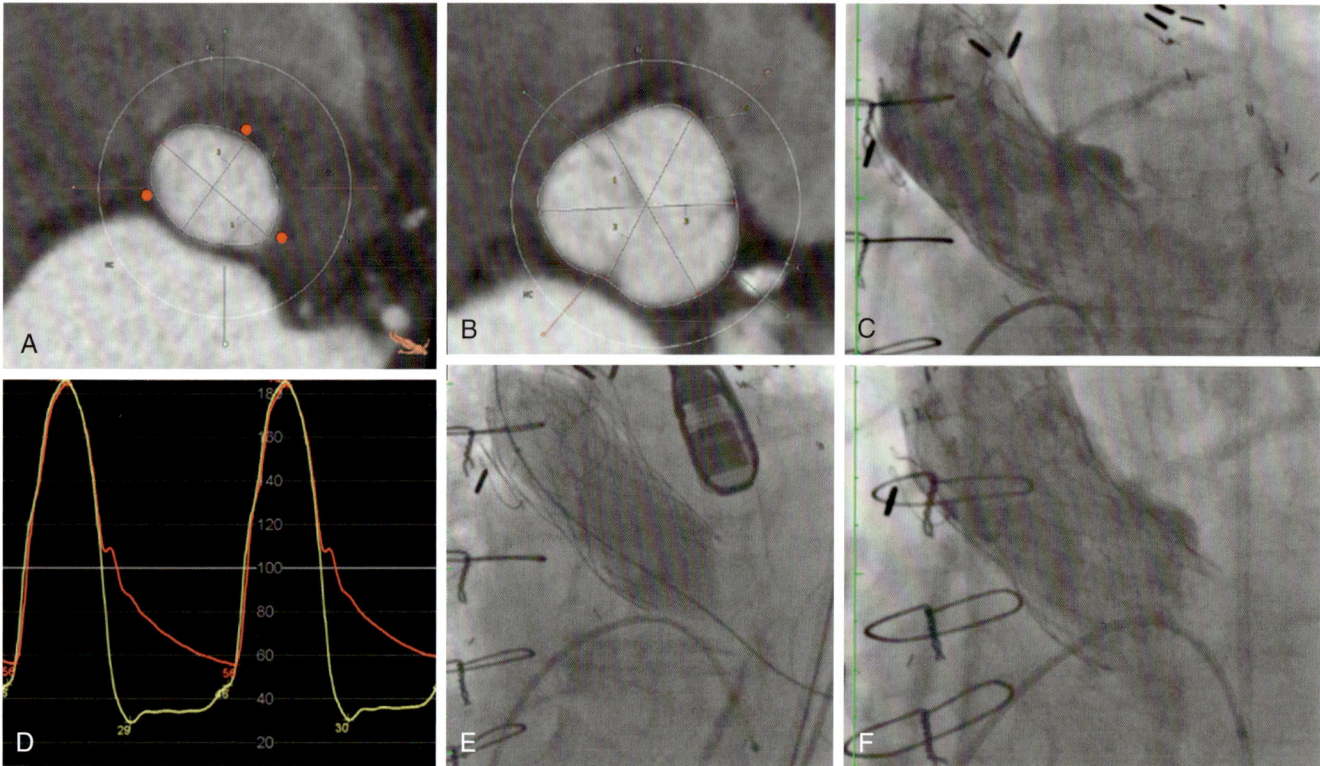

Fig. 54.6 **Residual aortic regurgitation treated with balloon postdilation.** The aortic annular perimeter was 74.1 mm and the perimeter-based diameter 23.6 mm (A). The mean width of the sinus of Valsalva was 29.9 mm, indicating that a 29-mm CoreValve (B) would be suitable for this procedure. After deployment of the 29-mm CoreValve, there was moderate to severe residual aortic regurgitation related to an underexpanded portion of the frame in the noncoronary portion of the annulus (C). Hemodynamics were consistent with moderate to severe aortic regurgitation with equalization of the aortic and left ventricular end-diastolic contours (D). A 24-mm True balloon was inflated (E), which lowered the degree of residual aortic regurgitation to mild (F). (Adapted from Gleason TG, Reardon MJ, Popma JJ, et al. 5-Year outcomes of self-expanding transcatheter versus surgical aortic valve replacement in high-risk patients. *J Am Coll Cardiol*. 2018;72[22]:2687–2696.)

cardiovascular mortality, and major stroke were 36.6%, 26.2%, and 5.1%, respectively.[21] Between 1 and 2 years, the incremental all-cause mortality, cardiovascular mortality, and major stroke rates were 12.3%, 7.9%, and 0.8%, respectively, illustrating the overall morbidity of the patients enrolled in the study.[21] Multivariate predictors of all-cause mortality at 2 years included the presence of coronary artery disease, admission from an assisted living center, and an STS PROM greater than 15%.[21] The frequency of moderate or severe paravalvular regurgitation was unchanged between the first and second years (4.3% at 1 year, 4.4% at 2 years).[21]

CoreValve High-Risk Clinical Trial

High-risk patients are those who have a greater than 10% risk of 30-day mortality with surgery.[22] In the CoreValve High Risk pivotal trial, 795 patients were randomized to CoreValve TAVR or surgical aortic valve replacement (SAVR) at 45 high-quality surgical centers in the United States.[23] The rate of death from any cause at 1 year was significantly lower in the TAVR group than in the SAVR group (14.2% vs. 19.1%), with an absolute reduction in risk of 4.9% (upper boundary of the 95% confidence interval [CI], –0.4; $P < .001$ for noninferiority; $P = .04$ for superiority).[23] Although the mortality benefit with TAVR over SAVR was maintained at 2 years,[24] mortality rates at 5 years were not different in the two groups (55.3% for TAVR and 55.4% for SAVR) (Fig. 54.7).[25] Major stroke rates were 12.3% for TAVR and 13.2% for SAVR. Aortic regurgitation remained more frequent in patients treated with CoreValve compared with SAVR at 5 years (Fig. 54.8). Nevertheless the hemodynamic valve performance remained superior for TAVR at 5 years (mean aortic valve gradient: 7.1 ± 3.6 mm Hg for TAVR and 10.9 ± 5.7 mm Hg for SAVR) (Fig. 54.9), and no clinically significant valve thromboses were observed. Freedom from severe structural valve deterioration was 99.2% for TAVR and 98.3% for SAVR ($P = .32$); freedom from valve reintervention was 97.0% for TAVR and 98.9% for SAVR ($P = .04$).[25]

The CoreValve High Risk Clinical Trial also provided the first glimpse into the complication tradeoffs that occurred with TAVR and SAVR.[26] Within 0 to 3 days, the major vascular complication rate was significantly higher with TAVR than with SAVR ($P = .003$),[26] whereas life-threatening or disabling bleeding ($P < .001$), encephalopathy ($P = .02$), atrial fibrillation ($P < .001$), and acute kidney injury ($P < .001$) were significantly higher with SAVR.[26] Procedural complications unique to TAVR included coronary occlusion in 0.5% of patients and TAVR dislodgements in 2.8% of patients.[26] Procedural complications unique to SAVR included aortic dissection in 0.8% of patients and injury to other heart structures in 2.0% of patients.[26]

The difference in the mortality rate between TAVR and SAVR was evident only during the recovery period (31 to 120 days); 15 patients undergoing TAVR and 27 patients undergoing SAVR died during this period.[27] This mortality difference was largely driven by higher rates of technical failure, surgical complications, and lack of recovery in the 31 to 120 days following surgery,[27] in contrast to deaths between 0 and 30 days, where the

CHAPTER 54 Self-Expanding Transcatheter Aortic Valve Replacement

TABLE 54.1 30-Day Outcomes With Self-Expanding Transcatheter Aortic Valve Replacement

Author	No. of Pts	Valve	Risk	Age, Years	STS, %	Death, %	All Stroke, %	≤Trace, %	Mild, %	Mod, %	PPM, %
								\<colspan Aortic Regurgitation\>			
Popma et al.[19]	489	CoreValve	Extreme	83.2 ± 8.7	10.3 ± 5.5	9.8	All: 4.0 Major: 1.9	41.8	43.0	15.3	24.6
Reardon et al.[31]	150	CoreValve	Extreme—Alternative access	81.8 ± 8.2	10.1 ± 5.6	9.5	All: 5.4 Major: 3.0	33.6	31.0	7.0	18.2
Adams et al.[23]	394	CoreValve	High risk	83.2 ± 7.1	7.31 ± 3.0	2.8	All: 4.5 Disabling 1.2	54.9	36.6	7.7	19.8
Reardon et al.[28]	864	CoreValve, Evolut	Intermediate	79.9 ± 6.2	4.4 ± 1.5	2.8	All: 3.4 Disabling: 2.2	35.7	35.9	3.2	25.9
Thyregod et al.[29]	145	CoreValve	Low	79.2 ± 4.9	2.9 ± 1.6	2.1	All: 1.4	23.4	61.3	14.5	34.1
Barbanti et al.[224]	10,822	Sapien 3: 5423, 45.9 Lotus: 3007, 25.4 Evolut-R: 1603, 13.6 Acurate: 1314, 11.1 Jena Valve: 345, 2.9 Portico: 130, 1.1	Variable	82.1 (81.4–82.9)	NR	2.2	All: 2.6 Disabling: 0.9	NR	NR	1.6	16.2
Bagur et al.[203]	20	Symetic Acurate	Intermediate	82.7 ± 7	4.7 ± 2.3	0	All: 0	75	25	0	5.3
Mollmann et al.[205]	89	First-in-Man Acurate Neo	High risk	83.7 ± 4.4	6.8 ± 4.1	3.4	Major: 2.2	95.1		4.9	11.5
Kim et al.[206]	1000	Acurate	Variable	81.1. ± 5.2	6.6 ± 7.5	1.5	Disabling: 2.3	50.4	46.0	3.4	9.9
Husser et al.[207]	622	Sapien 3	Variable	81 ± 6	NR	1.9	2.4	NR	NR	1.9	15.5
	311	Accurate		81 ± 6	NR	2.3	1.9	NR	NR	4.8	9.9
Jatene et al.[208]	49	Acurate	Variable	82.4 ± 5.4	6.1 ± 2.8	4	0	NR	NR	4	6
	56	CoreValve		82.3 ± 7.7	5.6 ± 3.3	11	4	NR	NR	12	25
	67	Sapien XT		83.1 ± 6.3	6.7 ± 4.9	4	2	NR	NR	4	11
Popma et al.[30a]	1468	CoreValve, Evolut R, or Evolut PRO	Low	74 +/- 5.9	1.9% +/-0.7%	0.5%	All: 3.4% Disabling: 0.7%	60.3%	36.1%	3.5%	17.4%

PPM, Permanent pacemaker; *STS*, Society of Thoracic Surgeons 30-day surgical mortality risk score.

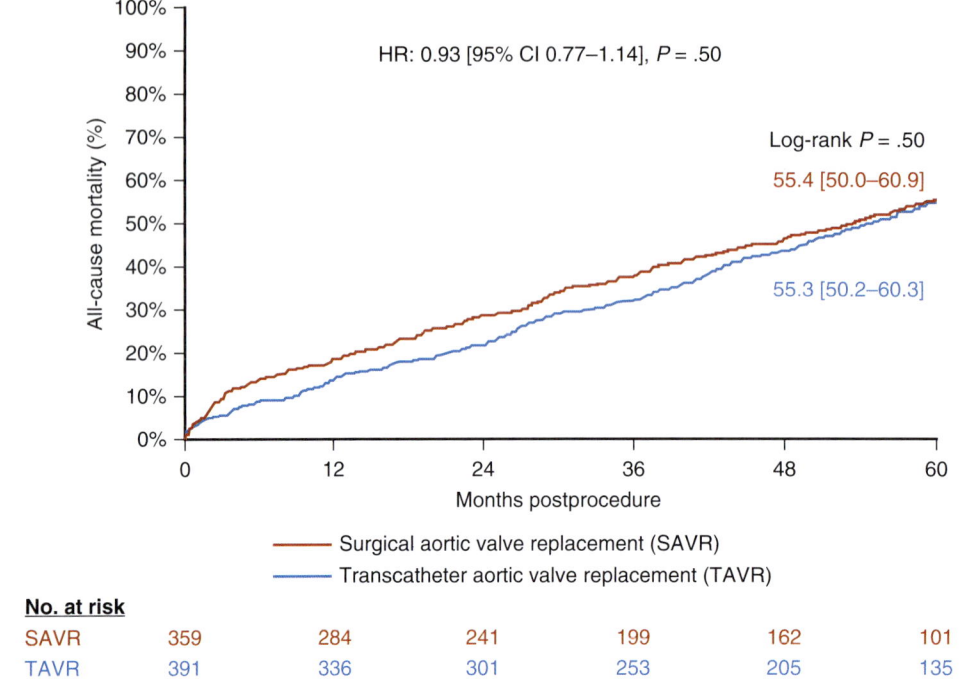

Fig. 54.7 Self-expanding-transcatheter aortic valve replacement versus surgical aortic valve replacement in high-risk patients: all-cause mortality to 5 years. *CI,* Confidence interval; *HR,* hazard ratio. (Adapted from Gleason TG, Reardon MJ, Popma JJ, et al. 5-Year outcomes of self-expanding transcatheter versus surgical aortic valve replacement in high-risk patients. *J Am Coll Cardiol.* 2018;72[22]:2687–2696.)

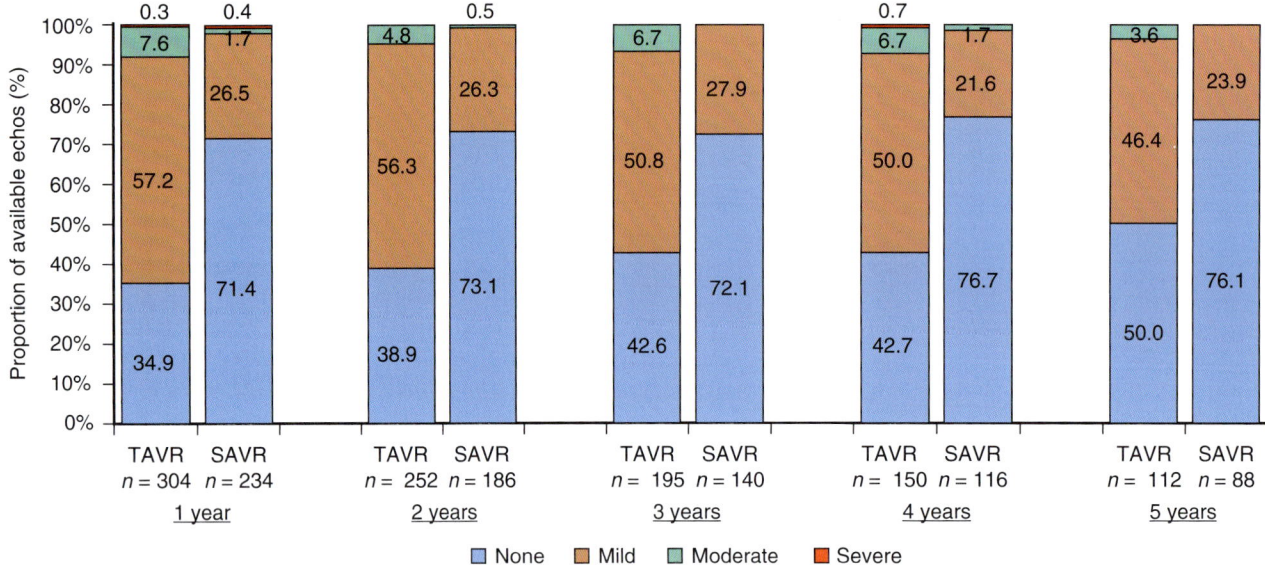

Fig. 54.8 Occurrence of aortic regurgitation through 5 years after transcatheter aortic valve replacement *(TAVR)* and surgical aortic valve replacement *(SAVR)*. Total aortic regurgitation reported by the investigational sites through 5 years for patients in the TAVR and SAVR groups. (Adapted from Gleason TG, Reardon MJ, Popma JJ, et al. 5-Year outcomes of self-expanding transcatheter versus surgical aortic valve replacement in high-risk patients. *J Am Coll Cardiol.* 2018;72[22]:2687–2696.)

causes of death were more technical failures in the TAVR group and lack of recovery in the SAVR group.[27] It is apparent that the incremental mortality benefit of TAVR over SAVR is most profound in frail and disabled patients.

CoreValve Intermediate Risk Clinical Trial

Moderate- (or intermediate-) risk patients are those who have an estimated surgical risk greater than 3% to 10%.[22] In the Surgical Replacement and Transcatheter Aortic Valve Implantation (SURTAVI) randomized study of 1746 patients who were deemed at intermediate risk for surgery, the estimated incidence of the primary end point using Bayesian analysis was 12.6% in the TAVR group and 14.0% in the SAVR group; posterior probability of non-inferiority was greater than 0.999.[28] This novel approach provided an interim analysis of the study before all patients had reached their 24-month end point based on simulations of the estimation of the posterior probability of a credible estimate of expected event rates

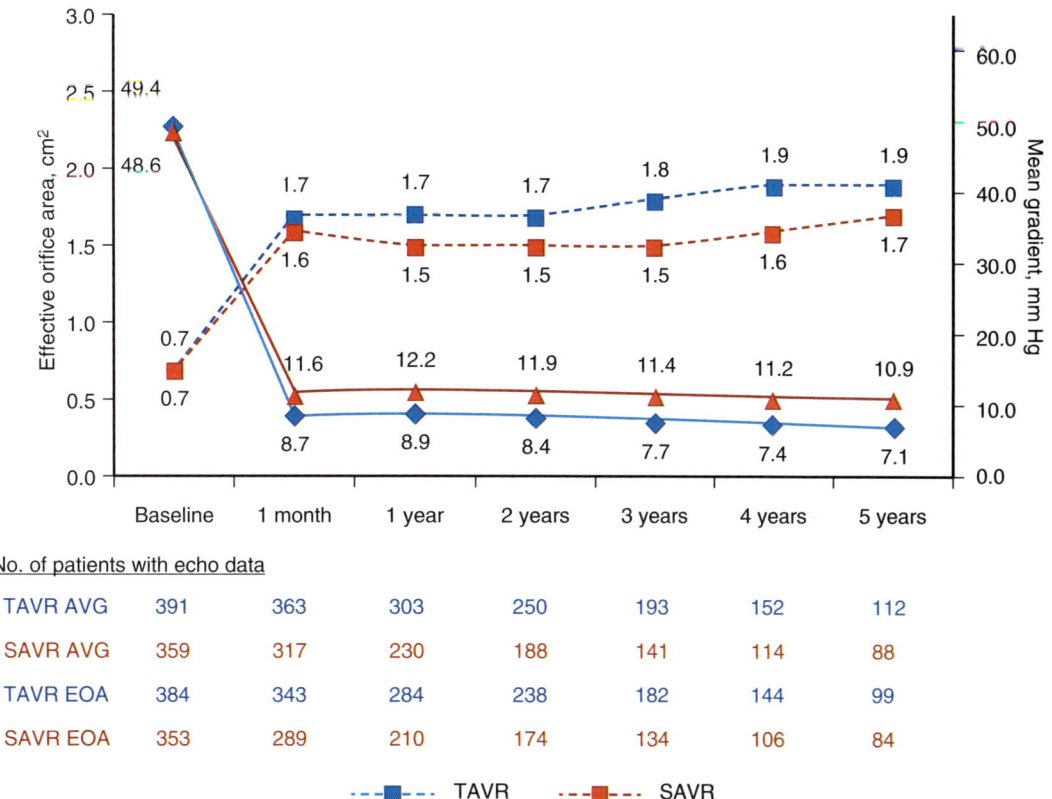

Fig. 54.9 Forward-flow hemodynamics through 5 years for patients in the transcatheter aortic valve replacement *(TAVR)* and surgical aortic valve replacement *(SAVR)* groups. Site-reported aortic valve effective orifice area *(dotted lines)* and mean gradient *(solid lines)* over time for patients in the TAVR *(blue lines)* and SAVR *(orange lines)* groups. TAVR was associated with a significantly larger effective orifice area and significantly smaller mean gradients at each time point compared with SAVR (all $P < .01$). *AVG,* Aortic valve gradient; *EOA,* effective orifice area. (Adapted from Gleason TG, Reardon MJ, Popma JJ, et al. 5-Year outcomes of self-expanding transcatheter versus surgical aortic valve replacement in high-risk patients. *J Am Coll Cardiol.* 2018;72[22]:2687–2696.)

(Fig. 54.10). SAVR was associated with higher rates of acute kidney injury, atrial fibrillation, and transfusion requirements, whereas TAVR had higher rates of residual aortic regurgitation and need for pacemaker implantation.[28] TAVR resulted in lower mean gradients and larger aortic valve areas as compared with SAVR. Structural valve deterioration at 24 months did not occur in either group.[28]

CoreValve Low-Risk "All Comers"

The Nordic Aortic Valve Intervention Trial (NOTION), a randomized clinical trial, compared TAVR with SAVR in an all-comers patient cohort.[29] A total of 280 patients 70 years of age or older with severe aortic valve stenosis and no significant coronary artery disease were randomized 1:1 to TAVR using a self-expanding bioprosthesis or SAVR[29]; the mean age was 79.1 years and 81.8% of patients were deemed to be at low risk.[29] The primary end point—death, stroke, or myocardial infarction within 1 year—was similar in the two groups (13.1% in TAVR vs. 16.3% in SAVR patients; $P = .43$ for superiority).[29] Compared with SAVR patients, TAVR patients had more conduction abnormalities requiring pacemaker implantation, larger improvements in effective orifice area, more total aortic valve regurgitation, and higher New York Heart Association (NYHA) functional class at 1 year. Surgery patients had more major or life-threatening bleeding, cardiogenic shock, acute kidney injury (stage II or III), and new-onset or worsening atrial fibrillation at 30 days than did TAVR patients.[29] Two-year results from the NOTION trial demonstrate the continuing safety and effectiveness of TAVR in lower-risk patients.[30]

Evolut Low Risk Trial

The Evolut Low Risk Trial was a randomized non-inferiority trial in which TAVR with a self-expanding bioprosthesis was compared to SAVR in patients who were at low surgical risk,[30a] defined as a predicted surgical mortality of no greater than 3% at 30 days. A total of 1468 patients were randomized to TAVR with a self-expanding bioprosthesis or SAVR in 86 centers worldwide. The primary endpoint, a composite of death or disabling stroke, was observed less frequently in the TAVR arm (5.3%) than the SAVR arm (6.7%) with a Bayesian analysis yielding a posterior probability of noninferiority of >0.999. The TAVR arm, compared to the SAVR arm, also demonstrated a lower incidence of disabling stroke (0.5% vs. 1.7%), bleeding complications (2.4% vs. 7.5%), acute kidney injury (0.9% vs. 2.8%), atrial fibrillation (7.7% vs. 35.4%), but had a higher incidence of moderate or severe aortic regurgitation (3.5% vs. 0.5%) and pacemaker implantation (17.4% vs. 6.1%.) In this study, patients assigned to TAVR also carried an advantage in hemodynamics at one year compared with SAVR patients with aortic valve gradients of 8.6 mmHg with TAVR versus 11.2 mmHg with surgery and effective orifice areas of 2.3cm2 with TAVR versus 2.0cm2 with SAVR.

Along with its counterpart in balloon-expandable TAVR,[30b] the Evolut Low Risk Trial is expected to lead to a Class I indication in the next iteration of practice guidelines, and represents a paradigm-shift in the treatment of patients with valvular heart disease. This is anticipated to have a large impact in the lives of thousands of low-risk patients with severe aortic stenosis who will likely soon have a treatment option that does not include open heart surgery.

SECTION V Structural Interventions

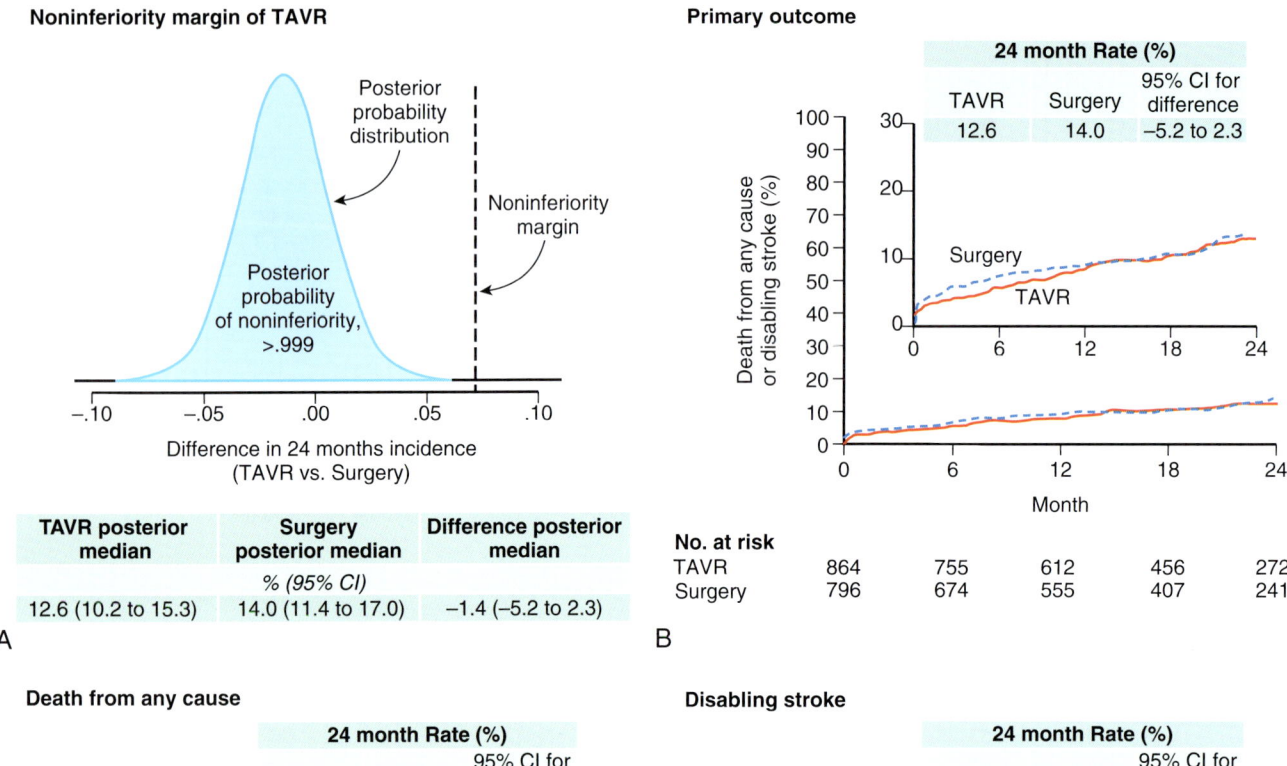

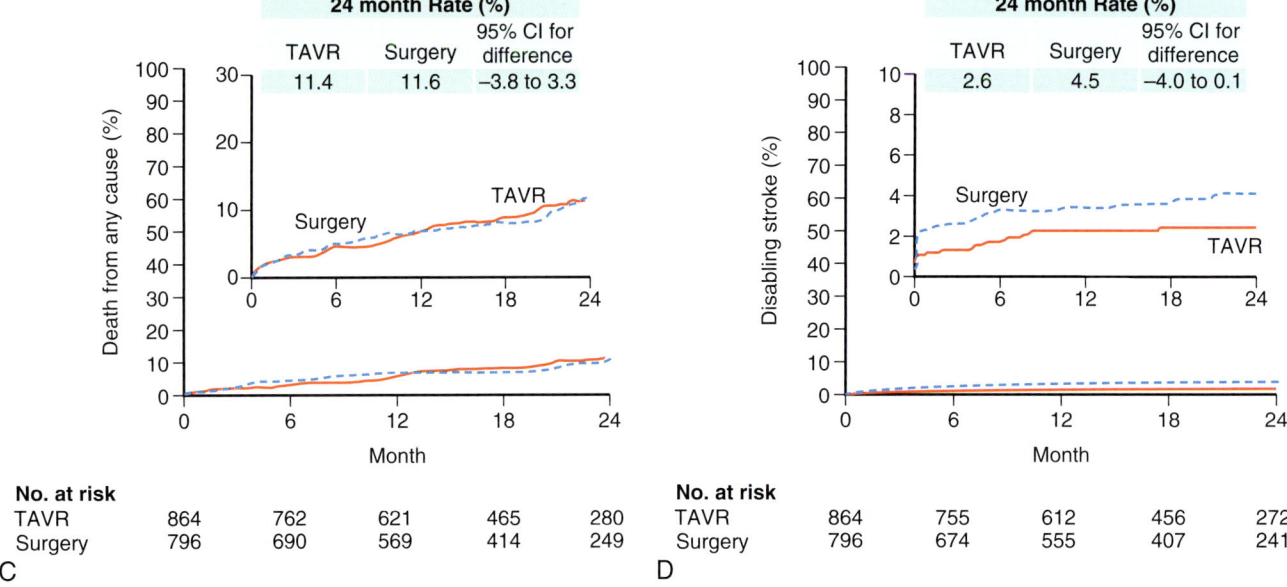

Fig. 54.10 Noninferiority analysis and time-to-event curves for the primary end point. In this Bayesian analysis, the posterior probability distribution for the difference in the primary end point (death from any cause or disabling stroke at 24 months) between patients who underwent transcatheter aortic valve replacement *(TAVR)* and those who underwent surgical aortic valve replacement (SAVR) confirmed that the noninferiority margin for TAVR was met (A). Also shown are time-to-event curves for the primary end point (B), death from any cause (C), and disabling stroke (D), findings that were similar in the two groups. In Panels B, C, and D, the insets show the same data on an enlarged *y*-axis. *CI,* Confidence interval. (Adapted from Reardon MJ, Van Mieghem NM, Popma JJ, et al. Surgical or transcatheter aortic-valve replacement in intermediate-risk patients. *N Engl J Med.* 2017;376(14):1321–1331.)

COREVALVE EXPANDED-USE REGISTRIES

Alternative Access

Alternative access was designed for patients in whom the IF anatomy precludes transfemoral (TF) access. The initial CoreValve Alternative Access study enrolled 150 patients with prohibitive IF anatomy who were treated with the CoreValve transcatheter heart valve delivered by way of the subclavian artery or a direct aortic approach using a sternotomy or right parasternal approach.[31] The death or major stroke rate was 15.3% at 30 days and 39.4% at 12 months, which was favorable compared with the expected outcome without treatment in this patient group. The individual rate of all-cause mortality and major stroke was 11.3% and 7.5% at 30 days and 36.0% and 9.1% at 12 months.[31] After TAVR, the effective aortic valve area was 1.82 ± 0.64 cm² at 1 month and 1.81 ± 0.51 cm² at 12 months. The mean aortic valve gradient was 9.7 ± 5.8 mm Hg at 30 days and 9.5 ± 5.7 mm Hg at 12 months.[31] A more recent report of the direct aortic approach with contemporary surgical techniques has shown improved results.[32]

A total of 202 patients were treated via subclavian access in the CoreValve Clinical Trials and Continued Access Registry and were propensity-matched with patients treated with TF access.[33] Significant differences in procedural outcomes include less post-TAVR balloon dilation (17.9% vs. 26.7% in TF patients, P = .03) and more general anesthesia (99.0% vs. 89.6% in TF patients, P <.001). There were no differences in procedure time (57.8 ± 45.3 vs. 57.5 ± 32.1 min in TF patients, P = .94) or procedural success between groups (P = .89). Event rates at 30 days or 1 year were also similar.[33] Percutaneous subclavian access is becoming increasingly popular. Additional alternative access approaches have included CoreValve implantation from a right thoracotomy,[34,35] suprasternal access,[36–38] transcarotid access,[39–41] and, more recently, a transcaval approach (Fig. 54.11).[42] Alternative access is used in less than 10% of cases owing to a reduction in the sheath profile with current-generation TAVR prostheses.

Failed Surgical Valves

Supra-annular TAVR devices may have particular value in patients with surgical valve failures.[43,44] In a prospective series that evaluated the use of CoreValve in 233 patients with symptomatic surgical valve failure deemed unsuitable for reoperation,[45] surgical valve failure occurred due to stenosis (56.4%), regurgitation (22.0%), or a combination (21.6%).[45] TAVR was then attempted in 227 patients; it was successful in 225 (99.1%). The all-cause mortality rate was 2.2% at 30 days and 14.6% at 1 year; major stroke rate was 0.4% at 30 days and 1.8% at 1 year.[45] Moderate aortic regurgitation occurred in 3.5% of patients at 30 days and 7.4% of patients at 1 year.[45] The rate of new permanent pacemaker implantation was 8.1% at 30 days.[45] The mean valve gradient was 17.0 ± 8.8 mm Hg at 30 days and 16.6 ± 8.9 mm Hg at 1 year.[45] Factors significantly associated with higher mean aortic gradients at discharge were surgical valve size, stenosis as the modality of structural valve failure, and surgical valve prosthesis-patient mismatch (PPM) (all P < .001) (Fig. 54.12).[45] The CoreValve or Evolut-R transcatheter valves may be particularly beneficial in patients with smaller surgical valves[46] with or without associated fracture of the underlying surgical valve (see Fig. 54.10).[47,48] In the Valve-in-Valve International Data registry (VIVID) registry, 162 patients with surgical valve failure were treated with either the CoreValve or Portico bioprosthesis.[49] CoreValve was associated with a larger effective orifice area (1.67 cm² vs. 1.31 cm²; P = .001), lower mean gradient (14 ± 7.5 vs. 17 ± 7.5 mm Hg; P = .02), and lower core laboratory-adjudicated moderate-to-severe aortic insufficiency (4.2% vs. 13.7%; P = .04) compared with Portico.[49] High implantation of the self-expanding bioprosthesis may optimize the postprocedural residual gradient (Fig. 54.13).[50]

End-Stage Renal Disease

In a series of 96 patients with end-stage renal disease at extreme risk for surgery (mean STS PROM, 16.2% ± 8.4%) who were treated with the self-expanding CoreValve, the rate of all-cause mortality or major stroke at 1 year was 30.3%; the rate of all-cause mortality was 5.3% at 30 days and 30.3% at one year.[51] New permanent pacemakers were needed in 26.8% of patients.[51] Importantly, sustained reductions (mean gradient 9.33 mm Hg) in the mean aortic valve gradients were documented at 1 year.[51]

Primary Aortic Regurgitation

Patients with aortic regurgitation at high risk for surgery present a unique challenge for TAVR owing to the absence of calcification for stabilization and larger annular diameters. A series of 26 patients undergoing treatment with CoreValve were prospectively followed.[52] Compared with patients with aortic stenosis, patients with aortic regurgitation were significantly younger (mean age 73 ± 10 vs. 82 ± 6 in aortic stenosis patients, P = .02) and had a higher incidence of severe pulmonary hypertension (sPAP > 60 mm Hg, 31% vs. 10% in aortic stenosis patients, P = .007).[53] Device success was lower in the aortic regurgitation group (79% vs. 96% in the aortic stenosis patients, P = .006).[52] At 1 month, patients treated for aortic regurgitation had a higher overall mortality (23% vs. 5.9% in aortic stenosis patients; odds ratio 4.22 [3.03 to 8.28], P < .001).[52] Results were consistent at 12 months: overall mortality (31% vs. 19% in aortic stenosis patients, hazard ratio 2.1 [1.5 to 4.41], P < .001).[52] Considering the ominous prognosis of these patients when treated medically, TAVR may be a reasonable choice in some. Problems with the early use of the self-expanding CoreValve have been mitigated with the use of new generation self-expanding bioprostheses that allow recapture with suboptimal positioning, better oversizing, procedural improvement with rapid pacing, and better sealing with a pericardial wrap.[53]

Low-Gradient Aortic Stenosis

To evaluate the use of the CoreValve in patients with low-gradient aortic stenosis, patients were stratified by left ventricular ejection fraction: low-gradient normal (≥50%) ejection fraction, and low-gradient, low (<50%) ejection fraction who did not respond to dobutamine (defined by generating a mean gradient above 40 mm Hg and/or velocity greater than 4.0 m/s, "nonresponders"). These patients were compared with extreme-risk patients from the U.S. Pivotal and Continued Access Study who had either low resting gradient, low ejection fraction and responded to dobutamine ("responders"), or a high resting gradient or velocity.[54] At 30 days, patients with low-gradient/low left ventricular ejection fraction (nonresponders and responders) had significantly higher rates of all-cause mortality or major stroke, all-cause mortality, and cardiovascular mortality than either high- or low-gradient normal ejection fraction patients.[54] At 1 year, only the responders had higher rates of these outcomes in comparison with the other three groups.[54] When all four subgroups were pooled, both decreasing mean gradient and stroke volume index were associated with increased mortality.[54] The most important finding in this study was that the preprocedural mean gradient was the only hemodynamic independent predictor of 1-year mortality (Fig. 54.14).[54]

Bicuspid Aortic Valve Disease

Patients with bicuspid aortic valve disease present a particular challenge for TAVR owing to the asymmetry (Fig. 54.15) of the commissures and calcification (Fig. 54.16) of the raphe.[55,56] Although bicuspid aortic valve disease has typically been an exclusion for clinical trials, more recent work has demonstrated the value of TAVR bioprostheses in this setting (Kochman, 2014 #446).[57] In some settings, valve selection based on "supra-annular" rather than "annular" sizing may be more useful for valve stabilization during deployment.[58] In a two-center series of 77 patients with bicuspid aortic valve disease, efficacy was evaluated by postprocedural valve function as mean gradient, peak velocity, effective orifice area, and moderate or greater paravalvular leak.[59] Procedural success was high in patients with bicuspid valves as well as those with tricuspid valves (98.7% vs. 99.1% in those with tricuspid valves).[59] There were no significant differences between groups in valve hemodynamics after TAVR, pacemaker implantation rate, or procedural complications.[59]

SECTION V Structural Interventions

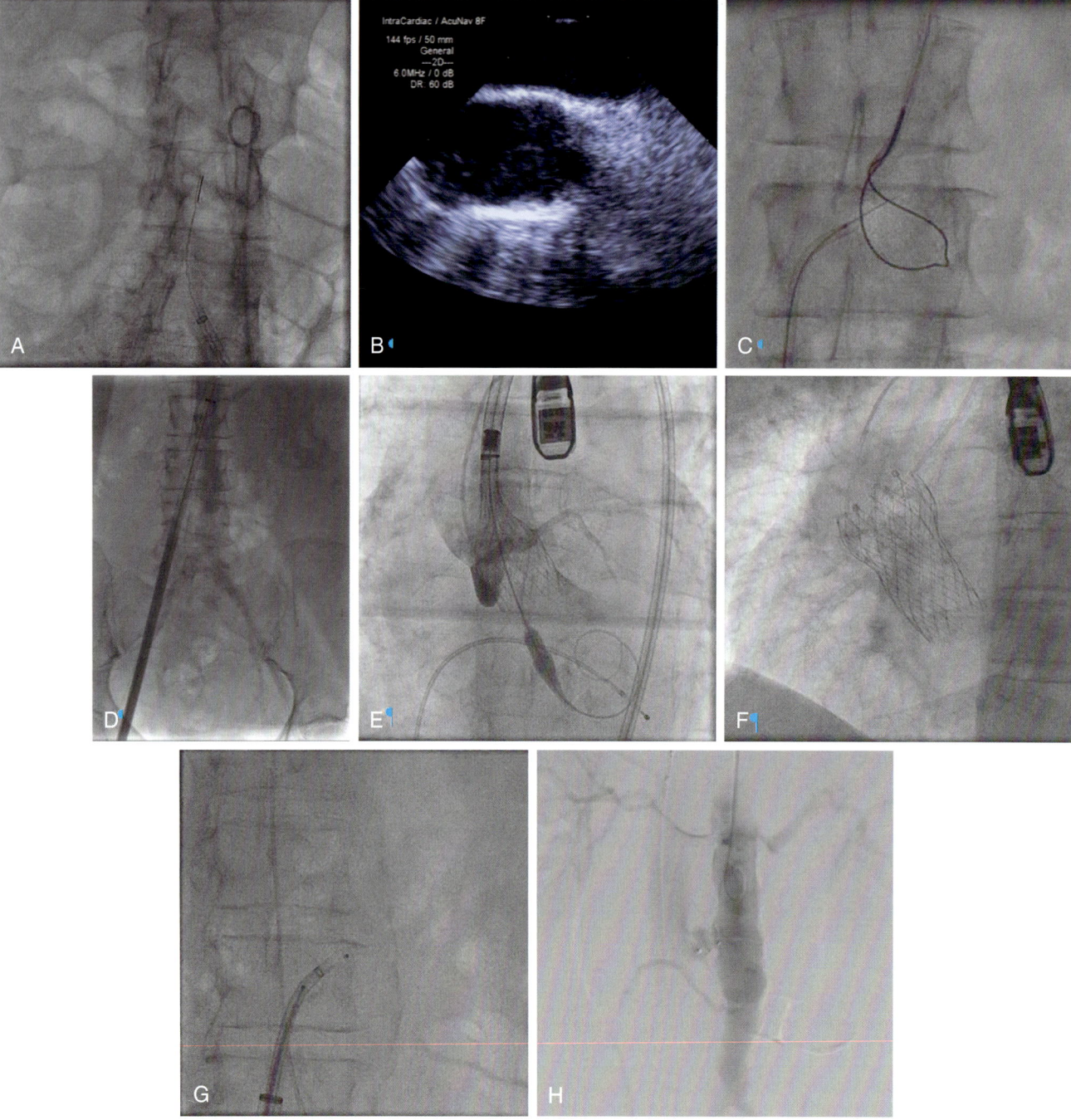

Fig. 54.11 Transcatheter aortic valve replacement (TAVR) via the transcaval venous approach for patients with severe peripheral artery disease. (A) An intracardiac echocardiogram (ICE) probe in the distal inferior vena cava (IVC) adjacent to a pigtail catheter in the aorta. (B) ICE images demonstrating the IVC at the top of the image and the aorta below it, identifying an appropriate site for cava-aortic puncture by minimizing the distance between the IVC and the aorta. In addition to preprocedure computed tomography images and intraprocedure angiography, ICE can assist in finding the optimal site for cava-aortic vascular access above the iliac bifurcation and below the renal vasculature, often overlying the L3 vertebra. (C) An electrified guidewire in the IVC is directed into a snare in the abdominal aorta. (D) A large-bore sheath is advanced from the IVC into the aorta over the guidewire. (E and F) TAVR is deployed in the standard fashion, as previously described. (G) An off-label patent ductus arteriosus (PDA) closure device is deployed across the cava-aortic fistula site. (H) Final digital subtraction angiography demonstrates minimal residual aortocaval shunt. Many patients have some residual shunting at the conclusion of the procedure, but the majority of fistulas are believed to close at 30 days postprocedure.

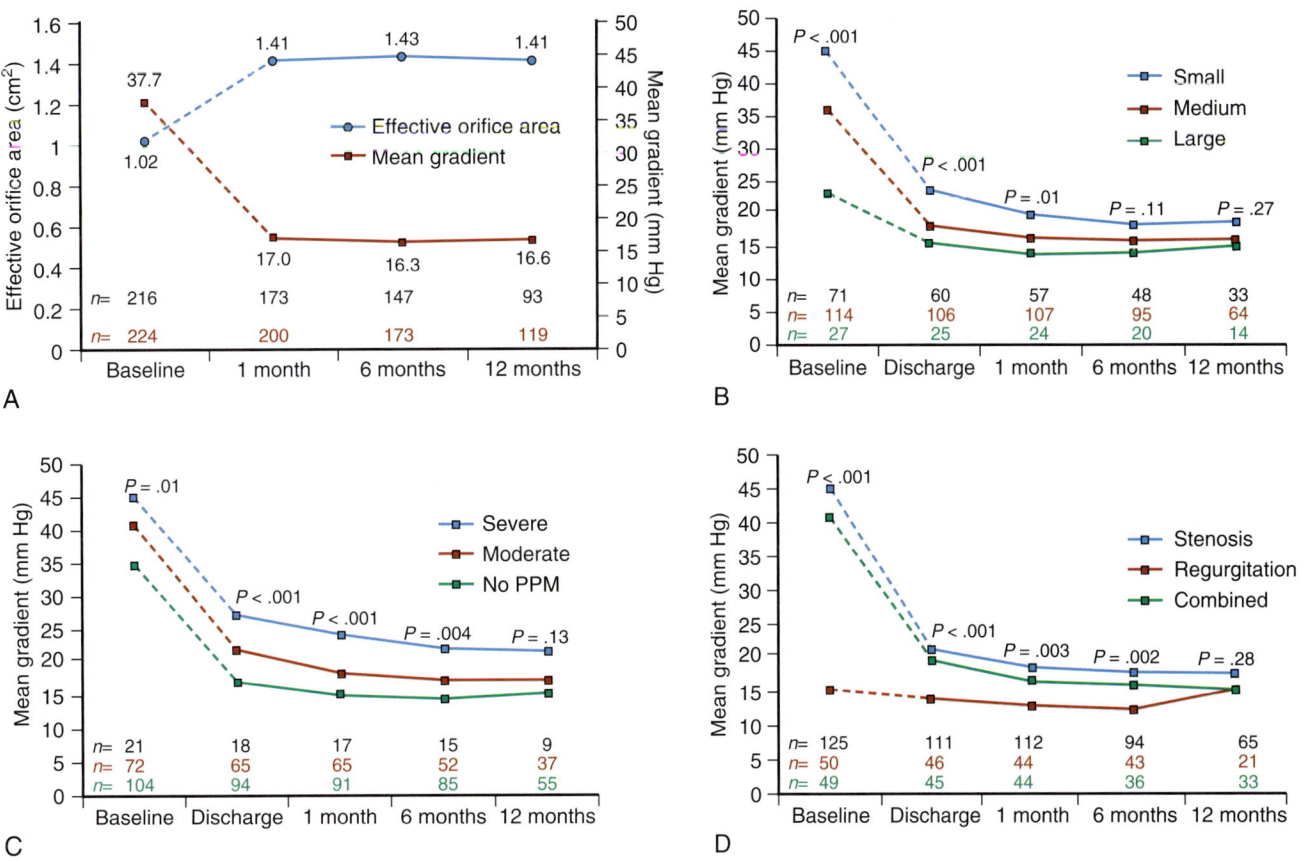

Fig. 54.12 Echocardiographic findings at 1 year in patients undergoing self-expanding transcatheter aortic valve replacement for surgical valve failure. (A) The effective orifice area and mean aortic gradients over time. The change from baseline to discharge was statistically significant ($P < .001$) for both effective orifice area and mean gradient in a corresponding paired analysis. (B) The mean aortic valve gradient according to surgical valve size showed higher gradients with smaller valve size, but these relationships were not significant after 1 month. The mean aortic valve gradient by (C) the degree of surgical valve prosthesis-patient mismatch (SV-PPM). (D) The modality of surgical valve failure (SVF) showed that more severe SV PPM and modality of SVF are associated with higher gradients through the first 6 months postprocedure. The dashed line indicates site-reported data at screening; all follow-up data are core lab reported.

A large registry series has provided further insights into the outcomes of patients with bicuspid aortic valve disease.[56,60,61] In one cohort of 561 patients with bicuspid aortic stenosis who were compared with 4546 patients with tricuspid aortic stenosis, patients with bicuspid aortic stenosis had more frequent conversion to surgery (2.0% vs. 0.2%) than those with tricuspid aortic valve disease; $P = .006$) and a significantly lower device success rate (85.3% vs. 91.4% than patients with tricuspid aortic valve disease; $P = .002$). Within the group receiving early-generation devices, patients with bicuspid aortic stenosis receiving the self-expanding device had more frequent aortic root injury (4.5% vs. 0.0% for tricuspid aortic stenosis; $P = .015$) when receiving the balloon-expanding device and moderate-to-severe paravalvular leak (19.4% vs. 10.5% for tricuspid aortic stenosis; $P = .02$). Among patients with new-generation devices, however, procedural results were comparable across different prostheses. The cumulative all-cause mortality rates at 2 years were comparable between patients with bicuspid and tricuspid aortic stenosis (17.2% vs. 19.4% in patients with tricuspid disease; $P = .28$).[60,61] Another iteration of this publication described the outcomes of patients with first- and second-generation devices in more detail.[61] Of 301 patients, 199 (71.1%) were treated with early-generation devices (i.e., Sapien XT, CoreValve) and 102 were treated with new-generation devices (i.e., Sapien 3, Lotus).[61] Moderate or severe paravalvular leak was significantly less frequent with new-generation compared with early-generation devices (0.0% vs. 8.5%; $P = .002$), which resulted in a higher device success rate (92.2% vs. 80.9%; $P = .01$).[61] There were no differences between early- and new-generation devices in stroke (2.5% vs. 2.0%; $P > .99$), life-threatening bleeding (3.5% vs. 2.9%; $P > .99$), major vascular complications (4.5% vs. 2.9%; $P = .76$), stage 2 to 3 acute kidney injury (2.5% vs. 2.9%; $P > .99$), early safety end points (15.1% vs. 10.8%; $P = .30$), and 30-days all-cause mortality (4.5% vs. 3.9%; $P > .99$).[61] An additional single-arm study in low-surgical-risk patients with bicuspid aortic valve disease treated with the Evolut bioprosthesis is ongoing.

Transcather Valve Therapies Registry "Real World Outcomes"

Between January 2014 and April 2016, a total of 9616 patients underwent TAVR with a self-expanding prosthesis with data entered in the Transcather Valve Therapies (TVT) Registry. Compared with patients treated with CoreValve TAVR, those who received Evolut-R TAVR had a lower STS-PROM score ($8.0 \pm 5.4\%$ vs. $8.7 \pm 5.3\%$; $P < .001$), more IF access (91.6% vs.

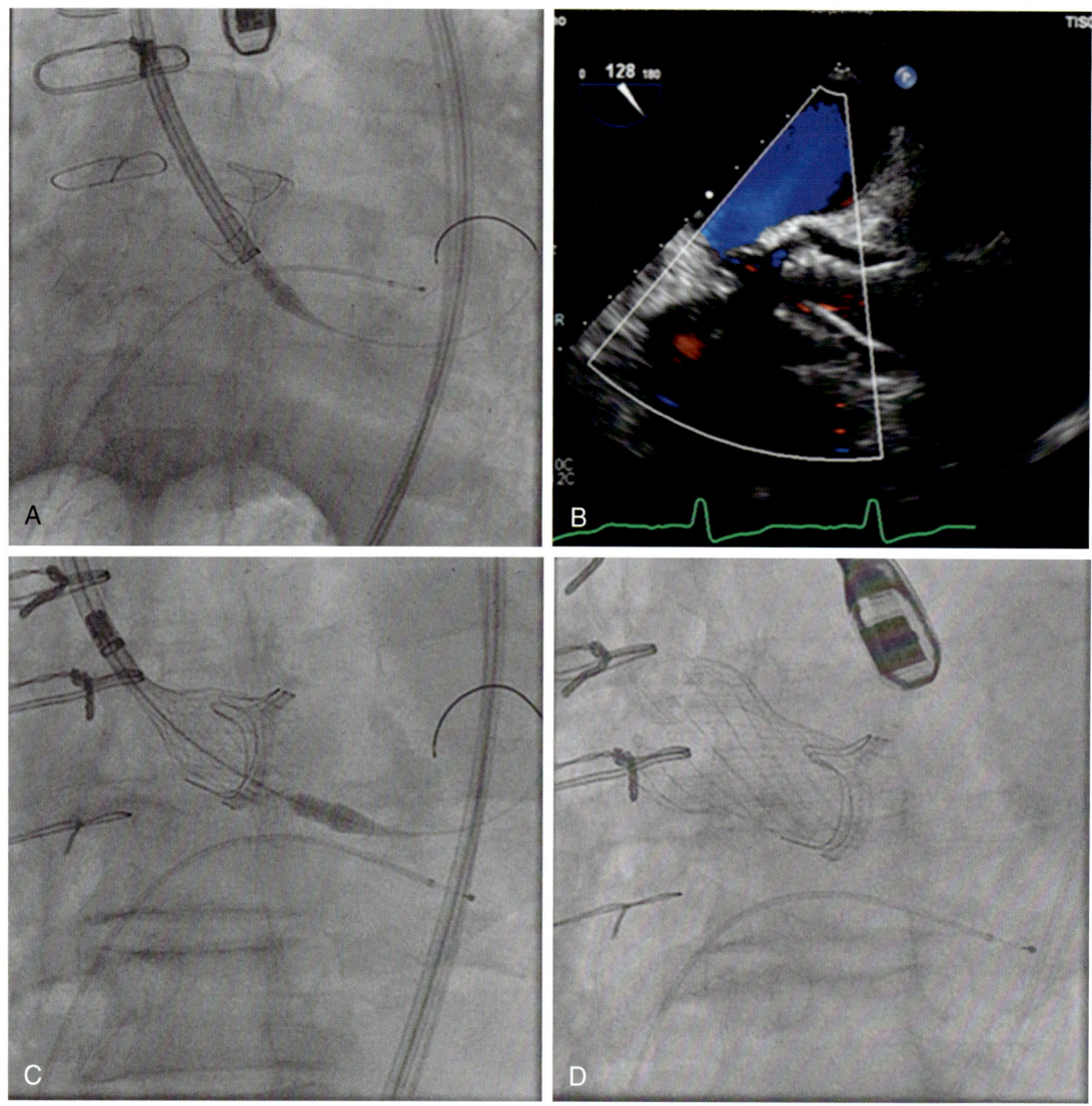

Fig. 54.13 CoreValve classic for surgical aortic valve failure. Valve-in-valve transcatheter aortic valve replacement for a failed surgical aortic valve bioprosthesis. (A) Fluroscopy of the initial positioning of the TAVR across the failed surgical bioprosthesis prior to deployment. (B) Transesophageal echocardiographic image of a partially deployed valve. This valve was repositioned to sit less deep into the left ventricular outflow tract. (C) The repositioned valve, now at the appropriate depth and well positioned relative to the failed surgical bioprosthesis. (D) Final angiographic result. (Adapted from Deeb GM, Chetcuti SJ, Yakubov SJ, et al. Impact of annular size on outcomes after surgical or transcatheter aortic valve replacement. *Ann Thorac Surg*. 2018;105(4):1129–1136.)

89.2%; $P < .001$), and more frequently had conscious sedation (27.4% vs. 12.7%; $P < .001$).[62] With Evolut-R TAVR, there was less need for a second prosthesis (2.2% vs. 4.5%; $P < .001$), less device migration (0.2% vs. 0.6%; $P = .01$), a lower incidence of moderate/severe paravalvular regurgitation (postprocedure, 4.4% vs. 6.2%; $P < .001$), and a shorter median hospital stay (4.0 vs. 5.0 days; $P < .001$).[62] Patients treated with Evolut-R TAVR had greater device success (96.3% vs. 94.9%; $P = .001$).[62] At 30 days, Evolut-R patients had both lower mortality (3.7% vs. 5.3%; $P < .001$) and less need for a pacemaker (18.3% vs. 20.1%; $P = .03$).[62]

COMPLICATIONS AFTER SELF-EXPANDING TRANSCATHETER AORTIC VALVE REPLACEMENT

Predictors of Mortality

Early and late mortality rates after TAVR are primarily related to underlying patient comorbidities, frailties, and disabilities. In an analysis of all patients enrolled in the high- and extreme-risk CoreValve clinical trials, the overall mortality rate was 5.8% at 30 days and 22.8% at 1 year.[63] Home oxygen use, assisted living, albumin levels below 3.3 g/dL, and age greater than 85 years predicted death at 30 days.[63] Home oxygen use, albumin levels below 3.3 g/dL, falls within the previous 6 months, STS PROM score greater than 7%, and a severe (≥ 5) Charlson comorbidity score predicted death at 1 year.[63] A simple scoring system created on the basis of these multivariate predictors effectively stratified risk at 30 days and 1 year into low-, moderate-, and high-risk subsets (Fig. 54.17).[63] This score showed a threefold difference in mortality rates for the low- and high-risk subsets at 30 days (3.6% and 10.9%, respectively) and 1 year (12.3% and 36.6%, respectively).[63] The 1-year mortality model was more stable than the 30-day model (C-statistics 0.79 vs. 0.75).[63] These factors may be useful for risk calculation when futility is discussed with patients being considered for TAVR.

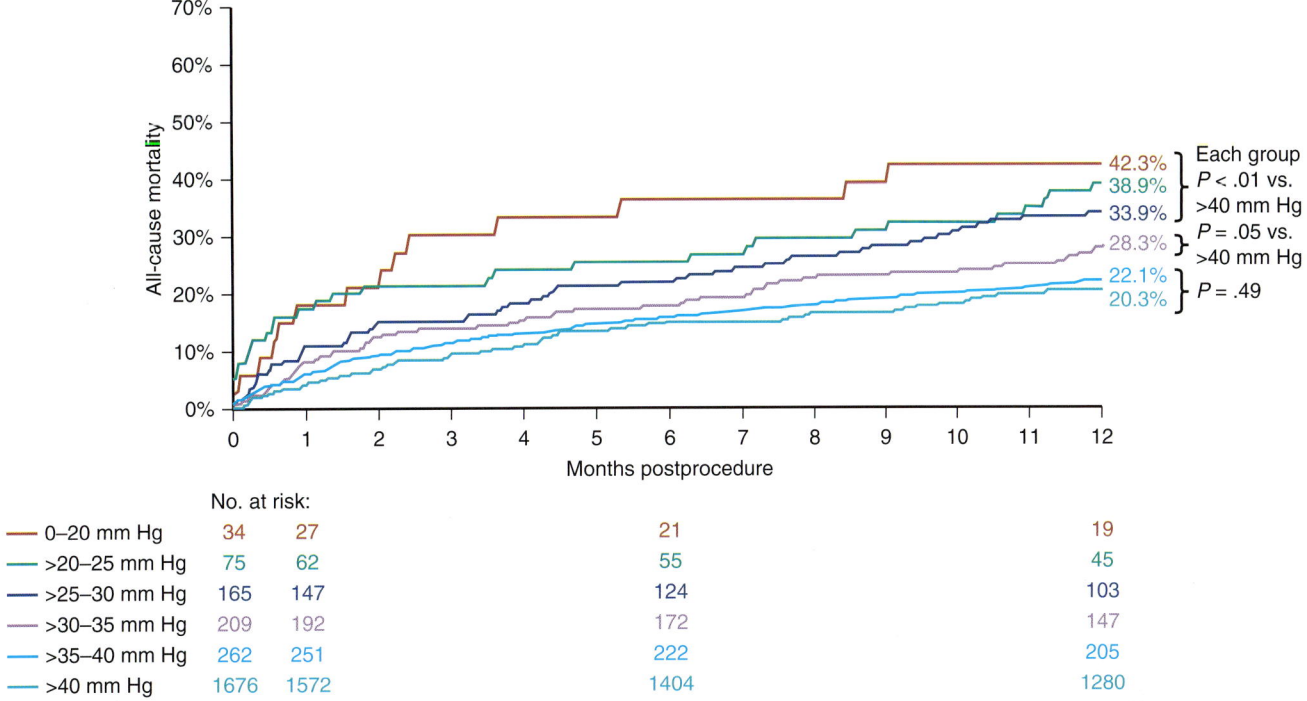

Fig. 54.14 Association of baseline gradient and all-cause mortality at 1 year. Patients with the lowest baseline mean gradient had the highest 1-year all-cause mortality. The group with gradients greater than 40 mm Hg was set as the reference, and each other group was compared with it. Groups with gradients of 0 to 20 mm Hg, greater than 20 to 25 mm Hg, and greater than 25 to 30 mm Hg were significantly different from the reference group (gradient >40 mm Hg) ($P < .01$), whereas the group with gradients greater than 30 to 35 mm Hg trended toward a significant difference ($P = .05$). There was no difference between the group with gradients greater than 35 to 40 mm Hg and the reference group.

Neurologic Injury

Neurologic injury is a known complication and limits the overall benefit of TAVR,[64] most often due to the release of embolic debris during the procedure.[65] In the CoreValve high-risk randomized study, the 30-day, 1-year, and 2-year stroke rates were 4.9%, 8.7%, and 10.9%, respectively, for TAVR and 6.2%, 12.5%, and 16.6%, respectively, for SAVR ($P = .46$, .11, and .05, respectively).[66] All-cause mortality in patients with a major stroke was 83.3% for TAVR and 54.5% for SAVR at 2 years ($P = .29$).[66] Late major stroke was disproportionately higher (23.8% at 2 years) among patients with poor IF access randomized to SAVR. Peripheral vascular disease, falls within 6 months, severe aortic calcification, and high (≥ 5) Charlson score predicted 1-year stroke after TAVR.[66] The impact of stroke using the National Institute of Health Stroke Scale (NIHSS) and Mini-Mental State Examination (MMSE) scores trended higher after SAVR than after TAVR. Lack of DAPT during and after TAVR was associated with early stroke.[66] The impact of major stroke after TAVR or SAVR is associated with a greater than 50% 1-year mortality rate (Fig. 54.18).[66]

In patients enrolled in the intermediate-risk Safety and Efficacy Study of the Medtronic CoreValve System in the Treatment of Severe, Symptomatic Aortic Stenosis in Intermediate Risk Subjects Who Need Aortic Valve Replacement (SURTAVI) Trial, the rates of 30-day stroke and postprocedural encephalopathy were higher after open chest surgery (SAVR) compared with TAVR (5.4% vs. 3.3%; $P = .031$; and 7.8% vs. 1.6%; $P < .001$, respectively).[67] At 12 months, the rate of stroke was not different between SAVR and TAVR (6.9% vs. 5.2%; $P = .136$).[67] Early stroke and early encephalopathy resulted in an elevated mortality at 12 months in both treatment groups.[67] Quality of life (QOL) after an early stroke was significantly lower in SAVR versus TAVR patients at 30 days and was similar at 6 and 12 months.[67]

TAVR patients enrolled in the CoreValve Pivotal Trials had a 1-year stroke rate after TAVR of 8.4%. Analysis of the stroke hazard rate identified an early phase (0 to 10 days; 4.1% of strokes) and a late phase (11 to 365 days; 4.3% of strokes).[68] Baseline predictors of early stroke included a NIHSS score greater than zero, prior stroke, prior transient ischemic attack (TIA), peripheral vascular disease, absence of prior coronary artery bypass surgery, angina, low body mass index (<21 kg/m^2), and falls within the previous 6 months.[68] Significant procedural predictors were total time in the catheterization laboratory or operating room, delivery catheter time in the body, rapid pacing used during valvuloplasty, and repositioning of the prosthesis.[68] Predictors of stroke between 11 and 365 days were small body surface area, severe aortic calcification, and falls within the previous 6 months. There were no significant imaging predictors of early or late stroke.[68] Neuroprotective devices have been developed and may be useful for reducing the incidence of stroke after TAVR.[69]

Post–Transcatheter Aortic Valve Replacement Aortic Regurgitation

Determination of the etiology of aortic regurgitation after CoreValve placement is an important factor in assessing both its significant and its treatment.[16,17,20,70–106] Significant aortic regurgitation due to paravalvular leaks is uncommon after Evolut TAVR; it is primarily related to low positioning of the Evolut frame, incomplete expansion of the frame into the eccentrically shaped annulus, rigidity of the underlying aortic annulus due to

SECTION V Structural Interventions

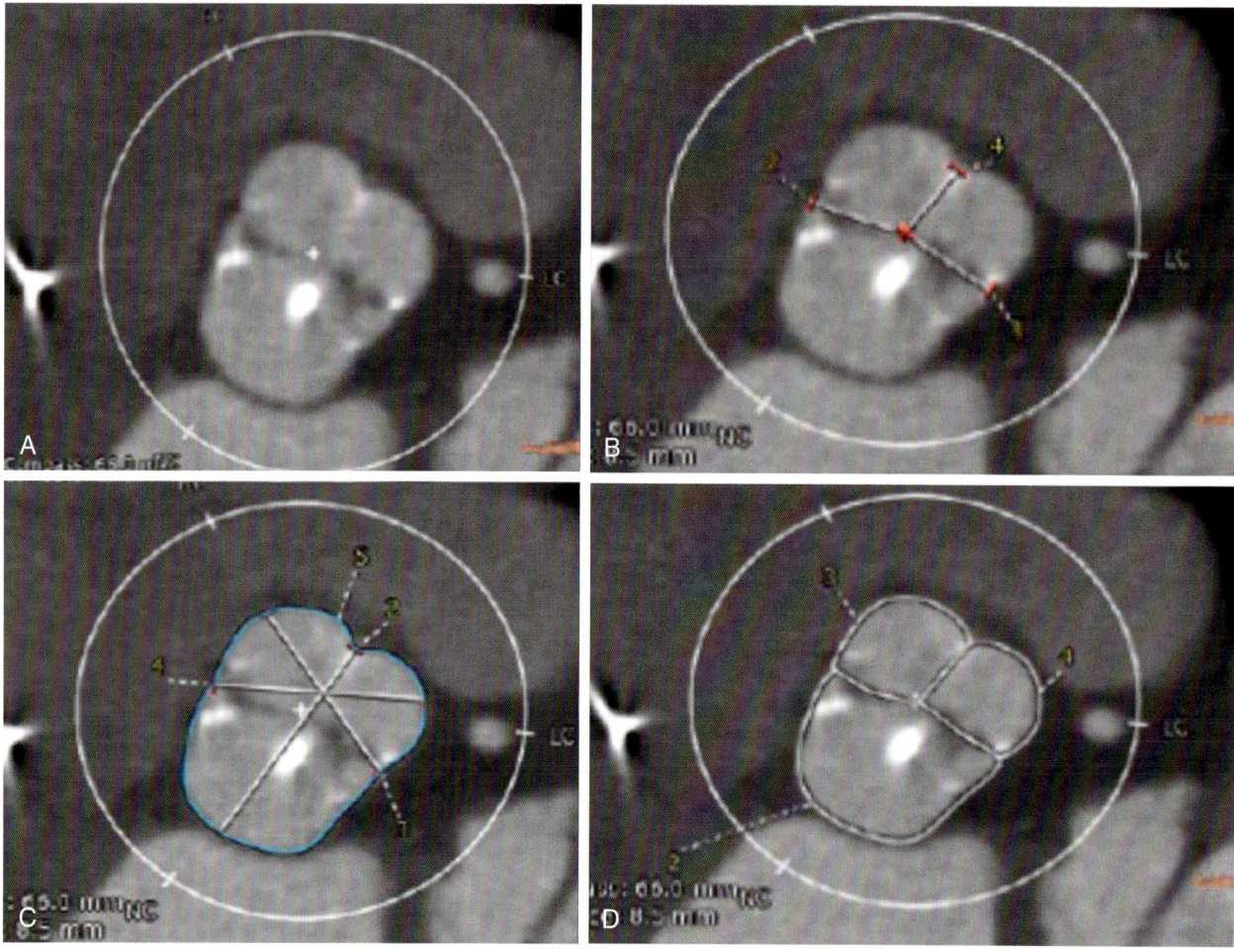

Fig. 54.15 Parameters for the assessment of leaflet asymmetry. (A) Tripost bicuspid aortic stenosis with a raphe of the left and right coronary cusps. Quantification of leaflet width (B), sinus of Valsalva width (C), and sinus area (D); these provide an estimate of the asymmetry of the noncoronary sinus relative to the combined right and left coronary cusps. (Adapted from Popma JJ, Ramadan R. CT Imaging of bicuspid aortic valve disease for TAVR. *JACC Cardiovasc Imaging.* 2016;9[10]:1159–1163.)

calcium, or undersizing of the valve relative to aortic annular size. When the Evolut frame is underexpanded, postdeployment valvuloplasty may be useful; when the Evolut frame is positioned too low after deployment, retraction of the frame loops using a retrieval snare may allow appropriate positioning within the annulus. Higher degrees of postimplantation aortic regurgitation (≥2+) have been associated with worse clinical outcomes, including low cardiac output, respiratory failure, delirium, new left bundle branch block, and in-hospital death. Moderate to severe aortic regurgitation improved in over 80% of patients in the first year after CoreValve implantation, likely due to annular remodeling with computed tomography (CT)–based valve sizing. Lower rates of paravalvular regurgitation have been observed with the Evolut-R and Evolut-PRO devices. Oversizing of the self-expanding prosthesis will lower the rate of paravalvular regurgitation.[6,104]

Vascular Access Complications

Due to the relatively large (14- to 18-Fr) sheaths required for TF aortic valve placement, a number of vascular complications may occur during self-expanding TAVR. Vascular complications can be predicted by high sheath-to-femoral artery ratios, vessel calcification, and female gender.[107,108] The development of major vascular complications after TAVR is an important predictor of early mortality.[108] Type A ascending aortic dissection is an uncommon (<0.5%) complication,[109] most often due to the separation of the self-expanding Nitinol capsule from the catheter nosecone in highly angulated aortic arches, particularly with early-generation CoreValve and Evolut-R systems. In the setting of resistance when the Evolut is being passed around the arch, reorientation of the catheter by 90 degrees in the descending aorta or using an extra-stiff guidewire will minimize the risk of this complication. Assessment of the IF access diameters using noninvasive imaging, such as CTA or vascular ultrasound, will permit appropriate vessel preparation with dilators or balloon angioplasty and allow placement of a 14-Fr (Evolut-R, minimal diameter 5.0 mm) or 16-Fr (Evolut-PRO or Evolut-R, 34 mm, minimum diameter 5.5 mm) sheath. In the event of iliac disruption, Viabahn-covered stents may be used.[110] More commonly, vascular complications develop at the site of common femoral artery arteriotomy. Most clinical centers now used a combination of two ProGlides placed in a "preclosure manner"; but in the event of failure, "crossover" balloon percutaneous transluminal angioplasty, covered stent placement,[111] or surgical closure may be required.[112] Caution should be used in the placement of a covered stent across the profunda due to potential vessel compromise.

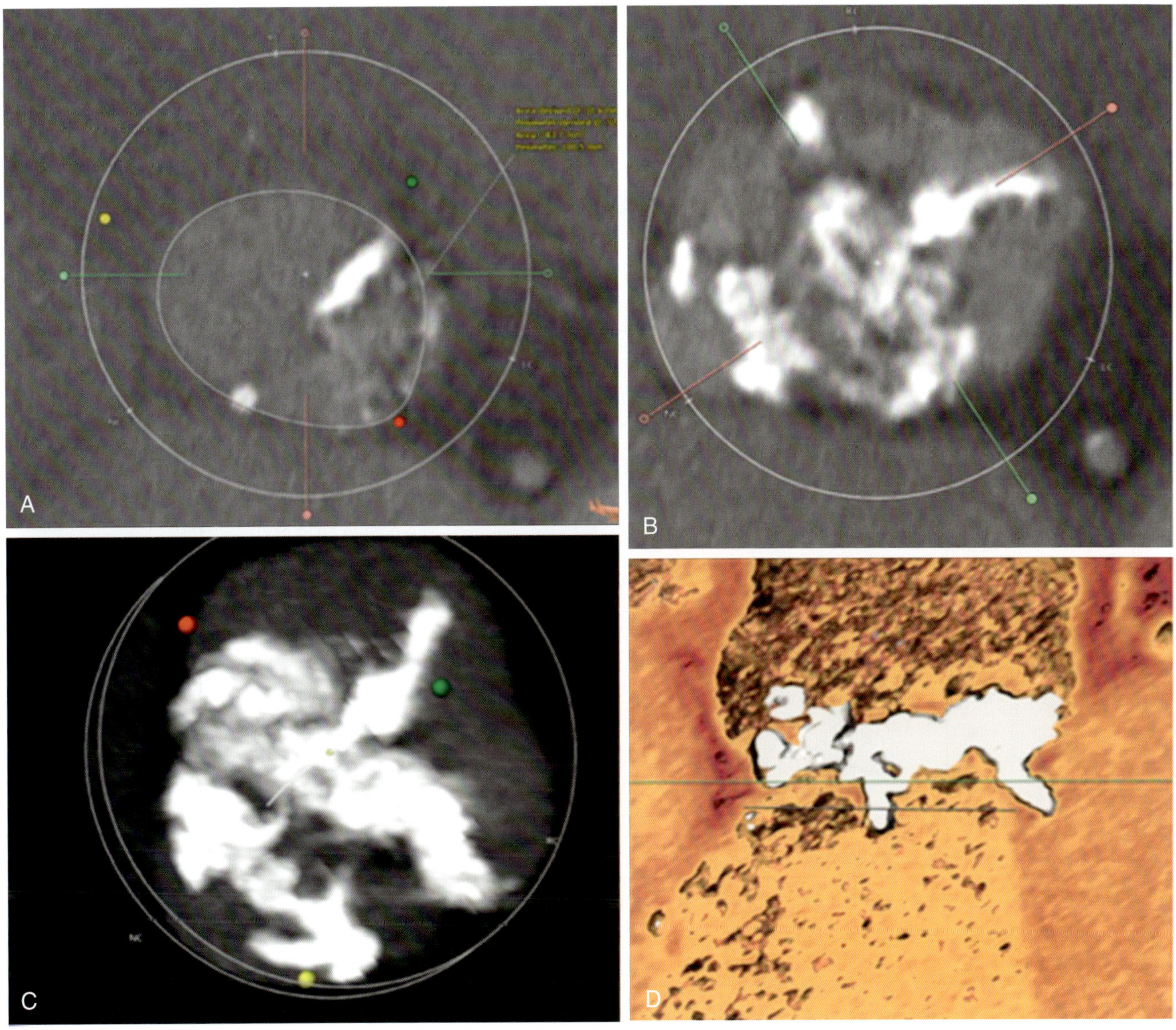

Fig. 54.16 Calcification of the bicuspid raphe. (A) Multidetector computed tomography (MDCT) cross section of the basal portion of the sinus of Valsalva demonstrating a calcified raphe between the right and left coronary cusps. (B) Higher in the midportion of the aortic sinus of Valsalva, a continuation of the calcified raphe is seen. (C) "Hockey puck" view of the bicuspid valve shows fusion of the raphe and nodular calcification of the fused leaflets and the noncoronary cusp. (D) Volume rendering of the aortic annulus shows extensive calcification and fusion of the left and right raphe. The area derived diameter of this case was 31.2 mm; the patient was successfully treated with a 29-mm SAPIEN 3 device, underscoring the difficulty of assessing TAVR sizing in the presence of bicuspid aortic valve disease. (Adapted from Popma JJ, Ramadan R. CT Imaging of bicuspid aortic valve disease for TAVR. *JACC Cardiovasc Imaging.* 2016;9[10]:1159–1163.)

Conduction System Disturbances

Owing to the location of the atrioventricular node and origin of the left bundle adjacent to the junction of the right coronary and noncoronary cusps, irritation of the membranous septum due to TAVR can affect atrioventricular conduction. A new intraventricular conduction defect (QRS complex duration greater than 100 ms) or bundle branch block occurs in up to 40% of patients after self-expanding TAVR but may resolve in up to 50% of patients within 30 days after the procedure. Preoperative conduction system disease, membranous calcification, and the depth of implant[113] are independent predictors of PPM.[114–153]

Conduction disturbances and heart block occur in up to 25% of patients after CoreValve TAVR placement but may be lower in patients treated with the Evolut-R and Evolut-PRO devices. This is likely due to a less extensive outward force at the LVOT, better positioning with retrievable Evolut, and a protective pericardial wrap that may lessen irritation of the membranous septum. Although there have been few studies to suggest late-term detriment in patients undergoing permanent pacemaker placement, pacemakers may result in less improvement in left ventricular function in patients with preexisting impaired left ventricular ejection fraction.

Coronary Artery Occlusion

Coronary occlusion after CoreValve TAVR is a rare (<1%) occurrence.[154–170] CTA has shown that the distance between the

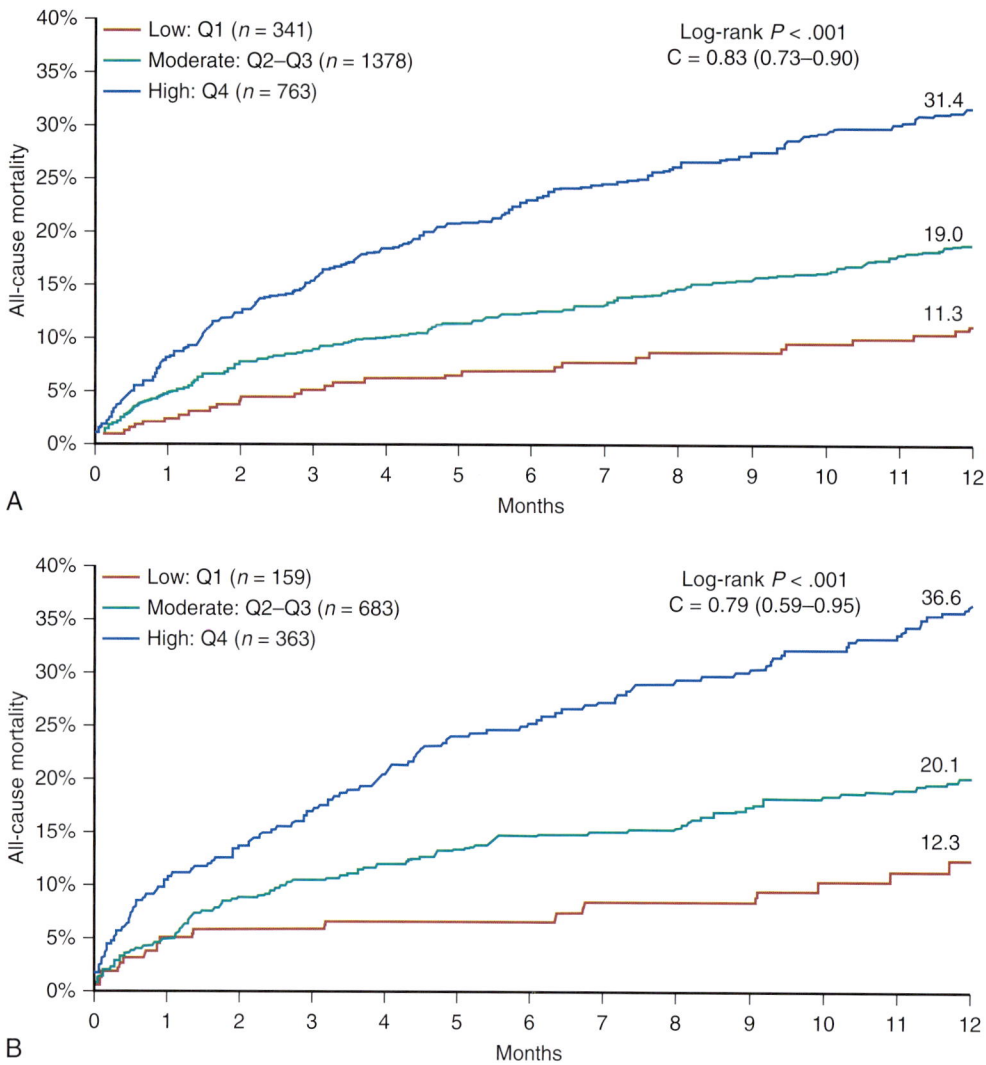

Fig. 54.17 Mortality risk score for transcatheter aortic valve replacement: impact of frailty and disability on outcome. A mortality risk score was derived using a subset of patients called the derivation cohort; this risk score was then tested in another subset of patients called the validation cohort. (A) Kaplan–Meier estimates of 1-year mortality rates for the derivation cohort by risk score. (B) Kaplan–Meier estimates of 1-year mortality rates for the validation cohort by risk score. The risk score showed a threefold difference in mortality rates for the low- and high-risk subsets at 1 year, with a more stable C-statistic than that seen at 30 days.

aortic annulus and the coronary arteries is reduced in patients with aortic stenosis, likely due to longitudinal remodeling of the aortic root in patients with degenerative aortic stenosis. As the degenerative native aortic valve is not removed but is circumferentially displaced after TAVR, patients with a narrow SOV and low origin of the native coronary arteries may be predisposed to coronary occlusion from displacement of the native valve during TAVR. Coupled with the constrained CoreValve frame diameter in the region of the coronary ostia, and better preprocedural screening using aortography and CTA screening to ensure an adequate SOV width and height, the frequency of coronary occlusion is now rare. In the unlikely occurrence of coronary occlusion, rescue percutaneous coronary intervention can be performed to reestablish coronary perfusion (Fig. 54.19).

Acute Kidney Injury

Acute kidney injury after TAVR may result from exposure to contrast during the procedure, hypotension during valve deployment, or particulate embolization from the aorta and aortic valve during deployment, among other factors. Acute kidney injury, defined by an increase equal to or greater than 0.3 mg/dL in serum creatinine within 72 hours, occurs in 15.8% to 20% of patients after TAVR, although severe kidney injury requiring renal replacement therapy is uncommon (<2%). Acute kidney injury occurs more often in women, with baseline renal insufficiency, general anesthesia, and transfusion of three or more red blood cell (RBC) units within 72 hours after TAVR[171]; it is associated with an increase in early[172] and late[171] mortality.

Leaflet Thickening and Thrombosis

A number of reports have demonstrated the presence of thrombus involving the leaflets of transcatheter aortic valves.[173–180] In a systematic microscopic and macroscopic pathologic analysis of self-expanding CoreValve transcatheter aortic valves removed at autopsy or surgically from the CoreValve U.S. Pivotal Trial of extreme- and high-risk patients, a total of 21 cases—with a median implant duration of 17.0 days (range 0 to 503 days)—were evaluated.[181] No valve frame fracture was observed and severe paravalvular gaps were uncommon. Inflammation and thrombus in the valve frame were minimal, but neointimal growth

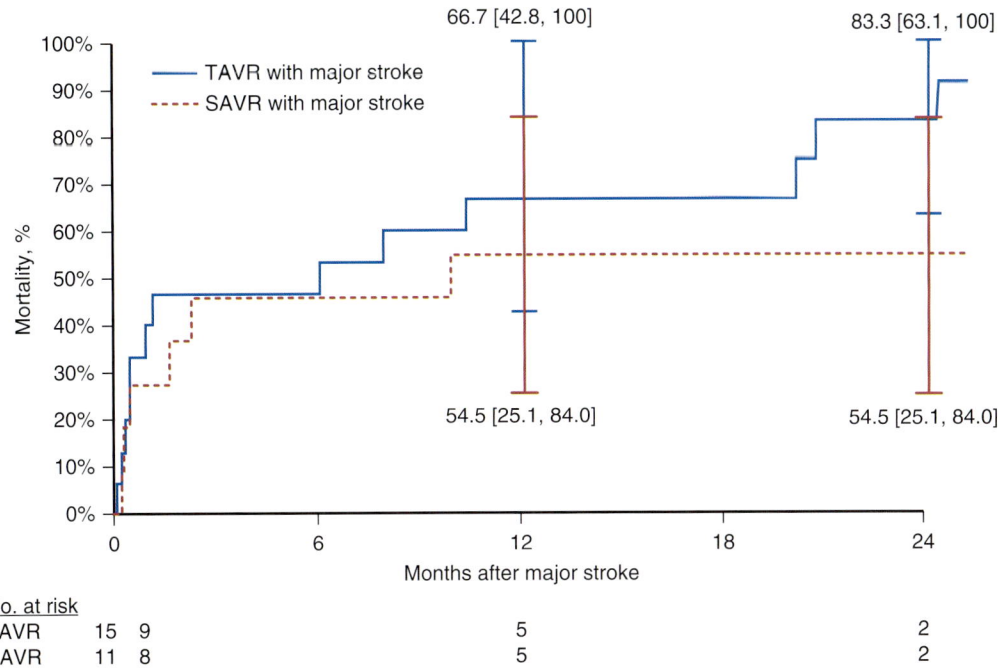

Fig. 54.18 Kaplan–Meier estimates of mortality after major stroke following transcatheter aortic valve replacement *(TAVR)* or surgical aortic valve replacement *(SAVR)*. Patients with major stroke within 30 days of TAVR or SAVR in the high-risk pivotal trial followed for 2 years. This time-to-event analysis assigned the day on which the stroke event occurred as day 0. (Adapted from Gleason TG, Schindler JT, Adams DH, et al. The risk and extent of neurologic events are equivalent for high-risk patients treated with transcatheter or surgical aortic valve replacement. *J Thorac Cardiovasc Surg*. 2016;152[1]:85–96.)

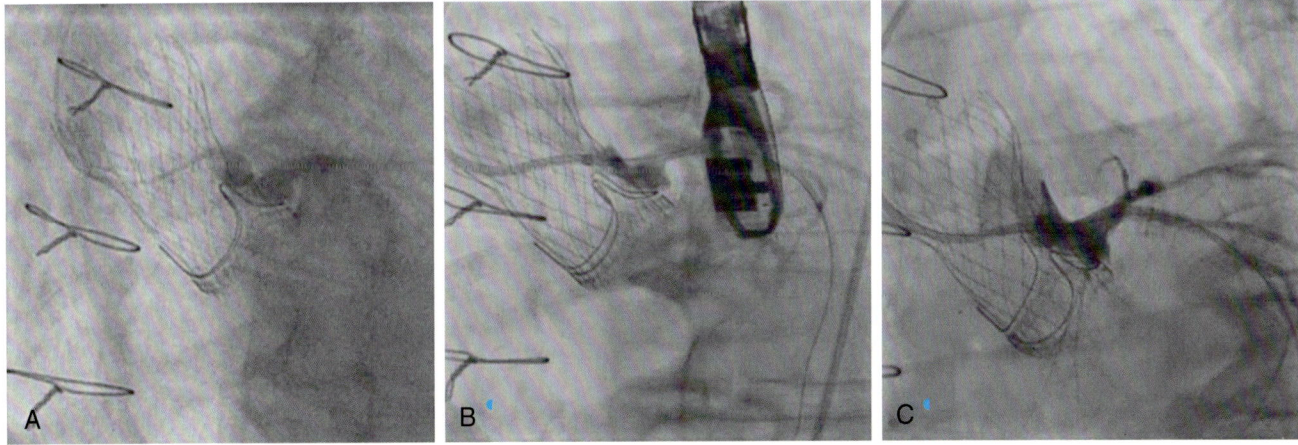

Fig. 54.19 Coronary obstruction after transcatheter aortic valve replacement in a patient with surgical valve failure. An elderly man developed chest pain and acute pulmonary edema after valve-in-valve transcatheter aortic valve replacement (TAVR) was performed. (A) Coronary angiography demonstrated partial obstruction of the left main coronary artery due to impingement of the old surgical bioprosthetic valve leaflet. (B) Since angioplasty equipment would not deliver past the heavily calcified leaflet, laser atherectomy was performed. (C) Final angiography result, demonstrating a patent "snorkel" stent into the left main coronary artery through a wire-frame cell of the TAVR's supporting structure.

increased overtime. Symptomatic valve thrombosis was observed in 1 patient (5%) and subclinical moderate leaflet thrombus was observed in 4 additional patients (19%). Inflammation of the leaflets was mild, whereas structural changes were minimal, and patient had infective endocarditis.[181] Pannus or leaflet calcification were not observed.[181]

Makkar and colleagues evaluated the computed tomographic images of 55 patients in a clinical trial of TAVR and from two single-center registries that included 132 patients who were undergoing either TAVR or implantation of surgical aortic valve bioprostheses.[179] Reduced leaflet motion was noted on CT in 22 of 55 patients (40%) in the clinical trial and in 17 of 132 patients (13%) in the two registries.[179] Reduced leaflet motion was detected among patients with multiple bioprosthesis types, including transcatheter and surgical bioprostheses.[179] Therapeutic anticoagulation with warfarin, as compared with DAPT, was associated with a decreased incidence of reduced leaflet motion (0% and 55%, respectively, $P = .01$ in the clinical trial; and 0% and 29%, respectively, $P = .04$ in the pooled registries).[179] In patients who were reevaluated with follow-up CT, restoration of leaflet motion was noted in all 11 patients who were receiving anticoagulation and in 1 of 10 patients who were not receiving anticoagulation ($P < .001$).[179] There was no significant difference in the incidence of stroke or TIA between patients with reduced leaflet motion and those with normal leaflet motion in the clinical trial (2 of 22 patients and 0 of 33 patients, respectively; $P = .16$).[179]

PREDICTORS OF OUTCOME

Women

Increasing information has accumulated regarding outcomes in women undergoing TAVR. The Women's INternational Transcatheter Aortic Valve Implantation (WIN-TAVI) registry was a multinational, prospective, observational registry of women undergoing TAVR for aortic stenosis.[182] Between January 2013 and December 2015, a total of 1019 women were enrolled (mean age, 82.5 ± 6.3 years, mean STS PROM 8.3% ± 7.4%).[182] TAVR was performed via TF access in 90.6% and new-generation devices were used in 42.1%.[182] In more than two-thirds of cases, an Edwards SAPIEN 23-mm (Edwards Lifesciences, Irvine, CA) or Medtronic CoreValve 26-mm or smaller (Medtronic Inc., Minneapolis, MN) device was implanted.[182] Outcomes include all-cause mortality (3.4%), stroke (1.3%), major vascular complications (7.7%), and life-threatening bleeding (4.4%.)[182]

Another registry compared the outcomes of 1708 women and 1979 men treated with self-expanding CoreValve devices.[183] At baseline, women tended to be slightly older and to be more frail, but they had fewer cardiac comorbidities, higher left ventricular systolic function, less coronary artery disease, and fewer previous strokes.[183] All-cause mortality was 5.9% for women and 5.8% for men at 30 days ($P = .87$) and 24.1% and 21.3%, respectively, at 1 year ($P = .08$).[183] The incidence of stroke was 5.7% in women and 4.0% in men at 30 days ($P = .02$) and 9.3% and 7.7%, respectively, at 1 year ($P = .05$).[183] Women had a higher incidence of bleeding, including more life-threatening bleeds and a greater incidence of major vascular complications than men at 30 days.[183] Similar findings were found in a German registry comparing the outcomes of women and men.[184]

Women at high risk for surgery seem to do particularly well with TAVR compared with SAVR. In the CoreValve High Risk randomized trial, a total of 353 women were enrolled with 183 assigned to TAVR and 170 assigned to SAVR.[185] TAVR-treated women experienced a statistically significant 1-year survival advantage compared with SAVR-treated women (12.7% vs. 21.8%; $P = .03$). The composite all-cause mortality or major stroke rate also favored TAVR-treated women (14.9% vs. 24.2% in SAVR-treated women; $P = .04$).[185]

Prior Coronary Artery Bypass Surgery

To evaluate the relative benefit of TAVR and surgery in patients with prior coronary artery bypass surgery, the results of the high-risk CoreValve randomized trial were reviewed. The 226 patients enrolled in this trial all had prior coronary artery bypass graft surgery.[186] At 1 year, all-cause mortality was 9.6% for TAVR versus 18.1% for SAVR ($P = .06$); cardiovascular mortality was 7.0% for TAVR versus 13.8% for SAVR ($P = .09$).[186] No differences were seen for stroke. The SAVR group had longer ICU and hospital stays, an increased incidence of acute kidney injury, life-threatening or disabling bleeding, and major adverse cardiac and cerebrovascular events ($P < .05$), whereas pacemaker implantation and paravalvular regurgitation were greater with TAVR at all time points.[186] Similar findings were found in the FRANCE-2 Registry.[187]

Chronic Lung Disease

The prevalence and severity of chronic lung disease (CLD) was determined at baseline in high- and extreme-risk patients with aortic stenosis from the CoreValve U.S. Pivotal Trial.[188] A favorable health benefit was defined as alive with a Kansas City Cardiomyopathy Questionnaire Overall Summary (KCCQ-OS) score equal to or greater than 60 and stability (<10-point decrease) or improvement in the KCCQ-OS from baseline. CLD was present in 55% (20% mild, 13% moderate, 22% severe) of the 1030 patients studied. All-cause mortality was higher in patients with moderate and severe CLD at 1 year (19.6% mild, 28.1% moderate, 26.9% severe CLD vs. 19.2% non-CLD; $P = .030$) and 3 years (44.8% mild, 53.0% moderate, 51.9% severe vs. 37.7% non-CLD; $P < .001$).[188] NYHA functional class improved in more than 80% of patients with CLD at 1 and 3 years.[188] All patients had a nearly 20-point improvement in KCCQ-OS at 1 and 3 years.[188] However, only 43.3% of patients with CLD had a favorable health benefit at 1 year and 22.5% at 3 years.[188]

CLINICAL CONTRAINDICATIONS

Clinical contraindications to CoreValve placement include sepsis; active endocarditis; recent myocardial infarction or cerebrovascular accident; left ventricular or atrial thrombus; uncontrolled atrial fibrillation; or severe mitral, pulmonary, or tricuspid regurgitation. Relative precautions would include active gastritis or peptic ulcer disease, uncontrolled bleeding diathesis, symptomatic carotid artery disease, or abdominal or thoracic aortic aneurysm.

POTENTIAL ADVANTAGES OF SELF-EXPANDING TRANSCATHETER AORTIC VALVE REPLACEMENT

Hemodynamic Performance

The supra-annular CoreValve design resulted in sustained reduction in aortic valve gradients and improvements in effective orifice areas compared with surgery.[189] See Fig. 54.20 for details on post-procedure hemodynamics. PPM is an important predictor of outcome after traditional surgical AVR and TAVR.[190] In the CoreValve High Risk randomized study, the incidence of severe PPM in the surgery group at 1 year was 25.7% versus 6.2% in the TAVR group ($P < .0001$).[191] Left ventricular mass index regression at 1 year was 6.8% for TAVR and 15.1% for SAVR in patients with severe PPM.[191] At 1 year the rate of all-cause mortality and acute kidney injury were significantly greater in all patients (TAVR + SAVR) with severe PPM compared with no severe PPM (20.6% vs. 12.0% [$P = .0145$] for death and 19.2% vs. 8.5% [$P = .0008$] for acute kidney injury).[191] A number of studies have demonstrated recovery of left ventricular function after TAVR.[20,192-196]

IMPROVEMENTS IN QUALITY OF LIFE

An extensive amount of work has been performed to evaluate the health status in patients undergoing CoreValve TAVR. In the 471 extreme-risk patients enrolled in the CoreValve study, there was substantial improvement in both disease-specific and generic health status measures, with an increase in the KCCQ-OS of 23.9 points (95% CI 20.3 to 27.5 points) at 1 month, 27.4 points (95% CI 24.2 to 30.6 points) at 6 months, and 27.4 points (95% CI 24.1 to 30.8 points) at 12 months.[197] Nonetheless, 39% of patients had a poor outcome after TAVR.[197] Baseline factors independently associated with poor outcome included wheelchair dependency, lower mean aortic valve gradient, prior coronary artery bypass grafting, oxygen dependency, very high predicted mortality with

Normal reference values for the CoreValve and Evolut R valves by native annular diameter quintiles at 30 days						
Quintiles	≤22.8 mm	>22.8–24.5 mm	>24.5–25.9 mm	>25.9–27.6 mm	>27.6–41.5 mm	P Value for Trend
CoreValve						
EOA, cm^2	1.71 ± 0.55 (166)	1.80 ± 0.53 (141)	1.92 ± 0.48 (167)	1.94 ± 0.52 (165)	2.06 ± 0.66 (160)	< .001
EOAi, cm^2/m^2	1.03 ± 0.33 (166)	1.02 ± 0.30 (141)	1.04 ± 0.29 (167)	1.01 ± 0.30 (165)	1.07 ± 0.36 (160)	.34
Mean gradient, mm Hg	9.01 ± 4.06 (180)	8.96 ± 4.71 (151)	8.75 ± 3.99 (179)	9.16 ± 4.50 (170)	8.75 ± 3.61 (171)	.75
DVI	0.59 ± 0.15 (172)	0.55 ± 0.13 (145)	0.54 ± 0.11 (173)	0.53 ± 0.12 (167)	0.55 ± 0.14 (170)	.001
Quintiles	≤22.3 mm	>22.3–≤23.2 mm	>23.2–≤24.7 mm	>24.7–≤26.2 mm	>26.2–≤30.2 mm	P Value for Trend
Evolut R						
EOA, cm^2	1.66 ± 0.42 (53)	1.82 ± 0.43 (38)	1.98 ± 0.56 (62)	1.98 ± 0.59 (49)	2.56 ± 0.77 (53)	< .001
EOAi, cm^2/m^2	0.99 ± 0.27 (53)	1.09 ± 0.26 (38)	1.10 ± 0.32 (62)	1.06 ± 0.34 (49)	1.29 ± 0.37 (53)	< .001
Mean gradient, mm Hg	7.94 ± 3.10 (58)	6.91 ± 2.58 (43)	7.66 ± 2.94 (63)	8.53 ± 3.49 (56)	6.40 ± 3.34 (57)	.21
DVI	0.61 ± 0.11 (57)	0.61 ± 0.14 (41)	0.61 ± 0.15 (63)	0.56 ± 0.14 (51)	0.58 ± 0.15 (55)	.07

Values are mean ± SD (n). Trend test P value from generalized linear modeling with quintiles as independent ordinal variable.

Fig. 54.20 Predicted gradients by annular size. *EOA,* Effective orifice area; *EOAi,* effective orifice area index; *DVI,* Doppler velocity index. (Adapted from Hahn RT, Leipsic J, Douglas PS, et al. Comprehensive echocardiographic assessment of normal transcatheter valve function. *JACC Cardiovasc Imaging.* 2019;12[1]:25–34.)

SAVR, and low serum albumin.[197] These results were sustained 3 years after the procedure.[47] In an additional analysis of 2830 patients who underwent TAVR in the CoreValve U.S. Pivotal Extreme and High Risk trials, 31.2% experienced a poor outcome at 6 months following TAVR (death, 17.6%; very poor QOL, 11.6%; QOL decline, 2.0%) and 50.8% experienced a poor outcome at 1 year (death, 30.2%; poor QOL, 19.6%; QOL decline 1.0%).[198]

In patients randomized in the U.S. Pivotal Extreme High Risk study to TAVR or SAVR, disease-specific and general health status improved substantially for both treatment groups.[199] At 1 month, there was a significant interaction between the benefit of TAVR over SAVR and access site.[199] Among surviving patients eligible for IF access, there was a clinically relevant early benefit with TAVR across all disease-specific and generic health status measures.[199] Among the non-IF cohort, however, most health status measures were similar for TAVR and SAVR, although there was a trend toward early benefit with TAVR on the Short-Form 12 Questionnaire's physical health scale.[199] There were no consistent differences in health status between TAVR and SAVR at the later time points. A formal economic analysis on the basis of individual, patient-level data from the CoreValve U.S. High Risk Pivotal Trial was performed.[200] Relative to SAVR, TAVR reduced initial length of stay an average of 4.4 days, decreased the need for rehabilitation services at discharge, and resulted in superior 1-month QOL.[200] Index admission and projected lifetime costs were higher with TAVR than with SAVR (differences of $11,260 and $17,849 per patient, respectively), whereas TAVR was projected to provide a lifetime gain of 0.32 quality-adjusted life-years ([QALYs]; 0.41 life year [LY]) with 3% discounting.[200] Lifetime incremental cost-effectiveness ratios were $55,090 per QALY gained and $43,114 per LY gained.[200] Sensitivity analyses indicated that a reduction in the initial cost of TAVR by approximately $1650 would lead to an incremental cost-effectiveness ratio below $50,000/QALY gained.[200]

LOTUS VALVE

The Lotus Aortic Valve Replacement System (Boston Scientific, Natick, MA; Fig. 54.21A) is a bioprosthetic valve consisting of three bovine pericardial leaflets mounted into a braided Nitinol frame that can be delivered via a TF approach.[201] The valve is fully repositionable and retrievable prior to detachment, does not require rapid pacing for deployment, and has an adaptive seal that minimizes paravalvular regurgitation. It has been evaluated in the REPRISE (REpositionable Percutaneous Replacement of Stenotic Aortic Valve through Implantation of LOTUS Edge Valve System) family of trials. The REPRISE III trial was conducted in 912 patients with high or extreme risk and severe, symptomatic aortic stenosis at 55 centers in North America, Europe, and Australia between September 22, 2014, and December 24, 2015.[201] Participants were randomized in a 2:1 ratio to receive either an Lotus valve or the self-expanding CoreValve bioprosthesis.[201] The primary safety composite end point at 30 days occurred in 20.3% of the Lotus valve patients and 17.2% of CoreValve patients. At 1 year, the primary effectiveness composite end point occurred in 15.4% with the Lotus valve and 25.5% with the CoreValve.[201] The 1-year rates of moderate or severe paravalvular leak were 0.9% for the Lotus valve and 6.8% for CoreValve.[201] The Lotus valve had higher rates of new pacemaker implants (35.5% vs. 19.6%; $P < .001$) and valve thrombosis (1.5% vs. 0%) but lower rates of repeat procedures (0.2% vs. 2.0%), valve-in-valve deployments (0% vs. 3.7%), and valve malpositioning (0% vs. 2.7%).[201]

SYMETIS ACURATE NEO

The Acurate Valve (Boston Scientific, Natick, MA; see Fig. 54.21C) is a self-positioning self-expanding valve placed by either a transapical[202,203] or TF route. It has a unique design comprising three stabilization arms that allow the trileaflet porcine pericardial valve to maintain coaxiality while being deployed. The Acurate Valve is deployed from the top (within the SOV)

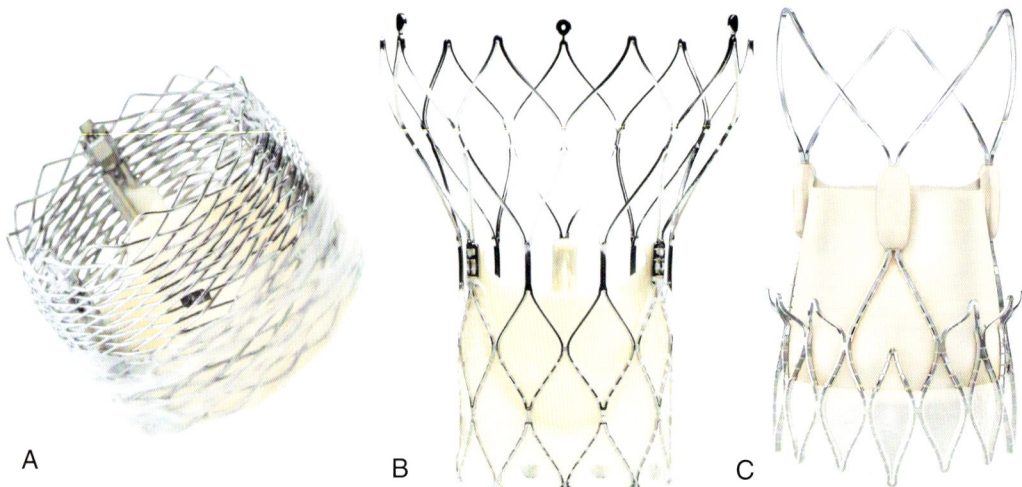

Fig. 54.21 Images of additional self-expanding and mechanical expanded transcatheter valves. (A) LOTUS Edge aortic valve system. (B) Portico transcatheter aortic valve replacement. (C) ACURATE *neo* aortic valve system. ([A and C] ©2019 Boston Scientific Corporation or its affiliates. All rights reserved. [B] Portico is a trademark of Abbott or its related companies. Reproduced with permission of Abbott, © 2019. All rights reserved.)

followed by the bottom (at the level of the annulus) with a minimum protrusion of the frame in the left ventricular outflow tract. This feature is particularly useful in patients with prior mitral valve prostheses.[203] The supra-annularly placed porcine leaflets provide low gradients and the pericardial skirt prevents aortic regurgitation. The stent body is not covered and minimizes the risk of coronary obstruction with low coronary arteries near the annulus.[204] Currently its sizes range from 23 to 27 mm.

A series of studies have been reported in high-risk patients who were treated with the Symetis Acurate transcatheter aortic valve.[203] After the Accurate Neo obtained a CE Mark in 2014 based on a first-in-man series of 89 patients,[205] a large prospective postapproval registry enrolled 1000 patients at 25 European centers who were followed for 1 year after TAVR.[206] Patients were deemed at high risk for SAVR (mean age, 81.1 ± 5.2 years; STS PROM, 6.6 ± 7.5%). At 1 year, 8.0% of patients had died, 2.3% had had disabling strokes, and 9.9% had permanent pacemaker implantations. The mean effective orifice area was 1.84 ± 0.43 cm^2, the mean gradient was 7.3 ± 3.7 mm Hg, and a greater than mild paravalvular leak (PVL) was observed in 3.6% of patients.[206] Later, a comparative analysis was performed of 1121 high-risk patients treated at three centers with matching of 2 patients treated with a Sapien 3 (n = 622) for each patient treated with Accurate Symetis (n = 311).[207] In-hospital complications were comparable between Symetis patients and Sapien 3 patients, including stroke (1.9% vs. 2.4%; P = .64), major vascular complications (10.3% vs. 8.5%; P = .38), or life-threatening bleeding (4.2% vs. 3.7%; P = .72).[207] Although there was more PVL in patients treated with Symetis (PVL moderate or greater, 4.8% vs. 1.8% in Sapien 3 patients; P = .01), elevated gradients and the need for a permanent pacemaker were lower in Symetis patients.[207] Thirty-day mortality was similar in the two groups.[207] A similar comparative analysis with Acurate NEO, CoreValve, and Sapien XT confirmed a lower need for a permanent pacemaker for the Acurate Symetis (6%) compared with the CoreValve (25%) and Sapien XT (11%; P = .013).[208]

The Acurate Neo has also been used in patients with native aortic valve regurgitation.[209] In a series of high-risk surgical patients undergoing TAVR due to pure aortic regurgitation and no or minimal leaflet calcification[210] the Acurate Neo was effective in correcting the aortic regurgitation in 19 of 20 patients. Prostheses were oversized based on the perimeter-derived annular diameter, with a tendency to oversize in cases of borderline annuli.[209] Device success was obtained in 90% of patients, and 1 patient (5%) underwent a valve-in-valve procedure.[209] At discharge, aortic regurgitation was absent in 14 patients (70%), mild in 5 patients (25%), and moderate in 1 patient (5%).[209] At 30-day follow-up, there was no mortality, no stroke, and 3 patients (15%) had received a permanent pacemaker.

PORTICO VALVE

The Portico THV (St Jude Medical, Minneapolis, MN; see Fig. 54.21B) is a self-expanding Nitinol prosthesis with bovine pericardial leaflets and a porcine pericardial sealing cuff that can be delivered via a TF, transaortic, subclavian, or transapical approach.[152,210–222] The valve is repositionable and resheathable, allowing for a greater degree of manipulation prior to valve deployment. Its positioning does not require rapid ventricular pacing. Initial data show successful device implantation in all patients and the ability to recapture. Its hemodynamic profile is similar to those of the other newer prosthesis with a postprocedural mean transvalvular gradient of 10 mm Hg and aortic regurgitation severity of mild or less in 90% of the patients. The Portico trial is currently enrolling in the United States and will compare the PORTICO valve with other commercially available valves in the high-risk and inoperable cohorts utilizing a TF or alternative access approach.

JENA VALVE

The JenaValve (JenaVAlve, Munich, Germany) consist of a self-expanding Nitinol stent designed to be placed in the subcoronary position with leaflets made of porcine root valve tissue fitted with an porcine pericardial skirt. It is placed via a transaortic route and has a set of "feelers" that allows the valve to be implanted in the correct orientation without coronary obstruction. Sizes range from 23, 25, and 27 mm. Results from a pivotal trial demonstrated procedural success of 89.6%, CVA rate of 3%, and 30-day mortality of 7.6%. No patients had severe paravalvular aortic regurgitation, and mild or trace was seen in 86.4%.

OTHER VALVE PROSTHESES

Numerous other TAVR prostheses are currently being evaluated. The self-expanding New Valve Technology (Hechingen, Germany) Allegra valve has completed a first study in humans.[223]

KEY REFERENCES

1. Nishimura RA, Otto CM, Bonow RO, et al. 2017 AHA/ACC Focused Update of the 2014 AHA/ACC guideline for the management of patients with valvular heart disease: a report of the American College of Cardiology/American Heart Association task force on clinical practice guidelines. *Circulation.* 2017;135(25):e1159–e1195.
4. Popma JJ, Reardon MJ, Khabbaz K, et al. Early clinical outcomes after transcatheter aortic valve replacement using a novel self-expanding bioprosthesis in patients with severe aortic stenosis who are suboptimal for surgery: results of the evolut R U.S. Study. *JACC Cardiovasc Interv.* 2017;10(3):268–275.
17. Toggweiler S, van Schie B, Zuber M, et al. Natural course of paravalvular regurgitation after implantation of the self-expanding corevalve: insights from serial TEE measurements. *J Invasive Cardiol.* 2015;27(9):435–440.
19. Popma JJ, Adams DH, Reardon MJ, et al. Transcatheter aortic valve replacement using a self-expanding bioprosthesis in patients with severe aortic stenosis at extreme risk for surgery. *J Am Coll Cardiol.* 2014;63(19):1972–1981.
22. Nishimura RA, Otto CM, Bonow RO, et al. 2017 AHA/ACC Focused Update of the 2014 AHA/ACC Guideline for the management of patients with valvular heart disease: a report of the American College of Cardiology/American Heart Association task force on clinical practice guidelines. *J Am Coll Cardiol.* 2017;70(2):252–289.
28. Reardon MJ, Van Mieghem NM, Popma JJ, et al. Surgical or transcatheter aortic-valve replacement in intermediate risk patients. *N Engl J Med.* 2017;376(14):1321–1331.
30a. Popma JJ, Deeb GM, Yakubov SJ, et al. Transcatheter aortic-valve replacement with a self-expanding valve in low-risk patients. *N Engl J Med.* 2019;380:1706–1715 Popma JJ, Deeb GM, Yakubov SJ et al. Transcatheter aortic-valve replacement with a self-expanding valve in low-risk patients. *N Engl J Med.* 2019;380:1706-1715.
69. Bagur R, Solo K, Alghofaili S, et al. Cerebral embolic protection devices during transcatheter aortic valve implantation: systematic review and meta-analysis. *Stroke.* 2017;48(5):1306–1315.
169. Sultan I, Siki M, Wallen T, et al. Management of coronary obstruction following transcatheter aortic valve replacement. *J Card Surg.* 2017;32(12):777–781.

Additional references available online at expertconsult.com.

中文导读

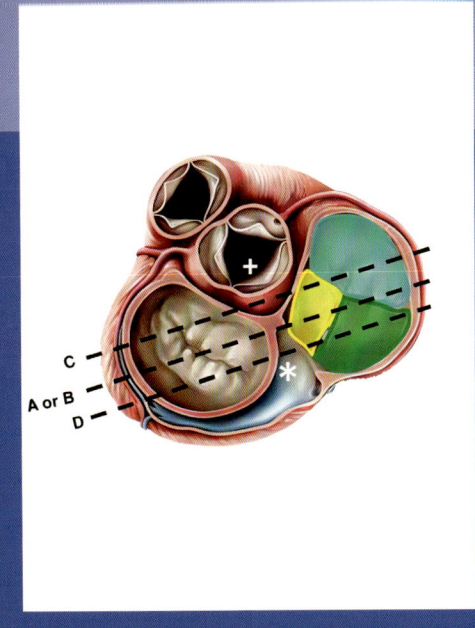

第55章
经导管瓣中瓣植入术

　　外科或经导管心脏瓣膜置换术是治疗心脏瓣膜疾病的主要方法，手术采用的人工心脏瓣膜分为机械瓣膜和生物瓣膜两类。其中，生物瓣膜是由动物或人体组织加工制成的人工心脏瓣膜。与植入机械瓣膜比较，植入生物瓣膜的患者无须长期抗凝治疗，因此，生物瓣膜在瓣膜置换手术中的应用比例呈上升趋势。然而，生物瓣膜的使用寿命有限，随着生物瓣膜使用率和患者预期寿命的增加，瓣膜衰败的发生率逐渐升高。虽然外科治疗生物瓣膜衰败的临床结局较前已有一定改善，但手术的并发症和死亡率仍相对较高。与外科再次开胸手术相比，经导管瓣中瓣植入术有创伤小、操作风险低等优势。研究表明，经导管瓣中瓣植入术可以显著改善患者的功能状态和生活质量。在经导管主动脉瓣或二尖瓣瓣中瓣植入术前应进行综合临床及影像学评估，以识别有冠状动脉开口闭塞或左室流出道梗阻等风险的患者。

　　本章详细介绍了经导管主动脉瓣及二尖瓣瓣中瓣植入术的术前评估、手术技术，以及临床结局。本章内容有助于读者掌握经导管主动脉瓣及二尖瓣瓣中瓣植入术的操作技术要点，以及了解该领域的前沿研究进展。

吕俊兴　张洪亮

章节要点

- 只要患者的生存时间足够长，所有瓣膜组织均会发生衰败。从人工心脏瓣膜植入到瓣中瓣手术的平均时间约为8年。
- 与外科再次开胸手术相比，经导管瓣中瓣植入术创伤较小，操作风险较低。
- 瓣中瓣植入后，患者的功能状态和生活质量常常有显著改善。
- 应充分了解外科瓣膜，以确定经导管植入瓣膜的类型、大小和位置。
- 冠状动脉开口闭塞是主动脉瓣瓣中瓣植入中一个必须注意的问题，可以通过综合筛查识别有风险的患者。
- 外科主动脉瓣生物瓣膜较小的情况下，残余狭窄是一个风险事件。
- 在二尖瓣瓣中瓣植入中，左室流出道梗阻是一个风险事件。
- 详细筛查可以识别大多数高风险患者，进而采取不同策略来降低风险。
- 目前在环中瓣手术方面相关经验有限，临床结局不理想。
- 瓣中瓣植入术可能使血栓形成和早期再狭窄的风险增加，术后可以考虑采用抗凝治疗。

55 Percutaneous Transcatheter Valve-in-Valve Implantation

Dale J. Murdoch, John G. Webb

KEY POINTS

- All tissue valves will fail if the patients live long enough. The average time from implant to valve-in-valve procedures has been approximately 8 years.
- Valve-in-valve procedures are less invasive and often lower risk than redo open-heart surgery.
- Improvements in functional status and quality of life are often dramatic.
- A detailed knowledge of surgical valves is required to choose the correct type, size, and position of transcatheter heart valve.
- Coronary ostial occlusion is a significant concern with aortic valve-in-valve implants. However, screening can identify patients at risk.
- Residual stenosis is a risk in the setting of small surgical aortic bioprostheses.
- Left ventricular outflow tract obstruction is a risk with mitral valve-in-valve implants.
- Screening can identify most patients at increased risk and various strategies are available to mitigate these risks.
- Experience with valve-in-ring procedures is limited, and outcomes have been less favorable.
- Valve-in-valve procedures may carry an increased risk of thrombosis and early restenosis; postprocedural anticoagulation should be considered.

BACKGROUND

The surgical replacement of heart valves is now routine, with over 275,000 valves implanted worldwide each year.[1,2] Mechanical prosthetic valves constructed from nonbiologic materials have the advantage of excellent durability but require lifelong anticoagulation. Biologic prosthetic valves, fashioned from animal or human tissue, do not require long-term anticoagulation and have thus been increasingly chosen by implanting cardiac surgeons and patients. In the United States, bioprostheses accounted for 79% of all surgical aortic implants between 2002 and 2010, with the highest rates in older, higher-risk patients.[3] Rates continue to increase, likely in part due to the availability of a valve-in-valve (ViV) option when these valves fail.

All bioprosthetic valves will fail eventually.[4] However, most valves last long enough, given the limited life expectancy of patients receiving them. The reported incidence of aortic or mitral valve deterioration requiring reintervention is high: 20% to 30% at 10 years and over 50% at 15 years.[5] The actual incidence of structural valve deterioration is likely higher. The mean age of surgical valves treated in the Valve-in-Valve International Data (VIVID) registry was only 8 years.[6] The limited durability of these valves, the significant increase in the proportion of bioprosthetic valves implanted, and improved life expectancy have led to an increasing incidence of surgical valve failure.[2] These patients are often at elevated risk for redo open-heart surgery due to advanced age, comorbidities, and postsurgical adhesions. Although the outcomes associated with redo surgery continue to improve, surgical mortality remains between 3% and 23% in various series,[7,8] and morbidity remains substantial.

Transcatheter aortic valve replacement (TAVR) is an emerging standard of care for many patients with severe native aortic stenosis.[9] The rapid evolution of transcatheter heart valve technology has transformed aortic valve replacement into a minimally invasive percutaneous procedure that is often performed under local anesthesia and with minimal morbidity. The success of TAVR and the clinical needs of high-risk patients with degenerative surgical prostheses has driven the introduction of ViV procedures; as a result, the transcatheter deployment of heart valves within previously implanted surgical bioprosthetic valves in the aortic, mitral, tricuspid and pulmonary positions is becoming increasingly common.

SURGICAL BIOPROSTHETIC HEART VALVES

Tissue heart valves were first utilized as transplanted cadaveric valves (allografts) in the early 1960s; subsequently, in the late 1960s, Carpentier introduced "bioprosthetic" valves made of porcine or bovine tissue (xenografts) and metallic frames.[10] Modern tissue valves are usually made of bovine pericardial tissue or porcine valve leaflets, although some allografts are still used.

Stented surgical heart valves consist of (1) a stent frame composed of metal alloys or polymers; (2) a sewing ring allowing fixation within the valve annulus or above it (supra-annular); and (3) three valve leaflets, which are sewn to the stent frame (either internally or externally). Stented "sutureless" surgical heart valves, modeled on transcatheter valve platforms, have recently been introduced.

Stentless valves eliminate the reduction in the annular area caused by a stent frame, thus increasing the effective orifice area.[11] Most stentless valves utilize porcine root tissue, although homografts as well as pericardial tissue may be used.[12] Stentless valves represent a challenge for ViV implantation as the lack of a rigid frame presents a problem for the fixation and fluoroscopic visualization of a transcatheter heart valve (THV).

SIZING

The size of an implanted bioprosthetic valve has significant implications for hemodynamic performance, likely mode of failure, and options for surgical or transcatheter therapy at the point of failure. Unfortunately the labeling of surgical heart valves lacks standardization across manufacturers[13]; frequently valves labeled as being of the same size will have different internal and external dimensions. Generally labeled valve sizes refer to the external dimension of the valve frame and/or sewing ring, whereas internal dimensions are 1 to 4 mm smaller.

In-depth knowledge of a surgical heart valve's characteristics is required to perform ViV procedures. Tables of valve dimensions published by manufacturers are useful[14] but may not represent the true internal dimensions, which is vital for selection of an appropriately sized THV. A ViV smartphone application will list a large range of commonly used surgical and transcatheter valves—with descriptions, images, dimensions, photographic and fluoroscopic images—along with guidance on sizing and positioning.[15] For each valve, stent's internal diameter as reported by the manufacturer is listed, along with a "true ID," which takes into account the reduction in internal diameter due to the leaflet tissue.[16] This easy-to-use application is vital for the planning of ViV procedures and reduces much of the confusion associated with the sizing of surgical valves.

The model and its labeled size should routinely be obtained from an operative report. When these are unavailable, measurements from transesophageal echocardiography (TEE) or computed tomography (CT) imaging may be helpful. In addition, pannus formation or leaflet calcification may help guide the choice of THV and procedural strategies.

HISTORY

Transcatheter native aortic valve implantation was initially performed via a transvenous transseptal approach in 2002.[17] However, retrograde transfemoral arterial access quickly became the preferred delivery approach,[18,19] with alternative access routes (apical, subclavian, carotid, caval, and aortic) currently being reserved primarily for patients with iliofemoral arterial disease.[20]

ViV proof of concept was demonstrated in animal models via a transatrial approach by Boudjemline et al. in 2005, followed by others in 2007.[4,21,22] Reports of the first human ViV procedures were published in 2007 by Wenaweser et al. and by Webb.[4,23] Subsequently large case series and reviews documented procedural advances and the reproducibility of the procedure.[14,24–26] Simultaneously, ViV implants were shown to be feasible and reproducible in the aortic, mitral, tricuspid, and pulmonary positions via a variety of delivery approaches.[14]

Subsequently the ViV International Data Registry investigators documented the rapidly growing international clinical experience. This work added tremendously to the understanding of the possibilities and limitations of the procedure.[27–29] Most recently, two large prospective clinical trials have documented excellent clinical, hemodynamic, and quality-of-life outcomes out to 1 year with both the balloon- and self-expandable SAPIEN XT and CoreValve THV systems.[30,31]

AORTIC VALVE-IN-VALVE PROCEDURE

Preprocedural Planning

To make sure that a ViV procedure will be safe and effective, careful patient evaluation and selection is required. Patients with failing bioprosthetic aortic valves frequently have multiple comorbidities, and attention to detail in the initial assessment can help to avoid potential pitfalls. A clear understanding of the initial cardiac surgery is required. The surgical report and history can provide necessary information such as the specifics of the surgical valve implanted (manufacturer, model, size), concomitant surgery (root replacement, coronary reimplantation, bypass grafts), and procedural complications.

The possibility of prosthetic valve endocarditis must be considered carefully in any patient presenting with bioprosthetic valve dysfunction, particularly in patients with aortic regurgitation (AR). Risk factors include AR, prior endocarditis, early valve dysfunction, fever, chills, anorexia, and weight loss.[32]

Echocardiography

Transthoracic echocardiography (TTE) is the cornerstone of the noninvasive evaluation of prosthetic heart valves.[33] However, TEE is sometimes required prior to ViV procedures.[2] Structural valve deterioration (SVD) can be defined in four stages (0 to 3), with SVD stage 0 being no significant change from immediate postimplantation assessment and stage 3 being severe stenosis and/or regurgitation.[34] Stage 2 with combined stenosis and regurgitation and stage 3 should prompt consideration of intervention. Severe patient-prosthesis mismatch (PPM), defined as indexed effective orifice area (EOA) ≤0.65 cm^2/m^2 for nonobese patients (body mass index [BMI] <30 kg/m^2) and indexed EOA ≤0.60 cm^2/m^2 for obese patients (BMI ≥30 kg/m^2), predisposes to early SVD and is associated with increased postprocedural gradients after ViV TAVR and reduced patient survival at 1 year.[35]

Angiography

The presence of obstructive coronary artery disease that might require revascularization should be excluded. Aortic root angiography can be particularly helpful in assessing the risk of coronary obstruction, as shown in Fig. 55.1. A useful technique is to find the fluoroscopic projection that (1) is perpendicular to the plane of the surgical valve and (2) superimposes the two valve posts (purposely positioned by the surgeon) on either side of the left coronary ostium.[36] In cases where aortography is not available, examination of the routine left anterior oblique cranial left coronary injection can often provide similar information.

Computed Tomography

Currently the risk of coronary ostial occlusion is more often assessed by CT (discussed later).

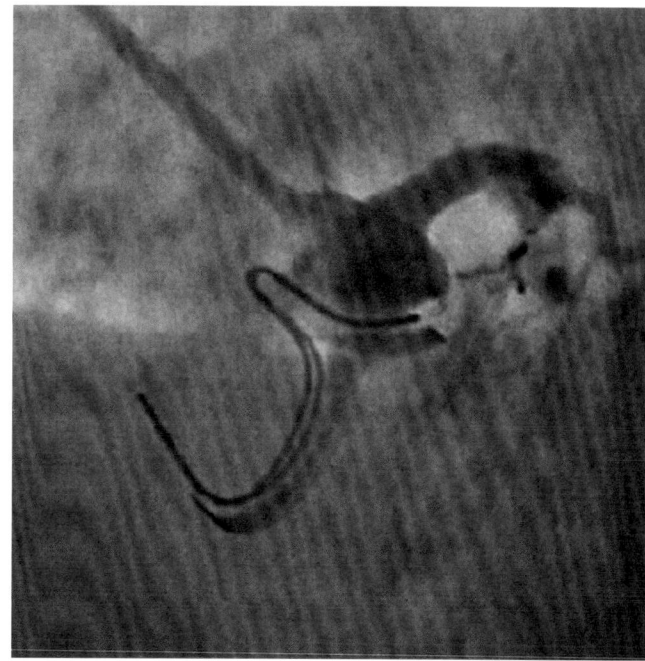

Fig. 55.1 Selective left main coronary artery injection perpendicular to the frame of the surgical bioprosthesis with adjacent posts overlapped can help in assessing the risk of coronary occlusion.

Angiographic imaging of the iliac and femoral arteries can be performed to evaluate the feasibility of a transfemoral approach for ViV implantation. Currently CT angiography is more often utilized. CT assessment of annular dimensions is the standard for native TAVR but is less useful for assessing degenerated surgical valves provided that accurate documentation of the implant size can be obtained. Sizing information is usually provided for aortic allografts, but CT assessment and sizing is recommended given the difficulty in measuring cadaveric human valves and because annular calcification is often significant.

MULTIDISCIPLINARY HEART TEAM ASSESSMENT

Patients assessed for ViV TAVR should be discussed by the heart team, similar to other patients under consideration for THV and high-risk or complex procedures.[9] Assessment of patient frailty can be made with specific tools, such as the essential frailty tool set[37]; such assessments can predict short- and medium-term outcomes and help in the allocation of limited resources.

CORONARY OBSTRUCTION

The first reported case of coronary obstruction resulting from an aortic ViV procedure occurred in 2011.[38] Since then it has become apparent that the risk of coronary occlusion with ViV procedures may be much higher than that seen with native valve TAVR. In one large registry of over 6000 patients, coronary obstruction occurred in 2.5% of ViV cases, as compared to 0.6% in native valve cases (P = .045).[39] Similarly, in an early VIVID registry report of 1612 aortic ViV procedures, coronary occlusion occurred in 37 patients (2.3%).[40] That aggressive screening can reduce the risk of coronary obstruction is evidenced by the much lower rates of coronary obstruction seen in the large PARTNER 2 SAPIEN XT and CoreValve US Expanded Use Study of 0.8% and 0.9%, respectively.[30,31]

The predominant mechanism of coronary obstruction in ViV TAVR is displacement of the surgical tissue leaflets toward the coronary ostia.[40,41] For ViV TAVR, the greatest risk occurs when there is a noncapacious aortic root and narrow sinotubular junction: the surgical valve leaflets are just a few millimeters from the coronary ostium and displacement by the THV causes coronary obstruction. The angulation of the surgical bioprosthetic valve is also important; tilting of the surgical valve toward the coronary ostium may cause occlusion even if there is a spacious aortic root. Risk factors for coronary obstruction with ViV TAVR are listed in Table 55.1.

The Vancouver approach for the assessment of coronary obstruction risk utilizes CT imaging to create a "virtual transcatheter valve to coronary ostium distance (VTC)".[41] For stented surgical valves, if the level of the coronary ostia is above the stent posts, the risk of coronary occlusion is almost zero and no further evaluation is required. If the coronary ostia lie below the stent posts, VTC assessment is recommended. THV implantation is simulated on the CT data by superimposing a cylinder within the surgical valve. A circular ellipse is created on the basal ring of the surgical valve and the cylinder extended toward the coronary ostia, corresponding to the height of the planned THV. The distance between the left and right coronary ostia and the virtual THV can then be measured to estimate risk of coronary occlusion. In VIVID registry data, 90% of patients with coronary ostial occlusion and CT data had a VTC of ≤4 mm, suggesting that this may be used as a cutoff figure (area under the curve: 0.943; P < .001).[40]

Current experience suggests that patients at risk of coronary obstruction with aortic ViV implantation can be routinely identified before the procedure. The question then becomes whether to reconsider other options, such as redo surgery or medical management, or to mitigate the risks of coronary obstruction. Various approaches may be considered to either reduce the risk of coronary occlusion or manage coronary occlusion should this occur. The risk of coronary obstruction may be reduced if outward displacement of the surgical valve posts and leaflets is minimized by avoiding oversizing, overexpansion, and postdilation of the THV. Splitting of the surgical valve leaflets to reduce the risk of left main coronary obstruction has recently been described (the Bioprosthetic or native Aortic Scallop Intentional Laceration to prevent Iatrogenic Coronary Artery obstruction [BASILICA] procedure). Should coronary obstruction occur, options might include emergent stenting or surgical bypass, often requiring cardiopulmonary support. A repositionable THV (e.g., EvolutR, Lotus) might offer the theoretical advantage of being removable should obstruction be recognized prior to release. Where the risk of coronary obstruction is high, a relatively routine approach has been to place a coronary stent at the ready in the coronary artery prior to THV implantation. The stent can then be withdrawn to the coronary ostium if needed. Although this can be helpful in establishing coronary patency, the durability of aorto ostial stenting in the presence of an obstructive bioprosthetic leaflet is questionable.

AORTIC VALVE-IN-VALVE PROCEDURE

ViV TAVR can be performed in a cardiac catheterization laboratory or hybrid operating room with either general or local anesthesia. Recent years have seen a strong trend toward the use of sedation and local anesthesia. Balloon dilation of degenerative aortic bioprostheses carries a significant risk of embolization, stroke, or acute severe AR.[42] Predilation is best avoided when possible, although valvuloplasty may sometimes be required for retrograde crossing of a severely stenotic and calcified bioprosthesis.

SELECTION OF A TRANSCATHETER HEART VALVE

There are key differences in the construction and delivery of balloon-expandable, self-expanding, and mechanically expanding THVs—differences that may affect the technical and clinical outcomes related to different devices. Photographs and fluoroscopic examples are shown in Fig. 55.2. The VIVID registry[27] found no difference in the occurrence of death or stroke between the transfemoral implantation of balloon-expandable and self-expanding valves at 30 days or 1 year. However, elevated postprocedural gradients and PPM were observed more often with balloon-expandable than self-expanding valves (average mean gradient 19.4 vs. 13.5 mm Hg, respectively), with a hazard ratio for an elevated postprocedural gradient of 1.87 (95% CI 1.21 to 2.9; P = .005). This difference may be related to the intraannular leaflet positioning of the SAPIEN XT THV as opposed to the more supra-annular leaflet positioning of the self-expanding CoreValve.[43]

Despite this theoretical advantage, the large-core lab-adjudicated Partner 2 ViV and CoreValve US Expanded Use studies found no significant differences in transvalvular gradients

TABLE 55.1 Risk Factors for Coronary Obstruction With Valve-in-Valve Transcatheter Aortic Valve Implantation

Stented surgical bioprosthesis with externally mounted leaflets
Stentless surgical bioprosthesis
Distance from low virtual transcatheter valve to coronary ostium, ≤4 mm
Narrow sinus of Valsalva diameter
Balloon postdilation of transcatheter aortic valve implantation
Coronary artery bypass graft to left coronary system (protective)

(the average mean gradients at 30 days were 17.1 and 17.0 mm Hg, respectively).[38,39] Perhaps this was the result of inclusion of a number of smaller surgical bioprostheses in the CoreValve study or of the frequent failure to achieve supra-annular positioning.

Small numbers of implants with other valve systems have been reported, including the Lotus (Boston Scientific), Acurate Neo (Boston Scientific), Portico (Abbott Vascular), JenaValve (JenaValve), and Inovare (Braile Medica) THVs.[44–48]

POSITIONING AND DEPLOYMENT OF A TRANSCATHETER HEART VALVE

The guiding principles of THV positioning within a surgical bioprostheses include (1) excluding the leaflets of the failed bioprosthetic valve from the neo-orifice, (2) securely fixing the THV frame to prevent embolization, and (3) positioning the THV leaflets relatively high in the aorta so as to maximize the effective orifice area (Fig. 55.3). Exclusion of the failed leaflets requires that the THV extend from the tips of the bioprosthetic valve posts to the annular ring. The level of the sewing ring generally presents the narrowest dimension within a bioprosthetic valve and forms a neoannulus for anchoring the THV.[49] Other components of the bioprosthetic valve, such as the posts and leaflets, are to some degree flexible and contribute little to securing the THV. Therefore it is important that some portion of the THV be within and extend slightly below the bioprosthetic ring. Since the pressure gradients acting on the THV dominate during diastole, a THV outflow larger than the bioprosthetic ring will aid in fixation. It is important to note that the sewing ring may or may not be radio-opaque and that the relationship between the sewing ring and a radio-opaque valve stent varies, particularly for annular and supra-annular surgical valves. It is important to be familiar with the fluoroscopic appearance of the THV, surgical valve, and their combination to ensure success with ViV procedures; the example photographs, radiographs, and video files in the ViV smartphone application are an invaluable resource.

Positioning the THV as high as possible within the failed bioprosthetic valve is important to maximize expansion of the THV leaflet, minimize gradients, and maximize valve orifice area (Fig. 55.4). Although this observation is speculative, low implantation resulting in intra-annular constrained leaflets may predispose to leaflet thrombosis or reduced durability. In vitro and in vivo hemodynamic assessment of Sapien XT and CoreValve placement has confirmed that optimal performance is achieved by

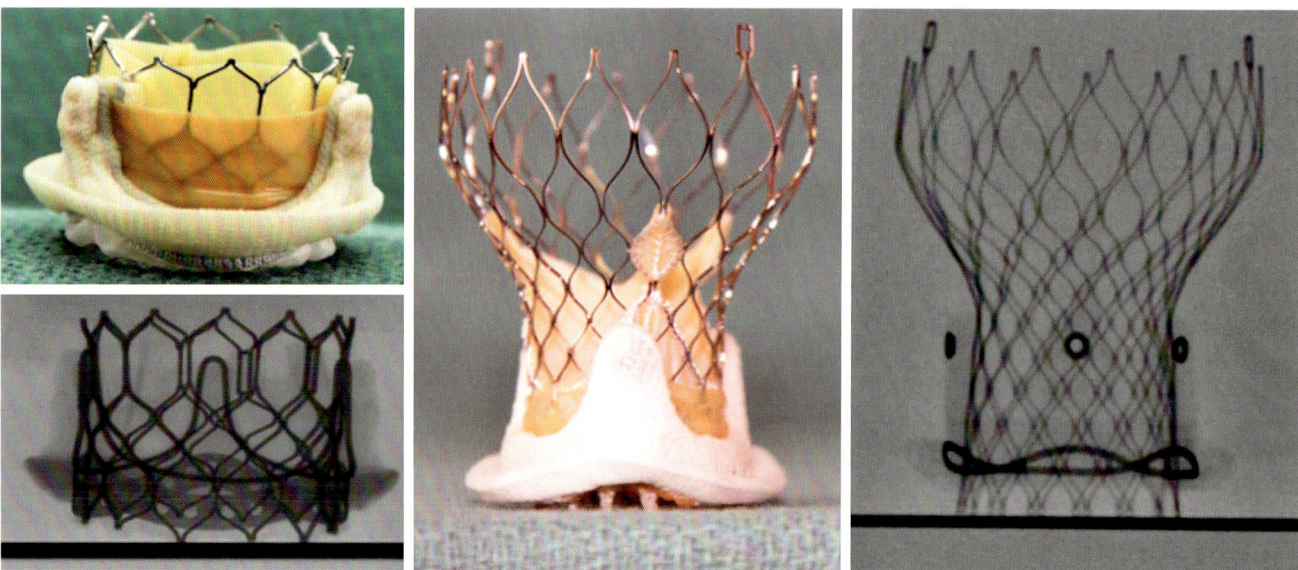

Fig. 55.2 Edwards SAPIEN 3 THV implanted in Carpentier Edwards Perimount surgical heart valve *(left)*; Medtronic CoreValve implanted in Medtronic Hancock II surgical heart valve *(right)*. (Adapted from Valve in Valve smartphone application (v.2.0) by Dr. Vinnie Bapat.)

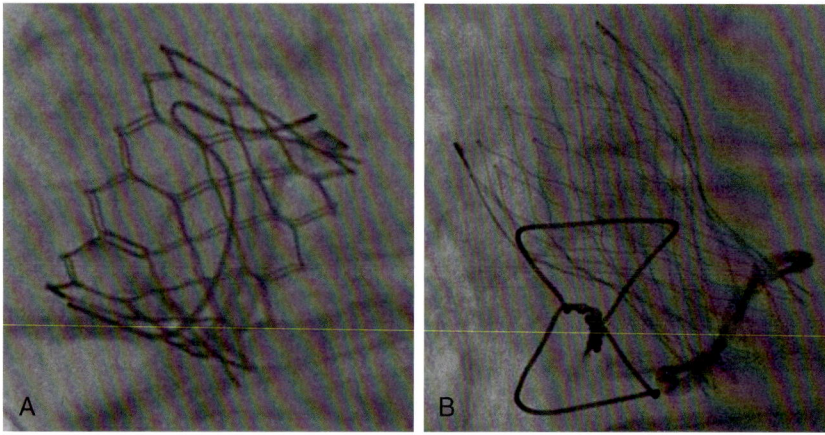

Fig. 55.3 Fluoroscopic image showing optimal positioning after deployment of (A) a SAPIEN 3 and (B) an Evolut R valve.

placing the THV leaflets above the neoannulus of the surgical valve.[28,50] In an analysis from the VIVID registry, high implantation was associated with significantly lower rates of elevated gradients in comparison with low implantation. Optimal implantation depth for the CoreValve Evolut was defined as 0 to 5 mm and for SAPIEN XT 0 to 2 mm. A more recent analysis reports similar findings for the newer SAPIEN 3 THV.

POSTDILATION

Conventional balloon valvuloplasty after THV deployment may be performed to improve transvalvular gradients in cases where underexpansion of the THV is observed.[30] Although postdilation may result in displacement of the bioprosthetic leaflets and posts and expansion of the THV outflow, expansion of the THV at the level of the constraining surgical valve ring is typically minimal.

Only recently has it has been established that very aggressive high-pressure dilation has the potential to deform, fracture, or crack many surgical valves, allowing for more complete THV expansion. Ex vivo studies demonstrate that most currently implanted bioprosthetic valves yield at 8 to 26 atm.[51,52] Balloon fracture appears to disrupt the internal valve frame, allowing distention without tearing the sewing cuff or causing protrusion of fragments. Notable exceptions are the Medtronic Hancock II and St. Jude Trifecta bioprosthetic valves, which typically do not fracture at achievable pressures.

Small case series have demonstrated the feasibility of dilating Mitroflow, Perimount, Magna and Magna Ease, Biocor Epic and Epic Supra, and Mosaic surgical valves.[53,54] Noncompliant valvuloplasty balloons (True, VIDA, or Atlas Gold dilation catheters [BARD PV, Tempe, AZ]) are typically sized 1 to 3 mm larger than the true internal diameter of the surgical valve. Success may be recognized by obliteration of the waist of the contrast-filled balloon (Fig. 55.5). To date complications have been infrequent, with most patients experiencing a marked reduction in transvalvular gradients.[54]

OUTCOMES AFTER AORTIC VALVE-IN-VALVE PROCEDURES

In the 10 years since the introduction of ViV procedures, procedural and clinical outcomes have steadily improved. Initially, patients undergoing ViV were at high risk of surgical reintervention, with multiple comorbidities. Despite this, patients undergoing

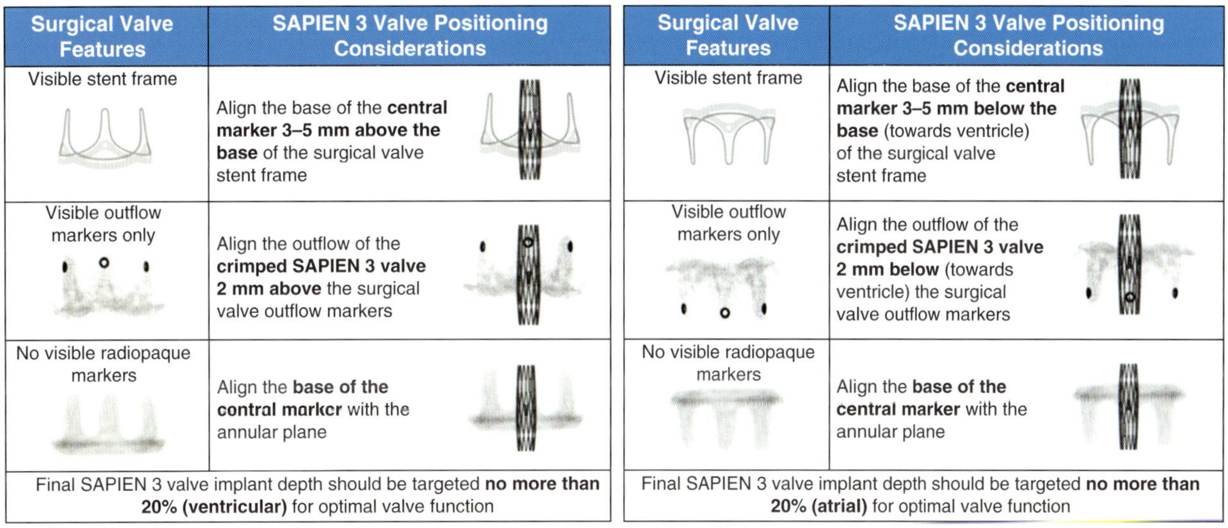

Surgical Valve Features	SAPIEN 3 Valve Positioning Considerations		Surgical Valve Features	SAPIEN 3 Valve Positioning Considerations	
Visible stent frame	Align the base of the **central marker 3–5 mm above the base** of the surgical valve stent frame		Visible stent frame	Align the base of the **central marker 3–5 mm below the base** (towards ventricle) of the surgical valve stent frame	
Visible outflow markers only	Align the outflow of the **crimped SAPIEN 3 valve 2 mm above** the surgical valve outflow markers		Visible outflow markers only	Align the outflow of the **crimped SAPIEN 3 valve 2 mm below** (towards ventricle) the surgical valve outflow markers	
No visible radiopaque markers	Align the **base of the central marker** with the annular plane		No visible radiopaque markers	Align the **base of the central marker** with the annular plane	
Final SAPIEN 3 valve implant depth should be targeted **no more than 20% (ventricular)** for optimal valve function			Final SAPIEN 3 valve implant depth should be targeted **no more than 20% (atrial)** for optimal valve function		

Fig. 55.4 Recommended positioning of the SAPIEN 3 valve in the aortic position *(left)* and the mitral position *(right)*.

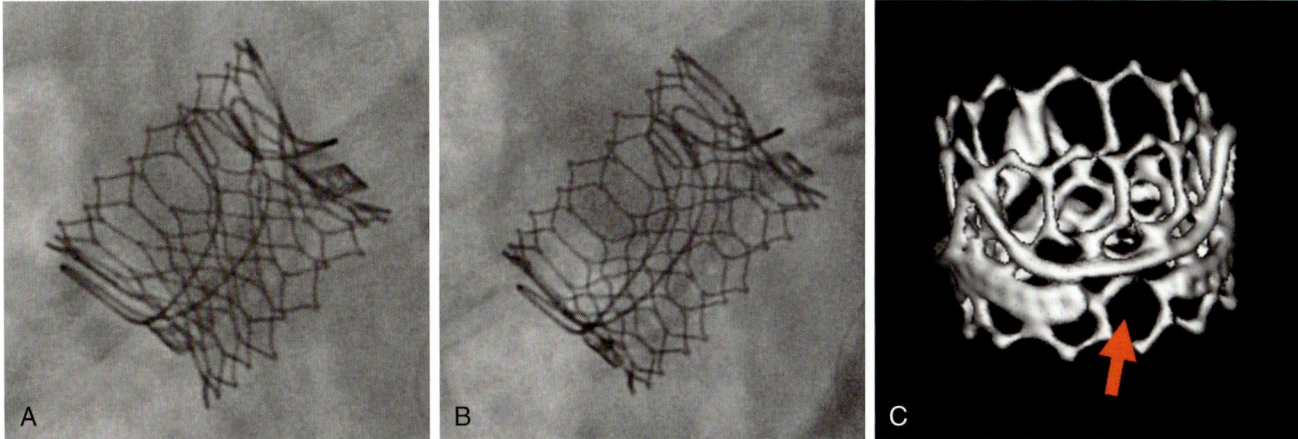

Fig. 55.5 Fractured surgical valve. An underexpanded SAPIEN 3 valve deployed in a Perimount surgical valve (A); improved THV expansion after high-pressure noncompliant balloon inflation (B), with fracture of the surgical valve demonstrated on computed tomography (C, *arrow*).

ViV TAVR in the initial VIVID registry report had lower 30-day mortality (7.6%) than expected by Society of Thoracic Surgeons mortality prediction scores (STS-PROMs) (9.8% [interquartile range, 7.7% to 16%]). One-year survival was 83.2% in this cohort, with reduced survival in patients with stenosis as the mode of failure (76.6%) and small (≤21-mm) valves (74.8%).

Recent prospective registries enrolling patients with balloon-expandable or self-expanding THVs show improvements in 30-day and 1-year survival despite similarly elevated STS-PROMs of approximately 9%. In the PARTNER 2 ViV Registry, all-cause mortality was 2.7% and 12.4% at 30 days and 1 year, respectively.[30] In the CoreValve US Expanded Use Study, all-cause mortality was 2.2% and 14.6% at 30-days and 1 year, respectively.[31]

Improvements in functional status and quality-of-life measures with aortic ViV are dramatic. In the PARTNER 2 ViV registry, 89.2% of patients reported New York Heart Association (NYHA) class I and II symptoms at 1 year compared with 9.9% at baseline, and significant improvements were observed in the Kansas City Cardiomyopathy Questionnaire (KCCQ) and 6-minute walk-test (6MWT) regardless of bioprosthesis size or residual gradient (Fig. 55.6).

PPM and elevated residual gradients are common after ViV procedures. In the VIVID registry reporting outcomes on over 900 patients, severe PPM (defined as an indexed EOA of <0.65 cm^2/m^2) was present in 24.6% and elevated residual aortic valve gradients (>20 mm Hg) in 27.9% of patients.[55] Stented surgical valves, higher BMI, and implantation of intra-annular Sapien-type THVs were identified as independent predictors of PPM. However, neither severe PPM nor elevated gradients had an association with Valve Academic Research Consortium (VARC) II–defined outcomes or 1-year survival.

Rates of complications differ slightly between native TAVR and ViV procedures. Malpositioning and/or valve embolization has been more common in ViV cases[2] and may be related to regurgitation as the mode of surgical valve failure, radiolucent surgical valves, and inexperience. The rate of malpositioning has markedly decreased in contemporary studies: in the 365-patient PARTNER 2 SAPIEN XT study, embolization did not occur.[30]

Stroke, which was once a major clinical concern,[56] is now less common, occurring in 0.9% to 2.7% of contemporary aortic ViV procedures.[30,31,57] Clinically significant AR is infrequent with ViV procedures, with moderate or greater AR reported in 1.9% (balloon-expandable) to 7.4% (self-expanding) at 12 months.[30,31]

MITRAL VALVE-IN-VALVE PROCEDURES

Transcatheter mitral ViV (MVIV) and valve-in-ring (ViR) replacement has emerged as a less invasive and very successful alternative in patients at high risk of morbidity or mortality with redo surgery. Procedures are performed in a cardiac catheterization laboratory or hybrid operating room with general anesthesia and TEE guidance. Transseptal procedures are performed using femoral venous access and a transseptal puncture with antegrade access to the mitral valve. Transapical procedures are performed through a small lateral thoracotomy and direct apical puncture. Although apical access may provide a more straightforward route to the mitral valve, the trade-off is the morbidity associated with a thoracotomy and apical injury. Although the bulk of early experience was with transapical access, less invasive transseptal access is increasingly favored. The great majority of procedures to date have been performed with Sapien-type balloon-expandable valves, although there is limited experience with other valves originally designed for aortic implantation.

Mitral bioprostheses are larger than their aortic counterparts and therefore often well suited to ViV procedures. Mitral annuloplasty rings and bands are more problematic. Rings may be flexible (bands), semirigid or rigid, complete, or incomplete, and D-shaped or saddle-shaped. Although flexible and semirigid rings/bands may circularize with implantation of a THV, rigid rings will not. THV implantation in a noncircular ring typically results in a deformed and incompletely expanded valve with instability, paravalvular regurgitation, and reduced durability. Additional challenges include THV positioning, anchoring, sizing, and sealing, with adverse outcomes related to paravalvular regurgitation, valve embolization, left-ventricular outflow tract (LVOT) obstruction, and requirement for surgical intervention.[58] Not surprisingly complication rates and 1-year mortality are higher with ViR procedures (28.7% or ViR vs. 12.6% for ViV).[44] Currently ViR procedures are recommended only for experienced operators and patients at prohibitive surgical risk.

Preprocedural Planning

Consideration of MVIV begins with a detailed history of prior mitral valve surgery, comorbidities, and onset of current symptoms; the possibility of endocarditis, thrombosis, or paravalvular leaks as the cause of mitral valve dysfunction is also considered. Careful review of the operative notes should include valve model and size as well as concomitant procedures such as anterior mitral leaflet resection, left atrial appendage excision, or interatrial septal patch repair.[45]

Routine TTE will usually define the cause of mitral valve dysfunction (stenosis, regurgitation, or mixed) and whether regurgitation is transvalvular, paravalvular/para-ring, or both. TEE may be necessary. When there is both transvalvular and paravalvular/para-ring regurgitation, combined THV implantation and paravalvular leak closure may be considered, but large paravalvular leaks or dehiscence of the sewing ring necessitate surgical intervention.[59]

Cardiac CT is increasingly used to assess the risk of LVOT obstruction, a rare but potentially fatal complication of MVIV. A simulated THV is placed in the intended implant position and the area of the "neo-LVOT" can thus be assessed. Although the acceptable ranges for neo-LVOT are undefined, a value of >2.5 cm^2 is associated with a low risk of LVOT obstruction and a value <1 cm^2 is associated with high risk.[45,46] Other factors associated with LVOT obstruction include a small LVOT and left ventricular cavity, an acute mitral-aortic angle, an elongated, thick or severely calcified anterior leaflet, and VIR procedures.

Sizing

Choice of THV for MVIV/ViR procedures is determined by the surgical prosthesis, with useful guidance provided by the mitral

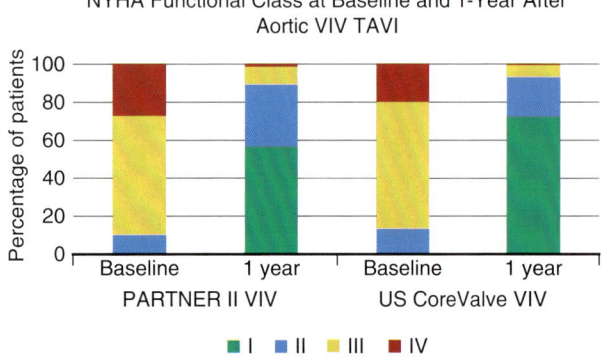

Fig. 55.6 Improved functional class 1 year after valve-in-valve (ViV) implantation in the PARTNER II ViV and US CoreValve ViV studies. *NYHA*, New York Heart Association; *TAVI*, transcatheter valve implantation.

ViV app. Generally the THV should be slightly larger than the surgical valve in internal dimensions, aiming for a conical deployment with the ventricular aspect of the THV flared: there is a greater pressure differential between the left ventricle (LV) and left atrium compared with the LV and aorta, and migration of a THV into the left atrium has been observed after undersized and cylindrical deployment.

Outcomes

Procedural and clinical outcomes have been reported in a number of small case series.[48,60–62] Recently Yoon et al. reported on a large multicenter series of 248 patients comprising 176 ViV and 72 ViR procedures.[44] Patients were generally at high risk with redo surgery (STS predicted risk of mortality 9% to 18%). The bulk of procedures were performed with balloon-expandable Sapien THVs performed via transapical or transvenous-transseptal access.

Currently outcomes are much more favorable and predictable with ViV as compared with ViR procedures. Device-related and procedural success rates, as per the Mitral Valve Academic Research Consortium (MVARC) definitions, are 96.0% versus 83.3% and 79.5% versus 58.3%, respectively. ViR procedures are associated with more frequent second-valve implantation, reintervention, and death.[44] Mitral gradients and areas are typically good (mean 6.0 mm Hg and 2.1 cm^2, respectively), although patients undergoing ViR procedures are more likely to have equal to or greater than moderate residual mitral regurgitation (19.4% vs. 6.8%). Clinical improvement in functional status was profound, with up to 90% reporting NYHA class I and II symptoms at 30 days.[60] One-year all-cause mortality was 16.9%, with advanced age and ViR procedures identified as risk factors in a multivariable analysis.

TRICUSPID AND PULMONARY VALVE IN VALVE PROCEDURES

ViV procedures have been performed in bioprosthetic valves in the tricuspid and pulmonary positions with excellent procedural and clinical success.[63–65] Details are beyond the scope of this chapter.

LONG-TERM DURABILITY

One-year outcomes for aortic ViV procedures have been reported in the large PARTNER VIV (SAPIEN XT) and US CoreValve series.[30,31] Early improvements in mean transaortic gradient and aortic valve area are maintained, with no reports of transvalvular AR. Clinical benefits with improvement in NYHA functional class and quality-of-life measures were sustained at 1 year.

Limited outcomes data exists beyond 1 year. Ye et al. reported their 8-year experience with ViV procedures in 73 patients (42 aortic, 31 mitral) with a median follow-up of 2.5 years.[62] At 2 years, 82.8% of aortic and 100% of mitral patients were NYHA functional class I or II. Estimated survival rates in this high-risk first-in-human series were 79.5%, 69.8%, and 40.5% at 2, 3, and 5 years, respectively. For aortic procedures, small surgical valve size (19 and 21 mm labeled size) was associated with reduced survival. Late structural deterioration of the THV was observed in 1 patient (1.4%) and valve thrombosis in 4 (5.6%). In a series of 23 consecutive transapical mitral ViV cases, survival was 100% at 30 days and 90.4% at a median follow-up of 2 years.[66] No structural valve deterioration was observed, although the authors comment that the durability of ViV THVs is currently unknown and early degeneration may be expected in cases of elevated gradients and when underexpansion is substantial.[2,67]

THROMBOSIS RISK AND ANTICOAGULATION

There is an increasing awareness that tissue leaflet thrombosis may be more common than previously appreciated, particularly in the setting of ViV implants.[68] Leaflet thrombosis is most often subclinical, involving a single leaflet, but may cause increased transvalvular gradients, early structural degeneration, or an increased risk of cerebrovascular events.[69,70] "Four-dimensional" volume-rendered CT is considered the gold standard for diagnosis, although artifacts generated by THV and surgical stent frames may be problematic.[71] TEE is less sensitive but can be diagnostic, as can a trial of anticoagulation.

From CT registry data, subclinical leaflet thrombosis is present in 7% to 13% of patients after TAVR.[70,72] Clinical aortic ViV thrombosis, typically associated with increased gradients, has been reported in 7.6% to 11.6% of patients at a median of 101 days post-procedure.[68,73]

Predictors of leaflet thrombosis include decreased left ventricular ejection fraction, an increase aortic valve gradient, and large THVs.[70,72] Computational flow models suggest that risk factors include increased blood residence time on valve leaflets (a nidus for thrombus formation), reduced cardiac output,[74] and intra-annular THV leaflets.[75]

Patients treated with anticoagulation (vitamin-K antagonist or novel oral anticoagulant) appear to be less likely to have leaflet thrombosis, leading some to recommend liberalized indications for routine anticoagulation. Early anticoagulation is typically successful in reducing increased gradients, although long-term therapy may be necessary. When the diagnosis is unclear, a trial of anticoagulation may be diagnostic.

SUMMARY

When surgical bioprosthetic heart valves fail, transcatheter ViV procedures can often provide a desirable alternative to redo surgery, with excellent functional and quality-of-life outcomes. Risks common to other transcatheter valve procedures, such as vascular injury and stroke, are increasingly infrequent. Malposition and paravalvular regurgitation are increasingly rare except in the setting of mitral ViR procedures. The risk of coronary obstruction with aortic implants is higher than with native aortic valve implant, but patients at risk can be identified with careful CT screening. Hemodynamic function is generally excellent. However smaller surgical aortic bioprostheses remain a significant concern due to the risk of THV underexpansion and residual aortic stenosis. Durability remains an area of uncertainty, although outcomes to date appear adequate for patients in whom the risk of redo surgery is high.

KEY REFERENCES

4. Webb JG. Transcatheter valve in valve implants for failed prosthetic valves. *Catheter Cardiovasc Interv*. 2007;70(5):765–766.
15. Bapat V. Valve-in-valve apps: why and how they were developed and how to use them. *EuroIntervention*. 2014;10(suppl U):U44–U51.
22. Walther T, Falk V, Dewey T, et al. Valve-in-a-valve concept for transcatheter minimally invasive repeat xenograft implantation. *J Am Coll Cardiol*. 2007;50(1):56–60.
27. Dvir D, Webb JG, Bleiziffer S, et al. Transcatheter aortic valve implantation in failed bioprosthetic surgical valves. *JAMA*. 2014;312(2):162–170.
28. Simonato M, Webb J, Kornowski R, et al. Transcatheter replacement of failed bioprosthetic valves: large multicenter assessment of the effect of implantation depth on hemodynamics after aortic valve-in-valve. *Circ Cardiovasc Interv*. 2016;9(6):pii:e003651.
30. Webb JG, Mack MJ, White JM, et al. Transcatheter aortic valve implantation within degenerated aortic surgical bioprostheses: PARTNER 2 valve-in-valve registry. *J Am Coll Cardiol*. 2017;69(18):2253–2262.
31. Deeb GM, Chetcuti SJ, Reardon MJ, et al. 1-Year results in patients undergoing transcatheter aortic valve replacement with failed surgical bioprostheses. *JACC Cardiovasc Interv*. 2017;10(10):1034–1044.

34. Dvir D, Bourguignon T, Otto CM, et al. Standardized definition of structural valve degeneration for surgical and transcatheter bioprosthetic aortic valves. *Circulation*. 2018;137(4):388–399.
41. Blanke P, Soon J, Dvir D, et al. Computed tomography assessment for transcatheter aortic valve in valve implantation: the vancouver approach to predict anatomical risk for coronary obstruction and other considerations. *J Cardiovasc Comput Tomogr*. 2016;10(6):491–499.
44. Yoon SH, Whisenant BK, Bleiziffer S, et al. Transcatheter mitral valve replacement for degenerated bioprosthetic valves and failed annuloplasty rings. *J Am Coll Cardiol*. 2017;70(9):1121–1131.
49. Bapat V, Adams B, Attia R, et al. Neo-annulus: a reference plane in a surgical heart valve to facilitate a valve-in-valve procedure. *Catheter Cardiovasc Interv*. 2015;85(4):685–691.
52. Allen KB, Chhatriwalla AK, Cohen DJ, et al. Bioprosthetic valve fracture to facilitate transcatheter valve-in-valve implantation. *Ann Thorac Surg*. 2017;104(5):1501–1508.
62. Ye J, Cheung A, Yamashita M, et al. Transcatheter aortic and mitral valve-in-valve implantation for failed surgical bioprosthetic valves: an 8-year single-center experience. *JACC Cardiovasc Interv*. 2015;8(13):1735–1744.
66. Cheung A, Webb JG, Barbanti M, et al. 5-year experience with transcatheter transapical mitral valve-in-valve implantation for bioprosthetic valve dysfunction. *J Am Coll Cardiol*. 2013;61(17):1759–1766.
70. Chakravarty T, Sondergaard L, Friedman J, et al. Subclinical leaflet thrombosis in surgical and transcatheter bioprosthetic aortic valves: an observational study. *Lancet*. 2017;389(10087):2383–2392.

中文导读

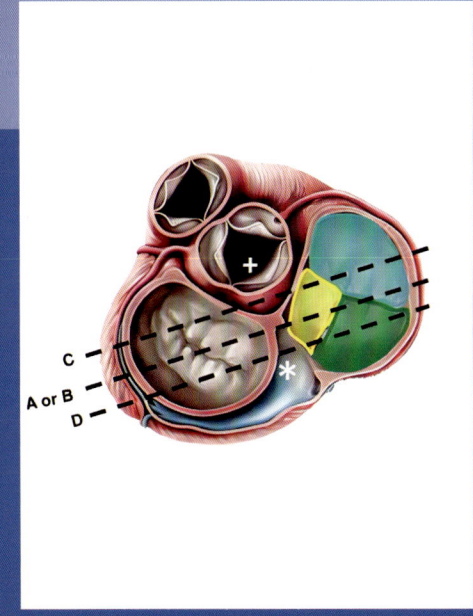

第56章
肺动脉瓣介入治疗

  无论是获得性的还是先天性心脏病所造成的孤立性肺动脉瓣功能障碍，在临床上都可以没有症状，并可以长期耐受。在西方国家中获得性肺动脉瓣疾病很少见，大多与风湿热、感染性心内膜炎和类癌综合征等疾病有关。在先天性心脏病中，瓣膜功能障碍是许多解剖缺陷的表现，也是一些早期修复策略的常见继发后果。

  除传统外科手术之外，经皮肺动脉瓣成形术对孤立的肺动脉瓣狭窄及慢性肺动脉瓣反流的疗效明确。经皮肺动脉瓣植入术更是除了传统右心室流出道重建手术外，已成为介入手术的重要手段。

  本章内容将深入探讨这项革命性技术的临床应用，包括详细介绍经皮肺动脉瓣成形术、经皮肺动脉瓣植入术的临床背景及适应证，并针对Melody和Sapien两款主流瓣膜的设计组成、详细规格参数、作为右心室流出道功能障碍的非手术治疗方案的适应证、技术，以及经皮肺动脉瓣植入术患者的临床预后进行全面讨论，并详细总结了肺动脉瓣介入治疗的干预时机、最新的研究结果和当前尚未解决的临床问题，为未来研究提供了明确的方向。

吕俊兴　张洪亮

章节要点

- 经皮肺动脉瓣成形术是所有中度以上孤立性肺动脉狭窄患者的一线治疗。
- 即使是危重的新生儿肺动脉狭窄，简单有效的球囊扩张术也是一个疗效确切的解决方案，并能有效避免未来的医疗干预需求。
- 经皮肺动脉瓣植入术适用于右心室至肺动脉导管功能不全的患者，以及特定补片功能不全或重建流出道的病例。
- 用于右室流出道小于22 mm的Melody和用于小于29 mm的Sapien两种支架瓣膜，已被批准在美国国内和国外使用。
- 经皮肺动脉瓣植入术是在患者全身麻醉的情况下进行的，通常采用股静脉路径。该手术能有效改善早期症状和缩小右心室容积。
- 植入时，瓣膜移位、外科移植体破裂或冠状动脉受压可能会使经皮肺动脉瓣植入术变得复杂；通过仔细评估解剖结构和确保正确的手术流程，这些情况应该是可以避免的。
- 经皮肺动脉瓣植入术已经成为常规临床实践的一部分，在过去的十年中，全世界有超过8000例手术，其延长了通道的寿命，并可能减少先天性心脏病患者在其一生中所需要的手术次数。

56 Pulmonary Valve Interventions

Robert Wagner, Ingo Daehnert, Philipp C. Lurz

KEY POINTS

- Percutaneous pulmonary valvuloplasty is the first-line treatment for all patients with more than moderate isolated pulmonary stenosis.
- Even in critical neonatal pulmonary stenosis, simple efficacious balloon dilatation can provide a definitive solution and avoid the need for future medical intervention.
- Percutaneous pulmonary valve implantation (PPVI) is suitable for patients with dysfunctional right ventricle–to–pulmonary artery conduits and for dysfunctional patch reconstructed outflow tracts in selected cases.
- Two stent-mounted valves, the Melody for right ventricular outflow tracts of less than 22 mm and the Sapien for those less than 29 mm, are approved for use within and outside the United States.
- PPVI is performed with the patient under general anesthesia, and a femoral approach is typically used. The procedure results in early symptomatic improvement and reduction of right ventricular volumes.
- PPVI can be complicated by device displacement, homograft rupture, or coronary artery compression at the time of implantation; these should be avoidable by careful assessment of anatomy and correct prestenting procedures.
- PPVI has become part of routine clinical practice, with more than 8000 procedures performed worldwide in the past decade. It prolongs conduit life and may reduce the number of operations required by patients with congenital heart disease during their lifetimes.

INTRODUCTION

Isolated pulmonary valve dysfunction, whether acquired or in the context of congenital heart disease, can be clinically asymptomatic and tolerated for a long time.[1] In Western countries, acquired pulmonary valve diseases are rare and mostly related to conditions such as rheumatic fever, infective endocarditis (IE), and carcinoid syndrome. In cases of congenital heart disease, valve dysfunction is a primary component of many anatomic defects and a common secondary consequence of several early repair strategies.

Isolated valvar pulmonary stenosis (PS) is a common heart defect in approximately 6% of neonates with congenital heart diseases.[2] However, the reported incidence varies widely. To complicate matters further, the condition may develop or retreat with age. After Morgagni first reported a cyanotic patient with PS and atrial septal defect in 1761 ("De Sedibus et Causis Morborum"), it took until 1982 to introduce an effective interventional treatment strategy for isolated PS besides surgical treatment.[3]

Nowadays, percutaneous pulmonary valvuloplasty is the first-line treatment for patients with more than moderate isolated or critical neonatal PS. Implemented by the experienced interventionalist, a simple efficacious balloon dilatation can provide a definitive solution and avoid the need for future medical intervention.

Increasing knowledge about potential harmful effects of chronic pulmonary regurgitation has made surgical revision of the right ventricular outflow tract (RVOT) a frequently performed operation in this population.[4] Typically, most patients require several repeat operations during their lifetime to halt the detrimental effects of valvular dysfunction. Since the techniques of percutaneous pulmonary valve implantation (PPVI) were first described by Philipp Bonhoeffer and colleagues more than a decade ago and as there have been 4500 implants in the United States since the original Investigational Device Exemption (IDE) study began in 2007,[5] the procedure has gained worldwide acceptance and has become a routine interventional procedure.[6]

Several devices have been investigated for purposes of interventional pulmonary valve implantation. Initially, Melody transcatheter pulmonary valve (Medtronic, Minneapolis, MN) obtained European and American regulatory approval. Later, Edwards Sapien valve (Edwards Lifesciences LLC, Irvine, CA) was successfully implanted in pulmonary position in 2006[7] and received U.S. Food and Drug Administration (FDA) approval for pulmonic procedures in early 2016.

This chapter explores the clinical applications of this revolutionary technology. Indications, patient selection, updated clinical results, and future directions of pulmonary valve interventions are discussed.

PERCUTANEOUS PULMONARY VALVULOPLASTY

Background and Clinical Indications

Isolated PS is third only to ventricular and atrial septal defect in its prevalence and can also occur in up to 50% of patients with other congenital cardiac defects. There are no convincing gender-related differences or differences between racial groups. Although most cases are isolated, a recurrence rate of up to 3% has been described in siblings and autosomal dominant pedigrees have also been reported.[8] PS is a characteristic cardiac finding in Noonan syndrome (dysplastic valve type), syndromes which phenotypically overlap with the Noonan syndrome including the LEOPARD, Alagille syndrome, and Williams syndrome. PS may also occur in patients with congenital rubella (Gregg syndrome) or most often in carcinoid syndrome in cases of acquired disease. The condition may be broadly divided into three categories: neonatal critical stenosis, dome-shaped, and dysplastic (10% to 15% of cases) stenosis. Neonatal critical stenosis is characterized by high-grade stenosis causing right ventricular (RV) failure, cyanosis, and duct-dependent pulmonary circulation. Successful balloon pulmonary valvuloplasty can be achieved in most cases irrespective of the nature of the stenosis. However, dysplastic valves may show variable results.[9] In the case of the dome-shaped valve, the valvular tissue is not thickened, the arterial walls are normal, and the annulus is usually within normal size (Fig. 56.1). However, the commissures are fused with the three resultant fibrous raphes extending from the level of the sinotubular junction, over the surface of the valve to a central orifice. Occasionally, this process occurs in a bicuspid valve (two raphes) or in an asymmetric tricuspid valve leading to an eccentric orifice. A typical finding is poststenotic dilatation of the main pulmonary artery (PA) that sometimes involves the left PA. In contrast, the dysplastic valve is characterized by severely thickened myxomatous valve leaflets with "cauliflower"-like changes affecting the distal tips. The valve's annulus is mostly hypoplastic. Supraannular narrowing is more common than poststenotic dilatation.

Beyond the neonatal period, most patients with PS are asymptomatic. The right ventricle and atrium are usually able to compensate over a long time and maintain resting cardiac output. Typical symptoms are exercise intolerance with breathlessness and fatigue. With advancing age, RV compliance falls, and cyanosis may once again appear in cases of open interatrial communications (foramen ovale, atrial septal defect) due to right-to-left shunting. Chest pain, syncope, and sudden death rarely occur. Besides clinical features (ejection systolic murmur, systolic click, splitting of second heart sound) diagnosis is based on electrocardiography (right atrial enlargement), chest x-ray (prominent pulmonary segment, RV enlargement, variable calcification in older patients, pulmonary hypoperfusion), and transthoracic echocardiography. Echocardiography permits prior visualization of the nature of the valvar stenosis and assessment of the peak instantaneous systolic gradient by continuous-wave Doppler measurements. Table 56.1 represents the therapeutic strategy with respect to severity of the valve's stenosis.[10] In neonates there may be a patent arterial duct with left-to-right shunt and RV dysfunction with high-grade tricuspid regurgitation (TR). A critical PS requires emergency intervention with balloon valvuloplasty to reduce mortality irrespective of the measured gradient.[11]

PROCEDURAL TECHNIQUE

Percutaneous pulmonary valvuloplasty can be performed under conscious sedation or general anesthesia from a transfemoral approach. Fifty to 100 IU/kg heparin in children, or a standard dose of 5000 IU in adults, is administered routinely at the beginning of the procedure and repeated as required. A full aseptic technique is used. Broad-spectrum intravenous antibiotics are not given routinely for isolated balloon valvuloplasty. Standard right heart catheterization techniques are used to assess PA and RV pressures, to perform a pullback gradient, and to characterize the outflow tract anatomy with angiography favorably obtained from a lateral projection. Careful measurement of the valve's annulus is made at this stage to inform subsequent catheter selection. After placing an end-hole catheter into a distal PA, an exchange wire (0.018- to 0.035-inch) is passed through this into a side-branch artery or through the duct into descending aorta in neonatal cases. This may optimize maneuverability of the balloon catheter. The diameter of the balloon catheter should be approximately 130% (120% to 150%) of the measured valvular annulus.[9,12,13] After balloon preparation and advancing it over the guidewire, it should reach a position such that the stenotic pulmonary valve rests at the midpoint of the balloon (Fig. 56.2). Partial inflation is useful to confirm correct positioning prior to subsequent complete inflation of 10 to 15 seconds and full waist obliteration.

TABLE 56.1 Classification of the Severity of Pulmonic Stenosis and Its Relationship to Therapeutic Strategy

Degree of Severity	Peak Doppler Gradient (at Rest)[a]	Interventional Therapy[b]
Mild	<40 mm Hg	No
Moderate	40–60 mm Hg	May be indicated
Severe	>40 mm Hg	Indicated

[a]In symptomatic patients and neonates with duct-dependant pulmonary circulation irrespective of gradient.
[b]Irrespective of symptoms.[10,15,113]

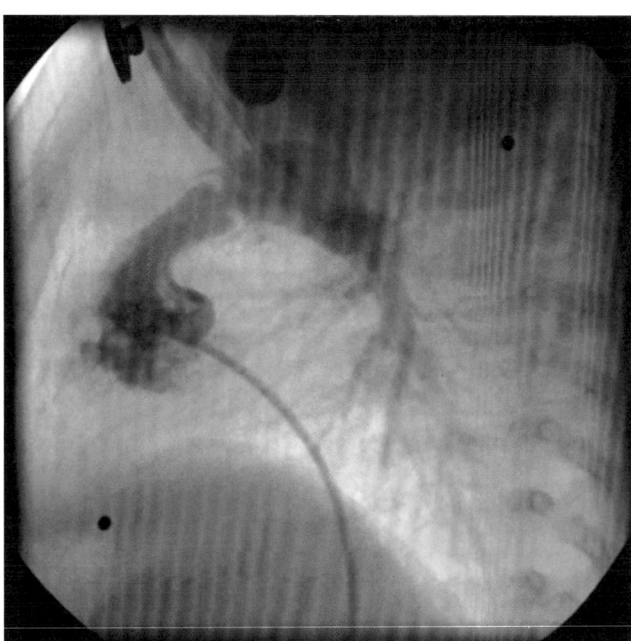

Fig. 56.1 Angiography of the right ventricular outflow tract in a neonate with critical pulmonary stenosis. Fluoroscopy shows the dome-shaped, high-grade stenotic valve.

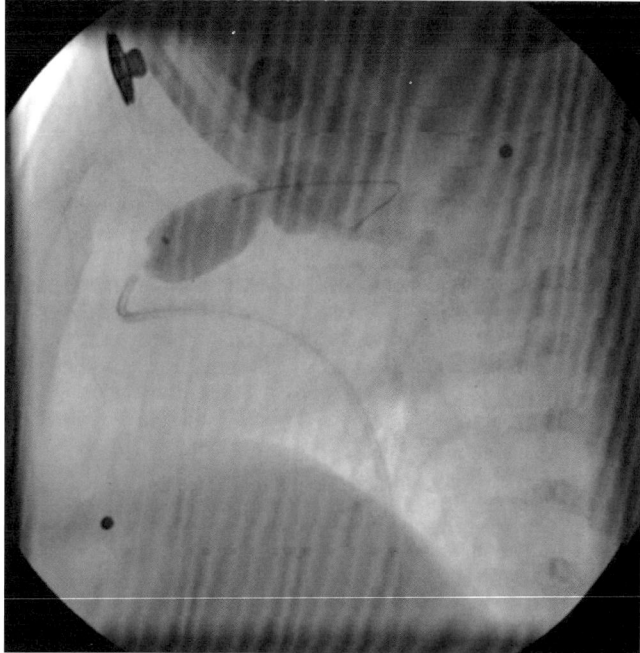

Fig. 56.2 Balloon inflation in a favored position with the stenotic pulmonary valve resting at the midpoint of the balloon.

Repeated gradient measurements and angiographies confirm the results. In adults or patients whose pulmonary valve annulus exceeds 18 to 19 mm, a double-balloon technique is preferred.

RESULTS AND OUTCOME

In general, percutaneous pulmonary valvuloplasty is an effective treatment strategy with a favorable long-term outcome irrespective of age.[10] With 95% after 5 years, 88% after 10 years, and even 84% after 20 years, freedom from reintervention after percutaneous pulmonary valvuloplasty (mostly for restenosis, less for regurgitation) is comparable to the reintervention after surgical valvuloplasty (mostly for regurgitation).[14] Outcomes in patients with dysplastic valves are more variable with a higher reintervention rate.[9]

Major complications include rupture of the RVOT and cardiac tamponade and injury to the tricuspid valve. If applied by experienced interventionalists, only mild pulmonary regurgitation will be apparent in most cases; however, moderate or severe insufficiency can occur. In this situation, a PPVI could be considered (see later). Minor complications (venous thrombosis, hemorrhage, transient arrhythmia, risk of infection or reaction to contrast) appear as often as in other comparable procedures. After successful relieving of high-grade stenosis, dynamic infundibular obstruction with resulting hypotension and hypoxia is a particular risk in the young patient. If it occurs, fluid boluses, β-blocker infusion, and/or prostaglandin infusion to maintain ductal left-to-right shunting can stabilize the situation. Mortality of the percutaneous approach to relieve PS is even low in neonates (0% to 0.5%).[15,16]

PERCUTANEOUS PULMONARY VALVE IMPLANTATION

Background and Clinical Indications

Over the past decades, advances in cardiac surgery, interventional procedures, intensive care, and noninvasive imaging have led to a substantial increase in life expectancy for many patients with congenital heart disease. This challenging, heterogeneous population of patients who were treated by corrective, semicorrective, or palliative surgical procedures, sometimes decades ago, is growing inexorably. Comparing birth registries for the years 1950–59 and 1990–99, the life expectancy of patients with congenital heart disease expressed by 18-year survival rates has increased from 10% to 70%.[17]

Studies have shown that the number of adult patients with congenital heart disease are similar to those for the pediatric population and will continue to grow.[18] For approximately 20% of these adults and children, late after neonatal repair of complex congenital heart disorders, such as tetralogy of Fallot, pulmonary atresia, persistent trunk, or D-transposition with RVOT obstruction, RVOT dysfunction manifesting as an obstructive lesion or as pulmonary regurgitation becomes clinically evident.

Surgical pulmonary valve replacement using valved homograft or porcine (e.g., Medtronic Hancock) and bovine xenograft conduits (e.g., Medtronic Contegra) helps to treat RVOT dysfunction. Undeniably the most frequent mode of repeat operation in patients with congenital heart disease, surgical pulmonary valve replacement is a safe procedure and is performed with low morbidity and mortality rates.[4] However, an important drawback is the limited life span of the conduits. Due to growth-related undersizing and degeneration of the conduit causing obstruction or pulmonary regurgitation, conduit life span is approximately 10 years.[19–22] Most patients must undergo several open heart procedures during their lives that raise potential risks for bleeding, adhesions, and sternal or cutaneous related complications.

To minimize the number of open heart operations, delaying surgical interventions for as long as possible has been the strategy of choice. This policy risks delaying necessary treatment beyond the point of no return, when RV dysfunction, impaired exercise capacity, and increased risk of sudden cardiac death, which can result from chronic adverse RV loading conditions,[23–25] may be irreversible.

The correct timing for surgical pulmonary valve replacement is unknown and remains a highly controversial issue among cardiologists who take care of children and adults with congenital heart disease.[4,26] Using magnetic resonance imaging (MRI), attempts have been made to establish RV volume thresholds as predictors of outcome after conduit placement. Cutoff points for RV end-diastolic volumes (EDV) have been reported, with some suggesting end-diastolic values of 150 to 170 mL/m² [26–30] and end-systolic volumes of 85 to 90 mL/m² [29,30] above which normalization of RV dimensions is less likely after pulmonary valve replacement. However, the impact of the timing of pulmonary valve replacement on RV function, exercise performance, and particularly, long-term survival remains undefined.[31] Recently, after analysis of our cohort, we proposed QRS duration of <150 ms as valuable predictor of favorable outcome of RV remodeling after PPVI, because it represents electrical and mechanical functions of the right ventricle.[32]

To postpone and potentially reduce the number of operations patients have to undergo throughout their lives, transcatheter stent implantation into stenotic conduits has been carried out,[33–36] although bare-metal stenting can potentially convert a pressure overload due to obstruction into a volume overload due to free pulmonary incompetence. With the introduction of percutaneous valve implantation, a nonsurgical technique has become available. It enables treatment of RVOT obstruction as well as regurgitation or mixed states of RVOT dysfunction. This minimally invasive method can potentially avoid open heart surgery for RVOT dysfunction in children and adults by restoring acceptable RV loading conditions.

Since the first description of a percutaneously implanted heart valve in 2000,[6] more than 10,000 PPVIs have been performed worldwide.[37–39] The Melody device became commercially available in Europe and Canada in 2006. It was certified by Conformité Européenne (CE) in 2006 and approved by the FDA for clinical use in the United States in 2010, making the new percutaneous strategy available to a broader population.

PPVI is performed to prolong the life span of conduits from the right ventricle to the pulmonary artery (RV-PA) and therefore postpone open heart surgery in children and adults with congenital heart disease. Over the past 10 years, increasing operator experience with PPVI has resulted in improved safety, efficacy, and outcomes, including freedom from transcatheter or surgical reintervention for pediatric or adult patients who underwent this procedure.[31,40–47]

Indications, technical aspects, and early and late results of PPVI using the Melody valve and the Sapien valve as nonsurgical treatment options for RVOT dysfunction are reviewed in the following sections.

Devices and Delivery Systems
Melody Transcatheter Pulmonary Valve

The Melody transcatheter pulmonary valve is composed of a segment of bovine jugular vein with a central valve (Figs. 56.3 and 56.4) sutured inside an expanded platinum-iridium stent. The currently used Cheatham platinum stent (CP Stent CP8Z34, NuMed, Hopkinton, NY) is 34 mm long; it can be crimped to minimum of 6 mm in diameter and reexpanded up to 22 mm. It consists of an eight-crown zigzag pattern with six segments along its length that are reinforced at each strut intersection with a gold weld. The venous segment is attached to the frame by continuous 5-0 polypropylene sutures around the entire circumference at the inflow and outflow and also discretely at each strut intersection. The suture is clear for all points except the outflow line,

SECTION V Structural Interventions

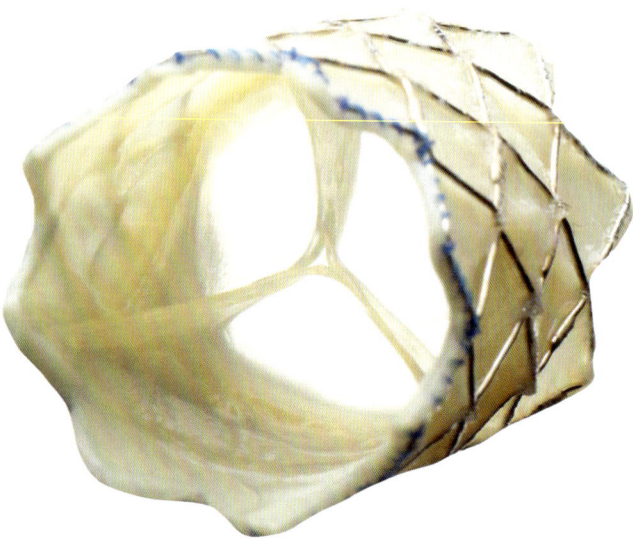

Fig. 56.3 Melody transcatheter pulmonary valve in an oblique view. Notice the *blue line* that identifies the outflow end of the device. (Courtesy Medtronic, Minneapolis, MN.)

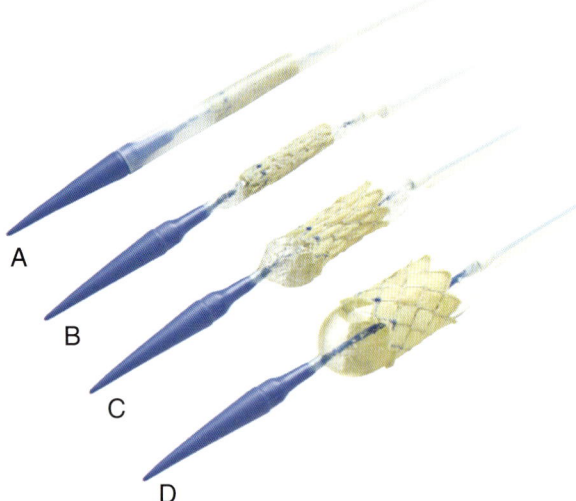

Fig. 56.4 Melody device and its delivery system. (A) Crimped device on the delivery system with a retractable sheath covering the device to protect it during the delivery. (B) Retracted sheath. (C) Deployment of the *i*nner balloon (*i*ndigo access). (D) Deployment of the *o*uter balloon (*o*range access). (Courtesy Medtronic, Minneapolis, MN.)

which is blue to signify the outflow end of the device. The valve is packaged and sterilized in a solution containing 1% glutaraldehyde and 20% isopropyl alcohol (see Fig. 56.3). The delivery system (Ensemble, Medtronic) contains a balloon-in-balloon (BiB) deployment design.

The Ensemble delivery system (Medtronic) contains a BiB deployment design. At its distal end, the valved stent is front-loaded and crimped (see Fig. 56.4). The system is available with outer balloon diameters of 18, 20, and 22 mm to fit different outflow tract diameters. To avoid incorrect implantation and potential failure, the tip of the delivery system is blue to correspond to the outflow suture of the device as described previously.

The body of the system is composed of a one-piece, 22-Fr Teflon sheath containing a braided-wire, elastomer-reinforced lumen. The retractable sheath that covers the stented valve during delivery is pulled back just before deployment. Contrast can be delivered through the retracted sheath from a side port to confirm positioning of the device before deployment. The proximal portion of the system has three ports, one for the *g*uidewire (*g*reen), one to deploy the *i*nner balloon (*i*ndigo), and one to deploy the *o*uter balloon (*o*range) (see Fig. 56.4). Technical details regarding the Melody valve are summarized in Table 56.2.

Sapien Pulmonic Transcatheter Heart Valve

The Edwards Sapien XT valve is radiopaque and made of a trileaflet bovine pericardial valve that is sewn by hand into a stainless steel stent (14 or 16 mm long) (Fig. 56.5). A fabric polyethylene terephthalate sealing cuff covers the proximal part of the stent and is designed to prevent paravalvular leakage. The valve tissue is fabricated from three equal sections of bovine pericardium that have been preserved in glutaraldehyde to crosslink the xenograft tissue and preserve its flexibility and strength.

The device was initially designed for aortic valve replacement and obtained certification for PPVI later.[48] Currently, the successor of the Sapien valve, the Sapien XT, is commercially available in 23-, 26-, and 29-mm-diameter sizes and is crimped onto the designated balloon delivery system (Retroflex).

In 2013, the third generation of the Retroflex III delivery system (Edwards Lifesciences) was FDA approved. It consists of a balloon catheter and a deflectable guiding catheter. The system requires a 22-Fr sheath (for the Sapien XT 23-mm valve) or 24-Fr hydrophilic sheath (for the Sapien XT 26-mm and Sapien XT 29-mm valve) (see Fig. 56.5). According to the manufacturer's data, improvements in design (e.g., Edwards eSheath, Edwards Lifesciences) offer smaller sheath sizes for the 23-mm valve (16 Fr), the 26-mm valve (18 Fr), and the 29-mm XT model (20 Fr).[49] The guiding catheter has a control handle on the catheter hub, which can be rotated to deflect the catheter passing through the tricuspid aperture to the RVOT. The Retroflex III system also contains a retractable nose cone catheter, which facilitates atraumatic delivery. Technical details regarding the Sapien valve are summarized in Table 56.2.

Patient Selection Criteria

Clinical Criteria

Clear-cut guidelines do not exist for treating RVOT dysfunction caused by obstruction or regurgitation. This issue is slightly less complex in the setting of RVOT obstruction because patients with significant obstruction tend to develop symptoms early. According to the 2010 European Society of Cardiology (ESC) and Association for European Pediatric Cardiology (AEPC) guidelines for the management of grown-up congenital heart disease[50] including indications for surgical intervention or PPVI in patients with RV-PA conduits, patients with RVOT obstruction should be treated if the gradient exceeds 60 mm Hg or with symptoms due to RVOT obstruction regardless of the RVOT gradient.

In the clinical setting, indications for PPVI can be adapted from the indications for RVOT bare-metal stenting.[34] In cases of RV pressure overload due to RVOT obstruction, symptomatic patients should undergo PPVI if the RV systolic pressure exceeds 65% of systemic pressures. In the absence of symptoms, patients should undergo treatment if RV pressures exceed 75% of systemic pressures as estimated by echocardiography and noninvasive blood pressure measurement.[40]

Pulmonary regurgitation can be clinically asymptomatic and be tolerated for a long time. When to intervene is the subject of ongoing discussions. It is common sense to base the indication criteria for transcatheter or surgical treatment

TABLE 56.2 Currently Available Systems for Percutaneous Pulmonary Valve Implantation

	Melody Transcatheter Valve	Sapien XT Transcatheter Heart Valve
Manufacturer	Medtronic Inc., Minneapolis, MN	Edwards Lifesciences LLC, Irvine, CA
Regulatory approval	CE 9/2006 FDA 01/2010	CE 2/2011 FDA 6/2014 (aortic) FDA 2/2016 (pulmonic[a])
(Tissue) characteristics	segment of bovine jugular vein with a central valve hand-sewn inside a stent	trileaflet bovine pericardial valve hand-sewn inside a stent
Stent type	Cheatham platinum stent (NuMED CP Stent CP8Z34) Length 34 mm Expandable up to 22 mm	stainless steel stent length of 14 or 16 mm
Available sizes	18, 20, 22 mm (depending on the favored Ensemble delivery system)	23, 26, 29 mm
Delivery system	Ensemble (Medtronic, Minneapolis, MN) with balloon-in-balloon (BiB) deployment design	Edwards Retroflex III containing a balloon catheter and a deflectable guiding catheter
Sheaths for implantation	One-piece 22-Fr Teflon sheath	(16 Fr[b]) 22 Fr for 23-mm valves (18 Fr[b]) 24 Fr for 26-mm valves (20 Fr[b]) 24 Fr for 29-mm XT valves

[a]For use in pediatric and adult patients.
[b]Data given for the Edwards eSheath.[49]
Technical comparison of the commercially available devices for TPVI: the Melody device and the Sapien XT Transcatheter Heart Valve as nonsurgical treatment options for right ventricular outflow tract dysfunction. *CE,* Conformité Européenne marking; *FDA,* U.S. Food and Drug Administration; *TPVI,* transcatheter pulmonary valve implantation.

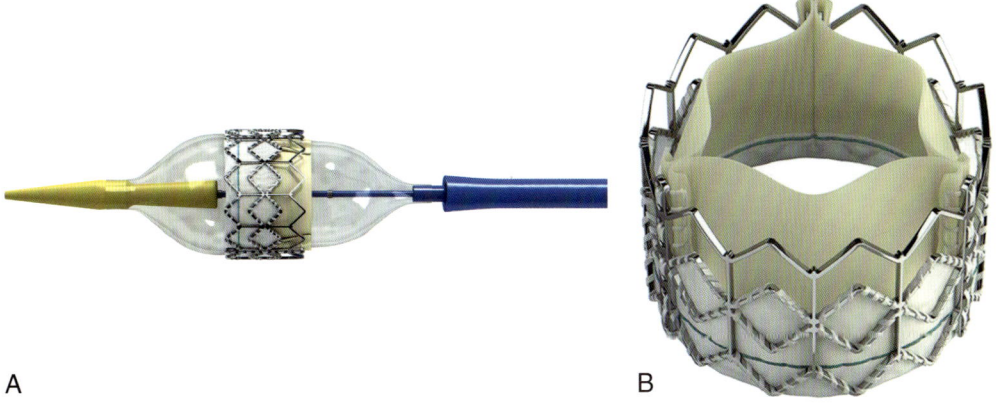

Fig. 56.5 (A) Top view of the Sapien pulmonic transcatheter heart valve. (B) The Retroflex III delivery system. (Courtesy Edwards Lifesciences LLC, Irvine, CA. Edwards, Edwards Lifesciences, RetroFlex, RetroFlex II, RetroFlex 3, RF3, Edwards SAPIEN, SAPIEN, SAPIEN XT and SAPIEN 3 are trademarks of Edwards Lifesciences Corporation.)

on a combined assessment of MRI-derived RV end-diastolic volume, end-systolic volume and systolic function, cardiopulmonary exercise testing (as an objective measure of the patient's exercise capacity), and atrial or ventricular dysrhythmia.[29] According to the 2010 ESC recommendations of the ESC grown-up congenital heart disease task force, PPVI may be indicated if the patient has severe pulmonary regurgitation (assessed by echocardiography or MRI) and one of the following: severe RV dilation, severe RV dysfunction, symptoms, or impaired exercise capacity.[50]

In 2011 the American Heart Association (AHA) stated, "It is reasonable to consider the percutaneous pulmonary valve replacement in patient with RV-PA conduits with moderate to severe pulmonary regurgitation or stenosis provided the patient meets inclusion/exclusion criteria for the available valve." The AHA writing committee recommended this procedure based on class IIa evidence (evidence level B).[51]

There is no absolute lower age limit, but an adequate body size (e.g., weight >20 kg) is required to accommodate femoral placement of the introducer.[24] Table 56.3 summarizes clinical indications for Melody and Sapien PPVI.

Preprocedural Assessment

To establish clinical indication criteria, all patients undergo a standardized assessment protocol. For screening, echocardiography is performed to determine the RVOT gradient and to semiquantitatively assess the severity of pulmonary regurgitation. Echocardiography is also used to estimate RV pressure (tricuspid valve regurgitant jet) and the RV to systemic pressure ratio (noninvasive blood pressure measurements) but may not be able to equal MRI in the assessment of RV function even when incorporating deformation analysis.[52] Therefore, as a crucial part of the assessment, patients undergo cardiac MRI unless contraindicated. We define RV dilatation in the context of pulmonary regurgitation as severe when the indexed RV end-diastolic volume is >150 mL/m^2 or the RV to LV end-diastolic ratio is >1.7. Indexed RV end-systolic volume and MRI-derived estimation of RV ejection may be included in decision making as published by Alvarez-Fuente.[29] It is of note that ventricular volume derived on MRI can differ by more than 15% depending on whether RV trabeculations are included in the volume or whether end-diastolic and end-systolic volumes are defined by the endocardial outline in each of the short-axis cine images, excluding RV trabeculations. In our practice, RV trabeculations are excluded when volumes are calculated. MRI also allows accurate quantification of pulmonary regurgitation using PA flow measurements, providing a calculated pulmonary regurgitation fraction. Objective exercise capacity is assessed by cardiopulmonary exercise testing on a bicycle using a ramp protocol. A peak oxygen uptake of less than 65% of predicted is considered as a significant impairment in exercise capacity. Appearance of inducible dysrhythmia is even likely on peak exercise levels or recovery from it. Finally, surface electrocardiograms (ECG) and Holter ECG monitoring are performed to detect dysrhythmia and define QRS duration as important predictors of favorable RV remodeling in our setting.[32]

Morphologic Criteria

Size and shape of the implantation site, also called the *landing zone*, and its anatomic relation to the coronary arteries are decisive morphologic criteria. They must be correct when considering patients as candidates for PPVI.

Size and Shape of the Implantation Site

The Melody device cannot be dilated to a diameter of more than 22 mm. Patients with nondilated conduits between the RV and PA of 22 mm or less offer an ideal environment for PPVI with this device. In contrast, native or patched outflow tracts after surgical repair for tetralogy of Fallot tend to be dilated and too large (>22 mm) and therefore do not provide a secure landing zone for Melody valves. In these cases, or if the conduit size at surgical implantation is at least 18 mm but no larger than 29 mm with significant discrete narrowing, the Sapien valve may be used for treatment.[7,49,53–55]

In our experience, the RVOT shape after prestenting is important because of the engineered nature of sutured pericardial tissue. Optimal valved stent function in Sapien procedures is guaranteed by a circular RVOT shape. In PPVI procedures with the Melody valve, the RVOT shape has much less impact on the hemodynamic outcome.

Studying the patient's operative reports in detail and, unless contraindicated, using MRI before the procedure helps to understand the anatomy of the outflow tract and to avoid implantation failure (Fig. 56.6). Cine MRI can determine the maximal and minimal dimensions of the RVOT and its shape throughout the cardiac cycle. Preprocedural three-dimensional (3D) reconstructions of the outflow tract further improve the understanding of the anatomy. It also allows to create reliable 3D roadmaps for RVOT interventions when using novel software solutions for fusing fluoroscopy images with MRI or computed tomography scans, as proposed by the Berlin and Poland groups.[56] If there is doubt about the reliability of MRI-derived measurements, balloon sizing of the RVOT at the time of catheterization is recommended and is discussed later (Fig. 56.7). The minimal diameter for PPVI is not less than 16 mm to avoid unacceptable residual gradients. Rare exceptions to this rule include cases in which 3D imaging and echocardiographic assessment suggest that sufficient space is available to deploy a valve to a reasonable diameter.

Assessment of Coronary Artery Anatomy

Coronary artery anatomy varies according to the type of congenital heart defect and is affected by surgical reinsertion into the aorta. In some cases, one or more of the relevant coronary artery branches are near the main PA. This configuration exposes patients who undergo RVOT interventions to the risk of fatal coronary artery obstruction due to expansion of the RVOT.[34,57]

The course of proximal coronary arteries in relation to the RVOT must be assessed before percutaneous valve deployment. Some centers prefer 3D whole heart MRI reconstruction to assess the anatomic relationship of the coronary arteries and the proposed implantation site (Fig. 56.8). We recommend selective coronary angiography and particularly aortic root angiography and simultaneous high-pressure balloon inflation within the landing zone (discussed later) at the time of catheterization in all patients to rule out the risk of coronary compression (Fig. 56.9).

Exclusion Criteria

The exclusion criteria result from the aforementioned and are adapted from the 2010 ESC and AEPC guidelines for the management of grown-up congenital heart disease: (1) evidence of risk of coronary compression; (2) central vein occlusion or significant obstruction; and (3) active or high risk for systemic infection

TABLE 56.3 Clinical and Morphologic Requirements for Percutaneous Pulmonary Valve Implantation

Clinical indications in the context of RV pressure overload or pulmonary stenosis:
  RV systolic pressure >65% of systemic pressure in symptomatic patients
  RV systolic pressure >75% of systemic pressure in asymptomatic patients
Clinical indications in the context of RV volume overload or pulmonary regurgitation:
  Severe pulmonary regurgitation on echocardiography or MRI and One or more of the following:
- Severe RV dilatation >150 mL/m^2 or the RV/LV end-diastolic ratio of >1.7 *and/or*
- Rapidly progressive RV dilation and/or
- Severe RV dysfunction and/or
- Symptoms and/or
- Sustained atrial or ventricular arrhythmia and/or
- Impaired exercise capacity (<65% compared with normal peak oxygen consumption)

LV, Left ventricular; *MRI*, magnetic resonance imaging; *RV*, right ventricular.

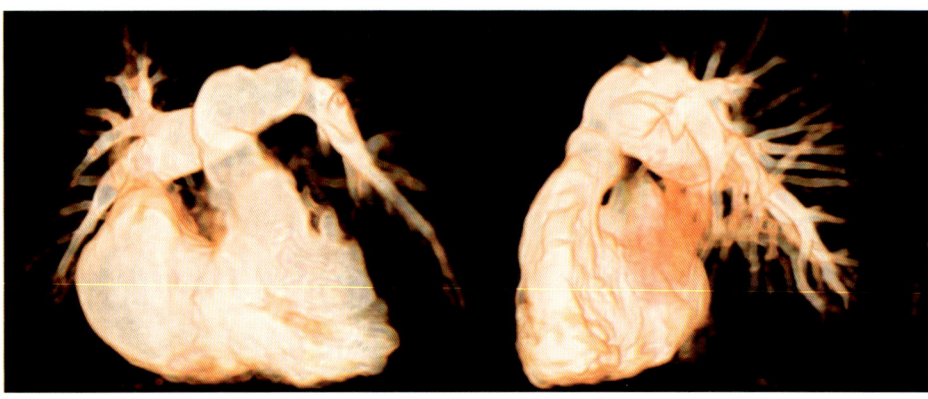

Fig. 56.6 Noninvasive, three-dimensional right ventricular outflow tract reconstruction by magnetic resonance tomography was performed in a patient with pulmonary atresia with an intact ventricular septum after repair by pulmonic homograft implantation. The patient had ventricular outflow tract dysfunction before percutaneous pulmonary valve implantation.

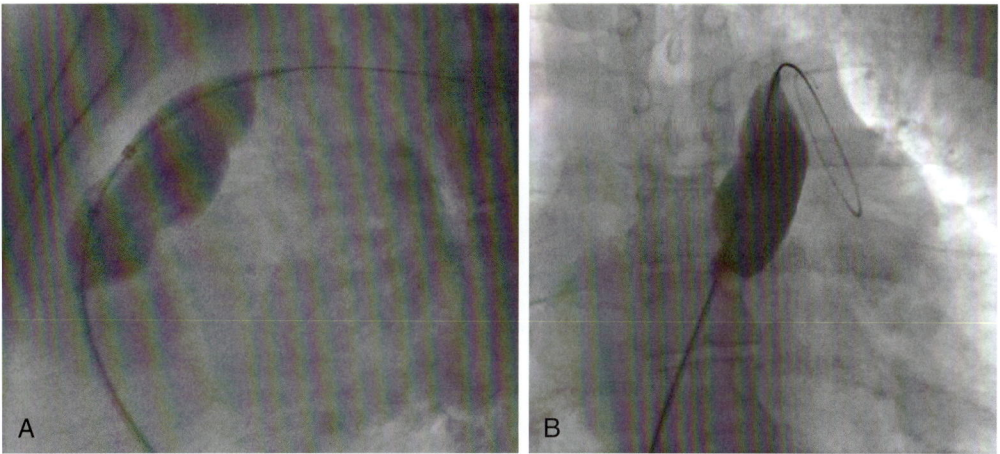

Fig. 56.7 Balloon sizing for the right ventricular outflow tract. Fluoroscopy shows the balloon sizing maneuver from 90-degree (A) and 0-degree (B) left anterior oblique views.

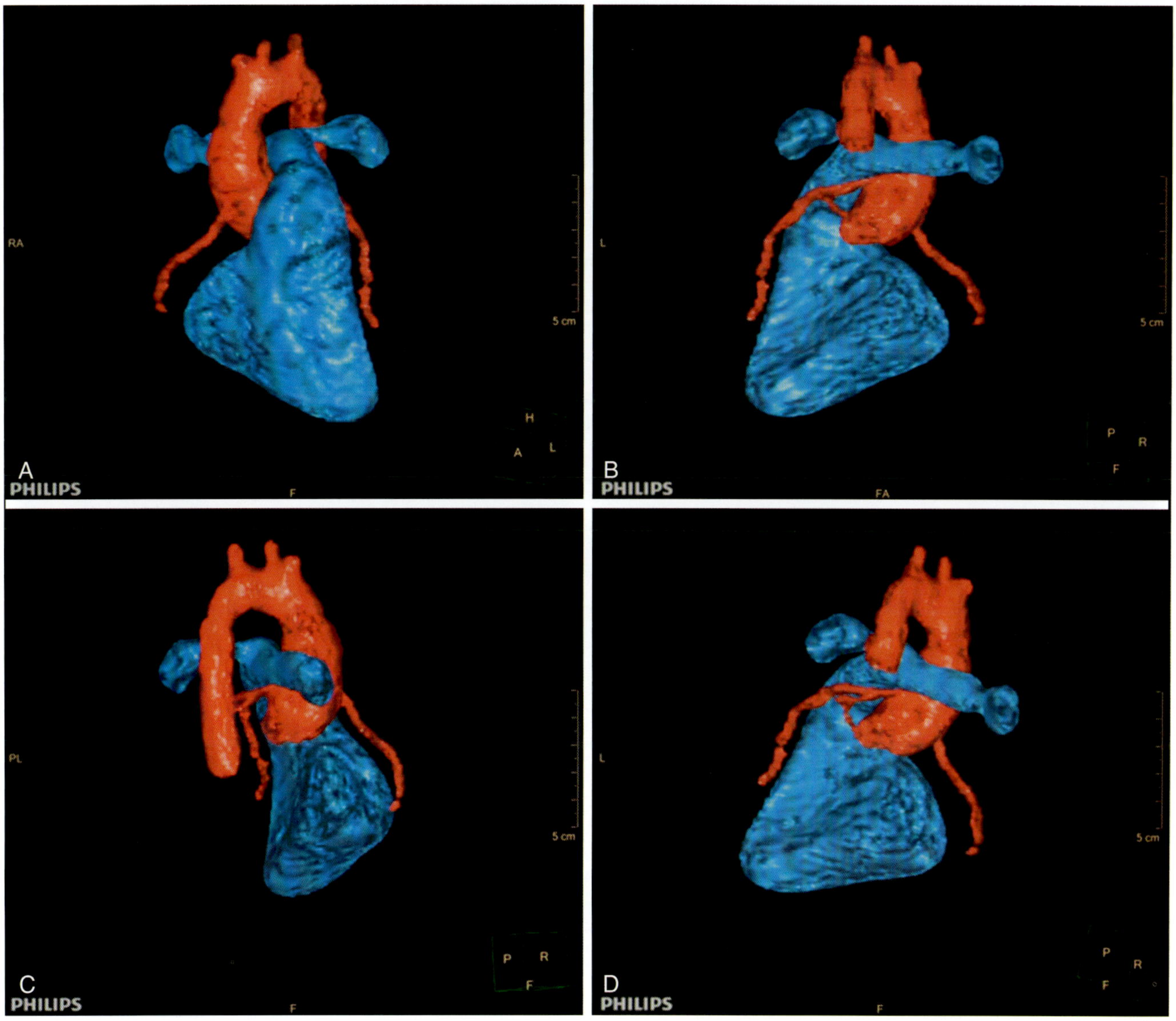

Fig. 56.8 Noninvasive, three-dimensional, whole heart imaging magnetic resonance tomography focused on the relation of the dysfunctional RVOT to the coronary arteries. (A) The anterior view. (B) The posterior view. (C and D) The oblique views (the right heart and pulmonary artery and branches in *blue*, the ascending aorta and coronary arteries in *red*, left heart is virtually removed to avoid overlay).

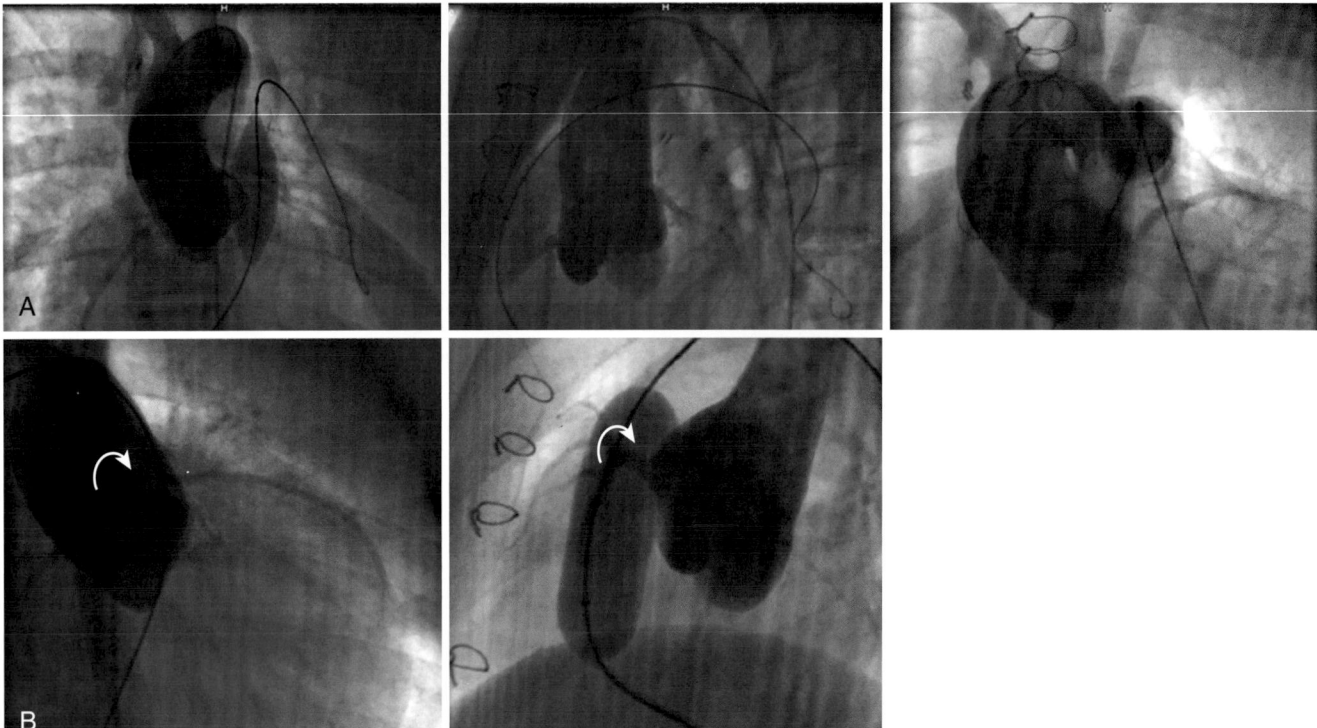

Fig. 56.9 Assessment of risk for coronary compression. (A) The 0-degree and 90-degree left anterior oblique (LAO) and 0-degree with 45-degree caudal angulation aortic root angiograms show high-pressure balloon inflation within the eligible landing zone, which is performed to rule out coronary compression. (B) The 0-degree and 90-degree LAO aortic root angiograms show compression of the left anterior descending coronary artery *(arrow)* during balloon inflation in the conduit. The procedure was therefore abandoned in this patient, and no percutaneous pulmonary valve implantation was performed.

(such as endocarditis, intravenous drug abuse). Open heart surgery should be preferred when additional interventions are reasonably considered (such as tricuspid valve repair, coronary artery bypass, arrhythmia surgery).

Procedure

Laboratory Setup

PPVI should be performed in a catheterization laboratory with a monoplane or, preferably, biplane fluoroscopy setup. Procedures must be performed under sterile conditions meeting the standards for surgical valve implantations. Autotransfusion kits (e.g., pleural drainage kits, cell saver) should be available in cases of acute bleeding. Although simultaneous surgical backup is not required, PPVI should be performed at institutions with a (congenital disease) surgical program. Ideally, the surgical team has access to and experience with extracorporeal circulation equipment.

PPVI is usually performed using general endotracheal anesthesia, although use of conscious sedation is feasible. Peripheral, central venous, and 5-Fr arterial line access is needed for continuous hemodynamic monitoring and anesthesia management. Femoral access is preferred because it allows an easier working position in the catheterization laboratory. Preparation of both groins for vascular access allows a quick change in case of problems. Jugular vein access can also be obtained if required. Use of a 10-Fr sheath (maximum) for initial venous access is appropriate.

Recommendations include aseptic technique meeting surgical standards, initiation of effective heparinization at the beginning of the procedure (50 to 100 IU/kg of heparin in children or a standard dose of 5000 IU in adults, repeated as required), and a single dose of broad-spectrum intravenous antibiotics for endocarditis prophylaxis.

Hemodynamic Assessment

Right heart catheterization is performed using standard techniques to assess pressures and saturation levels. Routine measurements are made for the RV, PA, and aorta, and additional measurements (e.g., branch PAs) are made as appropriate. To provide a stable position before advancing the delivery system, a stiff guidewire is positioned in a distal branch PA. In an endeavor to maintain the guidewire's tip at the level of the diaphragm, the operators must not interfere with the tricuspid valve chordae.

PA (biplane) angiography is performed using appropriate catheters. The catheter's tip should be placed just beyond the expected position of the pulmonary valve to allow assessment of the proposed landing zone and estimation of pulmonary regurgitation.

Morphologic Assessment

Assessing the suitability of the size and shape of the landing zone is a crucial part of preparation before the final PPVI procedure. Invasive morphologic assessment during catheterization is often necessary, especially in cases of borderline dimensions derived by MRI. Distensibility of the site can be assessed only by balloon interrogation and is therefore strongly recommended in cases of expected high distensibility of the RVOT (i.e., patch-extended or native outflow tracts). Soft sizing balloon catheters are commonly used for balloon interrogation. They should be partially inflated when positioned distally to the supposed landing zone and then slowly retracted across the RVOT back into the RV. The use of biplane orthogonal fluoroscopy allows accurate 2D measurements.

The anterior-posterior imaging plane with cranial tilt is ideal for visualizing the pulmonary bifurcation and distal end of the stented valve. The anterior-posterior cranial view with or without left anterior oblique angulation is used to assess the bifurcation. The lateral plane visualizes the anterior chest and landing zone for the transcatheter pulmonary valve and seems to be the ideal view during stent positioning.

The risk of coronary compression should be minimized before implanting a Melody or Sapien valve. The preferred stepwise approach includes noninvasive, 3D whole heart MRI to judge the proximity of the proximal coronary arteries to the RVOT (see Fig. 56.8). For all patients at the time of catheterization, aortic root and selective coronary artery angiography should be performed along with simultaneous high-pressure balloon inflation in the landing zone and selective coronary angiography (see Fig. 56.9).[34,40,57] If evidence of coronary artery compression is found, the procedure must be abandoned.

Device Setup

Before implantation, preparations include checking and removing the manufacture's identification label and flushing, crimping, and loading the valved stent onto the delivery system. The valved stent should be repeatedly flushed to remove residues of the glutaraldehyde preservative and to test leaflet function.

The device is then crimped before being front-loaded onto the delivery system. The blue stitching on the distal portion of the device must match the blue portion of the delivery system (*the carrot*), which is then verified by an independent observer to guarantee correct device orientation. Further crimping is performed while advancing the sheath carefully over the device during saline flushing through the side port to exclude air bubbles from the system and facilitating uncovering of the device (see Fig. 56.4).

Device Implantation

After removing the angiography catheter, the femoral vein may be dilated to 22 or 24 Fr.

The delivery system is introduced into the access site and advanced into the landing zone under fluoroscopic guidance. The tip of the guidewire must be seen at all times. If its position has been lost, advancement of the delivery system must stop because the risk of peripheral vascular rupture is high when trying to push the wire back into position while carrying the delivery system. The delivery system can be safely removed and repositioned as long as the valve is at least partially covered.

The operator must reestablish a stable wire position with the use of catheters before advancing the delivery system. Coordination between first and second operator is necessary to safely advance the system into the desired position. Pushing the system in the groin moves it forward or backward; turning is impossible. Driving the wire will determine how the delivery system's end moves up to the landing zone. After the most distal part of the delivery system has passed the landing zone, the wire should be first straightened in the right atrium (the loop keeps the tricuspid valve open) before continuing the implantation process. The outer sheath is retracted, uncovering the stented valve, which sometimes results in forward movement. Because there are no radiopaque markers on the outer sheath, complete uncovering of the delivery system can be confirmed only by checking the double markers placed on the proximal portion of the system (i.e., balloon shaft). It must be completely uncovered before balloon inflation. Contrast injection into the side arm of the delivery system can offer further confirmation.

Deployment of the Melody valve is achieved by hand-inflating the *i*nner (*i*ndigo) balloon. After confirmation of the position, the *o*uter (*o*range) balloon is inflated to complete deployment. The inner balloon is then deflated, followed by deflation of the outer balloon while recording the deflation.

The delivery system is removed with great care through the implanted valve to avoid leaflet damage. Sheath closure should not be attempted before careful and slow withdrawal of the balloon and delivery system into the inferior vena cava. Repeat angiography of the RVOT can rule out extravasations for confirmation of valvar competence. The RV pressure and RV-PA pressure gradient are measured to assess the outcome. After removing all catheters and the venous sheath, hemostasis is achieved with a single Z-stitch on the skin over the venous access and with manual compression of the arterial access.

Periprocedural Interventions

Predilation of the Landing Zone. Over time, RVOT anatomy evolves in response to the repair strategies and RV-PA conduits used. Besides the hemodynamic problems related to stenosis, aberrant anatomy may challenge cannulation when using a large delivery system. Predilation of heavily calcified or tortuous conduits can facilitate passage and positioning of the system (e.g., Mullins high-pressure balloon, NuMed Inc., and/or Atlas high-pressure balloon, C.R. Bard Inc., Murray Hill, NJ). Some operators believe predilation of stenotic conduits optimizes the hemodynamic result. In our view, the most significant benefit of predilatation is the fact that it provides an ideal assessment of the anatomy. The location of the waist of the balloon, if present, represents the most rigid part of the implantation site and depicts the optimal landing zone for the valved stent. However, aforementioned advantages of predilatation have to be counterbalanced with the risk of RVOT or RV to PA graft rupture. Boudjemline et al. report a rupture rate of 9% in the latter.[59] Notably, severe bleeding due to rupture is rare, with an incidence of approximately 2%.[59] Partial rupture of an RV-to-PA graft during valve implantation is a common finding. Although this complication has no clinical consequence in the majority of cases due to the covered nature of the stent, this could lead to severe bleeding if caused by predilatation. Unfortunately, it is still not completely understood which patients and RVOTs are at risk for this complication. Possible risk factors include heavy calcification and homografts, and patients treated in "lower-volume" centers are at risk for conduit rupture during RVOT interventions prior to PPVI.[59] We believe that the decision for predilatation has to be made individually in each patient, taking the possible advantages and disadvantages into account.

Prestenting of the Landing Zone. Prior to PPVI, prestenting with bare-metal stents may be helpful. Observational studies have found that prestenting the conduit before PPVI is associated with a lower risk of developing Melody stent fractures.[60] Furthermore, Cardoso presented a meta-analysis including data from 360 patients and five studies indicating that prestenting of the RVOT prior to PPVI was not only associated with a significant reduction in the overall incidence of stent fractures but also with a lower incidence of stent fractures associated with loss of stent integrity (types II and III stent fractures) and a significant reduction in the need for reinterventions.[61] Therefore prestenting of the conduit before PPVI has become standard practice in most centers. It provides an unmistakable landmark for correct valve positioning and can produce superior immediate hemodynamic results because it enhances rigidity of the landing zone.[42,45] On multivariable retrospective risk factor analysis for the development of stent fractures during follow-up, it appears that a more dynamic RVOT, as seen in a noncalcified RVOT or noncircumferential homografts, is associated with the occurrence of stent fractures.[61] This information supports the superior use of prestenting to support the implantation site prior to PPVI. An additional bare stent within the RVOT should improve the rigidness of the RVOT and thereby potentially reduces the risk of stent fractures. Randomized trials are needed to confirm the effectiveness of prestenting in prevention of stented-valve fractures.[60]

For prestenting with bare-metal stents, the balloon-expandable IntraStent (Max LD, EV3, Plymouth, MN) can be used on a BiB dilation catheter (BiB catheter, NuMed). They are chosen because they have smaller nominal balloon diameters than those subsequently used in the PPVI delivery system. This approach leaves some degree of residual outflow tract obstruction but reduces the risk of conduit rupture and facilitates safer anchoring of the valved stent.

Typically, an uncovered stent is used if obstruction ("jailing") of the origin of a pulmonary branch artery is expected after deployment of the preimplantation stent. Covered bare-metal stents (e.g., CP stent, NuMed) are preferred in small conduits that require dilation to diameters larger than their original sizes. This approach can reduce the risk of bleeding due to conduit rupture.

The optimal timing of prestenting in relation to definitive PPVI is unknown. Some centers allow stent ingrowth for 2 or 3 to 6 months,[39] especially if inadequate sealing by covered stents is expected. In our experience, a combined procedure and a two-stage procedure are valid options. For the latter, temporal free pulmonary regurgitation after prestenting is well tolerated in most patients (Fig. 56.10).

Although Sapien valve stent fracture in either aortic or pulmonic position has not been described, prestenting before Sapien PPVI is preferred because of the short length (14 to 16 mm) of the valve and better stability.[49,55,62,63] Prestenting with a covered stent could also prevent paravalvular leak due to the relatively short sealing skirt within a geometrically complex and potentially tortuous RV to PA pathway.[64]

Postdilation of the Valved Stent. According to the Medtronic guidelines, postdilation of the valved stent is indicated if there is a gradient of more than 20 mm Hg caused by the valve's diameter; preimplantation or postimplantation residual valve stenosis should be ruled out or treated separately when applicable.[58] Long-term follow-up data from the U.S. IDE Melody trial recently found a residual RVOT gradient of >20 mm Hg is related to a significant shorter freedom from reintervention and reoperation during a 7-year follow-up,[47] which has previously been reported by our group.[40] Therefore an aggressive approach to a residual RVOT obstruction is required to improve the long-term outcome after PPVI.

Although forceful opening of the stenotic implantation site could be achieved by aggressive predilatation or by postdilatation of the bare-metal stent following prestenting, we believe that high-pressure postdilatation to a maximum balloon size of 24 mm after implanting the Melody device is the safest option with regard to conduit rupture. Ultra-high-pressure balloons such as the Mullins-X ultra-high-pressure dilation catheter (NuMed) or Atlas PTA dilation catheter (C.R. Bard Inc.) are suitable.[58] Multiple postimplantation dilations can be considered in cases of residual gradients to achieve further expansion of the device and optimize the hemodynamic result without damaging the bovine venous valve.[40]

Results

Immediate Hemodynamic Outcome

The hemodynamic outcome after PPVI in the largest published report using the Melody[5,37,40,42,45,47] or the Sapien device[49,53,54,62] is summarized in Table 56.4.

Significant reductions in RV pressure, RVOT gradient, and ratio of RV to systemic pressure were demonstrated with both devices. Diastolic pulmonary arterial pressures rise after deployment, indicating restoration of valvar competence.[37,40,54] Angiography before and after insertion shows a significant reduction in pulmonary regurgitation in most patients. Paravalvar leaks after the procedure occur in approximately 2% of the interventions.[45] Data from the Melody Registry involving 40 international centers that treated more than 1000 patients by PPVI were reviewed.[65] Invasively measured RV systolic pressure fell from 62 ± 18 mm Hg to 43 ± 12 mm Hg ($P < .0001$), and percentage of patients with RVOT regurgitation of greater than grade 2 decreased (49% to 1%, $P < .0001$).[65]

Immediate Procedural Complications

Several single-center and multicenter trials consistently reported a low periprocedural complication rate using the Melody pulmonic valve. The London experience with 155 patients[40] and the U.S. Melody valve trial that enrolled 124 patients[5] found similar procedural complication rates of 6%. Smaller trials showed an overall early complication rate of up to 11%.[46] Analysis of the Melody Registry data found a major procedural complication rate of 2.7% and minor complication rate of 11.9% for 1003 Melody procedures.[65] Major procedural complications related to Melody PPVI include homograft rupture (2.2%), perforation of branch PAs or guidewire injury to the PA (1.7%), damage to the tricuspid valve (1.6%), device dislodgment (0.5%), compression of coronary arteries (0.3%), and PA obstruction (0.3% in the London experience).

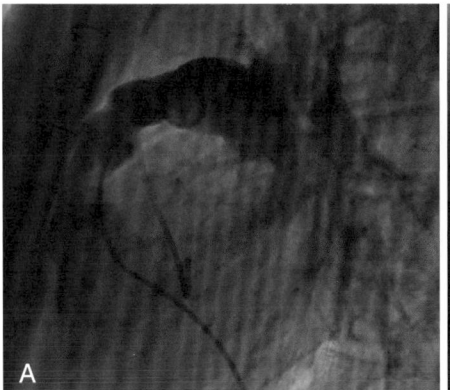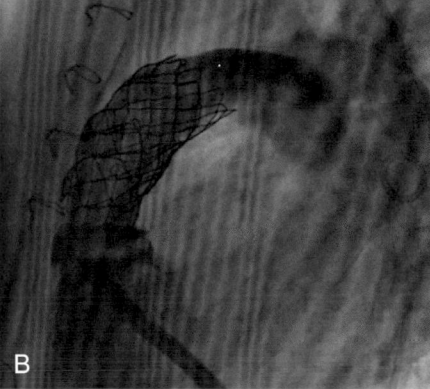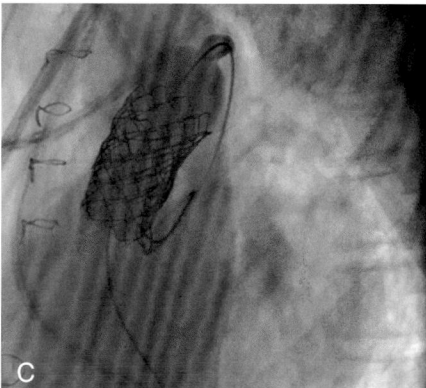

Fig. 56.10 Two-staged procedure with prestenting before transcatheter pulmonary valve implantation. A two-stage procedure with prestenting of a mixed dysfunctional xenograft (A) was performed to allow ingrowth of the right ventricular outflow tract (RVOT) stents (B) before percutaneous pulmonary valve implantation with a Melody valve was performed 3 months later (C). The temporally free RVOT regurgitation after prestenting was accepted.

TABLE 56.4 Hemodynamic Outcome Immediately After Percutaneous Pulmonary Valve Implantation

Parameter[a]	U.S. Melody Valve Trial (n = 124)		London Melody Experience (n = 151)		Munich/Berlin Melody Experience (n = 102)		Philadelphia Melody Experience (n = 104)		Early Sapien Experience (n = 7)		Intermediate Sapien Experience (n = 36)		Latest Sapien Experience (n = 25)	
	Before	After	Before	After	Before	After	Before	After	Before	After	Before	After	Before	After
RV systolic pressure (mm Hg)	65	41[b]	63	45[c]	NA	NA	72	47[c]	NA	NA	55	42[c]	61	39[c]
Peak RV to PA gradient (mm Hg)	37	12[b]	37	17[c]	37	14	39	11[c]	NA	NA	27	12[c]	39	9[c]
RV to systemic pressure (%)	0.74	0.42[b]	0.69	0.45[c]	0.62[c]	0.36[c]	NA	NA	0.78	0.39[c]	0.60	0.40[c]	0.64	0.36[c]

[a]Invasively measured pressures and gradients were reported before and after percutaneous pulmonary valve implantation in the largest trials (n > 100) of the Melody[5,37,40,42] and Sapien implants[53-54,62] in the pulmonary artery (PA) position. In all studies, a profound improvement in right ventricular (RV) to systemic pressure ratio in response to PPVI was seen (P = .001, P < .001). Some data were not available (NA). All parameters are expressed as medians. PPVI, Percutaneous pulmonary valve implantation.
[b]P = .001.
[c]P < .001.

Early phase 1 results from an international multicenter clinical trial of Sapien PPVI in 36 patients demonstrated successful valve deployment in 97%, but 7 patients (20.5%) experienced adverse events.[54] The major complication was device dislodgment. Homograft rupture occurred in none of the patients. All of the Sapien patients underwent prestenting (33.3%) or periprocedural stenting procedures (66.6%). Recently, Haas et al. confirmed these data with a multicenter, observational registry trial.[49]

Intervention-related coronary compression is a well-described complication in the setting of bare-metal stenting of the RVOT.[34] Approximately 3.5% to 6% of patients who are candidates for PPVI have coronary artery anatomy that increases the risk of coronary obstruction.[45,47] Several reports have described this potentially catastrophic complication,[66,67] which is strongly associated with early procedural death.[42]

Although coronary compression is avoidable in most patients, it remains a complex issue, and ruling out the risk for this complication is one of the most difficult steps in preprocedural planning for PPVI. Using a stepwise approach can minimize the risk. In case of doubt about the risk of coronary compression, we recommend abandoning the Melody or Sapien valve procedure. In experienced hands, careful technique and attention to the recommended instructions for use help to avoid fatal complications.

Follow-Up and Outcomes

Clinical Consequences

The success of PPVI depends on device function during follow-up. Short- and medium-term results of PPVI with the Melody or Sapien valve are thought to be similar, although more data are available for the former. Long-term outcome data for both valved stents are not yet available.

The overall mortality rate for PPVI during follow-up procedures was 0% to 5% and was not related to the device itself. Failure of the Melody or Sapien device may be related to malfunction of the stent or sewn valve. Although failure of the valve leading to pulmonary regurgitation occurs rarely and only in the context of endocarditis,[68-71] the most common reason for reoperation and reintervention is repeat stenosis of the stent portion of the device. Restenosis of the stent can be caused by late recoil or loss of radial strength of the device due to stent fractures.

We have demonstrated rates of freedom from reoperation of 93% ± 2%, 86% ± 3%, 84% ± 4%, and 70% ± 13% and rates of freedom from transcatheter reintervention (second PPVI or balloon dilation) of 95% ± 2%, 87% ± 3%, 73% ± 6%, and 73% ± 6% at 10, 30, 50, and 70 months, respectively (median follow-up of 28 months).[72] Initially, the most common reason for reintervention was occurrence of the hammock effect, in which the venous wall of the bovine valve hangs into the stented valve's lumen.[73] This effect occurred with the first design of devices that had only proximal and distal sutures. After device modification with sutures placed at all struts of the stent, no further cases of the hammock effect have been seen.

Stent fractures currently represent the most common reason for reintervention after Melody implantation. Without prestenting the RVOT, stent fractures occur in 20% to 21%[5,40] of valve placements, compared with 5% to 16% of cases after prestenting.[42,46] Nordmeyer and colleagues reported a stent fracture rate of 11%.[65]

In the U.S. Melody trial,[5] the rate of survival free from RVOT reintervention was 95.4% ± 2.1% at 1 year and 87.6% ± 4.5% at 2 years. The rate of freedom from a second PPVI was 96.9% ± 2.0% at 1 year and 90.4% ± 4.4% at 2 years. The rate of freedom from pulmonary valve dysfunction was 93.5% ± 2.4% at 1 year and 85.6% ± 4.7% at 2 years. By multivariable Cox regression analysis, a higher mean RVOT gradient on discharge echocardiography and younger age were associated with shorter freedom from transcatheter pulmonary valve dysfunction. The association between high RVOT gradients on echocardiography after PPVI and increased risk for reintervention draws a parallel to the London findings that a residual RVOT gradient of more than 25 mm Hg (invasively measured) results in higher rates of reintervention during follow-up.[40] It is thought that aggressive postprocedure dilation should be performed, especially in very stenotic conduits, to improve the long-term outcomes for these patients.

Data are available from the major four short- and medium-term observational studies with a total of more than 450 patients with 1 to 5 years of follow-up.[5,40,42,46,74] The rate of freedom from valve dysfunction or reintervention was approximately 94% at the 1-year follow-up assessment. The patients who did not require reintervention had consistently mild or less pulmonic valve regurgitation at the 1-year follow-up. Pulmonary regurgitation decreased from median values of 16% to 27% to 1% to 2%. Median peak velocity over the RVOT was 1.9 to 2.7 m/s at three 1-year echocardiographic follow-up. Nordmeyer and coworkers reported preliminary but promising Melody Registry data with a rate of 92.5% for 1-year freedom for all case events and 94.2% for PPVI-related events.[65]

There are no comparison studies with conventional surgery regarding pulmonary valve replacement by Sapien valves. Data on function of the Sapien valve are limited and available from smaller short- and medium-term observational studies with a total of fewer than 100 patients with RV-PA conduits,[53,54] these conduits and native RVOT,[55] or native RVOT interventions only.[75] In the largest series of 36 patients (Congenital Multicenter Trial of Pulmonic Valve Regurgitation Studying the Sapien Interventional Transcatheter Heart Valve [COMPASSION]) involving only patients with RV-PA conduits, successful valve deployment was achieved in 33 of 34 attempts.[54] In cases of native RVOT dysfunction after transannular repair of tetralogy of Fallot, a successful valve implantation was achieved in nine of 10 eligible patients.[75] The COMPASSION trial reported an early complication rate of 7 of 34 deployed valves primarily due to device migration (three cases, with two requiring surgical retrieval). Other complications included pulmonary hemorrhage (two cases), ventricular fibrillation (one case), and stent migration (one case).

In the report by Boone and colleagues of seven patients with a median follow-up of 10 months (range, 30 days to 3.5 years), no stent fractures were described.[53] In this series, recatheterization was necessary in one patient 9 months after the initial implantation due to restenosis of the bare-metal stent. The rate of freedom from reintervention at 6 months of follow-up was 97% in the COMPASSION trial, and one patient underwent elective placement of a second valve due to conduit-induced distortion of the initial implant. Haas and colleagues demonstrated a significant reduction of the RVOT-to-PA gradient, reduction in RV systolic pressure, and an increase in diastolic pulmonary pressure from 6.3 to 14.5 mm Hg, which was a sign of tremendously decreased pulmonary regurgitation with freedom from reintervention after 6 months.[55]

The same group analyzed current data of a multicenter, observational registry including 46 patients with Sapien PPVI.[49] Successful valve deployment was achieved in 43 of 46 attempts. They account for rates of periprocedural complication of 6.5% (device malefaction in one and device dislodgement in two other patients) and adverse events in 10.9% (bleeding in one and arrhythmias in four other patients). No stent fractures were observed again in a follow-up time of up to 2 years.[49]

However, studies including more patients with longer follow-up times are required to assess performance of the Sapien device in the pulmonary position.

Nature and Management of Stent Fractures

Stent fractures may lead to stent embolization and especially to restenosis.[40] Observational data suggest that prestenting reduces the risk of stent fracture.[59,76] Prestenting the conduit with a bare-metal stent before PPVI is therefore standard practice in most centers. Stent fractures most commonly affect one or more struts, do not impact stent integrity (type I), and have no significant hemodynamic effect.[61] In cases of radiologic evidence of multiple strut fractures and increased RVOT velocity (measured by echocardiography), the fractures do impact stent integrity and can lead to restenosis (type II).

Implantation of a second device within the index device (i.e., valve-in-valve procedure) is indicated and can be performed successfully.[77,78] This strategy relieves RVOT obstruction effectively, enhances stent integrity, and minimizes the risk of stent embolization. Technically, the second PPVI procedure corresponds to the initial implantation. The first valved stent provides a perfect landmark for positioning the second device, facilitating the valve-in-valve procedure.

There has been only one reported case of device embolization into the PA. Stent disintegration resulted from stent fractures (type III).[61] This complication is avoidable as long as stent fractures are diagnosed quickly and a valve-in-valve procedure is performed. Stent fractures are significantly associated with dynamic RVOTs, as seen in noncalcified RVOT or noncircumferential homografts.[79] This information is useful for patient counseling and confirms the prestenting strategy to support the landing zone before PPVI. To detect stent fractures and plan reinterventions, patients must be closely followed after PPVI with repeated chest radiography and echocardiography.

Valved Stent Endocarditis

IE after PPVI has been observed in approximately 1% to 5% of patients during 1- to 5-year follow-up.[42,68–71,76,80–82] The Melody Registry preliminary data reveal a 1-year post-PPVI rate of 2.7%.[65] At first glance, the rate of endocarditis after PPVI seems to be similar to the observed rate of endocarditis after surgical RVOT reconstruction, which ranges from approximately 0% to 5% of patients during 1- to 4-year follow-up. Uebing et al. reviewed available data in a meta-analysis with an overall IE incidence of 4.3% per patient year after Melody PPVI.[83] However, Villafañe and coworkers found the risk of endocarditis is underestimated.[71] Trials directly comparing the incidence of endocarditis with the two techniques were lacking until van Dijck et al. were the first to report on different incidence of IE after PPVI or surgical graft implantation for RVOT dysfunction.[81] The group presented data suggesting similar incidence rates of IE following Melody valve and Contegra implantation, both being significantly higher compared with homograft implantation for RVOT dysfunction. Other groups supported these concerns.[84,85] In theory, higher flow velocities across the Melody valve or Contegra conduit compared with laminar flow patterns in homografts may contribute to different IE rates and may well be as important as differences in valve structure or tissue characteristics.[83] This is attributed to the fact that jet lesions are known to cause endothelial damage that is suspected to play a major role in the pathogenesis of IE.[71] Factors predisposing to endocarditis reported in the literature include prior episodes of endocarditis,[40,68,69] male gender,[68] multiple stents,[68] dental treatment,[40,68] previous fungal infection,[40] and septic wounds.[40,68] Relevant residual or progressing RV-PA gradients (e.g., due to stent fracture) were related to an increased risk of endocarditis as turbulence flow patterns across the valve can predispose to endothelial damage and thrombus formation with subsequent infection.[69,71,83] Villafañe and colleagues recommend early surgical treatment in the setting of restenosis or regurgitation and in patients with no clinical improvement in response to medical treatment.[71] McElhinney and coworkers suggest that Melody valve replacement is not required during the acute treatment as long as there is no involvement of the valve system.[69]

It is notable that IE was not detected during the early postprocedural period in any of the mentioned studies.[81] The earliest case has been reported by our group at 1.9 months post implantation.[86] We reported on a case of blood-culture proven *Staphylococcus aureus* endocarditis after Edwards Sapien valve implantation, indicating that all patients with prosthetic valves, including those who have undergone either Melody or Sapien PPVI, are considered among those at highest risk for endocarditis, and therefore prophylaxis against bacterial endocarditis is strongly recommended for risk procedures.[81,83,87,88]

According to our clinical experience, stented valve endocarditis could be treated by ESC or AHA guidelines adopted long-term antibiotic therapy in a reasonable number of cases.[47] Although blood cultures are negative in a number of patients because of previous antibiotic treatment and combined transthoracic and transesophageal echocardiography is positive in three of four patients, modified Duke criteria should be used for diagnosis of stented valve endocarditis.[39] Additional techniques such as intracardiac ultrasound and nuclear medical scanning 18F-marked fluorodeoxyglucose or technetium-99-labled leukocyte positron-emission tomography/computer tomography (18F-FDG/99m-Tc PET/CT) could help in decision making in unclear cases.[39,70]

Continued analysis of data from recent trials may shed more light on the heatedly debated issue of IE following PPVI.[89]

Functional Outcome

Several studies have shown a significant improvement in the New York Heart Association (NYHA) functional class after PPVI.[5,37,40,46,49] Improvement has largely been maintained for the duration of follow-up, irrespective of the type of lesion (i.e., predominantly stenosis or predominantly regurgitation).[45]

Gillespie and McElhinney observed that even patients who were in NYHA class I before intervention frequently report better performance of daily routines and improved exercise tolerance after intervention.[45] The 7-year follow-up post Melody trial found an improvement of NYHA functional class that changed significantly from before implantation to 1 year ($P < .001$) after, but there was no difference from 1 year to subsequent follow-up time points up to 7 years.[47] Hager et al. were the first to report on improvement of quality of life 6 months after PPVI, which remained in a 5-year follow-up.[74]

Due to a variety of factors, exercise cardiopulmonary function is frequently abnormal in patients with complex congenital heart disease and is often assessed to guide decision making about interventions in patients with RVOT dysfunction. Peak oxygen consumption related to body weight ($\dot{V}O_2$/kg) and other metabolic parameters such as ventilatory efficiency and anaerobic oxygen consumption have been evaluated in studies of patients undergoing pulmonary valve replacement.[41,90–92] Exercise testing data show that patients with a predominantly stenotic lesion had a different response to PPVI compared with patients with a predominantly regurgitant lesion. Only patients with a predominantly stenotic lesion showed an improvement in peak $\dot{V}O_2$/kg.

It is assumed that significant RVOT obstruction limits augmentation of cardiac output, which is elicited by exercise, reducing exercise capacity. Our group demonstrated that reduction of the RVOT gradient was the only independent predictor of improved exercise capacity early after PPVI.[41] Pulmonary regurgitation may be reduced to a minimum (as a percentage and an absolute value) at peak exercise and may not be the limiting factor for cardiac output augmentation during exercise. This may reflect the shortening of diastole and reduced pulmonary vascular resistance during exercise.[41] By relieving only pulmonary regurgitation without improving the RV ejection fraction, peak $\dot{V}O_2$/kg may not be affected much in this subgroup, explaining differences in exercise capacity for the two groups. Recently, we reported on the ability to recover from exercise as described by VO_2 and VCO_2 decay after maximal exercise. Recovery from exercise after PPVI improves in both groups (predominant stenosis vs. predominant regurgitation). These findings could explain the symptomatic improvement observed in patients with predominant regurgitation despite the lack of increased maximal exercise capacity and might have implications for how we measure procedural success.[93] Cheatham et al. found that the maximum workload achieved increased from a median of

105 W (15 to 338 W) before PPVI to 121 W (27 to 271 W) at the 1-year evaluation ($P = .01$). The improvements remained stable at 2 and 3 years of follow-up.[47] Despite the fact that there were no significant changes in the percentage of predicted peak oxygen consumption (percent VO_2max) in the overall population, the ratio of minute ventilation to carbon dioxide production at the anaerobic threshold (Ve/VCO_2) improved early after PPVI and remained stable in accordance to the data by Batra.[94]

Functional and morphologic MRI with analysis of biventricular function and calculation of great vessel blood flow is performed before and within 1 month after PPVI. The data are mixed regarding changes in the RV ejection fraction after pulmonary valve replacement. Some studies found no change,[5,42] and others reported improvements in the acute period or short term.[44,90,91] We found an improvement in the effective RV stroke volume in patients with predominantly PS (40.6 ± 11.0 vs. 46.8 ± 8.0 mL/m^2, $P < .001$) and with a predominantly regurgitant lesion (37.1 ± 6.2 vs. 44.7 ± 7.5 mL/m^2, $P < .001$).[41] In the stenotic subgroup, improvement resulted from a decreased RV end-systolic volume and enhanced RV ejection fraction after relief of the pressure overload. In contrast, the RV ejection fraction remains unchanged in the regurgitant subgroup, with improvement in the RV and LV effective stroke volume due to abolishment of pulmonary regurgitation (reduction in pulmonary regurgitation fraction as assessed by MRI: 39.0% ± 8.6% vs. 3.0% ± 4.7%, $P < .001$). As in the surgical series of pulmonary valve replacement, relief of the RV volume overload resulted in a reduction in RV end-diastolic volume and the total RV stroke volume in patients with predominantly pulmonary regurgitation.[24,26]

Remarkably, there is no further reduction of RV size or improvement of RV function on MRI and exercise capacity parameters 1 year after PPVI compared with the early functional outcome.[92] The impact on RV diastolic function under conditions of RV dysfunction has not been addressed. Our group has begun examining tissue Doppler and speckle tracking echocardiography, as well as MRI-derived T1 mapping data and dynamic intracardiac pressure-volume analysis prior to treatment of RVOT dysfunction. The ideal timing of a surgical or percutaneous RVOT intervention remains unknown because long-term data are lacking. However, functional results suggest treating patients with pulmonary regurgitation before the onset of RV dysfunction or impaired exercise capacity. Some authors propose to perform earlier stenting of the RVOT under conditions of regurgitation. Performing presenting procedures in a "window of opportunity" after RVOT reconstruction or replacement by conduits with significant regurgitation, but undilated RVOT might arrest the increase of RVOT dimension. This approach could fix the RVOT to dimension capable for subsequent PPVI.[30] Debates on this approach are ongoing. Long-term data are needed.

Because of the right-to-left ventricular interaction, an important physiologic consequence of RV enlargement and dysfunction is secondary left ventricular dysfunction in some patients, which can influence exercise capacity. The impact of PPVI on left ventricular systolic and diastolic function is not trivial. Improved systolic function due to PPVI as estimated by the ejection fraction on myocardial velocity imaging has been reported in several studies.[41,90] Improvement in left ventricular diastolic function has also been reported.[31,72,91]

A meta-analysis that included data from three multicenter studies and 300 patients described the impact of Melody PPVI on TR. Concomitant and significant TR without a primary disease of the valve itself is often seen in patients with RVOT dysfunction due to pressure and/or volume overload (functional TR). It improves in 65% to 83% of cases after PPVI and remains stable over 5 years of follow-up.[95,96] This could extend surgical indications to patients with concomitant TR and dysfunctional RVOT suitable for PPVI.[95] Intended repair of TR should be postponed after PPVI.[96]

Extended Indications, New Valve Designs, and Future Directions

Approximately 15% of patients with dysfunction of the RVOT are eligible for the approved implantable valves.[48,97] Many patients are poor candidates because of their small physical size, limited vascular access, or the size and shape of the RVOT. It is not surprising that PPVI has moved beyond the original indications for off-label use in conditions with less than ideal hemodynamic and anatomic circumstances.

Case series report of effective and safe PPVI in patients with pulmonary hypertension[31] or failed bioprosthetic valves.[37] Most patients with RVOT dysfunction had patch enlargement of the RVOT as part of the initial surgical repair strategy. This clinical challenge prompted novel and sometimes creative approaches to treat RVOT failure using existing interventional pulmonic valve technology. Reports have described PPVI in native, stent-augmented RVOTs, which provided a landing zone that was nondistensible or could not distend beyond 22 mm for the Melody or 26 mm for the Sapien device.[43,61]

A small case series by Cheatham and coworkers described implantation or postimplantation dilation for the Melody valve using a 24-mm balloon.[98] This approach appeared not to compromise valve function, and it may effectively expand the pool of eligible patients.[98]

Patients with RVOT dysfunction with a predominantly regurgitant lesion and an enlarged outflow tract may not be eligible for PPVI. Several treatment strategies, including Melody valve implantation into the branch PAs[99,100] or anchoring by a bare-metal stent implanted across the main PA into a pulmonary branch ("jailing"), have been described as potential options.[101] A hybrid approach combining intraoperative PPVI with simultaneous conduit[102] or native RVOT downsizing[103] or direct exposure of the RV or RVOT (i.e., bailout procedure after a failed percutaneous attempt) showed feasibility.[104]

Innovative, experimental technologies include infundibular reducer devices,[105] nitinol self-expanding covered stents for RVOT downsizing (Edwards Altera device)[103] and alternative percutaneous valves such as the low-profile Colibri heart valve (Broomfield, CO),[73] and the Venus P Valve (Venus Medtech, Shanghai, China) (Fig. 56.11).[106–108] In 2010, Schievano et al. reported on feasibility of implantation of a novel self-expanding Medtronic Native Outflow Tract device (Medtronic Inc.).[109] Further adaptations, focusing on patients' RVOTs, led to the design of Medtronic's new valve for PPVI, the Harmony Transcatheter Pulmonary Valve (Medtronic Inc.) (see Fig. 56.11).[110] The new valve consists of a self-expanding frame of nitinol struts (nickel-titanium alloy). Porcine pericardial tissue valve is sewn into the center portion of the polyester-covered asymmetric, "hourglass" frame shape (diameters: proximal 42 mm, valve housing 22 mm, distal 34 mm).[110] The shape should facilitate valve's stabilization even in an oversized, dilated, and distorted RVOT.[39,110,111] The expanded valve reaches 55 mm in length with an outer diameter of 23.5 mm at the valved section. For implantation, a 25-Fr coil loading catheter delivery system is used. It comes with an integrated sheath and loading funnel that collapses the valve to facilitate mounting on the delivery system. During deployment, the retractable sheath helps to control self-expansion.[111,112] Currently, the Harmony valve is available for investigational use only. Recently, the first clinical study results became available.[111,112] The nonrandomized, prospective study enrolled 66 subjects in three sites in the United States and Canada of whom 20 received Harmony PPVI. The authors deemed high procedural success, safety, favorable acute device performance, and promising early clinical outcomes with preserved valvular function at a 6-month follow-up.[112] In January 2017, the prospective multicenter trial *"Medtronic Harmony Transcatheter Pulmonary Valve Clinical Study"* (NCT02979587) started enrolling.

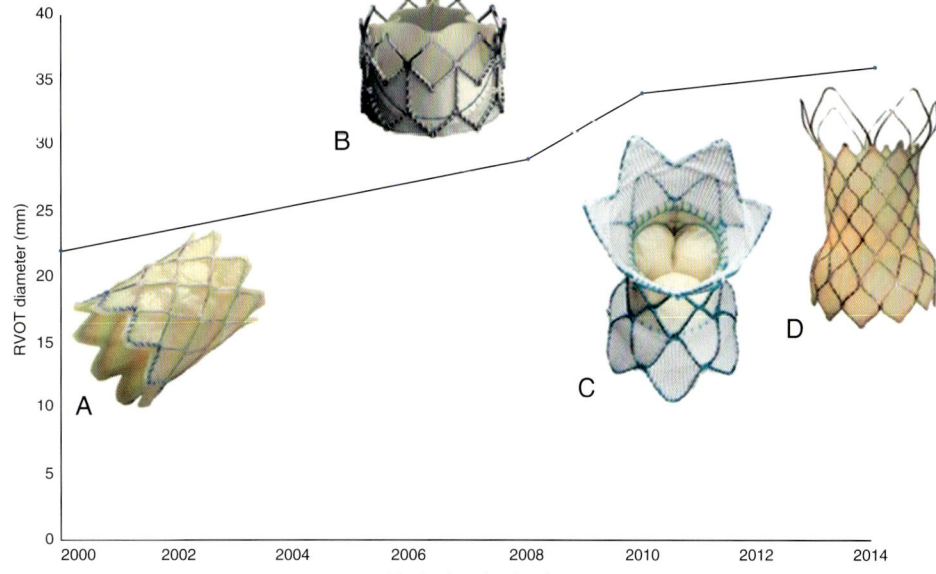

Fig. 56.11 Evolution of percutaneous pulmonary valve implantation. (A) Melody valve (Medtronic), balloon-expandable, max. diameter 22 mm. (B) SAPIEN XT valve (EdwardsLifesciences), balloon-expandable, max. diameter 29 mm. (C) Harmony valve (Medtronic), self-expanding, inflow diameter 34 mm, outflow diameter 42 mm. (D) Venus P-valve (Venus Medtech), self-expanding, max. diameter 36 mm. *RVOT,* right ventricular outflow tract.

New technical developments will offer nonsurgical treatment alternatives to a much broader patient population.[39,73,97]

KEY REFERENCES

5. McElhinney DB, Hellenbrand WE, Zahn EM, et al. Short- and medium-term outcomes after transcatheter pulmonary valve placement in the expanded multicenter US melody valve trial. *Circulation.* 2010;122(5):507–516. https://doi.org/10.1161/CIRCULATIONAHA.109.921692.

6. Bonhoeffer P, Boudjemline Y, Saliba Z, et al. Percutaneous replacement of pulmonary valve in a right-ventricle to pulmonary-artery prosthetic conduit with valve dysfunction. *Lancet.* 2000;356(9239):1403–1405. https://doi.org/10.1016/S0140-6736(00)02844-0.

29. Alvarez-Fuente M, Garrido-Lestache E, Fernandez-Pineda L, et al. Timing of pulmonary valve replacement: how much can the right ventricle dilate before it looses its remodeling potential? *Pediatr Cardiol.* 2016;37(3):601–605.

31. Lurz P, Bonhoeffer P, Taylor AM. Percutaneous pulmonary valve implantation: an update. *Expert Rev Cardiovasc Ther.* 2009;7(7):823–833. https://doi.org/10.1586/erc.09.57.

38. Petit CJ. Pediatric transcatheter valve replacement: guests at our own table? *Circulation.* 2015;131(22):1943–1945. https://doi.org/10.1161/CIRCULATIONAHA.115.016709.

40. Lurz P, Coats L, Khambadkone S, et al. Percutaneous pulmonary valve implantation: impact of evolving technology and learning curve on clinical outcome. *Circulation.* 2008;117(15):1964–1972. https://doi.org/10.1161/CIRCULATIONAHA.107.735779.

45. Gillespie MJ, McElhinney DB. Transcatheter pulmonary valve replacement: a current review. *Current Pediatrics Reports.* 2013;1(2):83–91. https://doi.org/10.1007/s40124-013-0013-9.

47. Cheatham JP, Hellenbrand WE, Zahn EM, et al. Clinical and hemodynamic outcomes up to 7 years after transcatheter pulmonary valve replacement in the US melody valve investigational device exemption trial. *Circulation.* 2015;131(22):1960–1970. https://doi.org/10.1161/CIRCULATIONAHA.114.013588.

49. Haas NA, Carere RG, Kretschmar O, et al. Early outcomes of percutaneous pulmonary valve implantation using the Edwards SAPIEN XT transcatheter heart valve system. *Int J Cardiol.* 2018;250:86–91. https://doi.org/10.1016/j.ijcard.2017.10.015.

50. Kenny D, Hijazi ZM, Kar S, et al. Percutaneous implantation of the Edwards SAPIEN transcatheter heart valve for conduit failure in the pulmonary position: early phase 1 results from an international multicenter clinical trial. *J Am Coll Cardiol.* 2011;58(21):2248–2256. https://doi.org/10.1016/j.jacc.2011.07.040.

54. Sabate Rotes A, Bonnichsen CR, Reece CL, et al. Long-term follow-up in repaired tetralogy of fallot: can deformation imaging help identify optimal timing of pulmonary valve replacement? *J Am Soc Echocardiogr.* 2014;27(12):1305–1310. https://doi.org/10.1016/j.echo.2014.09.012.

61. Cardoso R, Ansari M, Garcia D, et al. Prestenting for prevention of melody valve stent fractures: a systematic review and meta-analysis. *Catheter Cardiovasc Interv.* 2016;87(3):534–539. https://doi.org/10.1002/ccd.26235.

63. Wilson WM, Benson LN, Osten MD, et al. Transcatheter pulmonary valve replacement with the Edwards Sapien system: the toronto experience. *JACC Cardiovasc Interv.* 2015;8(14):1819–1827. https://doi.org/10.1016/j.jcin.2015.08.016.

64. Kim DW. Off-label, on-target: transcatheter pulmonary valve implantation with the SAPIEN valve. *JACC Cardiovasc Interv.* 2015;8(14):1828–1830. https://doi.org/10.1016/j.jcin.2015.09.011.

73. Kenny D, Hijazi ZM. The evolution of transcatheter pulmonary valve replacement. *Expert Rev Cardiovasc Ther.* 2013;11(7):795–797. https://doi.org/10.1586/14779072.2013.811970.

74. Hager A, Schubert S, Ewert P, et al. Five-year results from a prospective multicentre study of percutaneous pulmonary valve implantation demonstrate sustained removal of significant pulmonary regurgitation, improved right ventricular outflow tract obstruction and improved quality of life. *EuroIntervention.* 2017;12(14):1715–1723. https://doi.org/10.4244/EIJ-D-16-00443.

76. McElhinney DB, Cheatham JP, Jones TK, et al. Stent fracture, valve dysfunction, and right ventricular outflow tract reintervention after transcatheter pulmonary valve implantation: patient-related and procedural risk factors in the US Melody Valve Trial. *Circ Cardiovasc Interv.* 2011;4(6):602–614. https://doi.org/10.1161/CIRCINTERVENTIONS.111.965616.

83. Uebing A, Rigby ML. The problem of infective endocarditis after transcatheter pulmonary valve implantation. *Heart.* 2015;101(10):749–751. https://doi.org/10.1136/heartjnl-2014-307287.

92. Lurz P, Nordmeyer J, Giardini A, et al. Early versus late functional outcome after successful percutaneous pulmonary valve implantation: are the acute effects of altered right ventricular loading all we can expect? *J Am Coll Cardiol.* 2011;57(6):724–731. https://doi.org/10.1016/j.jacc.2010.07.056.

112. Bergersen L, Benson LN, Gillespie MJ, et al. Harmony feasibility trial: acute and short-term outcomes with a elf-expanding transcatheter pulmonary valve. *JACC Cardiovasc Interv.* 2017;10(17):1763–1773. https://doi.org/10.1016/j.jcin.2017.05.034.

Additional references available online at expertconsult.com.

中文导读

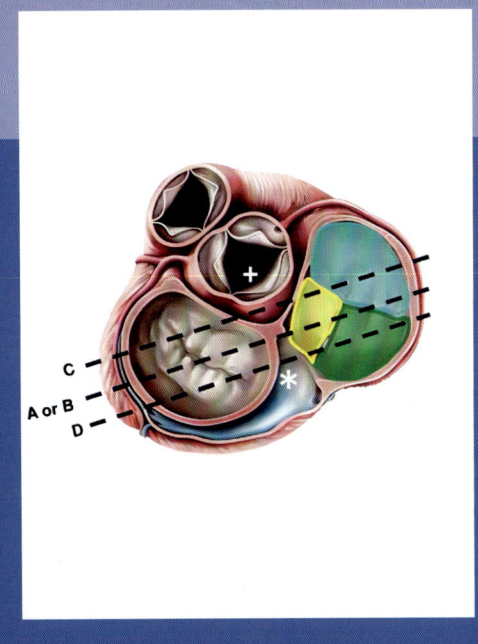

第57章
经皮三尖瓣修复

  三尖瓣最常发生的病变为功能性三尖瓣反流，多继发于左心系统疾病、肺动脉高压或心房颤动。由于三尖瓣结构复杂、变异性较大，缺乏标准的三尖瓣成像技术和三尖瓣反流分级标准，以及对三尖瓣病变的病理生理和自然病程缺乏认知，三尖瓣病变长期被忽视。因主动脉瓣或二尖瓣疾病进行外科手术的患者中需同期进行三尖瓣手术的比例高达60%，而且目前发现功能性三尖瓣反流是外科手术、经皮介入治疗和心力衰竭患者死亡的重要独立预测因子。本章节首先介绍了三尖瓣的解剖结构、三尖瓣关闭不全的病理生理机制和超声成像技术；然后介绍了目前经导管治疗三尖瓣关闭不全的方法、临床证据，以及操作方法，主要包括缘对缘修复技术、瓣膜重新对合装置、瓣环成形装置、植入腔静脉瓣膜等。对于三尖瓣生物瓣膜衰败或三尖瓣成形环失败的患者，可进行经导管瓣膜植入。

张洪亮　吴永健

章节要点

- 功能性三尖瓣重度反流的临床负担是巨大的，对于外科修复/置换风险高的患者仅可进行经导管治疗。
- 与二尖瓣相比，三尖瓣结构复杂、异质性大（瓣叶数量和瓣下结构）。
- 经皮三尖瓣缘对缘修复临床经验最多，大型随机对照临床研究正在进行。
- 很多模拟外科修复/置换的经导管技术正在早期研发和临床试验阶段。

57 Percutaneous Tricuspid Valve Repair

Gagan D. Singh, Jason H. Rogers

KEY POINTS

- The clinical burden of severe functional tricuspid regurgitation can be substantial, with limited transcatheter options for those at prohibitive risk for surgical repair/replacement.
- The tricuspid apparatus is complex and far more heterogeneous (with respect to number of leaflets and the associated subvalvular apparatus) than the mitral valve.
- Percutaneous tricuspid valve edge-to-edge repair carries the most clinical experience, with larger-scale randomized trials under way.
- Many additional transcatheter technologies that mimic surgical repair/replacement techniques are under varying stages of early development and clinical testing.

INTRODUCTION

In the contemporary era, there has been a relative explosion of interest in the design, development, and clinical dissemination of transcatheter technologies for aortic, mitral, and pulmonic valve disease. Many of these transcatheter techniques mimic established surgical approaches that have been performed for decades. The tricuspid valve (TV), often referred to as the "forgotten valve," has historically been understudied owing to its substantial anatomic variations and attributable disease processes and that most symptomatic tricuspid regurgitation (TR) is due to secondary or functional TV disease. Indeed, contemporary series report concomitant TV surgery in up to 60% patients undergoing surgery for primary left-sided aortic or mitral valve (MV) disease.[1] Hence significant TV disease is usually a surrogate for advanced-stage left-sided disease. When this is unaddressed during index surgical intervention for left-sided disease, patients experience increased morbidity and mortality.[2] With the burgeoning field of transcatheter technologies for aortic and MV disease, it is clear that those patients with concomitant and untreated TV regurgitation carry a less favorable long-term prognosis.[3,4] Therefore considerable interest has now shifted to the development of transcatheter technologies that allow for the treatment of TR to be performed in conjunction with or staged with transcatheter aortic or MV intervention. This chapter reviews the TV anatomic complex and the clinical relevance of surgical approaches; it also offers an update on transcatheter technologies in practice and in development for symptomatic TR.

THE TRICUSPID VALVE COMPLEX

The classic description of the TV complex says that it consists of three leaflets (anterior, posterior, and septal), the chordae tendineae, two discrete papillary muscles, the fibrous tricuspid annulus, and the right atrial (RA) and ventricular myocardium (Fig. 57.1). Successful valve function depends on the integrity and coordination of these components. However, considerable variability exists in the number of leaflets, papillary muscles, location of scallops or indentations, annular geometry, and the array of the chordae tendineae.[5–7] More recent anatomic reviews debate which is the largest TV leaflet—anterior versus posterior (Fig. 57.2).[5–7] The septal leaflet is the smallest and arises medially directly from the tricuspid annulus above the interventricular septum. The anterior papillary muscle provides chordae to the anterior and posterior leaflets, and the medial papillary muscle provides chordae to the posterior and septal leaflets. The septal wall gives chordae to the anterior and septal leaflets (there is no formal septal papillary muscle, as with the anterior and posterior papillary muscles). In addition, there may be accessory chordal attachments to the right ventricular (RV) free wall and the moderator band.

The overall length of the TV leaflets varies; however, the circumference of the anterior and posterior leaflets are of equal length. The anterior leaflet is the most mobile, whereas the septal leaflet is the least. The posterior leaflet is the shortest, with multiple scallops; anatomically it may not be clearly separated from the anterior leaflet in approximately 10% of the population. Additionally, anatomic landmarks of the leaflets vary considerably with one notable exception: the commissure between the septal and posterior leaflets is usually located near the entrance of the coronary sinus (CS) into the RA.

The tricuspid annulus has a complex three-dimensional structure, which differs from the more symmetric "saddle-shaped" mitral annulus. In an effort to better understand the shape and movement of the healthy and diseased tricuspid annulus, Fukuda et al.[8] performed a real-time three-dimensional transthoracic echocardiographic (TTE) study. They examined 15 healthy

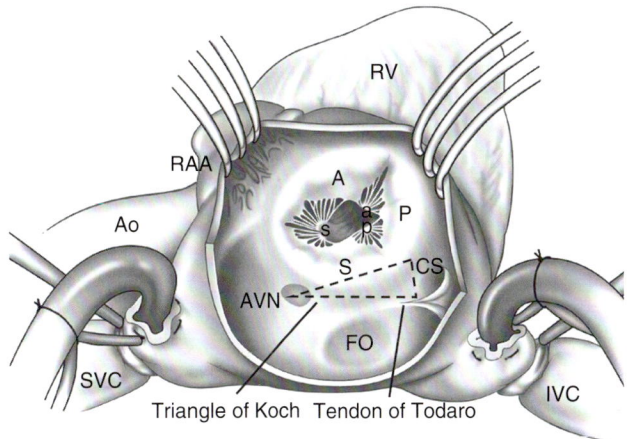

Fig. 57.1 Surgical perspective of the tricuspid valve complex. The tricuspid valve consists of three leaflets: anterior *(A)*, posterior *(P)*, and septal *(S)*. There are two main papillary muscles, anterior *(a)* and posterior *(p)*. The septal papillary muscle *(s)* is rudimentary, and chordae tendineae arise directly from the ventricular septum. Relevant adjacent structures include the atrioventricular node *(AVN)*, coronary sinus *(CS)* ostium, and tendon of Todaro, which form the triangle of Koch. *Ao,* Aorta; *FO,* foramen ovale; *IVC,* inferior vena cava; *SVC,* superior vena cava; *RAA,* right atrial appendage; *RV,* right ventricle. (Reproduced with permission from Rogers JH, Bolling SF. The tricuspid valve: current perspective and evolving management of tricuspid regurgitation. *Circulation.* 2009;119:2718–2725.)

subjects and 16 patients with functional TR (FTR); 75% had moderate to severe TR. The tricuspid annulus was mapped throughout the cardiac cycle and reconstructed on a computer workstation. Patients with FTR generally had a more planar annulus, which was dilated primarily in the anterior (along RV free wall) direction, resulting in a more circular shape as compared with the elliptical shape in healthy subjects.

Because the small septal wall leaflet is fairly fixed, there is little room for movement if the free wall of right ventricular/tricuspid annulus should dilate. Dilation of the tricuspid annulus therefore occurs primarily in its anterior aspect, which can result in significant FTR as a result of leaflet malcoaptation (Fig. 57.3). Other important factors influencing the degree of TR include right ventricular preload, afterload, and right ventricular systolic function. The influence of intravascular volume status and underlying right ventricular function on TV function stems from the fact that the tricuspid annulus is very dynamic and can change markedly with loading conditions. Even during the cardiac cycle, there is an approximately 19% reduction in annular circumference ($\approx$30% reduction in annular area) with atrial systole.[9]

The TV leaflets are generally supported by two papillary muscles (anterior and posterior), with 20% of the population having a third (septal). The anterior is the largest, with a complex array of chordae supporting the anterior and posterior leaflets. The posterior papillary muscle can subdivide into two to three segments giving off chordae to the posterior and septal leaflets. A moderator band, if present, usually connects to the anterior papillary muscle. Finally, chordae can arise directly from the interventricular septum to the anterior and septal leaflets or the RV free wall to the anterior and posterior leaflets.[6]

Other important anatomic structures involved with the TV complex, especially as it relates to potential transcatheter targets, are the superior and inferior venae cavae (SVC and IVC), atrioventricular node (AVN), right coronary artery (RCA), and CS. In humans, the origin of the SVC is located posterior to the RA appendage and adjacent to the interatrial septum. The origin of the IVC is formed anteriorly and superiorly by the eustachian valve (or its remnant). The tendon of Todaro serves as the posterior border of the triangle of Koch, with the anterior border being the CS. The triangle is completed more medially by the AVN (see Fig. 57.1).[10] Surgeons will use these anatomic landmarks to locate the AVN when they are performing either suture- or ring-based annuloplasty or TV replacement (discussed later); these landmarks may become important for transcatheter technologies that mimic these surgical approaches.

PATHOPHYSIOLOGY OF TRICUSPID INSUFFICIENCY

The prototypical patient with TR often has annular dilation and right ventricular enlargement, which is often due to left heart failure from myocardial or valvular causes, right

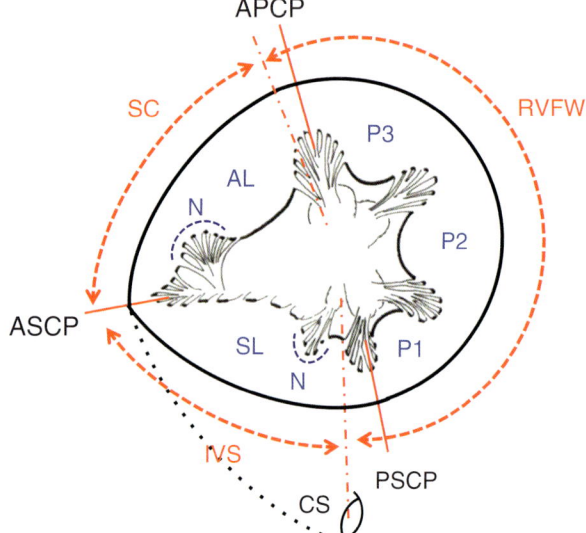

Fig. 57.2 Schematic diagram of the surgeon's view of the tricuspid valve. The posterior leaflet's annulus should be as long as the other two leaflet annuli. *AL,* Anterior leaflet; *APCP,* anteroposterior commissural point; *ASCP,* anteroseptal commissural point; *CS,* coronary sinus; *IVS,* interventricular septum; *N,* notch; *P1,* posterior leaflet 1; *P2,* posterior leaflet 2; *P3,* posterior leaflet 3; *PSCP,* posteroseptal commissural point; *RVFW,* right ventricular free wall; *SC,* supraventricular crest; *SL,* septal leaflet. (Reproduced with permission from Kawada N, Naganuma H, Muramatsu K, et al. Redefinition of tricuspid valve structures for successful ring annuloplasty. *J Thorac Cardiovasc Surg.* 2018;155:1511–1519,e1.)

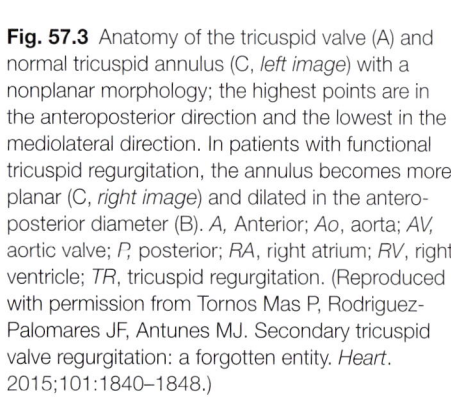

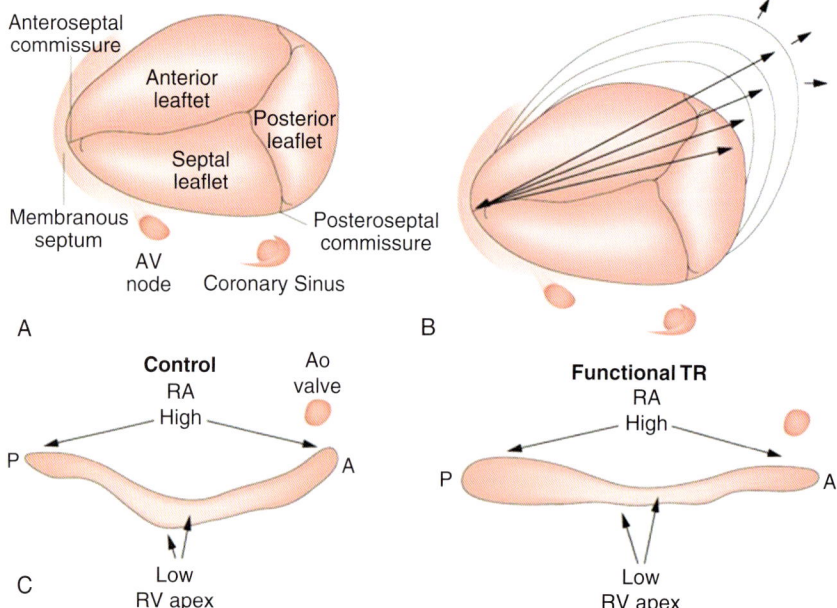

Fig. 57.3 Anatomy of the tricuspid valve (A) and normal tricuspid annulus (C, *left image*) with a nonplanar morphology; the highest points are in the anteroposterior direction and the lowest in the mediolateral direction. In patients with functional tricuspid regurgitation, the annulus becomes more planar (C, *right image*) and dilated in the anteroposterior diameter (B). *A,* Anterior; *Ao,* aorta; *AV,* aortic valve; *P,* posterior; *RA,* right atrium; *RV,* right ventricle; *TR,* tricuspid regurgitation. (Reproduced with permission from Tornos Mas P, Rodriguez-Palomares JF, Antunes MJ. Secondary tricuspid valve regurgitation: a forgotten entity. *Heart.* 2015;101:1840–1848.)

TABLE 57.1 Etiologies of Tricuspid Regurgitation

SECONDARY (75%)

Left heart disease (left ventricle dysfunction or valve disease) resulting in pulmonary hypertension

Any cause of pulmonary hypertension (chronic lung disease, pulmonary thromboembolism, left-to-right shunt)

Interatrial or interventricular shunt resulting in left-to-right shunting

Any cause of RV dysfunction (myocardial disease, RV ischemia/infarction, idiopathic)

Permanent atrial fibrillation

Isolated annular dilation (idiopathic tricuspid regurgitation)

PRIMARY (25%)

Rheumatic

Myxomatous—seen in up to 40% of patients with myxomatous mitral valve degeneration

Congenital (Ebstein anomaly, TV dysplasia, ventricular septal defect–related TV tethering)

Endocarditis (bacterial, marantic)

Endomyocardial fibrosis

Carcinoid

Traumatic (blunt chest injury, laceration)

Iatrogenic (pacemaker/defibrillator lead, RV biopsy)

Drug-induced disease (anorectic drugs, fenfluramine, phentermine, pergolide).

Ischemic heart disease affecting the RV with papillary muscle dysfunction or rupture.

RV, Right ventricular; *TV*, tricuspid valve.

TABLE 57.2 Emphasis of Echo Assessment of Right-Sided Valves.

Publication	Number of Pages Devoted to		
	MV + AV	TV + PV	Ratio
2003 — ASE Native Valve Regurgitation	11	5.5	2:1
2008 — ASE Native Valve Stenosis	15	4	4:1
2009 — ASE Prosthetic Valves	10.5	5.5	2:1
2014 — ACC/AHA Valve Disease	36	6	6:1
2017 — ASE Native Valve Regurgitation	27	15	2:1

ACC/AHA, American College of Cardiology/American Heart Association; *ASE*, American Society of Echocardiography; *AV*, aortic valve; *MV*, mitral valve; *PV*, pulmonic valve; *TV*, tricuspid valve.

ventricular volume and pressure overload, dilation of cardiac chambers, and at times permanent atrial fibrillation. This form of regurgitation is referred to as secondary or functional in etiology (functional TR, or FTR). With progressive dilation of the ventricle and annulus, there is failure of leaflet coaptation (loss of coaptation length) and an increase in tenting height. Less common causes of TV pathology include rheumatic or congenital heart disease, endocarditis, leaflet tear/prolapse, chordal rupture, papillary muscle rupture, or myxomatous degeneration of the TV (Table 57.1).

With isolated TR, patients may experience fatigue and decreased exercise tolerance as a result of decreased cardiac output. They may also experience the classic symptoms of "right-sided heart failure" from elevated RA pressures, such as ascites, congestive hepatopathy, peripheral edema, decreased appetite, and abdominal fullness. The assessment of intravascular volume status in a patient with severe TR can be difficult because of the pulsatile jugular venous pressure on physical examination. Atrial fibrillation is common as a result of RA enlargement.

IMAGING AND QUANTIFICATION OF TRICUSPID INSUFFICIENCY

The TV is arguably the most difficult valve to visualize and to assess quantitatively. Some of this difficulty is due to the variable anatomy of the TV complex. Until recently, there has been a deficit of clinical research focused on how to standardize qualitative and quantitative TV imaging. With renewed interest in the TV as a potential target for transcatheter techniques, there are now more guidelines and review articles attempting to standardize imaging of the TV (Table 57.2).[7,11] An in-depth review of the qualitative and quantitative TTE and transesophageal echocardiographic (TEE) assessment of TR are beyond the scope of this chapter. However, the following paragraphs offer a brief review the role of TTE and an overview of the TEE imaging planes needed to identify the specific TV leaflets required for transcatheter therapies.

For TTE, multiple thoracic windows with slight adjustments are needed to identify all three leaflets of the TV (Figs. 57.4–57.6). With this methodology, all three leaflets can be reproducibly seen on every patient. Adjunctive assessment of TV pathology requires careful assessment of IVC diameter and collapsibility, RV systolic pressure, and hepatic vein flow reversal.

Further interrogation with TEE is usually warranted, particularly for intraprocedural guidance. None of the guidelines have offered standardized TEE views to assess the TV leaflets. Our standard approach consists of obtaining dedicated sweeps along coaptation zones in the midesophageal, commissural, and transgastric views. The midesophageal view allows one to sweep the TV as the probe is advanced and retracted (Fig. 57.7). Starting in the esophagus, once the TV is encountered in the zero-degree omniplane, first the septal and anterior leaflets are usually identified; as the probe is pushed further in, the view changes to one that includes the septal and posterior leaflets (Video 57.1). Even in the midesophageal view, it can be difficult to ascertain which leaflets are being viewed. With a slight antero- and/or retroflex at the zero-degree omniplane in the midesophageal view, if the aortic valve comes in and out of view, the image will be of the anterior and septal leaflets. On the other hand, if one retroflexes and the CS comes in and out of view, the posterior and septal leaflets will be seen (Fig. 57.8).

After the midesophageal sweep, a commissural view of the TV is attempted. The goal of this view is to obtain a cross section of the TV and attempt to capture the anteroseptal and anteroposterior commissure. This is generally obtained in the midesophageal position with the omniplane at 50 to 60 degrees. This view will generally aim to provide the aortic valve and the septal, anterior, and posterior leaflets all in the same image. An x-plane is then obtained from this image; starting medially to laterally, one can see the anteroseptal coaptation, anterior septoposterior coaptation, and finally the anteroposterior coaptation (Video 57.2).

Finally, perhaps the best imaging plane from which to visualize all three TV commissures is the transgastric short axis. This view is generally achieved by advancing the TEE probe into the stomach with substantial anteroflexion. Once the TV is in view, slight adjustments in the omniplane at zero or 180 degrees will allow one to achieve this commissural view (Fig. 57.9). In the transgastric view, the omniplane can also be changed to 90 degrees and the long axis of the RV is visualized. Additional anteroflexion at this point will enable visualization of the posteroseptal coaptation

SECTION V Structural Interventions

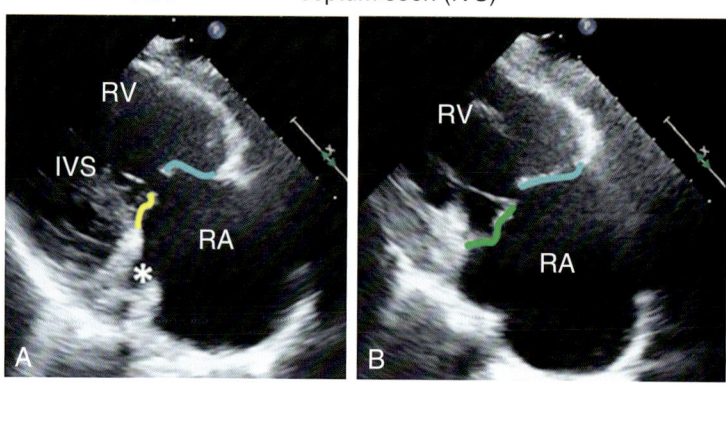

Fig. 57.4 Transesophageal echocardiographic parasternal inflow views. From the parasternal long-axis (*LAX*) view, the transducer is angled inferiorly and to the right (toward the right hip) to produce the parasternal inflow view. (A) If the coronary sinus ostium (*) or the muscular interventricular septum (*IVS*) is seen, the leaflets imaged are the anterior (*blue*) and septal (*yellow*) leaflets. (B) With the transducer angled more acutely inferiorly and to the right with no IVS seen, the anterior (*blue*) and posterior (*green*) leaflets are imaged (with no septal leaflet). *LV*, left ventricle; *RA*, right atrium; *RV*, right ventricle. (From Hahn RT. State-of-the-art review of echocardiographic imaging in the evaluation and treatment of functional tricuspid regurgitation. *Circ Cardiovasc Imaging.* 2016;9(12):e005332.)

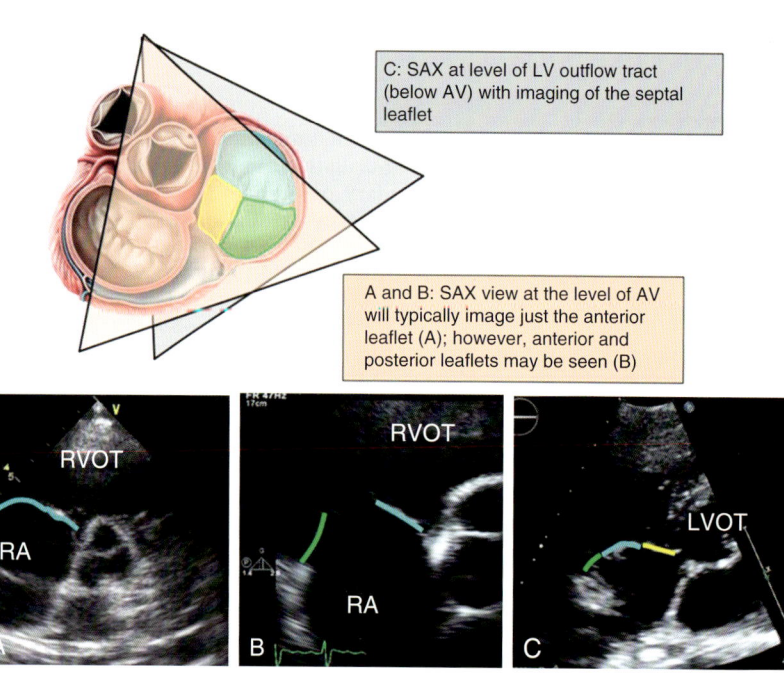

Fig. 57.5 Transesophageal echocardiographic parasternal short-axis (*SAX*) views. (A) From the SAX view at the level of the aortic valve (*AV*), a single anterior leaflet is typically imaged. This is in part because of the lower (apical) position of the septal leaflet. (B) As the lateral portion of the annulus dilates and loses its saddle shape, the anterior and posterior leaflets may be imaged. (C) As the transducer is angled toward the left ventricular outflow tract (*LVOT*), the septal leaflet may be seen. *LV*, Left ventricle; *RA*, right atrium; *RVOT*, right ventricular outflow tract. *Blue*, Anterior leaflet; *green*, posterior leaflet; *yellow*, septal leaflet. (From Hahn RT. State-of-the-art review of echocardiographic imaging in the evaluation and treatment of functional tricuspid regurgitation. *Circ Cardiovasc Imaging.* 2016;9(12):e005332.)

plane and retroflexion will provide the anteroposterior coaptation plane (Fig. 57.10).

The use of three-dimensional (3D) echocardiography has become critically important as an adjunct to structural heart interventions and no longer requires mental reconstruction of multiple two-dimensional images. We generally position/orient the 3D en face view of the TV in the same orientation as the "surgeons view." The aortic valve and the septal leaflets are positioned on the left, with the anterior leaflet at the 12- to 3-o'clock position, and the posterior leaflet positioned from the 3- to 6-o'clock position (see Fig. 57.7).

Future advances in echocardiographic imaging will make transcatheter TV interventions more accessible and feasible for standard clinical use. Numerous technologies are in development that will allow real-time high-resolution 3D images to be obtained from an intracardiac imaging probe that can be positioned in the RA, perhaps eliminating the need for TEE and general anesthesia.

CHAPTER 57 Percutaneous Tricuspid Valve Repair

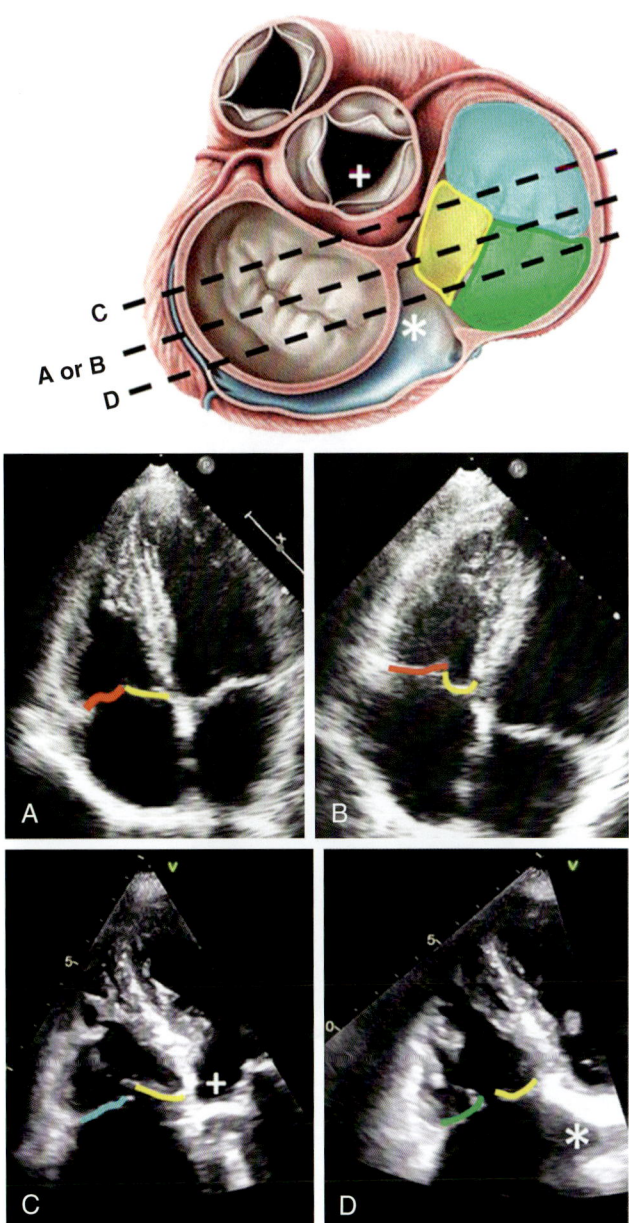

Fig. 57.6 Transesophageal echocardiographic apical four-chamber views. From the four-chamber views of the right ventricle (A and B), the septal leaflet can be clearly identified; however, the opposing leaflet can be the anterior or posterior leaflet *(red line)*. Angling the transducer anteriorly, so that a portion of the aorta (+) is imaged (C), will image the septal and anterior leaflets. Angling the transducer posteriorly, so that a portion of the coronary sinus (*) is imaged (D), will image the septal and posterior leaflets. *Blue,* Anterior leaflet; *green,* posterior leaflet; *yellow,* septal leaflet. (From Hahn RT. State-of-the-art review of echocardiographic imaging in the evaluation and treatment of functional tricuspid regurgitation. *Circ Cardiovasc Imaging.* 2016;9(12):e005332.)

TRANSCATHETER APPROACHES TO TRICUSPID REGURGITATION

There are a variety of technologies with varying mechanisms for reducing TR that are under preclinical and clinical evaluation. The main categories of transcatheter approaches for TV repair consist of (1) edge-to-edge repair techniques analogous to the MitraClip system (Abbott, Santa Clara, CA), (2) intravalvular coaptation devices, and (3) annuloplasty devices. In addition, caval valve implantation (CAVI) has been performed in an effort to reduce the effects of TR without necessarily impacting the TV complex itself. Finally, de novo transcatheter TV replacement has also recently been performed. Although there has been considerable interest in the development of these technologies, no one device or system has emerged as a leading approach owing to the complexity of the TV complex, its associated structures, and difficulty with durable TR reduction. Some of the global challenges for transcatheter-based devices include the following:

1. The tricuspid annulus is in close proximity to the RCA and damage or interaction with annuloplasty-based devices can occur.
2. The annular and leaflet tissue is more fragile and thinner than the MV, leading to potentially greater chances of dehiscence and tearing, particularly with annuloplasty-based devices.
3. Due to chordal density, tricuspid subvalvular maneuvering of catheter-based devices carries a greater risk of entanglement than it does for the subvalvular mitral apparatus.
4. Catheter navigation within the RA via fluoroscopy and TEE guidance is not straightforward, since the RA size, angle of the IVC to the tricuspid annulus, tricuspid annular shape, and number of tricuspid leaflets are all highly variable.
5. Standardized imaging of the TV and TR grading remains a challenge, although renewed interest in this topic[7] may resolve such issues in the future.
6. Imaging of the TV complex with intracardiac catheters present can be suboptimal due to substantial shadowing.

Despite the challenges, the interventional community continues work to define and refine the TV technologies, their role in the treatment of TR, and the clinical outcomes from their implementation. The following text outlines the major devices in the field of transcatheter TV technologies, their current state of development, and their stage of clinical application.

Transcatheter Edge-to-Edge Repair of the Tricuspid Valve

A dedicated first-generation steerable guide catheter (SGC) and a clip delivery system (CDS) for the TV has been developed (tricuspid valve repair system [TVRS]) and is in use for an early feasibility trial (Evaluation of Treatment With Abbott Transcatheter Clip Repair System in Patients With Moderate or Greater Tricuspid Regurgitation [TRILUMINATE] Clinical Trial, NCT03227757). However, more than 300 cases of edge-to-edge repair of the TV with the traditional MitraClip System have been performed.[12] The main differences between the TVRS and the commercial MitraClip systems are shorter working lengths of both the guide catheter and the CDS to allow ease of navigation within the RA. As widespread commercial availability for a dedicated TVRS is at least 3 to 5 years away, the remainder of this section describes only edge-to-edge repair of the TV using the standard MitraClip system.

Summary of Clinical Evidence

Both European and U.S. registries have confirmed that residual TR after transcatheter MV repair is associated with increased mortality.[13,14] Over the past 5 years several independent centers and one large multicenter registry have confirmed the safety and feasibility of TV edge-to-edge repair with the MitraClip system.[12] Procedural success was not consistently defined but the one common definition appears to be placement of a single clip with at least a one-grade reduction in TR. Based on this definition, procedural success is reportedly 91% to 97% without any major complications. Surprisingly, with clip placement and with as little as a single-grade reduction in TR, registry reports indicate improvement in New York Heart Association (NYHA) grade at discharge and an improved 6-minute walk test (6MWT)

1061

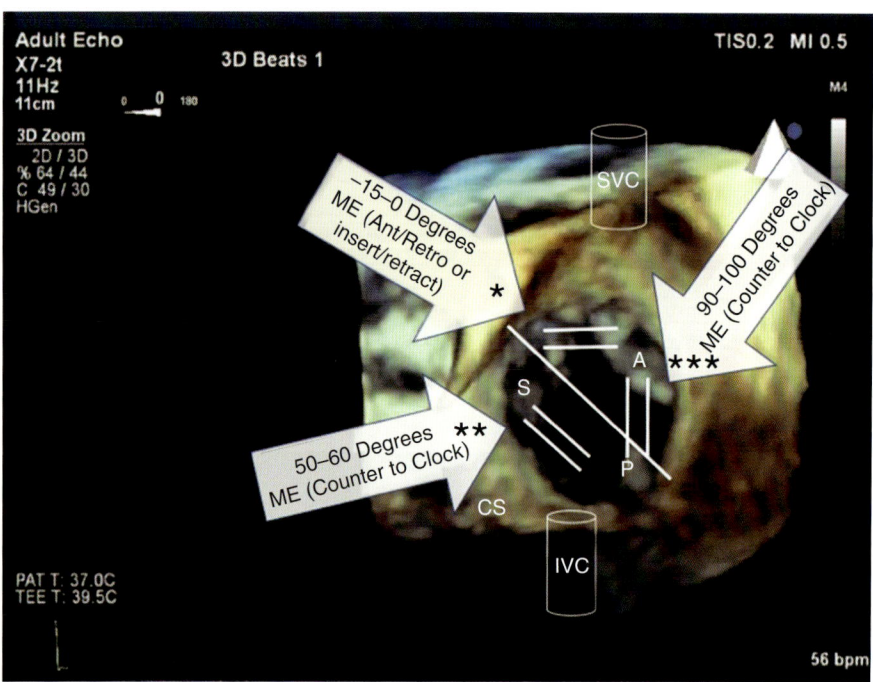

Fig. 57.7 Reconstructed three-dimensional transesophageal echocardiographic *(TEE)* en face view of the tricuspid valve demonstrates the two-dimensional TEE planes needed to see the individual commissural planes. Notice that to see the anteroseptal commissural plane *(A)*, the TEE omniplane is generally placed somewhere between –15 and 0 degrees with some mild anteroflexion or retroflexion; as the probe is inserted or retracted, the view will change from commissure to the central valve (*). If the omniplane is changed to approximately 50 to 60 degrees, this will enable visualization of the posteroseptal commissural plane *(S)* with slight counter- or clockwise rotation of the TEE probe as needed (**). Finally, with the omniplane at 90 to 100 degrees, the anteroposterior commissural plane *(P)* can be seen with counterclockwise adjustments as needed (***). *Ant,* Anteroflex; *CS,* coronary sinus; *IVC,* inferior vena cava; *ME,* midesophageal; *Retro,* retroflexed; *SVC,* superior vena cava.

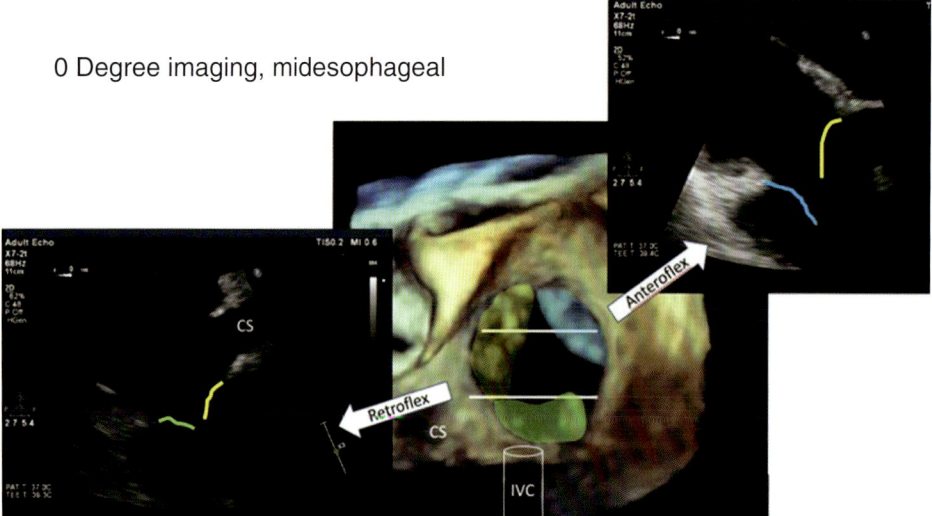

Fig. 57.8 *(Central panel)* Three-dimensionally reconstructed en face view of the tricuspid valve (TV). Left and right panels: Two-dimensional transesophageal echocardiographic (TEE) views of the TV leaflets. During screening TEE, it can be difficult to ascertain which of the TV leaflets is being imaged. One solution is to start neutral in the midesophageal view and advance until the TV leaflets are encountered. A slight anteroflexion or retraction will bring the aortic valve in and out of view, confirming that the TV leaflets being images are the septal *(yellow)* and anterior *(blue)* leaflets *(right panel)*. Conversely, the TEE probe can be retroflexed; as the CS comes in/out of view, this confirms that the septal *(yellow)* and posterior leaflets *(green)* are being imaged *(left panel)*. *CS,* Coronary sinus; *IVC,* inferior vena cava; *TEE,* transesophageal echocardiography; *TV,* tricuspid valve.

at 30 days.[12] These nonrandomized data are all that is available to the interventional community thus far with respect to edge-to-edge repair of the TV. The TRILUMINATE early feasibility study is a 25-center 75-patient global trial to evaluate the dedicated TVRS system (shorter working length of the SGC and CDS) for symptomatic moderate or severe TR. Enrollment for the early feasibility trial has completed with a pivotal (randomized) trial slated to begin in late 2019/early 2020. Additionally, there is a global registry of edge-to-edge repair of the TV with the off-label use of MtiraClip under way to describe procedural characteristics and outcomes of this approach.

Procedural Approach

There are two general approaches for using the commercial MitraClip system for TV repair. The first is the classic approach whereby the CDS is inserted into the SGC in a standard fashion. The alternate approach refers to the "miskey" technique where the CDS is rotated counterclockwise 90 degrees prior to being inserted into the SGC (Fig. 57.11). Most operators have now shifted to using the miskey technique, and this is what is described in several series and reviews[15,16]; however, it remains an area under active investigation.

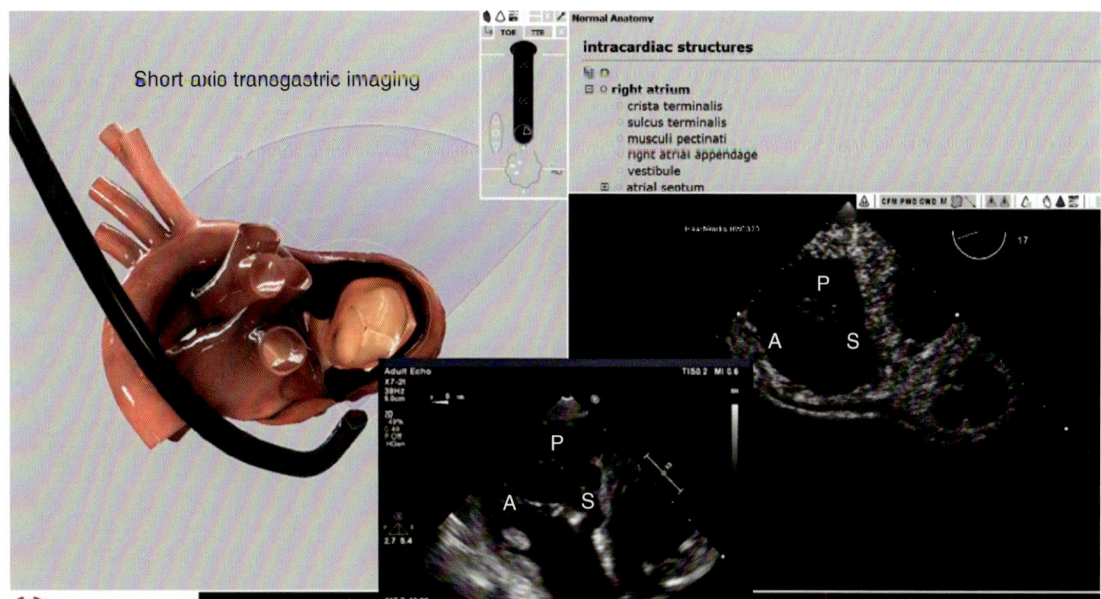

Fig. 57.9 Simulated images show positioning of the TEE probe and the imaging plane being acquired on the left panel. The simulated transgastric plane being acquired is shown on the right panel. An example from a recent patient is shown in the bottom inset, where all three commissures are identified. *A*, Anterior; *P*, posterior; *S*, septal.

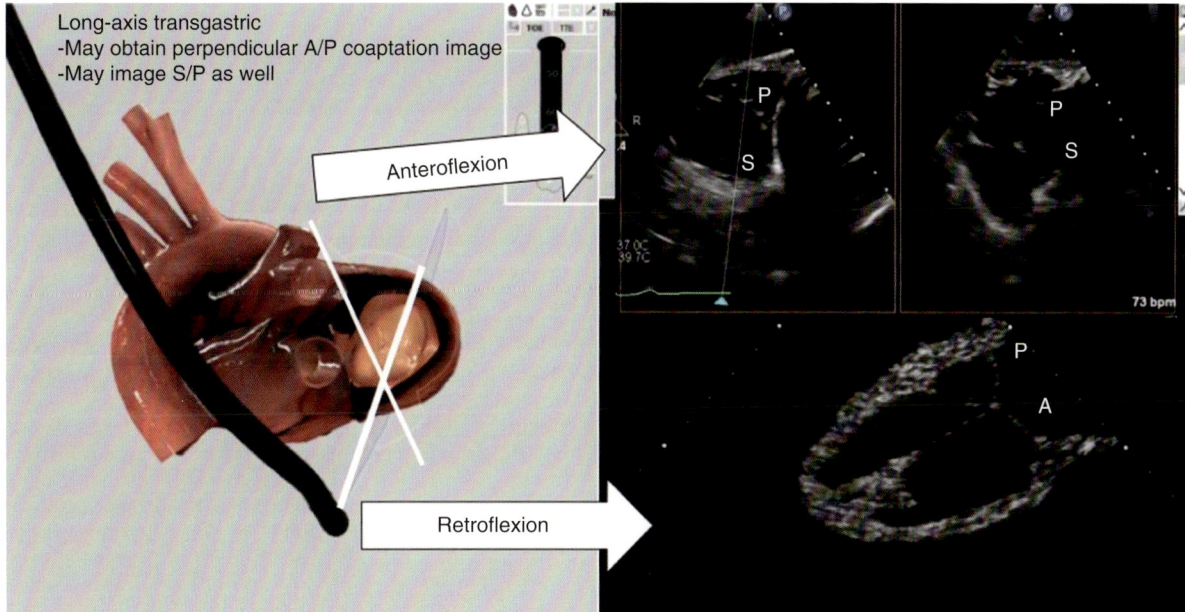

Fig. 57.10 Simulated transesophageal echocardiographic (TEE) positioning and images of the long-axis transgastric views are shown in the left panel. Generally once image acquisition has been achieved, a slight retroflextion will enable visualization of the anterior and posterior leaflets *(bottom right panel)*. Anteroflexion and slight retraction of the TEE probe at this point can enable visualization of the septal and anterior leaflets. *A*, Anterior; *P*, posterior; *S*, septal.

The steps for patient preparation, venous access, device nomenclature, and initial device maneuvering have been described previously.[17] For TV edge-to-edge repair, after venous access has been obtained, the SGC is inserted over a wire and into the RA. After the wire and dilator have been removed, the CDS is inserted into the SGC "miskeyed" 90 degrees counterclockwise (see Fig. 57.11). The entire SGC system is now rotated so that the plus/minus knob on the SGC is pointed down, facing the floor. The next step is to achieve straddle, which is generally done with slight retraction of the SGC and counterclockwise rotation to create more space, allowing the tip of the advancing CDS to move away from vital structures. These steps are performed under a combination of TEE and fluoroscopic guidance to avoid injuring vital intracardiac structures. As full straddle is achieved, the entire system is now generally pointing in the direction of the RA/SVC junction. At this stage, the "A" knob is applied on the CDS as the SGC is rotated clockwise. The clockwise rotation allows the system to face the TV annulus and the A knob application brings

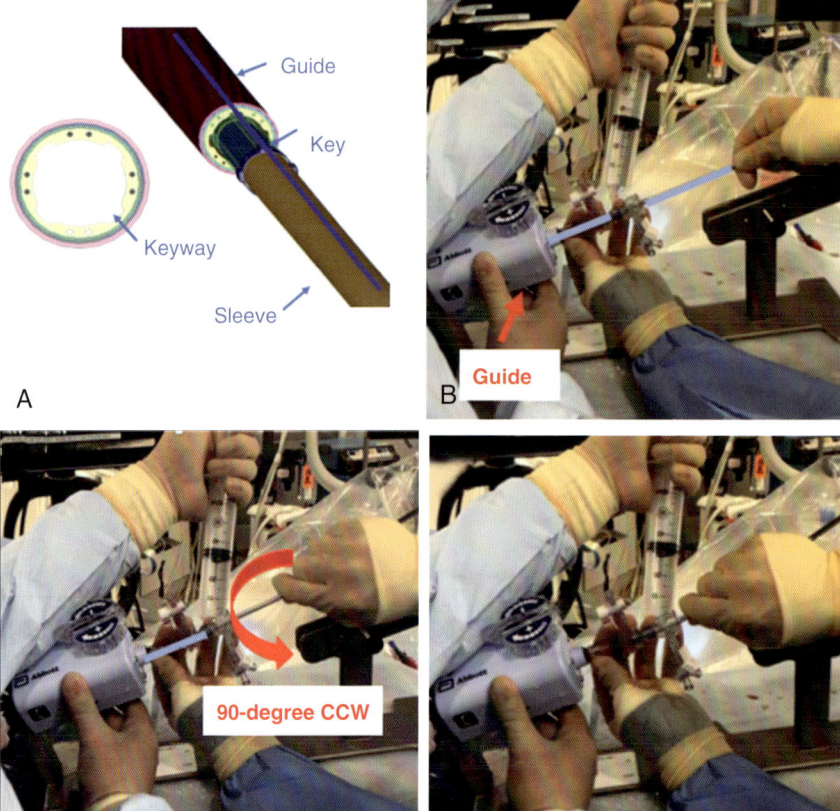

Fig. 57.11 "Miskey" steps using the MitraClip NT for tricuspid valve edge-to-edge repair. (A) Diagram demonstrating the cross section of the MitraClip guide catheter with four distinct grooves ("keyway") that will allow insertion of the clip delivery system (CDS) only in certain orientations. (B) During initial insertion, there are blue marker lines on both the steerable guide catheter (SGC) and the CDS. For mitral valve edge-to-edge repair, the blue lines are aligned and the CDS is advanced into the SGC. (C) For tricuspid valve edge-to-edge repair, once the blue lines have been aligned before insertion, the CDS is rotated 90 degrees counterclockwise and then advanced (CDS) into the SGC (D). *CCW*, Counterclockwise.

the clip down to the TV. Due to substantial variability, operators will need to advance/retract the system, clockwise/counterclockwise rotate SGC, or add plus/minus knob as needed based on real-time TEE imaging. Once the clip has successfully reached the paravalvular plane, the clip arms are opened and 3D TEE imaging is performed to orient the clip arms to be perpendicular to the intended coaptation plane. Next, the clip is partially closed and advanced into the RV under 2D TEE guidance. It is important to advance to a position just below the leaflets and not to maneuver the clip arms too much, as the risk of entanglement is much higher with the TV. Multiple imaging views can then be sought (discussed earlier in the imaging section) to assess for grasping and leaflet insertion. Simultaneous TEE use is critical in positioning and placing the clips; however, intracardiac echo (ICE) imaging may be needed to confirm adequate leaflet insertion.[18] We have used adjunctive ICE in cases where 2D TEE is unable to definitively confirm leaflet insertion (Fig. 57.12). Once leaflet insertion has been fully confirmed, the clip is tightened, TR reduction is assessed, the clip is detached, and the CDS is removed in the reverse order of its entry. Additional TV clips are placed as needed. Once the final clips have been deployed, the SGC and CDS systems are removed and hemostasis is achieved in a manner that has previously been described.[17]

Limitations and Challenges

The tricuspid leaflets are quite thin in patients with FTR. Multiple grasps in the same location without tightening of the clip may result in leaflet tearing and worsening TR. One should spend a significant amount of time scrutinizing leaflet insertion prior to grasping and minimize the number of grasps.

Supravalvular alignment is critical, and advancing the clip into the RV while maintaining this alignment (can be done using 2D TEE and fluoroscopy) is paramount. If a misaligned grasp does occur, once the clip is released, there can be substantial distortion of the leaflet coaptation plane and overall TR may worsen. The complex chordal and papillary muscle structure of the TV makes intravalvular manipulation of the CDS risky. We suggest careful supravalvular alignment by 3D TEE, minimal change of that alignment during RV entry, entry into RV with clip arms partially closed, and opening clip arms and retracting at the moment the leaflets are cleared by the clip arms. If or when entanglement does occur, it is important to reverse the minimal number of steps that may have been performed. In the worst-case scenario, if the clip cannot be freed, it can be deployed within the chordal structures. Excessive force for removal may result in chordal tear. In many cases, due to severe annular dilation, there is minimal (if any) leaflet coaptation. Gentle manual anterior chest compression provides extrinsic pressure on the TV annulus; it can bring the leaflets closer and reduce TR (Fig. 57.13). Anecdotally, some have suggested that this may lead to better leaflet insertion. In our experience, the leaflets do indeed come together, but the entire CDS/SGC system is shifted as well, leading to a grasp location different than the intended site and resulting in unpredictable TR reduction.

Intravalvular Coaptation Device: The FORMA Repair System

The FORMA repair system (Edwards Life Sciences, Irvine, CA) is a tricuspid spacer designed to occupy the effective regurgitant orifice area of centrally directed FTR with reduction in

CHAPTER 57 Percutaneous Tricuspid Valve Repair

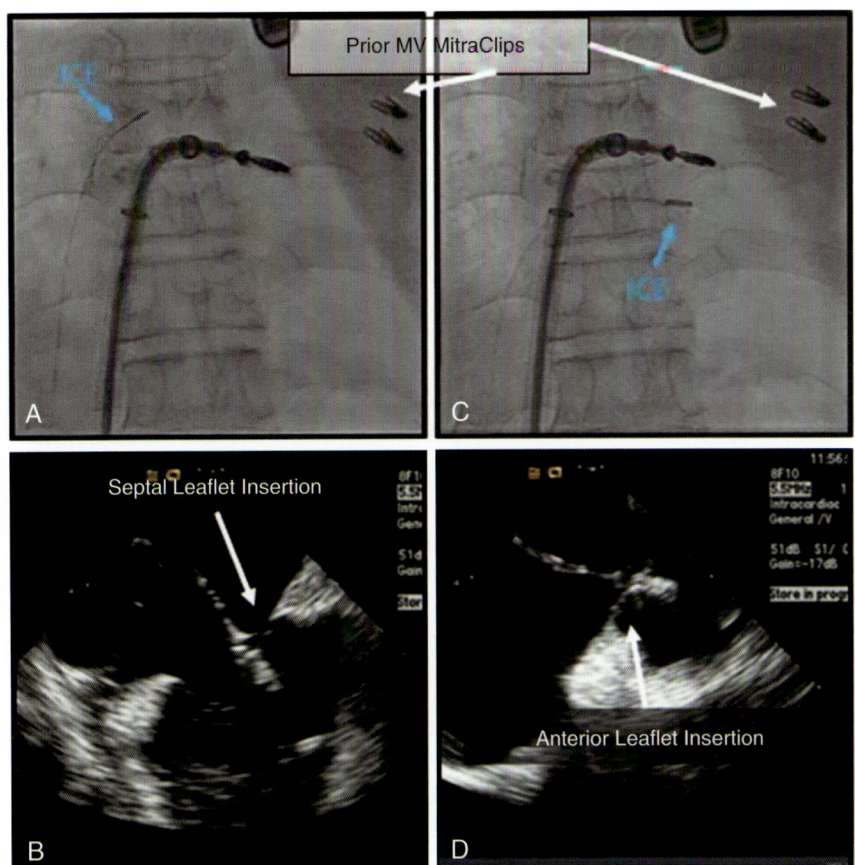

Fig. 57.12 Fluoroscopic (A and C) and intracardiac echo (ICE) (B and D) images from an edge-to-edge repair using the MitraClip system. Since leaflet insertion via transesophageal echocardiographic (TEE) was challenging to assess in this case, an ICE catheter was inserted via contralateral femoral venous access. The ICE catheter was initially advanced high in the right atrium and anteroflexed (A), which allowed visualization of adequate septal leaflet insertion (B). However, clear insertion of the anterior leaflet could not be seen. The ICE catheter was then navigated to below the clip and further retroflexed (C), allowing the operator to "look up" at the anterior leaflet insertion (D). *MV*, Mitral valve.

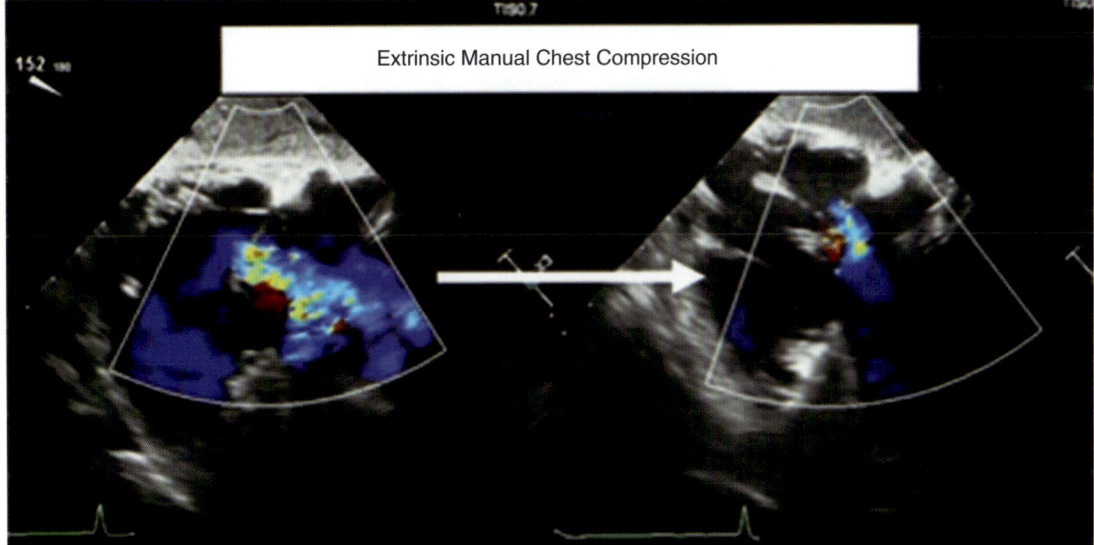

Fig. 57.13 Transthoracic echocardiographic parasternal right ventricular inflow view. The image on the left shows severe tricuspid insufficiency; with extrinsic manual sternal compression, the insufficiency has decreased substantially, indicating that annular dilation and malcoaptation as the main mechanism for tricuspid regurgitation in this patient.

jet severity by providing a prosthetic surface for the TV leaflets to coapt against. The device consists of a self-expanding foam spacer and a rail that is anchored to the RV apex (Figs. 57.14 and 57.15). The spacer is positioned across the annulus using real-time TEE guidance. It can be easily positioned in the atrial/ventricular direction once the RV anchor has been placed. Coaptation diameters of 12 and 15 mm are currently available. The spacer length is 42 mm; it is fixed to the RV apex using a six-pronged nitinol anchor designed to minimize the risk of perforation.

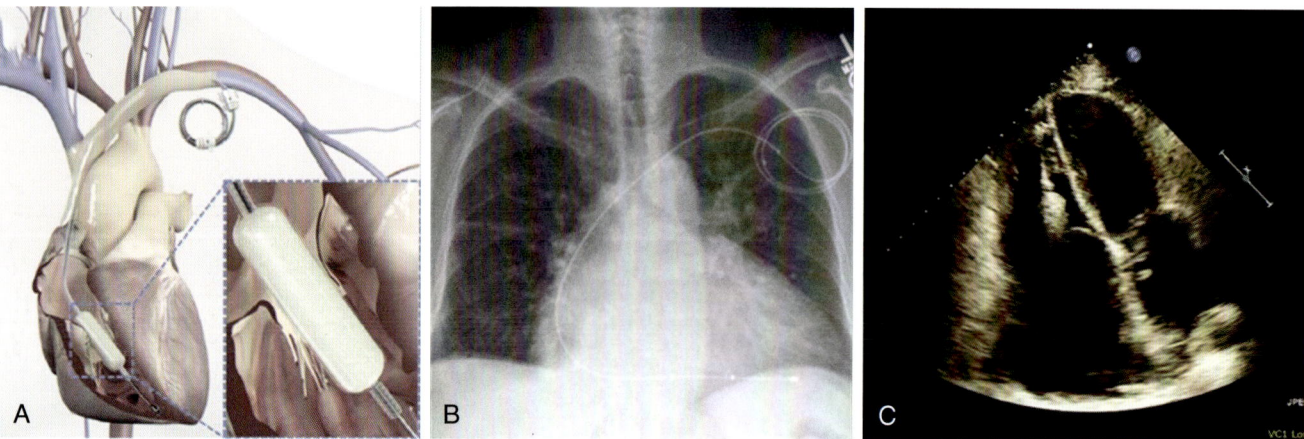

Fig. 57.14 Panel A shows schematic representation of the FORMA™ spacer system. Despite annular dilation with the spacer in place, the TV leaflets would now coapt against the prosthetic material of the spacer, creating a seal during systole and minimizing tricuspid regurgitation. Panel B is a plain x-ray of the chest showing the proximal rail buried in the subcutaneous tissue of the left upper chest; the course of the rail and spacer is similar to that of a standard pacemaker or defibrillator lead. Panel C is a transthoracic echocardiogram showing the spacer in place with the tricuspid valve leaflets coapting against the leaflets.

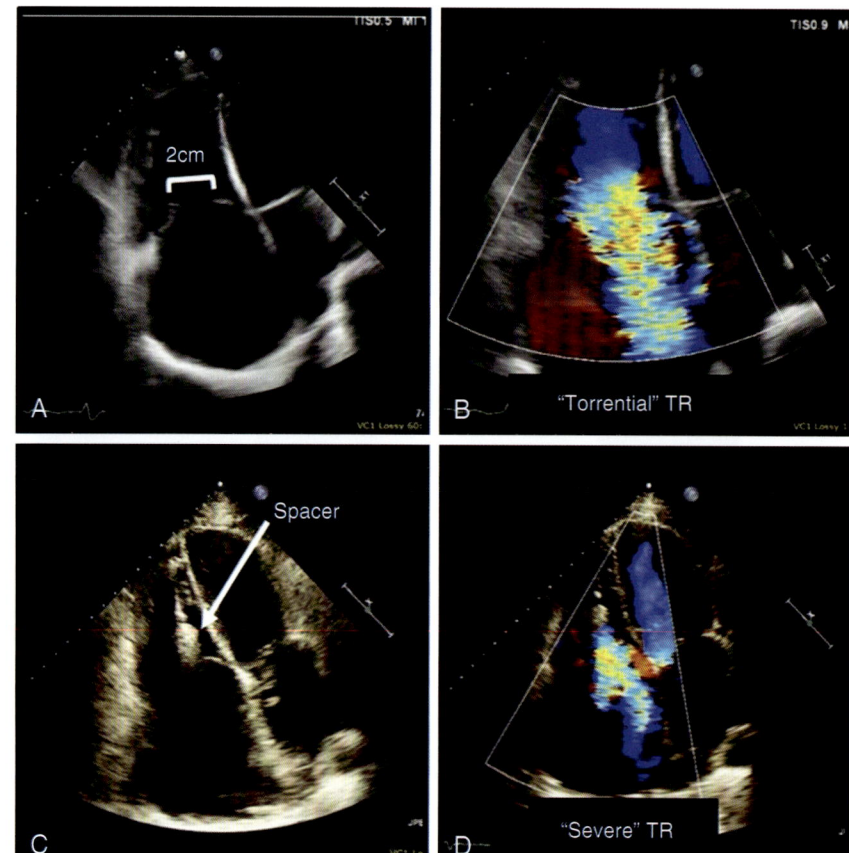

Fig. 57.15 Panels A to D are representative two-dimensional transthoracic echocardiographic images from a patient who underwent FORMA spacer implantation. (A) Shows a 2-cm coaptation gap resulting in torrential tricuspid regurgitation *(TR)* (B). However, 3 months after spacer implantation (C), the residual TR would still be categorized as severe (D). However, in comparison to the preimplant condition (B), there is a substantial reduction in TR, with the patient reporting improved New York Heart Association class and exercise tolerance.

Summary of Clinical Evidence

To date, data on 18 patients undergoing FORMA spacer implantation have been reported.[19] Their average age was 76 years, and 72% of enrollees were female. All patients had NYHA class II to IV symptoms with elevated brain natriuretic peptide. Successful device implantation, defined as implantation of the spacer resulting in reduction in TR by at least 1 grade without a need for surgical conversion or procedure death, was 89%. Although the 1 year mortality on follow-up was 0%, substantial morbidity was reported in the form of transient ischemic attacks (TIAs), rehospitalization for heart failure, minor gastrointestinal bleeding events, acute kidney injury, and device thrombosis, and 27% of patients experienced nondevice related infection. At 1 year,

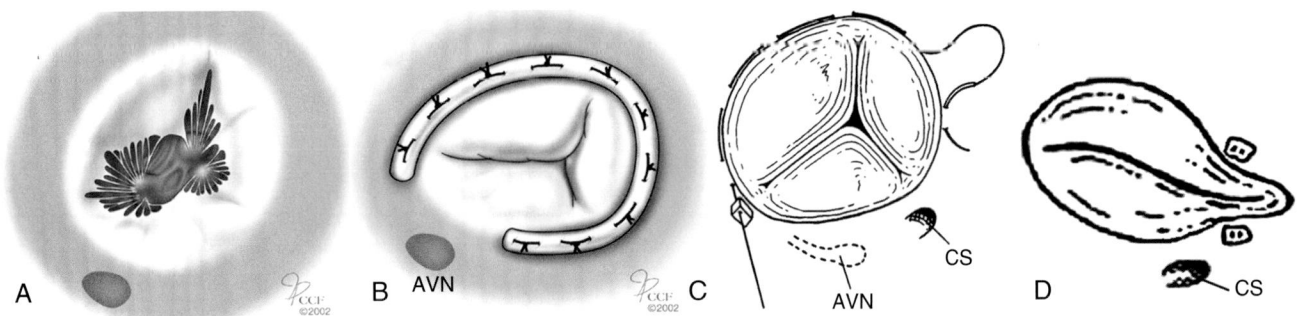

Fig. 57.16 Predominant surgical repair techniques for functional tricuspid regurgitation (FTR). The main surgical approaches for correcting FTR in the presence of a dilated annulus are shown. (A) Dilated tricuspid annulus with abnormal circular shape, failure of leaflet coaptation, and resultant tricuspid regurgitation (TR). Note that in FTR, dilation occurs primarily along the mural portion of the tricuspid annulus, above the right ventricular free wall. (B) Rigid or flexible annular bands are used to restore a more normal annular size and shape *(ovoid)*, thereby reducing or eliminating TR. The open ring shown spares the atrioventricular node *(AVN)*, thus reducing the incidence of heart block. (C) DeVega-style suture annuloplasty in which a purse-string suture technique is used to partially plicate the annulus and reduce annular circumference and diameter. (D) Suture bicuspidalization is performed by placement of a mattress suture from the anteroposterior to the posteroseptal commissures along the posterior annulus. *CS,* Coronary sinus. (Reproduced with permission from Rogers JH, Bolling SF. The tricuspid valve: current perspective and evolving management of tricuspid regurgitation. *Circulation.* 2009;119:2718–2725.)

nearly all patients reported improvement in NYHA class, reduction in hospitalization for heart failure, and improvement in the 6MWT from 256 ± 103 to 328 ± 82 m (P = .04). At 1 year, improvements in objective echocardiographic assessment of TR and RV function and size were less robust without any change in effective regurgitant orifice area, RV function, RV systolic function, IVC diameter, and RA volume. Based on the current extent of data, the FORMA spacer device for the treatment of TR for malcoaptation or noncoaptation appears to be safe, with improved symptoms at 1 year despite modest efficacy in reducing TR parameters by echocardiography.

There are two international registries for ongoing clinical and echocardiographic assessment of outcomes after FORMA implantation. A larger trial, called SPACER (tricuSPid trAnsCatheter rEpaiR system) has been launched for the assessment of outcomes after FORMA implantation. The estimated enrollment comprises 75 patients, and the primary outcome assessed will be the cardiac mortality of the as-treated cohort at 30 days compared with a literature-derived performance goal based on high-risk surgical outcomes for tricuspid repair/replacement.

Procedural Steps

Insertion of the FORMA spacer system requires the use of fluoroscopic and TEE guidance. Generally the left axillary vein (accessed either percutaneously or via cutdown) is utilized and a large-bore sheath is inserted into place; 20 Fr for a 12-mm device and 24 Fr for a 15-mm device. A pigtail is advanced into the RV and right ventriculography is performed to locate the tricuspid annular plane and the location on the RV apex that is perpendicular to the RV annulus. Next, a steerable delivery catheter is advanced into the RV and the distal anchor (connected to a rail) is deployed through the steerable catheter. The steerable catheter is removed over the externalized rail. Next, the spacer is tracked over the rail and into position as assessed by TEE and fluoroscopy. The device is then secured proximally with excess rail length coiled and buried into the subcutaneous tissue. The device can be fully retrieved throughout the entire procedure or up to several months later, similar to the removal process for pacemaker leads.[20]

Annuloplasty-Based Devices

There are two general annuloplasty-based surgical approaches for the treatment of FTR (Fig. 57.16). The first consists of suture annuloplasty whereby the annular size is reduced by using a purse-string suture technique along with pledgets to partially plicate the annulus, reduce annular size, and increase coaptation of the leaflets. The prototypical example of this technique is the De Vega annuloplasty.[21] Another example results in bicuspidization of the TV by placing a mattress suture from the anteroposterior to the posteroseptal commissure along the posterior annulus (Kay annuloplasty). The overall durability of suture-based annuloplasty is inferior to the use of rigid annuloplasty rings. Many patients with suture-based annuloplasty will develop recurrent FTR from progressive annular dilation or tissue dehiscence owing to the relative friability of the tissue. The other main surgical approach for the treatment of FTR consists of using a rigid prosthetic partial ring. Many of these prosthetic rings are partial so as to spare suturing in the vicinity of the AV node. Rings with a rigid backbone are thought to be effective and durable by reducing annular diameter and improving leaflet coaptation. Semirigid or flexible annuloplasty bands may allow for more physiologic motion of the annulus during the cardiac cycle but are felt not be as durable as their more rigid counterparts.[22]

Transcatheter annuloplasty-based strategies for TR reduction attempt to mimic the surgical approach. The two main categories of the percutaneous approaches consist of (1) complete annuloplasty systems versus (2) incomplete annuloplasty systems. Current complete annuloplasty systems consist of the Cardioband (Edwards Lifesciences, Irvine, CA), IRIS (Millipede Medical, Santa Rosa, CA), minimally invasive annuloplasty (MIA) (Micro-Interventional Devices, Inc., Newton, PA), and transatrial intrapericardial tricuspid annuloplasty (TRAIPTA). Percutaneous technologies that provide incomplete annuloplasty are the TriCinch (4Tech, Galway, Ireland) and Trialign (Mitralign, Tewksbury, MA). All transcatheter annuloplasty (complete or incomplete) devices for FTR have sparse clinical data to support their efficacy, durability, and safety (Table 57.3).

TABLE 57.3 Annuloplasty-Based Devices for Treatment of Functional Tricuspid Regurgitation

	Ring-Based Annuloplasty				Suture-Based Annuloplasty	
	Cardioband	**IRIS**	**MIA**	**TRAIPTA**	**Trialign**	**TriCinch**
Description	Anchors are delivered through a flexible catheter. Once all anchors are fixed, tension is applied, thereby reducing annular dimensions.	Helical anchors attach to annulus and sliders are actuated to reduce annular size.	Two proprietary Polycor anchors connected by MyoLast elastomer are compliant and self-tensioning once deployed.	A suture is placed circumferentially in the atrioventricular groove. Delivery is via a puncture into the pericardium via the right atrial appendage. Annular reduction is by direct extrinsic compression.	Two polyester pledgets are delivered in efforts to "bicuspidize" the TV. Delivery is via the right internal jugular vein.	Second-generation device contains a proprietary anchor delivered to the anterolateral annulus via direct puncture into the pericardium. The anchor is tethered to a self-expanding stent positioned in the inferior vena cava via a Dacron band.
Current clinical status	TRI-REPAIR $n \pm 30$	Direct surgical implants only, $n = 2$	First-in-man implants, $n = 2$ STTAR trial, $n = 2$	First-in-man implants, $n = 5$	SCOUT I. SCOUT II. $n \pm 50$	First-generation device ($n \pm 30$) trial completed. Second-generation device trial under way.
Clinical results	Reduction in quantitative and qualitative measures of TR. Reduction in annular dimensions.	Elimination of TR and reduction in annular dimensions.	Up to 9 implants required to create 270-degree ring pattern. Effects on TR and annular dimensions not publicly available. Procedural time <1 h.	Procedural success achieved in four of five patients. One patient died of intractable heart failure; another sustained an acute coronary injury.	100% acute implant success with reduction in TR and annular dimensions. Risk of midterm dehiscence and RCA damage with first-generation device.	Second generation: 7 patients with successful implantation without adverse events. First generation: risk of hemopericardium, anchor detachments, and RCA injury.

MIA, Minimally invasive annuloplasty; *RCA*, right coronary artery; *SCOUT*, Percutaneous Tricuspid Valve Annuloplasty System for Symptomatic Chronic Functional Tricuspid Regurgitation Trial; *STTAR*, study of transcatheter tricuspid annular repair; *TR*, tricuspid regurgitation; *TRAIPTA*, transatrial intrapericardial tricuspid annuloplasty; *TRI-REPAIR*, TrIcuspid Regurgitation RePAIr With CaRdioband Transcatheter System; *TV*, tricuspid valve. Adapted from Aboulhosn J, Cabalka AK, Levi DS, et al. Transcatheter valve-in-ring implantation for the treatment of residual or recurrent tricuspid valve dysfunction after prior surgical repair. *JACC Cardiovasc Interv*. 2017;10:53–63.

Cardioband

The Cardioband system is a direct annuloplasty band currently commercially available in Europe for the treatment of functional mitral regurgitation. Available in various sizes, the band is inserted with a 25-Fr guide catheter via femoral venous access. A combination of fluoroscopic and TEE guidance is used to fix helical anchors around the annulus. Once in position, the annuloplasty band is cinched, thereby reducing the annular dimensions. To date, at least 10 patients have undergone Cardioband implantation in the TV under compassionate use with an annular reduction up to 45% and a 70% reduction in effective regurgitant orifice area (EROA), with excellent safety profile. A Confirmite Europeene (CE) mark study (TrIcuspid Regurgitation RePAIr With CaRdioband Transcatheter System [TRI-REPAIR] 1 Clinical Trial, NCT 02981953) is currently under way.[22]

IRIS

IRIS is a complete semirigid adjustable annuloplasty ring. Surgical and catheter-based implants have been performed for the treatment of functional mitral regurgitation (FMR). The catheter-based device for FMR is currently delivered via a 24-Fr delivery catheter. Once the helical anchors have been inserted into the annulus using a combination of fluoroscopy, TEE, and ICE, interlocking actuators are tightened, thereby reducing the annular dimensions. Of the nine surgical implants, two cases had both mitral and TV implants. In both patients, FTR was reduced to zero with an average 36% reduction in tricuspid annular diameter. A transcatheter delivery system for the TV is currently in clinical development.[22]

Minimally Invasive Annuloplasty and Transatrial Intrapericardial Tricuspid Annuloplasty

The MIA mechanism of FTR reduction is based on a proprietary compliant and self-tensioning implant using a series of anchors and an elastomer. The catheter-based device provides a customizable number of implants deployed to the target annulus. The device is delivered via a 12-Fr sheath with an end deflector allowing for device deployment in a 270-degree ring pattern (sparing the AV node). Two surgical human implants have been reported.[22] Two patients have been enrolled with the catheter-based delivery system in the study of transcatheter tricuspid annular repair (STTAR) Trial. The procedure is reportedly reproducible and is completed in less than an hour under imaging guidance. It leaves a minimal footprint, thereby preserving physiologic function and future options for intervention.

The TRAIPTA device (Fig. 57.17) is a hybrid complete annular reduction device but requires access to the pericardial space. The RA appendage is punctured and a custom-shaped device is delivered via a 12-Fr catheter. The implant is premounted on a delivery loop that encircles the AV groove. A circumferential suture is then

CHAPTER 57 Percutaneous Tricuspid Valve Repair

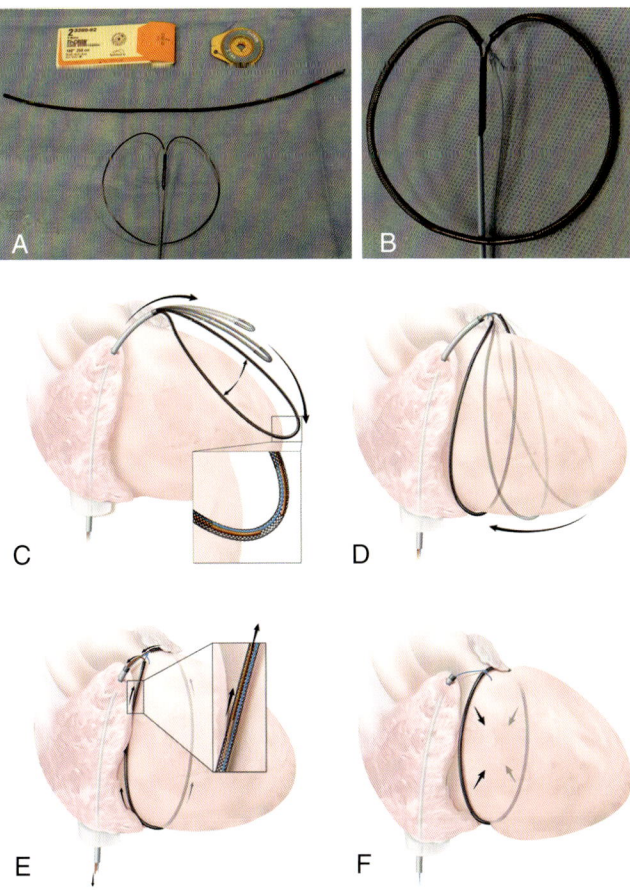

Fig. 57.17 (A) Braided suture (packaging and spool), transatrial intrapericardial tricuspid annuloplasty (TRAIPTA) implant, and delivery device. (B) TRAIPTA implant loaded onto delivery device. The suture is housed within the hollow TRAIPTA implant with a pretied Roeder sliding knot. (C) The system is advanced into the pericardium through the right atrial appendage. (D) The nitinol delivery device ensures that the system opens into a loop inside the pericardium and reaches the atrioventricular groove. (E) The delivery device is withdrawn. (F) The implant is tightened. (Reproduced with permission from Rogers T, Ratnayaka K, Sonmez M, et al. Transatrial intrapericardial tricuspid annuloplasty. *JACC Cardiovasc Interv*. 2015;8:483–491.)

adjusted to achieve TR reduction and reduce the annular dimensions. The RA appendage puncture is sealed using an occluder-like device.[23] Data from animal implants are encouraging, and first-in-man human implants have been reported with procedural success achieved in four out of the five implants for secondary mitral regurgitation.[24] The implant results in reverse left ventricle (LV) and RV remodeling and suggested electrical remodeling (reversion of atrial fibrillation). However, one patient experienced a myocardial infarction from coronary branch occlusion as a result of the implant and another died of intractable heart failure.[24] Additional clinical data are clearly needed to further clarify the role of this device.

Trialign

The Trialign system is a novel 14-Fr catheter-based system delivered via the right internal jugular vein; it is designed to replicate the Kay suture-based annuloplasty system. After venous access has been obtained via the right internal jugular vein through two separate punctures (one ventral and another lateral placed 2 cm apart), an articulating system delivers two pledgets to the anteroposterior and septoposterior commissures; these are cinched down and locked using a dedicated plication locking device, thus effectively plicating the posterior leaflet. If needed, an additional pair of pledgeted sutures can be placed. Additionally, a guide catheter via arterial access is used to engage, opacify, and assess the RCA intraprocedurally owing to potential injury as a result of the implant. The early safety and feasibility trial enrolled 15 patients. All patients had successful implantation, with 1 patient experiencing iatrogenic injury to the RCA requiring percutaneous coronary intervention. At 30 days, there was a 20% pledget detachment/dehiscence rate with the remaining patients having significant reductions in annular dimensions, EROA, and LV stroke volume. Additionally, patients experienced improved NYHA grade, 6MWT, and quality-of-life (QOL) assessments.[25] A larger trial (Safety and Performance of the Trialign Percutaneous Tricuspid Valve Annuloplasty System [SCOUT II]) of 60 patients is currently in progress.

TriCinch System

In an effort to mimic the Kay suture-based annuloplasty procedure, the TriCinch system cinches the anteroposterior commissure, thereby reducing the annular dimensions and improving TR parameters. The system consists of an 18-Fr steerable delivery system into the RA via the femoral vein. The system is directed toward the anteroposterior annulus. The first-generation system used an anchor clinically delivered directly into the tricuspid annulus. However, the next-generation system utilizes a proprietary anchor that is delivered to the pericardium after a controlled puncture into the pericardium from the RA. First, the puncture is made and the extracardiac (intrapericardial anchor) is deployed. At this stage, the anchor is preattached to the delivery system and a cable tethered to a much larger constrained self-expanding stent. The self-expanding stent is positioned in the IVC while tensioning the anchor, thereby reducing the septal-lateral annular dimension. Once adequate reduction has been achieved, the self-expanding IVC stent is deployed and the applied tension fully maintained. An early first-in-man trial with the current-generation pericardial anchor is under way. A clinical trial from the first-generation device was completed but reports of hemopericardium and anchor dehiscence necessitated device redesign.[22]

Caval Valve Implantation

CAVI is a technique designed to leave the tricuspid complex untouched but to reduce the unwanted effects of FTR on the body, thereby alleviating symptoms. The caval valves are deployed in an orientation such that the valves close during ventricular systole, thus limiting reversal of flow in the SVC and IVC. However, normal anterograde flow continues during ventricular diastole. This technique has the theoretical advantages of applying catheter-based valve implantation at a distance from vulnerable intracardiac structures (e.g., AV node, annulus, pericardium, RCA), absence of any footprint within the RA or RV, and not interfering with preexisting pacemaker or defibrillator leads.

The largest clinical trial to date was a multicenter registry of 25 patients demonstrating feasibility, safety, and acute hemodynamic effectiveness. A combination of self-expanding and balloon-expandable valves was utilized. This therapy, with successful implantation in 92% of the cohort, translated into improvement in acute hemodynamic improvement and subacute (30 day) improvement in NYHA class. However, 1-year mortality was high at 63%, albeit in a cohort of patients with an average Society of Thoracic Surgery (STS) score of 14.[26]

Although determinants of clinical candidacy for CAVI remain unclear, some have advocated that adequate RV function is required to derive clinical benefit.[27] In patients with advanced right-sided heart disease, there may not be adequate RV function to generate a substantial FTR jet, hence it is unclear if these patients would benefit from CAVI. On the other hand, in addition to severe RV dysfunction, these patients also have severe RV dilation with large malcoaptation distances. Even in the presence of severe RV dysfunction, the large malcoaptation distances

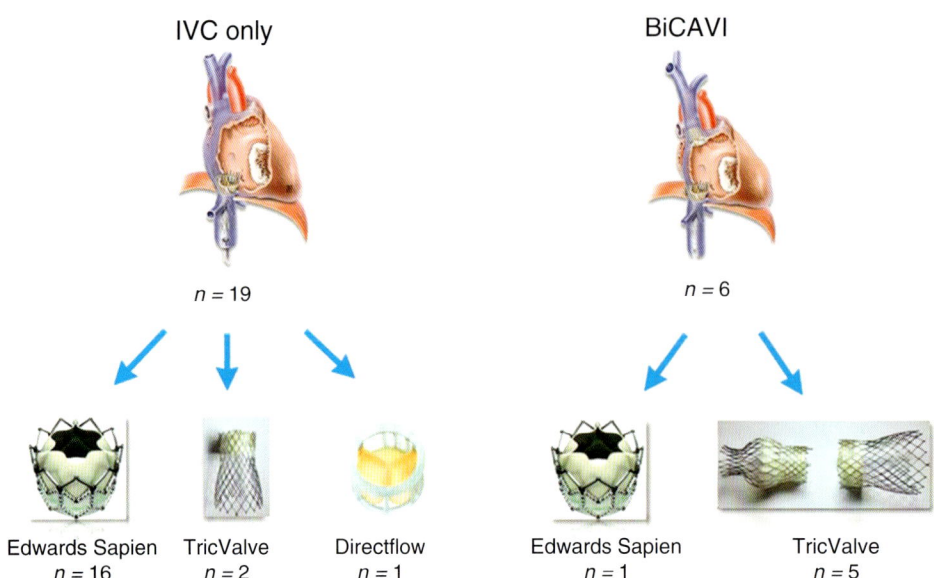

Fig. 57.18 Caval valve implantation. Procedural characteristics. The total number of valves implanted in this study was 25.[27] Patients were treated with single-valve implantation (n = 19; 76.0%) or bicaval valve implantation (n = 6; 24.0%). Balloon-expandable valves (Sapien XT or Sapien 3: n = 17; 78.3%) or self-expandable valves (TricValve: n = 7; 21.7%; Directflow: n = 1; 4.0%) were used for either single inferior vena cava *(IVC)* or bicaval valve implantation *(BiCAVI)*. One case was treated by IVC—the only implantation of a direct-flow medical valve prosthesis (Direct Flow Medical, Santa Rosa, CA). When self-expandable valves were used, different techniques of IVC landing zone preparation and downsizing were required, such as prestenting with one or more self-expandable stents (n = 16) or surgical banding (n = 2), depending on the local heart team's decision. (From Lauten A, Figulla HR, Unbehaun A, et al. Interventional treatment of severe tricuspid regurgitation: early clinical experience in a multicenter, observational, first-in-man study. *Circ Cardiovasc Interv*. 2018;11:e006061.)

result in "wide open" FTR; hence, even these patients may benefit from CAVI. Regardless of underlying RV function and coaptation distances, the presence of symptoms directly attributable to the TR jet is needed.

Anatomically, the portion of the IVC that crosses through the diaphragm is constrained by fibrous tissue that resists the dilation experienced by the remainder of the infradiaphragmatic IVC. Hence this "landing zone" serves as an optimal and reliable site for CAVI. Conversely, no such constrained fibrous tissue exists for the SVC as it joins the RA. Indeed, massive dilation of the SVC can lead to atrialization and a wide taper of the SVC as it enters the RA, making valve implantation difficult. It is not surprising that the largest series to date of CAVI comprises a vast majority of patients with IVC implants alone (Fig. 57.18).[26,27] In some cases where the size of the intradiaphragmatic IVC or SVC may be too large, some operators have prestented these segments with large-diameter balloon-expandable stents followed by valve implantation.[27]

TRANSCATHETER TECHNIQUE FOR DEGENERATED TV BIOPROSTHESIS

The vast majority (>85%) of TV surgical procedures occur for patients with concomitant surgeries for other primary indications, specifically during left-sided surgery such as coronary artery bypass grafting, MV replacement/repair, and aortic valve replacement.[28] Not surprisingly, patients with degenerated TV bioprosthetic (BioP) valves or with recurrent TR after surgical annuloplasty have become an important target for transcatheter intervention. Hence, in appropriately selected patients, valve-in-valve (ViV) or valve-in-ring (ViR) with the Edwards Sapien valve, currently U.S. Food and Drug Administration, or the Melody Transcatheter Pulmonary Valve, has been performed with an off-label intent.

Surgical treatment of FTR with ring annuloplasty is generally the preferred approach. However, in patients with failed prior repair or severe RV dilation and/or leaflet tethering, a repair may be inadequate and TV replacement is required. Alternatively, patients with primary TR (e.g., history of endocarditis or primary congenital disease) will undergo TV replacement. No large series has ever provided the true durability of these bioprosthesis with convincing accuracy. Nevertheless, degenerated bioprostheses (bioprosthesis stenosis or regurgitation) are commonly encountered in clinical practice. For these patients, reoperation for TV disease can be associated with substantial surgical risk. A transcatheter in the surgical ViV procedure for these patients can be an effective treatment strategy with very little risk to the patient.

Summary of Clinical Evidence

The Valve-in-Valve International Data (VIVID) registry provides the most contemporary outcomes in patients undergoing TV-ViV. A total of 156 patients were enrolled in this multinational registry between 2008 and 2015 to undergo TV-ViV. The vast majority (60%) of these patients underwent Melody valve implantation with the etiology of their original implant related to primary congenital TV disease. Patients undergoing Sapien ViV implantation tended to have more acquired TV disease necessitating TV replacement. In nearly all patients (90%), the TV-ViV was performed under general anesthesia via the transfemoral route (69%); the remaining access sites were transjugular (28%), with very few procedures performed via thoracotomy and a RA surgical window (3%). Procedural success was 98%, with only one patient having moderate paravalvular leak (PVL) and <5% having mild PVL; in all cases no further intervention was needed for the PVL. Thirty-day mortality was 0.03%, with >85% of patients reaching NYHA class I or II.[29] A more recent paper reports outcomes of TV-ViV with use of the Sapien S3 in five consecutive patients performed under

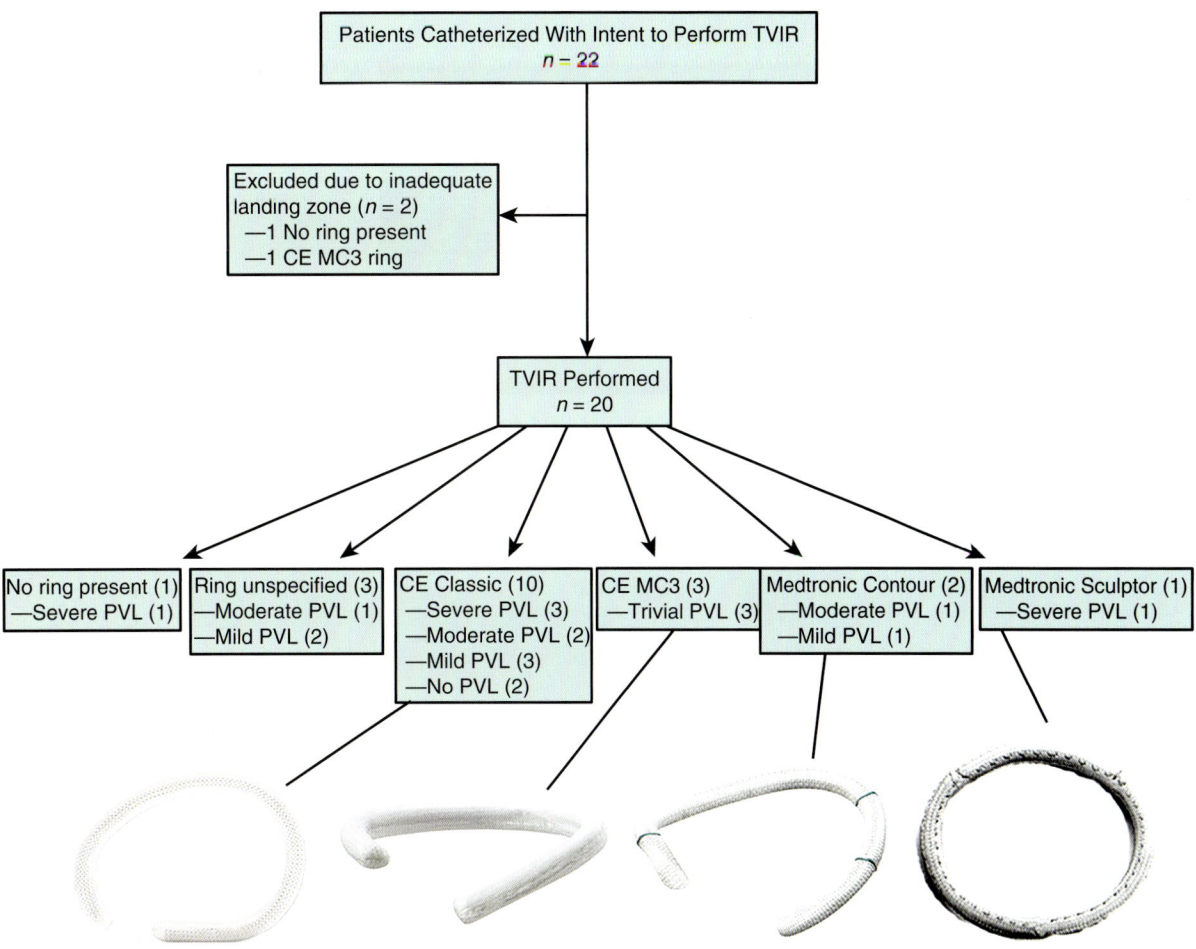

Fig. 57.19 Types of surgical rings used and incidence of paravalvular regurgitation after transcatheter valve replacement. Tricuspid annuloplasty data specifying type of annuloplasty ring and presence and degree of paravalvular leak *(PVL)* following transcatheter tricuspid valve-in-ring *(TVIR)* implantation. The numbers in parentheses indicate the number of patients for the given type of ring and grade of PVL. *CE MC3,* Carpentier-Edwards MC 3. (Reproduced with permission from Aboulhosn J, Cabalka AK, Levi DS, et al. Transcatheter valve-in-ring implantation for the treatment of residual or recurrent tricuspid valve dysfunction after prior surgical repair. *JACC Cardiovasc Interv*. 2017;10:53–63.)

conscious sedation. All patients had a 29-mm Sapien S3 valve successfully implanted without rapid pacing. There was no in-hospital or 30-day mortality and no patients with PVL. All patients were discharged on aspirin and Plavix.[30]

The procedure of TV-ViR is also a supported in the literature by a small series of 22 patients all with partial (incomplete) semirigid or rigid rings. Procedural success was 91%, with the Sapien valve being most commonly used. There was no procedural mortality; however, 90% of the implanted patients had some PVL arising from the "incomplete" area of the partial ring (Fig. 57.19). All patients with moderate to severe (30%) disease required intervention for the PVL consisting of device-based closure or redo surgery.[31]

Valve-in-Valve Procedural Steps Using the Edwards Sapien S3

As in every structural procedure, preprocedural planning for TV-ViV is paramount. During initial clinic evaluation, in addition to establishing the presence of severe and limiting right-sided heart failure symptoms, surface echocardiography should confirm the presence of severe BioP tricuspid stenosis (TS) or TR. Additionally, the original surgical operative report or valve card should be obtained to confirm the manufacturer and size of the bioprosthesis implanted. Using the ViV app for mitral bioprosthesis, the size of the recommended ViV implant can be obtained. We also perform an electrocardiographically-gated computed tomography (CT) scan of the chest for formal reconstruction (Fig. 57.20A) of the BioP TV and confirm the working dimensions of the BioP valve (diameters, area, and perimeter). If the recommended valve falls in between two sizes (26 vs. 29 mm), it important not to oversize too much as this would leave a substantial residual gradient. Our recommendation is that if the ViV app suggests either of the two sizes, we rely heavily on CT reconstruction and pick the Sapien implant size that is closest to the reconstructed dimensions.

The procedural setup is otherwise similar to that of a MV-in-valve procedure. We generally recommend that the patient be placed under general anesthesia, although the procedure has been performed under conscious sedation.[30] We next obtain femoral venous access and either one or two Proglides (Abbott) are used in a PreClose technique to secure the venotomy and ultimately an 8-Fr side arm sheath is put into place. On the contralateral groin, we will also have percutaneous arterial and venous access should the patient decompensate and necessitate placement on extracorporeal membrane oxygenation. Next, we will advance a standard Swan-Ganz catheter and obtain preprocedural right-sided pressures. Once in the RV an additional catheter (e.g., multipurpose catheter) can be advanced into the RA trans-TV gradients in cases

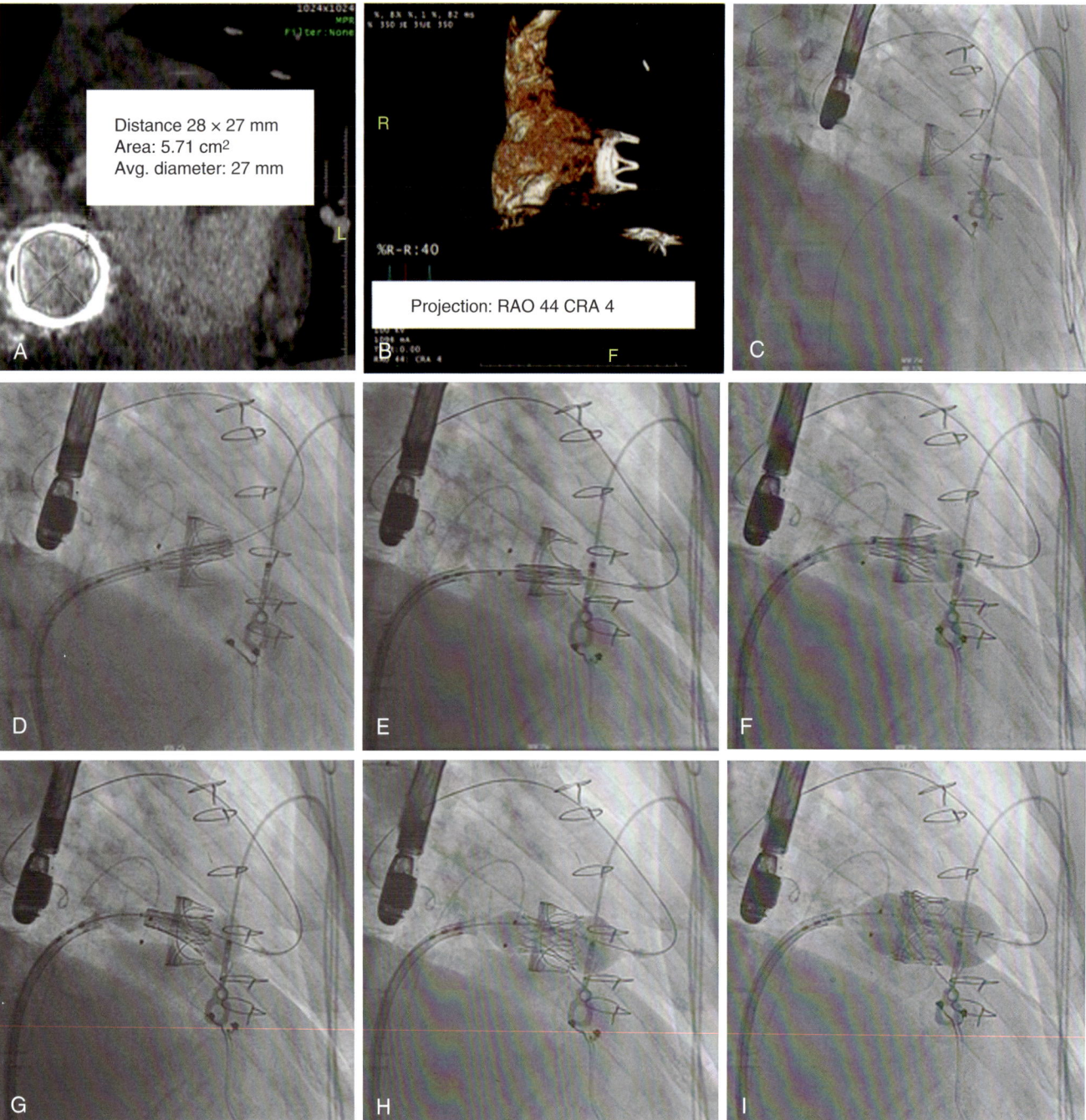

Fig. 57.20 This panel represents a series of images from a tricuspid valve–valve-in-valve (TV-ViV) procedure. The patient had a prior 27-mm Edwards Perimount valve implanted for tricuspid valve (TV) endocarditis. The patient presented with symptomatic right-sided heart failure with severe bioprosthetic TV stenosis. Preprocedural ECG-gated computed tomography (CT) demonstrated average diameters of 27 mm (A) and the valve-in-valve (ViV) app recommended implantation of either a 26- or 29-mm Sapien S3 valve. CT reconstruction also confirmed a planar (i.e., deployment) angle of right anterior oblique *(RAO)* 44 and cranial *(CRA)* 4 (B). After right heart catheterization was performed, the rail was exchanged out for a 0.035-inch stiff wire (e.g., Cook Extra Stiff Wire) (C). Next, the venous sheath was upsized to the transcatheter aortic valve replacement sheath and the Sapien S3 system (26 mm) was advanced across the bioprosthetic TV (D). Based on the ViV app outflow, the distal posts of the bioprosthetic valve should align with the leading edge of the Sapien S3 valve (D). However, there was misalignment between the Sapien valve and the bioprosthetic valve (D). Next, after using a combination of microadjustments of the 0.035-inch wire and the Edwards commander system, the Edwards Sapien valve was better aligned (E). Next, the balloon was slowly inflated only partially and additional microadjustments could be performed (F, G, and H) before fully expanding the valve (I).

of BioP TS. Ultimately the Swan-Ganz catheter is directed up into the left or right pulmonary artery. We then use an exchange-length 0.025-inch guidewire to remove the Swan-Ganz catheter and still maintain wire position to the pulmonary artery. A 5-Fr multipurpose catheter is then carefully advanced over the wire and into the pulmonary artery. The 0.025-inch guidewire is removed and exchanged for a 0.035-inch support wire (e.g., Cook Extra support wire, Amplatzer and others) and the multipurpose catheter is removed (see Fig. 57.20C). We next exchange the venous access sheath for an Edwards expandable access sheath. The valve is prepped on the back table as per manufacturer specifications and reverse-mounted (as compared with aortic valve delivery) on the Commander delivery catheter. The Sapien valve is advanced through the sheath and into the IVC under standard protocol as previously described, followed by retraction of the balloon into the undeployed valve to fully "mount" the valve. Next the image-intensifier is positioned so the fluoroscopic view is in plane with the valve; this is usually an RAO view with slight cranial-caudal projection. Then the mounted valve is advanced and positioned through the BioP valve with slight adjustments as needed (see Fig. 57.20D).

Unlike deployment for the aortic, pulmonic, or mitral positions, RV pacing for TV-ViV deployment is not possible. Options can include pacing the RA, but with higher atrial rates the AVN becomes refractory and heart block may develop. Others have reported pacing a floppy 0.035-inch wire that has been placed into the LV or inserting a temporary pacemaker through the CS and into a lateral ventricular branch; however, in many cases pacing may not be required. Unlike the left side of the heart, the right ventricular pressures are generally lower, and once the balloon begins to expand, there is no substantial motion of the Sapien valve as it is being deployed. Hence, TV-ViV can often be performed without rapid pacing.

The most technically challenging part of this procedure is positioning of the Sapien valve. As the valve expands, it shortens from the inflow side while the outflow side remains unchanged in position. If the patient's degenerated bioprosthesis has radiographic posts (see Fig. 57.20), positioning of the Sapien valve becomes easier as the outflow (ventricular) side of the Sapien valve must be aligned with the radiographic posts of the degenerated bioprosthesis. Once positioning is achieved (see Fig. 57.20E), the balloon is partially inflated, and this will still allow for coordinated micro-adjustments to the guidewire and the Commander catheter to ensure accurate final positioning before the balloon in fully inflated to deploy the Sapien S3 valve (see Fig. 57.20F-I). If the degenerated bioprosthesis does not have posts and only a central radioopaque wire is noted, positioning is a bit more challenging but still possible. Generally we recommend relying on positioning recommendations from the ViV app. The middle balloon marker on the Sapien valve and central wire on the degenerated BioP valve will serve as radiographic markers and positioning should be achieved in the manner described earlier, but taking these two radio-opaque landmarks into account. Once the Sapien valve has been deployed, the delivery system is removed, final trans-TV gradients are recorded, and the venotomy is secured with the previously deployed ProGlide devices. Medical therapy after ViV consists of systemic anticoagulation with warfarin over the long term, although others have reported the use of dual antiplatelet therapy alone.[32]

Valve-in-Ring Procedural Steps

The procedural steps for ViR are not that different from the ViV procedure described earlier. Venous access, creation of a rail, advancement, and mounting of the valve are similar to the steps for the previously described ViV procedure. It is important to align the ring so that the fluoroscopic view provides no parallax and the valve is positioned so the middle radiographic balloon marker is in position. Because of the nature of the incomplete ring and less material to "grab onto," there is a greater chance of device malposition and/or embolization.[29] PVL around an incomplete ring will require sealing with an occluding vascular plug. Unlike ViV, which has been shown to be performed safely under conscious sedation and without TEE, the ViR procedure should generally be performed under general anesthesia with TEE owing to the risk of device malposition and the high risk of PVL and potential need for catheter-based closure.

CONCLUSION

The most common manifestation of TV disease is FTR from left-sided heart disease, pulmonary hypertension, or long-standing atrial fibrillation. Generally considered benign and ignored from an anatomic, pathophysiologic, natural history, and imaging standpoint, it has now clearly become evident that FTR is an important independent predictor of mortality in the surgical, percutaneous, and heart failure population. There has been a large shift in the community to understand the interplay in the pathogenesis of symptomatic FTR. Most of these patients have had prior sternotomies or have comorbidities that preclude surgical intervention. The field of percutaneous TV therapies has rapidly expanded and is continuing to evolve.

Although edge-to-edge repair therapy is now the standard percutaneous approach for MV disease and has been applied for the treatment of FTR, its efficacy and durability for TV disease is unknown and under investigation. There are a variety of annuloplasty (direct and indirect) based catheter devices under active investigation, each with its strengths and limitations; however, it is still too early to determine which will become the clinically dominant approach. As described earlier, CAVI is a treatment strategy that reduces the untoward symptoms of FTR but does nothing to reverse or address the underlying pathology. Finally, for the group of patients with prior TV replacement, ViV appears to be a relatively straightforward and efficacious procedure.

It is an exciting time for our patients and percutaneous TV therapies as we improve our understanding of the valve and the symptoms associated with its diseased state. In the future, we expect to see improved design and application of the therapy and larger-scale clinical trials to answer the questions of efficacy and durability in appropriately selected patients.

KEY REFERENCES

1. Alqahtani F, Berzingi CO, Aljohani S, et al. Contemporary trends in the use and outcomes of surgical treatment of tricuspid regurgitation. *J Am Heart Assoc*. 2017;6(12):e007597.
2. Rodes-Cabau J, Hahn RT, Latib A, et al. Transcatheter therapies for treating tricuspid regurgitation. *J Am Coll Cardiol*. 2016;67:1829–1845.
4. Orban M, Besler C, Braun D, et al. Six-month outcome after transcatheter edge-to-edge repair of severe tricuspid regurgitation in patients with heart failure. *Eur J Heart Fail*. 2018;20:1055–1062.
6. Rogers JH, Bolling SF. The tricuspid valve: current perspective and evolving management of tricuspid regurgitation. *Circulation*. 2009;119:2718–2725.
7. Hahn RT. State-of-the-art review of echocardiographic imaging in the evaluation and treatment of functional tricuspid regurgitation. *Circ Cardiovasc Imaging*. 2016;9(12). e005332.
10. Ancona F, Agricola E, Stella S, et al. Interventional imaging of the tricuspid valve. *Interv Cardiol Clin*. 2018;7:13–29.
12. Taramasso M, Hahn RT, Alessandrini H, et al. The international multicenter trivalve registry: which patients are undergoing transcatheter tricuspid repair? *JACC Cardiovasc Interv*. 2017;10:1982–1990.

13. Kalbacher D, Schafer U, von Bardeleben RS, et al. Impact of tricuspid valve regurgitation in surgical high-risk patients undergoing MitraClip implantation: results from the TRAMI registry. *EuroIntervention*. 2017;12:e1809–e1816.
15. Tang GHL. Tricuspid clip: step-by-step and clinical data. *Interv Cardiol Clin*. 2018;7:37–45.
17. Singh GD, Rogers JH. Mitral regurgitation. In: Kern MJ, Sorajja P, Lim MJ, eds. *The Interventional Cardiac Catheterization Handbook*. 4th ed. Philadelphia: Elsevier; 2018. 362–288.
19. Perlman G, Praz F, Puri R, et al. Transcatheter tricuspid valve repair with a new transcatheter coaptation system for the treatment of severe tricuspid regurgitation: 1-year clinical and echocardiographic results. *JACC Cardiovasc Interv*. 2017;10:1994–2003.
22. Mangieri A, Lim S, Rogers JH, et al. Percutaneous tricuspid annuloplasty. *Interv Cardiol Clin*. 2018;7:31–36.
32. Latib A, Mangieri A. Transcatheter tricuspid valve repair: new valve, new opportunities, new challenges. *J Am Coll Cardiol*. 2017;69:1807–1810.

 Additional references available online at expertconsult.com.

中文导读

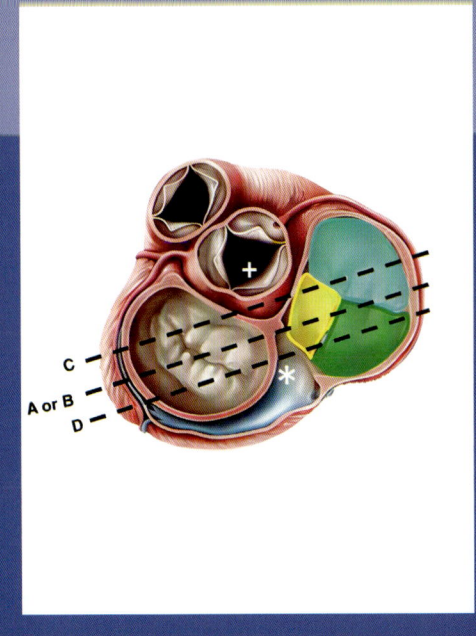

第58章
肥厚型心肌病

　　肥厚型心肌病诊断目前主要依靠超声心动图和MRI，部分患者存在梗阻性疾病，梗阻的严重程度取决于患者的负荷程度和肾上腺素能状态。

　　对有症状的患者应予以合理有效的治疗与管理，要及时评估患者心源性猝死的风险程度，对于高危人群应考虑使用植入式心脏复律除颤仪，药物治疗中β受体阻滞剂是治疗肥厚型心肌病的首选药物。

　　对于经最佳药物治疗但仍有症状的患者，肌切除术是首选治疗方法。肌切除术在经验丰富的中心死亡率可低于1%，最常见的并发症是左束支传导阻滞。当患者受限于本身的解剖结构、并发症、个人意愿或落后的医疗资源时，经皮室间隔酒精消融术提供了一种很好的替代治疗策略，可以减轻流出道梗阻症状，提高运动耐力。室间隔消融后并发症发生率较低，可与室间膈肌切除术相媲美，而合理筛选患者，尤其注意患者的解剖细节是手术成功的必要条件。

　　总之，肥厚型心肌病是一种复杂的遗传性疾病，具有多种异质性和临床表现，管理肥厚型心肌病患者应侧重于5点：①控制心力衰竭症状；②评估心源性猝死风险及予以合理的风险管理；③治疗心房颤动；④治疗符合侵入干预指针存在左室流出道梗阻的患者；⑤筛查家庭成员。

段振娅　吴永健

章节要点

- 肥厚型心肌病是一种与多种不同基因突变相关、临床表现变异很大的疾病。
- 部分患者存在梗阻性疾病，梗阻的严重程度取决于患者个体的负荷程度和肾上腺素能状态。
- 超声心动图和MRI主要用于诊断。
- 对有症状的患者进行医疗管理作为初始干预，心源性死亡高危人群应考虑植入式心脏复律除颤器。
- 对于经最佳药物治疗但仍有症状的患者，如果有经验丰富的手术团队，肌切除术是首选治疗方法。
- 当个别患者不适合接受肌切除术时，经皮室间隔酒精消融术提供了一种很好的替代治疗策略，合理筛选患者，尤其注意患者的解剖细节是手术成功的必要条件。

58 Hypertrophic Cardiomyopathy

Grant Henderson, Samir R. Kapadia

KEY POINTS

- Hypertrophic cardiomyopathy is a disease process that varies broadly in its clinical presentation and has been associated with many different genetic mutations.
- Obstructive disease is present in a subset of patients, where the severity of obstruction varies depending on loading conditions and adrenergic state in the individual patient.
- Imaging with echocardiography and magnetic resonance imaging are primarily used to make the diagnosis.
- Medical management is indicated in symptomatic patients as an initial intervention. Patients at high risk for sudden cardiac death should be considered for an implantable cardioverter-defibrillator.
- If an experienced surgical team is available, myectomy is considered to be the treatment of choice in good surgical candidates when symptoms persist despite optimal medical therapy.
- Alcohol septal ablation provides an excellent treatment option when surgical myectomy is not thought to be optimal for an individual patient. Careful attention to anatomic details and appropriate selection of patients are requisites for procedural success.

INTRODUCTION

By virtue of the broad variability in its phenotypic expression, hypertrophic cardiomyopathy (HCM) is a unique cardiovascular condition with a potential for the development of clinical symptoms during any phase of life.[1-7] The genetic foundation of HCM has been directly related to abnormalities of the genes encoding the cardiac sarcomere unit and may result in a complex disease phenotype that encompasses a spectrum of clinical and pathologic presentations. In the past, the nomenclature regarding HCM was often misleading. *Idiopathic hypertrophic subaortic stenosis* or *hypertrophic obstructive cardiomyopathy* (HOCM) typically described only a subset of patients with this disorder. With improved understanding of the clinical heterogeneity of this process, *hypertrophic cardiomyopathy* appears to be a more appropriate descriptive term.[8]

The rapid demystification of the genetic underpinnings of HCM has greatly expanded understanding of this entity. HCM is inherited in an autosomal dominant fashion, with more than 12 genes identified as being involved in the phenotypic manifestation.[9-11] Two of those genes (*MYH7* and *MYBPC3*) account for approximately half of the known cases of familial HCM.[9] Traditionally, the diagnosis of HCM has been primarily clinical, involving the use of echocardiography to evaluate for certain characteristic features such as asymmetric septal hypertrophy or systolic anterior motion of the mitral valve (SAM) with left ventricular outflow tract (LVOT) obstruction. Although there have been dramatic advances in understanding of the genetic predisposition for this disease state, the utility of genetic study for the absolute diagnosis remains preliminary. However, the future holds promise that genetics will become a more reliable tool for establishing and confirming this diagnosis.[12] The use of genotyping in risk stratification is also evolving.

Given the heterogeneity of the disease process even within the same family, its clinical course and long-term outcomes differ significantly. Therefore management strategies span the range from close outpatient follow-up to surgical remodeling of the myocardium. HCM appears to be an evolving process in some patients, and the phenotype changes with age. This presents a challenging dilemma in terms of grasping the clinical course of this disorder. Consequently, therapeutic strategies need to be individualized for each patient.

EPIDEMIOLOGY

The prevalence of this genetic disorder is estimated at 0.16% to 0.29% (≈1:625 to 1:344 individuals) in the general adult population,[9] making it one of the more common cardiac genetic disorders known. No distinct ethnic or geographic pattern of distribution has been identified. Estimating prevalence of the disease based on imaging evidence of left ventricular hypertrophy (LVH) alone may be misleading, as phenotypic expression of the underlying genetic mutations may not occur until later in life.[13,14] The clinical heterogeneity of this disorder plays into the difficulty in establishing a diagnosis. Often, the presentation lacks the classic features on echocardiography, and coexisting diagnoses that can cause myocardial hypertrophy, such as arterial hypertension and aortic stenosis, may also be present. HCM is a disease process that is known to evolve with age, and the development of LVH has been observed to occur more frequently with advancing age.[15-17] This can make diagnosis of HCM challenging and suggests that repeat evaluation at periodic intervals may be required to establish a diagnosis. Although it is not routinely accounted for in general practice, it is not uncommon to see patients with HCM in tertiary referral centers.

NATURAL HISTORY OF THE DISEASE

The heterogeneity of HCM lies not only in its varied presentations but also in its natural history in the patient population. Taking all patients with HCM into account, the disease is actually relatively benign; nearly two-thirds of patients with HCM have normal lifespans and minimal or no morbidity. However, the spectrum of disease also includes a subset of patients with severe, life-limiting symptoms including heart failure, arrhythmias, syncope, chest pain, and sudden death.[18-20]

Attempts to understand the links between genotype, phenotype, and natural history have yielded only limited clinical associations. Selection bias played a significant role in the initial attempts to characterize patient outcomes. Earlier studies from tertiary referral centers implied ominously high annual mortality rates of 3% to 6%; however, this work was limited by a significant referral bias.[1] More recent data from regional and community-based centers suggested an annual mortality rate of approximately 1.5%, and mortality has been reduced to 0.5% per year with introduction of implantable cardiac defibrillators (ICDs) to the HCM population.[21] However, in selected populations, the annual mortality rate may be as high as 5% to 6%, particularly in those symptomatic patients who are eventually referred to larger centers.[1,22,23]

The clinical course of the HCM population is often difficult to predict and poses a challenge to clinicians. Some genotype-phenotype correlations are being revealed, though the clinical usefulness of these correlations is not yet clear. For example, there is evidence that clinical phenotypes caused by the two most common HCM genes (*MYH7* and *MYBPC3*) cause more cardiomyocyte hypertrophy and less risk of systolic dysfunction than those caused by genes affecting thin myofilament proteins (e.g., *TNNT2*).[24,25]

The most feared and least predictable clinical manifestation is sudden cardiac death (SCD), particularly in the younger population. More commonly, patients develop symptoms such as angina, syncope, or exertional dyspnea. These symptoms can become progressively worse over time, and such patients can progress toward end-stage heart failure with failure of the left ventricle (LV). HCM patients may also develop atrial fibrillation (AF), putting them at risk for embolic strokes. Many HCM patients remain asymptomatic and have a comparably normal life expectancy. However, at some point even they are at risk for the development of SCD or AF. The challenge for clinicians is to closely monitor those who eventually develop symptoms and to offer timely therapy when it is indicated.

CLINICAL PRESENTATION

Although the spectrum of clinical presentation in HCM is large, most patients are actually asymptomatic and are diagnosed as the result of a murmur on examination, an abnormal electrocardiogram (ECG), or unexplained LVH discovered by echocardiography. The complex pathophysiologic interplay among LVOT obstruction, diastolic dysfunction, myocardial ischemia, arrhythmias, and mitral regurgitation typically results in the presenting complaints of exertional dyspnea, chest discomfort, syncope or near syncope, and SCD. Symptomatic patients who will have an adverse clinical course typically follow one of several pathways: (1) those at high risk for SCD; (2) progressive symptoms of exertional dyspnea and chest pain associated with presyncope or syncope in the setting of preserved LV function; (3) development of progressive congestive heart failure due to severe LV remodeling, which results in systolic dysfunction; and (4) consequences of supraventricular or ventricular arrhythmias such as AF or ventricular tachycardia (VT).[26-28]

SCD is the most common source of mortality attributable to HCM, despite occurring in only a small minority of identified HCM patients (~5%).[29] In addition, SCD is the single leading cause of cardiovascular death among young people as well as the most common cause of mortality in competitive athletes.[30] It is most commonly observed in asymptomatic children and young adults, and it appears that there is no advanced age at which the risk of SCD becomes negligible.[31] Whereas SCD is the most feared and dramatic complication of HCM, those at high risk for SCD actually constitute only a small fraction of the disease spectrum, and much effort has been devoted to the premorbid identification of this subset of patients.[32,33] Currently identified risk factors for SCD include prior cardiac arrest or sustained VT, family history of SCD, unexplained syncope or near syncope, LV thickness greater than 30 mm, hypotensive response during exercise stress testing, and nonsustained VT on Holter monitoring (Table 58.1).[32,34-39] In addition, an LVOT gradient greater than 30 mm Hg has been associated with an increased risk of SCD, progression to heart failure, and morbidity related to arrhythmia, including stroke.[40,41] However, an incremental increase in the subaortic gradient above 30 mm Hg has not been demonstrated to impart any additional risk. It is uncommon for HCM patients to suffer SCD without at least one of the aforementioned risk factors (<3%), though risk of SCD does not differ with respect to number of risk factors present.[32] There does appear to be a subset of HCM patients without the aforementioned conventional risk factors who are at risk for SCD, underscoring the importance of identifying additional markers of risk. In this regard, it has been shown that extensive late gadolinium enhancement (LGE) by cardiac magnetic resonance imaging (CMRI) is associated with increased risk of SCD in HCM, including in patients without traditional risk factors. LV apical aneurysm, elevated LVOT gradient, and end-stage heart failure with systolic dysfunction and ventricular remodeling may represent other SCD risk factors.[29,42] It has been suggested that the etiology of SCD in this population is related to the development of complex ventricular tachyarrhythmia,[43,44] often during mild to moderate physical exertion and with a circadian predilection for the early morning hours.[45]

TABLE 58.1 Risk Factors for Sudden Cardiac Death

Spontaneous sustained VT
Multiple prolonged or repetitive episodes of nonsustained VT (>3 beats at rate of >120 beats/min) on ambulatory monitoring
Family history of cardiac arrest or SCD
Prior personal history of cardiac arrest
Unexplained syncope (especially if exertional)
Abnormal response to exercise stress testing (especially hypotension)
LV thickness >30 mm
Younger age[a]
Late gadolinium enhancement of >15% LV mass on cardiac magnetic resonance imaging[a]
LV apical aneurysm[a]
End-stage hypertrophic cardiomyopathy (left ventricular ejection fraction <50%)[a]

[a]Direct relationship with SCD less well established.
CHF, Congestive heart failure; *LV*, left ventricle; *LVOT*, left ventricular outflow tract; *SCD*, sudden cardiac death; *VT*, ventricular tachycardia.

Chest pain, both typical and atypical in character, is a common feature in HCM and has been reported in up to 80% of patients in this population.[46] In many cases, angiography reveals normal coronary arteries. Despite this finding, numerous studies incorporating nuclear single-photon emission computed tomography (SPECT), positron emission tomography (PET), and magnetic resonance imaging (MRI) technologies have demonstrated significant reversible and nonreversible myocardial perfusion defects in this subset of patients, including autopsy findings of myocardial infarction in up to 15% of such patients.[46-50]

Collectively, these data have led to a mounting body of evidence suggesting that microvascular dysfunction may have a pivotal role in the development of myocardial ischemia and infarction in this group. The etiology of microvascular dysfunction is probably multifactorial and due in part to arteriolar medial hypertrophy, which results in reduced luminal diameter, impaired coronary vasodilatory response, and a supply-demand mismatch due to an abnormally thickened ventricle.[51] In addition, early work has suggested that evidence of microvascular dysfunction, as demonstrated by PET, is an independent predictor of increased mortality and may portend a worse prognosis years before the development of clinical deterioration.[47,52]

Syncope in patients with HCM is not an uncommon phenomenon and has a diverse array of possible etiologies, making the exact determination of mechanism challenging. Whereas it is regarded as an ominous prognostic sign and a known risk factor for SCD in the younger population, syncope in the adult population has not been independently associated with premature death, and recurrent episodes are rarely reported in patients who have suffered SCD.[27,53,54] Arrhythmic sources of syncope may be supraventricular (e.g., AF or flutter) or ventricular (e.g., VT or fibrillation). Hemodynamic mechanisms of syncope all result in a sudden and severe reduction in cardiac output that may involve ischemia, outflow tract obstruction, or severe diastolic dysfunction. Additionally, it has been suggested that activation of LV baroreceptors due to elevated intracavitary pressures may induce reflex hypotension and a consequent syncopal episode in a selected subgroup of patients.[55]

Heart failure—as manifested by a symptom complex of exertional dyspnea, orthopnea, and progressive fatigue—is most commonly encountered in adult patients with HCM, but it has been described in the juvenile population as well.[1] Usually, in the setting of preserved systolic function, symptoms are most commonly the consequence of diastolic dysfunction due to an abnormally thickened and noncompliant ventricle.[56] The combined influence of other variables such as ischemia, AF, and mitral regurgitation may also play a significant role in the development of hemodynamic decompensation in this population. A smaller number of patients with HCM and heart failure may have significantly reduced LV systolic function and chamber enlargement. It is important to recognize this subset of patients, given the potential alteration in therapeutic strategy.[27]

AF complicates the course of approximately 20% of patients with HCM and is associated with an increased risk of heart failure–related death.[36] The risk seems to be substantially greater in the subset of patients with outflow tract obstruction or an earlier onset of arrhythmia (<50 years of age). Advanced age, left atrial enlargement, and congestive symptoms are independently linked with the development of AF. Although it is strongly associated with an increased risk of fatal and nonfatal stroke, AF does not appear to be a risk factor for the development of SCD, and approximately one-third of patients have no long-term sequelae from this arrhythmia.[36]

Severe functional deterioration due to dyspnea, chest pain, palpitations, or pulmonary edema may complicate the course of the chronically affected. This is most likely caused by the loss of atrial contraction, reduction in diastolic filling time, and exacerbation of underlying ischemia.[56]

The nature of the clinical presentation may also be affected by a particular patient's age or gender. In contrast to their younger counterparts, older adult patients with HCM often develop marked symptomatology at an advanced age (>55 years), have lesser degrees of LVH usually confined to the septum, and have a dynamic subaortic gradient due to restricted excursion of the often anteriorly displaced mitral leaflets and posteriorly directed septal motion.[57] Whereas HCM seems to have a male predominance, female patients often are diagnosed at a later age, are more symptomatic, and are at a greater risk of death due to heart failure or stroke.[58]

DIAGNOSIS

Echocardiography

Given its safety and ubiquity, two-dimensional echocardiography is the most common method for establishing the clinical diagnosis of HCM via identification of a thickened, nondilated LV in the absence of comorbidities known to cause such a degree of LVH (i.e., hypertension, aortic stenosis, or physiologic hypertrophy of athletes).[56,59] Although LVH was classically thought to involve primarily the ventricular septum, its morphologic expression is extremely heterogeneous, and virtually any pattern of thickening may be observed.[60] In addition, there are significant differences in the pattern of hypertrophy between young and elderly patients. Elderly patients are often found to have an *elliptical* ventricular cavity with hypertrophy predominantly of the basal septum. In contrast, younger patients (<55 years) often have a crescent-shaped ventricular cavity associated with diffuse hypertrophy of the interventricular septum.[61]

Whereas a maximal wall thickness greater than 15 mm is the traditional echocardiographic benchmark for HCM, the degree of hypertrophy exhibits considerable variability (with a mean thickness of approximately 22 mm).[59,60] It is important to realize, however, that lack of characteristic LVH (>15 mm) on echocardiographic examination *does not* exclude the presence of an HCM gene mutation.[24,62] Therefore serial echocardiographic assessment may be necessary for adequate identification of suspected carriers, especially in the younger population, in whom the development of LVH may be delayed until after puberty.[56]

LVOT obstruction is observed in approximately two-thirds of patients with HCM and is usually dynamic in nature.[63] Subaortic obstruction is due to SAM of the anterior mitral leaflet, which results in mitral-septal contact during midsystole. Obstruction may not be present under resting conditions but can be provoked by pharmacologic (i.e., amyl nitrite) or physiologic (i.e., Valsalva) maneuvers. Significant mitral regurgitation frequently accompanies SAM owing to distortion of the valvular apparatus and malcoaptation of the anterior and posterior leaflets (Figs. 58.1 and 58.2).

Primary abnormalities of the mitral valve and associated structures are also commonly observed in HCM, including leaflet elongation, papillary muscle hypertrophy, and abnormal origins or insertions of papillary muscles.[56] Mitral regurgitation is also observed in up to 30% of patients who do not demonstrate obstructive physiology; it is primarily caused by leaflet prolapse, chordal rupture, or trauma resulting in calcification or fibrosis.[15] Less commonly, a midcavitary gradient is formed because of the anomalous insertion of the anterolateral papillary muscle directly onto the anterior mitral leaflet or an exaggerated proliferation of midventricular papillary musculature coming into apposition with the ventricular septum.[64]

Whereas the threshold for therapeutic intervention has traditionally been a gradient of greater than 50 mm Hg, it has been demonstrated that the presence of a resting LVOT gradient of 30 mm Hg or greater is an independent predictor of death from heart failure or stroke, progression of heart failure symptoms, and reduced functional capacity as well as SCD.[10] It is important not to misinterpret the Doppler spectral display of mitral regurgitation as an LVOT gradient, given its frequent presence in the setting of obstruction and its close spatial orientation to the LVOT. In the setting of SAM, mitral regurgitation is usually posteriorly directed into the left atrium and is often difficult to distinguish from LVOT flow. It is most useful to sweep anterior to posterior with continuous Doppler imaging to distinguish these two flows.

Given the magnitude of LVH associated with HCM, it is not surprising that more than 80% of patients have evidence of diastolic dysfunction by echocardiogram. This is manifested by reduced maximal flow velocity in early diastole, an increase in isovolumic relaxation time, and an increased atrial contribution to ventricular filling.[65] These findings are similar in patients with and without an LVOT gradient or cardiac symptoms, suggesting that diastolic dysfunction may be an earlier clinical manifestation in the spectrum of this disease process. Several studies have suggested that the presence of significant diastolic dysfunction by transthoracic or tissue Doppler echocardiography implies an increased risk of cardiac arrest, VT, or progression to significant cardiac symptoms.[66]

Electrocardiography

ECG findings in HCM are extremely heterogeneous, and most patients (>90%) have demonstrable abnormalities.[56,67,68] However, no pattern is highly specific for the condition, and the presence of a normal tracing does not imply absence of the disease state.[67] Increased voltages consistent with LVH and early

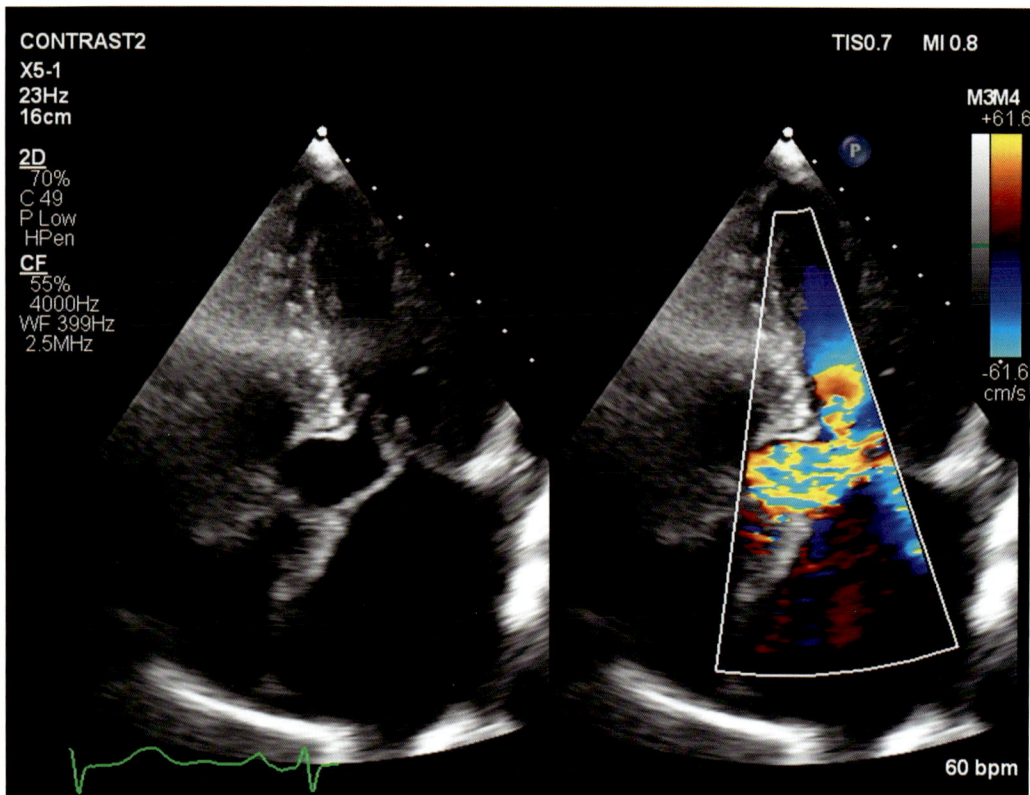

Fig. 58.1 Posteriorly directed mitral regurgitation accompanying systolic anterior motion of the anterior mitral leaflet in hypertrophic cardiomyopathy, visualized with two-dimensional and Doppler echocardiography.

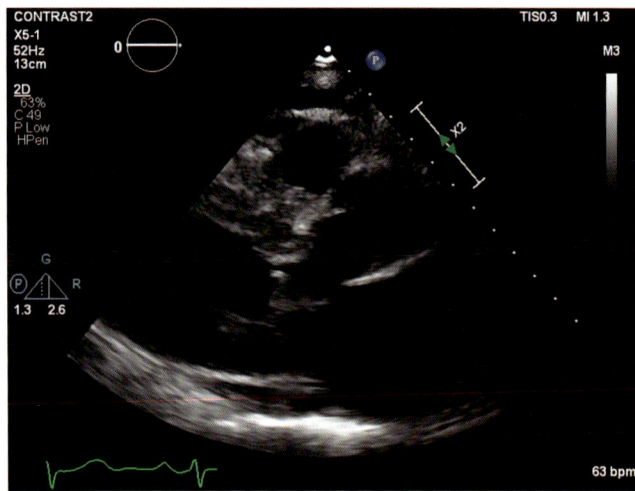

Fig. 58.2 Systolic anterior motion of the mitral valve visualized with two-dimensional echocardiography in the parasternal long axis.

repolarization abnormalities are most commonly encountered; left axis deviation, left atrial enlargement, T-wave inversion, and nonspecific ST-segment abnormalities are also frequently observed. The degree of LVH by ECG does not appear to correlate with the magnitude of hypertrophy when assessed by echocardiography.[17]

In a subset of Japanese patients with hypertrophy primarily limited to the ventricular apex, giant T-wave inversions were frequently seen in the anterior leads; these are often termed Yamaguchi disease.[69] Pathologic Q waves, often in the inferolateral leads, may be observed in up to 50% of patients with known HCM. Although it is not apparent on the surface ECG, approximately one-third of patients have delayed His-Purkinje conduction on formal electrophysiologic studies, possibly owing to strain on the anterior fasciculus, which lies within the hypertrophied ventricle.[68]

Magnetic Resonance Imaging

In comparison with traditional echocardiography, CMRI offers the advantages of superior resolution with precise morphologic characterization, enhanced tissue contrast capability, and production of three-dimensional images.[70,71] As a result, CMRI can better detect areas of hypertrophy that are not well visualized or are missed by traditional echocardiography. Particularly in patients with atypical hypertrophy of the anterolateral free wall, CMRI is a powerful adjunctive tool in the diagnosis of HCM.[71] Besides more accurate and reliable measurements of LV wall thickness, CMRI is superior to traditional echocardiography in identifying patients with LV apical aneurysm, which confers higher risk of adverse clinical outcomes.[72]

Through delayed hyperenhancement techniques, CMRI has demonstrated that asymptomatic patients with HCM frequently have patchy foci of myocardial scarring at the junction of the interventricular septum and the right ventricular free wall. Furthermore, scarring is limited to the areas of abnormal hypertrophy, and the degree of scarring is proportional to the magnitude of hypertrophy, whereas wall thickening was inversely related.[48] In addition, a greater extent of hyperenhancement has been positively associated with high risk for SCD and with progressive disease.[73]

CMRI also allows for better characterization of papillary muscle insertion and orientation. It is not uncommon to see hypertrophic, displaced, or distorted papillary muscles contributing to the obstruction or to mitral valve dysfunction. Assessment of mitral valve anatomy may be critical before the treatment plan for relief of obstruction is chosen, because patients with mitral valve anomalies are best treated with the use of myectomy rather than ablation. Considering all these facts, CMRI is a valuable adjunctive imaging modality for the diagnosis of HCM.

Exercise Echocardiography

Exercise echocardiography has been shown to be an important and safe component of the comprehensive evaluation of patients with HCM, particularly in those patients without a resting LVOT gradient. A patient's clinical course, and likelihood to progress to New York Heart Association (NYHA) functional class III or IV heart failure, can be predicted based on the presence or absence of an exercise-provoked LVOT gradient. Furthermore, in symptomatic HCM patients without a resting LVOT gradient, exercise echocardiography can be used to predict response to therapies such as surgical myectomy and alcohol septal ablation.[74]

Catheterization and Hemodynamics

Given the wealth of hemodynamic and anatomic data that can be derived noninvasively by echocardiography, cardiac catheterization is not required for the diagnosis of HCM. Catheterization is often used, however, if noninvasive imaging is of insufficient quality to quantify the degree or location of obstruction, to evaluate for coronary disease before a planned surgical therapy (i.e., myectomy or pacemaker implantation), or if anginal symptoms that may be attributable to ischemia are present in older patients.

The coronary arteries in patients with HCM are usually normal and typically of large caliber. Quite different from intramyocardial "bridging," compression of the left anterior descending (LAD) coronary artery may be observed during systole due to contraction of the hypertrophied ventricle, which results in a "sawfish" appearance.[75] Ventriculography may demonstrate systolic cavity obliteration, varying degrees of mitral regurgitation, and occasionally the hypertrophied septum prolapsing into the LVOT. Direct measurement and localization of the gradient is easily obtained by passing a multipurpose catheter into the apical portion of the LV and slowly withdrawing it while continuously monitoring the pressure waveform. Use of a wire via a guide catheter often results in increased control during the pullback and a more accurate determination of the level of obstruction. Contrary to what is observed in aortic stenosis, the gradient is noted before the aortic valve is crossed. This same technique can be performed using simultaneous aortic and LV pressure waveforms to allow side-by-side comparison.

The gradient in HCM is characteristically labile and various pharmacological and physiologic maneuvers may be employed to accentuate the obstruction in the catheterization laboratory, similar to those used with echocardiography. The term *postextrasystolic potentiation*,[76,77] or *Brockenbrough-Braunwald-Morrow sign*, refers to the augmentation of LV pressure with a concomitant decrement in aortic systolic and pulse pressures as a result of increased LVOT obstruction in the cardiac cycle that follows a premature ventricular contraction. Postextrasystolic increase in the gradient between LV and aorta is also seen with aortic stenosis, but, unlike the case in HCM, the pulse pressure (stroke volume) does not decrease. This is because in aortic stenosis, the larger stroke volume of the postextrasystolic beat leads to a higher gradient with no change in the severity of obstruction (Fig. 58.3).

Genetic Overview

HCM is the result of mutations in genes primarily encoding sarcomeric proteins that regulate contractile, regulatory, and structural functions; they are inherited in an autosomal dominant manner.[9,11,78] More than 1400 mutations involving 20 or more genes have been described, the most common of which include the cardiac troponins T, C, and I; cardiac myosin-binding protein C; cardiac β- and α-myosin heavy chains; myosin ventricular essential and regulatory light chains; cardiac α-actin; and titin.[9,79] Whereas most of these mutations are missense, resulting from substitution of an incorrect amino acid, deletions, insertions, and splice-site mutations are also well described.[80]

Several nonsarcomeric mutations that produce phenotypes similar to HCM have been identified. *PRKAG2* affects the regulatory subunit of the adenosine monophosphate (AMP)-activated protein kinase and may result in preexcitation, progressive conduction system abnormalities, and mild ventricular hypertrophy due to aberrant accumulation of glycogen within the myocyte.[80,81] Mutations of 2α-galactosidase or acid-α1,4-glucosidase (both of which are lysosome-associated membrane proteins) frequently result in multisystem glycogen storage disease and may also cause extreme LVH associated with ventricular preexcitation and mental retardation.[82]

There is great phenotypic heterogeneity among carriers of the same mutations, in part because of the effect of modifier genes and environmental factors.[9] Whereas it has long been known that many young carriers do not demonstrate the morphologic characteristics of the disease state until after adolescence, it has now been demonstrated that phenotypic expression of LVH can be delayed into late adulthood owing to incomplete penetrance of mutations involving cardiac myosin-binding protein C or troponin T.[83] The majority of studied HCM cases have involved familial mutations, but sporadic cases are also well described and may constitute a significant proportion of the population. Recent work involving the systematic molecular screening of known HCM cases has demonstrated that two mutations (*MYBPC3* and *MYH7*) account for the majority of familial cases. Mutations were detected in up to 60% of sporadic cases.[11] These data imply that a relatively limited screening process may be sufficient to identify the culprit gene in most familial cases and that identifiable mutations are responsible for most sporadic cases.

Given the fact that a number of studies have identified specific genetic mutations (Table 58.2) seemingly associated with a worse clinical prognosis and higher rates of SCD, there was initial enthusiasm that genetic testing could prospectively identify patients at higher risk for premature death. However, significant limitations, including selection bias, the small number of included familial cohorts, low frequency of specific gene mutations, and variability of the phenotypic product, have hindered most genotype-phenotype correlation studies.[9,84] Therefore because of the numerous genetic and environmental influences affecting the phenotypic product, there remains a great deal of clinical heterogeneity associated with specific mutations, making accurate risk stratification based on genetic analysis alone impractical at this time.

Despite the questionable practicality of using genetic testing for risk stratification, it remains an important part of clinical management in at least two scenarios for HCM patients. First, HCM patients should be screened for known causal mutations in the event they have first-degree relatives who may be affected by the disease. If a known pathogenic mutation is discovered in the patient, family members may be screened for the same mutation, thus elucidating their risk of developing clinical manifestations. This in turn can guide planning of follow-up examinations and discussions regarding participation in competitive sports for family members of affected patients. Second, patients with atypical clinical features can undergo genetic testing to evaluate for a nonsarcomeric genetic mutation (causing so-called "phenocopy" conditions). Recognition of these diseases is important as natural history varies from that of HCM and additional management strategies may be available (e.g., enzyme replacement therapy in Fabry disease).[85]

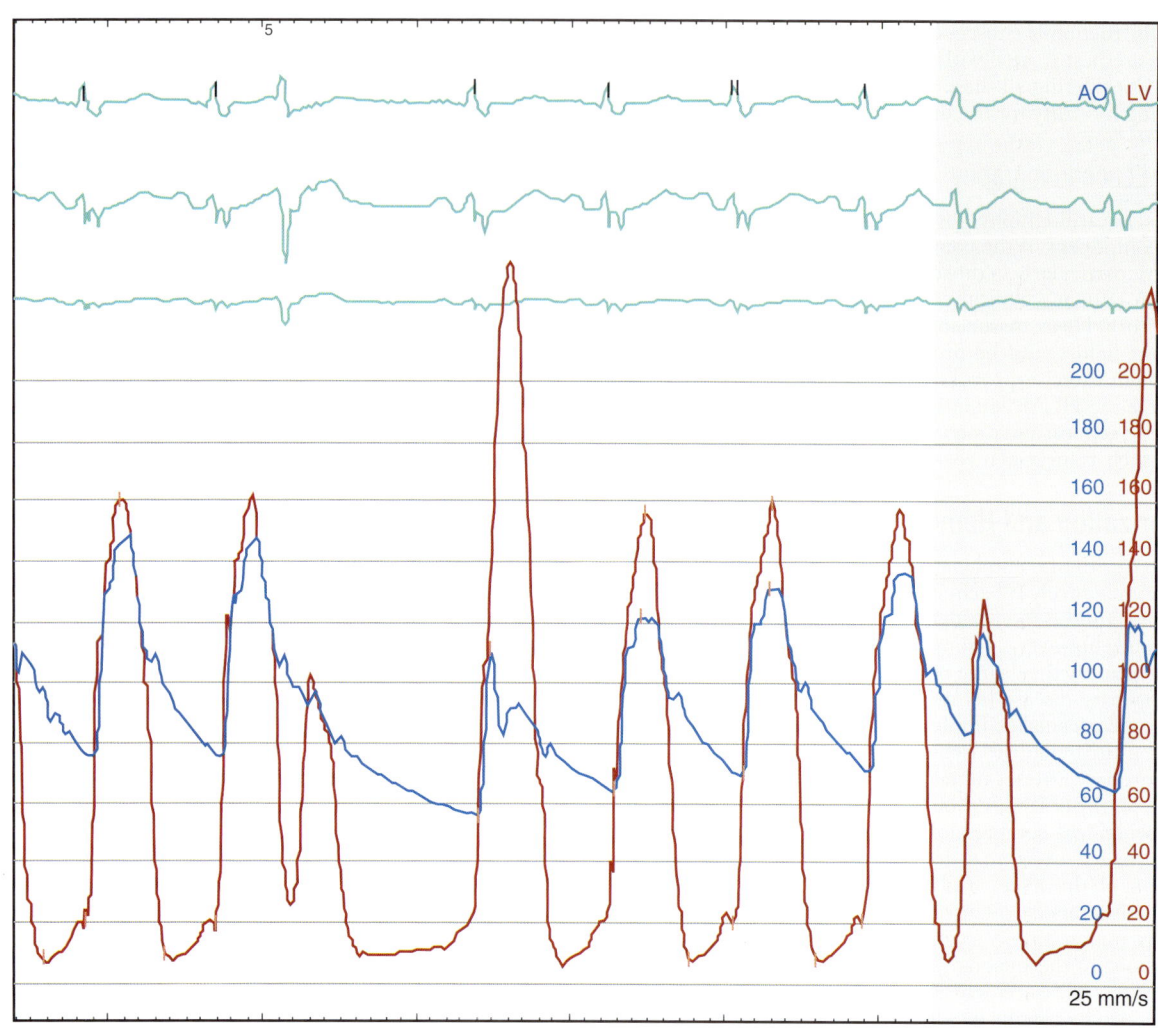

Fig. 58.3 The Brockenbrough–Braunwald–Morrow sign, signifying postextrasystolic potentiation of the left ventricular outflow tract gradient. An increase in left ventricular systolic pressure is accompanied by a decrease in the arterial pulse pressure, due to exacerbation of the dynamic outflow gradient after increased diastolic filling time after a premature ventricular contraction in a patient with hypertrophic cardiomyopathy. The red tracing represents left ventricular pressure, and the blue tracing represents aortic pressure. *Ao*, Aorta; *LV*, left ventricle.

TABLE 58.2 Established Causal Genes in Hypertrophic Cardiomyopathy

β-Myosin heavy chain 14q12 *MYH7* 30–40
Myosin binding protein C 11q1 *MYBPC3* 30–40
Cardiac troponin T 1q32 *TNNT2* 15–20
Cardiac troponin I 19q13.4 *TNNI3* 1–5
α-Tropomyosin 15q22.1 *TPM1* 1–5
Myosin essential light chain 3p21 *MYL3* <1
Myosin regulatory light chain 12q24.3 *MYL2* <1
Cysteine and glycine rich protein 3 11p15.1 *CSRP3* rare
Actin 15q14 *ACTC1* rare

Modified from Marian AJ, Braunwald E. Hypertrophic cardiomyopathy: genetics, pathogenesis, clinical manifestations, diagnosis, and therapy. *Circ Res*. 2017;121(7):749–770. https://doi.org/10.1161/CIRCRESAHA.117.311059.

TREATMENT

Medical Therapy

Medical therapy should be considered the initial therapeutic approach for the treatment of symptoms arising from the numerous pathophysiologic processes constituting HCM. Because of the relatively small number of cases, pharmacologic therapy for HCM is largely based on expert opinion, clinical experience, and retrospective observational analyses. Although patients with LVOT obstruction make up the greatest proportion of the symptomatic population, a significant number of patients without obstruction may also suffer the consequences of diastolic dysfunction, such as heart failure, angina, and AF.[1,56] Given the increasing use of early genetic and echocardiographic screening of athletes and affected families, it has become apparent that a significant percentage of phenotypically affected patients are entirely asymptomatic for an extended time. The available data also suggest that this population does not warrant empirical therapy until and unless symptoms develop.[56] Historically, the pharmacologic treatment of HCM has been limited to β-blockers, verapamil, and disopyramide.

Pharmacotherapy

β-Adrenergic Receptor Blocking Agents

β-Blockers have traditionally been the drugs of choice for the treatment of HCM. This may stem from the fact that the physiologic effects of these agents are well suited to address much of the problematic pathophysiology encountered in this population. Their negative chronotropic effect results in increased diastolic filling time, which reduces left atrial pressure and may improve congestive symptoms related to diastolic dysfunction. This is especially true in cases complicated by supraventricular arrhythmias such as AF. The negative inotropic effect of these agents results in reduced myocardial oxygen consumption with a resultant decrease in anginal symptoms.

Although there is no convincing evidence that β-blockers effectively reduce *resting* LVOT gradients, prior work and a large amount of clinical experience suggest that these agents reduce provocable gradients as well as substantially improving disabling symptoms related to exertion.[86,87] This is supported by data demonstrating an inverse relationship between peak oxygen consumption (VO$_2$) and degree of LVOT obstruction during cardiopulmonary exercise testing.[88] As a result, β-blockers as a class are the favored agents for patients with *latent* outflow tract obstruction.

The first agent initially used for the treatment of HCM, propranolol, has largely been replaced by newer-generation, longer-acting, nonselective β-blocking agents including atenolol, bisoprolol, and metoprolol.[87] Given the significant heterogeneity in clinical symptomatology, even within the same patient at different times in the disease course, it is important to individualize the titration of therapy based on current symptoms, resting heart rate (goal of 50 to 60 beats/min), exertional capacity, and the presence of untoward side effects.

Verapamil

Functioning both as a negative inotrope and a negative chronotrope by blocking the intracellular migration of calcium ions, the nondihydropyridine calcium channel blocking agent verapamil produces symptomatic improvement in patients with HCM through increased diastolic filling time and enhanced diastolic ventricular relaxation without negatively affecting systolic function and while ensuring reduced myocardial oxygen consumption.[56,89,90] In addition, verapamil has been shown to increase absolute myocardial blood flow during pharmacologic stress testing while also reducing ischemic burden and improving exercise tolerance in the asymptomatic patient population.[91,92] These effects may result from verapamil's enhanced vasodilatory properties, which are more pronounced than those seen with β-blockade and may well explain this agent's superior efficacy in patients with chest pain.

Whereas verapamil has classically been used in both obstructing and nonobstructing disease, caution should be exercised in initiating this agent in symptomatic patients with large resting gradients owing to well-documented reports of severe hemodynamic decompensation resulting in cardiogenic shock and pulmonary edema.[56,87]

Approximately 5% of patients with HCM will progress to an end stage characterized by impaired systolic function and symptoms of heart failure. Standard therapy for congestive heart failure—including diuretics, cautious use of vasodilators, β-blockers, avoidance of calcium channel blockers, and possibly digoxin—should constitute the pharmacologic regimen in these patients.[1,56] In symptomatic patients, it is common clinical practice to initiate therapy with β-blockers rather than verapamil. Should the patient be intolerant of side effects (i.e., fatigue, depression, or impotence), or if symptoms persist despite adequate titration of the medication, consideration should be given to changing (or adding) therapy to verapamil.[56] At present, no data suggest that combination therapy is more effective than either a β-blocker or verapamil alone.

Disopyramide

Disopyramide, a class IA antiarrhythmic agent, has a side-effect profile that includes a negative inotropic effect with reduced contractility and a reflexive increase in systemic vascular resistance, both of which have made it an attractive agent for the treatment of HCM for more than 30 years. Although it appears to have little or no effect on diastolic function, disopyramide has been shown to effectively reduce the outflow obstruction resulting from SAM, with improved symptomatic control in patients with resting gradients for whom other forms of therapy have failed.[93,94] Because of the possible potentiation of supraventricular arrhythmias such as AF and case reports of QT prolongation leading to torsades de pointes, close supervision and monitoring are essential during the initiation of this therapy.[95] Other side effects of disopyramide are primarily related to its anticholinergic properties; they include dry mouth (32%), urinary retention (14%), constipation (11%), and, rarely, hypoglycemia. The anticholinergic effects of disopyramide can be managed safely with the use of pyridostigmine, a cholinesterase inhibitor.[87]

Amiodarone

Previous data suggested that amiodarone may reduce the risk of SCD and improve survival in selected high-risk patients who have nonsustained VT on Holter monitoring.[96] However, later reports suggested that amiodarone may improve a patient's symptom score and functional status but may also be proarrhythmic and thus lead to an *increased* risk of SCD due to ventricular arrhythmia.[97,98] In contrast, more recent data indicate that lower-dose amiodarone (200 mg/day) in high-risk patients with recurrent nonsustained VT is not associated with any increase in cardiovascular mortality.[37] Amiodarone has been demonstrated to be effective for the treatment and prevention of ventricular arrhythmias in patients with HCM.[99] There is, however, substantial observational evidence and expert consensus opinion suggesting lack of efficacy in preventing SCD with antiarrhythmic drugs, including amiodarone, in HCM patients, and thus amiodarone should not be used for the sole indication of preventing SCD.[29,100] Selection of which patients are appropriate for chronic, long-term empirical therapy with this agent, especially considering its attendant side-effect profile, may be impossible to specify until more definitive trial data become available.

Dual-Chamber Pacing

Dual-chamber pacing, as a less invasive alternative to surgical septal myectomy, was met with initial enthusiasm in the early 1990s, when several observational and uncontrolled studies demonstrated a significant decrease in outflow gradient, reduced symptomatology with improved quality of life, and homogenous redistribution of myocardial perfusion reserve.[101,102] Although the exact mechanism is unclear, it has been proposed that activation of the right ventricular apex results in a dyssynchronous contraction of the septum with a reduction in outflow tract obstruction in the short term and a positive ventricular remodeling effect in the long term.[103] However, subsequent randomized controlled crossover trials comparing DDD-mode with AAI-mode pacing demonstrated a significant placebo effect in regard to sustained symptomatic relief and quality-of-life assessment, little improvement in functional capacity, and a more modest reduction in outflow gradient in most patients compared with the earlier uncontrolled trials.[104,105]

Of importance, a subpopulation of older adult patients (age >65 years) was objectively measured to have both symptomatic and clinical benefit as a result of DDD pacing.[104] During the same period, a randomized trial did demonstrate a significant improvement in exercise tolerance, symptom score, and LVOT gradient in patients with symptoms refractory to drug therapy and with resting gradients greater than 30 mm Hg.[105] Therefore there may be subsets of patients in whom dual-chamber pacing is of some symptomatic or clinical benefit. However, no data suggest that dual-chamber pacing effectively reduces the risk of SCD in this patient population.[101,104]

Further work suggests that the reduction in LVOT gradient depends on optimal timing of the atrioventricular interval, with too short an interval interfering with diastolic filling and left atrial emptying and too long an interval resulting in ineffective reduction of outflow obstruction.[106] Taking this into account, recent nonrandomized, observational data have demonstrated a significant reduction in symptoms, improved functional capacity, and consistent reduction in LVOT gradient when serial echocardiographic assessment was used to optimize the atrioventricular interval, pacing rate, and mode settings in patients using DDD pacemakers.[107] This may constitute the foundation for further randomized trials in this area.

Whereas data comparing dual-chamber pacing with surgical septal myectomy have demonstrated improvement in both groups in regard to functional status, a significantly greater reduction in LVOT gradient, improved subjective symptom status, and increased overall exercise duration was reported in patients who underwent myectomy.[108] Therefore, although it is not considered a primary therapeutic modality for most patients with symptomatic HCM, it has been suggested that the use of dual-chamber pacemakers may be reasonable in certain subsets of patients, including older adult patients averse to more invasive therapies and patients in whom pharmacotherapy is limited owing to bradycardia.[56,59]

Implantation of an Implantable Cardiac Defibrillator

Ventricular fibrillation or tachycardia is the primary mode of SCD in patients with HCM. Given the success of ICDs in reducing arrhythmic mortality in patients with coronary artery disease and a reduced ejection fraction, there has been an increasing interest in using the ICD for prevention and treatment of HCM-related arrhythmic death.[109] Although randomized data are lacking, a multicenter, retrospective trial demonstrated that implantation of an ICD in patients classically considered to be at high risk for SCD resulted in appropriate device intervention and aborted SCD in almost 25% of the enrolled patients over a 3-year period.[44] Patients in whom the device was implanted for primary prevention purposes experienced appropriate intervention at a rate of 5% annually, compared with patients who received the device after cardiac arrest or sustained VT, in whom appropriate intervention was noted at a rate of 11% annually. Based on these results, it has been suggested that ICD implantation is reasonable, should be considered in patients with one or more risk factors for SCD, and is warranted in patients with a prior history of cardiac arrest or sustained VT.[56]

Device selection should be based primarily on individual patient preference and characteristics. Dual-chamber devices have the advantage of atrial sensing and pacing functions and the ability to discriminate supraventricular from ventricular arrhythmias, resulting in a reduction in the number of inappropriate interventions. However, the dual-chamber devices have a higher potential for complications (usually related to the transvenous lead systems) than do single-chamber devices.[110]

According to the most recent guidelines from the American College of Cardiology and American Heart Association (ACC/AHA), ICD implantation is recommended for patients with prior documented cardiac arrest, ventricular fibrillation, or hemodynamically significant VT (class I). In addition, it may be reasonable to consider an ICD in patients with HCM under the following circumstances[56]:

- Sudden death presumably caused by HCM in one or more first-degree relatives (class IIa)
- Maximal LV wall thickness 30 mm or greater (class IIa)
- One or more recent, unexplained syncopal episodes (class IIa)
- Nonsustained VT (particularly before 30 years of age), in the presence of other SCD risk factors (class IIa)
- Abnormal blood pressure response to exercise, in the presence of other SCD risk factors (class IIa)

It may be reasonable to consider ICD implantation in high-risk children with HCM, based on unexplained syncope, massive LV hypertrophy, or a family history of SCD, after taking into account the relatively high rate of complications of long-term ICD implantation (class IIa).

The usefulness of ICD is uncertain in specific scenarios, especially when only one risk factor is present. The usefulness of ICD implantation is considered uncertain in patients with HCM who have isolated bursts of nonsustained VT in the absence of other SCD risk factors (class IIb). Likewise, the usefulness of ICD implantation is uncertain in patients with an abnormal blood pressure response to exercise in the absence of other risk factors (class IIb). ICD implantation is not recommended as a routine strategy in patients who have no indication of increased risk for SCD (class III). In addition, ICD implantation in patients with HCM in the absence of clinical manifestations of HCM is potentially harmful and should not be performed (class III). Furthermore, ICD placement as a strategy to permit patients with HCM to participate in intense competitive athletics is not recommended (class III).[56]

Among those who meet indications for ICD placement, single-chamber devices are reasonable in younger patients who do not need atrial or ventricular pacing (class IIa). Dual-chamber ICD implantation should be considered for patients with sinus bradycardia or paroxysmal AF (class IIa). Among patients with HCM who meet indications for ICD implantation, dual-chamber ICD may be reasonable in those with an LVOT gradient greater than 50 mm Hg and significant heart failure symptoms who may benefit from right ventricular pacing (most commonly patients older than 65 years of age) (class IIa). In addition, ICD implantation should be considered in all patients with NYHA class III to IV symptoms on maximal medical therapy and an ejection fraction of 50% or less who do not have any other indication for an ICD (class IIb).[56]

Surgery

Patients with resting or provocable gradients greater than 50 mm Hg who continue to experience significant functional limitation (i.e., NYHA class III to IV) due to limiting symptoms of exertional dyspnea, chest pain, or recurrent syncope despite maximal medical therapy may be considered candidates for surgical therapy.[56,85] Surgical therapy is not currently recommended for patients who are without significant outflow tract obstruction, for those who have relatively mild symptoms with obstruction, or to treat associated complications of this condition (e.g., AF, syncope) alone.[56]

There has been a significant evolution in the spectrum of surgical therapy for HOCM designed to effectively reduce outflow tract obstruction, from the original isolated septal myotomy performed by Cleland[111] in the 1960s to the more modern and widely employed Morrow myectomy[112] in combination with mitral valve repair or even replacement in selected patients. The "gold standard" septal myectomy, described by Morrow, is performed via an aortotomy so that the proximal septum is approachable via the aortic valve. Between 5 and 15 g of myocardial tissue is resected, from the base of the aortic valve to a region distal to the mitral leaflets, such that the area of mitral-septal contact that results in SAM is removed and the LVOT is enlarged.[112,113] Because it is of critical importance to correctly identify the involved portion of the ventricular septum and to resect enough myocardium to relieve the outflow tract gradient, most experienced centers employ transesophageal echocardiography (TEE) to assist in localizing the desired region for resection and to monitor the effect of resection on the gradient intraoperatively.[114]

Despite its more aggressive nature, an alteration in the classic Morrow procedure has been described in which an extended myectomy is combined with partial excision and mobilization of the papillary muscles, which results in amelioration of the outflow tract obstruction, reduced tethering of the subvalvular mitral structures, and a more individualized surgical resection depending on the extent and location of the patient's LVH.[114,115] In patients with specific comorbidities, such as AF or coronary artery disease, myectomy may be combined with adjunctive surgical procedures such as the maze procedure to treat AF or coronary bypass grafting in a single, efficient procedure.

Mitral valvular abnormalities, such as elongated and flexible leaflets, substantially contribute to the degree of outflow tract obstruction in an important minority of patients. These patients often benefit from mitral valve plication at the time of myectomy to more effectively reduce the degree of outflow tract obstruction that results from SAM and to reduce the associated mitral regurgitation.[113,114] Mitral valve replacement is typically reserved for patients with significant primary valvular abnormalities such as myxomatous degeneration leading to mitral valve prolapse or regurgitation.[116]

The modern-day septal myectomy procedure carries a relatively low operative risk due to continued technical refinement, with a cumulative operative mortality rate of less than 1% in very experienced centers.[117,118] It is important to note, however, that the risk accompanying surgical myectomy is dependent on the experience of the center performing the procedure. An analysis of 6386 patients who underwent surgical myectomy at 1049 U.S. hospitals between 2003 and 2011 showed that outcomes varied significantly between those centers in the top tertile of procedural volume (3.8% surgical mortality rate) and those in the bottom (15.6% surgical mortality rate).[119] Left bundle branch block (LBBB) after myectomy is understandably very common because of the location of the procedure. Complete heart block requiring implantation of a permanent pacemaker is more recently a rare complication, as is iatrogenic formation of a ventricular septal defect.[116,120]

A conclusive reduction in long-term mortality after myectomy has yet to be demonstrated in a randomized controlled fashion. However, nonrandomized multicenter observational data (as well as a wealth of clinical experience) suggest that this procedure results in significant improvement in a patient's functional capacity, heart failure symptoms, quality of life, and possibly even life expectancy.[1,113] In addition, reduction of the outflow tract gradient usually results in amelioration of SAM of the mitral apparatus and the resultant mitral regurgitation.[113,114,121,122]

Septal Ablation

Percutaneous septal ablation was introduced by Sigwart in 1995 in an effort to provide an alternative treatment strategy to relieve outflow tract obstruction in symptomatic patients who do not wish to undergo the more invasive surgical myectomy, who are suboptimal surgical candidates due to comorbidities, or who are located in areas without sufficient surgical expertise.[123] Through selective infusion of 100% ethanol into either the first or second septal perforator arteries, the septal ablation technique attempts to mimic the effect of the more traditional Morrow myectomy by inducing a controlled infarct in the basal portion of the hypertrophied septum, resulting in scarring, thinning, and akinesis and leading to a significant reduction in the LVOT gradient and SAM of the mitral valvular apparatus (Fig. 58.4).[123,124] Despite the paucity of large-scale randomized controlled trials documenting the long-term outcome of these patients, short-term observational

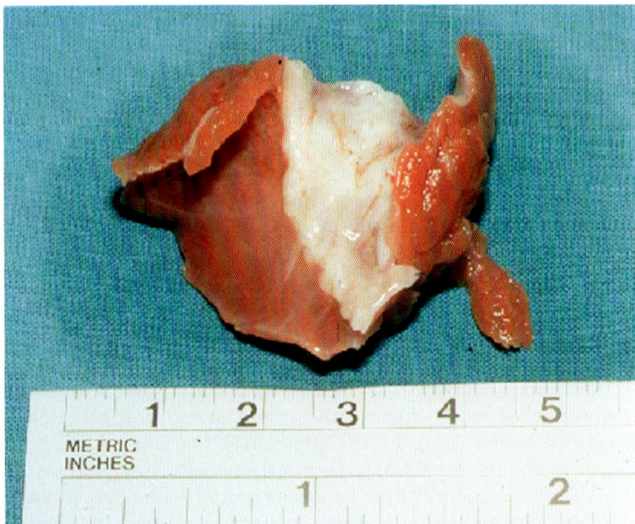

Fig. 58.4 Pathology specimen of the basal interventricular septum in a patient with hypertrophic cardiomyopathy several years after an alcohol septal ablation demonstrates fibrosis and scarring.

TABLE 58.3 Patient Selection Criteria for Alcohol Septal Ablation

Severe heart failure symptoms (i.e., New York Heart Association class III-IV) despite maximal medical therapy
Septal thickness >18 mm
Subaortic gradient >50 mm Hg (resting or with provocation) due to mitral-septal contact
Absence of papillary muscle or mitral valvular anomalies (i.e., anomalous papillary muscle insertion)
Absence of significant coronary arterial disease
Compatible septal perforator branch arterial anatomy
Relative contraindications to surgical myectomy (i.e., age, comorbidity)[a]

[a]Relative contraindication to surgical myectomy is a controversial selection criteria not uniformly followed.

studies have demonstrated a significant reduction in LVOT gradient, often a rapid reduction in limiting symptoms, improved exercise tolerance after ablation, and a mortality rate equal to or less than that of surgery at 1% to 4%.[125,126] The short-term success of this procedure combined with its obviously less invasive nature, wider availability, and association with shorter hospital stays has led to a dramatic increase in its use over the past 20 years.[127]

It is very important to carefully screen all patients being considered for septal ablation and to select those patients who will realize maximum benefit from the intervention (Table 58.3). As in the case of patients recommended for the traditional myectomy, the ACC and European Society of Cardiology (ESC) guidelines recommend that selection criteria include patients with septal hypertrophy (ideally greater than 18 mm and less than 30 mm), dynamic LVOT obstruction with a gradient greater than 50 mm Hg (either at rest or with provocation), and severely limiting heart failure symptoms (i.e., NYHA functional class III to IV) despite maximal medical therapy.[56,59] A thorough search for abnormalities that are better addressed surgically is essential before proceeding with catheter-based septal ablation. Such abnormalities include anomalous papillary muscle insertion into the mitral valve, an anatomically abnormal mitral valve with a long anteroposterior leaflet, coexistent coronary artery disease, primary valvular disease (aortic or mitral), and subaortic membrane or pannus, none of which would be adequately addressed by septal ablation.[56,59,127,128] Abnormally elongated and flexible anterior mitral leaflets resulting in an anterior location of the coaptation line and outflow tract obstruction also are not correctable via catheter-based techniques and require surgical myectomy with plication.[15]

Procedural Technique

Given the fact that most cases of HCM are diagnosed noninvasively with echocardiography and, often, no invasive hemodynamic studies have been performed before ablation, many operators reconfirm the presence of significant LVOT obstruction by positioning an end-hole catheter in the ventricular apex and recording a slow pullback under fluoroscopic guidance. Alternatively, simultaneous measurement of the ascending aortic and intracavitary pressures may be obtained via the placement of an ascending aortic catheter and an end-hole catheter as described earlier. If an LVOT gradient is not confirmed under basal or resting conditions, provocation with amyl nitrate or the Valsalva maneuver may be attempted.[129] Failure to confirm a significant gradient after these maneuvers should prompt the operator to further pursue alternative etiologies for the patient's symptom complex.

Standard diagnostic coronary cineangiography is performed as a first step to clearly define the patient's anatomy and to evaluate for concomitant atherosclerotic disease. Once this is completed, attention is turned to selection of the appropriate septal perforator branch through which to perform the ablation. To best view the anatomy of the septal branches as they course through the basal interventricular septum, the camera should be positioned in the right anterior oblique (RAO) posteroanterior (PA) cranial view or PA cranial view. From the RAO cranial view, the distance from the left coronary cusp to the first septal perforator can be measured, allowing for a reference as the operator continues with the procedure. It is also important to determine the septal vessel's course along the septum (i.e., on the right or left side), using the left anterior oblique (LAO) projection. At times, septal anatomy may vary such that one subdivision runs along the left side of the septum and another runs along the right. Selection of the left-sided subdivision is optimal for the ablation, because there is a reduced likelihood of inducing complete heart block during ethanol infusion. Most septal perforators arise from the LAD, although substantial anatomic variation has been described in which the vessels may arise from the left main trunk, the ramus intermedius, the left circumflex artery, diagonal branches, or even a branch of the right coronary artery.[129]

A temporary transvenous pacemaker is placed in advance as a prophylactic measure in case of the development of complete heart block during, or in days after, the ablation. Because heparin will be used for anticoagulation during the procedure, care should be taken to minimize the risk of bleeding during pacemaker insertion. After successful placement of both the temporary pacemaker and the arterial sheath, heparin is administered to achieve an activated clotting time of 250 to 300 seconds to prevent thrombosis in guide catheters and on wires.

After angiographic identification of the septal arteries, close attention must be given to vessel size, angulation, and the distribution of myocardial territories served by the given vessel. Angulation of the septal vessels, either at the origin from the primary vessel (e.g., the LAD) or at the bifurcation of a larger septal artery, is an important consideration in vessel selection. Vessels with angulations greater than 90 degrees are often technically challenging and result in difficulty passing the balloon into the selected vessel, with frequent prolapse of the wire into the mid-LAD.[129] Specialized techniques using catheters that allow control of the distal angle (Venture Catheter, St. Jude Medical, St. Paul, MN) may be useful in these circumstances.

There is substantial variation in the distribution of blood flow supplied by the septal perforators in patients with HCM compared with the unaffected population. In both autopsy and angiography studies, it has been demonstrated that the first septal artery may provide blood flow to regions other than the targeted basal septum (including the right ventricle); it may supply the basal septum incompletely and share this responsibility with a second septal branch, or it may subtend a substantially larger distribution of myocardium than would be expected.[129,130] Therefore an intimate knowledge of the myocardial distribution of blood flow supplied by the selected septal branch is essential to accurately target the correct area for ablation and to avoid infarction of an unanticipated region or an oversized infarction of the septum itself. This is most commonly accomplished during the procedure by the selective injection of dye under cine guidance and the concomitant use of transthoracic echocardiography (TTE) using injectable contrast material (see later discussion).

After angiographic assessment of the septal anatomy, a guide catheter providing extra support (such as a 6- or 7-Fr XB catheter) is used to engage the left main trunk. Subsequently, a 0.014-inch extra support wire with a soft tip is passed into the selected septal perforator branch, most commonly the first septal perforator (Fig. 58.5A). A short angioplasty balloon, usually 1.5 to 2 mm in diameter and 10 mm in length, is passed over the guidewire and into the septal branch. Difficulty in passing the balloon may be resolved by use of a stiffer guidewire to provide greater support for balloon placement. Care must be taken to seat the balloon deeply enough into the septal artery and to fully expand the balloon to ensure that the injected ethanol is not refluxed in to the LAD. Conversely, if the balloon is placed too deeply into the septal vessel, the injected ethanol may spare the basal portion of the septum, resulting in an unsuccessful procedure (Figs. 58.5B and C and 58.6).

It is essential at this point to verify the distribution of myocardium being supplied by the selected vessel, given the substantial degree of variability in the cardiac anatomy in this patient population. This can be accomplished by traditional angiography or TEE, with the aid of echocardiographic contrast. After correct positioning, as described earlier, the operator inflates the balloon (typically to 10 to 12 atmospheres) to occlude the perforator, and 1 to 2 mL of contrast material is injected to assess the full extent of myocardium supplied by the chosen vessel. Contrast should be injected slowly so as to mimic the anticipated alcohol infusion. Extreme caution should be taken to verify that the infused contrast material does not reflux into the LAD or into other coronary arteries (e.g., the posterior descending artery), thus possibly exposing a large amount of unintended myocardium to damage when the ethanol is infused. Aggressive contrast infusion may overwhelm collateral vessels and create an inferior LV wall infarction.

After angiographic confirmation of septal occlusion, further assessment of the septal distribution is obtained via contrast echocardiography (Fig. 58.7). After careful inspection of the septum in the apical long-axis, four-chamber, and parasternal long-axis views, 1 to 2 mL of contrast is injected into the septal branch through a tuberculin-type syringe. Because Albumex, a first-generation echocardiographic contrast agent, is no longer available in many countries, second- and third-generation agents are currently used. These agents have proved to be suboptimal because they traverse the capillary beds rapidly and produce a large amount of echocardiographic "shadowing" from the opacified ventricles. Therefore it is important to dilute these agents before injection. In our laboratory, the contrast vials are typically opened 10 to 15 minutes before the time of expected use so as to decrease their potency. The contrast is then further diluted with sterile saline in a 1:10 mixture at the time of injection.

Pulsed-wave Doppler echocardiography is the imaging method of choice in using the diluted contrast material to avoid destruction of the microbubbles with the higher-frequency continuous-wave ultrasound. This procedure allows the operator to verify that the chosen vessel primarily supplies the proximal

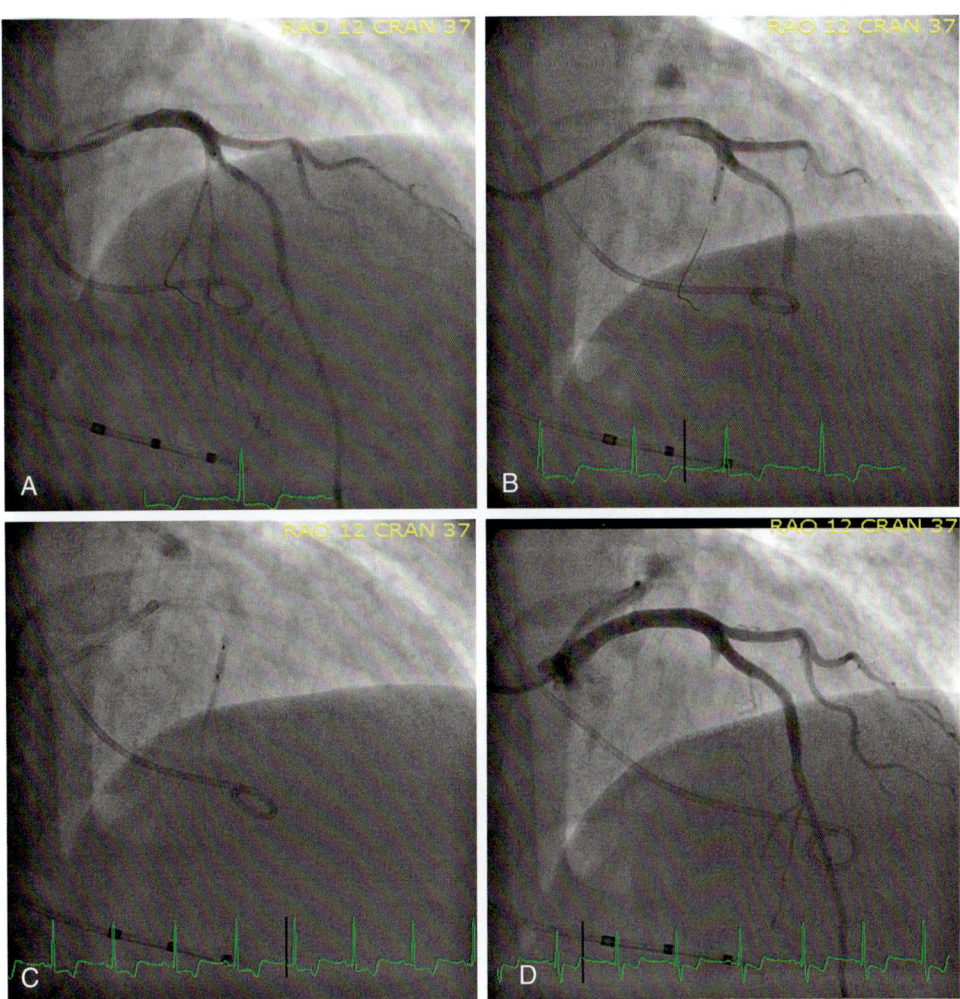

Fig. 58.5 Fluoroscopic images during alcohol septal ablation in a patient with hypertrophic cardiomyopathy. (A) The first septal perforator branch of the left anterior descending (LAD) artery is visualized in the right anterior oblique *(RAO)* cranial *(CRAN)* view. A support wire and short angioplasty balloon are advanced into the septal perforator. (B) The balloon is inflated in the proximal portion of the septal perforator branch, and occlusion is confirmed angiographically with contrast injection. (C) Occlusion of the perforator is confirmed by ensuring there is no reflux of contrast into the LAD. (D) Postprocedural angiography reveals obliteration of the septal perforator branch and integrity of the LAD and remaining coronary circulation.

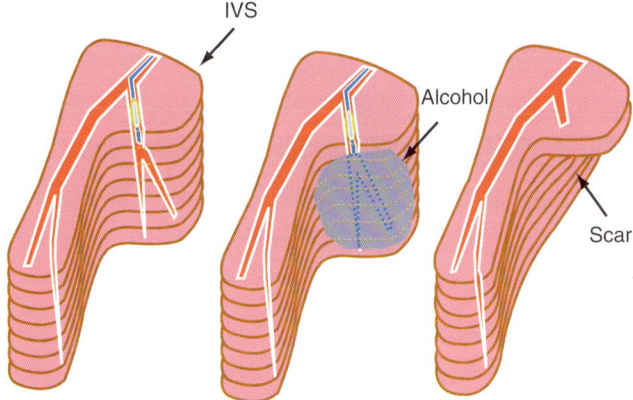

Fig. 58.6 Schematic overview of the alcohol septal ablation procedure depicts the resultant basal septal scar and enlargement of the left ventricular outflow tract. If the balloon is placed distally, the anterior septum is not ablated, which can result in a suboptimal result. *IVS,* Interventricular septum.

interventricular septum and not portions of the inferior wall, LV papillary musculature, or right ventricular free wall via the moderator band.[129,131] Ideally, contrast material will appear in the basal portion of septum responsible for the greatest extent of septal-mitral contact. Appearance of contrast in the distal septum or other regions of myocardium is a contraindication to ethanol infusion, because it can result in infarction of an undesired territory or an infarction of unanticipated size.

As a final method of ensuring that the desired area of myocardium has been selected, it is recommended that the operator document a greater than 30% reduction in the LVOT gradient during balloon inflation. A rather rapid reduction in gradient can be observed with prolonged balloon occlusion of a septal perforator branch. Such an observation suggests that the correct septal distribution has been targeted for ablation.[129,132] Before proceeding with ethanol injection, it is essential to confirm that the balloon has not migrated during this process and that the previously placed temporary pacemaker continues to have a suitable pacing threshold. This is easily done by fluoroscopic verification and injection of another 1 to 2 mL of contrast agent through the guide catheter.

After confirmation of proper balloon positioning, the operator may proceed with ethanol injection. Whereas most experienced centers use between 1 and 3 mL of desiccated ethanol, this volume may be adjusted based on the appearance of the septal anatomy and the degree of contrast washout.[129,133–135] Research has documented similar midterm hemodynamic outcomes with reduced complication rates, especially the requirement for a permanent pacemaker, when smaller amounts of ethanol (1 to 2 mL) are used.[136] If there is rapid contrast washout due to collateralization of the septal branch, the rate and volume of ethanol infusion should be reduced to prevent the alcohol from escaping to undesirable areas of myocardium via the collaterals.[125,129]

The ethanol is injected into the vessel over a 1- to 5-minute period with the balloon remaining inflated. During the initial infusion, continued monitoring of the resting gradient is essential

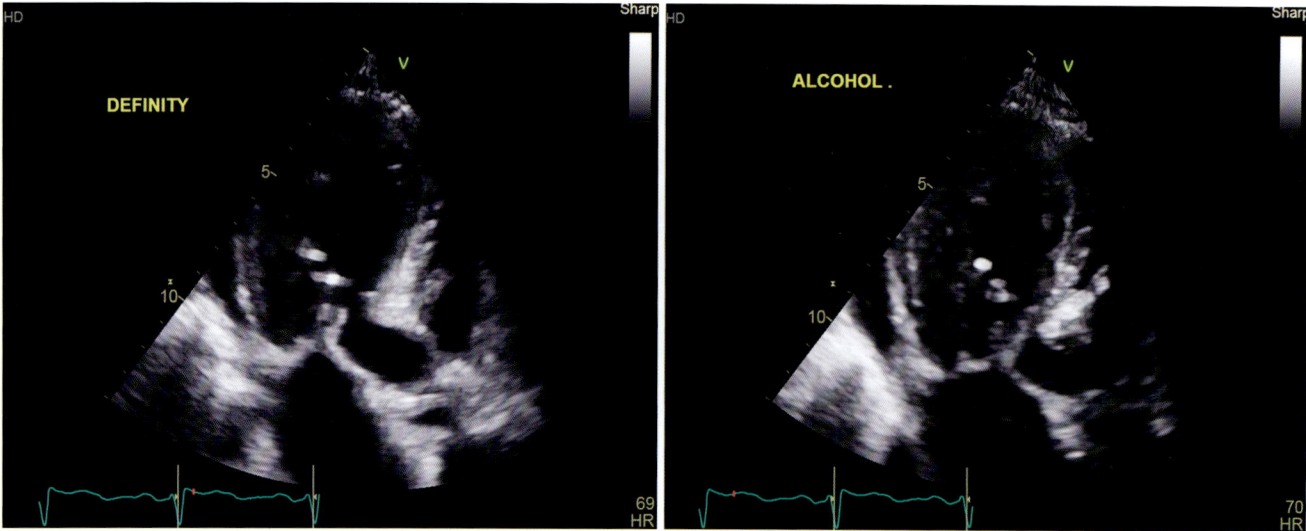

Fig. 58.7 Contrast echocardiography used during alcohol septal ablation procedure. *Left,* Apical three-chamber view after injection of echocardiographic contrast material into the first septal perforator branch reveals the territory of myocardium supplied by this vessel. *Right,* Alcohol is infused into this vessel, causing expected infarction of the basal interventricular septum. *HD,* High definition; *HR,* heart rate.

to judge the efficacy of the procedure. In general, a reduction in the LVOT gradient to less than 30 mm Hg in the setting of a resting gradient greater than 50 mm Hg, or a greater than 50% reduction of a provocable gradient, is considered indicative of a successful procedure in the catheterization laboratory (Figs. 58.7 58.8 and 58.9).[129]

Before the balloon is disengaged from the septal vessel, it is recommended that the guidewire be placed again into the septal branch for smooth removal of the balloon and maintenance of access across the left main trunk and the LAD. As a final step, angiography of the LAD and septal vessels is performed to verify the integrity of the coronary circulation. Phasic flow may be observed in the injected septal branch immediately after the ablation, although total occlusion is frequently observed (see Fig. 58.5D). Postprocedural care should take place in a coronary intensive care unit for 48 hours after ablation to allow for the rapid identification and treatment of possible complications. The amount of induced myocardial tissue destruction often results in elevation of the enzyme creatinine phosphokinase (CPK) to levels between 800 and 1200 U/L, although this is variable depending on the amount of alcohol injected, vessel size, and the method of enzyme measurement.[135] The transvenous pacing wire may be discontinued 48 hours after the procedure if there is an absence of bradyarrhythmia or heart block that would require continued observation or a permanent pacemaker. In most centers, the patient is transferred to a regular nursing floor for another 48 to 72 hours to observe for postprocedural complications before discharge.

The complication rate after septal ablation is relatively low and is comparable to that of septal myectomy. Since right bundle-branch block (RBBB) occurs in approximately half of patients treated with alcohol septal ablation, the risk of complete heart block after ablation is highest in patients with pre-existing LBBB; conversely, most patients after myectomy develop LBBB> The long-term results from a multinational alcohol septal ablation registry show that 89% of patients, after alcohol septal ablation, are in NYHA class I or II, the mean decrease of LVOT was 76%, and the 30-day mortality rate was 1%.[85,137]

A recent meta-analysis of all studies that have been done comparing outcomes in patients with alcohol septal ablation and those undergoing surgical myectomy that have been followed for a mean duration of at least 3 years revealed variable rates of pacemaker requirements in different cohorts (0% to 22% following

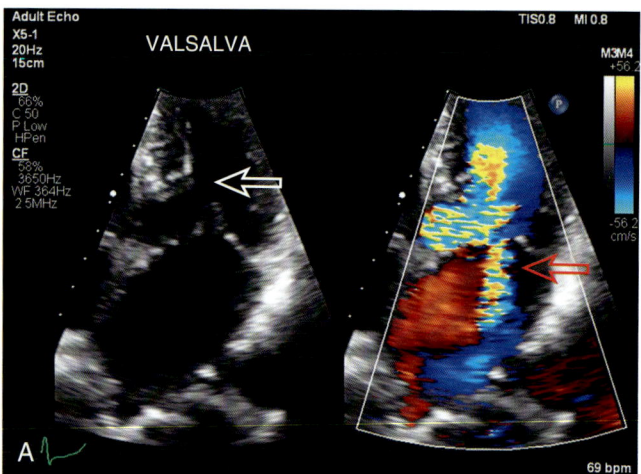

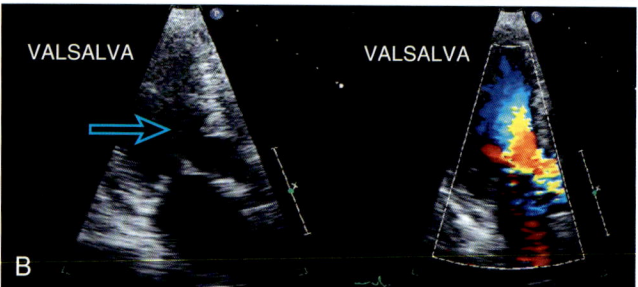

Fig. 58.8 Two-dimensional and Doppler echocardiography before and after alcohol septal ablation in a patient with hypertrophic cardiomyopathy. (A) Systolic anterior motion of the mitral valve is noted with Valsalva *(white arrow)* with resultant posteriorly directed mitral regurgitation *(red arrow)* preprocedurally. (B) After alcohol septal ablation, significantly less anterior motion of the mitral valve is noted during systole *(blue arrow)* resulting in less mitral regurgitation.

alcohol septal ablation, compared with 0% to 13% following myectomy). Overall, however, permanent pacemaker implantation was performed after alcohol septal ablation in 10% of the 2791 total patients compared with 4.4% after myectomy.[127,138]

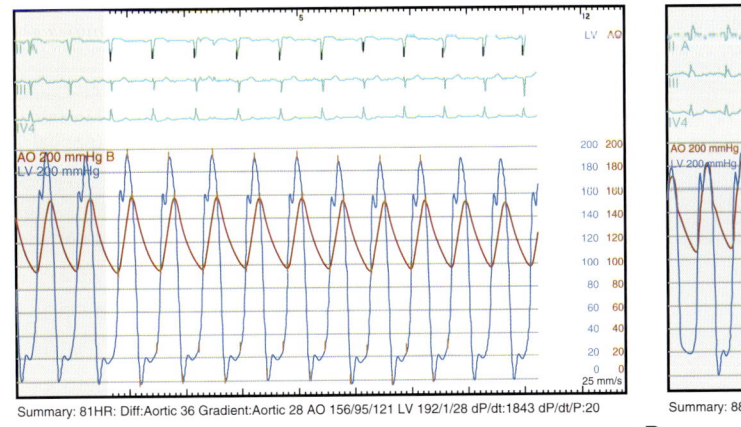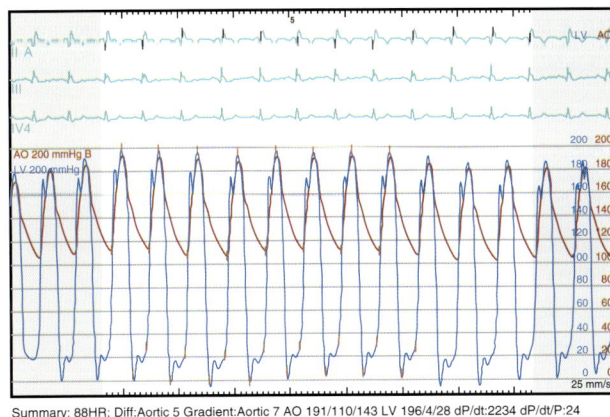

Fig. 58.9 Hemodynamics of a patient with hypertrophic cardiomyopathy before (A) and after (B) alcohol septal ablation. A significant reduction in left-ventricular *(LV)* to aortic *(AO)* pressure gradient is recorded postprocedure. Red tracing represents aortic pressure, and blue tracing represents left ventricular pressure.

The presence of a preexisting LBBB and a rapid bolus injection of ethanol during ablation have both been positively correlated with an increased incidence of high-degree atrioventricular block requiring permanent pacemaker implantation.[139] Extravasation of alcohol into the LAD during infusion is a rare but catastrophic complication that often results in a large infarction of the middle to distal anterior wall and is clearly associated with increased mortality. Coronary dissection caused by the extra support guidewire or the catheter has been reported in rare instances. Tamponade due to perforation of the right ventricular apex during insertion of a transvenous pacing wire or during interatrial septal puncture for periprocedural hemodynamic monitoring has also been reported. Overly extensive infarction of the interventricular septum as a result of too generous a quantity of infused alcohol or too rapid an infusion rate during ablation can result in a ventricular septal rupture.[129]

Ventricular arrhythmias can be seen both during and up to 48 hours after the procedure, but this complication is rare and usually does not require prolonged therapy. Unlike myectomy, septal ablation results in the formation of a large intramyocardial scar that may serve as substrate for future malignant ventricular arrhythmias. There has been some conjecture that this could result in an increased risk of late arrhythmic mortality, especially in younger patients undergoing ablation.[134] However, this hypothesis has yet to garner substantial evidentiary support. Patients should be observed closely for recurrence of symptoms or any arrhythmia. ICD implantation should be considered if there is evidence of nonsustained VT, but this is extremely rare. Objective assessment of functional capacity using exercise testing is appropriate for monitoring these patients. Repeat alcohol ablation may be considered if symptoms recur and an appropriate septal perforator is available for injection. If repeat ablation is not feasible, surgical myectomy may need to be considered in this group.

Despite the increased number of septal ablation procedures performed worldwide, there remains a paucity of randomized controlled trials. Existing data suggest that septal ablation and surgical myectomy have similar success rates in both short and longer terms (Table 58.4).[138,140] A meta-analysis demonstrated that, after adjusting for preprocedural gradient, the reduction in gradient after the procedure is similar in the two modalities.[141]

Both procedures have advantages and associated complications, underscoring the importance of careful patient selection and consideration of comorbidities before an intervention is chosen (Fig. 58.10). Given that ablation commonly produces a pattern of RBBB, patients with a preexisting LBBB are at very high risk of complete heart block after the procedure.[141] In addition, it has been suggested that female gender, first-degree atrioventricular block, and an increased volume of injected alcohol are additional risk factors for postprocedural complete heart block.[142] In contrast, myectomy produces a LBBB and less commonly requires permanent pacing. Myectomy can result in mild to moderate aortic insufficiency in up to 10% to 20% of patients but rarely leads to an adverse outcome.[143] By the nature of the procedure, ablation results in a permanent scar in the interventricular septum, and there remains some concern that this may serve as substrate for future ventricular arrhythmias, although this has not as yet been objectively documented.

As would be expected, ablation results in a reduced length of stay compared with myectomy and substantially contributes to an overall reduction in cost. Mortality is relatively low with both interventions and approaches 1% in experienced centers.[138] Several meta-analyses have also shown similar postprocedural outcomes, with no difference in long-term mortality between ablation and myectomy.[138,141] In summary, either surgical myectomy or alcohol ablation may be selected as a viable treatment option in symptomatic patients with LVOT obstruction. Which therapy should be selected is a complex decision that must be made only after taking into consideration the patient's clinical situation.

CONCLUSIONS

HCM is a complex genetic disease with multiple heterogeneous phenotypes and clinical manifestations. Because of the considerable heterogeneity of the disease and the lack of randomized controlled trials in this arena, HCM is variably managed across the world. The management in any patient with HCM should ideally focus on the following aspects:

- Control of heart failure symptoms
- Assessment of the risk of sudden death and appropriate risk management
- Treatment of AF
- Management of LVOT obstruction using invasive techniques, when indicated
- Screening of family members

Although the current guidelines provide an important framework that helps in evaluation and treatment of HCM, the unique characteristics and preferences of each patient should play a vital role in the decision-making and management strategies.

TABLE 58.4 Outcomes from all studies comparing surgical myectomy with alcohol septal ablation with a mean follw-up duration of at least 3 years and meta-analyses comparing myectomy with alcohol septal ablation.

Study	n (Myectomy/Ablation)	Mean Follow-Up (Years)	Mean Age (Years)	LVOT Gradient Postprocedure (mm Hg)	Periprocedural Mortality (%)	All-Cause Mortality (Annual %)
Agarwal et al.[141] (meta-analysis)	380/326	–	55/49	SMD 0.45 (favors myectomy)	–	–
ten Cate[144] 2010	91/40	5.4/6.6	54/49	8/–	2.2/0	1.8/0.8
Sorajja et al.[136]	177/177	5.7/5.7	63/62	13/–	1.1/0.6	2.5/2.4
Steggerda 2014[145]	161/102	5.1/9.1	59/56	19/10	1.2/2.0	1.5/2.2
Vriesendorp 2014[146]	316/250	6.3/7.9	58/52	10/9	1.6/1.2	1.9/2.0
Samardhi 2014[147]	47/23	3.6/3.8	57/48	–	1.3/1.1	1.5/1.4
Sedehi 2015[148]	52/171	3.2/13.7	56/47	–	0/0	1.5/0.9
Liebregts et al.[138] (meta-analysis)	2013/2791	6.2/7.4	56/47	–	1.3/1.1	1.5/1.4
Yang 2015[149]	22/37	3.0/3.0	46/45	–	0/0	1.5/0.9

LVOT, left ventricular outflow tract; *SMD*, standardized mean difference; *SMD*, standardized mean difference.

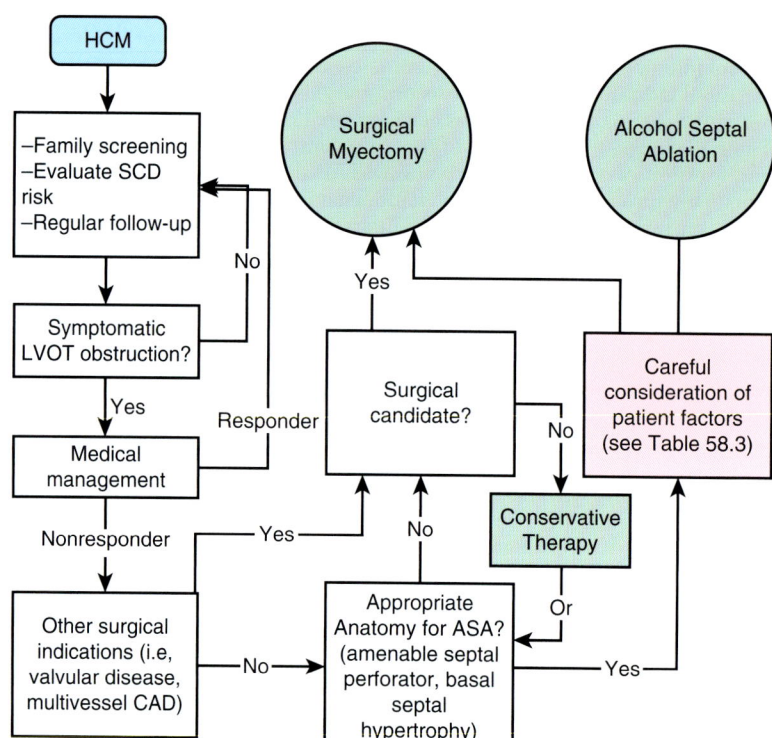

Fig. 58.10 Flowchart outlining management strategies for patients with hypertrophic cardiomyopathy. *ASA*, Alcohol septal ablation; *CAD*, coronary artery disease; *HCM*, hypertrophic cardiomyopathy; *LVOT*, left ventricular outflow tract; *SCD*, sudden cardiac death.

Despite significant improvement in the understanding of disease pathophysiology in the last few decades, there are considerable knowledge gaps that need to be addressed to improve care in this patient population. Long-term data on alcohol septal ablation will define its precise role in relation to myectomy in the management of medically refractory HCM. In addition, establishment of referral systems that facilitate the treatment of HCM at centers of excellence would be critical in optimal management. Improvements in risk stratification for SCD will more accurately identify patients with HCM at risk for SCD. Development of subcutaneous and leadless ICD systems will likely reduce complications and lower the threshold for device implantation in young patients. The role of genetic testing will also become clearer as genotyping becomes cheaper and more accessible. Further research is needed for a more thorough understanding of the genetic basis of this disease and to develop greater and more widespread clinical utility of genotyping in HCM.

Acknowledgments

We thank Dr. Gus Theodos, Dr. Shikhar Agarwal, and Dr. Matthew "Casey" Becker for their contributions to earlier versions of this chapter.

KEY REFERENCES

1. Maron BJ. Hypertrophic cardiomyopathy: a systematic review. *JAMA*. 2002;287(10):1308–1320. http://www.ncbi.nlm.nih.gov/pubmed/11886323.
2. Braunwald E, Lambrew CT, Rockoff SD, et al. Idiopathic hypertrophic subaortic stenosis. I. A description of the disease based upon an analysis of 64 patients. *Circulation*. 1964;30(suppl 4):3–119. http://www.ncbi.nlm.nih.gov/pubmed/14227306.
7. Maron BJ, McKenna WJ, Danielson GK, et al. American College of Cardiology/European Society of Cardiology clinical expert consensus document on hypertrophic cardiomyopathy. A report of the American college of cardiology foundation task force on clinical expert consensus documents and the European society of cardiology committee for practice guidelines. *J Am Coll Cardiol*. 2003;42(9):1687–1713. http://www.ncbi.nlm.nih.gov/pubmed/14607462.
32. Elliott PM, Poloniecki J, Dickie S, et al. Sudden death in hypertrophic cardiomyopathy: identification of high risk patients. *J Am Coll Cardiol*. 2000;36(7):2212–2218. http://www.ncbi.nlm.nih.gov/pubmed/11127463.
39. Watkins H. Sudden death in hypertrophic cardiomyopathy. *N Engl J Med*. 2000;342(6):422–424. https://doi.org/10.1056/NEJM200002103420609.
56. Gersh BJ, Maron BJ, Bonow RO, et al. 2011 ACCF/AHA guideline for the diagnosis and treatment of hypertrophic cardiomyopathy: executive summary. *J Am Coll Cardiol*. 2011;58(25):2703–2738. https://doi.org/10.1016/j.jacc.2011.10.825.
59. Authors/Task Force members, Elliott PM, Anastasakis A, et al. 2014 ESC guidelines on diagnosis and management of hypertrophic cardiomyopathy: the Task Force for the Diagnosis and Management of Hypertrophic Cardiomyopathy of the European Society of Cardiology (ESC). *Eur Heart J*. 2014;35(39):2733–2779. https://doi.org/10.1093/eurheartj/ehu284.
74. Rowin EJ, Maron BJ, Olivotto I, et al. Role of exercise testing in hypertrophic cardiomyopathy. *JACC Cardiovasc Imaging*. 2017;10(11):1374–1386. https://doi.org/10.1016/j.jcmg.2017.07.016.
76. Brockenbrough EC, Braunwald E, Morrow AG. A hemodynamic technic for the detection of hypertrophic subaortic stenosis. *Circulation*. 1961;23(2):189–194. https://doi.org/10.1161/01.CIR.23.2.189.
89. Bonow RO, Dilsizian V, Rosing DR, et al. Verapamil-induced improvement in left ventricular diastolic filling and increased exercise tolerance in patients with hypertrophic cardiomyopathy: short- and long-term effects. *Circulation*. 1985;72(4):853–864. http://www.ncbi.nlm.nih.gov/pubmed/4040821.
103. Nishimura RA, Trusty JM, Hayes DL, et al. Dual-chamber pacing for hypertrophic cardiomyopathy: a randomized, double-blind, crossover trial. *J Am Coll Cardiol*. 1997;29(2):435–441. http://www.ncbi.nlm.nih.gov/pubmed/9015001.
117. Krajcer Z, Leachman RD, Cooley DA, et al. Mitral valve replacement and septal myomectomy in hypertrophic cardiomyopathy. Ten-year follow-up in 80 patients. *Circulation*. 1988;78(3 Pt 2):I35–I43. http://www.ncbi.nlm.nih.gov/pubmed/3409517.
118. Merrill WH, Friesinger GC, Graham TP, et al. Long-lasting improvement after septal myectomy for hypertrophic obstructive cardiomyopathy. *Ann Thorac Surg*. 2000;69(6):1732–1735. 6 http://www.ncbi.nlm.nih.gov/pubmed/10892916.
119. Qin JX, Shiota T, Lever HM, et al. Outcome of patients with hypertrophic obstructive cardiomyopathy after percutaneous transluminal septal myocardial ablation and septal myectomy surgery. *J Am Coll Cardiol*. 2001;38(7):1994–2000. http://www.ncbi.nlm.nih.gov/pubmed/11738306.
124. Lakkis NM, Nagueh SF, Dunn JK, et al. Nonsurgical septal reduction therapy for hypertrophic obstructive cardiomyopathy: one-year follow-up. *J Am Coll Cardiol*. 2000;36(3):852–855. http://www.ncbi.nlm.nih.gov/pubmed/10987610.
125. Faber L, Meissner A, Ziemssen P, et al. Percutaneous transluminal septal myocardial ablation for hypertrophic obstructive cardiomyopathy: long term follow up of the first series of 25 patients. *Heart*. 2000;83(3):326–331. http://www.ncbi.nlm.nih.gov/pubmed/10677415.
138. Liebregts M, Vriesendorp PA, Mahmoodi BK, et al. A systematic review and meta-analysis of long-term outcomes after septal reduction therapy in patients with hypertrophic cardiomyopathy. *JACC Heart Fail*. 2015;3(11):896–905. https://doi.org/10.1016/j.jchf.2015.06.011.
141. Agarwal S, Tuzcu EM, Desai MY, et al. Updated meta-analysis of septal alcohol ablation versus myectomy for hypertrophic cardiomyopathy. *J Am Coll Cardiol*. 2010;55(8):823–834. https://doi.org/10.1016/j.jacc.2009.09.047.

 Additional references available online at expertconsult.com.

中文导读

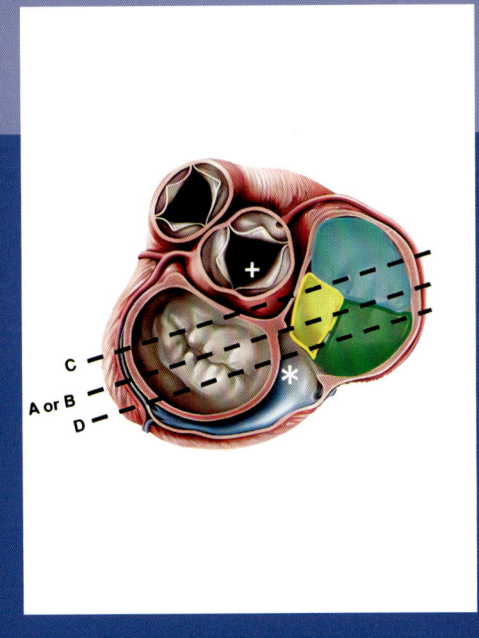

第59章
经皮球囊心包切开术治疗心包积液和心脏压塞

  心包穿刺是针对心包积液患者的诊断和治疗方法,对于部分患者,尤其是恶性心包积液的患者,存在复发的情况。对于置管引流3～5天后引流量仍超过50 mL/24 h的患者,须考虑更积极的治疗方法,包括心包内注射硬化剂、放疗、化疗、经皮球囊心包切开术、心包开窗术。其中经皮球囊心包切开术侵入性小,相对简单、安全,可作为心包开窗术的替代方案。

  本章节详细介绍了皮球囊心包切开术的操作及注意事项。经皮球囊心包切开术需要在导管室进行,患者处于局麻和轻度镇静状态,经剑突下入路置入球囊扩张导管,在透视引导下确保球囊精确定位于跨心包壁层的位置,进行2～3次球囊充气使心包形成足够的开口,抽出大部分心包积液,留置引流管以确定手术有效性及是否出血。术后24小时无明显心包引流(50 mL)后拔除导管,定期复查超声心动图,行胸部X线检查以监测引流心包积液引起的胸腔积液(通常为左侧)情况。注意术前需除外出血风险高的患者,围术期建议预防性应用抗生素。

  心包积液并不是经皮进入心包腔的先决条件,心包腔内经导管诊断和介入技术的发展得到了推动,目前已经越来越普遍,包括心外膜标测和消融、心包内给药、心包腔内超声心动图、心包镜引导下的活检和经皮左心耳结扎术。

王　真　吴永健

章节要点

- 心包穿刺是一种经导管从心包中抽出液体的手术，其适用于心脏压塞、大量心包积液（通常>2 cm）、有症状的中度心包积液（10~20 mm）或需要液体用于明确诊断的患者，也可用于对治疗效果欠佳的化脓性、结核性或肿瘤性心包积液的引流。
- 即使没有明显的心包积液，也可以在透视引导下使用钝头针经剑突下入路安全地进入心包腔。
- 经皮球囊心包切开术是一种创伤性较低的心包开窗术的替代方法，是一种有效的治疗复发性、游离性和血流动力学不稳定的心包积液的方法，特别是与肿瘤性疾病有关的心包积液。
- 经皮球囊心包切开术包括在心导管室的透视引导下，利用球囊导管建立心包壁层窗口。
- 心包腔内的经导管诊断和介入技术已经越来越普遍，包括但不限于心外膜标测和消融、心包内给药、心包腔内超声心动图、心包镜检查。

59 Percutaneous Balloon Pericardiotomy for Patients With Pericardial Effusion and Tamponade

Hani Jneid, Andrew A. Ziskind, Igor F. Palacios

KEY POINTS

- Pericardiocentesis is a catheter-based procedure in which fluid is aspirated from the pericardium. It is indicated in patients with cardiac tamponade, for large pericardial effusions (usually >2 cm), for moderate effusions (10 to 20 mm) in symptomatic patients, or if the fluid is needed for diagnostic purposes; it is also used to drain purulent, tubercular, or neoplastic effusions in patients who are resistant to treatment.
- The pericardial space can be safely entered with a blunt-tipped needle using a subxiphoid approach under fluoroscopic guidance even in the absence of a significant pericardial effusion.
- Percutaneous balloon pericardiotomy (PBP) is a less invasive alternative to surgical pericardial window and is an effective therapy for recurrent, free-flowing, and hemodynamically significant pericardial effusions especially if associated with neoplastic disease.
- PBP consists of creating a parietal pericardial window with a balloon catheter under fluoroscopic guidance in the cardiac catheterization laboratory.
- Catheter-based diagnostic and interventional techniques in the pericardial space have become increasingly common and include but are not limited to epicardial mapping and ablation, intrapericardial delivery of therapies, intrapericardial echocardiography, and pericardioscopy.

INTRODUCTION

The clinical presentation of patients with pericardial effusion varies. Some are completely asymptomatic, but others develop pericardial tamponade and cardiovascular collapse. Pericardiocentesis is a catheter-based technique that uses a needle to aspirate the pericardial fluid, usually under fluoroscopic or echocardiographic guidance.

Percutaneous balloon pericardiotomy (PBP) is a relatively novel catheter-based technique that is gradually replacing the more invasive surgical pericardial window procedure. The improved techniques for percutaneous access to the pericardial space and the adjunctive use of pericardioscopy provide additional opportunities for the use of this space in diagnostic and interventional techniques. As a result, novel pericardial interventions—such as epicardial mapping and ablation, percutaneous pericardial biopsy (PPB), intrapericardial therapy, and intrapericardial echocardiography—are rapidly evolving.

PERICARDIAL EFFUSION AND TAMPONADE

The normal pericardium is a fibroelastic sac composed of visceral and parietal layers separated by a thin layer (25 to 50 mL) of straw-colored fluid.[1] The normal pericardium has a steep pressure-volume curve; it is distensible when the intrapericardial volume is small but gradually becomes inextensible when the volume increases.[1] The intrapericardial pressure depends on the relationship between the absolute volume of a pericardial effusion, speed of fluid accumulation, and pericardial elasticity. The clinical presentation is related not only to the size of the effusion but also to the rapidity of its accumulation.

Pericardial effusion may result from a variety of clinical conditions (Table 59.1). Among medical patients, malignant disease is the most common cause of pericardial effusion with tamponade.[1,2] Pericardial tamponade is a clinical syndrome with defined hemodynamic and echocardiographic abnormalities that result from the accumulation of intrapericardial fluid and impairment of ventricular diastolic filling.[1,3] The ultimate mechanism of hemodynamic compromise is the compression of cardiac chambers due to increased intrapericardial pressure.

In all cases of cardiac tamponade, initial treatment consists of removing pericardial fluid by prompt pericardiocentesis and drainage.

Autopsy and surgical studies have shown that myocardial or pericardial metastases are found in approximately 50% of patients who have cardiac tamponade due to malignancy.[3-7] Although the short-term survival of patients with cardiac tamponade depends primarily on its early diagnosis and relief, long-term survival depends on the prognosis of the primary illness regardless of the intervention performed.[4,5,8]

PERICARDIOCENTESIS

Indications

Pericardiocentesis is the technique of catheter-based aspiration of pericardial fluid.[1,3] It is used to diagnose and treat patients with pericarditis complicated with pericardial effusion, cardiac tamponade, and effusive-constrictive pericarditis.

Many asymptomatic patients with large effusions but no hemodynamic compromise do not require pericardiocentesis unless there is a diagnostic need for fluid analysis. In a prospective study with long-term follow-up of patients with large, idiopathic, chronic pericardial effusions, Sagrista-Sauleda and colleagues[9] concluded that the pericardial effusions were usually well tolerated for long periods by most patients with severe tamponade; however, they can develop unexpectedly at any time. Although pericardiocentesis was effective in resolving these effusions, recurrences were common, prompting the study authors to recommend referral of patients with recurrences for pericardiectomy.[10]

When cardiac tamponade occurs, the emergency drainage of pericardial fluid by pericardiocentesis is lifesaving therapy for a patient who would otherwise develop pulseless electrical activity and cardiac arrest. Pericardiocentesis can relieve tamponade, obtain fluid for appropriate analysis, and assess hemodynamics before and after pericardial fluid evacuation to exclude effusive-constrictive pericardial effusion. In one series of 205 consecutive

TABLE 59.1 Causes of Pericardial Effusion and Tamponade

IDIOPATHIC CASES
Infections
    Viral
    Bacterial
    Fungal
    Others
Metabolic disorders
    Uremia
    Myxedema

COLLAGEN AND OTHER AUTOIMMUNE DISORDERS
Systemic lupus erythematosus
Rheumatoid arthritis
Rheumatic fever
Dressler syndrome
Others

NEOPLASTIC DISORDERS
Primary
Pericardial metastasis
Local invasion
Volume overload
Chronic heart failure

MISCELLANEOUS DISORDERS
Chest wall irradiation
Cardiotomy or thoracic surgery
Adverse drug reaction
Aortic dissection
After myocardial infarction
Trauma

From Jneid H, Maree AO, Palacios IF. Pericardial tamponade: clinical presentation, diagnosis and catheter-based therapies. In Parillo J, Dellinger PR, eds. *Critical care medicine*. 3rd ed. St. Louis: Mosby; 2008.

patients undergoing pericardiocentesis at Mayo Clinic, 16% were found to have effusive-constrictive pericarditis.[11]

Pericardiocentesis is an essential technique to be mastered by interventional cardiologists as it may be needed when coronary artery perforation (CAP) occurs during percutaneous coronary interventions (PCIs). In a case series of 150 CAPs from a single center (2005 to 2016), pericardiocentesis for tamponade was required for 48.0%, predominantly for Ellis type 3 CAP.[12] Coronary perforation can occur with higher frequency as a complication of chronic total occlusion (CTO) PCI. In a contemporary dataset of 2097 CTO PCIs performed in 2049 patients (2012 to 2017), CAP occurred in 85 patients (4.1%), of whom 12 (14%) experienced tamponade requiring pericardiocentesis.[13]

Elective pericardiocentesis is contraindicated for patients receiving anticoagulation, those with bleeding disorders, or cases of thrombocytopenia with platelet counts less than 50,000/μL. Pericardiocentesis is also ill-advised when the effusion is very small or loculated.[1,3] Preoperative *controlled* pericardiocentesis is safe and effective in patients with acute type A aortic dissection who have critical cardiac tamponade.

Technique

Pericardiocentesis was traditionally performed using a subxiphoid approach under electrocardiographic (ECG) and fluoroscopic guidance (Fig. 59.1A).[3] Traditionally, pericardiocentesis has been performed in the cardiac catheterization laboratory.[3] Fluoroscopic guidance is vastly enhanced by using a 90-degree true lateral projection (right lateral is preferred to reduce operator radiation exposure). The use of contrast and simultaneous right heart catheterization and hemodynamic monitoring has been proposed by some authors to enhance the efficacy of the procedure and also in the early diagnosis of effusive and constrictive pericarditis. Echocardiography-guided pericardiocentesis was introduced at the Mayo Clinic in 1979, and the use of ultrasound guidance has now become the standard of care. The procedure is now also performed in the noninvasive laboratory, intensive care unit, or at bedside under echocardiographic guidance.

Pericardiocentesis is based on the Seldinger technique of percutaneous catheter insertion. After local anesthesia has been administered to the skin and deeper tissues of the left xiphocostal area, the pericardial needle is connected to an ECG lead. The needle is advanced from the left of the subxiphoid area while aiming toward the left shoulder. This is usually done under fluoroscopic or echocardiographic guidance, but blinded procedures can be undertaken in emergencies. Often, a discrete pop is felt as the needle enters the pericardial space. When ST-segment elevation is observed on the ECG lead tracing, it signifies that the needle has touched the epicardium and should be withdrawn slightly until the ST-segment elevation disappears (see Fig. 59.1B). After the pericardial space has been entered, a stiff guidewire is introduced into the pericardial space through the needle, which is then withdrawn. A catheter is then inserted into the pericardial sac over the guidewire (see Fig. 59.1C). The drainage catheter typically has an end hole and multiple side holes. Intrapericardial pressure is measured by connecting a pressure transducer system to the intrapericardial catheter. Pericardial fluid is then removed, and samples of pericardial fluid are sent for appropriate biochemical, cytologic, bacteriologic, and immunologic analyses for diagnostic purposes. The first sample is usually reserved for microbiologic studies.

In cases of pericardial tamponade, aspiration of fluid should be continued until clinical and hemodynamic improvement occurs. The catheter is frequently left in place for continuous drainage and as a route to instill sclerosing or chemotherapeutic agents when needed. The catheter is secured to the skin using sterile sutures and covered with a sterile dressing. The success rate of pericardiocentesis is greater and the incidence of complications improves with increasing size of the effusion.

With the increasing need to access the pericardial space (discussed later), especially in patients with no pericardial effusion ("dry taps"), variations in the technique have been developed. For example, a microneedle or a 17-gauge Tuohy needle (Pajunk Medical Systems, Norcross, GA) containing a curved tip can be introduced using the subxiyphoid approach while observing its track fluoroscopically in the lateral projection. This reduces the risk of inadvertent right ventricular puncture.

Complications

Potential complications of pericardiocentesis include a heart or coronary vessel laceration, sometimes causing fatal consequences. Puncture of the right atrium or ventricle with hemopericardial fluid accumulation, arrhythmias, air embolism, pneumothorax as well as puncture of the peritoneal cavity or abdominal viscera have been reported. Acute pulmonary edema may infrequently occur when the pericardial tamponade is decompressed too rapidly.

The right xiphocostal, apical, right-sided, and parasternal approaches are also used for pericardiocentesis. The right xiphocostal approach is associated with a higher incidence of right atrial and inferior vena cava injury. Puncture of the left pleura and the lingula occurs more frequently with the apical approach,

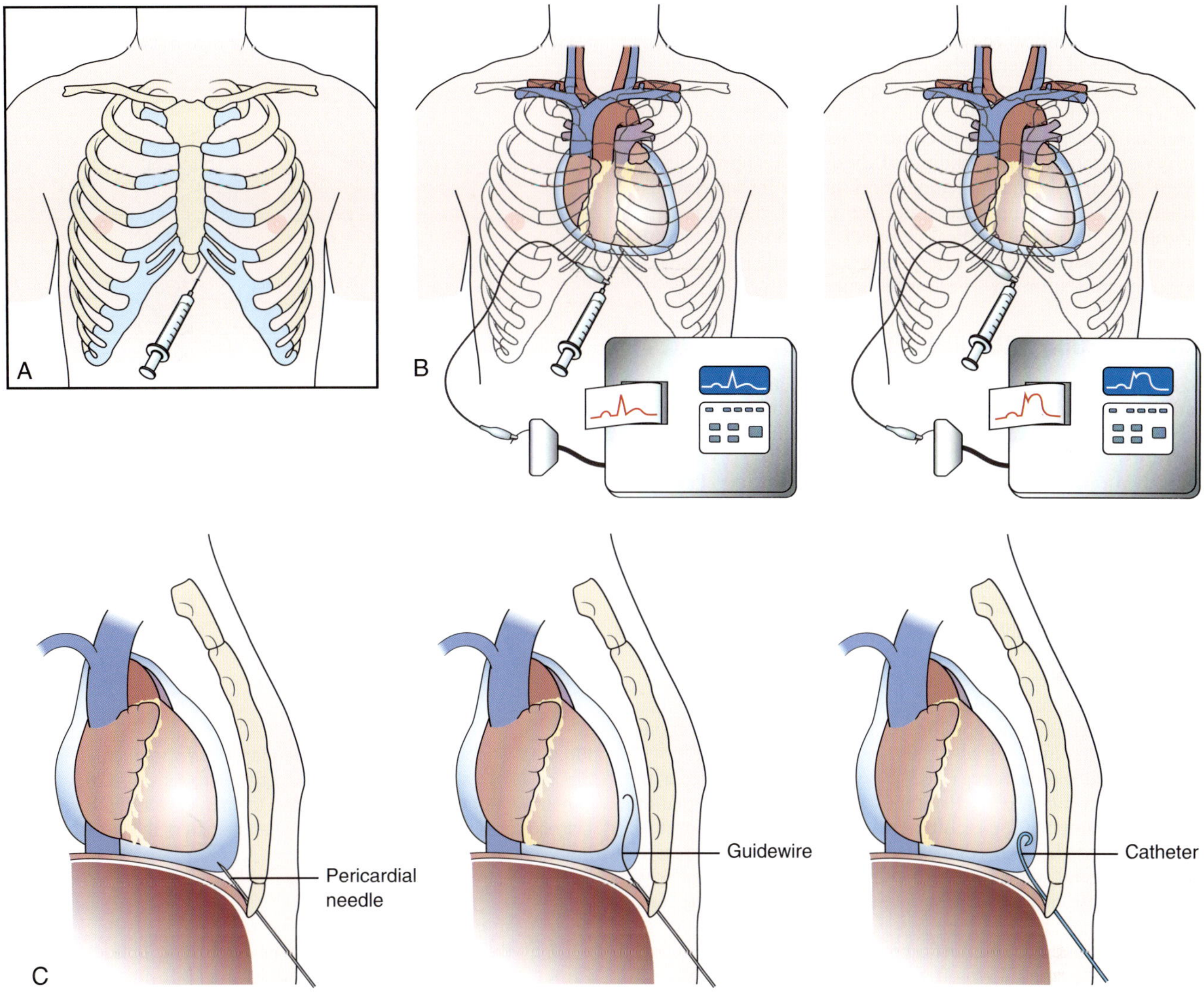

CHAPTER 59 Percutaneous Balloon Pericardiotomy for Patients With Pericardial Effusion and Tamponade

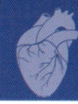

Fig. 59.1 (A) Diagrammatic representation of a pericardiocentesis procedure using the subxiphoid approach. (B) The pericardial needle is connected to an electrocardiographic (ECG) lead. The needle is advanced from the left of the subxiphoid area, aiming toward the left shoulder. ST-segment elevation is seen on the ECG lead tracing when the needle touches the epicardium. The needle should be retracted slightly until the ST-segment elevation disappears. (C) After the pericardial space has been entered with the pericardial needle, a guidewire is introduced in the pericardial space through the needle. The needle is removed, and a catheter is inserted over the guidewire anteriorly or inferiorly into the pericardial sac. (Modified from Jneid H, Maree AO, Palacios IF. Pericardial tamponade: clinical presentation, diagnosis and catheter-based therapies. In Parillo J, Dellinger PR, eds. *Critical care medicine*. 3rd ed. St. Louis: Mosby; 2008.)

and puncture of the left anterior descending artery and the internal mammary artery is more common with the parasternal approach. Echocardiographically guided pericardiocentesis is a safe and effective technique. In a cohort of 1127 therapeutic echocardiographically guided pericardiocenteses performed in 977 patients at the Mayo Clinic (1979 through 1998), the procedural success rate was 97% overall, with a total complication rate of 4.7%.[10] Echocardiography may be especially useful for patients with loculated effusions; unlike pericardiocenteses performed in the cardiac catheterization laboratory, the left chest wall is often used with echocardiographically guided pericardiocenteses. Novel safer techniques are emerging, including pericardiocentesis using continuous ultrasonographic guidance with a 7-cm micropuncture needle[14] or computed tomography–guided pericardiocentesis for high-risk patients (e.g., presence of pericardial adhesions, temporary pacing wires, or vascular conduits).[15]

Postprocedural Management

Pericardiocentesis may not completely evacuate the effusion in most cases because active secretion and bleeding into the pericardial space may continue.[1,3] The pericardial catheter should be left in place for 24 to 72 hours after initial fluid evacuation until the total daily drainage is 50 mL or less.

The patient is admitted for continuous monitoring and assessment of the rate of pericardial drainage. The pericardial space should be drained every 8 hours and the catheter flushed with heparinized saline. Systemic antibiotics—usually first-generation cephalosporin for empiric coverage of Gram-positive bacteria—are administered for the duration of the catheter stay. Based on the cause of the effusion, the patient's clinical and hemodynamic condition, and the amount of fluid drained, the pericardial catheter is usually removed within 72 hours or decisions for additional therapy are then contemplated.

Echocardiography can be used to monitor the resolution of the pericardial effusion and signs of cardiac compression before catheter removal. Patients who continue to drain more than 50 mL/24 hours after 3 days of standard catheter drainage should be considered for more aggressive therapy. Reaccumulation of the pericardial fluid is particularly common in patients with malignant pericardial effusions. Additional therapeutic approaches to prevent pericardial fluid reaccumulation include intrapericardial instillation of sclerosing agents and the use of chemotherapy, radiotherapy, PBP, and surgical pericardial window. Reaccumulation of fluid with recurrence of cardiac tamponade is considered an absolute indication for a pericardial window.

PERCUTANEOUS BALLOON PERICARDIOTOMY

For many patients with a pericardial effusion and tamponade, standard percutaneous pericardial drainage with an indwelling pericardial catheter is sufficient to avoid recurrence. Recurrences after catheter drainage have been reported for 14% to 50% of patients with pericardial effusion and tamponade.[5,16–18] Patients who continue to drain more than 50 mL/24 hours after 3 to 5 days of standard catheter drainage are considered for more aggressive therapy. Several approaches are available to prevent the reaccumulation of pericardial fluid, including intrapericardial instillation of sclerosing agents, chemotherapy, and radiation therapy.[19,20] A surgically created pericardial window may provide an alternative for the treatment of pericardial effusions,[21,22] but morbidity and late recurrences are common.[8,23,24]

The use of a subxiphoid surgical pericardial window has been advocated as primary therapy for malignant pericardial tamponade based on the high initial success in relieving tamponade[23–28] and an acceptable recurrence rate.[24] However, it is associated with high morbidity rates.[8,21–28] Patients with advanced malignancy and cardiac tamponade are often poor candidates for surgical therapy. Because life expectancy is already limited, the increased length of hospital stay associated with a surgical procedure may compromise the quality of these patients' remaining lives. The malnutrition and chemotherapy associated with advanced malignancy increase the risk of infection and other perioperative complications. It is preferable to offer a less invasive alternative.

Palacios and colleagues[29] proposed PBP as a less invasive alternative to the surgical pericardial window procedure. With this technique, a pericardial window and adequate drainage of pericardial effusion can be done percutaneously with a balloon catheter (Fig. 59.2). Since their initial report of eight patients, the multicenter PBP registry investigators have reported data on more than 130 patients.[30]

Technique

The PBP technique is relatively simple and safe. It is performed in the catheterization laboratory with the patient under local anesthesia and mild sedation with intravenous narcotics and a short-acting benzodiazepine. There is minimal discomfort. Patients may be candidates for PBP if they have undergone prior pericardiocentesis and have persistent catheter drainage. PBP also may be done as a primary therapy at the time of initial pericardiocentesis. For those who have previously undergone standard pericardiocentesis using the subxiphoid approach, a pigtail catheter has typically been left in the pericardial space for drainage. For patients who continue to drain more than 50 mL/24 hours after 3 to 5 days, PBP is offered as an alternative to a surgical procedure.

The subxiphoid area around the indwelling pigtail pericardial catheter is infiltrated with 1% lidocaine. A 0.038-inch guidewire with a preshaped curve at the tip is advanced through the pigtail catheter into the pericardial space (Fig. 59.3A). The catheter is then removed, leaving the guidewire in the pericardial space. The location of the wire should be confirmed by its looping within the

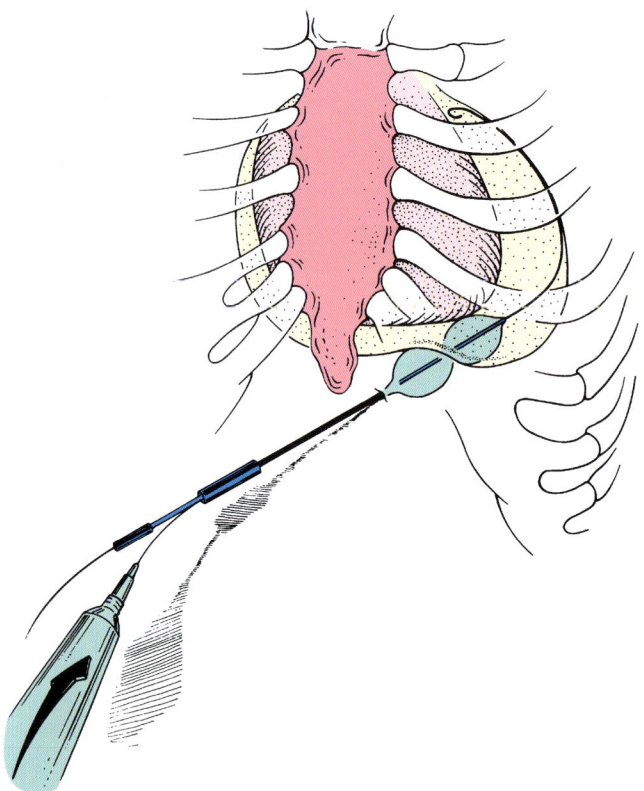

Fig. 59.2 Percutaneous balloon pericardiotomy technique. (From Ziskind AA, Pearce AC, Lemmon CC, et al. Percutaneous balloon pericardiotomy for the treatment of cardiac tamponade and large pericardial effusions: description of technique and report of the first fifty cases. *J Am Coll Cardiol.* 1993;21:1–5.)

pericardium. After predilation along the track of the wire with a 10-Fr dilator, a 20-mm-diameter 3-cm-long balloon dilation catheter is advanced over the guidewire and positioned to straddle the parietal pericardium. Care should be taken to advance the proximal end of the balloon beyond the skin and subcutaneous tissue. Precise localization of the balloon is accomplished by gentle inflation to identify the waist at the pericardial margin. The balloon is inflated manually until the waist produced by the parietal pericardium disappears (see Fig. 59.3B and C). If the pericardium is apposed to the chest wall, as indicated by failure of the proximal portion of the balloon to expand, a countertraction technique should be used in which the catheter is withdrawn slightly and then gently advanced while the skin and soft tissues are pulled manually in the opposite direction. This maneuver isolates the pericardium for dilation (Fig. 59.4).

Fluoroscopic imaging using multiple views (preferably biplane fluoroscopy) helps to ensure correct positioning of the balloon, which should be straddling the parietal pericardium (Fig. 59.5). At the operator's discretion, 5 to 10 mL of radiographic contrast material may be instilled into the pericardial space to help identify the pericardial margin. Two or three balloon inflations are then performed to ensure the creation of an adequate opening in the pericardium. Although transthoracic and transesophageal echocardiography may provide additional guidance to some aspects of the procedure, it is our experience that the balloon cannot be imaged adequately with echocardiography to identify the waist at the site of the pericardial margin.[31]

The balloon dilation catheter is then removed, leaving the 0.038-inch guidewire in the pericardial space. A new pigtail catheter is then advanced over this guidewire and placed in the pericardial space. If PBP is being performed at the time of primary

CHAPTER 59 Percutaneous Balloon Pericardiotomy for Patients With Pericardial Effusion and Tamponade

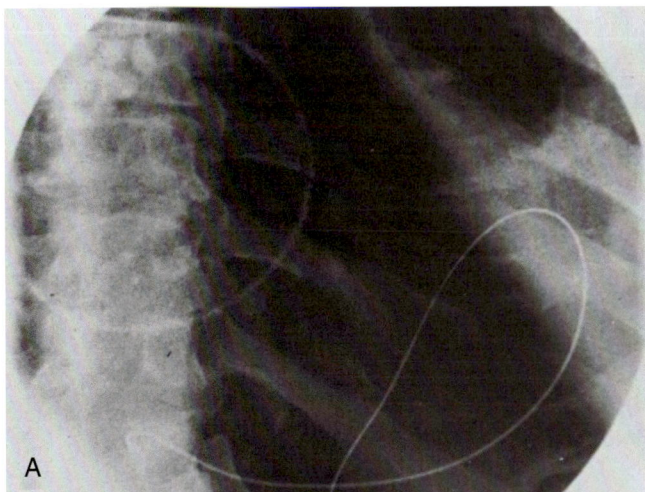

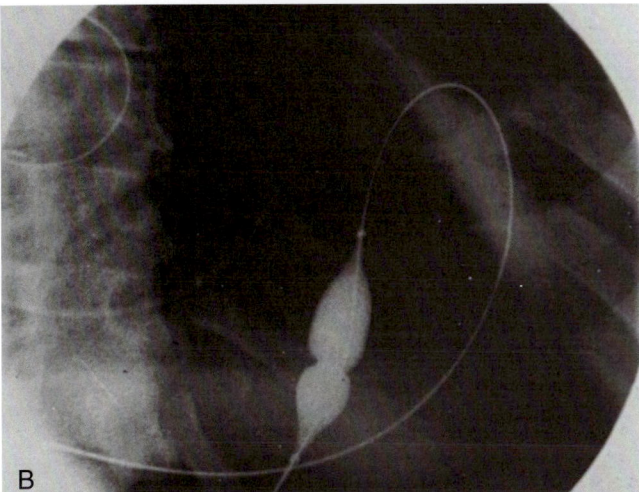

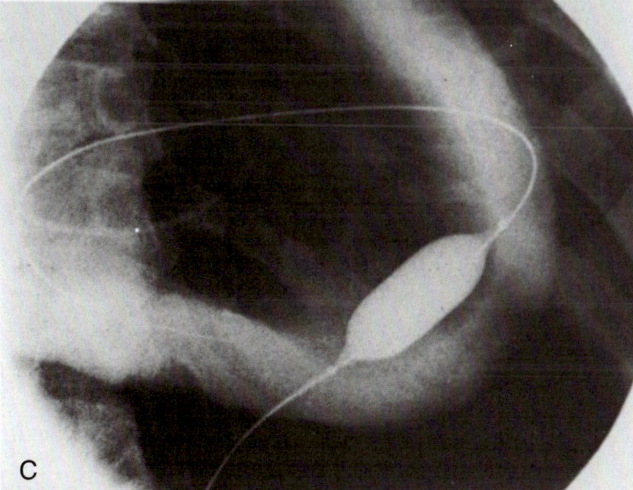

Fig. 59.3 Anteroposterior fluoroscopic images. (A) The 0.038-inch guidewire has been advanced through the pigtail catheter and can be seen looping freely in the pericardial space. (B) As the balloon is inflated manually, a waist is seen at the pericardial margin. (C) The waist disappears with full inflation of the balloon as the pericardial window is created.

pericardiocentesis, the pericardium is entered using a standard subxiphoid approach and a drainage catheter is inserted into the pericardial space. After the pericardial pressure has been

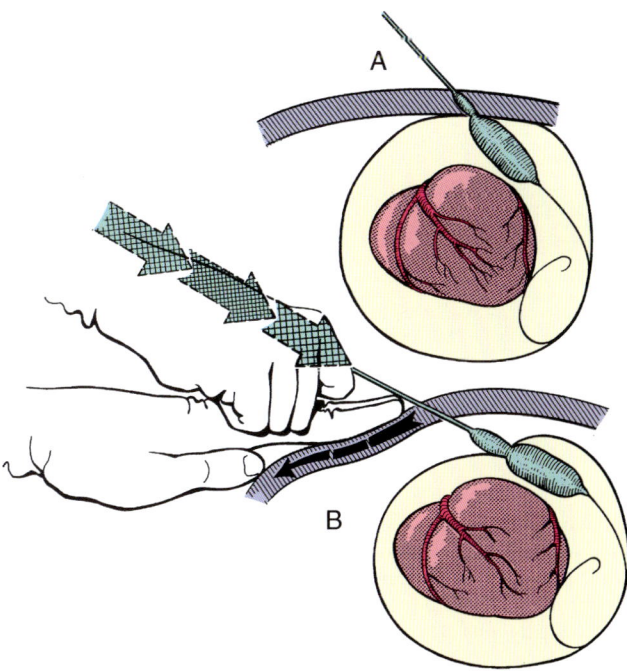

Fig. 59.4 Countertraction technique to separate the pericardium from the adjacent chest wall shown in a transverse view from below. (A) Initial trial inflation of the balloon demonstrates trapping of the proximal portion of the balloon in the chest wall structures. (B) Simultaneous traction on the skin and pushing of the balloon catheter results in displacement of the pericardium away from the chest wall, allowing proper inflation to occur. (Modified from Ziskind AA, Burstein S. Echocardiography vs. fluoroscopic imaging [letter]. *Cathet Cardiovasc Diagn.* 1992;27:86.)

measured, most of the pericardial fluid should be withdrawn, which reduces the volume remaining to pass into the pleural space.

Technical variations of the subxiphoid technique have included dilation of two adjacent pericardial sites, use of the apical approach,[32] use of an Inoue balloon catheter,[32–34] use of double balloons,[35] use of a combination of one long and one short balloon,[36] and use of an 18-mm dilating balloon to facilitate introduction of a 16-Fr chest tube into the pericardial space.[37] Other investigators have attempted laparoscopic pericardial fenestration,[38,39] used a cutting pericardiotome,[40] or implanted a pericardioperitoneal shunt.[41] Thoracoscopic techniques have been developed to create a larger pericardial window, with low morbidity rates compared with those for open surgical techniques.[42] With this technique, adequate long-term drainage may be provided and specimens for pathologic study obtained.[38,43]

Postprocedural Management

After the PBP procedure, the patient is returned to a telemetry floor. The pericardial catheter should be aspirated every 6 hours and flushed with heparinized saline (5 mL of 100 U/mL). Pericardial drainage volumes should be recorded, and the catheter should be removed after there has been no significant pericardial drainage (50 mL) for 24 hours.

At the time of the catheter removal, there is often evidence on the chest radiograph of a new or increasing pleural effusion. Follow-up two-dimensional transthoracic echocardiography is performed approximately 48 hours after removal of the pericardial catheter. Data are being collected on immediate removal of the pericardial catheter after PBP to facilitate early discharge. However, leaving the pericardial catheter in place may provide a measure of safety by allowing monitoring to determine whether

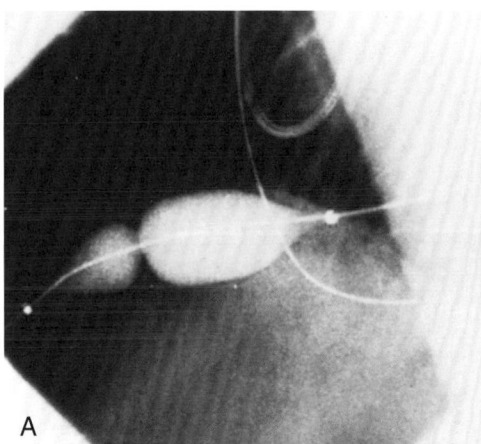
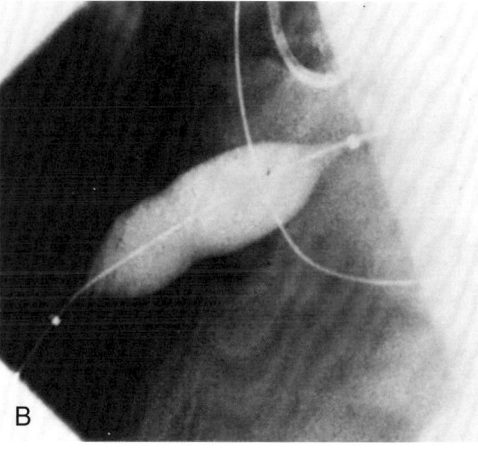

Fig. 59.5 Lateral fluoroscopic image of balloon inflation. (A) A waist is seen at the pericardial margin. (B) It disappears with full inflation.

the window is effective and whether bleeding is occurring. Periodic postprocedural echocardiography can be used to check for reaccumulation of pericardial fluid. Chest radiography should be performed to monitor the possible development of a pleural effusion (usually left) caused by drainage of the pericardial fluid.

Mechanism

The precise mechanism by which PBP works remains unclear. We assume that balloon inflation results in localized tearing of the parietal pericardial tissues, creating a communication of the pericardial space with the pleural space and possibly with the abdominal cavity.[44,45] The use of a flexible fiberoptic pericardioscope introduced over the guidewire after PBP has demonstrated a pericardial window freely communicating with the left pleural space (Fig. 59.6).[46]

Chow and colleagues supported this finding with their postmortem studies of balloon dilation, in which they used an Inoue balloon inflated to a maximum diameter of 23 mm.[47] Balloon dilation produced, without tearing, a smooth, oval pericardial window measuring 18.8 ± 16.4 mm. Histologic analysis revealed fragmentation and breakage of the elastic and collagenous fibers in the connective tissue bordering the pericardial sites.[47]

We have demonstrated passage of pericardial fluid from the pericardial space to the pleural space in some patients after PBP by manually injecting 10 mL of radiographic contrast material through the pericardial catheter. However, the ability to visualize free exit of contrast from the pericardial space does not appear to correlate with procedural success. Sugimoto and colleagues studied 28 patients who underwent surgical subxiphoid pericardial window procedures followed by tube decompression; 93% experienced permanent relief.[48] Postoperative echocardiograms demonstrated thickening of the pericardium-epicardium with obliteration of the pericardial space. Autopsy data that confirmed this fusion were available for four patients. The study authors concluded that the success of the subxiphoid pericardial window procedure depended on the inflammatory fusion of the epicardium to the pericardium, not on maintenance of a window.[48] Based on this surgical experience, it is unlikely that the PBP window remains open indefinitely. It is also possible that PBP, by leading to more effective pericardial drainage and maintaining a fluid-free pericardial space for a prolonged time, may permit autosclerosis to occur.

Results

Evidence-Based Literature

Palacios and coworkers reported the initial results of PBP in 8 patients with malignant pericardial effusion and tamponade.[29]

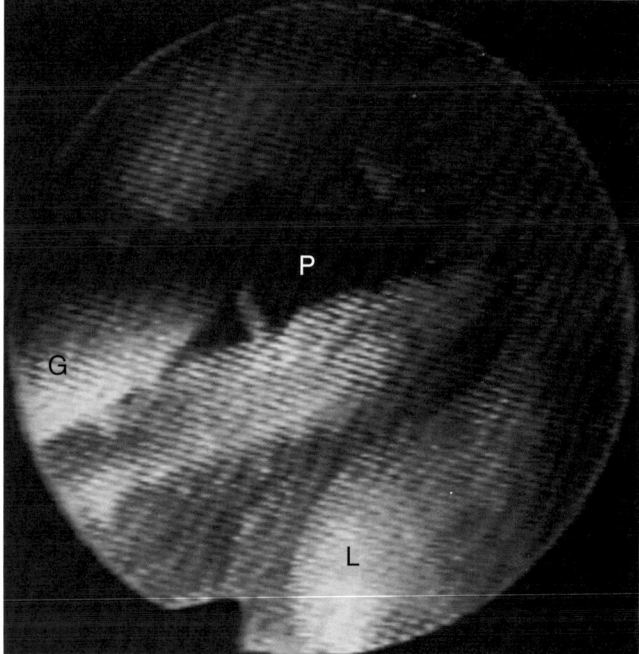

Fig. 59.6 Pericardioscopic view of the balloon pericardiotomy site. The scope has been withdrawn over a guidewire to visualize the external pericardial surface. This figure demonstrates direct communication of the pericardial window with the left pleural space. G, Guidewire; L, lung in left pleural space immediately outside the pericardium; P, pericardial window created by balloon dilation.

The technique was successful in all patients. There were no immediate or late complications related to the procedure and no patients had recurrence of pericardial tamponade or pericardial effusion after a mean follow-up of 6 ± 2 months.

The PBP technique has been studied in a multicenter registry to evaluate its therapeutic effectiveness and risks systematically. Data on 130 patients undergoing PBP from 1987 to 1994 in 16 centers have been analyzed.[30,46] In this cohort of 130 patients, the mean age was 59 ± 13 years, 52% were men, 69% had cardiac tamponade, and 58% had had a prior pericardiocentesis procedure performed. Of these patients, 85% had known malignancy (mostly lung cancer). PBP was defined as successful if there was no recurrence of pericardial effusion on echocardiographic follow-up and if no complications occurred that required surgical exploration or a surgical pericardial window. PBP was successful in 111 (85%) of 130 patients, with no recurrences of pericardial effusion or tamponade during a mean follow-up of 5.0 ± 5.8 months. Five cases were considered failures because of pericardial bleeding, and those patients underwent surgical windowing. Thirteen patients had recurrence of pericardial effusion (mean time to recurrence was 53 ± 65 days). Of those 13 patients, 12 underwent surgical pericardial procedures but six had a subsequent recurrence. Minor complications occurred in 11 patients (13%); the most common was fever. No patient had documented bacteremia or positive pericardial fluid cultures. After PBP, thoracentesis or chest tube placement was required in 15% of patients with preexisting pleural effusions, compared with 9% of patients without preexisting pleural effusions. Recently Irazusta and colleagues reported their single-center contemporary experience with 40 PBP procedures performed in 35 patients, the majority of whom had confirmed metastatic disease. In all cases, the procedure was successful; there were no acute complications, and the procedure was well tolerated at the first attempt.[49]

Technical Considerations

Echocardiographic and Chest Radiographic Qualifications

Echocardiography should be performed before PBP to rule out loculated pericardial fluid. If pericardial fluid is not free flowing, a surgical approach should be considered. If the chest radiograph reveals evidence of a large pleural effusion before PBP, this issue is less clear.

If a left effusion is moderate or large before PBP, the chance of needing thoracentesis is high, and PBP should be performed only if the cardiac benefits outweigh the risks of thoracentesis or chest tube placement. Patients with marginal pulmonary mechanics, such as those who have undergone pneumonectomy, should be evaluated with caution because the development of a left pleural effusion may compromise their remaining lung function.

Prophylactic Antibiotic Administration

Febrile episodes were documented six times in the first 37 patients, although no patient had documented bacteremia or positive pericardial drainage cultures. Beginning with the 38th patient, prophylactic antibiotic therapy was initiated and continued until the catheter was removed. No febrile episodes were seen in 49 subsequent patients. It is unclear whether this was related to prophylactic antibiotics, a random effect, or more extensive operator experience with a concomitant decrease in procedural time and catheter manipulation.

Bleeding Risk

The risk of bleeding from the pericardiotomy site appears to be increased in patients with platelet or coagulation abnormalities. PBP should be avoided in patients with uremic pericardial effusions or when coagulation parameters cannot be normalized (i.e., refractory coagulopathy or thrombocytopenia). In patients at high risk for bleeding, a surgical procedure under direct visualization may be safer.

Fluoroscopic Guidance

Attempts to guide balloon placement by transthoracic or transesophageal echocardiography have been disappointing. Although the dilating balloon can be visualized, it is not possible to distinguish proper placement (with a discrete waist) from entrapment of the proximal balloon in the soft tissues and ineffective pericardial dilation. We have found fluoroscopic guidance to be particularly essential to the countertraction technique and think that it should be mandatory for PBP.[31]

Risks of Cardiac and Pulmonary Injury

Because PBP is not performed until successful access to the pericardial space has been obtained and the guidewire is seen to be freely looping within the pericardium, the risks of cardiac injury are usually small. If the right ventricle is inadvertently entered and the balloon advanced, the results may be catastrophic. In the emergency setting it may be prudent to stabilize the patient with pericardiocentesis and leave a catheter in place for elective PBP under more controlled conditions.

Pleural Effusion

Development of a large pleural effusion after PBP is a significant concern. A left pleural effusion develops in most patients within 24 to 48 hours of the procedure (Fig. 59.7). In most cases the pleural effusion resolves, presumably because of the greater resorptive capacity of the pleural surfaces.

Thoracentesis or chest tube placement was required in 15% of patients with preexisting pleural effusions compared with 9% of those without preexisting pleural effusions in the multicenter PBP registry. It is likely that some patients have a large volume of fluid flow from the pericardial to the pleural space, but in many cases it is difficult to determine whether the effusion results from drainage of fluid from the pericardial space or from the progression of concomitant pleural disease. For this reason it is desirable to remove most of the pericardial fluid before creating the PBP window so as to limit the potential volume of fluid that can immediately move to the pleural space.

Duration of Catheter Placement

Most patients have a drainage catheter left in the pericardial space to monitor fluid output after the procedure. It is typically removed when pericardial drainage is less than 50 mL/24 hours. It may be possible to perform PBP without leaving a pericardial catheter in place, permitting an even shorter hospital stay and further decreasing the risk of infection.

Management of Balloon Rupture

Balloon rupture at the time of PBP can occur as a result of the combination of a large balloon, excessive inflation pressure, and an inelastic pericardium. Uncommonly, balloon rupture may be accompanied by catheter fracture because excessive resistance limits withdrawal. Our experience suggests that the frequency of balloon rupture can be minimized with proper technique, particularly the use of countertraction to isolate the pericardium, thereby avoiding dilation of the adjacent nonpericardial tissues.[31] Hemiballoon dislodgment sometimes occurs. Block and Wilson have described a technique to retrieve it by placing a second pericardial catheter, snaring the guidewire, and using a second catheter to pull the balloon fragment back.[50]

Adjunctive Diagnostic Approaches

Although patients with pericardial effusion may have a history of malignancy, malignancy is the cause of the effusion in only 50% of them.[1,4] Although cytologic analysis of the pericardial fluid may aid in the diagnosis, pericardial tissue is not routinely obtained by PBP for pathologic analysis, as is the case during a surgical pericardial window procedure. To address this need, a percutaneously introduced pericardial bioptome has been successful in providing tissue of diagnostic quality.[30] With the use of an aggressive serrated-jaw bioptome (Boston Scientific, Natick, MA) (Fig. 59.8A) that is advanced though an 8-Fr vascular introducer, multiple samples can be obtained from the posterolateral aspect of the parietal pericardium (see Fig. 59.8B). This technique remains investigational.

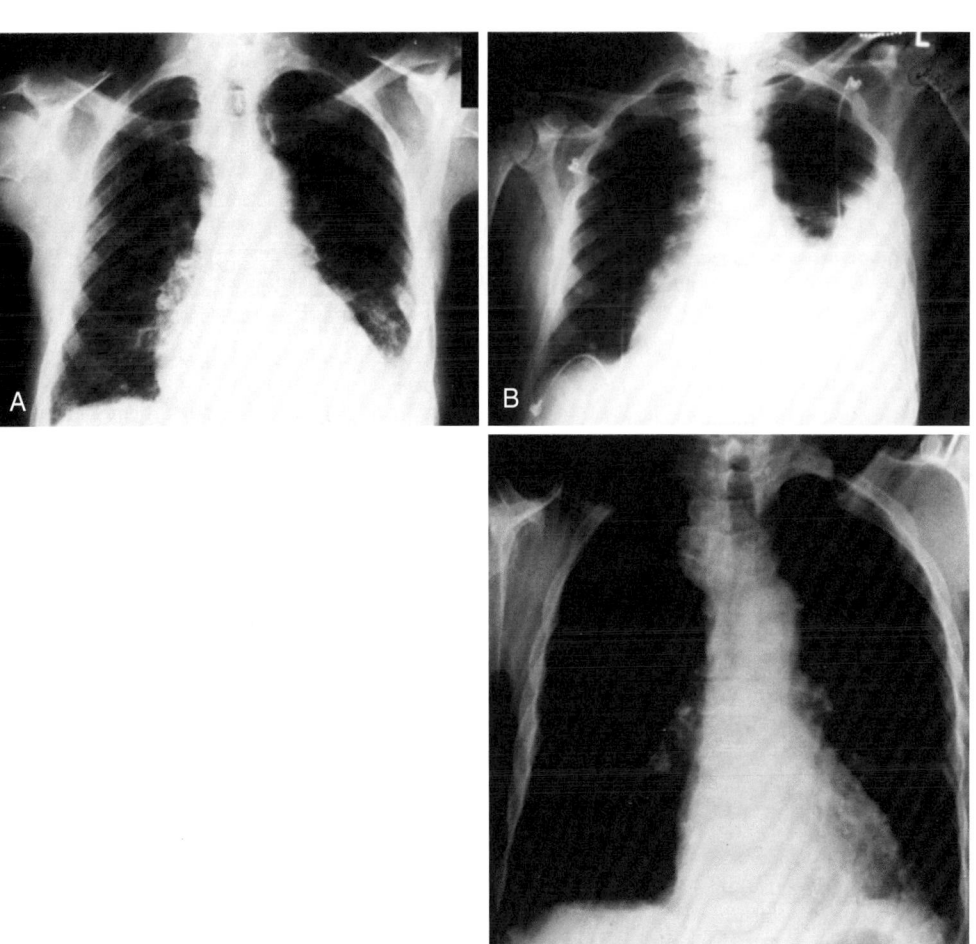

Fig. 59.7 Posteroanterior chest radiographs. (A) At admission, the radiograph shows an enlarged cardiac silhouette. (B) At 24 hours after percutaneous balloon pericardiotomy, a new left pleural effusion is seen. (C) One month later, complete resolution of the left pleural effusion is apparent. (From Palacios IF, Tuzcu EM, Ziskind AA, et al. Percutaneous balloon pericardial window for patients with malignant pericardial effusion and tamponade. *Cathet Cardiovasc Diagn.* 1991;22:244–249.)

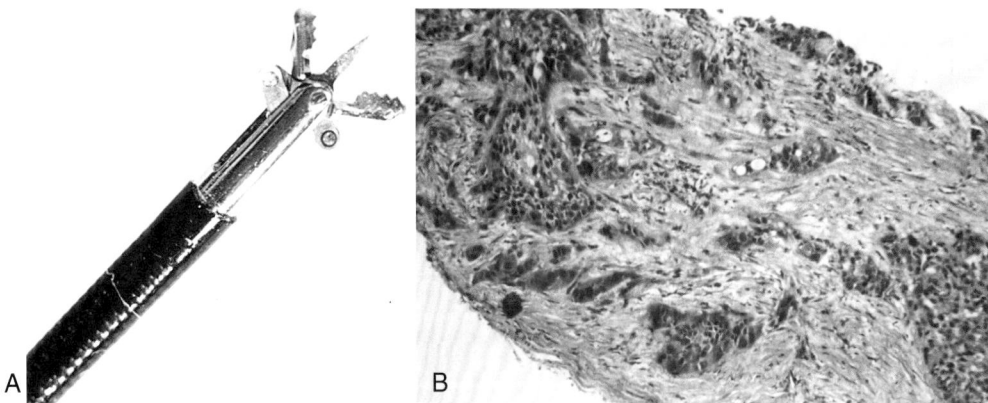

Fig. 59.8 (A) Pericardial bioptome with a center needle and aggressive serrated-jaw configuration. (B) Percutaneous pericardial biopsy specimen from a patient with newly diagnosed lung cancer. It contains sheets of squamous cell carcinoma. Malignant cells are seen trapped in the fibrin of the inflammatory exudate. (From Ziskind AA, Rodriguez S, Lemmon C, et al. Percutaneous pericardial biopsy as an adjunctive technique for the diagnosis of pericardial disease. *Am J Cardiol.* 1994;74:288–291.)

Summary

PBP offers a nonsurgical alternative for the management of pericardial effusion. PBP is particularly useful for critically ill patients with advanced malignancy and limited survival for whom it is desirable to avoid the risks and discomfort of anesthesia and surgery. PBP appears to palliate malignant pericardial disease successfully for the duration of their survival.

The decision to perform PBP rather than pericardiocentesis with or without sclerotherapy may depend on patient and institutional variables. PBP should be considered if pericardial fluid recurs after primary pericardiocentesis. In institutions with an aggressive surgical approach to malignant pericardial disease, this less invasive alternative to a surgical pericardial window may be considered for the primary treatment of malignant cardiac tamponade. In contrast, pericardiocentesis alone, without PBP

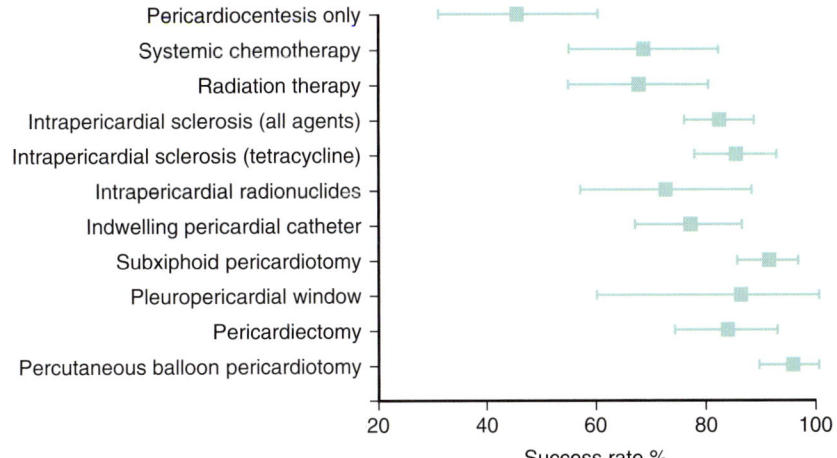

Fig. 59.9 Success rates with 95% confidence intervals (bars) for various treatment modalities for malignant pericardial effusions. (From Vaitkus PT, Herrmann HC, Le Winter MM. Treatment of malignant pericardial effusion. JAMA. 1994;272:272.)

at that time, is preferred if the cause of the pericardial fluid is unknown.

Samples of pericardial fluid should be sent for cell counts, cytologic analysis, culture, and special stains to assist with the diagnosis. Simple pericardiocentesis is also preferred if uremic platelet dysfunction or other coagulation abnormalities exist or there is the possibility of bacterial or fungal infection that could be spread to the pleural space.

The immediate and late results of PBP for patients with malignant pericardial effusion appear to be similar to those of surgical pericardiotomy. However, the role of PBP in the management of nonmalignant pericardial disease remains unclear. It is possible that PBP could be used for the treatment of pericardial effusions caused by viral infection, HIV-related disease, hypothyroidism, collagen vascular disease, and idiopathic effusions. PBP was reported with favorable results in a series of pediatric patients with nonmalignant effusions.[51] Additional long-term follow-up is needed on larger numbers of patients to clarify the role of this procedure in nonmalignant pericardial disease.

Vaitkus and colleagues performed a meta-analysis of prior studies in which the treatment of malignant pericardial effusions was defined as successful if the patient survived the procedure, the symptoms did not recur, and no other interventions directed at the pericardium were required regardless of the length of survival.[52] Success rates for the various treatments are shown in Fig. 59.9. Because no randomized data are available comparing the efficacy of PBP with that of a surgical or thoracoscopic pericardial window or with catheter drainage and sclerotherapy, procedures combining the use of PBP and sclerotherapy have not been done.

NOVEL CATHETER-BASED INTERVENTIONS IN THE PERICARDIAL SPACE

The use of percutaneous intervention techniques in the pericardial space has been progressively increasing and now encompasses multiple disciplines in cardiology. Many factors have contributed to the emergence of these techniques. Epicardial catheter mapping and ablation in the electrophysiology laboratory have opened a new horizon in cardiac electrophysiology. The pericardial space has been recognized as a natural drug receptacle, with many investigators attempting to exploit it as a reservoir to deliver therapeutic substances.[53] The latter include the intrapericardial instillation of drugs such as triamcinolone after electrophysiologic procedures to prevent pericarditis or steroids to treat incessant pericarditis, or other drugs such as tetracyclines, antiarrhythmics, and chemotherapeutic agents.

Epicardial Mapping and Ablation

Epicardial scar-related reentry has been recognized as an important cause of ventricular tachycardia, especially in patients with nonischemic cardiomyopathy. It was initially adopted in patients with Chagas cardiomyopathy. Now it is recognized that almost 30% to 60% of patients with nonischemic cardiomyopathy may need an epicardial approach to increase their long-term freedom from ventricular arrhythmias. Other forms of cardiac disease where epicardial ablation may play a role include arrhythmogenic right ventricular cardiomyopathy, as well as hypertrophic cardiomyopathy and cardiac sarcoidosis (although the latter two may have mid myocardial scars and may need a combination of endocardial and epicardial ablation). Other infrequent but clinically significant arrhythmias, such as supraventricular tachycardias and idiopathic ventricular tachycardia, also possess epicardial foci that cannot be ablated except from the epicardium.

Catheter-based intervention techniques in the pericardial space gained momentum after invasive cardiologists realized that pericardial fluid is not a prerequisite for a safe percutaneous entry into the pericardial space. Sosa and colleagues[54] were the first to show that the pericardial space can be safely entered with a blunt-tipped needle using a subxiphoid approach under fluoroscopic guidance. In their seminal work in 1996 in patients with Chagas disease,[54] they advanced an epidural needle toward the right ventricular apex until a slight negative pressure was felt, and they confirmed the needle position by small injections of contrast to delineate the cardiac silhouette. They established the feasibility and safety of epicardial mapping in patients with Chagas disease and recurrent ventricular tachycardia, one of whom underwent a successful epicardial circuit ablation.[54]

Epicardial mapping and ablation were subsequently adopted by several interventional electrophysiologists.[55] Sosa and colleagues[56] then performed epicardial mapping to guide endocardial and epicardial ablation in a series of 10 consecutive patients with ventricular tachycardia and Chagas disease. Epicardial mapping in that study enabled the detection of an epicardial circuit in 14 of 18 mappable ventricular tachycardias and helped guide endocardial ablation in four patients and epicardial ablation in six. The same approach was also attempted successfully in patients with recurrent ventricular tachycardia after myocardial infarction, demonstrating that postinfarction pericardial adherence does not preclude epicardial mapping and ablation.[57]

It has since become clear that failure of endocardial ablation can reflect an epicardial arrhythmic substrate, which can be safely treated by epicardial mapping and ablation using the percutaneous pericardial technique. In one series of 48 patients with prior

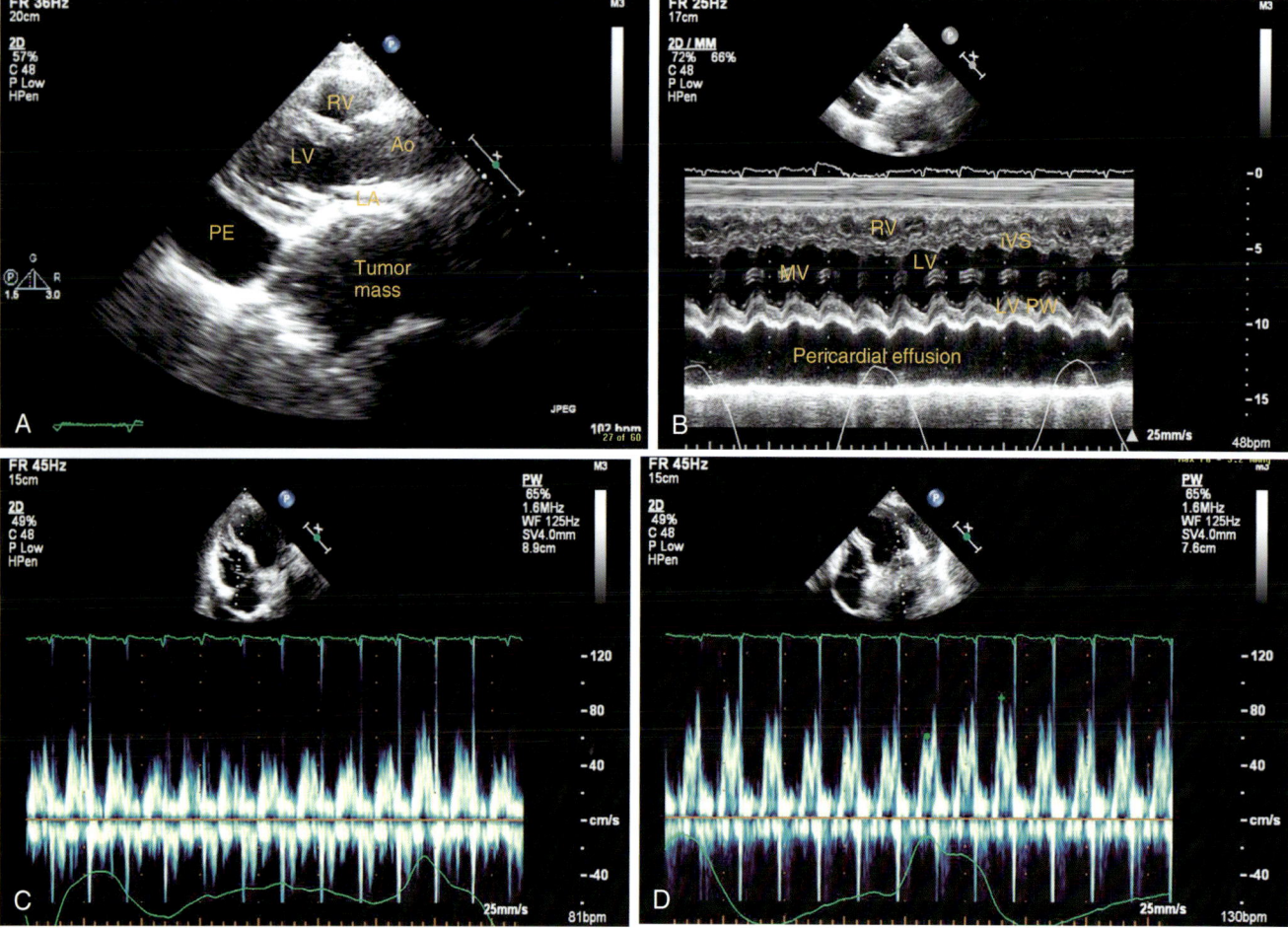

Fig. 59.10 (A) Parasternal long-axis view shows a large pericardial effusion located predominantly posteriorly and adjacent to a tumor mass in a patient diagnosed with lung cancer. The left atrium appears very small due to extrinsic compression by the tumor. (B) M-mode view of the pericardial effusion measuring 4.2 cm in its maximal diameter. (C) Marked respiratory variation in the inflow velocities across the tricuspid valve suggests increased intrapericardial pressure. (D) Marked respiratory variation in mitral inflow E velocities (>25%) suggests cardiac tamponade. *Ao*, Aorta; *IVS*, interventricular septum; *LA*, left atrium; *LV*, left ventricle; *LVPW*, left ventricular posterior wall; *MV*, mitral valve; *PE*, pericardial effusion; *RV*, right ventricle.

unsuccessful endocardial ablation, Schweikert and colleagues[58] showed that epicardial instrumentation and ablation can provide a safe and effective alternative strategy.

In addition to the subxiphoid approach for pericardial puncture (i.e., from the epicardial surface of the heart), other investigational approaches have been studied. Mickelsen and colleagues examined, in an experimental model, the transvenous access to the pericardial space for epicardial lead implantation for cardiac resynchronization therapy.[59]

Intrapericardial Echocardiography

Intrapericardial echocardiography is another example of a promising catheter-based technique in the pericardial space. Rodrigues and coworkers[60] introduced phased-array ultrasound transducers into the pericardial space of seven goats, using 10-Fr steerable catheters that were advanced by the transthoracic subxiphoid approach. They were then able to obtain detailed images of cardiac structures. This promising approach may help establish the relative positions of the ablation catheters and may facilitate epicardial ablation in the electrophysiology laboratory.

Several devices are being studied for safe and effective percutaneous access to the pericardial space. An example is the PerDUCER (Comedicus, Columbia Heights, MN), which has provided efficient, safe, and effective pericardial access in the normal or minimally abnormal pericardial space.[61,62]

Percutaneous Pericardial Biopsy

PPB was described in 1988 by Endrys and colleagues,[63] who reported a series of 18 patients undergoing pericardial biopsy using an endomyocardial bioptome inserted through an 8-Fr, 40-cm Teflon sheath with a curved tip and multiple side holes.[63] Endrys and colleagues allowed air to enter the pericardium to delineate the visceral and parietal pericardial layers; they obtained an average of eight samples per patient with no complications. They therefore showed that PPB could be safely performed using conventional invasive cardiology techniques.[63]

Because the floppy nature of the bioptome made it difficult to direct it to the appropriate site in the pericardial cavity, a modified technique using the distal portion of a 9-Fr right Judkins coronary guiding catheter was adopted to target pericardial biopsy sites.[64] Ziskind and colleagues subsequently used a special pericardial bioptome with a central needle and serrated jaws to perform pericardial biopsy.[30] They also maintained separation of the visceral-pericardial layer by avoiding complete evacuation of

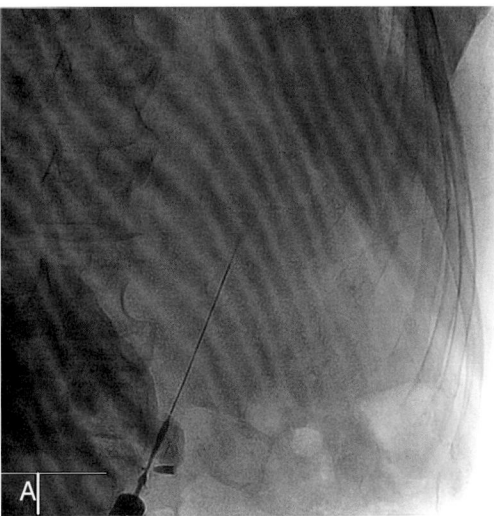 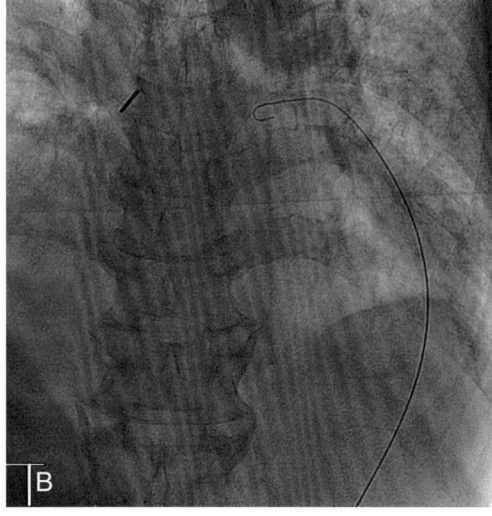

Fig. 59.11 (A) The pericardial space is accessed by the subxiphoid approach using a micropuncture kit in a patient with a large pericardial effusion. Injection of iodinated contrast material into the pericardial space confirmed the intrapericardial location. Subsequent transthoracic echocardiographic imaging with a bubble study further confirmed pericardial access. (B) A 0.035-inch guidewire is positioned in the pericardial space; a draining catheter is subsequently advanced over the guidewire to evacuate the effusion (Video 59.1).

pericardial fluid at the beginning of the procedure and therefore avoided instilling air into the pericardial cavity.[30] Selig and colleagues described a modified PPB technique using echocardiographic guidance without fluoroscopy.[65]

In summary, the PPB technique is safe and feasible in the cardiac catheterization laboratory. It is less invasive than surgical biopsy, can easily be modified to obtain tissue samples from pericardial masses, and has increased the diagnostic yield of pericardiocentesis and pericardial fluid analysis.

Pericardioscopy

Pericardioscopy can further help in the management of various pericardial pathologies by better visualization of the tissue, thus assisting focused biopsies, intrapericardial instillation of drugs, or implantation of epicardial leads.

Seferovic and associates[66] reported their experience with the use of pericardioscopy to assist pericardial biopsy and demonstrated the diagnostic value of pericardial biopsy to be significantly improved by pericardioscopy-guided extensive sampling. Their study included 49 patients with large pericardial effusions undergoing parietal pericardial biopsy. In 12 patients (group 1), pericardial biopsy was guided by fluoroscopy and obtained three to six samples per patient. In 22 patients (group 2), four to six pericardial biopsies per patient were obtained by pericardioscopic guidance using a 16-Fr flexible endoscope. In group 3, extensive pericardial sampling (18 to 20 samples per patient) was performed, guided by pericardioscopy in 15 patients. Sampling efficiency was better with pericardioscopy (group 2, 84.9%; group 3, 84.2%) compared with fluoroscopic guidance (group 1, 43.7%; $P < .01$). Pericardial biopsy in group 3 had higher diagnostic value than that in group 1 for revealing a new diagnosis (40% vs. 8.3%; $P < .05$) or establishing the cause (53.3% vs. 8.3%; $P < .05$). For group 2, pericardial biopsy had a higher yield in establishing the cause than that for group 1 (40.9% vs. 8.3%; $P < .05$). No major complications were observed in this study.

Percutaneous Left Atrial Appendage Suture Ligation

Percutaneous left atrial appendage (LAA) suture ligation is an alternative to oral anticoagulation for stroke prevention in patients with atrial fibrillation. The Lariat procedure[67] to percutaneously close the LAA depends on the ability of the operator to safely access and work in the pericardial space in a patient who usually has no pericardial effusion. It is performed in patients who have suitable LAA anatomy amenable to Lariat ligation.

A 13.5-Fr soft-tipped sheath is introduced into the pericardial space and a transseptal puncture is performed by means of the femoral vein by standard techniques. A magnet-tipped, 0.025-inch guidewire is advanced into the anterior aspect of the LAA. A magnet-tipped 0.035-inch wire is then advanced into the pericardium through the pericardial sheath to form a connection with the magnet-tipped wire in the LAA, over which the Lariat snare is advanced and closed at the mouth of the LAA using transesophageal echocardiography and fluoroscopic guidance. The preloaded suture is released from the snare and tightened with the suture-tensioning device. The snare is removed, and the suture is cut using a suture cutter. The pericardial sheath is exchanged for a drain, which is left in place for at least 4 to 6 hours or more if needed.

Price and colleagues[68] reported the results of the multicenter U.S. registry inclusive of 154 consecutive patients undergoing LAA ligation with the Lariat device at eight sites. Device success was achieved in 94% of patients, with an 86% procedural success rate and 10% major complication rate. Significant pericardial effusion occurred in 10.4% of patients after the procedure.

CONCLUSIONS

Pericardial effusion is caused by myriad conditions; it can complicate acute pericarditis and chronic effusive constrictive pericarditis or result in acute cardiac tamponade (Fig. 59.10). Pericardiocentesis (Fig. 59.11) serves as a diagnostic and therapeutic modality in patients with pericardial effusions. PBP is an effective therapy for recurrent, free-flowing, and hemodynamically significant pericardial effusions, especially those associated with neoplastic disease. Catheter-based diagnostic and interventional techniques in the pericardial space have become increasingly common and include epicardial mapping and ablation, intrapericardial delivery of therapies, intrapericardial echocardiography, pericardioscopy-guided biopsy, and percutaneous LAA suture ligation.

KEY REFERENCES

1. Jneid H, Maree AO, Palacios IF. Pericardial tamponade: clinical presentation, diagnosis and catheter-based therapies. In: Parillo J, Dellinger PR, eds. *Critical care medicine*. 3rd ed. St. Louis: Mosby; 2008.
3. Jneid H, Maree AO, Palacios IF. Acute pericardial disease: pericardiocentesis and percutaneous pericardiotomy. In: Mebazaa AGM, Zannad FM, Parillo J, eds. *Acute Heart Failure*. London: Springer; 2008.
9. Sagrista-Sauleda J, Angel J, Permanyer-Miralda G, et al. Long-term follow-up of idiopathic chronic pericardial effusion. *N Engl J Med*. 1999;341(27):2054–2059.
11. Kim KH, Miranda WR, Sinak LJ, et al. Effusive-constrictive pericarditis after pericardiocentesis: incidence, associated findings, and natural history. *JACC Cardiovasc Imaging*. 2018;11(4):534–541.
12. Lemmert ME, van Bommel RJ, Diletti R, et al. Clinical characteristics and management of coronary artery perforations: a single-center 11-year experience and practical overview. *J Am Heart Assoc*. 2017;6(9):pii: e007049.
14. Lakhter V, Aggarwal V, Bashir R, et al. Pericardiocentesis under continuous ultrasonographic guidance using a 7 cm micropuncture needle. *J Invasive Cardiol*. 2016;28(10):397–402.
15. Melvan JN, Madden D, Vasquez JC, et al. Computed tomography-guided pericardiocentesis: an alternative approach for accessing the pericardium. *Heart Lung Circ*. 2016;25(7):725–728.
29. Palacios IF, Tuzcu EM, Ziskind AA, et al. Percutaneous balloon pericardial window for patients with malignant pericardial effusion and tamponade. *Cathet Cardiovasc Diagn*. 1991;22(4):244–249.
46. Ziskind AA, Pearce AC, Lemmon CC, et al. Percutaneous balloon pericardiotomy for the treatment of cardiac tamponade and large pericardial effusions: description of technique and report of the first 50 cases. *J Am Coll Cardiol*. 1993;21(1):1–5.
49. Irazusta FJ, Jiménez-Valero S, Gemma D, et al. Percutaneous balloon pericardiotomy: treatment of choice in patients with advanced oncological disease and severe pericardial effusion. *Cardiovasc Revasc Med*. 2017;18(5S1):S14–S17.
54. Sosa E, Scanavacca M, d'Avila A, et al. A new technique to perform epicardial mapping in the electrophysiology laboratory. *J Cardiovasc Electrophysiol*. 1996;7(6):531–536.
56. Sosa E, Scanavacca M, D'Avila A, et al. Endocardial and epicardial ablation guided by nonsurgical transthoracic epicardial mapping to treat recurrent ventricular tachycardia. *J Cardiovasc Electrophysiol*. 1998;9(3):229–239.
68. Price MJ, Gibson DN, Yakubov SJ, et al. Early safety and efficacy of percutaneous left atrial appendage suture ligation: results from the U.S. Transcatheter LAA Ligation Consortium. *J Am Coll Cardiol*. 2014;64(6):565–572.

Additional references available online at expertconsult.com.

中文导读

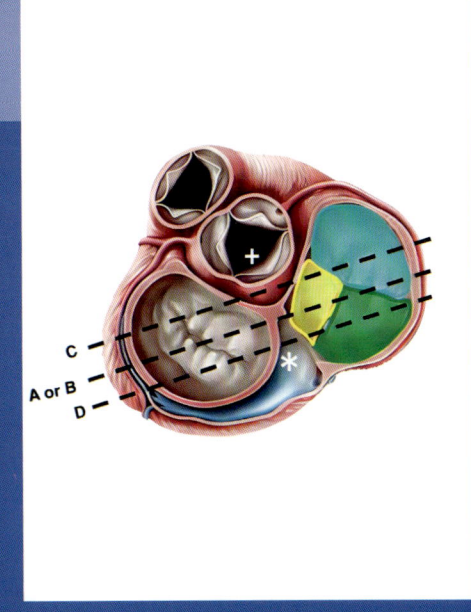

第60章
先天性心脏病的经导管治疗

　　经导管介入治疗技术可用于先天性心脏病的缺损封堵和狭窄扩张形成。本章节总结了先天性心脏病经导管介入治疗的现状，包括瓣膜狭窄、肺动脉狭窄、主动脉缩窄、房间隔缺损、动脉导管未闭等；详细介绍了经皮肺动脉瓣和主动脉瓣球囊成形术、肺动脉和主动脉狭窄的球囊扩张支架植入术、房间隔缺损和动脉导管未闭封堵术，以及经导管肺动脉瓣置换术的适应证、技术操作要点、即刻和长期效果、并发症、目前存在的问题及相应推荐。经皮肺动脉瓣球囊成形术适用于有严重肺畸形的新生儿和任何年龄中心排血量正常，伴有孤立性肺瓣膜狭窄且静息收缩压峰值梯度>40 mmHg的患者。

　　经皮主动脉瓣球囊成形术适用于瓣膜融合导致流出道梗阻的先天性主动脉瓣狭窄患者，不适用于瓣膜环发育不良或瓣膜小叶钙化的患者。肺动脉支架植入是大多数肺动脉狭窄患者的标准一线治疗方法。经皮封堵治疗已成为解剖条件合适的继发孔型房间隔缺损和动脉导管未闭的首选治疗方式。主动脉支架是治疗主动脉狭窄的有效方式，对年龄较小的儿童应尽量避免植入支架，而对老年患者植入带膜支架更安全。经导管肺动脉瓣置换术可以改善功能失调性右室流出道的狭窄和反流。

谷　喆　吴永健

章节要点

- 基于导管的治疗可用于多种先天性结构性心血管缺陷。
- 球囊扩张可缓解先天性肺或主动脉瓣狭窄患者的阻塞。如果瓣膜发育不全或钙化，这种治疗可能是不够的。
- 球囊扩张支架可有效缓解先天性肺动脉狭窄；对于成长中的儿童来说，晚期支架再扩张可能是必要的。
- 主动脉缩窄可用球囊扩张支架治疗；覆膜支架可以为主动脉脆弱的老年患者提供重要的安全优势。
- 经导管封堵器可安全有效地治疗继发孔型动脉间隔缺损或动脉导管未闭。
- 经导管肺动脉瓣置换术对于右心室至肺动脉导管或生物假体肺动脉瓣功能不良的患者是有效的治疗，如法洛四联症术后患者。

60 Transcatheter Therapies for Congenital Heart Disease

Bryan H. Goldstein, Wendy Whiteside, Jeffrey D. Zampi, Russel Hirsch

KEY POINTS

- Catheter-based therapies are available for a wide variety of congenital structural cardiovascular defects.
- Balloon dilation provides relief of obstruction for patients with congenital pulmonary or aortic valve stenosis. This therapy may not be adequate if the valve is hypoplastic or calcified.
- Congenital pulmonary artery stenosis can be effectively relieved with balloon-expandable stents; late stent redilation may be necessary in a growing child.

- Coarctation of the aorta can be treated with balloon-expandable stenting; covered stents may provide an important safety advantage for older patients with a fragile aorta.
- Transcatheter occlusion devices are available to safely and effectively treat a secundum-type arterial septal defect or a patent ductus arteriosus.
- Transcatheter pulmonary valve replacement is effective therapy in patients who have a dysfunctional right ventricle–to–pulmonary artery conduit or a bioprosthetic pulmonary valve, as in postoperative tetralogy of Fallot.

INTRODUCTION

This chapter summarizes the current state of the art of transcatheter therapy for structural congenital heart disease (CHD). It discusses catheter-based therapies that are available for some of the more common congenital defects, including semilunar valve stenosis, pulmonary artery (PA) stenosis, coarctation of the aorta, secundum atrial septal defect (ASD), and patent ductus arteriosus (PDA). New developments in transcatheter pulmonary valve replacement (TPVR) are also reviewed.

Percutaneous balloon valvuloplasty provides effective treatment in patients with congenital pulmonary or aortic valve stenosis. Surgical valvotomy for congenital semilunar valve stenosis has been replaced by these interventional catheterization techniques in most pediatric centers. Balloon-expandable stenting is standard therapy for most patients with PA stenosis. These arterial lesions often are elastic in nature—a characteristic that makes balloon angioplasty alone a less successful intervention. Coarctation stenting is an effective therapeutic intervention for selected patients with coarctation of the aorta. Transcatheter occlusion devices provide a safe, highly effective therapy for a secundum ASD or a PDA and constitute the treatment of choice for these defects. Finally, TPVR is currently routine therapy for selected patients with a dysfunctional right ventricle–to–pulmonary artery (RV-PA) conduit or bioprosthetic pulmonary valve (BPV); this remarkable new intervention can replace reoperation and is therefore an important therapeutic option for many patients.

PULMONARY BALLOON VALVULOPLASTY

Pulmonary valve stenosis is a common disorder, accounting for approximately 8% of congenital cardiac defects.[1] Except for neonates with critical pulmonary stenosis, patients with untreated pulmonary valve stenosis often survive well into adulthood.[2] However, when more than mild obstruction to right ventricular (RV) outflow is present, pulmonary valve stenosis should be relieved to prevent progression of obstruction,[3] RV hypertrophy, myocardial fibrosis, and dysfunction. Left untreated, significant pulmonary valve stenosis eventually produces clinical symptoms such as fatigue, dyspnea, and exercise intolerance. These long-term sequelae can be avoided if pulmonary valve stenosis is treated in childhood. Nevertheless, treatment is indicated at any age if hemodynamically significant pulmonary stenosis is documented. Since its introduction in 1982 by Kan and associates,[4] percutaneous balloon valvuloplasty has been shown to provide substantial relief of right ventricular outflow tract (RVOT) obstruction in patients with valvular pulmonary stenosis. Balloon pulmonary valvuloplasty can be performed safely and is minimally invasive. It is therefore regarded as the treatment of choice for patients with moderate to severe isolated pulmonary valve stenosis.

In congenital pulmonary valve stenosis, the valve leaflets are thickened and the commissures are fused to varying degrees. The lines of commissural fusion may appear as two or three raphes extending from the valve annulus to a small central orifice.[5] During childhood and young adulthood, the pulmonary valve leaflets are typically supple, doming upward during systole (Fig. 60.1). In older adults, pulmonary valve calcification may occur and may lead to diminished leaflet mobility. A less common form of pulmonary stenosis has been referred to as *pulmonary valve dysplasia* or *dysplastic pulmonary valve* syndrome.[5,6] It often occurs as a familial trait or as part of Noonan syndrome. A dysplastic pulmonary valve is characterized by thick, cartilaginous valve leaflets with poor mobility. The pulmonary valve annulus is often hypoplastic, and there may be little or no commissural fusion.

In isolated pulmonary valve stenosis, balloon dilation reduces the degree of valvular obstruction by separating fused commissures or by tearing the valve leaflets themselves.[7,8] Patients with severe pulmonary valve dysplasia with hypoplasia of the annulus and absence of commissural fusion may have minimal improvement after balloon valvuloplasty.[9] However, because a spectrum of pulmonary valve dysplasia exists, some patients with this disorder may derive substantial benefit from the balloon valvuloplasty procedure.[10]

Indications for Intervention

In contrast to balloon aortic valvuloplasty, the indications for intervention in balloon pulmonary valvuloplasty have been relatively constant over time and closely correlate with the surgical indications for valvuloplasty. In addition, the peak instantaneous pressure gradients measured by echocardiography correlate more closely with resting peak systolic gradients in the catheterization laboratory. For this reason, most physicians refer patients for catheterization and balloon valvuloplasty once the echocardiographic peak instantaneous pressure gradient is 40 mm Hg or

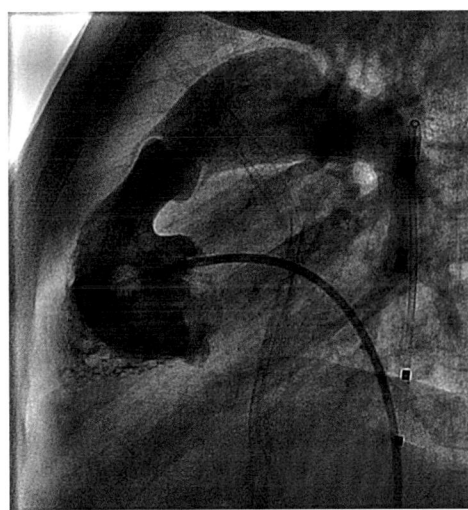

Fig. 60.1 Lateral right ventricular angiogram in a child with congenital pulmonary valve stenosis. The valve is thickened and domed in systole. There is poststenotic dilation of the main pulmonary artery.

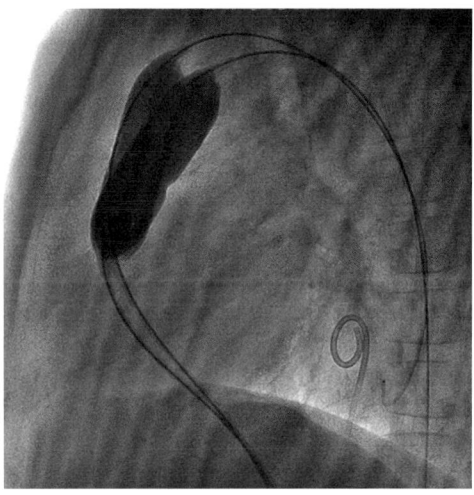

Fig. 60.2 Double-balloon pulmonary valve dilation in a child with pulmonary valve stenosis. Two balloons may be used if a single-balloon catheter requires a sheath that is thought to be too large for the child's femoral vein or if the valve annulus is too large for a single balloon.

higher or symptoms develop. The current recommendations for performing balloon pulmonary valvuloplasty are as follows[11]:

- Critical pulmonary stenosis, defined as pulmonary stenosis in a cyanotic infant requiring a PDA to provide adequate pulmonary blood flow
- Resting catheterization peak systolic ejection gradient or echocardiographic peak instantaneous pressure gradient 40 mm Hg or greater
- Resting catheterization or echocardiographic gradient less than 40 mm Hg in the setting of RV dysfunction or symptoms

For patients with a dysplastic pulmonary valve who meet these criteria, balloon valvuloplasty is an acceptable option, although the results may not be satisfactory, as discussed later.

Other indications for balloon pulmonary valvuloplasty that are not discussed in this text include treatment for pulmonary atresia with an intact ventricular septum but without RV-dependent coronary circulation and as a palliative procedure for patients with cyanotic CHD associated with pulmonary stenosis (e.g., tetralogy of Fallot [TOF]).

Technique

Balloon pulmonary valvuloplasty is usually performed with a percutaneous transfemoral venous approach. Right heart catheterization documents the severity of the lesion. RV angiocardiography is performed to confirm the nature of the lesion and to measure the diameter of the pulmonary valve annulus. Typically, the lateral projection is best suited to this purpose. Once the decision is made to proceed with valvuloplasty, an end-hole catheter is advanced to the left PA. The left PA provides better wire and balloon stability than a right PA position. We recommend crossing the tricuspid valve with a balloon-tipped catheter, whenever possible. This helps to prevent positioning of the catheter and wire between tricuspid valve cords and lowers the risk of tricuspid valve injury during balloon valvuloplasty. An exchange-length guidewire is advanced to the distal left PA, and the end-hole catheter is removed. The balloon valvuloplasty catheter is then inserted over the exchange wire. A balloon valvuloplasty catheter is used whose inflated balloon diameter is approximately 15% to 25% larger than the pulmonary valve annulus diameter. Balloon oversizing improves valvuloplasty effectiveness, and injury to the pulmonary valve annulus is unlikely when balloons smaller than 140% of the annulus's diameter are used.[12,13]

If the pulmonary valve annulus exceeds 25 mm or if the single-balloon catheter required is too large for safe introduction into a patient's femoral vein, we recommend a double-balloon technique, with two balloons positioned across the valve and inflated simultaneously (Fig. 60.2). The effective dilating diameter of two equal-sized balloons can be calculated based on cross-sectional area or on circumference. The sum of the balloon diameters by the circumference method is 120% of the equivalent single-balloon diameters, and by the area method it is 130%. Therefore the operator first selects the optimal single-balloon size, multiplies this diameter by 1.2 or 1.3, and then selects two balloons whose diameters are half of that product. Once inserted, the balloon valvuloplasty catheter is advanced across the valve and positioned with the valve at the midportion of the balloon. Partial balloon inflation, with a mixture of saline and contrast, is helpful to determine the precise location of the valve on the balloon. Care should be taken to avoid inflating the balloon across the tricuspid valve, which can result in tricuspid valve injury.

The valvuloplasty balloon or balloons are then inflated by hand until the waist produced by the valve on the balloon disappears. The period of balloon inflation is kept as brief as possible to minimize obstruction to RV outflow. Typically, three or four balloon inflations are performed with minor adjustments in balloon position to ensure adequate dilation of the pulmonary valve. After the dilation is completed, the valvuloplasty catheter is withdrawn and replaced with a diagnostic catheter. The residual RVOT gradient and cardiac output are measured to document the effectiveness of the procedure. A repeat RV angiogram may be performed if necessary to document the degree of subvalvular infundibular narrowing (which may be increased immediately after valvuloplasty) present at this point (Fig. 60.3).

Infants

Newborns and infants with critical pulmonary stenosis or atresia are frequently critically ill and hypoxemic (because of a right-to-left atrial shunt) and may have associated hypoplasia of the RV and tricuspid valve (Fig. 60.4). Because of these factors, in addition to the presence of severe RVOT obstruction, it is a technical challenge to successfully catheterize the PA and properly position a valvuloplasty balloon across the RVOT in these infants.[14–18] In infants with critical pulmonary stenosis, we prefer to perform the procedure with the child receiving prostaglandin E_1 infusion, for

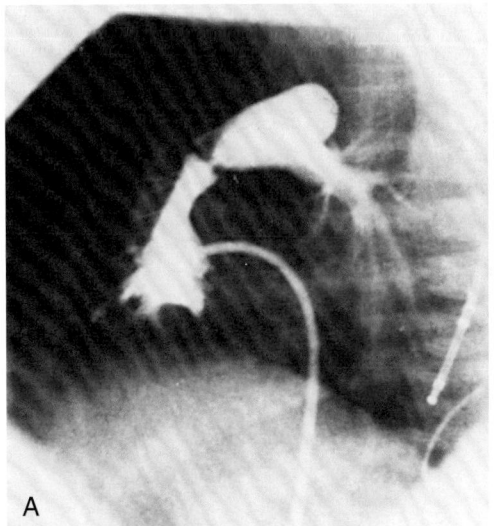
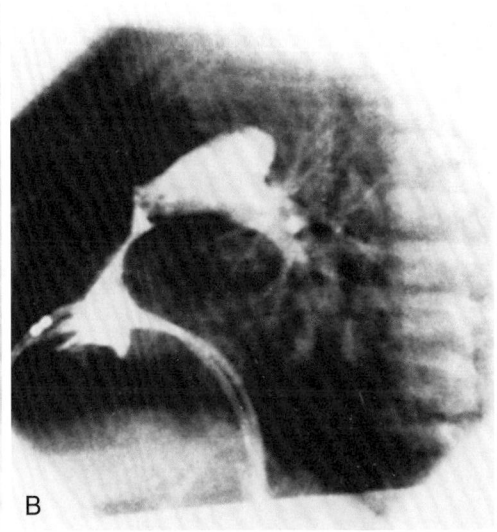

Fig. 60.3 Lateral right ventricular angiogram before (A) and immediately after (B) valvuloplasty in an infant with pulmonary stenosis. There is marked systolic narrowing of the right ventricular infundibulum after valvuloplasty that was not present before the procedure. Such dynamic infundibular narrowing may account for some residual gradient that may be measured immediately after the procedure and typically improves with time.

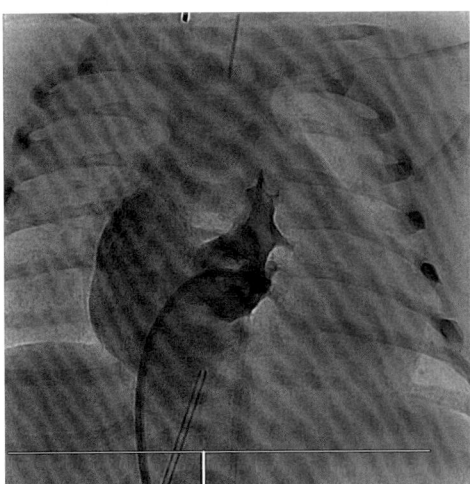

Fig. 60.4 Anteroposterior right ventricular angiogram in a newborn with pulmonary valve atresia and right ventricular hypoplasia. The right ventricle is small, and its outflow tract is evident immediately beneath the imperforate pulmonary valve. There was significant tricuspid regurgitation.

three reasons: first, the infant is in a more stable hemodynamic state during the procedure; second, a left-to-right ductal shunt maintains pulmonary blood flow during balloon occlusion of the RVOT; and third, the presence of a PDA allows the exchange guidewire to be positioned across the pulmonary valve and into the descending aorta, a course that facilitates catheter exchanges and subsequent valve dilation.

Acute Results

In patients with isolated pulmonary valve stenosis, percutaneous balloon valvuloplasty can be expected to provide excellent relief of obstruction (Fig. 60.5). Numerous studies have clearly documented significant acute reduction in the peak systolic pulmonary valve gradient to 30 mm Hg or less (i.e., mild residual stenosis). In their landmark 1982 report, Kan and colleagues reported the acute effects of valvuloplasty in an 8-year-old child with pulmonary stenosis.[4] The procedure decreased the peak gradient from 48 to 14 mm Hg and was performed without significant complications. Other studies have confirmed this initial observation that valvuloplasty provides impressive gradient relief acutely.[12,14–16,19–24]

The largest published clinical series of balloon pulmonary valvuloplasty was reported by the Pediatric Valvuloplasty Registry.[19] This registry reported the acute results of pulmonary valvuloplasty performed in 784 patients between 1981 and 1986. Overall, balloon dilation resulted in an acute decrease in the peak systolic pressure gradient from 71 to 28 mm Hg. The residual pressure gradients immediately after valvuloplasty were ascribed in part to subvalvular infundibular obstruction related to RV hypertrophy. Effectiveness of the procedure was not related to age (the series included 35 adults older than 21 years), but a larger residual gradient was observed in patients with a dysplastic pulmonary valve. The Pediatric Valvuloplasty Registry described five major complications (0.6%), primarily confined to infancy. There were two procedure-related deaths (0.2%), and in one neonate RVOT perforation and tamponade occurred. Two children developed severe tricuspid regurgitation related to injury to the tricuspid valve apparatus. Minor complications included femoral venous thrombosis, hemorrhage, and transient arrhythmias.

Several other studies have shown similar results, including data from the Congenital Cardiac Catheterization Project on Outcomes (C3PO),[23] which included 211 cases from eight institutions between 2007 and 2010. The overall procedural success rate was 91%, with 88% of patients obtaining a reduction in the valve gradient to less than 25 mm Hg. The independent risk factors for procedural failure on multivariate analysis were the presence of supravalvular stenosis and evidence of a dysplastic pulmonary valve. Only one patient had a life-threatening adverse event (ventricular fibrillation). Although the overall rate of adverse events was 12%, most of these were mild; only 3% of patients experienced a more severe adverse event. An important finding of this study was that 6% of neonates and 2% of adults required reintervention.

Adults

Several reports have described the successful application of percutaneous balloon valvuloplasty for treatment of adults with pulmonary valve stenosis.[20,22,25–36] Table 60.1 summarizes the pertinent clinical and hemodynamic data from 14 publications describing the acute results of pulmonary valvuloplasty in adolescents and adults. Pulmonary valvuloplasty has been performed successfully in patients as old as 84 years. In most published cases, a single-balloon technique has been used. However, when a 20- to 25-mm-diameter balloon was insufficient, the double-balloon technique has often been necessary.

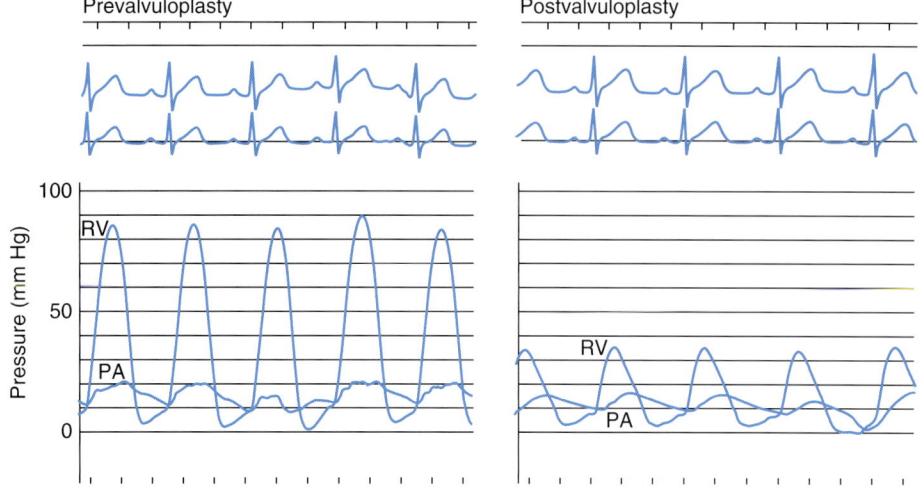

Fig. 60.5 Simultaneous right ventricular *(RV)* and pulmonary artery *(PA)* pressure recordings before and immediately after pulmonary valve dilation in a 15-month-old boy with severe pulmonary stenosis. The right ventricular systolic pressure was reduced from 86 to 36 mm Hg. The pulmonary valve systolic gradient decreased from 66 to 20 mm Hg (pressure recordings were made on the same scale).

TABLE 60.1 Summary of Published Reports of Pulmonary Valvuloplasty in Adults

Study	No. of Patients	Age Range (Year)	Balloon Technique	Peak Systolic Gradient (mm Hg) Before	After
Tentolouris et al.[25]	1	84	Double	70	34
Herrmann et al.[26]	8	23–66	Single	66	22
Sherman et al.[27]	4	48–67	Single (3) Double (1)	109	38
Al Kasab et al.[22]	12	21–37	Double	86	28
Fawzy et al.[28]	8	21–45	Double	107	36
Flugelman et al.[29]	1	62	Single	260	90
Presbitero et al.[30]	3	21–45	Single	130	29
Park et al.[31]	3	24–40	Double	108	51
Cooke et al.[32]	1	61	Single	105	13
Leisch et al.[33]	6	21–59	Single	78	38
Shuck et al.[34]	1	23	Single	30	2
Pepine et al.[20]	1	59	Single	130	30
Chen et al.[35]	53	13–55	Single	191	38
Taggart et al.[36]	40	18–82	Single (12) Double (8)	54	22

In these reports, balloon valvuloplasty acutely reduced the peak systolic gradient by 60% to 65%, from a range of 53 to 260 mm Hg before the procedure to 2 to 90 mm Hg after valvuloplasty. In most cases the peak systolic gradient immediately after valvuloplasty was in the mild range (20 to 40 mm Hg). In one report, there was a significant improvement in New York Heart Association (NYHA) classification in adults 30 days after valvuloplasty.[36] Therefore the available data clearly indicate that percutaneous balloon valvuloplasty provides effective therapy in adults as well as in children with congenital pulmonary valve stenosis. Balloon valvuloplasty appears to be effective even in the oldest patients, in whom valve calcification may be present.[25]

Long-Term Results

Long-term studies of balloon pulmonary valvuloplasty have confirmed that the benefits of this procedure are durable and comparable to the results of surgical valvotomy.[24,37–41] In several studies, the degree of residual stenosis remained low (<40 mm Hg, less than the current indications for intervention).[24,37–39,41] In the Pediatric Valvuloplasty Registry, 16% of patients required reintervention with either repeat valvuloplasty or surgical valvotomy during a follow-up period of 8.7 years.[38] Independent risk factors for a suboptimal late outcome included small valve annulus diameter, higher early residual gradient, smaller ratio of balloon-to-annulus diameter, and earlier year at initial intervention. This is similar to what we have found in our own long-term follow-up data.[39]

Pulmonary insufficiency, typically mild to moderate, is a common late complication of balloon pulmonary valvuloplasty and is likely more common in smaller patients at the time of valvuloplasty.[24,40–42] Resultant RV dilation correlates with the degree of pulmonary insufficiency.[40,41] However, pulmonary valve replacement, even in patients who develop RV dilation, has typically not been required for these patients.[41] In a study we performed comparing patients undergoing balloon valvuloplasty to an age-matched cohort of surgical patients,[39] although the residual gradient was slightly less after surgery (16 vs. 24 mm Hg, respectively; $P = .01$), the surgical group had significantly more pulmonary valve insufficiency and late ventricular arrhythmias.

In one study,[40] mild or moderate pulmonary regurgitation was associated with impaired exercise capacity, specifically lower peak oxygen consumption, when compared with lower amounts of regurgitation (85% ± 17% vs. 96% ± 16% of predicted; $P = .03$). In the same study, RV dilation (end-diastolic volume z score >2) was present in 40% of the study group, and the indexed end-diastolic volume of the RV correlated with the pulmonary regurgitation fraction ($R = .79$; $P < .001$). These results suggest that relatively modest amounts of pulmonary regurgitation may result in long-term RV dilation and reduced exercise tolerance. Alternatively, these results may simply reflect the severe nature of the pulmonary stenosis in these patients before intervention and the aggressive balloon dilation procedures required: median age at intervention was 0.2 years; median RV-to-aorta pressure ratio was 110% before valvuloplasty; and median balloon-to-annulus diameter ratio was 1.3 (range 1.0 to 2.0).

Therefore late follow-up data document excellent long-term results after percutaneous pulmonary balloon valvuloplasty and support the use of this procedure as the treatment of choice for patients with isolated valvular pulmonary stenosis.

Complications

Beyond infancy, percutaneous balloon pulmonary valvuloplasty is a very safe procedure. In the Pediatric Valvuloplasty Registry, the only two deaths occurred in infants with critical pulmonary stenosis, and the single case of perforation and tamponade occurred in an 8-day-old neonate.[19] Minor complications were primarily related to vascular injury or hemorrhage and were also much more common during the first 12 months of life. Overall, the Pediatric Valvuloplasty Registry reported a 1.2% to 1.8% frequency of major complications and a 4.8% frequency of minor complications in 168 infants. In contrast, in 656 children and adults, the frequency of major complication was 0.8% and the frequency of minor complication was 1.7%.

In the C3PO study of 211 balloon pulmonary valvuloplasty procedures in the current era across several institutions,[23] the overall adverse event rate was 12%, and most of these (79%) were of low severity. Again, neonates were more likely to experience adverse events (19% vs. 6%). In the overall cohort, the most common type of adverse event was transient arrhythmias and conduction abnormalities, which were seen in 5% of patients.

There have been no reports of long-term arrhythmias after valvuloplasty. Valvuloplasty may cause injury to the femoral vein, especially when the procedure is performed in infancy. As discussed earlier, the mild pulmonary valve insufficiency commonly seen after pulmonary valvuloplasty, although perhaps not entirely benign,[40] is rarely of clinical importance and may be less severe than after surgical valvotomy.[39]

Conclusions and Recommendations

Percutaneous balloon pulmonary valvuloplasty is the treatment of choice for children and adults with isolated congenital valvular pulmonary stenosis. Valvuloplasty successfully reduces significant RVOT obstruction, with a residual gradient that is usually in the trivial to mild range (i.e., <30 mm Hg). Follow-up studies have documented long-term effectiveness, with little restenosis. Late pulmonary insufficiency is common and may cause RV dilation, but need for pulmonary valve replacement is atypical. Pulmonary valvuloplasty is indicated in neonates with critical pulmonary stenosis and in patients of any age with isolated pulmonary valve stenosis whose resting peak systolic pressure gradient exceeds 40 mm Hg in the presence of a normal cardiac output.

AORTIC BALLOON VALVULOPLASTY

Aortic valve stenosis accounts for 4% to 6% of all cases of CHD.[43] Left ventricular (LV) outflow tract obstruction elicits LV hypertrophy and myocardial fibrosis, which may eventually lead to LV

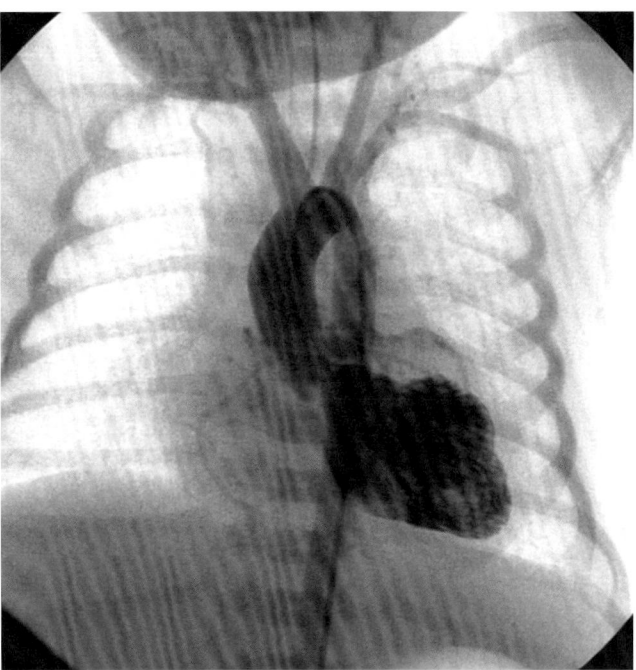

Fig. 60.6 Anteroposterior left ventricular angiogram in a newborn with critical aortic valve stenosis. The aortic valve leaflets are thickened, and there is severe left ventricular dysfunction.

dysfunction and congestive heart failure. Unlike most cases of congenital pulmonary valve stenosis, congenital aortic stenosis tends to progress over time.[38,44]

Successful percutaneous balloon valvuloplasty in children with congenital aortic valve stenosis was first reported in 1984 by Lababidi and colleagues.[44-46] Balloon valvuloplasty typically reduces the LV outflow tract obstruction to the mild range, and at most centers, it is the treatment of choice for children with congenital aortic stenosis who require intervention. In the past 30 years, there have been a few changes to the technique but considerable debate on the indications for percutaneous intervention.

Indications for Intervention

The current recommended indications for aortic valvuloplasty reflect the 2011 scientific statement from the American Heart Association.[11] The gradient criteria listed are resting peak systolic gradients measured in the catheterization laboratory with the patient sedated. Extrapolation to echocardiogram-derived Doppler peak instantaneous pressure gradients or mean gradient is not reliable, especially in the setting of aortic insufficiency.[47] In addition, given the impact of general anesthesia on systemic blood pressure, resting gradients should be obtained under light conscious sedation whenever possible.

Infants

Aortic balloon valvuloplasty is indicated for infants with critical aortic stenosis, which is defined as isolated aortic stenosis with either depressed LV systolic function or evidence of ductal dependency to maintain adequate cardiac output. Infants with critical aortic stenosis typically have severe congestive heart failure and shock with profound LV dysfunction (Fig. 60.6). Notably, the gradient across the aortic valve does not reflect the degree of aortic stenosis because of poor ventricular function and low antegrade flow across the aortic valve.

Children and Young Adults

In isolated valvular aortic stenosis, aortic balloon valvuloplasty is indicated in children with either of the following:

- Resting peak systolic gradient 50 mm Hg or greater
- Resting peak systolic gradient 40 mm Hg or greater if there are any symptoms (e.g., anginal chest pain, syncope) or ischemic changes on either resting or exercise electrocardiography (ECG)

Less well-established indications are:

- Resting peak systolic gradient 40 mm Hg or greater without symptoms or ischemic ECG changes in a patient who plans to become pregnant or to participate in competitive sports
- Resting peak systolic gradient less than 50 mm Hg in heavily sedated or anesthetized patients if the echocardiographically derived mean gradient is more than 50 mm Hg

Aortic valvuloplasty is not indicated in patients with a resting peak systolic gradient of less than 40 mm Hg who are without symptoms or ischemic ECG changes, nor in patients with severe insufficiency who have a surgical indication for aortic valve repair or replacement.

Technique

Percutaneous aortic valvuloplasty is usually performed from a retrograde transarterial approach, although the antegrade transseptal approach can also be used. In infants, alternative approaches include the carotid artery and the umbilical artery (see later discussion). We prefer the retrograde approach and use a transseptal catheter for continuous LV pressure monitoring throughout the procedure. After the transseptal puncture is accomplished, heparin is administered to increase the activated clotting time (ACT) to approximately 250 to 300 seconds. The aortic stenosis gradient is measured before angiography, with simultaneous ventricular and aortic pressure recordings. Alternatively, a single catheter with both end and side holes can be used to simultaneously measure the LV and aortic pressures. Aortic root and LV angiography are helpful to determine the baseline aortic insufficiency and measure the aortic valve annulus.

Once the decision has been made to proceed with balloon valvuloplasty (see indications described previously), a balloon with the proper diameter is chosen. This diameter is based on the aortic valve annulus diameter, which can be measured by echocardiography or by angiography. Typically, the balloon diameter is 90% to 100% of the aortic valve diameter. Unlike pulmonary balloon valvuloplasty, oversized balloons are not used for aortic valvuloplasty because they have been shown to increase the risk of injury to the aortic valve and annulus.[48] The single-balloon technique, as opposed to the double-balloon technique (which requires two arterial access points) is chosen primarily after consideration of the femoral arterial size to minimize the risk of femoral arterial injury. In our experience, a double-balloon technique is rarely needed until the aortic annulus is larger than 25 mm.

The balloon or balloons are inflated until the waist produced on the balloon by the valve is relieved (Fig. 60.7). Balloon inflation is kept as brief as possible to minimize arterial hypotension during the procedure. To minimize balloon movement during inflation, which has been suggested to cause increased aortic insufficiency during valvuloplasty, rapid ventricular pacing may be performed via a venous access site to temporarily lower stroke volume.[49,50] A recent randomized trial comparing results of valvuloplasty with or without rapid ventricular pacing in older adults with degenerative aortic valve disease did not demonstrate any immediate difference in the degree of aortic insufficiency. This study did not examine late postvalvuloplasty aortic insufficiency, and owing to the specific population studied, it does not necessarily inform the

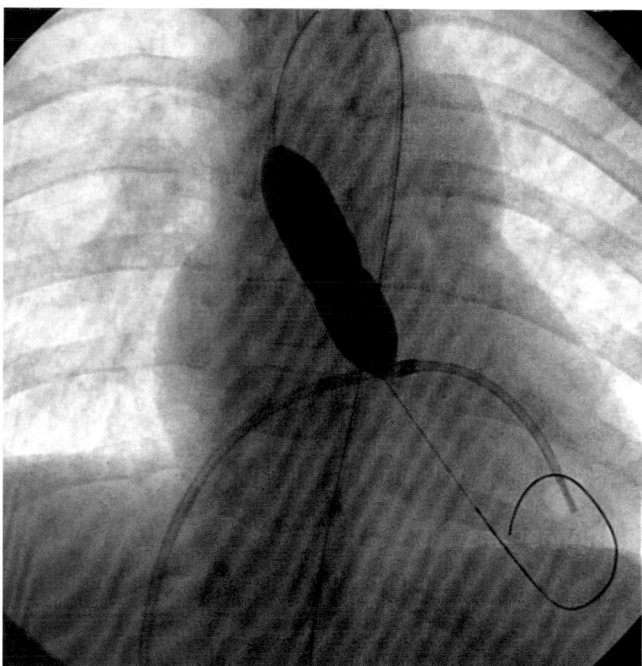

Fig. 60.7 Balloon dilation in a child with severe aortic valve stenosis. The waist produced by the valve annulus on the balloon is evident. Ventricular pressure was monitored throughout the procedure by a catheter placed in the left ventricle through a transseptal puncture.

practice of routine balloon aortic valvuloplasty in children and young adults.[51] After valvuloplasty, repeat measurements of LV and aortic pressures and aortic root angiography are performed to quantify the residual aortic stenosis gradient and degree of resultant aortic insufficiency.

Newborn Critical Aortic Stenosis

In newborns with critical aortic stenosis, prostaglandin E_1 infusion is initiated to maintain patency of the ductus arteriosus and support cardiac output. Intravenous inotropic support, and occasionally extracorporeal membrane oxygenation support, may be required to stabilize the patient before the procedure. Often, a transumbilical approach (Fig. 60.8) is used to spare the infant's femoral artery (which may be required for future percutaneous valve dilation procedures).

The carotid artery[52] and transvenous antegrade[53] approaches have also been reported as means to avoid femoral artery injury in small infants. The carotid approach can be accomplished by a cutdown procedure or by percutaneous access with ultrasound guidance. This route provides a relatively direct access to the aortic valve and is especially useful in low birth weight neonates with critical aortic stenosis. A single-balloon technique is used with a single inflation. In contrast, McElhinney and colleagues[52] reported starting with smaller balloons and performing serial dilations with progressively larger balloons until the desired degree of relief was obtained.

Rapid ventricular pacing is not necessary to stabilize the balloon during inflation given the depressed LV function. The most challenging aspect of the procedure is often crossing the aortic valve. Special care must be taken to avoid perforation of an aortic valve leaflet (by crossing with a very soft wire), because severe aortic insufficiency due to leaflet tear is poorly tolerated.

Acute Results

Since its first description, the effectiveness of balloon valvuloplasty in children and adolescents with congenital aortic valve stenosis has been clearly demonstrated, and the results have proven comparable to those of surgical valvotomy.[43,47,53-61] The Pediatric Valvuloplasty Registry,[53,59] historically the largest series of balloon aortic valvuloplasty procedures for congenital aortic stenosis, reported the acute results of 630 balloon valvuloplasty procedures in 606 children (age 1 day to 18 years) at 23 institutions between 1984 and 1992. The procedure usually produces an immediate 60% decrease in peak systolic gradient across the aortic valve (Fig. 60.9).[53] The mortality rate was 2.4% and was primarily limited to newborns; there were no deaths in patients older than 3 months of age. A recent study using data from the National Cardiovascular Data Registry (NCDR) Improving Pediatric and Adult Congenital Treatments (IMPACT) registry showed similar results in a cohort of 1026 patients undergoing isolated balloon aortic valvuloplasty.[55] Successful valvuloplasty, defined as a reduction in the aortic valve gradient to less than 35 mm Hg and mild or less aortic insufficiency, was reported in approximately 71% of patients with noncritical aortic stenosis and approximately 63% in patients with critical aortic stenosis. Interestingly, the overall 30-day mortality rate for the entire cohort was 2.4%, with a much higher rate seen in neonates with critical aortic stenosis, identical to the results from The Pediatric Valvuloplasty Registry.[55]

Severe aortic regurgitation is uncommon. Vascular complications have been limited primarily to neonates and young infants and have diminished in recent years with the development of lower-profile sheaths and catheters.

Traditionally, a good procedural result was a residual aortic valve gradient of 20 to 40 mm Hg,[48,55-61] with little to no worsening of the aortic insufficiency. In single-center series, some degree of aortic insufficiency is common after aortic balloon valvuloplasty, and several studies have shown that the degree of aortic insufficiency, like the degree of aortic stenosis, progresses over time.[62-66] It is less clear how procedural technique (including the use of rapid ventricular pacing), and patient selection affect both the occurrence and the progression of aortic insufficiency after valvuloplasty.

Long-term follow-up data of 509 and 272 patients who underwent valvuloplasty at single institutions revealed relatively high rates of aortic reintervention and aortic valve replacement.[64,66] In the study by Brown and colleagues,[63] a very interesting finding was that patients with residual gradients less than 35 mm Hg and with moderate or severe aortic insufficiency immediately after dilation were no more likely to require late aortic valve replacement than patients with residual gradients greater than 35 mm Hg with mild insufficiency. These data suggest that a more aggressive balloon valvuloplasty to obtain lower residual gradients, even at the cost of creating more aortic insufficiency, may be better for patients in the long term. Similar results were found in the other large follow-up study.[65] However, there are limitations to generalizing the results of a single-center experience, especially when the primary outcome measures of aortic reintervention and aortic valve replacement are highly dependent on timing of referral.

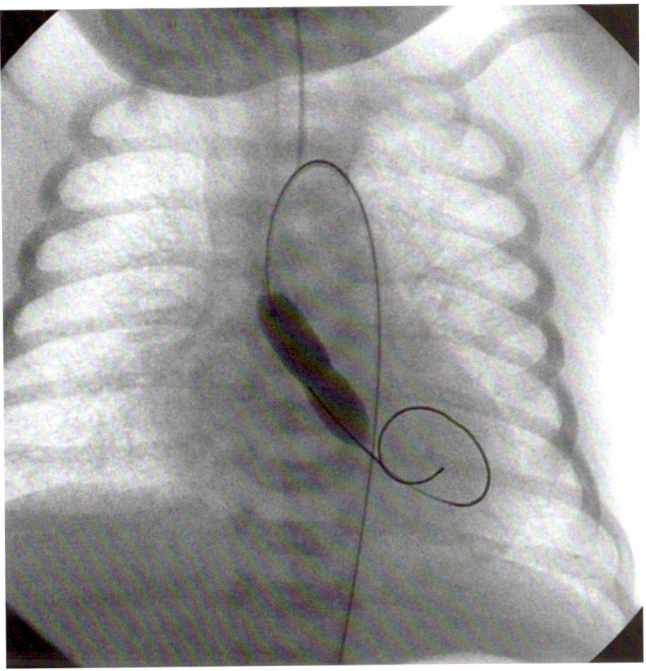

Fig. 60.8 Balloon dilation in a newborn with critical aortic stenosis (same patient as in Fig. 60.6). The catheter was introduced through the umbilical artery, thereby avoiding potential femoral artery injury in a newborn with low cardiac output.

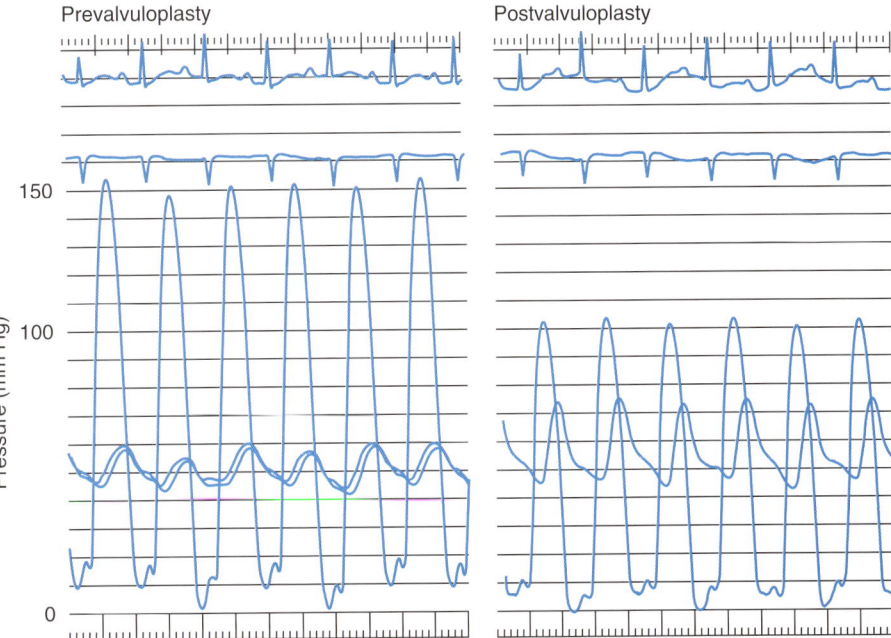

Fig. 60.9 Aortic and left ventricular pressure tracings in an 11-day-old infant with critical aortic stenosis, measured before and immediately after balloon dilation. The peak systolic gradient decreased from 96 to 29 mm Hg. Notice the improved aortic pulse pressure after valvuloplasty, which is indicative of an improved cardiac output. (From Beekman RH, Rocchini AP, et al. Balloon valvuloplasty for critical aortic stenosis in the newborn: influence of new catheter technology. *J Am Coll Cardiol*. 1991;17:1172–1176.)

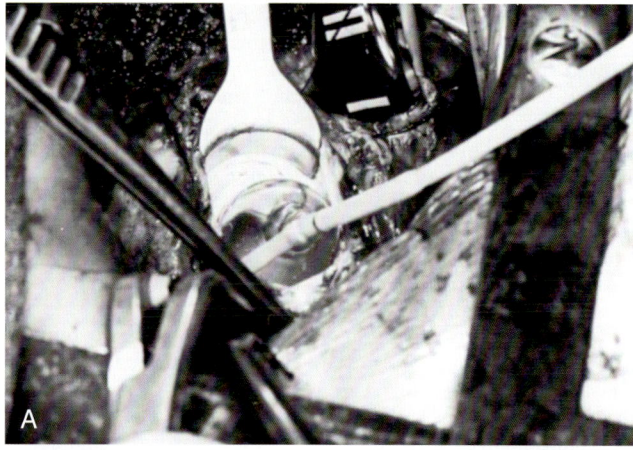
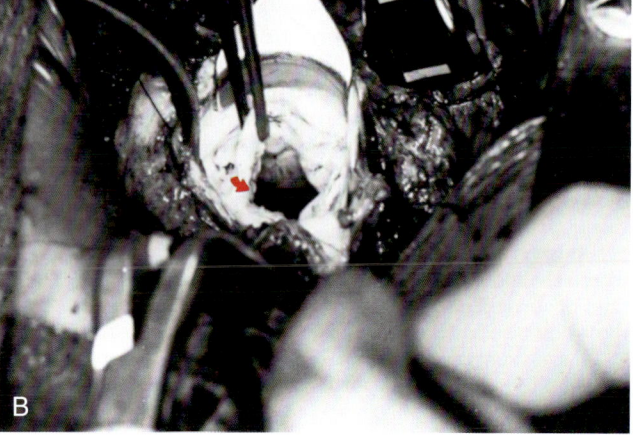

Fig. 60.10 The mechanism of balloon aortic valvuloplasty is demonstrated during surgery in an 18-year-old woman with congenital aortic valve stenosis. A 20-mm balloon had been inflated across the valve (A), producing a 3- to 4-mm tear across the line of commissural fusion *(red arrow)* (B). The valve leaflets are thick and dysplastic.

Timing of referral across the United States is largely influenced by era, surgeon preference, and heterogenous practice variation even within institutions.

The effectiveness of balloon dilation, in terms of both acute success and long-term freedom from reintervention, likely relates to the underlying morphologic substrate.[66] If a technically adequate balloon dilation fails to achieve a satisfactory hemodynamic result in a patient with congenital aortic valve stenosis, a more complex diagnosis is suggested; such patients may be found to have annular hypoplasia or valve leaflet calcification. Most congenitally stenotic aortic valves are bicuspid, involving a single central or eccentric commissure with a variable degree of fusion of its edges. The valve leaflets themselves are thickened but are rarely calcified in childhood. In older patients and in children with prior valve surgery, the leaflets may calcify, becoming less mobile and less amenable to balloon dilation. In congenital aortic valve stenosis, as in pulmonary valve stenosis, balloon valvuloplasty reduces the degree of stenosis by separating valve leaflets along the lines of commissural fusion (Fig. 60.10). In marked contrast, balloon valvuloplasty has proven to be much less successful in older patients with calcific aortic stenosis.[67–71] In these patients, the aortic valve stenosis is acquired, primarily as a result of calcium deposition within the leaflets, and little or no commissural fusion is present.[72,73]

Based on the Pediatric Valvuloplasty Registry, several other factors are associated with suboptimal results during balloon aortic valvuloplasty. A suboptimal result is defined as failure to perform the valvuloplasty (which occurred in 4.1% of registered patients), an immediate residual gradient of 60 mm Hg or more, an LV systolic pressure exceeding the aortic systolic pressure by 60% or more, mortality, or major morbidity.[61] Overall, a suboptimal outcome was reported for 17% of the 630 valvuloplasty procedures. Independent predictors for a suboptimal outcome included age younger than 3 months, a greater predilation systolic gradient, a balloon-annulus diameter ratio of less than 0.9, the coexistence of an unrepaired coarctation, and earlier year of the procedure. The effect of the balloon-annulus diameter ratio has been thoroughly evaluated, and the optimal ratio was found to be between 0.90 and 0.99. Smaller ratios were associated with an increased risk of suboptimal gradient relief. Larger ratios were associated with a greater risk of aortic insufficiency after valvuloplasty.

Critical Aortic Stenosis

In newborns with critical aortic stenosis, balloon aortic valvuloplasty has proven to be remarkably successful, with results comparable to those of surgical intervention at several premier institutions.[53,74–76] The Congenital Heart Surgeons Society reported the results of intervention in 110 neonates with critical aortic stenosis from 18 institutions.[75] Balloon aortic valvuloplasty was the initial procedure in 82 patients and surgical valvotomy in the remaining 28. Relief of aortic stenosis was significantly better in the balloon valvuloplasty group (gradient reduction of 65% ± 17% and median residual gradient of 20 mm Hg vs. 41% ± 32% and 36 mm Hg in the surgical group), although there was also a trend toward more aortic insufficiency in the balloon group. Early mortality was 18%, with no difference between groups.

In a study from our center,[74] 30 neonates were assigned to balloon valvuloplasty and 17 to surgical intervention on an intent-to-treat basis; early mortality was 13% in both groups. Early mortality was 14% in a series of 113 neonates treated with balloon aortic valvuloplasty, with approximately one-third of survivors requiring repeat intervention within 1 year.[54] Echocardiographic estimates of valve thickness or mobility have not correlated with valvuloplasty success in neonates.

Long-Term Results

Percutaneous balloon valvuloplasty and all other forms of therapy for congenital aortic valve stenosis should be regarded as palliative therapeutic procedures. As is the case after surgical aortic valvotomy,[77] late restenosis (5 to 20 years) should be expected after a successful balloon dilation procedure. As stated earlier, we caution against comparing follow-up peak instantaneous gradients determined by Doppler echocardiography against catheter-based measurements of peak systolic gradient obtained immediately after valvuloplasty because a false impression of restenosis may be obtained from echocardiography-derived assessments of valve gradients.[47]

Several studies have examined aortic restenosis requiring reintervention during middle- and long-term follow-up, including a prospective study examining the intermediate effectiveness of balloon valvuloplasty at our institution.[52,64,66,78–82] The recent study by Maskatia and coworkers represents the largest series of patients with 20-year follow-up data.[64] The rate of survival free from any aortic reintervention was 89% at 1 year and steadily declined to 27% at 20 years. Similarly, the rate of survival free from aortic valve replacement was 47% at 20 years. Predictors of reintervention and aortic valve replacement included a higher postvalvuloplasty gradient, whereas a higher grade of acute aortic insufficiency was associated only with shorter time to aortic valve replacement. Long-term mortality was low (88% survival at 20 years), and the highest hazard for death was during the first year after valvuloplasty. These results are similar to what has been found in other long-term follow-up studies.[66]

Critical Aortic Stenosis

Neonates with critical aortic stenosis appear to have a substantially higher risk of restenosis and progressive aortic insufficiency after balloon valvuloplasty: the reintervention-free survival rate has been approximately 50% at 5 years,[54,75,76] with aortic valve replacement or surgical repair of aortic insufficiency required in approximately 50% of patients at 10 years.[54,75]

Studies have found significant abnormalities during exercise testing and cardiac magnetic resonance imaging (MRI) in patients who have undergone aortic valvuloplasty.[83-85] This underscores the importance of ongoing medical supervision, particularly for patients who require intervention early in life.

Complications

Percutaneous balloon aortic valvuloplasty is a relatively safe procedure, and mortality is rare outside of early infancy.[55] Early mortality after balloon valvuloplasty in neonates has ranged from 13% to 18%; 15-year mortality has ranged between 5% and 28%.[55,64,75,76] These data compare favorably with the surgical experience, in which morbidity and mortality rates have been relatively high in neonates with critical aortic stenosis. Other complications reported in the Pediatric Valvuloplasty Registry were rare and included potentially life-threatening arrhythmias, cardiac perforation, and mitral valve injury. As described in detail earlier, valvuloplasty-induced aortic valve insufficiency may be an important complication of the procedure, but its relative incidence and importance in long-term patient outcomes is controversial.[64,85]

Femoral artery injury, thrombosis, and occlusion were relatively common in the past, particularly in infants, but their incidence has improved with current low-profile sheaths and angioplasty catheters.[86] We prefer not to exceed a 4-Fr exit profile in neonatal femoral arteries and to use the transumbilical approach for neonatal critical aortic stenosis if possible. Newer, 3-Fr sheaths are commonly used in infants who weigh less than 4 kg. Because future transfemoral valvuloplasty procedures (for restenosis) are likely to be necessary in these patients, femoral artery access should be preserved if at all possible.

A more recently recognized complication of neonatal aortic balloon valvuloplasty is aortic wall injury, in particular the creation of an intimal flap.[87] This diagnosis is made by angiography, echocardiography, or direct observation by the surgeon or pathologist. The complication was found in 28 (15%) of 187 procedures performed over a 23-year period, with no change in frequency over the study period. In one instance, a flap in the proximal ascending aorta extended into a coronary artery ostium, causing death, and another patient died suddenly at home. Multivariate analysis showed that aortic wall injury was more likely in patients with severe ventricular dysfunction at the time of the procedure, in procedures with greater numbers of balloon dilation attempts, and in procedures supervised by less experienced interventional staff.

Current Controversies

Several reports have compared the outcomes of aortic balloon valvuloplasty and surgical valvotomy for neonatal and infant congenital aortic stenosis.[79,80] Citing improved gradient reduction, a lesser degree of resultant aortic insufficiency, and less need for reintervention during follow-up, these authors have questioned the use of aortic balloon valvuloplasty as first-line therapy in infants and children. Again, retrospective, single-center studies are subject to several important limitations, probably the most important of which is center-related biases and the generalizability of the results to all patients.

The technique for aortic balloon valvuloplasty has improved over time with innovations such as rapid ventricular pacing and lower-profile catheters and sheaths. In addition, understanding of the relative importance of residual aortic stenosis and resultant aortic insufficiency is changing with time. Surgical valvotomy has additional long-term risks that are just beginning to be understood, including the impact of cardiopulmonary bypass and circulatory arrest on neonatal and infant neurodevelopment. Predicting which patients (i.e., which valves) would most benefit from aortic balloon valvuloplasty versus surgical valvotomy or repair is likely the next most important step to ensuring the highest quality of care in these challenging patients.

Fetal Intervention

Balloon valvuloplasty for fetuses with aortic stenosis for the purpose of preventing the development of hypoplastic left heart syndrome is currently well reported and appears to improve the chance of a biventricular circulation when successful. Currently, research focuses on accurately identifying fetuses at risk for this progression, developing techniques for in utero intervention, reducing the risks of technical failure and of fetal demise, and predicting which fetuses are most likely to benefit from intervention.[88-90]

Conclusions and Recommendations

Percutaneous balloon aortic valvuloplasty provides effective palliative treatment for congenital valvular aortic stenosis in infants, children, and young adults. At most pediatric cardiology centers, it is the treatment of choice. Valvuloplasty successfully reduces the peak systolic aortic stenosis gradient to the 20- to 40-mm Hg range, a result that compares favorably with open surgical valvotomy. Aortic insufficiency is not significantly increased in most patients. Mortality is uncommon and has been limited to critically ill neonates and young infants.

We recommend balloon valvuloplasty for patients whose resting peak systolic pressure gradient exceeds 50 mm Hg, for those whose resting peak gradient exceeds 40 mm Hg in association with symptoms or ischemic ECG changes, and for patients with heart failure and low cardiac output regardless of gradient. Balloon valvuloplasty is effective in neonates, children, and young adults with congenital aortic valve stenosis in whom commissural fusion is the primary anatomic cause of outflow obstruction. The procedure is less likely to be effective in patients with a hypoplastic valve annulus or with valve leaflet calcification.

BALLOON-EXPANDABLE STENTING FOR PULMONARY ARTERY STENOSIS

PA stenosis occurs commonly in patients with CHD. It is encountered as an isolated lesion in patients with arteriopathies such as Williams or Alagille syndrome or as a feature of complex CHD (e.g., TOF) both before and after surgery. Balloon angioplasty of PA stenosis or hypoplasia has yielded mixed results. Numerous reports document an immediate success rate of only 60% to 70% after balloon angioplasty of this lesion,[85-87] with restenosis rates in follow-up as high as 35%.[87]

Failure of angioplasty alone is often related to elastic recoil of the PA. These observations have led to the application of stent therapy to treat PA stenosis or hypoplasia. Since Mullins and colleagues first reported the use of balloon-expandable stents in the PAs and systemic veins in 1988,[88] transcatheter stenting has become the treatment of choice for many patients with PA stenosis and has demonstrated excellent early and long-term effectiveness.

SECTION V Structural Interventions

Technical Considerations

PA stenosis is considered significant when the measured gradient across the area of stenosis is greater than 20 to 30 mm Hg, the RV pressure is greater than one-half to two-thirds of systemic pressure due to distal obstruction, or there is relative flow discrepancy of greater than 35%/65% to each lung.[91] In low pulmonary flow states such as palliated single-ventricle lesions, gradients may be much lower, and the subjective angiographic appearance instead may determine the need for intervention.

When considering stent use in pediatrics, the wide range of patient sizes and the somatic growth over time of the majority of this patient population complicate stent choice in many anatomic positions. Stents are generally considered permanent structures, unless removed surgically. Implantation of large stents at adult size, or with the potential for redilation to adult size over time, is well accepted, safe, and widely described. However, in infants and small children, stent implantation is often considered more of a palliative option because these stent sizes lack growth potential over time and will require later surgical intervention for transection/removal.[91] Despite this, data evaluating PA interventions from a multicenter prospective registry, the C3PO study, found that 46% of all stent implantations used smaller, premounted stents.[92] Use of these stents was more common in younger patients and in nonelective or emergent cases and provides evidence of the relatively widespread use of small- and medium-diameter stents within the pediatric population in current practice. Recently, increasing attention has been focused on intentional stent fracture with ultra-high pressure balloon angioplasty, to create a complete longitudinal fracture to allow a small stent to expand beyond its maximal diameter and accommodate normal vessel growth.[93,94] In addition, there is currently much ongoing research on biodegradable stents for use in pediatric patients, such that a small stent placed in a child could be thought of as a temporary structure that would degrade over time and could later be replaced by a new larger stent with adult sized potential.

There are no stents developed specifically for use in pediatric patients with CHD, and therefore the majority of stents used in this setting represent off-label use of coronary and peripheral stents developed for adult purposes.[89,95,96] Technological advances have allowed stents and balloons to be delivered on lower profile systems; however, access site limitation is still a real consideration in pediatrics. Ideally, large stents, which ultimately can be dilated to a diameter of 18 mm, are appropriate for use in the PAs of a patient who can accommodate the appropriate delivery sheath. In some smaller patients, the internal jugular vein may accommodate a larger sheath than is possible with the femoral venous approach. In addition, a hybrid surgical approach, either with direct stent placement during cardiac surgery or via sternotomy and sheath placement in the main PA, can allow for placement of larger stents in smaller patients.

The balloon size chosen for stent implantation is typically up to three times the narrowest vessel dimension, not to exceed the dimension of the adjacent normal vessel. Although it is usually recommended that vessel side branches not be "jailed" in the process of stent placement, if jailing is necessary to address the stenosis, the use of an open cell stent can allow for later angioplasty through the stent struts to reopen these side branches in the event of restricted flow. In very proximal branch PA stenosis or distal main PA stenosis, techniques such as the simultaneous implantation of bilateral proximal PA stents[90] ("kissing stents") or implantation of a single stent crimped onto two balloons, extending from the main PA into both the proximal branch PAs ("bifurcating" or "flowering" stent), may be used.[97]

New imaging technologies such as rotational angiography and three-dimensional (3D) reconstruction can be useful in some cases of PA stenosis. This technology can augment traditional biplane angiography and allow for more complete understanding of the 3D anatomy of the stenotic area, can help to determine ideal angles for profiling an area of stenosis, and can be used as a roadmap to guide stent placement (Fig. 60.11; Videos 60.1 and 60.2).

Acute and Intermediate Outcomes

Early clinical studies of PA stenting used the Palmaz (Cordis, Bridgewater, NJ) stainless steel balloon-expandable stent (Figs. 60.12 and 60.13).[98–101] A multiinstitutional study of percutaneous stenting in the pediatric population was reported by O'Laughlin and colleagues in 1993.[98] A total of 121 Palmaz stents, 80 for branch PA stenosis, were implanted in 58 patients, most of whom

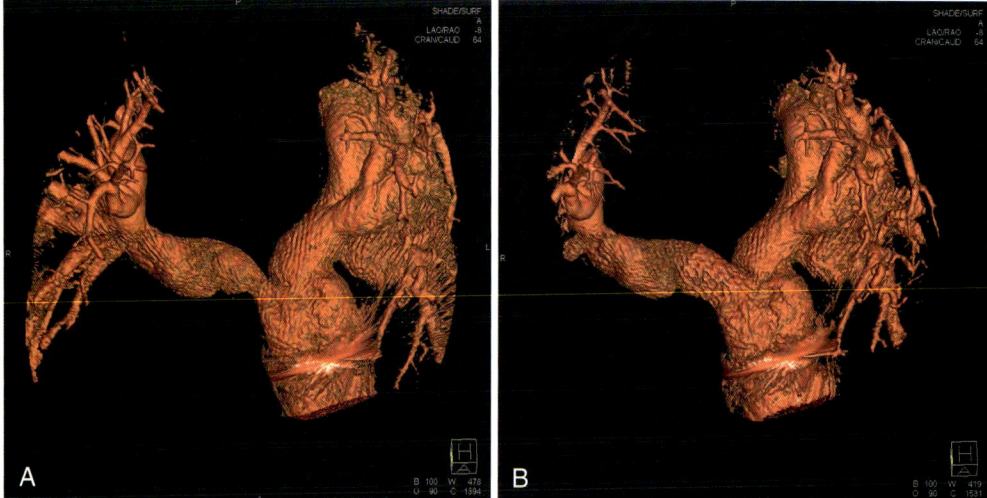

Fig. 60.11 Three-dimensional (3D) reconstruction of 64-slice computed rotational angiogram (CRA-64) performed on a 15-year-old boy with tetralogy of Fallot obtained after complete repair and placement of a 25-mm Hancock valved conduit, with proximal right pulmonary artery (RPA) stenosis before (A) and after (B) RPA stenting. These single views of the 3D reconstruction displayed at 8-degree left anterior oblique (LAO-8) profile the proximal RPA stenosis well. (See also Videos 60.1 and 60.2.) (Courtesy Dr. Aimee Armstrong, University of Michigan, Ann Arbor.)

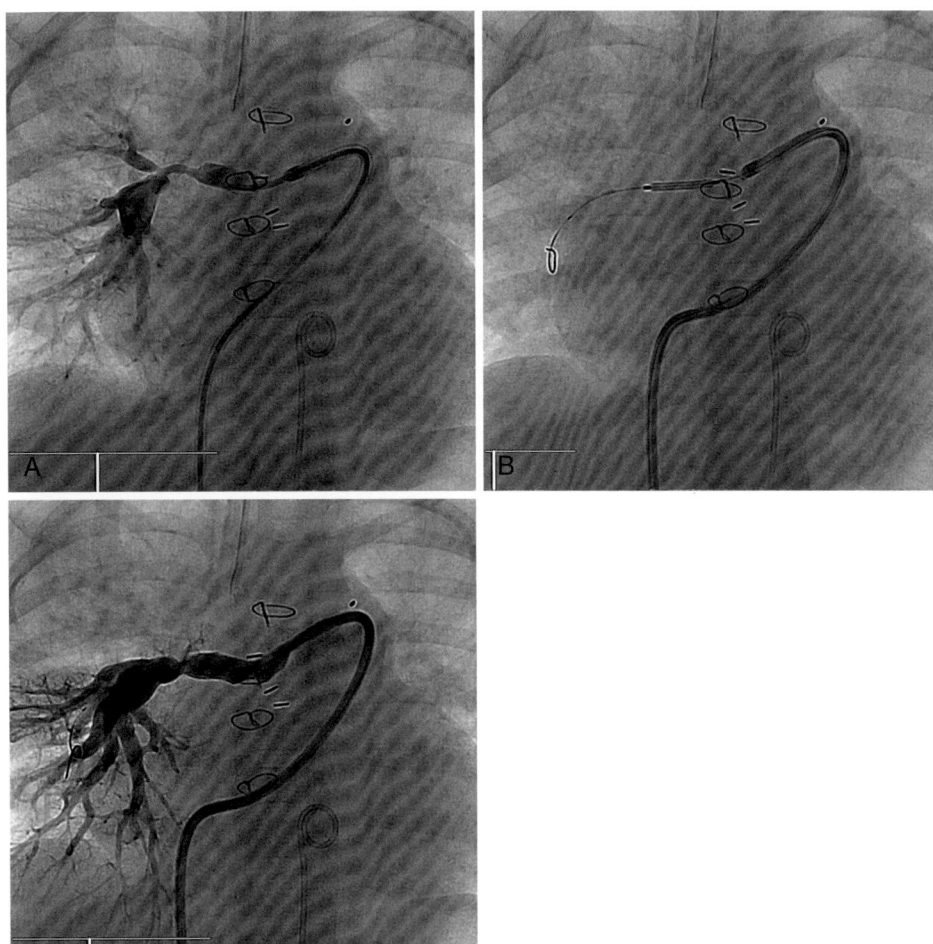

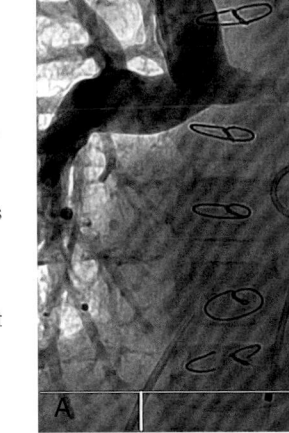

Fig. 60.12 Anteroposterior pulmonary artery angiograms before (A), during (B), and after (C) right pulmonary artery stenting in a 5-month-old infant after repair of pulmonary atresia and ventricular septal defect. There is severe proximal right pulmonary artery stenosis before stenting. After stent implantation, there is improvement in the stenosis, but a small upper lobe branch has been jailed.

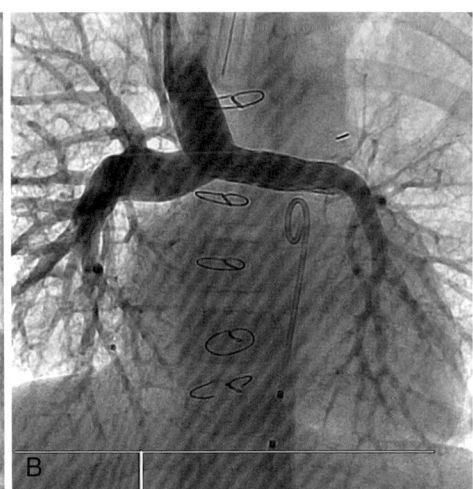

Fig. 60.13 Anteroposterior pulmonary artery angiograms obtained before and after left pulmonary artery stenting in an infant with hypoplastic left heart syndrome and left pulmonary artery hypoplasia. (A) Before stenting, there is diffuse hypoplasia of the proximal left and central pulmonary artery. (B) After stenting with two balloon-expandable stents, there is significant improvement in the pulmonary artery diameter and flow. The patient has a bidirectional Glenn shunt (superior vena cava–to–pulmonary artery anastomosis).

had undergone repair of TOF. In this series, stenting resulted in an increase in PA diameter from 4.6 to 11.3 mm, with an immediate decrease in RV systolic pressure. A follow-up cardiac catheterization was performed in 25 patients 8 months after stenting, and restenosis was identified in only one patient. The clinical benefits derived from PA stenting in children, including alleviation of symptoms and deferral of surgical intervention, were further validated in a large single-institution series by Fogelman and associates.[99] The largest series of PA stenting in children was reported by McMahon and colleagues in 2002.[102] Over a 12-year period, 664 Palmaz stents were implanted in 338 patients, most with a diagnosis of repaired TOF; the mean age was 12.2 years. After stenting, the systolic pressure gradient across the stenosis decreased from 41 to 9 mm Hg, and the mean diameter of the stented vessels more than doubled. With improved techniques and increased experience, morbidity and mortality decreased significantly during the second half of this series.

The adverse events associated with PA angioplasty and stenting collected in the C3PO registry were reported by Holzer and coworkers.[92] From 2007 to 2009, 1315 cases of PA rehabilitation were performed in 969 patients, 495 (38%) of which involved stent placement. The authors found an adverse event rate of 22%, with high-severity (moderate, major, or catastrophic) events in 10%. There was no significant difference between stent placement and standard balloon angioplasty alone. There were two procedure-related deaths (0.015%). The most common adverse events were reperfusion injury/endotracheal tube bleeding in 40 patients (12% of the adverse events), heart block in 37 patients (11%), confined vascular tears in 23 patients (7%), and stent malposition/embolization in 21 patients (6%). Unconfined tears occurred in nine patients (3%), and aneurysm formation occurred in five patients (2%). Independent risk factors for a high-severity adverse event included hemodynamic vulnerability, age less than 1 month, use of cutting balloons for angioplasty, and operator experience of less than 10 years.

Long-Term Outcomes

The longest follow-up series was reported in 2009 by Law and colleagues,[103] who described the long-term outcome of children who were originally enrolled in the Investigational Device Exemption (IDE) PA stent trial approved by the U.S. Food and Drug Administration (FDA) between 1989 and 1992. Their data, with a mean follow-up time of 13.2 ± 2.3 years, confirmed the lasting hemodynamic benefits in these children and documented the feasibility of late stent redilation. Although nonobstructive neointimal proliferation was seen almost universally, clinically important in-stent restenosis was uncommon. Repeated stent dilation in these patients was primarily indicated to accommodate somatic growth. There were no late complications. Despite this and many studies reporting a low rate of late in-stent restenosis, a 2014 study by Hallbergson and coworkers used a more defined criterion for restenosis (>25% narrowing of contrast-filled lumen–to–stent diameter), reported an incidence of 24%.[104] These authors found that patients with TOF who had multiple aortopulmonary collaterals, Williams syndrome, or Alagille syndrome had the highest incidence of in-stent restenosis; no association was found with stent type.

As previously mentioned, it is important that stents implanted into the PAs of children can be safely and effectively redilated to a larger diameter as the child grows. Reports from several institutions confirm the experimental observations that PA stents can be safely redilated to a larger diameter.[98,99,101,103–106] In 2003 Duke and colleagues[106] reported safe and effective stent redilation in 12 children with PA stenosis. Redilation was required because of a combination of patient growth and neointimal proliferation. Redilation increased the PA stent diameter to beyond its initial implantation size and effectively decreased the systolic gradient. These authors found neointimal proliferation to be precipitated by overdilation of stents at the time of implantation, in agreement with the practice of placing stents at a size that is no larger than the size of the normal adjacent vessel.

Conclusions and Recommendations

Experimental and clinical data from several centers indicate that balloon-expandable stenting provides an effective form of therapy for many patients with PA stenosis or hypoplasia. Because balloon angioplasty alone is initially unsuccessful in as many as 30% to 40% of patients, stenting is currently considered standard first-line therapy for most children with PA stenosis. If at all possible, implanted stents should have the capacity for later redilation with somatic growth. In infants and small children, in whom larger stents may be difficult to implant due to access site limitations, a hybrid approach for implantation should be considered. If implantation of a small stent is required, an understanding that these stents will require later surgical intervention or intentional fracture is necessary, but this should not preclude the use of stent therapy if clinically necessary.

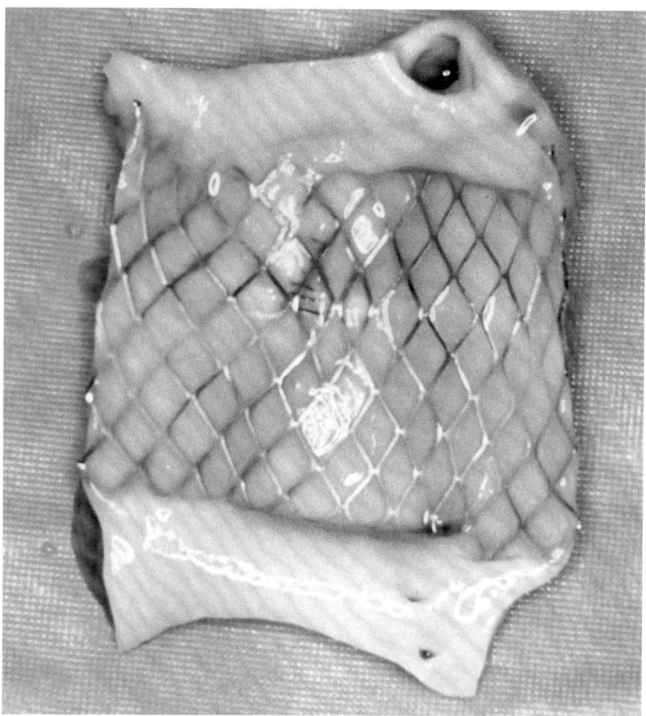

Fig. 60.14 Aortic stent explanted 6 weeks after stenting of an experimental coarctation in a canine model. The Palmaz P-308 stainless steel stent is almost completely covered with a thin layer of neointima. The sutures used to create the experimental coarctation are evident.

BALLOON-EXPANDABLE STENTING FOR COARCTATION OF THE AORTA

Coarctation of the aorta accounts for 8% to 10% of all CHD. For seven decades, surgical repair has been a conventional therapy for patients with a native (unoperated) or recurrent postoperative coarctation. Coarctation balloon angioplasty has been available since the mid-1980s, but its effectiveness has been diminished by higher rates of restenosis and aneurysm formation in up to 35% of patietnts.[107] As a result, in the late 1980s, balloon-expandable stenting emerged as the preferred transcatheter therapy for coarctation (Fig. 60.14). A stent's radial strength opposes elastic aortic wall recoil and may improve vessel integrity, thereby decreasing the risk of aneurysm formation at the dilation site. The availability of covered stents may provide an even safer therapy for coarctation in patients with a vulnerable aortic wall (e.g., Turner syndrome) and in older adults.

Technical Considerations

Stent therapy can benefit patients who have a native unoperated coarctation or a recurrent postoperative coarctation with equal effectiveness (Figs. 60.15 and 60.16). Most interventionalists attempt to limit stenting to older children and adolescents so as to maximize initial implant diameter and minimize arterial access site complications and the need for later stent redilation after somatic growth has occurred. Stent placement for native or recurrent coarctation of the aorta is indicated in patients who have a peak systolic ejection gradient greater than 20 mm Hg or a gradient of less than 20 mm Hg with associated systemic hypertension or LV dysfunction.[91]

Mild coarctation (i.e., resting systolic gradient <20 mm Hg) posed a therapeutic dilemma in the past because it was generally thought that the benefits did not outweigh the risks of surgery. However, more recent data suggest that mild coarctation may be associated with long-term rest and exercise hypertension and

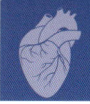

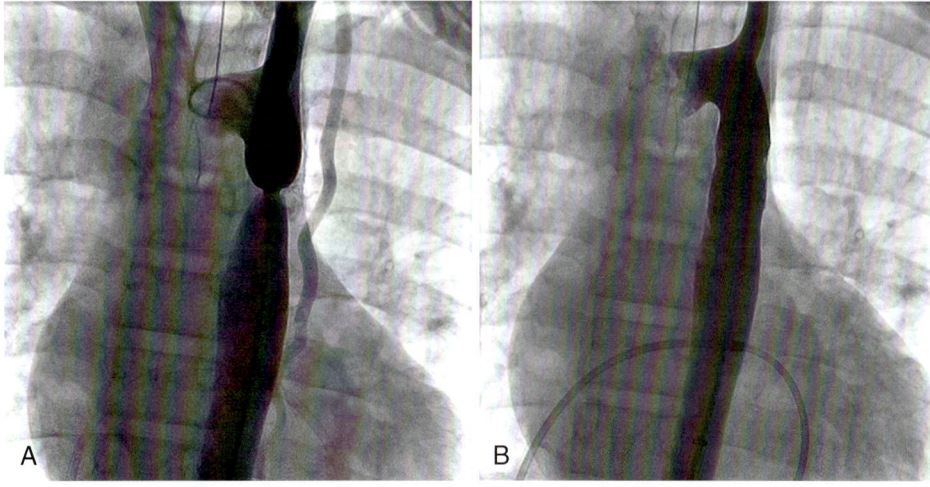

Fig. 60.15 Anteroposterior aortograms obtained before and after stenting in a 14-year-old teenager with a discrete native (unoperated) coarctation of the aorta. (A) Before stenting, there is a severe stenosis, and a systolic gradient of 41 mm Hg was measured. (B) After stenting with a balloon-expandable stainless steel stent dilated to a diameter of 16 mm, the pressure gradient is entirely eliminated.

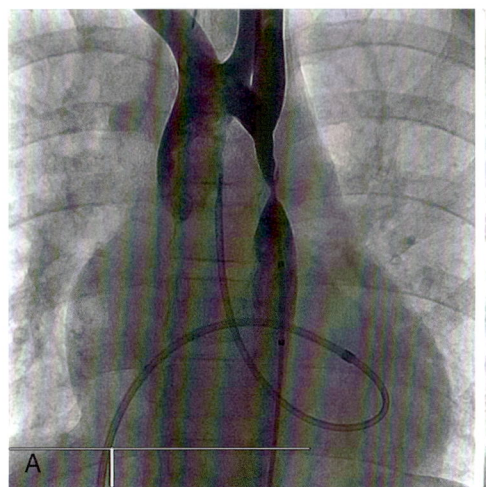
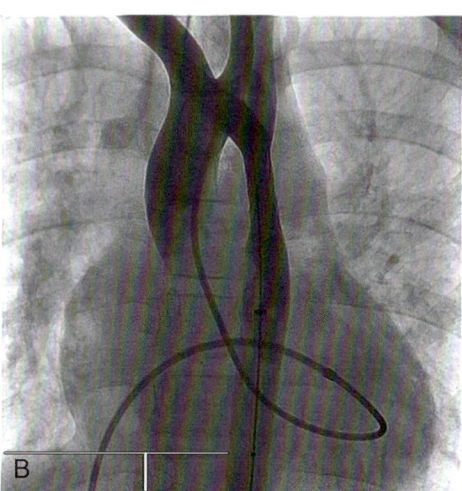

Fig. 60.16 Anteroposterior aortograms obtained before and after stenting in an 11-year-old child with a severe native coarctation of the aorta. (A) Before stenting, there was a severe stenosis that measured approximately 2 mm in diameter. (B) After the coarctation was stented with a bare-metal stainless steel stent intentionally dilated to a subtherapeutic diameter (8 mm) in an attempt to avoid undue aortic wall trauma, the gradient decreased from 31 to 10 mm Hg.

perhaps LV hypertrophy and diastolic dysfunction. Marshall and colleagues[108] reported the results of stent treatment in 33 patients with mild native or residual coarctation. At follow-up catheterization after stent placement, LV end-diastolic pressure had decreased significantly, from 17 to 14 mm Hg. Although larger clinical studies with longer follow-up periods are necessary, these data do suggest that there may be a place for nonsurgical intervention for mild degrees of coarctation.

Transcatheter stent therapy may also provide a reasonable treatment strategy for anatomic variations of coarctation that pose difficult surgical dilemmas. For example, hypoplasia of the transverse aortic arch is responsible for residual obstruction in a small proportion of patients after surgical coarctation repair. These lesions can be difficult to manage surgically because the operative procedure may require a period of hypothermic circulatory arrest. Pihkala and colleagues[109] reported the successful use of stent therapy in four children with transverse arch hypoplasia. Successful stenting in infants with complex aortic arch obstruction after the Norwood operation for hypoplastic left heart syndrome has also been described.[110,111] In these infants, an antegrade approach via the femoral vein or a carotid cutdown may be used to avoid femoral artery injury while allowing for implantation of a relatively large-sized stent with larger diameter potential to accommodate somatic growth. Imaging of the aortic arch with rotational angiography and 3D reconstruction can be of great value in visualization of complex or atypical coarctation anatomy (Fig. 60.17; Video 60.3).

In most reported series, balloon-expandable bare-metal stents have been used with good clinical effect and an overall good

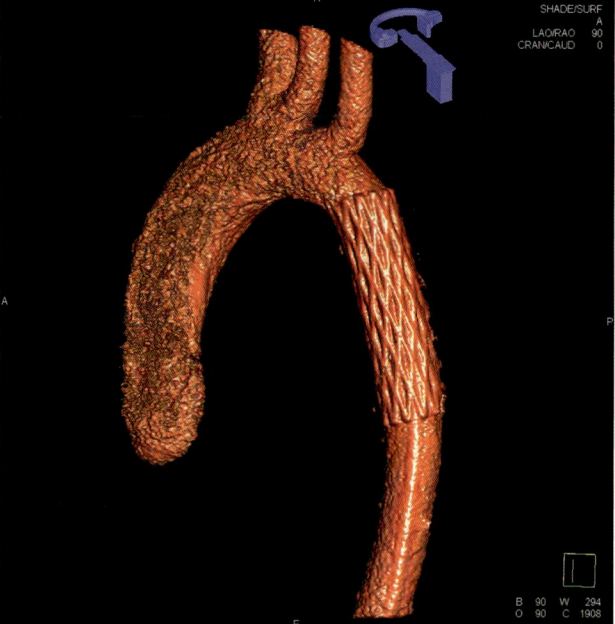

Fig. 60.17 Three-dimensional reconstruction of rotational angiogram performed on a 10-year-old boy with mild transverse arch hypoplasia, and long-segment coarctation of the aorta distal to the left subclavian artery after placement of a Palmaz 4010 stent (see also Video 60.3). (Courtesy Dr. Jeffrey Zampi, University of Michigan, Ann Arbor.)

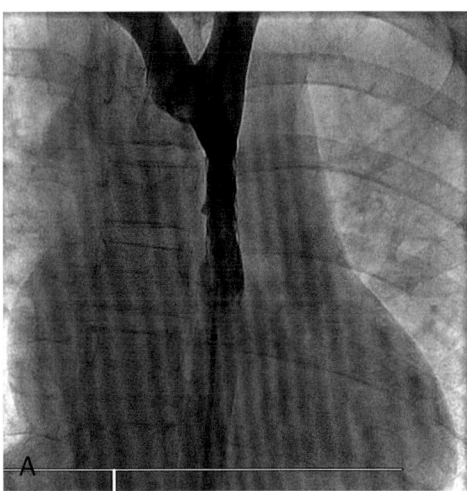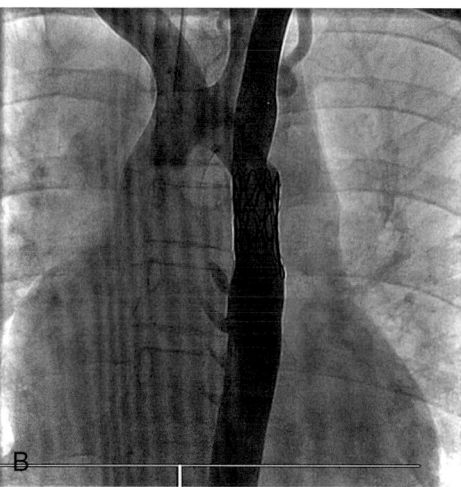

Fig. 60.18 Anteroposterior aortograms obtained before and 10 months after bare-metal stenting of a severe coarctation (same patient as in Fig. 60.16). (A) The initial angiogram demonstrates a small saccular aneurysm on the medial aspect of the stented area. (B) After stenting with a covered Cheatham platinum (CP) stent under compassionate use approval, the aneurysm is excluded and the residual coarctation stenosis is relieved. Reflux of contrast material into several intercostal arteries is evident.

safety profile but still with a 1% to 4% risk of acute aortic wall injury. In October 2017 the covered Cheatham platinum (CCP) stent (NuMed, Hopkinton, NY) received FDA approval for use in aortic coarctation (Fig. 60.18). This stent, consisting of a bare-metal stent covered in its entire length with an expandable sleeve of expanded polytetrafluoroethylene (ePTFE), may be particularly effective in stenting of complex coarctation anatomy and in patients in whom the aortic wall is more fragile (e.g., arteriopathies, advanced age).[112,113] With the use of covered stents, more complex and tighter coarctation can be treated with lower rates of complications.[114,115]

Clinical Outcomes

Numerous clinical studies in the past two decades have documented the effectiveness and relative safety of transcatheter stenting of coarctation of the aorta in both pediatric and adult populations.[108,116–123] A prospective, observational, multiinstitutional study carried out by 36 centers from the Congenital Cardiovascular Interventional Study Consortium (CCISC) compared the safety and efficacy of stent placement with that of balloon angioplasty and surgery for native coarctation of the aorta in patients weighing more than 10 kg.[124] Although all three arms of the study showed significant improvement in follow-up resting systolic blood pressure and coarctation gradient, the stent group achieved a lower gradient compared with the angioplasty group. Of the three, the stent group had the lowest likelihood of any complication (2.3% vs. 9.8% for angioplasty and 18.1% for surgery). In particular, aortic wall injury was significantly greater on follow-up imaging in the angioplasty group (21.4%) compared with the stent group (3.1%), primarily because of an increased risk of aneurysm formation. Stent patients were more likely to require a planned reintervention, primarily for stent redilation as part of a staged approach or secondary to patient somatic growth. There was no difference in unplanned reinterventions between the treatment groups. Although these results must be interpreted with some caution given the nonrandomized nature of the study, the findings suggest that stent therapy may be the lowest-risk intervention available to this patient population.

The largest series of coarctation stenting to date was reported in 2007 by Forbes for the CCISC.[119] In that multiinstitutional study, 627 stents were placed in 555 patients for native (52.3%) or recurrent postoperative coarctation. The median age was 15 years, and the median weight was 56.4 kg. A successful treatment outcome was achieved in 97.9% of procedures, with the systolic gradient decreasing from 32 to 3 mm Hg acutely. Complications occurred in 14.3% of procedures and included aortic wall injury (intimal tear, dissection/rupture, and aneurysm) in 3.9%, stent migration in 5%, and cerebral vascular accident in 0.7%. Acute aortic aneurysm formation was observed in six procedures (1.1%). Two patients (0.4%) with severe aortic wall injury were sent emergently to surgery but experienced severe neurologic injury and later died. Acute aortic wall complications were associated with performance of prestenting balloon angioplasty (odds ratio [OR], 4.18), location of coarctation in the abdominal aorta versus the isthmus or transverse aorta (OR, 5.74), and age greater than 40 years (OR, 2.95). At intermediate follow-up (median of 12 months), approximately one-quarter of patients in the CCISC study underwent additional aortic arch imaging, with identification of an abnormality in 29% of patients.[118] These abnormalities included aneurysm (9%), intimal tear/dissection (3%), stent fracture (4%), and stent reobstruction (11%). The authors identified an increased risk of aortic wall pathology in follow-up if the ratio of balloon diameter to coarctation diameter exceeded 3.5, but they found no association between age and late development of aortic wall pathology.

The immediate outcomes of covered stent placement for coarctation of the aorta were reported as part of the Covered Cheatham-Platinum Stents for Prevention or Treatment of Aortic Wall Injury Associated with Coarctation of the Aorta Trial (COAST) II. This multicenter, single-arm trial used the CCP stent for 158 patients with coarctation for either prevention, in high-risk patients, or treatment of preexisting aortic wall injury. Patients identified as high risk included those with a nearly atretic descending aorta, genetic syndromes associated with aortic wall weakening, or advanced age of 60 years or older. There was complete coverage of the site of aortic wall injury in 92% of patients. The remaining patients had minor endoleaks which did not require additional intervention. Serious adverse events occurred in 8% with access site complications occurring most frequently. Although use of CCP clearly has benefit in certain patient populations, it is unclear at this time whether CCP are superior to bare-metal stents for all patients. In 2014 Sohrabi et al. described the first randomized trial comparing bare-metal and CCP stents in patients with native coarctation.[125] Complication rates were similar between groups, but patients undergoing CCP stent implantation experienced a higher occurrence of pseudoaneurysm formation.[125] This association is not completely clear, and continued study of these two stent types compared with each other is necessary.

Data on long-term outcomes of stent implantation for aortic coarctation are limited, with the longest reported follow-up being 15 years.[114,122,126–128] Butera and associates[114] reported their long-term, single-center experience using both bare and covered stents in patients with coarctation. Recoarctation occurred as a result of neointimal hyperplasia, somatic growth, or stent fracture. In the bare-metal stent group, over a median follow-up period of 81.7 months, 23.9% of patients required reintervention due to restenosis, at a mean of 49.4 months from initial stent placement. Three patients (4.5%) required reintervention with covered stent implantation due to late aneurysm formation. There was a 100% success rate with reintervention. The covered stent group had a similar reintervention rate (22.4%) at an earlier mean follow-up time of 18.4 months. Three of 15 of these patients underwent staged redilation due to the severity of the initial lesion, and this may have contributed to the earlier time at reintervention in this group. Independent risk factors for reintervention included complex lesions, use of a balloon smaller than 14 mm in diameter for initial stent delivery, and an immediate poststent residual gradient of more than 10 mm Hg. Neointimal hyperplasia was present in 8.4% at follow-up, with a similar incidence in the two stent groups. Stent fracture was more common in the bare-metal group (5%), and the majority of these patients required reintervention due to restenosis. Somatic growth as a cause of reintervention was significantly associated with age younger than 15 years and use of a balloon diameter smaller than 14 mm at initial stent implantation.

Another long-term issue with patients after coarctation repair is systemic hypertension. Many studies have found that patients with coarctation continue to exhibit elevated blood pressure after their initial intervention or develop hypertension over time, even in the setting of a good anatomic result of intervention.[116,123] Holzer and coworkers[122] reported the intermediate and long-term follow-up results (up to 60 months) in patients included in the multiinstitution CCISC study. Twenty-three percent of patients continued to have systolic blood pressure greater than the 95th percentile, 9% had an upper-to-lower limb blood pressure gradient greater than 20 mm Hg, and 32% were taking antihypertensive medications. Eighty percent of patients studied a mean of 5.3 years after stent implantation for coarctation also exhibited abnormally elevated exercise blood pressure response.[128]

Lifelong surveillance for these patients, even after successful anatomic relief of coarctation, is therefore warranted for regular assessment of blood pressure, monitoring with cross-sectional imaging for late development of aneurysm formation or recurrent coarctation, and assessment of ventricular systolic and diastolic function.

Conclusions and Recommendations

Coarctation stenting is an effective approach to native and postoperative recurrent coarctation of the aorta. Most pediatric interventionalists limit stent implantation for coarctation to large children and adolescents to avoid the need for aortic stent redilation after somatic growth in a smaller child. Stent implantation is a promising intervention for more difficult variations on coarctation anatomy, particularly transverse arch hypoplasia, arch obstruction after the Norwood operation, and mild degrees of coarctation that have not warranted surgery in the past. In older adults in whom the aortic wall is friable, covered stents may provide a safer alternative because of the increased risk of aortic wall injury with coarctation dilation. Longer-term follow-up studies are necessary to more precisely define the late risks of stent restenosis, aortic aneurysm formation, the safety of late stent redilation after somatic growth in children, and blood pressure response to exercise in the face of a rigid, stented aortic segment.

TRANSCATHETER CLOSURE OF THE SECUNDUM ATRIAL SEPTAL DEFECT

ASDs result from deficient development of the intraatrial septum. The exact position of the defect is determined by the specific area that fails to develop and is traditionally described in anatomic terms.

Sinus venosus defects result from abnormal development of either the superior or inferior horns of the sinus venosus and are located superiorly or inferiorly along the posterior margin of the atrial septum. Superior sinus venosus defects frequently have associated anomalous drainage of the right upper pulmonary vein.

Primum ASDs result from deficiencies of the septum secundum, frequently as part of the complex of maldevelopment of the endocardial cushions (atrioventricular canal [AVC] defects). In the most severe form (complete AVC), the primum defect is part of a complex that includes an inlet ventricular septal defect (VSD) and a common atrioventricular valve. In the least severe form, the primum ASD defect is associated with a cleft in the anterior mitral valve leaflet.

Secundum ASDs result from deficiencies of the central portion of the atrial septum, the septum primum. These defects, usually in the region of the fossa ovalis, may be extensive in size, varied in shape, and often multiple in number (fenestrated atrial septum). It is secundum type defects, often with substantial peridefect margins and positioned some distance from other vital structures, that lend themselves well to percutaneous device closure. Further discussion in this section will focus on secundum ASDs.

Physiology

ASDs represent one of the most common forms of isolated acyanotic CHD.[129] Although the left atrial pressure is typically higher than that in the right atrium, flow across the atrial septum is determined in large part by the end-diastolic pressure within each ventricle, in turn reflective of relative ventricular compliance. The net size of the atrial level shunt is thus only in part dependent on the size of the ASD. Elevation of either LV or RV systolic pressure in the face of ventricular outflow tract obstruction will not impact atrial level shunting if ventricular relaxation is not adversely impacted.

With persistence of atrial level shunting, the right atrial and ventricular end-diastolic volumes are chronically increased, and both atrial and ventricular dimensions increase accordingly.[129] Additional RV volume will result firstly in delayed pulmonary valve closure compared with the aortic valve (causing the clinical sign of the fixed, split second heart sound), and a flow murmur across a normal pulmonary valve (identical to that of pathologic pulmonary valve stenosis, but without an ejection click).[130]

The additional pulmonary blood flow is well tolerated in most cases but, in rare cases, can lead to pulmonary hypertension and pulmonary vasoocclusive disease. Ultimately, Eisenmenger type physiology will prevail, at which point shunt flow will be right to left, and the patient will become cyanotic.[131–133] That pathologic end point should not be confused with right-to-left shunting resulting from a decrease in RV compliance with long-standing RV dilation. This latter scenario carries a substantially better prognosis than pulmonary vasoocclusive disease and can be diagnosed either on the basis of relatively normal RV and PA pressures determined by echocardiography or at cardiac catheterization.

CLINICAL PRESENTATION AND DIAGNOSIS

ASDs are typically asymptomatic during the first two decades of life. Diagnosis is most often made after detection of a murmur, indistinguishable from that of pulmonary valve stenosis, or with auscultation of a fixed split-second heart sound.[130] Infrequently, infants or children may present with failure to thrive or other more overt signs of congestive heart failure or recurrent lower respiratory tract infections. Later, in the third and fourth decades, if previously undiagnosed, symptoms may include undue fatigue, increased dyspnea on exertion, and a frequent sensation of palpitations.[129,133]

The electrocardiogram (ECG) may be normal early in childhood or at any age if right atrial enlargement (RAE) or right ventricular dilation (RVD) have not yet occurred. As those changes progress, typical ECG changes with right axis deviation, RAE, and RVD become more clearly apparent.

Echocardiography (transthoracic echocardiography [TTE] or transesophageal echocardiography [TEE]) remains the mainstay of diagnosis.[134] In standard long-axis views, the first indication of an ASD may be dilation of the anteriorly located right ventricle (RV). In short-axis views, that dilation may again be noted, especially in the region of the infundibulum. In four-chamber views, both the RA and RV will be seen to be dilated. However, the ASD is best seen and evaluated in both long- and short-axis subcostal views. These views allow for complete evaluation of the total septal length and provide excellent visualization of the defect margins. Color-flow mapping is of great importance. This allows determination of the direction of flow across the defect (left to right versus right to left) and provides further assessment to exclude the possibility of multiple defects (Fig. 60.19). Occasionally, poor acoustic windows may preclude clear TTE images. This is more likely in the adult patient, in the presence of obesity, or with chronic lung disease. At those times, elective TEE should be performed to confirm the diagnosis and prior to further discussion regarding possible defect closure and repair.[135]

Echocardiography is also invaluable in achieving a noninvasive measure of RV and PA pressures. Excessive elevation of right-sided pressures should introduce some caution prior to proceeding with defect repair, especially if there is color-flow evidence of right-to-left shunting across the ASD. Other causes of pulmonary vascular disease should be excluded before attributing the cause to an ASD.

Treatment and Outcome

Surgical repair has long been the mainstay of treatment for ASDs.[132,133,136] However, over the past two decades, substantial advances have been made with percutaneous closure devices. At this time, initial attempt at percutaneous closure of appropriate secundum ASDs are considered standard of care.[137-139] Currently in the United States, two devices are approved for use by the FDA Amplatzer Septal Occluder (Abbott Laboratories, Abbott Park, IL) and the Gore Cardioform Septal Occluder (W. L. Gore and Associates, Flagstaff, AZ).[140,141] Although different in design and construction, the principles of function, deployment, and follow-up are similar (Figs. 60.20 and 60.21). After deployment, both devices are designed to have two discs separated by a central core or waist. One disc is positioned on the left atrial side of the defect, with the core or waist straddling the defect, and the other disc opposed to the atrial membrane from the right atrial side of the atrial septum. The devices have intrinsic recoil that opposes both discs to each other, holding the devices in place on the atrial septum.

Irrespective of the device used, defect sizing is required prior to deployment. Reliance may be made on the TTE measurements with an empiric factor adjustment (e.g., 115% of the TTE measurement). However, most operators continue to rely on balloon sizing of the defect before choosing a particular sized device.[138,139] That is accomplished with a large, compliant balloon inflated across the atrial septum, with the narrowest area ("stretched diameter" or "waist") measured with angiographic calibration (Fig. 60.22). The current recommendation is to use a "stop-flow" technique for defect sizing. Once the sizing balloon is positioned across the atrial septum, it is slowly inflated while careful observation is maintained with TEE or intracardiac echocardiography (ICE). As soon as color flow across the defect is arrested, no further inflation occurs, and an angiographic measurement of that balloon waist size is used to choose the appropriately sized closure device. This technique is used to avoid

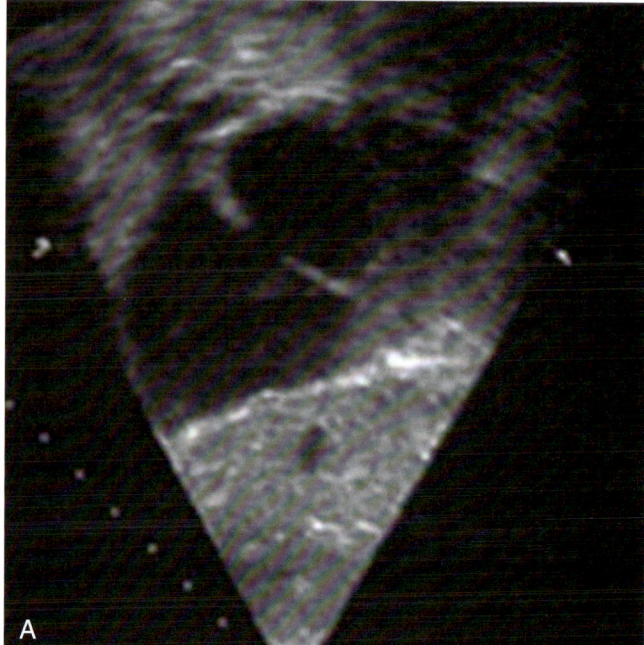
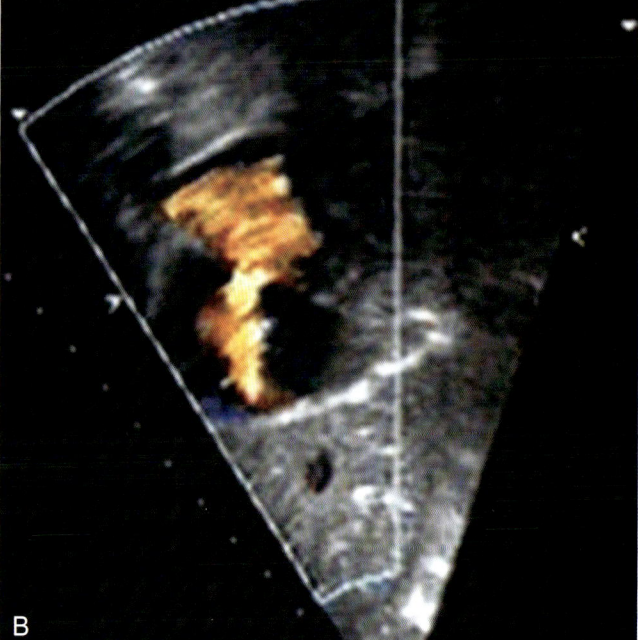

Fig. 60.19 Subcostal short-axis transthoracic echocardiographic images show a secundum atrial septal defect in two dimensions (A) and with color flow-mapping (B). The defect is central in the septum and has excellent margins for device support.

oversizing of the closure device, the main factor thought attributable to both early and late erosions of closure devices.[142]

Both devices are deployed through a delivery sheath that typically extends from the femoral region, although other access sites have been used. The left atrial disc is initially deployed and the device retracted back onto the atrial septum with both fluoroscopic and echocardiographic guidance. The remainder of the device is then deployed within the right atrium, so that the waist or core of the device straddles the defect. The delivery cable remains attached to the device until the time of release and can be used to retract the device if positioning is not acceptable (Fig. 60.23). Even after release, the devices can be retrieved with various intravascular snares if that should become necessary.

To ensure adequate device deployment, echocardiographic imaging is used in addition to fluoroscopy.[134] The majority of pediatric institutions continue to use TEE, but ICE has increased in popularity. This avoids the necessity of general anesthesia in most patients, but an additional femoral venous access site is required for positioning of the ICE probe within the right atrium. Deployment of the devices using echocardiography alone has also been described.[135] Three-dimensional echocardiographic imaging is frequently used with device placement.[143] This modality provides an en face view of the septum allowing the interventionalist to better appreciate the true shape and size of the defect. Whichever echocardiographic modality is used, it is imperative to ensure that atrial septal device tissue is noted to be present between the left and right atrial device discs in all different plains to ensure proper and safe device deployment prior to release from the delivery cable.

Percutaneous device closure has proven effective in repairing ASDs, with minimal morbidity and no effective mortality. Closure rates are comparable to surgery over similar time periods (97% to 99% at 12 months), but procedural morbidity is considerably lower.[137,143,144] Percutaneous closure avoids the necessity of a sternotomy, cardiopulmonary bypass, and mediastinal and chest-tube drainage but does have the disadvantage of some limited exposure to ionizing radiation. However, fluoroscopy times are typically brief, and low dose adjustments can be used. The risk of device embolization is also small and, in most cases, related to operator inexperience. The incidence of this complication is in the region of 0.1%.[138,139] The majority of acute complications have been related to rhythm disturbances, in most cases atrial flutter or other intermittent supra-ventricular tachycardias, and rarely complete heart block.[145] However, these complications are also rare, occurring less than 1% of the time. Thrombus formation on the device, with distal embolization is of great concern, justifying the recommendation for aspirin therapy until device endothelialization has occurred.[144,146] Collective review of this potential problem, including evaluation of various generations of early septal occluder devices reveals a low incidence (54 patients over a 14-year period).

Cardiac erosion with possible hemodynamic compromise, particularly by the Amplatzer Septal Occluder, is the most significant short- and long-term complication of percutaneous ASD closure.[147,148] The incidence appears to be low (<0.11%), according to both the manufacturer and published data and, in the majority cases, is related to device oversizing.[147] Deficiency of the retroaortic rim, with resulting need to position the device in a manner that straddles the aorta, may also be a risk factor.[149] Deficiency of that rim or oversizing of the device may cause either aortic compression or direct impingement of the wall of the aorta by either left or right atrial margins of the device (Fig. 60.24). In addition, oversizing of the device or placement of a device that is too large to be accommodated by the total septal length could cause part of the superior margin of the left atrial disc to abut against the roof of the left atrium. Continuous rocking motion of the device against either the aorta or the atrial wall may result in erosion. If any of these findings become apparent either during device deployment or after complete deployment, the device should be withdrawn, and attempts to reposition or resize the device should be made. Despite those attempts, if those findings persist, the device should be removed.[149]

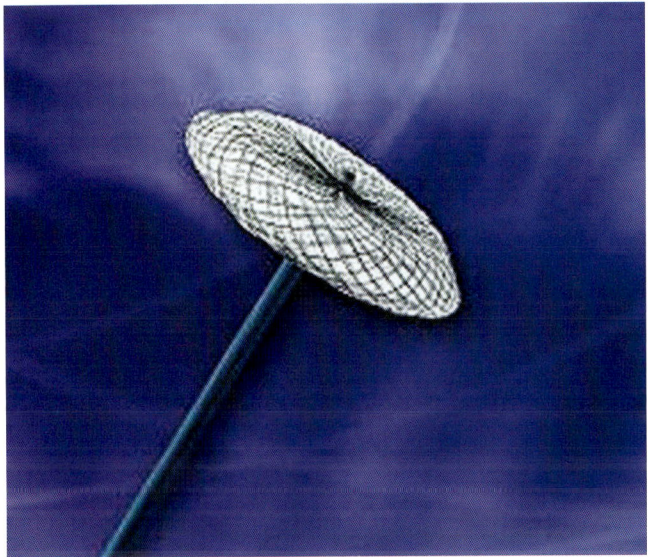

Fig. 60.20 Amplatzer septal occluder. The device is constructed from an alloy of nickel and titanium. The two atrial discs are separated by the central waist. In this photograph, the tethering cable, covered by the delivery sheath, remains attached to the device. (Courtesy AGA Medical, Golden Valley, MN.)

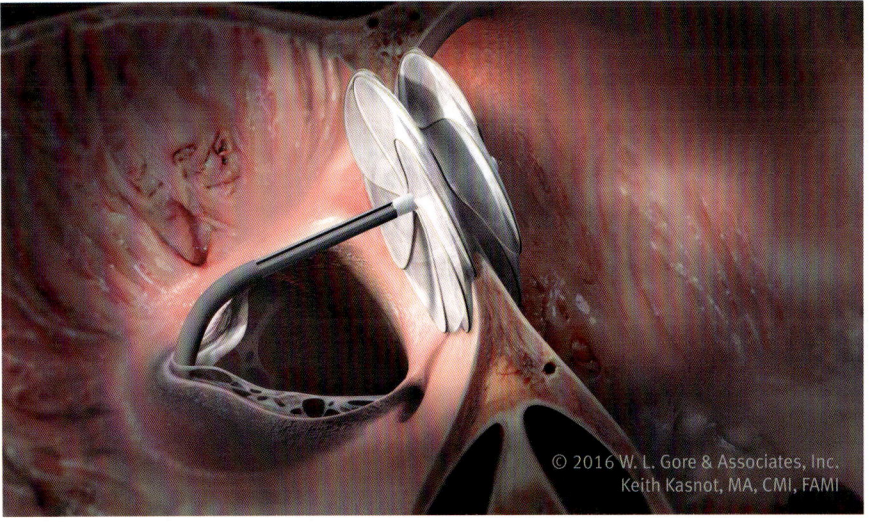

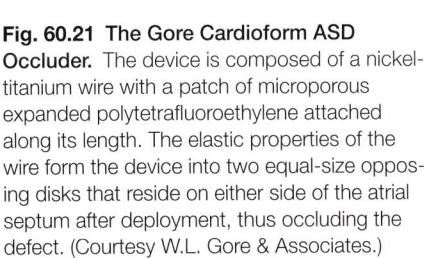

Fig. 60.21 The Gore Cardioform ASD Occluder. The device is composed of a nickel-titanium wire with a patch of microporous expanded polytetrafluoroethylene attached along its length. The elastic properties of the wire form the device into two equal-size opposing disks that reside on either side of the atrial septum after deployment, thus occluding the defect. (Courtesy W.L. Gore & Associates.)

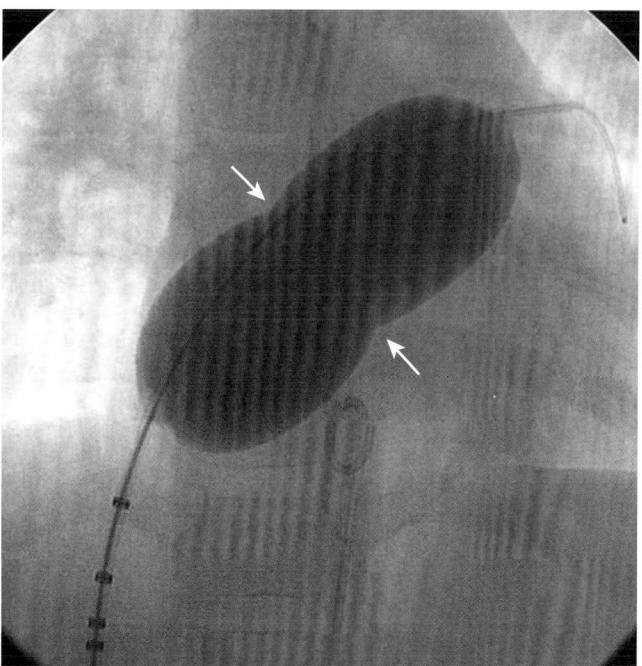

Fig. 60.22 Still frame of an angiogram demonstrating inflation of the balloon sizing catheter across the atrial septum. The indentations on the balloon *(white arrows)* indicate the stretched margin of the atrial septal defect. That diameter is measured, and an appropriately sized septal occluder is chosen accordingly.

Follow-Up

An echocardiogram should be performed within 24 hours of ASD device closure, to exclude the presence of a pericardial effusion. After device implantation, patients should remain on aspirin for at least 6 months, during which time complete device endothelialization occurs. Bacterial endocarditis prophylaxis prophylaxis is also recommended during that period and should be continued if residual atrial level shunting is apparent at the time of the 6-month echocardiogram. After that, follow-up should be at least on an annual basis, with echocardiography obtained during those visits. The right atrial and ventricular dimensions return to normal within 6 months if no significant atrial level shunting remains.[150]

TRANSCATHETER CLOSURE OF THE PATENT DUCTUS ARTERIOSUS

Introduction

The ductus arteriosus is a muscular artery that extends from the undersurface of the aortic arch to the roof of the main PA but mostly directed to the left. Although some degree of anatomic variation does occur (such as with a right aortic arch, when the ductus arises from the base of the left innominate artery), the relationship is generally consistent. It provides a vital function during fetal life, allowing blood that has entered the main PA via the RV to be redirected into the aorta. At birth, with an increase in arterial oxygen content and a decrease in circulating prostaglandins, the ductus arteriosus spasms and later becomes fibrotic with permanent closure. This occurs usually by 5 to 7 days in full-term infants but may not occur until 3 weeks. Persistence of the ductus arteriosus after that time occurs between 1 in 2500 to 1 in 5000 live births.[151,152] After closure, the ductus arteriosus has no further significance, unless associated with a right aortic arch and aberrant origin of the left subclavian artery. Those anatomic associations result in a vascular ring that could prove clinically significant with airway compromise or feeding difficulty in infancy.

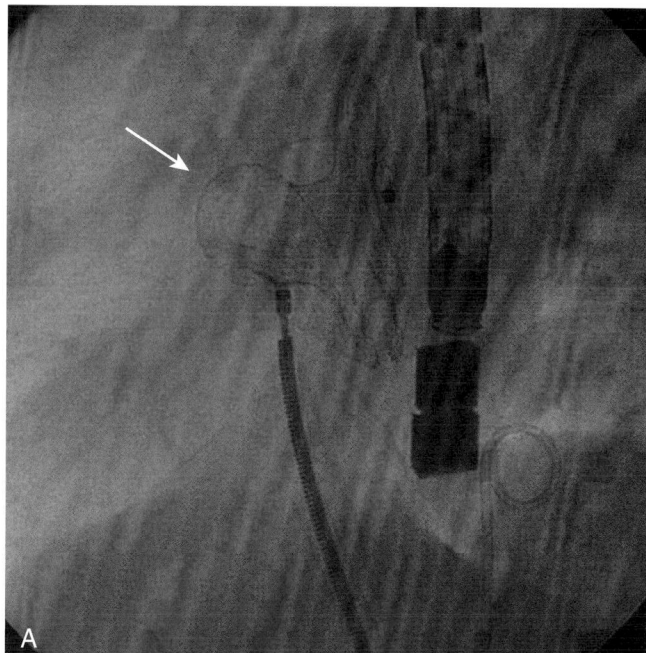

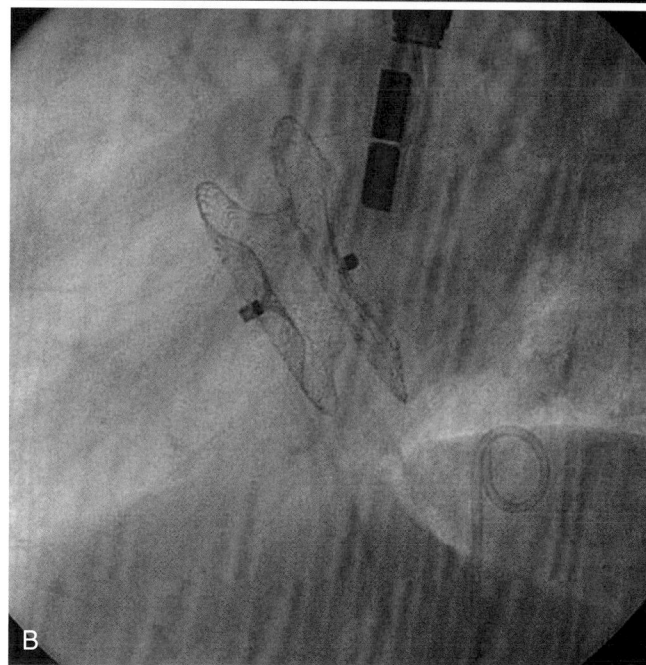

Fig. 60.23 Still-frame lateral image (A) demonstrates full deployment of an Amplatzer Septal Occluder with the cable still attached. Distortion of the superior margin of the right atrial disk of the device *(solid white arrow)*, resulting from downward tension by the delivery cable, is typical at this stage of deployment. Retraction and redeployment of the device is easily achieved while it is still attached to the delivery cable. A transesophageal echocardiographic probe is visible in the image. (B) Still-frame lateral image after release of the Amplatzer Septal Occluder from the delivery cable. The septal occluder immediately assumes the typical position, with the right and left atrial disks parallel to each other.

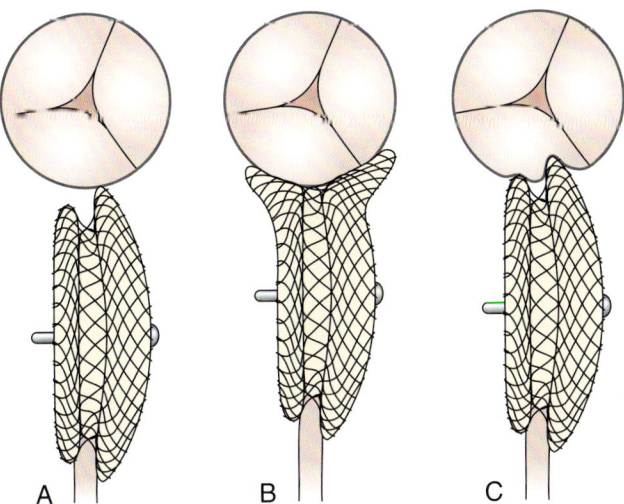

Fig. 60.24 Diagram demonstrates different relations of the Amplatzer Septal Occluder to the aorta after deployment. (A) Close proximity, possibly touching. (B) Straddling the aortic root. (C) Distortion of the aorta, which may increase the risk of erosion.

Physiology

Discussion regarding the influence of the PDA on the physiology of the neonate, particularly with regard to prematurity and hyaline membrane disease, is beyond the scope of this text. This discussion will thus be confined to the effect of the PDA on older children and adults, where the impact is similar.

The main factors contributing to the effects of a PDA are the size of the vessel, and relative resistance of the systemic and pulmonary vascular beds. When small, the hemodynamic effect is negligible, with flow occurring only during systole and limited by the resistance of flow through the narrow ductus. As the PDA increases in size, flow through the PDA will continue to be left to right as long as the pulmonary vascular resistance is lower than that of the systemic vascular bed (even in the presence of a completely unrestrictive vessel). Under those circumstances, PA pressures are equal to aortic, and the flow is left to right during both systole and diastole. With persistent shunting through a large ductus, the left atrium and ventricle become increasingly volume loaded and dilated. Furthermore, owing to this increased runoff into a lower resistance pulmonary vascular bed, the aortic pulse pressure (difference between the aortic systolic and diastolic pressures) will widen considerably. With continued LV dilation, wall stress and end-diastolic pressures will continue to increase, in turn increasing myocardial oxygen requirement. With the decrease in aortic diastolic pressure, coronary perfusion pressure can at times become narrowed. However, although theoretically important, this is usually of little clinical concern and the presence of coronary ischemia with only an isolated PDA has not been described.

Similar to other shunt lesions that expose the pulmonary vascular bed to persistently high pressure and flow situations, large PDAs could ultimately result in the development of pulmonary vascular occlusive disease.[153] At that time, flow direction across the PDA will reverse and Eisenmenger physiology will prevail.[154] Development of those changes will depend on the ductal size and duration of its presence, resistance to flow across the vessel, and individual patient susceptibility.

Clinical Presentation and Diagnosis

In infancy and childhood, the clinical presentation of PDA may vary from completely asymptomatic to the full spectrum of congestive heart failure. Symptoms may thus be completely absent but could include failure to thrive, dyspnea, poor feeding, and excessive perspiration. In older children, adolescents, and adults, congestive symptoms are less likely. It is not uncommon for the diagnosis to be suspected when an incidental murmur is heard during a well-child examination. Rarely, patients undiagnosed in infancy may present with symptoms of endocarditis, or pulmonary vascular-occlusive disease if the PDA is sufficiently unrestrictive.

Clinical signs may be absent if the PDA is small and hemodynamically insignificant. However, with increasing size of the PDA, more typical clinical features become apparent. The pulse pressure may be wider than expected (by palpation and blood pressure measurement), and a murmur of variable grade and duration may be auscultated. If the PDA is small, flow may occur only during systole, and a systolic regurgitant murmur will be present. In the larger PDA, flow will occur throughout the entire cardiac cycle, and the more typical multiphasic continuous machinery murmur will be present. As with all left-to-right shunt lesions, if flow is substantial, a middiastolic tricuspid flow murmur may also be audible. These clinical features will remain the same if the PDA is sufficiently stenotic. However, if the PDA offers little resistance to flow and PA pressures remain significantly elevated over time, the murmur may become diminished and disappear altogether as pulmonary vascular resistance increases to systemic levels. At that point, with Eisenmenger physiology present, flow across the PDA will become right to left and measured oxygen saturations in the lower extremities will be lower than those in the upper extremities.[155]

Confirmation of the diagnosis relies on echocardiography. The PDA is well seen in many different views, but the parasternal short axis, immediately above the level of the pulmonary valve, is ideal. If the PDA is small, 2D imaging may not be helpful; in those cases, color-flow mapping in the main PA reveals the flow occurring in an opposite direction to the antegrade PA flow. Caution should be used to avoid confusing a pulmonary insufficiency color jet from that of the PDA. Doppler interrogation of the ductal flow can also help in determining the degree of stenosis across the PDA and in estimating the PA pressure.

Treatment and Outcome

During the past three decades, percutaneous therapy for the patient with an isolated PDA has become standard of care at most institutions in the United States.[156] With the newer generation of vascular closure devices, this has currently also extended to treatment of significant PDAs in the premature, low-weight neonate or those patients in the early infancy with particularly large, hemodynamically important lesions. These small, flexible devices deliver through microcatheters and have substantially extended the age and size in which PDA closure is currently attempted.[142,157,158]

When necessary, surgical PDA repair is performed in most cases via the left lateral thoracotomy approach. Usually, the PDA is identified, tied off, and ligated. A left-sided chest tube drain remains in place for a brief period after surgery, and hospitalization, although usually brief, may extend for 3 to 4 days. The most significant, but fortunately rare, complications include damage to the recurrent laryngeal nerve, and inadvertent ligation of the left PA or descending aorta (the latter with often catastrophic effects if not immediately identified).[159,160] There is low but not unexpected morbidity from wound and skin infections. Pain and discomfort are not insignificant, and in most cases opioid analgesics are required in the first 24 hours. There is also a low incidence of vascular recanalization, but that may be dependent on surgical technique.

Transcatheter device closure of the PDA has currently been available for close to 30 years. Different methods have been

SECTION V Structural Interventions

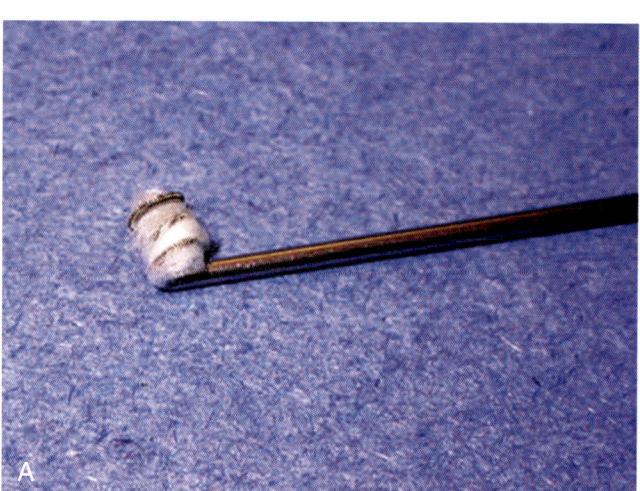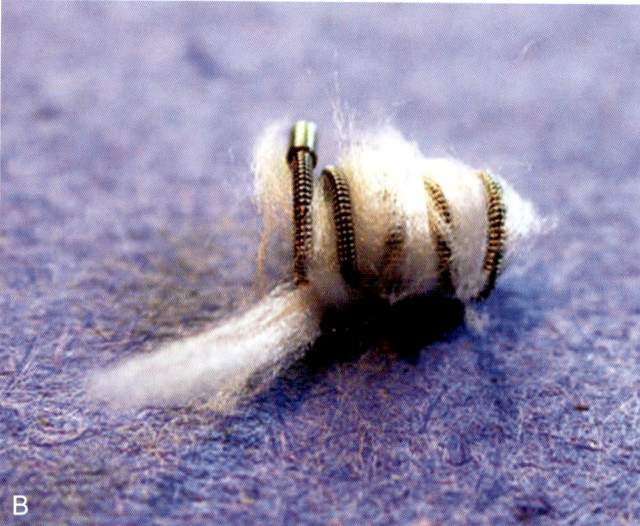

Fig. 60.25 Partial (A) and full (B) extrusion of a Gianturco coil from its delivery sleeve. The coil has polyester fibers attached that promote thrombosis once deployed.

available during this time, but with evolution of device technology and operator technique, two categories of devices are currently in use: coils and occluder devices. Given the differences in their design and delivery, these will be discussed separately.

Coils

Stainless steel Gianturco coils (Cook, Bloomington, IN) of various thickness, lengths, and loop diameters were initially available for general vascular occlusion (Fig. 60.25).[161–163] The application of these coils for small PDA closure began in the early 1990s, and since then, different techniques for their safe delivery and variations on the initial design and delivery have occurred. In general, after basic angiography of the PDA is complete, an appropriate-sized coil is chosen. The PDA deemed ideal for coil closure should narrow significantly along its course (to less than 2 mm), be sufficiently long to accommodate the multiple loops of the coil, and have a sufficient aortic ductal diverticulum. In that way, the loops of the coil on the aortic end of the PDA do not cause flow disturbance in the proximal descending aorta once deployed. Gianturco coils are delivered in a retrograde manner from the aortic end. Once the delivery catheter (typically a right coronary artery or similar shaped catheter) has crossed the PDA, approximately two-thirds of a loop of coil is extruded beyond the catheter tip (within the main PA) by an appropriate diameter pusher wire. The entire catheter-coil complex is then slowly withdrawn until the partially extruded coil is seen to "catch" on the PA wall. At that point, the catheter is then retracted back over the pusher wire into the aorta, with the coil held statically in place. As the catheter is withdrawn, the body of the coil straddles the length of the PDA, until completely extruded from the delivery catheter, when it springs back into the aortic ductal diverticulum and coils appropriately. With correct delivery, approximately two-thirds of the coil should remain on the pulmonary end of the PDA, a portion of the coil straddles the narrowest section of the vessel, and the remainder of the coil is tightly looped within the aortic ampulla. Repeat angiography is performed at a variable time after delivery to confirm appropriate placement and complete closure.

The risk of coil embolization has resulted in modifications, both of coil design and delivery method. Detachable coils (Cook) used a screw mechanism on a modified Gianturco coil that allowed repositioning and retrieval if initial positioning was incorrect.[163,164] However, that modification did not completely alleviate the risk of coil embolization after deployment. Snare

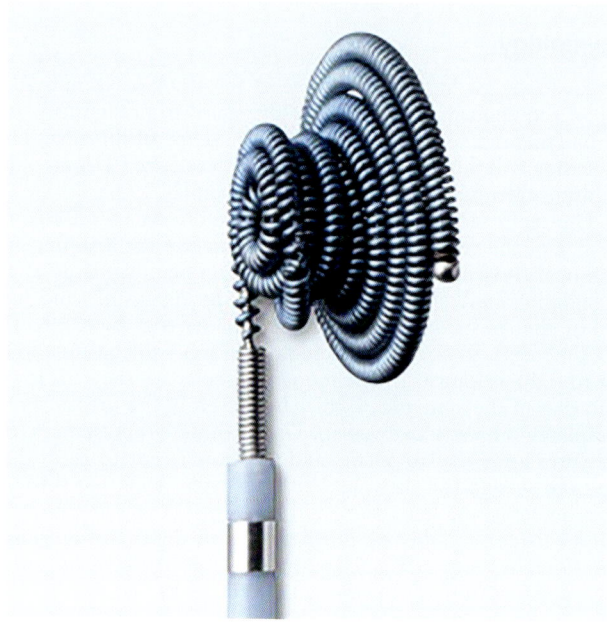

Fig. 60.26 The Nit-Occlud PDA occlusion device. The device consists of a preformed coil in a conical shape and is designed to be positioned in the aortic ductal ampulla, with a section of coil that straddles the patent ductus arteriosus and a smaller countercoil that resides in the pulmonary ductal ampulla after release. (Courtesy PFM Medical, Cologne, Germany.)

techniques to control coil delivery have also been described.[165] Once the initial loop of coil is advanced into the main PA, and prior to the retraction of the delivery catheter back into the aorta, a goose neck–type snare is positioned on the coil to maintain control at the time of delivery. While successful in experienced hands, a greater coordination between the primary catheterizer and the assistant is necessary. Some difficulty loosening the snare from the coil after complete delivery may also result in displacement after an initial apparently successful coil deployment. That technique is currently rarely required with the advent of the Nit-Occlud PDA closure device (pfm medical, Cologne, Germany). This device is a further modification of a detachable coil but has a unique cone-shaped morphology that is available in different

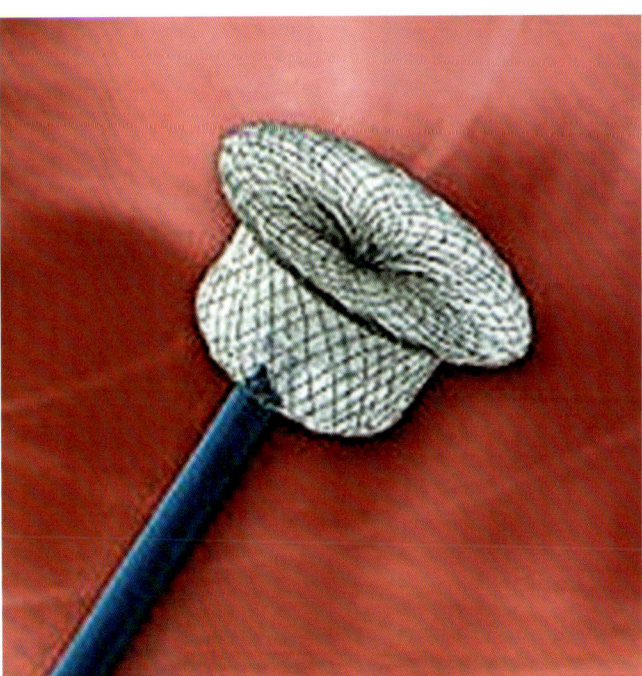

Fig. 60.27 Amplatzer Duct Occluder I. The device is constructed from an alloy of nickel and titanium. The larger end with the cap is designed to be placed on the aortic end of the patent ductus arteriosus, within the ductal diverticulum. The other end tapers slightly and houses the screw thread for placement of the delivery cable. This image shows the device attached to the delivery cable and the delivery sheath. (Courtesy AGA Medical, Golden Valley, MN.)

sizes and lengths (Fig. 60.26). The device is typically deployed in the descending aorta with a tethering cable passed antegrade from the pulmonary side. The body of the device is extruded into the descending aorta. The extruded device and delivery catheter are then retracted until the body of the closure device is lodged within the ductal ampulla. The delivery catheter is then withdrawn back across the ductal vessel, deploying the remainder of the device, but maintaining control. Confirmatory angiography can then be performed, and if the position is acceptable, the device is released from the tethering delivery cable. Until that point, the device can be easily retracted and redeployed if necessary.[166,167]

Previously, multiple, simultaneous coil deployment had also been used for closure of large PDAs.[168,169] However, with the advent of the newer duct occluder devices and plugs, this is largely of historical significance.

In general, coil occlusion has been successful in occluding small PDAs with closure rates between 95% and 100% at 2 years.[170,171] Duct size has been shown to be the single most important factor in predicting complete early and late closure. Small, residual shunts early after attempted closure has raised the prospect of persistent hemolysis with resulting anemia.[172] In most cases, this resolves within 72 hours, and if not, a repeat catheterization with further coil placement may be necessary. Early experience with coil occlusion was also associated with the concern for mild stenosis of the left PA or descending aorta.[173] However, with refinement of technique, and appropriate patient selection for coil placement this is less of clinical concern in the current era of PDA closure.

Duct Occluder Devices

Currently, the only noncoil device approved in the United States by the FDA is the Amplatzer Ductal Occluder family of devices (ADO I and ADO II; Abbott Laboratories).[174,175] The ADO I is a cone-shaped device which tapers from a larger circumference rimmed edge ("cap"). This device is designed to deliver through a sheath via the antegrade venous approach and has a delivery cable that remains attached until release (Fig. 60.27). The cable can also be used for retraction and repositioning of the device if necessary. Once the delivery sheath has been placed across the PDA and in the proximal descending aorta, the larger, aortic end with the "cap" is advanced out of the aortic end of the sheath. The device and sheath complex are then pulled back with the "cap" positioned on the side wall of the aorta or within the ductal diverticulum. At that point, the delivery cable and device are kept exactly in place and the sheath retracted to deploy the remainder of the device within the body of the PDA. Prior to final release, repeat angiography is performed to ensure adequate positioning of the device. This is performed with unscrewing of the delivery cable from the device (Fig. 60.28).

This device has proven to be highly effective in closing larger PDAs, with rates exceeding 98% at 6 to 12 months after closure.[167,174] The complication profile for this device has also been low, with few serious side effects. Similar concerns regarding left PA or aortic coarctation apply, but in practice, this has not been of particular concern.[174,176,177] Patient selection is important in avoiding those complications, and this device should be avoided when the PDA is less than 1 to 1.5 mm in the narrowest diameter or the PDA is an aortopulmonary window type defect with no obvious ampulla. Under those circumstances, a modification of device delivery can be used, with positioning of the aortic cap within the PDA itself and not against the side wall of the aorta. Hemolysis occurring immediately after delivery of Amplatzer occluder devices has also been rarely described but has either been self-limiting or resolved with coil placement within the device.[175]

The ADO II is a "biconical" modification of the original device. It is manufactured from a thinner-bore nitinol mesh and is able to be delivered through smaller guide catheters. The softer nature of the device allows improved conformation on both the aortic and pulmonary ends of the ductus, making it more suitable for smaller patients.[177,178]

FDA approval of other vascular occlusion plugs (Amplatzer Vascular Plug [AVP] I, II, and IV; Abbott Laboratories) has also widened the spectrum of devices available for PDA closure.[112,140] These plugs are available in multiple different sizes and, although mostly applicable in smaller patients, are on occasion suitable for use in adult-sized patients. Ductal closure rates with these devices appear similar to that of other available means.[167,175] The Micro-Vascular Plug (Medtronic Medical, Fridley, MN) has further expanded the device repertoire and, although used mainly in the small neonate and infant age group, may also have occasional application in ductal closure in older indicicuals.[178]

Follow-Up

Anticoagulation is not required after PDA occlusion with either coils or other devices. SBE prophylaxis remains indicated for at least the first 6 months and as long as residual PDA shunting is present. Follow-up echocardiography should be performed at least 6 months after PDA closure; thereafter, if no murmur is present, further testing is no longer necessary.

TRANSCATHETER PULMONARY VALVE REPLACEMENT

Disruption, removal, and replacement of the native pulmonary valve are common to a number of palliative and reparative surgeries for treatment of CHD. Placement of an RV-PA or RVOT conduit is common in surgical palliation of some forms of TOF, transposition of the great arteries, truncus arteriosus, and aortic valve disease treated with the Ross procedure. Even more commonly, in "typical" TOF with pulmonary stenosis, surgical

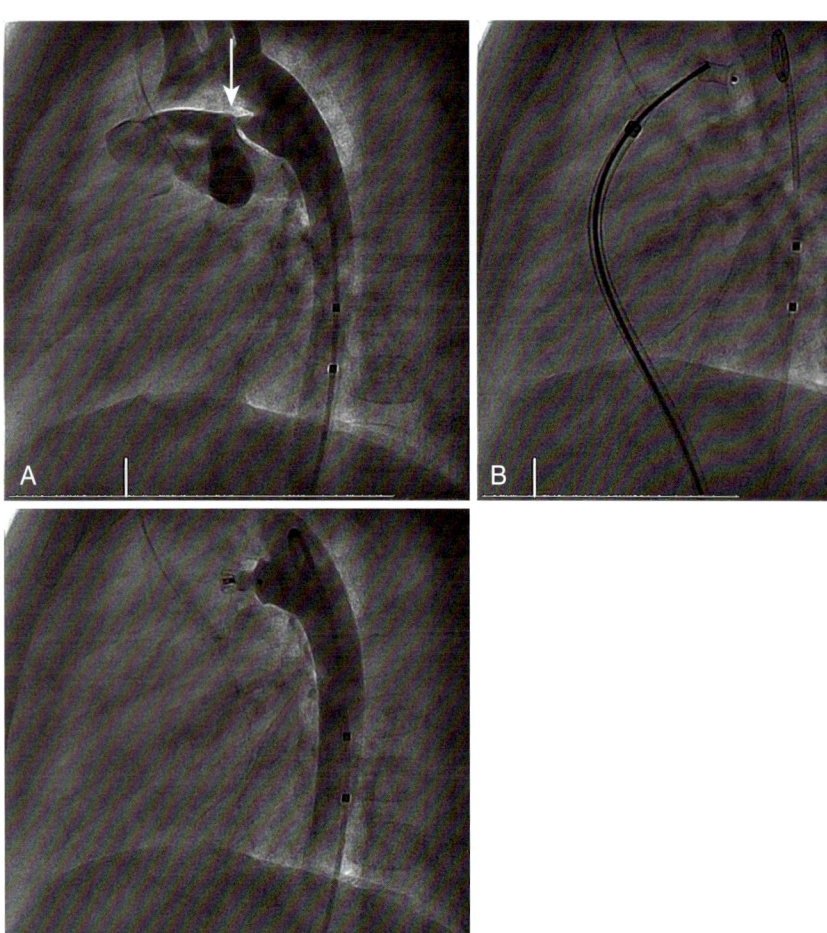

Fig. 60.28 (A) Still-frame angiogram of a moderate-size patent ductus arteriosus (PDA). The moderate PDA *(solid white arrow)* with a well-formed ductal diverticulum is noted. (B) The device has been deployed within the PDA but remains attached to the delivery cable. Retraction and redeployment are still possible at this point. (C) Still-frame angiogram demonstrating a small amount of residual flow passing through the device. This resolves within the first 24 hours after deployment as thrombosis occurs within the ductal occluder.

palliation involves enlargement of the pulmonary valve annulus with a transannular patch; this results in long-term pulmonary valve incompetence, which can be associated with late RV dilation and dysfunction. Over the past two decades, there has been increasing clinical emphasis on restoration of pulmonary valve function with pulmonary valve replacement before the development of irreversible RV dilation and dysfunction. Common long-term limitations to both the RV-PA conduit and BPV include recurrent stenosis and regurgitation. There is strong evidence that such dysfunction can be associated with exercise intolerance, arrhythmias, RV dysfunction, and an increased risk of late sudden death.[157,158] There is also evidence to show that intervention on a dysfunctional RV-PA conduit or BPV can halt or even reverse the risk of these adverse outcomes.[159–179] The long-established standard of care for clinically important RV-PA conduit or BPV stenosis or regurgitation is reoperation involving cardiopulmonary bypass and its attendant risks. Such patients face a lifetime of repeat RVOT operations.[180,181]

TPVR within an existing dysfunctional RV-PA conduit or BPV is currently an established and standard-of-care therapy. The goal of this therapy is to prolong the interval between surgical RVOT interventions (either RV-PA conduit or BPV replacement), with the intention to reduce the total number of open heart operations required over the lifetime of a patient. A second goal is to reduce the overall time during which a patient lives with some degree of clinically important RVOT dysfunction (valvular stenosis or insufficiency). TPVR was first introduced in the year 2000 by Bonhoeffer and colleagues.[182,183] This technology was subsequently acquired by Medtronic (Minneapolis, MN) and marketed as the Melody transcatheter pulmonary valve and the Ensemble

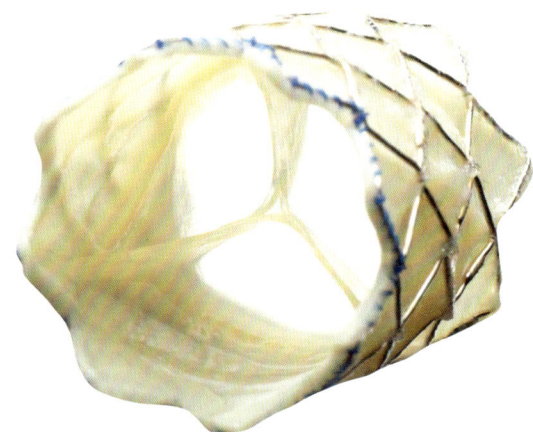

Fig. 60.29 The Medtronic Melody transcatheter pulmonary valve consists of a bovine jugular venous valve sutured onto a 28-mm balloon-expandable stent. (Courtesy Medtronic, Minneapolis, MN.)

delivery system (Figs. 60.29 and 60.30). In 2010, based on the results from the U.S. pivotal trial, Medtronic received Humanitarian Device Exemption (HDE) approval from the FDA to market the device in the United States. Based on effectiveness data from three distinct prospective clinical trials, the FDA granted premarket approval (PMA) to Melody in 2015, making Melody TPV the first device to transition from HDE to PMA pathways in the agency's history. Melody TPV is currently approved for

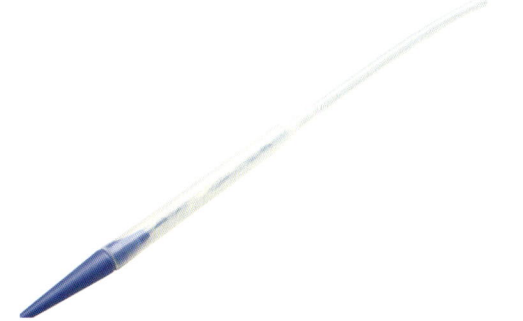

Fig. 60.30 The Medtronic Ensemble transcatheter valve delivery system is designed to percutaneously deliver the Melody valve. It consists of a 16-Fr delivery catheter with a 22-Fr distal pod that encloses the crimped Melody valve. (Courtesy Medtronic, Minneapolis, MN.)

implantation in the dysfunction RV-PA conduit or BPV. As of June 2018, more than 13,000 Melody valves have been implanted in more than 300 centers worldwide. The Edwards SAPIEN XT transcatheter heart valve (Edwards Lifesciences LLC, Irvine, CA) has FDA approval for TPVR in the dysfunctional RV-PA conduit.[184] Edwards' third-generation transcatheter heart valve, the SAPIEN 3, is currently under investigation for TPVR. Once approved, the S3 will be the preferred choice for TPVR given its design improvements over the second-generation valve, adding a skirt to reduce paravalvar leaks and offering a lower profile more flexible delivery system. However, at this point the Edwards' valves remain unsheathed (uncovered) during delivery across the right heart, which is disadvantageous when crossing the tricuspid valve and existing RVOT hardware.

Over the latter half of the past decade, there has been increasing interest in the performance of TPVR within the native (or patch-augmented) RVOT which includes approximately 80% of the overall cohort of patients with postoperative RVOT dysfunction. Although some native RVOT substrate provides an adequate "landing zone" (typically a region of true or relative stenosis) for TPVR with existing balloon-expandable technology, many patients with native RVOT dysfunction have a dilated, large, and dynamic RVOT that will not accept existing commercial valves. To address this potentially rather large CHD population, both Medtronic and Edwards have purpose-built devices in clinical trial. The Medtronic Harmony TPV system is a porcine pericardial tissue valve mounted on a novel self-expanding nitinol frame stent with polyester covering, to be deployed via a 25-Fr catheter with retractable sheath. More than one stent design will be necessary to treat the majority of this population; the first design has demonstrated favorable early results.[185] The Edwards Alterra Adaptive Present is an alternative approach to treatment of the dysfunctional native RVOT. Alterra, a novel self-expanding covered nitinol stent, will be delivered by a custom 16-Fr compatible sheathed delivery catheter, and contains a central rigid landing zone. Following placement of this adaptive present, the operator may place a standard 29-mm SAPIEN 3 valve within the Alterra landing zone, to complete a two-step TPVR process.

Physiology

RVOT obstruction is common in native and repaired CHD. Patients who undergo surgical repair that involves the placement of an RV-PA valved conduit or BPV require long-term monitoring (including echocardiography and cardiac MRI) to detect recurrent RVOT dysfunction, specifically stenosis or regurgitation, which eventually occurs in most. The physiology of conduit or BPV stenosis is similar to that of native pulmonary valve stenosis. There is an increase in RV systolic pressure directly related to the severity of the stenosis and the RV stroke volume. This elevated RV systolic pressure stimulates myocardial hypertrophy and, over time, fibrosis. Eventually, if it is not relieved, severe stenosis will result in RV systolic and diastolic dysfunction. If there is an associated atrial-level communication, the patient will become cyanotic as a right-to-left atrial shunt develops in response to the decreased RV compliance associated with progressive myocardial hypertrophy and fibrosis. Similarly, the physiology of conduit or BPV insufficiency can be compared with that of native pulmonary valve insufficiency. It results in an increased volume load on the RV that causes dilation and can eventually lead to the development of systolic and diastolic dysfunction. If left untreated, RV-PA conduit stenosis and insufficiency can each also lead to LV dysfunction secondary to septal shift and adverse ventricular/ventricular interactions.[186]

Clinical Presentation and Diagnosis

Patients with postoperative RVOT stenosis or insufficiency may be detected early by the presence of a systolic or diastolic murmur, respectively, often without symptoms. As conduit dysfunction progresses in severity or duration, patients may report exercise intolerance and shortness of breath with modest aerobic exercise.[157] Eventually, with progressive RVOT dysfunction, patients may develop right-sided heart failure. RV dysfunction is known to increase the risk of late arrhythmia and sudden death.[158] Echocardiography and cardiac MRI (or computed tomography [CT] angiography in the setting of a contraindication to MRI) are the noninvasive diagnostic studies of choice for assessment of RVOT anatomy. For RVOT stenosis, Doppler peak systolic gradients lower than 30 mm Hg are considered mild and those between 30 and 50 mm Hg are moderate (in the face of normal RV systolic function). For RVOT insufficiency, cardiac MRI is the imaging modality of choice to quantify RV systolic and diastolic volumes and biventricular systolic function.

Studies with cardiac MRI show that RV size and function can predict which patients may benefit from intervention for a dysfunctional RVOT.[187,188] Intervention is probably indicated for an RVOT with stenosis and/or regurgitation if the RV ejection fraction is diminished or if RV diastolic volume exceeds 160 to 180 mL/m^2. Geva and colleagues showed that all patients who had an RV end-systolic volume greater than 95 mL/m^2 had evidence of RV dysfunction by MRI.[186] Studies of patients with repaired TOF have found that elevation of B-type natriuretic peptide correlates with RV size, ejection fraction, diastolic function, and exercise capacity.[189]

Once the decision has been made that a dysfunctional postoperative RVOT warrants intervention, the feasibility of TPVR must be evaluated. Although TPVR had previously been recommended only for RV-PA conduits that were 16 mm or larger in diameter at surgical implantation, this is no longer an absolute indication. Smaller conduits may be dilated to larger diameter, recognizing that risk of wall disruption exists.[190] Likewise, TPVR is currently being performed in younger and smaller patients in lieu of surgical conduit revision.[191] Valved homograft or heterograft conduits are equally suitable for TPVR. Precatheterization evaluation typically includes cardiac MRI to evaluate the anatomic dimensions of the surgical RVOT,[192,193] the anatomy of the more distal PA, and the size and function of the RV. Cardiac MRI also can provide valuable information regarding the proximity of the RVOT to the coronary arteries. This is critical information because RVOT rehabilitation before or during valve implantation can occasionally cause coronary artery compression, occasionally with fatal results.[194,195]

Patients with significant RVOT stenosis (uncommon) or insufficiency (common) after repair of TOF using a transannular patch who have not undergone surgical PVR are increasingly candidates for TPVR. Some centers have recently demonstrated occasional success with TPVR in this population using the

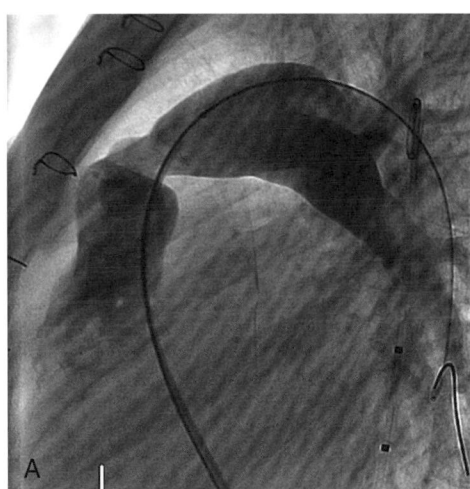 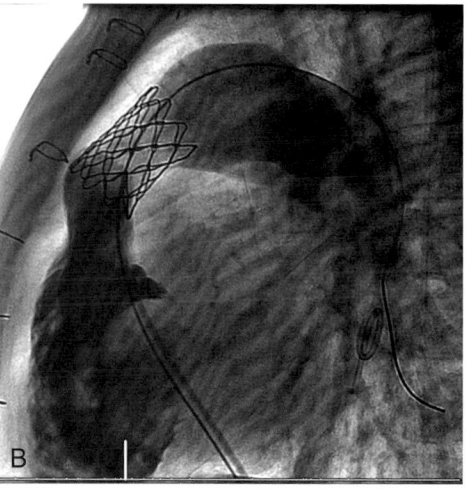

Fig. 60.31 Lateral angiograms in a 10-year-old boy 8 years after a Ross procedure following aortic valve endocarditis. (A) Before Melody valve implantation, there is significant stenosis and regurgitation of the right ventricle–to–pulmonary artery (RV-PA) homograft. (B) After Melody valve implantation, there is relief of the stenosis, and Doppler echocardiography documents only trace valve regurgitation.

Melody TPV, although this approach is limited by the relatively small maximal size of that device.[196] More frequently, operators are using the 29-mm SAPIEN XT or SAPIEN 3 valve (the latter of which is off-label as this is currently approved only for TAVR) for TPVR in the native RVOT cohort. However, even with availability of the 29-mm SAPIEN valves, the native RVOT frequently exceeds the maximal diameter of this currently available balloon-expandable technology. The self-expanding Medtronic Harmony TPV system and Edwards Alterra Adaptive Present are each under clinical trial at present and are expected to significantly shift the landscape, which is currently weighted heavily towards surgical PVR, in the treatment of large-diameter native RVOT insufficiency.

Treatment and Outcomes

In the United States, there are two FDA-cleared option for TPVR: the Medtronic Melody TPV and the Edwards SAPIEN XT transcatheter heart valve. The Melody TPV is a trileaflet bovine jugular venous valve that has been treated and preserved with glutaraldehyde and sutured into a 34-mm-long platinum-iridium stent (see Fig. 60.29). The stent is covered throughout its length by venous tissue. The valve is supplied in two versions: a 20-mm valve, which is indicated for dilation from 18 to 20 mm, and a 22-mm valve for dilation from 18 to 22 mm. With Melody, the diameters refer to the balloon diameter, which is the final valve *inner* diameter. Experience has suggested that these valves also function well at smaller implant diameters and to be expandable up to 24 mm, but these implant diameters are not listed on the FDA-cleared instructions for use.[197] Melody TPV implantation is performed with the 22-Fr sheathed Ensemble delivery system on an 18-, a 20-, or a 22-mm outer balloon catheter with a balloon-in-balloon design to facilitate a more controlled deployment (see Fig. 60.29). The SAPIEN XT is a trileaflet bovine pericardial tissue valve that has been treated by the "ThermaFix" process and sutured within a cobalt-chromium frame. The valve is available in 23-, 26-, and 29-mm versions (Outer Diameter) and are delivered via the NovaFlex+ deflectable delivery system. With SAPIEN, the diameters refer to the final valve *outer* diameter.

Technique

TPVR is most commonly performed from a femoral venous approach, but the internal jugular venous approach has also been used successfully, as have other central venous and hybrid perventricular strategies, when indicated. After baseline hemodynamic measurements are obtained, RV angiography is performed to assess RV function, the anatomy of the RVOT, and the branch PAs; all are important for determining the valve implantation site and the need for concomitant procedures (e.g., branch PA rehabilitation).

Although there are a number of approaches to the procedure, existing RVOT stenosis is typically treated with a combination of serial ultra-high-pressure angioplasty and large-diameter bare-metal stent implantation. Covered large-diameter stent implantation may also be used, following approval of the covered CP stent for aortic and, more recently, RVOT use.[198] It is important to establish that there will be no coronary artery compression with RVOT rehabilitation before the implantation of any stent. Therefore, during balloon angioplasty of the RVOT, the spatial relationship of the RVOT and coronary arteries is assessed with aortography or selective coronary angiography.[198] Once the possibility of coronary compression is ruled out, the RVOT is rehabilitated to the desired TPVR implant diameter, with placement of large-diameter bare-metal or covered stents (frequently several telescoped within one another for added radial strength). Early data suggested that inadequate conduit preparation (prestenting) resulted in an increased incidence of TPVR stent fracture and valve dysfunction, prompting a shift in approach to more comprehensive RVOT preparation.[199,200,202] An existing BPV, in contrast to an RV-PA conduit, only occasionally requires placement of a preparatory bare-metal stent because the BPV itself typically prevents compressive forces from interacting with the TPV when it is placed in a "valve-in-valve" fashion.[203]

After RVOT preparation, and with an ultrastiff exchange wire positioned in a distal PA, the TPV is serially rinsed in normal saline baths to adequately dilute the gluteraldehyde solution. The TPV is then either hand- or device-crimped onto the delivery system. In the case of Melody, the valve is then loaded into a self-sheathing mechanism. In the case of SAPIEN the valve is crimped onto the catheter shaft and then loaded onto the balloon after introduction into the inferior vena cava. In either case, it is of vital importance to be certain that the TPV is oriented properly on the delivery balloon (implanting the valve "upside down" will cause complete RVOT obstruction that could be fatal). A formal intraprocedural "time out" at this step is recommended to ensure and document that the TPV is properly oriented on the delivery system before implantation. The delivery system is advanced over the ultrastiff guidewire into the target implant site within the RVOT. Once it is in the desired position and the delivery system has been modified to the valve deployment configuration, the TPV is implanted with inflation of the implantation balloon(s). The balloon is then deflated and the delivery system is withdrawn over the guidewire. Repeat hemodynamic measurements and angiography are performed to document the immediate outcome (Figs. 60.31 and 60.32). If significant residual stenosis is present

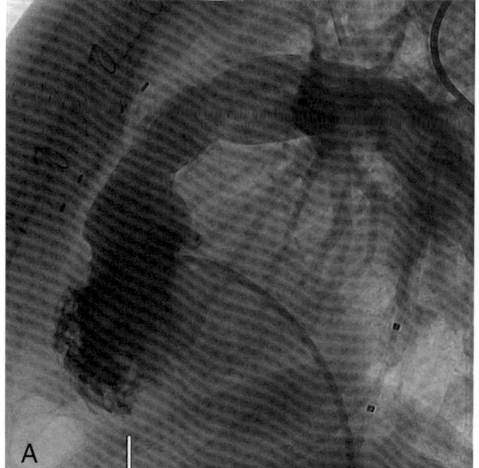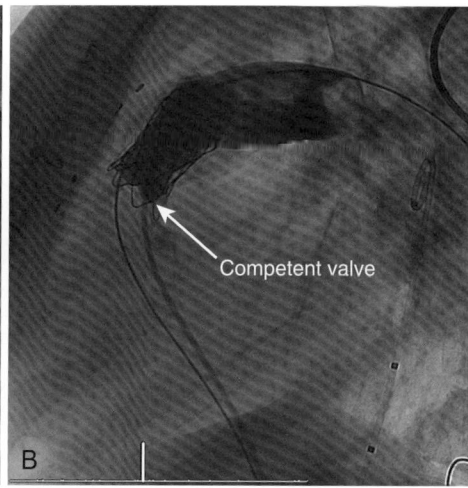

Fig. 60.32 Lateral angiograms in a 14-year-old girl who had undergone a Rastelli procedure for complex transposition. Two years earlier, she had undergone bare-metal stenting of the right ventricle–to–pulmonary artery (RV-PA) homograft for stenosis but was left with free regurgitation (A). After Melody valve implantation (B), there is no residual conduit stenosis or regurgitation (white arrow).

or a paravalvular leak is noticed, a high-pressure balloon can be used to postdilate the TPV within the RVOT. Adequate RVOT preparation before TPVR typically obviates this need. It is recommended that the patient be anticoagulated, most commonly with heparin, throughout the procedure. Variations on the technique described here, particularly prestenting of a stenotic conduit before Melody valve implantation, have become widespread. Evidence suggests that prestenting of the RV-PA conduit with at least one bare-metal stent (in some cases, multiple stents) before TPVR may improve the hemodynamic outcome and decrease the incidence of late Melody stent fracture.[199,200,202]

Although a number of the techniques previously detailed apply to the nonstenotic, native (patch-augmented) RVOT with pulmonary insufficiency, some approaches differ. In this case, relief of preexisting RVOT obstruction is not necessary. Instead, ensuring an adequate landing zone is critical. Following baseline hemodynamic and angiographic assessment, interrogation of the potential stent (TPV) landing zone is performed. Usually with the assistance of rapid RV pacing to promote balloon stability, a compliant large-diameter balloon (such as the Amplatzer sizing balloon II, Abbott, St. Paul, MN) is inflated within the RVOT, to evaluate for a persistent balloon waist, suggestive of a noncompliant tissue ridge. Coronary arteries may also be assessed with this balloon inflated in the RVOT. If an adequate landing zone is present for the TPV available to the operators, proceeding with TPVR may then occur, with or without the use of a large diameter balloon expandable stent first implanted. Use of a prestent in this case serves to "test" the adequacy of the landing zone, especially beneficial in borderline cases, as well as to prevent reinforce the TPV. It is recognized that this procedural approach will shift dramatically following approval of a self-expanding native RVOT TPV.

As experience with this procedure continues to grow, new techniques and changes in the device will undoubtedly occur to continue to make TPVR safer, more successful, and applicable to a larger range of RVOTs and patients.

Results

After an initial report on the first 34 patients, McElhinney and colleagues reported the short- and medium-term follow-up results from the expanded U.S. Melody valve trial in 136 patients over a period of almost 30 months.[204,205] This study evaluated the safety, procedural success, and short- and medium-term effectiveness of the Melody valve in patients with dysfunctional RV-PA conduits or BPVs. TPVR was attempted in 124 (91%) of 136 patients; of the remaining 12 patients, TPVR was not attempted in 6 because there was evidence of coronary artery compression during provocative testing. Melody valve implantation was successful in 123 of the 124 attempts (conduit rupture occurred in one patient, necessitating emergent surgical conduit replacement). Among the cohort with a primary TPVR indication of pulmonary stenosis or mixed pulmonary stenosis and pulmonary regurgitation, the median peak RV-PA pressure gradient was acutely reduced from 43.5 to 14 mm Hg. Pulmonary regurgitation was graded as none or trivial in all patients immediately after TPVR. The RV end-diastolic volume, as measured by cardiac MRI, demonstrated substantial reduction at the 6-month follow-up, whereas the RV ejection fraction was not changed. Although medium-term follow-up was limited, no patient had evidence of moderate or severe pulmonary regurgitation at 1 or 2 years of follow-up. Most patients remained in NYHA class I at 2 years. Improvements in cardiopulmonary exercise capacity were modest.[205] Freedom from recurrent RVOT intervention was 95.4% at 1 year and 87.6% at 2 years, which closely matched freedom from valve dysfunction (93.5% and 85.6% at 1 and 2 years, respectively). Ten of the 11 patients requiring RVOT reintervention received transcatheter therapy (90% received a second Melody implant, all in the presence of stent fracture with associated RVOT obstruction).

Since that time, investigators have reported the experience with Melody TPV implantation in 120 patients enrolled in the multicenter U.S. postapproval study.[206] In that study, TPV was implanted in 100 patients, with a 98.0% procedural success rate. Acceptable hemodynamic function was found in 96.7% of patients with evaluable data at 6 months. At 1-year follow-up, there were two patients who required surgical conduit replacement, no patients who required catheter-based reintervention, and no pulmonary insufficiency worse than mild.

Importantly, long-term results of a prospectively enrolled cohort have been reported.[207] Five-year freedom from TPV reintervention and explantation was 76 ± 4% and 92 ± 3%, respectively. In the patients who were alive and reintervention free, the median follow-up gradient was unchanged from early post-TPV replacement, and all but one patient had mild or less pulmonary regurgitation. Ten-year outcome data are anticipated in the near future.

Subsequent reports have demonstrated Melody TPV efficacy in patients with bovine jugular vein conduits,[208] in surgical BPV,[209] following the Ross procedure,[210] and in the rarer LV-to-PA conduit following palliation of corrected transposition of the great arteries,[211] among other subpopulations.

Limited published data exist describing experience with the Edwards Sapien XT valve.

Complications

TPVR has proven to be safe, with a procedural mortality of less than 0.2%.[212] Acute complications typically relate to RV-PA conduit injury (ranging from mild tear with associated pseudoaneurysm formation to frank conduit rupture with life-threatening hemorrhage), distal guidewire PA injury, or, more commonly, catheterization-related adverse events such as vascular injury or arrhythmia.[204] The Pulmonary Artery Repair with Covered Stents (PARCS) trial to evaluate the use of covered stents in the RVOT for treatment of clinically relevant conduit injury has been completed, with results anticipated to be published in the near future.[213] Coronary artery compression is identifiable during provocative testing and is therefore avoidable, but stent- and valve-related coronary artery compression has been described, occasionally with catastrophic results. Coronary compression can be anticipated in approximately 5% to 6% of TPVR candidates and is more common in patients with abnormal coronary artery anatomy.[195]

Given the limited published data following SAPIEN TPVR, the following discussion focuses exclusively on the Melody TPV. The most common complication in follow-up of Melody TPVR has been Melody stent fracture. In the expanded U.S. experience of 150 patients, freedom from Melody stent fracture was 77% at 14 months and 60% at 39 months, although this study included an early cohort where prestent implantation could not be performed.[199] Among all patients enrolled in North American and European prospective Melody TPV trials, at 3-year follow-up, freedom from any stent fracture and major stent fracture was 74 ± 3% and 85 ± 2%, respectively, and freedom from RVOT reintervention was 85 ± 2%. Placement of a prestent at the TPV implantation procedure was associated with longer freedom from stent fracture and RVOT reintervention than was no prestent.[214] These data have strongly shifted clinical practice toward the placement of RVOT stents before Melody valve implantation.

Endocarditis following TPVR is uncommon but not rare and may occur regardless of TPV type implanted. A number of studies have contributed to our understanding of an annualized rate of TPV-related infective endocarditis (IE) of approximately 2% to 3%, reflecting the relatively unprotected position of the TPV in the right heart.[207,214,215] Clinical outcomes in the setting of TPV-related IE reflect the lag time to diagnosis and the pathogenic organism, with *Staphylococcus aureus* being the worst player.

CONCLUSION

Similar to advances in transcatheter aortic valve replacement, the availability of TPVR is a remarkable advance for many CHD patients. This technology provides a transcatheter intervention for the dysfunctional RVOT that has the ability to ameliorate both stenosis and regurgitation. Studies have shown that TPVR improves RV hemodynamics and extends the lifespan of the existing RVOT. Currently, a decade in, outcomes data demonstrate excellent effectiveness and low complication rates, with sustained relief of pulmonary stenosis and pulmonary insufficiency. The ongoing hazard of IE remains a considerable risk for patients who will have a biologic prosthesis in place in the RVOT for more than half a century, in many cases. Importantly, we are on the cusp of commercial availability of two distinct purpose-built devices for TPVR in the native (patch-augmented) RVOT, which will substantially increase the population of patients eligible for this innovative and minimally invasive therapy.

KEY REFERENCES

10. Rocchini AP, Beekman RH. Balloon angioplasty in the treatment of pulmonary valve stenosis and coarctation of the aorta. *Tex Heart Inst J*. 1986;13:377–385.
11. Feltes TF, Bacha E, Beekman RH, et al. Indications for cardiac catheterization and intervention in pediatric cardiac disease: a scientific statement from the American Heart Association. *Circulation*. 2011;123:2607–2652.
37. McCrindle BW, Kan JS. Long-term results after balloon pulmonary valvuloplasty. *Circulation*. 1991;83:1915–1922.
52. McElhinney DB, Lock JE, Keane JF, et al. Left heart growth, function, and reintervention after balloon aortic valvuloplasty for neonatal aortic stenosis. *Circulation*. 2005;111:451–458.
53. Rocchini AP, Beekman RH, Ben Shachar G, et al. Balloon aortic valvuloplasty: results of the valvuloplasty and angioplasty of congenital anomalies registry. *Am J Cardiol*. 1990;65:784–789.
64. Maskatia SA, Ing FF, Justino H, et al. Twenty-five year experience with balloon aortic valvuloplasty for congenital aortic stenosis. *Am J Cardiol*. 2011;108:1024–1028.
66. NHLBI Balloon Valvuloplasty Registry Participants. Percutaneous balloon aortic valvuloplasty: acute and 30-day follow-up results in 674 patients from NHLBI Balloon Valvuloplasty Registry. *Circulation*. 1991;84:2383–2397.
87. Kan JS, Marvin WJ, Bass JL, et al. Balloon angioplasty for branch pulmonary artery stenosis: results from the valvuloplasty and angioplasty of congenital anomalies registry. *Am J Cardiol*. 1990;65:798–801.
89. Mullins CE, O'Laughlin MP, Vick GW, et al. Implantation of balloon-expandable intravascular grafts by catheterization in pulmonary arteries and systemic veins. *Circulation*. 1988;77(1):188–199.
93. Holzer RJ, Gauvreau K, Kreutzer J, et al. Balloon angioplasty and stenting of branch pulmonary arteries: adverse events and procedural characteristics. Results of a multi-institutional registry. *Circ Cardiovasc Interv*. 2011;4(3):287–296.
109. Marshall AC, Perry SB, Keane JF, et al. Early results and medium-term follow-up of stent implantation for residual aortic coarctation. *Am Heart J*. 2000;139:1054–1060.
113. Tzifa A, Ewert T, Brzezinska-Rajszys G, et al. Covered Cheatham-platinum stents for aortic coarctation. *J Am Coll Cardiol*. 2006;47:1457–1463.
119. Forbes TJ, Moore P, Pedra CAC, et al. Intermediate follow-up following intravascular stenting for treatment of coarctation of the aorta. *Catheter Cardiovasc Interv*. 2007;70:569–577.
138. Cowley CG, Lloyd TR, Bove EL, et al. Comparison of results of closure of secundum atrial septal defect by surgery versus Amplatzer septal occluder. *Am J Cardiol*. 2001;88:589–591.
145. Berger F, Vogel M, Alexi-Meskishvili V, et al. comparison of results and complications of surgical and Amplatzer device closure of atrial septal defects. *J Thorac Cardiovasc Surg*. 1999;118(4):674–680.
148. Amin Z, Hijazi ZM, Bass JL, et al. Erosion of Amplatzer septal occluder device after closure of secundum atrial septal defects: review of registry of complications and recommendations to minimize future risk. *Catheter Cardiovasc Interv*. 2004;63:496–502.
160. Bove EL, Kavey RE, Byrum CJ, et al. Improved right ventricular function following late pulmonary valve replacement for residual pulmonary insufficiency or stenosis. *J Thorac Cardiovasc Surg*. 1985;90(1):50–55.
177. Pass RH, Hijazi Z, Hsu DT, et al. Multicenter USA Amplatzer patent ductus arteriosus occlusion device trial: initial and one-year results. *J Am Coll Cardiol*. 2004;44(3):513–519.
183. Bonhoeffer P, Boudjemline Y, Saliba Z, et al. Percutaneous replacement of pulmonary valve in a right-ventricle to pulmonary-artery prosthetic conduit with valve dysfunction. *Lancet*. 2000;356(9239):1403–1405.
196. Morray BH, McElhinney DB, Cheatham JP, et al. Risk of coronary artery compression among patients referred for transcatheter pulmonary valve implantation: a multicenter experience. *Circ Cardiovasc Interv*. 2013;6(5):535–542.
205. McElhinney DB, Hellenbrand WE, Zahn EM, et al. Short- and medium-term outcomes after transcatheter pulmonary valve placement in the expanded multicenter US Melody valve trial. *Circulation*. 2010;122:507–516.
208. Cheatham JP, Hellenbrand WE, Zahn EM, et al. Clinical and hemodynamic outcomes up to 7 years after transcatheter pulmonary valve replacement in the US melody valve investigational de-vice exemption trial. *Circulation*. 2015;131(22):1960–1970.

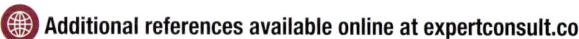 Additional references available online at expertconsult.com.

中文导读

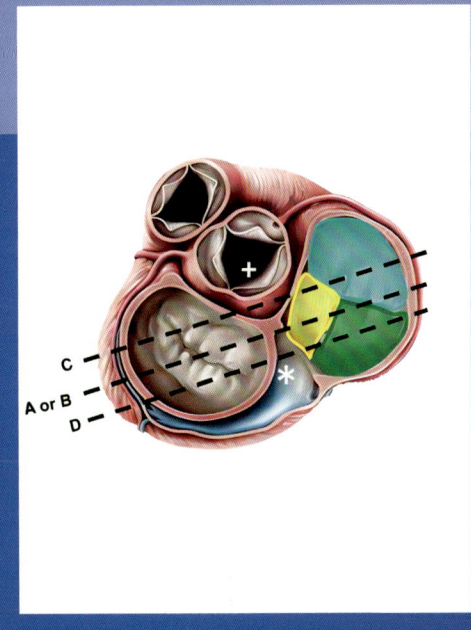

第61章
缺血性心脏病的干细胞治疗

急性心肌梗死导致的缺血性心肌病带来大量慢性心力衰竭患者，调节心肌梗死边缘区心肌是减轻心力衰竭症状和改善患者预后的重要靶点之一。干细胞移植治疗可改善血流灌注和心功能、减少左心室扩张、降低心绞痛发作频率，以及改善心力衰竭再梗死住院率和存活率等。干细胞治疗策略包括：分化细胞移植、干细胞动员和干细胞移植。其中干细胞移植是目前研究最全面的且有临床获益的治疗策略，涉及从自体或筛选良好的异体骨髓中取出干细胞，然后将其注入心肌梗死区。关于这些策略将如何向前推动并在预防（梗死期患者的治疗）或治疗（心力衰竭患者的治疗）心功能不全方面带来临床效益，仍存在一系列挑战。

胚胎干细胞和诱导多能干细胞能生成心肌细胞，未来自体心肌细胞再生可能会实现。提高干细胞治疗整体效益的策略包括干细胞类趋化因子、细胞因子策略，以及细胞片技术和可注射水凝胶等。干细胞可用于治疗慢性胸痛，但提高干细胞移植后存活率仍是一个关键研究问题。

本章总结了当前干细胞治疗的现状，正在进行的干细胞治疗研究及其发现的临床和科研意义，并讨论该领域未来可能的发展方向。

谢慕蓉　吴永健

章节要点

- 再灌注治疗的发展引起大量患者进展为慢性心力衰竭。调节心脏组织是减轻心力衰竭症状和改善患者预后的下一个重要前沿干预措施。
- 总体而言,该领域尚缺乏大规模研究提供强有力的循证证据,但多个子课题进行小规模研究的时代已经过去了。
- 细胞治疗可以改善心功能,但并不一定能降低电传导或引发心律失常的风险。
- 多种给药治疗策略和设备已进入临床研究领域。
- 从胚胎干细胞和诱导多能干细胞中生成心肌细胞表明,自体心肌细胞再生在未来可能实现。
- 最近的临床数据表明,自体细胞治疗心力衰竭可能比异体细胞治疗更有效。
- 学者们对通过调节干细胞来提高干细胞治疗整体效益的策略越来越感兴趣。
- 学者们对于再生疗法相关的分子机制有了更深入的了解,从而产生了新的治疗策略。
- 越来越多的临床证据表明,干细胞可用于治疗慢性胸痛。

61 Stem Cell Therapy for Ischemic Heart Disease

Vishal Dahya, Kevin H. Silver, Marc S. Penn

KEY POINTS

- Advances in reperfusion therapy have led to the development of a large population of patients with chronic heart failure. Modulation of cardiac tissue is the next great frontier to lessen symptoms of heart failure and improve patient outcomes.
- In general, the field has failed to demonstrate robust results in large scale studies. The time for small studies with multiple subgroups is past.
- Improvements in cardiac function with cell therapy do not necessarily imply improvements in electrical conduction or arrhythmogenic risk.
- Multiple delivery strategies and devices have entered the clinical realm.
- The generation of cardiac myocytes from embryonic stem cells and induced pluripotent stem cells suggests autologous cardiac myocyte regeneration may be possible in the future.
- Recent clinical data suggest that autologous cell therapy may be more efficacious than allogeneic cell therapy for heart failure.
- There is growing interest in strategies to modulate stem cells to enhance the overall benefits of stem cell therapies.
- There is greater understanding of the molecular mechanisms associated with regenerative therapies leading to novel treatment strategies.
- There is growing clinical evidence concerning the use of stem cells to treat chronic chest pain.

INTRODUCTION

The many efforts to maximize therapy for patients with acute myocardial infarction (AMI) have yielded significant benefits. Beginning first with thrombolytic therapy for AMI, and more recently with the wide availability of primary percutaneous coronary intervention (PCI) for ST-elevation myocardial infarction (STEMI), the mortality rates of this devastating ischemic event has decreased from almost 15% in clinical trials in the late 1980s[1] to less than 5% in recent primary PCI trials.[2] Prior to these advances, ischemic heart disease was the leading cause of chronic heart failure (CHF). Although further improvements in reperfusion are needed, the current advances have led to the growing epidemic of CHF, with many patients surviving what in the past might have been fatal events.

With these advances, the prevalence of congestive heart failure has increased dramatically over the preceding decade, with currently more than 10% of the United States population older than 65 years of age carrying the diagnosis. Although the mechanisms are still under investigation,[3,4] the development of CHF following myocardial infarction is more than just the loss of contractile tissue; it is also partly determined by the ventricular remodeling that occurs in response to myocardial necrosis.[5] The inflammatory response to myocardial necrosis leads to infarct expansion, dilatation of the left ventricle (LV) cavity, and replacement of cardiomyocytes with fibrous tissue.[3,5] Furthermore, the remodeling process results in an infarct border zone that is ischemic and may drive inflammation and further adverse remodeling.[6] Treatment of this border zone is at least one target of cardiovascular regenerative therapies because increasing the contractile reserve of the border zone is correlated with improved ventricular remodeling.[6,7] Currently available therapies to alter the remodeling process and the progression to CHF remain limited, and death rates from CHF continue to rise. Based on current trends, the problem is predicted to increase to greater than 6 million people by the year 2030.

The increasing burden of CHF has been addressed with pharmacologic therapy, which in some can delay and improve the morbidity and mortality of CHF; electrical therapy including cardiac resynchronization therapy; left ventricular remodeling surgery; and mechanical therapy, with the recent approval of the first left ventricular assist device for destination therapy. In terms of pharmacologic therapy, the noteworthy PARADIGM-HF trial (a multicenter, randomized study to evaluate the efficacy and safety of LCZ696 compared to Enalapril on morbidity and mortality in patients with CHF and reduced ejection fraction) demonstrated a long-sought benefit for the combination of angiotensin-neprilysin inhibition with sacubitril-valsartan. This combination of high-dose valsartan with neprilysin inhibition was found to be superior than enalapril in reducing the risk of death and heart failure hospitalizations.[8] Whether these greater benefits will be seen in clinical benefit or will be seen with additional pharmacologic strategies is of great debate.

To address the increasing prevalence of CHF, over the past 15 years cardiovascular medicine has taken great interest in the potential of regenerative therapies; more specifically, in stem cell therapies to prevent and treat cardiac dysfunction, since this approach, unlike all others, has the opportunity to address the underlying problem—loss of cardiac myocytes due to ischemic death. Although there was much excitement and fanfare in the beginning, the field has found the need to address many challenges. That said, there is progress and hope to improve patient outcomes in the future.

APPROACHES TO CELL THERAPY

The field of cell transplantation for the treatment of left ventricular dysfunction following ischemic injury continues to make significant progress, currently with dozens of studies completed and meta-analyses that continue to suggest overall benefit to those patients treated compared with controls.[9–12] The goal has not changed—define a cell type that possesses the capacity to incorporate into the recipient myocardium and that will be able to survive, mature, and electromechanically couple to each other and to native cardiac myocytes.

The field began with differentiated cell transplantation (Fig. 61.1A); the goal was to functionally achieve myoplasty through the transplantation of autologous skeletal myoblasts that would engraft into injured myocardium in patients with chronic ischemic heart failure.[13] Another strategy that has been implemented

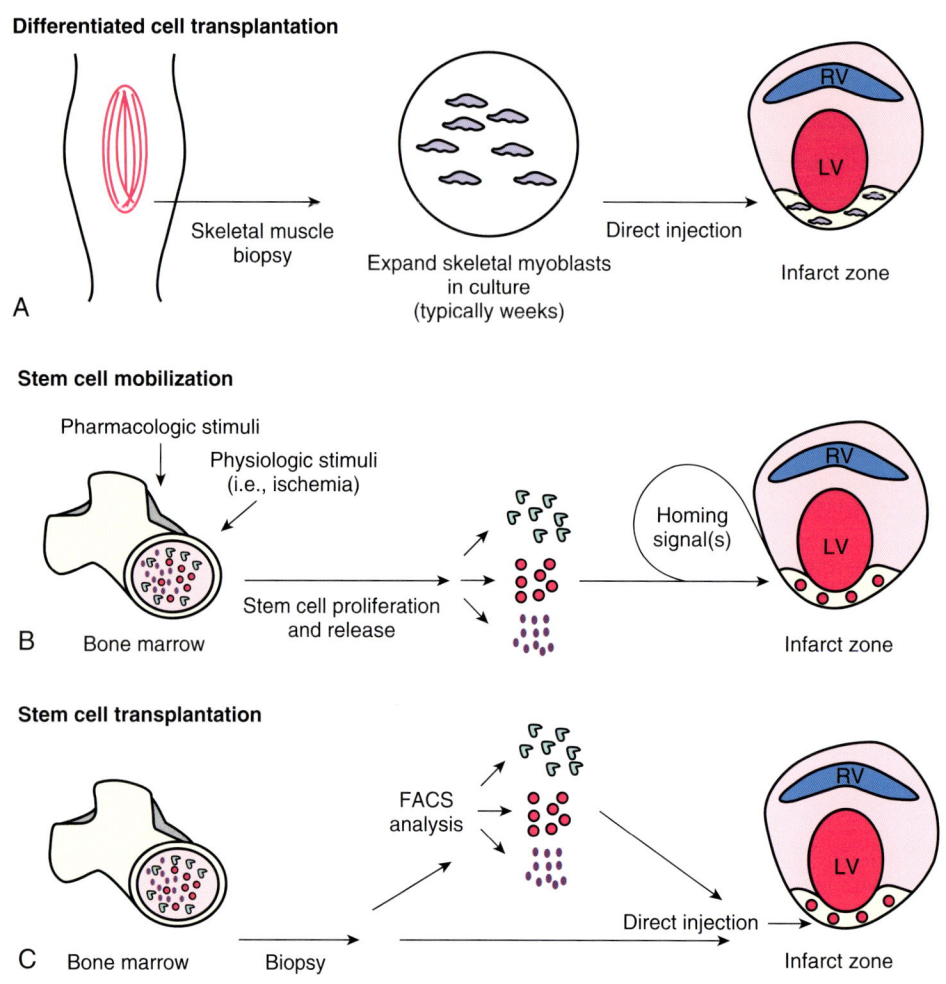

Fig. 61.1 Schematic diagram of (A) differentiated cell transplantation, (B) stem cell mobilization, and (C) stem cell transplantation strategies of cell therapy for the treatment of cardiac dysfunction. *FACS,* Fluorescence-activated cell sorting; *LV,* left ventricle; *RV,* right ventricle.

in clinical studies is stem cell mobilization (see Fig. 61.1B), which involves the pharmacologic mobilization of a patient's own bone marrow cells into the blood stream, homing of these stem cells to engraft into areas of myocardial damage, and then directing the engrafted stem cells to differentiate into cardiac myocytes and vascular structures that fully integrate with the native myocardium. By far the most comprehensively studied strategy to date that has shown some benefits is stem cell transplantation (see Fig. 61.1C) that involves the removal of stem cells from the bone marrow of the patient (autologous) or a well-screened donor (allogeneic) and then injection of the whole bone marrow or a selected population of bone marrow-derived stem cells into the infarct zone. Questions abound as to how these strategies will move forward and lead to clinical benefit in preventing (treatment in patients in the periinfarct period) or treating (treatment in patients with CHF) cardiac dysfunction. In this chapter we attempt to summarize the current state of knowledge, inform the reader of studies that are ongoing and what their findings may mean, and discuss where the field may be moving.

Differentiated Cell Transplantation

The goal of differentiated cell transplantation is the substitution of scarred myocardium with living viable cells ultimately leading to overall improvement of myocardial function. A number of cell types, including smooth muscle cells and skeletal myoblasts, have been studied as potential candidates for differentiated cell transplantation. The value of these cell types is born out of their accessibility and their ability to be expanded in vitro prior to transplantation.

Arguably the first strategy of cell therapy for CHF was cardiac myoplasty (cardiomyoplasty). During this procedure the heart was wrapped in skeletal muscle that was then paced to increase contractility of the weakened heart.[14–16] It was recognized that there was engraftment of skeletal muscle in the epicardial layers of the heart[17,18] which we currently recognize was the ingrowth and engraftment of skeletal myoblasts.[19]

Following these observations, the early preclinical and clinical studies with skeletal myoblasts set the stage for the potential benefits associated with the delivery and engraftment of exogenous cells into the heart to prevent and treat cardiac dysfunction. We learned that exogenous cells could engraft into the heart and that the engraftment of skeletal myoblasts could lead to clinical benefit, including inducing reverse remodeling of the left ventricular remodeling.[20–22] We further learned the importance of mechanical coupling of exogenous cells to the cellular milieu of the heart.[23] Skeletal myoblasts do not integrate into the electrical syncytium of the myocardium and have been shown in animal studies to induce slow conduction,[24] increase risk of reentrant rhythm,[25] and increase premature ventricular contractions and ventricular tachycardia in patients.[13]

Significant knowledge was gained through studies of skeletal myoblasts (SKMB); however, because of limitations due to arrhythmogenic potential and lack of vascular growth, SKMB for prevention and treatment has been appropriately largely abandoned.

Myocardial Regeneration

Since the turn of the century, a significant body of literature has rewritten the once strong-held belief that the heart cannot repair itself. We have learned that following myocardial infarction in humans, there is a transient mobilization of stem cells and expression of stem cell homing factors that recruit these cells to the heart.[26,27] Human female hearts transplanted into males were found to have cardiac myocytes and vascular structures that stained positive for the Y chromosome, suggesting that these cells originated from the stem cells of the transplant recipient.[28] Unfortunately, these studies demonstrate that stem cell engraftment and differentiation into cardiac myocytes is an infrequent event (0.02% cardiac myocytes, 3.3% endothelial cells). However, these studies do suggest that the normal physiologic response to myocardial injury is mobilization of stem cells, "homing" of these cells to the damaged myocardium, and differentiation of at least some of these stem cells into cardiac myocytes. Furthermore, if this natural repair mechanism can be potentiated, clinically meaningful myocardial regeneration may be achievable.

The excitement surrounding the use of stem cells is based on the unique biologic properties of these cells and their capacity to self-renew and regenerate tissue and organ systems. Fig. 61.2 groups different stem cell populations of interest in myocardial regeneration based on their cardiogenic potential. While once it was believed that all stem cell populations listed in Fig. 61.2 could differentiate into cardiac myocytes,[29,30] it is currently quite clear that, although many of these cell populations may lead to improved cardiac function,[29,31] virtually no adult stem cell can differentiate into cardiac myocytes. Arguably the one unmanipulated adult cell population that may hold the ability to differentiate into adult cardiac myocytes is cardiac stem cells (CSCs).[32,33] All cells that have pluripotent to totipotent potential, such as embryonic stem cells (ESCs) and induced pluripotent stem cells (iPS), have been shown to generate adult cardiac myocytes.[34–36]

Bone Marrow-Derived Mononuclear Cells

The transplantation of adult stem cells to the infarct-related vessel or via endocardial injection has progressed to the point where data from randomized controlled trials are now becoming available for patients with AMI (Table 61.1) and CHF (Table 61.2). The first randomized stem cell trial for patients with AMI was the Bone Marrow Transfer to Enhance ST-Elevation Infarct Regeneration-1 (BOOST) trial.[32] These trials for AMI can be summarized as follows:

- Patient populations of interest have mostly focused on patients with first STEMI and presumed normal LV function at baseline
- All patients underwent primary PCI with restoration of antegrade flow
- Bone marrow harvest was done on the day of stem cell infusion
- Varied cell preparation approaches have been used with cell dosing based on CD34+ cell number
- Cells were infused down the infarct-related vessel either by direct infusion or using stop-flow technique
- Baseline and follow-up measurements of LV function consisted of LV gram, cardiac magnetic resonance imaging (MRI), or echocardiography

As seen in Table 61.1, this strategy does not always result in a significant increase in cardiac function; however, the majority of trials have demonstrated a significant increase in cardiac function ranging from 2% to 6%. Importantly in some trials the early benefits seen with cell therapy were lost with subsequent follow-up, suggesting that infusion of bone marrow mononuclear cells accelerates healing of the heart but may not further improve.[37]

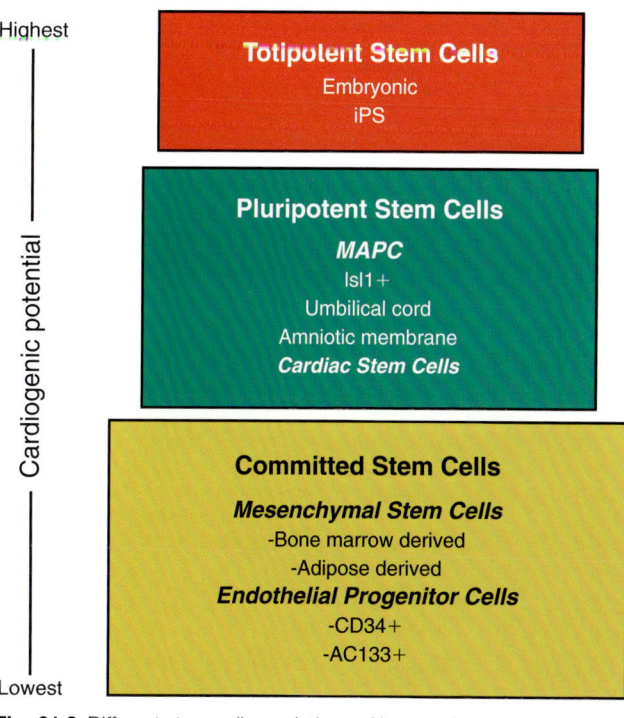

Fig. 61.2 Different stem cell populations of interest for myocardial repair stratified by the differentiation capacity of the given populations. *iPS*, Induced pluripotent stem cells; *MAPCs*, multipotent adult progenitor cells.

By far the most important stem cell AMI study to date is the Reinfusion of Enriched Progenitor Cells And Infarct Remodeling in Acute Myocardial Infarction (REPAIR-AMI) study.[38] This study continues to show improvement in cardiac function, as well as trends in benefit for clinical parameters, including hospitalization for heart failure reinfarction and survival. At the 4-month time point, the treated population had an increase in ejection fraction (EF) of 6% compared with baseline, whereas the control population exhibited only a 2.5% increase. In more recent follow-up studies, these benefits and evidence of decreased clinical events have been maintained out to 2 and 5 years after treatment.[39] The REPAIR-AMI study remains the benchmark against which all AMI studies are compared. Importantly, the success of the REPAIR-AMI study has led to the BAMI study (The effect of intracoronary reinfusion of bone marrow-derived mononuclear cells [BM-MNCs] on all-cause mortality in AMI, http://www.bami-fp7.eu). BAMI is the first study for stem cell treatment in patients with AMI that is powered to determine a mortality benefit. A planned total of 3000 patients will be enrolled, and the control group will receive standard of care without sham or placebo infusion. This landmark study will define the future of BM-MNC transplantation for the treatment of AMI for years to come.

In the United States, there are completed AMI BM-MNC studies that were designed and executed by the Cardiovascular Cell Therapy Research Network. These studies have largely failed to meet predefined end points. The Transplantation in Myocardial Infarction Evaluation (TIME)[40] study randomized patients between cells and placebo and treatment 3 or 7 days after primary PCI. The LateTIME[41] (a phase II, randomized trial evaluating the safety and effect of administration of BM-MNCs 2 to 3 weeks following AMI) study randomized between cells and placebo at 2 to 3 weeks after primary PCI. Whether the findings were negative because the cell preparation was devoid of functional benefit or because there are no signals for stem cell homing into the heart 2 to 3 weeks post-AMI[26] is unknown because the same cell preparation

TABLE 61.1 Stem Cell Transplantation in Acute Myocardial Infarction

Study	# Patients/ Placebo Control	Cell Type	Delivery Method	Time After Infarct	Baseline LV Function	Comments
Chen[117]	69/Yes	BM-derived MSCs	Intracoronary	18.4 ± 1.5 days	49%–53%	Improvement in perfusion, cardiac function and decreased LV dilation. No increase in restenosis noted
BOOST[118,119]	60/Yes	BM-derived mononuclear cells	Intracoronary	4.8 days	50%–51%	Six months after MI, increase in EF (6.7%) in patients who received BM cells compared with 0.6% in optimal medical management. Controls caught up, benefit not lost at 18 months
ASTAMI[120]	100/Yes	BM-derived mononuclear cells	Intracoronary	5–8 days	46%	Noted chest pain and/or EKG changes with infusion. No improvement 6 months after cell stem cell infusion
REPAIR-AMI[38]	204/Yes	BM-derived mononuclear cells	Intracoronary	4 days	47%–48%	Modest improvement in EF 4 months after stem cell infusion (5.5% with stem cells vs. 3.0% for placebo). For EF <49% at baseline, improvement was 7.5% with stem cells vs. 2.5% for placebo
Janssens[68]	66/Yes	BM-derived mononuclear cells	Intracoronary	4 days	46%–49%	First randomized, placebo-controlled blinded study for cell therapy at the time of AMI. No benefit seen
Yousef[121]	62/No	BM-derived mononuclear cells	Intracoronary	7 days	51%	Registry control group. Improved LV function and quality of life and mortality out to 5 years
Hare[70]	53/Yes	MSC (allogeneic)	Intravenous	1–10 days	53%	Trend towards improvement in LV function in AMI. Evidence of decreased arrhythmia in treated patients
Penn[66]	28	MAPC (allogeneic)	Adventitial	2–5 days	43%	Registry control. Significant improvement at 50M dose
TIME Trial[122]	120/Yes	BM-derived mononuclear cells	Intracoronary	3 or 7 days	36%	No benefit of BM-MNC delivery 3 or 7 days after AMI
LATETIME[123]	87/Yes	BM-derived mononuclear cells	Intracoronary	14–21 days	36%	No benefit of BM-MNC delivery 2–3 weeks after AMI
REGENT[124]	200/Yes	BM-derived mononuclear cells	Intracoronary	1 day	35%–39%	No significant improvement of LVEF or volumes. No differences in major cardiovascular event between groups
SWISS-AMI[125]	200/No	BM-derived mononuclear cells	Intracoronary	5–7 or 21–28 days	35%–40%	Did not find improved LV function measured by CMR after early or late transplantation.
FINCELL[126]	80/Yes	BM-derived mononuclear cells	Intracoronary	2.5–3 days	60%	First study showing that intracoronary stem cell therapy is safe after thrombolytic therapy and associated with improvement of global EF
HEBE[127]	200/No	BM-derived mononuclear cells	Intracoronary	3–8 days	41%–43%	No improvement in regional or global systolic function
PRESERVE-AMI[106]	161/Yes	BM-derived CD34+ cells	Intracoronary	7–11 days	37%	Primary end point of improvement in myocardial perfusion not met but did find dose-dependent improvement in LVEF and infarct size

AMI, Acute myocardial infarction; *BM*, bone marrow; *BM-MNC*, bone marrow-derived mononuclear cell; *CMR*, cardiac MRI; *EF*, ejection fraction; *EKG*, electrocardiogram; *LV*, Left Ventricle; *MAPCs*, multipotent adult progenitor cells; *MSCs*, mesenchymal stem cells.

TABLE 61.2 Stem Cell Transplantation in Chronic Heart Failure

Study	# Patients/ Placebo Control	Cell Type	Delivery Method	Time After Infarct	LV Function	Comments
Tse[128]	8/No	BM-derived mononuclear cells	Stem cell transplantation (NOGA-guided catheter-based intramyocardial injection)	Severe ischemic heart disease	Unchanged	Despite no change in EF, an improvement in target wall thickening and wall motion was seen by MRI. No acute procedure-related complications were seen
Seiler[129]	21/Yes	Stem cells mobilized from the BM	GM-CSF, first dose intracoronary then SC for 2 weeks	Chronic ischemia	Unchanged but decreased ischemia	Stem cell mobilization to induce angiogenesis as assessed by improved coronary collateral blood flow following 2 weeks of daily GM-CSF administration
Assmus[130]	75/Yes with crossover	Circulating progenitor cells (CPCs) or BM-derived mononuclear cells (BMCs)	Intracoronary infusion	Ischemic cardiomyopathy	Improved with BMC only	Baseline EF ~40% 2.9% improvement with BMC −1.2% without therapy −0.4% with CPC
Perin[131]	21/Yes, non-randomized	BM-derived mononuclear cells	NOGA-guided intramyocardial injection	Severe ischemic cardiomyopathy	Improved	
Schaefer[37]	10/No	BM-derived mononuclear cells	Catheter-based intramyocardial delivery	Chronic ischemia	Unchanged but decreased ischemia	Decreased stress-induced ischemia and CCS Angina Score
FOCUS[132]	92/Yes	BM-derived mononuclear cells	NOGA-guided intramyocardial injection	Ischemic cardiomyopathy	Unchanged	No benefit observed in LVESVi, MVO2, or reversible defects
POSEIDON[133]	30/No	Allogeneic and autologous MSCs	Endocardial	Ischemic cardiomyopathy	Unchanged	Not placebo controlled and underpowered but equivalence of safety for allo vs. auto
MYSTAR[134]	60/No	BM-MNCs	Intracoronary/ intramyocardial	Ischemic cardiomyopathy	Improved	First study to investigate combined application of stem cell therapy. Significant Improvement in infarct size and LV function
STAR-Heart[135]	391/No	BM-MNCs	Intracoronary	Chronic ischemic cardiomyopathy	Improved	Largest clinical trial of intracoronary BM-MNC transplantation. Improved hemodynamics, LV function, and exercise capacity
SCIPIO[136]	23/No	CSCs	Intracoronary	Severe ischemic cardiomyopathy	Improved	On average showed approximately 9% increase in LV function
CADUCEUS[48]	31/No	CDCs	Intracoronary	Severe ischemic cardiomyopathy	Improved	Significant decrease in myocardial scar by MRI
CHART-1[60]	271/Yes	CPCs	Endocardial	Ischemic cardiomyopathy	No change	No significant clinical benefit and no difference between serious adverse events
ALLSTAR[52]	134/Yes	CDCs	Intracoronary	Ischemic cardiomyopathy	No change	Did not reduce infarct size or improve LV volumes
ESCORT[105]	6/No	ESCs	Fibrin patch delivered epicardially	Severe ischemic cardiomyopathy	Improved	All patients symptomatically improved with increased systolic motion
ixCELL-DCM[61]	109/Yes	BM-derived MSCs (propagated)	Endocardial	Severe dilated ischemic cardiomyopathy	No change	Decrease in mortality and cardiac hospitalizations but no improvement in cardiac function

BM, Bone marrow; *CCS*, canadian cardiovascular society; *CDCs*, cardiosphere derived cells; *CSCs*, cardiac stem cells; *EF*, ejection fraction; *ESCs*, embryonic stem cells; *GM-CSF*, granulocyte macrophage colony stimulating factor; *LVESVi*, left ventricular end systolic volume index; *LV*, left ventricle; *MNC*, mononuclear cell; *MRI*, magnetic resonance imaging; *MSCs*, mesenchymal stem cells; *MVO2*, myocardial oxygen consumption; *SC*, subcutaneous.

failed in the TIME trial. This negative experience by the network highlights the importance of validating the functional reparative potential of the cell processing protocol in not only animal studies but also against proven human cell preparations such as those developed by Dimmeler and colleagues.[38] The network is currently focused on the combination of autologous CSCs and autologous mesenchymal stem cells (MSCs) (Combination of Mesenchymal and c-kit Cardiac Stem Cells As Regenerative Therapy for Heart Failure [CONCERT-HF], ClinicalTrials.gov—NCT02501811). The combination of these stem cells populations has been shown to increase the paracrine expression of SDF-1,[42] the overexpression of which has been directly shown to improve cardiac remodeling in severe LV dysfunction.[43] Although it may appear relatively unsophisticated to simply add more cells, this study will at least generate additional data on c-kit+ stem cells alone, as they were used in the SCIPIO (Stem Cell Infusion in Patients with Ischemic cardiomyOpathy) trial.[44]

NOVEL AUTOLOGOUS STEM CELL INDICATIONS AND TYPES

Several groups have taken open-minded approaches on either the indication or approach to improve patient outcomes with cardiovascular disease. The Adult Autologous CD34+ Stem Cells (ACT34) study focused on patients with chronic myocardial ischemia.[45,46] In this placebo-controlled study, patients received granulocyte colony stimulating factor (G-CSF) mobilization followed by apheresis and isolation of CD34+ cells. These cells were injected via an endoventricular approach using the NOGA catheter. The 1-year follow-up data for this patient population revealed sustained benefit of the 6-month findings of a decrease of 5.6 angina events per week and a doubling of exercise treadmill time compared with baseline. These data verify in the clinical setting the preclinical findings that stem cell–based cardiac repair results in significant and sustained enhanced tissue perfusion. Disappointingly the phase III Efficacy and Safety of Intramyocardial Autologous CD34+ Cell Administration in Patients With Refractory Angina (RENEW) study (ClinicalTrials.gov—NCT01508910) was stopped prematurely by the sponsor, leaving this population of patients to wait for future cell therapies; however, a recently published meta-analysis of all the studies done with CD34+ stem cells derived from G–CSF-mobilized leukopaks demonstrates clear benefit of vasculogenic stem cells in chronic angina with decreased frequency of symptoms at each time point.[47] Exercise capacity was also shown to be improved in this meta-analysis with improvement of total exercise time by 30 to 50 seconds across the 3- to 12-month time frame. These results are in parallel with another meta-analysis, which was done in 2016 to evaluate the effects of cell therapy on refractory angina. This analysis found that patients treated with cell therapy had a significant decrease in number of anginal episodes and antianginal medications accompanied by improvements in Canadian Cardiovascular Society (CCS) classes and exercise tolerance.[47]

Two different trials focused on the utility of autologous myocardial-derived stem cells on patients with evolving ischemic-induced myocardial remodeling or ischemic cardiomyopathy. The CADUCEUS[48] (CArdiosphere-Derived aUtologous Stem CElls to Reverse ventricUlar dysfunction, ClinicalTrials.gov—NCT00893360) trial generated autologous cardiosphere-derived cells (CDCs) and the SCIPIO (Cardiac stem cells in patients with ischaemic cardiomyopathy)[44] (Clinicaltrials.org—NCT00474461) trials isolated autologous CSCs. Based on relative dosing of stem cells in preclinical trials, it would appear that CSCs may be the most potent of all the adult stem cells.[49] If true, then CSC or CDC may be the best cells to implement for stem cell transplantation (see Fig. 61.1). The CADUCEUS trial delivered autologous CDC down the infarct-related vessels in stable patients within 1 year of an AMI and low EF. In the SCIPIO trial, CSCs were isolated from atrial tissue obtained at the time of coronary artery bypass surgery. These CSCs were cultured, and after sufficient propagation the cells were injected into injured myocardium through a percutaneous approach. The CSC population was infused into coronary artery on average 3 to 4 months after open heart surgery.[44] Just as adipose-derived stem cells can be rapidly harvested from adipose tissue,[50,51] it may become possible to rapidly isolate CSCs from the left atrial appendage in the operating room or endomyocardial biopsies in sufficient number to allow for meaningful myocardial support. The CADUCEUS group showed a benefit with autologous CDC, whereas the recent ALLSTAR (ALLogeneic Heart STem Cells to Achieve Myocardial Regeneration) trial[52] using allogeneic CDC failed to demonstrate any benefit, with no reduction in infarct size or improvement left ventricular volumes measured by MRI (Late Breaking Clinical Trials, AHA Scientific Sessions 2017). Whether ALLSTAR, in contrast to CADUCEUS, failed to demonstrate a decrease in myocardial scar because of the allogeneic source of the cells is unknown. However, given these results, in settings such as CHF where treatment can be scheduled, the results suggest that at least for now the focus should be on autologous cells. Thus far, data from the SCIPIO trial demonstrated varied but on average an approximately 9% increase in cardiac function. The field awaits future studies with autologous CSCs.

Mesenchymal Stem Cells and Multipotent Adult Progenitor Cells

Stromal progenitor cells comprise less than 0.05% of the adult bone marrow. MSCs and multipotent adult progenitor cells (MAPCs) form subpopulations of bone marrow stromal progenitor cells that maintain the ability to differentiate along multiple lineages.[30,53] MSCs can be immunoselected via cell surface CD45 negativity and cultured through as many as 40 population doublings before attaining senescence. In general, the benefits observed with MSCs following cell transplantation at the time of myocardial infarction may have little to do with the cell itself, but rather how factors secreted by the MSCs alter the tissue microenvironment. This so-called paracrine effect of MSCs has been demonstrated,[54] showing that injection of the supernatant of MSC cultures at the time of the myocardial infarction results in similar benefits that have been associated with MSC transplantation. We have demonstrated that SDF-1 released by MSCs results in the recruitment of CSCs to the infarct border zone, as well as inhibits cardiac myocyte death through the binding of SDF-1 to CXCR4-expressing cardiac myocytes in the infarct border zone.[55,56] Other groups have demonstrated that the benefits of MSCs are due to the release of miRNA-containing exosomes which have been shown to assist in cellular preservation and engage in resisting degradation.[32,33] Studies have also shown that these exosomes are also involved in cardiovascular disease as biomarkers and have emerged as being beneficial in ischemic cardiac disease treatment.[34–36]

Several strategies are being studied to improve the function of MSCs for the treatment of CHF. Both involve harvesting of bone marrow-derived MSCs and growing them under conditions that optimize their effects. The first effort has focused on inducing a cardiopoietic program within the MSCs.[57,58] This elegant work has detailed pathways that optimize the cardiac potential of adult MSCs. The findings of the C-Cure (Cardiopoietic stem Cell therapy in heart failURE) trial showed that these cardiopoietic MSCs have the potential to improve cardiac function (EF increased 7% with cells compared with 0.2% in placebo), decrease end-systolic volume (16 mL relative to placebo), and improve 6-minute walk distance.[59] Unfortunately, in the larger phase III CHART-1 (Congestive Heart Failure Cardiopoietic Regenerative Therapy) trial these cardiopoietic MSCs failed to meet their primary end point and show significant clinical benefit.[60]

The second approach in clinical development is a proprietary cell culturing system developed by Aastrom Biosciences in which adherent cells are propagated for 2 weeks in an enclosed system. The ixCELL DCM (Transendocardial Injection of ixmyelocel-T in Patients with Ischemic Dilated Cardiomyopathy) phase II trial delivered these cells via endocardial injection in patients with ischemic and nonischemic cardiomyopathy. This trial demonstrated a decrease in mortality and cardiac hospitalizations, in the absence of any clear benefit in cardiac function.[61] Due to the lack of improvement on cardiac performance, whether the improvement in clinical outcome was random or a reflection of delivery of the cell product remains to be determined.

MAPCs are stromal cells derived from the bone marrow and are able to differentiate into endothelial, epithelial, and mesenchymal cell types.[62] They can be expanded in culture for more than 80 population doublings and still maintain their pluripotency by differentiating into most somatic cell types.[62] Whether these multipotent stem cells exist in vivo or are the result of serial cell passages in culture remains to be determined. However, the demonstration that multipotent cells can be significantly expanded and their reparative and immunomodulation properties hold the potential for benefit in cardiovascular disease,[63] stroke (ClinicalTrials.gov-NCT01436487), graft versus host disease, and other pathologies.

Both MSCs and MAPCs have been shown to lead to decreased cardiac myocyte cell death, decreased infarct size, and improved cardiac remodeling and function in rodent[64] and porcine models[65] of AMI. Each of these cell types has entered the clinical realm, with MSC clinical trials entering the phase III arena.

The MAPC phase I trial was a dose ranging study in which 20, 50 and 100 million MAPCs were delivered to patients with first-time STEMI with postprimary PCI EF of 45% or less.[66] In contrast to BM-MNC or MSC trials, the MAPC phase I trial used catheter-mediated adventitial delivery of the MAPCs using the MercatorMed Systems Cricket Catheter 2 to 5 days after primary PCI. As shown in Fig. 61.3, as the balloon is inflated on this catheter a single needle is deployed that goes through the medial layer of the infarct related artery delivering the MAPCs to the adventitia. In preclinical studies, once in the adventitia, the MAPCs distribute through the infarct zone.[65] The delivery of MAPCs resulted on average in an absolute increase in EF of greater than 12% in those patients with baseline EF of less than 45%.[66] As in other studies, in patients with EF greater than 45% no significant improvement was observed.[67,68]

The ease of delivery of MAPCs with the MercatorMed Systems Cricket Catheter with respect to clinical workflow after PCI has led to the development of a clinical study to investigate the utility of stem cell delivery in non-STEMI (NSTEMI). NSTEMI has a higher 1-year mortality than STEMI,[69] likely due to the fact that patients with NSTEMI have a greater likelihood of prior AMI and impaired EF. MAPCs in this setting have the potential to decrease infarct expansion, as well as through its immunomodulatory effects (i) decrease adverse remodeling that may be initiated by an ischemic event in an impaired ventricle and (ii) decrease risk of additional plaque rupture along the coronary tree. This trial is ongoing and thus far has demonstrated the feasibility of delivering stem cells at the time of coronary intervention. Whether this leads to a measurable improvement in myocardial perfusion awaits completion of the trial.

From an interventional perspective, it is interesting to compare the loss of efficacy in the translation of MSCs and MAPCs from preclinical studies to human studies. The efficacy of the intravenous delivery of MSCs went from a relative increase of approximately 80% in rats to 10% at the high dose of MSCs in the phase I trial.[55,70] For MAPCs, the improvement in EF fraction in a porcine AMI model was approximately 38% and was

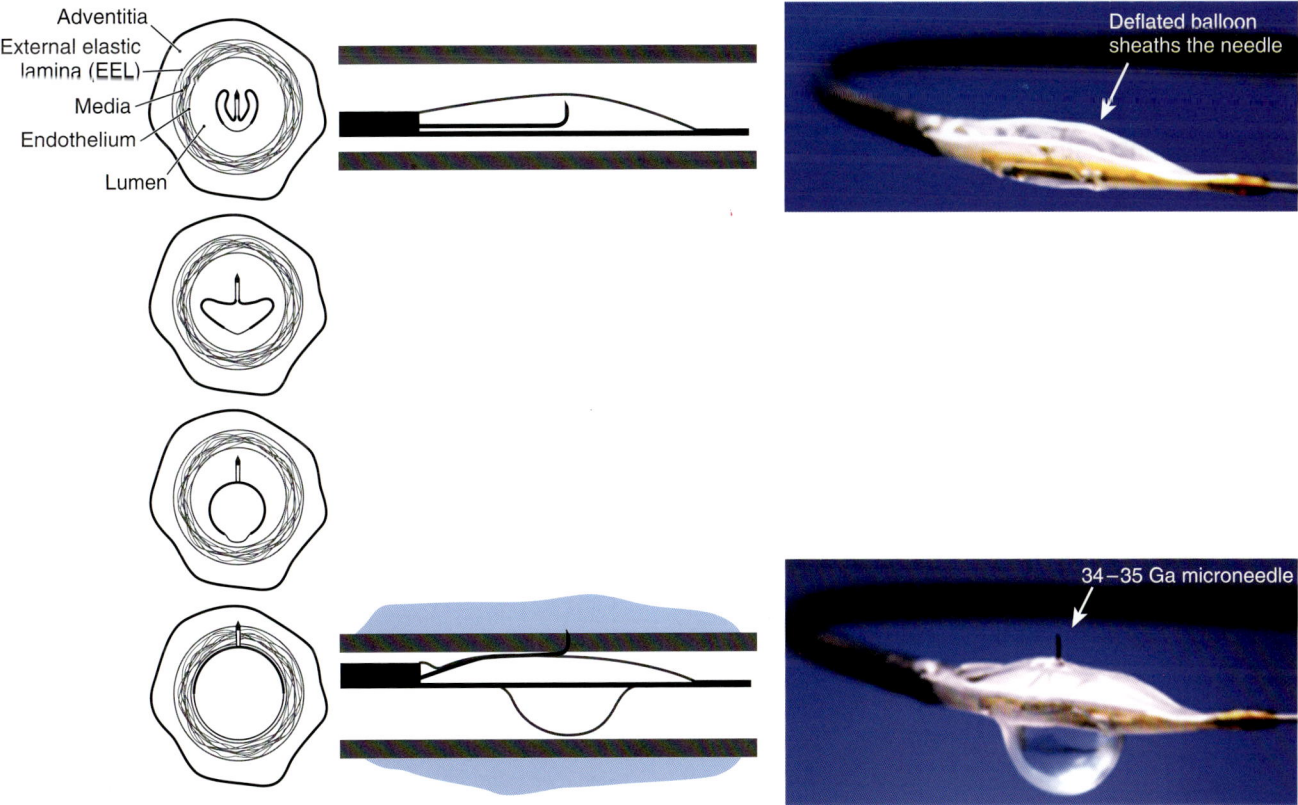

Fig. 61.3 Schematic representation of microneedle catheter–mediated delivery to the coronary adventitia and photographs of deflated and inflated Mercatormed Cricket Catheter.

approximately 35% in the phase I trial.[65,66] Although the consistency in effect in the MAPC trial could be due to the cells, it is more likely that the difference in translation was due to delivery method. In the MAPC trial, the cells were delivered to the adventitia in similar fashions avoiding the atherosclerotic intima of the diseased coronaries. In contrast, the efficiency of delivery of MSCs to the myocardium in patients with coronary artery disease could have been inhibited compared with that observed in rodents which have nondiseased arteries. The aforementioned Cricket catheter continues to offer an intriguing strategy for delivery of stem cells to the infarct region immediately following primary PCI, obviating the need for complex delivery systems or additional procedures in the catheterization laboratory.

OTHER STRATEGIES FOR DELIVERY OF STEM CELLS TO THE MYOCARDIUM

Studies have continued to attempt to define the optimal delivery strategy for stem cells, given the difficulty with degradation of cells prior to delivery using established methods. A developing method of stem cell delivery to the heart is cell sheet technology in which donor cells are contained in a cell sheet which allows them to preserve their cell surface proteins and extracellular matrix. The cell sheet, which is either monolayer or multilayer, is placed onto the epicardial heart surface at the area of ischemia.[71-73] This delivery method is thought to be superior to the intracoronary or intravenous methods because it does not require cell dissociation and there is significantly less trauma to both the donor cells and to the treated myocardium. Another emerging method of cell delivery for tissue regeneration is injectable hydrogels, which are hydrophilic polymers that act as structural support scaffolds to deliver cells to the epicardial surface.[6,7] An example of a hydrogel that has been recently used in murine myocardial models is fibrin glue, which is made by mixing fibrinogen and thrombin and results in a biocompatible glue that can be placed directly on the cardiac patch of stem cells which will then adhere to the infarcted myocardium. Multiple studies have showed that injectable hydrogels have been successful in improving the cell transplant survival, reducing infarct expansion, and preserving cardiac function.[74,75]

Cardiac Regeneration

As discussed previously, there is little evidence that adult stem cells result in regeneration of lost cardiac myocytes. It is likely that regeneration of cardiac myocytes and myocardial structures will require ESCs, cardiac myocytes generated from iPS, or gene therapy to induce local directed differentiation.[76,77] ESCs are continuously replicating cell lines derived from an embryonic origin isolated from the blastocyst inner cell mass.[78] The properties of ESCs include derivation from the preimplantation or periimplantation embryo, prolonged undifferentiated proliferation with conditional constraints, and the ability to form tissues derived from all three germ layers. When they are properly cultured, ESCs expand at a rapid rate and group to form embryoid bodies that have the ability to differentiate into a wide variety of specialized cells, including cardiomyocytes. A recent study used human ESC-derived cardiomyocytes in infarcted hearts of primates, which demonstrated significant improvement in left ventricular function assessed by cardiac MRI. The treated hearts were also found to have remuscularization of infarcts, which led to a significant reduction in scar size.[79]

Adult somatic cells have recently been shown capable of being differentiated into cardiac myocytes through the intermediate step of generating iPS or directly.[80,81] Transplantation of these cells leads to engraftment of cardiac myocytes in the infarct zone and improvement in cardiac function and remodeling. How these cells will ultimately translate into the clinic is as yet unclear. Undoubtedly, optimal translation will require scaffolds and biologics to optimize vascularization, integration, and workload of these contractile networks.

To date, there are no published clinical data for the delivery of significant numbers of cardiac myocytes to treat patients with CHF. There remains much excitement for the future of these cells, but for now autologous iPS-derived cardiac myocytes have shown significant utility for understanding the mechanisms associated with arrhythmias and cardiomyopathies.[82,83]

STEM CELL–BASED CHEMOKINE AND CYTOKINE STRATEGIES

An early focus of clinical trials for stem cell–based repair of the myocardium was based on cytokine-mediate mobilization of the marrow space using G-CSF and granulocyte macrophage-CSF (GM-CSF).[58] There is overall little evidence that stem cell mobilization of the marrow space in the periinfarct period with G-CSF leads to a significant change in cardiac function or remodeling.

One potential explanation for the failing of G-CSF mobilization in clinical trials is that mobilized hematopoietic stem cells are unable to home due to dysfunctional CXCR4 (the SDF-1 receptor) expression. G-CSF mobilizes stem cells via the degradation of CXCR4, thus releasing the stem cell from its anchor in the bone marrow. There is increasing evidence that the stem cell-mobilizing agent AMD3100—an antagonist to the CXCR4 receptor—induces stem cell mobilization that leads to improvement in cardiac function in preclinical models.[84] Interestingly, early use of AMD-3100 leads to stem cell mobilization but does not lead to persistent inhibition of CXCR4 binding in the myocardium,[84] whereas persistent AMD3100 administration leads to mobilization of stem cells yet no improvement in cardiac function. These data suggest a potential important role for cardiac CXCR4 expression in myocardial response to stem cell–mediated repair.

The bone marrow naturally releases stem cells into the blood stream on a daily basis. The concept of cytokine-based stem cell mobilization is to increase the number of circulating stem cells at the time the heart is signaling to recruit them. Thus, although G-CSF and AMD3100 induce stem cells to enter the blood stream, if the heart is not signaling to recruit them to the injured myocardium no benefit will be realized.[26,85] Initially we, and now others, have taken the opposite approach—prolong the period of time that the heart signals to recruit stem cells to the injured myocardium and take advantage of the fact that there are always circulating stem cells present in the blood stream.

Several years ago we defined stromal cell-derived factor as a stem cell homing factor to injured tissues.[26] We have demonstrated that if one prolongs SDF-1 signaling in the myocardium either via the delivery of MSCs, which express SDF-1 at baseline, or enhanced SDF-1–expressing MSCs, there is significant preservation of cardiac myocytes and cardiac function.[55] We have demonstrated that the reestablishment of SDF-1 expression through the delivery of SDF-1 plasmid to a model of ischemic cardiomyopathy leads to remodeling of the scar and improvement in EF.[86]

Based on these data and those from porcine models, SDF-1 gene transfer is currently under clinical development. In a phase I open-label dose escalation study, SDF-1 plasmid (JVS-100) was delivered via 15 endocardial injections using a helical injection catheter.[6] Fifteen injections of 1 mL per injection to the infarct and infarct border zone delivering 5, 15, or 30 mg total were performed. The trial demonstrated a dose-dependent improvement in 6-minute walk distance and NT-proBNP (N-terminal prohormone of brain natriuretic peptide), as well as neovascularization of the infarct border zone and stabilization of ventricular size and function in the higher two doses.[6] The utility of transient SDF-1 overexpression in CHF is being demonstrated in the randomized, blinded, and placebo-controlled 93 patient STOP-HF (St Vincent's Screening TO Prevent Heart Failure) trial in which the 4 months of high-dose JVS-100 led to a statistically significant 30-mL reduction in left ventricular end-systolic volume in high-risk patients with ischemic cardiomyopathy.[43] SDF 1 overexpression was also being studied in ischemic cardiomyopathy using retrograde infusion via the coronary sinus in the RETRO-HF (Study to Evaluate the Safety and Efficacy of JVS-100 Administered to Adults With Ischemic Heart Failure) trial. This was the first trial implementing retrograde infusion as a strategy for delivering a biologic, and, although delivery was achieved, no benefit was observed with the delivery of SDF-1 plasmid via this route.

The direct overexpression of SDF-1 prepares and induces the myocardium to engraft circulating stem cells[87]; it has similarly been shown that preparing the heart prior to stem cell infusion increases the efficacy of the procedure. In the CELL WAVE (Combined Extracorporal Shock Wave Therapy and Intracoronary Cell Therapy in Chronic Ischemic Myocardium) trial, the investigators used shock wave therapy directed at the heart to induce myocardial expression of SDF-1 and VEGF in patients with chronic ischemic cardiomyopathy. Twenty-four hours later patients underwent bone marrow harvest and intracoronary infusion of autologous bone marrow cells. This study showed that only patients who received the combination of shock wave therapy with autologous bone marrow infusion had improvement in EF, whereas shock wave or cell infusion alone had no effects.[87]

Increasing the survival of transplanted stem cells continues to be a critical issue with this therapy, and one proposed strategy is to precondition them with agonists such as growth hormone–releasing hormone[88] and angiotensin receptors. This was studied by Xu et al. with stimulation via angiotensin II type 2 receptor, the main peptide in the renin-angiotensin system, which is critical in cardiac remodeling after acute infarction. These preconditioned stem cells reduced cardiomyocyte apoptosis and inflammation, and this led to improvement in cardiac function after transplantation.[89] Alternatively, researchers have also exposed stem cells to different stressors to enhance their therapeutic efficacy and to prepare them for the strenuous environment of the ischemic myocardium. Stressors that have been recently studied include hypoxia, oxidative stress, and heat shock.[90,91] In 2015, the CHINA-AMI (Safety and efficacy of intracoronary *h*ypoxia-precond*i*tioned bone marrow mono*n*uclear cell *a*dministration for *a*cute *m*yocardial *i*nfarction patients) trial by Hu et al. tested the hypoxia preconditioning hypothesis in human patients and sought to assess the safety of intracoronary transplantation for AMIs. Results of this study found significant improvement in left ventricle volumes and postinfarct perfusion defects.[92] Heat shock therapy has also been used in the preconditioning process and is becoming more popular because studies have shown significant improvement in stem cell survival. A study by Feng et al. found that transplantation of these heat shock–treated stem cells into ischemic myocardium reduced apoptosis, improved global cardiac function, and attenuated fibrosis.[26] These studies are an excellent example of the execution of a clinical trial to test an important hypothesis and increase our understanding of the factors associated with success of cell therapy.

ELECTRICAL EFFECTS OF CELL THERAPY

Although the field is moving forward in trying to identify strategies that either preserve or improve cardiac function in patients at the time of AMI or with CHF, it is becoming clear that the mechanical and electrical effects of cell therapy are independent.[21,25] We have previously demonstrated that SKMB or MSCs (1 million of each cell type) delivered in the periinfarct period to the myocardium results in similar improvements in cardiac function; however, when these hearts undergo an electrophysiology study with the introduction of extrasystoles, the rate at which ventricular tachycardia is induced is significantly different depending on the cell type the animal received.[25] Animals that received SKMB were always inducible for ventricular tachycardia. As noted in Table 61.1, multiple studies have suggested an increased incidence of ventricular tachycardia in patients who received SKMB. This could be a spurious result due to the fact that all the patients in these trials have a history of myocardial infarction; however, while SKMB do express connexin 43 in culture, they do not express connexin 43 after transplantation, and SKMB do not electrically couple with the native myocardium.[25] The establishment of connexin 43 expression in SKMB has been shown to decrease the arrhythmogenic risk of SKMB. These data coupled with the clinical data to date demonstrating a decrease in clinical measures of arrhythmia in patients who received intravenous MSCs following AMI[70] suggest stem cell therapy could expand its potential clinical indications from simply improving cardiac function to decreasing reentry. Multiple studies have shown that ESCs are able to differentiate into multiple different cardiomyocytes which have distinctive characteristics including nodal like, atrial like, and ventricle like.[93,94] A 2012 study by Shiba et al. revealed that implanted ESCs into infarcted myocardium improved cardiac function and significantly reduced incidence of ventricular arrhythmia. The stem cells were also genetically encoded with a fluorescent signal to show that the grafts did beat synchronously with the host myocardium 4 weeks posttransplantation.[95]

As such, one could contemplate a trial where, instead of inducing further LV injury to interrupt a reentrant circuit, specific stem cells could be injected into the mapped circuit to reverse the area of slow conduction or remodeling the size of the scar. The safety associated with cell therapy justifies advancement of the approach into novel indications and trial designs that could address clinical populations with unmet needs.

FUTURE DIRECTIONS AND CONTROVERSIES

The field of stem cell therapy for the treatment of cardiovascular disease is continuing to make significant strides at the molecular level. The understanding of the role of exosomes and miRNAs in stem cell–mediated[96] repair is a significant advancement over the prior attempts at identifying proteins[97] that ultimately did not translate to clinical fruition. Clinically, for patients with ischemic heart disease, the only real progress has been in the area of chronic chest pain, where several randomized double-blind clinical trials demonstrated clear evidence of clinical benefit.[98] The meta-analysis of these trials[47] showing clear benefit and the recent U.S. Food and Drug Administration (FDA) regenerative medicine advanced therapy designation for this indication offer the real hope that we will see stem cell therapies benefiting ischemic heart disease patients in the near future. The following future directions of the field have been stratified into distinct focuses: relevant basic science and clinical science. Within each focus there are clear critical issues which need to be addressed in order to advance the field to prevent or treat cardiac dysfunction and improve outcomes in patients with heart disease.

Bench Investigation

Questions in the setting of basic science can generally be divided into two areas. The first question focuses on defining the molecular mechanisms associated with adult stem cell–based repair of the heart. As we have shown with SDF-1 over the past decade and a half, defining the molecular mechanisms associated with stem cell–based repair can lead to novel targets for therapy, insights into the biology of tissue healing,[99–101] and deliver to the clinical scientists novel agents for investigation. Although promising for heart failure, unfortunately the blind assumption by the uninformed that a therapeutic that works in one indication will work in another has led to the failed development of SDF-1 at this time (ClinicalTrials.org—NCT02544204, Late Breaking Clinical Trials, ACC 2018).

The growing interest in exosomes and the miRNA that they contain as a therapeutic modality offers new lines of investigation. Whether the therapeutic will ultimately be the exosome, miRNA, or strategies that increase exosome release and function[102] remains to be seen but offers an exciting and more clinically translatable druglike strategy then the use of stem cells themselves.

The second question is whether we can truly achieve cardiogenesis. There are little data that unmanipulated cardiac myocytes will divide and regenerate themselves following myocardial injury. Potential approaches to achieve cardiogenesis include:

- Genetic manipulation of cardiac myocytes to achieve cardiac myocyte proliferation as has been shown in engineered murine.[103,104]
- The introduction of in vitro generated cardiac myocytes from embryonic of iPS, the feasibility of which was shown by the recent publication of the ENCORE (Transplantation of Human Embryonic Stem Cell-Derived Cardiovascular Progenitors for Severe Ischemic Left Ventricular Dysfunction) trial using allogeneic ESC-derived cardiac myocytes.[105]
- Pharmacologic strategies to induce recruitment and directed differentiation of stem cells in vivo following myocardial infarction remain to be seen.

Clinical Investigation

There have been limited advances in cell therapy trials over the past 4 years, especially in the academic arena outside of the studies on chronic chest pain.[47] Excitingly, the PRESERVE-AMI study showed a dose-dependent improvement in cardiac function suggesting a druglike effect of the mobilized CD34+ stem cells in patients with recent AMI.[106] The field is maturing such that it is clear that the field can no longer advance on the execution of small underpowered studies.[107] It should be noted that editorials on studies that some in the field find encouraging and important progress, such as the PRESERVE-AMI, have suggested that these same studies should be recognized as further failures of cell therapy.[108] These failures have led some to suggest that we must be cautious with the current forms of cell therapy and revisit the call to consider increasing our attention towards cardiac regenerative medicine.[109,110] This movement towards regenerative medicine was discussed in a recent review article which concluded that advancements in biotechnology will eventually lead to the creation of "organ-on-a-chip models" which could mimic in vitro heart models, thus allowing researchers to expedite their investigations into the reparative properties of stem cells on advanced disease models[111]; however, such an approach may limit the understanding of the effects of the systemic endogenous stem cell pool on tissue repair.

The bench to beside to bench paradigm is alive and well in the field and is the most likely avenue to bring advances in clinical populations than the overhyped academic efforts that have plagued the field.[112]

As reviewed previously, an important question that needs to be addressed in the clinical realm is whether stem cell therapy will have significant benefit in patients with NSTEMI. All the trials to date have focused on patients with first STEMI with normal cardiac function prior to their ischemic event. Although this study population has been critical to demonstrate proof of concept and biologic effect, it is not the clinical population that is most at risk of adverse cardiac events. Furthermore, as many in the field are well aware, the number of STEMI continues to decline. Ultimately, if adult stem cell therapy is going to have a significant impact on patient outcomes, the therapy needs to be transitioned to patients with ischemic cardiomyopathy prior to their index event and who present with NSTEMI.

Strategies Beyond Simple Stem Cell Treatment That Could Move the Field Forward

Given the significant issue of stem cell survival after transplant, researchers have begun genetic modification trials in an attempt to overexpress cytoprotective genes. A cytoprotective protein that has shown promise in animal models is heme oxygenase-1 (HO-1), which, when induced, has been reported to be anti-inflammatory and antiapoptic.[91,113] A recent study revealed that induction of HO-1 can attenuate myocardial ischemia.[114] Overexpressing genes that code for antiapoptosis factors is another example of genetic modification to help sustain stem cell survival. Alternatively, animal trials have used protein kinase B, which plays a key role in multiple cellular processes, including cell proliferation and survival.[115] The constitutive overexpression of protein kinase B in a rat model of ischemic injury has been shown to reduce infarct size, inhibit cardiomyocyte death, and improve in left ventricular function.[116] Rodent stem cells have similarly been engineered to overexpress protein kinase B and transplanted these into ischemic rate myocardium. This not only had improved stem cell survival, but they also reduced adverse cardiac remodeling and enhanced regeneration of myocardial tissue leading to normalization of cardiac function.[30] It is likely that the next generation of stem cells that will enter clinical development for CHF will be modified to enhance stem cell paracrine function through the enhanced release of exosomes and the miRNA contained within. Conversely, strategies implementing direct gene therapy to the myocardium bypassing the stem cell completely is entirely possible as well. Fundamentally, as we have championed for almost two decades, stem cell therapy is a means to an end of defining novel biology that will lead to the development of novel drug therapy. The field continues to develop along that continuum.

CONCLUSIONS

The field of adult stem cell therapy for the prevention and treatment of cardiac dysfunction continues to make progress. The balance of data suggests that there is a therapeutic effect; the bench science is coalescing around some common themes for mechanism of action. The question remains regarding what the therapy will look like when it is optimized. Given the growing prevalence of patients with congestive heart failure and myocardial infarction combined with the economic burden of congestive heart failure, the potential human and societal benefits continue to be great.

 Additional references available online at expertconsult.com.

中文导读

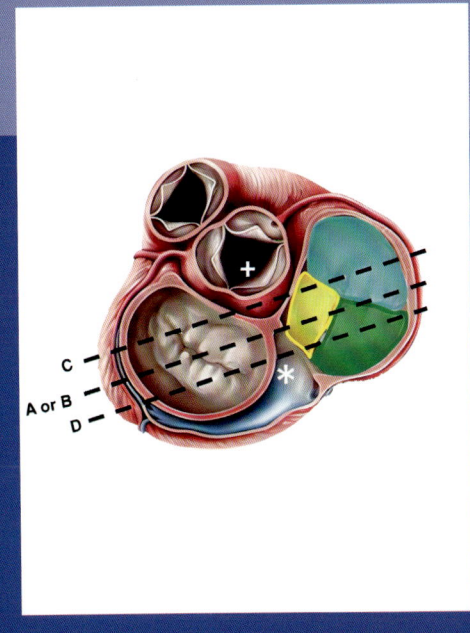

第62章
瓣周漏的经皮介入治疗

  瓣周漏是外科心脏瓣膜置换术后常见的并发症之一,其发生率为5%~17%。瓣周漏的主要临床表现为充血性心力衰竭和机械性溶血。经食管超声心动图联合3D超声是评估瓣周漏的重要影像学方法,可以对瓣周漏的位置和大小进行评估,同时可以用于介入治疗的术中指导。对于严重瓣周漏或药物治疗效果欠佳的患者,其治疗方案包括外科手术治疗和经皮介入治疗。与介入封堵相比,外科手术修补的并发症发生率更高。成功的经皮介入治疗可显著改善患者的临床症状及溶血性贫血。经皮主动脉瓣瓣周漏封堵术多采用主动脉逆行途径,经皮二尖瓣瓣周漏封堵术常常采用房间隔穿刺途径,新的技术如双导丝技术为瓣周漏的介入封堵拓宽了新思路。介入治疗相关的并发症包括瓣叶受损、卒中、血胸、封堵器栓塞和房间隔穿刺相关的并发症。

  本章节系统阐述了二尖瓣和主动脉瓣置换术后瓣周漏的评估方法,以及经皮介入封堵治疗的适应证和临床结局。

杨　城　吴永健

章节要点

- 人工心脏瓣膜置换术后瓣周漏的发生率为5%~17%。
- 超声心动图在二尖瓣和主动脉瓣瓣周漏的评估中发挥着重要作用。
- 外科手术修复是有效的，但与介入封堵相比，其并发症的发生率明显更高。
- 经皮瓣周漏封堵术是可行且安全的，其远期疗效与外科手术相当。
- 症状的改善和溶血性贫血的缓解及远期预后取决于瓣周漏修复或封堵的完整性

62 Percutaneous Treatment of Paravalvular Leak

Mario J. Gössl, Paul Sorajja

KEY POINTS

- Paravalvular regurgitation (leak) affects 5% to 17% of all surgically implanted prosthetic heart valves.
- Echocardiography is pivotal in the evaluation of both mitral and aortic paravalvular leaks.
- Surgical repair is effective but has significantly higher complications rates compared with a percutaneous approach.
- Percutaneous paravalvular leak closure is feasible and safe with long-term outcomes comparable to a surgical approach.
- Resolution of symptoms and hemolysis as well as long-term survival depend on completeness of defect closure with either approach.

INTRODUCTION

Percutaneous paravalvular closure with an Amplatzer ductal occluder device was first described in 2004 by Kort et al. in a 3–month-old infant who had undergone atrioventricular valve replacement with a 19-mm St. Jude mitral prosthesis in 2004 at 6-weeks of age.[1] Before that the only transcatheter closing techniques described were coil occlusions[2,3] and the double umbrella device.[4]

Paravalvular regurgitation due to an abnormal communication between cardiac chambers affects 5% to 17% of all surgically implanted prosthetic heart valves (both mechanical- and bioprostheses, with an estimated 500 to 10,200 cases annually).[5,6] The most common etiologies for paravalvular regurgitation are tissue friability, annular calcification, or infection; patients can present with symptoms of congestive heart failure, hemolytic anemia, or both. In this chapter, we will present appropriate assessment and indications for current percutaneous strategies to close and clinical outcomes of mitral and aortic paravalvular leaks (PVLs).

ASSESSMENT OF PARAVALVULAR LEAKS

When a patient with a history of aortic- or mitral-valve replacement presents with heart failure symptoms and is found to have a new systolic (mitral PVL) or diastolic (aortic PVL) murmur, a transthoracic echocardiogram is key in the initial workup (Figs. 62.1 and 62.2A and B). Assessment of metallic mitral valve prostheses may be difficult due to shadowing from the prosthesis into the left atrium, which can obscure the regurgitation signal (see Fig. 62.1). However, a thorough Doppler assessment can help confirm regurgitation as the major culprit.[7]

If the PVL is deemed severe and aggressive medical management fails, there are two management options: (A) surgical reoperation, which usually carries a significant mortality risk, or (B) a percutaneous closure of the PVL.

Due to an increased morbidity and mortality, reoperation is often avoided, especially if the underlying paravalvular tissue is friable (active endocarditis, steroid use) or heavily calcified. This notion is supported by Said et al., who recently reported the Mayo Clinic experience of 206 mitral reoperations for PVL between 1995 and 2015 (10% had an attempted percutaneous closure).[8] Early mortality was 5%; survival at 1, 5, and 15 years was rather low, with 83%, 62%, and 16%, respectively. Recurrence occurred in 43 (21%) patients, and reoperation was required in 19 (9%) patients. Multivariate analysis revealed advanced New York Heart Association (NYHA) class, active endocarditis, chronic steroids, previous coronary artery bypass grafting, baseline creatinine above 1.5, postoperative need for dialysis, and residual PVL ($P < .0001$) to be predictors of late mortality. Medical therapy (including standard heart failure management and repeated blood transfusions n cases with hemolysis) can help with symptoms but will not prevent progressive heart failure from volume and/or pressure overload, nor the need for the frequent administration of blood products.

The next step in the workup should include a transesophageal echocardiogram (TEE). The advantage of this approach is less shadowing of mitral valve prostheses and thus a more defined view on the location and approachability of the PVL. The two-dimensional (2D) echocardiogram is routinely combined with three-dimensional (3D) imaging, which further facilitates procedural planning (Fig. 62.2).

Despite a circular or oval appearance on 3D TEE, many PVLs follow a serpiginous track, rather than being cylindrical. Thus on the echocardiographic images, the left atrial orifice of the defect may appear large (see Fig. 62.2) but the actual size of the track may be much smaller, requiring a smaller closure device than initially estimated. The serpiginous nature of the track can also make crossing of the leak with interventional equipment difficult.

OUTCOMES

Outcomes for percutaneous PVL closure have been reported by several high-volume centers of excellence. The first reports were published by the groups at Lennox Hill Hospital New York and Mayo Clinic Rochester. Ruiz et al. reported a retrospective review of 57 percutaneous PVL closure procedures in 43 patients between April 2006 and September 2010 (38 paramitral and 11 paraaortic leaks, some with multiple procedures).[9] Successful closure was achieved in 89% of paramitral leaks (68% biological, 32% mechanical) and 73% of paraaortic leaks (55% biological, 45% mechanical). A total of 28 out of 35 patients improved by at least one NYHA functional class (eight by two functional classes, and two by three functional classes). The percentage of patients requiring blood transfusions and/or erythropoietin injections postprocedure decreased from 56% to 5%. The survival rates for patients at 6, 12, and 18 months after PVL closures were 91.9%, 89.2%, and 86.5%, respectively. These data showed that percutaneous repair of aortic and mitral valve PVLs is a viable option, but mortality in this high-risk patient population (mean Society for Thoracic Surgeons (STS) risk score 6.7 ± 5.48) remains high with up to >35% after 3 years. These data demonstrate the potential for durable clinical efficacy, which is dependent on residual regurgitation.

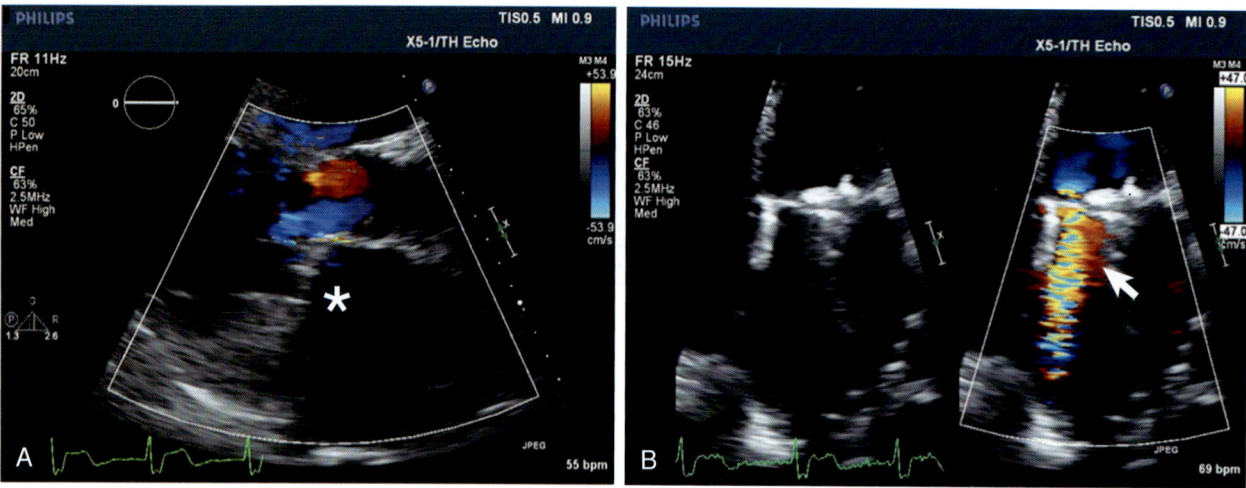

Fig. 62.1 Parasternal view (A) of the mitral valve prosthesis. The paravalvular leak is not visible in this view (*). In the four-chamber view (B) the medial paravalvular leak becomes visible (arrow). Even here, however, fine manipulations of the ultrasound probe were necessary to find the best color Doppler signal.

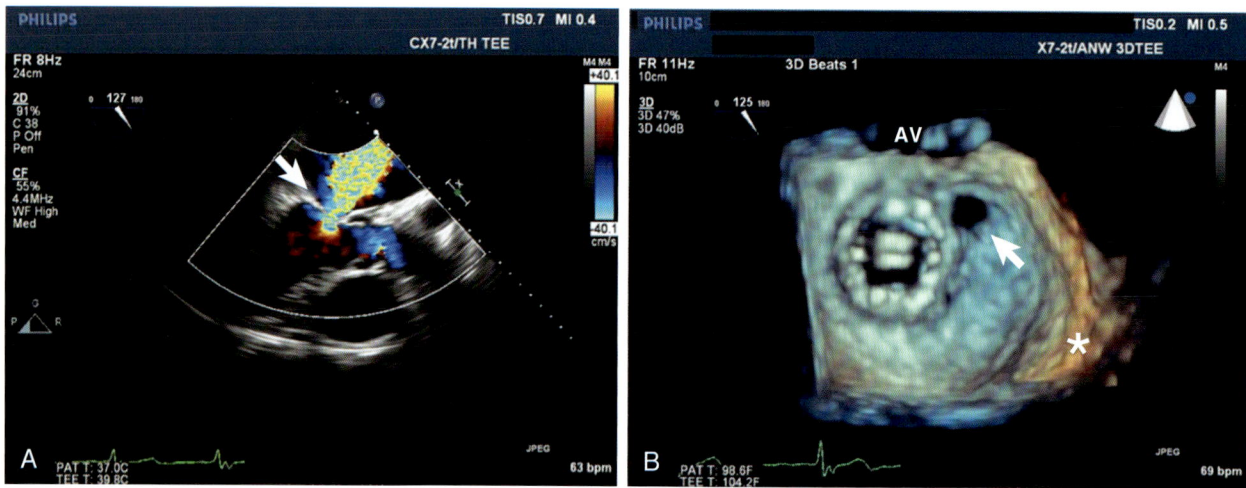

Fig. 62.2 Two-dimensional images (A) and 3D images (B) of the paravalvular leak (arrow), which reveal an anteromedial location of the paravalvular leak (the interatrial septum (*) as well as the aortic valve [AV] serve as anatomical markers for orientation purposes). The orifice of the paravalvular leak measured 7 to 8 mm in diameter.

Sorajja et al.[10] published the first prospectively collected acute and 30-day outcome data of 115 patients who underwent PVL closure at Mayo Clinic from February 2004 to September 2010 (15% of patients had multiple defects). Using strict criteria, closure was successful (i.e., ≤1+ residual regurgitation) in 77% of patients. The 30-day complication rate was 8.7% (sudden and unexplained death, 1.7%; stroke, 2.6%; emergency surgery, 0.9%; bleeding, 5.2%). Two devices embolized during the procedure and were retrieved without sequelae. No procedural deaths occurred, but two (1.7%) patients died by 30 days. The 3-year follow-up data (median follow-up was 11 months, range: 1 to 85 months) of the entire cohort demonstrated a 3-year estimate for survival free of all-cause mortality of 64.3%. Survival did not significantly differ for patients with no (69.9%), mild (62.4%), or moderate or severe (58.1%) residual regurgitation, before and after multivariate adjustment. The 3-year estimate of survival free of death or need for cardiac surgery was 63.7%, 59.0%, and 30.9% ($P = .01$), respectively.[11] Symptom improvement was confined to those patients who had no or only mild residual regurgitation after PVL closure, indicating near complete closure should be the goal of therapy. Hemolytic anemia was difficult to resolve and persisted in 14 of 29 survivors without an obvious relation between the degree of residual regurgitation and incidence of persistent hemolytic anemia.

More recently, Smolka et al. showed the importance of completeness of PVL closure in the setting of hemolysis.[12] In a limited study group of 116 patients (roughly 43% had signs of hemolysis), percutaneous PVL closure effectively reduced hemolysis if at least 90% reduction of PVL cross-sectional area was achieved.

Persistent hemolytic anemia has been shown to be an independent predictor for poor survival and need for cardiac surgery. Recently the Mayo Clinic authors updated their long-term outcome data, with a median follow-up length of 2.04 (0.7 to 4.9) years.[13] The longer follow-up led to a more differentiated outcome dependent on completeness of PVL closure. Alkhouli et al.[13] showed that of 231 patients with percutaneous PVL repair between 2006 and 2017, survival at 3 years was 61% in patients who had ≤ mild residual PVL and 47% in patients with higher grade of residual PVL ($P = .002$). Repeat surgical interventions were also more likely in patients with >mild residual PVL (6% vs. 17%; $P = .004$).

Similar results have been reported by Calvert et al., a combined UK and Ireland center of excellence experience (20 centers,

2004–15, 259 patients, median follow-up of 110 [7 to 452] days).[14] The one factor independently associated with major adverse cardiovascular events (MACE) was again the degree of persisting leak (>mild) at follow-up (hazard ratio [HR] 3.01; $P = .002$). In the Spanish HOLE registry (SpanisH real wOrld paravalvular LEaks closure), 469 patients at 19 centers were included.[15] The use of the Amplatzer III device (not available in the United States) and operator experience were independent predictors of procedural success in mitral PVLs; for aortic PVLs the only predictor of procedural success was the leak size (≥10 vs. <10 mm). The overall major adverse events rate (death or emergency surgery or stroke) at 30 days was 5.6%; the only predictor for combined adverse events was NYHA functional class IV (HR 4.2 [1.42 to 12.34]; $P = .009$).

Redo percutaneous PVL closure is associated with high complication rates. A limited study by Al-Hijji analyzed 16 redo PVL procedures at Mayo Clinic and compared them to successful first attempt procedures.[16] Procedural success was 75% (vs. 85% in the 1st attempt group); 30-day MACE was 12.5% in the redo group, compared with 4.2% in the age- and sex-matched patients who underwent PVL closure for the first time ($P = .35$).

While various devices for PVL closure have been used, none of these are U.S. Food and Drug Administration approved for this purpose. Commonly used devices off-label include the Amplatzer Septal Occluder, Duct Occluder, and Muscular Ventricular Septal Defect Occluder (St. Jude Medical, St. Paul, MN). These devices are woven from a larger-caliber nitinol mesh, resulting in a stiffer device with a higher profile, and may be associated with a greater risk of accelerating hemolysis. Our lab still prefers the Vascular Plug II as the primary device for PVL closure.

TRANSCATHETER CLOSURE VERSUS SURGICAL REPAIR

There are multiple reports comparing long-term results of transcatheter closure versus surgical repair. Zhang et al. analyzed outcomes of 87 consecutive patients with symptomatic PVL who received either transcatheter ($n = 46$) or surgical ($n = 41$) treatment at Shanghai Chest Hospital between January 2009 and December 2015.[17] Transcatheter closure was safer (MACE 56% vs. 17%; $P < .001$) and more cost-effective, but 13% of cases showed aggravation of hemolysis. The overall 5-year survival rates after transcatheter and surgical repair, however, were similar at 74% and 72%, respectively ($P = .45$).

Wells et al. analyzed 114 patients (56 underwent transcatheter closure, 58 underwent surgical repair) from 2017 to 2016.[18] There were no differences in the primary end point of a composite of death, reintervention for PVL, or readmission for congestive heart failure–related symptoms at 1 year (33.9% vs. 39.7%; $P = .53$) or 1-year survival (83.9% vs. 75.9%; $P = .28$). The largest data set come from the Mayo Clinic. Alkhouli et al. analyzed 381 patients who underwent transcatheter ($n = 195$) or surgical ($n = 186$) treatment of mitral PVL between 1995 and 2015. Technical success was higher (95.5% vs. 70.1%; $P < .001$), and in-hospital death occurred less often in the surgical group (3.1% vs. 8.6%, $P = .027$). After risk adjustment, however, there was no significant difference in long-term survival between patients who underwent surgical versus transcatheter treatment of PVLs.

Angulo-Llanos reviewed a one-center experience of percutaneous PVL procedures between years 2008 and 2014 ($n = 51$) and compared them to a cohort of surgical patients ($n = 36$) with a mean follow-up 785 days.[19] There were no differences in survival free from the composite end point (death from all causes and need for hospital readmission due to cardiovascular causes), according to the treatment received. However, after propensity score analysis in-hospital mortality was higher in the surgical group (30.6% vs. 9.8%, odds ratio 6, $P = .01$) and clinical improvement was higher in the percutaneous group (71.4% vs. 36.4%, $P = .002$).

Practice Guidelines

The current joint American Heart Association/American College of Cardiology guidelines for the management of valvular heart disease[20] give percutaneous PVL closure a IIA indication (reasonable approach) in patients with significant paravalvular regurgitation and symptoms NYHA III to IV who are high-risk surgical candidates, have a suitable anatomy, and undergo the procedure at a center with expertise. The European Society of Cardiology guidelines from 2012 on the management of valvular heart disease recommend reoperation if PVL is related to endocarditis, leads to hemolysis requiring repeated blood transfusions, or is associated with severe symptoms (class IC).[21] Transcatheter closure may be considered in selected cases in which reintervention is deemed high risk or is contraindicated. With regard to hemolysis related to the PVL, haptoglobin appears to be too sensitive and lactate dehydrogenase more closely related to the severity of hemolysis.

Percutaneous closure of the PVL is contraindicated when there are signs of active infection or there is significant dehiscence involving more than one-third of the valve ring.

GENERAL TECHNIQUES

Paramitral Defects

Paramitral leaks account for about 80% of PVL closures[9,10] and can be approached in a variety of ways. We favor an antegrade approach via a transseptal puncture. Real time 3D TEE is used for guidance of both the transseptal puncture as well as device deployment. For medially (especially postero-medially) located paramitral leaks, we prefer a high and posteriorly directed transseptal puncture so that there is enough room to maneuver within the left atrium. PVLs in other locations are usually readily accessed with standard transseptal punctures. Biplane fluoroscopy can be an additional, very helpful imaging tool. The PVL can be crossed in a right anterior oblique (RAO) view left anterior oblique (LAO) view of the valve, which provides the operator with a 3D understanding of wire position and direction.

Our standard equipment includes a 7- or 8-Fr Mullins dilator (with or without Mullins sheath), a standard transseptal needle, a preshaped guidewire (e.g., Inoue or Safari large curve), an Agilis small or medium curl steerable sheath (St. Jude Medical, Maple Grove, MN), a 0.035-inch, stiff j-tipped exchange length Glidewire (Terumo Medical Corp., Somerset, NJ), and a 5-Fr 125-cm multipurpose coronary catheter telescoped into a 6-Fr multipurpose coronary guiding catheter. For medially located leaks, we prefer the small curve Agilis sheath.

After the transseptal puncture and introduction of the Agilis-multipurpose-wire assembly into the left atrium, we steer the Agilis sheath towards the PVL using TEE and fluoroscopy imaging for guidance (Fig. 62.3). Once the defect is crossed with the Glidewire, both coronary catheters are advanced through the defect (Fig. 62.4). If crossing the defect with the catheters proves to be difficult, we choose a smaller catheter (i.e., a 4-Fr hydrophilic shuttle sheath, Cook Medical) to cross the defect or additional support; it may be necessary to exteriorize the wire that was used to cross the PVL. When using the transseptal approach, the wire can be exteriorized via the contralateral femoral artery (Figs. 62.5 and 62.6) or via the left ventricular apex. If the PVL cannot be crossed via the transseptal approach, a retrograde aortic (<2% occurrence) or transapical approach (10% occurrence) can be used.

Paraaortic Leaks

Paraaortic leaks account for about 20% of PVL closures and can almost always be approached via a retrograde aortic approach

(Fig. 62.7). Compared to paramitral leaks, paraaortic leaks tend to be smaller, and thus simultaneous or sequential closure device deployments are seldom necessary. Wire anchoring may still be necessary if multiple closure devices are planned to be placed. Except for posteriorly located leaks, for which TEE is preferable, transthoracic echocardiography is sufficient to guide the percutaneous closure of anteriorly located paraaortic leaks. Alternatively, intracardiac echocardiography can be used, but the experience with this imaging modality during PVL closure is limited. For adequate preprocedural planning, it may be beneficial to obtain computed tomographic images of the leak location, width, and length.

Crossing of the paraaortic leak with a 0.035-inch, stiff Glidewire is facilitated using a telescoped 125-cm 5-Fr multipurpose coronary catheter and 6-Fr multipurpose guide, respectively. Alternatively, if initial steering of the Glidewire into the defect is difficult, an Amplatzer left 1 coronary catheter can be used. If crossing of the defect is smooth, an anchor wire may not be necessary, otherwise the defect is crossed with a catheter and the Glidewire exchanged for a stiffer wire (e.g., a 0.032-inch Amplatzer extra-stiff exchange length guidewire).

PVLs after transcatheter aortic valve replacement (TAVR) can be approached in a similar fashion. Wiring the leak, however, may be somewhat more challenging, especially with current self-expanding valves (Evolute, CoreValve); often, a slightly higher crossing point within the valve's stent structure is necessary to facilitate smooth advancement of delivery catheters.[22] Since most para-TAVR leaks are small, crossing of the defect with a 5-Fr glide catheter and delivery of an AVP 4 may be sufficient and/or the only feasible option.

SPECIFIC TECHNIQUES

Double Wire—Simultaneous Deployment for Paramitral Leaks

A 20-Fr, large-bore, venous sheath to minimize blood loss from the groin access is useful. After crossing the defect with an initial 6-Fr multipurpose guide, two 0.032-inch exchange length Amplatzer extra-stiff wires are placed within the left ventricle (LV) (with a formed curve to match LV size) and the guide is removed. Using both wires, two appropriately sized delivery catheters (either the same size or one bigger and one smaller) can be advanced across the defect. The wires are removed, and the Amplatzer devices loaded and deployed in a simultaneous fashion.[23]

Anchor, Single Wire Technique—Sequential Deployment

If the operator estimates that the defect is not large enough for two simultaneous delivery catheter placements, but too large for one closure device, only one 0.032-inch exchange length Amplatzer extra-stiff wire will be placed within the LV cavity. A 6-Fr multipurpose guide will accept only a relatively small AVT II; hence replacing the guide with a Cook Shuttle catheter, which has a larger internal diameter, is often necessary. Leaving the wire within the delivery catheter allows deployment of an AVP II without losing access to the LV. After deployment of the AVPII, the delivery catheter is removed and placed back over the Amplatzer 0.032-inch wire only, leaving the AVP II wire outside the delivery catheter. Using this remaining rail, an appropriately sized delivery catheter can be used to recross the defect (along the 0.032-inch Amplatzer wire). This technique can be used even if three or more devices are needed. The anchor technique is also useful if the operator fears losing access across the defect during attempts of closure device deployment.[24]

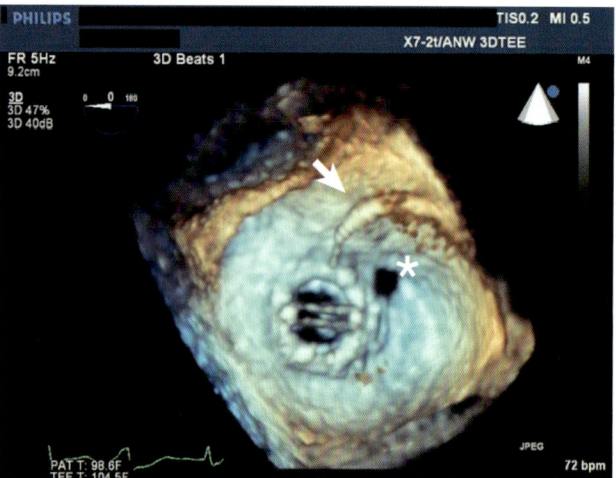

Fig. 62.3 Agilis catheter *(arrow)* after transseptal puncture, steering toward the anteromedial paravalvular leak (*).

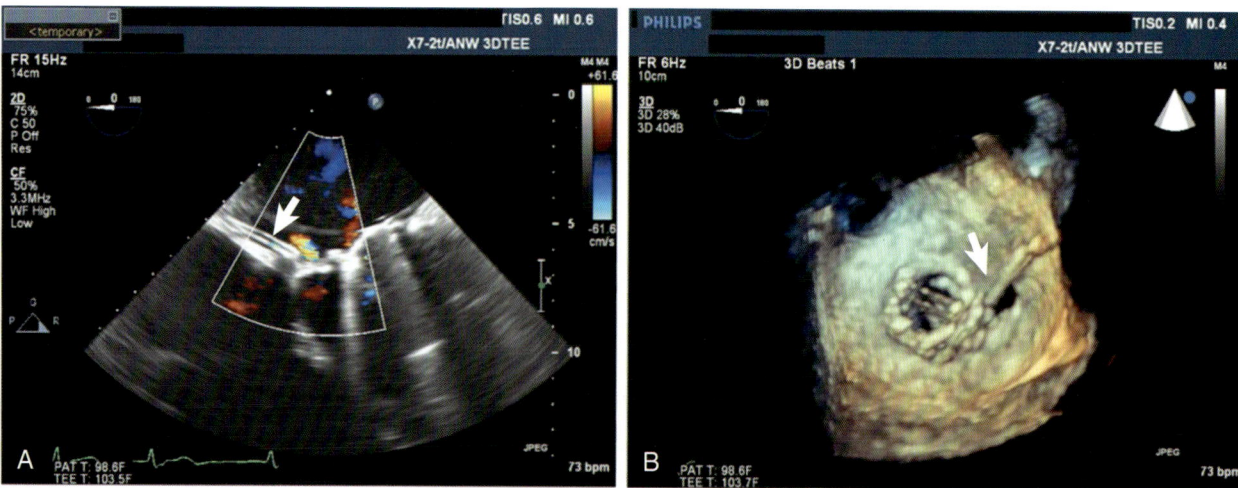

Fig. 62.4 The defect is successfully crossed with the wire and guiding catheters. (A) The two-dimensional view (*arrow* indicates the catheter crossing the paravalvular leak). (B) The catheter crossing the leak in three-dimensional *(arrow)*.

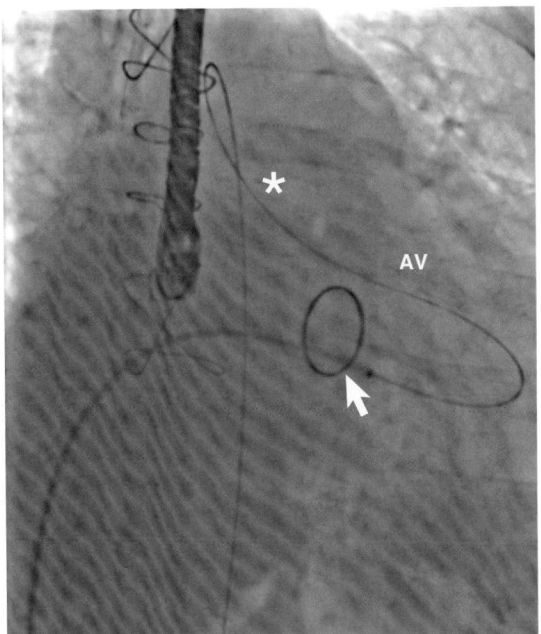

Fig. 62.5 Venoarterial rail. The figure shows a fluoroscopic picture of our patient. The Glidewire (*) is steered through the paravalvular leak (arrow) and the aortic valve (AV) and eventually exteriorized via the contra-lateral femoral artery.

Modified Anchor Technique—Single or Sequential Deployment Using an Arteriovenous Rail

If a more stable rail is needed for device deployment, a small modification of the anchor technique can be used. The Glidewire used to cross the defect is snared and exteriorized to the contralateral femoral artery creating an arterio-venous rail. Exteriorization is achieved by sending the Glidewire into the ascending aorta and capturing it there with a snare device (e.g., EnSnare, Hatch Medical, Duluth, GA). The arterio-venous Glidewire rail can be used similarly to the 0.032-inch Amplatzer anchor wire described in the previous section.

The AVP II and other closure devices may change their configuration once released by counterclockwise rotation of the delivery wire. It is, therefore, pivotal to "wiggle" the device by careful but determined pushing and pulling on the delivery wire and/or sheath. This push-pull maneuver also ascertains that the closure device does not slip into the left atrium or LV after release.

With taller patients, we prefer to use 100- or 110-cm long Shuttle sheaths, as 90-cm long sheaths may be too short.

SPECIAL SITUATIONS

Sewn or patched interatrial septa can be very difficult to cross with standard transseptal equipment. Occasionally, application of surgical cautery or radiofrequency energy is needed to facilitate crossing. At times, left ventricular apical puncture may be required for paramitral leak closure, either as the primary access or for wire exteriorization. After assessing the coronary anatomy with left coronary angiography (usually in an LAO cranial and an RAO caudal view) and determining the best puncture site and trajectory with transthoracic echocardiography, we use a 5-Fr/10-cm long paracardiocentesis needle (OneStep, Merit Medical, UT) to access the left ventricular cavity. If smaller caliber sheaths (4 or 5 Fr) are used, closure of the apical puncture site is not necessary. Larger sheaths (6- to 7-Fr) may be necessary, especially if a snaring device like the EnSnare is being used for wire exteriorization. In those instances, the apical puncture is closed with a 6-mm Amplatzer ductal occluder. Alternatively, a small surgical apical window (similar to transapical TAVR/transcatheter mitral valve repair procedures) can be considered for direct visualization of the apical puncture and better bleeding control.

COMPLICATIONS

Procedure-related complications include valve leaflet impingement, stroke, hemothorax, device embolization, and complications associated with transseptal puncture. External coronary artery compression when placing closure devices around the mitral ring is theoretically possible, but we have not observed it. A feared complication is the obstruction of a tilting-disk valve leaflet or the impingement of a mechanical or bioprosthetic valve leaflet during device deployment. With proper angulation, mechanical valve obstruction/leaflet impingement is easily recognized with fluoroscopy. Obstruction or impingement of bioprosthetic leaflets may be more difficult to recognize, but echocardiographic evidence of sudden valvular regurgitation or an increased transvalvular gradient are important indices for this complication. Albeit rare, device interference with a valve leaflet opening and closing mechanism can occur after device release due to tilting of the closure device. In this instance, the closure device can be pulled through the defect or retrogradely with a snare or a long, flexible bioptome.

In the rare instance that the closure device embolizes, retrieval attempts using snares or bioptomes can be undertaken. Devices typically embolize past the carotid arteries and lodge at the aortic bifurcation or common iliac arteries. Unless the embolized device is stretched by simultaneous proximal and distal snares, 8- to 10-Fr sheaths are necessary for safe retrieval.

Paraaortic leak closure may lead to coronary artery ostia obstruction. Aortography or selective coronary angiography may be needed to assess ostial clearance, especially if the PVL is located in close proximity to a coronary ostium and the ostial height is low (<10 mm).

Posterolateral paramitral leaks are located close to the left atrioventricular groove. Device closure in this location could theoretically lead to circumflex coronary artery obstruction.

Strokes are often hemorrhagic in nature, related to transitions of the anticoagulation regimen; we have not observed thromboembolic strokes. Careful attention to catheter flushing and adequate anticoagulation with an activated clotting time of 250 to 300 seconds are key in preventing thromboembolic complications.

When it is necessary to perform a left ventricular apical puncture for wire stabilization, a hemothorax may occur. Coronary artery injury, chest wall artery bleeds, as well as leaks through the Amplatzer 6-mm vascular plug used for closure of the apical puncture, are possible reasons for this complication. We perform left coronary artery angiography before and after puncture (RAO caudal and LAO cranial views) to assess the coronary anatomy at the apex and guide the apical puncture with echocardiography and fluoroscopy to avoid coronary artery severing. If a coronary artery laceration is diagnosed, it can be treated with immediate embolization with coils. Chest wall bleeds and vascular plug leaks are harder to assess or predict, and our lab does not use Floseal (Baxter, California) due to possible compound embolization into the ventricular cavity/systemic circulation. Creating a minimal left thoracic window for a safe apical puncture under direct visualization is another option. Bleeding from common sources like the intercostal muscles and the chest wall can potentially be avoided, and bleeding complications, as well as patient discomfort, are thus further minimized.

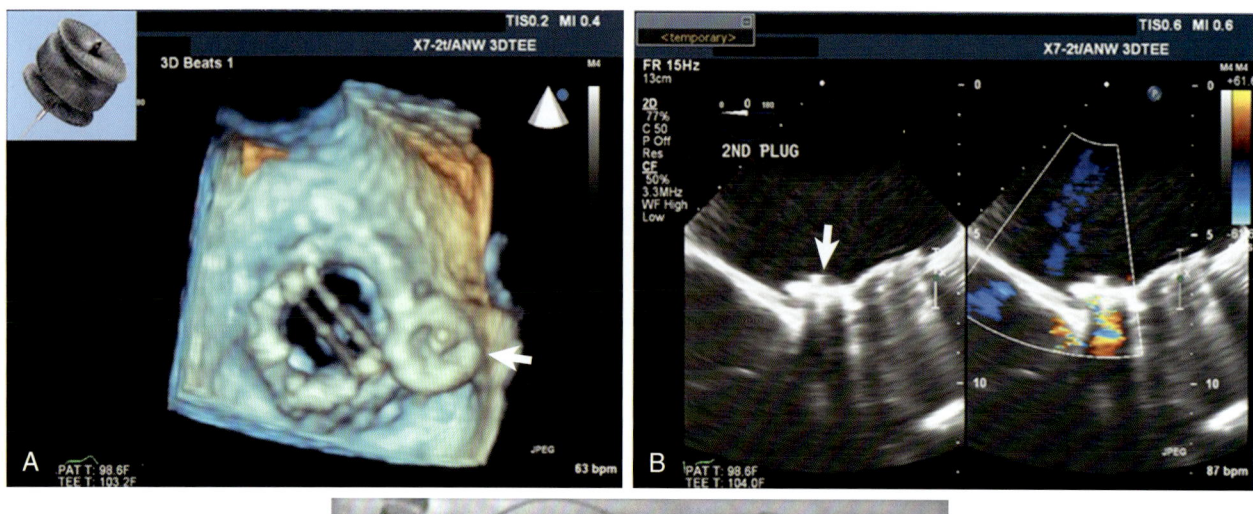

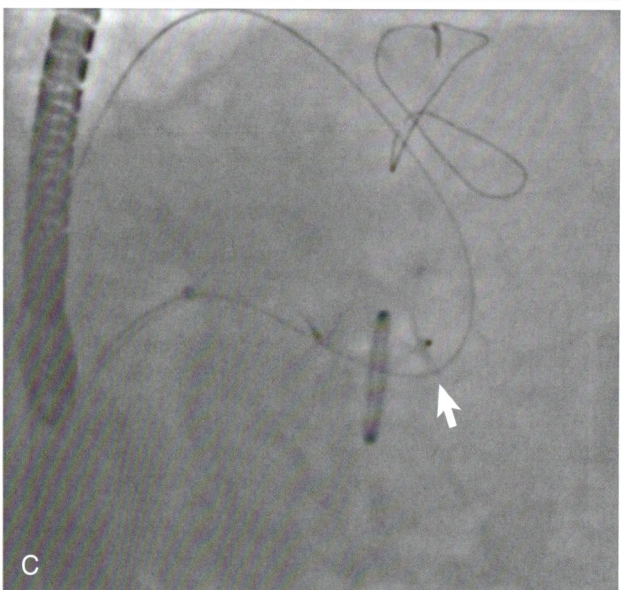

Fig. 62.6 (A) The successfully deployed AVP II within the former paravalvular leak *(arrow)* is shown, with a photograph of an AVP II vascular plug (St. Jude Medical) shown in the left upper corner. (B) The vascular plug in two-dimensional echocardiography *(arrow)* is shown. (B) The color Doppler image demonstrates no significant regurgitation through the paravalvular leak. (C) The deployed vascular plug *(arrow)* under fluoroscopy is shown.

FOLLOW-UP

We generally recommend 81 mg daily aspirin for 6 months (unless otherwise indicated) and clopidogrel for 3 months. Endocarditis prophylaxis is recommended for 6 months. In the particular case of a patient with severe coronary artery disease and permanent atrial fibrillation, we preferred to avoid triple antithrombotic therapy, and we elected to use warfarin with low dose aspirin. Surveillance transthoracic echocardiograms are performed before hospital discharge and on first routine clinical follow-up.

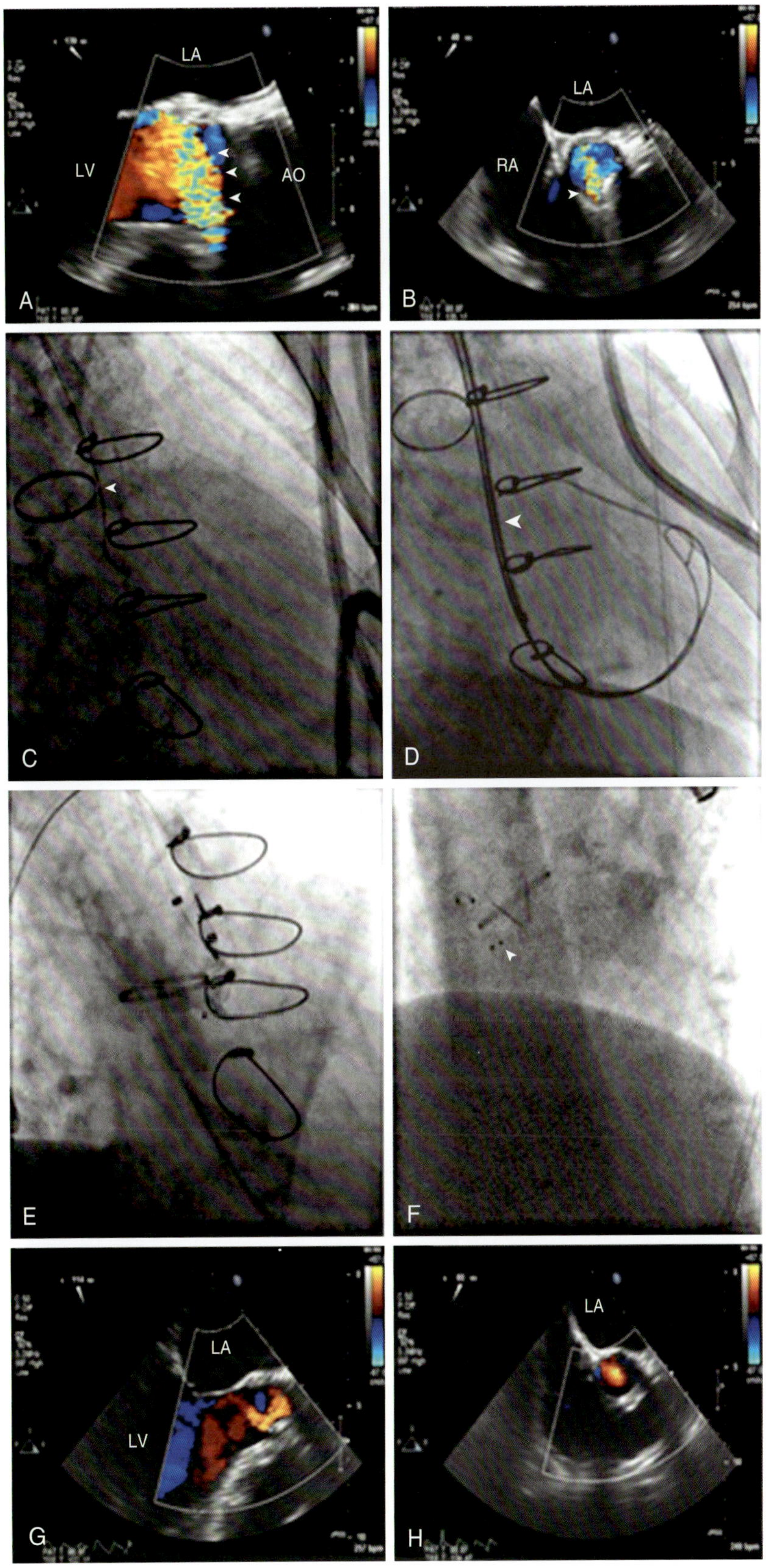

Fig. 62.7 Transesophageal echocardiography demonstrates severe anterior paravalvular regurgitation *(arrowheads)* in a long-axis (A) and short-axis view (B). (C) An AL-1 diagnostic catheter, placed from the right femoral artery, is steered toward the defect, which is then crossed with a 260-cm, angle-tipped, extra-stiff Glidewire *(arrowhead;* Terumo, Ann Arbor, MI). (D) Over the Glidewire, a 90-cm, 8-Fr Flexor Shuttle *(arrowhead;* Cook Medical, Bloomington, IN) is passed into the left ventricle, followed by placement of two 0.032-inch extra-stiff Amplatz wires. Over these two wires, two separate 6-Fr Flexor Shuttle sheaths are advanced into the left ventricle. The distal retention discs of two 10-mm AVP-2 plugs (St. Jude Medical, St. Paul, MN) are extruded in the left ventricle, followed by retraction and apposition against the left ventricular side (E) and deployed (F, *arrowhead*). The final view is chosen to demonstrate normal prosthetic leaflet motion. Postprocedural transesophageal echocardiography in long-axis (G) and short-axis views (H) demonstrates mild residual regurgitation. *AO,* Aorta; *LA,* left atrium; *LV,* left ventricle; *RA,* right atrium.

KEY REFERENCES

1. Kort HW, Sharkey AM, Balzer DT. Novel use of the Amplatzer duct occluder to close paravalvar leak involving a prosthetic mitral valve. *Catheter Cardiovasc Interv*. 2004;61(4):548–551.
8. Said SM, Schaff HV, Greason KL, et al. Reoperation for mitral paravalvular leak: a single-centre experience with 200 patients. *Interact Cardiovasc Thorac Surg*. 2017;25(5):806–812.
9. Ruiz CE, Jelnin V, Kronzon I, et al. Clinical outcomes in patients undergoing percutaneous closure of paraprosthetic paravalvular leaks. *J Am Coll Cardiol*. 2011;58(21):2210–2217.
10. Sorajja P, Cabalka AK, Hagler DJ, et al. Percutaneous repair of paravalvular prosthetic regurgitation: acute and 30-day outcomes in 115 patients. *Circ Cardiovasc Interv*. 2011;4(4):314–321.
11. Sorajja P, Cabalka AK, Hagler DJ, et al. Long-term follow-up of percutaneous repair of paravalvular prosthetic regurgitation. *J Am Coll Cardiol*. 2011;58(21):2218–2224.
14. Calvert PA, Northridge DB, Malik IS, et al. Percutaneous device closure of paravalvular leak: combined experience from the United Kingdom and Ireland. *Circulation*. 2016;134(13):934–944.
15. Garcia E, Arzamendi D, Jimenez-Quevedo P, et al. Outcomes and predictors of success and complications for paravalvular leak closure: an analysis of the SpanisH real-wOrld paravalvular LEaks closure (HOLE) registry. *EuroIntervention*. 2017;12(16):1962–1968.
17. Zhang Y, Pan X, Qu X, et al. Comparison of transcatheter and surgical treatment of paravalvular leak: results from a 5-year follow-up study. *Catheter Cardiovasc Interv*. 2017. [Epub ahead of print.].
19. Angulo-Llanos R, Sarnago-Cebada F, Rivera AR, et al. Two-year follow up after surgical versus percutaneous paravalvular leak closure: a nonrandomized analysis. *Catheter Cardiovasc Interv*. 2016;88(4):626–634.
22. Waterbury TM, Reeder GS, Pislaru SV, et al. Techniques and outcomes of paravalvular leak repair after transcatheter aortic valve replacement. *Catheter Cardiovasc Interv*. 2017;90(5):870–877.
23. Gossl M, Rihal CS. Percutaneous treatment of aortic and mitral valve paravalvular regurgitation. *Curr Cardiol Rep*. 2013;15(8):388.
24. Binder RK, Webb JG. Percutaneous mitral and aortic paravalvular leak repair: indications, current application, and future directions. *Curr Cardiol Rep*. 2013;15(3):342.

Additional references available online at expertconsult.com

中文导读

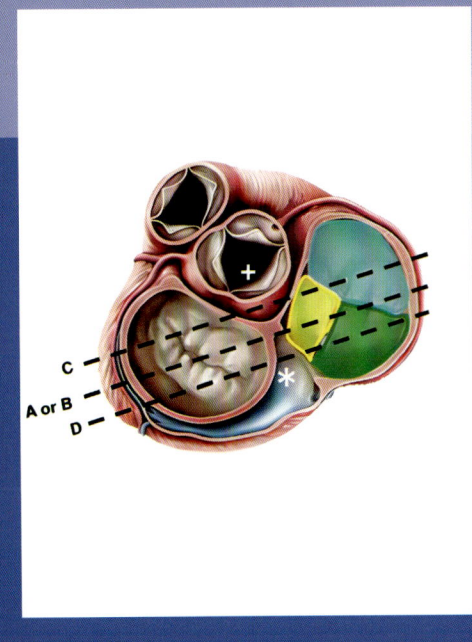

第63章
心力衰竭介入治疗

　　心力衰竭是一个日益严重的公共卫生问题，患者反复出现临床症状，生活质量差，给个人及社会造成了巨大负担。心力衰竭和介入心脏病学领域的融合促进了心力衰竭介入治疗的发展，干预措施通常针对原发性或继发性瓣膜病、左心室扩张或病理生理重塑、左心房和肺动脉压力升高或心排出量减少，以改善心脏结构、功能和血流动力学。本章节详细介绍了心力衰竭介入相关治疗方法包括经导管主动脉瓣置换术、经皮二尖瓣修复术（MitraClip经皮治疗）、经皮或杂交心室分割或重建、心房分流术和植入式血流动力学监测仪，阐述了它们的治疗原理、应用前景和研究现状。其中，除了经导管主动脉瓣置换术、MitraClip和CardioMEMS心力衰竭系统的肺动脉压力监测外，大多数介入性心力衰竭设备仍在研究中。即便如此，我们相信心力衰竭介入治疗新领域的未来将大有可为。

杨　城　吴永健

章节要点

- 尽管目前有较为完备的指南指导药物和电生理设备治疗，但许多心力衰竭患者的症状仍频繁发作，治疗效果仍然不佳。亟须新的治疗方法来改善患者的临床状况和预后。
- 心力衰竭的某些病因可以通过介入设备进行治疗，这一发现拓展了心力衰竭介入治疗领域的出现。
- 心力衰竭干预靶点包括原发性或继发性瓣膜病、左心室扩张或病理生理重塑、左心房高压、肺动脉高压和心排血量减少。
- 干预措施包括经导管主动脉瓣置换术、经皮二尖瓣修复术、经皮或杂交心室分割或修复术、心房分流术设备和植入式血流动力学监测仪。
- 除了经导管主动脉瓣置换术、经皮二尖瓣修复术（如MitraClip系统）和肺动脉压力监测（如CardioMEMS系统），大多数设备仍在研究中，以用于心力衰竭患者。
- 严重主动脉瓣狭窄是心力衰竭的潜在可逆原因。经导管主动脉瓣置换术改善症状并延长存在心力衰竭和中、高手术风险严重主动脉瓣狭窄患者的生存率。
- 功能性二尖瓣反流导致进行性心力衰竭的恶性循环，几种经皮二尖瓣修复和置换方法的初步发现令人鼓舞。
- 前壁心肌梗死后病理性左室重构导致进行性心力衰竭。经皮或杂交心室分割或重建设备旨在恢复更正常的椭圆左心室几何形状，减少心室容积，降低舒张末期压力，改善症状和预后。
- 左心房和肺动脉压力升高会增加心力衰竭的风险，心房间分流装置可以降低收缩性和舒张性心力衰竭患者的左心房压力，改善血流动力学和症状。
- 植入式血流动力学监测仪可以指导药物治疗的改变，以降低左心房和肺动脉压力，减少心力衰竭住院的发生率。
- 介入心脏病学和心力衰竭领域的融合可以进一步指导心力衰竭患者的治疗。

63 Interventional Heart Failure

Scott M. Lilly, William T. Abraham

KEY POINTS

- Despite current guideline-directed drug and electrophysiologic device therapies, many heart failure patients remain highly symptomatic, and outcomes remain poor. New therapies are needed to improve patients' clinical status and outcomes.
- Several causes of heart failure are amenable to interventional device-based therapies, an observation that led to emergence of the field of interventional heart failure.
- Interventional heart failure targets include primary or secondary valve disease, left ventricular dilation or pathophysiologic remodeling, elevated left atrial and pulmonary artery pressures, and reduced cardiac output.
- Interventions include transcatheter aortic valve replacement (TAVR), percutaneous mitral valve repair, percutaneous or hybrid ventricular partitioning or restoration, interatrial shunt devices, and implantable hemodynamic monitors.
- With the exception of TAVR, percutaneous mitral valve repair (e.g., MitraClip system), and pulmonary artery pressure monitoring (e.g., CardioMEMS system), most devices remain under investigation for use in heart failure patients.
- Severe aortic stenosis is a potentially reversible cause of heart failure. TAVR improves symptoms and prolongs survival of patients with heart failure and severe aortic stenosis at intermediate and higher surgical risk.
- Functional mitral regurgitation contributes to the vicious cycle of progressive heart failure, and preliminary findings for several percutaneous approaches to mitral valve repair and replacement are encouraging.
- Pathologic left ventricular remodeling after anterior myocardial infarction leads to progressive heart failure. Percutaneous or hybrid ventricular partitioning or reconstruction devices aim to restore a more normal elliptical left ventricular geometry and reduce ventricular volume, reducing end-diastolic pressure, and improving symptoms and outcomes.
- Elevated left atrial and pulmonary artery pressures increase the risk of heart failure, and interatrial shunt devices can lower left atrial pressure and improve hemodynamics and symptoms in systolic and diastolic heart failure patients.
- Implantable hemodynamic monitors can guide changes in pharmacologic therapies to accomplish reductions in left atrial and pulmonary artery pressures, reducing the incidence of heart failure hospitalizations.
- Convergence between the fields of interventional cardiology and heart failure is needed to guide the application of therapies for these patients.

INTRODUCTION

Heart failure is a growing public health problem. An estimated 5.1 million Americans have heart failure, and 825,000 new cases are diagnosed each year in the United States.[1] By the year 2030, the U.S. prevalence of heart failure is expected to exceed 8 million people.[2] Beyond these numbers, heart failure imposes an enormous burden on patients, caregivers, and the health care system.

New approaches are needed to improve the clinical status and outcomes of heart failure patients. Despite current drug and electrophysiologic device therapies, many patients have moderate to severe symptoms, a poor quality of life, and substantial limitations in exercise capacity. They are also at considerable risk for heart failure–related morbidity (e.g., hospitalization) and mortality.[3] Heart failure is the primary diagnosis in more than 1 million hospital admissions annually in the United States.[1] It is also associated with the highest rate of hospital readmissions compared with all other medical and surgical causes of hospitalization.[4] In 2012, due in large measure to the high rates of hospitalization and rehospitalization, the U.S. total economic burden from heart failure was estimated at $31 billion.[1]

The convergence of the fields of heart failure and interventional cardiology has produced a discipline called *interventional heart failure*. Although the term may be applied to virtually any invasive procedure performed in heart failure patients (e.g., diagnostic coronary angiography, percutaneous coronary intervention, invasive assessment of hemodynamics), it is more commonly reserved for the application of invasive therapeutic procedures intended to improve the clinical status and outcomes of heart failure patients.

Interventions usually target primary or secondary valve disease, left ventricular dilation or pathophysiologic remodeling, elevated left atrial and pulmonary artery pressures, or reduced cardiac output to improve cardiac structure, function, and hemodynamics. Myocardial ischemia is excluded from this list of interventional heart failure targets because coronary revascularization has not proved a beneficial heart failure therapy,[5] although it may be useful for the treatment of symptomatic angina in heart failure patients.[3]

Interventional heart failure procedures and devices include transcatheter aortic valve replacement (TAVR), percutaneous mitral valve repair (i.e., MitraClip percutaneous therapy), percutaneous or hybrid ventricular partitioning or restoration, interatrial shunt devices, and implantable hemodynamic monitors. With the exception of TAVR, MitraClip, and pulmonary artery pressure monitoring with the CardioMEMS heart failure system, most interventional heart failure devices remain under investigation in heart failure patients.

At least one form of neuromodulation (i.e., renal denervation) may be considered an interventional heart failure procedure when applied to the treatment of these patients, but it is not discussed in this chapter. Other forms of neuromodulation, including baroreflex activation therapy,[6,7] vagal nerve stimulation,[8,9] spinal cord stimulation,[10] and phrenic nerve stimulation,[11,12] involve the implantation of pulse stimulators and stimulation leads, and they are considered to be surgical or electrophysiologic interventions.

TRANSCATHETER AORTIC VALVE REPLACEMENT

Heart failure in patients with aortic stenosis carries a grave prognosis. If the aortic valve is not replaced, patients with heart failure due to aortic stenosis have a 2-year mortality rate of 50%.[13] In the setting of aortic stenosis, heart failure results from left ventricular hypertrophy with diastolic dysfunction or left ventricular dilation with systolic dysfunction, or both. Because heart failure results from the excess afterload caused by aortic stenosis, aortic valve replacement often leads to symptom improvement and a favorable outcomes, especially when the preoperative gradient across the aortic valve is high or a good contractile reserve has been demonstrated when the gradient is low.[14]

Aortic valve replacement is recommended in patients with severe aortic stenosis and symptomatic heart failure with an aortic velocity of 4.0 m/s or greater or a mean pressure gradient of 40 mm Hg or higher.[15] In asymptomatic patients, valve replacement is indicated when the left ventricular ejection fraction (LVEF) is less than 50%. In patients with an LVEF less than 50%, a calculated valve area less than 1.0 cm^2 but not meeting velocity or gradient criteria, low-flow, low-gradient severe aortic stenosis must be suspected. In these patients, a low-dose dobutamine stress study should be performed. If the study shows an aortic velocity of 4.0 m/s or greater, or a mean pressure gradient of 40 mm Hg or higher at any dobutamine dose, aortic valve replacement is recommended.[15] Few data are available regarding TAVR for patients with low surgical risk and patients with bicuspid aortic valves. Therefore, surgical aortic valve replacement is currently recommended for these patient subgroups. Surgical aortic valve replacement in patients with a reduced LVEF can significantly improve or normalize the LVEF and improve survival.[16,17]

An alternative to surgical aortic valve replacement in patients at intermediate or higher surgical risk is TAVR.[18] The Placement of Aortic Transcatheter Valves (PARTNER) trial compared TAVR with standard therapy in high-risk patients with severe aortic stenosis and cardiac symptoms, including a cohort of patients who were not considered to be suitable candidates for surgery (i.e., Cohort B). Of the patients randomized in Cohort B, 93% exhibited New York Heart Association (NYHA) class III or IV symptoms at baseline, compatible with an advanced degree of heart failure. TAVR significantly improved the NYHA class ranking compared with ongoing medical therapy alone. In this cohort, there was a statistically significant 45% reduction in death from any cause for patients treated with TAVR compared with medically treated patients.[19] These benefits were sustained at 2 years.[20]

Data from PARTNER Cohort A (i.e., TAVR vs. surgical aortic valve replacement) demonstrated significant improvement in LVEF with TAVR (from $35.7 \pm 8.5\%$ to $48.6 \pm 11.3\%$, $P < .0001$), comparable to that seen with surgical aortic valve replacement.[21] In addition, mortality did not differ between those assigned to TAVR compared with surgical valve replacement through 5 years of follow-up.[22]

These observations were extended in intermediate surgical risk groups in two large trials, PARTNER II (employing the Edwards SAPIEN valve) and Safety and Efficacy Study of the Medtronic CoreValve System in the Treatment of Severe, Symptomatic Aortic Stenosis in Intermediate Risk Subjects Who Need Aortic Valve Replacement (SURTAVI) (Medtronic CoreValve). These trials established comparable mortality and improvements in quality of life in patients with severe aortic stenosis undergoing surgical and TAVR.[23,24] A consistent finding across all contemporary TAVR trials is a higher rate of pacemaker implantation, and greater residual paravalvular leak than that observed with surgical valve replacement. However, as technical experience, procedural efficiencies, and device improvements are realized, these rates have declined, and the ancillary benefits of TAVR (shorter length of stay, cost) may eventually make this approach standard of care.

Today, TAVR is a reasonable option for the treatment of symptomatic heart failure in patients with severe aortic stenosis at intermediate or higher surgical risk. The Edwards SAPIEN and Medtronic CoreValve are TAVR devices with U.S. Food and Drug Administration (FDA) approval. Numerous alternative TAVR devices are under investigation. In addition, as the procedural risks from TAVR continue to decline, additional populations that may benefit are being evaluated. Among these are patients with severe symptomatic aortic stenosis and low surgical risk scores, as well as patients with moderate aortic stenosis and symptoms of heart failure. These trials will collectively inform the management of aortic stenosis across the risk and severity spectrum, and stand to considerably change the approach to aortic valve disease in large populations.

PERCUTANEOUS MITRAL VALVE REPAIR

Functional mitral regurgitation is common in patients with ischemic and nonischemic dilated cardiomyopathy. Some degree of functional mitral regurgitation usually exists in these patients, and 50% of heart failure patients with an LVEF of less than or equal to 35% exhibit moderate or severe functional mitral regurgitation.[25,26]

The cause of functional mitral regurgitation in dilated cardiomyopathy is complex but usually is related to increased left ventricular sphericity and apical and posterior displacement of papillary muscles.[27,28] The severity of functional mitral regurgitation in heart failure is an independent predictor of poor outcome. For example, severe functional mitral regurgitation is associated with a twofold increase in the mortality rate for patients with ischemic and nonischemic cardiomyopathy.[29]

After functional mitral regurgitation ensues in the setting of heart failure, it contributes to a vicious cycle of progressive left ventricular dilation or dysfunction and worsening of the functional mitral regurgitation (Fig. 63.1). Several heart failure therapies can break this vicious cycle and reduce the severity of functional mitral regurgitation by promoting reverse remodeling of the left ventricle. Examples include evidence-based β-blockers and cardiac resynchronization.[30,31] These therapies significantly reduce left ventricular volumes, improve the left ventricular sphericity index (i.e., restore the normal elliptical geometry of the left ventricle), increase the LVEF, and reduce functional mitral regurgitation. They also significantly reduce morbidity and mortality rates for heart failure patients.

Targeting functional mitral regurgitation to break the vicious cycle of progressive heart failure and worsening functional mitral regurgitation (see Fig. 63.1) may also improve patients' clinical status and outcomes. Evidence to support this idea is lacking, and carefully conducted, prospective, randomized, controlled trials that address this issue are needed.

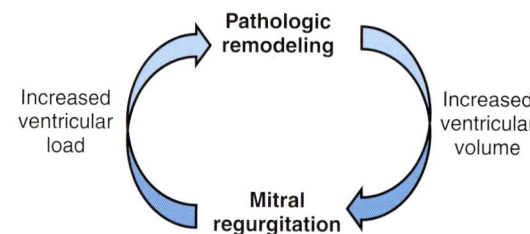

Fig. 63.1 Pathologic left ventricular remodeling leads to increased left ventricular volume with an increase in left ventricular sphericity and apical and posterior displacement of the papillary muscles, resulting in functional mitral regurgitation. Functional mitral regurgitation increases the left ventricular load, resulting in additional left ventricular dilation and dysfunction.

In the absence of definitive evidence, heart failure guidelines offer only a very weak recommendation (i.e., class IIb) for valve surgery for severe functional mitral regurgitation.[3] Many heart failure specialists do not refer these patients for surgical valve repair with ongoing pharmacologic therapy and, if indicated cardiac, resynchronization therapy, constituting the mainstay of treatment for functional mitral regurgitation in heart failure. Physicians are reluctant to refer heart failure patients with severe functional mitral regurgitation for surgical valve repair because of a lack of proof of efficacy and concerns about surgical morbidity and mortality.

Catheter-based alternatives to surgical mitral valve repair have been developed. A percutaneous approach to mitral valve repair using the MitraClip system (Abbott) is approved for the treatment of degenerative mitral regurgitation (Fig. 63.2A). The device is intended for the percutaneous reduction of significant symptomatic mitral regurgitation (≥3+) due to a primary abnormality of the mitral apparatus (i.e., degenerative mitral regurgitation) in patients who are at prohibitive surgical risk for mitral valve surgery.

The feasibility of the percutaneous approach using the MitraClip system was demonstrated in the first Endovascular Valve Edge-to-Edge Repair Study (EVEREST I). This was followed by EVEREST II, a randomized, controlled trial that enrolled patients who had an indication for and could undergo mitral valve surgery.[32] The trial enrolled patients with degenerative (73%) and functional (27%) mitral regurgitation. The study demonstrated the superior safety of the MitraClip device compared with mitral valve surgery, although the degree of mitral regurgitation reduction was somewhat less and the rate of subsequent mitral valve surgery was higher in the MitraClip group.

Despite the difference favoring surgery, reduction in left ventricular size was demonstrated in the MitraClip and surgery groups, and similar improvements were seen in both groups for NYHA class ranking and quality of life scores. Shorter intensive care unit time, shorter overall hospital length of stay, and a lower requirement for nursing or rehabilitation care after hospitalization were seen with MitraClip compared with mitral valve surgery.

Given the modest size of the EVEREST II trial (i.e., 60 device roll-in patients, 184 patients randomized to the device, and 95 control subjects) and the relatively low percentage of functional mitral regurgitation patients enrolled, the study was not considered to be a definitive test of percutaneous mitral valve repair in functional mitral regurgitation. EVEREST II selected patients with functional mitral regurgitation who could be randomized to surgical valve repair or replacement, rather than treated with standard optimal medical treatment.[3] The Cardiovascular Outcomes Assessment of the MitraClip Percutaneous Therapy for Heart Failure Patients with Functional Mitral Regurgitation (COAPT) trial was preformed to address these issues.

The COAPT trial enrolled 614 patients with heart failure, moderate-severe or greater mitral regurgitation, and symptomatic despite goal-directed medical therapy. Importantly, this is a population of patients in whom surgical therapies have not had a demonstrable benefit in mortality or heart failure–related hospitalization. Participants were randomized to MitraClip with medical therapy, or continued medical therapy alone. Patients who received MitraClip therapy had fewer heart failure hospitalizations at 24 months (primary end point; 36% device arm, 68% medical therapy alone, $P < .001$). Additionally, overall mortality was lower at 24 months in patients who received MitraClip (29% vs. 46%, $P < .001$).[33] Based on these observations, MitraClip was approved by the FDA in March 2019 for the treatment of moderate-severe or greater mitral regurgitation in patients with heart failure.

The original MitraClip was partly modified (Mitraclip NT) to permit broader opening of the clip. This change was undertaken in an effort to make the procedure more efficient, permit the grasping of leaflets with a wider range of anatomies (e.g., more significant prolapse), and to reduce the risk of single leaflet detachment. The MitraClip NT device is now available for commercial use.

Other percutaneous mitral valve repair technologies have also recently entered clinical trials. One of these, like MitraClip, is similarly based on the concept of re-apposing an anterior and posterior leaflet during systole to limit the degree of mitral regurgitation. The PASCAL device (Edwards Lifesciences; Fig. 63.2B and C) differs from MitraClip, in that it has a central spacer adjoined to two clasps with a deeper and wider grasping area. It is currently undergoing a safety and performance evaluation within the CLASP trial. The goal is to include 120 patients with moderate to severe mitral regurgitation and NYHA II or greater heart failure on appropriate medical therapy. Estimated study completion is in August 2021.

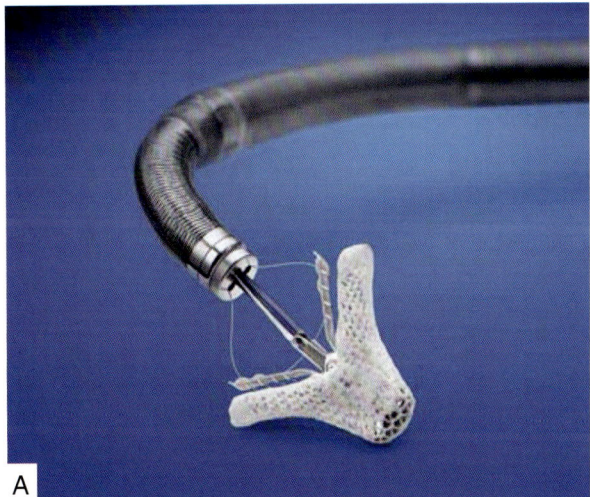
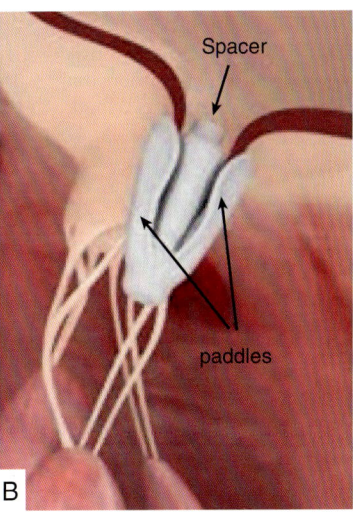
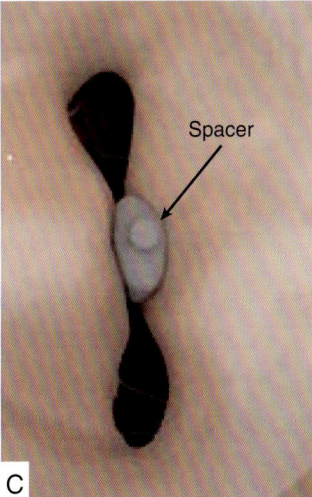

Fig. 63.2 (A) The MitraClip system approach is derived from the edge-to-edge surgical procedure for mitral valve repair. The MitraClip system replaces suturing with a clip to join the free edges of the opposing leaflets at the site of regurgitation. (B and C) The PASCAL device has a central spring, two clasps, and a broader and deeper grasping capacity. (A, Courtesy Abbott Vascular, Santa Clara, CA; B and C, Courtesy Edwards Lifesciences, Irvine, CA.)

While MitraClip and PASCAL are based on leaflet repair, other devices have been established around the concept of annuloplasty, and reside either in the coronary sinus, or secured to the mitral annulus via anchors or pledgets, that can be "cinched" to reduce the medial-lateral mitral annulus dimensions. A number of these strategies are currently in clinical trials. Whether or not direct leaflet repair strategies, in tandem with a percutaneous mitral annuloplasty, will result in outcomes that better approximate surgical mitral valve repair (which generally includes an annuloplasty ring in tandem with leaflet repair) is an intriguing hypothesis.

Complete transcatheter mitral valve replacement platforms have also been developed. The Edwards SAPIEN valve was approved for use in the mitral position in degenerated mitral bioprosthesis, an approval based on registry data demonstrating acceptable safety and efficacy of *off-label* SAPIEN valve use in this position. Other dedicated transcatheter mitral valves have entered into clinical trials for native mitral valve disease. These devices are currently implanted in a hybrid fashion, with an interventional cardiologist and cardiothoracic surgeon via a transapical route. The development of mitral valve replacement devices that can be reliably delivered via transseptal access is ongoing, and will reduce the complexity and procedural recovery for these patients. These trials, in aggregate, will inform future decisions about the management of functional mitral regurgitation in heart failure.[33]

PERCUTANEOUS TRICUSPID VALVE INTERVENTIONS

With the development of effective and commercially approved devices to treat aortic and mitral valve disease percutaneously, there has been a renewed interest in therapies that might benefit patients with tricuspid valve disease. Functional tricuspid regurgitation is common, and generally related to pulmonary hypertension and/or left sided heart valve disease. Surgery for isolated tricuspid valve disease has not been routinely undertaken—in part because of uncertainty regarding populations that benefit, and the degree of comorbidities that generally accompany significant tricuspid valve disease. However, the advent of percutaneous valve therapies have raised the possibility of "beating-heart" procedures, perhaps without general anesthesia, that may enable us to identify the patients appropriate for therapy, and the timing within which to undertake it.[34]

Devices for percutaneous tricuspid interventions have generally followed the prototypes of mitral devices, and include those meant to reappose adjoining leaflets (MitrClip in tricuspid position, "TriClip") and those meant to reduce annular dimension (TriCinch, TriAlign). Other approaches have been described, including the implantation of a transcatheter aortic valve in a degenerated tricuspid prosthesis or in the inferior vena cava to mitigate the hepatic and edematous sequelae of tricuspid valve disease.[35] Preclinical and first-in-man experience has been reported for many of these devices, with larger scale randomized trials forthcoming.

The largest experience with percutaneous tricuspid intervention has been accomplished using the MitraClip in the tricuspid position. Compassionate use in a series of 64 patients was reported, with severe, predominantly (88%) functional tricuspid regurgitation. Implant success was high (97%), and immediate reduction of ≥1 grade was accomplished in 91%. There were no procedural deaths or major complications, although 5% did not survive the hospitalization.[36]

PERCUTANEOUS OR HYBRID VENTRICULAR PARTITIONING OR RESTORATION

The effects of reducing ventricular volume and improving ventricular geometry through surgical ventricular restoration on ischemic heart failure have been reviewed elsewhere.[37] The Reconstructive Endoventricular Surgery Returning Torsion Original Radius Elliptical Shape to the Left Ventricle (RESTORE), an international registry of 1198 heart failure patients after anterior myocardial infarction, suggested that surgical ventricular restoration improved ventricular function and could be effective therapy in the treatment of ischemic cardiomyopathy.[38] However, the randomized, controlled Surgical Therapies for Ischemic Congestive Heart Failure (STICH) trial failed to confirm these results.[39]

The reasons for the failure of the STICH trial are uncertain, but the nature and risks of the surgical procedure itself and the technique used for ventricular reconstruction may have limited its effectiveness. The study authors postulate that "the lack of benefit seen with surgical ventricular reconstruction is that benefits anticipated from surgical reduction of left ventricular volume (i.e., reduced wall stress and improvement in systolic function) are counterbalanced by a reduction in diastolic distensibility."[39]

Minimally invasive percutaneous or hybrid approaches to ventricular restoration have been developed. A catheter-based approach using the Parachute device shows promise for the treatment of heart failure in patients with remote anterior myocardial infarction.[40] The Parachute device is constructed of an expanded polytetrafluoroethylene (ePTFE) membrane stretched over a nitinol conical frame (Fig. 63.3). It is deployed into the apex of the left ventricle to partition off damaged myocardium. The device reduces wall stress in the upper chamber by changing the left ventricular geometry and reducing volume. The compliant Parachute replaces stiff or rigid scar and provides an outward

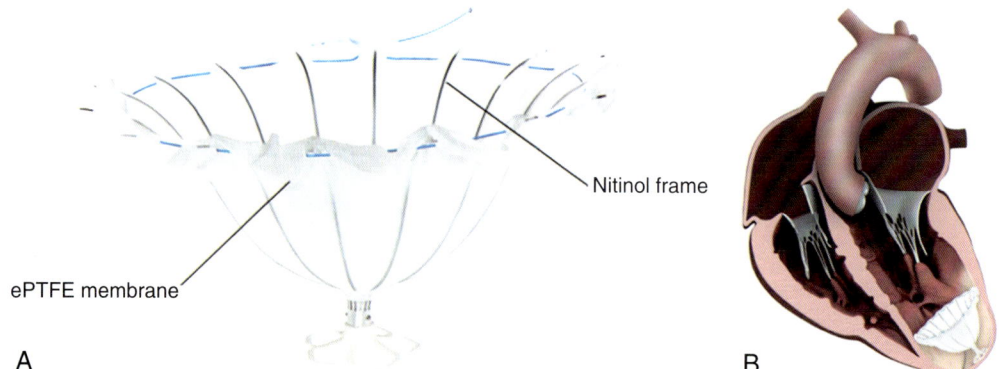

Fig. 63.3 (A) The Parachute device is constructed of an expanded polytetrafluoroethylene *(ePTFE)* membrane stretched over a conical nitinol frame. (B) The device is deployed in the damaged apex of the left ventricle, where it reduces wall stress in the upper chamber by changing left ventricular geometry and reducing volume. (Courtesy CardioKinetix, Menlo Park, CA.)

force with the anchors to aid in diastolic filling. It improves diastolic compliance, which reduces end-diastolic filling pressures.

The safety, feasibility, and preliminary clinical efficacy of the Parachute device were demonstrated in a small observational study, the Percutaneous Ventricular Restoration in Chronic Heart Failure Patients (PARACHUTE) trial.[41] Subsequent findings have suggested improved clinical outcomes for patients implanted with the Parachute device.[42] A multicenter, randomized, controlled trial (PARACHUTE IV) was designed to evaluate the possibility of percutaneous ventricular restoration using the Parachute device.[43] The study randomly assigned 478 patients with NYHA class III or IV ischemic heart failure, akinetic or dyskinetic left ventricular wall abnormality, and an LVEF between 15% and 35% to optimal medical therapy (i.e., control group) or optimal medical therapy plus implantation of the Parachute device. The primary end point was death or rehospitalization for worsening heart failure. This study was terminated before completion, due to an apparent excess of stroke and myocardial infarction in the treatment group. The Parachute device retains Conformité Européenne (CE) mark approval in Europe.

A minimally invasive approach to left ventricular reconstruction using the Revivent system (Bioventrix, San Ramon, CA) is being investigated.[44,45] The Revivent system is composed of internal and external anchors made up of titanium bars covered by polyester cloth (Fig. 63.4). The internal anchor is deployed in the right ventricular side of the myocardial septum, and the external anchor over the left ventricular free wall. This creates the ability to plicate the scarred left ventricle. The procedure is performed in hybrid fashion through the internal jugular vein (for internal anchor) in addition to a mini-thoracotomy (for external anchor), without the need for cardiopulmonary bypass. Preliminary observations include reductions in left ventricular volume, increased LVEF, and an increase in 6-minute walk test (6MWT). The BRAVE-TC (BioVentrix Registry Assessment of Ventricular Enhancement for the Revivent TC) trial is currently recruiting up to 100 subjects, with anticipated 5-year follow-up to assess the safety of this device. The ALIVE (American Less Invasive Ventricular Enhancement) trial is randomized 2:1 device to control, with the intent of enrolling 120 patients. The primary end points of the ALIVE trial include LV volume reduction, NYHA class, ejection fraction, quality of life, 6MWT, and rehospitalization at 12 months.

INTERATRIAL SHUNT DEVICES

Elevated intracardiac and pulmonary artery pressures are associated with poorer outcomes for patients with chronic heart failure, regardless of ejection fraction.[46,47] Excursions of left atrial pressure into an elevated range are a strong predictor of adverse clinical events.[47] Chronically lowering these pressures reduces the risk of heart failure related hospitalizations.[47,48]

Although lowering intracardiac and pulmonary artery pressures may be successfully accomplished in some patients with pharmacologic therapies, some patients are refractory to these therapies or poorly tolerate them. Pharmacologic therapies also may not fully address the dynamic increase in left atrial pressure during heart failure exacerbations or during exercise.[49]

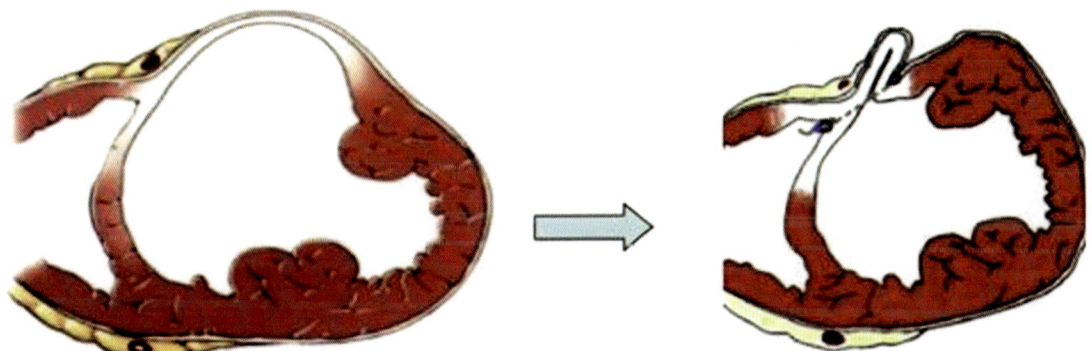

Fig. 63.4 The Revivent system. Two anchors, one deployed on the right ventricular side of the septum, and the other over the left ventricular free wall. They are secured by an internal anchor allowing ventricular plication without the need for cardiopulmonary bypass. (Courtesy BioVentrix, San Ramon, CA.)

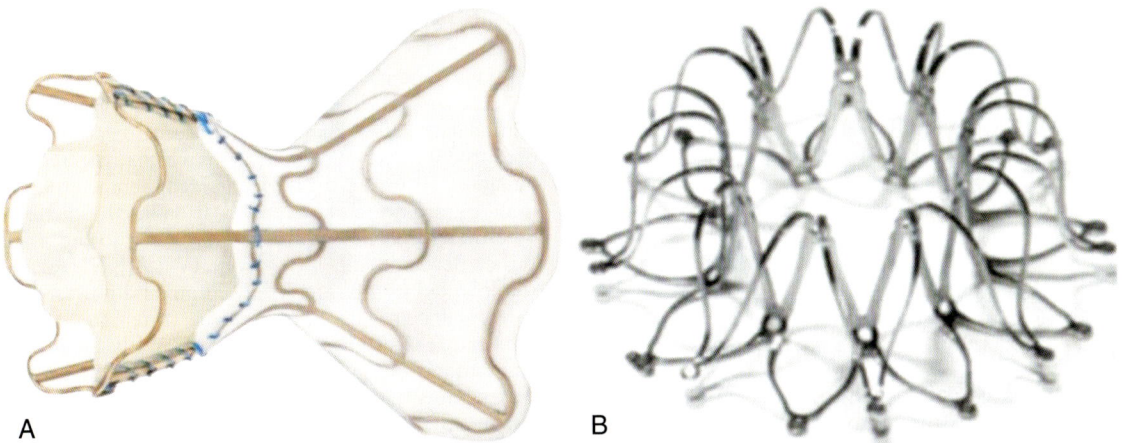

Fig. 63.5 (A) Unidirectional (valved) left-to-right interatrial shunt device. (B) Open left-to-right interatrial shunt device. (A, Courtesy V-Wave Medical, Hod HaSharon, Israel; B, Courtesy Corvia, Tewksbury, MA.)

A small interatrial shunt may reduce left atrial pressure and limit left atrial pressure increases during exercise and heart failure exacerbations. Evidence in support of this notion comes from patients with mitral valve stenosis and coexisting atrial septal defect. They have fewer symptoms than mitral valve stenosis patients with an intact septum.[50] Conversely, closure of an atrial septal defect in patients with left ventricular failure may worsen heart failure symptoms.[51]

Two devices for the creation of an interatrial shunt are being investigated for the treatment of heart failure (Fig. 63.5), and the early clinical experience has been good.[45,46] The V-Wave device (V-Wave Ltd, Or Akiva, Israel) is a trileaflet porcine tissue valve housed in a nickel titanium frame.[52] The initial implantation was reported in a patient with NYHA class III heart failure and an LVEF of less than 35%. Implantation was associated with a pulmonary artery to systemic (ascending aorta) blood flow ratio (Qp/Qs) of 1.17, improvement in the NYHA class, quality of life score, and exercise capacity at 3 months.[53] These findings are consistent with those reported in a pilot study of 10 patients, and the large animal preclinical studies that preceded human utilization. A larger trial that included heart failure patients with preserved ($n = 8$) and reduced ejection fraction ($n = 30$) was undertaken, and outcomes were recently reported. Procedural success (device implant) was achieved in all patients. There were significant improvements in functional class at 3 and 12 months, without changes in left or right ventricular function. There was, however, a reduction or absence of left to right atrial flow identified in 50% of participants, related to neointimal thickening and consequent fusion of the valve commissures. Importantly, functional improvement, morbidity, and mortality improvements were observed in those with patent shunts. A second-generation device has been created without a central valve, and histological studies have revealed no significant pannus infiltration at 6 months.[54,55]

The InterAtrial Shunt Device (IASD; Corvia Medical Inc., Tewkesbury, MA) consists of a nitinol device (outer diameter 19 mm) inserted percutaneously via a 16-Fr venous approach into the interatrial septum, producing a permanent 8 mm atrial septal communication. REDUCE LAP-HF (REDUCe Elevated Left Atrial Pressure in Patients with Heart Failure) was a phase I, open-label nonrandomized trial that evaluated the safety and performance.[56,57] Within this trial, 68 patients were enrolled (average ejection fraction 57% and mean rest pulmonary capillary wedge pressure [PCWP] 17 mm Hg). The co-primary end points of the study were reduction of PCWP at rest and exercise, along with evidence of left-to-right shunt on echocardiography. IASD placement was successful in 66 of 68 patients (97%). There were no major adverse events. After 6 months, IASD system implantation was associated with reduced rest or exercise mean PCWP in most participation (71%). The follow-up to the REDUCE LAP-HF trial randomized ($n = 44$) to device placement versus a sham procedure (REDUCE LAP-HF I).[58] At 1 month, the IASD resulted in a greater reduction in PCWP compared to the sham procedure ($P = .028$ accounting for all stages of exercise). A larger scale trial (REDUCE LAP-HF II) has initiated recruitment with the enrolment goal of 380 patients.

Other interatrial shunt devices have been created, and are being investigated for heart failure and pulmonary hypertension. Among these, the atrial flow regulator (AFR) has a small but growing experience in pulmonary hypertension and congenital heart disease.[59-61]

IMPLANTABLE HEMODYNAMIC MONITORS

Another approach to chronically lowering left atrial and pulmonary artery pressures is the use of an implantable hemodynamic monitor to guide changes in pharmacologic therapy. The CardioMEMS heart failure system was approved by the FDA on the basis of the CardioMEMS Heart Sensor Allows Monitoring of Pressure to Improve Outcomes in NYHA Class III Heart Failure Patients (CHAMPION) trial.[48,59] The pulmonary artery pressure sensor consists of a coil and a pressure-sensitive capacitor encased in a capsule. It is implanted into a branch of the pulmonary artery using a specialized delivery system during a right heart catheterization. It has no battery and is powered by a radiofrequency signal from outside of the body. Pressure data are transmitted wirelessly to a secure website, where physicians and nurses can view discrete data or pressure trends graphed longitudinally over time.

The CHAMPION trial randomized 550 NYHA class III heart failure patients with reduced or preserved LVEF to a treatment group for which investigators had access to daily pulmonary artery pressure measurements and used them to guide therapy or to a control group for which investigators had no access to daily pulmonary artery pressure measurements and managed patients using standard of care heart failure monitoring. During the first 6 months after randomization, there was a 28% reduction in the risk of heart failure hospitalizations for the treatment group compared with the control group ($P < .00002$). During the entire single-blinded follow-up period, averaging more than 15 months, the treatment group demonstrated a significant 37% decrease in the rate of heart failure hospitalizations compared with the control group. Therapy guided by the CardioMEMS system reduced the risk of heart failure hospitalizations for systolic and diastolic heart failure patients.[48,59] These effects were later corroborated in the control group, when providers were permitted open access to device measurements. CardioMEMS is approved by the FDA for patients with NYHA III heart failure, with at least one heart failure admission in the preceding 12 months. Postapproval observational data suggest that the efficacy of this form of ambulatory monitoring continues to be associated with reductions in heart failure admissions and overall heart failure costs.[60,61]

Systems for the direct measurement of left atrial pressure are under investigation. These devices have the advantages of directly conveying left atrial pressure without the assumptions inherent in surrogate indices (pulmonary artery diastolic pressure, PCWP). The HeartPOD system (Abbott) consists of an implantable sensor lead coupled to a subcutaneous antenna coil, a patient advisory module, and remote access by clinicians through a secure computer-based data management system. The sensor lead is implanted using a transvenous approach and transseptal crossing of the interatrial septum, placing the tip of the sensor system lead in the left atrium.[62,63] Observations from a pilot study in which patients served as their own controls demonstrated a significant reduction in the annualized rate of heart failure hospitalizations.[47] The Left Atrial Pressure Monitoring to Optimize Heart Failure Therapy (LAPTOP-HF) trial assessed the safety and efficacy of this device in patients with NYHA III heart, a related hospitalization in the preceding 12 months or elevated B-type natriuretic peptide. Patients were randomized to device implantation and pressure-guided therapy, or optimal medical therapy with a reminder module. There were concerns regarding the frequency of procedural related complications which prompted early trial termination. However, the device-guided therapy group did exhibit a trend toward decreased overall heart failure hospitalizations.

Other direct left-atrial pressure monitoring systems are in earlier development. One device (V-LAP; Vectorious Medical) is implanted in the interatrial septum and powered remotely via a wearable belt. The TITAN device (Integrated Sensing Systems Inc.) requires surgical implantation, and has completed first-in-man studies among patients undergoing left ventricular assist device implantation.[60] These devices will likely further establish a fundamental role for outpatient intracardiac pressure monitoring in heart failure, and clarify whether or not direct left atrial pressure compared with pulmonary artery pressure measurements are incrementally helpful in heart failure outcomes.

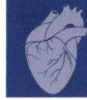

CONCLUSIONS

We are entering an era in which interventional cardiologists and heart failure specialists will work hand in hand to offer patients novel devices to improve their clinical status and outcomes. The devices can enhance cardiac structure, function, and hemodynamics. Many of these devices remain under investigation, but even if only a few succeed, the future of this new field of interventional heart failure will be bright.

KEY REFERENCES

3. Writing Committee M, Yancy CW, Jessup M, et al. 2013 ACCF/AHA guideline for the management of heart failure: a report of the American College of Cardiology Foundation/American Heart Association Task Force on practice guidelines. *Circulation.* 2013;128:e240–327.
8. Premchand RK, Sharma K, Mittal S, et al. Autonomic regulation therapy via left or right cervical vagus nerve stimulation in patients with chronic heart failure: results of the ANTHEM-HF trial. *J Card Fail.* 2014;20:808–816.
9. Zannad F, De Ferrari GM, Tuinenburg AE, et al. Chronic vagal stimulation for the treatment of low ejection fraction heart failure: results of the NEural Cardiac TherApy foR Heart Failure (NECTAR-HF) randomized controlled trial. *Eur Heart J.* 2015;36:425–433.
15. Nishimura RA, Otto CM, Bonow RO, et al. 2014 AHA/ACC guideline for the management of patients with valvular heart disease: executive summary: a report of the American College of Cardiology/American Heart Association task force on practice guidelines. *Circulation.* 2014;129:2440–2492.
22. Mack MJ, Leon MB, Smith CR, et al. 5-year outcomes of transcatheter aortic valve replacement or surgical aortic valve replacement for high surgical risk patients with aortic stenosis (PARTNER 1): a randomised controlled trial. *Lancet.* 2015;385:2477–2484.
23. Reardon MJ, Van Mieghem NM, Popma JJ, et al. Surgical or transcatheter aortic-valve replacement in intermediate-risk patients. *N Engl J Med.* 2017;376:1321–1331.
32. Feldman T, Kar S, Elmariah S, et al. Randomized comparison of percutaneous repair and surgery for mitral regurgitation: 5-year results of EVEREST II. *J Am Coll Cardiol.* 2015;66:2844–2854.
33. Patel A, Bapat V. Transcatheter mitral valve replacement: device landscape and early results. *EuroIntervention.* 2017;13. AA31–AA9.
34. Kapadia S, Krishnaswamy A, Tuzcu EM. Percutaneous therapy for tricuspid regurgitation: a new frontier for interventional cardiology. *Circulation.* 2017;135:1815–1818.
58. Feldman T, Mauri L, Kahwash R, et al. Transcatheter interatrial shunt device for the treatment of heart failure with preserved ejection fraction (REDUCE LAP-HF I [Reduce Elevated Left Atrial Pressure in Patients With Heart Failure]): a phase 2, randomized, sham-controlled trial. *Circulation.* 2018;137:364–375.
61. Desai AS, Bhimaraj A, Bharmi R, et al. Ambulatory hemodynamic monitoring reduces heart failure hospitalizations in "Real-World" clinical practice. *J Am Coll Cardiol.* 2017;69:2357–2365.

 Additional references available online at expertconsult.com.

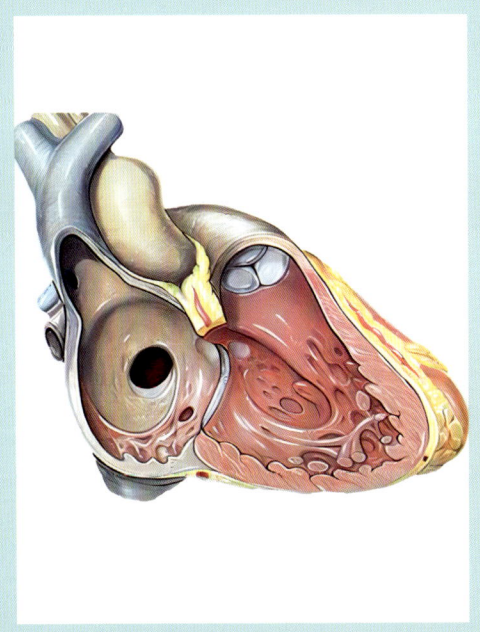

SECTION VI

第六部分

Evaluation of Interventional Techniques

介入治疗技术的评估

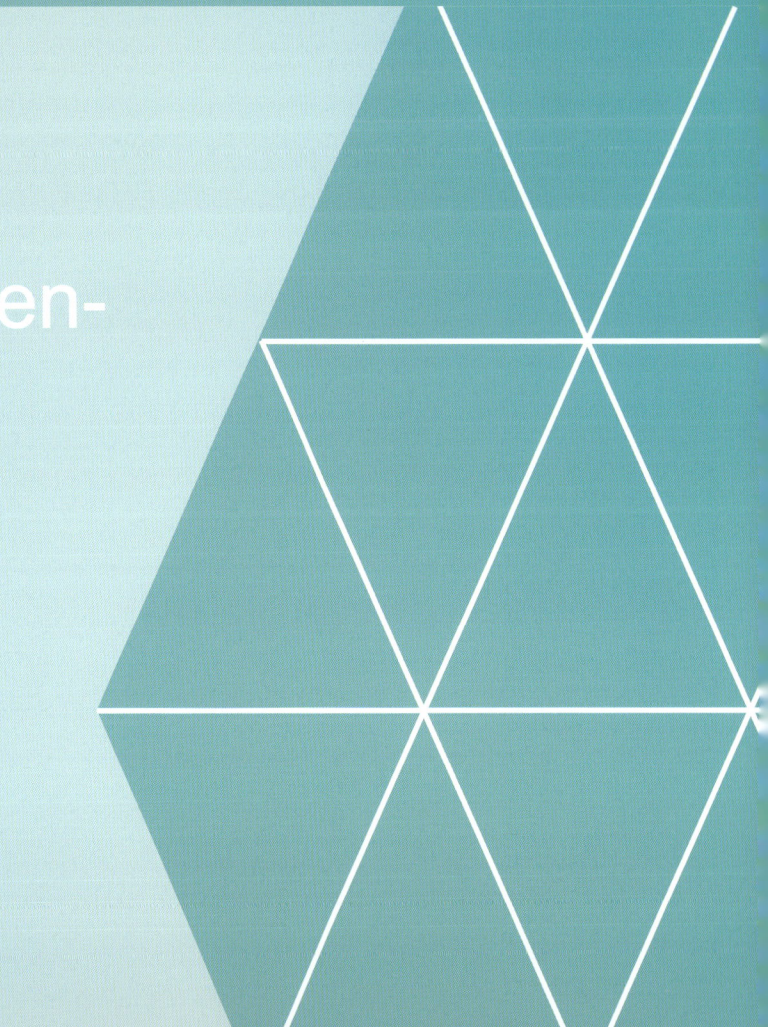

中文导读

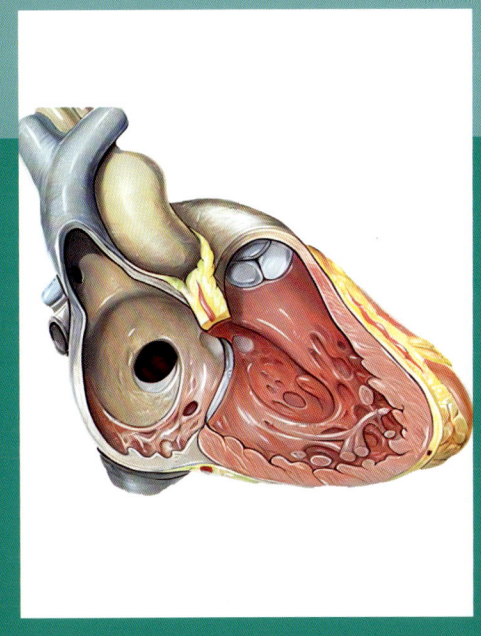

第64章
冠状动脉造影的定性、定量评估

　　经导管冠状动脉介入治疗在过去30年发展迅速，彻底改变了冠状动脉疾病的治疗格局。作为经皮冠状动脉介入治疗的基础，冠状动脉造影可以提供冠状动脉病变基线形态、血管狭窄严重程度、血流灌注状态，以及术后疗效等相关数据，为术者治疗决策、患者预后转归提供依据。在此基础之上，近年来多项研究显示冠状动脉量化评估为我们更清晰地阐释了冠状动脉不同形态病变及其发病机制、药物治疗和介入治疗作用机制，以及介入术后并发症的诱发因素，有助于进一步优化治疗决策。

　　本章分析讨论了既往用于经皮冠状动脉介入治疗患者风险分层的传统标准，以及已经广泛应用的多种评分体系，如SYNTAX评分，被证实其对于复杂病变治疗决策具有良好的预测价值。同时分析介绍了对于心肌血流灌注及微循环的新型评估方法，可更为精确预测急性心肌梗死患者预后转归；介绍了目前已在介入术后早期及远期疗效评估中广泛应用的冠状动脉造影量化评估方法，其可以协助探究新型药物及器械对于冠状动脉介入治疗的获益机制。本章条理清晰地向读者介绍了冠状动脉造影定性及量化评估的机制、应用现状及临床进展，相信会给读者在这一新兴领域带来更多的收获。

王玮玮　吴永健

章节要点

- 对于冠状动脉病变的深入了解是评估经皮冠状动脉介入治疗术后近远期风险的重要工具。
- 综合了解血管通畅率、潜在冠状动脉病变形态的累计积分，为评估预后提供了相关依据。SYNTAX评分作为冠状动脉病变的量化评估工具，为冠状动脉多支病变患者进行经皮冠状动脉介入治疗或冠状动脉旁路移植术的术式选择提供了重要依据。
- 冠状动脉长病变、血栓负荷较重、大隐静脉桥血管毁损、重度迂曲病变、重度成角病变，以及慢性闭塞性病变，属于经皮冠状动脉介入治疗高危险且介入失败率较高类型。
- 在急性冠状动脉综合征患者中，心肌血流评估和心肌灌注分级可以良好预测ST段抬高型心肌梗死患者预后及转归；同时可预测非ST段抬高型心肌梗死患者不良事件。对比定性评估，量化评估可以更好评价新型药物及器械对于ST段抬高型心肌梗死患者的治疗效果。
- 尽管冠状动脉造影是经皮冠状动脉介入治疗手术前后评估病变严重程度的"金标准"，但是由于受到病变形态及血流复杂性、病变部位入口及出口角度、狭窄段长度等因素影响，中度狭窄（40%~70%）病变需要更充分的评估方式，如血流储备分数。
- 通过可靠、可重复的量化评估方法，可以协助探究新型药物及器械对于冠状动脉介入治疗的获益机制。新型量化评估技术可以通过呈现三维影像清晰描绘闭塞性病变和分叉病变。
- 通过量化评估药物涂层支架或金属裸支架植入术后冠状动脉狭窄程度及管腔内径损失，可以预测冠状动脉再狭窄。

SECTION VI Evaluation of Interventional Techniques

64 Qualitative and Quantitative Coronary Angiography

Michael L. Chuang, Alexandra Almonacid, Jeffrey J. Popma

KEY POINTS

- An enhanced understanding of coronary lesion complexity remains a valuable tool for estimating early and late procedural risk after percutaneous coronary intervention (PCI).
- Aggregate scores that consider the vessel patency and underlying lesion morphology provide the most relevant information for estimating outcome. The SYNTAX trial score, a quantitative assessment of the extent of coronary artery disease, has proven a valuable tool for identifying appropriate patients for multivessel PCI or coronary artery bypass grafting.
- Longer lesions, thrombus-containing lesions, degenerated saphenous vein grafts, severe tortuosity and angulation, and chronic total coronary occlusions hold the highest risk for procedural failure with PCI.
- In the setting of acute coronary syndromes, assessment of myocardial blood flow and myocardial perfusion grade is useful in predicting prognosis for patients with ST-segment elevation myocardial infarction (STEMI) and may be valuable in predicting events in patients with non–ST-segment elevation myocardial infarction. Quantitative rather than qualitative indices are preferred to assess the value of new drugs and devices in STEMI patients.
- While coronary angiography is standard for assessing lesion severity before and after PCI, physiologically intermediate (40% to 70%) lesions require assessment using adjunct modalities, such as fractional flow reserve, due to the complexity of lesion morphology and flow, entrance and exit angles, and stenosis length that are difficult to quantify using qualitative lumen interpretation alone.
- Reliable and reproducible methods of quantitative assessment of lesion severity have provided important insights into the mechanisms of benefit of new drugs and devices in patients undergoing coronary intervention. The use of novel quantitative programs has yielded three-dimensional imaging methods for precise characterization of total occlusions and bifurcation disease.
- Late clinical restenosis can be predicted by the quantitative measurement of percent diameter stenosis and late lumen loss in patients undergoing drug-eluting and bare-metal stent placement.

INTRODUCTION

Percutaneous coronary intervention (PCI) has evolved dramatically over the past three decades, fundamentally altering the management of ischemic coronary artery disease (CAD). Bare-metal stents (BMS) and drug-eluting coronary stents (DES) are used in more than 95% of PCI procedures. Coronary arteriography is a fundamental component of PCI, providing prognostic information about baseline lesion morphology and severity, quantification of anterograde perfusion, and adequacy of the final result. Although conventional visual angiography has formed the cornerstone of clinical decision making for patients undergoing cardiovascular interventions, quantitative analyses of procedural and late angiograms have elucidated the therapeutic mechanisms of new devices and drugs and identified the factors predisposing to procedural complications, thrombosis, and restenosis, improving patient selection for these procedures.

The standard criteria used to stratify the baseline procedural risk of patients undergoing PCI are reviewed in this chapter. These criteria have been modified since the availability of DES, and several predictive scores (e.g., SYNTAX trial score) have provided useful tools for deciding between multivessel PCI and coronary artery bypass grafting (CABG) in patients with complex CAD. Newer methods to assess myocardial perfusion beyond coronary flow that provide important prognostic information for patients with acute myocardial infarction (AMI) are discussed. The quantitative angiographic methods used for evaluating early and late procedural outcome after PCI are outlined, including the value of these indices as surrogates for clinical outcome in novel stent studies.

QUALITATIVE ANGIOGRAPHY

Calculation of the procedural risk for PCI begins with accurate assessment of the complexity of the baseline coronary anatomy. Predictors for an adverse procedural outcome after balloon angioplasty were identified in early series, but a standardized approach to the assessment of lesion morphology in patients undergoing PCI was lacking until the late 1980s. Refinement of these criteria was necessary after the introduction of coronary stents in order to estimate procedural risk, particularly with the continued availability of CABG.

American College of Cardiology/American Heart Association Task Force, Society for Cardiac Angiography and Interventions, and Mayo Clinic Criteria for Lesion Morphology and Risk Stratification

A joint task force of the American College of Cardiology (ACC) and American Heart Association (AHA) in 2005 established criteria to estimate procedural success and complication rates after balloon angioplasty based on the presence or absence of specific high-risk lesion characteristics.[1] Although these criteria were developed based solely on the task force's clinical impressions (Table 64.1), their estimates of procedural success and complications closely correlated with the procedural outcomes demonstrated in patients undergoing multivessel balloon angioplasty.[2] Chronic total occlusion, high-grade stenosis, stenosis on a bend of

TABLE 64.1 American College of Cardiology/American Heart Association Characteristics of Type A, B, and C Coronary Lesions

Type A lesions: high success rate (≈85%), low risk
Discrete (<10 mm)
Concentric
Readily accessible
Nonangulated segment (<45 degrees)
Absence of thrombus
Little or no calcium
Less than totally occlusive
Not ostial in location
Smooth contour, no major side branch
No side branch involvement
Type B lesions: moderate success rate (60%–80%), moderate risk
Tubular (10–20 mm long)
Eccentric
Moderate tortuosity of proximal segment
Bifurcation lesion requiring double guidewire
Some thrombus
Moderate to heavy calcification
Total occlusion <3 months old
Moderately angulated (45–90 degrees)
Irregular contour
Type C lesions: low success rate (≈60%), high risk
Diffuse (>20 mm long)
Excessive tortuosity of proximal segment
Extremely angulated segment (>90 degrees)
Total occlusion >3 months old
Inability to protect major side branches
Degenerated vein grafts with friable lesions

Modified from Ryan TJ, Faxon DP, Gunnar RP, et al. Guidelines for percutaneous transluminal coronary angioplasty: a report of the American College of Cardiology/American Heart Association Task Force on Assessment of Diagnostic and Therapeutic Cardiovascular Procedures (Subcommittee on Percutaneous Transluminal Coronary Angioplasty). *J Am Coll Cardiol.* 1988;12:529–545.

TABLE 64.2 Definitions of Preprocedural Lesion Morphology

Variable	Definition
Eccentricity	Stenosis with one of its luminal edges in the outer one-fourth of the apparently normal lumen
Irregularity	Lesion ulceration, intimal flap, aneurysm, or sawtooth pattern
Ulceration	Small crater consisting of a discrete luminal widening in the area of the stenosis but does not extend beyond the normal arterial lumen
Aneurysmal dilation	Segment of arterial dilation larger than the dimensions of the normal arterial segment
Sawtooth pattern	Multiple, sequential stenotic irregularities
Lesion length	Measured shoulder to shoulder in an unforeshortened view
Discrete	Lesion length <10 mm
Tubular	Lesion length 10–20 mm
Diffuse	Lesion length >20 mm
Ostial location	Origin of the lesion within 3 mm of the vessel origin
Lesion angulation	Vessel angle formed by the centerline through the lumen proximal to the stenosis and extending beyond it and a second centerline in the straight portion of the artery distal to the stenosis
Moderate	Lesion angulation >45–90 degrees
Severe	Lesion angulation >90 degrees
Bifurcation	Medium or large branch (>1.5 mm) originates within the stenosis, and the side branch is completely surrounded by stenotic portions of the lesion to be dilated
Lesion accessibility	
Moderate tortuosity	Lesion is distal to two bends ≥75 degrees
Severe tortuosity	Lesion is distal to three bends ≥75 degrees
Degenerated SVG	Graft characterized by luminal irregularities or ectasia comprising >50% of the graft length
Calcification	Readily apparent densities within the apparent vascular wall at the site of stenosis
Moderate	Densities seen only with cardiac motion before contrast injection
Severe	Radiopacities seen without cardiac motion before contrast injection
Total occlusion	TIMI grade 0 or 1 flow
Thrombus	Discrete, intraluminal filling defect with defined borders that is largely separated from the adjacent wall; contrast staining may or may not be seen

SVG, Saphenous vein graft; *TIMI,* thrombolysis in myocardial infarction.

60 degrees or more, and occlusion location in vessels with proximal tortuosity were associated with adverse outcomes.[2] The most complex lesion morphologies (i.e., type C lesions) were associated with less satisfactory procedural outcomes.[3,4] Definitions for these variables are provided (Table 64.2).

With the improved outcomes associated with the use of coronary stents, contemporary composite risk scores were proposed.[5,6] The Society for Cardiac Angiography and Interventions (SCAI) Registry evaluated 61,926 patients (of whom 74.5% received stents) from the ACC National Cardiovascular Data Registry and classified their lesions in four groups: non-type C, type C, non-type C occluded, and type C occluded (Table 64.3).[5] These simplified criteria provided better discrimination for success or complications than the ACC/AHA original classification with a C-statistic of 0.69 for success using the ACC/AHA original classification system, 0.71 using the modified ACC/AHA system, and 0.75 for the SCAI classification.[5]

The Mayo Clinic risk score was constructed by adding integer scores for eight morphologic variables, and it was compared with the ACC/AHA risk score for 5064 patients undergoing PCI, of whom 183 (4%) experienced an adverse event (e.g., death, Q-wave myocardial infarction, stroke, emergency CABG).[6] The Mayo Clinic risk score offered significantly better risk stratification than the ACC/AHA lesion classification for the development of cardiovascular complications, whereas the ACC/AHA lesion classification was a better system for determining angiographic success.[6]

SYNTAX Score

The SYNTAX score was developed during the Synergy Between Percutaneous Coronary Intervention With Taxus and Cardiac Surgery (SYNTAX) trial to classify patients according to the complexity and extent of CAD.[7,8] A lesion is defined as significant when it causes a greater than 50% reduction in luminal diameter by visual assessment in a vessel that is more than 1.5 mm in diameter.[8] A multiplication factor of 2 is used for nonocclusive lesions, and a factor of 5 is used for occlusive lesions, reflecting the difficulty of the percutaneous treatment.[8] Up to 12 lesions are identified within the coronary tree, and each lesion is assessed for its severity, including total occlusion (with appropriate characterization) and side branches and their size.[8]

Each lesion is also weighted by its contribution to the myocardial bed that it supplies.[8] In a right-dominant system, the right coronary artery supplies approximately 16% and the left coronary

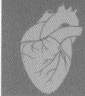

TABLE 64.3 SCAI Classification of Class I Through IV Lesions

TYPE I LESION[a]
1. Does not meet ACC/AHA criteria for type C lesion
2. Patent

TYPE II LESION
1. Meets any of the following criteria for type C lesion:
   - Diffuse (>2 cm long)
   - Excessive tortuosity of proximal segment
   - Extremely angulated segments >90 degrees
   - Inability to protect major side branches
   - Degenerated vein grafts with friable lesions
2. Patent

TYPE III LESION
1. Does not meet ACC/AHA criteria for type C lesion
2. Occluded

TYPE IV LESION
1. Meets any of the following criteria for type C lesion:
   - Diffuse (>2 cm long)
   - Excessive tortuosity of proximal segment
   - Extremely angulated segments (>90 degrees)
   - Inability to protect major side branches
   - Degenerated vein grafts with friable lesions
2. Occluded

[a]Highest success rate expected, lowest risk.
ACC/AHA, American College of Cardiology/American Heart Association; *SCAI*, Society for Cardiac Angiography and Interventions.
Modified from Krone R, Shaw R, Klein L, et al. Evaluation of the American College of Cardiology/American Heart Association and the Society for Coronary Angiography and Interventions lesion classification system in the current "stent era" of coronary interventions (from the ACC National Cardiovascular Data Registry). *Am J Cardiol*. 2003;92:389–394.

artery supplies 84% of the flow to the left ventricle, of which 66% is supplied by the left anterior descending artery and 33% is supplied by the left circumflex coronary artery. These factors have been included in the weight given to each segment.

Lesions are further graded by their complexity, including multiple tandem lesions, morphology of total occlusions, bifurcation and trifurcation involvement, aortoostial location, diffuse disease and small vessels, severe tortuosity, length greater than 20 mm, heavy calcification, and thrombus.[8,9] An online algorithm (http://www.syntaxscore.com) automatically sums each of these features to calculate the total score.

The SYNTAX score is an important prognostic tool for risk stratifying patients with multivessel disease who are being considered for coronary revascularization. Its predictive value was assessed for 1292 lesions in 306 patients who underwent PCI for three-vessel disease in the Arterial Revascularization Therapies Study Part II.[10] The rate of major adverse cardiac and cerebrovascular events at 370 days was 27.9% in the highest tertile of SYNTAX score and 8.7% in the lowest SYNTAX tertile (hazard ratio = 3.5, P = .001).[10] By multivariable analyses, the SYNTAX score independently predicted outcome and the risk of major adverse cardiac and cerebrovascular events. Compared with the modified ACC/AHA lesion classification scheme, SYNTAX score showed a better discrimination ability and goodness of fit.[10]

The SYNTAX score has been used to predict outcomes for patients enrolled in DES studies.[11,12] In an analysis of 819 patients with left main CAD who underwent revascularization in two Italian centers, the outcomes of patients undergoing PCI and CABG were studied. In patients with a SYNTAX score of 34 or less, the 2-year mortality rates were similar for CABG and PCI (6.2% vs. 8.1%, P = .461).[11] Among patients with a SYNTAX score greater than 34, those treated with CABG had lower mortality rates than those treated with PCI (8.5% vs. 32.7%, P < .001).[11] A similar correlation of the SYNTAX score and surgical outcome was not found for patients undergoing CABG.[13,14]

The value of the SYNTAX score in predicting clinical outcomes has been investigated and validated in other clinical settings, including patients who underwent primary PCI for ST-segment elevation myocardial infarction (STEMI) or non–ST-segment elevation myocardial infarction (NSTEMI).[15] The SYNTAX score is advocated in European and U.S. revascularization guidelines to risk-stratify patients with complex CAD to the most appropriate revascularization modality.[16,17]

Determining risk based purely on anatomic descriptions without the addition of clinical variables is an important limitation of the SYNTAX score. Patients with equivalent scores may have very different outcomes because of different comorbidities. To address this limitation, attempts have been made to combine clinically based scores with the SYNTAX score. The SYNTAX score II was developed to optimize decisions about the revascularization strategy.[18] It was developed and validated on the basis of a core model consisting of the anatomic SYNTAX score, age, creatinine clearance value, left ventricular ejection fraction, unprotected left main disease, peripheral vascular disease, female sex, and chronic obstructive pulmonary disease. The combination of clinical variables and the SYNTAX score has the best discriminatory value for patients undergoing multivessel PCI.[19,20]

In an effort to further integrate clinical and angiographic variables into a combined risk score, the Acute Catheterization and Urgent Intervention Triage Strategy–Percutaneous Coronary Intervention (ACUITY-PCI) trial included six factors: insulin-treated diabetes, renal insufficiency, baseline cardiac biomarker elevation or ST-segment deviation, bifurcation lesion, small vessel or diffuse CAD, and extent of CAD.[21] The ACUITY-PCI score had the best discrimination, calibration, and index of separation compared with other risk scores.[21] In a comparative analysis of 2094 patients enrolled in the ACUITY Study, the SYNTAX score; combined clinical variables plus SYNTAX score (CSS); new risk stratification (NERS) score; age, creatinine, and ejection fraction (ACEF) score; Global Registry for Acute Coronary Events (GRACE) score; and Thrombolysis in Myocardial Infarction (TIMI) study score were compared for their risk assessment of 1-year mortality, cardiac mortality, myocardial infarction, target-lesion revascularization (TLR), and stent thrombosis for patients with non–ST-segment elevation acute coronary syndromes undergoing PCI.[22] In this analysis, scores incorporating clinical and angiographic variables (i.e., CSS and NERS) showed the best balance between discrimination and calibration.[22]

Risk Assessment Using Specific Lesion Morphologic Criteria

Despite the value of risk scores in estimating aggregate procedural risk, they have several limitations when applied to individual patients. Identification of lesion characteristics, such as eccentricity, irregularity, angulation, and tortuosity, is limited by substantial interobserver variability. Agreement with ACC/AHA classification was found for only 58% of lesions in one series, with disagreement by two classification grades identified for almost 10% of lesions.[2] Similarly, the SYNTAX score suffers from the interobserver variability inherent in visual estimation of disease severity. The weighted κ value for the interobserver reproducibility of the SYNTAX score was 0.45, whereas the intraobserver weighted κ value was 0.59.[9]

Rather than a composite score, the description of individual morphologic features may be more predictive of early and late outcomes after PCI. Some ACC/AHA morphologic features are associated with complicated procedures (e.g., thrombus, saphenous vein graft [SVG] degeneration, angulated segments), whereas others are associated with unsuccessful but uncomplicated procedures (e.g., chronic total occlusions, diffuse disease).

Irregular Lesions

With the advent of coronary stents, the prognostic importance of irregular lesions has been diminished substantially, although identification of an irregular plaque on angiography suggests an acute coronary syndrome and intracoronary thrombus. Semiquantitative and quantitative measurements of lesion irregularity were developed in the early 1990s to better characterize lesion morphology in patients with acute coronary syndromes, but these methods have not found clinical utility independent of other clinical risk factors.

In 65 patients referred for first ACS, intravascular ultrasound (IVUS) was performed prior to any intervention. IVUS identified 224 lesions, including 115 plaque ruptures, whereas angiography identified 49 suspected plaque ruptures, with a 40% sensitivity and 97% specificity; positive and negative predictive values of angiography for plaque rupture were 96% and 61%, respectively.[23] Proximal coronary location, a wide cavity, and counterflow rupture were strong predictors of correct angiographic diagnoses, enabling four specific angiographic patterns to be identified using three-dimensional (3D) IVUS plaque rupture reconstruction.[23] An aneurysmal or ulcerated lesion was one of several components of a stent thrombosis risk score.[24]

Angulated Lesions

Vessel curvature at the site of maximum stenosis should be measured in the most unforeshortened projection using a length of curvature that approximates the balloon length used for coronary dilation. Although balloon angioplasty of highly angulated lesions is associated with an increased risk of coronary dissection, in the era of coronary stenting, the greatest impediment of angulated lesions is the inability to deliver the stent to the stenosis and straighten the arterial contour after stent placement, which may predispose to late stent fracture. Newer stent designs have leveraged conformability for angulated vessels to provide less vessel straightening after deployment. Prior to the understanding of the deleterious of late scaffold thrombosis, one of the potential advantages of bioresorbable scaffolds had been less vessel straightening than conventional metallic stents, particularly as the scaffold is resorbed over time.[25]

Lesion Calcification

Coronary artery calcium remains an important marker for coronary atherosclerosis. Conventional coronary angiography has limited sensitivity for the detection of smaller amounts of calcium and is only moderately sensitive for the detection of extensive lesion calcium (60% and 85% sensitivity for three- and four-quadrant calcium, respectively).[26] Coronary calcification reduces the compliance of the vessel and may predispose to dissection at the interface between calcified plaque and normal wall after balloon angioplasty.[27] Coronary calcification also reduces the ability to cross chronic total occlusions, and in severely calcified lesions, stent strut expansion is inversely correlated with the circumferential arc of calcium.[26] Patients treated with sirolimus-eluting stents who had lesion calcification had higher TLR rates than those who did not.[28,29] A pooled analysis of seven trials of first- and second-generation DES identified severe calcification as an independent predictor of poor outcome after PCI.[30]

Rotational atherectomy or other ablative technologies are the preferred pretreatment method in patients with severe lesion calcification, particularly ostial lesions; calcium ablation facilitates the delivery and expansion of coronary stents by creating microdissection planes within the fibrocalcific plaque. Even with these contemporary methods, moderate or severe coronary calcification is associated with reduced procedural success and higher complication rates, including stent dislodgment. A novel device, the Diamondback 360 Orbital Atherectomy System (Cardiovascular Systems, St. Paul, MN), used centrifugal action of a diamond-coated crown to modify calcified lesions in a series of 443 patients with severe calcification to facilitate stent placement; stent delivery was successful in 97.7% of cases.[31] In less severely calcified lesions, no difference in the restenosis rate was found after paclitaxel-eluting stent implantation in calcified or noncalcified vessels.[32] Calcification in SVGs usually occurs within the vessel wall rather than the lesion and is associated with older graft age, insulin-dependent diabetes, and a history of smoking.[33] Calcified lesions were an independent predictor of stent thrombosis in one series.[34]

Degenerated Saphenous Vein Grafts

SVGs degenerate over time, with 25% occluding within the first year after coronary bypass surgery[35] and 50% developing occlusion within 10 years after surgery, often necessitating repeat revascularization, although these rates have been improved with aggressive lipid lowering therapy. SVGs are the most common site for a culprit lesion in patients with acute coronary syndromes after CABG[36] and account for 6% of all PCIs.[37] PCIs for SVG lesions have been associated with a worse late outcome compared with native vessel interventions.[4,38,39] The SVG plaques are particularly prone to distal embolization.[38] The risk of embolic complications appears to be related to the degree of overall graft degeneration and the length and bulkiness of the lesion.[40] The risk of embolization may be reduced with the use of excimer laser atherectomy[41,42] and with the use of undersized balloons.[43]

Embolic protection devices (EPDs) have been associated with improved angiographic and clinical outcomes in percutaneous SVG interventions.[40] In the landmark Saphenous Vein Graft Angioplasty Free of Emboli Randomized (SAFER) trial, use of a distal balloon occlusion EPD was associated with a decrease (9.6% vs. 16.5%) in the 30-day composite outcome of death, myocardial infarction, emergency CABG, or TLR compared with no embolic protection.[44] Subsequent noninferiority comparisons have demonstrated similar benefit with proximal occlusion and distal filter EPD, with the benefit limited to reduction in periprocedural myocardial infarction.[45,46] When feasible, the use of EPDs during SVG PCI has been given a class I recommendation in the ACC/AHA PCI guidelines.[16] One exception may be in patients treated for in-stent restenosis (ISR), for which embolic protection may not be required.

Restenosis and TLR rates are lower with DES compared with BMS in SVG interventions, even though mortality and stent thrombosis rates are similar.[47] Self-expanding stents made with expanded polytetrafluoroethylene (ePTFE) provide no additional advantage over noncovered balloon-expandable stents in the development of early complications or late restenosis.[48,49]

Thrombus

Conventional angiography is relatively insensitive for the detection of coronary thrombus, but large thrombus may be visualized in up to 15% to 30% of patients undergoing PCI for acute coronary syndromes.[50] Angiographic thrombus is usually identified by the appearance of discrete, intraluminal filling defects within the arterial lumen, and it is associated with a 6% to 73% incidence of ischemic complications after PCI.[50] A large thrombus burden is an independent predictor of stent thrombosis in patients with STEMI treated with DES,[51] and it may be managed with intensive anticoagulation therapy before PCI to reduce periprocedural complications.[52]

Primary PCI-related complications of thrombus-containing lesions are distal embolization and thrombotic occlusion, and the risk of angiographic thrombus complications is related to the size of the coronary thrombus. Routine rheolytic thrombectomy provides no benefit in patients with AMI,[53] although it may be useful for patients with a large thrombus burden. Several aspiration catheters have been investigated in patients with AMI and large thrombus burden, but a meta-analysis of three randomized trials involving >18,000 patients undergoing PCI found no difference between PCI with routine aspiration thrombectomy and PCI alone for recurrent myocardial infarction, stent thrombosis, heart failure, or target-vessel revascularization.[54]

Traditionally, the extent of coronary thrombus has been determined using the semiquantitative TIMI thrombus grade (TTG). A novel method to assess intracoronary thrombus burden uses the discrepancy of luminal areas assessed with edge detection and video densitometry and measured with the Cardiovascular Angiography Analysis System II.[55] Thrombus remains an important predictor of outcome after PCI.[3]

Ostial Location

Ostial lesions begin within 3 mm of the origin of the coronary artery, and they are classified as aortoostial or non aortoostial lesions. Balloon angioplasty of ostial lesions is limited by suboptimal procedural outcome, primarily due to technical factors such as difficulties with guide catheter support, lesion inelasticity precluding maximal balloon expansion, and early vascular recoil limiting the acute angiographic result. Debulking techniques such as directional and rotational atherectomy improve compliance of the aortoostial lesion but have had limited effect on preventing late restenosis. Ostial lesions have been associated with higher rates of TLR after DES placement.[29,56]

DES have become the default therapy for most aortoostial lesions, although there are unique challenges of stent placement in the aortoostial location, such as protrusion of the stent into the aorta precluding subsequent injection catheter engagement, stent compression, and avulsion of the stent struts into the aorta when devices such as cutting balloon angioplasty are used to treat ISR.

Aortoostial lesions remain associated with higher failure rates than non aortoostial lesions.[54] Isolated non aortoostial stenoses of the left circumflex and left anterior descending coronary arteries[57] and ostial side branch bifurcation lesions are also effectively treated with DES,[54,58] but they pose unique challenges regarding vessel wall geometry, adequate ostial branch coverage (particularly for a narrow angle with the adjacent branch), and plaque shifting causing compromise of the parent or adjacent branch vessels. Whereas stent protrusion into the parent vessel of less than 1 mm is usually well tolerated, greater stent protrusion precludes treatment of the parent branches.[58] Stent fractures have been reported, with more advanced stenting techniques used to treat the parent vessel and ostial side branch stenoses.

Long Lesions

Lesion length may be estimated quantitatively as the shoulder-to-shoulder extent of atherosclerotic narrowing greater than 20%, although many clinicians estimate lesion length based on the identification of a normal-to-normal segment, which is usually longer than the length obtained with quantitative methods. Conventional balloon angioplasty of long lesions has been associated with reduced procedural success, particularly when the segment is diffusely diseased (e.g., >20 mm long), primarily because of the more extensive plaque burden in long lesions.

Stents improve late outcomes compared with balloon angioplasty, but stent and lesion length remain the most important predictors of restenosis in the stent era.[59] Coronary stents have been used to treat suboptimal angiographic results (i.e., spot stenting) and dissections after balloon angioplasty of longer lesions, although the "full metal jacket" stent approach to diffuse disease is associated with a higher recurrence rate in the absence of complete stent expansion, particularly in smaller vessels. Overlapping sirolimus-eluting stents provide safe and effective treatment for long coronary lesions.[60] However, stent length >35 mm remains a risk factor for restenosis and the need for revascularization.[61] Longer stented lesions were associated with stent thrombosis in one series.[34]

In a contemporary analysis of 10,004 patients undergoing surveillance, binary restenosis was detected in 2643 (26.4%) patients.[62] Use of a first-generation DES or BMS (odds ratio [OR] = 0.35) and use of a second-generation DES or first-generation DES (OR = 0.67) were independent predictors of lower rates of restenosis. On multivariate analysis, smaller vessel size (OR = 1.59 for each 0.5-mm decrease), total stented length (OR = 1.27 for each 10-mm increase), complex lesion morphology (OR = 1.35), diabetes mellitus (OR = 1.32), and history of bypass surgery (OR = 1.38) were independently associated with restenosis and were similar across the spectrum of stent devices.[62]

Bifurcation Lesions

Bifurcation lesions are common (up to 20% of all PCIs), and their percutaneous management is associated with higher rates of restenosis and thrombosis compared with nonbifurcation lesions.[63] The risk of side branch occlusion in bifurcation lesions is related to the extent of atherosclerotic involvement of the side branch and geometry of the carina.[64]

Several classification systems have been proposed (Fig. 64.1).[65–68] The Medina classification is the most commonly used and characterizes stenoses in the proximal parent vessel (0 = no disease; 1 = disease), distal vessel (0 = no disease; 1 = disease), and side branch (0 = no disease; 1 = disease). For example, a bifurcation lesion that involves the proximal and distal parent vessel and a side branch with a greater than 50% diameter stenosis is designated Medina 1,1,1, whereas a bifurcation lesion involving only the proximal parent vessel is designated Medina 1,0,0.[66]

One stent usually is preferable to two stents in the parent vessel and side branch.[69,70] If two stents are planned for the parent vessel and side branch due to complex bifurcation disease, several stenting techniques are possible, including simultaneous kissing stents, crush and double-kissing (DK) crush, culotte, T, and T-and-protrusion (TAP) stenting. Common to all of these strategies is a final kissing balloon inflation in the parent vessel and side branch,[71,72] although a sequential two-step dilation of the branch vessel followed by the parent vessel may also be suitable.[73] There is no consensus on which techniques are the optimal treatment strategy for bifurcation lesions.[74,75]

The origin of the side branch rather than the parent vessel is the most common location of failure (recurrence) after bifurcation stenting,[76] and one study of Medina 0,0,1 bifurcation lesions suggested that a two-stent strategy was associated with lower rates of clinical restenosis than a single-stent strategy.[77] Other studies have suggested that the DK crush technique is superior to Culotte stenting for left main CAD[78] and native vessel bifurcations.[79]

Dedicated bifurcation stents were developed to provide adequate vessel coverage and side branch access,[67,80–86] but they have been challenged with their higher profile and difficult delivery. A specifically designed side-branch stent has shown favorable results.[87–90] Drug-eluting balloons have been used in bifurcation lesions with mixed results.[91]

The angiographic analysis of bifurcation lesions is a challenging task. Although the visual assessment of these lesions is inaccurate, the standard quantitative coronary angiography (QCA) packages designed for single lesions cannot overcome the complexities of the bifurcation lesions.[92,93] In an effort to address this shortcoming, dedicated bifurcation QCA algorithms have been developed, such as the Cardiovascular Angiography Analysis System (Pie Medical Imaging, Maastricht, The Netherlands) and QAngio XA (Medis, Leiden, The Netherlands).[93–95] In a survey

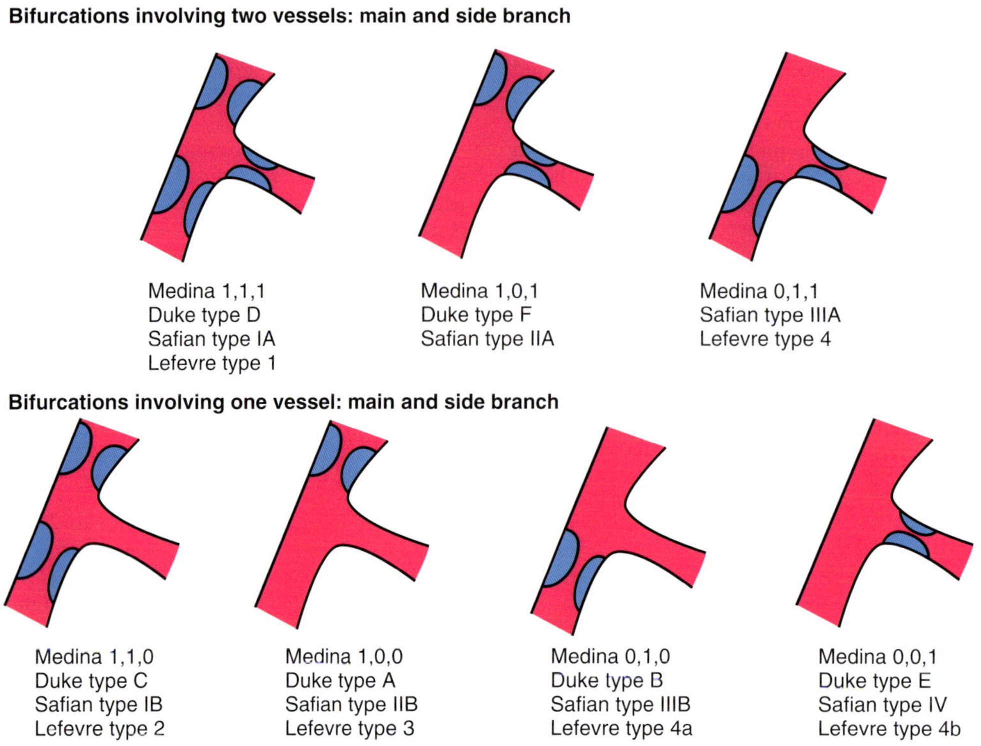

Bifurcations involving two vessels: main and side branch

Medina 1,1,1
Duke type D
Safian type IA
Lefevre type 1

Medina 1,0,1
Duke type F
Safian type IIA

Medina 0,1,1
Safian type IIIA
Lefevre type 4

Bifurcations involving one vessel: main and side branch

Medina 1,1,0
Duke type C
Safian type IB
Lefevre type 2

Medina 1,0,0
Duke type A
Safian type IIB
Lefevre type 3

Medina 0,1,0
Duke type B
Safian type IIIB
Lefevre type 4a

Medina 0,0,1
Duke type E
Safian type IV
Lefevre type 4b

Fig. 64.1 Schematic classification systems for types of bifurcation stenoses.

of experts in the field of bifurcation PCI, accuracy and precision of visual estimates of stenosis severity in phantom bifurcation lesions varied greatly and was less precise compared with the dedicated QCA algorithms, justifying the use of these software packages in clinical and research practice.[96]

Total Occlusion

Total coronary occlusion is identified as an abrupt termination of the epicardial vessel; anterograde and retrograde collaterals may be helpful in quantifying the length of the totally occluded segment. Coronary occlusions are common findings[97] and often lead to the decision to perform coronary bypass surgery rather than PCI in the setting of multivessel disease.[98,99] The success rate for recanalization depends on the occlusion duration and on certain lesion morphologic features, such as bridging collaterals, occlusion length >15 mm, and the absence of a nipple to guide wire advancement. Although newer technologies have been used to recanalize refractory occlusions,[100,101] better guidewires and operator and wire techniques have accounted for much of the improvement in crossing success.[102] Simultaneous coronary injections are sometimes useful for identifying the length of the total occlusion (Fig. 64.2). After the occlusion has been crossed, coronary stents have been used to provide the best long-term outcomes.[103] DES usually are preferred to BMS.[104]

The optimal technique for coronary revascularization is determined using four angiographic parameters: location of the proximal cap, occlusion length, existence of branches and size and quality of the target vessel at the distal cap, and suitability of collaterals for retrograde techniques.[105] On the basis of these four characteristics, there has been a substantial improvement in the ability of the operator to secure access to the coronary vessel.[105]

A key component to the assessment of total occlusion is definition of the collateral grades that provide blood flow to the jeopardized myocardium.[106] The Rentrop classification system includes Rentrop grade 0 (no filling), grade 1 (small side branches filled), grade 2 (partial epicardial filling of the occluded artery), and grade 3 (complete epicardial filling of the occluded artery). Anatomic collaterals summarized by the 26 potential pathways were consolidated into four groups: septal, intra arterial (bridging), epicardial with proximal takeoff (atrial branches), and epicardial with distal takeoff.[107] The size of the collateral connection can be quantified as group 0 (no continuous connection between donor and recipient artery), group 1 (continuous threadlike connection ≤0.3 mm), or group 2 (continuous small, branchlike collateral through its course ≥0.4 mm).[107]

Angiographic Complications After Percutaneous Coronary Intervention

Although the frequency of angiographic complications during PCI has been reduced substantially with the use of coronary stents, untoward effects resulting from disruption of the atherosclerotic plaque and embolization of atherosclerotic debris, thrombus, and vasoactive mediators still occur during 5% to 10% of PCIs (Table 64.4).

Coronary Dissection

Plaque fracture is an integral component of balloon angioplasty, although significant vessel wall disruption resulting in reduced anterograde flow and lumen compromise is a relatively uncommon occurrence (≈3%).[108] The National Heart, Lung, and Blood Institute (NHLBI) coronary dissection criteria categorize the severity of coronary dissection after PCI (see Table 64.4), with the prognostic implications of the coronary dissection depending on extension into the media and adventitia, axial length, existence of contrast staining, and effect on anterograde coronary perfusion. It is sometimes difficult to assess the angiographic residual lumen in the setting of coronary dissection because of the frame-to-frame lumen diameter changes seen with two-dimensional (2D) imaging. IVUS or optimal coherence tomography may provide a more accurate reflection of the lumen's circumference.[109–111] Dissections resulting in a residual stenosis area of 60% or greater

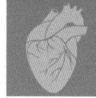

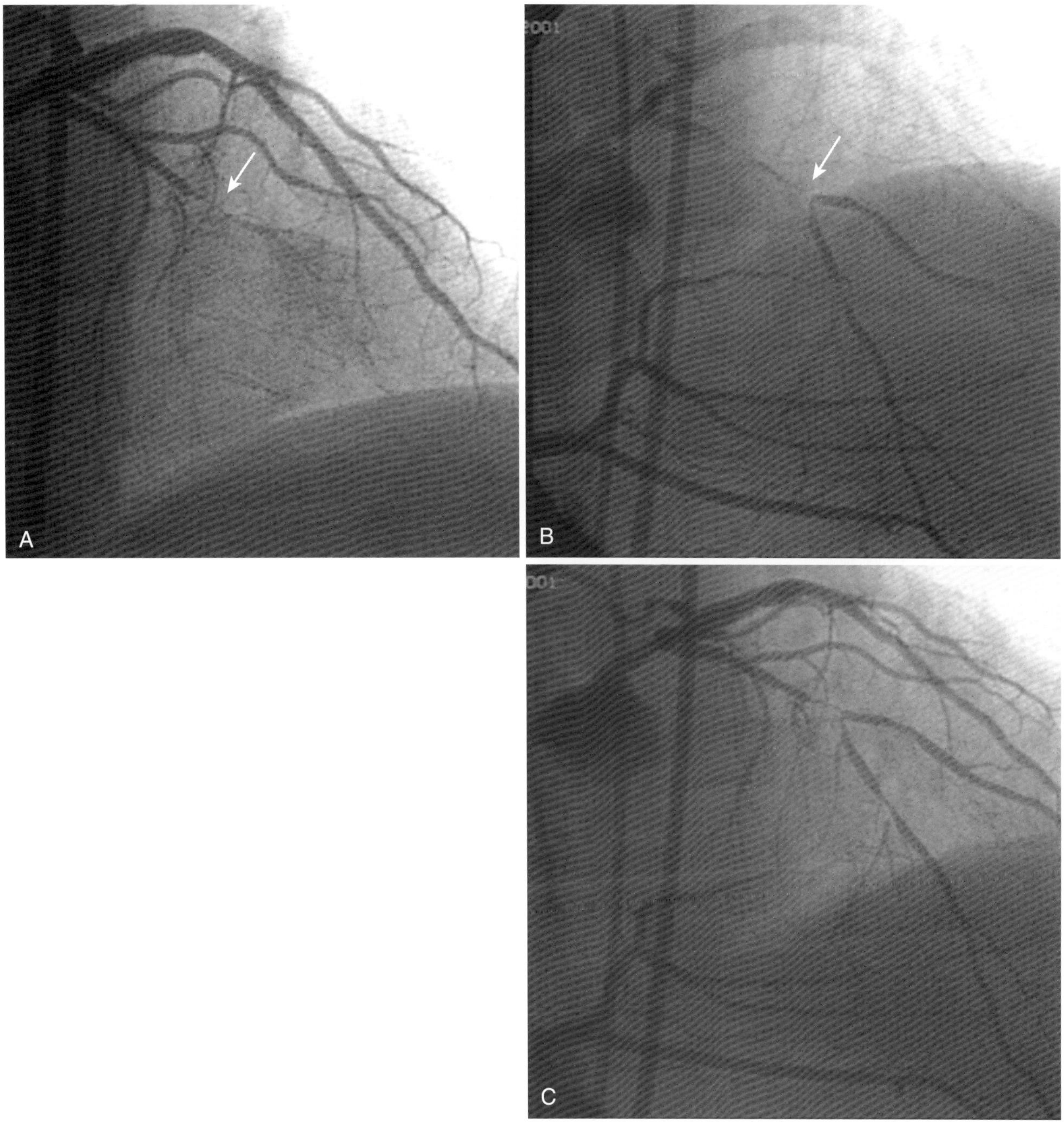

Fig. 64.2 Simultaneous coronary injections to visualize contralateral collaterals. (A) A total occlusion of the middle left anterior descending (LAD) artery is visualized by contrast injection in the left coronary artery *(arrow)*. The distal portion of the LAD is not visualized. (B) Injection of the right coronary artery shows right-to-left collaterals that fill the LAD to the point of occlusion *(arrow)*. (C) Simultaneous injection of the left and right coronary arteries provides sufficient visualization of the total occlusion to allow wire crossing.

by IVUS[109] and those extending to more than 5 to 10 mm in axial length are associated with a worse prognosis. A residual coronary dissection is an independent predictor of stent thrombosis.[63]

No-Reflow Phenomenon

Reduced flow during PCI, also known as the no-reflow phenomenon, is defined as a reduction in anterograde flow despite a patent lumen at the site of PCI.[112] It occurs during 1% to 5% of PCIs. The no-reflow phenomenon is a strong predictor of mortality after PCI.[113] It is more common (15%) during primary angioplasty for AMI.[114] Predictors include a higher plaque burden, thrombus, lipid pools seen by IVUS, higher lesion elastic membrane cross-sectional area, preinfarction angina, and TIMI flow grade 0 on the initial coronary angiogram.[115–118]

Compared with aspirates obtained from patients without the no-reflow phenomenon, aspirates obtained from patients who developed no-reflow contained more atheromatous plaque and significantly more platelet and fibrin complex, macrophages, and cholesterol crystals.[119] The 30-day mortality rate was significantly higher (27.5%) for patients with combined slow-flow and no-reflow phenomenon than for patients with normal coronary

TABLE 64.4 Complications After Percutaneous Coronary Intervention

Variable	Definition
Abrupt closure	Obstruction of contrast flow (TIMI grade 0 or 1) in a dilated segment with previously documented anterograde flow
Ectasia	Lesion diameter greater than the reference diameter in one or more areas
Luminal irregularities	Arterial contour that has a sawtooth pattern consisting of opacification but not fulfilling the criteria for dissection or intracoronary thrombus
Intimal flap	Discrete filling defect in apparent continuity with the arterial wall
Thrombus	Discrete, mobile angiographic filling defect with or without contrast staining
Dissection[a]	
A	Small radiolucent area within the lumen of the vessel
B	Linear, nonpersistent extravasation of contrast
C	Extraluminal, persisting extravasation of contrast
D	Spiral-shaped filling defect
E	Persistent lumen defect with delayed anterograde flow
F	Filling defect accompanied by total coronary occlusion
Length	Measured end to end for type B through F dissections
Staining	Persistence of contrast within the dissection after washout of contrast from the remaining portion of the vessel
Perforation	
Localized	Extravasation of contrast confined to the pericardial space immediately surrounding the artery and not associated with clinical tamponade
Nonlocalized	Extravasation of contrast with a jet not localized to the pericardial space, potentially associated with clinical tamponade
Side branch loss	TIMI grade 0, 1, or 2 flow in a side branch >1.5 mm in diameter that previously had TIMI 3 flow
Coronary spasm	Transient or permanent narrowing >50% when a <25% stenosis was previously identified

[a]National Heart, Lung, and Blood Institute classification system for coronary dissection.
TIMI, Thrombolysis in Myocardial Infarction.

blood flow after PCI (5.3%; $P < .001$).[114] Intracoronary or intragraft nitroprusside,[120] adenosine,[121] verapamil,[122,123] and nicardipine[124] and aspiration of atherosclerotic debris have each been used to correct the no-reflow episode.

Distal Embolization

Periprocedural myonecrosis provides clinical evidence of distal particulate embolization during PCI. Angiographic distal embolization is migration of a filling defect or thrombus that distally occludes the target vessel or one of its branches.[125] It occurs in approximately 10% of patients with AMI undergoing PCI. Embolic complications occur more often in patients with AMI and in patients undergoing balloon angioplasty of SVG lesions, particularly those with a recent occlusion.

Coronary Perforation

Coronary perforation is an uncommon (<1%) complication of PCI that is associated with significant morbidity and mortality.[126–130] Coronary perforations are uncommon in patients undergoing balloon angioplasty (0.1%) compared with patients undergoing atheroablative therapy (1.3%, $P < .001$).[127,131] Perforation due to coronary guidewires may manifest late after the procedure.[132] Initial management strategies include prolonged balloon inflation, reversal of anticoagulation, and in refractory cases, use of polytetrafluoroethylene (PTFE)-covered stents.[133–135]

Prognosis after coronary perforation depends on the extent of extravasation into the pericardium.[131] A classification scheme has been developed based on the angiographic appearance of the perforation. Type I perforations have an extraluminal crater without extravasation, type II perforations contain pericardial or myocardial blushing, and type III perforations have a diameter equal to or greater than 1 mm with contrast streaming and cavity spilling.[131] Type I perforations were associated with no deaths and cardiac tamponade occurred in 8% of patients, type II perforations were associated with no deaths and cardiac tamponade occurred in 13% of cases, and type III perforations were associated with a higher mortality risk and other adverse events.[131,136,137]

Coronary Spasm

Coronary spasm is a transient or sustained reduction in the diameter stenosis by more than 50% in an arterial segment with insignificant (<25%) baseline narrowing. Although coronary spasm may occur in approximately 5% of cases, its frequency has been reduced with the routine use of coronary vasodilators such as nitroglycerin and calcium channel blockers. Wire straightening of the vessel can mimic coronary spasm.

Abrupt Closure

Abrupt closure during coronary intervention is defined as an abrupt cessation of coronary flow to TIMI grade 0 or 1. It occurs during 3% to 5% of balloon angioplasty procedures. Abrupt closure may be caused by coronary dissection, embolization, or thrombus formation within the vessel. Its incidence has been markedly reduced with the availability of coronary stents.[138]

Stent Thrombosis

The Academic Research Consortium has proposed criteria for the timing and definitions used to document stent thrombosis in clinical studies. Timing of stent thrombosis is defined as acute (<24 hours), subacute (24 hours to 30 days), late (30 days to 1 year), and very late (after 1 year).[139] The categories of definite stent thrombosis, probable stent thrombosis, and possible stent thrombosis have been proposed as a more inclusive and

TABLE 64.5 Academic Research Consortium Stent Thrombosis Definitions

Event		Definition
Definite		
	Angiographic confirmation	TIMI flow grade 0 with occlusion originating in or within 5 mm of the stent in the presence of a thrombus *or*
		TIMI flow grade 1, 2, or 3 originating in or within 5 mm of the stent in the presence of a thrombus
		Plus at least one of the following criteria within the last 48 h:
		• New acute onset of ischemic symptoms at rest (typical chest pain lasting >20 min)
		• New ischemic electrocardiographic changes suggesting acute ischemia
		• Typical rise and fall in cardiac biomarkers
	Pathologic confirmation	Evidence of recent thrombus within the stent determined at autopsy or by examination of tissue retrieved after thrombectomy
Probable		Unexplained death within the first 30 days, irrespective of the time after the index procedure
		Myocardial infarction that is related to documented acute ischemia in the territory of the implanted stent without angiographic confirmation of stent thrombosis and in the absence of another cause
Possible		Unexplained death >30 days after intracoronary stenting

TIMI, Thrombolysis in myocardial infarction.

standardized way to characterize the occurrence of this event in patients undergoing stent implantation (Table 64.5).

The incidence of BMS thrombosis within 30 days of the procedure is less than 1%. Predictive factors for stent thrombosis include persistent dissection of NHLBI grade B or higher after stenting, greater total stent length, and a smaller final minimal lumen diameter within the stent.[140] DES administered with longer durations (3 to 6 months) of dual antiplatelet therapy have stent thrombosis rates similar to those found with BMS,[141,142] although premature discontinuation of dual antiplatelet therapy has been associated with higher stent thrombosis rates (6% to 29%) with the use of first-generation DES.[143,144]

Other factors that predispose to stent thrombosis are diabetes, prior brachytherapy, bifurcation lesions with two stents, AMI, renal failure, lower ejection fraction, and longer stent length.[143,144] One concern is the occurrence of very late (>1 year) stent thrombosis with the use of a DES[145] due to inflammation from the stent.[146,147] The likelihood has been substantially reduced with the use of second- and third-generation DES. The estimated incidence of very late stent thrombosis ranges from 0.2% to 0.6% per year up to 3 years after stent placement. Long-term dual antiplatelet therapy may not completely prevent stent thrombosis.[142] A lower stent thrombosis rate has been found for second-generation DES,[148-150] and a shorter duration of dual antiplatelet therapy has been recommended for newer stents.

Restenosis Pattern

When ISR occurs after BMS implantation, the risk of recurrence can be predicted by the pattern of restenosis.[151,152] Using the Mehran classification system, pattern I includes focal (<10 mm long) lesions, pattern II is defined as an ISR >10 mm within the stent, pattern III includes an ISR >10 mm extending outside the stent, and pattern IV is a totally occluded ISR.[151] Pattern I can be classified further by the location of the restenosis: Ia, at the stent articulation (for early generation stents) or gap between stents; Ib, at the edge of the stent; Ic, within the stent; and Id, multifocal.[151]

The need for recurrent TLR increased with increasing ISR class, from 19% to 35%, 50%, and 83% in classes I through IV, respectively ($P < .001$).[151] Restenosis after DES implantation usually is more focal than after BMS placement,[153] and with the sirolimus-eluting stent, it is more commonly seen at the margin of the stent due to balloon injury that is not covered with the stent.[154]

Late Aneurysm Formation

Late vessel wall expansion of greater than 20% after PCI is called a coronary artery aneurysm or, more precisely, a pseudoaneurysm. Aneurysms are rare findings after balloon angioplasty, atheroablation, and coronary stenting.

Coronary artery aneurysms most likely arise from tears or dissection and incomplete healing that compromises vessel wall integrity and results in vessel wall expansion. Coronary artery aneurysms are seen after <1% of DES placements, and their cause in this setting may be related to expansion of all three layers of the arterial wall due to inflammation, the effects of cytostatic or cytotoxic drugs, or malapposition of the stent struts.[155,156] Rarely, coronary artery aneurysms can become infected, requiring surgical intervention.[157,158]

Coronary Perfusion

Evaluation of pharmacologic and mechanical methods to reperfuse coronary occlusions in patients with STEMI is supported by the development of a reproducible angiographic method to assess the degree of coronary recanalization achieved with these therapies. The TIMI flow grade classification characterizes the extent of coronary recanalization in patients with STEMI treated with systemic thrombolytic agents and in patients with NSTEMI and unstable angina (Table 64.6).[159] The TIMI frame count[160] and the TIMI myocardial perfusion grade were developed to further quantify anterograde flow and assess distal microvascular perfusion.[161]

Thrombolysis in Myocardial Infarction Flow Grade Classification

The TIMI flow grade system is a valuable tool for assessing the efficacy of reperfusion strategies in patients with STEMI and for identifying patients at higher risk for an adverse outcome with acute coronary syndromes or undergoing PCI. Several thrombolytic trials have identified an important relationship between the 90-minute TIMI flow grade after thrombolysis and clinical outcome.[162] In the Global Utilization of Streptokinase and Tissue Plasminogen Activator for Occluded Coronary Arteries (GUSTO) angiographic substudy, the mortality rate for patients with TIMI grade 2 flow (7.4%) was similar to the mortality rate for those with TIMI grade 0 or 1 flow (8.9%). In contrast, the mortality rate was lowest (4.4%) for patients with TIMI grade 3 flow.[162]

TABLE 64.6 Thrombolysis in Myocardial Infarction Flow Grade Classification

Grade	Definition
3 (complete reperfusion)	Anterograde flow into the terminal coronary artery segment through a stenosis is as prompt as anterograde flow into a comparable segment proximal to the stenosis. Contrast material clears as rapidly from the distal segment as from an uninvolved, more proximal segment.
2 (partial reperfusion)	Contrast material flows through the stenosis to opacify the terminal artery segment, but contrast enters the terminal segment perceptibly more slowly than more proximal segments. Alternatively, contrast material clears from a segment distal to a stenosis noticeably more slowly than from a comparable segment not preceded by a significant stenosis.
1 (penetration with minimal perfusion)	A small amount of contrast flows through the stenosis but fails to fully opacify the artery beyond.
0 (no perfusion)	No contrast flow through the stenosis

Modified from Sheehan FH, Braunwald E, Canner P, et al. The effect of intravenous thrombolytic therapy on left ventricular function: a report on tissue-type plasminogen activator and streptokinase from the Thrombolysis in Myocardial Infarction (TIMI) Phase I Trial. *Circulation*. 1987;72:817–829.

TABLE 64.7 Thrombolysis in Myocardial Infarction Myocardial Perfusion Grades

Grade	Definition
3	Normal entry and exit of dye from the microvasculature. There is a ground-glass appearance ("blush") or opacification of the myocardium in the distribution of the culprit lesion that clears normally and is gone or is mildly or moderately persistent at the end of the washout phase (approximately three cardiac cycles), similar to an uninvolved artery. Blush that has only mild intensity throughout the washout phase but fades normally is also classified as grade 3.
2	Delayed entry and exit of dye from the microvasculature. There is a ground-glass appearance or opacification of the myocardium in the distribution of the culprit lesion that is strongly persistent at the end of the washout phase (i.e., dye is strongly persistent after three cardiac cycles of the washout phase and does not diminish or only minimally diminishes in intensity during washout).
1	Slow entry of dye into, but failure to exit the microvasculature. There is a ground-glass appearance or opacification of the myocardium in the distribution of the culprit lesion that fails to clear from the microvasculature, and dye staining is seen on the next injection (≈30 s between injections).
0	Failure of the dye to enter the microvasculature. There is minimal or no ground-glass appearance or opacification of the myocardium in the distribution of the culprit artery, indicating lack of tissue-level perfusion.

Despite these important associations, the TIMI classification system has several limitations. Substantial observer variability has been seen for the TIMI flow grade, with the best agreement between the angiographic core laboratory and clinical centers occurring when the artery is graded as open or closed (TIMI grade 0 or 1 flow; $\kappa = 0.84$).[160] Observer agreement is only moderate when assessing TIMI grade 3 flow ($\kappa = 0.55$) and is poor in the assessment of TIMI grade 2 flow ($\kappa = 0.38$). The lack of concordance for determining TIMI flow grade was also shown between experienced angiographic core laboratories.

Another limitation of the TIMI flow grade is that it provides ordinal values rather than continuous values, limiting its statistical power in clinical trials. Although the TIMI flow grade has classically compared flow in the infarct-related vessel to flow in the normal, nonculprit artery, flow in the non infarct-related artery in patients with STEMI is not truly normal compared with flow in patients without STEMI.[163] Difficulties in reproducibly assessing myocardial flow relative to other vessels (e.g., right coronary artery, total occlusions of the contralateral vessel) led some investigators to modify the definition of TIMI grade 3 flow to include opacification of the distal coronary artery within three cardiac cycles.[164] The three cardiac cycle definition of TIMI grade 3 flow results in an absolute rate increase of approximately 10% compared with the original definition.[165] Accordingly, more quantitative measures of anterograde flow were developed.

Thrombolysis in Myocardial Infarction Frame Count

The TIMI frame count (TFC) provides a quantitative assessment of the number of frames required for dye to reach standardized distal landmarks, and it may provide a more objective and precise method of estimating coronary blood flow than the TIMI flow grade.[160] The first frame used for TIMI frame counting is the cineframe in which a column of dye touches both borders of the coronary artery and moves forward, and the last frame is the cineframe in which dye begins to enter (but does not necessarily fill) a standard distal landmark in the artery. The standard distal landmarks for epicardial vessels are the first branch of the posterolateral artery for the right coronary artery, the most distal branch of the obtuse marginal branch in the dye path through the culprit lesion in the circumflex system, and the distal bifurcation, which is also known as the *moustache*, *pitch fork*, or *whale's tail*, in the left anterior descending coronary artery. These frame counts are corrected for the longer length of the left anterior descending coronary artery by dividing the TFC by 1.7 to arrive at the corrected TIMI frame count (CTFC).

The CTFC provides several advantages over TIMI flow grades. The CTFC is quantitative rather than qualitative, objective rather than subjective, and a continuous rather than a categorical variable. Observer variability is substantially less with TFC measurements compared with TIMI flow grades.[160] Although it was traditionally assumed that basal flow in nonculprit arteries in the setting of AMI after thrombolysis was normal, use of the CTFC has shown that basal flow in the uninvolved artery is abnormal.[163]

Thrombolysis in Myocardial Infarction Myocardial Perfusion Grade

Epicardial flow does not necessarily imply tissue-level or microvascular perfusion. These findings led to the development of the TIMI myocardial perfusion grade (TMPG; Table 64.7 and Fig. 64.3), which is a multivariate predictor of mortality in AMI.[161] The TMPG permits risk stratification even within epicardial TIMI grade 3 flow. Despite achieving normal TIMI grade 3 flow after reperfusion therapy, patients with diminished microvasculature perfusion (TMPG 0 or 1) have a persistently elevated mortality rate of 5.4% compared with patients with both TIMI grade 3 flow and TMPG 3, who have a mortality rate less than 1%.[161]

The TIMI flow grades and TMPGs can be combined to identify a group of patients with very low or very high mortality risks after STEMI. Patients with both TIMI grade 3 flow and TMPG 3 flow had a mortality rate of 0.7%, whereas patients with both TIMI grade 0 or 1 and TMPG 0 or 1 flow had a mortality rate of 10.9%. Another approach to assess myocardial perfusion is to use digital subtraction angiography (DSA) to quantitatively

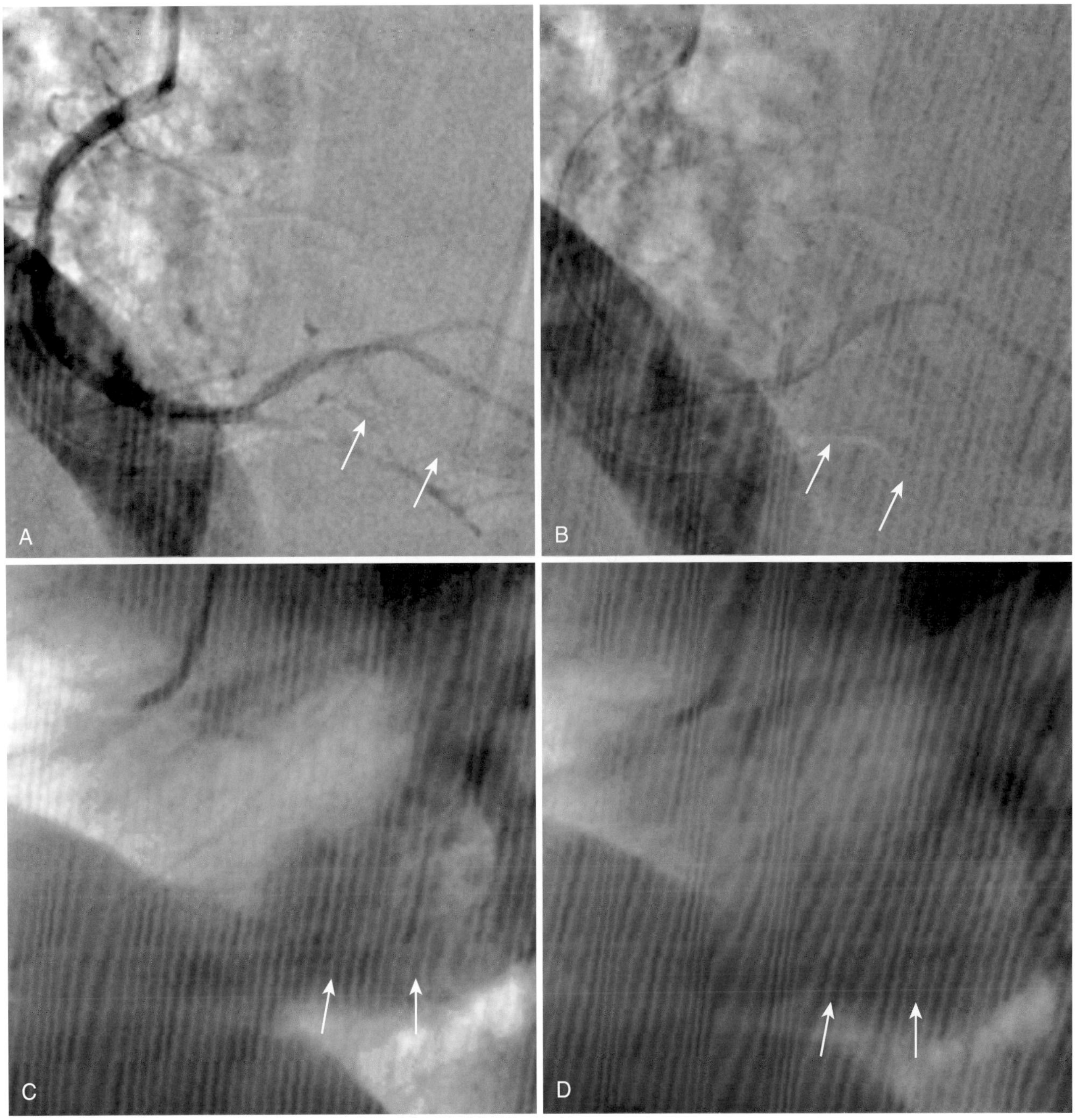

Fig. 64.3 Thrombolysis in Myocardial Infarction myocardial perfusion grade using digital subtraction angiography. Perfusion grade 0 is characterized by the absence of the typical ground-glass filling *(arrows)* of the distal vascular bed during coronary injection (A) and washout (B). Perfusion grade 1 is demonstrated by persistent contrast staining *(arrows)* at the beginning (C) and end (D) of the coronary injection.

characterize the kinetics of dye entering the myocardium during contrast angiography. DSA is performed at end diastole by aligning cineframe images taken before dye fills the myocardium with those taken at the peak of myocardial filling to subtract the spine, ribs, diaphragm, and epicardial artery. A representative region of the myocardium that is free of overlap by epicardial arterial branches is sampled to determine the increase in the grayscale brightness of the myocardium when it first reached its peak intensity. The circumference of the myocardial blush is measured using a handheld planimeter.

The number of frames required for the myocardium to first reach its peak brightness is converted into time (seconds) by dividing the frame count by 30 (for images acquired at 30 frames per second). The rate of rise in brightness (grayscale change per second) and the rate of growth of blush in circumference (centimeters per second) can then be calculated. Using DSA, microvascular perfusion was reduced in AMI patients compared with normal patients, as demonstrated by a reduction in peak brightness (grayscale peak), the rate of rise in brightness, the blush circumference, and the rate of growth of the blush circumference.[165]

Coronary Flow Velocity

Absolute flow velocity can be measured using PCI guidewire velocity.[166] With this technique, the guidewire tip is placed at the coronary landmark after PCI, and a Kelly clamp is placed on the

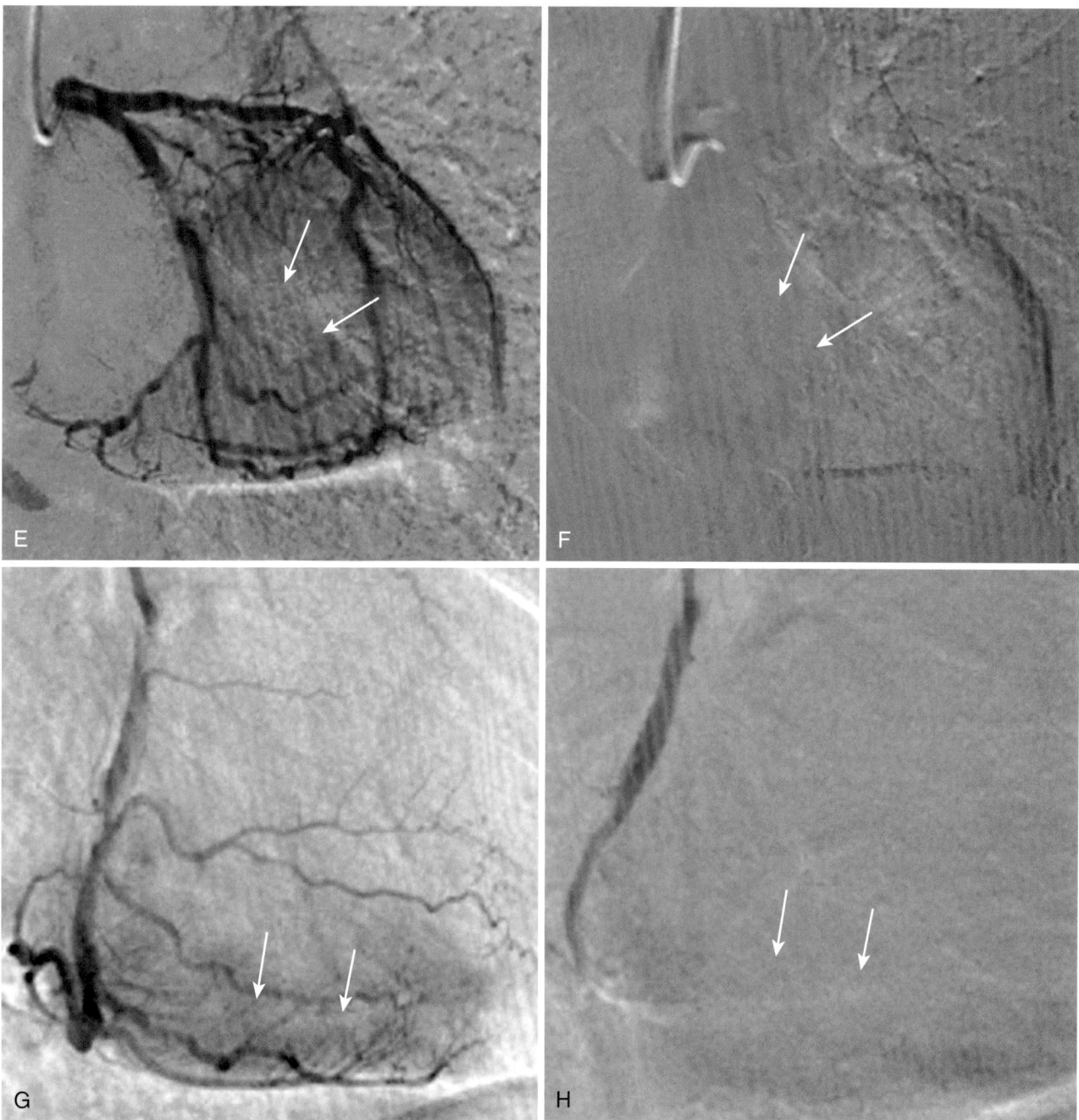

Fig. 64.3, Cont'd Perfusion grade 2 is manifested by a very prominent contrast appearance *(arrows)* at the end of coronary injection (E) that washes out at the end of the contrast injection (F). Perfusion grade 3 is shown as a normal ground-glass appearance *(arrows)* of the distal vascular bed at the end of the contrast injection (G) that washes out at the end of the injection (H).

guidewire at the point at which it exits the Y-adapter. The guidewire tip is then withdrawn to the catheter tip, and a second Kelly clamp is placed on the wire where it exits the Y-adapter. The distance between the two Kelly clamps outside the body is measured as the distance between the catheter tip and the anatomic landmark inside the body. Velocity (cm/s) may be calculated as this distance (cm) divided by TFC (frames) multiplied by the film frame speed (frames per second). Flow (mL/s) may be calculated by multiplying velocity and the mean cross-sectional lumen area (square centimeters) along the length of the artery to the TIMI landmark.

QUANTITATIVE CORONARY ANGIOGRAPHY

QCA is most commonly performed using automated arterial contour detection, although video densitometry and digital parametric imaging have also been tried with limited success. Whereas online QCA is somewhat cumbersome to use in the catheterization laboratory, offline QCA has proved to be valuable for research investigation in determining the effect of new drugs and devices on lumen dimensions early and late after PCI. For clinical decision making about intermediate lesions, neither trained visual estimates nor online quantitative angiography is a substitute for precise physiologic measurements of stenosis severity, such as fractional flow reserve or coronary Doppler measurements.[167]

Nonquantitative Estimates of Lesion Severity

Virtually every interventionalist visually estimates angiographic stenosis severity, although the estimations are of limited value for research studies because of substantial interobserver variability. Blinded review of angiograms by experienced cardiologists found that the average visual estimate of percent diameter stenosis was 85% before PCI (vs. 68% using quantitative methods) and 30% after PCI (vs. 49% using quantitative methods); these differences correspond to a 200% error in the estimation of percent diameter stenosis.[168] Visual estimates of stenosis severity also result in some values (e.g., 90% to 99% diameter stenosis) that are physiologically untenable for anterograde flow. Inherent visual overestimation and underestimation of stenosis severity can be overcome by retraining the clinician's eye.

A more quantitative approach to the assessment of lesion severity uses handheld or digital calipers to estimate quantitative diameters and percent diameter stenosis. Angiographic images are magnified, and calibration is performed by measuring the known dimensions of the diagnostic or guiding catheter using digital calipers. The observer then visually identifies the lumen border using the calipers, and a calibration factor is obtained to determine absolute coronary dimensions. Properly applied, this method appears to correlate weakly with automated edge-detection algorithms. If caliper measurements are obtained from nonmagnified images, the correlation with automated edge-detection algorithms is less accurate.

Computer-Assisted Quantitative Coronary Angiography

QCA was initiated almost 35 years ago by Brown and colleagues,[169] who magnified 35-mm cineangiograms obtained from orthogonal projections and hand-traced the arterial edges on a large screen. After computer-assisted correction for pincushion distortion, the tracings were digitized, and the orthogonal projections were combined to form a 3D representation of the arterial segment, assuming an elliptical geometry. Although the accuracy and precision were enhanced compared with visual methods, the time needed for image processing limited clinical use of this method.

Several automated edge-detection algorithms were then developed and applied to directly acquired digital images or to 35-mm cinefilm digitized images using a cine-video converter. Subsequent iterations of these first-generation devices used enhanced microprocessing speed and digital image acquisition to render the end-user interface more flexible, and they substantially shortened the time required for image analysis.

QCA is divided into several distinct processes, including film digitization (when applicable), image calibration, and arterial contour detection (Fig. 64.4).[170] For estimation of absolute coronary dimensions, the diagnostic or guiding catheter usually serves as the scaling device. A nontapered segment of the catheter is selected, and a centerline through the catheter is drawn. Linear density profiles are then constructed perpendicular to the catheter centerline, and a weighted average of the first and second derivative functions is used to define the catheter edge points. Individual edge points are then connected using an automated algorithm, outliers are discarded, and the edges are smoothed. The diameter of the catheter is used to obtain a calibration factor, which is expressed in millimeters per pixel. The injection catheter dimensions may be influenced by whether contrast or saline is imaged within the catheter tip and by the type of material used in catheter construction. As high-flow injection catheters have been developed, more quantitative angiographic systems have been using contrast-filled injection catheters for image calibration.

The automated algorithm is then applied to a selected arterial segment. Absolute coronary dimensions are obtained from the minimal lumen diameter (MLD) reference diameter, and from these, the percent diameter stenoses are derived. For most angiographic systems, interobserver variabilities are 3.1% for percent diameter stenosis and 0.10 to 0.18 mm for MLD for cineangiographic readings. Interobserver variabilities are slightly higher (<0.25 mm) for repeated analyses of the digital angiograms due to the slightly lower resolution compared with cineangiography. The two most commonly used QCA systems are described in the following sections.

Cardiovascular Angiography Analysis System

The Cardiovascular Angiography Analysis System (Pie Data Medical B.V., Maastricht, The Netherlands) is a QCA system developed for offline cineangiographic analysis (see Fig. 64.2). The edge-detection algorithm incorporates an optional correction for pincushion distortion. Its edge detection uses a weighted (50%) sum of the first and second derivatives of the mean pixel density, and it applies minimal-cost criteria for smoothing of the arterial edge contours. In addition to reporting an interpolated reference diameter and an MLD, subsegment analysis provides mean, minimum, and maximum subsegment diameters. Specific reporting algorithms have been developed for DES, for patients undergoing radiation brachytherapy, and for those undergoing peripheral intervention.

Coronary Measurement System

Specific features of the Coronary Measurement System (CMS, Medis, Leiden, The Netherlands) include two-point, user-defined centerline identification; arterial edge detection using a weighted (50%) sum of the first and second derivatives of the mean pixel density; arterial contour detection using a minimal-cost matrix algorithm; and an interpolated reference vessel diameter. One limitation of the minimal-cost algorithm used with the first-generation CMS system (and the Cardiovascular Angiography Analysis System II system) has been its inability to precisely quantify arterial lumen contours characterized by abrupt changes.

The CMS-GFT algorithm (Medis, Leiden, The Netherlands) is not restricted in its search directions, incorporating multidirectional information about the arterial boundaries for construction of the arterial edge that is suitable for the analysis of complex coronary artery lesions. Specific reporting algorithms have been developed for bifurcation lesions (Fig. 64.5), for DESs (Fig. 64.6), for patients undergoing radiation brachytherapy (Fig. 64.7), and for those undergoing peripheral intervention.

Factors Contributing to Variability Using Quantitative Coronary Angiography

Variability associated with measurements of MLD and reference diameter is affected by several factors, including the biologic differences among lumen diameters (e.g., reference vessel size, vasomotor tone, thrombus), inconsistencies in radiographic image acquisition parameters (e.g., quantum mottling, out-of-plane magnification, foreshortening), and variations in angiographic measurement (e.g., frame selection, factors affecting the edge-detection algorithm; Table 64.8). These factors should be controlled to improve the overall diagnostic accuracy of QCA.

Biologic Variability

Studies that include a wide range of vessel sizes have more biologic variability in vessel diameter (reflected in the standard deviation of the measurements) than those that are more restrictive in their inclusion criteria. Vasomotor tone may also affect the reference vessel size, resulting in distal vasoconstriction and vasospasm that dynamically affect the arterial diameter in paired

SECTION VI   Evaluation of Interventional Techniques

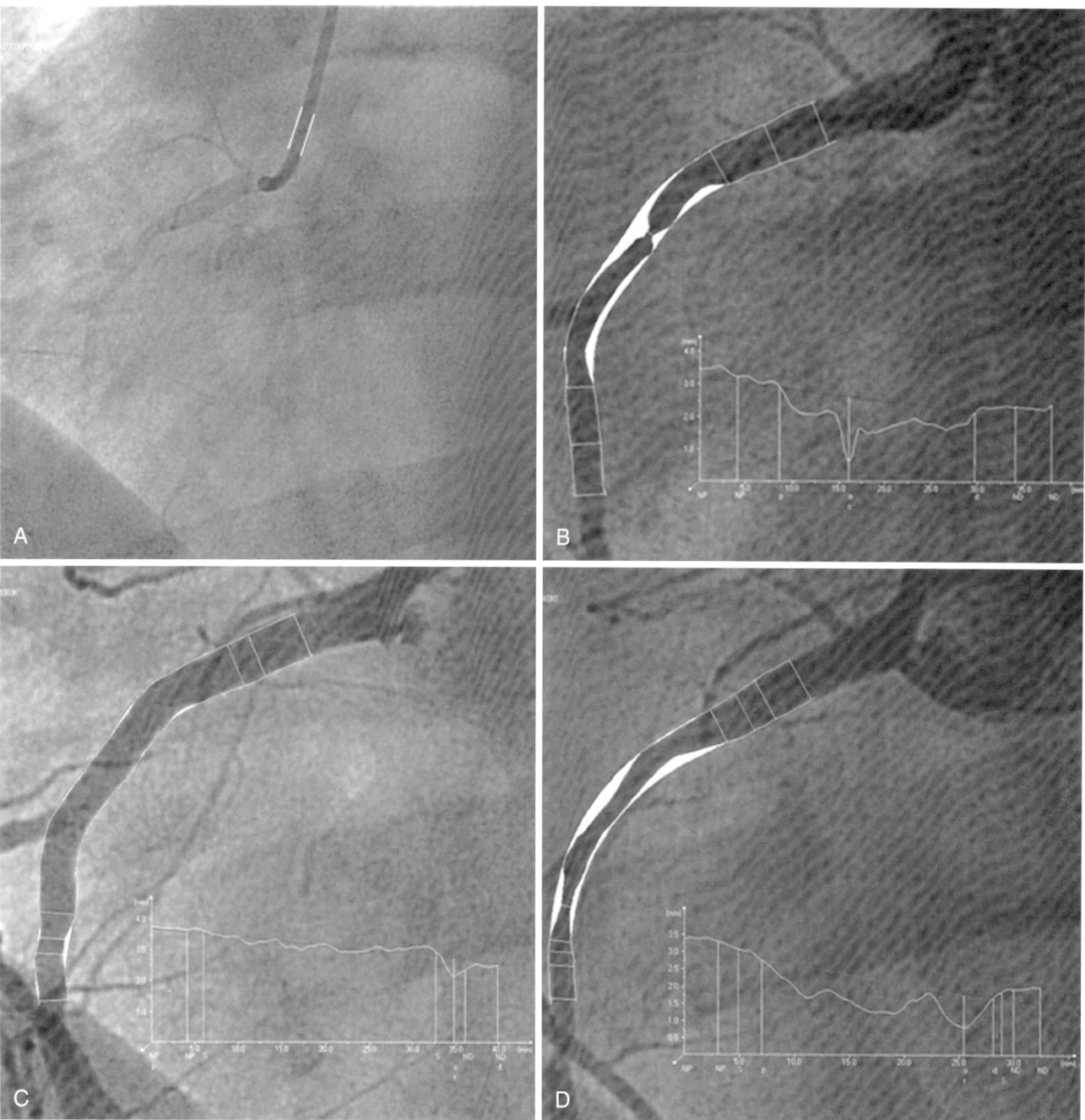

Fig. 64.4 Quantitative coronary angiography. (A) Image calibration is performed using the nontapered portion of the injection catheter as the calibration source. (B) The automated edge detection algorithm (Coronary Measurement System, Medis, Leiden, The Netherlands) is applied to the arterial contour, and the minimal lumen diameter is identified. A diameter function profile curve *(insert)* shows the diameters of the vessel along the length of the analysis segment. (C) After coronary stent placement, the identical length of artery is analyzed to assess lumen improvement. (D) At the time of angiographic follow-up, the location of late lumen loss along the length of the analysis segment is identified.

measurements. Transient maximum coronary vasodilation may be achieved with intracoronary (50 to 200 μg), intravenous (>10 μg/min), or sublingual (0.4 to 0.8 mg) nitroglycerin.

Acquisition Variability

Acquisition factors that affect variability include cardiac and respiratory motion artifact, vessel foreshortening, inadequate filling of the coronary artery (i.e., streaming), overfilling of the aortic cusp with contrast, and failure to separate overlapping branch vessels from the stenosis.[171] These factors may lead to overestimation or underestimation of lesion severity. Out-of-plane magnification and pincushion distortion may also contribute to small errors in angiographic imaging.

For sequential studies, use of the identical angiographic imaging laboratory allows replication of the x-ray generator, tube, and image intensifier parameters. With the introduction of digital imaging and archiving, image compression has raised potential

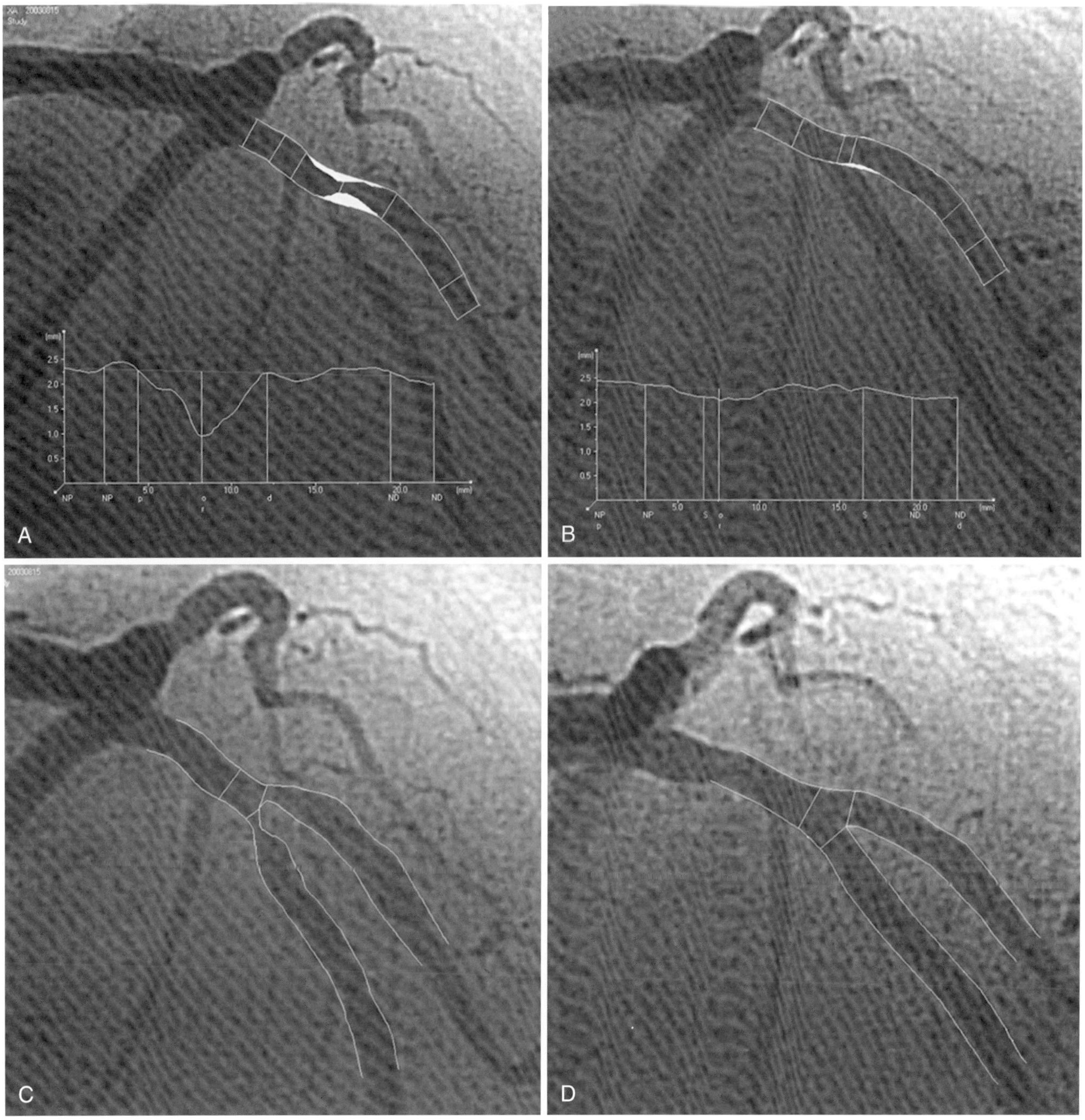

Fig. 64.5 Bifurcation quantitative analysis. Quantitative angiographic analysis of bifurcation lesions is complicated by the difficulty in identifying the minimal lumen diameter at the site of vessel branching. Three methods of bifurcation analysis have been employed. The first is conventional quantitative angiography separately applied to each branch (A, before intervention; B, after intervention). The second method is application of the edge algorithm to both branches (C, before intervention; D, after intervention). The third method is beginning analysis at the ostium of the branch (E, before intervention; F, after intervention).

problems with the quality of image quality for analysis. The Digital Imaging and Communications in Medicine (DICOM) 2:1 Joint Photographic Experts Group (JPEG) lossless compression has become the industry standard for image storage and transfer. It requires approximately 500 megabytes of storage for each imaging study.

The effect of image compression and decompression on image quality was evaluated by a joint task force of the American College of Cardiology and European Society of Cardiology using JPEG images at compression ratios of 1:1 (uncompressed), 6:1, 10:1, and 16:1.[172] Intraobserver analysis showed significant systematic and random errors in the calibration factor at JPEG compression ratios of 10:1 and higher, and they should not be used in QCA clinical research studies.[172] Similar issues exist for the analysis of S-VHS video tapes, which have substantial loss of image resolution. Flat-panel image acquisition does not affect the quality of QCA.[173]

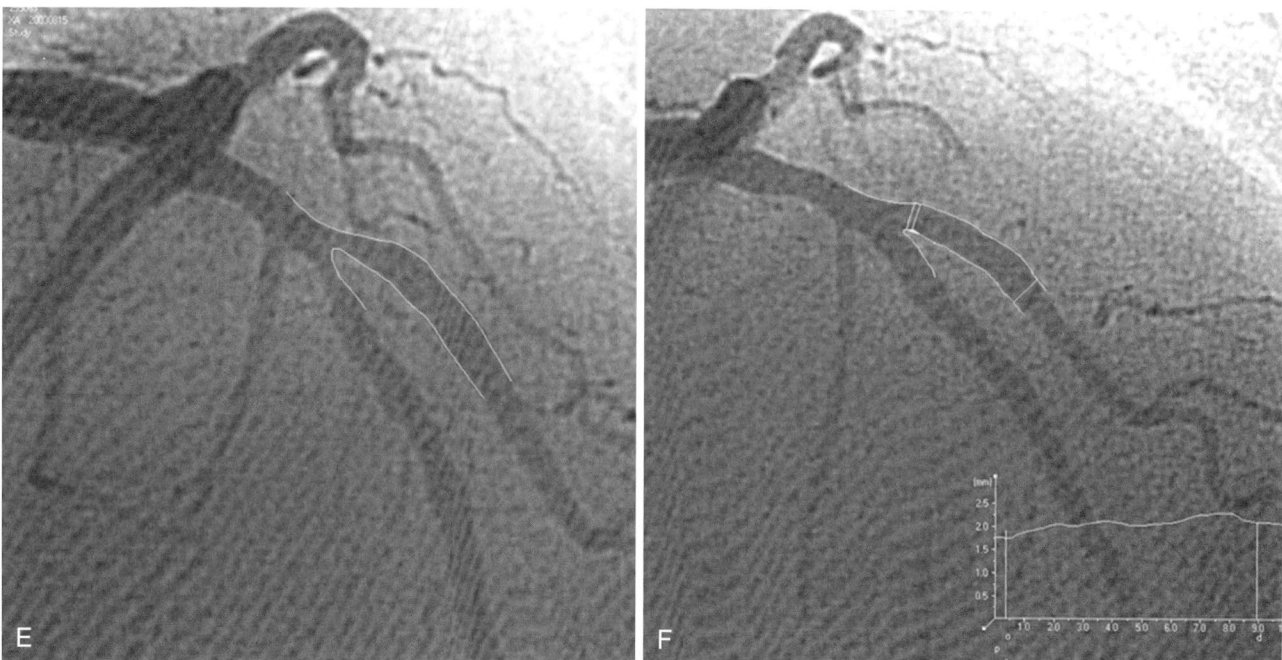

Fig. 64.5, cont'd

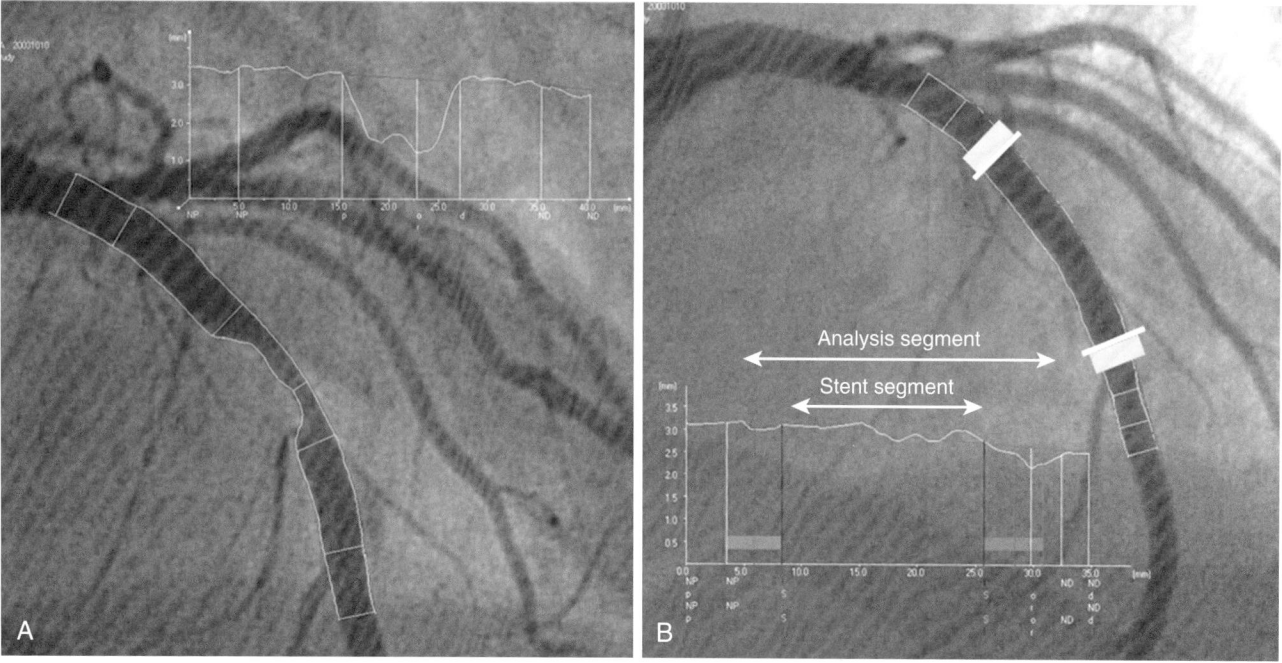

Fig. 64.6 Drug-eluting stent quantitative angiographic analysis. (A) Quantitative angiography is performed on a focal stenosis in the midportion of the left anterior descending coronary artery. (B) After placement of a drug-eluting stent, the proximal and distal portions of the stent are identified *(solid bars)*. A 5-mm proximal and distal edge is also analyzed *(shaded boxes)*. From these measurements, the minimal lumen diameters within the stent (stent segment) and within the region of analysis (analysis segment) are identified.

Measurement Variability

Analysis of two or more orthogonal projections permits a more accurate assessment of the physiologic significance of lesion severity, although a second, technically suitable projection in many cases is unavailable due to vessel foreshortening, overlap, and poor image quality. If orthogonal projections are not available, analyses of the worst-view projection may provide sufficiently accurate information for clinical studies. Herrington and colleagues[174] used a components-of-variance model to show that the process of acquiring and performing QCA on selected cineframes accounted for 57% of the total measurement variability, whereas day-to-day variations in the patient, procedure, and equipment accounted for 30% of total variability. Frame

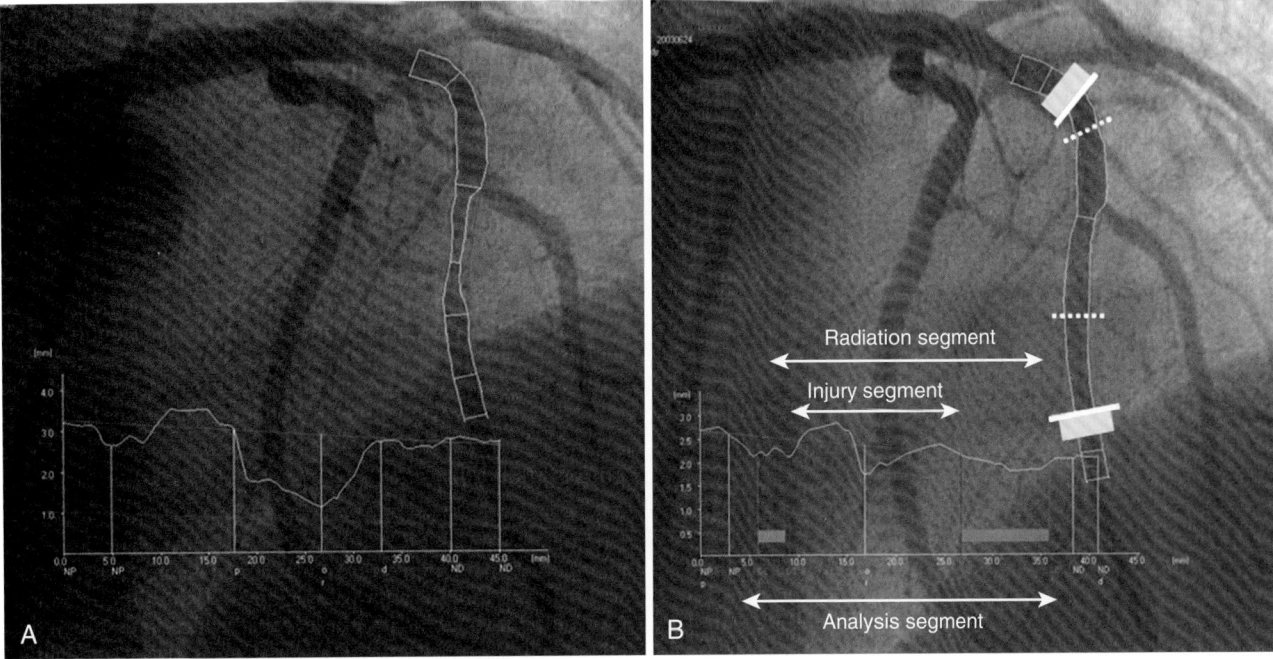

Fig. 64.7 Brachytherapy analysis. (A) Quantitative angiography is performed on a focal stenosis in the midportion of the left anterior descending coronary artery. (B) After balloon angioplasty, the proximal and distal portions of the balloon injury are identified *(dotted lines)*. After radiation brachytherapy, the proximal and distal portion of the radiation injury are identified *(solid lines)*. A 5-mm proximal and distal edge of the radiation zone is also analyzed *(shaded boxes)* to identify the edge effect. From these measurements, the minimal lumen diameters within the segment of balloon injury (injury segment), the segment of radiation injury (radiation segment), and the region of analysis (analysis segment) are identified. The shaded portion in the diameter function profile curve *(insert)* represents the region of the artery that was treated with radiation but was not injured with the balloon.

TABLE 64.8 Correctable Sources of Imaging Error During Acquisition

Source of Error	Potential Corrections
BIOLOGIC VARIATION IN LUMEN DIAMETER	
Vasomotor tone	Nitroglycerin, 100–200 μg intracoronary every 10 min
VARIATIONS IN IMAGE ACQUISITION	
Single Studies	
Vessel motion	
Cardiac	End-diastolic/end-systolic cine frame
Respiratory	Breath hold
Vessel foreshortening	Obtain multiple angiographic projections
Insufficient contrast injection	Use 7- or 8-Fr, large, high-flow catheters
Branch vessel overlap	Obtain multiple angiographic projections
Pincushion distortion	Image objects in center of image
Sequential Studies	
X-ray generator (pulse width/beam)	Repeat study in same imaging
X-ray tube (focal spot/shape/tube current)	Repeat study in same imaging
Image intensifier (magnification/resolution)	Repeat study in same imaging
Differences in angles and gantry height	Record gantry height/angle/skew on worksheet
Image calibration	Use measured catheter diameter
ERRORS IN IMAGE ANALYSIS	
Electronic noise	Recursive digitization and frame averaging
Quantum noise	Spatial filtering of digital image data
Automated edge-detection algorithm	Minimize observer interaction
Selection of reference positions	Interpolated or averaged normal segment
Identification of lesion length	Use of side branches, other landmarks
Frame selection	End-diastolic frame showing worst view

selection accounted for the remaining 13% of total variability. When direct digital angiography is performed and random errors associated with noise in the cine-video pathway are eliminated, frame selection may be a much more important contributor to overall measurement variability. Frame selection has been associated with substantial interobserver variability, and the frame demonstrating the sharpest and tightest view of the stenosis should be used.

Core laboratory reproducibility of various angiographic parameters may affect sample size calculations for various studies.[175] In a repeated (over 1 year) comparison of five quantitative parameters (e.g., MLD, ejection fraction) and six qualitative parameters (e.g., TMPG, TTG), MLD and ejection fraction were the most reproducible, yielding the smallest sample size calculations, whereas percent diameter stenosis and centerline wall motion require substantially larger trials.[175] Of the qualitative parameters, all except TIMI flow grade gave reproducibility characteristics yielding sample sizes of many hundreds of patients. Reproducibility of TMPG and TTG was only moderately good within and between core laboratories, underscoring an intrinsic difficulty in assessing them.[175]

Automated QCA systems have differences in the preferred method of calibration, location of the arterial border, construction of its contour, use of minimal-cost or smoothing algorithms, and selection of normal reference segments. Edge-detection algorithms that identify the arterial edge using a 50% weighted threshold of the first- and second-derivative extrema may produce systematically larger reference and obstruction diameters than those using a 75% weighted value (weighted toward the first-derivative extremum) or the first-derivative extremum itself. These systematic differences may also affect the accuracy and reproducibility of the absolute and relative angiographic measurements. Each angiographic core laboratory should independently determine its own variabilities during the performance of QCA studies, potentially permitting standardization of techniques among different core laboratories.

Quantitative Angiographic Indices

Lumen Improvements After Percutaneous Coronary Intervention

Early and late angiographic results after PCI have been described using a number of QCA criteria. Coronary stents provide a superior residual lumen compared with balloon angioplasty, but they may result in higher amounts of late intimal hyperplasia and late lumen loss than is seen after balloon angioplasty. The net balance is that stents provide a larger late angiographic result.

Angiographic Success

The change in MLD that occurs immediately after PCI is called the acute gain (mm), and the loss of MLD that occurs during the follow-up period is the late loss (mm). Relative changes that occur in the percent diameter stenosis are provided by the following relationship: % diameter stenosis = (1 − [MLD/reference vessel diameter]) × 100.

Traditionally, angiographic success after PCI has been defined as achievement of a <50% residual diameter stenosis,[1] which is most often associated with ≥20% improvement from the baseline diameter stenosis and symptom improvement. With the advent of coronary stents and the determination that stent thrombosis is associated with a suboptimal initial angiographic result, a more contemporary definition of angiographic stenting success is attainment of a less than 20% residual diameter stenosis within the stent, although higher (up to 30%) inflow or outflow diameter stenosis may exist due to residual plaque at the stent margins. Although the documented disparity between visual and quantitative estimates of angiographic success remains a challenge for self-reporting registries that describe procedural outcomes, there has been documented improvement in angiographic success rates over the past decade with the widespread use of coronary stents.[176]

Binary Angiographic Restenosis

Several binary criteria have been used to describe angiographic restenosis after PCI. Binary angiographic restenosis is best defined as a ≥50% diameter stenosis at follow-up, although other dichotomous criteria have been used (e.g., loss of <50% of the initial gain, MLD loss of ≥0.72 mm). Binary angiographic restenosis after DES placement may occur within the stent (i.e., ISR), within the 5-mm margins of the stent (i.e., edge restenosis), or within the segment between the proximal and distal reference segments (i.e., in-segment or in-lesion restenosis).

Late Lumen Loss

The long-term success of PCI can be measured by several QCA parameters. Serial QCA studies have shown that there is an approximately 0.5-mm reduction in lumen diameter that develops within 3 to 6 months after balloon angioplasty, although angiography cannot differentiate whether this reduction in lumen diameter results from intimal hyperplasia or arterial remodeling or constriction. Lumen loss after balloon angioplasty follows a near-Gaussian distribution. Because there is little or no arterial remodeling after BMS placement, late lumen loss after stent placement primarily results from intimal hyperplasia, and angiographic estimates of volumetric percent volume obstruction correlate well with intravascular ultrasound measurements of intimal hyperplasia.[177] Several technical factors may compromise the ability of late lumen loss to characterize overall reductions in lumen diameters, including calibration errors at the time of postprocedural or follow-up assessments and the relocation of the MLD between the postprocedural and follow-up examinations.[178] The distribution of late lumen loss after placement of DES is unlike the distribution of late lumen loss after BMS placement, with a narrowing variance (i.e., standard deviation) due to the reduced tissue growth and a rightward skew of the late-lumen-loss histogram.[179]

The patient-based relationship between late lumen loss and TLR was examined in 1314 patients with de novo lesions who were treated with BMS or paclitaxel-eluting stents.[180] Analysis found that the relationship between late lumen loss and TLR was monotonic and curvilinear, with the likelihood of TLR not exceeding 5% until the analysis segment late loss was >0.5 mm, and did not exceed 10% until late loss was >0.65 mm.[180] At lower magnitudes of late lumen loss, there was a very small incremental increase in the occurrence of TLR. With higher degrees of late lumen loss, the relationship of late loss and TLR was steep and almost linear.[180] The rate of TLR was related to median late loss and measures of its statistical distribution. TLR increased with the lack of homogeneous biologic response, manifested by greater variance (i.e., higher standard deviations) and a greater right skew of the late-lumen-loss histogram.[180]

To correct for the rightward skew and to develop better predictive models of restenosis, an optimized power transformation was applied to data from patients enrolled in two sirolimus-eluting stent trials to predict binary angiographic restenosis rates and compare them with observed restenosis rates.[179] The mean in-stent late loss was 0.17 ± 0.45 mm after sirolimus-eluting stent placement and 1.00 ± 0.70 mm after BMS placement. If a normal distribution was assumed, late loss accurately estimated in-stent binary angiographic restenosis for the BMS (predicted 35.4% vs. observed 35.4%) but underestimated the binary restenosis rate in the sirolimus-eluting stent arm (predicted 0.6% vs. observed 3.2%). Power transformation improved the reliability of the estimate in the sirolimus arm (predicted 3.2% vs. observed 3.2%).

Another study did not confirm the value of the power transformation as a predictor of binary angiographic restenosis.[181]

To formally evaluate four potential angiographic surrogate markers for TLR by applying well-defined criteria of surrogacy to an extensive database of randomized DES trials, Pocock and colleagues analyzed 11 multicenter, prospective, randomized stent trials enrolling 5381 patients with a single treated lesion and follow-up angiography.[182] Based on four surrogate criteria, late loss and percent diameter stenosis strongly predicted the risk of TLR, with in-segment percent diameter stenosis being the most highly predictive (C-statistic = 0.95). Whereas late loss as a surrogate was dependent on vessel size, percent diameter stenosis was independent of vessel size. Differences in TLR rates for BMS and DES were fully explained statistically by their differences in late loss and percent diameter stenosis. However, because of the curvilinearity of the logistic model, trials comparing two effective DES can have significant differences in mean late losses and percent diameter stenosis but negligible expected differences in TLR risk. Others have suggested a stronger relationship between late loss and TLR for comparative DES trials,[183] but whether late lumen loss will serve as a meaningful surrogate end point in DES comparative trials remains controversial.

Limitations of Quantitative Coronary Angiography

The ability of QCA to accurately detect the presence and severity of coronary atherosclerosis is limited by several factors. Compensatory arterial dilation occurs during the early stages of coronary atherosclerosis, resulting in a preserved coronary lumen despite significant coronary atherosclerosis. Routine coronary angiography can accurately measure the arterial lumen but is relatively insensitive for the detection of arterial wall atherosclerosis, circumferential plaque distribution, vessel wall calcification, and lumen dimensions after stent implantation.

Coronary angiography is limited to a lesser extent by radiographic factors, such as cardiac motion, pincushion distortion, and quantum mottling. Most analytic systems have difficulty discriminating values <1.0 mm due to the limitations of radiographic imaging of small objects (e.g., veiling glare, point spread function). Newer methods incorporating adaptive simultaneous coronary border detection have been developed to more accurately assess smaller vessel dimensions. Interpretation of 2D angiographic views can be affected by foreshortening and overlapping of vessels, leading to inaccurate measurements, particularly in tortuous vessels.[184]

Three-Dimensional Imaging

Some commercial software systems have developed 3D reconstruction of a coronary artery by fusing two or more orthogonal angiographic images to address some of the limitations associated with 2D QCA.[185,186] The 3D QCA yields a more accurate depiction than standard 2D QCA of intermediate lesions using fractional flow reserve as the reference standard.[187] Validation of 3D QCA against IVUS in small studies has shown good correlation between the two in assessing vessel geometry, especially assessment of segment length.[188,189] In an analysis of patients with left main stenosis, 3D QCA was better than 2D QCA in identifying a significant left main stenosis when using IVUS as the gold standard.[190] Given these results, 3D QCA reconstruction is proving to be a promising tool for clinical and research applications in interventional cardiology.

KEY REFERENCES

5. Krone R, Shaw R, Klein L, et al. Evaluation of the American College of Cardiology/American Heart Association and the Society for Coronary Angiography and Interventions lesion classification system in the current "stent era" of coronary interventions (from the ACC-National Cardiovascular Data Registry). *Am J Cardiol*. 2003;92:389–394.
6. Singh M, Rihal CS, Lennon RJ, et al. Comparison of Mayo Clinic risk score and American College of Cardiology/American Heart Association lesion classification in the prediction of adverse cardiovascular outcome following percutaneous coronary interventions. *J Am Coll Cardiol*. 2004;44:357–361.
8. Sianos G, Morel MA, Kappetein AP, et al. The SYNTAX score: an angiographic tool grading the complexity of coronary artery disease. *EuroIntervention*. 2005;1:219–227.
9. Serruys PW, Onuma Y, Garg S, et al. Assessment of the SYNTAX score in the Syntax study. *EuroIntervention*. 2009;5:50–56.
11. Capodanno D, Capranzano P, Di Salvo ME, et al. Usefulness of SYNTAX score to select patients with left main coronary artery disease to be treated with coronary artery bypass graft. *JACC Cardiovasc Interv*. 2009;2:731–738.
13. Holzhey DM, Luduena MM, Rastan A, et al. Is the SYNTAX score a predictor of long-term outcome after coronary artery bypass surgery? *Heart Surg Forum*. 2010;13:E143–E148.
18. Farooq V, van Klaveren D, Steyerberg EW, et al. Anatomical and clinical characteristics to guide decision making between coronary artery bypass surgery and percutaneous coronary intervention for individual patients: development and validation of SYNTAX score II. *Lancet*. 2013;381:639–650.
26. Mintz GS, Popma JJ, Pichard AD, et al. Patterns of calcification in coronary artery disease. A statistical analysis of intravascular ultrasound and coronary angiography in 1155 lesions. *Circulation*. 1995;91:1959–1965.
32. Moussa I, Ellis SG, Jones M, et al. Impact of coronary culprit lesion calcium in patients undergoing paclitaxel-eluting stent implantation (a TAXUS-IV substudy). *Am J Cardiol*. 2005;96:1242–1247.
51. Sianos G, Papafaklis MI, Daemen J, et al. Angiographic stent thrombosis after routine use of drug-eluting stents in ST-segment elevation myocardial infarction: the importance of thrombus burden. *J Am Coll Cardiol*. 2007;50:573–583.
67. Lefevre T, Louvard Y, Morice MC, et al. Stenting of bifurcation lesions: classification, treatments, and results. *Catheter Cardiovasc Interv*. 2000;49:274–283.
68. Movahed MR. Quantitative angiographic methods for bifurcation lesions: a consensus statement from the European Bifurcation Group. Shortcoming of the Medina classification as a preferred classification for coronary artery bifurcation lesions in comparison to the Movahed classification. *Catheter Cardiovasc Interv*. 2009;74:817–818.
151. Mehran R, Dangas G, Abizaid A, et al. Angiographic patterns of in-stent restenosis. Classification and implications for long-term outcome. *Circulation*. 1999;100:1872–1878.
161. Gibson C, Cannon C, Murphy S, et al. Relationship of TIMI myocardial perfusion grade to mortality following thrombolytic administration. *Circulation*. 2000;101:125–130.
165. Gibson CM, Cannon CP, Murphy SA, et al. Relationship of the TIMI myocardial perfusion grades, flow grades, frame count, and percutaneous coronary intervention to long-term outcomes after thrombolytic administration in acute myocardial infarction. *Circulation*. 2002;105:1909–1913.
166. Gibson CM, Dodge JT, Goel M, et al. Angioplasty guidewire velocity: a new simple method to calculate absolute coronary blood velocity and flow. *Am J Cardiol*. 1997;80:1536–1539.
179. Mauri L, Orav EJ, O'Malley AJ, et al. Relationship of late loss in lumen diameter to coronary restenosis in sirolimus-eluting stents. *Circulation*. 2005;111:321–327.
180. Ellis SG, Popma JJ, Lasala JM, et al. Relationship between angiographic late loss and target lesion revascularization after coronary stent implantation: analysis from the TAXUS-IV trial. *J Am Coll Cardiol*. 2005;45:1193–1200.
182. Pocock SJ, Lansky AJ, Mehran R, et al. Angiographic surrogate end points in drug-eluting stent trials: a systematic evaluation based on individual patient data from 11 randomized, controlled trials. *J Am Coll Cardiol*. 2008;51:23–32.
183. Mauri L, Orav EJ, Candia SC, et al. Robustness of late lumen loss in discriminating drug-eluting stents across variable observational and randomized trials. *Circulation*. 2005;112:2833–2839.

 Additional references available online at expertconsult.com.

中文导读

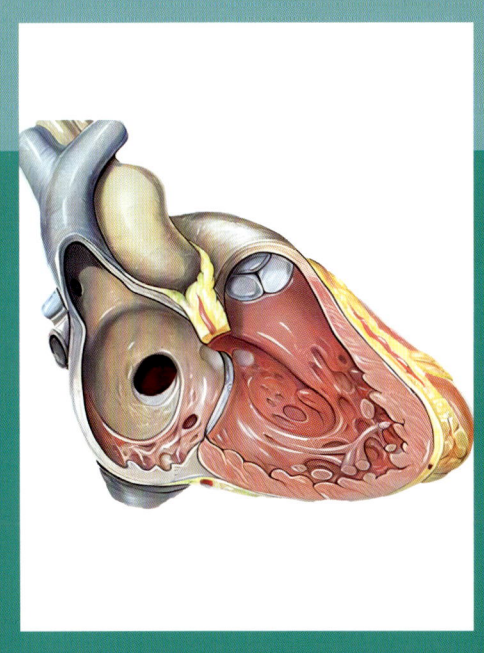

第65章
血管内超声

　　随着腔内影像学的快速发展，血管内超声作为冠状动脉造影的重要补充手段已经被广泛应用。血管内超声技术能清晰显示血管壁结构、精确测量管腔面积、辨认斑块成分组成及预测病变进展速度，已经成为临床实践和科学研究不可缺少的工具。本章节阐述了血管内超声的基本成像原理、操作要领、图像判读，以及临床应用。

　　血管内超声作为介入术者的"眼睛"，在冠状动脉手术中起到辅助决策作用，包括术前病变性质评估、术中支架尺寸选择，以及术后支架优化评价。血管内超声对斑块的评估主要包括定量和定性分析，前者可以测量病变长度和管腔面积，后者可以判断斑块组成，包括脂质池、纤维化及钙化。通过血管内超声评估可以决定病变所需支架的长短和大小，而术后血管内超声评价则可以提供支架膨胀程度，以及并发症的早期识别。随着临床应用的需求及成像技术的不断迭代，许多基于血管内超声的衍生物，包括虚拟组织学功能、血管内超声—近红外光谱分析组合、血管内超声—光学相干断层成像系统等，能够提供更多的信息。当代介入治疗不仅需要解剖学评价，更强调血管功能学的结果。未来，血管内超声技术将继续开发血管功能学测量，实现解剖学和功能学一体化评价，更好地辅助术者为患者提供个性化精准治疗。

胡祥铭　吴永健

章节要点

- 血管内超声是第一个直观显示血管壁动脉粥样硬化或其他病理变化的临床影像学方法。
- 血管内超声核心技术改进能够产生高分辨率图像，提供便捷操作。
- 血管内超声为血管生物学过程提供重要的参考，如斑块负荷程度、血管重塑和再狭窄。
- 面对复杂或难以解释的血管造影情况时，血管内超声作为一种实用工具，可以用于选择恰当的介入治疗策略，优化血运重建的结局。
- 目前处于探索阶段的一些先进技术可能会进一步提高血管内超声在介入心脏病学的研究和临床领域的实用性，特别是在需要复杂治疗来改善血管功能的情况下。

65 Intravascular Ultrasound

Yasuhiro Honda, Peter J. Fitzgerald, Paul G. Yock

KEY POINTS

- Intravascular ultrasound (IVUS) was the first clinical imaging method to directly visualize atherosclerosis and other pathologic conditions within the walls of blood vessels.
- Improvements in core IVUS technology have allowed for higher-resolution images and greater operator convenience.
- IVUS has provided significant insights into biologically mediated processes of the vasculature, such as the extent of plaque burden, vascular remodeling, and restenosis.
- IVUS is a practically useful tool in clarifying situations in which angiography results are equivocal or difficult to interpret, selecting the appropriate catheter-based intervention, and optimizing the results of revascularization procedures.
- Advanced technical developments currently being explored may further enhance the usefulness of IVUS in both research and clinical arenas of interventional cardiology, particularly with sophisticated therapeutic technologies to modify local vascular biology.

INTRODUCTION

Intravascular ultrasound (IVUS) was the first clinical imaging method to directly visualize atherosclerosis and other pathologic conditions within the walls of blood vessels. Because the ultrasound signal is able to penetrate below the luminal surface, the entire cross section of an artery—including the complete thickness of a plaque—can be imaged in real time. This offers the opportunity to gather diagnostic information about the process of atherosclerosis and to directly observe the effects of various interventions on the plaque and arterial wall.

The first ultrasound imaging catheter system was developed by Bom and colleagues in Rotterdam in 1971 for intracardiac imaging of chambers and valves.[1] In the early to mid-1980s, several groups began work on catheter systems designed to image plaque and facilitate balloon angioplasty and other catheter-based interventions. The first images of human vessels were recorded by Yock and colleagues in 1988, with coronary images produced the next year by the same group and by Hodgson and colleagues.[2] The intervening period has seen rapid technical improvements of the systems, with significant enhancement in image quality and miniaturization of the imaging catheters.

IMAGING SYSTEMS AND PROCEDURES

Basic Principles

IVUS imaging systems use reflected sound waves to visualize the vessel wall in a two-dimensional, tomographic format, analogous to a histologic cross section. These systems use significantly higher frequencies than noninvasive echocardiography, achieving greater radial resolutions at the expense of limited beam penetration. The resolution, depth of penetration, and attenuation of the acoustic pulse by tissue are dependent on the geometric and frequency properties of the transducer. Current IVUS catheters used in the coronary arteries have center frequencies ranging from 20 to 60 MHz, providing theoretical lower limits of resolution (calculated as half the wavelength) of 39 and 13 μm, respectively. In practice, the radial resolution is at least two to five times poorer (i.e., 40–150 μm) and is determined by factors such as the length of the emitted pulse and the position of the imaged structures relative to the transducer. There are two basic catheter designs, based on solid-state or mechanical approaches (Fig. 65.1). Both types of catheters generate a 360-degree, cross-sectional image plane that is perpendicular to the catheter tip.

Solid-State Dynamic Aperture System

In the solid-state approach, the individual elements of a circumferential array of transducer elements, mounted near the tip of the catheter, are activated with different time delays to create an ultrasound beam that sweeps the circumference of the vessel. As the number of elements has increased, there have been progressive improvements in lateral resolution. Complex miniaturized integrated circuits in the catheter tip control the timing and integration of the transducer activation and route the resulting echocardiographic information to a computer, where cross-sectional images are reconstructed and displayed in real time. One of the technical advantages of the multielement approach is the ability to manipulate the beam electronically—achieving, for example, the ability to focus at different depths.

The current solid-state coronary catheter system (Philips, San Diego, CA) has 64 transducer elements arranged around the catheter tip and uses a center frequency of 20 MHz. The latest coronary catheters in a rapid-exchange configuration are 3.5 Fr in scanner diameter and thus compatible with a 5-Fr guide catheter. Larger intracardiac echocardiography (ICE) or peripheral imaging catheters are produced in both over-the-wire and rapid-exchange configurations. As an exception, a phased-array catheter (8 or 10 Fr) for ICE imaging (Siemens Healthcare, Erlangen, Germany) uses a different technology, adapted from transesophageal echocardiography, which provides a sector ultrasound image with capabilities of color/spectral Doppler and real-time three-dimensional imaging. The catheter is compatible with multiple-frequency imaging (5 to 9 MHz) so that the operator can determine the desired trade-off between resolution and penetration (up to 15 cm).

Mechanically Rotating Single-Transducer System

In the mechanical approach, a single transducer element is rotated at 960 to 5400 rpm inside a protective sheath at the distal tip of a catheter, via a flexible torque cable that is spun by an external motor drive unit attached to the proximal end of the catheter. Images from each angular position of the transducer are collected by a computerized image array processor, which synthesizes a cross-sectional ultrasound image of the vessel. Mechanical IVUS systems are commercially available from several manufacturers in slightly different configurations. Currently available coronary imaging catheters operate at a center frequency of 40, 45, or 60 MHz with a distal crossing profile of 2.6 to 3.2 Fr, compatible

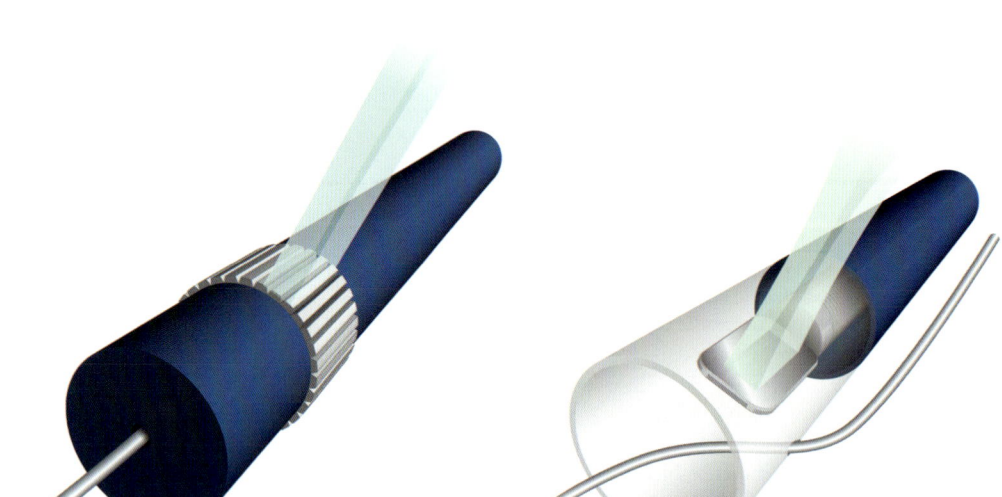

Fig. 65.1 Diagrams of the two basic imaging catheter designs: solid-state (A) and mechanical (B) approaches.

with 6-Fr (Philips; Boston Scientific Corporation, Natick, MA; Infraredx, Burlington, MA; ACIST Medical Systems, Eden Prairie, MN) or 5-Fr guide catheters (Philips; Boston Scientific; Terumo Corporation, Tokyo, Japan). Larger catheters with lower center frequencies are also available for intracardiac and peripheral imaging.

The catheters are advanced over a standard guidewire using a short rail section located distal to the protective sheath at the catheter tip. To improve the trackability and pushability, one manufacturer (Terumo) provides an imaging catheter with a second, long-rail section located proximally in addition to the standard short-rail section at the catheter tip. Unlike the solid-state catheter that incorporates the transducer assembly surrounding the guidewire lumen, the fact that the guidewire runs outside the catheter, parallel to the imaging segment, results in a shadow artifact in the mechanical IVUS image (the guidewire artifact).

Head-to-Head Comparisons

Mechanical systems have traditionally offered advantages in image quality compared with the solid-state systems because of their higher center frequencies and the larger effective aperture of a transducer element. In particular, near-field resolution is excellent with mechanical catheters, and digital subtraction of the ring-down artifact is not required. In addition, a stationary outer sheath of mechanical catheters allows the transducer to be moved through a segment of interest in a precise and controlled manner.

Conversely, the longer rapid-exchange design of the solid-state catheter may track better than the short-rail design of the mechanical systems in complex coronary anatomy. The distance of the transducer from the catheter tip is shorter than that of mechanical systems, which may also be beneficial in IVUS-guided intervention with chronic total occlusion (CTO) lesions. The solid-state catheter includes no moving parts and therefore is free from nonuniform rotational image distortion (NURD) (Fig. 65.2D). This artifact can occur with mechanical systems when bending of the drive cable interferes with uniform transducer rotation, causing a wedge-shaped, smeared image to appear in one or more segments of the image. This may be corrected by straightening the catheter and motor drive assembly, lessening tension on the guide catheter, or loosening the hemostatic valve of the Y-adapter.

Overall, technical improvements are continuously being made in both systems, and good-quality images can be achieved with either of them in most cases. With both systems, serial cross-sectional images can be reconstructed into a longitudinal display mode, and both still frames and video images can be digitally archived on local storage memory or on a remote server in accordance with Digital Imaging and Communications in Medicine (DICOM) standard. Either system can be installed directly into the cineangiogram system, enabling operators to quickly and easily incorporate IVUS interrogations into their interventional procedures.

Imaging Procedures

Before IVUS imaging, an intravenous injection of 5000 to 10,000 units of heparin or equivalent anticoagulation should be administered (an activated clotting time of >250 seconds is recommended). Intracoronary nitroglycerin (100 to 200 μg) should also be routinely administered before delivery of the IVUS catheter to induce maximal vasodilation and prevent vasospasm. The image integrity of the IVUS system should be checked before the catheter is inserted. Mechanical catheters require a saline flush before insertion to eliminate any air in the protective sheath. Incomplete flushing can leave microbubbles adjacent to the transducer, resulting in poor image quality once the catheter is inserted (see Fig. 65.2A). With a solid-state catheter, the catheter tip is first positioned in the aorta or a large proximal coronary vessel (not adjacent to any vessel wall) so that the ring-down artifact (a "halo" surrounding the catheter) can be electronically subtracted from the image before the catheter enters the coronary artery. If a significant ring-down artifact is observed with a mechanical catheter, microbubbles within the protective sheath may be suspected, requiring repeated saline flush procedures until the artifact is removed (see Fig. 65.2A).

The technique for delivering IVUS catheters is similar to that used for standard angioplasty or stent catheters. The imaging element is advanced at least 10 mm distal to the area of interest over a standard 0.014-inch angioplasty guidewire, and the length of the target vessel is systematically scanned by retracting the transducer within the protective sheath (mechanical system) or by withdrawal of the entire catheter (solid-state system). Automated pullback devices withdraw the imaging element at a steady

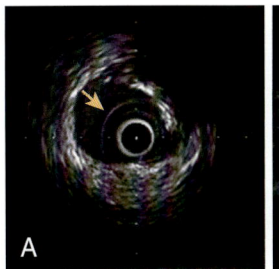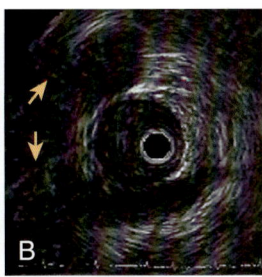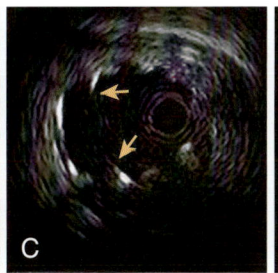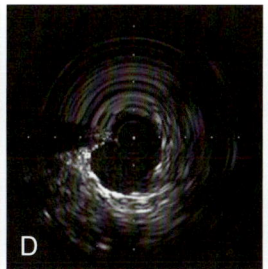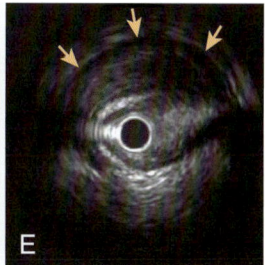

Fig. 65.2 Common image artifacts. (A) A "halo" or a series of bright rings immediately surrounding the mechanical intravascular ultrasound catheter *(arrow)* is usually caused by air bubbles that need to be flushed out. (B) Radiofrequency noise *(arrows)* appears as alternating radial spokes or random white dots in the far-field. The interference is usually caused by other electrical equipment in the cardiac catheterization laboratory. (C) "White cap" artifacts caused by side lobe echoes *(arrows)* originate from a strong reflecting surface, such as metal stent struts or calcification. Smearing of the strut image can lead to the mistaken impression that the struts are protruding into the lumen, potentially interfering with area measurements and the assessment of apposition, dissection, and so on. (D) Nonuniform rotational distortion (NURD) results in a wedge-shaped, smeared appearance in one or more segments of the image (between 9 and 4 o'clock in this example). (E) A "wrinkling" (or "accordion") artifact is caused by an artificial vessel kink associated with intravascular instrumentation (a guidewire or imaging catheter); this results in an abrupt change of arterial dimensions with external compression by a heterogeneous or low-echoic structure *(arrows)* partially surrounding the artery.

rate, which allows accurate axial registration of each cross section for serial studies or precise longitudinal distance measurements. Conventional IVUS systems offer a pullback rate of 0.5 or 1.0 mm/s, whereas higher image acquisition rates of the latest generation systems allow faster pullback at up to 9 mm/s (Terumo) or 10 mm/s (ACIST Medical Systems). Recent technological advances also allow coregistration of the ultrasound image with contrast angiography, providing precise localization of the ultrasound findings on the angiogram. Unless the patient complains of chest discomfort or myocardial ischemia is suspected, image acquisition is recommended to include the distal vessel, the lesion site, and the entire proximal vessel back to the aorta. Accurate evaluation of the aortoostial segment requires that the guide catheter be disengaged slightly from the ostium.

Safety

As with other interventional procedures, the risks of spasm, dissection, and thrombosis exist when intravascular imaging catheters are used. Early multicenter studies documented complication rates of 1% to 3%, including transient spasm as the most frequently reported event. Major complications, such as dissection, thrombosis, and abrupt closure with "certain relation" to IVUS, were identified in fewer than 0.5% of the cases. These studies were performed with first-generation catheters in the early 1990s, and it is likely that the incidence of spasm and other complications is substantially lower with the current generation of catheters. No acceleration in the progression of atheroma or allograft vasculopathy of arteries previously imaged by IVUS (compared with noninstrumented arteries) has been reported.[3,4]

IMAGE INTERPRETATION

Three-Layered Appearance of Arterial Wall

The interpretation of IVUS images relies on the fact that the layers of a diseased arterial wall can be identified separately. In muscular or transitional arteries, such as the coronary, iliofemoral, renal, and popliteal systems, relative echolucency of the media compared with the intima and the adventitia gives rise to a three-layered (bright-dark-bright) appearance (Fig. 65.3). The lower ultrasound reflectance of the media is caused by the presence of less collagen and elastin than in the neighboring layers. Because the intimal layer reflects ultrasound more strongly compared with the media, a spillover effect, known as "blooming," may be seen at the intima-media border. This results in a slight overestimation of the thickness of the intima and a corresponding underestimation of the medial thickness. Conversely, the media can appear artifactually thick when ultrasound signal attenuation occurs within the intimal layer. Compared with the intima-media border that may not be correctly delineated, the media-adventitia border, corresponding to the external elastic membrane (EEM), is accurately rendered because a step-up in echo reflectivity occurs at this boundary and no blooming appears. The adventitia and periadventitial tissues are similar enough in echoreflectivity that a clear outer adventitial border cannot be defined.

Several deviations from the classic three-layered appearance are encountered in practice. In truly normal coronary arteries from young patients, echoreflectivity of the intima and the internal lamina may not be sufficient to resolve a clear inner layer. This is particularly true when the media has a relatively high content of elastin. At the other end of the spectrum, patients with a significant plaque burden may have thinning of the media underlying the plaque, often to the degree that the media is indistinct or undetectable in at least some part of the IVUS cross section. This problem can be exacerbated by the blooming phenomenon. However, even in these cases, the inner adventitial boundary (at the level of the EEM) is usually identifiable. For this reason, the plaque-plus-media cross-sectional area (CSA) is adopted as a surrogate measure for plaque CSA alone. Adding in the media represents only a tiny percentage increase in the total CSA of the plaque.

Image Orientation

The determination of image orientation within the artery is another important aspect of image interpretation. The IVUS beam penetrates beyond the artery, providing images of perivascular structures including the pericardium, the myocardium, and the cardiac veins. Because these structures have a characteristic appearance when viewed from various positions within the arterial tree, they provide useful landmarks with regard to longitudinal and cross-sectional image orientation (Fig. 65.4).[5] The pericardium appears as a bright and relatively thick layer with varying degrees of "spokelike" reverberations created by the interwoven fibrous strands. The myocardium is often viewed on the side opposite to the pericardium as a variable pattern of homogenous, low-echoic gray-scale signals.

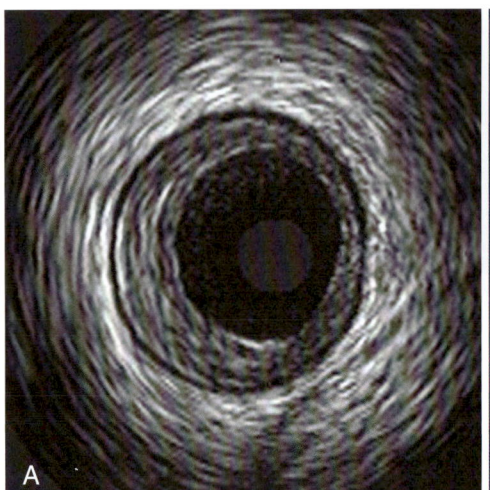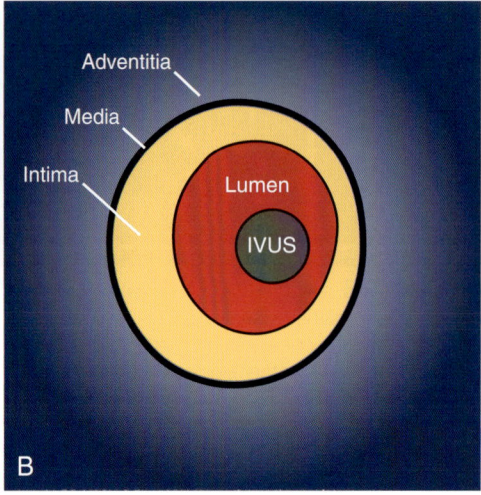

Fig. 65.3 Intravascular ultrasound image (A) and schematic diagram (B) demonstrate the classic three-layered appearance of the intima (plaque), the media, and the adventitia. In many cases the media is difficult to resolve clearly in some portion of the image, but in this particular image, it stands out in all sectors. Notice the speckled appearance of the blood within the lumen, particularly near the luminal border. *IVUS*, Intravascular ultrasound.

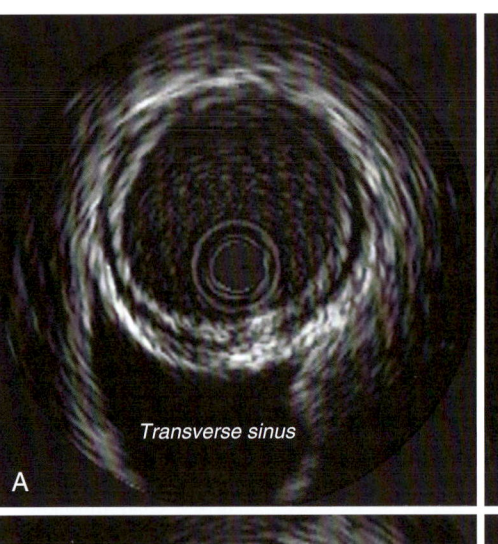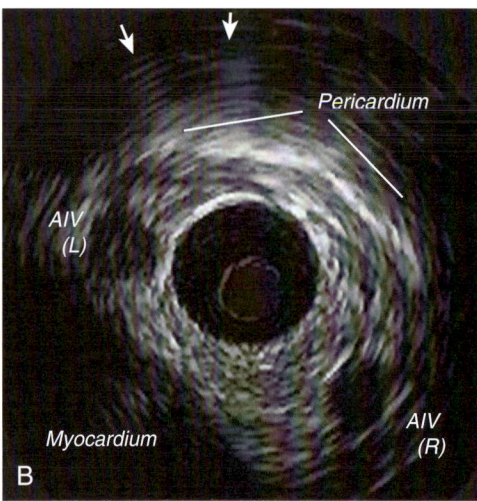
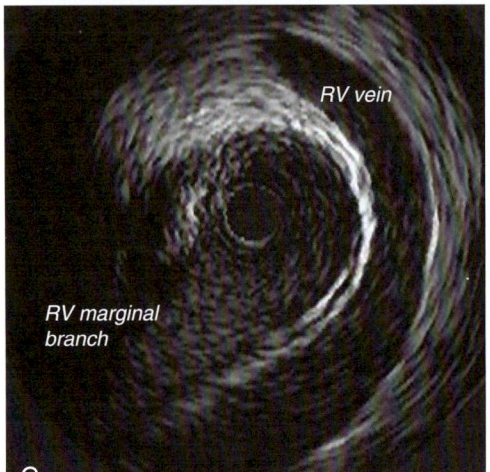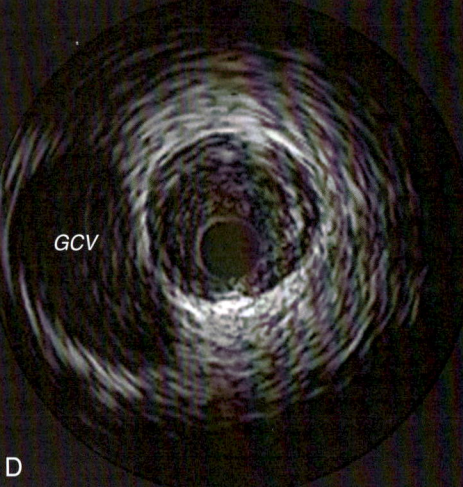

Fig. 65.4 Perivascular landmarks. (A) In the proximal portion of the left main coronary artery, a clear echo-free space filled with pericardial fluid, called the transverse sinus, is found adjacent to the artery, immediately outside the left lateral aspect of the aortic root. (B) In this distal cross section from the left anterior descending (LAD) coronary artery, the right *(R)* and left *(L)* branches of the anterior interventricular vein *(AIV)* are seen to straddle the coronary artery. The pericardium appears as a typical bright stripe with rays emitting from it *(arrows)*. (C) At the level of the middle right coronary artery, the veins arc over the artery, typically at a position just adjacent to the right ventricular *(RV)* marginal branches. (D) The great cardiac vein *(GCV)*, running superiorly to the left circumflex (LCx) coronary artery, appears as a large, low-echoic structure with fine blood speckle. Recurrent atrial branches emerge from the LCx artery in an orientation directed toward the GCV, whereas the obtuse marginal branches emerge opposite the GCV and course inferiorly to cover the lateral myocardial wall.

By default, current IVUS systems display the cross-sectional image as viewed from the ostium of the coronary artery tree looking distally into the vessel. Therefore in the left anterior descending (LAD) artery, the left circumflex (LCx) artery and the diagonal branches should emerge approximately 90 degrees counterclockwise from the pericardium, whereas septal branches typically emerge on the side opposite the pericardium (i.e., on the myocardium side). The distal LAD is accompanied by one or two anterior interventricular vein (AIV) branches, which run parallel to the LAD for a variable distance.

In the LCx artery, the great cardiac vein (GCV) runs superior to the LCx in most cases and immediately inferior to the left auricle. Therefore, viewed from the LCx, the recurrent arterial branches emerge in an orientation directed toward the GCV. In contrast, the obtuse marginal branches emerge opposite the GCV and course inferiorly to cover the lateral myocardial wall.

Unlike other epicardial coronary arteries typically accompanied by parallel venous structures, the proximal and middle right coronary artery (RCA) segments show a unique vein appearance: the vein arc crosses around the RCA in a "horseshoe" pattern, often at a position adjacent to the right ventricular (RV) marginal branches. The RV branches commonly have a geographic relationship with the pericardium similar to the diagonal branches of the LAD (approximately 90 degrees counterclockwise from the pericardium). The recurrent atrial branches typically emerge opposite the RV marginal branches.

Longitudinal image orientation facilitates accurate stent implantation in terms of optimal stent edge positioning, whereas cross-sectional image orientation is important particularly in terms of the guidewire direction in the treatment of CTO lesions. In off-line IVUS analysis, accurate longitudinal and cross-sectional orientation is essential for linking images of different phases of the same lesion in detail. The cross-sectional image orientation as presented on the screen can vary between serial imaging runs. The combination of perivascular landmarks and branching patterns allows the experienced operator to identify the vessel and the segment from the IVUS image alone; this can then provide a reference to the actual orientation of the image in space.

Quantitative Measurements

Unlike coronary angiograms, IVUS has an intrinsic distance calibration, which is usually displayed as a grid on the image. Electronic caliper (diameter) and tracing (area) measurements can be performed at the tightest cross section and at reference segments located proximal and distal to the lesion. The reference segment is typically selected as the most normal-looking cross section (i.e., largest lumen with smallest plaque burden) occurring within 10 mm of the lesion with no intervening major side branches.

In principle, all ultrasound measurements should be performed at the leading edge of boundaries because of the higher accuracy and reproducibility compared with those at the trailing edge.[6] For vessel measurement, the interface between the media and the leading edge of adventitia that corresponds to the EEM is used. In cross sections with large plaque burden or significant calcification, the circumference of EEM may not be fully identifiable because of ultrasound signal attenuation or acoustic shadowing. Extrapolation from the closest identifiable EEM border is acceptable only if the attenuation or acoustic shadowing involves a relatively small arc (<90 degrees). For lumen measurement, the interface between the lumen and the leading edge of the intima is used. Stagnant blood flow or the use of higher-frequency IVUS can increase the intensity of blood speckle, which may obscure the blood-tissue interface on a still image. A review of moving images can help to identify the true lumen border. During the procedure, saline can be injected through the guide catheter to reduce blood speckle. Metal struts of stents are seen as bright focal points in a circular-arrayed pattern on the IVUS scan, and stent measurement is performed at the leading edge of stent strut in the same way as in the nonstented segment.

Vessel and lumen diameter measurements are important in everyday clinical practice, where accurate sizing of devices is needed. All diameter measurements are performed relative to the center of mass (i.e., through the center point of the vessel or lumen) rather than the center of the IVUS catheter. The maximum and minimum diameters (i.e., the major and minor axes of an elliptical cross section) are the most commonly used dimensions. The ratio of maximum to minimum diameter defines a measure of symmetry.

Area measurements of vessel, lumen, and stent are performed with computer planimetry, using the interfaces of the leading edges. Plaque CSA (i.e., plaque-plus-media CSA) is calculated as the difference between the EEM and lumen CSAs. The ratio of plaque to EEM CSA is variously termed percent plaque area, plaque burden, or percent cross-sectional narrowing. Neointimal hyperplasia within the stent has low echoreflectivity at follow-up IVUS imaging, and its area is calculated as the difference between the stent and lumen CSAs. With motorized pullback, area measurements can be added to calculate volumes using Simpson's rule. For standardized data expression, the volume is presented as a volume index or average area, calculated as the absolute volume divided by the length of the analyzed segment.

Arterial remodeling is a bidirectional vessel response represented as the increase or decrease in vessel size that occurs during the development of atherosclerosis. In clinical settings, direct evidence of remodeling can be derived from serial changes in the EEM CSA in two or more IVUS measurements obtained at different times. In single-time-point studies, measurements of reference sites are used as a surrogate for the original vessel size before the artery became diseased. The reference segments used for such purpose should be measured without any major intervening side branches. Classification of arterial remodeling includes positive (or adaptive) remodeling, no or intermediate remodeling, and negative (or constrictive) remodeling. A remodeling index (the ratio of the EEM CSA at the lesion site to that at the reference site) as a continuous variable may also be used, in combination with the categorical classifications (positive remodeling = remodeling index >1.0 or 1.05; negative remodeling = remodeling index <1.0 or 0.95).[7]

Plaque Composition on Gray-Scale Intravascular Ultrasound

Early changes of atherosclerotic disease ("fatty streaks") are too thin to be visualized with IVUS. As plaque continues to develop, it can be detected with IVUS because it has different acoustic properties, depending on the composition of the plaque (Fig. 65.5). Regions of calcification are recognized as an intensely bright, echoreflective interface that creates a dense shadow more peripherally from the catheter, a phenomenon known as acoustic shadowing. This acoustic shadowing, often accompanied by "reverberations" (regularly spaced arcs behind the initial bright interface), precludes determination of the true thickness of a calcium deposit as well as visualization of any deeper tissue. Calcium deposits are described qualitatively as superficial or deep, according to the leading-edge location of the acoustic shadowing within the inner versus outer half of the plaque-plus-media thickness. The arc of calcium can be measured in degrees with the use of an electronic protractor centered on the lumen.

Densely fibrous tissue also appears as bright (echoreflective) on the ultrasound scan and can cause signal attenuation or partial acoustic shadowing. The extent of shadowing depends on the thickness and density of the fibrotic component, as well as the transducer power. Fatty plaque has less echoreflectivity than fibrous plaque due to extensive lipid infiltration. The brightness of the adventitia can be used as a gauge to discriminate predominantly fatty from fibrous plaque: an area of plaque that appears darker than the adventitia is considered fatty. In some cases with an image of extremely good quality, IVUS may identify the presence of a lipid pool from the appearance of a dark region within the plaque. However, the sensitivity and specificity of gray-scale IVUS for the detection of lipid accumulations are both relatively low. False channels within the plaque can give a similar appearance, and occasionally, shadowing from an adjacent calcified or fibrous region can mimic the appearance of a lipid pool.

Advanced Tissue Characterization

Radiofrequency Ultrasound Signal Analysis

Because visual interpretation of conventional gray-scale IVUS images is limited in the precise detection and quantification of specific plaque components, several advanced signal analysis techniques have been developed and introduced into the research and clinical arenas. One commercialized approach is

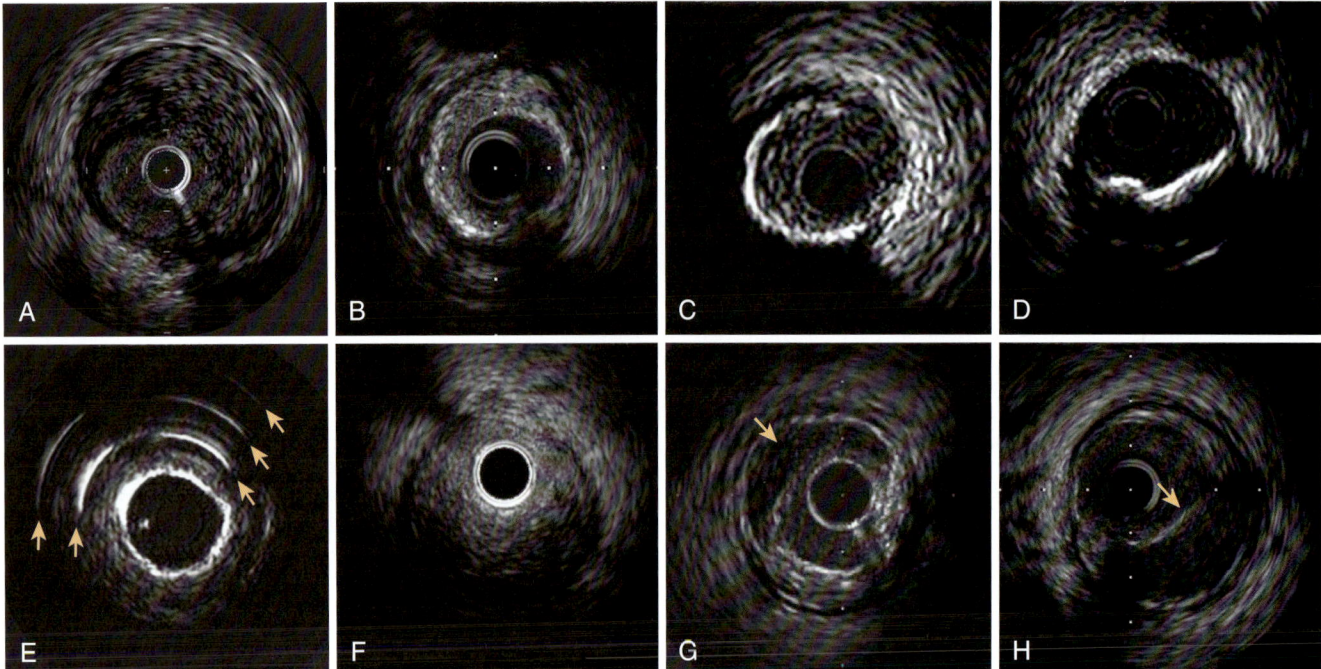

Fig. 65.5 Plaque characterization by gray-scale intravascular ultrasound. (A) Fatty plaque. (B) Fibrous plaque. (C) Deep calcification. (D) Superficial calcification. (E) Circumferential, "napkin-ring" calcification with multiple arcs of reverberation *(arrows)*. (F) Large plaque burden with deep ultrasound signal attenuation (despite absence of bright calcium) suggesting fibroatheroma with a necrotic core or pathologic intimal thickening with a lipid pool. (G) Plaque with a large low-echoic region suggesting a lipid pool *(arrow)*. (H) Ruptured (ulcerated) plaque with a remnant of a fibrous flap *(arrow)*.

to identify tissue components using computer-assisted analysis of raw radiofrequency (RF) signals in the reflected ultrasound beam.[8] This RF-IVUS analysis is based on the fact that greater information is contained in the backscattered ultrasound signal than is revealed by the conventional amplitude-based image presentation alone.

One system (IB-IVUS, Terumo) simply uses integrated backscatter (IB) values, calculated as the average power of the backscattered ultrasound signal from a sample tissue volume, to differentiate tissue types. Two other systems use spectral RF analyses with a classification tree algorithm developed from ex vivo coronary datasets (Virtual Histology [VH], Philips) or a pattern recognition technique based on the degree of spectral similarity between the backscattered signal and a reference library of spectra from known tissue types (iMap, Boston Scientific). All systems generate color-mapped images of the vessel wall, with a distinct color for each plaque component category (Fig. 65.6).

When combined with automated pullback and border detection techniques, these systems can provide a quantitative assessment of each tissue category over a three-dimensional coronary artery volume. All systems have demonstrated a correlation of IVUS-determined plaque compositions with corresponding histopathology of coronary specimens.[8] Current technical limitations include limited spatial resolution (100 to 250 μm); no classifications for thrombus, blood, or intimal hyperplasia; and potential errors caused by poor ultrasound penetration through extensive calcification.

Intravascular Ultrasound Combined With Near-Infrared Spectroscopy

Spectroscopy determines chemical compositions based on the analysis of spectra induced by interaction of light with tissue materials. Among the various spectroscopic techniques, the diffuse reflectance near-infrared spectroscopy (NIRS) is the frontrunner, showing the ability to identify the lipid component of atherosclerotic plaques in clinical settings. The commercially available coronary spectroscopy system (Makoto Imaging System, Infraredx) incorporates a dual-modality imaging catheter that provides simultaneous IVUS and NIRS imaging for coregistered acquisition of structural and compositional information. The 3.2-Fr imaging catheter is 6-Fr guide compatible and is configured similarly to conventional mechanical IVUS catheters in a rapid-exchange design with a protective outer sheath, except for an NIRS probe mounted adjacent to an extended bandwidth IVUS transducer. Unlike other light-based imaging techniques, this system does not require removal of blood from the imaging field.

The light reflected from tissue is analyzed by a spectrometer. With the use of a diagnostic algorithm, the processed data are color coded and displayed in a two-dimensional map of the vessel called a "chemogram" with the spatial (circumferential and longitudinal) information (see Fig. 65.6E). The current system is specifically designed for the detection of lipid-rich plaque, which is exhibited yellow on the chemogram, and a color scale from red to yellow indicates increasing algorithm probability of a lipid component of the vessel wall. The chemogram data are also laid in a halo surrounding the cross-sectional IVUS image in real time (see Fig. 65.6D). A summary of the results for each 2-mm section of artery is displayed as a block chemogram and is also portrayed in the central catheter artifact of the cross-sectional IVUS image. A lipid core burden index (LCBI) is computed as the fraction of valid pixels within the scanned region that exceed a lipid probability of 0.6, multiplied by 1000. In addition to a total LCBI of a given vessel segment, the maximum value of LCBI for any of the 4-mm subsegments, termed as maxLCBI$_{4\,mm}$, is often used to define a large lipid-core plaque in the segment. The accuracy of NIRS has been validated in coronary autopsy specimens and subsequently in vivo.[9,10]

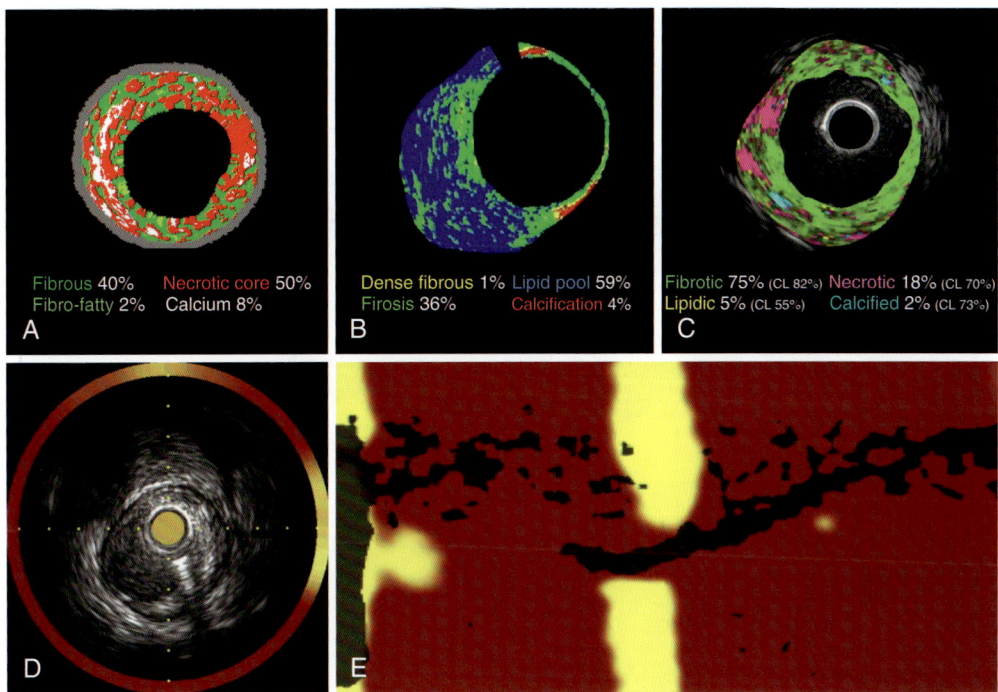

Fig. 65.6 Examples of plaque characterization by radiofrequency intravascular ultrasound (RF-IVUS) analyses and near-infrared spectroscopy (NIRS). (A) Virtual Histology system (Philips). Plaque components are determined by analyses of spectral RF signals with a classification algorithm. (B) Integrated backscatter (IB)-IVUS (Terumo). (C) iMap (Boston Scientific). Classification of tissue is made based on the degree of similarity between the sample and a reference frequency spectrum. This method enables confidence level *(CL)* assessment of each plaque component. (D) NIRS-IVUS. Spectroscopy data are laid in a halo surrounding the cross-sectional IVUS image in real time. A color scale from red to yellow indicates increasing algorithm probability of lipid content. (E) A chemogram (a two-dimensional map of spectroscopy data). The x-axis represents millimeters of pullback in the artery, and the *y*-axis represents degrees of rotation.

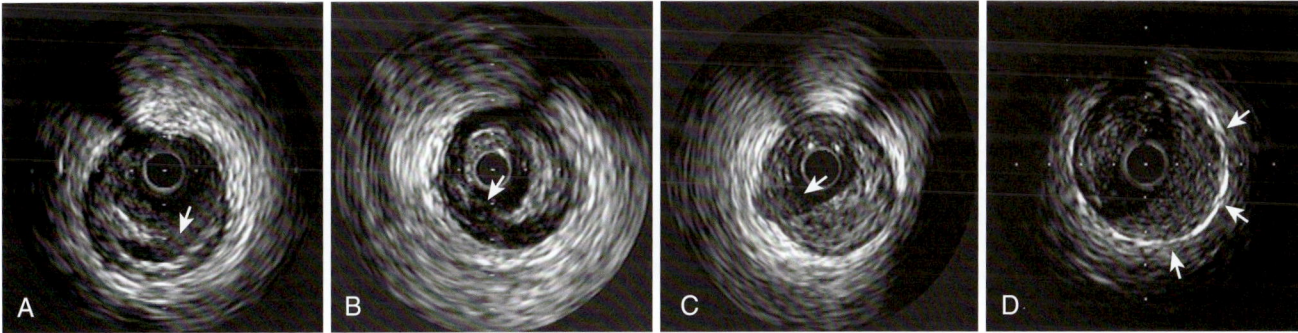

Fig. 65.7 Four examples of dissection. (A) A superficial (intimal) dissection *(arrow)* starting at 6 o'clock and extending clockwise. The dissection flap does not extend far into the lumen. (B) A deeper (medial) dissection *(arrow)* with a flap that extends into the lumen may compromise flow or precede abrupt closure. Injection of contrast in this setting can demonstrate free fluid flow behind the flap to better define the extent of tear. (C) Eccentric plaque with a deep (adventitial) dissection *(arrow)* at 8 o'clock that penetrates the external elastic lamina and extends into the adventitia. (D) Intramural hematoma *(arrows)* appears as an accumulation of blood within the medial space, displacing the internal elastic membrane inward and the external elastic membrane outward.

DIAGNOSTIC APPLICATIONS

Abnormal Lesion Morphology

Dissection appears as a fissure or separation within intima or plaque (Fig. 65.7). The severity of a dissection can be quantified according to depth (intimal, medial, or adventitial) and extent (circumferential and longitudinal). Intrastent dissection is another type of dissection, characterized as separation of neointimal hyperplasia from stent struts.

Intramural (intravascular) hematoma is recognized as an accumulation of blood within the medial space that displaces the internal elastic membrane inward and the EEM outward (Fig. 65.8G). On the IVUS image, it is observed typically as a homogenous, hyperechoic, crescent-shaped area, but it may have a heterogeneous or layered appearance when contrast dye or saline is trapped in the false lumen. Entry and exit points may or may not be observed.

Extramural (extravascular) hematoma is visualized outside the arterial wall. It manifests with an irregular shape and an echodim pattern due to the dilution of red blood cell concentration and dissemination through an echogenic adventitia or perivascular tissue (see Fig. 65.8H). Extramural hematoma is most often realized after an interventional procedure, such as atherectomy or

SECTION VI Evaluation of Interventional Techniques

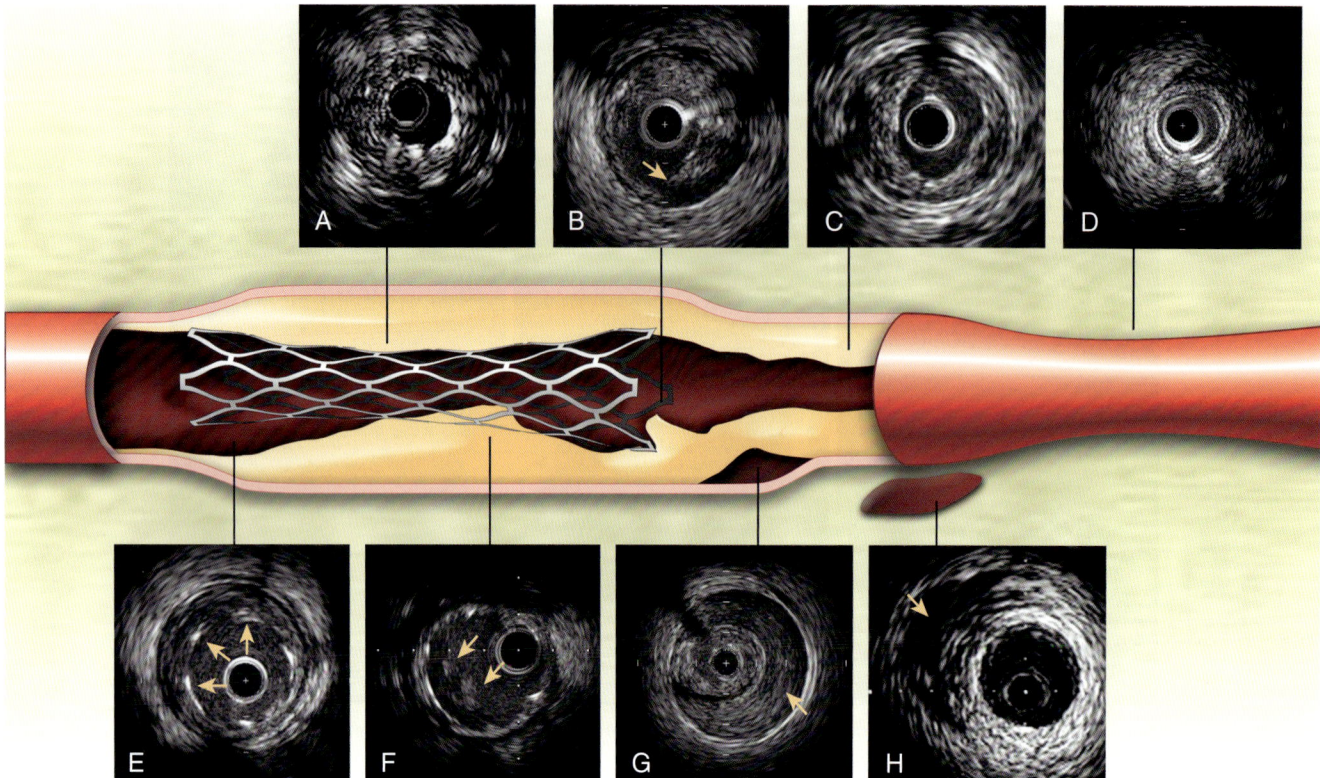

Fig. 65.8 **Problems with stent deployment detected by intravascular ultrasound (IVUS).** The diagram indicates the locations of the cross sections shown in the IVUS images. (A) Incomplete expansion relative to the ends of the stent and the reference segments. (B) An edge dissection with a disruption of plaque *(arrow)* at the stent margin. (C) Significant residual plaque burden at the segment uncovered by the stent. (D) Spasm at the adjacent nonstented segment. (E) Incomplete apposition, in which there is a gap between a portion of the stent *(arrows)* and the vessel wall. (F) Tissue protrusion (plaque prolapse, thrombus, or both) *(arrows)* within the stent. (G) Intramural (intravascular) hematoma detected as an accumulation of blood within the medial space *(arrows)* starting from the edge of the stent. (H) Extramural (extravascular) hematoma *(arrow)* visualized as an irregularly shaped, echodim pattern in the perivascular tissue.

recanalization of CTO lesions, and requires careful attention to antithrombolytic and antiplatelet treatment.

True aneurysm is defined as having an intact vessel wall and a maximum lumen area 50% larger than the proximal reference. In contrast, pseudoaneurysm shows a loss of vessel wall integrity and damage to adventitia or perivascular tissue.

Thrombus is typically recognized as an intraluminal mass, often with a layered, lobulated, or pedunculated appearance (see Fig. 65.8F). Acute thrombus may appear as a relatively echodense mass with speckling or scintillation, whereas old organized thrombus often has a darker ultrasound appearance. Thrombus is also more likely than soft plaque to have the appearance of blood flow in microchannels. However, none of these IVUS features is pathognomonic for thrombus, and slow blood flow, air bubbles, stagnant contrast, and echolucent plaque should be considered as differential diagnoses. Injection of contrast or saline may disperse the stagnant flow from the lumen, often allowing differentiation of stasis from thrombus.

Unstable Plaque
Gray-Scale Intravascular Ultrasound

By gray-scale IVUS, morphologic features associated with clinical instability or high risk for cardiovascular events after percutaneous coronary intervention (PCI) include noncalcified plaque with ultrasound attenuation, an echolucent zone within plaque, and scattered spotty calcification. In particular, echo-attenuated plaque (or attenuated signal plaque, defined as the absence of the ultrasound signal behind plaque that is either hypoechoic or isoechoic to the reference adventitia but contains no bright calcium) likely represents either fibroatheroma with a necrotic core or pathologic intimal thickening with a lipid pool (see Fig. 65.5F).[11]

Plaque rupture is diagnosed when a hypoechoic cavity within the plaque is connected with the lumen and a remnant of the ruptured fibrous cap is observed at the connecting site (see Fig. 65.5H). Ruptured plaques are often eccentric, less calcified, large in plaque burden, positively remodeled, and associated with thrombus. In patients with acute coronary syndrome (ACS), multiple plaque ruptures are frequently detected by three-vessel IVUS examination, suggesting that ACS is associated with pancoronary destabilization. However, lumen compromise and clinical symptoms likely depend on the severity of the original or coexisting stenosis or on thrombus formation, not solely on plaque rupture.

Extensive positive remodeling has also been shown to correlate with unstable plaque. Culprit lesions responsible for ACS typically exhibit extensive positive remodeling. Multiple clinical studies have also shown that preinterventional positive remodeling or large plaque burden assessed by IVUS predicts unfavorable acute- and long-term outcomes after PCI. Pathology studies support this clinical IVUS finding by demonstrating that lesions with positive remodeling frequently exhibit large, soft, lipid-rich plaques with increased inflammatory cell infiltrate. A

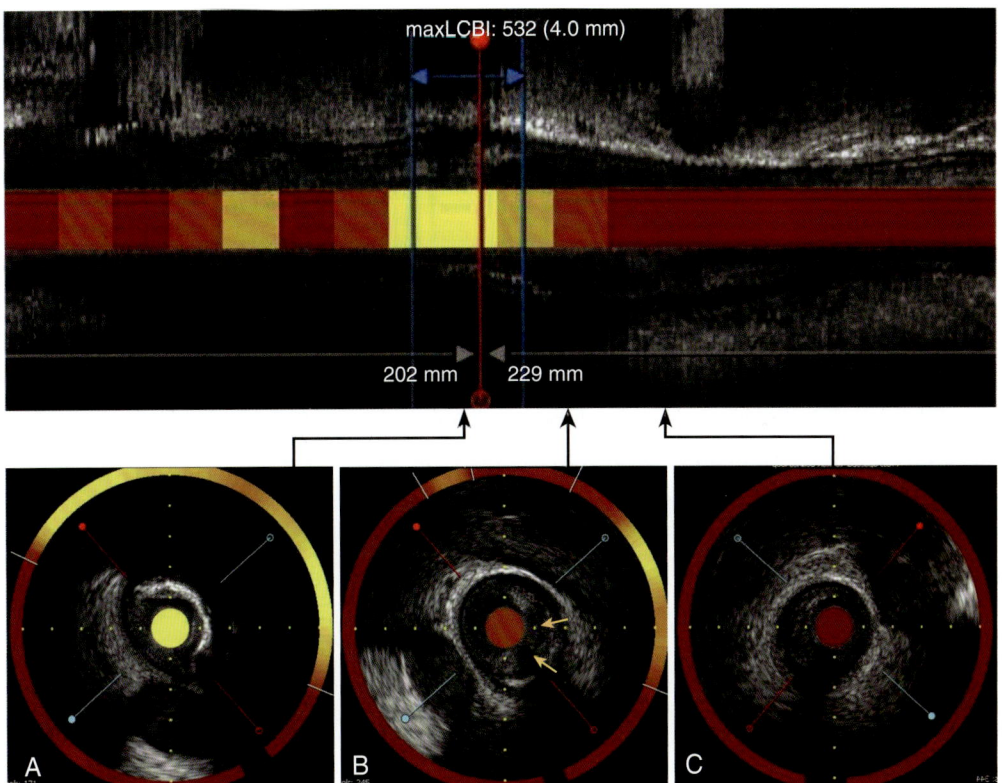

Fig. 65.9 An example case of lipid-core plaque detected by near-infrared spectroscopy (NIRS) intravascular ultrasound (IVUS). The patient developed an acute coronary syndrome 5 months after deferral of intervention for an intermediate lesion in the left anterior descending artery, based on fractional flow reserve calculated as 0.81. NIRS-IVUS at the event revealed a lipid-core plaque (maxLCBI$_{4\,mm}$, 532) (A) and plaque rupture *(arrows)* (B) immediately proximal to the minimum lumen area site (C).

clinical study with the combination of IVUS and optical coherence tomography has also linked positive remodeling with thinning of the fibrous cap in serial coronary examinations.[12]

Advanced Tissue Characterization

A number of clinical studies have indicated that plaque vulnerability, as determined by RF-IVUS (large lipid or necrotic core, or thin-cap fibroatheroma [TCFA]), is related to unstable lesion characteristics, clinical presentations, and future adverse events. Among them, the Providing Regional Observations to Study Predictors of Events in the Coronary Tree (PROSPECT) trial, one of the largest natural history trials, prospectively used three-vessel imaging with VH-IVUS in 697 patients with ACS.[13] In this trial a fibroatheroma (defined by VH-IVUS as the presence of >10% confluent necrotic core) was classified as a TCFA if more than 30 degrees of the necrotic core abutted the lumen in three or more consecutive frames. Multivariate analysis identified three baseline IVUS characteristics that independently predicted events at 3 years: (1) plaque burden greater than 70% (hazard ratio [HR] 5.03); (2) VH-determined TCFA (HR 3.35); and (3) minimal luminal area (MLA) less than 4.0 mm^2 (HR 3.21). Major adverse cardiac events (MACEs) occurred in 18% of those lesions with all three of these characteristics and in fewer than 1% of lesions with none of them. These results were replicated in several other prospective trials in which VH-determined TCFA was again associated with an increased occurrence of cardiac events.[14,15]

Identification of lipid-core plaque by NIRS-IVUS may also help to identify vulnerable atherosclerosis (Fig. 65.9). A higher prevalence of lipid-core plaque in patients with ACS has been reported compared with those with stable angina.[16] Another study revealed that most culprit lesions of ST-segment elevation myocardial infarction (STEMI) are characterized by a large, often circumferential lipid-core plaque concentrated at the culprit site.[17] In this study, a maxLCBI$_{4\,mm}$ greater than 400 was found to be a signature of plaques causing STEMI. In a study of early coronary artery disease, NIRS-IVUS also demonstrated a higher lipid content in the vascular wall in patients with endothelial dysfunction than in those with normal endothelial function.[18] With respect to the long-term prognostic value of NIRS-derived LCBI for future clinical outcomes, several small prospective registries have reported that presence of large lipid-core plaque detected by NIRS was associated with an increased risk of future MACE.[19–22] Currently, two large, prospective, multicenter studies are ongoing to confirm the ability of NIRS-IVUS to predict long-term coronary events, including the PROSPECT-II trial (900 ACS patients) and the Lipid-Rich Plaque (LRP) study (1500 patients with ACS or stable angina). The ongoing PROSPECT-II trial also includes a substudy cohort that is being randomized to everolimus-eluting bioresorbable vascular scaffold versus guideline-determined medical therapy for plaque stabilization.

Serial Monitoring of Disease Progression or Regression

The ability of IVUS to quantify arterial wall disease in a precise and reproducible manner allows serial evaluation of atherosclerotic plaque or transplant vasculopathy for the assessment of disease progression or regression. In serial studies for this purpose, the same IVUS system (in terms of catheter type, imaging console, and pullback device) should be used for serial imaging procedures at baseline and follow-up in a given patient. The use of automated pullback is mandatory for accurate axial registration of analysis segments. Some investigators recommend electrocardiogram (ECG)-gated image acquisition with a dedicated pullback device or software-based ECG-gated frame analysis of IVUS images obtained with a conventional pullback device, although the exact impact of these approaches on the outcomes of clinical studies has not been documented. A certain length of untreated coronary segment (typically 30 to 50 mm) is preselected for serial analyses using anatomic landmarks such as major side branches. Volume data are often normalized by pullback length (expressed as mean area) or by vessel size (expressed as percent volume) for comparative analysis.

The change of the intima or the plaque volume measured by IVUS has been increasingly used as a surrogate end point in clinical trials of the natural history of atherosclerosis and transplant vasculopathy and in monitoring the results of pharmacologic interventions such as lipid lowering. Relying on angiographic assessment alone for accurate evaluation of disease progression or regression is extremely challenging, particularly with a diffuse extent of disease and a variable degree of arterial remodeling. One pending question is whether disease progression or regression measured by gray-scale IVUS effectively reflects an increased or decreased risk of future cardiovascular events. Although several clinical trials suggest a significant association, a discrepancy between the imaging end point and clinical outcome has also been implied in some studies.[23–26] Clinical trials using IB-IVUS or VH have demonstrated stabilization of plaque composition by antiatherosclerotic agents, despite lack of change in total plaque volume observed by conventional IVUS measurement.[27,28] The Reduction in Yellow Plaque by Intensive Lipid-Lowering Therapy (YELLOW) trial, a prospective, randomized, single-center trial to determine the impact of statin therapy on intracoronary plaque lipid content assessed by NIRS, also demonstrated significant reduction of lipid content in obstructive lesions after short-term (7 weeks) intensive statin therapy.[29] Advanced tissue characterization techniques may supplement the simple plaque quantification by gray-scale IVUS, thereby enhancing the usefulness of IVUS-defined end points in the evaluation of new pharmacologic therapies.

Cardiac Allograft Vasculopathy

Cardiac allograft vasculopathy (CAV) is a major cause of long-term morbidity and mortality after heart transplantation and is characterized by various combinations of coronary intimal thickening and pathologic vessel remodeling. Compared with angiography, IVUS can directly visualize the arterial wall structure, offering a more sensitive method to detect CAV.

The prognostic value of IVUS in CAV has been well demonstrated in clinical studies. In particular, maximum intimal thickness (MIT) has been widely used as a surrogate marker for long-term outcomes in multiple studies where a rapid increase in MIT (≥0.5 mm during the first year after transplantation) was associated with significantly increased risk of all-cause death, myocardial infarction (MI), and subsequent development of angiographically severe CAV.[30,31] More recent studies demonstrated that modern IVUS analysis (e.g., paradoxical vessel remodeling, attenuated-signal plaque progression, periarterial small vessels) enhances the prognostic value of IVUS for better patient risk stratification.[32–34]

Myocardial Bridging

Myocardial bridging (MB) is a common congenital coronary anomaly that is located most frequently in the LAD. Although most patients are presumed asymptomatic, MB can cause typical or atypical angina, arrhythmia, or MI, most likely because of direct compression effects on the MB segment or accelerated atherosclerosis in the segment proximal to the MB. In vivo diagnosis of MB has traditionally been made with coronary angiography, based on the characteristic "milking" effect. For this reason, MB can be underdiagnosed in patients who have weak systolic arterial compression. IVUS can detect MB with much greater sensitivity, both by functional assessment (systolic arterial compression) and by a characteristic echolucent band (halo) appearance partially surrounding the artery. In a consecutive series, MB was identified by IVUS in 23% of 331 patients, whereas angiography alone detected MB in only 3%.[35] A histopathologic study demonstrated that the characteristic halo on the IVUS image of MB corresponds to muscle tissue overlying the coronary artery.[36] The direct assessment of muscle tissue by IVUS regarding length, thickness, and location, in combination with a functional measurement of systolic arterial compression, may provide prognostic information in specific patients, and determine the indication and strategy of treatment, especially when unroofing surgery is considered (7% to 9% of symptomatic MB patients may require surgery due to refractory angina despite medical treatment).[37,38]

INTERVENTIONAL APPLICATIONS

Angiographic Lesion Ambiguity

Preinterventional IVUS has been used to clarify situations in which angiographic findings are equivocal or difficult to interpret, especially in ostial lesions or tortuous segments in which the angiogram may not lay out the vessel well for interpretation. Particularly, in the assessment of left main coronary artery (LMCA) disease, angulations, calcification, or spasm in this location can lead to poor catheter engagement and confounded angiographic interpretation (Fig. 65.10). Several investigators have demonstrated that a high percentage of patients with angiographically normal LMCA are seen to have disease by IVUS. Conversely, another IVUS study demonstrated that fewer than half of the angiographically ambiguous LMCA lesions had significant stenosis.[39] This was especially true for ostial LMCA disease, in which only 36% of the lesions had a significant stenosis and 41% had plaque burden less than 50% as assessed by IVUS. Therefore patients with LMCA disease merit IVUS or physiologic assessment before a blind decision about treatment strategy is made, because the result of detailed evaluation can dramatically alter management and prognosis.

At bifurcation lesions including distal LMCA disease, the extent of side-branch involvement can be difficult to assess by angiography alone, and the decision to pursue revascularization or protection of the side branch is often dependent on ambiguous demonstration of these complex lesions. The combination of plaque and carina shift after balloon dilatation or stenting may cause severe narrowing or occlusion of a side branch, particularly in the presence of preexisting ostial disease. Conversely, the ostium of a jailed side branch can falsely appear stenosed on coronary angiography. This "pseudo" side-branch encroachment is caused by spasm, flow disturbance, or dye streaming due to jailing of the branch orifice by the stent. Although the true or pseudo encroachment may be identified by looking across from the parent artery into the ostium of the branch, accurate assessment requires direct IVUS imaging of the side branch.

Intermediate Lesions

Intermediate coronary lesions identified by angiography (40% to 70% angiographic stenosis) represent a challenge for revascularization decision making. Several physiologic studies have demonstrated that a considerable number of intermediate lesions referred for elective interventions are in fact hemodynamically insignificant and can be successfully managed with medical treatment alone. In early studies of proximal coronary lesions, MLA measured by IVUS demonstrated reasonable correlations with results from physiologic assessments. The ischemic MLA

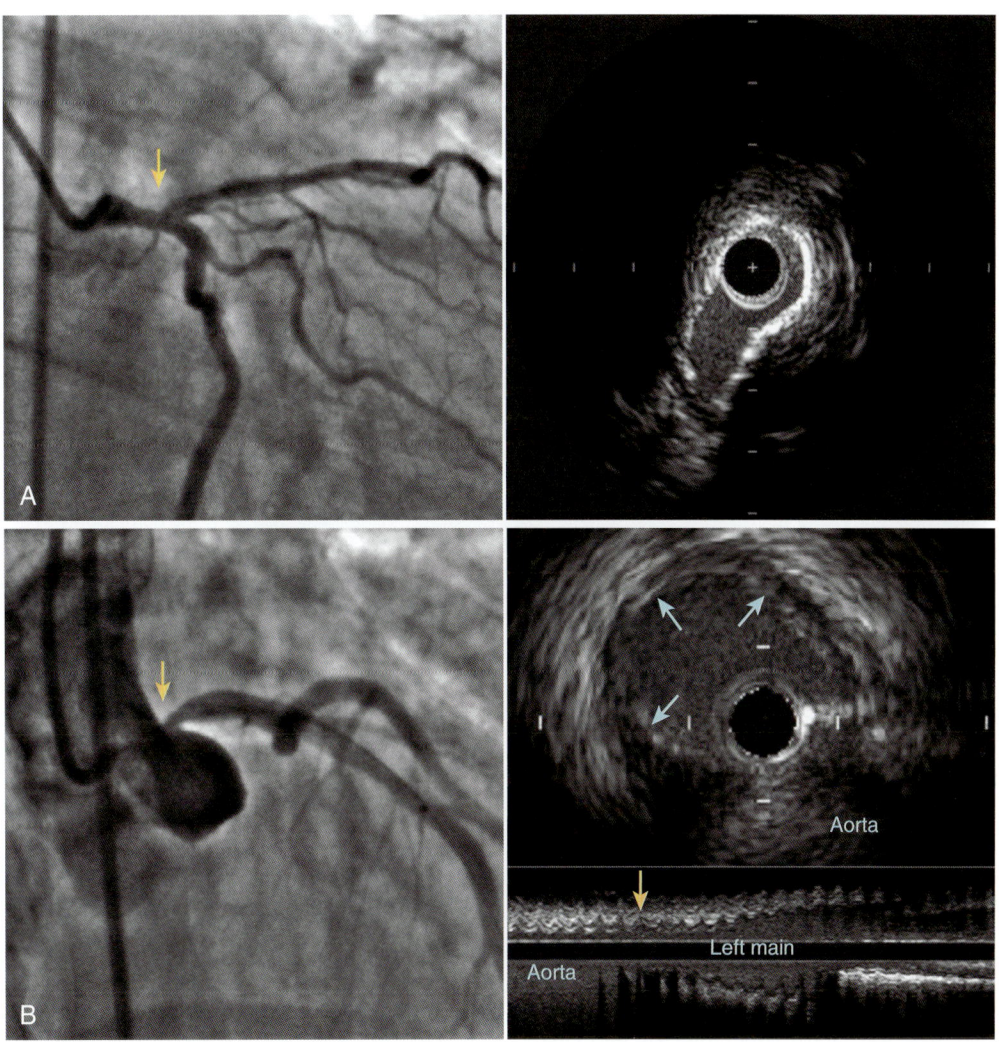

Fig. 65.10 Two examples of left main coronary artery (LMCA) assessment by intravascular ultrasound (IVUS). (A) A moderate stenosis *(orange arrow)* is observed at the distal LMCA segment by angiography *(left)*. IVUS reveals a significant lumen narrowing with napkin-ring superficial calcification at the corresponding segment *(right)*. (B) A significant stenosis *(orange arrow)* at the orifice of the LMCA is suspected by angiography *(left)*. IVUS demonstrates reverse vessel tapering of the corresponding segment *(orange arrow)* with only mild plaque accumulation *(blue arrows) (right)*.

threshold was identified as 3.0 to 4.0 mm² for major (non-LMCA) epicardial coronary arteries based on physiologic assessment with coronary flow reserve, fractional flow reserve (FFR), or stress scintigraphy. Among patients with intermediate coronary lesions in whom intervention was deferred based on IVUS findings (MLA >4.0 mm²), only 2.8% had target-lesion revascularization, and the composite event rate was 4.4% at up to 2 years.[40]

Later studies expanded the study population to encompass a wide variety of lesions and indicated that the diagnostic accuracies and optimal MLA cutoff values can vary depending on lesion location, vessel size, and the amount of myocardium supplied by the target vessel.[41-43] Overall, a meta-analysis of 11 clinical studies comparing IVUS and FFR identified the best MLA cutoff value to define the functional significance as 2.61 mm² in non-LMCA trials.[44] However, the pooled sensitivity and specificity of MLA were only 0.79 (95% confidence interval [CI] 0.76 to 0.83) and 0.65 (95% CI 0.62 to 0.67), respectively. Recent prospective multicenter trials also reported limited correlations between IVUS and FFR,[43] indicating IVUS-measured MLA is only one of many factors affecting coronary flow hemodynamics. In addition to the factors described previously, one inevitable limitation of IVUS-determined anatomic variables in estimation of physiologic significance is the inability to factor the information on downstream myocardial viability and blood supply from collaterals.

Compared with non-LMCA lesions, the IVUS-determined MLA appears to have better accuracy to predict significant FFR in LMCA lesions (MLA cutoff = 5.35 mm²; pooled sensitivity, 0.90, and specificity, 0.90, in the meta-analysis previously cited),[44-47] presumably due to relatively fewer variations in this location with respect to vessel anatomy and the amount of downstream myocardial burden. The clinical safety of deferred revascularization based on the IVUS-MLA was evaluated in a prospective multicenter study in which the predefined IVUS criterion of an MLA equal to or greater than 6 mm² was used for patients with intermediate LMCA disease. In this study, cardiac death and event-free survival were both comparable in the deferred versus the revascularized group over a 2-year follow-up period.[48] Another study group also confirmed the safety of IVUS-guided deferral of revascularization for intermediate LMCA disease but used a larger MLA cutoff value (7.5 mm²), which was predetermined based on the lower range of normal LMCA MLA in their clinical

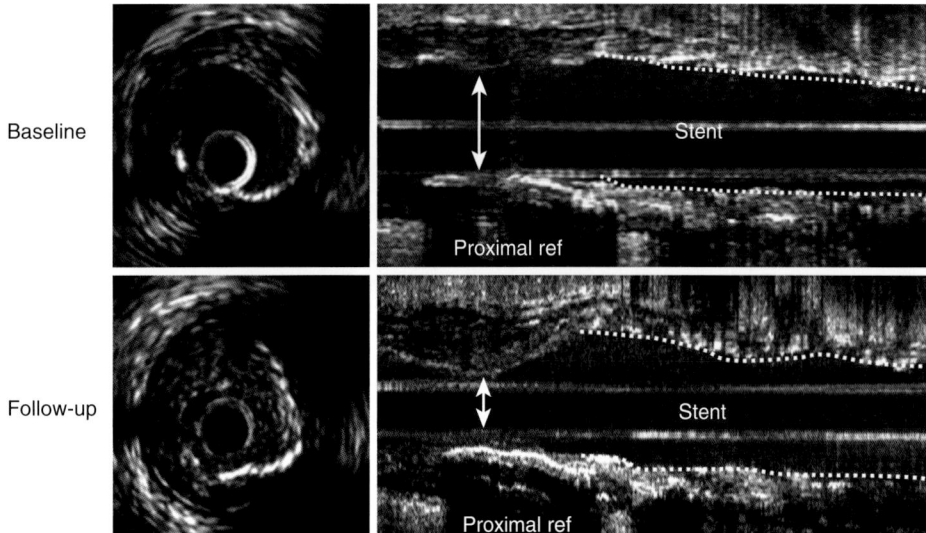

Fig. 65.11 **Proximal disease development 8 months after implantation of a drug-eluting stent.** The new stenosis at the proximal stent margin was primarily caused by plaque proliferation despite minimal neointimal hyperplasia observed inside the stent *(lower images)*. Baseline intravascular ultrasound shows a significant residual plaque at the corresponding uncovered segment *(upper images)*.

database.[49] However, in practice, the judgment should be made in conjunction with other information, such as the presence of diabetes[50] and plaque burden at the MLA site,[51] aside from direct FFR measurement.

Preinterventional Plaque Assessment

Preinterventional IVUS imaging is useful in determining the appropriate catheter-based intervention strategy. With current IVUS catheters, most significant stenoses can be safely imaged before intervention, providing detailed information about the circumferential and longitudinal extent of the plaque, and the character of the tissue involved. When observed by IVUS, angiographically hazy lesions represent a spectrum of morphologies, including calcium, dissection, thrombus, and excessive plaque burden with extreme remodeling. In particular, the presence, location, and extent of calcium can significantly affect the results of intervention (see Fig. 65.5). After balloon angioplasty, dissections are often observed at the junction of calcified and noncalcified plaque, where shear forces from dilation are high. For lesions with extensive superficial calcium, plaque modification through the use of rotational atherectomy may be required before balloon dilation or stent implantation. Conversely, even for lesions with significant calcification on fluoroscopy, IVUS may find the calcification to be distributed in a deep portion of the vessel wall or to have a calcium arc of less than 180 degrees. In these cases, stand-alone stenting is usually adequate to achieve lumen expansion large enough for a drug-eluting stent (DES).

Evaluation of plaque composition by preinterventional IVUS may also predict the occurrence of distal emboli during balloon dilation or stenting that may result in the "slow-flow" or "no-reflow" phenomenon leading to periprocedural MI. In gray-scale IVUS, predictive findings include large plaque burden with non calcium-related, ultrasound signal attenuation (particularly when the echo attenuation is equal to or greater than 5 mm in axial length), a large low-echoic region suggesting a lipid pool, and thrombus-containing plaque (see Fig. 65.5).[52,53] Studies with IB-IVUS, VH-IVUS, or NIRS-IVUS also demonstrated that the amount of lipid or necrotic core at preintervention was related to findings suggesting distal emboli.[54–59] Identification of high-risk plaques may help in selecting lesions suitable for distal protection devices,[60,61] although the optimal IVUS criteria for lesions that may most benefit from this strategy are yet to be defined.[62]

Selection of Device Size and Length

When assessed by IVUS, angiographically "normal" reference segments for PCI have a plaque burden of 35% to 51%. Precise measurements of vessel size and lesion length by IVUS can guide the optimal sizing of devices to be used. IVUS-guided balloon sizing was first systematically pursued by the Clinical Outcomes with Ultrasound Trial (CLOUT),[63] followed by a randomized multicenter study (the Balloon Equivalent to Stent [BEST] study) in which the nominal balloon size chosen was the closest size to the media-to-media diameter measured at the lesion site, and inflation pressure was determined based on the compliance curve to attain the target diameter.[64] In a contemporary DES trial of complex lesions (Angiography Versus IVUS Optimization [AVIO]), the size of the postdilation balloon was selected based on the average of the media-to-media diameters at multiple sites within the stented segment.[65] The precise vessel size measurement is also critically important for size selection of self-expanding stents or full-bioresorbable coronary scaffolds because undersizing of these devices is not amendable once they are deployed in the lesion.

Assessment of true lesion length by IVUS dictates the exact length of stent necessary to appropriately scaffold a lesion. Numerous IVUS studies of DES have identified greater reference plaque burden as an independent predictor of subsequent stent edge restenosis or thrombosis (Fig. 65.11).[66–70] The Impact of Stent Deployment Techniques on Clinical Outcomes of Patient Treated With the CYPHER Stent (STLLR) trial also demonstrated that geographic miss had a significant negative impact on both clinical efficacy and safety at 1 year after DES implantation.[71] Complete coverage of reference disease is currently recommended; however, longer stent length has also been reported to be independently associated with DES restenosis and thrombosis. On-line IVUS guidance can facilitate the determination of appropriate stent length for anchoring the stent ends in relatively plaque-free vessel segments while minimizing stent length for complete lesion coverage. One practical approach was proposed in a single-center registry in which stepwise IVUS criteria (plaque burden <50% as the primary target zone) were used to determine the optimal landing zone for DES.[72]

Common Stent Problems at Deployment

Postinterventional IVUS can identify several stent deployment issues (see Fig. 65.8). Incomplete stent expansion (or stent underexpansion) is defined as inadequate expansion of a portion of the stent compared with the distal and proximal reference dimensions; this may occur, for example, where dense fibrous or calcified plaque is present. Incomplete stent apposition (ISA) or stent malapposition occurs when part of the stent structure is not fully in contact with the vessel wall; this is defined by IVUS as one or more struts clearly separated from the vessel wall, with evidence of blood speckle behind the strut in a segment not associated with any side branches. Isolated ISA observed immediately after deployment usually is not directly linked to adverse clinical events, provided that the lumen is large enough to preserve blood flow. On the other hand, significant ISA possibly increases local flow disturbances, delays healing, or increases the potential risk for stent deformation at subsequent procedures. An early clinical study demonstrated an unexpectedly high percentage of these IVUS-detected stent deployment issues, even after angiographically successful results. These observations led to the concept of the high-pressure stent deployment technique currently used.

After stent implantation, IVUS may reveal tears at the edge of the stent (or edge dissections) in 8% to 20% of the cases. These tears have been attributed both to shear forces created at the junction between the metal edge of the stent and the adjacent, more compliant tissue, and to the effect of balloon expansion beyond the edge of the stent (the "dog-bone" phenomenon). Minor, non flow-limiting edge dissections do not appear to impact on late angiographic in-stent restenosis (ISR).[73,74] In fact, when imaged at follow-up, 75% were healed—a frequency similar to that seen after balloon angioplasty.[75] In contrast, significant residual dissections can lead to an increased risk of MACE after DES implantation, especially with a small effective lumen CSA at the segment containing the dissection.[76] Therefore a practical strategy is to make a determination from the IVUS image as to whether the tear is likely to be flow limiting. If this is the case, an additional stent is placed to cover this region. By angiography, tears are typically recognized as haziness at the stent edge. However, when investigated by IVUS, angiographic hazy lesions can represent a spectrum of abnormal anatomic morphologies and periprocedural complications, such as calcium, dissection, thrombus, hematoma, spasm, and excessive residual plaque burden at the reference segment (see Fig. 65.8). The etiology of persistent haziness can be precisely defined by IVUS because it has higher sensitivity than contrast angiography for detecting abnormal entities in the vessel wall. In addition, IVUS can demonstrate the precise location and severity of these findings.

Optimization of Stent Expansion

There is compelling evidence that procedure-related factors are important contributors to the development of both restenosis and thrombosis after stent implantation, regardless of stent type. In particular, stent underexpansion represents the most consistent risk factor across clinical IVUS studies. In the bare-metal stent (BMS) era, the predicted risk for restenosis was reported to decrease 19% for every 1-mm^2 increase in minimum stent area (MSA).[77] IVUS studies of BMS thrombosis also reported extremely high incidences of stent underexpansion (52% to 78%) in patients with early (acute or subacute) stent thrombosis.[78,79] This finding was subsequently replicated in DES studies (42% to 85% in patients with early thrombosis).[66,69,80,81]

Several investigators have evaluated the predictive value of IVUS-determined MSA for ISR in various types of stents. With receiver operating characteristic (ROC) analysis, the optimal diagnostic thresholds of MSA that best predict long-term stent patency were reported to be 5.0 to 5.7 mm^2 for DES and 6.4 to 6.5 mm^2 for BMS.[82-85] IVUS-determined MSA remains an independent predictor of restenosis (odds ratio [OR] 0.48 to 0.77), irrespective of DES type, including sirolimus-, paclitaxel-, zotarolimus-, and everolimus-eluting stents.[84,86]

In bifurcation lesions, both inadequate postprocedural MSA and increased neointimal hyperplasia are the major mechanisms of restenosis in the side-branch ostium. In a series of cases of unprotected LMCA disease treated with single- or two-stent strategies, the MSA cutoffs that best predicted subsequent restenosis were 5.0 mm^2 (ostial LCx), 6.3 mm^2 (ostial LAD), 7.2 mm^2 (within the polygon of confluence zone), and 8.2 mm^2 (LMCA).[87] Stent underexpansion was again identified as an independent predictor for MACE at 2 years (adjusted HR 5.56; 95% CI 1.99 to 15.49; P = .001), and the MACE-free survival rate was significantly lower in patients with underexpansion (observed at one or more segments) compared with no underexpansion (90 ± 3% vs. 98 ± 1%; log-rank P = .001).

Unlike BMS, the relative benefit of obtaining a larger MSA to ensure a greater "safety margin" for an unexpected amount of neointima (the "bigger is better" theory) can significantly vary among DES types, depending on the variability of subsequent neointimal proliferation. In addition, given the wide variety of clinical backgrounds, patient risk factors, lesion morphologies, and disease complexities in clinical practice, it is unlikely that a single prespecified MSA end point could be effectively applied to all target lesions. Nevertheless, the ability of IVUS to assess the results of stent implantation more precisely than angiography significantly contributes to enhanced clinical judgment for individual patients. The utility of IVUS to ensure adequate stent expansion cannot be overemphasized, particularly if there are clinical risk factors for DES failure (e.g., diabetes, renal failure).

Guidance for Complex Interventions

IVUS is useful in several aspects during complex interventions such as PCI on distal LMCA lesions, as discussed previously, and CTO lesions.[88-91] In lesions with abrupt-type occlusion, the entry point at the CTO ostium is often difficult to identify by angiography. If there is a side branch located near the entrance of the CTO, the IVUS catheter can be inserted into the side branch to examine the target for wire penetration. In addition, the IVUS catheter may possibly be inserted into the subintimal space to determine the direction of the true lumen; however, this procedure requires careful catheter manipulation because of the potential risk of enlarging the subintimal space. A true lumen is surrounded by all three layers of the vessel (i.e., intima, media, and adventitia). Side branches may provide another clue as they should communicate with the true but not with the false lumen. Prior to stenting after successful wiring through a CTO lesion, IVUS can also help to confirm the distal guidewire position within the true vessel lumen.

In PCI on CTO lesions, the solid-state catheter is often preferred because the distance of its transducer from the catheter tip is shorter than that of mechanical systems (10 vs. 20 to 33 mm, respectively). For this type of application, a shorter-tip solid-state catheter (2.5 mm tip-to-imaging distance) is also available (Eagle Eye Platinum ST, Philips). The longer monorail design of solid-state catheters may also offer better trackability and less frequent catheter trapping, which can occasionally be caused by separation of the IVUS catheter and guidewire, within the complex lesion anatomy. Finally, as with other interventional procedures, proper balloon and stent sizes as well as acute complications can accurately be evaluated by IVUS. Particularly, intramural or extramural hematoma (or perforation) can occur during the CTO procedure. Early detection and precise assessment of these conditions are crucial for safe and effective treatment of patients with CTO lesions.

Stent Problems at Follow-Up

Restenotic Lesions

The primary mechanism of restenosis can be accurately identified by IVUS, and it significantly affects the treatment strategy

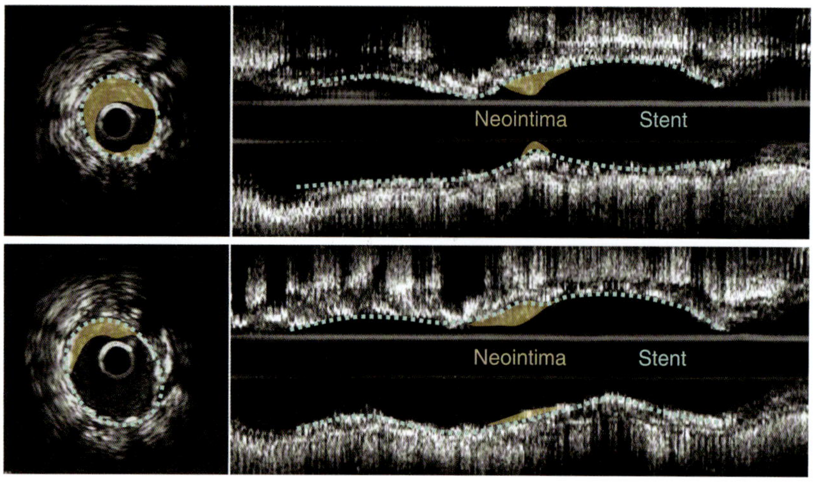

Fig. 65.12 Drug-eluting stent (DES) restenosis resulted primarily from stent underexpansion. Preinterventional intravascular ultrasound *(upper images)* revealed significant stent underexpansion at the midsegment with only a small amount of focal neointimal hyperplasia. This type of in-stent restenosis can be successfully treated with mechanical optimization by balloon dilation *(lower images)* and may not require additional DES implantation within the original restenotic stent.

in patients with restenotic lesions. In nonstent interventions, the majority of late lumen loss is caused by negative arterial remodeling (a decrease in EEM-CSA); only approximately a quarter of the late loss is caused by tissue proliferation. In contrast, late loss in stented lesions is primarily caused by neointimal proliferation rather than by chronic stent recoil. However, initial stent underexpansion can result in clinically significant lumen compromise, even with minimal neointimal hyperplasia (Fig. 65.12).[92] An IVUS study of ISR lesions after BMS demonstrated that 20% of lesions had an MSA of less than 5.0 mm², and an additional 4.5% had other mechanical problems that contributed to restenosis.[93] In most of these cases, stent underexpansion or other mechanical problems were not suspected angiographically at the time of reintervention. An IVUS study of DES restenosis also reported that 21% of ISR lesions had an MSA of less than 5.0 mm² at the MLA site, 38% of which were not associated with significant neointimal hyperplasia.[94] For this type of ISR, mechanical optimization is the first priority, and IVUS can be helpful to differentiate mechanical issues from exaggerated neointimal proliferation that may truly require DES implantation within the original restenotic stent.

For DES treatment of ISR, early clinical studies suggested a hypothesis that full DES coverage of the original stent might be important for the prevention of recurrent restenosis. However, this aggressive optimization strategy has been associated with several clinical issues and may not be feasible in every case. In a retrospective IVUS study of BMS restenosis treated with sirolimus-eluting stents, 77% of the uncovered BMS segments maintained adequate lumen patency at follow-up.[95] Therefore as long as the original BMS is well expanded and has a segment with sufficient lumen area, conservative coverage with DES can be a clinical option (the "spot stenting" strategy). Another study from the TAXUS trials evaluated follow-up IVUS results in patients who did not require revascularization at 9 months.[96] At 3 years, revascularization was required in 4.9% of paclitaxel-eluting stents and 6.7% of BMS. Multivariate analysis identified MLA at 9 months as a significant predictor of later revascularization for both stent types. Several investigators have used advanced tissue characterization techniques of IVUS to assess atherosclerotic changes of instent neointima (so-called neoatherosclerosis),[97–100] although the validity of this application and its clinical implications are yet to be established.

Late-Acquired Incomplete Stent Apposition

With serial IVUS performed immediately after the procedure and at follow-up, ISA can be classified as baseline or late acquired (Fig. 65.13). At follow-up, baseline ISA may have resolved or may persist; therefore ISA observed at follow-up could be either persistent baseline ISA (persistent ISA) or newly developed ISA in a segment in which struts were completely apposed to the vessel wall at baseline (late-acquired ISA [LISA]).

Despite optimal angiographic results with high-pressure balloon dilatation, baseline ISA can be observed with IVUS in 8% to 30% of DES recipients. This morphologic abnormality primarily results from selection of an undersized stent, stent underexpansion, or insufficient stent conformability in calcified or complex-shaped lesions (the so-called mechanical ISA).

LISA was first brought into the spotlight in intracoronary brachytherapy trials (9.3% average incidence by IVUS). However, subsequent IVUS studies have revealed that it also occurs in up to 5% to 6% of balloon-expandable BMS recipients. In DES, the incidence of LISA varies significantly among different DES types and patient populations. In elective stenting, clinical trials of second-generation DES showed lower incidences of LISA, particularly in phosphorylcholine-coated zotarolimus-eluting stents (0.4% in the ENDEAVOR-I to IV trials), compared with reports of 8% to 13% in patients treated with first-generation sirolimus- or paclitaxel-eluting stents.[101] Higher incidences were observed in more complex studies enrolling patients with acute MI or CTO, and in those treated with atherectomy before stenting. A meta-analysis of seven randomized trials reported that the risk of LISA in patients with a DES was four times higher than in those with a BMS (OR 4.36; 95% CI 1.74 to 10.94; P = .002).[102]

LISA primarily results from structural vessel wall changes that occur during the follow-up period ("biologic ISA"), in contrast to "mechanical ISA" seen with initial stent deployment. The most commonly reported mechanisms for LISA are "dissolution of thrombus" present at the baseline and "regional positive vessel remodeling" disproportional to persistent plaque area change.[103] Although thrombus dissolution can be seen in patients with any type of stent deployed for treatment of thrombus-containing lesions, abnormal positive vessel remodeling is observed more frequently in patients who received a DES or brachytherapy. With regard to vessel remodeling, incompletely apposed struts are seen primarily in eccentric plaques, and the gaps develop mainly on the disease-free side of the vessel wall.[104] The combination of mechanical injury at stent implantation and biologic injury by DES components may predispose the vessel wall to chronic, pathologic dilatation in the setting of little underlying plaque.[105]

Theoretically, long persistence of incompletely apposed DES struts might be associated with delayed reendothelialization, allowing fibrin and platelet deposition. A significant gap or aneurysm formation can also reduce local blood flow, promoting platelet adhesion and the coagulation cascade. However, it

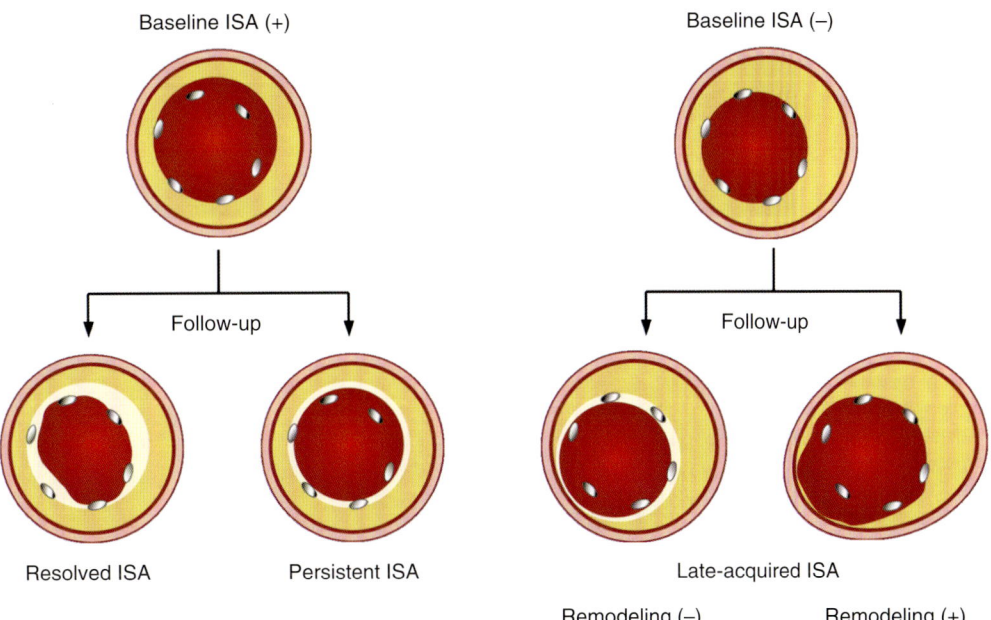

Fig. 65.13 Classification of incomplete stent apposition *(ISA)*. Baseline ISA can either resolve (resolved ISA) or remain (persistent ISA) at follow-up. Late-acquired ISA without vessel expansion is typically seen in thrombus-containing lesions, whereas late-acquired ISA with focal, positive vessel remodeling is more characteristic with brachytherapy and drug-eluting stents.

is still debatable whether LISA independently contributes to the occurrence of stent thrombosis. Most clinical trials have failed to show a prospective association between LISA and later thrombotic events, whereas multiple IVUS studies have demonstrated that LISA is frequently observed in lesions of late DES thrombosis.[105,106] This discrepancy may represent a multifactorial process of late DES thrombosis involving several other factors or pathways. In addition, most prospective studies were underpowered to detect a possible relationship of LISA with rare thrombotic events. A literature-based meta-analysis suggested a significantly higher risk of late or very late DES thrombosis in patients with late (persistent or late-acquired) ISA compared with those without late ISA (OR 6.51; $P = .02$).[102] However, careful interpretation is still required because of the inherent limitations of literature-based analyses of heterogeneous studies.

Another methodologic issue with respect to the clinical relevance of LISA is lack of appropriate grading or classification. Reported LISA is a spectrum ranging from tiny incomplete apposition to extensive aneurysm formation, and LISA associated with late thrombosis is often at the extreme end of this spectrum. Finally, the late development of ISA may simply represent a pathologic process within the arterial wall, such as chronic inflammation with endothelial dysfunction weakening the vessel structure rather than serving as a direct cause of thrombosis.[105] To accurately identify LISA posing a risk for future events across the spectrum, a better understanding of this phenomenon is essential.

Strut Fracture

Stent strut fracture is not a rare phenomenon in peripheral artery stenting (it occurs in up to 65% of cases of femoropopliteal stenting) and can also occur after DES implantation in coronary lesions (Fig. 65.14). By angiography, strut fracture is diagnosed as complete or partial separation of the stent at follow-up where there had been contiguity of the stent at baseline. By IVUS, strut fracture is defined as longitudinal strut discontinuity and can be categorized on the basis of its morphologic characteristics as strut separation, strut subluxation, or strut intussusception (Fig. 65.15).[101] Another recently proposed classification focuses on potential mechanisms of the strut fracture, categorizing them on the basis of the presence (type I) or absence (type II) of aneurysm at the fracture site.[107] Studies using angiography or IVUS have reported the incidence of DES fracture to be between 0.8% and 7.7%; ISR or stent thrombosis occurred at 22% to 88% of these cases.[101,106]

Theoretically, strut fracture in DES can reduce the local drug dose delivered to the arterial wall, as well as affecting the mechanical scaffolding of the affected lesion segment. In addition, the irregular edge of the fractured struts may chronically stimulate the vessel wall during cardiac movement. Conversely, deployment of long and rigid stents in angulated lesions with hinge motion can lead to significant alteration of local physiology, so that the strut fracture may help to restore the original dynamic state, at least in some cases. The exact incidence and clinical implications of strut fractures remain to be further investigated in large clinical studies.

Impact of Intravascular Ultrasound Guidance on Long-Term Outcomes After Stenting

Numerous clinical studies have provided evidence for the long-term benefits of IVUS in both BMS and DES implantation. In the DES era, the clinical impact of IVUS guidance was assessed for complex lesions (e.g., unprotected LMCA, bifurcation, long lesions) and in unselected patient populations.[108] The largest randomized controlled trial was the Impact of Intravascular Ultrasound Guidance on Outcomes of Xience Prime Stents in Long Lesions (IVUS-XPL), which randomized 1400 patients with long coronary lesions to receive IVUS-guided or angiography-guided everolimus-eluting stent implantation.[109] In this study the IVUS guidance resulted in a significantly lower MACE rate at 1 year (2.9% vs. 5.8%; HR 0.48; 95% CI 0.28 to 0.83; $P=.007$), driven by a lower risk of ischemia-driven target-lesion revascularization in IVUS-guided stent implantation (2.5% vs. 5.0%; HR 0.51; 95% CI 0.28 to 0.91; $P=.02$). The largest prospective multicenter registry (8582

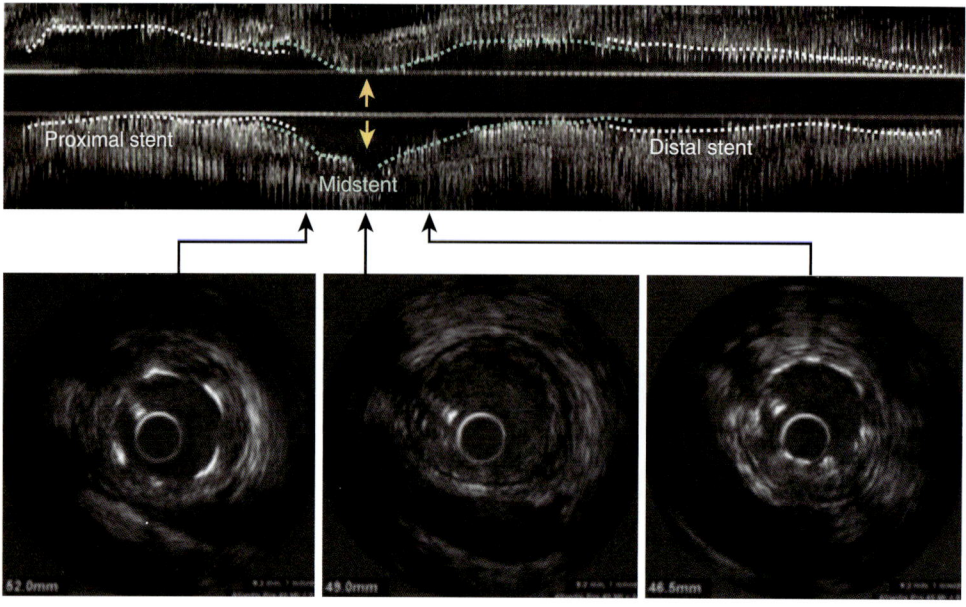

Fig. 65.14 Stent strut discontinuity (fracture) observed 8 months after deployment of three overlapping drug-eluting stents. On the cross-sectional intravascular ultrasound (IVUS) image *(bottom row, middle image)*, an abnormal paucity of stent struts, not seen at baseline, was detected at a portion of the midstent. The longitudinal IVUS image *(top)* shows an acute-angled bend at the corresponding segment *(arrows)*. However, in this particular case, the stent fracture (complete separation type) was not associated with increased intimal hyperplasia.

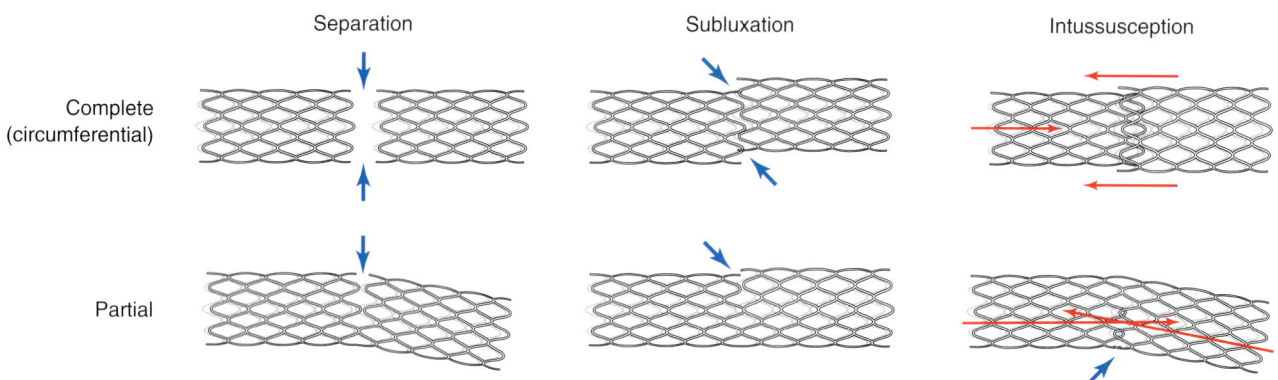

Fig. 65.15 Stanford classification of stent strut fracture. By intravascular ultrasound, strut fracture is defined as longitudinal strut discontinuity and can be categorized on the basis of its morphologic characteristics. *Blue and red arrows* represent stent fracture and resulting movement of the stent segments, respectively.

patients) including unselected patients treated with second-generation DES was the Assessment of Dual Antiplatelet Therapy With Drug-Eluting Stents (ADAPT-DES),[110] in which IVUS guidance was significantly associated with lower incidences of definite or probable stent thrombosis (0.7% vs. 1.5%, P = .002), MI (3.5% vs. 5.6%, P < .0001), and ischemia-driven target-lesion revascularization (4.8% vs. 6.0%, P = .02) at 2 years.

On the other hand, controversial results were also reported in some IVUS-guided stent trials. This discrepancy may have resulted, in part, from underpowered study design, differing procedural end points for IVUS-guided stenting, or various adjunctive treatment strategies that were used in these trials in response to suboptimal IVUS findings. Overall, two meta-analyses of clinical BMS studies have demonstrated that IVUS-guided stenting significantly lowers long-term angiographic restenosis and target-lesion or -vessel revascularization, with a neutral effect on death and nonfatal MI compared with an angiographic optimization.[111,112] More recently, 11 meta-analyses of IVUS-guided DES studies have also indicated that IVUS guidance can offer significantly lower rates of restenosis, mortality, MI, stent thrombosis, revascularization, and MACE compared with angiographic guidance alone.[108]

In most DES studies, IVUS-guided stent optimization was performed based on the individual operator's discretion. In contrast, the majority of the BMS trials used prespecified IVUS criteria for optimal stent expansion. It is also noteworthy that IVUS guidance appears to contribute to reduced hard end points (death, MI, or thrombotic events) in DES implantation, whereas improved restenosis and revascularization rates represent predominant benefits of IVUS-guided BMS implantation.

Bioresorbable Scaffolds

The IVUS appearance of polymeric bioresorbable scaffolds (BRSs) is considerably different from that of metallic stents, owing to the penetration of ultrasound beam through the polymer material. Specifically, IVUS often identifies the BRS strut as double-layered bright stripes, suggestive of endoluminal and abluminal strut surfaces (Fig. 65.16). In certain circumstances, this typical double-layered appearance of the BRS struts can be compromised on IVUS images, resulting in a single-layered presentation similar to metallic stents, which is attributable not only to its lower axial resolution than light-based imaging but also to the other intrinsic properties of ultrasound, such as blooming effects and the incident-angle dependence. Closely adjacent struts may also be difficult to identify separately because of sidelobe artifacts from the neighboring struts. In this context, higher-resolution 60-MHz IVUS can offer significantly improved visualization of BRS struts compared with conventional IVUS.[113]

Most BRS devices have unique mechanical properties compared with conventional metallic stents (e.g., relatively thick struts and

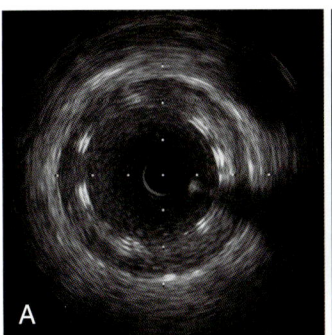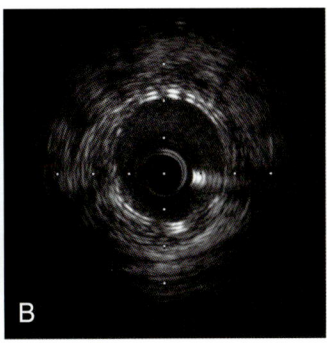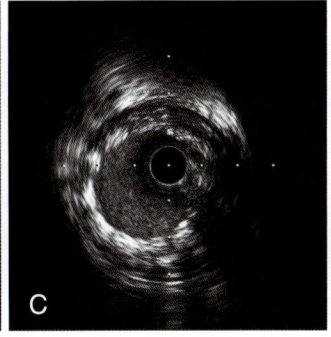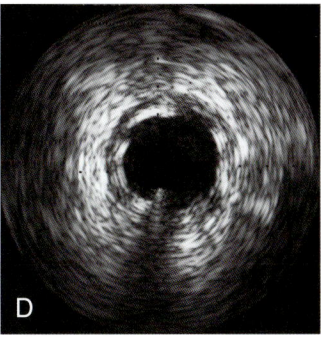

Fig. 65.16 Various presentations of polymeric bioresorbable scaffold (BRS) on intravascular ultrasound (IVUS) image. IVUS often identifies the BRS strut as double-layered bright stripes (suggestive of endoluminal and abluminal strut surfaces) (A and B), although this typical appearance can be compromised as a single-layered strut presentation (C and D), depending on the design of BRS, the IVUS system used, and the location and angle of the struts relative to the transducer. Unlike metallic stents, nonuniform strut distribution is observed frequently in BRS (B).

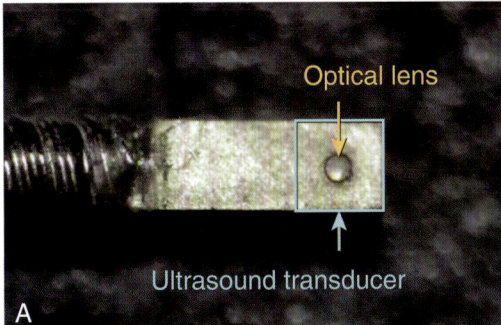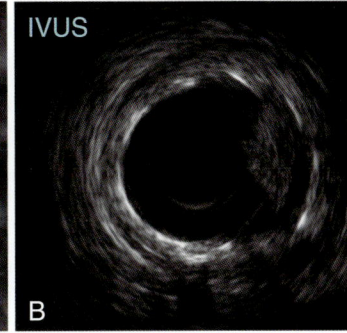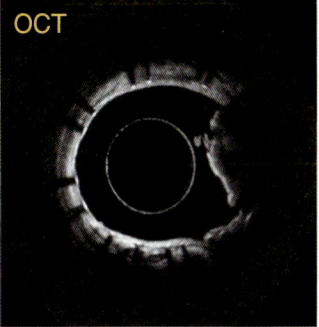

Fig. 65.17 Synergy of intravascular ultrasound *(IVUS)* and optical coherence tomography *(OCT)* technologies. (A) A 3-Fr rotational hybrid IVUS-OCT imaging catheter built using a 40-MHz ultrasound transducer with embedded OCT imaging fiberoptics (Novasight Hybrid System, Conavi Medical). A collinear alignment of the two probes allows the IVUS and OCT beams to travel in the same direction, providing precise coregistration of IVUS and OCT images. (B) Representative coregistered IVUS and OCT images of a coronary artery acquired simultaneously with the hybrid imaging catheter. Inside a previously implanted stent, IVUS shows thrombus or dissected neointima at 2 to 4 o'clock. OCT suggests the in-stent mass as red thrombus, characterized by typical high backscattering and signal attenuation. Thin neointimal coverage over the stent struts delineated on OCT is also not well resolved on IVUS, whereas IVUS visualizes the entire vessel wall that cannot be assessed with OCT due to its limited signal penetration.

expansion limits), so that accurate evaluation of lesion characteristics and vessel size prior to implantation is considered essential to guide appropriate lesion preparation, to avoid severe vessel-device size mismatch, and ultimately to achieve optimal scaffold expansion and apposition. In particular, a higher rate of scaffold thrombosis and association with inadequate scaffold expansion were reported in multicenter, observational studies, as well as recent meta-analyses of the Absorb Bioresorbable Vascular Scaffold (Abbott Vascular, Santa Clara, CA), which has the largest clinical experience in patients with complex lesions.[114–117] Multiple studies have reported that postprocedural nonuniform scaffold expansion, device-vessel mismatch, and implantation in small vessels were associated with adverse clinical events.[118–120] Although IVUS has clear advantage over angiography in precise evaluation of the target-vessel size and deployed BRS within the lesion, exact clinical utilities of IVUS-guidance in BRS implantation are yet to be established.[121]

SUMMARY AND FUTURE PERSPECTIVES

IVUS has evolved into an indispensable tool for research and clinical purposes, with mounting evidence supported by large-scale clinical trials. Although recent advances in intravascular optical coherence tomography currently allow rapid assessment of microscopic details of coronary surface structures, the demand for IVUS remains high because of its ability to provide a more complete picture of the vessel wall due to the greater tissue penetration of the ultrasound signal and its practical usefulness (i.e., no need for blood clearance) for real-time procedural guidance and assessment of treatment effects.

The latest-generation IVUS systems have enabled significant enhancement in image quality by using higher center frequency or extended bandwidth technology. Current technical efforts are also aimed at the development of hybrid devices. One such example is an IVUS-guided reentry catheter system (Pioneer Plus, Philips) that integrates a nitinol needle into a solid-state IVUS imaging catheter. This device is designed to facilitate the reentry of a guidewire into the true lumen from the subintimal space in peripheral CTO intervention. Potential synergy of different technologies may also include a combination of two diagnostic modalities. For instance, integration of IVUS and optical coherence tomography into one imaging catheter, which combines the advantages of ultrasound- and light-based imaging technologies, has recently received U.S. Food and Drug Administration (FDA) 510(k) clearance (Novasight Hybrid System, Conavi Medical, Toronto, Canada) (Fig. 65.17). Three-dimensional coronary artery reconstruction by fusion of biplane coronary angiography and IVUS is also being developed. This technology can provide detailed assessment of the arterial wall and plaque morphology with endothelial shear stress distribution in the coronary artery. Similarly, gathering anatomic and functional information, by combining IVUS and pressure and/or flow sensors, may represent one of the future directions for comprehensive assessment of coronary lesions. Finally, forward-looking IVUS technologies are actively being explored, and one commercial intracardiac imaging system (Foresight, Conavi Medical) has received FDA 510(k) clearance as a new potential option for guiding transseptal puncture, electrophysiology procedures, or catheter-based interventions for structural heart disease. Although these new technologies are yet to mature, the advances of diagnostic modalities will enable us to better understand the pathophysiology of cardiovascular disease and could help to realize the ultimate goal of delivering the most effective treatment to individual patients with truly low rates of complications.

Acknowledgments

We acknowledge all the former and current coworkers at the Stanford Cardiovascular Core Analysis Laboratory for their scientific contributions; Shinjo Sonoda, MD, Atsushi Takagi, MD, and Brian K. Courtney, MD, MSEE for their image courtesy; and M. Brooke Hollak, RN for her review and editing advice.

KEY REFERENCES

5. Fitzgerald PJ, Yock C, Yock PG. Orientation of intracoronary ultrasonography: looking beyond the artery. *J Am Soc Echocardiogr*. 1998;11(1):13–19.
6. Mintz GS, Nissen SE, Anderson WD, et al. American College of Cardiology Clinical Expert Consensus Document on Standards for Acquisition, Measurement and Reporting of Intravascular Ultrasound Studies (IVUS). A report of the American College of Cardiology Task Force on Clinical Expert Consensus Documents. *J Am Coll Cardiol*. 2001;37(5):1478–1492.
13. Stone GW, Maehara A, Lansky AJ, et al. A prospective natural-history study of coronary atherosclerosis. *N Engl J Med*. 2011;364(3):226–235.
21. Oemrawsingh RM, Cheng JM, Garcia-Garcia HM, et al. Near-infrared spectroscopy predicts cardiovascular outcome in patients with coronary artery disease. *J Am Coll Cardiol*. 2014;64(23):2510–2518.
61. Hibi K, Kozuma K, Sonoda S, et al. A randomized study of distal filter protection versus conventional treatment during percutaneous coronary intervention in patients with attenuated plaque identified by intravascular ultrasound (in press). *JACC Cardiovasc Interv*. 2018;11(16):1545–1555.
76. Kobayashi N, Mintz GS, Witzenbichler B, et al. Prevalence, features, and prognostic importance of edge dissection after drug-eluting stent implantation: an ADAPT-DES intravascular ultrasound substudy. *Circ Cardiovasc Interv*. 2016;9(7):e003553.
78. Cheneau E, Leborgne L, Mintz GS, et al. Predictors of subacute stent thrombosis: results of a systematic intravascular ultrasound study. *Circulation*. 2003;108(1):43–47.
87. Kang SJ, Ahn JM, Song H, et al. Comprehensive intravascular ultrasound assessment of stent area and its impact on restenosis and adverse cardiac events in 403 patients with unprotected left main disease. *Circ Cardiovasc Interv*. 2011;4(6):562–569.
88. Sumitsuji S, Inoue K, Ochiai M, et al. Fundamental wire technique and current standard strategy of percutaneous intervention for chronic total occlusion with histopathological insights. *JACC Cardiovasc Interv*. 2011;4(9):941–951.
91. Galassi AR, Sumitsuji S, Boukhris M, et al. Utility of intravascular ultrasound in percutaneous revascularization of chronic total occlusions: an overview. *JACC Cardiovasc Interv*. 2016;9(19):1979–1991.
93. Castagna MT, Mintz GS, Leiboff BO, et al. The contribution of "mechanical" problems to in-stent restenosis: an intravascular ultrasonographic analysis of 1090 consecutive in-stent restenosis lesions. *Am Heart J*. 2001;142(6):970–974.
101. Honda Y. Drug-eluting stents. Insights from invasive imaging technologies. *Circ J*. 2009;73(8):1371–1380.
108. Mintz GS. Intravascular ultrasound and outcomes after drug-eluting stent implantation. *Coron Artery Dis*. 2017;28(4):346–352.
109. Hong SJ, Kim BK, Shin DH, et al. Effect of intravascular ultrasound-guided vs angiography-guided everolimus-eluting stent implantation: the IVUS-XPL randomized clinical trial. *JAMA*. 2015;314(20):2155–2163.
110. Witzenbichler B, Maehara A, Weisz G, et al. Relationship between intravascular ultrasound guidance and clinical outcomes after drug-eluting stents: the assessment of dual antiplatelet therapy with drug-eluting stents (ADAPT-DES) study. *Circulation*. 2014;129(4):463–470.

 Additional references available online at expertconsult.com

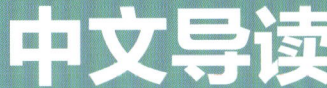

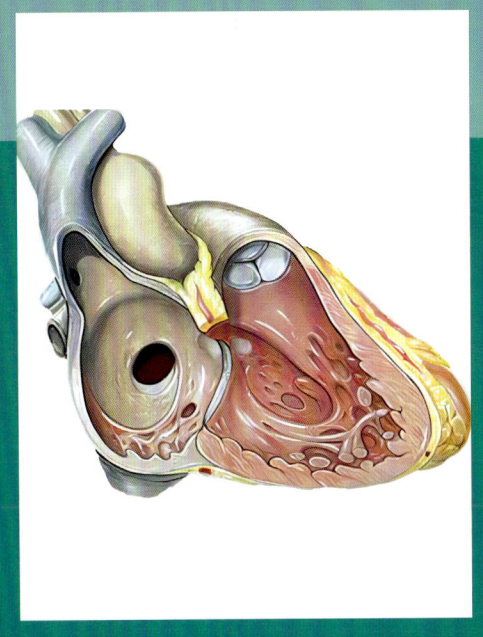

第66章
冠状动脉粥样硬化的动态演变：从动脉粥样硬化形成到易损斑块再到斑块消退

心血管疾病是导致死亡的首位病因，死亡率仍在持续增长，预计2030年之前，全球心血管疾病年死亡人数将超过2360万。冠状动脉粥样硬化性心脏病是一类可以长期无症状的疾病。这种疾病特点提示我们应该早期诊断和治疗，避免患者从无症状进展至急性冠状动脉综合征，从而减少死亡率，改善患者预后。本章节详述了冠状动脉粥样硬化的整个自然病程、转归，粥样硬化斑块的类型，促进动脉粥样硬化的机制（血脂、炎症、自身免疫应答等）。20世纪90年代，AHA根据动脉粥样硬化病变的组织学组成和结构提出了动脉粥样硬化病变分类方法。氧化低密度脂蛋白与炎症是动脉粥样硬化的主要机制。"易损"斑块的特征是薄纤维帽（厚度<65μm）、大坏死核心和巨噬细胞浸润增加，这三个特征定义了薄帽纤维动脉粥样硬化斑块。冠状动脉腔内影像和冠状动脉CT的使用，可早期发现"易损"斑块，针对这些高危人群的强化治疗，可以预防未来不良心血管事件的发生。冠状动脉腔内影像技术（血管内超声、光学相干断层成像）用于评估斑块脂质含量和纤维帽厚度，从而反映斑块稳定程度及炎症水平。减少斑块负担和炎症是治疗及稳定心血管疾病的主要措施，目前的他汀类药物、PCSK9抑制剂、直接抗炎症治疗（卡纳基努单抗）、其他治疗[如n-3脂肪多不饱和酸、接种血管内皮酪氨酸激酶（TEK）疫苗]等被证实可稳定甚至逆转冠状动脉粥样硬化斑块的过程。

叶蕴青　吴永健

章节要点

- 在全球范围内，心血管疾病是死亡的主要病因，2013年造成超过1730万人死亡。
- 急性冠状动脉血栓形成的机制已经很清楚，包括斑块破裂、侵蚀和较少见的钙化结节。
- 冠状动脉造影、冠状动脉CT和冠状动脉腔内成像与组织病理学的结合创造了薄帽纤维动脉粥样硬化斑块的概念。
- 仅凭形态学特征不足以识别可能破裂的薄帽纤维动脉粥样硬化斑块。薄帽纤维动脉粥样硬化斑块大部分稳定，只有少数发生破裂，并且大多数是完全无症状的。
- 急性冠状动脉事件风险作为一个以高风险或易损斑块为中心的简单因果原则，已转变为一个涉及斑块负担、全身性疾病和炎症的复杂模型。
- 减少斑块负担和炎症是导致疾病稳定和斑块消退的有效措施。

66 The Dynamic Spectrum of Coronary Atheroma: From Atherogenesis to Vulnerable Plaque to Plaque Regression

Pedro R. Moreno, Carlos A. Gonzalez Lengua

KEY POINTS

- Globally cardiovascular disease (CVD) is the leading cause of death, accounting for greater than 17.3 million deaths per year in 2013.
- The mechanisms involved in acute coronary thrombosis are well established and include of plaque rupture, erosion, and less frequently, calcific nodules.
- The correlation of coronary angiography, coronary computed tomography angiography and intracoronary imaging with histopathology created the concept of the thin-cap fibroatheroma (TCFA).
- Morphologic features alone are not enough to identify a TCFA that is likely to rupture. Most of them stabilize, only the minority rupture, and most of the rupture events are totally asymptomatic.
- Acute coronary event risk as a simple cause-and-effect principle centered on high-risk or vulnerable plaques has shifted to a complex model involving plaque burden, systemic disease, and inflammation.
- Reducing plaque burden and inflammation are effective measurements that lead to disease stabilization and plaque regression.

THE DYNAMIC NATURE OF CORONARY ATHEROMA: FROM ATHEROGENESIS TO PLAQUE REGRESSION

Globally cardiovascular disease (CVD) is certainly the leading cause of death, accounting for greater than 17.3 million deaths per year in 2013. This number that is expected to grow to greater than 23.6 million by 2030.[1–4] Deaths attributable to ischemic heart disease increased by an estimated 41% from 1990 to 2013.[5] Just in the United States alone, an estimated 16.5 million people have coronary heart disease (CHD), with approximately 1 million developing either new or recurrent events.[3,6]

Coronary atherosclerosis is a condition that remains asymptomatic over decades. Therefore, the natural history of the disease offers an opportunity for early diagnosis and therapy. Prevention of the transition from asymptomatic disease to acute coronary thrombosis may reduce mortality. In fact, the incidence of ST-segment elevation myocardial infarction (STEMI) in the United States and Europe has reduced 25% in the last 8 years.[7,8]

The mechanisms involved in acute coronary thrombosis are well established and include plaque rupture, erosion, and less frequently, calcific nodules.[9] The correlation of coronary angiography, coronary computed tomography angiography (CCTA), and intracoronary imaging with histopathology created the concept of the thin-cap fibroatheroma (TCFA).[7–13] The enthusiasm associated with this concept was the focus of several years of research and even clinical trials. However, the dynamic nature of this disease proved the hypothesis wrong. Morphologic features alone are not enough to identify a TCFA that is likely to rupture. Many stabilize and become thick cap fibroatheromas (ThCFA). Only the minority rupture. However, most of the rupture events are totally asymptomatic.[14] Therefore, conceptualizing acute coronary event risk as a simple cause-and-effect principle centered on high-risk plaques has shifted to a complex model involving plaque burden, systemic disease, and inflammation.[7,15] Most importantly, control of these factors will lead to disease stabilization and plaque regression.

This comprehensive review will cover a wide spectrum of the disease, from atherogenesis to plaque regression. The chapter is divided in five major topics as follows:

1. Atherosclerotic lesion classification and mechanisms of plaque progression
2. Vascular remodeling and thin-cap fibroatheroma
3. The myth of the "vulnerable plaque" and the transition to atherosclerotic disease burden
4. Intracoronary imaging
5. Mechanisms of plaque regression

Although primarily devoted to interventional cardiologists, the first two topics (pathophysiology) are also written for clinicians interested in the field. They summarize two decades of effort in understanding this fascinating but simultaneously fierce disease.

ATHEROSCLEROTIC LESION CLASSIFICATION

The human arteries have three layers; the innermost layer, called *tunica intima*, consists of a single layer of endothelium, basal lamina, subendothelial layer, and internal lamina. The middle layer, the tunica media, consists of layers of smooth muscle cells (SMCs) and extracellular matrix, also known as *elastic lamellas*. The outer layer is a rather thin layer of connective tissue, vasa vasorum, lymphatic vessels, and nerve fibers, and it is called the *tunica adventitia*.[16]

The primary event that triggers lesion formation is an abnormal accumulation of atherogenic plasma derived lipoproteins in the arterial intima.[17] This abnormal accumulation of lipoproteins initiates a pathological cell reaction involving oxidation, inflammation, and neovascularization that result in the lesion formation.[17,18] In the 1990s the American Heart Association (AHA) published a series of reports from the committee on vascular lesions of the council on arteriosclerosis lead by Herbert C. Stary MD; they proposed a practical classification of the atherosclerotic lesions according to their histological composition and structure (Fig. 66.1, Table 66.1).[19–22]

SECTION VI Evaluation of Interventional Techniques

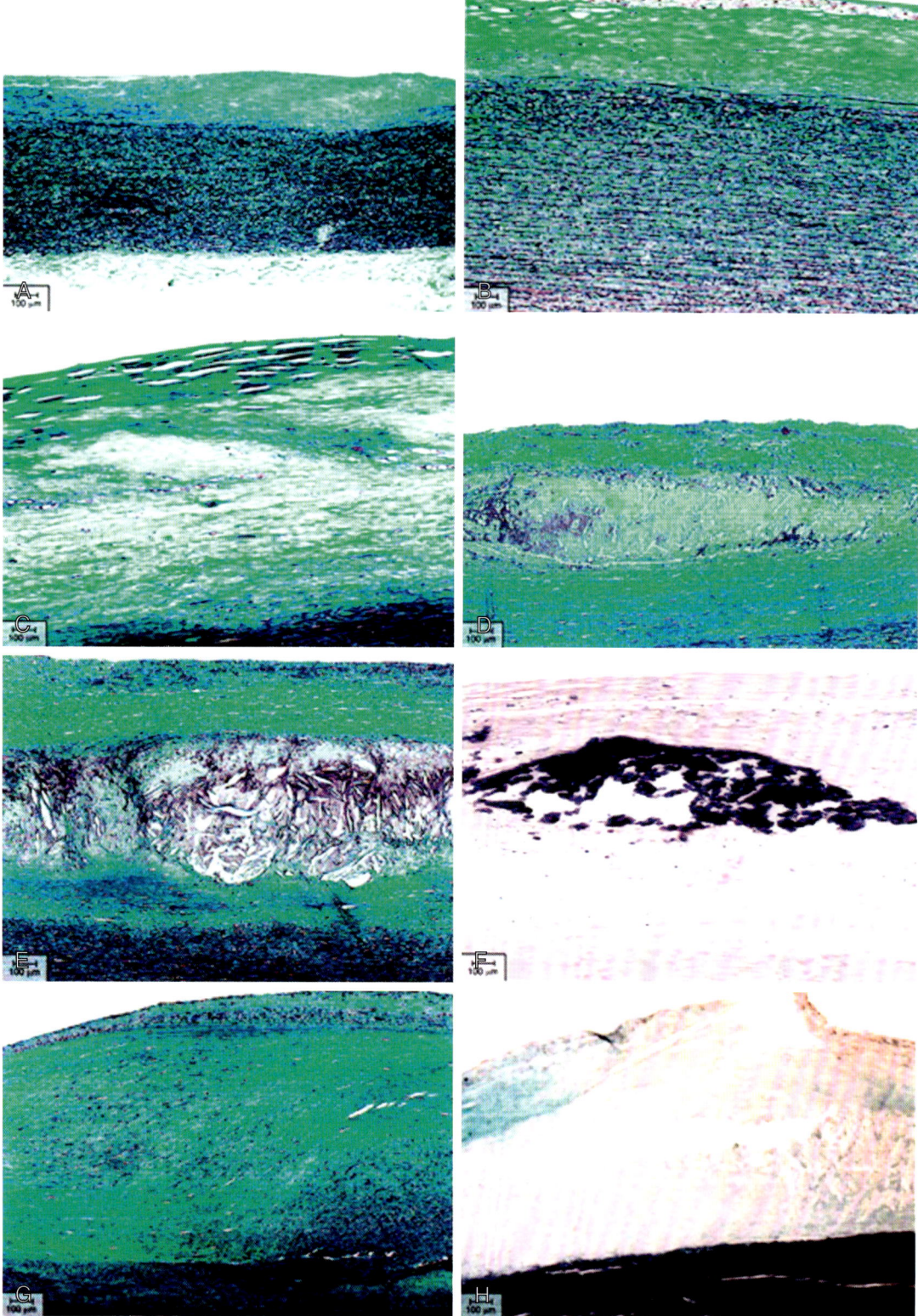

Fig. 66.1 Histological examples according to AHA classification. (A) Class I (nonspecific intimal thickening). (B) Class II (fatty streak). (C) Class III (preatheroma). (D) Class IV (atheroma). (E) Class Va (fibroatheroma). (F) Class Vb (calcific plaque). (G) Class Vc (fibrotic plaque). (H) Class VI (disrupted plaque). (A–E and G) Elastic trichrome stain. (F and H) Hematoxylin-eosin stain. *AHA,* American Heart Association. (From Moreno PR, Purushothaman KR, Fuster V, et al. Intimomedial interface damage and adventitial inflammation is increased beneath disrupted atherosclerosis in the aorta implications for plaque vulnerability. *Circulation.* 2002;105[21]:2504–2511.)

TABLE 66.1 American Heart Association Classification of Atherosclerotic Plaque

Type of Lesion	Composition	
Type I	Initial lesion with macrophage foam cells	Clinically silent, growth mainly from lipid accumulation, earliest onset as soon as first decade of life
Type II	Fatty streak, intracellular lipid accumulation in multiple foam cell layers	
Type III	Preatheroma: intra and extra cellular lipid accumulation	
Type IV	Atheroma: formation of the lipid core	Clinically silent or symptomatic, type IV lesions growth mainly from lipid accumulation, type V and VI growth from accelerate smooth muscle increase, collagen increase, hematoma and thrombosis.
Type Va	Fibroatheroma: lipid cored and fibrotic layers	
Type Vb (Type VII)	Calcific plaque: lipid core, fibrotic layers and calcium deposition	
Type Vc (Type VIII)	Fibrotic plaque: fibrous layers of connective tissue without significant lipid accumulation	
Type VI	Complicate lesion: type IV or V plaques with disruption of the surface, hemorrhage-hematoma or thrombosis	

Type I lesions are microscopically detectable lipid accumulations in the intima with a small group of macrophage containing lipid droplets (macrophage foam cells); this happens particularly in regions of intima with adaptive thickening or atherosclerosis prone regions.[17]

Type II lesions consist of fatty streaks or spots in the intima with adjacent layers of foam cells and T lymphocytes.[17]

Type III lesions or intermediate lesions are the preatheroma lesions. They are characterized by accumulation of extracellular lipid pools that lie just below layers of macrophages and macrophage foam cells. These lipid pools replace intercellular matrix proteoglycans and fibers and drive SMCs apart.[17]

Type IV lesions, or atheroma, consist of dense, well-defined accumulations of extracellular lipid in the intima (lipid core), microscopical macrophages, macrophage foam cells, and lymphocyte, concentrated in the lipid core formation.

Type V lesions often lead to an increase of the vessel external boundary without any significant narrow of the lumen (positive remodeling).[19] When a prominent fibrous connective tissue has formed around the lipid core, the lesions are considered type V lesions. If the fibrous connective tissue is part of the lipid core, the lesion is called *fibroatheroma* or *type Va lesion*. When the lipid core or other regions of the lesion are calcified, it is referred as *type Vb* (also called *type VII lesion* in a later review). A type V lesion without a lipid core or minimal lipid accumulation is called *fibrotic* or *type Vc lesions* (also called *type VIII lesion* in a later review).[19]

Type VI lesions are a complex disease, including plaque rupture, erosion, or intraplaque hemorrhage.

Mechanisms of Plaque Progression

Oxidized Low-Density Lipoprotein and Inflammation in Atherogenesis

Oxidized low-density lipoprotein (oxLDL) cholesterol is avidly taken up by macrophages via scavenger receptors, producing a cytoplasm overloaded with lipid droplets. As the inflow of oxLDL continues, it leads to extracellular lipid accumulation in the matrix of the plaque and cell death.[20] Distribution of oxLDL plays a pivotal role in plaque growth according to mathematical models based on physical laws.[21] Similarly, preclinical experimentation has demonstrated how oxLDL isoforms are associated with TCFA, depending on the predominant type of molecule and their induction of macrophage apoptosis.[22] The necrotic core is formed by apoptosis of lipid-laden macrophages, foam cells, and erythrocytes.[23] Active collagen dissolution by metalloproteinases contributes to core expansion, which plays a major role in plaque rupture.[24]

In the aorta, the necrotic core area corresponds to 40% of the total plaque area in the TCFAs and up to 50% in rupture plaques.[25] However, other studies of coronary arteries show necrotic areas of as little as 24% and 34% in TCFAs and ruptured plaques, respectively.[26] Core composition may influence the propensity for plaque rupture and thrombosis. An increased ratio of free cholesterol to esterified cholesterol with oxidized cholesterol increases the likelihood of thrombosis by interacting with the oxLDL (lectin-like) receptor 1 (OLR1), a cell surface receptor for oxLDL, and enhancing the expression of tissue factor.[23,27–30]

Finally, oxLDL triggers an inflammatory response that activates hypoxia inducible factor alpha (HIF-1α) in monocytes.[31,32] HIF-1α is a key transcriptional regulator responding to hypoxia and activating genes, which promote angiogenesis, among them vascular endothelial growth factor (VEGF). This proangiogenic effect of oxLDL provides the link between hyperlipidemia, inflammation, and angiogenesis in atherosclerosis.[31]

Monocyte-Macrophages and T Cells in Atherosclerosis

Once the inflammatory response is trigger by the lipoproteins, especially oxLDL, it provokes entry of bone-marrow derived monocytes into the intima.[33] Then, monocytes differentiate into macrophages, which are the major inflammatory cells involved in the progression of atherosclerosis.

Initially, macrophages were classified as proinflammatory/proatherogenic (M1), and antiinflammatory/antiatherogenic (M2). Nevertheless, recent evidence suggests that the microenvironment may be fundamental in directing the cell into morphologically and functionally distinct phenotypes.[34] It is the complex milieu of atherosclerosis that determines macrophage differentiation.

In progressing lesions, macrophages take on a proinflammatory phenotype (previously called M1).[34–36] This abnormal accumulation of inflammatory macrophages and dendritic cell activation is driven mainly by Interferon γ and other proinflammatory cytokines.[37] Migration and activations of other immune cells may also contribute, including natural killer and T2 helper lymphocytes, platelets, mast cells.[37] The proinflammatory macrophage releases proinflammatory cytokines (tissue necrosis factor α [TNF α], interleukin-1β [IL-1β], interleukin [IL]6, nitric oxide synthase [NOS], reactive oxygen species [ROS], leukotrienes, and matrix metalloproteinases [MMPs]), which leads to more inflammation, lesion growth, and tissue destruction.[35]

Counterbalance of Macrophage Inflammation and Postinflammatory Response

In normal circumstances, a postinflammatory response is carried out by cells that counterbalance the inflammatory process, promoting tissue repair. This postinflammatory response is driven mainly by regulatory T cells (Tregs).[37] Tregs execute their antiinflammatory response by targeting naïve and effector CD4+ and CD8+ T cells. In addition, dendritic cells and macrophages may also contribute to this response via CD25.[34] This action is mediated by competitive binding of IL-2 to on effector T cells and promoting antiinflammatory cytokines like IL-10.[34,37]

Resolution of Inflammation

Resolution of inflammation is probably the most important step to restore homeostasis and induce plaque stabilization. Antiinflammatory macrophages (previously called M2) are fundamental in this process.[37] Resolving macrophages will promote tissue repair by efferocytosis, transforming growth factor β (TGFβ),

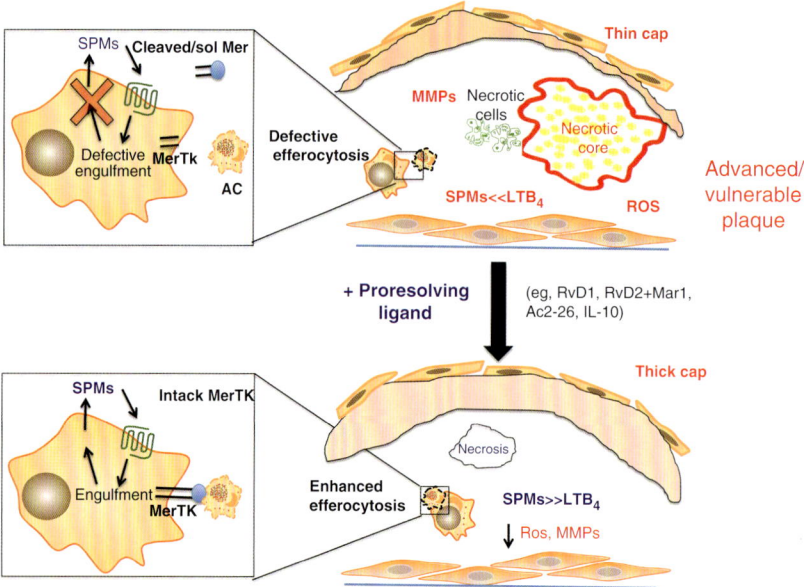

Fig. 66.2 Specialized proresolving mediators *(SPMs)* reduce lesion necrosis and enhance efferocytosis, fibrous caps, and the SPM/leukotriene (LT) ratio. Top panel: Key features of advanced plaques include large necrotic cores, thin fibrous caps, increased oxidative stress, and a dysregulated activation of matrix metalloproteinases *(MMPs)* and defective efferocytosis. New results indicate that advanced plaques also have an imbalance in an important receptor for efferocytosis and has recently been linked to the biosynthesis of SPMs. Cleavage of *MerTK* results in decreased efferocytosis and decreased SPMs. Bottom panel: When SPMs (or other proresolving ligands) are administered to mice with ongoing atherosclerosis, several key features of advanced plaques, like necrosis and oxidative stress, are markedly reduced. SPM administration also increases fibrous cap thickness and efferocytosis and restores the SPM/LTB4 ratio. RvD1 enhanced lesional efferocytosis in part because of its ability to limit MerTK cleavage. *AC*, apoptotic cell; *IL-10*, interleukin-10; *LTB4*, leukotriene B4; *ROS*, reactive oxygen species. (From Fredman G, Tabas I. Boosting inflammation resolution in atherosclerosis: the next frontier for therapy. Am J Pathol. 2017;187[6]:1211–1221.)

IL-10, annexin A1, and inflammation-induced endogenous lipids, called *specialized pro resolving meditators*.[38,39]

Efferocytosis, or the removal of short-lived apoptotic bodies from the atheroma, mediates resolution of inflammation.[40] Efficient clearance of apoptotic cells prevents secondary or postapoptotic cellular necrosis. Efferocytosis triggers an antiinflammatory response through the induction of TGFβ, IL-10, and other antiinflammatory cytokines[41]

Defective Efferocytosis

Impaired removal of short-lived apoptotic bodies decreases macrophage efflux from the atheroma, leading to secondary necrosis, macrophage apoptosis, and the release of prothrombotic factors, inflammatory chemokines, and collagenases (Fig. 66.2).[42]

Defective efferocytosis is due to multiple factors mostly led by an excessive local proinflammatory environment, age, intracellular energy metabolism, gut microbiota, genetic, and epigenetic factors.[41,43–45] Defective efferocytosis leads to lipid accumulation exceeding macrophage scavenger capacity, apoptosis, and secondary necrosis. MMPs release and tissue factor expression, triggering plaque rupture and atherothrombosis (Figs. 66.3 and 66.4).[28,37,46]

Vasa Vasorum Neovascularization

Atherosclerotic neovascularization evolves early in atherogenesis as a defense mechanism against hypoxia and oxLDL deposition in the tunica intima.[47] In early and advanced disease, the neovessels may play a defensive role, allowing lipid removal from the plaque through the adventitia and leading to hypoxia resolution and plaque regression. However, in the absence of proper hypoxia resolution, chronic inflammation, oxidized lipids, and proteases will further promote angiogenesis.

Neovessels can serve as a pathway for leukocyte recruitment to high-risk areas of the plaque, including the cap and the shoulder. Expression of vascular cell adhesion molecule 1 (VCAM-1), intracellular adhesion molecule 1 (ICAM-1), and E-selectin is two- to threefold higher in neovessels compared with the arterial luminal endothelium, confirming the pivotal role of neovessels as a pathway for leukocyte recruitment in human coronary plaques.[48]

Neovessels are characterized by a single layer of neo-endothelium. There is no tunica media or pericytes to stabilize these neovessels. Therefore, they are highly susceptible to injury by cytotoxic agents (e.g., oxidized lipids, oxidative stress).

Inflammation as a Promoter of Plaque Neovascularization

Angiogenesis is stimulated by inflammatory cells. For instance, apoptotic microvesicles at the submicrometer level found in atherosclerosis plaques are highly proangiogenic by regulating CD40L and are produced mostly by macrophages.[49] Histologic evidence has documented atherosclerotic neovascularization as a pathway for macrophage infiltration in advanced, lipid-rich plaques (LRPs; Fig. 66.5).[50] Neovessel content was significantly increased in plaques with severe inflammation associated with increased macrophage and T-lymphocyte infiltration.[51] Ruptured plaques exhibited the highest degree of neovascularization.[52] Further analysis of plaque angiogenesis in diabetic patients documented a complex morphology, including sprouting, red blood cell (RBC) extravasation, and perivascular inflammation.[53]

In summary, plaque neovascularization is initially a defense mechanism (physiological angiogenesis) to provide oxygen and to remove lipid from the plaque. It may eventually fail, leading to extravasation of RBCs, perivascular inflammation, and intraplaque hemorrhage (pathological angiogenesis) (Fig. 66.6).[54]

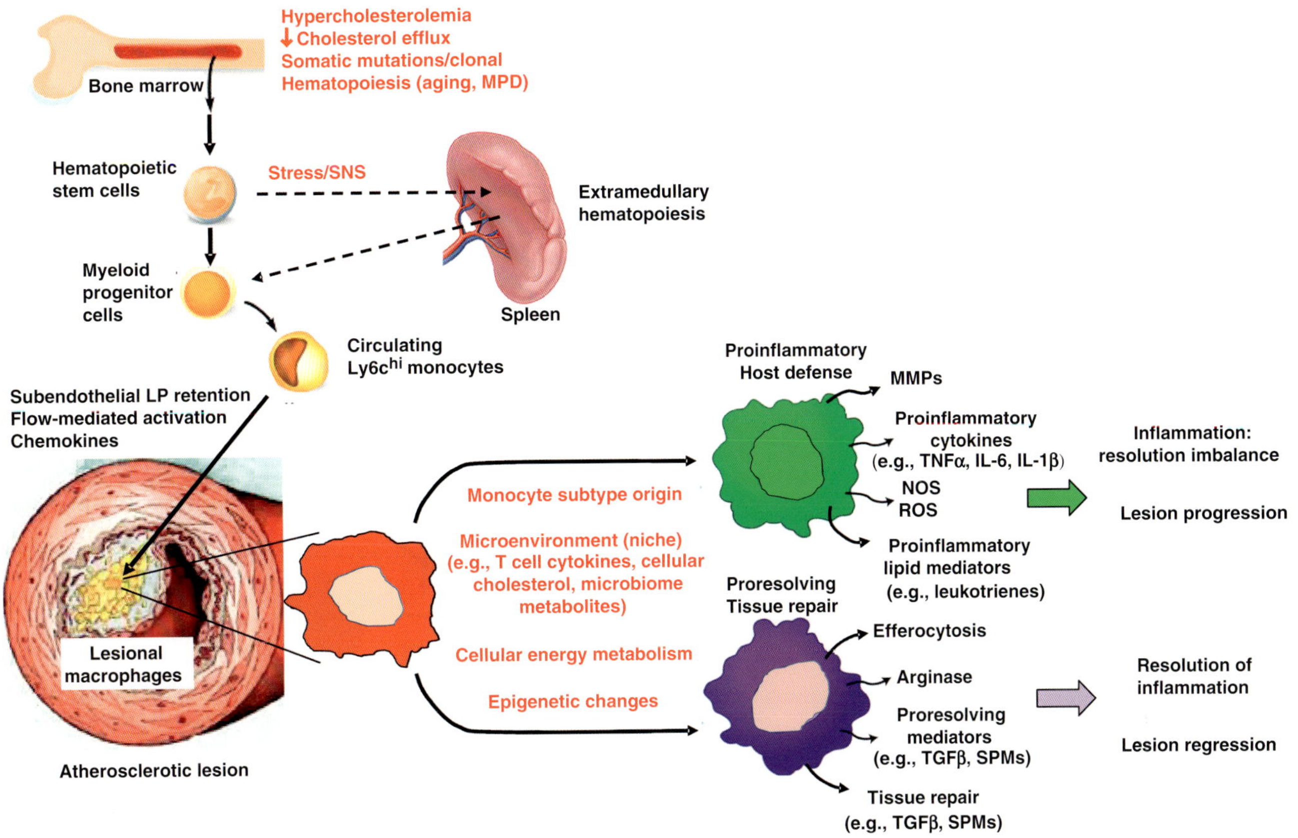

Fig. 66.3 Regulation of innate immune processes related to monocyte-macrophages in atherosclerosis. The major subpopulation of monocytes that contribute to atherosclerosis progression are Ly6c^{hi} monocytes, which enter lesions in response to subendothelially retained apolipoprotein-B-containing lipoproteins (*LPs*) and subsequent chemokine release by activated endothelial cells. After differentiation into macrophages, these myeloid cells undergo a variety of phenotypic changes under the influence of the factors listed in the figure. Those macrophages on the inflammatory end of the spectrum secrete proteins and carry out processes that promote atherosclerosis progression, whereas those on the resolution end of the spectrum promote lesion regression. *IL-1β*, Interleukin-1β; *IL-6*, interleukin-6; *MMPs*, matrix metalloproteinases; *MPD*, myeloproliferative disease; *NOS*, nitric oxide synthase; *ROS*, reactive oxygen species; *SNS*, sympathetic nervous system; *SPMs*, specialized proresolving mediators; *TGFβ*, transforming growth factor-β; *TNFα*, tissue necrosis factor α. (From Tabas I, Lichtman AH. Monocyte-macrophages and T cells in atherosclerosis. *Immunity.* 2017;47[4]:621–634.)

Intraplaque Hemorrhage

Angiogenesis injury may result in extravasation of RBCs into the plaque, also known as intraplaque hemorrhage. These events generate accumulation of cholesterol and the formation of cholesterol crystals, fibrin deposition, release of hemoglobin, heme and iron ions promoting local oxidative stress, lipid peroxidation, and sustained inflammatory burden.

Compared with nonhemorrhagic atheromas, hemorrhagic plaques have lower levels of epidermal growth factor (EGF), placental growth factor (PGF), and angiopoietin 1, and increased levels of VEGF.[55,56] OxLDL, ROS, and other inflammatory mediators induce rapid lysis of the extravasated erythrocytes, releasing lipid and free hemoglobin to the atheroma.[57] Extracorpuscular hemoglobin induces a Fenton reaction, leading to activation of ROS, inhibition of nitric oxide, and activation of MMPs.

Defense Against Intraplaque Hemorrhage

To counteract oxidative stress, macrophages stimulate the production of Heme oxygenase-1 and ferritin. Heme oxygenase-1-mediates heme oxidation, resulting in the formation of biliverdin, carbon monoxide, and redox-active iron (Fe^{2+}). These molecules exert a potent antiinflammatory effect. However, in advanced lesions, ferritin expression can increase heme oxidation and the production of higher amounts of pro-oxidant Fe^{3+},[57] which oxidizes lipids, leading to endothelial cytotoxicity.[58]

Extracorpuscular hemoglobin stimulates monocyte-macrophage differentiation in a nonfoamy macrophage called M(Hg), which has athero-protective functions.[36] M(Hg) is involved in phagocytosis of erythrocytes and hemoglobin clearance mediated by mannose receptor and CD163, a scavenger receptor for the hemoglobin–haptoglobin complex.[36]

Haptoglobin Genotype

The haptoglobin gene *(HP)* has two codominant alleles (*HP*1* and *HP*2*). The haptoglobin gene cluster resides at chromosome 16q22. The protein products of the two *HP* alleles are structurally different, and the cardiovascular effects of the polymorphisms play a major role in patients with diabetes mellitus (DM).[59] Multiple independent epidemiologic studies examining incident CVD have demonstrated that individuals with DM who are homozygous for the *HP*2* allele have a risk of cardiovascular events four to five times higher than those who are homozygous for the *HP*1* allele.

The mechanism by which the homozygous *HP*2* genotype regulates inflammation and enhances plaque vulnerability is by decreasing haptoglobin clearance. This is explained in part by a defective CD163 receptor in macrophages.[60] Similarly, persons

SECTION VI Evaluation of Interventional Techniques

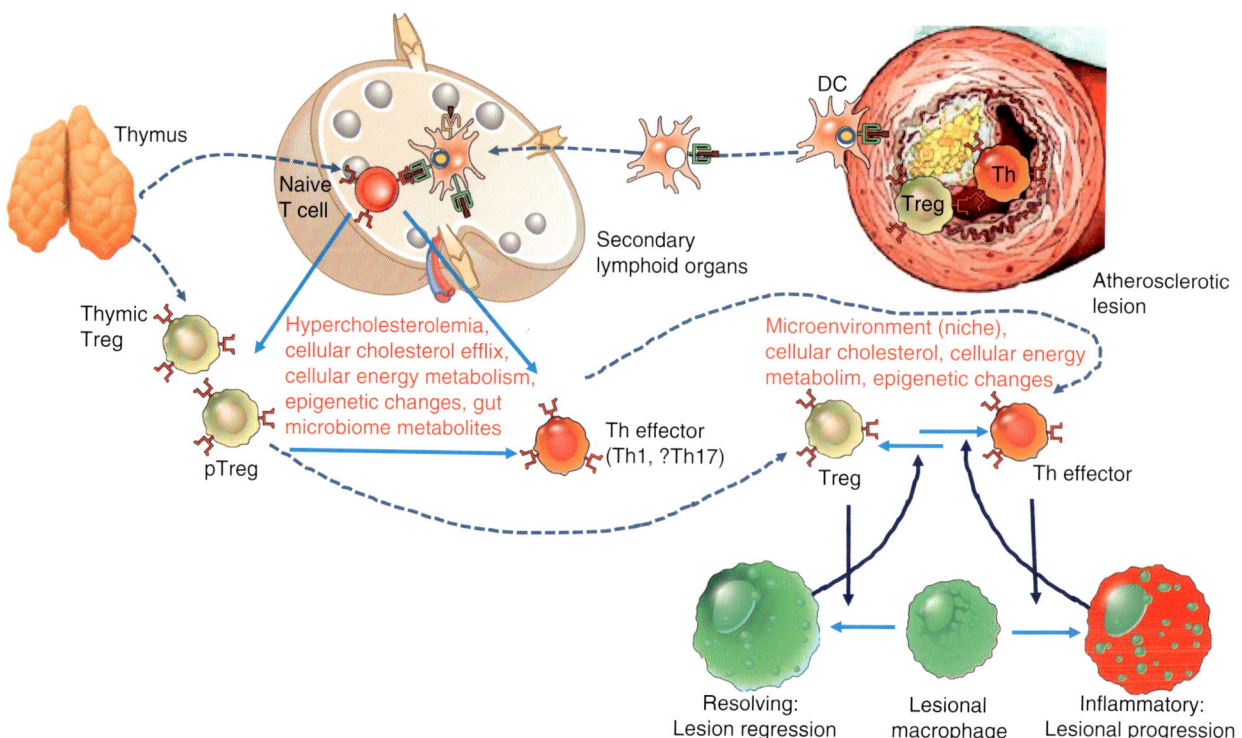

Fig. 66.4 Regulation and impact of adaptive immune processes related to T cells in atherosclerosis. T lymphocyte responses that affect atherosclerosis include a balance between inflammatory effector T (Teff) cells, mainly interferon-γ-producing T helper (Th) cells, and antiinflammatory regulatory T cells (Treg). Treg and Th cells migrate into developing atherosclerotic lesions and modulate the local inflammatory microenvironment, in large part by influencing macrophage phenotypes. Conversely, resolving or inflammatory macrophage phenotypes can shift the plaque T cell balance toward Treg and Th phenotypes, respectively. Change in the balance between Treg and Th cells could reflect phenotypic plasticity by permitting redifferentiation between regulatory and inflammatory phenotypes. DC, Dendritic cell. (From Tabas I, Lichtman AH. Monocyte-macrophages and T cells in atherosclerosis. Immunity. 2017;47[4]:621–634.)

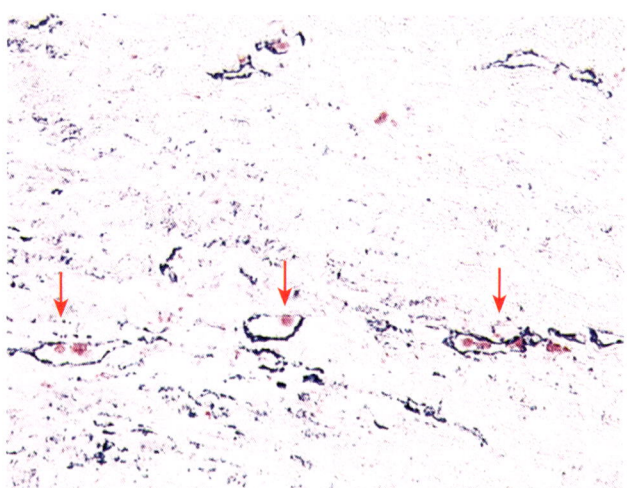

Fig. 66.5 Histologic evidence of atherosclerotic neovascularization as a pathway for macrophage infiltration in human aortic plaques obtained at autopsy. Bicolor, contrasting immunohistochemical technique reveals microvessels in cross sections (arrows), identified with the monoclonal endothelial cell marker CD34 linked to a blue chromogen, and inflammatory cells, identified with a combined macrophage and T-cell marker (CD68-CD3) linked to a red chromogen. (From Fuster VM, Moreno PR, Fayad ZA, et al. Atherothrombosis and high-risk plaque, part I: evolving concepts. J Am Coll Cardiol. 2005;46:937–954.)

homozygous for the *HP*2* allele have a higher inflammatory cell content, greater level of neovascularization, and higher MMP levels in the atheroma (Fig. 66.7).[61,62] Detection of TCFAs should include identification of intraplaque hemorrhage, iron deposition, RBC membranes, and hemosiderin deposits in macrophages. In patients with DM, genotyping may offer additional prognostic value.

Macrophage Interaction Between Iron and Cholesterol Homeostasis

The M(Hb) up-regulates ATP-binding cassette (ABC) transporters, increasing cholesterol efflux to apo A-I. This crucial pathway emphasizes the importance of iron homeostasis in directing cholesterol handling by macrophages (Fig. 66.8).[36] Nevertheless, recurrent intraplaque hemorrhage, enhanced oxidative stress, hemoglobin/heme accumulation, and proinflammatory microenvironment frequently overpower vascular and immunologic defensive mechanisms and irreversibly promote plaque progression toward instability and rupture.[57]

VASCULAR REMODELING AND THIN-CAP FIBROATHEROMA

As a defense mechanism, the vessel wall can expand significantly to harbor large atheromas without obstructing the lumen (Fig. 66.9). Also known as *remodeling*, this process is linked to high-risk atherosclerosis. The remodeling process promotes higher stress at the level of the fibrous cap, which makes plaques more prone

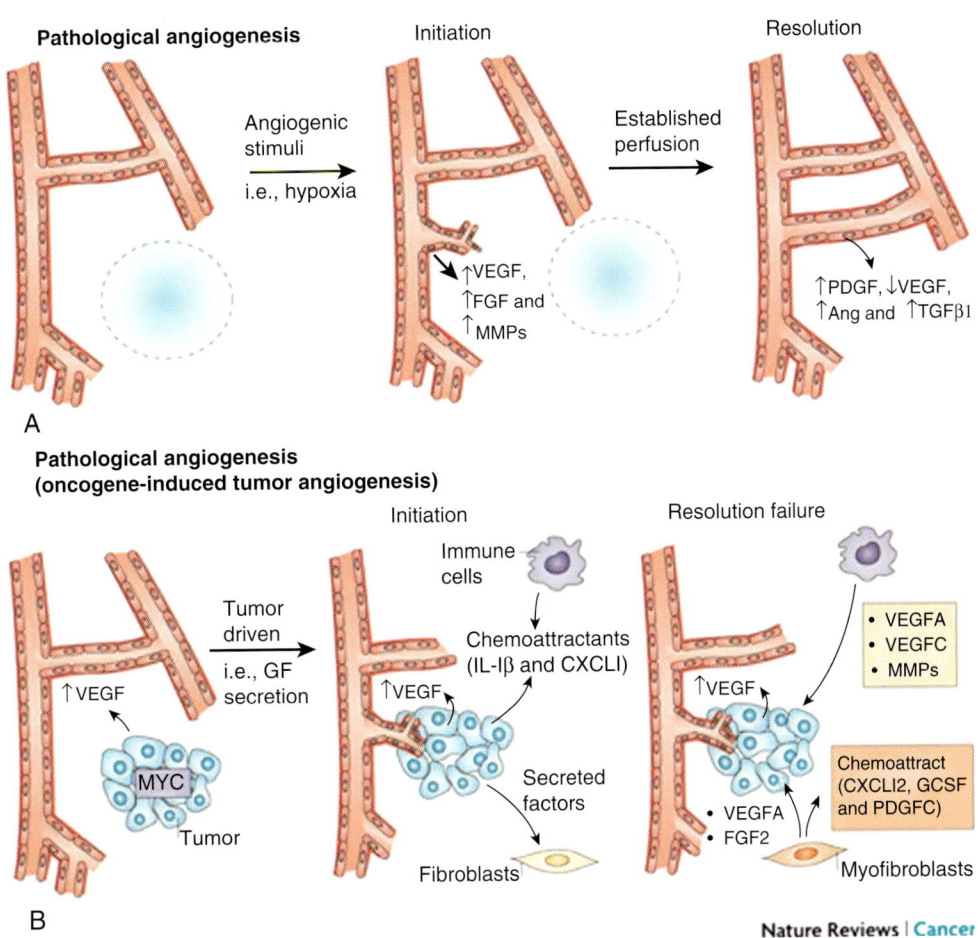

Fig. 66.6 (A) During physiological angiogenesis, stimuli such as hypoxia can trigger the angiogenesis cascade. In the initiation phase, an increase in endothelial cell-derived growth factors *(GFs)* such as vascular endothelial growth factor A *(VEGFA)* and fibroblast growth factor *(FGF)* cause vessel destabilization and initiate vessel sprouting and endothelial cell proliferation. Matrix metalloproteinases *(MMPs)* facilitate the remodeling of the extracellular matrix (ECM) and increase the biological availability of ECM-sequestered growth factors. On new vessel establishment and perfusion, VEGF levels decline, and the resolution phase ensues coincident with a rise in platelet-derived growth factor *(PDGF)*, angiopoietins *(Ang)*, and transforming growth factor-β1 *(TGFβ1)* expression responsible for the recruitment and stabilization of mural cells and vascular smooth muscle cells around the newly formed vessel. (B) Under pathological conditions, such as oncogene-driven tumor angiogenesis, tumor-secreted VEGFA can initiate the angiogenesis cascade. Tumor cells such as those driven by the MYC gene result in increased expression of soluble factors that are responsible for activating resident fibroblasts and for attracting immune cells. These stromal cell types are capable of sustaining the angiogenic process through the secretion of vascular growth- and inflammation-promoting factors, resulting in a failure to resolve the angiogenesis cascade. *CXCL1*, C-X-C motif chemokine ligand 1; *GCSF*, granulocyte colony stimulating factor; *IL-1β*, interleukin-1β. (From Chung J, Lee J, Ferrara N, et al. Targeting the tumor vasculature: insights from physiological angiogenesis. *Nat Rev Cancer.* 2010;10[7]:505–514.)

to rupture and clinical events. Cilla and associates[63] compared the geometric and physical properties of the different types of plaque remodeling (Fig. 66.10). The mechanisms responsible for remodeling involve an inflammatory process at the base of the plaque at the intimomedial junction, which leads to digestion of the internal elastic lamina and compromise of the tunica media and adventitia. Several studies have shown increased expression of MMPs in the intimomedial interface of remodeled plaques.[64–66] Disruption of the internal elastic lamina is associated with medial and adventitial inflammation, and evidence suggests that MMP10 plays a regulatory role in atherosclerosis progression by influencing plaque inflammation and vascular remodeling.[67] Burke and colleagues also demonstrated that marked expansion of the internal elastic lamina occurred in plaque hemorrhage with or without rupture.[68]

The clinical relevance of remodeling was pioneered by Schoenhagen and coworkers, who studied 85 patients with unstable coronary syndromes and 46 patients with stable coronary syndromes by using intravascular ultrasound (IVUS) before percutaneous coronary intervention (PCI).[69] The remodeling ratio (RR) is the area of the external elastic membrane at the lesion divided by the same area at the proximal reference site. Positive remodeling was defined as an RR value greater than 1.05, and negative remodeling was defined as an RR value less than 0.95 (Fig. 66.11). The RR was higher at target lesions in patients with acute coronary syndrome (ACS) than in patients with stable angina. Positive remodeling was more common in ACS cases (51.8% vs. 19.6%), whereas negative remodeling was more common in chronic stable angina cases (56.5% vs. 31.8%), confirming the histopathologic associations between plaque remodeling and vulnerability.[69]

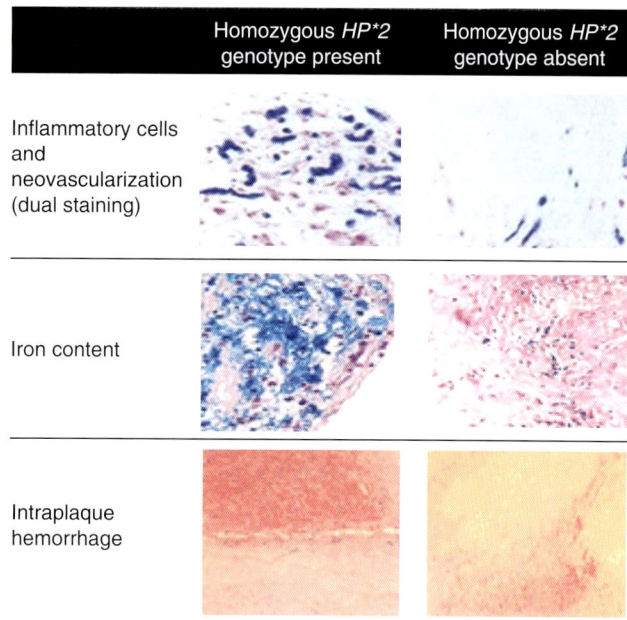

Fig. 66.7 Histologic analysis of plaques from diabetic patients homozygous for the HP*2 allele (left) were compared with control plaques (right). HP*2 plaques had a higher inflammatory cell content, higher degree of neovascularization, and higher level of intraplaque hemorrhage. (Courtesy Dr. K. Raman Purushothaman, Mount Sinai Hospital, New York, NY.)

The Concept of Thin Cap Fibroatheroma

Early in atherogenesis, the nascent fatty streak evolves into a transitional lesion or preatheroma. Death of macrophages, hypoxia, extravasation of erythrocytes, and free cholesterol replace lipid pools to form necrotic cores. Disease progresses through necrotic core expansion by active digestion of collagen, reducing the rim of fibrous tissue separating the core from the lumen forming the fibroatheroma. When macrophage-derived collagenolytic activity ruptures the cap of the fibroatheroma, the highly thrombogenic core is exposed to circulating blood and triggers thrombosis.[25,70] When quantified by ocular micrometry, all ruptured plaques are characterized by a thin fibrous cap, (<65 μm in thickness), a large necrotic core, and increased macrophage infiltration.[71] These three characteristics defined the TCFA (Fig. 66.12).[70,71]

Clinical Significance of the Thin-Cap Fibroatheroma

Pioneering studies by Ambrose and Fuster in 1988 described the baseline angiographic characteristics of lesions that produce acute myocardial infarctions (AMIs).[13] The investigators found that lesions evolving to complete occlusion had a mean percent diameter stenosis of 48% (Fig. 66.13). Many studies have reproduced these findings, supporting the concept that most lesions responsible for AMI evolve from nonobstructive disease.[72] However, contrary to those early publications, subsequent postmortem studies of subjects dying from cardiac arrest or AMI indicated that the percent luminal area stenosis at sites of thrombus was ≥75% in two-thirds of cases,[73] the mean stenosis of likely culprit

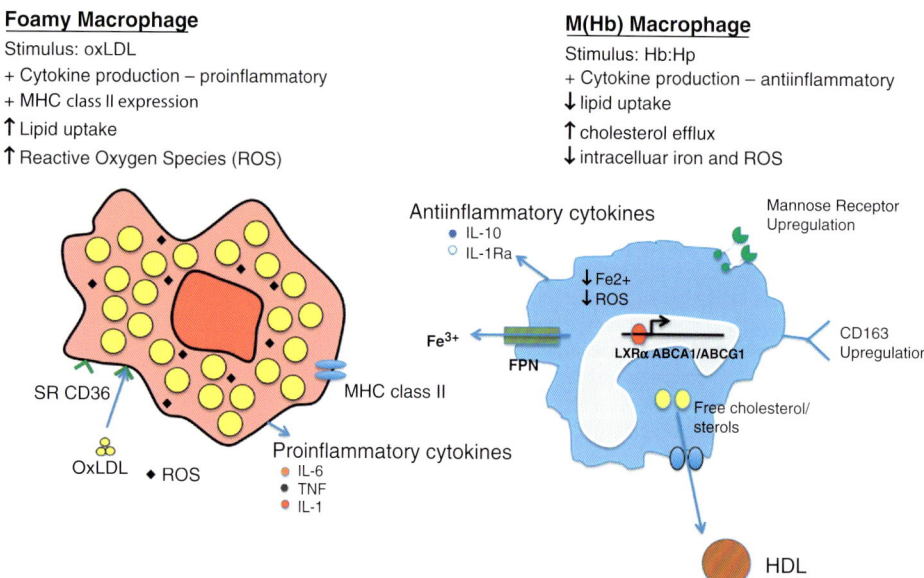

Fig. 66.8 Macrophage diversity in human atherosclerosis during intraplaque hemorrhage, exposure of monocytes to hemoglobin:haptoglobin complex (Hb:Hp) directs human monocytes into a hemoglobin-stimulated macrophage (M(Hb)) differentiation program characterized by up-regulation of CD163 and mannose receptors, increased expression of antiinflammatory cytokines and the iron exporter ferroportin (FPN), which decreases intracellular iron. The latter reduces reactive oxygen species (ROS), which activates liver X receptor α (LXRα)–mediated transcription of ATP-binding cassette (ABC) transporters. This program is distinct from macrophage foam cells, which demonstrate greater expression of the scavenger receptor (SR) CD36, uptake of oxidized low-density lipoprotein (oxLDL), ROS, and production of proinflammatory cytokines. HDL, High-density lipoprotein; IL, interleukin; MHC, major histocompatibility complex; TNF, tumor necrosis factor. (From Finn AV, Nakano M, Polavarapu R, et al. Hemoglobin directs macrophage differentiation and prevents foam cell formation in human atherosclerotic plaques. J Am Coll Cardiol. 2012;59:166–177.)

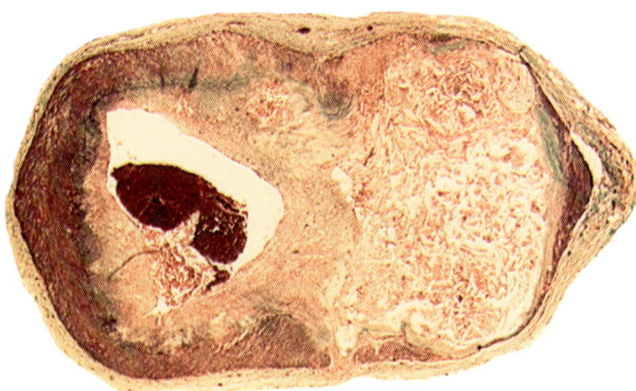

Fig. 66.9 Large human thrombotic plaque in the left main coronary artery shows extensive remodeling and a large necrotic core. (Courtesy Dr. K. Raman Purushothaman, Mount Sinai Hospital, New York, NY.)

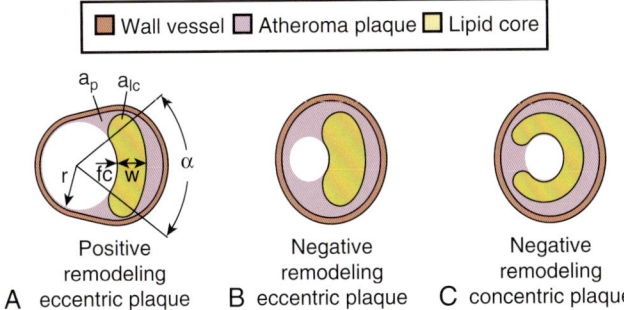

Fig. 66.10 Idealized cross-sectional models and geometric parameters: Fibrous cap thickness *(fc)*, lumen radius *(r)*, lipid core area *(alc)*, lipid core width *(w)*, lipid core angle *(α)*, and atheroma plaque area *(ap)*. (A) Positive arterial remodeling. (B) Negative arterial remodeling with an eccentric atheroma plaque. (C) Negative arterial remodeling with a concentric atheroma plaque. (From Cilla M, Pena E, Martinez MA, et al. Comparison of the vulnerability risk for positive versus negative atheroma plaque morphology. *J Biomech.* 2013;46:1248–1254.)

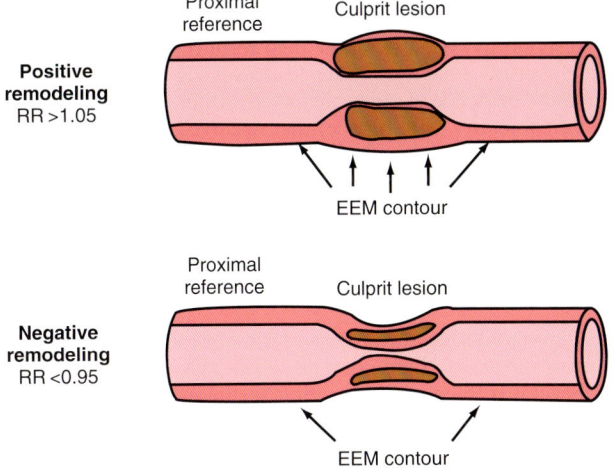

Fig. 66.11 Diagram explains the direction of positive and negative remodeling. *EEM,* External elastic membrane. (Modified from Schoenhagen P, Ziada KM, Kapadia SR, et al. Extent and direction of arterial remodeling in stable versus unstable coronary syndromes: an intravascular ultrasound study. *Circulation.* 2000;101:598–603.)

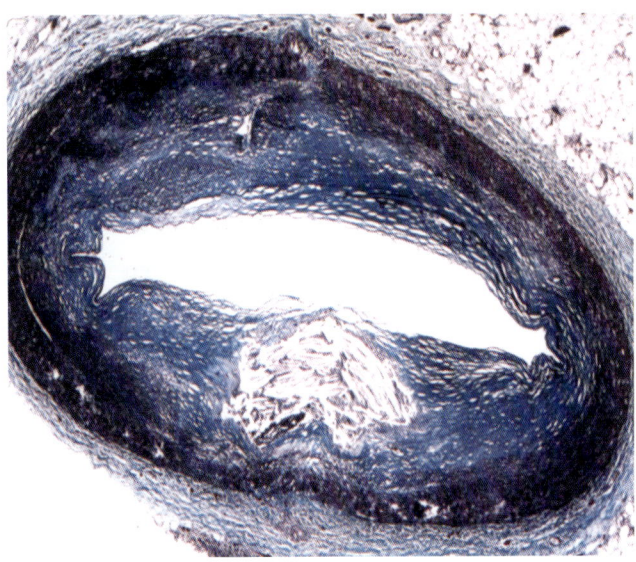

Fig. 66.12 Thin-cap fibroatheroma is characterized by a very thin fibrous cap and a large necrotic core (trichrome stain). (Courtesy Dr. K. Raman Purushothaman, Mount Sinai Hospital, New York, NY.)

lesions causing MI was greater than 90%,[74] and only about 10% of culprit lesions had a diameter stenosis of less than 50% after thrombus removal (Fig. 66.14).[75]

These findings were later corroborated by IVUS and optical coherence tomography (OCT) studies, which clarified that the early angiography studies did not take into account the interval progression of lesion severity that may have occurred before coronary thrombosis.[76,77] Despite this new evidence that challenged and defeated the old premise, this topic remains a source of controversy.[78]

Large Plaque Burden and the Expansion Hypothesis

The plaque expansion hypothesis highlights the correlation between plaque volume and acute events (Fig. 66.15). This hypothesis also reconciles differences in percent diameter stenosis of ruptured plaques responsible for ACS (severely obstructed lesions) and nonobstructive TCFAs.

The hypothesis that larger plaque volume is associated with more vulnerable phenotypes was postulated by Narula and colleagues after detailed analysis of 295 coronary plaques from patients who died suddenly.[28] The investigators reported that 70% of culprit lesions with plaque rupture were determined to be obstructive by angiography, with a percent diameter stenosis greater than 75%, whereas this was observed in only 40% of the specimens classified as TCFAs (see Fig. 66.14). If TCFA is a predecessor of ruptured plaques, TFCA must undergo a significant expansion of the plaque burden before rupture.[79] Furthermore, recurrent cycles of plaque rupture and healing lead to increased plaque volume and stenosis.[80] Therefore, plaque expansion may be responsible for the transition of nonobstructive TCFA to thrombosed, stenotic ruptured plaques.

Natural History of High-Risk Coronary Atheroma

To evaluate the natural history of this disease, a total of 697 patients with ACS underwent three-vessel coronary angiography and grayscale and radiofrequency assessment, also known as *intravascular ultrasound* and *intravascular ultrasound with virtual histology (IVUS-VH)* analysis. This natural history study, also known as the PROSPECT trial, documented symptomatic progression from nonobstructive to obstructive disease in 11.6% of patients at 3.4 years.[76] However, most of these events were rehospitalizations

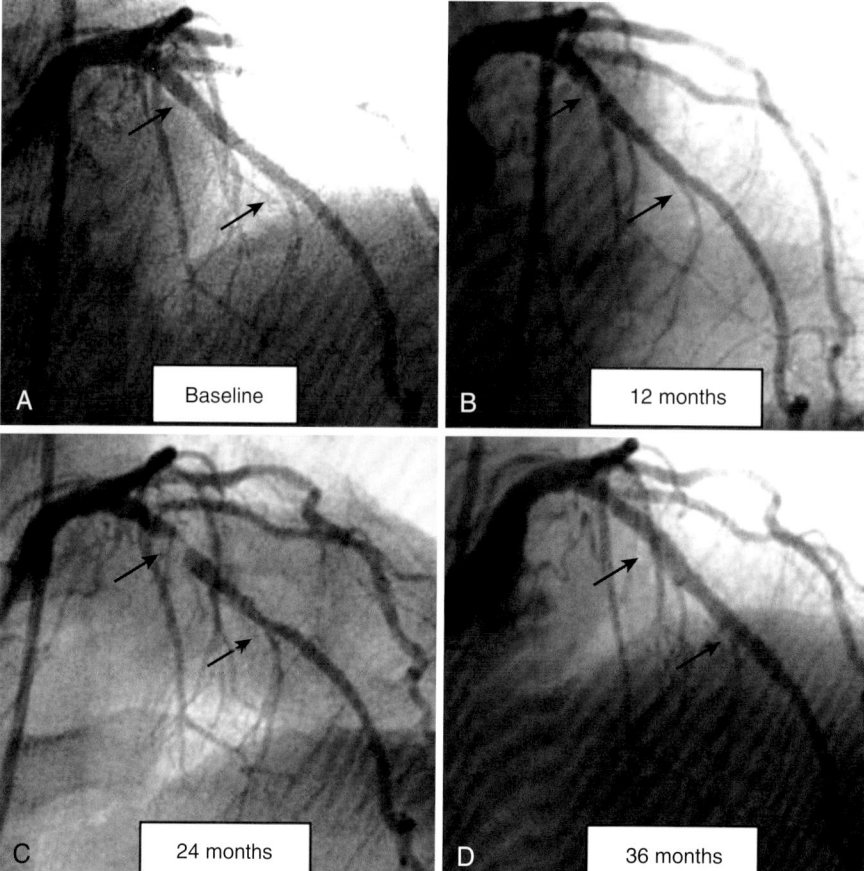

Fig. 66.13 Sequential coronary angiograms of the left anterior descending coronary artery were performed at 12-month intervals. Rapid progression from nonobstructive and asymptomatic to severely obstructive and symptomatic fulfills the clinical definition of high risk plaques. (A) Normal vessel seen by angiography. (B) Nonobstructive, asymptomatic coronary disease in the proximal segment *(arrows)*. (C) Obstructive, symptomatic coronary disease with acute coronary syndrome *(arrows)*. (D) The degree of stenosis is 10% to 20% 12 months after local therapy with a stent (36 months after the baseline angiogram). (Courtesy Mount Sinai Medical Center Cardiac Catheter Laboratory, New York, NY.)

for progressive angina. Cardiac death or AMI affected only 4.9% of the population. Three independent variables predicted these events: a plaque burden of 70% or greater (hazard ratio [HR] = 5.03, $P < .001$), a minimal luminal area of 4 mm² or less (HR = 3.21, $P = .001$), and IVUS-VH–derived TCFA morphology (HR = 3.35, $P < .001$). Plaques exhibiting all three features had an HR up to 11.05 ($P < .001$). Nevertheless, the prevalence of these high-risk plaques was only 4.2%.[76]

The PROSPECT trial supported the idea that high risk plaques are composed by specific anatomic features, and are associated with mild or "soft" events rather than death and AMI.

THE MYTH OF THE "VULNERABLE PLAQUE" AND THE TRANSITION TO ATHEROSCLEROTIC DISEASE BURDEN

The mechanism by which atherosclerotic plaques lead to major cardiovascular events is complex, difficult to predict, and remains a major ongoing challenge.[15,81] Initially, comprehensive risk approaches such a Framingham score or the atherosclerotic CVD risk score were developed with the aim to identify those patients at high risk.[7,82] More recently, with the use of intracoronary imaging and coronary CT, much effort has focused on finding that single "vulnerable" plaque that will identify high-risk individuals who will benefit from intensive treatment to prevent adverse cardiovascular events.[83]

The enthusiasm associated with this concept has been the focus of years of research and clinical trials. However, the dynamic nature of this disease proved the hypothesis too broad. Morphologic features alone are not enough to identify a TCFA that is likely to rupture.[7] Many stabilize and become ThCFA.[84] Only the minority rupture and most of the rupture events are totally asymptomatic.[84] Finally, the positive predictive value of TCFA was as low as 4%.[14]

Therefore, conceptualizing acute coronary event risk as a simple cause-and-effect principle centered on high-risk plaques has shifted to a complex model involving plaque burden, systemic disease, and inflammation.[7,15] Most importantly, control of these factors will lead to disease stabilization and plaque regression.

High-risk plaques are predominately asymptomatic and harmless in most cases. They can manifest simultaneously in multiple segments, highlighting a proinflammatory milieu that may respond to systemic rather than focal therapies. Moreover, plaque rupture does not always lead to ACS, and prior studies have found evidence of old healed areas within the atheroma (i.e., fibroinflammatory lipid plaque) that occurred without causing a clinical event.[26] These and other limitations seriously challenge the vulnerable plaque (VP) hypothesis, and the current clinical approach therefore employs systemic therapy as a preventive tool for all patients and imaging for a few (Fig. 66.16).

INTRACORONARY IMAGING

Ideally, we could measure the resolution of inflammation by the reduction of plaque lipid content and thickening of the fibrous cap. Several intracoronary imaging techniques have been proposed to characterize plaque composition at this level. Every imaging technique should have appropriate validation using histology. Proper histologic validation must include accurate assessment of the degree of histomorphologic components, including fibrous cap thickness, shear stress pattern, necrotic core area, macrophage area, positive remodeling, and vasa vasorum neovascularization. This histologic validation must involve linear regression analysis. The validation process should be confirmed in animal models before human application.[85] Most importantly,

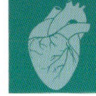

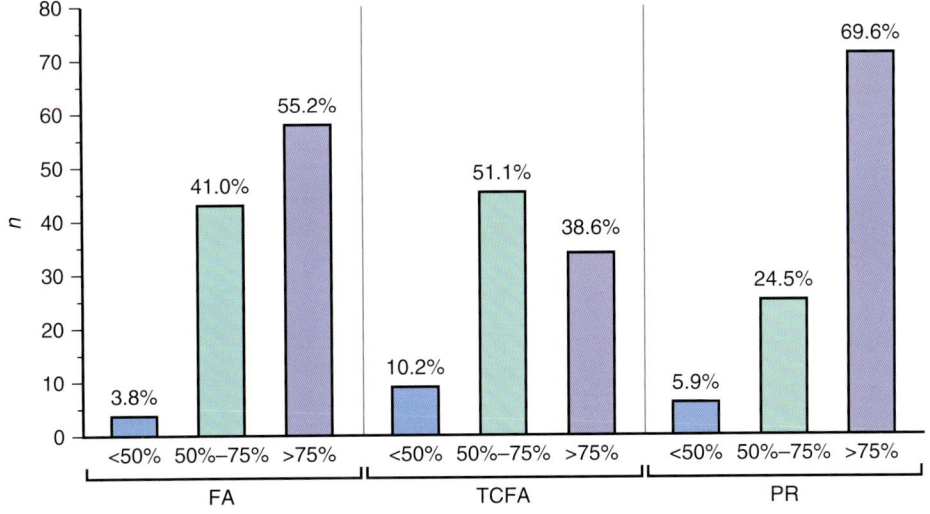

A

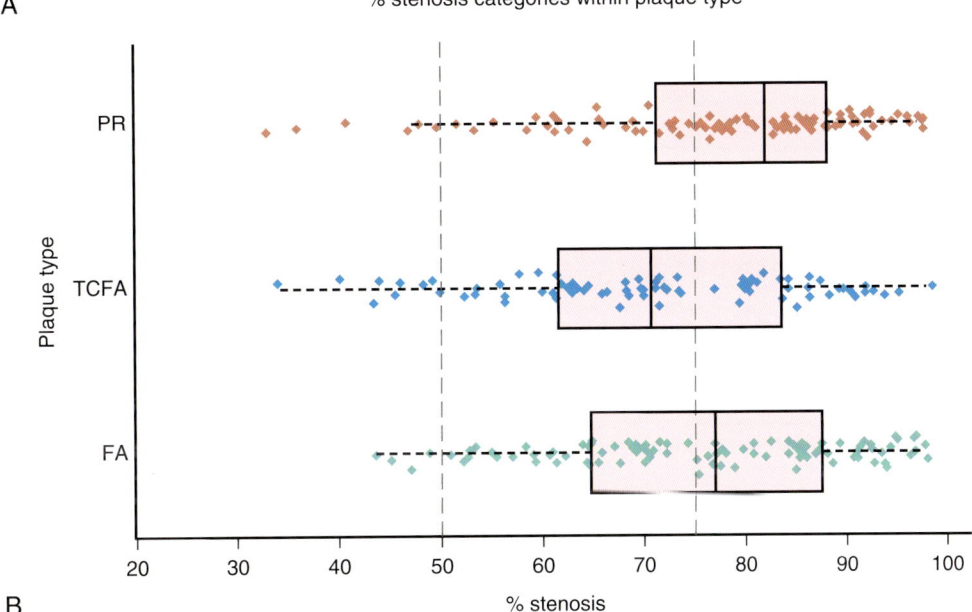

B

Fig. 66.14 Luminal obstruction in cases of fibroatheroma *(FA)*, thin-cap fibroatheroma *(TCFA)*, and plaque rupture *(PR)* with various degrees of percent diameter stenosis. The bar graph (A) and plot diagram (B) show a greater than 50% cross-sectional vascular area stenosis in most PRs and TCFAs. The distribution indicates that TCFAs may further enlarge before plaque rupture. The plot diagram shows numeric data through the lower, median, and upper quartiles. The whiskers represent the sample minimum and sample maximum observations. The pink boxes and their divisions indicate median and interquartile range (lower and upper quartiles).

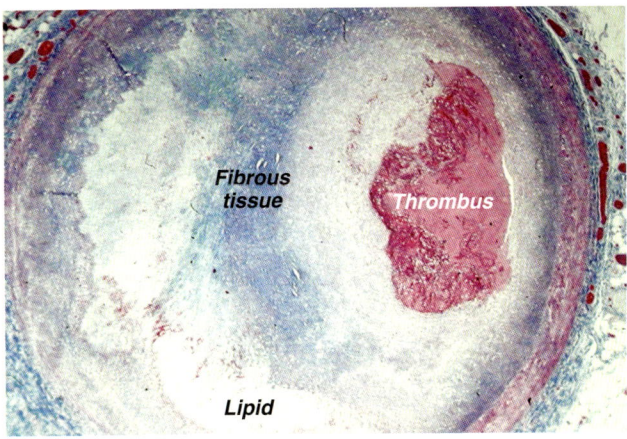

Fig. 66.15 Plaque erosion. In the cross section of a coronary artery containing a stenotic atherosclerotic plaque with an occlusive thrombosis superimposed, the endothelium is missing at the plaque-thrombus interface, but the plaque surface is otherwise intact. Trichrome stain renders the thrombus red, the collagen blue, and the lipid colorless. (Courtesy Dr. Erling Falk, Aarhus, Denmark.)

a prospective natural history study of each technique must validate prognostic, clinical implications.

Current intracoronary techniques to characterize plaque composition include IVUS, virtual histology (VH), intravascular OCT, and near-infrared spectroscopy (NIRS). Table 66.2 summarizes these techniques, the component detected, and their resolution or accuracy. The interventionalist must understand the potential and discern the limitations of these techniques before considering them for clinical use.

Intravascular Ultrasound

Unlike angiography, IVUS allows visualization of the disease in the vessel wall and provides cross-sectional and longitudinal images of atherosclerotic plaques in vivo.[86] IVUS is based on transmitting and receiving high-frequency sound waves from tissue through a low-profile catheter (≈1 mm), reaching a radial resolution around 200 μm. IVUS is safe, quick, and easy.

IVUS allows identification of hemodynamically significant lesions that may be underestimated by angiography, particularly in nonocclusive plaques with positive remodeling. IVUS delineates the degree of calcification, plaque burden, and arterial remodeling. It uses the amplitude of the backscattered ultrasound

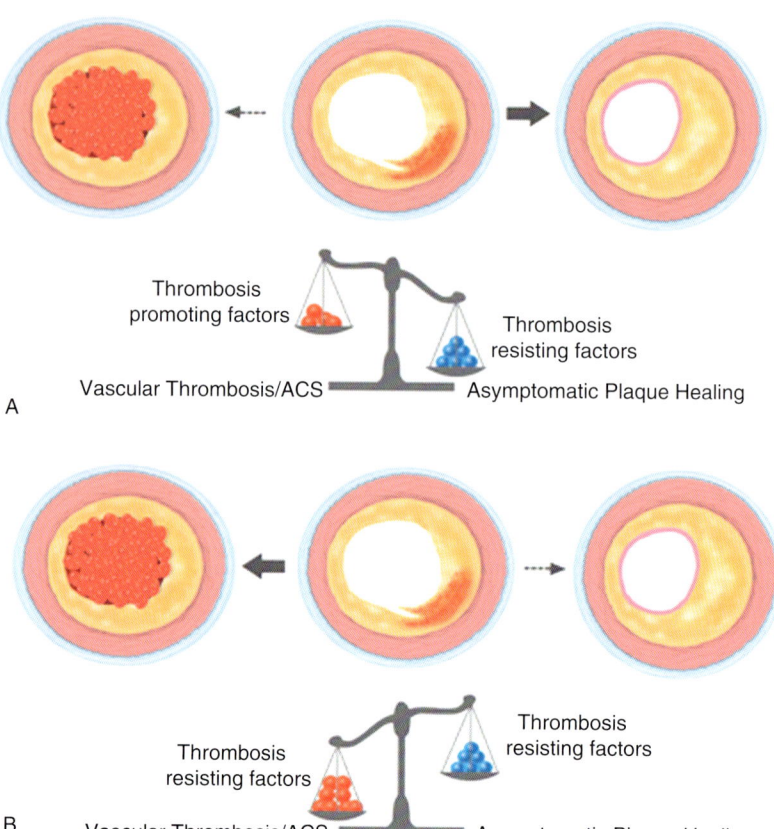

Fig. 66.16 Fate of ruptured coronary atherosclerotic plaques according to thrombotic milieu. The hypothesized interplay of prothrombotic and thrombosis resisting and containing factors that presumably determine the outcome of a ruptured coronary atherosclerotic plaque is shown. (A) In the most common scenario, small thrombus formation associated with plaque rupture is contained and vascular occlusive thrombus is inhibited. (B) In the less common scenario of several prothrombotic factors coinciding (e.g., inflammatory state, large lesion plaque burden, vasoconstriction, circadian rheological changes), local thrombosis associated with plaque rupture cannot be contained, and clinically significant vascular thrombosis occurs, triggering an acute coronary syndrome *(ACS)*. The constellation of factors leading to these different outcomes is unknown. (From Arbab-Zadeh A, Fuster V. The myth of the "vulnerable plaque": transitioning from a focus on individual lesions to atherosclerotic disease burden for coronary artery disease risk assessment. *J Am Coll Cardiol.* 2015;65[8]:846–855.)

TABLE 66.2 Summary of Intracoronary Techniques to Characterize Plaque Composition

Technology	Component Detected	Resolution/Accuracy (μm)
IVUS	Remodeling, plaque burden, calcium	100–250
IVUS with virtual histology	Necrotic core, calcium, collagen	480
OCT	Necrotic core, fibrous cap thickness, macrophages	5–20
Near infrared spectroscopy	Necrotic core	NA

IVUS, Intravascular ultrasound; *NA,* not applicable; *OCT,* optimal coherence tomography.

signal to differentiate highly echogenic components such as calcium and dense fibrous tissue from echolucent tissue, such as lipid and necrotic core. However, it cannot clearly differentiate between fibrous and fatty plaques.[87] Grayscale IVUS is an isolated technology not optimal to characterize plaque composition.

Several studies have reported the IVUS characteristics of culprit lesions and the presence of multiple ruptured plaques in patients with acute coronary events.[86,88] The evaluation of long-term outcomes of high-risk plaques arbitrarily defined as plaques with rupture, lipid core, dissection, or thrombus was performed. Multiplicity of high-risk plaques in the nontarget vessels (HR = 2.2; 95% confidence interval [CI] 1.4 to 3.4; P = .001) was the only independent predictor of long-term critical events. DM and ACS were significantly associated with the multiplicity of high-risk plaques.[89]

Because the IVUS resolution is lower than that needed to detect TCFAs, efforts at quantifying cap thickness with IVUS always overestimate the values compared with those provided by histology. With IVUS, ruptured plaques show thinner caps than nonruptured plaques (Fig. 66.17).[90] However, when ruptured plaques are histologically evaluated, the mean cap thickness is about 8 to 10 times lower than the resolution of IVUS (23 ± 19 μm in the coronary and 34 ± 16 μm in the aorta).[91] The significant overestimation of cap thickness is related to poor axial resolution, which means that no IVUS-related technology can detect TCFAs.[90]

IVUS can detect the necrotic core with a sensitivity of 46% and a specificity of 97%. Several studies using an integrated backscatter approach have attempted to improve these results.[92] A prospective study demonstrated that 93% of clinical events were associated with plaques with large, echolucent areas, a surrogate of the necrotic core, suggesting a prognostic value for IVUS.[93] Similarly, some studies have proposed the attenuation of the echo signal inside the plaque as being indicative of large necrotic cores, but no histologic validation has corroborated this finding. Although IVUS provides useful information about plaque echogenicity, we conclude that the exact sensitivity and accuracy needed to identify necrotic cores is unclear, and the resolution may not be sufficient to properly quantify this important feature of advance atherosclerotic plaques.[87]

Contrary to fibrous cap thickness, IVUS is an excellent tool for detecting remodeling, a major feature of advance atherosclerotic plaques.[94] IVUS-identified arterial remodeling increased understanding of the paradox of lumen and plaque size in high-risk plaques (i.e., large plaques can appear to be nonobstructive on angiography), leading to the realization that ruptured plaques are larger than nonruptured plaques.[88] No other imaging modality can show remodeling better; IVUS is considered the standard for detecting remodeling in vivo.[94]

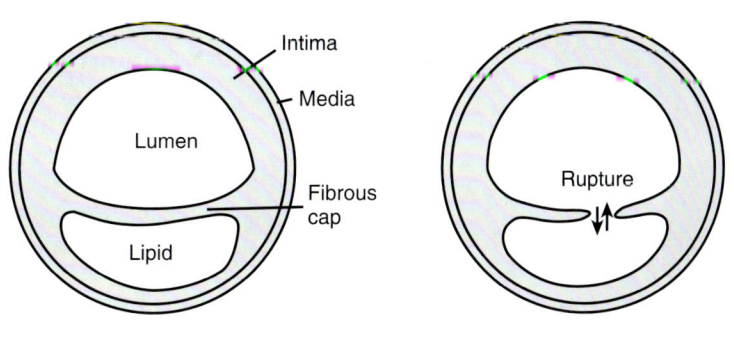

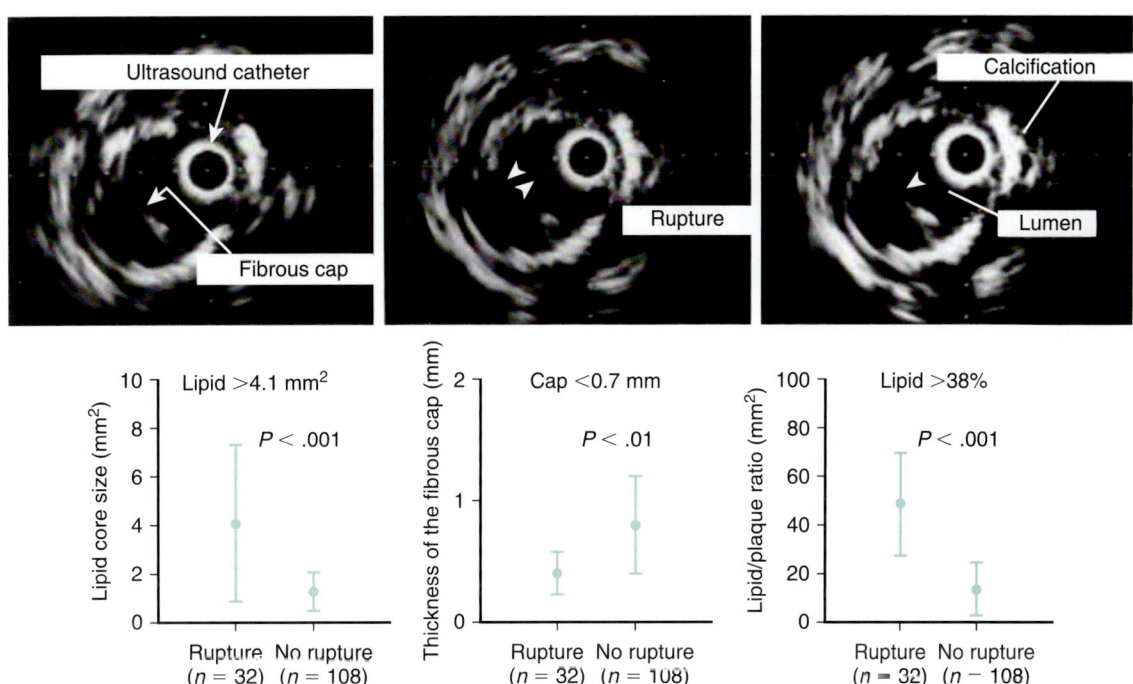

Fig. 66.17 Diagrams show nonruptured and ruptured plaques. Intravascular ultrasound images highlight the fibrous cap and a large echolucent area under the cap, suggesting a large necrotic core. The graphs describe lipid area, cap thickness, and lipid percent area in ruptured versus nonruptured plaques. (Modified from Ge J, Chirillo F, Schwedtmann J, et al. Screening of ruptured plaques in patients with coronary artery disease by intravascular ultrasound. *Heart*. 1999;81:621–627.)

Efforts to detect flow within the plaque and identify neovascularization (i.e., functional neovessels) were performed using contrast agents. Intravascular injection of microbubbles (i.e., small, encapsulated air or gas bubbles or albumin microspheres) can boost the Doppler signal from blood vessels. Microbubbles can help in visualizing flow in smaller vessels, even at the capillary level, as has been shown by contrast-enhanced echocardiography (CEE).[95] Direct visualization of atherosclerotic plaque microvessels using CEE was successfully done by Staub et al. in carotid plaques. This has been validated with histology in animal models and in humans.[96,97] In coronary arteries, IVUS-CEE has successfully identified plaque neovessels with spatiotemporal changes and enhancement-detection techniques (Fig. 66.18).[98]

To improve resolution, an IVUS prototype using harmonic imaging with transmission of ultrasound at 20 MHz (fundamental) and detection of contrast signals at 40 MHz (second harmonic) was developed to identify adventitial neovessels in rabbit models.[99] However, vasa vasorum detection of coronary atherosclerosis with IVUS imaging is still evolving for clinical use.

Another important feature of atheromatous lesions that are prone to rupture and can be properly identified with IVUS are high-risk calcifications such as *calcified nodules*. This was demonstrated by Lee and colleagues by analyzing sequential pathologic specimens in 856 sections from 29 coronary arteries from autopsies.[100] A carefully matched, ex vivo IVUS analysis found that calcified nodules had several features that distinguished them from nonnodular calcifications: a convex shape of the luminal surface of calcium (100% vs. 16.0%, $P < .001$), protrusion with a convex shape of the luminal surface (94.1% vs. 9.7%, $P < .001$), irregular luminal surface (64.7% vs 11.6%, $P < .001$), and irregular leading edge of calcium (88.2% vs. 19.0%, $P < .001$). Calcium nodules can protrude through and rupture the fibrous cap, becoming thrombogenic and leading to ACS, as reported by autopsy data.[9]

IVUS data about calcified nodules can provide useful prognostic information. This was shown by Xu and colleagues by performing a subgroup analysis of the PROSPECT study that included 699 patients with ACS.[101] Of these patients, 314 had nonculprit calcific nodules after imaging the three major coronary arteries. When correlated with coronary angiography, heavy calcification was seen in only three cases, whereas 35 and 19 had moderate calcification and hazy calcification, respectively. No calcification was seen in 257 patients. Characteristics of patients with nonculprit lesions and calcific nodules included older age, higher incidence

SECTION VI Evaluation of Interventional Techniques

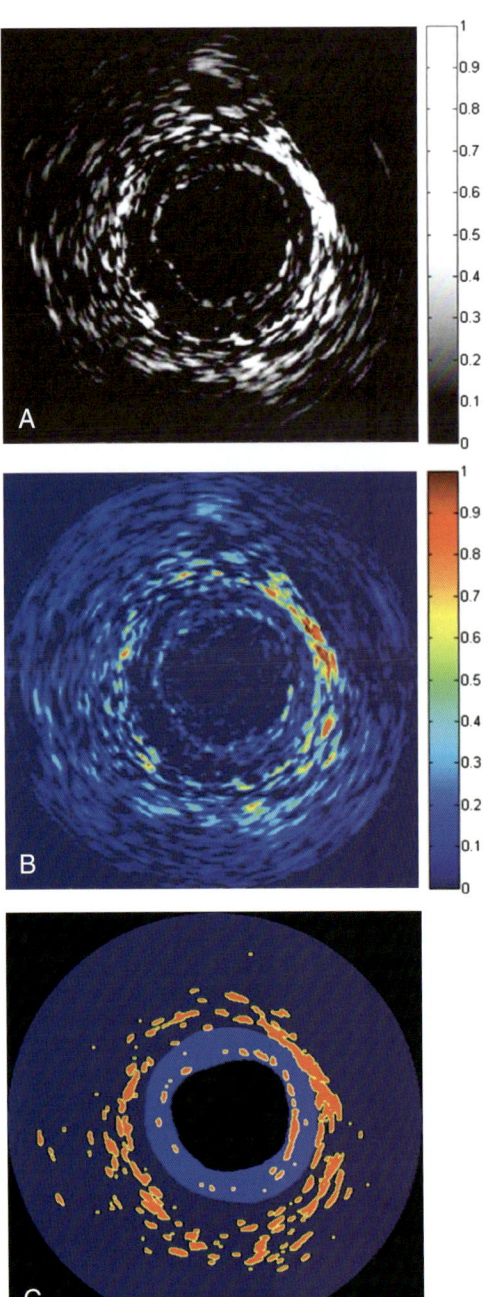

Fig. 66.18 Differential intravascular ultrasound images identify the vasa vasorum and show the postinjection signals subtracted from the baseline signals. (A) Black and white image. (B) Color-coded version of A. (C) Threshold needed to show most significant areas of enhancement. (Modified from Vavuranakis M, Kakadiaris IA, O'Malley SM, et al. Images in cardiovascular medicine. Detection of luminal-intimal border and coronary wall enhancement in intravascular ultrasound imaging after injection of microbubbles and simultaneous sonication with transthoracic echocardiography. *Circulation.* 2005;112:e1–e2.)

Detection of plaque inflammation in the fibrous cap requires a resolution of 10 to 20 μm to identify macrophages. Because IVUS resolution is 10 to 20 times lower, it cannot detect macrophages in atherosclerotic plaques.

Virtual Histology

Considering the significant limitations of IVUS, Nair and Vince at the Cleveland Clinic studied the ultrasound scattered reflection wave as an alternative to improve tissue characterization.[102,103] The backscattered reflection wave is received by the transducer and converted into voltage. This voltage is known as *backscattered radiofrequency data*.

Using a combination of previously identified spectral parameters of the backscattered ultrasound signal, the researchers developed a color-coded classification scheme and constructed an algorithm to determine plaque composition in vivo. A color assigned to each component was displayed on the IVUS image (Fig. 66.19). Four major plaque components were tested: fibrotic tissue (*dark green*), fibrofatty tissue (*yellow-green*), calcific-necrotic core (*red*), and dense calcium (*white*). The Movat pentachrome–stained histologic images identified homogeneous regions, representing each of the four plaque components (Fig. 66.20).

The unit of analysis (i.e., *box*) was initially composed of 64 backscattered radiofrequency data samples 480 μm long.[102] The algorithm developed was then validated ex vivo, with sensitivities and specificities between 79% and 93% for the four plaque components.[102] The initial studies were performed in ex vivo human coronary specimens with a 30-MHz, 2.9-Fr, and mechanically rotating IVUS catheter (Boston Scientific, Natick, MA). The initial catheter approved by the U.S. Food and Drug Administration (FDA) was a 20-MHz device (Eagle Eye Gold, Volcano, San Diego, CA). The catheter was upgraded with a 45-MHz transducer that is available for clinical practice. In vivo validation studies have shown positive results.[104]

VH gained significant attention with the PROSPECT trial.[76] IVUS-VH–derived TCFAs were associated with increased adverse cardiac events (HR = 3.35, $P < .001$). Most important, the highest-risk lesions (HR = 11.05, $P < .001$) were a conglomerate of several features, including a greater than 70% plaque burden, low minimal luminal area, and TCFA morphology. Isolating TCFAs by using VH may not be enough to categorize lesions as VPs. Use of VH also has been questioned by some studies that reported a poor correlation between IVUS-VH findings and histology for certain atheroma features in animal models,[105,106] and for VH findings and clinical presentations of patients with ACS.[107]

It would be ideal to perform a prospective study randomizing patients with high-risk plaques documented by VH or other modalities to receive medical or invasive therapies, although the large number of patients needed and the increased costs may limit the ability to test this hypothesis. The PROSPECT ABSORB trial is an investigator-initiated, multicenter, randomized clinical trial that is designed to test the ability of the ABSORB Bioresorbable Vascular Scaffold plus guideline-directed medical treatment to safely increase the luminal diameter of high-risk plaques compared with medical treatment alone.

The PROSPECT trial results were reproduced in the VH-IVUS in Vulnerable Atherosclerosis (VIVA) study.[108] The prospective study included 170 patients with stable angina or ACS with elevated cardiac biomarkers who were referred for PCI. They underwent three-vessel IVUS-VH before PCI and after PCI of the culprit vessel and were followed for up to 3 years. The composite primary end point of total MACEs included death, myocardial infarction (MI), and unplanned revascularization, and nonrestenotic MACEs included a combined end point of death, MI, and unplanned revascularization, excluding in-stent, restenosis-driven events.

of hypertension, and chronic kidney disease. Calcific nodules were located superficially in 91% of the patients and proximally in 55%, and one-third of the patients had at least one calcific nodule. Calcified nodules in nonculprit coronary segments in patients with ACS were prevalent, and their distribution correlated with areas associated with thrombotic events, but the rates of major adverse cardiovascular events (MACEs) were lower for lesions with calcified nodules than those without them during 3 years of follow-up.

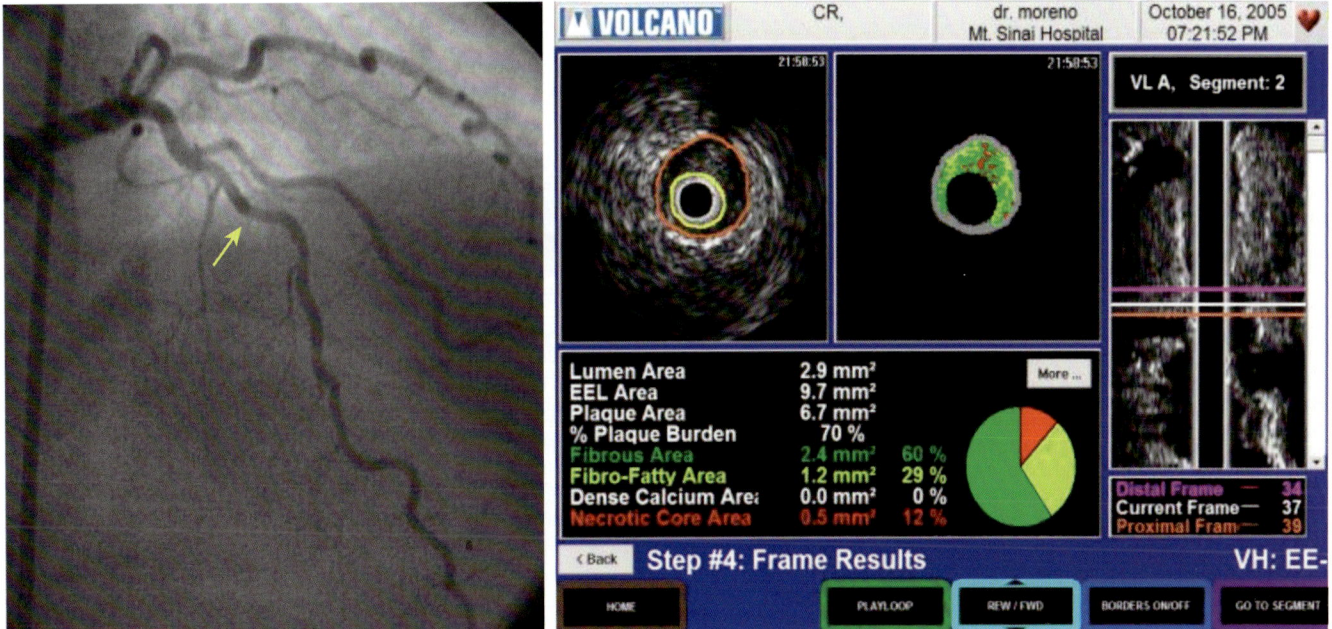

Fig. 66.19 Color-coded reproduction of virtual histology intravascular ultrasound plaque composition displayed in vivo in the catheter laboratory. *Arrow* on angiogram indicates the cross section imaged. *EEL,* External elastic lamina; *VLA,* Vessel lumen area.

A total of 30,372 mm of IVUS-VH data were analyzed, including 1096 plaques that were classified by IVUS-VH. From these, 19 lesions resulted in MACEs, including 13 nonculprit lesions and 6 culprit lesions (Fig. 66.21). Whereas the PROSPECT study was based in analyzing and following individual plaques,[76] the VIVA study assessed the association between IVUS-VH–based plaque classification and nonrestenotic MACEs on a whole-patient scale. These studies highlight the association between IVUS-VH–derived TCFAs and MACEs, confirming that this technology can identify plaques likely to cause adverse clinical events. VH also can be used to identify several features of TCFAs, including fibrous cap thickness, necrotic core area, plaque inflammation, and degree of positive remodeling.

Evaluation of cap thickness by IVUS-VH is limited. In their initial publication, Nair and Vince commented on the limitations: "The window size currently applied for selection of regions of interest and eventual tissue map reconstructions is 480 μm in the radial direction. Detection of thin fibrous caps (≤65 μm below the resolution of IVUS) is compromised, restricting the detection of 'vulnerable atheromas.'"[102] As a result, lesions with a fibrous cap thickness greater than 65 μm are incorrectly classified as TCFAs and perhaps overestimated. With an axial resolution of 250 μm, the method is insufficient to determine fibrous cap thickness.

Investigators have proposed a classification of IVUS-VH–derived TCFAs.[109] They have been defined as plaques with a rich necrotic core (>10%), without evident overlying fibrous tissue, and with a percent plaque volume of 40% seen on at least three consecutive images. These histologic features identify TCFAs that are prone to rupture. As also defined by histology, IVUS-VH–derived TCFAs cluster around the proximal segments of the arteries, are more often associated with positive remodeling, and are more frequently found in patients with ACS than those with stable angina.[110,111] Sawada and coworkers evaluated the ability of IVUS-VH and OCT to detect TCFAs in the same coronary lesions. IVUS-VH was very effective in detecting the absence of TCFAs. However, IVUS-VH diagnosed only half of the TCFAs compared with OCT.[112]

An initial concern was about the accuracy of using IVUS-VH–derived TCFAs to serve as surrogates for high-risk plaques and the prognostic value they could provide. This concern was mostly addressed by the PROSPECT trial, which highlighted the value of IVUS-VH–derived TCFAs. The concept was reinforced by a publication by Kubo and colleagues, which addressed the natural history of IVUS-VH–derived TCFAs in 99 patients undergoing PCI who were followed for 12 months with serial evaluations of coronary vasculature using IVUS-VH.[84] Of the 20 IVUS-VH–derived TCFAs seen at baseline, 15 (75%) healed: 13 (65%) became thick-cap fibroatheromas, and 2 became fibrotic plaques (10%). Only 5 (25%) remained unchanged. The investigators also reported the occurrence of 12 new IVUS-VH–derived TCFAs that developed during the follow-up period: 6 from pathologic intimal thickening and 6 from TCFAs identified at baseline. No acute coronary events resulting from the initially identified or newly formed IVUS-VH–derived TCFAs occurred during the follow-up period.[84]

IVUS-VH was initially developed to identify calcific necrotic cores. However, the incidence and degree of calcification in necrotic cores varies, and necrotic cores without calcification may not be properly identified.[10] Most advanced atherosclerotic lesions have some degree of necrotic core. IVUS-VH is used to validate the presence or absence of a necrotic core and determine the necrotic core area (mm^2) and percent of total plaque area.[113] A PROSPECT substudy reported that plaques with large areas of attenuation on grayscale analysis are associated with a large amount of IVUS-VH–detected necrotic core and are markers of fibroatheromas (i.e., TCFAs or thick-capped fibroatheromas).[114]

Despite the cumulative clinical evidence and proposed clinical applications for IVUS-VH, proper validation of necrotic core areas with histology using linear regression analysis has not been performed in humans and probably never will be. Limited studies have attempted to identify the correlations between necrotic core areas by using IVUS-VH with histology in a porcine model, and they demonstrated that IVUS-VH was unreliable in terms of necrotic core assessment.[105,106]

Many pathologic studies have established that necrotic core areas from patients with ACS are larger than those from patients with chronic stable angina.[26] Conversely, fibrous plaque areas (i.e., collagen) were significantly smaller in patients with ACS.[25]

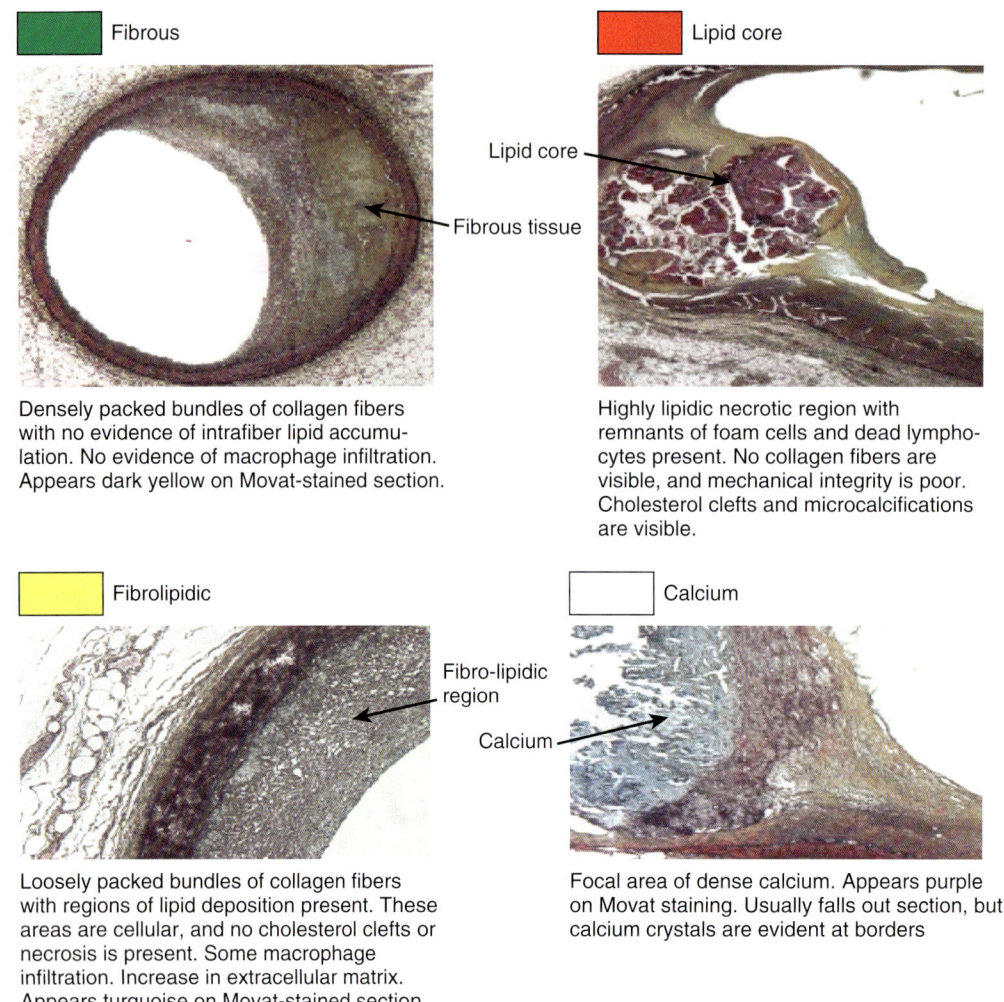

Fig. 66.20 Definitions of the plaque components visualized with virtual histology intravascular ultrasound. (Courtesy Dr. D.G. Vince, Cleveland Clinic Lerner Research Institute, Cleveland, OH.)

Surmely and associates concluded that data on plaque composition obtained by IVUS-VH contradict previously published histopathologic data.[107] However, Rodriguez-Granillo and colleagues identified larger necrotic areas in ruptured plaques and in nonculprit lesions from patients with ACS.[115] Validation with histology in cases of carotid atherosclerosis showed a diagnostic accuracy of 99.4% for TCFAs, 96.1% for calcified TCFAs, 85.9% for fibroatheromas, 85.5% for fibrocalcific atheromas, 83.4% for pathologic intimal thickening, and 72.4% for calcified fibroatheromas.[116] In a prospective study of 16 patients who underwent PCI, IVUS-VH analysis was correlated with assessment of coronary atherectomy specimens. Correlation coefficients ranged from 0.90 to 0.97 for plaque components.[117]

Detection of macrophages in the fibrous cap requires a resolution of 10 to 20 μm. Because IVUS-VH resolution is at least 10 to 20 times lower, it is impossible for it to detect plaque inflammation in vivo.

As previously stated, IVUS is an excellent tool for detecting positive remodeling, and IVUS-VH preserves this advantage. Positive remodeling is related to large necrotic core areas, which are more frequently seen in patients with ACS. Conversely, plaques with negative or constrictive remodeling are associated with smaller necrotic core areas, which usually are seen in patients with chronic stable angina. Studies have evaluated IVUS-VH–derived necrotic core areas in plaques with positive and negative remodeling and found smaller necrotic core areas in positively remodeled plaques.[88] However, some investigators have demonstrated contradictory data, with strong correlations between large IVUS-VH–derived necrotic core areas and positive remodeling.[114]

Vasa vasorum neovascularization and intraplaque hemorrhage require highly sophisticated technology and cannot be identified with IVUS-VH. Because of contradictory findings for the identification of necrotic core areas and remodeling, it impossible to determine the value of IVUS-VH–derived plaque composition in clinical practice.

Optical Coherence Tomography

OCT is a high-resolution intravascular imaging technique commonly used. Among the invasive modalities, OCT provides the highest resolution (5 to 20 μm).[118] This resolution translates into sensitivity and specificity values between 92% and 100% for all components of TCFAs[119] and produces superb images (Fig. 66.22). Optical frequency domain imaging (OFDI) allows high-speed comprehensive imaging, scanning up to 5 cm with a single contrast flush (Fig. 66.23).[120]

As the use of OCT has grown in clinical practice; guidelines have been developed for its application in the identification of plaque rupture, fibrous cap erosion, intracoronary thrombus, and TCFA location.[121–123] OCT can predict the no-reflow phenomenon in patients with large lipid cores who undergo PCI

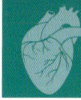

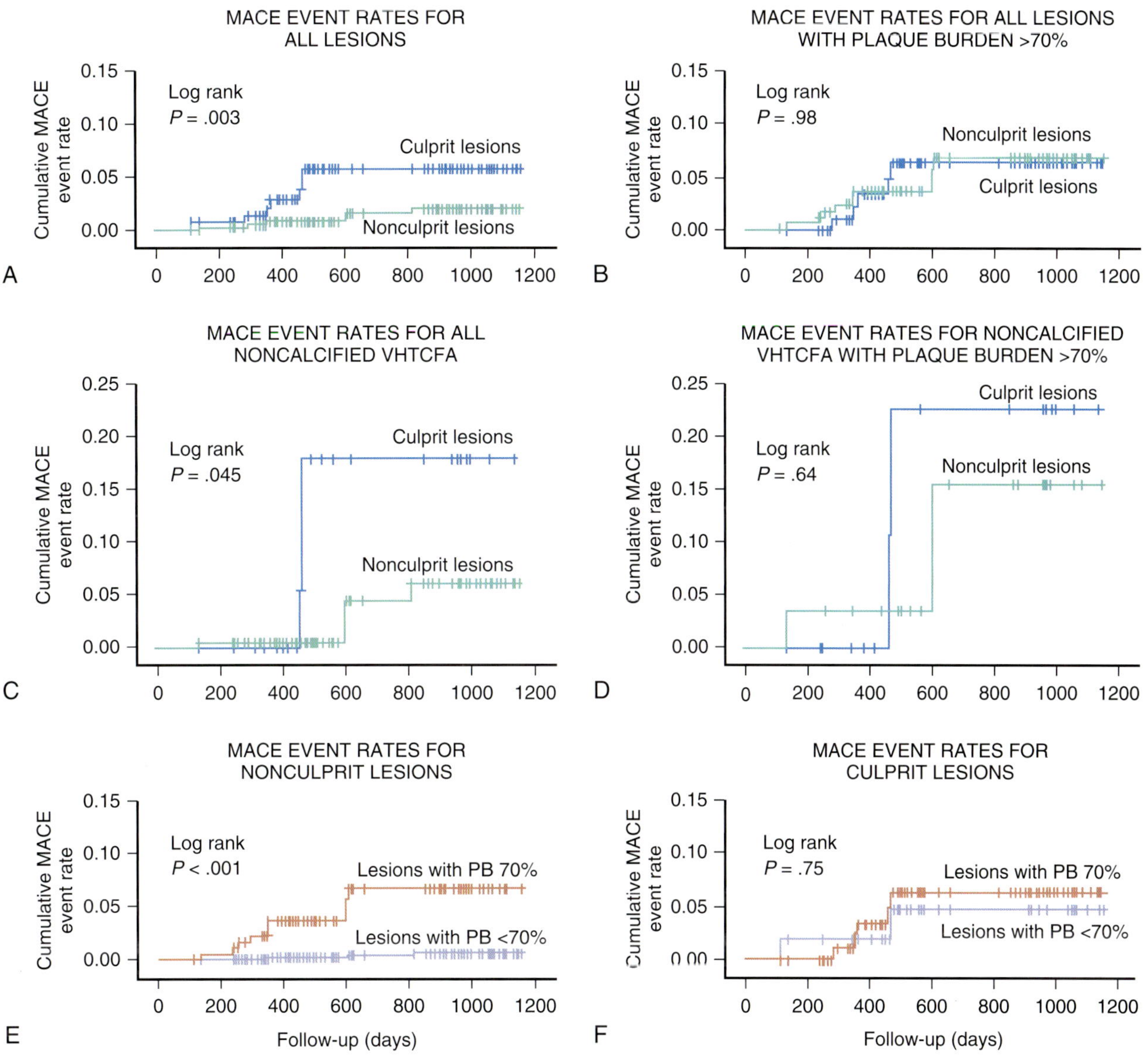

Fig. 66.21 Kaplan–Meier plot of the cumulative major adverse cardiac event *(MACE)* rates in the VH-IVUS in Vulnerable Atherosclerosis (VIVA) study. (A) All lesions. (B) Lesions with a plaque burden *(PB)* greater than 70%. (C) Noncalcified, virtual histology intravascular ultrasound thin-capped fibroatheromas *(VHTCFAs)*. (D) Noncalcified VHTCFAs with a PB greater than 70%. (E) Nonculprit lesions. (F) Culprit lesions.

for ACS.[124] OCT can identify several high-risk plaque characteristics, including eccentric plaque distribution, concave lumen shape, intimal laceration, ruptured plaque, microchannels, lipid pools, or a large lipid pool covered with a thin fibrous cap, macrophage accumulation, calcium deposition, and luminal thrombus (Fig. 66.24 and 66.25).[125,126]

Fig. 66.26 compares OCT with IVUS-VH for the detection of TCFAs. OCT can be used to detect several features of TCFAs, including fibrous cap thickness, necrotic core area, plaque inflammation, degree of positive remodeling, plaque neovascularization, and intraplaque hemorrhage.

OCT is the only imaging tool with enough resolution to identify fibrous cap thickness of 65 μm or less. This was demonstrated with histologic studies using proper linear regression analysis ($r = 0.89$; Fig. 66.27). In vivo studies showed that fibrous cap thickness was lowest in patients with AMI, intermediate in patients with unstable angina, and highest in patients with chronic stable angina (Fig. 66.28).[127] OCT can be used to estimate the incidence of TCFAs according to the clinical syndrome.

OCT has allowed researchers to identify levels of cap thicknesses that are associated with various clinical presentations. For instance, Yonetsu and colleagues demonstrated that the critical cap thickness associated with ACS was lower than 80 μm based on analysis in vivo of 266 lesions from 103 patients with ACS and stable angina.[128] In addition to measuring fibrous cap thickness, OCT can identify plaque rupture, fibrous cap erosion, and thrombosis more accurately than other imaging modalities, including IVUS and angioscopy. This was demonstrated by Kubo and associates, who studied patients with ACS and assessed fibrous cap thickness after statin treatment.[129]

OCT also can identify the mechanisms that lead to plaque thrombosis.[130] It provides direct evidence of cap discontinuity with a clear cavity created inside the plaque; it can also assess the type of thrombus formation after plaque erosion or rupture, including differentiation between red and white thrombus; and detect calcium in the atheroma as a protruding calcification, calcified nodule, or superficial calcium deposition.[130] Fig. 66.29 compares intracoronary imaging modalities for assessment of plaque rupture.

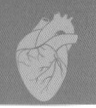

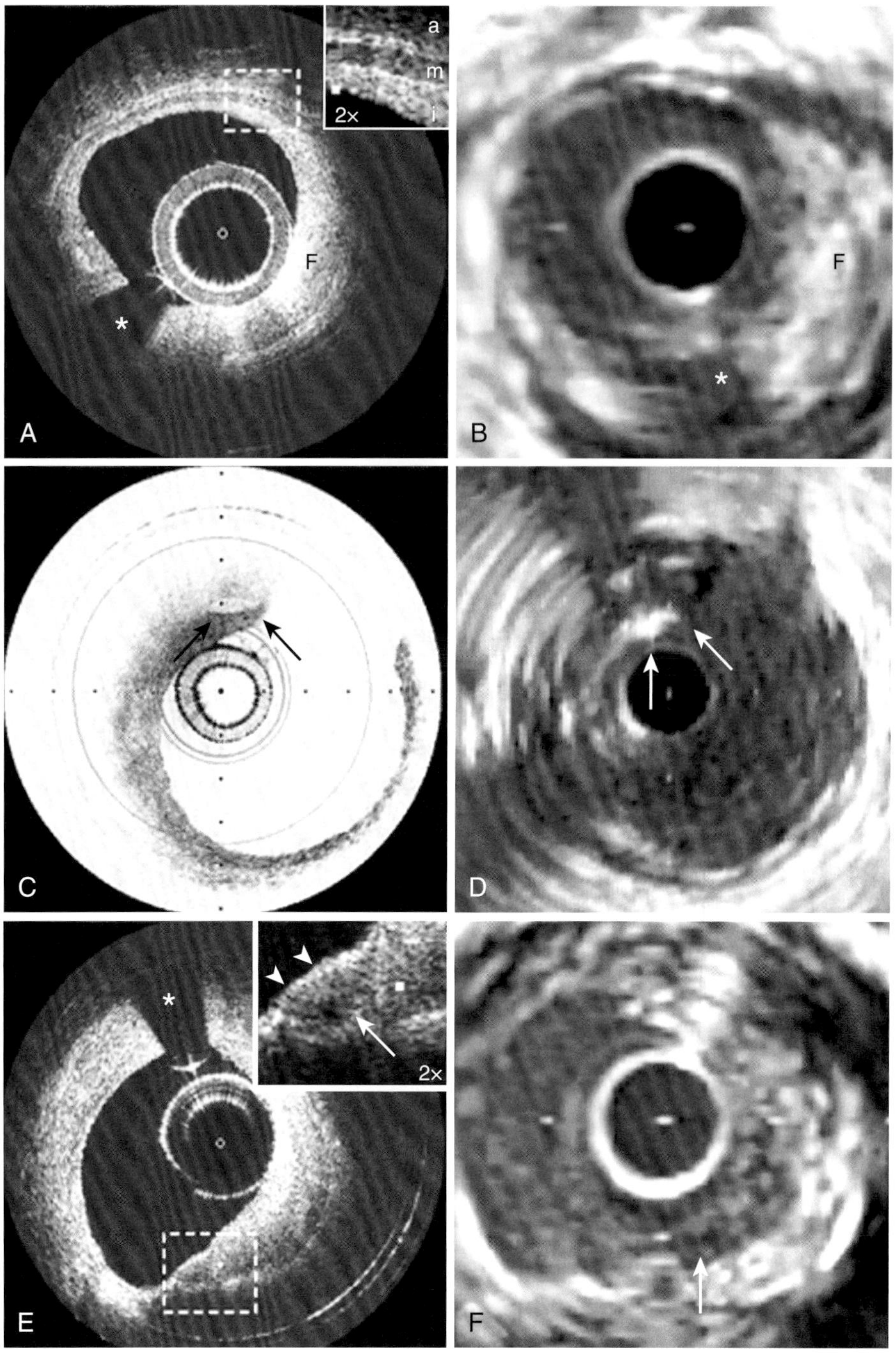

SECTION VI Evaluation of Interventional Techniques

Fig. 66.22 In vivo optical coherence tomography (OCT) images of various coronary plaque types *(left column)* are compared with corresponding intravascular ultrasound (IVUS) images *(right column)*. (A) From 9 o'clock to 2 o'clock, the three-layer structure (*a*, adventitia; *i*, intima; *m*, media) of a typical intimal hyperplasia is shown by OCT, along with a magnified area *(inset)*. A homogeneous, signal-rich pattern indicates the fibrous plaque (F), which is partly obscured by a guidewire artifact *(asterisk)*. (B) Fibrous plaque (F) on the IVUS image poor region surrounded by sharp borders represents calcific plaque *(arrows)*. (D) On the IVUS image corresponding to C, calcium is easily identified, but the strong signal obscures the structure in front of the calcium deposit, and a back-shadow artifact obscures that behind the deposit. (E) In a lipid-rich plaque, a signal-poor region *(arrow in inset)*, surrounded by diffuse borders and separated by a thin cap *(arrowheads in inset)*, is consistent with a thin-cap fibroatheroma. The asterisk indicates a guidewire artifact. (F) The intravascular ultrasound image corresponding to E suggests a superficial echolucent region *(arrow)*. (Modified from Low AF, Tearney GJ, Bouma BE, et al. Technology insight: optical coherence tomography—current status and future development. *Nat Clin Pract Cardiovasc Med*. 2006;3:154–162, quiz.)

The lipid pool and the necrotic core are signal-poor components and are therefore diffusely delineated with respect to the surrounding tissue. The LRP can be recognized by large areas of ill-defined, signal-poor regions that are evident to the naked eye. (Fig. 66.25 shows a simplified algorithm OCT interpretation.) This lipid pool is quantified by measuring the lipid arc (i.e., maximal degree of lipid pool) or by the number of quadrants involved on a particular cross-sectional OCT image.[131] When the cap is thick and the signal is strong, the operator can tell that the signal is coming from a fibrotic plaque, mostly composed of collagen. OCT can identify LRPs according to the characteristics of the signal described previously. This classification of the plaque moderately correlates with IVUS-VH for necrotic core identification.[129]

Linear correlations of human coronary plaque collagen were performed, and regression plots of OCT and measured collagen showed a correlation value of 0.475 ($P < .002$) and predictive values for collagen between 89% and 93%.[132] Nevertheless, OCT does not validate necrotic core areas as effectively as it does cap thickness and collagen, and further experimentation is warranted to achieve better necrotic and lipid tissue evaluation.[133,119]

Results from a study performed in the Thorax Center, Rotterdam, the Netherlands, demonstrated how vessel wall components, including necrotic cores and macrophages, can be distinguished by their optical properties with good histologic correlation.[134] Another study identified large necrotic cores as predictors of luminal stenosis from nonobstructive lesions when analyzed by OCT.[126]

OCT resolution allows proper identification of plaque inflammation (i.e., macrophage accumulation) in atherosclerotic plaques.[118] The first correlation in vitro was performed by Tearney and coworkers, who identified multiple strong backscatter

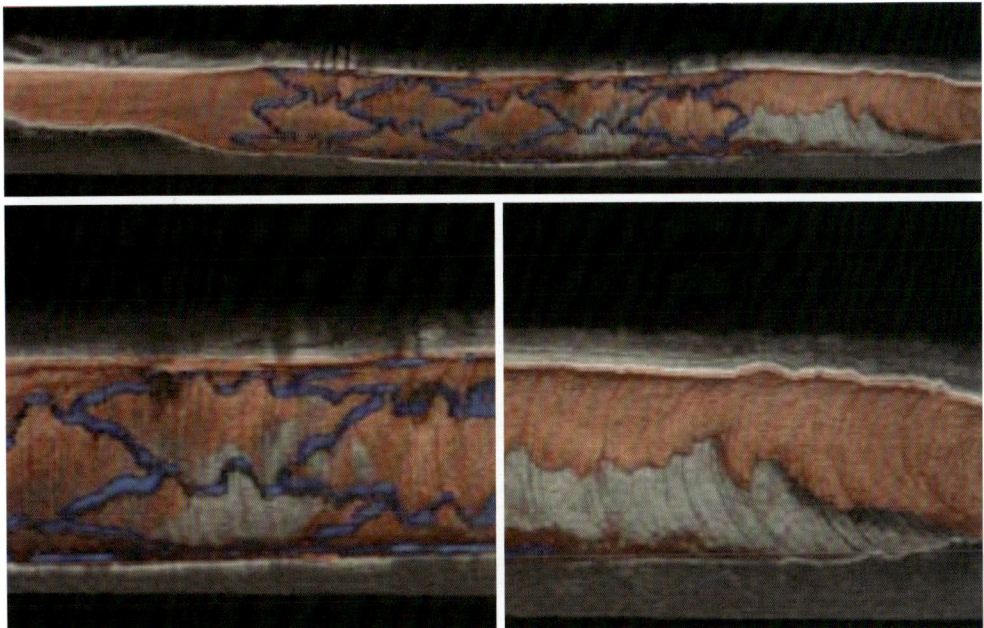

Fig. 66.23 In vivo optical frequency domain imaging of a coronary stent deployed in a porcine model shows normal endothelium *(red)*, dissections induced by the balloon during stent deployment *(white)*, and stent struts *(blue)*. (From Bouma BE. New insights from OCT, polarization-sensitive OCT, and the emergence of OFDI. *Presented at the Transcatheter Therapeutic Intervention [TCT] meeting.* Washington, DC; 2006.)

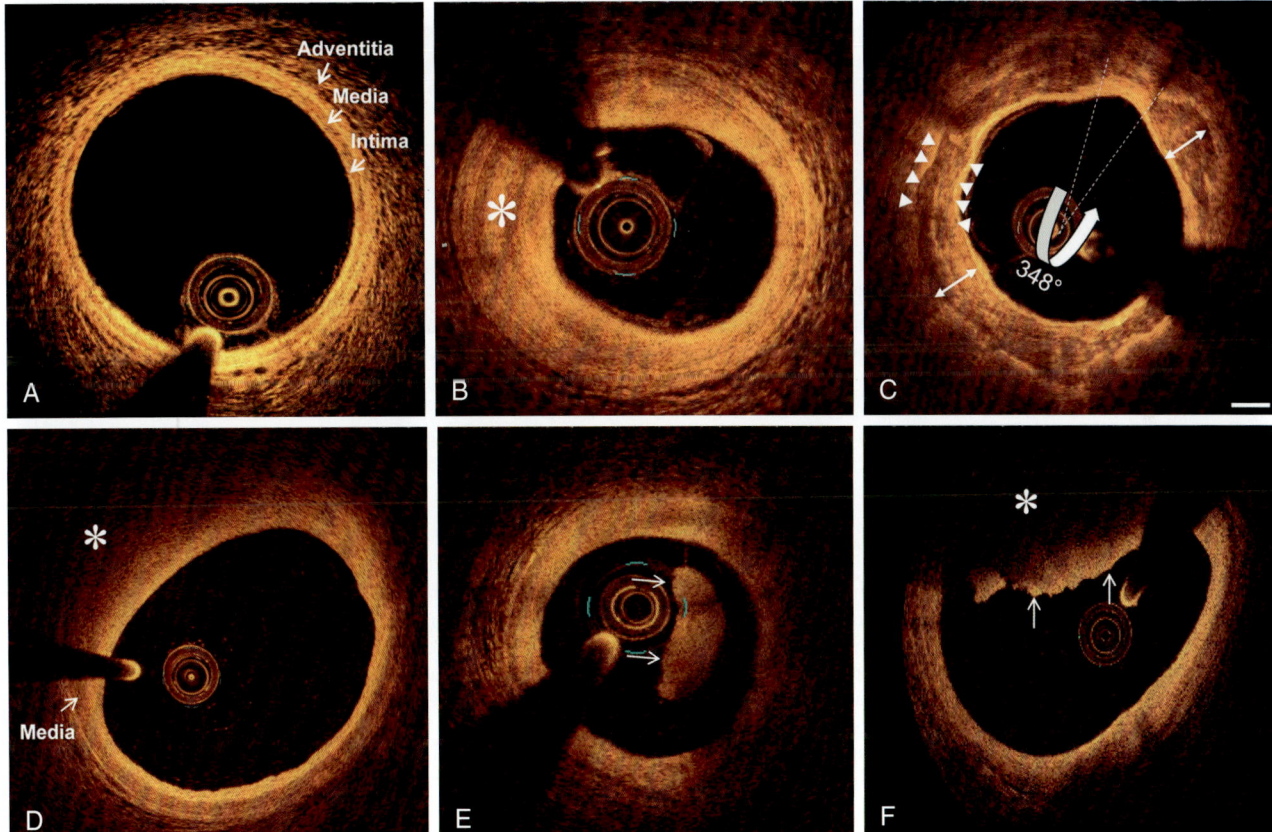

Fig. 66.24 Common morphologies detected on intracoronary optical coherence tomography. (A) Normal artery: the bright-dark-bright 3-layered appearance corresponding to intima, media, and adventitia is visualized in the entirety of the vessel circumference. (B) Fibrous plaque: note homogeneous, signal-rich regions *(asterisk)*. (C) Calcific plaque: characterized as a signal-poor region with sharply delineated borders *(arrowheads)*. Analysis of calcification depth *(double arrows)* and arc (measured at 348 degrees) is feasible in most cases with optical coherence tomography. (D) Lipid-rich plaque: characterized as a signal-poor region with poorly defined borders *(asterisk)*. Note that because of light attenuation, the media is not visible beyond the lipid content of the plaque. (E) White thrombus: mass floating within the lumen *(arrows)* that is platelet and white blood cell rich with minimal optical coherence tomographic signal attenuation. (F) Red thrombus: mass floating/attached to the luminal surface *(arrows)* that is rich in red blood cells and therefore highly attenuates the optical coherence tomographic signal, casting a shadow on the vessel wall behind the mass *(asterisk)*. (From Ali ZA, Karimi Galougahi K, Maehara A, et al. Intracoronary optical coherence tomography 2018: current status and future directions. *JACC Cardiovasc Interv.* 2017;10[24]:183–223.)

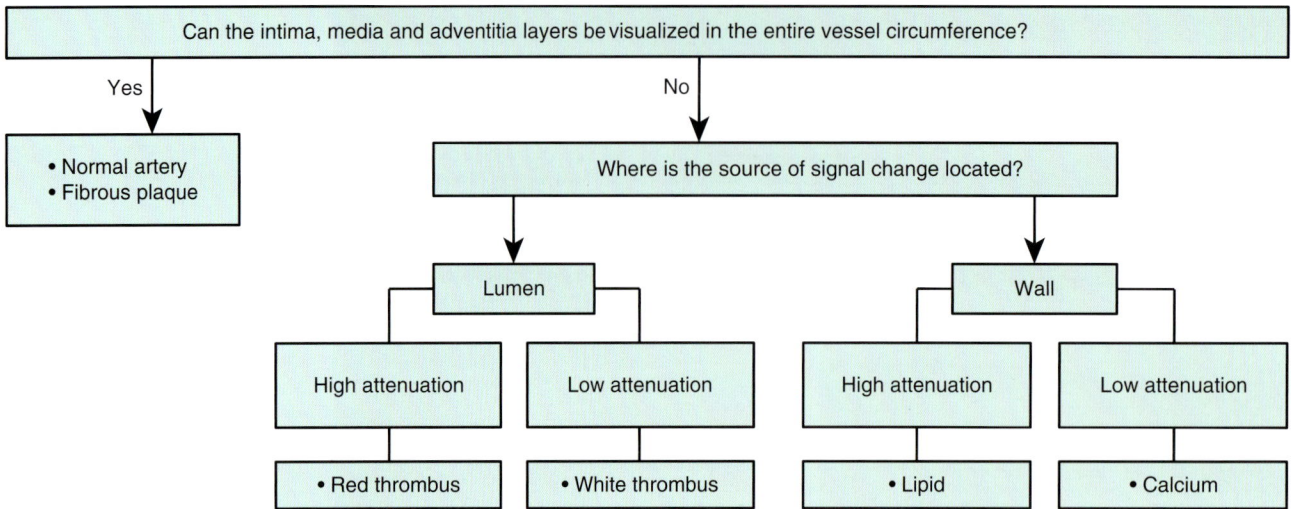

Fig. 66.25 Simplified algorithm for interpretation of optical coherence tomographic images in the native coronary arteries. This algorithm is useful in describing native coronary lesions, with the understanding that many lesions have a mixed appearance and contain more than one pathological morphology mentioned in the schematic. (From Ali ZA, Karimi Galougahi K, Maehara A, et al. Intracoronary optical coherence tomography 2018: current status and future directions. *JACC Cardiovasc Interv.* 2017;10[24]:183–223.)

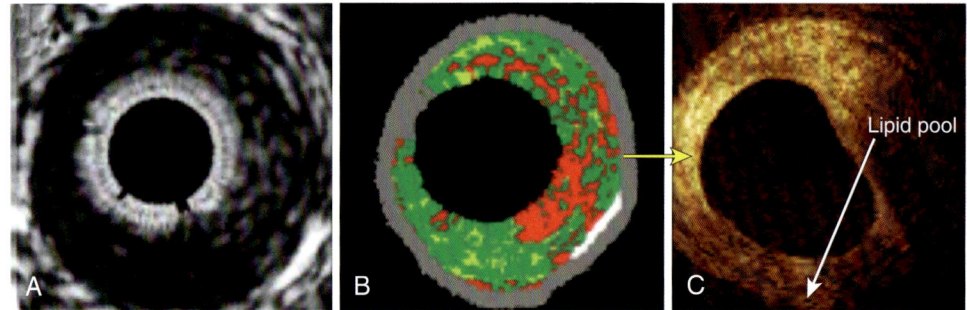

Fig. 66.26 A thin-cap fibroatheroma is imaged in vivo by three different invasive modalities. (A) Conventional intravascular ultrasound imaging. (B) Virtual histology intravascular ultrasound (IVUS-VH). (C) Optical coherence tomography (OCT). The yellow arrow from B to C corresponds to the matching cross-sectional frame of the same arterial segment by IVUS-VH (B) and OCT (C). (From Sawada T, Shite J, Garcia-Garcia HM, et al. Feasibility of combined use of intravascular ultrasound radiofrequency data analysis and optical coherence tomography for detecting thin-cap fibroatheroma. *Eur Heart J.* 2008;29:1136–1146.)

reflections from caps with abundant macrophage infiltration, resulting in a relatively high OCT signal variance.[135] The signal variance was processed with the use of logarithmic transformation (Fig. 66.30). Linear regression analysis showed correlations for raw and logarithmic OCT-derived and immunostained macrophages of 0.84 ($P < .0001$) and 0.47 ($P < .05$), respectively. In vivo studies showed increased macrophage density in ruptured plaques from patients with ACS (in culprit and nonculprit lesions) compared with nonruptured plaques from patients with chronic stable angina (Fig. 66.31).[136] OCT also can assess the content of macrophages located in the fibrous cap and enabled correlation of this macrophage density with the peripheral white blood cell count.[137]

OCT has limited plaque penetration; the depth is reduced to 2 to 3 mm. It is therefore not possible to image beyond the internal elastic lamina, and OCT cannot assess the diameter of the vessel to calculate the remodeling index, plaque volume, or plaque in deep layers of the vessel.[138] To this significant limitation of OCT, the difficulty of differentiating calcium from lipid in larger plaque burden vessels, limited visualization of structures underneath red thrombus due to shadowing effect from its high attenuation characteristic, distinguishing tissue protrusion from thrombus, and recognizing various artifacts need to be added.[138]

OCT is the gold standard for quantifying neovascularization and the effects of novel antiangiogenic therapies in common diseases such as age-related macular degeneration, extrafoveal choroid neovascularization, and proliferative diabetic retinopathy.[139] However, the number of studies specifically assessing atherosclerotic neovascularization or intraplaque hemorrhage is limited.

A study by Kitabata and colleagues proposed the use of OCT to identify intraplaque structures that may represent neovessels. These *microchannels* were defined as no-signal, tubuloluminal structures without a connection to the vessel lumen seen on three consecutive cross-sectional OCT images (Fig. 66.32). The investigators reported that plaques with microchannels displayed characteristics of vulnerability, including plaque rupture, positive remodeling, and thin fibrous caps, compared with plaques without these structures. A later study reported that the microchannels identified by OCT were markers of progression from nonobstructive to obstructive plaques[126] and that they were associated with unstable clinical syndromes.[140] However, histologic validation of the structures observed with in vivo OCT imaging has not been done.[140,141]

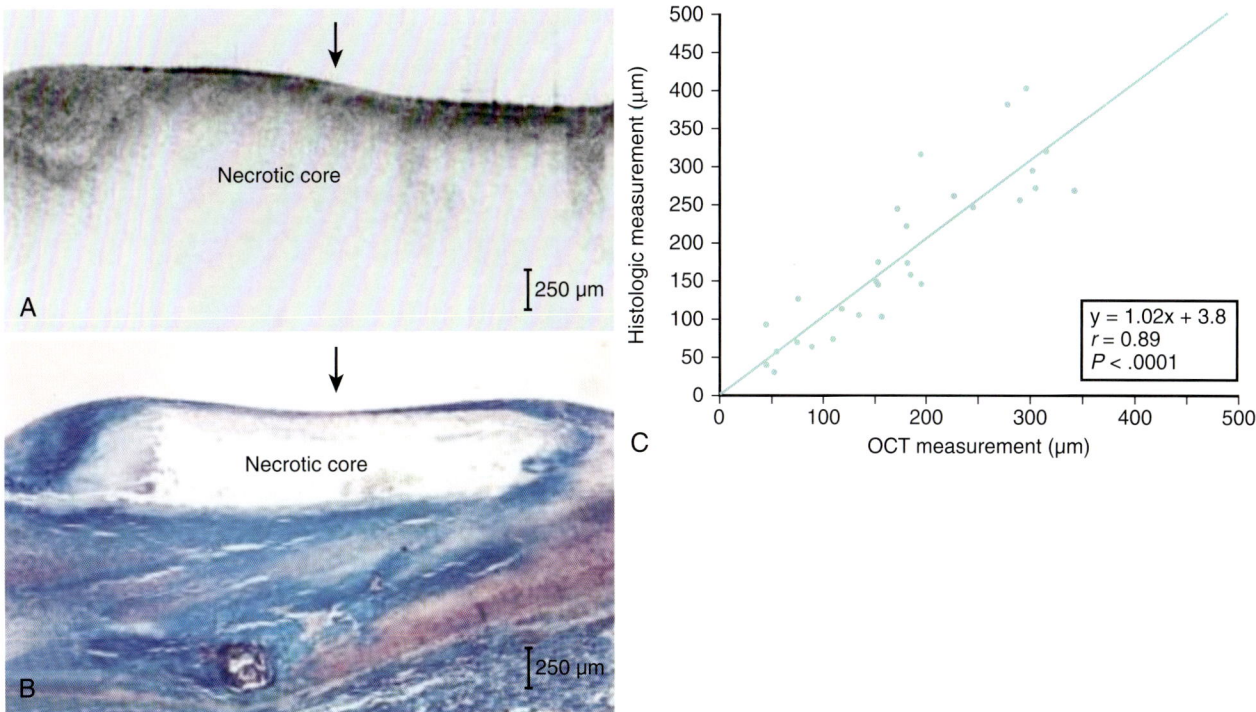

Fig. 66.27 Optical coherence tomography *(OCT)* evaluation of fibrous cap thickness. (A) Minimal fibrous cap thickness was 44.1 μm by OCT *(arrow)*. (B) Minimal fibrous cap thickness was 40.4 μm by histologic measurement *(arrow)*. The necrotic core is visualized underneath the fibrous cap. (C) Linear regression analysis shows an excellent correlation between OCT and histologic measurements in 29 human atherosclerotic plaques. (From Jang IK. Optical coherence tomography: studies of MGH. *Presented at Transcatheter Cardiovascular Therapeutics (TCT) meeting*. Washington, DC; September 24–28, 2002.)

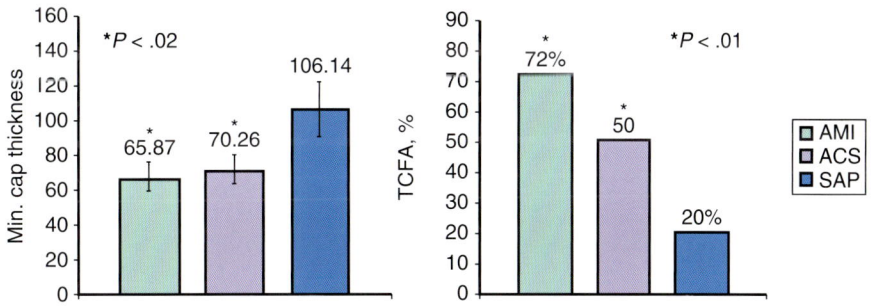

Fig. 66.28 In vivo quantification of fibrous cap thickness by optical coherence tomography. Cap thickness was lowest in patients with acute myocardial infarction *(AMI)*, intermediate in patients with acute coronary syndrome *(ACS;* unstable angina and non-ST segment elevation myocardial infarction), and highest in patients with chronic stable angina pectoris *(SAP)*. As a result, the incidence of thin-cap fibroatheroma *(TCFA)* is highest in those with AMI and lowest in those with SAP. (From Jang IK, Tearney GJ, MacNeill B, et al. In vivo characterization of coronary atherosclerotic plaque by use of optical coherence tomography. *Circulation.* 2005;111:1551–1555.)

Near-Infrared Spectroscopy

Spectroscopy is a nondestructive optical technology with the ability to analyze the chemical composition of plaque components.[142] After irradiation of tissue with a laser beam, scattered photons are acquired to identify specific features of plaque vulnerability. Plaque components such as calcium and cholesterol have specific absorption and reflectance patterns of light, producing a pattern that is converted into an image. This modality is important for the identification of the necrotic core, fibrous cap, and inflammation.[143]

Two modalities are being evaluated for intravascular detection of high-risk plaques: near-infrared and Raman spectroscopy. Both techniques have good correlations with histologic analyses of coronary and aortic tissue.[144] However, the complexity of signal analysis may force investigators to focus on only one or two features of plaque vulnerability.

The physicochemical characteristics of lipid and calcium and their shift patterns make Raman spectroscopy highly sensitive for plaque detection. However, only a few photons are recruited into the Raman shift, providing poor tissue penetration and a low signal-to-noise ratio. Backscattered noise can also decrease signal

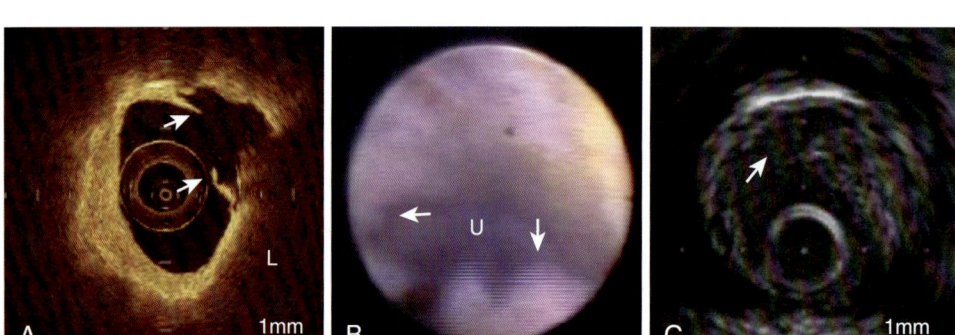

Fig. 66.29 Fibrous cap rupture during acute coronary syndrome assessed by various invasive modalities. (A) Optical coherence tomography demonstrates a lipid-rich area *(L)* and a fibrous cap discontinuation *(arrows)* that protrudes into the lumen. (B) Angioscopy shows a yellow lesion with cap disruption *(arrows)* and ulceration *(U)*. (C) Intravascular ultrasound shows an eccentric plaque rupture at the shoulder *(arrow)*. (From Kubo T, Imanishi T, Takarada S, et al. Assessment of culprit lesion morphology in acute myocardial infarction: ability of optical coherence tomography compared with intravascular ultrasound and coronary angioscopy. *J Am Coll Cardiol.* 2007;50:933–939.)

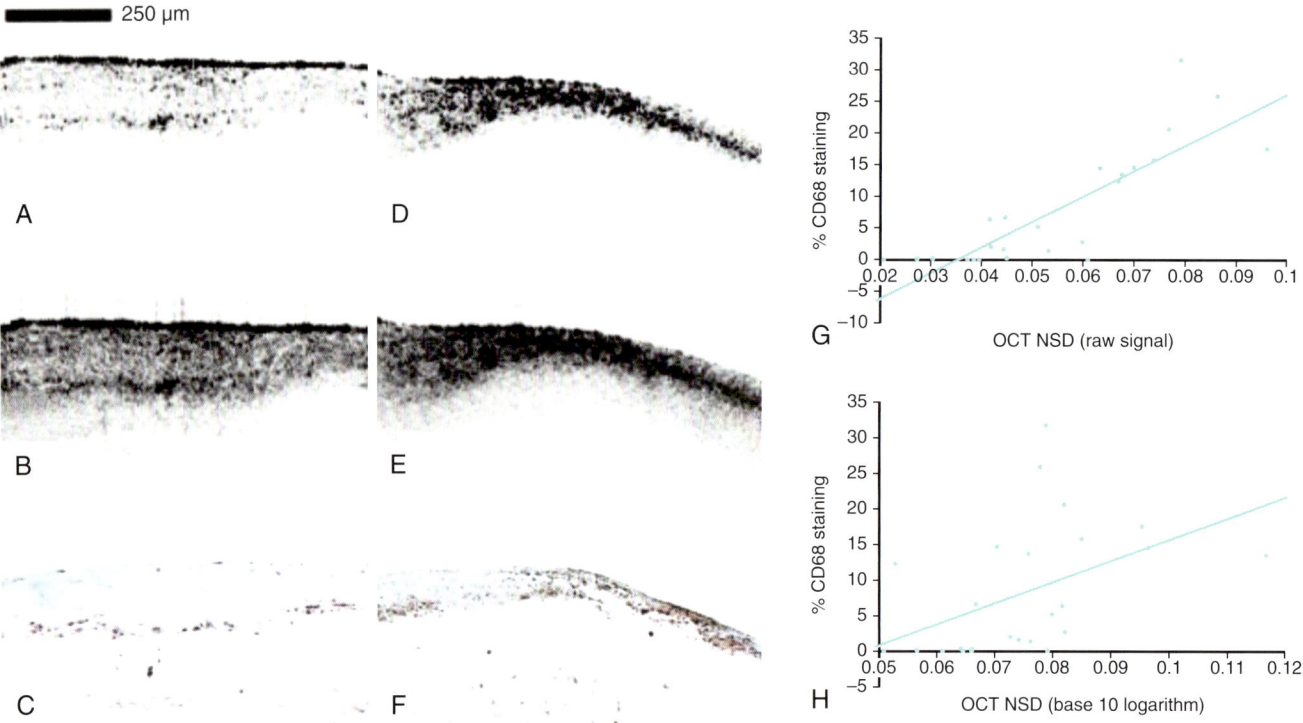

Fig. 66.30 Raw (A) and logarithm base 10 (B) optical coherence tomography *(OCT)* images of a fibroatheroma with a low density of macrophages within the fibrous cap. (C) Corresponding histology for A and B (CD68 immunoperoxidase stain, ×100). Raw (D) and logarithm base 10 (E) OCT images of a fibroatheroma with a high density of macrophages within the fibrous cap. (F) Corresponding histology for D and E (CD68 immunoperoxidase stain, ×100). Correlations are shown between the raw (G) and logarithm base 10 (H) OCT signal (normalized standard deviation *[NSD]*) and CD68 percent area staining *(diamonds,* NSD data; *solid line,* linear t). (From Tearney GJ, Yabushita H, Houser SL, et al. Quantification of macrophage content in atherosclerotic plaques by optical coherence tomography. *Circulation.* 2003;107:113–119.)

quality and limit imaging interpretation. Newer technologies in combination with IVUS have improved image quality by increasing signal acquisition.[145]

NIRS measures diffuse reflectance signals with the use of near-infrared light. The spectrometer emits light onto a substance and measures the light that is reflected over a wide range of optical wavelengths, which are processed as a spectrum, applied to an algorithm that predicts the probability of high-risk plaque, and displayed on a chemogram. The main objective of NIRS is quantification of the necrotic core. The result is reported on a scale of 1 to 999, called the *lipid core burden index (LCBI)*. Because of this feature, NIRS has the potential for becoming the standard for necrotic core evaluation.[146]

The NIRS system was evaluated in 106 patients undergoing PCI in a multicenter study, with encouraging results.[147] The investigators compared in vivo imaging with autopsy NIRS signals by

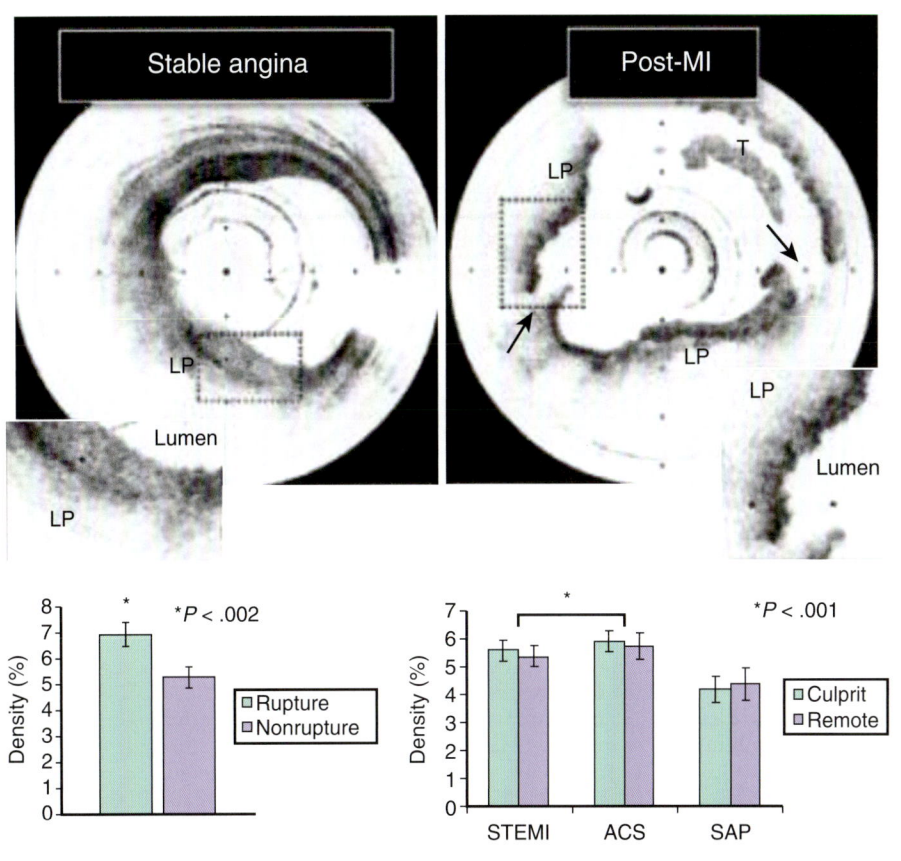

Fig. 66.31 Optical coherence tomography images of plaques from patients with stable angina *(upper left)* and after myocardial infarction *(MI) (upper right)*. Increased signal area is seen at the fibrous cap after MI *(detail)*, highlighting areas of increased macrophage density. The *black arrows* denote areas of fibrous cap rupture. Lower left, Increased macrophage density in ruptured *(green bar)* compared with nonruptured *(purple bar)* plaques. Lower right, Macrophage density in culprit *(green bar)* and remote *(purple bar)* plaques from patients with ST-elevation myocardial infarction *(STEMI)*, acute coronary syndrome *(ACS)*, and stable angina pectoris *(SAP)*. Macrophage density is higher in culprit and remote plaques from patients with STEMI and ACS compared with SAP. *LP*, Lipid pool. (From MacNeill BD, Jang IK, Bouma BE, et al. Focal and multi-focal plaque macrophage distributions in patients with acute and stable presentations of coronary artery disease. *J Am Coll Cardiol.* 2004;44:972–979.)

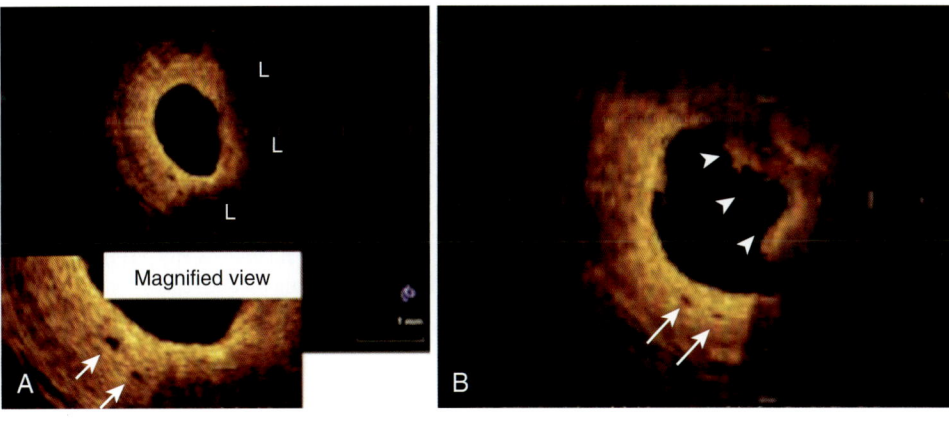

Fig. 66.32 Microchannels representing plaque neovascularization. (A) Eccentric, lipid-rich plaque (L) with microchannels *(arrows on inset)*. (B) Intracoronary thrombus *(arrowheads)* and two additional microchannels *(arrows)*. (Modified from Kitabata H, Tanaka A, Kubo T, et al. Relation of microchannel structure identified by optical coherence tomography to plaque vulnerability in patients with coronary artery disease. *Am J Cardiol.* 2010;105:1673–1678.)

using multivariate analysis. They found that NIRS appropriately identified lipid core–containing plaques in vivo. NIRS can be performed without replacing the blood in the vessel, but it can detect only one characteristic of advance atherosclerotic plaques, offering no input on the superficiality of lipid cores or fibrous cap thickness.

Catheters that combine NIRS with IVUS provide complementary data for evaluation of atherosclerosis by combining assessment of plaque burden, plaque composition, and vascular remodeling.[148] Multiple-imaging technology has shown excellent correlation with adverse cardiac events,[149] similar to that reported by the PROSPECT trial.[76] The combination of a catheter providing IVUS for determining plaque burden and minimal luminal area and NIRS for evaluating necrotic core content offers a more comprehensive assessment of the high-risk lesion.[150] This has been proved by correlating NIRS findings with clinical findings in various clinical scenarios, including STEMI,[148] periprocedural MI,[148] and cardiac arrest survivors.[151]

For patients with STEMI, Madder and colleagues reported a 5.8-fold higher maximum LCBI (4 mm) in culprit lesions compared with nonculprit plaques.[148] Large LCBI scores were reported for 95% of culprit lesions. The investigators identified a threshold (maxLCBI$_{4\,mm}$ > 400) for detecting culprit segments during STEMI with 85% sensitivity and 98% specificity. Similar results were reported by Erlinge and coworkers at the Transcatheter Cardiovascular Therapeutics meeting in 2013.[152] In patients surviving cardiac arrest, plaques with a large LCBI score were responsible for the clinical event.[151] Accumulated evidence suggests that large necrotic core lesions appear to be the most relevant substrate for life-threatening ACS.

Studies have found that plaques with large LCBI scores determined by NIRS are associated with increased risk of periprocedural AMI after PCI.[150,153] Plaques with a very large LCBI scores may benefit from placement of an embolic protection device (e.g., filter) to prevent distal embolization and reduce the incidence of periprocedural MI. This is the rationale of the Coronary Assessment by Near-Infrared of Atherosclerotic Rupture-Prone Yellow (CANARY) trial, and it will soon be known whether spectroscopy is a useful tool in the catheter laboratory for identifying a lipid core plaque that is at high risk of rupturing during therapy and causing complications.

NIRS in combination with IVUS has been shown to accurately detect high-risk plaques compared with OCT.[154] Roleder and associates evaluated 60 patients undergoing coronary angiography. OCT and combined NIRS-IVUS were done on 76 identical coronary segments. When OCT was used to define TCFAs based on a fibrous cap measuring less than 65 μm, the lesions exhibited positive remodeling, a higher plaque burden, a higher plaque volume, a smaller cross-sectional area, and longer plaque lengths, whereas NIRS revealed a greater LCBI score for 2-mm segments. OCT had greater accuracy for identifying TCFAs with an LCBI score higher than 315 and a remodeling index higher than 1.046.[154]

Most clinical data on NIRS come from cross-sectional studies, and there are few studies regarding its application for evaluation of the natural history of high-risk plaques with prospective follow-up. Accrued data appear to support the plaque expansion hypothesis, and it would be of great utility to assess the natural history and prognosis of lipid-rich atheromas with greater than 70% plaque burdens because of their potential for increasing MACEs during follow-up.

The ongoing PROSPECT II trial hopes to address these issues.[155] It is an investigator-initiated, multicenter, prospective registry for assessing the ability of intracoronary NIRS to identify nonflow-obstructing high-risk plaques that ultimately promote coronary events. This trial is recruiting 900 patients with ACS at 20 hospitals in Sweden, Denmark, and Norway. After patients undergo PCI of all culprit and obstructive lesions, three-vessel IVUS plus NIRS imaging will be performed to assess the proximal 6 to 8 cm of each coronary artery. The follow-up period will be at least 3 years, with assessment of secondary outcomes related to the safety and efficacy of bioabsorbable stents. Patients who have lesions with greater than 70% stenosis will be randomized to bioabsorbable stenting plus optimal medical therapy or to optimal medical therapy alone to assess a primary safety end point. Although still listed as recruiting, the study is planning to end enrollment in December 2019. Abbott withdrew the first-generation bioabsorbable stents in late 2017 and is no longer recruiting patients; the fate of this secondary end point remains unknown.[156]

The LRP study is an ongoing, multicenter clinical trial that is recruiting 9000 patients with ACS from centers in the United States, Europe, and Japan to evaluate the role of LCBI in predicting future MACEs. The LRP study will test whether a nonobstructive LRP documented by IVUS plus NIRS is associated with new coronary events within 24 months.[157] These study designs will help evaluate potential therapies for the prevention of cardiac events in patients with obstructive plaques with high-risk features.

NIRS can be used to follow patients after therapy. The YELLOW trial documented plaque regression after aggressive medical therapy with statins. In the YELLOW trial, 87 patients with stable CAD and multivessel disease underwent staged drug-eluting stent implantation for a significant secondary lesion (fractional flow reserve [FFR] <0.8), randomized to intensive statin therapy with rosuvastatin 40 mg a day versus standard statin therapy after the primary lesion was treated. The primary end point was the change in the extent of LRP, defined as the 4 mm long segment with the maximum LCBI (4 mm) of the secondary lesion between baseline and 6 to 8 weeks, as assessed by NIRS. High-intensity statin significantly decreased the lipid content in the plaque, especially in the setting of large amount of lipidic plaque at baseline. Interestingly, neither the plaque burden as assessed by IVUS nor the severity of the lesion as assessed by FFR changed.[158] This provocative finding could suggest that regression is not merely a reversal of progression, but instead involves emigration of the maladaptive macrophage infiltrate, followed by initiation of a stream of healthy, normally functioning phagocytes that mobilize necrotic debris and all other components of advanced plaques.[159,160] In this setting, NIRS might be a clinically useful index of plaque compositional change in the assessment of residual high-risk LRPs in statin-treated patients, compared with conventional plaque estimation by IVUS and physiological measurements by FFR, especially when co-registered to IVUS assessment of plaque burden that is now possible in a single catheter (Fig. 66.33 and 66.34).[158,160] Nevertheless, current commercialization limitations have made this technique unavailable for clinical use.

MECHANISMS OF PLAQUE REGRESSION

Multiple animal and human studies have documented plaque regression in both early and advanced atherosclerotic plaque.[161] For example, in apolipoprotein E (ApoE) deficient mice with hypercholesterolemia and atherosclerotic plaques, a rapid regression of atherosclerotic was induced by liver-directed gene transfer of ApoE (ApoE encoding adenoviral vectors), which reduces the cholesterol level to the wild type.[162] Also, when plaque-bearing aorta from the ApoE deficiency mice were transplanted into wild-type mice and exposed to low level of cholesterol, a regression of the atherosclerotic plaque was observed.[163]

Resolution of inflammation plays a crucial role in plaque regression. Macrophage plaque egression through perivascular lymphatic system is dependent on chemokine receptor 7 (CCR7).[164] The molecular mechanisms involved the liver X receptor (LXR) and the MERTK engulfment receptor responsible for the high density lipoprotein (HDL)-dependent reverse cholesterol transport.[165] Atorvastatin and Rosuvastatin promote clusters of differentiation CD68 cell emigration, increasing transcriptional activity and chromatin organization at the CCR7 promoter.[166] Marked inhibition of macrophage recruitment from circulating monocytes was achieved by significant reductions in endothelial adhesion molecules.[167] As a result, suppressed monocyte recruitment, rather than CCR7 efferocytosis, may be the predominant mechanism in plaque regression. In the absence of macrophage egression, local proliferation of M2 macrophages may be responsible for the clearance of apoptotic cells and TGFβ–mediated collagen synthesis.[168]

Plaque regression is intimately related to the HDL pathway. However, human studies documenting plaque regression show minimal or no changes in HDL-C plasma levels. Furthermore, successful pharmacologic efforts to increase HDL-C (up to 70%) showed no benefit.[169] Rather than HDL-C plasma levels, it is the HDL function through ApoA1 that likely drives the benefits of HDL.[170]

Finally, resolution of inflammation also involves the removal of Hb, haptoglobin, and iron after intraplaque hemorrhage. This pathway may be intimately ligated to the reverse cholesterol transport pathway, through the LXR.[171] The LXRα was reported to dominate the M(Hb) macrophage,[36] whereas LXRβ is required for iron-handling capacity in the Mhem macrophage.[172] Cholesterol removal and iron metabolism may interact within the same macrophage.[34]

Statin and Plaque Regression

Corti and associates were the first to document the eccentric pattern of plaque regression after aggressive lipid therapy.[173] Many studies have confirmed this observation (Fig. 66.35).[122,123] Lipid is the main plaque component that can be reversed with therapy, and the eccentric pattern of plaque regression suggests an effective reverse lipid transport system through the deeper layers of the vessel wall, which is probably mediated by vasa vasorum neovascularization.[124]

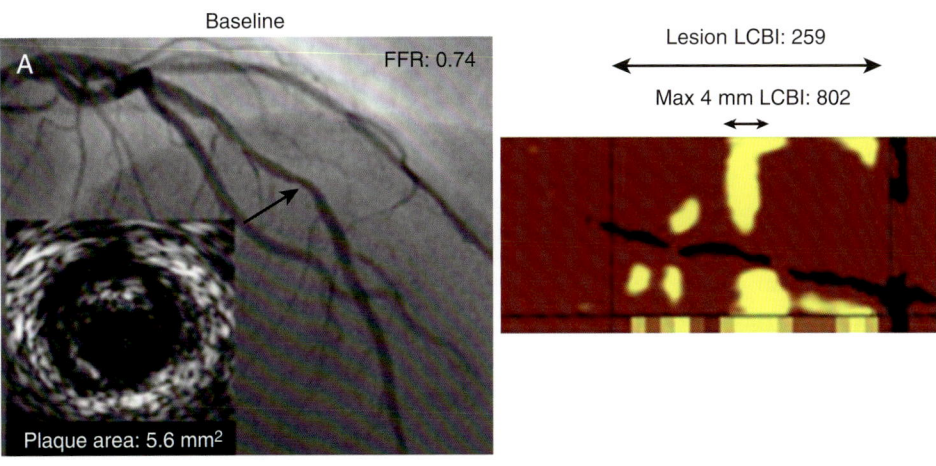

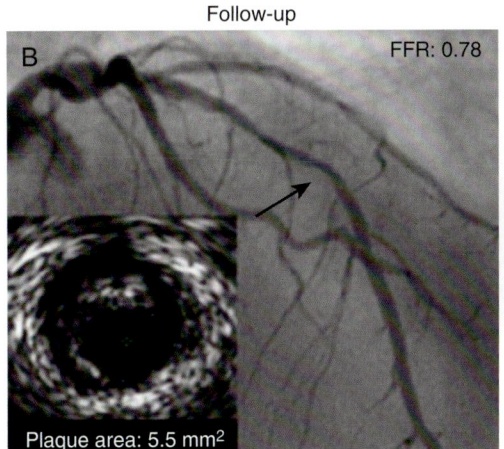

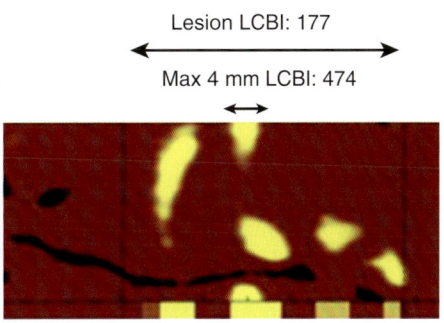

Fig. 66.33 Angiography, intravascular ultrasound (IVUS, *insets*), fractional flow reserve *(FFR)*, and near-infrared spectroscopy images of a severely obstructive lesion (A) before and (B) after 7 weeks of aggressive lipid-lowering therapy. Significant reductions occurred in the lipid core burden index *(LCBI)* without angiographic or intravascular ultrasound changes. (From Kini AS, Baber U, Kovacic JC, et al. Changes in plaque lipid content after short-term intensive versus standard statin therapy: the YELLOW trial (reduction in yellow plaque by aggressive lipid-lowering therapy. *J Am Coll Cardiol.* 2013;62:21–29.)

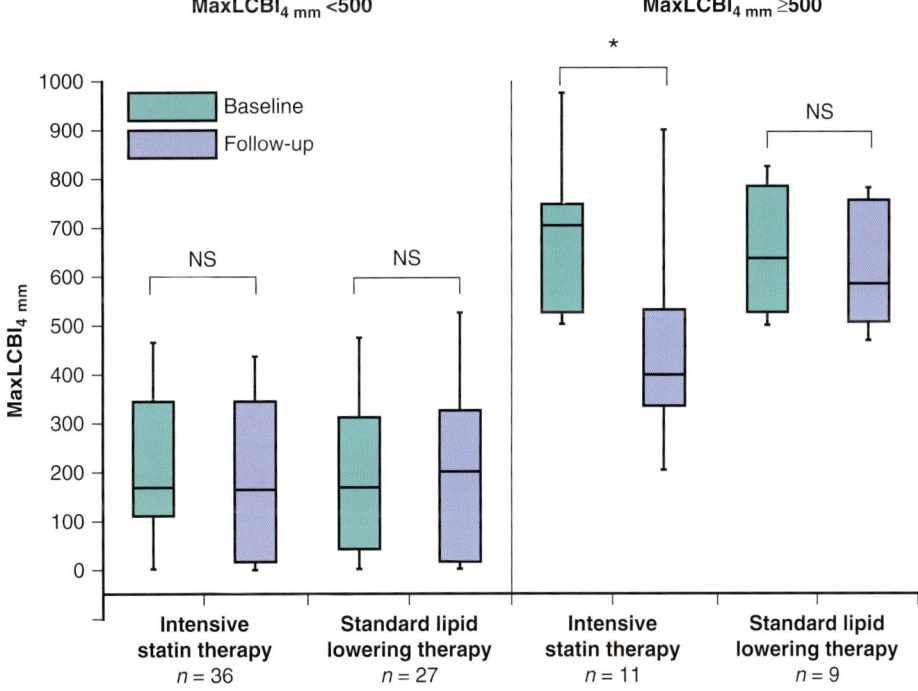

Fig. 66.34 Change in the extent of lipid contents within coronary plaques from baseline to follow-up (mean, 7 weeks) evaluated by serial near-infrared spectroscopy *(NS)* analysis. Lipid-rich plaque regression was identified in plaques having large lipid contents at baseline *(maxLCBI$_{4\ mm}$ ≥500)* receiving intensive statin therapy. *P = .004. (From Dohi T, Maehara A, Moreno A, et al. The relationship among extent of lipid-rich plaque, lesion characteristics, and plaque progression/regression in patients with coronary artery disease: a serial near-infrared spectroscopy and intravascular ultrasound study. *Eur Heart J Cardiovasc Imaging.* 2015;16[1]:81–87.)

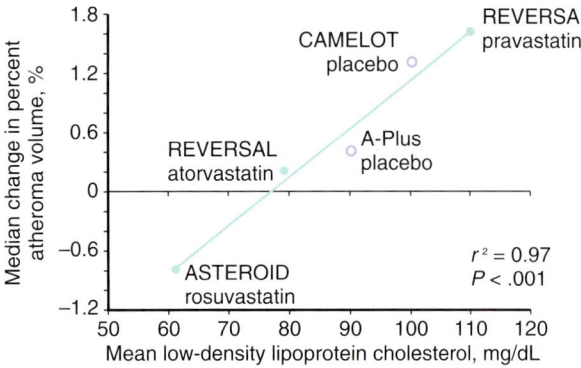

Fig. 66.35 Relationship between mean low-density lipoprotein cholesterol levels and median change in percent atheroma volume for several intravascular ultrasound trials.

Statins reduce cholesterol levels via competitive inhibition of hydroxymethylglutaryl (HMG) CoA reductase blocking the biosynthesis of cholesterol, reducing the intracellular level of cholesterol. In the hepatocyte, this lower level of intracellular cholesterol procedure increases expression of LDL receptor promoting plasma uptake of LDL.[174]

Although a key component of the statin effect, reduction of cholesterol is not the only mechanism of cardio protection mediated by statin; multiple properties such as reduction of inflammation, thrombogenicity, vasa vasorum neovascularization, and endothelial dysfunction have been described.[175]

Statins are antiinflammatory and reduce inflammatory cytokines and adhesion molecules, acting on both the innate and adaptive immune responses.[176] Statins decrease inflammatory cytokines such as IL-6, IL-8, and monocyte chemoattractant protein 1 (MCP-1).[177] Statins reduce MMP-1, MMP-3, and MMP-9 from both SMCs and macrophages in a rabbit model, which was reduced by both geranylgeranyl pyrophosphate (GGPP) and mevalonate.[178]

In the adaptive immune system, statins have effects on T-cell differentiation. Simvastatin reduced the differentiation of the proinflammatory IL-17 helper T cells (Th17) and enhanced the production of Tregs in a geranylgeranylation-dependent manner.[179]

Intensive statin therapy has produced a significant decrease in coronary events in patients with stable disease (i.e., Trending to New Targets [TNT] and Incremental Decrease in Events Through Aggressive Lipid Lowering [IDEAL] trials) and in patients with ACS (i.e., Aggrastat to Zocor [A to Z] and Pravastatin or Atorvastatin Evaluation and Infection Therapy–Thrombolysis in Myocardial Infarction 22 [PROVE IT–TIMI 22] trials). Statins have reduced the incidence of coronary death, AMI, and heart failure, independent of recurrent infarction.[180,181] Early intensive statin therapy for ACS was associated with clinical benefits that became evident after 4 to 12 months, including a decrease in serum VEGF levels, which probably represents an attenuation of plaque angiogenesis.[182,183] In the Effect of Rosuvastatin on Intravascular Ultrasound-Derived Coronary Atheroma Burden (ASTEROID) trial, aggressive therapy with rosuvastatin led to an absolute regression of atheroma volume (Fig. 66.36).[184]

The beneficial effects of statin therapy on plaque regression and stabilization have been documented many times with OCT, angioscopy, MRI, and IVUS-VH.[173,185]

Despite the tremendous value of statin therapy, patients have a 22% recurrent event rate within 2 years and demonstrate resistance to systemic therapy, as confirmed in the PROVE IT trial.[186] Even the best combination of systemic therapies does not successfully prevent all episodes of plaque rupture and thrombosis.

Nonetheless, intravascular imaging studies have demonstrated significant plaque regression with statin use.

One study included 1039 patients with coronary disease who underwent IVUS at baseline and after 104 weeks. They were randomized to atorvastatin (80 mg) or rosuvastatin (40 mg).[187] At 104 weeks, the percent atheroma volume (PAV) decreased by 0.99% (95% CI −1.19 to −0.63) in the atorvastatin group and by 1.22% (95% CI −1.52 to −0.90) in the rosuvastatin group ($P = .17$). The normalized total atheroma volume (TAV) was more favorable for patients receiving rosuvastatin compared with those on atorvastatin: −6.39 mm^3 (95% CI −7.52 to −5.12) compared with −4.42 mm^3 (95% CI, −5.98 to −3.26; $P = .01$). Plaque regression was induced in most patients in both groups: 63.2% of the patients receiving atorvastatin and 68.5% of the patients receiving rosuvastatin for PAV ($P = .07$), and 64.7% and 71.3%, respectively, for TAV ($P = .02$). Evidence of changes in plaque composition with plaque regression induced by high dose statin can be seen in shorter periods of time, as documented in the 6 to 8 week follow-up period of the YELLOW trial, including combinations of intravascular modalities, including FFR, NIRS, and IVUS.[158]

Finally, the YELLOW II trial documented the effect of high dose statin in plaque morphology, cholesterol efflux, macrophage functionality, and gene expression in peripheral blood mononuclear cells.[188] High-dose statin increases the thickness of the TCFAs, reduces the prevalence of TCFA from 20% to 7%, and increases cholesterol efflux by enhancing macrophage functionally documented by upregulation of genes *SQLE*, *DHCR24*, *FADS1*, *LDLR*, *ABCA1*, and *ABCG1*, which play critical biological functions related to cholesterol metabolism, signals transduction pathways, inflammation, and statin metabolism (Fig. 66.37).[188]

Proprotein Convertase Subtilisin/Kexin Type 9 Inhibitors and Plaque Regression

Proprotein convertase subtilisin/kexin type 9 (PCSK9) is an enzyme that binds to the LDL receptor in the hepatocyte membrane, leading to degradation of the LDL receptor and consequently reducing LDL liver uptake and increasing LDL plasma level.[189]

Two monoclonal antibodies that block the PCSK9 enzyme are available in the United States (Alirocumab and Evolocumab). These antibodies bind free plasma PCSK9 and promote degradation of the enzyme resulting in higher number of LDL receptor in the hepatocyte membrane, increasing the capacity to remove LDL from the circulation.[190]

PCSK9 inhibitors are capable of lowering LDL-C by as much as 60% in patients on statin therapy and 70% in patients not taking statin; they also decrease inflammation, oxidative stress, thrombosis, plaque burden, and improve cardiovascular outcomes.[191-193]

PCSK9 affects coronary plaques via several pathways, although its proinflammatory effect is driven mainly through the nuclear factor (NF)-κB expression. This NF promotes the release of inflammatory cytokines, chemokines, and adhesion molecules such as IL-1β, IL-12, IF-γ, VCAM1, and ICAM-1, leading to monocyte recruitment and expansion of the necrotic core.[191,194] In addition, PCSK9 can enhance the thrombotic substrate in atherosclerotic plaques by upregulating tissue factor (Table 66.3, Fig. 66.38).[195]

Plaque Regression and PCSK9 Inhibitors

The Glagov trial by Nicholls et al. was a multicenter double-blind, placebo-controlled randomized clinical trial of 968 patients with CAD that compared statin alone versus statin plus Evolocumab. After 78 weeks, the group of Statin plus Evolocumab achieved a

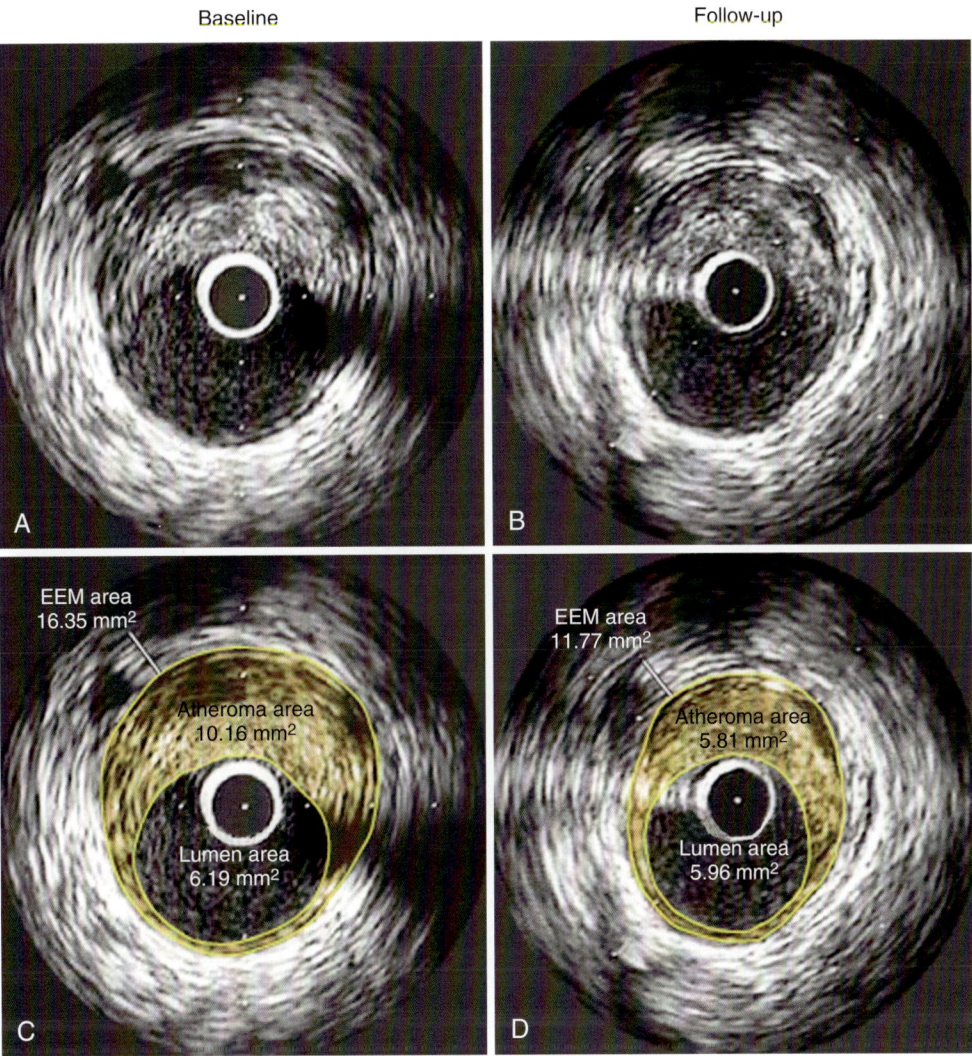

Fig. 66.36 (A and B) Baseline and follow-up intravascular ultrasound images of a single coronary cross-section after 24 months of rosuvastatin treatment. (C and D) Measurements superimposed on the same cross-sections demonstrate the reduction in atheroma area. *EEM*, External elastic membrane. (From Nissen SE, Nicholls SJ, Sipahi I, et al. Effect of very high-intensity statin therapy on regression of coronary atherosclerosis: the ASTEROID trial. *JAMA*. 2006;295:1556–1565.)

60% reduction of LDL level compared with the statin/placebo group; the primary end point of change in PAV was statistically significant in favor of Evolocumab, with a decrease of 0.95% compared with an increase of 0.05% in the placebo group. A greater number of patients experienced plaque regression in the Evolocumab group (64.3% vs. 47.3%). Despite all these positive findings, plaque progression was noted in 35.7% of the patients, despite the use of statin and PCSK9 inhibitors (Figs. 66.39 and 66.40). Extensive evidence from large randomized clinical trials have shown the efficacy in primary and secondary prevention of clinical events with the use of PCSK9.[196,197]

Direct Antiinflammatory Therapy

Recently, the CANTOS trial confirmed the direct role of inflammation in atherothrombosis, independent of the LDL level.[198] This study was a large randomized, double-blind, placebo-controlled clinical trial that included patients with prior history of MI and high-sensitivity C-reactive protein levels. The patients were randomized to placebo and three different doses of a fully human monoclonal antibody targeting IL1β (Canakinumab). IL1β is a proinflammatory cytokine that plays multiple roles in the development of atherothrombotic plaque, including the induction of procoagulant activity, the promotion of monocyte and leukocyte adhesion to vascular endothelial cells, and the growth of vascular smooth-muscle cells.[35] Patients taking Canakinumab showed a reduction of high-sensitivity C-reactive protein and IL-6 levels. Most importantly, these patients showed a statistically significant reduction in nonfatal MI, any nonfatal stroke, or cardiovascular death. In addition, patients taking Canakinumab had higher rates of infection-related mortality and lower incidences of cancer.[198]

Additional Therapies

The n-3 fatty polyunsaturated acids may provide stabilizing effects through the regulation of adhesion molecule expression, proinflammatory and proangiogenic growth factors secreted by the endothelium, and attenuation of the nuclear factor NF-κβ system.[199] Nishio and coworkers studied 49 nonculprit TCFAs from 30 patients with dyslipidemia who were not receiving treatment.[200] These patients were randomized to receive 1800 mg/day of eicosapentaenoic acid (EPA), plus a statin or a statin only. The statin dose was adjusted to achieve an LDL target of less than 70 mg/dL. Post-PCI assessment and OCT were performed at the 9-month follow-up. The investigators reported features of plaque stabilization, such as a higher increase in plaque thickness and greater decrease in lipid arch and lipid pool by OCT in patients receiving EPA plus a statin, compared with those receiving a statin alone.

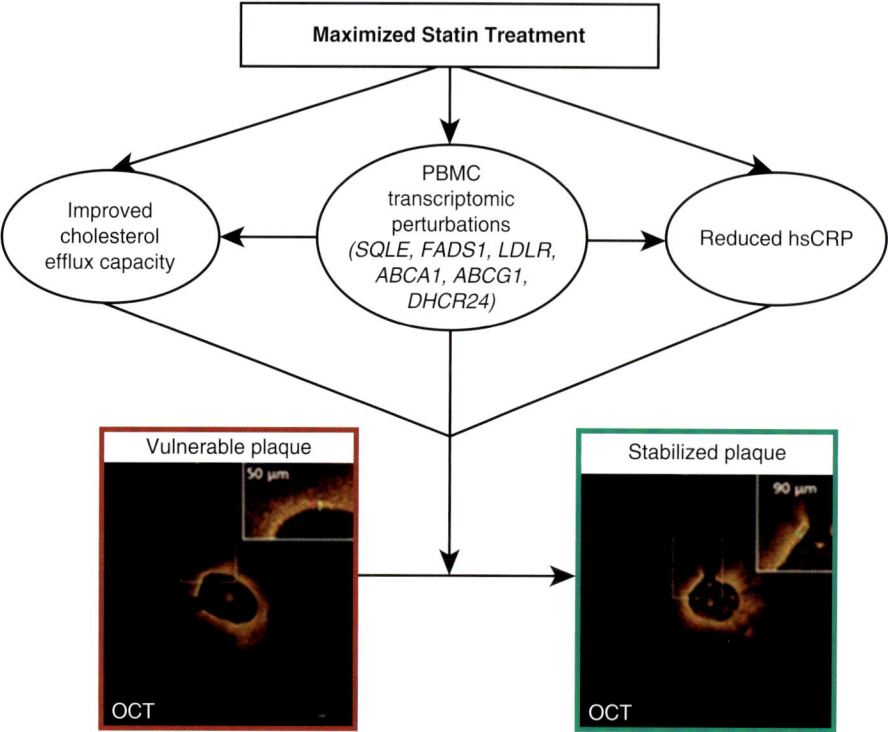

Fig. 66.37 High-intensity statins and intracoronary imaging, cholesterol efflux, and transcriptome perturbations. In patients with stable coronary artery disease, we detected a significant increase in fibrous cap thickness of obstructive coronary lesions by optical coherence tomography *(OCT)*, enhancement of cholesterol efflux capacity *(CEC)*, reduction in high-sensitivity C-reactive protein *(hsCRP)* level, and significant perturbations in the peripheral blood mononuclear cell transcriptome after 8 to 12 weeks of rosuvastatin 40 mg daily. Improved macrophage CEC and reduced hsCRP contributed to plaque stabilization independently of changes in serum cholesterol. Furthermore, the significant transcriptomic perturbations related to cholesterol synthesis, regulation of fatty acid unsaturation, cellular cholesterol uptake, efflux, and inflammation may cooperate in determining statin's beneficial effects on plaque stabilization. *PBMC,* Peripheral blood mononuclear cell. (From Kini AS, Vengrenyuk Y, Shameer K, et al. Intracoronary imaging, cholesterol efflux, and transcriptomes after intensive statin treatment: the YELLOW II study. *J Am Coll Cardiol.* 2017;69[6]:628–640.)

TABLE 66.3 NF-B Pathways Exerted by Proprotein Convertase Subtilisin/Kexin Type 9

Effect	PCSK9 Enzyme	PCSK9 Inhibition
Inflammation	Proinflammatory response by interleukin-1β, interleukin-12, and interferon-γ	Reduced monocyte recruitment Attenuated oxLDL–induced expression of proinflammatory chemokine synthesis and secretion
Necrotic core	Increased necrotic core fraction	Decreased macrophage and necrotic core content Inhibited oxLDL–induced apoptosis (via downregulation of caspase-9 and caspase-3 and improved Bax–Bcl-2 ratio) Reduced oxLDL–induced apoptosis of human endothelial cells
Proliferation	SMC proliferation and remodeling of extracellular matrix via NF-B pathway activation (I B and cyclin-dependent kinase inhibitors p21 and p27)	Increased SMC and collagen content
Activation of thrombotic pathway	Upregulation tissue factor and increase of thrombotic potential of atherosclerotic plaques by NF-B pathway	NA
Platelet activation	Increase platelet count and platelet crit	NA

TABLE 66.3 NF-B Pathways Exerted by Proprotein Convertase Subtilisin/Kexin Type 9—cont'd

Effect	PCSK9 Enzyme	PCSK9 Inhibition
Effect on oxLDL and LOX-1 (the major oxLDL receptor on endothelial cells, also present in arterial SMCs)	Positive-feedback loop between LOX-1 and PCSK9 LOX-1 is a potent mediator of atherogenesis (increased immunoreactivity)	Inhibits atherogenesis in hypercholesterolemic states by disrupting LOX-1 expression; LOX-1 inhibition reduces the state of oxidative stress, mitochondrial DNA damage, and NLRP3 inflammasome activation in macrophages
LDL receptor degradation	Reduced hepatic and macrophage LDL receptor levels with subsequent increase of LDL cholesterol levels and activation of LDL oxidation	Increased LDL receptor density
ApoER-2 degradation	Increased M1 macrophage phenotype. Increased M1 macrophage responses (migration, generation of reactive oxygen species, antibody-dependent cell cytotoxicity, and phagocytosis). Polyinosinic–polycytidylic acid– or interferon–induced production of proinflammatory cytokines, COX-2 expression, NF-I B , STAT1, and further activation of NF-B	Reduced monocyte recruitment
Lipoprotein(a) internalization	Reduced lipoprotein(a) internalization by hepatic HepG2 cells and primary human fibroblasts LDL receptor is a PCSK9-regulable clearance receptor for lipoprotein(a)	Dose-related reductions in lipoprotein(a) levels, greater in patients receiving statins

ApoER-2, Apolipoprotein E receptor-2; *COX-2*, cyclooxygenase-2; *LDL*, low-density lipoprotein; *LOX-1*, lectin-like oxidized low-density lipoprotein receptor-1; *NA*, not available; *NF-B,* nuclear factor-B; *NF-I B,* nuclear factor-B inhibitor; NLRP3 = NACHT, LRR, and PYD domains–containing protein 3; *oxLDL*, oxidized low-density lipoprotein; *PCSK9*, proprotein convertase subtilisin/kexin type 9; *SMC*, smooth-muscle cell; *STAT1*, signal transducer and activator of transcription.
(From Navarese EP, Kolodziejczak M, Kereiakes DJ, et al. Proprotein convertase subtilisin/kexin type 9 monoclonal antibodies for acute coronary syndrome: a narrative review. *Ann Intern Med*. 2016;164[9]:600–607.)

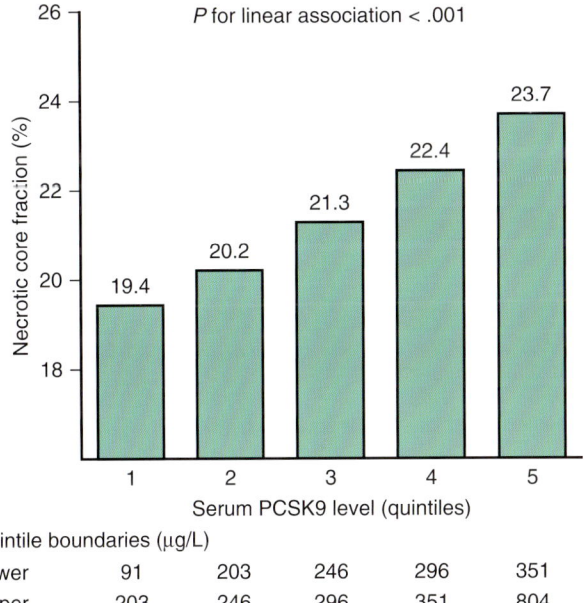

Fig. 66.38 Association between serum proprotein convertase subtilisin/kexin type *(PCSK9)* level and fraction of coronary plaque that consists of necrotic core tissue. (From Cheng JM, Oemrawsingh RM, Garcia-Garcia HM, et al. PCSK9 in relation to coronary plaque inflammation: results of the ATHEROREMO-IVUS study. *Atherosclerosis*. 2016;248:117–122.)

Another method to achieve plaque stabilization is the potentiation of reversal cholesterol transport system. This therapeutic alternative has been proposed to promote cholesterol efflux from macrophages by activation of the ABC transporters ABCA1 and ABCG1.[47,201]

In the search for systemic therapies, other approaches are being studied. For instance, preclinical data have demonstrated that vaccination against endothelial tyrosine kinase (TEK, formerly called TIE2), the angiopoietin receptor, promotes the formation of smaller atherosclerotic plaques with a more stable phenotype.[202] Similarly, both animal and human experiments have demonstrated that the selective inhibition of lipoprotein-associated phospholipase A_2 reduces its plasma activity and is associated with a decrease in plaque and necrotic core areas.[203,204]

Other therapies targeting pathways involved in TCFA formation include inhibition of MMP activity by doxycycline, which appeared to be as effective as simvastatin in reducing the incidence of plaque rupture in a cholesterol-fed rabbit model of atherosclerosis.[205] Similarly, the use of β-blockers decreased shear stress and the plaque vulnerability index seen in transgenic models of atherosclerosis.[206]

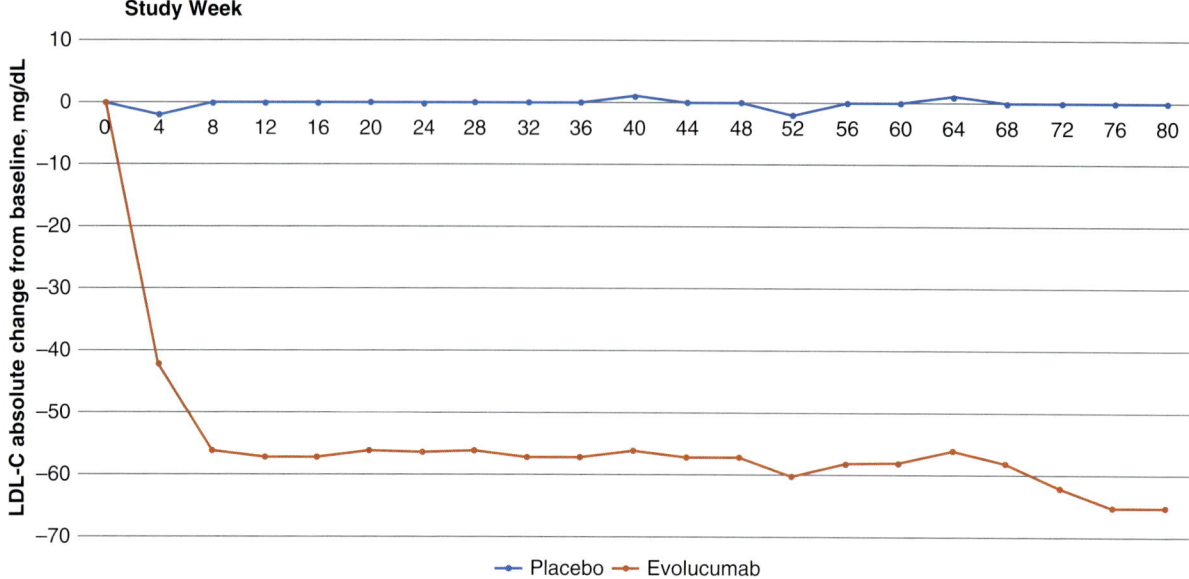

Fig. 66.39 Effect of evolocumab on progression of coronary disease in statin-treated patients. *LDL-C*, Low-density lipoprotein. (From Nicholls SJ, Puri R, Anderson T, et al. Effect of evolocumab on progression of coronary disease in statin-treated patients: the GLAGOV randomized clinical tripal. *JAMA*. 2016;316[22]:2373–2384.)

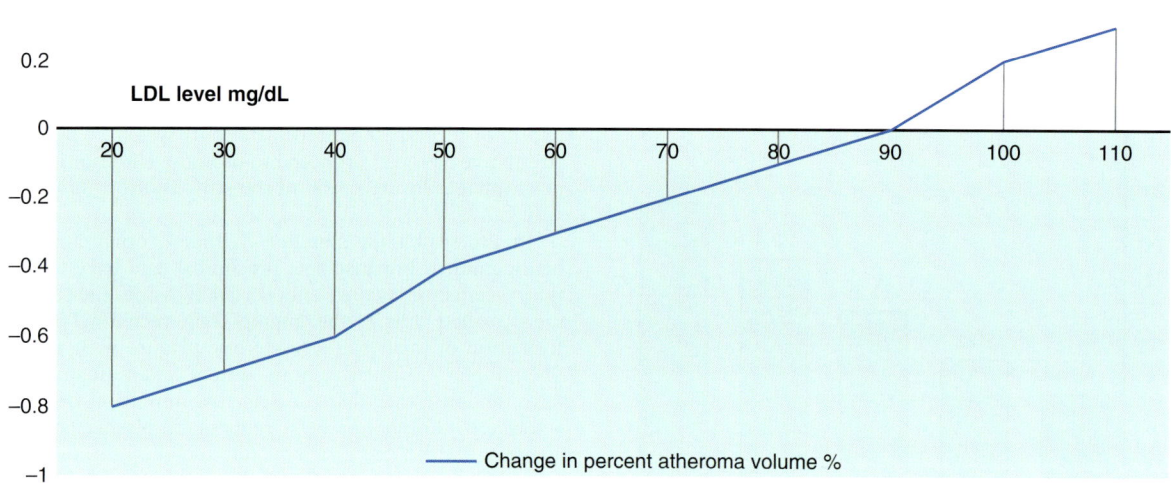

Fig. 66.40 Post hoc analysis examining the relationship between achieved low-density lipoprotein *(LDL)*-C level and change in percent atheroma volume. (From Nicholls SJ, Puri R, Anderson T, et al. Effect of evolocumab on progression of coronary disease in statin-treated patients: the GLAGOV randomized clinical trial. *JAMA*. 2016;316[22]:2373–2384.)

KEY REFERENCES

3. Benjamin EJ, Blaha MJ, Chiuve SE, et al. Heart disease and stroke statistics 2017 update: a report from the american heart association. *Circulation*. 2017;135(10):e146–e603.
7. Arbab-Zadeh A, Fuster V. The myth of the "vulnerable plaque": transitioning from a focus on individual lesions to atherosclerotic disease burden for coronary artery disease risk assessment. *J Am Coll Cardiol*. 2015;65(8):846–855.
9. Virmani R, Kolodgie FD, Burke AP, et al. Lessons from sudden coronary death: a comprehensive morphological classification scheme for atherosclerotic lesions. *Arter Thromb Vasc Biol*. 2000;20:1262–1275.
12. Motoyama S, Kondo T, Sarai M, et al. Multislice computed tomographic characteristics of coronary lesions in acute coronary syndromes. *J Am Coll Cardiol*. 2007;50:319–326.
14. Narula J, Kovacic JC. Putting TCFA in clinical perspective. *J Am Coll Cardiol*. 2014;64(7):681–683.
19. Stary HC, Chandler AB, Dinsmore RE, et al. A definition of advanced types of atherosclerotic lesions and a histological classification of atherosclerosis atherosclerotic lesion types advanced by histology type IV lesions. *Circulation*. 1995;92(5):1355–1374.
23. Moreno PR. Vulnerable plaque: definition, diagnosis, and treatment. *Cardiol Clin*. 2010;28:1–30.
25. Moreno PR, Bernardi VH, Lopez-Cuellar VH. Macrophages, smooth muscle cells, and tissue factor in unstable angina. Implications for cell-mediated thrombogenicity in acute coronary syndromes. *Circulation*. 1996;94 SRC:3090–3097.
26. Virmani R, Burke AP, Farb A, et al. Pathology of the vulnerable plaque. *J Am Coll Cardiol*. 2006;47:C13–C18.

28. Narula J, Nakano M, Virmani R, et al. Histopathologic characteristics of atherosclerotic coronary disease and implications of the findings for the invasive and noninvasive detection of vulnerable plaques. *J Am Coll Cardiol*. 2013;61(10):1041–1051.
34. Tabas I, Bornfeldt KE. Macrophage phenotype and function in different stages of atherosclerosis. *Circ Res*. 2016;118(4):653–667.
36. Finn AV, Nakano M, Polavarapu R, et al. Hemoglobin directs macrophage differentiation and prevents foam cell formation in human atherosclerotic plaques. *J Am Coll Cardiol*. 2012;59:166–177.
42. Tabas I. Macrophage death and defective inflammation resolution in atherosclerosis. *Nat Rev Immunol*. 2010;10:36–46.
48. Brien KD, McDonald TO, Chait A. Neovascular expression of E-selectin, intercellular adhesion molecule-1, and vascular cell adhesion molecule-1 in human atherosclerosis and their relation to intimal leukocyte content. *Circulation*. 1996;93:672–682.
64. Tabas I. Consequences and therapeutic implications of macrophage apoptosis in atherosclerosis: the importance of lesion stage and phagocytic efficiency. *Arter Thromb Vasc Biol*. 2005;25:2255–2264.
76. Stone GW, Maehara A, Lansky AJ, et al. A prospective natural-history study of coronary atherosclerosis. *N Engl J Med*. 2011;364(364):226–235.
78. Niccoli G, Stefanini GG, Capodanno D, et al. Are the culprit lesions severely stenotic? *JACC Cardiovasc Imaging*. 2013;6(10):1108–1114.
84. Kubo T, Maehara A, Mintz GS, et al. The dynamic nature of coronary artery lesion morphology assessed by serial virtual histology intravascular ultrasound tissue characterization. *J Am Coll Cardiol*. 2010;55(15):1590–1597.
108. Calvert PA, Obaid DR, Sullivan M, et al. Association between IVUS findings and adverse outcomes in patients with coronary artery disease: the VIVA (VH-IVUS in Vulnerable Atherosclerosis) study. *JACC Cardiovasc Imaging*. 2011;4:894–901.
128. Yonetsu T, Kakuta T, Lee T, et al. In vivo critical fibrous cap thickness for rupture-prone coronary plaques assessed by optical coherence tomography. *Eur Heart J*. 2011;32:1251–1259.
129. Kubo T, Imanishi T, Takarada S. Assessment of culprit lesion morphology in acute myocardial infarction: ability of optical coherence tomography compared with intravascular ultrasound and coronary angioscopy. *Am Coll Cardiol J*. 2007;50:933–939.
138. Ali ZA, Karimi Galougahi K, Maehara A, et al. Intracoronary optical coherence tomography 2018: current status and future directions. *JACC Cardiovasc Interv*. 2017;10(24):183–223.
142. Moreno PR, Muller JE. Detection of high-risk atherosclerotic coronary plaques by intravascular spectroscopy. *J Interv Cardiol*. 2003;16(3):243–252.
158. Kini AS, Baber U, Kovacic JC, et al. Changes in plaque lipid content after short-term intensive versus standard statin therapy: the YELLOW trial (reduction in yellow plaque by aggressive lipid-lowering therapy). *J Am Coll Cardiol*. 2013;62(1):21–29.
161. Moreno PR, Kini A. Resolution of inflammation, statins, and plaque regression. *JACC Cardiovasc Imaging*. 2012;5(2):178–181.
172. Boyle J, Johns M, Kampfer T, et al. Activating transcription factor 1 directs Mhem atheroprotective macrophages through coordinated iron handling and foam cell protection. *Circ Res*. 2012;110:20–33.
184. Nissen SE, Nicholls SJ, Sipahi I, et al. Effect of very high-intensity statin therapy on regression of coronary atherosclerosis: the ASTEROID trial. *JAMA*. 2006;295:1556–1565.
186. Cannon CP, Braunwald E, McCabe CH, et al. Intensive versus moderate lipid lowering with statins after acute coronary syndromes. *N Engl J Med*. 2004;350:1495–1504.
187. Nicholls SJ, Ballantyne CM, Barter PJ, et al. Effect of two intensive statin regimens on progression of coronary disease. *N Engl J Med*. 2011;365(22):2078–2087.
188. Kini AS, Vengrenyuk Y, Shameer K, et al. Intracoronary imaging, cholesterol efflux, and transcriptomes after intensive statin treatment: the YELLOW II study. *J Am Coll Cardiol*. 2017;69(6):628–640.
192. Sabatine M, Giugliano R, Wiviott S, et al. Efficacy and safety of evolocumab in reducing lipids and cardiovascular events. *N Engl J Med*. 2015;372(16):1500–1509.
198. Ridker PM, Everett BM, Thuren T, et al. Antiinflammatory therapy with canakinumab for atherosclerotic disease. *N Engl J Med*. 2017;377(12):1119.

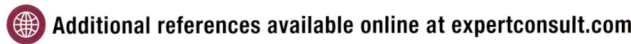 Additional references available online at expertconsult.com.

中文导读

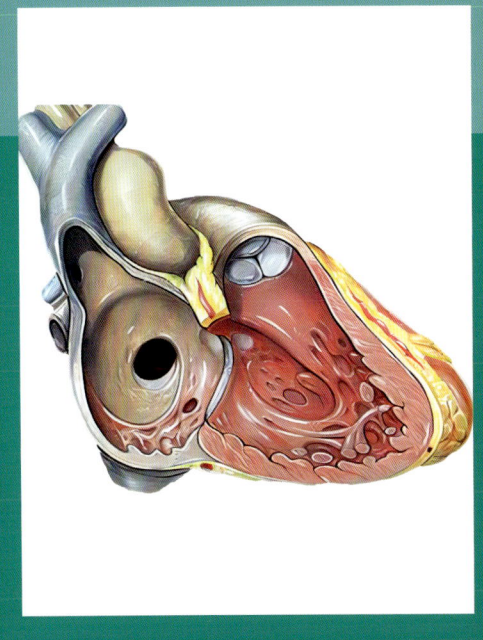

第67章
光学相干断层成像

　　光学相干断层成像能生成极高轴向分辨率的血管结构图像,并对血管结构进行与病理学结果高度一致的定量评估。光学相干断层成像可以精准识别纤维斑块、脂质斑块、钙化斑块、血栓、泡沫细胞聚集等病变;可实现对斑块进展或逆转,以及冠状动脉支架置入后血管反应的精准监测。光学相干断层成像回撤时的自动边缘检测,可以实时测量冠状动脉最小管腔面积(MLA)及最大狭窄程度,为经皮冠状动脉介入治疗手术规划提供更精确的参考数据。而光学相干断层成像引起的瞬时ST段抬高、心动过缓、冠状动脉痉挛等发生率极低,且易于处理。

　　目前光学相干断层成像主要临床应用场景包括:冠状动脉粥样硬化评估、支架置入评估、支架失败的评估、指导经皮冠状动脉介入治疗手术规划。光学相干断层成像的普及不仅仅是对冠状动脉粥样硬化评估、管理的革新,同时也将加深甚至更新行业对于冠状动脉粥样硬化这一疾病的理解。在国内光学相干断层成像的应用尚处于雏形阶段,而随着光学相干断层成像技术的持续迭代,这一技术或许将带领整个冠状动脉领域进入新的篇章。

张宇轩　吴永健

章节要点

- 光学相干断层成像是一种基于导管的新型影像技术，其应用于光纤技术，以获取独特的微观血管特征，可为医者提供实时的冠状动脉全层析视野，以及精准的测量。

- 光学相干断层成像在一部分患者中具有不可替代的作用，包括冠状动脉病变较复杂的患者（急性冠状动脉综合征、长病变、需用双支架的分叉病变、钙化血管等），以及冠状动脉造影模糊病变的患者。光学相干断层成像可以为这部分患者提供快速的、即时的冠状动脉病变分布情况及影响程度，从而指导精确的经皮冠状动脉介入术。得益于光学相干断层成像独特的属性及其出色的轴向分辨率，一些曾经因冠状动脉造影与血管内超声局限性而无法胜任的任务，现在可以轻松地实现：病变延续长度与钙化厚度的测量、血栓及后续引起急性冠状动脉综合征罪犯病变的识别、支架失败原因的确定，以及指导更加精准高效的冠状动脉内介入术等。

- 粥样硬化斑块具有很多特征，如纤维帽、血栓、血管新生、脂质池，以及巨噬细胞聚集等，光学相干断层成像能可靠地对这些特征进行定性、定量分析，并与病理学"金标准"保持高度一致的水准，将早期冠状动脉病变与严重病变区分开来。另外，急性冠状动脉综合征患者的光学相干断层成像数据还可以提示急性冠状动脉综合征发病机制，进而影响后续治疗策略。除此之外，光学相干断层成像提供的斑块特征定性、定量数据，还可应用于展现正在进行药物干预的患者斑块实时的稳定性，进而提示药物的有效性。

- 光学相干断层成像提供精确的血管结构，可指导经皮冠状动脉介入治疗策略，比如支架长短、尺寸及支架着陆区；频域光学相干断层成像系统如今可以在数秒内将较长的冠状动脉节段可视化，以提供相较其他横断面成像更完整的血管轴向图像，从而实现更高效的经皮冠状动脉介入治疗手术规划。此外，光学相干断层成像独特的自动边缘检测将提供即时的冠状动脉狭窄定位、定性，病变长度，参考管腔/血管维度，以提示合适的支架尺寸及长度选择。

- 目前血管内成像的一大局限性在于，光学相干断层成像的影像无法与冠状动脉造影的即时成像信息相匹配。光学相干断层成像的图像融合将解决这一问题，融合技术将实现光学相干断层成像图像与造影管腔轮廓的同时、同步匹配，从而将光学相干断层成像完全融入经皮冠状动脉介入治疗的操作流程中。

- 术者在床旁即时获取、分析光学相干断层成像的图像，有助于实现光学相干断层成像的日常临床应用。此外，支架贴壁不良或膨胀不全的自动可视化，将极大程度地优化支架的置入效果。

- 支架定位于复杂病变处时（如分支处双支架置入），可能发生支架变形或错位，因此需要置入后在适当的范围内重新调整支架位置，而光学相干断层成像的三维重建技术可出色地指导这一过程。

67 Optical Coherence Tomography

Giulio Guagliumi, Lorenz Räber, Kunihiro Shimamura, Takashi Akasaka

KEY POINTS

- Optical coherence tomography (OCT) is an innovative catheter-based imaging technology that uses light and fiberoptic technology to obtain unique details of the vessels on a microscopic scale. OCT provides real-time, full tomographic views of the coronary arteries with accurate measurements.
- OCT is an efficient method to rapidly map the extension and type of coronary artery disease, guiding precise percutaneous coronary interventions (PCIs) in complex patient and lesion cohorts (i.e., acute coronary syndromes, long lesion, bifurcations to be treated with two stent strategy, calcified vessels) or in presence of angiographic ambiguity. Because of its unique properties and high axial imaging resolution, OCT is able to overcome many of the limitations of coronary angiography and intravascular ultrasound (IVUS), including assessment of extension and thickness of calcium, identification of thrombus and thereby the responsible lesion for acute coronary syndromes, detection of causes of stent failure, and addressing more precise and effective coronary interventions.
- OCT can reliably detect and quantify atherosclerotic plaque characteristics (fibrous cap thickness and integrity, thrombus, neovessels, lipid pool, macrophage accumulations), thus differentiating early-stage coronary lesions from advanced ones, with close correlation with pathology. Identification of the underlying etiology in acute coronary syndrome patients (atherothrombotic: ruptured plaque, eroded plaque, calcified nodules; nonatherosclerotic: spontaneous coronary dissections, embolic disease, spasm, external compression) based on OCT features may prompt different treatment regimens. In addition, OCT provides quantitative indices that can be used to assess the effectiveness of novel pharmacologic interventions on plaque stabilization.
- Based on accurate vessel mapping, a procedural plan during PCI, including stent length, size, and landing zone, can be generated. Recent OCT (FD-OCT) systems produce a clear visualization of long coronary segments within a few seconds, with a more complete picture of the longitudinal vessel involvement (long view), which is a better guide for PCI compared with standard cross-sectional methods. Automatic lumen detection border allows for immediate identification of the site and severity of coronary stenosis, lesion length, and reference lumen and/or vessel dimensions, for appropriate stent sizing and length.
- A major limitation of the current practice of intracoronary imaging is that the information is not immediately correlated with the images obtained by the coronary angiography. OCT coregistration enables real-time, point-to-point, correspondence between OCT imaging and the angiographic lumen contour, leading to full integration of OCT into PCI workflow.
- Direct tableside control of OCT acquisition and analysis by the operator enables the use of OCT in daily practice, and automatic visualization of stent struts malapposition and stent underexpansion facilitates stent optimization.
- Three-dimensional (3D) reconstruction of OCT images after complex stent positioning (i.e., dual stents in bifurcation, or provisional stent across a large side branch that needs to be recrossed) may facilitate rewiring in the appropriate cell to avoid stent distortion and/or strut malapposition.

INTRODUCTION

Optical coherence tomography (OCT) is an innovative real-time, tomographic imaging modality able to assess and display vascular structure at very high resolution (axial resolution from 10 to 15 μm), providing close correlation with pathology. OCT delivers near-infrared light to the wall of the coronary artery through small-diameter optical fibers. The light that illuminates the vessel is absorbed and reflected (backscattered) by the structures in the tissue to different degrees. Different tissue types have different optical characteristics and the wavelength was selected so that lipid-rich tissue can be differentiated from fibrous and calcified tissue. This feature makes OCT especially useful for following plaque progression and regression and the vascular response to coronary stent implantation, including neoatherosclerosis deposits. Although OCT resolution is not sufficient to distinguish individual cells (including regenerating endothelium), OCT is able to measure the density of cellular aggregates and to provide information about their composition. For example, the OCT imaging signal characteristics observed in ex vivo coronary arteries in the presence of accumulated foamy macrophages (high signal intensity with high attenuation, sharp shadowing, and rapid changes from frame to frame) have been demonstrated to correlate with foam cell density,[1] whereas in preclinical model, fibrin deposition on stent struts, as detected by light microscopy and scanning electron microscopy (SEM), has specific attenuation properties by OCT.[2] Recent data also indicate that OCT can measures the collagen and smooth muscle cell in atherosclerotic plaques.[3] The current generation of OCT systems has significantly improved the signal-to-noise ratio, with superior near-field image quality and faster acquisition. The lumen profile, displayed at the end of a fast (2 to 3.5 seconds) pullback and based on automatic lumen detection border in every frame, provides immediate identification of the minimal luminal area (MLA) and the maximum degree of stenosis for a more accurate planning of the percutaneous coronary intervention (PCI) procedure. OCT may be used at different times as part of diagnostic and interventional procedures, before and after stent implantation (Fig. 67.1). Quantitative measurements of lumen, stent, and neointimal areas obtained by OCT are highly reproducible among different assessors and corelabs.[4,5]

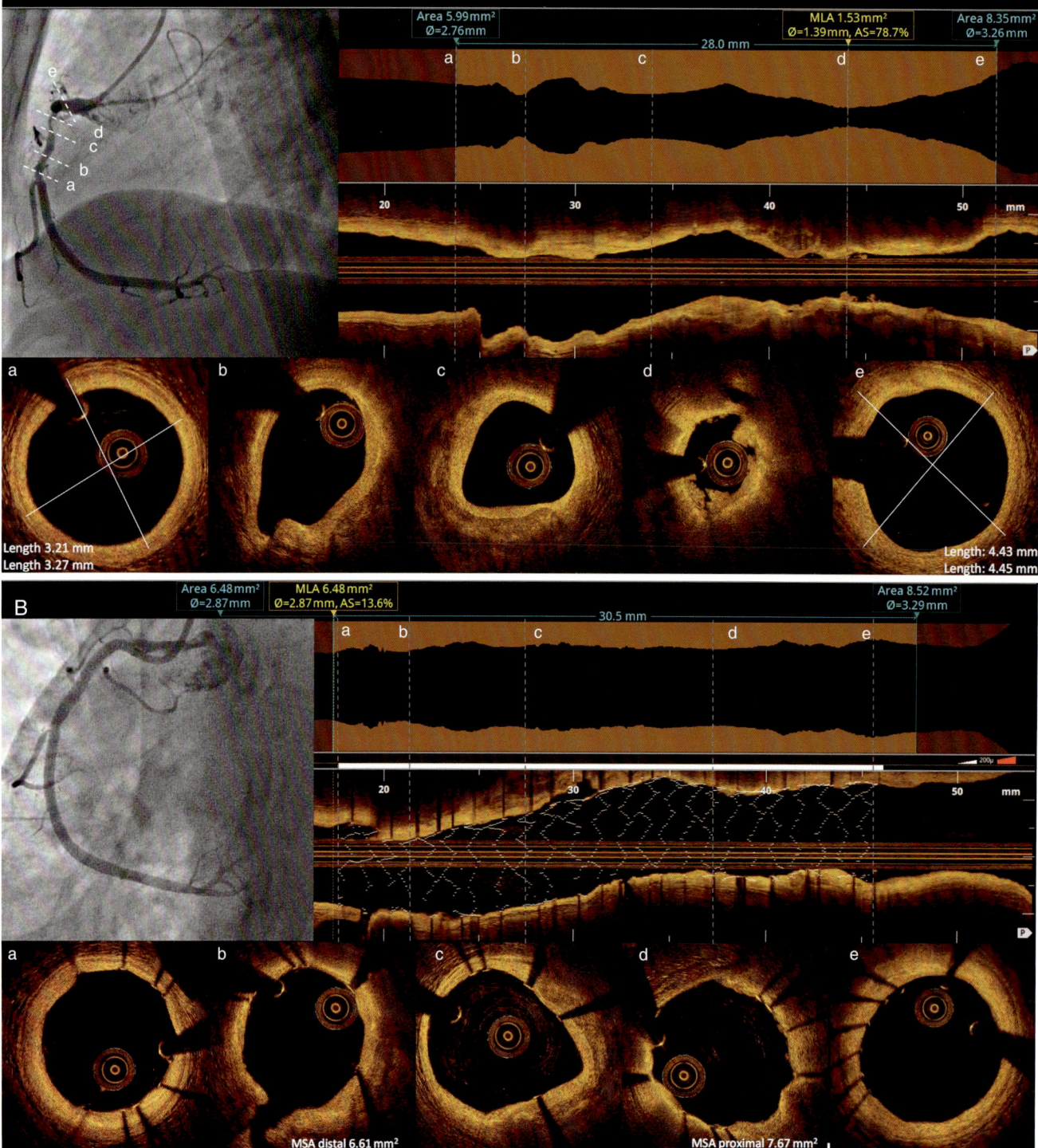

Fig. 67.1 Clinical use of optical coherence tomography (OCT) for stent optimization. Preprocedural OCT pullback performed to assess a severe lesion in the proximal-mid right coronary artery (A). Automated lumen profile detection (upper part of panel A) displayed a long lesion (28 mm, from a to e), with a minimal lumen area *(MLA)* of 1.53 mm (d) and an area stenosis (%AS) of 78.7%. OCT cross-sectional images showed different plaque types along the lesion: a fibrocalcific plaque (A-b and A-c) and a lipid-rich plaque with thrombus (A-d). Distal reference segment (A-a) with visible external elastic lamina (EEL) (rope) across the entire sections with a mean EEL diameter of 3.24 mm *(dotted lines)*. Proximal reference segment (A-e), with a mean EEL diameter of 4.44 mm. According to the smallest mean EEL diameter of the landing segments (distal reference), rounded down to the nearest 0.25 mm, a 3.0-mm stent diameter was selected. In case of stent sizing based on lumen approach, the mean distal reference diameter (2.76 mm A-e lumen profile) shall be rounded up to nearest 0.25 mm, and thus a 3.0-mm stent would be also selected. OCT pullback performed after stent implantation (B). An MLA of 6.48 mm² without stent edge dissection (B-a and B-e) and/or stent malapposition *(white apposition bar* from B-a to B-e) were detected. To assess the stent expansion, the stented segment was divided in two halves. The minimum stent area *(MSA)* at proximal stent was 7.67 mm² (B-b) with a proximal reference area of 8.52 mm² (B-d), resulting in 90% of stent expansion. The MSA at distal stent segment was 6.61 mm² with a distal reference area of 6.48 mm², resulting in a 103% stent expansion.

PHYSICAL PRINCIPLES OF OPTICAL COHERENCE TOMOGRAPHY IMAGING

The ability of OCT to create tomographic cross-sectional images of a vessel is based on optical interference of near-infrared light.[6] Light is emitted and collected back from the tip of a small-diameter optical fiber that rotates rapidly inside a transparent sheath of the catheter. For longitudinal scanning of the vessel, a drive motor unit on the table pulls back the fiber as it rotates within the sheath. The collected light carries information about the depth-resolved backscattering reflectivity of the tissue structures at the illuminated spot. Unlike ultrasound, in which the depth information can be resolved by measuring the time-of-flight of acoustic reflections, light is too fast to resolve depth information by direct measurement of photon time-of-flight. To overcome this property, the collected light is combined with a reference light beam to generate lower-frequency optical interference signals. These modulated interference signals can be measured with electronic components and digitally decoded to generate an optical backscattering profile of the tissue at the illuminated spot (A-scan). Multiple backscattering profiles are collected as the catheter core rapidly rotates within the vessel. These profiles are then represented in a two-dimensional (2D) image, the OCT B-scan frame displayed to the user.

In current Frequency-Domain OCT (FD-OCT), interference signals generated by an interferometer at various wavelengths are mathematically processed by Fourier transformation to determine the amplitudes of reflections returning from different depths. As in magnetic resonance imaging, the frequency of the recorded signal encodes position in the image.

The current generation of commercial OCT systems have a high image acquisition rate (158 to 180 frames/s), with a ranging depth of 4.6 to 5 mm in tissue. A pullback length of 75 up to 150 mm is obtained in 2 to 3.5 seconds at maximum pullback speed of 40 mm/s.

IMAGE ACQUISITION

The current generation of OCT systems improved image quality and significantly increased the speed of image acquisition by a factor of 10 compared with early generation systems. OCT uses a contrast flush (3 to 4.5 mL/s depending on vessel size) to clear the blood column and allow a clear path for the light beams to be emitted, reflected, and detected.[7] Imaging catheters are designed for rapid exchange over a 0.014-inch guidewire delivery, with a crossing profile of 2.4 to 2.8 Fr, compatible with 6-Fr or larger guiding catheters. Because of the very high speed of the pullback, OCT has the ability to scan longer segments of artery without need to occlude the vessel, resulting in minimal ischemic electrocardiographic changes and no major arrhythmias during imaging acquisition.[8]

The safety of use of OCT in current clinical practice (including patients presenting with ST-elevation myocardial infarction [STEMI] and/or stent thrombosis) has been repeatedly demonstrated.[9,10] Recently, Van der Sijde and colleagues reported the safety of intracoronary imaging (intravascular ultrasound [IVUS] and OCT) in more than 3600 consecutive diagnostic or interventional procedures (1142 performed with OCT and 2476 performed with IVUS). Invasive imaging-related complications, such as transient ST elevation, bradycardia, coronary spasm, thrombus formation, dissection, or stent deformation, were infrequent (OCT: n = 7, 0.6%; IVUS: n = 12, 0.5%; P = .6) and easily treatable. No major adverse events, prolongation of hospital stay, or enduring patient harm were observed.[11]

ARTIFACTS

Artifacts can be detected in all types of imaging, including OCT. Some artifacts are common to OCT and IVUS, whereas others are unique to the OCT imaging systems. Nonuniform rotational distortion (NURD) is caused by increased friction on the rotating components of the catheter during image acquisition and results in circumferential imaging loss or shape distortion (Fig. 67.2B). Data on bench tests have shown fewer NURD artifacts with OCT compared with IVUS.[12] The sew-up artifact results from rapid artery or imaging wire movement during single-frame imaging formation, leading to single-point misalignment of the luminal border (see Fig. 67.2A). Increased friction and deformation on the rotating components of the catheter, mainly caused by tortuous segments of coronary arteries or narrow calcified lesions, may result in coexisting multiple artifacts. The fold-over artifact is more specifically related to the new generation of FD-OCT devices. It is the consequence of "phase wrapping" or "aliasing" along the Fourier transformation when structure signals are reflected from outside the system's field of view (see Fig. 67.2F). Eccentric catheter position may affect OCT images differently before and after stent implantation. Tangential signal dropout due to eccentric catheter position adjacent to the luminal wall can lead to misinterpretation of lesions, generating a false impression of thin-cap fibroatheroma (TCFA), even giving the impression of a ruptured plaque under certain circumstances (see Fig. 67.2E).[13] In stented coronary arteries, eccentric catheter position may distort the image of the struts at distance from the scanning fiber as a result of the longer distance between each A-line and reduced lateral resolution.[6]

All cross-sectional images (frames) obtained with a pullback need to be initially screened for quality assessment and should be excluded from analysis if any portion of the image is out of the screen or if the image had poor quality caused by residual blood, artifacts, or reverberation (see Fig. 67.2).

IMAGE INTERPRETATION AND USE

OCT tissue characterization is based on signal intensity (backscattering) and signal attenuation.[14] The high resolution of OCT allows superb definition in the near field with precise bordering of the intima and media within the coronary arterial wall. In normal coronary artery, the intima appears as a signal rich layer nearest to the lumen, whereas the media is visualized as a signal-poor middle layer that encircles the vessel (three-layer structure) (Fig. 67.3A). The ability to evaluate subtle intimal thickening in vivo allows detection of the early phase of coronary atherosclerosis and monitoring of the plaque progression over time (see Fig. 67.3B). The OCT measurements of the intimal thickness are well correlated with findings on histologic examination.[15] Yabushita and coworkers developed objective OCT imaging signal criteria for differentiating distinct components of atherosclerotic tissues.[16] In their histology-controlled OCT study of 357 autopsy segments from 90 cadavers, calcified plaques appeared as signal-poor region (i.e., low backscattering) with low attenuation (signals behind can be appreciated) and with very sharp border zones (Fig. 67.4F); lipid-rich plaques, covered by a fibrous cap were characterized by a hyperintense internal layer (high backscattering), an underlying signal-poor layer with indefinite borders (high attenuation) and no other structures visible deeper in the arterial wall (see Fig. 67.4D); fibrotic plaques were seen as homogenous layers with high signal intensity (high backscattering) and low attenuation so that signals behind (e.g. media, adventitia) can still be detected. Validation tests revealed good intraobserver and interobserver reliability (κ = 0.83 to 0.84), as well as excellent sensitivity and specificity: 71% to 79% and 97% to 98%, respectively, for fibrous plaques, 95% to 96% and 97% for fibrocalcific plaques, and 90% to 94% and 90% to 92% for lipid-rich plaques. These definitions formed the basis for the in vivo assessment of plaque components and were subsequently endorsed by a Consensus Document on standardization and validation.[17] Using these definitions, Kawasaki and colleagues reported that

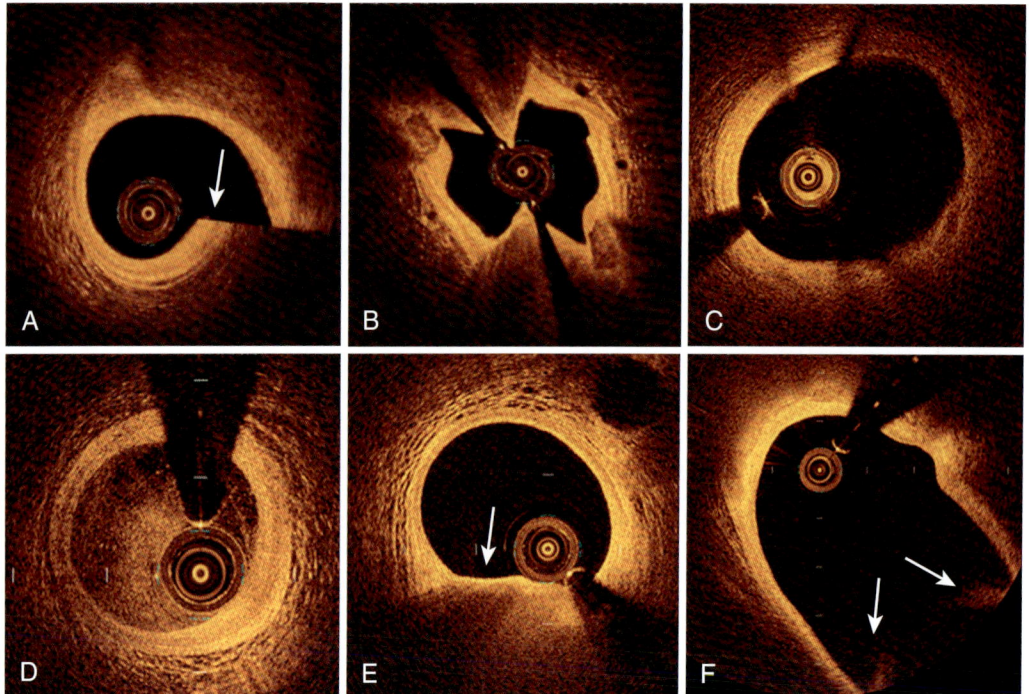

Fig. 67.2 Artifacts with optical coherence tomography. Increased friction and deformation on the rotating components can result in (A) seam line motion artifact, 3 o'clock, (B) nonuniform rotational distortion—focal image loss or shape distortion, and (C and D) artificial attenuation due to blood contamination of catheter or vessel, (E) tangential signal dropout, and (F) fold-over artifact.

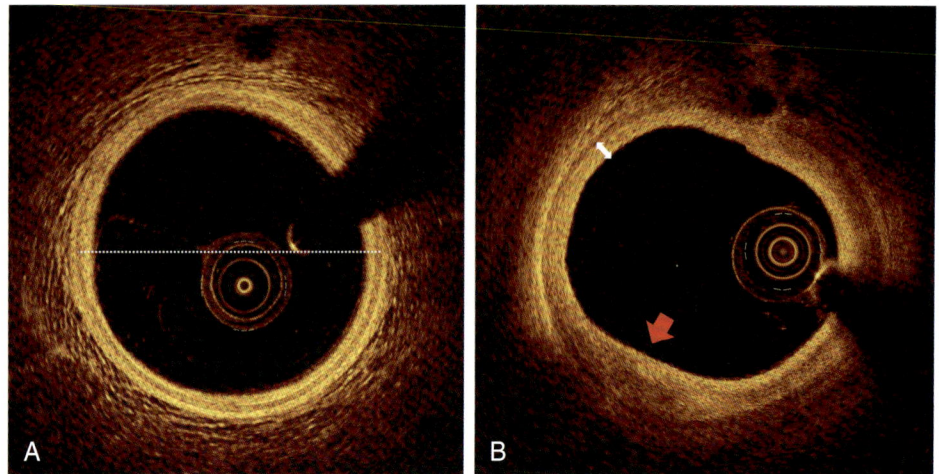

Fig. 67.3 Normal Coronary artery and early plaques in optical coherence tomography. (A) Normal/healthy vessel wall. Uniform three-layered structure composed of tunicae intima, media, and adventitia. Intima is a bright area, whereas the intermediate layer (rope) can be seen as a low-intensity area, encircling the vessel. Internal and external elastic lamina (EEL) can be detected. Visible EEL underneath a plaque can be used for plaque type identification (see Fig. 67.4) and during percutaneous coronary interventions as additional information for stent sizing based on reference landing segments (see Fig. 67.1). When applying an EEL-based approach, more than 180 degrees of EEL (in consecutive or opposite quadrants) should be visible at the selected landing sites, down-rounding the stent diameter to the smallest (usually the distal) EEL reference. (B) Intimal thickening, the first manifestation of coronary atherosclerosis *(red arrow),* appears as a homogeneous signal rich lesion without significant signal attenuation. The EEL remains visible and measurable.

OCT provided better separation of coronary plaque constituents than integrated backscatter or conventional IVUS.[18] For fibrotic plaques, the sensitivities were 98%, 94%, and 93%, respectively, and the specificities were 94%, 84%, and 61%. For calcified plaques, the sensitivities were 100%, 100%, and 100%, and the specificities were 100%, 99%, and 99%, respectively. For lipidic plaques, the sensitivities were 95%, 84%, and 67%, and the specificities were 98%, 97%, and 95%, respectively.

Distinguishing the three main tissue types from each other has a primary role in planning the PCI strategy in terms of lesion

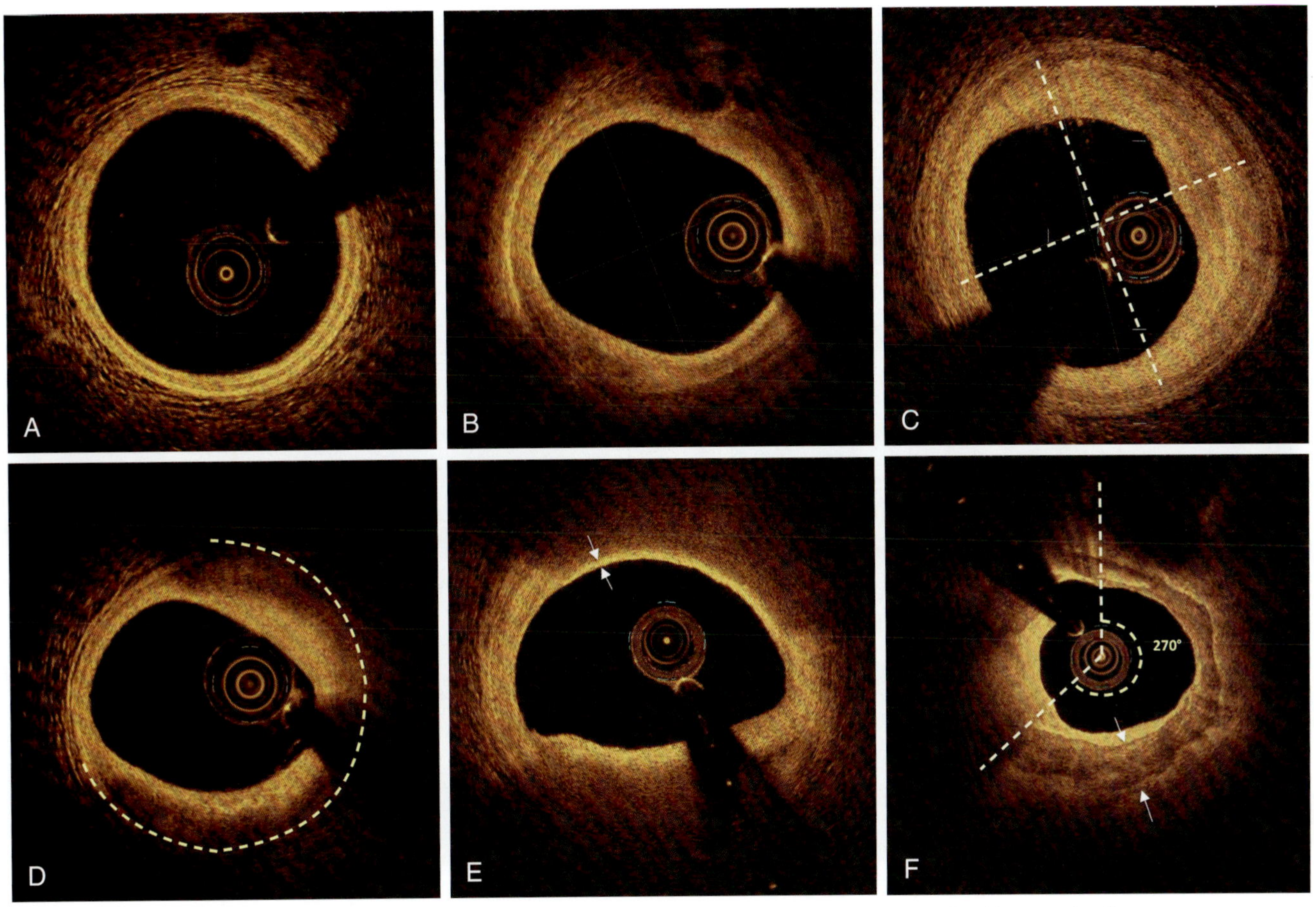

Fig. 67.4 Coronary plaque detection in optical coherence tomography. (A) Normal/healthy vessel wall. Uniform three-layered structure composed of intima, media, and adventitia. (B) Intimal thickening, with visible external elastic lamina (EEL). (C) Fibrous plaque, with concentric intimal thickening and homogeneous signal-rich appearance. EEL encircled the entire cross section. Two EEL diameters were perpendicularly measured *(dotted lines)*. (D) Lipid-rich plaque (from 11 to 8 o'clock). Lesion with lipid pool are identified as signal-poor region with poorly delineated borders, high signal drop-off (from 11 to 8 o'clock, *dotted line*) and no visible EEL behind. (E) Thin cap fibroatheroma. Lipid plaque with a cap thickness of less than 65 μm (fibrous cap thickness = 60 μm, *arrows*). (F) Severe calcific plaque, identified as a signal heterogeneous region with low attenuation, clear delineated borders but invisible EEL. Large angle (>270 degrees from 12 to 8 o'clock) of superficial thick calcification (maximum calcium thickness 680 μm, *arrows*).

preparation and optimal stent results, as the presence of large calcifications (e.g. >180 degrees, thickness >0.5 mm, length >5 mm), is a relevant predictor of poor stent expansion,[19] whereas lipid-rich tissue may increase the risk of plaque embolization and of no-reflow phenomenon. Furthermore, careful evaluation of the landing zone to avoid stent edge positioning in a segment with significant residual disease (i.e., >50% plaque burden) and especially in a lipid-rich plaque with a large lipid arc (>185 degrees) may reduce the stent edge recurrences.[20]

OCT detection of the external elastic lamina (EEL) can be used as a practical tool for assessing plaque composition and eventually appropriate stent size selection.[21] If EEL (rope) and adventitia (mesh) are visualized in a cross-sectional image, overlying normal tissue (three layered) or fibrous plaque (high intensity) can be anticipated. Conversely, if EEL cannot be seen underneath a plaque and OCT signal changes across the vessel wall (without evidence of thrombus into the lumen), high attenuation identifies a lipid plaque, whereas low attenuation and clear border recognize a calcified plaque (see Fig. 67.4).

During PCI, the knowledge of the composition of the vessel wall at the landing zones may be relevant to avoid geographical miss and select appropriate stent sizing. The threshold required to make EEL-based decisions is the visualization of at least 180 degrees of EEL at cross-sectional level. In the ILUMIEN III randomized controlled trial, the EEL identification at the reference segments was possible in 84% of the PCI cases. Local sites EEL identification was similar with OCT and IVUS, whereas core lab assessment found slightly better EEL visualization with IVUS. OCT-guided PCI using a specific EEL-based stent optimization strategy was noninferior to IVUS-guided PCI for achieving minimum stent area (MSA) and resulted in superior stent expansion and procedural success compared with angiography-guided PCI.

Unlike IVUS, coronary thrombus can be easily detected by OCT in various clinical settings, including acute coronary syndromes (ACSs) and stent thrombosis. A close correlation with pathology was demonstrated in 108 coronary arterial segments at postmortem examination.[22] White thrombus is imaged as a homogeneous, signal-rich, irregular mass with low-backscattering attenuation, whereas red thrombi are irregularly shaped, mural or luminal masses protruding into the lumen, characterized by high-backscattering attenuation and signal-free shadowing. Using a measurement of OCT signal attenuation within the thrombus, Kume and colleagues demonstrated that a cutoff value of 250 μm in the half-width of signal attenuation can differentiate

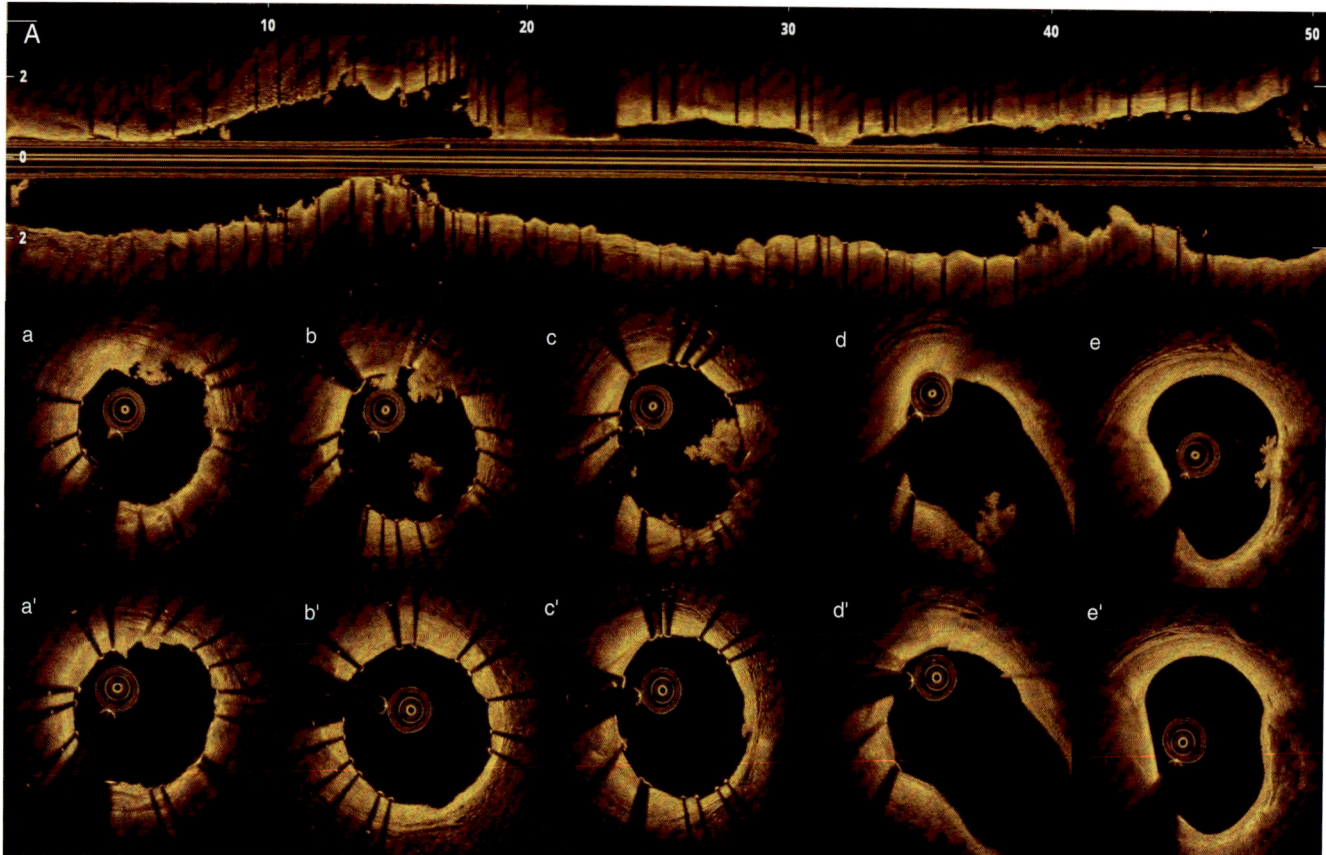

Fig. 67.5 White thrombus forming during percutaneous coronary intervention (PCI). Optical coherence tomography (OCT) pullback performed immediately after stent implantation. Multiple small intraluminal protruding masses, irregular in surface (thrombi), were detected by OCT inside and outside the stented segment (longitudinal view A and multiple cross-sectional images (A-a to A-e). White thrombus is characterized by a signal-rich mass, with no or low attenuation, protruding into the lumen. Anticlotting time (ACT) immediately measured was in the effective range recommended during PCI (280 seconds). According to the ACT result, and the accuracy of OCT in detecting new thrombus forming, IIb/IIIa receptor inhibitors were injected as dual intravenous bolus. A few minutes after the second bolus injection of IIb/IIIa receptor inhibitors, an OCT pullback was performed, revealing the complete removal of thrombus (corresponding a′ to e′ sections).

white from red thrombi with high sensitivity (90%) and specificity (88%). Thrombus detection may have important clinical implications, including identification and characterization of culprit plaque in patients presenting with ACS and unclear angiography,[23] identification of thrombus forming acutely during PCI (Fig. 67.5), and monitoring of mechanical and/or pharmacologic interventions for thrombus removal.[24] Various type of thrombus may require different approaches and interventions (Fig. 67.6).

Among various plaque components with clinical impact, macrophage accumulation plays a major role to trigger progression and instability of atherosclerotic coronary lesions. Autopsy series have shown that the thin caps of ruptured plaques are heavily infiltrated by macrophages. Given the close proximity to the lumen and its unique axial resolution, OCT enables detection of the pool of foamy macrophages confined to the luminal surface of the plaque.[25] Macrophages are identified in OCT images by the presence of high-intensity, signal-rich, linear or confluent punctuate regions (bright spots) accompanied by high attenuation and confirmed in adjacent consecutive frames. Tearney and associates tested ex vivo the ability of OCT to assess macrophage distribution within the fibrous cap. A high degree of positive correlation was reported between OCT signals and histologic measurements of fibrous cap macrophage density ($r < 0.84$, $P < .0001$). A range of OCT signal standard deviation thresholds (6.15% to 6.35%) yielded 100% sensitivity and specificity for identification of caps containing greater than 10% CD68 staining (see Fig. 67.6). Concerns have been raised about the specificity of bright-spot signals with intense attenuation in identifying macrophages. OCT may fail to discriminate macrophages from cellular fibrous tissue, calcium-fibrous tissue interfaces, microcalcifications, or cholesterol crystals.[26]

A milestone document on standardization, validation, and reporting for OCT, published by the International Working Group for Intravascular Optical Coherence Tomography, provides basic notions for collecting and interpreting imaging data with a high standard of quality and reliability.[17]

ACCURACY IN OPTICAL COHERENCE TOMOGRAPHY MEASUREMENTS

Postfixation and frozen measurements in excision tissues are not easily comparable to in vivo assessment because of possible changes in arterial optical properties caused by technical preparation and tissue shrinkage.[27] The processes of dehydration, paraffin embedding, sectioning, and staining result in a reduction of the circumference by approximately 19% ± 5% and a reduction in wall thickness of 18% ± 2%. Furthermore, backscattering of OCT signals due to fixation of cross-linked collagen may

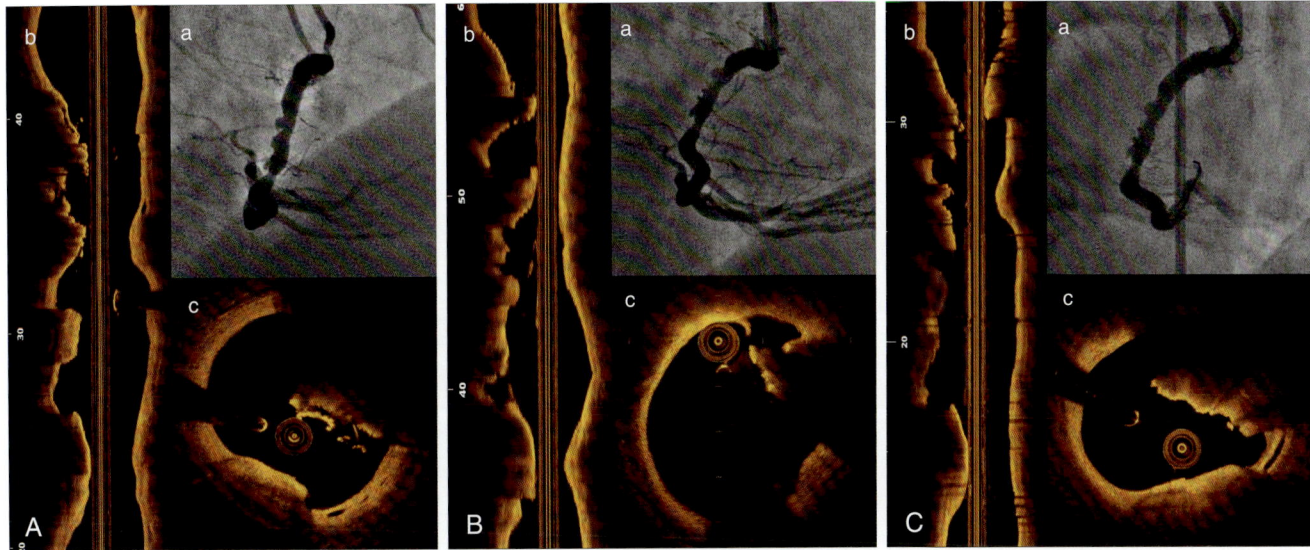

Fig. 67.6 Difficult removal of an organized red thrombus. The patient was admitted due to unstable angina. Coronary angiography (CAG) showed a moderate stenosis in the mid segment of right coronary artery (A-a) with multiple irregularities of the lumen profile, and no intraluminal filling defects. Optical coherence tomography (OCT) pullback displayed the presence of multiple intraluminal protruding masses, with surface irregularities (red thrombus A-c), impeding the vision of the underlying vessel wall. No clear ruptured plaque was identified. Red thrombus is detected by OCT as a high-backscattering protrusion with signal-free shadowing behind. Manual thrombus aspiration was attempted, without significant thrombus removal (A-b longitudinal view). Intravenous heparin infusion was started and maintained for 3 more days. Despite fewer irregularities being observed in the CAG lumen profile (B-a), no significant effects of de-thrombosis were seen in OCT with persisting red thrombi (B-b and c). Manual thrombus aspiration was performed again but was totally ineffective in thrombus removal (CAG, C-a: and OCT C-b and c). These two examples (Figs. 67.5 and 67.6) attest the role of OCT in potentially guiding therapeutic interventions.

enhance the delineation between lumen and vessel wall, compared with in vivo lumen measures, resulting in an artificial increase of reflectivity. The gap in lumen dimensions observed between OCT and histology findings in nonstented coronary segments was less clear when the arteries were treated with metallic stent implantation, with approximately 6% greater stent area and 10% greater luminal area by OCT across all stent types.[28]

In measurements of lumen diameter and luminal area, there is a good in vivo correlation between OCT and IVUS.[29,30]

To clarify differences in measures among current imaging techniques, a prospective, multicenter study comparing quantitative coronary angiography (QCA), IVUS, and OCT (Optical Coherence Tomography Compared with IVUS in a Coronary Lesion Assessment Study [OPUS-CLASS]) was performed by Kubo and colleagues in 100 patients and in a phantom model.[31] OCT accurately measured the MLA compared with the actual phantom, whereas IVUS significantly overestimated the MLA and was less reproducible than OCT ($P < .001$ vs. OCT). In the clinical study the minimal lumen diameter (MLD) measured by QCA was significantly smaller than that measured by OCT or IVUS ($P < .001$), and the MLA measured by IVUS was significantly greater than that measured by OCT, demonstrating that more accurate measurements of the coronary lumen may be achieved by using OCT compared with IVUS or QCA. In summary, compared with IVUS, OCT systematically underestimates the lumen dimensions by approximately 10%. This has clinically relevant consequences when MLA cutoffs for treatment decisions are considered, because previous validation versus fractional flow reserve (FFR) was mainly derived from IVUS studies (e.g., assessment of lesion significance in left main [LM] disease).

Reproducibility of OCT lumen and length measurements was evaluated by Fedele and associates.[32] In their study, OCT measurements were taken twice at intervals of 5 minutes in 25 patients undergoing coronary angiography. The per-segment and per-frame analyses proved to have excellent reproducibility with high correlation for intraobserver and interobserver measurements and intrapullback assessments of both lumen area and segment length ($R \geq 0.95$ and $P < .001$ for all).

A semiautomated contour-detection software that traces lumen boundaries of the longitudinal (L-mode) view is used for measurements in current generation OCT systems. The software automatically shows the cross-sectional areas calculated at all frames of the pullback as a graph superimposed on the longitudinal view. This lumen contour function enables quick and precise comparison of the automatically detected MLA with the reference areas over the entire length of the vessel imaged by the pullback (Fig. 67.7). A good correlation ($r = 0.99$) between manual and quantitative, fully automated three-dimensional (3D) lumen contour detection methods has been demonstrated.[33]

In spite of the technical ameliorations in optics, rapid imaging acquisition, automatic lumen detection and measurements (enabling use in daily practice), the adoption of OCT by cardiovascular centers remains extremely heterogeneous, ranging from routine use in Japan to more selective or occasional use in most other countries.[34] An expert consensus document on clinical use of intracoronary imaging organized by the European Association of Percutaneous Cardiovascular Interventions (EAPCI) appraises current evidence on clinical indications and provides consensus opinion regarding patients or lesions most likely to derive clinical benefit from an imaging-guided intervention, key parameters that characterize optimal stent results, and areas that warrant further research (i.e., algorithm standardization for PCI guidance) (Fig. 67.8).[35]

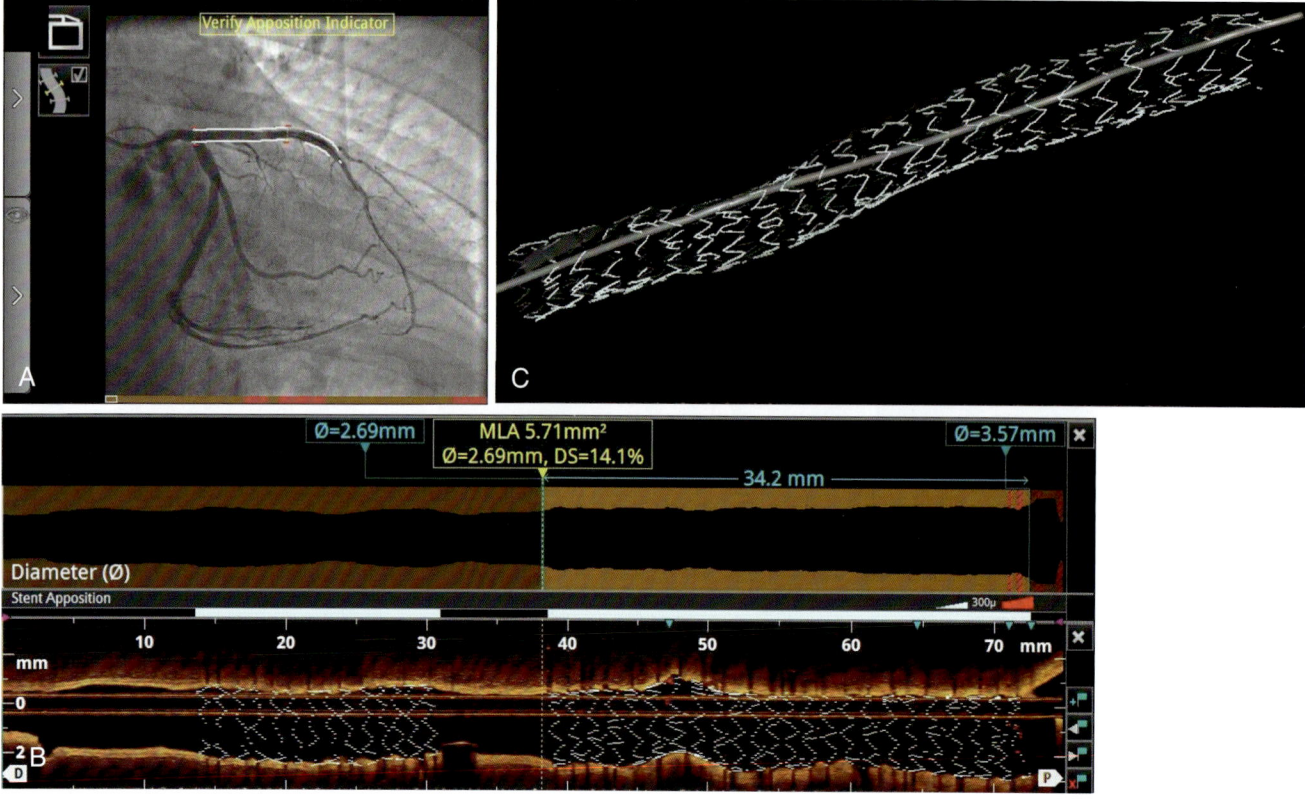

Fig. 67.7 New stent rendering system. After stent implantation, optical coherence tomography (OCT) can detect stent strut automatically. An angio-coregistration image showed there were two stents implanted in left anterior descending artery (A, *white lines*). Longitudinal OCT images revealed that two stents were implanted (B). Struts which were within 300 μm from the lumen were shown as *white dots* and struts which were more than 300 μm away from the lumen were shown as *red dots*. Three-dimensional reconstruction image also could show the stent (C). *MLA*, minimum lumen area.

CURRENT CLINICAL APPLICATION

Assessment of Coronary Atherosclerosis

Rupture of vulnerable plaque is responsible for approximately two-thirds of thrombotic coronary events. Histological features of vulnerable plaque include a large lipid core with a superimposed thin fibrous cap (cap thickness <65 μm), and an accumulation of macrophages localized at the subsurface of the fibrous cap. Because OCT has a near–histological degree of resolution, many in vitro and in vivo studies have been done to validate the capability of OCT to visualize these risky plaque features (Fig. 67.9).[36–38]

Kubo and colleagues used OCT, IVUS, and angioscopy in 30 consecutive patients with acute myocardial infarction (AMI) to assess the ability of each imaging method to detect the specific characteristics of vulnerable plaque.[37] OCT was superior in detecting plaque rupture (73% compared with 40% for IVUS and 43% for angioscopy; $P = .021$), erosion (23%, 0%, and 3%, respectively; $P = .003$), and thrombus (100%, 33%, and 100%, respectively; $P < .001$). Intraobserver and interobserver variability of OCT yielded acceptable concordance for these characteristics ($\kappa = .61$ to .83).

Because fibrous cap thickness in most ruptured plaques is less than 65 μm, the resolution required for their identification should be at least 50 μm.[38] OCT is the only available imaging technique with sufficient resolution to directly detect TCFAs.[39] Kume and coworkers examined the reliability of OCT in measuring fibrous cap thickness.[40] In 35 lipid-rich plaques from 38 human cadavers, a good correlation was observed between OCT cap thickness and histologic measures ($r = 0.90$; $P < .001$). New semiautomated software may allow one to increase the reproducibility of cap thickness measurements.[41] Jang and associates analyzed OCT images of 57 patients with stable angina pectoris (SAP), ACS, or AMI.[42] The AMI group more often had a thinner cap, more lipid, and a higher percentage of TCFA (72%, compared with 50% for the ACS group and 20% for the SAP group; $P = .012$). Using OCT, Tanaka and colleagues investigated the relationship between culprit lesion morphology and the patient's activity at the onset of ACS.[43] TCFA was a lesion predisposed to rupture in both rest onset and exertion-triggered ACS, whereas plaque rupture in those with fibrous caps thicker than 65 μm was strictly related to exertion level. Fujii and associates performed a prospective OCT analysis of all three major coronary arteries to evaluate the incidence and predictors of TCFA in patients with AMI and SAP.[44] Multiple TCFAs were observed more frequently in AMI patients than in SAP patients (69% vs. 10%; $P < .001$). In the entire cohort, multivariate analysis revealed that the only independent predictor of TCFA was AMI (odds ratio [OR] 4.12; 95% confidence interval [CI] 2.35 to 9.87; $P = .02$).

OCT has also demonstrated the ability to identify nonruptured plaque underlying coronary thrombosis.[45,46] Increasing attention has been paid to plaque erosion, histologically characterized by luminal thrombus and denudation of the endothelium, without evidence of fibrous cap disruption.[47] Because the resolution of OCT is insufficient to visualize endothelial cells, in vivo evidence of erosion remains indirect, based on the presence of thrombus and absence of fibrous cap rupture, an approach likely leading to some imprecision (Fig. 67.10). In an OCT observational study including 139 consecutive ACS cases, patients with erosion at the

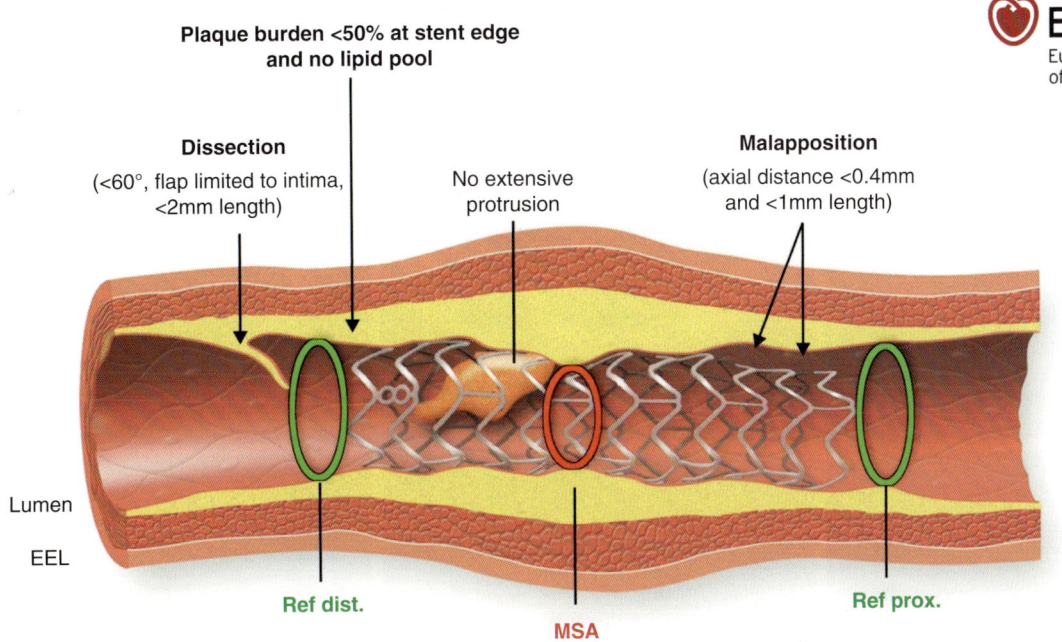

Fig. 67.8 Summary of postpercutaneous coronary intervention optimization targets for intravascular ultrasound *(IVUS)* and optical coherence tomography *(OCT)*. The most relevant targets to be achieved following stent implantation are shown. These include optimal stent expansion (absolute as well as relative to reference lumen diameter); avoidance of landing in significantly diseased vessel segments (atherosclerotic burden >50% of circumference or lipid-rich tissue); avoidance of large areas of stent malapposition; iregular tissue protrusion/dissections. Indications provided reflect the consensus of this group. Some are based on consistent and robust prospective data (e.g., stent expansion, landing zone) and others are less established (e.g., stent malapposition). *EEL,* External elastic lamina; *MSA,* minimum stent area. (From Räber L, Mintz GS, Koskinas KC, et al. Clinical use of intracoronary imaging. Part 1: guidance and optimization of coronary interventions. An expert consensus document of the European Association of Percutaneous Cardiovascular Interventions. Endorsed by the Chinese Society of Cardiology. *Eur Heart J.* Published online May 22, 2018. https://doi.org/10.1093/eurheartj/ehy285. Published on behalf of the European Society of Cardiology by permission of the Oxford University Press.)

culprit site had significantly improved major adverse cardiovascular events (MACEs) compared with plaque rupture throughout a mean follow-up of 32 months (erosions 14.0% vs. cap rupture 39.0% $P = .001$).[48]

Plaques with superficial calcific nodules are also assumed prone to rupture. An OCT study conducted by Lee and colleagues in 889 de novo culprit lesions (48% of patients presenting with ACS) demonstrated that calcific nodules were seen in 4.2% of all lesions.[49] In lesions with severe calcification (maximum calcium arc >180 degrees), 30% of ACS culprit lesions contained a calcific nodule, and the presence of calcific nodules was associated with ACS presentation independently of other vulnerable plaque morphologies.

Impact of Optical Coherence Tomography on Treatment Strategy in Acute Coronary Syndrome Patients

Culprit Plaque Morphology

In patients presenting with ACS (STEMI, non-STEMI [NSTEMI], unstable angina), data derived by OCT on culprit plaque (residual stenosis, plaque morphology) after thrombus removal have been used to decide different invasive strategies. Two observational studies suggest possible conservative treatment strategy (i.e., without stenting, guided by OCT).[50,51] The conservative strategy used manual thrombus aspiration and/or additional treatment with antiplatelet agents (glycoprotein IIb/IIIa inhibitor [GPI]), aspirin, clopidogrel or prasugrel, without stenting (see Fig. 67.10). If effective reperfusion and optimal thrombus regression were achieved on angiography, stenting was postponed allowing more time for the antithrombotic regimen to work, as determined by the results of a second angiogram and OCT.[50] The trigger for stenting was residual stenosis in the culprit lesion greater than 70% or evidence of large plaque prolapse. Only 62% of the patients received stent implantation. During a minimum follow-up period of 12 months, only one nonfatal myocardial infarction occurred, and only one additional stent implantation was performed for angina. The authors concluded that medical management without stents is safe and feasible in OCT-selected patients presenting with ACS and large thrombus burden, possibly reducing the risk of no-reflow phenomena in this setting. OCT revealed culprit lesion characteristics that were not disclosed by angiography and facilitated treatment decisions.

A prospective, proof of concept, single-center study performed in China, demonstrated that patients with ACS caused by plaque erosion detected by OCT can be successfully managed

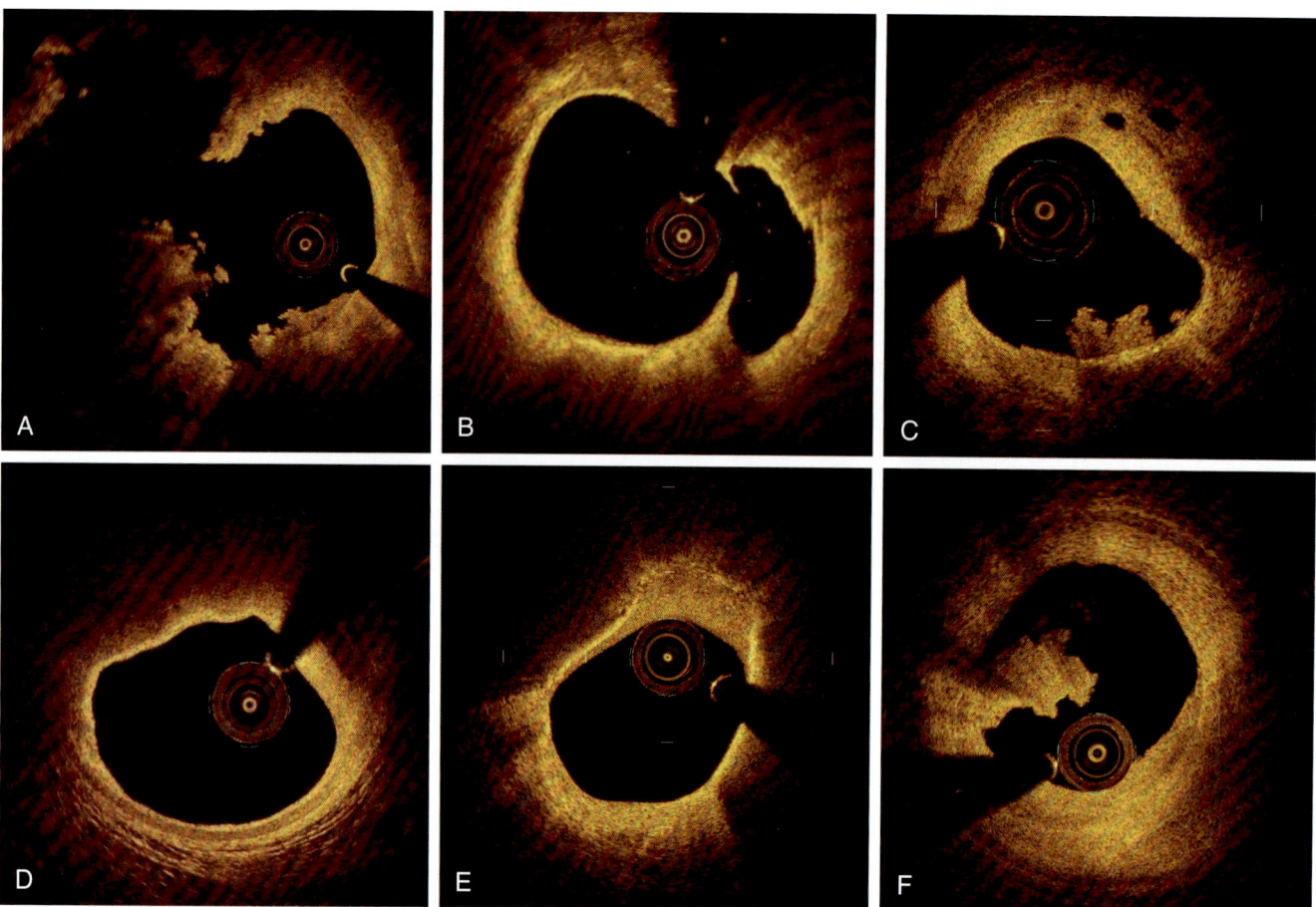

Fig. 67.9 Vulnerable plaque features. (A) Plaque rupture (from 9 to 12 o'clock) and protruding luminal thrombus (from 7 to 9 o'clock). (B) Plaque rupture is visualized as fibrous cap discontinuity which gives entrance to a cavity in communication with the vessel's lumen. Ruptured plaques usually have an extensive lipid core and a thin fibrous cap. The fibrous cap is typically thinnest at the site of rupture, and the plaque cavity indicates loss of lipid core due to the rupture. (C) Erosion with large lumen and multiple white protruding thrombi (from 5 o'clock to 6 o'clock) attached to a plaque with intact fibrous cap. (D) Thin-cap fibroatheroma with lipid-rich plaque and a cap thickness of less than 65 μm (9 to 12 o'clock). (E) Macrophage infiltrations are seen as a signal-rich, confluent or punctuate region that exceeds the intensity of background speckle noise (from 9 to 12 o'clock and from 2 to 4 o'clock). (F) White thrombus (8 to 9 o'clock) is visualized as intraluminal, protruding tissue with low attenuation and low backscattering of the optical signal.

by manual thrombectomy and/or GPIs followed by antiplatelet therapy (aspirin and ticagrelor) without stenting.[51] Among those 55 patients who revealed an angiographic stenosis of less than 70% following thrombus aspiration, antithrombotic therapy was provided without stenting. Thrombus volume was significantly decreased (−94.2%) and thrombus area was reduced by more than 50% in 78% of patients within 1 month. Minimal flow area increased from 1.7 to 2.1 mm². At 1-year follow-up the majority (92.5%) of patients treated with aspirin and ticagrelor without stenting remained free from MACEs, with a further decrease in thrombus volume between 1 month and 1 year.[52] Patients without residual thrombus were more frequently treated with GPI during the acute phase and had a lower thrombus volume at baseline.

Several caveats apply to such a treatment strategy. First, the reliable identification of the culprit plaque phenotype is not always possible, especially in patients presenting with STEMI, due to the amount of remaining thrombus which frequently obscures the underlying culprit plaque.[53] Second, these studies were underpowered for the clinical end point and did not include a control group treated with current-generation drug-eluting stents (DESs), which have been proven to be effective in treating STEMI due to eroded plaque by serial OCT observations.[54] Third, low-flow area and lethal bleeds were observed in these studies. Considering the possible impact on clinical, logistic, and legal aspects, these studies should be considered as hypothesis generating and need an adequately powered prospective randomized controlled study prior to application in daily routine.

Culprit Lesion Identification

Sometimes in patients presenting with STEMI/NSTEMI, the delineation of the culprit lesion can be challenging due to discordant clinical and angiographic findings, no identifiable lesion on angiography, or multiple potential culprits. The final common pathway of all the culprit plaques is thrombus, better identified by OCT than by IVUS (Fig. 67.11). Patients with myocardial infarction and nonobstructive fluoroscopic coronary artery disease, or with coronary artery spasm almost always show some form of atherosclerosis rather than normal arterial segments (microthrombi with/without lesions with an intact fibrous cap are the major abnormal morphologic findings detected by OCT) (Fig. 67.12).[55] These lesions have a more benign natural history than plaque ruptures. Additional OCT imaging may be useful to recognize the mechanism of ischemia and guide pharmacological and interventional decisions.

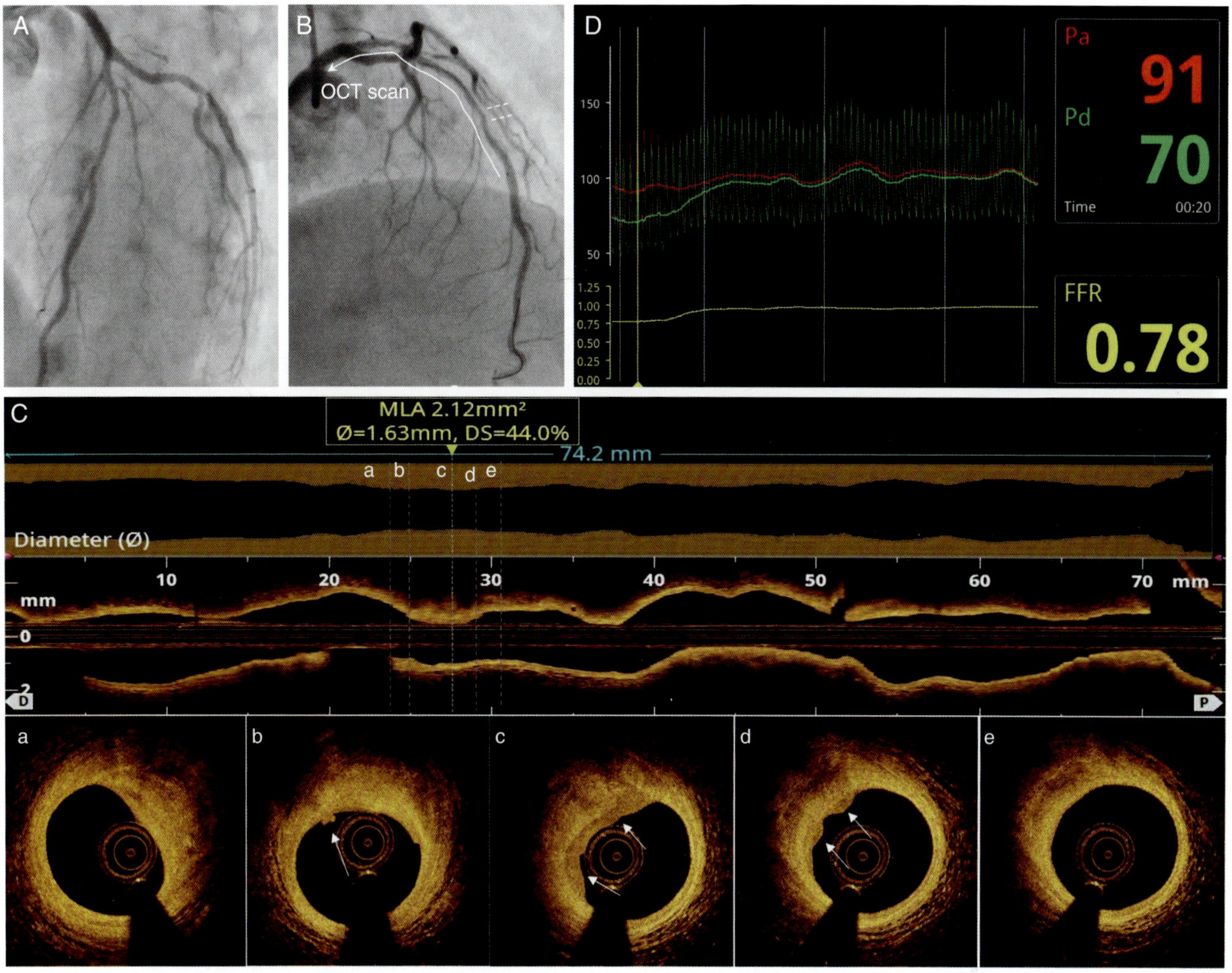

CHAPTER 67 Optical Coherence Tomography

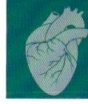

Fig. 67.10 Identification of culprit plaque in acute coronary syndrome and guidance for treatment. A 54-year-old female was admitted for non–ST-elevation myocardial infarction showing positive cardiac troponin and severe hypokinesis of the anterior wall. Coronary angiography demonstrated an intermediate stenosis in mid left anterior descending artery (LAD) with borderline fractional flow reserve (FFR) findings (A, B and D). Optical coherence tomography (OCT) longitudinal image also revealed intermediate stenosis, minimum lumen area (MLA) 2.12 mm² (C). OCT cross-sectional images showed fibrous plaque without intimal disruption (C-a to C-e) and thrombus (C-b to C-d, *white arrow*) indicating that the culprit lesion is plaque erosion. Patient was treated with optimal medical therapy including dual antiplatelet inhibition. No clinical events were observed at 1 year follow-up.

Spontaneous coronary artery dissection (SCAD) is an increasingly recognized cause of nonatherosclerotic ACS. SCAD can be misdiagnosed on coronary angiography, especially when it results in a diffuse stenosis with intramural hematoma compressing the true coronary lumen. Accurate diagnosis of SCAD is key because of differences in management compared with atherosclerotic disease. Success rate of revascularization is lower in SCAD, and, whenever possible, a conservative management strategy is indicated in patients with thrombolysis in myocardial infarction (TIMI) 3 flow in the infarct related artery. OCT allows direct visualization of intimal discontinuity, dissection flap and intramural hematoma.[56] However, since potential harm may be caused by the manipulation of the catheter within a dissected artery, it is advisable to avoid OCT imaging in suspected SCAD involving distal segments or small coronary arteries.

The most important role of OCT imaging may be in the guidance of percutaneous treatment, if required by ongoing, uncontrolled ischemia and or hemodynamic instability. By revealing the site of intimomedial flap, the longitudinal extent of the intramural hematoma, the position of the wire within the distal true lumen, and the stent apposition (Fig 67.13), OCT-guided PCI for SCAD resulted in favorable clinical outcomes, similar to other ACS etiologies.[57]

High-Risk Nonculprit Plaques

The ability of OCT to predict plaque instability over time is less established although clinically relevant.

Prospective studies are still needed to define which morphologic features of the plaque are associated with negative clinical outcome. Uemura and colleagues prospectively studied the ability of OCT to predict the natural history of nonsignificant coronary plaques (NSCPs). Fifty-three consecutive coronary artery disease patients with clinical indication for PCI and an additional nonobstructing coronary lesion (percent diameter stenosis <50%) at baseline angiogram were followed to evaluate the progression of NSCPs.[58]

Thirteen (18.8%) out of 69 lesions showed progression on angiography at 7-month follow-up. Several plaque characteristics detected by OCT were predictive of progression: intimal laceration (61.5% in those plaques with progression vs. 8.9% in those without progression; $P < .01$), presence of

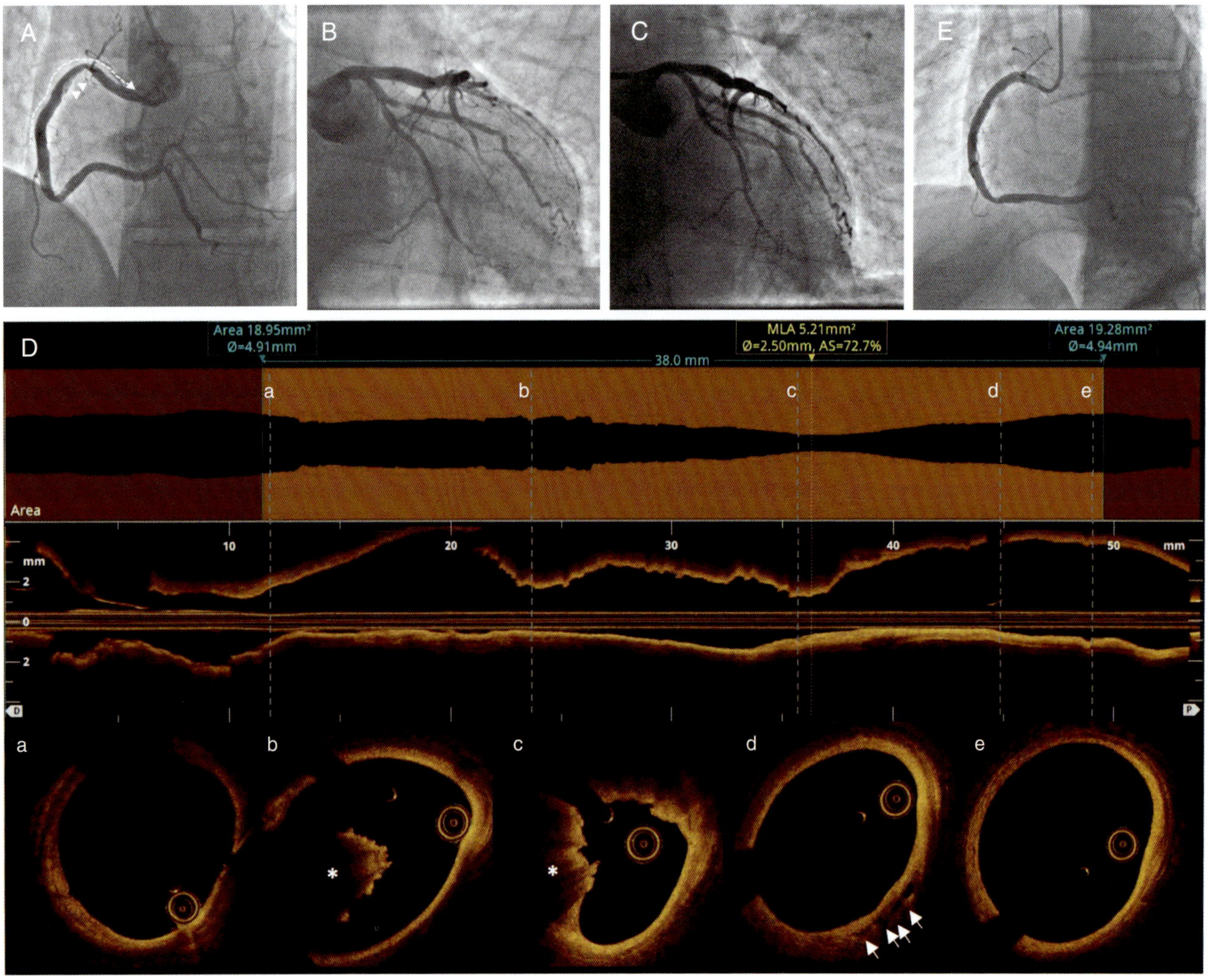

SECTION VI Evaluation of Interventional Techniques

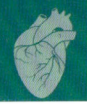

Fig. 67.11 Identify the morphology of non–ST-elevation myocardial infarction. A 60-year-old male admitted to the hospital because of acute chest pain. ECG revealed no significant ECG change with slightly positive cardiac troponin. Coronary angiography revealed moderate stenosis with contrast filling defect in the proximal portion of right coronary artery (RCA) (A, *arrow head*) and severe stenosis in the proximal portion of obtuse marginal branch (OM) (B). At first, everolimus-eluting stent (EES) 2.5/15 was implanted into OM based on the lesion severity (C). Then, optical coherence tomography (OCT) pullback was performed from the mid portion of RCA (A, *dotted arrow*) A red thrombus was observed protruding into the lumen on top of a lipid rich plaque (D-b and D-c, *asterisk*) with TCFA and microvessels (D-d, *white arrow*). According to the OCT imaging data, the culprit lesion was correctly identified and an EES 4/38 mm was implanted to the proximal portion of RCA (E). *AS*, Area stenosis; *MLA*, minimal luminal area; *TCFA*, thin-cap fibroatheroma.

microchannels (76.9% vs. 14.3%; $P < .01$), lipid pools (100% vs. 60.7%; $P = .02$), TCFA (76.9% vs. 14.3%; $P < .01$), macrophage images (61.5% vs. 14.3%; $P < .01$), and intraluminal thrombi (30.8% vs. 1.8%; $P < .01$). Regression analysis revealed TCFA and microchannel images to be strong predictors of disease progression, each with an OR of approximately 20. The luminal diameter of the stenosis was not predictive of plaque progression.

Cross-sectional studies of risk stratification by OCT have also been published. Yonetsu and associates reported a study of 266 coronary plaques identified on angiography.[59] A reliable measure of cap thickness was obtained in 188 (70.7%). The thickness of the fibrous cap was an independent predictor of plaque rupture, and the cutoff thickness for plaque rupture prediction was estimated to be less than 67 μm, in line with the data described by histology.

Finally, Guo and associates performed a cross-sectional study to evaluate the characteristics of coronary plaques associated with coronary thrombosis.[60] They included 42 patients with coronary plaque rupture detected by OCT in 216 native coronary artery lesions. Plaques were divided into those with thrombus (64% of coronary plaques) and those without thrombus. Ruptured plaques with thrombus had significantly thinner fibrous caps than those without thrombus (57 vs. 96 μm; $P = .008$).

The Relationship between coronary plaque morphology of the left anterior descending artery and long term clinical outcome (CLIMA) study investigated the predictive value of four OCT-based criteria to predict 1-year cardiac death or myocardial infarction in patients with nonsignificant proximal left anterior descending artery stenosis presenting for a clinically indicated angiography.[61] The four prespecified OCT criteria included a MLA <3.5 mm², lipid arc >180 degrees, cap thickness <75 μm, and the presence of macrophages. A total of 1004 patients were included, and these criteria were present only in a minority of 36 patients (3.6%). At 1 year, cardiac death or myocardial infarction occurred in 18.9% of patients fulfilling all four criteria and in 3% of the remainder (hazard ratio [HR] 7.54; 95% CI 3.1 to 18.6; $P < .001$).

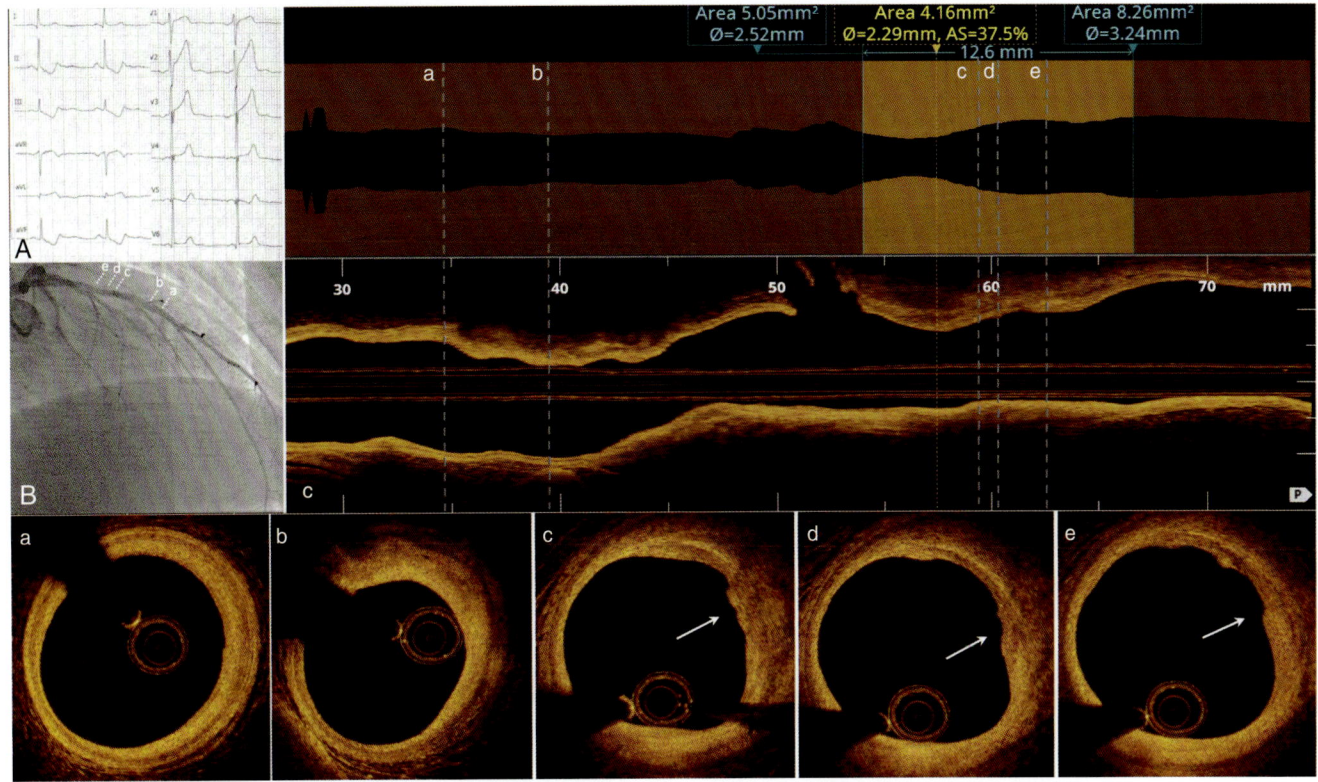

Fig. 67.12 Optical coherence tomography findings in myocardial infarction with nonobstructive coronary artery. A 45-year-old male was admitted with acute chest pain. ECG revealed ST elevation in the precordial leads (A) with positive cardiac troponin and akinesia in the anterior wall. The coronary angiography showed no obstructive coronary artery disease (B). Optical coherence tomography (OCT) longitudinal view showed only minor atherosclerotic plaques of fibrous tissue, without significant lumen reduction or clear thrombus deposition (C-a to C-e). However, clear irregularities of the intimal surface were detected in consecutive cross-sectional views (C-c to C-e, *white arrows*).

Optical Coherence Tomography to Monitor Reversal of Plaque Vulnerability

Due to the ability to measure fibrous cap thickness at different time periods, OCT can be used to monitor the impact of lipid-lowering agents on advanced coronary plaques (Fig. 67.14). An OCT study conducted by Takarada and coworkers demonstrated that statin therapy in patients with hyperlipidemia significantly increased the thickness of the fibrous cap (from 151 ± 110 μm to 280 ± 120 μm; $P < .01$) at 9 months' follow-up.[62]

In a prospective study of 42 patients with stable angina reported by Hattori and coworkers, statin therapy resulted in an increase in fibrous cap thickness when compared with dietary modification alone (52 ± 32 μm vs. 2 ± 22 μm, $P < .001$).[63]

In the EASY-FIT (Effect of AtorvaStatin therapY on FIbrous cap Thickness in coronary aterosclerotic plaque as assessed by optical coherence tomography) study, 70 patients with unstable angina were randomly assigned to either atorvastatin 20 mg or 5 mg, and OCT was serially performed in nonculprit plaques at baseline and 12 months.[64] The increase in fibrous cap thickness by means of OCT was greater in the higher-intensity statin group as compared with the low-dose statin group (69% vs. 17%; $P < .001$), and the change in cap thickness correlated with the reduction in low-density lipoprotein-C ($R = -0.450$; $P < .001$).

Nakamura and colleagues demonstrated in patients with STEMI that the proportion of TCFA observed in the culprit vessel decreased significantly from baseline to 9 months' follow-up in the high-intensity statin therapy group (26.4% vs. 9.7%; $P < .01$) compared with the lower-intensity statin therapy group (38.9% vs. 25%; $P = .18$).[65] In the Integrated biomarker and imaging study (IBIS-4), 153 nonnfarct-related arteries of 83 STEMI patients were assessed by OCT, and serial changes of cap thickness, macrophage accumulations, and lipid pool angle were assessed at baseline and 12 months' follow-up.[66] Minimum fibrous cap thickness as assessed using a semiautomated software increased from 64.9 ± 19.9 μm to 87.9 ± 38.1 μm ($P = .008$). Macrophage line arc decreased from 9.6 ± 12.8 degrees to 6.4 ± 9.6 degrees ($P < .0001$), and mean lipid arc decreased from 55.9 ± 37 degrees to 43.5 ± 33.5 degrees. In a lesion-level analysis ($n = 191$), 9 of 13 TCFAs at baseline (69.2%) regressed to non-TCFAs. Although it remains to be proved whether stabilizing morphometric plaque characteristics improves clinical outcome, OCT represents a unique tool for the in vivo monitoring of the impact of pharmacotherapy on advanced coronary plaques.

In summary, OCT can be used to evaluate morphologic features of atherosclerotic plaques and attempt risk stratification of rupture or progression according to specific morphologic characteristics. However, it is still unknown which patients undergoing diagnostic or interventional procedures should be screened for early detection of high-risk plaque and which changes in therapeutic management might occur after such accurate evaluation.

STENT ASSESSMENT

Given the large number of stents implanted each year, the exceptional technical evolution, and the major remaining issues of stent failure and thrombosis, OCT plays a very significant role for immediate and long-term stent assessment. OCT may contribute at various stages of stent placement: mapping the vessel disease before implantation, optimizing the stent deployment,

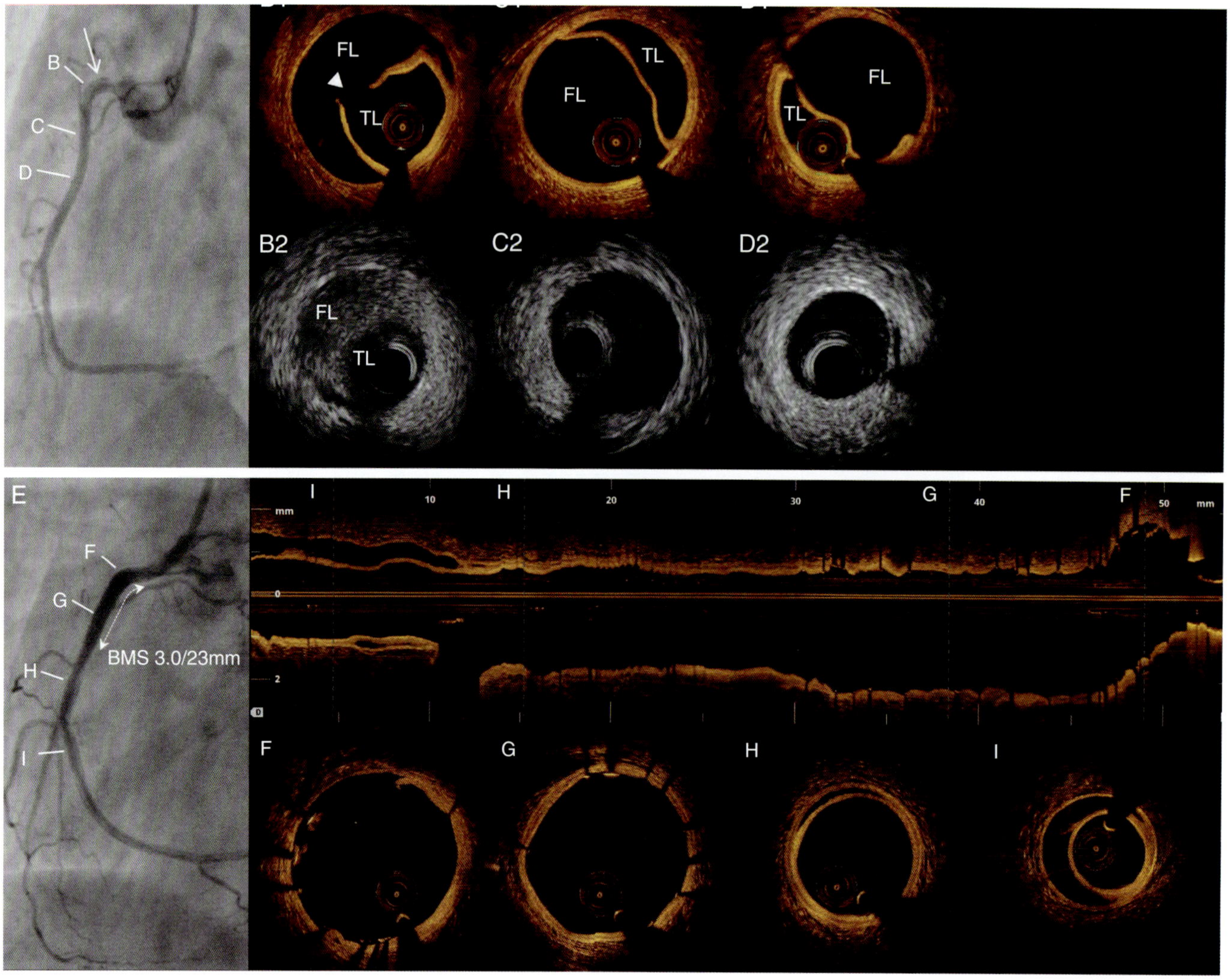

SECTION VI Evaluation of Interventional Techniques

Fig. 67.13 Identification of spontaneous coronary artery dissection and percutaneous coronary interventions guidance. A 43-year-old female was admitted due to recurring chest pain. ECG revealed an inverted T wave in lead II, III, aVF with positive cardiac troponin. Coronary angiography showed thrombolysis in myocardial infarction 2 grade flow with the contrast staining in proximal right coronary artery (A, *white arrow*). Optical coherence tomography (OCT) clearly depicted true lumen (B1 to D1, *TL*), false lumen (B1 to D1, *FL*), and the entry point compared with intravascular ultrasound (IVUS) (B2 to D2). Moreover, OCT identified the wire was segmentally passing through false lumen (B2), which IVUS did not clearly visualize (C2). After confirming the recrossed wire in the true lumen by OCT, bare metal stent *(BMS)* (3.0/23 mm) spot stenting, which covered the entry point of intimal tear, was preformed with OCT guidance. After stent implantation, the contrast staining disappeared (E) and OCT showed the entry point of intimal tear and false lumen were closed (F and G) and false lumen decreased distally to the stent (H and I).

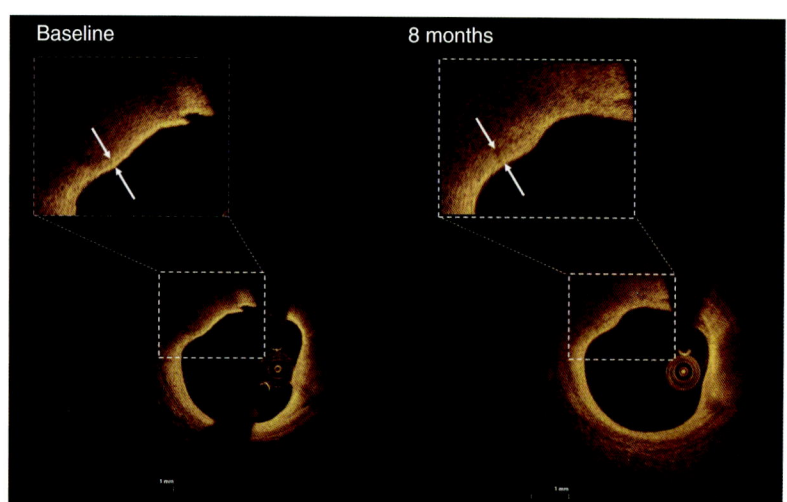

Fig. 67.14 Impact of lipid-lowering agents on advanced coronary plaques. A 55-year-old male was admitted with inferior ST-elevation myocardial infarction. Primary PCI was performed at the culprit lesion in mid right coronary artery. TCFA was observed at nonculprit-sites. High-intensity statin therapy (atorvastatin 80 mg od) was started and recommended in follow-up. OCT performed at 8 months follow-up demonstrated a significant increase of the minimum fibrous cap thickness at nonculprit lipid plaque (from 110 to 310 μm), with lumen enlargement (7.63 to 8.50 mm^2) compared with the baseline. *OCT,* Optical coherence tomography; *PCI,* percutaneous coronary intervention; *TCFA,* thin-cap fibroatheroma.

CHAPTER 67 Optical Coherence Tomography

quantifying the degree of stent coverage, and evaluating the mechanisms of delayed healing and thrombus formation.[67]

OCT can be used as an adjunct to PCI:

1. Preprocedure
   - To establish the real extent and severity of the atherosclerotic disease and choose the appropriate stent size and length (see Fig. 67.1)
   - To carefully assess the landing zone to avoid lipid-rich plaque or TCFA sitting at the stent edges
   - To establish the presence, type, and distribution of coronary calcium that may impact on stent expansion (i.e., circumferential distribution, length, and thickness of calcium) and eventually to guide a more aggressive lesion preparation (Fig. 67.15)
   - To establish the 3D anatomy and plaque distribution in complex lesion settings (i.e., bifurcation: plaque distribution at flow divider or limited to the opposite vessel wall; carina characteristics; length, angle prone to displacement with risk of side-branch occlusion).

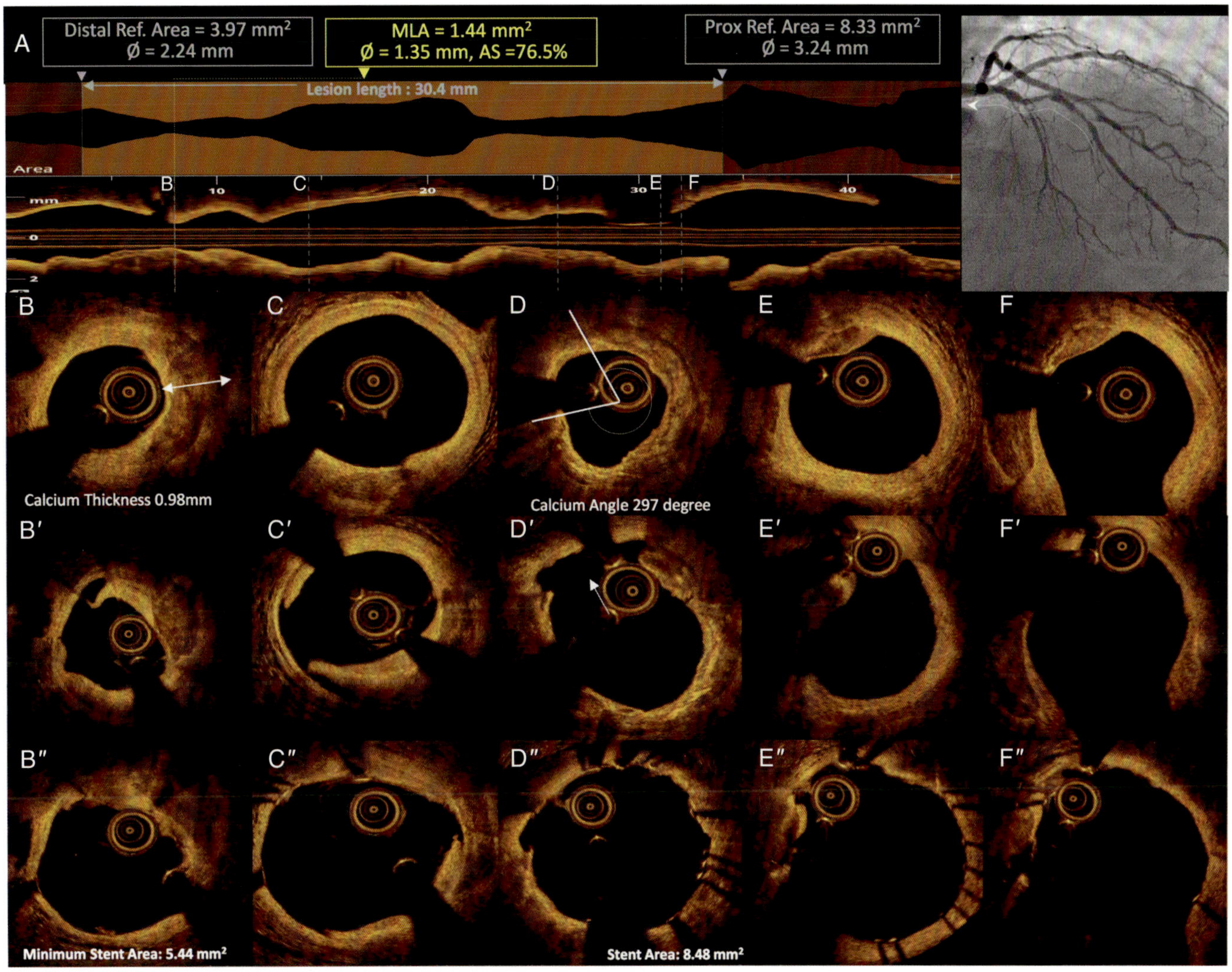

Fig. 67.15 Role of calcium fracture for stent expansion. Preprocedural optical coherence tomography (OCT) pullback *(dotted arrow)* was performed from mid to proximal left anterior descending artery (A). Longitudinal image (A) and cross-sectional images (B–F). OCT images showed multiple fibrocalcific lesions with mild (0 to 180-degree arc) (B, C, E, and F) to severe calcification (>270-degree arc) (D). Longitudinal image revealed there were multiple lesions in the distal and proximal segments. Different types of calcification were shown. There was focal calcification in the distal segment (B and C), and superficial or protruding calcium in the proximal segment (D, E, and F) Multiple calcified lesions were observed with different degrees of circumferential vessel involvement (mild 0–180-degree arc: B,C,E and F; severe >270-degree arc: D) and calcium thickness (B, 980 μm). Maximum calcium angle 297 degrees (D), maximum calcium thickness 0.98 mm (B), and calcium length 28.4 mm were combined to calculate a calcium score to assess the possible risk of stent underexpansion. A calcium score of 4 predicted a suboptimal stent expansion, suggesting an aggressive lesion preparation. According to the OCT assessment, scoring balloon was used on multiple calcified plaques. After lesion preparation, OCT images showed the expanded vessel with cracks of the calcified segments (D′, *arrow head*) and limited dissection (B′ to F′). Two everolimus-eluting stents (3.0/15 and 3.5/18 mm) were implanted with minimum overlap and postdilated with noncompliant balloons (3.0/15 mm, 22 atm. in the distal stent and 3.5/15 mm, 22 atm. in the proximal stent). Severe calcified segment (D) was expanded to 8.48 mm² (D″). Minimum lumen area was 5.44 mm² and the Expansion Index was 1.07. *AS,* Area stenosis; *MLA,* minimal luminal area.

2. Immediately after stent implantation
    - To document full stent apposition and adequate expansion
    - To confirm the full coverage of the diseased segment
    - To unmask relevant edge dissection, tissue protrusion, and remaining thrombus, which may significantly impact the patient outcome[68]
    - To guide the adequate cell rewiring toward major side branches with novel 3D imaging software (Fig. 67.16).[69]

Thresholds that should lead to corrective measures were recently published in an international consensus document.[35]

3. Stent/scaffold observed at follow-up
    - To disclose and measure the degree of stent strut coverage by tissues (quantitative analyses)
    - To assess causative mechanisms of stent failure, including excessive growing tissue, differentiated by optical properties (e.g., backscatter intensity and attenuation) in restenosis and neoatherosclerosis (Fig. 67.17)
    - To discover late malapposition, peristrut cavities, and local signs of toxicity in DESs or dismantling processes in bioresorbable scaffolds
    - To possibly individualize the treatment of stent failure based on causative mechanisms.

Despite more accurate information provided by high-resolution intracoronary imaging on stent positioning, mentally mapping the planned stent position from imaging to fluoroscopy remains challenging and time consuming. Direct translation of a desired stent implantation position from imaging to coronary angiography would result in more precise lesion coverage and stent placement. Co-registration of OCT imaging with coronary angiography allows a real-time point-to-point correspondence between angiographic and intracoronary images, automatically matched and displayed on an operational monitor of the CathLab, to avoid operator misjudgement (Fig 67.18). The basic principle of this system consists of tracking the radiopaque lens marker of the OCT catheter on the angiographic cine acquired during the OCT pullback.[70]

Principle of Stent Imaging

Metallic stent struts are strong reflectors of light and appear as bright points along the circumference of the vessel. Because light cannot penetrate the metallic strut, a shadow is generated behind. Therefore light reflection from the luminal surface of the metal does not provide a direct measurement of strut thickness. The luminal surface of the strut is expected to be found in the middle of the blooming, so half of the blooming value should be used as standard for calculation. When strut-level analysis is performed,

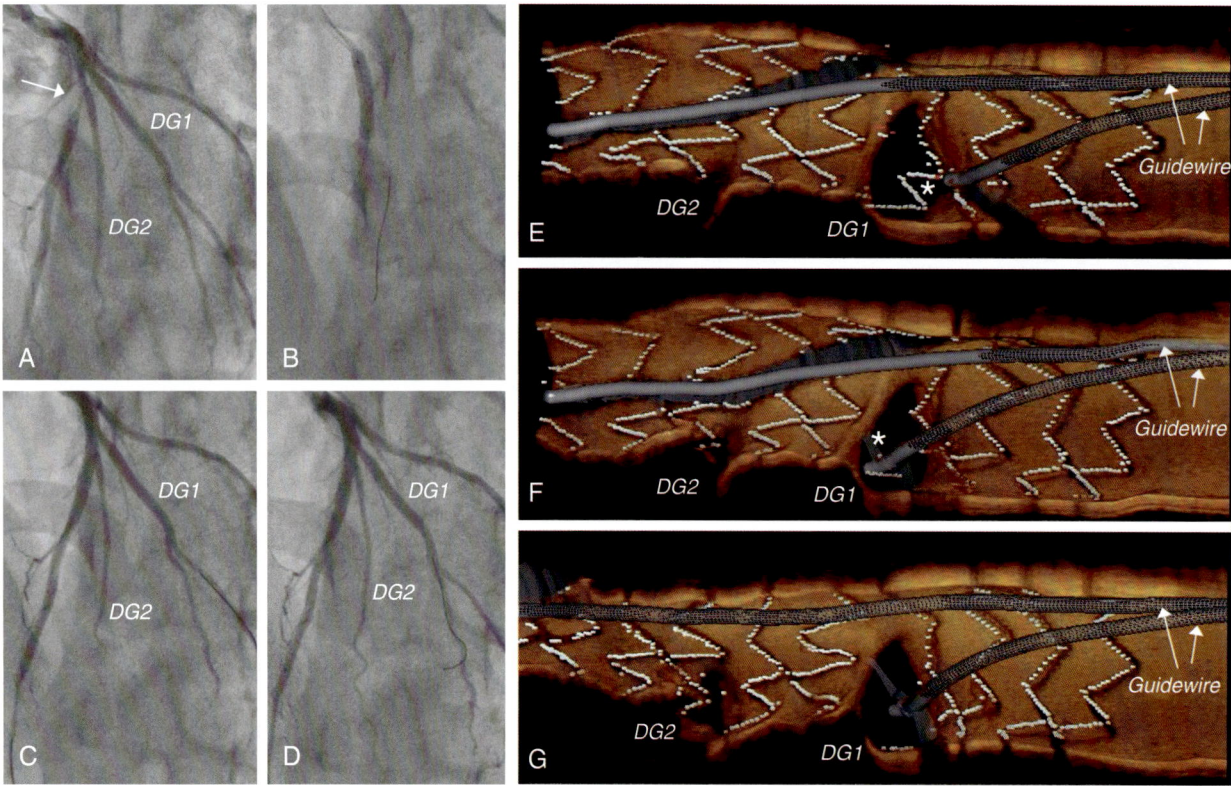

Fig. 67.16 Three-dimensional (3D) guidance for guidewire-recrossing into the appropriate cell and optimization in bifurcation lesion. Coronary angiography (CAG) showed severe bifurcation stenosis of the proximal left anterior descending artery (LAD), first diagonal *(DG1)* and second diagonal *(DG2)* (A, *white arrow*). A provisional side-branch stenting was performed with a biodegradable polymer sirolimus-eluting stent 3.5/18mm (B). A cell wire recrossing was performed to open the stent struts toward the major side branch (DG1). While CAG was unable to reveal which stent cell was re-crossed (C), 3D-OCT bifurcation software clearly displayed the guidewire crossing into a proximal small cell (E, asterisk), with a risk of major stent distorsion. After guidewire cell recrossing, 3D-OCT showed that the guidewire was crossing into a more favorable cell (F, *asterisk*). Kissing balloon technique (noncompliant balloon 3.0/12 mm in LAD, semicompliant balloon 2.5/15 mm in DG1, 8 atm.) was performed. Final CAG showed good stent expansion with appropriate dilation of ostial DG1 (D). Final 3D-OCT showed optimal opening of jailed DG1 (G).

the center of the luminal surface of the strut blooming is determined for each strut, and its distance to the lumen contour of the vessel wall is automatically calculated.

The monochromatic peak wavelength of the OCT is differently reflected, refracted, and absorbed by biodegradable polymeric scaffolds compared with the metallic struts. Because a larger amount of the OCT light energy is transmitted through the polymeric struts, only part of it is reflected at the endoluminal and abluminal sides of the struts, generating a visible optical frame border. As a consequence, the vessel wall can be imaged through the struts without any major signs of attenuation, and its luminal area can be readily measured behind the polymeric struts.[71]

Optimal Versus Suboptimal Stent Implantation
Strut Apposition

For accurate evaluation of stent apposition, the stent surface must be measured from the center of the stent reflection.[72] Incomplete stent apposition (ISA), synonymous with malapposition, is defined as separation of the strut from the lumen border by a distance greater than the width of the stent strut according to each stent specification.[73] ISA can be addressed at a cross-sectional level, expressed as number and length of consecutive cross sections with ISA together with area and volume measurements, or at a strut level, expressed as maximum distance of ISA at each strut. Acute malapposition can be readily displayed by OCT immediately after stent deployment, whereas the detection of persistent or late malapposition requires comparison of images obtained immediately after stent implantation with corresponding (sister) images at follow-up.

By using serial OCT, Ozaki and colleagues demonstrated that ISA observed at follow-up after implantation of a sirolimus-eluting stent was more frequently derived from acute malapposition without neointimal growth, rather than acquired late due to positive vascular remodeling.[74] Similar findings were reported by Inoue and associates with the use of current-generation DESs.[75] Acute malapposition ≥380 μm remained persistent more frequently over lipid or calcified plaque than over fibrous plaques (lipid, 13.4%; calcified, 18.2%; fibrous, 4.2%; lipid vs. fibrous, P = .001; calcified

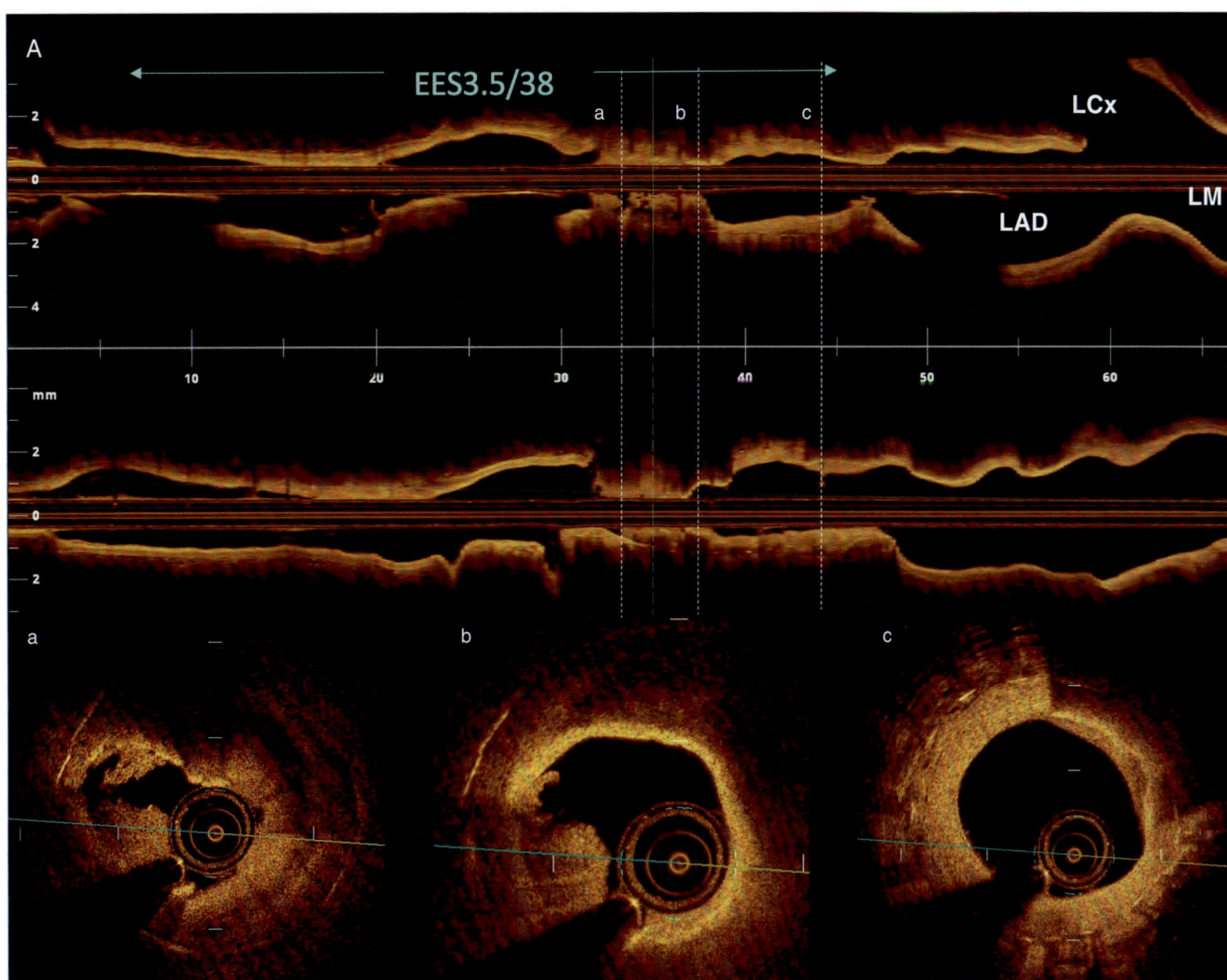

Fig. 67.17 Late stent thrombosis 1 year after everolimus-eluting stent *(EES)* implantation. Optical coherence tomography pullback was performed in left anterior descending artery *(LAD)* for late stent thrombosis of a current generation drug-eluting stent *(EES)* (A). Cross sectional images revealed lipid laden neoatherosclerosis with thrombus (A-a and A-b), and lipid laden neoatherosclerosis with macrophage infiltration (A-c). *LCx,* Left circumflex artery; *LM,* left main.

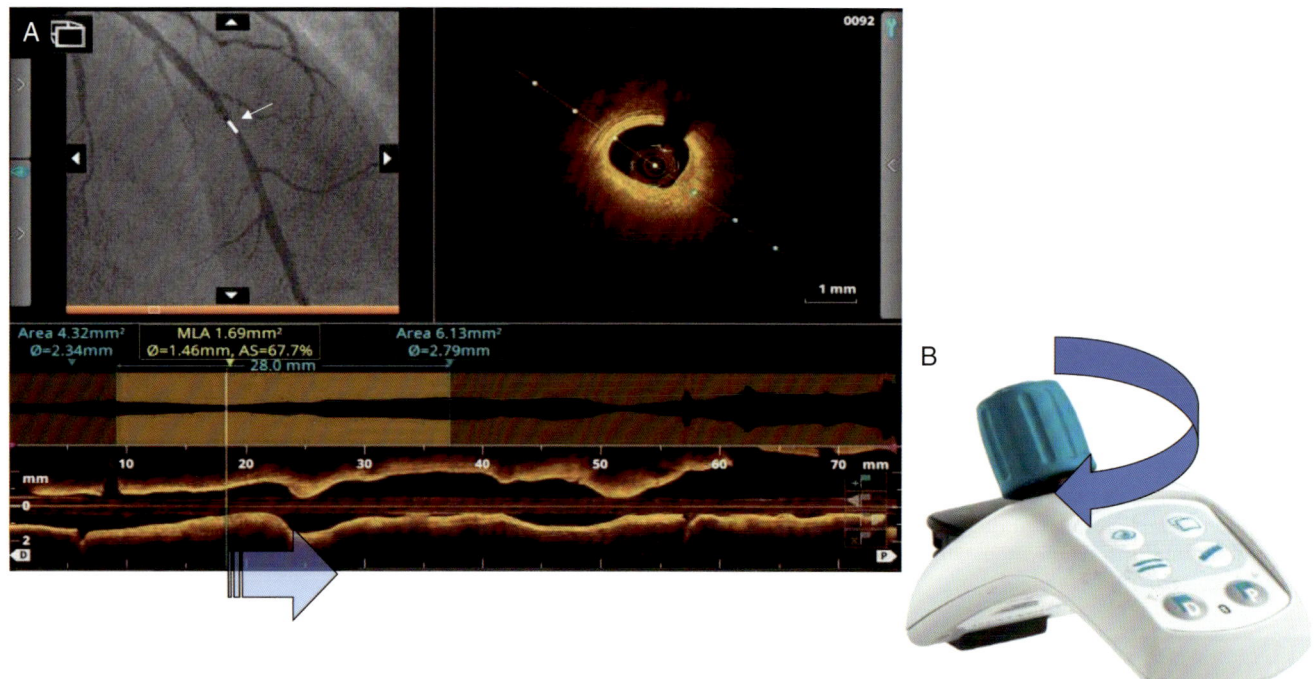

Fig. 67.18 Angio-coregistration and tableside controller for imaging navigation. Angio-coregistration image shows the position of optical coherence tomography sector as a white mark on the angiogram (A, *white arrow*) and the corresponding cross-sectional OCT image. The Tableside Controller may be used to position the cursor by turning the handle clockwise or counter clockwise. When the controller is turned clockwise (B), the position of the cursor moves to the right (A, *blue arrow*). *AS,* Area stenosis; *MLA,* minimal luminal area.

vs. fibrous, $P = .02$) and was associated with the presence of thrombi at follow-up (Fig. 67.19). Therefore the persistence of malapposition was influenced by both the amount of malapposition at stent implantation and the underlying nature of the treated plaque.

Kubo and colleagues showed that ISA (47% vs. 18%), dissection (40% vs. 16%), and tissue protrusion (58% vs. 20%) immediately after stent implantation are more often detected by OCT than by IVUS.[76] This superiority has been recently confirmed by the data collected in the ILUMIEN III randomized controlled trial (RCT).[21] Major malapposition, defined as a strut distance greater than 0.2 mm from the lumen border with stent underexpanion, was more common after both IVUS- and angiography-guided PCI than OCT-guided PCI (21%, 31%, and 11%, respectively, $P < .02$ and $P < .0001$). Major untreated edge dissections, defined as greater than 60 degrees in arc and/or 3 mm in length, were significantly more common after IVUS-guided PCI and angiography-guided PCI than OCT-guided PCI. Optimization of strut apposition under OCT guidance may enhance early strut coverage after DES implantation.[77]

With the systematic use of OCT in daily practice, suboptimal results including stent malapposition, remaining thrombus, plaque prolapse, and edge dissection are observed more frequently than expected.[21] Gonzalo and coworkers evaluated the reproducibility of these findings with OCT.[4] The reproducibility of edge dissection, tissue prolapse, in-stent dissection, and strut malapposition detected by OCT was 100% ($\kappa = 1.0$). However, minor abnormalities detected by OCT might not always require additional treatment. Kawamori and associates studied such abnormalities immediately after stent implantation and at follow-up.[78] In most cases, limited stent malapposition, plaque prolapse, or minor edge dissections substantially improved or resolved at follow-up.

Edge Dissection

A comprehensive analysis of OCT edge dissections was reported by Chamié and colleagues.[79] Qualitative and morphometric assessments at the stent edges revealed that dissections were frequently associated with remaining plaques (TCFA and lipid-rich lesions) at the landing zone and with the technique of implantation, suggesting some geographic mismatch as the main causative factor. They concluded that dissections with longitudinal length <1.75 mm, fewer than two concomitant flaps, flap depth of less than 0.52 mm, and flap opening of less than 0.33 mm and not extending into the media have favorable outcomes and can be left untreated. Similar findings were reported by Radu and coworkers using serial OCT after DES implantation to assess the morphology, healing response, and clinical outcomes of angiographically silent OCT edge dissections.[80] Angiographically silent dissections were not associated with acute stent thrombosis or restenosis during follow-up of up to 1 year and, in almost all cases, resulted in a complete sealing.

Presence of residual plaque burden, extensive lateral (>60 degrees) and longitudinal dissection (>2 mm), involvement of deeper vessel layers (tunicae media and adventitia), and localization distal to the stent increase the risk for adverse events (Fig. 67.20).[35]

Prati and colleagues reported a clinical benefit of OCT guidance in correcting stent abnormalities by optimizing decisions during PCI (the Centro per la Lotta contro l'Infarto-Optimisation of Percutaneous Coronary Intervention [CLI-OPCI] study).[81] The adjunctive information obtained by OCT resulted in significantly lower 1-year cardiac mortality (1.2% vs. 4.5%; $P = .010$), combination of cardiac death and myocardial infarction (6.6% vs. 13.0%; $P = .006$), and combination of all composite MACEs (9.6% vs. 14.8%; $P = .044$). Furthermore, the CLI-OPCI registry assessed the impact of OCT findings of suboptimal stent deployment in 1002 lesions (832 patients).[82] In-stent minimum lumen area <4.5 mm²

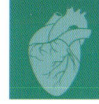

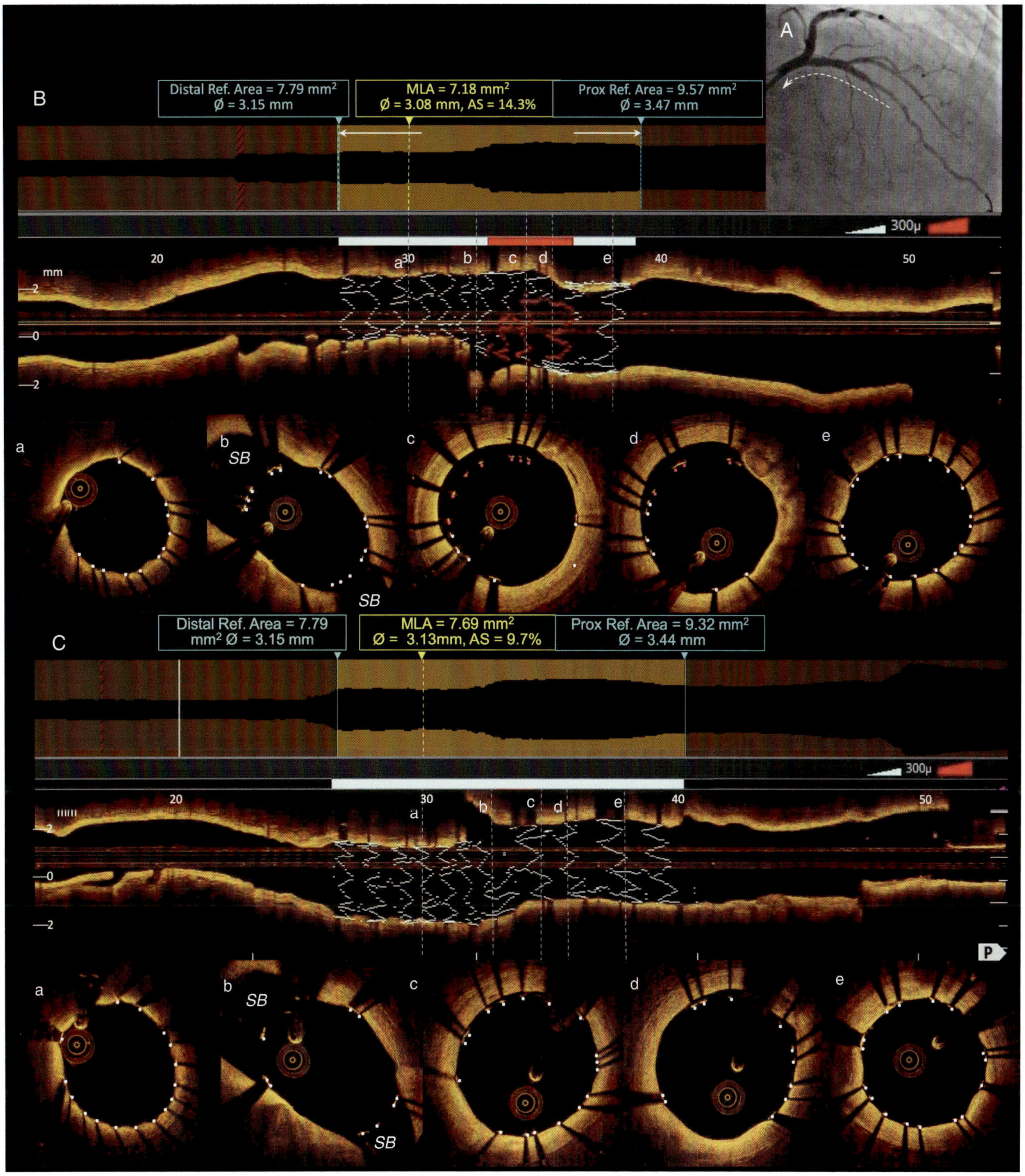

Fig. 67.19 **Role of optical coherence tomography (OCT) in detecting and correcting stent strut malapposition.** OCT pullback (A, *dotted arrow*) performed immediately after a provisional stent implantation (3.5/12 mm) in proximal left descending coronary artery, with good angiographic result. Automatic strut detection (a,b,c,d,e) identified each strut in the cross sections and displayed them with different colors accordingly to stent-wall apposition (complete apposition is visualized as *white dots* whereas remaining major malapposition is visualized as *red dots*), with a threshold set at 300 μm of distance. Similar data were displayed with the same colors in the longitudinal view through the apposition bar and the stent rendering. Automated stent rendering OCT images revealed completely apposed struts at distal and proximal stent segments (B-a, B-b, and B-e). Conversely, a large area of consecutive malapposed struts was observed (B-c and B-d) at midportion of the stent. According to the OCT results, postdilatation with 4.0 mm noncompliant balloon was added. OCT pullback revealed well apposed stent (C). Malapposed struts were improved by postdilatation (C-c and C-d). *AS*, Area stenosis; *MLA*, minimum lumen area; *SB*, side branch.

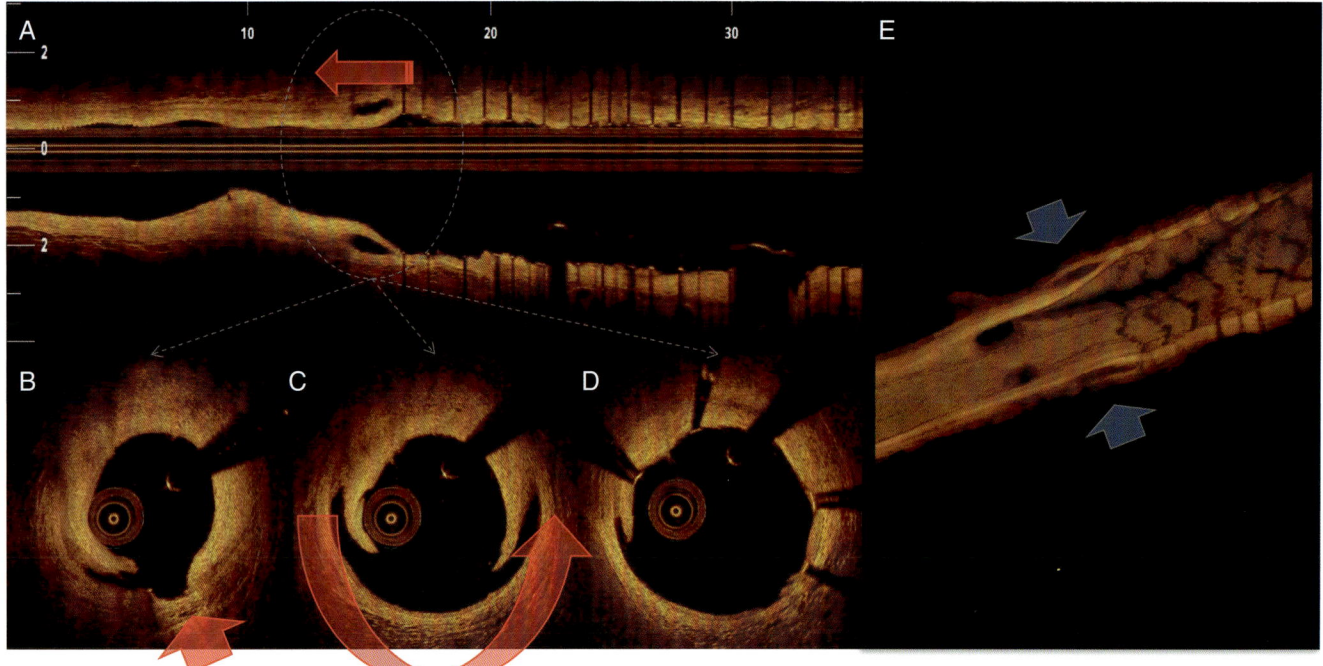

Fig. 67.20 Assessment of edge dissection. Optical coherence tomography (OCT) pullback was performed just after stent implantation. In the cross-sectional images a dissection involved the media layer (B, *red arrowhead*). Its lateral extension was greater than 60 degrees (C, *red arrow*). The extent of the dissection, as detected in the longitudinal view, was superior to 2 mm. According to the OCT images, this was a major dissection requiring additional stent implantation. Three-dimensional reconstruction clearly showed the position of edge dissection (E, *gray arrows*).

(HR 1.64, P = .040), dissection >200 μm at the distal stent edge (HR 2.54, P < .001), and reference lumen area <4.5 mm² at either distal (HR 4.56, P < .001) or proximal site (HR 5.73, P < .001) was associated with an increased risk of MACE at 1-year follow-up (59.2% vs. 26.9%; P < .001).

Strut Coverage

Histopathology obtained from autopsy cases highlights delayed healing and incomplete endothelial coverage as predictors of late stent thrombosis after DES implantation.[83] Unlike bare-metal stents (BMSs), which develop circumferential coverage with an average thickness of 500 μm or more, easily measured by IVUS and angiography, the smaller amount of neointimal growth after DES implantation is largely under the limit of resolution of these imaging techniques. Preclinical studies have demonstrated a close degree of correlation between OCT, light microscopy, and SEM in detecting coverage in DES.[2] In particular, all struts completely covered by FD-OCT were also fully covered by SEM.

The time course of tissue coverage after stent implantation is different according to stent type. In BMSs, normal neointima was observed 6 months after stent implantation. Conversely, at a later phase during an extended period of 5 years or longer, neointima undergoes various OCT signal changes with increased neovascularization, late lipid infiltration up to plaque disruption, and, eventually, thrombus formation.[84] In DESs, OCT performed at different time points demonstrated a higher rate of uncovered stent struts compared with BMSs, ranging from 15% to 20% at 3 months to 0% to 5% at 2 years, and a higher degree of heterogeneity in coverage.[85,86] However, different DES devices have different rates of coverage and uneven neointima response, possibly related to the polymer characteristics and specific drug kinetics.[72] Despite the fact that neointimal coverage in DES may progress over time, previous midterm OCT studies have shown that uncovered stent struts in first-generation DESs decreased but did not disappear in 6 to 12 months.[87,88] More recent OCT data on current-generation DESs (biolimus-zotarolimus and everolimus-eluting) have shown less heterogeneity, a higher degree of coverage, and a low rate of malapposition compared with first-generation DESs across all indications, including STEMI, supporting the better-observed clinical outcome.[89]

The optimal time for assessing DES coverage remains to be defined. Early assessment of strut coverage is challenged by the more difficult separation between fibrin and neointima tissues. Optical density of stent strut coverage, measured with novel optical frequency domain imaging, revealed that fibrin-covered struts had lower signal density than mature neointima tissue. Densitometric analysis may be a promising method for characterization of early stent tissue coverage. A novel OCT-based method to discriminate between fibrin and thrombus is near-infrared fluorescence OCT molecular imaging, which reliably detects fibrin as compared with neointima following injection of a fibrin-targeted agent.[90] By use of this catheter-based technology, an animal study suggested that DESs showed a greater fibrin deposition and fibrin persistence at day 7 and 28 as compared with BMSs. At the later time point (28 days), 18.6% ± 10.6% of OCT-covered stent struts remained fibrin positive. This technique is currently under clinical investigation. Longer time intervals (6 to 13 months) might be more useful for measuring the rate of strut coverage and the progression of the lesions. The extent of strut coverage has been used as a surrogate variable of outcome in numerous OCT trials, based on pathology studies and recent stent thrombosis registries, identifying strut coverage as an independent predictor of stent failure and very late stent thrombosis.[10,91,92] However, the clinical relevance of measuring the completeness of stent coverage has not been fully demonstrated, because there are no sufficiently powered prospective studies investigating the association between the presence and degree of uncovered struts with stent thrombosis. Recently, the DETECT-OCT trial (Determination of the Duration of Dual Antiplatelet Therapy by the Degree of the Coverage of The Struts on Optical Coherence Tomography) investigated the clinical effects of a tailored dual antiplatelet therapy (DAPT) duration based on the degree of uncoverage.[93] Specifically, in patients with <6% uncovered stent struts at 3 months, DAPT was stopped prematurely and in those with >6%, DAPT was continued for 12 months. Due to the inclusion of low-risk patients, clinical events were exceedingly rare, and the study remained inconclusive. Although the percentage of uncovered stent struts may provide prognostic information, it is unlikely that an invasive screening to detect uncovered struts will ever become routine in view of the added risks, high costs, and unclear clinical consequences. Strut coverage must be interpreted with caution because OCT cannot detect endothelial cells or their functionality. Furthermore, the composition of the material covering stent struts (whether cellular or noncellular in nature) remains incompletely addressed by current-generation OCT.

ASSESSMENT OF STENT FAILURE

There are multiple causes of stent thrombosis or restenosis, all coming into very similar angiographic views (occluded vessel or tight in-stent lesion). The use of intravascular imaging (IVUS or OCT) to assess mechanisms of stent failure is recognized by the existing guidelines, with the same level of evidence (class IIa, level C.).[94]

OCT is far superior to IVUS in the assessment of causative mechanisms of in-stent thrombosis or restenosis, as IVUS cannot assess stent strut coverage, differentiate neointima from neoatherosclerosis, or accurately reveal thrombus.

Because of the small size of the catheters, OCT may reach and cross difficult lesions, including severe ISR or in-stent thrombosis, provided an effective flow has been reestablished before the pullback.

In-Stent Restenosis

OCT provides an in vivo characterization of the tissue involved in in-stent restenosis (ISR). Gonzalo and colleagues evaluated the morphologic characteristics of ISR by OCT in 24 patients (DES, 84%; BMS, 16%).[95] The ISR tissue was classified based on optical pattern characteristics (homogeneous, heterogeneous, or layered), signal backscatter (high vs. low), presence and type of microvessels (peristruts vs. intraintimal), lumen shape (regular vs. irregular), and presence of abnormal intraluminal material. Tissue structure was layered in 52%, homogeneous in 28%, and heterogeneous in 20%. The predominant optical pattern was backscattering, found in 72% of cases. This classification has been adopted in studies addressing OCT findings and the treatment of ISR.

OCT studies assessing ISR were able to detect a new pathologic entity of late stent failure, neoatherosclerosis. The current concept and knowledge of in-stent neoatherosclerosis evolved quite recently, based on accurate histopathologic and OCT tissue assessment. Neoatherosclerosis is recognized by pathology as clusters of lipid-laden foamy macrophages within the neointima, with or without a necrotic core, neovessels, and microcalcifications.[96] Pathology and OCT studies have demonstrated that neoatherosclerosis is more common and occurs earlier in DES compared with BMS, with significantly more TCFA (Fig. 67.21D).[97,98] Despite the outstanding details provided by OCT, current systems may be limited as to proper evaluation of the entire spectrum of qualitative characteristics of the neointima. Consequently, the definitions of lipid-laden neointima used in OCT publications may differ, from a signal-poor region with invisible struts to neointima with a diffuse border and high-attenuation signals.[86,99] Intraintima neovascularization or calcification, or both, were frequently observed by OCT in presence of neoatherosclerosis.[100] Sometimes, neointima with echolucent layers mimics or partially overlaps advanced OCT patterns of neoatherosclerosis.[101]

Characterization of neoatherosclerosis by OCT also provides some prognostic data and is useful to guide the most appropriate therapeutic strategy for patients with stent failure. Indeed, neoatherosclerosis, characterized by a large amount of lipid and TCFAs, frequently manifests with an ACS and is associated with more periprocedural myocardial infarction.[102] Therefore the soft composition of neoatherosclerotic tissue detected by OCT may suggest a different treatment strategy compared with the fibrotic tissue of conventional ISR.[103]

Stent Thrombosis

In patients with stent thrombosis, OCT may detect and measure with a high degree of accuracy, the rate and distribution of uncovered and malapposed struts, the heterogeneity of the in-stent vascular response, and eventually the formation of de novo atherosclerotic lesions within the stented segment. In addition, OCT allows quantification of the completeness of thrombus removal after manual or mechanical thrombus aspiration and eventually suggests additional antithrombotic treatments.

Through better mechanistic understanding of the processes involved, OCT may allow tailored and more effective treatments of stent thrombosis. In patients presenting with late and very late stent thrombosis, Guagliumi et al. demonstrated a significantly higher percentage of uncovered struts and higher number of sections with >30% uncovered struts compared with uneventful matched imaging control patients.[104] The length of the segment with consecutive uncovered struts was the only OCT predictive factor for stent thrombosis at multivariate analysis. More recently, Taniwaki and coworkers reported OCT results in 64 patients presenting with very late DES (first and current generation) thrombosis.[91] The most frequently observed findings were strut malapposition (34.5%), neoatherosclerosis (27.6%), uncovered struts (12.1%), and stent underexpansion (6.9%). Interestingly, uncovered and malapposed struts were significantly more frequent in stented regions with thrombus compared with regions without thrombus (HR 8.26; 95% CI 6.82 to 10.04; $P < .001$ and HR 13.03; 95% CI 10.13 to 16.93; $P < .001$, respectively). Similarly, the maximal length of malapposed or uncovered struts (3.4 mm; 95% CI 2.55 to 4.25; vs. 1.29 mm; 95% CI 0.81 to 1.77; $P < .001$), but not the maximum malapposed distance, was greater in thrombosed compared with nonthrombosed segments.

Two large cohorts of patients with stent thrombosis have been prospectively recruited in Europe since 2011 in two different registries, the Prevention of Stent Thrombosis by an Interdisciplinary Global European Effort (PRESTIGE) and Morphological Parameters Explaining Stent Thrombosis assessed by OCT (PESTO).[10,92] In PRESTIGE, 217 patients presenting with early ($n = 62$, 28.6%) and late/very late stent thrombosis ($n = 155$, 71.4%) underwent immediate OCT. The underlying stent type was a new-generation DES in 50.3%. Stent underexpansion (stent expansion index <0.8) was observed in 44.4% of the cases. The predicted average probability (95% CI) that any frame had uncovered (or thrombus-covered) struts was 99.3% (96.1 to 99.9), 96.6% (92.4 to 98.5), 34.3% (15.0 to 60.7), and 9.6% (6.2 to 14.5) and malapposed struts was 21.8% (8.4 to 45.6), 8.5% (4.6 to 15.3), 6.7% (2.5 to 16.3), and 2.0% (1.2 to 3.3) for acute, subacute, late, and very late stent thrombosis, respectively. The most common dominant finding adjudicated for acute stent thrombosis was uncovered struts (66.7% of cases); for subacute stent thrombosis, was uncovered struts (61.7%) and underexpansion (25.5%); for late stent thrombosis, was uncovered struts (33.3%) and severe restenosis (19.1%); and for very late stent thrombosis, the most common dominant finding was neoatherosclerosis (31.3%) and uncovered struts (20.2%). The

SECTION VI Evaluation of Interventional Techniques

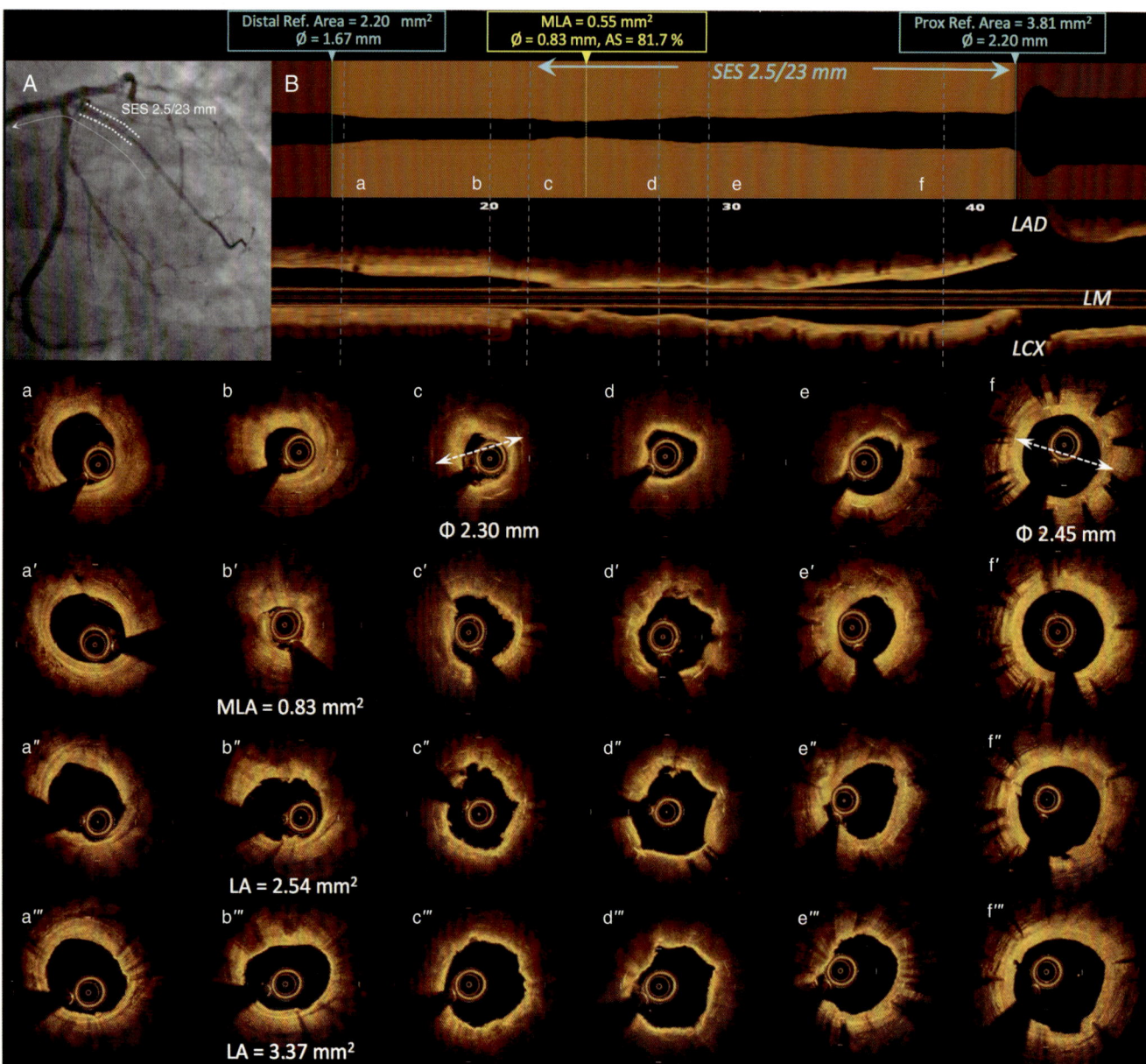

Fig. 67.21 **Guidance for the treatment of stent failure.** The patient was admitted with lateral acute myocardial infarction. Coronary angiography (CAG) showed total occlusion in the stented segment (7 years after sirolimus-eluting stent *[SES]* 2.5/23 mm implantation) in the proximal ramus. After thrombus aspiration optical coherence tomography (OCT) pullback was performed (A, *dotted arrow*). OCT images (B, longitudinal view) after thrombus aspiration showed significant diffuse in-stent tissue growth with an MLA (B, automatic detection lumen, *yellow dotted line*) of 0.55 mm^2. OCT cross-sectional images demonstrated diffuse neoatherosclerosis with in-stent calcium deposits (b), layered neointima (c), and lipid-laden neoatherosclerosis making invisible struts (d and e) in a partially underexpanded stent (c, stent diameter measured from visible struts was 2.3 mm^2). OCT images after 2.5-mm noncompliant balloon dilatation demonstrated large amount of remaining neointima (b' to e'). A more aggressive dilation with a 2.5-mm scoring balloon was performed obtaining larger in-stent lumen area (a" to f"). Adjunctive 3.0-mm drug-coated balloon dilation allowed better stent expansion, with limited remaining intrastent tissue and larger final minimum lumen area *(MLA)* (3.37 mm; a''' to f'''). *AS*, Area stenosis; *LA*, lumen area; *LCx*, Left circumflex artery; *LM*, left main.

PESTO multicenter French registry frequently (69%) used a two-step approach (i.e., initial dethrombosis with thrombus aspiration and GP IIb/IIIa receptor inhibitors, followed by deferred intracoronary imaging L). Use of OCT identified an underlying morphologic abnormality in 97% of cases, whereas the origin of stent thrombosis could be identified with certainty by angiography in only 12% of cases.

BIORESORBABLE VASCULAR SCAFFOLDS

The only bioresorbable scaffold with sufficient scientific evaluation in adequately powered studies and U.S. Food and Drug Administration (FDA)-approved device is the ABSORB BVS 1.1, which was retracted from the market in 2017 by the manufacturer in response to increased rates of target-vessel myocardial infarction and scaffold thrombosis. OCT has proven to be useful for monitoring the resorption process over time, for guiding scaffold implantation, and importantly to understand mechanisms of scaffold failures.[105,106] The material properties of polymeric struts (approximately 160 μm thick) allow for less overexpansion (i.e., ≤ 0.5 mm), and thus precise scaffold sizing according to OCT has a much higher priority than with metallic DESs. Underexpansion and malapposition were correlates of early and late scaffold thrombosis and therefore relevant targets to avoid by implementation of OCT-guided optimization.[107] Overexpansion may lead to scaffold fractures, a prothrombotic finding only visible by postprocedural OCT. The frequency of scaffold thrombosis occurring beyond the first year after implantation was fourfold higher as compared with metallic DESs.[108] OCT used in the largest registry of patients with very late scaffold thrombosis provided unique insights into failure mechanisms that were never observed in metallic DESs.[109,110] Scaffold fragments located in the vessel lumen (so-called late scaffold discontinuity) were identified as the leading cause (43%) of thrombosis (Fig. 67.22). This phenomenon is likely the consequence of the bioresorption-induced scaffold fragmentation leading to acquired malapposition in absence of a sufficient encapsulation in neointimal tissue. Other bioresorbable scaffolds received CE approval but were not evaluated in RCTs. In the absence of such data, the EAPCI consensus group on the clinical use of intracoronary imaging highly recommends the evaluation of any scaffold failure by OCT so that potential safety issues can be detected in a timely manner. In addition, any new bioresorbable device should undergo prospective evaluation by OCT according to the consensus group.

OCT-GUIDED STENT PROCEDURES: IMPACT ON CLINICAL OUTCOME

The use of OCT in PCI and in patients with stents has been demonstrated to be safe and effective for providing additional information. Although consistent clinical evidence suggests the superiority of IVUS-guided PCI particularly in complex lesions (e.g., long lesions or chronic total occlusions),[111] no single study powered for clinical outcomes compared OCT-guided versus angiography-guided PCI. Notwithstanding, two larger studies suggested noninferiority of OCT when compared with IVUS in terms of guiding PCI; the ILUMIEN III trial demonstrated noninferiority of OCT versus IVUS with respect to poststenting MLD, and the OPINION (optical frequency domain imaging vs. intravascular ultrasound in percutaneous coronary intervention) trial showed noninferiority with respect to the primary clinical end point of target-vessel failure in patients undergoing PCI with a second-generation DES.[112] In the OPINION trial, target-vessel failure occurred in 21 (5.2%) of 401 patients undergoing OCT-guided PCI, and 19 (4.9%) of 390 patients undergoing IVUS-guided PCI (HR 1.07, upper limit of one-sided 95% CI 1.80; $P_{noninferiority}$ = .042). With 89.8% angiographic follow-up, the rate of binary restenosis was comparable between OCT-guided PCI and IVUS-guided PCI (in-stent: 1.6% vs. 1.6%, P = 1.00; and in-segment: 6.2% vs. 6.0%, P = 1.00).

At least three major clinical settings that hold the highest risk of PCI failure and negative outcome might reap large benefits from the immediate use of OCT: complex interventions such as bifurcation (including distal LM disease) requiring advanced operative techniques,[113] ACSs, and stent failure.

Bifurcation lesions and related stent procedures are actively investigated with OCT because of the angiographic ambiguity in detecting complex tridimensional anatomy at the branching points.[114] Adjunctive OCT imaging may provide crucial information in planning and optimizing treatment, because two stent bifurcation techniques have repeatedly been associated with adverse cardiac outcomes and represent one of the guideline-endorsed risk factors for ischemic outcomes. OCT performed before the procedure can provide unique data on carina type, plaque distribution at the ostium (risk of side-branch occlusion after main branch stenting), lipid-rich plaque in adjacent segments (to decide on stent length), calcium arc and thickness (for adjunctive lesion preparation), assessment of stent diameter based on accurate proximal and distal reference size (relevant as the main branch tapers after the take-off of a side branch). Furthermore, in bifurcation lesions, OCT was able to identify the proximal rim at the ostium of the side branch as the region more likely to contain TCFA.[115,116] After stent placement, OCT may evaluate stent expansion, rule out edge dissection and intramural hematoma, detect strut malapposition, and guidewire position in stent cell recrossing (3D high-resolution software) to avoid abluminal rewiring, stent deformity, or accidental stent crush (see Fig. 67.17).[114] In bifurcation lesions, OCT scanning of both main and side branches is recommended when a two-stent technique is chosen (Fig. 67.23). The clinical significance of these OCT actionable imaging findings in complex bifurcation lesions treated with stents is under active investigation in large, prospective, multicenter RCTs (OCT Optimised Bifurcation Event Reduction [OCTOBER], ILUMIEN IV studies).

OCT can be used to assess and guide certain nonostial LM coronary artery disease interventions, provided there is adequate blood clearing (LM shaft not very short in length and not very large in diameter), as artifacts or incomplete frames may be detected in the proximal segment of LM, whereas the LM bifurcation is perfectly evaluated by OCT.[117,118] However, in this setting, cutoff lumen areas are not validated yet for OCT.

A multicenter, randomized study comparing OCT-guided PCI with angiography-guide PCI in 240 patients with NSTEMI ACS (The multicenter, randomized Does Optical Coherence Tomography Optimize Results of Stenting [DOCTORS]) proved that OCT-guided PCI was associated with higher postprocedural fractional flow reserve than PCI guided by angiography alone.[119] OCT use led to a change in procedural strategy in 50% of the patients in the OCT-guided group, mainly driven by the optimization of stent expansion without a greater number of stents or an increase in periprocedural myocardial infarction or kidney dysfunction. The findings of the DOCTORS study strengthen the evidence in favor of a potential benefit of OCT to guide PCI in patients with ACS.

UPCOMING TECHNOLOGIES

Interpretation of current images is limited to the evaluation of gray-scale signals and identification of individual plaque constituents is inferred from visual interpretation of recorded OCT images that requires individual experience. However, multiple tissue constituents can generate similar OCT imaging features. Methods for automated images analysis and OCT hardware modifications that can improve contrast based on structural tissue properties (structural anisotropy of tissue constituents via polarization-sensitive OCT) have been incorporated into a current clinical OCT system with evidence of improved tissue type characterization of atherosclerotic plaques.[3,120,121] Moreover, Tearney and colleagues reported on a new type of micro-OCT (μOCT) that enables imaging of the 3D microstructure with resolution improved by an order of magnitude of 10 (axial resolution ≤1 μm and a lateral resolution ≤2 μm in tissue), compared with the current OCT systems. μOCT uses a very broad bandwidth light source and common-path SD-OCT technology and provides clear pictures in cadaver of cellular and subcellular features associated with atherogenesis, thrombosis, and responses to coronary stents.[122,123] This outstanding level of resolution may dramatically improve evaluation of lesion vulnerability to anticipate the risk of plaque rupture and eventually passivate the

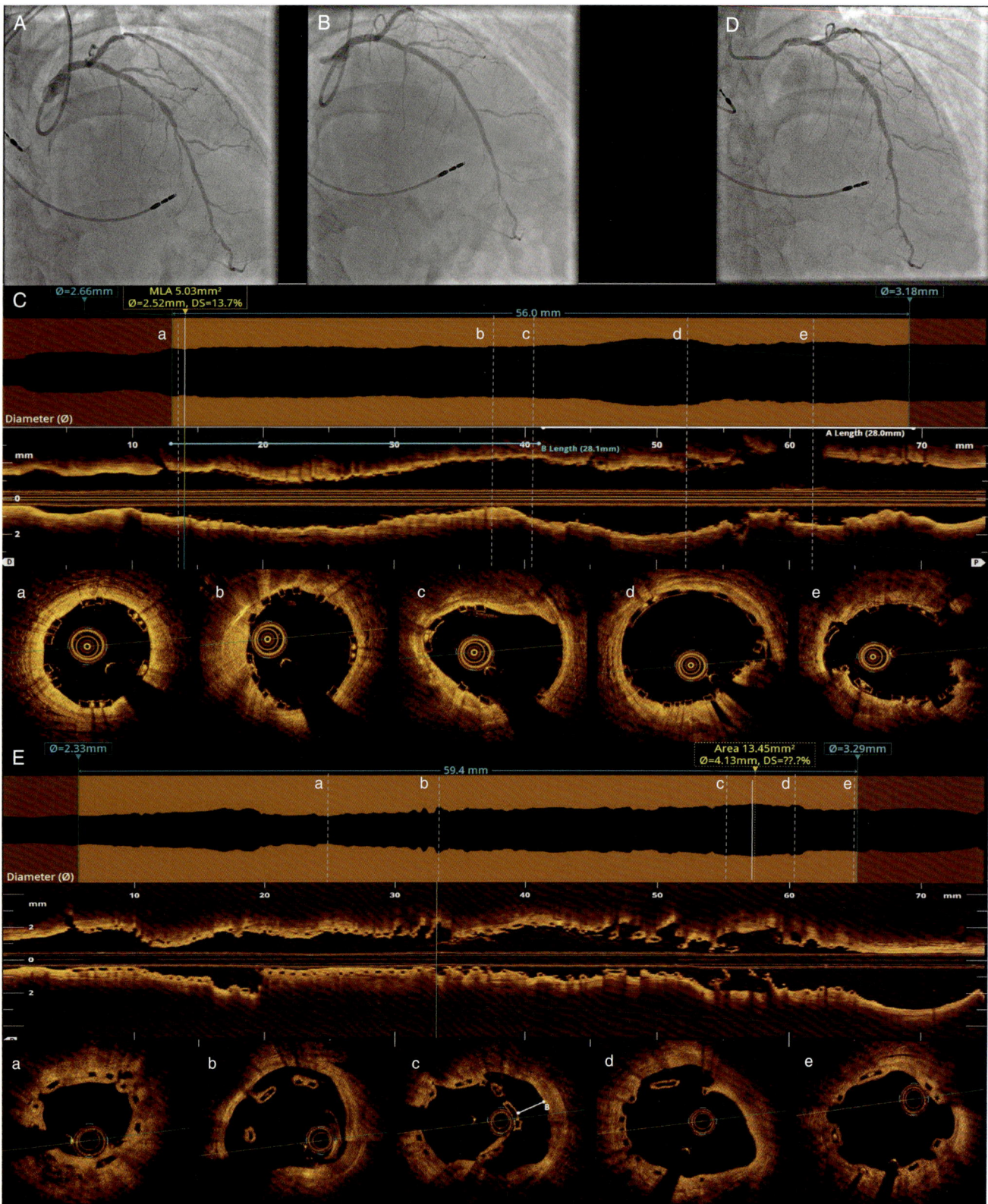

Fig. 67.22 **Late acquired malapposition and scaffold discontinuity after bioresorbable vascular scaffold (BVS) implantation.** A 60-year-old male was readmitted to the hospital 12 months after dual bioresorbable scaffold implantation (BVS 3.5/28 mm and BVS 3/28) in a long lesion of the left anterior descending artery (A) with an optimal acute angiographic (B) and OCT result (C-a to C-e). In-scaffold large lumen area (MLA 5.03 mm²) and no malapposition was obtained at scaffold implantation. Elective follow-up with CAG (D) and OCT (E) was performed at 1 year. In cross-sectional images, evagination (E-a and E-e) and large areas of malapposed struts (E-b, E-c, and E-d) were observed with possible discontinuity of the scaffold structure (longitudinal view). The malapposed maximum distance was 1.0 mm (E-c) *(white line)*. *DS,* diameter stenosis; *MLA,* minimal luminal area.

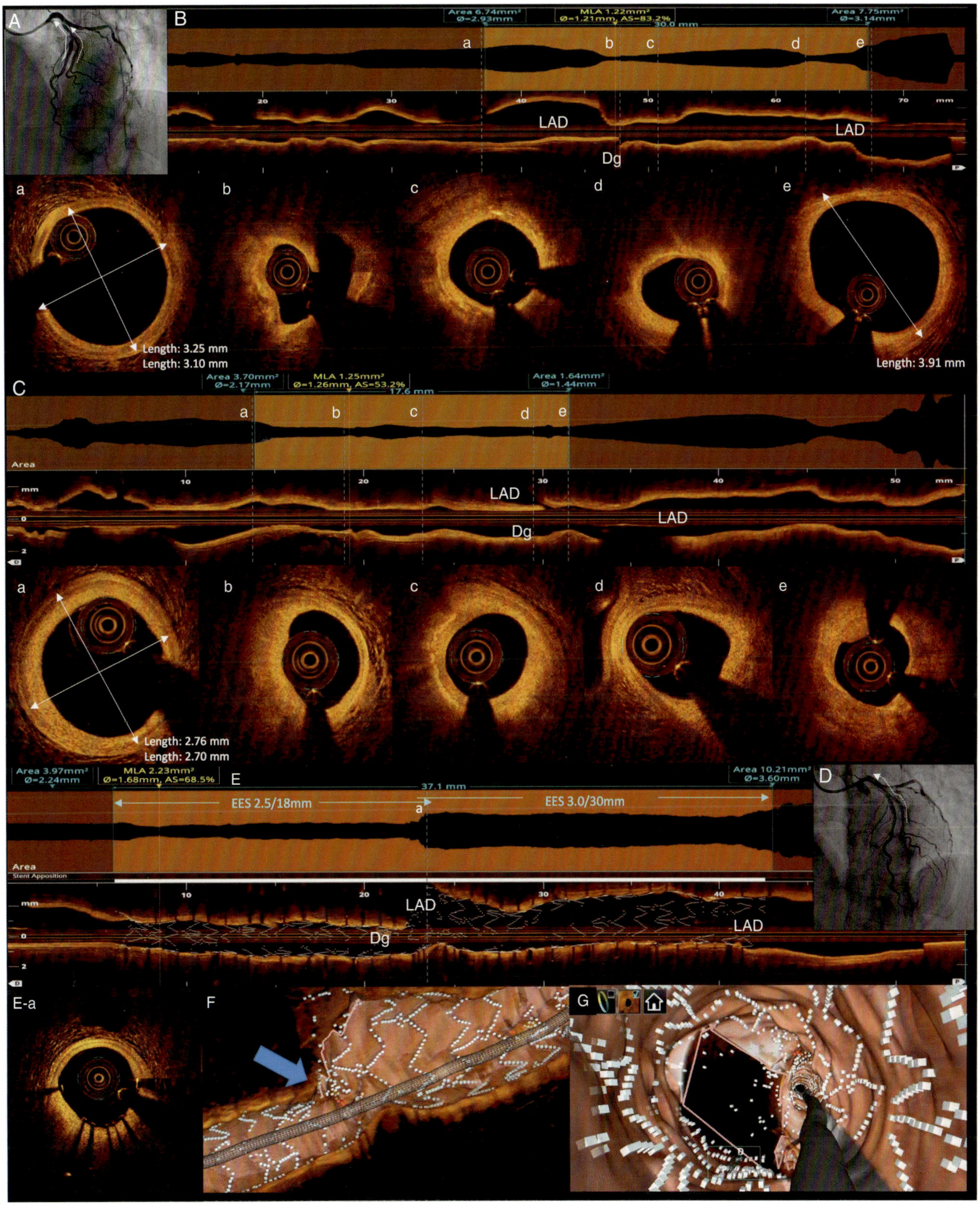

CHAPTER 67 Optical Coherence Tomography

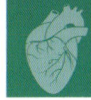

Fig. 67.23 Bifurcation lesion treated with two-stent and double-kissing crush tecqnique (DK crush), under OCT guidance. A 61-year-old female was admitted with unstable angina. Coronary angiography (A) showed a severe stenosis at the proximal segment of the left descending anterior coronary artery *(LAD)*, involving the bifurcation with a first large diagonal branch *(Dg,* Medina 1,1,1 classification). A DK-crush technique with two-stent implantation was selected to treat the LAD-Dg bifurcation. To achieve an optimal stent result in this complex patient and lesion setting, optical coherence tomography (OCT), co-registered with coronary angiography, was used as guidance during the stent procedure. OCT pullbacks were performed from the distal to proximal portion of LAD (A, *arrow*) and from the distal portion of Dg to proximal portion of LAD (A, *dotted arrow*) to obtain complete assessment of plaque type, distribution, and landing zone with precise measurements of stent length and size. OCT images from LAD (B) showed a long multifocal severe stenosis (B, automatic lumen detection border from a to e, length 30 mm). A normal distal landing zone for the stent was detected (B-a) and measured for lumen and external elastic lamina (EEL) diameters (B-a, *arrows,* mean 3.18 mm). In cross-sectional images calcified plaque and lipid plaque components (B-b, B-c, and B-d) were detected, as well as, the EEL diameter at proximal landing site was measured (B-e, 3.91 mm). OCT pullback from Dg (C) showed severe stenosis from the ostium of Dg to the middle of Dg. Cross-sectional images revealed lipid-rich plaque (C-b, C-c, and C-d). At the bifurcation, segment a fibro-calcific plaque was observed (C-d) , suggesting more aggressive focal lesion preparation, performed with scoring balloon. The mean EEL length of the distal reference segment of Dg was 2.73 mm. According to the OCT results, first everolimus-eluting stent *(EES)* 2.5/18 was implanted from the Dg (C-a) into the LAD with minimal protrusion, then crushed and recrossed by the guidewire in a proximal cell. Then EES 3/30 mm (based on the mean EEL diameter measured at the distal reference of LAD [B-a]) was implanted using the DK-crush stenting technique in LAD. Final OCT pullback was performed from Dg to LAD (D, *arrow*) after high pressure EES implantation showed optimal stent apposition (E, *white bar*) but remaining stent underexpansion in Dg (E, automatic detection lumen border; *yellow dotted line* to locate the underexpanded stent with an MLA of 2.23 mm2; E-a corresponding cross-sectional view). Based on the mean EEL of the distal reference segment (C-a, 2.75 mm), a 2.75/12-mm noncompliant balloon was used at high pressure to finally obtain the complete stent expansion without residual stenosis. Three-dimensional reconstruction image showed minimally crushed struts with full strut apposition at bifurcation segment (F, *blue arrow*). Three-dimensional flythrough image showed full opening of the stent struts toward the Dg and no ostial side-branch obstruction (G). *AS,* Area stenosis; *MLA,* minimal luminal area.

TCFA. In addition, OCT identification of plaque cellular components, such as inflammatory cells, is likely to be improved by 3D microstructure visualization. These advances may improve identification of lipid pool and accuracy in measuring of overlying fibrous cap thickness with new possibilities to assess and potentially treat plaques at high risk for future coronary events.

Future Advances in Optical Coherence Tomography

Some expected advances in intravascular OCT technology are improved imaging speed and usability, automated image classification and enhanced visualization, incorporation of alternative optical contrast sources, and OCT-combination devices. Improvements in light-source sweep rates will enable faster rotational and pullback rates and provide physicians with the ability to capture a high-density scan of the entire coronary artery between consecutive heartbeats, minimizing motion artifacts and reducing further the volume of contrast injected to displace blood during image acquisition. Clinical usability of OCT systems will be improved by features such as robust catheter autocalibration, debris-insensitive connectors, self-synchronizing flush and acquisition, and integration with existing catheter laboratory systems and networks.

New algorithms will recognize and avoid residual blood, guidewire reflections, and other structures that may appear to be part of the vessel wall. Interpolation across side branches will be accomplished by imposing continuity of the inner surface of the vessel across neighboring frames.

To provide functional information and a wider range of classifiable tissue types, future OCT systems will incorporate alternative optical approaches such as polarization sensitivity, Doppler/phase sensitivity, and spectral sensitivity to both endogenous and exogenous sources of contrast (spectrally tunable optical nanoparticles). Other intravascular diagnostic devices that provide complementary information, such as ultrasound, absorption spectroscopy, fluorescence spectroscopy, and Raman spectroscopy, may be engineered to reside alongside OCT in the same catheter probe. IVUS and OCT imaging using a single catheter may enable visualization of tissue microstructure in superficial layers of the artery wall at the same time as the deeper layers of the artery for evaluation of plaque burden and vessel remodeling. The combination of OCT with near-infrared, Raman, or other spectroscopic techniques will further improve the discrimination among tissue constituents in complex atherosclerotic lesions allowing for detailed analysis of the cellular and biochemical composition to identify plaque at risk of future clinical events. Advanced image processing algorithms will be developed to classify tissue types.[124]

Concurrent data collection from these modalities will expand the structural and functional information available to the cardiologist and should guide development and clinical use of novel cardiovascular therapies.

CONCLUSIONS

OCT enables real-time, full tomographic, in situ visualization of vessel microstructure with a unique high axial resolution. Previously unrevealed details on atherosclerotic plaque architecture and stent vascular response can be easily observed and quantified and would accelerate the understanding of coronary artery disease formation and treatment. Advances in the technology of OCT (angio-coregistration, automatic detection of the essential measurement to guide PCI, including visual rendering of stent apposition) have improved the ease of use and broadened the application of OCT from a research diagnostic tool toward an established technique for guiding complex coronary procedures.

Acknowledgments

The authors thank Keisuke Satogami, MD (Department of Cardiovascular Medicine, Wakayama Medical University, Wakayama, Japan); Paolo Canova, MD (Department of Cardiovascular, ASST Papa Giovanni XXIII, Bergamo, Italy) for their help with the figures; Maoen Xu, MD, Tao Chen, MD and Lijia Ma, MD (Department of Cardiology, the Second Affiliated Hospital of Harbin Medical University, Harbin, China) for providing the case used in Fig. 67-22; Kostantinos Koskinas, MD (Department of Cardiology, Bern University Hospital, Bern, Switzerland) for his help with the references; Antonio Sorropago, MD (Univerity of Milano-Bicocca, Milan, Italy), Francesco Moretti, MD (University of Pavia, Pavia, Italy) and Francesca Fenili for assistance with manuscript preparation and revision.

KEY REFERNCES

5. Gerbaud E, Weisz G, Tanaka A, et al. Multi-laboratory inter-institute reproducibility study of IVOCT and IVUS assessments using published consensus document definitions. *Eur Heart J Cardiovasc Imaging*. 2016;17:756–764.
10. Adriaenssens T, Joner M, Godschalk T, et al. Optical coherence tomography findings in patients with coronary stent thrombosis: a report of the PREvention of late stent thrombosis by an interdisciplinary global european effort (PRESTIGE) consortium. *Circulation*. 2017;136:1007–1021.
11. van der Sijde JN, Karanasos A, van Ditzhuijzen NS, et al. Safety of optical coherence tomography in daily practice: a comparison with intravascular ultrasound. *Eur Heart J Cardiovasc Imaging*. 2017;18:467–474.
17. Tearney GJ, Regar E, Akasaka T, et al. Consensus standards for acquisition, measurement, and reporting of intravascular optical coherence tomography studies: a report from the international working group for intravascular optical coherence tomography standardization and validation. *J Am Coll Cardiol*. 2012;59:1058–1072.
19. Fujino A, Mintz GS, Matsumura M, et al. A new optical coherence tomography-based calcium scoring system to predict stent underexpansion. *EuroIntervention*. 2018;13:e2182–e2189.
31. Kubo T, Akasaka T, Shite J, et al. OCT compared with IVUS in a coronary lesion assessment: the OPUS-CLASS study. *JACC Cardiovasc Imaging*. 2013;6:1095–1104.
35. Raber L, Mintz GS, Koskinas KC, et al. Clinical use of intracoronary imaging. Part 1: guidance and optimization of coronary interventions. An expert consensus document of the european association of percutaneous cardiovascular interventions: endorsed by the chinese society of cardiology. *Eur Heart J*. 2018. https://doi.org/10.1093/eurheartj/ehy285.
45. Jia H, Abtahian F, Aguirre AD, et al. In vivo diagnosis of plaque erosion and calcified nodule in patients with acute coronary syndrome by intravascular optical coherence tomography. *J Am Coll Cardiol*. 2013;62:1748–1758.
51. Jia H, Dai J, Hou J, et al. Effective anti-thrombotic therapy without stenting: intravascular optical coherence tomography-based management in plaque erosion (the EROSION study). *Eur Heart J*. 2017;38:792–800.
54. Saia F, Komukai K, Capodanno D, et al. Eroded versus ruptured plaques at the culprit site of STEMI: in vivo pathophysiological features and response to primary PCI. *JACC Cardiovasc Imaging*. 2015;8:566–575.
64. Komukai K, Kubo T, Kitabata H, et al. Effect of atorvastatin therapy on fibrous cap thickness in coronary atherosclerotic plaque as assessed by optical coherence tomography: the EASY-FIT study. *J Am Coll Cardiol*. 2014;64:2207–2217.
68. Prati F, Romagnoli E, Gatto L, et al. Clinical impact of suboptimal stenting and Residual Intrastent Plaque/Thrombus Protrusion in patients with Acute Coronary Syndrome: the CLI-OPCI ACS substudy (centro per la lotta contro l'infarto-optimization of percutaneous coronary intervention in acute coronary syndrome). *Circ Cardiovasc Interv*. 2016;9. https://doi.org/10.1161/CIRCINTERVENTIONS.115.003726.
69. Okamura T, Nagoshi R, Fujimura T, et al. Impact of guidewire re-crossing point into stent jailed side branch for optimal kissing balloon dilatation: core lab 3D optical coherence tomography analysis. *EuroIntervention*. 2018;13:e1785–e1793.
74. Ozaki Y, Okumura M, Ismail TF, et al. The fate of incomplete stent apposition with drug-eluting stents: an optical coherence tomography-based natural history study. *Eur Heart J*. 2010;31:1470–1476.
79. Chamié D, Bezerra HG, Attizzani GF, et al. Incidence, predictors, morphological characteristics, and clinical outcomes of stent edge dissections detected by optical coherence tomography. *JACC Cardiovasc Interv*. 2013;6:800–813.
86. Guagliumi G, Shimamura K, Sirbu V, et al. Temporal course of vascular healing and neoatherosclerosis after implantation of durable- or biodegradable-polymer drug-eluting stents. *Eur Heart J*. 2018;39:2448–2456.
91. Taniwaki M, Radu MD, Zaugg S, et al. Mechanisms of very late drug-eluting stent thrombosis assessed by optical coherence tomography. *Circulation*. 2016;133:650–660.
96. Otsuka F, Vorpahl M, Nakano M, et al. Pathology of second-generation everolimus-eluting stents versus first-generation sirolimus- and paclitaxel-eluting stents in humans. *Circulation*. 2014;129:211–223.
104. Guagliumi G, Sirbu V, Musumeci G, et al. Examination of the in vivo mechanisms of late drug-eluting stent thrombosis: findings from optical coherence tomography and intravascular ultrasound imaging. *JACC Cardiovasc Interv*. 2012;5:12–20.
113. Lassen JF, Burzotta F, Banning AP, et al. Percutaneous coronary intervention for the left main stem and other bifurcation lesions: 12th consensus document from the European Bifurcation Club. *EuroIntervention*. 2018;13:1540–1553.

Additional references available online at expertconsult.com.

SECTION VII

第七部分

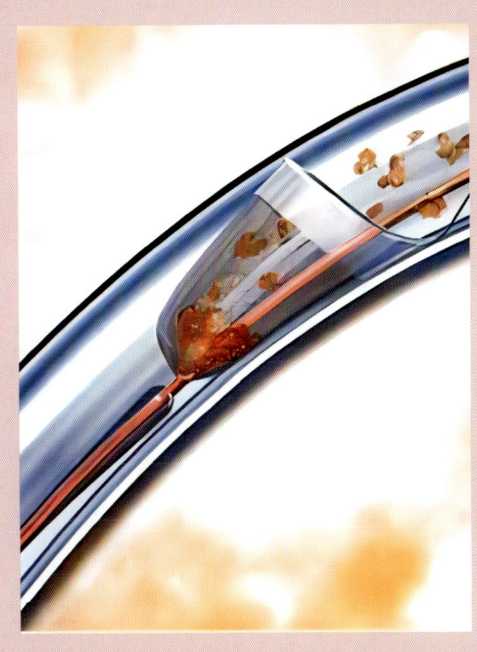

Outcome Effectiveness of Interventional Cardiology

介入心脏病学的疗效

中文导读

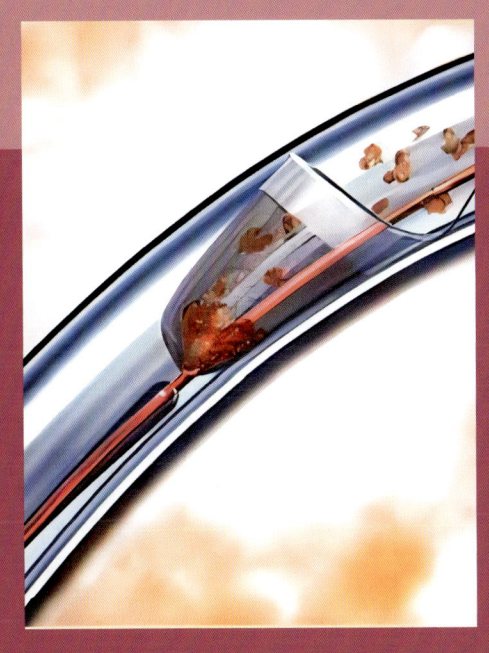

第68章
介入心脏病领域的卫生经济学

　　卫生经济学评价着眼于临床、人文、经济结果，为决策者提供关于医疗干预措施投入产出的重要信息，在介入性心脏病方面的公共卫生领域、技术评估领域、临床决策领域及卫生投资领域发挥重要作用。卫生经济学全面评价常见的3种方式为：成本—效果分析、成本—效用分析和成本—效益分析。

　　成本—效果分析与成本—效用分析在评价经济性方面最为广泛应用，评价指标主要有增加生命年或质量调整生命年。卫生经济评估常需分析长期成本产出，甚至患者终身，因此需将不同时间点的成本效益换算为同一时间点的成本效益，故需评估贴现或贴现率。卫生经济学研究主要有3种类型：借助Markov模型进行成本—效益分析、观察性研究、随机对照研究。卫生经济学效果的阈值选择，需政策制定者在综合判断多项研究、不同干预方式等基础上决定。

　　本章节对包括急性冠状动脉综合征、结构性心脏病等不同病种，阐述了传统药物治疗、介入治疗、冠状动脉搭桥等不同治疗方法，另外在抗栓治疗及不同用药等介入心脏病学方面，进行卫生经济学多方位的评估分析论述。

王　媛　吴永健

章节要点

- 卫生经济学非健康结局等价性的全面评价方式有三种：成本—效果分析、成本—效用分析和成本—效益分析。

- 成本—效果分析与成本—效用分析在评价经济性方面最为广泛应用，但成本—效益分析较少被应用。

- 成本—效果分析及成本—效用分析评估某治疗或措施的每一健康收益单位所耗费的成本。健康收益常通过增加生命年或质量调整生命年衡量。

- 经济评估通常有时间范围限制。通常情况下，需评估全生命时长，评估未来成本和健康效益。未来成本和健康收益的权重常与它们发生的时间相关，且未来成本和健康收益的权重多小于当前成本和健康收益。

- 卫生经济学研究主要有3种类型：借助Markov模型进行成本—效益分析、观察性研究、随机对照研究。

- 虽然从科学角度而言，在评估某治疗方法是否具有成本效益时，应使用成本—效果可接受曲线，但当政策制定者寻求一个基准来比较不同治疗方法和不同研究时，常需要阈值。

SECTION VII Outcome Effectiveness of Interventional Cardiology

68 Medical Economics in Interventional Cardiology

Zaher Fanari, Sandra Weiss, William S. Weintraub

KEY POINTS

- There are three forms of full economic evaluations that do not assume equivalence of health outcome: cost-effectiveness analysis (CEA), cost-utility analysis (CUA), and cost-benefit analysis (CBA).
- Both CEA and CUA are widely used to decide whether a medical intervention is economically attractive, whereas CBA is used much less.
- CEA and CUA assess the incremental costs for a therapy or strategy to produce an incremental unit of health benefit; health benefits are traditionally assessed as either the number of added life-years (LYs) or quality-adjusted life-years (QALYs).
- Economic assessment is usually assessed over a time horizon. Typically, a lifetime horizon is used and that requires assessing both the future costs and health benefits. Future costs and health gain are commonly weighted in relation to the time at which they occur, and usually future costs and health effects receive less weight than present ones.
- Medical cost studies generally fall into one of three categories: cost-effectiveness simulations using Markov models, observational studies, and randomized controlled trials (RCTs).
- Although from a scientific standpoint cost-effectiveness acceptability curves should be used when assessing whether a treatment is cost effective, a requirement for threshold usually arises when policy makers seek a benchmark to compare different treatments and judge different studies.

INTRODUCTION

Health care costs are increasing steadily in the developed world, due in part to the development of new and more expensive medical technologies and treatments.[1] The field of interventional cardiology has undergone tremendous changes over the past 10 years, with expansion in diagnostic and therapeutic tools used in coronary interventions, as well as the introduction of new catheter-based interventions for noncoronary cardiac conditions. Although percutaneous coronary intervention (PCI) remains among the most common major medical procedures in the United States, data suggest that the volume of PCI is declining or at least that there will be minimal growth in the near future.[2-4] On the other hand, there is significant expansion in the volume of noncoronary interventions, including peripheral arterial and structural heart disease interventions, with a concomitant increase in the involvement of interventional cardiologists in these procedures.[5]

The changes in the field, the aging population, and the limitations on resources and reimbursements the Patient Protection and Affordable Care Act have engendered make understanding basic concepts on medical economics a necessity. The goal of this chapter is to provide an overview of the basic concepts of medical economics and show the available evidence of economics in different aspects of interventional cardiology.

MEDICAL ECONOMICS: CONCEPTS AND METHODS

Basic Concepts/Terminology

A fundamental concept of economics is that resources are limited and can never satisfy all societal wants, and therefore when resources are used for health care, they are lost for other potential uses, such as education, infrastructure, or the environment. Thus we should think of cost not merely as money required to provide a particular good or service but rather as the opportunity cost, where it represents the consumption of the society's resources required to produce that good or service, that could have been used for other purposes.[1]

Because opportunity cost remains more a fundamental concept rather than a real measurement tool, other metrics for cost are necessary. The typical accounting price that is used in the regular market, which adds a reasonable amount of profit to the cost of production, is not clearly applicable in the U.S. medical field, due to cost shifting of many other expenses (e.g., bad debts, rejected payment by third parties, fee for services including employee salaries, cost of maintenance, and expansion of services).[6] The addition of these cost-shifting fees distorts the relationship between U.S. medical charges and medical resource consumption. Therefore U.S. medical charges should not be used as a surrogate for medical costs in research and policy evaluations.[6]

Other cost concepts used in medical economics include average cost, marginal cost, incremental cost, induced cost, and indirect cost. Average cost is overall cost per unit (i.e., the total costs divided by the total number of units of production). Marginal cost is the cost of producing one additional (or one less) unit of product, such as PCI or coronary bypass surgery. This concept excludes costs that do not vary as a direct function of production (termed fixed costs), such as the cost of the interventional laboratory or operating room facilities. Incremental cost is defined as the extra costs associated with an expansion in activity of a given service. Incremental cost is particularly useful in focusing on costs of shifting groups of patients from one diagnostic or therapeutic strategy to another and is essential in economic evaluations. For example, when a hospital is starting a transcatheter aortic valve replacement (TAVR) program, the incremental cost will adjust for the cost of hiring specialists who perform this procedure or training an existing interventional cardiologist, hiring a TAVR coordinator, training the catheterization lab staff about the procedure, and the cost of any new equipment and/or adjustment to the existing catheterization lab or operating room. Induced cost (or savings) is the cost of the tests or therapies added or averted as a consequence of some initial management decision, resource use, or both. For example, interventions that may cause more complications will increase (induce) use of resources, whereas an intervention that decreases complications or resource use may reduce (save) cost.[6]

Medical Economics Terminology

Overall, economic evaluations provide vital information to decision makers on both the inputs and outcomes of a health or medical intervention compared with available alternatives.[7] These types of analyses build on the results of clinical effectiveness studies but go beyond them to include a broader view of clinical, humanistic, and/or economic outcomes.[8] Clinical outcomes are medical events that are considered meaningful by medical professionals. Humanistic outcomes include a broad array of intangible personal attributes, typically self-reported by patients, such as quality of life and even spiritual well-being.[7] Economic outcomes represent the consumption and production of resources and their monetary value from the perspective of a decision maker.[7] A full economic evaluation is a study that provides a comparison of one or more interventions/approaches of interest to a defined standard of care, especially the cost of each intervention/approach in relation to the effects (or benefits or returns) of each. Comparing only investment costs between interventions or approaches is considered a partial economic evaluation.[9]

Cost Measurement

A thorough economic evaluation should completely account for all relevant costs. Such an evaluation does not include only the cost of the new treatment or test but also accounts for the costs of concomitant therapy, the costs of treating any complications, and the costs of subsequent events. For example, a new treatment for acute coronary syndrome might increase bleeding but reduce stent thrombosis and/or recurrent myocardial infarction (MI) and therefore the risk and cost of readmission. Therefore a fair evaluation would account for the extra cost of increase bleeding, as well as the potential cost savings of recurrent MI.[1]

The time frame for the economic evaluation needs to be long enough to encompass all costs resulting from a particular intervention, because subsequent and long-term clinical complications may be decreased or increased by a treatment or test. Although some therapies may pay for themselves with immediate savings, others may have higher initial costs but later significant savings. Therefore it is crucial for every economic evaluation to have sufficient scope to account for all relevant costs, including both early and late adverse events.[1] As costs may accrue over a lifetime, a lifetime time horizon will be the most inclusive. However, this may not always be feasible.

Evaluation of Procedure and Hospital Cost

Evaluation of the true cost of a specific procedure and the associated hospital stay is a very challenging process. In practice, obtaining the detailed data about individual resources being consumed for an intervention and adding up these costs to perform marginal or incremental cost analysis (the bottom-up approach) are difficult and often impractical. Performing a true bottom-up cost analysis (microcosting analysis) is a complex, time-consuming process that requires identification of all the inputs into a health care service and the assignment of an appropriate cost to each. Furthermore, even if this process was achievable for simple treatments, it becomes more complex when considering complex interventional procedures such as a PCI and very complicated when accounting for the entire hospital stay from admission to discharge.[1] Therefore most U.S. cost studies start with an aggregated measure of costs, such as can be obtained from hospital or physician bills (a top-down analysis).

To overcome this complexity, cost data in the United States are obtained mainly by one of two approaches: The first approach involves converting hospital charges (taken from the hospital bill) to costs using the ratios of costs to charges (RCCs) included in each hospital's annual Medicare Cost Report. This report is built based on annual reporting of every hospital to the Centers for Medicare and Medicaid Services (CMS) that includes details of expenses for direct patient care, overhead, capital equipment, and so forth related to billed charges. Although the Medicare RCCs are not designed for research, it still provides a moderately standardized means of estimating cost across hospitals in the United States. In addition, costs calculated with the RCC method are used to recalibrate diagnosis-related group (DRG) weights by CMS. Therefore this method provides a valuable tool for multicenter cost research. However, this approach has several limitations. First, this approach does not separate out overhead and most other fixed costs and therefore provides only an estimate of average rather than marginal cost, so it may overestimate potential cost savings. Second, due to the complexity of the instructions for reporting to CMS, hospitals may choose to interpret the instructions differently, resulting in significant variability in uncovering hospitals' actual costs. Finally, the RCCs themselves are an average of all cost-charge relationships from hospital revenue centers, such as the radiology, pharmacy, or laboratory departments; therefore the Medicare whole hospital-level RCCs may not be particularly accurate in converting these charges to costs to reflect individual patient resource consumption. In addition, this method is limited to hospitals using standardized methods of billing, applicable to most but not all U.S. hospitals and to no hospitals outside the United States. Finally, physician costs are not included in this approach.[6]

The second approach depends on calculating the hospital and intervention costs from reimbursement rates for DRGs reported to the CMS by hospitals. This approach also has several limitations. First, it is not sensitive to variations in resource-use intensity within a DRG, as DRG reimbursement rates represent the "average" cost for a particular diagnosis/procedure among all patients in that DRG. Second, the CMS decides in many cases not to increase reimbursement to cover the costs of new technology; therefore the cost of these new technologies may not be well reflected in the DRG.[6] However, this approach does not require collection of hospital bills and, with some assumptions, can potentially be applied to any hospitalization in any health care system, therefore simplifying its use. By assigning DRGs to hospitalizations within studies where DRGs from the hospital bill is not available, this approach can be used for international studies. However, assigning costs to a DRG for hospitalization in international studies is complicated and controversial.[6,10]

Many studies estimate costs by counting only big-ticket items used (e.g., number of diagnostic cardiac catheterizations, PCIs, or coronary artery bypass graftings (CABGs); days in the intensive care unit [ICU]; total hospital length of stay) and assigning a unit price to each item. The resulting linear formula: Total cost = Σ price × quantity is simple and inexpensive to use (which makes it desirable in clinical research); however, this approach suffers from some significant downsides. First, the source of cost weights is often acquired from available unrelated economic sources external to the resource data being analyzed and therefore of uncertain quality. Second, the appropriate set of big-ticket items necessary to estimate costs accurately by this method has never been rigorously defined. For example, some studies, especially multicenter clinical trials, may use the more easily obtained total hospital length of stay instead of defining specific ICU and non-ICU hospital lengths of stay that may be more representative of accurate cost. Third, most studies treat big-ticket items similarly to preserve the desired simplicity, although they are not necessarily homogeneous. For example, by using payments by the DRG, an uncomplicated single-vessel PCI would typically be assigned the same price as a complex three-vessel PCI or complex graft intervention that was complicated by abrupt closure, while the true costs of these procedures are, in fact, substantially different.[6]

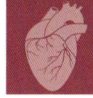

Evaluation of Physician Costs

Evaluating physician costs also has serious challenges. This estimation is also made by one of two approaches. The first approach depends on acquiring the "fee for service" bills from physicians' offices. This approach had several limitations. First, most patients receive services from several physicians and collecting these bills from multiple offices is a far more complicated process than collecting hospital bills. Second, due to multiple services with different costs and reimbursements in physicians' offices, cost-shifting process is used to cover for unreimbursed and underreimbursed services without the detailed report of real costs that is required by hospitals when they practice cost shifting. Therefore using "fee for service" bill is not an accurate reflection of the true market price for physician services.[6]

To overcome the limitation of using the physicians' bill, another approach uses the Medicare Fee Schedule based on the resource-based relative-value scale (RBRVS).[11] An estimation of physician costs can be created using available data from the American Medical Association Physician's Current Procedural Terminology (CPT). This approach is not ideal, but it has the advantage of being more objective and consistent and might represent the best available U.S. national measure of the economic value of physician work.[11]

Factors That Impact Cost Assessment

The different perspectives of patients, providers, health payers, and society will lead to different assessment of cost. Although patients may consider only out of pocket or copayment costs, health payers may consider the cost of the procedure, associated hospital cost, and whether the medication used is generic or nongeneric. Providers may consider cost in relation to the health benefit for an individual patient and then weigh it against public health implications of this procedure. When assessing the cost of a health service, ideally it should assess not only the immediate cost of the strategy but also consider the overall society perspective, which ultimately rests with all stakeholders in society. Societal costs include the hospital costs, physician fees, outpatient testing, and outpatient drug therapy costs, but also nonmedical direct expenses (e.g., transportation to the medical facility, child care, housekeeping) and the economic impact of lost productivity because of illness.[6,10]

However, total societal cost cannot be measured effectively because each component is measured by a proxy. To eliminate some of this uncertainty, payer costs are often measured instead. However, payer costs do not represent the complete spectrum of the societal costs. CMS uses DRGs to pay hospitals regardless of the cost of service to the provider, whereas private insurance may use a different scheme to pay providers. Payments may therefore have significant variability between payers.[10]

Furthermore, time effects are important to medical cost analyses because either inflation or deflation will change the cost of a procedure. A common approach to deal with this is to pick a base year and then use the medical inflation rate to deflate all costs in subsequent year to the base year.[6,10,12]

Another important factor in determining cost is related to geography. The costs of material and labor inputs to medical care can vary substantially from one part of the United States to another and between large urban university hospitals to small rural community hospitals, creating true differences in cost for medical services according to geography that needs to be adjusted. Several geographic adjustment indices are available, including the Medicare area wage index (for adjusting DRG reimbursement) and the Medicare Fee Schedule geographic adjustment factor.[6,10,12] International studies are yet more complex.

Analysis Methods

Several forms of economic evaluations can be performed, and each differs based on the selection and measurement of health outcomes. Although the term "cost effectiveness" is frequently used for all medical economic analyses, cost-effectiveness analysis (CEA) is only one type of assessment. The most basic form of economic evaluation is called a cost-consequence study, which is simply a table that lists the individual economic and health outcomes of alternative interventions. A more advanced but still basic economic form is called cost identification studies that measure only the investment cost of interventions and are used to provide the data needed to better design future studies that consider both the economic and health outcomes of two or more alternative therapies. A more advanced form of economic analysis is called cost minimization analysis (CMA), which differs from cost identification in assuming equivalence in health outcomes among alternative therapies and examines economic outcomes. So even though it examines only economic outcomes, in practice under the assumption of equivalence, a CMA is a form of full economic evaluation.[7]

There are three forms of full economic evaluations that do not assume equivalence of health outcome: CEA, cost-utility analysis (CUA), and cost-benefit analysis (CBA). The definitions and differences between these three forms are summarized in Table 68.1.[7] Both CEA and CUA are widely used to decide whether a medical intervention is economically attractive, whereas CBA is used much less because it requires measuring all health-related benefits of an intervention or approach in monetary terms without emphasis on either the longevity or quality of the lives involved.[7]

The primary goal of CEA is to evaluate different health care intervention options in common terms so that policy and other decision makers can be informed of the most efficient method of producing extra health benefits from among the alternative ways that health care dollars can be distributed. In both CEA and CUA

TABLE 68.1 Types of Full Economic Assessment

	Cost-Effectiveness Analysis	Cost-Utility Analysis	Cost-Benefit Analysis
Definition	A form of economic-efficiency analysis in which costs are valued in monetary terms and health benefits are valued in natural units.	A variant of cost-effectiveness analysis in which the health benefits are expressed in a scale that incorporates both longevity and patient preferences (utilities) for the health states produced.	A form of economic-efficiency analysis in which both the costs and outcomes (health benefits) are valued in monetary terms.
Unit of Health Outcomes	Natural units (e.g., the number of added life-years (LYs)	Summary measure in quality of life units (e.g., quality-adjusted LYs [QALYs])	Summary measure in monetary units (o.g., U.S. dollars)
Results	Cost-effectiveness ratio (C1 – C2) / (HB1 – HB2)	Cost-utility ratio (C1 – C2) / (QALY1 – QALY2)	Net benefits (B1 – B2) – (C1 – C2) or (B1– B2) / (C1 – C2)

B1, Monetary value of health outcomes of alternative 1; *B2*, monetary value of health outcomes of alternative 2; *C1*, total costs of alternative 1; *C2*, total costs of alternative 2; *HB1*, health benefit of alternative 1; *HB2*, health benefit of alternative 2; *QALY1*, quality-adjusted life-years of alternative 1; *QALY2*, quality-adjusted life-years of alternative 2.

the metric used to assess incremental cost effectiveness is the incremental cost-effectiveness ratio (ICER). An ICER is defined as the ratio of incremental costs to incremental health benefits or ICER = (C1 − C2) / (HB1 − HB2), where C1 and C2 are cost for treatment 1 and 2, respectively, and HB is the health benefit of treatment 1 and 2, respectively.[1]

ICER is a ratio that has a distribution because there is uncertainty in both cost and effectiveness measurements. When patient-level data are available, it is possible to consider the uncertainty in both cost and effectiveness due to the play of chance (i.e., stochastic error). To examine the confidence intervals of cost and effectiveness due to the play of chance, an approach called bootstrap analysis is widely used.[13] It depends on sampling both the cost and effectiveness distributions concurrently which allows for multiple estimates of the ICER to be made, plotted as a pictorial four quadrant distribution (Fig. 68.1): (1) Quadrant A: the new therapy is more effective and more costly than the previous standard; (2) Quadrant B: the new therapy dominates the standard, being more effective and less expensive; (3) Quadrant C: the new therapy is less effective and less expensive; and (4) Quadrant D: the new therapy is dominated by the standard, being less effective and more expensive. The dots represent the individual estimations of the ICER from the dual bootstrap analysis.

The ICER defines the cost that should be assumed for gaining one unit of output. In other words, if one of the alternatives is the usual practice, then it will tell us how much it will cost to gain a unit of outcome when moving from the usual practice to the alternative. The health benefit may be measured in any sensible unit, such as number of MIs averted, but most economics use the conventional option of measuring clinical benefits as either the number of added life-years (LYs) or quality-adjusted life-years (QALYs).[1,14] Both of these approaches require estimation of life expectancy with and without the intervention being considered.

Although LYs are conceptually simple because its estimation depends only on survival, many therapies are used primarily to improve quality of life rather than to increase longevity, and therefore a broader measurement of QALYs is needed. To estimate QALYs, it is first necessary to estimate utility. Utility is defined as the relative desirability of a particular health outcome or health state, assessed as the preference of a rater (typically a patient or a member of the general public) for that outcome relative to the defined and extreme alternatives (e.g., death, excellent health). Every health state will have a unique utility. In health care economics, utility is generally scaled from 0 to 1, with a utility of 0 for death and 1 for perfect health and functioning. The relationship between utility and cost can be assessed by CUA with the use of QALYs, which is life expectancy multiplied by utility. The value of 1 year of life in excellent health would be represented by 1.0 QALY (i.e., 1 life-year multiplied by a utility of 1).[1]

Utility Assessment

Utility may be measured by patient preference methods or by surveys that have been mapped to patient preference methods. Theoretically, the best direct measure of utility is the "standard gamble" method because it assesses both overall quality of life and risk aversion. However, this measure is complex to obtain and may not be practical to administer in large trials.[15] Most economic analyses derive utilities from surveys (e.g., EQ-5D or the Health Utilities Index). Using this approach, patient health states are defined by a number of explicit domains such as physical functioning and pain. Then, previously measured utility weights from patients (i.e., those with the condition of interest) or the general public (i.e., those who are at risk for getting the condition of interest) are assigned to each possible health state.[1,7]

Time Horizon and Discounting

The time horizon of an analysis reflects the length of time over which clinical health benefits and costs should be considered and included in the analysis. The time frame should be the same for both the clinical outcomes and costs. Although the time for many trials may be limited to either short or intermediate time horizon secondary to limitations related to budgets and enrollment, the evaluation of cost effectiveness from the societal perspective requires applying a long-term or lifetime time horizon.[16]

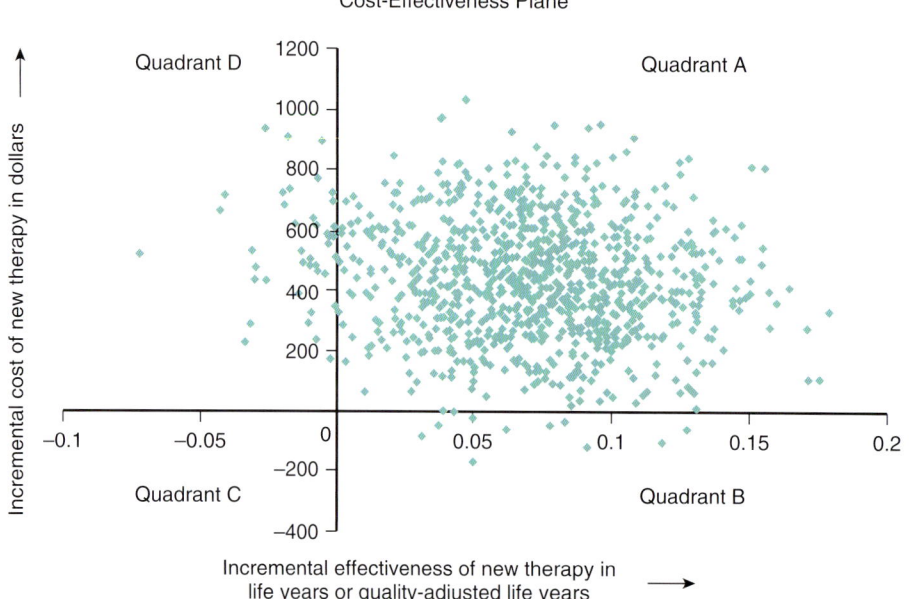

Fig. 68.1 Distribution of cost effectiveness. In quadrant A, the new therapy is more effective and more costly than the previous standard. In quadrant B, the new therapy dominates the standard because it is more effective and less expensive. In quadrant C, the new therapy is less effective and less expensive. In quadrant D, the new therapy is dominated by the standard because it is less effective and more expensive. Dots represent individual estimations of the incremental cost-effectiveness ratio from the dual bootstrap analysis.

Assessing the cost effectiveness over a lifetime horizon requires assessing both the future costs and health benefits. Future costs and health gain are commonly weighted in relation to the time at which they occur, and usually future costs and health effects receive less weight than present ones. This process is called discounting.[17]

The idea behind discounting comes from the assumption that money available or spent now is more valuable than money available or spent in the future, because money available now can be put to immediate use. Because costs are discounted, the benefits of health interventions must also be discounted. It is important to emphasize that discounting is not an adjustment for inflation, which is a separate consideration. As even in the absence of inflation, most individuals would prefer to have an equivalent health benefit or money now as opposed to in the future. The discount rate captures this time preference. When data regarding costs are derived from different years, older costs are usually inflated to their equivalent values in more recent years so that there can be a consistent economic basis. If future medical inflation costs rise uniformly, then future purchasing power for health care remains the same, and there is no need to adjust for medical inflation.[17]

Sensitivity Analysis

Even in the most carefully conducted cost-effectiveness studies, considerable uncertainty may remain regarding the parameters used to measure costs and health effects. This uncertainty is in addition to accounting for the play of chance with bootstrap analysis, which is not sufficient to account for any additional uncertainty or bias. To identify and assess the degree to which uncertainty in the parameter could affect the overall results, CEAs usually perform multiple evaluations in which one or more of the parameters are varied across reasonable ranges. The ranges reflect intrinsic variability or regional variation. As an example, the cost of diagnostic cardiac catheterization may be cheaper in some institutions or health care delivery settings compared with others; thus to determine the cost effectiveness of PCI in stable coronary artery disease (CAD), the cost of PCI could be varied over a range to determine the maximal cost at which it remains cost effective. This process (termed "sensitivity analysis") allows for a reasonable appraisal about the parameters that are most important in the analysis and the stability of the reference case results.[16]

Sensitivity analyses have typically assessed the effect varying selected parameters related to cost effectiveness one at a time. A more contemporary approach called Monte Carlo simulation permits all parameters to be varied simultaneously. These sophisticated analyses yield a cost-effectiveness acceptability curve, which accounts for uncertainty in all model estimates. The end result is that the curve displays the likelihood that a new intervention will have a cost-effectiveness ratio that falls below a particular societal "willingness to pay." (See Benchmarks in Economic Analysis later.)[16]

DATA SOURCE FOR ECONOMIC ANALYSIS AND DECISION MAKING

Medical cost studies generally fall into one of three categories: cost-effectiveness simulations using Markov models, observational studies, and randomized controlled trials (RCTs).

Simulation With Markov Models

Many economic analyses are developed as simulations. Simulations most commonly involve the construction of a decision tree to model the prognosis of a patient subsequent to the choice of a management strategy. Markov model is one of the widely used models in cost-effective analysis because it represents a convenient way of modeling prognosis for clinical problems with ongoing risk. The model assumes that the patient is always in one of a finite number of states of health referred to as Markov states (Fig. 68.2). The introduction of the presumed intervention will cause some of the patients to move to another Markov state. The transition from one state to another will represent the events of interest and the time of this transition is referred to as Markov cycles. By assigning a utility to each health state and running the model for health cycles until death, we can calculate cumulative QALYs. Similarly, costs are accumulated during the Markov cycles. The incremental costs of an intervention compared with a previous standard divided by the incremental benefits yield an ICER. Markov models are often informed by the medical literature, often including randomized clinical trials when available for the issue being considered.

For example, patients with stable CAD who undergo CABG may move from being disabled by angina to being well, staying disabled, or dying (see Fig. 68.2). Obviously, patients who die will not move to another state, whereas disabled or well patients may move from one health state to another. Assuming that the incremental utility of the well state is 1.0 and the dead state is 0, and if we assign a presumed incremental utility of 0.6 to the disabled states, and that the patient spends on average 2.5 cycles in the well state and 1.25 cycles in the disabled state before entering the dead state, the utility assigned would be (2.5 × 1) + (1.25 × 0.6), or 3.25 quality-adjusted cycles. This number is the quality-adjusted life expectancy of the patient.[18]

Cost-Effectiveness Analysis With Patient Level Data

Observational cost studies include both descriptive series without an intrinsic comparison group and nonrandomized treatment comparisons. Descriptive cost studies are useful when data about cost are not readily available in the literature and are usually used to make sample size projections for RCTs or to inform cost effectiveness and other health policy studies (in conjunction with appropriate sensitivity analyses). Observational comparison data can be helpful in estimating the real-world cost outside the restrictions or requirements of an RCT but usually require statistical techniques to adjust for treatment selection bias and bias that may be related to the variation of medical costs over time, among different geographic locations, and among different practice settings.

The second major approach to economic evaluation is to measure economic cost as an end point in an RCT. The strengths of this approach are (1) using prospective, complete data collection, (2) a well-defined protocol that measures directly the economic and clinical outcomes with few assumptions and little simulation, (3) random assignment to eliminate treatment selection bias, (4) concomitant collection of economic and clinical data that

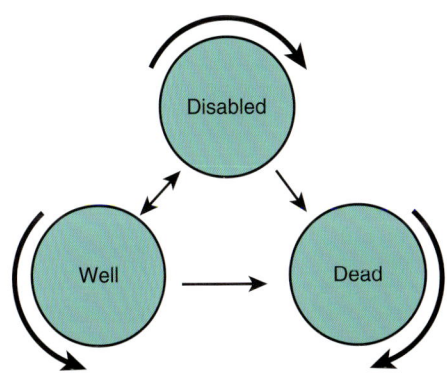

Fig. 68.2 Different health states. Movement among Markov states of health.

alleviates any concerns about inconsistencies among data sources, and (5) collection of patient level data permitting estimation of stochastic error. A potential disadvantage is that RCTs mandate protocol-driven care that can deviate from usual clinical practice (i.e., extra protocol-driven angiography or mandated office follow-up visits) and distort resource use patterns and make them unsuitable for economic analysis. Another limitation is related to the high selection criteria of patients involved in the trial, which may make the cost analysis not applicable to the general population. Clinical trials will generally have a time frame of weeks to several years. If the time horizon for CEA is lifetime, then survival, utility, and cost must be estimated beyond the time frame of measured data.[6,10,12]

Benchmarks in Economic Analysis

One of the major challenges in health care is that individual patients (and their physicians) wish to obtain all the health benefits that are available from modern medical technology. However, for society as a whole, resources are not adequate to meet this need for every individual, which forces difficult and potentially divisive choices. There is no absolute standard that can be applied to assess how much a certain society is willing to pay for medical care.[19,20]

This willingness to pay may be better understood by constructing a cost-effectiveness acceptability curve (Fig. 68.3), in which a range of ICER willingness-to-pay thresholds are displayed on the x-axis, and the y-axis indicates the probability that the new therapy has an ICER below this threshold. The curve can be constructed from Markov model simulations or from patient level data. Using this curve, we can estimate what can be acceptable for a treatment. Points A, B and C represent increasing willing-to-pay thresholds. Point A is the lowest, and there is a low probability of the new therapy being considered cost effective. Point C is the highest willingness-to-pay threshold, with the highest probability of the new therapy being cost effective. Point B is in between.

Although from a scientific standpoint cost-effectiveness acceptability curves should be used when assessing whether a treatment is cost effective, a requirement for threshold can arise when policy makers seek a benchmark to compare different treatments and judge different studies. In general, wealthier countries may be willing to pay more (i.e., accept a higher threshold) for a given treatment than poorer countries.[1,21] In the United States, cost-effectiveness ratios <$50,000 per LY or QALY gained is frequently regarded as economically attractive.[1] Conversely, a cost-effectiveness ratio of >$100,000 per added LY or QALY is frequently regarded as economically unattractive. The range between these two benchmarks is the gray zone in which there is no consensus on whether a treatment is economically acceptable.[1] However, assigning the same ICER threshold for different treatment in a wide range of diseases and different burden of these diseases may not be reasonable. Some countries may assign a general threshold for most cases but allow for a higher threshold for treatments that relieve considerable burden of illness (i.e., "the rule of rescue"). For example, in the Netherlands, the average acceptable ICER is approximately €20,000, but an ICER of €80,000 per QALY will be acceptable for illnesses associated with a considerable disease burden.[22] Similarly in Great Britain, the limit of acceptable ICER varies between £20,000 and £30,000 depending on the burden of the disease.[23]

MEDICAL ECONOMICS OF CORONARY INTERVENTIONS IN STABLE CORONARY ARTERY DISEASE (TABLE 68.2)

Therapeutic strategies for stable CAD are optimal medical treatment (OMT) and revascularization with either PCI or CABG. In the setting of stable CAD, both OMT and revascularization strategies have similar efficacy regarding prevention of MI and death.[24–26] However, the impact of these different strategies on patient quality of life and the cost of these options vary substantially in the short and long term. Medical therapy carries the lowest initial cost, but it is usually less effective in relieving angina.[25] However, this initial cost savings may be offset by the potential increased rate of repeated utilization and subsequent clinical interventions, including hospitalizations and additional revascularization. Similarly, the initial cost of PCI is usually lower than that of CABG; however, the need for potential repeat revascularization may increase the cost of the PCI strategy long term.

This section will discuss the comparative cost effectiveness of OMT with revascularization strategies, as well as among different revascularization strategies including comparing different techniques used in PCI.

Cost Effectiveness of Medical Therapy Versus Revascularization

Medical therapy for stable CAD witnessed significant improvement over the past few decades. This was mirrored by similar improvements in PCI techniques with the introduction of bare-metal stents (BMSs) and drug-eluting stents (DESs), as well as improved CABG techniques with increased use of the left internal mammary artery (LIMA) as a surgical conduit and the less invasive off-pump CABG (OPCABG) and minimally invasive keyhole techniques (minimally invasive direct coronary artery bypass grafting [MIDCAB]).

The Medicine, Angioplasty, or Surgery Study (MASS-II) trial that randomized 611 patients to either PCI or OMT showed a lower incidence of the primary outcome, the composite of overall mortality, Q wave MI, or refractory angina in CABG when compared with PCI and medical therapy with no significant difference between the latter two at 5 years.[24] A CEA of MASS II showed that the event-free costs were significantly favoring OMT versus PCI ($9071 OMT vs. $19,967 PCI; $P < .01$) and versus CABG ($9071 OMT vs. $18,263 CABG; $P < .01$) and CABG versus PCI ($18,263 CABG vs. $19,967.00 PCI; $P = .01$). In addition, the event-free plus angina-free costs significantly favored OMT versus PCI ($16,553 OMT vs. $25,831 PCI; $P = .04$), and versus CABG ($16,553 OMT vs. $24,614 CABGP < .001$); there was no difference between CABG and PCI ($25,831 PCI vs. $24,614 CABG; $P > .05$).[27]

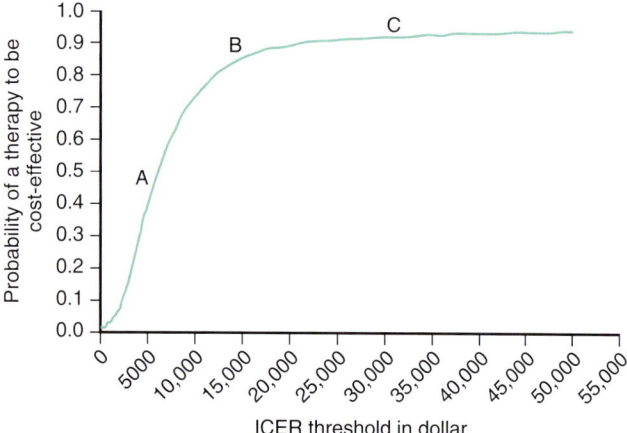

Fig. 68.3 Cost-effectiveness acceptability curve. Points A, B, and C represent increasing willingness-to-pay thresholds. Point A is the lowest, and there is a low probability of the new therapy being considered cost effective. Point C is the highest willingness to pay threshold with the highest probability of the new therapy being cost effective. Point B is in between. *ICER*, Incremental cost-effectiveness ratio.

The Bypass Angioplasty Revascularization Investigation 2 Diabetes (BARI 2D) trial randomized 2368 patients with both type 2 diabetes and heart disease to undergo either prompt revascularization with OMT or OMT alone.[26] There was no significant difference in the rates of death between patients undergoing prompt revascularization and those undergoing medical therapy. As for freedom from major cardiovascular events, although there was no difference between patients undergoing PCI and OMT, CABG was associated with fewer major cardiovascular events when compared with medical therapy.[26] CEA of BARI 2D trial showed that revascularization was associated with significantly higher costs compared with medical therapy. The 4-year costs were higher with both CABG ($80,900 CABG vs. $60,600 OMT; $P < .0001$) and PCI ($73,400 PCI vs. $67,800; $P < .02$). Using the $50,000/LY benchmark, OMT was more cost effective than PCI ($600/LY), whereas CABG was probably more cost effective than OMT ($47,000/LY).[28]

The Clinical Outcomes Utilizing Revascularization and Aggressive DruG Evaluation (COURAGE) trial that randomized 2287 patients with stable CAD to either PCI with OMT or OMT alone showed that PCI was not associated with any reduction in the risk of death, MI, or other major cardiovascular events when added to optimal medical therapy.[25] Furthermore, COURAGE showed that although PCI was associated with an incremental benefit for the first 12 to 24 months in the key domains of physical limitations, frequency of angina, and quality of life, that benefit disappeared by 36 months.[29] A CEA of COURAGE showed that PCI was associated with an added cost of approximately $10,000 per patient, without significant gain in LYs or QALYs. The ICER gained with PCI varied from just over $168,000 to just under $300,000 per LY or QALY gained and was therefore considered not cost effective.[30]

Cost Effectiveness of Percutaneous Coronary Intervention Using Drug-Eluting Stents Versus Coronary Artery Bypass Grafting in Stable Multivessel Disease

The first randomized controlled data to compare PCI with DES and CABG came from the Synergy between PCI with Taxus and Cardiac Surgery (SYNTAX) trial,[31] which showed that PCI with the paclitaxel-eluting TAXUS stent was associated with significantly higher rates of major adverse cardiovascular and cerebrovascular events (MACCEs) at 5 years in comparison with CABG (37.3% for DES vs. 26.9% for CABG; $P = .002$), in large part secondary to an increased rate of MI (9.7% DES vs. 3.8% CABG and target-vessel revascularization (TVR) (25.9% DES vs. 13.7% CABG, $P < .001$).[31]

The CEA of the SYNTAX trial showed that although CABG was associated with an initial $10,036 per patient higher hospitalization cost, over 5 years follow-up costs were higher with DES-PCI as a result of more frequent hospitalizations, revascularization procedures, and higher medication costs.[32] Over a lifetime horizon, CABG in patients with multivessel disease and SYNTAX score >22 remained more costly than DES-PCI, but the ICER was favorable ($16,537 per QALY gained). On the other hand, in patients with left main disease or a SYNTAX score of 22 or less, DES-PCI was economically dominant compared with CABG.[32]

Subsequently, the Future Revascularization Evaluation in Patients with Diabetes Mellitus: Optimal Management of Multivessel Disease (FREEDOM) trial showed higher incidence of the composite of death, MI, and stroke in diabetic patients undergoing PCI with DESs when compared with CABG at 5 years (26.6% DES vs. 18.7% CABG; $P = .05$), with a significantly higher incidence of TVR with PCI as early as 1 year (12.6% DES vs. 4.8% CABG; $P < .001$).[33]

TABLE 68.2 Medical Economics of Different Revascularization Strategies

Authors/Study	Comparator Groups	Type of Analysis	Results
Hlatky et al.[28]/BARI 2D	Patients with both type 2 diabetes and heart disease managed by either prompt revascularization (PCI or CABG) with OMT or OMT alone	Patient-level, RCT-based analysis	The 4-year costs were higher with both CABG ($80,900 CABG vs. $60,600 OMT; $P < .0001$) and PCI ($73,400 PCI vs. $67,800; $P < .02$). Using the $50,000/LY benchmark, OMT was more cost effective than PCI ($600/LY), while CABG was probably more cost effective than OMT ($47,000/LY)
Weintraub et al.[30]/COURAGE Trial	Patients with stable coronary artery disease managed by either PCI with OMT or OMT alone	Patient-level, RCT-based analysis	PCI was associated with an added cost of approximately $10,000 per patient, without significant gain in LY or QALY. The ICER gained with PCI varied from just over $168,000 to just under $300,000 per LY or QALY gained and was therefore considered not cost effective.
Cohen et al.[32]/SYNTAX trial	PCI using DES versus CABG in multivessel CAD or left main	Patient-level, RCT-based analysis	CABG in patients with multivessel disease and SYNTAX score >22 remained more costly than DES-PCI, but the ICER was favorable ($16,537 per QALY gained). On the other hand, in patients with left main disease or a SYNTAX score ≤22, DES-PCI was economically dominant compared with CABG
Magnuson et al.[34]/FREEDOM trial	PCI using DES versus CABG in patients with multivessel CAD and diabetes	Patient-level, RCT-based analysis	Although the cumulative 5-year costs were still higher with CABG ($3641 per patient), CABG was projected to be a more economically attractive option in comparison to PCI with DES, with substantial gains in both life expectancy and quality-adjusted life expectancy (ICER <$10,000 per LY or QALY gained)
Zhang et al.[36]/ASCERT trial	PCI versus CABG in MEDICARE multivessel CAD	Markov model on observational patients data	At 4 years, the average total costs were higher for CABG by $7825 ($32,428 CABG vs. $24,623 PCI). Unlike the RCT data, over a lifetime, the average total costs were higher for CABG by $6105 ($88,125 CABG vs. $82,020 PCI). However, using the common threshold of $50,000, CABG will often be a cost-effective strategy with an ICER of $48,135 per LY gained

ASCERT, American College of Cardiology Foundation/Society of Thoracic Surgery Database Collaboration on the Comparative Effectiveness of Revascularization Strategies; *BARI 2D*, Bypass Angioplasty Revascularization Investigation 2 Diabetes; *CABG*, coronary artery bypass grafting; *CAD*, coronary artery disease; *COURAGE*, Clinical Outcomes Utilizing Revascularization and Aggressive DruG Evaluation; *DES*, drug-eluting stent; *FREEDOM*, Future Revascularization Evaluation in Patients with Diabetes Mellitus: Optimal Management of Multivessel Disease; *ICER*, incremental cost-effectiveness ratio; *LY*, life-year; *OMT*, optimal medical treatment; *PCI*, percutaneous interventions; *QALY*, quality-adjusted life-year; *RCT*, randomized controlled trial; *SYNTAX*, Synergy Between Percutaneous Coronary Intervention With TAXUS and Cardiac Surgery.

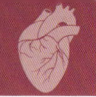

SECTION VII Outcome Effectiveness of Interventional Cardiology

CEA of the FREEDOM trial showed that initial procedural costs were higher with CABG ($8622 per patient). Over the next 5 years, even accounting for higher follow-up costs with PCI, the cumulative 5-year costs were still higher with CABG ($3641 per patient). However, when the analysis extended the modest gains in survival with CABG during the trial period to a lifetime horizon, CABG was projected to be the more economically attractive option in comparison with PCI with DES, with substantial gains in both life expectancy and quality-adjusted life expectancy (ICER <$10,000 per LY or QALY).[34]

Results from real-life registries demonstrated similar results. The American College of Cardiology Foundation/Society of Thoracic Surgery Database Collaboration on the Comparative Effectiveness of Revascularization Strategies (ASCERT) trial compared 86,244 Medicare patients who underwent CABG with 103,549 Medicare patients who underwent PCI and showed that although there was no significant difference in mortality between the groups at 1 year (6.24% CABG vs. 6.55% PCI; relative ratio [RR] = 0.95; 95% confidence interval [CI] 0.90 to 1.00) CABG was associated with a lower mortality rate at 4 years (16.4% CABG vs. 20.8% PCI; RR = 0.79; 95% CI 0.76 to 0.82).[35]

CEA of the ASCERT study[36] showed that in the first year, CABG was more costly and less effective than PCI with a higher cost by $10,951 during the initial hospitalization and by $9906 at the end of first year.[36] At 4 years, the average total costs were still higher for CABG by $7825 ($32,428 CABG vs. $24,623 PCI). Unlike the RCT data, over a lifetime, the average total costs were higher for CABG by $6105 ($88,125 CABG vs. $82,020 PCI). However, using the common threshold of $50,000, CABG will often be a cost-effective strategy with an ICER of $48,135 per LY gained (LYG).[36] Although ASCERT was large, with almost 200,000 patients, it was not randomized and thus subject to treatment selection bias, which can affect both clinical and economic outcomes.

In summary, although CABG is associated with higher initial and short-term costs, it seems to be a cost-effective long-term option compared with DESs, especially for high-risk patients with high angiographic complexity (SYNTAX score >32) or diabetes.

MEDICAL ECONOMICS OF CORONARY INTERVENTIONS IN ACUTE CORONARY SYNDROME (TABLES 68.3 AND 68.4)

Medical Economics of Reperfusion in ST-Elevation Myocardial Infarction

The management of ST-elevation MI (STEMI) witnessed major changes after the introduction of PCI. Although thrombolysis

TABLE 68.3 Medical Economics of Antiplatelet Therapy

Authors/Study	Comparator Groups	Type of Analysis	Results
Mahoney et al.[49]/ PCI-CURE Trial	Placebo vs. long-term clopidogrel in non–ST-ACS	Patient-level, RCT-(substudy) based analysis	Clopidogrel was associated with a higher average cost at 1 year of $253–$423. For patients who underwent PCI, the difference was less substantial and ranged from $155 lower to $90 higher with Clopidogrel. Clopidogrel proved to be a very attractive option with ICER of $2856–$4775 per LY without PCI and $935 per LY in the early PCI subgroup
Mahoney et al.[51]/ TRITON-TIMI-38	Clopidogrel vs. Prasugrel post-PCI in moderate- to high-risk ACS	Patient-level, RCT-based analysis	More than 14.7-month follow-up, prasugrel was associated with a net savings of $221 per patient when compared with clopidogrel. This saving was attributed to the lower rate of rehospitalizations involving PCI. Prasugrel was associated with life expectancy gains of 0.102 years (95% CI [0.030–0.180]), primarily because of the decreased rate of nonfatal MI. Prasugrel was shown to be an economically attractive strategy with an ICER of $9727 per life-year gained. However, this comparison was done between prasugrel and "brand" rather than "generic" clopidogrel
Nikolic et al.[53]/ PLATO Trial	Clopidogrel vs. ticagrelor post-PCI in moderate- to high-risk ACS	Patient-level, RCT-based analysis	Even though ticagrelor use was associated with higher costs of €362, that was balanced by a QALY gain of 0.13 compared with generic clopidogrel at 1 year. Therefore, the use of ticagrelor was an economically attractive option with an ICER of €2753 per QALY gained and €2372 per LY gained

ACS, Acute coronary syndrome; *CURE-PCI,* PCI substudy of the Clopidogrel in Unstable angina to prevent Recurrent Events trial; *ICER,* incremental cost-effectiveness ratio; *LY,* life-year; *MI,* myocardial infarction; *PLATO Trial,* The Study of Platelet Inhibition and Patient Outcomes; *PCI,* percutaneous coronary intervention; *QALY,* quality-adjusted life-year; *RCT,* randomized controlled trial; *TRITON-TIMI-38,* Trial to Assess Improvement in Therapeutic Outcomes by Optimizing Platelet Inhibition with Prasugrel Thrombolysis in Myocardial Infarction.

TABLE 68.4 Medical Economics of Antithrombotic Use in Acute Coronary Syndrome

Authors/Study	Comparator Groups	Type of Analysis	Results
Pinto et al.[58]/ ACUITY Trial	Non-ST ACS patients managed by UFH/enoxaparin plus a GP IIb/IIIa inhibitor, bivalirudin plus a GP IIb/IIIa inhibitor, or bivalirudin alone.	Patient-level, RCT-based analysis	Despite the higher drug cost of bivalirudin, the cumulative hospital stay costs were lowest with bivalirudin monotherapy (mean difference range: $184–$1081, P < .001 for overall comparison) with cost savings extending out to 30 days (mean difference range: $123–$938, P = .005). This saving was primarily due to less major and minor bleeding with bivalirudin ($8658/event and $2282/event, respectively).
Schwenkglenks et al.[60]/ HORIZONS-AMI trial	Early presentation STEMI (<12 h) managed by PCI and either heparin plus a GP IIb/IIIa inhibitor or bivalirudin alone.	Patient-level, RCT-based analysis	The use of bivalirudin alone was associated with a lifetime savings of £267 (£12,843 bivalirudin vs. £13,110 heparin + GP IIb/IIIa). Probabilistic analysis showed that bivalirudin use was associated with higher quality-adjusted survival at lower costs, suggesting that bivalirudin alone may be dominant with cost effectiveness being better than £20,000 per QALY gained.

ACS, Acute coronary syndrome; *ACUITY,* Acute Catheterization and Urgent Intervention Triage strategY; *GP IIb/IIIa,* glycoprotein IIb/IIIa; *HORIZONS-AMI,* Harmonizing Outcomes with Revascularization and Stents in Acute Myocardial Infarction; *ICER,* incremental cost-effectiveness ratio; *LY,* life-year; *PCI,* percutaneous coronary intervention; *QALY,* quality-adjusted life-year; *RCT,* randomized controlled trial; *STEMI,* ST-elevation myocardial infarction; *UFH,* unfractionated heparin.

was considered the mainstay therapy early on, primary PCI has become the standard of care currently based on multiple trials that compared the two strategies.

An economic analysis of the Comparison of Angioplasty and Pre-hospital Thrombolysis in Acute Myocardial Infarction (CAPTIM) trial showed that although there was no difference in 1-year outcomes between the two reperfusion strategies, costs were lower for primary PCI. The thrombolysis strategy in this trial included the use of rescue PCI, as needed.[37] Similarly results of the Swedish Early Decision reperfusion Study (SWEDES) trial and a subsequent Norwegian study showed that although there was no difference in clinical outcomes, primary PCI was a more cost-effective strategy. The SWEDES trial showed that PCI was associated with higher initial costs due to procedure and medication costs, but this was offset by lower hospitalization costs. Early discharge of low-risk patients who received primary PCI also helped to reduce total costs of care.[38,39]

Importantly however, primary PCI has been shown to be the cost-effective strategy only if resources are readily available. For example, in a hospital with an existing catheterization lab with night and weekend coverage that admits 200 patients with acute MI each year, PCI was associated with cost savings of <$30,000/QALY compared with thrombolysis.[40] On the other hand, if the hospital did not have the available resources, the cost to build a new catheterization lab, staff the lab with night call, and accept initial low volumes was not cost effective. In fact, transporting every patient from non–PCI-capable hospitals to PCI-capable facilities was more cost effective with $2750 saving per QALY.[41]

Medical Economics of Early Invasive Versus Early Conservative Strategies in Patients With Non-ST Elevation Acute Coronary Syndrome

The expansion of PCI use led to a gradual shift in the management of non-STEMI (NSTEMI) as well. Although initially many patients were treated only medically with intervention reserved for those with recurrent ischemia, a more aggressive approach with early revascularization started to emerge as an alternative choice. The timing of the procedure also shifted over time. This time shift can be seen with the change in the definition of an early invasive strategy in more contemporary trials comparing early invasive and conservative approaches (7 days in Fragmin and Revascularization during Instability in CAD II [FRISC II] [2000] vs. 2 days in Treat Angina with Aggrastat and Determine Cost of Therapy with an Invasive or Conservative Strategy [TACTICS-TIMI 18] [2001]).

The FRISC II trial compared an early invasive with an early noninvasive strategy in 2457 patients with unstable CAD. The results showed that the early invasive strategy was associated with a significant reduction the composite of death or MI (10.4% vs.14.1%; P = .005). There were also reductions in readmission (37% vs. 57%; P < .001) and revascularization after the initial admission with the early invasive strategy (7.5% vs. 31%; P < .01).[42]

The economic analysis of FRISC II showed that at the end of 1 year, the early invasive strategy was associated with a $3511 (23,876 Swedish Koruna [SEK]) higher cost compared with the noninvasive arm. The ICER for choosing the invasive instead of the noninvasive strategy was high, with $206,470 (SEK 1,404,000) per avoided death and $94,852 (SEK 645,000) per avoided death or MI.[43] However, it should be noted that what was called an early invasive approach in this trial was not associated with an early intervention. In contrast, the intervention was done within 1 week and was associated with a longer hospital stay (12 days vs. 8 day).

More consistent with current practice, the TACTICS-TIMI 18 trial randomized 2220 patients with unstable angina/NSTEMI to either an early invasive strategy with routine catheterization and revascularization as appropriate within 4 to 48 hours, or to a conservative, or a "selective invasive" strategy, with catheterization performed only if the patient had objective evidence of recurrent ischemia or a positive stress test. All patients were provided with appropriate medical therapy. The early strategy was associated with a significant reduction in the composite of death and MI (7.3% vs. 9.5%; odds ratio [OR] = 0.74; 95% CI 0.54 to 1.00; P < .05).[44]

Economic analysis of the trial showed that the early invasive arm had higher initial costs ($15,714 vs. $14,047) but lower follow-up costs out to 6 months ($6098 vs. $7180) with similar cumulative 6-month costs ($19,780 vs. $19,111). Therefore the early invasive strategy was shown to be cost effective with an estimated ICER of $13,000 per LYG.[45] These data showed that adapting an early invasive approach with the intervention specifically done in the first 48 hours was an economically attractive option.

Medical Economics of Antiplatelet Therapy

Medical Economics of P2Y$_{12}$ Receptor Antagonists

The benefit of dual antiplatelet therapy (DAPT) was established with data showing that the combination of aspirin and ticlopidine was associated with greater platelet inhibition than aspirin alone in patients with CAD treated with PCI.[46] However, ticlopidine use was associated with many side effects. Subsequently, clopidogrel, a P2Y$_{12}$ receptor antagonist, was studied in multiple clinical trials and proved to be an effective option for DAPT with fewer side effects than ticlopidine. However, the use of clopidogrel was still associated with substantial interpatient variability and a delayed onset of action. The reduced pharmacologic response in some patients to clopidogrel was associated with increased risk for adverse clinical events, including MI and stent thrombosis. This limitation of clopidogrel led to the introduction of the more potent antiplatelets, prasugrel, and ticagrelor, as alternatives to clopidogrel.[47]

Several trials have evaluated the economics of using oral P2Y$_{12}$ receptor antagonist after PCI. The PCI-CURE substudy of the Clopidogrel in Unstable angina to prevent Recurrent Events (CURE) trial showed that the use of clopidogrel was associated with a 31% reduction in cardiovascular death or MI (P = .002).[48] CEA of CURE-PCI showed that clopidogrel was associated with a higher average cost at 1 year of $253 to $423. For patients who underwent PCI during the initial hospitalization, the difference was less substantial and ranged from $155 lower to $90 higher with clopidogrel. Clopidogrel proved to be a very attractive option with ICER of $2856 to $4775 per LY without PCI and $935 per LY in the early PCI subgroup.[49]

Although clopidogrel was established as both a clinically effective and cost-effective strategy for PCI, the role of the novel adenosine diphosphate (ADP) receptor antagonists remained in question. The Trial to Assess Improvement in Therapeutic Outcomes by Optimizing Platelet Inhibition with Prasugrel Thrombolysis in Myocardial Infarction (TRITON-TIMI-38) randomized 13,608 patients with moderate-to-high-risk acute coronary syndrome (ACS) to receive either prasugrel or clopidogrel at the time of PCI. The study showed that prasugrel use was associated with a significant reduction in the combined end point of cardiovascular death, nonfatal MI, or nonfatal stroke (9.9% prasugrel vs. 12.1% clopidogrel; P < .001), as well as a significant reduction in urgent TVR (2.5% vs. 3.7%; P < .001) and stent thrombosis (1.1% vs. 2.4%; P < .001). However, patients receiving prasugrel had significantly higher rates of major bleeding (2.4% prasugrel vs. 1.8% clopidogrel, P < .03).[50]

CEA of the TRITON-TIMI-38 trial showed that over 14.7 months' follow-up, prasugrel was associated with a net savings of $221 per patient when compared with clopidogrel. This saving was attributed to the lower rate of rehospitalizations involving PCI. Prasugrel was associated with life expectancy gains of 0.102

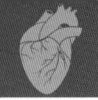

SECTION VII Outcome Effectiveness of Interventional Cardiology

years (95% CI 0.030 to 0.180), primarily because of the decreased rate of nonfatal MI. Prasugrel was shown to be an economically attractive strategy with an ICER of $9727 per LYG.[51] However, this comparison was done between prasugrel and "brand" rather than "generic" clopidogrel. Considering that, it remains likely although not proven that prasugrel is an economically attractive alternative.

The study of Platelet Inhibition and Patient Outcomes (PLATO) randomized 18,624 patients with moderate-to-high-risk ACS to receive either ticagrelor or clopidogrel upstream or at the time of PCI. The study showed that the use of ticagrelor was associated with a significant reduction in the composite of death from vascular causes, MI, or stroke (9.8% of ticagrelor vs.11.7% clopidogrel; hazard ratio [HR] = 0.84; 95% CI 0.77 to 0.92; $P < .001$). Furthermore, the use of ticagrelor was associated with no increased risk of major bleeding (11.6% ticagrelor vs.11.2% clopidogrel; $P = .43$).[52]

Economic evaluation of PLATO showed that even though ticagrelor use was associated with higher costs of ₡362, that was balanced by a QALY gain of 0.13 compared with generic clopidogrel at 1 year. Therefore the use of ticagrelor was an economically attractive option with an ICER of ₡2753 per QALY gained and ₡2372 per LYG.[53]

In summary, the use of clopidogrel as a second antiplatelet agent in addition to aspirin is attractive both clinically and economically, with further clinical and economic advantages to both ticagrelor and prasugrel as alternatives to clopidogrel.

Medical Economics of Antithrombotic Use in Acute Coronary Syndrome

The benefit of using unfractionated heparin (UFH) in addition to antiplatelet therapy in reducing the incidence of death and recurrent MI in the setting of ACS has been well established.[54,55] However, the use of UFH is associated with an unpredictable anticoagulant response secondary to its neutralization by protein binding and activated platelets. Furthermore, the discontinuation of UFH is associated with increased incidence of cardiac events.[56] Therefore several studies were preformed to demonstrate the benefit of more predictable anticoagulation using direct thrombin inhibitors.

Medical Economics of Antithrombotic Therapy Use in Non-STEMI Acute Coronary Syndrome

The Acute Catheterization and Urgent Intervention Triage strategY (ACUITY) trial randomized 13,819 patients with ACS to one of three antithrombotic regimens: UFH or enoxaparin plus a glycoprotein (GP) IIb/IIIa inhibitor, bivalirudin plus a GP IIb/IIIa inhibitor, or bivalirudin alone. The results showed that bivalirudin alone when compared with heparin plus GP IIb/IIIa inhibitor was associated with a noninferior rate of the composite of death, MI, or unplanned revascularization (7.8% vs. 7.3%, respectively; $P = .32$; RR= 1.08; 95% CI 0.93 to 1.24) and significantly reduced rates of major bleeding (3.0% vs. 5.7%; $P < .001$; RR = 0.53; 95% CI 0.43 to 0.65). There was no difference in any of the outcomes between the use of UFH or enoxaparin plus a GP IIb/IIIa inhibitor and that of bivalirudin plus a GP IIb/IIIa inhibitor.[57] Economic evaluation of the U.S. cohort of the ACUITY trial showed that despite the higher drug cost of bivalirudin, the cumulative hospital stay costs were lowest with bivalirudin monotherapy (mean difference range: $184 to $1081, $P < .001$ for overall comparison) with cost savings extending out to 30 days (mean difference range: $123 to $938, $P = .005$). This saving was primarily due to less major and minor bleeding with bivalirudin ($8,658/event and $2,282/event, respectively).[58]

In summary, in the setting of the medical management of NSTEMI ACS, the use of more predictable anticoagulation with bivalirudin is associated with cost saving when compared with UFH. During PCI, the use of bivalirudin alone seems to be a more attractive option than the combined use of UFH or enoxaparin with GP IIb/IIIa inhibitors.

Medical Economics of Antithrombotic Therapy Use in STEMI

The Harmonizing Outcomes with Revascularization and Stents in Acute Myocardial Infarction (HORIZONS-AMI) trial randomized 3602 patients with STEMI who presented within 12 hours after the onset of symptoms and who were undergoing primary PCI to treatment with heparin plus a GP IIb/IIIa inhibitor or to treatment with bivalirudin alone. Similar to the findings in ACUITY, the use of bivalirudin alone was associated with reduced 30-day rate of net composite of major bleeding and major adverse cardiovascular events, including death, MI, TVR, and stroke (9.2% vs. 12.1; RR = 0.76; 95% CI 0.63 to 0.92; $P = .005$), lower rate of major bleeding (4.9% vs. 8.3%; RR = 0.60; 95% CI 0.46 to 0.77; $P < .001$), lower 30-day cardiac death (1.8% vs. 2.9%; RR = 0.62; 95% CI 0.40 to 0.95; $P = .03$), and death from all causes (2.1% vs. 3.1%; RR = 0.66; 95% CI 0.44 to 1.00; $P = .047$).[59] Economic evaluation of the HORIZONS-AMI trial showed that the use of bivalirudin alone was associated with a lifetime savings of £267 (£12,843 bivalirudin vs. £13,110 heparin + GP IIb/IIIa). Probabilistic analysis showed that bivalirudin use was associated with higher quality-adjusted survival at lower costs, suggesting that bivalirudin alone may be dominant with cost-effectiveness being better than £20,000 per QALY gained.[60]

This finding was unique in that HORIZONS-AMI did not use a treatment arm with heparin alone. It stands to reason that heparin monotherapy may be as effective, if not more effective than bivalirudin monotherapy at a decreased cost. The How Effective Are Antithrombotic Therapies in Primary PCI (HEAT-PPCI) trial that randomly assigned 1917 patients undergoing emergency angiography to either UFH or bivalirudin showed that the use of bivalirudin compared with heparin alone was associated with higher incidence of the primary composite outcome of death, MI, CVA, and TVR (8.7% bivalirudin vs. 5.7% UFH; RR = 1·52, 95% CI 1.09 to 2.13; $P = .01$) without changing the incidence of major bleeding (3.5% bivalirudin vs. 3.1% UFH; RR = 1·15, 95% CI 0.70 to 1.89; $P = .59$).[61] The cost analysis of this trial has not been reported; however, UFH use would be expected to be more cost effective and even dominant to bivalirudin giving that UFH use is associated with lower cost and better outcomes without increasing the risk of complications.

MEDICAL ECONOMICS OF PERIPHERAL VASCULAR INTERVENTIONS (TABLE 68.5)

Admissions for peripheral arterial disease (PAD) have been increasing and are currently responsible for approximately 20% of all U.S. hospital admissions. Data analysis of more than 2 million hospital admissions for PAD between 2001 and 2007 showed that the choice of treatment has dramatically changed, with a 78% increase in endovascular procedures, and a concomitant decrease in open bypass and amputations.[62] That trend was associated with a change in the distribution of cases among different specialties involved in performing them. Between 1998 and 2005, there was a sixfold drop in peripheral procedures performed by interventional radiologists (5.6% of all cases in 2005), with a threefold increase for interventional cardiologists (29% of all cases), and a twofold increase for vascular surgeons (43% of all cases).[63] The number of interventional laboratories that have the capability to do peripheral vascular interventions is growing rapidly, with many fellowship programs currently offering additional training in these techniques. Advances in technology, uses of BMS and atherectomy, and intravascular imaging had helped to increase

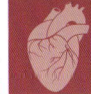

TABLE 68.5 Medical Economics of Peripheral Vascular Interventions

Authors/Study	Comparator Groups	Type of Analysis	Results
Bradbury et al.[70]/ BASIL Trial	Patients with severe limb ischemia due to infrainguinal disease managed by either a surgery-first or an angioplasty-first strategy	Patient-level, RCT-based analysis	For the first year, the hospital costs associated with a surgery-first strategy were $8469 higher ($34,378 bypass vs. $25,909 PTA). However, at the end of the 5-year follow-up and secondary to increased costs subsequently incurred by the need for repeat revascularization including surgery in the PTA patients, this difference decreased to $5521 ($45,322 bypass vs. $39,801 PTA) and was no longer significant. Although the bypass strategy was associated with better survival, it was not economically attractive with an ICER of $184,492 per QALY gained.
Kearns et al.[75]/ British Economic Evaluation	Patients with intermittent claudication and critical leg ischemia managed by PTA with no bail-out stenting, PTA with bail-out DES, DCB, primary BMS, primary DES, endovascular brachytherapy, stent-grafts and cryoplasty	Markov model on observational cohort using British economic evaluation	The cost and QALY were favorable for DCB over all other strategies in both intermittent claudication group (cost: £12,668 vs. £13,032–£17,578 and QALY: 6120 vs. 5931–6081) and critical limb ischemia (cost: £49,890 vs. £54,775–£58,097 and QALY 3402 vs. 2988–3297). The probability of DCB being cost-effective was at least 58.3% for patients with intermittent claudication and at least 72.2% for patients with critical leg ischemia.
Pietzsch et al.[76]/ US Medicare and German Economic Evaluation	Patients with intermittent claudication and critical leg ischemia managed by BMS, DES, or DCB compared with PTA alone	Markov model on combined cohort of 13 trials using U.S. Medicare and German economic evaluation	The drug-eluting strategies had a lower projected budget impact over 24 months compared with BMS and PTA in both the U.S. Medicare (DCB: $10,214; DES: $12,904; PTA $13,114; BMS $13,802) and German public health care systems (DCB €3619; DES €3632; BMS €4026; PTA €4290).

BASIL, Bypass versus Angioplasty in Severe Ischemia of the Leg; *BMS*, bare-metal stent; *DES*, drug-eluting stent; *DCB*, drug-coated balloon; *ICER*, incremental cost-effectiveness ratio; *PTA*, percutaneous transluminal angioplasty; *QALY*, quality-adjusted life-year; *RCT*, randomized controlled trial.

success and reduce complications.[19] It is estimated by industry that peripheral interventions will grow an average of 8% per year over the next 4 years.[4,5]

Cost Effectiveness of Noninvasive Therapy

The use of antiplatelet agents was shown to be effective in reducing the risk of vascular occlusion in a wide range of patients with PAD. A meta-analysis of 8000 patients from 46 randomized trials of antiplatelet therapy versus control and 14 randomized trials comparing one antiplatelet regimen with another showed that antiplatelet therapy produced a highly significant ($P < .0001$) reduction in vascular occlusion, with the largest absolute reductions among patients at highest risk of occlusion and smaller but still significant absolute reductions among lower risk patients. In addition, antiplatelet therapy in patients with PAD produced a significant 25% reduction ($P = .002$) in the incidence of vascular events (nonfatal MI, nonfatal stroke, or vascular death).[64]

The Clopidogrel for High Atherothrombotic Risk and Ischemic Stabilization, Management, and Avoidance (CHARISMA) trial that originally randomized 15,603 patients with either clinically evident cardiovascular disease or multiple risk factors for cardiovascular disease to receive clopidogrel plus low-dose aspirin or low-dose aspirin alone showed no significant difference in the composite of MI, stroke, or cardiac death.[65] However, a subgroup analysis including 9478 patients with manifest cardiovascular disease (prior MI, stroke, or symptomatic PAD) showed a significant reduction in the incidence of the composite of cardiovascular death, MI, or stroke with the use DAPT (7.3% vs. 8.8%; HR = 0.83, 95% CI 0.72 to 0.96; $P < .01$) as well as a reduction in hospitalizations for ischemia (11.4% vs. 13.2%; HR = 0.86; 95% CI 0.76 to 0.96; $P = .008$).[66] Economic evaluation of this subgroup showed that DAPT use was associated with $2607 higher cost with projected life expectancy increased by an average of 0.072 years. Therefore the use of DAPT appeared to be an economically attractive option with ICER of $36,343 per LYG.[67]

Vasoactive agents including cilostazol, naftidrofuryl oxalate, pentoxifylline, and inositol nicotinate are used for symptomatic relief in patients with intermittent claudication. A review and analysis of the results of 26 RCTs showed that both naftidrofuryl oxalate and cilostazol appear to be effective treatments with significant improvement in the logarithm mean of maximal walking distance from 0.181 to 0.762 and 0.108 to 0.337, respectively, for this patient population. However, naftidrofuryl oxalate seemed to be the only treatment that is likely to be considered cost effective with ICER of approximately £6070 per QALY gained when compared with no vasoactive drug, whereas cilostazol was associated with ICER of greater than £ 20,000 per QALY gained when compared with no vasoactive drug.[67]

Cost Effectiveness of Percutaneous Transluminal Angioplasty Versus Bypass Surgery

The first data on the comparative cost effectiveness of percutaneous transluminal angioplasty (PTA) versus bypass surgery comes from the Revascularization for Femoro-popliteal Disease trial that studied the impact of both strategies on men older than 65 with disabling claudication or chronic critical limb ischemia secondary to femoropopliteal stenosis. Initial angioplasty increased quality-adjusted life expectancy by 2 to 13 months in patients with disabling claudication and by 1 to 4 months in patients with chronic critical ischemia and resulted in decreased lifetime expenditures compared with bypass surgery in both groups. Using a maximum threshold cost of US$50,000 per QALY gained, PTA was cost effective when compared with vein bypass for lesions that could be treated with a better than 30% 5-year patency.[68]

The Bypass versus Angioplasty in Severe Ischemia of the Leg (BASIL) trial randomized 452 patients with severe limb ischemia due to infrainguinal disease to receive either a surgery-first or an angioplasty-first strategy. After 1 year, the two strategies did not differ significantly in amputation-free survival (71% bypass vs. 68% PTA; adjusted HR = 0.73, 95% CI 0.49 to 1.07).[69] However, 5-year follow-up of the BASIL trial showed that bypass surgery was associated with better overall survival (47% bypass vs. 41% PTA; adjusted HR = 0.61; 95% CI 0.50 to 0.75; $P < .009$) and a nonsignificant difference in amputation-free survival

(38% bypass vs. 37% PTA; adjusted HR = 0.85; 95% CI 0.5 to 1.07; P = .108).[70] Economic assessment showed that for the first year, the hospital costs associated with a surgery-first strategy were $8469 higher ($34,378 bypass vs. $25,909 PTA). However, at the end the 5-year follow-up and secondary to increased costs subsequently incurred by the need for repeat revascularization including surgery in the PTA patients, this difference decreased to $5521 ($45,322 bypass vs. $39,801 PTA) and was no longer significant. Although the bypass strategy was associated with better survival, it was not economically attractive with an ICER of $184,492 per QALY gained.[70]

Consistent with the previous disparate economic findings, clinical practice in this patient population remains quite variable with regards to angioplasty versus bypass selection.

Cost Effectiveness of Technological Advances in Endovascular Interventions

Although PTA alone was originally introduced as a treatment alternative to surgical revascularization, subsequent development of stent technology has demonstrated a lower incidence of target-lesion revascularization (TLR).[71-73] More recently, drug-coated balloons (DCBs) have emerged as a revascularization strategy that holds the promise of reducing TLRs further, while avoiding stent-related risks such as ISR and stent fracture and maintaining all therapeutic options for subsequent intervention.[74]

There are two studies that compared the economics of all three modalities. The first study was a British economic evaluation of the cost effectiveness comparing PTA with no bail-out stenting, PTA with bail-out DESs, DCBs, primary BMS, primary DESs, endovascular brachytherapy, stent-grafts, and cryoplasty in patients with intermittent claudication and critical leg ischemia. The cost and QALY were favorable for DCB over all other strategies in both intermittent claudication group (cost: £12,668 vs. £13,032 to £17,578 and QALY: 6120 vs. 5931 to 6081) and critical limb ischemia (cost: £49,890 vs. £54,775 to £58,097 and QALY 3402 vs. 2988 to 3297). Using £100,000 as a higher cut-off for calculation, the use of DCBs seemed to be more economically attractive by having both lower lifetime costs and greater effectiveness. The probability of DCBs being cost effective was at least 58.3% for patients with intermittent claudication and at least 72.2% for patients with critical leg ischemia.[75]

Another economic analysis was performed on a cohort of 2406 patients from 13 trials comparing the economic impact of the use of BMS, DES, or DCB compared with PTA alone based on the 2013 reimbursement rates of the U.S. Medicare and the German statutory sickness fund perspectives. Results showed a TLR rate of 14.3%, 19.3%, 28.1%, and 40.3% for DCB, DES, BMS, and PTA, respectively. The drug-eluting strategies had a lower projected budget impact over 24 months compared with BMS and PTA in both the U.S. Medicare (DCB: $10,214; DES: $12,904; PTA $13,114; BMS $13,802) and German public health care systems (DCB €3,619; DES €3,632; BMS €4,026; PTA €4,290).[76] Unfortunately, although DCBs constitute a cost-effective option, their use in the United States may be affected by recent changes in CMS reimbursements for both inpatient and outpatient catheterization laboratories.

MEDICAL ECONOMICS OF STRUCTURAL CARDIAC INTERVENTIONS (TABLE 68.6)

Structural heart disease is the field of interventional cardiology that may well witness the greatest growth in the next 10 years.[5] The field of structural interventional cardiology was first developed with transcatheter valvuloplasty of the mitral valve followed by the introduction of closure devices of atrial septal defects (ASDs) and patent foramen ovale (PFO).[20] Importantly, the recent introduction of TAVR and the development of new transcatheter techniques to manage mitral regurgitation promises an expected growth of 30% in the volume of structural procedure over the next decade.[5] This estimated growth is based on the expected increase in incidence of aortic and mitral valve disease in the future due to aging of the population in addition to greater penetration of these methods to reach broader populations. Analysis based on three large population-based epidemiologic studies showed that the prevalence of aortic and mitral valve disease in the population was estimated to be 2.5% but ranged from less than 1% for those younger than 54 years old to 4% to 8% by age 65 to 74 and 12% to 14% older than age 75.[77]

The approval of the Edwards Sapien valve (Edwards Lifesciences, Irvine, CA) in 2007 and the CoreValve (Medtronic, Minneapolis, MN) shortly thereafter in Europe lead to the performance of more than 60,000 TAVR procedures outside of the United States in 2011.[4] In the United States, the Edwards valve was approved in 2011 and the CoreValve was approved in 2014. The TAVR volume grew from 4627 per year in 2012 to 24,808 TAVR per year in 2015, and it is expected to grow more after TAVR was approved for intermediate-risk patients.[78] In light of this, we turn now to a specific discussion of the medical economics of percutaneous structural interventions.

Transcatheter Versus Surgical Closure of Secundum Atrial Septal Defects in Adults

Transcatheter ASD closure was shown to be a feasible option for the management of secundum ASD in adults.[79] Outcome analysis of a cohort of 718 ASD closures performed between 1988 and 2005 that included 383 surgical ASD closures and 335 transcatheter ASD closures showed no difference in mortality at 5 years between the two strategies (5.3% transcatheter vs. 6.3% surgical; P = 1.00), but transcatheter intervention was associated with a higher reintervention rate at 5 years (7.9% vs. 0.3%, P = .0038).[79] Cost effectiveness on this cohort showed that the 5-year cost of surgical closure was $15,304 versus $11,060 for the transcatheter alternative. At 5 years, transcatheter closure was marginally more effective than surgery (4.683 ± 0.379 LY versus 4.618 ± 0.638 LY).[80] So it seems that whenever feasible, transcatheter ASD closure seems to be a dominant strategy over surgical closure.

Medical Economics of Transcatheter Aortic Valve Replacement

It is estimated that 3.4% of the population older than 75 years has severe aortic stenosis, with 350,000 patients in the United States alone.[81] Forty percent of these patients do not get surgical intervention secondary to being considered either inoperable or at very high surgical risk. TAVR was developed as an alternative for surgical valve replacement. TAVR treats aortic stenosis by displacing and functionally replacing the native valve with a bioprosthetic valve delivered on a catheter (Edward Sapien) or trileaflet porcine pericardial valve on a self-expanding nitinol frame (CoreValve) through the femoral artery (transfemoral approach, TF-TAVR) or the left ventricular apex (transapical placement, TA-TAVR). It is estimated that there are approximately 102,558 TAVR candidates in North America and 189,836 TAVR candidates in Europe.[81]

Cost Effectiveness of Transcatheter Aortic Valve Replacement Versus Medical Therapy in Inoperable Patients

Symptomatic severe aortic stenosis in the absence of definitive treatment leads to progressive symptoms, functional decline, and death.[82] In patients who are considered not candidates for surgical aortic valve replacement (SAVR), medical therapy was not

TABLE 68.6 Medical Economics of Structural Heart Disease Interventions

Authors/Study	Comparator Groups	Type of Analysis	Results
Reynolds et al.[83]/ PARTNER B trial	TAVR vs. medical therapy in inoperable patients	Patient-level, RCT-based analysis	TAVR was associated with a mean cost of $42,806 for the initial procedure and $78,542 for the hospitalization. Follow-up costs through 12 months were lower with TAVR compared with standard therapy ($29,289 vs. $53,621). The cumulative 1-year costs remained higher with TAVR ($106,076 vs. $53,621). TAVR use was associated with ICER of $50,200 per LY gained and $61,889 per QALY gained.
Watt et al.[84]/ PARTNER B trial	TAVR SAPIEN vs. medical therapy in inoperable patients	Markov model for an estimated 10-year time horizon (same patient cohort as above)	TAVR was cost effective at 24 months with ICER of £18,500 ($31,450) per QALY gained.
Reynolds et al.[87]/ PARTNER A trial TF Cohort	TF-TAVR SAPIEN vs. SAVR in high-risk patients	Markov model on RCT patient data.	TF-TAVR overall admission costs were not significantly different from SAVR ($73,219 TAVR vs. $74,067 SAVR) and the 12-months costs were marginally lower for TF-TAVR (mean difference of −$1250; 95% CI −$18,132 to $13,867). TF-TAVR was economically dominant compared with SAVR in 55.7% of replicates with an ICER of $50,000/QALY gained in 70.9%.
Reynolds et al.[87]/ PARTNER A trial TA Cohort	TA-TAVR SAPIEN vs. SAVR in high-risk patients	Markov model on RCT patient data.	TA-TAVR total admission costs are higher than SAVR ($90,919 TA-TAVR vs. $79,024 SAVR). The 12-month cost was slightly higher with TA-TAVR ($100,504 TA-TAVR vs. $98,434 SAVR) with a mean difference of $2070 (95% CI −$9960 to $13,499). TA-TAVR was economically dominated by SAVR in the base case and economically attractive in only 7.1% of replicates
Reynolds et al.[89]/ US CoreValve trial	TAVR CoreValve vs. SAVR in high-risk patients	Markov model on RCT patient data.	The index admission and projected lifetime costs were higher with TAVR than with SAVR (differences $11,260 and $17,849 per patient, respectively), whereas TAVR was projected to provide a lifetime gain of 0.32 QALY (0.41 LY with 3% discounting). Lifetime ICER were $55,090 per QALY gained and $43,114 per LY gained.
Cohen et al.[91]/ PARTNER II and the SAPIEN S3i registry	TF-TAVR SAPIEN XT and S3 vs. SAVR in intermediate-risk patients	Markov model on combined RCT and registry patient cohort	The cost of the index hospitalization was more than $4000 less with TAVR than with SAVR. The total cost of TAVR through 1-year follow-up was $15,511. The cost post discharge out to 1 year was more than $11,000 less per TAVR patient. Projected over estimated remaining years of life, TAVR yielded a cost savings of $9692 per patient, as well as a 0.27-year gain in QALY.
Reynolds et al.[94]/ EVEREST II Trial.	Severe MR patients undergoing MitraClip vs. Surgical Mitral repair or replacement.	Markov model on RCT patient data.	Economic assessment using the study price of $18,000 showed that the clip strategy reduced costs by $2200/patient, making MitraClip economically dominant. But using a European sales price of $26,200, the overall costs were higher with the clip strategy by $6192 and the ICER ratio was unfavorable (>$400,000 per QALY gained). In a sensitivity analysis limited to patients with acute procedural success, the QALY gain was larger, the cost-offsets with the clip was greater, and cost effectiveness was more favorable (dominant at a MitraClip price of $18,000 and around $54,000 per QALY gained at a price of $26,200)

CI, Confidence interval; *EVEREST,* endoVascular Edge-to-Edge Repair Study; *ICER,* incremental cost-effectiveness ratio; *LY,* life-year; *PARTNER trial,* Placement of Aortic Transcatheter Valves trial; *QALY,* quality-adjusted life-year; *RCT,* randomized controlled trial; *SAVR,* surgical aortic valve replacement; *TAVR,* transcatheter aortic valve replacement; *TA,* transapical; *TF,* transfemoral.

effective in slowing the expected outcomes. The introduction of TAVR offered an alternative for this patient population.

The evidence supporting the use of TAVR in patients with severe aortic stenosis who are not surgical candidates comes from cohort B of the Placement of Aortic Transcatheter Valves (PARTNER) trial that randomized 358 patients with aortic stenosis who were not considered to be suitable surgical candidates to either medical management (inclusive of balloon valvuloplasty) or TAVR. The trial found an impressive absolute 20% reduction in 1-year mortality for TAVR compared with standard therapy in this population (30.7% TAVR vs. 50.7% standard therapy; HR = 0.55; 95% CI; 0.40 to 0.74; P < .001). However, TAVR was associated with a higher incidence of major strokes (5.0% vs. 1.1%, P = .06) and major vascular complications (16.2% vs. 1.1%, P < .001).[82] An economic evaluation of the PARTNER B cohort showed that TAVR was associated with a mean cost of $42,806 for the initial procedure and $78,542 for the hospitalization. Follow-up costs through 12 months were lower with TAVR compared with standard therapy ($29,289 vs. $53,621). The cumulative 1-year costs remained higher with TAVR ($106,076 vs. $53,621). TAVR would increase discounted life expectancy by 1.6 years (1.3 quality-adjusted LYs) at an incremental cost of $79,837. TAVR use was associated with ICER of $50,200 per LYG and $61,889 per QALY gained.[83]

On the other hand, a cost stimulation model based on the same cohort for an estimated 10-year time horizon showed that TAVR was cost effective at 24 months with ICER of £18,500 ($31,450) per QALY gained.[84] So even though TAVR in this group was associated with a considerable increase in cost, it was still associated with what might be considered an acceptable ICER per LY and a potentially acceptable ICER per QALY over time.

The recent U.S. trial evaluating the Medtronic self-expanding CoreValve compared with standard therapy in extreme risk

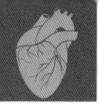

SECTION VII Outcome Effectiveness of Interventional Cardiology

patients has yielded similar improvement in outcomes with significant reduction in the incidence of death and stroke (26.0% CoreValve vs. 43.0% standard therapy; $P < .0001$).[85] An economic analysis of CoreValve in this population is unavailable.

Cost Effectiveness of Transcatheter Aortic Valve Replacement Versus Surgical Aortic Valve Replacement in High-Risk Patients

Because TAVR offered a less invasive approach for aortic valve replacement, the question of its applicability and effectiveness in high-risk surgical patients came to the forefront. Cohort A of the PARTNER trial tried to answer this by randomizing 699 high-risk patients with severe aortic stenosis to undergo either TAVR (by either a transfemoral or a transapical approach) or SAVR. The results showed that TAVR was noninferior to SAVR in the primary end point of death at 1 year (24.2% TAVR vs. 26.8% SAVR; $P = .44$). The rates of major stroke were not statistically different at 1 year (5.1% TAVR vs. 2.4%, SAVR; $P = .07$). At 30 days, major vascular complications were significantly more frequent with TAVR (11.0% TAVR vs. 3.2% SAVR; $P < .001$), whereas adverse events including major bleeding were more frequent after SAVR (9.3% TAVR vs. 19.5% SAVR, $P < .001$).[86]

CEA of cohort A of the PARTNER trial compared SAVR with both TF-TAVR and TA-TAVR. In the TF-TAVR cohort, the overall admission costs were not significantly different between groups ($73,219 TAVR vs. $74,067 SAVR) and the 12-month costs were marginally lower for TF-TAVR (mean difference of –$1250; 95% CI –$18,132 to $13,867). Both life expectancy and quality-adjusted life expectancy were slightly higher with TF-TAVR, making TF-TAVR economically dominant compared with SAVR in 55.7% of replicates with an ICER of $50,000/QALY gained in 70.9%.[87]

On the other hand, in the TA-TAVR cohort, the total admission costs remained higher, with TA-TAVR ($90,919 TA-TAVR vs. $79,024 SAVR). The 12-month cost was slightly higher with TA-TAVR ($100,504 TA-TAVR vs. $98,434 SAVR), with a mean difference of $2070 (95% CI –$9960 to $13,499). Life expectancy was similar for the TA-TAVR and SAVR groups, whereas quality-adjusted life expectancy tended to be less with TA-TAVR. Secondary to these, TA-TAVR was economically dominated by SAVR in the base case and economically attractive in only 7.1% of replicates. In summary, although TF-TAVR seems to be an economically attractive alternative to SAVR in high surgical risk patient, that was not the case for TA-TAVR.

Data from the U.S. trial evaluating the Medtronic self-expanding CoreValve comparing CoreValve TAVR to SAVR in high-risk patients also showed CoreValve use to be associated with significant reduction in mortality (14.2% CoreValve TAVR vs. 19.1% SAVR; $P < .001$ for noninferiority; $P = .04$ for superiority).[88] CEA of CoreValve showed that the index admission and projected lifetime costs were higher with TAVR than with SAVR (differences $11,260 and $17,849 per patient, respectively), whereas TAVR was projected to provide a lifetime gain of 0.32 quality-adjusted LYs (0.41 LYs with 3% discounting). Lifetime ICERs were $55,090 per QALY gained and $43,114 per LYG.[89]

Transcatheter Aortic Valve Replacement Versus Surgical Aortic Valve Replacement in Intermediate-Risk Patients

SAVR used to be the standard of care for patients with severe aortic stenosis and intermediate surgical risk. The PARTNER II trial comparing TAVR and SAVR outcomes in patients with intermediate risk for surgery showed that the rate of death from any cause or disabling stroke was similar in the TAVR group and the surgery group ($P = .001$ for noninferiority). At 2 years, the Kaplan-Meier event rates were 19.3% in the TAVR group and 21.1% in the surgery group (HR in the TAVR group, 0.89; 95% CI 0.73 to 1.09; $P = .25$). In the transfemoral-access cohort, TAVR resulted in a lower rate of death or disabling stroke than surgery (HR, 0.79; 95% CI 0.62 to 1.00; $P = .05$), whereas in the transthoracic-access cohort, outcomes were similar in the two groups.[90] CEA of PARTNER II and the SAPIEN S3i registry showed the cost of the index hospitalization was more than $4000 less with TAVR in the S3i registry than with SAVR. The total cost of TAVR through 1 year of follow-up averaged $80,977, which was $15,511 less than the $96,489 for SAVR. The cost post discharge out to 1 year was more than $11,000 less per TAVR patient, driven by sharply lower rates of both cardiovascular and noncardiovascular hospitalizations, as well as a greater than 50% reduction in days spent in rehabilitation centers and skilled nursing facilities, compared with SAVR patients. Projected over estimated remaining years of life, TAVR with the Sapien 3 valve yielded a cost savings of $9692 per patient compared with SAVR, as well as a 0.27-year gain in quality-adjusted LYs.[91]

The Surgical or Transcatheter Aortic Valve Implantation (SURTAVI) trial comparing self-expanding TAVR to SAVR showed that at 24 months, TAVR was noninferior to SAVR regarding death or any disabling stroke (12.6% TAVR vs. 14.0% SAVR; 95% CI 5.2% to 2.3%; posterior probability of noninferiority > .999).[92] Surgery was associated with higher rates of acute kidney injury, atrial fibrillation, and transfusion requirements, whereas TAVR had higher rates of residual aortic regurgitation and need for pacemaker implantation. CEA of this trial is expected in the near future.[92]

Cost Effectiveness of Percutaneous Mitral Valve Repair

Data comparing percutaneous mitral valve repair with surgical mitral valve surgery comes from the EndoVascular Edge-to-Edge Repair Study (EVEREST) II trial that randomly assigned 279 patients with moderately severe or severe (grade 3+ or 4+) mitral regurgitation in a 2:1 ratio to undergo either percutaneous repair with the MitraClip (Abbott Laboratories, Lake Bluff, IL) or conventional surgery for repair or replacement of the mitral valve. Results showed that surgical repair was associated with higher freedom from death, from surgery for mitral-valve dysfunction, and from grade 3+ or 4+ mitral regurgitation at 12 months (55% MitraClip vs. 73% mitral surgery; $P = .007$). This was mainly due to increased need for definitive surgery following use of the MitraClip (20% MitraClip vs. 2% surgery). There was no difference in death (6% in each group) or freedom from grade 3+ or 4+ mitral regurgitation (21% MitraClip vs. 20% surgery). Patients' quality of life improved from baseline to 12 months in the two study groups, yet surgery was associated with a transient decrease in the quality of life at 30 days.[93]

CEA of EVEREST II showed that the potential cost effectiveness of MitraClip compared with mitral valve surgery varied depending primarily on MitraClip price and acute procedural success. Economic assessment using the study price of $18,000 showed that the clip strategy reduced costs by $2200/patient, making MitraClip economically dominant. However, using a clip price of $26,200 (approximate European sales price), the overall costs were higher with the clip strategy by $6192 and the ICER ratio was unfavorable (>$400,000 per QALY gained). In a sensitivity analysis limited to patients with acute procedural success, the QALY gain was larger, the cost-offsets with the clip was greater, and cost effectiveness was more favorable (dominant at a MitraClip price of $18,000 and around $54,000 per QALY gained at a price of $26,200).[94] In summary, it seems that MitraClip may be an economically reasonable option if the equipment cost falls over time.

Economic Burden of Interventional Cardiology

A recent study comparing health care spending in the United States and 10 other high-income European countries showed

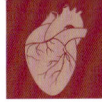

CHAPTER 68 Medical Economics in Interventional Cardiology

that the United States spends almost twice as much on medical care compared with any of these other countries, without achieving better outcomes.[95] This cost discrepancy is driven in part by the differences of procedures volumes and costs, as well as pharmaceutical, imaging, and administrative costs.[96] Although physician compensation is higher in the United States compared with other European countries, that is due, at least in part, to a longer work hours and higher patient volume per physician in the United States. Therefore higher U.S. physician compensation is not directly responsible to this significant difference in health care costs. Nonetheless, physicians are responsible for ordering tests, devising treatment plans including medication and procedural choices, and making final decisions on both admissions and discharges.[96] Interventional cardiologists, in their quest to deliver what they perceive as the best care to their patients, bear some responsibility for driving up the U.S. health care costs. Physicians in most cases do not know the costs of their interventions, do not pay these costs, but presumably benefit from performing high volumes of these costly procedures.[96] Although bringing costs under control is beyond what physicians can accomplish, they do have a critical role to play.

One of the major challenges in health care is that individual patients (and their physicians) wish to obtain all the health benefits that are available from modern medical technology. However, for society as a whole, resources are not adequate to meet this demand for every individual, which forces difficult and potentially divisive choices. There is no absolute standard that can be applied to assess how much a certain society is willing to pay for medical care.[19,20] Although it is difficult, physicians need to accept their partial responsibility as a factor in the U.S. health care cost crisis and participate in solving it. This can start by educating physicians about the cost and the cost effectiveness of their therapeutic options. Physicians must remain patient advocates but can choose wisely, and work with all stakeholders in society to include cost effectiveness in developing health care policy and guidelines.[97,98]

KEY REFERENCES

19. Fanari Z, Weintraub WS. Cost-effectiveness of medical, endovascular and surgical management of peripheral vascular disease. *Cardiovasc Revascular Med*. 2015;16(7):421–425.
20. Fanari Z, Weintraub WS. Cost-effectiveness of transcatheter versus surgical management of structural heart disease. *Cardiovasc Revasc Med*. 2016;17(1):44–47.
28. Hlatky MA, Boothroyd DB, Melsop KA, et al. Economic outcomes of treatment strategies for type 2 diabetes mellitus and coronary artery disease in the Bypass Angioplasty Revascularization Investigation 2 Diabetes trial. *Circulation*. 2009;120(25):2550–2558.
30. Weintraub WS, Boden WE, Zhang Z, et al. Cost-effectiveness of percutaneous coronary intervention in optimally treated stable coronary patients. *Circ Cardiovas Qual Outcomes*. 2008;1(1):12–20.
34. Magnuson EA, Farkouh ME, Fuster V, et al. Cost-effectiveness of percutaneous coronary intervention with drug eluting stents versus bypass surgery for patients with diabetes mellitus and multivessel coronary artery disease: results from the FREEDOM trial. *Circulation*. 2013;127(7):820–831.
36. Zhang ZEF, Kolm P, Grau-Sepulveda M, et al. Cost-effectiveness of revascularization strategies: a preliminary study from ASCERT. *Circulation*. 2012;126:A18630.
43. Janzon M, Levin LA, Swahn E. Cost-effectiveness of an invasive strategy in unstable coronary artery disease; results from the FRISC II invasive trial. The Fast Revascularisation during InStability in Coronary artery disease. *Eur Heart J*. 2002;23(1):31–40.
45. Mahoney EM, Jurkovitz CT, Chu H, et al. Cost and cost-effectiveness of an early invasive vs conservative strategy for the treatment of unstable angina and non–ST-segment elevation myocardial infarction. *JAMA*. 2002;288(15):1851–1858.
49. Mahoney EM, Mehta S, Yuan Y, et al. Long-term cost-effectiveness of early and sustained clopidogrel therapy for up to 1 year in patients undergoing percutaneous coronary intervention after presenting with acute coronary syndromes without ST-segment elevation. *Am Heart J*. 2006;151(1):219–227.
53. Nikolic E, Janzon M, Hauch O, et al. Cost-effectiveness of treating acute coronary syndrome patients with ticagrelor for 12 months: results from the PLATO study. *Eur Heart J*. 2013;34(3):220–228.
58. Pinto DS, Stone GW, Shi C, et al. Economic evaluation of bivalirudin with or without glycoprotein IIb/IIIa inhibition versus heparin with routine glycoprotein IIb/IIIa inhibition for early invasive management of acute coronary syndromes. *J Am Coll Cardiol*. 2008;52(22):1758–1768.
75. Kearns BC, Michaels JA, Stevenson MD, et al. Cost-effectiveness analysis of enhancements to angioplasty for infrainguinal arterial disease. *Br J Surg*. 2013;100(9):1180–1188.
83. Reynolds MR, Magnuson EA, Wang K, et al. Cost-effectiveness of transcatheter aortic valve replacement compared with standard care among inoperable patients with severe aortic stenosis: results from the placement of aortic transcatheter valves (PARTNER) trial (Cohort B). *Circulation*. 2012;125(9):1102–1109.
84. Watt M, Mealing S, Eaton J, et al. Cost-effectiveness of transcatheter aortic valve replacement in patients ineligible for conventional aortic valve replacement. *Heart*. 2012;98(5):370–376.
87. Reynolds MR, Magnuson EA, Lei Y, et al. Cost-effectiveness of transcatheter aortic valve replacement compared with surgical aortic valve replacement in high-risk patients with severe aortic stenosis: results of the PARTNER (Placement of Aortic Transcatheter Valves) trial (Cohort A). *J Am Coll Cardiol*. 2012;60(25):2683–2692.
89. Reynolds MR, Lei Y, Wang K, et al. Cost-effectiveness of transcatheter aortic valve replacement with a self-expanding prosthesis versus surgical aortic valve replacement. *J Am Coll Cardiol*. 2016;67(1):29–38.
94. Reynolds MR, Galper B, Apruzzese P. Cost effectiveness of the MitraClip compared with mitral valve surgery: 12-month results from the EVEREST II randomized controlled trial. *J Am Coll Cardiol*. 2012;60:B229. [abstract].
98. Garrison LP. Cost-effectiveness and clinical practice guidelines: have we reached a tipping point?—an overview. *Value Health*. 2016;19(5):512–515.

 Additional references available online at expertconsult.com.

中文导读

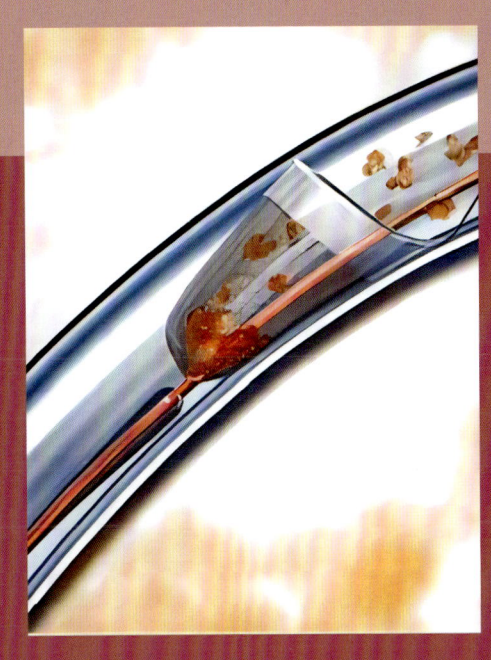

第69章
介入心脏病学医疗质量

　　医疗质量的评估和改进是每个医疗从业者、管理者的重要工作。介入心脏病学是近几十年来心脏病学内发展最快的领域，对介入心脏病学的医疗质量评估和改进更是得到越来越多的关注。20世纪90年代，最早应用于工业界的"持续质量改进"被引入医疗界。目前，"持续质量改进"已成为所有医疗机构的一项核心活动。这些基础的医疗质量控制系统同样适用于介入心脏病学。

　　高水平的质量是每个人都希望得到的医疗服务。但何为高质量的医疗，患者、医师、付款人和政府三方可能有不同的看法。患者往往更重视他们与医师的互动和时间，而不是重视遵守实践指南等问题。相比之下，付款人和政府机构可能更重视对绩效指标的遵守，以及减少不必要的程序和费用。按照美国医学研究所的报告，医疗质量被定义为"以符合当前专业知识的方式，为个人和人群提供的医疗保健系统、服务和用品以增加实现预期健康结果可能性的程度"。无论介入心脏病专家如何定义医疗质量，都需要一个医疗质量评估体系，以不断改善医疗结果。

　　本章从医疗质量管理的结构、进程和结果三个方面介绍如何构建好介入心脏病学或者心脏导管室的医疗质量管理框架，以及如何在临床指南的指导下在医疗过程和结果上评估医疗质量，并通过评估不断改进医疗质量。

姚　晶　吴永健

章节要点

- 由于州和联邦政府的规定越来越多，患者可以直接获得有关医疗质量的公开信息，以及医疗支付者对成本效益的压力，心导管室的医疗服务正在受到密切关注。
- 美国提高医疗质量的努力始于150多年前，2010年的《患者保护和可负担医疗法案》中纳入了公开报告等新举措。
- Donabedian三要素包含的结构、过程和结果，提供了一个评估医疗质量的概念框架。导管室人员应了解相关的结构要素、过程和结果。
- 每个导管室都应该制定一个质量框架，以确保每个患者每天都能在正确的程序、正确的执行下得到正确的结果。
- 该框架应包括构成质量基石的具体要素和活动。
- 公开报告增加了透明度，可以将报销与医疗质量挂钩。为了减少意外结果，如避免治疗高风险患者、增加公众对结果的理解等，公开报告有必要逐渐改进。

69 Quality of Care in Interventional Cardiology

Jennifer A. Rymer, Manesh R. Patel, Sunil V. Rao

KEY POINTS

- Owing to increasing state and federal regulations, direct patient access to publicly available information about the quality of care, as well as pressures from payers for cost-efficiency, the delivery of care in the cardiac catheterization laboratory is being examined closely.
- Efforts to improve the quality of medical care in the United States started more than 150 years ago, and new initiatives such as public reporting were incorporated into the Patient Protection and Affordable Care Act of 2010.
- Donabedian's triad of three domains—structure, process, and outcomes—provides a conceptual framework for evaluating the quality of medical care. Catheterization laboratory personnel should understand the existing structural elements, processes, and outcomes.

- Each catheterization laboratory should develop a framework of quality to ensure that the right patient gets the right procedure with the right execution and the right outcome on a daily basis.
- The framework should include the specific elements and activities that constitute the building blocks of quality.
- Public reporting increases transparency and is part of the proposed mechanisms to tie reimbursement to the quality of care. An increasing focus on how to improve public reporting is necessary in order to decrease unintended consequences—such as avoiding treatment of high risk patients—and increase public understanding of the results.

Quality is everyone's responsibility.

W. Edwards Deming[1]

INTRODUCTION

Interventional cardiology has grown rapidly since its inception more than 30 years ago. Invasive cardiovascular procedures have become the cornerstone for the evaluation and management of many cardiovascular diseases, especially coronary artery disease. Since the start of interventional cardiology, there have been efforts to measure and evaluate the quality of care.

Considerable attention has been focused on the cardiac catheterization laboratory because these procedures are widely used, easily identified with claims data, expensive, and associated with important complications. Attention continues to intensify because of increasing state and federal regulations, requests for public reporting of hospital and physician data, consumer pressures for care of the highest quality, and pressure from payers for cost-efficient care and the appropriate use of diagnostic cardiac catheterization and percutaneous coronary interventions (PCIs). There is also growing awareness that the quality of health care is compromised by preventable medical errors, the absence of evidence-based standards in many areas, lack of emphasis on disease prevention, patients' inadequate personal responsibility for maintaining their health, and disparities in health care delivery related to race, gender, income, and insurance status.

Numerous government and private agencies in the United States have been involved in the developing measurements of quality and disseminating data (Table 69.1). Report cards on cardiac operations and PCIs for hospitals and individual physicians exist in some states.[2,3] Interest in these reports continue to increase as data have emerged showing that patients fail to receive up to 45% of the tests and treatments recommended by evidence-based guidelines.[4] In an attempt to promote quality and improve outcomes, pay-for-performance programs, in which providers receive financial incentives for achieving certain benchmark goals in patient care, were developed.[5] With payment reform and Centers for Medicare and Medicaid Services (CMS) demonstration projects such as bundled payment care initiatives, there will be increasing focus on the efficient delivery of percutaneous procedures as part of a complete episode of care over a specified time period (e.g., 30 to 90 days).[6]

Although there are no formal national standards with which to judge the quality of cardiac catheterization laboratories, some states have used clinical practice guidelines and expert consensus documents published by the American College of Cardiology Foundation (ACCF), the American Heart Association (AHA), and the Society for Cardiovascular Angiography and Interventions (SCAI) to develop standards of quality.[7-9] Although these documents were never intended to serve as state or national standards, they have become the de facto basis for licensure regulations imposed by state health departments in an attempt to improve quality. To understand the current status of efforts to improve quality in the cardiac catheterization laboratory, it is helpful to examine some of the major events that comprise the history of efforts to improve the quality of health care in the United States.

EFFORTS TO IMPROVE QUALITY IN U.S. MEDICINE

Despite concerns about the state of American medicine, there have been profound improvements during the past 150 years. The American Medical Association (AMA) was founded in 1847, in part to address the disorganized and poor quality of health care in the United States. As a precursor of future efforts, the American College of Surgeons established the Hospital Standardization Program in 1917, promoting five basic patient care standards and surveying health care organizations to determine their acceptability for accreditation. In 1952, several other organizations collaborated with the American College of Surgeons to form the Joint Commission on Accreditation of Hospitals, now called The Joint Commission.[10]

A structure for organizing quality standards in health care was proposed by Avedis Donabedian in 1966 with the publication of an article that provided a broad definition of quality. It recommended evaluations in three areas: structure, process, and outcome.[11] This format was widely adapted and is still in use today.

During this early period, quality was often assessed by random chart audits or outcome-oriented chart surveys to evaluate metrics such as the use of blood products in surgical cases. Audit requirements were later minimized in favor of hospital-wide quality

SECTION VII Outcome Effectiveness of Interventional Cardiology

TABLE 69.1 Organizations Involved in the Assessment of Quality Care

Organization	Mission, Goals, and Focus	Website
Agency for Healthcare Research and Quality (AHRQ)	Lead federal agency charged with improving the quality, safety, efficiency, and effectiveness of health care for all Americans	www.ahrq.gov
National Guideline Clearinghouse (NGC)	An initiative of AHRQ that is a public resource for evidence-based clinical practice guidelines	www.guideline.gov
Centers for Medicare and Medicaid Services (CMS)	Host for Hospital Compare, which reports the process of care, risk-adjusted outcomes, and patient satisfaction measures for all hospitals in the United States	www.medicare.gov/hospitalcompare
CMS	Host for Physician Compare, which helps consumers find and choose physicians and other health care professionals enrolled in Medicare and will report several provider metrics in the future	www.medicare.gov/physiciancompare
Department of Health and Human Services (DHHS)	Provides links to hundreds of sites on the internet that contain reliable health care information and links to many government and nongovernment sources of information on health care quality	www.healthfinder.gov
The Joint Commission	Provides accreditation to hospital and other health care facilities; provides quality care and hospital quality measures for public reporting through the ORYX reporting program	www.jointcommission.org
National Committee for Quality Assurance (NCQA)	A private, 501(c)(3) not-for-profit organization dedicated to improving health care quality; operates the Healthcare Effectiveness Data and Information Set (HEDIS), a tool used by more than 90% of America's health plans to measure performance on important dimensions of care and service	www.ncqa.org
The American Health Quality Association (AHQA)	An educational not-for-profit national membership association dedicated to health care quality through community-based, independent quality evaluation and improvement programs	www.ahqa.org
National Quality Forum (NQF)	Sets national priorities and goals for performance improvement and endorses national consensus standards for measuring and publicly reporting on performance	www.qualityforum.org
American Medical Association (AMA)	AMA-sponsored Physician Consortium for Performance Improvement (PCPI) enhances quality of care and patient safety through development, testing, and maintenance of evidence-based clinical performance measures and measurement resources for physicians	www.ama-assn.org
American College of Cardiology Foundation (ACCF)	In collaboration with other professional organizations, develops clinical practice guidelines, expert consensus documents, and other quality programs, including Guidelines Applied in Practice (GAP) to assist with guideline application in clinical practice and Hospital to Home (H2H), an effort to improve the transition from inpatient to outpatient status for those with cardiovascular disease	www.cardiosource.org
American Heart Association (AHA)	In collaboration with other professional organizations, develops clinical practice guidelines, expert consensus documents, and other quality programs, including Get With the Guidelines, a hospital-based quality improvement program to ensure consistent treatment according to evidence-based guidelines, and Mission:Lifeline, a national, community-based initiative to improve systems of care for patients with ST-elevation myocardial infarction	www.my.americanheart.org
The Leapfrog Group	A voluntary program organized by large employers to promote big leaps in health care safety, quality, and customer value	www.leapfroggroup.org

assurance programs designed to detect care that was thought to be outside acceptable standards. Physician profiles reflecting the number of procedures performed, indications, and complications were compared with grouped data from similar physicians to identify outliers in the hope that they could be persuaded to change their practice habits by colleagues, the hospital, or other agencies.[12]

About 1990, a technique developed primarily for industry, called *continuous quality improvement* (CQI), was advocated by The Joint Commission. Compared with quality assurance programs, CQI tries to improve overall performance rather than merely to identify poor performers.[13-15] CQI has become a central activity for all health care organizations.

As efforts by the medical profession to improve quality were maturing, state and federal agencies were becoming interested in regulating health care, developing standards, and promoting high-quality medical care. By the late 1800s, many states required physician licensure and mandated educational standards for physicians. The National Board of Medical Examiners was founded in 1915 to provide a nationwide examination that licensing authorities could accept and use to judge candidates for licensure.

As the medical field expanded and specialty training became available, it was recognized that some type of certification process for specialists was necessary. To establish a uniform system, the American Board of Medical Specialties was formed in 1933. There are now 24 specialty boards that certify physicians, and this process has evolved to one of continuous professional development and lifelong learning through a Maintenance of Certification program requiring ongoing measurement of six core competencies.[16] Controversy has accompanied the Maintenance of Certification program, and it continues to evolve as several groups attempt to determine the optimal strategy.[17]

One of the first federal quality initiatives was the formation of the U.S. Food and Drug Administration (FDA) in 1906. With the enactment of Social Security in 1935 and Medicare in 1965, the federal government became more involved in setting requirements for the delivery of health care funded by federal dollars.

To monitor the care of Medicare patients, Congress enacted rules called *Conditions of Participation*, which required hospitals to provide certain services and conduct reviews to determine the appropriateness of hospital admissions. In 1972, amendments to the Social Security Act created the Professional Standards Review Organization program to promote hospital efficiency and eliminate unnecessary hospital use. This program failed to meet expectations and was unpopular because many thought that it emphasized cost containment rather than quality.[12] It was abandoned and replaced by other peer review organizations.[18]

At the same time, substantial changes in hospital reimbursement occurred, with a shift to a cost-per-case system based on assignment to a diagnosis-related group (DRG). The peer review organizations were responsible for validating correct assignment to a DRG and for monitoring hospital admissions, readmissions, surgical procedures, complications, and hospital deaths. Peer review organizations emphasized quality but focused more on outcome metrics than structure and process metrics, and they were not without their critics.[19]

As the amount of Medicare spending increased, the federal government became more involved in monitoring and controlling payments to physicians and hospitals. Before 1989, physician payments for services within the Medicare program were based on usual and customary charges for services by similar physicians in the previous year. Substantial changes in Medicare payments to physicians occurred as a result of the Budget Reconciliation Act of 1989, which redirected payments based on costs rather than charges. Costs were determined for the actual work involved, the overhead required to provide the service, and malpractice costs, with all three elements further adjusted for geographic differences in cost. This caused major changes in practice patterns, which had both positive and negative effects on the quality of care.

Additional federal funding led to the formation of the Agency for Health Care Policy and Research, which had a turbulent history and narrowly escaped being eliminated in 1995, only to be reauthorized in 1999 with a new mandate and new name: the Agency for Healthcare Research and Quality (AHRQ). Many other initiatives and programs were developed by professional organizations and government agencies over the next 10 years, with various degrees of success.

Several initiatives were proposed as part of the Patient Protection and Affordable Care Act (PPAHA public law 111 to 148) of 2010. In addition to sweeping changes in the delivery of health care, several provisions in this legislation specifically targeted the quality of health care, including establishment of a Patient-Centered Outcomes Research Institute, formation of a Medicare Innovation Center with $10 billion to fund payment reform and quality improvement pilots, and development of new systems linking payment to the quality of outcomes. The initiatives in the PPAHA and other progressive efforts promoted a major transformation of the American health care delivery system through the realignment of payment incentives to reward quality rather than quantity of care.

It is important for interventional cardiologists to understand this history as they interact with many parts of the developing quality infrastructure, such as The Joint Commission, board certification, maintenance of certification, increased transparency from public reporting, and payment reforms.

QUALITY IN INTERVENTIONAL CARDIOLOGY

But even though Quality cannot be defined, you know what Quality is.

Robert M. Pirsig[20]

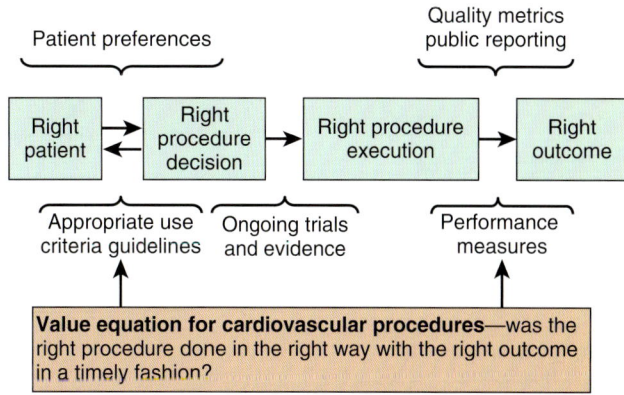

Fig. 69.1 Conceptual model and quality framework for high-quality interventional procedures.

Definition

A high level of quality is something everyone wants in health care, but it is not easily defined. Patients, physicians, payers, and government have different perspectives on the elements that contribute to high-quality health care. Patients frequently place greater emphasis on the interaction and time they have with their physician than on issues such as adherence to practice guidelines. In contrast, payers and government agencies are likely to place more emphasis on adherence to performance measures and on reductions in unnecessary procedures and costs.

The potential to deliver high-quality care in the cardiac catheterization laboratory centers on the core values promoted by the Institute of Medicine (IOM). In its report *Crossing the Quality Chasm*, quality is defined as "the degree to which health care systems, services, and supplies for individuals and populations increase the likelihood for desired health outcomes in a manner consistent with current professional knowledge."[21] The IOM further states that health care should be safe, effective, evidence based, timely, equitable, and patient centered.

Several definitions of quality have been proposed, reflecting the complexity of the health care system and its heterogeneous stakeholders. The RAND Corporation defines quality care as "providing patients with appropriate services in a technically competent manner, with good communications, shared decision making, and cultural sensitivity."[22]

An increasingly popular operational definition of quality is based on error reduction and the recognition that there are three major types of errors in health care: underuse, overuse, and misuse.[23] *Underuse* is the failure to provide a medical intervention when it is likely to produce a favorable outcome for a patient. *Overuse* is the use of a test or therapy even though its benefits do not justify the potential harm or costs. *Misuse* occurs when a therapy or diagnostic test is used in the wrong way or for the wrong purpose.

However quality is defined for interventional cardiologists, a structure for evaluating and measuring quality is needed to continually improve patient care (Fig. 69.1).[24] The structure suggested provides a framework of quality into which recognized building blocks of quality can be placed and used in everyday workflow. These building blocks include specific elements and activities:

- Quality and case reviews are performed on a regular basis by all members of the patient care team in the catheterization laboratory (e.g., cardiologists, nurses, technologists) and by cardiac surgeons, noninvasive cardiologists, and others if necessary.

SECTION VII Outcome Effectiveness of Interventional Cardiology

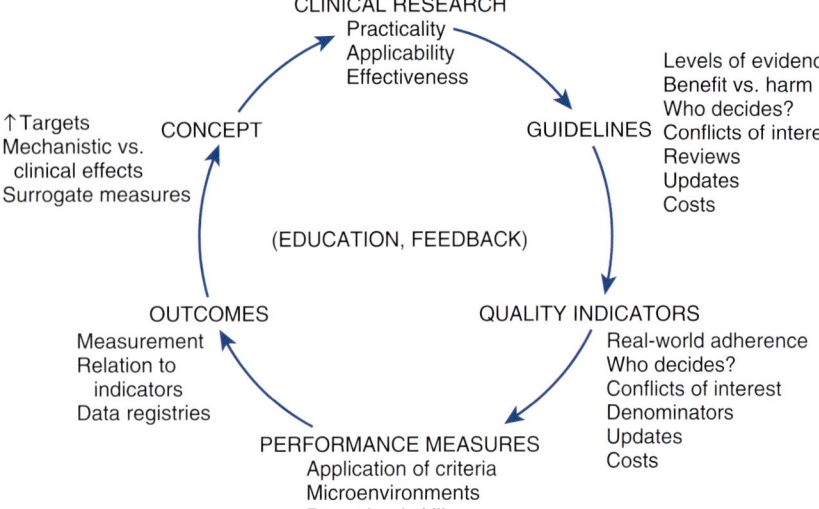

Fig. 69.2 Model for the integration of quality into the cycle of therapeutic development. Concepts from the basic research laboratory eventually lead to clinical studies. After well-conducted clinical research is completed, clinical practice guidelines are developed, leading to quality indicators and then performance measures intended to elevate the level of care and improve patient outcomes. (From Califf RM, Peterson ED, Gibbons RJ, et al. Integrating quality into the cycle of therapeutic development. *J Am Coll Cardiol.* 2002;40[11]:1895–1901.)

- Clinical practice guidelines, data standards, performance measures, and appropriate use criteria (AUC) are incorporated into daily practice.
- The CQI process is used as a tool to evaluate variations in practice and improve performance in the cardiac catheterization laboratory.
- Data are submitted to clinical registries such as the CathPCI Registry of the National Cardiovascular Data Registry (NCDR) to benchmark patient outcomes rather than using volume standards or administrative databases.
- Data from the NCDR and other local information are used to create dashboards for easy and understandable display of trends.

For invasive procedures, the decision to perform the procedure (i.e., right patient and right procedure) may be measured with AUC and clinical practice guidelines. A high-quality health care environment ensures that the patient is receiving the correct treatment for his or her condition. If the patient receives flawless and efficient delivery of the wrong treatment, high-quality care cannot exist. Patient preference is solicited as part of shared decision making along with the clinical recommendation. Execution of the right procedure is influenced by clinical practice guidelines, performance measures, and the best available evidence, but it also includes the operator's skill and experience as assessed by board certification and maintenance of certification, case reviews, and other peer review activities.

The right clinical result can be assessed by performance and outcome measures, some of which are publicly reported. In this fashion, the interventional practice of a facility and an operator may be evaluated, which provides the basis for determining the value of different practices.

Therapeutic Development and Quality

Quality in health care has its origin in the cycle of therapeutic development (Fig. 69.2).[25] The model starts with a hypothesis derived from basic scientific research, animal research, or other observations. It progresses to early clinical research with small, nonrandomized, and unblinded case series and eventually leads to a large, randomized, blinded, and well-designed clinical trial.

After one or more well-performed clinical trials provide clear information about a clinical question, the substrate is established for a clinical practice guideline. All available evidence and opinions are used to produce the clinical practice guidelines for medical conditions and therapeutic procedures (e.g., PCI guidelines).

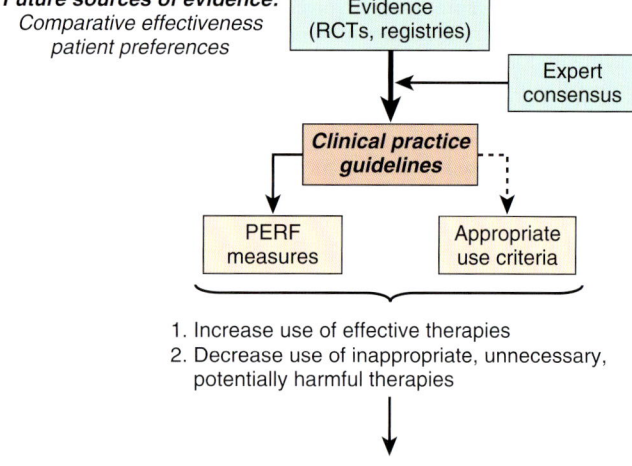

Fig. 69.3 The building blocks of quality. Performance measures and appropriate use criteria are derived from clinical practice guidelines. *PERF*, Performance; *RCT*, randomized controlled trial. (From Antman EM, Peterson ED. Tools for guiding clinical practice from the American Heart Association and the American College of Cardiology: what are they and how should clinicians use them? *Circulation*. 2009;119:1180–1185.)

The AUC and performance measures are then derived from clinical practice guidelines (Fig. 69.3).

JUDGING QUALITY IN INTERVENTIONAL CARDIOLOGY

The building blocks of quality fit into Donabedian's triad, a conceptual framework that has been used extensively.[11] The three domains (i.e., structure, process, and outcome) each identify a major area containing multiple metrics that can be assessed to determine the program's quality.

Structure

Structure refers to the physical components of health care delivery. For the cardiac catheterization laboratory, structural measures include the training, experience, and board certification of

TABLE 69.2 Structure, Process, and Outcome Measures in the Cardiac Catheterization Laboratory

STRUCTURAL INDICATORS

Personnel Indicators

Credentialing (training and certification) of physicians and staff
Reappointment criteria for physicians
Functioning peer-review process for operators
Staff development and continuing education

Equipment Indicators

Fluoroscopic image quality
Quality of stored images and stability of the image archive
Maintenance schedule for equipment
Evaluation of new equipment and disposables
Laboratory time lost or rescheduling because of equipment failure or problems
Electrical safety systems

ORGANIZATIONAL INDICATORS

Internal methods for tracking and comparing procedural data
Laboratory use (e.g., hours/day, procedures/laboratory/day, laboratory time/procedure)
Total full-time equivalents per procedure
Disposable equipment costs per procedure; total costs per procedure and per operator
Personnel costs per procedure
Delay time between procedures
Adherence to Occupational Safety and Health Administration (OSHA) guidelines
Procedure fluoroscopy and cine-angiography times
Radiation dosage to personnel
Radiation protection practices
Radiographic contrast use per case
In-hospital delays for procedures
Outpatient waiting times for procedures
Outpatient waiting times for procedure starts

PROCESS INDICATORS

Indications for procedures or adherence to appropriate use criteria
Indications for hospital admissions
Length of stay after procedures (i.e., total for laboratory and per physician)
Quality of angiographic studies
Quality (correctness) of study interpretation
Precautions for patients with renal insufficiency, contrast allergy, latex allergy, or other conditions

OUTCOME INDICATORS

Success rates for percutaneous coronary interventions
Risk-adjusted outcomes, especially mortality, emergency bypass surgery, and coronary perforation
Satisfaction surveys (e.g., patient, family, referring physician)
Frequency of coronary angiograms showing no significant disease

Modified from Heupler FA, Al-Hani AJ, Dear WE, et al. Guidelines for continuous quality improvement in the cardiac catheterization laboratory. *Cathet Cardiovasc Diagn.* 1993;30(3):191–200.

---

the physicians performing procedures; training and competency records for laboratory staff; adequacy of diagnostic, imaging, and therapeutic equipment including radiation safety; appropriate maintenance and calibration logs for equipment; educational opportunities for the staff; and internal methods used for tracking procedural data (Table 69.2).

To assess the knowledge base of interventional cardiologists, the American Board of Internal Medicine (ABIM) has administered an additional qualification examination for board certification in interventional cardiology since 1999. The maintenance of certification requirements is in evolution. Other requirements include maintenance of a valid certification in internal medicine or cardiovascular disease, documentation of adequate procedure volumes (e.g., 100 cases over 2 years), evidence of participation in a quality improvement project, and completion of self-evaluation modules for medical knowledge and practice performance. Hospitals and payers frequently adopt a requirement for board certification, but there are no data to prove that board-certified physicians provide a higher quality of care than those who are not board-certified. For other laboratory personnel, structural measures can include requirements for all technologists to be registered cardiovascular invasive specialists and to maintain certification in advanced cardiac life support.

Important structural components include education in the form of cardiac catheterization conferences, which provide a forum for discussing difficult management issues, and morbidity and mortality reviews as part of a peer review quality improvement program.[26] To be effective, these programs must emphasize improvement of performance rather than identifying individual physicians as potential one-time outliers. Collection of laboratory data with benchmarking against state or national data is important for assessing clinical outcomes. Examples include the NCDR's CathPCI Registry and the Acute Coronary Treatment and Intervention Outcomes Network-Get With The Guidelines (ACTION-GWTG) Registry of myocardial infarction.[27,28] Participation in these programs provides caregivers with standardized tools for data collection, including relevant data elements and definitions, and for the validated risk adjustment of patient outcomes, such as mortality rates. In addition to tracking outcomes, the data reports help to assess adherence to guidelines and performance measures and can serve as a focus for quality improvements within an institution.

Process

Process measures assess how the system works and how health care is delivered (see Table 69.2). An example in interventional cardiology is the door-to-balloon (DTB) time for patients with ST-elevation myocardial infarction (STEMI). To achieve an optimal DTB time, many steps spanning several hospital departments and services are necessary. The emergency department triages the patient with a possible STEMI, an electrocardiogram is obtained to confirm the diagnosis, and appropriate treatment is started. The interventional team is alerted, the cardiac catheterization laboratory is prepared, the patient is transported to the laboratory, and the culprit artery is opened.[29] A flaw in any step increases the DTB time and the possibility of not meeting the process measure.

Realizing that DTB times were suboptimal in many facilities, the Door-to-Balloon Alliance was launched in late 2006 with the goal of achieving a DTB time of 90 minutes or less for at least 75% of nontransferred patients.[30] Several process measures that improved DTB times were adopted and tracked, resulting in a significant improvement in national DTB times (Fig. 69.4).[31]

Other examples of process measures include collecting data to determine the appropriateness of performing a PCI or to enable the assessment of performance measures. Proper patient selection for PCI is receiving increasing scrutiny by all health care stakeholders because there is wide variation in its use (Fig. 69.5).[32] Assessing the appropriateness of a PCI involves understanding the patient's history, clinical presentation, and physical findings; noninvasive testing to determine ischemia severity; assessment of left ventricular function; and interpretation of coronary angiographic findings.

Outcomes

The third component of Donabedian's triad is *outcome*, which is the final product or result of previous actions. Outcomes are tangible measures such as procedural risk-adjusted mortality rates and other adverse outcomes such as vascular complications, bleeding, stroke, contrast nephropathy, cardiac tamponade, periprocedural acute myocardial infarction (AMI), and the rate of emergency coronary artery bypass grafting (CABG) (see

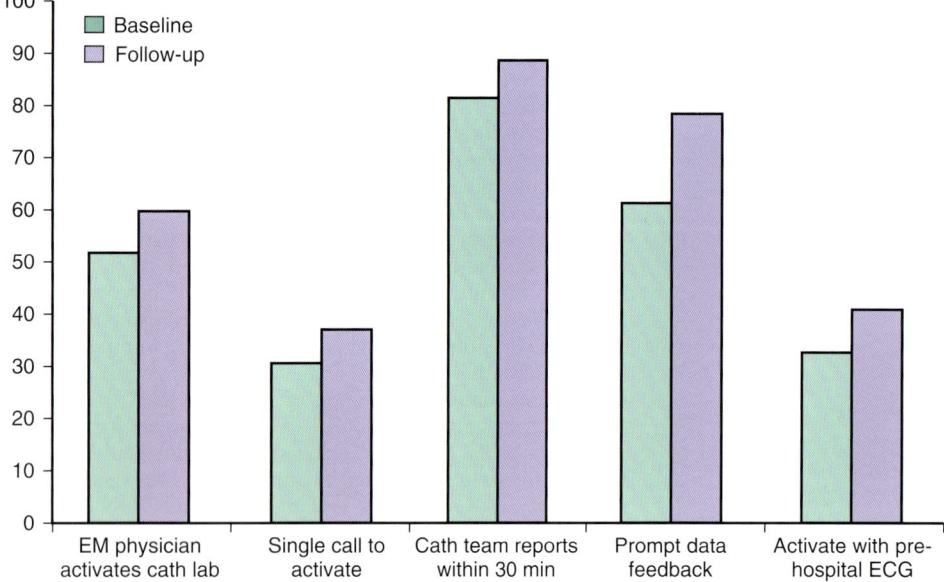

Fig. 69.4 Percentage of Door-to-Balloon Alliance hospitals reporting use of recommended strategies at baseline and in follow-up surveys. *Cath lab*, Catheterization laboratory; *ECG*, electrocardiogram; *EM*, emergency medicine. (From Bradley EH, Nallamothu BK, Herrin J, et al. National efforts to improve door-to-balloon time results from the Door-to-Balloon Alliance. *J Am Coll Cardiol*. 2009;54[25]:2423–2439.)

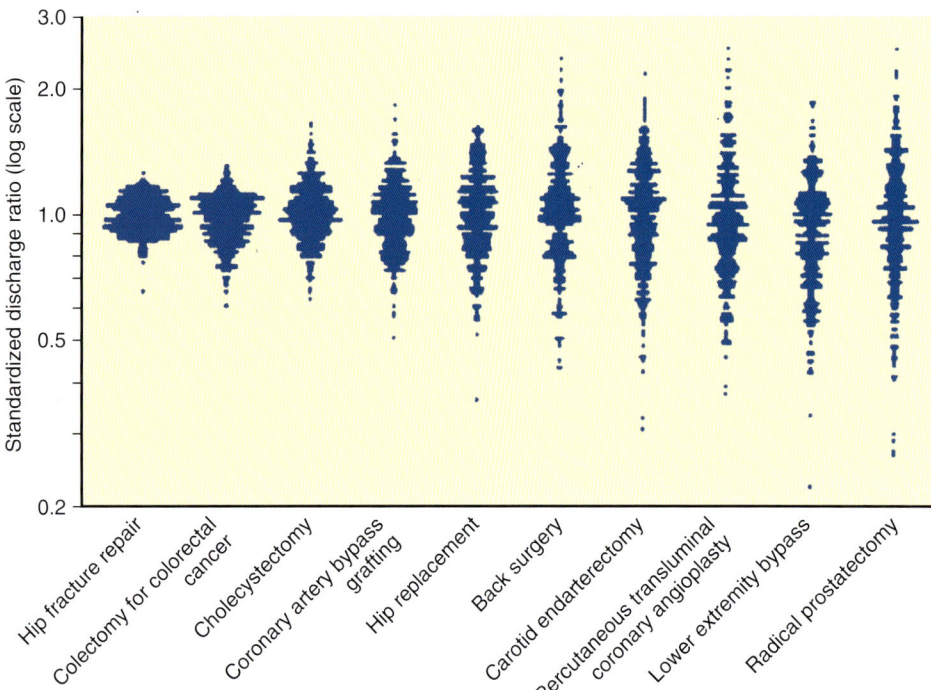

Fig. 69.5 Regional variations in 10 common surgical procedures are plotted. Each dot represents the ratio of the actual number of procedures performed to the average number in each of the 306 hospital referral regions in the United States. Little variation is seen per region for hip fracture repair *(far left)*. However, there is considerable and largely unexplained regional variation in the use of percutaneous transluminal coronary angioplasty. (From Center for the Evaluative Clinical Sciences. Dartmouth atlas of health care: cardiac surgery. www.dartmouthatlas.org/downloads/reports/Cardiac_report_2005.pdf. Accessed March 25, 2015.)

Table 69.2). The measurement of outcomes as quality indicators is attractive because of the implied association between outcome measures and hospital or physician performance. However, these tenuous associations can create challenges for accurate assessment. For example, the definition of a periprocedural AMI (i.e., any troponin level increase versus three or five times the baseline level) and the clinical significance of increased biomarker levels in the periprocedural period are subject to debate. Standardized protocols are needed for biomarker collection during the postprocedural period and for the interpretation of elevated biomarker levels in patients with acute coronary syndrome (ACS).

NCDR data have shown that only 26% of medical centers measure biomarkers after elective PCI, thus limiting use of the peri-PCI outcome measure.[33] Clinical data standards and definitions and standards for statistical models have been developed to help ensure consistency, but important issues remain.[34]

Many PCI-related adverse events—such as death or emergency CABG—are uncommon, especially when assessed at the operator level, because the total number of procedures annually is modest. For example, the 95% confidence interval for a 2% mortality rate for 100 PCI procedures is 0% to 7%. This is a wide range for judging whether the operator has a low or high mortality rate. Quarter-to-quarter or year-to-year outcome measures often vary widely when measured for a single center or operator.

Another important issue is risk adjustment. Factors other than the operator and facility influence outcome comparisons. Patient acuity, demographic features, and comorbid conditions affect the outcome independent of the quality of care provided.

TABLE 69.3 National Cardiovascular Data Registry CathPCI Risk Score System

Variable	Scoring Response Categories				Total Points[a]	Risk of Inpatient Mortality (%)
	<60 Years	≥60, <70 Years	≥70, <80 Years	≥80 Years		
Age	0	4	8	14	5	0.1
Cardiogenic shock	No	Yes	—	—	10	0.1
	0	25	—	—	15	0.2
Prior CHF	No	Yes	—	—	20	0.3
	0	5	—	—	25	0.6
Peripheral vascular disease	No	Yes	—	—	30	1.1
	0	5	—	—	35	2.0
Chronic lung disease	No	Yes	—	—	40	3.6
	0	4	—	—	45	6.3
GFR	<30	30–60	60–90	>90	50	10.9
	18	10	6	0	55	18.3
NYHA functional class IV	No	Yes	—	—	60	29.0
	0	4	—	—	65	42.7
PCI status (STEMI)	Elective	Urgent	Emergent	Salvage	70	57.6
	12	15	20	38	75	71.2
PCI status (no STEMI)	Elective	Urgent	Emergent	Salvage	80	81
	0	8	20	42	85	89.2
					90	93.8
					95	96.5
					100	98.0

[a]In the National Cardiovascular Data Registry (NCDR) risk prediction model for percutaneous coronary intervention mortality, points are assigned for the different variables, and the total number of points is used to predict the risk of inpatient mortality.

CHF, Congestive heart failure; GFR, glomerular filtration rate; NYHA, New York Heart Association; PCI, percutaneous coronary intervention; STEMI, ST-segment elevation myocardial infarction.

From Peterson ED, Dai D, DeLong ER, et al. Contemporary mortality risk prediction for percutaneous coronary intervention: results from 588,398 procedures in the National Cardiovascular Data Registry. J Am Coll Cardiol. 2010;55(18):1923–1932.

Risk adjustment for key clinical outcomes requires accurate and detailed clinical data and a rigorous risk-adjustment methodology to describe provider outcome measurements. Unfortunately, with a focus on risk adjustment, there is the potential for the gaming of outcomes by discharging patients early so that outcomes—such as contrast-induced nephropathy and in-hospital mortality—are not captured. A disproportionate emphasis on outcomes can result in clinical risk-averse behaviors.[35]

The NCDR was started in 1997 to help provider groups and institutions respond to increasing requirements to document the processes and outcomes of care in the cardiac catheterization laboratory. The NCDR is the most comprehensive outcomes-based data repository program in the United States, with seven hospital-based and one practice-based registry. More than 2200 hospitals nationwide participate in one or more of the NCDR registries, which collectively have amassed more than 15 million patient records.[28] Participation in some of the NCDR registries is required by several states and several payers.

Comprehensive data from the CathPCI Registry are provided to member institutions for internal quality assessment and improvement, and confidential data for individual operators are available through a secure portal. Using these data, risk-prediction models have been developed for PCI mortality and bleeding rates (Table 69.3).[36,37]

Outcome measures also include AUC. These criteria have been developed to determine whether coronary revascularization is a reasonable approach for a given clinical circumstance (Fig. 69.6).[38] Although acceptable indications in addition to AUC exist, measuring the degree of adherence to the clinical situations covered by the criteria is valuable for assessing the quality of patient selection. Application and assessment of appropriateness of care require collection of the relevant clinical variables. Because of evolving information about fractional flow reserve and revascularization from randomized controlled trials, the revascularization AUCs are updated every 2 to 3 years.

Outcome assessment often overlaps with and represents the aggregate effect of the other two components of the triad, structure and process. Improvement in the end product is therefore the ultimate measure of the overall success of medical care. Ideally, outcome assessment examines an isolated episode of care (i.e., a single PCI procedure) and includes a longitudinal follow-up assessment of the PCI. This may include the impact of care on indirect health-related measures such as patient satisfaction with the overall care process and quantification of the cost of the care delivery, including cost-effectiveness and cost-efficiency calculations.

BUILDING BLOCKS OF QUALITY
Clinical Practice Guidelines

The IOM defines *guidelines* as "systematically developed statements to assist practitioner and patient decisions about appropriate health care for specific clinical circumstances."[39] For almost 20 years, the AHA, ACCF, and subspecialty organizations have collaborated to develop clinical practice guidelines in cardiology. Guidelines can improve the quality of cardiovascular care and

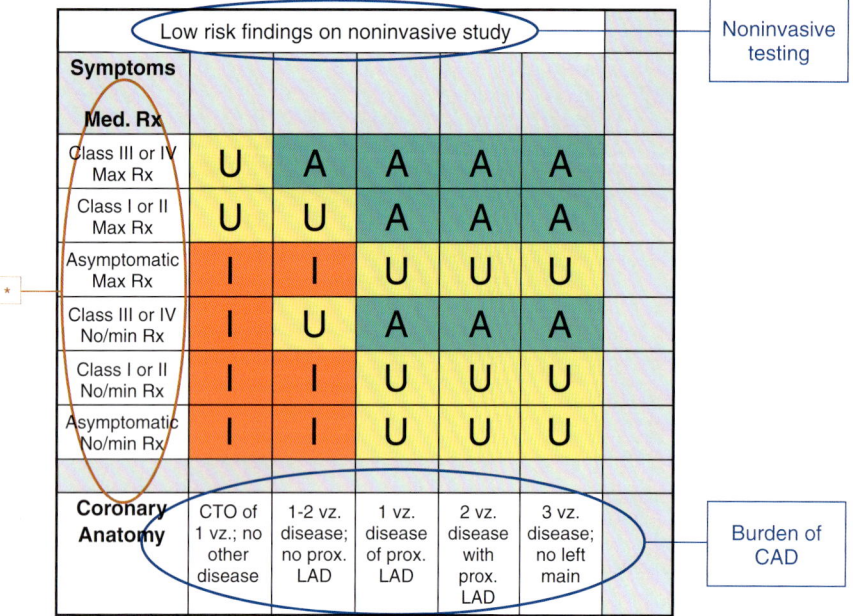

Fig. 69.6 Presentation of the coronary revascularization appropriate use criteria (AUC) for patients with low-risk findings on noninvasive studies. The burden of coronary artery disease is shown at the bottom of the table. The symptom class and degree of medical therapy is shown on the vertical axis. *A*, appropriate; *CAD*, coronary artery disease; *CTO*, chronic total occlusion; *I*, inappropriate; *LAD*, left anterior descending coronary artery; *Max*, maximal; *Med. Rx*, medical therapy; *Prox*, proximal; *U*, uncertain; *vz.*, vessel. (From Patel MR, Dehmer GJ, Hirshfeld JW, et al. ACCF/SCAI/STS/AATS/AHA/ASNC 2009 appropriateness criteria for coronary revascularization: a report by the American College of Cardiology Foundation Appropriateness Criteria Task Force, Society for Cardiovascular Angiography and Interventions, Society of Thoracic Surgeons, American Association for Thoracic Surgery, American Heart Association, and the American Society of Nuclear Cardiology Endorsed by the American Society of Echocardiography, the Heart Failure Society of America, and the Society of Cardiovascular Computed Tomography. *J Am Coll Cardiol*. 2009;53[6]:530–553.)

enhance the use of evidence-based therapies, leading to better patient outcomes, improved cost-effectiveness, and the identification of knowledge gaps that require further research.

After a thorough review of the evidence, guideline recommendations are developed with a designated level of evidence in a structured format (Fig. 69.7). To remain relevant and be embraced by clinicians, clinical practice guidelines must incorporate new evidence in a timely fashion. Guidelines are updated as new and important data are published. Guideline recommendations can be synthesized into algorithms, which can be used to develop quality indicators by specifying the clinical circumstances under which a technology or treatment should or should not be used. Class I and III guideline recommendations with level A evidence identify recommendations that can be considered for the development of a quality measure.

Unfortunately the process is not as straightforward as it seems because of the many treatment considerations for which reasonable uncertainty exists. A challenge to the development of quality indicators occurs in attempting to define which patients qualify for a particular indicator. In one study involving Medicare patients, less than half of all patients with an AMI qualified for a particular quality measure because of a long list of exclusions.[40] If a large number of patients are excluded from a particular quality measure, it may not be a meaningful reflection of the care provided by a physician or a facility. Determining how well a provider or an institution meets specified quality indicators is one way to gauge the quality of the health care delivered. Clinical practice guidelines and performance measures do not consider cost and value in their deliberations.[41]

Performance Measures

Performance measures are derived from clinical practice guidelines. A *quality indicator* is a variable, such as primary PCI performed in patients with STEMI within 90 minutes if PCI is immediately available. In contrast, *performance measures* must have a well-defined numerator and denominator and have appropriate and specified reasons to exclude patients from the tabulation within the measure.

Performance measure selection involves evaluating the strength of evidence supporting the measure, defining the importance of the outcome most likely to be achieved by adherence to it, and assessing the association between adherence to the performance measure and a clinically important outcome. Using the earlier example, the corresponding performance measure would be the proportion of eligible patients with STEMI who arrive at a PCI-capable hospital and receive primary PCI within 90 minutes of arrival. Guideline recommendations that clearly specify the patient population appropriate for a specified treatment or the optimal timing of a treatment are ideal for translation into performance measures.

A detailed description of the methodology for the selection and creation of American College of Cardiology and AHA (ACC/AHA) performance measures has been published.[42] Similar to quality measures, class I guideline recommendations identify potential patient care decisions that could be considered for a performance measure. Performance measures represent mandatory elements of clinical care, whereas failure to adhere to a performance measure represents inadequate or inferior care. "Ideal" performance measures should represent process, structure, or outcomes metrics that are important to patients or society, can be readily measured, are risk-adjusted for patient variability, and, most important, are modifiable through changes in practice. Other important attributes to consider in the development of a performance measure are the cost associated with implementing the measure, availability of reimbursement for the therapy or intervention, and the cost of collecting data required for the measure (Table 69.4).

Performance measures set a threshold for acceptable performance. This leads to questions regarding who determines the threshold and how the threshold level of performance is determined, because it is unlikely that 100% compliance will be achieved for every performance measure. One method of defining thresholds is to establish achievable benchmarks of care.[43] Adherence to a performance measure is determined in a large sample, and the rate of adherence in the top 10% of facilities or physicians is set as the achievable benchmark. Using this method avoids establishing unreasonable goals that might paradoxically lead to inappropriate actions to achieve the

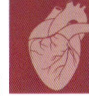

CLASS (STRENGTH) OF RECOMMENDATION	LEVEL (QUALITY) OF EVIDENCE‡

CLASS I (STRONG) — Benefit >>> Risk
Suggested phrases for writing recommendations:
• Is recommended
• Is indicated/useful/effective/beneficial
• Should be performed/administered/other
• Comparative-Effectiveness Phrases†:
  ○ Treatment/strategy A is recommended/indicated in preference to treatment B
  ○ Treatment A should be chosen over treatment B
	LEVEL A
	• High-quality evidence‡ from more than 1 RCTs
	• Meta-analyses of high-quality RCTs
	• One or more RCTs corroborated by high-quality registry studies

CLASS IIa (MODERATE) — Benefit >> Risk
Suggested phrases for writing recommendations:
• Is reasonable
• Can be useful/effective/beneficial
• Comparative-Effectiveness Phrases†:
  ○ Treatment/strategy A is probably recommended/indicated in preference to treatment B
  ○ It is reasonable to choose treatment A over treatment B
	LEVEL B-R (Randomized)
	• Moderate-quality evidence‡ from 1 or more RCTs
	• Meta-analyses of moderate-quality RCTs

	LEVEL B-NR (Nonrandomized) • Moderate-quality evidence‡ from 1 or more well-designed, well-executed nonrandomized studies, observational studies, or registry studies • Meta-analyses of such studies
CLASS IIb (WEAK) — Benefit ≥ Risk Suggested phrases for writing recommendations: • May/might be reasonable • May/might be considered • Usefulness/effectiveness is unknown/unclear/uncertain or not well established	**LEVEL C** • Randomized or nonrandomized observational or registry studies with limitations of design or execution • Meta-analyses of such studies • Physiological or mechanistic studies in human subjects
CLASS III: No Benefit (MODERATE) — Benefit = Risk (Generally, LOE A or B use only) Suggested phrases for writing recommendations: • Is not recommended • Is not indicated/useful/effective/beneficial • Should not be performed/administered/other	**LEVEL E** Consensus of expert opinion based on clinical experience when evidence is insufficient, vague, or conflicting
CLASS III: Harm (STRONG) — Risk > Benefit Suggested phrases for writing recommendations: • Potentially harmful • Causes harm • Associated with excess morbidity/mortality • Should not be performed/administered/other	

COR and LOE are determined independently (any COR may be paired with any LOE).

A recommendation with LOE C or E does not imply that the recommendation is weak. Many important clinical questions addressed in guidelines do not lend themselves to clinical trials. Although RCTs are unavailable, there may be a very clear clinical consensus that a particular test or therapy is useful or effective.

* The outcome or result of the intervention should be specified (an improved clinical outcome or increased diagnostic accuracy or incremental prognostic information).

† For comparative-effectiveness recommendations (COR I and IIa; LOE A and B only), studies that support the use of comparator verbs should involve direct comparisons of the treatments or strategies being evaluated.

‡ The method of assessing quality is evolving, including the application of standardized, widely used, and preferably validated evidence grading tools; and for systematic reviews, the incorporation of an Evidence Review Committee.

COR indicates Class of Recommendation; LOE, Level of Evidence; NR, nonrandomized; R, randomized; and RCT, randomized controlled trial.

Fig. 69.7 Classification of recommendations and level of evidence used in the American College of Cardiology Foundation and the American Heart Association clinical practice guidelines. Definitions of treatment recommendations and levels of evidence are shown. (From American Heart Association. Methodology manual and policies from the ACCF/AHA Task Force on Practice Guidelines. http://assets.cardiosource.com/Methodology_Manual_for_ACC_AHA_Writing_Committees.pdf. Accessed March 25, 2015.)

established goal. Table 69.5 lists current performance measures in cardiology.

There is interest in developing composite performance measures,[44] which combine two or more measures into a single index. Composite measures reduce the information burden by distilling the available indicators into a summary with which to examine multiple dimensions of performance and facilitate comparisons. The Society of Thoracic Surgeons developed and validated a composite measure for CABG comprising five process measures and six outcome measures, all of which are endorsed by the National Quality Forum (NQF) (Table 69.6).[45,46] The NQF has endorsed ACC/AHA and NCDR performance measures, potentially affecting future payment models. However, there are challenges to this approach. Details of an important individual measure can be diluted in the overall composite, and methods for deriving the composite must be transparent to prevent it from being perceived as a black box.

A detailed list of performance measures has been published for PCI.[47] Eleven measures encompassing the triad of structure, process, and outcome were identified; six are considered performance measures and five were recommended as quality metrics for self-improvement (Table 69.7). The measures identified as performance measures include comprehensive documentation of the indication for the procedures, assessment of candidacy for dual-antiplatelet therapy, postprocedural optimal medical therapy, patient referral to cardiac rehabilitation, regional or national PCI registry participation, and annual hospital PCI volume. Individual operator volume was identified as a quality metric. In addition to these measures, national agencies such as the CMS have identified potential outcome measures for PCI.

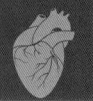

SECTION VII Outcome Effectiveness of Interventional Cardiology

TABLE 69.4 American College of Cardiology and American Heart Association Attributes for Satisfactory Performance Measures

MEASURES FOR IMPROVING PATIENT OUTCOMES
Evidence-based
Interpretable
Actionable

MEASURE DESIGN
Denominator precisely defined
Numerator precisely defined
Validity
    Face validity
    Content validity
    Construct validity
    Reliability

MEASURE IMPLEMENTATION
Feasibility
Reasonable effort
Reasonable cost
Reasonable time period for collection

Modified from Spertus JA, Eagle KA, Krumholtz HM, et al. American College of Cardiology and American Heart Association methodology for the selection and creation of performance measures for quantifying and quality of cardiovascular care. *J Am Coll Cardiol.* 2005;45(7):1147–1156.

TABLE 69.5 American College of Cardiology Foundation and American Heart Association Performance Measure Sets

Topic	Publication Date	Partnering Organizations
Chronic heart failure	2005	ACC, AHA: inpatient measures ACC, AHA, PCPI outpatient measures
Chronic stable coronary artery disease	2005	ACC, AHA, PCPI
Hypertension	2005	ACC, AHA, PCPI
ST- and non–ST-elevation myocardial infarction	2006	ACC, AHA
Cardiac rehabilitation	2007	AACVPR, ACC, AHA
Atrial fibrillation	2008	ACC, AHA, PCPI
Primary prevention of cardiovascular disease	2009	ACCF, AHA
Peripheral artery disease	2010	ACCF, AHA, ACR, SCAI, SIR, SVM, SVN, SVS
Percutaneous coronary intervention	2013	ACCF, AHA, SCAI, AMA

AACVPR, American Association of Cardiovascular and Pulmonary Rehabilitation; *ACC,* American College of Cardiology; *ACCF,* American College of Cardiology Foundation; *AHA,* American Heart Association; *ACR,* American College of Radiology; *PCPI,* AMA's Physician Consortium for Performance Improvement; *SCAI,* Society for Cardiovascular Angiography and Interventions; *SIR,* Society for Interventional Radiology; *SVM,* Society for Vascular Medicine; *SVN,* Society for Vascular Nursing; *SVS,* Society for Vascular Surgery.

TABLE 69.6 Individual Measures and Domains Included in the Society of Thoracic Surgeons Composite Score

OPERATIVE CARE DOMAIN
Use of at least one internal mammary artery graft

PERIOPERATIVE MEDICAL CARE DOMAIN
Preoperative beta blockers
Discharge beta blockers
Discharge antiplatelet medication
Discharge antilipid medication

RISK-ADJUSTED MORTALITY DOMAIN
Operative mortality

RISK-ADJUSTED MAJOR MORBIDITY DOMAIN
Prolonged ventilation (>24 h)
Deep sternal wound infection
Permanent stroke
Renal insufficiency
Reoperation

From O'Brien SM, Shahian DM, DeLong ER, et al. Quality measurement in adult cardiac surgery: part 2—statistical considerations in composite measure scoring and provider rating. *Ann Thorac Surg.* 2007;83 (4 suppl):S13–S26.

Outcome Measures

The ultimate goal of performance measures is to identify care opportunities that are likely to improve outcomes for patients and thereby the quality of care. Among interventional cardiologists there is general agreement regarding the outcome measures of importance, and they have been used in many trials. Death and freedom from major adverse cardiac events such as AMI, stroke, bleeding, and target-lesion or target-vessel revascularization are all important, relatively easy to quantify, and have been used in many trials. Improvements in symptoms and quality of life are also important but are more subjective and challenging to quantify, and collecting these data may involve additional cost and effort.

Many outcome measures require risk adjustment to compare outcomes at the provider level in a fair manner, but adjusting for the effects of comorbid medical conditions, severity of the underlying disease, and socioeconomic status is imperfect. This is a huge challenge when analyses are restricted to administrative claims data, which include data of inferior quality and lack the necessary clinical variables for risk adjustment. Because of the challenges in measuring outcomes, especially some long-term outcomes at the provider level, it is often easier to assess quality by adhering to performance measures as surrogates of actual quality on the assumption that a high level of adherence to performance measures results in better outcomes. In addition to traditional outcome measures, new measures—such as 30-day readmission after a PCI—have been implemented by CMS, with financial penalties imposed for high readmission rates; these measures are NQF-approved. Unfortunately, as recently shown in the congestive heart failure (CHF) population, reduction in readmissions through the CMS Hospital Readmissions Reduction Program (HRRP) has also resulted in increases in both 30-day and 1-year all-cause mortality rates.[48]

Appropriate Use Criteria

Although clinical practice guidelines provide a foundation for summarizing evidence-based cardiovascular care, there are many gaps in current knowledge and wide variations in practice patterns. The variability in the use of cardiovascular procedures raises questions of overuse or underuse. Realizing that clinical practice guidelines do not cover all possible clinical situations, AUC have been developed for cardiovascular imaging procedures and coronary revascularization.[49]

AUC should serve as a supplement to clinical practice guidelines and performance measures. They are intended to assist patients and clinicians but are not intended to diminish the acknowledged difficulty or uncertainty of clinical decision making and cannot substitute for sound clinical judgment and practice experience. The AUC allow assessment of use patterns for a

TABLE 69.7 2013 Performance Measures for Adults Undergoing Percutaneous Coronary Intervention

Performance Measure	Description[a]
Comprehensive documentation of indications for PCI[b]	Percentage of patients age ≥18 years for whom PCI is performed with comprehensive documentation of the procedure, which includes at a minimum the following elements: • Priority (e.g., acute coronary syndrome, elective, urgent, emergency, or salvage) • Presence and severity of angina symptoms (e.g., Canadian Cardiovascular Society classification system) • Use of antianginal medical therapies within 2 weeks before the procedure, if any • Presence, results, and timing of noninvasive stress test, fractional flow reserve, or intravascular ultrasound if performed • Significance of angiographic stenosis (i.e., quantitative or qualitative) on coronary angiography for treated lesion
Appropriate indication for elective PCI[c]	Percentage of patients age ≥18 years for whom elective PCI is performed in a native coronary artery who have an appropriate indication for the procedure suggesting that the overall benefits outweigh its risks
Assessment of candidacy for dual-antiplatelet therapy[b]	Percentage of patients age ≥18 years for whom PCI is performed who have documentation in the medical record that an assessment of candidacy for initiation and duration of dual-antiplatelet therapy was performed before the procedure
Use of embolic protection devices in the treatment of saphenous vein bypass graft disease[c]	Percentage of patients age ≥18 years for whom saphenous vein graft PCI is performed who received an embolic protection device during the procedure
Documentation of preprocedural glomerular filtration rate and contrast dose used during the procedure[c]	Percentage of patients age ≥18 years for whom PCI is performed who have preprocedural estimated glomerular filtration rate or an indication that the patient is on dialysis and the administered contrast dose documented in the catheterization report or procedure notes
Radiation dose documentation[c]	Percentage of patients age ≥18 years for whom PCI is performed who have the administered radiation dose documented in the catheterization report or procedure notes
Postprocedural optimal medical therapy composite[b]	Percentage of patients age ≥18 years for whom PCI is performed who are prescribed optimal medical therapy at discharge
Cardiac rehabilitation patient referral[b]	Percentage of patients age ≥18 years for whom PCI is performed who have been referred to an outpatient cardiac rehabilitation or secondary prevention program
Regional or national PCI registry participation[b]	Participation in a national or multisystem geographic regional PCI registry that provides regular performance reports based on benchmarked data
Annual operator PCI volume[c]	Average annual volume of PCIs performed by an operator over the previous 2 calendar years
Annual hospital PCI volume[b]	Annual volume of PCIs performed by a hospital over the previous calendar year

[a]Comprehensive information on these measures, including measure exceptions, is provided by the complete ACC/AHA/AMA-PCPI/NCQA/SCAI performance measurement specifications through the PCPI website (https://www.ama-assn.org/practice-management/payment-delivery-models/permissions-and-licensing-pcpi-measures).

[b]These measures are designated *performance measures*, which are process, structure, efficiency, or outcome measures that have been developed with ACCF/AHA methodology, including the process of public comment and peer review, and they have been designated as performance measures by the ACC/AHA Task Force on Performance Measures. Measures are intended for internal quality improvement and may be considered for purposes of public reporting or other forms of accountability.

[c]These measures are designated *quality metrics*, which are measures developed to support self-assessment and quality improvement at the provider, hospital, or health care system level. These valuable tools aid clinicians and hospitals in improving quality of care and enhancing patient outcomes but may not meet all specifications of formal performance measures and are therefore not appropriate for any use other than internal quality improvement.

PCI, percutaneous coronary intervention.

From Nallamothu BK, Tommaso CL, Anderson HV, et al. ACC/AHA/SCAI/AMA-Convened PCPI/NCQA 2013 performance measures for adults undergoing percutaneous coronary intervention: a report of the American College of Cardiology/American Heart Association Task Force on Performance Measures, the Society for Cardiovascular Angiography and Interventions, the American Medical Association-Convened Physician Consortium for Performance Improvement, and the National Committee for Quality Assurance. *J Am Coll Cardiol.* 2014;63(7):722–745.

test or procedure. Comparing use patterns across a large subset of a provider's patients can allow assessment of a provider's management strategies versus those of his or her peers. Ideally, measurement of the AUC in clinical practice would allow improvement of indications for procedures and stimulate discussions with patients as part of shared decision making.

The process of AUC development is well defined.[50] First, the AUC writing group combines specific clinical characteristics to create prototypical patient scenarios. Second, a technical panel is created from nominations by relevant professional societies, provider-led organizations, and health policy and payer communities. To preserve objectivity, the technical panels do not include a majority of individuals whose livelihood is tied to the technology under study. Third, the technical panel is provided with summaries of the relevant evidence from the literature and practice guidelines, and each member of the panel then independently assigns an appropriateness rating to each scenario. A numeric score is assigned to each scenario, with a score of 7 to 9 meaning *appropriate*, 4 to 6 meaning *may be appropriate*, and 1 to 3 meaning *rarely appropriate* indications to perform that test or procedure. Fourth, the technical panel meets as a group to discuss the initial ratings and the benefits and risks of the test or procedure in the context of the potential benefits to patients' outcomes, with an implicit understanding of the associated resource use and costs. After the group meeting, the individual panel members again rate each scenario for the final ranking. Fifth, the final appropriateness ratings are summarized using an established and rigorous methodology.[50]

The current terms of *appropriate*, *may be appropriate*, and *rarely appropriate* replaced the original terms of *appropriate*, *uncertain*, and *inappropriate* used in the RAND methodology.[51] The terminology was changed to provide a better characterization of the ratings in the context of real-world decision making and clinical uncertainty and to provide a better focus on the aim of the AUC in measuring overall clinical practice trends rather than adjudicating individual cases.

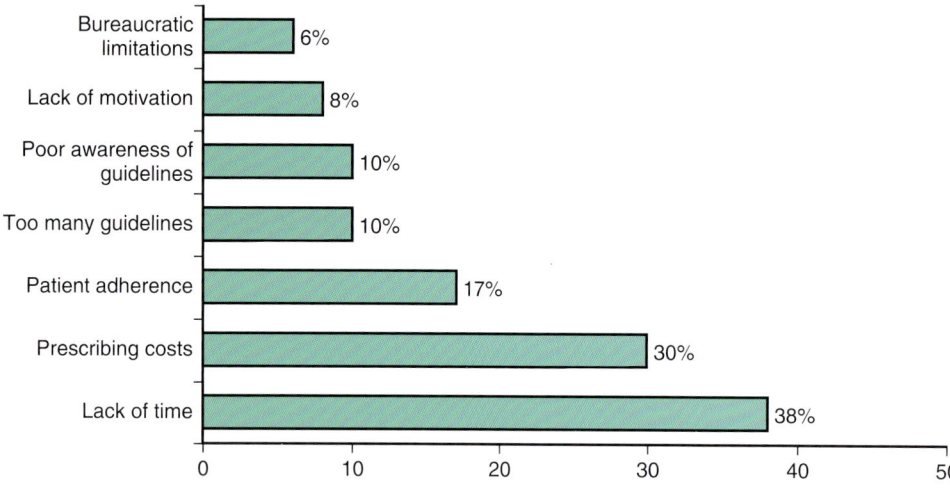

Fig. 69.8 Barriers cited by physicians that prevent guideline implementation. (Modified from Hobbs FD, Erhardt L. Acceptance of guideline recommendations and perceived implementation of coronary heart disease prevention among primary care physicians in five European countries: the Reassessing European Attitudes about Cardiovascular Treatment (REACT) survey. *Fam Pract*. 2002;19[6]:596–604.)

Recent Updates and Changes in Appropriate Use Criteria

There have been two recent updates to the AUC recommendations for stable ischemic heart disease (SIHD) and ACS.[52,53] For both documents, the terms *appropriate*, *may be appropriate*, and *rarely appropriate* continue to be used. For patients with SIHD, there continues to be an emphasis on using objective measures to better stratify patients who may be at low or intermediate risk and to better utilize intracoronary physiology testing to determine if PCI is warranted. There is also emphasis on ensuring that patients are on optimal medical therapy, including antianginals, prior to being treated with PCI. These recommendations come in large part from the goal of helping operators and providers to avoid offering invasive management to otherwise low-risk patients who have not been optimally managed with medications.

The AUC recommendations for ACS highlight several of the current controversies in ACS care and provides operator guidance. For instance, consideration of surgical revascularization in less acute ACS patients *may be appropriate* over potentially multivessel PCI.[38] To be consistent with the ongoing controversy of how to approach the nonculprit stenosis in an ACS patient, the ACS AUC recommendations state that nonculprit PCI at the time of primary revascularization *may be appropriate*. The only *rarely appropriate* rating in the updated AUC is for patients undergoing PCI with intermediate-severity nonculprit artery stenosis without further testing to determining the functional significance of the stenosis. Importantly, these criteria allow for clinical discretion for many clinical scenarios while also indicating where invasive management may and may not be appropriate.

Impact of Guidelines, Performance Measures, and Appropriate Use Criteria

Relatively few studies assess the extent to which guidelines are applied by clinicians in daily practice. Using data from the NCDR collected between 2001 and 2004, it was shown that 64% of patients undergoing PCI had a class I indication, 21% class IIa, 7% were class IIb, and 8% were rated class III.[54] The clinical success of a PCI was directly related to the class of indication. *Clinical success*, defined as less than 25% residual stenosis without MI, same-admission bypass surgery, or death, was attained for 92.8% of patients with a class I indication, 91.7% of those with a class IIa indication, 89% of those with a class IIb indication, and only 85.5% of those with a class III indication.

Unfortunately other studies have evaluated the extent to which guidelines are followed in clinical practice with disappointing results. For example, Lopes and colleagues examined a large cohort of patients from three randomized, double-blind clinical trials to determine whether patients with atrial fibrillation were being treated with antithrombotic therapy in accordance with accepted guidelines.[55] Only 13.5% of the patients in these trials were receiving indicated prophylactic antithrombotic therapy with warfarin. Similarly, data from the Worcester Heart Attack Study and the Global Registry of Acute Coronary Events (GRACE) show an increase in the use of guideline-recommended medications (i.e., β-blockers, angiotensin converting enzyme inhibitors, aspirin, and lipid-lowering agents) over time, but only about 60% of patients are receiving these medications.[56,57] These findings are not unusual, and other studies have documented that guideline recommendations are followed for a disappointingly small portion of inpatients and outpatients.[58]

Care providers may not be using guidelines to a greater extent in daily practice because of the sheer number of guidelines and their length, because they are comfortable with tried and true approaches to managing disease, because they desire to avoid standardized and rigid order sets that do not apply to all patients and are perceived as "cookbook" medical therapy, and because some patients have unique clinical issues with no specific guideline recommendations available, or, when available, the guidelines are based more on expert consensus than on data from multiple randomized trials.[59]

Tricoci and colleagues evaluated 16 current ACC/AHA guideline documents.[60] Of 2711 separate guideline recommendations, a median of 11% were based on level A evidence, compared with a median of 48% that were based on level C evidence; only 19% of class I recommendations were based on level A evidence. Expert consensus was used more frequently for imaging recommendations, whereas recommendations for revascularization procedures were more commonly based on level A or level B evidence.

These limitations exist in the United States and other countries. The Reassessing European Attitudes About Cardiovascular Treatment (REACT) survey obtained responses from 754 physicians, each with more than 10 years' experience, in five European countries to assess whether physicians' perceptions of coronary heart disease management matched their treatment practices and whether their perceptions of patients' awareness was an accurate reflection of their patients' understanding.[61] In the survey, physicians were asked to identify the most common barriers that prevented them from implementing guideline recommendations. The most common barrier, cited by 38% of the respondents, was lack of time (Fig. 69.8).

TABLE 69.8 Nonclinical Reasons for Recommending Cardiac Catheterization

Reason[a]	Frequently n (%)	Sometimes n (%)	Rarely n (%)	Never n (%)	Association With CSI (P Trend)
The patient is expected to undergo the procedure.	9 (1.5)	91 (15.6)	271 (46.4)	213 (36.5)	
Mean CSI	*51.5*	*49.7*	*49.8*	*49.9*	*0.99*
Colleagues would do so in the same situation.	22 (3.8)	134 (23.3)	240 (41.7)	180 (31.3)	
Mean CSI	*52.7*	*50.1*	*50.2*	*48.7*	*0.02*
You wanted to satisfy the expectations of the referring physician.	11 (1.9)	156 (26.9)	257 (44.2)	157 (27)	
Mean CSI	*52.6*	*50.0*	*49.3*	*50.3*	*0.90*
You wanted to prevent a possible malpractice suit.	16 (2.7)	123 (21.1)	245 (42.0)	200 (34.3)	
Mean CSI	*51.8*	*50.5*	*50.1*	*48.8*	*0.02*
Doing so would enhance the financial stability of your practice.	2 (0.3)	3 (0.5)	46 (7.9)	532 (91.3)	
Mean CSI	*49.7*	*55.9*	*51.1*	*49.7*	*0.22*

[a]Consider your own cardiac catheterization recommendations. A cardiologist sometimes recommends cardiac catheterization for other than purely clinical reasons. During the past 12 months, how often has each of these reasons led you to recommend cardiac catheterization for a patient?
CSI, cardiac intensity score.
From Lucas FL, Sirovich BE, Gallagher PM, et al. Variation in cardiologists' propensity to test and treat: is it associated with regional variation in utilization? *Circ Cardiovasc Qual Outcomes*. 2010;3(3):253–260.

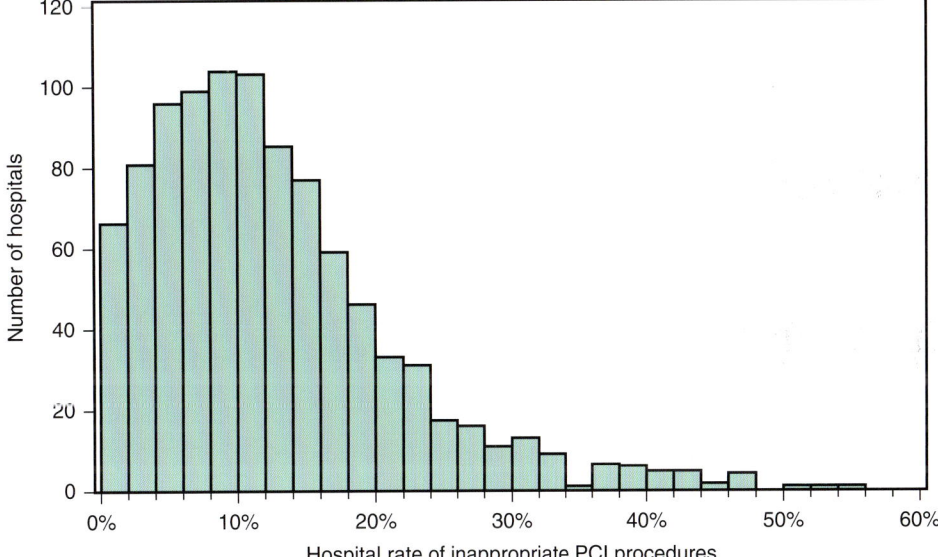

Fig. 60.9 Hospital-level variations in the rate of inappropriate percutaneous coronary intervention *(PCI)* procedures. (From Chan PS, Patel MR, Klein LW, et al. Appropriateness of percutaneous coronary intervention. *JAMA*. 2011;306:53–61.)

The potential effect of decision-maker bias regarding the recommendation for coronary artery revascularization has been examined.[62] Using the New York State database, the treatment decision (i.e., CABG, PCI, medical therapy, or no treatment) made by the cardiologist performing the cardiac catheterization was compared with the treatment recommendation from the relevant ACC/AHA guideline document. Guideline-supported indications for CABG applied to 13% of the study patients, indications for PCI applied to 59% of patients, and indications for CABG or PCI to 17% of patients. For the patients with an indication for CABG, the cardiologist recommended CABG for 53% and PCI for 34%. Among patients with indications for PCI, 94% were recommended for PCI, and among patients with indications for CABG or PCI, the cardiologist recommended PCI for 93% and CABG for 5%. Treatment recommendations also varied, depending on whether the catheterization laboratory did or did not offer PCI. These findings show the potential effect of decision bias on the application of guideline recommendations for coronary revascularization.

Considerable geographic variation in the use of PCI within the Medicare population has been documented in other large surveys (see Fig. 69.5).[32] Variation in cardiologists' propensity to make treatment recommendations is also affected by several nonclinical factors.[63] In a survey of 598 cardiologists, several nonclinical reasons to recommend cardiac catheterization, including protection from malpractice litigation, were identified (Table 69.8).

With the goal of improving outcomes for patients with cardiovascular disease, it is important to emphasize that some studies show a positive relationship between adherence to performance measures and clinical outcomes.[64] However, this relationship is not necessarily strong and does not completely explain all of the variations. An analysis of the National Registry of Myocardial Infarction (NRMI) database, showed that only 6% of the hospital-level variations in 30-day death rates after AMI could be attributed to differences in the use of performance measures.[65]

In 2011, Chan and associates reported the appropriateness ratings for more than 500,000 PCI procedures from the NCDR and documented that most urgent PCIs were appropriate, whereas approximately 12% of elective PCIs, comprising only 30% of the overall database, were deemed inappropriate.[66] However, there was substantial hospital-level variation in cases deemed inappropriate (Fig. 69.9). These data have increased the focus on developing systematic ways to capture the information needed for AUC reporting.

Contemporary studies that attempt to examine the impact of AUC on provider behavior are being performed.[67] In a multicenter, longitudinal, cross-sectional analysis of patients undergoing PCI between 2009 and 2014 at participating NCDR-CathPCI Registry hospitals, Desai and colleagues examine the number of patients undergoing inappropriate nonacute PCIs before and after the 2012 AUC for coronary revascularization. Although the volume of acute PCIs remained roughly the same from 2009 to 2014, the number of nonacute PCIs being performed dropped precipitously from 89,704 in 2010 to 59,375 in 2014. The number of inappropriate PCIs dropped from 21,781 to 7,921 over the study period, and the use of antianginals prior to PCI increased from 22.3% to 24.1% over the same time period ($P < .001$). However, the authors noted that hospital-level variation in the proportion of inappropriate PCIs remained persistent over the study period (median 12.6%, interquartile range 5.9% to 22.9% in 2014). Although the overall number of inappropriate PCIs declined, pockets of hospitals continued PCI practices not recommended by the 2012 AUC.

These data provide some early validation of the AUC and demonstrate opportunities to reduce the over- and underuse of coronary revascularization.[24] Unfortunately some payers are challenging and denying payment for individual cases rated "rarely appropriate" without an interactive review. This should be considered a misuse of the AUC, and the ACC and SCAI professional societies are providing leadership in responding to these types of challenges.

Best Practices

Best practices are processes are procedures that are generally accepted as being most effective, safe, and correct for commercial or professional procedures. The SCAI outlines best practices for pre-, intra-, and postprocedural management.[68] These best practice recommendations are updated every few years, with the last update performed in 2016. Best practice recommendations range from provider and institutional competence standards to the appropriate elements of the preprocedural history and physical.

The preprocedural preparation and evaluation of patients remains a large focus of the SCAI Best Practice Guidelines. The recommendations place a focus on careful consideration of individual patient risk factors, such as chronic kidney disease, risks of bleeding, ability to take antiplatelet therapy after PCI, and potential access site issues. Fig. 69.10 demonstrates the preprocedure checklist recommended as best practice for patients undergoing cardiac catheterization. Additional best practice recommendations include the process of procedural timeout, the appropriate procedural documentation that should exist, and the duties and responsibilities of the cardiac catheterization laboratory's physician director. Finally, the 2016 SCAI revision includes recommendations around how cardiac catheterization laboratories should prepare for potential emergencies, including protocols on how to alert cardiac surgical services for emergency procedures and how to obtain emergent echocardiography.

Quality Assurance and Continuous Quality Improvement

Quality assurance is a process based largely on the retrospective review of selected outcomes to determine discrepancies between practice and recommended standards of care.[69] It can be likened to inspecting the final product as it comes off the assembly line. Criteria are established to identify an acceptable product, and items not meeting these criteria are judged as flawed or damaged and rejected before leaving the factory. This process maintains a certain level of product quality, with only acceptable products reaching the market.

Applied to the clinical environment, quality assurance seeks to identify outliers in some aspect of clinical care. Identified outliers often provide an opportunity to improve, but if that fails, they can be denied further participation in clinical care (Fig. 69.11A). The structured quality assurance process may promote a level of defensiveness among health care providers because the process often focuses on determining who is at fault if something goes wrong—the so-called bad apple concept.[70]

The CQI process provides an alternative approach whereby specific problems are first identified, followed by the formulation of a solution by various stakeholders. This is validated by reevaluation of the process after the solution has been implemented (see Fig. 69.11B). For example, a facility may have an excessive number of patients with groin hematomas after PCI. Patients with hematomas are unhappy, have a prolonged hospitalization, and cost the facility more in resources. A CQI project could be initiated to reduce the number of patients with hematomas. It would require participation of all individuals involved, including physicians, catheter laboratory personnel, nursing staff in the recovery area, and others who interact with the patient. Each step in the process is carefully examined, opportunities for improvement are identified, and appropriate steps are taken to address defects in the process. The new process is initiated, and the results are assessed by determining whether the number of patients with hematomas has been reduced.

The CQI process has become a vital and expected component of a high-quality cardiovascular program with the goals of reducing variation and improving overall performance.[71] Several models for CQI exist. One model frequently used is the Plan-Do-Study-Act (PDSA) model; an alternative is the Focus-Analyze-Develop-Execute (FADE) model (Figs. 69.12 and 69.13). Many of these systems have been adopted from manufacturing and industry. The core actions of these models and most CQI programs include the following:

- Collection of data containing relevant patient variables that allow assessment of clinical processes, performance, and outcomes
- Feedback of performance and outcome information to the clinicians, with risk adjustment if necessary, and benchmarking of the data
- Implementation of appropriate interventions to reduce wasteful and inefficient variations in care and improve performance
- Use of an iterative process to assess the effectiveness of changes
- Answers to two questions: How am I doing compared with others? Am I getting better?

Despite the emphasis on the importance of CQI efforts, relatively few studies have formally examined the results or improvements in outcomes related to CQI. Moscucci and colleagues reported the results of a statewide CQI PCI initiative in Michigan.[72] It involved the use of a wide range of CQI strategies that relied on quarterly feedback reports to clinicians on their adherence to process and performance measures along with reports of crude and risk-adjusted outcomes. The program resulted in a demonstrable decrease in bleeding, transfusion requirements, vascular complications, and contrast use, which reduced the rate of contrast nephropathy. In a temporal observational study at the Mayo Clinic, Rihal and coworkers identified the benefit of CQI intervention for PCI delivery, showing improvements in clinical and economic outcomes.[73] In a recent analysis from the CathPCI Registry comparing the outcomes of patients in New York, a state with public reporting, with patients in Michigan, a state with CQI, Boyden and colleagues found that in a public reporting system there were fewer high-risk patients undergoing PCI and overall lower in-hospital mortality and other adverse events compared patients in a CQI state.[74]

Unfortunately there are several barriers to the implementation of CQI programs. Lack of hospital administrative and financial supports, the time and expense of internal data collection, and a deficit of physician leadership frequently hamper CQI efforts.[75]

Patient name	MRN	Procedure date

| Planned Procedure: (circle all that apply) | Diagnostic Cardiac Catheterization (L, R, simultaneous)
Coronary angiography
Left ventriculography
Intravascular Imaging/Hemodynamic Assessment (IVUS, OCT, FFR)
Possible PCI
Planned PCI
Other |

History and Physical Examination:		
Elective Outpatient Procedures: H&P documented within 30 days?	Yes	No
Inpatient Procedures: H&P documented within 24 hours of admission?	Yes	No
History of prior PCI or CABG: Yes No If yes, report/s obtained?	Yes	No
Stress test/LVSF assessment: Yes No If yes, report/s obtained?	Yes	No
Candidacy for DES:		
1. Major surgery in the past month or next year?	Yes	No
2. Is there any clinically overt or suspected bleeding?	Yes	No
3. Is patient on chronic anticoagulation (e.g., warfarin, TSOAC)?	Yes	No
4. Is there history of/anticipated medication non-adherence?	Yes	No
Allergies:		
1. Contrast: Yes No If yes, was the patient pretreated?	Yes	No
2. Aspirin: Yes No If yes, was the patient desensitized?	Yes	No
3. Heparin (HIT) Yes No If yes, consider alternative anti-thrombotic agents (DTI)		
4. Latex Yes No If yes, remove all latex products from procedural use		
Medications:		
1. Did patient take aspirin within the past 24 h?	Yes	No
2. Did patient take clopidogrel, prasugrel, or ticagrelor within the past 24 h?	Yes	No
3. Did patient take metformin within the past 24 h?	Yes	No
4. Did patient take sildenafil (or other PDE5 inhibitor) within the past 24 h?	Yes	No
5. Did patient receive LMWH within the past 12 h?	Yes	No
If yes for LMWH, time of last dose _____		
6. Did patient take anticoagulants	Yes	No
If yes, which agent _____ and when was last dose _____		
Informed Consent:		
Was informed consent obtained within 30 days?	Yes	No
Is there a healthcare proxy?	Yes	No
Is the patient DNR or DNI?	Yes	No
If Yes, was it revoked for procedure?	Yes	No
Sedation, Anesthesia and Analgesia:		
Are ASA and Mallampati Class documented?	Yes	No
Is there any contraindication to sedation present?	Yes	No
Risk scores applied?	Yes	No
Bleeding	Yes	No
CIN	Yes	No
Mortality	Yes	No
Laboratories and Studies:		
CBC and renal profile within 30 days (outpatient) or 24 h (inpatient)?	Yes	No
Hgb _____		
eGFR _____		
Was ECG performed within 24 h?	Yes	No
PT/INR performed within 24 h (for patients on warfarin)?	Yes	No
INR ≤1.8?	Yes	No
Urine/serum hcg in woman of childbearing age?	Yes	No
Does the patient require preprocedure hydration?	Yes	No
Preferred vascular access:	R L TR TF	
Same Day Discharge candidate?	Yes	No

Fig. 69.10 Society for Cardiovascular Angiography and Interventions preprocedure checklist for cardiac catheterization. (From 2016 SCAI Best Practices in the Cardiac Catheterization Laboratory. May 2016, Table 1.) *ASA*, American Society of Anesthesiologists; *CABG*, coronary artery bypass grafting; *CBC*, complete blood count; *CIN*, contrast-induced nephropathy; *DES*, drug-eluting stent; *DNI*, do not intubate; *DNR*, do not resuscitate; *DTI*, direct thrombin inhibitor; *ECG*, electrocardiogram; *eGFR*, estimated glomerular filtration rate; *FFR*, fractional flow reserve; *H&P*, history and physical; *hcg*, human chorionic gonadotropin; *Hgb*, hemoglobin; *HIT*, heparin-induced thrombocytopenia; *INR*, international normalized ratio; *IVUS*, intravascular ultrasound; *L*, left; *LMWH*, low molecular weight heparin; *LVSF*, left ventricular systolic function; *OCT*, optical coherence tomography; *PCI*, percutaneous coronary intervention; *PDE5*, phosphodiesterase type 5 inhibitor; *PT*, prothrombin time; *R*, right; *TF*, transfemoral; *TR*, transradial; *TSOAC*, target-specific oral anticoagulation.

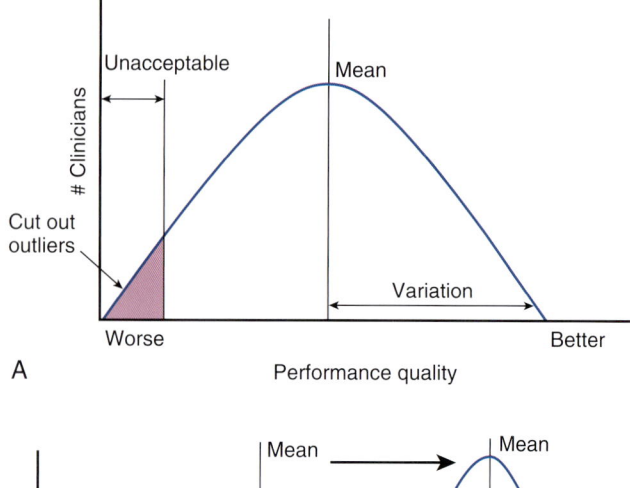

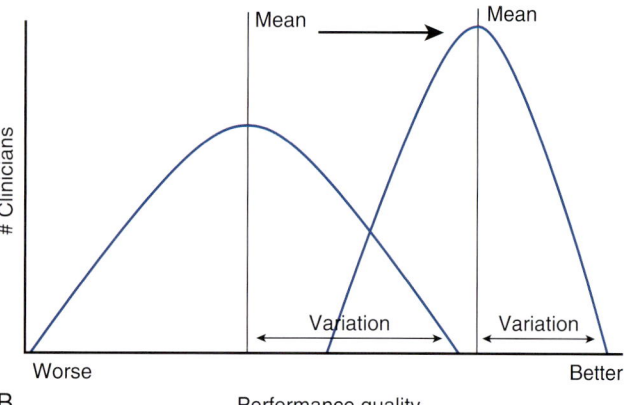

Fig. 69.11 (A) The goal of the quality assurance approach is to identify outliers that are unacceptable and should be excluded. (B) The goal of the continuous quality improvement approach is to identify opportunities for practice improvement and develop methods to respond to these opportunities, thus improving overall practice.

Benchmarking

Another essential building block of the quality framework is the process of benchmarking. A *benchmark* is a standard by which something can be measured or judged. Only by the collection of data can clinicians or hospitals compare, or benchmark, their care and outcomes with those of their peers and with national standards. Major strides in quality improvement require benchmarking coupled with changes in the systems of care as well as the engagement of local clinical leaders and administrative support.[76]

The NCDR was developed to assist facilities in the collection of data for use in benchmarking and quality improvement. Collection of laboratory data with benchmarking against state or national data is an important structural element in the assessment of clinical outcomes. Examples include the NCDR's CathPCI Registry, Acute Coronary Treatment and Intervention Outcomes Network–Get With the Guidelines (ACTION-GWTG) Registry of myocardial infarction, Society of Thoracic Surgeons Database, and Northern New England Cardiovascular Disease Study Group.[46,77,78] Participation in these programs provides caregivers with standardized tools for data collection, defined data elements and definitions, and validated risk-adjustment models for patient outcomes, such as mortality.

In addition to tracking outcomes, data reports help to assess adherence to guidelines and performance measure recommendations and can serve as a focus for quality improvements within an institution. The reports include regional benchmarking (i.e., comparison with similar hospitals) and national benchmarking against all participating facilities. Sample sections of a benchmark report from the CathPCI and ACTION-GWTG registries are shown in Figs. 69.14 and 69.15. Feedback with benchmarking is intended to

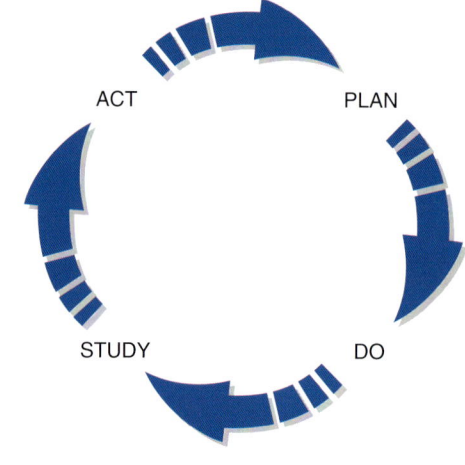

PLAN: Plan a change or test of how something works
DO: Carry out the plan
STUDY: Look at the results. What did you find out?
ACT: Decide what actions should be taken to improve

Fig. 69.12 The Plan-Do-Study-Act model for continuous quality improvement.

be used by hospitals and practices to target areas for improvement around which CQI efforts can be developed.[71] Benchmarking data are available to individual operators with their personal NCDR reports (i.e., dashboards) with relevant benchmarks.

Peer Review

One of the most challenging components of the quality framework is peer review. Catheterization laboratory directors are under increasing pressure to document the quality of care in their laboratories. Government agencies, aggregate purchasers of health care services, and accrediting organizations commonly request outcome data and other evidence of peer review activities.[79,80] Although representative of only a small number of operators, several highly publicized examples have pointed to the overuse of coronary stents, highlighting the need for local peer review.[81,82]

The primary goal of peer review is to improve patient care by analyzing physician performance and providing meaningful feedback to physicians.[83–85] The term *peer review* encompasses two clinical processes. Local peer review should occur in every laboratory as part of the quality framework. In that context, it is a patient-centered undertaking that should be positive, nonthreatening, and helpful to operators, but it should also identify and correct variations from accepted practice. Peer review programs should be individualized for each institution's catheterization laboratory and should remain flexible to accommodate change.[86]

Conflicts of interest are common among competing physicians, who may perceive a financial advantage to judging another physician's care adversely.[87] For peer review to be successful, there should be a formal method of oversight for perceived conflicts of interest within the peer review process. This can frequently be difficult, especially at smaller facilities. An independent facility accreditation process, such as that offered by Accreditation for Cardiovascular Excellence (ACE), may be helpful.[88] Court decisions have confirmed that physicians have a legal responsibility to perform peer review. Members of peer review committees and their activities are protected under state laws from discovery in lawsuits. Although antitrust laws cover peer review activities by a hospital medical staff, some actions that physicians or hospitals engage in may have an anticompetitive effect and violate federal antitrust laws. These laws prohibit efforts by one group of physicians to suppress competition from other physicians by preventing their entry into the relevant market (i.e., hospital) or excluding or restricting their professional activities.[89]

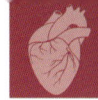

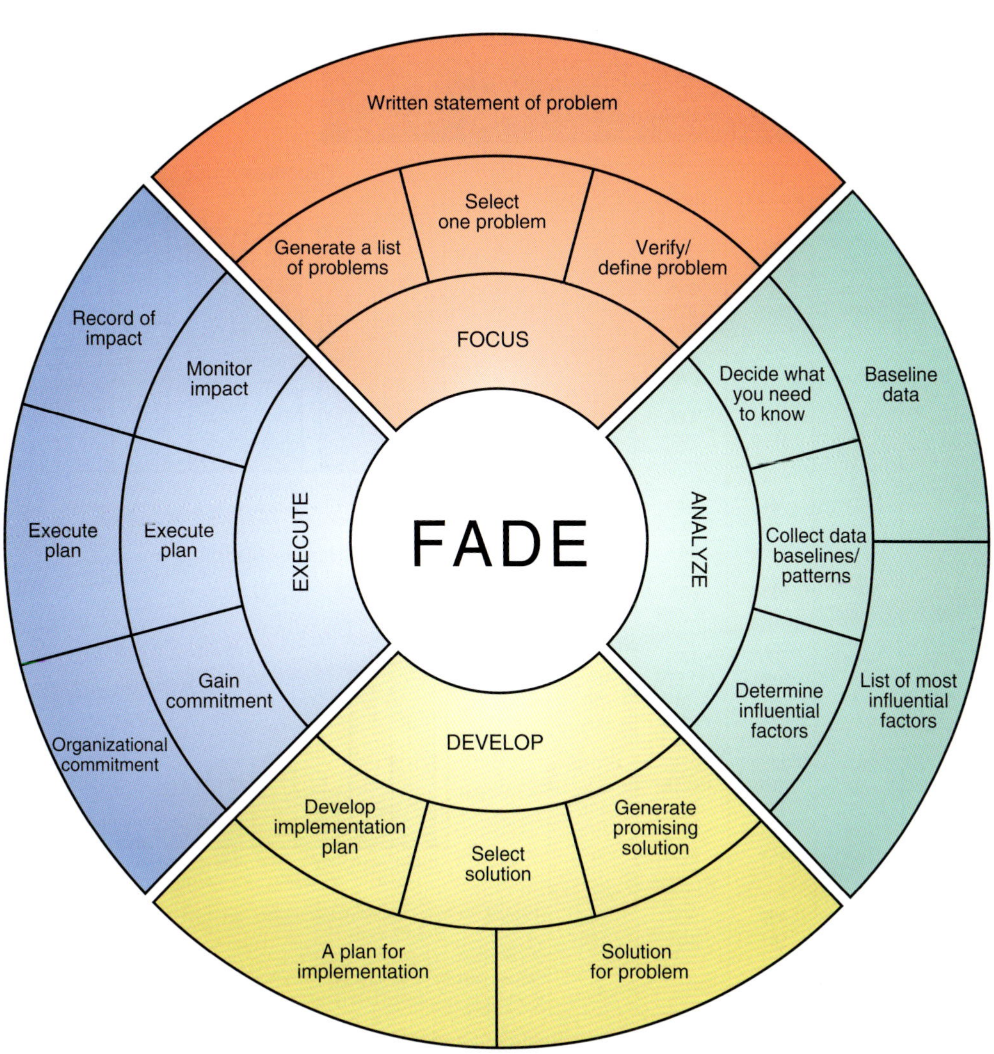

CHAPTER 69 Quality of Care in Interventional Cardiology

FOCUS: Define and verify the process to be improved

ANALYZE: Collect and analyze data to establish baselines, identify root causes and point toward possible solutions

DEVELOP: Based on the data, develop action plans for improvement, including implementation, communication, and measuring/monitoring.

EXECUTE: Implement the action plans, on a pilot basis as indicated.

EVALUATE: Install an ongoing measuring/monitoring system to ensure success.

Fig. 69.13 The Focus-Analyze-Develop-Execute *(FADE)* model is used to reduce variation and improve overall performance. (Courtesy Organizational Dynamics Institute, Wakefield, MA.)

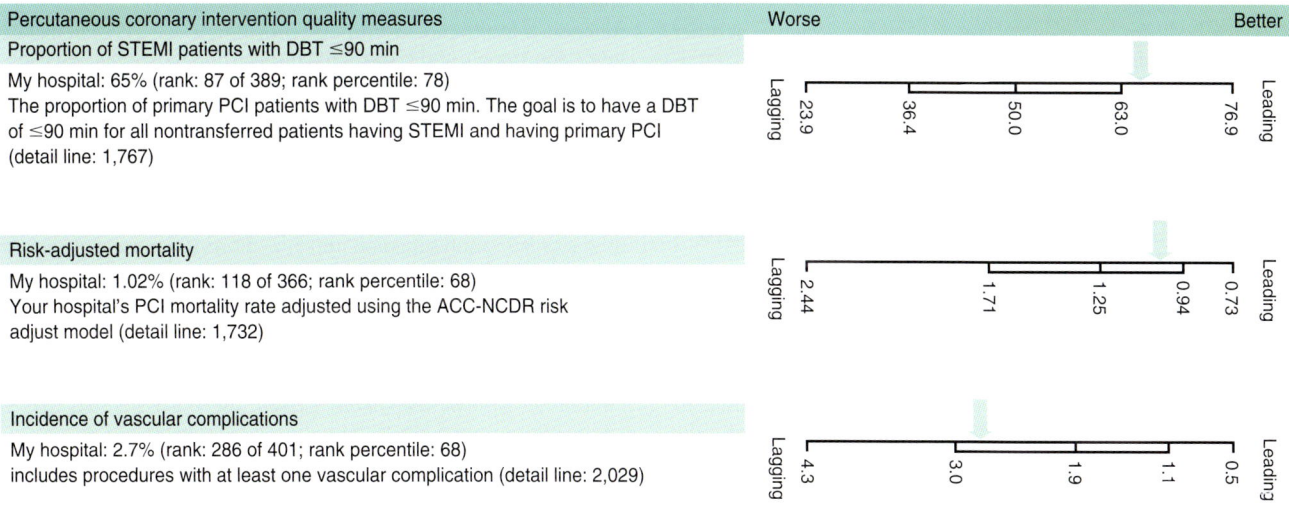

Fig. 69.14 Sample from the executive summary of a report from the CathPCI Registry, a source of cardiovascular data from the National Cardiovascular Data Registry *(NCDR)*.

1313

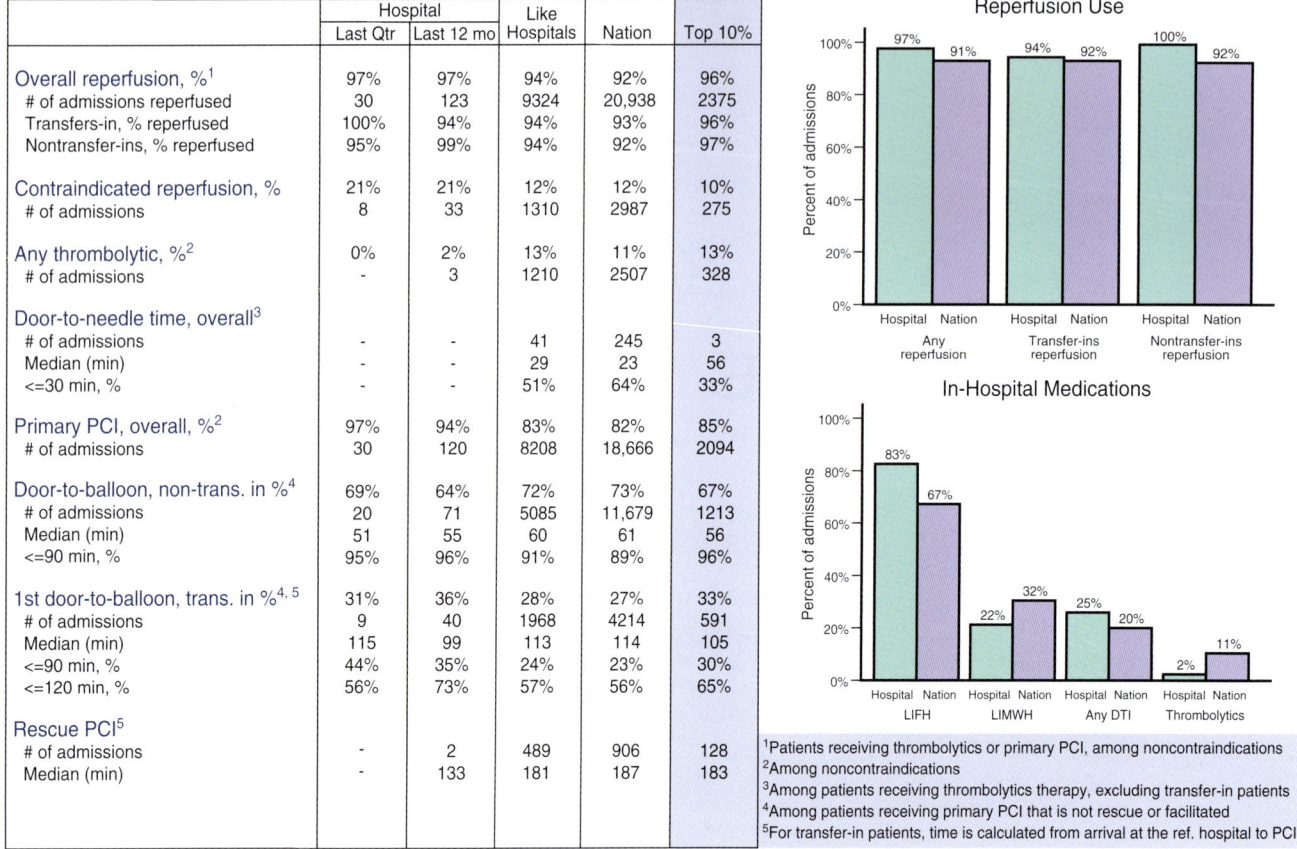

Fig. 69.15 Sample page of a report from the Acute Coronary Treatment and Intervention Outcomes Network–Get with the Guidelines *(ACTION-GWTG)* Registry. *DTI,* Direct thrombin inhibitor; *LMWH,* low molecular weight heparin; *PCI,* percutaneous coronary intervention; *Qtr,* quarter; *trans,* transfer; *UFH,* unfractionated heparin.

The second form of peer review (i.e., professional review activity) is specifically defined in federal law. It consists of an evaluation by the review bodies at hospitals, professional medical societies, or other entities to determine the professional competence of individual physicians through a formal review process that may result in restriction or termination of professional privileges and that requires due process.[90] Several publications from the SCAI define the best practices for this type of activity in the cardiac catheterization laboratory.[26,91–93]

DEVELOPING A QUALITY CULTURE IN THE CARDIAC CATHETERIZATION LABORATORY

Organizational Culture

Amid the escalating demands for high-quality health care, it is important to encourage a culture of quality in the cardiac catheterization laboratory. *Organizational culture* is the term used to describe the shared beliefs, perceptions, and expectations of individuals in organizations. Organizational culture can dramatically affect efforts to implement changes in procedures or processes.

Characteristics of organizational culture have been linked to financial performance, customer and employee satisfaction, and innovation. Supportive organizational cultures underlie successful initiatives of quality improvement, contribute to high levels of nursing care, job satisfaction, and patient safety[94,95] and help institutions adapt to rapidly changing health care demands while remaining competitive. Organizational culture is central to the operation and function of health care institutions, providing a shared vision that can guide appropriate and goal-directed social and individual behaviors.

Some aspects of organizational culture can have an opposite effect that undermines efforts for positive change. Many quality initiatives fail because of resistance to change, ingrained attitudes, lack of understanding, and poor communication. For success, the high-level leaders of an organization must focus on the mission and vision of the organization. Mission is a fundamental unit of culture, and failure to fulfill the organization's mission impedes efforts to improve quality. By focusing on the mission and embracing the role of advancing a quality culture, leaders can facilitate the dissemination of quality-oriented values throughout an organization. Four levels of intervention influence organizational culture: the individual, team or microsystem, organizational, and environmental levels.[96] In its landmark publication *Crossing the Quality Chasm*, the IOM asserted that all interventions must address these four dimensions.[21]

Physician Champions

Key to the development of a quality culture in the cardiac catheterization laboratory is the physician champion, who is an opinion leader, an agent of change, and a person who influences colleagues and friends. He or she is a respected individual who provides expert education, promotes a cause or a product, or gives support to staff for the diffusion and implementation of clinical practice guidelines, protocols, and research evidence. Physician champions are essential to a culture of quality and change. For example, a physician champion at a local institution can promote the increased use of radial access by educating colleagues, by helping others to become proficient in the procedure, or simply in leading by example.

In all cases the physician champion is perceived as a credible individual who has the ability to persuade others. He or she often influences other physicians to implement a new or revised process or guideline for quality improvement or to become physician champions themselves. The champion's role can be an invaluable tool for change within a health care organization. However, if the physician is unable or unwilling to engage in the tasks required to be effective, the role is not clearly defined, the sphere of influence is narrow, or institutional support is lacking, he or she will not be able to fulfill the expectations of the organization and change may not be implemented or sustainable.

Tools to Assist in Quality Improvement

The SCAI developed a quality improvement toolkit (QIT).[97] The SCAI QIT identifies routine meetings that help operationalize the activity of continuous quality improvement. Topics of these institutional conferences include morbidity and mortality, peer review of random cases, and selected interesting cases. Several hospitals have developed group meetings that address specific care processes, as for STEMI. At a minimum, cardiac catheterization laboratories should have peer review and morbidity and mortality conferences monthly to quarterly to ensure timely case reviews.

Operational improvements continue to translate quality initiatives into action in the cardiac catheterization laboratory. Preprocedural checklists, structured catheterization reports, and standardized data elements provide important adjuncts in the daily practice of invasive cardiology.[98] Real-time decision support tools such as electronic health records are easily integrated into the workflow. A structured time out before each procedure ensures proper patient identification, procedure confirmation, allergy assessment (including contrast and radiation thresholds), and other data collection.

PUBLIC REPORTING AND THE CARDIAC CATHETERIZATION LABORATORY

Effects of Reporting on Quality

Although the U.S. health care system is superior in many ways, it also has shortcomings, such as gaps in care, quality issues, and costs. Private sector employers and the federal government have seen an increasing portion of their revenue consumed by providing health care for employees and Medicare beneficiaries. This financial burden has pressured payers, who have pressured providers to accelerate efforts to improve quality.

Public reporting of physician, health plan, and institutional performance is used to steer patients to the best-performing providers and facilities on the assumption that they provide better and more cost-effective care. Patients are becoming more engaged in this process and seek public performance reports on providers and facilities. Public release of performance data improves the quality of care through greater transparency and accountability by health care providers.[99] According to the 2016 SCAI statement on public reporting, there are several key components of effective public reporting: (1) reported information must be important to the consumer; (2) credible information must be presented in a manner that is understandable by the public, (3) the information should stimulate consumers to act or change their behavior, and (4) the information should not generate false perceptions of an individual's or institution's quality of care.[100]

Public reporting of the results of cardiovascular interventions, especially by cardiac surgeons, is not new. Beginning in the mid-1990s, New York and Pennsylvania publicly reported cardiac surgery outcomes, and the Massachusetts Data Analysis Center (Mass-DAC) started a reporting program in 2002, as did California in 2003.[2,3,101,102] After its early years of operation, the New York program reported a reduction in the risk-adjusted mortality rate from 4.17% to 2.45%, with smaller yearly improvements thereafter.[103] The Pennsylvania CABG public reporting program documented a similar trend.[104] Recent data published by Waldo and colleagues have also demonstrated that those institutions identified as negative outliers by public reporting experienced significant reductions in in-hospital mortality (relative risk [RR], 0.83; 95% confidence interval [CI] 0.81 to 0.85), and to a lesser degree at nonoutlier institutions (RR, 0.90; 95% CI 0.87 to 0.92; interaction $P < .001$).[105] See Table 69.9 for a summary of current public reporting practices of four well-established state reporting programs.[100]

In evaluating public reporting programs, it is important to understand the data source and the distinction between administrative (claims) data and clinical data sources. For example, the Mass-DAC cardiac surgery reporting program uses clinical data from the Society of Thoracic Surgery database. In an important comparative study; cardiac surgery performance results based on clinical data were compared with performance results derived from administrative data during the same period. Considerable disparities were found in the results between the two data sets, which led to the conclusion that report cards using administrative data are problematic compared with those derived from audited and validated clinical data.[106] The same comparison was made within the New York cardiac surgery reporting program with similar conclusions.[107] The use of pure administrative data was inferior to that of clinical data in identifying outliers and assessing surgical outcomes.

At the national level, the CMS in collaboration with the Hospital Quality Alliance issues a web-based public report.[108] The following data are reported:

- Several process-of-care measures for patients with AMI, CHF, and other selected medical conditions and some surgical procedures
- Outcomes of care measures, including 30-day risk-adjusted mortality and readmission rates for MI, heart failure, and pneumonia
- Patients' hospital experiences, using information collected from the Hospital Consumer Assessment of Healthcare Providers and Systems (HCAHPS) survey
- The number (volume) of Medicare patients treated for certain illnesses or diagnoses
- Medicare inpatient hospital payment information

Large-scale public reporting efforts in cardiology and interventional cardiology have primarily focused on events such as AMI and CHF or on procedures such as CABG or PCI. Although some state programs report physician-level metrics, the confidence intervals around any point estimate are necessarily wide because of the small sample size for a single physician. Most public reporting has been at the facility level because greater statistical validity and larger denominators exist. Independent review of DTB time as a publicly reported measure of quality by the CMS showed that more than one-fourth of patients were excluded from hospital quality reports. The exclusion of this many patients demonstrates the potential disconnect among overall process improvement, public reporting, and reimbursement for quality measures.[109]

Meaningful programs rely on clinical data sources to avoid the pitfalls of administrative data and allow a robust risk adjustment of outcomes. In 2014, the NCDR launched a voluntary program for participants to publicly report clinically based hospital-level performance measures. Although the initial data release is limited to a few metrics from the CathPCI Registry, this will be expanded greatly over the next few years (Table 69.10). A pilot program in collaboration with CMS resulted in more than 350 hospitals' agreeing to post their 30-day readmission rates for PCI on the CMS website. More public reporting is expected in the future.

Potential Unintended Consequences of Public Reporting

Concern has been expressed that public reporting programs may lead to unintended consequences that could offset their benefits.[110,111] Although the early reduction in risk-adjusted mortality from CABG in the New York experience was touted as a success, another perspective subsequently emerged. Omoigui and colleagues reviewed 9442 isolated CABG operations performed from 1989 through 1993 at the Cleveland Clinic to assess referral patterns, case mix, and outcomes.[112] Patients referred to Cleveland from New York had a higher frequency of prior open heart surgery and were more likely to have New York Heart Association (NYHA) functional class III or IV heart disease compared with patients from Ohio, other states, and other countries. Their expected mortality rate was higher than that for other referral cohorts. The observed 5.2% mortality rate among patients referred from New York was significantly higher than that for any of the other referral sources, leading the study authors to speculate that the public reporting of outcome data in New York likely provoked the increased referral of high-risk patients out of state, explaining the reduction of CABG-related mortality rates in New York.

The public reporting of PCI data has a shorter history than that of cardiac surgery, but similar observations are being made. McCabe and colleagues recently reported the effects of New York public reporting policies on rates of PCI in patients with cardiogenic shock.[113] From concern that public reporting policies were leading to physician avoidance of performing PCI in higher-risk patients, the New York State Public Health Department decided to exclude patients with refractory cardiogenic shock from public reporting.[114,115] After the policy change, there was an increase in rates of PCI by 28%, compared with 9% for similar states over the same period (Fig. 69.16). Additionally, after the 2006 policy change, rates of adjusted in-hospital death decreased more significantly in New York (adjusted RR, 0.76; 95% CI 0.72 to 0.81; $P < .001$) compared with similar states (adjusted RR, 0.91; 95% CI 0.87 to 0.94; $P < .001$; interaction $P < .001$. The authors

TABLE 69.9 Summary of State Reporting

	New York (NY STATE)	Massachusetts (MASS-DEC)	Texas (THCIC)	Washington (COAP)
Basis for public reporting	Regulatory	Legislative	Legislative	Hospital Consortium Agreement
Year initiated	1991	2003	2009	2013
Public release level	Hospital and individual physician	Hospital	Hospital	Hospital
Outcome of interest	In-hospital/30-day mortality rate (1 year and 3 years cumulative), 30-day read missions	In-hospital mortality (30-day mortality to start w/2014 report)	In-hospital mortality and mean charges per case	In-hospital adjusted mortality, door-to-balloon time, proportion of appropriate use PCI
Risk adjustment method	RAMR	Hierarchical SMIR	RAMR	RAMR
Data source	Case-level clinical data	Case-level clinical data	Hospital inpatient administrative data	Case-level clinical data
Case stratification	Results reported for all cases and separately for Nonemergency cases	Stratified reports: STEMI/shock and No STEMI or shock	No stratification	Reported for MI and nonurgent separately
Latest report released	October 2015	October 2015	2015	June 2014
Data included in latest report	2010–12	2013	2012	2013
Number of PCI hospitals (latest report)	60	24	198	34
Number of PCI operators	390	~160	Not reported	Not reported
Number of PCIs	47,396 (2012) 152,579 (2010–12)	12,132	32,660	~12,000
Observed overall mortality	1%	1.57%	1.70%	1.90%
Data quality audit method	Audits of all cases of shock and stent thrombosis	Physician volunteers review all mortalities and high-ride covariates	No case-level audits	No case-level audits
Exclusions (year)	Refractory Cardiogenic Shock (2006)	Exceptional risk: simultaneous life-threatening condition (2009)	No public release of results for centers with <30 PCI cases	None
	Cardiac Arrest with Brain Injury (2010)		Rural hospitals not required to report	
Risk-adjustment refinement (year)	None	Compassionate use risk adjustment (2006): includes coma on presentation, STEMI with last remaining vessel	None	None

COAP, Clinical outcomes assessment program; *MASS-DEC*, Massachusetts data analysis center; *MI*, myocardial infarction; *RAMR*, Risk-adjusted mortality rates; *SMIR*, standardized mortality incidence rates; *STEMI*, ST-segment elevation myocardial infarction; *THCIC*, Texas healthcare information collection.

concluded that high-risk patients with cardiogenic shock were often not undergoing PCI in New York as a result of public reporting, and that the exclusion of these patients from the public reporting system resulted in higher rates of PCI treatment and better outcomes.

Concerns have also been raised about the public reporting of PCI data in Massachusetts.[116] This was indirectly confirmed by studying the risk profile of patients undergoing PCI at hospitals after they were identified as outliers in a public reporting program.[117] The risk profile of PCI patients at outlier institutions was significantly lower after public identification compared with nonoutlier institutions, suggesting that risk-aversive behaviors among PCI operators at outlier institutions was an unintended consequence of public reporting.

To minimize unintended consequences, other states, in addition to New York, specifically exclude extreme-risk and salvage patients. In the Massachusetts PCI registry (Mass-DAC), a compassionate use data element was added to capture these types of cases. In addition to concerns that the risk-adjustment methods currently available are suboptimal and do not include all relevant variables, there has been a suggestion that mortality rates must be adjudicated to determine whether they were procedure related or not. After further blinded review, about 80% of the deaths at one Massachusetts hospital were determined not to be directly related to the procedure but instead related to the natural history of disease in the patients.[116]

Payers have been focused on the cost profiling of physicians, and the accuracy of their methods has been questioned.[117] Fung and colleagues conducted a systematic review of the evidence that public reporting leads to an improvement in the quality of care.[118] They concluded that there was minimal evidence about the public reporting of individual provider data and practices and that a rigorous evaluation of many major public reporting systems was lacking. They found some evidence suggesting that public release of performance data stimulated quality improvement activity at the hospital level, but the overall effect of public reporting on effectiveness, safety, and patient-centered care remains uncertain.

The most compelling justification for public reporting of clinical outcomes is the public's right to know about the care they are likely to receive from hospitals and physicians. Transparency of information should allow patients to make better-informed decisions about their health care, but the reporting process must be accurate and fair. There is also growing interest in changing reimbursement models to be based on the quality rather than the quantity of care and on the development of quality measures approved by the NQF.

Improving Public Reporting

To examine how public reporting may be improved to more accurately assess quality of care, it is necessary to understand the current limitations in public reporting systems based on risk-adjusted mortality rates (RAMRs).[100] RAMR focuses entirely on mortality risk when PCI is performed, and is thus procedure-oriented

TABLE 69.10 National Cardiovascular Data Registry Measures for Public Reporting

Performance Measure	Source Registry	External Data	NQF Endorsed
Aspirin at discharge	CathPCI	No	Yes
Thienopyridine at discharge	CathPCI	No	Yes
Statins at discharge	CathPCI	No	Yes
PCI in-hospital risk-adjusted mortality (patients with STEMI and patients without STEMI)	CathPCI	No	Yes
30-Day all-cause risk-adjusted mortality (patients without STEMI or cardiogenic shock and patients with STEMI or cardiogenic shock)	CathPCI	Yes (CDC)	Yes
30-Day risk-adjusted readmission for PCI	CathPCI	Yes (CMS)	Yes

CathPCI, Subregistry of the National Cardiovascular Data Registry; *CDC*, Centers for Disease Control and Prevention; *CMS*, Centers for Medicare and Medicaid Services; *NQF*, National Quality Forum; *PCI*, percutaneous coronary intervention; *STEMI*, ST-segment elevation myocardial infarction.

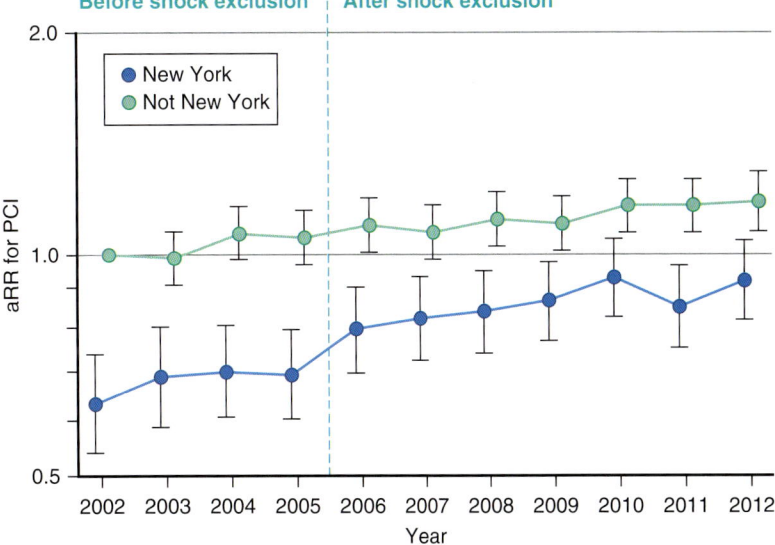

Fig. 69.16 Adjusted relative risk *(aRR)* of patients with cardiogenic shock and acute myocardial infarction receiving percutaneous coronary intervention *(PCI)* per year compared with non–New York states in 2002. (From McCabe JM, Waldo SW, Kennedy KF, et al. Treatment and Outcomes of Acute Myocardial Infarction Complicated by Shock After Public Reporting Policy Changes in New York. *JAMA Cardiol*. 2016;1:648–654.)

TABLE 69.11 2016 Society for Cardiovascular Angiography and Interventions Recommendations to Improve Public Reporting

In the future, PCI public reporting programs should:

- Transition from procedure based to disease-based reporting.
  - Include the risk-adjusted survival statistics for those patients undergoing PCI and those not undergoing PCI for a given presenting diagnosis.
- Deemphasize the importance of RAMR as a summary metric.
- Avoid rank ordering of programs based on RAMR point estimates.
- Patients suffering out-of-hospital cardiac arrest and those with preexisting DNR orders should be excluded from all public reports of PCI outcomes.
  - Adjudication of high-risk classification should be made at the local facility level.
- Hospital-specific risk adjusted mortality should be reported in two ways: including and excluding specific high-risk patient cohorts.
- Refrain from reporting physician-specific RAMR following PCI.
- Incorporate quality of care measures beyond RAMR (as shown in Table 69.6)

DNR, Do not resuscitate; *PCI*, percutaneous coronary intervention; *RAMR*, risk-adjusted mortality rates.

and not disease-oriented. This incentivizes risk-averse behaviors. Additionally, the reporting of RAMR, as previously mentioned, relies entirely on 30-day postdischarge mortality data from administrative sources and the National Death Index. As the median RAMR for PCI nationwide is 1.3%, it is a weak discriminator between programs because it is so low for most programs. Moreover, no analysis has ever shown that programs with lower RAMR demonstrate overall higher quality of care when compared with programs with higher RAMR. Finally, the consumer's ability to understand and appropriately assess quality of care based on statistical outcomes, such as RAMR, is likely to be limited and critically uninterpretable.

The 2016 SCAI recommendations provide guidance on how to improve the public reporting for PCI (Table 69.11).[100] To deincentivize avoidance of higher-risk cases, SCAI recommends including the risk-adjusted survival statistics both for patients undergoing PCI and those not undergoing PCI. In addition to excluding cardiogenic shock from public reporting, patients with out-of-hospital cardiac arrest and active do-not-resuscitate orders should not be included in public reporting outcomes. Additionally, instead of a focus on post-PCI RAMR, other measures should be included to assess quality of care, including the incidence of post-PCI contrast nephropathy, bleeding/vascular complications, and 1-year rates of revascularization. Measures such as patient satisfaction and operator caseload/institutional volume should also be accounted for. In the coming years, it is likely that public reporting of cardiovascular interventions will turn from a full focus on RAMR to the more comprehensive reporting of various quality measures.

CONCLUSIONS

Patients, payers, and physicians have interests in measuring and understanding the quality of interventional procedures. The goal is to measure and deliver the highest quality of care to patients undergoing invasive procedures. Current efforts to achieve this goal have fallen short, and important gaps exist in the ability to provide the highest quality of care for all patients. Implementing improvements in the quality of care is the next challenge in interventional cardiology. This goal is achievable if physicians and other members of the interventional care delivery team strive in their daily practice to ensure that the right patient gets the right procedure performed correctly, leading to the right outcome.

KEY REFERENCES

19. Rubin HR, Rogers WH, Kahn KL, et al. Watching the doctor-watchers: how well do peer review organization methods detect hospital care quality problems? *JAMA*. 1992;267(17):2349–2354.
21. Committee on Quality of Health Care in America. *Institute of Medicine. Crossing the Quality Chasm: A New Health System for the 21st Century*. Washington, DC: National Academy Press; 2001.
27. Brindis RG, Fitzgerald S, Anderson HV, et al. The American College of Cardiology-National Cardiovascular Data Registry (ACC-NCDR): building a national clinical data repository. *J Am Coll Cardiol*. 2001;37(8):2240–2245.
35. Resnic FS, Welt FG. The public health hazards of risk avoidance associated with public reporting of risk-adjusted outcomes in coronary intervention. *J Am Coll Cardiol*. 2009;53(10):825–830.
36. Peterson ED, Dai D, DeLong ER, et al. Contemporary mortality risk prediction for percutaneous coronary intervention: results from 588,398 procedures in the National Cardiovascular Data Registry. *J Am Coll Cardiol*. 2010;55(18):1923–1932.
38. Patel MR, Dehmer GJ, Hirshfeld JW, et al. ACCF/SCAI/ STS/AATS/AHA/ASNC 2009 appropriateness criteria for coronary revascularization: a report of the American College of Cardiology Foundation appropriateness criteria task force, Society for Cardiovascular Angiography and Interventions, Society of Thoracic Surgeons, American Association for Thoracic Surgery, American Heart Association, and the American Society of Nuclear Cardiology. *J Am Coll Cardiol*. 2009;53(6):530–553.
48. Gupta A, Allen LA, Bhatt DL, et al. Association of the hospital readmissions reduction program implementation with readmission and mortality outcomes in heart failure. *JAMA Cardiol*. 2018;3:44–53.
52. Patel MR, Calhoon JH, Dehmer GJ, et al. ACC/AATS/AHA/ASE/ASNC/SCAI/SCCT/STS 2016 appropriate use criteria for coronary revascularization in patients with acute coronary syndromes: a report of the American College of Cardiology appropriate use criteria task force, American Association for Thoracic Surgery, American Heart Association, American Society of Echocardiography, American Society of Nuclear Cardiology, Society for Cardiovascular Angiography and Interventions, Society of Cardiovascular Computed Tomography, and the Society of Thoracic Surgeons. *J Am Coll Cardiol*. 2017;69:570–591.
53. Patel MR, Calhoon JH, Dehmer GJ, et al. ACC/AATS/AHA/ASE/ASNC/SCAI/SCCT/STS 2017 appropriate use criteria for coronary revascularization in patients with stable ischemic heart disease: a report of the American College of Cardiology appropriate use criteria task force, American Association for Thoracic Surgery, American Heart Association, American Society of Echocardiography, American Society of Nuclear Cardiology, Society for Cardiovascular Angiography and Interventions, Society of Cardiovascular Computed Tomography, and the Society of Thoracic Surgeons. *J Am Coll Cardiol*. 2017;69:2212–2241.
62. Hannan EL, Racz MJ, Gold J, et al. Adherence of catheterization laboratory cardiologists to American College of Cardiology/American Heart Association guidelines for percutaneous coronary interventions and coronary artery bypass graft surgery. What happens in actual practice? *Circulation*. 2010;121(2):267–275.
65. Bradley EH, Herrin J, Elbel B, et al. Hospital quality for acute myocardial infarction: correlation among process measures and relationship with short-term mortality. *JAMA*. 2006;296(1):72–78.
66. Chan PS, Patel MR, Klein LW, et al. Appropriateness of percutaneous coronary intervention. *JAMA*. 2011;306:53–61.
67. Desai NR, Bradley SM, Parzynski CS, et al. Appropriate use criteria for coronary revascularization and trends in utilization, patient selection, and appropriateness of percutaneous coronary intervention. *JAMA*. 2015;314:2045–2053.
77. Brindis RG, Fitzgerald S, Anderson HV, et al. The American College of Cardiology-National Cardiovascular Data Registry (ACC-NCDR): building a national clinical data repository. *J Am Coll Cardiol*. 2001;37(8):2240–2245.
92. Klein LW, Uretsky BF, Chambers C, et al. Quality assessment and improvement in interventional cardiology: a position statement of the Society of Cardiovascular Angiography and Interventions, part 1: standards for quality assessment and improvement in interventional cardiology. *Catheter Cardiovasc Interv*. 2011;77(7):927–935.

93. Klein LW, Ho KK, Singh M, et al. Quality assessment and improvement in interventional cardiology: a Position Statement of the Society of Cardiovascular Angiography and Interventions, part II: public reporting and risk adjustment. *Catheter Cardiovasc Interv*. 2011;78(4):493–502.
100. Klein LW, Harjai KJ, Resnic F, et al. 2016 revision of the SCAI position statement on public reporting. *Catheter Cardiovasc Interv*. 2017;89:269–279.
105. Waldo SW, McCabe JM, Kennedy KF, et al. Quality of care at hospitals identified as outliers in publicly reported mortality statistics for percutaneous coronary intervention. *Circulation*. 2017;135:1897–1907.

 Additional references available online at expertconsult.com.

中文导读

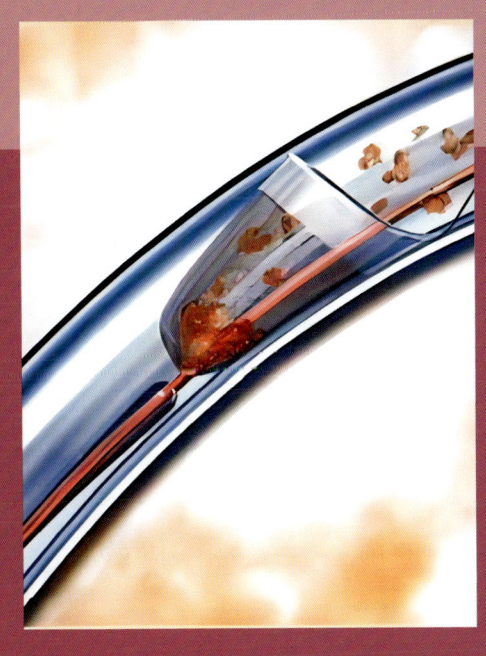

第70章
手术量和预后

研究表明手术的死亡率和手术量成反比，特别是对于高风险手术。高手术量的医院处理主要并发症及高风险手术的经验更为丰富，死亡率低。建议经皮冠状动脉介入治疗术者应该每年完成75例手术，每周至少完成2例，其中至少有1例经皮冠状动脉介入治疗，并且平均每月1例急诊经皮冠状动脉介入治疗（每年12例）；医院应该每周完成4例择期手术、每年200例，每月至少3例急诊经皮冠状动脉介入治疗（每年36例）。所有医院应进行手术分级管理，监督手术质量，低手术量的医师建议避免进行高风险手术。

王宇彬　吴永健

章节要点

- 在过去的30年,高风险手术的经验与结果呈负相关。
- 在冠状动脉介入时代,对医院病例量的要求为每周至少4例,对术者的要求为每周不低于1例。
- 手术量最低要求的标准对医师的影响很小(仅4%的患者到手术量小的医院就诊,仅7%的患者找手术量小的医师就诊),而相反手术量少的医院和医师占据很大的比例(27%的医院年手术量不超过200例,44%的医师年手术量不超过75例)。
- 充分考虑证据,研究应该充分包含手术量少的医院、事件率及统计学技术才具有代表性。
- 证据支持和患者的意愿迫使医学界为有经验的中心提供更多的人员、设备及资源。

70 Volume and Outcome

James G. Jollis, Margot M. Sherman Jollis

KEY POINTS

- An inverse relationship between experience and outcome for higher-risk procedures has been repeatedly demonstrated over the past 30 years.
- In the case of percutaneous coronary angioplasty, the minimum volume thresholds involve low numbers of fewer than four cases per week for hospitals and one case per week for physicians.
- The volume standards affect relatively few patients (4% of all patients undergo percutaneous coronary intervention [PCI] at low-volume hospitals and 7% are treated by low-volume physicians), but relatively larger numbers of operators (27% of hospitals and 44% of physicians perform fewer than 200 and 75 cases per year respectively).
- In considering the evidence, studies must be viewed according to representation by low-volume providers, event rates, and regression techniques.
- Supporting evidence and concern for patients compels the medical community to foster experienced interventional operators and facilities to the extent possible.

INTRODUCTION

A series of studies over 40 years have repeatedly identified a relationship between increased procedural volume and lower mortality, particularly for higher-risk procedures or patients.[1-18] The finding of better outcomes with increased experience seems rather obvious and, in isolation, should not engender much controversy. When the volume-outcome relationship is applied to health policy in a manner that suggests patients should avoid low-volume hospitals or physicians, passionate debate ensues. Fueled by intense policy interests, manuscripts that alternately support or refute volume standards continue to be published in the medical and health services research literature. This chapter will examine the volume-outcome relationship for coronary interventions in depth according to the strength of the evidence and the underlying reasons why study conclusions may vary despite consistency of the relationship. Based upon this review, a practical framework for public policy will be proposed.

To provide some perspective of the issue, one must first understand that the proposed volume thresholds represent very low numbers and impact relatively few patients. The relationship between worse outcome and low volume is most apparent among very low-volume operators. In the case of interventional cardiologist volume, an overall percutaneous coronary intervention (PCI) volume of 75 cases per year requires performance of fewer than two procedures per week, and a primary PCI volume of 12 involves treatment of one ST-segment elevation myocardial infarction per month. A hospital must perform four cases per week to reach a threshold of 200 elective PCI cases and three cases per month to reach a primary PCI threshold of 36 cases. With such low thresholds, low-volume providers treat relatively few patients. In the past, a reasonable gauge of the relative proportion of patients treated in low-volume institutions could be obtained from the National Inpatient Sample (NIS), a nationally representative cohort of patients of all ages treated at 20% of United States hospitals.[1] In response to concerns from members of the American College of Cardiology (ACC), researchers examined data from the National Cardiovascular Data Registry (NCDR) CathPCI registry, a more comprehensive dataset involving more than 90% of PCI procedures nationwide.[17] Data from the CathPCI Registry and the NIS indicate that only 4% of patients undergoing PCI are treated in hospitals with volumes less than 200 cases per year, yet the low-volume institutions treating these relatively few patients represent 27% of hospitals (Fig. 70.1).[19] National data from the CathPCI Registry indicate that, although 44% of physicians are considered low-volume operators, these operators perform only 10% of total PCIs.[17]

EVIDENCE FOR A VOLUME-OUTCOME RELATIONSHIP

The origins of the volume-outcome relationship date back to 1979 when Luft, Bunker, and Enthoven of Stanford University identified higher mortality at lower-volume hospitals for a number of surgical procedures, including open heart and vascular surgery.[2] Among 12 surgeries, the relationship was most evident among the higher-risk procedures, and their initial data identified a threshold of approximately 200 surgical procedures, greater than which procedural mortality decreased by 25% to 41%. In their initial work, the authors suggested that the observed relationships supported the regionalization of higher-risk procedures. Since the initial work, the volume-outcome relationship has repeatedly been demonstrated for a number of procedures and conditions.[12] Examining more than 3 million Medicare patients hospitalized at 4679 hospitals between 2004 and 2006 for acute myocardial infarction, congestive heart failure, or pneumonia, Ross and colleagues found those treated at lower-volume hospitals had significantly higher 30-day mortality. For acute myocardial infarction, the upper volume threshold was 610 cases, beyond which significant differences in mortality were no longer observed.

Volume standards for PCI were first introduced in the 1988 ACC/American Heart Association Guidelines.[20] Lacking empirical evidence regarding coronary angioplasty volume, the task force selected the threshold volume of 50 cases based upon the logic that one must golf about once per week to remain proficient and such an experiential relationship likely extended to coronary interventions. The publication of this standard unleashed a flood of concerns from approximately half of cardiologists performing angioplasty at the time who did not meet the one-case-per-week standard. Providers opposed to volume standards were concerned about restrictions to practice in the absence of empirical evidence of a volume-outcome relationship for PCI. They were also concerned that such standards would impede quality, low-volume physicians, and that annual volume standards did not take into account aggregate experience over a number of years.

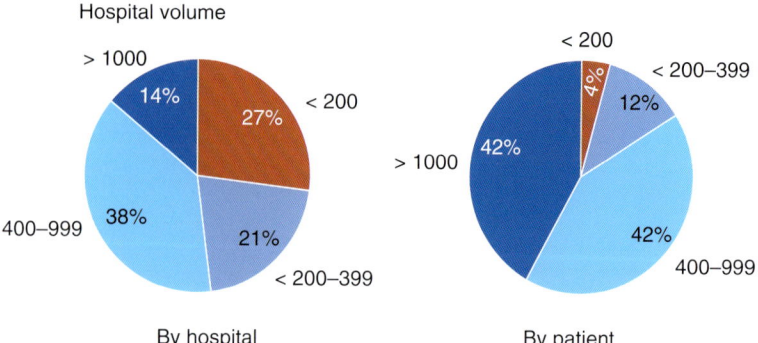

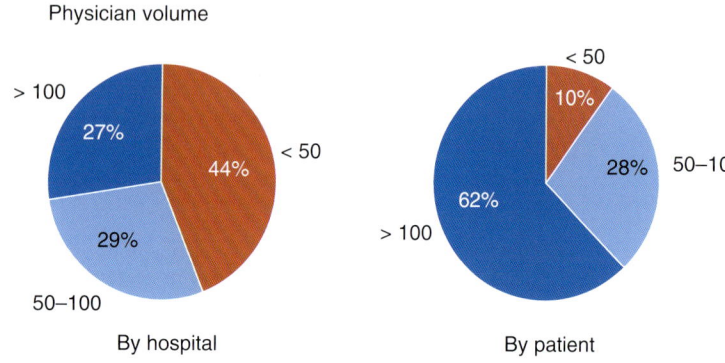

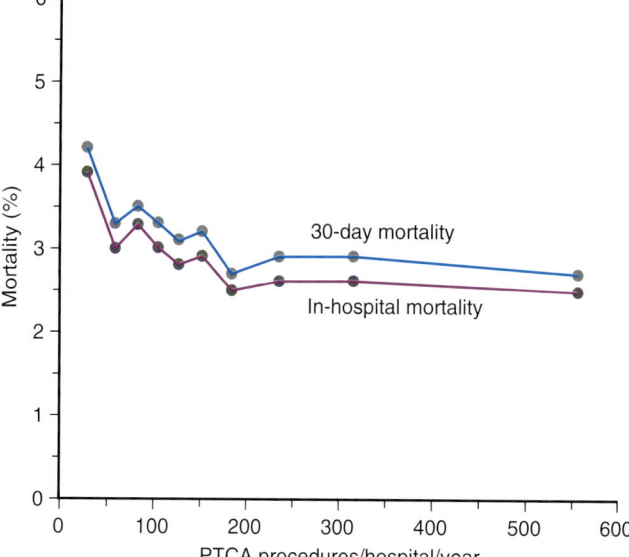

Fig. 70.1 Distribution of hospital and physician percutaneous coronary intervention (PCI) volume by hospitals, physicians, and patients. (Data from references Epstein AJ, Rathore SS, Volpp KG, et al. Hospital percutaneous coronary intervention volume and patient mortality, 1998 to 2000. *J Am Coll Cardiol*. 2004;43:1755–1762; Hannan EL, Wu C, Walford G, et al. Volume-outcome relationships for percutaneous coronary interventions in the stent era. *Circulation*. 2005;112:1171–1179; Fanaroff AC, Zakroysky P, Dai D, et al. Outcomes for PCI in relation to procedural characteristics and operator volumes in the United States. *J Am Coll Cardiol*. 2017;69(24):2913–2924; and Kontos MC, Wang Y, Chaudhry SI, et al. Lower hospital volume is associated with higher in-hospital mortality in patients undergoing primary percutaneous coronary intervention for ST-segment–elevation myocardial infarction. *Circ Cardiovasc Qual Outcomes*. 2013;6[6]:659–667.)

Fig. 70.2 Mortality for Medicare beneficiaries according to hospital volume. *PTCA*, Percutaneous transluminal coronary angioplasty. (From Jollis JG, Peterson ED, DeLong ER, et al. The relation between the volume of coronary angioplasty procedures at hospitals treating Medicare beneficiaries and short-term mortality. *N Engl J Med*. 1994;331:1625–1629.)

Empirical evidence supporting a volume-outcome relationship for PCI began to emerge in the 1990s. In a study of Medicare procedures, Jollis and colleagues found in-hospital mortality higher for those treated at low-volume hospitals at 3.9% than those treated at high-volume hospitals at 2.5%.[3] Among the 217,836 patients studied, the relationship between volume and outcome appeared J shaped, with the highest mortality for hospital volumes less than 100 Medicare procedures per year (Fig. 70.2). Because Medicare primarily involves patients older than age 65, a Medicare case volume of 100 represents an overall hospital volume of approximately 200 cases per year. For 19,594 patients undergoing elective PCI in 48 hospitals in the Society for Cardiac Angiography and Interventions registry, Kimmel found significantly higher mortality, emergency bypass, and major complications for patients treated at hospitals with volumes less than 400 cases per year.[4] In the New York State Coronary Angioplasty Reporting System, Hannan, Racz, Topol, and colleagues identified significantly higher risk-adjusted mortality for patients treated at hospitals with annual volumes less than 600.[5] Following the widespread adoption of coronary stents, repeat analyses of Medicare data by McGrath, Wennberg, and colleagues continued to identify higher mortality for low-volume hospitals. Evidence for a relationship between physician volume and outcome also emerged in related analyses, with both Jollis and Hannan identifying higher in-hospital mortality for physician volumes less than 75 cases per year.[5,6] Thus, with substantial compelling evidence, the PCI guidelines revised upward the minimum volume standards to 75 cases per year for physicians and 200 cases per year for hospitals.[21] The relationship continues to be observed in more recent data, including those from the NIS from 2005 to 2010, the German Drug Eluting Stent Registry, the Radial vs. femoral access for coronary intervention (RIVAL) trial, and the CathPCI Registry (Fig. 70.3).[14,17]

Between 2001 and 2014, there has been more than a 25% decline in the number of PCI procedures performed annually in the United States with corresponding declines in hospital and physician PCI volumes. In the NIS between 2005 and 2009, median operator volume has fallen from 53 to 33 per year and median hospital volume declined from 1024 to 693 per year.[22–24] In reformulating the clinical competency guidelines, the writing committee indicated that the majority of interventional cardiologists in the United States were not achieving the previously recommended threshold of 75 PCIs annually.[25] To remain relevant, these guidelines lowered the volume standard for physicians to "a minimum of 50 coronary interventional procedures per year (averaged over a 2-year period)."[25]

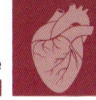

CHAPTER 70 Volume and Outcome

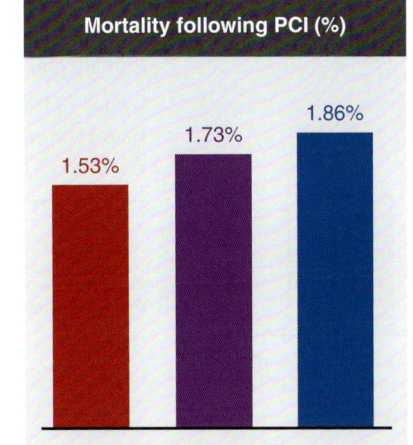

Fig. 70.3 In-hospital outcomes following percutaneous coronary intervention *(PCI)* by operator volume. (Adapted from Fanaroff AC, Zakroysky P, Dai D, et al. Outcomes for PCI in relation to procedural characteristics and operator volumes in the United States. *J Am Coll Cardiol.* 2017;69[24]:2913–2924.)

Since the original evidence was incorporated into updated guidelines, the volume-outcome relationship continues to be examined in contemporary studies. With improved technology and lower event rates, the question remains whether this relationship should continue to guide policy regarding hospital and operator volumes. To understand empirical evidence concerning the volume-outcome relationship, one must keep in perspective three basic concepts of observational research: frequency of the end point, representativeness of the sample, and regression analyses techniques. Considering evidence in light of these concepts, the relationship continues to be observed in higher-risk populations and samples with an adequate representation of low-volume providers.

The first consideration when evaluating empirical evidence is whether the study involves an adequate number of end points to observe a volume-outcome relationship. The relationship is most apparent in high-risk patients who are more likely to experience complications and death. In the first study of volume and outcome for coronary interventions, the greatest differences in mortality by volume were seen in the subset of patients with acute myocardial infarction, with mortality for low-, medium-, and high-volume hospitals of 8.1%, 7.1%, and 6.4%, respectively, compared with 1.3%, 1.2%, and 1.0% mortality for patients without myocardial infarction treated at low-, medium-, and high-volume hospitals.[3] Studies of acute myocardial infarction patients that include the universe of low-volume operators continue to provide persuasive evidence of a volume-outcome relationship. Srinivas and colleagues examined in-hospital mortality for 7321 patients undergoing primary PCI in New York State at 41 hospitals (volume range 1–172 primary PCIs per year) by 266 physicians (volume range 1–55 primary PCIs per year).[8] Risk-adjusted mortality was substantially lower for higher-volume hospitals at a volume threshold of 50 cases per year (≤50, >50 primary PCIs/year mortality 5.4%, 3.4%, odds ratio [OR] 0.58; 95% confidence interval [CI] 0.38 to 0.88) and for physicians at 20 cases per year (≤20, >20 primary PCIs/year mortality 4.2%, 2.9%, OR 0.63; 95% CI 0.44 to 0.91) (Fig. 70.4). Stratifying risk-adjusted mortality by hospital and physician volume, the highest mortality of 7.9% ($P = .01$) was seen for patients treated by low-volume physicians (<20 primary PCIs/year) practicing in low-volume hospitals (<50 primary PCIs/year), and conversely the lowest mortality of 2.8% was seen among patients treated by high-volume physicians (>20 primary PCIs/year) at high-volume hospitals (>50 primary PCIs/year). The stratified analyses showing an interaction between physician and hospital volume suggest that both physician and staff experience contribute to better outcomes. The most recent report from the NCDR for patients undergoing primary PCI, or PCI to treat ST-elevation myocardial infarction, continues to show higher mortality for lower-volume hospitals.[18] In-hospital mortality at low-volume hospitals (<36 cases per year) was 5.6%, compared with 4.8% mortality for high-volume hospitals (>60 cases per year), and the higher mortality remained statistically significant in adjusted models (OR 1.20; 95% CI 1.08 to 1.33; $P = .001$). Of interest from a public policy standpoint, low-volume hospitals were just as likely to be located in urban or suburban regions as higher-volume hospitals. These findings follow clinical intuition that experience is likely to be most important in managing complications and high-risk situations.

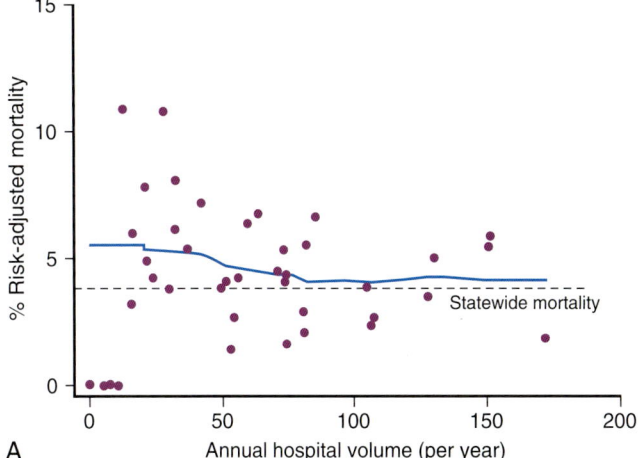

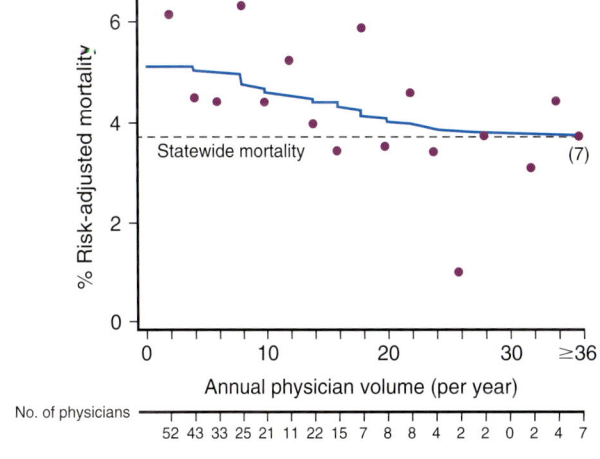

Fig. 70.4 Volume-outcome relationships for hospitals (A) and physicians (B) for primary percutaneous coronary interventions in New York State. (From Srinivas VS, Hailpern SM, Koss E, et al. Effect of physician volume on the relationship between hospital volume and mortality during primary angioplasty. *J Am Coll Cardiol.* 2009;53:574–579.)

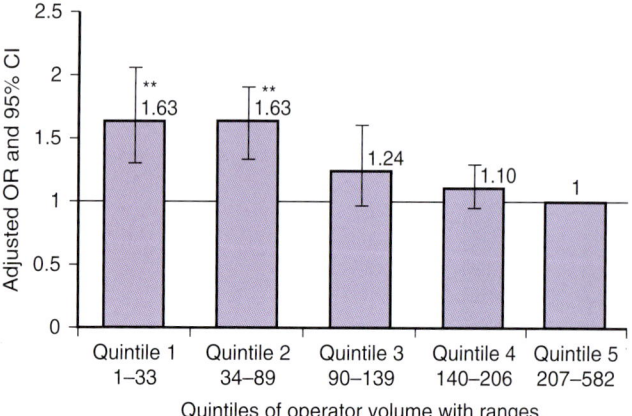

Fig. 70.5 Adjusted odds ratios *(OR)* for major adverse cardiovascular events with generalized estimating equations clustering modeling. ** *P* < .0001. *CI,* Confidence interval. (From Moscucci M, Share D, Smith D, et al. Relationship between operator volume and adverse outcome in contemporary percutaneous coronary intervention practice: an analysis of a quality-controlled multicenter percutaneous coronary intervention clinical database. *J Am Coll Cardiol.* 2005;46:625–632.)

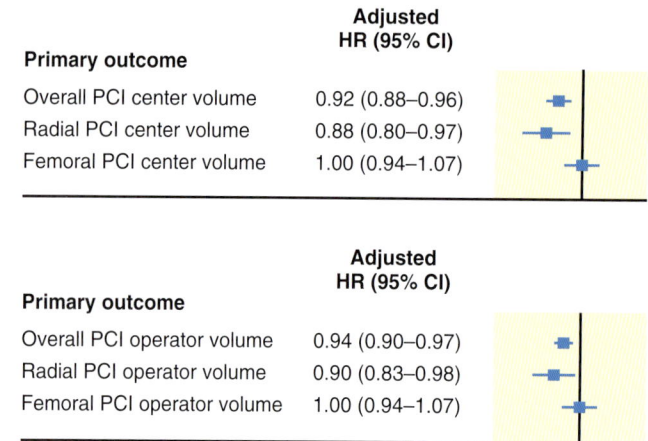

Fig. 70.6 Adjusted rate of death, myocardial infarction, stroke, or major bleeding (primary outcome) according to center and operator volume in the RIVAL (Radial vs. femoral access for coronary intervention) trial. *CI,* Confidence interval; *HR,* hazard ratio; *PCI,* percutaneous coronary intervention. (From Jolly SS, Cairns J, Yusuf S, et al. RIVAL Investigators. Procedural volume and outcomes with radial or femoral access for coronary angiography and intervention. *J Am Coll Cardiol.* 2014;63:954–963.)

Conversely, when adverse outcomes decline, the volume-outcome relationship is mitigated. Following the introduction of coronary stents, abrupt coronary artery closure and the need for urgent bypass surgery markedly decreased from 3.8% to 1.9% in Medicare patients.[3,7] Repeat analyses by McGrath, Wennberg, and colleagues found that the inverse relationship between volume and surgery was no longer apparent following the adoption of coronary stents. By combining end points, the ability of an observational study to observe a volume-outcome relationship increases. Moscucci and colleagues examined the composite end point of death, bypass surgery, stroke or transient ischemic attack, myocardial infarction, and repeat PCI for 18,504 patients treated at 14 Michigan hospitals participating in a quality improvement initiative.[9] Although individual complications were more common for low-volume physicians, the relationships did not reach statistical significance until combined as a composite end point (Fig. 70.5).

To understand empirical evidence, the second important consideration is whether the study population includes a representative sample of low-volume operators. Studies that include the universe of low-volume operators according to mandatory registries or hospital claims like the New York Coronary Angioplasty Reporting System, the NIS, or CathPCI consistently identify volume-outcome relationships, whereas those that rely on a voluntary participation by hospitals focused on quality improvement are less likely to include an adequate sample of low-volume providers sufficient to characterize the volume relationship. The most representative cohort of PCI patients involves the NIS cited earlier involving discharge records for a random sample of acute care hospitals that approximates a 20%- stratified sample of U.S. community hospitals.[22] The NIS includes all payers and thus includes patients younger than age 65. Examining 2,243,209 procedures performed between 2005 and 2010, Patel and colleagues found stepwise increase in mortality (*P* < .001) and complications (*P* < .001) according to annual physician volume quartiles (in-hospital mortality/complications >99 cases 0.6%/5.2%; 47 to 98 cases 0.9%/6.0%; 17 to 46 cases 1.2%/7.2%; 1 to 16 cases 1.7%/10.1%).[14]

Careful consideration of regression models represents a third important element of volume-outcome studies. Regression analyses simply examine the mathematical relationship between two variables according to a set of data points. As regression techniques become more complex, their presentation in manuscripts must be abbreviated to meet editorial requirements. Thus elaborate regression procedures have evolved into "black box" approaches to balancing comparisons. Without detailed presentations, readers are unable to assess whether regression techniques have overcome critical obstacles that limit their ability to reliably identify relationships of interest, namely confounding, multicollinearity, unmeasured risk, and model fit. Even the most sophisticated modeling techniques are limited by sample size and the potential for type II errors, incorrectly accepting the null hypothesis of no difference when a significant difference exist. Mortality differences by volume apparent in unadjusted data may lose their statistical significance in regression models as statistical thresholds are raised to satisfy probability assumptions. For example, Kumbhani and colleagues examined primary PCI volume and outcome for 29,513 patients directly presenting to 116 hospitals participating in the Get With The Guidelines (GWTG) registry.[26] Stratified by annual hospital primary PCI volume, there was a trend toward higher mortality for lower-volume institutions (<36 procedures 3.9%, 36 to 70 procedures 3.2%, and >70 procedures 3.0%). These differences were present despite the exclusion of patients treated in hospitals that submitted fewer than 30 patients and irrespective of the select nature of GWTG hospitals. Following adjustment in regression models, the mortality difference did not reach statistical significance (low-volume vs. high-volume, adjusted OR 1.3, *P* = .15). The study used generalized estimating equations, a technique that has become widespread over the past decade. This conservative approach accounts for the lack of independence of patients treated within the same hospital but requires larger samples or absolute differences to identify statistically significant findings compared to regression analyses that ignore "within-hospital" clustering. Generalized estimating equations raise the threshold for statistical significance, increasing the likelihood of a type II error. In viewing negative findings from regression-adjusted analyses such as the Kumbhani study, one must not confuse the "absence of proof" for "proof of absence." The RIVAL trial examined volume and outcome among 7021 patients treated in 158 hospitals using Cox proportional hazards regression models. The models adjusted for 14 demographic, clinical, and anticoagulation characteristics but did not account for the lack of independence of patients treated in the same hospital. With relatively fewer patients, the study identified significantly lower rates of the primary end point of death, myocardial infarction, stroke, or major bleeding among hospitals and operators with higher overall volumes and among providers with higher radial access volumes (Fig. 70.6).[14]

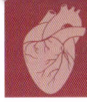

Public Policy Implications

As noted previously, those who argue against volume standards cite concerns about restricting high-quality, low-volume providers. Participation in national registries has been put forth as an alternative to minimal procedural volumes such that quality can be measured and ensured. Another advantage of this approach is that low-volume providers are incented to avoid high-risk patients, the patients for whom the volume-outcome relationship is most apparent. Unfortunately, registries lack statistical power to reliably identify quality, low-volume providers due to insufficient sample size. Low-volume hospitals and physicians have worse outcomes on average, and policies that broadly apply volume standards should avert procedural complications and deaths.

Although national guidelines have incorporated volume standards, the majority of decisions regarding physician and hospital practice occur at the local or state level irrespective of these guidelines.[25,27]

Interventional cardiologists are granted privileges at the hospital level, and hospitals have significant incentive to encourage all physicians to perform procedures in their facilities regardless of volume standards. The ability of hospitals to open and operate interventional cardiology programs is regulated at the state level and therefore standards vary widely. In many regions of the country, low-volume PCI programs are common and increasing in number despite national standards and empirical evidence. Coronary intervention represents a profitable activity from a hospital perspective, and hospitals have successfully lobbied many state governments to allow for an expansion of low-volume facilities.

With national declines in cardiac catheterization procedures since 2000, the need for continued expansion of PCI facilities is further called into question.[28] The necessity for additional hospitals and operators varies according to the elective or urgent nature of the procedure. Elective PCI procedures are relatively low risk and less subject to the volume-outcome relationship. However, the very nature of elective procedures allows for diversion of patients to higher-volume facilities, obviating the need for more PCI facilities. Whether volume standards should be strictly applied for primary PCI procedures represents a more challenging and uncertain policy question. The time-dependent relationship between device activation and survival coupled with extraordinarily long "first hospital door-to-device" times for patients requiring hospital transfer for acute intervention favor a broadening of the availability of primary PCI.[29,30] Particularly for patients presenting to rural hospital emergency departments where transport times to PCI facilities are longer than 30 to 40 minutes, a case can be made for expanding PCI facilities to rural areas. However, high-risk patients, including those with acute myocardial infarction, have the worst outcomes with low-volume providers, and a better strategy may involve reperfusion with fibrinolysis at the rural hospital, followed by transfer to a regional PCI facility. In addition, as noted in the CathPCI study of primary PCI, low-volume hospitals tend to locate in the same urban and suburban areas as their higher-volume counterparts, such that the expansion of PCI facilities does not significantly improve access for patients in rural locations.[18]

CONCLUSIONS

A relationship between lower-volume and worse outcomes has been established by sizeable and compelling empirical evidence over the past 40 years. This association is most apparent among high-risk patients and procedures. The strength of supporting evidence varies as a function of representation by low-volume providers, sample size, the number of outcomes of interest, and regression techniques. Although procedural volume represents only one facet of quality cardiovascular care, the supporting evidence and concern for patients compel the medical community to foster experienced interventional operators and facilities to the extent possible.

KEY REFERENCES

1. Epstein AJ, Rathore SS, Volpp KG, et al. Hospital percutaneous coronary intervention volume and patient mortality, 1998 to 2000. *J Am Coll Cardiol*. 2004;43:1755–1762.
2. Luft HS, Bunker JP, Enthoven AC. Should operations be regionalized? The empirical relation between surgical volume and mortality. *N Engl J Med*. 1979;301:1364–1369.
3. Jollis JG, Peterson ED, DeLong ER, et al. The relation between the volume of coronary angioplasty procedures at hospitals treating Medicare beneficiaries and short-term mortality. *N Engl J Med*. 1994;331:1625–1629.
5. Hannan EL, Racz M, Ryan TJ, et al. Coronary angioplasty volume outcome relationships for hospitals and cardiologists. *JAMA*. 1997;279:892–898.
6. Jollis JG, Peterson ED, Nelson CL, et al. Relationship between physician and hospital coronary angioplasty volume and outcome in elderly patients. *Circulation*. 1997;95:2485–2491.
8. Srinivas VS, Hailpern SM, Koss E, et al. Effect of physician volume on the relationship between hospital volume and mortality during primary angioplasty. *J Am Coll Cardiol*. 2009;53:574–579.
12. Ross JS, Normand SLT, Wang Y, et al. Hospital volume and 30-day mortality for three common medical conditions. *N Engl J Med*. 2010;362:1110–1118.
14. Jolly SS, Cairns J, Yusuf S, et al. RIVAL Investigators. Procedural volume and outcomes with radial or femoral access for coronary angiography and intervention. *J Am Coll Cardiol*. 2014;63:954–963.
17. Fanaroff AC, Zakroysky P, Dai D, et al. Outcomes for PCI in relation to procedural characteristics and operator volumes in the United States. *J Am Coll Cardiol*. 2017;69(24):2913–2924.
19. Dehmer GJ, Weaver WD, Roe MT, et al. A contemporary view of diagnostic cardiac catheterization and percutaneous coronary intervention in the United States: a report from the CathPCI Registry of the National Cardiovascular Data Registry 2010 through June 2011. *J Am Coll Cardiol*. 2012;60:2017–2031.
20. Ryan TJ, Faxon DP, Gunnar RM, et al. Guidelines for percutaneous transluminal coronary angioplasty: a report of the American College of Cardiology/American Heart Association Task Force on Assessment of Diagnostic and Therapeutic Cardiovascular Procedures. *Circulation*. 1988;78:486–502.
23. Riley RF, Don CW, Powell W, et al. Trends in coronary revascularization in the United States from 2001 to 2009: recent declines in percutaneous coronary intervention volumes. *Circ Cardiovasc Qual Outcomes*. 2011;4:193–197.
24. Desai NR, Bradley SM, Parzynski CS, et al. Appropriate use criteria for coronary revascularization and trends in utilization, patient selection and appropriateness of percutaneous coronary intervention. *JAMA*. 2015;314:2045–2053.
25. Harold JG, Bass TA, Bashore TM, et al. ACCF/AHA/SCAI 2013 update of the clinical competence statement on coronary artery interventional procedures: a report of the American College of Cardiology Foundation/American Heart to update the 2007 clinical competence statement on cardiac interventional procedures. *Circulation*. 2013;128:436–472.22.
26. Kumbhani DJ, Cannon CP, Fonarow GC, et al. Association of hospital primary angioplasty volume in ST-segment elevation myocardial infarction with quality and outcomes. *JAMA*. 2009;302:2207–2213.
28. Lloyd-Jones D, Adams RJ, Brown TM, et al. on behalf of the American Heart Association Statistics Committee and Stroke Statistics Subcommittee. Heart disease and stroke statistics—2010 update: a report from the American Heart Association. *Circulation*. 2010;121:e46–e215.
30. Jollis JG, Al-Khalidi HR, Roettig ML, et al. Regional systems of care demonstration project: American Heart Association Mission: lifeline(TM) STEMI systems accelerator. *Circulation*. 2016;134(5):365–374.

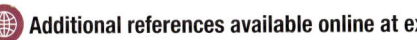

Additional references available online at expertconsult.com.